Oxford Textbook of

Trauma and Orthopaedics

Oxford Textbook of
Trauma and Orthopaedics

SECOND EDITION

Edited by

Christopher Bulstrode (Editor-in-Chief)

James Wilson-MacDonald
Deborah Eastwood
John McMaster
Jeremy Fairbank
Parminder J. Singh
Sandeep Bawa
Panagiotis D. Gikas
Tim Bunker
Grey Giddins
Mark Blyth
David Stanley
Paul H. Cooke
Richard Carrington
Peter Calder
Paul Wordsworth
Timothy W. R. Briggs

OXFORD
UNIVERSITY PRESS

OXFORD
UNIVERSITY PRESS

Great Clarendon Street, Oxford, OX2 6DP,
United Kingdom

Oxford University Press is a department of the University of Oxford.
It furthers the University's objective of excellence in research, scholarship, and education by publishing worldwide. Oxford is a registered trade mark of Oxford University Press in the UK and in certain other countries

First published 2000
Second published 2011
First published in paperback 2017

Impression: 1

Published in the United States of America by Oxford University Press
198 Madison Avenue, New York, NY 10016, United States of America

British Library Cataloguing in Publication Data
Data available

Library of Congress Cataloging in Publication Data
Data available

ISBN 978–0–19–955064–7 (Hbk.)
ISBN 978–0–19–876650–6 (Pbk.)

Printed and bound in China by
C&C Offset Printing Co., Ltd.

Acknowledgements

I would like to give special thanks to James Wilson-MacDonald, Deborah Eastwood, John McMaster, Jeremy Fairbank, and Parminder J Singh who worked unceasingly with me to bring this book to fruition. Their work was 'Above and Beyond the Call of Duty' and made the good parts of this book very good. I must take responsibility for the rest!

Thanks also to the team at Oxford University Press - Mandy Hill, Helen Liepman, Anna Winstanley, and Marionne Cronin, as well as to Gayathri Bellan for managing the project with courtesy and patience.

CJKB

Brief Contents

Contents

SECTION 3
The Spine

SECTION 4
The Shoulder

SECTION 5
The Elbow

SECTION 13
Paediatric Orthopaedics

Contributors

Joong Mo Ahn Department of Chemistry, University of Texas at Dallas, Dallas, USA

Philip M Ahrens Orthopaedic Department, Royal Free Hospital, London, UK

Amjid Ali Northern General Hospital, Sheffield, UK

Rouin Amirfeyz Trauma and Orthopaedics Department, Bristol Royal Infirmary, Bristol, UK

Howard An Department of Orthopaedic Surgery, Rush University Medical Center, Chicago, USA

Paul A Anderson Department of Orthopedics and Rehabilitation University of Wisconsin, Madison, Wisconsin, USA

William JS Aston Royal National Orthopaedic Hospital, Stanmore, UK

Roger M Atkins Department of Orthopaedics, Bristol Royal Infirmary, Bristol, UK

Inoshi Atukorala Department of Clinical Medicine, Faculty of Medicine, University of Colombo, Sri Lanka

R.D. Banerjee Cavendish Hip Fellow, Northern General Hospital, UK

Gordon Bannister Avon Orthopaedic Centre, Southmead Hospital, Westbury

John Bartlett Department of Orthopaedics, Austin Hospital, University of Melbourne, Melbourne, Australia

Alf Bass Orthopaedic Department, Royal Liverpool Children's Hospital (Alder Hey), Liverpool, UK

Sandeep Bawa Department of Rheumatology, Gartnavel General Hospital, Glasgow University Hospitals, Glasgow, UK

Maneesh Bhatia Consultant Orthopaedic Surgeon, Leicester, UK

Rej S Bhumbra Royal National Orthopaedic Hospital, Stanmore, UK

Gordon Blunn Institute of Orthopaedics and Musculoskeletal Science, London, UK

Mark Blyth Department of Trauma and Orthopaedics, Glasgow Royal Informary, Glasgow, UK

K Boffard Department of Surgery, Johannesburg Hospital, South Africa

Henry H Bohlman (deceased) University Hospitals Case Western Reserve, Cleveland, Ohio, USA

Pascal Boileau Department of Orthopedic Surgery and Sports Traumatology, Archet 2 Hospital, France

D Glynn Bolitho La Jolla, CA, USA

Steve Bollen Consultant Orthopaedic Surgeon, Bradford Teaching Hospitals Trust, Bradford, UK

O.M. Böstman Department of Orthopaedics and Trauma Surgery, University Central Hospital, Helsinki, Finland

John A Boudreau Department of Orthopaedic Surgery, St Louis University School of Medicine, Missouri, USA

Richard J Bransford Department of Orthopedic Surgery and Sports Medicine, University of Washington, Seattle, WA, USA

Timothy WR Briggs Royal National Orthopaedic Hospital, Stanmore, UK

L Renzi Brivio Center of Paediatric Orthopaedics, University of Verona, Italy

Colin Bruce Department of Orthopaedics, Royal Liverpool Childrens Hospital, Liverpool, UK

Elaine Buchanan Nuffield Orthopaedic Centre, Headington, Oxford, UK

Rachel Buckingham Nuffield Orthopaedic Centre, Headington, Oxford, UK

Christopher Bulstrode Nuffield Department of Orthopaedic, Rheumatological, and Musculo-skeletal Medicine, University of Oxford, John Radcliffe Hospital, Headington, Oxford, UK

Tim D Bunker Princess Elizabeth Orthopaedic Centre, Royal Devon and Exeter Hospital, Exeter, UK

Peter Burge Nuffield Orthopaedic Centre, Headington, Oxford, UK

Christopher M Caddy Department of Plastic and Reconstructive Surgery, Sheffield Teaching Hospitals NHS Foundation Trust, Sheffield, UK

Peter Calder The Catterall Unit, Royal National Orthopaedic Hospital, Stanmore, Middlesex, UK

Douglas A Campbell Leeds General Infirmary, Leeds, UK

Stephen R Cannon Royal National Orthopaedic Hospital, Stanmore, UK

Richard Carrington The Joint Reconstruction Unit, Royal National Orthopaedic Hospital, Stanmore, UK

Andrew Carr Nuffield Orthopaedic Centre, Headington, Oxford, UK

Lucinda J Carr Department of Neurology, Great Ormond Street Hospital, London, UK

Maurizio A Catagni Department of Orthopaedics and Ilizarov Unit, Lecco General Hospital, Lecco, Italy

E Chaloner Department of Vascular Surgery, Lewisham University Hospital, London, UK

Jens R Chapman Department of Orthopaedic Surgery, Harborview Medical Center, Seattle, USA

J Chell Department of Trauma and Orthopaedics, Queen's Medical Centre, Nottingham, UK

NMP Clarke Department of Orthopaedics, Southampton General Hospital, Southampton, UK

Charles R Clark Department of Orthopaedics and Rehabilitation, University of Iowa Hospitals and Clinics, Iowa City, USA

David Clark Department of Orthopaedics, Derbyshire Royal Infirmary, Derbyshire, UK

Colonel Jon Clasper Frimley Park Hospital Foundation Trust, Camberiey, UK

Glenn Clewer Prince Charles Hospital, Merthyr Tydfil, Wales, UK

Paul H Cooke Consultant Foot and Ankle Surgeon, Nuffield Orthopaedic Centre, Oxford, UK

Stephen Copeland Reading Shoulder Unit, Berkshire Independent Hospital, Reading, UK

Mike Craigen The Royal Orthopaedic Hospital, Birmingham, UK

Haemish Crawford Department of Orthopaedics, Starship Children's Hospital, Auckland, New Zealand

C Dall'Oca Department of Orthopaedics and Traumatology, Policlinico G.B. Rossi, University of Verona, Verona, Italy

Christopher J Dare

Evan M. Davies Consultant Orthopaedic Spinal Surgeon, Southampton University Hospitals; Child Health Department Surgical Spine Service, Southampton General Hospital, Southampton, UK

Mark S Davies London Foot and Ankle Centre, London, UK

Paul Rhys Davies University Hospital Llandough, Llandough, Penarth, UK

Tim Davis Department of Trauma and Orthopaedics, Queen's Medical Centre, Nottingham, UK

Thomas A DeCoster Department of Orthopaedics and Rehabilitation, The University of New Mexico, School of Medicine, Albuquerque, USA

SD Deo Department of Orthopaedics, Great Western Hospital, Swindon and Marlborough NHS trust, UK

Christopher Dodd Nuffield Orthopaedic Centre NHS Trust, Oxford, UK

James Donaldson Specialist Registrar, Royal National Orthopaedic Hospital Rotation London, UK

Simon Donell Consultant Orthopaedic Surgeon Norfolk and Norwich University Hospital, Norwich, UK

ND Downing Nottingham University Hospitals NHS Trust, Queens Medical Centre Campus, Nottingham, UK

Mark L. Dumonski Spine and Orthopaedic Surgery, Guilford Orthopaedic and Sports Medicine Center, Greensboro, NC USA

Roderick Duncan Department of Orthopaedics, Royal Hospital for Sick Children, Glasgow, UK

Deborah M Eastwood Consultant Orthopaedic Surgeon, The Catterall Unit, The Royal National Orthopaedic Hospital, Stanmore, Middlesex, UK

Georges El-Khoury Department of Radiology, University of Iowa Hospitals and Clinics, Iowa City, IA, USA

Roger Emery St Mary's Hospital, London, UK

David M Evans The Hand Clinic, Oakley Clinic, Windsor, UK

Jeremy Fairbank Nuffield Orthopaedic Centre, Headington, Oxford, UK

Najma Farooq Great Ormond Street Hospital for Children, London, UK

Julian Feller Epworth Richmond, Melbourne, Australia

Richard E Field Consultant Orthopaedic Surgeon and Director of Research, The South West London Elective Orthopaedic Centre, Epsom, Surrey, UK

Andrew Floyd Milton Keynes General Hospital, Eaglestone, UK

Brian JC Freeman Department of Spinal Surgery, Royal Adelaide Hospital, Adelaide, Australia

Lennard Funk Upper Limb Unit, Wrightington Hospital, Wigan, UK

Dominic Furniss Department of Plastic and Reconstructive Surgery, John Radcliffe Hospital, Oxford, UK

S Gaba Consultant Musculoskeletal Radiology, Leicester Royal Infirmary, University Hospitals of Leicester NHS Trust, Leicester, UK

Advait Gandhe Queen Alexandra Hospital, Portsmouth, UK

Brian Gardner Stoke Mandeville Hospital, Aylesbury, UK

Martin Gargan Department of Orthopaedics, Bristol Royal Hospital for Children, Bristol, UK

Gregory M Georgiadis Orthopaedic Trauma Services, The Toledo Hospital, Ohio, USA

Paul LF Giangrande Oxford Haemophilia and Thrombosis Centre, Churchill Hospital, Headington, Oxford, UK

Max Gibbons Nuffield Orthopaedic Centre, Headington, Oxford, UK

Grey Giddins Royal United Hospital, Bath, UK

Henk Giele Department of Plastic Surgery, John Radcliffe Hospital, Headington, Oxford, UK

Panagiotis D Gikas Institute of Orthopaedics and Musculoskeletal Science, Royal National Orthopaedic Hospital, Stanmore, Middlesex, UK

Andy Goldberg Royal National Orthopaedic Hospital NHS Trust, Stanmore, UK; The Institute of Orthopaedics & Musculoskeletal Science (IOMS), University College London, UK

Alastair Graham Department of Orthopaedic Surgery, Buckinghamshire Hospitals, High Wycombe, UK

Andrew C Gray Foothill's Medical Centre, Calgary, Canada

Michael Grevitt Nottingham University Hospitals NHS Trust, Queens Medical Centre Campus, Nottingham, UK

Ruby Grewal Department of Surgery, Hand and Upper Limb Center, University of Western Ontario, Canada

D Grinsell Department Surgery, University of Melbourne, St Vincent's Hospital, Australia

FS Haddad Consultant Orthopaedic Surgeon, University College Hospital, London, UK

R Handley Oxford Trauma Unit, John Radcliffe Hospital, Oxford, UK

Sammy A Hanna Sarcoma Unit, Royal National Orthopaedic Hospital, Stanmore, UK

Rajiv S Hanspal Rehabilitation Medicine, Stanmore Disablement Services Centre, The Royal National Orthopaedic Hospital, Middlesex, UK

Ian Harding Frenchay Hospital, Bristol, UK

Robert A Hart Department of Orthopaedics, Oregon Health and Science University, Portland, USA

Aresh Hashemi-Nejad Royal National Orthopaedic Hospital, Stanmore, UK

Stuart M Hay Robert Jones and Agnes Hunt Hospital, Shropshire, UK

Tim Hems Department of Orthopaedic Surgery, The Victoria Infirmary, Glasgow, UK

Philip Henman Great North Children's Hospital, Newcastle-upon-Tyne, UK

M Henry Department of Orthopaedics, Royal Infirmary of Edinburgh, Edinburgh UK

Anthony J Heywood Department of Plastic and Reconstructive Surgery, Stoke Mandeville Hospital, Aylesbury, Buckinghamshire, UK

Andreas F Hinsche Department of Orthopaedic and Trauma Surgery, Queen Elizabeth Hospital, Gateshead NHS Foundation Trust, Gateshead, UK

Jayme R Hiratzka Department of Orthopaedics and Rehabilitation, Oregon Health and Science University, Portland, USA

Brian J Holdsworth Department of Trauma and Orthopaedics, Queen's Medical Centre, Nottingham, UK

David Hollinghurst Great Western Hospital, Swindon, UK

Jon D Hop Holland, Michigan, USA

Andrew Howard Professor of Orthopaedic Surgery, Director of Spine Surgery and Spine Fellowship Program, Rush University Medical Center, Chicago

Benjamin J Hudson SpR Radiology, Norfolk and Norwich University Hospital, UK

Thomas Hughes ED Department, John Radcliffe Hospital, Headington, Oxford, UK

JS Huntley Department of Orthopaedics, Royal Hospital for Sick Children, Glasgow, UK

Jakub Jagiello Royal National Orthopaedic Hospital, Stanmore, UK

Andrew James Stobhill ACH Hospital, Glasgow, UK

Wingrove T Jarvis Department of Orthopaedics, Jackson Purchase, Medical Center, Mayfield, Kentucky, USA

Kassim Javaid Biomedical Research Unit, Nuffield Orthopaedic Centre, Headington, Oxford, UK

Bryn Jones Glasgow Royal Infirmary, Glasgow, UK

Nick Kalson Institute of Orthopaedics and Musculoskeletal Science, Royal National Orthopaedic Hospital, Stanmore, Middlesex, UK

Gregoris Kambouroglou Oxford Trauma Unit, John Radcliffe Hospital, Oxford, UK

John Keating Department of Orthopaedic Trauma, Royal Infirmary, Edinburgh, UK

Richard W Keen The Royal National Orthopaedic Hospital, Stanmore. Middx; University College London Hospitals, London, UK

Simon Kelley Department of Orthopaedics, Hospital for Sick Children, Toronto, Canada

Rashid Khan Department of Orthopaedics, Princess Alexandra Hospital, Harlow, Essex, UK

GJW King Department of Surgery, Hand and Upper Limb Centre, University of Western Ontario, Canada

Rohit Kotnis Nuffield Orthopaedic Centre, Headington, Oxford, UK

Deepak Kumar Chase Farm Hospital, Enfield, Middlesex, UK

Simon M Lambert Royal National Orthopaedic Hospital, Stanmore, Middlesex, UK

Ilana Langdon Royal United Hospital, Bath, UK

Loren L Latta Department of Orthopaedics, University of Miami, Miller School of Medicine, Florida, USA

Franco Lavini University of Verona, Verona, Italy

David Lawrie Aberdeen Royal Infirmary, Aberdeen, UK

Lisa Leonard Department of Orthopaedics, Brighton and Sussex University Hospitals Trust, Brighton, UK

Mui-Hong Lim Tan Tock Seng Hospital, Singapore

Chris Little Nuffield Orthopaedic Centre, Headington, Oxford, UK

William J Long Insall Scott Kelly Institute for Orthopaedics and Sports Medicine, New York, USA

Ahmad K Malik Orthopaedic Department, Royal Surrey County Hospital, Guildford, UK

Malgorzata Magliano Department of Rheumatology, Stoke Mandeville Hospital, Aylesbury, UK

S Naidu Maripuri Nevill Hall Hospital, Abergavenny, Wales, UK

JL Marsh Department of Orthopaedic Surgery, University of Iowa Hospital, Iowa City, USA

Will Mason Orthopaedics, Southampton University Hospitals Trust, Southampton, UK

Stuart JE Matthews Oxford Trauma Unit, John Radcliffe Hospital, Oxford, UK

Anthony McGrath SpR trauma and orthopaedics, Royal National Orthopaedic Hospital Stanmore, UK

John McMaster Oxford Trauma Unit, John Radcliffe Hospital, Oxford, UK

Ian McNab Nuffield Orthopaedic Centre, Headington, Oxford, UK

Eugene McNally Nuffield Orthopaedic Centre, Headington, Oxford, UK

Martin A McNally Nuffield Orthopaedic Centre, Headington, Oxford, UK

Philip McNee Nuffield Orthopaedic Centre, Headington, Oxford, UK

Henry McQuay Nuffield Department of Anaesthetics, John Radcliffe Hospital, Headington, Oxford, UK

RD Meek Department of Trauma and Orthopaedics, Southern General Hospital, Glasgow, UK

Yusuf Menda Department of Radiology, University of Iowa Hospitals and Clinics, Iowa City, IA, USA

Sergio Mendoza-Lattes Department of Orthopaedics and Rehabilitation, University of Iowa, Iowa City, Iowa, USA

Jonathan Miles The Royal National Orthopaedic Hospital, Stanmore, UK

Kerry R Mills Department of Clinical Neurophysiology, King's College Hospital, London, UK

Jo Mitchell Senior Orthotist, Nuffield Orthopaedic Centre, Oxford, UK

Berton R Moed Department of Orthopaedic Surgery, Saint Louis University School of Medicine, Missouri, USA

Khitish Mohanty University Hospital of Wales, Cardiff, UK

Paul Monk Nuffield Department of Orthopaedics, Rheumatology and Musculoskeletal Sciences (NDORMS), Nuffield Orthopaedic Centre, Oxford, UK

Fergal Monsell Department of Orthopaedics, Bristol Royal Hospital for Children, Bristol, UK

TR Morley Royal National Orthopaedic Hospital City OPD, London, UK

Wayne Morrison Department Surgery, University of Melbourne, St Vincent's Hospital, Australia

Andrew N Morritt Department of Plastic and Reconstructive Surgery, Sheffield Teaching Hospitals, NHS Foundation Trust, Sheffield, UK

Jacob Munro Department of Orthopaedic Surgery, Auckland City Hospital, Auckland, New Zealand

David Murray Nuffield Orthopaedic Centre, Headington, Oxford, UK

Ananda M Nanu Department of Orthopaedics, Sunderland Royal Hospitals, Newcastle upon Tyne, UK

Ali Narvani Reading Shoulder Unit, Royal Berkshire Hospital, Reading, UK

Colin Nnadi Spinal Unit, Nuffield Orthopaedic Department, Headington, Oxford, UK

Shahryar Noordin Department of Orthopaedics, Aga Khan University, Karachi, Pakistan

David Noyes Oxford Trauma Unit, John Radcliffe Hospital, Oxford, UK

John M O'Donnell Consultant Orthopaedic Surgeon, Mercy and Bellbird Private Hospitals, East Melbourne, Victoria, Australia

Michael J Oddy University College London NHS Foundation Trust, London, UK

Ben Ollivere West Suffolk Hospital, Suffolk, UK

JA Oni Nottingham University Hospitals NHS Trust, Queen's Medical Centre, Nottingham, UK

Hemant Pandit Nuffield Orthopaedic Centre, Headington, Oxford, UK

Martyn J Parker Department of Orthopaedics, Peterborough District Hospital, Peterborough, UK

J Mark Paterson Department of Orthopaedics and Trauma, St Bartholomew's and The Royal London Hospitals, London, UK

S Patil Department of Trauma and Orthopaedics, Southern General Hospital, Glasgow, UK

Delia Peppercorn North Hampshire MRI, North Hampshire Hospitals NHS Trust, Basingstoke, Hampshire, UK

Lars Peterson University Hospital of Coventry and Warwickshire, Coventry, UK

Nick Phillips Consultant Shoulder and Elbow Surgeon, University of Salford, UK

Clarissa Pilkington Department of Rheumatology, Great Ormond Street Hospital, London, UK

A Pohl Orthopaedic Trauma, Royal Adelaide Hospital, Australia

Rob Pollock Royal National Orthopaedic Hospital, Stanmore, UK

Matthew Porteous Department of Trauma and Orthopaedics, The West Suffolk Hospital NHS Trust, UK

DE Porter Senior Lecturer in Orthopaedics, University of Edinburgh, Edinburgh, UK

David Potter Northern General Hospital, Sheffield, UK

RA Preiss Department of Trauma and Orthopaedics, Southern General Hospital, Glasgow, UK

Amir A Qureshi Robert Jones and Agnes Hunt Orthopaedic Hospital, Shropshire, UK

S Rajasekaran Director and Head, Department of Orthopaedic and Spine Surgery, Ganga Hospital, Coimbatore, India

Manoj Ramachandran Department of Orthopaedics and Trauma, St Bartholomew's and The Royal London Hospitals, London, UK

F Rayan Department of Trauma and Orthopaedics, University College Hospital, London, UK

Peter Reilly Department of Orthopaedics, St Marys Hospital, Imperial College Healthcare, NHS Trust, UK

Jai Relwani Reading Shoulder Unit, Berkshire Independent Hospital, Reading, UK

Nicholas D Riley SpR,The Catterall Unit, Royal National Orthopaedic Hospital, Stanmore, UK

Simon NJ Roberts Robert Jones and Agnes Hunt Orthopaedic Hospital, Shropshire, UK

Andrew HN Robinson Orthopaedics, Addenbrookes Hospital, Cambridge, UK

Barry Rose Royal National Orthopaedic Hospital, Stanmore, Middlesex, UK

James H Roth Department of Surgery, Hand and Upper Limb Center, University of Western Ontario, Canada

Amir Salama Department of Orthopaedics, Heart of England trust, Birmingham,UK

Anish Sanghrajka SpR Dept of Orthopaedics and Trauma, St Bartholomew's and The Royal London Hospitals, London, UK

Tanaya Sarkhel Department of Orthopaedics and Trauma, Frimley Park Hospital Foundation Trust, Camberiey, UK

Augusto Sarmiento Miami, USA

Robert Savage Consultant Orthopaedic and Hand Surgeon, Royal Gwent Hospital, Newport, UK

Dietrich Schlenzka ORTON Orthopaedic Hospital, Helsinki, Finland

BW Scott Children's Orthopaedics, Leeds General Infirmary, Leeds, UK

Giles R Scuderi Insall Scott Kelly Institute for Orthopaedics and Sports Medicine, New York, USA

Philip Sell Department of Orthopaedics, Leicester General Hospital, Leicester, UK

TK Shanmugasundaram (Deceased 2008)

Shantanu Shahane Chesterfield Royal Hospital, Chesterfield, UK

Ryan Shulman Department of Medical Imaging, Royal Brisbane & Women's Hospital, Brisbane, Australia

Parminder J Singh Consultant Orthopaedic and Trauma Surgeon, Maroondah Hospital; Honorary Senior Lecturer for Monash University, Melbourne, Australia

Marco Sinisi PNIUnit, Royal National Orthopaedic Hospital, Stanmore, Middlesex, UK

John Skinner Royal National Orthopaedic Hospital, Stanmore, UK

David H Sochart North Manchester General Hospital, Manchester, UK

Mathew Solan Orthopaedics, Royal Surrey County Hospital, Surrey, UK

Tim Spalding University Hospital of Coventry and Warwickshire, Coventry, UK

Gavin Spence Evelina Children's Hospital, London, UK

Ben Spiegelberg Department of Colorectal Surgery, Hillingdon Hospital, Northwood, UK

Kesavan Sri-Ram Sarcoma Unit, Royal National Orthopaedic Hospital, Stanmore, Middlesex, UK

David Stanley Northern General Hospital, Sheffield, UK

JK Stanley Wrightington Hospital, Appley Bridge, UK

I Stockley Northern General Hospital, Sheffield, UK

John Stothard James Cook University Hospital, Middlesbrough, UK

Catherine Swales Nuffield Orthopaedic Centre, Headington, Oxford, UK

Amol Tambe Wrightington Hospital, UK

Simon Tan South Birmingham Trauma Unit, Selly Oak Hospital, Birmingham, UK

Andrew Taylor Department of Trauma and Orthopaedics, Queen's Medical Centre, Nottingham, UK

D Temperley Royal Albert Edward Infirmary, Wigan, UK

Tom Temple Department of Orthopaedics and Pathology, University of Miami Hospital, Miami, USA

Peter Templeton Children's Orthopaedics, Leeds General Infirmary, Leeds, UK

Sally Tennant Consultant Orthopaedic Surgeon, The Catterall Unit, The Royal National Orthopaedic Hospital, Stanmore, Middlesex, UK

DR Theile

Tim Theologis Nuffield Orthopaedic Centre, Oxford, UK

Simon Thomas Department of Orthopaedics, Bristol Royal Hospital for Children, UK

D Thompson Department of Neurosurgery, Great Ormond Street Hospital for Children, London, UK

Ian A Trail Centre for Hand and Upper Limb Surgery, Wrightington Hospital, Wigan, UK

SK Tucker Great Ormond Street Hospital for Children, London UK

Michael Uglow Department of Orthopaedics, Southampton General Hospital, Southampton, UK

Kelly Vince Orthopedic Surgery, Northland District Health Board, Whangarei Hospital, Whangarei, New Zealand

Andrew Wainwright Nuffield Orthopaedic Centre, Oxford, UK

Don Wallace Milton Keynes Hospital NHS Foundation Trust, Eaglestone, Milton Keynes, UK

Phil Walmsley Queen Margaret Hospital, Dunfermline, Scotland, UK

Michael Walton Department of Orthopaedics, Bristol Royal Hospital for Children, UK

David Warwick Orthopaedics, Southampton University Hospital, Southampton, UK

Duncan J Watkinson Department of Trauma and Orthopaedics, Queen Alexandra Hospital, Portsmouth, UK

John K Webb Nottingham University Hospitals NHS Trust, Queens Medical Centre Campus, Nottingham, UK, E Yeung

Krista E Weiss Harvard College, Cambridge, USA

Arnold-Peter C Weiss Harvard College, Cambridge, USA

Andy Williams Chelsea and Westminster Hospital, London, UK

John R Williams Trauma Unit, Newcastle General Hospital, Newcastle upon Tyne, UK

Adrian Wilson Department of Orthopaedics, North Hampshire Hospitals NHS Trust, Basingstoke, Hampshire, UK

James Wilson-MacDonald Nuffield Orthopaedic Centre, Oxford, UK

Roger Wolman Royal National Orthopaedic Hospital, Stanmore, UK

Paul Wordsworth Biomedical Research Unit, Nuffield Orthopaedic Centre, Headington, Oxford, UK

Zhiqing Xing Department of Orthopaedics and Rehabilitation, The University of New Mexico, School of Medicine, Albuquerque, USA

Eric Yeung Royal National Orthopaedic Hospital, Stanmore, London, UK

Amy B Zavatsky Department of Engineering Science, University of Oxford, Oxford, UK

SECTION 1

Fundamentals

1.1

Foundations of clinical practice

Thomas Hughes

Summary points

- Conscious and unconscious competency
- Clinical research and the placebo effect
- Trial design and the randomized controlled trial
- Critical review of the literature
- Clinical governance and audit
- Capacity and consent
- Principles of teaching and learning.

Introduction

This chapter aims to describe key knowledge that, while not directly involved in clinical work, is essential for expert clinical practice and therefore should be regarded as equivalent to basic sciences. Like the basic sciences, this knowledge underpins our clinical practice and guides us when faced with new situations.

Surgery and medicine rely on research and innovation to drive improvements in clinical practice. As an expert surgeon, you must know how to assess these innovations and be able to judge objectively whether or not you should incorporate any apparent improvements into your clinical practice.

What is the best treatment?

First do no harm

A common public assumption is that all medical treatment is beneficial. This may be a marker of the success of modern medicine, but some of the major advances of the last 50 years have been the acknowledgement that medical treatments cause harm as well as benefit, and the development of ways of quantifying the relative risks and benefits of treatments. The most recent manifestation of this trend is the current focus on patient safety—preventing harm to patients within the healthcare system.

Another recent trend is an increased focus on the patient as a consumer. There has been a shift towards healthcare provision structured around patient needs rather than simply providing the healthcare that healthcare workers think is best. There are costs and frustrations associated with this approach, but advantages in patient satisfaction and flexibility of healthcare provision. Healthcare evolves to solve patients' problems rather than the other way round.

For patients to be actively involved in their healthcare, they need to be informed consumers. Therefore part of the healthcare process is to educate the patient about the options available. Patients now have ready access to plentiful information, most of which is not peer reviewed, and may be covert advertising. This can result in health 'wants' being confused with health 'needs'. Surgical practice needs to evolve to meet these challenges.

The problem with structuring healthcare around patient demands is that healthcare, unlike buying a meal or holiday, does not usually result in an immediate objectively good or bad outcome. If you asked a *doctor* what treatment they would want from a surgeon, they would want a safe, experienced surgeon and anaesthetist operating in a good environment with motivated conscientious nursing staff. They would be in a fairly good position to judge this.

Patients have a limited number of surrogate measures on which to base their assessment of quality (current measures proposed to define 'good' healthcare in the United Kingdom (UK) include time on waiting list, hospital cleanliness, and 'nurse empathy'. Tables of operative results enable comparison of the quantity and timeliness of operations, but not necessarily the outcomes for the patients).

Box 1.1.1 Patients' questions you should be able to answer

- What is the best treatment?
  - How can you be sure?
- What does this test tell you?
  - How can you be sure?
- How can I be sure you make good clinical decisions?
- Why should I undergo this procedure?

Competence is being able to answer these questions, but expertise is demonstrated by the ability to defend your decision—to say why. This chapter aims to cover the foundation skills necessary for this expertise.

Government ratings may have little or no relationship to the outcomes that actually matter most to the patient or society, e.g. freedom from pain, employment, and good quality of life.

In trying to measure healthcare quality, there is a *technical* aspect (expertise, outcome), an *interpersonal* aspect (attitude, behaviour), and a *service* aspect (accessibility, environment). As patients usually cannot objectively judge the technical aspects, they tend to base their decisions on the interpersonal and service aspects, which are more amenable to measurement.

The technical aspects such as safety and competence tend to be taken for granted, which is unfortunate because the technical aspects are usually the major determinant of long-term outcome. Moreover, the really important outcomes are difficult to measure. For example, there is a long time lag between a poorly sited or poorly designed joint replacement and its ultimate failure. For these reasons, poor quality work can appear cost-effective if not evaluated carefully, and in a way that considers all costs.

In summary, healthcare quality measurement is vitally important, but often heavily flawed because of the temptation to use surrogate measures that are politically expedient or easy to measure, rather than concentrating on the outcomes that actually matter.

What does the patient want to know?

Performing an intervention such as an operation will have different results in different people. Humans are not linear predictable systems, which is probably why they have survived so long.

There are many different factors that contribute to the operative outcome: type of operation, preoperative function, risks from the operation, surgical skill, and risks from the anaesthetic. The contribution of these factors can be estimated from analysis of different populations of patients who all undergo the treatment, but this would ignore factors unique to that patient and that surgeon.

Imagine that you are the patient. You don't really care about all this. You want to know: 'Will *this* intervention, performed by *this* person, benefit or harm *me*, and by how much?' (Box 1.1.1).

To answer this, and be legitimately reassuring, it is necessary to demonstrate that:

- You and your anaesthetic and nursing team are safe and competent to carry out the operation and its aftercare
- The operation is appropriate for that patient and condition
- The likely risks are outweighed by the likely benefits.

Only when these conditions are fulfilled is the risk of harm to the patient minimized. Harm may occur in different forms: medical, financial, and social.

Medical harm

Medical harm is the harm directly resulting from the treatment, and may be physical or psychological.

The notion of medical harm has been crystallized in the minds of the UK public by cases such as Harold Shipman and paediatric cardiac surgery in Bristol. Harold Shipman was a general practitioner who murdered approximately 200 patients by giving lethal doses of opiates. Some cardiac surgeons in Bristol in the 1990s continued to perform complex paediatric operations despite overwhelming evidence of very poor results, heroically documented by an anaesthetist, Steven Bolsin, at great personal and professional cost.

Although these differ in being acts of active harm (Shipman) and passive harm (Bristol) in that Shipman set out to harm patients, but in Bristol the harm was not intended, both sets of events have been seen by the establishment as indicators of inadequate self-regulation by the medical profession. Steps such as revalidation and competence-based assessments have been introduced.

Revalidation is designed to identify poorly performing doctors and ensure that they are retrained. Revalidation is very expensive to perform if such assessments are to be both valid and reliable. Revalidation is likely to evolve to a system of re-taking one's exit exam every 5 years, as in the United States of America (USA).

Continuing Medical Education is an important part of ensuring continuing competence, but the providers of such education often have ulterior motives, and the end product (any benefit to patients) is not measured, just the process.

In addition to compulsory revalidation, league tables of mortality offer a superficial view of competence, and are being implemented for some surgical procedures in the UK, and have been available in the USA for some time.

As doctors, we need to recognize both the ageing of our knowledge, and the changing nature of our jobs. Specialties such as cardiothoracic and vascular surgery have changed completely in 10 years, and technology such as robotics will have an increasing role in trauma and orthopaedic surgery. It is likely that periodic retraining will be a normal expectation and will be written into job plans in the future.

Social harm

By medicalizing a normal human condition, it is possible to create 'diseases' where none previously existed. This is obviously good news if you have a product that cures the 'disease'. The widespread usage of antidepressants for a rather hazy definition of 'depression' medicalized many thousands of people who may have had no more than transient unhappiness. Direct-to-consumer advertising, allowed in some countries, encourages consumers to self-diagnose and approach doctors for specific branded products. These behaviours encourage expenditure on health 'wants' rather than health 'needs' which disadvantage the poor and less articulate and result in financial harm (see following section).

Back pain is an enormous social burden. In the UK, 50 million workdays are lost each year and 500 000 people are on long-term incapacity benefits for back pain. The advent of magnetic resonance (MR) scanning has enabled everyone to have a diagnosis, but it is likely that this validation of non-specific 'abnormalities' has not benefited patients or society.

Financial harm

There is direct financial harm to the patient and society in every illness through lost earnings and inability to participate in social activities. However, in a single healthcare provider system like the UK National Health Service (NHS), there is also an *opportunity cost* to every treatment.

For example, an opportunity cost occurs if one spends X pounds on drugs for Alzheimer's disease patients, then one cannot spend X pounds on hip prostheses. The decision about which treatment is the best option is laden with value judgements. Central questions are:

- Does the treatment work as claimed?
- What benefit does the patient or society gain from the treatment?

Box 1.1.2 Conscious competency—the development and ageing of knowledge (Figure 1.1.1)

One starts as a medical student, unaware of how much one does not know—the unconscious incompetent. An awareness of the breadth and depth of knowledge necessary gradually dawns over the course of medical school, making one conscious of one's incompetence. Through hard work, study, and practical experience in the early postgraduate years, conscious competence is achieved. As the knowledge becomes internalized and practice becomes automatic, we become the unconscious competent—we can do the job, but we don't always know why we do what we do.

The danger of unconscious competence is that it is easy for this to slip into unconscious incompetence—a process termed 'occupational senility'. Continuous Medical Education (CME)/postgraduate education helps us to find areas in which we are incompetent and remedy this. Educational skills such as teaching juniors and colleagues ensure that we remain aware of why we do what we do—nothing tests your understanding of a subject as well as having to explain it to someone else.

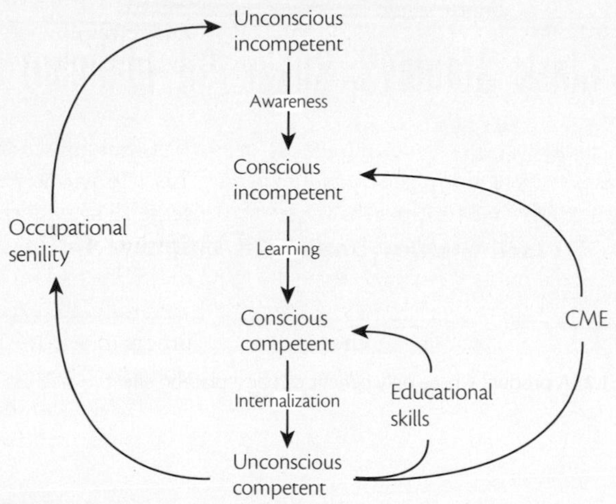

Fig. 1.1.1 Conscious competency.

Box 1.1.3 Medical business model

To understand the behaviour of device and pharmaceutical companies, it helps to understand their business model.

Developing and testing a new drug or device to the stage when it can be licensed is a calculated high-stakes gamble, costing more than US $1 billion for a new class of drug. There is a substantial risk that defects in the product may be found that will harm some patients. This can lead to not only the loss of the market for that product, but, if handled badly, major damage to the company that makes the product.

Patent laws for drugs and devices give the manufacturer 20 years' protection from other direct copying, although similar ('me-too') products may be allowed to compete. Unfortunately the time to develop and test medical products is rarely shorter than 10 years for a drug, although less for a device. The good news is that once a device/drug is approved for sale, it is generally cheap to manufacture and distribute.

The positive side of this business model is that it favours innovative companies, which should ultimately help patients. An unintended consequence is that once a company has a product licensed, any sales are effectively free money as the cost of production is very low, and the research and development has already been done—it is a 'sunk cost'—one that can never be recovered. This creates intense pressure to sell as much of the 'new' product as possible, whether or not it is a true advance compared to previous products.

From a company's point of view, it is vital to recoup its initial outlay in research and development as soon as possible, especially if there is a risk that the product may turn out not to be as good as everyone had previously thought, e.g. COX-2 inhibitors, ceramic joint replacements.

The pressure for sales results in an uneasy fusion of marketing and research in the later stages of development and testing. As these trials are industry sponsored, conflicts of interest may arise in the trial design and execution. One cannot be too sceptical when critically appraising such 'research'. Pharmaceutical companies spend twice as much on marketing as on research and development.

- What is the overall cost of the treatment, and what is the cost of not doing the treatment?

Performing these calculations necessitates value judgements on quality of life, which inevitably have a subjective element.

Engaging in futile or damaging treatment not only causes direct damage and waste, but also deprives another patient of an effective treatment. This makes the continuing presence of homeopathic hospitals funded by the NHS highly illogical, as anything that cannot prove superiority over placebo is just money diverted away from effective healthcare (Box 1.1.3).

Placebo

The placebo (Latin for 'I will please') effect is more than just what one attributes the apparent success of the 'snake oil' peddled by the quack. It is part of the psycho-social interaction that is present in any therapeutic interaction. It is heterogeneous, and has an interesting history.

The placebo effect appears governed by several factors, which appear additive:

- The patient: the patient's expectations of success influence the results, e.g. asthmatic patients experience symptomatic relief when using inert inhalers they believe to be bronchodilators
- The doctor: playing the role of an enthusiastic 'heroic rescuer' is associated with the highest placebo response, probably due to raising patient expectations. In alternative medicine, the lack of a scientific brake to this runaway enthusiasm goes some way to explain why ineffective treatments 'work'
- There is also likely to be a credibility factor: this can be exploited by looking like the 'consultant' in a private healthcare

advertisement—the usual cliché of being [male], avuncular, greying, white-coated, with some half-moon spectacles

- The doctor–patient interaction: patients with indeterminate symptoms respond better to positive behaviour and a definite diagnosis rather than uncertainty. If the patient has a significant investment, for example, by paying for the service, this is likely to increase their expectations of success
- The disease: chronic diseases with a fluctuating course, subjective symptoms with no objective pathology, anxiety, and common self-limiting diseases are all associated with a high placebo response
- Treatment and setting: tablets four times a day have a higher placebo effect than those twice a day (although possibly less compliance), and red tablets are more effective than white. Elaborate rituals and complex devices increase your chance of a good placebo effect, although this on its own does not justify an MR scan. Surgery itself has a marked placebo effect, demonstrated by the improvement experienced from a sham operation by Parkinson's disease sufferers in a stem-cell trial, and the efficacy of sham acupuncture.

It is sometimes argued that it does not matter what method is used, as long as the patient gets better. This sounds plausible, but if one is spending public funds on healthcare, one has a duty to ensure best value. Therefore treatments that cannot prove their effectiveness over a placebo should not be publicly funded.

By understanding and enhancing the placebo value in medicine, one can maximize patient satisfaction and the chances of patient compliance, both of which are likely to benefit your patient.

How do I know if I have done any good?

In the 1960s, prior to gastric acid-suppression drugs, gastric freezing was commonly performed. By freezing the gastric mucosa, acid-producing cells were damaged and acid formation was suppressed allowing the ulcer to heal and the patient was cured.

In an era where acid suppression drugs are cheap and effective, it is difficult to understand the disease burden of peptic ulceration to patients and society in general. It was found that reducing the temperature of the gastric mucosa to 5–10°C markedly reduced acid secretion. The exciting new technique of freezing the gastric mucosa was, in effect, a miracle cure for many patients.

In 1962, a trial of 24 patients by a past president of the American College of Surgeons showed that all had relief of symptoms of duodenal ulcers 6 weeks after having had a gastric freezing operation. More than 2500 gastric freezing machines were sold, and hundreds of thousands of freezings were carried out. Patient satisfaction was high, and a review of the procedure commented that 'the method is easy and the clinical results are astoundingly good'.

Although more than 100 articles about gastric freezing were produced in the following years, it was not until 1969 that a placebo-controlled trial of gastric freezing was published. This study, with approximately 75 patients in each arm had sufficient power to detect a 20% difference between the treatments, if one existed[1]. There was no difference between the treatment and control groups.

In short, a lot of time and energy and money had been expended on a placebo treatment. In addition active harm was done to patients—fatalities occurred in patients undergoing the treatment—and the financial harm was immense. Without the insight that properly conducted trials provide, doctors are little more than purveyors of snake-oil (Figure 1.1.2).

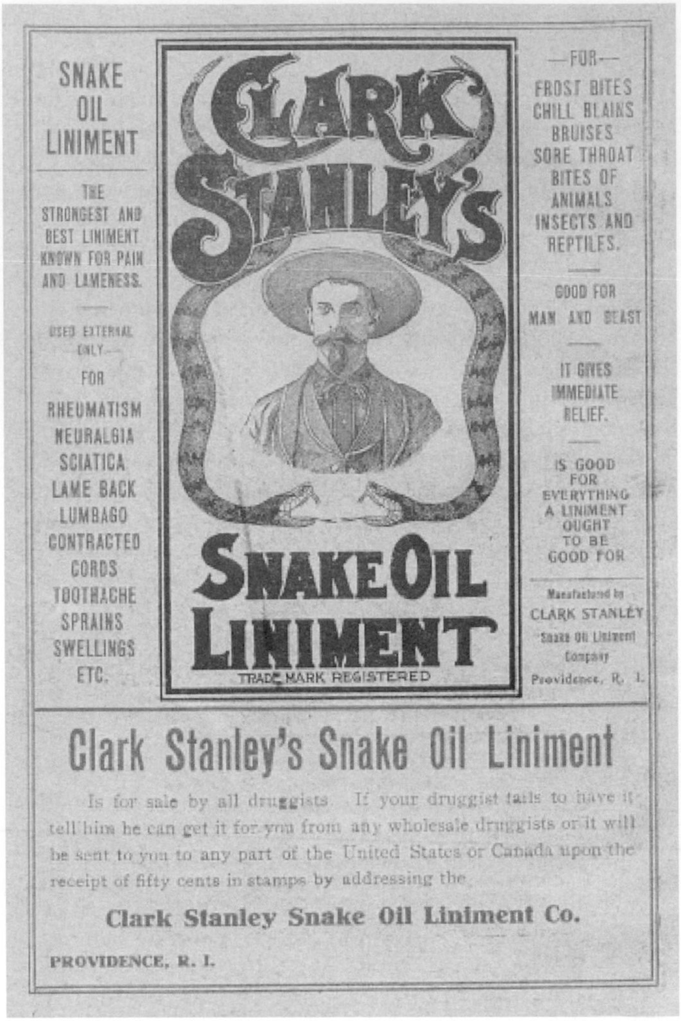

Fig. 1.1.2 A product whose only benefit can be a placebo effect.

Why do a trial?

To prove if one treatment is better than another. What sort of trial you do depends on what you are trying to prove:

- A *cohort* trial involves following groups of patients for a period of time and seeing what happens to them. For example, seeing how long different sorts of hip replacement last in different patients
- A *case–control* trial involves finding asymptomatic patients who match your symptomatic ones and seeing how they compare. For example, to understand the pathophysiology of osteoarthritis of the hip, you might find symptomatic patients and compare them with matched patients (age, weight, activity) who are not symptomatic
- A *controlled* trial is one where the active treatment (the one you are testing) is compared with either an inactive one (a placebo) or another sort of treatment, e.g. the current standard.

Comparing one sort of hip replacement with another would be a controlled trial

- A '*blinded*' trial is one where either the patient or the researcher does not know which treatment that patient is receiving. A '*double-blinded*' trial occurs when neither the researcher nor the patient knows which treatment the patient is receiving. Blinding reduces the risk of bias and this is an important part of trial design
- A *randomized* trial is one where the patients are randomly allocated to different treatments (Box 1.1.4). If one is going to do a trial, while the process of randomization is important; even more important is that the process by which patients are allocated is *concealed* from the researcher, e.g. sealed opaque envelopes.

Trial design

Trial design is more important than trial analysis: if the design of a trial is flawed, no amount of fancy analysis can remedy this. It is vital that you do some background reading and talk to someone with experience of trial design *before* you start collecting data. Any trial involving human subjects also needs ethical review before it can start.

A literature search should be performed to see whether anyone has already done the trial, but also to generate ideas about how best to perform the trial.

Box 1.1.4 Austin Bradford-Hill (1897–1991)

Sir Austin Bradford-Hill (Figure 1.1.3) pioneered the use of the randomized controlled trial in the assessment of streptomycin for the treatment of tuberculosis. Originally used in agricultural experiments, the randomized controlled trial is now the benchmark by which all interventional medical research is judged.

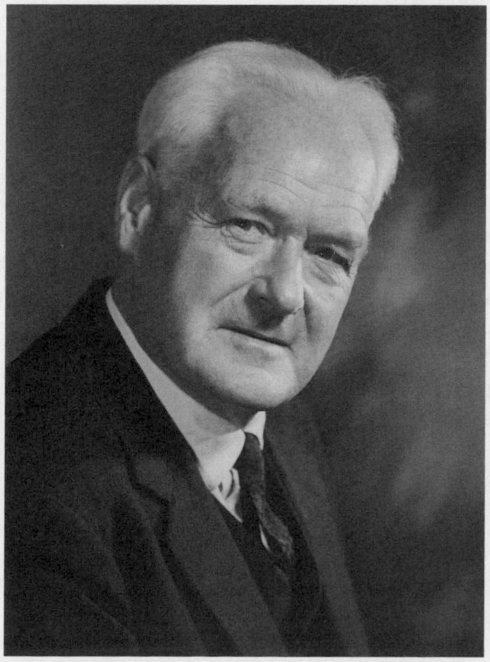

Fig. 1.1.3 Sir (Austin) Bradford ('Tony') Hill, by Godfrey Argent. © National Portrait Gallery, London.

When thinking about how many patients you will need for your trial, you need to consider incidence and prevalence. **Incidence** is the number of new cases of a condition, e.g. fractured neck of femur. **Prevalence** is the number of people with a condition at a particular point in time, e.g. back pain. If your disease is uncommon, recruiting a sufficient number of patients to be able to adequately power the study will be difficult.

Ethics and consent (Box 1.1.5)

Any trial will need ethical approval. All NHS Trusts and universities have a structure of ethics committee(s) for approving and monitoring clinical research. These committees are charged with ensuring that all research is of good quality and safeguards the rights of the patients and the reputation of the institution.

Informed patient consent is, excepting a few defined hyperacute situations, an essential component of any research, and the patient consent forms and accompanying information will be carefully scrutinized by the ethics committee.

Bias and confounding

Bias occurs when you fail to measure what you intend to/should measure. This may happen for a variety of different reasons—an example might be if you did a satisfaction survey of patients you saw in outpatients following hip surgery. You might achieve a very good satisfaction score, but by limiting your sample to those who are able to come to your outpatients, this may not be an accurate reflection of the true picture. Bias is therefore the inclusion of an error that distorts the trial in a non-random way (Box 1.1.6).

Confounding occurs when you fail to measure or spot an extraneous factor that accounts for your findings. Say you had a group of patients in whom you measured premature failure of hip prostheses and doughnut consumption, and found a strong relationship. Does this mean that doughnuts cause prosthesis failure? Or might it be that there is another variable that you have not measured that would explain this—a confounding factor?

Bias can be minimized by blinding, randomization, and concealment, but it is not always possible to randomize and blind in surgery.

Hawthorne effect

The Hawthorne effect is named after experiments done at the Hawthorne factory in the 1920s when factory workers were assembling relays for telecommunications equipment (Figure 1.1.4). Researchers looking for the optimal conditions for factory work increased the ambient light and found that production rates improved. They then reduced the ambient light and found that production rates improved again. Eventually the researchers deduced that the presence of the researchers was the over-riding influence on the workers' performance. Therefore the Hawthorne effect is that just by measuring something, one changes it. Having a

Box 1.1.5 Ethical principles

- Beneficence: do good
- Non-malfeasance: avoid doing harm
- Autonomy: respect for patients' wishes
- Justice: fairness.

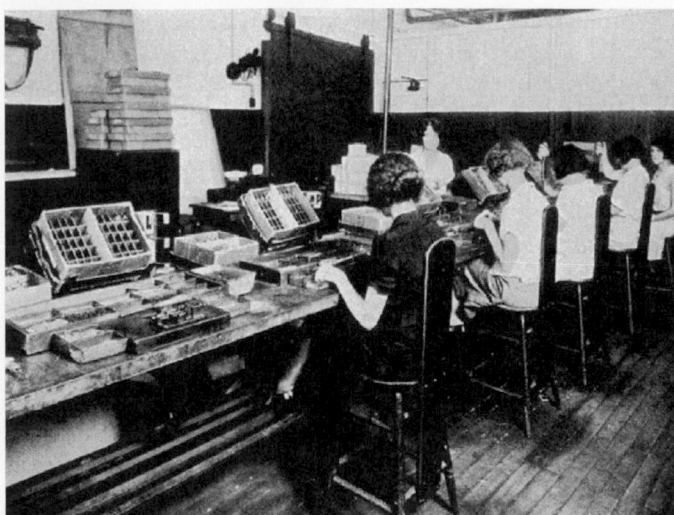

Fig. 1.1.4 Image of Hawthorne workers. From Gale, E.A. (2004). The Hawthorne studies – a fable for our times? *Quarterly Journal of Medicine*, **97**, 439–49.

control group ensures that the Hawthorne effect does not affect the results.

> The consumer of knowledge can never know what a dicky thing knowledge is until he has tried to produce it.
>
> F.J. Roethlisberger, investigator at Hawthorne.

Outcome measures

Objective or 'hard' outcomes, such as death, are preferred in research as there is little debate about their significance. Subjective or 'soft' outcomes, such as a change in a pain score, may not be valid or reliable across different populations of patients. If a validated measure of outcome is available, this makes design easier. If any of the measures used are in any way subjective, e.g. fracture angulation or code, it is best to have more than one independent observer and measure agreement between these observers.

If the 'hard' measure is rare or difficult to measure, then surrogate measures may be used. Death due to pulmonary embolism following joint replacement is quite rare, but using deep vein thrombosis (DVT) as a surrogate is fraught with difficulty as DVT is very common, but when limited to below the knee, does not seem to be associated with adverse outcomes.

Box 1.1.6 Common forms of bias

- **Selection** bias: the patients used may not be representative of the usual patient population group. The sickest patients are often excluded from trials
- **Observer** bias: there may be (unconscious) bias in the assessment by observers—minimized by blinding and concealment
- **Measurement** bias: flawed measurement may favour one group over another
- **Confirmation** bias: the tendency to look for factors that confirm rather than disprove our ideas
- **Publication** bias: trials with negative results are less likely to be published.

Where are all the randomized controlled trials in surgery?

The gold standard for pharmaceutical research is the double-blind placebo-controlled randomized controlled trial (RCT). RCTs are also the gold standard in surgery, and provide a definitive answer, e.g. for arthroscopic surgery in osteoarthritis. However, RCTs of any sort are uncommon in surgery. This is partly because in order to ensure the full placebo effect in the control group, one must perform a sham operation, and this is ethically and practically difficult. A pragmatic alternative is to randomize based on expertise—if there are two groups of surgeons available with expertise in variants of a surgical procedure, one can randomize patients between these two groups.

Another technique that is used to deal with the difficulty in conducting large RCTs is to use meta-analysis to combine the results of similar small trials.

Meta-analysis

In an ideal world, all medical and surgical practice would be based on evidence from well-conducted, multicentre, double-blinded, randomized placebo-controlled trials. Unfortunately such trials are very expensive to organize, and therefore are only performed to answer the most large-scale health questions, e.g. the CRASH (Corticosteroid Randomisation After Significant Head injury) and CRASH2 trials relating to the role of tranexamic acid in patients with major haemorrhage from trauma.

Meta-analysis is a structured review of all the trials relating to a particular research question. It is used when there are many small trials that relate to a research question, but none of them have the power to resolve the question on their own. The quality of evidence from each trial is weighted in a structured and predetermined way to allow a definitive assessment to be made. Meta-analysis may have the power to quantify benefit or harm that smaller trials may not be able to do, particularly if these effects are uncommon.

Careful judgement is necessary to combine the results of several trials in a way that does not prejudice the final result. The Cochrane Collaboration (Box 1.1.7) is an independent organization that organizes and validates meta-analyses of clinical questions.

Intravenous colloid

In the 1990s, intravenous colloid fluids, e.g. Haemaccel, Gelofusine were widely used for resuscitation as they were effective at improving a patient's blood pressure quickly, and the large protein molecules did not leak out of damaged capillaries as quickly as crystalloid. The downside of this is that once they did leak out, they tended to cause resistant tissue oedema, which is bad if the tissue involved is the brain.

In 1998 a meta-analysis performed by the Cochrane Collaboration suggested that colloids gave no benefit over crystalloid fluids, e.g. saline, and appeared to cause harm (up to 5% increase in mortality) in critically ill patients. This, together with their high cost (20 times that of crystalloid), are why colloids are not now used in resuscitation.

How can I use the medical literature to improve my practice?

The volume of medical literature is vast—there are more than 40 000 biomedical journals, and this number doubles every 20 years. The quality does not. How can you filter this soup of raw

Box 1.1.7 Archie Cochrane (1909–1988)

The Cochrane Collaboration (http://www.cochrane.org) is named after Professor Archibald Cochrane (Figure 1.1.5). Regarded as the father of evidence-based medicine, he firstly trained as a laboratory scientist, and then studied medicine before the Second World War.

Through his work on infectious disease he became interested in epidemiology and wrote an influential report on how to improve the NHS.

The report's stark logic championed the use of the RCT to ensure the best use of NHS funding. The book had a profound effect on medical thinking and policymaking.

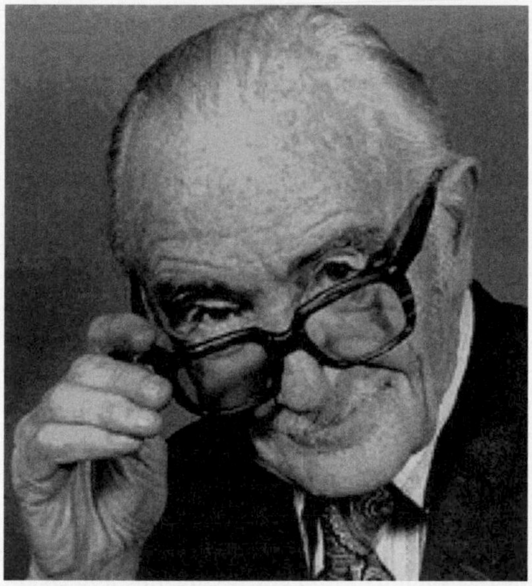

Fig. 1.1.5 Professor Archibald Cochrane.

data? How can you work out whether something is true or not? If true, can you apply this new knowledge to your daily practice?

The Bulstrode criteria for medical literature are short and sharp:

- *Do I understand it?* What is the author claiming?
- *Do I believe it?* Are there significant flaws in the design, execution, or analysis?
- *Do I care?* Is this relevant to my practice?

While the first and last of these depend on subjective judgements, the key skill is the ability to read a paper, spot flaws, and be able to judge whether it should change your clinical practice.

Professor David Sackett, one of the originators of evidence-based medicine, developed a set of criteria that expands on the Bulstrode criteria to help you evaluate whether a trial is valid and applicable to your practice (Box 1.1.8).

Box 1.1.8 Sackett's tests

Was the assignment of patients really random?

If patients were not assigned to treatment and control groups randomly, and/or the assignation not concealed adequately from those treating and assessing the patient, then it is likely that an unacceptable level of bias will be introduced.

Were all clinically relevant outcomes reported?

If, in a purely hypothetical situation, a new treatment centre starts up next to your hospital and its surgeon malaligns the hip prostheses, a subjective measure such as patient satisfaction on discharge might be good, but a measure of important long-term function such as return to employment or time to failure/revision might be poor.

Were the study patients similar to your own?

If the patients entering the study were markedly different from your own patients, it may be that the conclusions of the study might not be relevant to your situation. A shoulder reduction technique that has been validated on Japanese patients with an average body mass index of 20 may be less helpful when you are faced with a 200-kg Hell's Angel with their first dislocation.

Were the results clinically important?

If a difference was demonstrated by this treatment, was the difference large enough and important enough to justify changing your practice?

Is the therapeutic manoeuvre feasible in your practice?

It is necessary to think about whether the therapy being tested is viable in your clinical practice. Even if not, you may be able to plan to include it in a future service expansion.

Were all patients who entered the study accounted for at its conclusion?

If one was running a trial on behalf of a commercial sponsor, and some patients had inconvenient results, some people might be tempted to label these patients as 'lost to follow-up' and discount them from the analysis. Trials published now should include a CONSORT diagram: this is essentially a flowchart that demonstrates what happened to all the patients entered into the trial (http://www.consort-statement.org). Reputable trials are prospectively registered with published protocols (http://www.controlled-trials.com).

Evidence-based medicine

The conscientious, explicit and judicious use of current best evidence in making decisions about the care of individual patients.

The term 'evidence-based medicine' was coined by a group of physicians at McMaster University, Ontario, in the 1980s. The aim was to encapsulate the information search and analysis techniques that had been learned from epidemiology in a form that could be used at the bedside. Although this may seem like second nature now, this was in an era before the Internet, PubMed, Google Scholar, and online journals.

One of the problems in traditional medical practice is that doctors tend to carry on doing the things they were taught in medical school. One of the arguments against old-style medical school curricula was that it did not teach the skills for life-long learning.

The integration of the science behind 'evidence-based' practice into the medical school curriculum has ensured that future generations of doctors will be able to identify and challenge outdated or dangerous practice from an objective viewpoint.

Levels of evidence

With the many claims and counter claims of patients, healthcare providers, researchers, pharmaceutical and device manufacturers, one needs a league table to be able to work out which evidence trumps others (Table 1.1.1).

How can I ensure that this evidence is incorporated in practice?

It is all very well having found and assessed the best evidence, but you have been wasting your time if you cannot put it into practice. Approaching people and telling them that their practice is out of date and/or dangerous does not always result in the desired outcome (see Bristol, discussed under Medical Harm earlier).

Unless there is a pressing urgency, e.g. ongoing risk of significant harm to patients, it is necessary to prove that there is a problem with the current system. The way to do this is through audit. Audit is different from research in that audit is ensuring optimal usage of current knowledge, whereas research is about creating new knowledge.

An audit is performed to measure the organization's performance against agreed standard measures of performance. These might be international or national guidelines (e.g. National Institute for Health and Clinical Excellence, NICE), 'best practice', or College standards.

Guidelines are advisory summaries of evidence that are used to guide treatment. They are not supposed to be rigidly interpreted, but if one is going outside their advice, one should have good reasons. Protocols are designed to be rigid: they are standardized routines that can be used to streamline and minimize defects in a process. Both guidelines and protocols have inherent dangers in that they tend to stop people thinking about what they are doing, and may stifle innovation.

Any guideline or protocol must be both exhaustive and exclusive. It must cover all eventualities that will occur, and must reliably exclude other conditions that may look similar. Many protocols, elegantly simple in their first draft, can become so complex as to be unworkable when revised after testing. This is a measure of the inherent complexity within healthcare, which is why we need doctors who have the broad range of knowledge and skills to manage these problems, rather than just technicians.

> Make everything as simple as possible, but no simpler.
> Albert Einstein.

Audit

Audit is the process by which we ensure that we are meeting the standards that we set ourselves. Audit differs from research in that research is looking for new knowledge. Audit is about ensuring that present knowledge is being used in the most productive fashion. Audit may be used to generate and refine research questions, but is usually used in the context of a quality improvement framework.

Audit can be prospective, but is usually retrospective—at least in the first instance. For example, to audit time to theatre for open fractures, an easy way would be to collect all patients with a discharge diagnosis of open fracture. However, this would miss patients who had died or been transferred. A better way would be to prospectively collect the data on patients who come in through the Emergency Department with open fractures.

Types of audit:

- Basic clinical audit: throughput, morbidity, mortality, outcome, adverse events
- Patient audit: satisfaction survey
- Notes review
- Benchmarking: comparison between units e.g. TARN (Trauma Audit Research Network—http://www.tarn.ac.uk)
- National audits: e.g. *Trauma: Who cares?* (2007) (National Confidential Enquiry into Patient Outcome and Death, http://www.ncepod.org.uk)

Audit is an important part of Clinical Governance, being the way that clinicians measure their own performance against their peers,

Table 1.1.1 Levels of evidence for interventional studies

Level	Therapy
1a	Systematic review of similar RCTs
1b	Single RCT of good quality
1c	All or none (e.g. all treated patients cured/died)
2a	Systematic review of similar cohort studies
2b	Single cohort study
2c	'Outcomes' research; ecological studies
3a	Systematic review of similar case-control studies
3b	Single case–control study
4	Case-series, poor quality cohort, and case–control studies
5	Expert opinion or based on physiology or lab research

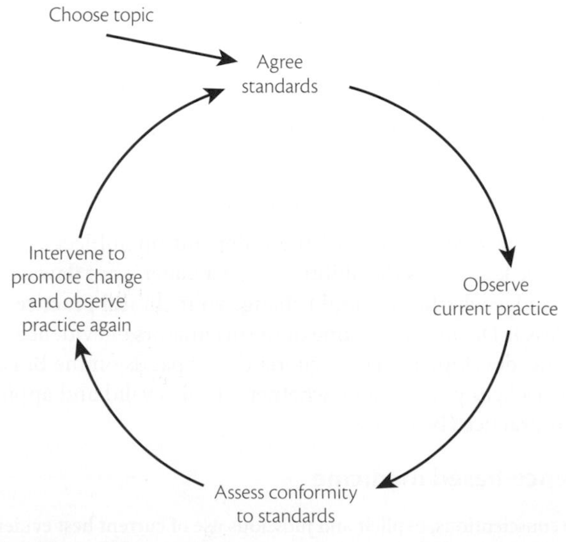

Fig. 1.1.6 The audit loop.

and also a structured way of demonstrating necessary service development. Audit data can be compared against agreed standards/national guidelines e.g. NICE/Scottish Intercollegiate Guidelines Network (SIGN)/'best practice' from the literature or College.

The most difficult part of the audit loop is usually making the change, and this is why audit usually takes place within the framework of Clinical Governance. This provides the oversight and a mechanism for pushing through the process changes necessary. If the audit requires a questionnaire, time spent researching the format and construction of questionnaires will substantially increase the quality of the information garnered.

Clinical Governance

This rather nebulous term is derived from the notion of Corporate Governance, used in business. Corporate Governance is the process of ensuring that the people who run the company (senior management) act in accordance with the interests of the people that own the company (the shareholders, represented by the Board).

Clinical Governance on the other hand means the process of showing that the work you do is as close to best practice as is feasible, and therefore is a quality assurance process. It was defined as:

> A framework through which NHS organisations are accountable for continuously improving the quality of their services and safeguarding high standards of care by creating an environment in which excellence in clinical care will flourish.
>
> Scally and Donaldson (1998).

From a clinician's viewpoint, Clinical Governance is important, as apart from clinical adverse incidents it is the only forum in which to demonstrate and resolve problems with clinical service delivery. Clinical Governance incorporates what were Morbidity and Mortality meetings, but should be proactive, identifying problems before they result in significant patient harm, incorporating best practice and a framework for service development/quality assurance.

Diagnosis and investigation

Your decision as to whether to offer a surgical solution to a patient's problem is based on clinical diagnosis and investigations. An expert should have insight into their own process of assessment, to be able to teach others but also to understand how and why things go wrong.

Clinical diagnosis

Much time, ink, and paper has been expended in pursuit of understanding the process of diagnosis. The short answer is 'we don't know'. However, some basic principles seem to be that:

- It takes about 10 000 hours to become an expert at something (chess, golf, orthopaedic surgery)
- Experts use pattern recognition to make diagnoses
- Teaching pattern recognition to non-experts will result in superficial expertise, but without the resilience and depth of knowledge to be able to deal with new situations safely
- Novices either work forwards from the history and examination, or backwards from diagnoses, or both. It may be that the ability to think through problems both forward and backwards is a precursor to expertise
- Problem solving is largely content-specific, i.e. being good at one clinical area does not necessarily imply that someone is good at another
- Clinical vignettes—examples of patients are integrated with the basic scientific knowledge and assembled by novices into mental models of diseases. This 'case-based learning' is not a substitute for hands-on learning, but may accelerate the rate of acquisition of mental models.

Clinical reasoning

> There is no such thing as clinical reasoning; there is no one best way through a problem. The more one studies the clinical expert, the more one marvels at the complex and multidimensional components of knowledge and skill that she or he brings to bear on the problem, and the amazing adaptability she must possess to achieve the goal of effective care.
>
> Norman (2005).

Why does clinical reasoning go wrong?

Research into clinical reasoning helps us understand some of the processes that underlie clinical decision-making.

- *Framing bias*: this is the context in which you see a patient. If you saw a patient with a hot swollen ankle in the Emergency Department, you might think of a fracture or septic arthritis, but in an outpatient clinic, a rheumatological condition would probably be your first thought

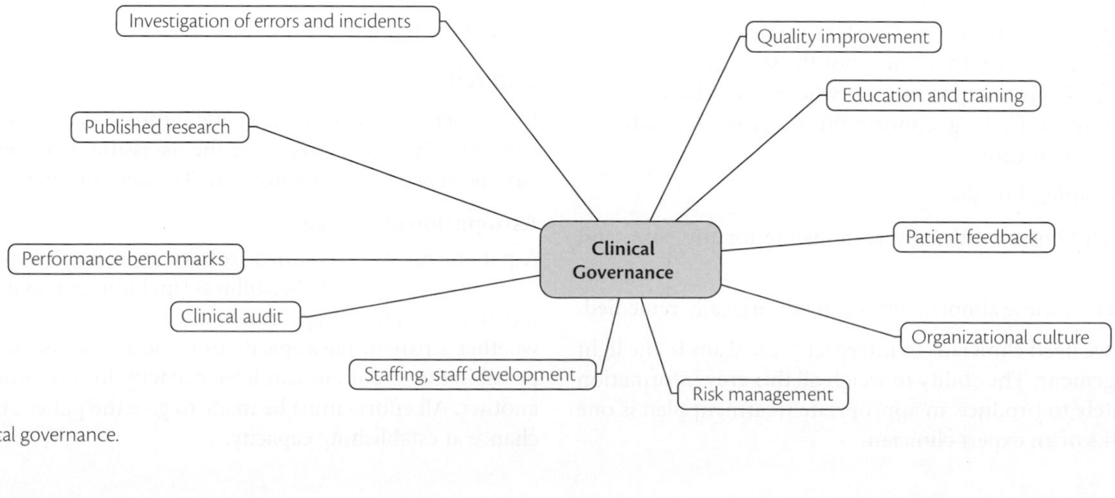

Fig. 1.1.7 Clinical governance.

- *Availability bias*: is all the information necessary to make the decision available?
- *Representativeness bias*: is the information used to make the decision representative of the true situation? We tend to over-weight information from sources we believe reliable and our cultural values may also affect the way we use information to make judgements
- *Anchor bias*: is the starting point for one's assessment rational. If one has seen two osteosarcomas in 1 week, this may alter your perception of the likelihood of further such cases, making you more likely to spot one, and may make overdiagnosis likely
- *Overconfidence*: this can be a response to the lack of certainty in a situation. If the risk inherent in a procedure is ignored because the person doing the procedure regards them as insignificant, this will flaw the consent process and make it invalid. The courts have made it abundantly clear that risk is what the patient perceives, not what the clinician thinks the patient perceives or should perceive.

If a trainee has persistent problems with poor clinical judgement, then this is usually handled through their training programme. If a colleague shows poor clinical judgement, this should be taken up through the Director/Divisional Director/Medical Director. If these avenues do not resolve the problem, in the UK there is the National Clinical Assessment Service, part of the National Patient Safety Agency (http://www.npsa.nhs.uk).

How do you use investigations?

As investigations have become more complex and are used earlier in the disease process, their flaws have become more apparent and caution is needed in interpreting the results. There are risks and benefits with all investigations but as the treating doctor, there is a duty of care to use them appropriately. Some tests may give misleading results if used in unsuitable groups of patients.

A patient with longstanding mechanical back pain has an MR scan of their back. An abnormality is noted but is perceived by the radiologist to be the result of normal wear and tear, but is mentioned in the report. The patient and their family may put pressure on the doctors because 'something must be done'. An operation may be performed that is both unsuccessful and/or has complications in the surgery, anaesthesia, or recovery period. Significant medical and financial harm has occurred to both the patient and society.

In this situation, the scan could be said to be a *false positive*—the scan implies that there is a significant abnormality that is responsible for the patient's pain, whereas in fact this is not the case. It could reasonably be argued that it was not the scan that was a false positive, but the diagnostic process as a whole. The MR scan may be very accurate at finding abnormalities. However, what is required is a scan that can:

- Find abnormalities, but also
- Predict which abnormalities are responsible for the pain, and further
- Predict which of these abnormalities can be surgically remedied.

This is why we need clinicians to interpret these scans in the light of clinical judgement. The ability to weigh all this grey information factors accurately to produce an appropriate treatment plan is one of the hallmarks of an expert clinician.

Both society and individuals seem far more tolerant of false positives than false negatives. It is seen as perfectly acceptable to provide too much treatment rather than not enough, whereas in reality both may result in similar rates of harm in the widest sense. A good, if politically charged, example of this would be screening for breast cancer:

> For every 2000 women invited for screening throughout 10 years, one will have her life prolonged. In addition, 10 healthy women, who would not have been diagnosed if there had not been screening, will be diagnosed as breast cancer patients and will be treated unnecessarily.
>
> Gotzsche and Nielsen (2006).

Such information is difficult to communicate to the public. By way of contrast, one does not have to open too many newspapers to find sensational reports of a catastrophic 'missed diagnosis': these are the opposite: the *false negative*.

These two situations, the false positive and false negative, can be put into a table together with the true positive and true negative (Table 1.1.2).

Table 1.1.2 Confusion matrix

		Reality	
		+	–
Test	+	True +	False +
	–	False –	True –

Apart from the cost, anxiety, and unnecessary investigation that a false positive test entails, there is another form of damage that of which an orthopaedic practitioner should be particularly aware. The radiation dose used in diagnostic testing, particularly in computed tomography (CT), is very large (Table 1.1.3).

The use of the 'scanogram' (CT head/neck/chest/abdomen/pelvis) in blunt trauma is associated with significant risks of lethal malignancy—approximately 1:500 for children and 1:3000 in adults. Patients have a right to understand the risks and benefits of investigations that are being performed, and the clinician has a duty to ensure they have access to information to make those choices.

Consent

Consent is the legal framework used to cover the agreement between a patient and a doctor to undertake a procedure. There are local rules for how consent is obtained and variation between different countries' legal frameworks; therefore general principles will be discussed.

Capacity

For consent to be informed a patient must have capacity to give this consent. The rules governing the assessment of mental capacity have been clarified in English law. The key components of this are:

Assumption of capacity

A patient must be assumed to have capacity, irrespective of age/disability/behaviour/beliefs/illness (including mental illness) or the fact that you may disagree with their decision. Each decision as to whether a patient has capacity must be a new assessment, and it is possible that a patient can have capacity in one situation but not another. All efforts must be made to give the patient the maximum chance at establishing capacity.

Table 1.1.3 Radiation doses from different procedures

Diagnostic procedure	Dose (mSv)	CXRs	Background radiation
XR limb	0.01	0.5	1.5 days
XR chest (PA)	0.02	1	2.4 days
XR lumbar spine	1.3	65	6 months
CT head	2.0	100	9 months
CT abdomen/pelvis	10	500	3.3 years
CT scanogram	40	1000	6.5 years

CT, computed tomography; CXR, chest x-ray; PA, posteroanterior; XR, x-ray.

Tests for capacity

The Mental Capacity Act (2005) uses four tests to establish capacity. The patient must be able to:

- *Understand* the information necessary for them to be able to take a rational decision about consent
- *Retain* the information long enough for them to be able to
- *Weigh* the information and be able to
- *Communicate* a decision about the consent to others.

If the doctor's opinion is that the patient lacks capacity to consent, and it is not an emergency, then medicolegal advice should be sought, through the hospital's usual channels.

Emergency situations

In an emergency, one may do what is necessary to preserve life and limb, but no more. Verbal consent should be sought, but is not essential.

Advance directives may still over-ride life-saving treatments, but only if they specifically include life-threatening situations.

Advance directives

Advance directives are now legally binding in parts of the UK. In an emergency, an advance directive may be over-ridden if the patient's condition is life threatening, unless the directive *specifically refers* to life-threatening condition being included, e.g. blood transfusion by Jehovah's Witnesses.

If there is doubt about a local situation, medicolegal advice should be sought.

Obtaining consent

Informed consent does not mean: 'sign here and I will do the operation'. Consent is a two-way process and may need to include negotiation about what will and will not be performed, and a frank discussion of the likely outcomes of these actions. Consent should include an understanding of what will occur if the operation does not take place.

Part of the process of negotiation is to manage the patient's expectations. If a patient has unrealistic expectations of surgery, this is the time to address this. Failure to understand the risks and likely outcomes is far more likely to lead to dissatisfaction and adverse outcomes for all concerned.

What risks need to be disclosed?

The notion of adequate risk disclosure has changed in the last few years from that of what a doctor deems necessary to what the patient deems necessary. The old legal definition of 'acceptable medical practice' (the Bolam test) being defined as acting 'in accordance with practice accepted by a responsible body of medical opinion' has been superseded by a patient-focused test—'what a reasonable patient would want to know' (Box 1.1.9).

Risks should be disclosed if the risk is more common than 1:1000, or is very serious—death or serious disability. The advice about risks must be recorded on the consent form. Risk should be numerically quantified and documented whenever possible. If a patient enquires about a specific risk they must be advised of the likelihood of this occurring.

Guidance on consent was published by the General Medical Council in 2008, which takes account of these changes and is freely available through their website (http://www.gmc-uk.org).

Communicating risk to patients

There are many examples of the public failing to understand medical risk or misinterpreting information, sometimes due to sensational or misreporting of the media, e.g. risks from MMR immunization.

Expression of risk in percentages is a good start, but may not be readily interpreted by patients with linguistic or educational barriers to understanding. Other approaches to help patients understand risk include the use of:

- *Crowd diagrams*: these are a visual representation of a population of patients with a condition and the number of positive/negative outcomes can be demonstrated by shading an appropriate number of these (Figure 1.1.8)
- *Number needed to treat* (NNT): as illustrated in the breast cancer screening example given earlier. This is an expression of the number of patients that need to be treated (or screened) to give

Box 1.1.9 Risk is defined by the patient, not the doctor

Chester v Afshar [2002]

A UK neurosurgeon consented a patient for a multilevel discectomy. Prior to this the patient had been clear that she had wanted to avoid surgery. The patient sustained cauda equina damage during surgery. The court found that the doctor had been negligent by not specifically warning the patient of the 1–2% risk of serious neurological damage, as this would have dissuaded the patient from surgery. The Law Lords commented:

> A surgeon owes a general duty to a patient to warn him or her in general terms of possible serious risks involved in the procedure. The only qualification is that there may be wholly exceptional cases where objectively in the best interests of the patient the surgeon may be excused from giving a warning...In modern law medical paternalism no longer rules and a patient has a prima facie right to be informed by a surgeon of a small, but well-established, risk of serious injury as a result of surgery.

Rogers v Witaker [1992]

An Australian ophthalmologist consented a patient for surgery. The patient specifically asked about the risk of damage to the 'good' eye, and was not told of this risk (approximately 1:14 000). Sympathetic ophthalmia occurred, making the patient blind. The doctor was found to be negligent.

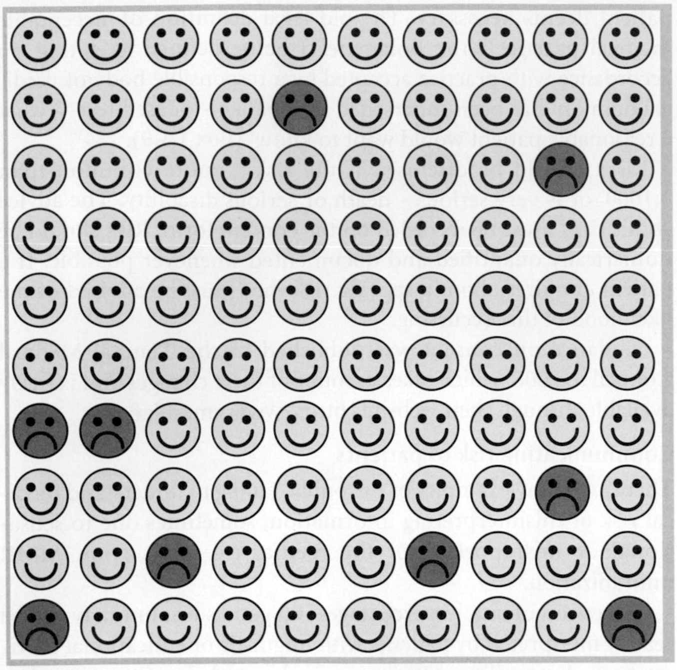

Fig. 1.1.8 Crowd diagram.

one unit of benefit/harm, e.g. NNT of primary repair for traumatic shoulder dislocation to prevent recurrent dislocation over 10 years is approximately 2. This means that two people have the operation to stop one person from having recurrent dislocations

- *'Bone age' or 'joint age'*: this describes the patient's condition by using an age-related comparison, e.g. 'You have the joints/bone density of an 80-year-old'. Although NNT appeals more to doctors rationalizing decision-making, it seems that presenting information in an age-related way personalizes the risk in a way patients can more easily understand.

Teaching and learning

As an expert clinician, you have a role and a duty to educate. You did not become an expert without the educational input of a large number of teachers. From Figure 1.1.9, as a conscious competent at the end of postgraduate training, you will be at the peak of your educational ability as a 'conscious competent'.

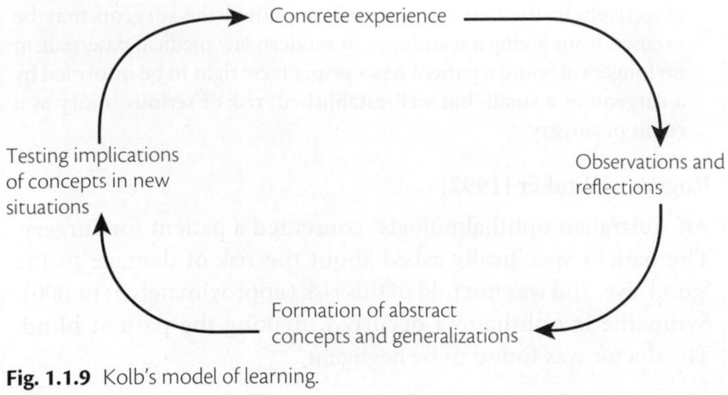

Fig. 1.1.9 Kolb's model of learning.

The danger is the ease of slipping into being an unconscious incompetent—you can do the job, but don't know why you are doing what you are doing. Regular teaching helps ensure that knowledge and skills are kept up to date. We can all remember inspirational teachers who appeared to effortlessly communicate complex ideas in a fun way. Good teaching does not just happen—it is the result of careful preparation of content, structure, and presentation, and the following section aims to help with this.

The model of learning developed by Kolb is helpful in considering medical teaching. Trainees are generally not short of concrete, i.e. real-life, experiences, but the trick is to teach in such a way as to build on these experiences and incorporate the theory and facts from textbooks into deeper knowledge.

When planning teaching, there should have some overall *aim* stated—what should the student be able to do/understand at the end? This aim can be broken down into component *goals*—specific chunks of learning that build together to achieve the aim. Telling students these aims and goals at the beginning of teaching helps them understand how the information is going to fit together into something that will be useful. This increases the chance that teaching becomes learning.

Practical skills

The most common teaching an orthopaedic surgeon will do is teaching practical skills, and for this it is helpful to have a minimal structure that helps organize how you transmit the information in a way in that is likely to be understood and retained.

- Explain
- Demonstrate
- Imitate
- Practice.

By explaining what you are going to do, and breaking it into stages, you allow the learner to look for the different stages when you put them together as a demonstration. The learner then imitates what you have demonstrated, and then practises this to a level of competence.

Feedback

When you are teaching practical skills it is important to be able to help the person you are teaching to improve. If you think back through your training, you will be able to think of times when this has not been done particularly well. A good acronym for this is PQRS:

- *Praise*: insist that the student identifies at least one thing they have done well
- *Question*: ask the student what they would do differently next time
- *Reflect*: ask the student and/or group to explore other ways of improving performance
- *Summarize*: the student should be able to identify one thing they have learned.

Small-group learning

While lectures are superficially efficient at teaching, the amount of learning is highly variable, and difficult for the lecturer to gauge.

Dividing large groups into small groups for teaching has many advantages:

- Uncertainty and lack of understanding are more likely to be voiced in a small group, and will be either corrected or voiced by the group
- Lazy people are forced to contribute. Quiet people are more likely to contribute (less of a problem with orthopaedic trainees)
- It is possible for the teacher to evaluate how much the student has understood
- It is possible to integrate other skills such as researching evidence and presentation skills.

Small-group teaching is initially quite challenging for many teachers as there is an implicit loss of control of the whole process, and there is a danger the whole thing goes wrong (very rare, providing the task is well structured).

Specific small-group techniques that may be useful are:

- *Problem-based learning*: give small groups of students a clinical problem to solve, and send them away to research it and produce a presentation based on their research for all the groups
- *Buzz groups*: when you are giving a lecture, create a task or activity that people do, initially on their own, and then discuss with their neighbour(s). Pick a few volunteers to find out the results and incorporate these back into your presentation. This acts as a break, wakes people up, allows you to test that they have understood what you are talking about, and allows you to incorporate the students' ideas into your teaching.

Bedside teaching

Bedside teaching is a particularly difficult skill to do well, yet is the one that has the most chance of inspiring students. A common complaint from students is that they rarely have the opportunity to examine patients with a senior doctor to guide them and give feedback.

Bedside teaching gives an opportunity for the expert to articulate their thought processes so that students may learn how an expert weighs different factors to make decisions. It provides an excellent opportunity to involve the patient both in decisions regarding their management and in the education process, and the evidence is that patients appreciate and enjoy this.

Crimes against PowerPoint

The ubiquity of electronic presentation using data projectors has spawned a number of habits that can detract from learning. There are a number of things that you can do to lessen the pain for the audience:

- The productive attention span is about 20 minutes. After this time do something different and interactive like using a buzz group activity
- Format your presentation in PowerPoint 97 and bring on a USB drive and CD, but also email it to yourself as a backup. Beware video in a presentation, as there are many different subformats which are usually incompatible. If you are planning to use video, it is safest to always take your own laptop
- The most readable format of projection text is white or yellow text on a dark background (blue or green). Red text may look good on a screen, but projects poorly. This is particularly important for people with poor vision/colour-blindness. Pure white backgrounds are tiring for the audience and should be avoided
- Use the 6 × 6 rule: do not put more than six lines of six words on each slide. This will prevent you just reading each slide, which is very annoying for the audience
- End with a 'take home message' summarizing your talk in *three* points in *nine* seconds and (approximately) *27* words. This is the 'sound bite' packaging of key information that you want people to remember from your presentation.

Assessment

Assessment is the term given to establishing whether the students have learned anything or not. Although this may sound obvious, care needs to be given to establishing the purpose of the assessment. Is the purpose:

- To rank the students in order of performance?
- To establish which students have reached a minimum standard of competence to go on in their training?

Training has generally moved away from the former towards the latter. Assessment should therefore be tied very closely to the curriculum: students should have a very clear idea of what is to be tested and the pass rate should be very high, as only the essentials—the core curriculum—must be tested, but they must be passed.

Teachers are always worried about examination materials, particularly practical (OSCE—objective structured clinical examination) stations getting out into the students' domain. This is going to happen anyway. The consequences of this can be minimized, and the effect harnessed by giving open access to certain assessment materials. For example, by publishing model OSCE stations with their marking schema, one ensures that the overall performance is much improved, this is: 'using the tail to wag the dog'.

Evaluation

A simple way of evaluating education is to use an anonymous questionnaire. Questionnaires need careful construction to ensure that you receive valid and reliable responses.

Summary

> Medicine is a science of uncertainty and an art of probability.
> Sir William Osler (1904).

This chapter has provided an overview of some of the key supporting skills for expert clinical practice. There is a limited amount of material that can be included in such a textbook as this, and therefore this chapter is little more than a dégustation menu.

The hope is that reading this chapter will equip the reader to go out and negotiate some of the uncertainties that will face them in everyday practice, and also to act as a roadmap for further reading for those who are looking for more information.

Further reading

Cochrane, A.L. (1972). *Effectiveness and Efficiency: Random Reflections on Health Services*. London: Nuffield Provincial Hospitals Trust.

General Medical Council (2008). *Consent: Patients and Doctors Making Decisions Together.* London: General Medical Council.

Gotzsche, P.C. and Nielsen, M. (2006). Screening for breast cancer with mammography. *Cochrane Database Systematic Reviews*, **4**, CD001877.

Mayer, T. and Cates, R.J. (1999). Service excellence in health care. *Journal of the American Medical Association,* **282**, 1281–3.

Norman, G. (2005). Research in clinical reasoning: past history and current trends. *Medical Education,* **39**, 418–27.

Portney, L.G. and Watkins, M.P. (2008). *Foundations of Clinical Research: Applications to Practice.* Upper Saddle River, NJ: Prentice Hall.

Robinson, W. (1974). Conscious competency – the mark of a competent instructor. *Personnel Journal,* **53**, 538–9.

Sackett, D.L., Haynes, R.B., and Tugwell, P. (1991). *Clinical Epidemiology: A Basic Science for Clinical Medicine.* Boston: Little, Brown.

Scally, G. and Donaldson, L.J. (1998). The NHS's 50th anniversary. Clinical governance and the drive for quality improvement in the new NHS in England. *British Medical Journal,* **317**, 61–5.

1.2

Classification and outcome measures

Hemant Pandit

Summary points

Classification is needed to:

- Plan treatment
- Communicate between clinicians
- Carry out research.

If it is to be useful it needs to be:

- Clear
- Reproducible
- Relevant.

Introduction

The field of trauma and orthopaedics is ripe with various classification systems and different outcome measures. It is important for a clinician to be conversant with them as they help in communication of ideas, sharing of opinion, and measurement of clinical outcomes. Many organizations perceive them as useful indicators of quality of practice, which is crucial in delivery of quality healthcare. In addition, the day-to-day practice needs to be open to external scrutiny, analysis, comparison for clinical improvement, legislation, and performance assessment by healthcare providers, healthcare system payers, and government and voluntary regulatory bodies. These reasons necessitate the availability of good classification systems and robust outcome measures.

Classification

Classification may be defined as a system whereby one can arrange or organize any number of people or things (seen as a division or a group) based on type, quality, characteristics, etc. (Box 1.2.1).

Box 1.2.1 Classification

- A system for organizing so that high-level decisions can be made
- Should be easy to use, reliable, reproducible, and clinically useful.

Any classification system should be clinically useful, reproducible, validated, easy to use, and, most importantly, have appropriate divisions to separate from each other all the (known) types or grades of the condition, it is meant to classify.

Biomedical studies are either experimental (the investigator assigned the exposures) or observational (investigator did not assign the exposures). An experimental study can be a randomized or a non-randomized controlled trial depending upon whether the allocation to a particular group was at random or not. An observational study can be analytical or descriptive depending upon whether there is a comparison group or not. The analytical studies can be further classified into cohort study (exposure precedes outcome), case–control study (outcome precedes exposure, e.g. identify an outcome and work backwards as to what might have caused the outcome), and a cross-sectional study (exposure and outcome occur at the same time).

Most reports of outcome in orthopaedics are observational studies. Whilst these studies give useful indications of outcome, in most cases they are open to a variety of bias. Bias may be defined as a non-random, systematic error in the design or conduct of a study that may result in mistaken inference about association or causation. In the orthopaedic literature, common types of bias include recall, selection, sampling, and publication bias.

Table 1.2.1 Classification of biomedical research reports

1. Longitudinal studies
A. Prospective
1. Deliberate intervention
a) Randomized (RCT)
b) Non-randomized
2. Observational studies
A. Prospective (deliberate intervention or observational)
B. Retrospective (deliberate intervention or observational)
3. Cross-sectional
A. Disease description
B. Diagnosis and staging
C. Disease process

Modified from Bailar and Mosteller (1986); Campbell and Machin (1993).

Box 1.2.2 Types of study

- Observational: good for creating hypotheses, weak for drawing conclusions
- Cohort: exposure precedes outcome
- Case–control: outcome precedes exposure
- Cross-sectional: simultaneous exposure and outcome.

The double blind, prospective, randomized clinical trial (RCT) is the gold standard of an experimental study design (Table 1.2.1). Randomization ensures that allocation to the comparison groups is unbiased. An RCT usually requires large numbers of patients whose diagnoses and severity grading is relatively similar (narrow entry criteria). Stirrat and colleagues in 1992 spelled out some of the problems that can arise with RCTs in surgery: 'Placebo operations are unethical. Blinding of the patient is usually difficult if not impossible. Surgical skills vary between surgeons and also the "learning curve" plays an important role when new operations are being compared to existing ones' (Box 1.2.2).

Outcome measures

Outcome measures are vital to the setting of standards of care and their measurement, as well as in the assessment of disease or injury severity. The British Paediatric Association Outcome Measures Working Group defines an outcome measurement as a subtype of health status measurement where changes in the measure are known (or at least believed) to be largely attributable to a health service intervention.

Outcomes can be binary (death), continuous (change in blood pressure), a count (number of episodes), or a score (knee society score, Oxford hip, knee, or shoulder score). Also, the outcome can be objective (mortality rate) or subjective (pain, quality of life). To assess outcomes, condition-specific and general questionnaires are widely available, but their sensitivity to change and validity is open to question (Box 1.2.4).

An outcome measure should be quick, simple to use, reliable, specific to the question being investigated, cost-effective, and applicable. In most cases, this 'ideal' instrument does not exist, although many measures have come into general use without meeting these criteria (Box 1.2.3).

Outcome measures may be broadly classified into those used to measure doctors' assessment, and those used to measure the patient's own assessment of their problem. In most cases, it is appropriate and perhaps necessary to record both types of outcome. These two measures tend to assess different aspects of a condition and should normally be presented as separate outcomes. In the past, patient-based outcome measures have been dismissed as being too unreliable (subjective test vs. objective data) but in fact these assessments tend to follow closely the main indication for the original indication.

Two essential requirements of an outcome measure are that it measures what it is supposed to and that this measure is made with the minimum of error. The former is called 'validity' and the latter 'reliability'. Content validity examines the ability of the instrument to measure all aspects of the condition for which it was designed so that it is applicable to all patients with that condition. One problem with increasing the content is that the reliability tends to decrease; however, validity at the expense of some reliability is the rule.

Another important issue with an outcome measure is 'agreement'. Various reliability coefficients are available. An intraclass correlation coefficient (ICC) should be used for continuous data to measure agreement between or within methods or raters. The Pearson correlation is based on regression analysis and is a measure of the extent to which the relationship between two variables can be described by a straight (regression) line. Pearson's product moment correlation coefficient tends to over-estimate the agreement and is unable to distinguish data when there is a systematic error. It is always worth plotting the results to find systematic biases when comparing data. The best way to plot the data is by placing the mean of points on the x-axis and the difference on the y-axis. This method has been extended by Altman and Brand for normally distributed data to include lines at two standard deviations above and below the mean line, these being termed the 'limit of agreement'.

If the instrument is being assessed for its reliability as a clinical test, then sensitivity, specificity should be used. These are derived from the proportions of a 2×2 table.

An outcome instrument should be able to detect changes with time and this is termed as 'responsiveness'. It is important to ensure that the instrument can detect a clinically important change, even if this is quite small. This has two implications—firstly the clinically important change should be and can be defined and secondly this change must be considered while designing an experiment so that power calculations can be made accordingly.

Outcome measures can be substantive (what one really wants to know) or surrogate (what one often ends measuring instead). For a substantive measure (e.g. time taken for an implant to fail), the follow-up is usually prolonged, and during the life of the study one tends to lose participants either due to withdrawal (by patient or surgeon) or due to an adverse event (death/physical or mental impairment) or inability to keep track of patient's movements (lost to follow-up). For these reasons, surrogate measures are commonly used in clinical practice. However, one has to remember that the

Box 1.2.3 Essential properties of 'good' outcome measures

- Validity
- Reliability
- Agreement
- Responsiveness.

Box 1.2.4 Outcome measures

- Binary, continuous, count, or score
- Objective vs. subjective
- Doctor-based vs. patient-based
- Needs validity, reliability, and reproducibility.

association between the surrogate and substantive outcome may be altered by the intervention and also unless the trial is powered to detect a difference in the substantive outcome, the effect of the intervention on the surrogate outcome may determine the clinical practice which can prove to be harmful.

Inclusion of health-related quality of life (HRQL) is increasing in popularity as an outcome measure after any intervention. There are two key dimensions to it: primary (physical, psychological, social, etc.) and additional (neuropsychological, personal productivity, pain, etc.). HRQL provides a method of measuring intervention effects as well as the effects of the untreated course of diseases, in a manner that may be helpful to both the investigator as well as the individual. Most outcome measures tend to assess one or more of HRQL.

Another commonly used measure in orthopaedics is 'survival analysis' (Box 1.2.5). This is important in studies where participants are entered over a period of time and therefore have various lengths of follow-ups. These methods permit the comparison of the entire survival experience during the follow-up and may be used for the analysis of time to any dichotomous response variable such as a non-fatal event or an adverse effect. The graphical presentation of the total survival experience is called the survival curve and the tabular presentation is called the life table. Two commonly used methods are Kaplan–Meier and Cutler–Edere method. For a Kaplan–Meier estimate, one needs to know the exact time of entry into the trial and also the exact time of the event or loss of follow-up. In this method, the follow-up period is divided into intervals of time so that no interval contains both deaths and losses. In addition, one makes two assumptions. Firstly, it is assumed that at any time patients who are censored have the same survival prospects as those who continue to be followed. Secondly, it is assumed that the survival probabilities are the same for the subjects recruited early and late in the study. For some studies, all that is known is that within an interval of time, a known number of deaths and losses occurred amongst the known number of participants at risk. In such cases, the Kaplan–Meier method can not be used. In the Cutler–Edere method, the assumption is made that the deaths and losses are uniformly distributed over an interval to overcome this problem.

For expressing survival data of a particular implant, the life-table method is usually used. In this method, generally the cumulative survival is calculated at regular time intervals (usually yearly).

Box 1.2.5 Survivorship analysis

- Allows study of patients who enter a study over a period of time
- Uses a life table to present results
- Relies on a valid end-point measure in terms of relevance and reliability
- Can be used for studying longevity of implants.

The life-table method has advantages as it reports number of implants followed, number of failures, loss to follow-up, and confidence intervals. Establishing patients who are lost to follow-up are important in interpreting a survival analysis. Each individual lost may have been a failure and may therefore have dramatically altered the final result of the analysis. This can be addressed by including a worst-case scenario calculation in all survival studies to display the possible results of the loss to follow-up on the study. Confidence intervals give some sense of uncertainty in the estimated treatment or intervention effect. In a survival study, wide confidence intervals suggest that the numbers at risk were small and the results must be treated with caution. The method of Peto is usually used to calculate confidence intervals.

This brief chapter can not summarize all the relevant classification systems and outcome measures used in trauma and orthopaedics. The reader should refer to standard orthopaedic textbooks for the same. An excellent in-depth critique on this subject is available in *Outcome Measures in Orthopaedics and Orthopaedic Trauma*, by Pynsent et al.

Further reading

British Paediatric Association (1992). *Outcome Measurements for Child Health.* London: British Paediatric Association.

Cutler, J.S. and Edere, F. (1958). Maximum utilization of the life-table method in analyzing the survival. *Journal of Chronic Diseases*, **8**, 699–713.

Kaplan, E.L. and Meier, P. (1958). Non-parametric estimation from incomplete observations. *Journal of the American Statistical Association*, **53**, 457–81.

Pynsent P., Fairbank J., and Carr A.J. (eds.) (2004). *Outcome Measures in Orthopaedics and Orthopaedic Trauma*, 2nd edn. London: Arnold.

1.3

The musculoskeletal system: structure and function

Parminder J. Singh and Rohit Kotnis

Summary points

- Structure of bone is comprised of cells, matrix, and water
- Bone consists broadly of three surfaces (periosteal, endosteal, and Haversian) and two membranes (periosteum and endosteum)
- The blood supply of bone is derived from four main routes (nutrient, metaphyseal, epiphyseal, and periosteal arteries)
- There are three main types of cells in bone (osteoblast, osteocyte, and osteoclast)
- The matrix is a composite material consisting of an organic and an inorganic component
- Two types of bone formation are intramembranous and endochondral ossification
- The skeleton is also involved in the vital homeostasis of calcium and phosphate.

Introduction

The human body is composed of cells and surrounding matrix. The cells are important in determining active functions of the tissues. The matrix determines the mechanical properties of the tissue and its structure is adapted to cope with the stresses it is exposed to. Tissues such as bone whose main function is support (a mechanical property) have a high ratio of matrix to cells. Tissues such as muscles (functional) are mainly cellular. This chapter describes the make up of bone and joints in more detail. In addition, the embryology and its role in calcium homeostasis is detailed.

Bone

Structure

Bone is tissue formed by the deposition of mineral within a collagenous framework. The mineral consists of hydroxyapatite and type I collagen (90%). The dry weight of bone is 70% mineral and 30% organic. The wet weight of bone is 70% mineral, 22% organic, and 8% water. The organic components of bone consist of 98% matrix and 2% cells.

Bone is a dynamic composite material whose structure is designed to cope with and respond to loading. It is continuously being resorbed and laid down, and this appears to serve two important functions. Firstly, it allows the skeleton to remodel in response to changes in demand and loading. Secondly, it prevents fatigue fractures developing under repetitive loading. At the microscopic level, bone consists of two forms: woven and lamellar.

Woven bone is considered immature bone or primitive bone and is normally found where rapid new bone formation occurs such as in the embryo and new born, fracture callus, and in the metaphyseal region of growing bone. Woven bone contains no uniform orientation of collagen fibres, which gives it isotropic mechanical properties. In other words, the mechanical behaviour of the woven bone is similar regardless of the direction of the applied forces. Lamellar bone begins to form one month after birth. By the first year, it is actively replacing woven bone as the latter is resorbed. By the age of 4 years, most normal bone is lamellar bone. Therefore, lamella bone is more mature bone that results from remodelling from immature woven bone. The collagen fibrils are arranged in parallel sheets called lamellae. The highly organized stress-oriented collagen of lamella bone gives it anisotropic properties; that is, the mechanical behaviour of lamella bone differs depending on the orientation of the applied forces.

Woven bone and lamellar bone are structurally organized into trabecular (spongy or cancellous) and cortical (dense or compact) bone. Trabecular bone is mainly found at the epiphysis and metaphysis and in cuboid bones such as the vertebrae. The surface area to volume ratio of trabecular bone is ten times that of cortical bone. Trabecular bones principally resists compressive forces and responds up to eight times faster than cortical bone.

Trabeculae are needed where there are tension forces. For example, the proximal end of the femur has large compressive forces on the medial side and tension forces on the lateral side where the abductor muscle inserts. Trabecular patterns designed to cope with compression fan out from the calcar up to the articular surface of the femoral head. On the lateral side, a second set of trabeculae at right angle to the first arch up and across from the lateral cortex to counter the tension forces (Figure 1.3.1). The line of the trabeculae appears to be partly determined genetically but is also modified by the loads passing through the bone. This response is known as Wolff's law and stated in simple terms says that bone responds to changes in the magnitude and direction of load by remodelling the shape and thickness of the cortex and of the trabecular pattern inside.

In contrast, cortical bone, which makes up 80% of the skeleton, is found in the diaphysis of long bones. Cortical bone is much

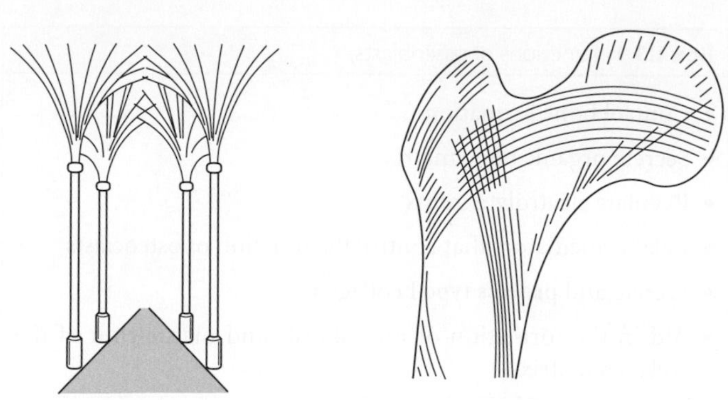

Fig. 1.3.1 The trabecular pattern of the neck of the femur is designed to provide maximum strength in the calcar where compression is greatest and through the top of the femoral neck where tension forces will be largest.

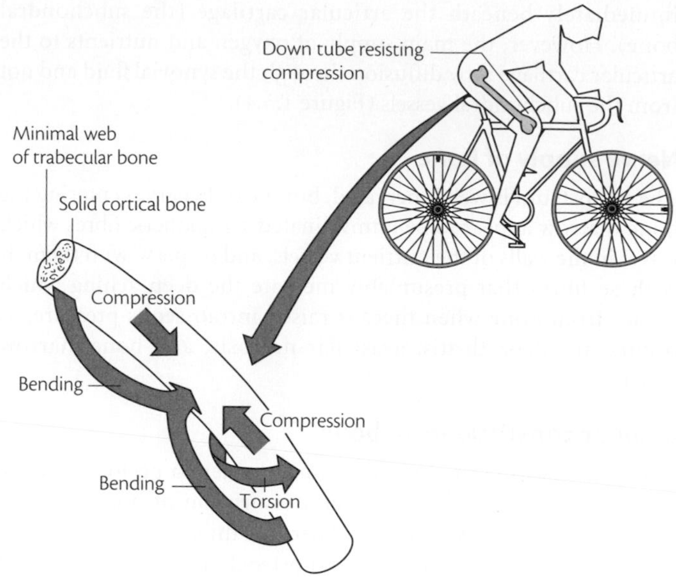

Fig. 1.3.2 Bone, like the tubing in the frame of a bicycle, is hollow and designed to be light yet resist bending, compression, and torsion forces.

stronger than cancellous bone and is subjected to bending and torsional forces as well as compressive forces. Cortical bone is made up of multiple layers of lamella bone and woven bone, with vascular channels located mainly in woven bone.

The basic unit of cortical bones is known as the Haversian system or osteon. This consists of concentric layers or lamellae surrounding a central Haversian canal. Haversian canals contain blood and nerves and communicate with the medullary cavity by Volkmann's canals. The capillaries in the central canal are derived from the principal artery of the bone or the epiphyseal and metaphyseal arteries. Each lamella consists of highly orientated, densely packed collagen fibrils which run in different directions. The collagen fibrils often interconnect with each other and between the lamellae which increases bone strength. Lamellae are lined with osteocytes which communicate via canaliculi. Osteons are major structural units of bone and are bound to each other by cement lines which define the outer boundary of each osteon. These thin layers of organic matrix mark sites where the resorption of bone stops and new bone formation begins. They separate, as opposed to bind, adjacent matrix lamellae.

Bone consists broadly of three surfaces (periosteal, endosteal, and Haversian) and two membranes (periosteum and endosteum). Periosteum covers the outer surface of bones except in the regions around synovial joints and is comprised of an outer fibrous and inner cambium layer. The inner layer contains cells that are capable of becoming osteoblasts and can also form hyaline cartilage. The outer layer has fewer cells and more collagen. It continues into the joint capsule and thereby connects one bone to another. Some ligaments and tendons insert into the outer layer. Periosteal cells can resorb and form bone in response to local stimuli. The periosteal blood vessels supply the outer third of the cortex. Sharpey's fibres anchor the periosteum to bone.

The central portion of long bones (the diaphysis) is mainly concerned with resisting compression and resisting bending and torsion and the shape approximates to a thin-walled tube (like a bicycle frame) (Figure 1.3.2). Muscles, tendons, and ligaments are bound firmly to the bone structure by fibre anchors deep in the cortex of the bone. These collagen anchors are cemented to the bone with hydroxyapatite (Figure 1.3.3).

Blood supply of bone

Bone is a highly vascular organ that receives up to 10% of cardiac output. The blood supply of bone is derived from four main routes (nutrient, metaphyseal, epiphyseal, and periosteal arteries). The arterial blood flow is centrifugal in direction (endosteum to periosteum). Venous blood flows in the opposite direction. Periosteal stripping of bone deprives it of venous drainage and collateral arterial supply. With aging, the periosteal blood supply diminishes in importance.

The blood supply to the epiphysis relies on penetrating vessels that ascend along the periosteal and perichondral layers and enter through the groove of Ranvier. The blood supply can be vulnerable to disruption following a physeal injury and can lead ultimately to avascular necrosis of the epiphysis. Following closure of the physis at skeletal maturity, anastomosis develops between the epiphyseal and medullary system.

The articular cartilage of the joint itself has no blood supply, but the epiphyseal vessels terminate in a capillary net in the bone

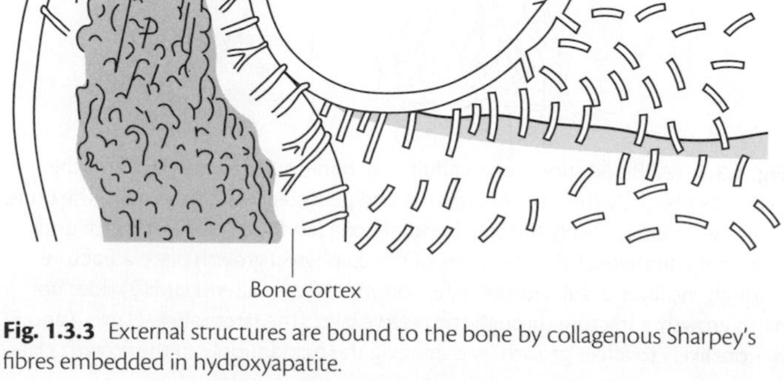

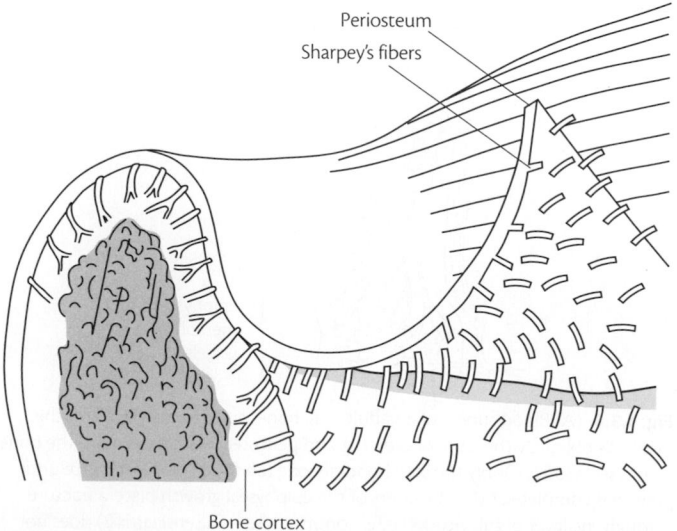

Fig. 1.3.3 External structures are bound to the bone by collagenous Sharpey's fibres embedded in hydroxyapatite.

immediately beneath the articular cartilage (the subchondral bone). However, the main supply of oxygen and nutrients to the articular cartilage is by diffusion through the synovial fluid and not from the subchondral vessels (Figure 1.3.4).

Nerve supply of bone

The periosteum is well innervated, but the only nerves entering the bone marrow appear to be unmyelinated sympathetic fibres which travel in the walls of the nutrient vessels, and disperse with them. It is these fibres that presumably mediate the deep aching which comes from bone when there is raised intraosseous pressure, as occurs in osteoarthritis, avascular necrosis, and bone marrow oedema.

Cellular constituents of bone

Bone cells assume specialized forms in order to perform diverse functions including formation and resorption of bone, mineral homeostasis, and repair of bone. There are three main types of cells in bone (osteoblast, osteocyte, and osteoclast) which are derived from different stem lines. Undifferentiated cells in the endosteum, periosteum, and Haversian canals differentiate into osteoblasts when stimulated.

Osteoblasts

Osteoblasts line the bone surface and produce matrix. Their shape is altered by their functional state: when active they resemble a cuboidal shape, and when in a static phase they adopt a flattened appearance. They possess hormone receptors for parathyroid hormone and a well developed endoplasmic reticulum. Osteoblasts have a variety of functions (see Box 1.3.1).

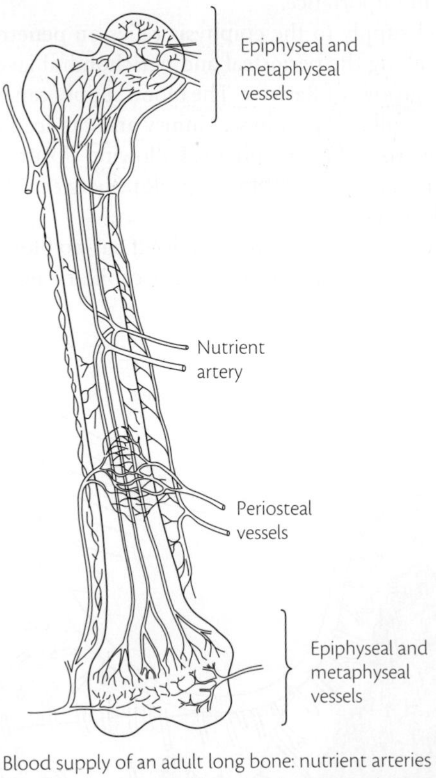

Fig. 1.3.4 (A) Blood supply of an adult long bone: nutrient arteries enter the diaphysis obliquely (because of growth), and periosteal vessels surround the bone; epiphyseal vessels supply the subchondral bone (and the epiphyseal plate until growth is completed). (B) The layers of the epiphyseal growth plate: a fracture through the layer of calcification (the common site—Salter–Harris 2) does not harm growth; a fracture through the reserve layer (the rarer Salter–Harris 4 and 5) is more likely to affect growth by damaging the blood supply to the growth plate.

Box 1.3.1 Functions of osteoblasts

- Control bone formation
- Secrete organic bone matrix
- Regulate electrolyte influx
- Release mediators that control the function of osteoclasts
- Secrete and process type I collagen
- Aid in the formation of microfibrils and maturation of the collagen matrix.

Osteocytes

Osteocytes make up more than 90% of the bone cells in the mature human skeleton and are surrounded by an organic matrix that can mineralize. They have a single nucleus and long branching cytoplasmic processes.

An osteocyte originates from an osteoblast and is, in effect, an osteoblast encased in calcified matrix. The canaliculi provide its nutrients and its metabolic activity is much reduced compared with osteoblasts.

Osteoclasts

These are bone lining cells responsible for bone resorption and resemble giant multinucleated cells. In contrast to the other bone cells, osteoclasts share a haematopoietic stem-cell precursor with cells of the monocyte family. These precursor cells may be found in the marrow or circulating blood. At their bone attachment, they possess a brush border which secretes lysosomal enzymes that degrade matrix components. Bone resorption creates Howship's lacunae in cancellous bone and cutting cones in cortical bone. Osteoclasts are rarely found in normal bone. On cancellous or periosteal surfaces, they create a depression referred to as Howship's lacuna. In dense cortical bone, they lead cutting cones that tunnel the bone creating resorption cavities.

Bone matrix

The matrix makes up 90% of the volume of lamellar bone and is a composite material consisting of an organic and an inorganic component. The inorganic component contributes 65% of wet weight of the bone. The organic component, principally collagen, gives bone its form and its ability to resist tension, while the inorganic or mineral component primarily resists compression. Demineralized bone is flexible, pliable, and fracture prone. The matrix serves two main mechanical functions (see Box 1.3.2).

Box 1.3.2 Functions of the matrix

- To prevent tissues from being torn apart (tension)—tensile forces predominate in tissues such as tendons and ligaments
- To stop tissues from collapsing (compression)—often found in bones and the intervertebral disc.

The main constituent of the matrix is water, which is held in equilibrium with the intracellular water by the osmotic pressure of the salts it contains. Where the matrix needs to resist compression, large hydrophilic feather-shaped molecules—proteoglycans—hold the matrix together (Figure 1.3.5).

Organic matrix

Collagens, predominantly type I, make up 90% of the organic matrix. The other 10% consists of glycoproteins and proteoglycans. Proteoglycans consist of a central protein core to which the negatively-charged glycosaminoglycans, either keratin sulphate or chondroitin sulphate, are attached. The negative charge attracts cations into the matrix to neutralize. A high osmotic pressure is created leading to the matrix continually attempting to draw in water. This will occur until it is resisted by tension arising in the fibrous network, leading to an equilibrium. However, to resist shear and maintain form requires the addition of collagen (Figure 1.3.6). There are also a small number of non-collagenous proteins that may influence matrix organization and bone mineralization. These include osteocalcin and osteonectin.

Structure of collagen

Collagen is the most common protein in the human body and consists of 19 different types. Common to all is a long triple helix made up of three helical alpha chains twisted around each other to form a superhelix. The structure allows collagen to resist stretching although it can be compressed easily. Collagen is laid down in bundles and layers wherever distraction forces may be significant (Figure 1.3.7) and can be thought of as being similar to the reinforcing steel rods found in concrete skyscrapers. The combination of an incompressible matrix (proteoglycans and water) with collagen creates a composite structure whose strength and mechanical properties far exceed those of its individual components. Depending on the arrangement of the collagen fibres, the matrix can specifically resist compression (articular cartilage), tension (the annulus of the intervertebral disc), and distraction (ligaments).

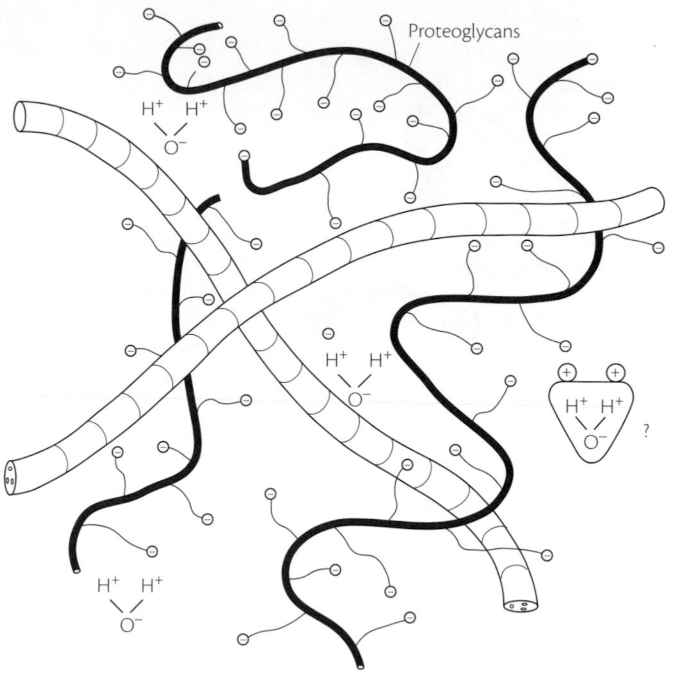

Fig. 1.3.6 Matrix consisting of hydrophilic proteoglycans, water, and collagen creating a tense structure which can resist multidirectional compression.

However, in order to resist bending, one further component is required in the composite—hydroxyapatite—a rigid crystal of calcium and phosphate (a form of ceramic), which converts a strong but flexible matrix into the rigid and unyielding structure of bone. The hydroxyapatite crystal is weak in tension but very strong in compression. When mixed into a composite it resists bending. The crystals are only 25μm long but are laid down in layers, creating bone, which for its weight is one of the strongest composite materials known.

Inorganic matrix

The inorganic matrix performs two essential functions (see Box 1.3.3).

Mineralization of bone

The formation of solid calcium phosphate in the organic matrix represents a phase transformation. Solid calcium phosphate first appears as a poorly crystalline apatite, whose crystallinity increases with time. Mineralization of bone collagen fibrils occurs in an organized fashion with progressive mineralization within hole zone regions in the collagen fibrils. Mineral continues to accumulate and gradually increases the density of the bone and its stiffness. The abnormal mechanical properties of bone in patients with osteomalacia or rickets illustrate its importance. In this group, the osteoid fails to mineralize, the bone weakens, and is more prone to skeletal deformities and pathological fractures. In osteoporosis there is a general reduction in bone mass. Thick trabeculae become

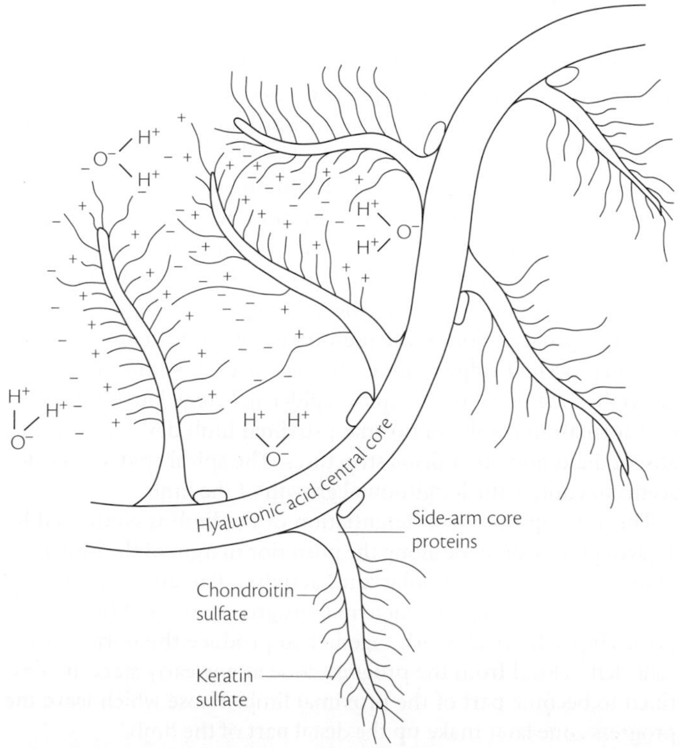

Fig. 1.3.5 Proteoglycans—long feathery molecules covered in negative charges which are highly attractive to water molecules (hydrophilic) and create the turgor pressure in the matrix.

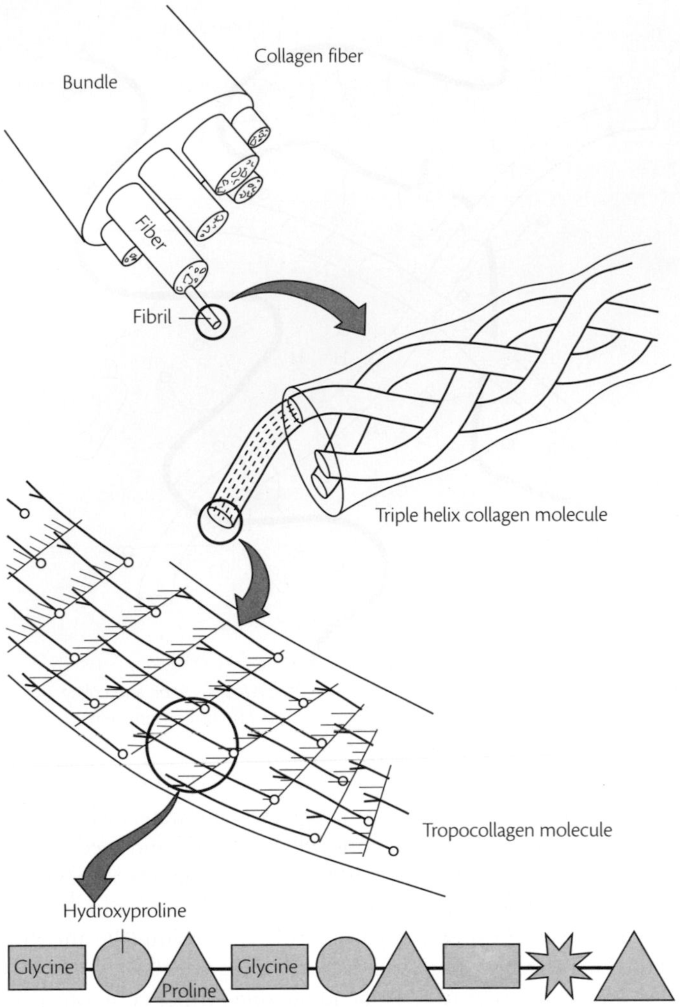

Fig. 1.3.7 Collagen—a triple helix of strands made from tropocollagen molecules. Each type of collagen has a characteristic repeating pattern of amino acids usually involving glycine, hydroxyproline, and proline. Collagen is very strong in tension.

thinner or may disappear altogether. The radiographic result is a coarsening of the main trabecular pattern. The reason for this paradox is that the main trabeculae may become slightly thinner in osteoporosis but do not disappear, but the small cross-trabeculae disappear and allow the main trabeculae to stand out even more clearly than before, making the bone look stronger rather than weaker on radiographs (Figure 1.3.8).

Box 1.3.3 Functions of the inorganic matrix

- An ion reservoir: about 99% of the body's calcium and 85% of phosphorus are associated with bone mineral crystals. Bone therefore helps in maintaining their extracellular fluid concentrations within ranges critical for normal physiological function, including nerve function and muscle contraction
- Gives bone most of its strength and stiffness: the calcium-phosphate crystals in the matrix create a rigid material able to withstand forces imparted by normal activity.

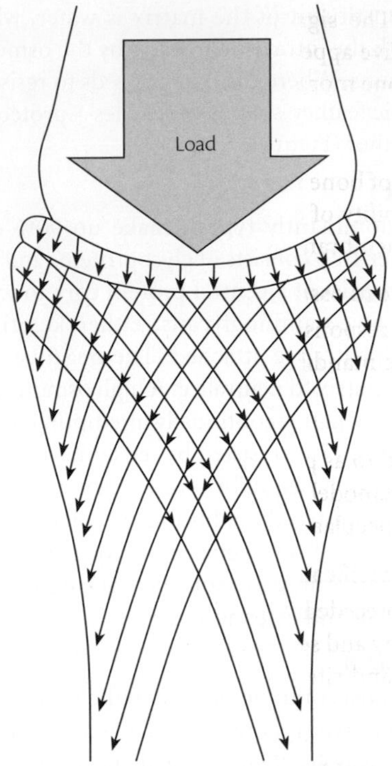

Fig. 1.3.8 In osteoporosis there is generalized loss of bone. The thick longitudinal stress-bearing trabeculae become thinner, and thin cross-bridging trabeculae disappear altogether. On radiography the loss of the cross-bridges enhances the definition of the longitudinal trabeculae, making the bone look stronger not weaker.

Embryology of the musculoskeletal system

The differentiation and organization of the embryo starts with the formation of the notochord during gastrulation. It is at this stage that ectoderm cells become programmed to form neural tissue. The signal to start forming the notochord appears to arise from a layer of dorsal mesoderm in contact with the ectoderm, which induces the ectoderm to infold and form the neural tube. The limb buds start to form shortly after this. They are produced by rapid division of mesoderm cells (the progress zone) which bulge out as a result of their fast growth. The thin layer of ectoderm lying over the end of the limb bud, called the apical epidermal ridge, seems to stimulate proliferation of the mesoderm beneath. Removal of this apical epidermal ridge at an early stage prevents limb formation altogether. Removal of the apical epidermal ridge late on in limb-bud formation results in normal proximal limb development but absent digits and other distal structures. The apical epidermal ridge seems to control the longitudinal growth of the limb.

The anteroposterior differentiation of the limb is controlled by an area of mesenchyme along the posterior margin of the limb bud, known as the zone of polarizing activity. The apical epidermal ridge, the underlying mesenchymal progress zone, and the zone of polarizing activity all work together to produce the normal limb. Cells left behind from the progress zone at any early stage are destined to become part of the proximal limb. Those which leave the progress zone later make up the distal part of the limb.

The gene controlling the ability of one group of cells to initiate differentiation in another is known as *Sonic Hedgehog* in humans. Activation of this gene in responsive cells seems to be mediated by retinoic acid. The signal sent out by the cells in which *Sonic Hedgehog* is active appears to be fibroblast growth factors 2 and 4, and possibly bone morphogenetic protein 2.

Formation of bone

The formation of bone tissue during development and in adult life is the responsibility of osteoblasts. The two types of bone formation are: intramembranous and endochondral ossification.

Intramembranous ossification

This process is responsible for forming the flat bones of the skull and parts of the mandible and clavicle. Precursor cells in vascular connective tissue enlarge, differentiate, and secrete thin strands of osteoid. Within a few days, mineralization commences and the tissue is referred to as primitive woven bone. Recognizable trabeculae form and remodel to mature lamellar bone. The fibrous tissue between the trabeculae is replaced by marrow.

Endochondral ossification

Ossification is preceded by a cartilage anlage or template. Cartilage cells hypertrophy and secrete matrix vesicles at a genetically predetermined time and site (primary ossification centre). The matrix calcifies and the chondrocytes die. Blood vessels enter the space and bring osteoblast precursors which differentiate and lay down mineralizing osteoid on the previously mineralized cartilage matrix. This method of laying down bone within a cartilage anlage is known as endochondral ossification and occurs almost everywhere in the human body apart from the skull and the clavicle (Figure 1.3.9).

As ossification of the primary centre commences, the periosteal sleeve lays an outer shell of bone which will become the cortex. In a long bone, this process starts in the centre of the diaphysis and spreads leaving only the bone ends as cartilage (epiphyses). At the junction of the cartilage and bone, the cartilage is organized to form a specialized structure referred to as the growth plate or physis. Osteocytes become incarcerated in rings of bone laid down around blood vessels, creating a pattern of interlinking rings with a Haversian canal running down the centre (Figure 1.3.10).

At differing times throughout the skeleton, secondary ossification centres are formed in the epiphyses in a similar fashion to the primary centres. Growth of the epiphysis occurs using endochondral ossification at the junction of the bone with the articular cartilage (secondary growth plate).

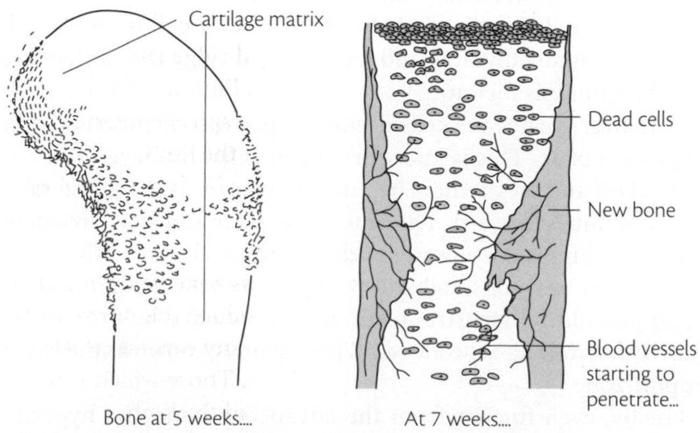

Fig. 1.3.9 Formation of bone at 10 weeks from a condensation of mesenchyme. This is followed by the formation of a cartilage model (anlage). The cartilage cells then die (apoptosis) and bone is laid down in place of the cartilage.

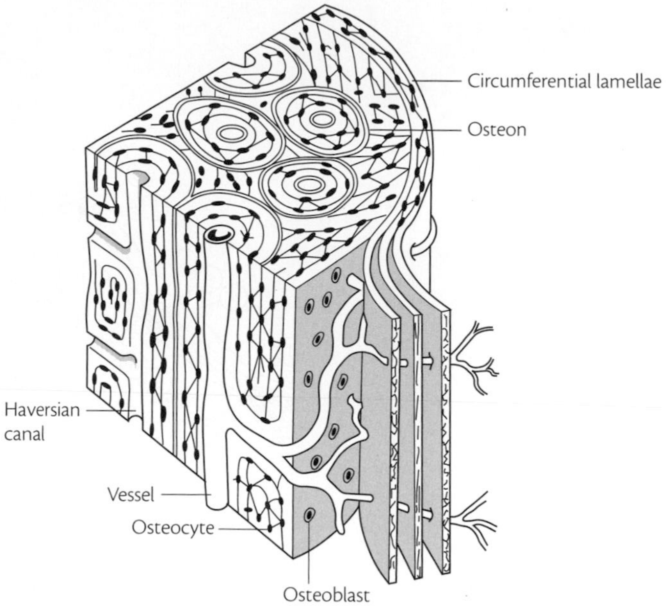

Fig. 1.3.10 Osteocytes become incarcerated in rings of bone laid down around blood vessels, creating a pattern of interlinking rings with a Haversian canal running down the centre.

The ossification of the bone spreads out from the ossification centres, each of which forms at a characteristic age and can be used to age skeletons by radiography. The last areas to ossify are the epiphyseal plates, where longitudinal growth of the bone will continue until adulthood (Figure 1.3.11). The diameter of bones also increases during growth through bone laid down under the periosteum. Remodelling may also continue on the inner cortex enlarging the diameter of the medulla in proportion to the dimensions of the rest of the bone.

In cortical bone, ossification continues in rings around each blood vessel. Each layer of bone laid down around the vessel has the collagen arranged at a certain orientation. The osteoblasts lay down collagen in organized lamellae to form an osteoid seam about 10mm thick. The next layer will have its collagen at a different orientation, creating a layered effect which is exceptionally strong. Ten to fifteen per cent of osteoblasts become incarcerated within the lacunae as osteocytces. In the centre of these sets of concentric rings the blood vessels flow in the Haversian canal (Figure 1.3.10).

The osteoid which has not yet been mineralized is about 10μm thick. Each layer of osteoid takes about 10 days to mineralize. An unusually thick layer of osteoid suggests that there may be a problem with bone mineralization such that it cannot keep pace with osteoblast activity (osteomalacia). In the adult there is a dynamic equilibrium between osteoclastic activity (resorbing bone) and osteoblastic activity (new bone being laid down) (Figure 1.3.12).

Remodelling

There are three main functions of remodelling (Box 1.3.4)

The control of remodelling is very precise. The amount of bone formed in each remodelling unit must precisely match that which has been resorbed. If this does not occur, the trabecular bone volume will change.

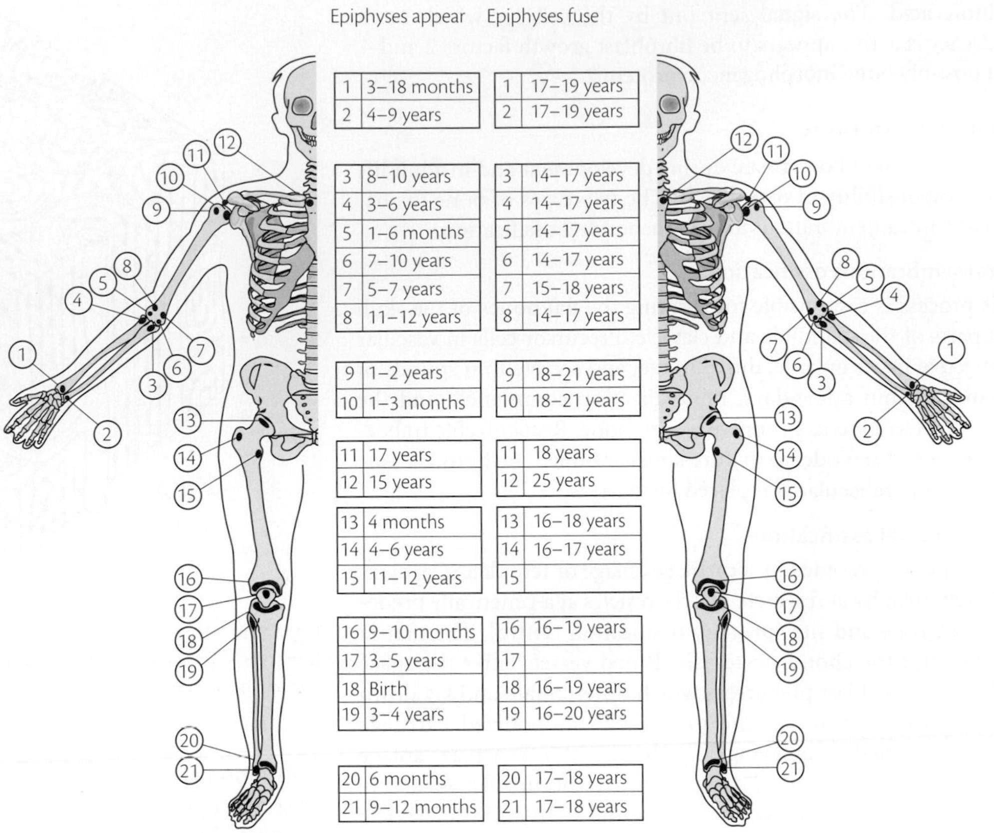

	Epiphyses appear	Epiphyses fuse
1	3–18 months	17–19 years
2	4–9 years	17–19 years
3	8–10 years	14–17 years
4	3–6 years	14–17 years
5	1–6 months	14–17 years
6	7–10 years	14–17 years
7	5–7 years	15–18 years
8	11–12 years	14–17 years
9	1–2 years	18–21 years
10	1–3 months	18–21 years
11	17 years	18 years
12	15 years	25 years
13	4 months	16–18 years
14	4–6 years	16–17 years
15	11–12 years	
16	9–10 months	16–19 years
17	3–5 years	
18	Birth	16–19 years
19	3–4 years	16–20 years
20	6 months	17–18 years
21	9–12 months	17–18 years

Fig. 1.3.11 Atlas of bone age. On the right side of the skeleton are the ages when centres of ossification first appear. On the left are the ages when the plates close. Sophisticated atlases can be used to calculate the age of a patient from the appropriate plain radiographs.

Both compact and cancellous bone are composed of individual basic multicellular units separated by cement (reversal) lines. This pattern is the result of bone remodelling activity involving organized groups of osteoclasts and osteoblasts. Osteoclasts are large multicellular structures with a large volume of cytoplasm. In cortical bone, following an activation stimulus, a group of osteoclasts form a cutting cone in the bone (a tunnel which is drilled into old bone) for up to 2.5mm. This resorption activity is followed by a short reversal phase when macrophages remove any debris. In the cavity created, osteoblasts line the walls of the cavity and lay down concentric lamellae of osteoid on the previously resorbed bone surface (Figure 1.3.13). The end result is the mature, mineralized, Haversial system (osteon) with a central vascular channel.

In cancellous bone, osteoclastic resorption to a depth of approximately 50μm occurs, followed by osteoblastic activity to replace the resorbed bone. The resultant bone packet is bounded by a cement (reversal) line and the trabecular surface.

There is a close link between the activity of the osteoclasts and of the osteoblasts, maintaining a constant mass of healthy bone and keeping the plasma levels of calcium and phosphate at the correct level. This linkage is probably mediated by cytokines which pass between the two cell types, osteoclasts (removing bone), and osteoblasts (rebuilding). If osteoclastic activity outstrips osteoblastic activity, a progressive reduction in bone mass occurs. This is known as osteoporosis. If this is rapid then plasma calcium and phosphate may rise (as in myeloma and other bone-lysing tumours). Excessive activity by the osteoblasts increases bone mass and removes calcium and phosphate from the plasma.

Bone growth and the epiphyseal plate

Growth plates consist of a series of histological layers which represent the stages that bone goes through when it is produced. At the front of the epiphyseal plate, there are relatively undifferentiated and quiescent reserve cells, ready to be activated and move the epiphyseal plate forward. This is the reserve cell layer. In this quiet area, the epiphyseal artery supplies nutrients to the growing epiphyseal plate. Immediately behind the resting cell layer are cells which are rapidly dividing and separating, driving the resting layer and the epiphysis forward.

This layer creates the cells needed to produce the matrix of the epiphyseal plate. This is known as the proliferative layer. Cells are budded off and they remain behind and mature as the proliferative layer continues forward. The cells grow larger and start producing matrix. Columns of cells are produced; those closest to the proliferative layer are still small and young, and those further back are larger and older (hypertrophied) and surrounded by the cartilage matrix that they have produced. This region is known as the hypertrophic zone.

Finally, even further from the advancing front, the hypertrophied cells start to die (apoptosis) and the cartilage matrix calcifies (the calcification layer). New blood vessels from the nutrient artery of the metaphysis grow into the back of this zone and from their

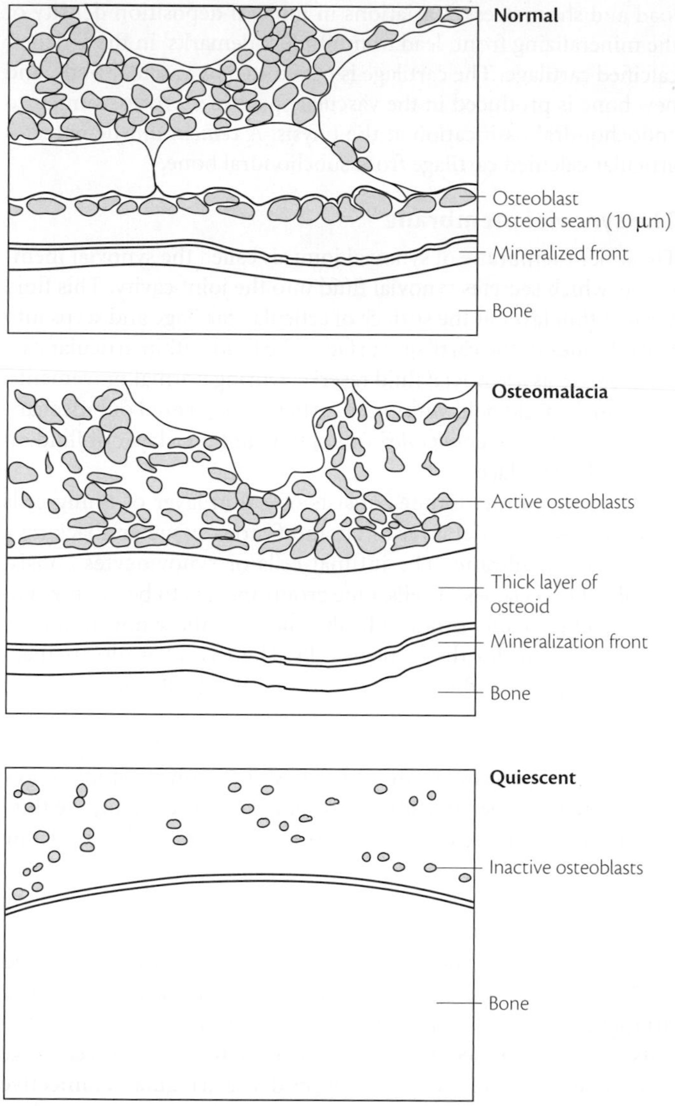

Fig. 1.3.12 Bone is normally in dynamic equilibrium, with old bone being removed and new bone constantly being laid down. Mature bone has a thin layer of osteoid on its surface, where mineralization of newly laid down osteoid has not yet occurred. In conditions where there is insufficient calcium, the layer of osteoid will be thickened because mineralization cannot keep up with the deposition of new osteoid. In elderly patients, bone activity may be reduced and the layer of osteoid may become very thin.

sides, cells appear which remove the calcified cartilage and start to lay down new endochondral bone.

From the orientation of the epiphyseal plate it can be seen that any fracture of the proximal side is, in effect, a simple fracture of new bone which can heal normally. Injury to the distal part of the epiphysis cuts off the blood supply to the cells about to create the next phase of the plate and effectively stops the plate's forward movement (Figure 1.3.14).

Box 1.3.4 Functions of remodelling

- Replacement/repair of old/damaged bone
- Reinforcement due to altered stresses
- Calcium homeostasis.

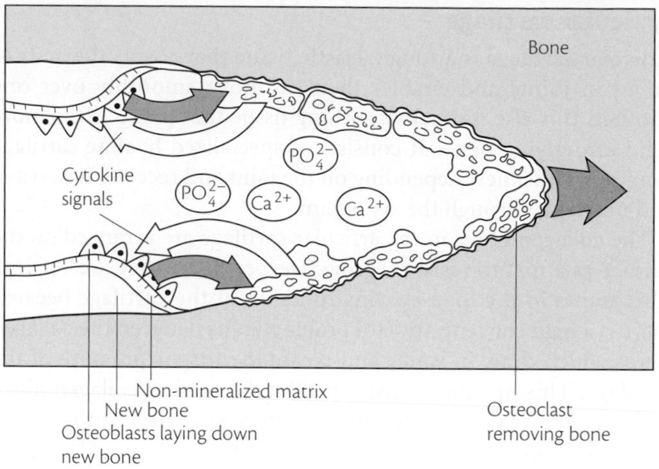

Fig. 1.3.13 A cutting cone in mature bone. Osteoclasts are cutting into old bone, resorbing as they go. Behind them, osteoblasts are laying down new bone communicating via cytokines.

Joints

Embryology

Joints initially appear in the embryo as condensations of mesenchyme. At around 8 weeks there appears to be a line along which cell death occurs. A cleft is created which develops into the joint. In the typical diarthrodial joint the cells around the cleft contribute to the synovium and articular cartilage.

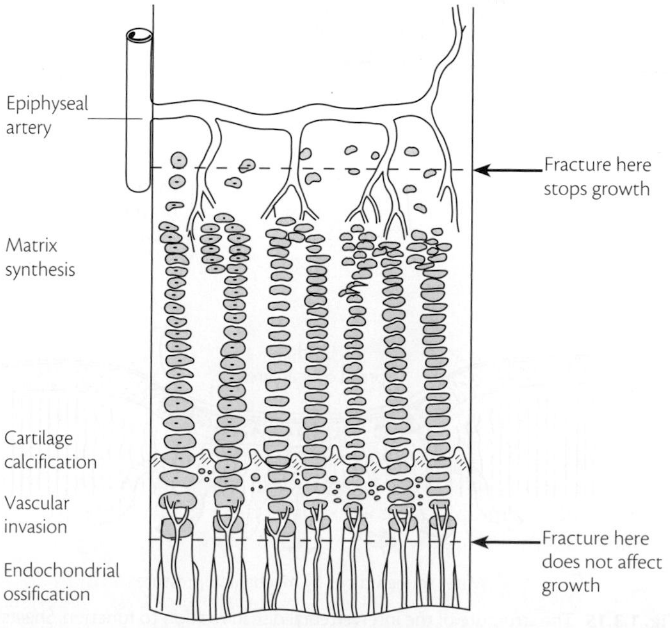

Fig. 1.3.14 Articular cartilage. The layers of collagen are oriented to resist the forces to which they are subjected. The surface layer is horizontal to resist shearing forces. The deeper layers are vertical to provide struts for the hydrostatic pressure which serves as a shock absorber.

Articular cartilage

Articular cartilage is a tough, elastic tissue that covers the ends of bones in joints and enables them to move smoothly over one another. It is also a shock-absorbing tissue that protects the more rigid underlying bone. It consists of specialized hyaline cartilage ranging in thickness depending on the joint and receives its oxygen and nutrients through the synovium.

The collagen fibres in the articular cartilage are arranged on the surface as a mat to resist shearing. Deeper down they are vertical. This assists in the load-bearing function of the cartilage because there is a high concentration of proteoglycans between the collagen fibres which draw in water and create the turgor pressure of the cartilage. This pressure constrained by the vertical collagen fibres converts articular cartilage into a hydroelastic suspension system which cushions and spreads load across its joint surface. The indentation of the outer layer of articular cartilage as a load moves across it squeezes out synovial fluid lying within the articular cartilage. This creates a fluid lubrication layer between the articular cartilage surfaces, which explains the low coefficient of friction of the articular surface (Figure 1.3.15).

Articular cartilage is mineralized at the junction between cartilage and bone. A mineralization front advances through the base of the hyaline articular cartilage at a rate which depends on cartilage load and shear stress. Variations in mineral deposition density of the mineralizing front, lead to multiple 'tidemarks' in the articular calcified cartilage. The cartilage is penetrated by vascular buds, and new bone is produced in the vascular space in a process similar to endochondral ossification at the physis. A *cement line* demarcates articular calcified cartilage from subchondral bone.

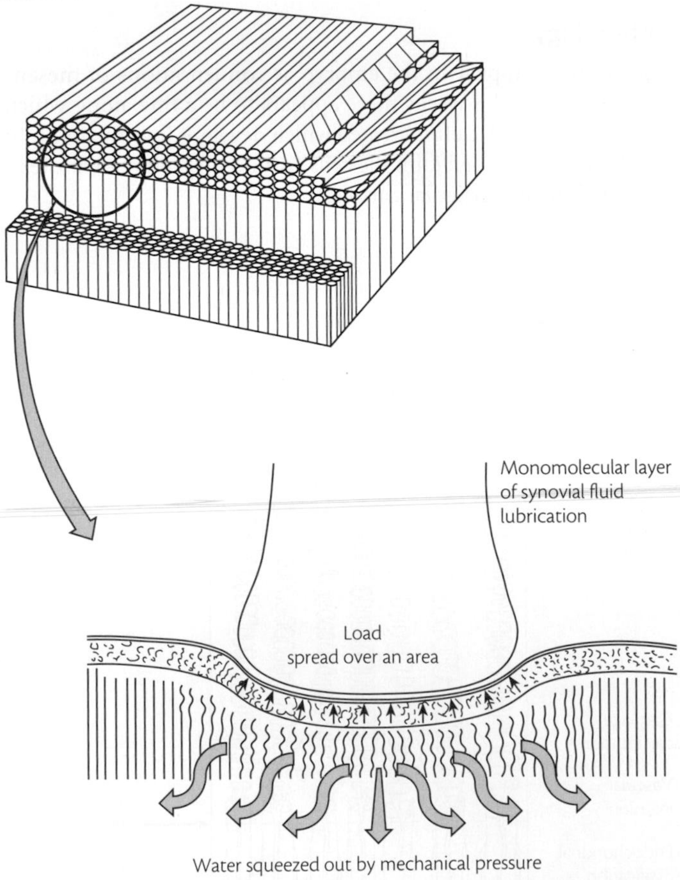

Fig. 1.3.15 The structure of the intervertebral disc in relation to function. Sheets of collagen laid in oblique sheets (like plywood) allow some movement but resist expansion. The central nucleus pulposus has a high concentration of proteoglycans that create a hydrostatic pressure which resists compression and acts as a shock absorber.

The synovial membrane

The inner membrane of synovial joints is called the synovial membrane, which secretes synovial fluid into the joint cavity. This fluid forms a thin layer at the surface of articular cartilage and seeps into irregularities in the cartilage surface. The fluid within articular cartilage serves as a synovial fluid reserve. During normal movements, the synovial fluid held within the cartilage is squeezed out mechanically (so-called *weeping lubrication*) to maintain a layer of fluid on the cartilage surface.

The synovial membrane consists of a thin layer of lining cells lying on a subintimal layer of fat and fibrous tissue and lacking a basement membrane. The intimal cells or synoviocytes consist mainly of two classes of cells. One group appears to be mainly synthetic and probably produce hyaluronate for the synovial fluid as well as nutrients for the cartilage cells. The second group are macrophage-type cells which clear detritus created by the movement of the joint.

Synovial fluid is made of hyaluronic acid and lubricin, proteinases, and collagenases. Synovial fluid exhibits non-newtonian flow characteristics. The viscosity coefficient is not a constant, the fluid is not linearly viscous, and its viscosity increases as the shear rate decreases.

Fibrocartilage

Fibrocartilage is the most common form of cartilage by weight and is characterized by a dense network of type I collagen commonly arranged parallel to tensile forces. Under the microscope, it consists of fibrous connective tissue arranged in bundles, with cartilage cells inbetween. The cells resemble dense irregular connective tissue but may be distinguished from them by their surrounding concentric striated area of cartilage matrix, their lacunae, and by their less flattened appearance.

Fibrocartilage is a tough material that provides high tensile strength and support and contains more collagen and less proteoglycan than hyaline cartilage. It is most present in areas subject to frequent stress such as intervertebral discs, the symphysis pubis, and the attachments of certain tendons and ligaments. In the annulus of the intervertebral disc, in combination with the proteoglycan rich nucleus pulposus, it provides a very strong load-bearing joint with a limited range of movement in all planes. The amount of fibrocartilage increases with age as hyaline cartilage transforms into fibrocartilage.

Calcium and phosphate homeostasis

The skeleton is also involved in the vital homeostasis of calcium and phosphate. Both ions are important for normal physiological function. Calcium is needed for neuromuscular conduction, especially in the myocardium and plays an important part in the clotting cascade. Phosphate ions have an equally important role as one of the ions that buffer the pH of the body fluids. Bone mineral homeostasis is tightly controlled by the synchronized action of the

Box 1.3.5 Ion homeostasis

- The intake may be disturbed (usually because of poor diet—dietary rickets)
- Regulation may be affected by inappropriate levels of parathyroid hormone, calcitonin, or vitamin D
- The kidneys may be unable to resorb calcium and/or phosphate so they are lost from the body (renal rickets)
- The bone may be destroyed and ions released by destructive processes (myeloma and other bone tumours).

vitamin D3 metabolites, parathyroid hormone, and calcitonin. These hormones regulate the dietary absorption of calcium, bone mineral resorption and deposition, and renal secretion and reabsorption of calcium and phosphorus.

Homeostasis of these ions can be influenced in four main ways (see Box 1.3.5).

Any disease process may affect more than one of these four causes of dysfunction, so that the final result in terms of whether the serum calcium is raised or reduced and whether the phosphate is affected in the same way or not depends on the actual disease and the body's response to it. However, if both calcium and phosphate are raised, their solubility product may be exceeded in which cases calcium phosphate may be deposited spontaneously in the tissues.

Further reading

Bostrom, M.P.G., Boskey, A., Kaufman, J.K., and Einhorn, T.A. (2000). Form and function of bone. In: Buckwalter, J.A., Einhorn, T.A., and Simon, S.R. (eds) *Orthopaedic Basic Science: Biology and Biomechanics of the Musculoskeletal System*, pp. 319–69. Rosemont, IL: American Academy of Orthopaedic Surgeons.

Buckwalter, J.A., Glimcher, M.J., Cooper, R.R., and Recker R. (1995). Bone biology, part I: structure, blood supply, cells, matrix and mineralization. *Journal of Bone and Joint Surgery*, **77A**(8), 1256–75.

Johnson, R.L., Riddle, R.D., and Tabin, C.J. (1994). Mechanism of limb patterning. *Current Opinion in Genetics and Development*, **4**, 535–42.

Tickle, C. (1994). On making a skeleton. *Nature*, **368**, 587–8.

1.4

Injury and repair

Parminder J. Singh and Rohit Kotnis

Summary points

- Types of injury—traumatic and overuse
- Importance of determining the energy involved in an injury
- The relevance of mechanical load curves
- Types of fracture healing—how and why they occur
- Healing in articular cartilage, tendon, ligaments, peripheral nerves, and brain tissues.

General concepts

The musculoskeletal system (also known as the locomotor system) provides the supporting framework for the human body, protects vital internal organs, and enables us to move in space through an arrangement of bones, ligaments, and articulations. The system consists of the human skeleton, made by bones attached to other bones with joints, and skeletal muscle attached to the skeleton by tendons.

Injury is damage caused to the structure or function of the body by an outside agent or force, which may be physical or chemical. Injury occurs when an acting force exceeds the elastic, plastic (hard tissues), viscoelastic (soft tissues), or endurance limits (stress, overuse) of a particular tissue (Box 1.4.1).

In a *traumatic injury*, the acting internal force (e.g. a contracting hamstring muscle tearing in a sprinter) or external force (e.g. a fall from a height causing a vertebral compression fracture) exceeds the strength of a normal tissue. A *pathological injury* occurs when a force of ordinary magnitude damages a tissue weakened by a pathological process (e.g. tumour /bone cyst).

A *stress* or *overuse injury* occurs after ordinary forces act repeatedly on normal tissues. Microinjuries are produced which do not have sufficient time to heal prior to the next submaximal event. The tissue fails after its endurance limit has been exceeded. In an overuse injury, the repeated impact produces a chronic inflammatory response (e.g. a tenosynovitis) which may prevent ultimate tissue failure by temporarily limiting the further use of an extremity.

Traumatic injuries

Mechanical trauma is the commonest cause of injury to the musculoskeletal system. These events are governed by Newton's second law of motion. This states that the force acting on a body is proportional to the product of the mass of the body and its acceleration (or deceleration).

Energy transmitted to the body is absorbed and dissipated through the bone and soft tissue envelope. Kinetic energy (KE) equals mass (m) × velocity (v) squared divided by two: $KE = mv^2/2$. Hence doubling the mass of a moving body will double its traumatizing kinetic energy, while doubling its velocity will quadruple the resulting traumatic impact. The kinetic energy imparted to an object can deform the object temporarily (elastic deformation) or permanently (plastic deformation), or cause its complete disruption (by exceeding the ultimate failure limit). A small part of the transmitted impact can be converted to thermal energy. If the impacting force exceeds the failure limit of the bone, it breaks.

Variables such as age and the rate at which loads are applied (strain rate) affect the resulting injury patterns. An example of how the relative strength of musculoskeletal tissues changes with age can be seen when a lateral force is applied to the knee joint in a child. This will most likely lead to a fracture through the epiphyseal plate or possibly a fracture of the adjacent tibial shaft. The same

Box 1.4.1 Types of mechanical deformation

- Elastic: measure of the stiffness of a material or its ability to resist deformation. (E = stress/strain in the elastic range of the stress–strain curve)
- Plastic: change in length after removing the load (before the breaking point in the plastic range)
- Ultimate strength: maximum strength obtained by the material
- Breaking point: point where the material fractures
- Viscoelastic material: exhibits stress–strain behaviour that is time rate-dependent. The deformation depends on the load and the rate at which the load is applied
- Endurance limit: the stress level below which a material will withstand cyclic stress indefinitely without exhibiting fatigue failure.

mechanism will tear the medial–collateral ligament in a young adult and cause a tibial plateau fracture in an older person. With higher loading rates, a bone appears stronger thus requiring more energy to fail. This also explains why a slowly applied load to a joint will probably lead to a bony avulsion, while at a faster loading rate an in-substance tear of the ligament is more common.

Injuries caused by firearms

Firearms can be divided into handguns, shotguns, and rifles. The barrels of most firearms have helical grooves imparting a spin to the bullet, which increases stability in flight and accuracy.

Velocity and kinetic energy

Velocity (distance divided by time) refers to the speed of a missile on exit. The muzzle velocity is the maximal velocity. Bullets with muzzle velocities below 1000 feet/s (305m/s) are considered 'low velocity'. This includes most rifles and shotguns. Bullets with muzzle velocities more than 1000 feet/s are considered 'high-velocity' firearms. Velocity on impact is important since tissue damage is proportional to a missile's KE. Because of its geometric progression, velocity is of greater importance than mass.

Ballistics is the science of the movement of a projectile through a firearm, the air, and into or through a target. The tissue destruction is determined by the dissipation of the energy upon impact (ΔKE). If the bullet or its fragments have remained within the target, the exit velocity is zero and complete energy transfer has occurred.

Maximizing tissue destruction

Secondary missiles are created when the KE is imparted to dense tissues (e.g. a tooth) which themselves become missiles. Cavitation is caused by the rapid expansion and elastic recoil of tissues impacted by a missile (Box 1.4.2). Cavitation is proportional to the density of the tissue, the velocity of the projectile, and KE on impact. The temporal cavity may exceed the missile diameter by a factor of five to ten, which may produce tissue destruction many centimetres beyond the missile path. One of the more harmful effects of cavitation is the resulting vacuum which sucks foreign bodies and organisms into the projectile's tract, an ideal situation for infection.

Clinical issues

When managing firearms injuries, ballistic information should be available (Box 1.4.3). A thorough physical evaluation with special focus on the neurovascular status must follow. Bullets may fragment and even change course in the body (for example, bouncing off the spine) so the search for injuries needs to be comprehensive. All firearm injuries involving vital structures and/or by high-velocity missiles must undergo evaluation and formal debridement in the operating room. This is frequently repeated at 24–48h.

Box 1.4.2 Side effects of cavitation

- Injuries to tissue remote from missile track
- Foreign bodies may be sucked into the wound
- Thorough and repeated debridement is vital.

Box 1.4.3 Relevant ballistic information

- Weapon type: calibre
- Distance: path of the bullet in the victim
- Presence, intensity, and location of powder burns (Figure 1.4.1)
- Number of bullets involved.

Musculoskeletal tissues: basic repair mechanisms

Tissues respond to injury

Most musculoskeletal tissues heal using three common phases: inflammation, repair, and remodelling. However, some structures (e.g. tendons) can heal using tissue-specific healing mechanisms. In contrast, some tissues (e.g. meniscus with *in situ* tears in the white zone) are incapable of repair.

The standard healing model: inflammation–repair–remodelling

Soft tissue injury can initiate a complex pathway of physical and biochemical changes. Healing progresses typically in four stages: haematoma, to inflammation, to proliferation, and finally remodelling (Box 1.4.4) Healing is most effective in well-vascularized tissues, and usually initiated from the tissues surrounding the injury site.

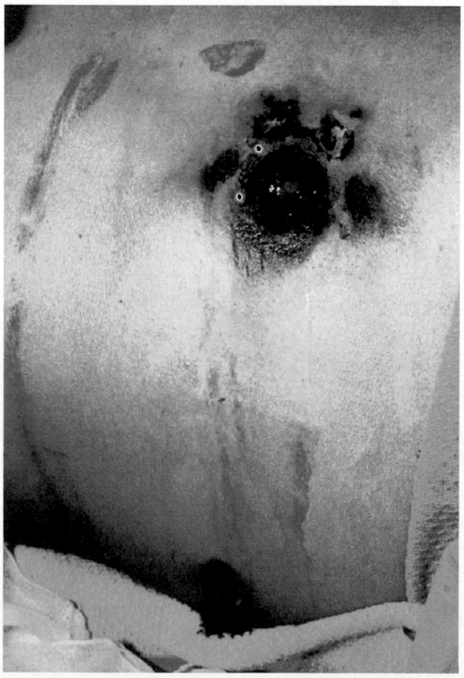

Fig. 1.4.1 M16 gunshot wound to the side of the chest of a soldier. The entrance wound is larger than the exit wound, and is identified by powder burns. Also see colour plate section.

Box 1.4.4 The standard healing model

- Haematoma: following injury, bleeding occurs in the zone of injury, followed by the formation of a primary platelet plug
- Inflammation: the dead tissue is phagocytosed by macrophages with the first week. The tissue is then replaced by granulation tissue
- Repair: granulation tissue replaced by tissue-specific matrix
- Remodelling: shape and structure optimized in response to stress. This continues for up to 18 months via realignment and cross linking of collagen fibres.

During haemostasis a primary platelet plug usually forms shortly after the injury. Secondary clotting occurs using fibrin and the coagulation cascade. Platelets release mediators that stimulate the next phase of healing.

During inflammation, the non-viable tissue is phagocytosed by macrophages within the first week. The end result is the formation of granulation tissue. Prostaglandins are actively involved in mediating this stage. Activation of the coagulation system and cytokines released by injured tissues attract polymorphonuclear leucocytes, monocytes, and T lymphocytes which remove necrotic material. They also release vasoactive mediators and activate growth factors and cytokines such as fibroblast growth factor, platelet-derived growth factor, and transforming growth factor-β (TGFβ). These attract cell migration, proliferation, and matrix differentiation.

Repair

The granulation tissue is replaced by a tissue-specific matrix which facilitates the ingrowth of undifferentiated pluripotent mesenchymal cells from surrounding muscle, periosteum, and marrow. These differentiate into tissue-specific cells such as osteoblasts, chondroblasts, myoblasts, and fibroblasts which fill the injury site with material closely resembling the original tissue.

Remodelling

In this phase, the disorganized repair tissue is optimized over several months under the guidance of local mechanical stresses. The result is tissue approaching the pre-injury status both structurally and functionally. However, scar tissue filling large defects contracts and this can be cosmetically unattractive or limit the movement of a limb.

Fracture mechanics and new bone formation

Structure and mechanical properties of bone

Normal bone is lamellar and is divided into cortical and cancellous bone. The mechanical properties of bone and its failure mechanisms directly derive from its composition and three-dimensional structure (Figure 1.4.2). Bone is a viscoelastic material and fractures are subsequently related to the magnitude of the force applied and its rate of application. This force is stored until breaking point and subsequently dissipated resulting in soft tissue damage.

Cortical bone has a slow turnover rate, a relatively high Young's modulus, and a higher resistance to torsion and bending than cancellous bone. Cortical bone is weakest in shear, weak in tension, and strongest in compression. Trabecular bone is less dense and undergoes increased remodelling related to the lines of stress (Wolf's law). It has a higher turnover rate, a lower Young's modulus, and a greater elasticity than cortical bone. Trabecular bone, with a much greater ability to deform plastically, is about four to 50 times weaker than cortical bone. By the fifth decade, progressive reduction in bone mass with changes in material properties reduces bone strength and modulus resulting in a greater susceptibility to fracture. This tendency is less severe in men because increased endosteal resorption is partially compensated by a concomitant

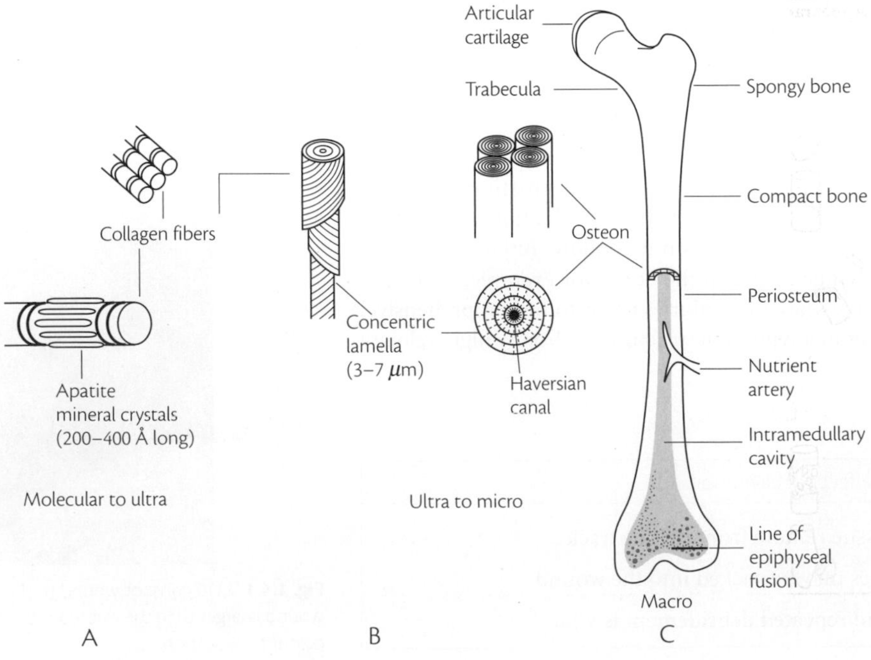

Fig. 1.4.2 The different structural levels of bone. A) The first level is a material composed of hydroxyapatite crystals embedded between collagen fibrils. B) The second level is an arrangement of the fibrils into sheets or lamellae with a preferred orientation. C) In long bones, the third level consists of an arrangement of lamellae into tubular osteons (or flat sheets), which form the basic structure of cortical and trabecular bone. Adapted from Katz, J.L. (1981). Composite material models for cortical bone. In: Cowin, S.C. (ed) Mechanical Properties of Bone, pp. 171–84. New York: American Society of Mechanical Engineers.

subperiosteal expansion. The loss in bone material with increasing age is partially counteracted by improved structural properties (increased polar moment of inertia).

Fracture mechanics

A fracture involves a breech in the continuity of bone. Injuries may be from indirect forces such as a twist. These are termed low-velocity injuries. With high-velocity injuries, the fractures may be highly fragmented and damage to the surrounding soft tissues much greater, compromising blood supply. The forces that bone has to withstand include compression, bending, and twisting. Bone is strongest in compression and weakest in tension. Compressive forces lead to fractures predominantly in cancellous bone (metaphysis). Transverse, oblique, and spiral fracture patterns primarily occur in diaphyseal bone. Failure commences with the formation of a small crack on the tension side. As this crack progresses to the neutral axis, and then to the convex side, a transverse fracture results (Figure 1.4.3).

Transverse fractures occur following a bending force and may be associated with a small extrusion wedge on the compression side. If the wedge is less than 10% of the circumference of the bone, the fracture is defined as simple transverse fracture. With larger extrusion fragments, the fracture is termed a wedge fracture. Oblique fractures are secondary to a bending force. The extrusion wedge remains attached to one of the main fragments. Spiral fractures result from indirect twisting injuries and may occur with a spiral wedge fragment.

Mechanisms of bone regeneration: overview

Fracture healing involves a complex series of events leading to restoration of bone to its pre-injury condition. Fracture repair is influenced by factors such as the mechanical and biological environment of the fracture site, motion at the fracture site, and stability.

Fracture healing and regeneration of new bone can principally occur by primary or secondary bone healing or distraction osteogenesis. The prerequisites for the type of fracture healing include the fracture gap size and the degree of motion between the two bone fragments.

Fracture healing

Fracture healing is a continuous process progressing from the initial fracture haematoma to, ultimately, bone remodelling. The most important factor is adequate blood supply.

Inflammation—formation of granulation tissue

Bleeding from the fracture site and disruption of surrounding tissues (periosteum, blood vessels, and muscles) results in a haematoma which may expand into the surrounding tissues. Soon after fracture, the blood vessels constrict, stopping any further bleeding The haematoma provides a source of haematopoietic cells capable of secreting growth factors. The fibrillar network of the haematoma serves as a scaffold for invading fibroblasts which become part of a composite matrix called granulation tissue (Figure 1.4.4). In the fracture thrombus, platelet-derived growth factor (PDGF) is released. Necrotic material releases cytokines which attract macrophages. Osteoclasts (derived from circulating monocytes) and their marrow precursors resorb bony debris and avascular bone ends. Cytokines also encourage vascular buds to form and begin to invade the fracture site. Examples of cytokines involved include fibroblast growth factor (FGF) which stimulates angiogenesis and TGFβ which initiates chondroblast and osteoblast formation. The fibroblasts replicate and form a loose aggregate of cells, interspersed with small blood vessels, known as granulation tissue. This is the perfused, fibrous connective tissue that replaces a fibrin clot.

Repair—formation of the fracture callus

During the repair phase, the fracture haematoma is replaced by soft callus consisting of fibroblasts, chondroblasts, and osteoblasts. A few days following the fracture, cells from the periosteum are

Fracture pattern	Appearance	Mechanism of injury	Location of soft-tissue hinge	Energy
Transverse	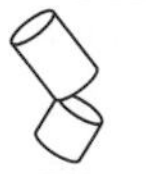	Bending	Concavity	Low
Spiral	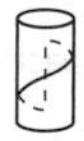	Torsion	Vertical segment	Low
Oblique transverse or butterfly	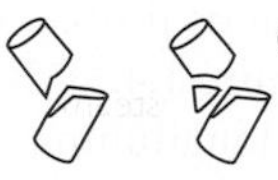	Compression + bending	Concavity or side of butterfly	Moderate
Oblique	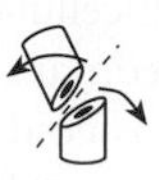	Compression + bending + torsion	Concavity (often destroyed)	Moderate
Comminuted	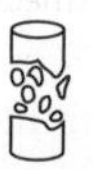	Variable	Destroyed	High
Metaphyseal compression	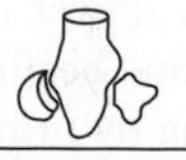	Compression	Variable	Variable

Fig. 1.4.3 Summary of long bone fracture mechanics. Reproduced from Gozna and Harrington (1982).

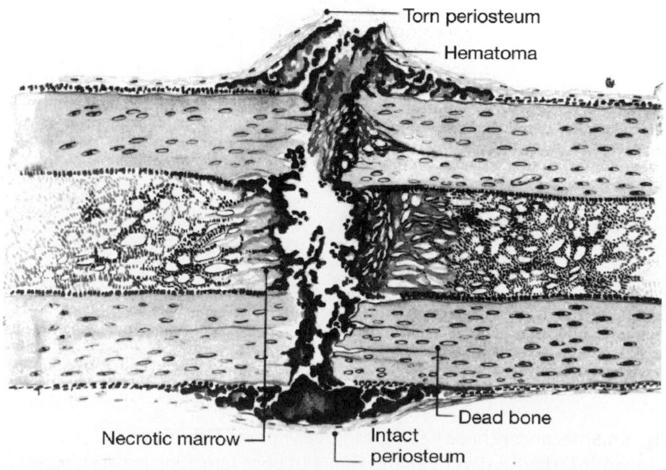

Fig. 1.4.4 Secondary bone healing: initial response after diaphyseal fracture. Periosteum remains intact over point of impact but is torn on opposite side. Hematoma forms on the periosteum and between fracture fragments. Bone ends and marrow adjacent to fracture site are necrotic. Reproduced from Cruess, R., Dumont, J. (1975). Fracture healing. *Canadian Journal of Surgery*, **18**, 403–13.

recruited, replicated, and transformed into specific cells. The periosteal cells proximal to the fracture gap develop into chondroblasts and form hyaline cartilage. The periosteal cells distal to the fracture gap develop into osteoblasts and form woven (immature) bone. The fibroblasts within the granulation tissue also develop into chondroblasts and form hyaline cartilage. This process forms the fracture callus. Eventually, the fracture gap is bridged by the hyaline cartilage and woven bone, restoring some of its original strength and stability. The callus strength and stiffness appears to be prerequisites for mineralization of the fibrocartilage and subsequent transformation to woven bone. Mineralization appears to be a two-step process. The glycosaminoglycans (inhibit mineralization) are counteracted by neutral proteoglycanases secreted by the chondrocytes. Calcium phosphate complexes released by chondrocytes and osteoblasts initiate callus mineralization.

The next phase is the replacement of the hyaline cartilage and woven bone with lamellar bone thereby restoring much, if not all, of the bone's original strength. The replacement process is known as endochondral ossification with respect to the hyaline cartilage and 'bony substitution' with respect to the woven bone. The lamellar bone begins forming soon after the collagen matrix of either tissue becomes mineralized. Vascular channels and osteoblasts penetrate the mineralized matrix. The osteoblasts form new lamellar bone upon the surface of the mineralized matrix. This new lamellar bone is in the form of trabecular bone.

The fibrinous to osseous callus transformation closely resembles enchondral ossification and typically occurs in the central healing zone. More peripherally, the cambium layer of the elevated periosteum generates woven bone using intramembranous ossification (Figure 1.4.5). This develops a circumferential bone sleeve, hard callus, conveying early and progressive stability to the fracture site.

Remodelling phase

This process begins during the middle of the repair phase and continues long after the fracture has clinically healed (up to 7 years). The remodelling process substitutes the trabecular bone with compact bone and allows the bone to assume its normal configuration and shape based on the stresses to which it is exposed (Wolff's law). The trabecular bone is first resorbed by osteoclasts, creating a shallow resorption pit known as a 'Howship's lacuna'. Then osteoblasts deposit compact bone within the resorption pit. Eventually, the fracture callus is remodelled into a new shape which closely duplicates the bone's original shape and strength.

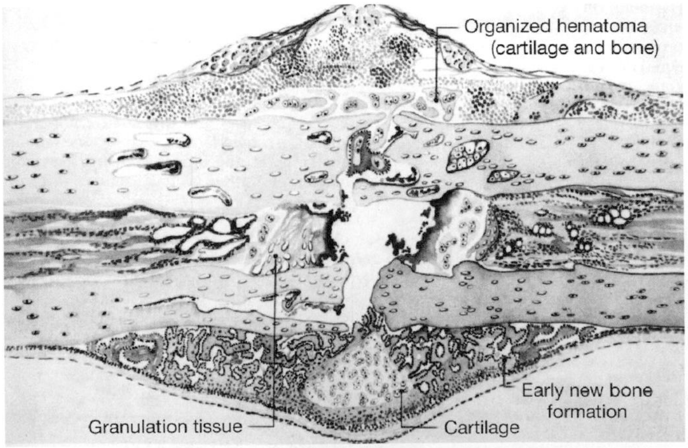

Fig. 1.4.5 Secondary bone healing: early repair phase. Organization of the haematoma. There is direct intramembranous bone formation between outer cortex and elevated periosteum; cartilage predominates in other areas. There is little callus formation between fracture fragments and in the marrow region. The exact mechanisms that govern callus formation are poorly understood.
Reproduced from Cruess, R., Dumont, J. (1975). Fracture healing. *Canadian Journal of Surgery*, **18**, 403–13.

Box 1.4.5 Repair phase of bone healing

- Fibroblasts, chrondroblasts, and osteoblasts invade granulation tissue
- Fibrous tissue is replaced by cartilage then bone to produce callus
- Bone healing from bone ends resembles endochondral ossification
- Bone healing from periosteum resembles intramembranous ossification.

Type of bone formation

Bone is formed via endochondral, intramembranous, and appositional ossification. With endochondral ossification, bone replaces the cartilage model. With intramembranous ossification, a cartilage precursor is not present. Undifferentiated mesenchymal cells differentiate into osteoblasts and deposit an organic matrix that mineralizes to form bone. Finally, with appositional ossification, osteoblasts align on the bone surface and lay down new bone.

Primary cortical healing occurs with rigid immobilization and anatomic reduction. With closed treatment of the fracture, endochondral ossification with periosteal bridging callus occurs. With rigidly fixed fractures (compression plate), direct osteonal or primary bone healing occurs without visible callus.

Primary bone healing

Primary or direct bone healing is characterized by the absence of formation of callus (which would otherwise be visible on x-ray). The prerequisites include anatomical reduction, absolute rigidity, and interfragmentary compression. Typically, primary bone healing usually occurs with a fracture gap of less than 2mm and motion at the fracture site of less than 1mm. With the development of anatomic reduction and stable fixation with metal plates and screws, the primary fracture healing was seen for the first time. The stability provided by the fixation allows early motion of adjacent joints allowing accelerated rehabilitation.

Primary bone healing is a continuous process of coupled bone resorption and bone formation (Figure 1.4.6). Bone remodelling units form parallel channels to the longitudinal axis of the bone and contain cutting cones lined by multicellular osteoclasts. Behind the cutting cone, the walls of the osteon are lined by osteoblasts which circumferentially appose new osteoid at the rate of about 1μm per day. Completion of a new osteon will take approximately 3–4 months.

The fracture site regains immediate stability with plate fixation, but fracture union usually occurs at a slower rate than would be seen under conditions of secondary bone healing. When comparing two identical fractures, one healing by primary and the other by secondary bone healing, the fracture that heals by secondary bone healing will initially be 66% stronger and 100% more rigid.

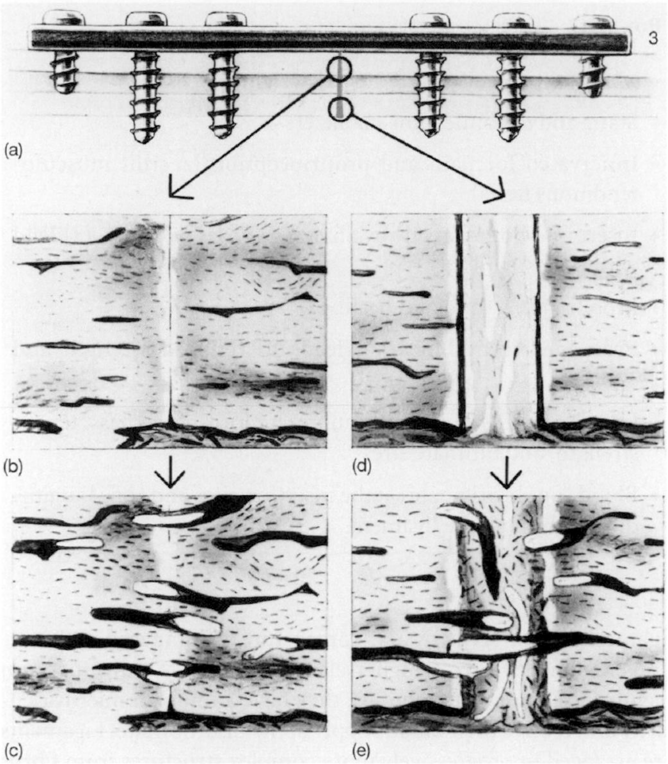

Fig. 1.4.6 Primary bone healing.

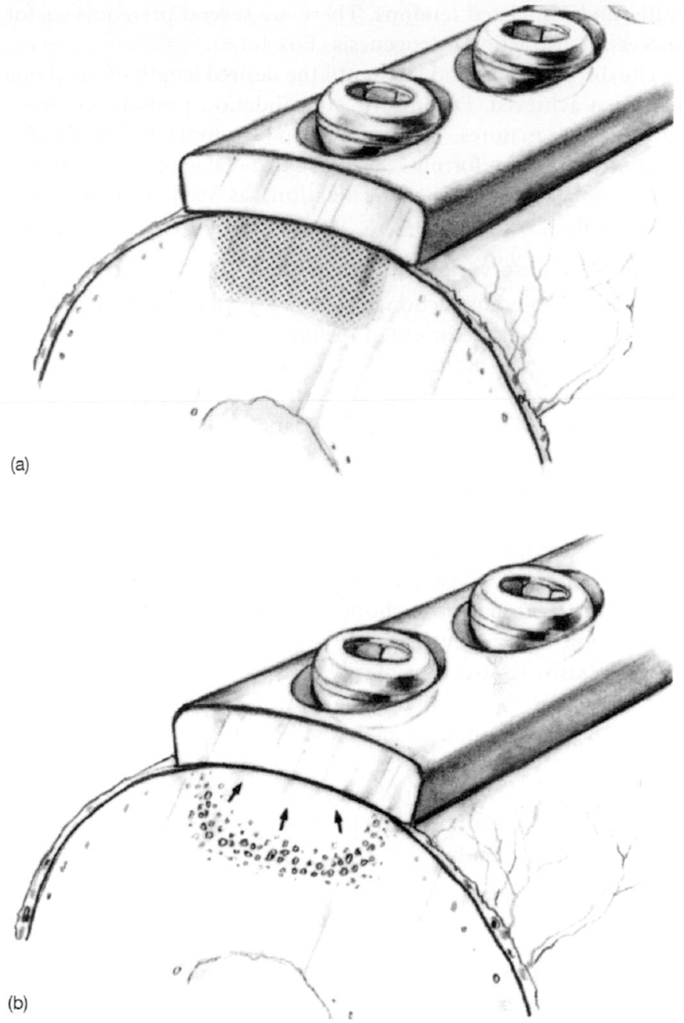

Fig. 1.4.7 Bone necrosis and remodelling after plate application. A) Application of a plate causes regional avascular necrosis under the implant. B) Within 3 months, bone metabolizing units advancing from the intact surrounding bone will remove the necrotic bone (initial porosis) and replace it with new lamellar osteons. Reproduced from Müller, M., Allgöwer, M., Schneider, R., et al. (1991). Basic aspects of internal fixation. In: Allgöwer, M. (ed), *Manual of Internal Fixation. Techniques Recommended by the AO-ASIF group*, 3rd edition, pp. 1–158. Berlin: Springer-Verlag.

Gap healing

Gap healing typically occurs with gap sizes less than or equal to 1mm. The process requires micromotion at the fracture site and occurs in three stages. In stage one, there is rapid filling of the gap with woven bone. Stage two involves Haversian remodelling of the avascular areas at the margins of the fracture edge. In stage three, remodelling of the woven bone to lamellar bone occurs and bridges the gap.

Plate effects

Plating of a fracture provides stability but does not guarantee a particular type of fracture healing. Tightly applied plates may lead to bone necrosis and/or stress shielding.

The bone necrosis directly underneath the implant is caused by the interruption of the periosteal blood supply and the plastic deformation distorting or obliterating the small intraosseous vessels. Plates remaining in place for prolonged periods alter the load-bearing requirements. The resulting stress-shielding effect is dependent on the rigidity of the construct and may lead to permanent reduction of bone cross-sectional area. For this reason, removal of a plate from a large bone should be managed by a period of partial weight bearing (Figure 1.4.7).

Neutralization plates protect the primary lag screw from bending, shear, and rotational forces.

A plate applied to the tension side of a bone achieves stability by axial compression, but also, because of its location on the tension side, bending forces are generated under load. This leads to increased axial compression. Such a plate is referred to as a tension band plate.

Secondary bone healing

Secondary bone healing is often seen with fractures managed with traction or cast. Secondary bone healing progresses through an inflammatory phase followed, within a few days, by a repair phase (several weeks to a few months), and finally a remodelling phase which may continue for several years.

Distraction osteogenesis

Ilizarov invented the technique of distraction osteogenesis in the 1950s. The procedure describes a process of new bone formation after the creation of an osteotomy using controlled gradual distraction of the bone ends. Optimally, intramembranous bone develops. If the process is disturbed (e.g. lack of stability), cartilaginous tissue or fibrous tissue forms and non-union may develop. In addition to bone formation, there are effects on the muscles, vessel walls, and associated tendons. There are several prerequisites for successful distraction osteogenesis (Box 1.4.6).

The distraction period lasts until the desired length of new bone has been achieved. During the consolidation period, the newly formed bone matures. The fixators can be removed when the distraction gap has uniformly consolidated and at least three new cortices have formed (neocorticalization) as seen on orthogonal radiographs.

Histological observations

After initiation of distraction, trabeculae form on both sides of the osteotomy which are oriented in line with the distraction force. The outer surfaces of the trabeculae are covered by a layer of osteoblasts. While the interzone is relatively avascular, the regions between the trabeculae contain abundant capillary blood supply. It appears that the interzone consists of undifferentiated mesenchymal cells which, under optimal conditions, directly transform into osteoblasts (intramembranous bone formation). Under less optimal conditions, chondroblasts or fibroblasts emerge. Depending on the conditions, consolidation of the regenerate may still occur, by a process similar to enchondral ossification. Alternatively, a fibrous non-union may develop.

The Ilizarov fixator is primarily used for bone lengthening and is particularly useful where deformity correction may also be required. In addition, the fixator can be used for the management of non-unions using compression (instead of distraction) and the acute management of complex fractures (e.g. tibial pilon fracture). With optimal conditions, bone formation is principally by intramembranous ossification.

Ligaments: injury and repair

Basic concepts

Ligaments are dense, highly organized connective tissue structures connecting bone to bone (Box 1.4.7) They are composed of cells (fibroblasts) and extracellular matrix principally of type I collagen (70% of the dry weight). They function by stabilizing joints and have embedded in them mechanoreceptors and free nerve endings. The sliding of collagen fibres over each other is key for changes in ligament length (growth and contracture). Compared with tendons, ligaments have a higher elastin content (e.g. ligamentum flavum). In contrast to tendons, they have a uniform microvascularity and receive their blood supply at the insertion site. Ligaments are arranged in progressively more complex structures from fibrils to fasciculi which have a predominantly parallel (collateral ligaments) or spiral (cruciate ligaments) organization.

Box 1.4.6 Prerequisites for distraction osteogenesis

- Fixator strong enough to provide stable fixation and eliminate torsion, shear, and bending
- Blood supply to osteotomy must be preserved—minimal soft tissue stripping/preserve periosteum
- Low energy corticotomy
- Distract at 1mm per day in steps of 0.25mm every 8h
- Osteogenic potential best where cancellous bone dominates—osteotomy through the metaphysis
- Latency period (no lengthening) of 3 days in young children and 5–10 days in adults
- Neutral fixation interval (no distraction) during consolidation
- Normal use of the extremity, including weight bearing (producing physiological loads).

Box 1.4.7 Characteristic of ligaments

- Mainly type I collagen (70% dry weight)
- Static and dynamic joint stabilizers
- Innervated for pain and proprioception (recruit musculotendinous units)
- Insert into bone directly by Sharpey's fibres or indirect (blend with periosteum)
- Mobilization stimulates healing
- Prolonged immobilization leads to reduced strength and elasticity
- Exercise results in increased ultimate force, thickness, tensile strength, and ultimate stress
- Blood supply originates at the insertion sites and runs longitudinally through the ligament.

Ligament insertion into bone represents a transition from one material to another and can be classified into two types: indirect insertion (more common) and direct insertion.

With indirect ligament insertion, superficial ligament fibres insert at acute angles into the periosteum and tend to be broader than direct insertions (e.g. tibial insertion of the medial collateral ligament of the knee). With direct insertions (e.g. femoral insertion of the medial collateral ligament of the knee), there are superficial and deep fibres. The deep fibres insert at right angles to bone and superficial fibres blend with the periosteum. The transition from ligament to bone occurs in four stages: ligament, to fibrocartilage, to mineralized fibrocartilage, to bone. Sharpey's fibres cross all four zones.

The tensile properties of ligaments are similar to those of tendons, with an initial toe region produced by the non-linear straightening of the crimped fibres. As elongation progresses, fibres become more parallel to the load. Ligaments exhibit viscoelastic properties such as creep, hysteresis, and stress relaxation. Clinically, this becomes relevant in anterior cruciate reconstruction where stress relaxation of graft materials may be observed in the initial hours after tensioning, and preconditioning may be appropriate prior to final tensioning. Many ligaments, such as the cruciates, have multiple bands of collagen fibres attached at different points of the insertion. This allows different components of the ligament to tighten with varying joint position.

Mechanisms of injury

Ligament sprains are the most common joint injuries. Three grades of severity are usually differentiated.

- Grade I disruption implies pain with stress, but no increase in laxity

- Grade II injuries produce a slight increase in laxity, but with a solid endpoint to stress
- Grade III injuries are complete disruptions of the ligament with significant laxity and an absence of a firm endpoint to stress.

In the knee, ligament injuries can be produced by contact (medial collateral disruption from a blow to the lateral aspect of the leg) or non-contact (anterior cruciate tears from varus internal rotation or valgus external rotation). The continued application of a deforming force will stress and injure secondary restraints, producing combined ligamentous disruptions. The most common mechanism of ligament failure is rupture of sequential series of collagen fibre bundles. Ligaments do not plastically deform. Mid-substance tears are more common in adults; avulsion injuries are more common in children. Avulsion typically occurs between the un-mineralized and mineralized fibrocartilage layers.

Healing of extra-articular ligaments

Healing occurs in three phases, a pattern similar to bone, and benefits from normal stress and strain across the joint. Immobilization adversely affects the strength (elastic modulus decreases) of an intact ligament and of a ligament repair. Immediately post injury, bleeding produces a fibrin clot. Within 3 days, macrophages, platelets, and neutrophils migrate to the injury site and release chemotactic, proteolytic and angiogenic factors. Early healing produces a disorganized cellular scar consisting primarily of type III collagen and proteoglycans. The proliferative scar formation slowly produces increased type I collagen. Remodelling takes place up to a year following injury. Mature ligament repair tissue only achieves 70% of the tensile strength of normal ligament tissue. The increased cross-sectional area of the repair tissue appears to compensate for this weakness. Increased tensile stress and early mobilization in the healing phase of a transected medial collateral ligament results in increased total collagen and improved histological organization. Therefore, operative repair is not always necessary.

Healing of intra-articular ligaments

Intra-articular ligaments do not display predictable healing. A fibrin clot is not produced after an anterior cruciate ligament injury, maybe because of synovial fluid interference. Repairs of mid-substance intra-articular ligament tears have rarely been successful and as a consequence such interventions have been replaced by primary or secondary reconstructions.

Injury and repair of articular cartilage

Basic concepts

The varieties of cartilage include: growth plate (physeal), fibrocartilage at tendon and ligament insertions, elastic (e.g. trachea), fibroelastic (e.g. menisci), and articular cartilage. Articular cartilage functions to reduce friction and distribute loads across joints. It is classically described as avascular, aneural, and alymphatic. Chondrocytes receive nutrients and oxygen from synovial fluid via diffusion through the matrix.

Composition

The tissue predominantly consists of water (65–80% of wet weight). Shifts of the retained water in and out of cartilage allow for surface deformation secondary to the stresses applied. In osteoarthritis, the water content may increase to account for 90% of weight. Increased water content results in increased permeability, reduced strength, and decreased Young's modulus of elasticity. In addition, water is involved in nutrition and lubrication. The primary mechanism responsible for lubrication during dynamic function is elastohydrodynamic lubrication. Here, deformation of articular surfaces and thin films of joint lubricates separates the surfaces. Other types of lubrication methods include: boundary, boosted, hydrodynamic, and weeping lubrication.

Collagen makes up 10–20% of the wet weight and type II collagen accounts for approximately 90–95% of the total collagen content. The cartilaginous framework which anchors the cartilage to the subchondral bone is responsible for tensile strength and shear stiffness. Cartilage consists of a limited number of chondrocytes (5% of wet weight) surrounded by extensive extracellular matrix consisting mainly of type II collagen and proteoglycans (10–15% of wet weight). Protein polysaccharides provide compressive strength. Proteoglycans are produced by chondrocytes and are composed of subunits of gylcosaminoglycans (GAGs). GAGs are bound to a protein core by a sugar bond to form an aggregan molecule. Charged hydrophilic groups on the proteoglycans hold water and produce the swelling pressure resulting in the ability of cartilage to resist compressive loads. Shear and compression squeeze water to the articular surface and thus diminish friction during joint motion. Other matrix components include adhesives (fibronectin, chondronectin) and lipids.

With aging, chondrocytes increase in size and no longer reproduce leading to a relative hypocellularity. Cartilage stiffness increases. The proteoglycans decrease in mass and size. Protein content increases and water content decreases. These changes lead to a reduced elasticity. The structure and layers of articular cartilage are described in Box 1.4.8.

Cartilage injury

Vascular–inflammatory tissue response to injury occurs only once the subchondral bone is penetrated, allowing distinction between superficial cartilage injuries which do not involve the

Box 1.4.8 Structure of articular cartilage

- Collagen network held in tension by hydrostatic pressure from proteoglycan surface
- Surface gliding layer (10–20%): tangential array of cells and collagen fibres inserted at right angles to each other. This zone has the greatest tensile strength
- Middle transitional layer (40–60%): obliquely arranged fibres
- Deep radial layer (30%): vertical fibres with increased chondrocyte volume. The collagen fibres are oriented perpendicular to the joint surface
- Tidemark; boundary between the calcified and uncalcified cartilage
- Basal zone: calcified cartilage linking to the subchondral bone (hydroxyapatite crystals anchor the cartilage to subchondral bone) forms a transitional zone of intermediate stiffness between cartilage and subchondral bone.

Box 1.4.9 Types of cartilage injury

- Superficial: vertical fissures (wedge-shaped defects) that rarely progress beyond the tidemark and subchondral bone
- Deep: penetrates subchondral bone resulting in haematoma, fibrin clot, and activation of inflammatory response. Fissuring of the calcified cartilage and then the subchondral bone can occur with secondary progression to fibrillation of the more superficial layers.

subchondral bone and deep cartilage injuries which do (Box 1.4.9, Figure 1.4.8).

Cartilage healing

The stages of cartilage healing are summarized in Box 1.4.10. Deep injuries may heal with fibrocartilage which is produced by undifferentiated marrow mesenchymal stem cells that differentiate into cells capable of producing fibrocartilage. Type I collagen is in abundance at 1 year post injury. For deep injuries, most of our knowledge stems from techniques such as drilling and puncturing the bed of osteochondral defects and abrasion chondroplasty. Here the calcified cartilage is penetrated or removed down to bleeding subchondral bone which is initially covered by a fibrin clot. This is followed by formation of hyaline cartilage (type II collagen) and later fibrocartilage (type I collagen). Superficial lacerations cause chondrocytes to proliferate but do not heal because cartilage is avascular.

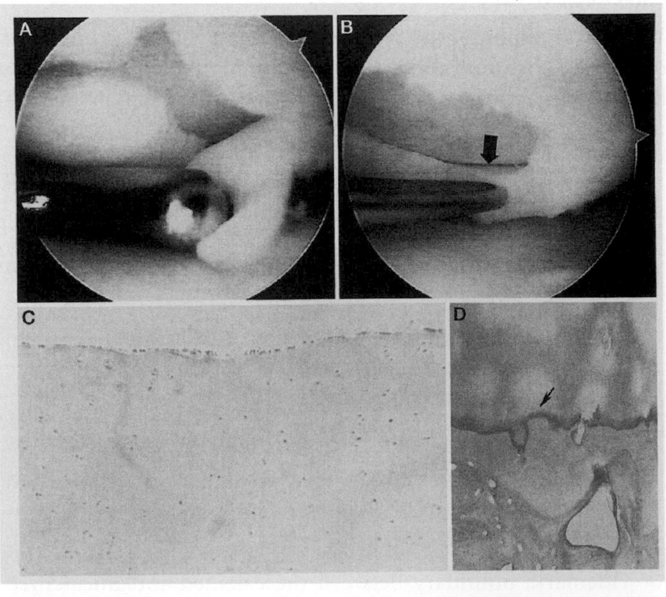

Fig. 1.4.8 A) Arthroscopic view of the medial femoral condyle in a 22-year-old female football player. The chondral delamination flap is identified at tip of probe. B) The same arthroscopic view after removal of the delamination flap. Further delamination (arrow) extends past the border. C) A histological section of the delamination flap in the same patient. The surface and superficial layers appear normal. D) A histological section of the delamination border from the same patient, demonstrating failure at the tidemark (arrow).

Box 1.4.10 Cartilage healing

- Superficial: chondrocyte proliferation and matrix production insufficient to repair the defect completely
- Deep: fibrin clot replaced by hyaline cartilage (type II collagen) and then by fibrocartilage (type I collagen)

Injury and repair of tendons

Structure and anatomy

Tendons are densely arranged tissues that connect and transmit loads from muscle to bone. They are structurally organized in order to resist high tensile forces and are composed of groups of collagen bundles (fascicles—composed of fibrils), separated by endotenon with surrounding epitenon (Box 1.4.11). The predominant cell type is fibroblasts. They are arranged in parallel rows in fascicles with surrounding peritenon (areolar tissue). The spindle-shaped fibroblasts mainly produce type I collagen and synthesize the connective tissue matrix precursors including elastin, and proteoglycans. Elastin is a protein found in small quantities within tendons (less than 1% dry weight). It enables tendons to undergo large changes in length without any permanent structural change. The water-binding capacity of proteoglycans, glycoproteins, and glycosaminoglycans influences the viscoelastic properties of tendons.

The collagen contains a high concentration of the amino acids glycine (33%), proline (15%), and hydroxyproline (15%). All types of collagen consist of three particular chains covalently cross-linked and combined with globular and non-helical structural elements to form a rigid triple tropocollagen molecule. In the extracellular matrix, collagen molecules become aligned head-to-tail and side-by-side in a quarter-staggered array (Figure 1.4.9) leading to a highly ordered and stable unit of microfibrils and fibrils.

Tendons surrounded by paratenon are referred to as vascular tendons. Those surrounded by a tendon sheath are called avascular tendons. The avascular tendons contained within synovial sheaths

Box 1.4.11 Structure of tendon

- Mainly type I collagen (85%)
- Small amounts of type III and IV collagen
- Fascicles held together by endotenon (permits longitudinal movement)
- Endotenon is continuous with periosteum—carries blood supply, lymphatics, and nerves
- Epitenon—peripheral to the endotenon
- Paratenon surrounds some tendons and functions as an elastic sheath to allow free gliding
- Peritendon—comprised of the epitenon and paratenon (Figure 1.4.10)
- Synovium surrounding some tendons is called tenosynovium (e.g. flexor tendons in hand).

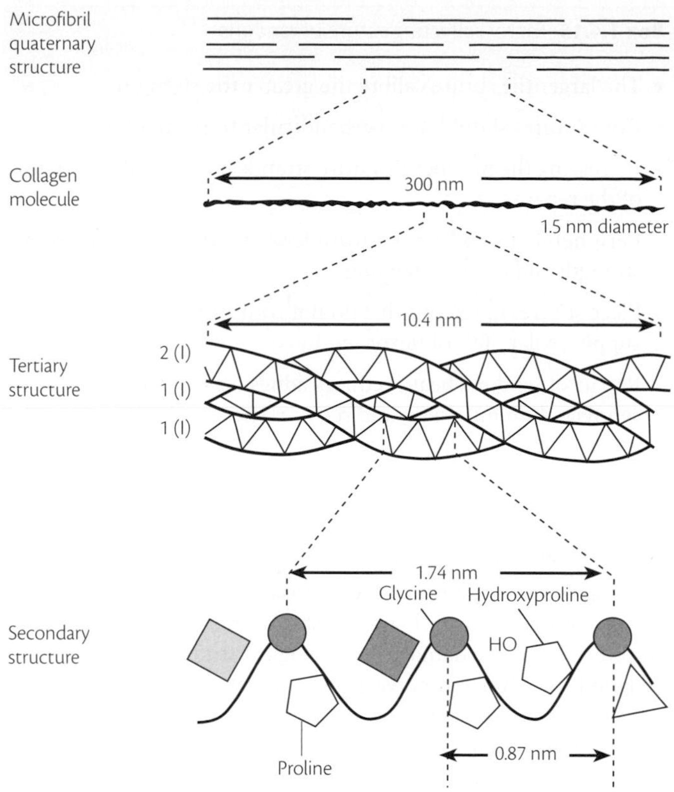

Fig. 1.4.9 Schematic drawing of the structural organization of collagen in the microfibril.

have mesotenons that function as vascularized conduits called vincula. In addition, both types of tendons have additional blood supply from vessels originating in the muscle and bone attachments.

Biomechanical properties

Tendons insert into bone via four transitional tissues: tendon, fibrocartilage, mineralized fibrocartilage (Sharpey's fibres), and finally to bone. Tendinous structures orient themselves along stress lines and possess one of the highest tensile strengths of all soft tissues. However, because of the low amount of ground substance, tendons resist shear and compressive forces poorly.

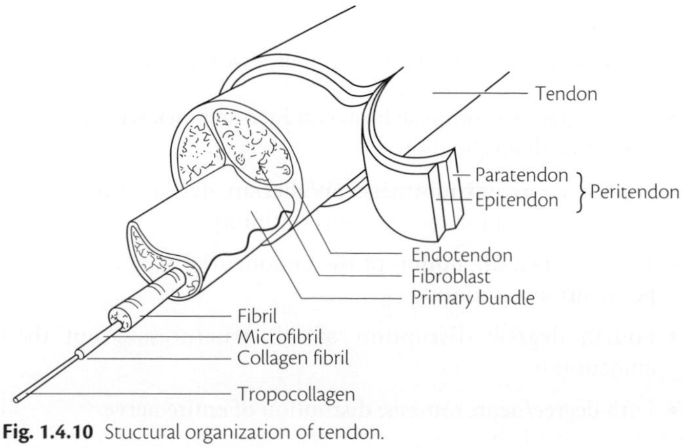

Fig. 1.4.10 Stuctural organization of tendon.

Box 1.4.12 Factors affecting biomechanical properties of tendons

- Exercise increases collagen fibril size and strength, ultimate tensile strength (UTS), and stiffness
- Immobilization decreases water content and proteoglycan concentration, UTS, and stiffness
- Anatomical location
- Collagen content of fibril and fibril diameter reduces with age leading to reduced UTS. The collagen cross linking increases with age leading to greater stiffness

Elongation of tendons is dependent on the force magnitude and the rate and duration of the force. With repetitive loading and unloading, their stress–strain curve moves to the right as the tendon becomes less stiff or more compliant. An increase in elongation, speed, and a higher strain rate moves the curve to the left, indicating increasing stiffness. This protects tendons from rupturing under very large eccentric forces. Tendons also exhibit creep. In an isometric contraction, tendon lengthening from creep allows the muscle to shorten over time. This increases muscle performance by decreasing fatigue.

Factors affecting the properties of tendons are described in Box 1.4.12.

Tendon injury

Indirect or direct trauma may lead to tendon injury. The former commonly manifests as an intrasubstance rupture or bony avulsion. The injury is influenced by anatomic location, vascular supply, skeletal maturity, and the magnitude of the applied force. Most indirect injuries are at the bone–tendon or muscle–tendon interface. This is related to tendons' ability to withstand high tensile forces. Mid-substance tendon rupture is often secondary to pre-existing pathological conditions and may be seen in chronic overuse injuries with repetitive microtrauma and incomplete healing. Common sites of degenerative change include the Achilles, patella, rotator cuff, and biceps tendons.

Tendon healing

Tendons have extrinsic and intrinsic healing potential. The extrinsic theory hypothesises that an inflammatory response by the surrounding tissues is involved. The intrinsic theory maintains that tendons possess an intrinsic capability to heal.

Healing continues in three phases: inflammatory, reparative or collagen-producing phase, and a remodelling phase (Box 1.4.13). In the inflammatory phase, cells from the extrinsic peritendinous tissues (synovial sheath, deep fascia, and periosteum) and intrinsic tissue of the epitenon and endotenon move into the injured area (first 48–72h) and remove cellular debris and collagen remnants. Granulation tissue is produced to bridge the defect. In the inflammatory phase, tendon repair strength is almost entirely dependent on the suture strength. In the reparative stage, fibroblasts are actively involved in collagen synthesis and resorption. The remodelling phase results in increased mechanical strength. Tension on the granulation tissue results in remodelling of fibre architecture; similar to Wolff's law for bone.

Box 1.4.13 Healing of tendons

- Inflammatory phase (to day 14): defect filled with fibrin clot, tissue debris, and fluid
- Reparative phase: collagen synthesis begins in first week (maximum at week 4)
- Collagen orientates over 4 weeks (perpendicular to the long axis of the tendon to parallel)
- The synovial sheath repairs in 3 weeks
- Remodelling (after 4 weeks): collagen production changes from type III to type I for 12 months.

Box 1.4.15 Factors affecting suture of tendons

- The larger the suture calibre the greater the strength
- Core sutures should pass perpendicular to the tendon
- Increasing the number of suture strands increases the strength of the repair
- Peripheral epitendinous suture leads to 10–50% increase in strength and reduces gapping
- Place sutures in regions that do not compromise tendon blood supply (volar 50% of flexor tendons)
- Repair of tendon sheath reduces adhesion formation, restores synovial fluid nutrition, and restores sheath mechanics.

Methods of improving tendon repair

The most important factor appears to be postoperative mobilization of tendon repairs. Rapid commencement of tendon gliding provides the stimulus for cellular activation of the epitenon (intrinsic response). Continued immobilization stimulates ingrowth of cells from the surrounding tissues (extrinsic response) leading to adhesions. An ideal postoperative protocol is one providing the greatest tensile stress across a repair and preventing gap formation or rupture of the repair. The ultimate goal is to restore immediate motion and stress to a tendon repair. Limiting factors include the strength of the repair, which is a factor in all locations of injury. The benefits of passive mobilization are characterized in Box 1.4.14.

Following suture principles increases strength of the repair (Box 1.4.15).

Nerve injuries and repair

Peripheral nerve anatomy

The peripheral nerve is a highly organized structure made of nerve fibres, blood vessels, and connective tissue. They possess peripheral processes named axons which are covered with a fibrous tissue called endoneurium. The axons group into nerve bundles called fascicles (smallest unit of a nerve), covered by a connective tissue layer named perineurium. Schwann cells support and surround the axons. Groups of fascicles are bound together by the epineurium, which provides a gliding surface. Fascicles are vascularized segmentally by epineurial vessels and each fascicle has a longitudinally-oriented perineurial and endoneurial microvascular system. Myelinated axons conduct action potentials rapidly, facilitated by nodes of Ranvier (gaps between Schwann cells).

Box 1.4.14 Consequences of passive mobilization of tendons

- Rapid recovery of tensile strength
- Fewer adhesions
- Improved excursion
- Better nutrition.

Classification of nerve injuries

Sharp lacerations result in nerve transactions whereas the energy transfer secondary to a blast, crush, or traction injury leads to unpredictable nerve damage. Neurological studies such as electromyography (EMG) and nerve conduction studies may be useful to document injury extent. Cortical evoked potential testing is the most accurate method. Seddon (1943) first described three types of nerve injury: neurapraxia, axonotomesis, and neurotomesis. Subsequently, Sunderland (1951) defined five severity degrees with two degrees lying between axonotomesis and neurotomesis (Box 1.4.16).

Healing of nerve injuries

Peripheral nerve injury results in death of the distal axons and Wallerian degeneration of myelin. Macrophages remove degraded myelin and axoplasm. Regeneration is dependent on nerve cell survival. The remaining Schwann cell tube serves as a guide for the sprouting axon. The distal nerve stumps and target organs facilitate axonal regeneration using neurotropic and adhesive factors. Within hours of injury, a regenerating axon produces multiple sprouts from the most distal intact node of Ranvier which enter the Schwann cell tubes. Eventually, only one axon is regenerated. Proximal axonal budding occurs approximately 1 month post injury and results in regeneration at a rate of about 1mm/day.

Box 1.4.16 Types of nerve injury in progressive order of severity

- First degree/neuropraxia: local conduction block secondary to segmental demyelination
- Second degree/axonotmesis: Wallerian degeneration with distal degeneration, epineurium continuity
- Third degree: disruption of the endoneurial tube and axon, perineurium continuity
- Fourth degree: disruption of all structures except the epineurium
- Fifth degree/neurotomesis: disruption of entire nerve.

Pain is the first modality to return. The final pathway to achieving nerve regeneration requires the plasticity or re-education of the central nervous system. The brain must undergo some re-education to interpret the stimulus correctly.

Nerve repair

Basic principles

Some basic principles are discussed in Box 1.4.17. Motor recovery is unlikely if there is lack of reinnervation by 18 months, and results are worse if repair is performed 6 months after the injury.

The following key concepts underpin successful nerve repair:

1) Microsurgical techniques with adequate magnification, instrumentation, and microsuture
2) Adequate exposure of both ends followed by debridement and resection of the damaged nerve section to minimize scar tissue formation
3) Reapposition of nerve ends tension-free with avoidance of extreme positioning of the extremity
4) Primary nerve repair should be performed whenever possible
5) Align fascicles accurately.

Accurate nerve alignment is critical for optimal outcome. The simplest method is using anatomical landmarks such as epineural blood vessels and fascicle arrangement. Electrical stimulation in the awake patient can help delineate motor and sensory fascicles in the proximal stump. Staining of the nerve ends using acetylcholinesterase (motor) and carbonic anhydrase (sensory) may be performed on sections of proximal nerve ends to identify sensory and motor fascicles of the proximal stump only.

Repair techniques

Three types of direct repair are available to the surgeon: epineural, group fascicular, and fascicular. Factors influencing results of nerve repair are summarized in Box 1.4.18.

- *Epineural repair* is used when internal topography of the nerve is unclear. Fascicles are aligned using fine monofilament suture under high-power magnification. Sutures are placed only through the epineurium to avoid bunching. Tension must be assessed after the repair and the extremity taken through a gentle range of motion
- *Group fascicular repair* is most useful in nerves with few groups and in partial lacerations where complete fascicular groups are lacerated. The fascicle groups are exposed by splitting the epineurium longitudinally. The largest identifiable fascicle group should be repaired first. The epineurium is finally repaired to minimize tension
- *Fascicular repair* is useful in partial lacerations and in nerves with few fascicles. The technique requires dissection of external and internal epineurium to expose the fascicles. Repair is effected using one or two sutures of 10-0 or 11-0 nylon placed in the perineurium.

Nerve grafts

Complex crush and blast injuries are best treated with nerve grafts. When there is no recovery after approximately 3 months, exploration and repair may be indicated. The success of grafting and sources of nerve graft are documented in Box 1.4.19.

Postoperative care

The site of the nerve repair, or the proximal and distal ends of a nerve grafts, are carefully documented. The extremity is immobilized in a position that relaxes all suture lines which may be maintained for 4 weeks. Regeneration is monitored by physical examination and electrical studies. As sensory axons may regenerate to sensory end-organs, the signal the brain receives may not correspond to the actual stimulation. The patient must be

Box 1.4.17 Principles of nerve repair

- Sharp lacerations should be explored and repaired
- Open injuries with nerve deficits: explore and nerve ends repaired or tagged for later repair
- Blunt closed injuries should be observed
- If no recovery in 3 months (lack of advancing Tinel, electrical studies), explore
- Delayed repair: contamination, lack of soft tissue cover, blast injury, or head injury prevent assessment

Box 1.4.18 Factors that influence success of repair

- Age: children do best (greater cerebral plasticity adapts well to new signals). Adults may improve up to 5years
- Level of injury: proximal injuries have poorer results because distal muscles becomes fibrotic before regenerated motor axons reach their target
- Type of nerve: mixed motor and sensory nerves have inferior recovery compared with primarily motor or sensory nerves—difficulty in alignment.

Box 1.4.19 Successful grafting procedures and sources of nerve graft

- Principles which provide good nerve healing:
  - Healed and supple wound
  - Well-vascularized recipient bed
  - Nerve ends must be free of scar tissue
  - Fascicular anatomy is recorded, and appropriately matched groups of fascicles connected with a nerve graft.
  - Grafts must be sutured tension-free in the correct anatomic alignment for success.
- Sources of graft:
  - Sural nerve provides 30–40cm of graft—tightly packed fascicles and little interfascicular tissue
  - Medial antebrachial cutaneous nerves
  - Terminal branch of the posterior interosseous nerve.

re-educated to interpret the new signal. Children accomplish this much more readily than older patients. Placing the cut nerve endings into a tube (silicone, biodegradable material, or vein) has demonstrated excellent results in pure sensory nerve injuries.

Proprioception

Proprioception gives us a sense of position and movement in relation to space, and initiates and coordinates the muscle functions that first stabilize a joint and then make it the fulcrum of a precise, coordinated motion. Deficits occur when afferent sensory nerve fibres are interrupted (injury or disease) and can affect entire limb function. Vision can be a substitute but is less effective in the lower than in the upper extremity. Proprioception relies on information from sensory, visual, and vestibular inputs. Based on afferent information, efferent stimuli are generated centrally. These stimuli activate agonistic and antagonistic muscle groups to reposition joints and extremity segments.

Sensory input derives from muscle spindles, Golgi tendon organs, Pacinian corpuscles, Meissner's corpuscles, and other receptors in muscles, tendons, ligaments, joints, and skin. The cell bodies of these nerve fibres are located in the dorsal root ganglia. From here, fibres connect to neurons relaying information centrally to the cerebellum, medulla, thalamus, and the cerebral cortex (Figure 1.4.11). Isolated injuries to ligaments, joints, muscles, or other end-organs results in a focal loss of feedback.

Head injuries: presentations and outcomes

Head injury is often associated with major musculoskeletal disruptions and cerebral lesions are commonly diagnosed late or managed inadequately. Head injuries are two to three times more common in males and have a higher incidence in summer months. The commonest mechanism of injury is motor vehicle accidents. Although many head injuries present similarly, they can be differentiated by the type of pathological lesion as follows.

- **Shearing/diffuse axonal injuries** Shearing is a consequence of acceleration, deceleration, and rotational forces which damages the brain by stretching and compressing fibre tracts; and moving the brain over bony prominences. Shearing and diffuse axonal injuries are rarely picked up on initial computed tomography (CT) scans. Magnetic resonance imaging (MRI) is the gold standard in detecting these injuries.
- **Contusions** These are bruises or haematomas on or close to the brain's surface. They commonly affect the frontal and temporal lobes. They may be asymptomatic or associated with severe neurological deficits and seizures.
- **Epidural haematoma** This refers to a collection of blood between the dura mater and the skull and occurs secondary to a tear of the middle meningeal artery. They can cause sudden compression of the brain and be fatal. Clinically, a short lucid interval is typical, followed by loss of consciousness.
- **Subdural haematoma** The bleeding occurs within the subdural space. Onset may be acute or, especially in the elderly, chronic. Chronic lesions are commonly caused by linear and rotational forces which tear the veins between the brain and the dura mater. Most subdural haematomas result in significant focal damage of the cortex and co-exist with brain contusions.

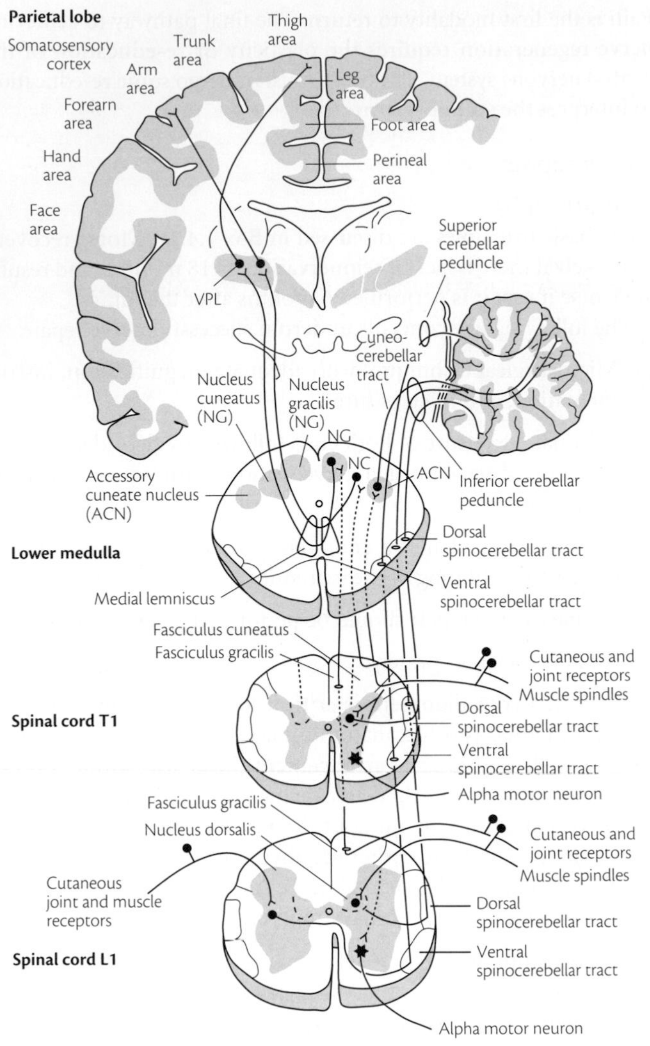

Fig. 1.4.11 The central nervous system pathways mediating proprioception and stereognosis. Note that the origin of the crossed ventral spinocerebellar tract is on the left side of the diagram and the origin of the other tracts in on the right. ACN, accessory cuneate nucleus; NC, nucleus cuneatus; NG, nucleus gracilis; VPL, thalamic nucleus ventral posterolateral.

- **Subarachnoid haemorrhage** Bleeding into the subarachnoid space is often caused by trauma but may occur spontaneously after rupture of a berry aneurysm. The bleeding is usually diffuse and does not cause a space-occupying lesion.
- **Intracerebral haematomas and brain displacement** These space-occupying lesions are often accompanied by swelling of surrounding brain tissues. They may cause life-threatening brain herniation following expansion.

Classification and assessment of head injuries

The Glasgow Coma Scale provides a score (in the range 3–15) to initially assess the likelihood of a brain injury. A score of 3 indicates that the patient is unresponsive. A score less than 9 must prompt an urgent evaluation of the airway. With a score of 15, the patient is alert, oriented, and able to follow commands. While the Glasgow Coma Scale is an excellent predictor of gross outcome, it is less reliable in predicting neurobehavioral outcomes. The most reliable predictor of neurobehavioral outcome is the duration of post-traumatic amnesia. When the patient has sustained post-traumatic amnesia of 24h or less, the head injury is classified as mild. If the post-traumatic amnesia lasts from 24h to 7 days, the head injury is considered moderate. Post-traumatic amnesia beyond 7 days indicates a severe head injury.

CT scans and MRI scans provide additional parameters to assess head injury. However, a patient with a very severe head injury may have negative initial findings on both CT and MRI scans.

In summary, the key factors that predict the severity of a head injury are as follows:

- The Glasgow Coma Scale score
- Duration of loss of consciousness or coma
- Duration of post-traumatic amnesia
- The nature and extent of the cerebral lesion as seen on CT or MRI.

Positive prognostic factors include high premorbid intelligence quotients and socioeconomic status, as well as a supportive family structure.

Clinical presentation: postconcussive syndrome

Neurobehavioral symptoms following head injuries are often missed because of inexperience or masking secondary to pain medication. Typical symptoms of postconcussive syndrome include inhibition, euphoria, emotional lability, confusion, memory disturbance, disturbance of social or occupational functions, concentration, and higher-order thought deficits.

Many head injuries have psychological sequelae such as irritability and agitation as well as exaggerated reactions to painful stimuli. Protracted malaise and depression may be the sequelae of a concomitant head injury. Diagnosis and management of many head injuries can be improved by consulting an experienced clinical neuropsychologist skilled in cognitivebehavioural techniques such as desensitization or hypnotherapy.

Acute and chronic higher cortical deficits due to head injuries

Acute deficits

Patients with significant head injuries are usually comatose or obtunded on presentation. With recovery, the level of cortical arousal becomes heightened and the mental status improves. Postcomatose patients, display moderate to severe global and diffuse deficits of cognitive function.

Influence of age

Adult patients may remain in a coma for long periods and only gradually recover their mental capabilities. Children tend to improve quickly or perish. Typical symptoms resulting from traumatic brain injury in adults are either absent or short-lived in the paediatric population.

Language functions

Most adult patients sustaining injury to the temporal lobe will experience severe aphasia, difficulties in comprehension, naming, repetition, reading, and writing. If children present with aphasic symptoms, recovery is often rapid. Complete mutism, which resolves in 1 or 2 weeks, may be pronounced. Similar differences have been observed with respect to visual and visuospatial dysfunction.

Psychiatric problems

Adults may suffer a range of psychiatric conditions, from mild anxiety disorders to psychosis. Children under 10 years of age frequently suffer attention-deficit disorders without the hyperactive component. Adolescents tend to experience depression, anxiety, and explosive behaviour.

Long-term deficits

Most neurobehavioral recovery occurs 12 months after injury. Improvement up to 3 years is not uncommon. Residual deficits usually involve attention and concentration, verbal and visual memory, and higher-thought processes including planning, problem solving, and strategy formation. Resolution of these symptoms is usually much more complete in the paediatric population.

Further reading

Allgower, M. and Spiegel, P. (1979). Internal fixation of fractures: Evolution of concepts. *Clinical Orthopaedics and Related Research*, **138**, 26–9.

Anderson, H. (1990). The role of cells versus matrix in bone induction. *Connective Tissue Research*, **24**, 3–12.

Blenman, P., Carter, D., and Beaupre, G. (1989). Role of mechanical loading in the progressive ossification of a fracture callus. *Journal of Orthopaedic Research*, **7**, 398–407.

Buckwalter, J. and Cooper, R. (1987). Bone structure and function. *Instructional Course Lectures*, **36**, 27–48.

Cruess, R. and Dumont, J. (1975). Fracture healing. *Canadian Journal of Surgery*, **18**, 403–13.

Ilizarov, G. (1989). The tension-stress effect on the genesis and growth of tissues: Part I. The influence of stability of fixation and soft tissue preservation. *Clinical Orthopaedics*, **283**, 249–81.

Ilizarov, G. (1989). The tension-stress effect on the genesis and growth of tissues: Part II. The influence of the rate and frequency of distraction. *Clinical Orthopaedics*, **283**, 249–81.

Katz, J.L. (1981). Composite material models for cortical bone. In: Cowin, S.C. (ed) *Mechanical Properties of Bone*, pp. 171–84. New York: American Society of Mechanical Engineers.

Kenwright, J., Richardson, J., Cunningham, J., *et al.* (1991). Axial movement and tibial fractures: a controlled randomised trial of treatment. *Journal of Bone and Joint Surgery*, **73-B**, 654–9.

Müller, M., Allgöwer, M., Schneider, R., *et al.* (1991). Basic aspects of internal fixation. In: Allgöwer, M. (ed), *Manual of Internal Fixation. Techniques Recommended by the AO-ASIF group*, 3rd edition, pp. 1–158. Berlin: Springer-Verlag.

Perren, S. (1979). Physical and biological aspects of fracture healing with special reference to internal fixation. *Clinical Orthopaedics and Related Research*, **138**, 175–96.

Seddon, H. (1943). Three types of nerve injury. *Brain*, **66**, 237–88.

Sunderland, S. (1951). A classification of peripheral nerve injuries producing loss of function. *Brain*, **74**, 491–516.

Wolff, J. (1892). *Das Gesetz der Transformation der Knochen*. Hirschwalk, Berlin.

1.5

Haemoglobinopathies

Paul L.F. Giangrande

Summary points

- Haemoglobinopathies are commonly inherited disorders of haemoglobin synthesis
- Thalassaemia is commonest around the Mediterranean countries and has skeletal manifestations due to massive marrow expansion with thinning of the cortex
- Sickle cell crises occur in homozygotes and are a result of venous occlusion causing avascular necrosis. Infection and exposure to cold can sometimes precipitate these painful events
- If surgery is needed blood cross-match must be carefully performed in advance, the theatre should be kept warm, and the hydration and acid/base balance of the patient monitored carefully.

Introduction

Haemoglobinopathies are inherited disorders of haemoglobin resulting from synthesis of abnormal haemoglobin molecules. In general, these conditions are encountered in people originating from tropical or subtropical areas, and it is believed that these conditions originally developed to confer protection against malaria. Although the management of these disorders is primarily the province of the haematologist, these conditions may be accompanied by orthopaedic and other surgical complications.

Sickle cell disease

This condition is due to a single mutation in the β-globin chain of the haemoglobin molecule: valine is substituted for glutamic acid at position 136. The abnormal haemoglobin is unstable and forms precipitates within the erythrocyte due to polymerization when deoxygenated. The gene is encountered predominantly in people of Afro-Caribbean origin, among whom the gene frequency may be as high as 5%. The gene is also found with a lower frequency among people of the Mediterranean region, Middle East, and Indian subcontinent. Carriers of this condition (sickle cell trait) have a mixture of both normal and abnormal haemoglobin (Hb A/S) but have no clinical problems. The term sickle cell disease applies to Hb S/S homozygotes, who have significant problems including recurrent episodes of painful 'crises'. These are due to intramedullary necrosis following occlusion of small vessels. Often there is no obvious precipitating cause, but it is recognized that infections, dehydration, and exposure to cold or low levels of oxygen can provoke crises. The most frequently involved areas are the knee, lumbosacral spine, elbow, and femur. Less often the ribs, sternum, clavicles, calcaneus, and facial bones are affected. Involvement of the facial bones may be associated with impressive facial swelling. Joint effusions are commonly seen when the knees or elbows are involved. The course of sickle cell disease is variable and many patients with sickle cell disease lead essentially normal lives punctuated by only occasional painful crises. However, in others the course can be much more serious with recurrent strokes such that bone marrow transplantation may be required in some cases.

Crises in bones and joints should be treated conservatively, with bed rest, maintenance of good fluid balance, and correction of hypoxia if the lungs are affected. Crises can be extremely painful, and opiate analgesics are usually needed. Extensive sickling within the lungs can be life threatening ('chest crisis'). This can initially present with cough, fever, and pleuritic chest pain, and a chest radiograph shows extensive infiltration of either one or both lung fields (Box 1.5.1).

Adults with sickle cell anaemia typically have a chronic haemolytic anaemia, with a haemoglobin level typically in the range of 7–10g/dL. The blood film is characteristic (Figure 1.5.1), with numerous irreversibly sickled cells (which are evident even in the absence of clinical problems), target cells, and normoblasts. The chronic haemolytic process results in consumption of folic acid, and oral supplementation is often required. Parvovirus infection in young children with sickle cell disease, and other haemolyic anaemias, can trigger the onset of a profound but transient drop in the haemoglobin level ('aplastic crisis').

Fetal haemoglobin is composed of paired α- and γ-chains, but by approximately 6 months of age production of β-chains replaces that of fetal γ-chains and this is when the first symptoms of the condition appear. Dactylitis ('hand–foot syndrome') is often the first manifestation of the condition: the digits of the hand or feet become painful, swollen, hot, and tender due to sickling within the bone. There are usually no radiologic changes during the acute episode, although subperiosteal bone formation may be seen a couple of weeks afterwards. Permanent shortening of the digits may occasionally result. Children born with sickle cell anaemia have a normal birth weight, but often exhibit delayed growth, reflected by delayed bone age on radiologic examination. Avascular necrosis of

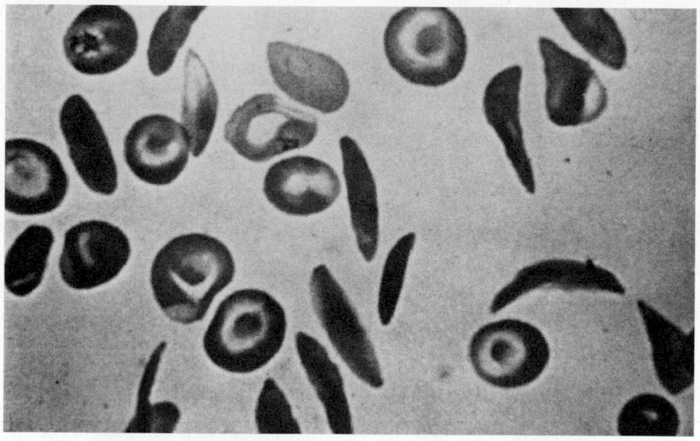

Fig. 1.5.1 Peripheral blood film from a patient with sickle cell anaemia, showing the typical hyperchromatic sickled cells as well as target cells.

the hip is a not infrequent complication in adolescents as well as adults, and may be bilateral. The risk is particularly high in individuals with haemoglobin SC disease, and this is believed to reflect the fact that these patients tend to have higher haemoglobin concentrations and thus the whole blood viscosity is higher. Total hip replacement may certainly be carried out, although the revision rate is quite high in these patients as the poor quality of the bone may result in early loosening of the prostheses. Osteonecrosis may also occur in other joints, such as the shoulder.

Repeated episodes of splenic infarction lead to loss of immune function with particular susceptibility to capsulated bacteria. Patients with sickle cell anaemia are particularly vulnerable to pneumococcal infections, and vaccination against both *Streptococcus pneumoniae* and *Haemophilus influenzae* as well as continuous prophylactic penicillin are important measures. Osteomyelitis due to *Salmonella* is also a recognized complication of sickle cell disease, involving the bones of the leg and axial skeleton in particular. Blood cultures may yield positive results, but needle aspiration of suspicious lesions is often required. There is a significant risk of vaso-occlusive stroke in patients with sickle cell anaemia, which may present as sudden onset of seizures, coma, visual disturbances, or hemiplegia. Gallstones formed from aggregates of bilirubin often form in sickle cell anaemia, as in other chronic haemolytic anaemias, and this may present as acute onset of abdominal pain. Leg ulcers are not infrequent in older patients, and tend to develop over the medial and lateral malleoli. These tend to heal very slowly, if at all, and skin grafts may be required. Early treatment of injuries to the area may prevent the development of such ulcers. Repeated infarction within the hypertonic environment of the renal medulla often results in recurrent episodes of painless haematuria. Eventually, the ability to concentrate urine is impaired, and patients are thus prone to dehydration. It is thus vital that particular attention be paid to fluid balance in patients with sickle cell anaemia who are hospitalized for any reason, particularly after surgery when oral fluid intake may be restricted.

Surgery in patients with sickle cell anaemia

Elective surgery in patients with sickle cell disease is generally safe, but it must be appreciated that despite optimal care there is a significant risk of perioperative complications such as precipitation of a sickling crisis (including acute chest syndrome or stroke), infection, or serious transfusion reactions. Patients with sickle cell disease do not tend to require regular transfusions to maintain a stable haemoglobin level. If they do require a blood transfusion for any reason, it should be borne in mind that these patients are at particular risk of developing red-cell antibodies after repeated transfusions (particularly against Kell and Duffy antigens) because of their different ethnic origin from the general donor population, and screening for such antibodies is thus particularly important before surgery to ensure that compatible blood can be made available in case of necessity. Certain measures can be taken in the setting of surgery to minimize the risk of provoking a sickle crisis:

- Keep operating theatre warm (at least 25°C)
- Ventilate with 100% oxygen before and after intubation or extubation
- Keep the patient warm in the recovery room
- Ensure adequate hydration at all times
- Monitor acid–base balance
- Pay particular attention to splints to ensure that peripheral circulation is not restricted.

A tourniquet can be applied in the case of procedures that require a bloodless field. The repeated postoperative use of a spirometer appears to reduce the risk of pulmonary complications, such as atelectasis or infection, presumably by promoting aeration throughout the lungs.

Thalassaemia

The thalassaemias are actually a group of haematological disorders in which a defect in the synthesis of one or more of the globin polypeptide chains is present, resulting in the formation of unstable aggregates of globin chains within erythrocyte precursors which are prematurely destroyed. A full classification of the thalassaemias is beyond the scope of this chapter, but the principal division is that between disorders involving the α-chain and the β-chain of the haemoglobin molecule. The prevalence of the genes for

Box 1.5.1 Complications of sickle cell disease

- Vascular occlusions in:
  - Bone marrow
  - Brain
  - Kidney
  - Lung
  - Retina
  - Spleen
- Aplastic crisis (parvovirus B19)
- Leg ulcers
- Gallstones
- Osteomyelitis
- Priapism.

thalassaemia is particularly high in Mediterranean countries (especially Greece, Italy, Cyprus, and North Africa), the Middle East, the Indian subcontinent, and South East Asia. Carriers of β-thalassaemia, the commonest form in European countries, have no clinical problems, apart from a mild and persistent microcytic anaemia with a haemoglobin typically in the range from 10–12g/dL.

Clinical and laboratory features

Severe anaemia becomes apparent at 3–6 months of age in β-thalassaemia major, and this is accompanied by massive enlargement of the liver and spleen due to excessive red cell destruction and extramedullary erythropoiesis. Examination of the blood film shows severe hypochromic, microcytic anaemia with reticulocytosis. Haemoglobin electrophoresis is required for definitive diagnosis: the hallmark of β-thalassaemia major is the absence of normal haemoglobin A, which is replaced by fetal haemoglobin (Hb F) together with some Hb A_2.

Skeletal changes in thalassaemia

In the absence of treatment with regular blood transfusions, there is marked expansion of the bone marrow to compensate for the ineffective erythropoiesis. This is associated with both osteoporosis and thinning of the cortex in the bones, which can result in pathological fractures. Striking features in untreated children include prominence of the parietal and frontal bones and protrusion of the maxillary bones, leading to malocclusion of teeth and orthodontic problems (Figure 1.5.2). Radiographs of the skull show a characteristic 'hair-on-end' appearance, due to widening of the diploë (Figure 1.5.3). Premature fusion of the epiphyses of the long bones, particularly the epiphysis of the proximal humerus, can result in shortening of the arms. Very occasionally, expansion of the haemopoietic tissue within spinal vertebrae leads to extrusion of marrow into the paravertebral area which can result in spinal cord compression. Decompressive laminectomy and even radiotherapy have been used in such cases to prevent permanent paralysis. Compression fractures of the vertebrae may also be seen (Box 1.5.2).

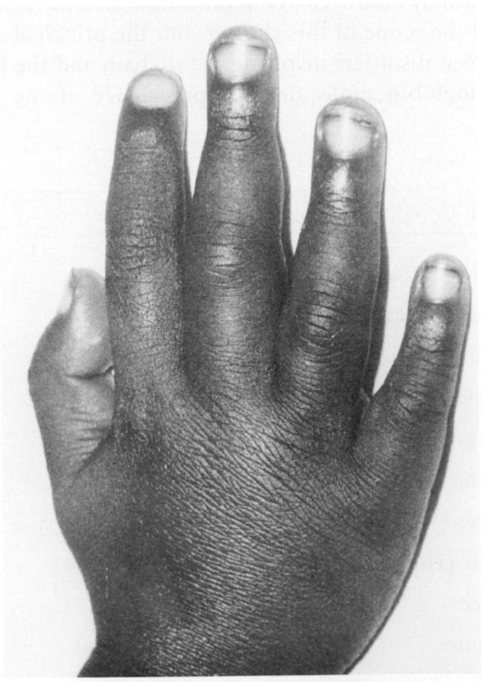

Fig. 1.5.2 Child with severe thalassaemia. Striking features in untreated children include prominence of the parietal and frontal bones and protrusion of the maxillary bones, leading to malocclusion of teeth and orthodontic problems.

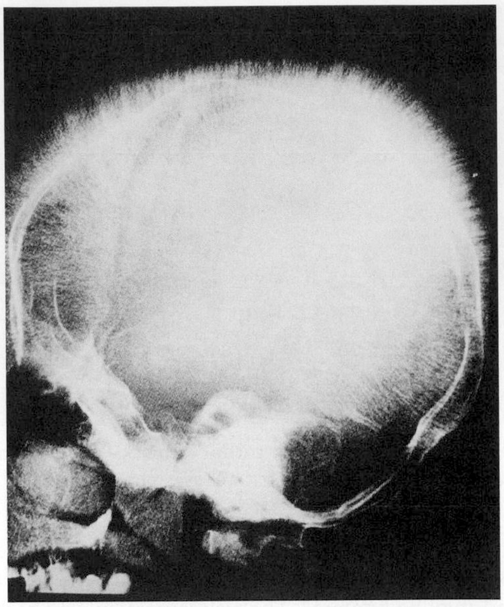

Fig. 1.5.3 Skull radiograph of a patient with severe thalassaemia. The typical 'hair-on-end' appearance is due to widening of the diploë.

Box 1.5.2 Thalassaemia: summary of key points

- Thalassaemia trait: chronic microcytic anaemia but no other significant problems
- Thalassaemia major: profound anaemia requiring regular blood transfusion
- Iron overload can result in:
  - Diabetes mellitus
  - Cardiac failure and arrhythmias
  - Cirrhosis
- Iron chelation therapy (e.g. with desferrioxamine) can delay onset of iron overload
- Many patients from developing world exposed to hepatitis and HIV after repeated blood transfusions
- Musculoskeletal complications can include:
  - Prominence of maxillary and frontal bones of skull, with dental malocclusion
  - Frontal bossing and 'hair-on-end' appearance on skull x-ray
  - Premature fusion of epiphyses
  - Spinal cord compression due to extrusion of hypertrophic bone marrow
  - Pathological fracture due to cortical thinning and osteoporosis.

Medical complications

Somewhat paradoxically, many of the serious medical complications seen in thalassaemia actually result from treatment of the condition. In contrast to sickle cell disease, people with β-thalassaemia major require regular blood transfusions. A programme of regular transfusions to maintain a haemoglobin level of 10g/dL will lead to regression of hepato-splenomegaly and skeletal changes. The skeletal changes described earlier are therefore unlikely to be seen by orthopaedic surgeons working in developed countries, where children are adequately treated from an early age. Splenectomy may occasionally be needed to reduce the requirement for blood transfusions, but this should be delayed until the patient is at least 6 years old because of the high risk of pneumococcal and other bacterial infections earlier in life. Pneumococcal vaccine should be given preoperatively in such cases, and prophylactic penicillin will be required after splenectomy. Patients should also be vaccinated against *Haemophilus influenzae.*

Regular blood transfusion eventually leads to iron overload, with deposition of iron in the tissues resulting in fibrosis. Iron overload may result in diabetes mellitus, cirrhosis, and cardiac complications such as arrhythmias or congestive cardiac failure. Subcutaneous infusions of the chelating agent desferrioxamine may postpone the onset of iron overload. Oral iron chelators such as deferasirox and deferiprone have become available in recent years. Some patients with thalassaemia (particularly those in the developing world) have also been exposed to viral infections such as hepatitis C or even HIV through blood transfusions.

Further reading

Angelucci, E., Barosi, G., Camaschella, C., *et al.* (2008). Italian Society of Hematology practice guidelines for the management of iron overload in thalassaemia major and related disorders. *Haematologica*, **93**, 741–52.

Bellet, P.S., Kalinyak, K.A., Shukla, R., Gelfand, M.J., and Rucknagel, D.L. (1995). Incentive spirometry to prevent acute pulmonary complications in sickle cell diseases. *New England Journal of Medicine*, **333**, 699–703.

Hernigou, P., Zilber, S., Filippini, P., Mathieu, G., Poignard, A., and Galacteros, F. (2008). Total THA in adult osteonecrosis related to sickle cell disease. *Clinical Orthopaedics and Related Research*, **466**, 300–8.

Issaragrisil, H.C., Piankigagum, A., and Wasi, P. (1981). Spinal cord compression in thalassemia: report of 12 cases and recommendations for treatment. *Archives of Internal Medicine*, **141**, 1033–6.

Lau, M.W., Blinder, M.A., Williams, K., Galatz, L.M. (2007). Shoulder arthroplasty in sickle cell patients with humeral head avascular necrosis. *Journal of Shoulder and Elbow Surgery*, **16**, 129–34.

1.6

Prevention of thrombosis in orthopaedic surgery

David Warwick

Summary points

- The risk–benefit of thromboprophylaxis in orthopaedic surgery remains unclear
- Some conditions, such as major trauma, carry a much higher risk than others, such as routine knee replacement
- Some patients appear to be genetically more predisposed than others
- In trials of efficacy of thromboembolism, the use of deep vein thrombosis as a surrogate endpoint for death from a pulmonary embolus may not be completely reliable
- There is a variety of mechanical and chemical methods available, each of which has real and potential advantages as well as real and potential dangers
- Even the length of time that a patient is at risk after major surgery is unclear
- Clinicians should adhere to guidelines where possible.

Introduction

Despite a huge literature base, thromboprophylaxis in orthopaedics remains controversial. The scale of the problem is disputed and the cost–benefit, risk–benefit, and practicality of any particular protocol is uncertain.

Areas of controversy

Do we need prophylaxis at all?

Against prophylaxis

Some surgeons question the very need for prophylaxis, citing very low death rates in series without routine prophylaxis (Box 1.6.1). With changes in orthopaedic practice (quicker surgery, regional anaesthesia, earlier mobilization) the problem of venous thromboembolism (VTE) appears to be receding. The rates of symptomatic VTE without prophylaxis are probably only in the region of 4% after joint replacement without prophylaxis and so there is much being spent, and a risk of bleeding complications being taken, for relatively small gain. No study has shown a longer-term risk of chronic venous insufficiency and pulmonary hypertension in orthopaedic patients who develop postoperative deep vein thrombosis (DVT) or pulmonary embolism (PE). The cost and potential risk of prophylaxis is thereby believed to be unjustified.

For prophylaxis

Even a low death rate, when multiplied by the very large number of procedures performed, represents a large number. Symptomatic DVT and PE are important outcomes; society will not tolerate avoidable risk and there is an estimated £68 million in litigation costs for VTE. On the balance of probability (the civil test for breach of duty), VTE can be reduced with prophylaxis. The cost of treating a symptomatic VTE is probably higher than routine thromboprophylaxis. A robust study to show, or exclude, chronic venous insufficiency after orthopaedic thrombosis has yet to be performed; until that study is available, the potential for this expensive and morbid complication should be avoided.

How strong is the evidence that prophylaxis works?

Against prophylaxis

There are no studies which show death can be reduced with prophylaxis, or that one modality is any better than another. This is because death is so rare that an adequate sample size cannot be accrued.

For prophylaxis

There is some evidence that heparins reduce death in surgery. There is compelling evidence that thromboprophylaxis substantially reduces symptomatic VTE. That is a worthwhile effect in

Box 1.6.1 Epidemiology

- Death still occurs even without thromboprophylaxis
- There is some evidence that thromboprophylaxis may prevent death or chronic venous insufficiency; there is good evidence that it reduces morbidity from symptomatic DVT and PE
- Thromboprophylaxis may be cost-effective depending on the modalities used
- There are few data on the morbidity of thromboprophylaxis as a result of increased bleeding.

itself; the pyramid of VTE means that a proportionate reduction in death can be logically adduced. Most fatal PEs have no warning from a symptomatic DVT; there is very strong evidence that asymptomatic DVT (the usual endpoint in clinical trials) is reduced by suitable prophylaxis.

Is chemical prophylaxis too dangerous?

Against prophylaxis

Unavoidable bleeding is unacceptable in a surgical patient—it carries a morbidity of its own and reflects on the surgeon's skill. Any chemical carries an intrinsic risk of bleeding. If that risk is similar to the risk of symptomatic VTE that it aims to prevent, nothing has been gained yet a healthcare resource has been spent. Anecdotal experience and many studies do show a higher rate of bleeding with chemicals than placebo.

For prophylaxis

There is no evidence that postoperative bleeding compromises the longevity of an implant. If a patient develops VTE in the postoperative phase, the required therapeutic anticoagulation invokes an even higher risk of bleeding. Bleeding is correlated with the administration of the chemical too close to surgery; guidelines which delaying the chemical until the risk of bleeding has evaporated, covering the interim with a mechanical method, should allow safe prophylaxis.

Is aspirin good enough?

For aspirin

It is cheap, easy to administer, and is used by a fair proportion of surgeons. There are studies to show it reduces the frequency of both radiological and symptomatic VTE. It is suitable for extended duration use because it is an oral agent. The American Academy of Orthopaedic Surgeons (AAOS) has recommended aspirin.

Against aspirin

It is mainly an antiplatelet rather than antithrombotic agent; the risk reduction achieved is far less than that with low-molecular-weight heparin (LMWH), fondaparinux, or newer oral agents. It carries a risk of gastrointestinal complications and bleeding, particularly in the elderly. The Pulmonary Embolism Prevention (PEP) trial showed no benefit for symptomatic VTE in the subgroup of total hip replacement (THR) and total knee replacement (TKR) patients. The death rate was the same in the placebo and the aspirin group. The AAOS guidelines only addressed PE which revealed a dearth of studies to show any benefit, let alone superiority, for aspirin. The National Institute of Health and Clinical Excellence (NICE) and the American College of Chest Physicians (ACCP) specifically advise against its use.

Are mechanical methods alone adequate?

For mechanical alone

These methods are inherently safe. Foot pumps are as effective as LMWH in the short-term for THR; intermittent pneumatic compression (IPC) appears effective in THR and TKR. Meta-analysis suggests that even simple TED (thromboembolic deterrent) stockings convey a significant risk reduction.

Against mechanical alone

Compliance by patient and ward staff, especially as the patient becomes increasingly mobile, limits the duration of use to a period that may be shorter than the patient's risk of thrombosis. VTE is not only promoted by venous stasis—activation of coagulation is an important aetiological factor which may persist beyond the period of venous stasis. There may be a protective effect with chemical prophylaxis from the cardiac mortality that accompanies joint replacement.

Pathogenesis

Major trauma and orthopaedic surgery predispose to VTE. Virchow's triad of altered blood components, venous stasis, and endothelial damage are all represented. The soft tissue exposure, bone cutting, and reaming induce systemic hypercoagulability and fibrinolytic inhibition. Patients may be relatively immobile after surgery. During hip replacement, femoral vein blood flow is obstructed by the manoeuvres required to expose the femoral canal and acetabulum. This may not only damage endothelium, in the proximal femoral vein, but also cause venous distension and thus endothelial damage distally, particularly in valve pockets, but also allow the concentration of clotting factors. Anterior subluxation of the knee and the vibration may cause local endothelial damage during knee replacement.

What is the risk?

Some orthopaedic procedures, such as minor upper limb surgery, probably carry no risk of thrombosis, whilst other procedures, such as complex lower limb trauma reconstruction or revision hip surgery, carry a particularly high risk.

Individual patients each have their own risk, determined by comorbidity (venous disease, obesity) and particularly by genetic predisposition. A previous PE or DVT is the strongest individual risk factor.

Fatal pulmonary embolism

With modern surgical and anaesthetic techniques, but without prophylaxis, the death rate from PE after hip replacement or knee replacement is probably around 0.2%; perhaps slightly higher after hip fracture. With 1.2 million arthroplasties per year in Europe, that equates to 2400 deaths—a huge problem. The death rate after other orthopaedic procedures is unknown, but fatal PE is occasionally seen after lower limb trauma and pelvic trauma; there are case reports after ankle fracture, knee arthroscopy, and even elbow replacement.

Symptomatic and asymptomatic pulmonary embolism or deep vein thrombosis

Symptomatic event rates are summarized in Table 1.6.1.

Other factors can increase an individual's personal risk (Table 1.6.2).

Chronic venous and pulmonary sequelae

The frequency of chronic venous insufficiency, an important longer-term outcome, is unknown. It is likely to be rare after asymptomatic thrombosis (the majority of thrombosis after orthopaedic surgery) but common after symptomatic thrombosis. Chronic pulmonary hypertension is a potential sequelae for those who survive a symptomatic PE.

Table 1.6.1 Risk of venous thromboembolism derived from International Consensus Statement* and ACCP guidelines**

Procedure or condition	Fatal PE	Symptomatic VTE	Asymptomatic DVT
Hip fracture	?1%	4%	60%
Hip replacement	0.2–0.4%	3–4%	55%
Knee replacement	0.2%	3–4%	60%
Knee arthroscopy	?	0.2%?	7%
Isolated lower limb trauma	?	0.4–2%	10–35%
Spinal surgery	?	6%	18%
Spinal cord injury	?	13%	35%
Major trauma	?	?	58%

DVT, deep vein thrombosis; PE, pulmonary embolism; VTE, venous thromboembolism.

*Nicolaides, A.N., Fareed, J., Kakkar, A.K., et al. (2006). Prevention and treatment of venous thromboembolism. International Consensus Statement (guidelines according to scientific evidence). *International Angiology*, **25**(2), 101–61.

Geerts, W.H., Pineo, G.F., and Heit, J.A. (2004). Prevention of venous thromboembolism: the seventh ACCP conference on antithrombotic and thrombolytic therapy. *Chest* **126, 338S–340S.

Outcome measures

No study could be large enough to directly show a reduction in fatal PE because it is so rare. Reduction in fatal PE is, of course, not the only purpose in thromboprophylaxis. Symptomatic DVT and PE are a cause of considerable cost (both medical and medico-legal) and are likely to cause longer-term sequelae (chronic venous insufficiency and pulmonary hypertension). Furthermore, fatal PE usually has no warning signs in the leg, so that reduction in asymptomatic DVT is itself an important goal of prophylaxis.

Table 1.6.2 Risk factors for thromboembolism

Malignancy	Acute medical illness
Recent thrombotic stroke (within 4 weeks)	Acute myocardial infarction (within 12 weeks)
Heart failure	Sepsis
Respiratory disease	Rheumatic heart disease
Inflammatory bowel disease	Nephrotic syndrome
Personal or family history of VTE	Age >60 years (risk rises linearly with age)
Dehydration	Obesity (body mass index >30)
Myeloproliferative disease	Drugs OCP/HRT, tamoxifen, chemotherapy
Major trauma to lower extremities	Inherited thrombophilia
Antiphospholipid syndrome	Paroxysmal nocturnal haemoglobinuria
Central venous catheter *in situ*	Smoking
Varicose veins	Immobility
Continuous travel of more than 3h approx. 4 weeks before or after surgery	Pregnancy; current or recent (within 6 weeks) any gestation

Until the past few years, almost all prophylaxis studies relied on radiological surrogates assuming that a reduction in DVT demonstrable by imaging would correlate with a reduction in symptomatic endpoints. There is evidence to support this. A reduction in symptomatic DVT of 66% with heparin after orthopaedic surgery has been correlated with a similar reduction in fatal PE; a reduction in radiological DVT correlates with a reduction in symptomatic VTE when given for a prolonged time after hip replacement and hip fracture. This correlation is self-evident, given that thromboembolism represents a pyramid of the same disease (Figure 1.6.1).

Most studies refer to hip and knee arthroplasty patients; there are far fewer data on other orthopaedic procedures.

General prophylactic measures (Box 1.6.2)

Early mobilization

There is a good physiological premise, although only weak circumstantial evidence, to encourage early mobilization.

Neuraxial anaesthesia

Anaesthetists are keen to use these techniques (spinal or epidural anaesthesia) as they reduce mortality and enhance perioperative analgesia. Furthermore, neuraxial anaesthesia also reduces the risk of VTE by about 50%, probably due to enhanced blood flow. Because of concerns that a spinal haematoma could develop with concomitant use of chemical prophylaxis and neuraxial anaesthesia, it is prudent to avoid giving neuraxial anaesthesia and chemical prophylaxis too close together. Local anaesthetic guidelines should be followed.

Surgical technique

Rough surgical technique will potentiate thromboplastin release. Prolonged torsion of the dislocated hip whilst reaming during hip replacement, or aggressive dorsal retraction of the tibia during knee replacement, inhibit venous return and damage the endothelium.

Tourniquet

There is no evidence that tourniquets promote thrombogenesis. The accumulation of clotting factors whilst the tourniquet is inflated is probably balanced by the fibrinolytic and valve-flushing hyperaemia on tourniquet deflation

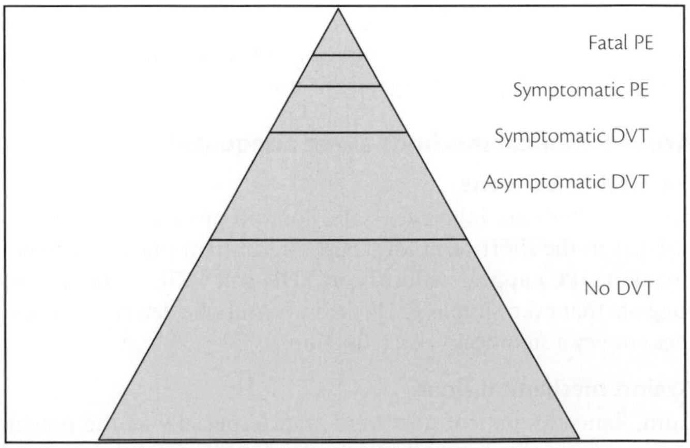

Fig. 1.6.1 The pyramid of venous thromboembolism.

Box 1.6.2 General prophylactic measures

- Early mobilization. No evidence in practice
- Neuraxial anaesthesia reduces VTE by 50% but precludes some types of chemical prophylaxis
- Gentle surgical technique. No evidence in practice
- Tourniquet—not thought to have any effect.

Secondary prophylaxis

This means that no prophylaxis is given around the time of surgery; an investigation (e.g. ultrasound or venogram) is performed some time after surgery and therapeutic doses of chemical are then given if the test is positive for a large clot; repeat screening for a small clot. Ultrasound is not too sensitive for small asymptomatic DVT and venography is too invasive. Thirty per cent of THR patients with a negative venogram 10 days after surgery will develop a DVT in the next 3 or 4 weeks. Major and even fatal VTE can occur within the first 10 days. Therapeutic doses of anticoagulant within the first 2 weeks of surgery invite a high complication rate. Prophylaxis is not so expensive whereas routine investigation and treatment of detected thromboses or later-emerging events is. This method of secondary prophylaxis is not recommended.

Mechanical methods (Box 1.6.3)

Advantages and disadvantages

Mechanical methods are intuitively attractive to orthopaedic surgeons, who have to balance risk and benefit in the perioperative period, as they carry no bleeding risk. The most recent meta-analysis (through the UK NHS Health Technology Assessment process) reviewed 17 graduate compression stocking (GCS) trials, 22 intermittent pneumatic compression (IPC) trials, and three foot pump trials. Of these, 14 trials were in hip and knee surgery. The review concluded a 72% odds reduction for mechanical methods alone. All mechanical methods have the disadvantages of expense and compliance. Furthermore, they are not practical for, nor is there evidence for, extended duration prophylaxis.

Graduated compression stockings

These are commonly used. To work, they must be properly woven, well-fitted, and remain in place. The evidence is sparse for efficacy after orthopaedic surgery, but a meta-analysis of other surgical studies suggests a modest benefit. There is no clear benefit for above-knee rather than below-knee stockings.

Box 1.6.3 Secondary prophylactic measures (mechanical)

- Compression stockings
- Intermittent compression devices
- Foot pumps
- IVC filters.

Intermittent pneumatic compression devices

These devices enhance venous flow and also have a fibrinolytic effect due to release of factors from the endothelium from compression. The peak venous flow varies with different devices: frequency of contraction; number of compartments; above- or below-knee design; inflation pressure. The ideal parameters have not been established; however, in general these devices are effective, with an overall risk reduction of about 26%.

Foot pumps

These devices empty the venous plexus in the sole of the foot rhythmically, so flushing out the deep leg veins. The foot should be level or slightly dependent so that the plexus can fill (pre-load) prior to it being emptied by the impulse. Stockings probably do not enhance flow. The efficacy will also depend on factors such as the pressure and frequency and the impulses. The risk reduction is probably similar to LMWHs in hip arthroplasty but the evidence for knee arthroplasty is less secure.

Inferior vena cava filters

These devices ('umbrellas') are inserted percutaneously through the femoral vein and are lodged in the inferior vena cava. They cannot prevent thrombosis in the leg, nor do they prevent embolism; they merely catch an embolus and prevents it from reaching the lungs. They are associated with a complication rate which includes death from proximal embolism and venous distension. Their role should be confined to the occasional case where anticoagulation is contraindicated yet the risk of embolism is high. The typical example would be a pelvic fracture transferred from one centre to another who has already developed a leg DVT yet needs a major surgical reconstruction.

Chemical methods (Box 1.6.4)

Advantages and disadvantages

Chemical methods such as LMWH, pentasaccharide, warfarin, direct thrombin inhibitors, and factor Xa inhibitors are effective in reducing the risk of VTE. They are generally easy to administer (tablet or injection) and can be used for an extended duration. Relative to the overall cost of surgery, they are fairly inexpensive.

These drugs all carry an inherent risk of bleeding—a risk which properly concerns orthopaedic surgeons.

Box 1.6.4 Secondary prophylactic measures (chemical)

- Aspirin: cheap but weak
- LMWH: definitely reduce symptomatic DVT. Safe if used carefully
- Warfarin: less good than LMWH and has side effects
- Pentasaccharides: at least equal effect as LMWH but not reversible. Bleeding concerns
- Anti-Xa inhibitors: as effective as LMWH but more practical as oral so can be used for a prolonged period. Not reversible.

Aspirin

Aspirin is familiar, cheap, available, and easy to use. However, it only has a weak antithrombotic effect (since it is an antiplatelet agent rather than an anticoagulant). The PEP trial (2000) showed a reduction of about a quarter for symptomatic VTE with aspirin compared with placebo, which is less than would be expected with LMWH (about two-thirds). It risks alternative complications (wound bleeding, transfusion, gastrointestinal bleeding). Although the AAOS recommend its use in THR and TKR, NICE and the two largest evidence-based consensus groups, ACCP and National Institute for Clinical Excellence (ICS), all specifically recommend against its use because if chosen as the sole prophylactic method, then patients are deprived of safer and more effective alternative mechanical and chemical methods. It is not even licensed for thromboprophylaxis in the United Kingdom (Table 1.6.3).

Low-molecular-weight heparins

This class of drugs is readily bio-available and has a wide window of safety; therefore monitoring is not required. There are several different types but they are all broadly similar. The drugs are relatively cheap and easy to administer by injection once or twice daily, depending on half-life. LMWHs have been very widely studied and are at least as effective as warfarin, compression devices, and foot pumps. They are more effective than unfractionated heparin and far more effective than placebo. There is little evidence that if used safely they cause bleeding. However, particular care (dose amendment or alterative therapy) should be taken in those with reduced renal function.

Warfarin

Used carefully, it is effective in reducing venographic DVT; fatal PE is exceedingly rare as a reported outcome. It can be continued for as long as the patient is at risk for an extended duration. Meta-analysis shows that it is not as effective as LMWH. Although warfarin is used widely in North America, it is generally regarded as obsolete in Europe (Table 1.6.3).

Pentasaccharide

These synthetic antithrombotic agents precisely inhibit factor Xa. Fondaparinux (Arixtra) is the first of this class to be widely studied and commercially available. It is excreted renally rather than metabolized by the liver. Because of its long half-life (15h) it can be administered by once-daily injection. The clinical trial programme shows that fondaparinux may be more effective than LMWH but may cause more bleeding. However, these differences may be least partly explained by differences in the proximity to surgery when the trial drugs were administered. The drug is not readily reversed and must be used carefully or avoided in those with poor renal function.

Table 1.6.3 Drawbacks of aspirin and warfarin

Drawbacks of Warfarin
◆ Needs regular monitoring, which is expensive and time consuming;
◆ If started too close to surgery or at too high a dose, there will be a risk of bleeding;
◆ If started judiciously – later and at a lower dose – there will be an interval of several days during which the patient will be unprotected at their most thrombogenic phase;
◆ Interaction with many drugs and alcohol.
◆ Not as effective as LMWH
Drawbacks of Aspirin
◆ Only weak antithrombotic effect so limited efficacy
◆ Weak evidence base
◆ GI bleeding, wound bleeding
◆ Not recommended by NICE, ACCP (but is by AAOS)
◆ Not licensed for Thromboprophylaxis in UK

Direct anti-Xa inhibitors and direct thrombin inhibitors

These drugs became available in 2008 and may transform thromboprophylaxis. They are given orally and have a broad therapeutic and safety window so that monitoring is not required. They offer a pragmatic solution to those who would otherwise need regular injections (LMWH, fondaparinux) or complex monitoring (warfarin). They are given after surgery and are continued for as long as the patient is at risk of VTE. The drugs are difficult to reverse. Presently, two are available: a. direct thrombin inhibitor (Dabigatran, Boehringer Ingelheim) and an anti-Xa inhibitor (Rivaroxaban, Bayer). Others are due to follow.

Combined methods

When to start chemical prophylaxis

Thromboprophylaxis involves a balance of risk and benefit, like most medical interventions. If an effective dose of chemical is administered too close to surgery, bleeding will occur. If the drug is given *before* surgery, it provides an anticoagulant remedy to peroperative thrombogenic factors (tissue thromboplastins and venous stasis). If the drug is given too long before surgery, the serum levels will be too low for any prophylactic effect; if given too close to surgery then surgical bleeding can be expected. The alterative is to give the drug *after* surgery. If given too close after surgery, the soft tissues and bone will still be vulnerable to bleeding side effects; if given too late after surgery, then although the risk of surgical bleeding is diminished, the thrombogenic process will be well-established before the drug can act. The drug now has to function as a therapeutic rather than a prophylactic (Figure 1.6.2). The drug has to be given 'just in time' to be effective yet to avoid bleeding.

Stacked modalities

There is a trend for so called 'stacked modalities' in which a mechanical method is used to cover the perioperative phase, with a drug then started only when the surgeon and anaesthetist feel that in that individual patient the bleeding risk has decayed.

Individualized flexible use of mechanical and chemical methods

In the late 20th century, there tended to be a conflict between chemical methods and mechanical methods. This dichotomy was inappropriate, as each has advantages and disadvantages. Furthermore, the obsession with evidence-based medicine tended to allow recommendations only if supported by a particular randomized trial or meta-analysis. However, the randomized trial is only as valid as the unitary hypothesis studied and generalizability

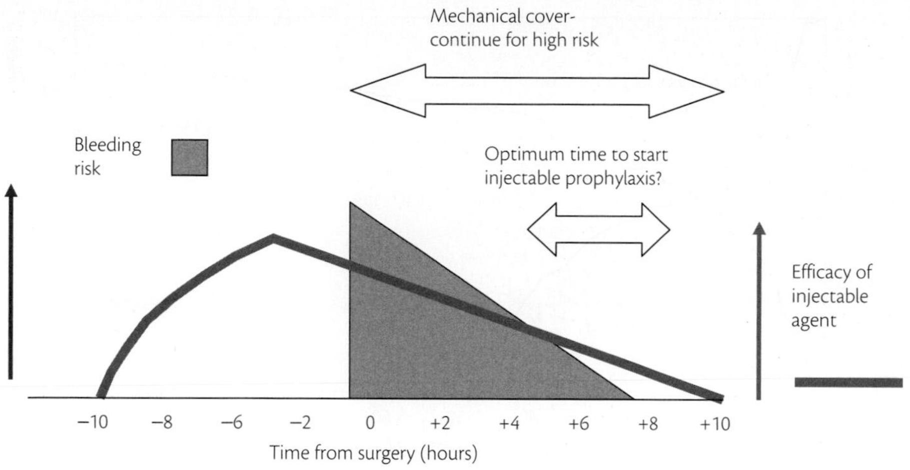

Fig. 1.6.2 'Just in time' prophylaxis.

is hampered by the exclusion criteria applied to the studied sample. Therefore, clinicians should regard randomized trials and meta-analyses as showing the general direction rather than constraining sensible practice. A pragmatic view would support a combination of mechanical and chemical methods.

Particularly high risk of thromboembolism

For these patients (e.g. with previous thrombosis, strong family history, or prolonged surgery), mechanical and chemical methods can both be used together for as long as possible.

Particularly high-risk bleeding

For these patients, a mechanical method should be used until the bleeding risk is lessened; an effective chemical can be safely started and continued for as long as there is a risk of thrombosis.

Uncertain delay to surgery

For these patients (e.g. hip fracture and major trauma), the mechanical method can be started as close to the moment of trauma as possible—in the Emergency Department—and continued until such time after surgery as the clinician feels that a drug can be safely commenced.

Lower risk of thrombosis

In these patients, the cost and risk of prophylaxis may not be justified at all. If prophylaxis is deemed necessary then a mechanical or chemical method could be used, whichever is judged safer and most cost-effective.

Box 1.6.5 General considerations

- Timing of start and end of thromboprophylaxis is a complex decision
- Prophylaxis should be continued for 2 weeks after knee replacement and 5 weeks after hip fracture and hip replacement surgery
- Stacking combines mechanical and chemical methods.

Duration of use

If prophylaxis is used, it should be given for an appropriate duration of time. The risk of thrombosis depends on many factors, such as the particular procedure performed, the likelihood of postoperative immobility, and the individual's inherited propensity to thrombosis. Thromboprophylaxis in the latter part of the 20th century was usually continued only whilst the patient remained in hospital. This was for pragmatic rather than scientific reasons. However, it is now apparent that the risk of thrombosis in hip or knee arthroplasty and hip fracture persists for much longer (Figure 1.6.3). Several sources show that half of symptomatic VTE after knee replacement and two-thirds after hip replacement and hip fracture occur beyond the second week. Randomized controlled trials clearly show that the risk of later symptomatic VTE can be reduced by about two-thirds if prophylaxis is continued for longer. The precise period depends on many factors, but current evidence supports 14 days for knee replacement and 4–5 weeks for hip replacement and hip fracture (Box 1.6.5). This is likely to be a cost-effective approach. Because patients are discharged from hospital sooner and sooner, then a system must be established to continue prophylaxis after discharge. The advent of the new oral agents which do not require monitoring will allow effective and practical extended duration prophylaxis.

Guidelines

There are now several authoritative guidelines available, based on a systematic literature review (Table 1.6.4). Guidelines should ensure that safe and effective prophylaxis is routinely given according to a protocol that has been accepted by the surgeons and anaesthetist, yet properly funded by the health system.

The guidelines have two common threads: to provide *effective prophylaxis without causing harm* and to use *risk assessment*. There are differences. In particular the AAOS guidelines only address PE and support the use of aspirin; the other guidelines address the spectrum of VTE and reject aspirin. The International Surgical Thrombosis Forum has suggested a model for the design and interpretation of guidelines in orthopaedics (Box 1.6.6).

In the author's institution, guidelines have been implemented which are consistent with existing guidelines, to provide effective

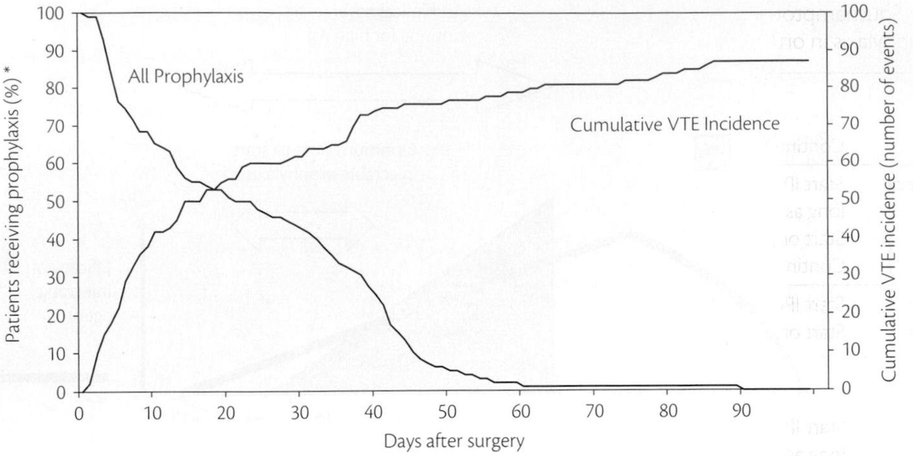

Fig. 1.6.3 Discrepancy between duration of prophylaxis and onset of symptomatic VTE. Reproduced from Warwick, D., Friedman, R.J., Agnelli, G., *et al.* (2007). Insufficient duration of venous thromboembolism prophylaxis after total hip or knee replacement when compared with the time course of thromboembolic events: Findings from the GLORY Global Orthopaedic Registry. *Journal of Bone and Joint Surgery*, **89-B**, 799–807.

prophylaxis yet avoid potential bleeding by using mechanical prophylaxis first, then switching to chemical (Table 1.6.5). It is likely that the LMWH will be replaced with an oral anti-Xa or direct thrombin inhibitor.

Future research

Individual risk analysis

Like so many other diseases in medicine, there is likely to be a genetic predisposition to both thrombosis and bleeding. Risk factor analysis should provide a clear understanding of those at greatest risk of thrombosis or bleeding; this would allow safe yet effective prophylaxis tailored to the individual's critical thrombosis period.

Duration of risk for venous thromboembolism

The duration of risk for any procedure, let alone individual, is not known. Does the risk rebound when prophylaxis is stopped?

Ideal mechanical–chemical combination

A combined approach seems sensible, but needs to be validated; the most effective, yet safe and affordable, protocol must be established.

Table 1.6.4 Guidelines for treatment and prevention of venous thromboembolism

Name	Coordinator	Reference	Year
NICE	UK Government	NICE	2007
AAOS	American Academy	AAOS	2007
International Consensus Statement	International Union of Angiology	Nicolaides et al.	2006
ACCP	American College of Chest Physicians	Geerts et al.	2004

Box 1.6.6 The ideal guideline: International Surgical Thrombosis Forum recommendation

For those with a demonstrable risk of thrombosis, thromboprophylaxis should be started with an effective dose as close to the thrombogenic insult as possible, without introducing a greater or equal risk of alternative complications, and continued until the risk of thrombosis has reduced to a clinically negligible rate, with due consideration of cost and practicality. Surgeons also should consider their own threshold of comfort between thrombosis and bleeding based on their patient's individual risk factors when deciding the safe proximity to surgery for chemical methods, i.e. before or after the trauma. Individual patients may have their own risk for thrombosis and bleeding as well as duration of risk for each. Initiation and duration of prophylaxis should therefore ideally be tailored. The ideal chemical agent should be both injectable and oral, reversible, have a wide therapeutic and safety margin, and be predictable in nearly all patients (elderly, renal impairment, liver impairment) without interaction and be monitored with simple coagulation tests in critically ill patients. The ideal mechanical method should be comfortable, quiet and cost-effective. The guideline should not constrain the surgeon or anaesthetist into a practice which is not available, practical, affordable or deliverable. All methods should have an acceptable compliance when handled by the patients themselves (e.g. self-administered pharmaceuticals, mechanical devices).

From Warwick, D., Dahl, O.E., Fisher, W.D. (2008). Orthopaedic thromboprophylaxis: Limitations of Current Guidelines. *Journal of Bone and Joint Surgery*, **90-B**, 127–32.

Role of new oral agents

A safe and effective oral agent will support simple protocols for extended prophylaxis in those with higher risk of VTE (e.g. day-case knee arthroscopy or plaster casts with additional risk factors).

Table 1.6.5 Southampton University Hospital Guidelines for thromboprophylaxis in orthopaedic procedures

Total hip replacement	Start IPC in recovery and continue for as long as tolerated Start oral anti-Xa/anti-thrombin on day after surgery Continue chemical for 5 weeks
Fractured neck of femur	Start IPC in Emergency Department and continue for as long as tolerated Start oral anti-Xa/anti thrombin on day after surgery Continue chemical for 5 weeks
Total knee replacement	Start IPC in recovery and continue for as long as tolerated Start oral anti-Xa/antithrombin or LMWH on day after surgery Continue chemical for 14 days
Major lower limb trauma	Start IPC in Emergency department and continue for as long as tolerated Start LMWH at 5pm daily once risk of bleeding from soft tissue, brain, spine, and surgery has been ruled out
Elective spinal surgery	Start IPC in theatre and continue until patient is fully mobile Read operation note to see if patient may be suitable for LMWH
Traumatic spines, pelvis, acetabulum	Ultrasound on arrival if transfer and no effective prophylaxis Start IPC if USS is negative. Discuss and document management with consultant if USS is positive Start LMWH minimum of 24h postoperatively and continue until mobile
Other surgery and trauma	Patient should be offered grade II compression stockings or IPC until mobile Risk assessment: give LMWH when bleeding risk has been ruled out if one or more risk factors

IPC, intermittent pneumatic compression; LMWH, low-molecular-weight heparin; USS, ultrasound scan.

Further reading

American Academy of Orthopaedic Surgeons (2007). *Clinical Guideline on Prevention of Pulmonary Embolism in Patients Undergoing Total Hip or Knee Arthroplasty.* Available at http://www.aaos.org/Research/guidelines/PE_guideline.pdf

Geerts, W.H., Pineo, G.F., and Heit, J.A. (2004). Prevention of venous thromboembolism: the seventh ACCP conference on antithrombotic and thrombolytic therapy. *Chest,* **126**, 338S–340S.

Lieberman, J.R. and Hue, W.K. (2005). Current concepts review – prevention of venous thromboembolic disease after total hip and knee arthroplasty. *Journal of Bone and Joint Surgery,* **87A**, 2097–112.

NICE (2007). *Venous thromboembolism: reducing the risk of venous thromboembolism (deep vein thrombosis and pulmonary embolism) in inpatients undergoing surgery.* Clinical Guideline 46. Available at http://www.guidance.nice.org.uk/CG46.

Nicolaides, A.N., Fareed, J., Kakkar, A.K., *et al.* (2006). Prevention and treatment of venous thromboembolism. International Consensus Statement (guidelines according to scientific evidence). *International Angiology,* **25**(2), 101–61.

PEP Trial Collaborative Group (2000). Prevention of pulmonary embolism and deep vein thrombosis with low dose aspirin: Pulmonary Embolism Prevention (PEP) trial. *Lancet,* **355**, 1295–302.

Warwick, D., Dahl, O.E., and Fisher, W.D. (2008). Orthopaedic thromboprophylaxis: Limitations of Current Guidelines. *Journal of Bone and Joint Surgery,* **90-B**, 127–32.

Westrich, G.H., Haas, S.B., Mosca, P., and Peterson M. (2000). Meta-analysis of thromboembolic prophylaxis after total knee arthroplasty. *Journal of Bone and Joint Surgery,* **82-B**, 795–800.

1.7

Pain and its control

Henry McQuay

Summary points

- The origin, transmission, and reception of chronic pain is not easy to understand
- The perception of pain is altered by mood and itself alters mood. There is, therefore, a close link between chronic pain and depression
- Although pain is subjective, pain scales and diaries can be used to provide reproducible measures of pain
- The choice of method of pain control is not simply a ladder. New stronger agents need to be added in, not substituted for weaker ones
- Neuropathic pain will require unconventional analgesics in combination.

Definition and classification of pain

Pain is an unpleasant sensory or emotional experience associated with actual or potential tissue damage, or described in terms of such damage. Chronic pain is pain which is still present after 3 months despite sensible treatment. Radicular pain is felt in the distribution of a nerve root, so that pain is felt in an area corresponding to one of the dermatomes down the arm or leg or round the trunk. It is typically caused by compression. Referred pain is felt superficially in the dermatome of an affected viscus or other deep structure innervated by that root. An example is pain felt in the left arm because of cardiac disease (Table 1.7.1).

The two major types of pain are nociceptive and neuropathic. Nociceptive is 'normal' pain, such as pain after an injury. Neuropathic pain is pain after nerve injury, and can be central (post-stroke pain) or peripheral (Box 1.7.1).

Pain sensation and transmission

The easiest way to think of pain in the nervous system is the idea of pain receptors and nerve cables dedicated to the transmission of pain signals. This model is a hard-wired, line-labelled system. For most acute pain and, indeed, in chronic nociceptive pain, this simple idea works well. The concept of specific cables whose transmission can be blocked is reinforced by everyday observations, for instance the ability to perform surgery painlessly by using a local anaesthetic block. But the inadequacy of this simple explanation is exposed in chronic pain, particularly with nervous system damage. The return of pain after an initially successful cordotomy, and the phenomenon of phantom limb pain are two examples. In a hard-wired, line-labelled system the pain should not recur after the cordotomy and amputees should not feel pain in the absent foot or hand because the receptors and the cables are no longer there. The ability of the nervous system to rewire is called plasticity. It is manifest in the return of pain after destructive procedures, and the concept of 'pain memory' in the spinal cord and brain has to be invoked to explain the phantom pain. Such phenomena mean that the simple view of a hard-wired, line-labelled system does not explain all that we see.

Pain perception can be amplified or damped by endogenous influences such as mood or endorphins, or exogenous factors, drugs given, or the circumstances of the injury. The classic scenario where pain is damped down is the injured soldier who continues, despite a shattered leg, to get themselves out of battle. Conversely a stubbed toe when you are tired and miserable is immeasurably more painful than the same injury on a morning when you are cheerful. In chronic pain it is sometimes very hard to disentangle depression from pain. Pain makes depression worse and depression makes pain worse. This pattern is all too familiar to those who manage pain. The thinking clinician needs to deal with both the pain and the depression. In chronic pain, distress and disability may also amplify the pain, and good pain relief will not improve disability. Under these circumstances expectations need to be realistic.

Box 1.7.1 Definitions in pain

- Chronic pain has been present longer than 3 months
- Radicular pain is caused by compression of a nerve
- Referred pain arises from a viscus but presents elsewhere
- Nociceptive pain is the normal pain after an injury
- Neuropathic pain arises from the nervous system itself.

Table 1.7.1 Types of pain with examples

Acute	1. Nociceptive	2. Neuropathic a. Peripheral	b. Central	3. Visceral	Combined
	Postop Burns 'Sprains & Strains'			'Stone' pain ulcer	
Intermittent/ incidental	Headache Migraine Osteoarthritis	Trigeminal neuralgia		Dysmenorrhoea Endometriosis Pelvic IBS Dyspepsia	Cancer (1,2,3)
Chronic	Rheumatoid arthritis Osteoarthritis FM Myofascial (e.g. neck-shoulder) Low back pain	Postherpetic neuralgia (PHN) Diabetic mono/poly neuropathy Nerve trauma	Spinal cord injury Central post stroke Multiple sclerosis Parkinson's disease	Pelvic	Cancer (1,2,3) LBP with radiculopathy (1,2a) Whiplash (1,2a)

Pain is necessarily subjective. It is what one human being reports to another. There may be few objective signs to judge the severity of reported pain and many patients have no obvious (visible) handicap (Box 1.7.1). The most important principle is that the patient and the doctor are best served if the doctor believes the patient's report. Their problems may be ill-understood, even disbelieved, at work and at home. Chronic pain changes people, affecting their personal and working lives, and ultimately their personalities. Often such changes are reversible with successful treatment. Much time and energy is wasted on procedures designed to 'catch the patient out'. Labelling patients as malingerers or the pain as psychogenic may be easier than admitting that there is no successful treatment.

Acute pain

In the peripheral nervous system most of the nociceptive signalling of thermal and mechanical stimuli comes from activation of polymodal nociceptors which are innervated by C-fibres. Tissue damage leads to the release of peptides and this inflammatory soup activates and sensitizes peripheral nerve endings, and causes vasodilatation and plasma extravasation. These fibres also respond to local chemical stimulation by becoming sensitized to chemical, thermal, and mechanical stimuli. The net result is swelling, pain, and tenderness. If the injury is repeated, the pain is amplified (Box 1.7.2).

The idea that the nervous system can change led to the idea of 'plasticity', a concept which has had a major impact in both acute and chronic pain. At its simplest, a memory of a pain is created and stored in the nervous system. Preventing such a memory being laid down led to the idea of pre-empting postoperative pain; any pain after the operation would be easier to treat if the memory had been minimized. It was hoped that any long-term sequelae, such as the phantom pain which can occur after amputation, could also be prevented. These were attractive ideas, but had little evidence to support them. One issue of importance for treatment of chronic pain is to determine at what level of the nervous system such memories might be stored. If the memory is stored at a 'central' level, then attacking the pain in the leg or arm where it originated might not do any good. However, the memory might be held centrally but require continued input from the periphery to sustain it. Attacking the pain in the leg or arm would then have some logic. This plasticity is evident after amputation or plexus avulsion, when phantom sensations in the 'absent' limb can be evoked by touch elsewhere, for example, touching the chin causing pain in the arm. The plasticity can be used to control symptoms. Looking at the good arm in a mirror produces the impression that you are looking at the 'absent' arm. Moving the good arm, and watching the reflection in the mirror of that good arm, may improve the phantom pain.

Many treatments or interventions are used to treat both acute pain and chronic pain. Not surprisingly, chronic pain has more twists and turns because its origins may be more complicated and because the nervous system can behave strangely if damaged or continuously bombarded by pain messages. The concept of plasticity has led to interventions coming in and indeed going out of fashion. For example, long-term measures, such as cutting the nerves thought to carry a particular pain message, are now no longer popular because the nervous system will 'rewire'. The pain may then be more difficult to manage than it was initially. Better drug control of difficult pain has also reduced the necessity for destructive procedures (Box 1.7.4).

Methods of measuring pain

Pain measurement is subjective, but if some simple rules are followed, pain measurement can be made to work well in research settings and, perhaps even more importantly, pain can be recorded along with vital signs as part of the normal clinical course (Box 1.7.3).

Box 1.7.2 Patient's perceptions of pain

- Varies between individuals
- It is best to believe the patient.

Box 1.7.3 Measuring pain

- Pain should be measured alongside other vital signs
- Patient diaries are best for chronic pain.

Research pain scales

The same pain scales tend to be used in acute and chronic pain. It is sensible in chronic pain to use pain scales in conjunction with disability and quality-of-life measures. It makes no sense to invent your own scale. It is far better to use proven tools. The IMMPACT group's publications make recommendations about choice of scale for measuring pain in different contexts.

Pain intensity and pain relief can be measured by either word categories or visual analogue (100-mm line) scale.

Categorical and visual analogue scales

For chronic work, when patients are recording over long periods, we tend to use diaries with categories, and ask about both pain intensity and pain relief. The clinician's global view is a notorious overestimate and should not be used.

Clinical practice pain scales

The argument for using pain charts as part of normal practice is to improve the quality of care. It is the fact of a chart rather than the form of the chart which is most important. Charting should be done together with vital signs (the fifth vital sign), and can then be used for both clinical care and for audit.

Problem areas

Two important groups of patients, children and the unconscious, present particular problems for pain measurement. With unconscious patients there is little alternative to using variations in vital signs, such as blood pressure rise, as a proxy for a report of increased pain. We do not know how well these proxies work. There are special scales for children over 3 years of age. Below 3 years of age, experienced staff interpreting crying and other behaviour is the best guide available (Box 1.7.4).

Box 1.7.4 Problems in pain management

- Plasticity leads to return of pain after cordotomy
- The brain has 'pain memory'
- Internal factors (e.g. emotional state) affect pain perception
- External factors can also have profound effects
- Depression increases pain; pain increases depression.

Treatment

Drugs are the mainstay of treating both normal (nociceptive) and neuropathic pain (Box 1.7.5). The menu of remedies also includes stimulation devices, from trancutaneous through to implanted stimulators, cognitive behavioural therapy (pain programmes), complementary techniques, and invasive methods from injection through to surgery designed to block transmission of the pain message (Figure 1.7.1).

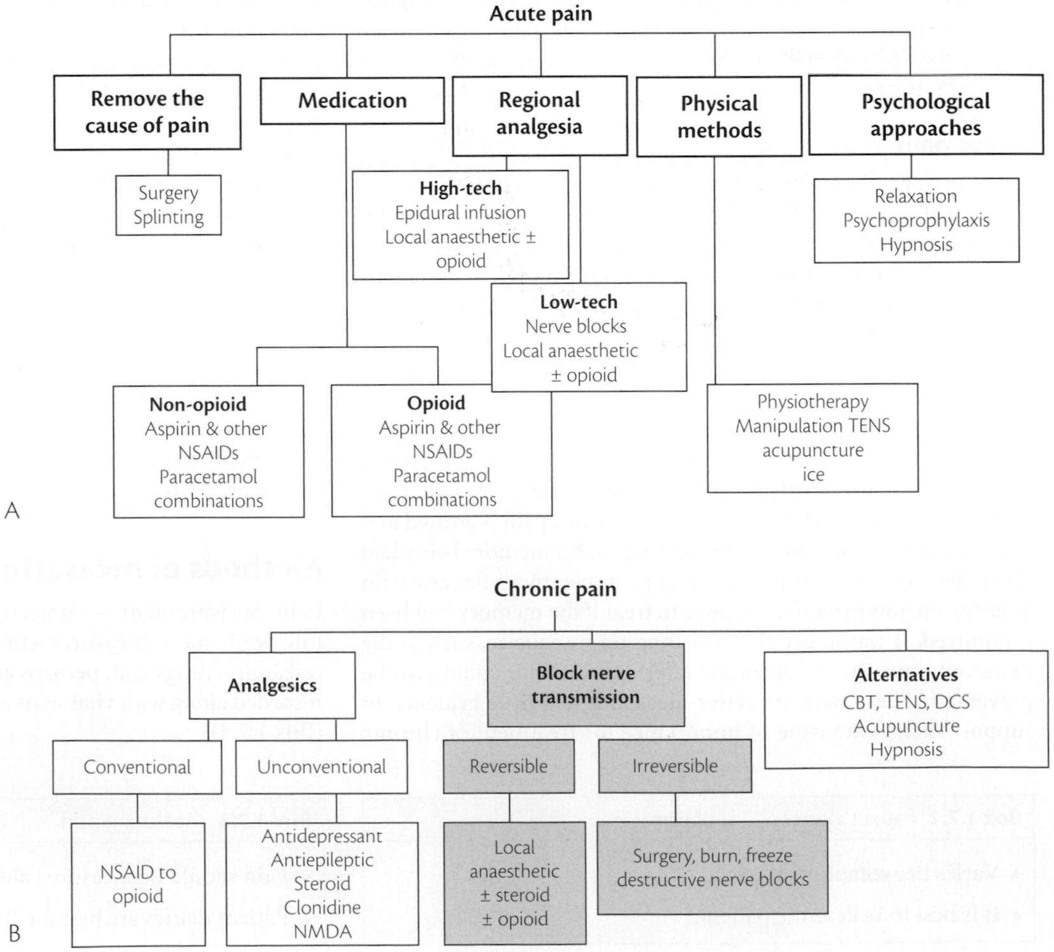

Fig. 1.7.1 Treatment options for acute (A) and chronic (B) pain.

Box 1.7.5 Principles of drug therapy for pain

- Start with safe first-line drugs
- Add in stronger drugs if necessary but continue first-line drugs
- Fit in with available drugs and specific patient requirements
- Be aware of local prejudices, e.g. NSAIDs in bone healing
- Consider best route of delivery.

Treating normal (nociceptive) pain

The basic algorithm for treating nociceptive pain, acute, chronic, or acute on chronic, is shown in Figure 1.7.2, derived from the pain 'ladder' which is widely used in palliative care. This ladder was formulated originally in the 1980s under the aegis of the World Health Organization (WHO). In its raw form, it captured the treatment care pathway for pain by representing increasing strengths of analgesia as further steps or rungs up the ladder. At the bottom rung, or step 1, is a non-opioid analgesic, usually paracetamol (acetaminophen); at step 2 a non-steroidal anti-inflammatory drug (NSAID) or a combination of minor opioid with paracetamol; and at step 3 addition of a strong opioid, morphine, by mouth or injection. This simple pathway has had enormous global impact in palliative care, even though the drugs used may vary in different countries.

This algorithm is as useful in trauma and orthopaedics as it is in palliative care. In acute pain, perioperative or traumatic, one is working right to left as pain decreases. In chronic pain the patient needs to use the three strengths of analgesic as the pain increases or decreases, the 'three pot' system. The 'basic' algorithm is thus the same across the different pain intensities, making teaching and implementation more effective, but the choice of particular drugs will vary locally with availability.

The visual presentation of the ladder differs from the original WHO palliative care ladder in two main ways, because we wanted to convey visually the principle of 'add rather than replace', by which we meant that if the pain becomes more severe you add a stronger analgesic to your other analgesic(s), rather than replacing a weaker one. The inversion of the diagram compared with the original, with the basic building block (step 1) at the top of the picture is to emphasize the 'add not replace' concept, because putting the step 1 drugs at the bottom of the algorithm makes it more likely that they will be overlooked and omitted in the management of moderate or severe pain.

Box 1.7.6 Routes of administration

- Patient-controlled analgesia gives patient control and avoids the risk of overdose
- Slow-release oral analgesics cover background chronic pain
- Quick release can then be used to control flares of pain.

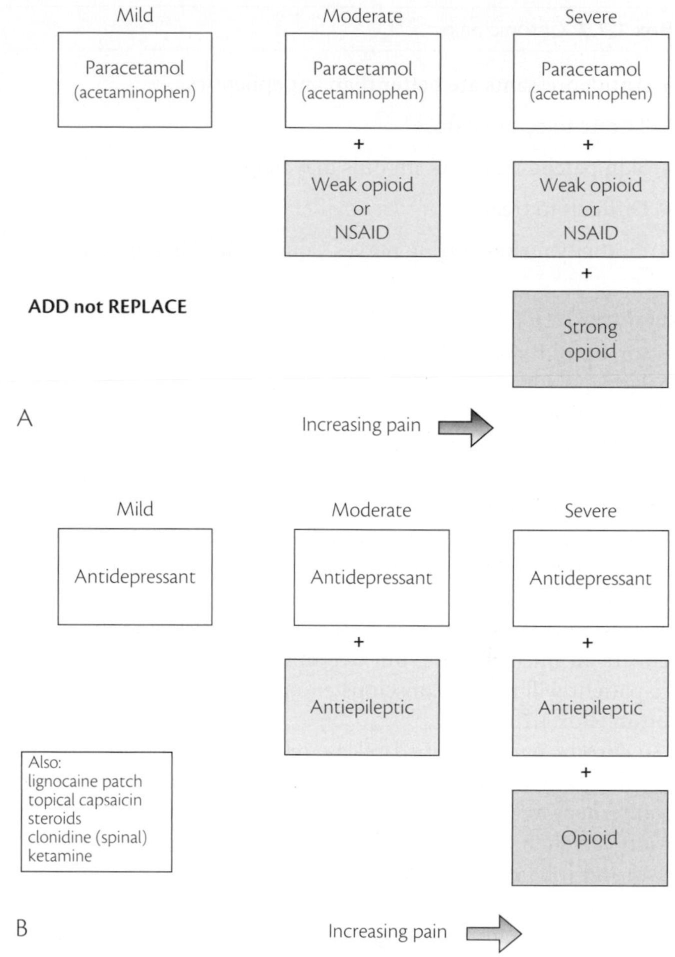

Fig. 1.7.2 Algorithms for analgesics in nociceptive pain (acute above, chronic below).

Fleshing out the detail of the drugs and the route of administration will vary for each of the drug choices, each section of the algorithm, and each of the pain intensities. The key concept is to keep as much in common as possible, while fitting in with available drug choice and clinical situation. For instance, lower starting doses might be used in older people. Some of the detail will rightly be determined by local custom and practice, and where the detail on the pathway is at variance with local belief, then there is a danger that the whole pathway loses credibility. A simple example is pain caused by a fractured bone and NSAIDs. When staff have been told not to use NSAIDs because they are said to impair bone healing, then including NSAIDs on the pathway damages the credibility of the whole plan. While many may doubt that NSAIDs have significant clinical impact on bone healing, the detailed algorithm will need to be subject to local variation to give it the local ownership which it needs if it is to be part of everyday clinical practice.

The step 2 drugs in the algorithm are the NSAIDs and the minor opioids, such as codeine. NSAIDs are powerful analgesics. Standard oral NSAID doses provide analgesia equivalent to that from intramuscular morphine (10mg). However, the adverse effects of NSAIDs at therapeutic doses limit their utility, particularly for extended use in chronic pain. In those for whom NSAIDs are contraindicated and paracetamol (acetaminophen) is not sufficient, a

Box 1.7.7 Chronic pain

- Antidepressants are better than antiepileptics
- Titrate to optimal dose
- Skin patches and oral steroids may help
- Difficult to treat
- Plasticity makes cutting nerves valueless in the long term

minor opioid should be added to the paracetamol to improve analgesia.

The choice of strong opioid will vary according to local availability, custom, and practice. While morphine is the gold standard, orally in chronic pain or by injection in acute pain, other formulations or alternative opioids are used. For example, when swallowing or gastrointestinal function is impaired, injected, sublingual, topical, nasal, or inhaled routes of administration may be better. In perioperative care, patients self-administer strong opioid via patient-controlled analgesia systems (PCA). Pressing the button delivers an injected dose, but overdose is made unlikely because the patient will not be conscious enough to continue to press the button (Box 1.7.6).

In chronic pain, modified-release oral formulations are convenient for patients, allowing the greater part of the daily opioid requirement to be taken just twice a day. A normal-release formulation can then be used to deal with flares of pain. Faster acting nasal and inhaled formulations are now being developed to give improved control of these flares, or 'breakthrough' pains.

These drug regimens may fail to control pain in some cases. It is estimated that in cancer pain 5–10% of patients need a different approach. Perhaps the most important change in the last 30 years is the realization that destructive invasive techniques rarely produce long-term benefit because the system eventually rewires, and the pain may be more difficult to manage than before. Reversible invasive techniques such as long-term epidural infusions using local anaesthetic, opioid, and other drugs such as clonidine can provide the necessary control, and can be withdrawn if the pain improves, without making the situation worse (Box 1.7.7).

Treating nerve damage (neuropathic) pain

Peripheral neuropathic pain can rarely be managed adequately over the long term with the conventional analgesics described earlier. An example in orthopaedics is complex regional pain syndrome

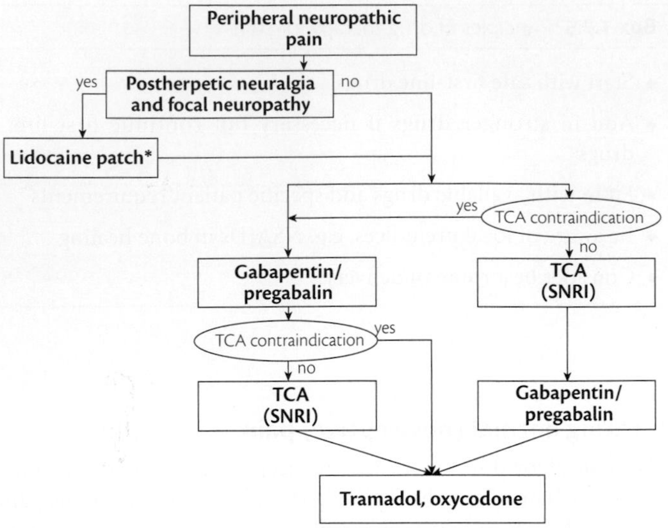

Fig. 1.7.3 Algorithm for analgesics in neuropathic pain. From Finnerup, N., Otto, M., McQuay, H., et al. (2005). Algorithm for neuropathic pain treatment: An evidence based proposal. *Pain*, **118**, 289–305.

(CRPS). The dose–response for opioids is shifted to the right in neuropathic pain compared to nociceptive pain, and response is often minimal. The reason remains a mystery.

The unconventional analgesics listed in Figure 1.7.1B are antidepressants and antiepileptics. Both classes of drugs have proved effective in a wide variety of neuropathic pain syndromes, and also in fibromyalgia and irritable bowel syndrome, which fall outside the usual lists of causes of neuropathic pain. An algorithm for drug management of neuropathic pain, using an analogous format to that for nociceptive pain, is shown in Figure 1.7.3.

Further reading

Finnerup, N., Otto, M., McQuay, H., Jensen T., and Sindrup S. (2005). Algorithm for neuropathic pain treatment: An evidence based proposal. *Pain*, **118**, 289–305.

Moore, A., Edwards, J., Barden, J., and McQuay, H. (2003). *Bandolier's Little Book of Pain*. Oxford: Oxford University Press.

Ramachandran, V.S. and Rogers-Ramachandran, D. (1996). Synaesthesia in phantom limbs induced with mirrors. *Proceedings of the Royal Society of London. Series B*, **263**(1369), 377–86.

Turk, D.C., Dworkin, R.H., Allen, R.R., *et al.* (2003). Core outcome domains for chronic pain clinical trials: IMMPACT recommendations. *Pain*, **106**, 337–45. Available at: http://www.immpact.org

1.8

Biomechanics

Amy B. Zavatsky

Summary points

- A knowledge of basic biomechanical principles is key to understanding and developing the practice of orthopaedic surgery
- Mathematical models can be used to calculate forces and strains in musculoskeletal tissues
- The musculoskeletal system is highly indeterminate
- It is important to know the mechanical properties of musculoskeletal tissues so that suitable replacements can be found
- Forces in the joints and muscles can be several times larger than the external loads applied to the body.

Introduction

Biomechanics is the application of the principles of mechanics and the techniques of engineering to the study of biological systems, including the human body. From an early date, one of the major areas of biomechanical study has been the musculoskeletal system or locomotor system. A knowledge of biomechanics is important not only for understanding existing orthopaedic practice, but also for designing new treatments, such as joint replacements and tissue-engineered bone or cartilage substitutes. This chapter explains how loads are transmitted by the tissues of the musculoskeletal system. Further information on a range of biomechanical applications in orthopaedics and on the basic principles of engineering mechanics can be found elsewhere.

Loads applied to the body

Ethical considerations and measurement difficulties mean that direct measurements of forces and strains in living human tissues are scarce. One alternative to direct measurement of forces is the creation and solution of a mathematical model of the system of interest. The particular body or mechanical system to be analyzed is isolated and all the forces or loads which act on it are defined clearly and as completely as possible. This isolation of the body of interest is accomplished by means of a 'free-body diagram', which is a diagrammatic representation of the isolated body showing all the forces applied to it both by mechanical contact and by body forces, such as those due to gravitational attraction. Only when a clear free-body diagram has been completed should mathematical relationships between the force quantities be written and solved (Box 1.8.1).

Figure 1.8.1A shows a man carrying a briefcase climbing some stairs. The system of interest is the man, and so he is drawn separately as the first step in constructing a free-body diagram (Figure 1.8.1B). All the forces acting on the man are then drawn as arrows (called 'vectors'); these represent the force magnitudes, directions, and points of application. A vector is usually written in boldface type (**F**) or with an arrow over it ($\vec{F}$).

When the area over which the force is applied is small compared with the other dimensions of the body, the force is considered to be 'concentrated' at a point. These are the types of force acting on the man's feet (labelled $\mathbf{F}_L$ and $\mathbf{F}_R$ in Figure 1.8.1B) and on the hand which he rests on the handrail (labelled $\mathbf{H}_L$ in Figure 1.8.1B). These particular forces are a good example of Newton's third law of mechanics (sometimes known as 'action and reaction'). The man's foot pushes against the stair with a certain force, and the stair pushes back on the foot with a force of the same magnitude and line of action, but in the opposite direction. The forces $\mathbf{F}_L$, $\mathbf{F}_R$, and $\mathbf{H}_L$ all have units of newtons (N) in the SI system.

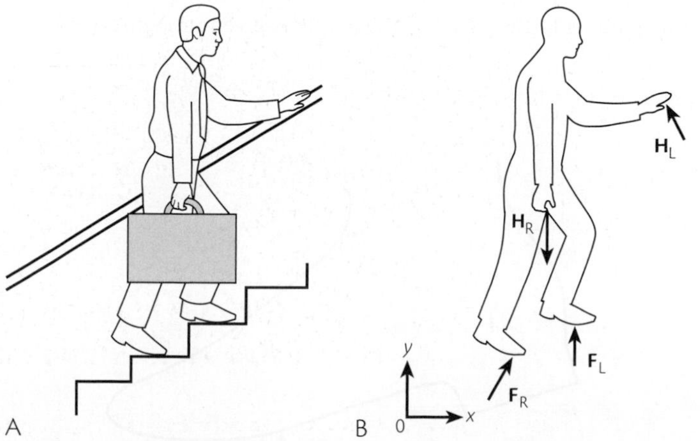

Fig. 1.8.1 A) A man climbing stairs. B) Free-body diagram of a man climbing stairs, excluding the force of body weight.

An arrow (labeled $\mathbf{H}_R$) indicates the downward force due to the weight of the briefcase which the man carries in his right hand. The force $\mathbf{H}_R = m_B\mathbf{g}$, where m_B is the mass of the briefcase in kilograms (kg) and **g** is the acceleration associated with the gravitational force of attraction (9.81m/s^2). Note that 1N = 1kg m/s^2. Note also that the force $\mathbf{H}_R$ acts downward.

'Distributed' forces are applied over an area, or they may be distributed over a volume. The weight of a body or body segment is the force of gravitational attraction distributed over its volume, but this is usually taken as a concentrated force acting through the centre of gravity of the body or the relevant body segment. The weight of the man (not included in Figure 1.8.1B) is equal to the mass of the man m_M (in kg) times **g**.

If, instead of the whole man, the bones, muscles, and joints of his feet were of interest, the non-uniform distributed forces (Figure 1.8.2), rather than the concentrated forces $\mathbf{F}_L$ and $\mathbf{F}_R$ (Figure 1.8.1B), would have to be considered. The distributed forces act over the area of contact between the man's feet and the stairs. The parts of these forces perpendicular to the soles of the man's shoes can be thought of as pressures; they have units of force per unit area, namely N/m^2 or pascals (Pa). Instrumentation has been designed to measure plantar pressure using either shoe insole devices or floor-mounted platforms and mats.

Pertinent dimensions should also be represented on the free-body diagram. In biomechanical studies, a wide variety of physical measurements are required, including not only body segment lengths and masses, centres of mass, and moments of inertia, but also locations of muscle origins and insertions, angles of pull of tendons, and lengths and cross-sectional areas of muscles. In the past, most of these measurements were made on cadavers, but now many subject-specific measurements can be made *in vivo* using plane radiography, computed tomography, or magnetic resonance imaging.

It is also usual to indicate a set of coordinate axes on the free-body diagram. For simplicity, only two dimensions will be considered in this example, and so in Figure 1.8.1B the axes *x* and *y* have been added. The *x* axis points to the right, and the *y* axis points upward. If a *z* axis were included, it would point out of the page. The origin O of this global coordinate system is fixed on the bottom stair.

Each force vector in Figure 1.8.1B could instead be drawn as the sum of two perpendicular vectors, one parallel to the *x* axis and one parallel to the *y* axis. An example is given in Figure 1.8.3A, in

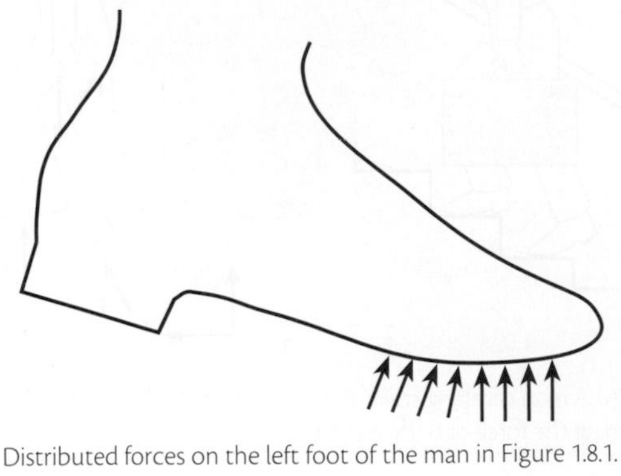

Fig. 1.8.2 Distributed forces on the left foot of the man in Figure 1.8.1.

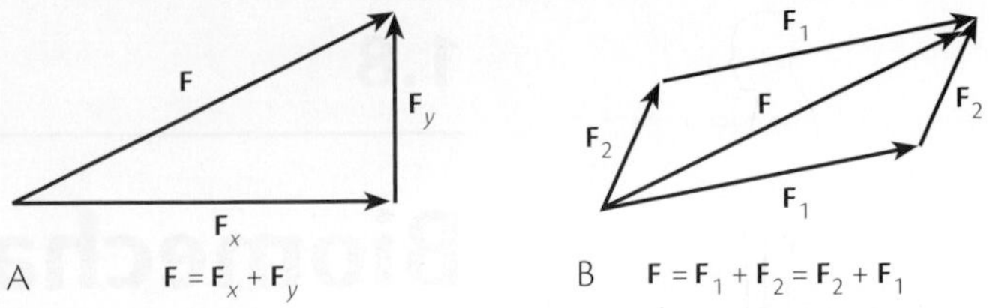

Fig. 1.8.3 The parallelogram law of vector addition. A) Perpendicular forces F_x and F_y add to give F. B) Forces F_1 and F_2 add to give F. Note that the order of addition is not important: $F_1 + F_2 = F_2 + F_1 = F$.

which $\mathbf{F} = \mathbf{F}_x + \mathbf{F}_y$. The absolute values of the two perpendicular vectors ($|\mathbf{F}_x| = F_x$ and $|\mathbf{F}_y| = F_y$) are known as the 'components' of the vector **F**. The graphical construction in Figure 1.8.3A is an example of the 'parallelogram law of vector addition', in which the resultant of two vectors is found by drawing each vector to scale and arranging them tip to tail. The resultant then connects the tail of the first vector drawn to the tip of the last vector drawn. The vectors to be added need not necessarily be parallel, nor does it matter in which order they are drawn (Figure 1.8.3B).

External loads applied to the body can often be measured accurately using force transducers which give an electrical signal proportional to the applied force. The device used to measure the ground reaction force ($\mathbf{F}_L$ or $\mathbf{F}_R$ in Figure 1.8.1B) is called a force plate or force platform (Figure 1.8.4). When a person walks or runs across the force plate, the force measured no longer simply equals body weight but is an indication of both the mass and the inertia of the body (Figure 1.8.5A,B). Figures 1.8.6A–C show how the components of the ground reaction force change over time during the stance phase of walking. Figure 1.8.6D shows a normal pattern of ground reaction force vectors as seen in the sagittal plane; this plot is known as a Pedotti diagram or a butterfly diagram.

Statics versus dynamics

When a body is in equilibrium (either stationary or moving at constant velocity, according to Newton's first law of mechanics), the resultant force and resultant moment acting on it are zero

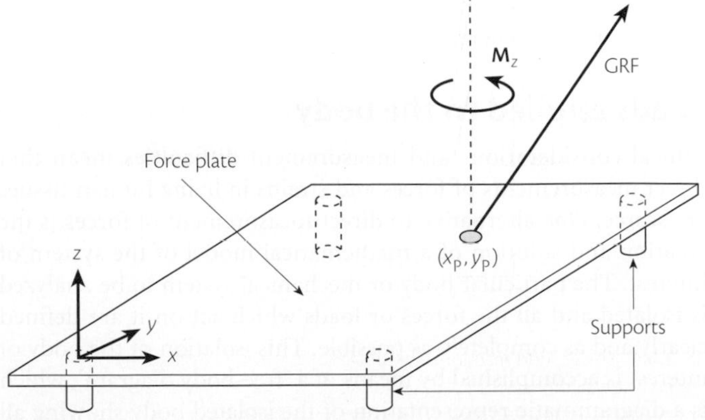

Fig. 1.8.4 The force plate. The ground reaction force (GRF), the free moment of rotation (M_z), and the centre of pressure (x_p, y_p) are shown. Note that the axis directions differ from those shown in Figure 1.8.1.

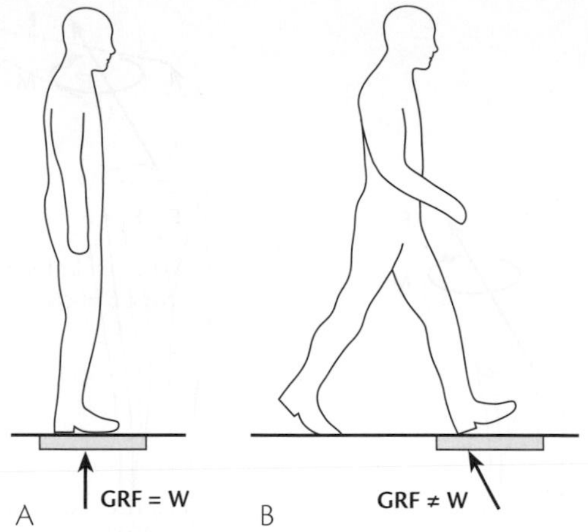

Fig. 1.8.5 A) A static measurement on the force plate. The ground reaction force (GRF) equals the man's weight (W). B) A dynamic measurement on the force plate during normal level walking. The ground reaction force (GRF) does not equal the man's weight (W).

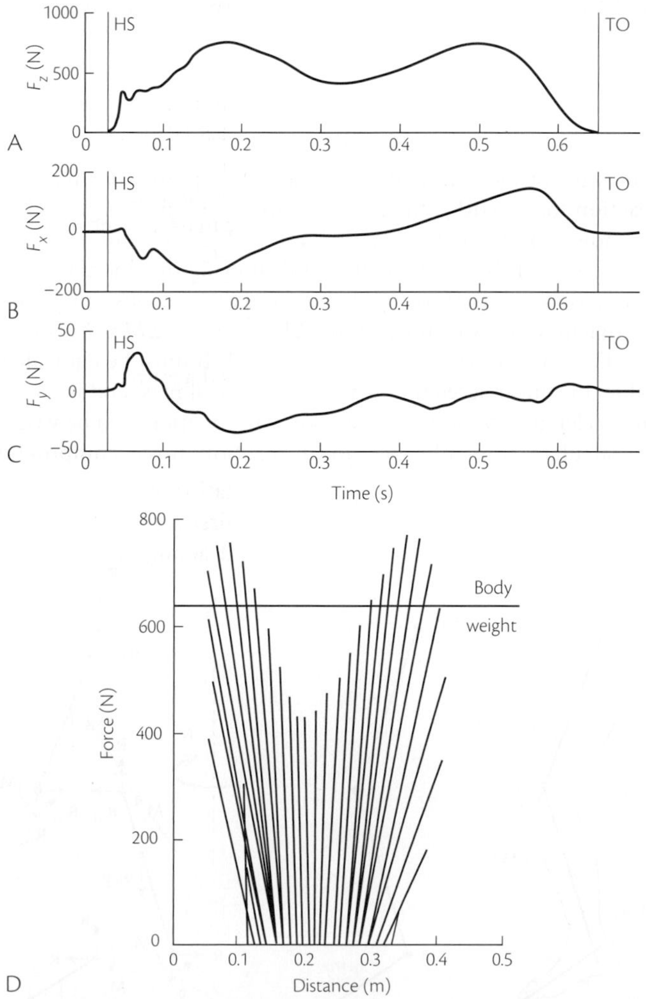

Fig. 1.8.6 The ground reaction force during the stance phase of normal gait. A) The vertical component F_z is positive upward. B) The fore–aft horizontal component F_x is positive forward. C) In this case the mediolateral horizontal component F_y is positive laterally. D) The pattern of ground reaction force vectors as seen in the sagittal plane. HS, heelstrike; TO, toe-off. Data courtesy of the Oxford Gait Laboratory, Nuffield Orthopaedic Centre NHS Trust, Oxford, UK.

Box 1.8.1 Steps in drawing a free-body diagram

- Isolate and draw the body or system of interest
- Draw as arrows all forces applied to it
- Add a coordinate system and pertinent dimensions
- Write the equations of motion or static equilibrium.

($\Sigma\mathbf{F} = 0$, $\Sigma\mathbf{M} = 0$). Moment is the term used to describe the tendency of a force to rotate a body about some axis. The magnitude of a moment **M** is proportional to the magnitude of the force **F** which causes it and to the moment arm *d*, which is the perpendicular distance from the axis about which rotation occurs to the line of action of the force, or $|\mathbf{M}| = |\mathbf{F}|d$, as shown in Figure 1.8.7A. The moment produced by two equal and opposite but non-collinear forces (**F** and –**F**) a distance *d* apart is known as a couple **C** with magnitude $|\mathbf{F}|d$ (Figure 1.8.7B). Notice that the sum of the two forces is zero since they are equal and opposite. There is no tendency for the forces to translate the body, but they do tend to rotate it. Moments and couples are vectors, and their directions are given by the 'right-hand rule' (Figure 1.8.8).

To check whether the sum of the forces acting on a body is zero, the force vectors must be summed either graphically using the 'parallelogram law' (Figure 1.8.3) or algebraically using the force components. For the moments acting on a body in two dimensions to be in equilibrium, the clockwise moments about any point must balance the counterclockwise moments about the same point.

Dynamics is the study of the motion of bodies under the action of forces. It involves the tendency of unbalanced forces to translate a body and the tendency of unbalanced moments to rotate a body. From Newton's second law, we know that $\Sigma\mathbf{F} = m\mathbf{a}$, or the acceleration of a particle (or of the centre of mass of a body) is proportional to the resultant force acting on it and is in the direction of the force. The constant of proportionality is the mass of the particle or body. Note that acceleration, like force, is a vector and has components in the *x*, *y*, and *z* directions. For moments in two dimensions, $\Sigma M_z = I\alpha$ where *I* is the moment of inertia (or tendency of the body to resist rotation) and α is the angular acceleration. The moment of inertia is usually referred to the centre of mass of the body or segment (Box 1.8.2).

Loads internal to the body

Before finding the forces acting in particular body tissues during activity, it is necessary to quantify the resultant force and moment

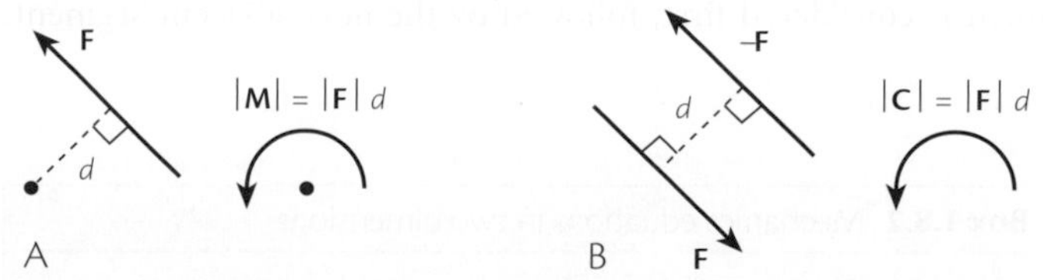

Fig. 1.8.7 A) The moment M of force F about a point. The length *d* is the moment arm of the force F. B) Two equal and opposite but non-collinear forces F form the couple C.

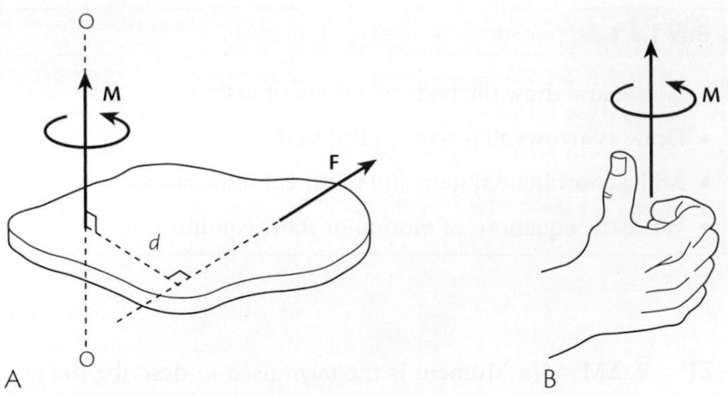

Fig. 1.8.8 The 'right-hand rule'. The moment M of force F about O–O is represented as a vector pointing in the direction of the thumb, with the fingers pointing in the direction of the tendency to rotate. Adapted from Meriam and Kraige (1993).

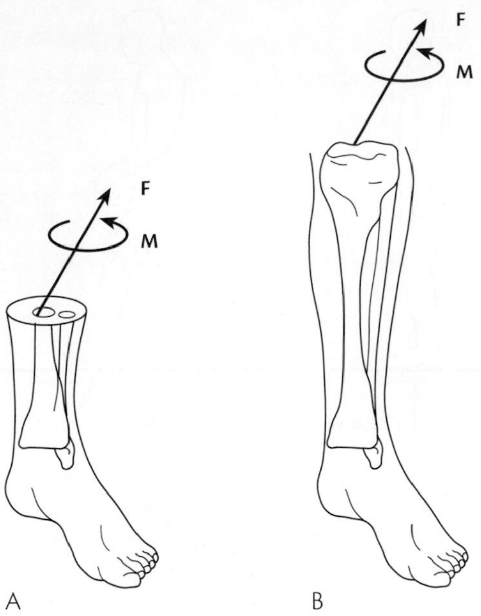

Fig. 1.8.9 Resultant force F and resultant moment M acting at a section (A) through the shank and (B) through the knee. Adapted from O'Connor (1991).

acting along a limb or at a joint. For static situations, this is relatively easy. A free-body diagram of the body is drawn and an imaginary slice taken through it at the section of interest. This imaginary slice may be through a bone shaft (Figure 1.8.9A) or through a joint (Figure 1.8.9B). A resultant force **F** and a resultant moment **M** act at this section, and they balance the external loads and segment weights. At a joint, these quantities are sometimes called the 'resultant joint force and moment' or the 'intersegmental force and moment'. The calculated resultant forces and moments at the sections shown in Figure 1.8.9 do not correspond to actual forces and moments, and they cannot be measured with transducers. They are abstract quantities that are often used not as final results but as inputs to a second step—determination of the distribution of these forces and moments among the structures of the body.

In dynamic situations, the body is usually divided into segments, and the forces, moments, and accelerations of each segment are considered separately. An example of a two-dimensional link-segment model of the lower limb is shown in Figure 1.8.10. The limb is divided into three segments (thigh, shank, foot), each with its own mass m_i and moment of inertia I_i (Figure 1.8.10A). In this simple model, the links are connected by pins. To draw a free-body of each segment, we disconnect the link-segment model at the joints and draw the resultant force and moment at each joint (Figure 1.8.10C). On the foot segment, the resultant joint force $\mathbf{R}_a$ at the ankle has two components, R_{xa} and R_{ya}. The resultant joint moment is $\mathbf{M}_a$. On the free-body diagram of the shank segment, $\mathbf{M}_a$ and the components of $\mathbf{R}_a$ are opposite in direction to those drawn on the foot segment. The same is true for the joint reaction force and moment at the knee, as shown on the free-body diagrams of the shank and thigh segments.

In link-segment models of the lower limb, the most distal segment is considered first, followed by the next adjacent segment, moving proximally. Figure 1.8.11A is a free-body diagram of the foot segment showing all the forces acting on it: the known ground reaction force (**GRF**), the known segment weight ($m_f\mathbf{g}$), and the unknown joint (ankle) reaction force ($\mathbf{R}_a$) and moment ($\mathbf{M}_a$). Figure 1.8.11B is a 'kinetic diagram' showing the 'inertial forces' $m_f\mathbf{a}_f$ and $I_f\alpha_f$ on the foot. We know from the previous section that, for dynamics in two-dimensions, $\Sigma\mathbf{F} = m\mathbf{a}$ and $\Sigma M = I\alpha$, so that the diagrams in Figures 1.8.11A and 1.8.11B must be equivalent. When the linear acceleration **a** of the centre of mass and the angular acceleration α_f of the foot are known, equations can be written to calculate the unknown joint reaction force components

Box 1.8.2 Mechanics equations in two dimensions

- Statics: $\Sigma F_x = 0, \Sigma F_y = 0, \Sigma M_z = 0$
- Dynamics: $\Sigma F_x = ma_x, \Sigma F_y = ma_y, \Sigma M_z = I\alpha$

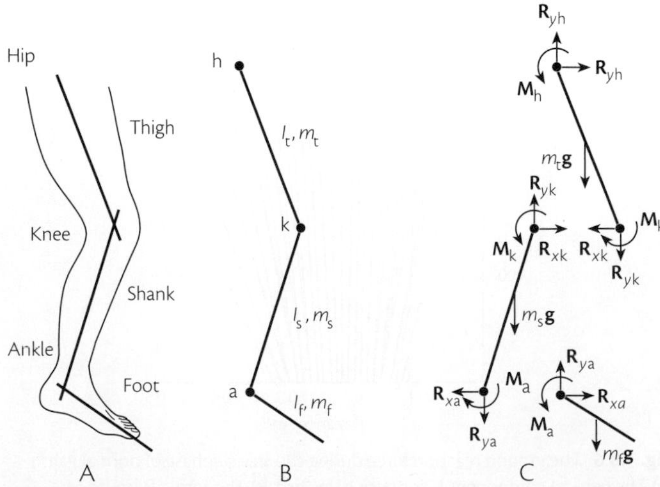

Fig. 1.8.10 A, B) A sagittal-plane link-segment model of the lower limb. Each link has a mass m_i and a moment of inertia I_i. (C) Free-body diagrams of the three links, each showing the segment weight and the intersegmental forces F_i and moment M_i. Adapted from Winter (1990).

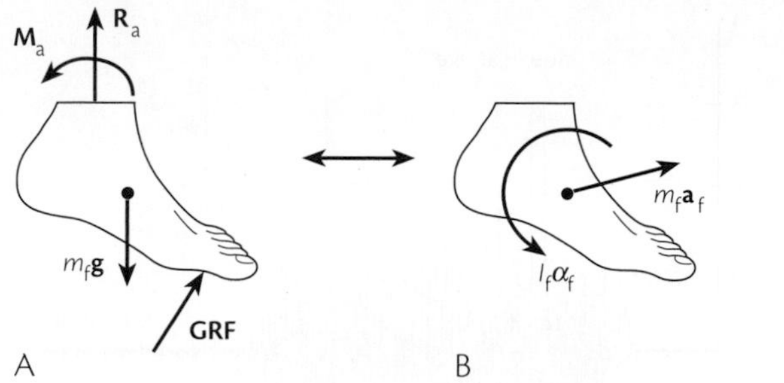

Fig. 1.8.11 A) Free-body diagram and (B) kinetic diagram of the foot during the stance phase of walking.

(R_{xa} and R_{ya}) and the joint reaction moment ($\mathbf{M}_a$). Once these are found, the equilibrium of the shank can be considered and, after that, the thigh.

The usual method for finding the accelerations needed for a dynamic analysis of a link-segment model is to measure the sequential positions of each segment and then to differentiate the position data with respect to time, once to obtain segment velocity and twice to obtain segment acceleration. Because measurement errors are magnified in the differentiation process, the position data must first be filtered to remove unwanted noise. Optoelectronic motion analysis systems (Figure 1.8.12) are commonly used to collect three-dimensional position data. A minimum of three markers is fixed to each body segment of interest, and the changing positions of the markers are recorded by at least two cameras. Some systems use reflective markers, while others use markers containing light-emitting diodes which flash on and off in sequence. A more detailed discussion of motion analysis systems can be found in books on gait analysis.

The problem of indeterminacy

In mechanics, a system is called 'determinate' if the number of equations describing it is the same as the number of unknown quantities (force, position, etc.) When there are more unknown quantities than there are equations, the system is called 'indeterminate' or 'redundant'. The musculoskeletal system is highly indeterminate. Figure 1.8.13 shows as an example a sketch of the knee with its known joint force $\mathbf{F}^k$ and joint moment $\mathbf{M}^k$. Also shown on the drawing are all the unknown forces at the knee: muscle forces $\mathbf{f}^m$, ligament forces $\mathbf{f}^l$, and forces $\mathbf{f}^c$ in the articular cartilage which result from contact between the tibia and the femur. With six equations of equilibrium in three dimensions, it is possible to solve for six unknown quantities. The problem is that there are far more than six unknown forces in Figure 1.8.13—the forces cannot be found using the equations of equilibrium alone. Methods to solve this 'problem of indeterminacy' involve either increasing the number of equations or decreasing the number of unknowns (Box 1.8.3).

Structures which carry load

Bone, muscle, tendon, ligament, and articular cartilage are the load-bearing tissues of the musculoskeletal system. Muscles produce force and are therefore thought of as 'active' tissues. Bones, tendons, ligaments, and articular cartilage are 'passive' structures, since they take up load only as needed to balance the external, inertial, and muscle forces and moments.

Muscle

As an 'active' tissue, a muscle generates force as a result of neural stimulation. It is possible to tell when a muscle is active by detecting the electrical signal or electromyogram (EMG) associated with its contraction. In most cases in orthopaedic biomechanics, electrodes placed on the skin (surface electrodes) are used for this measurement. The raw EMG signal varies in amplitude in a seemingly random way above and below a zero level (Figure 1.8.14). Unfortunately there is no simple relationship between the amplitude of the EMG signal and the force produced by a muscle.

In simulations in which muscle forces are prescribed, the simplest and most common model of muscle contraction dynamics is

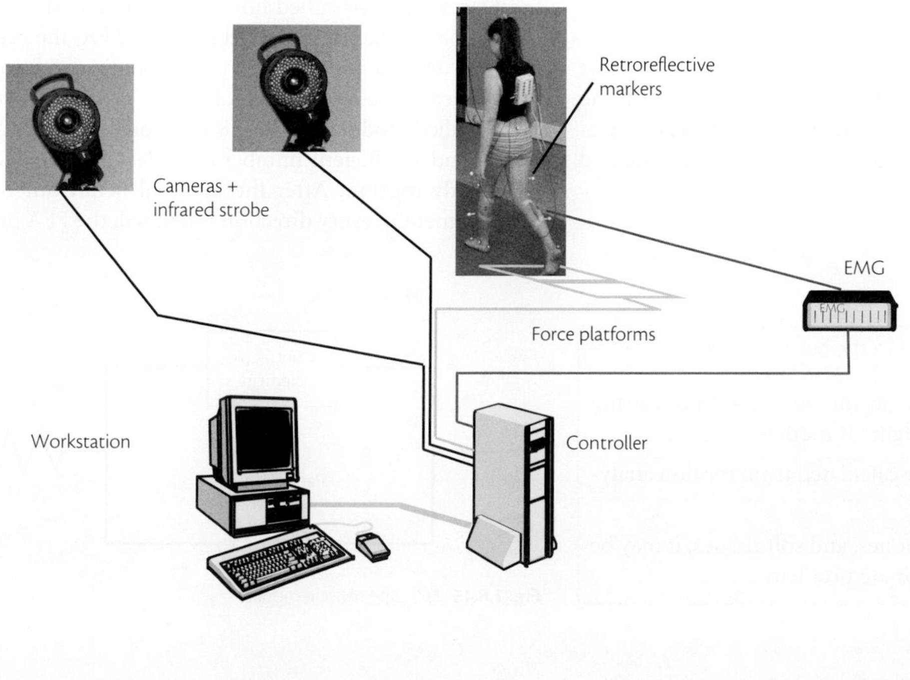

Fig. 1.8.12 Schematic diagram of a motion analysis system. Courtesy of the Oxford Gait Laboratory, Nuffield Orthopaedic Centre NHS Trust, Oxford, UK.

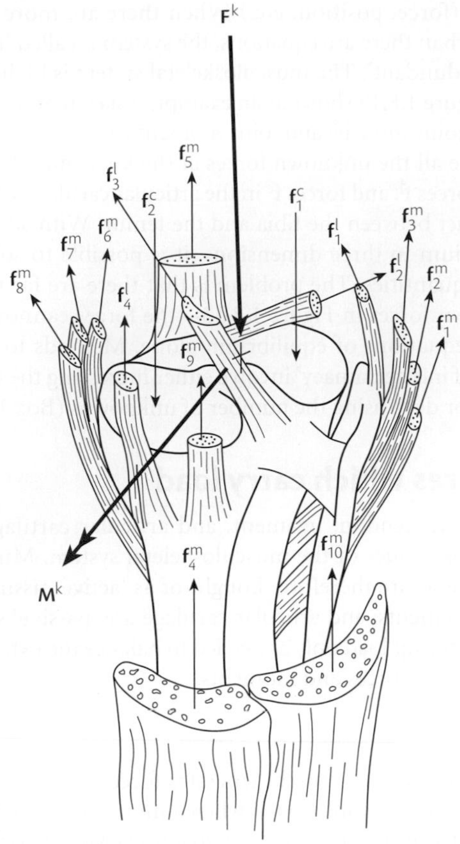

Fig. 1.8.13 The indeterminate force system at the knee. Reproduced from Crowninshield, Pope, and Johnson(1976).

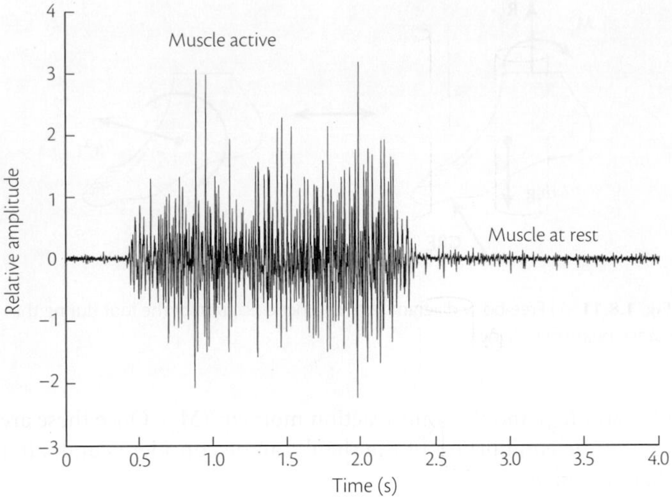

Fig. 1.8.14 An EMG signal from the flexor carpi radialis during clenching of the fist in a normal subject. Data collected with a surface electrode and sampled at 4 kHz. Periods of rest and activity are evident. Data courtesy of S. Taffler, Oxford Orthopaedic Engineering Centre.

the Hill-type model (Figure 1.8.15). The force produced by the contractile process is attributed to the 'contractile element' and depends on the muscle length, the velocity of contraction, and the muscle activation. Hill's equation is often modified and used to relate these parameters to muscle force. The passive resistance of the muscle to being stretched is represented by a spring, the 'parallel elastic element'. Total muscle force is then the sum of the active and passive elements. Some models include a series elastic element (not shown in Figure 1.8.15) next to the contractile element. The elasticity of the muscle tendon can be included in series with the muscle model (Figure 1.8.15). Storage of energy in the elastic elements is thought to be important in activities such as running and jumping.

Bone

The mechanical functions of the bones of the skeleton are to support and protect the tissues of the body and to function as a lever system on which the muscles can act. As a result of external forces and muscle forces, bones are subjected to all kinds of loading: tension, compression, bending, shear, torsion, and combinations of these (Figure 1.8.16). The idea that bone perceives and adapts to the forces applied to it is known as 'Wolff's law'.

Bone is difficult to model using the basic techniques of classical mechanics due to its complex geometrical and mechanical properties. For instance, the cortical and trabecular parts of bone are each made up of different proportions and arrangements of organic and inorganic material. As a result, the ability of bone to resist deformation varies throughout its substance.

Since the early 1970s, an advanced computer technique of structural stress analysis called finite-element analysis (FEA) has been used in biomechanics to model bone. In FEA, the geometry of the model is defined first. The model is then divided into a number of sections called 'elements', all of which are connected together at points called 'nodes' (Figure 1.8.17). Forces must be applied at the nodes, and a sufficient number of nodes must be fixed to prevent rigid-body motion. After the material behaviour or stiffness of every element in every direction is defined, the FEA program solves

Box 1.8.3 Calculating loads internal to the body

- Resultant forces and moments in the body are found using free-body diagrams and link-segment models
- Accelerations, if needed, can be calculated from motion analysis data
- To find the forces in muscles, bones, and soft tissues, it may be necessary to solve an indeterminate problem.

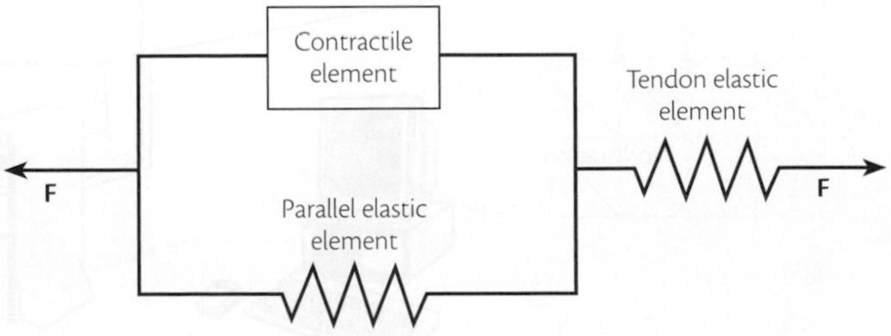

Fig. 1.8.15 Hill-type muscle model.

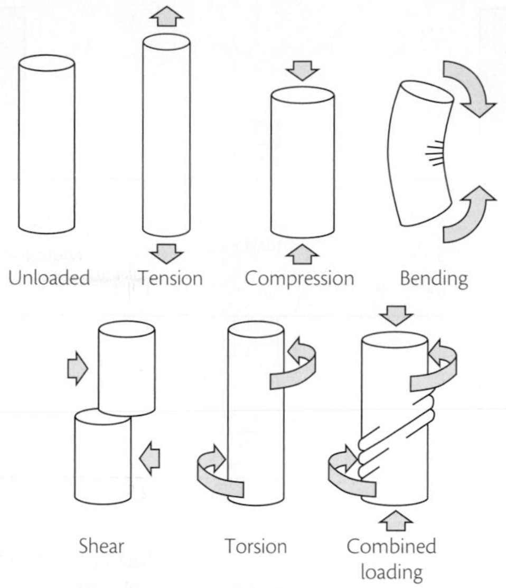

Fig. 1.8.16 The types of loads to which bone may be subjected. Reproduced from Nordin and Frankel (1989).

a large number of equations governing force equilibrium at the nodes to find the nodal displacements within the model. From these displacements, strains and stresses can be calculated.

FEA has been used to study the stresses in bones (Figure 1.8.18), fracture fixation, prosthesis design, and bone-implant interaction. The method is particularly useful for identifying areas of 'stress concentration' (high and sometimes unexpected increases in stress occurring near notches, sharp changes in geometry, or cracks) and 'stress shielding' (in which the load distribution between two materials with very different stiffnesses leads to one of them 'shielding' the other from stress). An example of the latter situation is the insertion of a metal joint replacement causing lower-than-normal stresses in the surrounding bone. This could lead to bone resorption in accordance with Wolff's law. Some FEA models now incorporate simulations of bone growth, repair, and remodelling. Although FEA is cheap compared with clinical, animal, or laboratory testing methods, the combination of FEA with experimental analyses is many times more powerful than the sum of their individual applications.

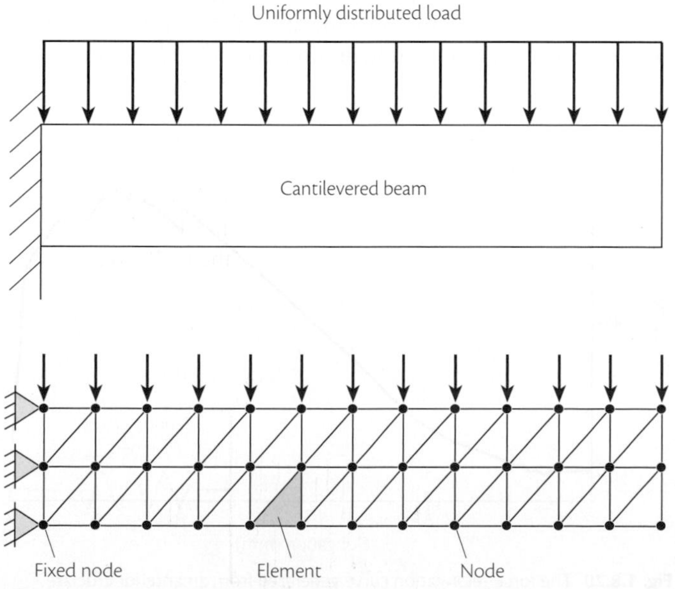

Fig. 1.8.17 A) A uniformly distributed load applied to a cantilevered beam. B) A simple finite-element model of the beam.

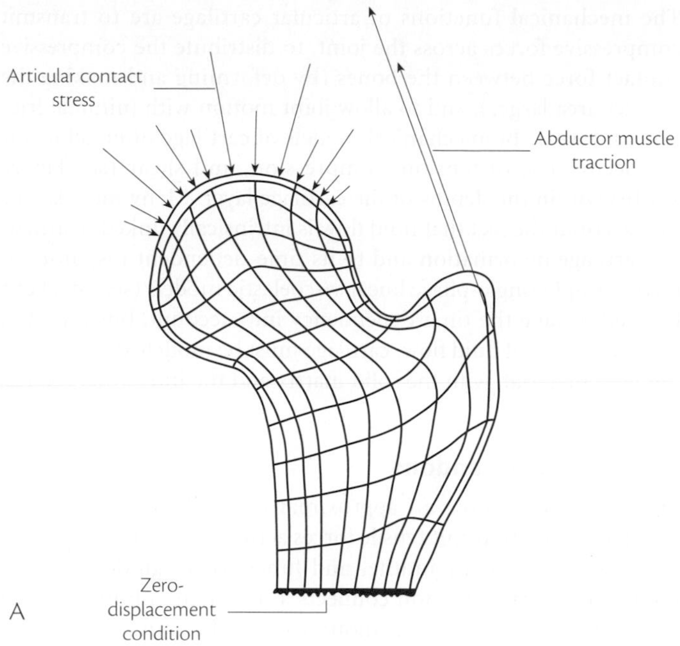

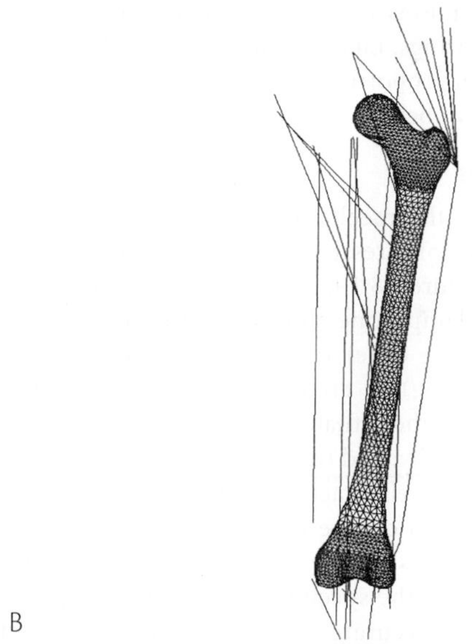

Fig. 1.8.18 A) Two-dimensional finite-element model of a coronal plane section of a proximal femur. Reproduced from Brown et al. (1980). B) Three-dimensional finite-element model of the femur. Lines of action of the major muscle group forces are shown. Courtesy of K. Polgar, Oxford Orthopaedic Engineering Centre.

Articular cartilage

The articulating surfaces of the bones in a synovial joint are covered with a thin layer of connective tissue known as articular cartilage.

The mechanical functions of articular cartilage are to transmit compressive forces across the joint, to distribute the compressive contact force between the bones (by deforming and making the contact area larger), and to allow joint motion with minimal friction and wear. Biomechanical models of cartilage often allow for the occurrence of tension, compression, and shear (see Figure 1.8.16) within the depths of the cartilage layer. Many models take into account the fact that fluid flow is intrinsically linked to articular cartilage deformation and to its time-dependent responses to loads. Simple single-phase linear viscoelastic models (see later) can be used to take the time-dependency into account, but for a full representation of fluid flow, cartilage must be modelled as at least a biphasic material, with the solid matrix and the interstitial fluid as the two phases.

Ligaments and tendons

Ligaments and tendons are approximately parallel-fibred collagenous tissues that transmit tensile forces across the joints. A ligament connects one bone to another and functions to guide and limit joint movement. A tendon connects a muscle to a bone across a joint, thereby causing joint motion when the muscle contracts. Tendons also store elastic energy. In models of the musculoskeletal system, ligaments and tendons are often modelled by a small number of tension-only springs. Like articular cartilage, ligaments and tendons contain a high proportion of water and so also exhibit time-and history-dependent behaviour under load.

Mechanical properties

Much information about the mechanical properties of tissues comes from tension and compression tests performed using a tensile-testing machine (Figure 1.8.19). The ends of the tissue specimen are held in special clamps, one attached to the rigid base of the testing machine and the other to a moving actuator (in a hydraulically-driven machine) or crosshead (in a screw-driven machine). The movement of the actuator/crosshead up or down is usually controlled electronically, and the load applied to the specimen is measured with a load cell attached to the testing machine. Deformation of the specimen can be measured by tracking the movement of the actuator/crosshead or by attaching an extensometer or strain gage directly to the specimen. In many cases, however, these methods are not accurate enough, and a non-contact optical method must be used. This typically involves recording on high-speed video the positions of reference marks placed on the specimen before the start of the test.

The output from any tension or compression test is typically a plot of applied load P versus specimen elongation Δl. Figure 1.8.20 shows a plot for a tensile test on a ligament. The 'structural properties' of the entire ligament can be found from such a graph. These include the stiffness (slope of the linear part of the curve), energy absorbed (area under the curve), and ultimate (maximum) load and elongation. These values depend, amongst other things, on the geometry of the tissue, such as its cross-sectional area and length, and on the properties of the tissue substance.

To study the 'mechanical properties' of the ligament tissue alone, it is necessary to calculate and plot a graph of stress versus strain. Stress σ is defined as the load P divided by the cross-sectional area A perpendicular to the load: $\sigma = P/A$. Strain ε is defined as the change in specimen length Δl divided by the original length l: $\varepsilon = \Delta l/l$. Mechanical properties such as the elastic modulus (slope of the linear part of the curve), strain energy density (area under the curve), and ultimate (maximum) stress and strain can be found from a graph of σ versus ε (Figure 1.8.21).

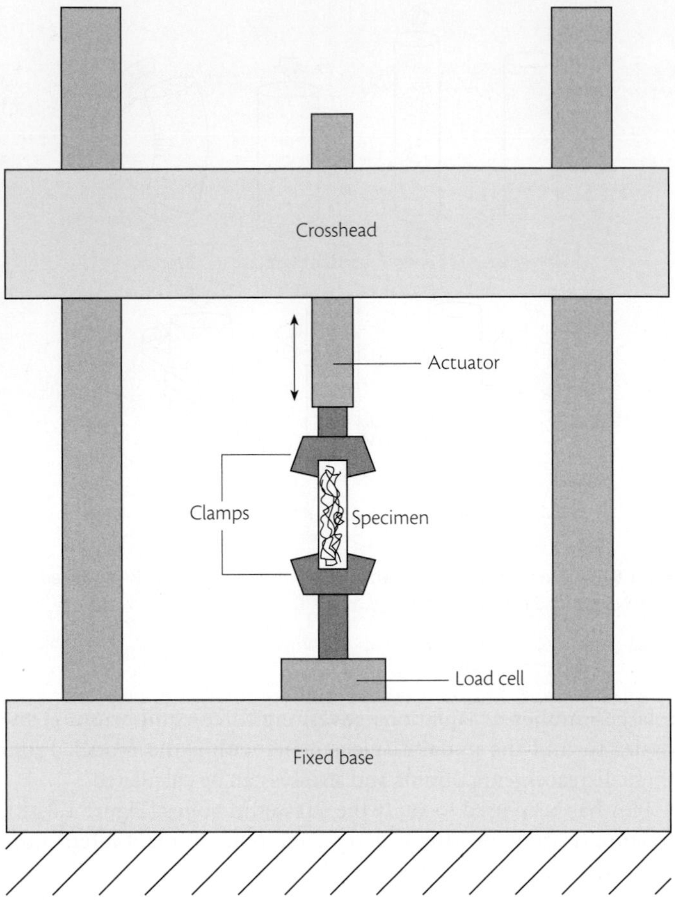

Fig. 1.8.19 Schematic diagram of a tensile-testing machine.

It is important to recognize that mechanical measurements on tissues are affected by experimental, biological, and external factors. Experimental factors include specimen orientation, strain rate, temperature, and tissue hydration. Biological factors are tissue

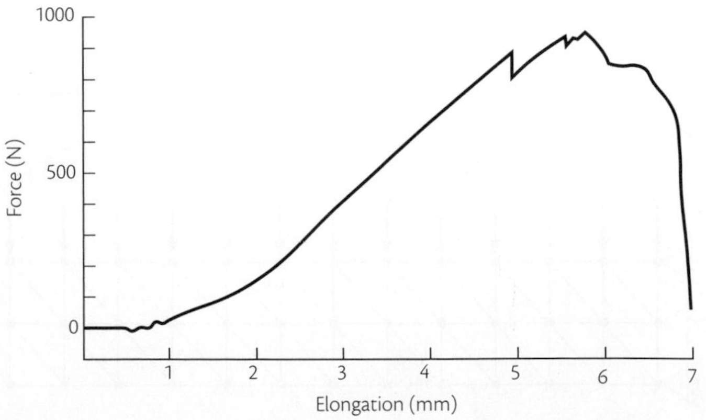

Fig. 1.8.20 The force–elongation curve generated from an anterior cruciate ligament tested in tension to failure. Reproduced from Carlstedt and Nordin (1989), based on data from Noyes (1977).

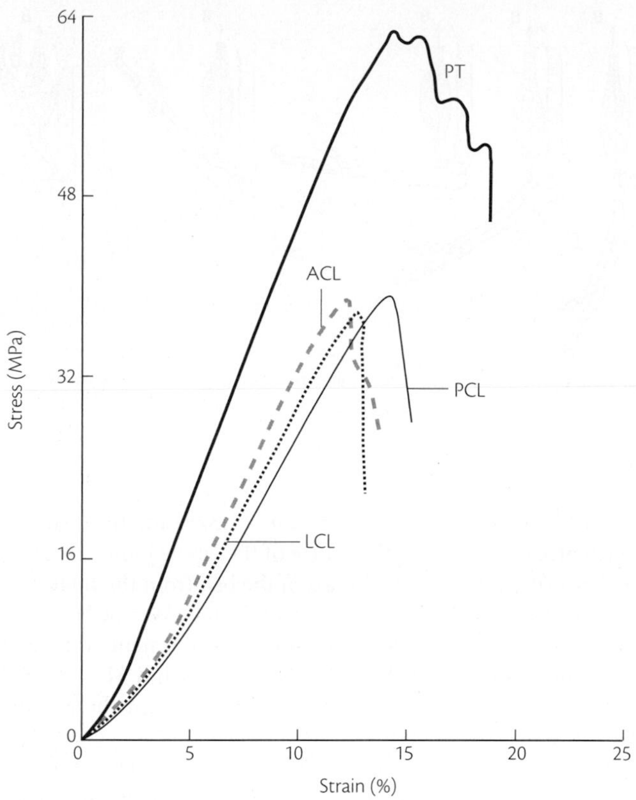

Fig. 1.8.21 Typical stress–strain curves for the patellar tendon (PT), anterior cruciate ligament (ACL), posterior cruciate ligament (PCL), and lateral collateral ligament (LCL) fascicle–bone units. Note the much larger elastic modulus and ultimate stress for the PT specimen. Reproduced from Butler et al. (1986).

maturation, age, immobilization, and exercise. Storage by freezing and sterilization are external factors.

Viscoelasticity

Almost all polymers (plastics) and all biological materials exhibit time-dependent or viscoelastic properties. Viscoelasticity is a mechanical behaviour involving both fluid-like (viscous) and solid-like (elastic) characteristics. The viscoelastic properties of soft tissues, in particular articular cartilage, have received much attention. The main features of viscoelasticity are shown in Figure 1.8.22. Stress relaxation (Figure 1.8.22A) is a decrease in stress in a material subjected to prolonged constant strain. Creep (Figure 1.8.22B) is an increase in deformation or strain that occurs when a constant load is applied. Hysteresis (Figure 1.8.22C) is a characteristic behaviour related to energy dissipation in which a material property plot follows a closed loop, i.e. the loading and unloading curves are not coincident. These features of the behaviour of biological materials are rarely taken into account in models of joints and limbs because the duration of the activity being studied is relatively short, the viscoelastic effects are secondary, or inclusion of such effects would make the models too difficult to solve.

Load transmission across joints

Here we use a simple, well-known example to illustrate some important points about the loads across joints. Consider the situation shown in Figure 1.8.23A in which a weight is held in the hand

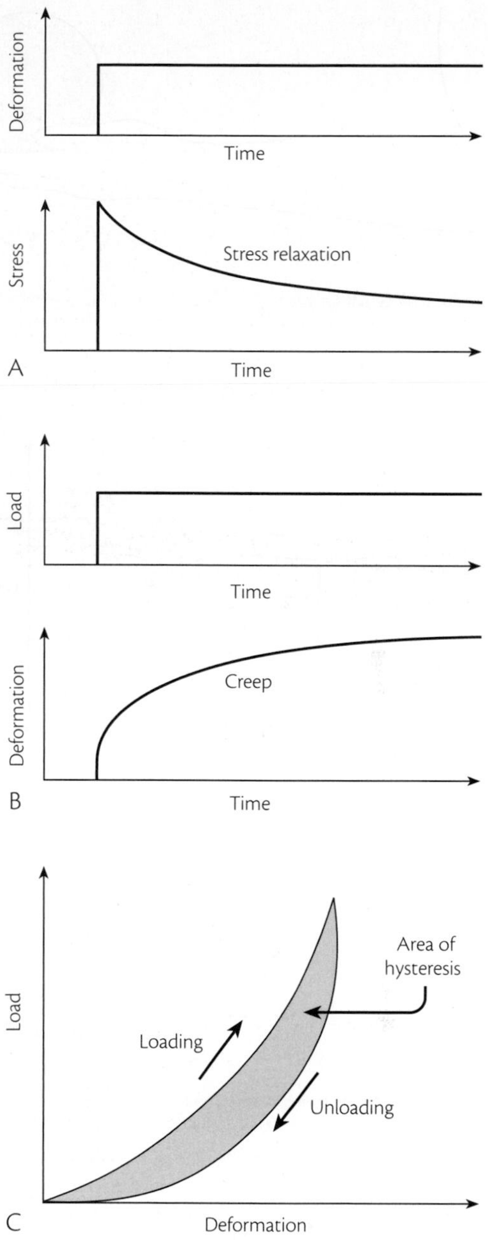

Fig. 1.8.22 A) Stress relaxation; B) creep; C) hysteresis.

Box 1.8.4 Mechanical loading of musculoskeletal tissues

- Although loaded primarily in tension and compression, the tissues of the musculoskeletal system can also undergo shear, bending, and torsion
- Due to their complicated shapes and non-uniform properties, it may be necessary to use FEA to model these tissues
- A tensile-testing machine can be used to measure both quasi-static and time-dependent mechanical properties of tissues.

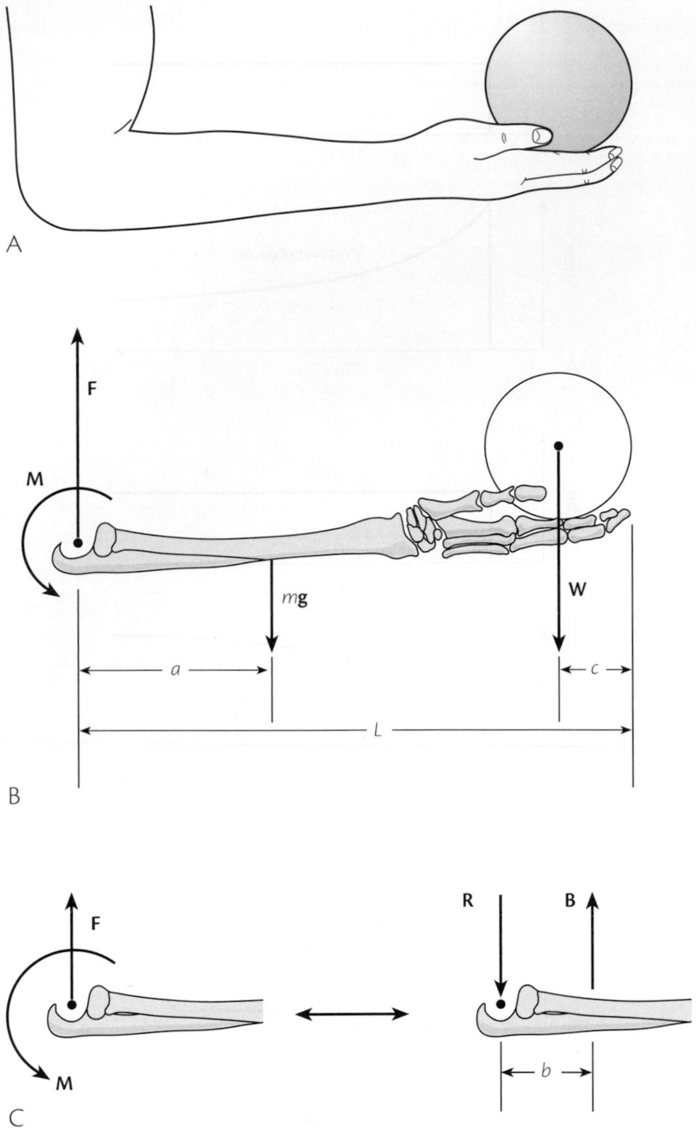

Fig. 1.8.23 A) A heavy ball is held in the hand with the elbow joint flexed to 90° and the forearm parallel to the ground. B) A free-body diagram of the situation shown in (A): W, weight of the ball; *mg*, weight of the forearm and hand; F, intersegmental force at the elbow joint; M, intersegmental moment at the elbow joint. C) Distribution of F and M amongst the relevant anatomic structures at the elbow joint: B, the biceps muscle force; R, the articular contact force. Reproduced from An et al. (1997).

with the elbow joint held fixed at 90° flexion and the forearm parallel to the ground. To find the forces transmitted by the anatomic structures at the elbow joint during this activity, it is necessary first to draw a free-body diagram of the forearm (Figure 1.8.23B) and to calculate the intersegmental force **F** and moment **M** at the elbow. In Figure 1.8.23B, the weight **W** of the ball and the weight *mg* of the forearm and hand both act downwards. In this example, it is obvious that the force **F** balances the forces **W** and *mg*, and so must act upwards, having a vertical component only. In addition, the moment **M** must be counterclockwise to balance the moments of **W** and *mg* about the centre of the elbow joint. Assuming that the arm belongs to a person of height 170cm and body mass 60kg, anthropometric tables can be used to estimate the length and mass

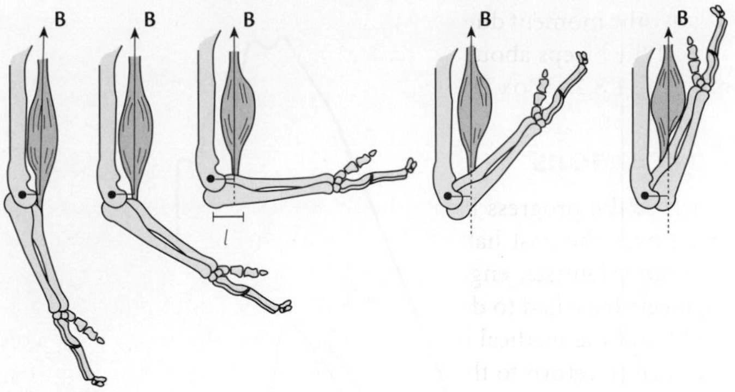

Fig. 1.8.24 The biceps (B) at various elbow flexion angles. Note the variations in the moment arm *l* of biceps. Reproduced from Leveau (1992).

of the forearm and hand ($L = 43$cm, $m = 1.3$kg) and the distance of their centre of mass from the centre of the elbow joint ($a = 29$cm). The position of the centre of mass of the ball from the fingertips is estimated to be $c = 9$cm. For this example, take W = 50 N.

Solving the equations for static force and moment equilibrium in two dimensions gives **F** = 62.75N upwards and **M** = 20.70Nm counterclockwise. To distribute **F** and **M** amongst the anatomic structures of the joint, a model of the elbow joint is needed. Figure 1.8.23C shows a simple model in which it is assumed that the biceps is the only muscle acting. For the elbow position in Figure 1.8.23A, it is assumed that the line of pull of the biceps is parallel to the humerus and that its insertion is $b = 4$cm from the centre of the elbow joint. It is also assumed that the elbow is a hinge (has a fixed axis of rotation) and that the articular contact force **R** acts vertically at this flexion angle. Using static equilibrium of force and moment in two dimensions (two equations, two unknowns) gives the biceps force **B** = 517N upwards and the joint reaction force **R** = 454N downwards.

It is important to note that the magnitudes of both **B** and **R** are larger than the magnitude of the external load **W**. The biceps force **B** is larger because its moment arm *b* is smaller than the moment arm of the external load ($L–c$). The joint reaction force **R** is larger than **W** because it must balance both **B** and **W**. That the muscle and joint reaction forces are larger than the external loads is true for most joints. Indeed, the joint reaction forces at the hip and knee can be several times body weight.

One further important point to note is that the moment arm of a muscle about a joint may change as the joint flexes. This obviously influences the force that it is necessary for a muscle to provide to

Box 1.8.5 Muscle forces and joint contact forces

- Due to their smaller moment arms about the joints, muscle forces are typically much larger than external loads
- Joint contact forces can also be rather large, since they must balance both external forces and muscle forces
- Moment arms of muscles may change as the joints they cross flex and extend.

balance the moment due to an external load. The changing moment arm of the biceps about the centre of the elbow joint is illustrated in Figure 1.8.24 (Box 1.8.5).

Conclusions

Much of the progress in the field of biomechanics that has been made over the past half-century has been due to collaborations between scientists, engineers, and clinicians. The scientists and engineers have had to delve into the anatomy and physiology textbooks and the medical literature, while the orthopaedic clinicians have had to return to the mathematics and physics that they studied years before. Both sides have benefited, along with many thousands of patients. This chapter has reviewed and explained some of the fundamental concepts and techniques involved in studying the biomechanics of the musculoskeletal system. It is hoped that clinicians have found this introduction useful and that they will be encouraged to explore the subject further.

Further reading

Bartel, D.L., Davy, D.T., and Keaveny, T.M. (2006). *Orthopaedic biomechanics: Mechanics and design in musculoskeletal systems.* Upper Saddle River, NJ: Prentice Hall.

Buckwalter, J.A., Einhorn, T.A., and Simon, S.R. (eds) (2000). *Orthopaedic Basic Science: Biology and Biomechanics of the Musculoskeletal System*, second edition. Rosemont, IL: American Academy of Orthopaedic Surgeons.

Meriam, J.L. and Kraige, L.G. (2007). *Engineering mechanics: Dynamics*, sixth edition. New York: John Wiley & Sons.

Nigg, B.M. and Herzog, W. (eds) (2007). *Biomechanics of the Musculo-skeletal System*, third edition. Chichester: John Wiley & Sons.

Nordin, M. and Frankel, V.H. (eds) (2001). *Basic Biomechanics of the Musculoskeletal System* third edition. Philadelphia, PA: Lippincott Williams & Wilkins.

1.9

Gait analysis

Christopher Bulstrode

Summary points

- Gait analysis tries to obtain reliable clinically relevant information from the way in which patients walk
- Each technique has its own specific advantages and disadvantages, but all to a greater or lesser degree 'interfere' with the patient's ability to walk
- As yet it remains mainly a research tool.

Introduction

The study of non-biological systems has been defined as 'hard' science and those of biological systems as 'difficult science'. This is because biological systems fluctuate. Gait analysis is the study of walking, a process made up of a multitude of complex fluctuating parameters. Each pace that we take is slightly different from the last, and your gait is different from mine. This means that some differences that we may observe are merely the result of biological variability, while other equally subtle ones may be diagnostic of abnormality.

Many techniques for performing gait analysis have been developed in an attempt to qualify (what is the problem?) and quantify (how bad is it?). Some of the techniques available are listed in Table 1.9.1. Any useful measurement of gait will strive to achieve the following (Box 1.9.1):

- **The observer principle** The equipment used to measure gait should not be so heavy and cumbersome that it interferes with the patient's ability to move freely, i.e. it should not in itself alter the gait
- **Sensitivity and specificity** It should reliably detect the differences in gait needed to make a diagnosis, while ignoring differences which are merely a result of inter- and intraindividual variability
- **Relevance** The differences that it measures should be valuable in making a diagnosis and in choosing treatment. The measurements needed to diagnose a knee with cruciate instability will be different from those needed to understand the problems of cerebral palsy
- **Reproducible** It should give the same result consistently every time the measurement is made. If possible these results should be independent of when or where the measurements were taken
- **Useable** It should not be too expensive and should not require a highly skilled operator to use or interpret results.

Clinical utility is the concept of addressing the question of whether the test measures things which cannot be measured in any other way, and whether these measures actually lead to new clinical decisions being made which are 'better' than those made using the old methodology.

So far, no system of gait analysis has come close to these basic requirements.

Equipment used for gait analysis (Table 1.9.1) can be classified into four simple groups (Box 1.9.2). Those which:

1) Measure the 'reaction force' which the patient has on their environment, e.g. foot pressure plates. These rely on having a force plate in the floor so the patient has to walk onto the plate
2) Record the translational movement and acceleration of limbs and how much joints bend. These rely either on putting markers on the patient which can be visualized from at least two

Box 1.9.1 Prerequisites of a good gait analysis system

- Measure without interfering
- Reliably distinguish normal from abnormal
- Valuable in deciding on appropriate treatment
- Give reproducible results
- Not cost too much.

Box 1.9.2 Types of gait analysis system

- Pressure plates
- Measure movement and bending of joints
- Record activity of muscles
- Measure energy expenditure.

directions so that a three-dimensional plot of the limbs can be made. Alternatively, sensors may be fitted onto the patient which measure joints bending or limbs accelerating

3) Electrical activity of muscles (myography). Records can be obtained either from needles inserted into the muscles (specific) or skin pads. Unfortunately there is little correlation between the amount of activity recorded and the power developed by a muscle
4) Overall energy expenditure. In very simple terms the 'better' the gait the less energy will be used to achieve an equivalent speed.

If a combination of these techniques is used, complex calculations can be performed using computers to calculate the forces passing through the patient's limbs and the body. From that it may even be possible to determine which muscle is contracting (or failing to relax) at each phase of the gait cycle. These calculations are complex and inevitably rely on some estimations (educated guesses). Any error in the data entered into the equations will be amplified by those calculations, so paradoxically the more complex the calculations the higher the chance of meaningless results being produced.

There are few conditions in which gait analysis is still considered as being of potential value in determining what treatment is most appropriate.

Table 1.9.1 Some measurement tools used in gait analysis

Stereo photographs
Video
Goniometers
Instrumented walkways
Accelerometers
Foot pressure pads
Electromyography (EMG)—surface electrodes and intramuscular electrodes
Oxygen consumption

Cerebral palsy

Myography can be used to determine whether muscles are active continuously or only during part of the gait phase. If muscles are found to be active through all phases of gait, then division or lengthening may improve gait but transfer will not. If, however, contraction only occurs during the swing phase of gait, then transfer may provide the best result. The situation is complicated by the fact that any change in the action of one muscle (by lengthening or transfer) may change the behaviour of other muscles.

Summary

To date, no method of gait analysis has proved invaluable in the assessment of a patient. No trials have yet demonstrated its benefit over simple clinical assessment. This may, in part, be because the surgical treatment options remain so crude in conditions such as cerebral palsy.

Further reading

Whittle, M.W. (2007). *Gait analysis: an introduction*, fourth edition. Oxford: Elsevier.

1.10

Imaging

Joong Mo Ahn, Yusuf Menda, and Georges Y. El-Khoury

Summary points

- Each modality of imaging—digital radiography, multidetector computed tomography (MDCT), magnetic resonance imaging (MRI), ultrasound, and nuclear medicine studies—has its own advantages and disadvantages
- Conventional radiography is the best for initial evaluation of a musculoskeletal problem
- MDCT rapid survey of multiple trauma patients is easily performed using the new high speed computed tomography scanners
- MRI is the imaging modality of choice for internal derangement of the knee and other soft tissue injuries
- Radionuclide bone imaging is most suitable for screening the whole skeleton for metastases
- Positron emission tomography is useful for identification of tumour, inflammation, and infection.

Introduction

There are a number of imaging modalities currently available to the practising orthopaedic surgeon, including digital radiography (DR), multidetector computed tomography (MDCT), magnetic resonance imaging (MRI), ultrasound, nuclear medicine studies, and studies where iodinated contrast is injected into the extremity joints, such as conventional arthrography or magnetic resonance arthrography.

Radiography

The radiographic examination is the best and most available imaging study for the initial evaluation of patients with orthopaedic problems. Generally, radiography should precede any complex imaging studies such as computed tomography (CT) or MRI.

X-rays used in medical imaging are either generated in x-ray tubes or emitted from radioactive isotopes. Those generated in x-ray tubes are used in radiography, fluoroscopy, and CT. X-rays emitted from radioactive isotopes are used in nuclear medicine and are called γ-rays. In the x-ray tube (Figure 1.10.1), x-rays are generated when a fast stream of electrons is suddenly stopped by the target or anode (positive terminal). The electrons originate on the negative terminal of the tube which is also known as the cathode or filament. The area of the target bombarded by electrons is known as the focal spot., which should be as small as possible, preferably 1 mm or less. The quantity of x-rays emitted from the x-ray tube is proportional to the number of electrons flowing from the filament (cathode) to the target (anode); this is measured in milliamperes (mA) and is preselected by the technologist. The quality, or penetrating properties, of the x-ray beam is determined by the energy of the electrons striking the target. This is determined by the kilovoltage setting (kV_p). Modern x-ray tube casings are designed with filters to remove the low energy radiation from the x-ray beam. Filtration is an essential technique utilized to change the composition and improve the quality of the x-rays beam. High-energy x-rays generate significant scatter radiation which results in foggy images and diminished tissue contrast on radiographs. The use of a fixed or a reciprocating (motorized) grid is the most commonly applied technique for controlling scatter in medical radiography.

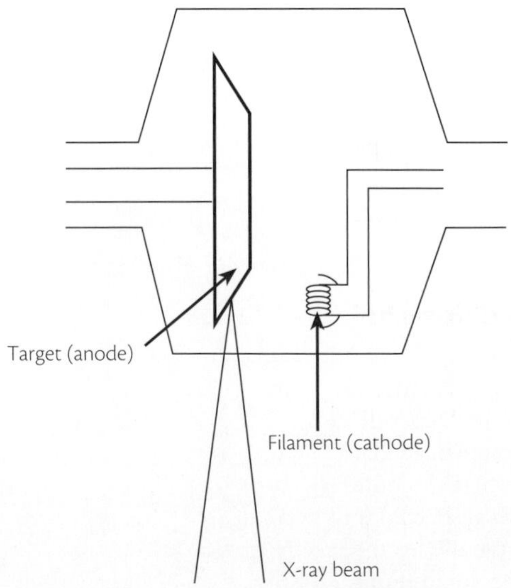

Fig. 1.10.1 Diagram of x-ray tube. Rotation of the anode increases the heat capacity of the tube and allows more x-rays to be generated.

X-Ray Machine design
◆ The anode (focal spot) is small to optimize definition
◆ Filters maximize useful imaging radiation
◆ Grids remove radiation scattering from tissues
◆ Quantity (mA) and energy (kV) are optimized for imaging task
◆ Shuttering down field size reduces radiation & improves image quality

Limiting the field size, or restricting the size of the beam to the area of interest achieves two very important objectives: it reduces scatter and cuts radiation to the patient.

Variations in tissue composition give rise to differences in how much of the primary x-ray beam is transmitted through the patient. Structures that stop much of the primary beam have high attenuation. Bone has high beam attenuation, whereas inflated lung has low beam attenuation, and appears dark on a radiograph, while bones appear white on the radiograph. Fat attenuates x-rays more than air, while water and soft tissues attenuate it more than fat but less than bone. These variations in the ability of the different tissues to attenuate the x-ray beam form the basis for tissue contrast on radiographic images.

A major problem with film as an x-ray detector in orthopaedics is related to the wide variation in extremity thickness, which may result in underexposure in one part and overexposure in another on the same radiograph. An alternative to the conventional radiographic film is the digital image or radiograph. Images can be manipulated to improve density and contrast, they can be enlarged or minimized; images can also be transmitted from station to station. The dose to the patient is reduced because the storage phosphor is more sensitive than the screen-film system; repeat exposures due to technical errors are also eliminated because the image contrast and density can be manipulated at the workstation.

Digital imaging vs Conventional films
◆ Improves contrast range
◆ Radiation dose to patients is reduced
◆ Assists storage

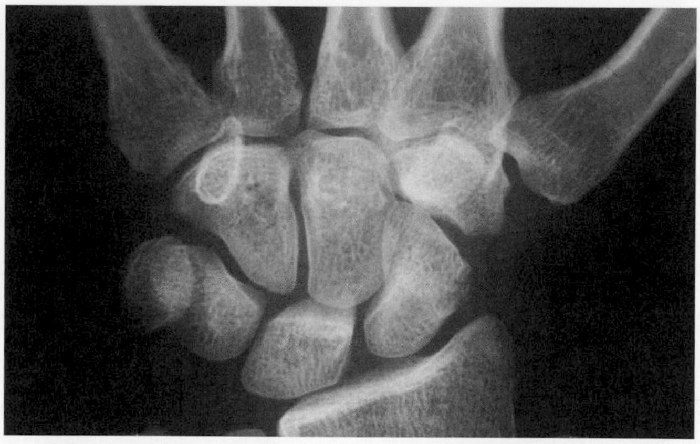

A

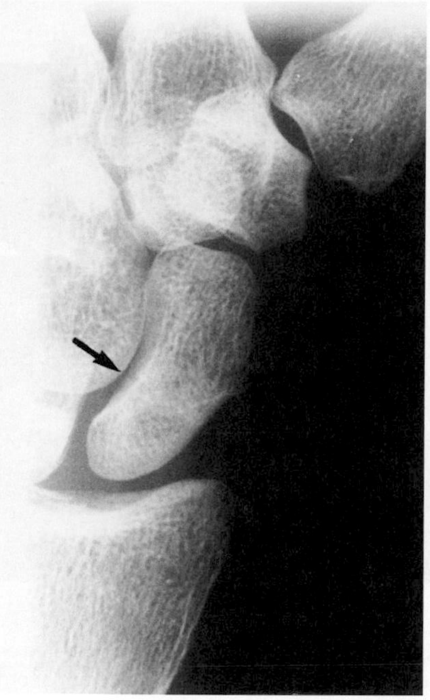

B

Fig. 1.10.2 Scaphoid view demonstrating a subtle fracture. A) The routine PA view of the wrist was unremarkable and showed no fractures. B) The scaphoid view, obtained by placing the hand and wrist in ulnar deviation along with 15 degrees of cephalad angulation of the x-ray tube, shows a subtle non-displaced fracture (arrow).

Radiographic techniques

For most orthopaedic problems, two orthogonal radiographic views of the structure under investigation are considered a basic requirement. Depending on the anatomical region, additional views are often needed. In the trauma setting, two orthogonal views may be difficult to obtain. When a non-displaced fracture of the navicular is suspected it is advantageous to put the long axis of the navicular parallel to the film (Figure 1.10.2). Small avulsion fractures at the dorsum of the triquetrum are best detected on mildly pronated lateral views of the wrist (Figure 1.10.3). The pisiform, pisitriquetral joint, and the hook of the hamate are best visualized on mildly supinated lateral views as well as carpal tunnel views (Figure 1.10.4).

Standing AP views of the knees are recommended for patients with osteoarthritis, to demonstrate the extent of articular cartilage loss (Figure 1.10.5). Many authorities believe that radiography for ankle injuries is overutilized, and several criteria have been suggested to limit unnecessary examinations; the Ottawa criteria are probably the best known.

It is not necessary for orthopaedic surgeons to know all the appropriate views that can be used. X-ray departments will arrange for appropriate views, provided that the diagnosis under consideration is clearly stated in the request form.

Neck pain can be initially evaluated with an anteroposterior (AP) and lateral views of the cervical spine. The American College of

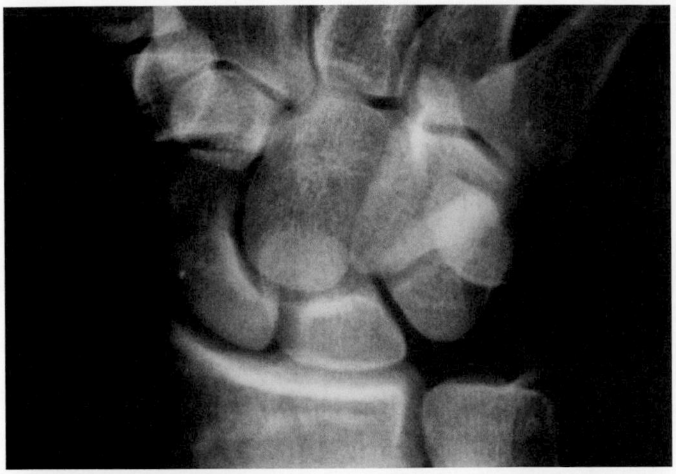

A

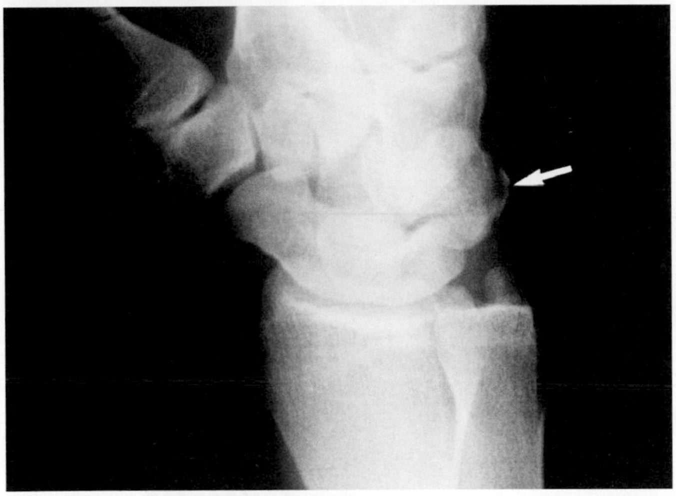

B

Fig. 1.10.3 Avulsion fracture of the triquetrum demonstrated on mildly pronated lateral view of the wrist. A) PA view of the wrist shows no abnormalities of the triquetrum. B) Mildly pronated lateral view clearly demonstrates the avulsion fracture of the dorsum of the triquetrum (arrow).

Radiology has developed appropriateness criteria for the use of imaging studies in the trauma setting. If the upper thoracic spine or lower cervical spine is obscured by the shoulders, a swimmer's view is usually quite helpful. For the lumbar spine, AP and lateral views are typically sufficient. Occasionally, oblique views are used to look for defects in the pars interarticularis, but these oblique views add significant radiation dose to the patient, increase the cost of the examination, and should not be used routinely.

Views
◆ For many conditions guidelines indicate when x-Rays are needed ◆ Two films at right angles are the usual requirement ◆ Some areas and problems have special views ◆ Radiographers will choose the most appropriate views for each diagnosis

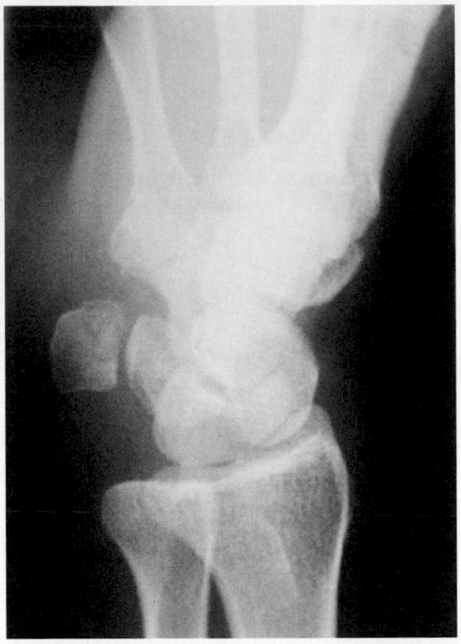

Fig. 1.10.4 Mildly supinated lateral view of the wrist demonstrates a pisiform fracture which was difficult to see on routine views.

Radiation protection

Gonadal shielding should always be used where appropriate, and care taken to minimize exposure to other patients and staff. Appropriate personnel radiation-monitoring devices should be worn by health professionals whenever there is a possibility of exposure to radiation.

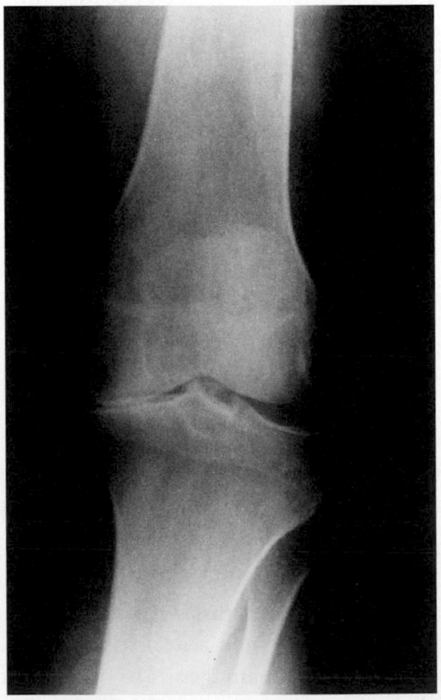

Fig. 1.10.5 Standing AP view of the left knee of a 70-year-old male showing marked narrowing of the joint space medially indicating almost total loss of cartilage. Varus deformity of the knee and mild lateral subluxation of the tibia are also present.

Multidetector row computed tomography (Box 1.10.1)

The introduction of helical CT and MDCT has transformed the value of CT in acquiring volumetric data sets, improving resolution and allowing very thin slices (0.3mm). It also enables reconstruction of images in any plane as well as three dimensions (Figures 1.10.6–1.10.8). Other advantages of MDCT are increased speed and increased total volume covered. This is valuable for multitrauma patients, with head, chest, spine, and abdominal injuries, as all can be scanned at the same time. The whole body from the head to below the hips can be imaged in less than 30s.

MDCT scanners currently generate hundreds or even thousands of images on each patient. It has, therefore, become impractical to print images or view studies one image at a time. Postprocessing workstations are now a necessity, and the task of interpreting CT studies from printed images has disappeared. Parallel advances in picture archiving and communication (PACS) technology have taken place, allowing real-time viewing, manipulation of large stacks of images, and distribution of images throughout the medical centre.

Box 1.10.1 Multidetector row computed tomography

- Allows rapid scanning of multiple areas
- High definition and low dosage
- Enables reconstruction of images in any plane
- Work stations enable rapid viewing of multiple images.

Magnetic resonance imaging (Box 1.10.2)

Magnetic resonance imaging (MRI) is now the primary imaging technique for internal derangement of the knee, disc disease, muscle and tendon injuries, early detection of osteonecrosis, and evaluation and staging of many soft tissue and bone neoplasms.

Physical principles

The basic principle of clinical MRI is that any nucleus with an unpaired proton or neutron, such as hydrogen atoms, will react to external magnetic fields. When a subject is placed in a strong magnetic field, some of the protons align with the magnetic field while spinning and precessing around the axis of the magnetic field. This is analogous to the wobble of a spinning top (Figure 1.10.9). Hydrogen atoms in different tissues (fat versus muscle) will have different constants and precess at different frequencies.

The equilibrium of spin alignment can be disturbed by applying a radiofrequency pulse at the frequency of precession. As the protons come back into alignment, they emit electromagnetic radiation in the radiofrequency spectrum that is collected and turned into magnetic resonance images.

Definitions

- **T_1 relaxation time** Also called longitudinal relaxation or spin–lattice relaxation time, T_1 relaxation time is a tissue-specific time constant. T_1 images depict anatomy well: fat is white, water is black
- **T_2 relaxation time** Also called transverse relaxation time or spin–spin relaxation time, this is also a tissue-specific time constant. T_2 images show pathology well. Fat is black, water white.

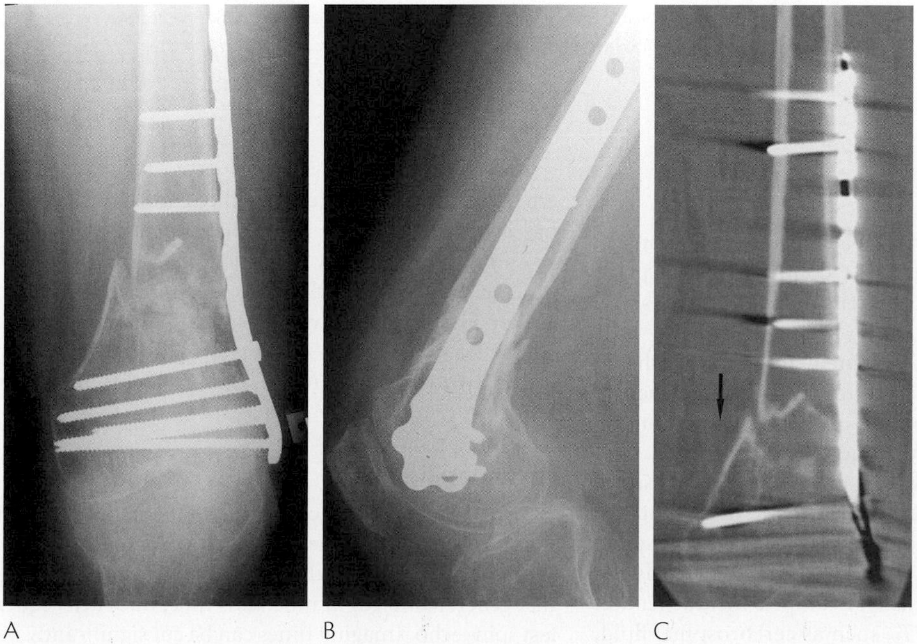

A B C

Fig. 1.10.6 Fracture non-union. A 56-year-old-male with left distal femur fracture treated with a LISS plate and screws. Patient continued to have pain several months after the surgical fixation. A, B) AP and lateral views of the distal left femur show good apposition and alignment of the fracture fragments. No complications are noted with the hardware. C) Coronal and sagittal CT reformations of the distal left femur show absence of bony bridging across the fracture gap (arrows). The diagnosis of non-union was made.

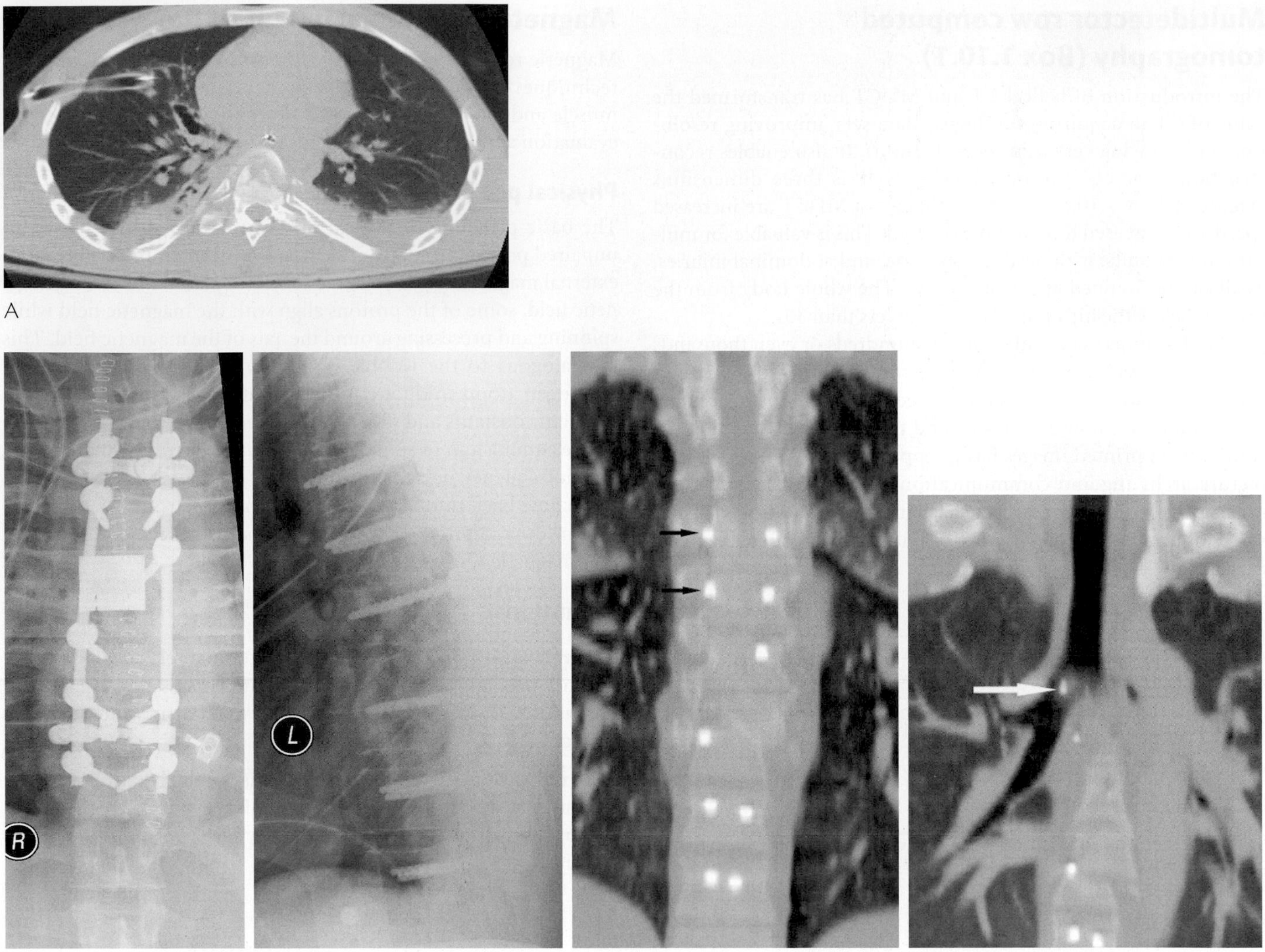

Fig. 1.10.7 Hardware malplacement. A 32-year-old male who was involved in a motor vehicle accident. A) CT of the thoracic spine revealed a fracture dislocation in the mid-thoracic spine. B, C) The fracture was treated emergently with pedicle screws and rods for stabilization. Postoperative AP and lateral views revealed no complications. D, E) Postoperatively the patient developed persistent cough and strider. Coronal CT reformations demonstrated that the superior two screws on the right side (arrows) are outside the vertebrae and the tip of the upper screw on the right is within the right main bronchus (white arrow).

Pulse sequences

A pulse sequence is a precisely defined pattern of radiofrequency pulses and listening intervals. The most commonly used pulse sequence in the study of the musculoskeletal system is the spin–echo sequence (Figure 1.10.10).

A spin–echo sequence can be T_1 weighted, accentuating the T_1 properties of tissue, or T_2 weighted, accentuating the T_2 properties of the tissue. In general, T_1-weighted sequences depict anatomy better and T_2-weighted images show pathology to advantage.

On T_1-weighted images, tissues with a short T_1 have high signal intensity and are bright (Box 1.10.3). An example of a substance with a short T_1 is fat. Tissues with long T_1, such as cerebrospinal fluid, have low signal intensity. On T_2-weighted sequences, tissues with a short T_2 have low signal intensity. Examples include tendon and ligament. Tissues with a long T_2, such as cerebrospinal fluid, are bright on T_2-weighted sequences. Inflamed, oedematous tissue has more extracellular water than normal and will therefore be lower in signal intensity on T_1-weighted images and will be higher in signal on T_2-weighted images than normal tissue. Most tumours appear relatively dark on T_1-weighted images, less than fat and similar to muscle. On T_2-weighted images, most tumours show increased intensity, but not usually as bright as cerebrospinal fluid.

Fast imaging

Conventional spin–echo images are the mainstay of MRI, but the T_2-weighted images take a long time to acquire and are susceptible to motion artefacts. Other pulse sequences have been developed that generate images in much less time; one such sequence is called fast spin–echo. Imaging times can be cut significantly because up to

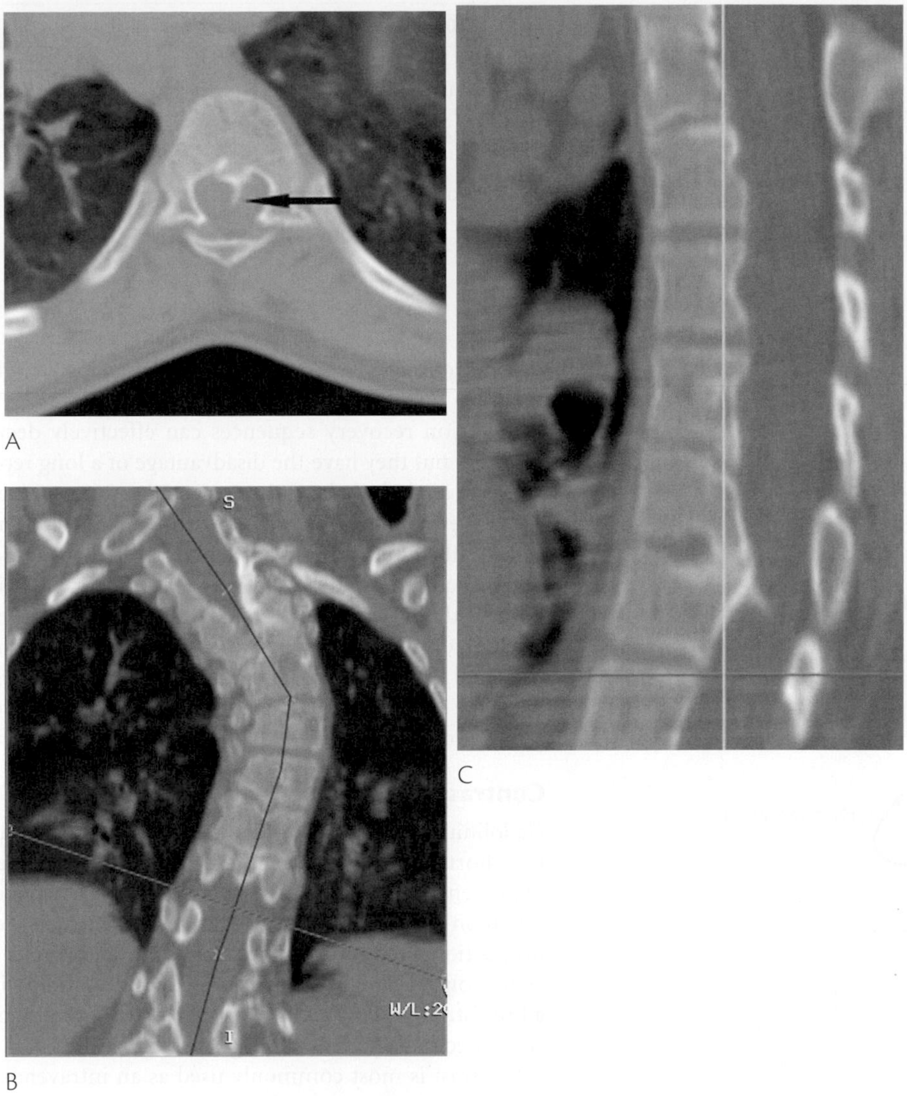

Fig. 1.10.8 Congenital scoliosis. A 10-year-old boy who is known to have congenital scoliosis now presenting to the paediatric orthopaedic clinic with difficulty walking and long track signs. A) Axial CT section through T11 shows a spike of bone projecting into the spinal canal (arrow). This was diagnosed as representing diastematomyelia. B). A coronal multiplanar reformation illustrates the multiple congenital vertebral anomalies in the upper thoracic spine along with severe scoliosis. The blue line illustrates the plane along which the curved planar reformation will electronically correct the scoliotic curve. C) A curved planar reformation straightens the spine and provides a better view of the diastematomyelia.

32 lines of the image can be acquired in a single repetition. Besides reducing time of acquisition, fast spin–echo images have less distortion of the image when hardware or metal is present in the scanned area (Box 1.10.4). One disadvantage to fast spin–echo sequences is that oedema is harder to detect than with spin–echo images.

Box 1.10.2 MRI

- Atoms with unpaired electrons align in a magnetic field
- They also spin and precess
- A radio signal disrupts the precession
- As the molecules return to their original orientation they emit a radio signal
- The source and strength of the signals allows a three-dimensional picture to be created.

Spin–echo T_2-weighted images have traditionally been used to detect oedema that is often present as a sign of many pathological processes. These T_2-weighted sequences are sensitive for detecting oedema because signal intensity of fat is low and signal intensity of water is high on T_2-weighted images. However, with fast spin–echo T_2-weighted images, the signal from fat is not suppressed and oedema can be masked. To overcome this limitation, methods to suppress the signal from fat are often employed.

Fat suppression

The two currently used methods of suppressing fat signal are frequency selective chemical presaturation and inversion recovery. Chemical presaturation is a technique that is applied to other sequences such as fast spin–echo, whereas inversion recovery is a pulse sequence itself, and cannot be combined with other sequences. When using chemical presaturation, the machine takes advantage of the fact that the hydrogen protons in fat have a slightly faster precessional rate than water hydrogen protons. By placing a very selective radiofrequency pulse that only deflects fat hydrogens

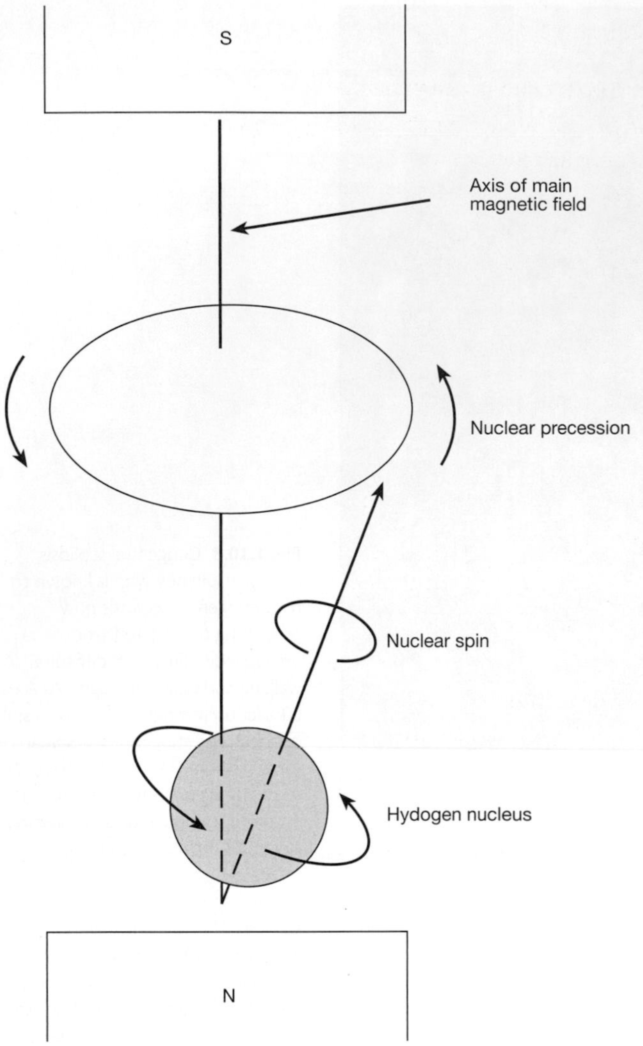

Fig. 1.10.9 Diagram of a hydrogen proton in an external magnetic field. Note that the nucleus has spin as well as precession around the main direction of the external magnetic field.

Box 1.10.3 T_1 and T_2 weighted images

- On T_1 fat is white, water black
- On T_2 cerebrospinal fluid is bright, tendons and ligaments are dark
- Tumours and inflammation are dark on T_1 and light on T_2 images.

immediately before the main pulse sequence, signals from fat can be nullified, and signals from all other tissues unaffected. This is usually used with fast spin–echo T_2-weighted sequences to increase the conspicuity of oedema or fluid. Chemical presaturation can also be used with T_1-weighted images after the administration of contrast. Increases in signal from contrast accumulation are more conspicuous when surrounding fat (bright on T_1-weighted images) is dark.

Inversion recovery sequences can effectively decrease signals from fat, but they have the disadvantage of a long repetition time, and take a relatively long time to acquire. Newer inversion recovery pulse sequences include a fast inversion recovery sequence, which still suppresses fat signal and is very sensitive for oedema, but is acquired rapidly, similar to fast spin–echo. One important point is that if fat suppression is desired for images obtained following contrast administration, chemical saturation should be used and inversion recovery avoided. Inversion recovery will suppress the signal changes caused by the contrast, whereas chemical saturation will not.

Contrast agents

Gadolinium is a transition element which has paramagnetic activity, shortening both the T_1 and T_2 relaxation times of nearby hydrogen nuclei. The T_1 shortening produces a higher (brighter) signal on T_1-weighted images. Enhancement of tissues is roughly proportional to blood flow to the tissue, and results in increased signal on T_1-weighted images. Therefore, following contrast administration, T_1-weighted sequences are typically obtained and compared to T_1-weighted images before contrast.

Contrast is most commonly used as an intravenous agent, but can also be instilled into joints, resulting in an MR arthrogram. This has been applied to the shoulder for improving the characterization and detection of labral abnormalities and in the knee for evaluating osteochondral fragments and postoperative menisci.

Clinical applications (Box 1.10.5)

Upper extremity

Tendon degeneration, tendinopathy, partial and full thickness tears of the rotator cuff all show-up as areas of increased signals on the T_2-weighted images. Fat suppression and magnetic resonance

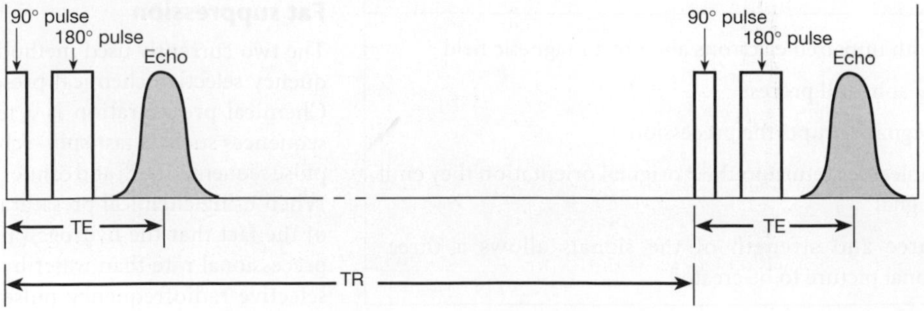

Fig. 1.10.10 Spin–echo pulse sequence. It consists of a 90-degree pulse followed by a pause, after which a 180-degree pulse is applied. Then after an additional pause, the receiver coil is set to listen to a signal (echo) emitted from the tissues; after a longer pause, the cycle is repeated.

Box 1.10.4 MRI modifications

- Fast imaging reduces metal artefact
- Chemical presaturation and inversion recovery suppress the fat signal
- Gadolinium concentrates in inflamed tissue and enhances signal.

Box 1.10.5 Clinical applications of MRI

- Rotator cuff is well visualized
- In the elbow MRI shows soft tissue and bone injury simultaneously
- MRI of the wrist requires high-resolution MRI and thin slices
- Damage to the triangular fibrocartilage is well visualized.

arthrography will increase the conspicuousness of cuff abnormalities (Figure 1.10.11).

MR arthrography extends the capabilities of conventional MRI because contrast solution distends the joint capsule, outlines intra-articular structures, and leaks into abnormalities.

By demonstrating the inferior labral–ligamentous complex, MR arthrography makes a major contribution to the evaluation of patients with suspected glenohumeral instability (Figure 1.10.12). Although MR arthrographic images have demonstrated greater than 90% accuracy in the detection of anteroinferior glenoid labral tears, diagnostic confidence may be further increased when the shoulder is images in abduction and external rotation (ABER). This involves flexing the elbow and placing the patient's hand posterior to the contralateral aspect of the head or neck. An anteroinferior glenoid labral tear that is non-displaced when the shoulder in a neutral position has a greater likelihood of being displaced from the glenoid rim and becoming more conspicuous when the shoulder is in the ABER position.

The multiplanar capabilities of MRI enable the elbow joint to be imaged in true sagittal and coronal planes, facilitating more accurate diagnosis of ligamentous injuries. The superior soft tissue contrast of MRI provides simultaneous evaluation of bone and soft tissue, allowing for assessment of all the static and dynamic stabilizers.

The use of MRI to evaluate the wrist has lagged behind that of larger joints, because of technical limitations of spatial resolution. Thin and contiguous slices are needed for adequate MRI of the wrist. Therefore, high-resolution MRI is essential to evaluate normal and abnormal features of the hand and wrist.

MRI or MR arthrography can localize and characterize tears of the triangular fibrocartilage complex (Figure 1.10.13), helping to identify those patients that would benefit from surgery. MR arthrography combines the advantages of arthrographic depiction of anatomic perforation with the direct visualization of marrow, cartilage, and soft tissues allowed by MRI and can be performed with single-, double, or triple-compartment injection.

Knee (Box 1.10.6)

MRI is an effective modality for diagnosing tears of the anterior cruciate ligament, and is also accurate for detection of meniscal tears. Normal menisci have low signal intensity on all pulse sequences, and tears are seen as linear increased signal that contacts a surface of the meniscus on two consecutive images. Another sign of meniscal tears is abnormal contour of the meniscus, with truncation being a sign of a displaced fragment (Figure 1.10.14). Following partial meniscectomy, retears are difficult to diagnose by MRI. Intra-articular contrast is a method to improve the characterization of the postoperative meniscus.

A tear of the anterior cruciate ligament can be shown on MRI by detecting abnormalities of the ligament itself, such as increased signal within the ligament, or by detecting secondary signs that the anterior cruciate ligament is torn (Figure 1.10.15). Primary signs include abnormal increased signal of the anterior cruciate ligament, and abnormal orientation of the ligament. Secondary signs

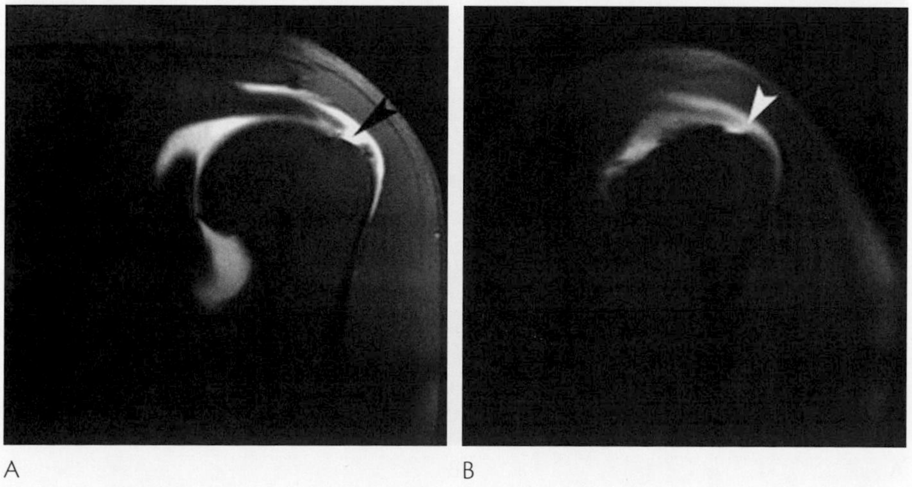

Fig. 1.10.11 Full-thickness rotator cuff tear. A 33-year-old man with shoulder pain after sliding and landing on his shoulder. A) Fat-suppressed oblique coronal T1-weighted MR arthrogram demonstrates a communicating defect (arrowhead) of the infraspinatus tendon, representing full-thickness tear. B) Fat-suppressed coronal T1-weighted MR arthrogram again shows detachment of the lower lamina from the styloid process of the ulna (arrowhead).

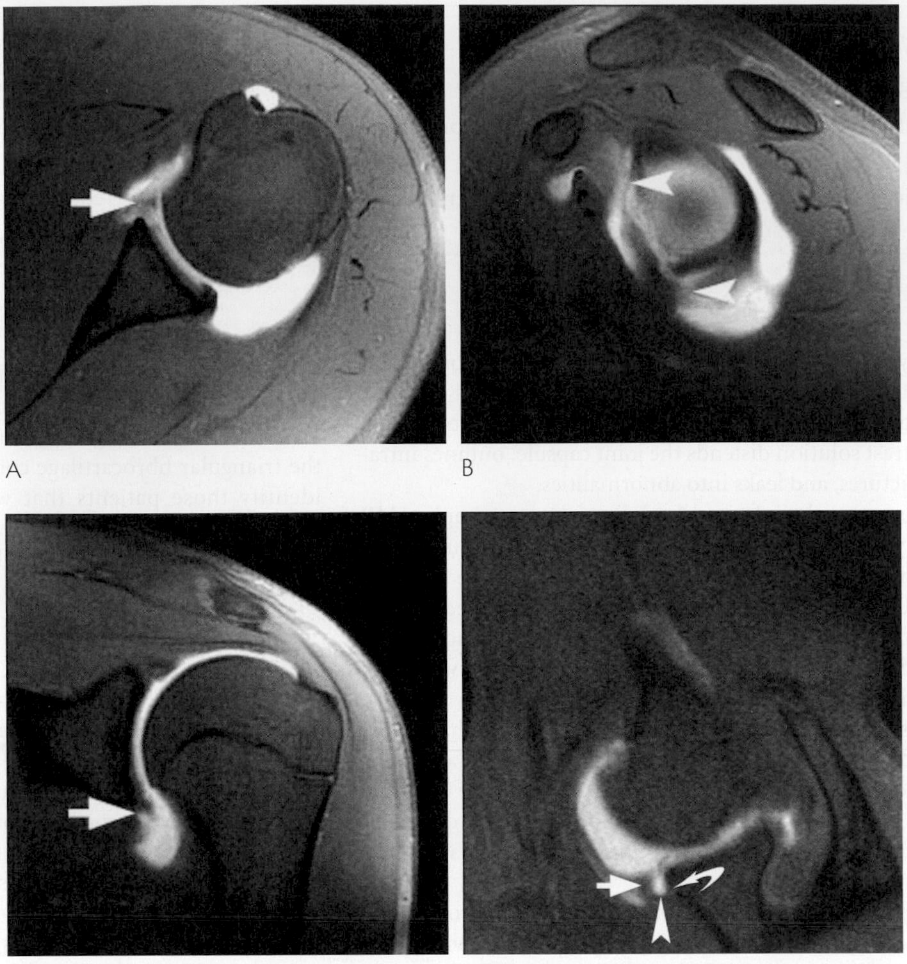

A B C D

Fig. 1.10.12 Glenohumeral instability. A 15-year-old boy who had dislocated his shoulder. A) Fat-suppressed transverse *T*1-weighted MR arthrogram demonstrates torn labrum (arrow). B) Fat-suppressed sagittal *T*1-weighted image shows Bankart lesion extending from 1 o'clock to 5 o'clock position (arrowheads). C) Fat-suppressed coronal *T*1-weighted image reveals detachment of the labroligamentous complex (arrow) from the glenoid. D) Fat-suppressed ABER (abduction external rotation) view reveals contrast material in a gap (arrowhead) between the periosteum and scapular neck (curved arrow), at the base of the anterior glenoid labrum. Note the presence of contrast material rounding the corner of the glenoid and passing through freely floating torn anterior glenoid labrum (arrow).

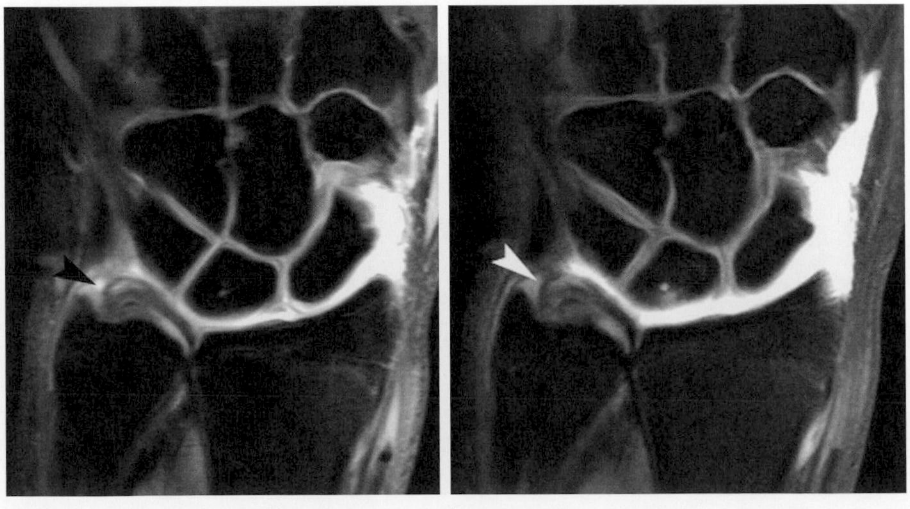

A B

Fig. 1.10.13 Triangular fibrocartilage complex tear. A 14-year-old girl with ulnar-sided wrist pain. A) Fat-suppressed coronal intermediate weighted MR arthrogram demonstrates defect and tear of the lower lamina of the triangular ligament from the styloid process of the ulna (arrowhead), indicating peripheral tear of the triangular fibrocartilage complex. B) Fat-suppressed coronal *T*1-weighted MR arthrogram again shows avulsion of the ulnar attachment of the triangular fibrocartilage complex (arrowhead).

Box 1.10.6 MRI and internal derangement of the knee

- Meniscal tears show linear abnormal signal in two consecutive slices
- Postmeniscectomy re-injury is hard to diagnose with enhancement
- Anterior cruciate damage can be diagnosed by primary and secondary findings
- Any change in signal in the posterior cruciate is abnormal
- Medial collateral ligament damage is well visualized
- Bone contusion and occult fractures show up well
- The patella tendon shows a bright area following damage.

result from laxity of the knee including anterior translation of the tibia, abnormal posterior position of the posterior horn of the lateral meniscus, and abnormal orientation of the posterior cruciate ligament such as hyperbuckling. A prior severe injury may show as bone contusions, medial collateral ligament injury, and haemarthrosis.

Any increase in signal in the posterior cruciate ligament is abnormal. Conversely, the anterior cruciate ligament often has some strands of increased signal within it, and this can be problematic for detecting subtle anterior cruciate ligament tears, and decreases the accuracy of MRI for evaluating partial anterior cruciate ligament tears. Medial collateral ligament injuries produce, abnormal signals both deep and superficial to the medial collateral ligament, and if the ligament is focally disrupted or not visualized at all, then complete tear is diagnosed.

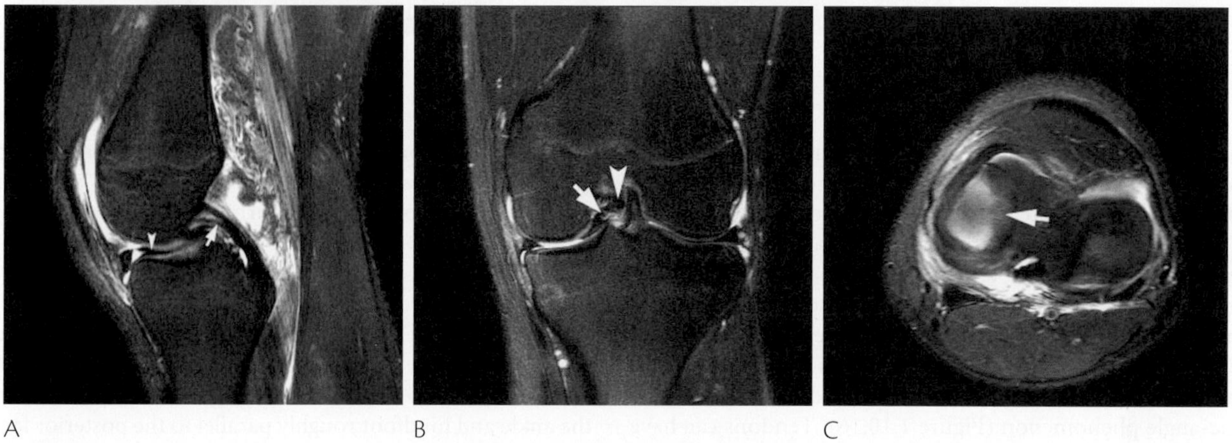

Fig. 1.10.14 Bucket-handle tear of the medial meniscus. A 17-year-old male wrestler with significant knee pain and locking. A) Fat-suppressed oblique sagittal *T*2-weighted sequence shows an abnormal band of low signal intensity (arrowhead) and double posterior cruciate ligament sign (arrow), representing bucket-handle tear. B) Fat-suppressed coronal *T*2-weighted image demonstrates a centrally displaced meniscal fragment (arrow) inferior to the posterior cruciate ligament (arrowhead). C) Fat-suppressed transverse *T*2-weighted image reveals a displaced fragment of the meniscus (arrow).

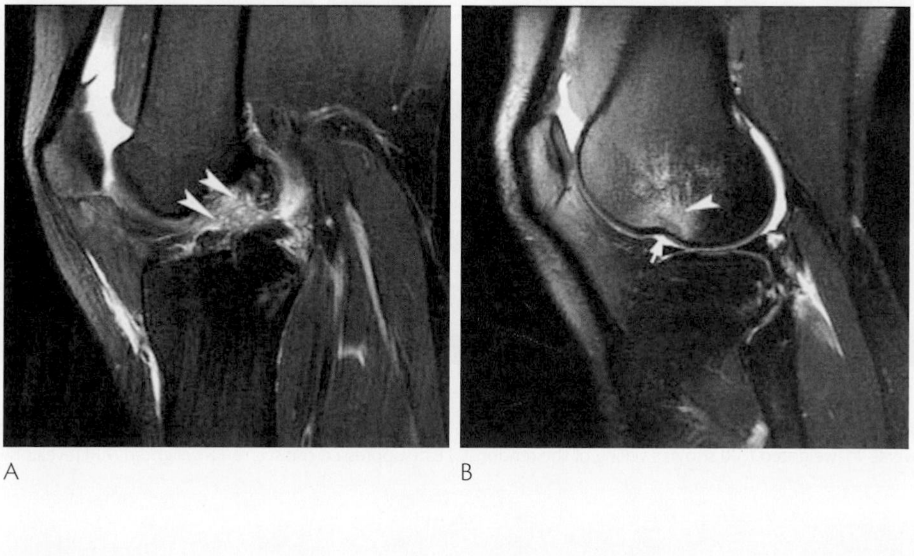

Fig. 1.10.15 Anterior cruciate ligament tear. An 18-year-old female volleyball player who fell on her left knee. A) Fat-suppressed oblique sagittal *T*2-weighted MR image demonstrates hyperintense and amorphous swelling of the torn anterior cruciate ligament fibers (arrowheads), indicating acute injury. B) Fat-suppressed oblique sagittal *T*2-weighted MR image, obtained at the level of the lateral femoral condyle, shows accentuation of the lateral notch (arrow) with associated hyperintense bone marrow edema (arrowhead), representing bone contusion caused by impaction with posterior tibial plateau.

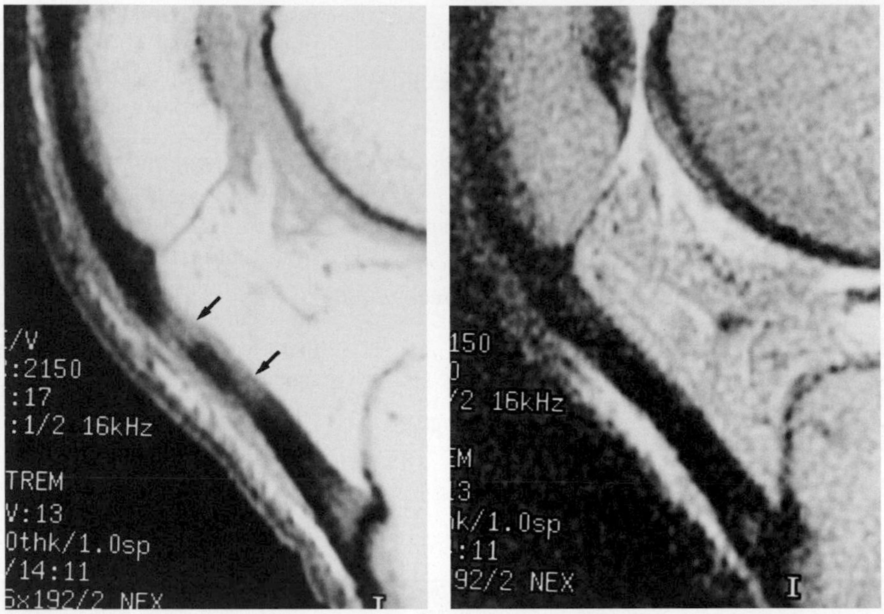

Fig. 1.10.16 Magic-angle artefact. A) Proton-density-weighted image of the patella shows patchy increased signal of the patellar ligament (arrows). The patient had no symptoms at this location. B) *T*2-weighted image shows normal signal intensity of the tendon, separating this artefact from patellar tendonitis.

In a patient with persistent pain following trauma in whom plain films are negative, MRI can show contusions or occult fractures. It can also be used to evaluate patients with suspected injury to the patellar ligament In patellar tendinitis or partial tearing, the ligament may show increased signal intensity on T_1-weighted, T_2-weighted, and proton density images; it also shows increased AP diameter proximally and the margins of the affected ligament become indistinct, especially posterior to the thickened segment.

One artefact that commonly occurs with musculoskeletal MRI is the magic-angle phenomenon (Figure 1.10.16). Tendons can have a falsely increased signal when they are oriented approximately 55 degrees out of the main magnetic field. The supraspinatus tendon, just proximal to its insertion on the greater tuberosity, commonly shows this artifact. Other tendons that commonly show magic-angle effects are the patellar ligament, the foot flexor tendons such as flexor hallucis longus, and, occasionally, the peroneal tendons. If increased signal is seen on a short echo time (TE) sequence, it is important to confirm the abnormality on a long TE sequence.

Ankle and foot

For the Achilles tendon, axial and sagittal planes are sufficient for evaluation (Figure 1.10.17). However, the other tendons that cross the ankle joint do not run in a straight course, but curve around the ankle and hindfoot roughly parallel to the posterior facet of the subtalar joint. Therefore, in order to image these tendons in cross-section, oblique imaging planes should be used. When studying the foot flexors and extensors, sagittal sequences are followed by oblique coronal sequences that are perpendicular to the posterior facet of the subtalar joint (Figure 1.10.18).

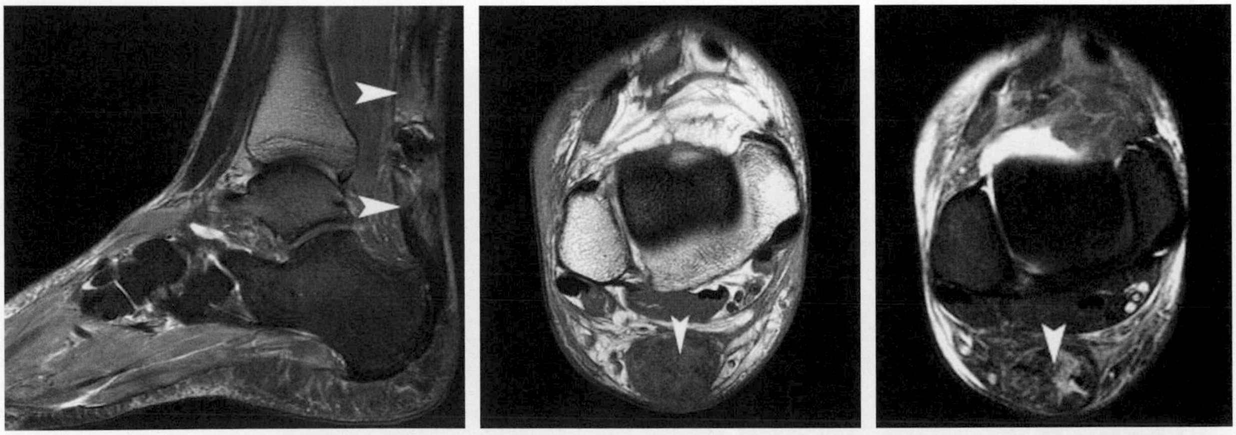

A B C

Fig. 1.10.17 Achilles tendon tear. A 35-year-old woman with heel pain. A) Fat-suppressed sagittal *T*2-weighted MRI demonstrates wavy appearance and discontinuity of the Achilles tendon (arrowheads). B) Transverse *T*1-weighted MRI shows swelling of the tendon. C) Fat-suppressed transverse *T*2-weighted MRI reveals hyperintense signal intensity within the tendon.

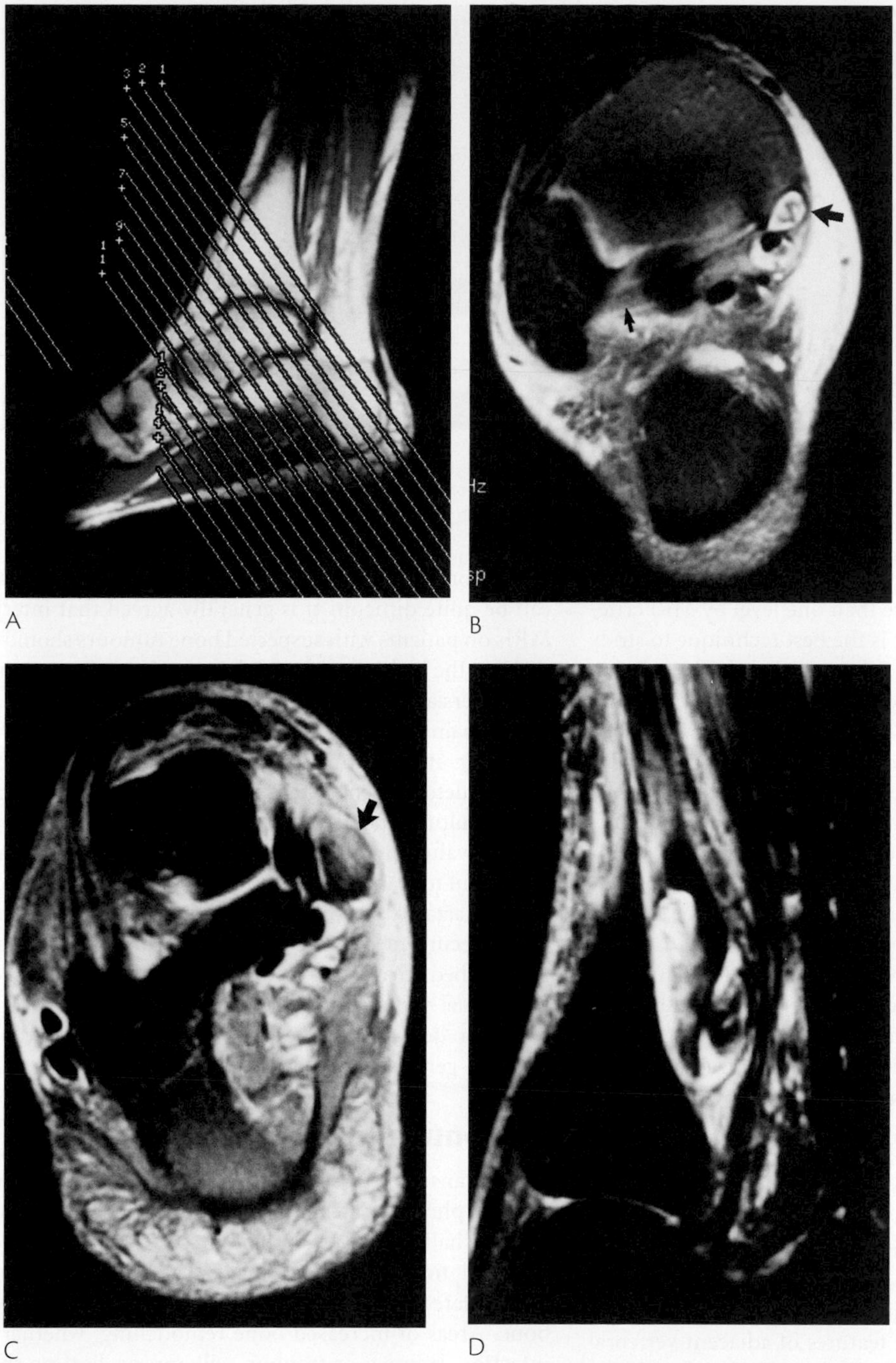

Fig. 1.10.18 Oblique coronal plane for hindfoot imaging. A) Lateral scout view during acquisition of a hindfoot MRI study shows the orientation of slices for oblique coronal imaging. Note that the slice orientation is perpendicular to the posterior facet of the subtalar joint. B) A 60-year-old patient with hindfoot pain following a fall. Oblique axial *T*2-weighted image showing debris in an otherwise empty tendon sheath of posterior tibial tendon (large arrow). Scan is at the level of posterior talofibular ligament (small arrow). C) Oblique *T*2-weighted image distal to (B) shows distal fragmented end of tendon (arrow). D) Sagittal inversion recovery image shows proximal end of tendon curled up at the musculotendinous junction.

Spine (Box 1.10.7)

From an orthopaedic standpoint, MRI is very useful for evaluating patients with possible disc disease, metastatic disease, congenital anomalies, and trauma.

MRI is very sensitive for detecting abnormal signal and morphology of intervertebral discs (Figure 1.10.19). Normally the disc is lower in signal intensity than vertebral bone marrow on T_1-weighted images, and higher in signal on T_2-weighted images. With disc degeneration, signal remains low on the T_2-weighted images.

While MRI is very sensitive for detecting abnormal discs, care must be taken when interpreting the study to correlate with the

Box 1.10.7 MRI of the spine

- Degenerate discs show clearly with decreased signal on T_2
- 38% of 'normal' patients may show disc abnormalities on MRI of the spine
- Metastases in the spine show complete marrow fat loss
- The oedema from acute fractures may mimic malignant infiltration
- Vertebral osteomyelitis shows as low signal on T_1, high on T_2.

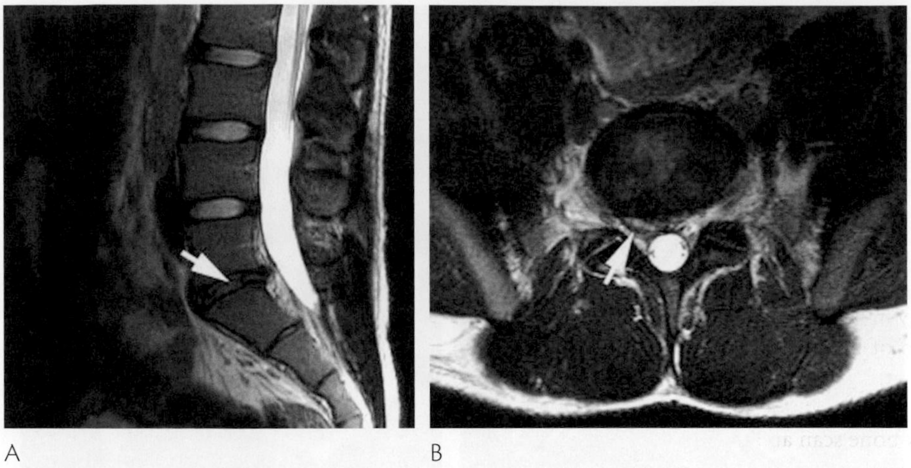

Fig. 1.10.19 Disc protrusion. A 20-year-old man with low back pain. A) Sagittal *T*2-weighted MRI demonstrates loss of signal intensity of the L5–S1 intervertebral disc (arrow), reflecting changes caused by degenerative disc disease. B) Transverse *T*2-weighted MRI, obtained at the level of the L5–S1 disc, shows right paracentral focal bulge of the disc (arrow), representing disc protrusion.

patient's symptoms. In an asymptomatic population, over one-third have disc abnormalities at more than one level by MRI criteria. MRI with contrast enhancement is the best technique to study individuals with the failed back syndrome, and differentiating recurrent disc herniation from epidural scarring following surgery.

For evaluating patients with suspected metastases to the spine, MRI is also the procedure of choice. It shows the extent of bony involvement, degree of compression of the cord, and extraspinal extension of the tumour. It is more specific than bone scan for characterizing metastatic deposits, and the entire spine can be surveyed in the right clinical setting. Metastases replace the normal fatty bone marrow and therefore appear as focal low-signal areas on T_1-weighted images. MRI is also helpful for distinguishing benign from metastatic aetiologies of compression fractures. If a part of the affected vertebral body marrow is intact, then the fracture is likely to be benign. Metastatic compression fractures typically show diffuse complete replacement of the marrow signal. One caveat to this rule is in the setting of acute compressions. The oedema associated with acute compression fracture leads to diffuse replacement of the marrow signal, and resembles metastatic deposit. In this setting, the best approach is to repeat the MRI in 6 weeks if the clinical suspicion for metastatic disease is low, or to biopsy the collapsed vertebra in the setting of higher suspicion.

Patients with vertebral osteomyelitis usually present with back pain. The typical plain radiographic features of adjacent vertebral endplate destruction with loss of intervertebral disc height may lag for several weeks. Often, the white blood cell (WBC) count and erythrocyte sedimentation rates are non-specific, and no fever is present. In this setting, MRI is a very sensitive method to detect vertebral osteomyelitis and discitis. The classic findings are adjacent vertebra with abnormal replacement of marrow signal with oedema, low signal on T_1-weighted and high signal on T_2-weighted images. The intervertebral disc usually shows increased signal on T_2-weighted images as well.

Neoplasms (Box 1.10.8)

For most tumours, there are no tissue-specific features on MRI that allow definitive diagnosis. Notable exceptions include lipoma and soft tissue haemangioma. The MRI appearance of a benign lipoma is characteristic. However, differentiating the low-grade liposarcoma from a benign lipoma with some internal septations can be quite difficult. It is generally agreed that interpretation of MRIs on patients with suspected bone tumours should not be done without the plain films at hand. Use of intravenous contrast is also controversial.

The main use of MRI in the evaluation of patients with tumours is staging and postoperative follow-up. MRI is superior to plain film for detecting the extent of disease for surgical planning. It can be difficult to separate peritumoural oedema from actual tumour. When evaluating a patient with primary bone malignancy, it is important to scan the entire extremity involved to detect any occult skip metastases. For the postoperative patient, MRI can be used to detect recurrent disease. However, haematoma or seroma in the surgical bed are often present and can make exclusion of recurrent or residual tumour difficult. Follow-up scans will typically show stable or decreasing size of seromas and haematoma whereas tumours generally increase in size.

Radionuclide bone imaging

Bone scans are most commonly done using technetium-99m labelled phosphonates (^{99m}Tc MDP, ^{99m}Tc HEDP). When ^{99m}Tc decays (half-life 6h), gamma rays are emitted, which are then detected to produce an image. ^{99m}Tc-labelled phosphonates accumulate preferentially in the mineral phase of newly forming bone. Areas of increased bone remodelling, whether it is due to infection, trauma, or tumour, will appear 'hot' on the bone scan compared to normal bones. Therefore bone scan abnormalities are usually not specific for a disease process. The primary strength of bone scans is its relatively high sensitivity when trying to rule out bone disease.

Box 1.10.8 MRI and tumours

- Low-grade lipomas can be difficult to distinguish from benign ones
- Tumour margins may be exaggerated by oedema
- Seroma in a tumour bed can mimic recurrence.

Bone scans are routinely done 3h after injection of ^{99m}Tc-labelled phosphonates. The 3-h interval allows clearance of the radiopharmaceutical from the soft tissue to reach optimal bone to soft tissue contrast. Planar whole body scans are ideal for screening of the entire skeleton. They may not, however, show the optimal contrast for lesion detection in the spine because of uptake in the normal parts of the vertebrae anterior and posterior to the lesion. Spinal lesions are significantly better detected with tomographic imaging (single photon emission computerized tomography, SPECT) because of the better spatial resolution. Exact localization of the abnormality in the vertebra on SPECT imaging also helps with differentiation of benign versus malignant lesions. To evaluate the blood flow and vascularity of a lesion, a three-phase bone scan is performed, which includes immediate flow and blood pool images followed by bone scan at 3h.

Tumour imaging (Box 1.10.9)

Although many bone metastases are lytic on x-rays, they stimulate osteoblastic activity and new bone formation. This accounts for the increased uptake of bone tracers in osseous metastases. The typical pattern is the presence of multiple focal areas of increased uptake predominantly in the axial skeleton.

Bone scans are more sensitive than x-rays in detection of metastatic bone disease, and are used for assessment of treatment response to chemotherapy and hormonal therapy. Primary malignant bone tumours generally demonstrate intense uptake of bone tracers. Osteosarcomas typically appear as areas of markedly increased uptake on the bone scan. Bone scan cannot be used to assess the extent of the Ewing sarcoma because the area of increased uptake is usually larger than the extent of the tumour. Bone scans in osteosarcoma and Ewing sarcoma are used to evaluate metastatic disease at initial staging and follow-up (Figure 1.10.20). Bone scans are of limited value in assessing response to neoadjuvant chemotherapy because of persistent increased uptake related to bone remodelling.

Many benign bone tumours also show intense uptake of the tracer on bone scan. Therefore bone scans cannot be used to differentiate between benign and malignant lesions. Bone scans can be used to screen for polyostotic disease in fibrous dysplasia and enchondroma.

Trauma and sports injuries (Box 1.10.10)

Bone scans are highly sensitive for diagnosis of occult fractures in patients with pain and a negative x-ray. Bone scans are done most frequently to evaluate fractures in the wrist, hips and spine, but become positive within 24h after any fracture in 90–95% of patients. In elderly patients, bone scans may only become positive after some time and repeat imaging at 72h is suggested if the initial bone scan is negative. Bone scans may remain positive for up to 3 years after a fracture.

Bone scans can be also helpful to evaluate post-traumatic complex regional pain syndrome, type 1 (CPRS-1; reflex sympathetic dystrophy). The typical pattern of CRPS-1 is diffuse increased bone tracer uptake of the involved extremity, most prominent in periarticular regions. The flow and vascularity may be increased in the initial phase of disease, but may be negative in the late phase of the disease after 60 weeks of onset of symptoms. Bone scans are also used in the management of heterotopic ossification. There is

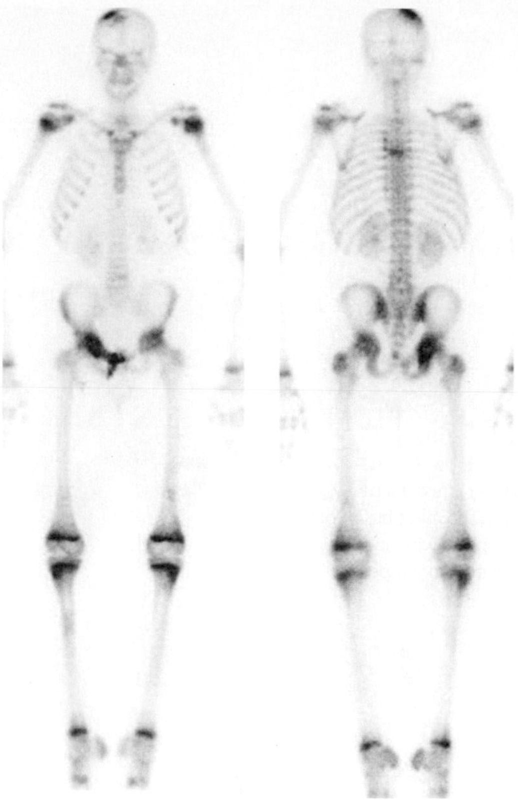

Fig. 1.10.20 Metastatic Ewing's sarcoma. Whole body bone scan shows multiple lesions with increased uptake in the right frontoparietal skull, left humeral head, thoracic spine, right acetabulum, left distal femur, and right proximal tibia. Note also the normal uptake in the growth plates in this adolescent.

Box 1.10.9 Bone scans for bone tumours and metastases

- More sensitive than plain x-rays in detecting metastatic disease
- The extent of an Ewing's sarcoma is exaggerated on bone scan
- Neoadjuvant chemotherapy also produces an abnormal scan
- Bone scans do not reliably distinguish benign and malignant tumours.

Box 1.10.10 Bone scans in trauma and sports injuries

- Bone scans may not become positive for up to 72h after trauma
- Shin splints and stress fractures are easily distinguished by bone scan
- Complex regional pain syndrome shows uptake especially around joints
- Heterotopic bone is 'hot' until it is mature
- Tomographic bone scan should be used for suspected spondylolysis.

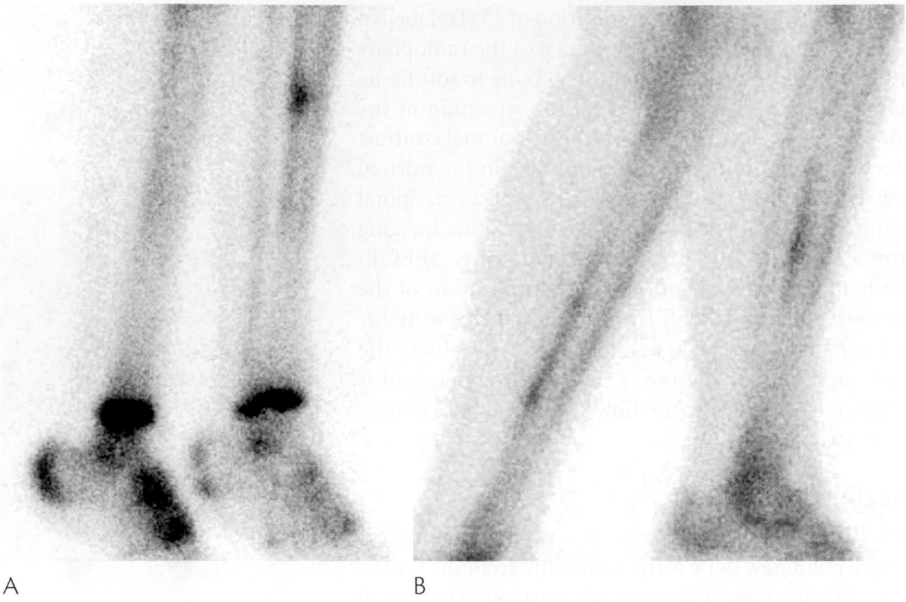

Fig. 1.10.21 A) Stress fracture with focal uptake in the mid tibia on bone scan. B) Shin splints with linear cortical uptake at the posterior aspect of both tibiae.

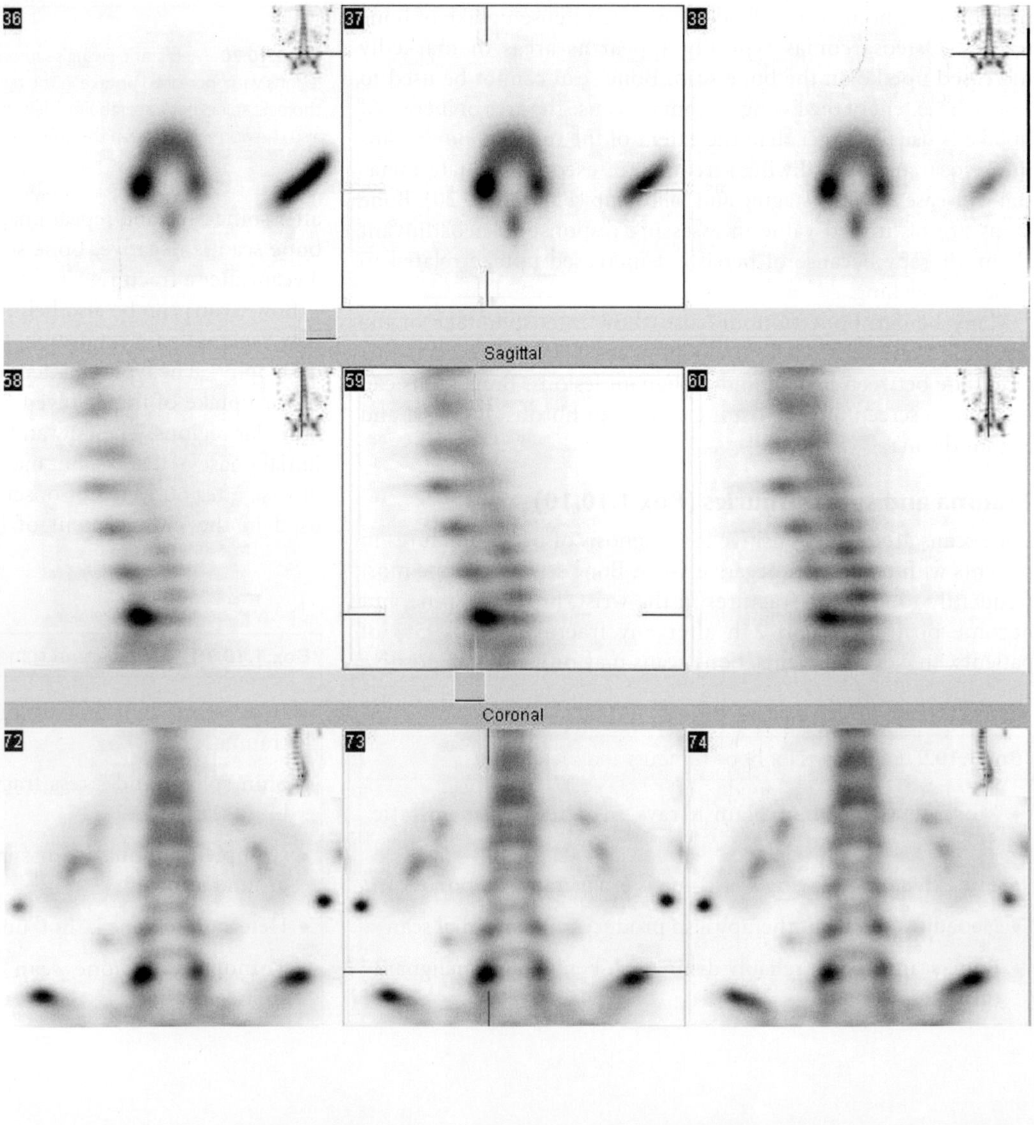

Fig. 1.10.22 Spondylolysis. Focal uptake consistent with right pars fracture at L5 on bone SPECT including transaxial, sagittal, and coronal tomographic images.

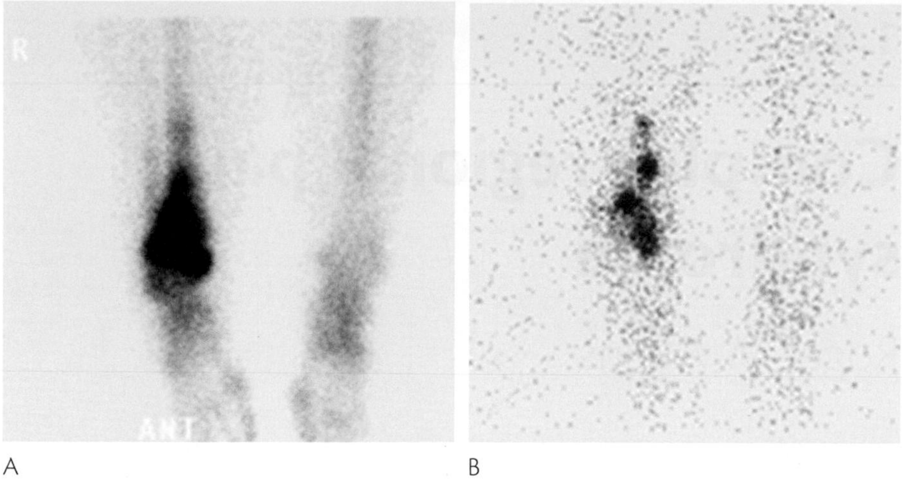

Fig. 1.10.23 Infected nonunion of the right distal tibia. A) Bone scan shows intense uptake which may be secondary to prior fracture or osteomyelitis. B) Simultaneous In-111 WBC scan demonstrates multiple foci of abnormal accumulation of labeled WBCs in the distal tibia, consistent with osteomyelitis.

intense soft tissue uptake of the radiopharmaceutical during formation of heterotopic ossification, but this normalizes or shows only mild uptake in mature heterotopic ossification.

Early stress fractures are not usually visible on plain radiographs. A negative bone scan excludes stress fracture lesions even in clinically suspected cases. The typical finding of a stress fracture on bone scan is focal fusiform increased uptake at the site of injury (Figure 1.10.21). Bone scintigraphy is also helpful to differentiate stress fractures from shin splints. The typical presentation of shin splints on the bone scan is a linear uptake along the posteromedial aspect of the middle third of the involved tibia (Figure 1.10.21).

A positive bone scan in the pars region indicates spondylolysis as the cause of low back pain and correlates with good outcome after fusion surgery. Tomographic images of bone scintigraphy (SPECT) of the lumbar spine need to be obtained as more than 50% of active spondylolysis may not be detected with routine planar bone scans (Figure 1.10.22).

Infection imaging

A three-phase bone scan is the initial test of choice for diagnosis of osteomyelitis after a negative/inconclusive x-ray. Increased bone tracer uptake reflecting bone remodelling may, however, also be seen after fracture, surgery and hardware placement. In these cases labelled WBC scans are used to complement bone scans.

Labelled WBCs, which can be labelled with ^{111}In or ^{99m}Tc, do not accumulate in fractures or sites of orthopaedic surgery in the absence of infection (Figure 1.10.23). Labelled WBCs, however, accumulate in normal bone marrow. If bone marrow distribution has changed secondary to surgery or prosthesis or if there is active marrow proliferation, such as seen in patients with diabetic arthropathy, the labelled WBC scan may show increased/asymmetric uptake in the absence of infection. Therefore labelled WBC imaging should be done in conjunction with a bone marrow scan to differentiate infection from changes in bone marrow.

Box 1.10.11 Positron emission tomography

- FDG uptake is enhanced in malignant cells
- PET can give false positives in some benign lesions.

Positron emission tomography (Box 1.10.11)

The most commonly used radiopharmaceutical in clinical positron emission tomography (PET) imaging is the glucose analogue 2-[^{18}F] fluoro-2-deoxy-D-glucose (F-18 FDG). FDG uptake is enhanced in the malignant cells because of the enhanced transport of glucose (increased number of glucose transporter proteins on cancer cells) and because of the inefficient use of glucose for energy generation in malignant cells. After FDG enters the cells it is phosphorylated in the same way as glucose but does not enter further metabolic pathways and therefore accumulates inside the cell. FDG uptake is not specific for tumours and can be also seen with infections and inflammation.

F-18 FDG decays by positron emission. The emitted positron has a very short range and readily captures an electron when it comes to rest, releasing two photons.

FDG PET has been used for diagnosis and grading of soft tissue sarcomas. FDG PET is also positive in most bone sarcomas. False positive PET is seen in a number of benign bone lesions including giant cell tumours, fibrous dysplasia, eosinophilic granuloma, chondroblastoma, aneurysmatic bone cysts, non-ossifying fibroma, and osteomyelitis.

Further reading

American College of Radiology (1995). Cervical spine trauma, Expert Panel on Musculoskeletal Imaging. In *ACR appropriateness criteria for imaging and treatment decisions*, p. MS2. Reston, VA: American College of Radiology.

Fishman, E.K., Wyatt S.H., Bluemke D.A., and Urban, B.A. (1993). Spiral CT of musculoskeletal pathology: preliminary observations. *Skeletal Radiology*, **22**, 253–6.

Jensen, M.C., Brant-Zawadzki, M.N., Obuchowski, N., Modic, M.T., Malkasian, D., and Ross, J.S. (1994). Magnetic resonance imaging of the lumbar spine in people without back pain. *New England Journal of Medicine*, **331**, 69–73.

Stiell, I.G., McKnight, R.D., Greenberg, G.H., *et al.* (1994). Implementation of the Ottawa ankle rules. *Journal of the American Medical Association*, **271**, 827–32.

1.11

Complex regional pain syndrome

Roger M. Atkins

Summary points

- Complex regional pain syndrome (CRPS) is a disabling chronic pain condition of unknown aetiology
- Traditionally it was thought to be rare; however, prospective studies demonstrate it to be common following both trauma and operative procedures involving the upper and lower limbs
- The condition is usually self-limiting over a maximum period of 2 years, although minor abnormalities may remain
- In a minority of cases it does not resolve and is responsible for severe chronic disability
- Treatment is aimed at functional restoration of limb function supported by pharmacological intervention.

Introduction

Complex regional pain syndrome (CRPS), previously termed reflex sympathetic dystrophy (RSD), consists of abnormal pain, swelling, vasomotor instability, contracture, and osteoporosis (Box 1.11.1). It used to be considered a rare, devastating complication of injury, caused by abnormalities in the sympathetic nervous system and seen mainly in psychologically abnormal patients. Modern research is altering this view radically.

Terminology

The International Association for the Study of Pain (IASP) has replaced the condition's many synonyms with CRPS, which avoids suggesting aetiology or site. The IASP have produced diagnostic criteria which have not been universally adopted and we have proposed a different approach which is more relevant for the orthopaedic surgeon (Box 1.11.2).These two sets of criteria are identical for diagnostic purposes within an orthopaedic context.

CRPS is subdivided into type 2, where there is a causative major nerve injury (the original causalgia described by Mitchell in American Civil War casualties), and type 1, where there is not (previously reflex sympathetic dystrophy or algodystrophy). This distinction is clinically important since in type 2 CRPS, treatment can be directed directly at the damaged nerve.

Clinical features

CRPS is a biphasic condition with early swelling and vasomotor instability giving way to late contracture and joint stiffness The hand and foot are most frequently involved, although the knee is increasingly recognized The elbow is rarely affected, whereas

Box 1.11.1 Features of CRPS

- Abnormal pain
- Swelling
- Vasomotor instability
- Contracture
- Osteoporosis.

Box 1.11.2 Suggested criteria for the diagnosis of CRPS within an orthopaedic setting

The diagnosis is made clinically by the finding of the following abnormalities:

- Neuropathic pain: non-dermatomal, without cause, burning, with associated allodynia and hyperpathia
- Vasomotor instability and abnormalities of sweating: warm, red, and dry; cool, blue, and clammy; or an increase in temperature sensitivity. Associated with an abnormal temperature difference between the limbs
- Swelling
- Loss of joint mobility
- Joint and soft tissue contracture.

These clinical findings are backed up by:

- Radiographic evidence of osteoporosis after 3 months
- Increased uptake on delayed bone scintigraphy early in CRPS.

Box 1.11.3 Timeline of CRPS

- Begins within 1 month
- Neuropathic pain replaces injury pain
- Early clinical features: swelling and vasomotor instability (initially hot, pink, and dry—then blue, cold, and sweaty)
- Late clinical features: contracture, atrophy, and joint stiffness. Nails pit, hairs break. Tendons trigger.

shoulder disease is common and the hip is affected in transient osteoporosis of pregnancy.

CRPS usually begins up to a month after the precipitating trauma. As the effects of injury subside, a new diffuse, unpleasant, neuropathic pain arises. Neuropathic pain occurs without a noxious stimulus and spontaneous or burning pain (causalgia), hyperalgesia (increased sensitivity to a noxious stimulus), allodynia (pain provoked by innocuous stimuli, such as gentle touch), and hyperpathia (temporal and spatial summation of allodynia) are common. Pain is unremitting, worsening, and radiating with time (Box 1.11.3).

Early phase

Vasomotor instability (VMI) and oedema dominate the early phase (Figure 1.11.1), although this is less marked with more proximal CRPS. Classically, initially the limb is dry, hot, and pink, later becoming blue, cold, and sweaty. In most cases there is merely an increase in temperature sensitivity. Oedema is marked and loss of joint mobility is due to swelling and pain.

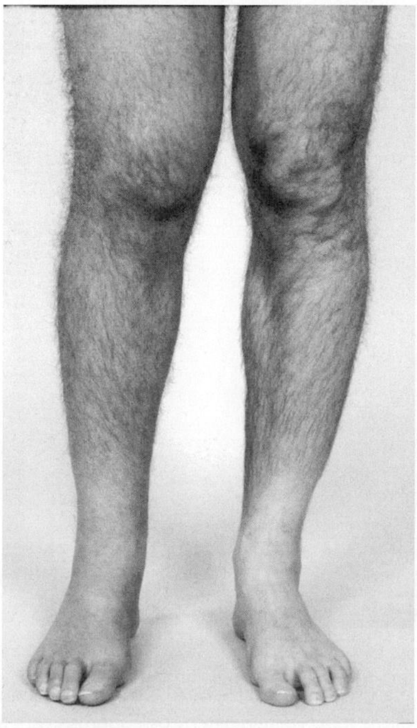

Fig. 1.11.1 A patient with early CRPS type 1 affecting the leg. Note the swelling of the leg and the discolouration of the shin.

Late phase

Passing into the late phase, VMI recedes, oedema resolves, and atrophy of every tissue occurs (Figure 1.11.2). The skin is thinned and joint creases and subcutaneous fat disappear. Hairs become fragile, uneven, and curled while nails are pitted, ridged, brittle, and discoloured brown. Palmar and plantar fascias thicken and contract simulating Dupuytren's disease. Tendon sheaths become constricted causing triggering and muscle contracture combined with tendon adherence leads to reduced tendon excursion. Joint capsules and collateral ligaments shorten and adhere, causing contracture.

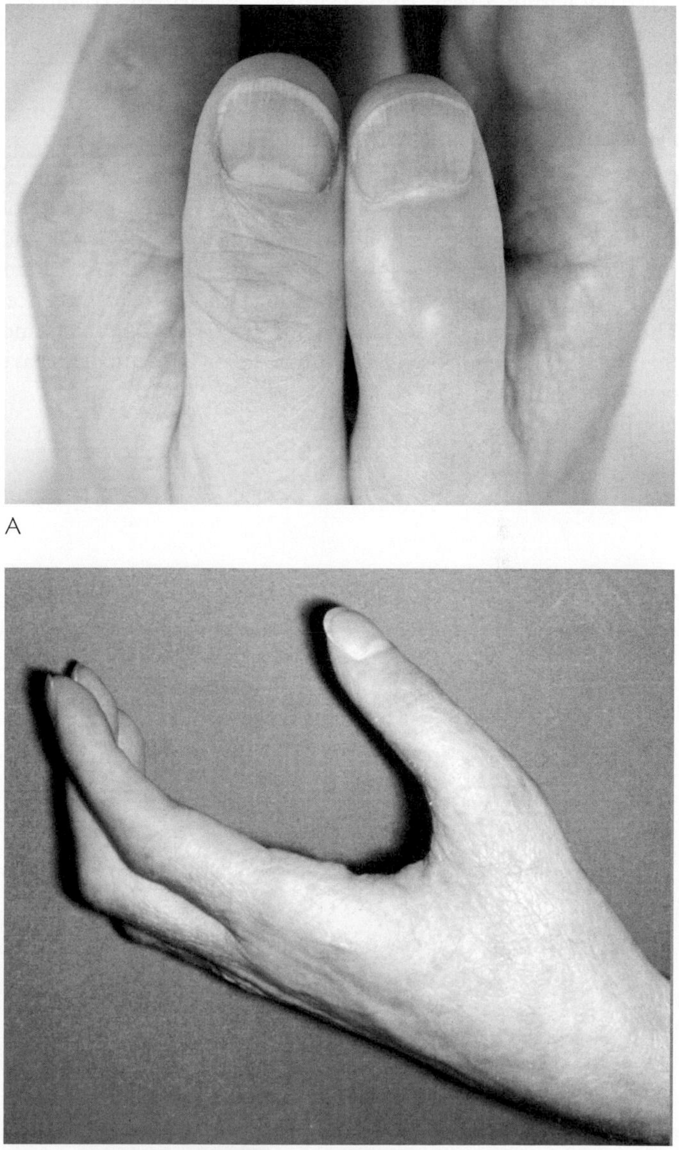

A

B

Fig. 1.11.2 The late phase of CRPS. A) Detail of the thumbs of a patient with late CRPS type 1 of the right hand. There is spindling of the digit, particularly distally. The nail is excessively ridged and is discoloured. B) The hand of a patient with late CRPS type 1. The patient is trying to make a fist. Note the digital spindling and extension contractures with loss of joint creases.

Bone changes

Bone involvement is universal with increased uptake on bone scanning in early CRPS (Figure 1.11.3). This is not periarticular, suggesting arthralgia but generalized and may not occur in children. Later, the bone scan returns to normal and there are radiographic features of rapid bone loss: visible demineralization with patchy, subchondral or subperiosteal osteoporosis, metaphyseal banding, and profound bone loss (Figure 1.11.4).

Incidence

Severe, chronic CRPS is uncommon and the prevalence is less than 2% in retrospective series. In contrast, prospective studies show that mild CRPS occurs after 20–40% of every fracture and surgery where it has been actively sought. Although these cases resolve substantially within a year, some features—particularly stiffness—remain, suggesting that CRPS may be responsible for significant long-term morbidity even when mild.

Aetiology

CRPS may occur after any particular trauma while an identical stimulus in a different limb does not cause it. The incidence is not changed by treatment method and open anatomic reduction and rigid internal fixation does not abolish it. It is unclear whether injury severity or quality of fracture reduction alters the incidence. There is, however, an association with excessively tight casts and there may be a genetic predilection. The following aetiologies have been proposed (Box 1.11.4):

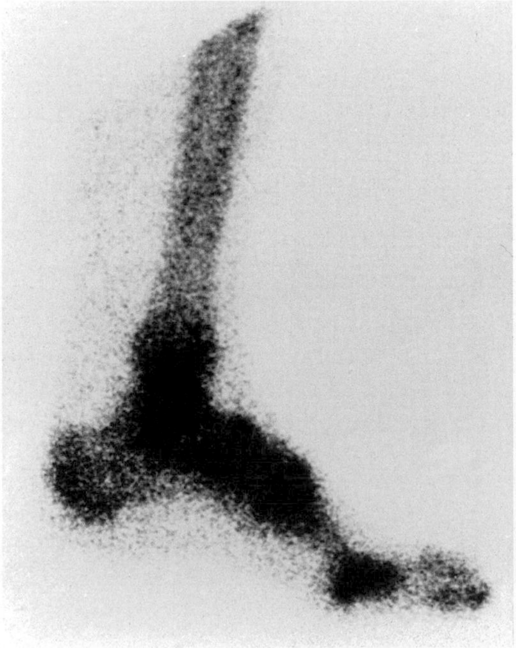

Fig. 1.11.3 Bone scan changes in CRPS. The delayed phase of a bone scan of a patient with early CRPS type 1 of the lower leg. There is increased uptake throughout the affected region. The bone scan will usually revert to normal after 6 months.

Psychological abnormalities

CRPS is not primarily psychological and most patients are psychologically normal. There is an association with antecedent psychological stress which probably exacerbates pain in CRPS, as in other diseases. It seems likely that the severe chronic pain of CRPS causes depression and that a 'Sudecky' type of patient who develops CRPS is at risk of a poor outcome because they will not mobilize in the face of pain.

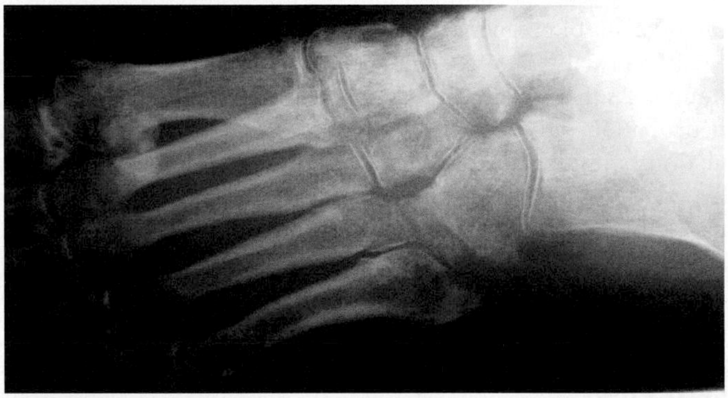

A

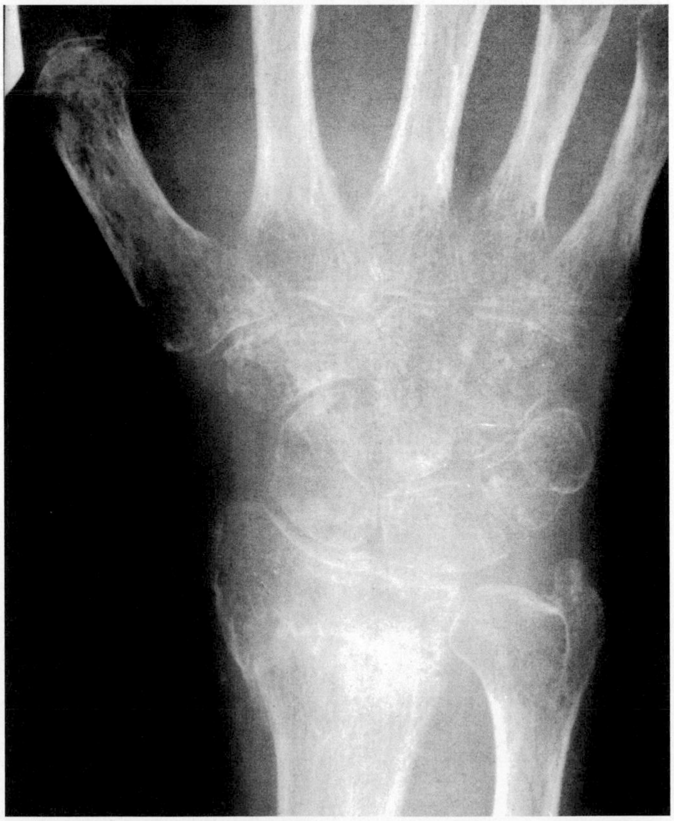

B

Fig. 1.11.4 Radiographic features of CRPS. A) Oblique radiograph of a patient with CRPS type 1 of the foot. There is patchy osteoporosis with accentuation of the osteoporosis beneath the joints. B) Profound osteoporosis in a patient with late severe CRPS type 1 affecting the hand.

Box 1.11.4 Epidemiology and pathogenesis of CRPS

- Up to 20–40% of all fractures if looked for carefully
- Usually resolves within 1 year
- Not affected by treatment, but tight casts may predispose
- Patients are psychologically normal.

Abnormal (neuropathic) pain

Pain is normally caused when a noxious stimulus activates high-threshold nociceptors. Neuropathic pain in CRPS occurs without appropriate stimulus and has no protective function. However, injured peripheral nerve fibres undergo cellular changes which cause usually innocuous tactile inputs to stimulate the dorsal horn cells via A-β fibres from low-threshold mechanoreceptors, causing allodynia in CRPS 2. Furthermore, axonal injury prevents nerve growth factor transport which is essential for normal nerve function. In CRPS 1, inflammatory mediators released by the initial trauma (and possibly retained due to a failure of free radical clearance), can sensitize nociceptors to respond to normally innocuous stimuli.

Sympathetic nervous system abnormalities

A number of features of CRPS suggest sympathetic nervous system (SNS) dysfunction (e.g. vasomotor and sudomotor disturbance); however, SNS activity is not usually painful. In CRPS, some pain (termed sympathetically maintained pain, SMP) is SNS dependent and is relieved by stellate ganglion blockade and worsened by noradrenalin injection. Furthermore, there is an abnormal difference in cutaneous sensory threshold between the limbs, which is reversed by local anaesthetic sympathetic chain blockade, while increasing sympathetic activity worsens pain. SMP is explained by the body's reaction to injury. After partial nerve division, injured and uninjured somatic axons express α-adrenergic receptors and sympathetic axons come to surround sensory neurons cell bodies in dorsal root ganglia. These changes make the somatic sensory nervous system sensitive sympathetic mediators.

Abnormal inflammation

CRPS is associated with inflammatory changes including macromolecule extravasation and reduced oxygen consumption. In animals, infusion of free radical donors causes a CRPS-like state and amputated human specimens with CRPS show basement membrane thickening consistent with overexposure to free radicals. These considerations suggest that CRPS is an exaggerated local inflammatory response to injury. In other words, CRPS represents a local form of the systemic free radical disease that causes adult respiratory distress syndrome and multiple organ failure after severe trauma. This concept is supported by evidence that the free radical scavenger, vitamin C, is effective prophylaxis against post-traumatic CRPS. An alternative explanation is a primary capillary imbalance causing stasis, extravasation, and consequent local tissue anoxia.

Immobilization

Undue immobilization has been proposed as the cause of CRPS and all features of CRPS, except pain, are seen after cast immobilization. CRPS is associated with an often overlooked abnormality of motor function, varying from weakness to incoordination and tremor. The best description is that in CRPS-1, patients find it difficult to initiate or accurately direct movement. Learned pain avoidance behaviour in response to allodynia may exacerbate changes of disuse since normal tactile and proprioceptive input are necessary for correct central nerve signal processing. In some patients, there is a central sensory confusion: in response to an apparently painful non-noxious stimulus, the patient cannot determine whether it is truly painful. The consequent impairment of integration between sensory input and motor output may be the major cause of CRPS.

Investigations and differential diagnosis

CRPS is a clinical diagnosis and there is no single diagnostic test which is definitive. The classic case is obvious and direct effects of trauma, fracture, cellulitis, arthritis, and malignancy are common alternative diagnoses. The patient is systemically well with normal general clinical examination, biochemical markers, and infection indices.

X-ray appearances and bone scans have already been discussed. Sudeck's technique of assessing bone density by radiographing two extremities on one plate remains useful. A normal bone scan without radiographic osteoporosis virtually excludes adult CRPS. Temperature difference between the limbs is greater in CRPS than other pain syndromes but this is not usually applied in an orthopaedic context. Magnetic resonance imaging shows early bone and soft tissue oedema with late atrophy and fibrosis but is not diagnostic.

Management

Proper scientifically constructed prospectively randomized blinded studies are few and uncontrolled investigations are particularly unreliable in CRPS. Most patients are sensible people, concerned at the development of inexplicable pain, but the occasional 'Sudecky' patient fares poorly and should be treated vigorously. Early treatment before contractures occur gives optimal results, so a high index of clinical suspicion must be maintained.

Modern CRPS treatment emphasizes functional rehabilitation of the limb to break the vicious cycle of disuse, rather than SNS manipulation. Initial treatment from the orthopaedic surgeon is by reassurance, excellent analgesia and intensive, careful physiotherapy avoiding exacerbation of pain. Non-steroidal anti-inflammatory drugs may be preferred to opiates. Immobilization and splintage are generally avoided, but if used, joints must be placed in a safe position and splintage is a temporary adjunct to mobilization. If the patient does not respond rapidly, a pain specialist should be involved and treatment continued on a shared basis. Second-line treatment is often unsuccessful and many patients are left with pain and disability. Further treatments include centrally-acting analgesic medications such as amitriptyline, gabapentin, or carbamazepine; regional anaesthesia; the use of membrane-stabilizing drugs such as mexiletine; calcitonin; sympathetic blockade and manipulation; desensitization of peripheral nerve receptors with capsaicin; transcutaneous nerve stimulation or an implanted dorsal column stimulator. A different approach including behavioural therapy may be necessary in children. Where the knee is affected, epidural anaesthesia and continuous passive motion may be appropriate (Box 1.11.5).

Box 1.11.5 Treatment of CRPS

- Vigorous physiotherapy to avoid contractures
- Good analgesia while avoiding pain
- Avoid splintage and immobilization
- Behavioural therapy may help, especially in children
- Surgery to release contractures is rarely needed and should not be rushed into.

The role of surgery is limited. Where CRPS is caused by a surgically correctable painful lesion, such as median nerve compression at the wrist, surgery should be undertaken cautiously in the presence of active disease. Surgery is rarely indicated to treat fixed contractures which usually involve all of the soft tissues. Surgical release must therefore be radical and expectations limited. Surgery for contracture should be delayed until the active phase of CRPS has completely passed and ideally there should be a gap of at least 1 year since the patient last experienced pain and swelling.

Amputation in CRPS should be approached with extreme caution because pain may continue.

Further reading

Butler, S. H. (2001). Disuse and CRPS. In: Harden, R.N., Baron, R., and Janig, W. (eds) *Complex Regional Pain* Syndrome, Vol. 22, pp. 141–50. Seattle, WA: IASP Press.

Van Hilten, J.J., Blumberg, H., and Schwartzman, R.J. (2005). Factor IV: movement disorders and dystrophy. Pathophysiology and measurement. In: Wilson, P., Stanton-Hicks, M., and Harden, R.N. (eds) *CRPS: Current Diagnosis and Therapy*, Vol. 32, pp. 119–37. Seattle, WA: IASP Press.

Veldman, P.H., Reynen, H.M., Arntz, I.E., *et al.* (1993). Signs and symptoms of reflex sympathetic dystrophy: prospective study of 829 patients. *Lancet*, **342**(8878), 1012–16.

1.12

Neuromuscular disorders

Tim Theologis

Summary points

- Neurological disorders can be sensory, motor, or a combination of the two
- Motor disorders may be flaccid or spastic, static or progressive
- Splints may improve function but are not proven to prevent contractures
- Botulinum toxin and tenotomy can be used to manage spasticity
- Osteotomies may be needed to manage rotatory abnormalities
- Sensory nerve abnormalities may cause Charcot joints.

Definitions and classification

A wide variety of conditions that affect the central nervous system, peripheral nerves, or muscle are included under the term neuromuscular disorders. A significant number of patients with these conditions may require orthopaedic treatment.

The anatomic distribution, neurological type, and severity of neuromuscular disorders also vary substantially. Neuromuscular disorders affecting the central nervous system present with an anatomical distribution depending on the affected area of the brain or spinal cord. They can, therefore, present as hemiplegia, paraplegia (diplegia), quadriplegia, or total body involvement (Box 1.12.1). Peripheral nerve diseases may affect the extremities only. Muscle conditions may affect proximal or distal muscle groups.

The neurological patterns also vary. Disorders affecting the central nervous system may present as paralysis, spasticity, dystonia, athetosis, or a mixture of these patterns. Sensory loss may accompany some conditions. Peripheral nerve conditions usually produce muscle weakness. Conditions affecting muscle also produce weakness which can be either generalized or confined to certain muscle groups.

Paralysis may be flaccid or spastic. Understanding of this, and of the aetiology of the development of secondary musculoskeletal deformities, is important. In flaccid paralysis, deformity is due either to the unopposed activity of antagonist muscle(s) or it is a flail deformity in which limb position is only the result of gravity. In spastic paralysis, the aetiology of deformity is due to abnormal overactivity of muscle groups. The interaction and balance between agonist and antagonist muscles are impaired, patterns are more complex, and the results of treatment less predictable. In mixed patterns or in the presence of athetosis or dystonia the results of surgical treatment are unpredictable and sometimes catastrophic.

It is important to understand whether the condition affecting the patient is static or progressive. Establishing an accurate diagnosis is the first step for this. Some conditions (e.g. acute onset of poliomyelitis) may be progressive for a short period of time and then become static later. Others (e.g. multiple sclerosis) progress periodically with long static periods in between. The result of orthopaedic treatment is more predictable in stable neurological conditions and after the patient has established a pattern and any compensations.

Evaluation

The majority of adult patients with neuromuscular disorders are referred to the orthopaedic surgeon after their diagnosis is established. A significant number, however, may be referred undiagnosed for an 'orthopaedic' deformity which may be the result of an underlying neurological condition. A high index of suspicion should therefore be present in order to avoid missing the diagnosis in these cases.

A thorough history and a detailed clinical examination are always the cornerstones of diagnosing and evaluating the neuromuscular patient. In particular, neurological examination including muscle power, sensation, and reflexes should be included. The range of

Box 1.12.1 Types of paralysis

- Static versus progressive
- Spastic versus flaccid
- Hemiplegia = one side
- Diplegia = both sides (typically worse in legs)
- Paraplegia = both legs, usually with sensory loss
- Quadriplegia = all limbs

movement of joints and any contractures should be recorded. The spine should always be examined. Specific tests should be performed as required: a positive Gower's test is indicative of muscular dystrophy. Difficulty grasping and releasing objects may indicate myotonia, while the development of cavovarus foot deformity may be the first sign of a hereditary motor sensory neuropathy. When assessing or planning treatment for conditions affecting the hand, two-point discrimination and stereognostic tests should be performed.

Treatment of the patient with neuromuscular disorders should be tailored to his or her personal needs. Some general guidelines may apply to most of these conditions but the neurological patterns and the severity of the conditions vary to the degree that an effort to apply strict treatment rules would be dangerous. While assessing a patient for orthopaedic treatment it is important to get to know their personal needs and to set a specific aim and target.

The aim of orthopaedic treatment of the adult patient with neuromuscular disorder may vary. In patients with severe scoliosis or painful hip dislocation, for example, the aim is to alleviate the pain. Improving the quality of life by offering a better sitting posture or better access for hygiene may be another aim. Correcting or preventing further progression of a deformity which is painful or produces a functional impairment may be necessary. Improving function may be a relative indication for treatment. This always carries the risk of an unpredictable negative result which may further compromise the already affected function of the patient. Such treatment should, therefore, always be discussed in depth. Finally, on rare occasions, patients may request orthopaedic treatment for cosmetic reasons. Treatment decisions are facilitated by a multidisciplinary team approach.

Treatment modalities

The role of the orthopaedic surgeon in the management of the patient with neuromuscular disease is limited. The number of patients who are candidates for surgery is also limited and selection should be done carefully. Conservative treatment including orthoses, splints, serial casting, and physiotherapy are used extensively to prevent joint contractures or control undesired movement (Figure 1.12.1). When orthoses are used to improve function, any benefit from these is evident and can be recorded. The use of the earlier mentioned treatment modalities to prevent contractures, however, would need extensive long-term studies to be documented. In fact, splinting, casting, and physiotherapy are all used for the prevention of contractures on an empirical basis. However, their functional use is important. The use of ankle–foot orthoses for a foot-drop or gastrocnemius spasticity, the use of walking aids, or standing frames is certainly valuable.

Postural management of the non-ambulatory patient, and particularly wheelchair design and type, is important to prevent pressure sores, and to maximize the patient's potential for mobility and communication. Seating arrangements may also provide some external support for patients with lack of head control, spinal deformity, or pelvic obliquity.

Nerve blocks with phenol or alcohol injections have long been used to control spastic muscle groups.

Intramuscular injections of botulinum toxin A are extensively used to control spasticity in several neuromuscular conditions, including multiple sclerosis, dystonia, spinal cord injury, and cerebral palsy. The toxin works by blocking the motor endplate for several months. New nerve ends sprout eventually and the muscle regains power.

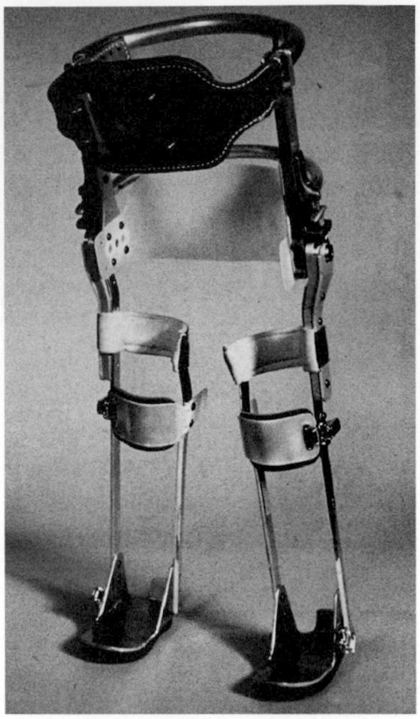

Fig. 1.12.1 Orthoses in neuromuscular disorders are used to improve function and prevent deformity.

Systemic drugs, such as baclofen, gabapentin, dantrolene, and diazepam, have also been used to control spasticity. More recently, intrathecal administration of baclofen through a continuous infusion using an implanted pump has been used to control lower limb spasticity.

Functional electrical stimulation of weak muscles has also been used to aid ambulation in patients with conditions producing paraplegia or hemiplegia. Results of longer-term studies are now emerging and these are encouraging (Box 1.12.2).

Surgical treatment of adult patients with neuromuscular disorders may include division or lengthening of tendons or muscles, transferring of tendons, neurectomy, bony operations including osteotomy, or joint fusion or excision. Lengthening or transferring tendons or muscles weakens the structure. This should be taken into account when planning such surgery, particularly in adults where weakness is a greater problem than in children because of the higher ratio of body weight to muscle power. Extensive

Box 1.12.2 Non-operative treatment of neuromuscular disease

- Splints
- Serial casting and physiotherapy
- Postural management in wheelchairs
- Nerve blocks with phenol and alcohol
- Intramuscular injection of botulinum toxin
- Systemic muscle relaxant drugs
- Functional electrical stimulation of muscles

procedures, such as the multilevel soft tissue releases in cerebral palsy, are well tolerated by children but are rarely performed in adults (Box 1.12.2).

Surgical treatment of specific conditions

The specific problems in a number of neuromuscular disorders more commonly seen in orthopaedic clinics are presented in Table 1.12.1. Some surgical procedures commonly required for these problems are also included to provide some general information although this list is by no means comprehensive. As mentioned earlier, orthopaedic surgery in neuromuscular disorders should be personalized and tailored to the needs of the specific patient. Some of the most common orthopaedic problems in adults with neuromuscular conditions are discussed in the following sections.

Central nervous system

Cerebral palsy (Box 1.12.3)

Despite the large number of publications on the treatment of children with cerebral palsy, little is written in the orthopaedic literature on the management of adults with the condition. While most hemiplegic patients maintain good mobility throughout life, the diplegics tend to deteriorate in their adult years. Their walking distance may diminish and they may present with joint contractures and a crouch gait. They often complain of knee and, more specifically, patellofemoral pain due to the increased loading of the joint. The persistent femoral anteversion and external tibial torsion that coexist, often referred to as 'malignant malalignment', are also responsible for the abnormal loading of the patellofemoral joint. Their frequently dysplastic hips may develop degenerative changes and become painful. Progressive foot deformity, usually planovalgus in diplegia and equinovarus in hemiplegia, and joint degenerative changes are also common.

Soft tissue surgery to eliminate joint contractures is not as effective in adult cerebral palsy as it is in children. This is partly due to the long-established intrinsic bone and joint deformities which commenced during the growing years. Extensive surgery in adult cerebral palsy also carries a high risk of compromising the patient's already limited ability to ambulate. The reason is the inevitable muscle weakness that follows any muscle or tendon lengthening and the postoperative immobilization in addition to any underlying weakness. Limited surgery to address specific problems is more desirable. Dysplastic and/or degenerative hips in ambulant patients may require reconstruction to improve coverage. Femoral varus derotation osteotomy, often combined with pelvic osteotomy or an acetabuloplasty, can be considered. Joint replacement surgery or arthrodesis has also been suggested for adult cerebral palsy. Operations which are often performed in childhood to correct stiff or crouch knee gait, such as hamstrings release with rectus femoris transfer, have not been reported in adults. Supracondylar extension femoral osteotomies can be used to correct severe knee flexion deformities. Foot operations to correct deformity or pain certainly have a place. Lengthening the tendon(s) responsible for the deformity and correcting the deformity with a bony operation is the principle usually followed. Subtalar or triple fusion may be necessary and this depends on the level of the deformity. A recent study in Norway showed that the most common procedures performed in adults with cerebral palsy were lower-limb soft tissue releases and foot deformity corrections.

Upper-limb surgery in adult cerebral palsy patients is rarely performed. Shoulder internal rotation deformity may be corrected with derotation osteotomy. Flexion deformity of the elbow may be improved by lengthening of the biceps and brachialis, but this involves the risk of loosing adequate elbow flexion power which may be more important functionally. Pronation of the forearm is usually due to spasticity of both the pronator teres and quadratus, and lengthening may be beneficial. The expected gain from these operations, however, is less in adults as the ideal age for this surgery is during the teenage years. Hand surgery requires candidates with reasonable intelligence, voluntary control, and sensation, including stereognosia, proprioception, and two-point discrimination. Dorsal transfer of flexor carpi ulnaris to the extensor digitorum communis to aid weak extensors, as well as fractional lengthening of the finger flexors to correct fixed deformities, have been described. Furthermore, operations to correct the thumb-in-palm deformity include release of the adductor and flexors, release of the first dorsal interosseous, and rerouting of the extensor pollicis longus. Joint contractures are not correctable, however, by soft tissue procedures if bone and joint deformity is present. Proximal row carpectomy and fusion of the wrist have been suggested for stabilization for cosmetic or functional purposes.

Non-ambulatory patients are at high risk of developing the triad of scoliosis, pelvic obliquity, and hip dislocation (Figure 1.12.3). These deformities are usually already established when patients reach skeletal maturity and those who require treatment may have received it during adolescence. Painful hip dislocation, affecting seating posture and hygiene and also associated with decubitus ulcers, can be a major problem in non-ambulant patients. However, it is unclear what percentage of untreated patients develop late pain or quality of life problems and reports are only limited. Femoral head excision or resection of the proximal femur has been suggested, but failure of these operations to alleviate pain leaves no surgical options for further management. Simple valgus proximal femoral osteotomy to alleviate the pressure on the femoral head may be a more sensible option. Arthrodesis in unilateral disease or reconstruction may be another option. Incomplete transiliac osteotomy combined with femoral varus-shortening derotation osteotomy appears to offer optimal results. Interposition arthroplasty using prosthetic material may offer salvage in difficult cases.

Knee flexion contractures in non-ambulatory patients are rarely a problem since they are functional in the sitting position. Finally, severe foot deformities may be responsible for skin pressure problems, either from the foot plate of the wheelchair or from underlying bones. Extensive soft tissue releases are usually sufficient for correction of the foot into a reasonable position that does not cause pressure problems.

Head injury and stroke

Adult patients who present to orthopaedic clinics after stroke or head injury are frequently hemiplegics. Equinus or equinovarus foot deformities are the most common problems (Figure 1.12.4). During their recovery period, they usually require a rehabilitation programme which may include casts or orthoses and nerve blocks or botulinum toxin injections.

The recovery period lasts about 6–12 months for stroke patients and 12–18 months for head injury patients. Surgery may then be considered for patients with equinus gait and reasonable ability for gait re-education. Tendon lengthening and transfer surgery based

Table 1.12.1 Treatment modalities

Category	Disorder	General features	Spine	Upper limb	Hip	Knee	Foot	Other	Comment
Central nervous system									
Cerebral palsy	Ambulators	Deterioration with time		Wrist flexion-pronation Thumb in palm *Tendon lengthenings* *Wrist fusion*	?Dysplasia *?Reconstruction*	'Stiff' or crouch plus pain? *Osteotomy*	Equinovarus or planovalgus *Bony corrections*	Rotational abnormalities *Osteotomies*	
	Nonambulators		Scoliosis Kyphosis *Spinal fusion*	Shoulder, elbow and wrist deformities	Dislocation *Proximal femoral valgus osteotomy* *Proximal excision* *THRFusion*	Flexion deformity *Posterior release or femoral osteotomy*	Any deformity *Soft-tissue correction*	Loose ability to walk at 20–25	Autosomal recessive
Friedreich ataxia	Spinocerebellar degeneration	Ataxia Areflexia Extensor plantar reflex	Scoliosis in all *Fusion of progressive curves in non-ambulators*				Cavovarus *TA and TP lengthening,* *?Triple fusion*	Myocardiopathy death at 30–40	Autosomal recessive
Cerebral vascular accident or head injury	Usually hemiplegia of adult onset	'Stable' pattern 6–12 months after onset		Shoulder, elbow and wrist deformities	'Stiff'	'Stiff' *EMG-based rectus release*	Equinus/varus *TA and TP lengthening Split TA transfer*	Toe clawing *Flexor tenotomies*	
Multiple sclerosis		±Ataxia Sensory loss Spasticity Sphincter disturbance	Back pain		Flexion deformity Adductor spasticity	Flexion deformity Quadriceps weakness	Equinus *As in CVA*		
Motor neuron disease	Bulbar palsy Amyotrophic lateral sclerosis Progressive muscular atrophy	Dysphagia Dysarthria Sphincters maintained	Head support	Atrophy of the small muscles of the hand			May present with foot drop	Weakness predominant Trunk and limb muscle fasciculation	Poor prognosis typically 3 years
Spine									
Spinal dysraphism		Hydrocephalus, Arnold–Chiari Latex allergy	Dysraphism, Tethered cord Congenital or developmental scoliosis *Spinal fusion*	Mild impairment may be present	Dislocation *Reconstruction rarely required in adults*	Fixed flexion or hyper-extension or instability (valgus thrust) *Release or osteotomy to fit orthosis*	Any deformity *Bony corrections* Ulcers, infection *Aggressive treatment*	Walking ability deteriorates with age	Prevention with folic acid
Spinal muscular atrophy	Severe (Werdnig–Hoffmann)	Never survive to adult age							Autosomal recessive
	Intermediate	Some survive to adult age	Progressive paralytic scoliosis *Spinal fusion*		Dysplasia *Reconstruction rarely indicated*			Proximal weakness	Autosomal recessive
	Mild (Kugelberg–Welander)	Usually survive and > 50% are mobile	Scoliosis rare		Rare contractures		Rare contractures	Proximal weakness	Autosomal recessive

Poliomyelitis	Chronic Postpolio syndrome	Weakness Fatigue	Scoliosis					Frequent falls	Discussed elsewhere No change in overall impairment
Tetraplegia/ paraplegia			*Spinal stabilization may be required*	Weight-bearing problems in paraplegia *Tendon transfers possible in tetraplegia*	Contractures Pressure sores *?Reconstruction or excision arthroplasty*	Flexion deformity	Any deformity *Soft-tissue balancing procedures*	High risk of fractures *?Treatment controversial*	
Neuropathies									
Hereditary motor and sensory neuropathies	Seven types (Charcot–Marie–Tooth disease corresponds to types I and II)	Demyelination or hypertrophy of peripheral nerves	Scoliosis (10%) *As in idiopathic scoliosis*		Dysplasia *?Reconstruction*		Cavovarus *Plantar release Os calcis steotomy Tibialis posterior transfer ?Triple fusion*		Autosomal dominant or recessive (depends on type)
Nerve/root compression or injury				Brachial plexus or peripheral palsy *Re-construction*			Foot-drop *TA or TP transfer based on EMG*		
Degenerative/ diabetic							Ulcers Charcot joints		
Muscular									
Muscular dystrophies	Duchenne	Survival into early adult life is increasingly likely	Scoliosis Spinal fusion			Contractures			X-linked
	Becker	Slowly progressive	Scoliosis *Spinal fusion*				Equinus/varus *TA lengthening ± TP transfer*		X-linked
	Emery-Dreifuss	Slowly progressive Mobile until 30–50 years of age	Restricted neck flexion Paraspinal muscle stiffness	Elbow flexion deformities			Equinus/varus *TA lengthening + TP transfer*		X-linked
	Facioscapulo-humeral	Slowly progressive Variable severity		Scapular winging *Soft-tissue or bony scapulo-thoracic fixation*				Infantile form more severe	Autosomal dominant
	Limb girdle	Variable onset and severity	?Scoliosis	Proximal weakness	Proximal weakness		Equinus		Autosomal recessive
Myotonias	Myotonic dystrophy	Delayed muscle relaxation Variable learning difficulties		Delayed release of hand grip			Hindfoot varus	Progressively worse through the generations	Autosomal dominant
	Congenital myotonic dystrophy	Hypotonia mental retardation	Scoliosis *Spinal fusion*				Club-foot *Serial casting May require surgery*		Autosomal dominant
	Myotonia congenita	Short episodes of muscle rigidity after rest						No deformities	Autosomal dominant or recessive

Table 1.12.1 (cont'd) Treatment modalities

Congenital myopathies	Nemaline	Hypotonia, variable severity and survivorship	Scoliosis or lordosis may be present	Proximal weakness				Proximal weakness, rare contractures	Autosomal dominant
	Central core	Hypotonia, slowly progressive	Kypho-scoliosis	Proximal weakness	Dislocation Contractures *Releases and/or reconstruction*	Flexion deformity *Release or osteotomy*	Club-foot or pes cavus *Bony correction*	Walking ability may be lost in adult years	Autosomal dominant
	Centronuclear or myotubular	Variable presentation	Scoliosis Lordosis	Winged scapula			Cavovarus	Proximal weakness, may loose ability to walk	Variable inheritance
	Fiber-type Disproportion	Not uniform entity—variable presentations	Scoliosis		Dislocation *Reconstruction*			May loose ability to walk	Variable inheritance
	Congenital muscular dystrophy	Weakness and stiffness						Joint contractures may be present *Soft-tissue releases*	
Polymyositis-dermatomyositis	Idiopathic, viral, or bacterial	Gradual onset of muscle weakness Characteristic skin rash						Joint contractures rarely need releases or tendon lengthenings	Cortico-steroids
Myasthenia gravis	Thymus antibodies inhibiting acetylcholine receptors	Easy fatigue after repeated muscle activity						Increased anesthetic risk	Anti-cholinesterase drugs Cyclosporin Thymectomy
Arthrogrypotic syndromes									
	Variable etiology	Multiple joint contractures	Scoliosis can be present: severity is variable	Shoulder internal rotation *Humeral osteotomy* Wrist flexion and ulnar deviation *Proximal row carpectomy*	Dislocation, flexion contractures	Flexion contractures or iatrogenic extension *Distal femoral osteotomy*	Clubfoot usually rigid *Talectomy Arthrodesis*	80%–90% long-term community ambulators Good social and professional adjustment	

TA, tibialis anterior; TP, tibialis posterior; EMG, electromyography; THR, total hip replacement; CVA, cerebrovascular accident.
[a]The most usual orthopedic treatment required is presented in italics.

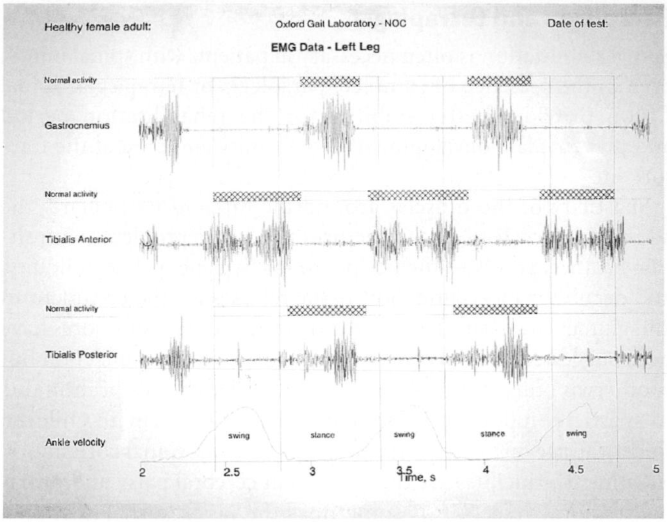

Fig. 1.12.2 Dynamic electromyography of gastrocnemius and tibialis anterior and posterior during gait is used to aid treatment decisions on tendon lengthening and transfer.

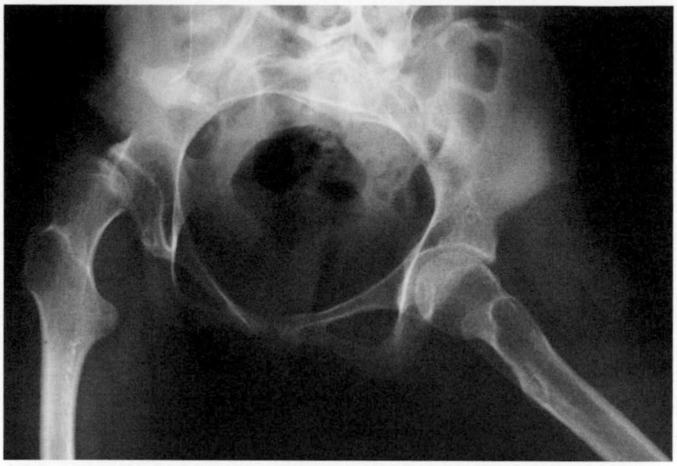

Fig. 1.12.3 Pelvic obliquity, wind-swept hips with subluxation/dislocation, and scoliosis are the most common orthopaedic problems of non-ambulatory patients with cerebral palsy.

on dynamic electromyography will eliminate spastic equinus in most patients and over half will be able to walk brace free and have improved knee and hip motion 1 year postoperatively (Figure 1.12.2). Painful toe deformities that pose problems with footwear may also require correction.

Stiff knee gait due to quadriceps spasticity and resulting in foot clearance problems may be treated with tenotomy of the rectus femoris in carefully selected patients. An increased risk of heterotopic ossification following hip surgery in stroke and head injury patients has been reported. Furthermore, stroke patients are at a higher risk of hip fracture.

Other central nervous system disorders

Patients with multiple sclerosis may present with lower-limb problems, usually as a result of spasticity. Muscle weakness and the presence of ataxia may complicate the problems further. The same principles for the management of foot problems as for stroke apply here and tendon balancing is the aim.

Adult patients with Friedreich's ataxia may present with stiff cavovarus feet that require correction. Triple fusion is required for these deformities and lengthening of tibialis posterior, and often the Achilles tendon should be performed to prevent recurrence of the deformity. Scoliosis also occurs in all patients with Friedreich's ataxia. Surgery while the patient is still ambulatory would compromise the ability to walk and should be postponed until they are confined to a wheelchair.

Patients with rapidly progressive motor neuron disease seldom require orthopaedic treatment but may present in orthopaedic clinics complaining of limb weakness, foot deformity (usually a foot-drop), or atrophy of the small muscles of the hand.

The spine

Spinal dysraphism (myelodysplasia)

Although a large number of children and adolescents with low thoracic, lumbar, or sacral myelodysplasia are ambulators, a large

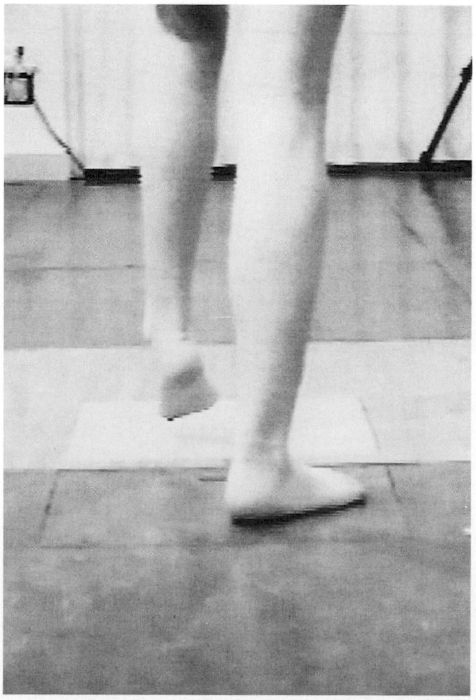

Fig. 1.12.4 Equinovarus foot in adult spastic hemiplegia due to head injury.

Box 1.12.3 Surgery for cerebral palsy

- Soft tissue releases work better in children
- Osteotomies in adults help manage rotatory and angular deformity
- Aim to release contractures without causing instability
- Balance muscles and joint alignment.

percentage of them lose the ability to walk later in adult life. Almost a third of patients with sacral-level spina bifida lose their ability for independent ambulation in adult life. Scoliosis, pelvic obliquity, hip dislocation, and knee contractures have been suggested as reasons for loss of ambulation. The level of the lesion, lower limb spasticity, the additional body weight, and the lack of sensation in the sole of the foot which leads to ulcers and deep infection are certainly some of the most important parameters.

Treatment of infection appears to be the most frequent orthopaedic treatment required for the adult myelodysplastic patient and toe, ray, Symes, or below-the-knee amputations are not infrequent.

Postpolio syndrome

The postpolio syndrome is the development of new neuromuscular symptoms, including fatigue or new muscle weakness, which may involve previously unaffected muscles and musculoskeletal complaints, usually muscle pain. Back injury, radiculopathy, compression neuropathy, and any other condition that could account for these symptoms should be first excluded. Patients' specific complaints usually include general fatigue, difficulty with motor control during walking, stair climbing, and transferring (Figure 1.12.5). The syndrome affects women more often than men and more severely affected by poliomyelitis patients are at higher risk. The prevalence of the condition is 28.5% of all paralytic poliomyelitis cases and it presents with a peak at 30–34 years after the acute illness.

New muscle weakness in poliomyelitis may be due to chronic overuse and degeneration of the surviving motor units. Nonfatiguing resistance exercise has, therefore, been suggested and results appear encouraging. Despite the new neuromuscular symptoms and functional changes the impairment status of the majority of patients remains unchanged.

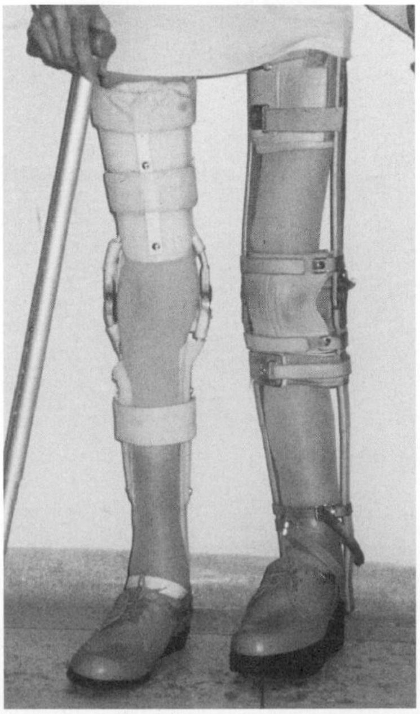

Fig. 1.12.5 Previously independent adult poliomyelitis patient who complained of fatigue and knee pain. She required knee–ankle–foot orthosis to maintain her ambulatory status.

Paraplegia and tetraplegia

Spinal stabilization is often necessary in patients with spinal injury, even in the presence of complete paraplegia or tetraplegia. Spinal fusion provides better stability for the rehabilitation period and prevents late development of deformity and pain at the fracture site.

Spasticity of the muscles around the hip and particularly the adductors, may lead to contractures that cause problems with sitting balance, access to the perineum for hygiene, pelvic obliquity, and decubitus ulceration. Soft tissue releases for the contractures and gluteus maximus flaps for the treatment of pressure sores have been suggested. Hip instability may occur following infection but is otherwise rare in the absence of dysplasia. Hip dislocation due to spasticity following spinal cord injury can occur in children under the age of 9 years and is very rare in adult spinal cord injury. Treatment principles are the same as in cerebral palsy and proximal femoral resection is sometimes the last resort. Functional electrical stimulation has been used in this field with some success.

If joint contractures secondary to muscle spasticity occur, surgical release may be necessary, particularly in patients who are able to stand or walk with the aid of orthoses. Lower extremity fractures are common in spinal cord injury patients because of the existing osteoporosis: their treatment remains controversial as both surgical and conservative treatment have advantages and disadvantages.

Neuropathies

Hereditary motor sensory neuropathies

The most common orthopaedic problem in these conditions is foot deformity, usually cavovarus (Figure 1.12.6). Hip dysplasia may be present and may become symptomatic and require treatment if coxa valga and subluxation are present. Scoliosis is also present in 10% of patients and follows the idiopathic pattern requiring bracing or arthrodesis of progressive curves.

The aggressiveness of treatment of cavovarus foot deformity depends on the rigidity of the deformity. Soft tissue procedures may include plantar release and lengthening of the Achilles tendon, with or without anterior transfer of the tibialis posterior tendon. The reasoning for the transfer is the fact that tibialis posterior is a major deforming force in the cavovarus foot and it weakens last in peripheral neuropathies. Soft tissue procedures are enough in the absence of fixed deformity. Coleman's block test determines whether the hindfoot varus is correctable or not. In the presence of uncorrectable varus, an os calcis osteotomy (displacement or wedge) is necessary. Uncorrectable cavus requires midfoot or basal metatarsal osteotomy. Early correction of the deformity with these soft tissue and simple bony procedures is preferable before skeletal maturity and results are satisfactory while long-term results of triple arthrodesis as salvage procedure for the late deformed and rigid foot is less satisfactory (Box 1.12.4).

Toe clawing is a frequent problem in these patients. Flexor tenotomy or flexor to extensor transfer for the lesser toes can be performed before the onset of fixed deformity. Fusion or interposition arthroplasty of the interphalangeal joints is necessary later. A Jones procedure, involving fusion of the interphalangeal joint and proximal transfer of the extensor hallucis longus to the neck of the first metatarsal, is indicated for the great toe deformity.

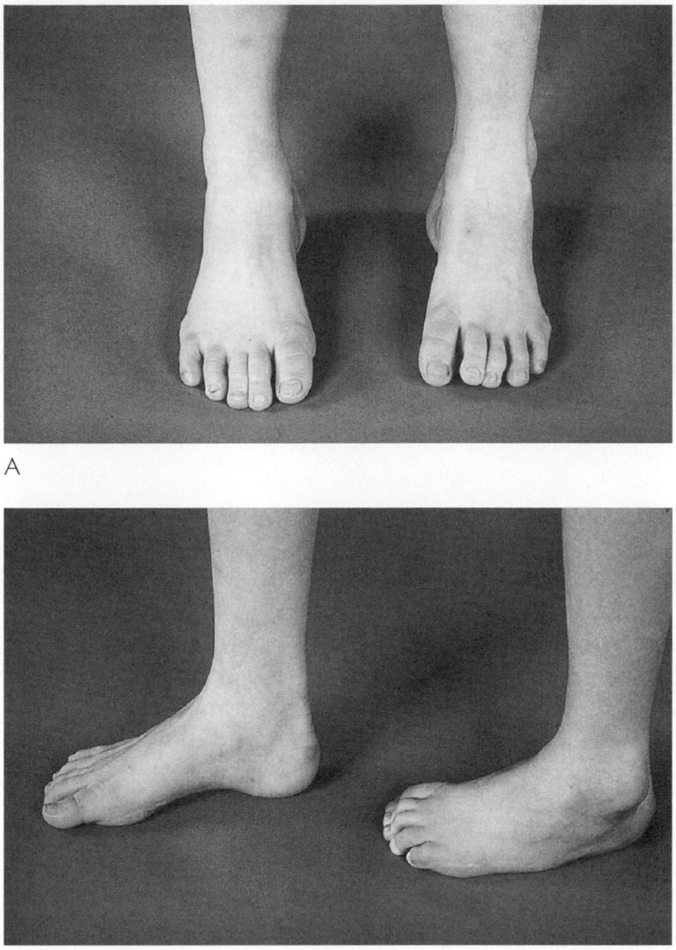

A

B

Fig. 1.12.6 Symptomatic cavovarus feet in a patient with Charcot–Marie–Tooth disease (type I hereditary motor sensory neuropathy).

Upper-extremity involvement occurs in two-thirds of these patients. Intrinsic muscle weakness, reduced sensation, and loss of dexterity are the main problems. Operative treatment is rarely indicated but may be performed to release contractures, or to lengthen or transfer tendons. Wrist fusion for stabilization may also be considered.

> **Box 1.12.4** Surgical options for foot deformities
>
> - Flexible deformity: plantar release and tibialis posterior tendon transfer
> - Rigid heel varus: calcaneal displacement osteotomy
> - Rigid plantarflexion of the first metatarsal: extension osteotomy of the first metatarsal
> - Rigid cavus: midtarsal osteotomy.

Traumatic and degenerative neuropathies (Charcot joint)

Nerve injury may be due to acute trauma or compression. This may involve nerve roots near the spinal cord, nerve stems as at the brachial plexus, and peripheral nerves. Nerve reconstruction after such injuries and tendon transfers and reconstruction after brachial plexus injuries is discussed elsewhere (see Chapters 12.26 and 6.9).

Foot-drop or loss of active dorsiflexion of the foot may be due to pathology at the peroneal nerve, sciatic nerve, or the fifth lumbar nerve root. A simple ankle–foot orthosis is recommended for early treatment in order to prevent a fixed plantar flexion deformity. If recovery of the nerve is not expected, tendon transfers may be considered. If the foot-drop is mainly due to peroneal muscle weakness while tibialis anterior maintains activity, a split lateral transfer of the tibialis anterior tendon can be considered. In the absence of tibialis anterior activity, anterior transfer of tibialis posterior may be considered and dynamic electromyography during gait may be useful to assess the activity of the muscle during the swing phase of gait.

Other conditions may cause peripheral neuropathies and diabetes is the most common. Diabetic ulcers are due to neuropathy, and prevention and patient education are effective. Musculoskeletal infection and joint neuroarthropathy (Charcot joint) can also be present in diabetes. Their differential diagnosis is based on clinical grounds and also on magnetic resonance imaging and scintigraphy.

Repetitive trauma to insensate joints, particularly the weight-bearing ones, can cause characteristic changes that define the neuropathic or Charcot joint. Changes include effusion, subluxation, and bone sclerosis, erosion, and destruction. Later, osteophytes, calcium deposits, osteochondritis, and periarticular fractures may be present. The development of characteristic Charcot changes often follows an injury that led to fracture or dislocation. If conservative treatment fails, surgery to arthrodese or replace the joint has been suggested but the failure rate is high because of the lack of sensation, and amputation may be necessary in some cases.

Myopathies

The various types of myopathies, their inheritance, and their clinical characteristics relevant to the orthopaedic surgeon are listed in Table 1.12.1. Only a few types of myopathy may require orthopaedic surgery in adulthood.

Further reading

Nagoya, S., Nagao, M., Takada, J., Kaya, M., Iwasaki, T., Yamashita, T. (2005). Long-term results of rotational acetabular osteotomy for dysplasia of the hip in adult ambulatory patients with cerebral palsy. *Journal of Bone and Joint Surgery*, **87-B**(12), 1627–30.

Pinzur, M.S., Sherman, R., DiMonte-Leine, P., *et al.* (1986). Adult-onset hemiplegia: changes in gait after muscle balancing procedures to correct the equinus deformity. *Journal of Bone and Joint Surgery*, **68-A**, 1249–57.

Shapiro, F. and Specht, L. (1993). The diagnosis and orthopaedic treatment of inherited muscular diseases of childhood. *Journal of Bone and Joint Surgery*, **75-A**, 439–54.

Shapiro, F. and Specht, L. (1993). The diagnosis and orthopaedic treatment of childhood spinal muscular atrophy, peripheral neuropathy, Friedreich ataxia and arthrogryposis. *Journal of Bone and Joint Surgery*, **75-A**, 1699–714.

1.13

Neuromuscular and skeletal manifestations of neurofibromatosis

Jeremy Fairbank

Summary points

- Neurofibromatosis type 1
- Single gene disorder
- Serious scoliosis
- Pseudoarthrosis of a long bone
- Hypertrophy of a part
- An unusual radiographic lesion of bone.

Introduction

Neurofibromatosis type 1 (NF-1) is one of the commonest single gene disorders (17q11.2) (1 in 3000–4000 live births). The gene product functions as an antitumour agent, a function suppressed in mutations. At least 40% of children with NF-1 have serious cosmetic or functional involvement of the musculoskeletal system. NF type 2 is particularly associated with acoustic neuromas (22q12.2), is much rarer (1 in 25 000), and has few, if any, musculoskeletal manifestations.

NF-1 presents to orthopaedic surgeons with spinal deformity; neurofibromas, and other tumours affecting the spinal cord and peripheral nerves; pseudarthrosis of long bones, especially the tibia; limb gigantism associated with plexiform neurofibromas; and pectus excavatum. Radiological manifestations of NF-1 frequently cause diagnostic difficulties, and may mimic other conditions. A rare but important association is with phaeochromocytoma, which should be considered before anaesthetizing anyone with NF-1.

Diagnosis

Consider NF when confronted by:

- Serious scoliosis
- Pseudoarthrosis of a long bone
- Hypertrophy of a part
- An unusual radiographic lesion of bone.

Check for a family history of NF-1. Look for cafe-au-lait spots. (The skeletal manifestations of the disease may precede the appearance of neurofibromas). There should be more than 6 spots with a diameter greater than15mm in children older than 5 years. Freckles appear in the axillae and groin later in childhood. Lisch nodules in the iris are diagnostic. These can only be seen with a slit lamp. Subcutaneous and nerve-based neurofibromas are common. There is an increased risk of developing brain tumours (especially optic glioma) and leukemia. Learning disability is common. About 2% of individuals with NF-1 also develop phaeochromocytoma. This should always be suspected in patients who are hypertensive.

Management of musculoskeletal problems

Pseudoarthrosis of long bones

Pseudoarthrosis appearing in any long bone in infancy is usually, but not always, associated with NF-1 (50–90%). The tibia is by far the most frequent (1 in 250 000 live births), but pseudoarthrosis has been observed in all of the other long bones. This is a very difficult condition to manage and beyond the scope of this text. At least six different patterns have been described (Boyd classification). Surgical treatments include: osteotomy; onlay grafts; bypass grafts; pedicle grafts; intramedullary rods; vascularized bone graft; electrical stimulation; bone transport; amputation, either as a primary procedure or as salvage.

Focal gigantism

Hypertrophy of a bone, digit, or an entire limb, combined with unusual lengthening or shortening of a bone can give serious cosmetic and practical problems. These require plastic and orthopaedic surgical expertise.

Spine

Spinal deformity occurs in about 5% of cases. Scoliosis may be indistinguishable from idiopathic scoliosis, or be dysplastic with short segment aggressive deformities with loss of part or all of the vertebral body that require surgical treatment. Kyphosis is commonly associated with dysplastic spines. This may present challenging problems for the surgeon, though not usually sufficient to damage the spinal cord unless there is dislocation of the spine or a large meningocoele. It is best to avoid resection of tumours associated with dysplastic curves. Other features are scalloping of the posterior margin of vertebral bodies; enlargement of the intervertebral foramina; pedicle defects; vertebral body dysplasia; dumb-bell tumours; dural ectasia (a saccular dilatation of the dura, sometimes with extensive protrusion of the dura out of the intervertebral foramen); lateral meningocele; and, rarely, intrathoracic meningoceles. Spinal tumours, both intra- and extradural are common and include neurofibromas, gliomas, meningiomas and schwannomas.

Plexiform neurofibromas

These are extensive tumours involving muscle and bone especially in the pelvis and lower limbs. They are difficult or impossible to resect. Many remain stable, but may become malignant. Magnetic resonance can be used to monitor size and shape. Positron emission tomography scanning seems a good method for identifying malignant change.

Radiographic features

NF-1 patients have a high frequency of skeletal involvement, sphenoid dysplasia is diagnostic. Bone deformities are caused by destruction by neurofibromatous tissue, aberrations of skeletal growth, abnormal development of body parts or systems, malignant bone tumours, intervertebral foramenal enlargement, cortical bone defects, bone cyst formation, bowing of long bones, and pseudoarthrosis of long bones.

Management

This is focused on the management of complications. This can be complex and challenging. Resection of individual tumors should be confined to those that are symptomatic.

Further reading

Fairbank, J. (1994). Orthopaedic manifestations of neurofibromatosis. In Huson, S. and Hughes, R. (eds.) *The Neurofibromatoses*. London: Chapman and Hall.

SECTION 2

Bone and Soft Tissue Tumours

2.1

Choice of surgery for tumour: Staging and surgical margins

Panagiotis D. Gikas and Timothy W.R. Briggs

Introduction

Bone and soft tissue tumours are rare and constitute less than 1% of all malignancies. Such tumours should, when possible, be treated at specialized tertiary centres where there is a dedicated multidisciplinary team of medical, nursing, and counselling services to manage these often difficult problems.

A poorly performed biopsy at a non-specialist centre is reported to be the major cause of error and failure of limb salvage in two review articles. Although the procedure itself is not complicated, the indications for using this technique, the choice of needle, the appropriate setting, the anatomic site, the distribution of tissue, and the potential need for adjuvant treatment all must be carefully considered prior to performing the biopsy. Needle biopsies should be viewed as surgical procedures and are associated with risks and hazards.

Important issues that must be considered when performing biopsies for suspicion of tumour include:

- Understanding the indications, based on clinical and radiographic information
- Obtaining appropriate staging studies
- Choosing the best biopsy technique: excisional versus incisional; closed versus open
- Performing the biopsy through an appropriate anatomic approach
- Obtaining representative, diagnostic tissue
- Careful handling of the biopsy specimen
- Avoiding complications.

Biopsies are best performed in specialist centres under the supervision of an orthopaedic surgical oncologist who will ultimately be responsible for the definitive care of the patient and who is working in close collaboration with an expert musculoskeletal radiologist and pathologist.

Staging for musculoskeletal tumours (Box 2.1.1)

Accurate preoperative surgical staging of musculoskeletal tumours is currently possible because of advanced imaging techniques, providing diagnostic information and helping clinicians in choosing the most appropriate treatment option for the patient. The aims of surgical staging are to determine the surgical margins of resection and to facilitate interinstitutional and interdisciplinary communication regarding treatment data and results.

There are two aspects to staging musculoskeletal tumours, namely clinical staging and pathologic grading. Clinical staging defines the local and systemic extent of the disease which is required in the planning of treatment to achieve both local and distal control. Clinical staging relies on a variety of imaging studies which not only pinpoint the anatomical location of the tumour but also serve as baseline indices for post-treatment comparisons. Pathologic grading categorizes tumours according to their predicted biological behaviour which may range from indolence to widespread metastasis (determined by a combination of features including cellularity, degree of pleomorphism, mitotic activity, necrosis, and infiltrative nature). Pathologic grading relies on biopsy of the tumour and therefore should follow clinical staging.

Plain radiography is the initial imaging modality in the evaluation of bone tumours. Some benign lesions have characteristic radiographic features that make biopsy unnecessary. Examples include fibrous cortical defects, bone islands, simple bone cysts, and bone infarcts. Radiographic features can also help in distinguishing malignant from benign bone lesions in many patients. The important radiographic signs for grading bone tumours are listed as follows, in order of priority:

- Pattern of destruction: geographic or not geographic, appearance of marginal interface zone
- Penetration of the cortex by the lesion
- Absence or presence of a sclerotic rim
- Absence or presence of the expanded cortical shell, as well as its extent.

In the staging of bone tumours, computed tomography (CT) scanning has a role in the detailed evaluation of local disease and in assessing the lungs for pulmonary metastases. It can be used to assess disease in areas that are not easily visualized with plain radiographs, such as the spine and pelvis.

Magnetic resonance imaging (MRI) (with or without contrast) is the modality of choice for imaging and staging of musculoskeletal tumours. Accurate depiction of the soft tissues allows sensitive detection of soft tissue extension and medullary involvement by a tumour.

Certain lesions have appearances that are usually characteristic enough for a diagnosis to be made based on MRI findings. Examples of such lesions include lipomas, superficial and skeletal muscle haemangiomas, benign neural tumours, periarticular cysts, haematomas, and pigmented villonodular synovitis.

MRI is increasingly used to assess tumour response to preoperative chemotherapy. This assessment is achieved by evaluating changes in a tumour's size, margins, signal intensity, and enhancement patterns. Moreover, MRI can be useful in differentiating tumour recurrence from chronic post-therapeutic changes.

Radionuclide bone scanning has a role in detecting metastases, skip lesions, lesion multiplicity, and postoperative tumour recurrence. Bone-forming, metastatic lesions in the lungs (e.g. osteosarcoma) are occasionally detected with bone scintigraphy.

Soft tissue masses and the soft tissue components of bony tumours may be visualized by using ultrasonography (US). The aim of ultrasonography in the evaluation of musculoskeletal lesions is to confirm the presence of a lesion, to determine if the lesion is cystic or solid, to assess the relationship of the mass to the surrounding structures (e.g. neurovascular bundle), to evaluate the vascularity of the mass, and to guide interventional procedures if indicated.

The role of angiography has largely been replaced by cross-sectional imaging modalities. Angiography can still have a preoperative role in decreasing tumour size by allowing embolization of feeding vessels and a postoperative role in decreasing haemorrhage, again through the embolization of tumour-supplying vessels.

Positron emission tomography (PET) scanning has been shown to have sensitivity similar to that of serial CT scanning and MRI for detecting lesions and for distinguishing postsurgical scarring from recurrent tumours. However, the specificity of PET is higher than that of serial CT scanning or MRI making it better in depicting residual/recurrent disease after treatment. The main disadvantage of PET scanning is the high cost of the equipment, therefore limiting availability.

Percutaneous needle biopsy is now standard practice. Given the increase in the use of CT and ultrasound for accurate needle placement, biopsy is now primarily a radiologist-led procedure.

Enneking system for surgical staging of malignant bone and soft tissue tumours

The Enneking system for the surgical staging of bone and soft tissue tumours is based on grade (G), site (T), and metastasis (M) and uses histological, radiological, and clinical criteria. It is the most widely used staging system and has been adopted by the Musculoskeletal Tumour Society. This system should be used for staging mesenchymal lesions only, because their biological behaviour differs from that of non-mesenchymal tumours (e.g. Ewing sarcoma, lymphoma, and leukemia).

Grade

Bone tumours are graded as follows:

- G0: benign lesion
- G1: low-grade malignant lesion
- G2: high-grade malignant lesion.

Surgical grade generally follows histological grade; however, a higher surgical grade may be applied if the radiographical features and clinical behaviour of a lesion indicate an aggressiveness that is incompatible with its benign histological features.

Site

The site and local extent of bone tumours are classified as follows:

- T0: a benign tumour that is confined within a true capsule and the lesion's anatomical compartment of origin (i.e. a benign intracapsular, intracompartmental lesion)
- T1: an aggressive benign or malignant tumour that is still confined within its anatomical compartment (i.e. an intra-compartmental lesion)
- T2: a lesion that has spread beyond its anatomical compartment of origin (i.e. an extracompartmental lesion).

Metastasis

Metastatic classification is as follows:

- M0: no regional or distant metastasis
- M1: regional or distant metastasis.

Under the Enneking system, malignant tumours are classified into stages I–III, with further subdivisions into A and B. Grade 1 and grade 2 tumours are stage I and stage II, respectively. T1 and T2 tumours are stage A and stage B, respectively. Tumours with distant metastasis are stage III (Table 2.1.1).

Enneking staging system for benign tumors

The Enneking staging system divides benign tumours into latent, active, or aggressive tumours (Table 2.1.2). Latent tumours are asymptomatic and are usually discovered incidentally. They reach

Table 2.1.1 Enneking system for the staging of malignant bone and soft tissue tumours

Stage	Grade	Site	Metastasis
IA	G1	T1	M0
IB	G2	T2	M0
IIA	G2	T1	M0
IIB	G2	T2	M0
III	G1 or G2	T1 or T2	M1

Table 2.1.2 Enneking system for staging of benign lesions

Stage	Description	Grade	Site	Metastasis
1	Latent	G0	T0	M0
2	Active	G0	T0	M0
3	Aggressive	G0	T1 or T2	M0 or M1

a stage of non-growth after a period of slow growth. Active tumours are mildly symptomatic and may be discovered if pathologic fracture occurs or if the tumour is associated with mechanical dysfunction. Active tumours usually grow steadily. Aggressive benign lesions grow rapidly and usually are symptomatic and tender on palpation.

Surgical margins (Box 2.1.2)

Surgery is the mainstay of treatment for musculoskeletal tumours. These tumours are surrounded by a non-tumorous reactive zone containing inflammatory cells and neo-vascular tissue. This pseudocapsule contains microscopic extensions of tumour which may be continuous with, or satellites of, the main tumour mass (Figures 2.1.1 and 2.1.2).

Intralesional margins imply a procedure which crosses the pseudocapsule and enters into the substance of the tumour. Often tumour tissue is removed piecemeal. Curettage is an example of intralesional surgery. Recurrence can be high with intralesional margins in incomplete curettages as macroscopic evidence of tumour remains after surgery. Intralesional margins are only used in benign tumours such as bone cysts, aneurysmal bone cysts, and giant cell tumours.

Marginal margins are those in which a tumour is removed in one piece and the plane of dissection passes through the pseudocapsule or reactive zone. Excisional biopsies or tumours which are shelled out are examples of surgery with marginal margins, and microscopic residual tumour may exist. Recurrent rates of malignant tumours are high after surgery with marginal margins if adjuvant chemotherapy is not used.

Wide margins include the entire tumour and its pseudocapsule or reactive zone and a cuff of normal tissue en bloc. During this procedure, tumour is never seen. Consensus has not been reached on the definition of what constitutes a cuff of normal tissue. In principle, the proximal or distal cut edge of normal muscle represents a wide margin if it is 5cm or more from the tumour border. Removal of bone at a similar distance beyond the tumour also constitutes a wide margin. Surgical margins which include the normal fascia surrounding the muscle of an intramuscular tumour are regarded as wide even though the absolute thickness of the muscle and fascial cuff may only be 1–2mm. Synovium or periosteum which covers the periosteal extension of a distal femoral tumour is regarded as an anatomic barrier and if excised en bloc with the tumour constitutes a wide margin even though again the thickness of the tissue may be 1–2mm.

Box 2.1.1 Staging—summary

- Clinical staging defines the local and systemic extent of the disease; it relies on a variety of imaging studies
- Pathological grading categorizes tumours according to their predicted biological behaviour; it relies on biopsy of the tumour and therefore should follow clinical staging
- The Enneking system for the surgical staging of bone and soft tissue tumours is based on grade (G), site (T), and metastasis (M) and uses histological, radiological, and clinical criteria.

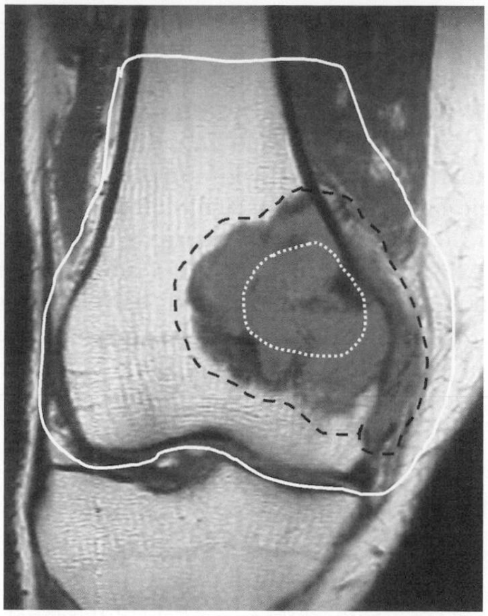

Fig. 2.1.1 Coronal MRI of distal femoral osteosarcoma with extraosseous extension of tumour. The intralesional margin (dotted line), the marginal margin (broken line), and the wide margin (full line) are indicated. A radical margin would be a resection of the entire tumour-containing compartment which would imply a total femoral resection.

Radical margins are achieved when the entire tumour-bearing compartment is removed en bloc. For bone sarcomas, radical margins include the en bloc removal of the bone of origin and the entire soft tissue compartment into which the tumour has entered. For soft tissue sarcomas, this includes anatomical fascia surrounding that compartment and bony borders when present. Radical margins are associated with the lowest risk of recurrence.

With limb-sparing surgery as the preferred technique, the majority of uncomplicated bone or soft tissue resections aim at complete uncontaminated surgical margins. The use of chemotherapy has improved the rate of local control in osteosarcoma while allowing

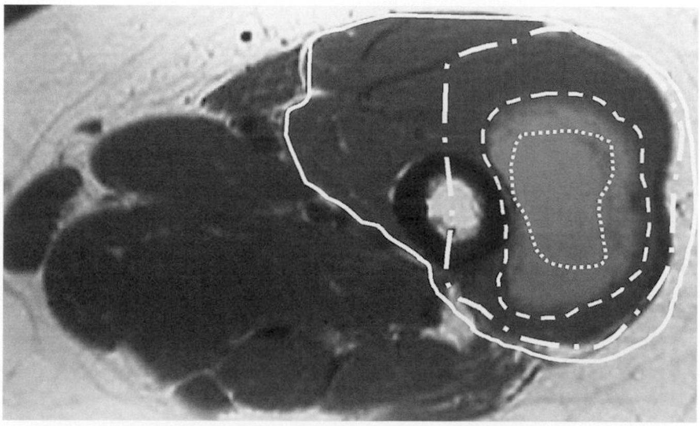

Fig. 2.1.2 Axial MRI of soft-tissue sarcoma of the thigh lying adjacent to the mid-diaphysis of the femur. The intralesional margin (dotted line), the marginal margin (broken line), and the wide margin (chain line) are all indicated. A radical margin (full line) would be a resection of the entire tumour-containing compartment, which in this case would mean a total quadriceps resection including a section of femoral diaphysis.

wide excisional limb-sparing surgery. Similarly, radiotherapy has had a major influence on decreasing the size of surgical margins in soft tissue sarcoma resections. Specifically, combination radiotherapy and marginal surgery has had the same results as surgery with wide margins alone, and the recurrence rates for surgery with wide margins combined with radiotherapy are similar for radical surgical margins alone. If vital neurovascular structures are adjacent to the tumour, marginal surgery may be selected and combined with adjuvant therapy. In selected tumours, such as those which are completely within a single muscle, or subcutaneous and not engaging the deep fascia, surgery with wide margins alone may be sufficient to achieve local control. Decisions regarding choice and combination of modalities need to be tailored to each case.

Biopsy techniques (Box 2.1.3)

Now that staging has been completed, the decision to perform a biopsy is considered. Plain radiographs of bone lesions are often diagnostic or can significantly narrow the differential and aid in determining whether or not a biopsy should be performed (i.e. a classic osteochondroma or osteoid osteoma needs no biopsy prior to excision).

Open incisional biopsy is the conventional method for obtaining a representative specimen and is considered to be the 'gold standard.' In carefully selected patients, closed needle or trephine biopsies are appropriate. This is a well established practice, with a reported accuracy of 78–97%. The site and method of approach must provide samples that are adequate for diagnosis and deliver them with the minimum amount of morbidity. Two attempts at percutaneous biopsy are justified. Percutaneous biopsy yield compares well with open biopsy and is more cost-effective. In experienced hands, percutaneous biopsy can be performed quickly, with less patient morbidity, and at a fraction of the cost of open surgical biopsies. Closed biopsies are ideal for difficult-to-access lesions in the vertebrae and pelvis and can be performed under CT or fluoroscopic guidance. Additionally, needle biopsies, when compared to open biopsies, lessen the risk of potential biopsy complications such as tumour spillage or haematoma and contamination, wound dehiscence, and infection. Finally, a needle biopsy tract is easier to excise en bloc with the final resection specimen. Different systems exist allowing percutaneous biopsy of musculoskeletal lesions:

- Fine needle aspiration (FNA) with a small, 18- to 23-gauge needle: FNA obtains a few cells for morphologic evaluation by a cytopathologist. Tissue is generally not available for further pathologic studies and is subject to sampling error. The architecture of the lesion is not preserved, making the diagnosis more difficult. FNA has been used successfully in select instances. The role of the cytopathologist in interpreting the sample is to decide whether the lesion is benign or malignant, primary, or metastatic. Thus, FNA is best employed to confirm suspected metastatic tumours, recurrent tumours at primary or metastatic sites such as lymph nodes, and, occasionally, suspected non-neoplastic conditions such as osteomyelitis
- Core needle biopsy with a cannulated, cutting trocar system to obtain a core of tissue
- Trephine system utilizing a stout, sharp bone cutting tool: the main advantage of core needle biopsy and trephine biopsy over FNA is the ability to preserve tissue architecture, facilitating both histological diagnosis and grading.

All biopsy tracts must be resected en bloc with the tumour at the definitive surgical procedure. Even needle biopsies can leave behind viable tumour cells that are a potential source for local recurrence, despite adjuvant treatment. Therefore, the skin puncture must be marked with India ink or a modest stitch so it can be identified later, even after weeks of neoadjuvant therapy.

CT guidance is used primarily for bone-based pathology and for deep soft tissue tumours that are beyond the focus of a standard ultrasound probe. CT also allows biopsy of smaller lesions with confidence and the final position of the needle can be reliably recorded. This is important for retrospective confirmation of needle position in non-diagnostic pathology reports. Ultrasound is suitable for superficial soft tissue lesions and for bone-based pathology such as osteosarcomas which commonly have a large extraosseous 'soft tissue' component at the time of presentation. The avoidance of critical anatomical structures within the biopsy field will affect the choice of guidance system and both CT and ultrasound may play a role. In certain centres, specialist biopsy-designed MRI is now available.

Box 2.1.2 Surgical margins—summary

- Musculoskeletal tumours are surrounded by a non-tumorous reactive zone (pseudocapsule)
- Intralesional margins imply a procedure which crosses the pseudocapsule and enters into the substance of the tumour
- Marginal margins are those in which a tumour is removed in one piece and the plane of dissection passes through the pseudocapsule
- Wide margins include the entire tumour and its pseudocapsule or reactive zone and a cuff of normal tissue en bloc
- Radical margins are achieved when the entire tumour-bearing compartment is removed en bloc.

Needle systems

Several needle systems have been devised for biopsies of the musculoskeletal system. In our unit we routinely use two needle types:

Jamshidi® needle

This cutting needle with a tapered end (aiding tissue retention) and a disposable trocar is used for lesions that are predominantly osteoblastic and centrally sited within bone, or for predominantly lytic or mixed intraosseous lesions that have an intact surrounding rim or cortex (Figure 2.1.3). It is unsuitable for soft tissue biopsy work.

Tru-Cut® or Temno® (preloaded) needles

These are predominantly used for extraosseous soft tissue specimens, or when cortical bone destruction allows access to the medulla (Figure 2.1.4). Hemorrhagic lesions may fail to produce a

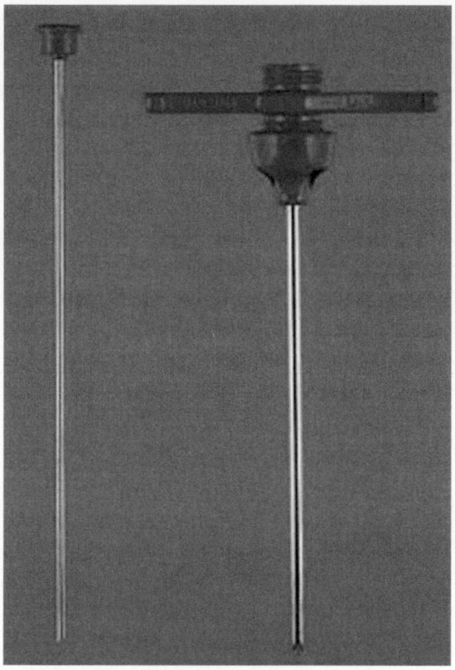

Fig. 2.1.3 A Jamshidi® needle system.

satisfactory core, but direction under ultrasound or CT guidance improves the diagnostic yield. Multiple specimens can be provided for the histopathologist.

Technique

Full aseptic conditions are observed in all cases, and the appropriate method of anaesthesia, depending on the age of the patient, is selected.

Having chosen the radiological technique that complements the percutaneous biopsy, a small stab incision is made with a No. 15 blade at the site of entry of the needle and the selected needle type inserted. Care must be taken in cases of suspected malignant but contained lesions not to take the needle beyond the point of natural tissue hold-up. For example, with a subperiosteal osteosarcoma contamination of the medulla from the biopsy must be avoided. In tumours close to joints it is imperative that the biopsy is located in such a way that the joint cavity is not contaminated by needle placement.

With all specimens care is taken to reduce tissue crush. Specimens should ideally be delivered fresh and unfixed to the histopathology department allowing imprint preparation to be made to ensure that lesional tissue is present in a sample. In cases of potential infective diagnoses, additional samples must be sent for microbiology examination.

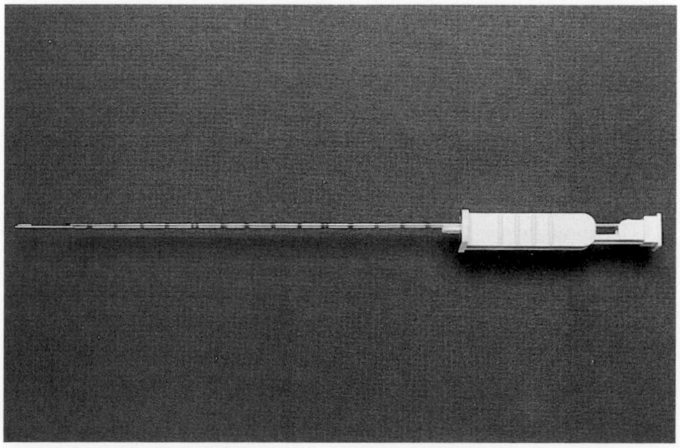

Fig. 2.1.4 A Tru-Cut® needle.

Complications

Any biopsy is a surgical procedure and is associated with potential risks and complications. A poorly executed or interpreted biopsy increases the risk of error in diagnosis, wound complication, and a potentially deleterious change in treatment course or outcome, including the need for a more complex resection or amputation, increased risk for local recurrence, or death. Because of the small sample size, needle biopsies are more subject to: 1) errors in diagnosis, particularly in grade of heterogeneous tumours; 2) anatomical misrepresentation resulting in obtaining non-diagnostic or indeterminate tissue; and 3) inability to perform research studies or special diagnostic studies such as cytogenetics or flow cytometry which may be necessary for definitive diagnosis, as is the case with small blue cell malignancies.

Therefore, when the diagnosis, based on needle biopsy, is in reasonable doubt having been reviewed by a specialist musculoskeletal pathologist, the clinician must proceed as though no biopsy had been performed. Frequently, this means repeating the biopsy, usually by the conventional open technique.

Conclusion

Optimizing surgical margins, and thus local control of tumour, requires accurate preoperative imaging of the tumour and surrounding anatomy. Surgical planning includes the selection of an appropriate position for the biopsy site. Improperly placed biopsy incisions may prevent the possibility of limb salvage surgery.

Needle biopsy of bone and soft tissue tumours is both safe and accurate when performed in a specialist centre. Radiologists are best placed to perform most biopsies as they have a number of imaging modalities at their disposal, enabling them to take the most appropriate tissue sample. The main disadvantage to pathologists is the small amount of tissue available.

Box 2.1.3 Biopsy techniques—summary

- Open incisional biopsy is considered to be the 'gold standard'
- Percutaneous biopsy yield compares well with open biopsy, is more cost-effective, with less patient morbidity, and at a fraction of the cost of open surgical biopsies
- All biopsy tracts must be resected en bloc with the tumour at the definitive surgical procedure
- Careful planning is necessary and good collaboration between surgeons, radiologists, and pathologists is crucial to avoid unnecessary/dangerous procedures.

Further reading

Enneking, W.F., Spanier, S.S., and Goodman, M.A. (1980). A system for the surgical staging of musculoskeletal sarcoma. *Clinical Orthopaedics and Related Research*, **153**, 106–20.

Mankin, H.J., Mankin, C.J., and Simon, M.A. (1996). The hazards of the biopsy; revisited. *Journal of Bone and Joint Surgery*, **78-A**, 656–63.

Saifuddin, A., Mitchell, R., Burnett, S., Sandison, A., and Pringle, J. (2000). Ultrasound guided needle biopsy of primary bone tumours. *Journal of Bone and Joint Surgery*, **82-B**, 50–4.

Springfield, D.S. and Rosenberg, A. (1996). Biopsy: complicated and risky. *Journal of Bone and Joint Surgery*, **78-A**, 639–43.

2.2

Amputations, endoprosthetic joint replacement, massive bone replacement, other alternatives

William J.S. Aston, Gordon Blunn, and Timothy W.R. Briggs

Summary points

- The aims of the bone tumour surgeon are to improve survival and maintain optimal function of the patient; this can be achieved by amputation or limb salvage
- Limb salvage provides no greater risk to the survival of the patient than with amputation
- Reconstruction after removal of the tumour is commonly achieved by using endoprosthetic replacements, autografts, or massive allografts
- Complications of limb salvage include infection and difficulties associated with soft tissue reattachment and coverage of the bone replacement.

Introduction

The aim of the bone tumour surgeon is to improve the survival and maintain optimum function for the patient. To achieve this, a segment of bone has to be removed and often surrounding soft tissues associated with the tumour are sacrificed aiming to achieve complete clearance of the tumour. The addition of adjuvant chemotherapy has greatly improved the outcome of this technique.

If limb salvage will not achieve tumour clearance then amputation should be undertaken. Survivorship and local recurrence rates in patients with osteosarcoma are similar for amputation and limb salvage.

Limb salvage may be undertaken by endoprosthetic replacement, massive bone replacement, or other alternatives which will be discussed later.

Amputation

Amputation of the affected limb is performed when limb-sparing surgery would leave inadequate resection margins to gain local control of disease and when resection would leave the limb useless due to sacrifice of the neurovascular bundle.

When comparing amputation to limb salvage the survival rates and local recurrence rates are similar and therefore limb salvage provides no greater risk to the survival of the patient than with amputation. Functional comparison between the two treatments has shown better function in the limb salvage group and less energy expenditure. If the amputation level is above the knee then limb reconstruction patients function better. Preservation of the knee joint has better results when compared to arthrodesis or rotationplasty.

Limb salvage

A number of issues need addressing when considering whether a patient is suitable for limb salvage and limb reconstruction. Patient considerations include the general health of the patient, the degree of metastatic disease and therefore the expected survivorship, and whether the patient wants to take on the risks associated with limb salvage. Surgical considerations include whether or not reconstruction to produce a functional limb is possible with regard to which muscles and neurovascular structures will be left after tumour clearance, whether the physes have fused, the age and size of the immature patient, and how much remaining bone will be left for fixation of the prosthesis/graft to the bone either with a stem, extracortical plates, or both. Limb salvage is more cost-effective when compared with amputation.

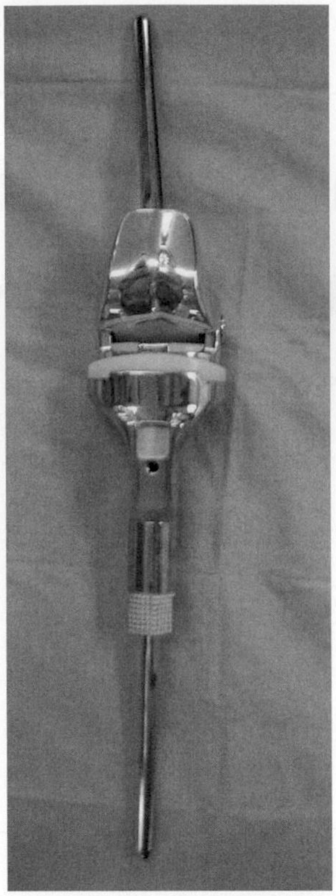

Fig. 2.2.1 A rotating hinge knee prosthesis and proximal tibial replacement (SMILES®, Stanmore Modular Individualised Lower Extremity System).

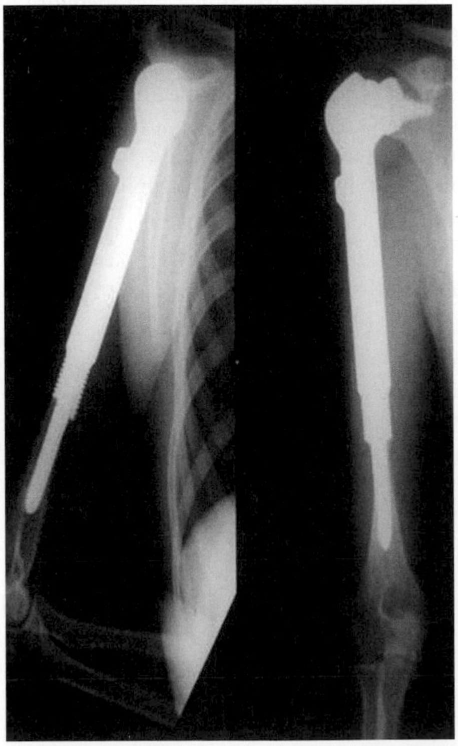

Fig. 2.2.2 Anteroposterior and lateral radiographs of the right humerus showing a proximal humeral replacement *in situ*.

Endoprosthetic replacement

Endoprostheses in the context of limb salvage for bone tumours have been used extensively since the 1970s in bone tumour centres. Endoprosthetic replacement usually involves replacing one or more joints with an associated segment of the adjoining bone (Figures 2.2.1 and 2.2.2). In some cases a joint-sparing procedure, with replacement of the intervening segment, may be possible, such as in the case of a diaphyseal replacement. Traditionally these prostheses have been custom made and more recently modular off-the-shelf systems have been developed. Custom-made replacements are used for specific cases or if a growing prosthesis is required in an immature patient.

Survivorship of endoprosthetic replacements

Survival of massive endoprostheses is not as good as primary arthroplasty. Ten-year survival with mechanical failure as the end point is 75% and for failure for any cause is 58%. The limb salvage rate at 20 years is reported as 84%.

Infection rates are high and comparable to other methods of massive reconstruction. Patients with significantly increased risk are those with pelvic or proximal tibial reconstruction, radiation therapy, and paediatric expandable prostheses. If the prostheses remain infection free and are strong enough to avoid mechanical failure then aseptic loosening becomes the main problem. Survival rates are different, depending on the anatomical location and are related to the patient's age and the amount of bone remaining after tumour resection.

Modes of failure and factors influencing failure

Aseptic loosening is more common in distal femoral and proximal tibial resections than the proximal femur. Another factor influencing the survival of distal femoral replacements is the amount of bone resected at the time of the operation. The removal of less bone increases the survival of the implant due to the decreased offset loading at the interface of the intramedullary stem with the bone. Taking all this into account the poorest outcomes, with regard to loosening, are in the under 20 age group, with greater than 60% resection of the femur.

Loosening secondary to osteolysis begins at the interface between the implant and the shoulder of the bone producing a reduction in the bone density and progresses towards the tip of the implant.

In order to combat this problem fixation has been augmented by collars allowing bone to integrate with the implant aiming to form a bony bridge and therefore a biological fixation. Collars have been made of sintered porous titanium beads and can be augmented with bone graft. Hydroxyapatite-coated collars (Figure 2.2.3) have been shown to provide more reliable bone integration in up to 70% of cases compared to no ingrowth recorded in non-grafted porous collars on a review of retrieval specimens at our institution. It was also shown that size of the radiolucent lines around the intermedullary cemented stem is inversely proportional to the amount of ingrowth on the collar. The risk of revision for aseptic loosening is reduced by 52% in distal femoral replacements when a rotating hinge is used compared to a fixed hinge design. In proximal tibial replacement the risk of revision at 10 years for aseptic loosening is 46% when using a fixed hinged design and reduced to 3% when using a rotating hinge.

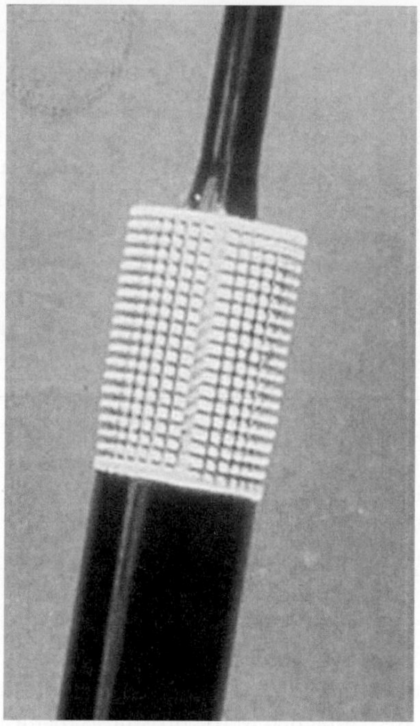

Fig. 2.2.3 A hydroxyapatite coated collar.

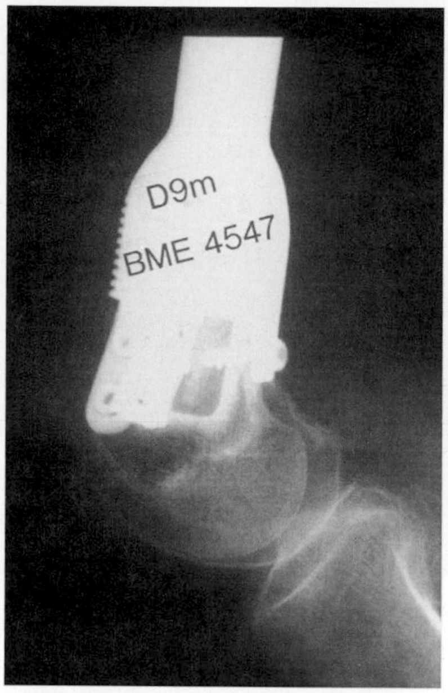

Fig. 2.2.4 A joint-sparing/diaphyseal femoral replacement.

Loosening can be reduced by the use of porous-coated uncemented intramedullary stems with additional stabilization with extramedullary plates and screws. In comparison to cemented intramedullary stems the incidence of aseptic loosening is reduced; however, other complications may arise, such as implant failure and bony resorption under the shoulder of the stem, potentially making revision more difficult. This has led to the use of partially-coated stems aiming to reduce stress protection and therefore bony resorption under the collar.

Pelvic replacements

Periacetabular tumour resection and reconstruction has become a viable alternative to hindquarter amputation. Often there is a long period from the onset of symptoms to diagnosis of tumours in this region and this makes extensive resections necessary. Complications related to the surgery are high (infection, dislocation) and reconstruction options include: arthrodesis, allografts, a saddle-type femoral prosthesis, or a hemipelvic reconstruction with a total hip replacement.

Diaphyseal/joint-sparing replacements

In some cases replacement of the diaphysis of a long bone is possible without replacement of the associated joint (Figure 2.2.4). In patients where complete excision of the bone tumour would leave an intact joint with only a very small segment of metaphyseal/diaphyseal bone, rather than sacrifice the joint some advocate the use of a joint-sparing prosthesis in selected patients. These prostheses use individualized methods of fixation of the segment close to the joint.

Growing prostheses

Large numbers of bone tumours occur in adolescents. Resection often necessitates excision of the epiphyseal growth plates particularly around the knee in the immature skeleton, causing subsequent leg length discrepancy with continuing growth. Extendible prostheses were first used in 1976.

There is an actively growing part which replaces the growth plate and a passively growing part which fixes the device on the other side of the joint to be replaced. Most designs have relied on a worm screw mechanism which is turned by a hexagonal screw driver inserted through a small incision. Apart from aseptic loosening, infection is the major complication of this type of implant. Secondary to the multiple surgical interventions infection rates of up to 40% have been published.

The major development in recent years is that of non-invasive growing implants (Figure 2.2.5). The worm screw mechanism is replaced by a gear box and magnet which is driven by electromagnetic induction, enabling lengthening of the limb with no anaesthetic, in much smaller increments and on a more regular basis. This negates the need for multiple repeat procedures and has been shown to decrease the rate of infection. It also reduces others complications such as loss of range of motion requiring physiotherapy, associated with lengthening in larger increments.

Revision of massive implants

Revision in this group of patients is unfortunately common and challenging when compared to primary arthroplasty. This is due to the relatively young population, for which the advent of chemotherapy has meant that a significant proportion of them can expect to outlive their implant. Functional limb salvage in these patients is therefore dependant on the longevity of the implant and the success of subsequent revision procedures. Options for revision are varied and highly tailored to the individual situation. The most common method of revision is the use of another massive prosthesis. Revision is technically challenging due to the loss of bone stock associated with the initial procedure and secondary to the mode of loosening. The implant design in this situation is crucial and may

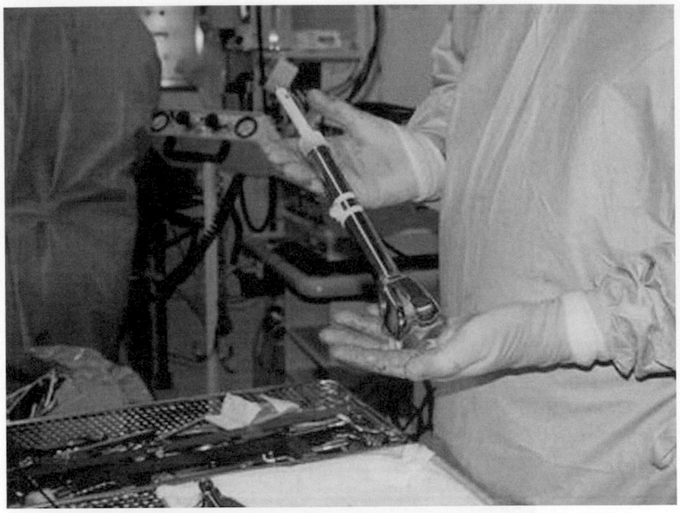

Fig. 2.2.5 A non-invasively growing distal femoral replacement.

be modified from the traditional stem fixation by extracortical plates with or without stem fixation, cortical and medullary screw fixation, fluted stems, and the use of hydroxyapatite.

Rotationplasty has been advocated for failed endoprosthetic reconstruction. Other options for revision include the use of allografts, arthrodesis, and amputation.

Massive bone replacement

An alternative to endoprosthetic replacement is the use of autografts and allografts for reconstruction. These grafts are fixed in position with plates or intramedullary nails.

Autografts

Autografts can be vascularized or not and most commonly are taken from the fibula. These have been used for all types of reconstruction. En bloc resection of the bone and tumour, then irradiation with 50Gy and then re-implantation with or without a vascularized fibula graft has also been advocated.

Allografts

Massive allografts have problems associated with their use, including infection, fracture, and early-onset osteoarthritis.

Other alternatives

These include tumour excision and arthrodesis of the joint with or without a graft and excision without any bony replacement such as the Tikhoff–Lindberg procedure. Rotationplasty has been described for the management of tumours around the knee. It involves excision of the tumour and the knee joint, rotation of the remaining tibia through 180 degrees, and fixation to the remaining femur, leaving the ankle joint at the level of the contralateral knee as the functional joint and enables prosthetic fitting. It has also been advocated as a revision procedure for failed limb salvage.

Distraction osteogenesis after excision of tumour has been used mainly in the tibia and around the knee, with good to excellent functional results.

Complications of limb salvage

These encompass all the complications associated with primary arthroplasty of the particular anatomical location, but at significantly increased rates. Most complications are associated with the soft tissue coverage of the implant and the musculature required to drive the prosthesis. One of the most challenging areas with regard to the soft tissues is around the knee. Commonly significant amounts of tissue have to be resected to enable tumour clearance, leaving the patient with a deficient extensor mechanism and a soft-tissue defect. The gastrocnemius rotation flap is commonly used to cover the defect around the knee and has been shown to significantly improve outcome with regards to the infection rate in proximal tibial replacement. Other solutions include myocutaneous latissimus dorsi free flaps.

Proximal tibial resection produces a deficient extensor mechanism by removing the tubercle. Current methods of reconstruction include turning down the middle third of the patella tendon with a central block of patella bone and attachment to the prosthesis by means of wires or plate and screw fixation into a hydroxyapatite-coated trough or simply a soft tissue reconstruction incorporating the patella tendon and a gastrocnemius flap. In other areas of the body tendons are reattached to the prosthesis by means of strategically placed suture holes through the prosthesis or to a prolene mesh placed around the prosthesis, such as around the shoulder girdle.

Resections around the proximal humerus produce a gross deficit in rotator cuff function and subsequently subluxation of the head of the prosthesis during movement can become a problem. To combat this, mesh reconstruction from the glenoid labrum to the shaft of the humerus can be used, or alternatively a captive glenoid component can be used. A stable construct should be the treatment goal in shoulder reconstruction, in order to enable effective function of the arm and hand.

Functional outcomes

Functional outcome is measured by three main scores to enable and standardize the assessment of function after limb salvage or ablative surgery in tumour patients. The Musculoskeletal Tumour Society (MSTS) score is filled out by the clinician and assigns values on a scale of 0–5 for pain, function, emotional acceptance, walking ability, use of supports, and gait. In the upper limb, gait, walking ability, and use of supports is replaced by hand positioning, manual dexterity, and lifting ability. The Toronto Extremity Salvage Score measures physical function and the Short Form 36 is used to represent the patient's perception of their mental and physical health. These two are filled out by the patient.

Further reading

Blunn, G.W., Briggs, T.W.R., Cannon, S.R., *et al.* (2000). Cementless fixation for primary segmental bone tumour endoprostheses. *Clinical Orthopaedics and Related Research*, **372**, 223–30.

Gupta, A., Meswania, J., Pollock, R., *et al.* (2006). Non-invasive distal femoral expandable endoprosthesis for limb-salvage surgery in paediatric tumours. *Journal of Bone and Joint Surgery*, **88-B**(5), 649–54.

Jaiswal, P.K., Aston, W.J.S., Grimer, R.J., *et al.* (2008). Peri-acetabular resection and endoprosthetic reconstruction for tumours of the acetabulum. *Journal of Bone and Joint Surgery*, **90-B**, 1222–7.

Jeys, L.M., Kulkarni, A., Grimer, R.J., Carter, S.R., Tillman, R.M., and Abudu, A. (2008). Endoprosthetic reconstruction for the treatment of musculoskeletal tumours of the apendicular skeleton and pelvis. *Journal of Bone and Joint Surgery*, **90-A**(6), 1265–71.

Rougraff, B.T., Simon, M.A., Kneisl, J.S., Greenberg, D.B., and Mankin, H.J. (1994). Limb salvage compared with amputation for osteosarcoma of the distal end of the femur. A long-term oncological, functional, and quality-of-life study. *Journal of Bone and Joint Surgery*, **76-A**, 649–56.

2.3

Benign tumours of soft tissues

Kesavan Sri-Ram, Anthony McGrath, Eric Yeung, Ben Spiegelberg, Nick Kalson, Barry Rose, Rob Pollock, and John Skinner

Summary points

- Ganglion cyst
- Intramuscular myxoma
- Myositis ossificans
- Nodular fasciitis
- Haemangioma
- Lipoma
- Cavernous lymphangioma
- Glomus tumour
- Neurofibroma
- Desmoid tumour
- Elastofibroma
- Schwannoma
- Synovial chondromatosis.

Ganglion cyst (Box 2.3.1)

A ganglion cyst is a benign cystic lesion which occurs around a joint but does not communicate with the joint cavity. However, there are other types of cystic lesions, which are similar to this soft tissue condition, which occur in the subperiosteal area, intraosseous compartment, intraneural space within the nerve sheath, and around the meniscus (usually lateral) of the knee. A ganglion cyst is the result of myxoid degeneration and softening of the fibrous tissue around a joint capsule or tendon sheath, which produces a swelling of the surrounding connective tissue.

Clinical presentation

Clinically they present with a cystic swelling over the dorsum or volar aspect of the wrist, but they can also occur on the volar aspect of fingers, dorsum of foot, around knee and ankle. They are usually painless but their presence over the joint often causes restriction in joint movement and an aching sensation. Sometimes they are associated with a history of minor trauma or repetitive use of the wrist and fingers.

Radiological features

Ultrasound is the main investigation to prove that it is a cystic lesion, and magnetic resonance imaging (MRI) can show that it is not connected to the joint, although this is rarely indicated.

In the intraosseous type, radiographs can show a round, well-defined osteolytic area with a thin rim of sclerosis. The cortex may be thin or expanded. MRI will show a high signal on T2-weighted images and low signal in T1-weighted images.

Pathological features

Macroscopically, a ganglion cyst is characterized by a yellow viscous, mucoid, jelly-like material surrounded by a thick fibrous capsule. There is no synovial lining. Microscopically there are fibroblast-like cells producing the mucoid ground substance. Macrophages are also found within the myxoid tissue.

Treatment and outcome

A ganglion cyst can be left untreated if it is asymptomatic. Often it can regress spontaneously. Aspiration and excision with debridement of the soft tissue bed are the main treatment options, but recurrence rates are high in both, especially aspiration. In intraosseous ganglion cyst, curettage with or without grafting can be used in symptomatic cases with few recurrence.

Intramuscular myxoma (Box 2.3.2)

Intramuscular myxoma is a benign soft tissue neoplasm which occurs in skeletal muscle. It is rare and tends to be more common

Box 2.3.1 Ganglion cyst

- Benign cystic lesion occurring around a joint but not communicating with the joint cavity
- Usually a cystic swelling over the dorsum or volar aspect of the wrist
- Ultrasound to confirm cystic nature if in doubt
- Mucoid contents with no synovial lining
- Aspiration; surgical excision but high recurrence rate.

in females. Although it is benign, it can grow to a large size, and can be mistaken for a soft tissue sarcoma. These lesions typically present late in adulthood, mostly around the age of 40. Typical locations are the buttock, thigh, lower leg, shoulder, and forearm. They are either encased within a muscle group, or attached only to the muscle fascia. These lesions tend to be mobile.

Clinical presentation

They tend to present as a firm painless soft tissue swelling, which usually grows slowly. Most intramuscular myxomas present as a solitary lesion, but in 'Mazabraud syndrome' multiple myxomas are associated with fibrous dyplasia.

Radiological features

As this is a soft tissue tumour, MRI scanning demonstrates the lesion clearly and in the majority of cases will confirm the diagnosis without the need of a biopsy. The tumour appears as a lobular mass within the skeletal muscle or muscular fascia. On T1-weighted images, a low intensity signal is seen, but on T2-weighted sequences a high intensity signal is returned (Figure 2.3.1). A recent radiological review suggested that in intramuscular myxoma, there is a peritumoural fat rim visible in T1 images on MRI, and the surrounding muscle shows increased signal intensity in T2-weighted or fluid-sensitive sequence. These can be the most reliable features to differentiate benign myxoma from other malignant sarcomas.

Pathological features

The myxoma usually appears like a soft translucent mass, with a thin rim of fibrous tissue around it, and lies against muscle or fascia. Histologically, myxomas consist of sparse, bland-appearing cells within a myxomatous matrix. The cells have small nuclei and no mitotic figures, and their appearance resemble fibroblasts.

Treatment and outcome

These lesions are usually treated with marginal excision. As they are easily separated from the muscle layer excision is usually complete and recurrence is rare.

Myositis ossificans

Myositis ossificans is an extraosseous non-neoplastic growth of new bone. It occurs most commonly in the second and third decades. It is uncommon in children (fewer than 7% of cases occur in the first decade), where it needs to be differentiated from myositis ossificans progressiva (see later section). The process is usually confined to muscle although involvement of tendon and

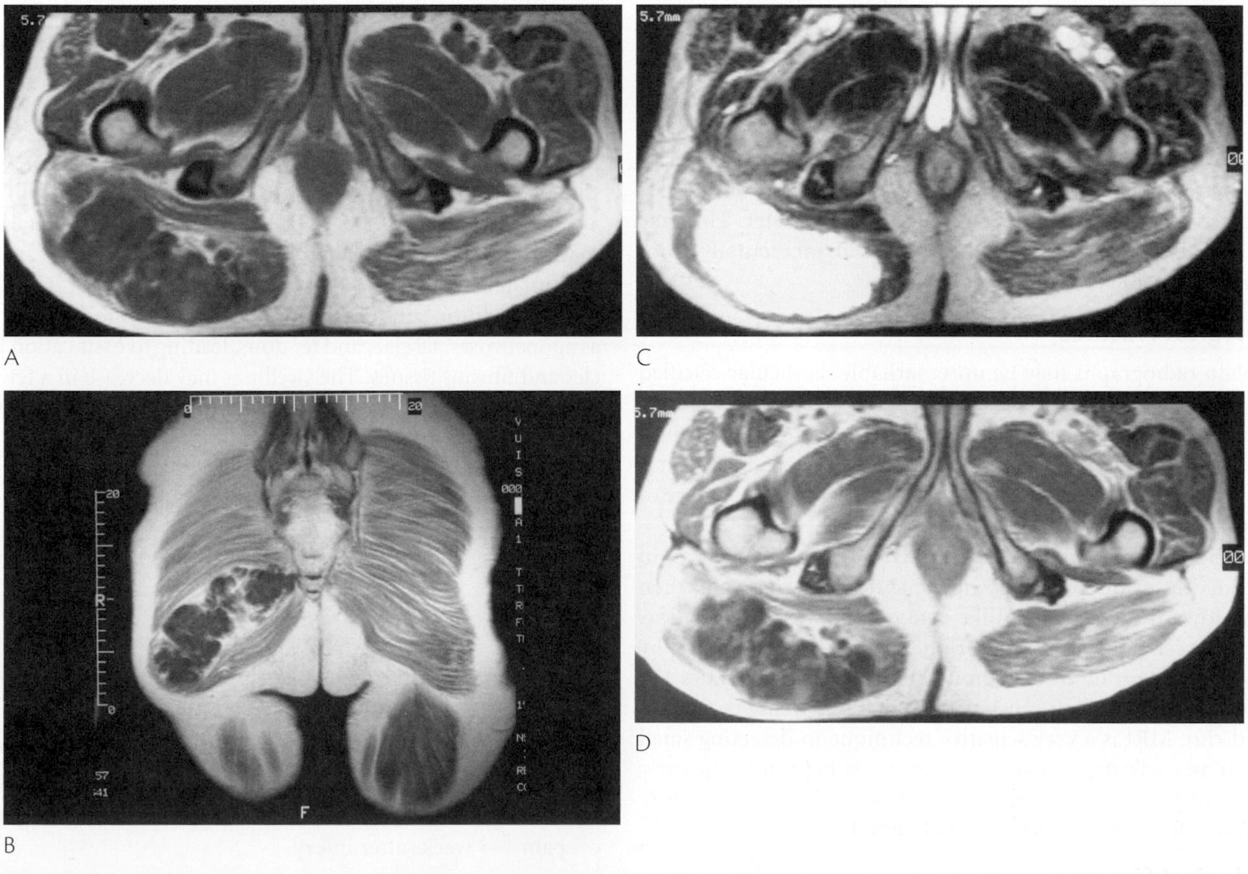

Fig. 2.3.1 MRI studies of an intramuscular myxoma of the gluteus maximus in a 61-year-old man. The patient presented with a history of a slowly enlarging painless mass in his right buttock. (A) Transverse T_1-weighted image (time of repetition, 600 ms, time of echo, 17 ms) of the pelvis shows a lobular low signal intensity mass within the gluteus maximus muscle. Notice that the mass is contained within the muscle fascia. (B) Coronal T_1-weighted image (time of repetition, 600 ms, time of echo, 17 ms) of the buttocks shows the extent of the lobular mass within the muscle. (C) Transverse T_2-weighted image (time of repetition, 2200 ms, time of echo, 80 ms) of the pelvis shows high signal intensity within the mass. This difference in signal intensity between T_1-weighted and T_2-weighted images is characteristic of myxomatous tissue. (D) Transverse T_1-weighted image (time of repetition, 600 ms, time of echo, 17 ms) following intravenous administration of gadolinium-based contrast material shows no enhancement of the central component of the mass. Minimal peripheral enhancement is seen at the interface with the surrounding skeletal muscle.

Box 2.3.2 Intramuscular myxoma

- Benign soft tissue neoplasm occurring in skeletal muscle; rare, typically presents late in adulthood, mostly over the age of 40
- Firm, painless soft tissue swelling
- MRI can demonstrate the nature of the soft tissue lesion clearly and confirm the diagnosis without the need of a biopsy
- Treated with marginal excision; recurrence is rare.

subcutaneous fat has been reported. The quadriceps and brachialis muscles are the sites most commonly affected (80%). Other sites affected include the intercostals, erector spinae, pectoralis muscles, glutei, small hand muscles, and the chest.

Myositis ossificans usually occurs in response to soft tissue trauma (75%). The history of trauma may be difficult to elicit. Proposed atraumatic mechanisms include non-documented trauma, repeated small mechanical injuries, extensive burns, immobilization due to coma/paraplegia, and injuries caused by ischaemia or inflammation (Box 2.3.3).

Clinical presentation

Myositis ossificans usually presents as a rapidly enlarging mass with significant pain 1–3 weeks after injury. The patient may have a swelling and the area may be warm. This acute phase is not generally associated with systemic symptoms, except in children who may feel unwell and tired. Blood tests may reveal an increased erythrocyte sedimentation rate and serum alkaline phosphatase. A subacute phase follows before the myositis matures, usually between 3–6 months, evolving into a painless, hard, well-demarcated mass averaging 3–6cm in greatest diameter. The condition may be asymptomatic and diagnosed incidentally from radiographs obtained for unrelated problems.

Radiological features

Early plain radiographs may be unremarkable. Follicular calcified density can be seen in the soft tissues from 3–6 weeks. By 6–8 weeks, calcification becomes sharply circumscribed, being seen around the periphery of the lesion (Figure 2.3.2). The periosteal reaction is that of benign lamination unlike the more aggressive appearance of osteosarcoma.

Serial radiographs show the zonal phenomenon of calcification first occurring in the periphery of the soft tissue mass and then working toward the centre, unlike osteosarcoma where calcification extends centrifugally to the periphery. Computed tomography (CT) scanning can be of enormous help as it demonstrates the mass with a central radiolucency surrounded by a dense peripheral calcified rim. MRI is a very sensitive technique in detecting small lesions at an early stage. Bone scans are most helpful in the early detection of myositis ossificans and are typically positive before bone mineralization is detected on radiographs.

Pathological features

Lesions may be classified by tissue site: the mass may be pedunculated (attached to the underlying bone by a stalk), in continuity with the periosteum, or intramuscular. Macroscopically, lesions have a well-circumscribed shell of bone and a soft red-brown centre.

Microscopically, there are three distinct zones, becoming apparent approximately 2 weeks following onset. These consist of a central undifferentiated zone, a surrounding zone of immature osteoid formation, and a peripheral zone with mature bone. Acutely, there is proliferation of undifferentiated mesenchymal cells. At approximately 2 weeks, osteoid production begins at the periphery and fibrous tissue begins to form around the shell. There is an irregular mass of immature proliferating fibroblasts at the lesion's centre. Moving peripherally, fibroblasts become more mature and structured, osteoblasts and islands of disorganized osteoid appear. Further peripherally, trabeculae of lamellar and woven bone are present with islands of chondroid tissue. Importantly, the lesion does not invade surrounding tissue.

Treatment and outcome

During the acute phase, treatment for myositis ossificans is conservative, as lesions become painless and may spontaneously reabsorb after 3–6 months. No pharmacological treatment is necessary. Indomethacin or other non-steroidal anti-inflammatory drugs (NSAIDs) may be used as an adjunct, although their efficacy has not been clearly established. A biopsy may be required if the lesion appears suspicious or without a history of trauma. Early surgery is contraindicated. In occasional cases, surgical excision is required, although success is limited. This should be performed once the lesion has matured, 12–18 months following onset. There have been a few isolated reports of malignancy occurring close to myositis ossificans. This is an extremely rare event and should not prompt the removal of lesions.

Myositis ossificans progressiva

Myositis ossificans progressiva is a rare (incidence $1/10^{-7}$), autosomal dominant disorder with equal sexual predilection. The average age of onset is 5 years. It is characterized by skeletal malformation and progressive, disabling heterotopic osteogenesis, which is ultimately fatal.

The condition produces painful swellings in the soft tissues such as aponeuroses, fasciae, and tendons, leading to ossification in muscles and fibrous tissues. The swellings may decrease in a few weeks, but joints affected become stiff. The most common sites affected are the sternocleidomastoid, and paraspinal muscle groups as well as the masticatory muscles, shoulder, and pelvic girdle muscles. Muscle groups not affected are the abdominal muscles, extraocular

Box 2.3.3 Myositis ossificans

- Extraosseous non-neoplastic growth of new bone; occurring most commonly in the second and third decades
- Extraosseous bone appears most commonly in response to soft tissue trauma (75%)
- Usually presents as a rapidly enlarging mass with significant pain 1–3 weeks after injury
- Follicular calcified density is observable in soft tissues at 2–6 weeks
- Treatment is conservative; lesions gradually spontaneously reabsorb after 3–6 months; NSAIDs may be used as an adjunct; if troublesome surgical excision only if lesion mature (12–18 months from onset).

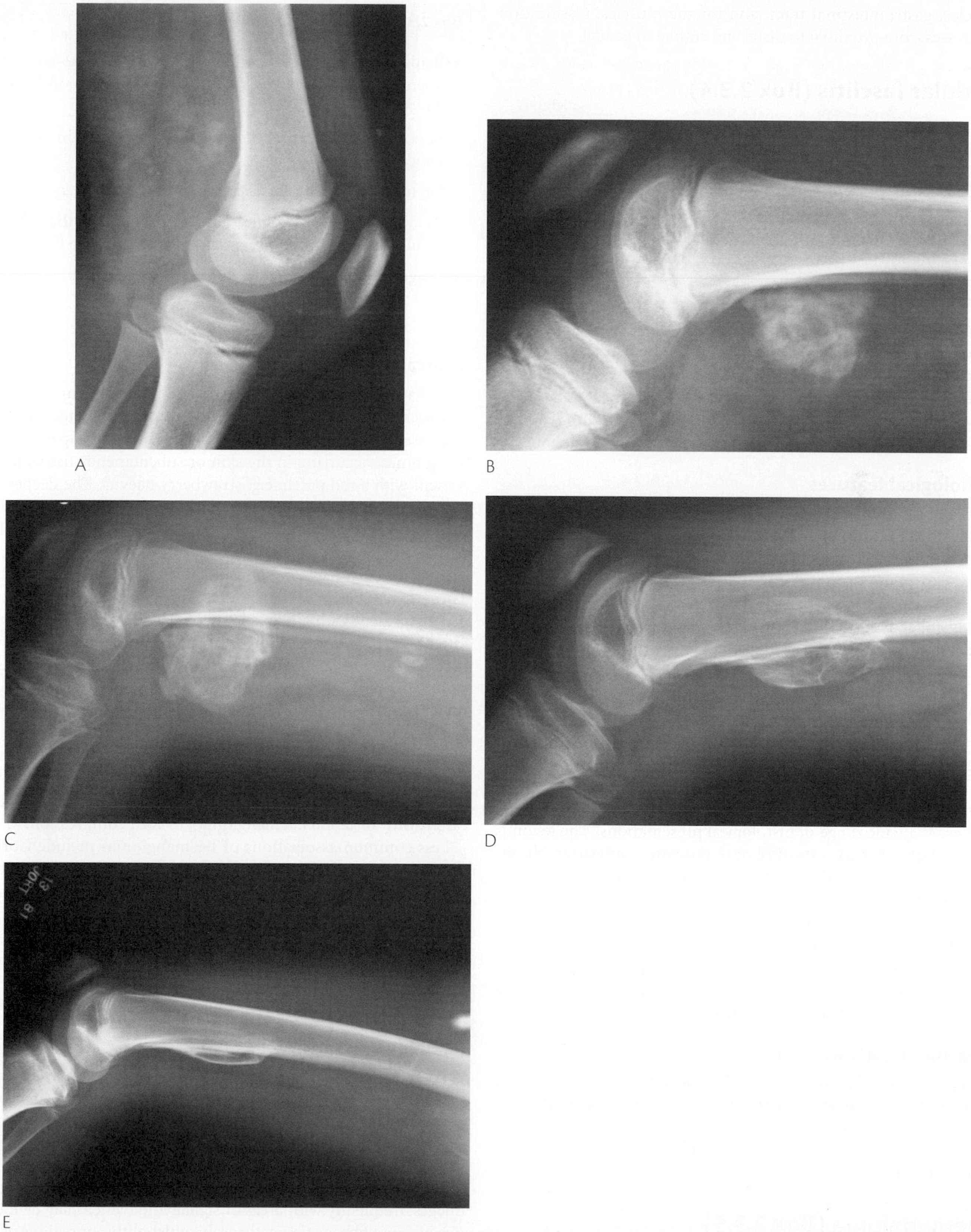

Fig. 2.3.2 A 10-year-old boy struck in the back of his knee with a hockey stick, presented 3 weeks later with an enlarging painful mass on the posterior aspect of his distal thigh. (A) Lateral radiograph of knee/distal thigh reveals a calcified mass, no periosteal reaction. (B) It was elected to follow and repeat the radiographs. Two weeks later, the mass is better defined, progressing to mineralization. Note the clear demarcation with underlying femoral cortex. (C) Ten years after the original injury further remodeling and resolution has occurred (D), (E).

muscles, gastrointestinal tract, and tongue muscles. Ossification progresses from proximal to distal and cranial to caudal.

Nodular fasciitis (Box 2.3.4)

Nodular fasciitis is a benign reactive process of the soft tissues related to fascia. It is also known as subcutaneous pseudosarcomatous fibromatosis, or proliferative fasciitis. It is frequently misdiagnosed as a sarcoma. It is most common between 20–40 years of age. Approximately 10% of lesions occur in children. It is rare in patients older than 60. The male to female ratio is equal and the cause is unknown.

Box 2.3.4 Nodular fasciitis

- Benign reactive process of the soft tissues related to fascia; frequently misdiagnosed as a sarcoma; most common between 20–40 years of age
- Lesions can be rapidly growing, usually within 3 weeks; patients may report pain
- No unique radiological features of nodular fasciitis
- Characterized by a proliferation of fibroblasts in the subcutaneous tissues, commonly associated with the deep fascia
- Diagnosis and treatment are by excisional biopsy.

Clinical presentation

Lesions are small (1–3cm) and solitary, and commonly arise in the upper limbs (46%), chest and back (20%), and in the head and neck (17%). Half of the lesions are located in the subcutaneous fascia, and the remainder is situated in deep fascia in relation to muscles, tendons, vessels, nerve sheaths, and periosteum. Patients may complain of pain or tenderness associated with the lesion.

Radiological features

There are no unique radiological features of nodular fasciitis. The higher fibrous components of the lesions make them hypoechoic relative to muscle when examined on ultrasonography. MRI findings vary depending on the histological characteristics of the lesion. Hypercellular lesions types can be seen as hyperintense lesions. Highly collagenous lesions return a hypointense signal on all MR images.

Pathological features

Nodular fasciitis is characterized by a proliferation of fibroblasts in the subcutaneous tissues and is also usually associated with the deep fascia. Three subtypes may be identified on the basis of location: subcutaneous, intramuscular, or fascial. It is frequently misdiagnosed as a neoplastic lesion.

There is a wide range of histological presentations. The lesion is richly cellular and consists of plump, immature-appearing fibroblasts arranged in irregular short fascicles. The size and shape of cells vary, but they have discrete nucleoli and abundant mitotic figures that are not abnormal. In early lesions, the cells are embedded in a rich mucopolysaccharide matrix with little collagen. Over time, the amount of collagen increases, especially in head and neck lesions in children. The lesion is not often encapsulated but is usually well demarcated from surrounding tissues.

Treatment and outcome

Both diagnosis and treatment are by excisional biopsy. Spontaneous regression and involution of lesions in response to steroid injections have been reported. There is an extremely low incidence of recurrence after resection (1–6%). Nodular fasciitis lesions do not develop metastases.

Haemangioma (Box 2.3.5)

A haemangioma is an abnormal proliferation of blood vessels that may occur in any vascularized tissue and accounts for 7% of all benign soft tissue tumours. There is debate as to whether these lesions are neoplasms, hamartomas, or vascular malformations.

Clinical presentation

Most haemangiomas are superficial and tend to occur in the head and neck region. They can be divided into intramuscular, synovial, and osseous according to location. The common superficial haemangiomas, occurring in the skin or subcutaneous tissue, usually present with a red patch, e.g. strawberry naevus. The deeper haemangiomas are less common and may present with pain and swelling. Visceral haemangiomas may cause organ dysfunction. They may also be noted incidentally, especially osseous haemangiomas.

Intramuscular haemangiomas occur most often in young adults. They often occur in the lower extremity, especially the thigh, and usually present with a palpable mass, with normal overlying skin. Often, the pain and swelling associated can be exacerbated with exercise and alleviated with elevation. Synovial haemangiomas are rare. In tendons, they usually present as a painless mass. In joints, they may present with pain, swelling, and sometimes mechanical symptoms. The knee is the commonest site, and the symptoms may mimic meniscal or ligamentous pathology. Osseous haemangiomas are usually incidental findings, but may present with pain and swelling. They may also present as pathological fractures or rarely, with vertebral haemangiomas, as cord compression.

Less common associations of haemangiomas include Gorham disease and Kasabach–Merritt syndrome. In Gorham disease there is massive osteolysis due to haemangiomas. Most patients are younger than 40 years and can present with dull aching pain or insidious weakness. In Kasabach–Merritt syndrome, there are coagulopathies due to trapping of platelets within large haemangiomas. These patients can present with diffuse petechial haemorrhages and ecchymosis in association with a large soft tissue mass.

Radiological features

With soft tissue haemangiomas, plain radiography may show soft tissue shadows and benign-appearing periosteal reaction or chronic cortical thickening and remodelling in adjacent bone. Small round calcified densities (phleboliths) within the soft tissue mass are diagnostic but not always present. On MRI, the imaging of choice, haemangiomas show increased signal on both T1- and T2-weighted images, frequently with areas of signal void, which may be indicative of dense fibrous tissue, thrombi, phleboliths, or regions of high flow (Figure 2.3.3).

With osseous haemangiomas, the plain radiographic features vary according to the lesion's anatomic location. In the skull, a lytic appearance, often with fine radiating striations, is seen. In the

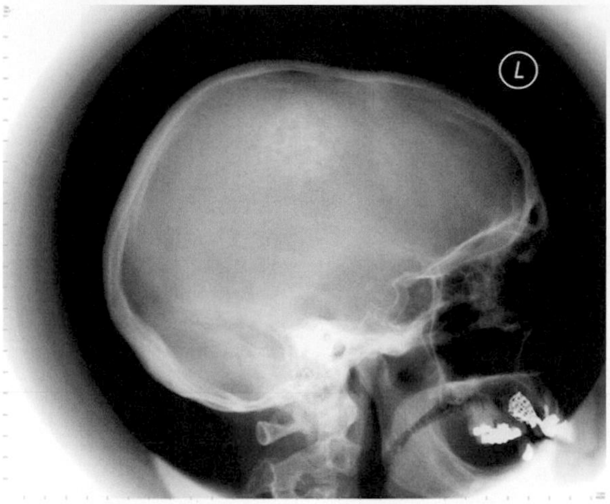

Fig. 2.3.3 Plain radiographic appearance of haemangioma affecting the skull.

vertebrae, there are parallel vertical trabeculae ('corduroy' appearance). In long bones, the appearances are less specific. CT is of limited use and on MRI there is increases signal on T1 and T2 images. Ultrasound is an excellent technique for diagnosing haemangiomas. Carried out by an experienced radiologist the lesion can be characterized, the vessels seen, the type of flow noted, and the compressibility of the lesion confirmed. If solid components are found, these will require further investigation.

Pathological features

Haemangiomas are benign lesions with increased numbers of blood vessels. They can affect numerous tissue types (individually or in combination), including skin, subcutaneous tissue, viscera, muscle, synovium, and bone, but they do not spread to avascular tissue such as cartilage. The aetiology remains unclear, although it is thought that excessive angiogenesis mediated by cytokines, such as basic fibroblast growth factor (bFGF) and vascular endothelial growth factor (VEGF), is responsible.

Histologically, haemangiomas are classified into capillary, cavernous, and arteriovenous, according to the calibre of the vessel involved. Capillary haemangiomas are characterized by a proliferation of capillary-sized vessels, lined by flattened endothelium forming small slit-like structures arranged in lobules. Microscopically, there is a proliferation of endothelial cells with numerous mitotic figures; mast cells are also seen, predominately in the involuting phase haemangiomas. Cavernous haemangiomas show dilated blood-filled vessels, also lined by flattened endothelium. Adventitial fibrosis and inflammation often results in a thicker vessel wall. Calcification is often seen. Arteriovenous haemangiomas contain larger vessels in the form of arteries and veins in close association.

Treatment and outcome

Observation is the appropriate treatment for the majority of haemangiomas. Biopsy is sometimes required to differentiate a soft tissue sarcoma especially if solid components are found on ultrasound examination. This can either be open or needle, but there is often excessive bleeding. Embolization can be of use especially in high-flow lesions and can provide symptomatic relief. It is often more useful as an investigation prior to surgery.

Box 2.3.5 Haemangioma

- Abnormal proliferation of blood vessels that can occur in any vascularized tissue
- 7% of all benign soft tissue tumours
- MRI is the imaging of choice
- Capillary, cavernous, and arteriovenous, according to the calibre of the vessel involved
- Observation for the majority of lesions with surgical excision in symptomatic cases
- No risk of malignancy, but recurrence after excision is common (10–50%).

Surgical excision can be considered for symptomatic haemangiomas. The osseous type tends not to require treatment unless associated with fracture. Steroids and radiotherapy are thought to be useful in Gorham disease. In Kasabach–Merritt syndrome, excision and adjuvant therapy with steroids, radiotherapy, interferon, and pentoxifylline have been used to control the disease.

The natural history of many haemangiomas is that of gradual fatty replacement, atrophy, and involution over time. There is no risk of malignancy, but recurrence after excision is common (10–50%). The more limited the extent of the disease, the more likely it is to be controlled by surgical excision.

Lipoma (Box 2.3.6)

Lipomas are the commonest benign soft tissue tumour, occurring in 1% of the population.

Clinical presentation

Lipomas are relatively uncommon in childhood, and tend to present in the fourth and fifth decades. They are usually subcutaneous, and can present at any site, including organs. They can present in multiple sites. They are uncommon around the face and hands and feet.

Their usual location lies between the skin and deep fascia. They have a soft fluctuant and lobular feel, and a well-defined edge. Lipomas are usually asymptomatic. Pressure symptoms and a mass effect will herald their presence if large in size (in that case the possibility of a liposarcoma should be considered).

Radiological features

For most subcutaneous lipomas, no imaging studies are required. If imaging is needed, MRI is the most helpful, especially with intramuscular lipomas (Figure 2.3.4). The tumour usually appears as a small homogeneous mass, although it may appear as a large inhomogeneous lesion with infiltrative margins. MRI does not, however, allow for a reliable distinction between a lipoma and a well-differentiated liposarcoma. Fat suppression sequences are mandatory to confirm that the lesion fully suppresses. If there are areas within the lesion that remain bright then a biopsy of these areas will be required prior to excision.

Pathological features

Lipomas are slow-growing, benign fatty tumours and consist of lobules of fat, with a surrounding capsule, which may becomes

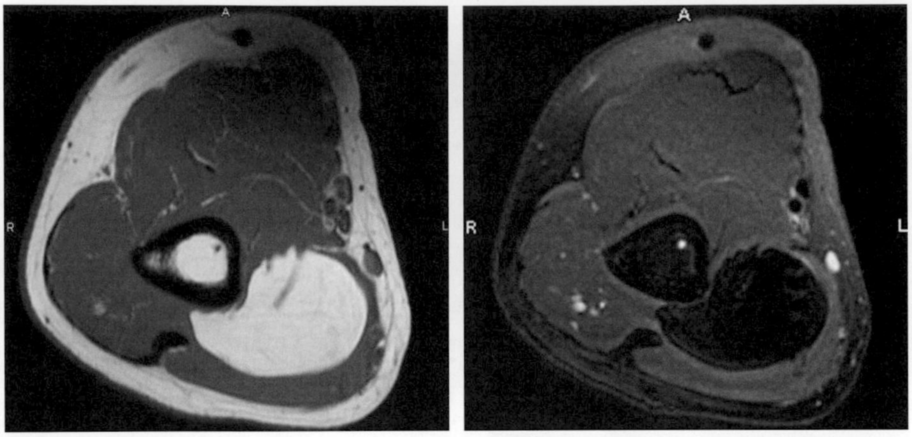

A B

Fig. 2.3.4 Lipoma of the right arm T1-weighted (A) and fat suppression (B) images.

tethered to adjacent structures. Atypical lipomatous tumours are considered to be well-differentiated liposarcomas. They have a predilection for local recurrence but do not generally metastasize.

Macroscopically, lipomas are multilobular masses with a yellow appearance. Microscopically, they have the same appearance as mature non-neoplastic adipose tissue. There are many variants including angiolipomas (mixture of mature fat cells and numerous branching vascular channels), spindle cell lipomas (consisting of mature adipocytes, small spindle cells, and bundles of mature collagen), pleomorphic lipomas (mixture of mature adipocytes, spindle cells, collagen, and bizarre 'floret-type' multinucleated giant cells), myxolipomas (myxoid transformation), fibrolipomas (septae of connective tissue), chondrolipomas (chondroid metaplasia), osteolipomas (osseous metaplasia), and myolipomas (presence of smooth muscle proliferation).

Treatment and outcome

As most lipomas are asymptomatic, surgical excision is usually for cosmetic reasons. If symptomatic, marginal excision can be carried out; the tumour is simply 'shelled out' with complete removal of the capsule in an extracapsular plane.

Recurrence is uncommon, but may occur if excision is incomplete. Lipomas rarely undergo sarcomatous change. Liposarcomas are malignant tumours that arise from adipocytes (the majority do not arise from pre-existing lipomas). They may recur locally and may metastasize. Fatty tumours of the retroperitoneum or in intramuscular locations should be considered to be potential liposarcomas until proven otherwise. The size of liposarcomas may vary considerably. The majority of tumours present between 5–15cm and extremely large retroperitoneal tumours have been reported.

Box 2.3.6 Lipoma

- Commonest benign soft tissue tumour (1% of population)
- If needed, MRI is imaging of choice
- Slow-growing, benign fatty tumours consisting of lobules of fat, with a surrounding capsule
- Surgical excision if symptomatic
- Rarely undergo sarcomatous change.

Cavernous lymphangioma (Box 2.3.7)

Lymphangiomas are uncommon, hamartomatous malformations of the lymphatic system that involve the skin and subcutaneous tissues. There are two main types: superficial lesions called lymphangioma circumscriptum (simple lymphangiomas) and deeper lesions which include cavernous lymphangiomas and cystic hygromas.

Clinical presentation

Cavernous lymphangiomas usually arise during infancy or early childhood with equal distribution between sexes. They are commonly found around the head and neck, and less so in the extremities. The lesions are located deep within the dermis, and usually present as painless swellings. The overlying skin is not affected. The consistency is one of a small rubbery nodule. They are usually small (1cm) but may be large enough to affect an entire limb. They tend to enlarge as the child grows, and episodic, or sometimes constant, pain is more likely.

Radiological features

Clinical assessment is usually sufficient for diagnosis. Plain radiographs may display any associated skeletal deformities. Contrast-enhanced MRI can help differentiate these lesions (no enhancement) with vascular lesions (which enhance). Imaging is also particularly helpful in respect to planning excision.

Pathological features

Cavernous lymphangiomas are often poorly demarcated between the skin and subcutaneous tissue, and they do not have a distinct capsule. They may extend along fascial planes between muscle groups and may lie within muscle septae.

Microscopically, the nodules in cavernous lymphangioma are characterized by large, irregular channels in the reticular dermis and subcutaneous tissue that are lined by a single or multiple layers of endothelial cells. An incomplete layer of smooth muscle often lines the walls of these malformed channels. The surrounding stroma consists of loose or fibrotic connective tissue with a number of inflammatory cells, and is usually variable. These tumours often penetrate muscle.

Treatment and outcome

Observation may be the most appropriate treatment. If symptoms are severe, or if the diagnosis is of doubt, excision biopsy forms the mainstay of treatment. The indistinct margins make complete excision difficult. Additional treatment modalities include the use of intralesional OK432 (Picibanil®, Chugai Pharmaceutical Co.) after excision. This sclerosing agent has had mixed results.

Lymphangiomas have a strong tendency for local recurrence unless they are completely excised. As they represent hamartomatous malformations, there is no significant risk of malignant transformation.

Glomus tumour (Box 2.3.8)

The glomus body is a specialized form of arteriovenous anastomosis found in the stratum reticularis. This anastomosis is surrounded by smooth muscle and glomus cells (modified smooth muscle cells). Glomus tumours are relatively uncommon benign neoplasms, arising from the arterial portion of the glomus body, differentiating to become glomus cells. These tumours have also been observed in extracutaneous locations that are not known to contain glomus cells. One explanation for this finding is that these tumors may arise from perivascular cells that can differentiate into glomus cells.

The incidence is unknown. Presentation can be at any age, but most commonly in the fifth decade. Two variants occur; solitary or multiple. The former is more common in women and the latter in men where it is usually inherited in an autosomal-dominant fashion.

Clinical presentation

Patients usually suffer from paroxysmal pain, exacerbated by cold temperatures. Multiple lesions often cause cosmetic concerns, but are less likely to be painful. Solitary lesions are usually blue or purple, small, and located in the periphery, e.g. subungual areas of the fingers and toes. Multiple lesions are subdivided into regional or localized, disseminated, and congenital plaque-like forms.

Special tests to aid diagnosis during examination include the Hildreth sign (disappearance of pain after application of a tourniquet proximally on the arm) and the Love test (eliciting pain by applying pressure to a precise area with the tip of a pencil or needle).

Malignant glomus tumours, or glomangiosarcomas, are extremely rare and usually represent a locally infiltrative malignancy. They are usually larger than 1cm and grow rapidly.

Radiological features

In certain locations, plain radiographs are of use. For example, in subungual lesions, there may be bony erosion. In finger-tip lesions, there may show an increased distance between the dorsum of the phalanx and the underside of the nail.

MRI is most helpful. The tumour appears dark as a well-defined mass on T1-weighted images and as a bright contrast enhancing mass on T1 post-gadolinium fat saturation images. Ultrasound may also be helpful.

Pathological features

Glomus tumours are benign and rarely show local infiltration. They arise from the arterial portion of the glomus body, or the Sucquet–Hoyer canal, which is an arteriovenous shunt in the dermis that contributes to temperature regulation.

Macroscopically, they are small (less than 1cm), well-circumscribed masses with a fibrous capsule. Solitary and multiple glomus tumours have distinct histopathological features. Solitary lesions appear mostly as solid well-circumscribed nodules surrounded by a rim of fibrous tissue, containing endothelium-lined vascular spaces surrounded by clusters of glomus cells. Multiple lesions are usually less well circumscribed and less solid-appearing. They appear similar to a haemangioma, and contain multiple irregular, dilated, endothelium-lined vascular channels that contain red blood cells. The vascular spaces are larger than those in solitary glomus tumours. Small aggregates of glomus cells are present in the walls of these channels and in small clusters in the adjacent stroma.

Glomangiosarcomas resemble benign glomus tumours. However, glomangiosarcomas have more atypia, pleomorphism, and mitotic figures, and they have an invasive growth pattern.

Treatment and outcome

Asymptomatic glomus tumours can be observed. Malignant transformation is extremely rare. Excision is required for those that are symptomatic and simply involves shelling out the tumour from its fibrous capsule. Other treatment approaches include argon and carbon dioxide laser therapy and sclerotherapy with hypertonic saline or sodium tetradecyl sulfate. These are probably helpful in the presence of multiple lesions.

The prognosis is excellent. Excision of painful lesions most often results in cure, with a low recurrence rate for solitary lesions. Recurrences are secondary to incomplete excision. Malignant glomus tumours are extremely rare and usually locally aggressive.

Box 2.3.7 Cavernous lymphangioma

- Hamartomatous malformations of the lymphatic system involving skin and subcutaneous tissues
- May extend along fascial planes between muscle groups; may lie within muscle septae
- Conservative treatment but perform excision biopsy if uncertain diagnosis
- High risk of local recurrence unless completely excised
- No risk of malignant transformation.

Box 2.3.8 Glomus tumour

- Most commonly seen in the fifth decade; solitary or multiple lesions
- MRI most helpful imaging modality
- Arise from arterial portion of the glomus body (an arteriovenous shunt in the dermis that contributes to temperature regulation)
- Surgical excision if symptomatic benign lesions; wide local excision for malignant lesions
- Low recurrence rate if complete excision.

Their overall prognosis is good when they are treated with wide excision. However, metastases do occur and are associated with a very poor prognosis.

Neurofibroma (Box 2.3.9)

Neurofibromas are benign tumours of fibrous and neural elements. They can occur in a peripheral nerve, but also in the skin or subcutaneous tissue. Lesions may be solitary or multiple. They affect both sexes equally, and tend to occur in young people (20–30 years).

Clinical presentation

Presentation is usually with a lump which may be painful, or with symptoms of a compressive neuropathy. Multiple neurofibromas are seen in von Recklinghausen's disease (neurofibromatosis-1; NF-1). This is an autosomal dominant condition, characterized by multiple skin nodules and café-au-lait patches, occurring in approximately one of 2500–3300 live births.

Three subtypes of neurofibroma exist, namely cutaneous, subcutaneous, and plexiform. Both cutaneous lesions and subcutaneous lesions are circumscribed and may be soft or firm. These nodules may be brown, pink, or skin coloured. Plexiform neurofibromas are non-circumscribed, thick, and irregular, and they can cause disfigurement by entwining important supportive structures. This subtype is specific for NF-1.

Radiological features

Plain radiography and CT are of limited use. On MRI, neurofibromas demonstrate low or intermediate signal on T1-weighted images and homogeneously bright signal on T2-weighted images. Heterogeneity on T2-weighted images is suggestive of malignant transformation

Pathological features

Neurofibromas consist of pale fibrous tissue with neural elements running into and through the tumour. They are composed of Schwann cells, fibroblasts, mast cells, and vascular components. Microscopically, neurofibromas are characterized by wavy, spindle-shaped nuclei and a loose mucinous stroma. The cells are arranged in short interlacing fascicles or bundles, and the intercellular environment is loose and myxoid, with thin wavy collagen fibres and inflammatory cells such as lymphocytes and mast cells.

Treatment and outcome

Excision is the treatment of choice when the symptoms of pain and/or paraesthesia become intrusive, or when the tumour enlarges. It is not possible to separate the tumour from nerve fibres; therefore, en bloc excision is performed if the nerve can be sacrificed. If not, intracapsular shelling out of the tumour can be performed, accepting the increased risk of recurrence.

Solitary neurofibromas rarely undergo malignant transformation. Follow up, particularly in patients with NF-1, is recommend as the risk is higher (reported between 2–30%). Any change, growth, or pain may be a sign of malignant transformation and a biopsy should be performed.

Box 2.3.9 Neurofibroma

- Benign tumours of fibrous and neural elements
- Presentation with painful lump, or with symptoms of compressive neuropathy
- Multiple neurofibromas seen in von Recklinghausen's disease (neurofibromatosis-1: NF-1)
- Three subtypes exist: cutaneous, subcutaneous, and plexiform (specific to NF-1)
- Malignant transformation is rare in solitary neurofibromas.

Desmoid tumour (Box 2.3.10)

Desmoid tumour was first described arising from the rectus abdominis muscle in postpartum women. It is now recognized that they can arise from any mesenchymal tissue. They are locally aggressive, but do not metastasize. They are also known as aggressive fibromatosis.

Desmoid tumours most commonly occur in women after childbirth. Peak incidence is between 25–35. Although desmoid tumours can arise in any skeletal muscle, they most commonly develop in the anterior abdominal wall and shoulder girdle.

Clinical presentation

Patients usually complain of a lump that slowly increases in size. Pain is often a late feature. There may be a history of local trauma, e.g. previous scar. Local pressure may cause other symptoms such as neurological dysfunction. The tumours are usually firm, smooth, and mobile, but may be adherent to surrounding structures. The overlying skin is usually unaffected.

Radiological features

CT and MRI are useful for both diagnosis and follow-up of desmoid tumours. In particular, MRI can demonstrate the extent of the tumour and also the relationship to adjacent structures. On MRI, these tumours are isointense to skeletal muscle on T1 images and hyperintense on T2 images (Figure 2.3.5). They also display septum-like internal inhomogeneity and a surrounding hypointense capsular band.

Pathological features

The cause of desmoid tumours is uncertain but may be related to trauma or hormonal factors. There may be a genetic association. Spontaneous regression of desmoid tumours has been observed following menopause.

Desmoid tumours often appear as infiltrative, usually well-differentiated, firm overgrowths of fibrous tissue, and they are locally aggressive. Macroscopically, these tumours are firm and white in appearance. The size varies considerably. Microscopically, desmoid tumours are composed of abundant collagen surrounding poorly circumscribed bundles of spindle cells.

Treatment and outcome

Surgical excision with wide local margins is the treatment of choice. Marginal excision is associated with recurrence. Achieving adequate excision of recurrent disease is difficult. Alternatives to excision include radiotherapy, medication (antioestrogens and prostaglandin inhibitors) and chemotherapy (e.g. vincristine, methotrexate, or doxorubicin). These are usually reserved for those

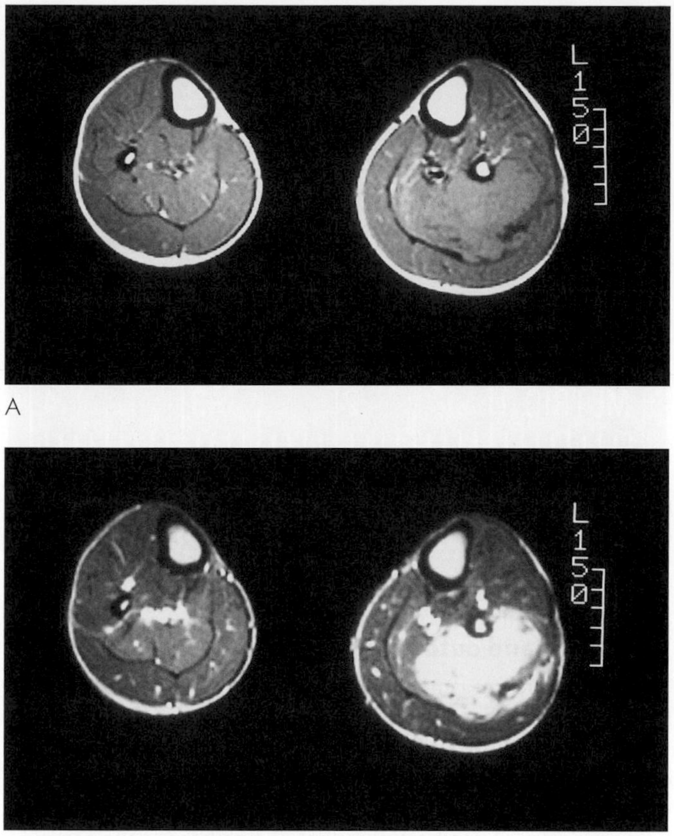

Fig. 2.3.5 T1-weighted (A) and T2-weighted (B) images of a large desmoids tumour in the proximal part of the leg in a 37-year-old woman. The lesion is isotense to skeletal muscle on T1 but hyperintense on T2.

who refuse or are unfit for surgery or as an adjunct to surgery when further excision would be technically difficult.

After surgery, MRI may be useful for monitoring recurrence. Local recurrence rates are reported to be as high as 70%, although some 'recurrences' may actually be metachronous disease. Malignant transformation is extremely rare, but may follow radiotherapy.

Elastofibroma (Box 2.3.11)

Elastofibroma is a rare, benign, slow-growing connective-tissue tumour that occurs most often in the subscapular area in elderly women, and was first described in 1961. They are usually solitary, and in up to one-third of cases, there is a family history of the same tumour suggesting a genetic predisposition.

Clinical presentation

Elastofibromas are usually located at the lower pole of the scapula, deep to the serratus anterior, and often attached to the periosteum of the ribs. There is normally a long history of swelling and pain. Often, they are detected incidentally during chest CT examinations. Less common sites include the deltoid muscle, ischial tuberosity, greater trochanter, olecranon, and thoracic wall.

Radiological features

Radiographs are usually normal, but may show a mass displacing the scapula (Figure 2.3.6). Ultrasound is helpful with an appearance consisting of arrays of linear strands against an echogenic background. However, the appearances can be similar to the surrounding muscle, making it difficult to detect. MRI shows a lenticular, unencapsulated, soft tissue mass with skeletal muscle attenuation interspersed with strands of fat attenuation. Smaller lesions are better seen with gadolinium enhancement.

Pathological features

The aetiology of this tumour remains unclear, although there is an increased prevalence in people who perform manual labor involving the shoulder girdle. It is uncertain as to whether elastofibromas are a true neoplastic process or a formation of reactive tissue in response to the local movements.

Macroscopically, the tumour is an ill-defined nodular mass with a white or grey glistening surface. Microscopically, they are dermal unencapsulated tumours composed of branched and unbranched elastic fibres, eosinophilic collagen bundles, and scattered fatty tissue. The elastic fibres have a degenerated, beaded appearance or are fragmented into small globules or droplets arranged in a

Box 2.3.10 Desmoid tumour

- Most commonly seen in women after childbirth
- Can arise in any skeletal muscle but seen most commonly in anterior abdominal wall and shoulder girdle
- Infiltrative, well-differentiated, firm overgrowths of fibrous tissue, that are locally aggressive
- Surgical excision with wide local margins is the treatment of choice to reduce risk of recurrence
- Malignant transformation is extremely rare.

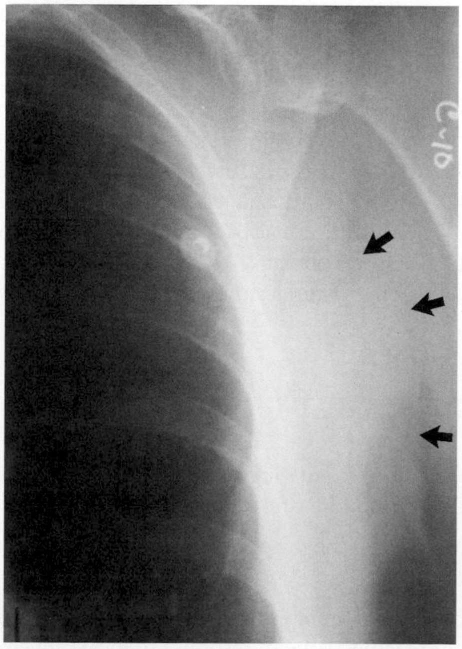

Fig. 2.3.6 Radiograph of the left chest wall in a 67-year-old male showing soft tissue fullness secondary to a large elastofibroma.

linear pattern. The interspersed spindle or stellate cells show a fibroblast-like appearance.

Treatment and outcome

Biopsy is usually required to confirm the diagnosis, although its characteristic location and radiological appearances are sometime sufficient. Complete surgical excision is the treatment of choice in symptomatic patients.

Recurrence after surgery is unusual. Spontaneous regression without treatment has also been observed.

Schwannoma (Box 2.3.12)

Schwannomas are benign, encapsulated tumours of the nerve sheath. They are seen in peripheral nerves and in the spinal roots, and are the commonest neurogenic tumour.

Clinical presentation

Schwannomas usually affect people aged 20–50 years. The prevalence is unknown. The lesion usually presents as a palpable mass or pain and paraesthesia (compressive neuropathy). The masses are slow growing, and may be present for several years before becoming symptomatic. Common locations for the tumours include the head, the flexor surfaces of the upper and lower extremities, and the trunk. The mass is usually mobile in the transverse plane and tethered along the axis of the nerve from which it arises. It is usually tender. Schwannomas are almost always solitary, but multiple lesions may be seen patients with neurofibromatosis type 1 (von Recklinghausen's disease).

Radiological features

Plain radiograph are generally not helpful, except in the case of the rare intraosseous lesions. The features are of a benign-appearing, well-circumscribed lesion. MRI is more useful. It usually shows a round or oval mass with a moderately bright signal on T1-weighted images and a bright, heterogeneous signal on T2-weighted images. The lesion enhances uniformly with gadolinium contrast. There is often a 'target' sign on T2-weighted images.

Pathological features

Their cells of origin are thought to be Schwann cells derived from the neural crest. These masses usually arise from the side of a nerve (Figure 2.3.7), are well encapsulated, and have a unique histological pattern. The capsule consists of epineurium. Microscopically, there are two distinct regions, known as Antoni A and B. The amount of each varies from lesion to lesion.

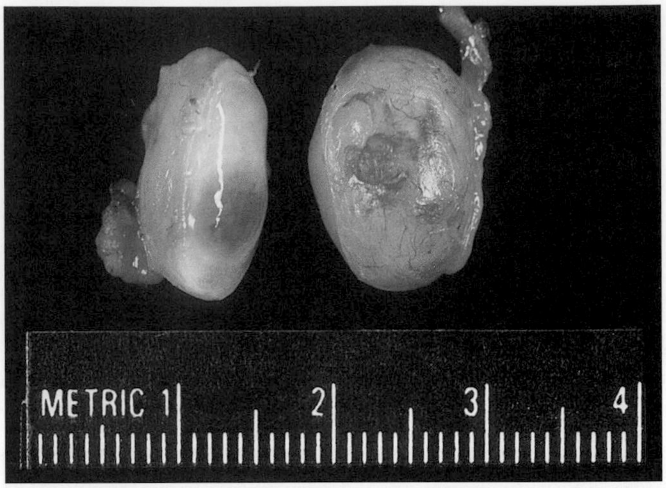

Fig. 2.3.7 Characteristic macroscopic appearance of a schwannoma as an encapsulated eccentric growth of the associated nerve. Also see colour plate section.

Treatment and outcome

These tumours are generally easily excised. The nerve is usually splayed out over the lesion. The lesion is excised marginally, and the nerve fibres are spared. Intralesional resection is warranted when complete resection would result in permanent neurologic deficit.

The most common complication is initial neurapraxia; however, neurologic deficit can be permanent, if significant neural tissue is excised. Generally, after resection patients experience complete and rapid relief of symptoms. Recurrence is unlikely following complete resection.

Synovial chondromatosis (Box 2.3.13)

Synovial chondromatosis is a rare benign condition in which foci of cartilage develop in the synovial membrane of joints, bursae, or tendon sheaths as a result of metaplasia of the subsynovial connective tissue. These ectopic foci of cartilage can result in painful joint effusions and the generation of loose bodies and mechanical symptoms.

Clinical presentation

Most patients are middle-aged, but it can be seen in children. Typically, a patient presents with monoarticular pain (most commonly the knee), swelling, stiffness, and symptoms of locking and giving way. The presence of a large effusion is not uncommon

Box 2.3.11 Elastofibroma

- Rare, benign, slow-growing connective-tissue tumour occurring most often in the subscapular area of elderly women
- Usually located at the lower pole of the scapula, deep to serratus anterior
- Uncertain if they represent a true neoplastic process or a formation of reactive tissue in response to local movement
- Surgical excision for symptomatic patients.

Box 2.3.12 Schwannoma

- Benign, encapsulated tumours of the nerve sheath (commonest neurogenic tumour)
- Palpable mass or pain and paraesthesia (compressive neuropathy); multiple lesions in NF-1
- 'Target sign' on MRI scan
- Cells of origin are Schwann cells; mass arises from the side of a nerve and is well encapsulated
- Marginal surgical excision sparing nerve fibres.

together with a restricted range of motion. The knee is affected in 60–70% of cases, with the shoulder, elbow, and hip being the next most commonly affected.

Radiological features

If loose bodies undergo ossification, they may be visible on plain radiographs, with two views of the affected joint (Figures 2.3.8 and 2.3.9). On MRI, cartilaginous nodules have intermediate signal intensity on T1-weighted images and high signal intensity on T2-weighted images. Intra-articular gadolinium increases the sensitivity for these lesions. This imaging is particularly helpful preoperatively, as it shows the extent of unmineralized as well as mineralized disease.

Pathological features

Synovial chondromatosis occurs as either a primary or secondary form. In primary synovial chondromatosis, there is ectopic cartilage in synovial tissue and loose bodies in the joint cavity with or without calcification (osteochondromatosis). There is no joint pathology. This is either synovial metaplasia or a true neoplasia. In secondary synovial chondromatosis, there is associated pathology, such as osteoarthritis, rheumatoid arthritis, osteonecrosis, osteochondritis dissecans, neuropathic osteoarthropathy, tuberculosis, or osteochondral fractures. Free chondral or osteochondral fragments formed by underlying disease implant into the synovium and induce metaplastic cartilage around them.

Treatment and outcome

Symptoms due to the acute inflammation can be treated with NSAIDs, as well as rest and thermal therapy. Patients with recurrent painful effusions, mechanical symptoms, or both, due to synovial chondromatosis refractory to conservative interventions are candidates for surgery. This can range from arthroscopic excision of loose bodies, with limited synovectomy to an open arthrotomy and total synovectomy. However, controversy exists regarding the benefit of synovectomy. In older patients with secondary disease, primary arthroplasty is an option.

The most common complications include stiffness and recurrence of mechanical symptoms due to loose-body generation. Recurrence from surgery is in up to 20% of cases. Aggressive postoperative physiotherapy is required to minimize joint stiffness. Transformation to synovial chondrosarcoma is rare.

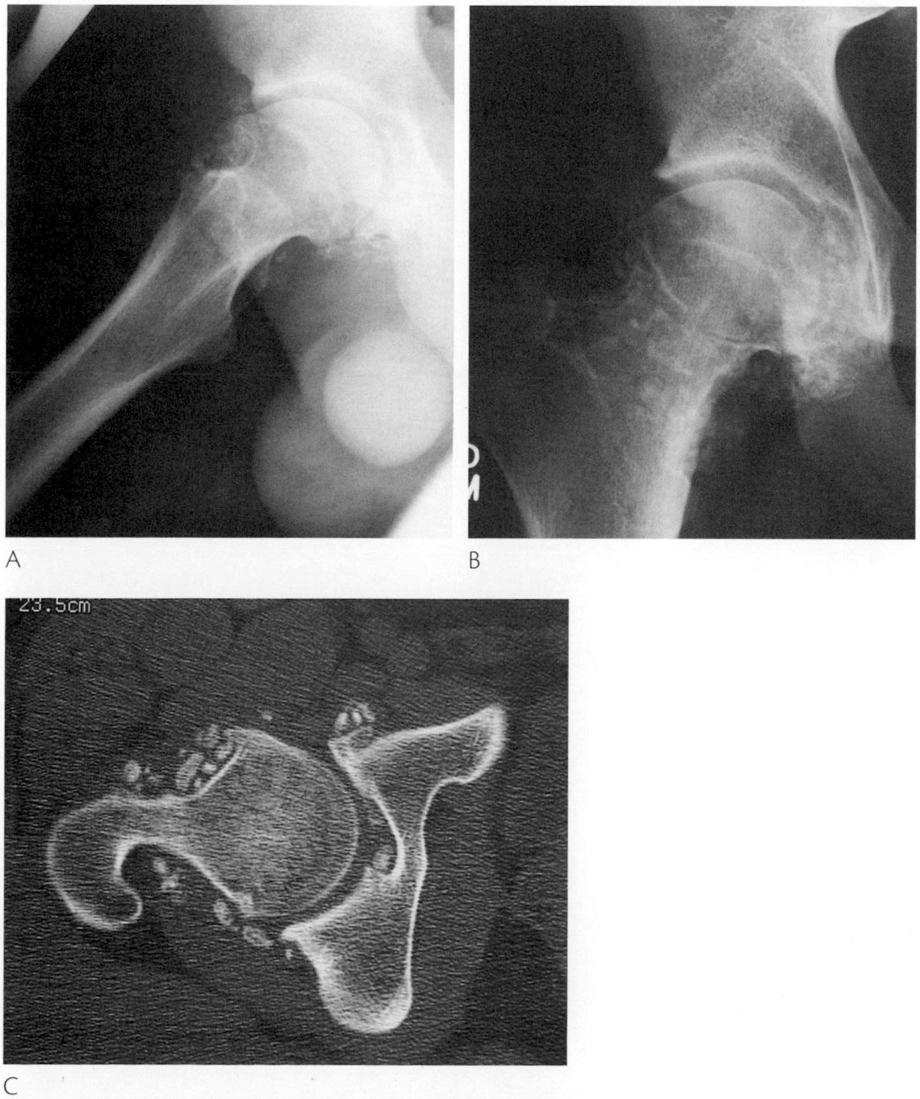

Fig. 2.3.8 Anteroposterior (A) and lateral (B) plain radiographs of the right hip and computed tomography scan (C) demonstrating multiple opacities consistent with synovial chondomatosis.

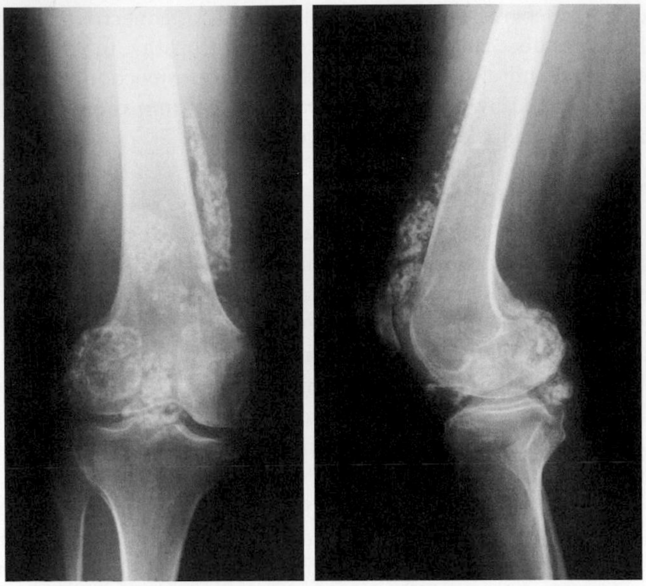

Fig. 2.3.9 Anteroposterior (A) and lateral (B) views of the right knee showing multiple opacities characteristic of synovial chondromatosis.

Box 2.3.13 Synovial chondromatosis

- Foci of cartilage develop in synovial membranes as a result of metaplasia of the subsynovial connective tissue
- Present with pain ± joint mechanical symptoms
- Primary or secondary
- Consider partial/complete synovectomy in resistant cases
- Rare transformation to synovial chondrosarcoma.

Further reading

Ferrari, A., Bisogno, G., Macaluso, A., *et al.* (2007). Soft-tissue sarcomas in children and adolescents with neurofibromatosis type 1. *Cancer*, **109**, 1406–12.

Matsumoto, K., Hukuda, S., Ishizawa, M., Chano, T., and Okabe, H. (1999). MRI findings in intramuscular lipomas. *Skeletal Radiology*, **28**, 145–52.

Rosenberg, A.E. (2008). Pseudosarcomas of soft tissue. *Archives of Pathology & Laboratory Medicine*, **132**(4), 579–86.

Stull, M.A., Moser, R.P. Jr, Kransdorf, M.J., Bogumill, G.P., and Nelson, M.C. (1991). Magnetic resonance appearance of peripheral nerve sheath tumors. *Skeletal Radiology*, **20**, 9–14.

2.4

Malignant tumours of soft tissues

Rej S. Bhumbra, Panagiotis D. Gikas, Sammy A. Hanna, Jakub Jagiello, and Stephen R. Cannon

Summary points

- Malignant vascular tumours of soft tissue
- Synovial sarcoma
- Malignant peripheral nerve sheath tumours
- Rhabdomyosarcoma
- Leiomyosarcoma
- Epithelioid sarcoma
- Clear cell sarcoma
- Malignant fibrous histiocytoma
- Chordoma.

Malignant vascular tumours of soft tissue

Three major categories of vascular tumours have been identified: benign lesions such as haemangiomas; tumours of intermediate malignancy (haemangioendothelioma); and highly malignant tumours (angiosarcoma). They are all very rare tumours accounting for less than 1% of soft tissue sarcomas.

Clinical presentation

The majority of haemangioendotheliomas are solitary lesions but may occur in association with other cutaneous vascular abnormalities such as those found in Klippel–Trenaunay or Mafucci's syndrome. The mass is usually painless.

The majority of angiosarcomas arise in skin. Associations exist with lymphoedema, trauma, and previously irradiated tissues. Lesions are often diffuse and can present late with ulceration and a nodular character.

Radiological features

Plain radiographs may demonstrate punctate calcification within the tumour, which can be encountered in any vascular lesion. Magnetic resonance imaging (MRI) may show high-flow signals of vascular structures. Angiography is useful as it may help to identify feeding vessels for preoperative embolization.

Pathological features

The vessel in which endotheliomas arise usually remains intact with the tumour developing within the lumen of the vessel.

Cutaneous angiosarcomas are usually well- or moderately-differentiated tumours that tend to form vascular-like structures infiltrating or dissecting irregularly into the dermis (unlike haemangiomas).

Treatment and outcome

Surgery with or without adjuvant radiotherapy is the mainstay of treatment. Angiosarcomas are generally more difficult to control locally because of their infiltrative nature.

The prognosis of haemangioendothelioma is comparatively good with more than 80% 5-year survival (lung and local lymph nodes being the commonest sites of dissemination).

Angiosarcomas are aggressive tumours with less than 20% 5-year survival. They commonly metastasize to the lung, liver, and spleen.

Synovial sarcoma (Box 2.4.1)

Synovial sarcoma is a rare and aggressive soft-tissue tumour, which accounts for 8–10% of all human malignant sarcomas diagnosed annually. Its peak incidence is in adults in their third to fifth decades of life, but it can also occur in children.

Clinical presentation

The most common mode of presentation is a deep-seated, painless mass. Periarticular regions in the extremities are especially affected. It is more common in the lower limb and appears to have a close association with tendon sheaths, bursae, joint capsules and in less than 10% of cases involves the articular surface. Invasion of adjacent bone is seen in 10–20% of cases, which is not as common as in other soft-tissue sarcomas. Other sites of involvement include the head and neck, trunk, lung, intestine, and retroperitoneum.

Radiological features

Plain radiography of synovial sarcomas reveals calcifications within the lesion in 30% of cases. Computed tomography (CT) scanning demonstrates heterogeneous lobulated masses with mixed cystic and solid appearances, which can be secondary to necrosis and/or haemorrhage. Thoracic CT scans are obtained to detect pulmonary metastases, and are an important part of the staging process.

MRI is the imaging modality of choice for diagnosing synovial sarcoma. The clear contrast between the lesion and normal tissues enables accurate assessment of tumour local invasion. It also is very valuable in revealing involvement of the neurovascular bundle and lymphatics. MRI is also excellent for surveillance and monitoring of the development of local recurrence after surgical resection, or sarcomatous changes secondary to radiation treatment.

Tumours appear sharply marginated, largely cystic or multiloculated with internal septations. Because of the cystic appearance and the well-defined margins, synovial sarcomas can be misdiagnosed on MRI.

Technectium-99m (^{99m}Tc) bone scans and positron emission tomography (PET) scans are obtained to screen for bony metastases. These can be either lytic or mixed in nature.

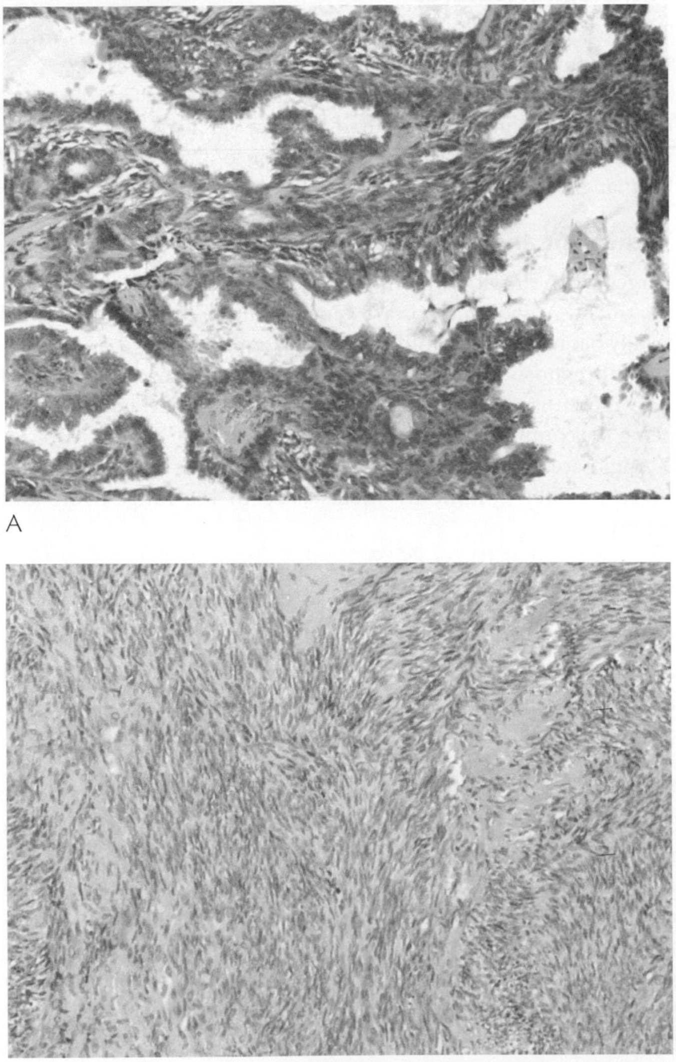

Fig. 2.4.1 A) Biphasic synovial sarcoma showing glandular-like spaces with an intervening spindle cell component (10×; H&E stain). B) Monophasic synovial sarcoma is composed of fascicles of spindle cells with ill-defined basophilic cytoplasm (10×: H&E stain). Also see colour plate section.

Pathological features

Histologically, synovial sarcomas are divided into three subtypes: biphasic, monophasic, and poorly differentiated. The biphasic type contains epithelial and spindle cell elements (Figure 2.4.1A). The monophasic contains only spindle cells (Figure 2.4.1B). The poorly differentiated type has areas of mono-biphasic morphology surrounded by poorly differentiated areas with high cellularity, pleomorphism, round cells, mitoses, and necrosis.

Ninety to 95% of synovial sarcoma cells are characterized by the presence of a translocation t(X:18). This seems specific to the disease, as it is not seen in other soft-tissue sarcomas, and this can be used as a good diagnostic tool.

Treatment and outcome

Complete surgical excision is the mainstay of treatment. The extent of resection has a significant bearing on the outcome. Local recurrence and metastases are common with contaminated surgical margins. Many authors have reported the use of radiotherapy as an aid to surgery to achieve local disease control, especially in cases with positive resection margins. However, its role after achieving complete excision has not been fully evaluated.

The use of chemotherapy remains a controversial issue, and its influence on survival is debatable. Some authors recommend its use for systemic disease control, especially in children, but other believe the use of multiple chemotherapy agents does not affect survival.

Overall survival for completely resected lesions ranges from 50–80% at 5 years, compared to 25–30% when there are distant metastases at the time of presentation.

Malignant peripheral nerve sheath tumours (Box 2.4.2)

These are a rare variety of soft-tissue sarcomas of ectomesenchymal origin. The World Health Organization (WHO) recommends the use of the term MPNST as a replacement for the terms malignant schwannoma, malignant neurilemmoma, and new ribbon sarcoma. They are commonly misdiagnosed because of their cellular origin and the histopathological similarities with other spindle cell sarcomas (leiomyosarcoma, rhabdomyosarcoma).

Clinical presentation

MPNST represent 10% of all soft-tissue sarcomas, affecting adults in their second to fifth decades of life. Patients with type 1 neurofibromatosis are, however, affected at an earlier age. The most common sites of occurrence include the sciatic nerve, brachial plexus, and sacral plexus. Other sites include the pelvis, retroperitoneum, and infratemporal fossa. They usually present as painful mass with a biologically aggressive behaviour.

Box 2.4.1 Synovial sarcoma

- 8–10% of all human malignant sarcomas
- Deep-seated, painless mass affecting predominantly periarticular regions
- 90–95% are characterized by the presence of a translocation t(X:18)
- Surgical excision ± adjuvant radiotherapy.

Radiological features

MRI of these tumours reveals inhomogeneous lesions with necrosis and haemorrhage. It is the imaging modality of choice as in all soft-tissue sarcomas, as it can reveal the nerve of origin and the relationship to adjacent structures.

Pathological features

Histological examination in most cases shows spindled cells with many nuclei, similar to Schwann cells. These are arranged in sweeping fascicles alternating with myxoid areas. Mitotic figures are frequent. Heterotopic islands of cartilage and bone can also be seen. Four subtypes are recognized in the literature and include: cartilagenous, epitheliod, glandular, and rhabdoid. Tumour cells in all four subtypes show positive staining for S100.

Treatment and outcome

Radical surgical resection is the treatment of choice. In extremity lesions, amputations should be considered when there is extensive involvement of surrounding structures, especially the neurovascular bundle, making excisions not feasible. These tumours are resistant to radiation and chemotherapy, but radiotherapy is still sometimes used in cases with contaminated surgical margins.

Local recurrence occurs in approximately 40% of MPNST cases, this being the highest local recurrence rate of any soft-tissue sarcoma. Survival at 5 years is 40–45%. Metastases occur in the lungs, bone, pleura, and retroperitoneum.

Rhabdomyosarcoma (Box 2.4.3)

Represents the most common soft-tissue sarcoma in children, accounting for 5–8% of all childhood cancers.

Clinical presentation

These are fast growing and highly malignant neoplasms, arising from rhabdomyoblasts. Lesions can arise in any part of the body except bone. The most commonly affected sites include the head and neck, extremities, genitourinary (GU) tract, trunk, orbit, and retroperitoneum. Approximately 90% of patients are younger than 18, with two age peaks (2–6 years—head and neck tumours; 14–18 years—extremities).

Radiological features

Plain radiographs usually reveal calcifications in lesions. CT scans are obtained to diagnose pulmonary and liver metastases. MRI is the main diagnostic tool and it reveals a clear definition of the mass and its invasion of adjacent structures. It is also very valuable in detecting local recurrence, and bone marrow metastases. The latter cases are usually associated with normal ^{99m}Tc and PET scans, which are insensitive to bone marrow infiltration when the bone cortex is intact.

Pathological features

Histologically, rhabdomyosarcomas are divided into four different subtypes according to the cells encountered in the tumour (Figure 2.4.2). These are embryonal, alveolar, spindle cell, and undifferentiated (anaplastic, pleomorphic).

The embryonal is the most common and affects children under the age of 15, occurring mainly in the head and neck. In the botryoid subtype of embryonal rhabdomyosarcoma, the cambium layer is characteristic, and contains a condensation of loose tumour cells below an epithelial surface. This usually affects the vagina and GU tract. The alveolar type is characterized by cells lining up along membranes resembling lung alveoli. This is more aggressive and affects the trunk and extremities. The spindle cell type has a fascicular, spindled, and leiomyomatous growth pattern and can demonstrate notable rhabdomyoblastic differentiation. In the undifferentiated type, no evidence of myogenesis differentiation is present.

Treatment and outcome

Treatment involves a combination of surgery, radiotherapy, and chemotherapy. Obtaining a 2-cm clear margin is recommended, and all cases are routinely given radiotherapy postoperatively. Chemotherapy is used in certain cases to shrink the tumour to aid later surgical resection. Common agents used include cyclophosphamide, adriamycin, and ifosfamide.

Patients with non-metastatic rhabdomyosarcoma have a survival rate of 70% at 5 years after combined modality therapy. In 14% of patients, metastases are present at the time of diagnosis, decreasing the survival rate to 20% at 5 years. The most common sites of distant lesions include the lungs and bone marrow.

Leiomyosarcoma (Box 2.4.4)

Leiomyosarcoma is an aggressive soft-tissue sarcoma derived from smooth muscle cells. These malignant tumours arise from mesenchymal cell lines.

Of all soft-tissue sarcomas, approximately 5–10% are leiomyosarcomas. The aetiology of this tumour is unknown. Leiomyosarcoma of soft tissue is thought to arise from the smooth muscle cells lining small blood vessels. Leiomyosarcoma can also arise directly from the viscera, including the gastrointestinal tract and uterus.

Box 2.4.2 Malignant peripheral nerve sheath tumours

- Represent 10% of soft tissue sarcomas
- Term encompasses malignant schwannoma, malignant neurilemmoma, new ribbon sarcoma
- Surgical excision; resistant to radio/chemotherapy
- High local recurrence rate (40%).

Box 2.4.3 Rhabdomyosarcoma

- Most common soft tissue sarcoma in children (5–8% of all childhood cancers)
- Fast growing and highly malignant neoplasms, arising from rhabdomyoblasts
- Neo-adjuvant chemotherapy + surgical excision + adjuvant radiotherapy
- Non-metastatic disease has 70% survival at 5 years.

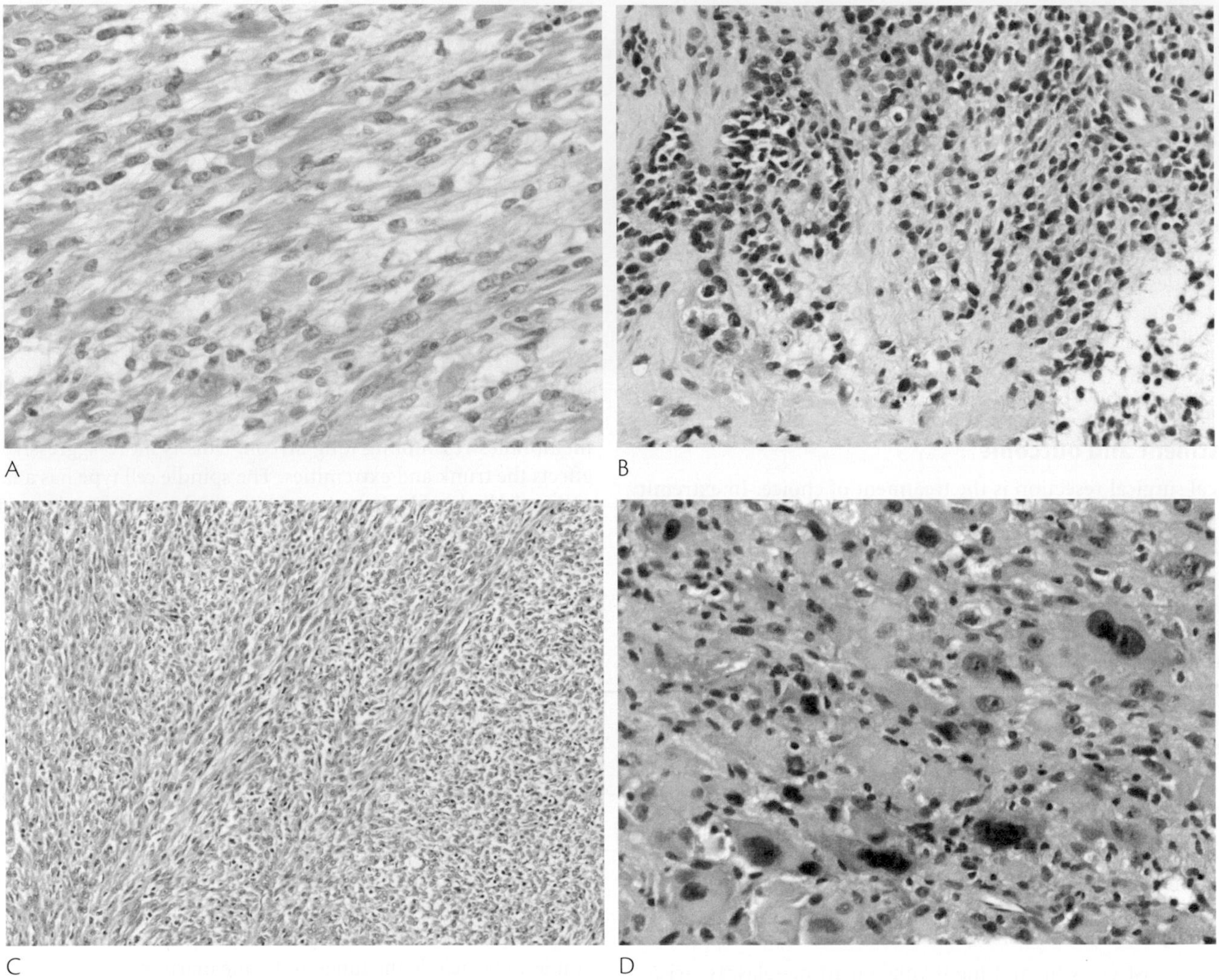

Fig. 2.4.2 A) Typical embryonal rhabdomyosarcoma featuring fascicles of elongated spindle cells with striking rhabdomyoblastic differentiation (20×; H&E stain). B) Typical features of alveolar rhabdomyosarcoma showing small round blue cells with focal rhabdomyoblastic differentiation (20×; H&E stain). C) Intertwining long fascicles of spindle cells with eosinophilic cytoplasm and prominent nucleoli characterize the spindle cell variant of rhabdomyosarcoma (10×; H&E stain). D) Pleomorphic rhabdomyosarcoma is characterized by large cells with pleomorphic nuclei and eosinophilic cytoplasm (20×; H&E stain). Also see colour plate section.

Clinical presentation

There are no specific clinical features diagnostic of leiomyosarcoma of soft tissue that distinguish these tumours from other soft tissue sarcomas. Women are affected more than men (2:1), with the disease typically occurring in the fifth and sixth decades of life. This gender distribution may reflect the proliferation of smooth muscle in response to oestrogen. It is a tumour of adulthood but it does account for about 6–7% of all childhood malignancies.

The most common site of involvement of leiomyosarcoma is the retroperitoneum, accounting for approximately 50% of occurrences. Presenting signs and symptoms for retroperitoneal tumours can include: an abdominal mass, pain, swelling, weight loss, nausea, or vomiting.

Leiomyosarcoma of somatic soft tissues, like other soft tissue sarcomas, often present as an enlarging, painless mass. However, when leiomyosarcoma arises from a major blood vessel, symptoms of vascular compromise or leg oedema may be present, as well as neurologic symptoms.

Approximately 15–30% of patients have metastatic disease at presentation. The most common metastatic site is the lung. Other common sites for metastases are the skin, bone, liver, and lymph nodes.

Radiological features

Initial imaging should include plain radiographs of the affected area, an MRI of the lesion, and a chest CT scan (to evaluate for the presence of metastatic disease).

MRI is the study of choice for the evaluation of the anatomic extent of the tumour, especially to adjacent structures. CT imaging is useful in evaluating the extent of retroperitoneal tumours.

Pathological features

While histologically similar, soft tissue leiomyosarcoma has classically been subdivided into three groups for prognostic and treatment purposes: leiomyosarcoma of somatic soft tissue; cutaneous leiomyosarcoma; and leiomyosarcoma of vascular origin.

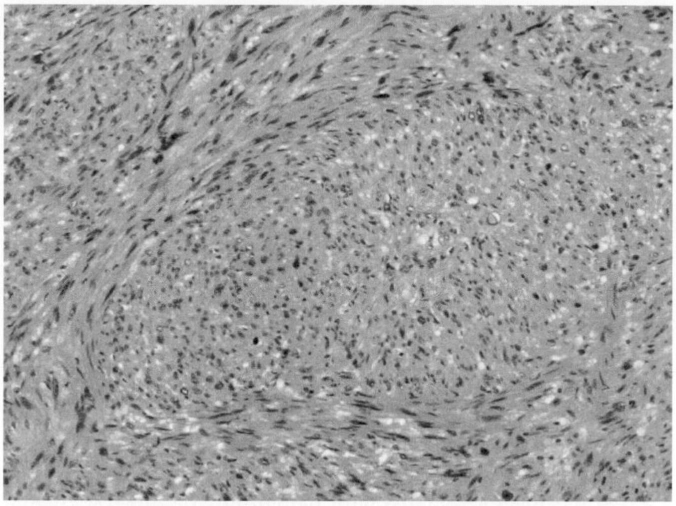

Fig. 2.4.3 Typical microscopic features of high-grade leiomyosarcoma characterized by intersecting fascicles of eosinophilic spindle cells (10×; H&E stain). Also see colour plate section.

There is little histological difference between leiomyosarcoma arising from deep, subcutaneous, or dermal sites or in association with vessels.

Leiomyosarcomas are typified by spindle cells with a centrally placed blunt-ended cigar-shaped nucleus and abundant cytoplasm, arranged in intersecting bundles (Figure 2.4.3). Greater nuclear eccentricity, hyperchromatism, atypia, and size accompany more poorly differentiated cells.

Treatment and outcome

Leiomyosarcomas are aggressive tumours that are often difficult to treat. The prognosis is poor, with survival rates among the lowest of all soft tissue sarcomas.

Surgical resection remains the only potentially curative treatment option. Five-year survival rates of 80% and 67%, respectively, in stages I and II, and of 12–50% in the more advanced stages. Tumours of the extremity have a better prognosis with greater than 60% survival at 5 years.

Adjuvant radiotherapy is indicated if the tumour is larger than 10cm or situated adjacent to neurovascular structures, which, if spared, necessitate a marginal resection. Chemotherapy comes into play as the primary treatment with inoperable tumours and may be a first line of treatment of choice in the case of lung disease. The two drugs most frequently used are doxorubicin and ifosfamide.

The prognoses of infants and young children tend to be better than those of adolescents and adults with similar diagnoses.

Box 2.4.4 Leiomyosarcoma

- 10% of all soft tissue sarcomas
- Most develop in the skin and deep soft tissues of the extremities and retroperitoneum
- 15–30% have metastatic disease at presentation
- Surgical resection ± adjuvant radiotherapy; chemotherapy for inoperable/metastatic disease

Epithelioid sarcoma (Box 2.4.5)

The term 'epithelioid sarcoma' was first coined by Enzinger in 1970. He described a group of hand sarcomas often confused with a chronic inflammatory process, a necrotizing granuloma, or a squamous cell carcinoma.

Clinical presentation

These represent the most common soft tissue sarcomas occurring in the hand in young adults. They mainly arise from the subcutaneous tissue, fascia, tendon sheaths, or joint capsule. The upper extremity is more commonly affected than the lower extremity. In many cases, patients present with a small, painless, ulcerating nodule on the extensor surface of the hand or forearm.

Radiological features

MRI is the imaging modality of choice to reveal the extent of local invasion and association with surrounding structures.

Pathological features

The histological features of epithelioid sarcoma include the presence of malignant cells which are epithelioid, spindled, or mixed in appearance. An abundance of chronic inflammatory cells is commonly encountered along the margins of tumour nodules, which can obscure the diagnosis in some cases.

Treatment and outcome

Radical resection and/or amputation are the treatments of choice. The role of radiotherapy and chemotherapy as adjuvant treatments is not very clear and has not yet been fully determined. Five-year survival in the literature ranges between 50–70%. Local recurrence and metastases, especially pulmonary, are common features of the disease. Routes of spread include the tendon sheaths, the fascia, and the lymphatic system.

Clear cell sarcoma (Box 2.4.6)

Clear cell sarcoma of tendons and aponeuroses is a rare and aggressive cancer, accounting for less than 1% of all soft tissue sarcomas. They are easily mistaken for malignant melanomas because of their histochemical and structural similarities. Many authors use the term 'malignant melanoma of the soft parts' to refer to these tumours.

Clinical presentation

They represent a distinct entity with a predilection for occurring in the tendons and aponeuroses of young adults. Eighty to 90% of

Box 2.4.5 Epithelioid sarcoma

- Most common soft tissue sarcomas occurring in the hand in young adults
- Chronic inflammatory cells are commonly found in lesions making diagnosis difficult
- Radical resection is the treatment of choice
- Local recurrence and pulmonary metastases are common.

lesions develop in the lower limb, with the ankle and foot being the commonest sites. Other sites include the knee, thigh, elbow, hand, head and neck, and trunk. They all exhibit an aggressive behaviour with a high incidence of local recurrence and metastases.

The commonest presentation is a painless, deep-seated mass, which is bound to adjacent tendons or aponeuroses.

Radiological features

Intralesional calcifications are rarely seen on plain radiography or CT scanning. MRI commonly reveals areas of necrosis and/or haemorrhage within the lesion.

Pathological features

Clear cell sarcomas are mainly made up of round or fusiform cells arranged in nests separated by fibrosclerotic bands or septa. Giant cells with more than 10–12 nuclei may also be encountered within the tumour mass. Tumour cells are mostly uniform and have vesicular nuclei containing prominent nucleoli and clear or pale staining cytoplasm. These tumours and malignant melanomas share similar histological characteristics and features, and both are positive for the protein S100, suggesting a close relationship between both entities. The site of occurrence is, however, different. The majority of cases are associated with a chromosomal translocation t(12:22)(q13: q12).

Treatment and outcome

The recommended treatment is a wide/radical excision or amputation if necessary, both with local lymph node clearance. The roles of adjuvant radiotherapy and chemotherapy are debatable, but used in many centres.

The prognosis is generally poor, with a 5-year survival rate of 60–70% after radical excision ± adjuvant treatments. This falls to 30% at 10 years. Local recurrence and metastases are common features, especially with a positive surgical margin. Metastases are usually to lymph nodes and the lungs. Less common sites include the skin, bone, and liver. Overall, 70% of patients develop metastases at some stage of the disease.

Malignant fibrous histiocytoma (Box 2.4.7)

Malignant fibrous histiocytoma (MFH), described by O'Brien and Stout in 1964, is the most common soft tissue sarcoma of late adult life accounting for 20–24% of soft tissue sarcomas.

Box 2.4.6 Clear cell sarcoma

- Rare and aggressive cancer; less than 1% of all soft tissue sarcomas
- Predilection for occurring in the tendons and aponeuroses in the lower limbs of young adults
- Painless, deep-seated mass, bound to adjacent tendons or aponeuroses
- Similar histological features to malignant melanomas
- Poor prognosis; 70% will develop metastases at some stage of the disease.

It is a heterogeneous tumour with respect to histology and prognosis with malignant cells of histiocytic origin. Early osseous invasion and metastases to regional lymph nodes is common. The term MFH is still in use, but is gradually being replaced by the term pleomorphic sarcoma.

Clinical presentation

MFH occurs more commonly in Caucasian patients. The male to female ratio is approximately 2:1. Peak incidence is in the fifth and sixth decades. Although rare in children, the angiomatoid subtype is the most frequently occurring variety in patients younger than 20 years.

MFH occurs most commonly in the extremities (70–75%, with lower extremities accounting for 59% of cases), followed by the retroperitoneum. Tumours typically arise in deep fascia or skeletal muscle.

MFH has been associated with hematopoietic diseases such as non-Hodgkin lymphoma, Hodgkin lymphoma, multiple myeloma, and malignant histiocytosis.

The most common clinical presentation is an enlarging painless soft tissue mass in the thigh, typically 5–10cm in diameter. Two-thirds are intramuscular. Retroperitoneal MFH usually presents with constitutional symptoms, including fever, malaise, and weight loss. This can be confused with infection or abscess presentation. MFH also occurs secondary to radiation exposure and may occasionally be seen adjacent to metallic devices, including total joint prostheses.

Radiological features

Plain radiographs are always indicated, reflecting the invasive nature of tumour. Bony lesions will show destructive changes with cortical erosion and a poorly defined, permeative margin. Other changes such as matrix mineralization are less common. CT typically reveals a non-specific, large, lobulated, soft tissue mass of predominantly muscle density, with nodular and peripheral enhancement of solid portions.

One should keep in mind that the diagnosis of MFH is made using histopathology, not by imaging; however, MRI remains invaluable for delineating tumour extent.

Pathological features

Uncertain histogenesis and numerous subtypes make MFH a rather controversial entity.

The tumour contains both fibroblast-like and histiocyte-like cells in varying proportions, with spindled and rounded cells exhibiting a storiform arrangement.

Five histologic subtypes have been described:

1) Storiform/pleomorphic (most common)
2) Myxoid
3) Giant cell
4) Inflammatory (usually retroperitoneal)
5) Angiomatoid.

Treatment and outcome

Early and complete surgical removal is indicated because of the aggressive nature of the tumour. Surgical excision with irradiation to residual local disease is the treatment modality of choice.

The sensitivity of MFH to radiotherapy and chemotherapy is poor, and evidence is lacking for adjuvant treatment.

Patients with low-grade, intermediate-grade, and high-grade tumours have 10-year survival rates of 90%, 60%, and 20%, respectively. Patients with tumours smaller than 5cm at presentation have survival rates of 79–82%. Patients with tumours larger than 10cm have survival rates of 41–51%.

The rate of metastasis varies with the histologic subtype from 23% (myxoid) to 50% (giant cell). Distant metastasis most commonly occurs to the lung (90%) and bone (8%) Resection with negative microscopic margins decreases the incidence of local recurrence.

The overall survival rate of patients with MFH ranges from 36–58% at 5 years; however, patients with retroperitoneal tumours have an overall 5-year survival rate of 15–20%.

Chordoma (Box 2.4.8)

Chordoma is a relatively rare malignant midline tumour strictly arising in the midline of the axial skeleton, primarily at its cranial and caudal ends. Chordomas are tumours derived from remnants of the primitive notochord. They often metastasize late and despite surgical resection, and adjuvant radiotherapy, recurrence is common.

Clinical presentation

Chordomas are tumours arising from remnants of the primitive notochord and are epithelial in origin. They are relatively rare (make up only 1–4% of primary malignant soft tissue tumours) slow growing, malignant neoplasms. Peak distribution is in patients aged 55–65 years. Males are affected twice as frequently as are females, with a preponderance of cases in the sacrococcygeal location.

Chordomas have a predilection for the ends of the spinal column. Approximately 50% of spinal chordomas originate in the sacrococcygeal area. Approximately 35% occur at the base of the skull near the spheno-occipital area, and 15% are found in the vertebral column. These lesions present clinically as destructive bony masses with extensive soft tissue involvement. They erode and impinge upon adjacent structures, giving rise to variable presentation.

In the cranial region, they can cause cranial nerve palsies, hydrocephalus, headaches, and torticollis.

Sacral chordomas are often missed at the initial presentation, with patients being symptomatic for several months or even years prior to being correctly diagnosed. Most patients have pain that is difficult to distinguish from mechanical back pain. Symptoms may include altered bowel habits, or a feeling of fullness in the rectal area. Physical examination must include a rectal examination to exclude a potential presacral mass.

Chordomas are locally aggressive but metastasis is relatively uncommon.

Radiological features

Plain radiographs do not provide sufficient information concerning the diagnosis or the planning of the surgical procedure and can often be obscured by bowel gas. Chordoma lesions are seen as midline lobular lesions, with areas of osteolysis, occasionally with expansion and osteosclerotic rimming. MRI scans are essential to map out the true extent of the tumour especially sagittal views of the whole of the sacrum (Figure 2.4.4).

Pathological features

Based on light microscopic morphology, chordomas have been divided into three subtypes: conventional, chondroid, and dedifferentiated. Grossly, conventional chordomas have a soft, tan, myxoid appearance with areas of haemorrhage. Immunochemistry is extremely useful for distinguishing chordoma from other tumours, especially chondrosarcoma.

Dedifferentiation or sarcomatous transformation occurs in 2–8% of chordomas and is associated with a poor prognosis.

Treatment and outcome

Definitive resection should always wait until a final pathological diagnosis is made. The mainstay of treatment is en bloc resection of the tumour with a wide margin, leaving a cuff of normal tissue.

Aggressive initial therapy improves overall outcome. Tumours detected and diagnosed early have a favourable prognosis if treated with a complete or en bloc excision. A complete excision may involve a combined anterior-posterior operation, vertebrectomy if the spine is involved, and subsequent stabilization. A permanent colostomy may be required and the patient may need intermittent self catheterization in the long term.

The importance of a complete excision is demonstrated by the longer disease-free period compared to that following an incomplete excision. In aiming to achieve a clear resection margin, sacrificing sacral nerve roots and excision of the rectum may be required.

Surgical resection margins are reportedly the most important predictor of survival and local recurrence with sacral chordomas. The findings suggest that obtaining wide surgical margins posteriorly, by excising parts of the piriformis, gluteus maximus, and sacroiliac joints, may result in better local disease control in patients with sacral chordoma.

Adjuvant radiotherapy must be given in the case of incomplete excision. Radiation therapy may also salvage some patients with local recurrence.

The 5-year and 10-year survival rates for conventional chordoma are approximately 50% and 25–30%, respectively. Survival rates appear to be influenced more by local tumour progression than by metastasis.

All three types of chordomas can metastasize, usually later in the course of the disease (except dedifferentiated chordomas, which can metastasize early). Vertebral body chordomas have a higher

Box 2.4.7 Malignant fibrous histiocytoma

- Most common soft tissue sarcoma of late adult life
- Occurs most commonly in the extremities (70–75%, with lower extremities accounting for 59% of cases), followed by the retroperitoneum
- Contains both fibroblast-like and histiocyte-like cells in varying proportions
- Surgical excision ± radiotherapy for residual disease
- Aggressive with survival rate between 36–58% at 5 years.

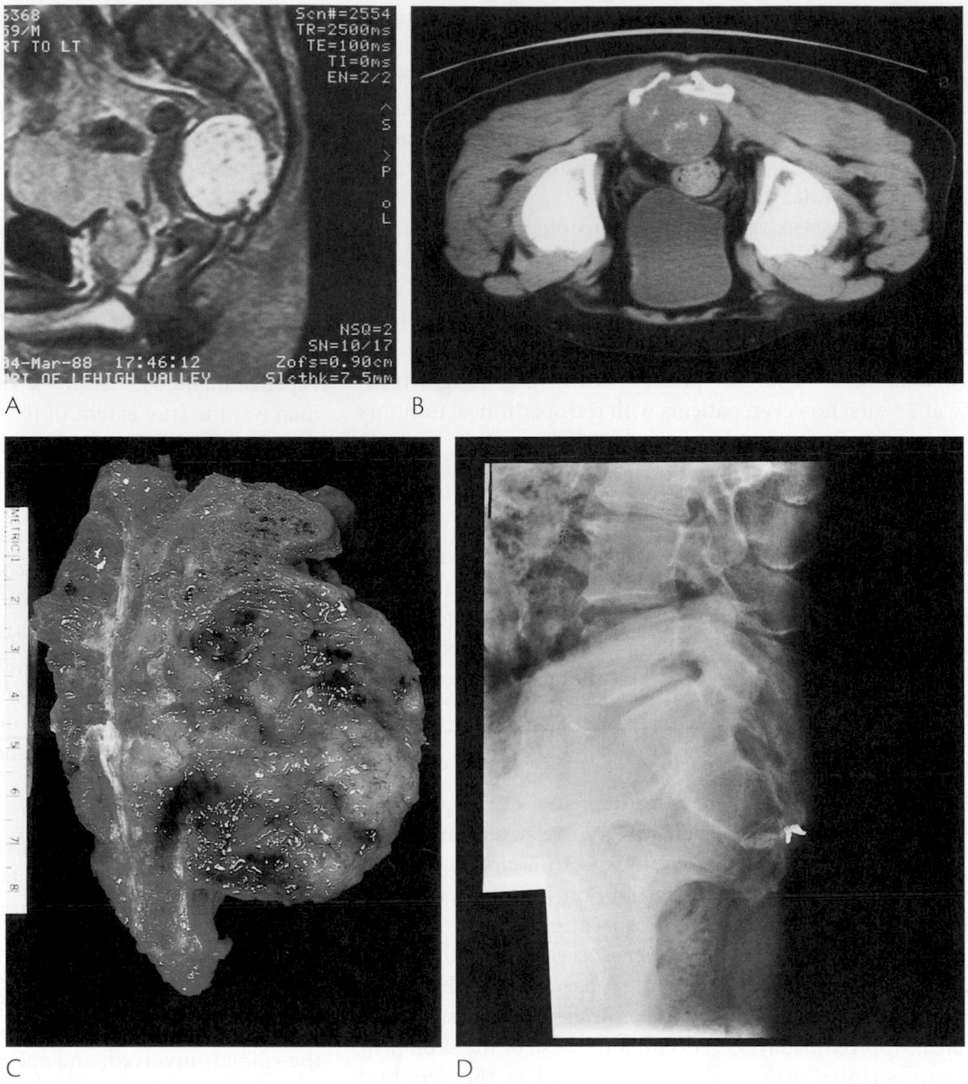

Fig. 2.4.4 A) Sagittal magnetic resonance imaging reveals a large anterior soft-tissue mass extending from the sacrum and abutting the rectum. B) A computed tomography scan reveals the residual calcification present throughout the chordoma. C) Gross resected specimen shows the extensive anterior soft-tissue mass. D) Postoperative lateral radiograph demonstrates the partial sacrectomy at the S2–3 level.

Box 2.4.8 Chordoma

- Develops from notochordal remnants
- Divided into three subtypes: conventional, chondroid, and dedifferentiated
- Locally aggressive but metastasis is relatively uncommon
- Usually present with pain and often cause neurological deficits
- Mainstay of treatment is en bloc resection of the tumour with a wide margin.

incidence of metastasis than do those arising in the clivus or sacrum.

Further reading

Ferrari, A., Gronchi, A., Casanova, M., *et al.* (2004). Synovial sarcoma: a retrospective analysis of 271 patients of all ages treated at a single institution. *Cancer*, **101**(3), 627–34.

Punyko, J.A., Mertens, A.C., Baker, K.S., *et al.* (2005). Long-term survival probabilities for childhood rhabdomyosarcoma. A population-based evaluation. *Cancer*, **103**(7), 1475–83.

Randall, R.L., Albritton, K.H., Ferney, B.J., *et al.* (2004). Malignant fibrous histiocytoma of soft tissue: an abandoned diagnosis. *American Journal of Orthopedics*, **33**(12), 602–8.

Sciubba, D.M., Chi, J.H., Rhines, L.D., and Gokaslan, Z.L. (2008). Chordoma of the spinal column. *Neurosurgery Clinics of North America*, **19**(1), 5–15.

Weiss, S.W., and Goldblum, J.R. (eds.) (2001). *Enzinger and Weiss's Soft Tissue Tumors*, 4th edn. Philadelphia, PA: Mosby-Harcourt.

2.5

Benign bone tumours

Anthony McGrath, Kesavan Sri-Ram, Eric Yeung, Ben Spiegelberg, Nick Kalson, Barry Rose, Rob Pollock, and John Skinner

Summary points

- Unicameral bone cyst
- Aneurysmal bone cyst
- Non-ossifying fibroma/fibrous cortical defect
- Bone island
- Fibrous dysplasia
- Osteochondroma
- Enchondroma
- Langerhans cell histiocytosis
- Chondroblastoma
- Giant cell tumour
- Osteoblastoma/osteoid osteoma
- 12.Periosteal chondroma.

Unicameral bone cyst (Box 2.5.1)

Unicameral bone cyst, (solitary bone cyst, simple bone cyst) (UBC) is a benign lesion characterized by a fluid-filled intramedullary cavity lined by a thin soft tissue membrane. It comprises between 3–5% of all primary bone tumours, with a 2:1 male predominance. Most UBCs occur in the proximal humerus and femur in young people aged 5–15 years, and in the ilium and calcaneum in older patients. The exact pathogenesis is still unclear.

Clinical presentation

Unicameral bone cysts are often asymptomatic, and discovered following an associated fracture. Other symptoms include localized tenderness, joint stiffness, swelling, and deformity or growth retardation if the cyst disrupts the epiphysis.

Radiological features

Plain radiographs are the investigation of choice for UBC (Figure 2.5.1). Typically they appear as a purely lytic lesion with a well-defined border and narrow zone of transition. They tend to occur centrally with some mild expansion of the bone but not breaching the cortex. The cortex is thinned and there is no periosteal reaction unless it is associated with a fracture. It is a unilocular lesion, but often appears multiloculated due to the prominent ridges on the cortical wall.

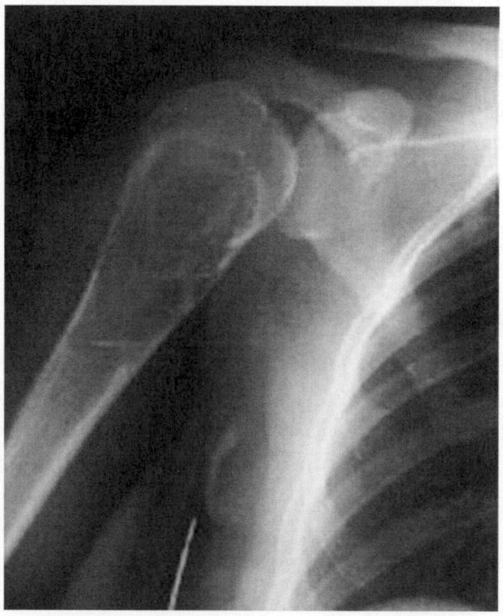

Fig. 2.5.1 Typical appearance of a proximal humeral unicameral bone cyst.

When a thinned cortical area fractures, the periosteum often remains intact, and the small fracture fragment can be seen within the base of the lesion (the fallen fragment sign) which is pathognomonic for a UBC with a fracture.

In young children, a UBC starts at the metaphysis adjacent to the epiphysis. As the bone grows, the lesion moves away towards the diaphysis. The lesion is classified as active when it is still within 1cm from the epiphysis, and latent when it is near the diaphysis.

Bone scan is often normal, and computed tomography (CT) shows only a fluid level. Intracystic septa can be demonstrated if radio opaque contrast is injected within the lesion. Magnetic resonance imaging (MRI) shows a bright fluid signal in T2-weighted images, and low signal in T1-weighted images.

Pathological features

Occasionally, a biopsy is taken to differentiate between UBC, aneurysmal bone cyst, and fibrous dysplasia. Grossly, the cortex is thin; the fluid is clear or yellow, with a fibrous membrane which lines the inner wall. Associated bleeding can be seen within the cavity if there is a fracture. Histological examination shows that the membrane consists of fibroblasts, with a cementum-like structure deep to it. This consists of strong eosinophilic and calcified material, surrounded by immature bone fragment, osteoclast-like giant cells, mesenchymal cells, and lymphocytes, but there would be no cellular atypia.

Treatment and outcome

Treatment is often non-operative. Small lesion in non-weight-bearing bone can be monitored regularly until skeletal maturity, but large cysts, or cysts at sites where there is high risk of fracture, should be treated. Operative management includes aspiration of the cyst followed by injection with either steroid or bone marrow, with recent studies suggesting that steroids may provide superior healing rates. Repeat injection may be required if there is no evidence of healing after 2 months. If it is not healing despite several injections, especially in the weight-bearing skeleton, curettage and bone grafting with or without internal fixation can be of benefit. Pathological fracture through the cyst often causes healing of the cyst after the fracture is united, probably due to an antiprostaglandin effect or decompression of the pressure of the cyst following the fracture.

More recently, injection of demineralized bone matrix and bone marrow had been shown to have good effect. In general, most patients will achieve an excellent outcome following any of the treatments.

Aneurysmal bone cyst (Box 2.5.2)

Aneurysmal bone cyst (ABC) is a locally destructive, expansile benign lesion. It is characterized by multiple loculations filled with blood and separated by fibrous septa. It accounts for about 2% of all primary bone tumours, and there is a slight female dominance of 3:2. It can arise as a primary lesion, or as secondary process associated with other lesions such as giant cell tumour, chondroblastoma, UBC, osteoblastoma, fibrous dysplasia, or even osteosarcoma.

ABC usually presents in the metaphysis of long bones, especially the proximal humerus, distal femur, and proximal tibia. It can also present in the ilium and in the posterior column of the vertebrae (accounts for 15–25%). Seventy-five per cent of patients present under the age of 20. It is postulated that ABCs arise from an increase of venous pressure secondary to some local circulatory compromise causing local haemorrhage.

Box 2.5.1 Unicameral bone cyst

- Proximal humerus and femur in young people aged 5–15years, ilium and calcaneum in older patients
- Often asymptomatic, pathological fracture common presentation
- Plain radiographs most useful: purely lytic lesion, well-defined border, narrow zone of transition
- Macroscopically: cortex is thin, fluid is clear or yellow, fibrous membrane lines inner wall
- Large cysts at high-risk sites should be treated: aspiration ± steroid injection; curettage + grafting ± internal fixation.

Clinical presentation

Most cases present with mild pain and swelling, but sometimes it can progress quite rapidly, mimicking malignancy. Spinal lesions can present with neurological symptoms. Pathological fracture, however, is not common (8–20%).

Radiological features

ABC appears as a destructive cystic lesion with bony resorption on plain radiographs (Figure 2.5.2). It is usually eccentric, with a narrow zone of transition and associated with cortical expansion. The growth plate is not normally breached, unless the ABC is secondary to a chondroblastoma or giant cell tumour.

Radiographic appearance is often seen in four phases:

1) Initial: small lytic lesion
2) Growth: rapid expansile growth, a 'blow-out' appearance
3) Stable: multiloculated cystic appearance, with thin outer cortex contained by the periosteum. Septation with fluid level can often be seen
4) Healing: ossification within the trabeculae of the lesion.

Bone scan shows a diffuse increased uptake in the periphery with a decreased central uptake. Angiography shows accumulation of contrast in the cavity, with hypervascularity in the periphery. CT and MRI can demonstrate the cavities and fluid level as well as delineating the lesion from the surrounding structures.

Pathological features

Macroscopically, ABC is a cystic lesion with septated cavities filled with blood. Microscopically, evaluation of the curetted tissue shows haemorrhagic tissue separated by cellular stroma. This stroma contains fibroblast, histiocytes, haemosiderin-packed macrophages, and osteoclast-like giant cells. There are numerous mitotic figures without atypical forms present in this stroma, and the vessels within them are quite dilated, probably contributing to the bleeding in

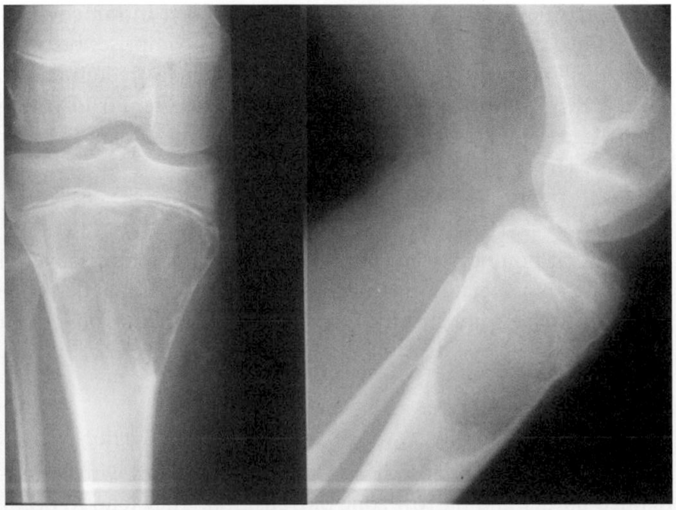

Fig. 2.5.2 Typical appearance of an aneurysmal bone cyst of the proximal tibia. A destructive cystic lesion is evident with thinning of the cortex but no breaching of the growth plate.

the cavities. A 'highly mineralized matrix with a chondral aura' lining the vascular area can be a diagnostic characteristic for ABC.

A solid variant of ABC has also been described. It has similar clinical and radiographic features to the cystic from, but lacking the cavernous spaces. The highly proliferative stromal cells appear very similar to giant cell tumour, which gives an impression that it may be a secondary ABC.

Treatment and outcome

Spontaneous healing is rare, and treatment is usually surgical. Curettage with or without bone grafting has been the acceptable method, together with various adjuvant therapies like phenol, liquid nitrogen and high-speed burring of the cavity wall, to reduce the recurrence rate. Recurrence rate of ABC following curettage with or without grafting has been shown to be about 20–30%, and reduced to about 10% with adjuvant therapy. Selective embolization of the feeding vessels prior to surgery can help to significantly reduce blood loss and should be used in large lesions. Resection of the expanded extremity of lesion, such as fibula or metatarsal, is another option.

Newer methods of minimally invasive introduction of demineralized bone and autologous bone marrow into the cysts, with no curettage has been used with some success. Percutaneous sclerotherapy using polidocanol has also been tried with some good results. Both of these methods have the advantage of avoiding open curettage, and hence reducing the risk of surgical morbidity. However, this does not provide tissue sample for definitive diagnosis and still has the potential for further cyst progression.

Non-ossifying fibroma/fibrous cortical defect (Box 2.5.3)

Fibrous cortical defects and non-ossifying fibroma are considered as abnormal developmental proliferations of fibrous tissue and histiocytes. Non-ossifying fibroma is larger, slightly different in radiological appearance, but is histologically identical. They are often termed as 'metaphyseal fibrous defects'. These lesions are common, and are present in over one-third of children under 14 years. Most are incidental findings. There is a slight male dominance of about 2:1.

Box 2.5.2 Aneurysmal bone cyst

- Usually presents in the metaphysis of long bones; 75% under age of 20
- Pain and swelling, pathological fracture uncommon; occasionally can progress rapidly mimicking malignancy
- Destructive cystic lesion with bony resorption on plain radiographs; usually eccentric, with narrow zone of transition and cortical expansion
- Macroscopically: cystic lesion with septated cavities filled with blood
- Spontaneous healing is rare, treatment usually surgical; curettage and bone grafting ± adjuvant therapy.

They commonly present in the metaphysis of lower limbs, such as distal femur, proximal/distal tibia, and fibula. Occasionally they can present in the humerus, clavicle, or ilium. Most of the lesions are solitary, but rarely can be multiple. A Jaffe–Campanacci syndrome had been described with multiple lesions, mental retardation, precocious puberty, congenital blindness, and kyphoscoliosis. The aetiology of these lesions is largely unclear.

Clinical presentation

Most of these lesions are completely asymptomatic. Large lesions can present with swelling, mild pain, or pathological fracture. There is no evidence to suggest that they can undergo malignant transformation.

Radiological features

On plain radiographs, fibrous cortical defects are usually in the metaphysis or diaphysis of long bones, they appear as eccentric radiolucent areas up to 2cm with a smooth margin and a thin sclerotic rim (Figure 2.5.3). The cortex can sometimes be eroded, but no periosteal reaction develops. Non-ossifying fibroma presents with similar features, but much larger in size, reaching to about 7cm. They can cause cortical expansion, and sometimes involve the whole width of thin bones, such as the fibula. Both lesions have their long axis parallel to the axis of the long bone, and are often found near the insertion of tendons, which suggests that stress or avulsion injury may contribute to the cause. With bone growth, they migrate from metaphysis to diaphysis. But when healing occurs, the sclerosis starts from the diaphyseal end towards the metaphysis.

The diagnosis of these lesions can usually be made by plain radiographs; bone scans only show increased uptake in the active healing phase or in pathological fractures. CT and MRI are not usually indicated.

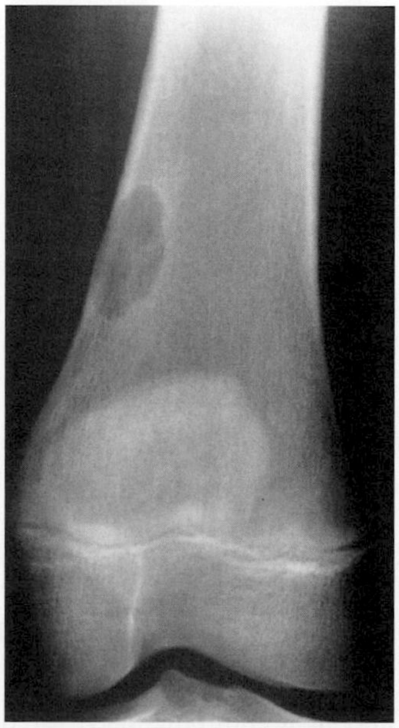

Fig. 2.5.3 Anteroposterior radiograph of the distal femur in a skeletally immature male. A well-circumscribed fibrous cortical defect is noted in the medial femoral cortex.

Pathological features

It is rare that any sample will reach the pathologist as no surgical treatment or biopsy is required. For those curetted samples which reach the pathology lab, the proliferative spindle cell stroma is intermixed with fibroblasts, collagen fibres, and histiocytes. Multinucleated giant cells are often present, and there is no cellular atypia. There is no reactive bone formation unless in the case of pathological fractures.

Treatment and outcome

Most of the fibrous cortical defects and non-ossifying fibromas regress and heal spontaneously, and no treatment is necessary. For those who present with pathological fracture, closed treatment is recommended to allow spontaneous union. The lesions that are at high risk of fracturing can be treated with close monitoring and modification of activity until they regress. Surgical treatment comprises curettage and bone grafting; more recently, demineralized bone matrix with bone marrow has been used with good results. Internal fixation is occasionally necessary if the pathological fracture is unstable or irreducible.

Bone island (Box 2.5.4)

Bone island, or enostosis, is a benign solitary area of mature lamellar bone within the cancellous bone. Found in about 1% of the population, predominantly adults, they have no gender predilection. They are predominantly found in adults, and rarely in children. In long bones they usually present in the epiphysis or metaphysis. The size of the bone island varies between 2–20mm, but occasionally they can be as large as 10cm. Any lesion larger than 2cm is termed 'giant bone island'.

Clinical presentation

Bone islands are asymptomatic, usually found incidentally, and should not cause pain. They can grow very slowly with time, enlarging about 30% over 20 years. Any bone island that is painful or grows more rapidly in size would suggest more aggressive disease.

Box 2.5.3 Non-ossifying fibroma/fibrous cortical defect

- Mostly found in children/young adults between 2–20, commonly present in the metaphysis of the lower limbs, such as distal femur, proximal/distal tibia and fibula
- Usually asymptomatic
- Metaphysis or diaphysis of long bones; eccentric radiolucent area, smooth margin, and thin sclerotic rim; cortex can sometimes be eroded, but no periosteal reaction develops; non-ossifying fibromas are much larger in size, reaching to about 7cm
- Multinucleated giant cells are often present; there is no cellular atypia
- Most regress and heal spontaneously; for those presenting with pathological fracture, closed treatment of the fracture is recommended to allow spontaneous union.

Osteopoikilosis is a rare condition consisting of multiple periarticular lesions, identical to bone island, throughout the skeleton.

Radiological features

Typically bone island can be diagnosed with plain radiographs, with the characteristic round or oval shape of high density within the cancellous bone (Figure 2.5.4). It is homogenous and blends into the native bone, giving a 'brush border'-like appearance. There is no bone destruction or periosteal reaction in the surrounding area.

Bone island is usually cold on bone scanning, but occasionally it can have increased uptake in the giant form. CT can demonstrate the benign morphology if plain radiographs are not enough to make the diagnosis.

Pathological features

Bone island rarely needs biopsy, but histologically it is an area of compact, mature lamellar bone with a well-developed Haversian system. Occasionally there is some woven bone present, with some increased osteoblastic activity and blood flow, indicating a degree of remodelling.

Treatment and outcome

Repeat radiographs can be used to monitor if the lesion is growing in size. If it enlarges more than 25% in 6 months, or 50% in 12 months, especially in the large ones (greater than 2cm), then it should be biopsied to exclude more aggressive lesions. Otherwise no treatment is required.

Fibrous dysplasia (Box 2.5.5)

Fibrous dysplasia is a slow-growing lesion where normal bone marrow is replaced by metaplastic woven bone and fibrous tissue.

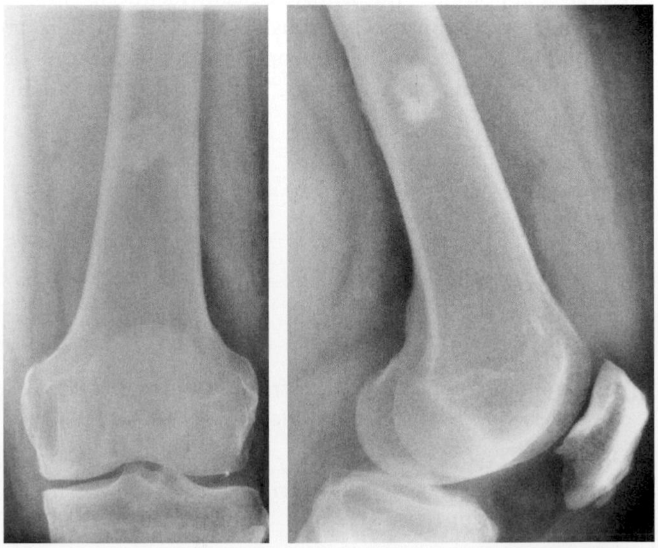

A B

Fig. 2.5.4 (A)This anteroposterior view of the distal femur in a 50-year-old male shows a typical bone island in the medullary canal. It was completely asymptomatic and discovered incidentally. (B) Lateral view. Note the radiating spicules of lesional bone blending into the surrounding native trabeculae.

Box 2.5.4 Bone island

- Can affect any bone, predominantly seen in adults
- Asymptomatic, incidental findings
- Diagnosed with plain radiographs; characteristic round or oval shape of high density within the cancellous bone
- Area of compact, mature lamellar bone with a well developed Haversian system
- No treatment required.

It may involve one (monostotic, 85% of the cases) or multiple bones (polyostotic 15%). They can be clustered around a single limb of the upper or lower extremity, or involve the whole skeleton. Certain syndromes, such as McCune–Albright disease and Mazabraud disease, have been associated with this lesion.

Fibrous dysplasia accounts for about 7% of all bone tumour or tumour-like conditions, and has no gender predilection. It can present at any age, but most lesions are found before 30 years of age as they are more active during growth. The most common locations are long bones, ribs, craniofacial, and pelvis.

A mutation of the Gsα gene has been found to be associated with fibrous dysplasia. It was first discovered in patients with McCune–Albright syndrome, and recent studies had shown that isolated fibrous dysplasia also has the mutated Gsα gene present. This gene mutation can lead to activation of adenylate cyclase within the cell, which increases cell proliferation but inappropriate differentiation, resulting in excessive production of disorganized fibrotic bone matrix.

Clinical presentation

The majority of monostotic lesions are asymptomatic, and are found incidentally during the investigation of other problems in the same region. Bone pain, stress fractures, and pathological fractures are the usual modes of presentation, especially on weight-bearing bones such as the femur.

Fibrous dysplasia can also present with a gradual deformity of the limb. The severity of the deformity depends on the age of the patient, the extent, the site of the lesion, or whether it is monostotic or polyostotic. The classic 'shepherd's crook deformity' of the proximal femur is characteristic of fibrous dysplasia. It is postulated that the deformity is secondary to the intermittent stress fractures through the dysplastic bone, and the bone then deforms with normal mechanical load. Other presenting symptoms and signs include limping, leg length discrepancy, tibial bowing, and exophthalmos associated with skull lesions.

Fibrous dysplasia is known to be associated with other conditions in certain syndromes. In McCune–Albright syndrome, polyostotic fibrous dysplasia is associated with precocious puberty and pigmented skin lesions. In Mazabraud syndrome, polyostotic lesions are associated with intramuscular myxoma. Oncogenic osteomalacia is a rare condition that is sometimes found in patients with fibrous dysplasia, symptoms of which are fatigue, joint pain, weakness, and fractures with an abnormal blood picture (hypophosphataemia, normocalcium, and increased alkaline phosphatase). Malignant transformation can occur in about 0.5%, but much higher (4%) in McCune–Albright syndrome.

Radiological features

On plain radiographs, fibrous dysplasia appears as a well-circumscribed diaphyseal lesion with a 'ground-glass' appearance (Figure 2.5.5). This is similar to cancellous bone, but more homogenous with no trabecular pattern. The lesions are usually in the centre of the medullary canal and are surrounded by a rim of reactive bone which fades into the surrounding cancellous bone. As the lesion replaces normal cortical and cancellous bone, the distinction becomes obscured. The bone diameter can expand as the lesion enlarges with its reactive rim of bone, and the cortex is slowly resorbed at variable rates, producing endosteal scalloping. There is, however, no periosteal reaction. As the lesion becomes quiescent after skeletal maturity, the rim of reactive bone is thicker and the lesion itself has a higher density.

Other variations of the classical appearance of fibrous dysplasia have also been described, with a cystic form (a radiolucent area with a sclerotic rim), pagetoid form with dense trabeculae-like pattern, or intralesional calcification indicating the presence of cartilage. Of note, the polyostotic form has similar appearance and variations as the solitary form.

Radionuclide bone scintigraphy can be used to show the extent of the disease. Isotope uptake is high in active lesions in young people, but reduces as the lesions mature. CT is the best investigation to show the characteristic of fibrous dysplasia, where the native cortex, reactive bone, and endosteal scalloping can be demonstrated clearly. The poorly mineralized area of abnormal bone also appears classical with CT. MRI can demonstrate the shape and size of the lesion, and returns a low signal intensity in T1- and T2-weighted images as they tend to have a lower water content.

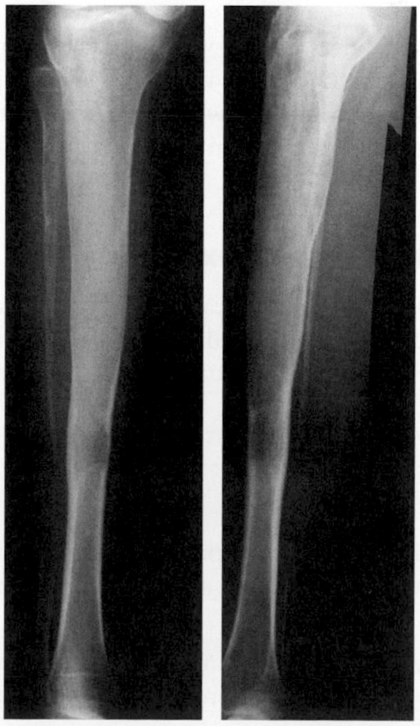

Fig. 2.5.5 A) Anteroposterior and (B) lateral radiographs of the tibia and fibula in a 20-year-old female with Albright's syndrome. Note the extensive involvement of the tibial medullary canal with mild cortical expansion. The classic ground-glass appearance is seen.

In the case of fracture with haemorrhage, or cystic changes, a more hyperintense signal on T2-weighted images is seen.

Pathological features

The gross appearance of the lesion shows a yellowish gritty fibrous tissue with some trabeculae of bone scattered throughout. The surrounding rim of bone is usually intact. Microscopically, the thin trabeculae of bone are surrounded by a fibrous stroma of spindle shape cells. The pattern of the trabeculae is haphazard. There is minimal osteoblastic rimming, unless it is associated with fracture, and there is no cellular atypia or pleomorphism.

Treatment and outcome

Asymptomatic lesions do not require any surgical treatment, but they will need to be monitored to assess for progression, risk of pathological fracture, deformity, or, rarely, malignant changes. Bisphosphonate therapy, especially pamidronate, has been shown to have some good effect in reducing bone pain, and also induce healing of the lesion with thickening of the cortex and ossification of the lesion.

Surgical treatment of fibrous dysplasia is indicated for symptom control, correction of deformity, fixation of fractures, and non-union of fractures. Curettage and bone grafting had been used to fill up the defects. In weight-bearing bones with a large defect, internal fixation with or without cortical grafting had also been shown to have good results. In severe bony deformity, osteotomy and internal fixation may be required to straighten and strengthen the skeleton. External fixation using monoaxial or circular frame has also reported good results, especially in severe deformity or shortening. Utilizing the circular frame technique, distraction osteogenesis has been shown to achieve good length correction. Autologous fibula strut grafting can also be used and can achieve good results.

Pathological fractures in non-weight-bearing bones can usually be treated non-operatively, but in the weight-bearing lower limb may require fixation. Patients with large lesions, or severe polyostotic disease, often require multiple surgeries for progressive deformities.

Osteochondroma (Box 2.5.6)

Osteochondromas are benign cartilaginous neoplasms found in any bone that undergoes enchondral bone formation. They account for 35% of benign bone tumours and 9% of all bone tumours. There is a higher incidence in male patients (3:1) and generally affects patients younger than 20 years old. The most common locations for solitary osteochondromas are the distal femur, proximal tibia, proximal humerus, and pelvis.

Box 2.5.5 Fibrous dysplasia

- Slow-growing lesion where normal bone marrow is replaced by metaplastic woven bone and fibrous tissue; usually seen before the age of 30
- Usually asymptomatic or can present with bone pain, stress fractures, pathological fractures, and gradual limb deformity
- Fibrous dysplasia appears as a well-circumscribed diaphyseal lesion with a 'ground-glass' appearance
- Surgical treatment indicated for symptom control, correction of deformity, fixation of fractures, and non-union of fractures.

Clinical presentation

The majority of patients are asymptomatic and the lesions are noted as incidental findings. Pain is usually caused by direct mass effect on the overlying soft tissue where it can cause irritation to surrounding tendons, muscle, or neurovascular structures and a bursa may form over the lesion. Pain can also indicate malignant transformation. The lesions tend to stop growing when a patient reaches skeletal maturity; increase in size of the lesion in adults is a sign of possible malignant transformation.

Hereditary multiple exostoses (HME) is an autosomal dominant condition that affects one in 50 000; it results in formation of multiple osteochondromas. If, in an affected family, an osteochondroma has not formed in a patient older than 12 the condition is unlikely to manifest itself. The condition is associated with short stature and long bone deformities particularly affecting the forearm and knee. Operative treatment is advocated to prevent and reduce progression of deformity and functional impairment.

Radiological features

Plain radiography is the modality of choice for identifying osteochondromas (Figure 2.5.6). They have the appearance of a pedunculated or sessile lesion with well-defined margins that blends imperceptibly with host bone. They usually point away from the growth plate, towards the diaphysis and are typically located at the metaphysis. Size varies from 2–15cm. Signs of malignant change can be fuzzy margins of the cartilage cap and the presence of lucent zones within the lesion. MRI can be useful in assessing for malignant change; in particular, the cartilage cap can be observed for irregularity and size. Normally the cap thickness decreases with age, therefore in adults with a cap greater than 1cm and pain, malignant transformation should be suspected.

Pathological features

Macroscopically, osteochondromas resemble cauliflowers, with a stalk that is continuous with the intramedullary bone topped by a cartilage cap. This cap is of varying thickness but reduces with age. Microscopically, osteochondromas derive from aberrant cartilaginous growth plate tissue which proliferates separate to the growth plate. This aberrant tissue remains subperiosteally where it may disappear or proliferate as an osteochondroma perpendicular to the growth plate. The cartilage cap is organized into a structure similar to the epiphysis and during skeletal growth the base of the cap undergoes enchondral ossification. Signs of malignant progression are an irregular surface to the cap with differing sizes of cartilage lobules and invasion into surrounding soft tissue. Malignant progression is usually to a low-grade chondrosarcoma.

Treatment and outcome

Treatment for an asymptomatic lesion is non-operative, the patient should be informed to return to clinic if the lesion becomes larger or painful. Resection of osteochondromas should be performed if it is symptomatic, displays suspicious features of malignant transformation, causes functional impairment, cosmetic deformity,

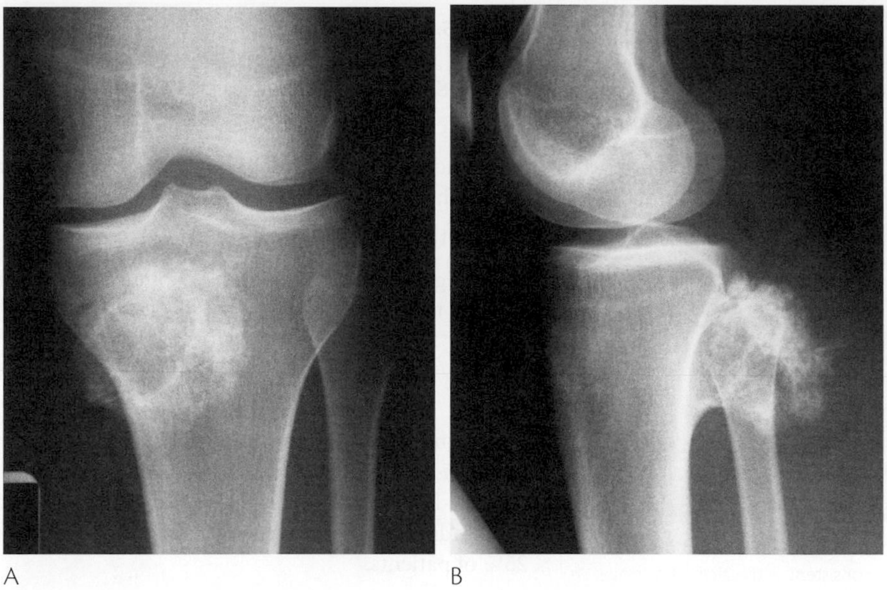

Fig. 2.5.6 Typical radiographic appearance of a proximal tibial osteochondroma (A) anteroposterior and (B) lateral views. Note the pedunculated lesion with well defined margins that blend imperceptibly with host bone.

or damages surrounding structures. During resection all of the cartilage cap and perichondrium should be removed to prevent recurrence.

Malignant transformation of solitary osteochondromas is rare and occurs in less than 1% of patients. However, patients with multiple lesions have a higher rate of malignant transformation of 5%. The local recurrence rate after resection of osteochondroma is less than 2%.

Enchondroma (Box 2.5.7)

Enchondromas are benign cartilaginous neoplasms, and usually present as solitary lesions in intramedullary bone. Enchondromas account for 12% of benign bone neoplasms. Solitary enchondromas are more common in patients aged 20–40 years and are often incidental findings; multiple enchondromas tend to affect 0–10 year olds. There is no sex predilection. Common sites for solitary lesions are the hands (especially the proximal phalanx) and feet, followed by humerus, femur, pelvis, and tibia.

Clinical presentation

Enchondromas are often incidental findings as they are generally asymptomatic; a growing lesion in the skeletally mature patient or pain in the absence of a fracture are generally highly suspicious for malignancy and should be further investigated.

Box 2.5.6 Osteochondroma

- Also known as osteocartilaginous exostoses
- Most common benign bone neoplasm
- Pedunculated or sessile lesions typically located at the metaphysis of long bones
- Treat surgically if symptomatic
- Malignant transformation of solitary osteochondromas occurs in 1%, patients with multiple lesions have a higher rate of 5%.

Multiple enchondromas can also occur in three distinct disorders:

1) *Ollier's disease*: a non-hereditary disorder where multiple enchondromas, identical radiographically to solitary lesions, are found in the metaphysis and diaphysis of long bones. It commonly has a unilateral distribution and causes limb deformity
2) *Maffucci syndrome*: a non-hereditary disorder, less common than Ollier's disease, in which multiple enchondromas are associated with haemangiomas
3) *Metachondromatosis*: a rare autosomal dominant disorder consisting of multiple enchondromas associated with osteochondromas.

Radiological features

Plain films reveal a long, oval, lytic lesion in the intramedullary canal; calcification within the lesion is common, often appearing as rings and arcs (Figure 2.5.7 and 2.5.8). Enchondromas tend to occupy the diaphyseal region in the short tubular bones and the metaphyseal region in longer bones. It can be difficult to distinguish between enchondroma and low-grade chondrosarcoma on plain x-rays; cortical breakthrough, soft tissue mass, deep endosteal scalloping of the cortex, location in the axial skeleton, and size greater than 5cm generally guide towards chondrosarcoma. CT scan is helpful to determine any endosteal cortical erosion; this modality is used at skeletal maturity to provide a baseline for future comparison.

Pathological features

Macroscopically, enchondromas are well-circumscribed lesions with discrete cartilage lobules measuring up to 1cm. Again they are difficult to tell apart from low-grade chondrosarcomas. Cytology is not helpful in determining between the two. Microscopically, enchondromas consist of multiple hyaline cartilage nodules separated by normal marrow with lamellar bone encompassing it, whereas low-grade chondrosarcoma consists of a mass of cartilage

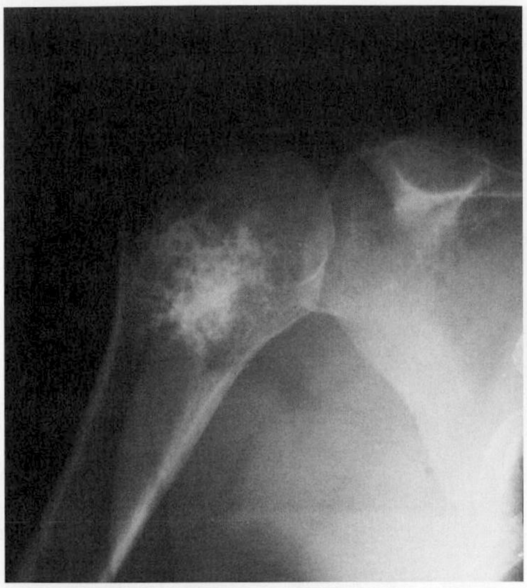

Fig. 2.5.7 Typical appearance of an enchondroma of the proximal humerus. Note the stippled calcifications and 'O-rings' consistent with calcified cartilage.

commonly permeating the marrow and trapping lamellar bone on all sides.

Treatment and outcome

Solitary enchondromas do not require surgical intervention but should be followed-up to monitor for malignant progression. Enlarging lesions in the skeletally mature or symptomatic patients should have intralesional curettage. Where malignant transformation is suspected, surgical treatment will vary from curettage to en bloc resection depending on the histological grade. Patients with multiple enchondromatosis should be monitored closely with regular follow-up clinics observing for symptomatic changes and cortical destruction in the lesions. Like solitary lesions, treatment depends on the histological grade of the tumour. Adjuvant therapy is not necessary.

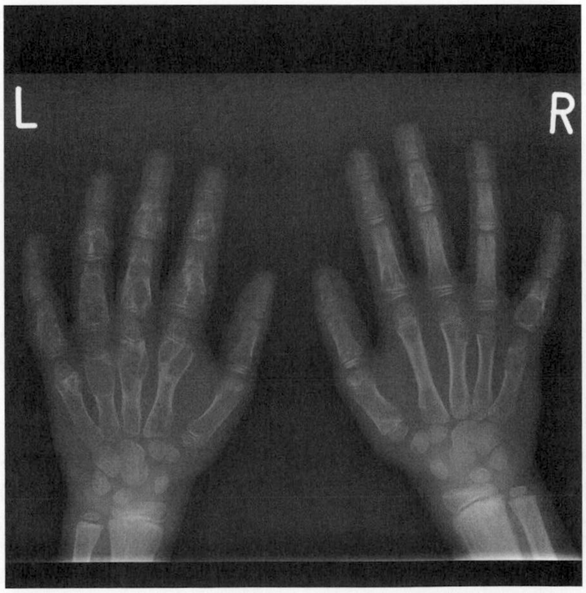

Fig. 2.5.8 Hand radiographs of a child with Ollier's disease (multiple enchondromas).

Box 2.5.7 Enchondroma

- Benign cartilaginous neoplasm; commonly incidental finding
- Most common type of hand tumour
- Difficult to differentiate from low-grade chondrosarcomas; combine histology with radiology for maximum information
- Treat if symptomatic
- Malignant transformation of solitary enchondromas is rare (less than 1%).

Malignant transformation of solitary enchondromas is rare (less than 1%). In patients who have had intralesional curettage for solitary lesions, recurrence rates are less than 5%. In multiple enchondromatosis, malignant transformation can occur in up to 25% of patients.

Langerhans cell histiocytosis (Box 2.5.8)

Langerhans cell histiocytosis (LCH) is a very rare disorder characterized by proliferation of Langerhans cells and mature eosinophils in any tissue of the body. The most commonly affected sites are the skeleton (70%), skin, and lymph nodes; occasionally the liver, spleen, lungs and bone marrow are involved. LCH affects males more than females (2:1) and is more common in children younger than 15 years old; it has an unknown aetiology.

Clinical presentation

LCH has been divided into three distinct groups ranging from mildest to more severe:

1) Eosinophilic granuloma: children aged 5–15 years. A benign proliferation of Langerhans histiocytes occurring in a unifocal or multifocal manner that commonly affects the skeletal system
2) Hand–Schuller–Christian: children aged 1–15 years. It is a chronic, multifocal infiltration classically presenting with a triad of a skull lesion, exopthalmos, and diabetes insipidus.
3) Letterer–Siwe disease: usually in infants less than 3 years old. The most malignant form, leading to widely disseminated clusters of Langerhans cells throughout the body. Characterized by fever, cachexia, otitis media, hepatosplenomegaly, skin rash, generalized multiple lesions, and a poor prognosis.

Radiological features

Imaging studies alone are rarely enough to be diagnostic, and frequently biopsy is needed. Lesions can vary from difuse osteopenia to focal, sharply-defined lesions. The classic radiographic findings of vertebra plana are enough to make a presumptive diagnosis without need for biopsy (Figure 2.5.9). They include: vertebral collapse, maintenance of disc spaces, lack of extraspinal spread, and lack of soft tissue mass. Respiratory involvement can be evident on plain films acutely as interstitial infiltrate in the mid zones and lung bases; older lesions show a honeycomb appearance. Patients with an apparent solitary lesion should be screened to rule out any further lesions with a bone scan.

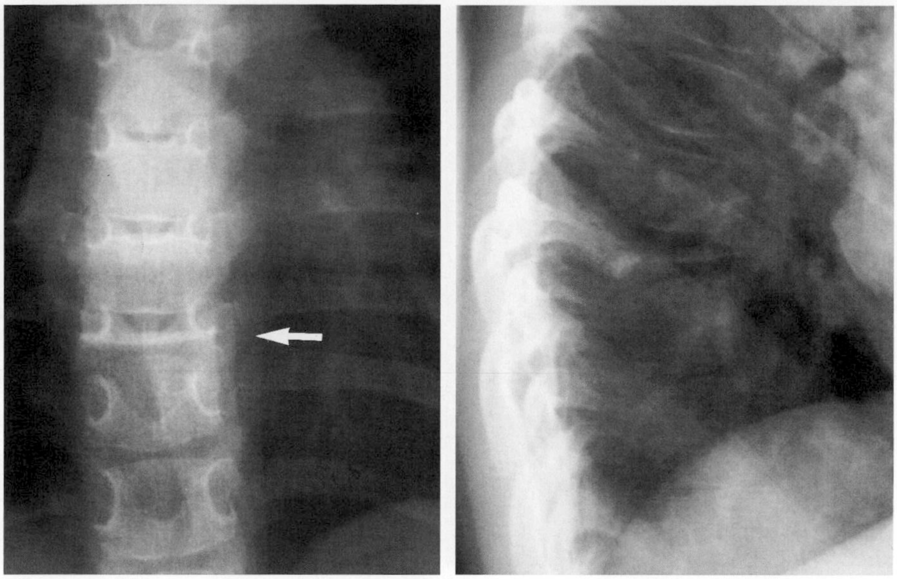

A B

Fig. 2.5.9 Langerhans cell histiocytosis of the spine causing vertebra plana in a 12-year-old boy. A) Anteroposterior and (B) lateral views showing collapse of T3.

Pathological features

Microscopic features can vary with different proportions of eosinophils and histiocytes from one lesion to another. Criteria to form a diagnosis are at least two of either: proliferation of eosinophilic histiocytes on light microscopy, demonstration of X bodies by electron microscopy, positive OKT6 immunological marker, or immunohistochemical reactivity for S100 protein.

Treatment and outcome

Solitary bone lesions can resolve spontaneously or after biopsy. Other treatment modalities that are used include injection of steroid and curettage with or without internal fixation with grafting. Cutaneous lesions respond well to PUVA (psoralen plus ultraviolet) treatment. Treatment of more widespread disease is with chemotherapy, a regimen of moderate dose methotrexate, prednisolone, and vinblastine is used.

Patients should be followed up for at least 5 years as even in isolated LCH recurrences can occur in as many as 10%.

Signs of a poor prognosis include: young age at the onset of disease, involvement of multiple organ systems, rapidity of disease progression, and especially liver, respiratory, or haematological dysfunction.

Box 2.5.8 Langerhans cell histiocytosis

- Very rare disorder characterized by proliferation of Langerhans cells and mature eosinophils into any tissue of the body
- Imaging studies alone are rarely diagnostic; frequently biopsy is needed
- Isolated bone lesions can be treated with curettage; more widespread disease will require systemic treatment
- Monitor for recurrence; poor prognosis if multiple organ involvement.

Chondroblastoma (Box 2.5.9)

It is a rare and distinct tumour, accounting for approximately 4% of primary benign bone tumours composed of immature chondroblasts within a scanty chondroid matrix. Chondroblastoma is located in epiphyseal secondary ossification centres. The tumour does not heal spontaneously, can behave aggressively, and has a low but real risk of metastasizing; surgical removal is required.

Clinical presentation

Most patients are males, with a peak incidence in the second decade of life. The commonest presenting symptom is pain with local tenderness and loss of function.

Examination usually reveals local tenderness, and can show reduced range of motion or fixed deformity in the joint adjacent to the lesion. Because of the lesions' proximity to joints, patients are commonly misdiagnosed as having intra-articular pathology such as labral or meniscal tears. When the proximal tibia or distal femur is involved an effusion may be detected in the adjacent knee joint.

Chondroblastoma most commonly occurs in the distal and proximal femur, the proximal humerus, and the proximal tibia.

Radiological features

Investigation with x-ray radiography should be performed, and chondroblastoma has a distinctive radiological appearance as a well demarcated lytic lesion with a thin sclerotic margin of increased bone density, almost always confined within the bone cortex (Figure 2.5.10). Occasionally the tumour breaches the cortex or has ill-defined margins; cortical destruction may be seen in aggressive tumours. Tumours are confined in epiphysis in 40% of cases; in the remainder of cases the tumour extends to the adjacent metaphysis.

MR and CT may be used to view the extent of the tumour and support the differential diagnosis. Because of the risk of metastasis, screening chest radiographs/CT scan should be performed on presentation.

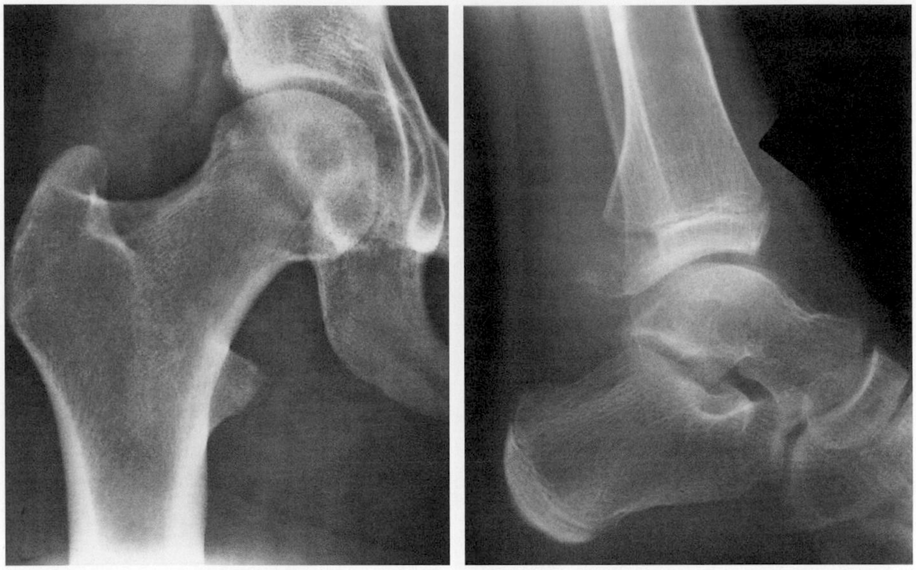
A B

Fig. 2.5.10 Anteroposterior view of the right hip in a 16-year-old female (A) reveals a poorly defined lytic lesion in the epiphysis. Lateral view of right ankle in a 12-year-old male (B) showing a destructive lytic lesion of the posterior epiphysis.

Central chondrosarcoma, chondroma, and low-grade chondrosarcoma resemble chondroblastoma and radiological and clinical examination does not give a definitive diagnosis; histological examination of surgical specimens is required.

Box 2.5.9 Chondroblastoma

- Principally affects adolescents in their second decade
- Occurs in epiphyses
- Contains chondroblasts and multinucleate giant cells
- Curettage or radiofrequency ablation.

Pathological features

Macroscopically, chondroblastoma is most often contained by the periosteum, forming a surrounding sclerotic rim. Tumours can invade the adjacent joint, often through intra-articular ligaments such as the ligamentum teres or cruciate ligament. Chondroblastomas are lobulated with pink haemorrhagic areas of soft tissue interspersed with grey-blue chondroid tissue. The chondroid tissue may or may not be calcified.

Microscopically, chondroblastoma has distinctive pathological features. The predominant cell type is round or polygonal chondroblasts with eosinophilic cytoplasm and grooved coffee-bean like or indented nuclei, together with multinucleated osteoclast-like giant cells.

Treatment and outcome

There is no accepted standard treatment for chondroblastoma. Curettage, either alone or with cryotherapy, or packing the cavity with bone graft or polymethylmethacrylate has been described.

En bloc resection with reconstruction may be necessary when there is extensive aggressive disease and intralesional excision would leave a large bony defect.

Radiation is not used due to the tumour's low sensitivity to radiation and possibility of inducing a secondary sarcoma.

Successful radiofrequency ablation of chondroblastoma under CT guidance in locations which are challenging to access surgically, such as the femoral head, provides an alternative therapeutic option, but care must be taken to avoid damage to adjacent hyaline cartilage.

Eighty to 90% of patients with chondroblastomas treated with curettage make a full recovery without recurrence or metastatic disease. A proportion of patients are left with residual pain and limited range of motion. Although a relatively high rate of recurrence has been reported, ranging from 8–21%, this may reflect inadequate treatment and re-curettage usually results in cure.

The rate of metastasis ranges from 0.8–6% and typically involves the lungs. Metastatic lesions have the same benign histology as the primary tumour. Malignant transformation, a controversial entity, is thought to occur in roughly 1% of chondroblastoma and is often resistant to resection. These patients have a poor prognosis.

Giant cell tumour (Box 2.5.10)

Giant cell tumour of bone (GCTB) is an aggressive and potentially malignant tumour that has been described as the most challenging benign tumour of bone. Its natural history varies widely, ranging from local bony destruction, local recurrence, to distant metastasis and malignant transformation.

GCTB accounts for 5% of all primary bone tumours and occurs most frequently in the distal femur, proximal tibia, proximal femur, proximal humerus, and the distal radius. Fifty per cent of lesions occur around the knee. It is slightly more common in females (ratio 1.5:1), usually presenting in the third and fourth decade of life. GCTB is more common in Asia and China, accounting for up to 20% of bone tumours, where it is also more common in men than women.

GCTB is a mesenchymal tumour originating from a neoplastic mononuclear fibrotic stem cell which coordinates the recruitment and activation of osteoclast-like giant cells, resulting in bone destruction.

Clinical presentation

Patients most often present with pain, local swelling, and warmth. Pathological fracture is the initial presenting feature in 15% of cases and is inevitable if presentation is delayed. Symptoms may be present for several months before presentation, by which time in one-third of cases the tumour exceeds half the bone diameter, has destroyed the cortex and reached the subchondral region.

Radiological features

The radiographic appearance of GCTB is of a purely lytic radiolucent lesion without matrix calcification located eccentrically in the epiphyseal region of the bone but often extending to the metaphysis (Figure 2.5.11). Most lesions have a blurred interface with surrounding bone. Cortical breakthrough and periosteal reaction may be seen. MRI has the benefit of illustrating soft tissue involvement. CT scanning can demonstrate mineralization and bony absence in the lytic region.

Because of the risk of metastasis, chest x-ray should be performed on diagnosis.

Pathological features

Grossly, GCTB is a lytic lesion, with the affected part of the bone expanded and the cortex thinned, or bridged in advanced cases. GCTB is typically red-brown due to haemorrhage, spongy, and friable. Cystic cavities, which may be filled with blood, are often seen. Microscopically GCT results from neoplastic growth of undifferentiated mesenchymal cells of bone. There are two predominant cell types, multinucleated giant cells and mononuclear stromal cells, typically uniformly arranged.

The histological composition of GCTB is complex and shares similarities with other bone lesions which contain multinucleate osteoclast-like giant cells; aneurysmal bone cyst, chondroblastoma, giant-cell rich variants of osteosarcoma, and osteoid osteoma.

Treatment and outcome

The surgeon must decide on three variables for treatment of GCTB: 1) whether to use intra-lesional curettage or en bloc resection; 2) whether to use adjuvant therapy, such as phenol; and 3) what material to use to fill the defect.

The morbidity of en bloc resection makes it inappropriate for most GCTB, which are most often in the epimetaphyseal region, where en bloc resection would involve the articular surface. Therefore, the standard treatment for most cases of GCTB is intralesional curettage with/without adjuvant therapy and filling with bone cement (polymethylmethacrylate, PMMA). Adjuvant therapy, such as phenol, hydrogen peroxide, and cryotherapy, aims to remove microscopic tumour that may remain after curettage through their thermal (liquid nitrogen, PMMA) or chemical (hydrogen peroxide, phenol) toxicity.

The increased understanding of the molecular pathogenesis of GCTB as an osteoclastic resorptive lesion has led to the trial use of bisphosphonates, which are antiosteoclastic, as an adjuvant therapy, with promising results.

En bloc resection is generally reserved for large, aggressive GCTB which have destroyed the cortex usually with a fracture. Tumours of the proximal femur and distal radius have a higher risk of local recurrence due to the difficult anatomy

Radiation is an alternative when tumour resection is not possible or incomplete, e.g. in the pelvis, sacrum, or vertebra, and resection will result in neurological or functional morbidity. However, it is important to remember that radiotherapy increases the risk of malignant transformation.

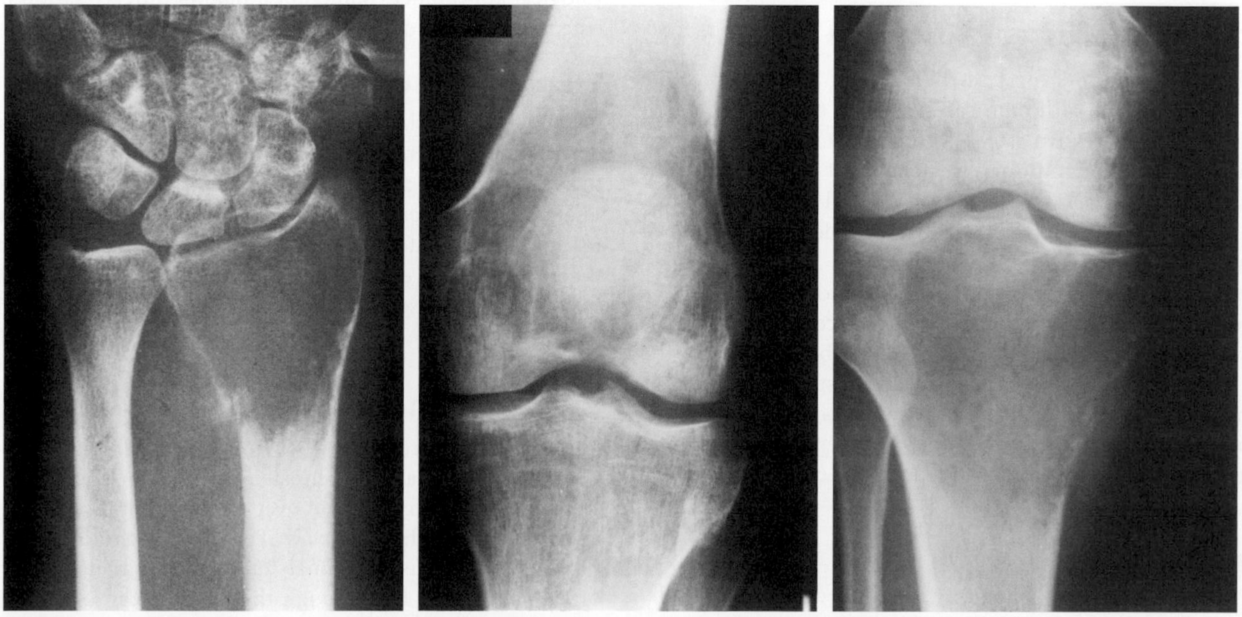

A B C

Fig. 2.5.11 Anteroposterior radiograph (A) of an aggressive giant cell tumour (GCT) in the distal radius of a 25-year-old male. Anteroposterior radiograph (B) of GCT of the distal femur in a 50-year-old male; note the thinning of the surrounding cortices. Anteroposterior radiograph (C) of an aggressive GCT of the proximal tibia in a 23-year-old female; the lesion has broken through the medial cortex.

Box 2.5.10 Giant cell tumour

- Benign lesion occurring predominantly around the knee; has metastatic potential
- Lytic radiolucent lesion without matrix calcification located eccentrically in the epiphysis
- Two cell types: multinucleated giant cells causing bone resorption and mononuclear stromal cells (neoplastic)
- Curettage with adjuvant treatment and cementation has lowest recurrence rate
- Metastasis is rare (2–3%) but has a poor prognosis if not removed surgically.

The overall outcome for GCBT in large series is a disease-free survival of greater than 85%. Although recurrence is not fatal in most cases, the morbidity after multiple procedures and rate of secondary arthritis can be high.

More mitotically active lesions are more likely to recur. Recurrent lesions are more likely to develop possibly life-threatening metastasis and patients with recurrences should, as part of the staging process, have a CT scan of the chest.

Malignant transformation is seen in less than 10% of cases but has a poor survival. Pulmonary metastasis is rare, affecting 2–3% of patients with benign GCBT. The pathology of tumours that metastasize is identical to those that do not. Survival is not compatible with persistent pulmonary lesions and nodules should be removed surgically. When this is not possible, whole lung radiotherapy is recommended. Malignant lesions should be treated like sarcomas.

Follow-up with radiographs of the primary site and chest should be for at least 5 years, as cases of recurrence and metastasis have been reported many years after treatment.

Osteoblastoma/osteoid osteoma (Box 2.5.11)

Osteoblastoma accounts for less than 1% of all primary bone tumours. It is benign, although rare variants, termed malignant osteoblastoma or aggressive osteoblastoma exist. The term osteoblastoma is reserved for tumours greater than 1.5cm in diameter; those smaller than 1.5cm diameter are termed osteoid osteoma. Males are twice as likely to be affected as females and 80–90% of patients are under the age of 30.

Osteoblastoma can affect any bone but the most common site is in the posterior elements of the spine, which accounts for approximately one-third of all osteoblastomas. Long tubular bones are the second most common site (34% of cases, most often the femur, tibia, and humerus). Tumours in long tubular bones usually occur in the diaphysis or metaphysis, and rarely in the epiphysis. Tumours in the spine almost always involve the posterior elements, and may involve the vertebral body as well.

Clinical presentation

Almost all osteoblastomas present with pain, which is generally mild but progressive. Other common complaints are gait disturbance, swelling, warmth and tenderness. The pain may not respond to non-steroidal anti-inflammatory drugs, unlike osteoid osteoma. When found in the spine, paresthesiae, paraparesis, or scoliosis may be the presenting complaint. Presentation is on average 6 months to 2 years after onset of symptoms. Less often, osteoblastoma presents with atypical clinical features, such as weight loss, night pain, epistaxis, tooth impaction, and aspirin overuse.

Radiological features

Radiological features are non-specific and include osteosclerosis, osteolysis, cortical thinning, and expansion of bone.

Osteoblastomas in the spine are well-defined expansile osteolytic lesions that are variably calcified or ossified, most often arising from the posterior elements (Figure 2.5.12). Long bone osteoblastoma on radiographs show cortical expansion, sometimes extending to cortical destruction, and often have a periosteal reaction. CT scanning is the most useful scanning modality for osteoblastoma, although it does not provide a definitive diagnosis.

Osteoid osteomas on plain radiographs can be classified as cortical, subperiosteal, or medullary in location. It is generally a round or oval well-circumscribed lesion with a radiolucent nidus.

Definitive diagnosis of osteoblastoma on radiographs alone is rarely possible; it is more likely that osteoblastoma will be included in a list of differential diagnosis, including chondroblastoma, osteosarcoma, ABC, chondrosarcoma, osteomyelitis, giant cell tumour.

Pathological features

Grossly, lesions are gritty, friable, and red to tan in colour. The tumour–bone interface is generally sharp, with a rim of reactive sclerosis. Microscopically the classic description of osteoblastoma is of long interanastomosing trabeculae of osteoid or woven bone undergoing varying degrees of calcification, some trabeculae are calcified, others are pink immature osteoid. Trabeculae are surrounded by a single row of osteoblasts. The intertrabecular stroma is a loose fibrovascular tissue with capillary proliferation, a few osteoclast-like giant cells, and spindle cells. Mitosis is seen in less than 10% of cells. Osteoblastomas are known for their range of histological appearances sometimes making differentiation between osteoblastomas and osteosarcomas difficult.

Treatment and outcome

Osteoblastomas should be removed to prevent or arrest bone destruction and remove pain symptoms. Treatment is surgical and includes curettage ± grafting. For small osteoid osteomas, radiofrequency ablation has been used successfully. For larger lesions wide resection is indicated; this can be difficult with spinal lesions and therefore aggressive intralesional excision with fusion and internal fixation may be used instead. Following complete removal of the tumour recurrence is uncommon.

Periosteal chondroma (Box 2.5.12)

Periosteal chondroma is a slow-growing benign lesion found within or underneath the periosteum of tubular bones. It is usually situated in the proximal end over the metaphysis, but may occur anywhere along the diaphysis. The most common sites are the proximal humerus, proximal femur, and small tubular bones of the hands and feet, though the tumour can occur in almost any bone.

It is uncommon, representing less than 1% of all bone tumours, but is three times more common than periosteal chondrosarcoma.

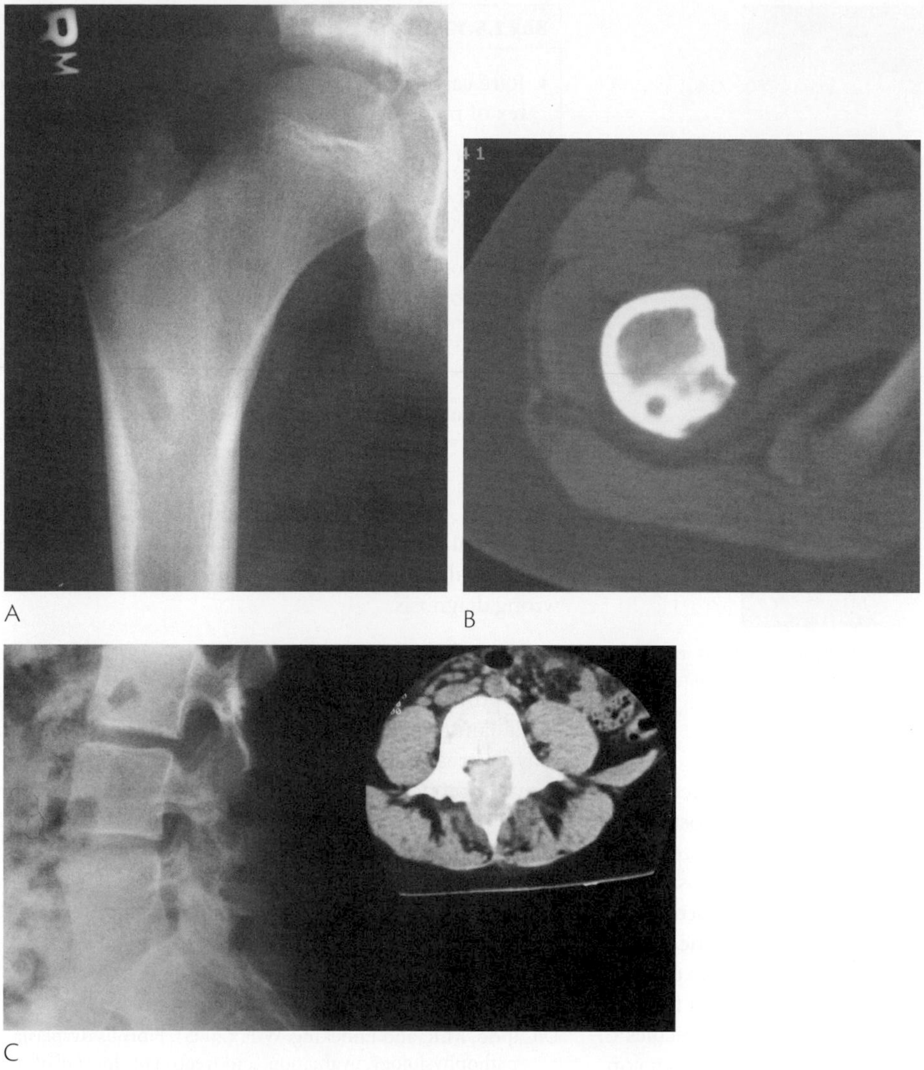

Fig. 2.5.12 A) Anteroposterior radiograph of the proximal femur showing a radiolucent lesion in a medullary location without extensive reactive sclerosis
B) Computed tomography scan localizes the nidus just inside the cortex in the subtrochanteric region of the femur. This lesion is consistent with an osteoid osteoma. C) Typical radiological appearance of osteoblastoma of the fourth lumbar vertebra in a 10-year-old child.

It is most common in men in the second decade of life, though can affect adults and children. Very occasionally multiple lesions are seen.

Clinical presentation

Pain and palpable swelling with local tenderness are the most common presenting symptoms, often with reduced function at the adjacent joint, although many lesions are non-painful and found incidentally on imaging performed for other reasons. One-third of cases are associated with a soft tissue mass, palpable swellings are non-tender and fixed to underlying bone. In contrast to enchondroma and osteochondroma, in which growth after skeletal maturity is cause for concern, continued growth of periosteal chondroma in adults occurs without malignant transformation and is not a worrying feature.

Box 2.5.11 Osteoblastoma/osteoid osteoma

- Benign neoplasm of bone that arises from osteoblasts
- 90% of patients under 30 years old; pain, often increasing over time
- Affects the long tubular bones and spine
- Expansile lesion with cortical thinning and periosteal reaction; variable ossification
- Radiofrequency ablation; curettage; wide resection for larger lesions.

Radiological features

On plain radiographs periosteal chondroma is seen as a sharply marginated, radiolucent, shallow, semi-lunar cortical concavity adjacent to the cortex, with scalloping as it erodes the cortex, and overhanging edges (Figure 2.5.13). There is variable calcification or the cartilaginous matrix, seen in roughly 50% of tumours and a sclerotic reaction of the cortex, which remains intact underlying the lesion. Focal calcification or ossification is seen in approximately one-third of tumours. Periosteal new bone forms buttresses overhanging the edges of the tumour. Lesions can have a blurred indistinct margin, or be surrounded by a thin cortical shell. Pathological fractures have not been reported. MRI is useful in the

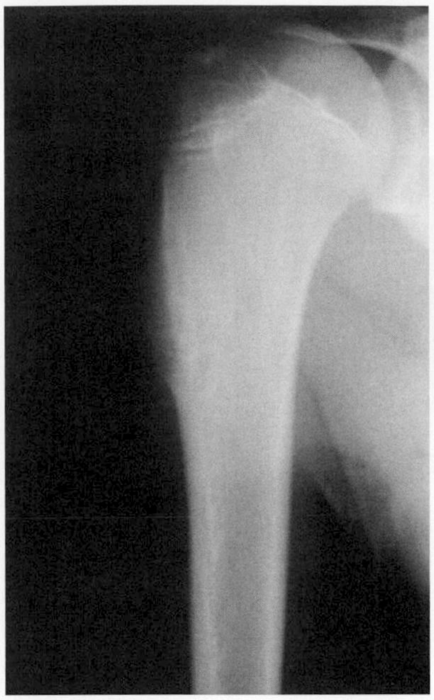

Fig. 2.5.13 Typical radiographic appearance of periosteal chondroma in a 15-year-old male. Note the scalloping of the underlying cortex and peripheral areas of 'buttressing' new bone arising from the mature cortex.

diagnosis of periosteal chondroma, showing a lobulated lesion bordered by a hypointense rim, indicating an intact periosteum.

Radiographs are helpful in differentiating from osteochondroma, periosteal osteosarcoma, and periosteal chondrosarcoma. Periosteal chondrosarcoma is round and shows popcorn calcification, is usually larger than 5cm, does not have a sclerotic reactive bone rim on its cortical side, and is primarily exophytic. Osteochondroma does not have a rim of bone separating it from the medullary cavity. Osteosarcoma shows perpendicular spicules of calcification, not seen in periosteal chondroma. Other benign conditions that can involve the periosteum should also be considered.

Pathological features

Grossly periosteal chondroma is covered by a thin shell of periosteum, is embedded in, and erodes the cortex without invading the medulla cavity. The lesion is composed of white-grey or blue, firm cartilagenous tissue. Tumours range from 1–10cm, but are usually less than 6cm in greatest dimension.

Histological examination shows a benign appearing lesion composed of hyaline matrix arranged in a lobular pattern with no atypical cellular elements. The matrix is separated by fibrous connective tissue or lamellar bone. Invasion of the surrounding soft tissues is not seen.

Box 2.5.12 Periosteal chondroma

- Rare cartilage lesion located between the periosteum and cortex of proximal long bones
- Affects adolescents predominantly
- Sharply marginated, radiolucent concavity adjacent to the cortex
- Histologically benign cartilage separated by fibrous connective tissue or lamellar bone
- Periosteal chondrosarcoma/osteosarcoma are the two most serious differential diagnoses
- Surgical excision if painful lesion.

Unusual and atypical findings can result in misdiagnosis so careful clinical and radiological examination is required to avoid a wrong diagnosis.

Treatment and outcome

Asymptomatic latent lesions may be managed by observation—malignant transformation has never been reported. Painful lesions may be treated with by en bloc or marginal excision, or interlesional curettage. The most effective treatment is en bloc resection, which prevents recurrence. Where the functional morbidity from resection is high, curettage should be performed, although recurrences have been reported. Bone grafting may be used with a large defect. Very few incidences of recurrence are recorded, estimated as less than 5%.

Further reading

DiCaprio, M.R. and Enneking, W.F. (2005). Fibrous dysplasia. pathophysiology, evaluation, and treatment. *Journal of Bone and Joint Surgery*, **87-A**, 1848–64.

Docquier, P.L. and Delloye, C. (2005). Treatment of aneurysmal bone cysts by introduction of demineralized bone and autogenous bone marrow. *Journal of Bone and Joint Surgery*, **87-A**, 2253–8.

Mirra, J.M., Gold, R.H., and Rand, F. (1982). Disseminated nonossifying fibromas in association with café-au-lait spots (Jaffe–Campanacci syndrome). *Clinical Orthopaedics and Related Research*, **168**, 192–205.

Suneja, R., Grimer, R.J., Belthur, M., *et al.* (2005). Chondroblastoma of bone: long-term results and functional outcome after intralesional curettage. *Journal of Bone and Joint Surgery*, **87-B**, 974–8.

Szendroi, M. (2004). Giant-cell tumour of bone. *Journal of Bone and Joint Surgery*, **86-B**, 5–12.

Unni, K.K. (1996). *Dahlin's Bone Tumours: General aspects and Data on 11087 cases*, 5th edn., pp. 24–45. Philadelphia, PA: Lippincott-Raven.

2.6

Malignant bone tumours

Rej S. Bhumbra, Panagiotis D. Gikas, Sammy A. Hanna, Jakub Jagiello, and Stephen R. Cannon

Summary points

- Chondrosarcoma
- Osteosarcoma
- Ewing's sarcoma
- Myeloma of bone
- Fibrosarcoma of bone or soft tissue
- Lymphoma of bone
- Malignant vascular tumours of bone.

Introduction

Primary malignant bone tumours account for 1% of cancer deaths. The incidence for the three most common excluding myeloma is only nine per million of population per year. As a result all primary malignant bone tumours are best managed at one of the five centres directly funded by The National Commissioning Group.

All such patients are managed by a multidisciplinary team and, where appropriate, entered into national and international trials aimed at improving survivorship and achieving maximum function.

Patients present with a variety of symptoms including pain, swelling, and loss of function. In children and adolescents, making a diagnosis of 'growing pains' must be a diagnosis of exclusion, and all clinicians should investigate thoroughly patients that complain of 'night pain'.

Patients presenting with malignant bone tumours usually have a mass which increases in size. This may happen slowly over a period of years or months or more quickly in a matter of weeks. These tumours are usually painless until the late stages. Any mass greater than 5cm in size that lies deep to the fascia and is increasing in size, should be investigated as a potential malignant tumour until proved otherwise. Again the management should involve a multidisciplinary team compromising the surgeon, and a radiologist, pathologist, oncologist, and radiotherapist. Again, for the best outcomes bone and soft tissue tumours are best managed in specialist centres.

Chondrosarcoma (Box 2.6.1)

Chondrosarcoma is a malignant tumour of cartilaginous origin, in which the tumour matrix formation is chondroid in nature.

Lesions are designated as primary when they arise de novo or as secondary when they occur within a pre-existing lesion such as an enchondroma or osteochondroma. The vast majority (greater than 85%) are primary central chondrosarcomas, designated as such based on their location centrally within the medullary cavity. A minority (up to 15%) of conventional chondrosarcomas develop from the surface of bone, most of them as a result of malignant transformation within the cartilage cap of a pre-existing osteochondroma. These are therefore called secondary peripheral chondrosarcomas. A minority (less than 1%) occur at the surface of bone, possibly of periosteal origin, and are designated periosteal chondrosarcoma. Their histology is similar to that of conventional chondrosarcoma.

Clinical presentation

Chondrosarcoma is the second most frequent primary malignant tumour of bone, representing approximately 25% of all primary osseous neoplasms.

The incidence rate of chondrosarcoma is dependent on patient age, peaking at eight cases per million of population in those aged 80–84 years. The incidence in children is low. Most tumours arise in patients older than 40 years. The exact cause of chondrosarcoma is not known. There may be a genetic or chromosomal component that predisposes certain individuals to this type of malignancy.

The following is a list of some benign conditions that may be present when chondrosarcoma occurs:

- Enchondromas
- Osteochondromas
- Multiple exostoses
- Ollier's disease
- Maffucci's syndrome: a combination of multiple enchondromas and angiomas.

A slight male predilection exists, with a male to female ratio of 1.5–2:1.

Tumours are predominantly located in the pelvis, femur, humerus, ribs, scapula, sternum, or spine. In tubular bones, the metaphysis is the most common site of origin. The proximal metaphysis is more frequently involved than the distal end of the bone. Chondrosarcoma is rare in the hands and feet and if it occurs, does so as a complication of a multiple enchondromatosis syndrome.

The most common symptom at presentation is pain, which is often present for months and typically dull in character. It may be worse at night and classically described as being relieved by taking anti-inflammatories. Local swelling may be present, and when the tumour occurs close to a joint, effusion may be present, or movement may be restricted. The average duration of symptoms prior to presentation is 1–2 years. The tumour occasionally presents as a pathological fracture.

Radiological features

The distinction between benign and malignant cartilaginous lesions can be difficult. For the distinction between enchondroma and central grade I chondrosarcoma, conventional radiography is not reliable. Dynamic contrast-enhanced magnetic resonance imaging (MRI) shows greater sensitivity, although an absolute distinction between benign and malignant cannot be made on radiological grounds alone.

The locations and radiographic appearances of the different chondrosarcoma subtypes are often characteristic, with the mineralized chondroid matrix as a punctate or ring-and-arc pattern of calcifications that may coalesce to form a more radiopaque flocculent pattern of calcification and aggressive features of endosteal scalloping and soft tissue extension (Figure 2.6.1).

Computed tomography (CT) and MRI are indispensable adjunct tools for optimizing tumour characterization. Evidence of a large unmineralized soft tissue mass associated with a lesion with radiological features indicative of a chondrosarcoma should raise the level of suspicion for dedifferentiation.

Pathological features

Central and peripheral chondrosarcomas are histologically similar, and for both, three different grades are discerned (grade 1 represents the least aggressive in terms of histological features, and grade 3 represents the most aggressive) which is at present the best predictor of clinical behaviour. Recurrence of low-grade chondrosarcoma bears the risk for tumour progression toward a

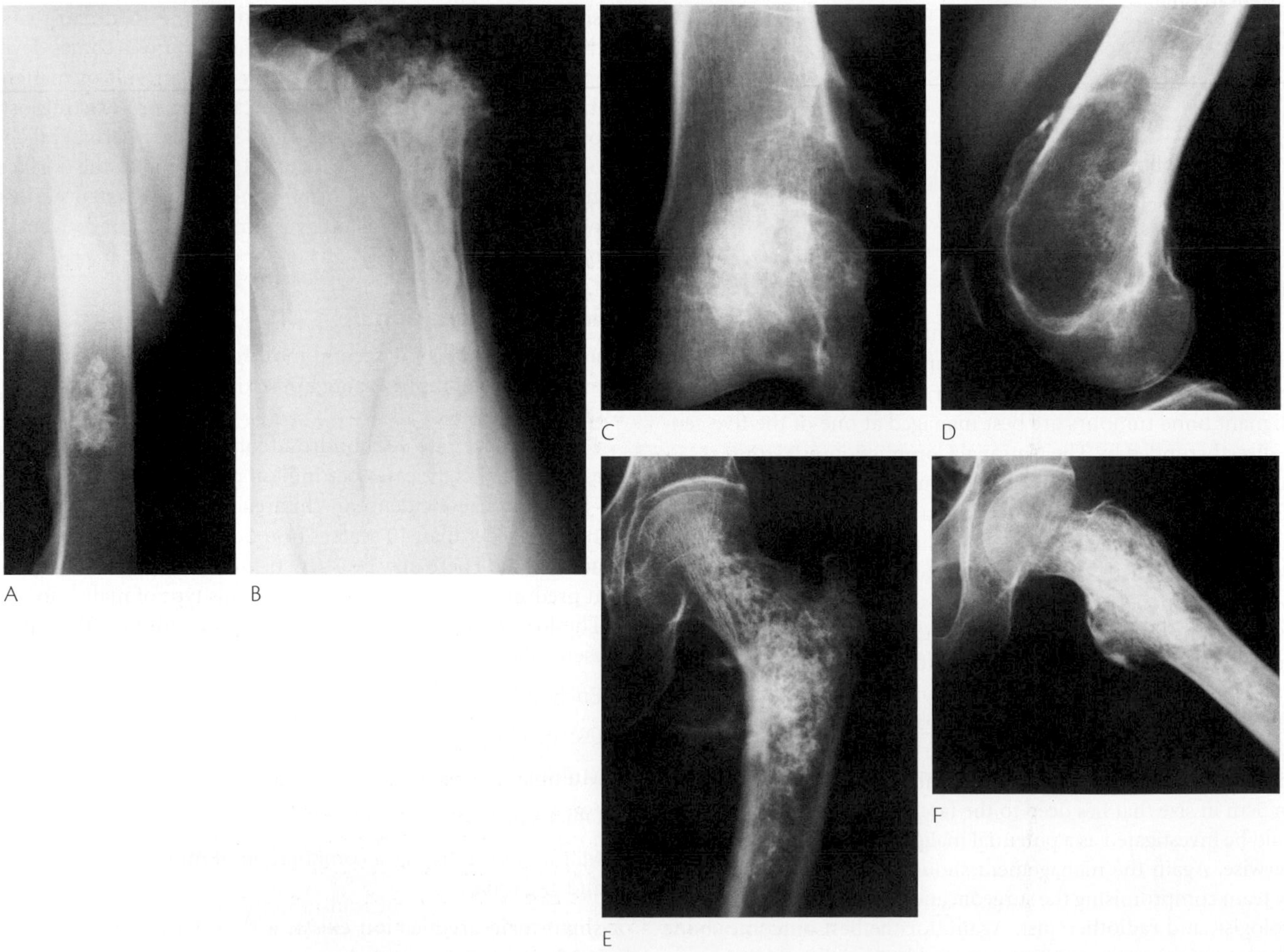

Fig. 2.6.1 Lateral radiograph (A) of the distal femur revealing a lytic lesion involving the metaphysis along with its calcification. There is cortical thickening and reactive periosteal changes. A coincidental traumatic fracture is seen above. Anteroposterior radiograph (B) of the left proximal humerus showing a large calcified tumour extending well down the medullary canal. Anteroposterior radiograph (C) of the right distal femur and knee joint showing a lytic destructive lesion with cortical thickening and marked bone destruction. Lateral view (D) showing the lytic destructive lesion. Anteroposterior (E) and lateral (F) views of a left proximal femoral chondrosarcoma. A large calcified lesion is evident with significant soft tissue extension.

higher grade or even dedifferentiation, with a severe adverse prognosis.

Central and peripheral chondrosarcomas differ at the molecular genetic level. The exostosin (EXT) genes, causing multiple osteochondromas, are involved in the origin of osteochondroma and peripheral chondrosarcoma. In contrast, in the far more common central chondrosarcoma, EXT is not involved, and the initiating event is still unknown.

In addition to conventional chondrosarcoma, several rare subtypes of chondrosarcoma are discerned, together constituting 10–15% of all chondrosarcomas. These include:

- Dedifferentiated chondrosarcoma (dismal prognosis)
- Mesenchymal chondrosarcoma (highly malignant lesion)
- Clear cell chondrosarcoma (low-grade malignant tumour).

Treatment and outcome

For all grades and subtypes of non-metastatic chondrosarcoma, complete surgical treatment offers the only chance for cure. Wide, en bloc excision is the preferred surgical treatment of intermediate- and high-grade chondrosarcoma cases. However, wide excision can lead to considerable morbidity and a demanding reconstruction, depending on the location. On the other hand, in low-grade chondrosarcoma, extensive intralesional curettage followed by local adjuvant treatment, for example, phenolization or cryosurgery (liquid nitrogen), and filling the cavity with bone graft or PMMA (polymethylmethacrylate) cement has promising long-term clinical results and satisfactory local control. In some cases of low-grade chondrosarcoma, intralesional excision may not be adequate, for example, because of large size or an intra-articular or pelvic localization. In these cases, wide resection remains the preferable choice for local therapy. Metastases are rare in low-grade chondrosarcoma of the long bones. In the case of soft tissue involvement in chondrosarcoma grade I, wide en bloc resection is recommended.

In patients with multiple exostoses the development of secondary peripheral chondrosarcoma is rare (assumed in the literature to be less than 2%) and usually presents after skeletal maturity. Complete surgical removal of the cartilage cap with the pseudocapsule has excellent long-term clinical and local results.

The prognosis for patients with dedifferentiated chondrosarcoma is still poor, despite adequate wide surgical resection and adjuvant systemic therapy.

Chondrogenic tumours are considered relatively radiotherapy (RT) resistant. RT can be considered in two situations: after incomplete resection, aiming at maximal local control (curative), and in situations where resection is not feasible or would cause unacceptable morbidity (palliative).

Chemotherapy is generally not effective in chondrosarcoma, especially in the most frequently observed conventional type and the rare (low-grade) clear cell variant. Chemotherapy is only possibly effective in mesenchymal chondrosarcoma, and is of uncertain value in dedifferentiated chondrosarcoma; both subtypes are rare and bear a poor prognosis.

The prognosis for chondrosarcoma depends on the grade of the lesion and the attainment of complete excision of the tumour. For lower-grade chondrosarcomas, prognosis is very good (90% 5-year survival) after adequate local control. There is a low incidence of pulmonary metastasis if the primary lesion is widely resected. Metastasis to other bones can occur, but is much less common. Dedifferentiated chondrosarcoma has a uniformly poor prognosis (less than 10% 1-year survival).

Box 2.6.1 Chondrosarcoma

- For conventional low-grade chondrosarcoma confined to the bone, intralesional curettage with local adjuvant therapy (phenol application/cryosurgery/cementation) is an option to decrease surgical morbidity
- For intermediate- to high-grade tumours, clear margins are necessary to prevent recurrence
- Poor response to radiotherapy/chemotherapy.

Osteosarcoma (Box 2.6.2)

Osteosarcomas can be subdivided into intramedullary, cortical (either on or in), or arising in pre-existing pathology. Intramedullary osteosarcomas include high- and low-grade osteosarcoma as well as telangiectatic osteosarcoma. Cortical lesions are subdivided into surface lesions, such as the parosteal and variable grade periosteal osteosarcomas or the rare intracortical osteosarcoma. Secondary osteosarcomas occur in pre-existing irradiated tissue beds, infection, infarction, Paget's, fibrous dysplasia, or other bony lesions. Less common lesions include multifocal osteosarcoma as well as soft tissue osteosarcoma.

Clinical presentation

Incidence is approximately five per million population, and three per million in those less than 20 years. Although described as bimodal, the majority of cases occur in the rapidly growing bones of children and young adults. Common sites for osteosarcoma are the metaphyses of the distal femur, proximal tibia, proximal humerus, proximal femur as well as the mandible. Despite micrometastases, which are common, patients tend not to be systemically unwell. Mass and pain are the most common presenting features.

Radiological features

Plain film evaluation confirms the extent of mineralized bone destruction, the osteolytic and blastic nature of the lesion, periosteal elevation, secondary ossification and soft tissue extension. Bone destruction is more extensive than films portray but the diagnostic sensitivity, cost, and widespread availability of radiographic plain film evaluation makes it a mandatory initial imaging modality (Figures 2.6.2 and 2.6.3).

MR evaluation is of major benefit to assess the extent of intra- and extraosseous tumour infiltration. It also enables tumour relationship to neurovascular structures to be determined, which affects limb-salvage decision-making during preoperative planning. Tumour can be separate from, in contact with, displacing, effacing partially or completely encasing the neurovascular bundle. If vasculature integrity needs further description appropriate angiography is requested.

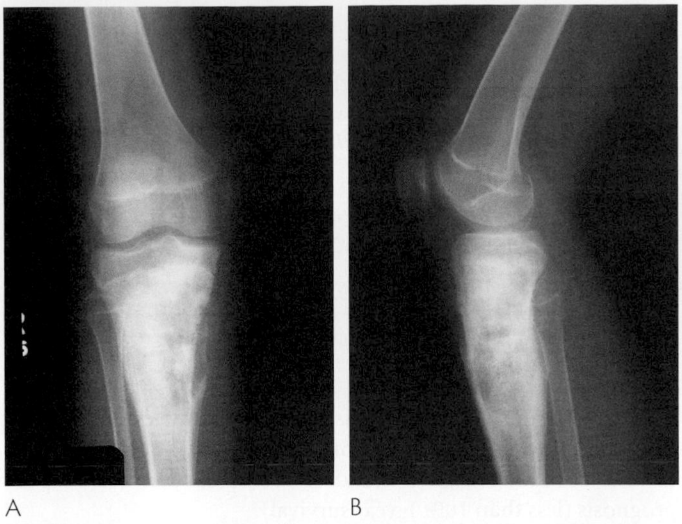

Fig. 2.6.2 Osteosarcoma of the proximal tibia in a 14-year-old female. A) Anteroposterior and B) lateral radiographs showing a mixture of ill-defined radiodense and radiolucent regions with periosteal new bone formation.

A bone scan and CT chest are used to detect multifocal sites and chest metastases respectively.

Pathological features

Conventionally osteosarcomas are mineralized centrally with more immature bone at the periphery. The heterogeneous behaviour of conventional osteosarcoma is represented in the cellular population. Most commonly mixed, cell type can also be predominantly osteo-, chondro-, or fibroblastic, affecting necrosis rates following chemotherapy. The presence of osteoid and malignant stromal cells is needed to diagnose osteosarcoma. Cells may have a lace, trabecular, or sheet-like pattern

High-grade intramedullary osteosarcoma

These constitute 80% of all osteosarcomas leading to the descriptive use of 'conventional' or 'classic'. They are the subtype upon which the majority of survivorship analyses are made. Most have penetrated the cortex and have an associated soft tissue mass, making this a stage IIB lesion. This more common subtype presents with CT detectable pulmonary metastases in 20% of patients.

Telangiectatic osteosarcoma

An aggressive, osteolytic, expansile lesion that can radiologically appear identical to an aneurysmal bone cyst. They contain fewer, but highly malignant cellular elements and account for 3.5–11% of osteosarcamatous cases.

Multifocal osteosarcoma

Affecting multiple bones significantly worsens the prognosis. It is rare, and detectable with whole-body bone scan or perhaps in the future, whole-body MRI. Metachronous lesions occur years after the primary lesion and are differentiated from recurrence by occurring at a different site. Multifocal lesions are in different bones. It is not yet discernable whether multicentric osteosarcoma represents multiple de novo tumours or multiple bone metastases within a narrow time window from a solitary bone primary site.

Skip metastases which are seen in 10% of lesions, are detectable in the same bone at the same time, but can be at differing stages of local bony destruction.

Parosteal osteosarcoma

Low-grade lesion classically over the posterior aspect of the distal femur or the proximal humerus. Differentiated from a sessile osteochondroma in that the osteosarcoma is on the bone surface and not in uniform continuity with the cancellous bone of the metaphysis. Seen more commonly in the third or fourth decade and slightly more so in females, with radiographic features of ossification and lobulation. Can be confused with synovial osteochondromatosis or myositis ossificans. Depending on the extent of bone involvement treatment is either by shark-bite resection or wide excision. Chemotherapy is only instituted if high-grade or de-differentiated areas are found on histological analysis.

Periosteal osteosarcoma

Unlike the other groups this tends to occur in the diaphysis of the long bones and consists mainly of chondroblastic cells. Ninety-five per cent involve the distal femur or proximal tibial meta-diaphysis. It is usually of intermediate grade, and typically arises from the anteromedial bone portion.

Secondary osteosarcoma

Classically arises in 1% of patients with Paget's disease. Its diagnosis can be expedited by appreciating that soft tissue extension, detectable on MRI, is the hallmark of malignant transformation. The advanced age of pagetoid patients makes chemotherapy less tolerable, significantly worsening the prognosis for these patients. Less than 5% of secondary osteosarcomas occur in irradiated bone.

Treatment and outcome

Chemotherapy and surgery form the mainstay of treatment. Limb salvage is usually possible in up to 80% of patients. Prior to the introduction of chemotherapy mortality from osteosarcoma was approximately 85%, even with radical resection or amputation. This is a representation of its propensity to micro metastasize early in its natural history. Chemotherapy kills the malignant cells and aims to improve patient survivorship and ultimately cure. Surgery compliments this by obtaining a margin negative resection, followed by bony and soft tissue reconstruction.

New chemotherapy protocols, with appropriate surgery, have produced an approximate 75% survival at 5 years. There is no difference in survival if chemotherapy is administered prior or post surgery. This is in accordance with the presence of non-detectable lung micro-metastases and the tumour cell's response to chemotherapy being ultimately responsible for the patient prognosis. Common chemotherapeutic agents include cisplatin, doxorubicin, ifosfamide, and methotrexate. Immunostimulants, immunotherapy, cytotoxic T-cells, and monoclonal antibody therapy treatments are ongoing but have yet to yield a reproducible and consistent survival improvement.

Surgical resection aims to achieve a complete tumour resection with an appropriate margin, without tumour spillage or neurovascular damage that may render a salvaged limb functionless. If this is not possible, amputation is considered. It is not a 'failure' to

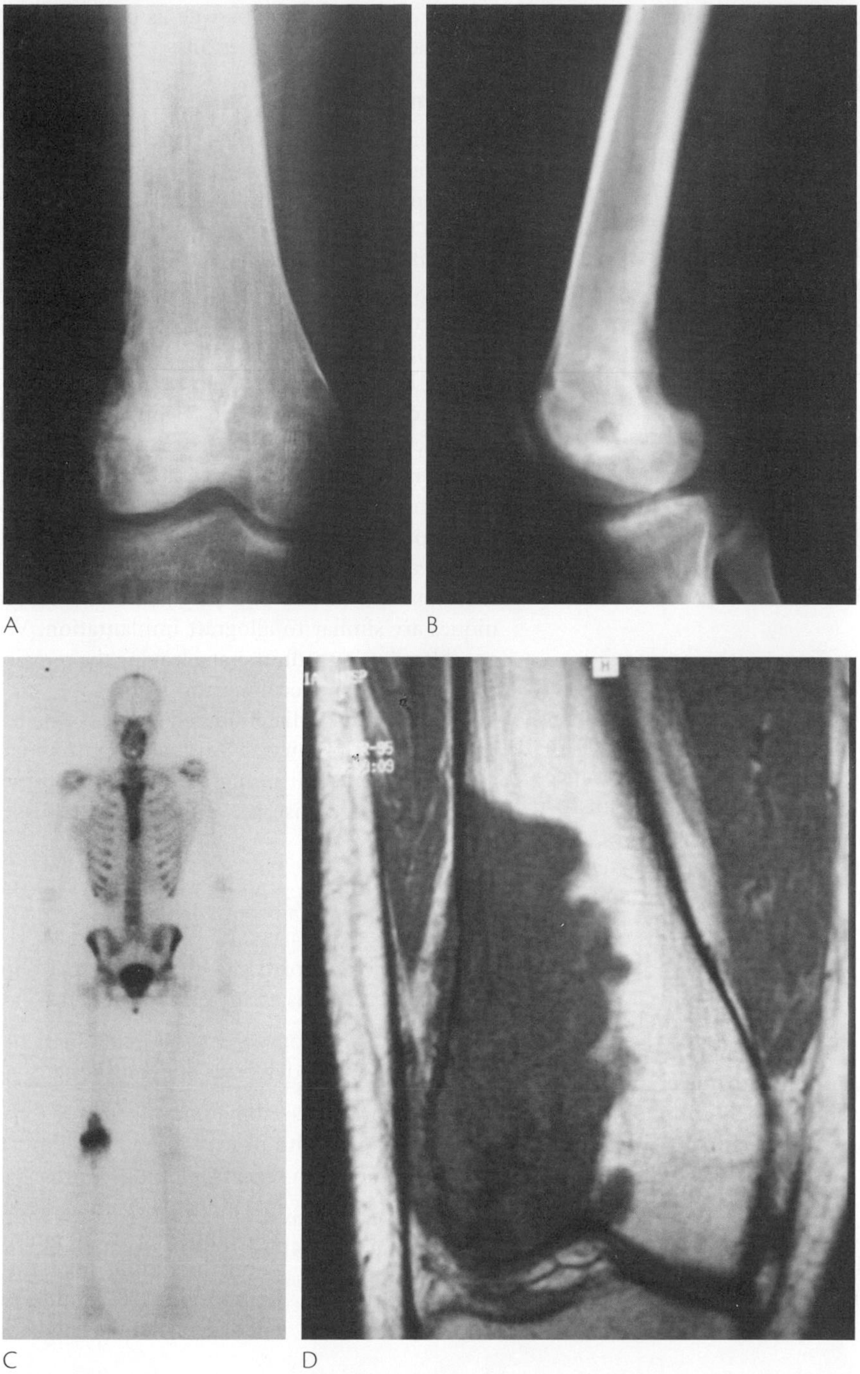

Fig. 2.6.3 Osteosarcoma of the distal femur. A) Anteroposterior and B) lateral plain radiographs revealing cloudy opacities and sclerotic regions. C) Bone scan showing increased uptake in the distal femur. D) MRI scan confirming the intramedullary extent of the tumour and a small soft tissue mass. No skip lesions were identified.

amputate and just as much careful preoperative planning, operative attention to detail, and postoperative care is warranted as any limb salvage operation.

The major factors associated with a bad prognosis in osteosarcoma are a poor response to chemotherapy (less than 90% necrosis), skip or pulmonary metastases (stage), and the tumour grade. Other poor outcomes are associated with large tumours, axial/pelvic and central tumours, older patients, and tumours in pre-existing pathological tissues. Patient survivorship for conventional osteosarcoma remains at 75% at 5 years. Of the total number of recurrences, approximately 5% occur after 5 years. Follow-up protocols vary but most patients need to be reviewed every 3 months

Box 2.6.2 Osteosarcoma

- Incidence is five per million population, and three per million in those less than 20 years
- Subdivided into intramedullary, cortical (either on or in), or arising in pre-existing pathology
- Chemotherapy and surgery form the mainstay of treatment
- Prognosis depends on response to chemotherapy (less than 90% necrosis), skip or pulmonary metastases (stage), and the tumour grade.

for the first 2 years, 6-monthly up to 5 years, and then yearly reviews can continue.

Ewing's sarcoma (Box 2.6.3)

Ewing's sarcoma is a cluster of tumours consisting of intra- and extraosseous Ewing's sarcoma, primitive neuroectodermal tumour (PNET), Askin's tumour (PNET of chest wall), periosteal Ewing's, and neuroepithelioma. Cell origin is primarily neural. The tumour is often aggressive but is usually chemo- and radiosensitive.

Clinical presentation

The incidence is approximately two per million, affects 5–20-year-olds and has an increased prevalence in Caucasians.

Ewing's sarcoma can present with localized features of pain, mass, and pathological fracture, as well as systemic constitutional symptoms of fever, weight loss, or malaise. The long bones, pelvis, vertebrae, ribs, or clavicle are most commonly affected, with the femur, tibia, humerus, and fibula involved in decreasing frequency. Like osteosarcoma, approximately 20% of patients present with metastatic disease.

Radiological features

Classically there is laminated periosteal 'onion-skinning' in the diaphysis of a long bone in association with a permeative moth-eaten bony radiolucent lesion (Figure 2.6.4). These appearances are also very similar to infection and with the raised inflammatory markers, can cause a delay in reaching the correct diagnosis.

MR describes extent of marrow infiltration, soft tissue extension, solid and necrotic tumour elements, cortical thickening, and periosteal reaction.

Pathological features

The absence of osteoid formation can produce liquid pus-like material on biopsy of the soft tissue component. Sheets of small, undifferentiated, round cells with prominent nuclei and poorly visualized cytoplasm make other lesions such as lymphoma, myeloma, histiocytosis, rhabmyosarcoma, metastatic neuroblastoma, small-cell osteogenic sarcoma, and mesenchymal chondrosarcoma all possible diagnoses. The Ewing's groups of tumours have a 95% sensitivity of surface expression of p30/32 MIC2 antigen and CD99. The t(11:22) translocation is found is 90% of patients. PNET is differentiated from Ewing's both histologically by Homer Wright rosettes as well as positive staining of the neural S100 marker with PNET lesions.

Treatment and outcome

Local, multicentric, and metastatic Ewing's sarcoma is treated with a combination of systemic (chemotherapy) and local (surgery with or without radiotherapy) therapies. Chemotherapeutic regimens include the use of actinomycin, cyclophosphamide, doxorubicin, etoposide, and ifosfamide. These have improved survivorship and have necessitated local control measures in the last 30 years. The treatment modality depends on the patient medical status, tumour location, and extent of spread.

Long bone lesions that can be resected safely are amenable to joint reconstruction. Pelvic lesions can present particular challenges, especially in the paediatric population. Open growth plates mean that resection with or without joint reconstruction can leave children with considerable pelvic girdle and lower limb deficits. Resection (or indeed complete hemipelvic disarticulation), extracorporeal radiotherapy, and re-implantation is possible given the radiosensitive nature of Ewing's sarcoma. Re-implantation techniques are similar to allograft implantation. Viable tumour cells are ablated using radiotherapy leaving the remaining scaffold available for host bone recolonization.

The presence of disseminated disease remains the most important factor in predicting survival. Approximate 3-year survival rates in patients with lung metastases on presentation are 40%, 70% in isolated disease, and 30% with disseminated disease.

Box 2.6.3 Ewing's sarcoma

- Incidence is approximately three per million, affects 5–20-year-olds and has an increased prevalence in Caucasians
- Classically radiographs show laminated periosteal 'onion-skinning' in the diaphysis of a long bone
- Treated with a combination of systemic (chemotherapy) and local (surgery with or without radiotherapy) therapies; generally chemo/radio sensitive
- Three-year survival rate in patients with lung metastases on presentation is 40%, 70% in isolated disease, and 30% with disseminated disease.

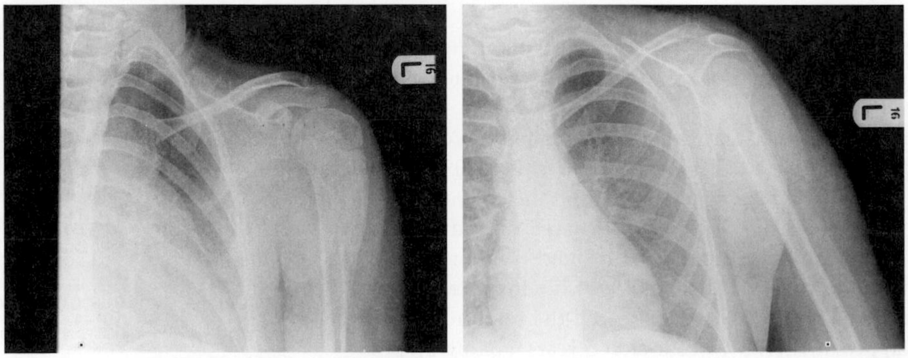

A B

Fig. 2.6.4 Typical radiographic appearance of Ewing's sarcoma of the proximal humerus: A) anteroposterior and B) lateral radiographs.

Any survivorship figures need to be interpreted with caution. Clearly small appendicular tumours have a completely different prognosis to large axial tumours or those located within the pelvis. Follow-up between both oncologist and orthopaedic surgeon follows the same regimen as for osteosarcoma.

Myeloma of bone (Box 2.6.4)

Myeloma of bone is of haematological origin and is managed primarily by haematological oncologists. Causes have been attributed to radiation exposure and a genetic predisposition. If isolated it is termed plasmacytoma or multiple myeloma if disseminated.

Lesions produce a neoplastic single clone proliferation of plasma cells that produce a monoclonal immunoglobulin. The orthopaedic team is involved in managing the plasma cell-induced osteolytic skeletal destruction and secondary bony structural failure. Other medical ramifications include hypercalcaemia, anaemia, renal failure, hyperviscosity syndrome, or recurrent bacterial infections.

Clinical presentation

With an incidence of four per 100 000 per year, multiple myeloma is the most common primary bone tumour in adults. It is primarily a disease of patients after their fourth decade, with the median incidence at age 65. It is more common in black patients presenting with fever, pain, or weakness. It can be asymptomatic. Additional orthopaedic presenting complaints include axial, thoracic, or appendicular limb pain as well as secondary effects such as spinal cord compression or pathological fracture.

Extramedullary plasmacytoma presents as a soft tissue mass.

Normocytic, normochromic anaemia is found at diagnosis in approximately 70% of patients. Leucopenia and thrombocytopenia are less common. Erythrocyte sedimentation rate is often raised. Urinary Bence Jones protein and an aberrant serum paraprotein (or M-protein) is found in 90% of patients at presentation. Plasma electrophoresis enables quantitative measurement to secure a diagnosis and disease monitoring.

Differential diagnoses include metastatic carcinoma, lymphoma, monoclonal gammopathy of unknown significance (MGUS), smouldering multiple myeloma (SMM), acute leukaemia, or POEMS (Polyneuropathy, Organomegaly, Endocrinopathy, M-protein, Skin anomalies) syndrome.

Minimal diagnostic criteria consist of more than 10% plasma cells in bone or a plasmacytoma plus one of serum or urine paraprotein or lytic bone lesions. The International Myeloma Working Group has staged the disease using B_2 microglobulin (MHC class I) levels as it is an overall marker for body tumour burden. Stage I is classified as a level less than 3.5mg/L, II lies between 3.5–5.5mg/L, and stage III more than 5.5mg/L.

Radiological features

Plain film evaluation demonstrates punched-out lytic lesions or fractures in 75% of patients at diagnosis (Figure 2.6.5). Technetium-99m-labelled bone scans are usually cold hence conventional radiographs are used for the detection of lytic lesions with *no surrounding sclerosis*. The lateral skull is classic for the 'pepper-pot' appearance. CT and MRI are more sensitive and may be useful when skeletal pain is atypical and radiographs show no abnormalities.

Pathological features

Histological analysis reveals large basophilic cytoplasmic plasma cells containing rounded or oval eccentric nuclei with clumped chromatin and a perinuclear halo.

Treatment and outcome

Most patients with focal plasmacytoma undergo surgery if feasible, radiation, and subsequent observation. Multiple myeloma presents challenges at multiple levels and care is targeted on disease control and suppression, the extent of which depends on the disease progression and patient status. The anaemia is managed with erythropoietin and bony destruction slowed by bisphosphonates.

Asymptomatic patients with low B_2 microglobulin levels are observed. Symptomatic patients receive chemotherapy and haematopoietic stem-cell transplantation.

Orthopaedic input is usually at the pre-, impending, or postfracture stage. Fracture union in the presence of pathological bone proceeds at varying rates in comparison to normal bone. Long, locked intramedullary nails form the mainstay of operative treatment.

Depending on the stage, median survival is 62 months for stage 1, 45 months for stage 2, and 29 months for stage 3 disease. Follow-up is with haematologists with a low threshold for orthopaedic consultation.

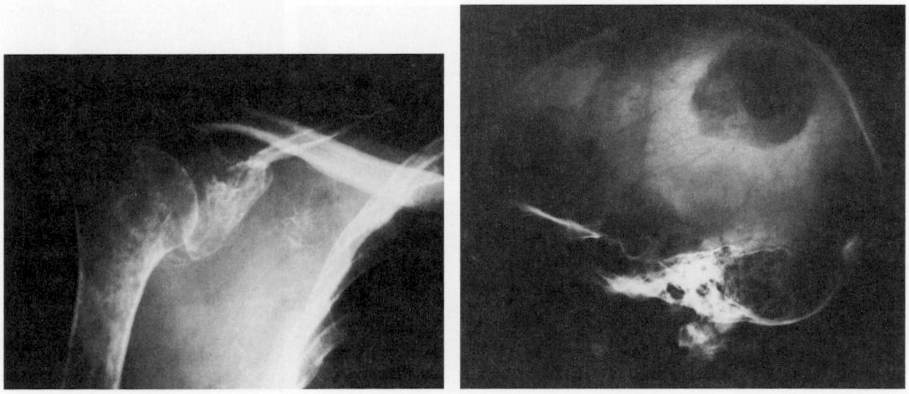

A B

Fig. 2.6.5 A) Anteroposterior view of the shoulder demonstrating multiple lytic punched-out lesions in the proximal humerus with thinning of the cortices. Note that the body of the scapula has been completely destroyed. B) Lateral view of the skull demonstrating multiple punched-out lesions that vary in size.

Box 2.6.4 Myeloma of bone

- Neoplasm of haematological origin
- Plasmacytoma if isolated or multiple myeloma if disseminated
- Plain films demonstrate punched-out lytic lesions or fractures in 75% of patients at diagnosis
- Patients managed by haematologists; orthopaedic input is usually at the pre-, impending, or post-pathological fracture stage.

Fibrosarcoma of bone or soft tissue (Box 2.6.5)

Fibrosarcoma is a tumour of mesenchymal cell origin that is composed of malignant fibroblasts in a collagen background. It can occur as a soft tissue mass or as a primary or secondary bone tumour. Fibrosarcoma was diagnosed much more frequently in the past; it is now more reliably distinguished histologically from similar lesions, such as desmoid tumours, malignant fibrous histiocytoma, malignant schwannoma, and high-grade osteosarcoma.

The two main types of fibrosarcoma of bone are primary and secondary. Primary fibrosarcoma is a fibroblastic malignancy that produces variable amounts of collagen. It is either central (arising within the medullary canal) or peripheral (arising from the periosteum). Secondary fibrosarcoma of bone arises from a pre-existing lesion or after radiotherapy to an area of bone or soft tissue. This is a more aggressive tumour and has a poorer prognosis.

Clinical presentation

Fibrosarcoma represents 10% of musculoskeletal sarcomas and less than 5% of all primary bone sarcomas.

Fibrosarcoma of bone usually affects the metaphysis of long bones in patients over 50 years of age. Presenting features include pain, mass effect, decreased range of movement, and fracture. Pre-existing pathological lesions or irradiated tissue needs to be considered with increased suspicion.

Fibrosarcoma of the soft tissues usually affects a wider age spectrum of patients than fibrosarcoma of the bone does, with an age range of 35–55 years. It often arises in the soft tissues of the thigh and the posterior knee. It is generally a large, painless mass deep to fascia and has an ill-defined margin.

Radiological features

Typically, an osteolytic, metaphyseal, eccentrically placed lesion associated with cortical destruction and soft tissue extension, with a marked absence of ossification or mineralization. MRI is the best

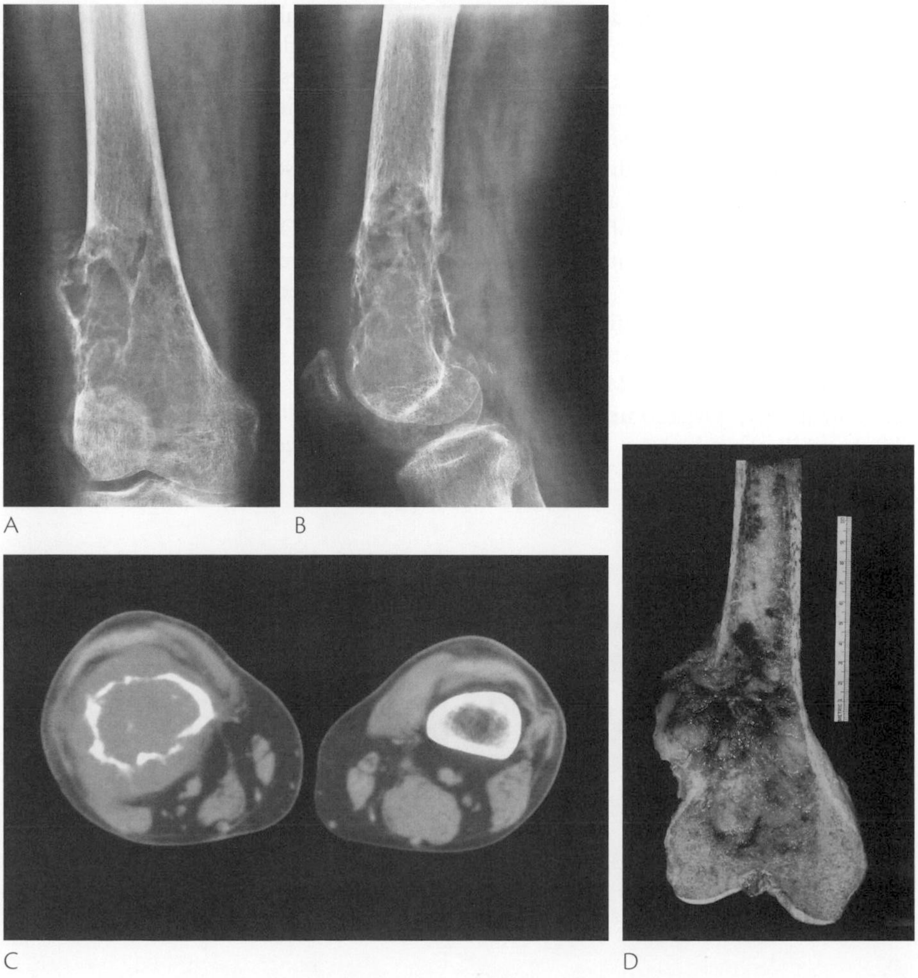

Fig. 2.6.6 Fibrosarcoma of the distal femur. A) Anteroposterior and B) lateral plain radiographs showing destructive lesion. A CT scan of the same patient (C) demonstrates that the tumour has broken through the cortex to form a soft tissue mass. Gross pathological specimen of the tumour (D).

modality for examining soft tissue masses and providing information about the local extent, lesion size, and involvement of the neurovascular structures. Fibrosarcoma of bone typically has extraosseous extension (Figure 2.6.6).

Pathological features

Well-differentiated forms have multiple plump fibroblasts with deeply staining nuclei in a rich collagen background. Intermediate-grade tumours have the typical herringbone pattern, showing the diagnostic parallel sheets of cells arranged in intertwining whorls. A slight degree of cellular pleomorphism exists.

High-grade lesions are very cellular, with marked cellular atypia and mitotic activity. The degree of cellularity, nuclear atypia, and pleomorphism are used to classify fibrosarcoma into grades 1–3. The higher grade 3 lesions are deemed to be malignant fibrous histiocytomas. In fact, some pathologists believe that the division between malignant fibrous histiocytoma, high-grade osteosarcoma, and fibrosarcoma may be artificial.

Treatment and outcome

Grade 1 lesions are managed operatively without chemotherapy. Grade 2 lesions involve chemotherapy and resection. Grade 3 lesions follow malignant fibrous histiocytoma/osteosarcoma regimens. Radiation is administered in palliative cases and incomplete resections.

If all grades are included, primary fibrosarcoma of the bone has a worse prognosis than osteosarcoma, with a 5-year survival rate of 65%. In high-grade primary fibrosarcoma, the 10-year survival rate is less than 30%. Secondary fibrosarcoma is associated with a very poor outcome, the survival rate at 10 years being less than 10%.

For congenital fibrosarcoma of bone in children, the prognosis (which is related to age and to time to diagnosis) is much better, with the disease having long-term survival rates of grater than 50%.

Soft tissue fibrosarcoma is associated with a 40–60% survival rate at 5 years. The infantile form has an even better 5-year survival rate, in excess of 80%.

Box 2.6.5 Fibrosarcoma

- Tumour of mesenchymal cell origin, composed of malignant fibroblasts in a collagen background
- 5% of bone sarcomas, usually affects the metaphysis of long bones in patients over 50 years of age
- Primary or secondary in a pre-existing lesion
- Grade 3 lesions are deemed to be malignant fibrous histiocytoma.

Lymphoma of bone (Box 2.6.6)

Primary lymphoma of bone (PLB) is a rare, malignant, neoplastic disorder of the skeleton. The vast majority of them are non-Hodgkin lymphoma (NHL), whereas primary Hodgkin lymphoma (HL) of bone is extremely rare.

Primary lymphomas of bone are uncommon malignancies (approximately 5% of primary malignant bone tumours and 5% of all cases of extra-nodal NHL). Comprehensive immunohistochemical studies are required to establish an accurate histological diagnosis of primary NHL of bone. Most cases of primary NHL of bone are classified as diffuse large B-cell lymphomas (DLBCL) in the World Health Organization (WHO) classification of haematological malignancies.

Clinical presentation

There is a marginal male preponderance. The incidence of disease is distributed fairly evenly in the second through to the eighth decades. Primary NHL of bone can arise in any part of the skeleton, but long bones (femurs, tibia) are the most common sites to be affected.

Patients with primary NHL of bone commonly present with local bone pain, soft tissue swelling, a mass, or a pathological fracture. Prolonged pain is the usual clinical symptom.

The WHO recognizes the following four groups of lymphoma involving bone:

1) A single primary bone site with or without regional nodes
2) Multiple bone sites but no visceral involvement
3) A bone lesion and involvement of multiple lymph node sites
4) Soft tissue lymphoma, with bone involvement detected by bone biopsy or marrow aspirate.

Groups 3 and 4 would most likely represent metastatic involvement of bone.

Radiological presentation

PLB tumours produce osteoclast-stimulating factors that cause lytic bone destruction (Figure 2.6.7). The most common radiographic features include:

- Permeative, lytic pattern of bone destruction (74%)
- Metadiaphyseal location (69%)
- Periosteal reaction (58%)
- Soft tissue mass (80–100%).

Sequestrum formation is a feature of PLB that can help to differentiate it from most other diagnostic possibilities. Sequestra have been reported in 11–16% of patients with PLB. Finally, involvement of adjacent bones is seen in 4% of cases.

After biopsy of the bone lesion confirms the diagnosis of lymphoma, CT scanning of the chest, abdomen, and pelvis is needed to exclude distant spread. The CT scan may be combined with positron emission tomography (PET), which is emerging as a possible modality for initial staging and follow-up. Technetium-99m (^{99m}Tc) bone scintigraphy also can be used to look for additional sites of involvement.

Pathological features

The clinical features and radiological findings of PLB are usually non-specific, with the diagnosis relying principally on tissue histology.

The Rappaport classification system (1956) was based on light microscopic appearance. The Ann Arbor staging system, developed initially for HL, has been widely applied to the NHLs. This staging system is based on anatomic location and does not involve histology. Due to the advances of immunohistochemical markers there are now a myriad of new classification systems.

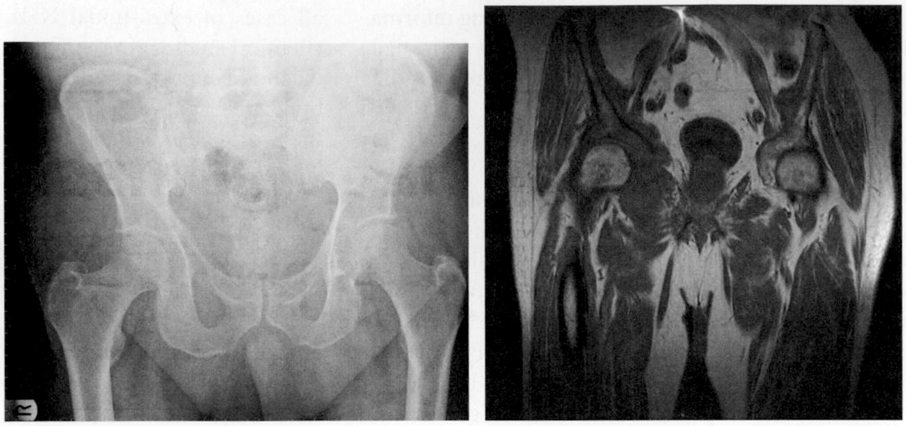

Fig. 2.6.7 Typical radiographic appearance of bone lymphoma affecting the right acetabulum: A) plain radiograph; B) MRI scan.

Treatment and outcome

Treatment for PLB often involves radiation therapy to control the tumour in the affected bone. In certain instances, surgical intervention for control of the primary bone lesion may be desirable or necessary. Several studies indicate that patients with primary NHL of bone have a favourable outcome, especially when treated by combined modality therapy.

Combined modality therapy includes a method of local control, usually radiation therapy, and a systemic treatment, usually combination chemotherapy. Recurrence at the initial primary site is uncommon. Late, distant soft tissue metastases to lung, liver, and brain account for most of the mortality and much of the morbidity.

Average survival is 19–27 months for low-grade lymphoma and less than 11 months for high-grade tumours.

Malignant vascular tumours of bone (Box 2.6.7)

Malignant vasoformative tumours are rare. Three variants of malignant vascular tumours of bone are commonly described: haemangioendothelioma (angiosarcoma), haemangiopericytoma, and epitheloid haemangioendothelioma.

Haemangioendothelioma/angiosarcoma

An uncommon malignant neoplasm characterized by rapidly proliferating, extensively infiltrating anaplastic cells derived from blood vessels and lining irregular blood-filled spaces. The term angiosarcoma may be applied to a wide range of malignant endothelial vascular neoplasms affecting a variety of sites. Angiosarcomas are aggressive and tend to recur locally, spread widely, and have a high rate of lymph node and systemic metastases. The rate of tumour-related death is high.

Box 2.6.6 Primary lymphoma of bone

- Most primary lymphomas of bone are B cell neoplasms (diffuse large B-cell lymphomas (DLBCL)
- Radiographic features include a permeative, lytic pattern of bone destruction
- Combined modality therapy includes a method of local control, usually radiation therapy, and a systemic treatment, usually combination chemotherapy.

Clinical presentation

Bone angiosarcomas appear most often in adults (second to seventh decades of life). Bone and soft tissue angiosarcoma are also reported to be more frequent in males. Thirty-three per cent affect the axial skeleton, 33% in long bones, and the rest in the small bones of the hands and feet.

These tumours can be multifocal, or multicentric, involving multiple bones of the same extremity. Pain is commonplace. Presentation features include:

- Pathologic fractures (10%)
- Other intrinsic characteristics of a malignant vascular proliferation (e.g., bleeding, thrombocytopenia, or intravascular disseminated coagulation)
- Compression of adjacent neurovascular structures which leads to pain.

Radiological presentation

A solitary lesion (60% of cases) presents as a destructive lytic mass with irregular borders or a mixed lytic–sclerotic pattern and occasional bony expansion. It has a distinctive pattern of soap-bubble lesions because it frequently extends up and down the bone. CT scan is helpful in illustrating the permeative, invasive character of the radiographic lesions and shows their multiplicity.

Pathological features

The main problem in the diagnosis of angiosarcoma is histopathological recognition. Microscopic findings include the presence of vascular spaces which are lined by atypical endothelial cells, with significantly increased numbers. Higher-grade lesions are more cellular and abnormal mitoses.

Treatment and outcome

Surgical resection and radiation therapy are the standard treatment for localized disease. Treat high-grade lesions as malignant bone neoplasms, with a combination of radical en bloc excision followed by radiotherapy and/or chemotherapy.

All angiosarcomas tend to be clinically aggressive, difficult to treat, and are often multicentric. They have a high local recurrence rate and metastatic potential. They are often misdiagnosed, leading to a poor prognosis and a high mortality rate. The reported 5-year survival rate is around 20%.

Haemangiopericytoma

Haemangiopericytomas are rare, typically low-grade sarcomas.

As with angiosarcomas the aetiology of haemangiopericytomas is largely unknown; they have been reported secondary to radiation, chemical exposure, and, rarely, burns or scars.

Haemangiopericytoma is a malignant tumour of mesenchymal origin that occurs in the extremities. Tumour typically spreads via haematogenous dissemination, primarily to the lungs. Metastatic disease is usually the cause of death.

Clinical presentation

Haemangiopericytomas primarily manifest as slow-growing, painless masses in the extremities, commonly the femur and proximal tibia. They can also occur in the pelvic fossa and the retroperitoneum.

Most documented cases occur within the third to fifth decades. They have been documented in children.

Additionally, 35% of skeletal tumours with oncogenic osteomalacia have been reported to be haemangiopericytomas. Oncogenic osteomalacia occurs with bone or soft tissue tumours and refers to the musculoskeletal symptoms of cramping and diffuse bone and muscle pain associated with electrolyte abnormalities, most notably hypophosphataemia.

Radiological features

With plain radiography, bony lesions predominantly present as intramedullary lytic masses. They may be well circumscribed, with a periosteal reaction or sclerotic border. They also may display cortical destruction, producing indeterminate borders with a honeycomb appearance. Findings of soft tissue haemangiopericytomas on plain films are usually non-specific. Bone scanning is indicated to exclude other sites of disease in patients who present with a bony haemangiopericytoma. MRI ± angiography should be used to distinguish between vascular malformations and tumours.

Pathological features

Haemangiopericytomas are neoplasms of pericytes that form solid sheets and nests around irregularly formed vascular channels. The vascular lining is normal and is composed of a single layer of non-malignant endothelial cells. Pericytes are of mesenchymal derivation and partially surround the endothelial cells of capillaries and small venules to assist blood flow regulation. These cells are located outside the connective-tissue compartment and are surrounded by their own basal lamina.

Box 2.6.7 Malignant vascular tumours of bone

- Three variants are commonly described: haemangioendothelioma (angiosarcoma), haemangiopericytoma, and epitheloid haemangioendothelioma of bone
- Aggressive lesions tend to recur locally, spread widely, and have a high rate of lymph node and systemic metastases
- Need aggressive surgical excision + adjuvant treatment (radiotherapy).

A diagnosis of haemangiopericytoma is made solely on the basis of architectural patterns exhibited histologically. Thus this type of tumour cannot be accurately distinguished from other neoplasms that have vascular characteristics, without such detailed histological information. The diagnosis of this tumour and evaluation of its clinical course remain complex challenges for tumour surgeons and histopathologists.

Treatment and outcome

Treatment of haemangiopericytomas is based on the grade of the sarcoma.

Low-grade bone tumours require surgical resection and are not usually treated with chemotherapy. High-grade bone tumours may be treated with chemotherapy, but because of the rarity of these tumours, the direct benefit of treatment is unknown.

Soft tissue haemangiopericytomas are treated with surgical resection and radiation therapy to decrease local recurrence.

Epithelioid haemangioendothelioma

A low- to intermediate-grade vascular tumour composed of epithelioid endothelial cells. Epithelioid haemangioendothelioma is an extremely rare vascular bone tumour with a slow growth and poor prognosis. It represents 1% of all vascular neoplasms and is locally aggressive. Other proposed terms have included 'sclerosing angiogenic tumour'.

Further reading

Edwards, C.M., Zhuang, J., and Mundy, G.R. (2008). The pathogenesis of the bone disease of multiple myeloma. *Bone*, **42**(6), 1007–13.

Flemming, D.J. and Murphey, M.D. (2000). Enchondroma and chondrosarcoma. *Seminars in Musculoskeletal Radiology*, **4**(1), 59–71.

Ludwig, J.A. (2008). Ewing's sarcoma: historical perspectives, current state-of-the-art, and opportunities for targeted therapy in the future. *Current Opinion in Oncology*, **20**(4), 412–18.

Siegel, H.J. and Pressey, J.G. (2008). Current concepts on the surgical and medical management of osteosarcoma. *Expert Review of Anticancer Therapy*, **8**(8), 1257–69.

Wafa, H. and Grimer, R.J. (2006). Surgical options and outcomes in bone sarcoma. *Expert Review of Anticancer Therapy*, **6**(2), 239–48.

2.7

Metastatic bone disease

Panagiotis D. Gikas and Timothy W.R. Briggs

Summary points

- Metastatic pathological fractures rarely unite, even if stabilized
- Never rush to fix a pathological fracture; traction or splintage will suffice while investigations are performed and surgical intervention discussed
- When surgery is indicated for spinal metastases, both decompression and stabilization are generally required
- Implants should allow immediate weight-bearing and last the lifetime of the patient
- Always use a multidisciplinary team.

Introduction

Bone is the commonest site for metastasis in cancer and is of particular clinical importance in breast and prostate cancers because of the prevalence of these diseases. At postmortem examination, 70% of these patients have evidence of metastatic bone disease. However, bone metastases may complicate a wide range of malignancies, resulting in considerable morbidity and complex demands on healthcare resources. Carcinomas of the thyroid, kidney, and bronchus also commonly give rise to bone metastases, with an incidence at postmortem examination of 30–40%. However, tumours of the gastrointestinal tract rarely (less than 10%) produce bone metastases.

Clinical presentation (Box 2.7.1)

This is typically in one of three modes:

- Acute admission with pathological fracture or neurological compromise
- Referral to clinic with unexplained musculoskeletal pain
- Referral from oncologist/breast care team (surgeon, radiologist, or oncologist).

Pain

Bone metastases are the most common cause of cancer-related pain. The pathophysiological mechanisms of pain in patients with bone metastases are poorly understood but probably include tumour-induced osteolysis, tumour production of growth factors and cytokines, direct infiltration of nerves, stimulation of ion channels, and local tissue production of endothelins and nerve growth factors. Although 80% of patients with advanced breast cancer develop osteolytic bone metastases, approximately two-thirds of such sites are painless.

Different sites of bone metastases are associated with distinct clinical pain syndromes. Common sites of metastatic involvement associated with pain are the base of the skull (in association with cranial nerve palsies, neuralgias, and headache), vertebral metastases (producing neck and back pain with or without neurologic complications secondary to epidural extension), and pelvic and femoral lesions (producing pain in the back and lower limbs, often associated with mechanical instability).

Hypercalcaemia

Hypercalcaemia most often occurs in those patients with squamous cell lung cancer, breast and kidney cancers, and certain haematological malignancies (in particular myeloma and lymphoma). In most cases, hypercalcaemia is a result of bone destruction, and osteolytic metastases are present in 80% of cases.

Secretion of humoral and paracrine factors by tumour cells stimulates osteoclast activity and proliferation, and there is a marked increase in markers of bone turnover. Several studies have established the role of parathyroid hormone-related peptide in most cases of malignant hypercalcaemia.

The signs and symptoms of hypercalcaemia are non-specific, and the clinician should have a high index of suspicion. Common symptoms include fatigue, anorexia, and constipation. If untreated, a progressive increase in serum calcium level results in deterioration of renal function and mental status. Death ultimately results from renal failure and cardiac arrhythmias.

Pathological fractures

The destruction of bone by metastatic disease reduces its load-bearing capabilities and results initially in microfractures, which cause pain. Subsequently, fractures occur (most commonly in ribs and vertebrae). It is the fracture of a long bone or the epidural extension of tumour into the spine that causes the greatest disability.

Compression of the spinal cord or cauda equina

Spinal cord compression is a medical emergency, and suspected cases require urgent evaluation and treatment. Pain occurs in most patients, is localized to the area overlying the tumour, and often worsens with activities that increase intradural pressure (e.g. coughing, sneezing, or straining). The pain is usually worse at night, which is the opposite pattern of pain from degenerative disease. There may also be radicular pain radiating down a limb or around the chest or upper abdomen. Local pain usually precedes radicular pain and may predate the appearance of other neurologic signs by weeks or months. Most patients with spinal cord compression will have weakness or paralysis. Late sensory changes include numbness and anaesthesia distal to the level of involvement. Urinary retention, incontinence, and impotence are usually late manifestations of cord compression. However, lesions at the level of the conus medullaris can present with early autonomic dysfunction of the bladder, rectum, and genitalia.

Spinal instability

Back pain is a frequent symptom in patients with advanced cancer and in 10% of cases is due to spinal instability. The pain, which can be severe, is mechanical in origin, and frequently patients are only comfortable when lying still.

Surgical management of metastatic bone disease (Box 2.7.2)

The role of the orthopaedic surgeon in the management of metastatic bone disease, always part of a multidisciplinary team, falls into three principal categories (British Orthopaedic Association Guidelines):

1) Prophylactic fixation of metastatic deposits where there is a risk of fracture
2) Stabilization or reconstruction following pathological fracture
3) Decompression of spinal cord and nerve roots and/or stabilization for spinal instability.

Any surgical procedure should provide immediate stability, allowing weight bearing and as a general rule the fixation should aim to last the lifetime of the patient. The surgeon must assume that the fracture may not unite and should aim to stabilize all lesions in the affected bone. Furthermore, if there is the slightest doubt as to the underlying pathology, and in particular where there is a solitary bony lesion, then further investigations including scintigraphy, magnetic resonance imaging scan of the lesion, and percutaneous bone biopsy should be carried out before definitive surgery. This allows the detection of primary bone neoplasms or solitary renal metastases (these have good prognosis and should be treated like primary bone tumours)

Box 2.7.1 Modes of clinical presentation—summary

- Musculoskeletal pain
- Pathological fractures
- Neurological complications (cauda equina compression/ spinal instability)
- Fatigue, anorexia, constipation secondary to hypercalcaemia.

Fracture risk assessment

Where fracture is likely to occur, then prophylactic fixation should be performed prior to the administration of radiotherapy. It is essential, therefore, to have a reliable method of predicting the risk of a pathological fracture occurring.

In an effort to provide a reliable and reproducible measure of the risk of pathological fracture, Mirels devised a scoring system which is a useful aid to fracture risk assessment (Table 2.7.1). For scores of eight or above, the risk of fracture is high and prophylactic fixation should be carried out prior to radiotherapy being administered.

Hip

Where destruction is limited to the femoral neck or head, a cemented hemiarthroplasty or total joint replacement is recommended as a primary procedure. Long stem femoral implants should be considered. Subtrochanteric fractures or lesions with limited bone loss are best stabilized by 'reconstruction' nails with locking screws up the femoral neck (Figure 2.7.1). This greatly reduces the risk of subsequent femoral neck fracture.

Pelvis and acetabulum

The majority of pelvic lesions are treated with prophylactic palliative radiotherapy alone. However, acetabular reconstruction with pins and cement can be carried out where there is an imminent risk of failure of the socket

Shoulder girdle and upper limb

Metastatic lesions or fractures of the scapula and clavicle are usually managed with radiotherapy alone. In the humeral head, significant destruction is, in most cases, best treated by hemiarthroplasty.

Shafts of major long bones (humerus, femur, tibia)

Intramedullary nailing is the procedure of choice with locking screws to give rotational stability and to prevent telescoping (Figure 2.7.2). Apart from the case of solitary renal metastases, the potential spread of tumour cells within the medulla by nailing is acceptable within the context of palliative treatment. The entire bone and operative site should be included in the postoperative radiotherapy field. Since these fractures are unlikely to unite,

Table 2.7.1 Mirels' scoring system for metastatic bone disease

Score	1	2	3
Site	Upper limb	Lower limb	Peritrochanteric
Pain	Mild	Moderate	Functional
Lesion	Blastic	Mixed	Lytic
Size (as seen on plain x-ray, max. destruction of cortex in any view)	<1/3	1/3–2/3	>2/3

Maximum possible score is 12; if lesion scores 8 or above, then prophylactic fixation is recommended *prior* to radiotherapy.

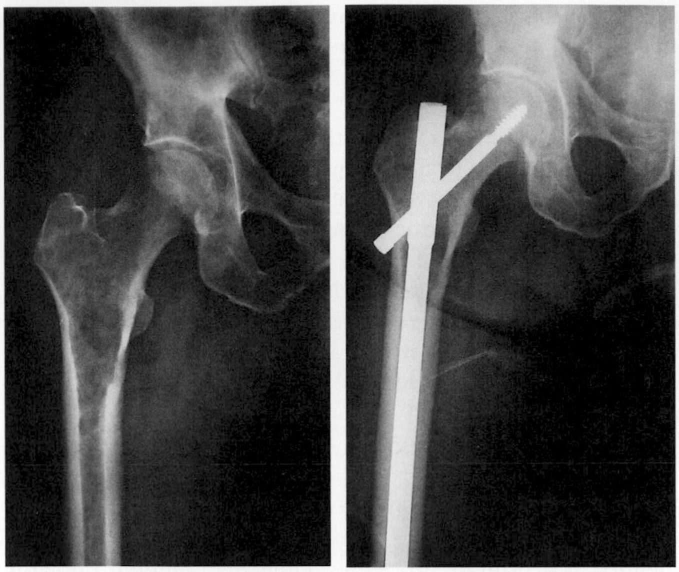

A B

Fig. 2.7.1 Anteroposterior views of right proximal femur (A) showing extensive metastatic destruction of subtrochanteric region and (B) after internal fixation with an intramedullary reconstruction nail.

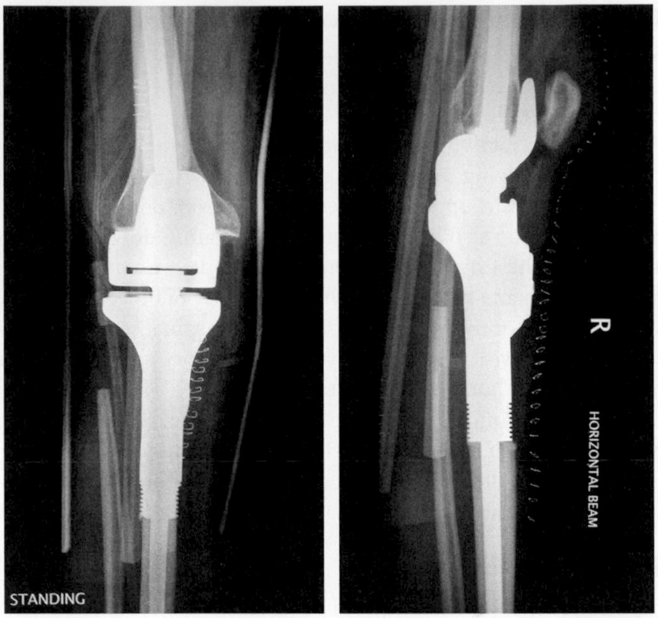

A B

Fig. 2.7.3 Anteroposterior (A) and lateral (B) views of right proximal tibia showing proximal tibial replacement with custom-made endoprosthesis for metastatic renal cell carcinoma.

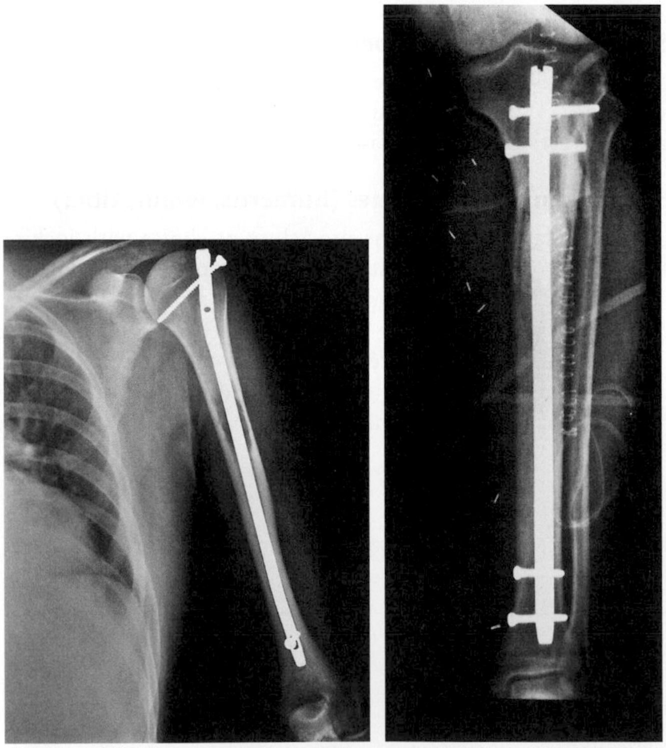

A B

Fig. 2.7.2 (A) Anteroposterior view of the left humerus showing interlocking intramedullary nail fixation for metastatic disease. (B) Intramedullary nail fixation for metastatic lesion of the proximal tibia (cement was also used).

load-bearing, rather than load-sharing, devices should be used, and solid nails, of a greater diameter than may be used for purely traumatic fractures, may be considered. Packing of major bone defects with methylmethacrylate bone cement is useful in maintaining stability in some cases. All of the lesions in the affected bone should be stabilized to minimize the risk of further surgery being required. Reconstruction nails, stabilizing the femoral neck, are recommended in the femur.

Endoprosthetic surgery

Extensive bone destruction at the metaphyses of major long bones is sometimes so great that reconstruction can only be achieved using custom or modular endoprostheses (Figure 2.7.3). However, major surgery such as this has to be balanced against the likely timeframe of survivorship of the patient.

Adjuvant therapy

Radiotherapy is generally palliative, and often given as a single fraction. It can produce effective bone healing and sclerosis and, when given prophylactically, can prevent pathological fracture occurring. It will not, however, cure pain of a 'mechanical' nature, and only 30–40% of pathological fractures will unite even after radiotherapy. It is recommended that following nailing or other surgical procedures in patients with metastatic bone disease, radiotherapy to the affected bone and operative field (unless field sizes are excessive) should be considered by the appropriate specialist within the context of the multidisciplinary team. The spinal cord is radiosensitive, and this may limit the scope for adjuvant treatment of the axial skeleton.

Box 2.7.2 Surgical management of metastatic bone disease—summary

- Prophylactic fixation of metastatic deposits when there is a risk of fracture
- Stabilization or reconstruction following pathological fracture
- Decompression of spinal cord and nerve roots and/or stabilization for spinal instability
- Use Mirels' scoring system for fracture risk assessment.

Endocrine therapy, bisphosphonates, and chemotherapy may all have a role in the management of patients with metastatic bone disease.

Treatment for spinal metastatic bone disease

Over the last two decades there has been considerable improvement in the implants available to manage structural deficiency of the spine, notably pedicle screws, cages, and plating or rodding systems. The objectives of surgery are:

- Maintenance of, or restoration of, spinal cord/nerve root function
- Preservation of, or restoration of, spinal stability
- Preservation of as many normal motion segments as possible.

Treatment of spinal metastatic disease may involve radiotherapy ± surgery:

Indications for radiotherapy

- No spinal instability
- Radiosensitive tumour
- Stable or slowly progressive neurology
- Multilevel disease
- Surgery precluded by general condition
- Poor prognosis
- Postoperative adjuvant treatment.

Indications for surgery

- Spinal instability evidenced by pathological fracture, progressive deformity, and/or neurological deficit
- Clinically significant neurological compression, especially by bone
- Tumour insensitive to radiotherapy, chemotherapy, or hormonal manipulation.

Conclusion

The prognosis for patients with metastatic bone disease is steadily improving. The orthopaedic surgeon should never assume that a lytic lesion, particularly if solitary, is a metastasis and appropriate tests should always be done to exclude a primary bone neoplasm. Management of metastatic bone disease should always be done in the context of a multidisciplinary team.

Further reading

British Orthopaedic Association and the British Orthopaedic Oncology Society (2002). *Metastatic Bone Disease: A Guide to Good Practice.* London: British Orthopaedic Association.

Coleman, R.E. (2006). Clinical features of metastatic bone disease and the risk of skeletal morbidity. *Clinical Cancer Research*, **12**(20 Pt 2), 6243s–6249s.

SECTION 3

The Spine

3.1

Cervical spine disorders

Howard An and Mark L. Dumonski

Summary points

- Degenerative cervical spine disorders may manifest clinically with axial neck pain, radiculopathy, myelopathy, or a combination of these clinical symptoms
- The findings on radiographs and MRI are pertinent if they correlate with the clinical symptoms
- The initial treatment for patients with degenerative cervical spine disorders is conservative, including non-narcotic analgesics, anti-inflammatory medications, exercise program, physiotherapy, and occasional injections
- Surgical indications include significant radicular pain despite conservative treatment, profound neurologic deficits, and presence of significant myelopathy
- Surgical treatment for cervical radiculopathy includes laminoforaminotomy, anterior cervical discectomy and fusion (ACDF), and artificial disk replacement, and surgical treatment for myelopathy includes anterior discectomy and/or corpectomy with fusion, posterior laminoplasty, and posterior laminectomy and fusion. The surgeon should be familiar with the specific indications as well as advantages and disadvantages of each procedure.

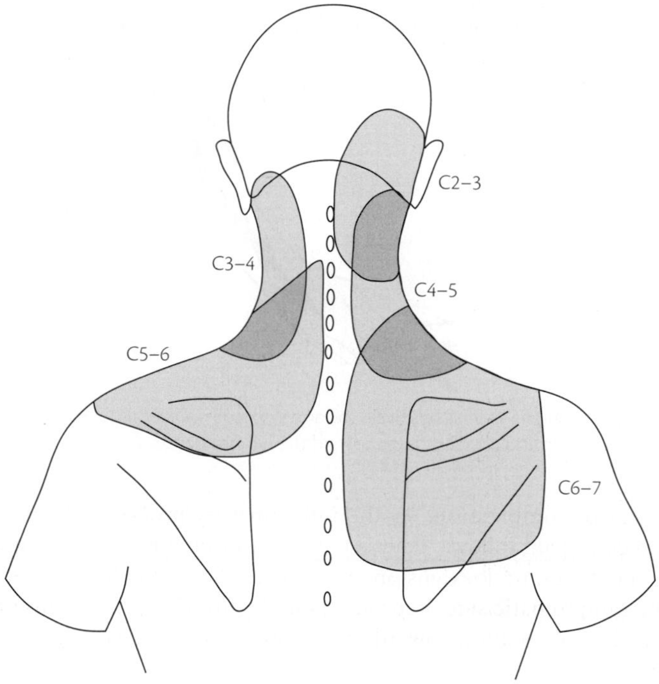

Fig. 3.1.1 A composite map of pain distribution from zygapophyseal joint injections. (Reproduced from Dwyer *et al.* (1990).)

Introduction

Degenerative disorders of the cervical spine may present as any combination of neck pain, radiculopathy, or myelopathy. A careful history and physical examination is essential, as each diagnosis requires different treatment options and prognoses. This includes proper interpretation of patients' complaints, a thorough physical examination, and an appropriate selection and review of diagnostic tests. In addition, various other aetiologies such as neoplastic, infectious, and inflammatory processes must be considered. This chapter will describe the history, physical examination, and treatment for degenerative disorders of the cervical spine.

History and physical exam

A patient presenting with degenerative cervical disc disease typically presents with axial neck pain, radicular symptoms, myelopathic symptoms, or a combination of any of these. Patients with axial neck pain may present with pain referred to the shoulder, upper arm, or interscapular area (Figure 3.1.1) and, if so, these symptoms should not be confused with radicular symptoms associated with nerve root involvement. These patients may also complain of neck stiffness, muscle spasm, or headache. Upper cervical radiculopathy involving the C3 or C4 nerve root may be confused with axial neck pain, as the pain is typically in the neck and the trapezius muscle. Occipitocervical pain, particularly with neck rotation in elderly patients, may be a sign of degenerative atlanto-occipital or atlanto-axial joint pain.

In the setting of degenerative disease, radicular symptoms may be caused by a herniated disc, chronic disc degeneration with osteophyte formation, or instability within the spinal motion segment. While most patients will present with signs and symptoms consistent with involvement of a single nerve root, multiple roots are occasionally involved. Paresthesias generally develop in the early

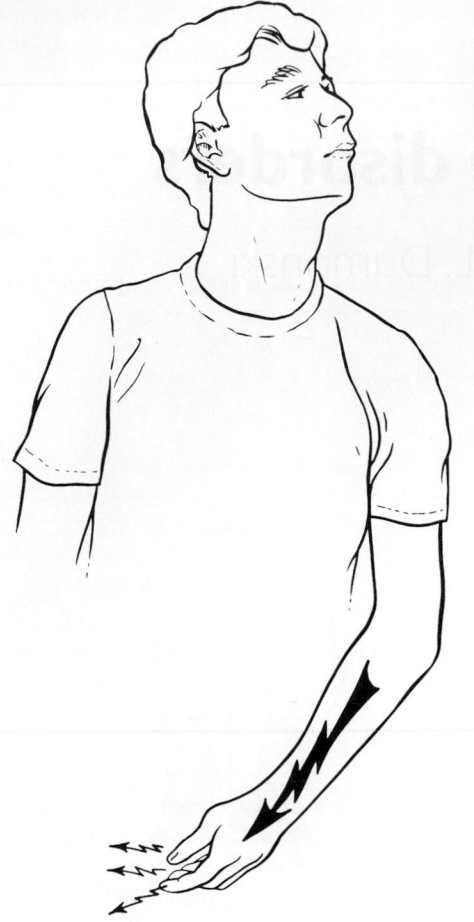

Fig. 3.1.2 Spurling's sign is positive if the arm symptoms are reproduced by hyperextension and lateral rotation toward the symptomatic side.

stages of compression. As the inflammatory process continues, radicular pain follows. Pain is typically exacerbated with Valsalva manoeuvres, neck extension, and when rotating the head toward the symptomatic side. Reproduction of pain with hyperextension and lateral rotation toward the symptomatic side is diagnostic

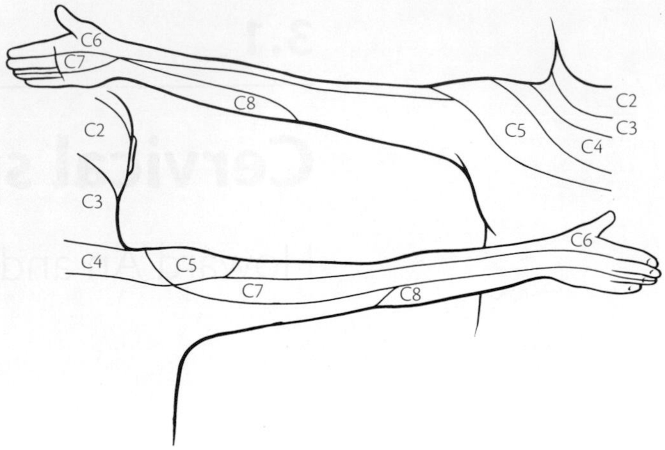

Fig. 3.1.3 Dermatomal distribution in the neck and the upper extremity.

and referred to as a positive Spurling's sign (Figure 3.1.2). This decreases the size of the intervertebral foramen, further impinging the involved nerve root. This can also be accomplished with axial compression, but the latter is less reliable. An additional reliable indicator of cervical radiculopathy is the shoulder abduction relief sign, in which the ipsilateral shoulder is abducted, relieving the tension of the effected nerve root. A positive finding corresponds to the relief of the radicular symptoms. Similarly, axial traction of the neck may relieve radicular symptoms, also by increasing the dimension of the neural foramina.

Each cervical nerve root has its own characteristic pain distribution and motor deficits (Figures 3.1.3–3.1.7). Compression of C3 or C4 will manifest with pain about the posterior neck, occiput, and over the trapezius muscle and shoulder. Occasionally, C4 radiculopathy is referred down the anterior superior chest. C5 radiculopathy typically radiates down over the shoulder to the lateral aspect of the proximal arm. Patients will complain of fatigue or frank weakness in shoulder abduction and overhead activities, as the deltoid is almost purely innervated by the C5 nerve root (while the biceps has duel innervation form both C5 and C6). The biceps reflex primarily indicates C5 pathology. C6 radiculopathy involves neck

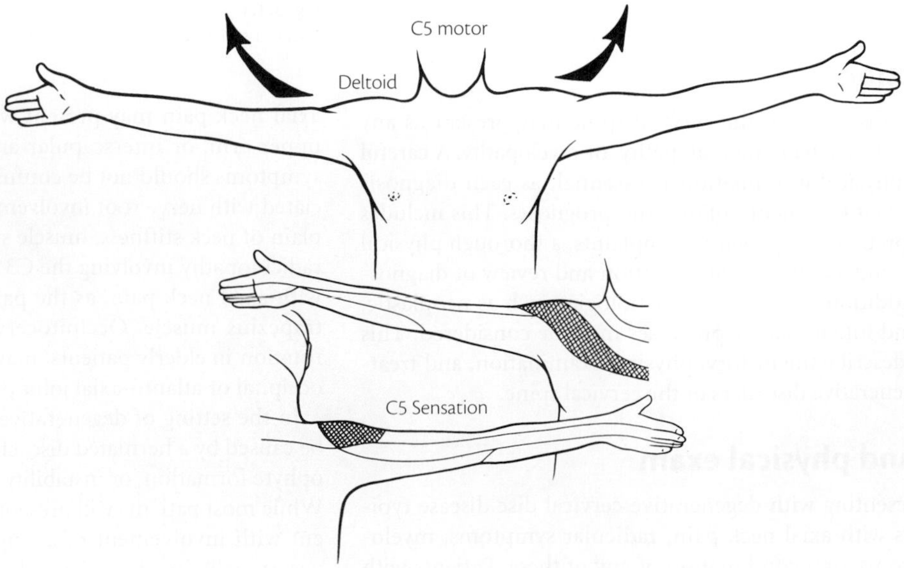

Fig. 3.1.4 C5 radiculopathy.

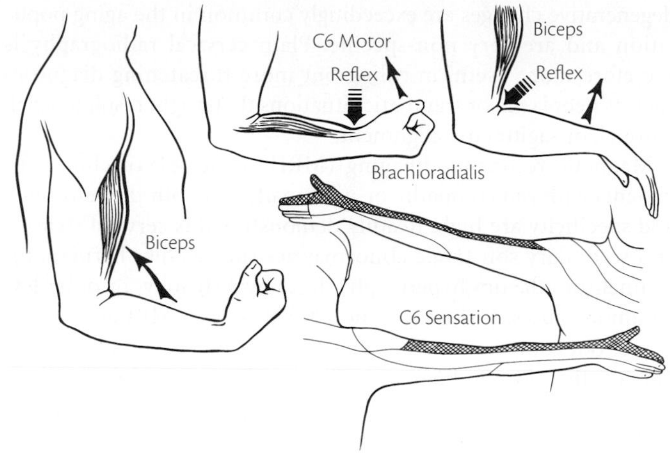

Fig. 3.1.5 C6 radiculopathy.

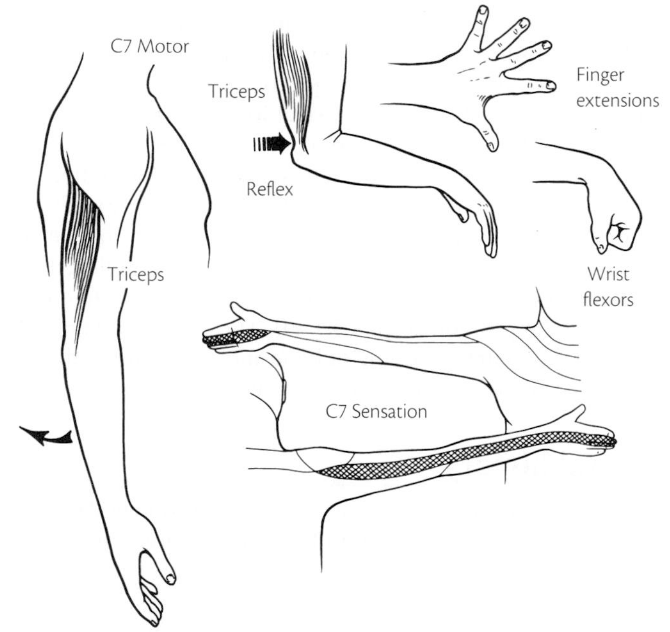

Fig. 3.1.6 C7 radiculopathy.

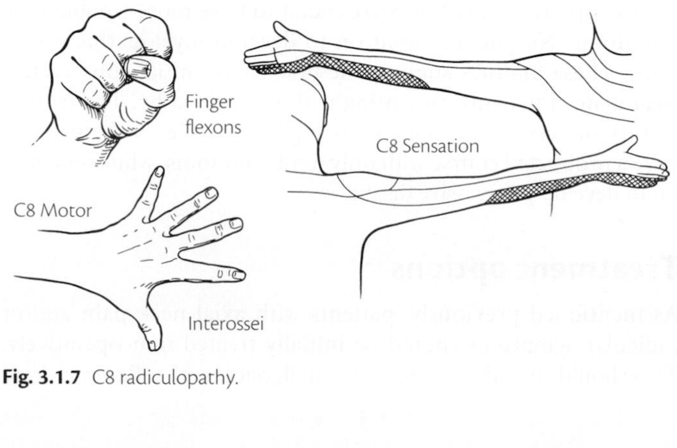

Fig. 3.1.7 C8 radiculopathy.

pain radiating across the biceps, anterior arm, the radial aspect of the forearm, and the dorsum of the thumb and index finger. Weakness affects the biceps and/or wrist extensors. The extensor carpi radialis longus and brevis are innervated by C6, while the extensor carpi ulnaris is primarily innervated by C7. Therefore wrist extensor weakness may reflect either C6 or C7 pathology. The brachioradialis reflex is most directly affected by C6 compression. C7 radiculopathy is associated with pain along the posterior shoulder and arm, posterolateral forearm, and the middle finger. However, involvement of the index and ring fingers, as well as the first web space, can also be seen. The triceps muscle is most commonly affected, resulting in weakness and a diminished reflex. Unlike shoulder weakness, however, weakness of the triceps muscle is an infrequent complaint, unless the patient uses the muscle repetitively. Patients with C8 radiculopathy describe pain along the ulnar border of the arm and forearm to the small finger, often involving the ulnar half of the ring finger. Motor deficits may be noted with abduction, adduction, and flexion of the fingers. Intrinsic muscle atrophy of the hand is frequently seen in chronic cases.

The symptoms of cervical myelopathy may include gait difficulties, decreased manual dexterity, paresthesias, urinary urgency or frequency, spasticity, or weakness. In contrast to cervical or lumbar radiculopathy, pain is not a common presenting symptom. The gait disturbance is an early presenting complaint and the symptoms are usually insidious and slowly progressive. The characteristic stooped wide-based gait of the elderly is a common end result. Complaints involving clumsy or numb hands suggest upper extremity involvement, which may occur concurrently with, or follow, gait changes. Manual dexterity deficiencies will often silently progress until the patients are surprised at the lack of their ability to complete routine activities of daily living. Hand weakness may also be present, which typically manifests as decreased grip strength. Patients may have coexistent cervical and/or lumbar stenosis, in which case the clinical presentation may manifest as both upper and lower motor neuron lesions.

There are multiple physical examination findings consistent with cervical myelopathy. The finger escape sign is tested by asking the patient to hold all digits of the hand in an adducted and extended position. A positive finding is elicited when the two ulnar digits fall into flexion and abduction within 30s. In the grip and release test, the patient is asked to form a fist and then release all digits into extension, then to rapidly repeat the sequence. If the patient is unable to perform this motion 20 times within a 10-s period, the test is positive. To perform the Oppenheim test, a sharp object is run along the crest of the tibia. Extension of the great toe is a positive finding. The Babinski sign is a specific indicator of cord compression and is also positive when the great toe extends. It is elicited by running a sharp object distally along the lateral border of the plantar aspect of the foot and medially across the metatarsal heads. A Hoffmann reflex is strongly indicative of cervical cord impingement. It is present when the fingers and thumb flex in response to rapid extension of the distal interphalangeal joint of the long finger. Patients with spinal cord compression at C6 may exhibit the inverted radial reflex where, by tapping the distal brachioradialis tendon, a diminished reflex is elicited with a reciprocal contraction of the finger flexors (Figure 3.1.8). L'Hermitte's sign refers to the perception of a generalized electric shock involving the upper and lower extremities as well as the truck with flexion of

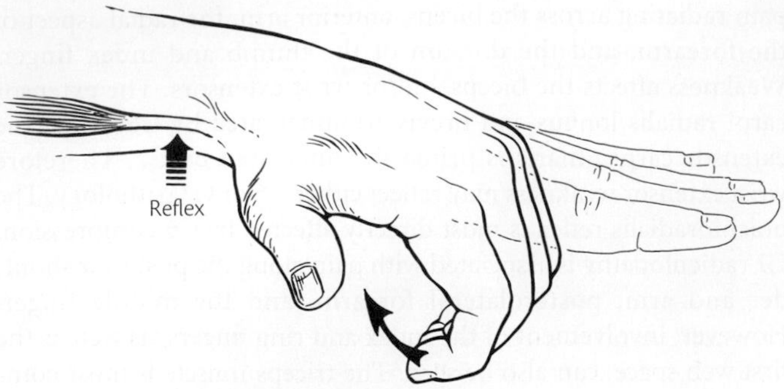

Fig. 3.1.8 Paradoxical brachioradialis reflex or inverted radial reflex: tapping the distal brachioradialis tendon elicits a reciprocal spastic contraction of the finger flexors.

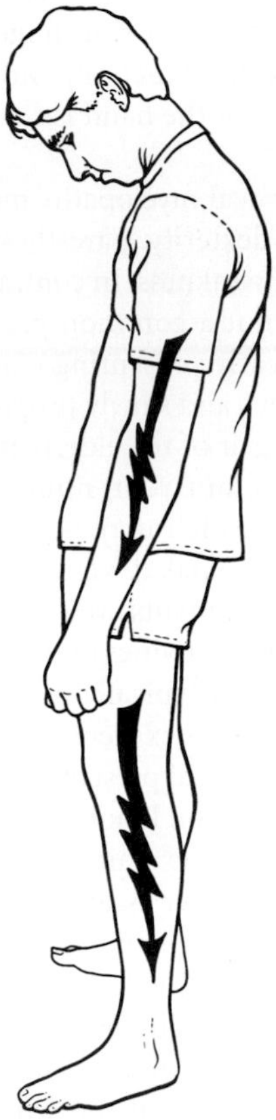

Fig. 3.1.9 L'Hermitte's sign: neck flexion or extension elicits electric shock sensation involving upper and lower extremities as well as the trunk.

the neck (Figure 3.1.9). The scapulohumeral, or Shimizu, reflex is a very sensitive test which is elicited by tapping the tip of the spine of the scapula. The test is positive if there is brisk scapular elevation with abduction of the humerus. Finally, clonus may appear several weeks following cord compression. A positive test is defined as more than two repetitive beats during sudden wrist or ankle dorsiflexion.

Diagnostic tests

Patients with symptomatology relating to their cervical spine are often initially sent for plain radiographic evaluation. However, degenerative changes are exceedingly common in the aging population and are very non-specific. Plain cervical radiography is therefore more useful in ruling out more threatening diagnoses such as neoplasm, or traumatic situations that might result in axial, coronal, or sagittal malalignment.

Magnetic resonance imaging (MRI) is the test of choice for patients with radiculopathy or myelopathy, as both the sensitivity and specificity are high. Readily demonstrated is cervical stenosis and secondary soft tissue abnormalities such as disc herniations, ligamentum flavum hypertrophy, facet hypertrophy, or other less common causes. It should be noted that there is MRI evidence of nerve root compression in as many as 19% of asymptomatic individuals, therefore radiographic abnormalities must be correlated with the patient's history and physical exam findings. In patients with long-standing cervical myelopathy, MRI may also reveal intrinsic cord pathology such as atrophy or oedema. Limitations of MRI are difficulty in distinguishing soft tissue versus bone as in ossification of the posterior longitudinal ligament (OPLL) and less accurate assessment of bony foraminal stenosis.

Computed tomography (CT) is also a non-invasive study and is better at demonstrating bony abnormalities, as cortical margins are much more distinct than those seen with MRI. Therefore, stenosis secondary to osteophytes, hypertrophy of the uncovertebral joints, or hypertrophy of the zygoapophyseal joints are readily demonstrated with CT imaging. While axial images are helpful, 45-degree oblique reconstruction views will better assess the foramina and bony foraminal stenosis. CT myelography is an invasive study that precisely demonstrates the degree of spinal cord deformation and mechanical blocks to the flow of cerebrospinal fluid. A filling defect of myelographic dye on an oblique projection is a typical finding of nerve root compression (Figure 3.1.10). The combination of MRI and CT gives accurate imaging of bone and soft tissue landmarks and makes myelography rarely needed clinically.

Natural history

The natural history of axial neck pain without neurological involvement is generally favourable and surgical intervention is not thought to result in better outcomes than conservative treatment measures. Non-operative treatment in patients with isolated neck pain is therefore recommended. The natural history of cervical radiculopathy was elucidated in a classic study published in 1963 by Lees and Turner. They conservatively followed 51 patients that initially presented with radicular pain. Of the ten patients with 10–19-year follow-up, three had only a single pain episode and no recurrence of symptoms, while three continued to have persistent mild symptoms. Only four were found to have more troublesome symptoms. No patients went on to develop myelopathic symptoms. These findings support the practice of initial conservative treatment in patients presenting with radiculopathy. The natural history of cervical myelopathy is highly variable. Some patients have a protracted course with only mild symptoms, while others go on to develop progressive disability.

Treatment options

As mentioned previously, patients with axial neck pain and/or radicular symptoms should be initially treated non-operatively. This should include non-narcotic analgesics, anti-inflammatories,

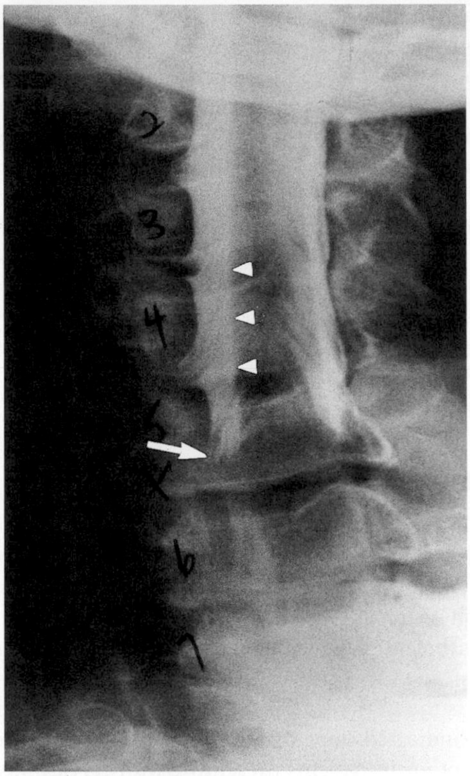

Fig. 3.1.10 A filling defect of myelographic dye on an oblique projection at C5 to C6 (arrow). This patient also has complete block of the dye due to stenosis of the spinal canal. The spinal cord is well outlined by vertical shadows in the dye column (arrowheads).

a soft collar, and progressive exercises. Physical therapy modalities such as heat and ultrasound may make the patient more comfortable, although it is unclear if this has any significant advantage over the natural history. In the setting of neck pain without neurological involvement, cervical fusion procedures offer unpredictable results and should generally be avoided. Some surgeons favour the use of discography and fusion but controversy exists regarding the specificity of cervical discograms and fusion for axial neck pain.

If radiculopathy is present, the same non-operative treatment should be given for 2–3 months. A brief course of systemic corticosteroids may help alleviate symptoms and allow the natural history to take its course. Steroid injections, either in the epidural space or targeted toward isolated nerve roots, may also be effective both from a diagnostic and a therapeutic standpoint. Traction is often helpful, as it allows a compressed nerve some temporary relief and likely promotes recovery. Care should be taken to avoid traction that results in extension of the patient's neck, which narrows the spinal canal and foramina, often resulting in increased symptoms. A cervical collar may be placed in the reverse position such that the narrow portion is anterior, leaving the neck in a slightly flexed position. In patients with radiculopathy, surgical intervention is indicated after several weeks of non-operative management (as outlined earlier) or if signs or symptoms worsen. The exception is the patient presenting with profound muscle weakness. These patients may need early intervention in order to maximize the chances of root recovery.

There is a minimal role for conservative treatment in patients with myelopathy. In patients with cervical stenosis and little or no significant myelopathy, conservative treatment or regular interval observation may be appropriate. As the natural history is that of slow stepwise deterioration, surgical intervention is generally required. Patients with mild to moderate symptoms can be expected to have a greater recovery of function, although some patients with severe symptoms can recover to a significant degree. It is important, however, that these patients understand that the surgical goal is to halt progression of their symptoms and that improvement is not predictable. If it is decided that both the cervical and lumbar spine require decompression, the cervical spine should be addressed first, followed by lumbar decompression at a later date.

Surgical techniques

Depending on a variety of factors, cervical disc disease can be approached either anteriorly or posteriorly. A patient with isolated radiculopathy (without significant neck pain) attributable to a lateral disc herniation or foraminal stenosis is typically treated posteriorly via a laminoforaminotomy (Figure 3.1.11). In this procedure, the medial 50% or greater of the ipsilateral facet joint is removed and the nerve root is decompressed under direct vision. Any anterior pathology that may be present need not be addressed as long as the extent of the nerve root is decompressed. Advantages of this approach are in the relatively low surgical morbidity and the fact that the motion segment is not destabilized (thus, a fusion procedure is avoided). Potential disadvantages include continued segmental degeneration, the possibility of incomplete decompression, and the inability to restore disc (and therefore foraminal) height. Anterior cervical discectomy and fusion (ACDF) is preferred in patients with radiculopathy or myelopathy associated with segmental kyphosis and significant neck pain. The spondylotic segment is distracted about 2mm, providing additional decompression of the foramen, which is then stabilized with bone graft

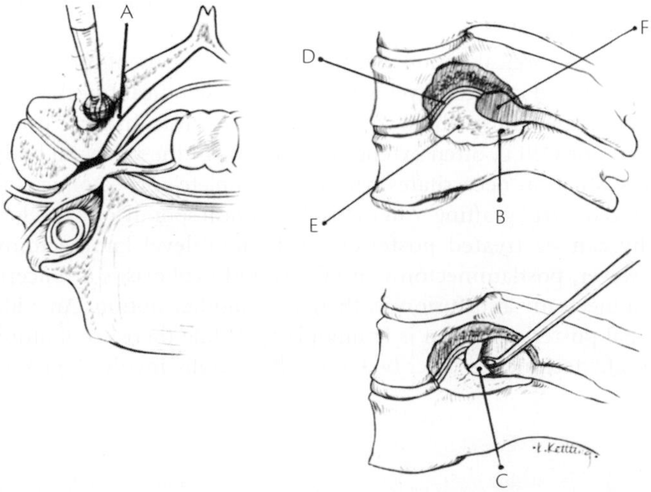

Fig. 3.1.11 A diagram showing posterior laminoforaminotomy technique: A, the lamina and the facet joint are thinned with a power burr; B, laminotomy may be enlarged with a Kerrison rongeur; C, extension of laminotomy laterally with a curette; D, the facet joint is thinned laterally to remove about 50 per cent of the joint; E, the remainder of the facet joint is removed using a curette; F, laminotomy defect.

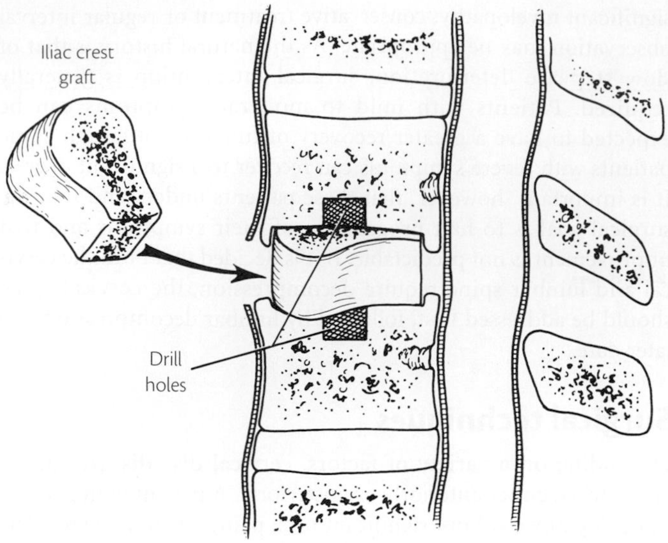

Fig. 3.1.12 Smith–Robinson tricortical iliac crest fusion technique. Following diskectomy, the interspace is distracted about 2 mm and the middle of the endplate is drilled to allow vascular flow to the graft. The graft is inserted about 2 mm countersunk from the anterior margin of the vertebral body.

(Figure 3.1.12). This approach typically directly addresses the compressive pathology on the cord or nerve root, restores disc (and foraminal) height, negates the possibility of repeat disc herniation, and minimizes the neck pain that might have been originating from the previously mobile segment. Disadvantages include the increased morbidity and operative time in harvesting autograft (allograft may also be used), decreased neck motion, complications related to plate utilization, possible non-union, and the possibility that a fused segment may accelerate adjacent segment degeneration. Cervical disc replacement is emerging as an additional treatment option for cervical radiculopathy. It offers many of the advantages associated with anterior neural decompression, while segmental motion is theoretically maintained. Early biomechanical and clinical studies are encouraging; however, long-term results are unknown.

Various surgical options are also available for patients presenting with isolated cervical myelopathy (without significant neck pain). These patients usually have cord compression from large osteophytes or OPLL, often extending posterior to the vertebral body. This situation necessitates partial or complete corpectomies followed by strut grafting. Alternatively, cervical spondylotic myelopathy can be treated posteriorly with multilevel laminectomy; however, postlaminectomy instability and kyphosis is a concern. Laminectomy and fusion is, therefore, another option. An additional posterior option is laminoplasty. While there are multiple specific techniques described, they all generally involve 'opening' the lamina of multiple levels in a trapdoor-type fashion, preserving the paraspinal musculature and facets. With this approach, motion is better maintained as compared to fusion procedures (but not entirely preserved) and the procedure is technically less demanding. A significant concern associated with laminoplasty procedures is the notion that it may result in increased postoperative neck pain in some patients. As a general rule, posterior approaches are preferred when decompression is required at more than three levels and when cervical lordosis is maintained. If there is two- to three-level involvement, an anterior approach is preferred. If a kyphotic deformity is present, an anterior approach is mandatory. If multilevel corpectomy and strut grafting is performed, a combined anterior and posterior approach should be considered to provide a biomechanically-sound posterior segmental fixation construct.

Conclusions

When evaluating patients with cervical degenerative conditions, it is essential to obtain a thorough history, provide a detailed physical examination, and obtain appropriate testing. With this information, the physician should be able to provide the vast majority of patients with a proper diagnosis and supply counselling on the natural history of the disease process. Most often, non-operative treatment is the preferred initial treatment and may be curative. Surgery is indicated only after an adequate trial of conservative management, or in patients presenting with cervical myelopathy. Various surgical approaches are available once surgery is decided upon, each approach having its own set of advantages and disadvantages. The ultimate decision should be based upon the patient's diagnosis and symptoms, the site of the primary pathology, the number of segments involved, the patient's sagittal alignment, and the surgeon's preference. Regardless of the diagnosis or surgical approach, patients must be made fully aware of the potential limitations of a proposed intervention, in addition to the benefits. Only then will the probability of a successful procedure from the standpoint of both the physician and the patient be optimized.

Further reading

Boden, S.D., McCowin, P.R., Davis, D.O., *et al.* (1990). Abnormal magnetic-resonance scans of the cervical spine in asymptomatic subjects. A prospective investigation. *Journal of Bone and Joint Surgery*, **72A**, 1178–84.

Gore, D.R., Sepic, S.B., Gardner, G.M., *et al.* (1987). Neck pain: a long-term follow-up of 205 patients. *Spine*, **12**, 1–5.

LaRocca, H. (1988). Cervical spondylotic myelopathy: Natural history. *Spine*, **13**, 854–5.

Lees, F. and Turner, J.W. (1963). Natural history and prognosis of cervical spondylosis. *British Medical Journal*, **2**, 1607–10.

Shimizu, T., Shimada, H., and Shirakura, K. (1993). Scapulohumeral reflex (Shimizu). Its clinical significance and testing maneuver. *Spine*, **18**, 2182–90.

3.2

Degenerative disease of the thoracic spine

Jayme R. Hiratzka, Robert A. Hart, and Henry H. Bohlman

Summary points

- Thoracic degenerative disease is an uncommon problem and is often misdiagnosed
- Posterolateral approaches such as transpedicular or lateral extracavitary reduce morbidity associated with thoracotomy while avoiding the risk of neurologic injury associated with posterior laminectomy
- Correct preoperative identification of level is crucial and requires specific imaging, such as full-length MRI or CT.

Introduction

Degenerative changes of the thoracic spine are common, and are probably universal by the age of 50. In most cases these are asymptomatic beyond some loss of physical height and an increase in thoracic kyphosis. Two main clinical entities exist: thoracic disc herniation and thoracic spinal stenosis.

Thoracic disc herniation

Introduction

This was first described in association with paraplegia. In practice, many thoracic herniations are asymptomatic. The difficulty is to find those that are clinically significant. This is made more difficult by the wide range of presenting symptoms.

As diagnostic imaging has progressed, surgical treatment for patients with severe persistent symptoms has also improved. Using a conventional laminectomy, it is difficult to obtain adequate disc removal without manipulation of the spinal cord. Over a third of patients were left with persistent symptoms or worsened neurological deficits when laminectomy alone was used. Since the 1980s, new techniques such as anterior (transthoracic) and lateral extracavitary decompression and expanded posterior approaches such as costotransversectomy or transpedicular resections have improved results and reduced complications. Advances in thoracoscopic techniques have led to reports of video-assisted minimally invasive approaches to the anterior thoracic spine.

Incidence

The annual incidence of symptomatic thoracic herniations has been estimated at one per million of the population (much less frequent than in the cervical or lumbar regions). A prevalence of 15–37% has been documented by both autopsy and imaging. Surgically treated thoracic herniations comprise only 0.15–4% of all disc surgeries.

Ninety-five per cent of thoracic disc herniations occur at or below the T6–T7 vertebral level. The remainder occur at any level. They mainly occur in the fourth and fifth decades in both sexes and require special care.

Aetiology

About 50% of cases are said to be traumatic. Recent research suggests that lumbar disc herniations are mainly of genetic origin, but no such research has been done on thoracic discs. Intradisc calcification is seen in up to 50% of patients. Scheuermann's kyphosis has been noted as an associated diagnosis. Neurological deficits secondary to these lesions are probably due to a combination of vascular disturbance and direct mechanical compression of the spinal cord. Approximately two-thirds of herniations are central, with the balance occupying a paracentral or lateral position. Intradural disc herniations have also been described.

Presentation and diagnosis

Symptomatic thoracic disc herniations can be associated with a variety of initial complaints. The array of attributed local and radiating pain symptoms can result in lengthy delays in diagnosis. Patients may present with prior workup and treatment for disorders including cholecystitis, renal colic, cardiac disease, endometriosis, and lumbar disc disease.

Examination

Neurological abnormalities are predictably limited to the lower extremities or bowel and bladder function. Upper motor neuron signs in the lower extremities such as clonus and Babinski reflexes may be found, particularly in patients with gait abnormalities, lower-extremity weakness, or bowel and bladder complaints. A concordant level of change in sensitivity to pinprick may be identified.

Abdominal reflexes may be absent. Differential diagnosis in patients with myelopathic symptoms should include systemic causes of upper motor neuron weakness, such as multiple sclerosis or amyotrophic lateral sclerosis. These can occur concomitantly with a thoracic disc herniation, and will contribute to a poor neurological outcome with surgical treatment.

Imaging

Plain radiographs should be obtained on all patients. These may demonstrate abnormalities such as disc calcification or narrowing of a disc space. Changes associated with Scheuermann's disease, such as end-plate irregularities, Schmorl's nodes, and vertebral body wedging, may also be present.

Computed tomography (CT) myelograms or magnetic resonance imaging (MRI) are definitive investigations. The frequent occurrence of thoracic disc herniations in asymptomatic patients requires careful correlation of clinical complaints with the radiological findings.

Identification of level

Identification of level is essential for patients being considered for surgical treatment, and this is not easy. This can be done either by a sagittal MRI showing both the sacrum and the herniation on a single cut, or by an anteroposterior topogram reconstructed from the CT scan to demonstrate the ribs at each level, allowing a precise count of thoracic and lumbar vertebrae. This is a critical aspect of presurgical preparation.

Treatment

The treating physician must establish that surgery holds a reasonable expectation of improvement for the patient (Box 3.2.1).

Problems and complications

Incomplete removal of the herniated disc fragments

It is our opinion that centrally located herniations with neurological deficits are best treated via an anterior thoracotomy approach. Adequate exposure for complete decompression of the spinal cord is difficult to achieve via a costotransversectomy or a transpedicular approach, particularly for calcified disc herniations, which can extend intradurally. These issues may contribute to the somewhat lower numbers of patients with complete neurological recovery and pain relief following posterior decompressions than for those undergoing transthoracic excision.

Wrong level

Identification of level is essential for patients being considered for surgical treatment. It is not always easy to identify the correct level from images. This can be done either by a sagittal MRI showing both the odontoid process and the herniation on a single cut, or by an anteroposterior topogram developed with the CT scan to demonstrate the ribs at each level, allowing a precise count of thoracic and lumbar vertebrae.

Pulmonary complications

Haemothorax and pneumothorax are recognized potential complications of a transthoracic approach.

Box 3.2.1 Decision and treatment in thoracic disc herniation from various studies

- 37% of asymptomatic volunteers have herniations demonstrable via MRI
- Of 55 patients with herniations, without motor deficit:
  - (15) 27% eventually underwent surgery
  - 77% of those treated non-operatively (31/40) returned to work
- Transthoracic decompression: ~90% of those treated do well
- Costotransversectomy/transpedicular approach: slightly less good outcomes
- Lateral extracavitary approach (LECA):
  - Significant improvement in pain and neurological status in 15/20 patients
  - 18/33 experienced at least one complication
- Minimally invasive version of LECA: limited results.

Thoracic spinal stenosis

Introduction

While stenosis of the lumbar spinal canal and intervertebral foramen is well recognized, thoracic spinal stenosis remains a comparatively rare entity. Like lumbar stenosis, thoracic spinal stenosis occurs when degeneration produces enlargement of structures surrounding the dural sac, with secondary compression of the neural structures. Compression may be posterior, from the ligamentum flavum and facet joint capsules, or anterior, from the intervertebral disc or posterior longitudinal ligament. Patients with congenitally narrow canals are particularly at risk for developing these problems.

Classification

Spinal stenosis may be developmental or acquired through degenerative processes. It may also occur at a stress riser above a previous spinal fusion (iatrogenic).

Presentation and diagnosis (Box 3.2.2)

Symptoms may vary from those of lumbar spinal stenosis due to the potential involvement of the spinal cord. However, lumbar spinal stenosis must still be considered in the differential diagnosis, as these patients may present with similar complaints and lumbar stenosis is much more common.

Box 3.2.2 Clinical presentation of thoracic spinal stenosis

- Sensory:
  - Stocking distribution of sensory changes
  - Activity related lower limb pain
  - Usually bilateral
- Motor:
  - Above T9—spastic paresis
  - Below T9—flaccid paresis
- Reflex: mixed response
- Bladder: 40% bladder dysfunction.

Sensory abnormalities of the lower extremities occur in virtually all patients, often in a stocking or other non-dermatomal distribution. Some patients demonstrate a thoracic sensory level. Activity-related lower-extremity pain or dysaesthesia is reported by the majority of patients, and 30–40% have bowel and bladder dysfunction. In one series, lesions above T9 tended to show spastic paresis whereas those with lesions in the region of T11–T12 have a flaccid paralysis.

Approximately 50% of patients demonstrate spasticity in the lower extremities, although there appear to be somewhat higher rates of paresis. This may be due to concomitant lumbar stenosis, with a secondary loss of lower-extremity reflexes.

Investigation

Diagnosis is confirmed by myelogram/CT scan or by MRI. It is important to determine whether the primary compression is due to anterior structures (e.g. ossification of the posterior longitudinal ligament or a herniated disc) or posterior structures (ligamentum flavum and facet capsule hypertrophy). As with a herniated thoracic disc, accurate determination of the spinal levels involved is critical. Complete three-dimensional imaging of the lumbar spine should be performed to ensure that a more caudal lesion is not present.

Management

Observational treatment may be sufficient for patients with myelopathy without incapacitating claudication or weakness. However, in most of the patients we have diagnosed with this condition, weakness and gait abnormality with or without lower extremity claudication is already present. We believe that these patients should be offered surgery aimed at decompression of the spinal cord.

The decision of whether to proceed with anterior or posterior decompression depends on the location of the spinal cord compression. Most of the patients described in the literature have posterior compression due to hypertrophy of the posterior structures, which can be treated by laminectomy. Careful technique is required, with the use of a burr to thin the posterior bone. The remaining soft tissue is then gently elevated off the dura with curettes and a small pituitary rongeur. Use of Kerrison rongeurs should be limited to the 1- to 2-mm punches in the areas adjacent to the facets and lateral to the cord. The decompression must be wide enough to include the medial aspects of the facet joints and must include all potentially compressive levels. Fusion of these patients is not generally required because of the stability provided by the thoracic cage.

Patients with anterior compression should be treated with anterior transthoracic decompression of involved segments.

Results

All series are small. About 70–80% will experience improvement or good resolution of neurological symptoms with adequate decompression. Patients can develop recurrent symptoms despite initially successful surgical treatment. This can be due to recurrent bone formation at the operated level or degeneration at additional spinal levels. Therefore, these patients require regular follow-up with reimaging of appropriate levels for recurrent symptoms.

Further reading

Abbott, K.H. and Retter, R.H. (1956). Protrusions of thoracic intervertebral disks. *Neurology*, **6**(1), 1–10.

Barnett, G.H., Hardy, Jr. R.W., Little, J.R., *et al.* (1987). Thoracic spinal canal stenosis. *Journal of Neurosurgery*, **66**(3), 338–44.

Capener, N. (1954). The evolution of lateral rhachotomy. *Journal of Bone and Joint Surgery*, **36B**(2), 173–9.

Epstein, N.E. and Schwall, G. (1994). Thoracic spinal stenosis: diagnostic and treatment challenges. *Journal of Spinal Disorders*, **7**(3), 259–69.

Hamilton, M.G. and Thomas, H.G. (1990). Intradural herniation of a thoracic disc presenting as flaccid paraplegia: case report. *Neurosurgery*, **27**(3), 482–4.

Hawk, W. (1936). Spinal compression caused by ecchondrosis of the intervertebral fibrocartilage: with a review of the recent literature. *Brain*, **59**, 204–24.

Larson, S.J., Holst, R.A., Hemmy, D.C., and Sanees, A. (1976). Lateral extracavitary approach to traumatic lesions of the thoracic and lumbar spine. *Journal of Neurosurgery*, **45**(6), 628–37.

Love, J.G. and Kiefer, E J. (1950). Root pain and paraplegia due to protrusions of thoracic intervertebral disks. *Journal of Neurosurgery*, **7**(1), 62–9.

Maiman, D.J., Larson, S.J., Luck, E., and El-Ghatit, A. (1984). Lateral extracavitary approach to the spine for thoracic disc herniation: report of 23 cases. *Neurosurgery*, **14**(2), 178–82.

Marzluff, J.M., Hungerford, G.D., Kempe, L.G., Rawe, S.E., Trevor, R., and Perot, P.L. (1979). Thoracic myelopathy caused by osteophytes of the articular processes: thoracic spondylosis. *Journal of Neurosurgery*, **50**(6), 779–83.

Muller, R. (1951). Protrusion of thoracic intervertebral disks with compression of the spinal cord. *Acta Medica Scandinavica*, **139**(2), 99–104.

Palumbo, M.A., Hilibrand, A.S., Hart, R.A., and Bohlman, H.H. (2001). Surgical treatment of thoracic spinal stenosis: a 2- to 9-year follow-up. *Spine*, **26**(5), 558–66.

Yonenobu, K., Ebara, S., Fujiwara, K., *et al.* (1987). Thoracic myelopathy secondary to ossification of the spinal ligament. *Journal of Neurosurgery*, **66**(4), 511–18.

3.3

Clinical presentations of the lumbar spine

Jeremy Fairbank and Elaine Buchanan

Summary points

- Classification of back pain has proved challenging
- This is important both for clinical practice and research
- MRI scanning is important for radicular pain but can be difficult in back pain patients as there is such a high incidence of asymptomatic abnormality.

Introduction

Low back pain is one of the most common presenting complaints in orthopaedic practice. Often the cause of the pain is not understood, and consequently the diagnosis and the explanations given to patients are inconsistent. This causes uncertainty and, in some cases, prolongation of symptoms. Back pain is sometimes the presenting complaint where there is serious underlying pathology. It may be difficult or impossible to distinguish these cases from the generality of back pain complaints. Progress has been made in our understanding of back pain complaints, and it is now possible to give a structured approach to management for which there is at least some evidence.

The principal objectives of the clinician are to identify those patients with serious underlying pathology, and to try to place the rest in clinical groups relevant to the available treatment options. Generally these are non-operative, and these methods are emphasized in the chapters in this section. Surgery has a definite role in the management of root pain, particularly in the presence of progressive neurological deficit or neurogenic claudication. The place of surgery in the management of some cases of back and referred pain, which has failed to respond to conservative management, is more controversial.

Classification

A number of clinical and pathologic classifications have been reported. We use a scheme elaborated in 1990 based on history, examination, and magnetic resonance imaging (MRI). Plain x-rays have little value in this area.

Fairbank–Hall (1990) classification

Type 1: 'simple' or 'non-specific' low back pain

This is the common type of back pain. Attacks occur acutely, and often for no obvious reason. Precipitating factors are often normal everyday events or actions. The vast majority of attacks will improve within 6 weeks, and are generally handled in family practice, by physiotherapists, chiropractors, or osteopaths. If the symptoms are prolonged or severe, specialist advice is sought. The majority of pain is felt in the lumbar spine, but there may be referral to buttocks or thighs, occasionally to the lower legs. Pain tends to be worst when sitting, and is often better with activity. Treatment is activity. Attacks are self-limiting, although they may be recurrent. Generally people will improve with or without intervention because the natural history is good. A whole variety of treatments can be helpful for pain relief and functional recovery. None of these, however, cure or prevent recurrence. Details of management can be found in Chapter 3.4.

Type 2: persisting back pain-related disability, 'chronic'

The interface between type 1 and type 2 is indistinct. Type 2 has chronic persistent symptoms that may/may not vary in severity. Often the onset is insidious and flare ups may be anticipated by the patient. The pain is back dominant and often refers into the thigh or even further down the leg depending on severity—so-called thermometer pain. It tends to be unresponsive to a wide variety of simple conservative management. There is a trend toward managing these patients in specialized rehabilitation programmes (see Chapter 3.4) based on cognitive behavioural principles. A small number of these patients may be suitable for spinal fusion or spinal stabilization. This is discussed in Chapter 3.6. Hall has further developed this scheme to distinguish patients who are likely to benefit from rehabilitation from those likely to benefit from pain management.

Type 3: root pain

These patients have back and leg pain in a dermatomal distribution with or without correlating neurological deficit. L5 can usually be distinguished from S1 in the distribution in the foot. L4 usually has a strong component of anterior thigh pain. In classical disc prolapse, the back pain precedes the leg pain, which eventually predominates. It is not usually possible to distinguish lateral recess stenosis from disc herniation clinically. Surgery provides quicker relief of leg pain and function, but not better long-term recovery. Management is discussed in Chapter 3.7.

Type 4: neurogenic claudication

Patients in this group present with walking-related back and leg pain. They are usually middle-aged or older, but it can occur in the young as well. These patients are intolerant of standing and walking, and relief is usually obtained by sitting, squatting, or lying. Often there is a flexed posture in walking and their symptoms are helped by any wheeled device such as a supermarket trolley or pushchair. In most, the symptoms do not deteriorate with time. Surgical management is an option for those with severe restriction of walking. Management is discussed in Chapter 3.8.

Type 5: 'Not classified above' (includes tumour, infection, vertebral collapse, deformity, inflammatory and chronic pain syndrome)

These patients have symptoms that do not fit easily in other groups. Any patients with unusual or persistent symptoms or pain which cannot otherwise be explained fall into this group. Sometimes it is clinically impossible to distinguish those patients with serious pathology, including infection and tumours from those without. The management of those with pain related to systemic pathologies is discussed in Section 2.

Diagnosis

History

Diagnosis is made mainly on the basis of history, and so time must be spent with patients listening to their complaints. This process may be aided by proformas and computer-based interview systems. As so much depends on the history, it is essential to give the patient time to tell their story and to listen to what they are saying. History-takers should bear the following points in mind when listening to their patients.

Age

Back pain is common from the age of 16 onwards. However, it is rarely severe in teenagers and tends to be most bothersome in our middle years (30–55). Serious pathology (infections and tumours) can occur in all ages but is more common in people outside this age range than within it. Therefore, patients presenting with back pain who are younger than 16 or older than 55 should be reviewed with particular care. Symptomatic disc prolapse is uncommon in teenagers and unusual over the age of 60. Neurogenic claudication is most common over age 60, unusual below the age of 40, but can occur even in teenagers with developmental spinal stenosis. Insufficiency fractures occur most often in those over age 70. Spondylolysis and spondylolisthesis may manifest themselves at any age, but they tend to cause back pain in patients under the age of 40 and neurogenic symptoms in older patients. Management is discussed in Chapter 3.17.

Pain pattern

Pain from a specific level in the spine (e.g. a metastasis) is usually referred about two segments distal to its source in the cranial part of the spine (Figure 3.3.1). The referral tends to be further from the source of the pain in the caudal part of the spine. This pain does not, in general, go to the front of the trunk or lower limb. Localization of the source level may be aided by percussion or palpation of the spine (although, curiously, pain from discitis, which is often severe, is not always exacerbated in this way).

The clinician should be familiar with the concepts of *referred pain* and *root pain*, and the distinction between them.

Referred pain is characterized by variation in distribution with severity: the worse the pain, the further it will felt down the lower limb ('thermometer pain'). Referred pain usually radiates posteriorly towards the knee, although in chronic cases it may go further down the leg. Referred pain is difficult, because it varies with sensitivity and is not associated with reliable clinical signs.

Root pain is usually dermatomal, although there are significant individual variations. Historically a variety of methods have been used to derive dermatome charts (Figure 3.3.2). Sometimes these can be confirmed by examination by light touch and pinprick testing. Root and referred pain can coexist. Some patients will have entirely root pain in a classical distribution without back pain. Pain felt on the front of the thigh, if it emanates from the spine, is generally from the L3 or L4 roots. L5 root pain usually radiates to the dorsomedial aspect of the foot. S1 root pain spreads to the lateral side and the sole of the foot. There are frequent variations of pattern in clinical practice. Coughing and sneezing tend to exacerbate root pain due to disc prolapse.

Patients with neurogenic claudication have difficulty in defining the site and nature of their symptoms. Some deny that they experience pain at all, preferring such terms as 'heaviness'. The distribution of this pain is a poor guide to the nerves involved. Bilateral lower-limb pain implies a central lesion. This may be central stenosis, a central disc prolapse, or a tumour affecting the cord, conus, or cauda equina.

The term 'myofascial pain' describes a wide variety of musculoskeletal symptoms. These have characteristic pain patterns which may be small and localized. One such syndrome has trigger points over the posterior iliac crest and an associated pain pattern. These pains may respond to a local anaesthetic injection. Copious literature on this topic can be found in rheumatological texts.

If a pain drawing is used to identify pain patterns, some will have widespread bodily symptoms. This could be related to systemic pathology (inflammatory, thyroid, etc.). If systemic pathology has been excluded and there is associated disability and distress, then chronic pain syndrome should be considered. This needs specialist management. Many clinicians have been caught out, dismissing a patient's symptoms of serious underlying pathology as psychogenic.

Pain from the hip is often confused with back pain. It is usually felt in the groin and/or over the greater trochanter. It can radiate over the front of the thigh to the knee. Occasionally it is felt just in the knee, notably in children. Uncommonly, hip pain is experienced in the buttock alone. Hip pain is usually exacerbated by getting out of a chair, as well as by walking, although in the early stages of osteoarthritis of the hip continued exercise can relieve pain after the initial painful movement. These symptoms can be fully evaluated by examining the hip. Gauvain's test, in which the extended leg is gently rolled by the examiner while the patient is lying and relaxed, produces either pain or involuntary ipsilateral abdominal contracture. Rotation in flexion or abduction may also reproduce hip pain.

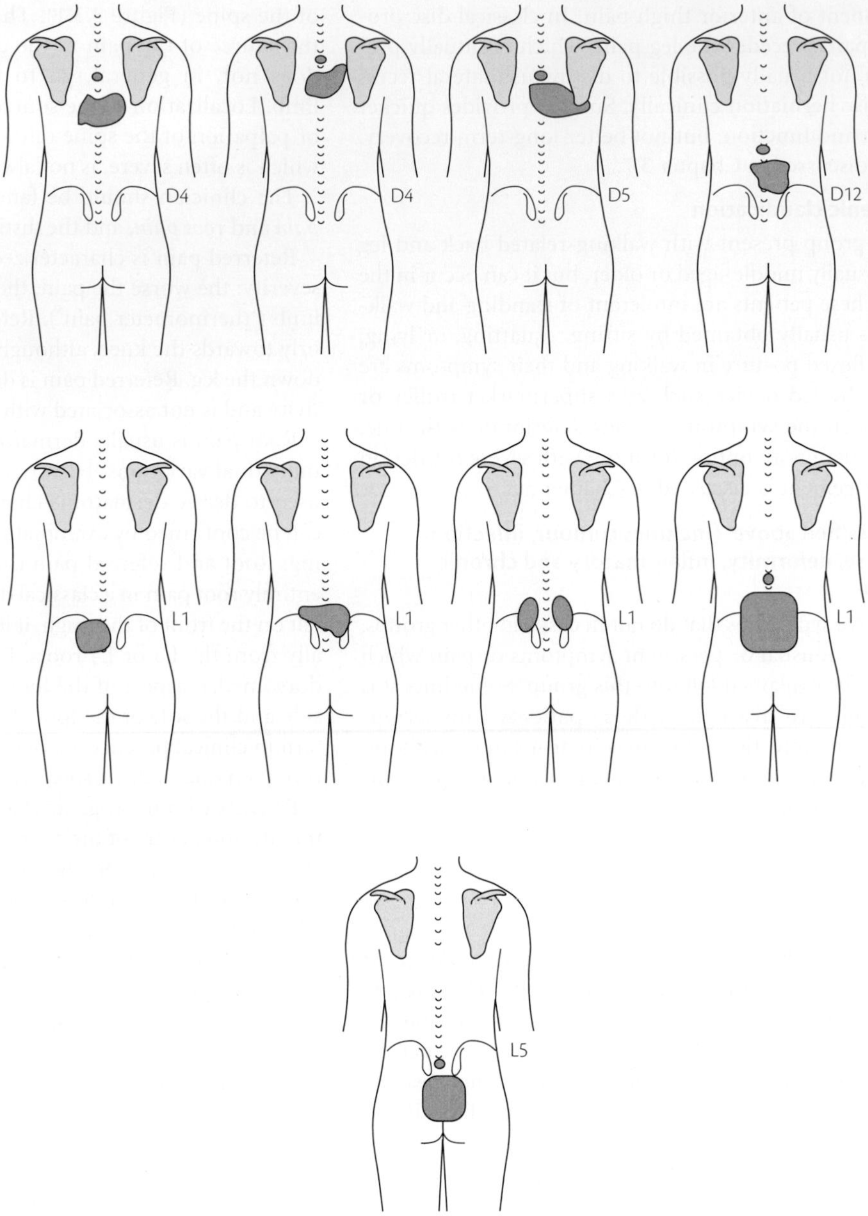

Fig. 3.3.1 Pain patterns arising from single vertebrae affected by fractures or metastases.

Diurnal and longer-term fluctuations in back pain

Night pain is common in degenerative spinal conditions so specificity is poor. However, it is also a feature of pain from fractures, metastases, and infections. It is the quality of the night pain that differs. Intractable pain at night necessitating the person to get out of bed, which is not responsive to pain relief, should raise suspicion of possible serious pathology. Especially if there are other red flags in the history.

Scoliotics tend to have fatigue pain which becomes worse through the day. Ankylosing spondylitis is characterized by severe and prolonged morning stiffness (all patients with back pain report morning stiffness to a greater or lesser extent).

Walking-related pain

Root pain is usually exacerbated by walking (and often just while standing still). Neurogenic claudication has a variable walking distance from day to day. The patient or spouse may notice a flexed posture during walking. Sometime it is easier walking up hill. Riding a bicycle may be easier than walking if severely restricted. Many patients find it much easier to walk while pushing a supermarket trolley or wheeled walker. It is often not possible for these patients to 'walk through' the pain as vascular claudicants can. Neurogenic claudication may be distinguished from vascular claudication by the duration of recovery. Vascular claudicants can usually carry on walking after 1–3min, whereas cauda equina claudication requires 5–20min for recovery.

Sitting-related pain

Many chronic back pain patients are intolerant of sitting; there are many theories related to this incriminating the disc, ligaments, muscles, and facet joints. Driving more than 1000 miles a week is a possible risk factor for chronic back pain. Sitting tends to relieve the pain of neurogenic claudication.

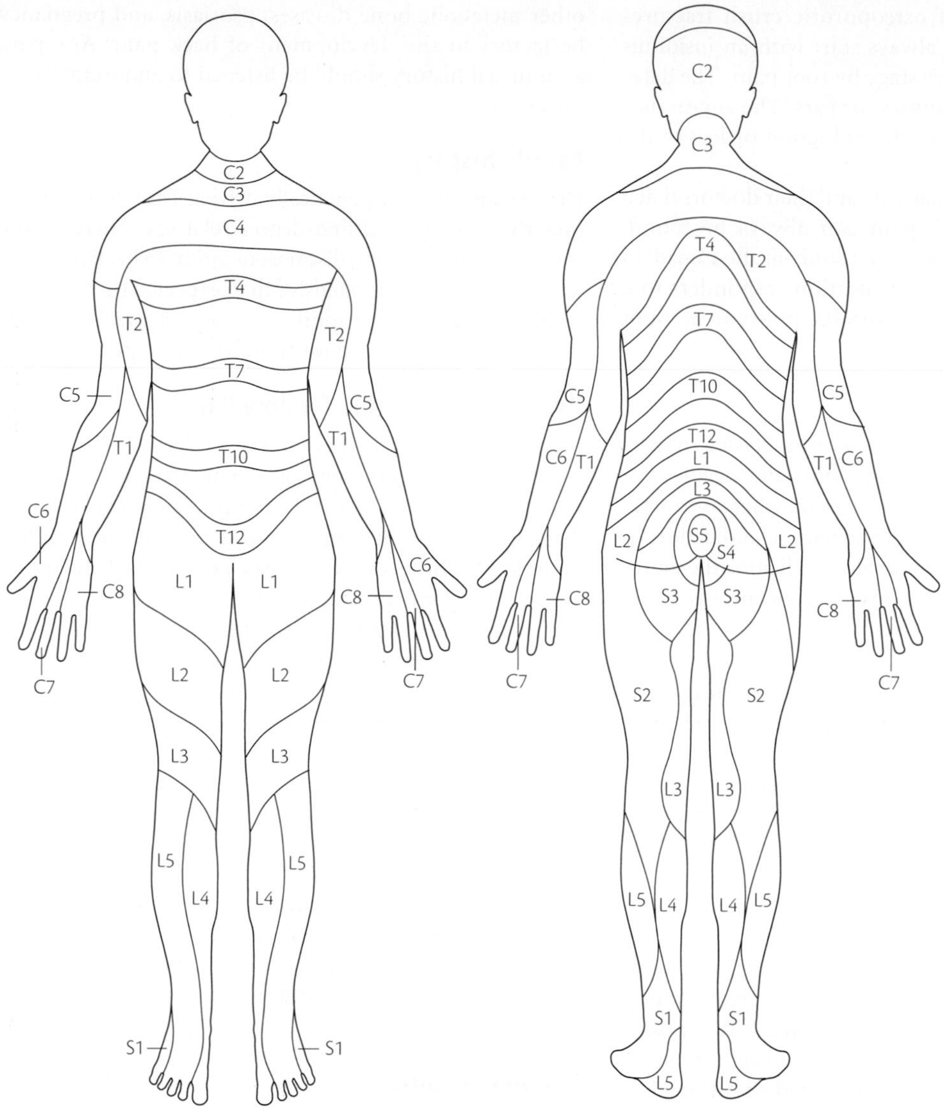

Fig. 3.3.2 Dermatome chart.

Gender

The overall incidence of back pain is similar in men and women. The prevalence of disc degeneration, disc prolapse, and lytic spondylolysis and spondylolisthesis is more common in males. Degenerative spondylolisthesis is more common in females.

Occupation

Back pain is common in the working age group regardless of employment status or occupation. Work is good for the health of those with back pain. Modern healthcare encourages the use of 'fit notes' rather than sick notes, i.e. establish what the person can do, and modified hours/duties to make work manageable. Heavy manual work is not as strong a factor as is often assumed. Disc degeneration is universal and largely driven by genetic factors. Individuals with more severe disc degeneration than their age-matched contemporaries are more likely to have back pain. Sitting and exposure to vibration are limited contributors to prevalence. Back pain undoubtedly presents more of a problem to members of social classes 4 and 5 because their work tends to be more physical and therefore harder to do with back pain. Social service payments depend on inability to work. The structure of workman's compensation systems has a profound effect on the incidence and duration of back pain disability. The longer an individual is off work, the less likely he or she is to return to work. There are also strong confounding factors, such as smoking and litigation following actual or perceived injury to the spine. Training in manual handling may be of importance in making work more comfortable. There is some evidence that fitness programmes in the working environment can lead to significantly shorter sickness absence. In modern work environments it is rare to find jobs at the extreme of the ergonomic envelope for spinal loads.

Onset of symptoms

The nature of the original onset of symptoms and how an attack starts is worth analysis. Type 1 pain usually starts acutely, frequently while performing normal activities. Often patients will admit that there was no obvious precipitating factor to an attack. Insufficiency fractures usually precipitate acute pain if they are symptomatic (only about 25% of osteoporotic crush fractures cause pain). Disc prolapse almost always start with an insidious onset of back pain followed at a later stage by root pain. The delay in onset of root pain varies from minutes to years. The appearance of the root pain may be accompanied by reduction or loss of the back pain.

There is an expectation amongst patients and their doctors that a precipitating cause for their back pain can always be found. Litigation may be a factor in this quest. In a study at the Canadian Back Institute, 70% of 6000 non-compensation responders to a questionnaire were unable to identify a specific injury to account for the onset of their symptoms.

Pain type

The words used to describe back pain are often culturally determined. Some descriptive terms, such as 'burning', 'pins and needles', or 'numbness', may be associated with radicular pain, whereas 'cramp' or 'ache' tends to relate to vascular, neurogenic claudication or referred pain. These terms may have some value in eliciting the source of pain in the individual, but they have resisted useful analysis.

Smoking

Smoking has been shown to be a risk factor in pseudarthrosis following spinal fusion. An association between smoking and disc degeneration has been established. The relationship to back pain, however, remains unclear. Heavy smokers often have poorer social circumstances and if employed have more physical occupations. It is likely that psychosocial factors will have greater predictive value for back pain related disability than smoking.

General medical questions

Some systemic conditions may present with back pain. Tuberculosis and other infections, metastases, lymphomas, pancreatitis, or a leaking aortic aneurysm can all cause pain in the back. Pain arising from metastases and from infection is frequently unremitting and may be worse at night. The patient should be asked about past history of cancer, weight loss, eating habits, disturbances of digestion, bowel and bladder function, night sweats, drugs, and allergies. Diabetes mellitus, hypothyroidism, osteoporosis, osteomalacia and other metabolic bone diseases, psoriasis, and pregnancy may all be factors in the development of back pain. Any patient with an unusual history should be listened to and examined with particular care.

Family history

Disc degeneration is genetically driven. Disc prolapse patients frequently have affected first-degree relatives. There is some epidemiological data linking disc degeneration to back pain, particularly if it is earlier or more extensive than expected by age. It is likely that response to pain has important genetic elements. Family patterns of psychosocial factors have an influence on perceived disability.

Psychosocial factors (yellow flags)

Listening to the patient is the most effective way of assessing the psychological component of a patient's history. Patients with strong psychosocial factors have the same range of pathologies as those who do not. It is the response to pain which differs, not the pathology. These should always be screened during back pain assessments. Psychosocial questionnaires are widely used and have been shown to add value. Examples can be found in *The Back Pain Revolution* (see 'Further reading'). In particular, high levels of disability, worklessness, and high healthcare utilization should raise concern. The structure of the social services payment system is an important factor in the rise in back pain disability in developed countries. Litigation over personal injury claims has long been recognized as having an important effect on treatment outcome and reported disability. For those with significant pain-related disability, a comprehensive biopsychosocial assessment by a clinician or multidisciplinary team is recommended as early as possible, and certainly before any surgical management is considered. Combined physical and psychological management has been shown to be effective in reducing disability, distress, medication usage, and healthcare utilization.

Further reading

Waddell, G. (2004). *The Back Pain Revolution*, second edition. Edinburgh: Churchill Livingstone.

3.4

Non-operative management of non-specific low back pain (types 1 and 2)

Jeremy Fairbank and Elaine Buchanan

Summary points

- Back pain is common
- Most attacks are self limiting
- Exercise and fitness programmes seem to be the most effective intervention
- CPP programmes are effective for chronic back pain and should be introduced early.

Introduction

Most people will experience back-dominant pain of a non-specific nature at some time in their life. The severity of the episodes varies within and between individuals. Persisting symptoms and recurrences are common. For the majority (type 1) the natural history is of improvement, in pain and function, over a few months regardless of intervention. Beyond this time the majority will no longer consult but will continue to experience back pain symptoms at a lower level. However, 7% will develop persisting back pain-related disability (type 2). For these, the resultant cost to the individual, healthcare, and society is significant.

There are many studies demonstrating that specific spinal structures, such as disc, facet joints, ligament, and muscle, can produce back pain. Symptoms from these structures are more severe in the back but may refer to the leg. Non-specific low back pain clearly has a physical basis. Many theories regarding specific pathologies exist, but none have stood up to the rigor of research. Furthermore, spinal imaging of asymptomatic people frequently demonstrates degenerative change. Despite extensive research, clinicians cannot identify specific back pain pathologies in the majority of people with back-dominant pain. Pain only explains 10% of the variance of back pain-related disability. There is emerging evidence from Hong Kong that disc degeneration earlier or more extensive than expected by age group has a relationship with back pain, but causation has not been established.

There is no known prevention or cure for low back pain. Evidence-based interventions can provide short-term benefit of small to moderate magnitude. The focus of intervention is symptom management, and prevention of persisting back pain-related disability. It may be that subgroups of non-specific low back pain respond differently to different interventions.

Initial management (type 1)

Patient/public education

From the outset it is essential that the person with back pain understands the normality, non-specific nature, good prognosis, and self-care options. An explanation, specifically addressing the concerns of the individual, reinforced by evidence-based patient information is reassuring and empowering for most. The back book is one such example, which is widely used in the United Kingdom. A large media campaign in Australia demonstrated sustained improvements in the population's back pain beliefs by providing positive messages about back pain.

Pharmacological symptom relief

Pharmacology is commonly used in an attempt to make back symptoms more manageable. Consideration needs to be given to the risks versus benefits. Compliance with medication is a problem and repeated review of effectiveness and side effects is essential. Guidelines consistently recommend regular paracetamol and/or non-steroidal anti-inflammatory (NSAID). For those with moderate/severe symptoms, weak opioids, tricyclic antidepressants, or muscle relaxants may add benefit. In those with the most severe symptoms, strong opioids may be required for pain relief. If the need for strong opioids persists, then an early, comprehensive, biopsychosocial assessment is strongly recommended.

Non-pharmacological symptom relief

There is evidence supporting the effectiveness of manual therapy (physiotherapy, osteopathy, or chiropractic) and the McKenzie method in reducing pain and disability. The effect sizes, however, are small to moderate. The profession delivering manual therapy seems to be less important than the competence of the individual clinician. For those who prefer non-pharmacological pain relief, acupuncture and massage have been shown to be effective. Ongoing treatment beyond a few months has not been shown to add any additional value.

Optimizing activity including work

Everyone with non-specific low back pain should be advised to remain active. All normal activities are good for back pain. When symptoms are severe, activity should be modified rather than stopped. There is no evidence that one type of exercise is superior to another. Compliance with exercise is likely to be improved if the recommended activity is enjoyable and practical for the individual. Back fitness programmes (supervised, individual, graded exercise delivered in groups) are cost-effective in improving functional ability.

The bothersomeness of back pain is greatest in the age group of the working population. Work is good for our health and can be therapeutic for those with back pain. Where work is difficult to maintain, short-term modified hours or duties may be helpful. It is important that any modification advised is accompanied by a planned progression, clear timescales, and progress reviews. Ergonomic work environments have been shown to improve comfort and satisfaction.

Biopsychosocial screening

Psychological factors are an important part of the low back pain experience. They contribute to the progression from type 1 to type 2 back pain and have been identified as important barriers to resolution.

For those who fail to return to normal activities by 4–6 weeks, a comprehensive biopsychosocial assessment is recommended. The predictive value of psychosocial factors, yellow flags (Box 3.4.1), has been demonstrated. Questionnaires combined with a detailed clinical interview explore the functional and emotional impact of back pain. Efficient screening will identify around 85% of those who will go on to develop persistent back pain-related disability. Establishing the level of risk is important, but engaging those at risk with biopsychosocial intervention is key to influencing their outcome.

Box 3.4.1 'Yellow flags' for biopsychological screening

- Unhelpful beliefs:
  - Activity will cause pain/injury
  - Recovery is not possible
  - Pain is caused by a serious health condition (cancer)
- Maladaptive behaviours:
  - Excessive use of medication, rest or passive interventions
  - Withdrawal from normal activities including work
- Compensation:
  - History of claims
  - Lack of financial incentive to return to work
- Diagnosis/treatment:
  - Conflicting diagnosis
- Iatrogenic diagnosis:
  - Leading to fear or catastrophizing
  - High healthcare utilization
  - History of failure to respond to intervention
- Emotions:
  - Fear of pain/disability
  - Depression and/or anxiety
  - Low self efficacy
- Family:
  - History of abuse
  - Over-/undersupportive family
  - Family history of pain related disability/worklessness
- Work:
  - Belief work is harmful
  - Unhappy/unsupportive work environment
  - History of excessive sick leave
  - Low job satisfaction.

Investigation

Spinal imaging is unlikely to change the diagnosis, management, or outcome in people with non-specific low back pain. Degenerative changes are commonly found and correlate with age, but only weakly correlate with pain and do not explain disability. It requires large epidemiological studies to show a relationship with earlier than expected or more extensive than expected disc degeneration. Imaging for reassurance has been shown to improve satisfaction, but not to achieve reassurance. There is morbidity associated with imaging non-specific low back pain. In addition, future healthcare costs are greater due to increased healthcare-seeking behaviour. Where systemic pathology is suspected, spinal magnetic resonance imaging (MRI) is highly sensitive and adds value in excluding this possibility. MRI is essential for surgical planning, in the small number of people who are being considered for spinal fusion, disc replacement, or other disc focused intervention.

Back pain treatments which are no longer recommended

Over the years, a wide variety of treatments for back pain have evolved. Internationally, there is consensus in back pain guidelines against the use of the following treatments (due to evidence of ineffectiveness, lack of effect, or lack of evidence of effectiveness): bed rest; exercise therapy; injection of therapeutic substances (epidural, facet injections); electrotherapy (interferential therapy, laser, short-wave diathermy, transcutaneous electrical nerve stimulation (TENS), ultrasound); lumbar supports, mattresses, or traction.

Management of persisting pain-related disability (type 2)

Persisting non-specific low back pain is common. Over time, most return to normal activities despite pain. In some (7%), pain has a dramatic impact on lifestyle and function and results in cognitive, emotional, and behavioural changes. It is the interaction between pain and psychology which differs, not the duration or pathology. There is strong evidence that structural changes have little meaning in the context of back pain disability. Pain behaviours are learnt and may be altered. Intervention aims to adjust behaviour and empower the person to cope better with the symptoms of back pain.

Recent evidence has demonstrated changes within the brain and raises the possibility of cortical reorganization and degeneration. Equally, this raises the possibility of reversing the process. As yet, the studies of the brain in people with type 2 back have small samples, which limit generalizability, but the findings are encouraging. Dorsolateral prefrontal cortex degeneration has been shown to correlate with level of depression. Animal studies have also demonstrated inflammatory and neuropathic alterations to dorsal horn of cord with degeneration of the inhibitory interneuron system. This has not been replicated in patients. Alteration to central pain memories has also been proposed.

For those who are at risk of persisting back pain-related disability, combined physical and psychological interventions (CPP) have been shown to be effective in reducing disability, distress, healthcare utilization, and improving return to work. Initially less intensive, CPP (<30h, often uniprofessional) provides good results for most. The more costly, higher intensity CPP (>60h) is best reserved for those who have a limited response to less intensive CPP (see Table 3.4.1).

Table 3.4.1 Content of Combined Physical and Psychological (CPP) intervention programmes

Low intensity CPP programmes (12–30h): unidisciplinary (cognitive behavioural principles)		**High intensity CPP programmes (>60h): interdisciplinary (cognitive behavioural therapy)**
Education	**Guided practice**	**Education and guided practice as listed +**
Pain mechanisms	Supervised exercise	Pain psychology
Effective pain control	Goal defined activities	Cognitive therapeutic methods
Healthy lifestyles	Activity scheduling	Graded exposure to feared activities
Functional goal setting	Applied relaxation	
Set back self management		
Return to work advice and links		
Communication skills		

Further reading

Linton, S.J. (2005). *Understanding Pain for Better Clinical Practice: A Psychological Perspective*. Edinburgh: Elsevier.

Linton, S.J. and Halden, K. (1998). Can we screen for problematic back pain? A screening questionnaire for predicting outcome in acute and subacute back pain. *Clinical Journal of Pain*, **14**, 209–15.

National Institute of Health and Clinical Excellence (2009). *Low back pain: early management of persistent non-specific low back pain. www.nice.org.uk/CG88*. London: NICE.

UK Beam (2004). United Kingdom back pain exercise and manipulation randomized trial: effectiveness of physical treatments for back pain in primary care. *British Medical Journal*, **329**, 1377–85.

Van Tulder, M., Becker, A., Bekkering, T., *et al.* (2004). *European guideline for the management of acute non-specific low back pain in primary care.* http://www.backpaineurope.org

Waddell, G. (2004). *The Back Pain Revolution*, second edition. Edinburgh: Churchill Livingstone.

3.5

Cauda equina syndrome

Jeremy Fairbank

Summary points

- Cauda equina syndrome is a devastating consequence of cauda equina compression
- The most common cause is a large disc herniation in the presence of a narrow vertebral canal
- Expeditious decompression can prevent the syndrome when some urinary function is preserved.

Introduction

Cauda equina is a well-known but rarely diagnosed condition. Untreated, the consequences of this syndrome for the patient are devastating. Poor results can occur even with expeditious treatment. It is a frequent cause of negligence litigation. It is important that clinicians are aware of its presenting features and the pitfalls surrounding diagnosis. Patients with severe back pain may go into retention because of severe pain without cauda equina syndrome (CES). It is sometimes difficult to distinguish the effects of severe pain from true cauda equina compression. If in doubt seek help and an emergency magnetic resonance scan. If the symptoms are of rapid evolution, this is a surgical emergency. If the onset is slow, it is more difficult, but an early magnetic resonance scan is very helpful in identifying the aetiology. Cauda equina compression can occur when there is a large, and particularly central, disc prolapse in association with a relatively narrow vertebral canal. CES may come on insidiously and incompletely. On other occasions, it may have an acute onset and profound deficit. Other causes of CES include: tumours, both primary and secondary; fractures where the lumbar canal is seriously distorted; infections with epidural pus; and haematomas, either spontaneous or as a complication of spinal surgery.

Clinical presentation

Symptoms

- Severe pain in the back and/or either one or both legs. Sometime there is not such severe pain, so be careful in excluding the diagnosis
- Unilateral or bilateral perianal numbness is a strong warning symptom of cauda equina compression. Altered sensation wiping the perineum is commonly noticed
- Urinary symptoms: these may range from frequency and nocturia, through to urgency and dribbling, to retention, and in some cases complete incontinence
- Faecal symptoms: these range from prolonged straining at stool to faecal incontinence
- Sexual: relates to loss of sexual sensation and, in males, impotence. This is not often a presenting feature but may be a feature of chronic onset. This is the major long-term symptom along with urinary incontinence

Signs

- Sensory: ranges from unilateral to bilateral alteration in perianal sensation to complete anaesthesia. The end of an unravelled paper-clip is a helpful aid to assess loss of pinprick sensation
- Motor: there are no reliable motor signs
- Reflex: there are no reliable reflex signs; often ankle reflexes are reduced or lost
- Anal tone: rectal examination will reveal poor or absent anal tone and loss of capacity to squeeze the examining finger.

Some literature suggests that surgery within 24h of onset is likely to be successful (>90% relief of symptoms) whilst surgery after 48h onset is likely to be a failure. It is likely that this is an oversimplification. Gleave and Macfarlane distinguished those patients with retention or retention and overflow (CESR) from those with bladder dysfunction (CESI)—the former do badly even with expeditious surgery. McCarthy and colleagues reviewed a larger series and were not able confirm this distinction. Indeed they were not able to relate time to surgery and outcome at all. Todd has presented evidence that timing does matter. DeLong et al in the largest meta-analysis to date support the distinction of CESI and CESR.

One issue is that it is sometimes difficult to identify when the clock starts 'ticking' at the onset of CES. This is important when negligence in diagnosis or treatment is alleged. Many believe that this is when 'autonomic' symptoms and signs occur (urinary incontinence or retention). Others will time it from onset of perianal numbness (usually but not always bilateral). In all events the patient should be warned that their recovery of autonomic function may well be imperfect. Most patients will have back pain indefinitely.

Management

- CES should be managed in secondary care
- Urgent imaging (magnetic resonance imaging, radiculogram or myelo-computed tomography can all be used) should be available within 8h of admission
- Urgent surgical treatment is needed by a surgeon familiar with or supervised by a surgeon experienced in these lesions (all neurosurgical units and orthopaedic units with trained spinal surgeons). Surgery should ideally be performed within 24h of onset of symptoms, but where onset is unclear or incomplete as soon as possible after diagnosis and imaging. Our current practice is to operate as quickly as feasible. If this means in the middle of the night when surgical skill may be worst, then the operation should wait until first thing in the morning
- Surgical decompression is by a bilateral laminectomy with discectomy (some surgeons use a unilateral discectomy but we do not recommend this).

Further reading

Ahn, U., Ahn, N., Buchowski, J., Garrett, E., Siebern, A., and Kostiuk, J. (2000). Cauda equina syndrome secondary to lumbar disc herniation: a meta-analysis of surgical outcomes. *Spine*, **25**, 1515–22.

DeLong, W.B., Polissar, N., and Neradilek, B. (2008). Timing of surgery in cauda equina syndrome with urinary retention: meta-analysis of observational studies. *Journal of Neurosurgery Spine*, **8**, 305–20.

Gleave, J. and Macfarlane, R. (1990). Prognosis for recovery of bladder function following lumbar central disc prolapse. *British Journal of Neurosurgery*, **4**, 205–9.

Jerwood, D. and Todd, N. (2006). Reanalysis of the timing of cauda equina surgery. *British Journal of Neurosurgery*, **20**(3), 178–9.

Lavy, C., James, A., Wilson-MacDonald, J., and Fairbank, J. (2009). Cauda equina syndrome. *British Medical Journal*, **338**, 936.

McCarthy, M., Aylott, E., Grevitt, M., and Hegarty, J. (2007). Cauda equina syndrome: factors affecting long-term functional and sphincteric outcome. *Spine*, **32**(2), 207–16.

Todd, N. (2005). Cauda equina syndrome: the timing of surgery probably does influence outcome. *British Journal of Neurosurgery*, **19**(4), 301–6.

3.6

Surgical management of chronic low back pain

Jeremy Fairbank

Summary points

- A very small proportion of back pain patients respond to surgical treatment
- Patient selection is poorly defined
- The rationale of treatment ranges from immobilization (fusion) to claimed restoration of normal movement (disc replacement and flexible fixation).

Introduction

Patients with chronic low back pain are frequently referred to orthopaedic surgeons. The majority of these patients do not require surgical treatment, and should be managed by non-operative means. A small proportion may benefit from surgical stabilization of the spine or disc replacement. This chapter is concerned with the rationale for this approach, investigation, surgical methods, and the results.

The surgeon and patient have to take a decision after weighing up the risks and benefits of the procedure (often hard to define) against the disability. Spinal fusion may be regarded as either an attempt to speed up the natural progress of degenerative changes towards a functional ankylosis or a prevention of progressive deformity or instability. The aim is to reduce the severity of back pain and improve functional ability.

The evidence on which to base these decisions is developing. Several randomized trials of spinal fusion have now been completed:

In Sweden, trials showed an outcome advantage of fusion over conventional physiotherapy, but could show no difference between three different surgical techniques. In Norway and in the United Kingdom, studies could show no advantage of surgery over intensive rehabilitation. These trials have caused controversy, especially in the United States, where there are high rates of surgery for back pain.

'Soft' fusion using a variety of posterior devices has been practised for 20 years, but no large trial completed. The rationale remains experimental, not least because of our poor understanding of intersegmental biomechanics in relation to pain. Many ingenious devices have been developed to alter these, but results are anecdotal. In the Spine Stabilisation Trial in the United Kingdom, there was a small subset of patients who had the Graf procedure. This was underpowered, and there was no obvious advantage seen in these patients of surgery over rehabilitation and they required more revision surgery. Surgery was quicker with fewer complications than spinal fusion.

Disc replacement has evolved in the last 30 years, with cohort studies only reported until two Food and Drug Administration-approved trials. The Charité study was against a BAK (Bagby and Kuslich) anterior cage procedure (now abandoned) that showed non-inferiority. The ProDisc study showed non-inferiority using an unvalidated version of the Oswestry Disability Index (http://www.mapi-institute.com/; email: contact@mapi-trust.org) over 360-degree fusion. Both these trials show a non-statistically significant advantage to disc replacement and it is likely that they were underpowered. No study against rehabilitation has been reported yet. Surgeons should consider the difficulties of selecting patients and the high risks of revision surgery before recommending this procedure.

Rationale

It is assumed that back pain may be generated from the low back by 'mechanical' means or through a source of 'inflammatory' agents (usually assumed to be the intervertebral disc) irritating neural tissues.

- Mechanical back pain is generated by movement, and may be controlled by rest or immobilization by external splintage (corsets, braces, plaster), or internal splintage (fusion, with or without internal fixation, or limitation of movement by special implants). In some cases there may be instability of the spine, actual or perceived, which can be controlled by spinal fusion
- Inflammatory pain may be managed surgically by excision of a whole disc, or at least a substantial part of it, and replacement of it by allograft or autograft bone, cages made of various materials containing bone, or artificial disc prostheses designed to replace either the nucleus or whole disc
- Both mechanical and inflammatory pain may be involved in patients with previous root decompression surgery.

Unfortunately, reality has not always followed expectation, and the results of treatment have varied considerably. Carragee used

Box 3.6.1 Indications for back pain surgery

- Where non-operative treatment has failed
- Where a clear rationale for surgery can be made supported by high quality evidence
- Where contraindications are excluded
- Where there is a clear understanding of the risks and benefits of intervention.

discography to identify 'best bet' patients for spinal fusion. Only 27% met his strict criteria of success compared with 72% of a control-spondylolisthesis group (Box 3.6.1).

Spinal instability

Spinal stability is a much abused term. There are at least four ways in which this can be conceived:

1) In mechanical terms, as summarized in White and Punjabi's (1990) definition of stability
2) In temporal terms, where symptoms wax and wane more or less predictably with time. Some patients report increasing frequency and duration of attacks of pain
3) In perceptual terms, where the spine feels unstable although no abnormal motion or position can be detected by conventional radiography
4) In postural terms, where the spine is unbalanced.

White and Punjabi defined stability as 'a condition of the spine under normal physiological loading where there is neither abnormal strain nor excessive or abnormal motion in the functional spinal unit'. The functional spinal unit is a motion segment, consisting of bone, disc, and bone, as well as its supporting joints, ligaments, and muscles. Instability is the loss of the ability of the spine under physiologic loads to maintain relationships between vertebrae in such a way that there is neither damage or subsequent irritation to the spinal cord or nerve roots and, in addition, there is no development of incapacitating deformity or pain from structural changes.

Perceived or functional instability is sometimes called 'instability syndrome'. The patient complains of giving way, getting stuck, a ratchety flexion in the spine, and, occasionally, a sensation of disconnection of the top of the body from the bottom. Panjabi has recently published a hypothesis based on the concept of a single trauma or cumulative microtrauma causing subfailure injuries of the ligaments and embedded mechanoreceptors leading to disturbed muscle control. Harris has suggested that mismatch between expected and actual proprioceptive information may be a potent source of 'distress' in the central nervous system, experienced as pain. There is a strong body of evidence suggesting proprioceptive dysfunction in chronic back pain patients.

Sagittal balance

Humans stand and walk best if they can keep their frame in balance, which means, when standing, the head is over the hips, which are in turn over the heels. In other words, the gravity line goes through the cervicothoracic junction and the lumbosacral joint. Deviations from this (usually forward) overload the posterior lumbar musculature and require compensatory hip extension and knee flexion. All may be well at skeletal maturity, but loss of balance may follow kyphosis due to disc degeneration and fractures. Imbalance has become increasingly recognized as an important cause of back pain. Surgery can be used to correct imbalance by osteotomy or facetectomy during fusion, but milder cases may well respond to rehabilitation and exercise.

Spinal stenosis

There is anecdotal evidence that adults with spinal stenosis have a long history of back pain. Arguably the flexed posture these individuals adopt may be a contributory factor to sagittal imbalance. There is experimental evidence that these individuals are at more risk of trouble with their backs if they have a disc prolapse.

Assessment of instability

A good history is essential. The 'ideal' patient for spinal fusion, may have some or all of the following characteristics: a nonsmoking 'normal citizen'; no litigation outstanding or other potential secondary gains from his or her pain; a clear history; and a crescendo of symptoms, but with pain-free or low pain intervals. Some patients with recurrent attacks of pain report prodromal symptoms preceding an attack. Surgeons have tried many methods to identify good responders: for example, a trial period in external splintage, or a rational response to discography. External fixation has also been tried, but has not proved popular because of complications and poor predictive ability. Flexion–extension radiographs have been used for many years, but their value is very limited. Standing views may be of value if the gravity line or whole body can be included. This approach remains experimental.

Confounding factors

Failures of the surgical approach can be attributed to two main areas: the patient and the surgical methodology.

The patient

A technically correct operation achieving a solid fusion may not relieve pain, and indeed it can make it worse. There may be a variety of reasons for this.

1) Patient selection. Often significant psychosocial factors contribute to the extent of pain-related distress and disability. Even the most experienced surgeons can be caught out. Some surgeons make use of psychological questionnaires to aid in the selection of patients, but there is no good study to show that using these methods improves results. Ideally a pain psychologist should identify the degree of psychosocial involvement before the surgeon embarks upon surgical treatment. Pain-related distress should be treated first
2) Poor recognition of sagittal imbalance
3) The wrong levels may be selected for surgery
4) Smoking cigarettes has been associated with a high pseudarthrosis rate in many studies
5) Involvement in litigation or worker's compensation has long been recognized as being associated with poor clinical results.

Surgical methodology

The objective of most procedures is to obtain a solid bony fusion, avoiding damage to the surrounding soft tissues. A wide variety of methods are available, and comparisons between them are difficult. Posterolateral fusions tend to be easier to perform, but are probably less reliable in terms of both fusion rates and in immobilizing a segment (or functional spinal unit). Interbody fusions, either from the back or from the front, are more likely to fuse with instrumentation, but are technically more difficult to perform, and carry a higher risk of complication. Spinal instrumentation has evolved rapidly, increasing in complexity and expense. It has been difficult to demonstrate that its use has any advantage. Some studies, but not all, suggest that the use of instrumentation increases the fusion rate. Unfortunately this is not necessarily accompanied by an improvement in clinical results. The evidence base would support the use of uninstrumented posterolateral fusion as the best option with lowest complication rate.

Discography

It is likely that a significant proportion of patients have discogenic or segmental pain. Proponents of this view use provocative discography to identify painful segments. Discography can identify segments where pain is reproduced by injection of saline into the disc and adjacent normal discs. It identifies patients with inappropriate responses (over-reaction to local anaesthetic or skin penetration by needle) and inappropriate or multilevel response to disc injection. The 'normal' disc is usually pain free when injected. There is a large literature on this, but many studies are flawed. Carragee's studies are a good starting point. He was able to demonstrate only a predictive value for discography of 50–60% in spinal fusion patients.

Use of instrumentation

The objective of treating these patients is to relieve symptoms and improve function. In theory this requires that a fusion be achieved. There is a close, but by no means total, correlation between fusion and pain relief.

There remains considerable uncertainty surrounding internal fixation. This may be unnecessary for a single-level posterior fusion, but may be useful if more than one level is involved. Certainly the experience with spinal fusion for scoliosis would support this view. Large trials are probably necessary to resolve these issues.

Further reading

Carragee, E.J., Lincoln, T., Parmar, V.S., and Alamin, T.A. (2006). Gold standard evaluation of the 'discogenic pain' diagnosis as determined by provocative discography. *Spine*, **31**(18), 2115–23.

Mirza, S.K. and Deyo, R. (2007). A systematic review of randomized trials comparing lumbar fusion surgery to nonoperative care for treatment of chronic back pain. *Spine*, **32**(7), 816–23.

Rossignol, M., Arsenault, B., Dionne, C., *et al.* (2007). *Clinic on low-back pain in interdisciplinary practice (CLIP) guideline.* Montréal: Direction de Santé Publique, Agence de la santé et des services sociaux de Montréal. http://www.santepubmtl.qc.ca/Publication/pdftravail/CLIPenglish.pdf

3.7

Management of nerve root pain (syn: sciatica, radicular pain)

Jeremy Fairbank

Summary points

- Radicular pain can be diagnosed clinically and confirmed by imaging
- Pain caused by disc herniation can be very severe, but often resolves without intervention
- Surgery is often successful if non-operative treatment fails.

Introduction

True nerve root pain has a lifetime prevalence of less than 5%. Lumbar-sacral nerve root pain radiates in the distribution of one or more dermatomes and may be associated with neurological deficits. Although back pain may coexist, the severity of the leg pain predominates. The most common cause is disc prolapse (also called herniation). The majority are at L4/L5 or L5/S1. However, other pathologies which have the potential to compress or irritate a nerve root include tumour, infection, or neuritis. It has become clear in the last few years that disc degeneration and the proportion of degenerate discs that is herniated is driven by genetic factors. Genetics explains 60% of the variance, with minimal contributions from environmental factors such as smoking and trauma. This means that family history should always be explored. There is evidence that mechanical compression of a nerve root results in sensory and/or motor deficits. The onset, duration, and extent of the pressure have been shown to be important. However, compression alone does not cause pain. Some degree of inflammation/irritation must exist for nerve to refer pain. The pathophysiology of nerve root pain is not fully understood. Research has explored the chemical effect of the nucleus pulposus coming into contact with a nerve root, in particular the dorsal root ganglion. A large number of inflammatory and signalling substances, including cytokines (especially tumour necrosis factor, TNF), nitric oxide, and nerve growth factor have been suggested to play a role. There may be an immunological element as well, as the nucleus is normally avascular. It is likely that mechanical and biochemical factors act together, altering intraneural permeability, intraneural blood flow, and nutrition, resulting in degeneration of nerve fibres and reduced nerve conduction.

Clinical features (Box 3.7.1)

Root pain caused by disc prolapse is usually preceded by back pain. The interval varies from a few minutes to years. Leg pain usually predominates in a dermatomal distribution. Pain is exacerbated by coughing and sneezing, walking, and standing. Night pain is common. Pain may be relieved by lying and flexing the spine. Root pain (sciatica) can be extremely severe, and associated with numbness and paraesthesia. Weakness may be experienced with poor push-off, flapping gait, and foot drop. The appearance of foot drop

Box 3.7.1 Features of root pain caused by disc prolapse

- Back pain precedes leg pain
- Leg pain usually predominates
- Leg pain is in a dermatomal distribution
- Pain is exacerbated by:
  - Coughing and sneezing
  - Walking and standing
  - Night pain is common
- Pain may be relieved by:
  - Lying
  - Flexing the spine
- Weakness may be experienced with:
  - Poor push-off
  - Flapping gait
  - Foot drop.

is sometimes associated with pain improvement. Perineal numbness, and associated bladder or bowel symptoms are important indicators of cauda equina syndrome but the latter may be associated with pain severity and analgesic intake.

Examination should include an assessment of sensation to both light touch and pinprick (the end of a paper-clip is effective). Straight-leg raising is restricted. I prefer to flex the hip and knee first, and then gradually and gently extent the knee. This allows assessment of hip pain, and is unfamiliar to experienced patients with illness behaviour. Weakness should be sought particularly in extension of the great toe and foot, foot eversion, and knee extension. Ankle and knee reflexes must be recorded.

Imaging is best done by magnetic resonance (MR). If this is unavailable or contraindicated, computed tomography or myelography may be used. Disc herniations are seen in up to 25% of normal scans, so it is essential to interpret the scan in light of the clinical picture. Large discs tend to respond better to treatment than small ones. Attention should be paid to the vertebral canal diameter. Small canals give more trouble than large ones. Look out for other contributing factors to nerve pain such as lateral recess and exit foramenal stenosis (Table 3.7.1).

Natural history

Nerve root pain caused by disc herniation usually gets better. Unfortunately the time scale is unpredictable. Clinical practice, observational data, and now some useful randomized controlled trials have given reasonably clear guidance on management. No non-operative treatment comes out better than natural history. However, explanation and analgesia, possibly combined with muscle relaxants, are important. Epidurals (either spinal or caudal) do not alter natural history, though the short-term relief of root pain may be convenient for some. Surgery may be indicated from 8 weeks from onset, unless there is evidence of cauda equina involvement or progressive neurological deficit, when surgery is indicated straight away. This is informed by a number of trials, including the SPORT study, and, most recently Peul and colleagues, who compared an early with delayed surgical strategy. All of these favour early surgery over non-operative care in the short/medium term. The patient has to weigh up the risks (persisting pain, nerve damage, cauda equina damage (rare but devastating), dural tears, and recurrence) against (90%) benefit of relief of nerve root pain but not back pain. Earlier studies give a recurrence rate of 10% in 10 years, but Peul and colleagues found 20% at 2 years. There is evidence from one trial that traditional disc space curettage produces inferior results to simple fragment removal. It should be emphasized that these trials are done on patients with clear-cut indications. In clinical practice this not always the case, and there are many studies showing poor outcome when the McColloch criteria are not met (see Box 3.7.2). He wrote in the first edition of this book the following:

Table 3.7.1 Results of a prospective but not randomized controlled trial of lumbar disc herniation

Time since surgery	Non-surgical results	Surgical results
1 year	60% better	92% better
4 years	No statistical difference between the two groups	
10 years	No difference between 4-year and 10-year follow-up (60% better)	

Data from Weber (1983).

Indications for discectomy

The prerequisite for any surgical procedure is a precise diagnosis in a patient who is positively motivated to recover from surgery. Not only must the clinical syndrome be obvious (Box 3.7.2), but there must also be a clearly defined, unequivocal lesion on imaging that corresponds, anatomically, with the clinical root level. Where MR imaging is readily available, it has become the imaging modality of first choice.

Strong indications for surgical intervention

- Bladder and bowel involvement, i.e. the cauda equina syndrome: in these patients an acute massive disc herniation causes bladder and bowel paralysis that probably requires immediate surgical excision for the best prognosis
- Progressive motor deficit: in the face of progressing weakness, it is wise to intervene early with surgical excision of the disc herniation.

Relative indications for surgical intervention

- Failure of conservative treatment is the most common reason for surgical intervention for the symptomatic lumbar disc herniation. Conservative treatment should last for at least 6 weeks and not more than 3–4 months, and result in improvement in the patient's symptoms and signs
- Very rarely, one will encounter a patient who does not respond to any form of pharmacological or physical pain control within a few days to a few weeks of the onset of sciatica. Their severe incapacitating pain merits urgent surgical consideration
- Conservative treatment can also fail in that the patient experiences recurrences of the sciatic syndrome
- Significant motor deficit with significant positive straight-leg raising test: if a patient has grade 3 (or less) motor strength with

Box 3.7.2 Clinical criteria for the diagnosis of a disc rupture causing acute sciatica*

1. Leg pain (including buttock pain and pain radiating below the knee) must follow a radicular distribution and be the dominant complaint when compared with back pain
2. Neurological symptoms (paraesthesia or weakness) should be present in a radicular distribution
3. Straight-leg raising must be significantly reduced
4. Neurological signs (motor, sensory, reflex, and wasting) should be present in a radicular distribution

* Three or four of the listed criteria should be clinically present to satisfy the clinical diagnosis of acute sciatica due to a disc rupture.

or without significant straight-leg raising reduction, surgery may be indicated. Weber has shown that these patients eventually recovered just as well with non-surgical intervention. Often these patients are in extreme pain and will not wait for the benefits of conservative care. Occasionally, these patients present with a history of severe pain which has resolved while the neurological deficit has increased. This rare patient is also a surgical candidate. Important points about surgical technique are made in Box 3.7.3.

Lumbar disc herniation in the adolescent patient

The young patient with a disc herniation is a special problem. Because of the high proteoglycan content of the discal material (responsive to chymopapain) and the prevalence of disc protrusions rather than disc extrusions in this age group, I recommend that the optimum treatment is chemonucleolysis rather than surgical intervention. Unfortunately chyomopapain is not currently available, although there are hopes that it may return to the market. Surgery can be effective but the recurrence rate is significantly higher than with chymopapain.

Recurrent lumbar disc herniation

The patient who has successful relief of sciatica after disc excision has a 5–20% chance of a recurrent disc rupture causing sciatica. Unfortunately, most recurrent disc herniations are at the same level and same side, and scar tissue from the previous surgery introduces a new element in diagnosis and treatment. Scarring 'tacks' down the dura to the back of the disc space so that a smaller amount of herniated nuclear material is capable of producing a significant amount of pain and neurological deficit in the relatively immobile nerve root. Because of the immobility of the scarred dura, transdural ruptures, although rare, can occur. Almost invariably the scar between the dura and the disc restricts migration of the recurrent disc fragments, i.e. on exploration they are routinely found opposite the disc space.

Determining the anatomic level by clinical assessment can be difficult because some neurological changes are residual from the prior lumbar disc herniation, and the dura may not simply be immobilized, it may be distorted from the scar tissue, leading to root involvement lower than usual for the level of the lumbar disc herniation (e.g. a recurrent L4–L5 lumbar disc herniation may affect a number of sacral roots).

Investigation can be difficult to interpret because of the scar tissue. It may be helpful to enhance the MR examination with gadolinium. The surgery is also difficult and prone to complications such as missed lesions, dural tears, and neurological damage. A basic principle in any repeat surgery is to gain as wide an exposure as possible.

Box 3.7.3 The principles of surgical intervention for symptomatic disc prolapse

- You are not performing disc surgery, you are decompressing a nerve root
- You must leave the nerve root freely mobile and undamaged
- You must leave behind as little scar as possible
- You must not create further instability in the motion segment.

Conclusion

Surgical discectomy and/or decompression to relieve sciatica is an operation with clear-cut indications and is usually followed by a high level of success. Microsurgical techniques facilitate the exercises but will not improve an overall success rate of 80–90%. In the end, the decision to operate on a patient with a lumbar disc herniation and/or lateral zone stenosis is largely dependent on patient preference and rarely on necessity. In the short term, however, surgery will result in less pain and improved function compared with conservative care.

Further reading

Peul, W., van den Hout, W., Brand, R., Thomeer, R., and Koes, B. (2008). Prolonged conservative care versus early surgery in patients with sciatica caused by lumbar disc herniation: two year results of a randomised controlled trial. *British Medical Journal,* **336**, 1355–8.

Weber, H. (1994). Spine update: the natural history of disc herniation and the influence of intervention. *Spine,* **19**, 2234–8.

Weinstein, J., Tosteson, T., Lurie, J., *et al.* (2006). Surgical vs nonoperative treatment for lumbar disk herniation. The Spine Patient Outcomes Research Trial (SPORT): a randomized trial. *Journal of the American Medical Association,* **296**, 2441–50.

Weinstein, J., Lurie, J., Tosteson, T., *et al.* (2006). Surgical vs nonoperative treatment for lumbar disk herniation: The Spine Patient Outcomes Research Trial (SPORT) observational cohort. *Journal of the American Medical Association,* **296**, 2451–9.

3.8

Management of neurogenic claudication and spinal stenosis

Jeremy Fairbank

Summary points

- Neurogenic claudication is a common symptom
- Back pain and leg pain occur with standing and walking
- Spinal stenosis may be developmental or acquired or a combination of both
- An important spinal differential diagnosis is loss of sagittal balance
- There are many causes, both medical and orthopaedic, that may contribute to difficulty with walking and poor outcomes from surgical treatment.

Introduction

Spinal stenosis was described in 1954 by Verbiest. It causes a syndrome that is usually easy to recognize. It includes difficulty with walking (neurogenic claudication). Once considered rare, it is now clear that this syndrome occurs frequently with advancing years. Verbiest recognized two forms: developmental and acquired. Developmental stenosis may be localized to a single level or involve the whole spine. It is almost universally present in achondroplasia. People with narrow canals are probably more likely to encounter trouble with back symptoms than those with wide canals, although the evidence for this statement is not robust. Acquired stenosis is associated with distortions of the spinal canal and exiting nerve root canals. This is secondary to disc degeneration causing narrowing of the disc space, disc bulges, and herniations. This in turn distorts facet joints, which degenerate and throw out osteophytes. The ligamentum flavum looses its elasticity and tends to crumple and thicken, occupying the vertebral canal and compressing the thecal sac and nerve roots. All of this is more marked when the lumbar spine is extended, particularly during standing and walking, and less marked when sitting or squatting. Many patients find they cannot lie on their back and have to sleep in a fetal position.

Clinical presentation

Generally symptoms develop gradually. Some just have back pain, but most have unilateral or bilateral leg symptoms. Most report pain, but some have difficulty in finding words to describe a sensation of heaviness, loss of function, or even giving way. Usually the pain appears after standing or walking for a time. The period may vary from day to day as does the severity. Relief occurs with sitting or squatting. Again this varies but may take 10m or more to recover—much slower than vascular claudication. Many are helped with walking aids such as a supermarket trolley. The main differential diagnoses are those conditions which affect walking and balance. Be especially alert to loss of sagittal balance.

Management

- Investigation is by imaging of the lumbar spine, usually with magnetic resonance imaging. Where this is unavailable, computed tomography or myelography are inferior substitutes. It is important to exclude other causes of claudication, such as peripheral vascular disease
- Non-operative treatment includes explanation, which can often be highly effective; simple analgesics such as paracetamol and sometimes non-steroidal anti-inflammatory drugs. One trial has supported the use of gabapentin; epidural steroids may help; walking aids including portable seats and all-terrain rollators with a seat fitted; light rucksacks (many find carrying shopping in bags increases their symptoms)
- Surgery involves decompressing the cauda equina, lateral recesses, and exit foramena, depending on the radiological anatomy, clinical symptoms, and signs. This can be achieved by a variety of techniques ranging from laminectomy to microdecompression. There is controversy concerning the use of fusion either with or without implants. Fusion is more commonly employed in the United States than elsewhere. It is more likely to be used if the patient has a degenerative spondylolisthesis. This condition most commonly occurs at L4/L5, and is much more frequent in women than in men
- There are a range of devices that can be inserted between the spinous processes to maintain the motion segment in flexion. The role of these devices and their duration of action remain controversial
- The outcome of surgery depends on comorbidity and age. Patients over 80 tend to have worse outcomes (but they also have

more comorbidity). As a rule of thumb, 70% of patients will have a good outcome. Even so, few will obtain the walking capacity of their fit contemporaries. Complication rates vary, but for decision making I tell patients 5% will be worse off and may regret the decision to proceed with surgery. This may be due to root damage, cauda equina damage, impaired vascularity, infection, and recurrence. It is not always possible to tell why outcome is poor in a particular case, but it is important to ensure that the decompression was complete. Loss of sagittal balance is sometimes a cause of poor outcome.

Further reading

Jansson, K-Å., Blomqvist, P., Granath, F., Németh, G. (2003). Spinal stenosis surgery in Sweden 1987-1999. *European Spine Journal*, **12**, 535–41.

Pratt, R., Fairbank, J., and Virr, A. (2002). The reliability of the Shuttle Walking Test, the Swiss Spinal Stenosis Questionnaire, the Oxford Spinal Stenosis Score, and the Oswestry Disability Index in the assessment of patients with lumbar spinal stenosis. *Spine*, **27**, 84–91.

Malmivaara, A., Slatis, P., Heliovaara, M., Sainio, P., Kinnunen, H., Kankare, J., et al. (2007). Surgical or nonoperative treatment for lumbar spinal stenosis?: A randomized controlled trial. *Spine*, **32**(1), 1–8.

Verbiest, H. (1954). A radicular syndrome from developmental narrowing of the lumbar vertebral canal. *Journal of Bone and Joint Surgery*, **36B**, 230–7.

3.9

Clinical presentation of spinal deformities

Jeremy Fairbank

Summary points

- Incidence 2–4/1000
- Idiopathic most common pattern
- Sagittal and coronal balance are critical for management of spinal deformity.

Introduction

This chapter gives an overview of the spectrum of spinal deformity, its classification, and the broad principles of management.

Historical review

Spinal deformity has been recognized at least since the Egyptian civilization. Various forms of external traction, bracing, and manipulation have been used to treat these deformities with doubtful benefit. It has been recognized that there are extraordinary deforming forces at work, particularly during growth.

Epidemics of tuberculosis and poliomyelitis in the developed world in the early part of the twentieth century precipitated considerable advances in the management of spinal deformity. Both poliomyelitis and tuberculosis are responsive to public health measures. This is not the case for other forms of scoliosis, despite school screening programmes in some countries. The cause or causes of adolescent idiopathic scoliosis, the most common form of scoliosis, remain elusive.

The convention is to describe the magnitude of curves by Cobb angle, and the direction of convexity (right or left). Scoliosis surgeons usually view erect radiographs as if seen from behind. Radiographs give a two-dimensional view of the spine. Scoliosis is a complex deformity involving rotation of the apical vertebrae out of the curve. This means that at the apex the vertebral body lies lateral to the tip of the spinous process. The experienced eye is familiar with this rotation, and it should be borne in mind when considering the nature and severity of the deformity.

A scoliosis is best seen with the patient bent forward sufficiently to place the apex of the curve on the skyline. If the spine is rotated, this is reflected in a rib hump in the thoracic spine or a loin hump in the lumbar spine (Figure 3.9.1). This is formalized into the Adams forward-bending test. Surface topography is useful for defining and monitoring the changing shape of the back during growth and after treatment. It can reduce the use of radiography, and may detect a deteriorating curve earlier than is the case with

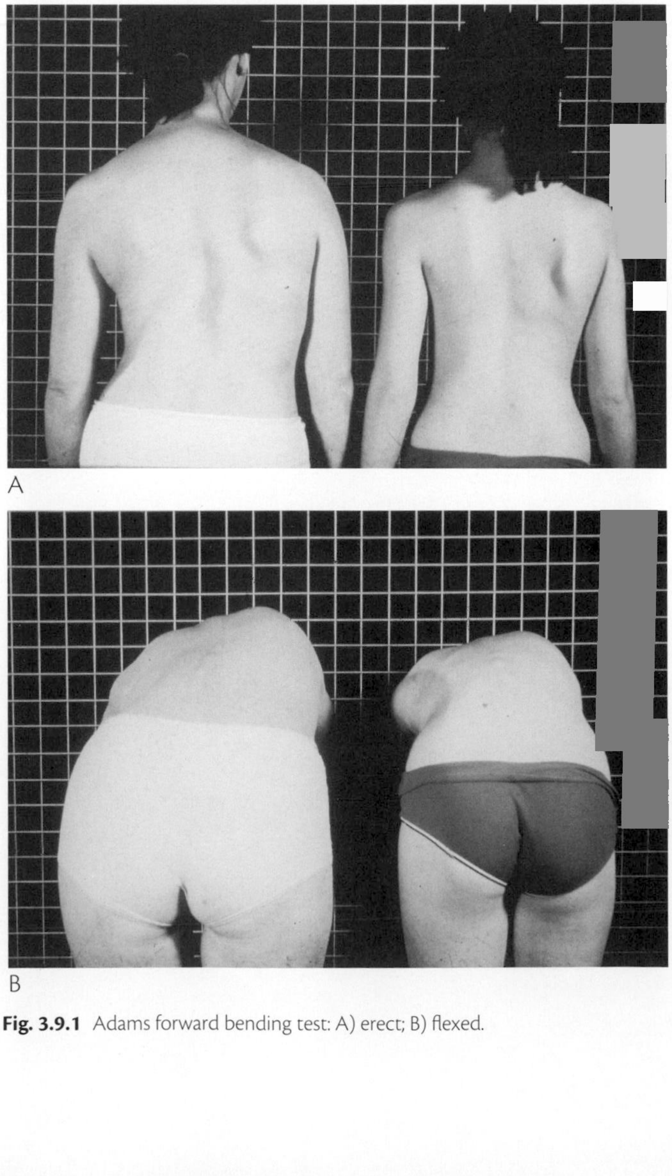

A

B

Fig. 3.9.1 Adams forward bending test: A) erect; B) flexed.

radiographs. A variety of commercial systems are in use, including ISIS2 (Figure 3.9.2), although there is no standard for data presentation. ISIS2 offers improved precision and sensitivity to change of rib hump measurements and truncal asymmetry.

Sagittal profile and the capacity to keep the head over the hips when standing still are crucial elements in understanding spinal deformity. The spine is usually lordotic at the apex of the curve. Some believe that the lordosis is the underlying cause of the curvature. Kyphosis is an important deformity which is sometimes more dangerous to the spinal cord than scoliosis (Box 3.9.1). The thoracic and sacral regions of the normal spine have physiological kyphosis, which in pathological situations can become excessive. The cervical and lumbar spines are normally lordotic. Loss of lordosis in both parts of the spine can be painful—the so-called flat-back syndrome. If any part of the spine becomes excessively kyphotic, without the capacity to compensate through lordosis, sagittal balance is affected. A localized kyphosis (kyphos or gibbus), for whatever reason, poses a particular threat to the spinal cord. Kyphosis can be assessed clinically by the same methods used for the assessment of scoliosis. Surgical treatment of kyphosis carries a higher risk to spinal cord function compared with surgery for scoliosis.

Clinical evaluation and examination

History

The history should establish the first identification of the deformity and its evolution. Family history is important. The obstetric history, childhood illnesses, and the onset of menarche (the first

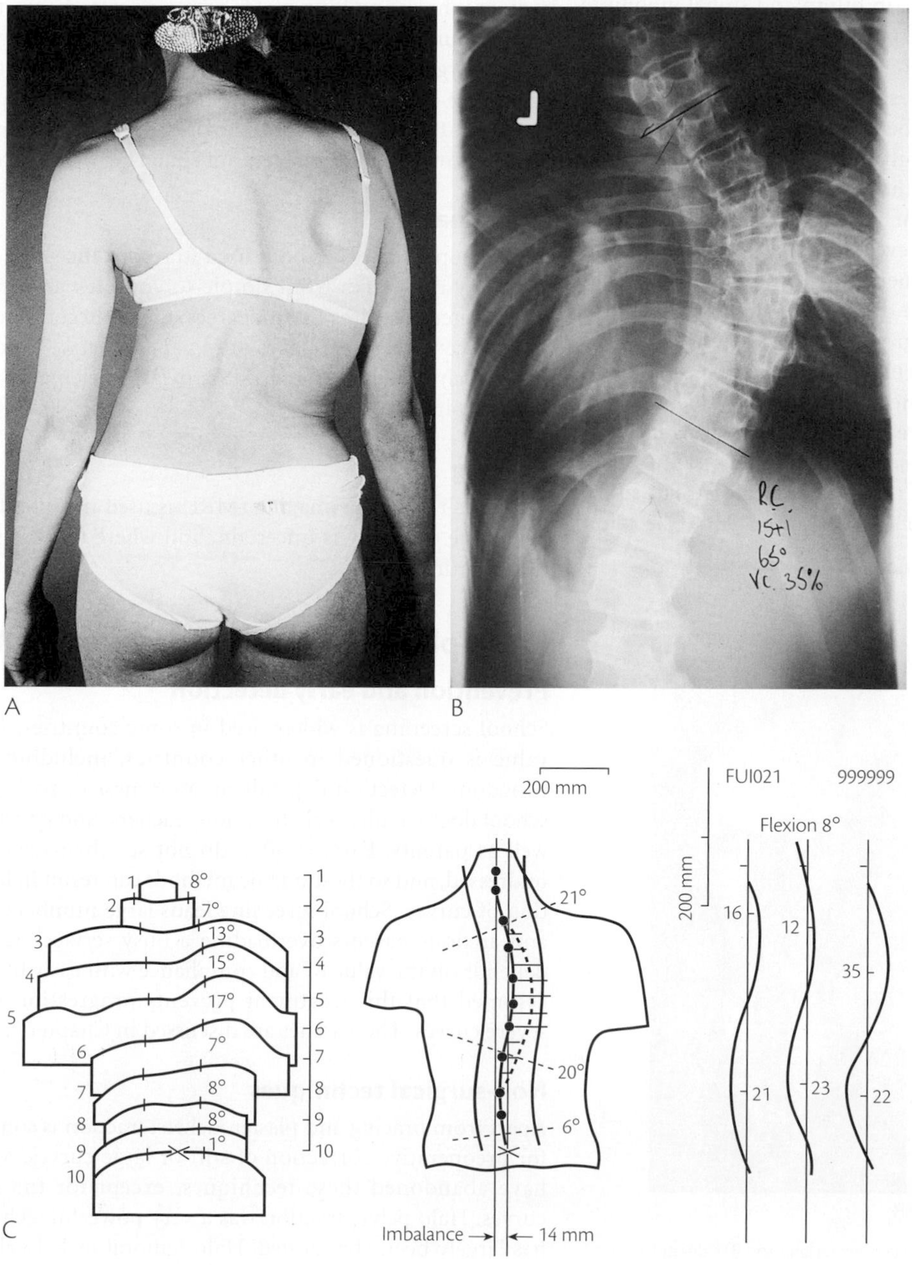

Fig. 3.9.2 (A) Patient with adolescent idiopathic scoliosis. B) ISIS2 scan and C) radiograph of patient in (A).

menstrual period), if relevant, should be reviewed. Many curves are painless, but night pain, rest pain, or fatigue pain should be identified. The patient should be checked for neurological and cardiopulmonary symptoms, and asked about analgesic usage and absence from school or work.

It is useful to establish how aware the patient is of the curve, as this may have a bearing on subsequent management. The distress that a curve causes to the patient and his or her family may be out of proportion to its severity.

Examination (Box 3.9.2)

The examination of scoliotic patients should be carried out with care. Adolescent females in particular are often unused to doctors and are embarrassed to undress. The parents or carers should be present if possible. Gowns may reassure the patient, but conceal vital signs.

Examine the undressed patient from behind while he or she is standing up. Then ask the patient to perform forward and side bending to review the shape of the rib hump and spinal mobility. Assess the level of the pelvis. If the pelvis is tilted, it is sometimes useful to use blocks to level it before assessing the spine. A plumb line from the vertebra prominens should fall through the natal cleft. Deviations from this should be recorded, with the direction measured in centimeters (trunk shift). Sagittal balance should be assessed to ensure the head is over the hips with knees extended.

Signs of puberty are useful for the assessment of growth potential. In girls, pubic hair and breast development occur at the start of the adolescent growth spurt, and menarche towards the end of it. In boys, pubic hair appears before the start of the growth spurt. Axillary hair appears at the end of growth in both sexes.

Note any deviations from the normal pattern of curve, and identify the site of any pain by asking the patient to point this out. It is important in the growing child to record height on a growth chart. Some also make regular records of sitting height and weight.

The whole skin should be seen to check for café au lait spots (neurofibromatosis type 1, Chapter 1.13) (Figure 3.9.3). Check for hairy patches, nevi, and dimples in the midline over the spine (present in spinal dysraphism). Note the presence and type of foot deformities, lower-limb asymmetries, truncal and breast asymmetries, skull/facial asymmetries, and handedness.

A neurological examination is important. Focus on evidence of long tract signs (reflexes and plantar responses), evidence of asymmetric muscle wasting, the presence of abnormal abdominal reflexes, posture, gait, and cranial nerve abnormalities.

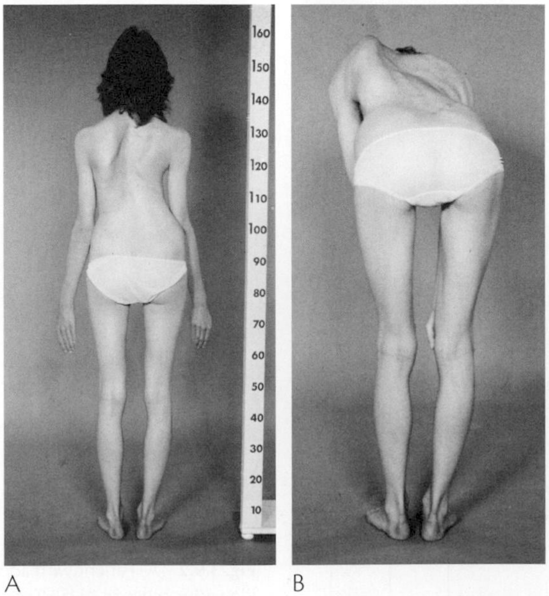

Fig. 3.9.3 A) Neurofibromatosis (note curve convex to left) and B) café-au-lait spots.

Investigations

Radiography

Radiography should be used with caution, particularly in the growing child. Low-dose regimens, fast films, and rare earth screens should be used. Eos claims to involve 10% of this exposure only (http://www.biospacemed.com/). Gonadal shielding can be used after an initial unprotected film. Erect anteroposterior and lateral radiographs, using long plates where necessary, are taken at the first encounter. Supine lateral bending films are only indicated just before surgery to help define the curve for instrumentation. Bone age can be determined by an anteroposterior radiograph of the left wrist, but the Risser sign and the presence of a vertebral ring apophysis provide a good indicator of spinal growth potential.

Spine shape

Surface topography has been used to record the shape of the back. A variety of devices from simple to complex are available. The scoliometer measures tilt in degrees; the body contour formulator is a device to transfer shapes onto paper. Surface topography systems, such as Quantec and ISIS2, measure elements not seen on radiographs.

Imaging

Magnetic resonance imaging (MRI) is used in patients with pain, where the aetiology is uncertain, and where there is suspicion of tumor or infection.

Principles of management (Box 3.9.3)

Prevention and early detection

School screening is widely used in some countries. However, its value is questioned in other countries, including the United Kingdom. Detection depends on awareness of scoliosis amongst school doctors, physical education teachers, and ballet teachers, as well as parents. Parents often do not see their teenage children undressed, and so these ad hoc methods can result in late presentation of curves. School screening leads large numbers of teenagers and anxious parents overloading a busy service. Screening also depends on the value of and compliance with early bracing, as it is assumed that this treatment prevents progression of the more severe curves. These issues are discussed in Chapter 3.14.

Non-surgical techniques

Apart from bracing and plaster jackets, traction is sometimes used for preoperative correction of stiff or large curves. Many centres have abandoned these techniques, except for the most severe curves. Halo pelvic traction was a very powerful technique which has largely been abandoned. Halo femoral or halo chair traction

Box 3.9.1 Kyphosis

- Angular kyphosis secondary to congenital hemivertebrae, tuberculosis, and occasionally fracture tends to progress, even after skeletal maturity, and will cause spinal cord compression
- In general, spinal cord compression due to kyphosis requires anterior decompression and stabilization. Some cases also require posterior fusion
- Surgical correction of kyphosis due to Scheuermann's disease is rarely indicated, and the result is not always rewarding
- Correction of kyphosis carries a significant risk to spinal cord function.

Box 3.9.2 Investigation

The spinal cord should be investigated (usually by MRI) in the following patients:

- Those with congenital scoliosis (20% have anomalies, including syrinx, cord anomalies, tumours, diastematomyelia)
- Those with abnormal skin markings over the spine or café au lait spots
- Those with early-onset idiopathic scoliosis and adolescents presenting younger than 11 years
- Those with painful scoliosis
- Probably all those having surgery.

is sometimes used in very severe curves. Preoperative Cotrel or dynamic traction is used still in some centres, but there is little evidence of efficacy.

Surgical techniques

Most techniques depend on obtaining a solid fusion. In posterior surgery, it is vital to destroy the apophyseal (facet) joints. Autologous bone graft is best, but allograft and artificial materials avoid problems with the bone donor site. Unfortunately there is a tendency for the rib hump to recur following fusion, whatever system is used, especially in the younger patient with growth potential. The common surgical techniques used in spinal deformity surgery are described in the rest of this section.

Epiphysiodesis and growing rods and titanium ribs

Epiphysiodesis has a limited place in the management of early-onset idiopathic scoliosis. It involves damaging convex growth plates with a view to preventing progression in the young child. Subcutaneous distraction rods can be distracted at regular operations, but there is a high incidence of complications. Other surgeons use a Luque 'trolley', where two rods are fashioned into a U-shape. These are placed with the bend at each end of the curve, and wired onto the laminae. In theory this allows the rods to slide on one another as the spine grows. Titanium ribs (VEPTR) are designed to serially distract the thorax to develop respiratory function.

Box 3.9.3 Scoliosis

The principles of management include the following:

- The greater the potential for growth, the greater the ultimate deformity is likely to be
- Periods of rapid growth are often associated with rapid deterioration of the curve
- Spinal fusion arrests spinal growth over the fused segment except, possibly, in younger patients, where a posterior fusion does not prevent continuing anterior growth (the crankshaft phenomenon)
- The 'rib hump' tends to deteriorate with growth, even after a successful spinal fusion
- Lung development (elaboration of alveoli) is completed by the age of 7 years. Thereafter the lungs only increase in capacity during normal growth
- In general, curves starting at an age of less than 7 years may become sufficiently severe to affect respiratory function
- Vital capacity is likely to be less than predicted (calculated from arm span) in curves with a Cobb angle greater than 70 degrees. Significant respiratory dysfunction only occurs in curves with Cobb angles greater than 100 degrees
- The cosmetic consequences of scoliosis mainly relate to the size of the rib hump, trunk imbalance, effects on the waistline and pelvic obliquity, and differences in shoulder height. These do not always relate clearly to the site or severity of the scoliosis
- In general, thoracic curves are not painful, although some patients (especially adults) complain of fatigue pain. Occasionally this is sufficient for them to opt for surgery. Continuous pain in a child or adolescent is an alarm signal for serious pathology
- Thoracolumbar and lumbar curves may well cause pain, especially in adults, which may be sufficient to warrant the risks of surgery. Pain is more likely when one vertebra translates laterally on the one below it and with loss of sagittal and coronal balance.

Costoplasty (thoracoplasty)

These procedures are designed to reduce the size of the rib hump by resecting, transposing, or even transplanting ribs, and are often used at the end of growth. The excised ribs sections can be used as bone graft.

Fusion in situ

This is used where correction is likely to cause spinal cord damage. In the past, prolonged decumbency on a plaster bed was used. Now a well-fitting plaster cast is the norm. A fusion *in situ* may result if a plaster cast is used (but by no means always), implants are removed because of evidence of spinal cord damage intraoperatively.

Harrington system

The Harrington system is a distraction rod with hooks at each end (Figure 3.9.4) widely used from 1950 to 1980. Good corrections can

Box 3.9.4 Curve progression

- Curves with Cobb angles greater than 30 degrees at skeletal maturity progress in adult life at a rate of up to 1 degree/year. There is considerable individual variation, but in general the larger the curve, the more it is likely to deteriorate
- All interventions should be viewed as a balance between risk and benefit against the probable outcome if the curve is left untreated
- The risks of inducing spinal cord damage up to and including paraplegia during and after surgery vary with different deformities. It is essential that these risks are discussed with patients and their families before embarking on surgical treatment
- The selection of implant and surgical approach depends on the skills of the surgeon (i.e. what he or she is accustomed to using) and what health service resources can afford. The best results depend on good technique and careful bone grafting. There is still considerable argument about the optimum implant. However, there is no doubt that an implant of some sort is required in most cases.

be obtained, but these may be partially lost before the fusion becomes solid. This technique has not been very successful in derotating curves. It has been enhanced with sublaminar wires (Figure 3.9.5)

Luque system

Eduado Luque of Mexico City was the first to promote the use of sublaminar wires. The rods can be contoured so that their lower ends are driven into the pelvis (Galveston technique, Mehdian technique). This is especially valuable in neuromuscular curves with pelvic obliquity. The Hartshill rectangle system uses sublaminar wires. This has been promoted for the fixation of all types of scoliosis, but it is difficult to use and fixation to the pelvis is unsatisfactoy. Now it used to supplement other systems particularly when bone quality is poor. A current sublaminar tape system (universal clamp) shows promise where bone quality is poor.

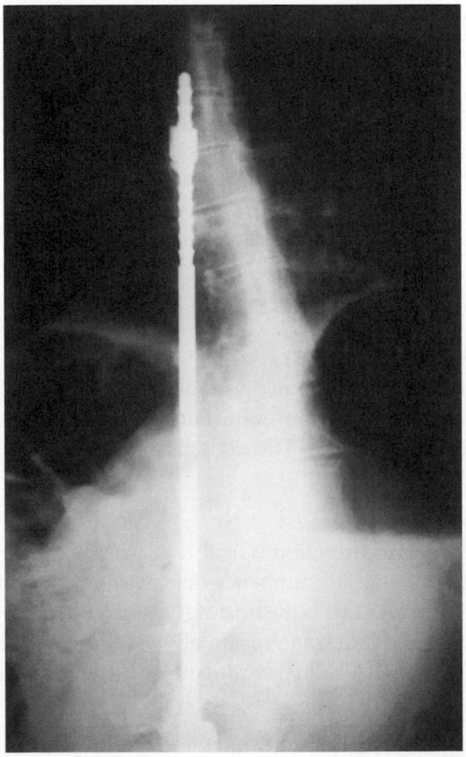

Fig. 3.9.4 A single Harrington rod used to stabilize the thoracolumbar spine.

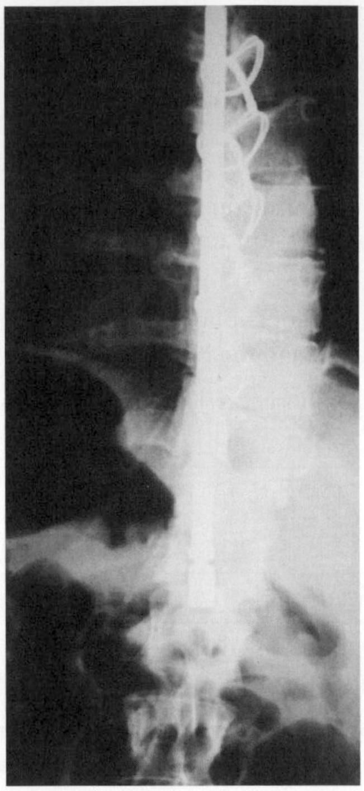

Fig. 3.9.5 Harrington rod used with sublaminar wires.

Double-rod systems

The Cotrel–Dubousset (CD) system was the first specifically designed for the treatment of adolescent idiopathic scoliosis. It depends on contouring a knurled rod in the concavity of the curve. This is secured by hooks and pedicle screws to the spine, and correction is obtained by rotating the rod so that its curve lies in the sagittal plane. A second rod is then placed on the convexity of the curve and secured to hooks and cross-links. This system is adaptable to a wide variety of applications. The Texas Scottish Rite Hospital (TSRH) and Isola systems uses similar techniques, but are engineered using a smooth rod.

The Universal Spine System (USS2) uses side-opening screws and hooks, and a smooth rod which allows the rod to be contoured into the shape required (Figure 3.9.6). The spine can then be pulled onto the rod, obtaining the correction (similar to the Luque method). Variations on these methods are constantly been developed but the extra gains in correction are obtained at high cost.

Anterior systems

The Dwyer system was the first system designed for anterior surgery and was a most important development. It uses titanium screws and staples, which are crimped onto a titanium cable placed in tension around the convexity of the curve. It risks kyphosing the spine. Zielke (VDS) system uses a 4-mm threaded rod which allows selective tightening of each level (not possible with the Dwyer

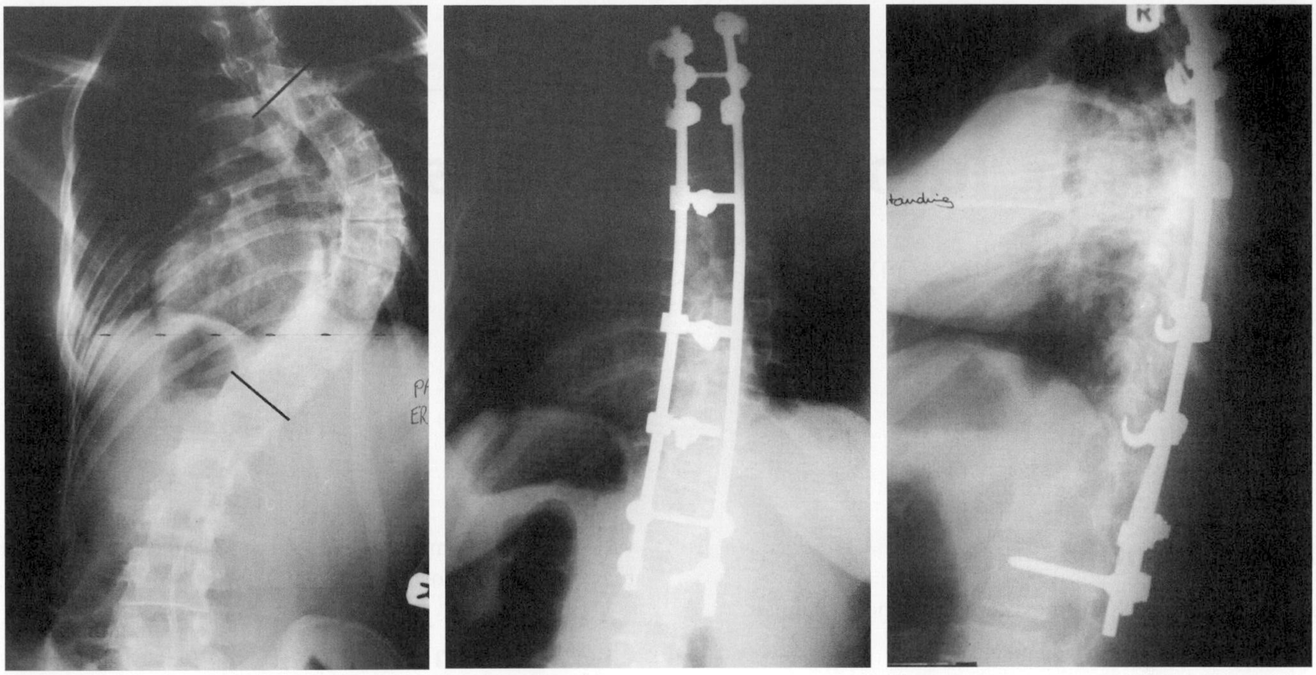

A B C

Fig. 3.9.6 Ultrasound scan for deformity correction. A) Preoperative 70-degree right thoracic idiopathic curve; B) postoperative anteroposterior view; C) postoperative lateral view.

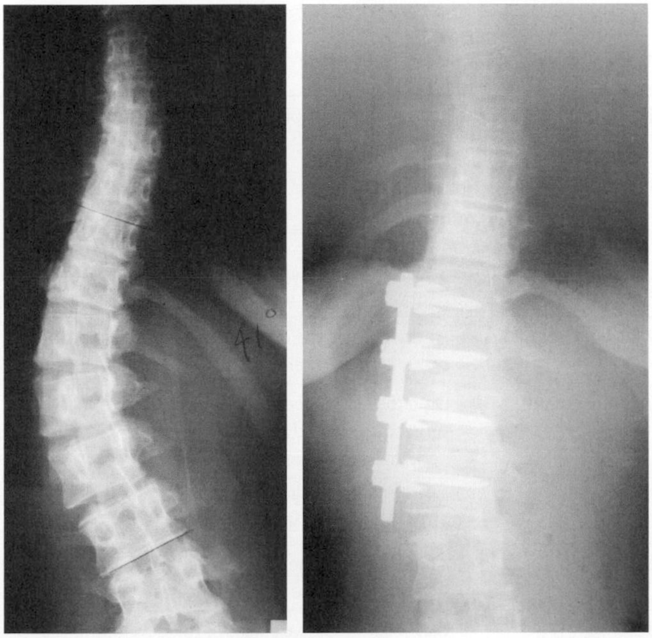

A B

Fig. 3.9.7 Ultrasound scan short-segment anterior fusion of the spine from T12 to L3 for thoracolumbar scoliosis.

system once the screw head has been crimped onto the cable) and a derotation device which allows superior correction. The disadvantage of this system is that the threaded rods are fiddly and the rod-tightening process is tedious. The rod fracture rate was 10–20%. The Webb–Morley system used a soft rod which is placed in tension like the Dwyer cable, but each screw can be individually adjusted. The TSRH system and latterly the USS2 have also been adapted to the front of the spine (Figure 3.9.7). Here it is possible to use a rod-rotation manoeuvre to obtain correction, as well as pulling the implants onto a prebent rod.

Risk management (Box 3.9.4)

Spinal surgery has become one of the leading specialities involved in litigation (second to obstetrics in the United Kingdom). Good practice and risk management should become second nature to a spine surgeon. Litigation often arises where patient's expectations of the outcome of a procedure are not matched to reality. The surgeon should give a reasoned account of the possible natural history of the condition (not always easy to do) and a careful explanation of the risks as well as the benefits of a procedure. Careful and regular record-keeping is essential, especially where difficult decisions are involved and when things are going wrong. The consent process is often prolonged, and may be aided by counselling by non-medical practitioners (we use experienced physiotherapists) and contact with other patients who have had similar procedures.

3.10

Idiopathic scoliosis

Jeremy Fairbank

Summary points

- Idiopathic scoliosis is the most common type of scoliosis
- It affects predominantly adolescent females
- Management depends on severity, cosmesis, and prognosis.

Introduction

Terms used in the discussion of scoliosis are defined in Table 3.10.1. Curve patterns are summarized in Table 3.10.2.

Incidence

About 80% of new cases of scoliosis have adolescent idiopathic scoliosis (AIS). Infantile and juvenile idiopathic scolioses comprise 0.5–4% and 7–10% respectively of all idiopathic scoliosis. In the 1950s the incidence of infantile idiopathic scoliosis in Europe was high compared with that in North America; current figures are comparable. Up to 10% of adolescents have minor scolioses of less than 10 degrees. The incidence of these small angles is equivalent in boys and girls. A Cobb angle of 10 degrees is generally accepted as the criterion above which a scoliosis exists. The larger the curve, the greater is the female-to-male ratio (Table 3.10.3).

Aetiology

The aetiology of idiopathic scoliosis remains elusive. Most work has focused on AIS, and it is clear that a complex and probably multifactorial process is involved. Naturally occurring scoliosis in vertebrates is seen almost exclusively in humans, although a number of animal models for the condition exist. There are many observed differences between convexity and concavity, but it is difficult to distinguish those factors that may be causing the curve from those that may result from it. Current thinking is that there is a defect of central processing or control which plays on a growing spine whose susceptibility to deformation varies from one individual to another. Girls may be more vulnerable to this process because they have a shorter and more rapid adolescent growth of spine than boys. Genetic studies have now identified areas of interest on various chromosomes that predispose to scoliosis and may prove to be the most important aetiological factor.

Classification

A spectrum of curve patterns has been classified, either to aid decisions of surgical management or (in one case) to define bracing decisions. There has been increasing interest in the sagittal as opposed to the coronal profile of the spine. Classification by surface

Table 3.10.1 Definitions and glossary

Scoliosis	Lateral curvature of the spine in an otherwise healthy person
Early onset scoliosis	
(Infantile)	0–3 years
(Juvenile)	3–10 years
Adolescent	> 10 years
Apical vertebra	At the apex of the curve, which is usually horizontal on an anteroposterior erect radiograph
Curve direction	Described by direction of convexity (note that spine surgeons frequently use radiographs as if seen from behind—the opposite of convention)
End vertebrae	Most tilted with respect to horizontal plane of erect radiograph above and below apical vertebra
Cobb angle	Angle between the apical vertebrae (an analogous system may be used for the measurement of kyphosis)
Risser sign	Classification of five stages of the development of the iliac apophysis on an anteroposterior film of the iliac crests (as seen on an anteroposterior radiograph of the spine). The apophysis develops from lateral to medial before fusing: 0, no apophysis; 1, 25%; 2, 50%; 3, 75%; 4, 100%; 5, closure
Lordosis	Reverse curve of spine (opposite of kyphosis)
Structural curve	A curve which does not correct on side-bending
Compensatory curve	A curve which does correct on side-bending

Table 3.10.2 Classification of curve patterns by anatomic site

Pattern	Anatomy	Apical vertebra direction	End vertebra/range	King classification of thoracic curves
Single major curve	High thoracic	T1 or T2 (rarely C7)		
	Thoracic	T4–6	Upper T4–6	Kings III (King IV pattern is 'long' thoracic curve extending into lumbar spine)
		Convex to right	Lower T11–L2	
	Thoracolumbar	T12–L1	Upper T8–10 Lower L3	
	Lumbar	L2		
			Upper T11–L1 Lower L4–5	
Major/minor curve	Major thoracic/minor lumbar	Usually right thoracic curve	Upper curve T4/5–T12 Lower curve T12–L4/5	King II
Double major curve	Thoracic/lumbar	Usually right thoracic curve	Upper T4/6–T10/12	King I
		Apex T7/8 and left lumbar, apex L1/2	Lower T10/12–L4/5	
	Thoracic/thoracolumbar	Apex T6/7; usually convex to right	Upper T4–T9/10	
		Apex T11/12; convex to left	Lower T9/10–L3	
	Thoracic/thoracic	Upper apex T3/4 convex to left lower apex within thoracic spine, convex to right (the upper curve is easily missed on conventional radiographs, and is structural on side-bending)	Upper T1/2–T5/6	King V
			Lower T5/6–T11/L2	
Multiple curve patterns		Usually short and there is little deformity		

topography is still poorly defined, although this is likely to be important in assessing outcome. The Cobb angle (the coronal profile of the spine) remains pre-eminent, although this angle is only one component of a complex change following treatment or observation.

A reliable method of classification is anatomical, describing the direction of the convexity of the curve and the level of the apical vertebra and is widely used whereas the King–Moe classification (Figure 3.10.1), which divides thoracic curves into five types, is now less used. Limitations of the King–Moe classification include poor reliability and the fact that only the coronal plane is considered and scoliosis is a three-dimensional deformity.

Lenke and coworkers have also developed a classification designed to help surgical decisions in response to dissatisfaction with the King–Moe system. This classification considers structural versus compensatory curves and introduces for the first time the sagittal plane and as important modifier. This system is now widely used but its complexity and poor reproducability often precludes day to day use in the clinical setting for all but the most common curve patterns.

Table 3.10.3 Prevalence of adolescent idiopathic scoliosis

Cobb angle	Prevalence	Female-to-male ratio
< 10°	100/1000	1:1
> 10°	20–30/1000	8:1
> 20°	3–5/1000	—
> 30°	2–3/1000	—

Natural history

There have been a number of retrospective reviews of untreated AIS, although most of these series are small. The detailed review by

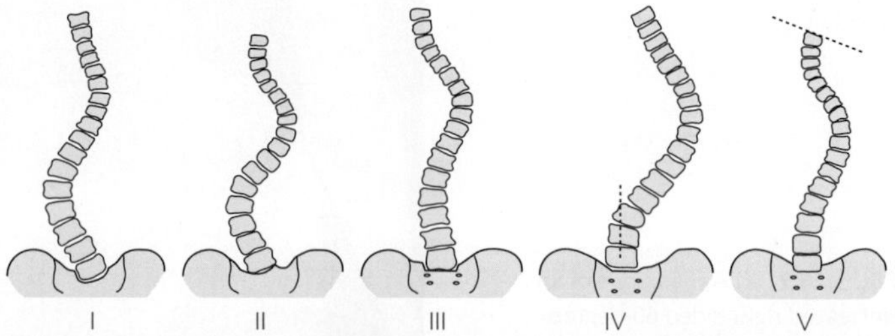

Fig. 3.10.1 King–Moe classification system for idiopathic scoliosis: type I, primary lumbar curve greater than the compensatory thoracic curve; type II, primary thoracic curve with compensatory lumbar curve; type III, short pure thoracic curve; type IV, long C-shaped thoracolumbar curve; type V, double thoracic curve with extension into cervical spine and compensatory lumbar curve.

Weinstein in 1999 is an excellent source for these. It is unlikely that further reviews of the natural history of this condition will be possible, as treatment is widely available. It might be self-evident that the more severe the curve at skeletal maturity, the more problems arise, but this accurate generalization is often wrong in individual cases. At one time it was claimed that curves did not progress in adults, but this is clearly not the case for curves greater than 30 degrees. Even so, progression is unpredictable with one adult progressing by 8 degrees and another by 80 degrees. An annual increment of 1 degree can be expected for curves greater than 40 degrees at skeletal maturity. Double curves, lumbar curves (without thoracic cage support), and curves in association with imbalance tend to progress more rapidly.

Cardiorespiratory function

This is not usually an issue in AIS, although an untreated early-onset curve may be bad enough to affect vital capacity. Curves of less than 70 degrees have no measurable effect on vital capacity. Significant reductions in vital capacity occur in curves greater than 100 degrees and, if severe enough, may eventually cause cor pulmonale and shortened life expectancy.

Cosmesis

This is a crucial consequence of AIS. Thoracic curves are associated with a rib hump dependent on the degree of rotation of the apical vertebra. The rib hump ranges from the trivial to the very conspicuous and often it is an oblique shoulder line or pelvis that causes a problem. The distress caused to the patient is very variable, and some will find the risks of surgery justified for very small humps. Others prefer to tolerate a deformity which can be concealed with appropriate clothing. The level of distress should not be underestimated (Figure 3.10.2). It is often the justification for prolonged non-operative treatment and much major surgery in this area. We studied the assessment of cosmesis and developed a scoring system which relates to assessment by independent reviewer. Patient perception may bear only limited relation to the severity of the curve. The Scoliosis Research Society Score attempts to quantify the cosmetic impact of the deformity allowing studies to be performed although little has been published in this important area.

Lumbar curves are usually less conspicuous than thoracic curves, although they can have an adverse effect on the waistline. Double curves tend to be inconspicuous, but are more prone to progression. Truncal imbalance may cause distress. Curve progression may be associated with loss of height in adults.

Pain

Back pain is common, and there is limited evidence that scoliosis is a major cause of back pain. Thoracic curves in general do not cause significant pain in adolescents, although some do experience apical pain. There is deterioration in the thoracic curve in some adults, especially during pregnancy, and they may experience significant pain.

Thoracolumbar and lumbar curves are more likely to cause back pain. Relief is often provided by lying and precipitated by standing or walking as the day goes on. This is one of the most common reasons for scoliosis surgery in adults, and occasionally in adolescents. Pain is more likely when translation (lateral subluxation) occurs, where one vertebra moves laterally on the one below. This may occur in both primary and secondary curves.

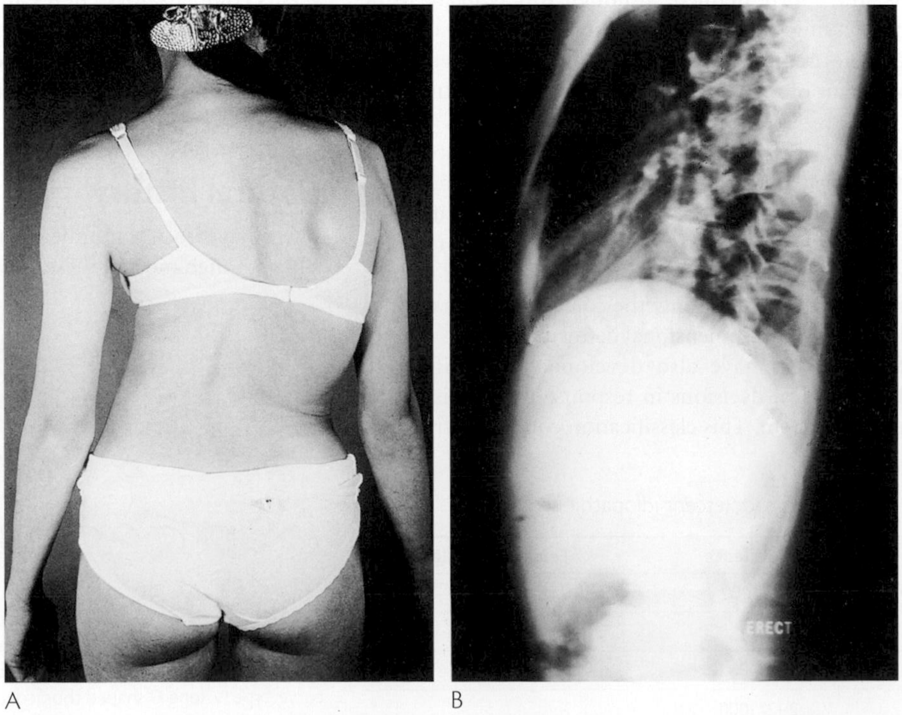

Fig. 3.10.2 A) Appearance of an untreated right-sided 60-degree thoracic curve. B) Lateral view of the thoracic spine showing the lordosis seen in idiopathic scoliosis. This is an important element in the cosmetic deformity.

Pregnancy

There is little evidence that the management of pregnancy should be altered in any way because of treated or untreated scoliosis. Epidurals may not be possible if the lumbar spine has been fused posteriorly. Pregnancy may be associated with additional curve progression, but studies have shown variable results.

Neurological problems

Spinal cord compression is a not a problem in untreated AIS. Secondary degenerative changes in the lumbar spine may cause root compression.

Progression during growth

Understanding the potential for progression is the key to management. The probability for progression depends on the following:

- Growth potential
- The severity of the curve
- The site of the curve.

Growth potential

A growth chart is the easiest way to see growth potential. Menarche is an important landmark for spinal growth, which occurs most rapidly in the first year premenarche. The Risser sign is the best radiological indicator of growth potential. If the iliac apophysis has not appeared, or has only just appeared, curves are more likely to progress (Risser 0 or 1; see Table 3.10.1).

Curve severity

The larger the curve at presentation, the more inevitable is progression. Sixty-eight per cent of curves in the range 20–29 degrees will progress in children with Risser signs of 0 or 1. Curves of over 30 degrees almost invariably progress if there is significant growth potential. Curves of over 50 degrees at skeletal maturity will progress during adult life with an annual increment of at least 1 degree. Some curves in the range 30–50 degrees will progress in adults.

Site of curve

Double curves are more likely to progress than single curves as are lumbar curves and thoracolumbar curves without thoracic cage support.

Management

Management options are observation, bracing, and surgery. Exercises and physiotherapy regimens are widely used but evidence for efficacy remains anecdotal. Plaster beds and localizer casts are of historical note.

Risks and benefits have to be carefully considered against the severity and potential for deterioration for each individual. The clinician has to be clear on the expectations of patients and their families, and on their capacity to comply with treatment. Careful counselling is essential, and this may require more than one visit to the clinic before treatment is initiated.

Initial assessment

A full history includes birth history, age of menarche, childhood illnesses, and family history. Symptoms of the curve, including pain and deformity, and how it originally was discovered should be noted. Pain, if present, needs a full evaluation. Commonly this may be fatigue or apical pain. The pain may be remote from the curve and, especially in adults, irrelevant to it. Pain severity is assessed by its effects on daily life and analgesic intake (if any). Sometimes there may be neurological symptoms of significance such as paraesthesia or numbness. Where relevant, a history of interventions is essential.

Examination

Height, weight, sitting height, and span should be recorded on a growth chart. Look at the facies, eyes, and palate. The shape and relative height of the shoulders should be noted, as well as the position of the scapulae. A plumb line from the vertebra prominens allows measurement of any truncal imbalance. Lordosis and kyphosis should be reviewed. Examination should include an assessment of the deformity and its flexibility. The forward-bending test allows assessment of the site and severity of any rib hump (see Chapter 3.9; Figure 3.10.1). Leg length, limb asymmetry, and foot deformities should be noted, and a full inspection of the skin for hairy patches, skin tethering or dimples, and café au lait spots should be performed. Look for evidence of joint laxity. A careful neurological examination should be carried out, paying particular attention to lower-limb reflexes and abdominal reflexes. Cord anomalies may occur without neurological signs or with very subtle signs. Assess the stage of puberty. Pubic hair appears in boys before their growth spurt. Axial hair appears when there is little or no spinal growth in both sexes.

Radiography

All efforts should be made to minimize exposure of the growing child to radiation. There is good evidence that excessive radiography in children increases cancer risk in later life. A request for imaging should be justified by a defined therapeutic gain in every case. The spine is assessed by standardized erect anteroposterior and lateral radiographs. Long cassettes should be used if available. Both views should ideally show the head to the proximal femur. Various techniques, including rare-earth screening, have been developed to minimize radiation requirements. Some centres have used coned lateral views of the lumbosacral junction to identify a spondylolysis, but the number of exposures needed to pick up each case is not justified. Supine anteroposterior bending or traction radiographs are needed to define the flexibility of the curve if surgery is impending, but not as part of curve monitoring. In some cases, such as small infants, supine radiographs are best. Comparable views are needed to detect progress.

Follow-up anteroposterior radiographs are widely used, unless the unit is equipped with a device to measure surface topography such as ISIS (see Chapter 3.9; Figure 3.10.2) or Quantec. There is some evidence, at least for ISIS, that curve progression can be identified earlier than radiography, as the 'rib hump' leads the development of the scoliosis. This method can significantly reduce radiation exposure.

If the curve is painful, of early onset (under 10 years), morphologically unusual or there is any evidence of neurological abnormality (e.g. hairy patch, dimple, absent abdominal reflex, or lower-limb or foot asymmetry), the spinal cord should be investigated. Many centres routinely perform magnetic resonance imaging (MRI) of the entire neural axis in the presence of any spinal deformity to rule out spinal dysraphism which is present in 3% of so-called 'idiopathic curves'. Before any surgery, MRI scan is mandatory. These abnormalities include Arnold–Chiari malformations, syrinx, tethered cord, and diastatomyelia. Computed tomography is rarely indicated in adolescent idiopathic scoliosis.

Counselling

Patients and their parents will need a careful explanation of the condition. In many cultures the majority of people have never have heard of the condition. Parents require reassurance that they have not failed in their duty of care to their child. Curves can appear remarkably quickly, so that large curves can present in families familiar with the condition and with a sibling already affected. It is worth checking siblings with a forward-bending test if they are available in the clinic. Parents may rarely see their teenage children's backs. Patients' organizations for scoliotics exist in many countries, and some families obtain considerable support and comfort from them (examples are http://www.sauk.org.uk; http://www.srs.org/). Many surgeons have systems in which their experienced patients counsel new ones, particularly those considering surgical treatment. This system needs to be monitored with care to prevent inaccurate or insensitive advice being given.

Treatment options

Treatment options are observation, bracing, or surgery. The surgeon needs to consider the natural history of the curve, and the aspirations and expectations of the patient and his or her family. Treatment places considerable demands on all family members. Some interventions are difficult to sustain in a dysfunctional individual or family. Generally the child or adolescent will decide which treatment option is chosen. If this different from the expectations of the rest of the family, long-term resentments can arise. The family practitioner needs to be kept closely informed of the clinician's advice.

Observation

Positive aspects

Generally this option is safe. A small curve with a low probability of progression is easy to monitor. The younger child with a small curve may need to be viewed every 4–6 months, depending on growth rate. The passage of time allows the family to absorb the implications of other treatment options.

Negative aspects

The timing of intervention, particularly bracing, may be difficult. In retrospect it is easy to see when treatment has been instituted too late.

Bracing

Many braces have been designed for the treatment of scoliosis. Controversy exists as to what a brace is actually doing (see Chapter 3.14).

Positive aspects

Much controversy surrounds brace treatment. There is one controlled trial comparing the patients of surgeons with a high threshold to bracing with those with a low threshold, which shows small but significant advantages in the treatment group. More recently, a meta-analysis of bracing and natural history papers came out in favor of bracing.

Negative aspects

Brace compliance may be poor. A review suggests that the full conventional regimen of wearing the brace for 23h per day is best. This is difficult for most teenagers, although younger patients usually comply better. Most regimens allow the brace to be removed for sports. Brace wearing from a very young age to adolescence is not usually needed. This regimen may be bitterly resented by the child, and can become a cause of emotional warfare between the child and his or her parents. Blame is then assigned if the regimen fails and surgery is required. Bracing compliance varies with culture and is much more difficult in hot countries. Some studies of brace compliance have cast doubt on how much the brace is actually worn (a conspiracy between children and their parents), while other studies show good accord between compliance and diary. Much depends on the quality of the brace maker and the support services for the families. Braces are expensive, and may need to be changed frequently in a rapidly growing child.

Surgery

The objective in most cases is to fuse the spine in the best possible position. In the past this was achieved using either plaster beds or localizer casts, and required prolonged immobilization (up to a year). These operations were dogged by high pseudarthrosis rates, and were confined to a few dedicated surgeons and patients. The first successful spinal implant was the Harrington rod, which was developed in Texas in the late 1940s and early 1950s during a horrendous poliomyelitis epidemic. Many other implant systems have followed.

Positive aspects

Modern surgical treatment allows early mobilization and often avoids the need for postoperative jacketing and bracing. The pseudarthrosis rate is low; indeed, it is now almost unheard of in AIS.

Negative aspects

This is major surgery with a small but significant risk of spinal cord damage. The Stagnara wake-up test was an important advance, but has been superseded by the clonus test and, more generally, by various forms of spinal cord monitoring. The wake-up test involves voluntary movement of the feet and hands during the surgery. The clonus test exploits the normal phenomenon that clonus can be elicited during the normal waking process. If it is absent, it suggests an interruption of the normal reflex pattern.

Spinal cord monitoring can be sensory, motor, or both. Sensory monitoring is easier and is widely used. Potentials evoked by peripheral nerve or distal spinal cord stimulation are detected by an epidural or cortical electrode. Motor evoked potentials are detected peripherally following magnetic transcranial stimulation or direct stimulation of the spinal cord. Anaesthetic techniques may have to be adjusted to make this possible.

None of these methods are foolproof. The incidence of complication is difficult to determine, although in the 1970s the Scoliosis Research Society collected data suggesting that the risk of paraplegia was 1%. This figure may be too high with current methods, although it is widely used by scoliosis surgeons when counselling their patients for surgery. Early infection is fortunately rare, although a high incidence of unexpected infection has been found with normally non-pathogenic organisms such as *Propionibacterium acnes* when rods are removed late for pain. Patients should therefore be warned of this late complication as part of the consent process.

Spinal instrumentation and spinal fusion

Preinstrumentation era

Up to the 1950s, none of the various attempts that had been made to develop implants for the stabilization of the spine had been successful. The majority of spinal fusions were obtained by prolonged immobilization in plaster beds or with the use of plaster localizer jackets. Spinal fusion was first described in 1911 by Hibbs and Albee independently in the United States. Fusion, usually using autograft, is an essential component of spinal surgery. If fusion is not used, or fails, the implants will inevitably fail eventually. In the 1940s Allen, in the United Kingdom, developed a bottle-screw device for the instrumentation of scoliosis.

Harrington rod era

This device was developed in Texas in Harrington's garage. It was the surgeon's response to the overwhelming poliomyelitis epidemics of the time, which resulted in aggressive and progressive spinal deformities in small children. It consists of a distraction hook, where the upper hook can be moved away from the lower hook on a ratchet. The hooks were initially placed under the laminas. It was immediately successful, although Harrington did not publish until he was sure of the results. Although some modifications were made to the system, it has remained a gold standard for subsequent spinal implants (Figure 3.10.3).

Anterior spinal surgery

Unfortunately, although impressive results were obtained with the Harrington rod, it was not ideal for treating the severe postpolio deformities. Again, it was this condition which, in the late 1960s, led Dwyer, in Australia, to develop his screw and cable system for use on the front of the spine. This was one of the first orthopaedic implants to be made of titanium. This approach revolutionized spinal surgery, although it was many years before anterior spinal surgery became widely adopted. Credit for this goes to Hodgson,

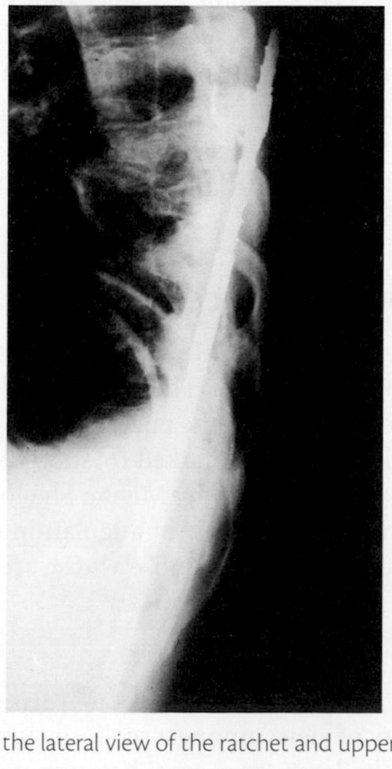

Fig. 3.10.3 Detail of the lateral view of the ratchet and upper hook of a Harrington rod.

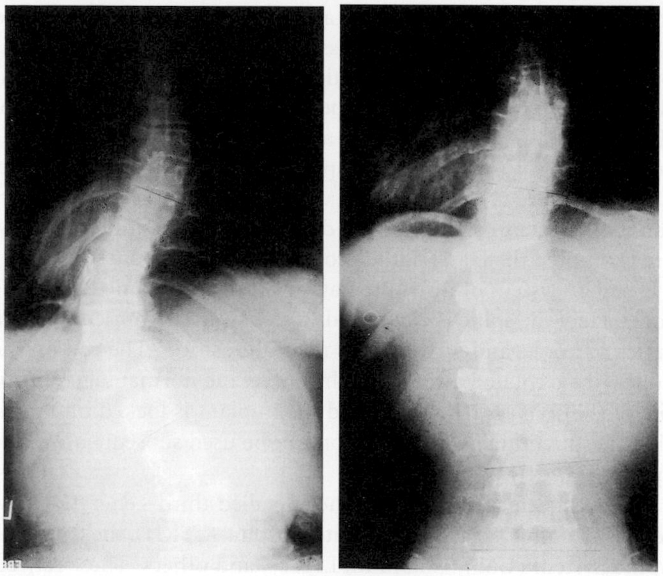

A B

Fig. 3.10.4 A) A left-sided thoracolumbar idiopathic scoliosis. B) The same curve treated by an anterior approach using a short-segment fixation (Webb–Morley implant).

a British expatriate surgeon in Hong Kong, who combined Dwyer instrumentation with the Harrington rod. The anterior approach proved to be a most effective method in the management of deforming spinal tuberculosis. Figure 3.10.4 shows the use of a Webb–Morley implant which evolved from the Dwyer system.

Segmental fixation

Once again it was poliomyelitis which precipitated Eduardo Luque of Mexico City to develop a technique based on an earlier Portuguese idea of sublaminar wires. The wires were passed under the lamina of each segment and over a pair of stainless steel rods, which were contoured to the desired shape of the spine. Each rod was bent at right angles at one end (L-rod). This proved to be a productive, economical, and powerful technique for the management of neuromuscular scoliosis. It has been used for all types of scoliosis.

It is a powerful method, but has gained a reputation for a high risk of spinal cord damage. This relates not only to the sublaminar wires, but also to the possibilities offered for overvigorous correction. The technique was modified by adapting it to Harrington rods. This allows the spine to be pulled onto a bent Harrington rod to obtain correction without too much distraction—the Harri–Luque technique. This depends on a modification of the Harrington rod where the rod locks into a square rather than a round socket in the lower hook. This has proved effective in the management of AIS, although it has been superseded by later methods.

Luque rods were also modified to allow pelvic fixation—the Galveston technique. This is still used in the management of neuromuscular curves. Another modification is the joining of the two rods into a rectangle. A variety of versions of this are available, including the Hartshill rectangle.

Double-rod systems

Cotrel and Dubousset (CD) in France developed a whole new concept of correction of scoliosis. Cotrel tried various modifications of the Harrington system including a link between the distraction rod on the concavity and a compression rod on the convexity. This produced a better correction of the curve. He came to realize that this had been obtained at the expense of increasing the rotation of the curve. Although others had appreciated this before, scoliosis surgeons began to realize the importance of rotation of the spine. Dickson in Leeds revitalized the concept of lordosis as an important component of the thoracic deformity of idiopathic scoliosis. He promoted the Harri–Luque concept on the contoured rod.

The CD system of instrumentation was the outcome of Cotrel's ideas. Here the spine is connected to a contoured knurled rod by a series of hooks and screws in its neutral position. The rod on the concavity is rotated away from the curve, the normal sagittal profile of the spine is recovered, and the implant is locked into position. Distraction and compression can be used subsequently. This system is widely used.

CD has been superseded by the so-called third-generation systems, including Texas Scottish-Rite Hospital (TSRH), the Universal Spine System (USS), Colorado, Legacy, and others. These rely on two rods and increasingly an emphasis is placed on apical translation and derotation with more advance rod connection mechanisms. The concave rod can be contoured and the spine is then pulled towards the rod. There is some evidence (notably for the USS system) that this method improves derotation compared with the CD system (Figures 3.10.5 and 3.10.6) although the benefit of more recent innovations and the use of pedicle screws in isolation are under evaluation.

The revolution in spinal implants has had some important consequences:

1) These powerful techniques probably increase the risks of spinal cord injury compared with a simple Harrington rod procedure; although in most cases the improved correction is self-evident. However, this is counteracted by improved techniques, reduced operative time, and state-of-the-art spinal cord monitoring techniques

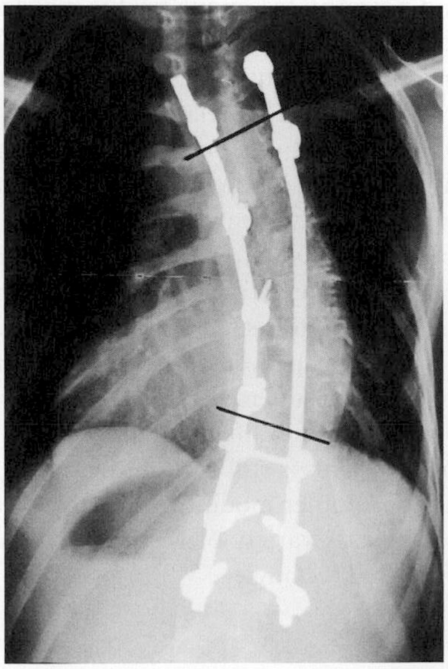

Fig. 3.10.5 A right-sided thoracic curve treated with a USS implant. Note the use of both hooks and screws.

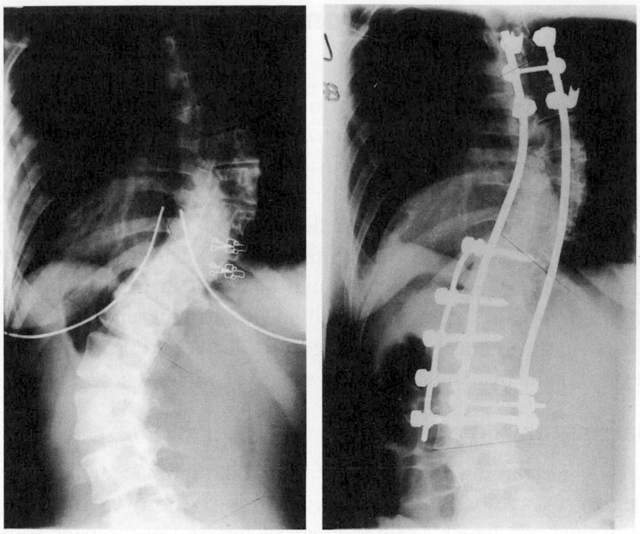

A B

Fig. 3.10.6 A) A double idiopathic curve (King I). B) The same curve treated with combined anterior instrumentation (Webb–Morley implant) and posterior USS instrumentation.

2) Pseudarthrosis has become an increasingly rare risk with the advances in surgical technique summarized previously. However, none of these techniques is possible without strict adherence to classical methods of spinal surgery. These include scrupulous subperiosteal dissection out to the tips of the transverse processes, excision of facet (apophyseal) joints, and bone grafting. Autologous bone is best, although other sources of bone can be used. It should be placed on laminas and transverse processes which have been carefully decorticated

3) Infection remains a matter of concern, particularly since the introduction of double-rod systems. In our practice, removing the implant (assuming that the fused area has united) usually cures late pain. There is some evidence of immunological suppression after major spinal surgery. There is also a strong suspicion that more metal increases the risk of infection. We, and others, have grown *Propionibacterium acnes* from cases developing pain several years after apparently successful surgery. At this stage removal of the metalwork resolves the problem (Figure 3.10.6).

Infantile idiopathic scoliosis

This condition is distinct from AIS. It is much less common, and is more frequent in boys than girls. The direction of the curve is more frequently to the left. Many of the curves improve or even resolve with observation. Curves with marked rotation are much less likely to resolve, as was demonstrated by Mehta. She found that a measurement reflecting the difference of angulation of the ribs at the apex of the curve was higher in those whose scoliosis progressed (Figure 3.10.7).

Conclusion

There is a diversity of views amongst scoliosis surgeons on decision management in the large 'grey area' between patients presenting

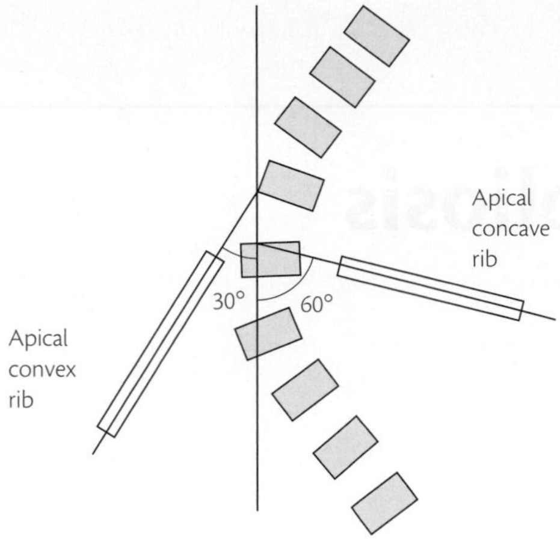

Fig. 3.10.7 Rib–vertebral angle difference (RVAD). In this example RVAD = 60 − 30 degrees = 30 degrees. If RVAD is greater than 20 degrees, the curve is likely to progress.

with small curves and little growth potential (where most parties agree that no intervention is needed) and large curves with much growth potential (where surgical intervention is beneficial). Honest discussion with the family is essential, with a careful weighing of risk and benefit of natural history versus intervention. Surgical treatment and bracing both carry serious risks. Future developments require large trials of operative and non-operative management, the development of outcome measures relevant to appearance and cosmesis, and the longer-term issues of pain and disability. Technology to assess surface topography needs further development to enable the effects of time and treatment to be presented to patients and their families.

Further reading

Hidalgo-Ovejero, A.M., García-Mata, S., Martinez-Grande, M., *et al.* (2000). Classification of thoracic adolescent idiopathic scoliosis. *Journal of Bone and Joint Surgery*, **82A**, 901.

Leroux, M.A., Zabjek, K., Simard, G., Badeaux, J., Coillard, C., and Rivard, C.H. (2000). A noninvasive anthropometric technique for measuring kyphosis and lordosis: an application for idiopathic scoliosis. *Spine*, **25**, 1689–94.

Mehta, M. (1972). The rib–vertebra angle in the early diagnosis between resolving and progressive infantile scoliosis. *Journal of Bone and Joint Surgery*, **54B**, 230–43.

Rowe, D., Berbstein, S., Riddick, M., Adler, F., Emans, J., and Gardner-Bonneau, D. (1997). A meta-analysis of the efficacy of non-operative treatments for idiopathic scoliosis. *Journal of Bone and Joint Surgery*, **79A**, 664–74.

Weinstein, S.L. (1999). Natural history of idiopathic scoliosis. *Spine*, **24**, 2592–605.

3.11

Congenital scoliosis and kyphosis

Jeremy Fairbank

Summary points

- Congenital scoliosis and kyphosis accounts for about 20% patients with spinal deformity
- Associated with other developmental anomalies of neuraxis, cardiovascular and urogenital systems.

Introduction

Congenital scoliosis and kyphosis are deformities of the spine in the coronal and sagittal planes caused by failures of formation or segmentation of the spine, or combinations of both. They are due to a combination of genetic and environmental factors (e.g. alcohol). The notochord appears to be a key structure in pathogenesis. The *Pax-1* gene is required for the formation of the ventral parts of the vertebrae during primary segmentation and border formation between structures of the vertebral column. Reduced or impaired *Pax-1* gene expression may lead to failure of segmentation (i.e. border formation) and subsequent vertebral fusions. Vertebral malformation is usually apparent on radiographs or on prenatal ultrasound examination. They are frequently related to other mesodermal and ectodermal anomalies, which often arise from the same segments. Cardiac anomalies are commonly associated with congenital scoliosis, which is often first identified from radiographs taken to manage the cardiac problem. At least 20% of cases of congenital scoliosis have anomalies within the vertebral canal, including syrinx formation, and a divided spinal cord. When this occurs, a diastematomyelia may be found. This is a sagittal fibrous or bony band dividing the vertebral canal, dural sheath, or spinal cord.

Embryology*

The body axis is established during gastrulation. Cells migrate through the primitive streak and the three layers of the embryonic disc are generated. At about 16 days, some cells pass through the anterior tip of the streak (called Hensen's node) to give rise to the notochord. The overlying ectoderm becomes the neural plate, later the neural tube. The paraxial mesoderm differentiates into 42–44 small epithelial spheres with central lumina (somites) in a craniocaudal sequence (Figures 3.11.1A and 3.11.2A). The first five (occipital) somites appear in stage 9 (about 20 days). The dorsolateral

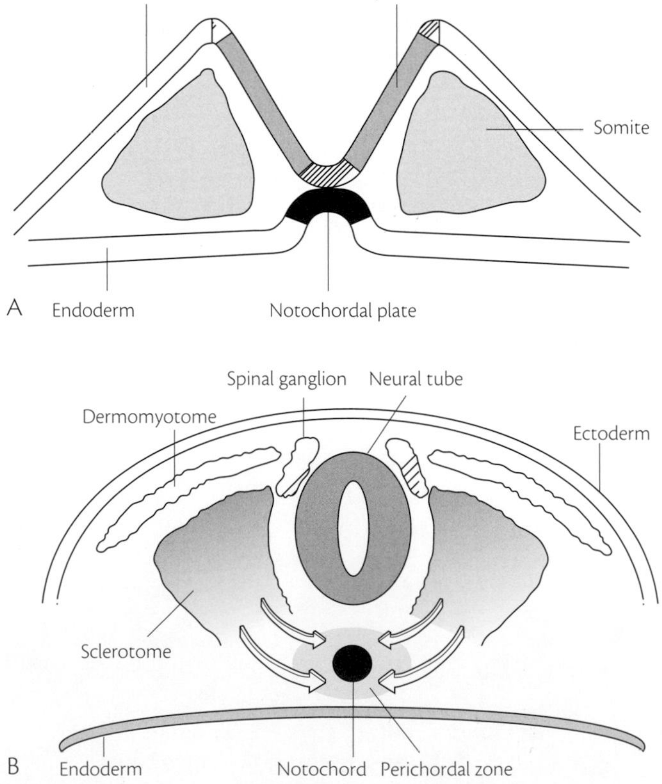

Fig. 3.11.1 Transverse scheme showing somitic development at 3–6 weeks. A) The neural plate develops folds on both sides as the paraxial mesoderm differentiates into somites. The notochordal plate is in close apposition to the closing neural plate. B) The dorsolateral parts of the somites form dermomyotomes, while the ventromedial parts lose their epithelial structure and form sclerotomes. Cells from these areas migrate to surround the notochord and form the perichordal zone.

* Based on chapters written for first edition by K.M. Dávid and H.A. Crockard.

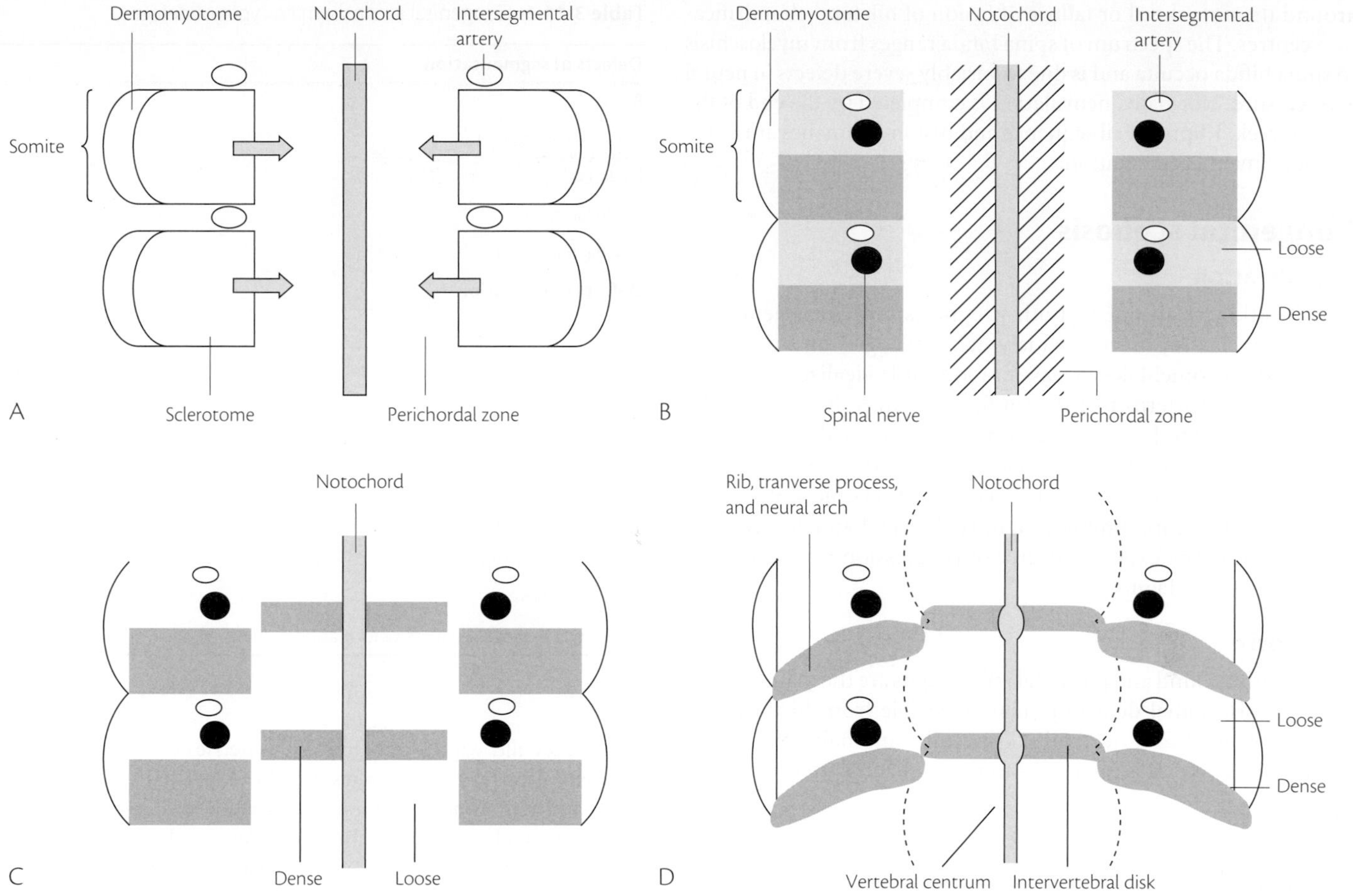

Fig. 3.11.2 Coronal scheme demonstrating the formation of the vertebral column. A) Sclerotome cells migrate towards the midline to form the perichordal zone. B) Cranial (low cellular density) and caudal (high cellular density) areas form the sclerotomes. The perichordal zone is still unsegmented. C) Dense and loose areas develop in the perichordal zone. D) The dense areas in the perichordal zone develop into intervertebral discs and the loose areas develop into vertebral centra.

parts of the somites retain their epithelial arrangement to form dermatomes and myotomes (giving rise to smooth muscle of the dermis and striated trunk musculature respectively). The ventromedial sclerotomes migrate toward the midline to surround the notochord and form the perichordal zone (Figure 3.11.1B).

The lateral part of each sclerotome shows a division to loose cranial and dense caudal halves in stage 13 (about 28 days) (Figure 3.11.2B). The loose cranial halves contain the spinal nerves, dorsal roots, ganglia, and the intersegmental vessels, while the dense caudal halves give rise to the lateral processes (ribs and transverse processes) and neural arches of the vertebrae.

At stage 14 (about 32 days), the perichordal zone also shows zones of high and low cell density axially (Figure 3.11.2C). The zone of high cell density contributes to the formation of intervertebral discs, whereas the low-density areas develop into the centra of the vertebrae. Two somites contribute to each vertebral body on both sides. The only deviation from this rule is the five occipital somites forming basiocciput, which becomes the clivus.

Chondrification of the vertebral column begins at 6 post-ovulatory weeks in the vertebral bodies and progresses dorsally and ventrally to the neural arches and rib anlagen.

The first signs of ossification are detectable at about 9 weeks and at birth there are three ossification centres for each vertebra, one for the vertebral body and one for each neural arch. Bony union between these primary ossification centres begins during early childhood. At puberty, secondary ossification centres (apophyses) appear at the tips of spinous processes and vertebral endplates. Atypical vertebrae (atlas, axis, and sacrum) show special patterns of ossification. The notochord expands in the area of discs forming the nucleus pulposus. The notochordal cells disappear by about 10 years. Axial position and vertebral phenotype along the embryonic axis is an early event controlled by the combinatorial expression of Hox genes.

Clinical significance

Common vertebral congenital anomalies are spina bifida, hemivertebrae, wedge vertebrae and fusions. Scoliosis involves deviation and rotation of vertebral bodies and congenital scoliosis may be caused by hemivertebrae and wedge vertebrae and by vertebral bars. Hemivertebrae have an absence of one chondrification centre or possibly lateral deviation of the notochord. A vertebral bar is a localized failure of segmentation. Posterolaterally it will result in progressive combination of lordosis and scoliosis. Anteriorly it will cause progressive kyphosis. Butterfly vertebrae (sagittal cleft vertebrae) are perhaps due to an inadequate amount of sclerotome cells around the notochord or failure of fusion of bilateral chondrification centres. The spectrum of spina bifida ranges from myeloschisis to spina bifida occulta and is due to variably severe defects in neural tube closure. Normally, neurulation is completed by the end of the fourth week. Klippel–Feil sequence and fusion anomalies are a failure of primary segmentation.

Congenital scoliosis

Classification

Classification is an aid to both prognosis and treatment. The McMaster classification is widely acknowledged and based on untreated outcome. Like all classifications, it is idealized and there will always be patterns that do not fit neatly into the scheme. The McMaster system does not encompass the similar defects seen in congenital kyphosis, nor the developmental anomalies of the posterior elements which may be mistaken for idiopathic scoliosis.

The main types are summarized in Table 3.11.1 and illustrated in Figure 3.11.3. The expected degree of progression for the various types is shown in Figure 3.11.4.

Diagnosis

Prenatal ultrasound and postnatal radiographs are the main method of diagnosis. Spinal deformity may be visible from birth. In the absence of significant deformity, congenital anomalies may come to light at any age. It is important to pay particular attention to the spine of a child with lower-limb asymmetries or foot deformities. Congenital vertebral anomalies may be associated with myelodysplasia and lumbosacral agenesis. They are also seen in the VATER (vertebral–anal–cardiac–tracheo–(o)esophageal–renal) syndrome, the Freeman–Sheldon syndrome, and Larsen's syndrome.

Table 3.11.1 Congenital scoliosis: main types of defect

Defects of segmentation
Bilateral
Block vertebra
Unilateral
Unilateral bar
Unilateral bar and hemivertebra
Defects of formation
Pseudarthrosis/agenesis
Hemivertebra
Unilateral complete failure of formation
Fully segmented
Semisegmented
Incarcerated
Unsegmented
Wedge vertebra
Unilateral partial failure of formation

Box 3.11.1 Management of congenital spinal deformity

- Image the spine in two planes
- A dorsal hemivertebra may threaten the spinal cord as the kyphosis develops
- An unsegmented bar or asymmetry of growth plates can progress malignantly and require early surgery
- MRI is an essential investigation.

Natural history

The majority of malformations occur in the thoracic spine or thoracolumbar junction. Those involving failure of segmentation in the cervical spine are usually known as the Klippel–Feil syndrome (Figure 3.11.5). Affected individuals have a short neck, a low posterior hairline, and limited neck movement. The malformations are associated with a wide variety of anomalies including facial asymmetry, cleft palate, ptosis, facial nerve palsy, deafness, torticollis,

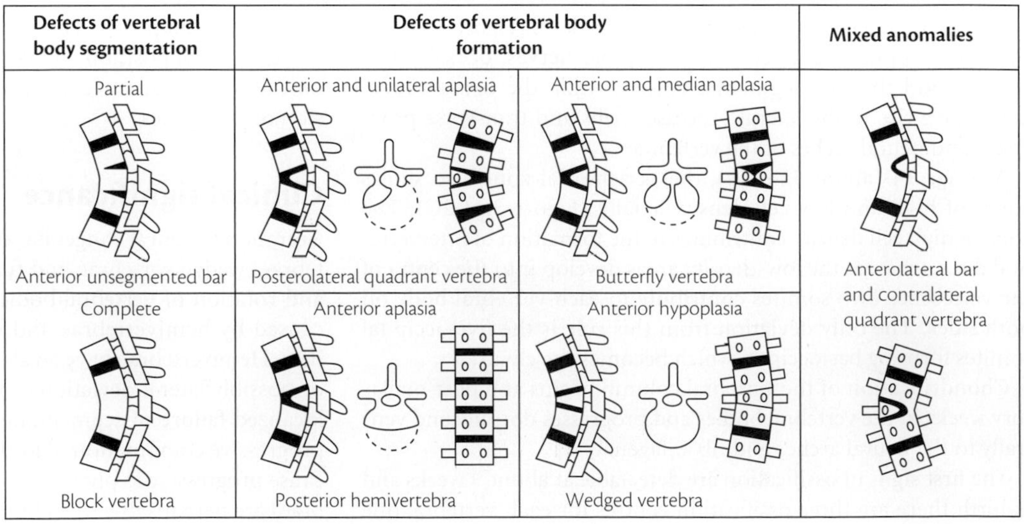

Fig. 3.11.3 Drawings showing the different types of vertebral anomalies that produce a congenital kyphosis or kyphoscoliosis.

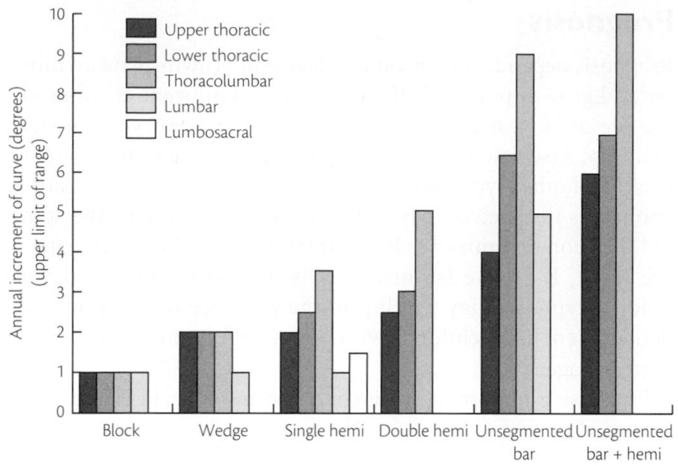

Fig. 3.11.4 Summary of the expected annual progression of the Cobb angle in patients with congenital scoliosis. (Data from McMaster and Ohtsuka (1982).)

webbing of the neck, thoracic scoliosis (both congenital and 'idiopathic' patterns), Sprengel's shoulder, a variety of cardiac anomalies, respiratory problems due to chest deformity, and abnormalities of central control. Up to 20% demonstrate mirror movements of the hands (synkinesia), which may be due to spinal cord anomalies; voluntary movement of one hand is associated with involuntary movement of the other. Thirty per cent of affected individuals have genitourinary tract anomalies. A hemivertebra at the lumbosacral junction causes a particularly severe deformity and requires early surgical treatment. Vertebral anomalies at the cervicothoracic junction usually cannot be corrected surgically, and require early fusion *in situ*. Occasionally there are anomalies separated by apparently normal vertebrae. Curves may develop above and below congenital anomalies, as well as the more usual pattern with the anomaly at the apex of the curve. Neurological deficit is very unusual in scoliosis, unless there is spinal cord anomaly or diastematomyelia. It is common in congenital kyphosis.

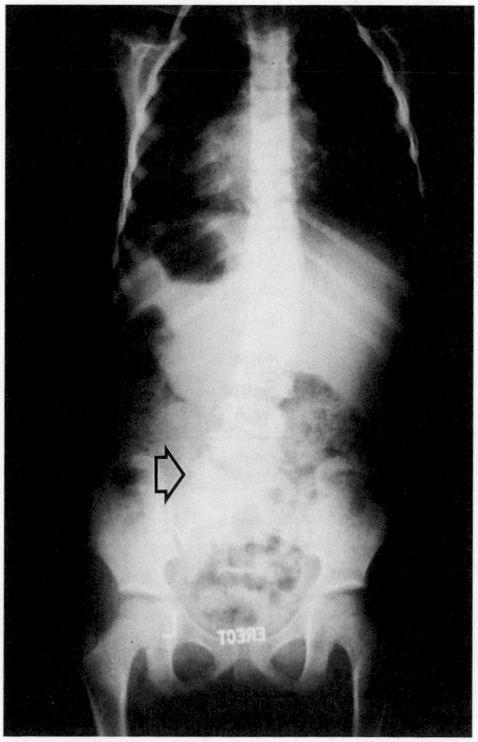

Fig. 3.11.5 L5 hemivertebra.

Congenital kyphosis

This may occur through failure of formation, failure of segmentation, and rotatory dislocation of the spine. Failure of formation may occur, very rarely with, or without dislocation of the vertebral canal. A dorsal hemivertebra will cause a kyphosis. This will be more severe if the vertebral body does not form at all. These are dangerous deformities, and usually progress and may cause spinal cord compression. This produces an insidious myelopathy, which may not be recognized until the deficit is profound. If left untreated, these deformities eventually cause a complete paraplegia. Therefore they require early surgery. An unusual, but particularly dangerous, pattern is when a congenital scoliosis is combined with a kyphotic element and dislocation of the canal. This requires fusion *in situ* at diagnosis.

Natural history

McMaster and Singh have published a series of 112 patients with congenital kyphosis. They distinguished 68 patients with type I kyphosis (failure of anterior formation of a vertebral body), 24 with type II (failure of anterior segmentation), and 12 with type III (mixed type). Eight were unclassifiable (Type IV). These anomalies can occur at any level in the spine, but 66% of all types had an apex between T10 and L1. All progressed during adolescence, but certain patterns were particularly dangerous.

Differential diagnosis

Infantile idiopathic scoliosis is diagnosed in the absence of recognized congenital malformations. Congenital scoliosis is seen in some rare syndromes such as spondylothoracic dysplasia (Jacko–Levin syndrome), the VATER association, Goldenhar syndrome, Russell–Silver syndrome, Williams syndrome, and rarely in common syndromes such as Down syndrome. Freeman–Sheldon syndrome and Larsen's syndrome may also have congenital spinal deformities.

Presentation

Cases may present throughout life, although the majority of severe cases will present in the first 2 years of life. Prenatal ultrasound identifies an increasing proportion of cases.

Cases are often spotted by the parents, and a low threshold for requesting spinal radiography is needed when there is clinical suspicion of spinal deformity. A common reason for referral to a spine surgeon is diagnosis from a chest radiograph taken during investigation of cardiac anomalies found at routine postnatal examination.

There may be anomalies of posterior elements that are undiagnosed. They may be found incidentally during surgery of 'idiopathic' scoliosis and risk surgical damage to the cord.

Associated anomalies

There is a high incidence of associated anomalies in children with congenital scoliosis, since this is a defect of development of both the mesoderm and the ectoderm. These include spinal, cardiac, and urogenital anomalies. Rib anomalies are commonly associated with the vertebral anomalies.

Spinal canal

Intraspinal anomalies include neurenteric and epidermoid cysts, lipofibromas, teratoma, absent or duplicated nerve roots, filum terminale thickening or tethering, bone or fibrous spurs (diastematomyelia), and diplomyelia. These are best identified by magnetic resonance imaging (MRI), which is an essential preoperative investigation.

Skin

Skin dimples, naevi, and hairy patches over the spine should be treated with suspicion. Masses due to lipomata or meningoceles, or the scars of closed meningoceles are also an indication for radiography. There is a probable relationship between spinal dysraphism and congenital scoliosis.

Lower limb

Any baby presenting with lower-limb anomalies or leg-length discrepancies should have the spine examined clinically, and probably radiologically. If a congenital scoliosis has been diagnosed, look for asymmetries of the legs and feet, and foot anomalies such as clubfoot, vertical talus, cavus foot, etc. Neurological examination should include looking for wasting of muscles and reflex alteration or asymmetry. Unexplained trophic changes in the skin of the foot may be manifestations of spinal cord dysfunction.

Cardiac anomalies

Approximately 10% of patients with congenital scoliosis have cardiac anomalies which range from minor to severe.

Urogenital anomalies

Renal tract anomalies are seen in 25–40% of cases. These may be identified by ultrasound or contrast radiography. Some are identified from spinal MRI scans. Less commonly there may be uterine or vaginal anomalies.

Prognosis

Prognosis depends mainly on the degree of growth-plate asymmetry and growth potential. If a child has a significant curvature by the age of 10 years, there is likely to be a large curve by skeletal maturity. Associated anomalies of the neurological system, cerebral palsy, and other syndromes may also influence prognosis. Cardiac anomalies themselves may not influence curvature of the spine, but the thoracotomies needed to treat them can be detrimental to the spine. If a wide laminectomy is needed to treat intracanal lesions, kyphosis may develop in the presence of a neurological deficit. Generally, children with congenital scoliosis are shorter than average.

Prognosis is important in this condition and given in Figure 3.11.6.

Box 3.11.2 Management of congenital scoliosis

- Curves showing strong asymmetry of growth plates are likely to progress, particularly if there is an unsegmented bar
- A majority of patients with congenital scoliosis tend to be short
- Growth in an area of deformity tends to increase the deformity rather than increasing height
- Associated anomalies may well affect prognosis
- Lung development continues to the age of 7 years, so that severe chest deformities before this age are associated with reduced pulmonary development. Respiratory function is significantly diminished in curves with Cobb angles greater than 70 degrees
- Congenital curves of less than 30 degrees by the age of 10 years are less likely to progress than those over 30 degrees
- MRI is essential.

	Type of congenital anomaly					
			Hemivertebra			
Site of curvature	Block vertebra	Wedged vertebra	Single	Double	Unilateral unsegmented bar	Unilateral unsegmented bar and contralateral hemivertebrae
Upper thoracic	< 1°–1°	* – 2°	1°– 2°	2°– 2.5°	2°– 4°	5°– 6°
Lower thoracic	< 1°–1°	2°– 2°	2°– 2.5°	2°– 3°	5°– 6.5°	6°– 7°
Thoracolumbar	< 1°–1°	1.5°– 2°	2°– 3.5°	5°– *	6°– 9°	> 10°– *
Lumbar	< 1°– *	< 1°– *	< 1°–1°	*	> 5°– *	*
Lumbosacral	*	*	< 1°–1.5°	*	*	*

No treatment required | May require spinal fusion | Require spinal fusion

Fig. 3.11.6 McMaster prognosis. (Data from McMaster and Ohtsuka (1982).)

Management (Box 3.11.1 and Box 3.11.2)

Plain radiography is essential for evaluating and monitoring the progress of the curve. Once the child can sit or stand, an erect whole-spine radiograph is best. In younger children, radiographs every 6 months are necessary to monitor the curve. Measurement of the Cobb angle is not very accurate (within 5 degrees at best), so that significant small changes may be missed. Close attention to the behaviour of the more aggressive patterns is essential, with regular and regularized radiographs. Older children can be monitored with surface topography where it is available. Plain radiography can usually be used to evaluate the bony anatomy and pedicle widening, and to identify ossified diastematomyelia.

MRI scanning of the spine, including the craniocervical junction, is essential in all patients with congenital scoliosis. If surgery is not contemplated, this investigation can wait until the child is old enough to cooperate with the investigation without a general anaesthetic. The object is to identify spinal anomalies. If any are found, the patient should be sent for advice from a neurosurgeon. Controversy exists on the advisability of surgical resection of spurs, dividing the filum of tethered cords, and drainage of cysts. Generally the threshold for surgery is lower where there is an actual or progressive neurological deficit.

In general, bracing does not have much to offer patients with congenital scoliosis. It can be used to buy time when surgery is threatened in a small child. However a 'wait and see' policy is usually ill advised.

Surgery should be attempted sooner rather than later, particularly in the malignant patterns and in hemivertebrae at the lumbosacral junction.

Surgical options

Fusion *in situ*

The simplest procedure is a posterior fusion *in situ*. Clearly, the earlier this is done, the smaller will be the curve and consequent deformity. Posterior fusion is usually appropriate for the cervicothoracic junction because the risk of obtaining anterior access at these levels is unjustified. Elsewhere in the spine this is usually combined with an anterior fusion. The posterior procedure alone does not prevent continuing anterior growth and the 'crankshaft phenomenon'. However, it is the safest option in the presence of spinal cord anomalies. This type of surgery may prevent progression, but does nothing for present cosmesis except that the brace can be removed once the fusion is established.

Posterior fusion with correction

It is sometimes possible to correct mobile curves associated with a congenital malformation with modern instrumentation systems. It is important that congenital anomalies of the spinal cord are identified preoperatively, as correction of the curve may cause paraplegia.

Epiphysiodesis

A convex growth arrest involves a combined anterior and posterior ablation of growth plates. Normally rib graft is available from the anterior approach.

The best result is an improvement in the curve. Otherwise there should be stabilization of the curve. If the curve progresses, then instrumentation and an extended fusion is needed.

Osteotomy

This is an option where there is a block vertebra or where a previous fusion *in situ* has been performed.

Vertebrectomy

This is the procedure of choice for treating an isolated hemivertebra, particularly at the lumbosacral junction.

VEPTR or titanium rib

This technique depends on expanding the thoracic cavity unilaterally or bilaterally. Serial lengthening is needed, followed by definitive fusion.

Management of spinal cord abnormalities

This is outside the scope of this book. Neurosurgical advice is essential.

Further reading

Campbell, R., Smith, M., Mayes, T., *et al.* (2004). The effect of opening wedge thoracostomy on thoracic insufficiency syndrome associated with fused ribs and congenital scoliosis. *Journal of Bone and Joint Surgery*, **86A**, 1659–74.

Marks, D., Sayampanathan, S., Thompson, A., and Piggott, H. (1995). Long-term results of convex epiphysiodesis for congenital scoliosis. *European Spine Journal*, **4**, 296–301.

McMaster, M. and David, C. (1986). Hemivertebra as a cause of scoliosis: a study of 104 patients. *Journal of Bone and Joint Surgery*, **68B**, 588–95.

McMaster, M. and Ohtsuka, K. (1982). The natural history of congenital scoliosis; a study of two hundred and fifty-one patients. *Journal of Bone and Joint Surgery*, **64A**, 1128–47.

McMaster, M. and Singh, H. (1999). Natural history of congenital kyphosis and kyphoscoliosis: a study of one hundred and twelve patients. *Journal of Bone and Joint Surgery*, **81A**, 1367–83.

3.12

Neuromuscular scoliosis

Jeremy Fairbank*

Summary points

- All children with neurogenic or myogenic conditions are at risk of developing scoliosis
- The more severe the involvement, particularly in those who cannot stand, the more likely is the curve to progress
- Surgery is the only effective way of treating these curves, and in general the earlier the better.

Introduction

Neuromuscular scoliosis is the term given to that group of scoliotic deformities associated with muscle weakness of any origin (in the past, the term paralytic was used to describe this group of scoliosis). Neuromuscular scoliosis is usually classified into neuropathic and myopathic disease. Neuropathic disorders responsible for neuromuscular scoliosis include upper motor neuron conditions such as cerebral palsy, spinocerebellar degeneration, syringomyelia, spinal cord trauma, and spinal cord tumours. Lower motor neuron lesions include spinal muscular atrophy (SMA), poliomyelitis, other viral myelitides, myelomeningocele, and trauma. Neuropathic abnormalities also include dysautonomia. Myopathic pathology includes muscular dystrophy, particularly Duchenne muscular dystrophy, the congenital myopathies, congenital hypotonia, myotonia dystrophica, and arthrogryposis.

This classification does not indicate the relative frequency of neuromuscular scoliosis or the frequency of surgical intervention. More important, it does not indicate the type of scoliosis. The surgical treatment depends on the type of scoliosis and the underlying disease, rather than on whether the underlying lesion is neuropathic or myopathic.

In neuromuscular scoliosis, a child already hampered by an underlying and usually incurable condition is further disabled by progressive deformity that aggravates the functional deficit, compromises cardiorespiratory function, and transforms a normal-looking child into one twisted and perhaps crouched in a wheelchair. While it is not preventable by any currently available methods, it is a serious problem that is worth recognizing early so that prompt assessment can be made and an optimal management protocol adopted. Historically, many of the developments in this area were based on experiences with polio, which was complicated by progressive spinal deformity in some cases. This was partly but not wholly explained by asymmetry of muscle tone and strength and partly by severity and extent of involvement. Many of the implant systems now used date back to the polio era.

Presentation and natural history

Scoliosis presents as visible deformity of the trunk, and physicians and therapists should be aware of its increased incidence in children with mental or physical disability. The first indication may be shoulder or pelvic obliquity, rib hump, visible spinal curvature or, in the case of non-ambulant patients, loss of sitting balance. Initial assessment must include careful physical examination with recording of side and site of deformity, trunk balance, height of rib hump and shoulder inequality, pelvic obliquity, leg-length discrepancy, general mobility, and levels of intelligence (school grade), and social independence. The appearance of the deformity should be documented by clinical photography and surface topography, and the nature of structural bony deformity determined by radiography. Radiographs should include erect anteroposterior and lateral views of the spine, either standing or seated as appropriate, and left wrist for indication of bone age. Scoliosis measurements are best made by the Cobb method. More detailed analysis such as magnetic resonance imaging (MRI) and computed tomography (CT) may be indicated in particular cases or where surgery is contemplated. Because of the more severe effects of spinal deformity on children whose muscle function is already compromised, respiratory and cardiac assessment are essential, as well as complete neurological evaluation. Figure 3.12.1 shows the clinical and radiological appearance of scoliosis in a 16-year-old boy who had suffered a traumatic paraplegia at the age of 4.

Because children with neuromuscular scoliosis frequently have other significant problems, the effect of their deformity must always be seen in its complete context and not considered in isolation. Severe scoliosis is an ugly deformity, but to describe this as 'cosmetic' should not belittle the patient's complaint. Other problems

* Based on chapters written for first edition by Frank E. Dowling and Charles Galasko

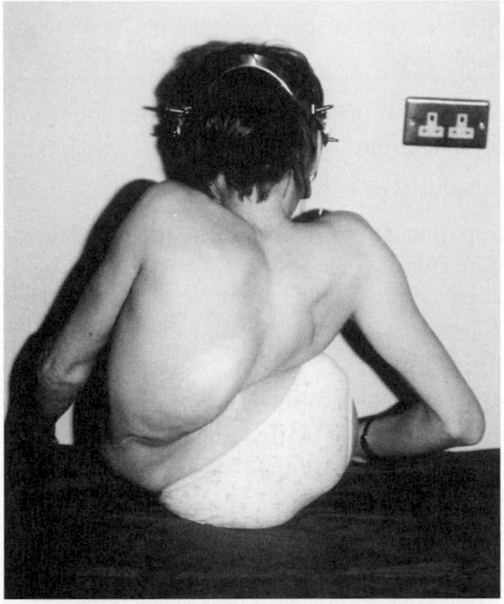

A

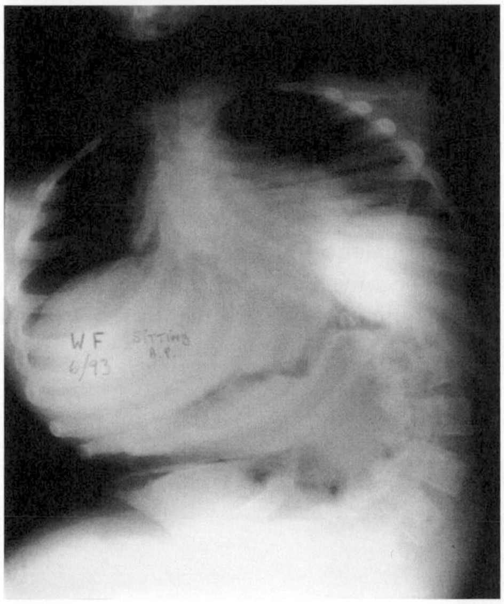

B

Fig. 3.12.1 A) Clinical photograph: neuromuscular scoliosis in a habitual wheelchair sitter. B) Seated anteroposterior radiograph.

include cardiorespiratory restriction, secondary to the mechanical inefficiency of deformed chest cage working with inadequate nerve and muscle structures. Patients with restricted ambulation may have increased difficulty as trunk imbalance increases and pelvic obliquity causes hip problems and apparent leg-length inequality. Pain is sometimes an issue and can be helped by surgery.

Non-ambulant patients confined mostly or exclusively to a wheelchair show a very distinctive curve pattern with a thoracolumbar apex and a long swinging C shape that includes an oblique pelvis, almost as if it were the last vertebra in the curve (Figures 3.12.1B and 3.12.2). This pelvic obliquity is difficult to measure accurately but is the source of a significant proportion of the ill effects of spinal deformity in this group. In addition to cardiopulmonary compromise and cosmetic effect, wheelchair sitters will lose the ability to sit unsupported as the pelvis becomes more

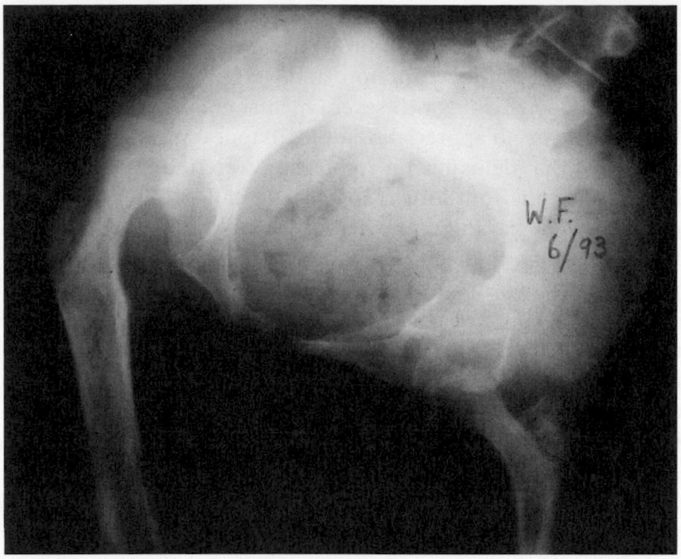

Fig. 3.12.2 Pelvic obliquity in a habitual wheelchair sitter.

oblique (Figure 3.12.1A). Thus, needing one hand for support in their activities of daily living, they are reduced to single-handed function and further disability. This may be manifest in increased difficulty in all functions such as transfer from bed to chair, self-catheterization, or merely a simple two-handed task such as eating or dealing cards. Skin ulceration is another and potentially fatal complication. While neural deficit always carries the risk of pressure sores around the buttocks, sacrum, and hips, this may be complicated by pelvic obliquity as its progression presents new areas of skin with greater or lesser underlying bony points to do the damage. Pain or discomfort means that sitting times or tolerance may diminish.

Neuromuscular kyphosis is less common but carries the similar cardiopulmonary and cosmetic complications. In addition, severe kyphosis entails the strong possibility of spinal cord compression, which is not generally the case with lateral curvature of the spine.

Prognosis in neuromuscular scoliosis is generally of steady progression during growth, more rapid during phases of growth spurt, and significant slowdown but not complete arrest at skeletal maturity. Morbidity or mortality may result from the scoliosis itself or from the underlying condition, and neither should be considered in isolation. Management decisions must be based on present deformity, pain or discomfort, projected progression, the implications of increased functional deficit of any sort, and life expectancy. In the end, it is an individual judgement call that should take into account the views of the patient and of all the carers involved with the child.

Management

Exercises and other physical manoeuvres and orthotics are ineffectual in controlling progression in neuromuscular scoliosis, and it is fruitless to burden children already disabled with further invasion of their lives. Surgery, on the other hand, has a longer history for this type of scoliosis than any other varieties. Because surgery offers the only effective method of improving a scoliotic deformity, the indications and counterindications, advantages and risks, should be well understood and discussed before a decision is made.

The aim of surgery is to reduce deformity, prevent progression, reduce pain and discomfort, preserve cardiorespiratory function, and maintain motor function and activities of daily living. Ten years ago, a child with severe mental and physical disability having little or no appreciation of their appearance, and mobility so limited that demands on respiration were minimal, will have had little to gain from surgery that was painful, major, and dangerous. This view has to be revisited in the face of other advances in medicine where these children are living longer and studies supporting intervention are published.

It should be remembered that scoliosis surgery is primarily a spinal fusion, the artificial stiffening of a spine that has been manually straightened to reduce the curve and its consequences. This is achieved by bone graft and metal implants. Improvements in posterior techniques have reduced the need for anterior procedures. An important objective is to prevent and treat pelvic obliquity. Bone grafting from the pelvis is much less needed as artificial agents to stimulate fusion become more widely available. Respiratory function improvement is not commonly found after these operations, but there may be reductions in respiratory infection rates. Ambulant patients may loose function after their spine is stiffened. The nature of this is not always easy to predict, but can include rolling on the floor, gait, transfers, self-catheterization, self-feeding, protecting pressure areas, and swimming (Figure 3.12.3).

Duchenne muscular dystrophy and spinal muscle atrophy

Severe curves in most types of scoliosis (e.g. idiopathic, congenital, and scolioses associated with cerebral palsy and spina bifida) are usually best treated by combined anterior and posterior surgery, but by the time patients with Duchenne muscular dystrophy (DMD) or SMA have developed severe curves, they are not fit for anterior spinal procedures. Progressive curves contribute to loss of forced vital capacity (FVC) (Figure 3.12.4). A 4–5% decrease in FVC occurs for every 10 degrees increase in curvature. In DMD progressive motor weakness accelerates FVC loss. There is some evidence that untreated scoliosis diminishes life expectancy. Progressive increase in pelvic obliquity often makes sitting uncomfortable and may make it impossible. Hips can dislocate or become painful.

Over 90% of patients with DMD develop a scoliosis when they become wheelchair bound at an average age of 9.5 years. Once the patient is in a wheelchair, the scoliosis progresses relentlessly to a C shape. This makes sitting uncomfortable and eventually results in loss of sitting balance. Activities of daily living, such as defecation, may become extremely difficult if a patient has a significant pelvic obliquity of 80 degrees or more (Figure 3.12.5).

Box 3.12.1 Three types of scoliosis occur in patients with neuromuscular disease

1. Collapsing curve that involves the entire spine and progressive pelvic obliquity
2. An idiopathic type curve
3. An idiopathic curve which subsequently develops into a collapsing curve.

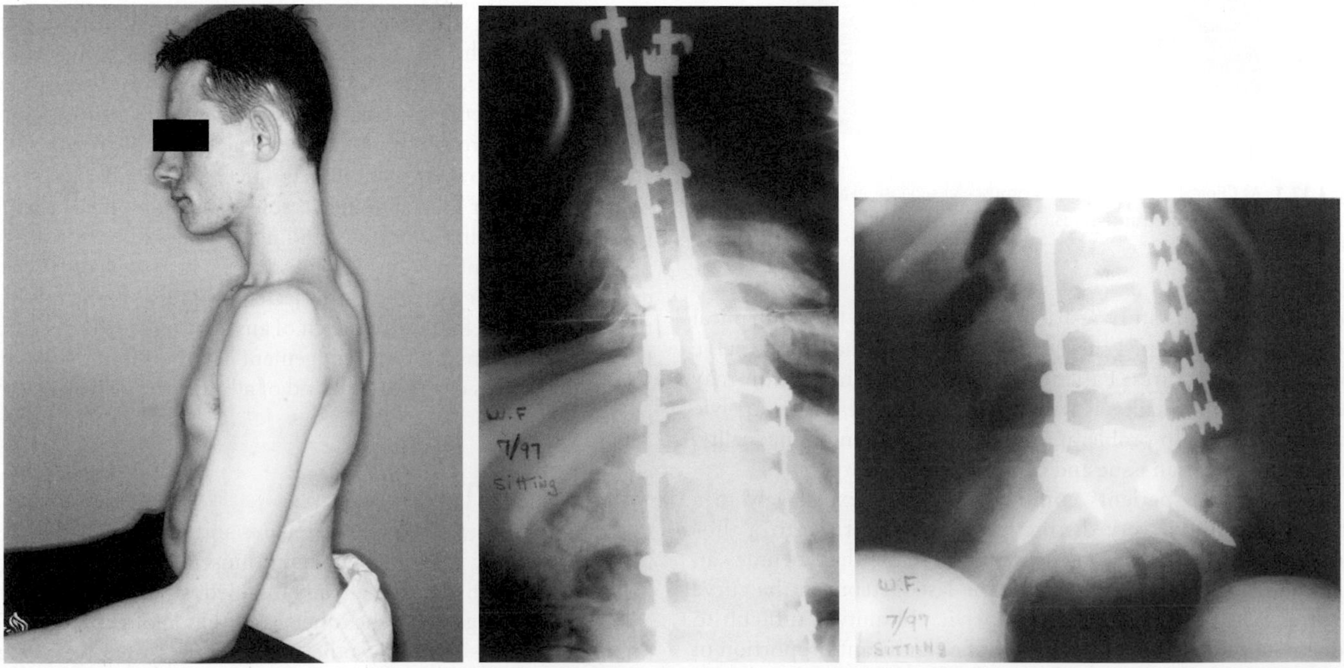

A B C

Fig. 3.12.3 A) Postoperative clinical photography, showing good cosmetic correction. B) Postoperative anteroposterior seated radiograph, showing correction, improved balance, and instrumentation. C) Postoperative view of leveled pelvis (cf. gross obliquity in Figure 3.12.2).

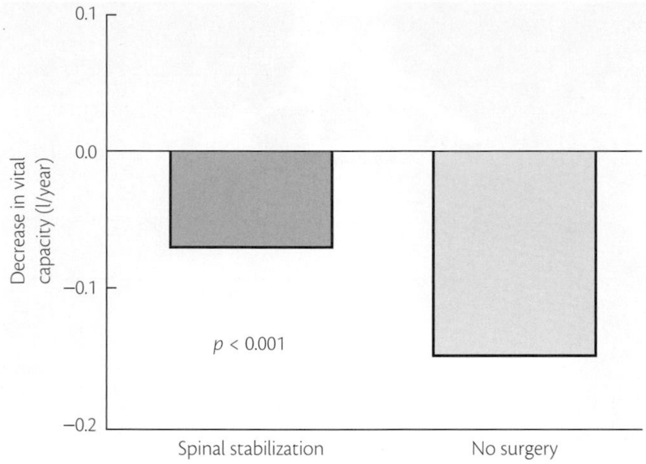

Fig. 3.12.4 The effect of spinal stabilization on forced vital capacity in patients with DMD. The annual reduction in vital capacity was significantly smaller in patients who underwent spinal stabilization compared with those who were fit for surgery but where the offer of surgery was declined ($p < 0.001$).

Delayed referral (or where the family will not accept surgery) will mean that a window of opportunity for surgical treatment is lost. Not all DMD cases get scoliosis and it may be that a lordotic spine is protective. There is accumulating evidence that corticosteroids can alter the natural history of DMD. Cardiomyopathy occurs especially in DMD and may restrict the treatment window for scoliosis surgery.

Patients with neuromuscular disease have multiple problems. A multidisciplinary team is essential (including, for example, paediatric neurologist, clinical geneticist, respiratory technician, paediatric cardiologist, paediatric anaesthetist, orthotist, physiotherapist, occupational therapist, and wheelchair and seating experts). From the spine point of view, 6-monthly erect radiographs and respiratory function tests are needed to monitor curve progression with expert input on cardiac function. If a curve starts to progress, then surgery should be considered sooner than later.

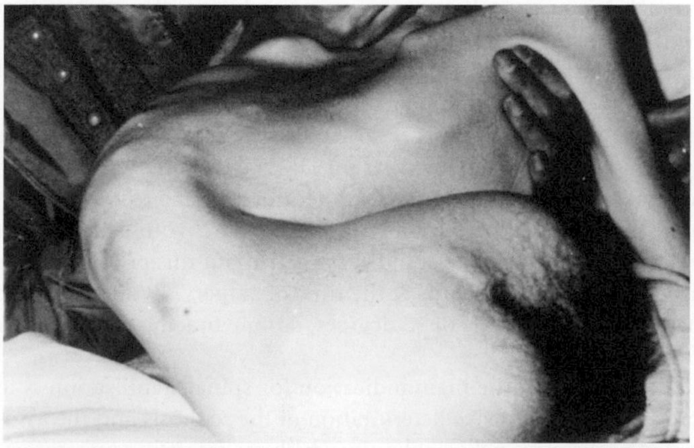

Fig. 3.12.5 Patient with DMD who was referred 6 months prior to death. The main reason for referral was difficulty with defecation. This is not surprising in view of the gross pelvic obliquity associated with the C-shaped collapsing scoliosis of the entire spine. The pelvis is almost vertical rather than horizontal.

Scoliosis in Duchenne muscular dystrophy

DMD is the most rapidly progressive and the most common childhood neuromuscular disorder. It is an X-linked condition and affects only boys. The gene locus is on the short arm of the X chromosome and has been isolated and sequenced. Deficiency of its product dystrophin affects skeletal, cardiac, and smooth muscle. It is a large gene and may display genetic, and hence clinical, heterogeneity. Parents are usually unaware of any problem in the first year of life. About 50% of patients present in the second year with walking and speech delay. They may also present with abnormalities of gait such as toe-walking, a tendency to frequent falling, reluctance to walk, or 'laziness'. The muscle weakness is relentlessly progressive. The ability to walk is lost on average at 9 years with a range from 6–12 years. Death usually occurs in the teens or early twenties, but life expectancy for some is slowly increasing with new methods of ventilatory support. It is characterized by progressive degeneration of skeletal muscle without an associated structural abnormality in the central nervous system.

Therapy through orthoses or seating

Attempts have been made to control the scoliosis by modifications of the wheelchair and the use of spinal orthoses. Although they may slow its progression, these measures do not prevent the development of a severe curve. Patients do not like orthoses as they lack the muscle power to pull away from any painful pressure area. Furthermore, the orthosis may diminish the already limited lung function in these patients. At best, spinal bracing only slows progression of the curve. Moulded seats can be useful for patients with cerebral palsy, particularly those with severe mental as well as physical disability, but patients with DMD and SMA find them too restrictive and prefer modular seating.

Therapy through standing and ambulation

It is possible to prolong ambulation in patients with DMD by the use of knee–ankle–foot orthoses (KAFOs). These are designed to hyperextend the hips, tightening the Y ligament to maintain the patient's balance and promoting lumbar lordosis. Swivel walkers and standing frames may also postpone scoliosis and reduce loss of respiratory function.

Surgical stabilization

Spinal surgery is indicated in patients with DMD when they have lost independent ambulation, they have developed an early scoliosis, and they are still fit for surgery. Ideally, the surgery should be carried out when the curve is approximately 20 degrees, but often it is not carried out until the curve is more extensive. Fitness for surgery depends on both lung function and cardiac function. Provided that they do not have a cardiomyopathy, it is safe to operate on patients with a forced vital capacity of less than 35% if the anaesthetist is skilled in the management of these patients.

The main role of surgery is to stabilize the spine, improve the existing scoliosis, prevent a deterioration in the curve, and improve any pelvic obliquity. Spinal stabilization gives patients better sitting balance for the remainder of their lives and allows them to

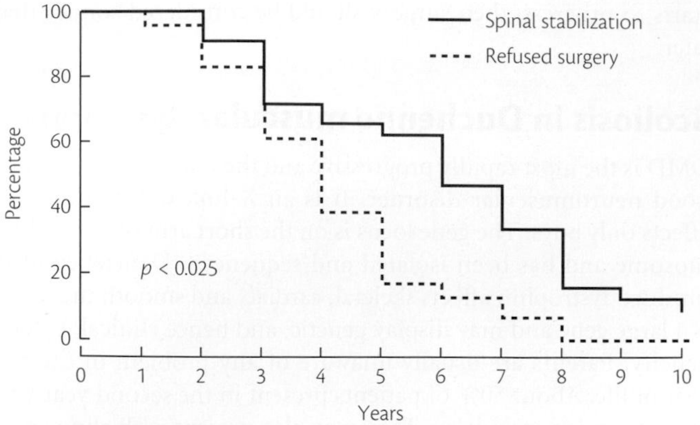

Fig. 3.12.6 Kaplan–Meier survival curve in patients with DMD. Both groups of patients were offered surgery. Time zero in the refused-surgery group was when they were offered surgery; in the spinal stabilization group it was when they underwent surgery. Patients who underwent surgery had a significantly longer survival than patients where surgery was declined ($p < 0.025$).

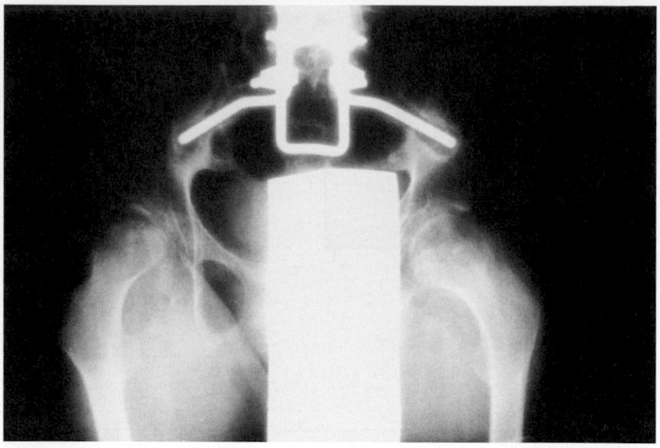

Fig. 3.12.7 A patient with DMD who developed significant bilateral pelvic pain following spinal stabilization. The radiograph shows osteolysis around the rods inserted into the pelvis. The pelvic portions of the rods were removed and there was no associated infection. Following this removal, the patient's pain settled completely.

continue to sit comfortably in a wheelchair until they die, usually from a respiratory infection. Mobile arm supports may be needed as holding spine in extension makes self-feeding more difficult. One study suggests that life expectancy is increased in those choosing surgical treatment over those who rejected it.

Postoperatively, patients are mobilized early. They start to sit in wheelchairs 3–5 days after surgery. The spinal fixation must be sufficiently strong to obviate the necessity for any postoperative spinal orthoses (Figure 3.12.6).

Scoliosis in spinal muscle atrophy

The spinal muscle atrophies are a group of hereditary proximal and symmetrical muscular atrophies associated with degeneration of the anterior horn cells of the spinal cord and in severe cases of the bulbar motor neuron. Inheritance is autosomal recessive. The disorders are caused by an abnormal or missing gene (survival motor neuron gene, SMN1). 3 types are recognized, determined by the age of onset and the severity of symptoms. Type I (Werdnig–Hoffman) is evident at birth or within a few months. Type II (juvenile or intermediate SMA) starts at age 6–18 months, and Type III (Wolhlfart–Kugelberg–Welander or mild SMA) at ages 3–15 years.

Natural history of spinal muscle atrophy

There is usually a period of apparently normal development followed by an insidious or occasionally relatively acute onset of weakness, and then a plateau during which the weakness remains relatively static. The age of onset is variable and is not an absolute guide to classification. It is associated with weakness of the respiratory muscles, and children with Type I usually die from intercurrent infection before the age of 3 years.

Scoliosis can occur very early (Figure 3.12.7) and develops in the vast majority of patients. It is the most serious deformity occurring in these patients, but dislocation of the hip occurs more frequently than in DMD. Surgery can improve the scoliosis and prevent progression. The immediate impact on respiratory function is probably neutral but it may well prevent progression. Standing with appropriate support is probably beneficial in reducing progression.

Management of scoliosis in spinal muscle atrophy

Because the onset of scoliosis is much earlier, the treatment is slightly different. Once the diagnosis has been made, patients should be persuaded to stand. In the mild group, standing must be encouraged and, if the disease progresses to the extent that the child loses his or her independent mobilization, KAFOs, swivel walkers, or standing frames should be prescribed, depending on the ability of the child to cope with these aids. Once the diagnosis of intermediate SMA has been made, KAFOs or a swivel walker should be provided. In the severe form of the disease, the patient will only be able to stand in a standing frame with trunk support.

Once the child has developed scoliosis, spinal orthoses are indicated to minimize the progression of the curve until he or she is old enough for surgery. Patients as young as 15 months may present with curves of 50–60 degrees or more. Bracing should be continued until the child is old enough for spinal surgery, ideally at least 12 years of age. If bracing or serial plaster jackets cannot control the progression of the curve, earlier surgery may be required. The type of procedure is the same as for DMD with spinal stabilization and facet joint fusion from the upper dorsal spine to the sacrum, and fixation to the sacrum or pelvis. The youngest patient with SMA on whom the author has carried out this procedure was aged 6 years and 9 months at the time of surgery. By that time she had developed a curve of 95 degrees, despite bracing and standing treatment.

As with DMD, the main indication for spinal stabilization is to prevent the progressive deterioration of the scoliosis and the associated progressive pelvic obliquity which makes sitting uncomfortable, if not impossible (Figure 3.12.8). In addition, there may be a positive benefit on lung function, but this is not the indication for surgery.

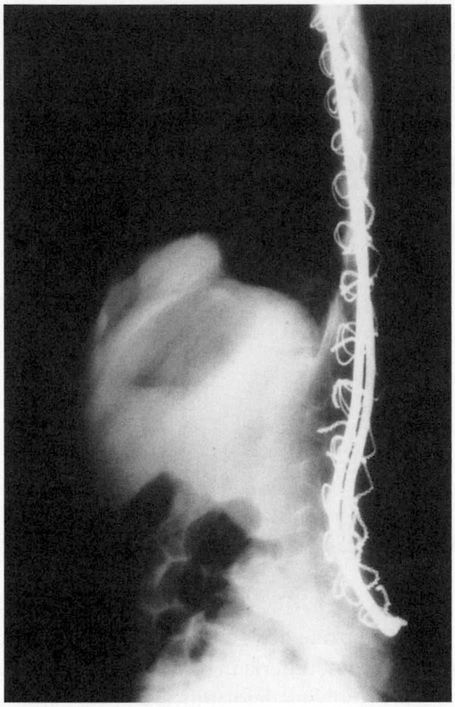

Fig. 3.12.8 Lateral radiograph following modified Luque spinal stabilization and fusion in a patient with DMD. A lumbar lordosis has been moulded into the rod. The rod used was an open rectangle, with the closed end wired to the sacrum and the open ends trimmed to length, depending on the height of the patient.

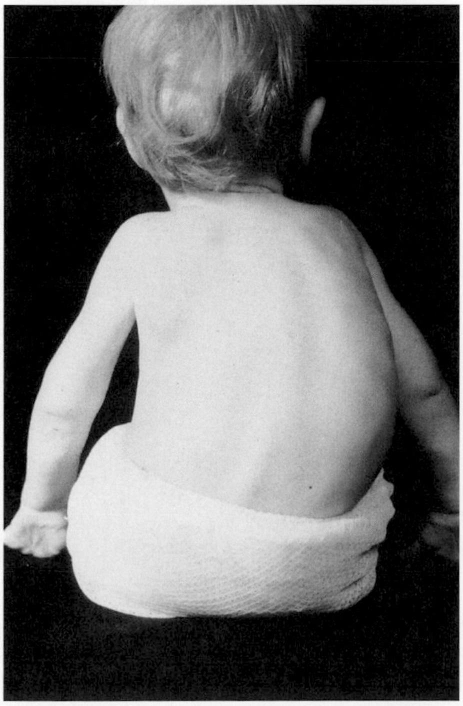

Fig. 3.12.9 Scoliosis can occur very early in SMA. This 15-month-old boy with the intermediate form had a curve of 53 degrees with associated pelvic obliquity.

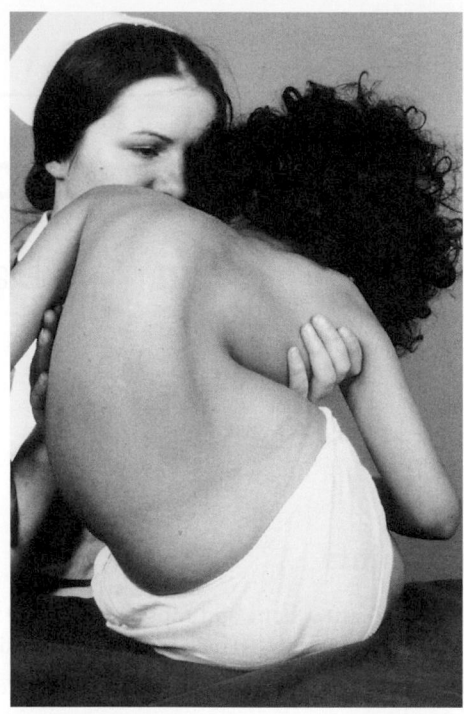

Fig. 3.12.10 A female patient with intermediate SMA who was referred when she was no longer fit for surgery. She has a typical C-shaped curve with marked pelvic obliquity and was unable to sit.

Summary

Neuromuscular scoliosis behaves differently from idiopathic scoliosis. It usually involves the entire spine and is associated with increasing pelvic obliquity that affects sitting balance, makes sitting uncomfortable, and may make sitting impossible. The increased pelvic obliquity may also predispose to dislocation of the hip. In DMD and SMA, the progressive scoliosis is associated with deterioration in lung function, in addition to the impaired lung function secondary to the disease process itself. The development of scoliosis is the most severe of the deformities than can occur in these patients because it has such a devastating effect upon their quality of life. Standing slows down the progression of the curve as well as the deterioration in lung function.

3.13

Syndromal scoliosis

Evan M. Davies

Summary points

- Syndromes which affect bone and muscle may affect the ability of the spinal column to stay balanced and lead to scoliosis
- Scoliosis associated with syndromes behaves differently from idiopathic scoliosis
- Intervention in syndromic scoliosis may require more complex intervention and multiagency support.

Introduction

Some syndromes have a high incidence of scoliosis. This occurs due to poor neuromuscular control, deficient soft tissue restraints, or dystrophic bone. The intrinsic strength of the spinal column is reduced and deformities have a higher prevalence rate, present earlier in life, and tend to have more serious progression potential.

It is important in syndromal spinal deformities to understand the patient's needs in a holistic way, and thus the spinal problems should not be divorced from the other, often much greater, needs of the child.

Early-onset progressive scoliosis

Although the development of all the conductive airways is complete at birth, only a relatively small number of respiratory bronchioles and alveoli exist. These multiply many times from the numbers present at birth to their full maturation by the age of 7 years. Restriction of the available space in the thoracic cavity can have a major effect on lung development. After birth until about the age of 7 years the effect is on the number of alveoli rather than the number of airways. Early-onset scoliosis under the age of 7 years, particularly in the first year or two of life, can result in serious future health problems.

Infantile progressive scoliosis

The great majority of infantile idiopathic scoliosis cases are benign and resolve without treatment. Twenty-five per cent do not resolve naturally; in most of these progression can be prevented by treatment or they can be made to resolve eventually. In 5% of infantile idiopathic cases the natural history is severe progression (Figure 3.13.1).

Parameters such as the size of the curve (Cobb angle) and the degree of transverse plane deformity (rib vertebra angle difference (RVAD)) are important criteria in distinguishing possibly progressive from possibly resolving deformities; clinical parameters are far more important. The overall child assessment is more important to assessing potential curve progression. The healthy well child with no significant comorbidities is likely to represent a fetal moulding that normally resolves when tone is fully developed. The neurologically challenged child with associated comorbidities is more likely to progress than the idiopathic scoliosis patient.

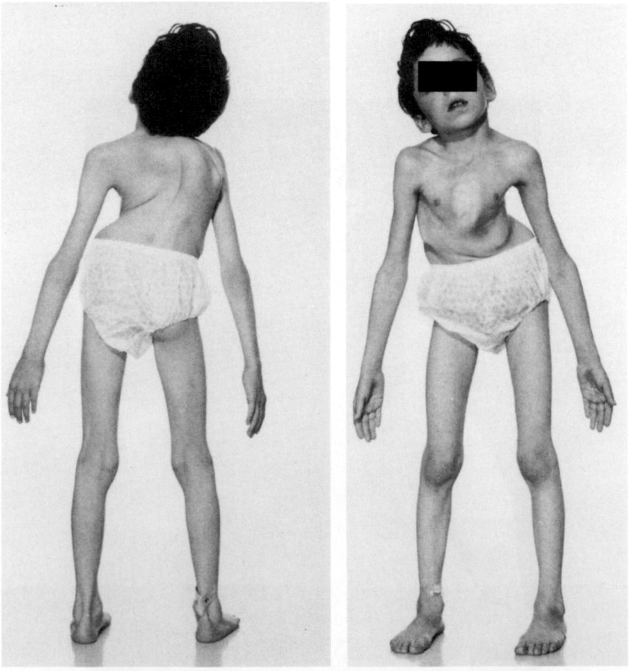

A B

Fig. 3.13.1 Infantile idiopathic malignant progressive scoliosis in a boy aged 8 years. Note the severe chest wall deformity which will have impaired alveolar multiplication.

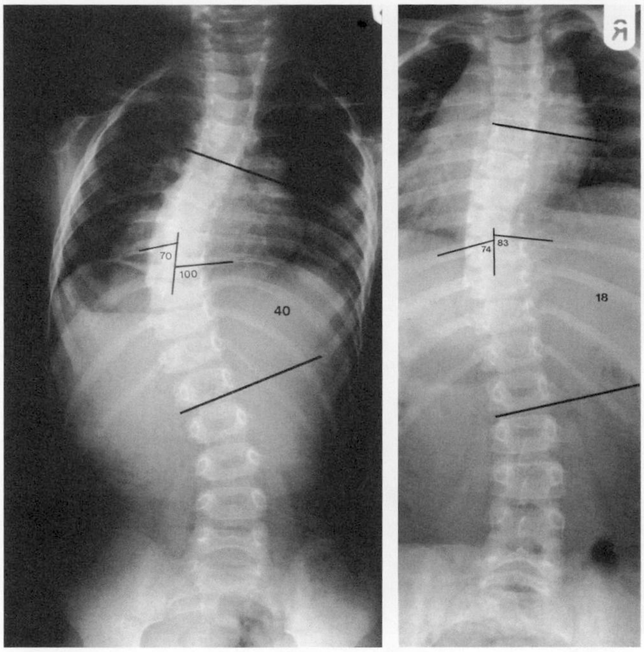

Fig. 3.13.2 A) Measuring the RVAD at the apex of a curve and measuring Cobb angle: the RVAD is in excess of 20 degrees and Cobb angle is in excess of 30 degrees, indicating progression. (b) The same patient 5 years later after serial EDF casting, showing a much reduced Cobb angle and RVAD. The deformity is now clinically resolving.

In addition to the geometric parameters measurable on a frontal spine film (Figure 3.13.2) (i.e. Cobb angle in excess of 30 degrees and RVAD in excess of 20 degrees), clinical assessment of curve stiffness is also important. The resolving curve tends to be flexible, but the progressive curve, particularly the malignant one, tends to be rigid. Resolving curves readily overcorrect, but progressive curves hardly change at all.

Males are affected more than females in a ratio of 3:2. Thoracic curves are more common, but other patterns are not unusual. Most thoracic curves are convex to the left. Right thoracic curves in females and double-structural curves seem to have greater progression potential.

The condition is thought to be due initially to moulding of the malleable infantile skeleton. This is supported by the fact that plagiocephaly, plagiothorax, palgiopelvy, bat ear, and tight sternomastoid are all correlated with the convex side of the scoliosis. There is a higher incidence of mental retardation, congenital hip dislocation, congenital heart disease, and inguinal hernias, and there is a definite familial trend. These additional clinical features strongly support the notion that early-onset progressive scoliosis is syndromal rather than idiopathic. This is confirmed by the association with chromosomal abnormalities.

Treatment

Non-surgical treatment

If the child is diagnosed and referred within the first year of life, conservative treatment can be effective at promoting resolution or preventing progression. The older the presentation, the more difficult it is to achieve these goals. Once the child reaches the age of 4 or 5 years, non-operative treatment is probably of no avail. Serial elongation–derotation–flexion (EDF) casts are applied under a light general anaesthetic every 2 or 3 months, with the precise frequency being determined by growth, hygiene, and the state of the cast. As the plaster hardens, pressure moulding of the spine is carried out to exert an untwisting effect. Windows are then cut in the back and front of the cast to allow vests to be changed whenever required and thus promote hygiene. Once the child has reached the age of 4 or 5 years, the deformity becomes too rigid to be influenced by external cast pressure. The child is then observed at intervals of 6 months. Curves can resolve over several more years, with the rotational component being the last part to disappear. Curves that have been prevented from progressing should clearly be observed regularly throughout the adolescent growth period. There is no evidence that bracing favourably influences the natural history of any form of scoliosis, least of all the early-onset type.

Surgical treatment

Surgery is indicated for cases that have resisted serial cast treatment. It can potentially do more harm than good. As with all structural scolioses, the problem is one of relative anterior spinal overgrowth and therefore a posterior fusion is contraindicated as it will create a tether that may lead to a crankshaft deformity and a worse outcome.

An anterior epiphysiodesis to prevent the anterior growth is essential to prevent further curse progression. The treatment options are then to continue with external splintage or use a posterior growth system (Figure 3.13.3). Posterior growth systems just distract the spine and they require reoperation and lengthening every 6 months in order to gain maximal spinal length. Alternatively the Luque trolley technique implants rods that distract over wires as the spine grows. The disadvantage of the trolley systems is that the spine is opened at all levels whereas the growing rods can be passed submuscularly. Premature growth arrest is possible if the whole spine is opened by a growing pseudarthrosis controlled by the rods occurs in the majority and prevents patients have as many surgeries as with a growth rod. Which ever system is used they have a high complication and reoperation rate requiring intense follow-up and management.

Thoracic insufficiency syndrome

Thoracic insufficiency syndrome (TIS) is used to describe the inability of the thorax to satisfactorily support lung growth, respiratory function, or spine development due to congenital and acquired chest wall, spine, and other syndromic deformities. This is associated with Jeune syndrome (asphyxiating thoracic dysplasia) or Jarcho–Levin syndrome (multiple vertebral and rib fusion anomalies. Traditional spinal arthrodesis will only worsen the pulmonary compromise associated with these conditions and will not correct the thoracic deformity. The titanium rib project developed by Campbell and Smith is an expandable device attached to the ribs and spine. This device is associated with an opening thoracic osteotomy. This device is lengthened 6-monthly until skeletal maturity. These surgeries have allowed thoracic wall expansion to improve lung development.

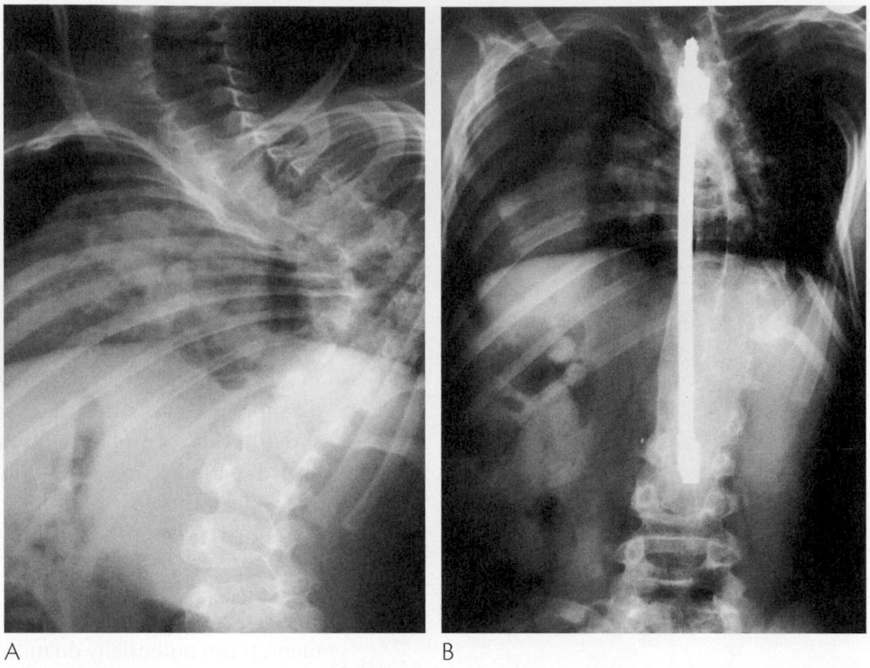

Fig. 3.13.3 A) Early-onset progressive scoliosis showing a right thoracic curve with substantial vertebral rotation. B) The same patient 10 years after anterior growth arrest and insertion of a posterior growing rod, showing solid fusion and a sustained correction.

Neurofibromatosis (see also Chapter 1.13)

There are two main sub-divisions, peripheral neurofibromatosis (NF-1) and central neurofibromatosis (NF-2). Spinal deformities are associated with NF-1 which is the common form of neurofibromatosis, with a prevalence rate of six per 1000. It has an autosomal dominant mode of inheritance with high penetrance but variable expressivity. There is a high mutation rate with many sporadic cases presenting as new mutations. The condition can affect all components of the musculoskeletal system, but the common clinical findings, are: nerve sheath tumours; café-au-lait spots; diffuse, soft tissue hypertrophy; subcutaneous nodules; bone hypertrophy; vascular malformation; congenital tibial pseudarthrosis; congenital shortening; osseous cysts; melorheostosis; and neuroendocrine tumours. Any two of the following are considered diagnostic:

- Positive family history
- Positive nodule biopsy
- Six café-au-lait spots measuring at least 1.5cm
- The presence of multiple nodules.

Spinal deformity in NF-1

Those individuals who are minimally affected clinically have deformity patterns which are indistinguishable from their idiopathic counterparts. Patients present with late-onset idiopathic-type scolioses or with late-onset idiopathic-type hyperkyphosis (Scheuermann's disease). Only careful clinical assessment of these criteria satisfies the diagnosis. These deformities can be managed in the same way as idiopathic deformities. Hyperkyphosis can be successfully treated orthotically.

The scoliosis affecting NF-1 patients is no different from idiopathic scoliosis itself; it is equally resistant to orthotic treatment. Only surgical treatment alters its natural history and the decision to treat is based on the same principles as idiopathic scoliosis. Preoperative magnetic resonance imaging (MRI) scanning is mandatory in order to detect any intracanal abnormalities which could produce neurological problems during surgery.

With NF-1 patients there is a tendency for deformities to reach unacceptable appearance earlier than with ordinary idiopathic scoliosis. The deformity is then at a higher risk of a crankshaft phenomenon if the deformity is only approached from posteriorly. Therefore it is appropriate to carry out an anterior discectomy and growth plate excision before posterior stabilization, in order to prevent late curve deterioration.

In severe NF-1 cases dystrophic bone changes may occur. In the axial skeleton, these include rib pencilling, enlarged intervertebral foraminae, and scalloped vertebral surfaces (Figure 3.13.4). The spinal deformities in severely expressed NF-1 are different. The curves tend to be short, sharp, and angular with a lot of rotation, while the kyphoses are also angular and tend to be in the thoracic or even cervical regions. The two often go together, with a lower thoracic lordoscoliosis and a high thoracic kyphosis above. These dystrophic types of deformity tend to develop at a much younger age and have much more progression potential. The degree of disfigurement produced by a deformity of considerable magnitude, often in association with short stature and other surface deformities, does provide indications for early surgical treatment. Because rapid progression of the dystrophic lordoscoliosis is inevitable, there is no sense in withholding surgical treatment. However, combined posterior and anterior surgery is essential, with the focus of attention on the front of the spine. Multiple discectomy with growth-plate ablation is a mandatory first stage (Figure 3.13.5). Definitive posterior instrumentation and fusion should be carried out in the older child, and some form of growing instrumentation should be provided for younger patients.

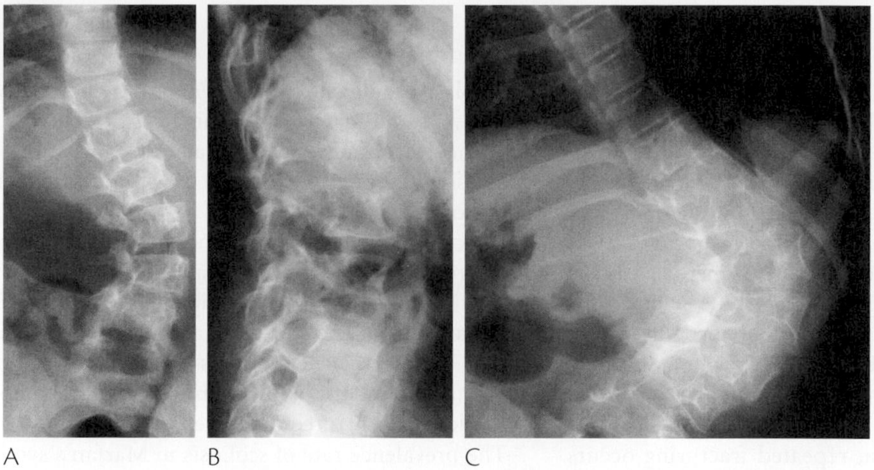

Fig. 3.13.4 A) The typical short sharp angular curve in association with von Recklinghausen's disease. B) Lateral radiograph demonstrating marked vertebral body scalloping and pronounced widening of the foraminae. C) Five years later showing severe progression. Again, note the vertebral scalloping and the pencilling of the twelfth rib on the concave side.

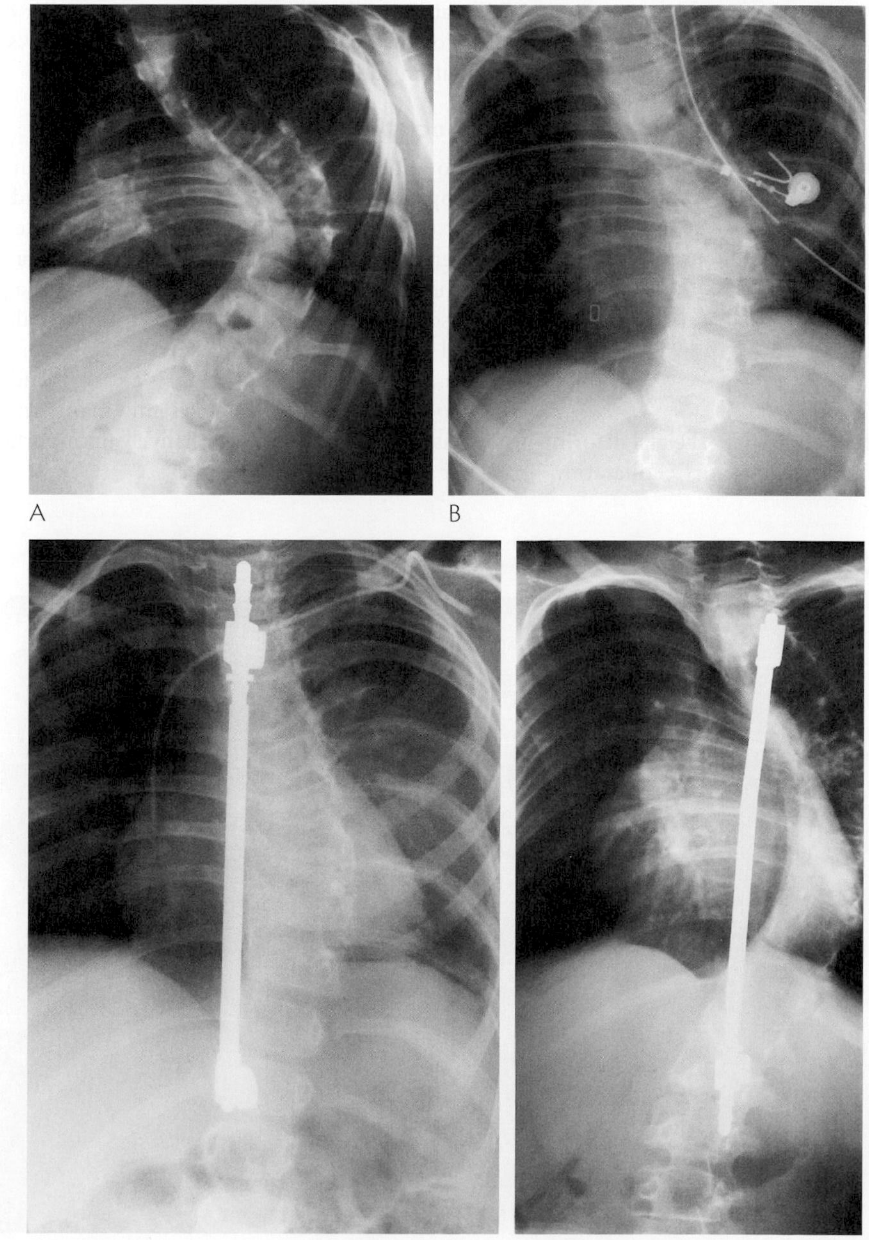

Fig. 3.13.5 A) Early-onset scoliosis in association with von Recklinghausen's disease. B) After anterior discectomy and growth plate excision. Note the correction that occurs when the front of the spine is shortened. C) The first growing rod. D) The last of many growing rods 10 years later showing a sustained correction and a solid fusion. Note that with growing rods it is often technically much easier to insert it upside down so that the ratchets are in the lumbar region.

Mesenchymal disorders

Osteogenesis imperfecta

Represents a group of disorders which arise from primary inherited defects in collagen synthesis with the common feature of bone fragility. The most common biochemical abnormality is defective synthesis of sufficient type I collagen. The diagnosis is usually made on the basis of the presence of blue sclerae or a positive family history. Floppy mitral valves and aortic incompetence are important complications. The disease may be sufficiently mild to resemble those changes seen in idiopathic juvenile osteoporosis.

In severe osteogenesis imperfecta, repeated fracturing occurs which may start *in utero*, thus producing gross deformity and considerable ambulatory disability. Death is not uncommon either at birth owing to the soft deficient skull or in the first 2 years of life as a result of respiratory infection. Blue sclerae and deafness are less common in severe disease.

Lateral spinal radiographic appearances show multiple compression fractures and biconcave vertebrae. Spinal deformities are rare in mild disease, with a prevalence rate no greater than in idiopathic scoliosis, but patients with severe disease invariably have a spinal deformity (Figure 3.13.6). These are of the two primary types—lordoscoliosis and kyphosis. Bracing can be of some benefit in kyphotic situations, although soft ribs can easily be deformed by the brace. Progressive deformity is difficult to manage because of the soft bone. Some form of segmental instrumentation is required to dissipate loads along with a profuse amount of allograft bank bone to facilitate a solid fusion.

Marfan's syndrome

A dominantly inherited disorder characterized by skeletal deformity, arachnodactyly, dislocated lenses, and aortic dilatation. Fibroblast-produced collagen is deficient and the soft tissue laxity thereby produced leads to joint hypermobility or dislocation, a tendency to hernias, aortic dilatation, and spinal deformity by increasing the intrinsic load on the spine consequent upon deficient soft tissue support.

Affected individuals are tall and thin, and the increase in stature is disproportionate. The fingers and toes are long and thin, and the palate is high and arched. Aortic incompetence, dissecting aneurysm, and mitral and tricuspid valve disease are the usual causes of death. The correct diagnosis is of extreme importance because many tall slim marfanoid patients present in scoliosis clinics and cardiology review is required after.

The prevalence rate of scoliosis in Marfan's syndrome is about 50% and the nature of the deformity is very similar to idiopathic scoliosis. The prevalence rate of kyphosis seems to be very small. Double-structural curves are more common in Marfan's syndrome. Treatment is along the same lines as that recommended for idiopathic scoliosis; for larger curves or earlier onset preliminary anterior discectomy should precede posterior segmental instrumentation and fusion (Figure 3.13.7).

Homocystinuria

The condition resembles Marfan's syndrome but can be differentiated by the presence of widened epiphyses and metaphyses, frequent osteoporosis of the spine, and in particular an increased incidence of thromboembolism. It is due to a deficiency of the enzyme cystathionine synthase. Homocystinuria patients generally have some degree of mental retardation, a malar flush, fair hair, dental crowding, large skull sinuses, and a narrow high-arched palate. The most serious problem is a strong tendency to thrombosis of both arterial and venous systems; in one series, two out of five serious thromboses followed relatively unimportant elective orthopaedic procedures.

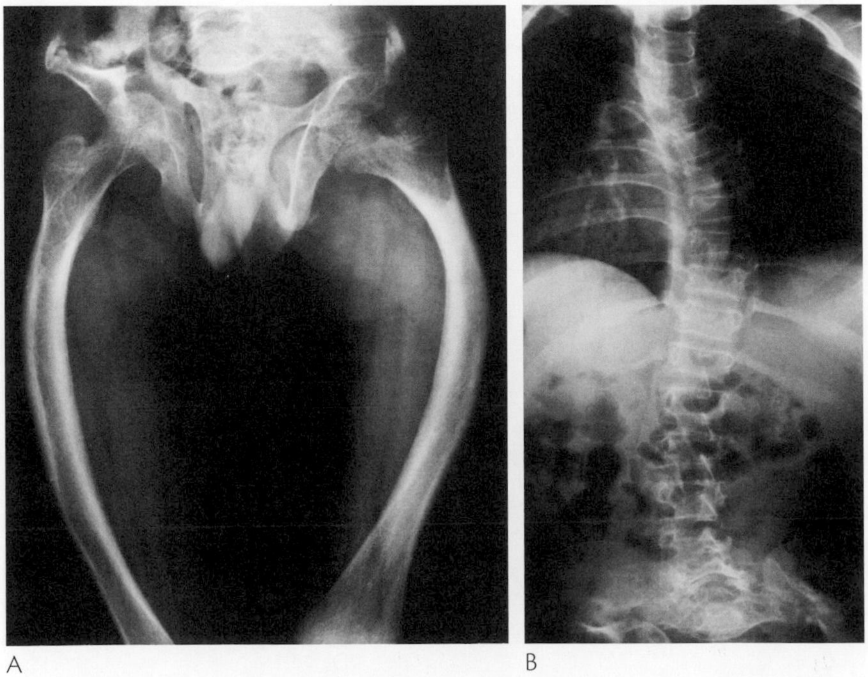

Fig. 3.13.6 A) Severe osteogenesis imperfecta with pelvic and leg deformity. B) These patients always have a scoliosis.

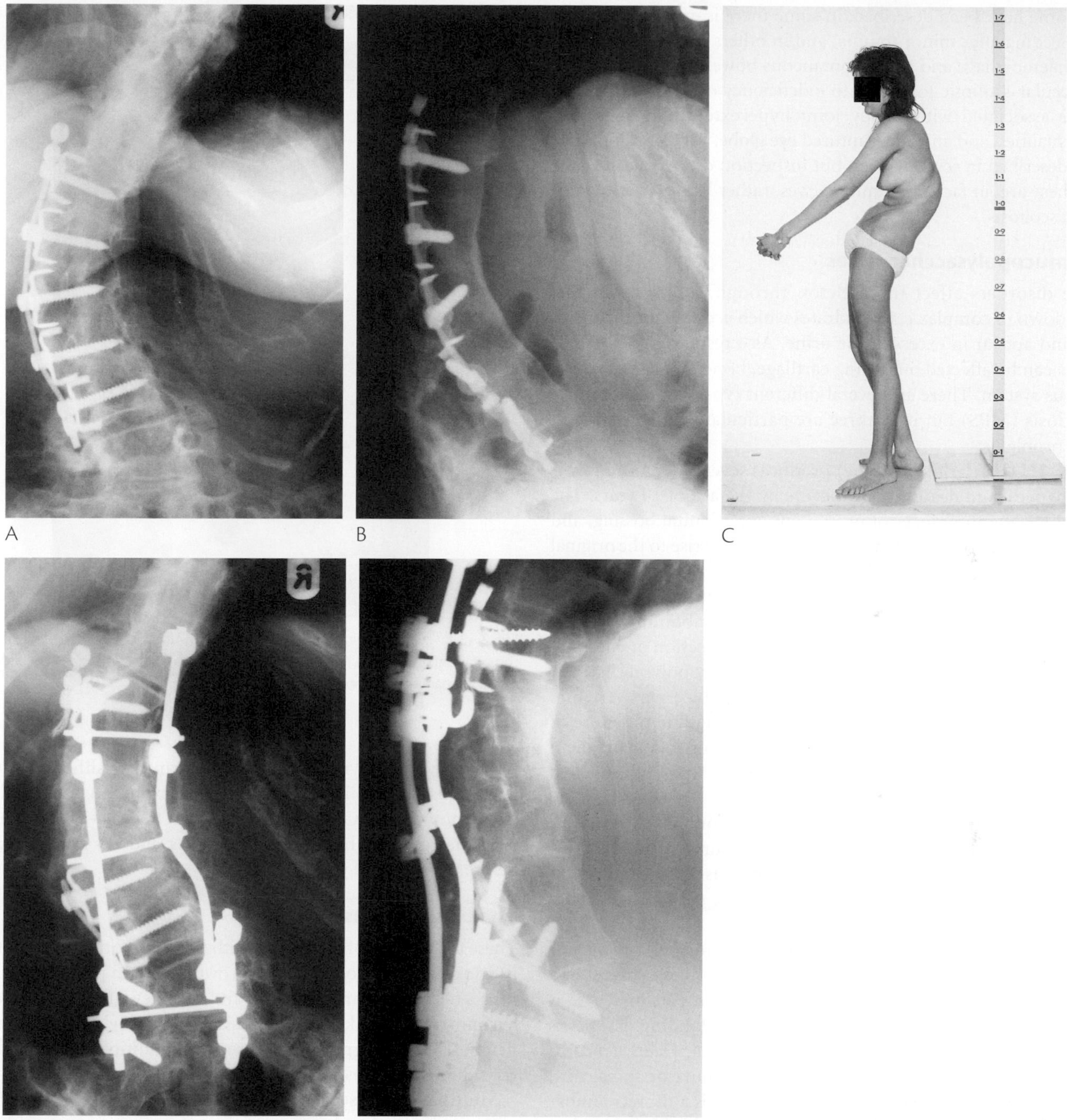

Fig. 3.13.7 A) Severe lumbar scoliosis in a girl with Marfan's syndrome treated 12 years previously by anterior Dwyer instrumentation. There is clearly a solid interbody fusion. B) Lateral radiographs showing that with time the fusion has bent into significant kyphosis. C) Sideways view of the patient showing a severe deformity which was also very painful. D) After two-stage spinal osteotomy and posterior instrumentation. E) Lateral radiograph 3 years postosteotomy showing an excellent correction of this difficult deformity. Her pain resolved.

There is platyspondyly on lateral spine radiographs and a 50% incidence of scoliosis on frontal radiographs, which appears to be similar to idiopathic scoliosis.

Congenital contractural arachnodactyly

This is an autosomal dominant condition characterized by contractures which are present at birth and tend to affect the proximal interphalangeal joints of the fingers, the elbows, the knees, and the ankles. Spontaneous improvement in these contractures always occurs. In addition, there is dolichostenomelia (long thin limbs), arachnodactyly, and abnormalities of the external ears. Scoliosis can occur; it is similar to idiopathic scoliosis and should be treated similarly.

Ehlers–Danlos syndrome

Excessively stretchable, fragile, and bruisable skin is also associated with loose-jointedness. A number of different types of Ehlers–Danlos syndrome have been described; in some there is excessive bruising and bleeding after minor trauma, and in others there is uncontrollable haemorrhage and even spontaneous bowel rupture. Type 6 is the occular-scoliotic form due to a deficiency of lysyl hydroxylase and is associated with floppy joint hyperextensibility, vascular abnormalities, and an easily ruptured eye globe. Severe scoliosis has been described in several series, but inspection of the data suggests that these are, in fact, fairly mild curves, rather like late-onset idiopathic scoliosis.

The mucopolysaccharidoses

These disorders affect the skeleton through failure of normal breakdown of complex carbohydrates which accumulate in the tissues and appear in excess in the urine. As a result many different tissues can be affected, including cartilage, bone, liver, and central nervous system. There are several different types of mucopolysaccharidosis (MPS) but only three are particularly associated with spine problems.

MPS 1H (Hurler's syndrome) produces severe mental and skeletal changes, and death usually occurs by the age of 10 years. The typical facial appearances of prominent eyes, frontal bossing, and coarse features with a flattened nasal bridge gave rise to the original description of gargoylism. There is abdominal enlargement due to hepatosplenomegaly. The fingers are stubby, the hands are broad, and the joints are stiff. There is an oblique acetabulum with subluxating hips. Death occurs from respiratory infection or coronary heart disease due to the accumulation of mucopolysaccharides. The spine is affected by a persistent infantile biconvex vertebral body shape and characteristic vertebral beaking due to failure of the anterosuperior corners of the vertebrae to form, making them hook-shaped. There is a characteristic kyphosis and the attached ribs are paddle shaped.

MPS II (Hunter's syndrome) is less common and milder than Hurler's syndrome, and affected individuals survive into the third decade. Only males are affected. Again, there is short stature with stubby fingers, stiffness, and contracture. The spinal changes are similar to Hurler's syndrome but less obvious.

MPS IV (Morquio's syndrome). There is normal intelligence and variable physical disability, but the major problems are a short-trunked stature with a height of not more than 120cm. There is joint and skin laxity, genu valgum, and corneal clouding. The pelvis is hypoplastic and there is epiphyseal dysplasia. Death tends to occur as a result of either cardiorespiratory failure or spinal cord compression. As with MPS I and MPS II, there is a thoracolumbar kyphosis with platyspondyly and anterior vertebral breaking but there are two additional major spinal problems in Morquio's syndrome: a thoracolumbar kyphosis (Figure 3.13.8) and atlanto-axial instability as a result of a deficient odontoid. The thoracolumbar kyphosis is associated with a barrel-shaped chest and prominent sternum to the point where premature fusion of the sternal segments with an immobile chest can lead to severe respiratory dysfunction.

If the kyphosis is not severe it can be braced, but if neurological symptoms develop then it must be treated by anterior dural decompression, strut grafting, and posterior metalwork neutralization as with any kyphosis producing cord compression.

C1–2 instability is common and, while there may be clear physical evidence of myelopathy, the neurological signs are often atypical with tiredness, weakness, vague leg pains, paroxysmal tachypnoea, respiratory arrest, syncope, and gait abnormality. Although some of these signs can be bilateral, they are often expressed unilaterally.

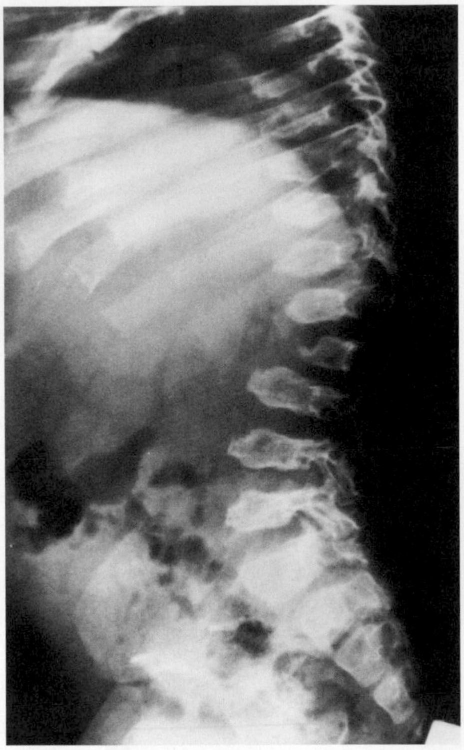

Fig. 3.13.8 Typical appearances of platyspondyly and a bullet-shaped thoracolumbar vertebra in Morquio's syndrome (MPS IV). There are similar lateral spinal appearances in spondyloepiphyseal dysplasia.

The notoriety of C1–2 instability is such that C1–2 fusion should be carried out prophylactically in all cases, and this implies surgery before the age of 10 years.

The bone dysplasias

These are a group of conditions with the common factor that there is disordered development and growth of some part of the skeleton. There are many of these and, as they are not frequently encountered. The Skeletal Dysplasia Society provides guides on the diagnosis and prognosis for these rare conditions and should be consulted when the diagnosis is considered.

Multiple epiphyseal dysplasia is characterized by short stature with significant involvement of the epiphyses of hips and knees. The hands are characteristically short with stubby fingers. The problem here is of irregular epiphyseal growth without normal endochondral ossification while bone modelling is normal. The femoral capital epiphysis is always involved in a severe Perthes disease-like process. Secondary osteoarthritis is common in early adult life. The spine can be involved in a process similar to Scheuermann's disease and responds to extension bracing. Significant scoliosis is not encountered.

Chondrodysplasia punctata (stippled epiphysis) is characterized by stippled epiphyses, extra-epiphyseal calcification, skin lesions, cataracts, mental retardation, short limbs, and short stature. The spinal stippling is caused by chalky deposits, and there are separate ossification centres for the body and posterior elements giving a characteristic separated appearance on a lateral radiograph

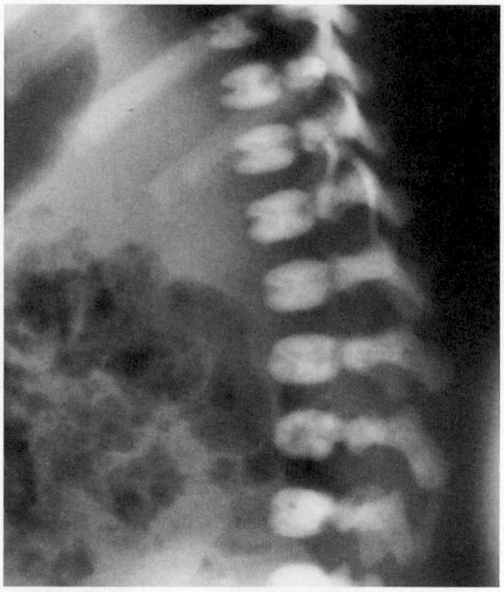

Fig. 3.13.9 Chondrodysplasia punctata. Note the separation of anterior and posterior elements and the chalky deposits.

(Figure 3.13.9). Spinal deformities, if present, are of the congenital variety with a recognizable anomaly at the curve apex.

Achondroplasia is a bone dysplasia with predominantly metaphyseal involvement and is an autosomal dominant condition with the great majority appearing as new mutations. The typical appearance is that of short limbs with short fingers on trident hands, a bulging cranium with a low nasal bridge, and characteristic pelvic changes with squaring of the iliac wings, more horizontal acetabulae, and widening of the upper femoral metaphysis with a short femoral neck.

There are two important effects on the spine in achondroplasia—spinal stenosis and a thoracolumbar kyphosis. Both can give rise to neurological problems. As with other dysplasias and the mucopolysaccharidoses, kyphosis is particularly prevalent and is due to a thoracolumbar anterior wedged bullet-shaped vertebra. This produces a local angular kyphosis (Figure 3.13.10) but, importantly, 90% of these kyphoses resolve spontaneously. Therefore the spine should be observed to allow the natural history to reveal itself. If the kyphosis persists and progresses to the point of neurological disability, anterior dural decompression and strut graft posterior metalwork is necessary.

The most common sites for a stenosis in the achondroplastic subject are the thoracolumbar or upper lumbar regions. The anteroposterior diameter of the spinal canal is particularly reduced. Less than half of achondroplastic individuals have symptoms or signs of spinal stenosis, and less than 20% exhibit objective neurological findings. Preoperative imaging determines the levels that require being decompressed. In the achondroplastic adult, adequate decompression can be carried out by undercutting so as not to jeopardize posterior facet joint stability bilaterally. In the immature spine even this degree of decompression can give rise to a progressive kyphosis and thus concomitant fusion is necessary (Figure 3.13.11). Sometimes preoperative imaging demonstrates a prolapsed intervertebral disk rather than bony canal stenosis as the offending problem.

The upper cervical spine can also be the source of neurological problems because the occipitalization of C1 in association with

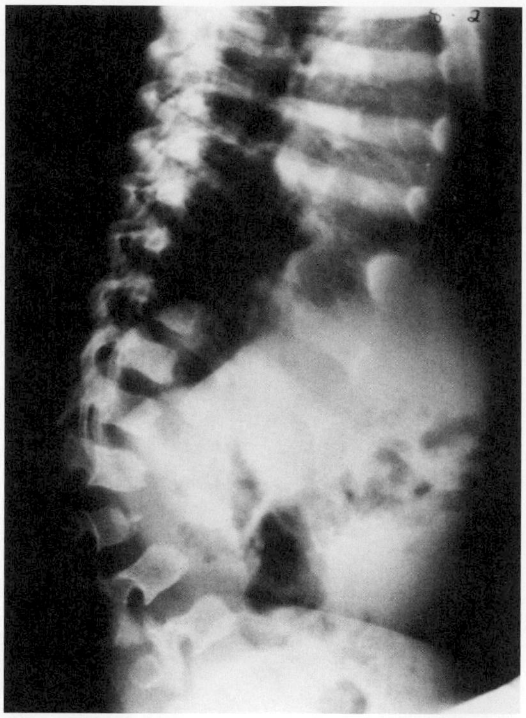

Fig. 3.13.10 A bullet-shaped thoracolumbar vertebra is common in skeletal dysplasias and is shown here in achondroplasia. Ninety per cent of these will correct spontaneously.

stenosis of the foramen magnum can give rise to secondary atlantoaxial instability. Fusion from C2 to the occiput in extension is required.

Spondyloepiphyseal dysplasia tarda is associated with mild dysplasia of vertebrae and large joints, with the hips and shoulders particularly affected. It is often confused with Morquio's syndrome. There is a small pelvis, a deep acetabulum, and a short femoral neck, but the distal epiphyses are not involved. The trunk is short with sternal protrusion and the vertebral changes are typical. There is platyspondyly, but the vertebral bodies are humped posteriorly, differentiating them from multiple epiphyseal dysplasia and MPS IV. Significant kyphosis is not the rule but may have to be dealt with by anterior decompression, strut grafting, and posterior metalwork. Mild kyphoses can benefit from extension bracing.

Spondyloepiphyseal dysplasia congenita is rare. The features of platyspondyly, Scheuermann-type changes of kyphosis, and bullet-shaped thoracolumbar vertebrae are more pronounced than in the tarda variety but can respond to extension bracing.

Diastrophic dysplasia is an autosomal recessive condition of short limbs, club-foot, joint contractures, and spinal deformity. A cystic swelling of the ear in the first few days of life later ossifies to produce the typical 'cauliflower ear' deformity. The first metacarpal is short, giving rise to the term 'hitch-hiker's thumb'. There are dysplastic epiphyses and the hips are particularly severely involved. The club-foot deformity, like early-onset progressive malignant scoliosis, is particularly resistant to correction. Height seldom exceeds 1m.

There are a number of important spinal problems in diastrophic dysplasia. Odontoid hypoplasia can give rise to atlantoaxial stability which may require fusion. The cervical spine is particularly

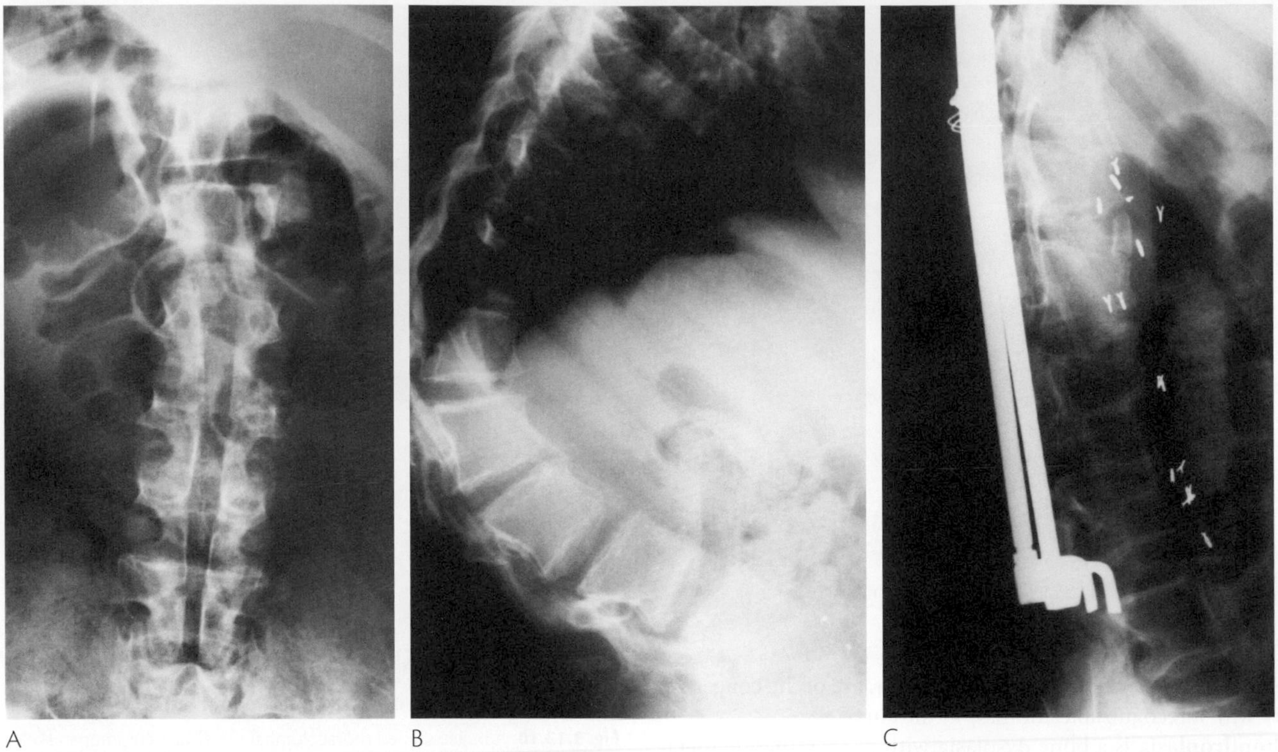

Fig. 3.13.11 A) A long decompression was carried out to correct developmental spinal stenosis in association with achondroplasia in a growing child but no concomitant fusion was performed. B) During adolescence a severe kyphosis developed which had tensioned the spinal cord with redevelopment of neurological signs. C) After anterior release and anterior and posterior fusion, the deformity was corrected and the neurological features resolved.

prone to the development of a kyphosis which can in its own right produce neurological problems and even death. Sometimes the kyphosis can improve spontaneously, and therefore the neurological situation should be closely monitored before prescribing anterior and posterior fusion. Scoliosis is common in dystrophic dysplasia but curvature seldom becomes severe. Because of the relatively young age of patients, anterior and posterior fusion is required. Spina bifida occulta is a virtually constant finding in either the neck or lumbar region, and if instrumentation is to be used then the tethering effect must be preoperatively excluded by MRI scanning prior to the application of metalwork.

Further reading

Mehta, M.H. (1972). The rib vertebra angle in the early diagnosis between resolving and progressive infantile scoliosis. *Journal of Bone and Joint Surgery Br*, **54B**, 230–43.

Moe, J.H. (1984). Harrington instrumentation without fusion plus external orthotic support for the treatment of difficult curvature problems in young children. *Clinical Orthopaedics and Related Research*, **185**, 34–45.

Moe's Textbook of Scoliosis and Other Spinal Deformities (1994). W.B Saunders

Kim, D.H., Betz, R.R., Huhn, S.L., Newton, P.O. (2008). *Surgery of the Pediatric Spine.* Thieme Medical Publishing.

Weinstein, S.L. (2001). The Pediatric Spine (2nd Edition). Lippincott Williams and Wilkins.

3.14

Brace treatment in idiopathic scoliosis: the case for treatment

Ian Harding

Summary points

- Brace treatment has best chance of success in younger children and those with smaller curves
- In most cases it can be expected to stop the curve becoming worse.

Introduction

To brace or not to brace is still a matter of debate. A large number of studies of this question are still being presented, with no less than 459 papers reported in Medline between 1966 and 1995. Most of these papers are retrospective and are open to criticism on various points. A meta-analysis has been published by Rowe and colleagues (1997). A recent cochrane review states that there is very low quality evidence in favor of using braces, making generalization very difficult. It suggests further prospective studies following Scoliosis Research Society Guidelines.

History

The first effective brace module for idiopathic scoliosis was the Milwaukee brace (Figure 3.14.1). This was molded individually. Module braces, such as the Boston brace (Figure 3.14.2), which are made from prefabricated plastic were then developed. The module is trimmed to the needs of the individual patient and fitted with pads to correct the curvature.

Indications

The indication for conservative treatment of idiopathic scoliosis is the possibility of influencing the natural history. This means that we must predict what will happen if the individual case is or is not treated. The natural development of idiopathic scoliosis is influenced by age, sex, stage of pubertal development, skeletal development (Risser sign), and the pattern and progression of the curves.

Bracing is ineffective in curves with a Cobb angle in excess of 50 degrees. To be effective, bracing should reduce the incidence of surgical treatment.

One study compared the effectiveness of brace treatment in adolescent idiopathic scoliosis with non-treated scoliosis cases, all with Cobb angles between 25–35 degrees. This supported the use of brace treatment in this subset of patients. Brace treatment is also supported by a meta-analysis which suggests that the 23-h regimen is better than shorter regimens.

The cosmetic appearance of the trunk is important. Another study showed a 41% improvement of the surface shape during brace treatment, although only a 9% improvement was seen radiographically. Brace treatment probably prevents progression of the Cobb angle, but some have reported improvement. Premenarchal children may have an increased risk of failure compared with older children.

Today, the indications generally suggested are as follows:

- A Cobb angle between 25–45 degrees
- A visible progression of 5 degrees observed during the previous 6 months

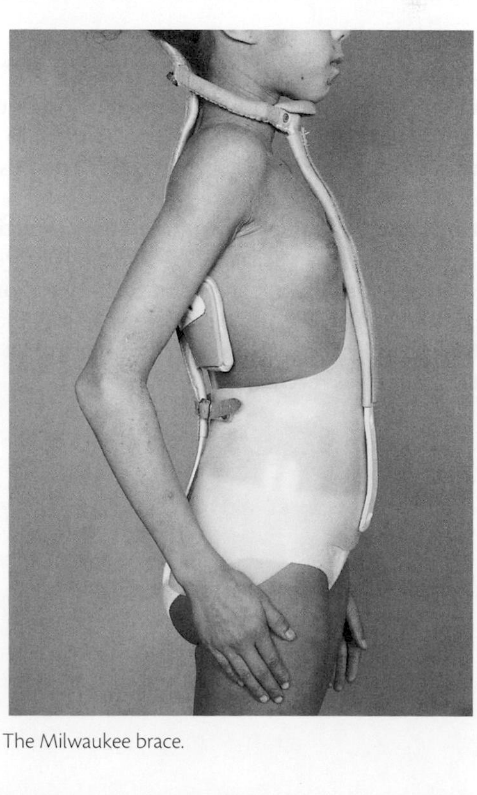

Fig. 3.14.1 The Milwaukee brace.

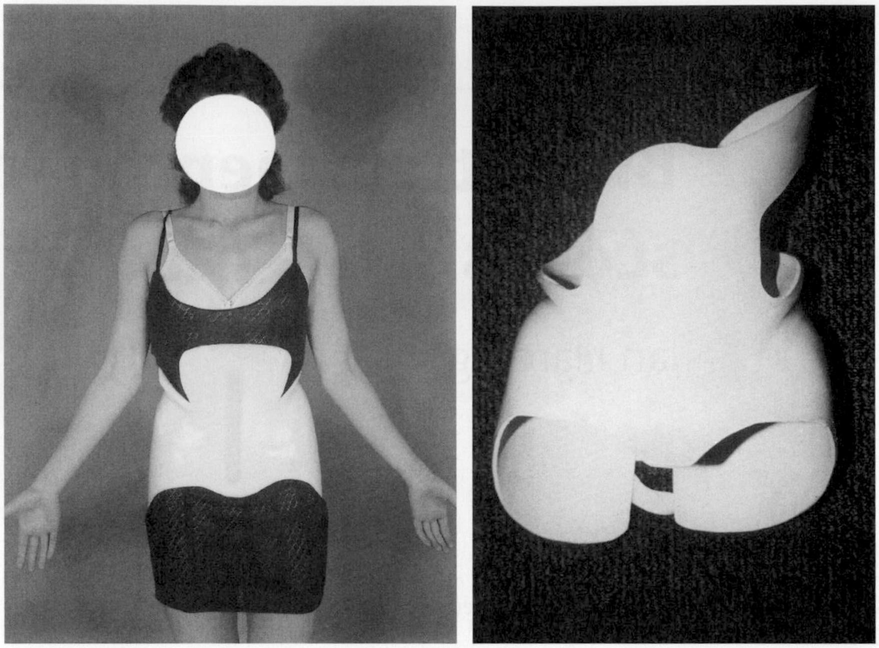

Fig. 3.14.2 The Boston brace.

- At least 1 year of growth remaining
- Risser sign, 0–3.

Effectiveness depends on compliance; full parental support and cooperation with the orthopedic surgeon, the physiotherapist, and the orthotist is essential. A sufficient number of cases must be treated annually to obtain optimum results. Many new non-rigid braces have entered the market place but the results are no more or less encouraging at this stage than the more traditional rigid braces.

Results of brace treatment

Brace treatment should prevent further progression of the curvature. Usually an improvement of 10–20% is reported. In rare cases the curvatures are almost completely corrected. The Boston brace is more successful than the Milwaukee brace.

The best results are obtained when the initial correction of the scoliosis in the brace is at least 50%. The poorest results are obtained when there is a hypokyphosis of the thoracic area of less than 20 degrees. The brace must be used for at least 20h a day. It is taken off for sporting activities. Brace treatment must continue until skeletal maturity is reached (Risser 4).

Weaning from the brace treatment must be carried out slowly over a period of 4–6 months. A slow correction loss is often seen after cessation of treatment. The end result is usually a few degrees less than the degree of the scoliosis seen before the start of the treatment. The maximal correction loss is observed within 2 years of the end of the weaning. A follow-up of 2 years has been found to be enough to predict failure.

The failure rates ranges up to 30%. The reasons for these variations are mainly different indications for bracing.

Conclusion

Brace treatment of idiopathic scoliosis may influence the natural history in some individuals and may reduce the number of patients requiring surgical treatment. Close monitoring is required.

Further reading

Dickson, R.A. and Weinstein, S.L. (1999). Bracing (and screening): yes or no? *Journal of Bone and Joint Surgery,* **81B**, 193–8.

Stefano, N., Silvia, M., Josette, B-S., *et al.* (2010). Braces for Idiopathic Scoliosis in Adolescents. *Spine*, **35**, 1285–93.

3.15

Iatrogenic spinal deformity

Paul Rhys Davies and John K. Webb

Summary points

- Laminectomy, especially in the growing child can lead to late kyphosis
- Various strategies are available to prevent this.

Introduction

Iatrogenic spinal deformity is an abnormal alignment of the spine which is caused by medical treatment.

Aetiology

There are three main causes of iatrogenic deformity:

1) Postdecompressive surgery
2) Post-thoracic surgery
3) Postirradiation.

Teratogenic events can lead to spinal maldevelopment *in utero.*

Postdecompressive surgery deformity

Adults

This is a relatively common complication of spinal surgery in adults. It is caused by excessive removal of the posterior elements of the spine and/or a failure to recognize lesser spinal deformity in the coronal or sagittal plane prior to surgery because sole reliance has been placed upon magnetic resonance imaging for preoperative assessment. Spondylolisthesis due to excessive facet (zygopophyseal) joint resection is the most common problem but lateral subluxation (especially at L4/5 and less so at L3/4). The integrity and orientation of the facet joints is critical to spinal stability. If more than 50% of the facet joint is excised, there is a significant risk of subluxation. This may precipitate spinal stenosis (see Chapter 3.8). The recognition of this complication by spinal surgeons has reduced the incidence of this complication. The identification of an underlying spinal deformity must be identified preoperatively so that the problem is not exacerbated by injudicious decompression.

Children

Multilevel laminectomies in children (usually for the treatment of spinal tumours) have a high incidence of late kyphosis. This occurs in up to 50% of children undergoing multilevel cervical laminectomy. The younger the child at the time of surgery, the more likely it is that deformity will occur. The facet joints are more horizontal in children than adults and therefore the risk of kyphosis is greater. In the young, the initial kyphosis may lead to anterior wedging of the vertebrae, resulting in further kyphosis. The posterior ligaments and the paraspinal musculature also play an important role in maintaining the sagittal profile of the spine. Disruption of these during major surgery may encourage kyphosis. Kyphosis is the most common deformity following multilevel laminectomy and is progressive with a risk of neurological deficit. The level of the surgery is important. The cervical spine is most at risk, followed by the thoracic spine (Figures 3.15.1 and 3.15.2). The lumbar spine is rarely affected.

Scoliosis rarely occurs following laminectomy and is usually caused by the pathology which precipitated the original surgery or its treatment. Scoliosis may be a presenting feature of a spinal tumour (Figure 3.15.3). Surgical excision of the tumour does not prevent progression of the curve.

Lordosis

Lordosis of the spine, producing a characteristic swan-neck deformity, may be seen following multilevel cervical laminectomy. Lordosis also occurs as a compensatory effect above an iatrogenic thoracic kyphosis and in the lumbar spine after extensive laminectomy.

Management

Prevention is the most effective method of treating this condition. Surgeons should try to preserve the posterior structures, especially the facet joints and ligaments. Liaison between the neurosurgeon and the orthopaedic spinal surgeon are important with prevention and appropriate primary surgery being preferable to revision surgery and stabilization. Laminoplasty (instead of laminectomy) has been shown to have a reduced incidence of kyphosis in the cervical spine in children. Instrumented spinal fusion at the time of surgery

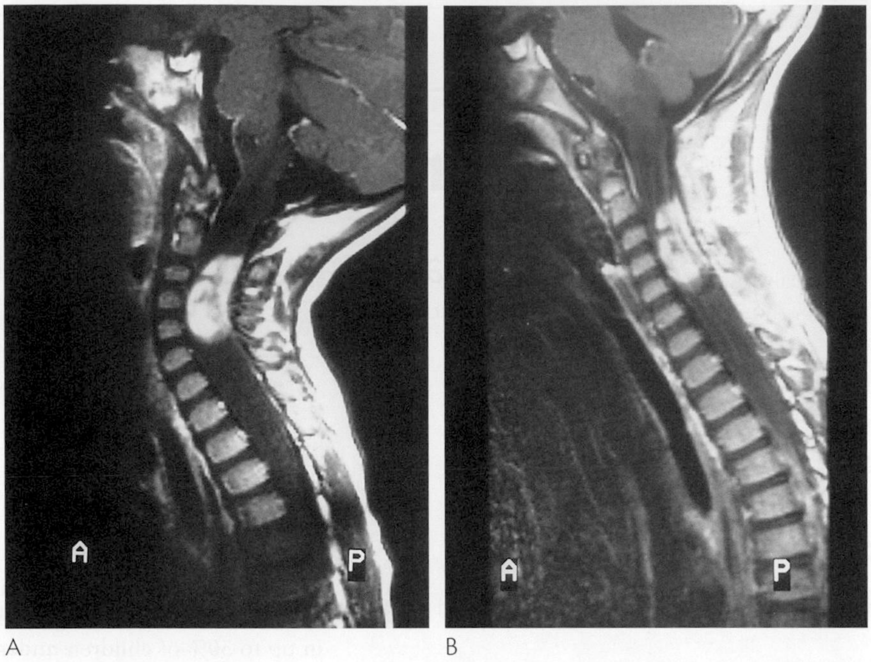

Fig. 3.15.1 A) Preoperative MRI of a 4-year-old girl who presented with an intradural tumour. She subsequently underwent C3–7 laminectomy. B) The postoperative MRI which demonstrates the loss of normal cervical lordosis. The patient developed a progressive cervicothoracic kyphosis which required correction and stabilization with ligament reconstruction.

may be appropriate; for example, in spinal stenosis with coexistent degenerative spondylolisthesis.

Long-term postoperative follow-up is mandatory, especially in the young patient at risk. External support by bracing or a halo-jacket may be helpful in preventing progression. If the deformity is progressive, *in situ* fusion or correction and fusion are the best approaches. A combined anterior and posterior approach will be necessary for correction of a kyphosis.

Ligament reconstruction has been described for postcervical laminectomy deformity. The theoretical advantage of this technique over fusion means that the growing child can gain some longitudinal growth and not be doomed to a shortened cervical spine.

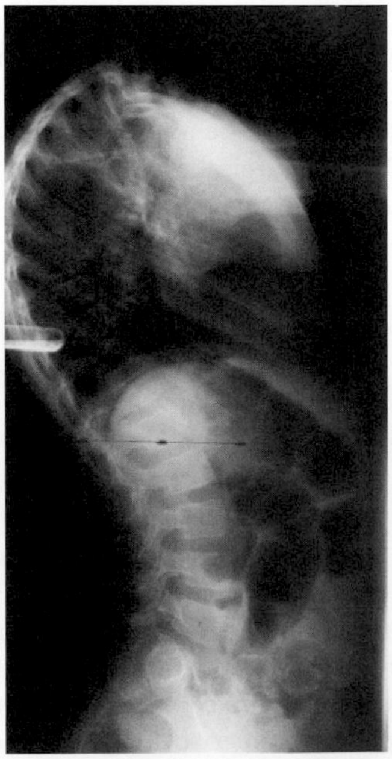

Fig. 3.15.2 A lateral thoracic spinal radiograph of a boy who presented with a thoracic cord astrocytoma. He subsequently underwent T3–7 laminectomy followed by radiotherapy. The radiograph shows that, following surgery, the patient developed a progressive thoracic kyphosis measuring 90 degrees from T2 to T12.

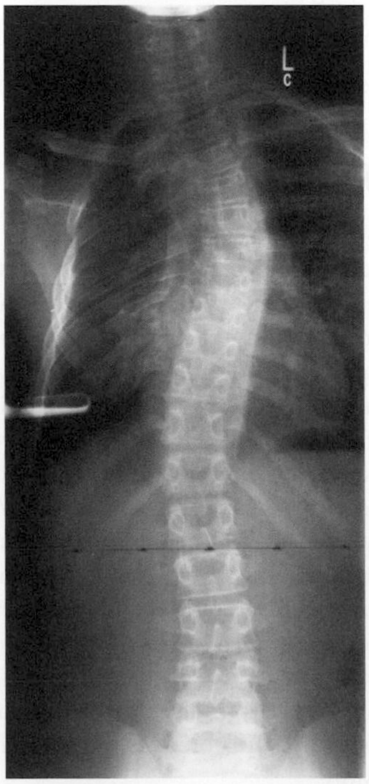

Fig. 3.15.3 A progressive scoliosis developed in this boy who had undergone thoracic surgery followed by irradiation for an intrathoracic tumour.

This may occur if the neck is fused at a young age, preventing further growth.

Post-thoracic surgery deformity

The removal of ribs in a growing child can destabilize the thoracic spine and lead to the development of scoliosis. The more ribs that are removed, and the closer the ribs are resected to the spine, the worse the resulting deformity. The curve deviates with the convex side to the side of the rib resection. In the developed world, the most common cause of thoracogenic deformity is the resection of multiple ribs for the treatment of malignancy. Elsewhere, tuberculosis is the main cause of this deformity.

Treatment

Conservative treatment is not usually possible. The absence of lateral ribs prevents the application of a brace to apply pressure to the spine. Instrumented correction and stabilization are required for progressive curves.

Postirradiation deformity

Radiotherapy is used as a treatment for childhood tumours, such as Wilms' tumour and neuroblastomas. The normal growth of the spine may be affected, leading to spinal deformity. The epiphysis is particularly susceptible to radiation damage. The first case of scoliosis induced by radiation was described by Arkin and colleagues in 1950. Skeletally immature patients who receive more than 1000cGy are at risk. The risk of deformity increases with the amount of radiation absorbed. Asymmetric radiation is more likely to lead to scoliosis and symmetric radiation may lead to a kyphotic deformity. In another study, it was noted that 59 out of 81 patients who had radiotherapy for Wilms' tumour developed a subsequent scoliosis.

The younger the patient at the time of exposure to radiation, the more risk there is of spinal deformity. Patients aged less than 2 years at the time of radiotherapy are particularly at risk.

Management

All paediatric patients undergoing spinal irradiation require follow-up by an orthopaedic surgeon or spine specialist until skeletal maturity. The principles for bracing or surgical management are the same as those for idiopathic deformity (Chapter 3.10). The risk of pseudarthrosis and infection is high, and healing may be prolonged if surgery is undertaken.

Conclusion

The importance of iatrogenic deformity lies in its recognition and prevention. This is certainly true for postlaminectomy deformity. Reducing the extent of surgery on the thoracic cage will decrease the risk of post-thoracotomy deformity. Radiation therapy is likely to generate spinal deformity, and these patients require vigilant follow-up. In adults, the most common deformity occurs as a result of a failure to fully appreciate the position of the spine preoperatively followed by injudicious decompressive surgery.

3.16

Kyphosis

Michael Grevitt and John K. Webb

Summary points

- Kyphosis may be a focal deformity limited to a few spinal segments or a more global problem involving the thoracolumbar spine
- The causes are myriad and reflect all the disease processes that affect bone
- As well as producing pain from disturbed sagittal balance, neurological complications can occur infrequently
- Conservative treatment in established kyphotic deformity has a limited role
- The aims of surgery are to correct the deformity, restore sagittal alignment and decompress the neural elements as required.

Introduction

There are many causes of a kyphotic deformity of the spine, and the incidence and prevalence varies with the population studied. Postinfectious kyphosis is more common in developing countries, whereas post-traumatic, congenital, and degenerative deformities predominate in Western cultures.

The thoracic spine has a normal posterior convex angulation which usually measures 40 degrees. There is a wide physiological variation, and the mean figure alters with the age and sex of the individual. During adolescence, males have a greater kyphosis than females. The mean thoracic kyphosis increases with age in both sexes and is most pronounced at a mean age of 13.8 years. Importantly, unlike the coronal plane where we are all identical, our sagittal profile is like a fingerprint and very individual. When a sagittal deformity occurs it may be well tolerated or poorly tolerated depending on the individual normal profile including the pelvic position and lower limbs.

Classification of kyphosis is summarized in Table 3.16.1, and the management of each type is discussed in detail in the following sections.

Table 3.16.1 Classification of kyphosis

Congenital
Type I: failure of segmentation
Type II: failure of formation
Type III: combined
Developmental
Scheuermann's disease
Postural round back
Inflammatory
Pyogenic spondylodiskitis
Tuberculous spondylitis
Ankylosing spondylitis
Rheumatoid arthritis
Metabolic
Osteoporosis
Osteomalacia
Post-traumatic
Iatrogenic
Post-laminectomy
Post-radiation
'Flatback' deformity
Neoplastic
Spinal metastases
Neurofibromatosis
Aneurysmal bone cysts
Osteochondrodystrophies

Congenital kyphosis

Winter proposed a classification of congenital kyphotic deformities in 1977. In type I, normal vertebral segmentation is absent, resulting in an anterior bone block. Type II results from defects in formation of one or more vertebral bodies, and type III is a combination of types I and II.

In Type I deformities, the anterior bone acts as a tether and the angulation increases with continued posterior growth. The severity depends on the length of affected spine and the growth differential between the anterior and posterior elements of the spine. Type II deformities range from mild to severe. Mild cases show failure of formation of variable portions of a single vertebra. In severe types there may be total absence of a vertebral body and multiple defects. They occur most commonly at the thoracolumbar junction and, if asymmetric, a kyphoscoliosis results. The deformity increases significantly with growth and may lead to paraplegia, most commonly in adolescence.

The natural history of congenital kyphosis is poor and there is no successful non-operative treatment. The surgical treatment depends on the type of anomaly, the age of the patient, and the magnitude of the deformity.

If detected early, type I deformities can be treated by posterior fusion alone (extending one vertebra above and below the segmentation defect). Although the deformity is not corrected, it will prevent any deterioration in the curve. If a significant deformity exists, anterior osteotomies of the unsegmented bar combined with posterior instrumentation will be required to achieve correction and stabilization.

Type II deformities are best treated by posterior fusion (between the ages of 1–3 years). Resultant anterior growth reduces the deformity. Above the age of 5 years the same treatment can be applied if the kyphosis is less than 50 degrees. Deformities greater than this require both anterior and posterior surgery. The principles of surgery are to release the anterior tethers (anterior longitudinal ligament, annulus, and cartilaginous vertebral anlage) and insert bone grafts to achieve solid fusion. Correction of the deformity can be achieved at the time of anterior surgery or when posterior instrumentation is used. When the deformity is associated with a paraparesis, preoperative magnetic resonance imaging (MRI) is required to define the site of compression and exclude a tethered cord. In these cases, the anterior procedure should include partial vertebral resection to decompress the cord and to provide adequate space for the cord to move forward when correction is performed.

Developmental kyphosis

Scheuermann's disease

This condition of unknown cause is often associated with kyphosis. Avascular necrosis of the ring apophyses, disc herniations through the endplate (Schmorl's nodes), excessive mechanical stress, and endocrine abnormalities have all been implicated in the pathogenesis.

The prevalence is approximately 1% of the general population and the female-to-male ratio is 2:1. The radiographic features of Scheuermann's disease are rarely seen before the age of 10, but most are apparent by 13 years of age.

Pain is the most common complaint (50%); it is usually intermittent and located over the apex of the curvature. Long-term studies of this group confirm that pain remains a problem, and they continue to be employed in less physical jobs than controls. Greater deformity is associated with poor lung function. The deformity and its location are also frequent complaints. A typical Scheuermann kyphosis is shown in Figure 3.16.1 and the radiological criteria for its diagnosis are given in Table 3.16.2.

There are atypical forms of Scheuermann's disease. One form has endplate irregularity, Schmorl's nodes, and disc-space narrowing without wedging or increased kyphosis. The other form has the clinical appearance of classic Scheuermann's kyphosis but without the vertebral body changes.

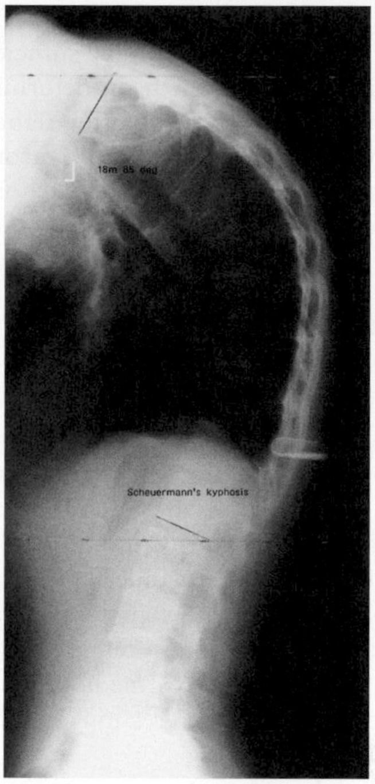

Fig. 3.16.1 Scheuermann's kyphosis: typical radiographic features in an 18-year-old male with an 85-degree deformity.

An increased incidence (30%) of spondylolysis and spondylolisthesis has been noted in patients with Scheuermann's disease, possibly due to the increased posterior element loading and lumbar hyperlordosis. Neurological complications, although rare, are well recognized; spastic paraparesis may develop secondary to the angular deformity alone or as a result of a herniated thoracic disc.

Management

The main indications for treatment are pain and deformity, especially in the growing child. The objectives are correction of the deformity and reduction of the progression of the kyphosis. Orthotic treatment has consisted of hypertension casts and Milwaukee braces. Correction of the deformity is readily achieved using these methods; the smaller the deformity, the greater is the correction. There is some loss of correction after cessation of treatment, but 69% maintain a useful improvement. Brace treatment is not recommended in skeletally mature individuals (whose vertebrae have no remodelling potential). Surgery may be indicated in deformities greater than 70 degrees and where orthotic treatment is unacceptable or has failed. Posterior correction and fusion have been associated with a high pseudarthrosis rate, which prompted the development of anterior instrumentation and strut grafting techniques. However, with deformities that correct to less than

Table 3.16.2 Criteria for diagnosing Scheuermann's kyphosis

Irregularity of the vertebral endplates
Narrowing of the intervertebral disk spaces
Three or more vertebrae with wedging of greater than 5°
A thoracic kyphosis exceeding 45°

70 degrees on hyperextension radiographs, posterior fusion alone, combined with modern implants, will be sufficient in the adolescent with potential anterior growth. In deformities greater than 70 degrees, additional release of anterior tethers and fusion is required. The latter can be achieved by thoracotomy or by using the thoracoscope. Most recently, even large deformities have been treated by modern instrumentation systems using posterior approaches alone.

Postural round back

This can be distinguished from Scheuermann's disease by the modest kyphosis (40–60 degrees) and accentuated lumbar lordosis. The deformity is mobile, and is easily and voluntarily correctable with no associated muscle contractures. Radiographs show normal vertebral morphology without endplate irregularity. This condition should not be diagnosed until after 13 years of age as Scheuermann's disease may not manifest itself before then.

Treatment follows the same principles as outlined for Scheuermann's kyphosis. Postural exercises may be sufficient in preadolescent children. Brace treatment should be commenced with radiographic evidence of progression or endplate changes.

Inflammatory kyphosis

Pyogenic spondylodiscitis

This is a common problem in developing countries, and is becoming increasingly prevalent in Western societies with an aging population, intravenous drug abusers, and the increased longevity of high-risk groups such as diabetics.

Staphylococcus aureus is the most common organism isolated (50–70%), and presenting symptoms may include fever, malaise, and back pain. There may be leucocytosis and raised erythrocyte sedimentation rate. However, atypical features are common and may include symptoms that lead to chest and abdominal investigations. In one series, the average period from first symptoms to diagnosis was 3 months. The radiographs may show intervertebral disc and adjacent endplate destruction (Figure 3.16.2).

In the absence of septicaemia, neurological deficit, or significant deformity, a tissue biopsy should be performed prior to antibiotic therapy. Tissue may be obtained by percutaneous methods or by transpedicular costotransversectomy or laminectomy. Surgery has a limited role and is indicated in the acute phase to decompress neural structures or for radical debridement in uncontrolled sepsis. In debilitated patients unfit for major surgery, drainage of a thoracic epidural abscess may be achieved via the thoracoscope. A less invasive approach may be adopted in the lumbar spine with minimal kyphosis. This involves application of a spinal external fixator to stabilize the adjacent motion segments and the installation of a suction–irrigation system in the intervertebral disc.

Cervical spine involvement is uncommon. Kyphosis may progress in the absence of pain. Surgical stabilization may be required with anterior and posterior surgery. Kyphosis may result from collapse of the disc space and vertebral destruction. Pain and progressive deformity are common sequelae. The principles of surgery in these cases are anterior radical debridement of all infected material, decompression of the dura, and bone grafting of the anterior column defect. During the latter process the sagittal contour of the spinal column is restored. Collapse of the graft may

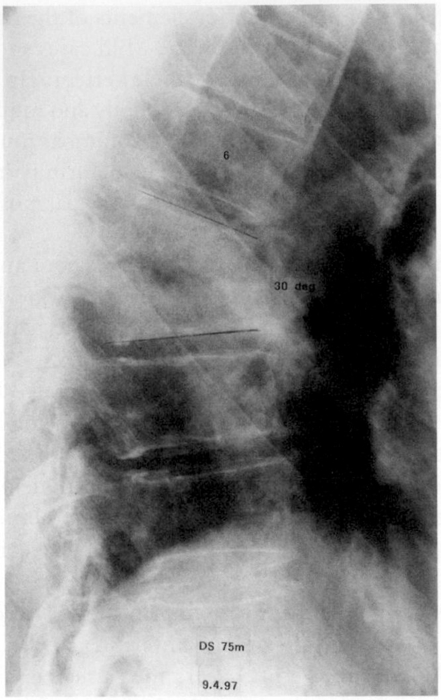

Fig. 3.16.2 Pyogenic spondylodiscitis: lateral radiograph of localized kyphosis resulting from Staphylococcus aureus spondylodiscitis and vertebral collapse of T7–8 in a 62-year-old diabetic man.

be prevented by wearing an orthosis, but modern pedicular/hook implant systems allow posterior stabilization without the need for postoperative bracing.

Tuberculous spondylitis

Tuberculosis remains a major health problem worldwide and a significant cause of acquired kyphosis (Figure 3.16.3). Its management is described in detail in Chapter 3.18.

Ankylosing spondylitis

This is a chronic inflammatory disease of unknown aetiology. It affects 0.02–2% of the general population, and is more common in males (2.4:1). Ankylosing spondylitis can be classified as an enthesopathy, i.e. inflammatory focus at the site of ligament or capsule insertion that produces reactive bone formation. Progressive endochondral ossification occurs which produces stiffness and ankylosis of the joints.

In the spine, ankylosis of the sacroiliac joints is followed by ossification of the interspinous and interlaminar ligaments, ankylosis of the facet joints, ossification of the annulus fibrosus, and syndesmophyte formation. This proceeds in a cranial direction and may involve the whole axial skeleton to produce characteristic radiographic appearances (bamboo spine). During the inflammatory episodes, pain is reduced by a flexed posture (which reduces facet joint pressure). This predisposes to development of kyphotic deformities in the cervicothoracic, thoracic, and lumbar spine. In severe cases, individuals are unable to stand upright, lose horizontal gaze, and develop a 'chin-on-chest' deformity. The functional limitations are exacerbated by flexion contractures or ankylosis of the hips.

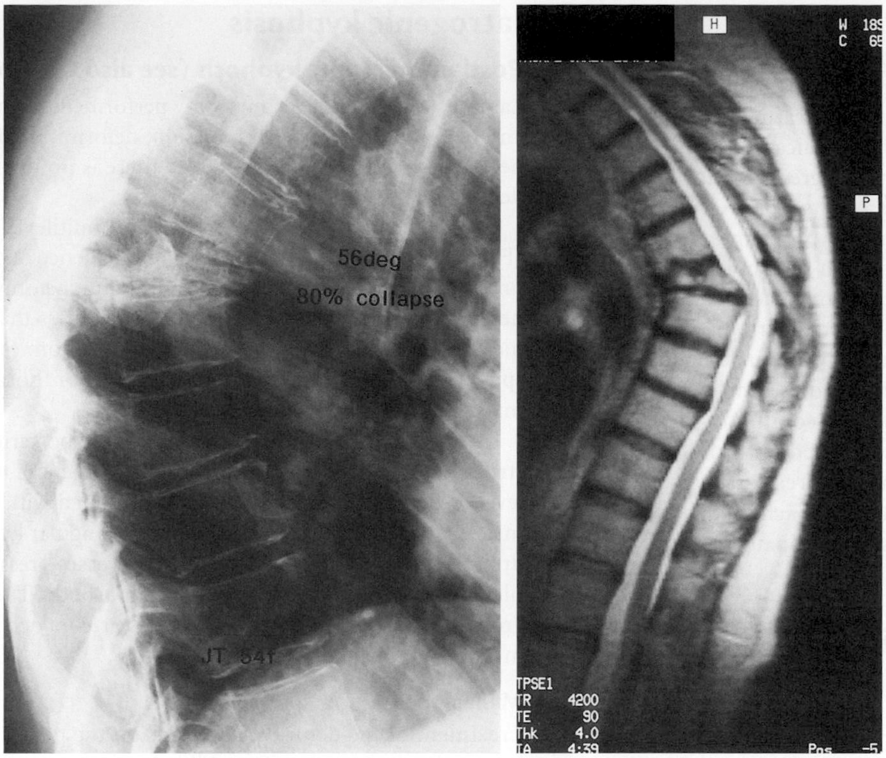

A B

Fig. 3.16.3 Post-traumatic kyphosis. A) Lateral radiograph of a T7 vertebral fracture in a 57-year-old woman treated conservatively 18 months previously. B) T_2-weighted MRI scan demonstrating cord compression.

Management

Modern conservative treatment emphasizes non-steroidal anti-inflammatory medication combined with regular exercise to maintain spinal mobility. Sleep in the supine position and on pillows is necessary to try to prevent kyphosis.

In most cases the problematic kyphotic deformity is located in the lumbar spine. It may be corrected by a lumbar osteotomy, first described by Smith-Peterson and colleagues in 1945. Other techniques have been described, but the general principle is acute angular correction of the spinal deformity below the conus medullaris thereby reducing the risk of neurological damage. The aim is to restore horizontal gaze and sagittal alignment of the spine so that C7 is centred over the sacrum. We currently favour the technique described by Thomasen in 1985. The lamina and pedicles of L3 are removed and the vertebral body is decancellized. Finally, an osteotomy of the posterior vertebral cortex is performed. Extension of the spine closes the osteotomy and creates an extension–compression fracture. The correction is held with pedicle screw instrumentation and the spine is formally arthrodesed. The screws should be inserted before the osteotomy is made. The advantages of this technique are that by shortening the spine, neural tension is avoided and the risks of aortic rupture reduced. Typical corrections of 30–40 degrees are achieved with this technique.

In severe thoracic kyphosis (with normal or increased lumbar lordosis and normal cervicothoracic alignment), multiple anteroposterior thoracic osteotomies are used to correct the deformity. In cases where the primary deformity is at the cervicothoracic junction, an extension osteotomy is performed. This is carried out at the C7–T1 level (below the entrance of the vertebral arteries in the transverse processes of C6) and uses the relatively capacious spinal canal at that level to obtain correction safely.

The final correction should achieve a balanced spine in the sagittal plane with the centre of gravity passing through the sacrum. Failure to do so risks the development of pseudarthrosis (due to tensile stress on the fusion mass) and progressive kyphosis above the stiff instrumented section (J.K. Webb, unpublished data).

Metabolic kyphosis

Osteoporosis and osteomalacia

Longitudinal studies demonstrate that kyphosis increases with advancing age. The kyphosis is more severe in women and is negatively correlated with bone mineral density.

The kyphotic deformity may be severe and result in sternal stress fractures and impingement of the costal margin on the iliac crest. Pulmonary complications are rare; an age-related decrease in vital capacity, especially when combined with a past history of cigarette smoking, is the usual cause of lung dysfunction in this group.

With rapidly progressive deformities it is important to exclude other conditions that mimic postmenopausal osteoporosis, such as spinal metastases, multiple myeloma, and endocrine disorders. A bone biopsy and quantitative histomorphometry is indicated in cases where osteomalacia is suspected.

The majority of affected individuals are asymptomatic, but some may complain of increasing deformity and back pain.

Management

Conservative treatment should be tried first; analgesics, anti-inflammatory agents, and extension exercises are prescribed. These measures may be supplemented with underarm orthoses.

Surgery may be indicated when there is incapacitating pain unresponsive to non-operative treatment, progressive deformity, and in the rare instance where paraparesis results from retropulsed bone from compression fractures. Technical problems arise from the porotic bone that provides poor fixation for implants. Additional problems are posed by the coincident chronic medical conditions that increase postoperative morbidity. An anterior release and thoracotomy are often poorly tolerated. The laminae maintain their strength longer than the vertebral bodies, and an alternative approach is shortening of the posterior column of the spine (by osteotomies and facetectomies) combined with multisegmental stabilization with alternate sublaminar wires and Mersilene tapes attached to Luque rods. Correction may be achieved, but the pseudarthrosis rate is greater than in cases of idiopathic juvenile kyphosis treated surgically.

Post-traumatic kyphosis

Kyphosis is a recognized common complication after thoracolumbar and lumbar fractures (Figure 3.16.3). Considerable controversy surrounds the treatment of these injuries, particularly burst fractures. The posterior column of the spine is a biomechanical concept that includes the bone and ligamentous structures dorsal to the posterior longitudinal ligament. It functions as a tension band; progressive kyphosis results from its damage when associated with anterior column injury (i.e. compression fractures). Identifying injury to the posterior column is often difficult; a widened interspinous gap or dorsal haematoma should be sought in the physical examination. Plain radiographs may show interspinous widening or laminar fractures. Posterior column injury may be inferred from the amount of damaged vertebral body, the spread of the fractured fragments, and the degree of corrected traumatic kyphosis. Soft tissue damage may be better visualized with modern MRI sequences.

A kyphotic deformity of 30 degrees is associated with an increased incidence of back pain. Progressive deformity may also result in late-onset paraparesis but as stated earlier in some individuals this may be well tolerated whereas in others it is not.

Management

The treatment of post-traumatic kyphosis is initially symptomatic; surgery is indicated where conservative treatment has failed or where there is neurological deficit. The goals of surgery are decompression of the spinal cord, correction of the deformity, and establishing spinal stability.

Posterior approaches (without transpedicular osteotomy) fail in the majority of cases; the bone graft is under tension, and pseudarthrosis and implant failure are common occurrences. Anterior approaches permit cord decompression and restoration of a solid anterior column to the spine. The correct sagittal alignment must also be obtained postoperatively. In moderate kyphosis this can be achieved in one procedure. In more severe deformities the anterior procedure may need to be combined with shortening of the posterior column by Smith-Peterson osteotomies and pedicle screw instrumentation.

Iatrogenic kyphosis

Postlaminectomy kyphosis (see also Chapter 3.15)

Laminectomies are less commonly performed during discectomies and nerve root canal decompression; deformities after these laminectomies are rare in adults where there is no pre-existing spinal deformity.

The incidence of deformity rises with multilevel laminectomies (Figure 3.16.4); one study reported an incidence of 46% in patients under 25 years of age who underwent laminectomy. Where laminectomies were performed in patients aged less than 15 years, the incidence of deformity was 46%; all laminectomies in the cervical spine or cervicothoracic junction and 36% of thoracic laminectomies were followed by kyphoses.

Removal of the tension band effect of the posterior ligamentous structures results in unopposed flexion moment of the spine at that level. When total facetectomies are combined with laminectomies in adults, it results in subluxation and an angular kyphosis. In children the increased bending moment increases pressure on the cartilaginous portion of the anterior vertebral body. There is decreased growth in this area and wedging of the vertebra occurs. This results in a long gradual kyphotic deformity.

Management

Treatment of the deformity depends on the pathology necessitating the laminectomies. The child should be carefully monitored and when kyphosis develops, a brace should be applied to control the deforming forces temporarily. Where the original diagnosis was a malignant tumour with poor prognosis, this should be the only treatment. If the prognosis is good, surgery should be recommended as prolonged brace treatment is ineffective.

Technical problems result from the deficient bone stock posteriorly, and isolated fusion in this area has a high pseudarthrosis rate.

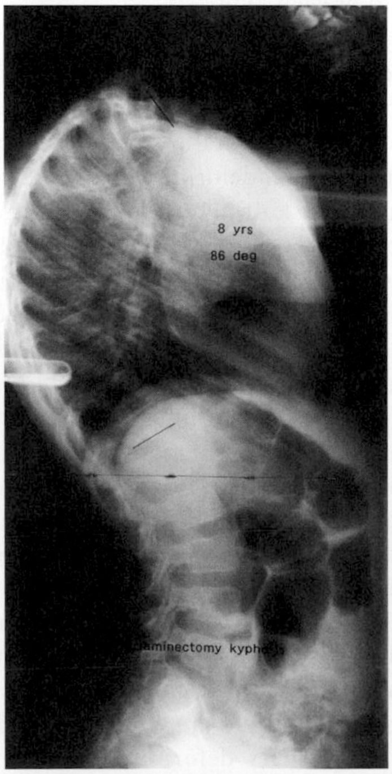

Fig. 3.16.4 Postlaminectomy kyphosis resulting 5 years after multilevel laminectomies for a spinal intramedullary tumour.

Continued posterior growth will cause further progression of the deformity. A combined approach is necessary. Anterior discectomies, correction of the deformity with strut grafting, and arthrodesis should be followed by posterior fusion carried into the normal lordotic segments. This may be performed as a single operation or as a staged procedure. Instrumentation may not be possible in these children, especially in the upper thoracic spine. A halo-cast should then be worn for 4 months.

Postradiation kyphosis

Radiotherapy for childhood malignancies (Wilms' tumour and neuroblastoma) may include the spine in the irradiated field. Radiation affects the epiphyseal plate of long bones and vertebrae, resulting in disturbance of metaphyseal remodelling and reduced longitudinal growth. Spinal deformity occurs with differential growth of the affected vertebrae. Vertebral endplate irregularities ('bone within bone' appearance) are common radiological features.

The threshold radiation dose for producing spinal deformity is 1000cGy; no spinal deformity has occurred with radiation below this level. Symmetric portals for irradiation produce a pure kyphosis; asymmetric fields produce either a scoliosis or a kyphoscoliosis. The younger the patient at the time of exposure, the greater is the risk; this is most marked in children aged less than 2 years. In one study of 81 patients who had received radiotherapy for Wilms' tumours, all but one subsequently developed a spinal deformity. Nineteen developed a kyphoscoliosis and two a kyphosis.

Management

Significant deformity is rare before the age of 10 years; curves may deteriorate during the pubertal growth spurt. There is no evidence for delayed skeletal maturation in these children. Orthotic treatment may be used for curves between 20–40 degrees, although there is no good evidence that orthoses produce permanent improvement.

Surgery is indicated for curves greater than 40 degrees or where a kyphotic deformity of more than 20 degrees exists at the thoracolumbar junction. The principles of fusion and the selection of fusion levels are the same as those for idiopathic scoliosis. Pseudarthroses and infections are more common in the irradiated spine; repeat bone grafting may be necessary at 6 months.

Neoplastic kyphosis

Spinal metastases

Skeletal metastases are present in 70% of patients with terminal cancer, and half of these have demonstrable spinal lesions. Most are asymptomatic, but progressive tumour infiltration of the vertebra may lead to collapse, kyphotic deformity, and pain. Up to 5% of these patients will also develop neurological deficits from compression by tumour or retropulsed bone or disc. In these instances radiotherapy is less effective and surgery may be indicated.

Decompression of the spinal cord, reconstruction of the anterior column, and restoration of sagittal alignment may all be achieved via an anterior approach. These patients are often cachetic and in poor general condition; using the earlier discussed principles, perioperative mortality rates of 30% have been reported.

In the past, surgical treatment for metastatic cord compression involved laminectomies. This approach was abandoned as the clinical results were poor. Adequate neural decompression was not achieved, and further cord damage occurred through the resultant spinal instability. A better appreciation of the need to restore the normal sagittal contour, more radical posterolateral decompression, and modern pedicle instrumentation have led to a resurgence of posterior surgery in spinal metastatic disease. This surgery is better tolerated, and the neurological and functional outcomes are comparable with the best reports of anterior decompression.

Further reading

Gill, J.B., Levin, A., Burd, T., and Longley, M. (2008). Corrective osteotomies in spine surgery. *The Journal of Bone and Joint Surgery Am*, **90**(11), 2509–20.

Lowe, T.G. (2007). Scheuermann's kyphosis. *Neurosurgery Clinics of North America*, **18**(2), 305–15.

Mundwiler, M.L., Siddique, K., Dym, J.M., Perri, B., Johnson, J.P., and Weisman, M.H. (2008). Complications of the spine in ankylosing spondylitis with a focus on deformity correction. *Neurosurgical Focus*, **24**(1), E6.

Munting, E. (2010). Surgical treatment of post-traumatic kyphosis in the thoracolumbar spine: indications and technical aspects. *European Spine Journal*, **19**, Suppl 1, S69–73.Epub 2009 Sep 11.

Potter, B.K., Lenke, L.G., and Kuklo, T.R. (2004). Prevention and management of iatrogenic flatback deformity. *The Journal of Bone and Joint Surgery Am*, **86A**(8), 1793–808.

Smith-Peterson, M.N., Larson, C.B., and Aufranc, O.E. (1945). Osteotomy of the spine for correction of flexion deformity in rheumatoid arthritis. *Journal of Bone and Joint Surgery*, **27A**, 1–11.

Thomasen, E. (1985). Vertebral osteotomy for correction of kyphosis in ankylosing spondylitis. *Clinical Orthopaedics and Related Research*, **194**, 142–52.

3.17

Spondylolisthesis and spondylolysis

Dietrich Schlenzka

Summary points

- Spondylolysis is a stress fracture of the vertebral arch. It may lead to vertebral slipping, spondylolisthesis.
- Spondylolysthesis is commonly lytic, isthmic, or degenerative.
- Spondylolysis and Spondylolysthesis can affect both children and adults.
- Most common symptoms are low-back pain and/or radiating pain. True neurologic deficit is rare
- Treating clinicians should be aware of the processes involved and the common consequences.
- The majority of symptomatic patients are treated non-operatively
- Operation is indicated in rare cases with neurologic deficit and in children or adolescents with a slip of 50 per cent or more
- Most common complications of surgery are nerve root compromise (especially in connection with slip reduction) and non-union.

Classification

Spondylolisthesis is the forward slip of a vertebra on another. The most common cause is *degenerative* spondylolisthesis which is seen in the older population as a result of disc and facet joint degeneration. In the young, the majority of vertebral slips are of the *isthmic* type in which an interruption (spondylolysis) or elongation of the pars interarticularis (isthmus) of the vertebral arch is present (Figures 3.17.1–3.17.3). *Dysplastic* spondylolisthesis develops because of congenital changes in the upper part of the sacrum and the vertebral arch of L5. Subluxation of the facet joints is always present in this form. True dysplastic spondylolisthesis is extremely rare. According to the classification of Newman and Wiltse (Table 3.17.1), additional types of spondylolisthesis are *traumatic* spondylolisthesis in acute fractures and *pathological* spondylolisthesis caused by infection or tumour destruction of parts of the vertebral arch. *Iatrogenic* spondylolisthesis after excessive resection of posterior vertebral elements should be added.

The Wiltse classification has been critisised rightly for being inconsistent and mixing aetiologic (e.g. dysplastic) and anatomic (e.g. isthmic) terms. As its inventors already realised, the distinction between isthmic and dysplastic forms is not always possible. And no specific treatment guidelines are derived. To overcome these shortcomings, improved classification systems have been proposed by Marchetti and Bartolozzi (1997) and Mac-Thiong and Labelle (2006). They are rather complex and do still not yet allow a clear scientifically based distinction between dysplastic and isthmic slips. Furthermore, their treatment recommendations are not validated in clinical series so far. For clinical decision making at present, the essential factors are the degree of slip, the sagittal alignment (lordosis/kyphosis) at the level of the slip, patient's age, and symptoms. In this context, it is of secondary interest whether a slip is to classify e.g. as dysplastic or not.

Spondylolysis is a fatigue fracture of the isthmus of the vertebral arch with the histological characteristics of a fibrocartilaginous pseudarthrosis. The lysis may heal, resulting in a normal or elongated isthmus (Figure 3.17.4).

Spondylolisthesis affects only humans. It has never been described in animals except in an experimental study.

Spondylolysis has never been found in a newborn. The youngest reported patient with spondylolisthesis reported in the literature was 3.5 months old, and a case reported of unilateral spondylolysis with 4-mm slip in a 10-month-old girl. In Caucasians the prevalence of spondylolysis is 4.4–5% at early school age. It increases during growth, and is 6–7.2% in adults. In some ethnic groups the prevalence is much higher (Alaskan Inuit, 32.9%; Japanese Aino, 41%). Isthmic spondylolisthesis is more common in males, but severe slips occur more frequently in females. Lumbar spondylolysis affects the fifth lumbar vertebra in 90% of cases, the fourth in 5%, and the third in 3%. Symptomatic spondylolysis is more likely if it occurs in the segments above L5. Spondylolysis may be present without vertebral slip. In most cases, however, it leads to spondylolisthesis. In the majority of individuals the slip is mild (10–20% of vertebral body length). The slipping occurs during the growth period, and slip progression is rare after growth is complete.

Risk factors for the progression of spondylolisthesis in young individuals are a high degree of slip and age before growth spurt.

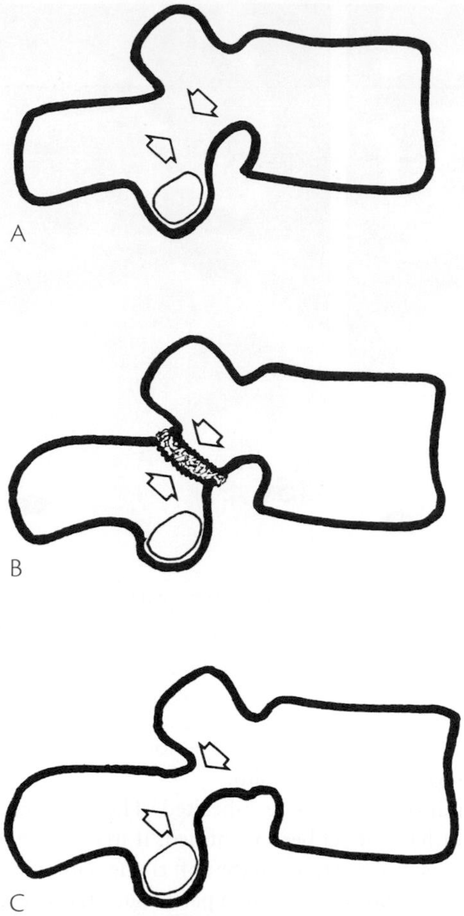

Fig. 3.17.1 A) Isthmus (pars interarticularis) of the vertebral arch (arrows). B) Isthmus defect (spondylolysis). C) Isthmus elongation.

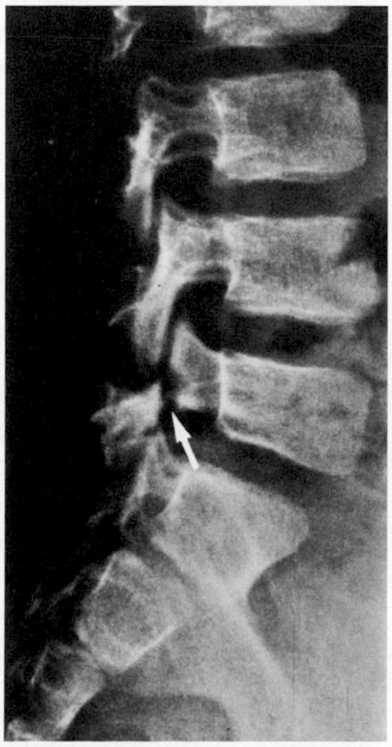

Fig. 3.17.2 Spondylolysis (arrow) of L5 on lateral radiograph.

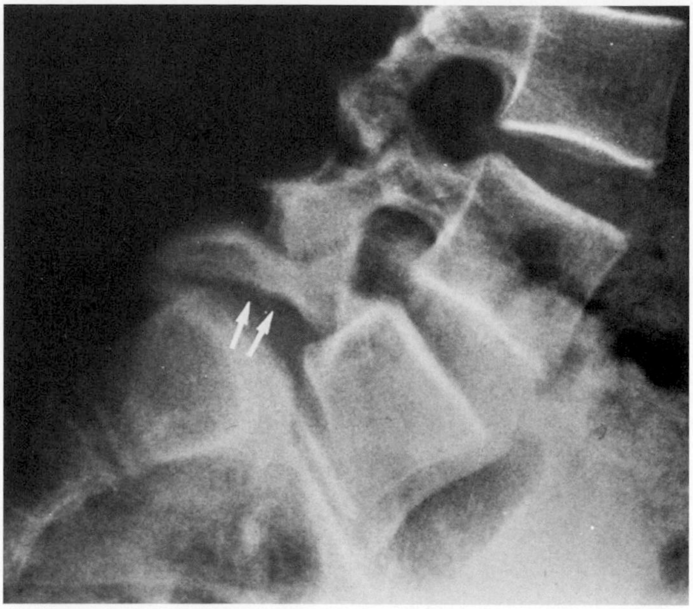

Fig. 3.17.3 Elongated isthmus (arrows) and L5 slip.

Table 3.17.1 Classification of spondylolisthesis

I	Dysplastic
II	Isthmic
	A Spondylolysis
	B Isthmus elongation
	C Acute fracture
III	Traumatic
IV	Degenerative
V	Pathologic
VI	Iatrogenic

The trapezoidal shape of the slipped vertebral body and rounding of the upper endplate of the sacrum are secondary changes.

According to Laurent and Einola (1961), slip is measured as the ratio of the sagittal slip to the sagittal length of the slipped vertebral body expressed as a percentage (Figure 3.17.5A). The lumbosacral kyphosis seen in more severe slip is assessed from the same radiograph and measured as the angle between the posterior border of the first sacral vertebral body and the anterior or posterior border of the fifth vertebral body (Figures 3.17.5B and 3.17.6A).

Aetiology

Spondylolysis is related to the erect posture of humans and to lumbar lordosis. A higher incidence has been found in individuals

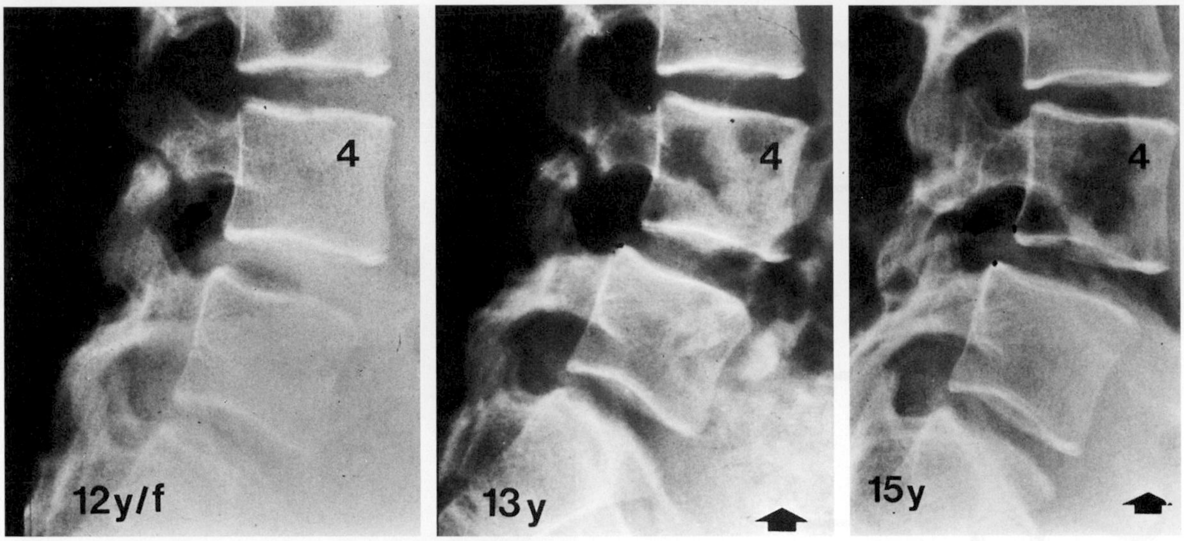

Fig. 3.17.4 Spontaneous healing of a spondylolysis. A) Symptomatic L4 lysis in a 12-year-old girl. B) One year later a mild slip is present and the patient is symptom free. C) After 3 years the lysis has healed, the isthmus is elongated, and the patient is symptom free.

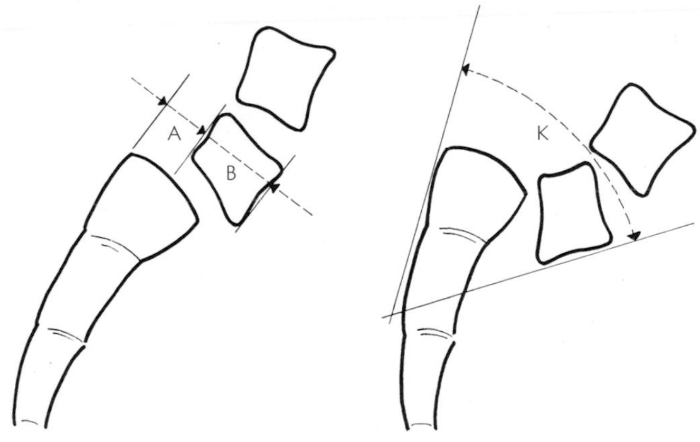

Fig. 3.17.5 A) Calculation of the amount of vertebral slip according to Laurent and Einola (1961): slip (%) = $A/B \times 100$. B) Measurement of lumbosacral kyphosis as the angle between the posterior wall of S1 and the anterior (or posterior) wall of L5.

practising sporting activities with repeated hyperextension movements of the lumbar spine and/or lifting (e.g. gymnasts, divers, javelin throwers, weight lifters, ballet dancers). The possible role of particular sagittal profiles and pelvic parameters (including elevated pelvic incidence) is emerging.

Marty et al (2002) found that individuals with spondylolisthesis have a higher pelvic incidence, a steeper sacral slope and a greater sacral kyphosis than control persons. The concept of abnormal pelvic morphology and disturbed spino-pelvic balance in spondylolisthesis is supported also by other authors. However, Huang et al (2003) could not confirm increased pelvic incidence as a predictor of slip progression. Based on an anthropological study, Whitesides et al. (2005) stated that increased pelvic incidence in spondylolisthesis appears to be secondary to changes in the sacral table angle (i.e. the angle between the superior endplate and the posterior wall of S1) caused by the slip.

The condition can also be inherited. The primary site of the inborn error has not yet been identified. It may in the bony structures (isthmus dysplasia), or in the soft tissues (intervertebral disc, ligaments), or in both leading to a particular sagittal profile with a high pelvic incidence and a high lumbar lordosis.

Disc degeneration

The disc below the slipped vertebra is pathological even in young individuals whether or not they have pain. Degeneration of the adjacent disc above the slipped vertebra is common in symptomatic patients. Symptomatic disc hernia at the level of the slip is rare in patients with isthmic spondylolisthesis.

Lumbar scoliosis

Lumbar scoliosis is seen as a secondary phenomenon to spondylolisthesis. 'Sciatic' scoliosis is due to pain and muscle spasm, and usually disappears after relief of symptoms. Structural ('olisthetic') curves are caused by rotational displacement of the slipped vertebra. Lumbosacral fusion is indicated if progression occurs (Figure 3.17.7).

Thoracic scoliosis in a patient with lumbar spondylolisthesis is managed as a separate entity according to the normal procedure for scoliosis management (see Chapter 3.10).

Natural history

The natural history of isthmic spondylolisthesis is benign in the majority of cases. The affected segment stabilizes itself. Even so, isthmic spondylolisthesis is the most important cause of low back pain and radiating leg pain in children and adolescents. The prognosis of back pain and working ability of adults with isthmic

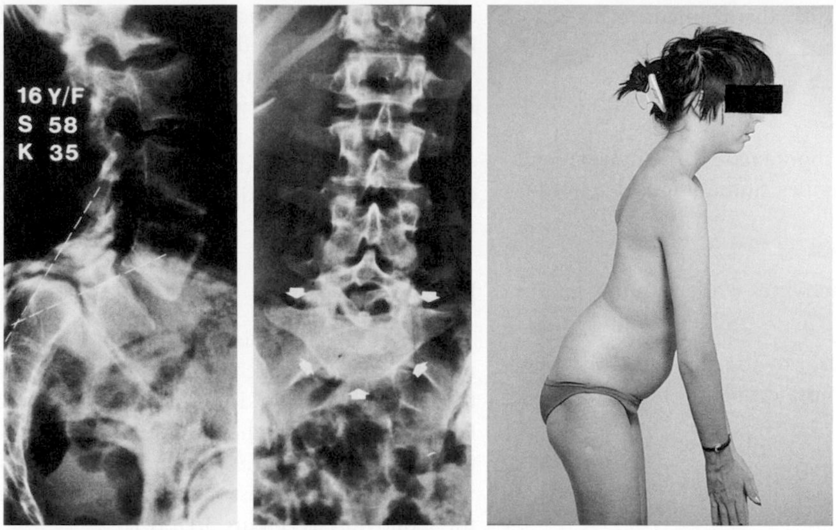

Fig. 3.17.6 Severe isthmic L5 spondylolisthesis in a 16-year-old girl. A) standing lateral radiograph, slip 85%, lumbosacral kyphosis 35 degrees; B) anteroposterior radiograph shows axial projection of L5 ('Napoleon's hat'); C) clinical appearance of the patient.

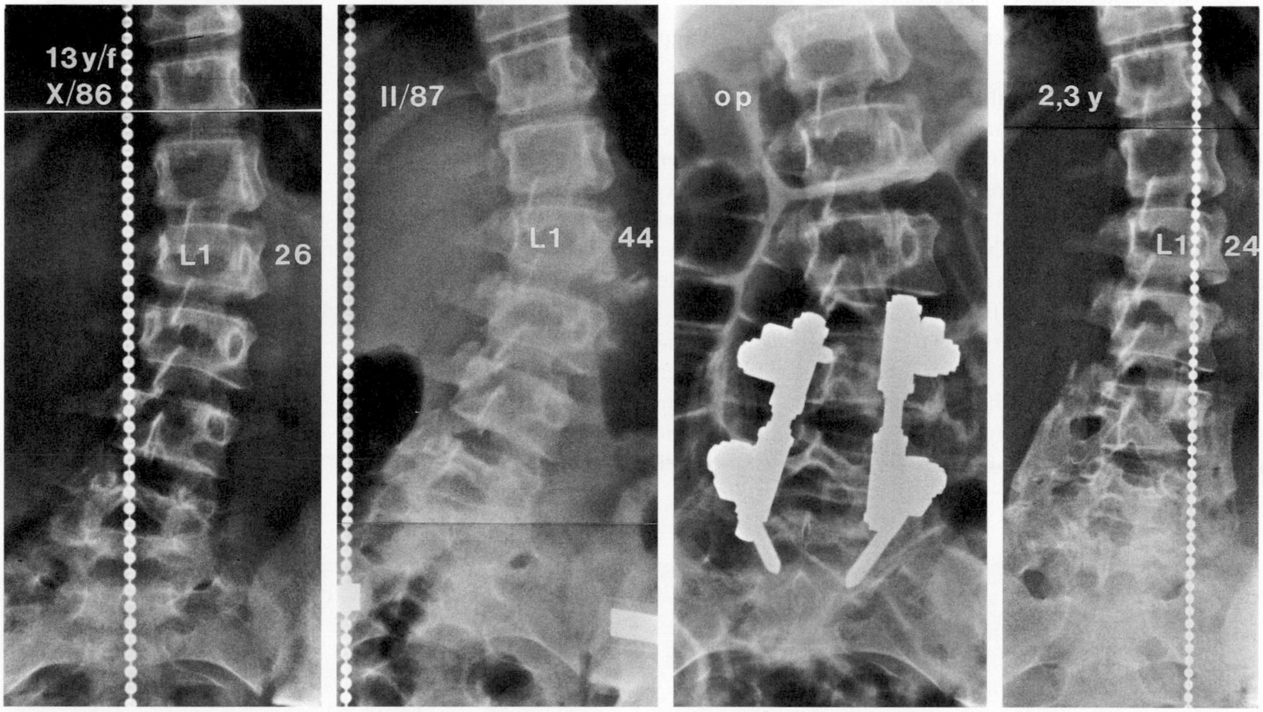

Fig. 3.17.7 Olisthetic scoliosis in a 13-year-old girl with sacralization of L5 and a pain-free 12% isthmic slip at L4. A) Cobb angle 26 degrees, Boston brace treatment started. B) Scoliosis progression to 44 degrees despite brace treatment, no slip progression. C) Instrumented posterolateral fusion of L3 to L5. The lateral tilt of L3 was fully corrected. D) A satisfactory result is seen 27 months after the operation: the Cobb angle is 24 degrees, fusion is solid, and implants are removed. The patient is free of symptoms.

spondylolisthesis is no different from the rest of the population. Back pain symptoms in adults are related to the following:

- Slip of more than 25%
- Spondylolysis at L4
- Early disc degeneration
- Low socioeconomic status
- High occupational loading of the back
- Severe psychosomatic stress symptoms.

There is no explanation yet as to why some people with spondylolysis or isthmic spondylolisthesis become symptomatic while the majority remain symptom free. It is also unknown why slips above L5 seem to cause relatively more pain symptoms than L5 slips. The proposed sources of the pain include the lytic defect itself, the intervertebral disc, and the ligaments. This is not yet resolved.

Presentation

The onset of the symptoms is often spontaneous. In young patients there is often a history of sports activities. Sometimes acute trauma is reported.

The main symptoms are as follows:

- Low back pain during physical activities while standing and/or sitting
- The pain radiates to the buttocks, to the posterior or lateral aspect of the thigh, and, rarely, more distally to the lower limb, ankle, or foot.

In severe slip (>50%) symptoms may include:

- Gait disturbances
- Numbness
- Muscle weakness
- Symptoms of cauda equina compression.

There is no direct relationship between severity of subjective symptoms and the amount of slip.

Gait and posture are normal unless radicular symptoms are present or the slip is severe. The mobility of the lumbar spine is free or decreased due to muscle spasm and pain. There is local tenderness during palpation and in most cases a step can be felt between the spinous processes at the level of the slip. Hamstring tightness is common in younger patients. The Laségue test is usually negative. Muscle power, reflexes, and skin sensation of the lower extremities are normal in the majority of patients.

In severe slips, the posture of the patient is abnormal (Figure 3.17.8). The sacrum is in a vertical position due to retroversion of the pelvis. There is a short kyphosis at the lumbosacral junction and a compensatory hyperlordosis of the lumbar spine, usually reaching up into the thoracic region. The spine is scoliotic and often out of balance. The patient is unable to extend hips and knees fully during standing and he or she walks with a typical pelvic waddle. The hamstrings are extremely tight and signs of neural impairment (muscle weakness, disturbances of skin sensation, incontinence) may be present. Astonishingly, even in very severe slips, neurological findings are rare and many patients are often free of pain despite significant posture changes and hamstring tightness.

Investigation

The vertebral slip is diagnosed from a plain lateral radiograph of the lumbar spine taken in standing position and centred on the lumbosacral junction. In most cases the lysis can be seen from the lateral radiograph. If there is doubt, oblique radiographs will show the defect (Figure 3.17.9). A computed tomography (CT) scan with tilted gantry is the most reliable imaging mode for demonstrating the spondylolysis (Figure 3.17.10).

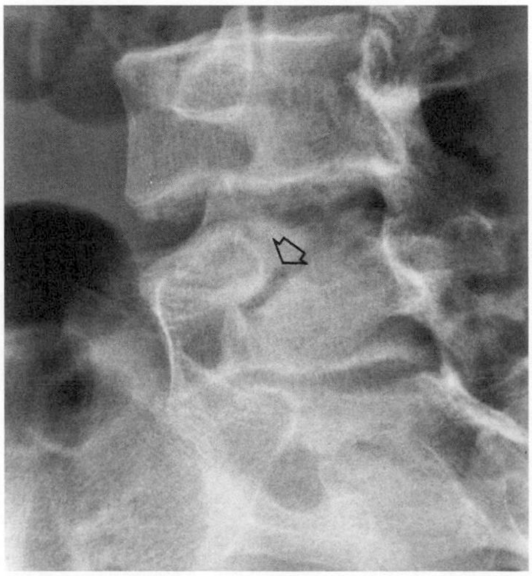

Fig. 3.17.9 Oblique radiograph of bilateral spondylolysis ('scotty dog's collar').

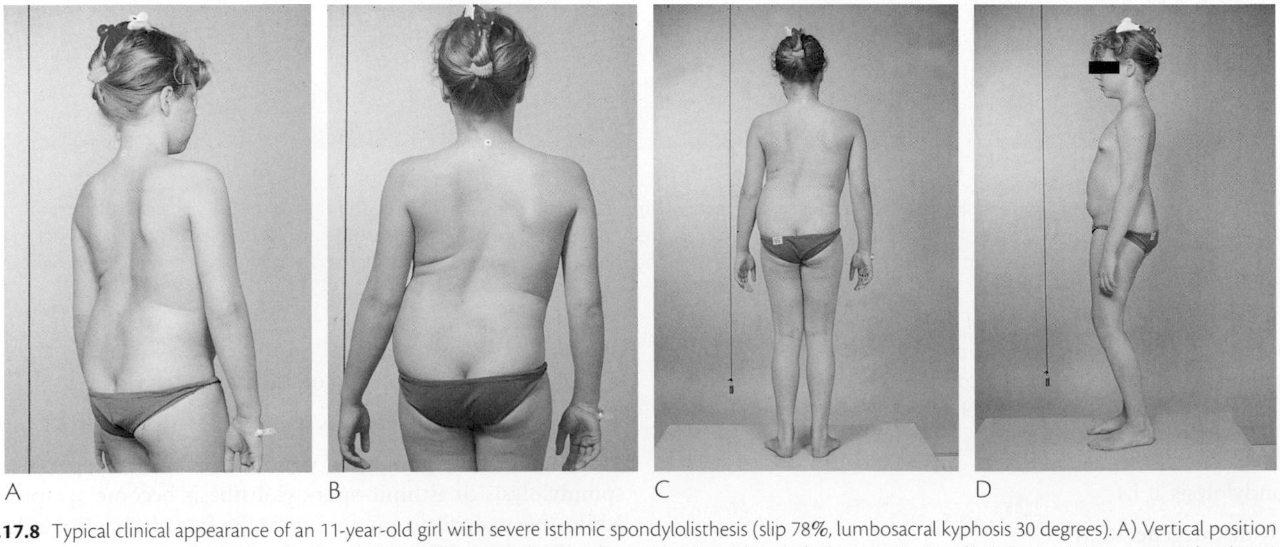

Fig. 3.17.8 Typical clinical appearance of an 11-year-old girl with severe isthmic spondylolisthesis (slip 78%, lumbosacral kyphosis 30 degrees). A) Vertical position of the sacrum due to retroversion of the pelvis, lumbosacral kyphosis, compensatory thoracic lordosis. B) and C) The spine is out of balance, and there is secondary 'sciatic' lumbar scoliosis. D) The patient is forced to stand with hips and knees flexed.

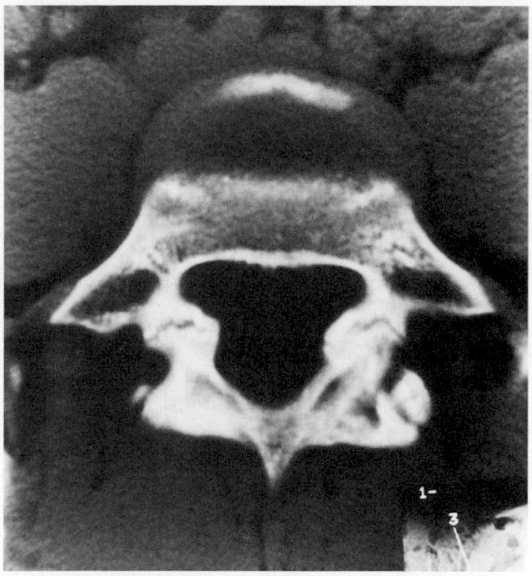

Fig. 3.17.10 CT scan of bilateral spondylolysis.

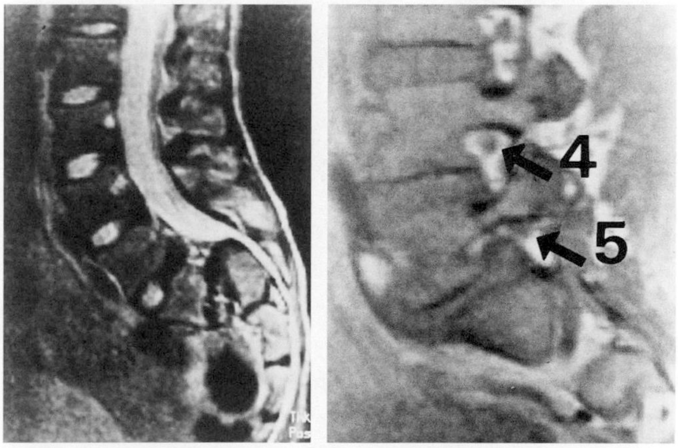

A B

Fig. 3.17.11 A) MRI of a 10-year-old girl with spondyloptosis. B) MRI of a 34-year-old female with mild isthmic L5 slip and severe radiating pain. Lateral disk hernia compressing the L5 root against the pedicle.

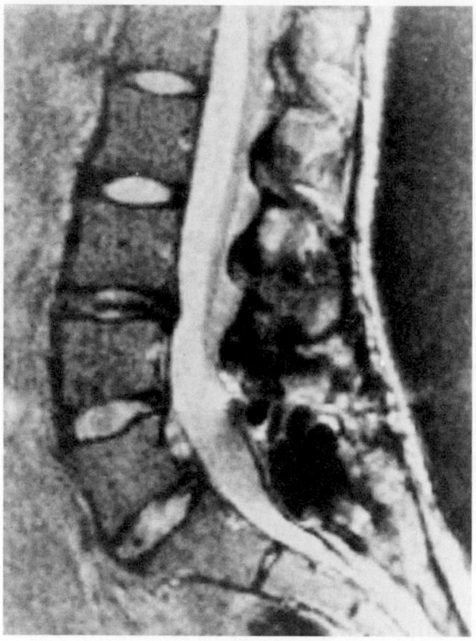

Fig. 3.17.12 Disc degeneration on MRI of a 20-year-old female 56 months after direct repair of a symptomatic L5 lysis. The patient has only mild low-back symptoms.

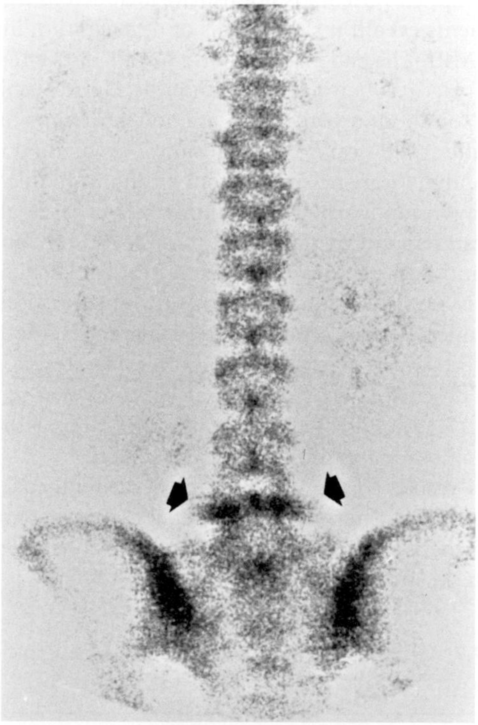

Fig. 3.17.13 Scintigraphy showing fresh traumatic spondylolysis in a 15-year-old boy.

Magnetic resonance imaging (MRI) demonstrates the shape of the spinal canal and possible compression of neural structures (Figure 3.17.11) and shows degenerative disc changes in and above the olisthetic segment (Figure 3.17.12). However, the clinical relevance of disc degeneration seen on MRI is unclear and therefore in this respect MRI is uncertain.

Technetium scintigraphy is used in patients where fresh (traumatic) spondylolysis is suspected with normal radiographs. The impending lysis may be seen in the scintigram (Figure 3.17.13). It also helps to judge the possible healing of the defect.

Electroneuromyography may be indicated in cases with clinical neurological signs. Discography can be used for preoperative assessment of the condition of the disc(s) above the slipped vertebra.

Management in children and adolescents

Symptomatic spondylolysis or mild spondylolisthesis (up to 25% slip) is treated non-operatively by decreasing the level of physical activities, strengthening of back and abdominal muscles, and sometimes a brace or plaster of Paris jacket.

At this stage it is very important to explain to the patient and his or her parents that the natural course of the condition is benign and that the symptoms resolve, usually after several months, without any special treatment. Sports players are advised to modify their training program to avoid pain-causing exercises. There is no reason to stop all physical activities. Younger patients before or during the growth spurt should be followed up with radiographs at 6- to 12-month intervals because of the risk of progression at this age.

Indications for operation in children and adolescents are:

- Pain unresponsive to non-operative measures
- A slip of more than 25% in a very young patient (even with minor symptoms) to prevent further slip progression
- Significant posture changes
- Gait disturbances
- Possible neurological changes in the severe slip.

The choice of operative procedure depends on the amount of slip and on the personal experience and preferences of the surgeon. Table 3.17.2 represents the author's policy and is used as a guideline for decision-making. The final decision is an individual one depending on the patient's skeletal maturity, gender, anatomical features of the slip, ability to cooperate, and the aspirations of the patient and his or her parents.

Uninstrumented segmental posterolateral fusion *in situ* using autogenous bone from the posterior iliac crest is the method of choice for cases with slip up to 50% (Figure 3.17.14). The segment above the slipped vertebra is not usually included in the fusion in young patients even if it shows signs of degeneration in discography or on MRI. The patient is mobilized 2 or 3 days after the operation wearing a soft brace for 3 months. Sports activities are forbidden for about a year. There are no restrictions on physical activities after solid healing of the fusion. This method is safe and effective, and there are no specific complications. In this young age group, bony fusion is achieved in almost 90% of cases, and subjective results are good or satisfactory in 82–96%. Symptoms disappear in most cases even when solid fusion is not achieved.

If there is a lysis without a slip or a very mild slip, direct repair of the isthmic defect is recommended. Different methods of internal fixation (screws, cerclage wires, butterfly plates, hook plates) have been described. The author prefers Scott's wiring technique (Figure 3.17.15). Postoperative immobilization with a plastic thoracolumbosacral orthosis is recommended for 3–6 months. Equivalent results to the results of posterolateral fusion can be expected in the mid-term. Schlenzka et al (2006) were not able to prove the benefit of direct repair in comparison to segmental fusion in a long-term study.

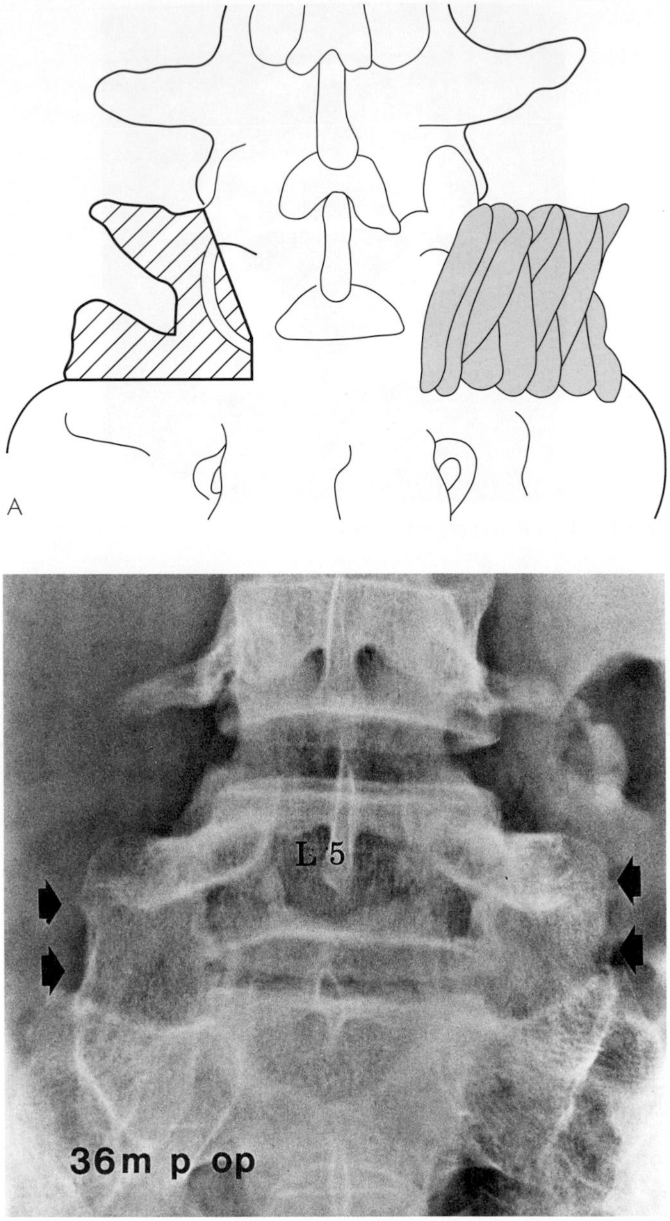

Fig. 3.17.14 A) Posterolateral fusion. B) Anteroposterior radiograph shows a bilaterally strong fusion mass 3 years after operation.

Table 3.17.2 Management of isthmic spondylolisthesis in children and adolescents

Slip (%)	Symptoms	Treatment
0–25	–	Follow-up
0–25	+	Conservative; posterolateral fusion; direct repair
> 25–50	±	Posterolateral fusion
> 50	±	Anterior fusion
> 50 + LS kyphosis	±	Combined fusion
100 (ptosis)	±	Reduction, combined instrumented fusion

LS, lumbosacral

If the slip exceeds 50%, the physiological lumbosacral lordosis decreases and a progressive kyphotic deformity develops. For biomechanical reasons, posterior or posterolateral fusion is not sufficient to prevent progression without anterior support. Anterior interbody fusion through a transperitoneal approach using autogenous tricortical iliac crest grafts is preferred (Figure 3.17.16). Combined anterior and posterolateral (circumferential) fusion is necessary to stop progression in slips with significant lumbosacral kyphosis (more than 10–20 degrees) (Figure 3.17.17). There is no need to include more than the olisthetic segment into the fusion. After anterior or combined procedures the patient is mobilized at the second or third postoperative day and wears a plastic thoracolumbosacral orthosis for 3–6 months. The clinical results of anterior and combined fusion in severe slip are comparable to the

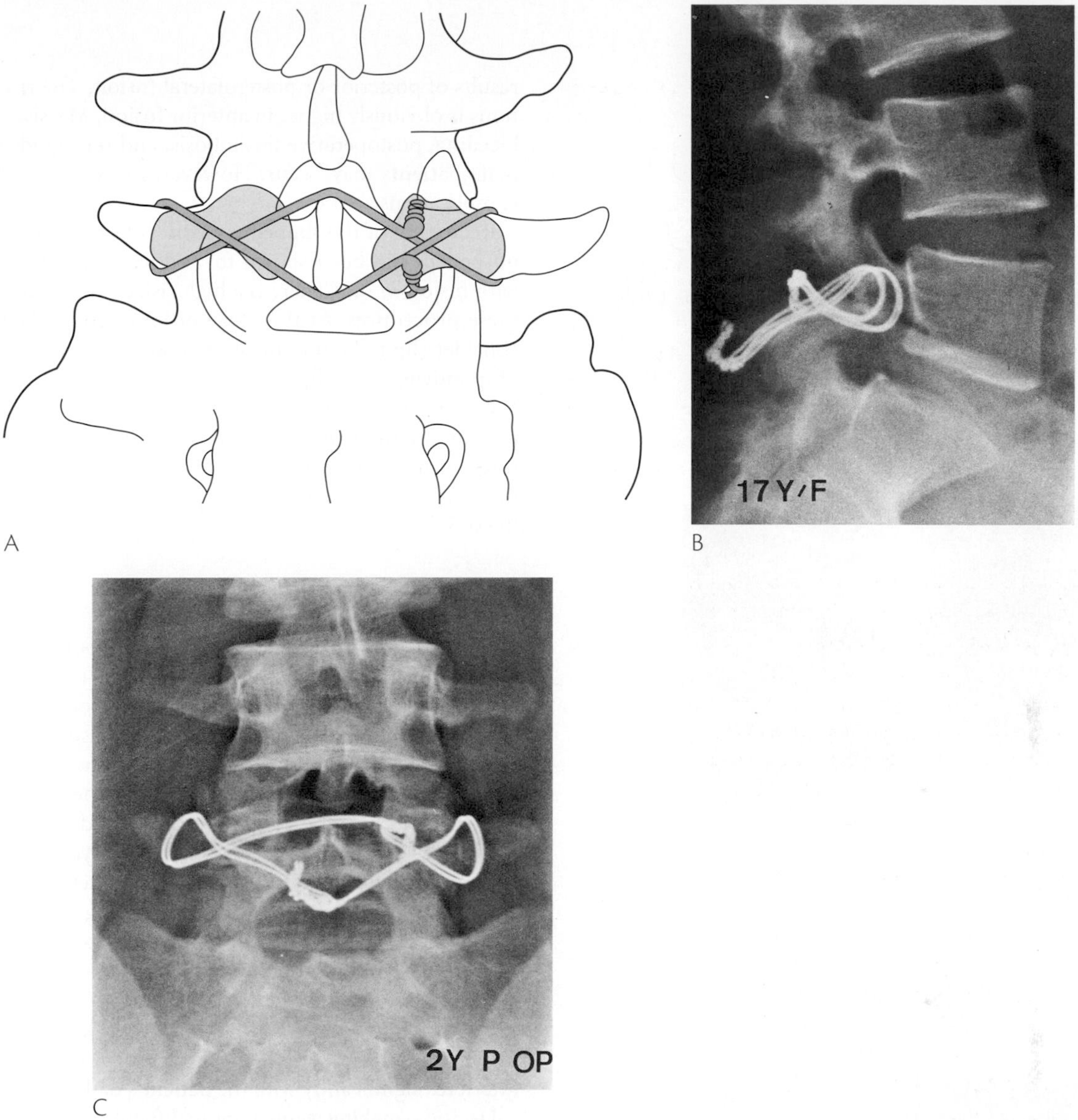

Fig. 3.17.15 A) Direct repair of the spondylolysis using cerclage wires according to Scott. B) Lateral and C) anteroposterior radiograph 2 years after operation.

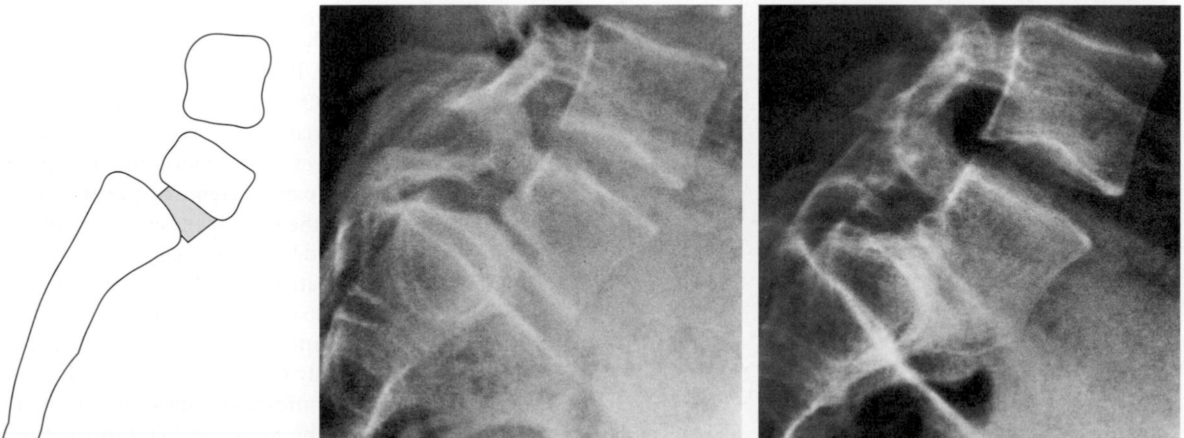

Fig. 3.17.16 A) Anterior interbody fusion. B) Preoperative radiograph of a 17-year-old boy with severe isthmic L5 slip (slip, 60%; lumbosacral kyphosis, 10°). C) Three years after uninstrumented anterior interbody fusion in situ there is no progression of the deformity.

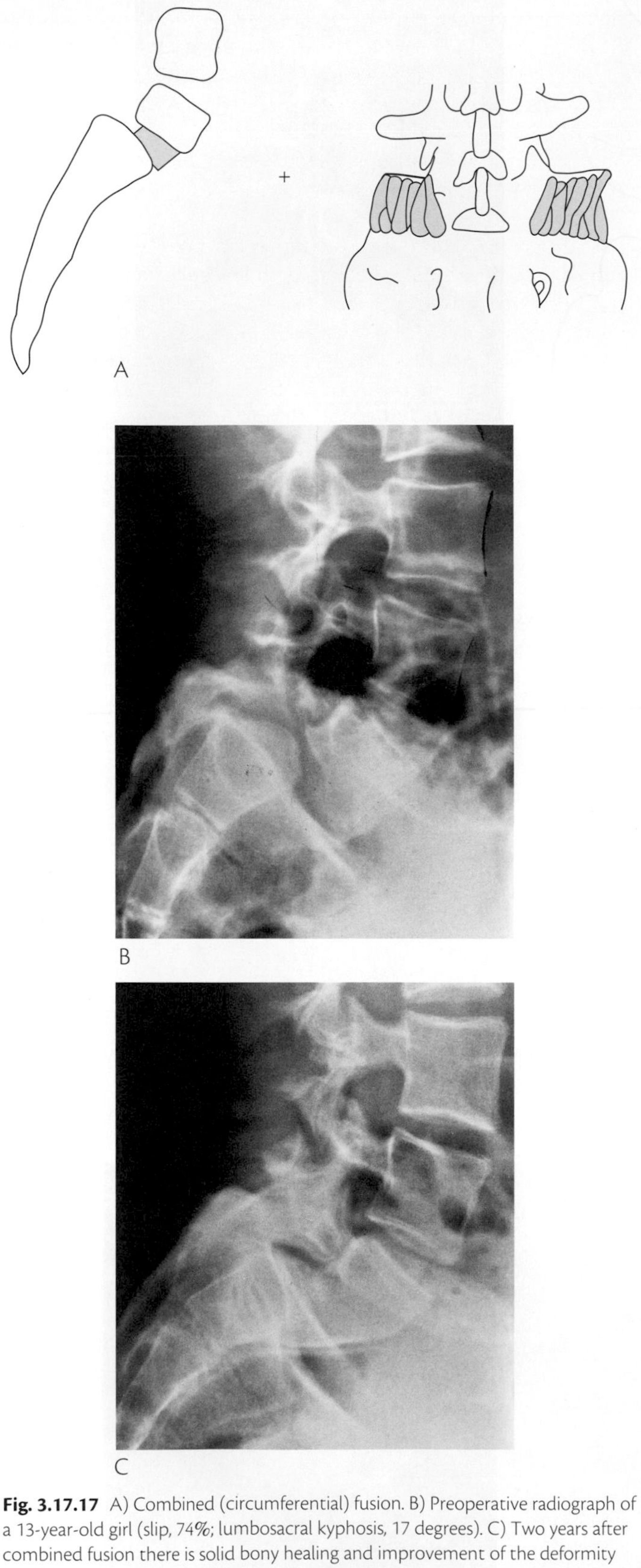

A

B

C

Fig. 3.17.17 A) Combined (circumferential) fusion. B) Preoperative radiograph of a 13-year-old girl (slip, 74%; lumbosacral kyphosis, 17 degrees). C) Two years after combined fusion there is solid bony healing and improvement of the deformity (slip, 52%; lumbosacral lordosis, 4 degrees).

results of posterior or posterolateral fusion. The risk of complications is obviously higher in anterior fusion. Massive intraoperative bleeding, postoperative thrombosis, and retrograde ejaculation in male patients may occur. However, in experienced hands these complications are rare.

Reduction of the slipped vertebra is technically possible. So far no benefit has been shown for reduction procedures compared with fusion *in situ*. There is a high risk of complications related to these procedures. At this stage of knowledge, the author would consider slip reduction in children and adolescents only for cases of spondyloptosis (slip of 100% or more).

Decompressive laminectomy is indicated in young patients only in rare cases where there is true impingement of neural structures. If decompression is performed during growth, segmental fusion always has to be added to prevent subsequent progression of the slip.

Management in adults

The primary treatment of a symptomatic spondylolysis or isthmic spondylolisthesis is non-operative. Load reduction, stabilizing exercises of abdominal and back muscles, local injections of steroids/local anaesthetics, physiotherapy, a soft brace, and pain-relieving drugs should be tried first. In some cases changes to the working environment of the patient may be necessary. It is very important to give the patient objective understandable information. One should not underestimate the psychological effect on a non-medical person of being told that a vertebral arch in his or her back has 'broken' and has caused 'slipping' of the vertebra. The natural history of this condition has to be explained to the patient with special emphasis on the benign course and the tendency of the process to self-stabilize in the long term.

Indication for operation is severe low back and/or radiating pain which does not respond to the measures described earlier and interferes significantly with the patient's daily activities.

Decision-making is much more difficult than in the treatment of young patients. The older the patient, the more likely it is that changes outside the lytic/olisthetic segment are responsible for the symptoms, i.e. one has to clarify whether the radiological finding of spondylolysis or isthmic spondylolisthesis is really the sole cause of the patient's symptoms. In addition to the patient's history and physical examination, a thorough analysis of all aspects of the individual case is mandatory. Pain analysis (pain drawing, visual analogue scale, Oswestry Questionnaire) and assessment of the patient's psychosocial situation are performed. Radiological investigations include flexion–extension views and discography to identify the actual source of pain. Diagnostic pars blocks can be very useful and may identify the spondylolysis as an isolated source of pain and pars repair could be considered.

The choice of the operative procedure depends on the results of the preoperative work-up. Posterolateral fusion augmented with transpedicular instrumentation (Figure 3.17.18) is performed in patients who suffer mainly from low back pain. If root symptoms are predominant, decompression (Gill's operation) is indicated. During this procedure the loose lamina and the pseudarthrotic tissue of the lysis are carefully removed bilaterally. The nerve roots have to be totally free after this resection. In some patients the roots are caught under the pedicle. Additional resection of the medial and inferior parts of the pedicle is necessary to achieve complete

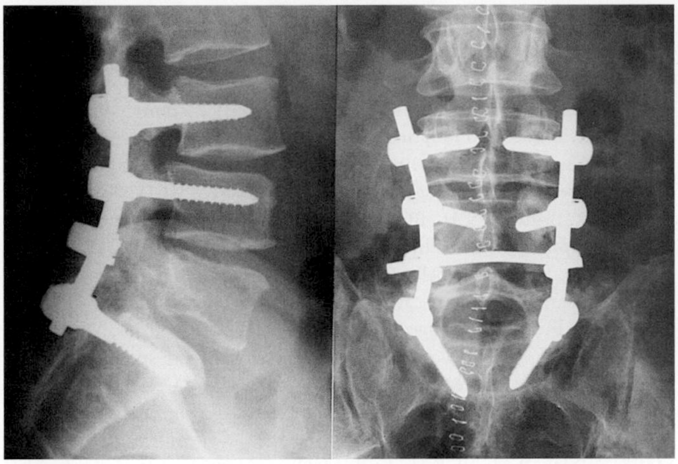

Fig. 3.17.18 Instrumented posterolateral fusion of L3 to the sacrum in a 47-year-old male with symptomatic isthmic L5 spondylolisthesis and degenerative olisthesis of L3.

nerve root decompression. Gill's operation alone is sufficient only if the olisthetic disc is severely degenerated and the segment is stable. Otherwise, instrumented posterolateral fusion is added.

The extension of the fusion proximally (one or more segments) depends on the condition of the segment(s) above the slipped vertebra.

Direct repair of the spondylolysis may be performed in young adults with symptomatic spondylolysis or mild slip if the condition of the disc is satisfactory on MRI investigation. The author uses this procedure in adults mainly at the L4 level because in the L5 slip the disc below is almost invariably abnormal.

Slip reduction is not usually indicated in adult patients. Adult patients with a severe slip (>50%) should be treated by decompression and instrumented fusion *in situ* to the sacrum. Sometimes the fusion will need to extend to L4 depending on the slip angle, the disc/facet status, and the slip angle.

In cases of spondyloptosis with severe symptoms and impairment of patient's posture, L5 vertebra resection and fusion of L4 onto the sacrum may be considered. This is a high-risk procedure and should be performed only by very experienced spine surgeons (Figure 3.17.19).

The results of operative treatment of isthmic spondylolisthesis in adult patients are as unpredictable as all low back pain operations. The literature is unhelpful because of different approaches to patient selection and the influence of the specific socioeconomic environment in different countries. One study reported a fusion rate of 88% after uninstrumented posterolateral *in situ* fusion and a clinical success rate of 55% in 45 adult patients. Risk factors for a poor outcome were compensation cases and pseudarthrosis. A trend towards unsatisfactory result was seen in males, middle-aged individuals, smokers, and patients with preoperative radicular symptoms. Another study used transpedicular fixation and achieved a 94% fusion rate. They reported numerous instrumentation-related complications (malposition of screws with and without neurological damage, screw loosening, and breakage). There is no evidence that the addition of interbody spacers would improve patients' outcome. Most of the complications were of no clinical importance, but the potential danger of implants is obvious. They should be used only by well-trained spine surgeons.

Conclusion

Spondylolysis occurs in 4.4% of children and about 6% in the adult population. In general it is a benign condition. The majority of individuals that develop mild or moderate isthmic vertebral slip

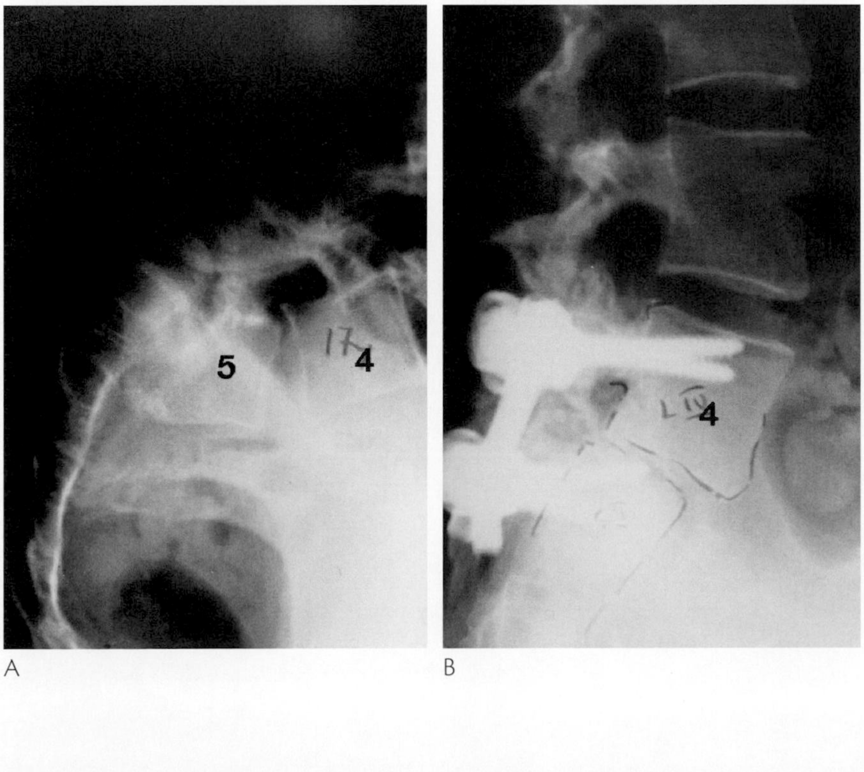

Fig. 3.17.19 A) Preoperative radiograph of a 17-year-old female after an unsuccessful attempt at fusion for severe slip at 13 years of age (slip, 100%; lumbosacral kyphosis, 60 degrees). B) Lateral radiograph after staged L5 vertebra resection, reduction using halofemoral traction, and instrumented fusion of L4 onto S1. (Operation performed by Dr T. Laine, ORTON Orthopaedic Hospital, Helsinki, Finland.)

remain free of symptoms for their whole life or show only mild symptoms.

In children and adolescents with mild slip, primary treatment of pain symptoms is non-operative. Young children before growth spurt need radiographic follow-up to check for progression. If the slip exceeds 25% in a child, segmental fusion should be considered. Uninstrumented posterolateral fusion is the method of choice for treatment of pain symptoms not responding to conservative measures in slips up to 50%. In severe slips (>50%) anterior or combined fusion is necessary to prevent further progression of lumbosacral kyphosis. The clinical results of *in situ* fusion in this age group are satisfactory in 80–90%. Slip reduction has not yet been shown to be superior to *in situ* fusion. It may be performed in cases with spondyloptosis and severe impairment of neurological function and sagittal malalignment of the spine.

In adults, careful analysis of the patient's problems is crucial to identify the source of pain and the importance of non-organic factors and the environment. If pain is moderate, non-operative treatment is indicated. If symptoms persist and interfere with daily activities, operation may be necessary. Decompression (Gill's operation) is indicated if radicular symptoms are dominant. Posterolateral spondylodesis augmented by transpedicular fixation leads to solid fusion in over 90% of patients. Subjective outcome depends very much on patient selection. Slip reduction is not indicated in adult patients. Vertebra resection may be considered in adult patients with severe subjective and objective symptoms due to spondyloptosis.

Further reading

Lamberg, T.S., Remes, V.M., Helenius, I.J., *et al.* (2005). Long-term clinical, functional and radiological outcome 21 years after posterior or posterolateral fusion in childhood or adolescence isthmic spondylolisthesis. *European Spine Journal*, **14**, 639–44.

Laurent, L.E. and Einola, S. (1961). Spondylolisthesis in children and adolescents. *Acta Orthopaedica Scandinavica*, **31**, 45–64.

Lenke, L.G., Bridwell, K.H., Bullis, D., *et al.* (1992). Results of in situ fusion for isthmic spondylolisthesis. *Journal of Spinal Disorders*, **5**, 433–42.

Mac-Thiong, J-M. and Labelle, H. (2006). A proposal for a surgical classification of pediatric lumbosacral spondylolisthesis based on the current literature. *European Spine Journal*, **15**, 1425–35.

Marchetti, P.G. and Bartolozzi, P. (1997). Classification of spondylolisthesis as a guideline for treatment. In: Bridwell, K.H. and DeWald, R.L. *The textbook of spinal surgery*. 2nd edn. Lippincott-Raven Publishers Philadelphia.

Molinari, R.W., Bridwell, K.H., Lenke, L.G. *et al.* (2002). Anterior column support in surgery for high-grade, isthmic spondylolisthesis. *Clinical Orthopaedics*, **349**, 109–20.

Poussa, M., Remes, V., Lamberg, T. *et al.* (2006). Treatment of severe spondylolisthesis in adolecence with reduction or fusion in situ: Long-term clinical, radiologic, and functional outcome. *Spine*, **31**, 583–90.

Schlenzka, D., Remes, V., Helenius, I. *et al.* (2006). Direct repair for treatment of symptomatic spondylolysis or mild isthmic spondylolisthesis in young patients: no benefit in comparison to segmental fusion after a mean follow-up of 14.8 years. *European Spine Journal*, **15**, 1437–47.

Fig. 3.17.3 Elongated isthmus (arrows) and L5 slip.

3.18

The infected spine

Jeremy Fairbank*

Summary points

- TB is the most common spine infection worldwide
- In the developed world, staphylococcal infections are more frequent
- Untreated these infections can cause paralysis or even death.

Introduction

It is known that spinal infections have afflicted humans since early times. Osteomyelitic changes affecting the spine have been demonstrated in skeletons from 4000 BC found in the Nile Valley and in Egyptian mummies.

Pathology

Classification is normally by the causative organism. Infective organisms may be pyogenic, granulomatous, or parasitic. Infection is usually either by direct implantation or secondary to a septic focus elsewhere in the body with spread into the vertebrae through Batson's plexus of veins or the segmental arteries. Infection may affect the vertebral body, the intervertebral disc, the epidural space, and the posterior elements, but most commonly involves the anterior and middle columns.

Pyogenic spinal infections

Pyogenic infections may present acutely or chronically. The presentation depends on the age of the patient, the immune response, and the infecting organism. Almost any infective organism can cause vertebral infection under suitable conditions. The most common by far is *Staphylococcus aureus*, but in a significant minority of cases there is *Escherichia coli*, *Proteus*, and streptococcal involvement. The mode of spread is usually from other septic foci via the vascular system. The most common site is in the lumbar spine and multiple vertebral involvement is usual. Infection may track along tissue planes, and without early control will cause secondary abscess formation and pointing at distant sites. The vertebral canal may be invaded by pus and granulation tissue either directly from the disc space or through the exit foramenae causing meningitis or transverse myelitis. If this occurs, recovery is uncommon. Retropulsion of bone or disc causes neural compromise, and destruction of vertebral body and discs causes local instability and deformity. However, with effective control, healing occurs with fusion of adjacent vertebrae.

Epidemiology

The incidence of pyogenic spinal infection is almost certainly increasing because of increased awareness, diagnostic improvements, and enlargement of the 'at-risk' group (HIV/AIDS, poor nutrition, the elderly, diabetes, and other comorbidity) Spinal infection represents 3–4% of all osteomyelitis, but the figure has been quoted as high as 16%. The population incidence is about 1 in 250 000. Spinal infection is involved in 10–11 per 10 000 hospital admissions for back pain. Epidural abscess is thankfully rare and represents about 1.2 per 10 000 hospital admissions.

Box 3.18.1 Populations particularly at risk include the following

- The elderly
- Intravenous drug users
- Immune deficiency states, including AIDS
- Rheumatoid arthritis
- Malignancy
- Spinal fractures and paraplegia
- Infective endocarditis
- Renal failure
- Sickle cell disease
- Chronic alcoholics.

* Based on chapters written for first edition by T.R. Morley, S. Rajasekaran, and T.K. Shanmugasundaram

Box 3.18.2 Clinical signs include the following

- Localized tenderness
- Muscle spasm and limitation of movement
- Local or distant fluctuant mass
- Sinus formation
- Occasional angular defect.

The presence of associated 'conditions' tends to delay diagnosis and there is a higher risk of neurological compromise. Direct spread of infection also occurs with stab wounds, gunshot wounds, and surgical trauma to the spine.

Clinical features

Localized constant pain, often at an unusual site and exacerbated by movement and percussion, is the most common feature, and there is associated muscle spasm. Most patients do not present with acute pyogenic signs. Fever is present in only about a third of cases.

Neurological deficits may be present and careful evaluation is vital, especially where there is pre-existing pathology. Neurological signs, which will depend upon the nature and site of the spinal infection, will be present in 15% of patients. Quadriplegia is a presenting feature in cervical spine involvement, and paraplegia in the thoracic spine. Lumbosacral involvement is more likely to produce single or multiple root deficits.

Primary extradural abscesses have a predilection for the thoracic spine. The usual presentation is a history of severe local unremitting pain with single root symptoms. There is a tendency for the epidural abscess to spread throughout the epidural space causing rapid onset of neurological deterioration and paraplegia.

Investigations

Laboratory investigations

The erythrocyte sedimentation ratio (ESR) is usually above 50mm/h, and C-reactive protein (CRP) and alkaline phosphatase may be raised. These tests are non-specific and may be difficult to evaluate, particularly in children and patients with rheumatoid arthritis. CRP is best for postoperative infection. The white cell count is raised in less than half of cases. Blood cultures when the patient is febrile are more reliable. Urine culture may be valuable if urethral manipulation is considered to be causative.

Imaging

Although plain radiography is imperative, it is of little value in early cases. Disc-space narrowing and occasionally paraspinal widening occurs after 2–3 weeks, and secondary bone changes may take up to 3 months to occur. The earliest changes are of loss of delineation of subchondral bone. Radiographic changes are progressive with time but may remain limited to the disc complex (Figure 3.18.1). Plain radiographs are not very useful in assessing response to treatment.

Nuclear studies

Technetium-99m bone scans can be positive as early as 2 days from the onset of symptoms; they have a high sensitivity (95%) but a lower specificity (75%). Positron emission tomography (PET) scanning is helpful but not widely available. Indium and gallium scans have proved less useful.

Computed tomography scanning

Computed tomography (CT) scanning (Figure 3.18.2) is useful for assessing the degree of bone destruction and examining the surrounding soft tissues.

Magnetic resonance imaging scanning

Magnetic resonance imaging (MRI) scanning has become the most important investigation. It has a sensitivity of 96%, about the same as radionuclear scanning, but has a higher specificity (up to 95%) (Figure 3.18.3).

Microbiology

The diagnostic 'yield' from needle biopsy is disappointingly low. A histological diagnosis is almost invariably positive, but less than 50% produce a positive culture, particularly when antibiotics have been used. Pus from needle biopsy of the primary focus or from more distant abscess cavities gives 80–90% successful culture.

Histology

Needle biopsy can provide confirmatory material especially when culture is negative.

Differential diagnosis

The most common differential is between infection and tumour. Haematomas may mimic epidural infection. Diagnosis of pyogenic infection within either the disc or the bony canal can be difficult after recent spinal surgery.

Non-operative treatment

The principles of non-operative treatment are rest and appropriate antibiotics. When the diagnosis is certain, the organism is known, and there are no progressive neurological features, non-operative treatment is indicated. Bed rest and intravenous antibiotics may be required initially with the acute presentation, and this should be continued until pain reduces and a response can be confirmed. The patient may then be mobilized in a brace and continue on oral antibiotics.

The length of time required on antibiotics is arbitrary and depends on the organism, its sensitivity, and the patient's clinical response. As a guide, intravenous antibiotics should be used for a period of 6–8 weeks followed by a similar period of treatment with oral antibiotics. Some recommend indefinite antibiotics to suppress infection. Serial ESR/CRP examination is usually of value and antibiotics should continue for a month after both symptoms and ESR have returned to normal. Radiographic and MRI evaluation is useful, but there is a distinct lag-time before healing can be confirmed.

Surgical management

Surgical management is indicated if there is a failure of conservative treatment, or the diagnosis and organism cannot be confirmed, or there is a significant neurological deficit, particularly when there is epidural spread. Mechanical instability may also be an indication for surgical management. The aims of surgery are to drain the abscess, make a definitive diagnosis, and decompress the neural tissue, either root or cord. Following this, it is necessary to achieve stability and rapid healing of the lesion by bone grafting

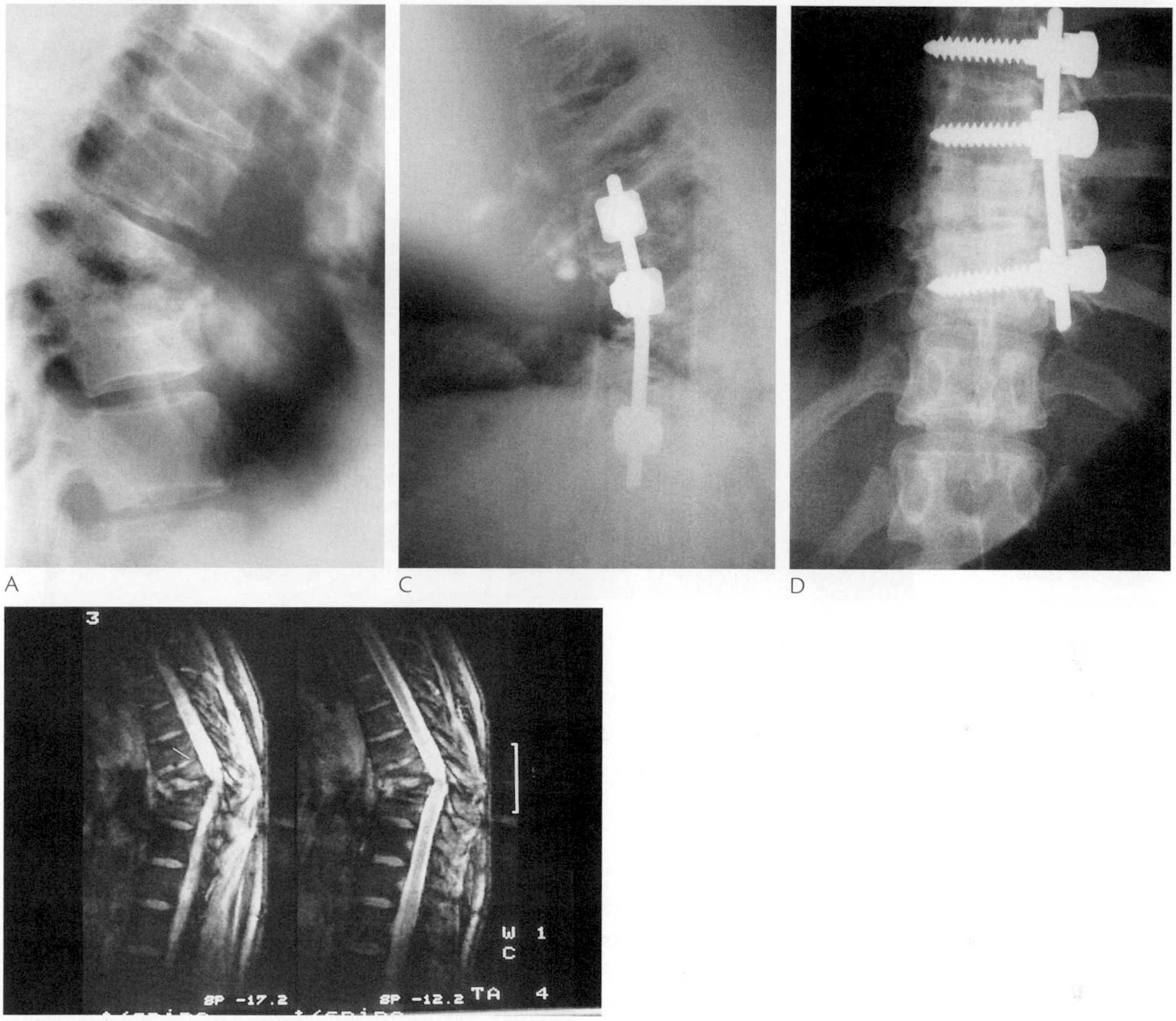

Fig. 3.18.1 A) Plain lateral radiograph of a 42-year-old drug abuser presenting with increasing pain and deformity in the thoracic spine. B) MRI showing typical vertebral destruction from *Staphylococcus aureus*. There is clearly cord compression. C) Anteroposterior and D) lateral radiographs following debridement, grafting, and internal fixation.

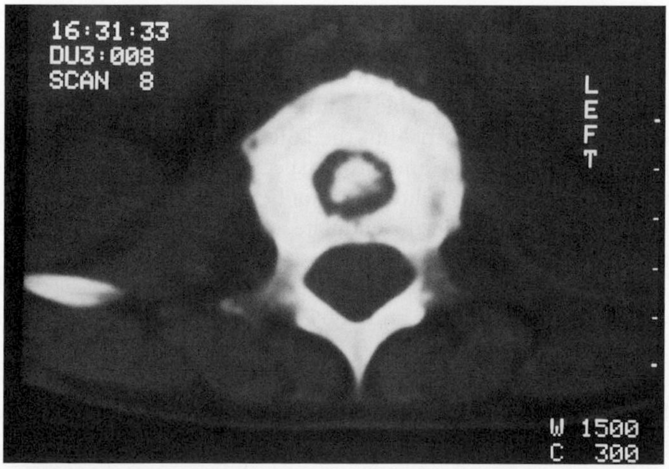

Fig. 3.18.2 A CT scan in a child with sickle cell disease reveals the infected site which had been missed at surgical exploration. The infecting organism was *Salmonella*.

and internal fixation. Surgery should always be directed to the area of pathology. Usually this involves an anterior approach to the spine. There is no place for decompressive laminectomy alone, which almost invariably produces instability, except in the rare cases of epidural abscess or where there is primary posterior involvement.

In the debilitated patient it is possible to drain an abscess by the posterolateral approach. It is difficult to achieve spinal stability by this approach, particularly if there has been significant vertebral destruction.

There is a significant mortality following surgery in the high-risk groups, where diagnosis has been delayed and destruction of soft tissue is extensive. Neurological recovery occurs in more than 80% of cases, particularly where there is neurological sparing preoperatively. Recovery may be delayed for many weeks, particularly in elderly patients.

Late deformity following pyogenic infection can present a formidable challenge. The neurological deficit which often accompanies

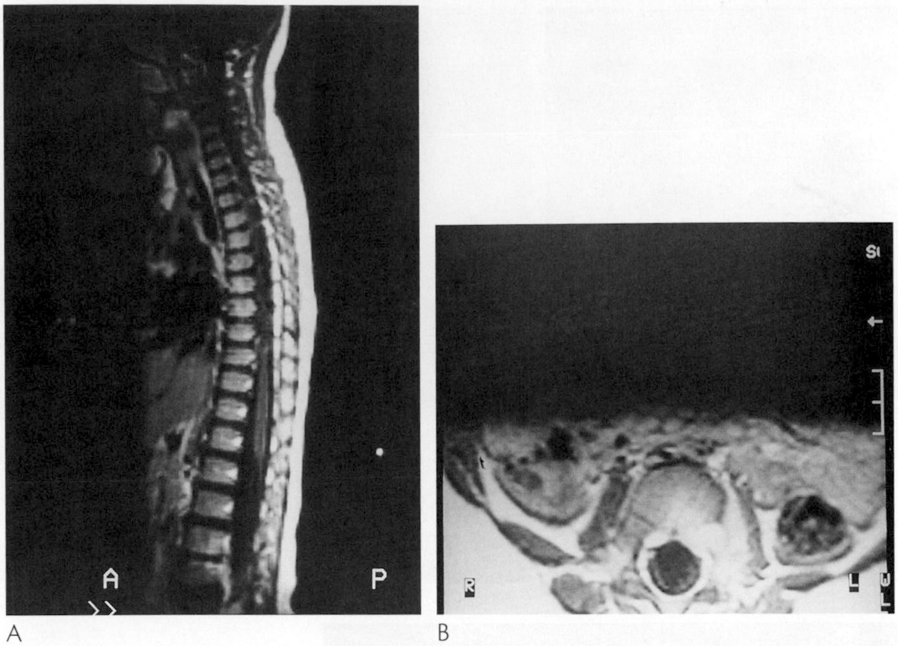

Fig. 3.18.3 MRI of a 9-month-old child with a pyrexial illness. The MRI shows bony destruction of the left pedicle of L5, with a soft-tissue extension. The organism was *Escherichia coli*.

severe deformity adds to the difficulty. Scarring in the neural canal and almost certainly long-standing vascular inadequacy makes correction and stabilization a high-risk procedure.

Discitis and postoperative infection

Although the term discitis was originally used solely for infection in children it has now come to describe any primary disc-space infection. There are two types of discitis, one occurring in children and the other occurring following endplate closure. In adults, haematogenous spread probably cannot occur through the intact endplate. Either an intradiscal procedure has been undertaken or there is a defect in the endplate.

Disc-space infection in children

Discitis in children is characterized by severe localized back pain and spasm, loss of disc-space height, and a raised ESR. In the pre-antibiotic era this condition was known as benign osteomyelitis, because discitis is usually self-limiting and heals without antibiotics to a bony ankylosis.

Children present with only mild toxaemia but with a constant well-localized back pain, muscle spasm, and stiffness. The child will often not weight-bear. Pain may be referred to the hips and upper thigh, particularly when the infection is in a lumbar disc. Delay in diagnosis is not uncommon. The white cell count is usually normal, but with a raised ESR or CRP. Blood cultures are usually negative. Initially there are no radiographic changes. After 2 weeks there is a progressive disc-space narrowing, and at about 2–3 months some endplate irregularity is apparent. Quite marked central erosions into the endplate may be produced.

MRI is usually diagnostic. Disc biopsy for culture and histology is usually unnecessary.

The mainstay of treatment is rest, initially strict bed rest, followed by mobilization in a well-fitting cast or brace as soon as the pain reduces, often after 2 or 3 days. Broad-spectrum intravenous antibiotics are usually given initially before progressing to oral treatment. This is despite the fact that it has been shown that this condition is usually self-limiting, even without antibiotics.

Surgery has a place only when pain persists, and in these cases there is often marked endplate destruction and sclerosis. Following curettage and grafting, healing is often rapid.

It is notable that late kyphosis rarely occurs in childhood discitis. However, in babies who develop vertebral infection in the first few months of life, vertebral destruction is rapid and is followed by the development of kyphosis (Figure 3.18.4).

Disc-space infection in adults

Disc-space infection can occur following any invasive procedure on the disc. The avascular disc is prone to low-grade infection with only a small innoculum but can almost certainly be minimized by prophylactic antibiotics.

Postdiscectomy discitis is characterized by the onset of severe back pain a few days after an invasive procedure. The pain is continuous and may be referred to the hips. Tenderness is well localized and there is considerable spasm of the back muscles. The white cell count is often normal but the ESR and CRP is raised. MRI is usually positive. Rest and broad-spectrum antibiotics may be required even if the condition cannot be confirmed with certainty. Late erosive changes in the endplate are seen on both MRI scans and radiography.

The natural history is of resolution over a period of weeks and occasionally months. About 50% fuse spontaneously within 2 years.

Postoperative infection

Spinal surgery involving implants carries an infection risk of 3–4%. We found 95% involved either *Propionibacteria* or *Staphylococcus aureus*. The remainder involve Gram negative organisms. Prophylactic antibiotics should always be used when implanting metal.

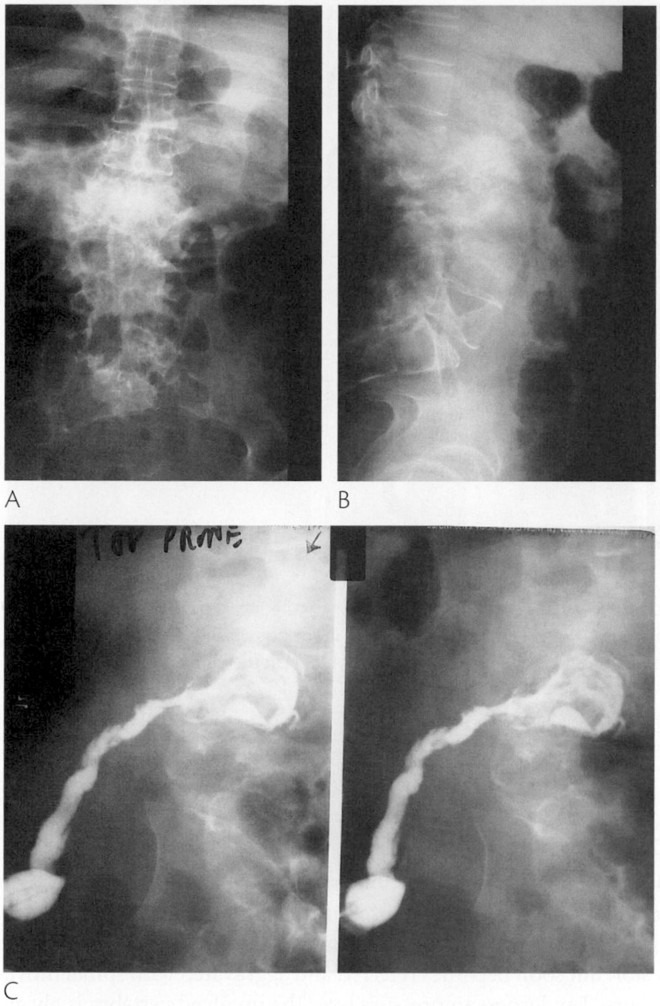

Fig. 3.18.4 Very extensive postoperative infection following spinal surgery. The sinogram shows a tract down to the spine and surrounding a methylmethacrylate vertebral body replacement.

Effective treatment implies early diagnosis and drainage. As with implants elsewhere, the wound is opened thoroughly, debrided, and thoroughly irrigated, and the metal is left in place until fusion has occurred. Intravenous antibiotics may be required for 6–12 weeks followed by oral therapy. Cure can only be obtained with removal of the implants.

Granulomatous infections of the spine

Granulomatous lesions are caused by organisms typified by the formation of a granuloma. The most common of these are tuberculosis and brucellosis, but fungi can also be a cause.

Tuberculosis

More than 30 million patients suffer from overt tuberculosis in the world today, of whom 2–3% have involvement of the skeletal system. Spinal tuberculosis accounts for roughly 50% of all cases. There are an estimated two million patients with active spinal tuberculosis in the world, and the numbers are likely to increase due to the poor economy and living standards of the developing nations, the increasing incidence of HIV-infected patients, and emergence of multidrug-resistant strains.

Pathology

The organism usually responsible for spinal tuberculosis is *Mycobacterium tuberculosis*. Pulmonary tuberculosis is found in less than 10% of patients (Figure 3.18.5A). The spread of infection is mainly via the arterial vascular channels and Batson's perivertebral venous plexus. More than 50% of lesions occur in the dorsolumbar region. Children show a higher incidence of cervical involvement than adults. About 5% of patients have skip lesions, which are separated by two or three normal vertebrae (Figure 3.18.5B).

The vertebral bodies are affected in the majority of the patients, but the appendices (pedicle, laminas, transverse process, or spinous process) are involved in less than 10%. Many types of body involvement are observed (Figure 3.18.6). Paradiscal infection is the most common type, especially in adolescents and young adults. The infection spreads through the epiphyseal arteries and there is narrowing of the disc space with involvement of the adjacent bodies. Disc-space narrowing is observed 2–3 months before any osseous changes are seen (Figure 3.18.6A).

Tuberculosis in children

Complete destruction of one or two vertebrae is more common in children below the age of 10 years. The anterior column deficit is enormous, and these children are specifically prone to severe deformity and late-onset paraplegia (Figure 3.18.6B). Posterior or the appendicial lesions may affect the pedicle, transverse process, laminas, or spinous process (Figures 3.18.7 and 3.18.8).

The natural history of spinal tuberculosis

The natural history of untreated spinal tuberculosis is one of continued destruction of the vertebral bodies and progressive deformity with potential for neurological deficit due to compression of the neural structures by caseous and infective granulation tissue. Specific antituberculous chemotherapy can arrest the progress of the disease at any stage and hasten the healing and consolidation of the focus.

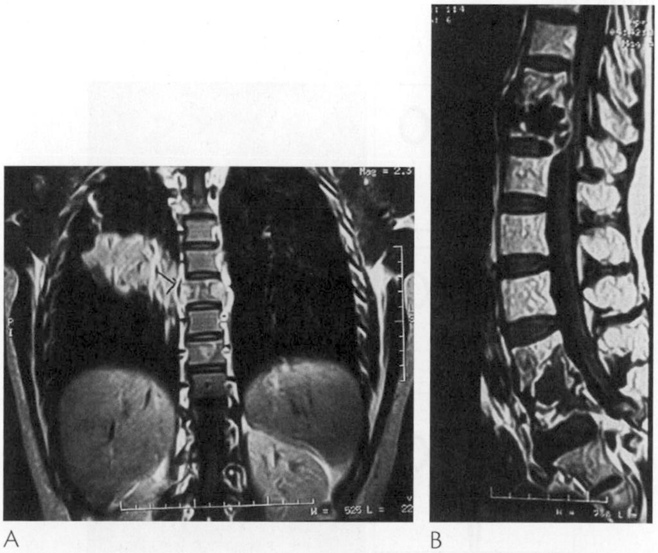

Fig. 3.18.5 A) MRI of an adolescent girl showing a tuberculous focus of infection at the mid-dorsal level together with a pulmonary lesion. B) Skip lesions are seen in about 5% of patients investigated using plain radiography and in about 15% when MRI is used.

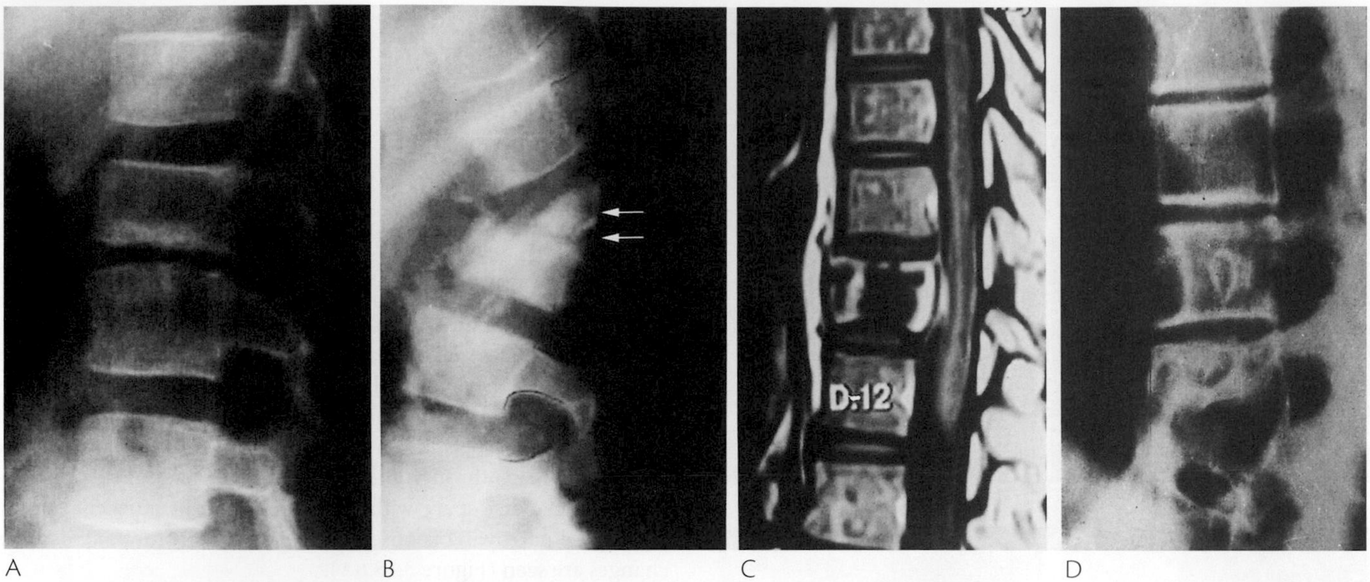

Fig. 3.18.6 The various types of body lesions seen commonly. A) Reduction of disc space with marginal erosions is the first sign of paradiscal lesion. B) Complete destruction of vertebral bodies can be seen, especially in children, and severe deformities occur. C) Body lesions with reduction in the body height and normal disc spaces can cause difficulty in differential diagnosis with metastasis and other neoplastic conditions. D) Anterior lesions show notching in the anterior margin without involvement of the whole body or the disc.

The disc is destroyed early in the course of the disease. The rate of bony fusion in spinal tuberculosis is high. In patients with severe disease, many vertebral bodies are destroyed and there is usually a severe collapse before contact of healthy bone can take place (Figure 3.18.9B). Deformity may progress to more than 60 degrees in about 5% of the patients, and there may be some neurological symptoms or signs in about 15–20%. Children who have a severe collapse of more then 90 degrees in the dorsal and the dorsolumbar vertebra are also prone to late-onset paraplegia in their second or third decade.

Clinical features

There is usually insidious, but sometimes acute onset of weight loss, loss of appetite, malaise, and evening rise of temperature, pain, and restriction of movement localized to the site of the lesion but soon becomes referred and aggravated with spinal movements. Tenderness to pressure over the involved vertebra is always present, and tapping on the spinous process causes referred pain. Deformity occurs as the involved vertebrae are softened. A retropharyngeal abscess causes difficulty in deglutition and phonation

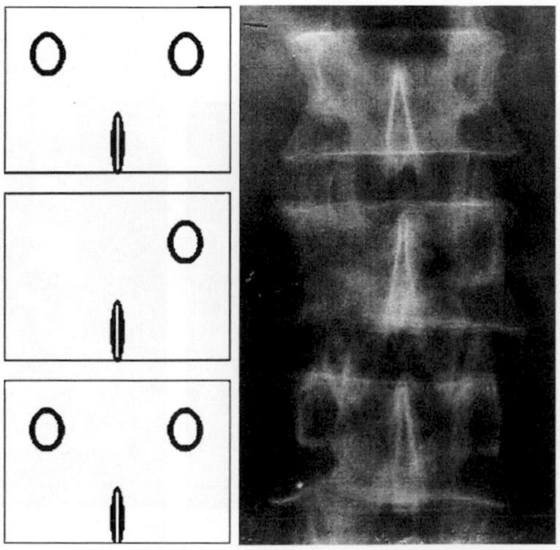

Fig. 3.18.7 In the anteroposterior radiograph of the spine a normal vertebra has two pedicles and a spinous process resembling the eyes and the beak of an owl. Destruction of a pedicle as shown in the figure leads to loss of a pedicle, resulting in the 'winking owl' sign.

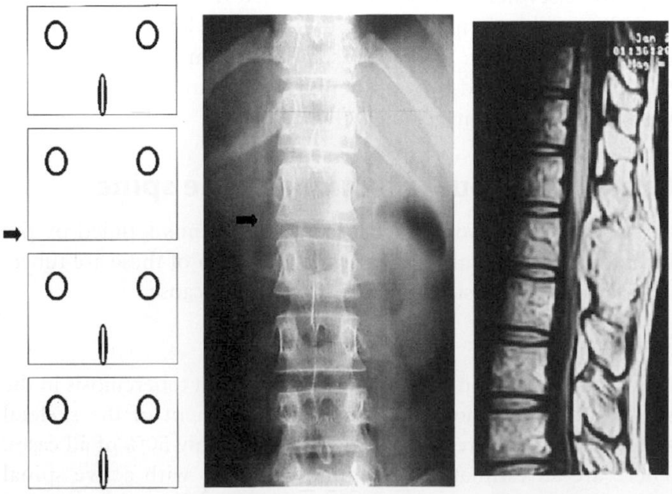

Fig. 3.18.8 A normal radiograph has two pedicles and a spinous process resembling the eyes and the beak of an owl. A tuberculous lesion of the spinous process of L1 vertebra has lead to the loss of the beak, resulting in a 'beakless owl' sign.

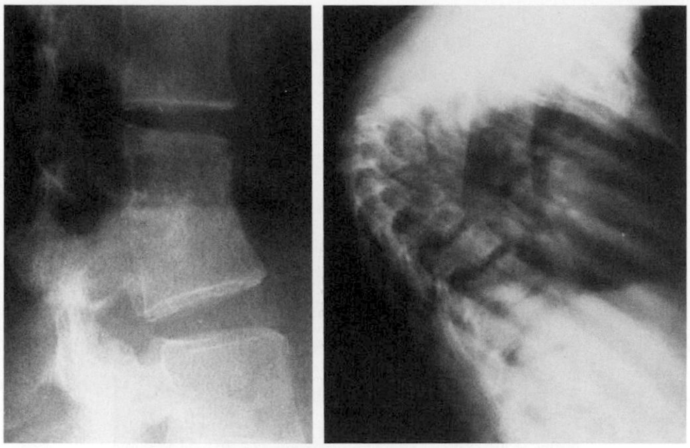

A B

Fig. 3.18.9 A) Paradiscal lesions with minimal destruction heal by bony fusion which is the hallmark of spinal tuberculosis. In patients with severe destruction and loss of several vertebral bodies a severe collapse has to occur before contact of healthy vertebra can occur and consolidate. B) The increase in deformity, especially in children, can occur over many years.

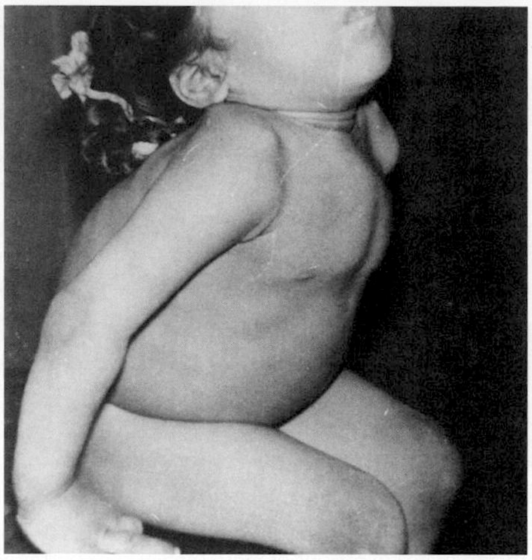

Fig. 3.18.10 A 4-year-old child with extensive involvement of the mid-dorsal region with spinal instability. There was severe pain even on minimal movement and the child had to support the trunk with both upper limbs to adopt a sitting posture.

(Figure 3.18.10A). A cold abscess is present in more than half of patients (Figures 3.18.11 and 3.18.12).

Thoracic paravertebral abscesses may spread into the extrapleural space or may rupture into the pleura, resulting in empyema or track backwards along the intercostal vessels and nerves onto the chest wall. In lumbar lesions, the majority of cold abscesses enter the psoas sheath and form a psoas mass in the groin, the pelvis, the gluteal region, or the posterior aspect of the thigh or the popliteal region.

Diagnosis

MRI is very useful for delineating the soft tissue masses in both the sagittal and coronal planes and for indicating the extent of the disease and the spread of the tuberculous debris (Figure 3.18.13). A relative lymphocytosis, an elevated ESR, and a positive tuberculin skin test are not infallible; skin test and ESR may be normal in more than 10% of patients. ESR may provide a rough guide for assessing response to therapy. Enzyme-linked immunoabsorbent assay (ELISA) for antibody to mycobacterial antigen-6 is also used in diagnosis and in differential diagnosis from other diseases such as brucellosis, typhoid, and syphylitic infections. CT is better for assessing bony destruction (Figure 3.18.14).

Treatment of uncomplicated spinal tuberculosis

Chemotherapy using antituberculous drugs is the mainstay of treatment. Chemotherapy has also made surgery more successful by drastically improving wound healing and reducing secondary wound infections. Surgery is helpful in managing deformity, neurological involvement, and non-response to chemotherapy (Figure 3.18.15). Unless there is an emergency, it is safer to perform a definite surgical procedure after chemotherapy for 3–4 weeks and adequate improvement of the nutritional status of the patient. Treatment is summarized in Table 3.18.1.

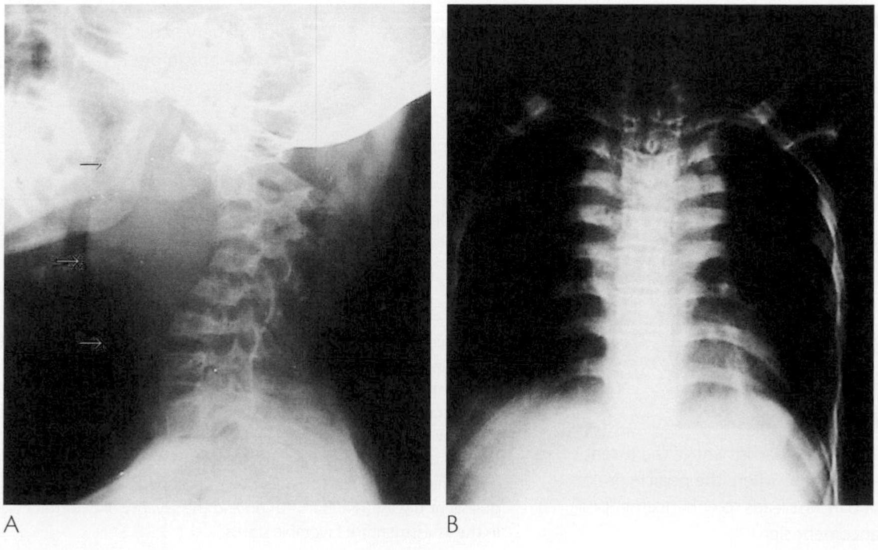

A B

Fig. 3.18.11 A) Lateral radiograph of the cervical spine showing abnormal kyphosis of the cervical vertebra due to the tuberculous focus at C1–2. Note the large prevertebral soft-tissue shadow indicating a large retropharyngeal cold abscess. This patient presented with dysphagia and had difficulty in breathing, requiring immediate intervention. The normal prevertebral shadow does not exceed more than 2–3mm and an increase must raise suspicion of retropharyngeal abscess.
B) A cold abscess in dorsal lesions usually collects in the paravertebral space and appears as a fusiform paravertebral shadow on anteroposterior radiographs.

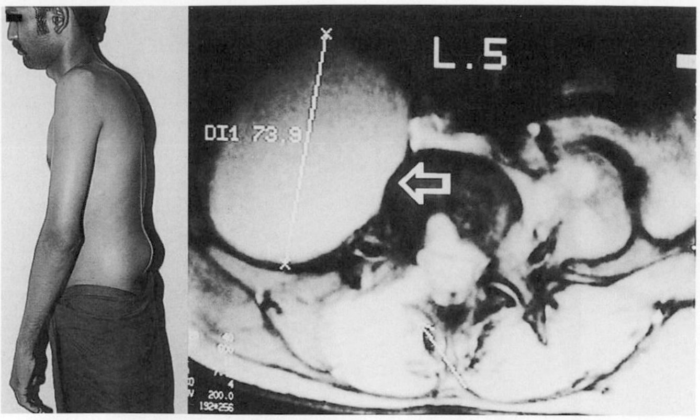

Fig. 3.18.12 A) Cold abscess in lumbar lesions can travel along the lumbodorsal fascia and present in the Petit's triangle. B) However, the abscess usually collects in the psoas sheath and huge collections of more than 1L are commonly seen.

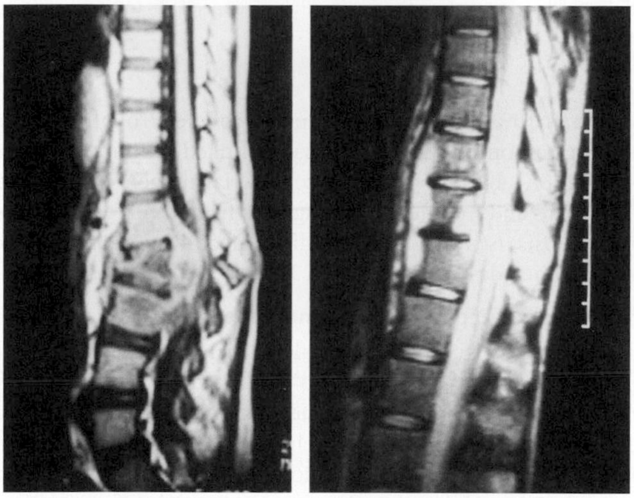

Fig. 3.18.13 MRI is superior to all other forms of investigations in demonstrating the anatomy of the spinal canal and the extent and cause of pressure over the neural structures. It demonstrates clearly whether compression is due to an abscess or to sequestration of the disc and necrotic bone into the spinal canal. Subligamentous spread of a paraspinal mass with involvement of contiguous vertebra strongly suggests a tubercular infection.

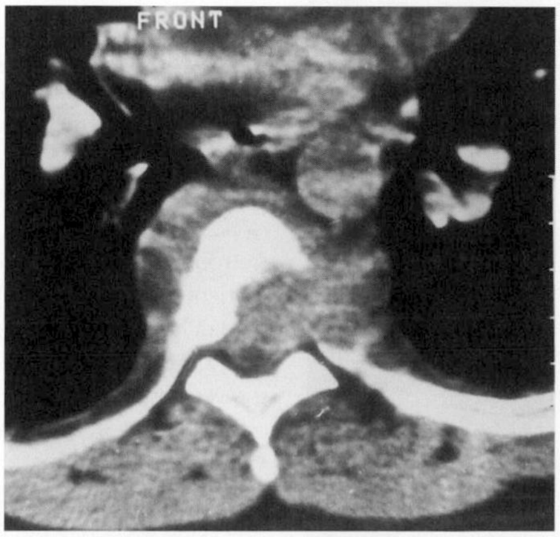

Fig. 3.18.14 A CT scan is very useful for the accurate assessment of the extent of bony destruction and the early identification of lesions where the pedicle or the posterior structures are involved. Injection of contrast leads to enhancement of the border of the paraspinal mass (rim-enhancement sign).

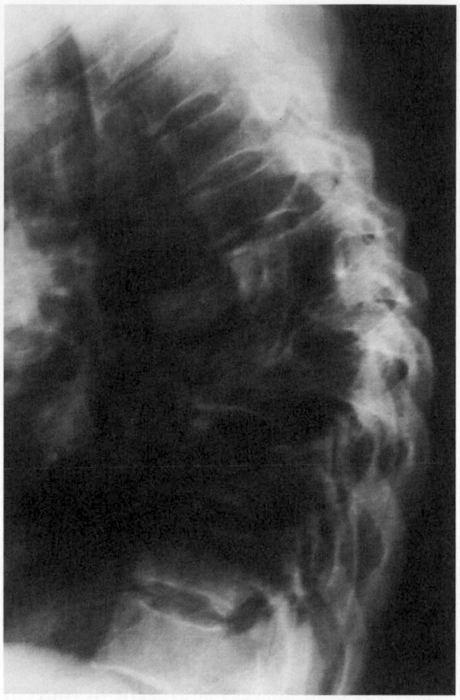

Fig. 3.18.15 Dorsal lesion with destruction of two vertebral bodies which has been debrided followed by anterior fusion using multiple rib grafts.

Table 3.18.1 Conclusions of MRC trials

Centers	Conclusions
Korea and Rhodesia	Ambulant outpatient chemotherapy treatment with isoniazid and PAS for 18 months was highly successful
	Daily addition of streptomycin not necessary
Korea	No extra benefit from rest in hospital for 6 months
Masan	No benefit from plaster jacket for first few months
Pusan	
Rhodesia	Debridement as a surgical procedure offered no advantage over ambulant chemotherapy
Rhodesia versus Hong Kong	Radical surgery had no advantage over ambulant chemotherapy in preservation of life and health and in achievement of favorable status
	Radical surgery may achieve favorable status quickly with earlier fusion and decreased tendency for progress in deformity
Madras, India	Short-course chemotherapy with daily isoniazid and rifampin for 9 months achieved higher rate (98 per cent) of favorable status than radical surgery (88 per cent) at 5 years

Inclusion criteria: patients with clinical and radiologic evidence of tuberculosis involving any vertebra from the first dorsal to the first sacrum and without neurologic involvement.

Exclusion criteria: presence of severe extraspinal disease (tuberculous or nontuberculous) or a previous history of antituberculous chemotherapy or surgical intervention.

Favorable status: no residual neurologic impairment, sinuses, clinically evident abscess, or impairment of physical activities due to the spinal lesion, and with radiologically quiescent disease. (NB Bony fusion and the severity of deformity were not considered in the assessment for favorable status.)

The current recommended daily dosage for the treatment of adults, with or without HIV infection, is 300mg isoniazid, 600mg rifampin (rifampicin), and 20–30mg/kg pyrazinamide. In this intensive phase, which lasts for 2 months, ethambutol (or streptomycin for children who are too young to be monitored for visual acuity) should be included when the severity of the lesion is extensive and there are complicating factors like neurological involvement, in patients from a population where there is a high primary resistance to isoniazid, and if there is a suspicion of drug resistance. After the intensive phase of 2 months, with either the triple-drug or the four-drug regimen, a continuation phase using isoniazid and rifampin can be continued for a period of 9–12 months.

Late deformity can occur in two distinct phases: the *active phase*, which includes the changes in the first 18 months when the disease is still active, and the *healed phase*, which includes all changes in deformity after cure has been achieved. The extent of the collapse and its progress during a long-term follow-up has been found to depend on the age of the individual, the level of the lesion, and the presence of spinal instability. Paraplegia due to tuberculosis has traditionally been divided into two groups: *early-onset paraplegia*, which occurs within the first 2 years of the onset of the disease, and *late-onset paraplegia*, which usually occurs after many years.

Brucellar spondylitis

Brucella is endemic in agricultural areas of the world, particularly where goats are common. *Brucella melitensis* is found in goat's milk, although other milk- producing animals can act as a reservoir. *Brucella abortus* and *B. suis* are present in about 30% of the cattle in the United Kingdom but rarely cause disease. Brucellar infections present in a similar way to tuberculosis. Spinal *Brucella* is mainly found in the lumbar region and multiple sites are common. Presentation may be relatively acute, particularly if *Brucella* causes a meningitis. *Brucella* can also cause a local sacral ileitis. Diagnosis depends on considering the possibility of brucellosis and on bacterial culture and serology. The usual treatment is chemotherapy with a range of antibiotics (tetracycline, streptomycin, and rifampin (rifampicin)). Chemotherapy should be maintained for at least 3 months and possibly longer, and even then the recurrence rate is high. Surgical management is limited to patients who fail to resolve, particularly if there is neurological compromise.

Fungal infections

Fungi may cause granulomatous lesions in the spine. Fungal infections include coccidioidomycosis blastomycosis, histoplasmosis, cryptococcosis, and aspergillosis. They all occur in endemic regions and are rarely seen in the United Kingdom except in cases of immunodeficiency. They are all difficult to identify and to treat.

Parasitic infections

Echinococcus is a very rare cause of spinal infection which presents with large expansile lytic lesions (hydatid cysts). Diagnosis is made by a positive complement fixation test as well as the typical radiological changes. Treatment is by radical surgery combined with mebendazole. Results are very poor with a high rate of recurrence and also a high rate of paraplegia.

Minimally infective organisms causing spinal infection

Salmonella typhimurium can cause spinal infection in endemic areas and typically in patients with concomitant sickle cell disease. Other *Salmonella* species can cause spinal infection in the immunosuppressed. Commensals such as *Serratia marcescens* and *Nocardia* have been reported as causing spinal infection. These organisms have little relevance except in the immunocompromised.

Further reading

Collins, I., Wilson-MacDonald, J., Chami, G., *et al.* (2008). The diagnosis and management of infection following instrumented spinal fusion. *European Spine Journal*, **17**, 445–50.

Tuli, S.M. (1997). *Tuberculosis of the Skeletal System*. New Delhi: Jaypee Brothers.

3.19

Cross-sectional imaging in spinal disorders

S. Gaba, Philip McNee, and Eugene McNally

Summary points

Disc Degeneration

- DDD - Multifactorial disease
- MRI is key imaging technique but cannot differentiate painful from painless degenerate disc
- Normal disc on T2W MRI has outer black annulus fibrosus and inner bright nucleus pulposus
- On T2W MRI DDD is dark and discitis is bright and but occasionally disc may be bright in DDD due to liquefied nucleus.

Degenerative disc disease

Disc degeneration is a multifactorial disease. There is a general misconception to consider degeneration as a part of the normal ageing process but many factors including mechanical, genetic, nutritional, and traumatic causes have all been implicated in its aetiology. Similar changes have been described in asymptomatic young individuals, further evidence that genetic factors play a significant role (Figure 3.19.1).

A wide spectrum of imaging techniques has been used to image low back pain. Plain film changes of degenerative disc disease (DDD) are a late finding. Computed tomography (CT) changes can be appreciated earlier, but only when the disc has bulged beyond its normal margins or when intradiscal gas or osteophytes have developed. Due to its ability to detect changes in the water content of the disc, magnetic resonance imaging (MRI) plays a principal role in identifying the degenerate disc and in differentiating other causes of pain; however, there are no reliable findings that help to differentiate the painful from the painless degenerate disc. Recent advances in MRI like functional T_2 mapping can also evaluate disc function.

The adolescent disc demonstrates three different anatomical areas on T_2-weighted (T2W) water-sensitive MRIs. There is a black outer zone of annulus fibrosus, a bright inner zone of the nucleus pulposus, and an intermediate zone, histologically representing a transition between the regular lamellae of the annulus and the more loosely packed nucleus. With increasing age, the ability of the nucleus to imbibe water decreases and there is a gradual loss of its bright signal. The early changes of disc degeneration parallel this change, but occur at a faster rate. Lumbar disc degeneration assessment is graded on the basis of MRI signal intensity on T2W mid-sagittal fast spin echo images, and distinction between nucleus and annulus, disc structure, and height. A grade 1 disc is homogenous, hyperintense, has normal height with a clear distinction between nucleus and annulus. A grade 5 disc is inhomogeneous, hypointense, with a collapsed disc space with loss of distinction between nucleus and annulus.

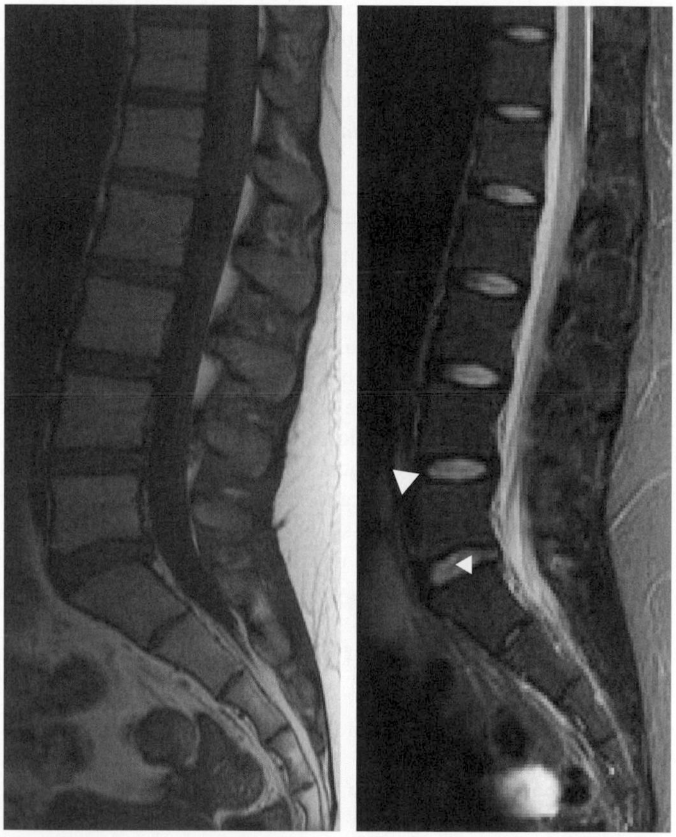

Fig. 3.19.1 Normal T1W (A) and T2W (B) sagittal images for lumbar spine. Short arrow shows annulus fibrosus and longer arrow points to the nucleus pulposus.

Cadaveric studies have shown that annular disruption is the decisive factor in disc degeneration. Annular tears, particularly radial tears are not necessarily a consequence of ageing. Annular tears can be radial, concentric, or transverse. A specific type, with a hyperintense round lesion surrounded by a black annulus has been called a high signal zone (HSZ) (Figure 3.19.2). There is some evidence that discs with HSZs are more likely to be symptomatic at discography. Other authors however, disagree. Annular tears are more conspicuous following gadolinium enhancement. On serial MRI of annular tears in lumbar discs, it has been suggested that hyperintensity on T2W MRIs and enhancement of annular tears do not indicate that the tear is acute in nature. With progressive DDD there is loss of vertical height, disc material bulges in all directions, and the facet joints sublux. The combination of these changes can narrow the spinal canal, lateral recesses, or exit foramina and cause nerve root compression.

The adjacent vertebral bodies also show changes in form of signal alteration (Table 3.19.1).

Type 3 endplate changes can be seen on plain films. Type 1 changes are non-specific and simply indicate marrow oedema (Figure 3.19.3).When present on both sides of a disc, which demonstrates low signal on T2W images, increased marrow water can usually be attributed to disc degeneration rather than tumour

Table 3.19.1 Types of degenerative (Modic) marrow changes

Endplate marrow change	T1W signal	T2W signal	Pathological change
Type 1	Decreased	Increased	Increase in water content
Type 2	Increased	Increased	Increase in fat
Type 3	Decreased	Decreased	Bony sclerosis

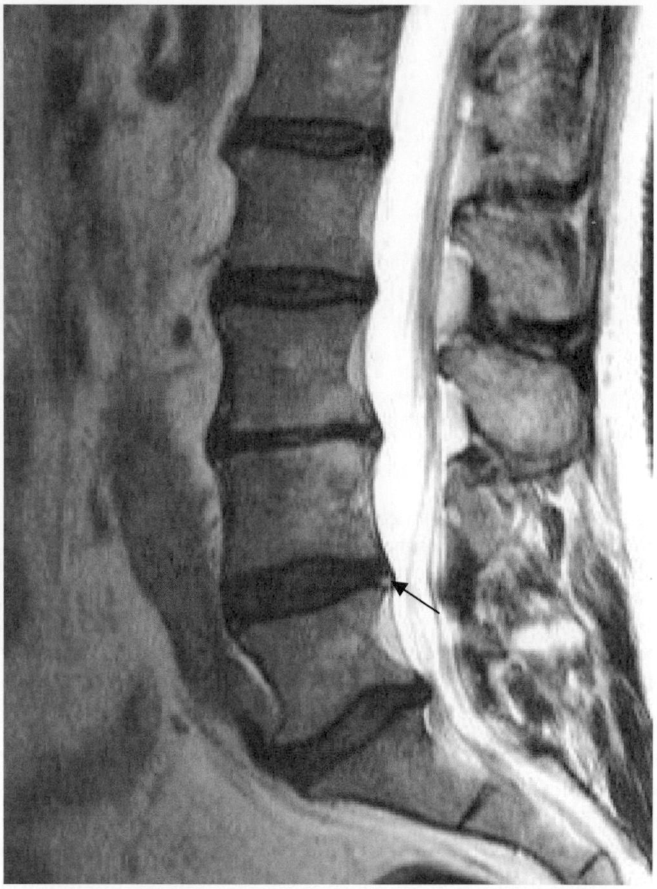

Fig. 3.19.2 Focal high signal (HIZ) in the posterior L4/L5 annulus (arrow) represents an annular tear.

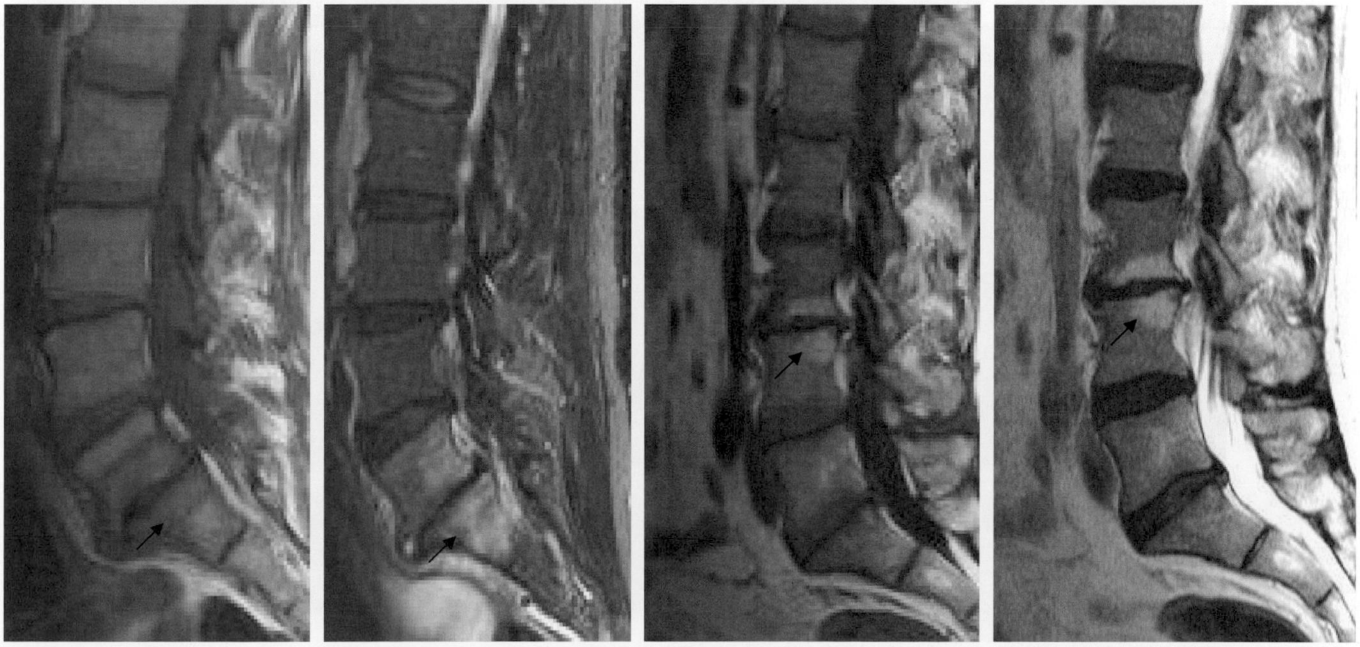

A B C D

Fig. 3.19.3 A) and B) Type 1 Modic change. Low signal endplate change on T1W and corresponding high signal on T2W (arrows) due to marrow oedema. C) and D) Type 2 Modic change. High signal endplate change on T1W and corresponding high signal on T2W (arrows) due to fatty marrow change.

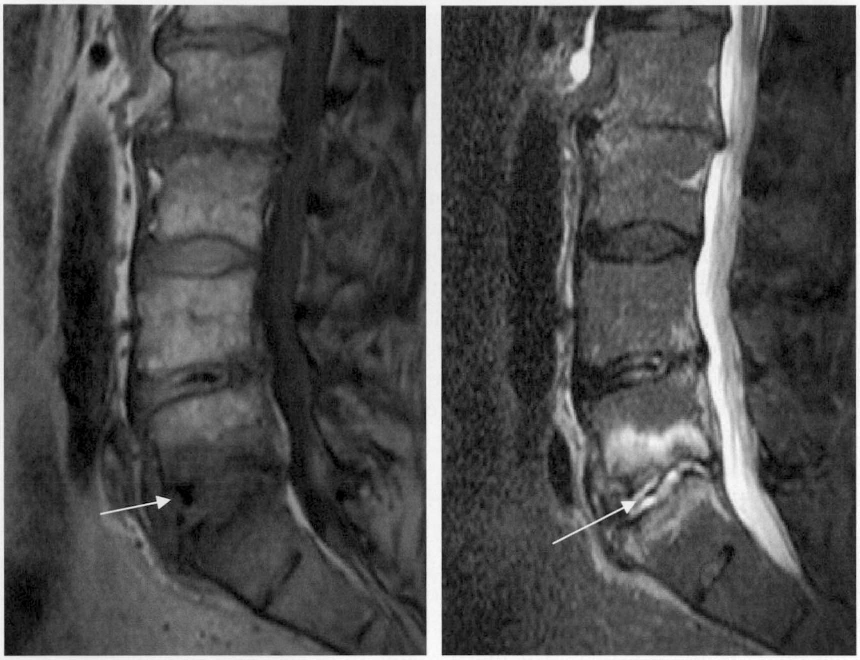

Fig. 3.19.4 A) T1W sagittal image demonstrates abnormal low signal in the L5/S1 disc (arrows) and endplates. B) T2W sagittal image shows corresponding high signal in the disc and endplate bone marrow oedema with a small prevertebral phlegmon.

or infection. Discitis is also associated with peridiscal marrow oedema however, in contradistinction to DDD, the infected disc has high signal on T2W images (Figure 3.19.4). In some cases of severe disc degeneration, the nucleus can become liquefied, and also return high signal on T_2. In these cases, differentiation from discitis can be more difficult. As many of the infections are low grade and inflammatory indices are often normal or only minimally elevated, enhancement of the vertebral body endplates following administration of gadolinium-labelled diamino-tetraethyl-pentaacetic acid (Gd-DTPA) may assist, but it is non-specific and can also occur after uncomplicated surgery. Simultaneous enhancement within the endplate, posterior annulus, and vertebral body itself is more specific for infection. The pattern of endplate changes may provide a clue, in that fatty type 2 changes are unlikely to persist adjacent to an actively infected disc. In other cases, biopsy may be required to exclude infection (Figure 3.19.5).

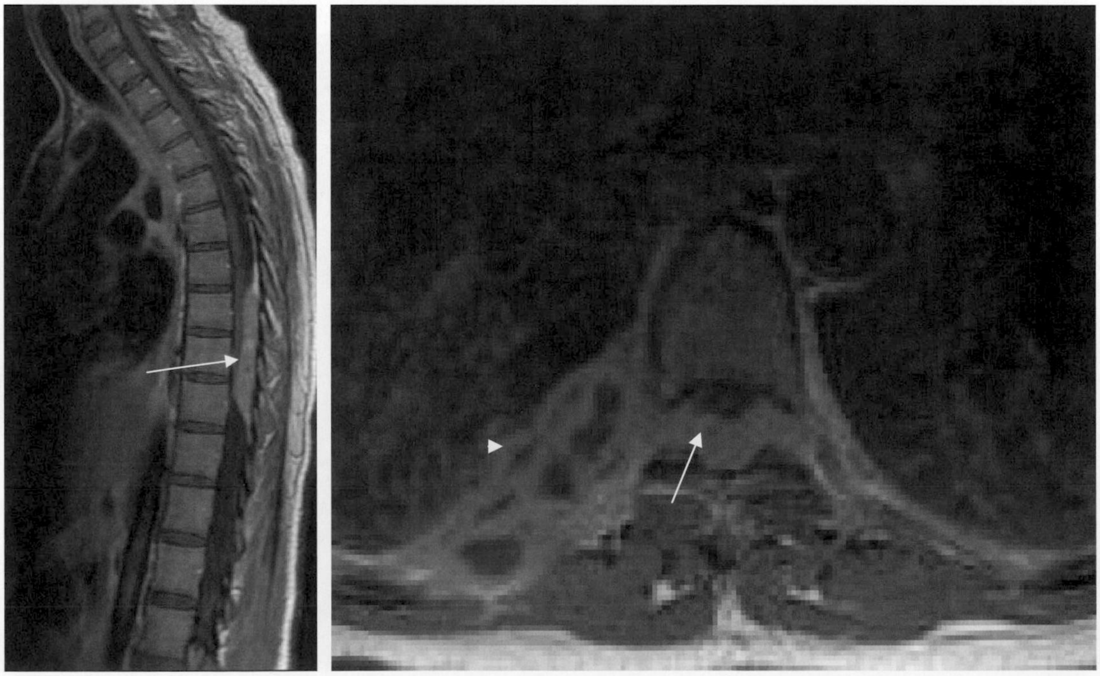

Fig. 3.19.5 A) Sagittal postcontrast T1W images shows enhancing epidural abscess in the mid thoracic region (arrow). B) Axial postcontrast T1W through lower thoracic region demonstrates right paravertebral (arrow head) and epidural abscess (arrow) with peripheral enhancement.

Disc prolapse

Annular disc degeneration may lead to annular tear and disc herniation. Disc herniation is most common at the L4/5 and L5/S1 levels. Plain radiographs have no role in the investigation of a patient with sciatica. Increasing use of non-ferromagnetic metalwork has improved the diagnostic capability of MRI after surgery as well. In the postfusion patient with radiculopathy, where implanted metal may interfere with both CT and MR interpretation, CT myelography may still have a role.

On MRI, disc prolapse is classified as disc herniation or disc bulge. If disc displacement in axial plane beyond the edges of the ring apophysis is less than 50% it is disc herniation and if more it is termed as disc bulge. Disc bulge is regarded as a degenerative process distinct from disc herniation.

Disc herniation is further subdivided on the basis of circumference, shape, and location. On the circumferential basis, localized displacement in axial plane beyond the edges of the ring apophysis is of two types: focal, if it is less than 25% and broad based, when the displacement is 25–50%.

On the basis of the shape it is classified as: protrusion, if the greatest distance in any plane, between the edges of the disc material beyond the disc space is less than the distance between the edges of the base of the herniated disc in the same plane (Figure 3.19.6); otherwise it is termed as extrusion. Extrusion can be referred to as sequestration if the displaced disc material has no continuity with the parent disc. Migration is a term used when the disc material is displaced away from the site of extrusion, irrespective of sequestration (Figure 3.19.7).

On the basis location, in the axial plane, it is classified as: central, subarticular (lateral recess region), foraminal (pedicle), and extra foraminal (far lateral). In sagittal plane it is categorized as discal, pedicular, supra- and infrapedicular. Nerve sheath tumours and facet synovial cysts can occasionally mimic disc extrusion or sequestration on MRI and may pose a diagnostic challenge.

A number of studies have emphasized that disc prolapse as revealed by MRI have been noted in asymptomatic individuals. In addition, the grade of disc degeneration or prolapse does not predict the clinical outcome. Furthermore, histologically proven degenerate discs with substantially decreased amount of nuclear material can still produce normal images on MRI.

Disc prolapse

- Plain radiograph has no role in patient with sciatica.
- MRI changes do not always correlate with symptoms.
- Disc prolapse nomenclature
- On MRI, nerve sheath tumours and facet joint cyst can occasionally mimic a sequestrated disc
- Spinal cord compression and spinal canal stenosis should be excluded on axial MRI images

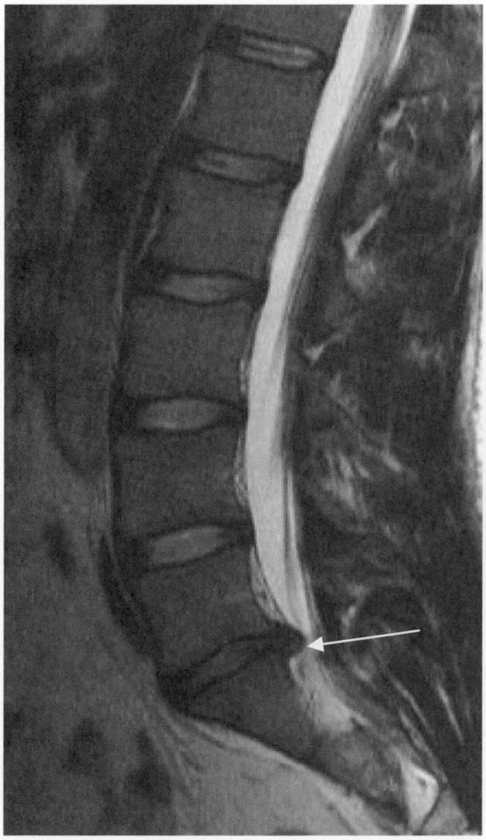
A

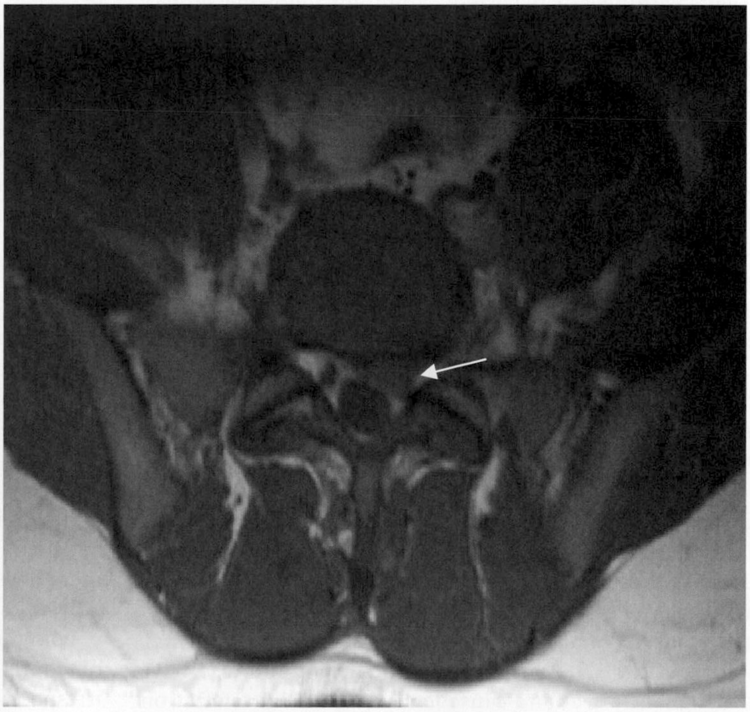
B

Fig. 3.19.6 Broad based L5/S1 disc protrusion: A) T2W sagittal; B) T1W axial. Left paracentral disc protrusion (arrows). The left S1 nerve root is not visible in the lateral recess. The right S1 nerve root is well visualized.

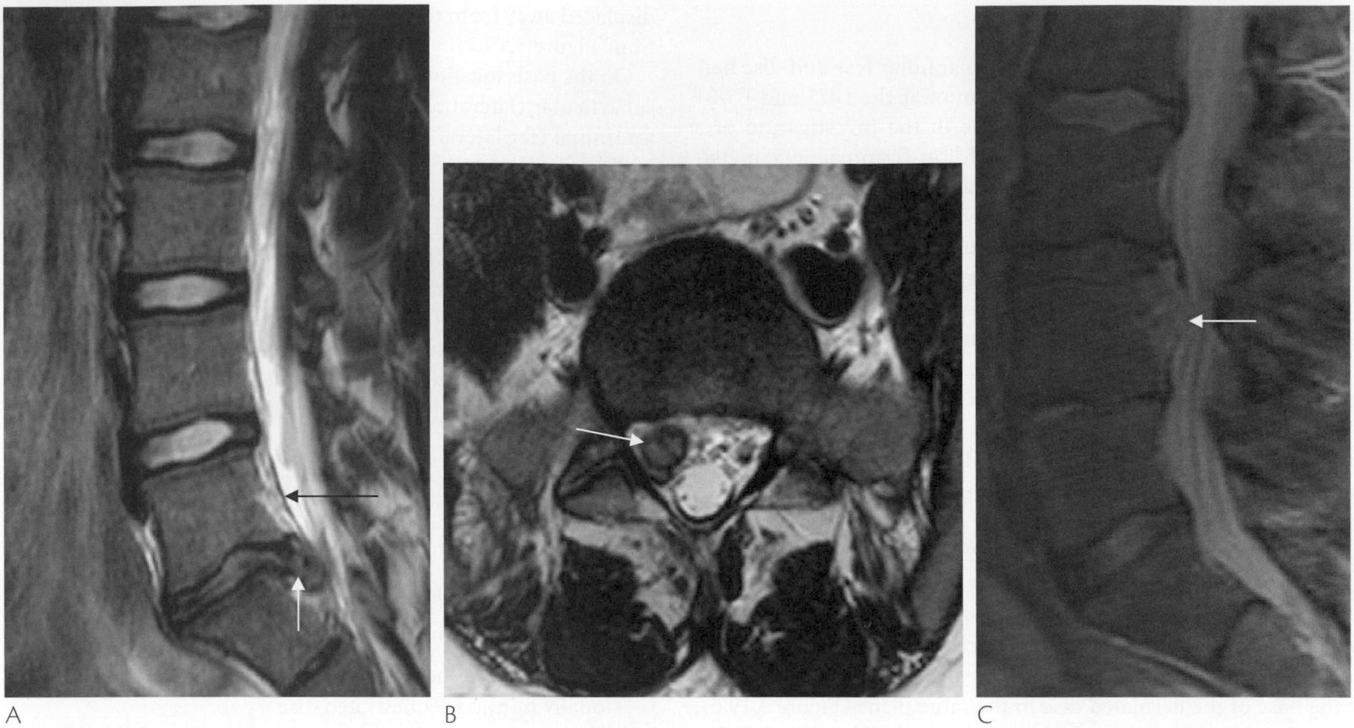

Fig. 3.19.7 Disc extrusion. A) T2W sagittal and B) T2W axial MRI demonstrate large L5/S1 disc extrusion (white arrow) elevating the PLL (black arrow). On axial image through the S1 vertebral body, disc appears to be sequestrated. C) Sequestered disc. Disc fragment (arrow) is noted posterior to the L4 vertebral body. It lacks continuity with the parent disc.

Imaging the postoperative spine

The patients with new or persistent symptoms following surgery (failed back syndrome) pose a difficult diagnostic dilemma. If symptoms persist or recur then images should be inspected to confirm that surgery was undertaken at the correct level and side. Thus, identification of lumbosacral transitional vertebra (LSTV) on MRI is very important. Disc bulge, protrusion, and spinal canal stenosis is nine times more common at the interspace immediately above LSTV. L5 can be readily identified on axial MRI as iliolumbar ligament always arises from the transverse processes of L5. If these points have been confirmed, persistent or new low back pain or recurrent sciatica following discectomy can be attributed to recurrent or residual disc material, epidural fibrosis or haematoma, discitis, arachnoiditis, or abscess (Figures 3.19.8 and 3.19.9).

Plain films are still used to assess spinal fusion, especially to assess metal discontinuity or fracture and displacement. Flexion and extension views can be used to assess vertebral stability. Cross-sectional CT imaging has largely superseded plain radiography as it can provide more detailed information. Implanted metal is not a contraindication to MRI or CT per se; however, depending on the metal used, paramagnetic artefacts, distortion, and beam hardening can obscure anatomic detail. In comparison to the steel implants, titanium metal implants cause fewer artefacts on CT as they have a low x-ray attenuation coefficient and also have less ferromagnetic affect and cause less susceptibility artefact on MRI. Ultrasound is utilized to diagnose, delineate the size and location of postoperative collections, and aspirate superficial collections. Where there is clinical suspicion of postoperative discitis, contrast-enhanced MRI is the imaging investigation of choice; however, in the early stages it may be difficult to discriminate between septic and aseptic discitis. Imaging findings must be correlated with the clinical picture and biochemical markers.

In persistent or recurrent radicular symptoms, the differential diagnosis is between recurrent disc material, neural irritation from epidural granulation tissue, and, rarely, residual disc material. It has been proposed that contrast-enhanced MRI is superior to MRI, CT, and myelography in discriminating recurrent disc from scar tissue. Where enhancement is used, it has been suggested that ionic MR contrast media, in comparison to non-ionic media, diffuses less readily into disc material and provides greater contrast with scar. The addition of fat-suppressed T_1 images and obtaining images immediately after the contrast injection may improve scar visualization. Residual disc may only show rim enhancement due to surrounding granulation tissue. The degree of enhancement of scar tissue is also dependent on its age and reaches a maximum by the first year. Disc enhancement may also be seen if imaging is delayed.

Gadolinium should not be regarded as mandatory to diagnose recurrent disc material. In equivocal cases, gadolinium enhancement does help, although it is important to appreciate that vascularized discs may enhance and dense fibrosis may not. The presence of epidural scar tissue on MRI does not necessarily indicate a poor outcome. Disc degeneration is a risk factor for recurrent herniation irrespective of its volume.

The MRI appearance of epidural haematoma depends on its age. In the early phase, the signal characteristic is that of fluid—low on T_1 and high on T_2. As it begins to deteriorate, methaemoglobin

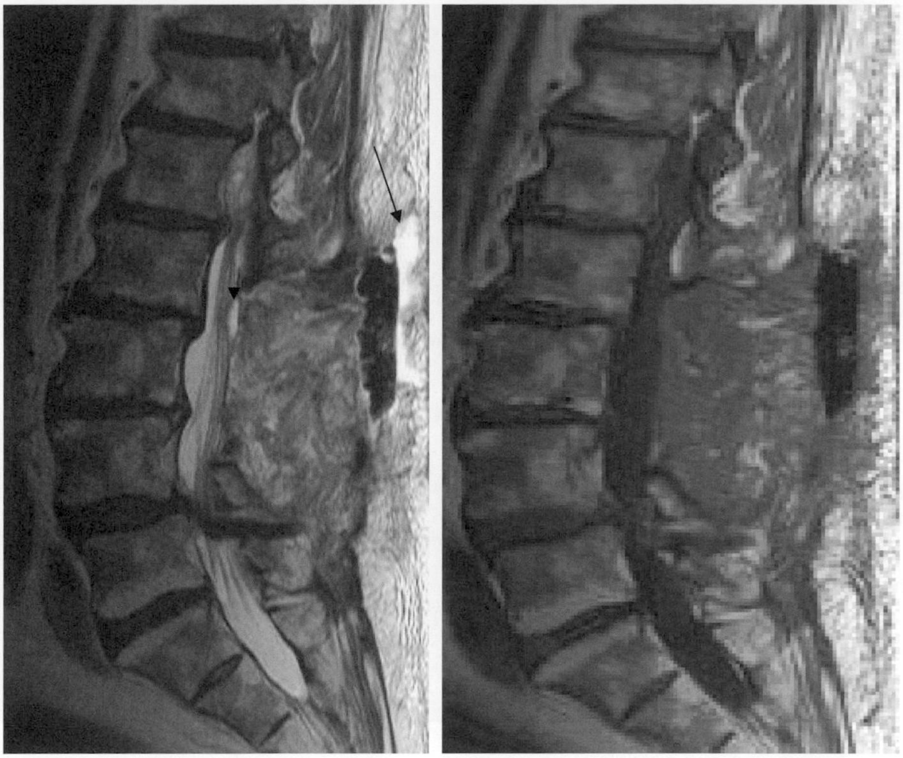

A B

Fig. 3.19.8 A) T2W and B) T1W sagittal images. Subcutaneous abscess (arrow) with an air fluid level in a patient with posterior spinal decompression surgery. Small epidural fluid collection (arrowhead).

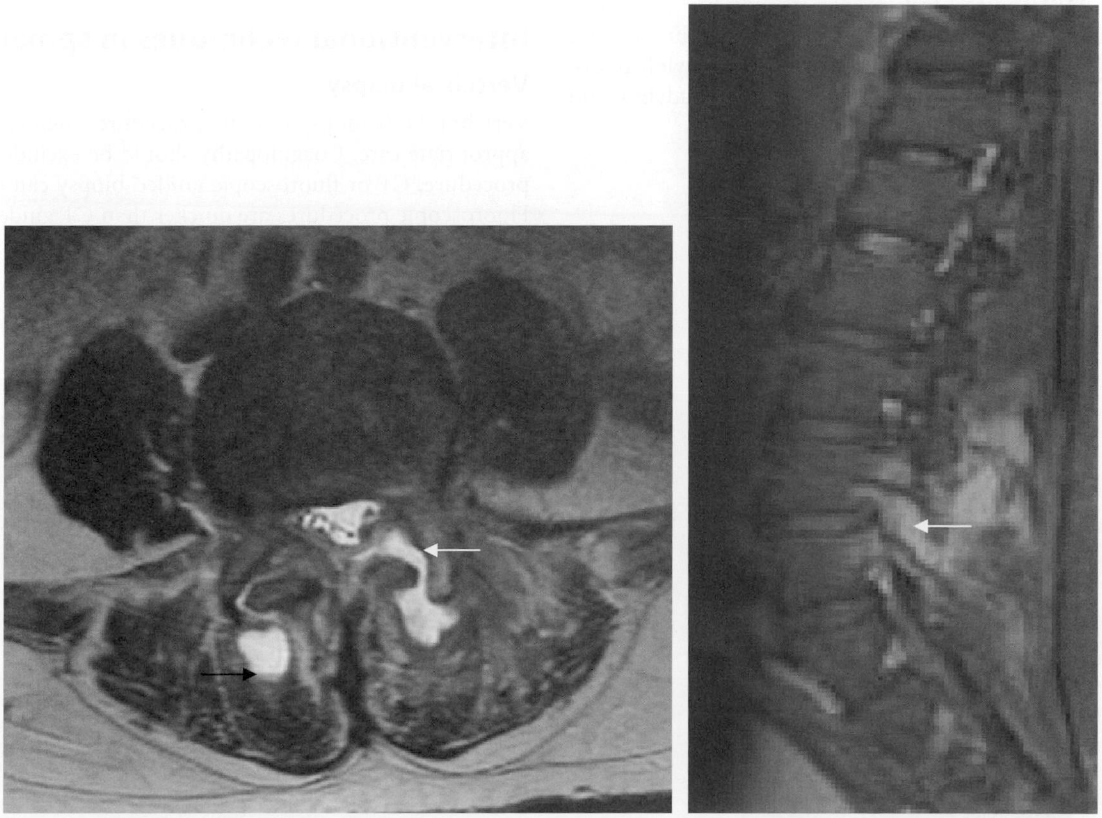

A B

Fig. 3.19.9 A) T2W axial and B) sagittal images. Bilateral facet joint (white arrow) septic arthritis with fluid and debris level (black arrow), in a patient with posterior spinal decompression.

release causes the signal on T_1 to increase. Finally, haemosiderin deposition causes the signal on T_2 to become low. In most cases, haematoma comprises several of these stages.

Other potential MRI findings in the failed back syndrome include arachnoiditis, seromata, and, rarely, pseudomeningocele. Arachnoiditis is diagnosed by the identification of one of several patterns. The most specific is clumping and agglutination of multiple nerve roots. Another pattern, termed the 'empty sac', occurs when the nerve roots adhere to the thecal sac itself, leaving an apparently empty cerebrospinal fluid space. This pattern can be seen in asymptomatic individuals, emphasizing the importance of clinical correlation.

Other conditions

The most common tumour encountered is the vertebral haemangioma. As these lesions contain both fat and fluid elements, its MRI appearances are usually typical; the lesion is bright on both T_1 and T_2 images (Figure 3.19.10). Metastases and myeloma may have variegated marrow appearance on MRI (Figure 3.19.11) (Table 3.19.2).

Spondylolisthesis is classified as degenerative, isthmus (spondylolytic) and dysplastic, traumatic, and pathological. Degenerative spondylolisthesis is commonly noted at L4/5 and isthmic is more often at L5/S1 (Figure 3.19.13). Axial loaded MRI may show dynamic degenerative spondylolisthesis, which may be missed on plain radiography or conventional MRI. A facet joint effusion of 1.5mm or more at L4/5 is suggestive of degenerative spondylolisthesis even if anterior translation is not noted on supine lumbar spine MRI. On MRI, indirect features of pars spondylosis are widening of the canal size and posterior vertebral wedging and are helpful in diagnosing pars defect in absence of spondylolisthesis. A full discussion of infection, tumour, ankylosing spondylitis, and spondylolisthesis is beyond the scope of this chapter.

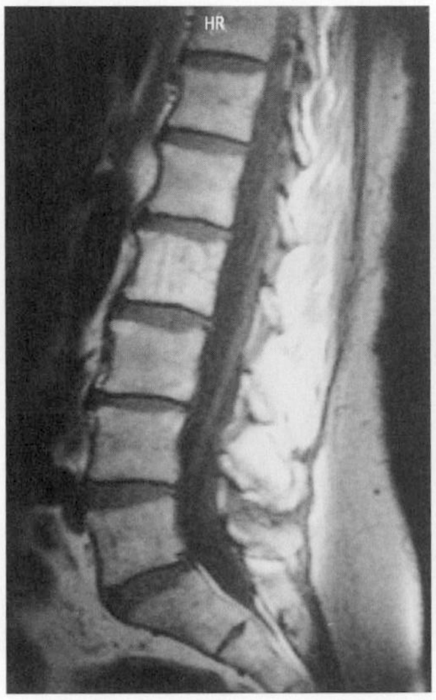

Fig. 3.19.10 Large haemangioma in L2 vertebral body. Increased (bright) signal on both T1 (Fig A) and T2W (Fig B) images due to fat content.

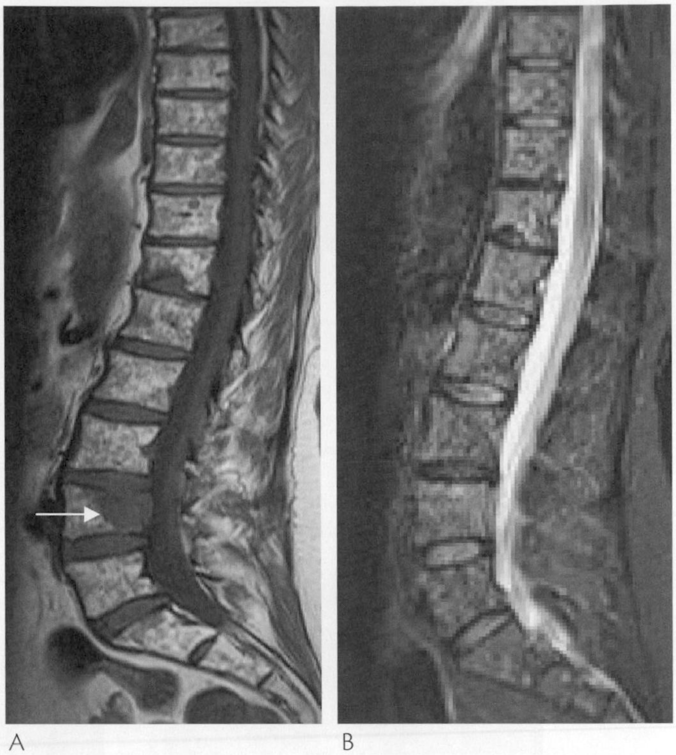

Fig. 3.19.11 Variegated appearance of bone marrow on both T1W and T2W sagittal images due to myeloma infiltration. Large focal myeloma deposit in L4 (arrow).

Interventional techniques in spinal disease

Vertebral biopsy

Vertebral body biopsy is a safe procedure when carried out with appropriate care. Coagulopathy should be excluded prior to the procedure. CT or fluoroscopic guided biopsy can be performed. Fluoroscopic procedures are quicker than CT guided procedures, but CT provides more accurate needle placement for smaller lesions (Figure 3.19.14).

Table 3.19.2 Differentiating features of benign and malignant vertebral collapse (Figure 3.19.12)

Imaging features of vertebral collapse	Benign	Malignant
Marrow signal	Band of normal marrow	Greater than 50% abnormal marrow
Multiplicity	Multiple. Similar patterns and ages	Multiple focal lesions, variable patterns
Pedicle involvement	Absent (other than oedema)	Present. Expansion
Presence of gas and linear fracture lines	Present	Absent unless coexistent degeneration is present
Soft tissue mass	Mostly absent. Small mass may be present in acute trauma	Often present. May be large
Convex bulge of the posterior cortex	Posterosuperior convexity. Sharply angled	Bulge involves whole of the posterior cortex

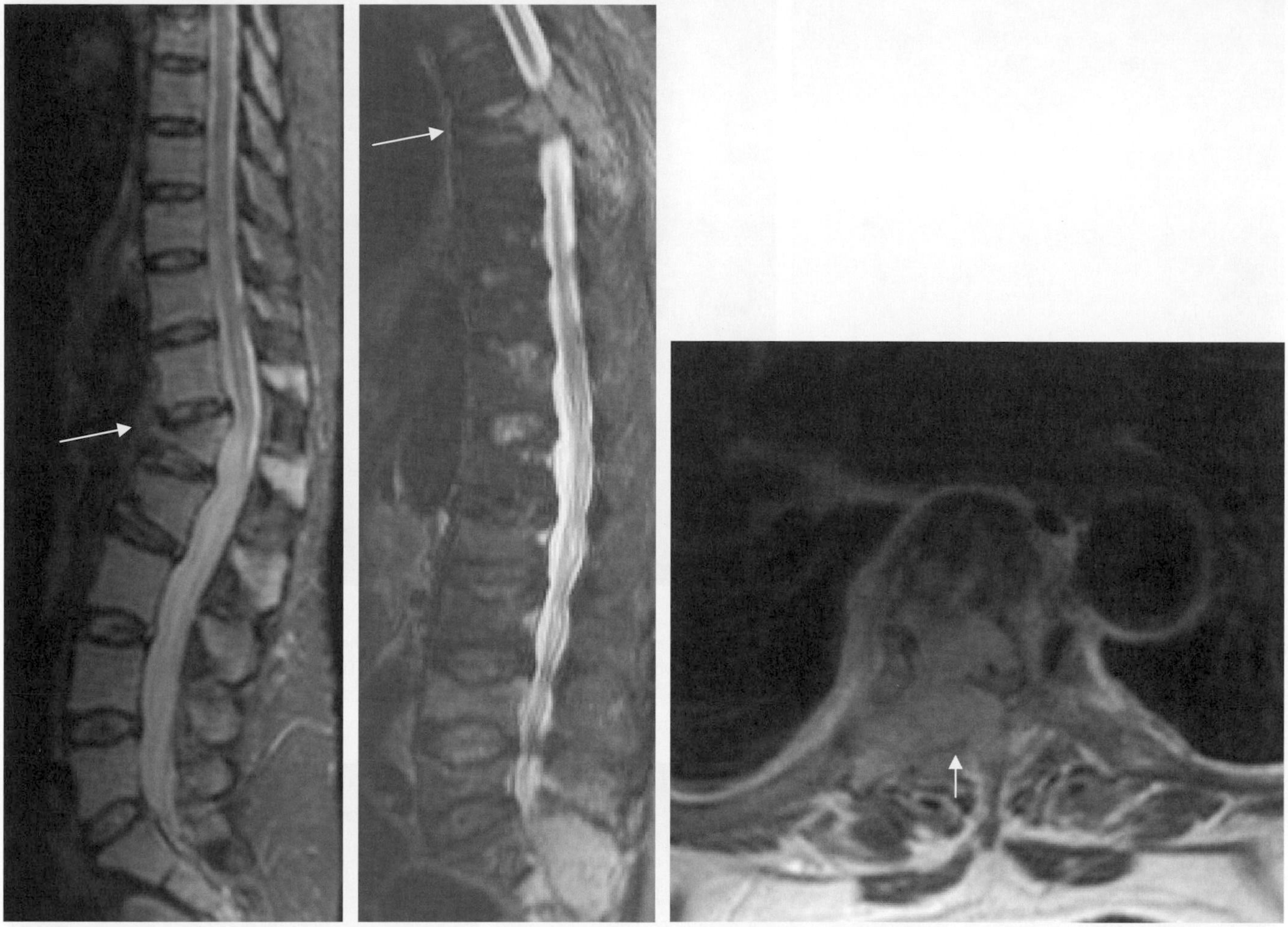

A B C

Fig. 3.19.12 A) Benign collapse of L1 vertebra (arrow) in patient with trauma. B) and C) Malignant collapse of D8 vertebra (arrow) with cord compression in patient with metastatic renal cell carcinoma. Bone expansion of the right pedicle and transverse process with large soft tissue mass leading to thecal and cord compression (arrow).

CT-guided core biopsy was found to be 93.3% accurate with highest accuracy rates for malignant lesions and false negative for benign, inflammatory, pseudotumoural and systemic pathologies. A negative biopsy in neoplastic lesions must be further confirmed with an open biopsy. Reported complications including infection, haematoma, and self-limiting neurapraxia are rare.

Intradiscal interventional procedures

Percutaneous access to the lumbar and thoracic discs is readily achieved via posterolateral and cervical discs via an anterolateral route under fluoroscopic control.

Discography

Statistics on lost man-hours and health costs in the patients with chronic disabling back pain show no evidence of abating despite a proliferation of surgical procedures and fusion devices. Part of the difficulty is patient selection, as routine imaging cannot confirm an abnormality as the definitive source of pain. This is where discography has a role. Discography can provide both anatomical and more importantly 'physiological' information on the source of pain, though false negatives and positives are the subject of much controversy (Figure 3.19.15).

Discography is most useful at differentiating painful from non-painful discs and should be regarded as a preoperative examination. Discography is valuable in selected patients with moderate loss of nuclear signal intensity and no other MRI features of DDD. Lesser roles include differentiating scar tissue from recurrent disc and confirming disc containment prior to percutaneous surgery. Pressure-controlled manometric discography can distinguish asymptomatic discs with grade 3 (Dallas Discogram Scale) annular tears from symptomatic discs.

Percutaneous intradiscal therapy

It is of two types, intradiscal electrothermal therapy (IDET) and percutaneous intradiscal radio frequency thermocoagulation (PIRFT). In the former, heat is generated electrically and in the latter through radiofrequency. These modalities are used in treatment of painful annular tears by coagulating the inflammatory tissue and the nerve endings, thus ablating pain. The treatment, however, is not permanent and, if successful, has to be repeated.

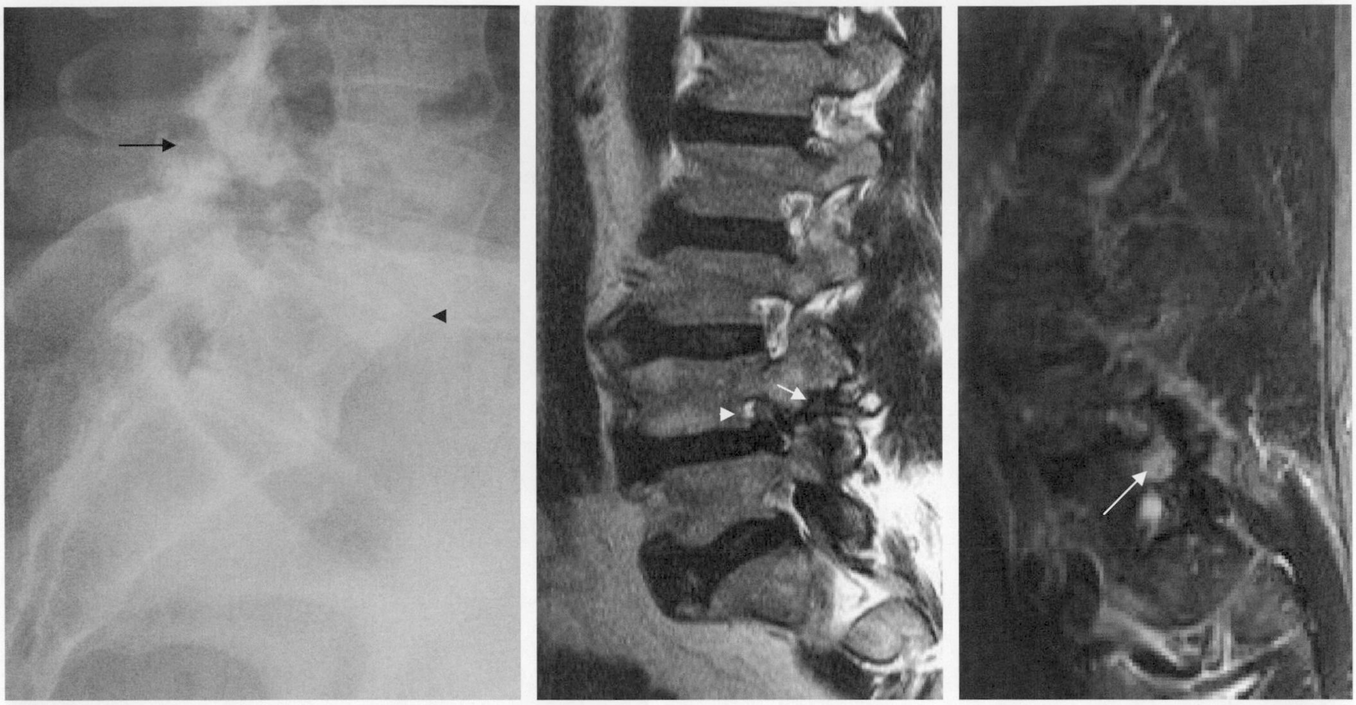

A B C

Fig. 3.19.13 A) Plain lateral x-ray lower lumbar spine demonstrates pars defect (arrow) at L4/5 with grade 1 spondylolisthesis (arrowhead). B) T2W sagittal image with chronic pars defect at L4/5 with oblique orientation of the neural foramen (arrowhead). C) Short T_1 inversion-recovery (STIR) sagittal image shows high signal in the region of pars due to stress change.

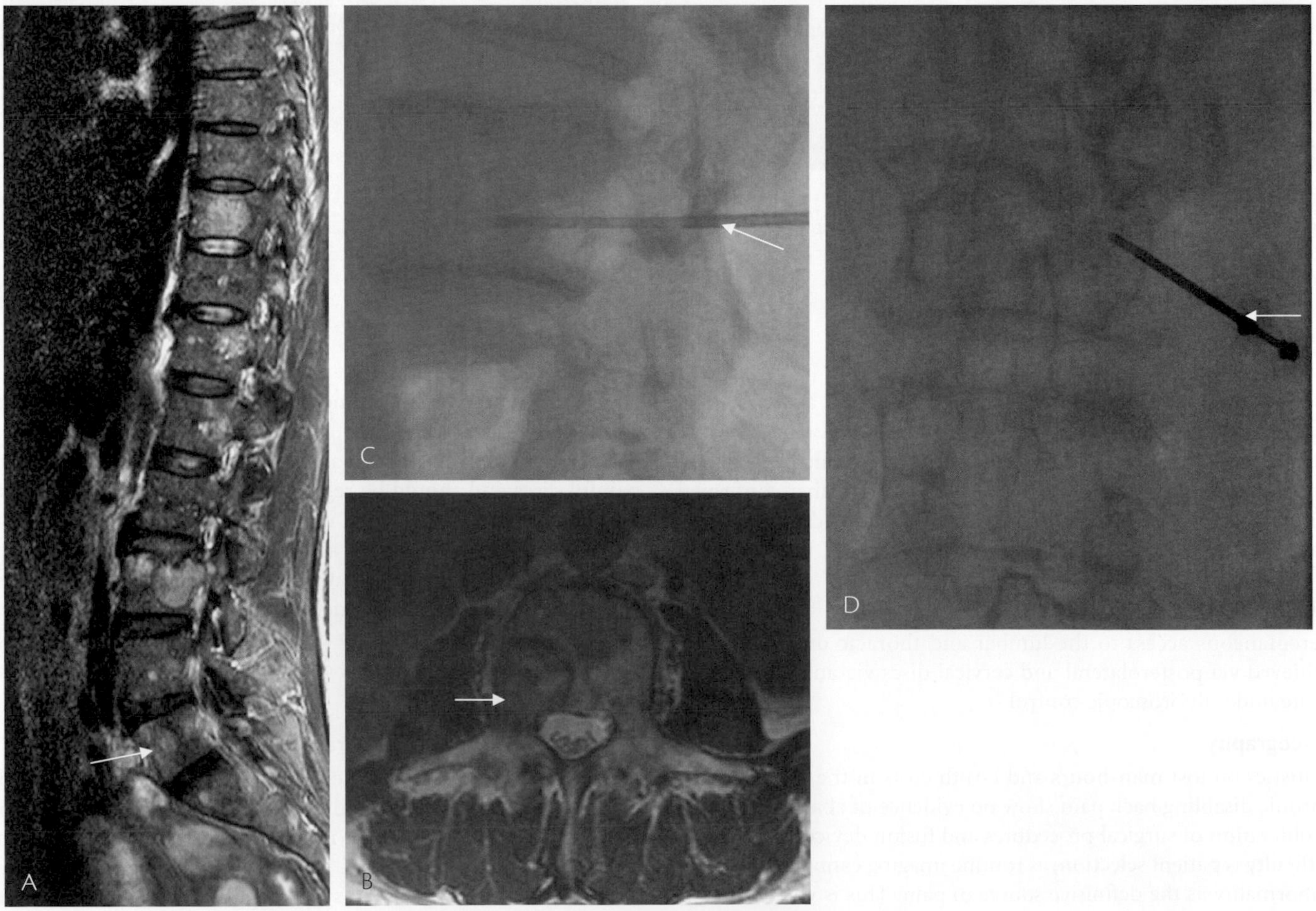

Fig. 3.19.14 A) STIR sagittal and B) T_2 axial MRIs demonstrate presence of metastatic lesions (arrows) in spine. C) and D) Fluoroscopic-guided transpedicular approach. Lateral and AP views demonstrate L3 vertebral biopsy using Bonopty biopsy system (arrows) in patient with carcinoma larynx.

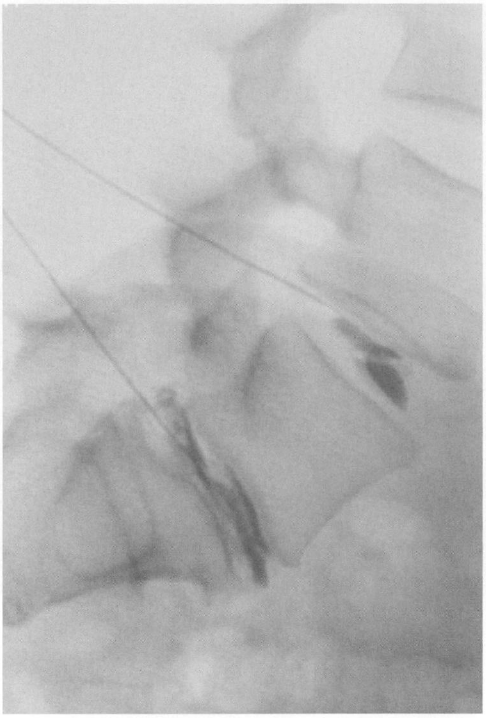

Fig. 3.19.15 Lateral lumbar discogram shows normal filling pattern of L4/5 disc and degenerate filling pattern of protruded L5/S1 disc with an annular tear.

In IDET a catheter is passed into the nucleus pulposus such that it lies along the inner margin of the annulus whereas in PRIFT the catheter is placed into the centre of the disc. Initial non-randomized studies suggested a favourable outcome for IDET but not for PRIFT. Various randomized controlled trials (RCTs) have suggested both favourable and unequivocal outcomes. A recent study, however, has shown that with application of strict selection criteria (patients with mild disc degeneration, annular tear proven on imaging, and pain on low-pressure discography), superior outcomes can be achieved with IDET.

Prolapsed discs that have failed to respond to conservative measures can be treated by a variety of intra- and extradiscal measures. Intradiscal treatment includes chemonucleolysis, percutaneous nucleotomy, and laser nucleotomy. All involve instrumentation of the nucleus pulposus and its removal by chemical dissolution, suction, or heat.

Chemonucleolysis helps in reducing turgidity in the nucleus and decreasing pressure on the nerve root. Significant improvement of outcome and reduction in recurrence rate has been demonstrated with an addition of 1000U of an intradiscal chymopapain following transforaminal endoscopic discectomy. Percutaneous laser disc decompression has made vaporization of a small area of the nucleus pulposus possible.

An alternative means of percutaneous disc excision is automated percutaneous lumbar discectomy. Dynamic stabilization system is useful to prevent progression of initial lumbar degenerative disc disease after nucleotomy for symptomatic prolapsed disc. According to NICE guidance (2006), the potential candidates for disc decompression using coblation are patients with contained disc leading to back and leg pain. Percutaneous endoscopic transforaminal lumbar discectomy (PELD) are also being performed for the herniated discs and forminoplastic PLED is considered to be an efficacious treatment option for soft migrated disc herniation.

Percutaneous facet joint injection

Facet joint arthritis is easily seen on axial CT or MRI sections. The appearances mimic changes of osteoarthritis elsewhere, with joint-space irregularity, osteophytes, and subarticular sclerosis. It is frequently identified in the asymptomatic population. There are no firm clinical signs confirming the facet as the source of the patient's symptoms. Injection of local anaesthetic and steroid into the facet has been used as both a diagnostic test and a therapeutic measure (Figure 3.19.16). There is moderate evidence of long- and short-term relief of lumbar facet joint pain by use of an intra-articular facet joint injection, medial nerve blockade, and neurotomy or rhizolyis. Occasionally, small synovial cysts can be identified arising from the facet joint. These can be intra- or extraspinal. Intraspinal lesions may present with neural compression (Figure 3.19.17). Imaging-guided cyst aspiration can be performed under fluoroscopic, CT, and MRI guidance. An interlaminar approach under fluoroscopic guidance has been used to puncture an intraspinal zygoapophyseal cyst to alleviate the radicular symptoms.

Each facet receives dual innervations from the median branches above and below. Median branch blockade is an alternative to facet blockade provided that both branches are injected. The target point is the elbow between the transverse and the superior articular process. Functional status improvement was noted in 82% of the patients with local anaesthetic nerve root block of the lumbar facet joint irrespective of steroid use. Rhizolysis (radiofrequency neurotomy) is similar to medial branch blockade but achieves more long-lasting results. Like IDET, this treatment is not permanent. If a satisfactory response to intra-articular facet injection is achieved,

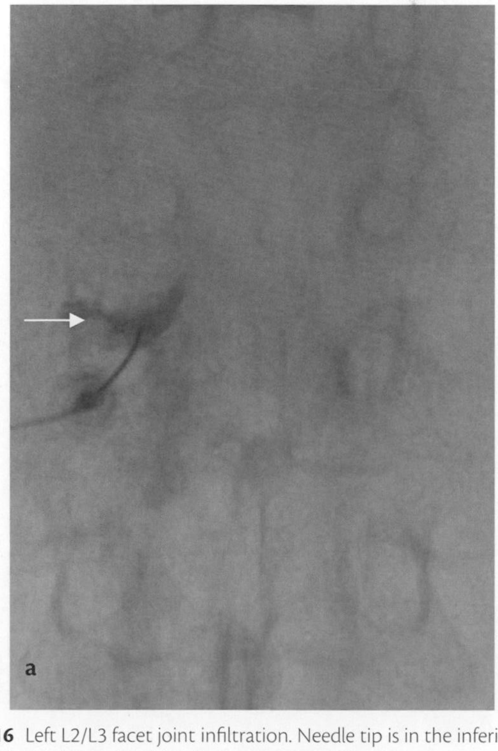

Fig. 3.19.16 Left L2/L3 facet joint infiltration. Needle tip is in the inferior recess of the facet joint and is outlined by the contrast (arrow).

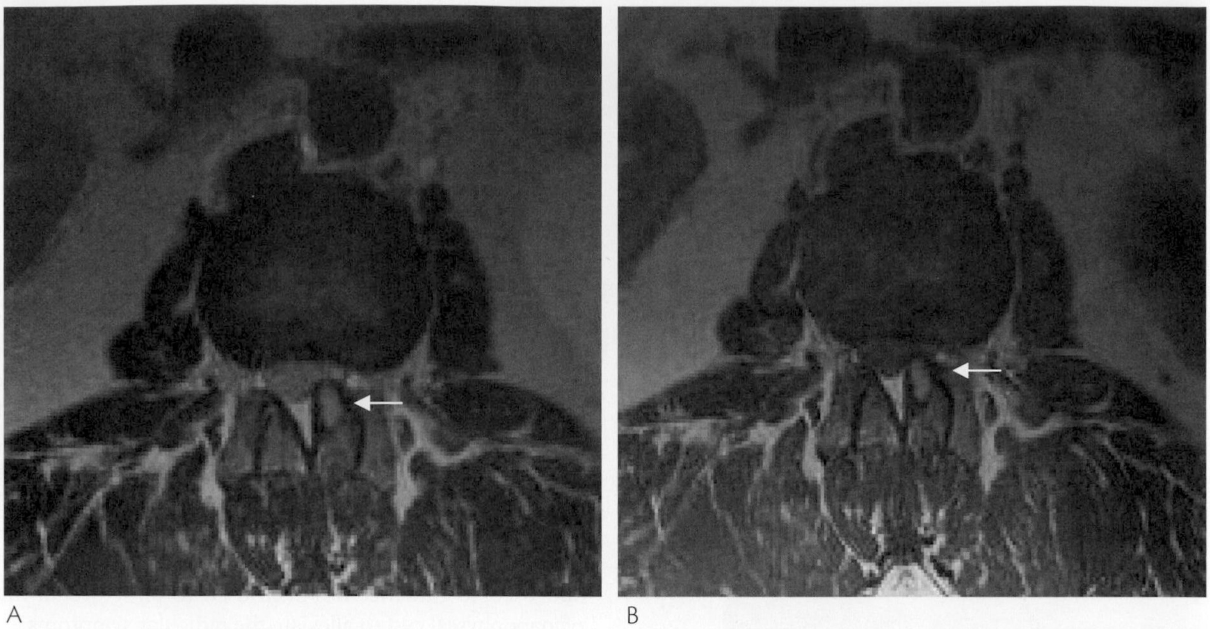

Fig. 3.19.17 Left L3/L4 intraspinal facet joint cyst (arrows). T2W (A) and T1W (B) axial MRIs show bright signal in the facet joint cyst suggesting presence of internal haemorrhage.

more long-term pain relief is gained by medial nerve neurotomy by radiofrequency ablation or cryoneurolysis.

Selective nerve root blockade

Multilevel disc degeneration and multiple root symptoms are common in older age groups. Images obtained in the recumbent position may underestimate the presence or degree of root impingement. Selective root blockade provides a means whereby an individual root can be anaesthetized and the subsequent effect on symptoms determined (Figure 3.19.18).

Vertebroplasty/kyphoplasty

Percutaneous vertebroplasty involves the injection of cement into a collapsed vertebral body, mainly for pain relief. Patient selection for both procedures should be performed with a multidisciplinary approach including spinal surgeon and radiologist. The principal

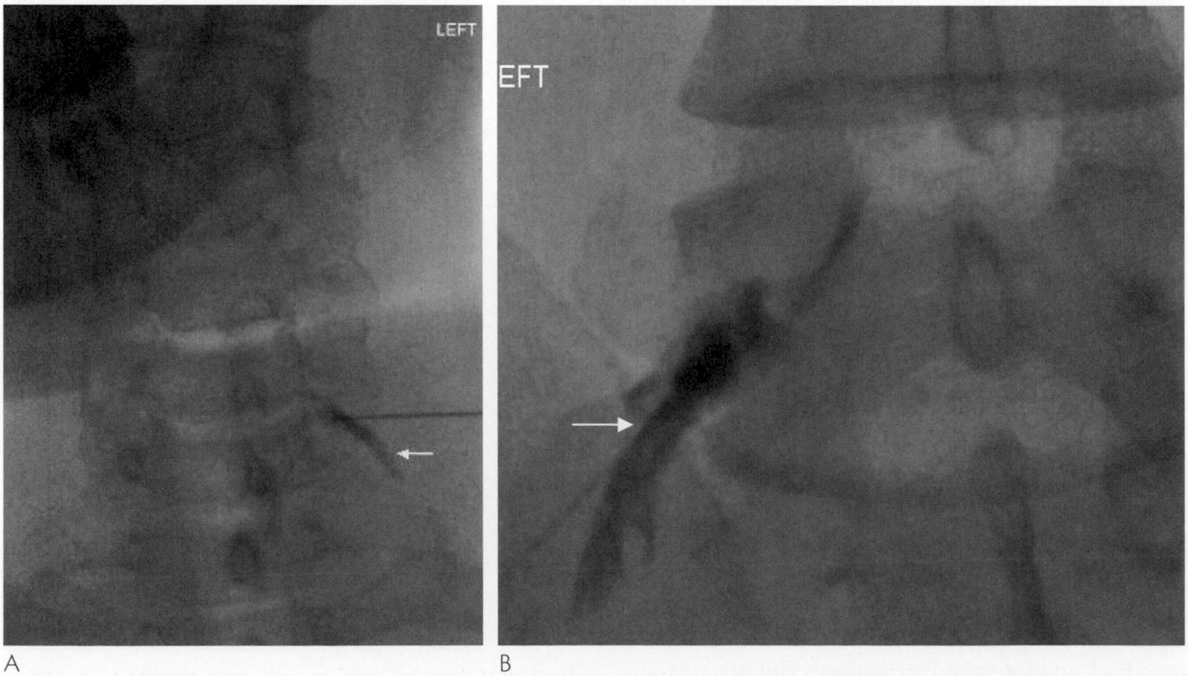

Fig. 3.19.18 A) Cervical root block. B) Lumbar root block. The contrast outlines the root sheath. Nerves are seen as a filling defect (arrows).

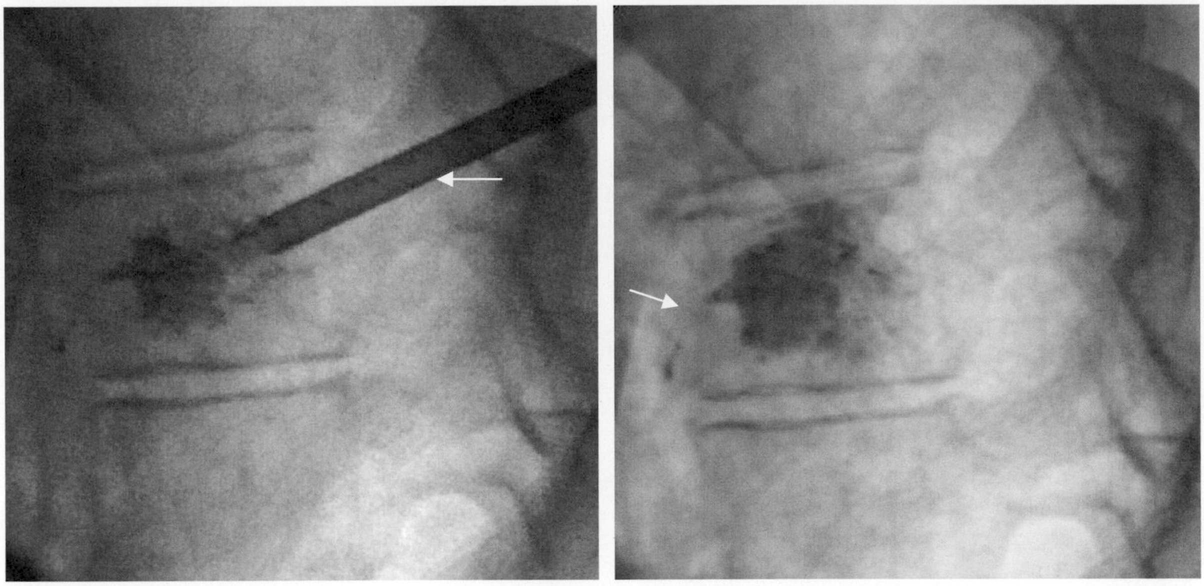

Fig. 3.19.19 A) Lateral fluoroscopic view demonstrates 11G vertebroplasty cannula (arrow) with cement filling the D12 vertebral body. B) Shows an excellent filling of the vertebral body and minor extravasation into the prevertebral vein (arrow).

indication is painful osteoporotic collapse. Indications also include malignant collapse and expansive intravertebral haemangioma. Vertebroplasty can be considered in patients with intractable pain due to vertebral fractures. It is contraindicated in coagulopathy. VERTOS and INVEST are two current multicentre RCTs that have yet to confirm a more favourable outcome with percutaneous vertebroplasty than conservative treatment.

The technique involves the injection of polymethylmethacrylate (PMMA) into collapsed vertebral bodies. The vertebral body is cannulated either by a direct posterolateral approach or via the transpedicular route. Once needles are positioned, cement is injected under pressure to support the vertebral body. Complications include extravasation of cement, which may lead to nerve or thecal compression (Figure 3.19.19).

A variation on this procedure is balloon kyphoplasty. This procedure is used to correct an angular deformity resulting from vertebral collapse. Following vertebral cannulation, a Teflon balloon is dilated under pressure within the vertebral body. Once the deformity has been corrected, the balloon is deflated and removed and the cavity is filled with cement.

Out of the two percutaneous vertebral augmentation techniques, vertebroplasty offers comparable pain relief but is safer as often only a unilateral approach is utilized, with fewer requirements of PMMA and without risk of adjacent level fracture.

Further reading

Modic, M.T. and Ross, J.S. (2007). Lumbar degenerative disc disease. *Radiology*, **245**, 43–61.

Pfirrmann, C.W., Metzdorf, A., Zanetti, M., Hodler, J., and Boos, N. (2001). Magnetic resonance classification of lumbar intervertebral disc degeneration. *Spine*, **26**, 1873–8.

Milette, P.C. (2000). Classification, diagnostic imaging, and imaging characterization of a lumbar herniated disc. *Radiologic Clinics of North America*, **38**, 1267–92.

Manchikanti, L., Singh, V., Falco, F.J., Cash, K.A., and Pampati, V. (2008). Lumbar facet joint nerve blocks in managing chronic facet joint pain: one-year follow-up of a randomized, double-blind controlled trial: Clinical Trial NCT00355914. *Pain Physician*, **11**, 121–32.

Uetani, M., Hashmi, R., and Hayashi, K. (2004). Malignant and benign compression fractures: differentiation and diagnostic pitfalls on MRI. *Clinical Radiology*, **59**, 124–31.

SECTION 4

The Shoulder

4.1

The clinical evaluation of the shoulder

Tim D. Bunker

Summary points

- History: onset event, radiation, exacerbation, night pain, functional deficit
- Examination: active and passive movement, impingement signs, instability tests
- Investigation: x-rays, ultrasound, CT and MR.

Clinical assessment

Diagnosis depends upon three lines of enquiry, all of which should concur for the case to be proven. The first line of enquiry is the history. Using questions and answers we develop a short list of two or three possible pathologies. This is then subject to rigorous analysis against known facts. Occasionally the inquisition will trigger a red flag (the crescendo pain of calcific tendinitis), or it leads into an area where mistakes in diagnosis can lead to tragic events (the missed secondary tumour in the humeral metaphysis). However, we must remember that patients are human, they forget, dissemble, and sometimes lie. So ask the same question in two different ways (for instance, 'have you had any illnesses?' followed by 'what tablets are you on?') and if the answers don't match you discard them or dig deeper.

The second line of enquiry is to examine the shoulder in a logical stepwise manner. But remember:

- That examination techniques may be *75% accurate*, or less
- Tests can *be confounded* (for instance, stiffness renders the impingement tests null and void)
- Some conditions can have a very similar examination profile to others, *they mimic* the other condition.

Fortunately pathology from the shoulder tends to fall into one of four areas: the stiff shoulder, the wobbly shoulder, pain on reach (the painful arc), and the remnants. Examination will at least get you into one of these four areas, and the first three have a specific forensic investigation that will prove the case.

So we come to the third line of investigation, and the most powerful, the forensics. In our case, radiology, ultrasound, magnetic resonance imaging (MRI), and arthroscopy. Rarely blood tests will be required. Stiff shoulders merit a radiograph; wobbly shoulders merit examination under anaesthetic and arthroscopy; and pain on reach merits an ultrasound. Forensics trumps the history and the examination.

Our problem is that we do not have unlimited time in outpatients. For this reason the hip surgeon goes to the forensics first, the radiograph of the hip, and then asks the patient about their symptoms. The shoulder surgeon has been hampered by the lack of forensics, but portable ultrasound can be performed rapidly in the clinic, and can give a firm diagnosis on those with pain on reach, and radiographs will sort out the stiff shoulders. Finally shoulder arthroscopy has come of age so that most shoulder conditions cannot only be identified but can also be treated arthroscopically.

Age is key to shoulder pathology. A useful aphorism is that 'all patients below the age of 40 have instability until proven otherwise', for instability is a condition of teens to thirties. Rotator cuff disease is a degenerative disease that starts to give pain on reach in the forties, tears of the cuff in the late fifties to sixties, and cuff arthropathy in the eighties (thus the aphorism 'Grey hair equals cuff tear). The Japanese call contracture (frozen shoulder) '50-year-old shoulder' for a reason, and if the letter states that the patient is 70 and has had a hip replacement then it is more likely that they have arthritis in the shoulder rather than a contracted (frozen) shoulder.

Observation

Dr Watson was a poor doctor for Holmes had to admonish him: 'Observe my dear Watson, don't just look!' Facts can be deduced as the patient enters the room, before a word is said or a hand shaken. Do they look biologically the same age as their chronology, younger or older? How are they dressed, for patients with stiffness or loss of reach can't pull sweaters over their heads, so will have clothes that button or zip up? How are they holding the shoulder? How protective are they? Is their neck held stiffly or moving normally? Remember the aphorism 'Grey hair equals cuff tear'. With increasing experience you may note subtle signs such as the oven burns from syringomyelia, the bossed clavicles of glenoid dysplasia, or the absent facial expression of the patient with fascioscapulohumeral dystrophy.

Introduce yourself whilst cautiously shaking their hand, and at the same time note whether they have the shoulder shrug of the patient with a massive cuff tear, the stiff shoulder of arthritis, Dupuytren's palmar contracture so often associated with contracted (frozen) shoulder, the engulfing hand of acromegaly, the rheumatoid hand of the rheumatoid shoulder, a weak grip, a strong grip, a tentative protective grip, a stiff shoulder, or a mobile shoulder.

The history

The problem with shoulders is that a history of true shoulder pain (pain felt over deltoid insertion), that has come on insidiously, is made worse by shoulder movement, that radiates down the radial border of the forearm, and that awakens the patient at night could come from *virtually any patient with any disorder* of the shoulder. Such a history would fit with a rotator cuff problem, a contracture (frozen shoulder), a calcific deposit, arthritis, or even instability. Even worse, since the majority of these problems are soft tissue problems, they won't show up on a radiograph. Quel horreur, what can we do? The answer is that the shoulder surgeon relies more upon the objective physical signs and provocative tests of the examination, and these guide him to the correct investigation. The history should not be dismissed, but it can be performed rapidly. As Cyriax said 'with the shoulder the history matters little; it is the examination that counts'.

Referred pain

The first purpose of the interview is to ascertain whether the pain is from the shoulder *or referred from another source.* True shoulder pain originates from the shoulder and radiates to the muscles of the arm, around the insertion of deltoid. Indeed many patients will say, 'It's not my shoulder doctor, it's my arm', and will vigorously rub the deltoid insertion when asked to show where the pain is. When severe, the pain will radiate down the radial border of the forearm to the wrist, occasionally to the thenar eminence. The pain may radiate into the supraspinatus fossa, beneath trapezius, but pain more central to this, or along the medial border of the scapula is far more likely to be referred from the neck. Shoulder pain is made worse by shoulder movement.

Alarm bells should ring in patients whose pain radiates into the hand, for this is the pattern of referred pain from the C6 and C7 nerve roots. Similarly, beware of the patient whose pain radiates to the ulnar side of the forearm, the axilla or the chest, for this is the radiation from the thoracic outlet, the lower trunks of the brachial plexus (C8, T1), or the C8 and T1 roots. In patients with such radiation, always suspect a neurological cause for their pain and perform a careful neurological examination.

Referred pain from the viscera (gall bladder to right shoulder and myocardium to left shoulder) is mentioned in every textbook, but search as I may I have yet to see such a case in a shoulder clinic, despite being responsible for the secondary care of 400 000 patients and the tertiary care of 3 million people for the last two decades.

Pain coming from the acromioclavicular joint and the sternoclavicular joints are better localized than glenohumeral joint pain. Patients will point to the acromioclavicular joint when that is the cause. Pain from the sternoclavicular joint is well localized and radiates out along the subcutaneous border of the clavicle.

True shoulder pain

Enquiries should be made into the generic qualities of the pain: the onset event, duration, severity, radiation, exacerbating features, and what treatments have been attempted so far and to what effect? But lots of pathologies share the same features of pain in the shoulder, so it is only really worth seeking those factors that are specific to certain pathologies. The nature of pain is rarely discriminatory in the shoulder.

- *The onset event*: note the date of onset and calculate the duration. Is the condition acute or chronic? Often shoulder pain comes on insidiously, but if there was an initiating event this is an important clue. How much energy was involved in the event? Enough to tear a degenerate cuff? Enough to cause a transient dislocation? Enough to cause a fracture? There are some pathologies that have a distinct onset. Acute calcific tendinitis has a sudden onset with such severity of pain that the patient takes themselves to the emergency department in the middle of the night. The patient with neuralgic amyotrophy awakens with severe burning pain in the arm, followed by weakness in various muscles around the shoulder. The rotator cuff tear has a sudden severe pain followed by a window of relief lasting some hours (the lucid interval), then severe pain from that night onwards
- *Night pain* is a common feature of shoulder disorders. This may vary from difficulty settling, to occasional awakening, to awakening every night, to arising at four in the morning as further attempts at sleep are impossible to the final stage of being exiled to the spare room for keeping their partner awake all night. These latter stages should trigger alarm bells, a radiograph should always be taken to exclude a metastatic deposit in the humeral neck or a calcific deposit. Analgesic consumption is important, the amount of consumption and need for opiates. Night pain will not give you a specific diagnosis *but it will influence your priority to treat.* For instance, the patient with a contracted (frozen) shoulder who has no night pain can be treated conservatively, but if the patient arises at four every morning as further sleep is impossible, consideration should be given to performing an arthroscopic capsular release
- *Pain on reach*: a functioning rotator cuff is essential to reach. Pain and weakness on reaching forward, upward, outward, or backward, in a mobile shoulder, is specific to rotator cuff disease. This pain is made worse with load such as lifting a kettle, or even a cup of tea, and the shoulder will fatigue with prolonged reach such as driving
- *Jerk pain*: a sudden minor wrench on the contracted capsule (frozen shoulder) brings disproportionate pain and tears to the eyes in contracted (frozen) shoulder. This is never mentioned in any textbook, but is a solid fact
- *Previous treatment*: previous steroid or local anaesthetic injection, administered to a specific site (cuff, acromioclavicular joint, or glenohumeral joint), may have alleviated their pain for a duration. This allows you to pinpoint the specific area of pathology.

The majority of patients will present with pain and can then be placed into one of three categories: stiff shoulders (arthritis and contracted (frozen) shoulder), wobbly shoulders (instability), and loss of reach (pinching, partial and full thickness tears of the rotator cuff), so we need two additional lines of questioning about stiffness and instability.

Stiffness

Stiffness limits function. Yet it is extraordinary how patients can adapt to stiffness in one shoulder. Neer showed how most activities can be performed as long as you have 150 degrees of flexion, 40 degrees of external rotation, and internal rotation to L2. The Stanmore functional triangle has been described as the ability to reach the mouth, the opposite axilla, and wipe the bottom. Less movement than this severely compromises the ability to maintain independent living. There are five main causes of stiffness.

1) The contracted (frozen shoulder). A slow onset of pain felt near the insertion of deltoid, with inability to sleep on the affected side, painful and restricted elevation and external rotation, with a normal radiographic appearance
2) Arthritis of the shoulder. A slow onset of true shoulder pain, a continuous background toothachy pain with intermittent exacerbations, a feeling of sticking, squeaking, or grinding, global stiffness, and radiographs showing arthritis. Often accompanied by a hip replacement!
3) Scarring following fracture. Global stiffness and pain with a fracture event and a radiograph demonstrating the fracture and its sequela
4) Stiffness associated with the late stages of a massive cuff tear. The patient, aged over 40 years, injures the shoulder, goes to the emergency department and has a radiograph that is normal, and is told that they have no bony injury. The pain continues such that they go to physiotherapy and have non-specific treatment without a diagnosis for some months until they are told that nothing can be done. Despite loss of power on elevation, loss of power into external rotation, and infraspinatus wasting, several more months pass by. The shoulder stiffens, particularly into internal rotation due to contracture of the posterior capsule. Carers are concerned and they have a second radiograph and are once more told that there is nothing wrong (with the radiograph). Months pass until eventually the patient sees a shoulder surgeon and an ultrasound in his clinic demonstrates a massive cuff tear. It is too late now to repair it! How many times must we hear this story?
5) Locked posterior dislocation. There is a traumatic event. A single anteroposterior radiograph is taken that demonstrates the light-bulb sign of locked posterior dislocation, but unfortunately no axillary radiograph is taken and the inexperienced emergency doctor fails to recognize the fact that the shoulder is dislocated. The shoulder is locked in marked internal rotation. The head is prominent posteriorly. This is a red flag situation. Those who have neglected to make the diagnosis thus far will be sued.

You, of course, will take the axillary radiograph and make the diagnosis.

As you can see all you need to make the accurate diagnosis in stiffness is a radiograph, *in two planes, and to interpret it correctly.*

Instability

At last we come to an area where the history is discriminatory. If the patient says their shoulder came out, it came out. This history can be pursued vigorously. Describe the first dislocation, how and when? Was this traumatic or atraumatic? Was it transient or locked out? Did it go back spontaneously, with a little help from bystanders, at hospital, under sedation, or under general anaesthetic? Was it secure afterwards, were they protective, did it redislocate, how, when, how many times, how was it then put back in?

Strangely, patients have little concept of the direction of dislocation, to be honest it is so painful they don't care, but if radiographs were taken with it dislocated this is helpful, as is the presence of a Hill–Sachs or reversed Hill–Sachs lesion at the time of the consultation.

Of course there is a group of patients with symptomatic subluxation, and atraumatic transient dislocation, for whom diagnosis can be difficult. Always suspect this as a cause of shoulder pain in anyone less than 40 years of age.

Some patients will helpfully show you they can dislocate the shoulder. Beware; this is a red flag situation. They may just have marked joint laxity with posterior positional dislocation, in which case they gently sublux on raising the internally rotated adducted shoulder and then get a clunk of relocation as the shoulder is abducted. But if they dislocate with the elbow at the side and a huge grin on the face, beware—this is a Polar III, muscle-induced dislocation that will be resistant to any surgical adventure. The history and examination for muscle patterning and Polar III instability is complex and will be described in detail in Chapter 4.7.

Neurological and other conditions

Finally, one of the joys of being a shoulder specialist is that patients will turn up outside the three boxes of stiff shoulders, wobbly shoulders, and loss of reach. These are the remnants, but no less important for being so. These cases are the neurological conditions: the winging scapulae, thoracic outlet syndromes, neuralgic amyotrophy, and a variety of nerve palsies. Then the curios: the Sprengel's shoulder, obstetric plexus palsies, glenoid dysplasias, muscular dystrophies, as well as disorders of the acromioclavicular and sternoclavicular joints. Finally come the nasties, for tumours do occur around the shoulder, primary tumours being rare, but the proximal humerus is a common site for secondary tumours. Thus the patient may present with weakness, loss of function, swelling, wasting, noises, and winging.

Weakness

Weakness can only come from three things: rupture of a tendon (common), muscle weakness (myopathy, extremely rare), or failure of motor enervation (nerve palsy, rare).

Weakness from tendon rupture

Weakness from a rotator cuff tear is common. The patient complains of inability to reach and will often say that they have to assist the arm, by holding the forearm with the opposite unaffected hand. Commonly the patient will have to assist to brush the hair, to wash, to brush the teeth, and to reach forwards. They will adapt and use tricks such as holding the elbow to the side whilst lifting, and will lean right forwards almost touching the floor to dress and undress. Wasting will be apparent. Usually the weakness is accompanied by pain.

The isolated rupture of long head of biceps occurs with a sudden painful event, is associated with bruising down the course of biceps (rotator cuff tears rarely bruise), and the patient notices a change in shape of biceps to the 'Popeye muscle'. This is painful when it occurs, but the pain settles within a few days, so the patient may present with weakness of elbow flexion and supination (using a screwdriver), although this is uncommon because the short head of biceps is intact. Weakness is more commonly seen in the rarer rupture of the distal tendon of insertion into the radial tuberosity.

Isolated ruptures of pectoralis major are subtler. There is a painful event in a 20-year-old man, who is a weightlifter or frequent gym user, who may or may not be on 'health food supplements' that may or may not contain nandrolone or some other androgenic steroid. There is a change of shape of the anterior axillary fold accompanied by bruising. There is weakness of pectoralis major.

Weakness from nerve palsy

Axillary nerve palsy is rare. It occurs after anteroinferior and inferior dislocations of the shoulder. There is decreased sensibility of the badge area of skin and weakness and wasting of deltoid. Muscle fasciculation may be seen. The injury is often a neurapraxia, but the nerve can be completely ruptured and require grafting.

Suprascapular nerve palsy is usually insidious in onset, presenting as a severe burning pain over the upper scapula accompanied by rapid wasting of infraspinatus (and supraspinatus although that is less obvious as it is covered by the healthy trapezius). It mimics cuff tear but the wasting is much more severe than seen with rotator cuff tears and has a more rapid onset. There is weakness and fatigue on reach.

Injuries to the long thoracic nerve and to the spinal accessory nerve lead to loss of scapula control and winging. Patients often complain that the 'shoulder blade sticks out'. It may press awkwardly against the seatback when seated on a chair. Partners and family members note the cosmetic asymmetry of the shoulder blade. There is a loss of the shoulder fulcrum and lifting is weak and limited.

Weakness from muscle dystrophy

Fascioscapulohumeral dystrophy (FSHD) is the rarest of the causes of shoulder weakness. Patients usually present from late teens through to late twenties with shoulder girdle weakness particularly in abduction and flexion. The facial muscles are weak leading to a loss of facial expression, and that weird symptom, inability to whistle! Strangely the deltoid muscle is often preserved leading to a 'Superman' appearance. The key to diagnosis lies in the affected chromosome 4q35.

Swelling and deformity

Occasionally patients complain of swelling. A swollen sternoclavicular joint is often noted by a perimenopausal female looking in the mirror. Swelling of the medial clavicle can occur in SAPHO (synovitis, acne, pustulosis, hyperostosis, and osteitis) syndrome or Garre's sclerosing osteomyelitis. The patient may notice a swelling over the acromioclavicular joint with the 'Geyser' sign where fluid herniates out of the top of the joint from a communication with a massive cuff tear. The massive bursal fluid swelling of cuff tear arthropathy disturbs the patient with this condition. Remember that tumours both benign and malignant occur around the shoulder.

Deformity may be a presenting complaint, usually in children and adolescents. The deformity of congenital pseudarthrosis of the clavicle, the bossed clavicle of primary glenoid dysplasia, the elevated scapula of Sprengel's shoulder, the 'waiter's tip position' of Erb's palsy. The absent pectorals of Poland's anomaly and the dimples of posterior positional dislocation are all infrequent findings in the shoulder clinic.

Examination

The examination is more revealing than the history. Most pathology will fall into one of three boxes: the stiff shoulder, the wobbly shoulder, and pain on reach (the cuff). Examination should be tailored to the pathology suggested by the history. For instance, if the history points towards a wobbly shoulder then the time available to you should be used for instability tests, rather than the more esoteric eponymous tests of the rotator cuff. In the real world time is limited.

A plethora of eponymous clinical signs have sprung up over the last two decades. However, few have weathered the tests of specificity and sensitivity to gain mandatory use in the examination. Beware that clinical signs can be confounded, particularly by stiffness. Thus the belly press sign, an enormously important sign of subscapularis dysfunction, can be confounded by stiffness into internal rotation, producing a false positive belly press sign. Inspection and palpation are common to all stems, but should not take long.

Inspection

Stand back and look at the profile of both shoulder girdles from the front. Is there asymmetry? Is one shoulder lower than the other? Is the posture slouched (common with thoracic outlet problems), are the scapulae protracted (gunslingers posture)? Is there asymmetry of deltoid bulk that is more pronounced than dominance should allow? Look from the side. Is the biceps' shape altered? Look from the back. Is there wasting of infraspinatus (rotator cuff tear or suprascapular nerve entrapment)? Is there any winging? Pay attention to old surgical scars. Are the scars stretched as occurs with instability, or are there any striaie on the skin?

Pay careful attention to the humeral head. Is it elevated or more prominent than it should be, for this will suggest a tear of the cuff? If, like Sherlock Holmes, you are observing rather than just looking, inspection will take a matter of seconds.

Palpation

The sternoclavicular and acromioclavicular joints are subcutaneous, and if the history has suggested that they are culpable, then they are easy to palpate. However, the glenohumeral joint line cannot be reached because the acromion covers the posterosuperior aspect, the coracoacromial ligament covers the anterosuperior aspect, and the conjoined tendon covers the anterior joint line. This only leaves the posterior joint line that lies beneath both deltoid and infraspinatus rendering palpation of the joint line impractical. Yet the greater tuberosity can be palpated easily. Since this is the site of most cuff pathology you may detect tenderness and even a 'sulcus and eminence' of the tear itself. Unless there is a lump or bump don't spend too much time palpating. But do place a hand on the shoulder as you move it for soft crepitus and catching may be felt from the cuff, squeaking from an arthritic joint surface, or even a clunk of subluxation or relocation in unstable shoulders.

Examination for stiffness

The examination for stiffness precedes all else, for if the joint is stiff no further examination is required—the patient needs a radiograph of the shoulder. Stiffness confounds the tests of rotator cuff dysfunction and so must precede them. Finally if the opposite of stiffness, excessive motion, is discovered then more attention must be placed on instability testing.

Active movement

Ask the patient to move the shoulder himself or herself—this is active motion. Using a single finger to guide and nudge the patient's arm into flexion will save you a great deal of time with verbal instruction. Patients do not understand instructions such as 'flex or abduct your shoulder'. Place your other hand over the shoulder as the patient moves so that you will detect the rhythm between scapulothoracic and glenohumeral motion, detect translation of the humeral head, and finally detect crepitus, creaking and clunking. *This means you have to examine one shoulder at a time, starting obviously with the normal side.*

See if there is a restriction in active movement (that is, the range that the patient can comfortably initiate and sustain), and then the passive movement (the limit to which you can move the shoulder when pain is abolished). Four movements will be assessed, forward elevation, external rotation, internal rotation, and cross body adduction. By convention zero degrees is the anatomical position with the arm to the side and the antecubital fossa pointing forwards.

Note the level at which active movement ceases. Now rather than cause the patient increasing pain by forcing the shoulder passively further up, ask the patient to stoop forward *(the bow test of Kolbel)* for this often eases their pain and allows you to assess their passive range without hurting them (Figure 4.1.1). With the arm supported by you in this position of maximum elevation, ask them to stand, and finally now ask them to lower the arm, whilst you pay particular attention to how the scapula moves. You will see, in patients with rotator cuff disease, that they lock the glenohumeral joint during descent through their painful arc, leading to pseudo-winging.

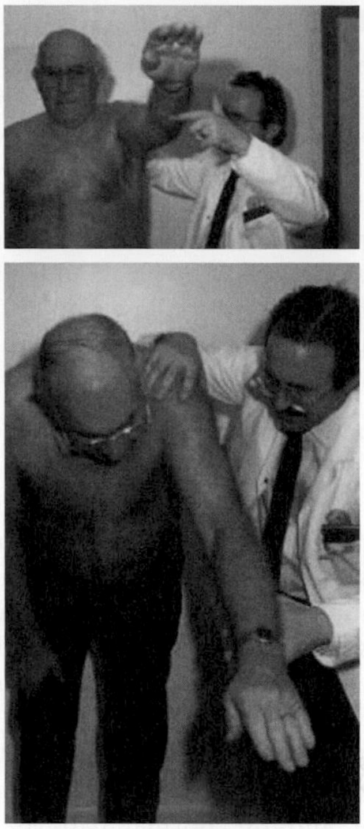

Fig. 4.1.1 Ask the patient to stoop forward (the bow test of Kolbel) for this often eases their pain and allows you to assess their passive range without hurting them.

Passive movement

If despite stooping the patient forward the shoulder will not move further, then we have a block to passive motion, true stiffness. Always note the quality of the end point of this movement. A leathery block to movement suggests a contracture. A firm bony end point is caused by osteophyte impingement in arthritis. An open end point—in other words, you know that the joint will move further but you dare not move it any more because of inordinate pain—is a red flag, it means either that there is a tumour or that the patient is exaggerating their symptoms.

Assess rotation both actively and passively. Beware for the shoulder is designed to position the hand accurately in space. Patients with little external rotation will cheat and abduct the arm in order to get the hand into position. (Remember that in every good detective story a few false clues are thrown in to see how clever you really are.) Keep the patient's elbow locked to the side when testing external rotation (Figure 4.1.2). Patients with rotator cuff disease have near normal external rotation, but painful restriction of internal rotation. Patients with frozen shoulder and arthritis have passive restriction of both external rotation and internal rotation. Internal rotation is measured by the vertebral level at which the thumb rests at maximum internal rotation reach. If the patient has marked restriction of elbow flexion (for instance, in rheumatoid disease) then vertebral level is not an accurate method of measurement.

If significant passive stiffness is discovered then no further examination is required. A radiograph is mandatory and this will be normal in contracture and abnormal in arthritis, massive end-stage cuff tear, and locked posterior dislocation. Remember that stiffness may nullify further testing by producing false positive results.

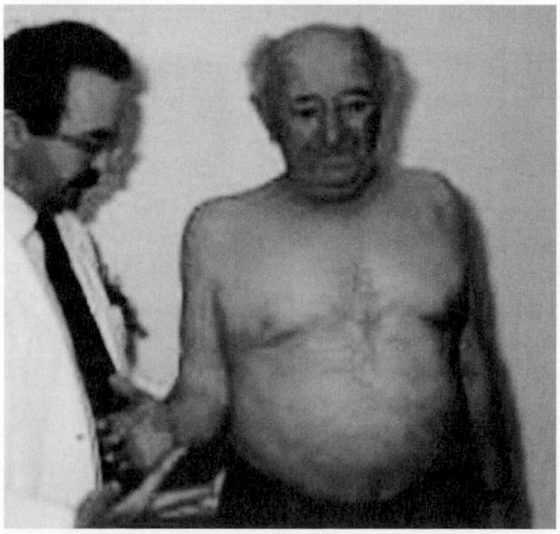

Fig. 4.1.2 Keep the patient's elbow locked to the side when testing external rotation.

Examination of the rotator cuff

To understand the clinical signs associated with rotator cuff disease you must first understand the anatomy and pathology of the rotator cuff. Most important is Professor Olivier Gagey's concept of the fibrous skeleton of the cuff. The supraspinatus tendon comes from the centre of its muscle belly and migrates to the anterior edge of the tendon footprint of insertion. This central oblique tendon is extremely strong and acts as a 'firebreak' to tears. The majority of tears start just behind this tendon insertion leading to the typical posterosuperior cuff tear. This concept is expanded in Chapters 4.2 and 4.3.

The posterior superior cuff

Neer's sign

This is the classic painful arc (Figure 4.1.3). Movement into the first 70 degrees of flexion is easy and pain free, but then as the footprint of the supraspinatus passes under the acromion, from 70–120 degrees, there is impingement between the surfaces and pain, and motion slows. As the footprint clears the under surface of the acromion, from 120 degrees to top pain eases and motion speeds up once more (Table 4.1.1).

Neer's test is to inject some local anaesthetic into the bursa, bathing the bursal side of the footprint of cuff insertion. This abolishes the impingement and the normal pattern of movement is restored.

Hawkins's sign

The arm is elevated in the scapula plane to 90 degrees. Now the elbow is flexed to a right angle and the arm is internally, and then externally rotated (Figure 4.1.4). Pain is seen to occur on internal rotation as the footprint of supraspinatus impinges against the anterior acromion. The sensitivity and specificity for Hawkins sign is 75%. It is one of the most useful tests of the posterosuperior cuff. Beware that passive limitation of internal rotation nullifies this test.

Table 4.1.1 Eponymous tests for the rotator cuff

Sign	Eponym	Tests
Painful arc	Neer	Supraspinatus
Impingement	Hawkins	Supraspinatus
Cuff tear	Jobe	Supraspinatus
ER lag sign	Hertel	Supraspinatus
ER lag	Hornblower	Supraspinatus
Belly press	Napoleon	Subscapularis
Lift off	Gerber	Subscapularis
IR lag sign	Hertel	Subscapularis
Bear hug	DeBeer	Subscapularis
SLAP	O'Brien	Biceps/SLAP
Thrower's	O'Brien	Biceps/subluxation
Resisted supination	Lafosse	Biceps wear
Shape	Popeye	Biceps rupture

ER, external rotation; IR, internal rotation; SLAP, superior labrum anteroposterior.

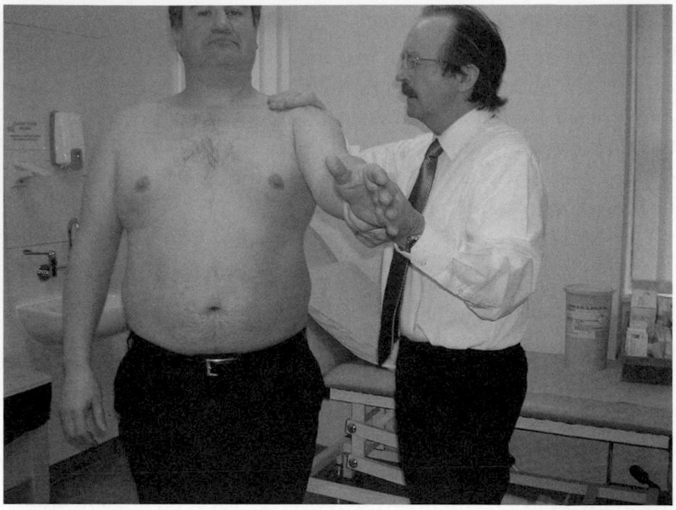

Fig. 4.1.3 Neer's sign. The first 70° of movement are normal and rapid. Above 70° the patient winces, slows down, and becomes protective.

Jobe's sign

The arm is brought up in the scapula plane with the elbow extended and the arm fully internally rotated such that the thumb points to the ground (the Australians call this the 'empty tinny test' for it is the position in which you test that your can of beer is finally empty) (Figure 4.1.5). The patient is asked to hold this position against resistance from the examiner. If there is damage to the supraspinatus insertion then pain will register with the patient. If there is a tear of supraspinatus the arm will be weak. The accuracy of Jobe's sign is 58%. It is another good test.

If either Neer's, Hawkins's or Jobe's signs are positive then you should move straight to the ultrasound examination (Figure 4.1.6). The ultrasound will show you whether there is a tear, give you its exact position, and a measure of its dimension, it is worth a thousand eponymous tests. However, there are many other tests of the posterosuperior cuff and it is pertinent that you have heard of them.

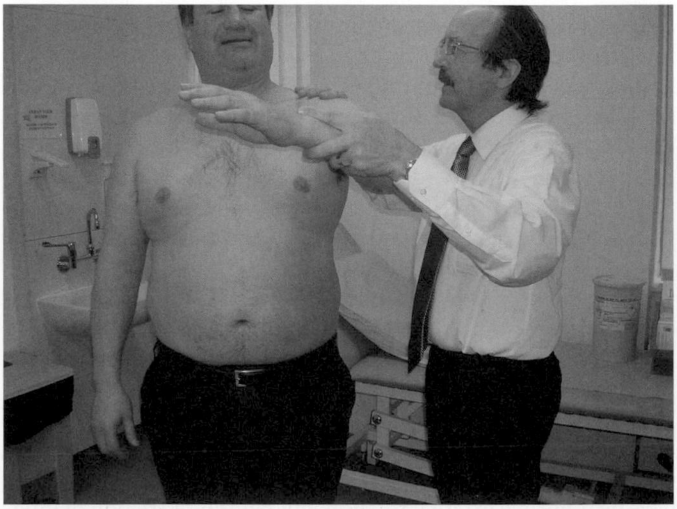

Fig. 4.1.4 Hawkins's sign. The arm is elevated in the scapula plane to 90 degrees. Now the elbow is flexed to a right angle and the arm is internally and then externally rotated.

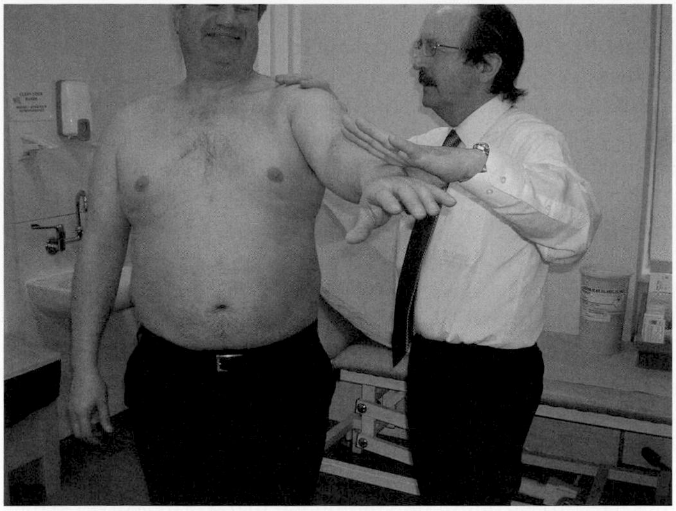

Fig. 4.1.5 Jobe's sign. The arm is brought up in the scapula plane with the elbow extended and the arm fully internally rotated such that the thumb points to the ground. (The Australians call this the 'empty tinny test' for it is the position in which you test that your can of beer is finally empty.) The patient is asked to hold this position against resistance from the examiner.

Lag signs

These depend on weakness of a segment of the cuff. They are the modern equivalent of the '*drop arm sign*'. The drop arm sign was a particularly barbaric way of looking at a patient with a massive supraspinatus tear. The examiner elevated the arm to 120 degrees in the full knowledge that, without a functioning cuff, the patient will find it impossible to maintain this position. The examiner then let go and the arm dropped to the side! Patients were not as amused by this test as their examiners!

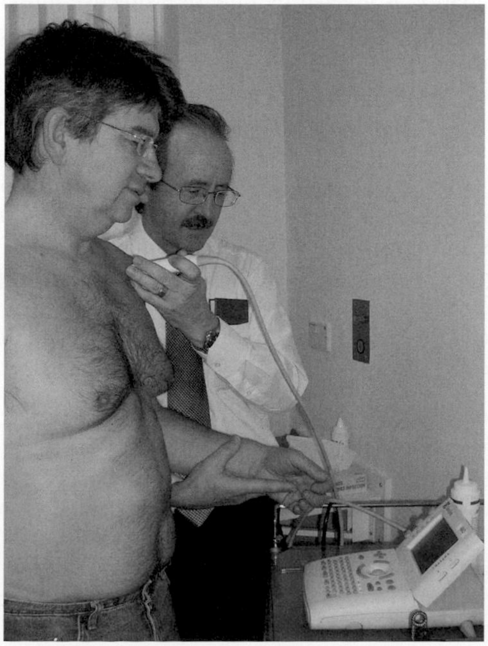

Fig. 4.1.6 Point-of-care ultrasound can be performed by the surgeon in the clinic.

The external rotation lag sign

This demonstrates that there is a significant tear in supraspinatus. Like the drop arm sign this depends on placing the arm into a position that needs a strong supraspinatus and then letting go. The examiner takes the affected elbow and supports the weight of the upper arm with the shoulder in 90 degrees of scapular elevation. Now, using their other arm, the examiner externally rotates the forearm into full external rotation. Maintaining this position against gravity depends upon an intact supraspinatus. Now the examiner lets go of the forearm. If the cuff is intact this position can be maintained by the patient, but if the cuff is torn then the forearm will drop by about 30 degrees, the external rotation lag. In real life there are problems with the test. The examiner must understand exactly what they are doing, as must the patient. Pain may interfere with the test. Stiffness will render it null and void. There is difficulty between assessing how much movement is recoil and how much is lag. It is poorly reproducible. It has a specificity of 63% and a sensitivity of 80%. It has been superseded by portable ultrasound.

Hornblower's sign

This is another lag sign. All military hornblowers must assume an identical position when blowing their horns. Otherwise they would look a mess! This position is with the hand at the lips and the elbow as high as it will go so that the arm, and forearm are parallel to the ground. This position can be maintained in the face of a torn rotator cuff. However, if the examiner now takes the hand, and fully externally rotates the forearm so that the forearm is now perpendicular to the ground we now have a position that can only be maintained with an intact cuff. Let go of the hand now and the forearm will drop, or lag, by 30 degrees. This test suffers from the same problems as the external rotation lag sign. It has been superseded by portable ultrasound.

The subscapularis

Tears of the anterosuperior cuff (subscapularis and biceps) are less common than those of the posterosuperior cuff. These tears start around the biceps pulley and the superior part of the insertion of subscapularis into the lesser tuberosity. Subscapularis has a multipennate tendon of insertion into the lesser tuberosity.

The belly press sign (Napoleon's sign)

This is the single most useful test of subscapularis function. The patient is asked to place the palm of the hand upon their abdomen. Now they are asked to keep the hand where it is and bring the elbow forward as far as it will go. If there is a complete tear of the subscapularis they will not be able to bring the elbow forwards. If they can pull the elbow forwards they are then asked to press the hand hard into the belly. If there is a partial tear of subscapularis they elbow will drop back (a lag sign) (Figure 4.1.7). Beware—if the shoulder is stiff a false belly press sign occurs, for instance, in patients with limited internal rotation from arthritis. Beware patients can cheat; in this case they flex the wrist pulling the elbow forwards, producing a false negative belly press sign. They must keep the wrist in a neutral position or the test is null and void. Finally, biceps problems can mimic subscapularis problems confounding the belly press sign.

The lift off test

This test is similar to the belly press sign, but is performed in more internal rotation. This means that the wrist must be placed on the

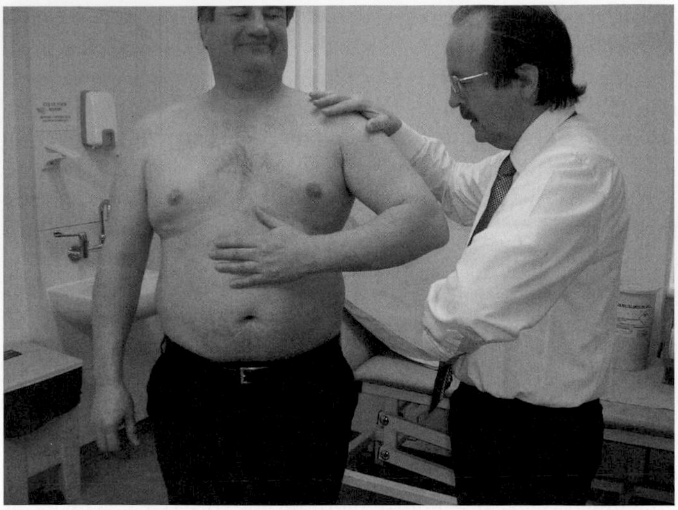

Fig. 4.1.7 The belly press sign (Napoleon's sign). This is the single most useful test of subscapularis function. The patient is asked to place the palm of the hand upon their abdomen. Now they are asked to keep the hand where it is and bring the elbow forward as far as it will go. If there is a complete tear of the subscapularis they will not be able to bring the elbow forwards. If they can pull the elbow forwards they are then asked to press the hand hard into the belly. If there is a partial tear of subscapularis they elbow will drop back (a lag sign).

small of the back, rather than on the abdomen. Now the patient is asked to actively increase the internal rotation by lifting the wrist away from the skin. The problem with this test is pain. Patients with cuff problems do not like placing the hand into internal rotation, and pain nullifies the test. Stiffness will also nullify the test.

Internal rotation lag sign

This is a modification of the lift off test. The arm is placed with the wrist on the small of the back. The examiner now takes the wrist and pulls it 5cm away from the skin. With an intact subscapularis, and no pain or stiffness, the patient should be able to maintain this position. However, if subscapularis is torn then the wrist will drop (lag) back onto the skin of the small of the back. Once again it is difficult to discriminate between recoil and lag, and has the same problems of pain and stiffness.

The biceps

There is not a good test for biceps! Biceps shape is important. All medical students know the 'Popeye sign' of a ruptured long head of biceps. However, you can have a complete intra-articular rupture of long head of biceps without a Popeye sign when the hypertrophied tendon jams in the sulcus, like a cork in a bottleneck. Between these two extremes the biceps can adopt subtle changes in shape.

Lafosse sign

This test is designed to isolate biceps by asking the patient to supinate the forearm against resistance. The examiner cradles the elbow with the shoulder held at about 40 degrees of scapular elevation. The examiner grips the patient's wrist and pronates the forearm, asking the patient to resist (supinate) this force.

O'Brien's test

This is designed to detect a SLAP (superior labrum anteroposterior) tear. It is performed similarly to the Jobe test, but with the arm held at 20 degrees inside the neutral position (across the body) and at 90-degree elevation, and full internal rotation. The patient is then asked to resist the attempts of the examiner to push the arm towards the ground.

Yergason only described his test in one patient, yet this test has been copied from textbook to textbook. Speed's test also has a low sensitivity and specificity. These tests are fully covered in Chapter 4.4

Examination for instability

First some definitions are needed. Laxity is defined as 'asymptomatic excessive translation'. This is to be differentiated from instability, which is defined as 'excessive translation that causes symptoms in the conscious patient'.

Start with some general observations. Does the patient, like Abraham Lincoln, have the appearance of Marfan's syndrome? Are they tall, thin, and have arachnodactyly? Do they have the rubbery skin of Ehlers–Danlos? More to the point, and more commonly, do they have striaei, one of the commonest markers of laxity? Do they have surgical scars that have stretched, another marker of laxity? A peculiar pit, or dimple, on the posterior aspect of the shoulder has recently been described as an association with posterior positional instability.

One of the dilemmas with examination of the unstable shoulder is that the patient will not let you! The art of examining the unstable shoulder is akin to horse whispering, you must first gain the trust of the patient. Like the abused horse the patient will have come across doctors before who have tried to dislocate their shoulder (the apprehension sign), have caused undue pain to their shoulder, and this shows in their eyes. Like the scared horse the whites of the patient's eyes will be showing, never releasing their laser-like concentration on what nasty trick you are about to do to them. Moreover they will be resistant to any movement of their shoulder, for they know that they live on the knife-edge of dislocation, one of the most painful conditions that can occur to the human frame. Why else do you think that the inquisitors used the rack to torture confessions from their victims? This resistance to examination leads to another chicken-and–egg conundrum for any examination is greeted by intense protective muscle spasm. This complicates any examination for abnormal muscle couples around the shoulder.

The examination starts by gaining the patients trust, and you do this by examining the *good shoulder first*, and gently. More can be gained by looking at the asymptomatic shoulder than the protected shoulder. Most patients with dislocation have a pair of loose shoulders already. This is true even of most traumatic dislocations (as has been shown by Cheng Wallace (2007) in a study of 215 professional rugby players), but more so for atraumatic and posterior positional dislocation. So the first thing to look for is *excessive mobility*, and the second thing *excessive translation* and finally *provocative testing* (Box 4.1.1).

Excess movement

Hyperlaxity

Laxity is a feature of youth! Stiffness is a feature of ageing. Children have been shown to have marked shoulder laxity. However, by the age of 18 (the commonest age for first-time dislocation) the extreme laxity of youth will have passed. The normal end point for external rotation is about 70 degrees. However external rotation of 85–95 degrees is clearly abnormal and this is termed '*hyperlaxity*'. It is a clear sign of shoulder laxity. The normal shoulder will

Box 4.1.1 Examination for instability

- Excess laxity:
  - Hyperlaxity (external rotation greater than 80 degrees)
  - Internal rotation (internal rotation above T5)
  - Beighton's score
  - Striae
  - Gagey's sign (lax inferior capsule)
- Excess translation:
  - Rowe forward
  - Rowe backward
  - Sulcus
  - Drawer tests
- Provocative:
  - Posterior jerk: posterior subluxation
  - Apprehension sign: anterior subluxation
  - Crank test: anterior subluxation
  - Jobe relocation test: anterior subluxation.

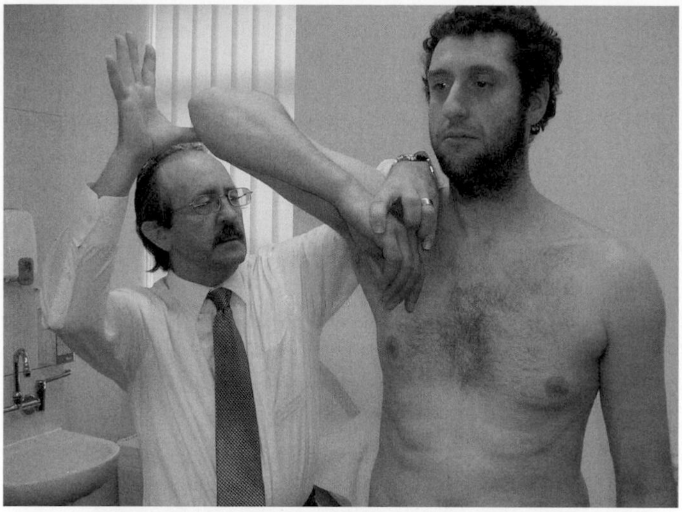

Fig. 4.1.8 Gagey's sign. This is a sign of excessive capacity or laxity of the inferior capsule. With the arm abducted to 90°, the elbow fully flexed and the hand captured and not allowed to move from that position, the elbow is pushed upwards, abducting the arm as fully as it can go. The looser the inferior capsule, the higher the elbow will go.

internally rotate to T7 (the lower border of the scapula); anything more is a sign of laxity.

Beighton score

The Beighton score is a useful objective guide to laxity. Wrist hyperflexion counts for two points, little finger hyperextension at the metacarpophalngeal joint a further two, elbow recurvatum another two, knee recurvatum a further two, and the final two come from the ability to stoop forward so as to place the palms of the hands flat on the floor. This gives a total out of ten points.

Gagey's sign

This is a sign of excessive capacity or laxity of the inferior capsule. With the arm abducted to 90 degrees, the elbow fully flexed and the hand captured and not allowed to move from that position, the elbow is pushed upwards, abducting the arm as fully as it can go. The looser the inferior capsule, the higher the elbow will go (Figure 4.1.8).

Excess translation

Now is the time to stress the joint and see if translation is excessive. Of course this depends on what is normal and the examiner can only gain an appreciation of that with experience. Massive muscular men may show no apparent translation, whereas tiny, size zero girls may demonstrate a fair degree of translation for the same applied force. The amount of translation is graded by convention as 0 for nil, 1 for normal translation, 2 for translation to the glenoid rim, 3 for subluxation, and 4 for dislocation. We will try to translate the joint forwards (Rowe test), downwards (sulcus sign), and backwards (posterior jerk test).

Rowe test

This is the single most useful test of the unstable shoulder. The key is to unpack the capsule of the joint so that it is at its very loosest, for in that state abnormal translation can be shown, that can never be revealed when the capsule is in its tightest configuration. This means getting the standing patient to lean forwards some 40 degrees. Then the patient lets the arm hang down limply. In this unpacked position the surgeon grips the humeral head in one hand and steadies the socket by firmly holding the scapula and clavicle in the other hand. Now the surgeon applies forward (Figure 4.1.9) and then backward translation to the joint. The degree of translation is graded 0–4. Clearly the asymptomatic side must be tested first.

Anterior drawer test

This test is analogous to the anterior drawer test of the knee. The test was first described by Gerber and Ganz in 1984; their description of the test is precise, but has been incorrectly copied into major textbooks. Like the Rowe test, the anterior drawer depends upon unpacking the capsule, positioning the shoulder with the capsule in its loosest configuration. The patient lies supine on the couch and the shoulder is held in the unpacked position of 70-degree flexion in the scapular plane, and neutral rotation. The patient's forearm is gripped in the examiner's axilla. One of the examiner's arms stabilizes the scapula whilst the other drives the humeral head forward and backwards (posterior drawer test). This is a good test but the examiner needs three hands and the patient has to lie down. The Rowe test is easier and quicker. Many textbook editors describe the test being done with the patient seated, and the arm at the side. In this position the capsule is firmly packed and translation will be markedly inhibited confounding the test.

Sulcus sign

Some patients have really loose shoulders. These patients will dislocate in one direction and sublux in the opposite direction; they are thus classified as having multidirectional instability. These patients can be seen to sublux inferiorly by pulling down on the arm, when a dimple will appear between the acromion and the top of the humeral head, the so-called 'sulcus sign' (Figure 4.1.10).

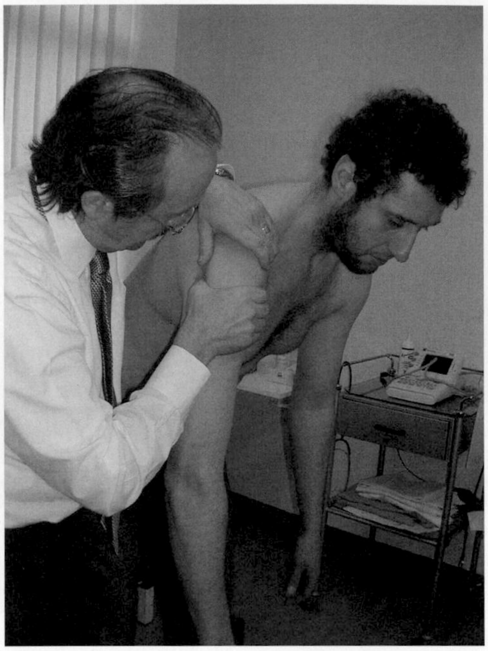

Fig. 4.1.9 Rowe test. This is the single most useful test of the unstable shoulder. The key is to unpack the capsule of the joint so that it is at its very loosest, for in that state abnormal translation can be shown, that can never be revealed when the capsule is in its tightest configuration. This means getting the standing patient to lean forwards some forty degrees. Then the patient lets the arm hang down limply. In this unpacked position the surgeon grips the humeral head in one hand and steadies the socket by firmly holding the scapula and clavicle in the other hand and then pushes the head forwards assessing the degree of abnormal translation.

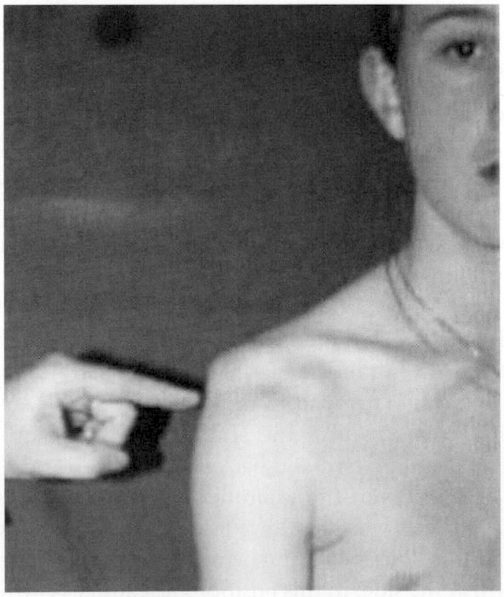

Fig. 4.1.10 These patients can be seen to sublux inferiorly by pulling down on the arm, when a dimple will appear between the acromion and the top of the humeral head, the so-called 'sulcus sign'.

Provocative tests

Posterior jerk test

Posterior instability is tested with the 'posterior jerk test'. This test is poorly described in standard textbooks. The arm is elevated in adduction and internal rotation, and the humeral head will gradually slip off the back of the glenoid; this is usually pain free. With the shoulder thus dislocated the arm is taken from adduction to abduction and the humeral head will suddenly relocate with a jerk; this is usually associated with pain (Figure 4.1.11).

The apprehension test

This is a crude test that mimics an anterior dislocation whilst the inquisitor observes the patient's psychological resistance and physical protective instincts towards the thing they most dread, dislocation of their shoulder. By the twenty-first century doctors should use such barbaric tests sparingly! The diagnosis should already be clear from the history, or emergency department records, or radiographs. The diagnosis of recurrent anterior dislocation is seldom difficult (unlike posterior positional dislocation). If there is some difficulty then the *Rowe test* is far more revealing and does not hurt. For the sake of completeness we will describe the test. The shoulder is brought up into 90 degrees of abduction and then progressively externally rotated. The normal shoulder can be fully externally rotated until a firm passive end point is reached, and it will cause no pain. However, this same manoeuvre in a patient who has recurrent instability will cause extreme apprehension, then pain, and will finally dislocate. Clearly if examining the patient awake, in the clinic, the examiner should stop at the stage of apprehension but there are two further extensions of this test. If the patient is not looking sufficiently apprehensive then the shoulder is cranked into more external rotation, the *crank test*. If the patient is looking sufficiently apprehensive then pressure is applied to the humeral head to translate it back into socket, and the flood of relief visible on the patient's face gives a positive relocation test, eponymously named after that kind Dr Jobe, the *Jobe relocation test*.

Neurological examination

If examination has revealed that the shoulder is not stiff, that the tests of the rotator cuff are normal, and that there is no evidence of instability, radiographs and POC ultrasound are normal then you have a problem; you are also going to run over the twenty minutes allotted to each patient. Turn to the chapter on examination of the cervical spine for further details.

The acromioclavicular joint

The acromioclavicular joint (ACJ) is subcutaneous, and therefore much easier to examine than the shoulder joint itself. It is rare for the ACJ to be the culprit if it is not tender along its anterior, superior, or posterior joint line. Instability can be seen if gross and the joint translates abnormally if it is unstable. Finally the joint can be stressed by torsion, elevating the shoulder into the high painful arc, or by compression (the scarf test), or 'cross-over test', or extension and adduction with resistance 'the half nelson or resisted extension test'. O'Brien's test described an active compression test with the upper limb flexed to horizontal at the shoulder with a little adduction. If the origin of the pain is in doubt, a small amount of lignocaine (1–2mL) can be injected directly into the ACJ and the tests repeated. The cross-over test and resisted extension test are most sensitive (77% and 72% respectively). O'Brien's test was found to have low sensitivity (41%) but high specificity (95%). A positive finding on all three tests, however, conferred an accuracy of 93% and probably renders a diagnostic injection test unnecessary.

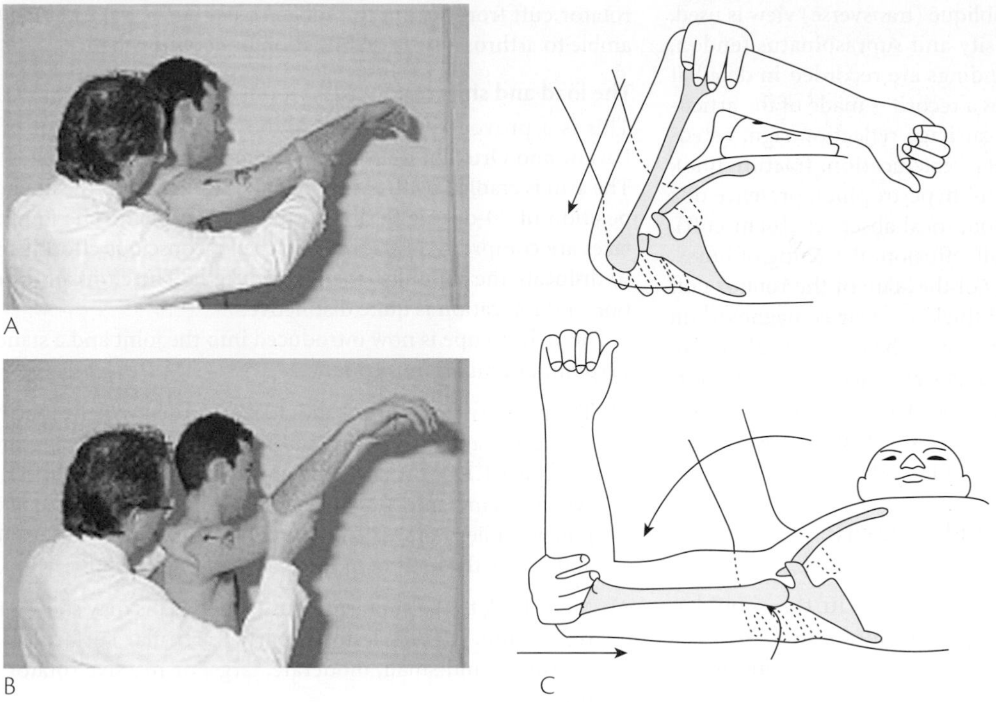

Fig. 4.1.11 Posterior jerk test. Posterior instability is tested with the 'posterior jerk test'. This test is poorly described in standard textbooks. The arm is elevated in adduction and internal rotation, and the humeral head will gradually slip off the back of the glenoid; this is usually pain free. With the shoulder thus dislocated the arm is taken from adduction to abduction and the humeral head will suddenly relocate with a jerk; this is usually associated with pain.

Investigation, the forensics

Plain radiographs

In the twenty-first-century rush to get scans, plain radiographs are often forgotten. This is a mistake. There are many things that are best seen on plain old-fashioned radiographs and these are fractures, calcific deposits, arthritis, tumours, and locked dislocations. All right you can see these on an MRI scan, but who has instant access to an MRI scanner in clinic? Besides, calcific deposits are far more difficult to see on MRI than on plain radiographs. A radiograph is the mandatory investigation for the stiff shoulder, and mandatory in any patient with a history of cancer (Box 4.1.2). The radiograph should be taken in the plane of the glenoid, which is 30 degrees to the sagittal plane of the body; this is the true AP of the shoulder.

Although cuff disease and instability are soft tissue diseases they may lead to secondary bone changes that can be seen on radiographs. Radiographs may show changes in the greater tuberosity in rotator cuff disease. These will range from irregularity of the bony footprint, sclerosis, pseudocysts, and eventually flattening of the tuberosity.

Changes may also occur at the anteroinferior acromion with sclerosis (sourcil sign) and spur formation within the footprint of the coracoacromial ligament. Less accurate is a reduction in the acromiohumeral distance, or a break in Shenton's line of the shoulder.

Secondary changes in instability are the Hill–Sachs lesion (best seen on a Stryker notch view or West Point view) and bony Bankart lesions (best seen on an axillary or Bernageau view).

ACJ arthropathy is most readily confirmed with a plain radiograph of the joint. This requires the x-ray beam to be tilted 20–30 degrees in a caudal direction and the voltage reduced to ensure that the ACJ is not obscured by the base of the acromion or over-exposed (Zanca view).

Box 4.1.2 Investigations

- Stiff shoulder: plain radiograph
- Wobbly shoulder: examination under anesthesia, arthroscopy
- Pain on reach: ultrasound.

Computed tomography scanning and computed tomography arthrography

Computed tomography (CT) scans are useful for surgical planning, particularly prior to fracture fixation and complex primary shoulder replacements. In continental Europe, CT is commonly used in the assessment of rotator cuff tears, particularly to assess fatty infiltration of the muscle belly (using the Goutallier classification) prior to surgery. CT arthrography can be used for rotator cuff disease and instability, but has been mainly superseded by MR arthrography (MRA).

CT is a useful modality for examining the sternoclavicular joint.

Ultrasound

In the clinic time is of the essence, so an abbreviated study is permitted, scanning in only three planes, as opposed to the 12 planes recommended in most radiological texts. An axial scan is first used to demonstrate the lesser tuberosity, subscapularis, biceps sulcus, and long head of biceps tendon. Secondly, an oblique coronal (or longitudinal) view is used to show the greater tuberosity and the supraspinatus. Finally, a saggittal oblique (transverse) view is used, demonstrating the greater tuberosity and supraspinatus tendon, rotator interval, and biceps. All findings are recorded in detail at the time. In each of the three planes a record is made of the articular appearance (normal, positive cartilage reflection sign, osteophytes), the bone (normal, irregular, calcification, fracture line), the collagen (normal, heterogeneous, hypertrophic), presence of a defect (rim-rent, cleft, delamination, focal absence, absent cuff), and the presence of an effusion (nil, effusion, flattening of bursa, bursal concavity). A firm diagnosis of the state of the rotator cuff and biceps is then recorded. A full thickness tear is diagnosed on sonography if the tendon is absent, or if there is a focal deficit. A combination of one or more indirect signs such as a bursal concavity, an effusion around the biceps, bony irregularity, or a positive cartilage reflection sign allow a judgement to be made by the surgeon of the presence of a supraspinatus tear.

Magnetic resonance imaging and magnetic resonance arthrography

MRI has revolutionized the field of imaging in the shoulder, because it can image the soft tissues. Unlike ultrasound, MRI can image through the bone, and it can image the bone, and it can image to depths of tissue that cannot be reached by high frequency ultrasound. It is therefore the imaging modality of choice for instability, as it will demonstrate labral abnormalities. Visualization of SLAP tears and Bankart tears are improved by MRA using gadolinium enhancement.

MRI is the imaging modality of choice for large rotator cuff tears where the degree of retraction under the acromion, and the degree of wasting and fatty infiltration of the muscle belly will determine whether the tear should be repaired, or whether repair is a forlorn hope. MRA is useful in demonstrating articular side partial tears.

MRI is not as good as CT for looking at bone yet it is the investigation of choice for avascular necrosis. MRI is the investigation of choice for lumps, masses, and tumours around the shoulder. MRI will demonstrate pathology that cannot be seen by ultrasound, such as labral cysts and ganglia.

However MRI is not without problems. The equipment is extremely expensive and far from portable! Patients do not like MRI. It is claustrophobic, noisy, and patient unfriendly. One-third of patients will not have a second MRI scan. It will demonstrate morphology, but not histology. It suffers from a phenomenon called the 'magic angle effect' that can produce false positive results. MRI is very bad at showing calcific deposits as these are dark, as is the tendon, so there is no contrast difference between the calcium and the tendon.

MRA suffers from the problem that it is invasive. Intra-articular injection of gadolinium is usually done under image intensifier control and local anaesthetic. This ramps up the degree of difficulty, often needing two radiology suites, careful timing, transfer from room to room, and the time of a skilled radiologist. On top of this patients do not like invasive diagnostic procedures.

Arthroscopy

Shoulder arthroscopy remains the gold standard forensic investigation for the shoulder. Not only can the inside of the glenohumeral joint be appreciated, but also the outside view of the rotator cuff from within the subacromial bursa. An essential preamble to arthroscopy is examination under anaesthetic.

The load and shift test

This is a provocative test, being the shoulder equivalent of the Barlow and Ortolani tests of the hip, or the pivot shift in the knee. The arm is cradled by the examiner and brought into the unpacked position of 70-degree flexion in the scapula plain. The joint surfaces are compressed (loaded) and then a conscious effort is made to dislocate the shoulder, then to reduce it. The clunk of dislocation and relocation is quite distinctive.

The arthroscope is now introduced into the joint and a standard 12-point examination is conducted.

1) The primary landmark of shoulder arthroscopy is the long head of biceps, and this is a good place to start the examination (Figure 4.1.12). Examine the anchor (SLAP tears), the tendon (vinculae, mesentery, ensheathed biceps, hourglass biceps), the pulley (pulley failure, partial tearing, subluxation, dislocation), and finally the tendon may have ruptured
2) Move back to the supraspinatus tendon. This may show a rim-rent lesion, PASTA lesions (partial articular surface tendon avulsion), and small, moderate, large, or massive rotator cuff tears
3) Next examine the rotator interval for angiogenesis and granulation tissue (contracted [frozen] shoulder), or widening (instability), the bumper sign (coracoid impingement), the comma sign (subscapularis rupture), and as a hiding place for loose bodies
4) Examine the middle gleno-humeral ligament. It can be variable in thickness or exhibit a Buford complex (cord-like with a high origin)
5) Examine the subscapularis for partial tears, HAGL (humeral avulsion of the glenohumeral ligaments) lesions, pulley lesions, or complete tears
6) Examine the labrum. This can show evidence of PSI (posterosuperior internal impingement), SLAP tears, ASI (anterosuperior internal impingement), Detrisac type 2 lesion, Bankart tear, Perthes lesion, ALPSA lesion (anterior labrum periosteal sleeve avulsion), bony Bankart lesion, inferior fibrillation, posterior fibrillation, and posterior Bankart lesion
7) Examine the glenoid surface with its central grey spot. There may be arthritic damage, anterior crevassing or cratering (instability), or a bony Bankart (reverse pear-shaped glenoid)
8) Come to the inferior glenohumeral ligament that may be stretched or torn. There may be a positive see through sign or a positive drive through sign (associated with instability). The inferior recess may be contracted or loose and is a favourite hiding place for loose bodies
9) Return to your starting point either taking the high road where you see the bare area, Hill–Sachs lesions, and the state of the articular surface, or the low road where you see the posterior labrum and posterior gutter
10) Now exit the glenohumeral joint and enter the loft-space of the subacromial bursa. Examine the roof for impingement signs,

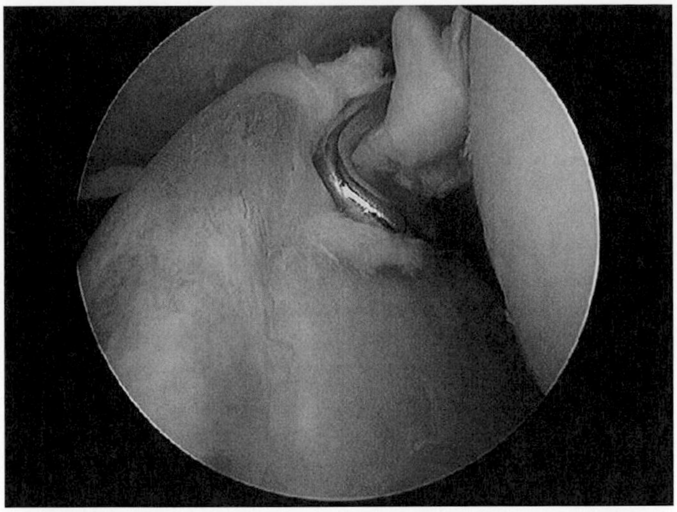

Fig. 4.1.12 Long head of biceps, the primary landmark of shoulder arthroscopy.

firstly scuffing of the coracoacromial footprint (Copeland–Levy A1); gross fibrillation (A2); loss of footprint and sclerosis (A3)

11) Examine the floor of the loft-space, the bursal surface of the rotator cuff. Is it normal? Examine for scuffing (B1), fibrillation and partial tearing (B2), or a full thickness rotator cuff tear (B3). Is there a plica?

12) Finally examine, ballotte, and palpate the under surface of the acromioclavicular joint and expose it if necessary.

The 12-point examination is thorough and should confirm the diagnosis. More detail can be sought from textbooks such as *Shoulder Arthroscopy* by Bunker and Wallace, which is available free on the Internet at sites such as http://www.shoulderdoc.co.uk. These days arthroscopy is rarely used for diagnosis alone, it is used for treatment, releasing contracted shoulders, decompressing impinging shoulders, repairing rotator cuff tears, and stabilizing the unstable joint. All of these will be covered in the ensuing chapters in this section.

Summary

Surgeons only need to know two things: when to operate and how to operate. When to operate is what this chapter has been about. Knowing when to operate involves establishing the diagnosis and the severity of the disease. However, despite the advances in clinical examination and the profusion of forensic examinations (radiographs, CT, ultrasound, MRI, MRA, and arthroscopy) that are now available to us, the diagnosis can remain elusive. *The surgeon must take in a vast amount of information, solve several simultaneous equations at once, discard the dissembling and lies, assemble the truths, seek concordance, check with forensics, and come to a solution.* Nobody said this was easy; it is why surgeons are carefully chosen, continuously examined, trained for 20 years, and prefer coastal navigation to football. Higher-level reasoning has always, and will always be the most important distinctive characteristic of the consultant surgeon.

As to how to operate, that will be covered in the following chapters.

Further reading

Al-Shawi, A., Badge, R., and Bunker, T. (2008). The detection of full thickness tears of the rotator cuff using ultrasound. *Journal of Bone and Joint Surgery*, **90B**(7), 889–92.

Farber, A., Castillo, R., Clough, M., Bahk, M., and McFarland, E.G. (2006). Clinical assessment of three common tests for traumatic anterior shoulder instability. *Journal of Bone and Joint Surgery*, **88A**(7), 1467–74.

Hegedus, E.J., Goode, A, Campbell, S., *et al.* (2008). Physical examination tests of the shoulder. *British Journal of Sports Medicine*, **42**(2), 80–92.

Hertel, R., Ballmer, F., Lambert, S., and Gerber, C. (1996). Lag signs. *Journal of Shoulder and Elbow Surgery*, **5**(4), 307–13.

MacDonald, P., Clark, P., and Sutherland, K. (2000). An analysis of the accuracy of the Hawkins and Neer subacromial impingement tests. *Journal of Shoulder and Elbow Surgery*, **9**(4), 299–301.

4.2

Pathology of cuff tears

Peter Reilly

Summary points

- Rotator cuff tears are common
- Aetiology complex and multifactorial
- Tendons deteriorate with age
- Posterosuperior tears are more common
- They evolve in a typical fashion
- Anterosuperior tears are less common.

Introduction

Rotator cuff pathology accounts for one-third of all shoulder referrals. Theories on aetiology are broadly divided into two camps: intrinsic (related to the tendons themselves) and extrinsic (related to factors external to the tendon). The relative significance of each of these factors has stimulated much debate and zealots defend their views with fervour! The aim of this chapter is to give a balanced review of the relevant literature, concluding that many factors are at work and the end result is tendon pathology.

Macroscopic structure

Structurally and functionally the rotator cuff should be considered as a complex of four muscles arising from the scapula whose tendons blend as they insert onto the humerus (Figure 4.2.1).

The supraspinatus inserts onto the superior facet of the greater tuberosity of the humerus. The greater supraspinatus muscle bulk anteriorly is reflected in an increased tendon thickness. Laterally the supraspinatus tendon passes under the acromioclavicular joint and the coracoacromial arch. The arch is formed by the anterior undersurface of the acromion and the coracoacromial ligament (CAL). The subacromial bursa reduces friction as the humeral head and supraspinatus tendon move relative to the arch.

The infraspinatus inserts onto the middle facet of the greater tuberosity. The teres minor is the smallest of the rotator cuff muscles, and attaches to the lowest facet of the greater tuberosity.

Posteriorly the supraspinatus tendon blends with the infraspinatus about 15mm proximal to the insertion and from this point cannot be separated by blunt dissection. The infraspinatus and teres minor merge proximal to the musculotendinous junction.

The subscapularis is a large triangular muscle, which originates from the subscapular fossa. The subscapularis tendon is visible inside the shoulder joint as it passes laterally through the oval foramen of Weitbrecht to insert onto the lesser tuberosity.

The long head of biceps lies in the interval between the subscapularis and supraspinatus tendons, passing through the glenohumeral joint from its origin, the supraglenoid tubercle, to the bicipital groove. Its synovial sheath is an extension of the articular capsule.

Microscopic structure

Clark and Harryman examined the detailed structure of 32 intact rotator cuffs. A five-layer structure to the supraspinatus and infraspinatus tendons was reported as follows: (superficial to deep) obliquely orientated fibres of the coracohumeral ligament (1mm thickness); parallel tendon fibres (3mm thickness); the tendinous fascicles then become smaller and less uniformly orientated (3mm thickness); loose connective tissue with some thick collagen fibres; and a thin continuous sheet of collagen fibrils (2mm thickness). The coracohumeral ligament extends posterolaterally and envelops the tendon. It has been suggested that this sandwiching effect may help to prevent tendon delamination.

Nakajima further considered the differences between the joint and bursal sides of the supraspinatus tendon as an explanation for intratendinous partial thickness tears. The tendon bundles were found to differ on both the joint side and the bursal side depending on the distance from the insertion.

At the tendon–bone interface a stepwise transition is seen. The stages of tendon, fibrocartilage, calcified fibrocartilage, and bone are thought to optimize the distribution of forces over the attachment site, which minimizes stress concentrations, and facilitates angular change.

Function of the rotator cuff

The rotator cuff is of prime importance in glenohumeral motion, ensuring that the humeral head is kept in contact with the glenoid. Three groups of muscles act on the shoulder joint: scapulohumeral, axioscapular, and axiohumeral. The first group consists of the rotator cuff, the dynamic stabilizers of the shoulder, and the deltoid, a prime mover. The axioscapular (including rhomboids

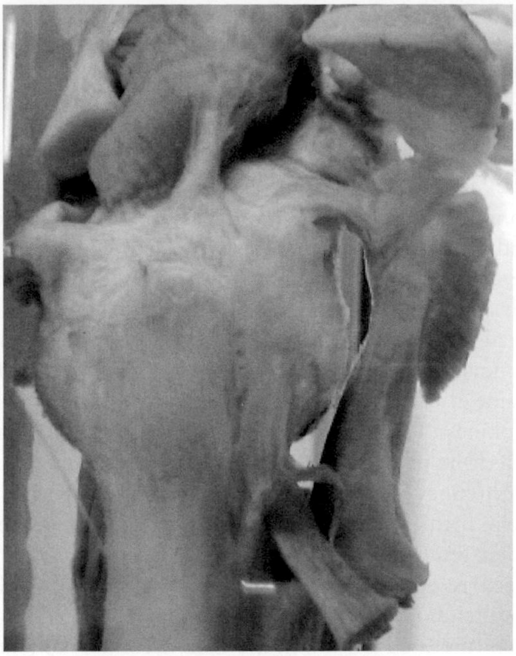

Fig. 4.2.1 The anatomy of the rotator cuff. Note the central oblique tendon of the supraspinatus forming the anterior column.

and serratus anterior) and the axiohumeral (latissimus dorsi and pectoralis major) are important in joint motion and force generation.

The supraspinatus is a humeral head compressor and arm abductor. The subscapularis is primarily an internal rotator, and infraspinatus an external rotator. Both these muscles compress the humeral head against the glenoid during abduction. Furthermore, the subscapularis acts a restraint to anterior displacement of the humeral head. Teres minor is an external rotator working in conjunction with infraspinatus.

During abduction the rotator cuff muscles hold the humeral head against the glenoid, countering the vertical shearing action of the abducting deltoid. The compressive force increases up to 90 degrees of abduction, beyond this it gradually reduces. At 90 degrees the resultant force of abduction and compression in an unloaded limb approximates to body weight.

The direction of the resultant force is not constant as the arm is abducted. This leads to alteration in the position of the humeral head relative to the glenoid. In the case of abduction in the scapular plane with neutral rotation, the force is initially directed downward to the inferior border of the glenoid. At between 30–60 degrees of abduction the high shear forces cause movement of the vector to the superior edge of the glenoid, and with further abduction this moves back to the centre.

Incidence

It has been shown that there is an incidence of 9.5 per 1000 of patients with shoulder pain presenting to primary care. Of these patients it was found that 74% had signs of impingement and 85% had evidence of painful or torn rotator cuffs. A recent systematic review looking, more specifically, at rotator cuff tears has shown that in an unselected cadaveric population the incidence of both partial and full thickness tears is 30.24%. The incidence of tears increases with age and many now consider this to be part of the normal ageing process.

Pathogenesis

In 1934 Codman put forward the theory that the cause of rotator cuff disease (RCD) was actually an intrinsic degeneration of the tendon, but subsequent opinion moved towards external factors being the main component in the aetiology. It was thought that mechanical compression of the tendons of the cuff caused the tendon to tear. Changes in the morphology of the structures surrounding the supraspinatus outlet were thought to cause stenosis and compress the cuff underneath the acromion leading to attrition. Currently consensus has drifted back towards Codman's original theory supporting a combination of repetitive microtrauma and age-related degeneration.

Intrinsic causes

A degenerated tendon is more likely to rupture than a normal tendon during physiological loading. Riley and colleagues have histologically examined supraspinatus tendons looking at the organization of the tendon collagen fibres and the appearance of the tendon fibroblasts. They showed that degenerative changes within the tendon increase with age, and more severe degeneration is associated with tendon damage. They also showed that there were changes in collagen composition and cross-links associated with the physiological loading conditions; however, there is a higher rate of collagen turnover in degenerate (ruptured) tendons. Within these degenerate tendons the expression of matrix metalloproteinase (MMP) enzymes (produced by tenocytes to mediate the matrix turnover) is altered, suggesting that tendon degeneration is an active, cell-mediated process. It was hypothesized that tendinopathy may result from an imbalance between synthesis and degradation of the tendon, perhaps due to failure to regulate specific MMP activities in response to repeated injury or mechanical strain.

The evidence for tendon degeneration has been further supported by the detection of highly sulphated glycosaminoglycans (GAGs) in inflamed supraspinatus tendon. These GAGs are associated with amyloid deposition. Others have shown that patients with chronic tears showed deposition of amyloid in 70% of tendons, compared to only 25% of those with acute traumatic tears. Amyloid has a fibrillar ultrastructure forming extensive antiparallel pleated sheets making it resistant to proteolytic digestion. Therefore once deposited in tissue it tends to remain and accumulate, ultimately leading to irreversible changes in the structure of the affected tissue.

Sano and colleagues looked at tendon thinning, the presence of granulation tissue, and partial thickness tears. They found that the more degenerate tendons were weaker. Degeneration was significantly greater in tendons that failed at their insertion.

There is evidence that granulation tissue itself may weaken the tendon insertion by inducing osteochondral destruction. The chemical mediators, interleukin-1 beta, cathepsin D, and MMP-1 were present at the insertions of 16 torn supraspinatus tendons but not in controls. Macrophages and multinucleated giant cells were found at the tear site.

Blood supply

It is likely that rotator cuff tendon vascularity, particularly in relation to the supraspinatus, is one of a number of intrinsic factors contributing to RCD.

The vascularity of the supraspinatus tendon has been a focus of interest since the time of Codman. He described the critical zone of the supraspinatus tendon, half an inch proximal to the insertion, which appeared anaemic and hypothesized that perfusion had a crucial role in tendon pathology.

He stated 'tears of the supraspinatus tendon had much to do with overuse of the arms in an abducted position without giving the tendons time to let their circulation do its duty'. Against this it has been suggested that the supraspinatus tendon blood supply is the same as the infraspinatus and consequently can not be responsible for the high rates of failure reported.

The majority of authors have concluded that the supraspinatus tendon blood supply differs from that of the other rotator cuff tendons. The critical zone of Codman probably represents a hypovascular area, caused by anastomosis of vessels originating from the greater tuberosity and the supraspinatus muscle belly. The tenuous vascularity of this area not only makes it more vulnerable to degeneration, but also modifies any attempts at repair.

Mechanical properties

Standard textbooks, books on surgical technique, and original research papers tend to promulgate an anatomically incorrect depiction of the torn supraspinatus. Illustrations in these texts portray supraspinatus as a homogeneous flat tendon, whereas in fact it is a distinctly heterogeneous tendon, a feature that has marked clinical relevance. Nakajima and Fukuda showed quite elegantly that the central tendon is markedly denser and stronger than the rest of the tendon on histological preparations of the supraspinatus tendon. They demonstrated how the central thick tendon migrates towards the anterior margin of the tendon as you move towards its insertion. Itoi confirmed this work and showed that the anterior third was by far the strongest with a strength to failure of 411N, the mid portion 152N, and the posterior third just 88N. Nakagaki et al. and Bigliani et al. supported this work and provided correct illustrations of the nature of the tendon. Others have shown how the superior (bursal side) of the tendon is twice as strong as the articular side. Gagey et al. introduced the concept of the fibrous frame of the rotator cuff. These workers performed three-dimensional reconstruction of magnetic resonance imaging scans and demonstrated the deep fibrous reinforcement of the supraspinatus that is the central oblique tendon. They showed how supraspinatus has one tendon, whereas subscapularis is multipennate and they show how the single tendon of supraspinatus inserts into the anterior extremity of the greater tuberosity. This pattern of migration of the central oblique tendon has been confirmed by Roh et al. This central oblique tendon (that we will term the *anterior column*), being the strongest part of supraspinatus, remains intact when all around it the tendon fails. In effect it acts as a *firebreak* and determines the pattern of posterosuperior rotator cuff tearing. From these observations a hypothesis was developed that there is a definite and progressive pattern of cuff tear extension that is determined by the special anatomy of this tendon. Understanding this pattern (Figure 4.2.2) allows the surgeon to predict which structures are contracted and need to be released, and to develop a plan to close the defect using fundamental surgical techniques such as rotationplasty, rather than treating each surgery as a lucky dip or magical mystery tour.

Extrinsic causes

Subacromial impingement is compression of the subacromial bursa and the supraspinatus tendon between the anterior acromion and the coracoacromial ligament superiorly and the humerus inferiorly.

A recent study has suggested that the subacromial bursa is a proinflammatory membrane that may be responsible for shoulder pain. Blaine et al. demonstrated the presence of various inflammatory cytokines (TNF, IL-1, IL-6, COX-1, and COX-2) in bursal specimens from patients with subacromial bursitis and RCD. Some of these cytokines (IL-1, IL-6) have been reported to play an important role in mediating the catabolism of collagen. It has been suggested that removal of the subacromial bursa, which is rich in Substance P receptors, is the key to pain relief in acromioplasty.

The peritendinous changes in RCD may be a secondary phenomenon. Increased tension in the CAL, secondary to tendinopathy, may stimulate new bone growth leading to the spur seen on radiographs, and this spur may cause more damage. Structural features such as lateral sloping of the acromion and glenoid version may also have an extrinsic effect in cuff degeneration.

This does not exclude the role of acromial morphology in the impingement syndrome. Bigliani et al. described three distinct types of acromion (types I–III, see Box 4.2.1). The relationship with full thickness cuff tears was recorded: 3% in type I, 24% type II, and in type III 73%. They studied 420 cadaveric scapulas and concluded that acromial morphology was not age dependent, but that spur formation was.

Position of the scapula may have an influence on the supraspinatus as it passes under the arch formed by the acromion and CAL. A forward scapula posture, caused by a combination of forward head posture and increased kyphosis, may cause an outlet stenosis and effectively squeeze the tendon as it passes through.

Recently the idea of *internal impingement* has surfaced. Some surgeons noted arthroscopically that patients with attrition of the posterosuperior labrum also had attrition of the posterosuperior cuff insertion, and that as the shoulder was maximally abducted and externally rotated (the ABER position) these areas contacted. This was termed PSI or posterosuperior internal impingement and may be the cause of shoulder pain in throwing athletes. Similarly an anterosuperior labral lesion has been seen alongside attrition of the biceps pulley and this has been termed ASI, or anterosuperior internal impingement.

Relevance of impingement to rotator cuff tears

Neer estimated that 95% of lesions of the rotator cuff were the end result of impingement. This is often quoted but generally accepted as historical and excessive. Neer's hypothesis was based on cadaveric and preoperative observations. It is not difficult to believe that direct attrition may occur on the bursal surface of the supraspinatus.

More recently support for impingement in the aetiology of cuff tears has come from two-dimensional finite element modelling of

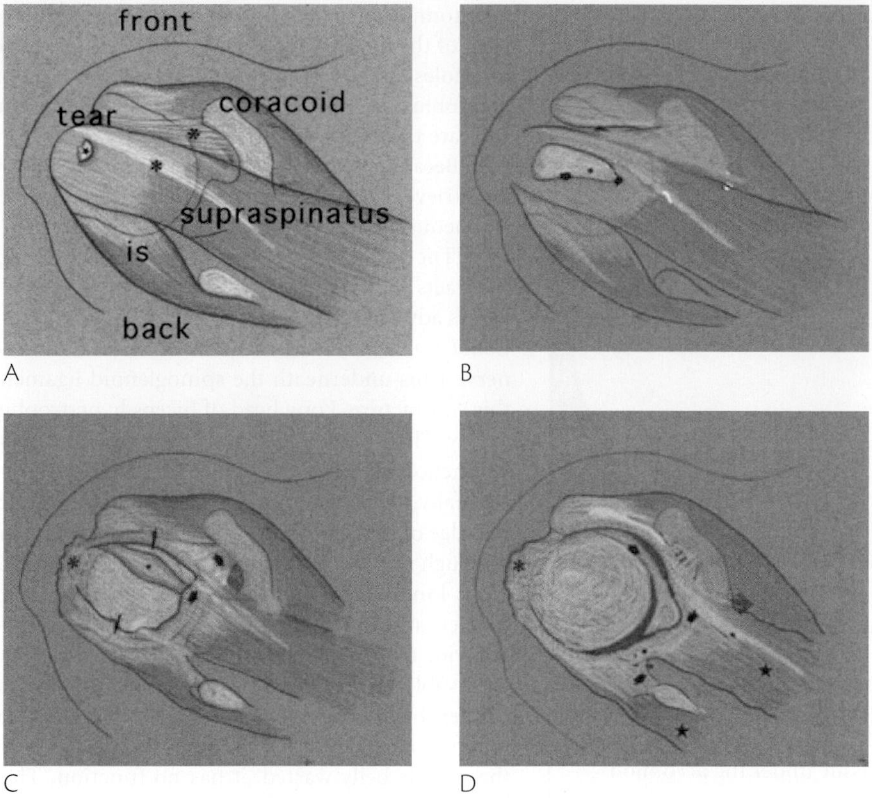

Fig. 4.2.2 The pattern of posterosuperior cuff tearing. See text for details.

the supraspinatus tendon. Impingement simulated by a 1-mm indentation on the bursal side of the tendon was found to be a stress riser in the area of the critical zone. Effects were found throughout the tendon, not just on the bursal side, which was thought to suggest a role for impingement in the aetiology of joint side tears.

Whatever the role of impingement in the aetiology of rotator cuff tears, acromioplasty does not appear to prevent their occurrence. Hyvonen et al. followed-up 96 shoulders without rotator cuff tears for 9 years after open acromioplasty and found 12 full thickness and seven partial thickness tears.

Genetics

Harvie et al. convincingly demonstrated that there is a genetic susceptibility to RCD. They have carried out a retrospective, cohort study of 205 patients with full thickness tears of the rotator cuff, using ultrasound to determine the prevalence of RCD in their siblings. They have shown that the relative risk of full-thickness tears in siblings versus controls was 2.42 and the relative risk of symptomatic full-thickness tears in siblings was 4.65. They suggest that the significant phenotypic expression is likely to occur at the level of the development of the ultrastructure of the tendon.

Box 4.2.1 Bigliani grade of acromial morphology

- Type I: flat, found in 17% of specimens
- Type II: curved, 43%
- Type III: hooked, 40% of which 14.2% had associated spur formation.

The pattern of rotator cuff tears

This chapter has shown how repeated tensile or compressive overload can cause changes within the ageing rotator cuff. Macroscopically this leads to the initiating event, which is the rim-rent lesion. The rim-rent lesion can be demonstrated by ultrasound or by arthroscopy (Figure 4.2.3). This lesion is constantly situated 7mm behind the biceps pulley just posterior to the insertion of the anterior column. Gradually the rim-rent peels further back off its footprint of insertion into the superior facet of the greater tuberosity. As it does so secondary reactive changes occur on the bone, which becomes sclerotic and nodular. These nodules appear on radiographs as tiny sclerotic rings and are often misreported as cysts, although tiny true cysts can also occur. Eventually the deep surface rim-rent will peel so far back that it emerges on the bursal side as a pinhole full thickness tear. This gradual enlargement of the deep surface partial thickness tear may take years to evolve. During this time the supraspinatus is weakened and its normal centring effect is lost. The head subluxes upward and secondary impingement occurs between the bursal surface of the cuff and the acromion.

These secondary reactive changes can be seen by placing an arthroscope into the bursa. The bursa becomes fibrillated, and then wears through and the bursal surface of the cuff becomes damaged and fibrillates—this is the impingement lesion of Neer. Reactive changes will occur on the acromion and have been classified into four grades by Uhtoff (see Box 4.2.2).

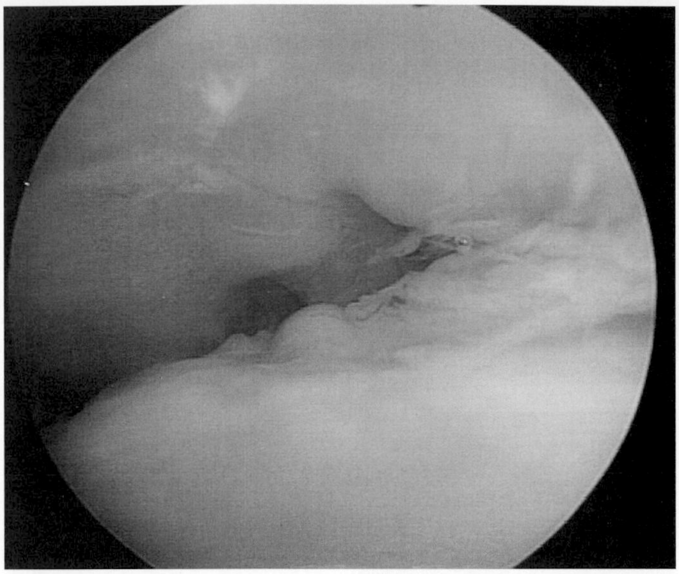

Fig. 4.2.3 The rim-rent tear is the first stage of the typical posterosuperior tear.

Box 4.2.2 Uhtoff grade of acromial pathology

- Firstly there is a loss of areolar tissue under the acromion
- Then the coracoacromial ligament and the fibrous pad that represents its footprint of insertion into the acromion thicken
- Thirdly there is fibrillation of the insertion of the coracoacromial ligament
- Finally there is eburnation of the undersurface of the acromion and loss of the footprint of insertion of the coracoacromial ligament.

Meanwhile the cuff tear extends, either slowly, or it may suddenly give with even mild trauma. Knowledge of the normal morphology of the tendon explains the pattern of tear exposed at surgical repair. Knowledge of the morphology of the capsule explains the contractures which occur, and that will need to be released during surgical reconstruction. We must always remember that the tendon and capsule merge and blend towards their combined insertion, and that for a full thickness tear to occur, both capsule and tendon must have dis-inserted. The tendon retracts, but the capsule contracts.

As the small tear extends into a moderate tear the anterior column, being so strong, acts as a firebreak and resists extension, and so instead of becoming a larger crescentic tear, the tear becomes asymmetric or L-shaped. At the same time the superior capsule, having dis-inserted contracts back towards the glenoid, pulling the cuff, with which it is merged, along with it. The coracohumeral ligament reinforces the superior capsule and, as this powerful thickening of the capsule contracts, it pulls the anterior column with it, towards the coracoid. This determines the releases that will be necessary for a small to moderate tear.

Now a singular event happens; at 3–5cm the tear extends over the North Pole of the humeral head, causing a buttonhole (boutonniere) situation. Just as in the proximal interphalangeal joint of the finger when a boutonniere lesion occurs, the joint button-holes up through the tear and the lateral slips get stretched out and sublux around the joint. In the case of the shoulder, the lateral slips are the anterior column to the front and infraspinatus to the rear. Because the infraspinatus has subluxed backwards and cannot be retrieved from under the acromion at surgery the surgeon may erroneously think that it too has torn, but this is hardly ever the case. The capsule at the junction of the supra- and infraspinatus contracts severely and it is the release of this *junctional scar* that allows advancement of supraspinatus in large cuff tears. This *junctional scar* is hidden under the acromion and the suprascapular nerve runs underneath the spinoglenoid ligament just medial to this contracture. Long head of biceps hypertrophies and may start to fray. The capsule continues to contract. The muscle bellies, being defunctioned, waste away.

Finally, the tear continues to extend and retracts right back to the edge of the glenoid rim. The anterior column may still be intact, although now very stretched. The anterior column uproots, uncovering long head of biceps, which now becomes painful, frays further, and can sublux or rupture. As the biceps pulley fails, the superior margin of subscapularis may tear and the humeral head now subluxes forward as well as upward. The capsule contracts further. Infraspinatus subluxes further back yet, contrary to popular opinion, rarely tears, although the tendon is stretched out and the muscle belly wasted, it has no function. The junctional scar becomes even thicker. This is the classic 'bald head tear'.

Arthritic change may now occur between the North Pole of the humerus and the acromion, as well as the surfaces of the humerus and superior pole of the acromion, which are maintained in a subluxed position. This arthritic change is called 'cuff tear arthropathy' and is the end stage of the spectrum of cuff disease. Two per cent of the population over the age of 80 will have cuff tear arthropathy.

Conclusions

The aetiology of supraspinatus tendon failure is multifactorial. Intrinsic and extrinsic factors combine, resulting in the high prevalence reported in cadaveric and radiological studies. These factors are intimately related to normal supraspinatus structure

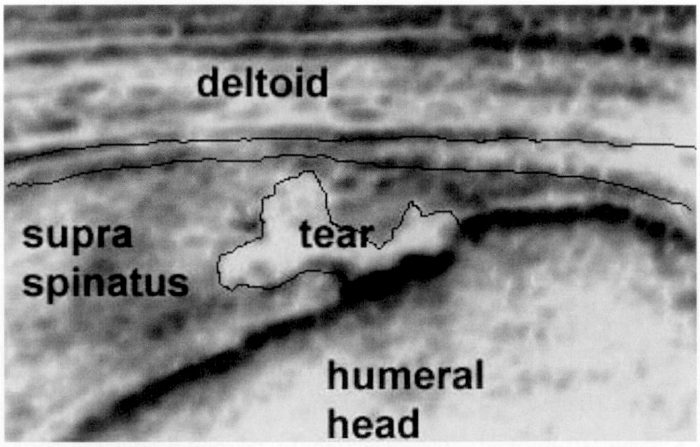

Fig. 4.2.4 Ultrasound scan of a tear originating on the articular side, the next stage from the rim rent.

and function. There is now a good body of evidence that RCD is an intrinsically initiated phenomenon, with the changes in the surrounding structures being a secondary feature. It is, however, simplistic to seek a single cause of rotator cuff failure; rather it is appropriate to consider how the pieces of a complex puzzle fit together.

Further reading

Brooks, C.H., Revell, W.J., and Heatley, F.W. (1992). A quantitative histological study of the vascularity of the rotator cuff tendon. *Journal of Bone and Joint Surgery*, **74B**, 151–3.

Burkhart, S.S. (1998). Biomechanics of rotator cuff repair: converting the ritual to a science. *Instructional Course Lectures*, **47**, 43–50.

Clark, J.M. and Harryman, D.T. 2nd (1992). Tendons, ligaments, and capsule of the rotator cuff. Gross and microscopic anatomy. *Journal of Bone and Joint Surgery*, **74A**(5), 713–25.

Codman, E.A. (1934). *The Shoulder. Rupture of the Supraspinatus Tendon and Other Lesions in or about the Subacromial Bursa.* Boston, MA: Thomas Todd.

Itoi, E., Berglund, L.J., Grabowski, J.J., *et al.* (1995). Tensile properties of the supraspinatus tendon. *Journal of Orthopaedic Research*, **13**, 578–84.

Nakajima, T. (1994). Histological and biomechanical characteristics of the supraspinatus tendon. *Journal of Shoulder and Elbow Surgery*, **3**, 79–87.

Neer, C.S. 2nd (1972). Anterior acromioplasty for the chronic impingement syndrome in the shoulder: a preliminary report. *Journal of Bone and Joint Surgery*, **54**(1), 41–50.

Uhthoff, H.K. and Sano, H. (1997). Pathology of failure of the rotator cuff tendon. *Orthopedic Clinics of North America*, **28**, 31–41.

4.3

Treatment of rotator cuff disease

Lennard Funk and Amol Tambe

Summary points

- Arthroscopic techniques have revolutionized the surgical management of rotator cuff disease
- Arthroscopic subacromial decompression (ASD) is accepted as a well established method for the treatment of symptomatic impingement after conservative treatment has failed
- Appropriate patient selection is paramount to a successful outcome
- Attention to detail including patient set-up, maintaining optimum fluid pressure and portal placement are essential to achieve successful outcome
- Erroneous diagnosis is the commonest cause of failure following ASD
- Thorough debridement of the subacromial bursa forms a key element of ASD. Aggressive bony resection with violation of deltoid origin can cause undesirable outcome
- Many large studies indicate good to excellent results for ASD in over 85% patients.

Rotator Cuff repair:

- Surgery for rotator cuff repair has evolved from open to mini-open to all arthroscopic
- Arthroscopic rotator cuff surgery can be challenging as cuff tears present in a variety of shapes and sizes with variable tendon quality
- Number of classifications exist for rotator cuff tears but it is important to understand the tear geometry to enable good repair
- Traumatic cuff tears in the active population causing functional loss, irrespective of the age of the patient, constitute an indication for rotator cuff repair
- Key principles in arthroscopic cuff repair include assessment of the tear, release and tendon mobilisation, secure attachment of the tendon to the prepared footprint and regaining movement and its control
- Number of portals are utilised for arthroscopic rotator cuff repair though most can be accomplished by the four portal technique
- Direct tendon to bone repair, margin convergence, single row and double row repair are some of the commonly used repair techniques
- Arthroscopic surgery has facilitated 'Accelerated rehabilitation programmes', which are gradually replacing the more traditional post-operative immobilisation protocols following rotator cuff repair.

Arthroscopic subacromial decompression

Arthroscopic resection and repair techniques have completely transformed our management of rotator cuff disease, and continue to evolve and improve. Arthroscopic subacromial decompression (ASD) is the operation of choice when dealing with primary subacromial impingement syndrome of the shoulder. A carefully taken history will reveal a patient aged between 40 and 50 years with pain on reach and exercise, difficulty getting to sleep but little awakening, a painful arc on elevation that interferes with recreation, yet the patient continues in their normal work routine. Clinical examination will show positive impingement signs. Investigations should include radiographs to look at the acromial shape and an ultrasound scan to exclude a rotator cuff tear. Local anaesthetic with or without steroid injections in the subacromial space (Neer's test) will further confirm the diagnosis and is a good predictor of the outcome of ASD.

Conservative treatment involves turning the dysfunctional cuff into a functional cuff again. Two facets need to be addressed: pain and function. The pain can be eased by injection of cortisone (in any form) into the subacromial bursa, and refraining from those activities that aggravate the condition (reach, sport, and overhead work). Therapists can then supervise muscle retraining, starting with scapular control, and then working on to glenohumeral control.

Indications for surgery

Indications for surgery are failure of proper conservative treatment, in the patient aged over 40 who has true impingement, which has been abolished temporarily by subacromial injection of local anaesthetic. While an impinging acromial spur is an indication for ASD, patients can present with impingement symptoms without bony spurs and require ASD (Figure 4.3.1). ASD is also indicated in secondary impingement after failed non-operative treatment including calcific tendinitis. It is important to ensure that the

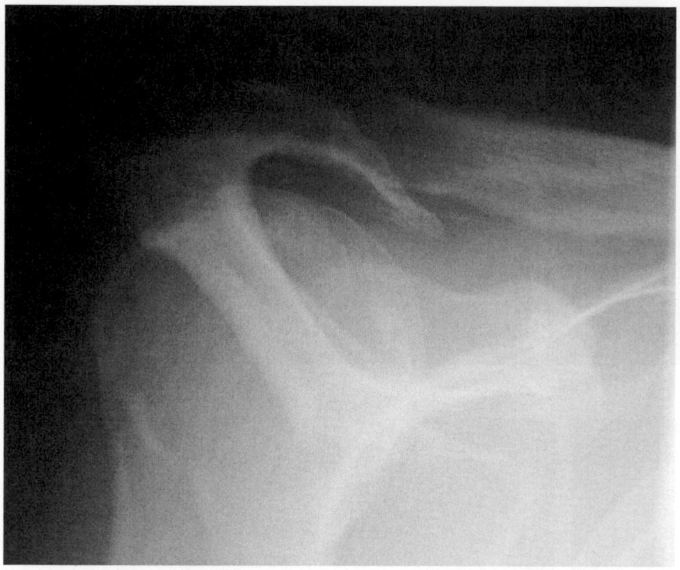

Fig. 4.3.1 Large acromial spur.

patient has full passive motion and no capsular stiffness when considering arthroscopic subacromial surgery. If they are stiff the diagnosis is wrong!

Contraindications

There are no absolute contraindications to ASD; however, the results of ASD in the following situations are usually poor and should be avoided:

- *Glenohumeral stiffness*: impingement should not be diagnosed in the presence of restricted motion
- *Secondary impingement as a result of instability*: subclinical instability is often seen in overhead athletes and can lead to subacromial impingement. The primary pathology must be dealt with before considering ASD
- *Hyperlaxity*: the results of ASD in patients with hyperlax joints are not as favourable and can be disappointing
- *Impingement secondary to a large os acromiale*: this type of impingement is a 'dynamic impingement' due to flexion of the os with deltoid contraction. Fusion of the os acromiale is unpredictable with failure of fusion in up to 50% of cases. Excision of the os, maintaining the deltoid insertion from the deltopectoral fascia, may be more appropriate but the evidence either way is poor.

History

Dr Harvard Ellman, who published his results in 1987, pioneered this technique and now this is the benchmark throughout the advanced world. In the properly selected patient, ASD should give excellent or good results in 88% of patients. These days there is no place for open decompression except as a method of exposure for open cuff repair. Open acromioplasty evolved from Neer's first description where a wedge of anterior acromion was removed using an osteotome, and ended with the two-stage Rockwood acromioplasty. In this technique the first stage was to remove the full thickness of the acromion that extends anterior to the acromioclavicular joint (ACJ). The second stage is to remove a wedge of anterior acromion extending from the initial cut and exiting the inferior surface of the acromion 1.5cm (three burrs' breadths) posterior to the anterior cut. This technique is now copied arthroscopically.

Impingement classification: Copeland–Levy

The Copeland and Levy classification is a useful descriptive arthroscopic grading system for impingement lesions on both the acromial and bursal surfaces ('kissing lesions') (Figure 4.3.2 and Figure 4.3.3).

Complications

The complication rates for ASD are very low, with reports ranging from 0.7–3%.

Complications of interscalene regional blocks and general anaesthesia are rare, but with increasing use are sometimes encountered. Interscalene blocks can cause a Horner's syndrome when the stellate ganglion is affected by the local anaesthetic, or a hemidiaphragmatic palsy if the phrenic nerve is anaesthetized.

Rarely, nerve compression problems have been reported with the lateral decubitus position, including superficial radial nerve compression, contralateral lateral femoral cutaneous nerve neuralgia, and contralateral peroneal nerve palsy. This is easily avoided with due diligence in positioning. Erroneous portal placement may make surgery more difficult. This is especially so when swelling due to fluid extravasation distorts the anatomical landmarks. Bleeding in the subacromial space during surgery can be troublesome and is caused by lacerating the acromial branch of the thoracoacromial trunk with the shaver. This vessel runs around the circumference of the acromion between the deltoid and the coracoacromial ligament. This can be controlled with electrocautery at the anterior acromial edge. Bleeding can also occur from the bone itself and this is controlled by increasing the pump pressure. An aggressive release of the anterior structures may release a portion of the deltoid as well, producing a deltoid sag anteriorly. ASD should not be performed in cuff-deficient shoulders as it can result in proximal migration of the humeral head and predispose to anterosuperior escape of the humeral head. If subacromial debridement is indicated, humeral escape can be minimized by leaving a portion of the coracoacromial ligament intact and performing a reverse acromioplasty or tuberoplasty. Wound infection is low in shoulder arthroscopy and reported to be less than 1%. Capsulitis with resultant stiffness in the shoulder is well documented post ASD.

Failure of treatment

Erroneous diagnosis leading to the failure of ASD is the most common complication of arthroscopic acromioplasty. Up to 50% of acromioplasty failures can be attributed to incorrect diagnosis. Other causes of failure after ASD are inadequate or excessive bone removal from the anterior acromion, scarring between the cuff and the acromion and the failure of rehabilitation.

Technique

Setup

Regional interscalene block with or without a general anaesthetic is commonly used in the beach chair or lateral decubitus position. It is essential to ensure the following:

- All pressure points are well protected
- Prolonged strong traction should be avoided (lateral decubitus)

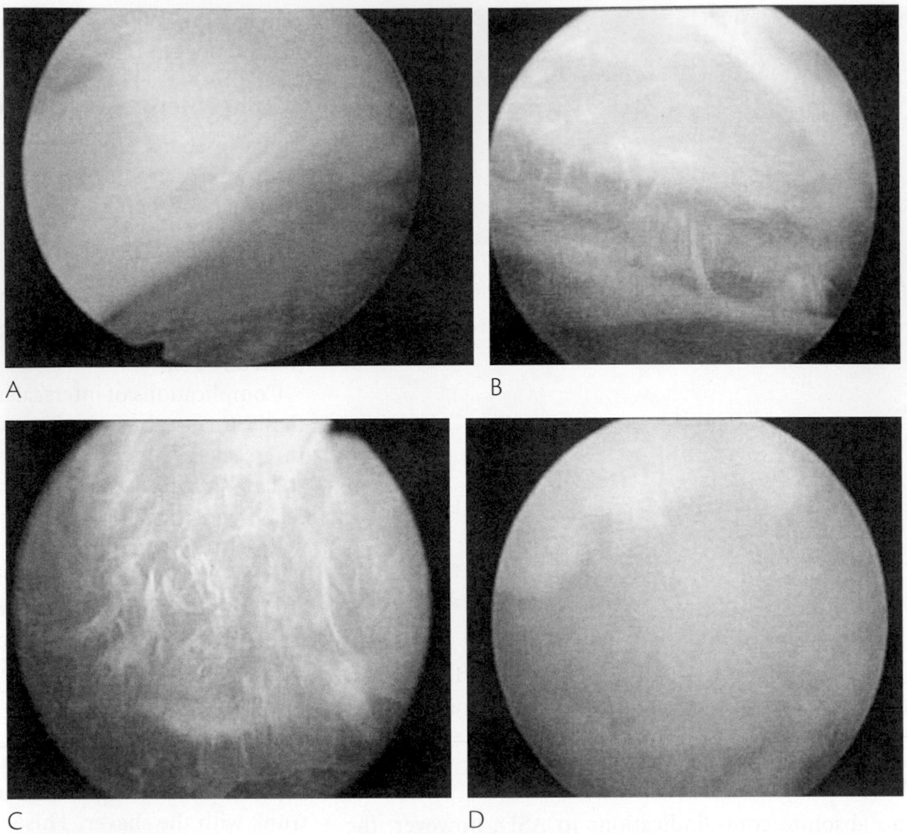

Fig. 4.3.2 Copeland and Levy impingement classification (Acromial side). A) A0 Normal - smooth surface; B) A1 Minor scuffing, or local inflammation; C) A2 Marked scuffing/ damage to acromial undersurface; D) A3 Bare bone areas. See also colour plate section.

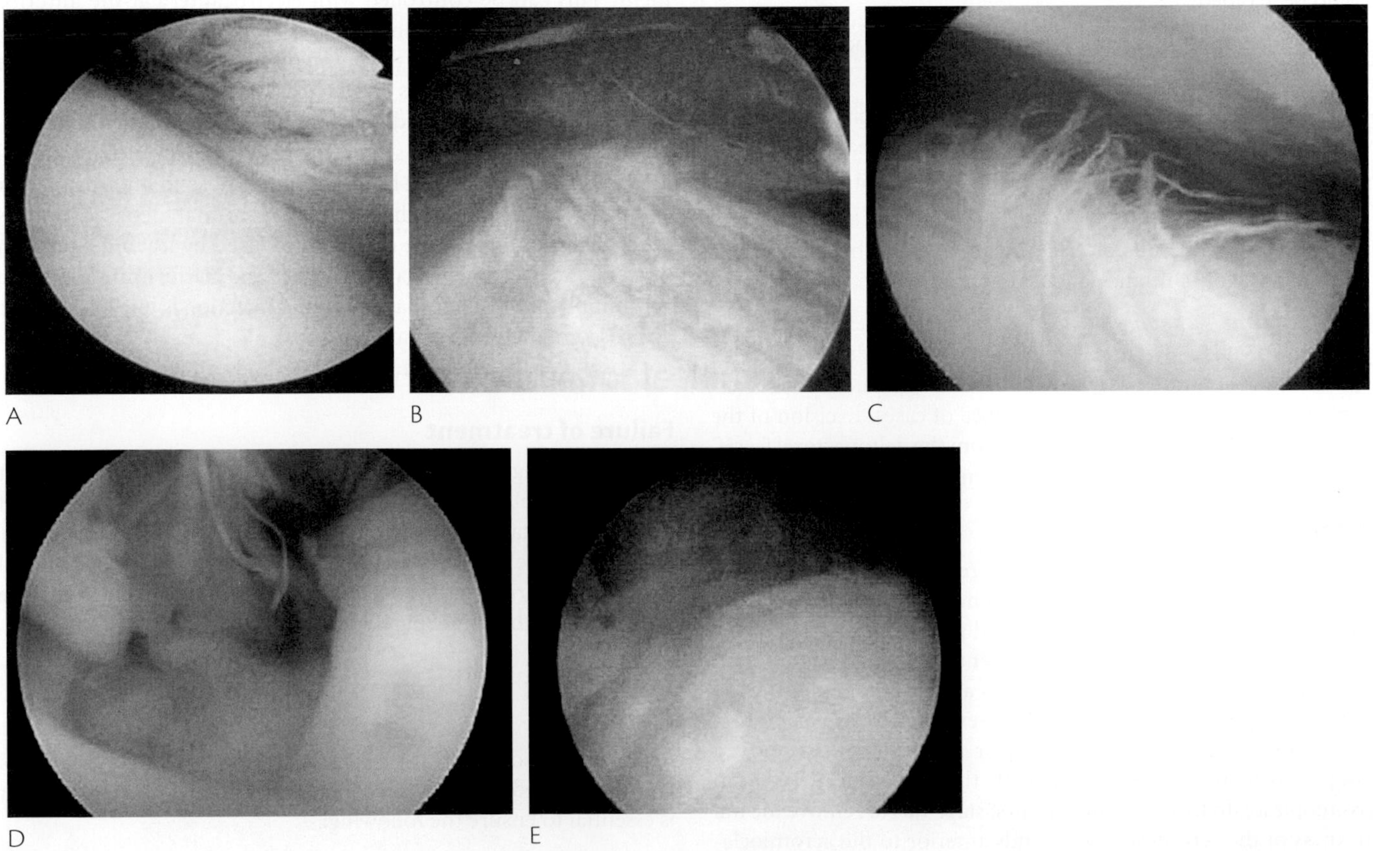

Fig. 4.3.3 Impingement classification (Bursal side). A) B0 Normal, smooth surface; B) B1 Minor scuffing; C) B2 Major scuffing of cuff, partial thickness tear; D) B3 Full thickness tear; E) B4 Massive cuff tear. See also colour plate section.

- Patient should be adequately warmed, usually with a warm air blanket
- Large saline usage can be reduced with good anaesthesia and control of bleeding with thermal radiofrequency.

Portals

It is useful to palpate and mark the outline of the lateral clavicle, acromion, scapular spine, the ACJ, and the coracoid with a marking pen. This helps in accurate portal placement.

Three portals are commonly used (Figure 4.3.4), in the following order:

1) *Posterior portal* is the common starting portal and is in the 'soft spot' of the shoulder—2cm below the posterolateral corner of the acromion and 2cm medial to this line. This gives the ability for a initial glenohumeral arthroscopy for the diagnosis of possible associated glenohumeral articular cartilage damage, labral tears, and the opportunity to assess the rotator cuff tear from its undersurface, along with the intra-articular long head of biceps tendon and subscapularis
2) *Anterior portal* is lateral to the coracoid process and below the coracoacromial (CA) ligament, at the level of the ACJ externally and within the rotator interval internally. This portal is used for instrumentation from anteriorly and can also be used for ACJ excision
3) *Lateral portal* is approximately 2cm posterior to the anterior lateral corner of the acromion and 4–6cm inferior to the lateral border of the acromion. It is best to create the portal using an outside-in technique with a spinal needle. This portal is used for instrumentation.

Glenohumeral arthroscopy

A systematic arthroscopy of the glenohumeral joint is performed, with palpation of structures via the anterior portal.

Bursoscopy

The subacromial space is entered via the posterior portal. To adequately classify the impingement the scope must be within the subacromial bursa. To ensure this, it is essential to withdraw the arthroscopic sheath completely out of the shoulder and whilst palpating the posterior edge of the acromion, direct the sheath and introducer upwards into the subacromial space. The undersurface of the acromion can be felt against the introducer tip and directing the tip towards the anterior and lateral aspect of the acromion will ensure correct placement of the scope, as this is the most capacious part of the bursa. We introduce the scope with the camera looking down on to the cuff and visualization of the white dome of the cuff confirms correct placement. Occasionally, inflamed and thick bursal tissue will obscure the view of the rotator cuff. In this situation, sweeping the introducer sheath in the bursa might help to break adhesions. The structures to be identified in the subacromial space are the CA ligament, the rotator cuff, and the anterior edge and the lateral edge of the acromion, as these will help orientation within the small space (Figure 4.3.5). The camera is then turned 180 degrees to look at the undersurface of the acromion. Before using the resector examine the opposing surfaces of the rotator cuff and the acromion for impingement lesions that are classified according to the Copeland– Levy classification system. The bursal surface of the cuff is examined for any tears.

Acromial resection

The lateral portal is created and used for soft tissue and bone resectors. ASD consists of subacromial bursectomy, CA ligament recession or resection, and anterior acromioplasty. Having assessed the impingement lesion, the subacromial bursa is debrided from the acromial undersurface and the surface of the rotator cuff. It is particularly essential to debride the posterior curtain of bursal tissue that can obstruct the view while working in the subacromial space. There is no need for a cannula in the lateral portal as it can sometimes restrict the movement of the shaver within the bursa. A soft tissue shaver or a radiofrequency wand can be used for soft tissue debridement. The wand provides the facility of coagulating any bleeders that might disrupt visualization. The CA ligament is peeled off from the acromial undersurface. Care is taken to preserve the deltoid muscle fibres. Using sweeping movements, the acromion is cleared to define the anterior spur. It is also important to carry this process laterally to clearly define the lateral bony edge of the acromion. Medially, the debridement is limited to the ACJ.

The CA ligament is released, rather than excised, as patients have complained of postoperative 'clicking' with excision of the ligament. It has been shown that the ligament regenerates and reattaches to the acromion over time. Bleeding from the acromial branch of the thoracoacromial artery may disrupt visualization and this can be controlled with fluid pressure management or electrocautery.

The amount of acromion resection can be determined by the amount of anterior acromion 'hanging' below the anterior deltoid

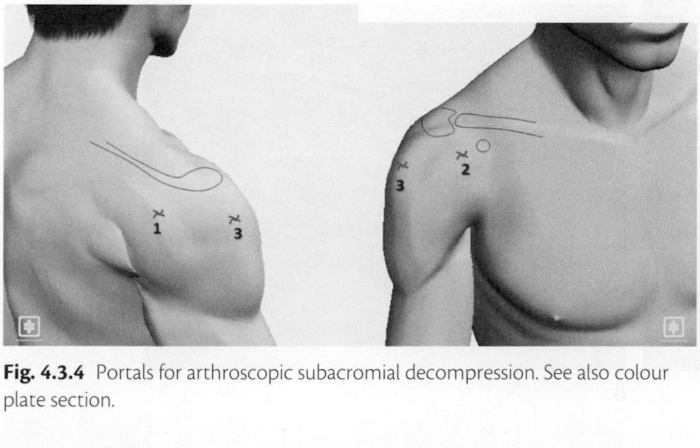

Fig. 4.3.4 Portals for arthroscopic subacromial decompression. See also colour plate section.

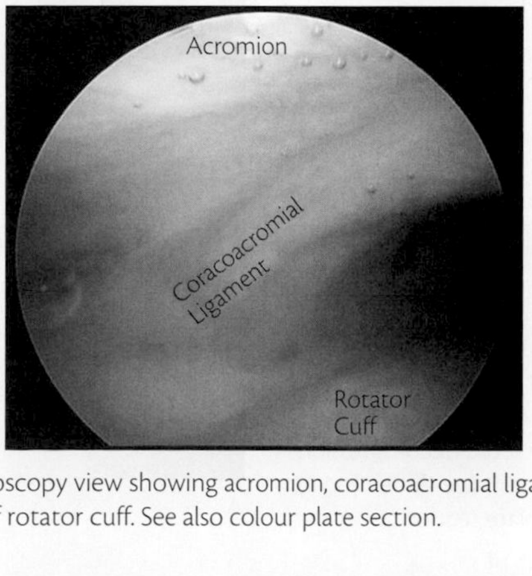

Fig. 4.3.5 Bursoscopy view showing acromion, coracoacromial ligament, and bursal surface of rotator cuff. See also colour plate section.

origin. This is assessed by placing the shaver tip between the anterior acromion and the deltoid (Figure 4.3.6).

Acromioplasty is performed by beginning laterally at the anterolateral corner of the acromion and progressing medially to the ACJ capsule. To achieve a flat acromion, more bone must be resected anteriorly than posteriorly. The anterior resection is progressively tapered posteriorly. The resection is carried out so as to have a smooth transition zone without bony ridges. The arthroscope is now switched to the lateral portal. The resector is introduced via the posterior portal and the sheath of the resector is laid flush against the posterior acromial undersurface. If an adequate decompression has been achieved the posterior undersurface can be used as a 'cutting block' to continue resection until satisfactory clearance is achieved (Figure 4.3.7).

Results

The results of ASD are good to excellent in over 85% of patients in many large studies. The better results are in studies where strict inclusion and exclusion criteria are used, excluding secondary impingements, stiff shoulders, rotator cuff tears, and workers' compensation cases.

ASD is accepted as a well-established method for the treatment of primary impingement syndrome. It allows the surgeon to evaluate the glenohumeral joint and address any intra-articular pathology at the same time. Patient selection on the basis of correct diagnosis of primary impingement syndrome is the key to a successful result. While the advantages of ASD are well documented, issues of a learning curve and adequacy of bone resection are pertinent.

Arthroscopic rotator cuff repair

In Chapter 4.2 we covered the pathomechanics of rotator cuff tears. In order to manage cuff tears we need to understand the pathology, nature of the tear, and the type of tear.

The operative approach for rotator cuff repairs has evolved from the classic open approach to a miniopen, or deltoid-sparing, approach, then finally to an 'all-arthroscopic' repair. This evolution has resulted from an improved understanding of rotator cuff

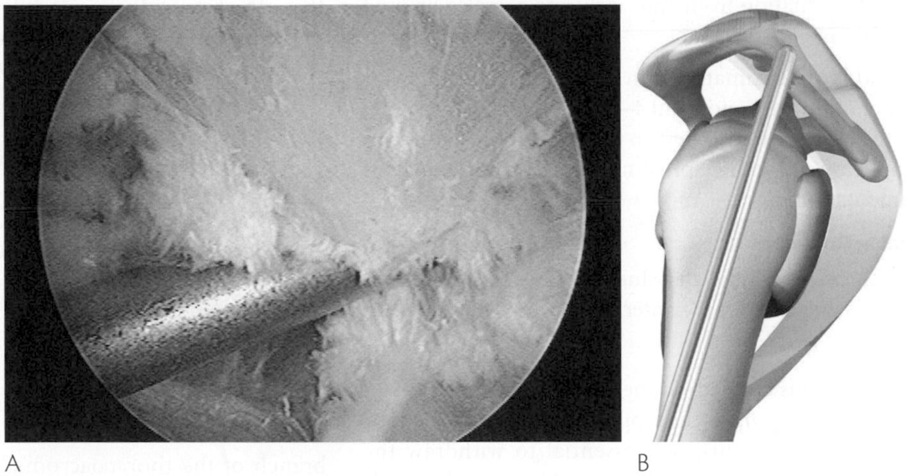

Fig. 4.3.6 Assessing resection level using shaver (scope and three-dimensional). See also colour plate section.

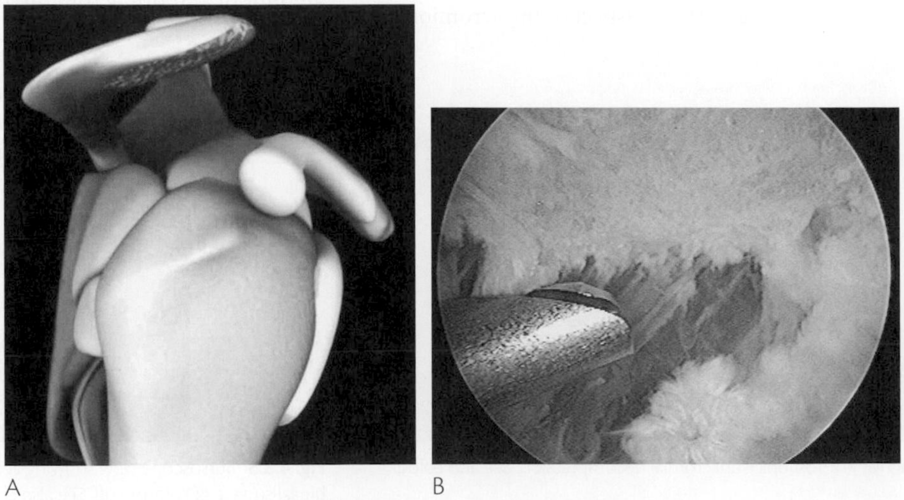

Fig. 4.3.7 Completed decompression images (scope and three-dimensional). See also colour plate section.

tear patterns and advancements in arthroscopic instrumentation and techniques. The ability to repair the rotator cuff without detachment of the deltoid is a tremendous benefit to the patient, offering decreased pain associated with the cuff repair, avoidance of complications related to deltoid reattachment, and optimization of the rehabilitation process.

Classifications

The key to understanding the pattern of rotator cuff tearing is the central oblique tendon (Figure 4.3.8), which runs from the middle of the muscle to the anterior leading edge of the tendon at its insertion. The most common cuff tears involve the supraspinatus and infraspinatus tendons. Such tear patterns are known as posterosuperior rotator cuff tears. *Posterosuperior cuff tears* originate behind the thickened anterior oblique cord of supraspinatus and extend posteriorly. The term *anterosuperior rotator cuff tear* is defined as a lesion of the cuff that includes full thickness tears of the supraspinatus, extending anteriorly to involve the rotator interval structures and potentially the subscapularis tendon.

In order to optimally manage rotator cuff tears it is essential to understand the tear pattern and be able to document this. Many classifications exist for various aspects of cuff pathology. The following classifications are some that have relevance in our clinical practice.

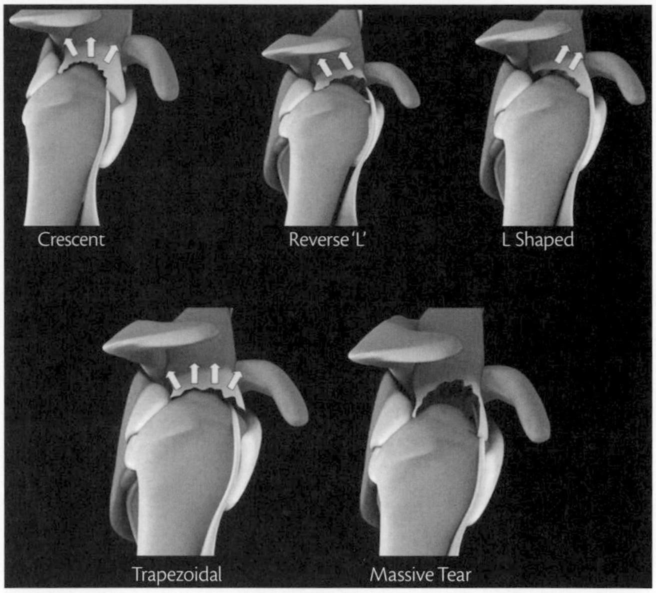

Fig. 4.3.9 Tear patterns (adapted from Ellman and Gartsman). See also colour plate section.

Tear size: Cofield classification of tear size

- Small: <1cm
- Medium: 1–3cm
- Large: 3–5cm
- Massive: >5cm.

Tear propagation pattern: Ellman and Gartsman classification (Figure 4.3.9)

- Crescent
- Reverse L
- L-shaped
- Trapezoidal
- Massive tear full thickness rotator cuff tears.

Cuff tear retraction in the frontal plane: Patte classification (Figure 4.3.10)

- Stage 1: proximal stump close to bony insertion
- Stage 2: proximal stump at level of humeral head
- Stage 3: proximal stump at glenoid level.

Topographic classification of rotator cuff tears in the sagittal plane: Habermeyer classification (Figure 4.3.11)

- Sector A: anterior lesions—subscapularis tendon, rotator interval and long head of the biceps tendon
- Sector B: central superior lesions—supraspinatus tendon
- Sector C: posterior lesions—infraspinatus and teres minor lesions.

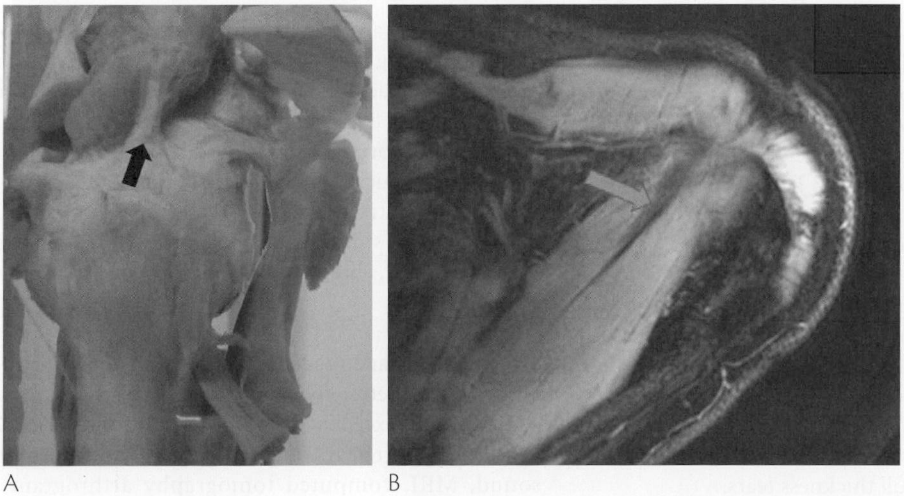

Fig. 4.3.8 Central oblique cord of supraspinatous (macroscopic, ultrasound, and arthroscopic views). See also colour plate section.

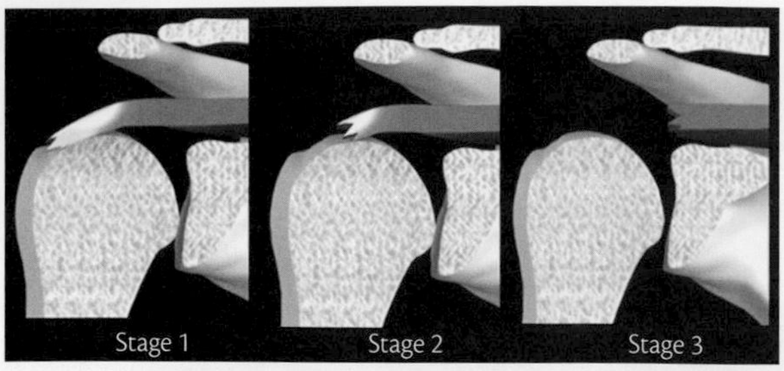

Fig. 4.3.10 Patte classification (adapted from Patte). See also colour plate section.

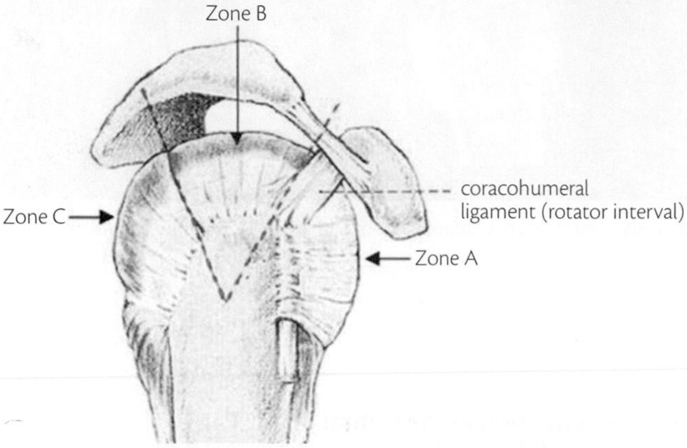

Fig. 4.3.11 Habermeyer classification (adapted from Habermeyer). See also colour plate section.
Source: Habermeyer, P., Magosch, P., and Lichtenberg. S. (2006). *Classifications and scores of the shoulder*, p. 19. Springer, Heidelberg, Germany.

Fatty muscle atrophy: Goutallier classification

- Stage 0: normal muscle
- Stage 1: some fatty streaks
- Stage 2: less than 50% fatty muscle atrophy
- Stage 3: 50% fatty muscle atrophy
- Stage 4: greater than 50% fatty muscle atrophy.

Indications

The presence of chronic degenerative cuff tears is well accepted and over 24% of patients over the age of 60 years will have an asymptomatic, full thickness, degenerative cuff tear. These people generally do not require a rotator cuff repair and have compensated for the functional loss of cuff muscles adequately. However, a traumatic episode with extension of the chronic tear may tip the balance and lead to weakness and pain. This group often do benefit from functional restitution.

Within the active population, no matter the patient's age, an active sporting individual with a traumatic rotator cuff tear is an indication for rotator cuff repair. A fully functional cuff is necessary to return to demanding functional activities. Rotator cuff tears also increase in size over time. Partial thickness tears have been shown to progress to full thickness tears, and small full thickness tears progress to large to massive full thickness tears.

Even prior to the imaging available now, Codman stated that in a traumatic cuff tear in an active patient:

> If such a syndrome is present I do feel that not only is exploration indicated but that it should be strongly urged, for immediate suture should be a simple and successful operation. Delay means retraction of the tendon and a much more serious problem.

The advent of advanced imaging in the form of magnetic resonance imaging (MRI) and ultrasound scans has made the diagnosis of the presence of a cuff tear easier, but not the ability to easily differentiate between a chronic degenerative tear and an acute traumatic tear. This still relies on good, sound clinical judgement.

The decision to proceed to a rotator cuff repair should be made prior to confirmatory imaging. Ultrasound can confirm the presence and size of the tear, along with associated pathology such as biceps involvement. MRI is useful to assess the quality of the rotator cuff muscles for muscle atrophy and fatty infiltration.

Muscle atrophy and fatty infiltration of the torn rotator cuff muscles has been shown to be associated with higher rates of failure of repair and poorer functional outcomes. There is also a correlation between muscle atrophy, fatty infiltration, and age; cuff tear size; and length of symptoms. However, rotator cuff muscle atrophy has also been shown to be a product of increasing age even in the absence of a tear. This should all factor into the decision-making process and prognostication, but one should not make a decision for surgery based on the muscle atrophy and fatty infiltration alone.

The indications for surgery are:

1) Active person (usually between the ages of 40–70 years)
2) Usually an episode of injury
3) Rotator cuff weakness and pain, which interfere with daily life
4) A proven rotator cuff tear on MRI or ultrasound.

Requirements for surgery:

1) Full passive range of glenohumeral motion
2) Surgeon with adequate skills, experience, and facilities
3) Postoperative rehabilitation
4) Compliant patient.

Contraindications

Absolute contraindications for arthroscopic rotator cuff repair include ongoing active infection and medical contraindications to appropriate anaesthesia. It should not be undertaken unless adequate facilities, equipment, and instruments are available and the surgeon appropriately skilled and trained in undertaking arthroscopic reconstructive shoulder procedures.

Relative contraindications include: significant glenohumeral arthrosis, joint stiffness, massive tears with significant retraction, muscle atrophy, and fixed humeral head elevation.

Results

The results of arthroscopic rotator cuff repair are equivalent to, and possibly better than, traditional open repairs. Most studies show good to excellent results in over 90% of cases. Cuff integrity has been reported to range from 71–94%, as assessed by ultrasound, MRI, computed tomography arthrogram or magnetic

Table 4.3.1 Results of arthroscopic rotator cuff repair for full thickness tears summarized

Author (year)	No.	Mean age (years)	Average follow-up (months)	Excellent and good clinical results	Cuff integrity (imaging method)
Wolf et al. 2004	96	57.6	78	94%	Not done
Bouileau et al. 2005	65	60	29	92%	71% (CTA)
Charousset et al. 2008	114	59.4	24	94%	75% (CTA)
*LaFosse et al. 2007	105	52	23	94%	89% (CTA)
*Huijsmans et al. 2007	264	59	22	91%	92% (ultrasound)

*Indicates studies with double-row rotator cuff repair technique only. CTA, computed tomography arthrogram.

resonance arthrogram. The variation in the literature is due to differences in patient selection, techniques, follow-up, and imaging methods. However, it is clear that the failure of repair integrity is associated with the following factors: tear size and retraction, advancing age, muscle atrophy, and fatty infiltration and quality of the tendon tissue.

Table 4.3.1 summarizes some recent large studies with results of arthroscopic cuff repair surgery of full thickness tears.

Most of the more recent studies appear to show that improved results can be obtained with double-row repairs, stronger anchors and sutures, and improved techniques. Advancements in our understanding of the cuff tear biology and developments in the field of orthobiologics may show further improvements in these results over the forthcoming years.

Principles

Bigliani described five factors that facilitate favourable results in rotator cuff repair surgery. These are:

1) Perform an adequate subacromial decompression
2) Maintain the integrity of the deltoid origin
3) Mobilize the torn tendons
4) Repair the tendons to bone
5) Carefully stage and supervise the rehabilitation programme.

Bunker described six principles:

1) Assess the cuff tear
2) Release the capsular contractures
3) Reintroduce healing biology
4) Reattach the tendon to its anatomical footprint
5) Protect the repair
6) Regain movement and its control.

These were described for open cuff surgery, but the principles are identical for arthroscopic repair. The only difference is the surgical approach.

Repair of the tendon only comprises one component of the factors listed. This highlights the importance of assessment of the tear retraction, pattern, and mobility; performing adequate releases to allow a repair without tension; and the biological preparation of the tendon and the bone for healing. 'Prior proper preparation prevents poor performance'!

Technique

Portals (Figure 4.3.12)

Portals are created in the following order, depending on their requirement:

1) *Posterior portal* for initial glenohumeral arthroscopy and later posterior instrumentation
2) *Lateral portal* is utilized for initial traction and debridement of the rotator cuff tendon edges. It is then used for preparation of the footprint area, the release of adhesions, and bursectomy. And viewing for a lateral '50-yard' view of the rotator cuff
3) *Superior lateral portal* is made outside-in, about 1cm lateral to the lateral border of the acromion. It is used for footprint preparation, tendon edge debridement and anchor insertion, and knot tying, obtaining a good 45-degree dead-man's angle for anchor insertion

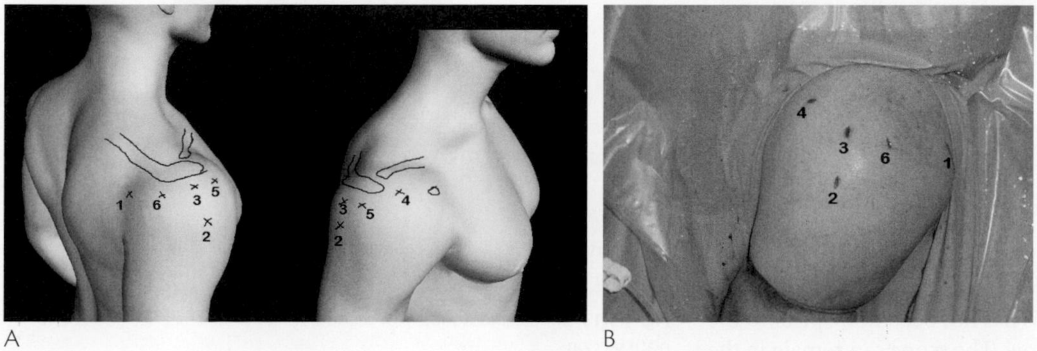

A B

Fig. 4.3.12 Portals for arthroscopic rotator cuff repair. See also colour plate section.

4) *Anterior portal* is used for instrumentation from anteriorly, suture passing through the anterior rotator cuff edges and biceps tenodesis. It can also be used for ACJ excision
5) *Anterior and posterior accessory lateral portals*: these portals are made about 1–2cm lateral to the anterolateral and posterolateral corners of the acromion. These portals can be used for additional anchor insertion, along with additional instrument passing and knot tying as necessary
6) *Neviaser portal* is very useful for suture passing in a retracted cuff tear. It is made in the triangle bordered by the clavicle anteriorly, scapula spine posteriorly and acromion laterally. It is also best made using an outside-in technique.

Small to moderate tears

- Most small to moderate-sized rotator cuff tears are of a crescent shape. These tears do not need much mobilization and can be directly repaired to the bone
- *Glenohumeral joint*: the tear is first examined from the glenohumeral joint via the posterior portal. The superolateral portal is then created to provide the ideal position for anchor insertion. The tendon edges can now be debrided via this portal and the humeral footprint area prepared
- *Bursa—anterior releases (and acromioplasty)*: the scope is then placed into the subacromial bursa via the posterior portal. The tear can be seen from superiorly now. Anterior bursal adhesions and the coracohumeral ligament can be released via the superolateral portal using a radiofrequency and/or a soft tissue shaver. The CA ligament is released off the acromion at this stage and the size of any acromial spur assessed. An acromioplasty can now be performed, although we prefer to leave this until after the cuff repair to avoid any bleeding from the exposed bone during repair
- *Bursa—lateral view, posterior releases*: the lateral portal is created and the scope moved to that portal. This gives a front-to-back panoramic view of the cuff and tear, known as the'50-yard' view. Posterior bursectomy and releases can now be performed via the posterior portal. The cuff is then reassessed for its mobility. It should reduce without any tension whatsoever
- *Bursa—anchor insertion*: an anchor can be inserted via the superolateral portal. It is preferential to use a cannula for this and insert the anchor at 45 degrees to the bone surface ('dead man's angle')
- *Suture passing and repair*: the anterior portal is now created for instrumentation and suture passing. For small tears, a suture passer can be passed from the anterior and posterior portals, retrieving sutures from the anchor. Simple suture repair, mattress repair, or a modified Mason–Allen (locking) repair can be performed. Our preference is for the last in this list, which provides a stronger repair than the other two. Careful suture management is essential here and some of the key points are:
  - Never have more than two suture limbs in a single portal
  - Ensure sutures are not twisted or caught in soft tissue before tying
  - Tie knots via the superolateral portal
- *Subacromial decompression*: if this has not been done prior to the cuff repair it can be performed now. The scope can remain in the lateral portal and the burr inserted via the posterior portal. A 'cutting block' technique can be used for the acromioplasty. Alternatively, the scope can be returned to the posterior portal and the acromioplasty performed via the lateral portal
- *Glenohumeral joint check*: the repair is then assessed from the glenohumeral joint, via the posterior portal. This is where restoration of the footprint can be assessed.

Double-row repair of small cuff tears (Figure 4.3.13)

For poor quality cuff tissue or to ensure a stronger repair with footprint restoration, a double-row repair can be performed. Suture bridge techniques with a medial and lateral anchor have simplified this. We prefer the technique described by Boileau (unpublished).

1) *Medial anchor*: a double-loaded anchor is inserted adjacent to the humeral articular surface through the superolateral portal. Both suture limbs of one suture strand are passed through the cuff anteriorly via the anterior portal. The two limbs of the other suture are passed through the cuff posteriorly via the posterior portal
2) *Medial row tying*: a suture limb of each strand is retrieved out of the superolateral portal. These are tied externally and the knot tucked down onto the cuff by pulling on the opposite suture limbs
3) *Lateral fixation (suture bridge)*: the free suture limbs are retrieved out of the superolateral portal. These are then passed through an anchor eyelet and the anchor inserted into the laterally. Anchors designed specifically for this purpose are ideal (e.g. PushLock ®, Arthrex; Versalok ®, Mitek).

Large tears

The technique for repairing large cuff tears depends on the tear pattern. Recognition of the correct tear pattern will help determine the most effective strategy for repair (Table 4.3.2). The principles and techniques apply equally for large and massive tears as for small tears (discussed earlier). Mobilization of the cuff may be required underneath the cuff, as well as above. Adequate cuff mobilization and preparation is the key to a good tension-free repair.

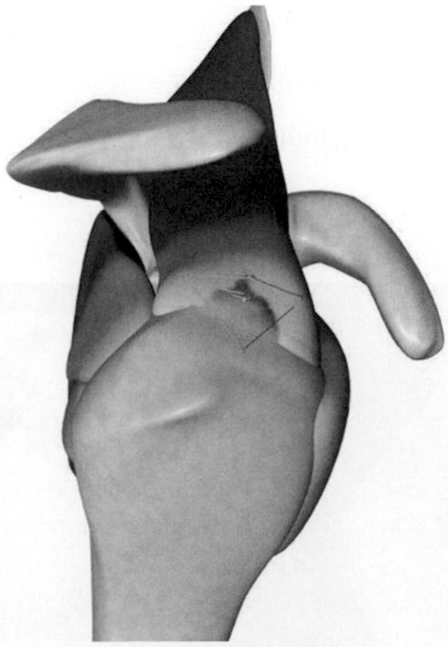

Fig. 4.3.13 Simple and double row techniques for small tears. See also colour plate section.

Table 4.3.2 Repair techniques

Crescent	Repair of free margin of cuff tendon directly to bone with suture from suture anchors
U-shape	Double-row repair, with suture bridge
V-shape	Side-to-side repair (margin convergence), then repair of the free lateral margin of the cuff tendon directly to the bone with sutures from an anchor
L-shape/ reverse L-shape	Anchor placement corresponding to the elbow of the 'L', followed by side-to-side sutures (if possible) and repair of the remaining lateral margin to bone with additional suture anchors. Or double-row repair centred over the elbow of the 'L'

Suture passing can be accomplished with numerous devices. Generally, there are three main categories:

1) *Cuff penetration and suture retrieval*: these instruments penetrate the cuff and retrieve the suture from the anchor. They should be passed through a portal remote and perpendicular to the viewing portal—generally the anterior, posterior, or Neviaser portal (e.g. CleverHook®, Mitek; PathSeeker®, Mitek; Arthro-Pierce®, Smith & Nephew)
2) *Suture shuttle relays*: a shuttle relay or suture is loaded through the instrument and passed through the cuff. The suture from the anchor is passed through the shuttle relay and passed back through the cuff (e.g. Spectrum system®, Conmed; Accu-Pass®, Smith & Nephew)
3) *Suture punches*: the original Caspari suture punch has evolved to many new forms. The anchor suture is loaded into the jaws of the punch. The tissue is grasped by the jaws and a modified needle pushes the suture through the cuff. This is done perpendicular to the cuff edges, usually via the lateral portals.

The majority of large tears can be repaired by margin convergence techniques or a double-row repair. We prefer a double-row repair wherever possible. Margin convergence cannot be performed if there is no adequate anterior cuff for side-to-side sutures. This is only present if the central oblique tendon of supraspinatus is not involved, i.e. anterosuperior tears. In these situations a double-row repair is preferred.

The long head of biceps is often involved in anterosuperior cuff tears and can be incorporated into the repair, as with open surgery. This is a 'dynamic' tenodesis.

Margin convergence (Figure 4.3.14)

The preparatory steps are the same as for a small tear, as listed earlier, but more extensive releases may be required. This can be achieved viewing from the lateral portal and mobilizing from the anterior, posterior, and superolateral portals.

Side-to-side (margin convergence) sutures are passed from the posterior to anterior portal, using a penetrating grasper or shuttle relay system. These are tied through the anterior portal, working from medial to lateral.

The tear is then converted to a small tear and this can then be repaired as a small tear with a suture anchor repair.

Double-row repair (Figure 4.3.15)

We prefer to use a simplified technique, which does not involve intra-articular knot tying. This is a modification of Boileau's two-anchor technique, using four anchors. This technique is suited to large C-shaped tears and some L tears.

Subscapularis

Arthroscopic repair of subscapularis (Figure 4.3.16) is technically feasible and results are as good as open repairs in the hands of suitably skilled and experienced surgeons. Subscapularis tears, similar to supraspinatus tears, originate on the articular side of the tendon and progress in a similar manner to other cuff tears. LaFosse has classified these on the basis of intraoperative evaluation and preoperative computed tomography scans (Table 4.3.3).

Type I–III lesions can be repaired from inside the glenohumeral joint, viewing from posteriorly and working from anteriorly. It is often useful to flex the shoulder to 90 degrees to improve visualization, and also externally rotate to improve access to the lesser tuberosity.

Table 4.3.3 Classification of subscapularis tears

Type	Lesion
I	Partial lesion of superior one-third
II	Complete lesion of superior one-third
III	Complete lesion of superior two-thirds
IV	Complete lesion of tendon but head centered and fatty degeneration classified as less than or equal to stage 3
V	Complete lesion of tendon but eccentric head with coracoid impingement and fatty degeneration classified as more than or equal to stage III

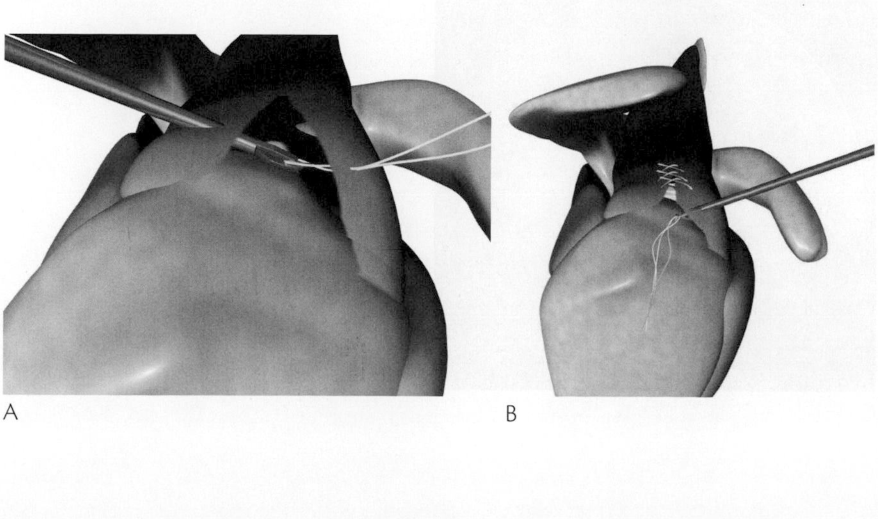

Fig. 4.3.14 Margin convergence techniques. See also colour plate section.

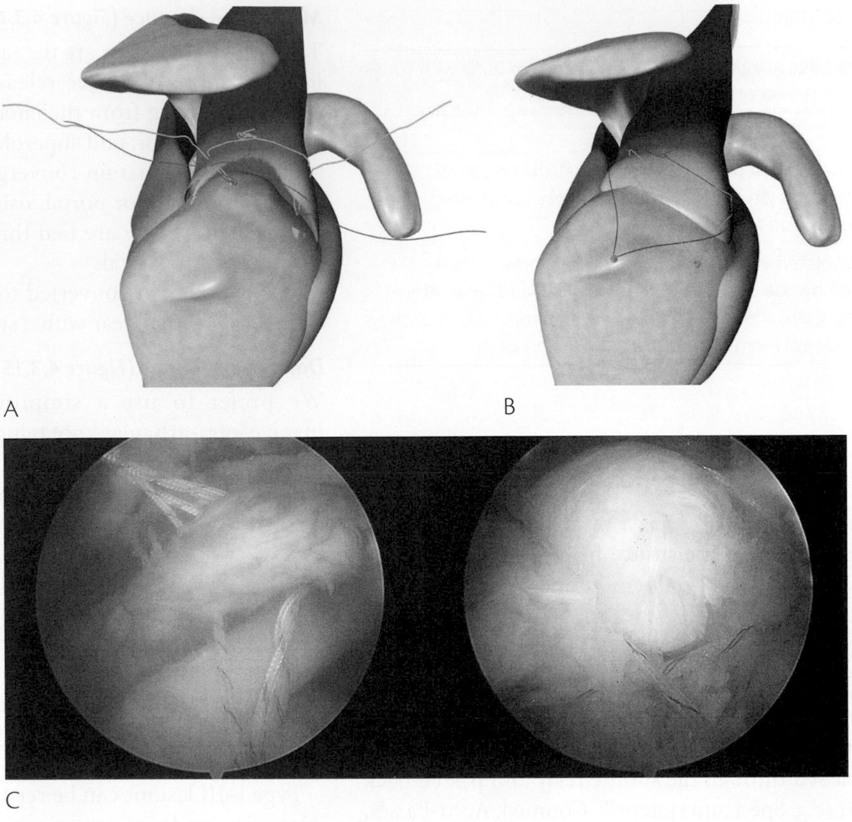

Fig. 4.3.15 Double-row technique for large tears. See also colour plate section.

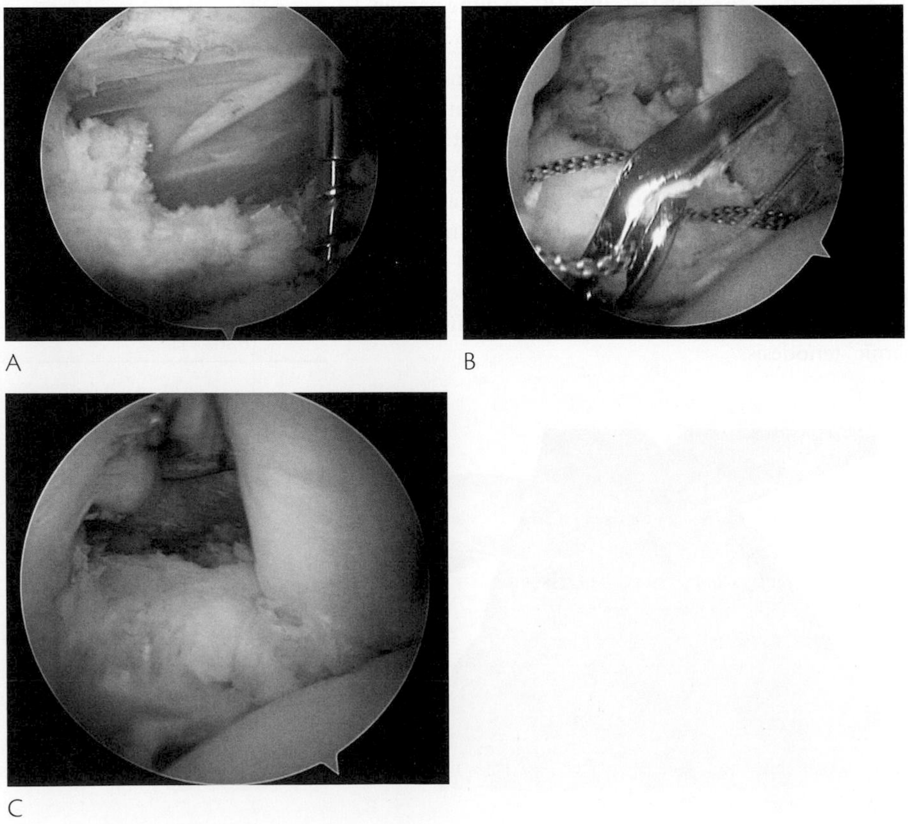

Fig. 4.3.16 Arthroscopic subscapularis repair. See also colour plate section.

In chronic tears, it might be difficult to easily identify the tendon edges. Using a radiofrequency probe the scarred tissue in the rotator interval can be debrided from lateral to medial, releasing the superior glenohumeral and coracohumeral ligaments from their humeral attachments, thus exposing and mobilizing the tendon. The scope can be moved to an anterolateral portal for an improved medial view and preparation continued. Often a second, more medial portal is required for anchor placement and suture passing. The coracoid and conjoined tendon should be identified before creating this portal and a spinal needle used to locate the safe placement lateral to the coracoid.

Repair of the tendon is performed from inferior to superior, with cuff suture-anchors in the lesser tuberosity. A footprint reconstruction can be achieved by using mattress sutures inferiorly and medially, followed by simple sutures laterally and superiorly.

The long head of biceps is often affected and is best managed with a tenodesis. This can be incorporated in the most superior suture anchor fixation. The suture-loop technique, popularized by LaFosse, ensures a strong fixation of the tendon.

Postoperative rehabilitation

Advances in our understanding of tendon healing and tendon responses to immobilization, along with developments in the field of shoulder rehabilitation, has allowed us to progress from the traditional enforced and prolonged periods of immobilization. Rehabilitation goals following surgery are to implement a continuum of exercises that restores optimal function while protecting the anatomic integrity of the injured or repaired tissues.

Rotator cuff repairs should not be performed under any tension and the tear should be assessed on-table through a range of motion (passive motion) confirming the security of the repair. The fixation should be rigid enough to allow this also (similar to fracture fixation surgery). There is evidence that moderate stresses can be placed on the suture line before the end of 3 weeks to improve collagen tissue healing and increased stresses within certain limits enhances healing and improves joint function.

New 'accelerated' rehabilitation programmes provide very low loads through the cuff as measured by electromyography. Each exercise combines passive motion, scapula control, core stability, and proprioception early postoperatively, thus establishing a better basis for strengthening later. The exercises allow a progression of intensity and load that is within the healing tissue's capabilities. Closed-chain exercises are an integral part of accelerated rehabilitation programmes. They can be started early and used throughout the rehabilitation process.

A key element in rehabilitation is the successful transition in the flow of exercises from the protected exercises of the acute phase to the functional phase. This can be achieved without complete immobilization. Accelerated rehabilitation promotes functional recovery and reduces postoperative pain, which allows patients an early return to desired activities. These exercises and protocols are available on the website http://www.shoulderdoc.co.uk. The protocol we use is shown in Box 4.3.1.

Box 4.3.1 'Accelerated Rehabilitation Protocol' following rotator cuff repair

Pre-op (Prehabilitation)

- Range of motion Exercises
- Maximise shoulder strength of deltoid, intact cuff muscles and scapula stabilisers.

Day 1 – 3 weeks

- Shoulder immobiliser abduction pillow (night use) – wean off as tolerated.
- Passive / Active Assisted ROM in all directions **as tolerated**
- Level 1 Exercises (<20% EMG), which combine and concentrate on proprioception, scapula setting and core stability. Closed chain exercises are incorporated.
- Wean off sling over 1-3 weeks, as tolerated.

3-6 weeks:

- **Do not force or stretch**
- Isometric exercises in neutral as pain allows – up to 50% maximum voluntary contraction
- Open Chain Exercises **as tolerated**
- (Level 2-3 Exercises)

6 weeks +:

- Progress to full active and resistance exercises in all ranges
- (Level 3Exercises)

	Milestones
4 Weeks	Passive ROM equal to pre op level
8 Weeks	Active ROM equal to pre op level

Return to functional activities

Driving	6 Weeks
Swimming	Breaststroke: 6 weeks Freestyle: 3 months
Golf	3 Months
Lifting	3 Months (Then guided by the strength of the individual patient)
Return to work	Sedentary job: 3 weeks Manual job: Guided by Surgeon

Acknowledgements

The senior author would like acknowledge his mentors who taught him the techniques and principles: Mr Stephen Copeland, Ofer Levy (Reading Shoulder Unit, UK), and Laurent LaFosse (Alps Surgery Institute, France).

Further reading

Bigliani, L.U. and Levine, W.N. (1997). Current concepts review – subacromial impingement syndrome. *Journal of Bone and Joint Surgery*, **79-A**, 1854–68.

Boileau, P., Brassart, N., Watkinson, D.J., Carles, M., Hatzidakis, A.M., and Krishnan, S.G. (2005). Arthroscopic repair of full-thickness tears of the supraspinatus: does the tendon really heal? *Journal of Bone and Joint Surgery*, **87-A**(6), 1229–40.

Bunker, T. (2002). Rotator cuff disease. *Current Orthopaedics*, **16**(3), 223–33.

Codman, E.A. (1934). *The Shoulder*. Brooklyn, NY: G. Miller & Company.

Cordasco, F.A. and Bigliani, L.U. (1997). The rotator cuff. Large and massive tears. Technique of open repair. *Orthopedic Clinics of North America*, **28**(2), 179–93.

Goutallier, D., Postel, J., Bernageau, J., Lavau, L., and Voisin, M.C. (1994). Fatty muscle degeneration in cuff ruptures. Pre- and postoperative evaluation by CT scan. *Clinical Orthopaedics and Related Research*, **304**, 78–83.

Huijsmans, P.E., Pritchard, M.P., Berghs, B.M., van Rooyen, K.S., Wallace, A.L., and de Beer, J.F. (2007). Arthroscopic rotator cuff repair with double-row fixation. *Journal of Bone and Joint Surgery*, **89-A**(6), 1248–57.

Lafosse, L., Brozska, R., Toussaint, B., and Gobezie, R. (2007). The outcome and structural integrity of arthroscopic rotator cuff repair with use of the double-row suture anchor technique. *Journal of Bone and Joint Surgery*, **89-A**(7), 1533–41.

Levy, O., Sforza, G., Dodenhoff, R.M., and Copeland, S.A. (2000). Arthroscopic evaluation of the impingement lesion: pathoanatomy and classification. *Journal of Bone and Joint Surgery*, **82-B**(Suppl. III), 233.

Matthews, L.S. and Blue, J.M. (1998). Arthroscopic subacromial decompression – avoidance of complications and enhancement of results. *Instructional Course Lectures*, **47**, 29–33.

Metcalf, M.H., Savoie, F.H., Smith, K.L., and Matsen F.A. III. (2002). 'Meta-analysis of the surgical repair of rotator cuff tears: a comparison of arthroscopic and open techniques.' Poster presentation at the Arthroscopy Association of North America 21st Annual Meeting, Washington, D.C. April 25–28, 2002.

Rockwood, C.A. Jr. and Lyons, F.R. (1993). Shoulder impingement syndrome: diagnosis, radiographic evaluation and treatment with a modified Neer acromioplasty. *Journal of Bone and Joint Surgery*, **75-A**, 409–24.

Sher, J.S., Uribe, J.W., Posada, A., Murphy, B.J., and Zlatkin, M.B. (1995). Abnormal findings on magnetic resonance images of asymptomatic shoulders. *Journal of Bone and Joint Surgery*, **77-A**(1), 10–15.

Yamaguchi, K., Tetro, A.M., Blam, O., Evanoff, B.A., Teefey, S.A., and Middleton, W.D. (2001). Natural history of asymptomatic rotator cuff tears: a longitudinal analysis of asymptomatic tears detected sonographically. *Journal of Shoulder and Elbow Surgery*, **10**(3), 199–203.

4.4

Biceps

Philip M. Ahrens

Summary points

- LHB pathology is a commonn cause of anterior shoulder pain
- Clinical evaluation and diagnostic imaging are both imprecise
- Isolated biceps pathology may be present in the younger athlete
- Degenerative biceps pathology is often associated with rotator cuff pathology
- Failure to treat concomitant LHB pathology is a cause for surgical failures in many other shoulder conditions

Introduction

The long head of the biceps tendon (LHB) is an enigmatic structure but is also an important cause of shoulder symptoms. Though its anatomy is well described, understanding of its surrounding restraints and structures such as the rotator interval are still being evaluated. More problematically for surgeons its function is still hotly debated, and poorly defined, leading to contention regarding potential surgical treatment.

This chapter will attempt to clarify the current understanding of the role and pathology of the LHB at the shoulder, and propose treatment strategies that are appropriate for the available evidence, and attainable for modern arthroscopic treatment modalities.

Anatomy

The LHB arises from the supraglenoid tubercle and the superior glenoid labrum. Its origin is, however, variable, and most anatomical studies have shown the labral origin to be more common. The intra-articular course is extrasynovial, and it exits the glenohumeral joint via the intertubercular (bicipital) groove, between the lesser and greater tuberosities, and carries a synovial reflection down within this groove.

At the point of exit from the joint a complex set of restraints exist. The 'biceps sling' comprising the superior glenohumeral ligament (SGHL), anterior band of the coracohumeral ligament, and capsule of the rotator interval, forms the anterior (or medial) restraint. The leading edge of the supraspinatus (anterior column) forms the posterior restraint. Failure of any of these structures may lead to instability. The course of the tendon within the bicipital groove is constrained, and vulnerable to many pathological abnormalities. At the inferior limit of the groove it passes beneath the tendon of the pectoralis major, before merging into the lateral muscle belly.

The intra-articular course of the tendon is oblique, variable depending on shoulder rotation and elevation, and is subject to significant shearing forces, which predispose the tendon to pathological changes.

The primary function of the biceps is at the elbow as a flexor and forearm supinator. The function of the long head at the shoulder is still unclear. Evolutionary change has rendered the LHB less functional at the shoulder in humans, and anatomical, biomechanical, neurophysiological, and radiological studies have produced conflicting results. The LHB contributes to 7–10% of abduction strength, but only with the humerus in external rotation. The head depressor effect of the LHB is also minimal, though more interest has recently been focused on its role as a secondary anterior stabilizer in the unstable shoulder.

Diagnosis

The clinical evaluation of LHB pathology is notoriously imprecise. Unfortunately current imaging investigations are only moderately more accurate, truly leaving dynamic arthroscopic diagnosis the gold standard investigation.

Clinical evaluation of the shoulder has been dealt with in Chapter 4.1, but there are certain specific points regarding diagnosis of LHB pathology that warrant further attention.

The history, typically, is of well-located, anterior shoulder pain that the patient can point to at the bicipital groove. This pain may radiate down the arm, along the biceps muscle belly, but can extend as far as the hand, usually along the radial border of the forearm towards the thumb. This referred pain needs to be distinguished from radicular pain of cervical origin. The painful clunk of a subluxing tendon is quite specific, but is an infrequent symptom. SLAP (superior labral tear from anterior to posterior) lesions may present with deep-seated pain on certain activities, or with pain associated with instability, or shoulder pain in a young patient with negative clinical signs of rotator cuff pathology.

Palpation of the tendon in the bicipital groove, classically described with the arm in 10 degrees of internal rotation, is a useful sign, but correlation with the contralateral shoulder is important. Clinical tests such as Speed's test, Yergason's test, and biceps instability test, are poorly validated, and a recent paper has reported sensitivity and specificity of 50–67% for palpation and Speed's tests in the diagnosis of partial thickness tears.

The clinical diagnosis of SLAP lesions is no easier. Many tests have been proposed, and many variations exist, the most widely defined being the O'Brien active compression test and the Biceps Load II. The AERS (abduction external rotation supination), Mayo shear, anterior superior SLAP test, and biceps tension tests are also commonly used.

Imaging

Plain radiography has a limited role in the diagnosis of LHB pathology. The two views that may show bony changes associated with arthritis, malunion of fractures, and loose bodies are the anteroposterior in external rotation and the Fisk view, an axial view centred on the bicipital groove.

Arthrography and computed tomography arthrography were the first imaging techniques to visualize the intra-articular tendon, but these have been largely superseded by ultrasound (US) and magnetic resonance imaging (MRI).

Both MRI and US can demonstrate the entire LHB tendon from origin to the musculotendinous junction, and gross pathology such as dislocation and rupture are well shown by both modalities. The spatial resolution, and dynamic capability of modern US now provides advantages in diagnosing partial tears, subtle dynamic instability, and the hourglass lesion. Unfortunately, studies have still only reported moderate accuracy of MRI (37% concordance with arthroscopic findings) and US (49% sensitivity). These findings are largely due to both techniques being poor at demonstrating partial thickness tears, which usually occur on the deep surface of the tendon.

Inflammation and intrinsic degeneration

As an intra-articular, but extrasynovial structure, the LHB is prone to tenosynovitis. The tendon is also subject to significant shearing forces in its oblique course though the glenohumeral joint. The forces acting on the tendon vary with arm position, notably rotation and elevation, though in the majority of functional positions the tendon bears upon the medial wall of the groove, that is, the lesser tuberosity and the biceps sling. Tenosynovitis is, by definition, an inflammatory condition and is reversible in the majority with conservative measures.

Tendinosis represents irreversible degenerate change within the tendon. This is commonly seen in association with subacromial impingement and degenerate rotator cuff disease. Progressive degenerate change may lead to 'hypertrophy', 'atrophy', and partial tendon tears and eventually rupture. Though the link between tendinosis and pain is less clear, partial thickness tears are often symptomatic and cause mechanical symptoms in the shoulder. These tears are usually on the deep surface of the tendon, often at the entry to the bicipital groove or within the groove itself, and therefore interfere with the smooth gliding of the tendon over the biceps pulley and within the groove.

Box 4.4.1 Pathology affecting the LHB

- Tenosynovitis (impingment)
- Tendinosis
- Partial tears/rupture
- Hypertrophy (hourglass)
- Instability
- Biceps anchor lesions (SLAP).

Rupture

Rupture of the LHB, often termed 'spontaneous', is a well-recognized clinical entity, producing the characteristic 'Popeye' sign of the descended lateral muscle belly. Males in their fifties and sixties, often with manual occupations, are most frequently affected, and often have no or only a short history of preceding symptoms. The rupture itself often heralds the resolution of symptoms, and many ruptures therefore never present to orthopaedic surgeons. The cosmetic deformity is also usually well tolerated in this patient population.

The functional deficit produced by rupture (and also by surgical tenotomy) is again only demonstrable at the elbow, with a loss of 20% of forearm supination strength and 8–20% of elbow flexion strength. This deficit is generally well tolerated in the elderly, but in the sporting population and manual workers may be more significant.

Hourglass biceps

The 'hourglass biceps' is a term describing mechanical entrapment of an enlarged or hypertrophic tendon within the glenohumeral joint on elevation. It is analogous to the bucket-handle meniscal tear or the triggering of a flexor tendon in the hand, leading to a loss of active and passive movement. The LHB glides passively into the bicipital groove on elevation of the arm, but enlargement of the tendon can block this excursion, and the tendon buckles and impinges between the humeral head and the superior glenoid. This leads to a loss of the terminal 10–20 degrees of elevation, often with associated discomfort. With time, tendon delamination and tears occur, though this phenomenon may also cause progressive damage to the tendon restraints, and tendon instability.

Instability of biceps

Dislocation of the LHB was the first recognized pathology of the LHB described in the first part of the nineteenth century. It remains one of the most common indications for surgical treatment of the LHB. Instability may be dynamic, defined as subluxation, or static, as in a fixed dislocation. The majority of instability is medial (anterior), though posterior (lateral) instability may occur with dislocations and supraspinatus tears. The failure of the biceps sling allows medial displacement of the tendon, which in turn causes abrasion of the LHB on the subscapularis tendon, first recognized by Walch as the 'hidden lesion', of a LHB dislocation and partial thickness, deep surface subscapularis tear.

Medial biceps instability has been classified by Walch (Figure 4.4.1) and may occur anterior to the subscapularis (the least

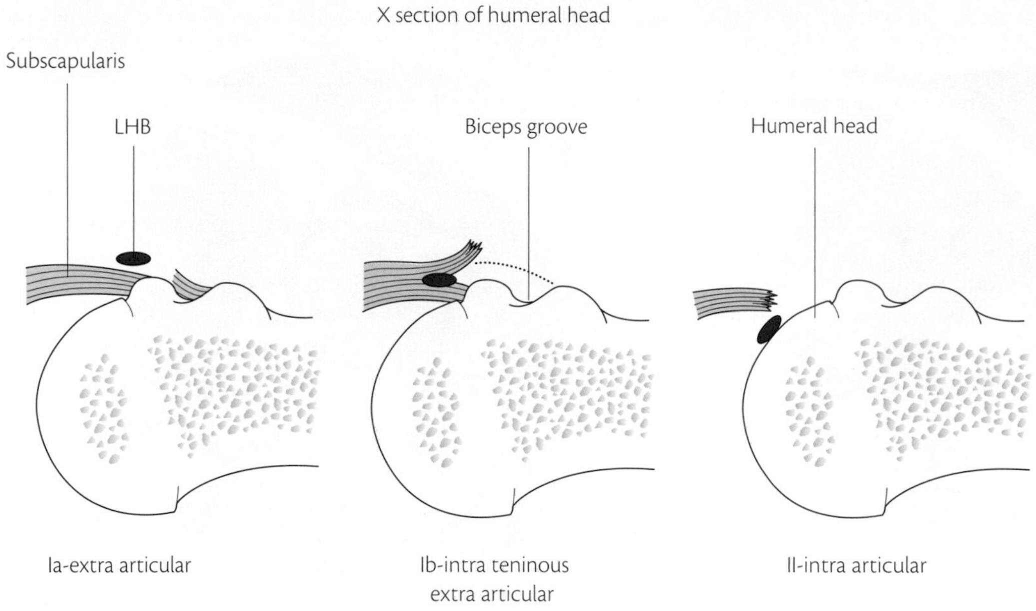

Fig. 4.4.1 Walch classification of biceps dislocation. Cross-section of humeral head.

common), into the substance of the tendon (partial subscapularis tear), or beneath the tendon a condition that has to be associated with a full thickness subscapularis tear.

The importance of lesser grades of instability is also now appreciated, especially in sporting injuries, and has been described to be present in up to 45% of arthroscopies for rotator cuff tears.

Sports injury

Anterosuperior internal impingement

Isolated LHB pathology is particularly important in the athlete. The overhead and throwing athlete are particularly vulnerable and instability, partial tears, and SLAP lesions are all common.

Anterosuperior internal impingement (ASI) is a novel diagnosis that has been brought to light by dynamic arthroscopic studies. At arthroscopy, abrasion is seen on the anterosuperior labrum, just in front of the biceps origin with a corresponding 'kissing' lesion at the LHB pulley. It is thought that these two structures shear against each other in the follow through phase of throwing when the arm is in adduction and internal rotation and rapidly decelerating. It is commonly seen in sports injuries but how to manage it remains contentious. At the present state of knowledge, the use of a sports physiotherapist to change the pattern of follow through may be the best management, but it is unpredictable.

Posterosuperior impingement

Another common condition in the athlete is posterosuperior impingement (PSI). This is a complex syndrome involving repetitive forced contact between the deep surface of the supraspinatus and posterior labrum and may lead to posterosuperior labral fraying, tears, and deep surface cuff pathology. A tight posterior capsule, anterior capsular laxity, and instability have all been implicated in its pathogenesis.

Superior labral anterior posterior lesions

It was only following the advent of shoulder arthroscopy that lesions of the superior labrum and biceps anchor were recognized. Snyder first described the 'SLAP' lesion in 1990, in relation to the throwing athlete, and it is now recognized as an important cause of shoulder dysfunction, and a common indication for surgery.

Snyder described four types of lesion, and although these have been expanded to include many subtypes and associated instability lesions, the original classification still describes the four major types of lesion well (Figure 4.4.2).

SLAP lesions may be produced either by the acceleration or deceleration phases of the throwing movement, as well as compression injuries with proximal displacement of the humeral head. There is also an overlap with anterior instability and superior extension of the classical Bankart lesion as well as posterosuperior impingement, which may lead to posterior SLAP lesions.

Type I SLAP lesions describe degenerative fraying of the superior labrum. They may be found prematurely in athletes, or in association with the normal ageing process. Anterosuperior fraying is most common in ageing, while posterosuperior fraying raises the possibility of PSI. Type II lesions are the most common lesions requiring surgical intervention. True bicipital/labral avulsions must be carefully distinguished from a mobile meniscoid labrum, which is a normal variant. Type III lesions are less common and the type IV lesion poses particular decision-making difficulties with respect to repair of the entire complex or labral repair and LHB tenodesis.

Surgery

Indications

The primary indications for surgical intervention in biceps pathology are mechanical lesion such as instability, entrapment,

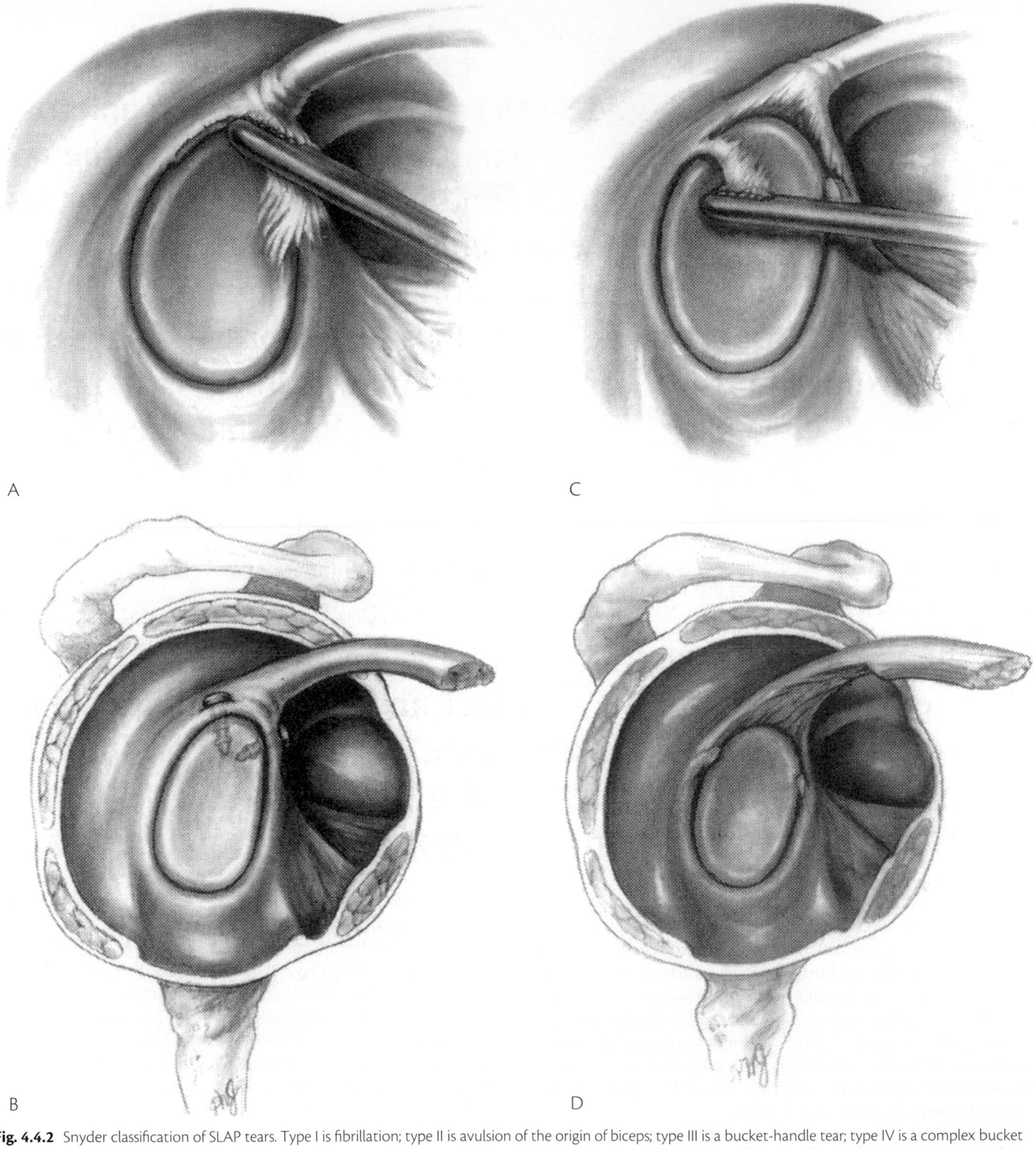

Fig. 4.4.2 Snyder classification of SLAP tears. Type I is fibrillation; type II is avulsion of the origin of biceps; type III is a bucket-handle tear; type IV is a complex bucket handle tear extending into the tendon. Reproduced from Snyder, S.J., Karzel, R.P., and Del Pizzo, W. (1990). SLAP lesions of the shoulder. *Arthroscopy*, **6**, 274–9, with permission from Elsevier.

and partial tendon tears. Secondary indications are refractory pain due to tenosynovitis and early tendinopathy, and treatment of concurrent rotator cuff disease, instability, and arthritis. Determining the relative contribution of the LHB to shoulder pain is difficult, but careful arthroscopic evaluation can prevent surgical failures due to missed LHB pathology.

A LHB rupture in a young patient or manual worker may also be an indication for early surgery, which should be performed within 6 weeks of rupture to be successful and restore strength.

Contraindications

As loss of the LHB from the shoulder has little, or no, consequences on shoulder function there are few contraindications for surgical intervention. Unnecessary intervention obviously subjects patients to the risk of the surgical procedure, but the possibility of neglecting bicipital pain must always be considered.

One contraindication to tenotomy is in the pseudoparalytic arm with anterosuperior escape due to a large rotator cuff tear. In this situation, active elevation will not be restored with a simple tenotomy. Tenotomy is also contraindicated in young active patients where a tenodesis should always be performed.

Tenotomy

Arthroscopic biceps tenotomy is the simplest, most reliable, and probably most common surgical intervention to the LHB. Releasing the tendon close to its origin allows the tendon to retract outside the glenohumeral joint, and will relieve bicipital symptoms at the shoulder effectively. This technique was popularized in the 1990s in Europe, and many studies have confirmed its effectiveness The limitations of this procedure are the cosmetic deformity often produced, a small incidence of persistent muscle belly cramping on activity, and the loss of elbow flexion and supination strength. It is of interest that not everyone who undergoes surgical tenotomy shows the cosmetic 'Popeye' sign after surgery. This is either due to the tendon still being held by vinculae, or, more commonly, a hypertrophied tendon retracts into the sulcus but then gets trapped there like a cork in a bottle.

Tenodesis

Open tenodesis was historically the treatment of choice for bicipital pathology. Many techniques were described, and many more have recently been described as arthroscopic techniques. There are broadly three groups of techniques: soft tissue techniques using suture fixation of the tendon to other tendons or the transverse humeral ligament; fixation of the tendon to bone using sutures and anchors; and fixation of the tendon within the bone of the proximal humerus (Figure 4.4.3). The first technique is evidently the simplest, and the last the most mechanically secure.

Box 4.4.2 Treatment options

- Physiotherapy
- Injection (US guided)
- Debridement ± subacromial decompression
- Tenotomy
- Tenodesis
- SLAP repair.

SLAP repair

The different classes of SLAP lesion require different surgical approaches. Type I lesions do not require intervention, or merely debridement if found in association with other pathology. Type II lesions require repair of both the superior labrum and biceps anchor. This is usually achieved with suture anchors placed anterior and posterior to the LHB origin. Type III lesions can usually be excised, though an attempt to repair very peripheral tears may be indicated. Finally the treatment of type IV tears will depend on the extent of damage to the biceps tendon itself. A combination of excision and repair may be used for the labral portion of the tear, and the decision between LHB tendon repair or tenodesis will depend on the extent of bicipital involvement both in terms of percentage cross-sectional tearing and extent of tear propagation along the length of the LHB.

Results of surgery

The results of surgery to the biceps tendon are difficult to assess due to the majority of series including associated rotator cuff repair, subacromial decompression, debridement, and stabilization procedures. There are a few papers, however, where isolated tenotomy, tenodesis, and SLAP repairs have been reported.

Isolated athroscopic tenotomy in patients with irreparable rotator cuff tears has been reported, with good results. Poor function of the teres minor is, however, associated with poorer results. Manou and colleagues in a small series showed that complementary acromioplasty did not confer additional benefit and Walch confirmed this finding if the preoperative acromiohumeral distance is less than 7mm. Indeed, a large cuff tear is a contraindication to

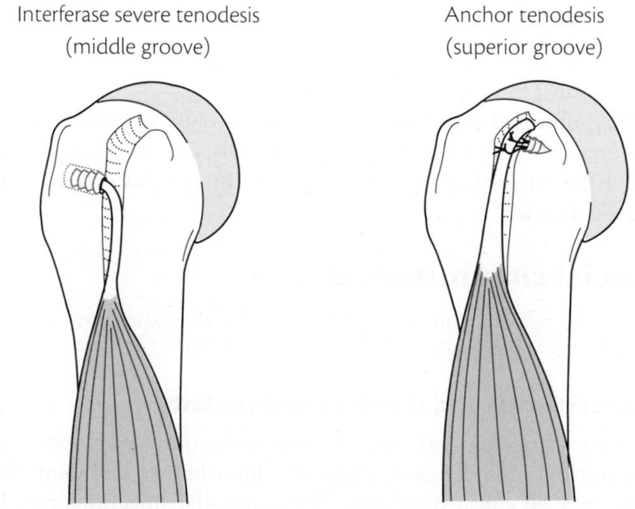

Fig. 4.4.3 Methods of fixation of the tendon during tenodesis.

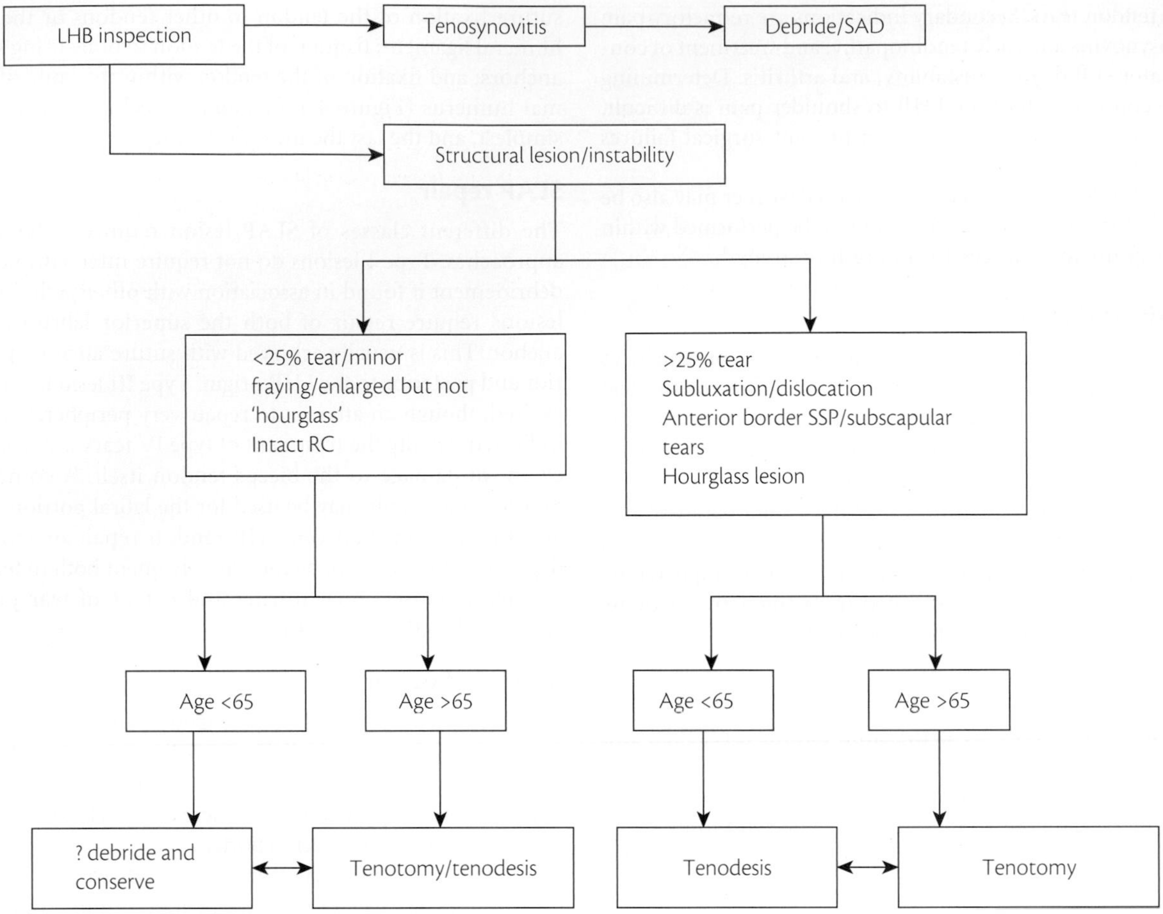

Fig. 4.4.4 Treatment algorithm. SAD, subacromial decompression.

releasing the coracoacromial ligament with anterior acromioplasty as this may lead to anterosuperior escape.

The results of isolated tenodesis have been reported both in the presence of advanced rotator cuff disease and for isolated LHB pathology. For the former group the results of tenodesis appear equivalent to tenotomy, and for the latter group 77% of patients could return to their sporting activities.

The published results of SLAP repair have been favourable but more variable. The heterogenicity of lesions, associated pathology, and different surgical approaches makes interpretation of the literature difficult.

Special circumstances

There are certain conditions, or procedures, apart from rotator cuff disease that warrants attention to the LHB.

Osteoarthritis and shoulder arthroplasty

Primary glenohumeral osteoarthritis commonly produces LHB symptoms. Osteophytes in the groove, loose bodies, and joint effusions may all cause symptoms. Intra-articular injections may be partially effective by addressing symptoms generated by the LHB. Both in arthroscopic treatment of early osteoarthritis and during joint replacement addressing the LHB by tenotomy or tenodesis is recommended.

Proximal humeral fractures and their fixation

The rational for treatment of the LHB in fractures and their fixation is similar to that of osteoarthritis. The LHB is frequently damaged at the level of the fracture and any degree of malunion affecting the bicipital groove, usually at its superior or inferior boundaries, will lead to poor gliding properties of the tendon. Persistent anterior shoulder pain following malunion should alert the surgeon to possible LHB pathology, and LHB tenodesis at the time of fracture surgery should always be considered.

Conclusion

The LHB is a fascinating structure. Recognition of its importance in generating shoulder symptoms is currently high, and much new research is emerging.

Further understanding of its role at the shoulder and clarification of the basic science of its pathology is needed before consensus on its treatment will be reached. Future advances will include further development of imaging techniques, particularly US, and scientific clinical results will guide treatment options, in particular in terms of surgical technique. Reconstructive procedures to stabilize the unstable tendon, and potentially repair tendon tears, which have to date proved unsuccessful, would be a great advance, and with the advance of arthroscopic techniques will hopefully be realistic goals in the near future.

Further reading

Ahrens, P.M. and Boileau, P. (2007). The long head of the biceps tendon and associated tendinopathy. *Journal of Bone and Joint Surgery*, **89B**(8), 1001–9.

Barber, F.A., Field, L.D., and Ryu, K.N. (2007). Selected instructional course lecture. Biceps tendon and superior labrum injuries: decision-making. *Journal of Bone and Joint Surgery*, **89A**, 1844–55.

Snyder, S.J., Karzel, R.P., and Del Pizzo, W. (1990). SLAP lesions of the shoulder. *Arthroscopy*, **6**, 274–9.

Walch, G., Boileau, P., Noel, E., *et al.* (1992). Impingement of the deep surface of the supraspinatus tendon on the postero-superior glenoid rim: an arthroscopic study. *Journal of Shoulder and Elbow Surgery*, **1**, 238–45.

Walch, G., Nové-Josserand, L., Boileau, P., and Lévigne, C. (1998). Subluxations and dislocations of the tendon of the long head of the biceps. *Journal of Shoulder and Elbow Surgery*, **7**(2), 100–8.

Walch, G., Edwards, B.E., Boulahia, A., Nové-Josserand, L., Neyton, L., and Szabo, I. (2005). Arthroscopic tenotomy of the long head of the biceps in the treatment of rotator cuff tears. Clinical and radiographic results of 307 cases. *Journal of Shoulder and Elbow Surgery*, **14**(3), 238–46.

4.5

Frozen shoulder

Tim D. Bunker

Summary points

- Frozen shoulder is caused by a contracture of the capsule
- Counterintuitively not all patients recover completely
- At arthroscopy spectacular angiogenesis is seen
- Pathology shows bands and nodules of type III collagen populated by fibroblasts and myofibroblasts
- Arthroscopic capsular release has improved the management of this condition.

Introduction

Codman coined the term frozen shoulder in 1934. He said it was difficult to define, but then went on to propose a definition which has not been bettered in 70 years. He stated '*this is a condition which comes on slowly with pain over the deltoid insertion, inability to sleep, painful incomplete elevation and external rotation, the restriction of movement being both active and passive, with a normal radiograph, the pain being very trying and yet all patients are able to continue their daily habits and routines*' (Box 4.5.1). The problem is that many of these features are shared by other common shoulder conditions such as rotator cuff disease. However, there is one clinical feature that distinguishes capsular contracture from all other conditions, restriction of passive external rotation in the face of a normal radiograph. There are only two pathologies that cause limited passive external rotation: firstly damage to the joint surface such as occurs in arthritis, head splitting fractures, and locked dislocation (all of which have an abnormal radiograph); and secondly contracture of the ligaments. Since the radiograph is normal this condition can only be due to contracture of the ligaments.

Codman stated, '*Even the most protracted cases recover with or without treatment in about two years*'. This statement has been repeated from text to text without any questioning of the evidence. It has led to the commonly held view that this is a benign condition that resolves completely. However, Simmonds stated 'complete recovery is not my experience' and DePalma stated' it is erroneous to believe that in all instances restoration of function is attained'. Shaffer et al. (1992) in a very detailed follow-up study found that at 7 years, 50% had mild pain, stiffness, or both. They found that 60% had measurable restriction of passive mobility and they concluded 'this made us question whether this is a benign self-resolving condition'. Griggs et al. who stated that 'even amongst the patients who were satisfied, a substantial number were not pain free' confirmed these findings. Ten per cent had mild pain at rest, and 27% had mild or moderate pain with activity. Forty per cent of the satisfied patients had abnormal shoulder function. Our own studies at 2–5 years showed that although 86% had an improvement in their level of pain, this did not mean that they had no pain. Only 53% had no pain, 33% had an occasional pain, and 14% had marked residual pain. These findings have been confirmed by the largest ever study from Oxford (Hand and Carr) on 273 patients followed for up to 20 years. Using a functional score they demonstrated that 40% of their patients had mild to moderate persistent symptoms at 7 years.

The arthroscopic appearance is spectacular. Firstly there is evidence of capsular contracture with a reduced joint volume. The capsule is thickened and difficult to penetrate with the arthroscope and the joint difficult to navigate due to capsular contracture. The spectacular feature is angiogenesis (Figure 4.5.1). This is most marked in the rotator interval area. As the disease progresses into the stiff and contracted phase, the angiogenesis declines and thick white scar can be seen and palpated within the capsule. The early studies of the pathology in capsular contracture of the shoulder showed dense collagen causing fibrosis and marked vascularity in the capsule. Lundberg made the first link between this condition and the other contractile diseases such as Dupuytren's disease,

Box 4.5.1 Codman's criteria for contracted (frozen) shoulder

- Condition comes on slowly
- Pain at deltoid insertion
- Inability to sleep
- Painful incomplete elevation and external rotation
- Restriction of movement being both active and passive
- The pain being very trying
- Yet patients continue in their daily habits
- Radiographs are normal.

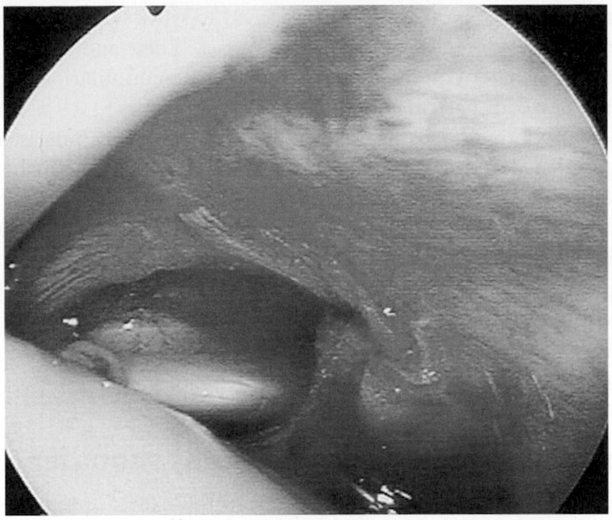

Fig. 4.5.1 The main arthroscopic finding in contracted (frozen) shoulder is angiogenesis. See also colour plate section.

when his histopathologist, Dr Norden, noted that the histology of the shoulder capsule showed compact or dense collagen with many cells that were fibroblasts. Hannafin et al. took biopsies at arthroscopy and showed that in the first phase of this disease there was a hypervascular appearance of the synovium with underlying normal capsular architecture; in stage two there was perivascular scar formation and extensive scar formation in the underlying capsule; and in the final phase extensive capsular fibroplasias. This was confirmed by Bunker and Anthony in 1995 where, using immunocytochemistry, the cells were shown to be mainly fibroblasts. These authors showed for the first time contractile myofibroblasts, the pathognomonic cell of contracture seen in such diseases as Dupuytren's contracture. These authors demonstrated a mass of type III collagen laid down in bands and nodules looking very similar to the histology of Dupuytren's disease (Figure 4.5.2). Further confirmation has come from Killian et al. (2001) who showed a significant increase in fibroblasts, and under electron microscopy a loss of collagen fibril order and fourfold increase in fibre diameter. In summary, all the histological evidence to date shows that this is a capsular contracture of the shoulder (Box 4.5.2). Edwards and Carr have recently examined the inflammatory cells that are to be found near the synovium and around the vessels and have shown the presence of T cells, B cells, and mast cells.

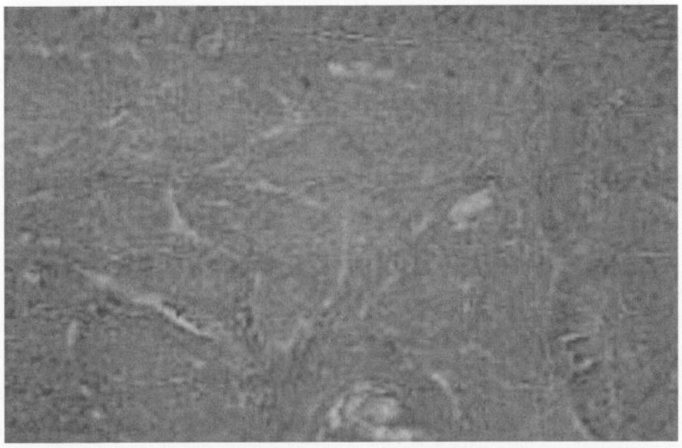

Fig. 4.5.2 The histology of contracted (frozen) shoulder shows nodules and bands of type III collagen with fibroblasts and myofibroblasts. See also colour plate section.

The question then arises as to why this should happen? What precipitates the angiogenesis, and what orders the fibroblasts to accumulate and lay down collagen? Cell messengers (cytokines and growth factors) control these cellular responses and several groups have looked at cell messengers in capsular contracture. Hamada, in Japan, has found increased levels of vascular endothelial growth factor (VEGF) in stiff shoulders that may account for the angiogenesis that is seen at arthroscopy. Rodeo et al. found raised levels of transforming growth factor (TGF) beta and platelet-derived growth factor (PDGF) and suggested that these may act as a perpetual stimulus to fibrosis. Bunker et al. found elevated levels of fibrogenic growth factors (FGF) and this work has been elegantly confirmed by Colville's group who took joint fluid from patients with capsular contracture and found that this tissue caused a 5000% increase in *in vitro* fibroblast proliferation compared with control groups.

On the cellular level, one may question why the scar that is laid down is not quickly remodelled as in normal healing? Bunker et al. looked at the question of remodelling that is mediated by MMPs (matrix metalloproteinases). They found an absence of MMP 14 and an elevation of the MMP inhibitor TIMP (tissue inhibitor of metalloproteinases). Hutchinson et al. actually treated patients with end-stage gastric cancer with marimastat, a synthetic TIMP, and found that within 4 months half their patients developed stiff shoulders and a quarter developed Dupuytren's disease. When the marimastat was stopped the disease regressed. These studies show a tantalizing future where this disease could be treated medically if the molecular basis is better understood.

There has been very little work done on the genetics of capsular contracture. Family studies are difficult to do on conditions where two-thirds of those affected outwardly appear to return to normal. Bunker et al. found that patients with capsular contracture had a normal karyotype, that is they were 46XY if male and 46XX if female, but the cells from the shoulder capsule showed some clonal chromosomal changes. These changes were numerical trisomy of chromosomes 7 and 8, a similar finding to that in other studies of Dupuytren's disease.

Treatment of contracted (frozen) shoulder

The search engine Google will give you 3 360 000 websites that promise a surgery-free instant cure for frozen shoulder.

Box 4.5.2 Histology of contracted (frozen) shoulder

- Type III collagen
- In nodules and bands
- Highly cellular
- Cells are fibroblasts and myofibroblasts
- Very vascular
- Nerve fibres present
- Few inflammatory cells found in periphery or around vessels
- Mast cells present.

These treatments range from herbal pastes applied to the feet to 12 weeks of osteopathic stretching, many with celebrity affidavits and newspaper cuttings attached!

Comparison of treatments is confounded by inadequate diagnosis, lack of controls, underpowered studies, and a failure to look at immediate results of intervention. These confounding factors apply equally to surgical as well as non-surgical studies.

Steroids have been shown in many randomized prospective controlled studies to have no benefit over home exercises. However, many papers can be criticized as they studied painful stiff shoulders, in other words primary and secondary frozen shoulder, so many of the patients would have had other shoulder disease. One paper performed arthrograms of the study group and 11 of 36 had cuff tears, yet were kept in the study! In one recent randomized controlled study (Ryans 2005) patients receiving steroid has less pain than the placebo group at 6 weeks, without any improvement in movement, but by 16 weeks both steroid and placebo showed no difference in any outcome measure. In another randomized placebo-controlled study (Carette et al. 2003), the groups receiving steroid had significantly better SPADI scores than placebo at 6 weeks, without any measurable improvement in movement, but by 12 months steroid and placebo were improved to a similar degree with respect to all measurable outcome measures.

Diercks and colleagues showed that intensive *physiotherapy* prolonged the natural history of the disease from 15 months to 24 months and achieved a lower Constant Score of 76 compared to 87 in the control group who did home exercises. Once again we must stress that what the patients want is not for their disease to be prolonged from 15 to 24 months, but for it to end *today*. The Ryans (2005) study showed that the physiotherapy groups had improved movement at 6 weeks over steroid or placebo, but more pain, and no measurable difference at 16 weeks. Similarly the Carette (2003) study showed no difference between physiotherapy and placebo at any stage of follow-up.

Joint distension with or without steroids has been examined in a number of studies. Most of these studies are flawed by small numbers (just eight patients in one group), confounded by giving distension, steroid, and physiotherapy at the same time, by repetitive treatments (weekly distensions for 6 weeks in one study), by a lack of control groups (no peer-reviewed study with controls), and outcomes being examined at up to 2 years when 90% of untreated patients should have an improvement in outcome at that stage.

Manipulation under anaesthetic has been the mainstay of surgical treatment for decades. There are many studies showing good and relatively rapid improvement. Sneppen et al. showed that 75% of their patients attained a near normal range of movement, 79% were relieved of pain, and 75% returned to work within 9 weeks. However, manipulation is not without risk. Loew and colleagues examined the collateral damage caused by manipulation. They found that four patients out of 30 had an iatrogenic SLAP tear following manipulation, three had a partial tear of subscapularis, and four had a detachment of the anterior labrum. No patient had a fracture, dislocation, or cuff rupture. They examined the pattern of tearing of the capsule, the expected and desired effect of manipulation, by dividing the glenoid rim into thirds. Twenty-four of the 30 had a tear of the anteroinferior third of the capsule, 11 of the superior third, and 16 of the posteroinferior capsule. All patients had a significant improvement in movement, flexion improving by 70 degrees and external rotation by 50 degrees.

Box 4.5.3 Treatment of contracted (frozen) shoulder

- Supervised neglect
- Physiotherapy
- Steroid injection
- Hydrodilatation
- Manipulation under anaesthetic
- Arthroscopic release.

Surgery for contracted (frozen) shoulder

Arthroscopic capsular release (ACR), in the hands of the expert shoulder surgeon, has transformed the management of capsular contracture. Ogilvie Harris and colleagues compared the results of manipulation versus arthroscopic release in their hands. Although both groups gained the same substantial improvement in range of motion, the arthroscopic group had significantly better pain relief and function, to the extent that twice as many were graded excellent. The following year, J.P. Warner (1996) showed a 49-degree increase in elevation, 42-degree increase in external rotation, and improvement in Constant Scores from 13 to 77/100. Harryman and Matsen published a year later (1997) and demonstrated rapid, excellent results. The range of motion went from 41% of the opposite side to 78% on the first postoperative day and 93% at the end of the study. Before surgery 6% could sleep and after, 73%. They were the first to show the dramatic speed of recovery following treatment, which is the very thing that patients want. Berghs et al. confirmed this with a dramatic improvement on day 1 post surgery in 36% and 88% improvement within 2 weeks. Pain improved from 3.6/15 to 12.6/15 and the partial Constant Scores from 20/75 to 62/75. There were no complications in three of these studies, but one transient axillary neurapraxia in the Harryman study. Arthroscopic release appears to show great promise for it delivers what the patient wants: relief of pain, undisturbed nights and improved function *today*, or if not today *this week*, in the majority of people, with minimally invasive, keyhole day-case surgery.

Indications

In the past surgeons treated the contracted shoulder with neglect and reassured patients that it would get better in 18 months, or 2 years. Is that what the patient wants? Well I would suggest you ask the patient. Patients would like to be free of their pain, able to sleep at night, and able to move their arm. And they would like it today, or tomorrow at the latest, but they do not want to suffer for a further 2 years. ACR gives them the opportunity of rapid relief (30% better on day 1 and 80% better by day 5).

The indication for ACR starts with a proven diagnosis of contracture (all other causes of stiffness excluded, radiographs normal), intrusive pain, and jerk pain by day, awakening by night, and stiffness leading to a significant loss of function, all of which is getting worse and not better.

As with any musculoskeletal disorder there is a spectrum of disease. Some patients have a very mild form of contracture that resolves rapidly, and some have a very severe contracture. The latter can be detected easily. Men, with insulin-dependent diabetes, severe Dupuytren's contractures, bilateral disease, external rotation tethered at minus 10 degrees, and failed previous manipulations, populate the severe end of the spectrum. The mild form is far more difficult to detect for with little stiffness it can be, and often is, confused with the impingement stage of rotator cuff disease. This confusion with impingement in the early stages of mild disease may be responsible for the good results obtained by fringe practitioners who amuse the patient whilst nature affects a cure. These people with mild disease will get better anyway, they probably will never be seen in a surgeon's clinic, and they need no interference. The majority of patients lie somewhere in between these extremes. For them the key indication for surgery is night awakening. ACR should be considered if the pain is severe enough to awaken the patient from sleep every night, or many times a night. When this is accompanied by intrusive stiffness and jerk pain the case for ACR is strong. At this stage the risks and benefits of surgery should be explained to the patient. The risks are those of general anaesthesia, failure to improve in 10%, and an infection risk of about one in 3000. The patient then makes their decision, but thanks to arthroscopy the days of nihilistic neglect for the contracted shoulder are over.

Contraindications to surgery

The contraindications to ACR are mild disease with no awakening, resolving disease, and the patient who is unfit for surgery. The surgeon must always bear in mind that in 90% of patients the pain eventually abates and the patient must never be placed in harm's way by the administration of anaesthesia, or by surgery.

Surgical lore dictates that it is an error to interfere during the early painful phase of the contracted shoulder, but is this true? Colville found that the converse was true and that patients did better the earlier that they were treated. Klinger et al. demonstrated effective treatment with ACR performed early in the disease process. In reality most patients are optimistic that the condition will resolve for the first 3 months, then go to their primary care physician who institutes conservative treatment for 3 months, and the patient only presents to the surgeon at around 6 months' duration when conservative treatment has failed. The author's preference is to operate on the severely symptomatic patient as soon as a definitive diagnosis is established, for ACR is the most effective and rapidly acting therapy, and the evidence is that no harm is done by intervening early.

Surgical lore also dictates that it is an error to intervene in diabetics, but is this true? Ogilvie-Harris (1997) showed that ACR was an effective treatment for the resistant diabetic frozen shoulder and this was confirmed by Massoud et al. (2002). Harryman and Matsen (1997) found no difference between the results of ACR in diabetics and non-diabetics. The evidence is that ACR is effective in diabetics.

Procedure

Arthroscopic release is, in reality, a combination therapy that consists of four elements: a washout, a variable release of the capsule, some surgeons inject cortisone, and most gently manipulate the joint. As yet there are no randomized controlled prospective studies that can prove which of the four elements of the procedure are the most important. Intuitively it would seem that the release is the most important element as the results are so much better than those of manipulation. There is also no doubt that the more radical the release the less need there is for any element of manipulation.

Whilst arthroscopic release is far easier than reconstructive surgery, such as arthroscopic cuff repair, it is not for the inexperienced. The capsule is very thickened and the joint space has a small volume. Entry into the joint can thus be difficult. The joint space is contracted, manoeuvrability is tricky, and the joint surfaces may be inadvertently damaged.

The patient must be told that they bear responsibility for the outcome of their surgery. All the surgeon is doing is releasing a joint that wants to stiffen and it is up to the patient to maintain the movement achieved at surgery. To this end they are shown Codman's stooping exercises and instructed that these should be *big and slow*, tai chi rather than karate! This can be supplemented by range of motion exercises as demonstrated by Rockwood using a stick, pulley, and TheraBand®.

Further reading

Berghs, B.M., Sole-Molins, X., and Bunker, T.D. (2003). Arthroscopic release of frozen shoulder. *Journal of Shoulder and Elbow Surgery*, **13**(2), 180–5.

Bunker, T.D. (1997). Frozen shoulder. In: Norris, T. (ed.) *Orthopaedic Knowledge Update: Shoulder and Elbow*, pp. 255–63. Rosemont, IL: American Academy Orthopaedic Surgery.

Bunker, T.D. and Anthony, P.P. (1995). The pathology of frozen shoulder. *Journal of Bone and Joint Surgery*, **77B**, 677–83.

Colville, J. (2007). Adhesive Capsulitis; Does timing of manipulation influence outcome? *Acta Orthopaedica Belgica*, **73**(1), 21–5.

Gerber, C., Espinosa, N., and Perren, T.G. (2001). Arthroscopic treatment of shoulder stiffness. *Clinical Orthopaedics and Related Research*, **390**, 119–28.

Harryman, D.T. II, Matsen, F.A. III, and Sidles, J.A. (1997). Arthroscopic management of refractory shoulder stiffness. *Arthroscopy*, **13**, 133–47.

Killian, O., Kriegsman, J., Berghauser, K., *et al.* (2001). Die frozen shoulder. *Der Chirurg*, **72**, 1303–8.

Rodeo, S., Hannafin, J., Tom, J., Warren, R., and Wieckicz, T. (1997). Immunolocalisation of cytokines and their receptors in frozen shoulder. *Journal of Orthopedic Research*, **15**, 427–36.

4.6

Calcifying tendinitis

Don Wallace and Andrew Carr

Summary points

- Calcifying tendonitis remains an enigmatic condition
- The pathology shows hydroxyapatite crystals lying in extra-cellular matrix vesicles
- There are two presentations, acute and chronic
- Acute episodes can be treated by analgesia and barbottage
- Chronic lesions can be treated conservatively, or by excision of the calcific deposit, arthroscopically or by barbottage.

Introduction

Periarticular calcification of the shoulder is frequently an incidental radiographic finding in asymptomatic patients. Some patients may have mild symptoms and a few will present with severe pain when these calcifications are undergoing resorption. The condition of formation and subsequent resorption of rotator cuff calcification is usually referred to as calcific or calcifying tendinitis. Although calcification may occur in the degenerate torn rotator cuff as a secondary process, the calcium deposition associated with calcifying tendinitis is transitory and does not lead to permanent damage of the involved shoulder.

Incidence

Estimates as to the incidence of rotator cuff calcification in the general population vary considerably with age and type of sample. Estimates vary between 2.7–8% of the population, but many of these are asymptomatic.

The distribution of calcific deposits within the rotator cuff has been well documented by several authors. Calcification within the supraspinatus is more likely to become symptomatic, probably because of subacromial impingement of the swollen area of tendon. Calcification is found in supraspinatus in 74–82% of symptomatic cases.

Calcifying tendinitis seems to be a disease of middle age with a peak incidence in the fifth decade, but rarely presents in the elderly. Therefore calcification must be self-limiting. In Bosworth's series almost 10% of deposits vanished in 3 years of follow-up.

Most authors found a higher incidence of calcification in females with an incidence range of 57–77%. The right shoulder is involved slightly more frequently and 13–24% of cases are bilateral. Although there have been reports of an association between periarticular shoulder calcification and calcification around the hip there is no evidence of any association of calcifying tendinitis with any systemic disorder of calcium metabolism or medical conditions such as diabetes or gout. With regard to the rotator cuff itself, there is no correlation between significant rotator cuff disease and calcifying tendinitis although partial cuff tears occasionally occur when a calcific deposit bursts into the subacromial bursa.

Although cuff tears are not associated with calcifying tendinitis, the edges of a torn degenerate cuff may show some calcification radiographically. This has a characteristic stippled appearance and should be considered a separate condition with a clinical course which reflects that of the underlying cuff disease.

Classification

Various classification systems for calcifying tendinitis have been proposed. In general, anatomical and radiological classifications have not been very helpful in directing management. Bosworth classified the deposits according to their size and thought that large deposits were more likely to become symptomatic. Deposits have also been classified by the quality of their radiographic appearance. DePalma classified the condition by the duration of symptoms at presentation into acute, subacute, and chronic forms. These probably represent different stages in the evolution of the disease process and the distinction between acute and chronic presentations does help plan initial management.

Pathology

Macroscopically the calcium deposits seen in calcifying tendinitis are usually encapsulated in the substance of the tendon and have a chalky white appearance (Figure 4.6.1) or sometimes a more liquid consistency like toothpaste when incised. Histologically, the deposits are multifocal and are separated by areas of fibrocartilage that are usually avascular. The tendon surrounding the deposits is frequently abnormal, showing evidence of fibrillation and thinning.

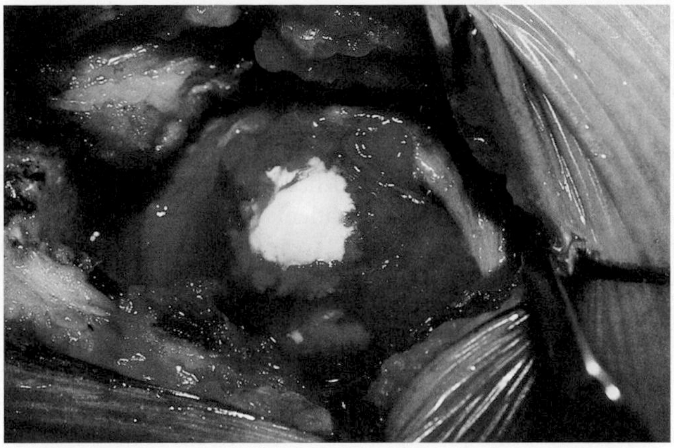

Fig. 4.6.1 Appearance of calcific deposit at surgery. The deltoid has been split and the subacromial bursa incised to reveal the chalky white deposit encapsulated in the supraspinatus tendon.

Under the electron microscope the calcium deposits appear as vesicle-like structures containing crystalline material. Chemical analysis has shown the crystals to consist of hydroxyapatite. Frequently there is a cellular reaction around the calcium deposits that may have a granulomatous appearance due to the presence of multinucleated giant cells. The deposits are often infiltrated by macrophages, polymorphs, and fibroblasts. Crystalline particles are often seen in the cytoplasmic vacuoles of the macrophages and giant cells indicating active phagocytosis of the calcified deposits. There is also frequently evidence of repair with fibroblasts and new capillary formation in the adjacent tendon.

The pathogenesis of these findings is unclear. Codman originally proposed that calcification occurred within a degenerate cuff, and there is experimental evidence to support a link between degeneration, mechanical disruption, and subsequent calcification of the tendon in rabbits. The self-resolving nature of the disease and the epidemiology observed in humans is, however, against a mechanical cause. An attractive theory of cyclical changes within an initially macroscopically normal tendon has been advanced by Uhthoff and Sarkar. They have suggested that the site of calcification initially undergoes transformation into fibrocartilage. Calcium crystals are then deposited in matrix vesicles that eventually coalesce to form deposits that gradually replace the fibrocartilage. After a variable resting period, spontaneous resorption of calcium occurs as vascular channels grow into the deposit and macrophages start to phagocytose the material. Phagocytosis is accompanied by the laying down of granulation tissue that is eventually remodelled to form normal tendon, thereby completing the cycle. The aetiology of the initiating fibrocartilagenous transformation in this cycle remains unexplained but tissue hypoxia might provide the initiating stimulus.

Clinical presentation

The initial formation of calcium deposits rarely causes significant symptoms. However, patients may be aware of vague discomfort in the shoulder for many months before an acute attack. This mild clinical presentation is referred to as chronic calcifying tendinitis. The pain is frequently referred over the outer aspect of the upper arm, particularly over the deltoid insertion. Patients frequently exhibit tenderness over the cuff insertion at the site of the deposit and may have a decreased range of elevation due to pain. A large deposit in the supraspinatus tendon can cause symptoms of subacromial impingement and patients may exhibit a painful arc and have a positive impingement signs.

The acute phase of calcifying tendinitis is usually very painful and associated with the resorption of the deposits. The clinical picture in many ways resembles that of a septic arthritis or acute gout. Patients complain of severe night pain and rest pain, and hold the affected shoulder in adduction and internal rotation. The patient resists any attempt at moving the shoulder and any movement elicited is likely to be scapulothoracic in origin. The shoulder is generally tender and warm to touch. The source of the severe pain in this acute condition is probably from within the tendon itself since there is little evidence of acute bursal inflammation either macroscopically or histologically. At surgery the calcified material often squirts out when incised and has a more liquid consistency than in the chronic situation. The probable mechanism of acute pain is therefore increased intratendinous pressure resulting from inflammation around the resorbing deposit. A more ill-defined fluffy appearance on radiograph, indicative of resorption, has been described in the acute situation.

Investigations

Deposits are usually easily seen on radiographs in the subacute or chronic phase (Figure 4.6.2). In the acute phase the calcification may be very difficult to visualize radiographically because of its diffuse nature. Acute calcifying tendinitis can, however, usually be distinguished clinically from other causes of severe shoulder pain. Magnetic resonance imaging is unhelpful as the calcified deposit and the tendon give the same dark signal. The white cell count and sedimentation rate are normal in calcifying tendinitis and frequently elevated in infection. Serum urate may be elevated in acute gout. In cases of doubt the glenohumeral joint should be aspirated to exclude an effusion.

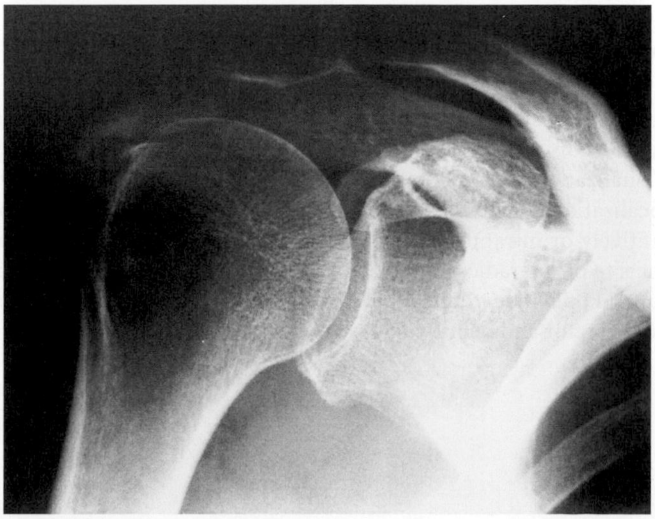

Fig. 4.6.2 Plain anteroposterior radiograph of the shoulder of a 53-year-old female with symptoms of subacromial impingement showing a large calcific deposit in the supraspinatus tendon.

Management

Acute calcifying tendinitis

The main priority in acute cases is pain relief. Opiate analgesia as well as anti-inflammatory medication is usually required. A subacromial injection of long-acting local anaesthetic (e.g. bupivicaine) is usually of benefit and some authors have advocated needling or barbottage of the deposit under ultrasound control following local anaesthetic infiltration to relieve pressure within the painful tendon, accompanied by lavage of the subacromial space.

Corticosteroids have an effect on reducing vascular proliferation and macrophage activity, so they may contribute to a prolongation of the resorption process despite providing transient symptomatic relief. In a comparison between steroid injection and local anaesthetic injection alone no significant difference in outcome was observed in one study. Therefore the use of corticosteroid is not recommended.

Chronic calcifying tendinitis

Cases of chronic or subacute disease usually respond to conservative measures consisting of local therapy including heat, ultrasound, and local anaesthetic injections into the subacromial bursa. Physiotherapy is useful in maintaining the range of motion of the glenohumeral joint. In resistant cases surgery is probably the most dependable way of dealing with large symptomatic deposits. The most commonly accepted indications for surgery are constant pain that interferes with the activities of daily living, and a failure to improve after 3 months of conservative treatment.

Surgical removal of calcium deposits gives good results in most series. Gschwend reported good or excellent results in 25 of 28 cases and DePalma reported 96% good results but the time taken to recover from surgery was quite long. Only 53% had recovered by 6 weeks and a further 30% took 10 weeks. At operation the question arises whether to perform an acromioplasty. Vebostad reported on 43 cases in which one of three procedures had been carried out: arthroscopic excision of the deposit, excision of the deposit, and acromioplasty alone. There was no difference in the results between the three groups with 80% having good or excellent results.

Arthroscopy

Arthroscopic techniques are now the gold standard for excision of calcific deposits with 90% success rates in many studies. However, arthroscopic excision of the deposit is technically demanding. Visualization of the deposit may be difficult and good preoperative localization is helpful with plain films or ultrasound either preoperatively or intraoperatively. Probing the tendon with a needle at the site of the radiographic deposits may produce an exudate that can aid operative localization. The deposit is debrided with a synovial resector and debris removed with suction.

Barbottage

The needling and subsequent irrigation and aspiration of chronic and subacute calcific deposits under radiographic control has been described. This technique is most useful when there is radiographic evidence of resorption of calcium (diffuse calcification) and is less effective at breaking up the hard chalky substance of a large well-defined lesion. Overall 75% of patients treated with this method were improved at a minimum of 1-year follow-up. This technique has also been reported under ultrasonic guidance, thereby avoiding the use of radiographic screening.

Another minimally invasive approach that has recently been reported is the use of a lithotripter to provide high-energy extracorporeal shock waves to calcifications within the rotator cuff. However, the technique appears to be less effective than barbottage or arthroscopic excision, often requires multiple treatments, and patients don't like it. Time will tell whether it may provide a useful alternative to surgery in the future for patients with well-localized deposits.

Summary

Most patients with calcifying tendinitis will have minimal symptoms and can be treated conservatively. The spontaneous resolution of the condition makes the evaluation of the various popular operative and non-operative treatments difficult. Patients who present with acute symptoms in the resorbing phase of the condition will have a good result if treated symptomatically but the treatment of subacute and chronic cases is less clear. There are no prospective randomized studies comparing different treatments, and these should be a priority of future clinical research. The pathological processes involved in the evolution of calcifying tendinitis continue to be unravelled but the initiating stimulus for the fibrocartilagenous metaplasia and the stimulus for calcium resorption remain elusive.

Further reading

Ark, J.W., Flock, T.J., Flattow, E.L., and Bigliani, L.U. (1992). Arthroscopic treatment of calcific tendinitis of the shoulder. *Arthroscopy*, **8**, 183–8.

Bosworth, B.M. (1941). Calcium deposits in the shoulder and subacromial bursitis: a survey of 12 122 shoulders. *Journal of the American Medical Association*, **116**, 2477–82.

Comfort, T.H. and Arafiles, R.P. (1978). Barbotage of the shoulder with image intensified fluoroscopic control of needle placement for calcific tendinitis. *Clinical Orthopaedics and Related Research*, **135**, 171–8.

Loew, M., Jurgowski, W., Mau, H.C., and Thomsen, M. (1995). Treatment of calcifying tendinitis of the rotator cuff by extracorporeal shock waves: a preliminary report. *Journal of Shoulder and Elbow Surgery*, **4**, 101–6.

Uhthoff, H.K. and Sarkar, K. (1990). Calcifying tendinitis. In: Rockwood, C.A. and Matsen, F.A. (eds.) *The Shoulder*, pp. 744–88. Philadelphia, PA: W.B. Saunders.

4.7

Instability

Simon M. Lambert

Summary points

- The fundamental principle or essence of the shoulder is concavity compression. Stability of the shoulder is the condition in which a balanced centralizing joint reaction force (CJRF) exists to maintain concavity compression of the glenohumeral joint whatever the position of the limb and hand.
- Instability is a symptom. It can be defined as the condition of symptomatic abnormal motion of the joint. It refers to a perturbation of concavity compression. It is not a diagnosis.
- Instability is the result of perturbations of structural factors and non-structural factors.
- The clinical syndrome of instability is a disturbance of one or more of these factors in isolation or together. The relative importance of each factor to the syndrome can change over time. The relationship between these factors is described by the Stanmore triangle.
- Both structural and non-structural factors can be perturbed by arrested or incomplete development (dysplasia) or by injury (disruption).
- The aim of treatment is the restoration of (asymptomatic) stable motion by restoration of the CJRF and so restoration of the condition of concavity compression.
- Management follows simple principles: surgery should be undertaken within the context of a well-considered rehabilitation program largely centred around optimizing rotator cuff function.
- Failures of management are often due to failure of or incomplete diagnosis, failure of healing, inadequate attention to patient- and pathology- specific rehabilitation programs, or insufficient attention to lifestyle considerations.
- Disrupted anatomy is restored, preferably by anatomic operations with predictably good outcomes. Dysplastic anatomy is augmented, often by non-anatomic operations with less predictable outcomes. Revision stabilizations are generally non-anatomic, and have higher failure rates.

Stability: definition

Stability of any articulation can be defined as *asymptomatic normal mechanical behaviour at rest and in motion.* It depends on structural integrity and intact neural control systems (afferent, efferent, and neuromuscular connections). For the glenohumeral joint (GHJ) stability is therefore the product of a functionally (not necessarily anatomically) intact rotator cuff, competent capsular and labral structures, a sufficient surface arc (or surface area) of contact between humeral head and glenoid, and an intact neuromuscular system comprising central and peripheral connections. Motion about the centroid of rotation and 'containment' of the humeral head on the size-mismatched glenoid is the result of concavity compression. This is generated by the centralizing joint reaction force (CJRF) of the rotator cuff (including the tendon of the long head of biceps, LHB), and is facilitated by the conformity of the glenoid/labral surface. Rotator cuff competence is a function of centrally-driven activation, and the strength and inertia of the cuff muscles. Shoulder joint position sense and motion are the product of right parietal cortical programming (the parietal 'reach region'), and visual, vestibular, and cervical afferent inputs. Mechanoreceptors in the capsulolabral structures, tendon, and muscle, and the gliding planes (acromio–coraco–deltoid, and scapulothoracic) maintain this activity.

Instability: definition

Instability is usefully defined as the condition of *symptomatic abnormal motion of the joint.* This universal definition combines the mechanistic view and the clinical perspective, and distinguishes the pathological state from the constitutional state of laxity, in which anatomical anomalies may exist, but which does not necessarily cause impairment of function. Since it is a symptom, the term implies recognition (a cerebral cortical event) of the abnormal motion (a difference in position, motion direction, or motion velocity has been identified). Thus 'instability' cannot be determined by examining the shoulder under anaesthetic (EUA). Laxity (looseness) of the GHJ can be determined by EUA either by comparison of the perceived abnormal with the perceived normal side or by reference to what is considered a normal range of laxity for the population.

Instability: aetiology

The relationship between the dominant factors in creating stability in the GHJ can be described by an equation (see Box 4.7.1).

Box 4.7.1 The stability equation

$$\text{Stability (CJRF)} = \text{RC}^{a} + \text{SAC}^{b} + \text{CLPM}^{c} + \text{NS}^{d}$$

where: a–d = proportional values of the factors: these vary from case to case; CJRF = centralizing joint reaction force; CLPM = capsulolabral proprioceptive mechanism; NS = neurological control mechanisms; RC = rotator cuff anatomy and function; SAC = surface arc of contact (surface area of contact).

Each factor varies in relevance to the individual patient, but several points are applicable:

- Everyone starts life with a rotator cuff, the anatomy of which varies very little (although subscapularis can vary in the 'height' of its attachment to the lesser tuberosity). The GHJ will remain stable in the partial absence of medial capsulolabral structures (for instance, after surgical release for frozen shoulder syndrome) providing the rotator cuff function is normal. The tendon of the LHB has a special role in linking rotator cuff activity, humeral head position, and overall upper limb position, particularly in activities requiring optimal close-packing of the shoulder and elbow. Many anomalies of the intra-articular tendon are described, and isolated rupture of the tendon does not lead to humeral head instability, provided the closely associated components of the rotator cuff remain intact. In contrast, senile rotator cuff rupture presents as superior GHJ instability
- The surface arc of contact or surface area of contact (SAC) can vary. The commonest reason for this is a bony Bankart lesion. Rarer causes are segmental dysplasia of the glenoid, congenital glenoid version anomalies, and humeral head defects (Broca or Hill–Sachs, and McLaughlin lesions)
- The capsulo-labral proprioceptive mechanism (CLPM) can vary considerably. The labrum can be absent, hypoplastic, or dysplastic, and ligament anomalies are well recognized in subjects with no instability. The incidence of ligamentous anomalies in patients with atraumatic structural instability is the same as the general population. Lax individuals do not appear to have a greater prevalence of anomalies of ligament morphology. However, they may have a greater joint volume, a more capacious joint, and more elastic ligaments than normal
- Neural control systems are readily deranged by central or peripheral neurological conditions. It is recognized that aberrant muscle activation or suppression contributes to GHJ instability, and diseases of the cerebellum and basal ganglia may present with shoulder instability, particularly of the scapulothoracic joint. It is not known if there are variations in the densities or function of mechanoreceptors in the capsule and labrum in patients with atraumatic structural and muscle-patterning instability (see later in this chapter).

The clinical syndrome of instability is a disturbance of one or more of these factors in isolation or together, and the relative importance of each factor to the syndrome can change over time. The pathologies causing instability comprise structural (RC, SAC, CLPM) and non-structural (NS) elements (Box 4.7.2 and Figure 4.7.1). The structural elements may be damaged by extrinsic force

Box 4.7.2 Structural and non-structural causes of GHJ instability are based on perturbation of the elements of the stability equation

$$\underbrace{\text{Stability (CJRF)} = \text{RC}^{a} + \text{SAC}^{b} + \text{CLPM}^{c}}_{\text{structural}} + \underbrace{\text{NS}^{d}}_{\text{non-structural}}$$

Note that the CLPM can be disturbed structurally (discontinuity or dysplasia), and non-structurally (deafferentation).

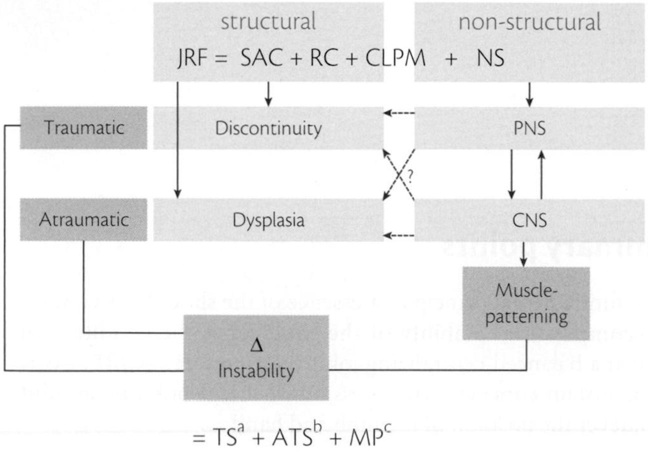

Fig. 4.7.1 The aetiology of GHJ instability. ATS, atraumatic structural factors(s); CNS, central nervous system; MP, muscle patterning (neuromuscular; PNS, peripheral nervous system; TS, traumatic structural factor(s)). *Notes:* 1) For any individual the diagnosis of GHJ instability may include one or more cause(s). For instance a hyperlax (dysplastic) individual who has had recurrent painful non-traumatic GHJ dislocations and who sustains a dislocation of the GHJ by the acute application of extrinsic force leading to disruption of the CLPM will have acquired a traumatic structural instability on a background of atraumatic instability: two pathologies are present in the one shoulder. 2) The eventual 'equation' of the diagnosis of instability for an individual can be defined as:

$$\text{Instability} = (\text{TS})^{a} + (\text{ATS})^{b} + (\text{MP})^{c}$$

where a,b,c are proportionality factors: not all individuals will have all elements present at presentation. However, pathology can change over time, and the importance of each factor in the instability diagnosis may change (see Figure 4.7.2). Thus treatment strategies may need to change.

(traumatic structural); acquire microtraumatic lesions over time (atraumatic structural); or be congenitally abnormal, or comprised of abnormal collagen. The non-structural elements can be congenitally abnormal or can be acquired over time as pertubations of neuromuscular control, particularly at periods of skeletal growth.

Classification: the Stanmore (instability) triangle

The combined concepts that structural (traumatic and atraumatic) and neurological system disturbances can cause instability, the observation that more than one pathology can be present in the shoulder at the time of diagnosis, and that pathology can change over time led Bayley to the classification of instability as a continuum of pathologies, which can be graphically displayed as a triangle (Figure 4.7.2). The polar pathologies are labelled types I (traumatic instability), type II (atraumatic instability), and type III

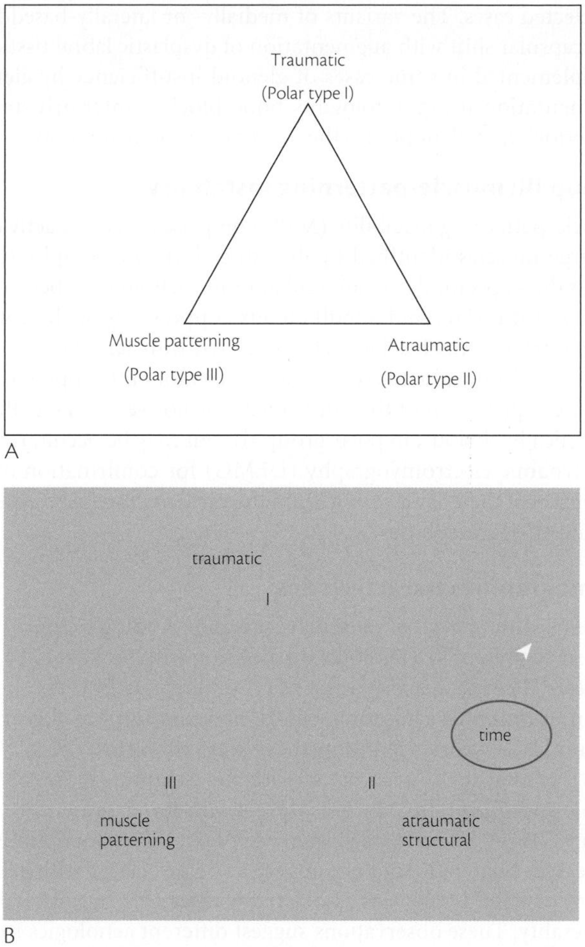

Fig. 4.7.2 A) The Stanmore classification of glenohumeral joint (GHJ) instability. *Notes:* 1) The space between any axis and the opposing apex represents the gradient of influence of the apical component in the instability. Thus, the energy of the injuring force (and so the mount of trauma) of the first GHJ dislocation increases as we progress from axis III–II towards polar group I. 2) The presence of clinically obvious aberrant muscle patterning increases as we progress from axis I–II to polar group III. 3) The incidence of structural abnormality increases as we progress from polar group III towards the axis I–II. 4) The intervening axes, joining neighbouring apices, describe the spectrum of instabilities which exist as compound conditions, i.e. trauma with atraumatic structural, atraumatic structural with muscle patterning, and so on. These axes are labelled as subsets I/II, II/I, etc. and describe the relative proportion of the contribution of each pathology to the overall diagnosis. This schema can therefore be used to describe any instability, and any combination of instabilities. The utility of the schema has been demonstrated by others (Gibson et al. 2004). B) Instability is also defined by the time or pattern of onset. The term 'chronic' is confusing: the definition of the term is unclear and we prefer not to use it. Thus 'acute' refers to the first event, 'recurrent' to the second and subsequent events, and 'persistent' to the locked condition. All temporal types are represented in the Stanmore system, so that, for instance, polar group I (traumatic structural) may have acute, recurrent, and persistent types. This is equally true for the two other groups. The evolution of instability over time (e.g. in response to treatment) can be mapped with the addition of a z-axis, representing time. The emergence of different patterns of instability over time is exemplified by the polar group I case following sports trauma in which the second dislocation occurs during a sneeze: the arm is not in the provocative position, but pectoralis major activity pulls the humerus off the glenoid. This case has migrated from pure polar type I to an interpolar group I/III. The treatment must take this into account: if surgery is undertaken and the aberrant PM activity goes undiagnosed the repair is imperilled. Rehabilitation of the inappropriate PM activation, with subscapularis activation/strengthening should precede capsulolabral repair in almost all cases.

(neurological dysfunctional or muscle patterning). Polar groups I and II and the axis I–II representing the spectrum between the two poles correspond to the TUBS-AMBRI classification which also allows for a spectrum of structural shoulder pathology but which does not admit those shoulders in which there is no structural (traumatic or atraumatic) cause for the instability. The characteristics for each polar group are given in Box 4.7.3. Jaggi has further subdivided polar group III into peripheral, central, positional, protective, and combination subtypes (personal communication). The interpolar spectrum describes dual pathologies in which traumatic, atraumatic and muscle-patterning factors play a variable role in the emergence of instability.

The clinical syndromes of glenohumeral joint instability

Group I (traumatic structural instability)

The traumatic structural group includes the TUBS (Traumatic, Unilateral, Bankart lesion present [in the anterior instability type], Surgery usually indicated) group but also includes the posterior traumatic instability characterized by the McLaughlin or Reversed Hill–Sachs lesion and posterior labral damage or locked posterior dislocation. Instability can thus be recurrent (acute or chronic) or persistent (acute or chronic). Luxatio erecta is a version of anterior instability, usually of the more elderly, and may be associated with infraclavicular plexopathy, and extensive bruising indicative of rupture of the circumflex vessels. In general shoulder clinics, acute recurrent anterior GHJ instability is the commonest form of instability. Assessment is based on the history of the initiating event, the

Box 4.7.3 Characteristics of the polar groups of the Stanmore classification

- Group I—traumatic structural:
  - Significant injury
  - Often a Bankart lesion
  - Usually unilateral
  - No abnormal muscle patterning
- Group II—atraumatic structural:
  - No history of acute injury (repetitive microtrauma)
  - Structural damage to articular surfaces
  - Can be unilateral
  - Not uncommonly bilateral
  - No abnormal muscle patterning
- Group III—muscle patterning:
  - No history of injury
  - No structural damage to articular surfaces seen at arthroscopy
  - Capsular dysfunction may be present
  - Abnormal muscle patterning observable (may be occult)
  - Often bilateral.

examination is discussed in Chapter 4.1 and investigation is best undertaken by magnetic resonance arthrography (MRA) or EUA and arthroscopy.

Treatment comprises, in principle, surgical intervention for most cases in which capsulolabral or rotator cuff disruption is evident. There remains controversy regarding the choice of open versus arthroscopic surgical techniques.

Group II (atraumatic structural instability)

In this group the incidence of ligamentous anomalies is the same as the population of traumatic instabilities. Within this group is the population defined as AMBRI (Atraumatic, often Multidirectional, often Bilateral, treated by Rehabilitation/physiotherapy)—in the original definition of AMBRI, surgical treatment by Inferior capsular shift is indicated if rehabilitation fails. This concept may be flawed: some patients will fall into the category of subgroup II/III and so will possess some neuromuscular control aberration. These patients may fail surgery because of the muscle-patterning behaviour, and may have a substantially greater probability of developing instability or postcapsulorrhaphy arthropathy if surgery is undertaken. The decision to operate should not be made on the basis of failed physiotherapy.

This group also contains a subgroup of individuals with benign hypermobility syndrome (of which Ehlers–Danlos syndrome is a variant), characterized by a Beighton score of greater than five out of a total possible nine points. Hypermobility may be limited to the upper limbs. These patients may present with pain rather than overtly abnormal displacements.

Anterior atraumatic instability is less common than posterior types. Posterior structural anomalies (including posterior glenoid dysplasia, excessive glenoid retroversion, glenoid hypoplasia, and medialized posterior capsular attachment) create the environment in which obligatory positional posterior displacement may occur during elevation of the arm in the sagittal plane. If abnormal clinically obvious muscle activation appears *at the onset* of this motion, then the diagnosis is modified to acknowledge the muscle patterning: the case is group II/III (peripheral subtype). If the muscular activation occurs *during* the motion, and appears to be provoked by the position of the arm at the shoulder, then the diagnosis is still II/III but with the suffix (protective subtype). If there is no clinically or electrophysiologically-proven aberrant muscle activation then the condition is labelled II (positional subtype).

Scapular dyskinesis is common, and reflects the attempt by the scapular postural muscles to maintain scapulohumeral homeostasis. Serratus anterior can be suppressed in some cases: the aberrant muscle activity now affects the scapular primarily. This represents a scapulothoracic (STh) type III condition. The total diagnosis is therefore STh(III)/GHJ(II).

Assessment of the structural diagnosis is by MRA and/or diagnostic arthroscopy. These are complementary, not alternatives; MRA is useful to look for capsular detachments, bony defects, and the bulk and quality of rotator cuff muscles (particularly subscapularis, for the anterior, and infraspinatus, for the posterior types), while arthroscopy is useful to look for the subtleties of internal lesions of occult instability: bicipital and deep surface cuff lesions, soft tissue Broca defects, internal impingement lesions, and external impingement lesions.

Treatment comprises rehabilitation, avoidance of activities promoting the instability, pain management, and surgical intervention in selected cases. The variants of medially- or laterally-based inferior capsular shift with augmentation of dysplastic labral tissue are complemented in some cases of glenoid insufficiency by glenoid augmentation using autologous bone blocks (anteriorly and/or posteriorly), or glenoplasty (the Scott posterior glenoplasty).

Group III: muscle-patterning instability

Muscle-patterning instability (MPI) comprises aberrant activation of large muscles identified by dynamic electromyography (latissimus dorsi, pectoralis major, and anterior deltoid have been characterized thus far) and simultaneous suppression of the rotator cuff (infraspinatus has been characterized thus far: whether suppression of infraspinatus reflects whole rotator cuff suppression or specific suppression of the infraspinatus is not yet clear). MPI can be clinically obvious, in polar group III, but may be occult, requiring dynamic electromyography (DEMG) for confirmation of the suspicion of the existence of MPI in the presentation (as in types II/III and III/II instabilities).

Demographic characteristics

Patients with abnormal muscular activation leading to 'pure' MPI appear to present in a trimodal distribution with peaks at 6, 14, and 20 years. The mean age at onset of symptoms was 14 years and the mean duration of symptoms before presentation was 8 years. In the under 10 years age group there were more females (71% vs 47%), greater laxity (estimated with the Beighton score, 63% vs 29%), and bilaterality (54% vs 42%), with fewer presenting with pain (17% vs 50%). As age increased laxity decreased and pain increased. Bilaterality did not appear to be associated with gender, laxity, or pain. Laxity was associated with gender but not pain or bilaterality. These observations suggest different aetiologies for the MPI in the three cohorts.

Bayley (2005) used DEMG in latissimus dorsi (LD), pectoralis major (PM), anterior deltoid (AD), and infraspinatus (IS) to evaluate the patterns of muscular activation in patients who clearly demonstrated, visibly or by palpation, apparently abnormal muscular activation immediately before and during dislocation of the GHJ in the outpatient clinic. These muscles were chosen because they were reliably accessible. Early pilot studies were expanded into a cohort study of over 1000 cases of glenohumeral instability (GHI) seen at the Royal National Orthopaedic Hospital, a tertiary referral centre, over a 22-year period (1981–2003), from which DEMG data were extracted. The results are summarized in Box 4.7.4.

MPI was diagnosed, clinically and/or electrophysiologically, in 494 shoulders (45% of the entire cohort of 1097 shoulders) of 386 patients. In 44% the MPI affected both shoulders. The dominant arm was affected more often in right-handed patients, the non-dominant more often in left-handed patients. The central neurological basis for these differences remains obscure. There were 323 shoulders with 'pure' MPI; 161 shoulders presented a mixed picture of MPI in addition to either traumatic or atraumatic structural causes for the instability.

The value of recognizing this form of instability is given by the success of specialist physiotherapy using biofeedback techniques versus conventional therapy for retraining abnormal muscle activity: 76% of patients had either no change or a deterioration of their condition with conventional therapy (including conventional strengthening exercises) compared with 61% of patients overall achieving improvement in their condition with specialist therapy.

Box 4.7.4 Characteristics of patients displaying aberrant muscle-patterning GHJ instability (MPI)

1) 52% of the entire cohort of patients with GHI had abnormal muscle activation (muscle-patterning, MP) during a standard set of movements
2) 47% of unidirectional GHI had MPI
3) 27.6% of anterior GHI had MPI, involving PM, or PM + LD coupled
4) 84.8% of posterior GHI had MPI, involving LD, or AD + suppressed IS coupled
5) 83.8% of multidirectional GHI had MPI, involving LD > PM > AD
6) 100% of inferior GHI had MPI, involving PM + LD coupled
7) One or two muscles were implicated in 88% of unidirectional and 92% of multidirectional MPI
8) Clinical impression of MPI instability was incorrect in 12% of cases
9) Clinical impression was correct but the wrong muscles were identified in 33%
10) Further abnormal muscles were identified by DEMG in 32.5% of cases.

The incidence of iatropathic arthropathy increases with inappropriate surgery in those with type III instability while no type III in which surgery was not performed developed arthritis.

Dynamic electromyography

Given the limitation that only four muscles have been studied in depth, the evidence strongly suggests that these, and perhaps other muscles, are implicated in many cases of instability. Inappropriate activity in PM, LD, and AD, with suppression of IS appear either singly or as couples in the generation of instability in shoulder with and without capsular collagen insufficiency. Whether suppression of IS reflects specific inappropriate inactivity in IS alone or reflects abnormal activation of the rotator cuff as a whole remains unknown.

DEMG provides additional information about abnormal muscle activation or suppression in subtle MPI in which clinical examination has a low specificity and sensitivity. DEMG was found to be most useful in patients presenting with pain, glenohumeral capsular insufficiency, and occult muscle patterning, categorized as the interpolar group II/III. Given that a chance of a successful outcome for rehabilitation of patients with MPI (symptoms abolished or controlled) was diminished fivefold for anterior and tenfold for posterior instability after inappropriate surgery in patients with MPI, it is clear that the identification of this specific cohort is important. These patients contribute to the failures of the AMBRI group after rehabilitation (if MPI has not been recognized). It is noteworthy that the pathology is not defined by direction but rather that the direction of instability is determined by the pathology.

In MPI rehabilitation is used as the first mode of treatment: there is usually a change in aberrant muscle activity within 6 months. Therapy has to go on for at least 2 years, possibly for cortical re-imprinting to be re-established There is a 25% recurrence rate within 2 years, needing 'top-up' therapy, including inpatient treatment in which a multidisciplinary approach is favoured. The value of specific suppression of specific muscles by injection of botulinum toxin is unclear in MPI.

Multidirectional instability

Multidirectional instability (MDI) is not a diagnosis but a symptom. Multidirectional *laxity* is assessed by EUA. It may be difficult to determine when a lax shoulder is centralized during EUA. Fluoroscopy is invaluable in such cases. An individual shoulder may have the same pathology (i.e. group I, II, or III pathology) causing instability in each of more than one direction, or more than one pathology (e.g. group I in one direction, and group II/III in the other direction), thus distinguishing 'simple' MDI from 'complex' MDI. The underlying diagnoses of the different directions of instability are distinguishable by the history, clinical observations, arthroscopy, and/or MRA (Figure 4.7.3) supplemented by DEMG where necessary. Each pathology is treated separately, with rehabilitation of MPI elements taking priority.

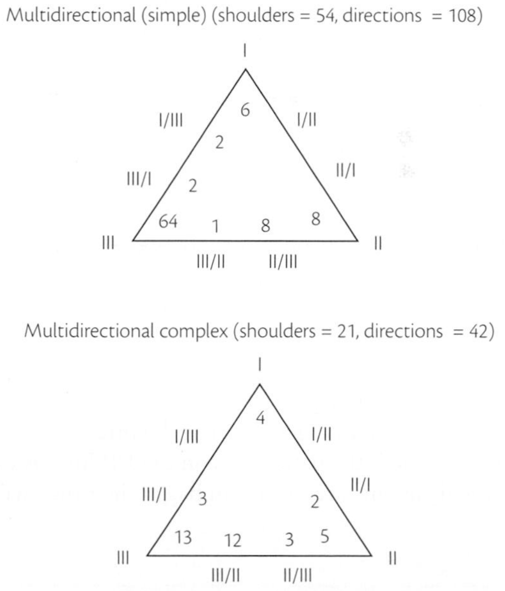

Fig. 4.7.3 Characteristics of multidirectional instability for a simple diagnosis (one type of pathology accounts for all directions of instability) or complex diagnoses (more than one type of instability pathology account for the several directions of instability). 'Single diagnosis' means that the pathology creating the instability in both or all directions is the same. 'Multiple diagnosis' means that the pathology of each direction of instability is different. It follows that the treatment of a case in the multiple-diagnosis MDI set is different for each direction: an inferior capsular shift might be the appropriate intervention for the II component, but the III (muscle-patterning) component should also be considered, and almost universally should be treated first. Many patients experience satisfactory return of sufficient stability with successful treatment of the III component (which is easier in the un-operated shoulder) and choose not to proceed to capsular surgery. The numbers refer to numbers of shoulders studied.

Management of glenohumeral instability

Having diagnosed the specific pathology (-ies), treatment is directed at each element in the instability syndrome. The pathology of instability can be expressed as a useful equation acting as a checklist to define the management strategy (Box 4.7.5). The aim of treatment is the restoration of (asymptomatic) stable motion by restoration of the CJRF, optimization of the angular range of stability, and so restoration of concavity compression. Management follows simple principles (Figure 4.7.4): surgery should be undertaken within the context of a well-considered rehabilitation programme largely centred around optimizing rotator cuff function. In general, disrupted anatomy is restored, preferably by anatomic operations with predictably good outcomes. Dysplastic anatomy is augmented, often by non-anatomic operations with less predictable outcomes. Revision stabilizations are generally non-anatomic, and have higher failure rates.

The surgical treatment of structural dislocation depends upon the pathology detected on plain radiographs, MRA, and arthroscopy. Of the structural elements the capsulolabral pathology (CLPM) is the most common. Structural SAC lesions are becoming more frequent due to the increasing professionalism of contact sports leading to bone damage to the glenoid. Finally rotator cuff (RC) structural damage is common in dislocation in middle and old age, and is more commonly recognized these days.

The labrum is often torn during traumatic dislocation. This can be the classic Bankart lesion, where the labrum tears from the bone along the anteroinferior quarter of the glenoid. A variety of Bankart variants have been described such as the ALPSA (anterior labrum periosteal sleeve avulsion) lesion and the Perthes lesion. The Bankart tear may extend into a SLAP lesion, or extend around the inferior glenoid, or even involve the entire circumference of the socket. These lesions will need to be released (as they often heal in an abnormal position), reduced to their proper position on the glenoid rim and re-attached using suture anchors to a freshened bed so that they can heal strongly in an effective position. Labral repairs for patients at the Polar I position can be done either arthroscopically or by classic open surgery through a deltopectoral approach.

The glenohumeral ligaments may stretch or tear, or avulse from the humeral surface as a HAGL (humeral avulsion of the glenohumeral ligaments) lesion. The ligaments may be thin, stretched, or elastic if the patient lies on the I/II line, as the majority do. If the ligaments are loose and baggy then they will need to

Box 4.7.5 The instability pathology equation

$$\text{Instability} = (\text{traumatic structural})^n + (\text{atraumatic structural})^n + (\text{neurological})^n.P.t$$

or

$$\text{Instability} = (\text{I})^n + (\text{II})^n + (\text{III})^n.P.t$$

where: n = proportionality coefficient (different for each patient); P = 'patient factors', e.g. epilepsy, athetosis, other dystonias; t = time.

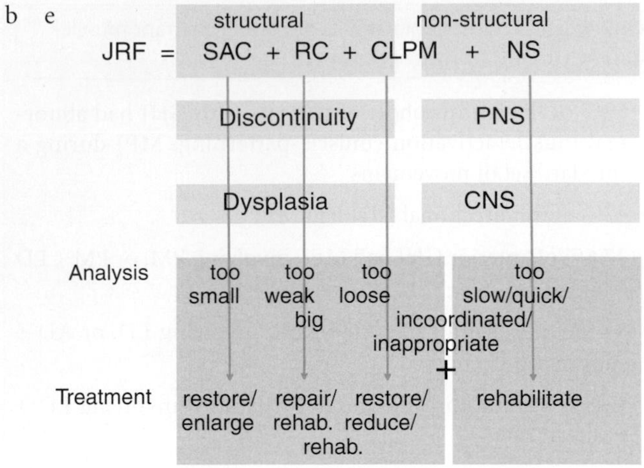

Fig. 4.7.4 Management strategies.

Notes: 1) Treatment includes interventions to restore anatomy to the near-normal state ('anatomical') and those which enlarge or augment surface area of contact, or reduce joint capacity ('non-anatomical'). 2) The rationale for the restoration (of humeral head surface contour) or augmentation (of glenoid surface area) of the angular range of stability is described by the following equation:

$$\text{Angular range of stability} = \frac{\text{glenoid arc length}}{\text{radius of humeral head}} \times \frac{360}{2\pi}$$

3) The risk of complications including failure to achieve stability increases for non-anatomical interventions. 4) Revision of non-anatomical operations for failure has a high rate of complications. 5) Rehabilitation takes priority: optimization of rotator cuff function frequently restores sufficient stability even in an anatomically-deranged joint.

repaired at the time of surgery. The capsule is often globally loose and may need to be tightened South to North and often East to West as well. At open surgery this is easy to do. The capsule is opened using a vertical capsulotomy and three sutures are placed to close the rotator interval. This will usually effect the necessary inferior capsular shift. As the capsulotomy is closed it can be overlapped East to West making sure that it is not overtightened. If more of a shift is required then a Neer T-shaped capsulotomy is performed. The rotator interval is closed and then a South to North double-breasting is performed to create a full and proper Neer inferior capsular shift. The vertical capsulotomy is then closed with as much double breasting East to West as required.

This is where things get difficult at arthroscopic surgery. All capsular shifts depend upon closing the rotator interval. If the interval is not securely closed then any South to North plication will merely open the rotator interval more, negating the effect of the capsular shift. Arthroscopic rotator interval closure can be performed, but is not easy, because the anterior working cannulae themselves take up most of the interval. To place more than one suture in the interval is more difficult still. To place three sutures in the interval arthroscopically is just showing off, very few surgeons have the requisite skill to do this. Double breasting is just not possible arthroscopically. This means that the further down the Polar I/II line towards the Polar II end becomes more and more difficult to perform arthroscopically.

If there is bone loss to the anteroinferior glenoid then this bone loss will need to be made good. This can not be done using a ligamentous repair and will need bone to be transferred to make up the SAC loss. The normal way to do this is a Bristow–Latarjet transfer of the coracoid process. This operation is performed using a deltopectoral approach. The musculocutaneous nerve must be exposed and protected throughout the procedure. The bone surfaces of the coracoid and the glenoid neck must be decorticated so that the coracoid will unite to the scapula. The coracoid is attached with one or two AO lag screws.

If the defect is larger than usual, too large for a coracoid transfer, then a tri-cortical bone block may be needed from the pelvic rim to make up the SAC defect.

In the middle aged to elderly patient the dislocation may be complicated by tearing of the rotator cuff itself. In these patients recurrent dislocation is not the long-term problem, it is the cuff tear itself, and this will need to be repaired.

Further reading

Bayley, J.I.L., Lewis, A., and Kitamura, T. (2005). The classification of shoulder instability. New light through old windows. *Current Orthopaedics*, **18**, 97–108.

Cofield, R.H. and Irving, J.F. (1987). Evaluation and classification of shoulder instability. With special reference to examination under anesthesia. *Clinical Orthopaedics and Related Research*, **223**, 32–43.

Malone, A.A., Jaggi, A., Lambert, S.M. *et al.* (2006). 'Demographic differences between structural and muscle-patterning instability.' Abstract at Proceedings of the 17th Annual Scientific Meeting, The British Elbow and Shoulder Society, Edinburgh, 31 May–2 June, 2006.

Thomas, S.C. and Matsen, F.A. III. (1989). An approach to the repair of avulsion of the glenohumeral ligaments in the management of traumatic anterior glenohumeral instability. *Journal of Bone and Joint Surgery*, **71A**, 506–13.

4.8

Surface replacement of the shoulder

Stephen Copeland and Jai Relwani

Summary points

- The design of the surface replacement arthroplasty has evolved over the past 20 years. From cemented prostheses such as the SCAN, to cementless prostheses such as the Copeland, the basic concept and design of the surface replacement favouring maximal bone preservation has remained constant.
- Indications and surgical technique have been refined over this period, the latest modification being the use of computer-assisted navigation to optimise the size and position the implant in situ.
- Surface replacement prosthesis has demonstrated clinical results at least equal to those of conventional stemmed prostheses.

Introduction

The only part of any prosthesis that is of use to the patient is the new, shiny joint surface. The patient is unaware of whether this surface is fixed by a stem or cement or whether it is a pure surface replacement.

Development of the Copeland surface replacement arthroplasty (CSRA) for arthritis began in 1979, with the first clinical use of the prosthesis occurring 7 years later, in 1986. In 1993, hydroxyapatite coating was introduced to allow biologic fixation with bony ingrowth. Simple instruments were designed to allow anatomic placement of the humeral head based on identifying the centre of the sphere. Once this point has been identified, the prosthesis can be positioned to replicate the original anatomic bearing surface, including version, offset, and angulation.

The basic concept and design of surface replacement was to remove as little of the bone stock as possible and not to broach the humeral shaft. Initial fixation was by a cementless press fit single peg of taper fluted design using a hydroxyapatite coating for osseointegration (Figure 4.8.1). The head was made of cobalt-chrome, and the glenoid component of ultra-high-molecular-weight polyethylene (UHMWP). The radius of curvature of the head and glenoid were designed to conform with each other. Eight head sizes replicate the original anatomic bearing surface, including version, offset, and angulation. The surface replacement prosthesis has demonstrated clinical results at least equal to those of conventional stemmed prostheses.

History

Zippel in Germany implanted two surface replacements that were fixed by a transosseous screw but no follow-up is recorded for these cases. Steffee and Moore in the United States were implanting a small

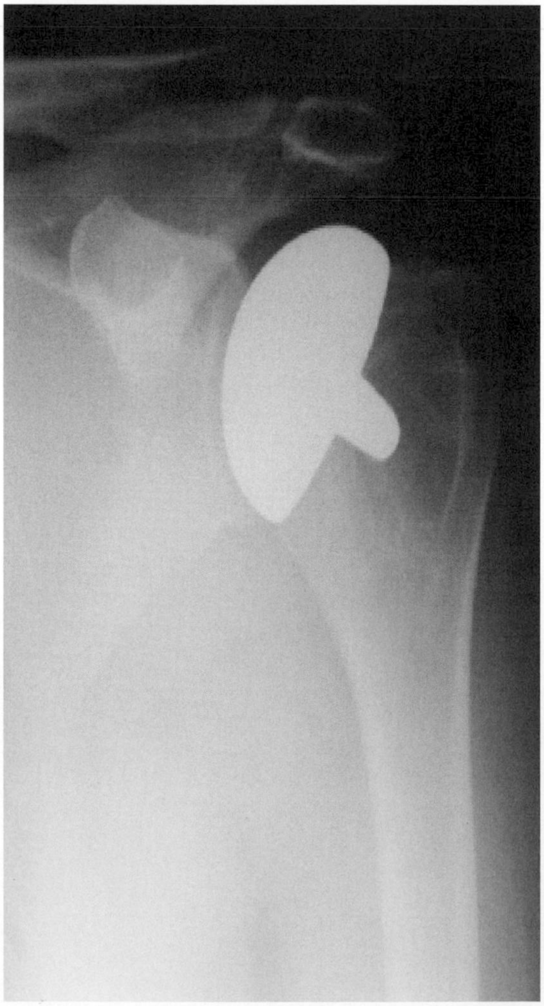

Fig. 4.8.1 The Copeland surface replacement arthroplasty is a surface replacement design with initial fixation from a short peg.

hip-resurfacing prosthesis into the shoulder and, in Sweden, in greater numbers, a surface replacement SCAN (Scandinavian) cup was being used as a cemented surface replacement. It was based on the same surface replacement philosophy that the CRSA was designed on.

Potential disadvantages of the glenoid and stemmed prosthesis

The most frequent shoulder arthroplasty performed is a stemmed cemented total shoulder replacement. However, there are certain disadvantages to this type of design. The most common component to fail is the glenoid component with a reported incidence of radiolucent lines on radiographs as high as 30% and a significant rate of late loosening of the glenoid component over time. Glenoid failure may be associated with significant bone loss and cause major problems when revision surgery is undertaken, sometimes making the revision 'impossible'.

Similar problems can occur with stemmed humeral components, albeit less frequently. The bone loss, however, can be very marked, and revision from a stemmed humeral implant can be extremely difficult, often requiring splitting the humerus to remove the stem and cement. This may result in perforation of the shaft and fractures. Fractures may also occur at the stem tip due to stress risers in the area (Figure 4.8.2), and are difficult to treat, especially in this elderly and infirm group of patients. In cementless stems, reaming of the bone can result in a fracture.

Deformities in the humeral shaft can occur with previous fractures and may pose a challenge getting a stemmed prosthesis past the deformed area. Similarly, it is not possible to use a stemmed implant in the presence of other metalware such as a nail or screw in the medullary cavity of the humerus. Although screws and nails can be removed, the stem of an elbow replacement coming up the shaft may preclude a stemmed shoulder replacement altogether.

An additional problem with stemmed fixation is that of 'pilot error'. It has been shown that approximately 30% of the unsatisfactory results after shoulder replacements are due to component malposition and that, if version is incorrect by more than 15 degrees, this can lead to a painful shoulder. Incorrect placement can and does occur, and removal and repositioning of a stem is a major reconstruction problem. One always has to bear in mind what would happen if the joint should fail and thus plan a backup or revision procedure.

There is no evidence to indicate why the humeral stem should extend half the length of the humerus, sometimes with the cement tracking down to the elbow. On the other hand, one needs only to resurface the damaged surface of the humeral head to achieve comparable results and function to the stemmed prosthesis.

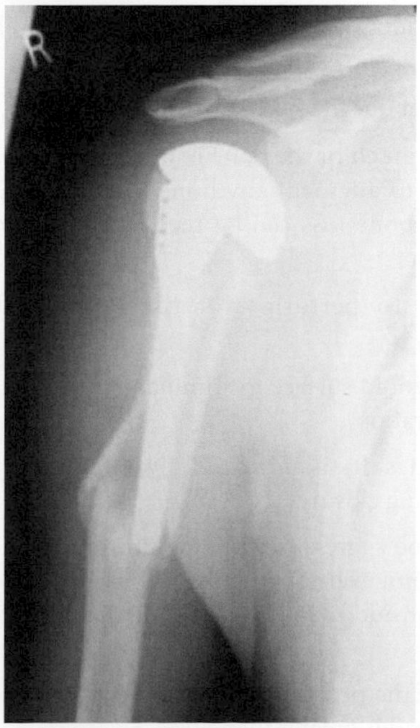

Fig. 4.8.2 Periprosthetic fracture of the humerus.

Potential advantages of the surface replacement (Box 4.8.1)

- The head is anatomically seated, restoring anatomical variations of version, offset, and angulation in each individual patient
- There is no requirement for intramedullary canal reaming or cementation, making it a less traumatic and safer procedure in an elderly patient given the lowered risk of fat embolus or hypotension
- There are no complications associated with an intramedullary canal previously filled with cement, fracture fixation devices, or a stem from elbow arthroplasty. If there is a malunion at the proximal end of the humerus with secondary osteoarthritis, the malunion can be left undisturbed, the tuberosities intact, and just the humeral articulation resurfaced
- Unlike stemmed prostheses, there is no stress riser effect that could result in a shaft fracture at the tip of the prosthesis
- Resurfacing can be used in congenital abnormalities of the humerus that do not permit the passage of standard intramedullary stemmed prostheses
- Revision surgery to a stemmed prosthesis or arthrodesis can be performed easily as there is no loss of bone stock and no cement to retrieve from within the humeral shaft.

Indications and contraindications

The commonest indication for surface replacement is arthritis, either degenerative or inflammatory. Other indications are mild avascular necrosis, instability arthropathy, post-trauma arthritis, post-infective arthritis, and arthritis secondary to glenoid dysplasia

Box 4.8.1 Advantages of surface replacement

- No stem constraints
- Allows simple accurate anatomical resurfacing
- Offset is correct
- Less invasive surgery
- No canal reaming
- No stress riser at end of stem
- Easier revision
- Bone stock conserving.

or epiphysis dysplasia. This prosthesis could be considered for Seebauer type I cuff tear arthropathy.

The best results are achieved in cases of osteoarthritis where the rotator cuff is intact. Conversely, suboptimal results are seen in individuals with cuff tear arthropathy and also in instances of post-traumatic arthritis. The surface replacement arthroplasty can be used in circumstances of moderate erosion of the humeral head, by bone grafting the defect. If there is more than 60% contact between the undersurface of the trial prosthesis and humeral head, after it has been milled, then it would be suitable for surface replacement. In other words, up to 40% of the humeral head surface area may be replaced by bone graft.

The contraindications for surface replacement arthroplasty include active infection, bone loss of the humeral head exceeding 40% of the surface, and acute fractures. Cases with an irreparable cuff tear would be suitable for the extended articular surface (EAS) replacement or a reverse shoulder arthroplasty.

Approximately 92% of our cases requiring shoulder arthroplasty receive a surface replacement. It is our opinion that surface replacement should be the standard prosthesis of choice for all cases, unless specifically contraindicated. *The question now is not when to use a surface replacement, but what are the limited residual indications for a stemmed implant?*

Hemiarthroplasty versus total shoulder arthroplasty using the surface replacement prosthesis

When deciding to do a hemiarthroplasty or a total arthroplasty, one must balance the possibility of longer-term glenoid wear and loosening in a total replacement with the possibility of late glenoid erosion in a hemiarthroplasty, necessitating conversion to a total replacement.

Our surface replacements had a 1% revision rate over 4 years. A survivorship analysis of the two groups in our series showed 97.1% survival of the hemireplacements and 81.7% survival of the total replacements. (Log rank test p = 0.0028). The total shoulders functioned slightly better, but revision rates were higher in the total shoulder group (18.3%) as compared to the hemiarthroplasty group (2.1%) (p <0.0001) (Figure 4.8.3).

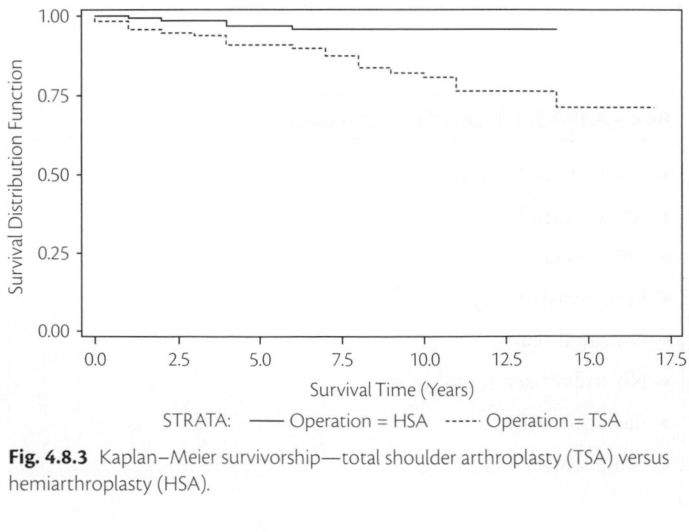

Fig. 4.8.3 Kaplan–Meier survivorship—total shoulder arthroplasty (TSA) versus hemiarthroplasty (HSA).

We perform and recommend hemiarthroplasty now as a general rule, with the glenoid being replaced only infrequently, in view of the long-term results in our series.

Surgical pearls (Box 4.8.2)

The detailed surgical technique is outside the scope of this chapter, but the reader is referred to its detailed description in the article by Copeland and colleagues for further information.

Results of surface replacement from other groups

Good clinical early results have been obtained with cups developed by Steffee and Moore (1984), and by Jónsson et al. (1986). Zippel in Germany implanted two surface replacements that were fixed by a transosseous screw but no follow-up is recorded for these cases. Rydholm and Sjögen from Sweden reported the results of the 'SCAN cup' in 1993 and 2003. Rydholm performed 84 SCAN cups, a hemispherical cemented cup, in 70 patients, and 72 cups in 59 patients were followed for 4.2 years (range, 1.5–9.9 years). The clinical results obtained showed 94% of the patients being pleased regarding pain relief and 82% reporting improved shoulder mobility. Shoulder function was significantly improved. Radiographs were analysed regarding the position of the cup, proximal migration of the humerus, and glenoid attrition during the follow-up period. Any

Box 4.8.2 Surgical pearls

- Confirm that patient position allows arm to extend and adduct adequately on table
- Have a low threshold for an acromioplasty and acromioclavicular joint excision
- Expose the junction of the head and anatomic neck adequately, a crucial step requiring removal of all osteophytes on the humerus
- Accurately identify the centre of the humeral head before proceeding
- If in doubt about the size, downsize
- Preserve as much of the bone reamings in the patient's blood as possible to augment any bone loss in the humeral head; up to 40% bone loss can be reconstituted during a surface replacement
- Remember to perform soft tissue release/balancing as necessary
- Drill the glenoid surface to stimulate bleeding and fibrocartilage regeneration
- Reconstruct soft tissues carefully, including repair of the deltoid during closure
- Do not be too aggressive with the acromioplasty and acromioclavicular joint excision in cases with poor or irreparable rotator cuff; consider using the deltopectoral approach in these cases
- Do not use the prosthesis in cases of fracture or if bone loss from the head is greater than 40%

change of the distance between the superior margin of the cup and the greater tuberosity and/or change of inclination of the prosthesis were regarded as signs of prosthetic loosening. With that definition, 25% of the cups were found to be loose at follow-up. Prosthetic loosening, however, had no bearing on the clinical result. Progressive proximal migration of the humerus in 38% of the shoulders and central attrition of the glenoid in 22% of the shoulders did not show any relationship to gain of mobility, pain relief, or functional ability. Of note, no central fixation peg was used for this cup. Long-term follow-up at 13 years included 54 cups in 46 patients (13 patients deceased, no revisions). Six cups had been revised 10 years (range, 5–16 years) after the index operation (four– for persistent pain, one for stiffness, and one for prosthetic loosening). Pain at rest on a 100-mm visual analogue scale was 15mm (range, 0–62mm) and pain on motion was 32mm (range, 0–85mm). Twenty-six (50%) could comb their hair (compared with 56% at first follow-up), 32 (62%) could wash their opposite axilla (90% at first follow-up), and 31 (60%) could reach behind (77% at first follow-up).

Alund et al. reported on 40 shoulder surface replacements for rheumatoid disease using the SCAN prosthesis. They reported one revision to total shoulder replacement, and 39 shoulders were followed up for a mean of 4.4 years (0.9–6.5 years). The median Constant score was 30 (15–79), mean proximal migration of the humerus 5.5mm (standard deviation [SD] 5.2mm) and mean glenoid erosion 2.6mm (SD 1.7mm). Proximal migration and glenoid erosion did not correlate with shoulder function or pain. Radiographic signs of loosening (changes in cup inclination combined with changes in cup distance above the greater tuberosity) occurred in one-quarter of the shoulders. At follow-up, 26 patients were satisfied with the procedure, despite poor shoulder function and radiographic deterioration.

Fink prospectively evaluated 45 Durom cups in 39 patients (30 women, 9 men) with rheumatoid disease. The average follow-up was 45.1 ± 11.6 months with a minimum of 36 months. Fifteen shoulders had an intact cuff (group A), 18 had a partial tearing or a repaired rotator cuff (group B), and 12 shoulders a massive cuff tear (group C). In group A rheumatic shoulders, the Constant score increased from 21.5 ± 9.6 points preoperatively to 66.1 ± 9.8 points at 36 months postoperatively; in shoulders of group B, from 19.6 ± 9.7 points preoperatively to 64.9 ± 9.6 points at 36 months postoperatively; and in shoulders of group C, from17.5 ± 8.7 points to 56.9 ± 9.8 points at the latest follow-up examination. All shoulders were pain-free at the latest examination. No complications, component loosening or changes of cup position were observed.

The Copeland Mark III prosthesis results

From 1993, the entire non-articular surface (implant–bone interface) of the glenoid and humeral components has been hydroxyapatite coated. The initial mechanical press-fit is thus followed later by a biological fix with bony ingrowth due to the hydroxyapatite coating. This is the current Mark III design. Between September 1993 and August 2002, 209 shoulders underwent surface replacement arthroplasty at our unit using the Mark III prosthesis with hydroxyapatite coating. Clinical and radiological outcome was assessed at an average duration of follow-up of 4.4 years. No evidence of radiolucency was seen in any humeral implant. Thomas et al. reported a 6.3% incidence of lucencies in their series using the Mark III implant. Asymptomatic non-progressive lucency of less than 2mm was seen in seven of the 29 glenoid components inserted, which did not require further treatment.

Six shoulders (2.8%) required revision surgery (one malposition of glenoid, two instability, and three painful arthroplasties). Using the Kaplan–Meier analysis, the probability that the implant would survive to the start of the tenth year after surgery was estimated to be 96.4%. The results of Mark III CSRA are comparable to conventional stemmed prostheses. There was no difference between hemiarthroplasty and total shoulder arthroplasty in terms of functional outcome. No hemiarthroplasty has been revised for component loosening.

Table 4.8.1 summarizes the results of surface replacement prostheses published thus far.

Table 4.8.1 Surface replacement prostheses studies

	Author				
	Copeland/Levy	**Thomas**	**Alund**	**Rydholm**	**Fink**
Implant	Copeland Mark 2 (pre-HA coating)	Copeland Mark 3	SCAN	SCAN	Durom
Indication	Mixed	Mixed	Rheumatoid	Rheumatoid	Rheumatoid
No. of replacements	103	48	39	72	45
Average age at surgery (years)	64.3	70	55	51	62.7
Follow-up (months)	60–120 (mean 80)	24–63 (mean 34.2)	24–72 (mean 52)	50–95 (mean 50)	45.1 ± 11
Mean preoperative Constant score	15.4	16.4	NA	NA	19.5
Mean postoperative Constant score	52.4	54	30	Not available but 92% of patients satisfied with pain improvement	62.6
Preoperative VAS	NA	NA	80 (median)		NA
Postoperative VAS	NA	NA	16 (median)	15–32 (mean)	NA
Radiologic lucent/lytic lines	5.1% (pre-HA coating)	6.3%	20%	25%	0%
Overall patients satisfied	93.9%	NA	83%	92%	94%

HA, hydroxyapatite; VAS, visual analogue score.

Revision surgery is greatly simplified having originally implanted a cementless surface replacement. At the time of revision of a surface replacement arthroplasty, the only bone lost is the bone that would have been removed had a stemmed prosthesis been used at the first operation. There is no need to remove a cemented stemmed prosthesis, which can be associated with loss of bone stock, perforation, and fracture of the humeral shaft. The preservation of bone facilitates revision to a stemmed prosthesis or to glenohumeral arthrodesis.

Conclusions

Surface replacement of the shoulder has been proven to be at least as successful as stemmed implants in the treatment of shoulder arthritis. The hydroxyapatite coating has been a major advance in reducing lucent lines and loosening. The bone-preserving nature of the implant allows it to be used in a most situations, including cases of deformity. If complications do occur, then they can be more easily treated, and the results of surface hemiarthroplasty appear to be comparable with stemmed hemiarthroplasty. The geometry and mechanics of the shoulder joint are now much better understood. It is no longer justifiable to continue with intramedullary (either cementless or cemented) fixation in a straightforward arthritic problem.

Future considerations

Future prostheses for the shoulder are likely to be of the bone-preserving nature. As materials improve, prosthesis wear will hopefully become less of a problem. Modern technology allows for more accurate preoperative planning. Computer assistance during surgery could translate this planning to a practical solution to optimize implant position and soft tissue balancing, which ultimately with improved materials should increase longevity of the prosthesis and improve function after shoulder arthroplasty. The next challenge facing us will probably be that of regenerating the surface!

Further reading

Boileau, P. and Walch, G. (1997). The three-dimensional geometry of the proximal humerus. Implications for surgical technique and prosthetic design. *Journal of Bone and Joint Surgery*, **79B**(5), 857–65.

Copeland, S. (2006). The continuing development of shoulder replacement: "reaching the surface". *Journal of Bone and Joint Surgery*, **88**(4), 900–5.

Gartsman, G.M., Roddey, T.S., and Hammerman, S.M. (2000). Shoulder arthroplasty with or without resurfacing of the glenoid in patients who have osteoarthritis. *Journal of Bone and Joint Surgery*, **82**(1), 26–34.

Jónsson, E., Egund, N., Kelly, I., Rydholm, U., and Lidgren, L. (1986). Cup arthroplasty of the rheumatoid shoulder. *Acta Orthopaedica Scandinavica*, **57**(6), 542–6.

Levy, O. and Copeland, S.A. (2001). Cementless surface replacement arthroplasty of the shoulder. 5- to 10-year results with the Copeland mark-2 prosthesis. *Journal of Bone and Joint Surgery*, **83B**(2), 213–21.

Levy, O. and Copeland, S.A. (2004). Cementless surface replacement arthroplasty (Copeland CSRA) for osteoarthritis of the shoulder. *Journal of Shoulder and Elbow Surgery*, **13**(3), 266–71.

Neer, C.S. (1974). Replacement arthroplasty for glenohumeral osteoarthritis. *Journal of Bone and Joint Surgery*, **56**(1), 1–13.

Torchia, M.E., Cofield, R.H., and Settergren, C.R. (1997). Total shoulder arthroplasty with the Neer prosthesis: long-term results. *Journal of Shoulder and Elbow Surgery*, **6**(6), 495–505.

4.9

Stemmed total shoulder replacement

Ian A. Trail

Summary points

- Stemmed shoulder replacement remains the gold standard for shoulder with an intact rotator cuff.
- The scarred capsule must be released before the implant is introduced.
- This chapter discusses the merits of total shoulder replacement versus hemiarthroplasty and the management of complications.

History

Gluck of Berlin was probably the first surgeon to implant a humeral head made from ivory. However, most people recount the story of Emile Pean and how he replaced the destroyed shoulder of a young Parisian in 1893. The implant was made of platinum and vulcanized rubber. The implant had no hope of survival in the face of active tuberculosis and was removed 2 years later, the patient surviving both operations.

Credit must be given to Charles Neer for giving us the first successful shoulder replacement. The Neer prosthesis was designed for the management of complex fractures and first used in 1955. Later Neer extended its use to rheumatoid and osteoarthritis of the shoulder. A high-density polyethylene glenoid component was soon added to the metal humeral implant. The original Neer prosthesis was so well designed that for three decades it remained the gold standard.

During the 1980s surgeons were realising that a greater range of implants was needed to replicate the patient's own anatomy. In particular, the diameter of the humeral head (at 48mm or 50mm according to manufacturer) was noted to overstuff the shoulder of small women whose native head size was 38–43mm. Thus the mono-block Neer implant was replaced by a number of modular implants. Specifically the stem and head of the humeral components were interchangeable, allowing a better fit to the patient's normal anatomy. However, the large head diameter was kept, the neck length being reduced, and this failed to solve the problem.

A decade later careful anatomical studies by Iannotti and co-workers in the United States, Roberts and Wallace in the United Kingdom, and Boileau and Walch in France led to the understanding of variable anatomy. In particular it was noted that the head diameter varied from 38–50mm, that the version of the shoulder was peculiar to the individual (and not a constant 30 degrees), but most importantly that the centre of the humeral head was not directly in line with the centre of the humeral shaft, giving us the concept of posterior and medial offset (Figure 4.9.1). A third generation of prostheses now came on the market with variable head diameters and the ability to offset the head on the prosthetic shaft, thereby replicating the patient's own anatomy more accurately. The price paid for this accuracy was increased complexity of the prosthesis (Figure 4.9.2).

Philosophy

There is no doubt that the philosophy of surgeons undertaking total shoulder replacement has changed over the years. Surgeons now understand that shoulder replacement is a soft tissue procedure as much as a bony one. A'soft tissue procedure' means optimizing rotator cuff function, releasing the contracted capsule, and repairing the subscapularis strongly enough to allow early movement with no risk of retear.

The aim of shoulder replacement has always been to alleviate pain, improve movement, increase function, and allow the patient to maintain their own independence. These benefits should be expected to last for a minimum of 10–15 years.

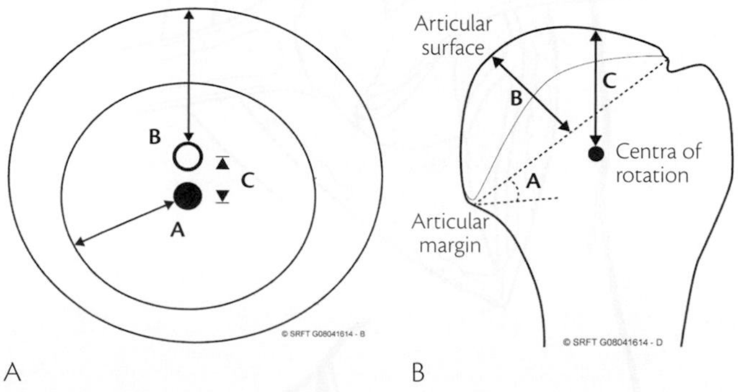

Fig. 4.9.1 Offset/intraversion, depth of head, and radius of curvature.

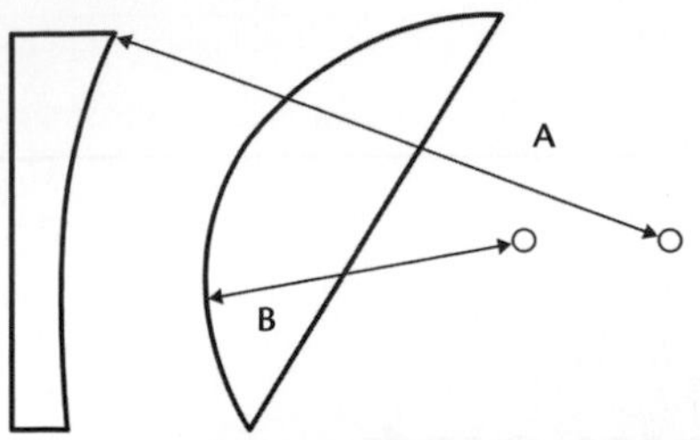

Fig. 4.9.2 Mismatched radius of curvature.

The implants used currently have a number of similarities and none can claim that their clinical outcome is any better than another. With regard to implant design there is now a move towards perfect anatomical replacement of the humeral head. This is possible with a surface replacement and increasingly it is so with stemmed implants. Whilst to date there is no evidence that this drive towards anatomical replacement has had any effect on clinical outcome, it has a beneficial effect on any glenoid component in so much that it seems to reduce migration and loosening and, as a consequence, improve longevity.

Whether a glenoid component should be inserted or not remains contentious. What can be said from a review of the literature is that any series comparing hemiarthroplasty (HA) to total shoulder replacement (TSR) does seem to indicate that total shoulders do better, at least in the short to medium term. With regard to whether a surface replacement or a stemmed humeral component should be used, there is no comparative data. It does not appear that humeral loosening of either a stemmed or a surface implant is significant. The only potential problem is the difficulty of access to insert a glenoid component with the head still in place if resurfacing is used (Figure 4.9.3).

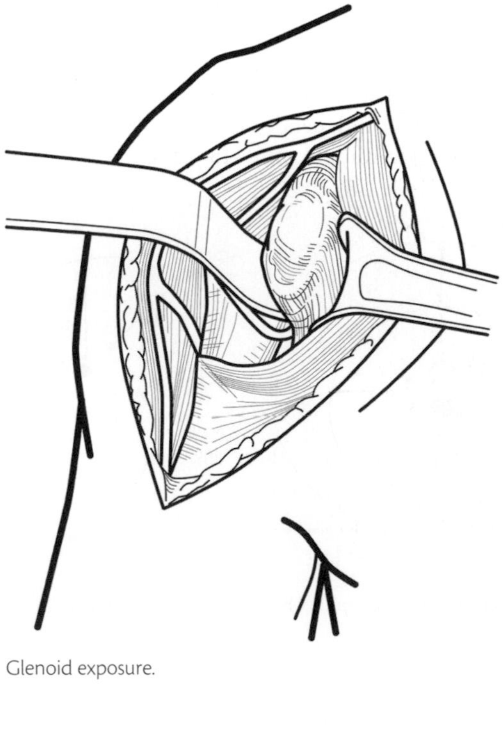

Fig. 4.9.3 Glenoid exposure.

Finally, the role of postoperative mobilization and therapy cannot be understated. It is crucial for any surgeon undertaking this type of surgery that they have access to an experienced network of therapists such that early and appropriate mobilization can start immediately after surgery.

Anatomy

The deltopectoral approach is standard for stemmed shoulder replacements. A skin incision is made over the deltopectoral groove along the line connecting the coracoid to the midpoint of the lateral aspect of the humerus (Figure 4.9.4). Three structures cross the deltopectoral interval: two arteries and one vein. The arteries are branches of the thoracoacromial trunk: the deltoid artery and the acromial artery. The acromial artery can be preserved, but the deltoid artery must be ligated and divided. The deltoid artery has two patterns. The commonest pattern gives off a large pectoral branch as it emerges from the thoracoacromial trunk, and then passes directly into the bulk of the deltoid muscle. The less common variant runs alongside the cephalic vein giving off a series of much smaller pectoral branches. This second pattern confuses the novice shoulder surgeon who incorrectly thinks that these are tributaries of the cephalic vein when actually they are branches of the variant deltoid artery. The deltopectoral interval is always developed medial to the cephalic vein, with preservation of its major tributaries leaving it on the deltoid muscle. The cephalic vein must never be taken off the deltoid. The cephalic vein should be preserved if possible. There is usually no need to release the deltoid muscle either proximally or distally although it is useful to free the undersurface of the muscles from the humerus and rotator cuff so that the head can be pushed back freely when it comes to exposing the glenoid. Be careful for the axillary nerve runs on the deep surface of the deltoid and can be entrapped in scar, particularly following fractures of the humeral neck. The terminal branch of the posterior circumflex artery sends a small anastomosing branch that enters the bone lateral to the insertion of pectoralis major, a vessel that can easily be torn whilst mobilizing deltoid.

Incising the clavipectoral fascia at the lateral edge of the conjoined tendon up to, or through, the coracoacromial ligament exposes subscapularis and the anterior capsule. It is often helpful to release the top half of the insertion of pectoralis major in order to gain a better exposure of the inferior capsule.

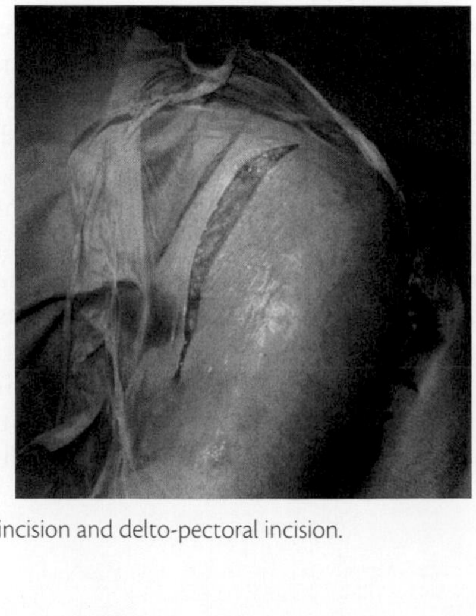

Fig. 4.9.4 Skin incision and delto-pectoral incision.

The subscapularis is incised at its insertion on the lesser tuberosity along with the subjacent capsule. The junction of the middle and lower third of the subscapularis is demarcated by the anterior circumflex vessels. These should be ligated or coagulated and divided. It is also important to leave a 1-cm stump of subscapularis/capsule for reattachment of the muscle to the humerus. Alternatively the lesser tuberosity can be osteotomized from the humerus, being reattached at the end by sutures or anchors (Figure 4.9.5).

Finally, as with all joint replacements, it is important to release contractures, particularly of the anterior and inferior capsule. Patients suffering with arthritis often suffer with significant stiffness resulting in marked contracture. It is only if these contractures are released that a significant improvement in range of motion be obtained. Plainly care must be taken when releasing the inferior capsule as this could result in damage to the axillary nerve. The latter will result in a deltoid paralysis, which is a catastrophe. Some surgeons actually dissect the quadrilateral space and place a silastic sling around the axillary nerve and its accompanying posterior circumflex artery and vein, whereas other surgeons make a point of seeing the neurovascular bundle so that it can be protected throughout the procedure. With the axillary nerve seen or placed in a protective sling the inferior capsule can be released, and this is the key to glenoid exposure and regaining a good range of movement postoperatively.

The superior capsule must now be released, including the coracohumeral ligament, and if necessary the long head of biceps (Figure 4.9.6).

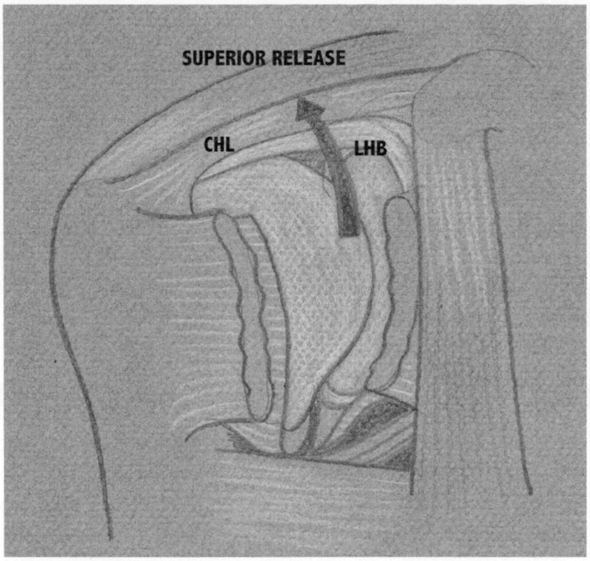

Fig. 4.9.6 Balancing the prosthesis.

Pathology

The principal indications for joint replacement in the shoulder are inflammatory/rheumatoid arthritis, degenerative joint disease, secondary osteoarthritis, avascular necrosis, and trauma. Added to this in a special category is cuff tear arthropathy.

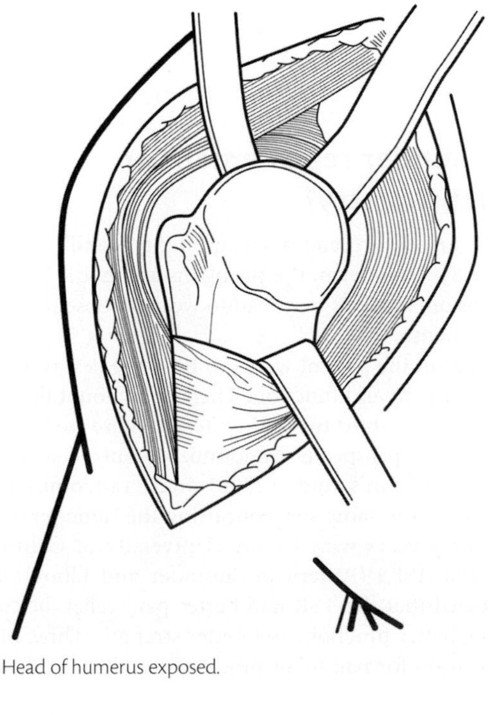

Fig. 4.9.5 Head of humerus exposed.

In rheumatoid or inflammatory arthritis the disease process is typically erosive with loss of bone and cyst formation. In this condition the glenoid can be markedly eroded anteriorly and superiorly. In addition there is often thinning of the rotator cuff with superior subluxation of the humeral head. Erosion of the glenoid may be of such severity that it is insufficient to support a glenoid component. Any bone cysts should be curetted and filled with either bone graft or cement. Again any soft tissue contracture should be released. Repair of the rotator cuff may not be feasible because the tendon tissue is so poor.

Degenerative joint disease can present with significant deformity of both the humeral head and glenoid. The glenoid is eroded posteriorly with posterior subluxation of the humeral head. The latter is often flattened anteriorly. Added to this there can be a number of large osteophytes surrounding the whole of the humeral head with loose bodies either inferiorly or posteriorly. Capsular contractures are common and will need to be released at surgery.

The treatment of patients with avascular necrosis of the humeral head can be rewarding at least in the short term. In most cases a HA is all that is required and good results can be expected. Patients are often relatively young and the soft tissues around the shoulder are well maintained. Because of their young age these patients may need regular and long-term follow-up as at some stage revision is likely.

Joint replacement in post-traumatic arthritis is probably the most difficult and is often unrewarding. The normal anatomy can be so distorted that the surgeon can experience significant difficulties navigating the joint. In these cases the glenoid may not be damaged and may not require replacement. Paramount to the success of the operation is reconstruction of the fractured tuberosities. These must be re-attached strongly to the humeral shaft in the correct anatomical location allowing movement to resume as soon as possible after surgery. If the tuberosity has to be osteotomized and reattached this can be both difficult and lead to diminished function.

The role of shoulder arthroplasty in acute trauma falls outside the remit of this chapter. Plainly an implant should only be used in cases that cannot be treated by open reduction and internal fixation or where there is a significant risk of avascular necrosis. Surgical techniques used are significantly different from those used in arthritis. Obtaining correct humeral length, alignment, and version are critical to success. Further difficulties arise from the fixation of the greater and lesser tuberosities to the prosthesis and humeral shaft. Bony union can also be unpredictable. Implant manufacturers have responded to these difficulties and their implants have been modified for use in the trauma scenario.

Indications and contraindications (Box 4.9.1)

Shoulder arthroplasty is indicated in all the earlier discussed clinical situations, in patients who are suffering sufficient pain, loss of movement, weakness, and reduced function. Pain remains the principal indication particularly if the patient is having difficulty sleeping and requires strong analgesia on a regular basis. Patients who undergo total shoulder arthroplasty do improve the range of motion of their shoulder, but surgeons should beware operating for this symptom in isolation. A patient with a stiff yet pain-free shoulder will not do as well as one with a painful yet mobile joint.

Before embarking on shoulder arthroplasty it is important to assess the status of the bone stock, not only of the humerus but especially the glenoid. Is there sufficient bone stock to support a glenoid component? This can be assessed by radiographs, particularly an axillary view, or by computed tomography scan. It is important to allow for any correction of deformity. Any deficit in the rotator cuff should also be assessed as this may affect outcome.

Patient motivation is an important factor in the success of the operation. The patient has to be committed to a surgical procedure and the lengthy postoperative rehabilitation programme. The patient must have a realistic expectation and an ability to follow advice as appropriate. The experience of the surgeon and supporting team, particularly physiotherapists, are vital factors. Finally, the least significant factor is the prosthesis itself.

The principal contraindication to surgery is lack of bone stock to support the prosthesis. This usually affects the glenoid side. If the deltoid muscle is not functioning then any arthroplasty will be unsuccessful. The better option here would be an arthrodesis.

Rotator cuff deficiency may cause difficulties. If the shoulder is concentric on the glenoid (Seebauer I) with a small tear (less than 2cm) a standard shoulder replacement is effective, but if the tear is large then a CTA head or a reverse shoulder can be used. If, however, the shoulder is subluxed upwards (Seebauer II) then a reverse implant should be used (Figure 4.9.7).

Infection is a definite contraindication. Infection will usually be encountered in the revision situation. Again this contraindication is not absolute in so much that two-stage surgery can often be successful. The first stage involves the removal of any metalwork or prosthesis and the debridement of soft tissues and bone. The second stage involves insertion of the prosthesis covered by appropriate antibiotics.

Finally, a neuromuscular disorder can make the outcome of TSR unpredictable. With good medical management in conditions such as epilepsy and Parkinson's disease the results of surgery can often be quite gratifying.

Box 4.9.1 Indications and contraindications for shoulder replacement

Indications

- Primary osteoarthritis
- Rheumatoid arthritis
- Avascular necrosis
- Post-traumatic arthritis
- Other inflammatory arthritides:
  - Psoriatic
  - Pigmented villonodular synovitis (PVNS)
  - Ankylosing joint disease
  - Synovial chondromatosis
- Secondary osteoarthritis:
  - Post-dislocation or dislocation surgery
  - Acromegalic arthropathy
  - Primary glenoid dysplasia
- Cuff tear arthropathy (CTA):
  - Seebauer type I selective hemiarthroplasty
  - Seebauer type II reverse polarity replacement.

Contraindications

- Active infection
- Paralytic dislocation
- Lack of bone stock.

Relative contraindications

- Previous infection
- Syringomyelia.

Total shoulder replacement or hemiarthroplasty?

The insertion of a glenoid component is still controversial (Figure 4.9.8). Long term, the problems are that HA may lead to glenoid erosion and TSR may lead to wear or loosening of the glenoid component.

In the interim the patient wants to have the best result in terms of pain, movement and function. There is no doubt that TSR wins out over HA in the short to medium term. There are four level-one evidence studies (prospective randomized controlled studies) that show this. Gartsman's study (2000) on 51 randomized patients, operated on by the same surgeon, using the same prosthesis and followed for 3 years with UCLA (University of California–Los Angeles) and ASES (American Shoulder and Elbow Surgeons) scores showed that the TSR had better pain relief, better patient satisfaction, better function, and better strength. Three of the HAs came to revision for painful glenoid erosion during the study, but

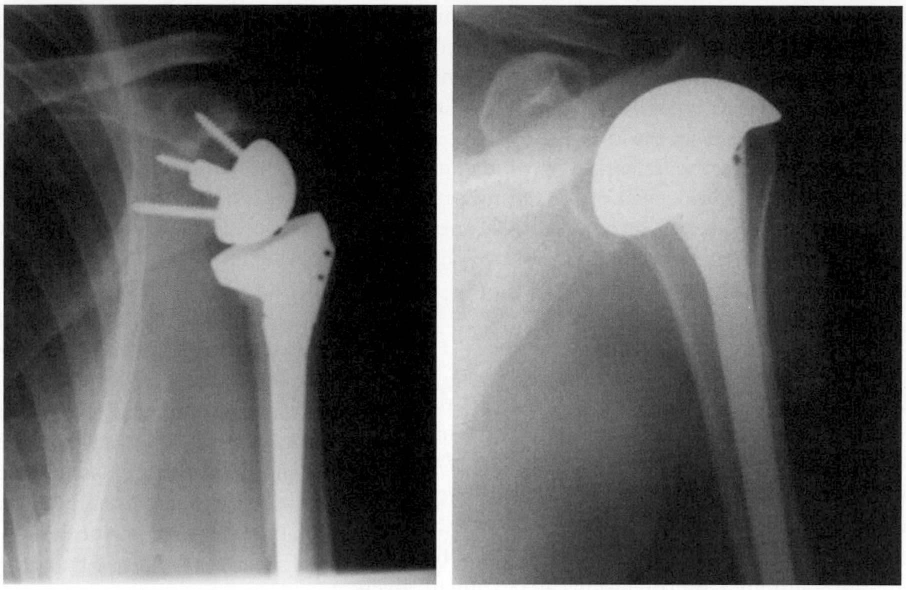

Fig. 4.9.7 Delta prosthesis (A) and CTA head (B).

none of the TSRs came to revision. Kirkley's study (2005) on 41 randomized patients also had three HAs come to revision for painful glenoid erosion during the study, but none of the TSRs were revised. The study by Sandow et al. (1998) on 32 randomized patients showed that the TSR group had significantly less pain, and the study by Jónsson (1998) on 49 randomized patients showed significantly better Constant scores for the TSR group. Of course all these studies suffered from low numbers so Kirkley did a meta-analysis (2005) combining these randomized studies and showed that the TSR group had significantly better pain relief, significantly better function, and better movement than the HA group (Figure 4.9.9).

There is also a lot of level 2 and 3 evidence (not randomized) that TSR fares better than HA. In our study (Haines and Trail 2006) on 124 patients, both groups improved significantly and equally, with a small trend towards better results for pain and movement in the TSR group but the major cause for revision was glenoid pain due to erosion in 12% of the HA group. The Tornier group (2003), in a study of 601 TSR compared to 89 HA, showed good to excellent results in 94% of the TSR group compared to 86% of the HA group, with the TSR group having better scores for pain, mobility, and activity, and their conclusion was that TSR was better than HA. Finally Bigliani and co-workers (2007) did a meta-analysis that included 23 non-randomized studies with 1952 patients and showed that the TSR group had significantly better pain relief, significantly better elevation, significantly better gain in elevation, significantly greater gain in external rotation, and significantly better patient satisfaction. There is no more to be said.

So what about the late results? Well there is no doubt about painful glenoid erosion following HA. It was bad enough for revision surgery in 12% of our study, 12% of Gartsman's study, and 12% of Kirkley's study. In Sperling and Cofield's long-term study 72% of the HA group had glenoid erosion on radiographs at 10 years.

And what of glenoid revision following TSR? Sperling and Cofield had a 97% survival of their glenoids at 10 years. In the Radnay and Bigliani meta-analysis of 1952 patients only 1.7% of

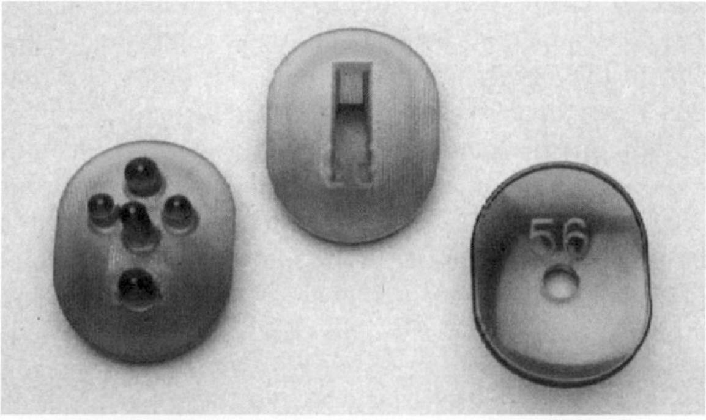

Fig. 4.9.8 Pegged and keeled glenoid components.

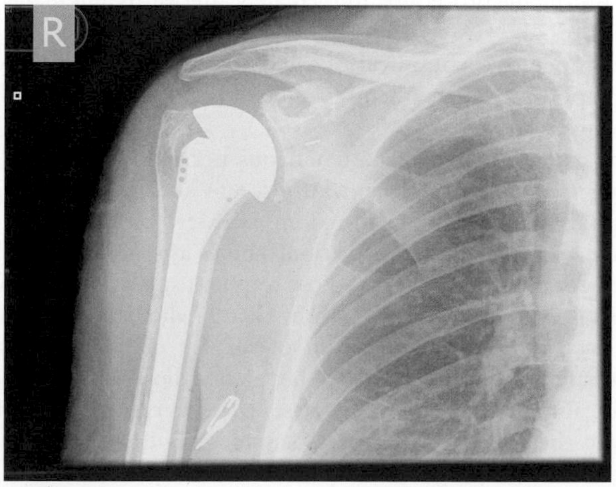

Fig. 4.9.9 Final position on x-ray.

sockets needed revision. In Bunker's study with a minimum 10-year follow-up there was a 94% survival for the glenoid. The TSR versus HA debate will continue to rumble on but evidence is now stacking up for the superiority of TSR in the short to medium term, and greater survival of TSR in the long term.

What is also of note is that improvements in glenoid component design, preparation of the glenoid, fixation including cementing techniques, and, interestingly enough, an anatomical humeral head replacement have resulted in a lower incidence of migration and loosening and potentially better long-term survival.

Results

Whilst it is difficult to prove, I have no doubt that the results of shoulder replacement continue to improve and certainly have become more reproducible. This is a testament to all of the surgeons who have helped develop prostheses as well as the techniques of surgery. With regards to the results themselves, these are now being reported from all corners of the globe. Generally these are extremely favourable, although interpretation can be difficult given the lack of standardization of outcome evaluation. In Europe the Constant score, and more recently the Oxford score, and in the United States the ASES score have been used. Unfortunately these are not interchangeable. As such it is probably more sensible to break the scores down into their various components, particularly pain relief, range of motion, strength, and finally function.

It is not possible to report on every single article that has been written on shoulder arthroplasty. As such I have chosen six with the largest numbers and the longest follow-up. These have been summarized in Table 4.9.1. As can be seen in most series the authors report extremely good pain relief and an average range of motion of between 100–110 degrees of abduction and 110–120 degrees of forward flexion; internal rotation to the buttock or lower lumber spine and an external rotation of 40–50 degrees. As a result of this there is a significant improvement in function. Perhaps more importantly authors are now reporting that these improvements continue for 10 or 15 years.

Complications

As with all joint replacements, whilst most patients can expect a good to excellent result some will get a complication. These can arise during the procedure, immediately afterwards and in the long term (Box 4.9.2).

Peri-operative complications include nerve or blood vessel injury, peri-prosthetic fractures, and, on occasion, implant-related problems.

The axillary and musculocutaneous nerves are always at risk during shoulder replacement. At a recent audit at Wrightington Hospital (Wigan, United Kingdom) we were able to identify 17 instances of neuropraxia of various nerves after shoulder arthroplasty. As all these patients had concomitant supraclavicular nerve blocks it was not possible to know clearly whether these injuries had occurred as a direct result of surgery or the block itself. Fortunately all these recovered although one took 12 months. More significant and permanent injuries, however, can occur, particularly to the axillary and musculocutaneous nerves. The axillary nerve can be damaged during an inferior capsular release. The musculocutaneous nerve lies on the undersurface of the short head of biceps and can be damaged when this muscle is retracted. Damage to either nerve can leave the patient with a significant functional deficit. It is therefore important that any damage should be identified at the time of surgery and rectified. Postoperative neuropraxia should be monitored, and if at 6 weeks there has been no improvement then electromyographs obtained. The latter will often distinguish between neuropraxia and definitive nerve damage. For the latter it is important that further exploration and nerve repair is undertaken as appropriate. Finally, later management might involve some form of tendon transfer.

Fortunately vascular injuries following TSR are rare. The author has seen two in over 17 years of consultant practice. As would be expected, diagnosis is relatively straightforward. Indeed if prompt help is summoned by way of vascular expertise including an arteriogram and bypass grafting, then a good outcome can be expected. It should also not be assumed that this compromise has occurred as a direct result of surgical trauma. In one case in the author's practice intraluminal occlusion was found quite distal to the surgical site. It was assumed that this was 'an accident waiting to happen' perhaps precipitated by external rotation of the arm. Whatever the circumstances the surgeon should not hesitate to seek urgent advice and must not prevaricate in the vain hope that things will improve spontaneously.

Periprosthetic fractures can include fractures of the glenoid but more commonly the humerus, the latter as a result of overzealous manipulation of the upper extremity during exposure, particularly external rotation, but also inadvertent reaming and finally impaction of the prosthesis. The commonest follows external rotation and takes the form of a spiral fracture. Plainly great care should be taken when the humeral head is exposed, particularly in patients with fragile bone. Management of this problem is fortunately relatively straightforward and involves the insertion of a longer-stemmed humeral component and the application of cerclage wires (Figure 4.9.11). It is, however, important that the stem of the humeral component extends beyond the end of the fracture by at least two diameters of the radius of the humerus. Interoperative fracture of the glenoid, however, would probably preclude the insertion of a glenoid component. Fixation should be attempted. In most circumstances this can be undertaken by the use of a lag screw.

Postoperatively there are two major complications: infection and instability. Infection after TSR is relatively uncommon with most published series reporting an incidence of between 1–2%. As with all arthroplasty, one must assume that the implant was contaminated at the time of surgery. Infection can present immediately after surgery or somewhat later (12 months after surgery). A number of factors increase the likelihood of infection, particularly previous surgery, diabetes mellitus, and systemic corticosteroids. Multiple organisms have been described, particularly *Propionibacterium acnes*, *Staphylococcus aureus*, and *Staphylococcus epidermidis* and even *Candida*. *P. acnes* is an acrotolerant anaerobic Gram-positive rod that is sensitive to clindamycin, erythromycin, tetracyclines, piperacillin, and penicillin G. It is sensitive to ultraviolet light. It is a commensal in the skin of the face and shoulder girdle, accounting for the incidence of acne in these sites. It is therefore a specific risk to shoulders and not to the hip and knee and is difficult to grow in the laboratory. In a significant number of cases no organism can be identified. Continuing antibiotic use or poor bacteriological techniques may account for this.

Table 4.9.1 Results of total shoulder replacements

Study	N				
Stewart and Kelly (1997)	58	RA	9.7 years	29/37 pain free	9 glenoids loose on x-ray
				Elevation 53–75°	9 humeral stems loose on x-ray
				→	
				ER 5–38°	
				→	
Norris and Iannotti (2002)	176	OA	3.8 years	Pain 73.9 15.5	7 glenoids loose
				→	
				Elevation 102–138°	5 cases of instability
				→	
				ER 14–45°	
				→	
Sperling et al. (2004)	78	Mixed	16.8 years	Pain 4.7 2.1	TSR
				→	
				Abduction 65–112°	3 glenoids loose
				→	
				ER 17–43°	2 infections
					Hemi
					2 humeral loosening
					1 infection
					2 glenoid wear
				→	→
Trail and Nuttall (2001)	105	RA	8.8 years	Flexion 61–78°	4 HHR TSR
				→	
				Abduction 47–67°	
				→	
				ER 16–36°	
				Kaplan–Meier at 8 years 92%	
Deshmukh et al. (2005)	320	mixed	14.0 years (subset)	Kaplan–Meier at 20 years 85%	3 cases of dislocation
				Revision as end point	2 infection
					4 perioperative fractures
				→	
Haines et al. (2005)	124	OA	Up to 11.6 years	Flexion 64–103°	2 cases of fractures at the shaft of the humerus
				→	
				Abduction 53–92°	1 case of instability
				→	→
				ER 11–39°	5 HHR TSR
				Kaplan–Meier at 12 years 90%	4 glenoids revised

ER, external rotation; HHR, humeral head replacement; OA, osteoarthritis; RA, rheumatoid arthritis; TSR, total shoulder replacement

Box 4.9.2 Complications of shoulder replacement

- Intraoperative:
  - Axillary or musculocutaneous nerve injury
  - Anterior or posterior circumflex artery injury
  - Incorrect implant position (version, offset, height)
  - Inadequate initial fixation
  - Glenoid or humeral fracture
- Postoperative:
  - Infection
  - Dislocation
  - Subscapularis failure (suture line)
  - (Deep vein thrombosis and pulmonary embolism are extremely rare)
- Long term:
  - Rotator cuff failure
  - Glenoid loosening
  - Glenoid erosion
  - Polyethylene wear.

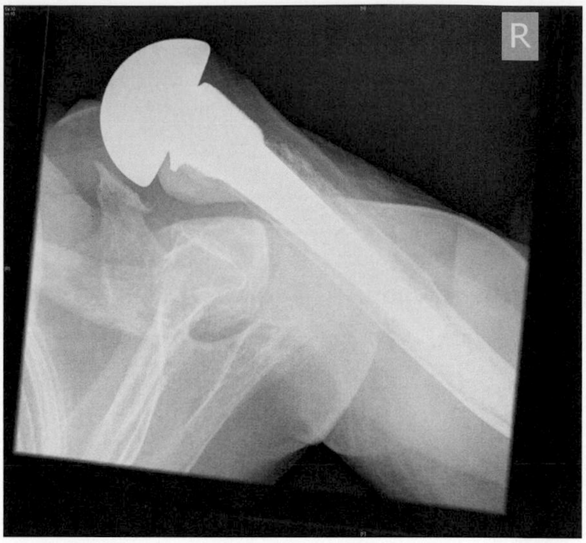

Fig. 4.9.10 Anterior subluxation of the humeral head.

The C-reactive protein (CRP) and white cell count (WCC) can be normal in 40% of revision cases where infection is later confirmed by biopsy. When infection has been confirmed either by clinical means, cultures, or blood tests, then two-stage revision surgery is the only remedial treatment. The first stage involves removal of the implant and the insertion of an antibiotic-loaded cement ball and stem which fits down the humerus like a HA or packing the space with gentamicin beads. The second stage is removal of the antibiotic-impregnated cement spacer and the reinsertion of a new prosthesis. In the author's experience this type of surgery is relatively successful. It seems to result in a resolution of the infection leaving the patient with a relatively pain-free and mobile shoulder joint.

The time interval between the two stages of surgery depends on the clinical situation but should be a minimum of 3 months. Prior to the second stage it is crucial that the patient's wounds have healed and that there has been no recurrence of infection. Added to this, blood parameters including erythrocyte sedimentation rate, CRP, and WCC should all be normal. If there is any uncertainty then an open biopsy of soft tissues and bones should be undertaken to exclude infection prior to the second stage.

The incidence of dislocation varies widely (Figure 4.9.10). In most cases it arises as a result of poor surgical technique, that is, malalignment of the components, particularly excessive humeral retroversion, excessive soft tissue release, or poor reconstruction. Version is variable but the average humeral retroversion is 21 degrees. Glenoid version has to be performed by naked eye, for it is difficult to measure even radiographically.

With regard to the soft tissues, release of contractures is key to the procedure but must not lead to damage of the rotator cuff or subscapularis. At the end of the procedure the subscapularis muscle should be firmly attached to the lesser tuberosity. Thereafter, therapy whilst allowing movement should protect this repair, at least in the early 4–6-week period after surgery.

In the author's opinion instability can be extremely difficult to treat. If revision surgery is contemplated this should involve an assessment of the alignment of the prosthesis and muscles around the shoulder. Whilst realignment of the humeral component is relatively straightforward, that of the glenoid can be more difficult. The removal of a cemented glenoid component can result with insufficient bone being left for the insertion of a second. Treatment is very difficult; the alternatives include insertion of a corticocancellous bone graft or impaction grafting technique where appropriate. The results of these are unpredictable and leaving the patient with a HA will not correct instability.

Instability can occur after failure of the subscapularis repair. Mobilization and reinsertion of the subscapularis can be successful. This can be reinforced by a pectoralis major transfer. Of all revision surgeries for instability however, in the author's experience, the most successful has been the revision of an anatomical shoulder replacement to a reverse implant. This can stabilize the shoulder but it relies on the presence of good glenoid bone stock to support the glenosphere.

Failure of the rotator cuff is common in the elderly patient a decade on from surgery. This can occur after minor trauma and result in the patient presenting with a sudden loss of movement, particularly abduction and external rotation. In the author's experience the clinical picture is usually typical. In the first instance treatment is often a course of physiotherapy. Cuff repair in the degenerate cuff of the 80-year-old following shoulder replacement is doomed to failure, and one way out may be revision to a reverse polarity replacement.

Loosening of the glenoid component, may be the current rate-limiting step in TSR (Figure 4.9.11). Glenoid lucent lines remain a concern. Historical papers report a high incidence of lucent lines, but these could be detected in the recovery room and were thus a sign of poor surgical technique. However, studies using modern cement techniques are also of concern. Mansat had lucent lines in 67%, but

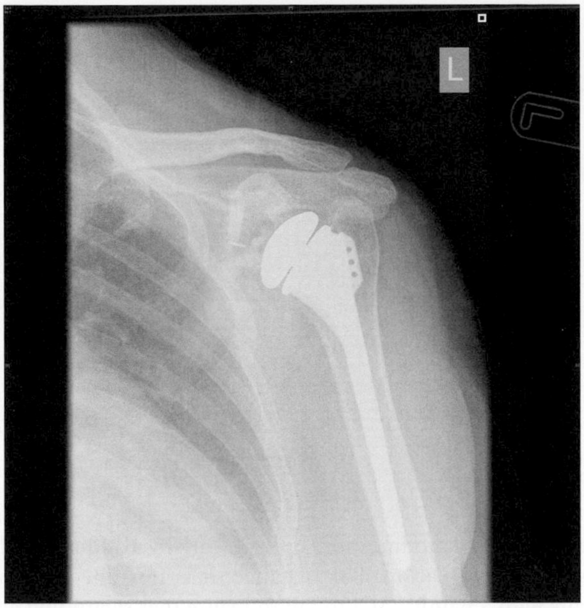

Fig. 4.9.11 Glenoid loosening.

complete lucent lines in only 35%, yet had no case of glenoid loosening and no revision for loosening. The Tornier multicentre group study had lucent lines detectable on day 1 in 60% of cases (a sign of poor technique) and 25% were progressive. The good news is that despite these high figures for lucent lines, glenoid revision rates are low with a figure of 1.7% in the meta-analysis of 1952 cases undertaken by Bigliani and co-workers.

When the glenoid loosens, management means revision surgery; the principal indication being pain. With the newer modular implant the ease of surgery has increased because the head can be separated from the stem of the humerus; this makes any approach to the glenoid easier to undertake. The removal of cemented monoblocks from the humerus, however, is notoriously difficult. Reconstruction of a glenoid relies on either the insertion of a corticocancellous graft or impaction grafting techniques. These are highly specialized and should only be undertaken in units familiar with these techniques. This type of surgery involves a significant amount of time, resource, and equipment. If reconstruction of the glenoid is not possible then the patient will have to be left with a HA.

Further reading

Bryant, D., Litchfield, R., Sandow, M., Gartsman, G.M., Guyatt, G., and Kirkley, A. (2005). A comparison of pain, strength, range of motion, and functional outcomes after hemiarthroplasty and total shoulder arthroplasty in patients with osteoarthritis of the shoulder. *Journal of Bone and Joint Surgery,* **87A,** 1947–56.

Deshmukh, A.V., Koris, M., Zurakowski, D., and Thornhill, T.S. (2005). Total shoulder arthroplasty: long-term survivorship, functional outcome, and quality of life. *Journal of Shoulder and Elbow Surgery,* **14,** 471–9.

Dines, J.S., Fealy, S., Strauss, E.J., *et al.* (2006). Outcomes analysis of revision total shoulder replacement. *Journal of Bone and Joint Surgery,* **88A,** 1494–500.

Haines, J.F., Trail, I.A., Nuttall, D., Birch, A., and Barrow, A. (2006). The results of arthroplasty in osteoarthritis of the shoulder. *Journal of Bone and Joint Surgery,* **88B,** 496–501.

Iannotti, J.P., Gabriel, J.P., Schneck, S.L., Evans, B.G., and Misra, S. (1992). The normal glenohumeral relationships. *Journal of Bone and Joint Surgery,* **74A,** 491–500.

Neer, C.S. (1955). Articular replacement for the humeral head. *Journal of Bone and Joint Surgery,* **37A,** 215–28.

Norris, T.R. and Iannotti, J.P. (2002). Functional outcome after shoulder arthroplasty for primary osteoarthritis: A multicenter study. *Journal of Shoulder and Elbow Surgery,* **11,** 130–5.

Qureshi, S., Hsiao, A., Klug, R.A., Lee, E., Braman, J., and Flatow, E.L. (2008). Subscapularis function after total shoulder replacement: results with lesser tuberosity osteotomy. *Journal of Shoulder and Elbow Surgery,* **17,** 68–72.

Sperling, J.W., Cofield, R.H., and Rowland, C.M. (2004). Minimum fifteen-year follow-up of Neer hemiarthroplasty and total shoulder arthroplasty in patients aged fifty years or younger. *Journal of Shoulder and Elbow Surgery,* **13,** 604–13.

Stewart, M.P.M. and Kelly, I.G. (1997). Total shoulder replacement in rheumatoid disease. *Journal of Bone and Joint Surgery,* **79B,** 68–72.

Trail, I.A. and Nuttall, D. (2002). The results of shoulder arthroplasty in patients with rheumatoid arthritis. *Journal of Bone and Joint Surgery,* **84B,** 1121–5.

4.10

Acromioclavicular joint

David Potter

Introduction

The acromioclavicular joint (ACJ) is the sole skeletal connection between the upper limb and the axial skeleton and provides both strength and stability to the shoulder. The three-dimensional alignment of the joint, particularly in the sagittal plane, is very variable which should be borne in mind, especially when trying to inject the joint. It is rare to find anyone older than 35–40 years of age without some evidence of degenerative change. The ACJ is also one of the most commonly injured joints of the body, accounting for 12% of all dislocations. Controversies regarding indications for surgical treatment of the joint, and the bewildering choice of procedures described, makes this small joint the subject of a disproportionate amount of debate and discussion amongst shoulder specialists.

Acromioclavicular joint arthropathy

Clinical presentation

There are two different groups of patients who present with arthropathy of the ACJ. The first patient is relatively young, in their twenties or thirties, usually male with a background of sporting injury or heavy manual work. Arthropathy in these patients can develop subsequent to a discrete, single episode of trauma to the shoulder or a history of taking part in a contact sport. Heavy manual work with a large amount of overhead lifting may contribute to the development of ACJ arthropathy. The early onset of arthropathy in this group may be related to premature damage to the intra-articular fibrocartilage disc in a similar model to that seen in the knee following meniscal injury.

The second group of patients suffering from the symptoms of ACJ arthropathy are middle-aged and may give a history of manual work or sport. However this is not consistent and presumably there is a constitutional element as with most other joints. The onset of symptoms can often be slow with long periods of minimal discomfort.

The clinical symptoms, signs, and investigations for ACJ pathology are dealt with in Chapter 4.1.

Initial treatment

The treatment of patients with mild to moderate arthropathy of the ACJ is non-surgical in the first instance. Advice can be given regarding activity modification, both at work by avoiding overhead tasks and in recreation. For instance, it is not uncommon for patients with a painful ACJ to fail to realise that swimming a mile three times weekly to keep fit is aggravating their arthritic ACJ. Regular analgesia and anti-inflammatory medication can also be discussed, although its effectiveness in the longer term is often not sustained.

Intra-articular injections of steroid are often advocated as an effective treatment of ACJ arthropathy. Whilst this is certainly worth trying in the patient without advanced arthropathy, it is the author's view that the beneficial effects are often not sustained. Placing the injection accurately can also be difficult and may be improved by the use of ultrasonography or fluoroscopy.

Surgical treatment

Surgery provides a safe and effective option if conservative treatment has failed, and in patients with severe arthropathy. The principle of surgery involves excising the distal end of the clavicle. Debate regarding whether the procedure is best done open or arthroscopically remains and also the optimal length of clavicle to excise.

Excision of the distal clavicle is usually attributed to Mumford whose name is attached to procedures such as the 'mini-Mumford' or 'arthroscopic Mumford'. According to the literature it is unclear whether Mumford or Gurd performed the first clavicle excision as they both published their techniques in 1941 in relation to the treatment of ACJ dislocation. Ellman was one of the first surgeons to describe arthroscopic excision of the distal clavicle in 1994 since when the arthroscopic technique has become popular.

Surgical anatomy

The ACJ is planar and has no inherent bony stability. Stability of the joint is therefore provided by the coracoclavicular ligaments and the ACJ ligaments with the joint capsule itself playing a minor role.

The conoid ligament inserts more medially on the conoid tubercle of the clavicle than the trapezoid ligament. Selective ligament sectioning work by Fukuda, has demonstrated that the conoid is responsible for constraining anterior and superior displacement of the clavicle, particularly under high load. The trapezoid ligament contributes less to vertical stability of the clavicle but help to stabilize the ACJ under axial compressive load.

The capsule of the ACJ is thickened superiorly and inferiorly to form discrete acromioclavicular (AC) ligaments. The superior ACJ ligament is more substantial and thicker (2–5mm) than the inferior ligament and provides rotational stability of the joint.

The lateral edge of the trapezoid ligament is 16.7mm ± 2.4mm from the articular surface of the clavicle. The medial edge of the trapezoid ligament is 28.2 ± 5.7mm from the end of the clavicle. Looking at the conoid ligament, this inserts on the clavicle between 33.5–49.7mm from the articular surface. There were no significant differences between men and women for the trapezoid ligament insertion although there was for the conoid insertion which was closer to the articular surface in women. The superior AC ligament inserts on the clavicle medially for 5.5mm ± 1.7mm in men and only 3.6mm ± 0.78mm in women. The acromial attachment of this ligament extended for 8.1mm in men and 4.7mm for women.

If we first consider open surgery, it is clear that in order to expose the distal clavicle, the superior AC ligament has to be incised and a limited amount of the delto-trapezial fascia has to be reflected. The minimum amount of bone that should be resected in order to abolish bone contact postoperatively has been shown by Branch to be 5mm. However, this will inevitably lead to loss of stability as the superior AC ligament is also lost and most surgeons recommend an excision of at least 10mm to avoid postoperative pain due to persistent posterior impingement of the clavicle on the acromion. As long as the excised segment is no more than 15mm, the trapezoid ligament should not be damaged.

Arthroscopic excision of the distal clavicle has the perceived advantages of avoiding the pain and potential morbidity of an open surgical exposure and allows resection of the clavicle without disrupting the deltotrapezial fascia. It is also said that arthroscopic excision preserves the superior AC ligament, leading to better preservation of rotational and horizontal stability, although this may not be the case given the evidence presented earlier. If the standard excision of 5mm of clavicle is carried out, this will almost certainly lead to complete detachment of the superior AC ligament in most patients, particularly females. If one wishes to preserve the clavicular attachment of the superior AC ligament it would seem more logical to excise no more than 3–4mm of bone from the clavicle and perhaps a similar amount from the acromion. A secondary advantage of an arthroscopic resection is the ability to perform glenohumeral inspection and treatment of occult pathology.

There are two approaches for arthroscopic ACJ resection: the direct and indirect methods. The common indirect approach involves exposing the ACJ through the subacromial bursa. The advantages of this technique are that the approach is familiar to the surgeon and that secondary impingement can be treated as appropriate. The direct approach involves establishing a viewing portal directly posterior to the ACJ with an anterior working portal; however, establishing a good view initially can be difficult.

Results of surgery

Surgical treatment of ACJ arthropathy is both effective and safe. There have been numerous series published giving results in patients having either open resection or arthroscopic resection.

Two studies have attempted to compare open with arthroscopic resection. Freedman et al. randomized 17 military recruits with ACJ pain into two groups; the first group underwent open ACJ resection whereas the second group underwent indirect arthroscopic resection. The only significant finding was that patients in the arthroscopy group had a better improvement in their pain score from baseline to 1 year postoperatively. They highlighted trends suggesting that the arthroscopy group had better results in all the parameters measured, including return to sports, subjective results, and objective shoulder assessment. However, the study groups were small and the authors acknowledge that their results should be interpreted with caution.

Flatow et al. also compared the results of open versus arthroscopic ACJ resection. Their study, however, was retrospective and looked at pain relief only and they did not make any objective assessment. The arthroscopic approach used in this study was the direct technique. They reported good pain relief in both groups, although pain relief occurred much sooner in the arthroscopy group, in fact 3.4 months earlier.

Complications of surgery and their treatment

Patients who have an unsatisfactory result following ACJ excision can be split into three groups: those who have persistent pain in the shoulder following good surgery; those patients with pain and/or instability as a result of excessive bone resection; and finally those patients who have pain due to inadequate resection. Clearly in the first group, the failure is with the initial diagnosis rather than a fault of the surgery and the patient must be reassessed and the correct cause of the symptoms established. This is unfortunately rather more difficult after surgery than before. Inadequate bone resection is an uncommon cause of failure of arthroscopic resection. The solution is revision surgery, although the surgeon must be cautious to avoid going too far the other way and resecting too much bone.

The second most common complication after an incorrect diagnosis is the patient with pain due to having had an excessive amount of bone resected from the distal clavicle. This problem is usually seen in patients who have had open surgery. Open surgery will defunction the stabilizing constraints of the AC ligaments. If the resection compromises the coracoclavicular ligaments as well then the patient may develop painful instability of the clavicle, which is quite miserable and difficult to treat. The patient may have the worst of all worlds, with impingement of the acromion against the resected clavicle in elevation, local soft tissue irritation caused by instability of the distal clavicle, and scapular fatigue caused by failure of the link between the clavicle and acromion or scapula—what could be called claviculoscapular dissociation. Stress views of the ACJ will show an increased width in the resection gap with load bearing, which can sometimes be quite dramatic. An x-ray or fluoroscopy of the ACJ with the upper limb fully elevated will sometimes demonstrate acromioclavicular impingement even if the joint space with the arm at rest is 1–2cm. Occasionally some of this group of patients will require revision reconstructive surgery. The author currently uses a semitendinosis free tendon graft that is used to restore stability to the ACJ through a figure-of-eight loop between tunnels in the acromion and distal clavicle. If the clavicle is also vertically unstable, a second loop is passed between the coracoid process and clavicle. Initial stability can be improved between the coracoid and clavicle by using a suture anchor, sling, or TightRope® (Arthrex) suture.

Acromioclavicular dislocations

Aetiology

Dislocations of the ACJ are common injuries, representing around 12% of all dislocations around the shoulder and 8% of all dislocation injuries of the body. By far the commonest mechanism of injury is a fall, landing directly on the tip of the shoulder. The joint can be dislocated as a result of a direct blow to the clavicle, this mode of injury producing some of the more unusual dislocation types as described subsequently.

Classification

AC dislocations are universally classified according to the system proposed by Tossy in 1963 and Allman in 1967. These initial classifications were amalgamated to describe the three most common types of dislocation. Three further dislocation patterns (IV, V, and VI) were added by Rockwood in 1984.

A grade I injury involves a partial disruption of the ACJ capsule and ligaments with no deformity or instability. A grade II injury involves complete disruption of the ACJ ligaments although the coracoclavicular ligaments are broadly intact and may be partially damaged. There may be some minor caudal displacement of the acromion although this is often not seen, particularly initially, as the intact coracoclavicular ligaments continue to provide vertical stability. On examination of the ACJ, there is usually some anteroposterior laxity of the joint due to the disruption of the ACJ ligaments. A grade III separation describes an injury in which there is complete disruption of both the ACJ ligaments and coracoclavicular ligaments. This is responsible for the typical ACJ dislocation as seen on radiographs and apparent on clinical examination. However, there is no appreciable posterior displacement of the clavicle and due to the contribution of the intact deltotrapezial fascia, the clavicle is not grossly unstable and there is usually not more than 100% displacement of the acromion relative to the clavicle. Grade IV and V injuries are relatively uncommon but occur in roughly equal proportions and it is important to differentiate them from the more common injuries as results with conservative treatment are often disappointing. A grade IV injury is similar to a grade III with complete tears of the AC and coracoclavicular ligaments, except that there is significant posterior displacement to the extent that the distal clavicle pierces the trapezius muscle and becomes button-holed in an irreducible manner. A grade V dislocation involves extensive separation of the deltotrapezial fascia normally attached to the distal clavicle. This allows significant displacement of the acromion on the clavicle and certainly more than 100% of the thickness of the distal clavicle. A grade VI injury is extremely rare and will never be seen by most shoulder specialists in their lifetime.

Examination and diagnosis

The diagnosis of an acute ACJ injury is not particularly difficult. The patient gives a history of acute pain in the shoulder following a fall or direct blow to the shoulder. The pain is sharp and localized to the tip of the shoulder. Examination of the patient reveals tenderness over the injured joint with or without the deformity associated with a dislocation. The distal clavicle should be located by direct palpation and an assessment made of vertical and AP stability. Alignment of the distal clavicle with the acromion should be ensured to avoid missing a grade IV injury. Plain radiographs are usually sufficient to confirm the diagnosis. A standard AP of the shoulder will be taken as part of a trauma series along with an AP view of the ACJ. These views will allow distinction to be made between grade II, III and grade V injuries. It should be borne in mind that due to pain, the patient with a grade V injury may be reluctant to allow the injured arm to hang and in supporting it, may reduce the separation seen on the AP view to resemble a grade III injury. In this situation, clinical examination will allow the correct grade to be diagnosed as these patients have significant vertical instability of the clavicle with no firm end-point. An axial view is essential to allow diagnosis of a grade IV injury in which the distal clavicle will be seen to lie posterior to the acromion. In more subtle injuries a magnetic resonance imaging (MRI) scan will show ACJ capsule disruption, surrounding oedema and possibly signal change in the region of the CC ligaments.

Treatment options

The treatment of grade I and II injuries is non-surgical and consists of symptom relief with analgesia and anti-inflammatory medication. The arm should be supported with an immobilizer and ice packs can be applied to the injured area. Generally speaking, for grade I injuries the symptoms will resolve in a couple of weeks and the patient can return to normal daily and sporting activities relatively quickly. Patients with grade II injuries often experience discomfort for longer, perhaps 4–8 weeks, although treatment is similar. There is no evidence to suggest that prolonged immobilization of grade II injuries facilitates a more prompt recovery or reduces the incidence of later onset pain and arthropathy. Patients should be warned that chronic discomfort is not unusual following a previous grade II injury and may require subsequent surgery.

At the opposite end of the spectrum, most doctors would recommend surgical treatment of grade IV, V, and VI injuries. As their classification suggests, these types of dislocation involve significant displacement with associated soft tissue disruption. Grade IV injuries if neglected or more commonly missed, are very painful, presumably due to the irritation of the trapezius by the distal end of the clavicle and can cause considerable late disability. Grade V injuries, whilst often not as painful initially, are associated with marked deformity due to the prominence of the distal clavicle under the skin. Contrary to popular belief, this deformity is largely caused by the weight of the upper limb pulling the shoulder downwards, with the clavicle remaining relatively undisplaced. Due to this loss or incompetence in the superior suspensory complex of the shoulder, the deltoid and periscapular muscles are required to work much harder than normal to support the upper limb, particularly when the patient is performing repetitive overhead activities. This often results in the patient experiencing fatigue pain located to the scapular region and chronic disability. The patient will complain of an inability to perform overhead activities, describing an aching or dragging sensation in the scapular region.

Whether to treat grade III injuries with surgery or not has been the subject of debate, discussion, and uncertainty for decades and it seems that a clear answer to this dilemma is no nearer than it was 20 years ago. Whilst it is true that most patients with a grade III injury cope perfectly well, both with the deformity and any minor discomfort, there are a minority who continue to be symptomatic and seek further treatment. This is apparent when reviewing the surgical treatment options available for reconstruction of the dislocated ACJ. Of course, if patients with grade III injuries never required surgery, it is unlikely that there would be so many different operations available for reconstruction described in surgical textbooks.

Results of conservative and surgical treatment of acromioclavicular joint dislocations

It is generally believed that grade I and II injuries to the ACJ are benign and patients do well once the initial pain of the injury has resolved. However, according to a review published by Shaw, post-traumatic arthritis is relatively common with 40% of patients reporting significant pain at 6 months post-injury and 14% reporting a high level of pain at a minimum of 1 year. Many of these patients ultimately required surgical treatment. Mouhsine et al. studied a group of 33 patients with grade I and II injuries managed conservatively. From this group nine patients required surgery for late ACJ symptoms (chronic pain).

The treatment of grade III injuries provides the most controversy of all ACJ separations and there have been hundreds of articles published on the subject. Dias and other authors have reported up to 50% of patients treated non-operatively will have residual symptoms of pain and weakness. Spencer has reviewed the literature on this subject and points out that there are in fact only nine papers that directly compare conservative treatment with some form of surgical management. Of course, the findings of some of these papers will be heavily influenced by the type of surgical procedure used during the study. Only three of these studies were performed prospectively. Perhaps the best known of all these studies is the work published by Bannister et al. in 1989. In this study 60 patients with grade III injuries were randomized to either standard conservative treatment or surgery with a Bosworth screw that was removed at 6 weeks. Forty-four patients were evaluated at 4 years post-injury. The results in the non-operative group showed 100% patients had good or excellent results; 84% of patients in the operative group had similar results with the remaining 16% fair. Five patients in the operative group had complications of their treatment including loss of reduction and metalwork problems. Despite reporting uniformly good results in the non-operative group, in fact four patients failed treatment and underwent surgery. Operated patients also took longer to return to work and sport. Despite stating that all patients in this study had grade III injuries, in fact 12 had displacement of more than 2cm which is much more likely to represent a grade V injury; these patients in Bannister's study did better with surgical treatment. Of course it may be argued that there may be potentially better surgical treatments available today than in the 1980s and more objective methods of assessing shoulder function may alter the results seen.

Surgical treatment of acute acromioclavicular joint dislocation

Over the years, there have been numerous different surgical techniques described for the treatment of acute grade III–VI ACJ dislocations. These include direct repair of the coracoclavicular ligaments, usually with some method of temporary stabilization of the joint, using sutures, tape, screws, or plates. Stabilization of the distal clavicle has also been advocated by transfer of the coracoacromial ligament, with or without excision of the distal clavicle, but this technique is more commonly used in the chronic situation. Currently, the preference seems to be towards reduction of the dislocation without formally repairing the disrupted coracoclavicular ligament, with indirect stabilization either with a hook plate, coracoclavicular screw, or using an arthroscopic technique to place sutures between the clavicle and coracoid process. The choice of technique depends on published results, the resources available to the surgeon and their expertise in open or arthroscopic surgery.

Applying a hook-plate to maintain reduction of the reduced ACJ is a relatively simple surgical procedure that has its advocates. The disrupted joint capsule can be repaired simultaneously with or without excision of the intra-articular disc. The plate will require removal at or around 3 months or earlier if there is evidence of osteolysis under the acromion. The hook is designed to be placed posterior to the ACJ and should therefore not interfere with healing or movement in the recovery phase. In a study from Salzburg the results in terms of shoulder function were significantly better in the surgical group, particularly when comparing pain and power. Surgical complications were seen in four of 28 patients with one haematoma, two superficial infections, and one plate eroding the acromion.

The use of a coracoclavicular screw for the treatment of an acute ACJ dislocation is widely attributed to Bosworth. Most surgeons would now use a partially threaded (16mm) 6.5-mm cancellous screw. It is imperative that the screw is placed centrally in the base of the coracoid process to minimize the possibility of pull-out and this can either be done with a conventional open approach or a percutaneous technique using a cannulated system and fluoroscopy. The thread of the screw should cross both cortices of the coracoid and the screw should not be tightened excessively as this will over-reduce the dislocation and lead to ACJ dysfunction. A disadvantage of this type of rigid fixation is that it must be removed before overhead movement of the upper limb can be allowed. Most surgeons would therefore plan to remove the Bosworth screw around 8 weeks after fixation, but there is a possibility of late displacement if the injured coracoclavicular ligaments have not fully healed by this stage.

Coracoclavicular sutures or slings are popular techniques largely because there is no requirement for hardware removal. Perhaps the simplest method within this type is to knot a Dacron® or PDS 5-mm tape over the clavicle after first passing it around the base of the coracoid. However, this does little to address anteroposterior instability of the clavicle and there is often subsequent loss in reduction as the knot slips or the sling lengthens slightly. Breslow performed a biomechanical study comparing a simple coracoclavicular suture loop passed under the coracoid with a suture fixed into the coracoid using a suture anchor. One proposed advantage of the suture anchor technique is that the suture is instantly fixed and stable on the coracoid when an anchor is used whereas when a suture loop is passed under the coracoid, some movement or slippage can occur, leading to laxity in the construct. Breslow concluded that a similar degree of stability can be achieved after coracoclavicular fixation using a suture anchor or suture loop. However, the use of a suture anchor eliminates the need to pass instruments under the coracoid which can be both difficult and risk neurovascular injury.

A novel technique using a TightRope® (Arthrex) suture (originally described by Wolf for the reconstruction of chronic acromioclavicular dislocations and subsequently adapted for use in the acute situation and described by Qureshi and Potter) has become popular over the last 3 years. It has all the advantages of the rigid coracoclavicular fixation of a Bosworth screw, with the benefit of flexibility as seen with the suture techniques. One major attraction is that the suture is placed using an arthroscopic technique, both ensuring accurate placement through the coracoid and minimizing disruption to the torn coracoclavicular ligament complex. Finally, as no rigid fixation is employed there is no need for hardware removal prior to a return to normal activities. To insert the TightRope® suture the base of the coracoid process is identified and debrided arthroscopically. A jig is then used to percutaneously drill a guide wire through the middle of the clavicle approximately 3cm from its distal end and then through the middle of the base of the coracoid. After the guide wire is over-drilled with a cannulated 4mm drill, the TightRope® suture is pulled through both holes. The suture is tied over a button on the superior surface of the clavicle after reducing the ACJ dislocation manually. At present there are no long-term results of this technique published although interim results have been presented. Clearly this technique requires healing of the coracoclavicular ligament complex to be successful; this is more likely if the dislocation is reduced and stabilized early. It is also not clear at this stage whether the reduced ACJ will become arthritic as a result of the initial dislocation, although secondary treatment of this problem is much easier than the options for reconstructing a symptomatic chronic dislocation of the ACJ. This technique is also very well suited to complex displaced fractures of the distal clavicle, particularly those involving the ACJ, which usually require surgical reduction but are very difficult to treat with conventional methods.

Surgical treatment of chronic acromioclavicular joint dislocation

Numerous surgical techniques have been described for the treatment of the chronic, symptomatic ACJ dislocation. It should be said that grade I and II injuries can also be troublesome for the patient and require surgery, although in the absence of significant instability, simple ACJ excision, either open or arthroscopic, is probably sufficient. It is often worthwhile excluding instability in these patients by performing a stress x-ray. Patients with a high-grade separation can complain of several different symptoms justifying surgery, such as local irritation from the prominent distal clavicle, impingement of the unstable joint in elevation, or scapular fatigue pain and weakness. Surgical procedures can be broadly grouped into those relying on a transfer of the coracoacromial ligament based on the Weaver–Dunn procedure; autogenous tendon graft procedures (anatomic coracoclavicular reconstruction); and reconstruction using synthetic ligament and dynamic muscle transfers.

The Weaver–Dunn procedure was originally described in 1972, and has become the 'gold-standard' of ACJ reconstruction. The procedure essentially involves detaching the coracoacromial ligament from the acromion and transferring it onto or into the resected distal end of the clavicle to provide stability. The original Weaver–Dunn technique is now usually modified to include augmentation of the repair to provide initial security, preventing subsequent displacement. The coracoacromial ligament is exposed prior to detachment by either splitting anterior deltoid or detaching anterior deltoid from the clavicle and anterior acromion, although the operation can be performed arthroscopically. Detaching the ligament with a small flake of bone from the acromion may promote healing of the transfer and certainly helps to prevent cut-out of the sutures used to secure the transfer. The ligament is placed into the canalized end of the clavicle and secured in place with sutures passed through drill holes in the clavicle. Perhaps not surprisingly, this transfer in itself has little strength in the early phase of healing. There are several ways in which the initial stability of a Weaver–Dunn repair can be improved, using coracoclavicular slings or sutures. Although it is the author's practice currently to use a PDS tape, the best biomechanical results are seen with a suture anchored into the base of the coracoid and tied through drill holes in the anterior half of the clavicle, which resists translation under a 100N cyclical load. The final construct at 246N is not as strong as the native coracoclavicular ligaments at 590N.

Increasing interest is being expressed in more anatomical reconstructions of the dislocated ACJ using tendon grafts. It has been noted that whilst a coracoacromial ligament transfer prevents superior migration, it is less good at resisting anteroposterior translation. This is not too surprising when one remembers that the coracoacromial ligament takes its origin from the tip of the coracoid and when transferred, inserts into the resected distal end of the clavicle. The native coracoclavicular ligaments of course arise from the base of the coracoid and insert into the undersurface of the clavicle some way from the distal end. With this in mind, surgical techniques have been described using autogenous tendon grafts including palmaris longus, flexor carpi radialis, gracilis, and semitendinosis. It has been the author's personal experience that there are both early failures associated with anatomical reconstructions using semitendinosis (usually due to the tendon cutting out of the clavicle tunnel) and late failures (mainly seen on the coracoid side and possibly related to failure of revascularization). It is also worth mentioning that harvesting a semitendinosis tendon graft can be associated with donor-site morbidity, which is particularly relevant when the surgical procedure is on the shoulder not the lower limb. It is the author's current practice to perform a modified Weaver–Dunn procedure for routine primary reconstructions and a semitendinosis tendon graft in revisions and when it is not possible to use the coracoacromial ligament.

Artificial ligament substitutes are not widely used, given the poor results previously seen in anterior cruciate ligament reconstruction in the knee, although following work by Wallace and Neuman, the 'Surgilig' technique is gaining interest. The procedure uses a polyester coracoclavicular sling looped under the coracoid and then fixed to the anterior clavicle with a small fragment screw and washer. It is suggested by the Nottingham unit that this procedure can be used for both acute dislocations as well as in revision.

Other conditions affecting the acromioclavicular joint

Distal clavicular osteolysis

Distal clavicular osteolysis was first described in 1936 and was thought to be secondary to a traumatic injury. In 1982, Cahill published a series of 45 male patients with clavicular osteolysis, suggesting repetitive microtrauma as the aetiology. All but one of his patients were weight-lifters. He noted the presence of micro-fractures in the subchondral bone in 50% of cases and proposed that repetitive overloading of the joint caused subchondral stress fractures and remodelling. There is certainly evidence of increased osteoclastic activity in many excised specimens. Patients present with pain localized to the ACJ and almost always give a history of regular and intense weight-training or overhead athletic activity. X-rays are often normal in the early part of the natural history and in cases where doubt exists as to the diagnosis, an isotope bone scan or MRI scan will be diagnostic. The condition is self-limiting with appropriate activity modification, although many young male patients are unwilling to cease their training activities. In these circumstances, Auge and Fischer have shown arthroscopic distal clavicle excision, gives good to excellent results in most patients.

Pseudodislocation of the distal clavicle

In children, the clavicle is surrounded by a thick periosteal sleeve that extends distally to the ACJ. A secondary ossification centre is present at the distal end of the clavicle that fuses with the clavicle at about the age of 19 years. Children and adolescents are much more likely therefore to fracture the distal clavicle than to dislocate the ACJ. The distal ossification centre is usually very difficult to visualize on a plain x-ray and the true diagnosis is often not appreciated. This type of injury is therefore often known as a pseudodislocation. Unless there is significant displacement, conservative management is usually recommended and there is often excellent remodelling. In markedly displaced injuries, open reduction is worthwhile, the clavicle being reduced and replaced back into the periosteal sleeve which is then repaired. Temporary stabilization is provided by a coracoclavicular screw or suture.

Rheumatoid arthritis of the acromioclavicular joint

The ACJ and subacromial bursa are said to be the primary sources of pain in 60% of patients who have rheumatoid arthritis and a painful shoulder. The symptoms as expected, consist of pain associated with swelling and tenderness over the joint. The radiological changes can be graded using the Larsen system from I to V. Treatment is best instigated by a rheumatologist initially to control the disease systemically. Localized disease in the ACJ can often be mediated by an intra-articular steroid injection and for advanced and resistant cases, ACJ excision as for degenerative arthropathy is effective.

Further reading

Allman, F.L. Jr. (1967). Fractures and ligamentous injuries of the clavicle and its articulation. *Journal of Bone and Joint Surgery*, **47A**, 780–4.

Bannister, G.C., Wallace, W.A., Stableforth, P.G., and Hutson, M.A. (1989). The management of acute acromioclavicular dislocation. *Journal of Bone and Joint Surgery*, **71B**, 848–50.

Mumford, E. (1941). Acromioclavicualr dislocation: a new operative treatment. *Journal of Bone and Joint Surgery*, **23A**, 799–802.

Richards, A., Potter, D., Learmonth, D., and Tennent, D. (2005). 'Arthroscopic stabilisation of acute distal clavicle fractures and dislocations using the Tightrope syndesmosis repair system.' Presented at the Annual Meeting of the Arthroscopy Association of North America, Vancouver, BC, May, 2005.

Rockwood, C., Williams, G., and Young, C. (1998). Disorders of the acromioclavicular joint. In: Rockwood, C. and Matsen, F.(eds) *The Shoulder*, 2nd edn., pp. 483–553. Philadelphia, PA: Saunders.

Tossy, J.D., Mead, N.C., and Sigmond, H.M. (1963). Acromioclavicular separations: useful and practical classification for treatment. *Clinical Orthopaedics and Related Research*, **28**, 111–19.

Weaver, J.K. and Dunn, H.K. (1972). Treatment of acromioclavicular injuries, especially complete acromioclavicular separation. *Journal of Bone and Joint Surgery*, **54A**, 1187–94.

4.11

The clavicle and sternoclavicular joint

Simon N.J. Roberts

Summary points

- Fractures and dislocations of the sternoclavicular joint are uncommon and often successfully treated non-operatively
- There are a number of poorly defined sclerotic, sometimes inflammatory, conditions with a predilection for the medial clavicle.

Introduction

The word clavicle is derived from the Latin clavicula, 'small key', which refers to the musical symbol of similar shape. It describes an unusual and interesting bone in its development, function, and the disorders to which it is susceptible. It is the only human long bone that forms by intramembranous ossification. Although the central ossification centre is the first in the body to form, and is responsible for longitudinal growth in the first 5 years of life, the medial and lateral centres, which appear between 12–19 years of age, are among the latest to fuse (22–25 years).

The clavicle is the only bony connection between the upper limb and trunk, forming unusual and incongruous synovial joints at either end, each with a fibrocartilaginous intra-articular meniscus. Medially, there is a saddle-shaped sternal articulation which includes a facet with the first rib in 25% of cases. Both joints are primarily stabilized by strong extra-articular ligaments rather than capsular condensations (Figure 4.11.1). These lie some distance from the joints themselves and act as pivots, enforcing a degree of translational movement. This shearing tends to occur in the two compartments of the sternoclavicular joint with predominantly anteroposterior movements occurring between the sternum and meniscus, and superoinferior movements in the lateral compartment. At rest, the interclavicular ligament helps the superior capsular ligament to produce shoulder 'poise', resisting the upward force on the medial clavicle produced by the weight of the arm pulling down from laterally, across the fulcrum of the first rib and rhomboid ligaments.

The medial clavicle and its sternal articulation appear uniquely susceptible to a number of rather unusual disorders, both traumatic and atraumatic, with a very confused terminology.

Whilst subcutaneous and easily amenable to clinical examination (see Chapter 4.1), imaging is difficult. The 40-degree upwards angle 'serendipity' plain radiograph is the most useful (Figure 4.11.2), but cross sectional imaging with side-to-side comparison will usually be required.

Traumatic conditions (Box 4.11.1)

Fractures and dislocations of the medial clavicle are rare, particularly by comparison with injuries to the shaft and lateral end, comprising less than 3% of injuries. Fractures are caused by high-energy compression and are almost always associated with multisystem trauma. Dislocations, however, may be entirely atraumatic anteriorly (very rarely posteriorly), especially in young adults with ligamentous laxity. In these cases, supportive treatment is usually successful, the results of open surgery poor, and the surgical risks high.

Acute anterior dislocation is caused by a blow to the front of a retracted shoulder with axial compression. Closed reduction under anaesthetic by scapular retraction over a bolster with direct pressure over the medial clavicle is usually (at least temporarily) successful, and may be maintained with a figure-of-eight sling, but redislocation is expected.

Acute posterior dislocation is much less common, caused by axial compression from a blow to the back of a protracted shoulder

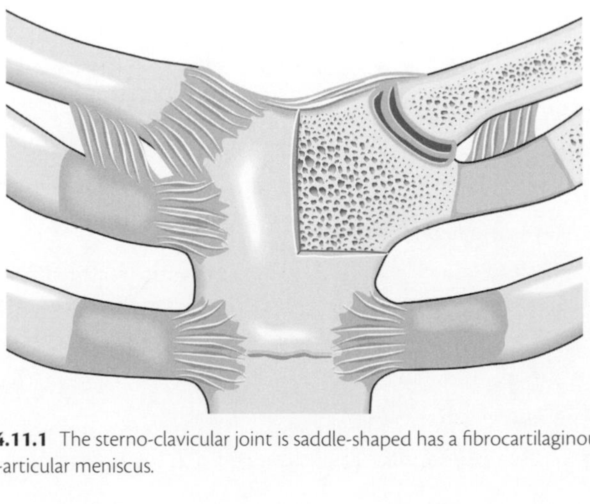

Fig. 4.11.1 The sterno-clavicular joint is saddle-shaped has a fibrocartilaginous intra-articular meniscus.

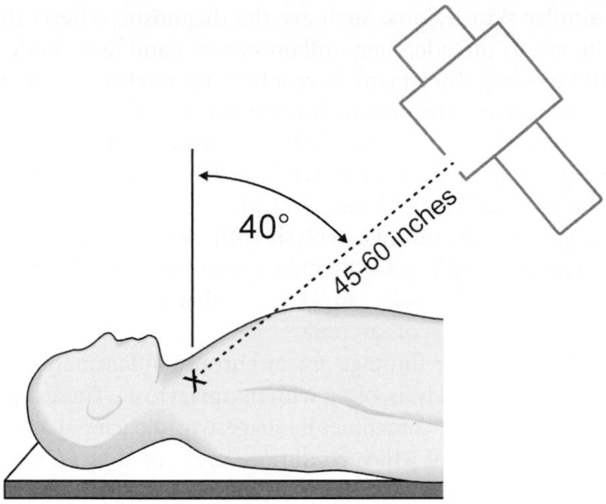

Fig. 4.11.2 Imaging is difficult. The 40-degree upwards angled 'serendipity' plain radiograph is the most useful, but cross-sectional imaging with side-to-side comparison will usually be required.

and may compress the structures of the neck. Closed reduction should be attempted, if necessary assisted by a towel clip, if within 7 days or so of injury, but intervention delayed longer than this is less likely to succeed and more likely to damage the adjacent vessels. Before skeletal maturity (NB 25 years!), the injury is often an occult physeal separation.

In chronic dislocations, the risks and benefits of surgery need to be carefully balanced. Preoperative imaging will include vascular studies. Excision arthroplasty is the preferred procedure with or without one of the stabilization procedures (with a thoracic surgeon on standby). Interosseous metalwork should never be used to maintain reduction in view of the risk of migration causing serious injuries including death.

Box 4.11.1 Traumatic disorders of the sternoclavicular joint

Dislocation

- Anterior:
  - Reducible
  - Likely to redislocate, but may be minimally symptomatic
- Posterior:
  - Likely to be reducible inside 1 week
  - More risk later
  - May cause neck compression
- Atraumatic: usually responds to symptomatic treatment.

Fracture

- Uncommon
- High-energy compression
- Associated with multisystem trauma.

Atraumatic conditions (Box 4.11.2)

The investigation and diagnosis of lesions of the medial clavicle is made more difficult by the confusing descriptions and nomenclature of the very large number of eponymous and acronymous conditions beloved of rheumatologists, which are characterized by a spectrum of local and systemic inflammatory and non-inflammatory features. Having excluded tumour and hamartoma, there are four possible aetiopathologies: inflammatory (auto-immune and idiopathic), infective (acute, chronic low grade, often multifocal, and recurrent), ischaemic (Friedrich's disease and radionecrosis), and degenerative.

Non-inflammatory conditions

Condensing osteitis of the clavicle was first described by Brower in 1974 and typically occurs unilaterally in women of late premenopausal years, sparing the sternoclavicular joint. It shares morphological and radiological features with osteitis of the ilium and pubis, and histologically, despite the title, there is a relative absence of inflammatory reaction. The features are often indistinguishable from aseptic necrosis, which is more usually described in

Box 4.11.2 Sclerotic lesions of the medial clavicle

Inflammatory

- Infection
- Septic arthritis
- Osteomyelitis
- Inflammation
- Chronic recurrent multifocal osteomyelitis of Garré
- Sternocostoclavicular hyperostosis (SCCH) syndrome
- Intersternocostoclavicular ossification
- SAPHO (synovitis, acne, pustulosis, hyperostosis, and osteitis) syndrome
- Chronic symmetric plasma cell osteomyelitis
- Chronic sclerosing osteomyelitis
- Primary chronic osteomyelitis
- Pustulotic arthro-osteitis
- Acne-associated spondylarthropathy
- Arthro-osteitis with pustulosis palmoplantaris
- Juxtasternal arthritis and enthesitis
- Pustulotic arthro-osteitis
- Tumorous osteomyelitis.

Non-inflammatory

- Condensing osteitis
- Avascular necrosis/post-radiation
- Osteoarthritis.

adolescents, has a similarly good prognosis, and also usually spares the sternoclavicular joint. Both disorders run a relapsing and remitting course, eventually clinically resolving. Both may be best described as a variant of osteochondrosis, and the interesting observation has been made that the clavicle, ilium, and pubis all have a fibrocartilage covering, perhaps explaining the predilection of the condition for these sites. Other suggestions have included mechanical compression and various endocrine changes.

Osteoarthritis tends to affect the dominant limb in perimenopausal women.

The prognosis is good for all of the listed conditions after a relapsing natural history with standard supportive measures that may include intra-articular steroid injections.

Inflammatory conditions

Arthritis

Sternoclavicular septic arthritis may occur with the same spectrum of organisms as other joints, but is characterized by an insidious onset and a tendency to abscess formation. The joint may also be involved in any of the inflammatory arthritides. Approximately 17% of patients with ankylosing spondylitis have radiological sternoclavicular changes.

Arthro-osteitis

In the presence of inflammatory changes extending into the medial clavicle, the terminology is a problem. There is a condition of low-grade inflammation of the medial clavicle that may be recurrent and multifocal (commonly symmetrical). It typically runs a relapsing and remitting course with a good overall prognosis. It was first described in children by Garré in 1893 without the help of any other investigations (just before the birth of radiography) as a chronic, relapsing, and multifocal condition, and is now considered related to a large number of other named non-suppurative inflammatory disorders (Table 4.11.1).

The sternocostoclavicular hyperostosis syndrome (SCCH) was described in middle-aged Japanese men by Sonozaki et al. as a separate entity, involving ossification of the periarticular ligaments of the sternoclavicular joint, and is probably related to diffuse idiopathic skeletal hyperostosis and ankylosing spondylitis. It has been associated with palmoplantar pustulosis in 60% of cases and also psoriasis, suggesting the connection with the SAPHO (synovitis, acne, pustulosis, hyperostosis, and osteitis) syndrome. It may be most appropriate to consider that the SAPHO syndrome is composed of several disorders that share some clinical, radiological, and pathological characteristics, even if the skin disorder is transient or not noticed. Even Tietze's syndrome has been associated with similar skin lesions. Such are the diagnostic criteria that it may be fair to include many inflammatory conditions under the SAPHO heading since many have a high prevalence of associated skin disorders and therapeutic immunosuppression is reported to be of benefit. On the other hand, the prevalence of sternoclavicular pathology in patients with systemic arthritis and palmoplantar pustulosis is nearly 50% (Figure 4.11.3).

Radiographically, mixed osteolysis with intense sclerosis is seen, often with periostitis, and the enlargement of the subcutaneous bone may become massive, suggesting a diagnosis of fibrous dysplasia, Paget's disease, or sarcoma.

Histologically, the findings are of chronic inflammation, with mixed new bone and lysis, often with plasmacytosis. These findings are variable, and may sometimes be suggestive of bacterial osteomyelitis. The question of which conditions are caused by an infective agent either in the lesion or elsewhere, and which are best treated by antibiotics and which by immunosuppression is important and has not been answered. It is a concern that *Propionibacterium acnes*, a common skin saprophyte found in the skin lesions of severe acne, has also been isolated from the bone and joint lesions of patients diagnosed as suffering from both SAPHO and Garré's disease, as have raised antistaphylolysin titres.

At one end of the spectrum of such disorders is frank osteomyelitis and at the other end, sternocostoclavicular hyperostosis. In between lies a less well-defined variety of musculoskeletal manifestations associated with plamoplantar pustulosis and seronegative arthropathy, perhaps best described as pustulotic arthro-osteitis.

A clinical diagnosis can often be made and biopsy is not always necessary (and in any case usually not helpful). Similarly, an isotope bone scan excludes synchronous lesions. Computed tomography is useful in delineating the extent of any hyperostosis. Magnetic resonance imaging is the investigation of choice for the sternoclavicular joint itself and the periarticular soft tissues. Laboratory tests will exclude metabolic bone disease and help with assessment of the systemic inflammatory response.

In addition to supportive measures, in the presence of inflammation, it would seem reasonable to combine rheumatological treatment of any systemic condition with a therapeutic trial of antibiotics. Although radiation therapy has been suggested for the hyperostotic syndromes it may also be a cause of the clinically similar radiation osteitis! Bisphosphonates have been used but there are few data at present on their effectiveness.

Surgery

In disease localized to the medial clavicle, whether traumatic, degenerative, or inflammatory, surgical excision may be expected

Table 4.11.1 Clinical features

Disorder	Age	PPP	Other sites	Chest wall	Inflammation
Garré; chronic recurrent multifocal osteomyelitis (CRMO)	<20	<40%	+/−	+/−	+
Sternocostoclavicular hyperostosis (SCCH, DISH, AS)	30–60	30–50%	+/−	+	+
Synovitis, acne, palmoplantar pustulosis, hyperostosis, osteitis (SAPHO)	Adults	+	+	−	+
Osteitis condensans claviculare (Brower)	Young women	−	−	−	−
Avascular necrosis (Friedrich)	Adolescents	−	−	−	−

PPP, Palmo plantar pustulosis.

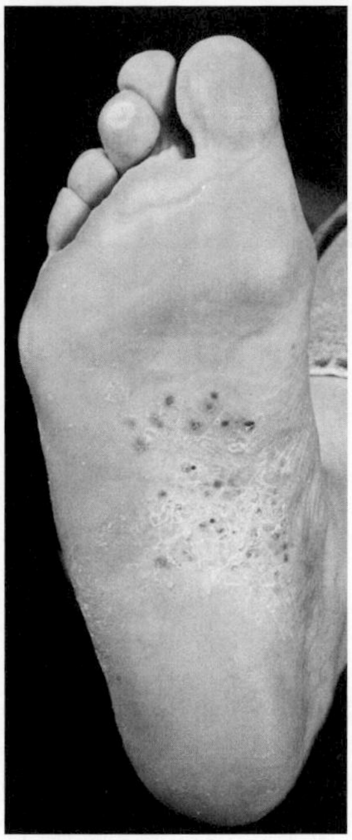

Fig. 4.11.3 The sternocostoclavicular hyperostosis syndrome (SCCH) was described by Sonozaki et al. It has been associated with palmoplantar pustulosis.

to be curative, but symptoms are usually not sufficiently disabling for patients to undergo the procedure. Good results have been described in small series in many of the discussed conditions following resection of the medial clavicle, but emphasize the importance of either retaining or reconstructing the costoclavicular ligaments.

Conclusion

The medial clavicle is affected by a number of interesting and slightly unusual conditions, many of which are relatively benign and require only supportive measures. There is collection of sclerotic disorders of the clavicle that may be categorized as either inflammatory or non-inflammatory on the basis of clinical, haematological, and radiological signs. In the presence of signs of inflammation, systemic upset, or remote signs, it may be difficult or impossible to exclude infection even on biopsy. In these patients, particularly in children, a trial of antibiotics is recommended. Fortunately, surgical excision of the medial clavicle is rarely necessary, but usually successful when needed.

Further reading

Bae, D.S., Kocher, M.S., Waters, P.M., Micheli, L.M., Griffey, M., and Dichtel, L. (2006). Chronic recurrent anterior sternoclavicular joint instability: results of surgical management. *Journal of Pediatric Orthopedics*, **26**(1), 71–4.

Brower, A.C., Sweet, D.E., and Keats, T.E. (1974). Condensing osteitis of the clavicle: a new entity. *American Journal of Roentgenology, Radium Therapy and Nuclear Medicine,* **121**(1), 17–21.

Garré, C. (1893). Ueber besondere formen und folgezustande der akuten infektisen osteomyelitis. *Beiträge zur Klinischen Chirurgie*, **10**, 257–65.

Kahn, M.F. (1995). Why the "SAPHO" syndrome? *Journal of Rheumatology*, **22**(11), 2017–19.

Levy, M., Goldberg, I., Fischel, R.E., Frisch, E., and Maor, P. (1981). Friedrich's disease. Aseptic necrosis of the sternal end of the clavicle. *Journal of Bone and Joint Surgery*, **63B**(4), 539–41.

Roberts, S.N.J. and Hayes, M.G. (2000). Sclerotic lesions of the clavicle. *CME Orthopaedics*, **2**, 44–7.

Sonozaki, H., Mitsui, H., Miyanaga, Y., *et al.* (1981). Clinical features of 53 cases with pustulotic arthro-osteitis. *Annals of the Rheumatic Diseases*, **40**(6), 547–53.

4.12

Disorders of the scapula

Roger Emery

Summary points

- Sprengel's deformity causes a high riding, fixed, hypoplastic scapula
- Sprengel's deformity may be associated with Klippel Fiel syndrome
- Winging of the scapula can be caused by trapezius palsy or serratus anterior palsy
- Trapezius palsy is usually due to damage to the spinal accessory nerve
- Serratus palsy is usually caused by damage to the long thoracic nerve
- Fascio-scapulo-humeral dystrophy presents with loss of scapula control from the late teens to the late twenties
- FSHD is autosomal dominant and linked to alteration of the 4q35 gene.

Evolution and comparative anatomy

When humans assumed the erect position, the shoulder evolved with the series of complex adaptive changes exchanging stability for mobility. In our amphibian ancestry the forelimbs evolved from the longitudinal lateral folds and pectoral fins. After the migration of spinal nerves and muscle buds, the nerve fibres repeatedly divided to form a plexus and different regions of muscle tissue often combined or segmented as function evolved. Cartilage rays called radicals arose between muscle buds to form a support structure, and the proximal portions of these radials coalesced to form basal cartilages, or basilia, of the primitive pectoral girdle. They migrated ventrally towards the midline anteriorly to form a ventral bar, the precursor of the paired clavicles, and projected dorsally over the thorax to form the precursor of the scapula. Articulations within the basilia developed at the junction of the ventral and dorsal segments. The basic mammalian pattern developed with articulations arising between a well-developed clavicle and sternum medially and a flat and fairly wide scapula laterally.

Four main variations of pectoral girdle are seen in mammals. Those adapted for running have lost their clavicle to mobilize the scapula further, and the scapula is relatively narrowed. Mammals adapted for swimming also lost their clavicle although the scapula is wider, permitting more varied function. The shoulder girdles modified for flying have a large, long, well-developed clavicle with a small, narrow, curved scapula. Finally, shoulders modified for brachiating (including humans) have developed a strong clavicle, a large coracoid process, and a widened strong scapula. Adaptations also seen in the erect posture were the relative flattening of the thorax in the anteroposterior dimension, leaving the scapula approximately 45 degrees to the midline and the evolution of the pentadactyl limb.

Embryological development

The limb buds, consisting of a core of mesenchyme and a covering layer of ectoderm, become visible at the beginning of the fifth week. By the sixth week of development the first hyaline cartilage models of the forelimb bones can be recognized, which will eventually form by endochondral ossification. An area, termed the interzone, which has not undergone chondrification is the precursor of the shoulder joint. The clavicle is the first bone in the body to begin to ossify. Subsequently the scapula, which at this time lies at the level of C4 and C5, also forms by intramembranous ossification. The interzone assumes a three-layer configuration, with a chondrogenic layer on either side of a loose layer of cells. At this time, the glenoid lip is discernible, although cavitation or joint formation has not occurred. The scapula undergoes marked enlargement at this time and extends from C4 to approximately T7.

Early in the seventh week the shoulder is well formed, with the middle zone of the three-layered interzone becoming progressively less dense with increasing cavitation. The scapula has now descended and spans from just below the level of the first rib and the fifth rib. The final few degrees of downward displacement occur later when the anterior rib cage drops obliquely downward. By the eighth week the upper limb musculature is well defined and the shoulder joint has the form of the adult glenohumeral joint.

Postnatal development

The postnatal development of the shoulder is mainly concerned with the appearance and progress of the secondary sites of ossification. The scapula at birth has its body and spine ossified by intramembranous ossification. The coracoid process has two, and occasionally three, centres of ossification. The first appears during the first year of life at the centre of the process with the second arising around the age of

10 years at its base. These two centres unite with the scapula around age 15 years. The acromion has two ossification centres which arise during puberty and fuse together around age 22 years. Failure of this fusion produces an os acromiale and may be present in up to 4.2% of the population. The glenoid fossa has again two ossification centres. The first appears at the base of the coracoid process around age 10 years and fuses around age 15 years. The second centre is a horseshoe shape arising from the inferior portion of the glenoid during puberty and forms the lower three-quarters of the glenoid. The vertebral border and inferior angle of the scapula each have one ossification centre, both of which appear at puberty and fuse around age 22 years.

Congenital elevation of the scapula (Sprengel's deformity)

Congenital elevation of the scapula is a rare congenital deformity first described by Eulenberg in 1863. Sprengel (1891) recognized that the deformity was caused by failure of the scapula to descend. In this condition the scapula lies high in relation to the thoracic cage and is usually rotated and hypoplastic (Box 4.12.1).

The disability is dependent on the severity of the deformity. In mild cases, the scapula is only slightly elevated and is slightly smaller than normal with minimal loss of function. In the severe cases it creates an ugly deformity with widening of the base of the neck. Occasionally the scapula can be so elevated that it almost touches the occiput and the patient's head is deviated towards the affected side. Abduction is decreased in these severe cases as the glenoid faces downwards.

Other congenital anomalies, such as scoliosis, cervical ribs, malformations of ribs, and anomalies of the cervical vertebrae (Klippel–Feil syndrome), are commonly present; rarely, one or more scapular muscles are partly or completely absent. Cervicothoracic spine and thoracic outlet radiographs are required to identify these structural changes particularly if surgical correction is considered. An omovertebral bone together with a very straight clavicle is found in between a third and half of patients.

Surgery is only indicated in severe deformities, after consideration of the age of the patient and the severity of any associated deformities. Corrective surgery is too major to consider before the age of 3 years. However, the earlier surgery is performed after this age the better are the results, because as the child grows the operation becomes more difficult and ultimately impossible. In children older than 8 years attempts to bring the scapula inferiorly to its normal level may seriously stretch and damage the brachial plexus. Limited resection of the prominent superomedial angle may be considered after this age. It must be made clear to the parents that the results of surgery are occasionally disappointing as the deformity is never simply elevation of the scapula alone, but always complicated by malformations and contractures of the soft tissues.

Box 4.12.1 Sprengel's deformity

- The scapula is high, rotated, and hypoplastic
- Disability is variable and relates to the degree of deformity
- Other congenital anomalies are often present: scoliosis, cervical ribs, and cervical vertebrae anomalies (Klippel–Feil syndrome)
- An omovertelual bar may be present
- Surgery is only indicated in severe cases between the ages of 3–8 years
- Techniques include extraperiosteal release, trapezius transfer, and osteotomy.

Numerous methods of lowering the scapula have been described to correct this deformity. Before addressing the scapula position, consideration should be given to morcellation of the clavicle on the ipsilateral side as in severe deformities it reduces the risk of brachial plexus palsy. Many techniques of lowering the scapula have been described.

Woodward (1961) described transfer of the origin of the trapezius muscle to a more inferior position on the spinous processes. This utilizes a more cosmetic midline approach from the spinous process of the first cervical to the ninth thoracic vertebra. The patient is placed prone and draped so that the shoulder girdle and arm can be moved freely. The skin and subcutaneous tissues are undermined laterally to the medial border of the scapula. The lateral border of the trapezius is identified distally and separated by blunt dissection from the underlying latissimus dorsi muscle. Then the fascial sheath of origin of the trapezius is released from the spinous processes by sharp dissection. The origins of the rhomboideus major and minor muscles are similarly freed and separated from the muscles of the chest wall. This sheet of muscles can be retracted laterally to expose any omovertebral bone or fibrous bands attached to the superior angle of the scapula. The omovertebral bone, any fibrous band, or contracted levator scapulae are freed, taking care not to injury the spinal accessory nerve, the nerves to the rhomboids, or the transverse cervical artery. The supraspinatus part of the scapula is usually deformed and should be excised with its periosteum thus releasing the levator scapulae. The scapula can be displaced inferiorly with the attached sheet of muscles distally until its spine lies at the same level as that of the opposite scapula. With the scapula in this position, the aponeuroses of the trapezius and rhomboids are reattached to the spinous processes at a more inferior level. Postoperatively a sling or Velpeau bandage is worn for 2 weeks.

An alternative and simpler method is to lower the scapula by osteotomy. The patient is placed semiprone with the affected side uppermost. A vertical incision is made over the medial border of the scapula. The scapula is exposed by incising the periosteum along the medial part of the origin of supraspinatus and infraspinatus, which can be swept laterally. An osteotomy is made 1cm from the vertebral border with an oscillating saw passing through the base of the spine (Figure 4.12.1). Mobility of the lateral part of the scapula is gained by removal of the medial strip of scapula above its spine. This also allows removal of fibrous bands and any omovertebral bone. Remaining fibrous bands on the inferior strip of medial scapula are also divided. The lateral part of the scapula can be protracted and lifted away from the chest wall so that a finger can be swept between subscapularis and the underlying ribs, ensuring that any adhesions or fibrous bands are divided. Once the blade of the scapula is completely mobile, the lateral portion is rotated downwards and stabilized with sutures passing through the periostium and bone to the remaining strip. This procedure requires a longer period of immobilization in a sling for 6 weeks.

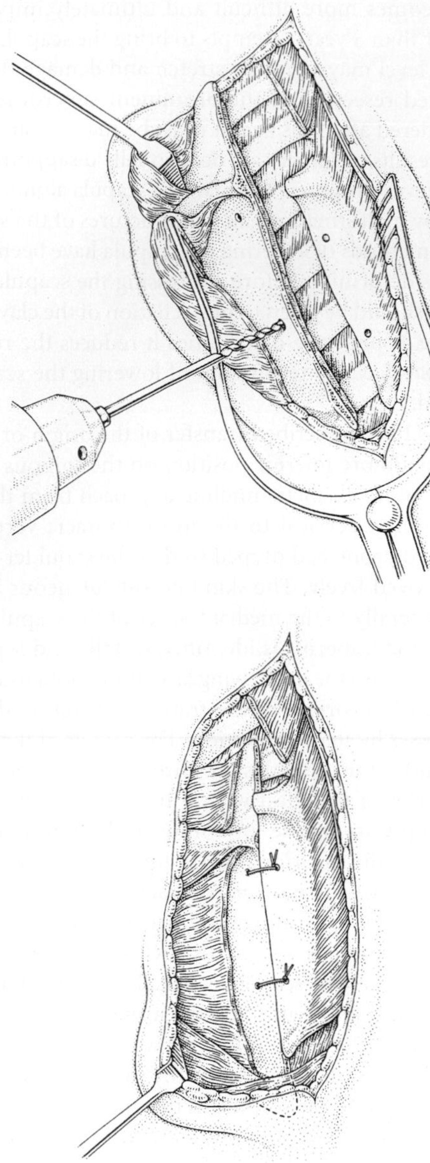

Fig. 4.12.1 Scapular osteotomy for Sprengel's deformity. Reproduced from Wilkinson, J.A. and Campbell, D. (1980). Scapular osteotomy for Sprengel's shoulder. *Journal of Bone and Joint Surgery*, **62-A**, 486–90.

The major complication following these procedures is the significant risk of brachial plexus palsy. This risk is higher in severe deformities particularly in the presence of a straight clavicle and deformed high first rib. The other recognized complication is damage to the spinal accessory nerve on the undersurface of the trapezius.

Winging of the scapula

Stability of the scapula is of paramount importance to efficient shoulder function. Paralysis or weakness of the scapular stabilizing muscles causes profound loss of function

It is of note that although we use the terms *protraction*, *retraction*, and *winging*, there can be few joints in the human body whose movement is so poorly defined (Box 4.12.2). We do not even have proper terms of reference regarding the range of motion of the scapulothoracic joint; somewhat surprising when we observe the remarkable range of movement maintained in patients who have undergone a glenohumeral arthrodesis. Observations are often focused on scapulothoracic rhythm, disturbance of which is a useful finding but usually reflects pathology arising from the glenohumeral or subacromial articulations rather than the scapula or its control.

Loss of trapezius function

The trapezius and levator scapulae support the entire weight of the upper extremity in the erect position (Figure 4.12.2A). In addition to their suspensory role they participate in a complicated muscle couple controlling scapulothoracic movement. The upper fibres of the trapezius and levator scapulae pull cephalad, whilst the lower fibres of the trapezius, acting with the rhomboids and the latissimus dorsi, pull the arm backwards (Figure 4.12.2B), allowing the upper fibres of trapezius to rotate the scapula.

The major cause of trapezius palsy is injury to the spinal accessory nerve (Box 4.12.2). Although the dangers of iatrogenic injury cannot be overstressed, it is important to appreciate that this palsy is commonly seen when the nerve is sacrificed during radical neck dissection for malignant disease. The ensuing disability can be so great that preservation should be encouraged if at all possible. The disability may be compounded by using the levator scapulae muscle to cover the carotid artery during this procedure. Not only is it the only other suspensory muscle, but it is also of great importance in late reconstruction of the shoulder girdle.

The spinal accessory nerve is the major nerve supply to trapezius. It exits the base of skull through the jugular foramen and passes obliquely through the sternomastoid muscle in its upper third before crossing the posterior triangle of the neck to enter trapezius. As it lies very superficially, it is vulnerable to injury and is at risk with even the simplest surgical operation in the neck region. The injury is usually not recognized at the time of surgery and the diagnosis is often delayed until the patient describes inability to abduct the arm without pain. Some of the palsies are due to neurapraxia and recover spontaneously. Electromyographic examination may be of help but if there is no recovery by 10 weeks the nerve should be explored. If the nerve is found in continuity lying in scar tissue, neurolysis may be successful, but if there is obvious discontinuity then suture or grafting is necessary. Should the repair be unsuccessful or not possible, surgical reconstruction with muscle transfers should be considered.

Box 4.12.2 Winging of the scapula

- Causes profound loss of shoulder function
- May be due to trauma of the long thoracic nerve, e.g. backpackers' shoulder
- May be involved in the postviral syndrome, neuralgic amytrophy
- Surgical reconstruction with tendon transfers is possible.

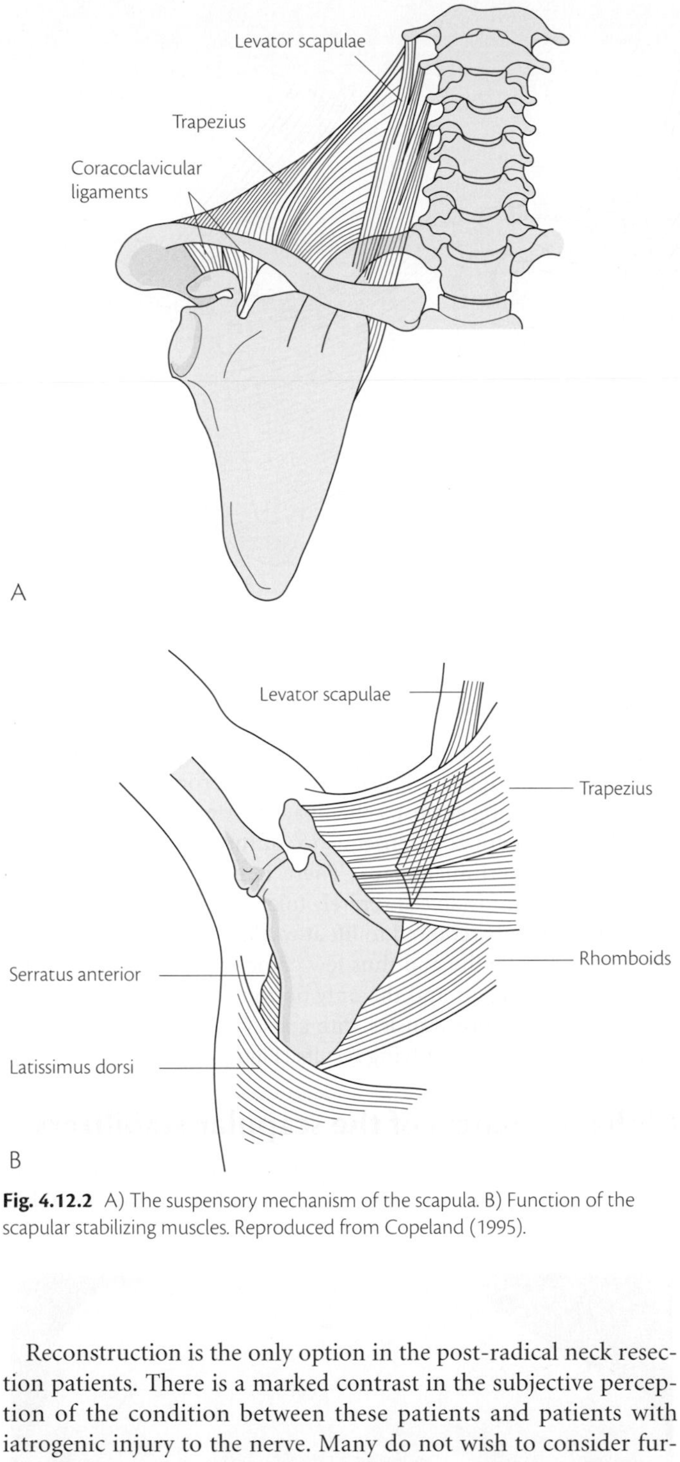

Fig. 4.12.2 A) The suspensory mechanism of the scapula. B) Function of the scapular stabilizing muscles. Reproduced from Copeland (1995).

Reconstruction is the only option in the post-radical neck resection patients. There is a marked contrast in the subjective perception of the condition between these patients and patients with iatrogenic injury to the nerve. Many do not wish to consider further surgery and have insufficient disability to require reconstruction. The degree of disability is extremely variable which may be partly due to the dual innervation from C2 and C3 (occasionally C3 and C4) in some patients. The indications are usually not precise and depend on the activity level, age, and life expectancy of the patient.

The cause of pain in these patients may be uncertain. It is important to try and ascertain the mechanism in order to plan treatment. Pain from neurologic denervation and adhesive capsulitis may be a factor in the early phase. Ptosis of the scapula may cause discomfort by a brachial plexus traction radiculitis. More commonly the pain appears to be due to fatigue and functional impingement (Figure 4.12.3).

The procedures to restore the function of the scapulothoracic articulation must address not only the winging, but also the ptosis due to loss of the scapular suspension mechanism. The complex nature of force couples makes substitution of even one muscle acting in a single plane difficult. The Eden–Lange tendon transfer of levator scapulae and the rhomboids (Figure 4.12.4A) is probably best for near-normal. These three muscles are used to replace the upper, middle, and lower portions of the trapezius respectively.

The alternative procedures, originally used in patients with facial nerve paralysis in which the spinal accessory nerve was used as a motor for the facial muscles, have significant disadvantages. Dewar and Harris (1950) transferred the levator scapulae insertion laterally to substitute for the upper trapezius, and used a fascial sling in place of middle and lower parts of trapezius (Figure 4.12.4B). The slings were passed from the vertebral border of the scapula to the spinous processes of the second and third thoracic vertebrae. Unfortunately, these slings used in this procedure and the many variations described tend to stretch with time. If soft-tissue reconstruction fails, the only other option is limited to scapulothoracic fusion. This procedure has also been suggested as an option as a primary procedure in cases where heavy demands are anticipated. Conservative treatment has not been found successful other than treating concomitant adhesive capsulitis.

Loss of serratus anterior function

On elevation of the arm as the upper fibres of trapezius rotate the scapula, the serratus anterior assists by rotating the scapula forwards and maintaining the vertebral border of the scapula in firm apposition with the chest wall in all positions (Figures 4.12.2 and 4.12.3). Paralysis of this muscle may limit active elevation, but more frequently presents as deformity with fatigue pain on elevation of the arm. The fine tuning of scapula movement is of paramount importance in shoulder performance. In many vigorous shoulder activities the scapula is positioned so that the glenoid centre line and axis of the humeral head are closely aligned, for example, in a boxer's punch, bench press, throwing action, and

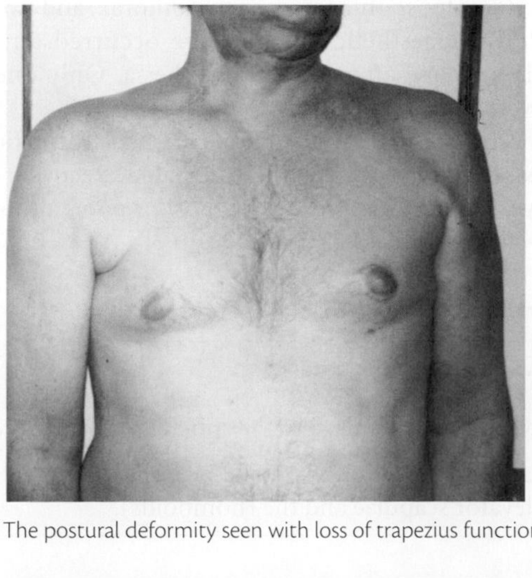

Fig. 4.12.3 The postural deformity seen with loss of trapezius function.

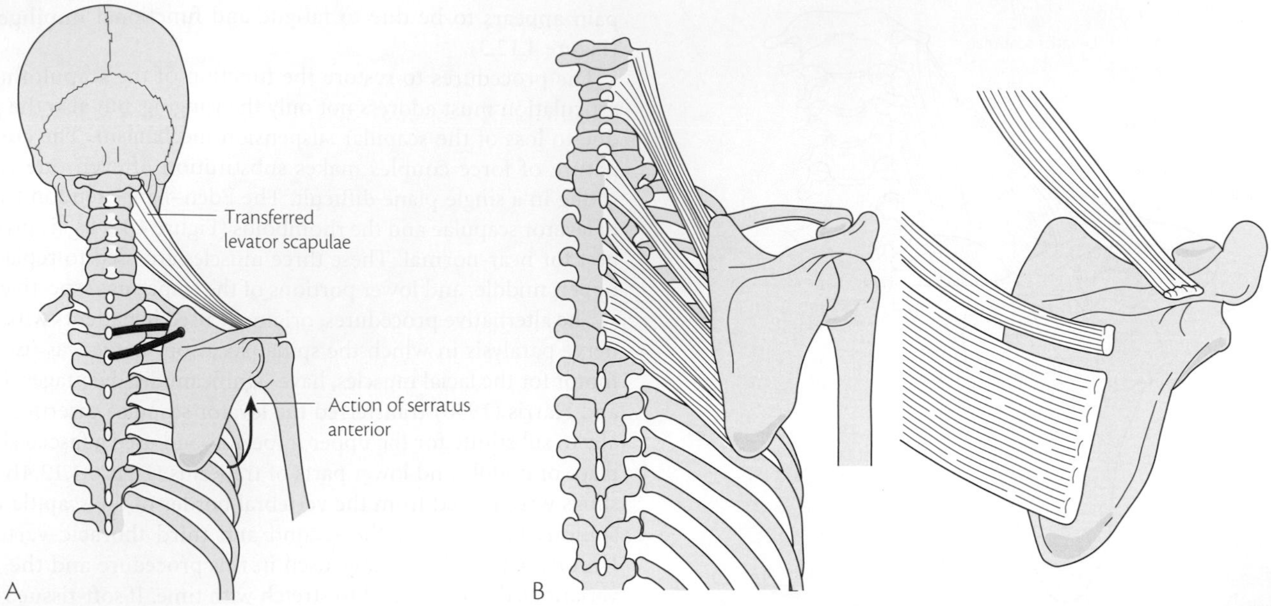

Fig. 4.12.4 The principles of muscle transfer for the loss of trapezius function. A) The Eden–Lange procedure. B) The Dewar and Harris procedure. Reproduced from Copeland (1997).

tennis shot. It is easy to demonstrate the effect of fatigue if the glenoid centre line and humerus are not aligned. Try maintaining the arm or lifting an object with the scapula deliberately retracted. With the scapula correctly protracted, the glenohumeral joint stabilizes with ease, making more muscle action available for power.

Long thoracic nerve palsy is the major cause of serratus anterior weakness. This nerve is formed from the roots of C5, C6, and C7 immediately after leaving their intervertebral foramina. It runs collaterally to the main brachial plexus and is often spared in traction lesions. The cause of long thoracic nerve palsy is often difficult to explain, but may follow viral illness, carrying objects on the shoulder, open iatrogenic injury in the axilla, lying on the operating table, and long periods of anaesthesia. It is also described after recumbency for a prolonged period of time and immunization, but these causes are rarely encountered in clinical practice. Kauppila and Vastamäki (1995) presented 27 cases of iatrogenic causes. These occurred during seven operations for first rib resection, four mastectomies with axillary clearance, two scalenotomies, two surgical procedures for spontaneous pneumothorax, and two infraclavicular plexus anaesthetic blocks. Nine occurred after general anaesthesia and one after spinal anaesthesia. Only one of these cases recovered spontaneously.

Palsies occurring after closed trauma are usually traction lesions and spontaneous recovery can be anticipated. Recovery is usually seen by 1 year. After this time the prognosis is poor, although some cases may still recover at 2–3 years.

Box 4.12.3 Loss of trapezius function

- Usually caused by damage to the spinal accessory nerve
- Surgical reconstruction is possible (the Eden–Lange transfer of the levator scapulae and the rhomboids).

The major problem is pain with difficulty in lifting the arm and lifting weights (Figure 4.12.5). Discomfort from the prominent scapula when sitting against a chair back is common. The shoulder may also be painful as a consequence of functional impingement within the subacromial space. There is little useful treatment; braces are uncomfortable and rarely tolerated, but may be of value in selected patients required to lift at work. Many patients learn to live with the disability and thus few come to surgery. There is no place for nerve repair and the only option is surgical reconstruction. Pectoralis major transfer with a fascia lata graft to the lower pole of scapula gives gratifying results (Figure 4.12.6).

Global weakness of the scapular stabilizers

Generalized weakness of the scapular stabilizers is commonly seen with many injuries and conditions affecting the shoulder.

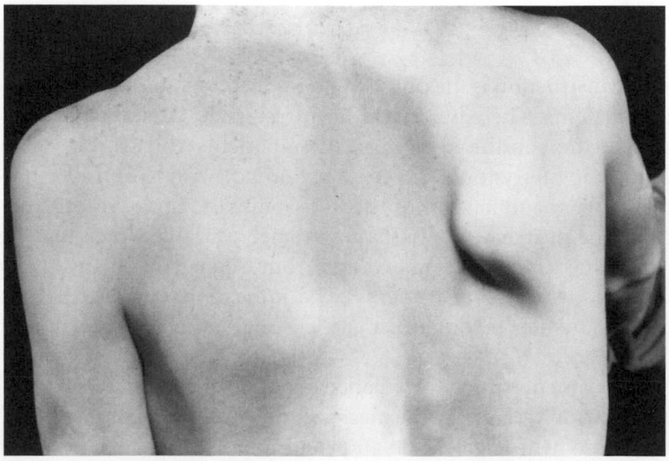

Fig. 4.12.5 Winging due to long thoracic nerve palsy. Reproduced from Copeland (1997).

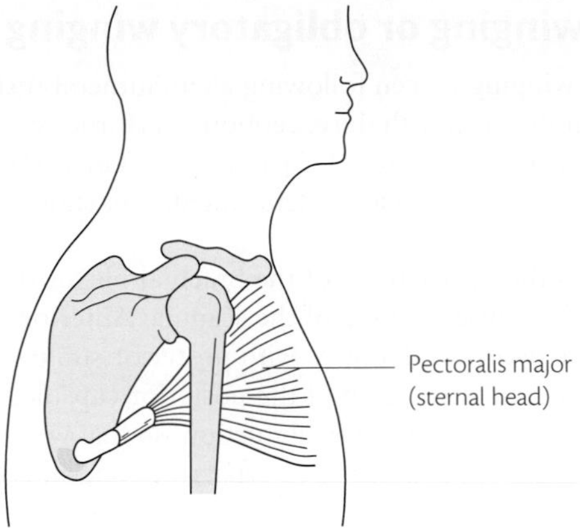

Fig. 4.12.6 Transfer of pectoralis major with fascia lata graft for serratus anterior palsy.

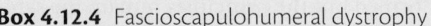

Box 4.12.4 Fascioscapulohumeral dystrophy

- Autosomal dominant inheritance
- Unilateral presentation with slow development of both shoulders
- Scapulothoracic fusion improves function.

Careful examination will often demonstrate minor winging even in the absence of stiffness of the glenohumeral joint. When the weakness is severe, the imbalance as a consequence of relatively greater strength of deltoid pulling up the scapula causes winging on elevation of the arm. Duchenne showed this mechanism of winging of the scapula in his treatise *Physiology of Motion* (Figure 4.12.7). This is the situation in muscular dystrophies affecting the muscles of the scapula.

Muscle dystrophies should be suspected in cases of atraumatic onset of weakness and atrophy occurring in first and second decade. The most common type is fascioscapulohumeral dystrophy (FSHD; Landouzy–Déjerine disease) (Box 4.12.4). A positive family history is common, as this is an autosomal dominant condition with sporadic cases appearing very occasionally. Recent genetic linkage studies have mapped the FSHD gene to chromosome 4q35. On presentation it is usually unilateral, with the other side not developing until months or even years later. Involvement of the facial muscle may be detected early, with the child's inability to whistle or blow out candles on the birthday cake. This condition has a variable muscle involvement and prognosis. There is usually good life expectancy and slow deterioration. The deltoid is spared but loses its stable origin and tilts the scapula rather than raising the humerus. The cosmetic appearance due to the selective muscle loss is characteristic and may cause difficulty with clothing (Figure 4.12.8).

In this condition, muscle involvement is global, precluding muscle transfer. If the function of the deltoid muscle is preserved and the disability is severe, scapulothoracic fusion should be considered. This operation recreates the stable origin by anchoring the scapula to the fourth, fifth, and sixth ribs. This procedure was described by Copeland and Howard in 1978. There are many

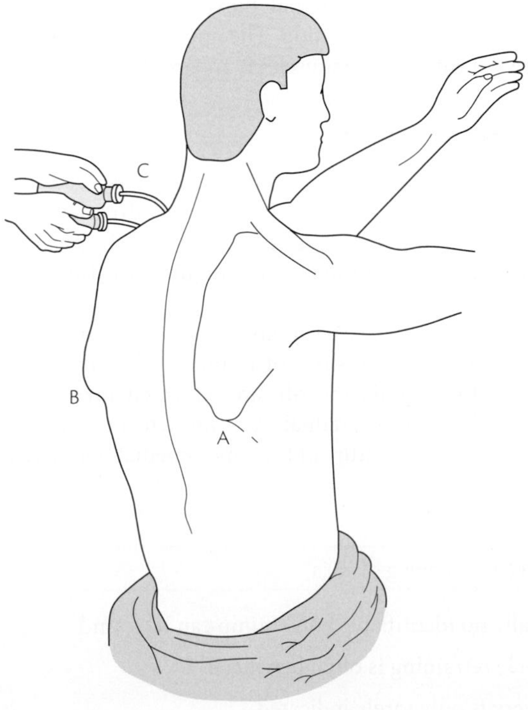

Fig. 4.12.7 Illustration from Duchenne's *Physiology of Motion* (1959, W.B.Saunders) showing faradic stimulation creating winging of the scapula.

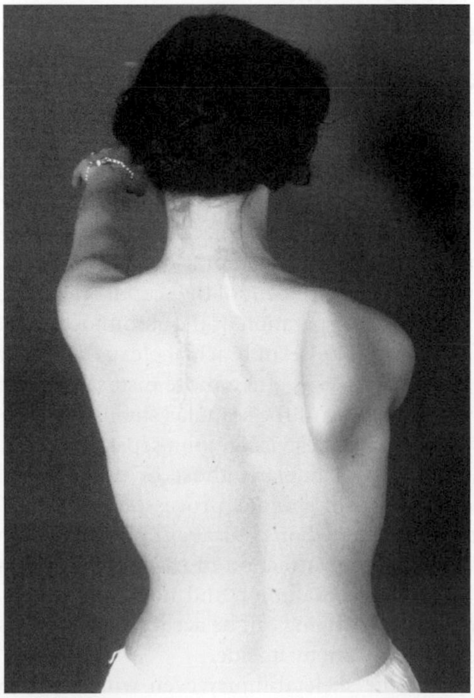

Fig. 4.12.8 Typical appearance of facioscapulohumeral dystrophy. Reproduced from Copeland, S.A. and Howard, R.C. (1978). Thoracoscapular fusion for facioscapulohumeral dystrophy. *Journal of Bone and Joint Surgery*, **60-B**, 547–51.

technical variations performed but the principles remain the same. The results in 11 shoulders were reported with an average range of 90 degrees of flexion and 100 degrees of abduction. There was no deterioration with time and the vital capacity was preserved. The most frequent complication reported is stress fracture, which is treated by immobilization in a sling.

Scapulothoracic fusion

The patient is initially placed supine to harvest sufficient corticocancellous bone graft from the iliac crest. The patient is then moved into the prone position with the arm free and supported on an adjustable stool.

An incision is made along the medial border of the scapula. The atrophied muscles on the deep and superficial surfaces of the scapula are stripped laterally for at least 2cm. The subjacent three ribs (usually the fourth, fifth, and sixth) are exposed by subperiosteal dissection. Retractors are placed under the ribs to protect the pleura. Corticocancellous grafts are placed between each rib and the scapula. Three to four screws are inserted taking care that they do not protrude into the pleura. Chips of bone are packed between the grafts. The shoulder should be fused and held in 50 degrees of abduction and 30 degrees of forward flexion with sufficient internal rotation to place the hand in front of the mouth.

A spica cast or shoulder brace is worn for 3 months. The abduction is reduced slowly over a week by adjusting the brace or replacing the spica with foam wedges.

An alternative method of fixation is with Luque wires through drill holes in the scapula. A pelvic reconstruction plate on the posterior surface can be incorporated to increase the strength of fixation. This method allows early mobilization and a sling rather than a spica.

Loss of the scapular suspensory mechanism

The ligamentous structures, that is, the conoid and trapezoid parts of the coracoclavicular ligaments, are important static suspensory structures and constraints to scapular movement. They not only prevent the scapula from dropping but also prevent posterior displacement of the clavicle and protraction of the scapula (Figure 4.12.1).

An injury commonly not recognized is described by Rockwood and Matsen and termed 'scapulothoracic dissociation'. This results from violent lateral displacement of the scapula causing disruption of the soft tissues with separation of the acromioclavicular joint or fracture of the clavicle. Vessel or brachial plexus damage may occur with these injuries. There is also a more discrete type of injury in which there is stretching of the scapular stabilizers usually associated with type IV acromioclavicular joint separations and displaced clavicular fractures, particularly those of the lateral third. The increased distance from spinous processes to medial border of scapula can be appreciated on clinical examination or on the chest radiograph. Similarly, protraction of the scapula with soft-tissue stretching is seen with malunion and non-union of the clavicle. The protraction and winging can be accentuated by resisted external rotation with the arm by its side.

Restoration of the skeletal injury even with repair of the disrupted ligaments may be insufficient to correct the deformity, and specific rehabilitation of the scapular muscles must be stressed.

Pseudowinging or obligatory winging

Obligatory winging is seen following glenohumeral fusion. This is rarely of significance, with the exception of arthrodesis for brachial plexus injury. In some cases of C5 and C6 root avulsion, the upper part of serratus anterior may be denervated. This should be assessed prior to surgery.

Injuries to the upper roots of the brachial plexus during childbirth may also cause winging of the scapula. Anterior contracture and capsular tightness develops with posterior subluxation of the humeral head and stretching of the posterior capsule. The glenohumeral joint becomes fixed in abduction, so that when the shoulder is forced into adduction and external rotation, superior winging due to the contracture occurs—known as the scapular sign of Putti.

An abduction contracture of deltoid may cause secondary winging. This is not so rare and many cases are reported, so it should be looked for in clinical practice. It is often bilateral and usually affects the anterior part of deltoid. Two types occur; congenital or secondary to multiple intramuscular injections. The treatment is by release of fibrous bands and manipulation. A defect in deltoid may result and require closure by transfer of posterior deltoid anteriorly. Displacement of the scapula and pseudowinging may be seen with large subscapular osteochondromas.

Voluntary winging

Rowe (1988) described four patients with voluntary winging. A more common appearance of winging is seen in cases of habitual or voluntary glenohumeral instability. In this situation the ability to sublux the shoulder requires winging of the scapula to destabilize the glenohumeral joint. The role of the scapula in this poorly understood condition is well demonstrated by observing the persistent muscle activity of the muscles controlling the scapulothoracic movement after brachial plexus anaesthesia blocked in patients with severe dysfunction. The importance of addressing the task of re-educating these muscles is apparent.

Snapping scapula

Presentation with a tactile and acoustic clunk localized at the superomedial corner of the scapula is not infrequent. This phenomenon, termed a snapping scapula, is usually encountered in the third decade and normally only requires treatment if painful (Box 4.12.5).

A variety of causes have been reported but the condition remains poorly understood. A history of trauma is not uncommon, but fractures of the scapula and ribs are extremely rare causes. More commonly the onset is gradual. A prominent Luschka's tubercle, excessive forward curvature of the superomedial border, exostoses,

Box 4.12.5 Snapping scapula

- Usually no identifiable bony bump can be found
- Muscle retraining is often beneficial
- Surgery is only rarely indicated.

or tumours are potential skeletal causes. These identifiable causes are comparatively rare and the majority of patients present with poor posture with sagging of the shoulder girdle such that the superomedial corner descends and impinges on the chest wall.

Plain radiographs, including a carefully positioned lateral view, will exclude an exostosis or obvious bony cause. Computed tomography is of limited value and difficult to interpret. Occasionally narrowing between the superomedial corner and the chest wall can be demonstrated in comparison to the contralateral side. Magnetic resonance imaging has little place, with the exception of defining the rare cases of tumor.

The treatment is usually non-operative; careful assessment and correction of abnormal posture is essential. The snapping or grating often disappears when the scapula is passively elevated and retracted. This can be demonstrated to the patient and is helpful in increasing the patient's understanding of the rehabilitation programme. Before abandoning these measures in favour of surgery it is important to consider the natural history and the not infrequent association with psychological stress. It is interesting to note that very few cases fail to resolve with time. However, this can be a disabling condition and can be relieved by surgical resection of the superomedial scapula. Some authors advocate arthroscopic resection, but since the surgical landmarks are few, and important nerves are close by, this technique should be left to a few superspecialists.

Further reading

Bigliani, L.U., Compito, C.A., Duralde, X.A., and Wolfe, I.R. (1996). Transfer of the levator scapulae, rhomboid major and rhomboid minor for paralysis of the trapezius. *Journal of Bone and Joint Surgery*, **78A**, 1534–40.

Copeland, S.A. and Howard, R.C. (1978). Thoracoscapular fusion for facioscapulohumeral dystrophy. *Journal of Bone and Joint Surgery*, **60B**, 547–51.

Harper, G.D., McIlroy, S., Bayley, J.I.L., and Calvert, P.T. (1999). Arthroscopic partial resection of the scapula for snapping scapula—a new technique. *Journal of Shoulder and Elbow Surgery*, **8**, 55–7.

Kauppila, L.I. and Vastamäki, M. (1995). 'Iatrogenic serratus anterior paralysis: long-term outcome in 26 cases.' Presented at 6th ICSS Meeting, Helsinki, 27 June–1 July, 1995.

Richards, R. and McKee, M.D. (1989). Treatment of painful scapulothoracic crepitus by resection of the supero-medial angle of the scapula. *Clinical Orthopaedics and Related Research*, **247**, 111–16.

Wilkinson, J.A. and Campbell, D. (1980). Scapular osteotomy for Sprengel's shoulder. *Journal of Bone and Joint Surgery*, **62A**, 486–90.

4.13

Reverse geometry replacement

Duncan J. Watkinson and Pascal Boileau

Summary points

- RSR provides a unique tool for patients with cuff tear arthropathy
- RSR is a useful tool for fractures, tumours, and revision of shoulder replacements
- However RSR comes with specific complications such as scapular notching and acromial fractures
- The 10 year results of RSR show that prosthetic loosening is no more frequent than with anatomical prostheses.

Introduction

Conventional shoulder arthroplasty has been extremely successful in many forms of arthritis. The aim is to resurface the arthritic joint, but also to restore joint biomechanics. Deficiency of the soft tissues, and in particular of the rotator cuff, is therefore a major problem. Contractures can be released, the subscapularis can be lengthened, but an irreparable cuff tear is by definition an insurmountable obstacle to restoring normal biomechanics.

Whilst a tear is the most common cause of cuff dysfunction, there are other situations where the proximal humeral anatomy is distorted and the cuff is either physically or functionally compromised. These include certain fractures and fracture sequelae, as well as certain revision situations. In all of these cases poor active elevation and an unstable centre of rotation secondary to a deficient cuff cannot be corrected by a conventional shoulder prosthesis.

Historical perspective

Neer recognized the challenge posed by arthrosis associated with massive irreparable cuff tears and suggested that it was realistic to pursue 'limited goals rehabilitation'. The limited results of *hemiarthoplasty* in this setting have been confirmed by several other authors who reported inconsistent pain relief and small improvements in active elevation.

Conventional *total shoulder arthroplasty* fared no better, as superior eccentric loading of the glenoid component by the unstable humeral head increased the risk of premature loosening, the so-called rocking horse phenomenon.

In the early 1980s, a number of *constrained shoulder prostheses* were introduced. Increased constraint stabilized the centre of rotation, but at the expense of premature aseptic loosening, and most never progressed beyond the experimental. This same lesson had already been learned with excessively constrained prostheses in other joints.

In 1985, Grammont introduced a revolutionary design of *semi-constrained reverse geometry total shoulder replacement (RSR)*. The idea of reversing the ball and the socket was not new. However, previous designs had sought to preserve the shoulder's anatomical centre of rotation by using a glenoid component shaped like a chess pawn, with a small head offset from the glenoid base-plate by a neck. Grammont's prosthesis, the Delta, used a large hemispherical glenoid component applied directly to the surface of the glenoid in order to minimize torsional stresses, yet stabilize the centre of rotation and optimize range of movement.

This design has progressed well beyond the experimental and its popularity has encouraged a number of imitations, each striving to 'improve' on the original design.

Biomechanics

Intact rotator cuff

Shoulder elevation is a rotatory movement requiring a muscular moment to overcome the moment resulting from the weight of the arm. In practice, this is provided by the deltoid and the supraspinatus, but the initial forces produced by the deltoid when the arm is alongside the body are predominantly vertical shear. It is the role of the rotator cuff to oppose this upward force and stabilize the centre of rotation, in order to convert a vertical linear force into a rotatory movement. A useful analogy is of a person standing on the edge of a cliff holding a ladder on a rope that is secured to a rung halfway down its length. If they pull on the rope, the ladder will simply slide up the cliff. However, if they place their foot on the top rung of the ladder and then pull on the rope, the ladder will swing away from the cliff.

The situation is, however, a little more complex than this. The cuff does not simply oppose the vertical component of the deltoid, but also generates compressive forces that help to stabilize the centre of rotation in the sagittal as well as in the coronal plane. Furthermore, the deltoid itself also generates compressive forces as elevation increases, and beyond 60 degrees these compressive forces exceed its vertical shear force, thus diminishing the role of the cuff.

Deficient rotator cuff

Post defined a massive rotator cuff tear as measuring 5cm or more in the sagittal plane. This is, however, a somewhat arbitrary figure, and a massive tear is perhaps more usefully defined as one involving at least two complete tendons. In practice, this means the supraspinatus plus the infraspinatus, and/or the subscapularis. Any remaining cuff is also likely to be degenerate, and its function may be further compromised by fatty degeneration of the muscle bellies.

Without a functional cuff, the unopposed upward force generated by the deltoid muscle causes the humeral head to migrate proximally and ultimately to abut the acromion. It is still a matter of some speculation why certain patients are able to maintain useful active elevation despite this biomechanical disadvantage, yet others are not and exhibit what has been termed pseudoparalysis. An intact coracoacromial arch should provide a fulcrum to stabilize the centre of rotation, so why do some patients lose active elevation? This may sometimes be explained by pain inhibition of the deltoid, yet pseudoparalysis is often painless. In these cases, upward migration of the humerus is probably sufficient to functionally lengthen and thus seriously weaken the deltoid. Furthermore, a massive cuff tear, particularly one involving subscapularis, may destabilize the centre of rotation of the shoulder in the sagittal as well as in the coronal plane. The humeral head may therefore sublux anteriorly as well as superiorly, thus diminishing the fulcrum provided by the acromion.

A massive cuff tear is often a gradual process of cuff wear rather than a sudden catastrophic failure of the cuff. This means that the bony surfaces have the opportunity to remodel, a process which can eventually lead to acetabularization of the glenohumeral joint (Figure 4.13.1). This adaptive process has been described by Hamada in five stages:

- *Stage 1*: a balanced cuff tear with no upward migration of the humeral head (acromiohumeral distance more than 6mm)
- *Stage 2*: upward migration of the humeral head without any secondary bony changes (acromiohumeral distance 5mm or less)
- *Stage 3*: remodelling of the subacromial space with erosion of the undersurface of the acromion and the greater tuberosity
- *Stage 4*: glenohumeral narrowing in addition to stage 3, with predominantly superior erosion of the glenoid
- *Stage 5*: collapse of the humeral head in addition to stage 4 (this corresponds to true cuff tear arthropathy as described by Neer).

Principles of reverse geometry shoulder replacement

As mentioned earlier, previous attempts at RSR had used a glenoid component shaped like a chess pawn in order to restore the centre of rotation to its anatomical location (Figure 4.13.2A). This meant that the upward force of the deltoid was applied to the head of the glenoid component, and the neck of the component provided a lever arm. The end result was the application of excessive torsional forces to the glenoid base-plate causing early loosening. What is more, the small size of the glenoid head meant that impingement between the components limited the potential range of movement. Broström published the only series in the literature for this type of design (the Kessel prosthesis). Pain relief was achieved in 90%, but average active elevation was only 35 degrees and the reoperation rate was 26%.

Grammont was therefore facing a formidable challenge. His prosthesis needed to stabilize the centre of rotation in the absence of a functional cuff, restore a functionally weakened deltoid, optimize the range of movement allowed by the prosthesis, yet avoid premature loosening.

The crucial element of his design was a large hemispherical glenoid component applied to the glenoid *without a neck* (Figure 4.13.2B). This had the following consequences:

- The centre of rotation was medialized, thus minimizing torque on the glenoid component
- The humerus was displaced medially and distally, thus retensioning the deltoid
- Impingement between the components was minimized, thus optimizing range of movement.

Medialization of the centre of rotation

The use of a hemispherical component applied directly to the glenoid means that the centre of rotation is at the bone–prosthesis interface. There are therefore no torsional forces applied to this interface as there were with designs that used a neck to preserve a more anatomical (lateral) centre of rotation (Figure 4.13.2C).

Displacement of the humerus

The humeral component articulates under the glenoid hemisphere, which means that the humerus is displaced medially and distally relative to its normal position. In the normal shoulder the middle fibres of the deltoid course around the greater tuberosity, giving the shoulder its rounded contour. The tuberosity effectively acts as a cam, increasing the tension in the deltoid muscle as well as altering the angle at which it acts on the humerus. Medial displacement of the humerus removes this cam effect and the deltoid has a more linear course between the acromion and its humeral insertion, effectively lengthening the muscle. It is therefore vital that the humerus is also displaced distally, not only to restore the deltoid tension that was lost as a result of the deficient cuff (and the consequent upward migration of the humeral head), but also to compensate for this effective lengthening of the deltoid. Clinical measurements have demonstrated that mean lengthening of the upper limb following RSR is 1.5cm.

Component impingement

As has been well documented in hip arthroplasty, rotation around a small sphere is typically limited by impingement between the components. In the shoulder, scapular rotation can compensate to a degree for limited glenohumeral movement, but the use of a large glenoid hemisphere maximizes component excursion. Furthermore, in the absence of a neck on the glenoid component, a larger hemisphere also reduces the risk of impingement between the humeral

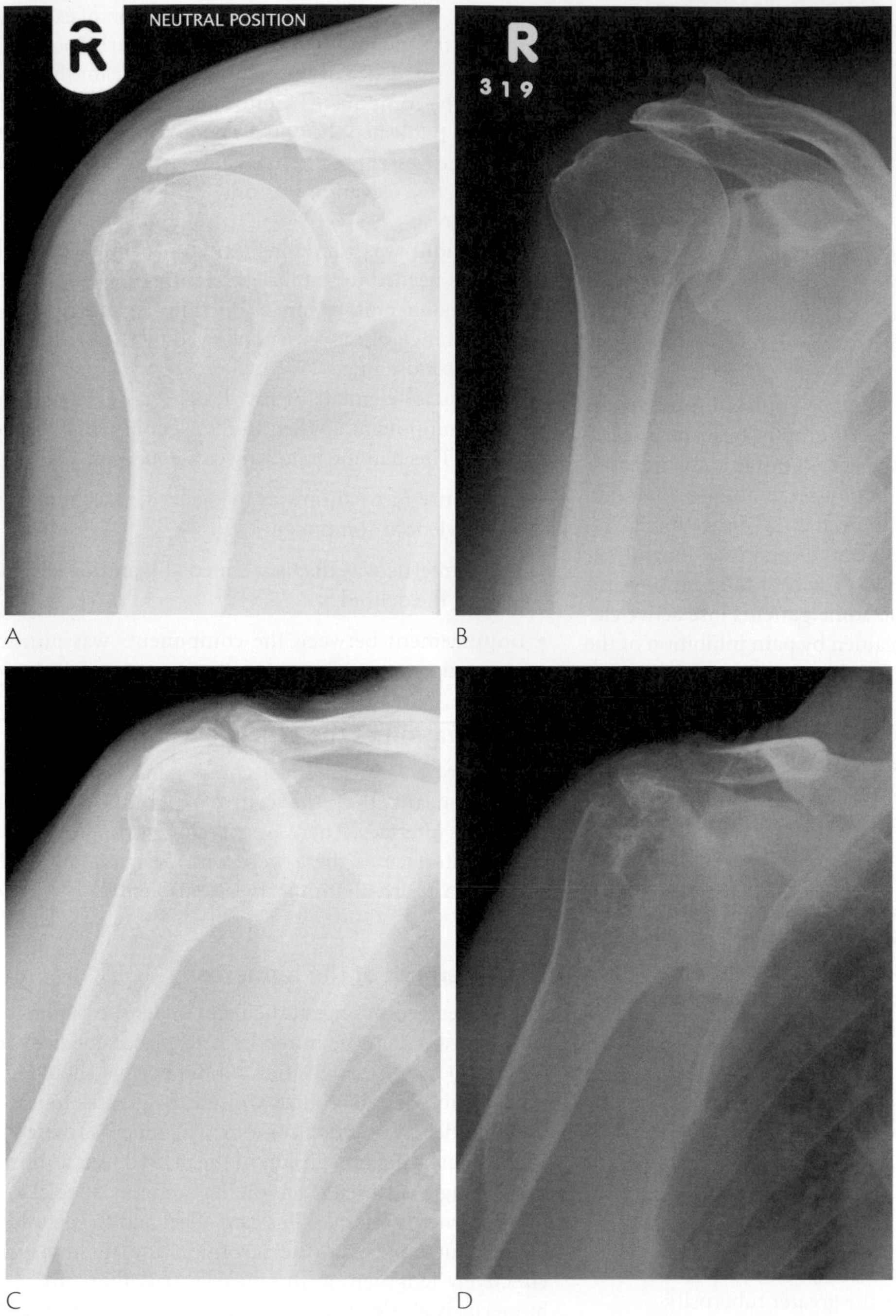

Fig. 4.13.1 Hamada classification of massive cuff tears (stage 1 not shown). A) Stage 2. B) Stage 3. C) Stage 4. D) Stage 5.

cup and the inferolateral aspect of the scapula. This will be discussed later on the subject of scapular notching.

Minimizing aseptic loosening

The most important factor in minimizing the risk of premature loosening of the glenoid is medialization of the centre of rotation and the attendant abolition of torsional forces at the bone–prosthesis interface. However, particularly during the earlier stages of elevation, the glenoid component is nevertheless subjected to significant shear forces that may also jeopardize glenoid fixation.

Grammont's first design for the glenoid component was a monoblock which fitted over and around the glenoid like a barrel and was fixed with cement. However this was rapidly abandoned in favour of the current design which provides superior fixation in the limited bone stock of the scapula and greater resistance to shear forces. The glenoid component now has two parts: the metaglene and the glenosphere.

The metaglene is a circular baseplate with a central pillar and a hydroxyapatite coating. Its fixation to the glenoid is augmented by two divergent screws whose heads lock into the plate, as well as two

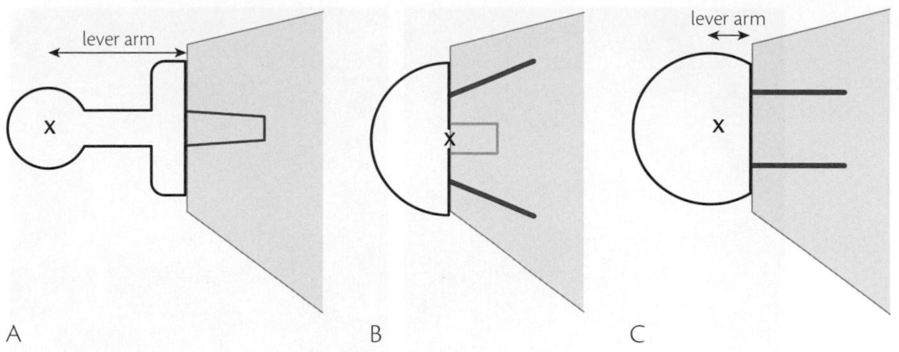

Fig. 4.13.2 Glenoid component design and centre of rotation (COR). 'X' marks COR. A) Old designs maintained a lateral COR. Deltoid force applied at COR induced excessive torque at bone–prosthesis interface and early loosening because of the resulting lever arm. B) Delta RSR places COR at the bone–prosthesis interface. Deltoid force applied at COR does not develop any torque because there is no lever arm. C) Use of a three-quarter hemisphere potentially reduces the risk of notching but at a price. COR is once again lateralized relative to bone–prosthesis interface and a (smaller) lever arm is reintroduced.

non-locking screws. Not only is the bone-stock limited by the shape of the scapula, but in many of these elderly patients the bone itself is of poor quality. The locking plate configuration therefore provides superior pullout strength as compared to a central peg alone, or to non-locking screws. The superior screw is aimed at the base of the coracoid and the inferior one into the inferior pillar of the scapula as these represent the thickest areas of bone in the scapula medial to the glenoid.

The hemispherical glenosphere fits over the metaglene and is fixed with a peripheral morse taper and a central countersunk screw.

On the humeral side a polyethylene cup is carried by a modular humeral component. The latter is composed of a stem and an epiphyseal component which may be cemented or uncemented. There is, however, very little evidence to support the use of the uncemented stem at present.

Indications

Massive irreparable cuff tear

The Delta RSR was originally designed for elderly patients with painful cuff tear arthrosis who had failed to respond to conservative measures. In essence this meant Hamada stages 3–5 (Figure 4.13.3). However, patients without bony changes (Hamada stage 2) who fail to respond to simpler surgical procedures such as arthroscopic debridement and biceps tenotomy may also benefit from RSR.

Whilst most authors agree that RSR should be reserved for patients over the age of 70 years, most series do include a number of patients who are younger than this. Those who still have active elevation above shoulder height despite cuff-tear arthrosis may obtain good results with a conventional hemiarthroplasty. In the presence of painful pseudoparalysis, the case for RSR in a patient under the age of 70 becomes stronger, but both surgeon and patient should be aware of the uncertain long-term results, and each case should be judged on its individual merits.

Revision surgery

RSR is indicated for revision cases where there is either significant distortion of the proximal humeral bony anatomy or a deficient rotator cuff. The most common situation where this is encountered is in a fracture hemiarthroplasty that has failed because of tuberosity non-union or malunion.

Fracture sequelae and acute fractures

Painful malunion or non-union of a three- or four-part proximal humeral fracture is another difficult surgical situation. Hemiarthroplasty alone cannot restore cuff function unless combined with osteotomy of the tuberosities, but the results of this are often disappointing and there is a high rate of tuberosity non-union. RSR offers a solution without the need for tuberosity osteotomy (Figure 4.13.4).

In the acute displaced four-part fracture, hemiarthroplasty remains the treatment of choice, but accurate and durable reconstruction of the tuberosities around the prosthesis can present a considerable challenge. Malposition, non-union, or migration of the tuberosities are significant risks and can seriously compromise results. RSR has been suggested as an alternative, particularly if the tuberosities are comminuted or osteoporotic as is often the case in the elderly.

Results

Cuff tears have a high prevalence in the elderly, but few cause sufficient symptoms to warrant a RSR. Furthermore even the original RSR, the Delta, is still quite a new prosthesis. Most series are therefore relatively small and follow-up is at best short to medium term.

Only five series with more than 20 patients have been published for the Delta RSR to date (Table 4.13.1). As one might expect, the results for primary reverse arthroplasty are significantly better than for revision surgery. In the largest series to date (Wall et al. 2007), elevation improved from 76 degrees to 142 degrees in the CTA group, but from 58 degrees to 118 degrees in the revision group. Constant score improved from 27.7 to 65.1 in the former versus 19.7 to 52.2 in the latter.

In the only published review of acute three- or four-part fractures treated with RSR, mean active elevation was 97 degrees despite secondary displacement of the tuberosities in 53%. Mean age/sex adjusted Constant score was 66%. Unlike hemiarthroplasty, clinical results were not influenced by tuberosity healing.

Whilst RSR has been shown to restore active elevation, active external rotation is not significantly improved. The main determinant of

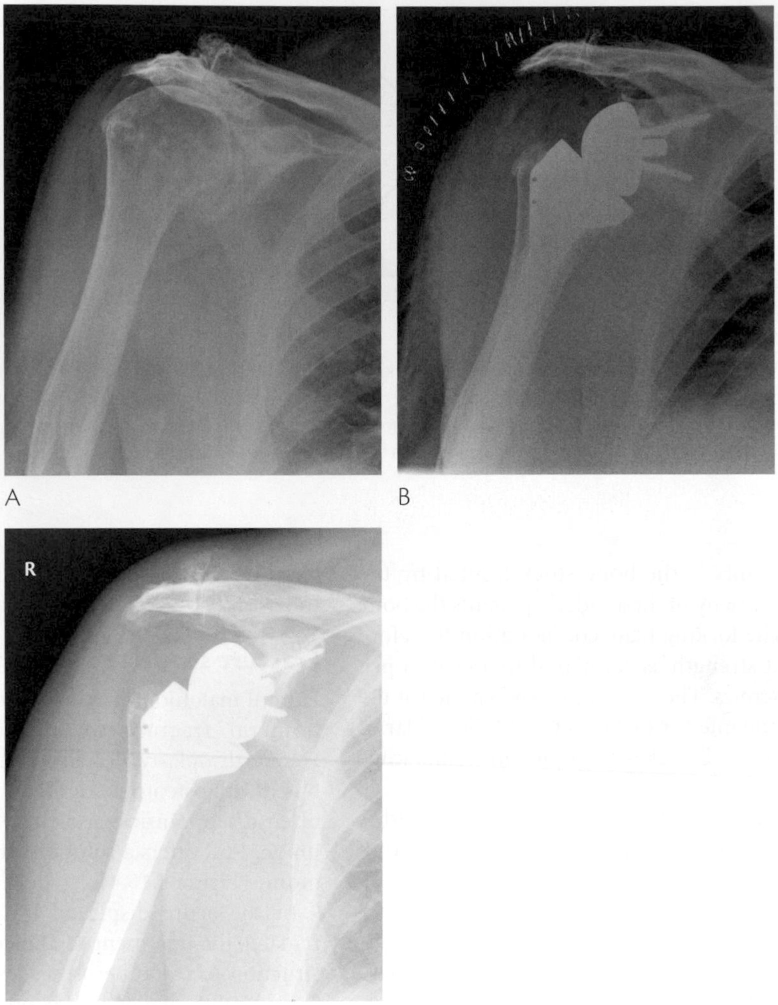

Fig. 4.13.3 Cuff tear arthrosis treated with Delta RSR. A) Stage 4 cuff tear arthrosis. B) Glenoid component positioned low with slight inferior overhang. C) No notch at 18 months.

postoperative active external rotation is therefore the preoperative condition of the posterior cuff. Latissimus dorsi transfer has been described in association with RSR. Active external rotation did not improve significantly with the arm at the side, but functional external rotation in the Constant score did. The authors argued that this resulted in a better ability to position the hand in space and thus superior function.

Survivorship analysis of a multicentre series of 80 cases demonstrated 10-year survival of 91% for revision and 84% for glenoid loosening, but only 58% for 'absolute Constant score <30' as an end point. Confidence intervals were, however, wide.

Complications

Reported complication rates range from 19–50%, but rates vary considerably between primary and revision cases. In the largest series to date, a complication rate of 13% was reported for primary surgery as opposed to 37% for revision cases. This large difference has been confirmed by others.

As well as the complications that affect conventional shoulder arthroplasty, there are three that appear to be a particular problem with the reverse design, namely notching, instability, and acromial fracture.

Notching

Whilst the absence of a neck on the glenoid component conveys great benefits, the reduced offset between the humerus and the scapula can also have a significant detrimental effect: impingement between the superomedial aspect of the humeral component and the lateral pillar of the scapula just below the glenoid. This commonly results in damage to the humeral cup and the appearance of a notch on the scapula. This has been reported in 44–68% of cases.

In many cases the notch is small and does not extend as far as the inferior screw, but it can extend to and even beyond this screw in up to 28% of cases (Figure 4.13.5). These larger notches are difficult to explain on the basis of physical impingement alone, and are probably due to osteolysis induced by polyethylene wear particles released from the damaged humeral cup.

The risk of notching may be reduced by inserting the glenoid component with a slight inferior overhang relative to the glenoid in order to minimize the physical impingement (Figure 4.13.3).

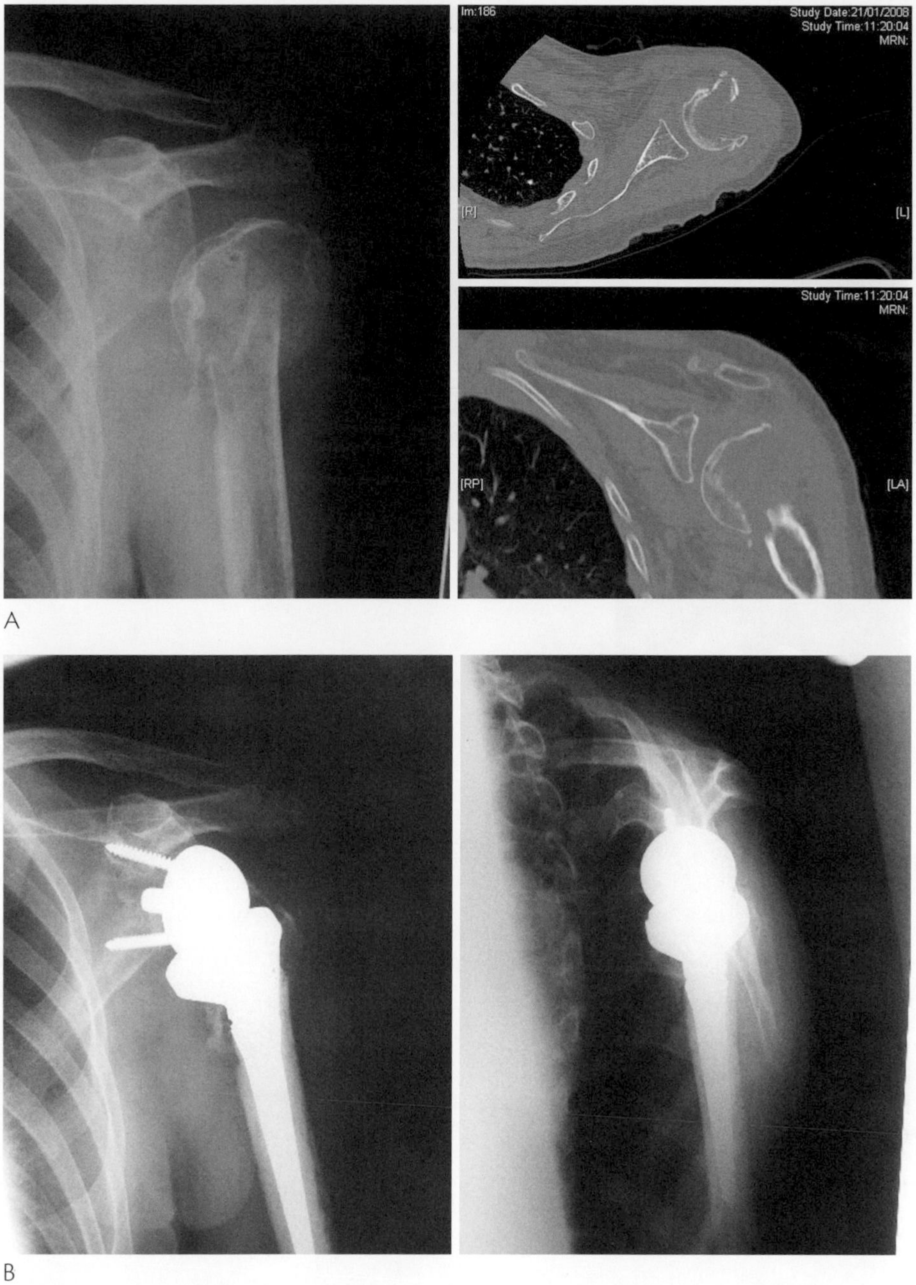

Fig. 4.13.4 Four-part fracture non-union treated with Delta RSR. A) Non-union with very poor bone quality. B) Delta RSR.

Table 4.13.1 Results of the Delta RSR (five largest published series)

Series	Pathology	No. in series	FU months	Active elevation (pre/post)	Constant score (pre/post)	Revision	Complications	Notch
Sirveau (2004)	CTA	80	44	73°/138°	22.6/65.6	4%	NA	65%
Werner (2005)	CTA, rev	58	38	42°/100°	29%/64%*	–	50%	
Boileau (2005)	CTA, rev, FS	45	40	55°/121°	17/58	13%**	24%	68%
Wall (2007)	CTA, rev, FS	240	40	86°/137°	23/60	3.5%	19.1%	50.7%
Bufquin (2007)	Fracture	43	22	NA/97°	NA/44	2%	28%	25%

*Age adjusted Constant score; **but 0% in the CTA group; CTA, cuff tear arthrosis; FS, fracture sequelae; rev, revision.

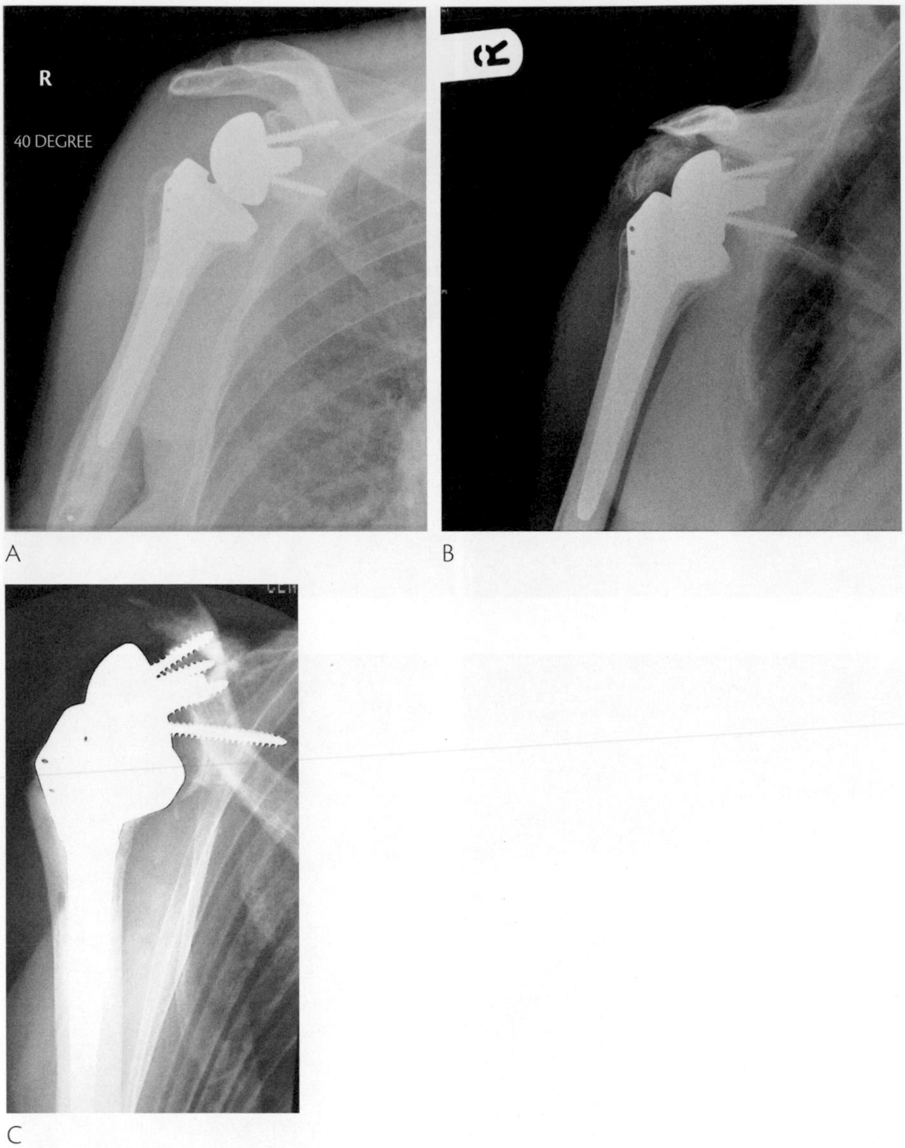

Fig. 4.13.5 Scapular notching. A) Minor notching. B) Moderate notching reaching inferior screw. C) Severe notching extending beyond inferior screw.

This has been confirmed in a cadaveric study and also a retrospective clinical study.

Despite the high prevalence of notching, loosening of the glenoid component has not been a significant problem to date, even with very large notches. It should be noted however that there are no long-term reviews in the literature and notching is arguably the greatest threat to long-term survival of RSR. Because of this, most authors recommend that RSR should be reserved for patients over the age of 70 at present.

Instability

In the absence of a functional cuff, a semi-constrained reverse prosthesis depends on deltoid tension to maintain compression between the congruent joint surfaces. Inadequate tension can cause instability that may be addressed by increasing the thickness of the humeral cup or adding a neck extension under the cup in order to increase deltoid tension.

Acromial fracture

At the other end of the spectrum, excessive deltoid tension can cause a fracture of an acromion that may have been eroded and weakened preoperatively by the action of the humeral head (Figure 4.13.6). However, such fractures are often asymptomatic and may present as incidental radiological findings.

The future of reverse geometry shoulder replacement

The Delta RSR has proved to be extremely popular as it offers a unique solution to a difficult orthopaedic problem. It has therefore

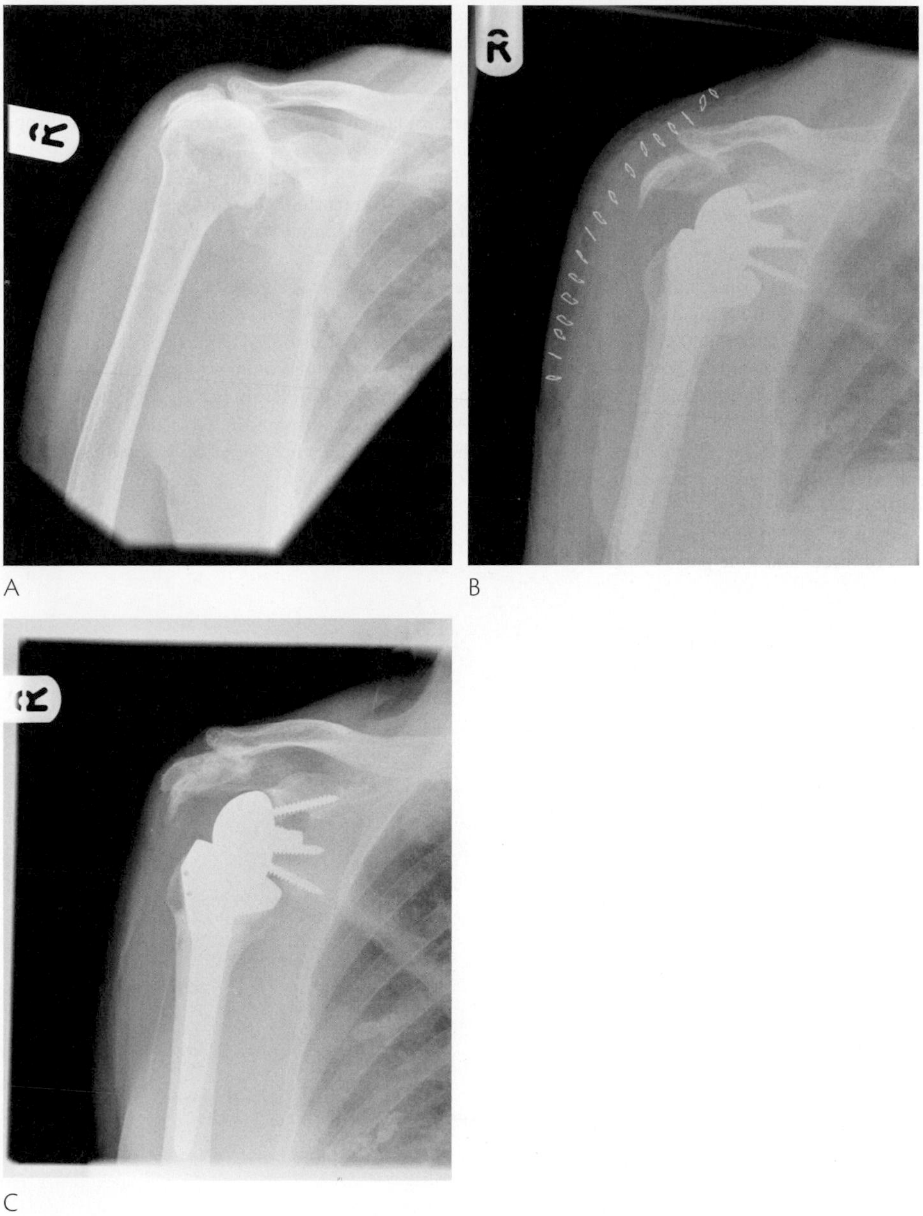

Fig. 4.13.6 Acromial fracture. A) Stage 4 cuff tear arthrosis with thinning of the acromion. B) Delta RSR. Acromion intact on postoperative film. C) X-ray at 3 months shows acromial fracture.

encouraged a number of imitations with a variety of purported improvements. Several of these prostheses are very close to the Delta with small changes designed essentially to improve ease of implantation. Only time will tell whether any of these small changes have any unforeseen side effects.

There are, however, some new reverse designs that have moved further away from the Delta concept, mainly in an effort to reduce notching. The danger is that these changes may sacrifice the principles which have made the Delta RSR successful. For example, one proposed solution has been to use a glenoid component that is between a sphere and a hemisphere. This may reduce the risk of impingement between the humeral component and the scapular neck, but it does so by lateralizing the centre of rotation relative to the bone–prosthesis interface, in effect reintroducing a neck onto the glenoid component (Figure 4.13.3C). Although the offset is not as great as on older unsuccessful reverse designs, it remains to be seen whether it creates sufficient torsional forces at the glenoid component–bone interface to induce premature loosening.

The Delta itself needs longer follow-up in order to determine whether notching is a threat to its survival. Furthermore, whilst it has been shown retrospectively that a low position of the metaglene is associated with a reduced incidence of notching, prospective studies are required to confirm that this can be reliably achieved and that notching can indeed be avoided or at least minimized.

Conclusion

Modern RSR has proved itself as a useful tool in the treatment of a number of conditions where conventional shoulder arthroplasty offers limited and uncertain results because of deficient cuff function.

It has been shown to provide reliable pain relief and also to restore active elevation, though active external rotation often remains limited. However, it is important to remember that only short- to medium-term results are available at present. Early loosening has not been a problem, but notching could potentially lead to failure in the longer term. Careful patient follow-up is therefore essential.

Further reading

Boileau, P., Watkinson, D.J., Hatzidakis, A.M., and Balg, F. (2005). Grammont reverse prosthesis: design, rationale, and biomechanics. *Journal of Shoulder and Elbow Surgery*, **14**(Suppl. 1), 147S–161S.

Boileau, P., Watkinson, D.J., Hatzidakis, A.M., and Hovorka, I. (2006). Neer Award 2005: The Grammont reverse shoulder prosthesis: results in cuff tear arthritis, fracture sequelae and revision arthroplasty. *Journal of Shoulder and Elbow Surgery*, **15**(5), 527–40.

Broström, L.Å., Wallenstein, R., Olsson, E., and Anderson, D. (1992). The Kessel prosthesis in total shoulder arthroplasty. A five-year experience. *Clinical Orthopaedics and Related Research*, **277**, 155–60.

Bufquin, T., Hersan, A., Hubert, L., and Massin, P. (2007). Reverse shoulder arthroplasty for the treatment of three- and four-part fractures of the proximal humerus in the elderly: a prospective review of 43 cases with a short-term follow-up. *Journal of Bone and Joint Surgery*, **89B**(4), 516–20.

Field, L.D., Dines, D.M., Zabinski, S.J., and Warren, R.F. (1997). Hemiarthroplasty of the shoulder for rotator cuff arthropathy. *Journal of Shoulder and Elbow Surgery*, **6**, 18–23.

Gerber, C., Pennington, S.D., Lingfelter, E.J., and Sukthankar, A. (2007). Reverse Delta III total shoulder replacement combined with latissimus dorsi transfer. A preliminary report. *Journal of Bone and Joint Surgery*, **89A**(5), 940–7.

Guery, J., Favard, L., Sirveaux, F., Oudet, D., Mole, D., and Walch, G. (2006). *Journal of Bone and Joint Surgery*, **88A**(8), 1742–7.

Hamada, K., Fukuda, H., Mikasa, M., and Kobayashi, Y. (1990). Roentgenographic findings in massive rotator cuff tears. *Clinical Orthopaedics and Related Research*, **254**, 92–6.

Neer, C.S., Watson, K.C., and Stanton, F.J. (1982). Recent experience in total shoulder replacement. *Journal of Bone and Joint Surgery*, **64A**(3), 319–37.

SECTION 5

The Elbow

5.1

Clinical evaluation of elective problems in the adult elbow

Amir Salama and Amjid Ali

Summary points

- History: presenting complaint; past medical history.
- Examination: inspection; palpation; movement; special tests.

Introduction

In the assessment of elbow problems a detailed history is essential. This should include information regarding the patient's age, sex, hand dominance, and occupation. In addition, a full description of the presenting complaint, previous elbow problems, the patient's hobbies or sporting activities, and previous medical history must also be recorded.

Presenting complaint

Most patients presenting with elbow disorders report pain usually associated with localized tenderness and/or reduced range of movement. They may also describe the inability to perform specific activities. It is important to document the duration of symptoms and exacerbating or relieving factors. The nature of the pain is important to document, whether this radiates or if there are any associated symptoms. These may include swelling, locking, or reduced range of movement. These symptoms usually occur in combination. The patient should be asked specifically about previous elbow problems and whether there is any history of trauma or surgical procedures. Pain in other joints is also relevant as the elbow may be part of a systemic illness, such as inflammatory arthropathy.

In common with other upper limb presentations it is important to ask about neck symptoms and any neurological symptoms in the upper limbs.

Past medical history

This should include a general past medical history to assess whether the patient would be suitable for surgery if this is required. It is also important to ask about current medication as this often indicates medical comorbidities that the patient may not initially have mentioned. Any family history should be noted as this may bring to light problems such as haemophilia or osteochondromatosis.

A social history must include details of the patient's occupation, sporting activities and hobbies, together with details of their alcohol intake and smoking history. All of these may impact on the underlying diagnosis, treatment options, and rehabilitation.

Examination

Inspection

The whole of both upper limbs must be exposed in order to compare the symptomatic and contralateral sides.

Before the patient is asked to do anything the posture of the upper limbs should be noted. At this stage it is also sensible to examine the axilla for scarring which may impact on upper limb function. The elbow should then be inspected for scars (traumatic or surgical), or obvious swelling which may be caused by inflammatory arthropathy, acute injury, or neoplastic lesions. There may also be evidence of psoriasis or paper-thin skin indicative of Ehlers–Danlos syndrome. Examination of the hands for evidence of intrinsic muscle wasting that may indicate ulnar nerve pathology is also essential.

Palpation

A systematic approach to palpation of the elbow will avoid missing relevant signs (Box 5.1.1).

Palpation is most easily performed with the patient sitting and the elbow at 90 degrees. Palpation of the lateral and anterior aspect is best carried out standing in front or to the side of the patient. Palpation of the medial and posterior aspect of the elbow is more comfortably undertaken by standing behind the patient with the shoulder slightly abducted.

It is suggested that palpation of the elbow begins on the lateral side. However, if the examiner feels that this may cause pain it is better to start on the medial side to prevent the patient becoming apprehensive and therefore making further evaluation of the elbow difficult. The lateral supracondylar ridge should be palpated and

Box 5.1.1 Palpation of the elbow

- Lateral:
  - Lateral supracondylar ridge
  - Lateral epicondyle and common extensor origin
  - Infracondylar recess
  - Radiocapitellar joint
  - Radial head
- Posterior:
  - Olecranon bursa
  - Bony anatomy
  - Triceps
- Medial:
  - Ulnar nerve
  - Medial epicondyle and common flexor origin
  - Medial supracondylar ridge
- Anterior:
  - Brachioradialis
  - Biceps tendon
  - Lacertus fibrosis
  - Brachial artery.

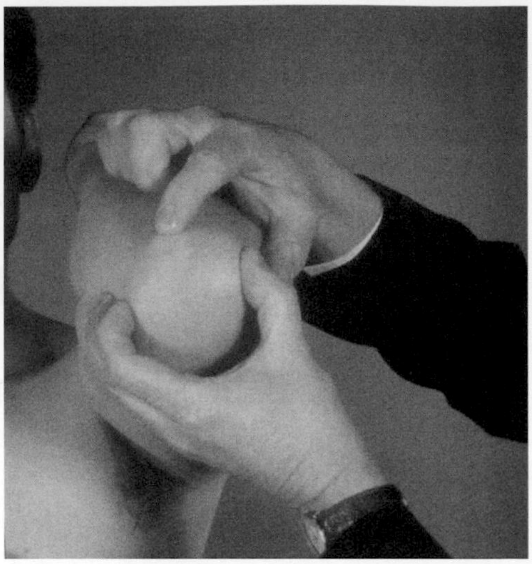

Fig. 5.1.1 With the elbow flexed the two epicondyles and the tip of the olecranon form an isosceles triangle. When the elbow is extended they form a straight line if the elbow is normally located.

any tenderness noted. Progress should be made down the ridge to the lateral epicondyle onto the common extensor origin and then down onto the lateral ligament complex.

The extensor carpi radialis longus can be assessed by resisted wrist extension with radial deviation and the extensor carpi radialis brevis by resisted wrist extension in neutral. Any pain reproduced may point the clinician towards a diagnosis of lateral epicondylitis. The infracondylar recess (recess between lateral condyle and radial head) should be palpated looking for an effusion (fluctuant swelling) or synovial hypertrophy (boggy swelling). The radiocapitellar joint should be palpated in conjunction with pronation and supination of the forearm, and flexion and extension of the elbow looking for subluxation or dislocation of the radial head, or radiocapitellar crepitus.

Palpation should then progress to the olecranon. Any tenderness or swelling may be indicative of an olecranon bursa. The relationship between the tip of the olecranon and the epicondyles should be assessed in both flexed and extended positions. In the extended position the condyles and the olecranon should form a straight line. With the elbow at 90 degrees these bony landmarks form an isosceles triangle (Figure 5.1.1). Any abnormality in this may indicate a previous fracture or congenital abnormality. Whilst palpating posteriorly the triceps should be examined under resistance in order to assess for a partial or complete rupture.

Moving towards the medial side the ulnar nerve should be palpated behind the medial epicondyle. Its presence should be noted and if it cannot be easily palpated in its usual location then palpation anterior or over the medial epicondyle may reveal a subluxed ulnar nerve (present in 10% of patients). Flexion and extension of the elbow whilst palpating the ulnar nerve may make this more obvious. Tinel's sign may be positive in cases of ulnar neuritis and if palpation does indicate ulnar nerve pathology at the elbow the examiner should carry out a neurological examination of the hand.

Palpation of the medial epicondyle and common flexors may reveal signs of medial epicondylitis (tenderness and reproduction of pain on resisted wrist flexion). Careful palpation may distinguish this from pronator syndrome, which would be indicated by tenderness over the belly of pronator teres.

Anteriorly the brachioradialis muscle, the biceps tendon, and lacertus fibrosis can be palpated. Palpation of a normal biceps tendon is relatively easy but after a rupture there may be quite a lot of swelling and tenderness which makes palpation more difficult. If this diagnosis is suspected then resisted flexion and resisted supination should be assessed. The lateral hook test involves the examiner's index finger being hooked under the distal biceps from the lateral side. In a normal tendon this is possible but in the ruptured tendon it is impossible to hook the tendon.

Movement

Movement of the elbow is best assessed with the patient standing. It is essential to compare both upper limbs.

With the arms by the side, alignment should be assessed with the elbow in full extension looking for any valgus or varus deformity (Figure 5.1.2). The carrying angle is on average 10 degrees in males and 15 degrees in females. A varus deformity is always abnormal and if present is usually the result of a childhood supracondylar fracture. A valgus deformity is due to loss of height of the lateral column which may be secondary to a previous fracture of the distal humerus or avascular necrosis of the capitellum. If a valgus deformity is present the ulnar nerve should be assessed as the patient may have tardy ulnar nerve palsy.

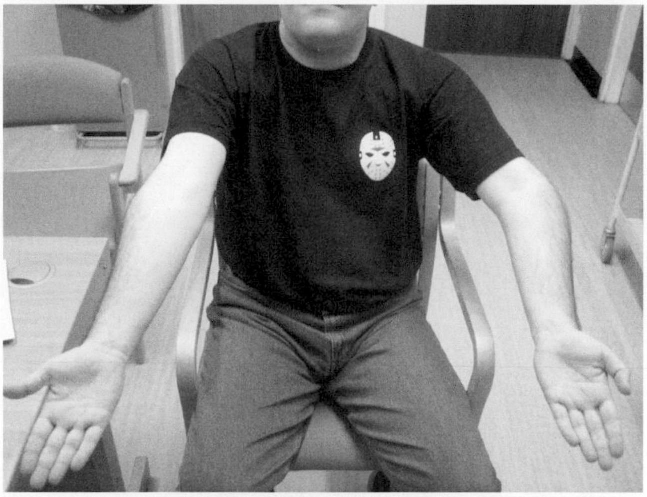

Fig. 5.1.2 Cubitus varus of the left elbow. The deformity is the result of malunion of childhood supracondylar humeral fracture.

If there is longstanding valgus or varus deformity then stability of the elbow should be assessed as instability secondary to attenuation of the ligaments may be present.

In a normal elbow, the carrying angle is valgus in extension but becomes varus in full flexion.

If the patient does not have any problems with the shoulders, elbow flexion and extension is best assessed with the shoulder at 90 degrees of abduction and with the forearm in full supination. The patient is then asked to fully extend and flex the elbow (Figure 5.1.3). This method will pick up even quite subtle loss of movement when compared to the normal elbow. To document the range of movement full extension is recorded as 0 degrees with full flexion being approximately 140 degrees. Hyperextension of up to 10 degrees is normal and is recorded as a negative integer, i.e. −10 degrees to 140 degrees.

If hyperextension is observed then the examiner should look for other signs of generalized ligamentous laxity and document this by recording the Beighton score.

Forearm rotation is assessed with the arms adducted to the side of the body and with the elbows at 90 degrees. If the patient is asked to extend the thumb then this can be used to gauge the range of movement. Normal supination is around 85 degrees with pronation around 80 degrees. If there is any discrepancy, the wrist must be examined as problems at the distal radioulnar joint may present with abnormal pronation and supination.

It is important to record both active and passive ranges of movement.

The power of different muscle groups around the elbow should be documented using the Medical Research Council grading system.

Provocative tests

The choice of provocative tests will be determined by the patient's history and examination (Box 5.1.2). After a complete examination of the elbow an examination should be carried out of the neck as this may be the source of radicular pain experienced around the elbow. Neurological examination of the upper limb should also be performed.

Lateral epicondylitis

Tenderness just anterior and superior to the lateral epicondyle around the origin of extensor carpi radialis brevis is suggestive of lateral epicondylitis. To confirm this, the examiner should ask the patient to extend the wrist against resistance (Figure 5.1.4) and also extend the middle finger to resistance. Both of these manoeuvres

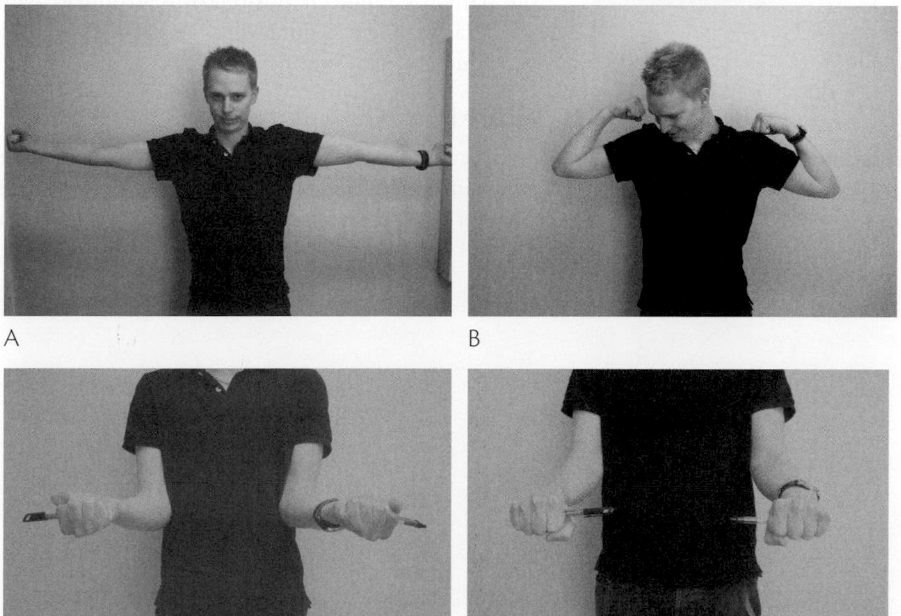

Fig. 5.1.3 Range of movement of the elbow. (A,B) Subtle loss of extension and flexion on the right elbow can be noticed. (C,D) Full pronation and supination.

Box 5.1.2 Provocative tests for elbow disorders
◆ Lateral epicondylitis: resisted wrist extension ◆ Medial epicondylitis: resisted wrist flexion ◆ Posterior elbow impingement: passive forced extension ◆ Anterior elbow impingement: passive forced flexion ◆ Instability: tests as described in Chapter 5.3.

should reproduce pain around the lateral aspect of the elbow if lateral epicondylitis is present. Passive volar flexion of the wrist with the elbow in full extension and the forearm pronated may also cause pain in the same region. It is often found that pinch grip is uncomfortable and may be weak. If the signs are positive for lateral epicondylitis a small amount of local anaesthetic can be injected around the origin of extensor carpi radialis brevis and resolution of the pain will confirm the diagnosis. Care must be taken not to inject the elbow joint as an intra-articular pathology may then be missed.

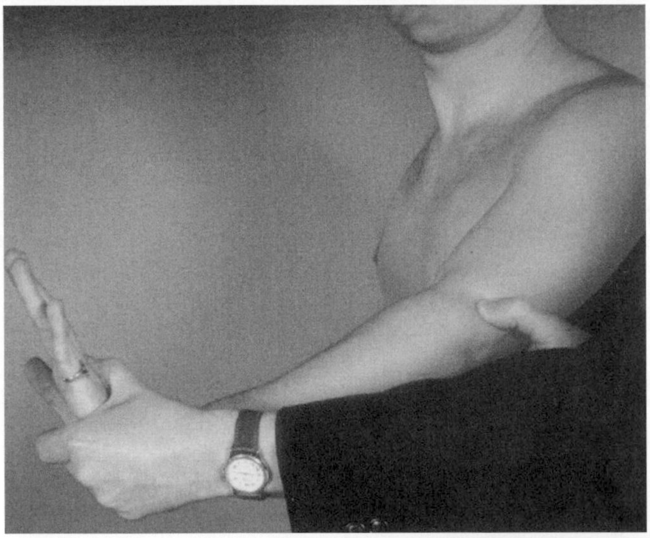

Fig. 5.1.4 Provocative test for lateral epicondylitis. Resisted wrist extension results in localized pain over the extensor origin.

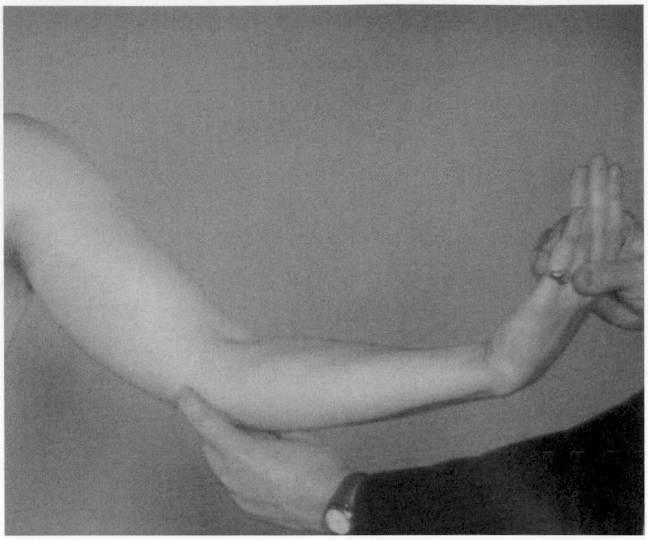

Fig. 5.1.5 Provocative test for medial epicondylitis. Resisted wrist flexion results in localized pain over the flexor origin.

Medical epicondylitis

There is tenderness localized to the origin of the common flexors at the medial epicondyle. The examiner should test flexion of the wrist against resistance (Figure 5.1.5) which should produce pain. Passive extension of the wrist with the elbow in extension may also reproduce symptoms.

Impingement

Anterior and posterior impingements are usually caused by osteophytic change on the coronoid and olecranon processes respectively. This can be tested by asking the patient to extend to just a few degrees short of the patient's full extension and then the examiner passively, gently but quickly, extends the elbow to the limit of the patient's range. If positive this produces pain posteriorly. A similar manoeuvre done with the patient's elbow in flexion will reproduce anterior impingement pain.

Elbow instability

Significant progress has been made in the understanding of elbow instability over the last few years. It is discussed in detail in Chapter 5.3 and therefore no further mention will be made here.

5.2

Lateral and medial epicondylitis

Nick Phillips

Summary points

- Most common in middle age.
- Classically ECRB affected laterally, Pronator teres and FCR medially.
- Histology is angiofibroblastic hyperplasia-tendinosis, not inflammation.
- Treatments include physical and injection therapy, as well as surgery.
- Concomitant ulna neuritis medially reduces success of surgery.

Introduction

Lateral and medial epicondylitis of the elbow are commonly referred to by the terms tennis and golfer's elbow respectively. Although originally described in tennis players and golfers, the overall incidence in the population is between 1–3%. This peaks in the fifth decade, affecting 10% of women and up to 19% of men. Only half of these will ever seek medical help.

The pathology of both lateral and medial epicondylitis involves the origins of the muscles, so the term 'epicondylitis' is inaccurate.

On the lateral side, extensor carpi radialis brevis (ECRB) is the site of the classical lesion, but sometimes the anteromedial edge of extensor communis and the deep surface of ECRL are involved. Medial epicondylitis usually involves the origin of pronator teres and flexor carpi radialis, but can occasionally affect flexor carpi ulnaris and even palmaris longus.

The classical report from Goldie in 1964 was the first to identify the pathology within the tendinous insertions of the lateral epicondyle, but the excised tissue showed no evidence of inflammatory activity. Subsequent analyses of excised specimens commonly showed both fibroblastic and vascular granulation tissue infiltration of normal tendon tissue. Similar histological changes have been identified in flexor carpi radialis and pronator teres on the medial side of the elbow. This has led to the term 'angiofibroblastic hyperplasia tendinosis'. As the degenerative process continues to affect the tendons, tears within the tendon substance can occur. Macroscopic tears are found in up to one-third of surgically treated cases. Complete tendon ruptures are rare.

The aetiology of epicondylitis is predominantly overuse of the forearm muscles. Lateral epicondylitis is related to activities that increase the tension, and thus the stress, of the wrist and finger extensors. Electomyographic studies in tennis players have revealed high levels of activity in ECRB during both the acceleration and early follow-through phases in ground strokes and during the cocking phase of the serve. The backhand stroke appears the more problematic, though only when executed with a single-handed action (two-handed strokes appear protective). Medially it is the overactivity of the wrist flexor and pronator muscles, as in golf and baseball pitching. Again, electromyogram recordings report high activity within the common flexor muscles at the point of contact with the golf ball.

History and clinical examination

The history of a suspected epicondylitis should include evaluation of sporting and occupational activity. Duration of symptoms, treatments received to date, and pre-existing comorbidities, such as cervical spondylosis, should be established. There is a significant incidence of concurrent lateral and medial epicondylitis, approaching 20% in those patients whose medial symptoms are treated surgically. Any history of morning stiffness or 'locking and catching' should alert the examiner to possible intra-articular pathology. Symptoms radiating into the extensor muscles of the forearm, provoked by supination and (less often) pronation, suggest radial tunnel syndrome or posterior interosseous nerve (PIN) entrapment.

Examination should establish the site of tenderness over the epicondyle, or more commonly just anterior to the prominence of the

Box 5.2.1 Histological changes in lateral and medial epicondylitis

- Fibroblastic change
- Vascular granulations
- 'Angiofibroblastic hyperplasia tendinosis'.

epicondyle, distal to the insertion of the tendon. Laterally, radiocapitellar pathology may be suspected if pain occurs when the forearm is rotated with a gripped hand (such as using a screwdriver). Tenderness over the course of the radial nerve, or pain on resisted forearm rotation suggests a PIN lesion. Five per cent of patients may have concurrent lateral epicondylitis and PIN entrapment.

Medial epicondylitis is associated with ulnar nerve neuropraxia in 23–61% of patients. Over half of those undergoing surgery for medial epicondylitis may have suffered with ulnar nerve symptoms. Less common is medial collateral ligament injury or insufficiency. Clearly the history is important as this may reveal sports such as baseball pitching or javelin throwing. Intra-articular pathology, such as post-traumatic or primary osteoarthritis, is an occasional cause of medial elbow pain.

Investigation

If clinical examination is not felt to be sufficiently diagnostic, various investigations may be used to help clarify the condition.

Plain radiographs show abnormal calcification in up to 20% of patients undergoing surgery for lateral epicondylitis. Diagnostic ultrasound may detect abnormalities within the ECRB tendon. Magnetic resonance imaging has also been shown to correlate well with a degenerate ECRB tendon as found at surgery. It may also detect subtle tears in the lateral ligament complex and subsequent posterolateral instability. Interestingly, infrared thermography appears to be a highly sensitive investigative tool, with specificity of between 94–100% for the assessment of unilateral and bilateral tennis elbow.

Treatment options

There are both non-operative and operative options available for treatment of epicondylitis.

Non-operative interventions

Non-operative interventions include rest, brace, physiotherapy, non-steroidal anti-inflammatory drugs, and injection therapy. It has been claimed that a combination of these treatments may offer a cure in up to 90% of patients with tennis elbow. However, significant inconsistencies exist in the literature with some authors claiming less than 25% success at 1 year.

Rest

Cessation of any painful or aggravating activity, the alteration of technique or equipment, or modification of workplace ergonomics may all help.

Brace

This is used to counteract the muscle forces of both contraction and tension. Braces ultimately reduce the tensile forces within the tendon and thus protect the damaged area. They must be non-elastic and are worn on the upper part of the forearm.

Physiotherapy

Classical deep friction manipulation over the extensor tendon and Mills manipulations, as described by Cyriax in the 1930s, continue to be offered as a means of treatment. They, however, prove of little long-term benefit to the majority of patients, with approximately 70% of patients suffering recurring symptoms. In comparative studies of corticosteroid injection versus physiotherapy versus 'wait and see' treatment, results based on patient satisfaction scores showed similar outcomes at 1 year for the conservative groups. The injection group had both a delayed recovery time and higher recurrence rates. Physiotherapy was superior to injection and 'wait and see' treatment at 6 weeks, but no difference was found at 1 year. The amount of time off work and the number of other treatments tried by the physiotherapy group was less over the study period.

Both low-power laser and high-voltage stimulation appear to be ineffective in providing a long-term cure. Ultrasound, whilst useful for diagnosing and tracking pathology in the tendons, appears to offer little therapeutic difference from placebo treatments.

Non-steroidal anti-inflammatory drugs

There are no studies to show these to be of use in the treatment of epicondylitis.

Injection therapy

Corticosteroid injections currently remain a popular choice for many physicians. The initial results are usually good, but the benefit may not last. It is important to emphasize that the pathology of tendinosis does not involve inflammatory cells, and it has been postulated that much of the benefit of the injection results from the disruption of fibrin within the tendon by the insertion of the needle. 'Dry needling', however, appears to have little increased therapeutic effect over placebo.

Recent reports suggest autologous blood injection or plasma spun down from a patient's own blood, has a significant effect on tendon healing and resolution of symptoms. The important components appear to be transforming growth factor beta and fibroblast growth factor. The technique is, however, time consuming and there are increased costs and greater potential exposure to blood products. One group reported 22/28 benefited from autologous blood injection at a mean follow-up of 9.5 months.

Operative interventions

Lateral epicondylitis

Surgical treatment falls into three basic categories:

- Release of the common extensor origin
- Resection of the degenerate or ruptured tendon with repair of the defect
- Thermal disruption of the diseased tissue within the tendon.

Release of the extensor tendon origin can be performed using either an open, percutaneous, or arthroscopic technique.

Box 5.2.2 Non-operative interventions: conservative treatment

- Rest
- Brace
- Physiotherapy
- NSAIDs
- Corticosteroid injections
- Autologous blood injections.

Approximately 80% of patients report good results following an open procedure and over 90% success is reported for a percutaneous release. Synovial fistulas from both the percutaneous and arthroscopic releases remain a concern (2% reported).

Resection of the degenerative part of the ECRB tendon with repair was described by Coonrad and Hooper in the 1970s and by Nirschl in the 1990s. Results match those obtained in the release studies and are successful in 77–85 %.

Thermal disruption of the degenerative tendon has recently been reported to be beneficial. The procedure, however, should not be performed under a local anaesthetic, as patients can experience considerable pain during the application of the probe's impulse whilst within the tendon (personal communication).

Medial epicondylitis

Surgical treatment falls into two categories:

- Release of the common flexor origin
- Resection of the degenerative tendon and repair.

There is no safe way to percutaneously release the common flexor origin because of the proximity of the ulnar nerve, so it is recommended to always release the origin through an open approach.

Results appear to be comparable from both procedures, with reported success rates between 87–97%. It is noted that concomitant ulnar neuritis decreases the chances of a successful surgical outcome to around 60%, leading some surgeons to recommend decompression of the ulna nerve as part of the operation. Transposition, however, should be reserved for cases where there is evidence of subluxation. Despite these considerations, symptomatic ulnar neuritis may persist in almost two-thirds of cases.

Postoperative rehabilitation following surgery

Postoperative management following surgery for lateral and medial epicondylitis varies from early mobilization as pain allows, to resting in a plaster backslab for 2 weeks. Progressive rehabilitation and grip strengthening is then undertaken. Some patients can return to sporting activities at 8–10 weeks, but most need longer to fully recover and rehabilitate. The average rehabilitation period is 4–6 months, although it is not uncommon for improvement to continue for a year.

Failure of operative treatment is uncommon, and other potential sources of pain and dysfunction should be considered if a patient fails to make a good recovery from surgery. Intra-articular causes such as secondary osteoarthritis, osteocartilaginous loose bodies, or synovial plicae may be present. Laterally, posterior nerve entrapment should be considered.

Complications are rare, and apart from local wound sensitivity, infection, and complex regional pain syndrome, the most common is instability, due to damage to the lateral ligament complex. Percutaneous and arthroscopic procedures have been associated with synovial fistulae.

Box 5.2.3 Operative interventions: surgical treatment

- Release of common extensor/flexor origin
- Resection of degenerate tendon and repair
- Thermal disruption of the degenerate tendon*

*Applies to the treatment of lateral epicondylitis.

Further reading

Bissett, L., Beller, E., Jull, G., Brooks, P., Darnell, R., and Vincenzino, B. (2006). Mobilisation with movement and exercise, corticosteroid injection, or wait and see for tennis elbow: randomised trial. *British Medical Journal*, **333**(7575), 939.

Connell, D.A., Ali, K.E., Ahmed, M., Lambert, S., Corbett, S., and Curtis, M. (2006). Ultrasound-guided autologous blood injection for tennis elbow. *Skeletal Radiology*, **35**(6), 371–7.

Coonrad, R.W. and Hooper, W.R. (1973). Tennis elbow—its course, natural history, conservative and surgical management. *Journal of Bone and Joint Surgery*, **55-A**, 117–82.

Edwards, S.G. and Calandruccio, J.H. (2003). Autologous blood injections for refractory lateral epicondylitis. *Journal of Hand Surgery*, **28A**, 272–8.

Goldie, I. (1964). Epicondylitis lateralis humen (epicondylalgia or tennis elbow). A pathogenetical study. *Acta Chirurgica Scandinavica, Supplementum*, 339.

Nirschl, R.P. and Pettrone, F. (1980). Medial tennis elbow—surgical treatment. *Orthopedic Transactions of the American Academy of Orthopedic Surgeons*, **7**, 298–9.

Nirschl, R.P. and Sobel, J. (1981). Conservative treatment of tennis elbow. *The Physician and Sports Medicine*, **9**, 42–54.

Roles, N.C. and Maudsley, R.H. (1972). Radial tunnel syndrome—resistant tennis elbow as a nerve entrapment. *Journal of Bone and Joint Surgery*, **54-B**, 499–508.

Verhaar, J.A. (1994). Tennis elbow—anatomical, epidemiological and therapeutic aspects. *International Orthopaedics*, **18**, 263–7.

5.3

Chronic instability of the elbow

Amir Salama and David Stanley

Summary points

- Posterolateral rotatory instability is the commonest following elbow dislocation
- Diagnosis is mainly clinical and by examination under anaesthesia
- Surgical treatment is the mainstay.

Introduction

Elbow instability is relatively uncommon in the general population. However, in the past few years it has received a lot of attention as the mechanism of elbow dislocation and types of elbow constraint have become much better understood.

Biomechanics of elbow dislocation

Elbow dislocations or subluxations typically occur as a result of a fall onto the outstretched hand. The elbow experiences an axial compressive force as the hand hits the ground and the elbow starts to flex. The body then rotates internally on the elbow (forearm rotates externally on the humerus) resulting in a supination moment at the elbow. A valgus moment also occurs as the mechanical axis passes through the lateral side of the elbow. This combination of valgus, supination, and axial compression during flexion is the mechanism responsible for subluxation or dislocation of the elbow (Box 5.3.1). It can be divided into three stages. In stage 1 the ulnar part of the lateral collateral ligament is disrupted. This results in posterolateral rotatory subluxation of the elbow, which reduces spontaneously. With additional disruption, the capsule tears anteriorly and posteriorly. The elbow in stage 2 instability is capable of an incomplete posterolateral dislocation in which the medial edge of the ulna rests on the trochlea such that a lateral radiograph gives the impression of the coronoid being perched under the trochlea (Figure 5.3.1A). This can be reduced readily with minimal force or by the patient self-manipulating the elbow. In stage 3, the coronoid and radial head are fully posterior to the trochlea and capitellum, respectively. Depending on the severity of tissue disruption in stage 3 (A, B, or C) the elbow will be stable in valgus (stage 3A), unstable in valgus (stage 3B), or grossly unstable except when flexed greater than 90 degrees after reduction (stage 3C). In stage 3C, the entire distal aspect of the humerus is stripped of soft tissues, rendering the elbow extremely unstable even in a cast (Table 5.3.1). The pathoanatomy of these stages of elbow dislocation represent a circle of progressive soft tissue disruption from the lateral to the medial aspect of the elbow (Figure 5.3.1B).

Constraints to elbow instability

The elbow has both static and dynamic constraints (Figure 5.3.2). The three primary static constraints are the ulnohumeral articulation, the medial collateral ligament, and the lateral collateral ligament, especially the ulnar part (the lateral ulnar collateral ligament). The secondary constraints include the radial head, the common flexor and extensor origins, and the capsule. The dynamic stabilizers include the muscles that cross the elbow joint and produce compressive forces across the joint. The anconeus, triceps, and brachialis are the most important muscles in this regard. If the coronoid process is fractured, the radial head becomes a critical stabilizer and must not be excised if the coronoid and the ligaments cannot be securely repaired.

Classification of elbow instability

Five criteria should be considered when evaluating elbow instability in order to help plan appropriate treatment:

1) The articulation(s) involved (ulnohumeral, radiohumeral, proximal radioulnar, or a combination)
2) The direction of displacement (posterolateral rotatory, valgus, varus, anterior, or varus posteromedial)
3) The degree of displacement (subluxation or dislocation)

Box 5.3.1 Forces causing elbow dislocation
◆ Valgus
◆ Supination
◆ Axial compression.

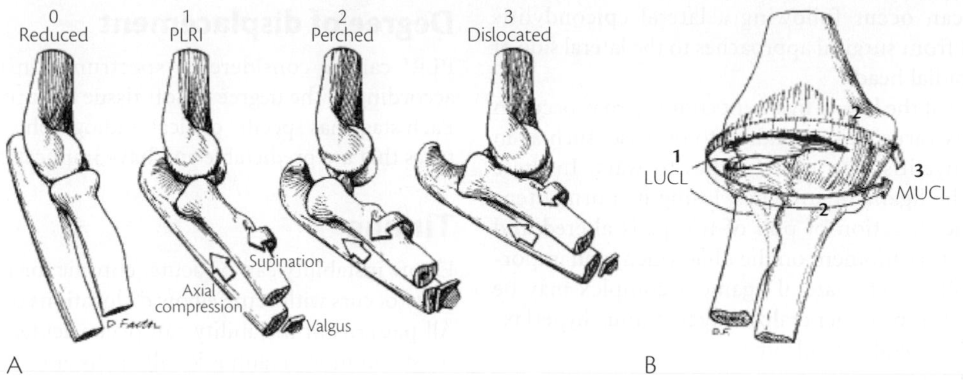

Fig.5.3.1 (A) Elbow instability is a spectrum from subluxation to dislocation. The three stages shown correspond with the pathoanatomic stages of capsuloligamentous disruption shown in Figure 5.3.1B. Reprinted with permission from O'Driscoll, S.W., Morrey, B.F., Korinek, S., and An, K.N. (1992). Elbow subluxation and dislocation. *Clinical Orthopaedics and Related Research*, **280**, 186–97. (B) Horri circle, Soft tissue injury progresses in a circle from lateral to medial in three stages correlating with those shown in Figure 5.3.2A. AMCL, anterior medical collateral ligament; LUCL, lateral ulnar collateral ligament.

4) The timing (acute, chronic, or recurrent), and

5) The presence or absence of associated fractures.

Articulation(s) involved

Two categories of elbow instability exist according to the articulation(s) involved: the hinge joint (the radius and ulna as a unit articulating with the humerus) and the proximal radioulnar joint leading to subluxation or dislocation of the radial head from the ulna. Dislocation of the radial head from the ulna is usually traumatic and often part of a Monteggia fracture-dislocation. Instability can also involve both joints in a combined fashion.

Direction of displacement/patterns of instability

Posterolateral rotatory instability

In posterolateral rotatory instability (PLRI) the radius and ulna rotate externally in relation to the distal humerus, leading to posterior displacement of the radial head relative to the capitellum. Here, the proximal radioulnar joint is intact and both forearm bones rotate as a single unit. This differentiates PLRI from isolated dislocation of the radial head, where the proximal radioulnar joint is disrupted and the ulnohumeral articulation is intact. It is usually posterolateral rather than direct posterior so that the coronoid can pass inferior to the trochlea. The main static constraints to posterolateral laxity are the lateral ligament complex, the radial head, and the coronoid process, with a smaller contribution from the common extensor origin.

Traumatic: as the lateral ligament is the first to be disrupted, PLRI is the most common instability seen following elbow dislocation. It represents a spectrum of instability (see Figure 5.3.1). The Horri circle (stage I to III) represents the soft-tissue disruption that occurs in a circular fashion from lateral to medial when the elbow dislocates. The lateral ligament is usually avulsed from its humeral origin. Radial head and capiteller fractures can contribute to loss of height on the lateral side of the elbow, loss of congruity, and slackening of the lateral ligament complex. Therefore every attempt should be made to preserve the radial head and capitellum in good alignment following fractures, and when excision is necessary, arthroplasty should be considered.

Damage to the lateral ligament complex may also be due to chronic attenuation or iatrogenic injury.

Table 5.3.1 Stages of soft tissue disruption

Stage 1	Disruption of LUCL
Stage 2	Disruption of the other lateral ligamentous structures and anterior and posterior capsule
Stage 3	Disruption of MUCL
3A	Partial disruption of MUCL
3B	Complete disruption of MUCL
3C	Distal humerus stripped of soft tissues with severe instability

LUCL, lateral ulnar collateral ligament; MUCL, medial ulnar collateral ligament.

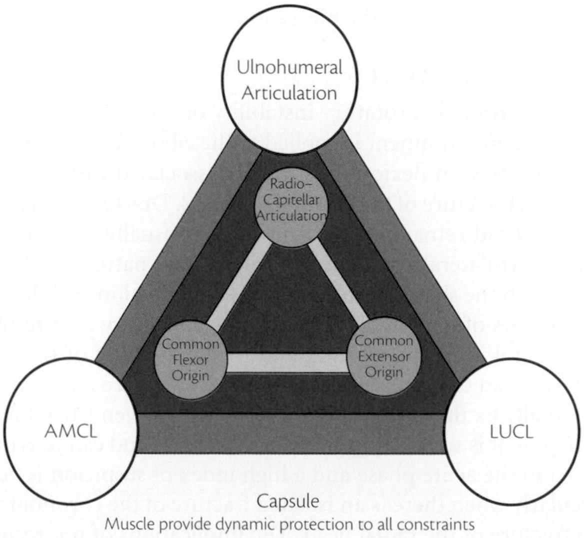

Fig.5.3.2 Primary and secondary constraints. Adapted from O'Driscoll, S.W., Jupiter, J.B., King, G.J.W., Hotchkiss, R.N., and Morrey, B.F. (2000). The unstable elbow. *Journal of Bone and Joint Surgery*, **82-A**(5), 724–38.

Iatrogenic: PLRI can occur following a lateral epicondylitis release, or may result from surgical approaches to the lateral side of the elbow joint and radial head.

Chronic attenuation of the lateral ligament complex may occur in long-standing cubitus varus and secondary to overuse, such as in patients with poliomyelitis who use crutches to walk. In these chronic conditions the ligament stretches, losing its normal tension. In addition, the direction of pull of triceps is altered and exerts an external rotatory moment on the ulna which is an important component of PLRI. The lateral ligament complex may be inherently lax in conditions of generalized ligamentous hyperlaxity, for example, Ehlers–Danlos syndrome.

Valgus

Valgus instability is seen in one of two varieties: post-traumatic or chronic overload. Post-traumatic valgus instability implies rupture of the media1 collateral ligament. It may be associated with disruption of the common flexor and pronator origin. Valgus instability is usually found in patients with radial head fractures that are associated with tears of the medial collateral ligament, or in patients with stage III elbow dislocations. The medial collateral ligament usually heals after elbow dislocation, perhaps because of the vascularity of the surrounding muscles.

In the throwing athlete, valgus instability can occur from repetitive microtrauma or overload that leads to attenuation or rupture of the anterior band of the medial collateral ligament.

Varus

Varus instability is attributable to disruption of the lateral collateral ligament complex and can be shown acutely in patients with elbow dislocations and in many patients with recurrent or chronic instability when this ligament fails to heal. As the forces across the elbow are principally valgus because of the anatomic alignment, it is not often subjected to varus stress and this pattern of instability may not be obvious.

Anterior

Anterior instability of the elbow is rare and typically is seen in association with fractures of the olecranon.

Varus posteromedial

Varus posteromedial rotatory instability occurs when a varus and internal rotation moment is applied to the elbow during axial loading of the elbow in flexion. It is usually associated with an anteromedial facet fracture of the coronoid process. Due to the varus force the radial head remains intact and there is usually an avulsion of the lateral collateral ligament. This instability pattern is clinically noticed with the shoulder in 90 degrees of abduction and the elbow in 90 degrees of flexion. This is a significant injury as it results in ulnohumeral joint incongruity and medial loading of the elbow, which can lead to premature arthritis. It is therefore recommended to internally fix the anteromedial coronoid fact even when the fracture fragment is small. This injury can be subtle and can pass unrecognized in the acute phase and a high index of suspicion is needed particularly when there is an isolated fracture of the coronoid without a fracture of the radial head. The implications of not recognizing this varus posteromedial rotatory instability are potentially devastating, as subsequent reconstructive options are difficult.

Degree of displacement

PLRI can be considered a spectrum consisting of three stages according to the degree of soft tissue disruption (see Figure 5.3.1). Each stage has specific clinical, radiographic, and pathological features that are predictable and have implications for treatment.

Timing

Elbow instability can be acute, chronic, or recurrent. Acute instability occurs with acute elbow dislocations or fracture-dislocations. All patterns of instability can occur acutely with PLRI being the most common. Traumatic valgus instability implies rupture of the medial collateral ligament and, usually, a fracture of the radial head. It is a distinct problem, separate from dislocation. Recurrent instability occurs when soft tissue healing after elbow dislocation is incomplete and is almost always PLRI. Chronic elbow instabilities present to the clinician as either chronic unreduced dislocations or fracture dislocations. Chronic dislocations, whilst infrequently seen in the developed world, are unfortunately still common in some developing countries and their management is challenging.

Associated fractures

When an elbow dislocation is associated with an elbow fracture(s) it is referred to as a complex dislocation. Fracture-dislocations most commonly involve the coronoid and radial head and are referred to as a terrible triad. This name has been coined since it often results in persistent instability, non-union, malunion, and proximal radioulnar synostosis. Other fractures include avulsion fractures of the lateral collateral ligament, impression fractures of the radial head or the posterior part of the capitellum, and olecranon fractures. The goal of management of fracture-dislocations of the elbow is to restore the osseous-articular restraints and convert the injury to a simple dislocation. This has been demonstrated to have a generally favourable long-term prognosis. The recognition of an anteromedial facet fracture of the coronoid as a distinct and important type of coronoid fracture makes an important addition to the Regan and Morrey classification, which is based on fragment size alone.

Box 5.3.2 Injury patterns in elbow instability

- Posterolateral rotatory: rupture of the ulnar part of the lateral collateral ligament
- Valgus:
  - Rupture of the medial collateral ligament
  - Often radial head fracture
- Varus: rupture of the lateral collateral ligament
- Anterior: fracture of the olecranon
- Varus posteromedial:
  - Anteromedial facet fracture of the coronoid process
  - Avulsion of the lateral collateral ligament.

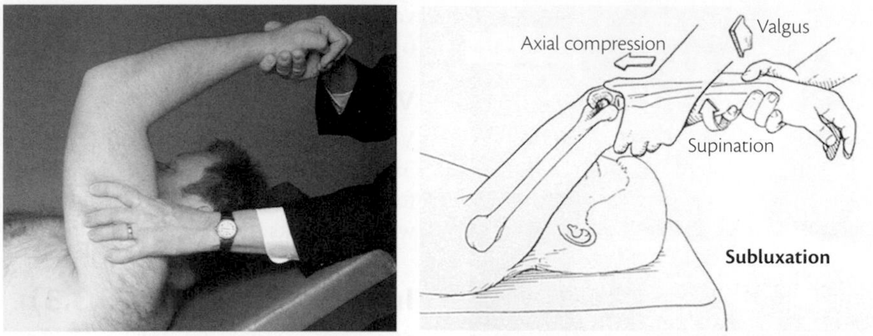

Fig.5.3.3 Lateral pivot shift (O'Driscoll). Patient supine, affected limb overhead. With forearm supinated, valgus and axial loading applied, elbow is flexed from full extension. In posterolateral rotatory instability as the elbow is flexed the radial head subluxes/dislocates and is seen as a prominence posterolaterally. With flexion beyond 40 degrees the radial head suddenly reduces with a palpable and visible clunk. The test is best done under general anaesthesia for radial head dislocation and relocation to be seen. When this manoeuvre is performed with the patient awake, the test is positive in presence of apprehension.

Evaluation of recurrent elbow instability (Box 5.3.2)

Posterolateral rotatory instability

PLRI is the commonest pattern encountered in clinical practice. In this type of instability patients may present with a spectrum ranging from vague symptoms in the elbow to frank recurrent posterolateral dislocation. Symptoms include: lateral elbow pain, recurrent clicking, popping, snapping, or locking of the elbow. The elbow position most typically associated with symptoms is approximately 40 degrees of flexion with the forearm in supination. The subluxation reduces on pronation. Symptoms are often brought on by activities such as pushing up with the arms when rising from an armchair or doing press-ups. These activities place the elbow in an unstable position of external rotation of the forearm with valgus and axial loading of the elbow. This in the presence of a previous history of dislocation or even an injury without dislocation suggests PLRI. A history of surgery on the lateral side of the elbow and a family history of ligamentous laxity should be sought. A thorough examination to identify signs of previous trauma or surgery, cubitus varus deformity, and range of movement is essential. Several clinical tests for PLRI have been described (see Table 5.3.1 and Figures 5.3.3–5.3.7) All these place the elbow in a position of maximal instability, with a combination of external rotation of the forearm, valgus, and axial loading, which try to reproduce either the symptoms or displacement of the radial head. It is important to look for coexistent valgus or varus instability as well as generalized ligamentous hyperlaxity.

Valgus instability

Valgus stress testing is performed with the forearm fully pronated so that PLRI is not mistaken for valgus instability.

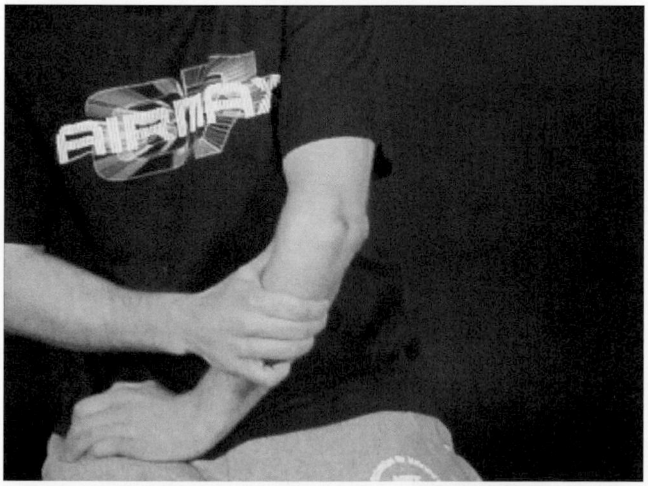

Fig.5.3.4 Patient performing his own drawer test. With the elbow flexed 40 degrees, anteroposterior force is applied to the radius and ulna with the forearm in external rotation. This aims to sublux the forearm away from the humerus on the lateral side, pivoting on the intact medial ligaments. Under general anaesthesia the radial head is seen dislocating, whereas with the patient awake apprehension occurs.

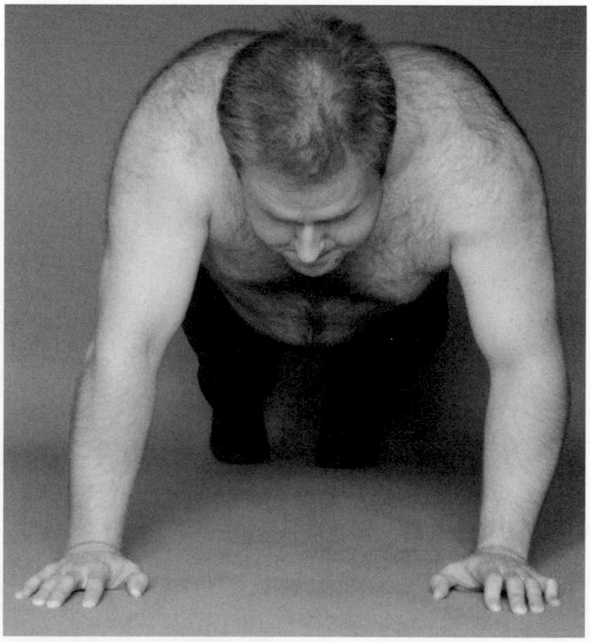

Fig.5.3.5 Floor push-up test (Regan). Patient pushes off the floor with elbows flexed 90 degrees, forearms supinated, and arms abducted. The test is positive if apprehension or radial head dislocation occurs as the elbow is extended.

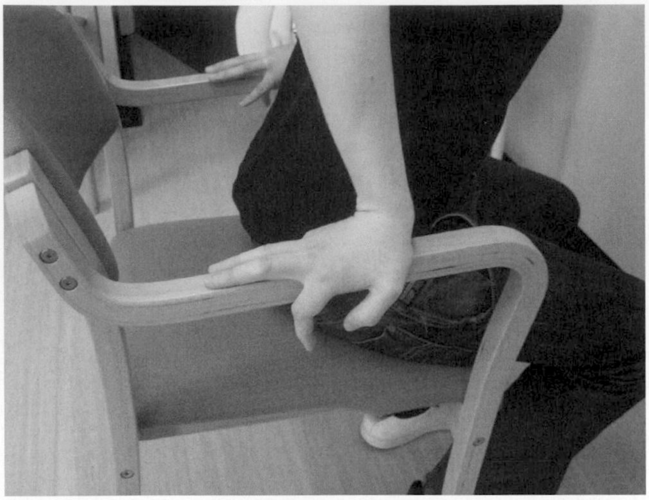

Fig.5.3.6 Chair push-up test (Regan). Patient pushes off from sitting position; causes apprehension or radial head dislocation on extension.

Forced pronation prevents PLRI because the intact medial soft tissues are used as a hinge or fulcrum. Clinical examination may elicit point tenderness distal to the medial epicondyle along the ulnar collateral ligament. The location of tenderness is important to differentiate ulnar collateral ligament injury from medial epicondylitis and flexor–pronator mass strains. Flexing the wrist and pronating the forearm to decrease traction on the flexor–pronator mass can assist in differentiating these entities although they may coexist. Palpating with the elbow in 50–70 degrees of flexion moves the flexor mass anterior to the ulnar collateral ligament, allowing direct palpation of the ligament. The milking manoeuvre (Figure 5.3.8) is performed by abducting the shoulder and flexing the elbow to 90 degrees and the thumb is pulled posteriorly to create a valgus stress on the elbow. Comparison is then made with the opposite elbow. Medial opening and pain signify a positive test.

Varus instability

Varus stress testing is easiest to perform with the shoulder fully internally rotated. Both valgus and varus stress testing are performed with the elbow in full extension and in 30 degrees of flexion which unlocks the olecranon from the olecranon fossa.

Investigations (Box 5.3.3)

Plain radiographs of the elbow are often normal but occasionally demonstrate an avulsion fracture of the origin or insertion of the lateral ligament complex. The presence of fractures of the radial head, coronoid process, and capitellum can be demonstrated as well as the presence of degenerative changes. Impression fractures of the radial head or the posterior part of the capitellum may also be seen. The drop sign—an ulnohumeral distance greater than 4mm on the plain lateral film of the unstressed elbow—may be present on immediate post-reduction lateral radiographs but usually disappears after muscle loading with mobilization. Concern is warranted only when the sign is still present on follow-up radiographs as it can be indicative of residual instability following elbow dislocation. It has been shown that properly performed magnetic resonance imaging (MRI) is sensitive and specific in demonstrating lateral collateral ligament pathology. However, PLRI is a clinical diagnosis, and the MRI should not be relied upon to make the diagnosis. Arthroscopic examination of the elbow may show posterior displacement of the radial head, an elongated lateral ligament complex, or widening of the lateral joint space. The diagnosis of PLRI remains a clinical entity with a combination of the history, active and passive apprehension tests, and examination of the elbow under anaesthesia. Apprehension is usually all that can be elicited when the patient is awake and general anaesthesia is needed

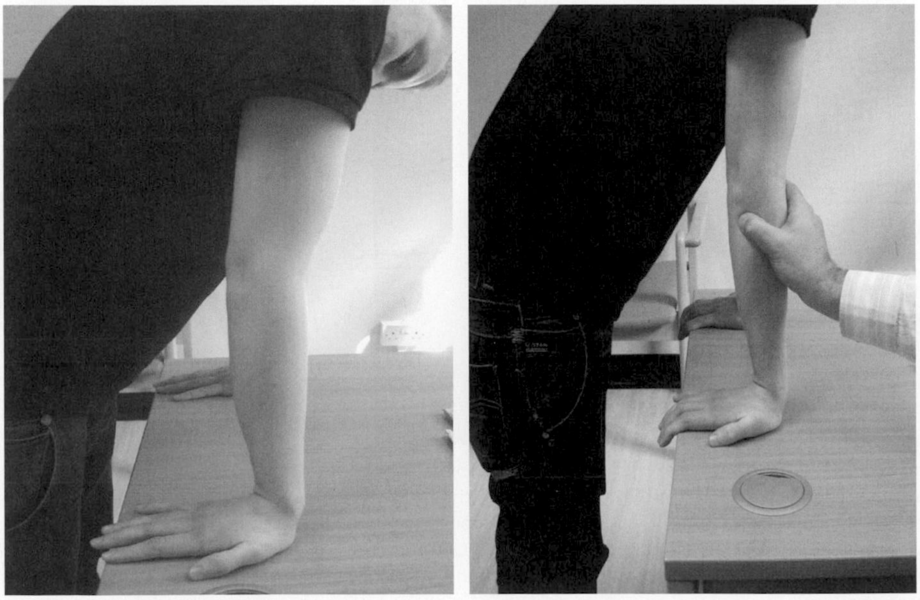

A B

Fig.5.3.7 Table-top test (Arvind). (A) Patient performs a press-up on the edge of a table with the forearm in supination. In the presence of instability, apprehension occurs. (B) Relocation test. The manoeuvre is repeated while the examiner's thumb presses on the radial head, preventing subluxation. The test is positive if thumb pressure relieves apprehension.

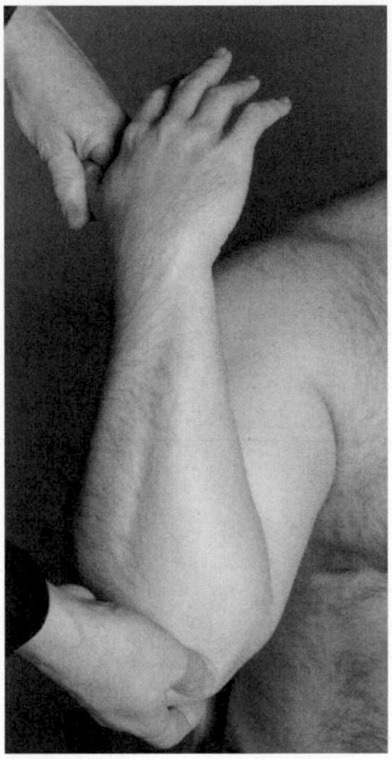

Fig.5.3.8 The milking manoeuvre.

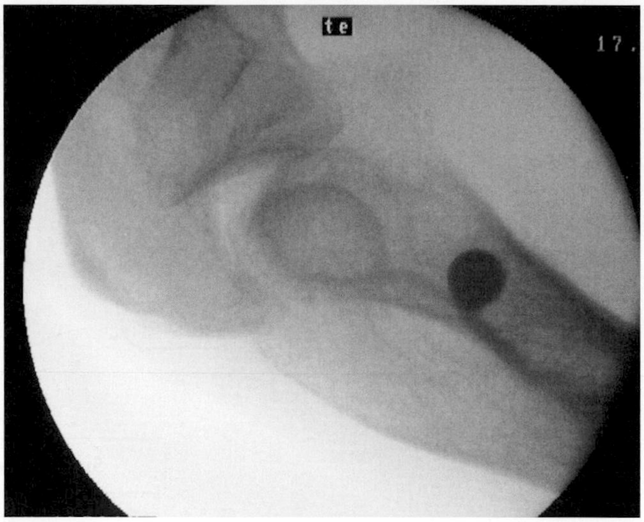

Fig.5.3.9 Screening during lateral pivot shift.

to demonstrate displacement of the radial head and/or dimpling of the soft tissue.

With the patient under general anaesthesia, examination should be performed for valgus and varus instability as previously described. Testing for valgus instability with the forearm in supination may give a false positive result in the presence of PLRI, and so this should be performed with the forearm in pronation. Inability to demonstrate varus instability does not imply that the lateral ligaments are intact, as the ulnohumeral articulation is the main constraint to varus. PLRI is tested using the pivot shift and posterolateral drawer tests. If these fail to demonstrate instability the elbow should be screened using the image intensifier and the test repeated to detect dislocation or subluxation of the radial head (Figure 5.3.9).

Management

Recurrent posterolateral rotatory instability

Treatment depends on the severity of the patient's symptoms. The ligament does not become stable over time, except possibly when a patient is seen in the very early stages. Conservative treatment by avoiding provocative activities and bracing to limit supination and valgus loading may be offered to some patients if surgery is declined. Surgical management is the standard and aims at reattaching, retensioning, or reconstructing the lateral ligament complex together with treating any bone deficiency of the radiocapitellar and ulnohumeral articulation by replacement of the radial head or coronoid reconstruction, and correcting any varus deformity of the humerus by osteotomy prior to ligament reconstruction. One or a combination of these may be necessary, depending on individual assessment and the underlying pathology.

Reattachment and retensioning of the lateral ligament complex with imbrication and advancement have been used, but reconstruction with a graft usually provides a more reliable construct. A tendon graft is used, with fixation achieved by bone tunnels, anchor sutures, or interference screws. The docking technique provides a stable construct and allows tensioning of the graft. Although an autograft of palmaris longus is commonly employed, the use of a strip of triceps tendon, semitendinosus, gracilis, plantaris, and synthetic ligaments have also been used. The latter is worth considering in cases of generalized ligament hyperlaxity. If both medial and lateral ligaments need to be reconstructed, a circumferential graft can be used and attached to both sides of the ulna. Arthroscopically-assisted repair of the avulsed lateral ligament complex has been described. Arthroscopic electrothermal shrinkage of the lateral ligament complex as the sole treatment for posterolateral elbow instability has also been used.

Valgus instability is usually treated in a similar fashion to ligament reconstruction procedures on the medial side of the elbow.

Results of surgery for ligament reconstruction

Generally if there is no degenerative arthritis and if the radial head is intact, approximately 90% of patients have a satisfactory outcome with no subsequent recurrent subluxation. If the radial head is excised or if there is degenerative arthritis of the ulnohumeral joint, the outcome is less satisfactory at between 67–75%. The results are not good in patients with generalized ligamentous laxity.

Box 5.3.3 Investigations for elbow instability

- Radiographs: fractures particularly anteromedial coronoid
- MRI: often reveals ligament injury
- Examination under anaesthesia:
  - Valgus instability
  - Varus instability
  - Pivot shift for posterolateral instability
  - Arthroscopic examination: reveals widening of lateral joint space and/or posterior subluxation of the radial head.

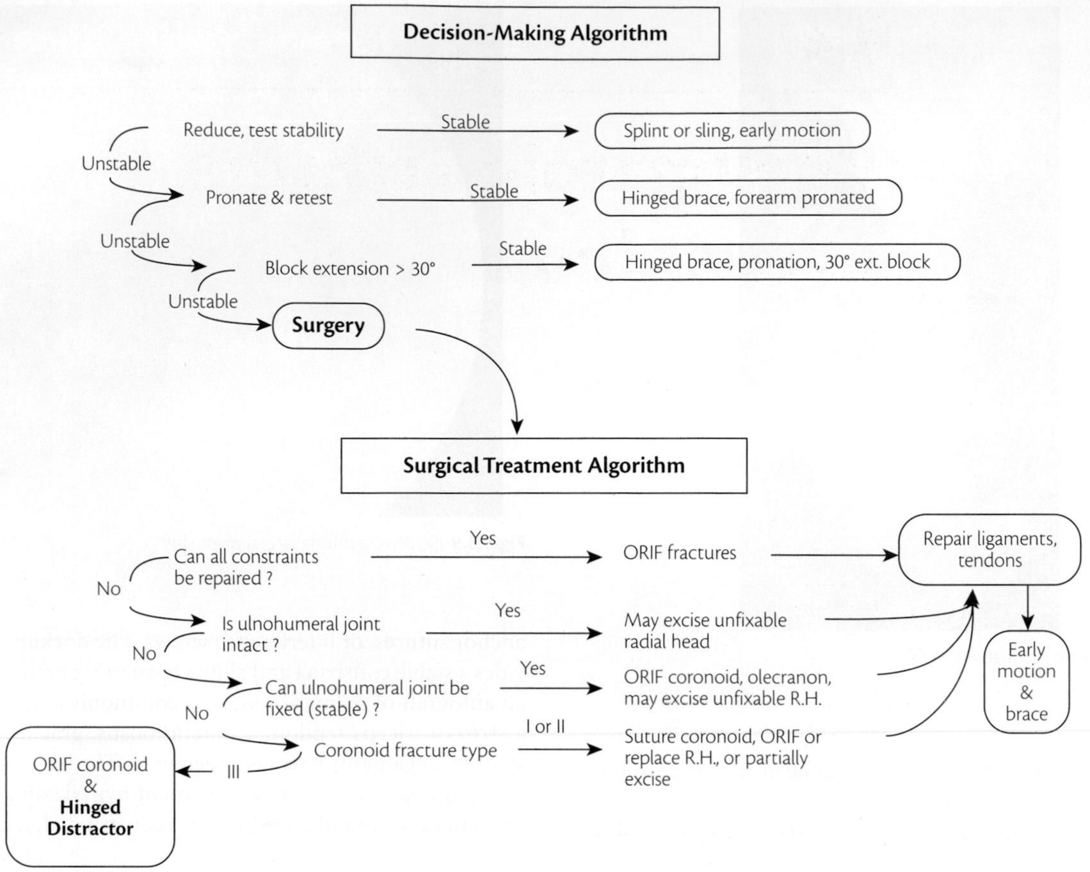

Fig.5.3.10 Chart showing the decision-making algorithm for acute dislocations and fracture-dislocations. The term stable implies functional stability, meaning that the elbow does not apparently subluxate in the functional arc of motion and appears reduced on plain radiographs. ORIF, open reduction and internal fixation; R.H., radial head. Reproduced with permission from O'Driscoll, S.W., Jupiter, J.B., King, G.J.W., Hotchkiss, R.N., and Morrey, B.F. (2000). The unstable elbow. *Journal of Bone and Joint Surgery*, **82-A**(5), 724–38.

Simple elbow dislocation and fracture dislocations

O'Driscoll described an algorithm that helps in decision-making once the elbow is reduced (Figure 5.3.10).

Subluxation or dislocation must be detected by careful examination throughout the comfortable range of motion and by radiographic examination, with anteroposterior and lateral radiographs made initially after the reduction and every 5–7 days for the first 3 weeks.

When the elbow is stable to valgus stress only with the forearm in pronation (that is, a stage-3A dislocation), the injury is treated immediately in a cast-brace that allows unlimited flexion and extension and holds the forearm in full pronation.

The presence of fractures usually changes the management, and almost always these fractures should be treated surgically. In general, the approach to the unstable elbow is to fix the bones internally and then repair the ligaments (particularly on the lateral side) so that early motion can be commenced.

Coronoid process fractures that are type I and type II (those involving 50% of the height of the coronoid process or less) should be fixed if the joint is subluxated or dislocated. Type III fractures (those involving more than 50% of the coronoid process) cause instability and must always be fixed.

Fractures of the radial head are best managed by internal fixation when technically possible. When the radial head is comminuted and has to be excised, prosthetic replacement is indicated if the elbow is unstable and cannot be rendered stable by ligament reconstruction alone.

Repair of an acute ligament injury is indicated in all fracture-dislocations requiring internal fixation of the radial head or the coronoid process, or both, and following reduction of a dislocation if gross instability does not allow early protected motion in a cast-brace without subluxation.

Further reading

O'Driscoll, S.W., Morrey, B.F., Korinek, S., and An, K.N. (1992). Elbow subluxation and dislocation. *Clinical Orthopaedics and Related Research*, **280**, 186–97.

O'Driscoll, S.W., Jupiter, J.B., King, G.J.W., Hotchkiss, R.N., and Morrey, B.F. (2000). *Journal of Bone and Joint Surgery*, **82-A**(5), 724–38.

5.4

Rheumatoid arthritis of the elbow

David Clark

Summary points

- 50% of RA patients have elbow involvement
- Females affected 3 times more than males
- Peak incidence 60-70 years of age
- Radiological severity assessed using the Larson radiological grading system
- No single test used to diagnose RA
- The management of RA requires a multidisciplinary approach
- Anti-TNF drugs are used when disease-modifying agent combinations have failed to control symptoms
- Intra-articular and intramuscular cortisone is an effective way of controlling flare-ups
- Total elbow arthroplasty is indicated in severe RA where there is failure of medical management to control symptoms
- 10 year survival rates of total elbow replacement between 80 % (unlinked) and 92 % (linked).

Introduction

Rheumatoid arthritis (RA) is the most common form of inflammatory arthritis and affects 3% of women and 1% of men. The classification criteria developed by the American Rheumatism Associated require four of the following:

- Morning stiffness
- Symmetrical arthritis
- Arthritis of three or more areas
- Arthritis of hand joints
- Rheumatoid nodules
- Positive rheumatoid factor
- Radiographic findings typical of RA.

The elbow is involved in 20–50% of patients with rheumatoid disease and, in the majority of cases, it is bilateral. Women are affected three times more commonly than men. The elbow is the first joint to be affected by RA in only 2.1–3% of cases. In the early stages, the synovitis causes pain and tenderness, especially over the radiohumeral joint line, with associated loss of elbow extension. Later, the whole elbow may become swollen and stiff. Finally, when bone destruction is severe, instability and capsular rupture result in a flail elbow (see Figure 5.4.1). Ulnar collateral ligament incompetence may cause valgus ulnar humeral instability and ulnar nerve dysfunction. Annular ligament incompetence can lead to radial head subluxation.

Pathophysiology

The aetiology in RA is unknown. The genetic predisposition, the involvement of activated immune cells, and the response to immunosuppressing therapy, all suggest the disease is immune mediated. The cell-mediated immune response (T cells that incite an inflammatory response) is initially against soft tissue (synovitis) and later, against cartilage (chondrolysis), and then bone (periarticular bone resorption). The pathological spectrum of RA spans across early disease when joints exhibit active synovitis without structural damage, to late disease when the joints may be mechanically damaged, mal-aligned, and unstable without persistent active synovitis.

RA is a rare disease in men under the age of 30 years. The incidence rises to peak at 60–70 years. In women, the prevalence of disease increases from the mid twenties to a fairly constant level at 45–75 years with a broad peak at 65–75 years. The genetic contribution in RA is around 15–20% and this can exert a significant effect on disease expression. The risk of RA in first-degree relatives is almost double that amongst the general population.

Radiological grading

The standard radiographic assessment of RA was proposed by Larsen and colleagues in 1977. He grades the disease into six stages (Figure 5.4.2).

- Grade O: normal
- Grade 1: slight abnormality—one or more of the following changes are present:
  - Periarticular soft tissue swelling
  - Periarticular osteoporosis and slight joint space narrowing
- Grade 2: definite early abnormality erosions (an obligatory sign and joint space narrowing is noted)
- Grade 3: medium destructive abnormality; erosions and joint space narrowing is more marked

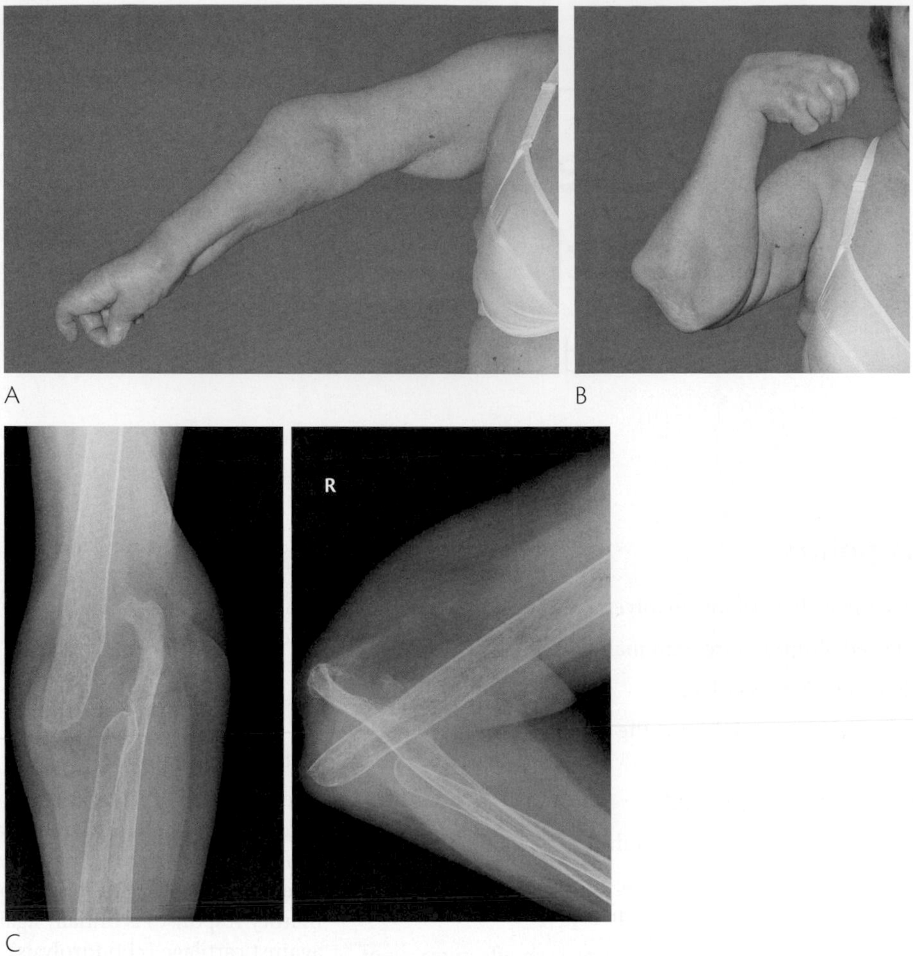

Fig.5.4.1 An example of a 72-year-old female patient with severe rheumatoid arthritis (Larsen grade 5) who has a painless elbow with a functional range of motion.

- Grade 4: severe destructive abnormality; marked erosion, joint space narrowing, bone deformation is also present
- Grade 5: mutilating abnormality. Original articular surfaces have disappeared, gross bone deformation is present.

Biomechanics

An understanding of the function and biomechanics of the elbow is important when considering the design and features of total elbow replacement. The main role of the elbow joint is to position the hand in space but a full range of movement of the elbow is not required for many activities of daily living. It has been shown in normal volunteers that most tests can be carried out with a 100-degree arc of flexion between 30–130 degrees, and a 100-degree arc of forearm rotation equally divided between pronation and supination. In patients with elbow RA the flexion arc is often well preserved until a late stage in the disease.

The other main role of the elbow joint is to act as a fulcrum for the forearm lever, and this stability is essential for normal strength and function. Increasingly, severe erosion of the subchondral bone of the elbow joint, due to RA, gives rise to varus/valgus and antero-posterior instability and thus weakness, because of the loss of the elbow joint as a stable fulcrum.

Many RA patients are unable to carry out the more demanding activities of daily living because of pain and weakness caused by reflex inhibition of adjacent muscles. One group found the average flexion strength of the elbow in rheumatoid patients tested at 90 degrees, was approximately 50% of the normal young adult. The activities of daily living, such as eating and dressing, can apply compressive loads of up to half of the body weight to the elbow and may be as high as three times body weight with certain actions, such as pushing up out of a chair or lifting heavy weights.

History and clinical examination (Box 5.4.1)

When assessing the elbow in a patient with RA, it is important to perform a thorough evaluation of the cervical spine, shoulder, wrist, and hand in both upper limbs, to determine if the patient's complaints are limited to the elbow or are more diffuse in nature. The age, occupation, hand dominance, and age of onset of RA should be assessed.

Isolated elbow involvement in RA is rare. It should be noted that associated wrist (distal radioulnar joint) pathology can contribute to loss of forearm rotation and limited shoulder abduction can prevent the ability to compensate for loss of pronation. Specific elbow problems that require assessment are pain, stiffness, swelling, instability, and ulnar nerve symptoms.

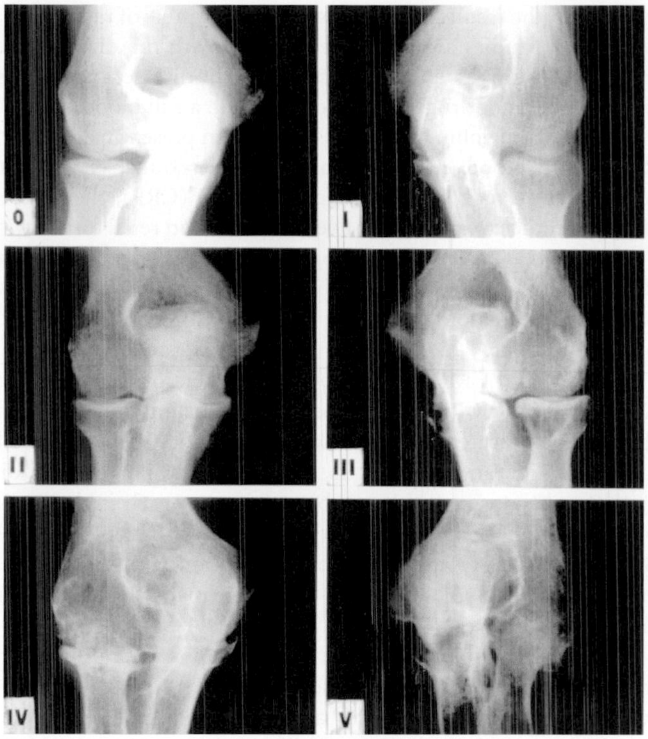

Fig.5.4.2 The Larson radiological grading of elbow rheumatoid arthritis

Pain arising in the joint is often diffuse in nature. It is commonly felt on the lateral side initially. To gauge the level of pain in the elbow an assessment of night and rest pain should be made together with the number of anti-inflammatory painkillers taken per day. In addition, an assessment of whether there is pain on certain specific activities of daily living is made, including washing, dressing, and lifting simple household objects, for example, the ability to lift a mug, kettle, or a pan.

Mild stiffness may hardly be noticed. If it is severe, it can be very disabling. The patient may be unable to reach to the mouth (loss of flexion), or to the perineum (loss of extension). Limited supination makes it difficult to carry large objects. It is very important to consider the function of the whole arm as a unit as well as the patient's age, occupation, and overall condition prior to forming a treatment plan.

An in-depth medical history is taken of age at onset of the RA, current drug treatment relating to anti-inflammatory drugs, disease modifying drug therapies, and specifically whether the patient is taking prednisolone or anti-tumour necrosis factor (TNF) therapies. An assessment of the extra-articular complications of RA should be made, specifically relating to pulmonary and cardiac symptoms and the neurological effects of peripheral entrapment of the ulnar nerve. It is important to assess the effects of the RA on other joints, particularly in the lower limb, and whether the patient has had or is awaiting total hip, total knee, or forefoot arthroplasty surgery. If surgery is being contemplated a general medical history must be taken to assess fitness for anaesthesia (diabetes, ischaemic heart disease, use of warfarin, lung pathology).

Finally, a social history is useful in noting where the patient lives (flat, a bungalow, or two storey house), who the patient lives with, the need for social service support and an assessment of mobility, particularly the use of walking aids.

Box 5.4.1 Rheumatoid elbow symptoms that require assessment

- Pain
- Stiffness
- Swelling
- Instability
- Ulnar nerve dysfunction.

Examination (Box 5.4.2)

General considerations include a rapid assessment of the patient's habitus and whether walking aids or a wheelchair are being used. The patient should be asked to undress to reveal the whole of the upper limb. Screening examination of the neck and shoulders should be made to assess range of movement and pain. Rheumatoid involvement of the neck or shoulder may make examination of the elbow difficult because of pain and stiffness.

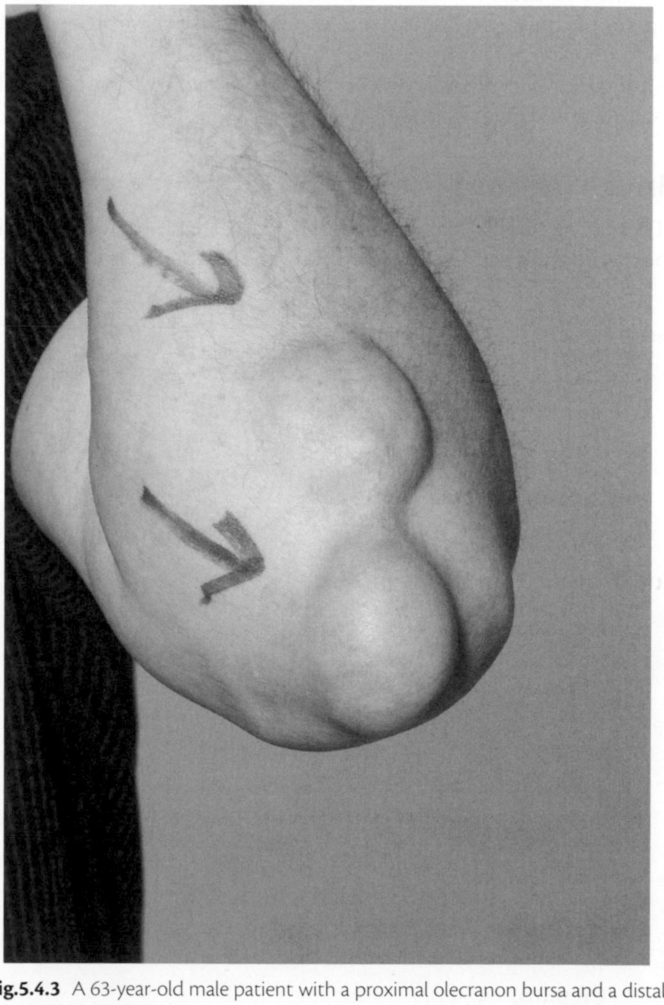

Fig.5.4.3 A 63-year-old male patient with a proximal olecranon bursa and a distal rheumatoid nodule.

Look

With both upper limbs exposed, the patient holds their arms by the side of the body with palms forward; this enables varus or valgus deformity at the elbow to be assessed. The patient then holds the arm out sideways at right angles to the body with palms upwards and elbows straight. An assessment of muscle wasting, swelling, lumps (Figure 5.4.3), surgical scars, and skin colour can be made.

Feel

The back of the elbow joint is palpated for warmth, subcutaneous nodules, synovial thickening, and fluid. Laterally, the joint line can be palpated for swelling and crepitus. The radial head should be assessed for tenderness, and to make sure it is properly aligned and not subluxed or dislocated. The ulnar nerve can be palpated behind the medial epicondyle and assessed for sensitivity and Tinel's test for cubital tunnel syndrome.

Move

Flexion and extension are compared on the two sides. Pronation and supination can be measured and compared with the elbows tucked into the sides and flexed to a right angle.

Rheumatoid nodules (Figure 5.4.3) occur in 30% of patients with progressive seropositive disease. These are most commonly subcutaneous and occur on the extensor surface of the elbow and especially around the olecranon. They are usually mobile but can be fixed to deeper tissues. In addition, they can be found in the spine, occiput, and other areas exposed to mechanical pressure. Nodules have a characteristic histology in that they are made up of a central area of fibrinoid necrosis surrounded by an area of palisading epithelial cells and fibrocytes.

Investigations (Box 5.4.3)

There is no single test to diagnose RA. Instead, the diagnosis is based upon many factors, including the characteristic signs and symptoms, the results of blood tests, and the results of radiographs. Laboratory studies are performed to help with the diagnosis, to monitor the progress and complications of the disease, and to assess the side effects of drugs. Blood tests include a full blood count to measure haemoglobin (anaemia is a common presenting feature of RA), white blood cell count and platelet count, erythrocyte sedimentation rate (ESR), C-reactive protein (CRP), rheumatoid factor, antinuclear antibodies, liver enzymes, and renal function.

Rheumatoid factor (immunoglobulin M) is detected by the Rose–Waaler assay and is positive in approximately 80% of RA patients. Rheumatoid factor may also be positive in a number of other conditions.

The ESR and CRP are non-specific markers of inflammation. A high ESR and CRP suggest the presence of inflammation, but they do not indicate the cause of this inflammation. The anticitrullinated peptide antibody test is more specific than rheumatoid factor for diagnosing RA. It may be positive very early in the course of the disease. The test is positive in 50–90% of patients with RA. Between 30–40% of people with RA have autoantibodies called antinuclear antibodies (ANAs). However, many healthy people also have a positive ANA test.

Plain anteroposterior and lateral radiographs are an important measure of disease progression (see Fig 5.4.1C). In established RA, radiographs are used to classify and monitor disease progression from osteoporosis, soft tissue swelling, periarticular cysts, joint space narrowing, alteration of joint architecture, and finally, gross joint destruction. About 15–30% of patients with RA will have radiographic changes in the first year. However, after the first 2 years of RA, more than 90% of people have changes on radiographs.

Magnetic resonance imaging (MRI) scans are more sensitive than radiographs for detecting the cartilage damage caused by RA. Therefore, MRI scans may be more effective than radiographs for detecting the early changes of RA.

In patients where the elbow joint is the first joint to present, aspiration of the joint for microscopy, Gram staining, crystals, and culture, may aid in the diagnosis by excluding other conditions

Box 5.4.2 Examination of the rheumatoid elbow

- Look:
  - Scars
  - Deformity
  - Muscle wasting
  - Rheumatoid nodules
  - Swelling
- Feel:
  - Rheumatoid nodules
  - Swelling
  - Tenderness
  - Ulnar nerve irritation
- Move:
  - Flexion/extension
  - Pronation/supination
  - Crepitus.

Box 5.4.3 Investigations in the diagnosis and assessment of the rheumatoid patient

- Blood investigations:
  - Full blood count and ESR
  - Rheumatoid factor
  - Anticitrullinated peptide antibody
  - Antinuclear antibody
  - CRP
  - Liver and renal function
- Radiographs:
  - Elbow
  - Cervical spine
- Elbow aspiration:
  - Occasionally indicated.

that may cause a swollen elbow. These include infection, gout, pseudogout, and other connective tissue diseases.

Treatment

The therapeutic goals are the control of synovitis and pain, maintenance of joint function, and the prevention of deformities. The management of RA requires a multidisciplinary team approach, usually headed by a rheumatologist and may involve the use of drugs, physical therapy, and sometimes surgery (Table 5.4.1).

Education by a clinical nurse specialist plays a vital role in helping patients understand their disease, and associated drug therapy. The management of RA has changed substantially over recent years with the emphasis now being on early diagnosis and aggressive early intervention with disease-modifying antirheumatic drug (DMARD) therapy. This approach has been shown to make a long-term difference to prognosis. Anti-TNF drugs are indicated in patients not responding to conventional DMARDs. The aim of initial drug therapy is to prevent disease deterioration as well as to alleviate pain.

A multidisciplinary team should be involved early and throughout the course of the disease. This involves specialist nurses who can take patients through the details of drug regimens, side effects, and monitoring requirements, and physiotherapists who can help with non-pharmacological pain relief, introduce appropriate exercise, and discuss the balance between activity and rest. Occupational therapists provide resting splints for painful joints, and aids which maintain function, independence, and employment.

The key role of all professionals in early RA is education. Evidence exists that educating patients with early RA is an independent predictor of good disease control.

Non-steroidal anti-inflammatory drugs (NSAIDs) represent first-line treatment in all types of arthritis, acting to decrease the synovial reactivity and alleviate pain and swelling. Disease-modifying drugs such as sulphasalazine, methotrexate, and azathioprine are used in mild, moderate, and severe disease. Some patients with mild disease may respond with symptom control to a single disease-modifying drug while those with poor prognosis disease may need early aggressive combination drug strategies (Box 5.4.4).

Table 5.4.1 Treatment options

Non-operative treatment	Operative treatment	
	Synovectomy	Total elbow arthroplasty
Activity modification	Open versus arthroscopic	Unlinked
Ice, heat	± radial head excision	Linked
Splinting		Convertible
NSAIDs		
Disease modifying agents (methotrexate, gold, sulphasalazine, infliximab)		
Steroids (intra-articular, intramuscular, oral)		

Box 5.4.4 Poor prognostic indicators in rheumatoid arthritis

- Young age
- Female
- Slow onset of disease
- Symmetrical upper extremity disease
- High level of disability at presentation
- Rheumatoid nodules present
- High titres of rheumatoid factor
- High ESR/CRP
- Early erosive changes on radiograph.

Methotrexate is now the most commonly used disease-modifying drug with a relatively high rate of response. Its risk of toxicity is reduced by the co-prescription of folic acid.

Unlike NSAIDs, the use of steroids slows the course of the disease. Over the short term, they exert a profound effect on the symptoms of RA but their long-term use is contraindicated due to their significant side effects.

TNF is a key cytokine in RA inflammation and damage. Over the past 5 years, drugs that block this cytokine (adalimumab, etanercept, and infliximab) have been introduced into clinical practice. Two of the drugs, adalimumab and etanercept are subcutaneous injections that can be self-administered; infliximab is given intravenously every 8 weeks after initial induction. These drugs have made a huge difference to the management of many patients with active disease who have failed to respond to conventional treatments. It is estimated that up to 5% of all RA patients may require such therapy. In the United Kingdom, anti-TNF therapies are restricted to patients with ongoing active disease who have failed to respond to at least two conventional disease-modifying drugs, where one is methotrexate.

It is important in early RA to monitor treatment response and modify therapy accordingly (Table 5.4.2). This requires a combination of subjective and objective assessment using a disease activity score, which is an amalgamation of the number of tender and swollen joints, the ESR, and a visual analogue score of the patient's overall health.

Surgical intervention

Surgery is indicated when appropriate non-surgical management has failed, giving rise to functional limitations due to pain or loss of motion (Table 5.4.3). It is important when surgery is being contemplated to preoperatively assess the cervical spine with radiographs and to be certain that the patient will be compliant with postoperative rehabilitation.

The primary aim of surgery on the elbow is to relieve pain and/or restore joint function.

- *Pain:* pain is the most common primary indication for elbow surgery. The pain relief is most predictable and complete after total elbow replacement

Table 5.4.2 Summary of drug therapy

Drug	Side effects	Monitoring	Surgery
NSAIDs	Gastrointestinal bleed, decrease renal function and bone healing. May increase INR	NA	Stop five half-lives before
Methotrexate	Nausea, neutropenia, thrombocytopenia	LFTs monthly	Continue
Sulphasalazine	Neutropenia, thrombocytopenia, nausea, depression	LFT/FBC 3-monthly	Continue
Azathioprine	Neutropenia, thrombocytopenia, nausea	FBC, LFTs monthly	Continue
Prednisolone	Osteoporosis, poor wound healing		In long-term users use high-dose hydro-cortisone to cover stress response to surgery
Anti-TNF	Reactivation of TB		Stop 14 days prior
	Deterioration of bronchiectasis		Discuss with rheumatologist
			Restart 14 days postoperatively

FBC, full blood count; FBS, [TBC]; INR, international normalized ratio; LFT, liver function test; NA, not applicable; NSAIDs, non-steroidal anti-inflammatory drugs; TB, tuberculosis; TNF, tumour necrosis factor.

- *Stiffness:* a range of movement of less than 100 degrees that does not allow the patient to reach the mouth or perineum is an indication for surgical intervention. In most instances, prosthetic joint replacement is effective at restoring a functional arc of motion
- *Instability:* instability often causes severe disability and pain. A linked total elbow replacement is effective treatment
- *Weakness:* total elbow replacement may improve strength by virtue of its elimination of the reflex inhibition associated with pain. This is a secondary benefit of surgery.

Synovectomy

Synovectomy with radial head excision is an accepted procedure for the early stages of RA (Larsen grades 1 and 2), with chronic synovitis and pain. Following synovectomy, the synovium initially regenerates normally, but with time it will generate back into rheumatoid synovial tissue.

Excision of the radial head was recommended by most authorities in the past but today the radial head is preserved if it is not severely involved in the disease process or causing pain with pronation or supination. The negative effect of radial head resection is to increase the loading of the ulnar compartment of the joint. In addition, resection of the radial head results in deterioration of the postoperative outcome from 70% to 45% during a 6-year period.

Previous synovectomy does not affect the results of total elbow replacement and can therefore be considered in the early, painful stages of rheumatoid destruction of the elbow joint. A lateral approach to the elbow is used and if the radial head is excised there is excellent exposure of the anterior compartment for synovectomy.

Lee and Morrey have reported arthroscopic elbow synovectomy results similar to those achieved by open synovectomy.

Review of the literature suggests up to 90% excellent pain relief for the first 2–5 years after surgery, with late results demonstrating deterioration over time with the success rates falling to 60% at 5–10 years. The largest study reviewed 171 rheumatoid elbows with synovectomy and radial head excision with failure defined as the need for revision surgery or significant pain. The study reported a 1-year survival rate of 85% and a 6.5-year survival rate of 45%.

Ulnar nerve compression at the elbow may at times also be an indication for synovectomy of the elbow, with or without neurolysis and nerve transposition.

Interpositional arthroplasty

Although at one time popular in Europe, this procedure is now rarely carried out in patients with RA. It is contraindicated in patients with significant joint destruction and gross loss of bony architecture. The primary indication is a young, active patient without an inflammatory arthritis, who has a severe post-traumatic arthritis associated with severe pain and limited motion, and is too young or active for total joint arthroplasty. The disadvantage of resection interposition arthroplasty in patients with RA is the risk of progressive bone loss with accelerated instability. This loss of bone may, in the long run, be such that reoperation by prosthesis is

Table 5.4.3 Summary of surgical indications

Early RA (Larson 1, 2); joint space preserved	→	Conservative treatment (NSAIDs—anti-TNF; DMA—physical Rx; steroids)	→	Painful radial head Painful synovitis	→	Synovectomy + radial head excision (open/closed)
Loss of joint space, good bone stock (Larson 3, 4)	→	Conservative treatment (NSAIDs—anti-TNF; DMA—physical Rx; steroids)	→	↑rest pain loss of function ↑pain with ADLs	→	Arthroplasty linked or unlinked
Larson vs flail arm	→	Conservative treatment (NSAIDs—anti-TNF; DMA—physical Rx; steroids)	→	Pain Loss of function	→	Linked arthroplasty

ADLs, [TBC]; DMA, disease modifying agents; NSAIDs, non-steroidal anti-inflammatory drugs; TNF, tumour necrosis factor.

rendered impossible. The method has slowly lost ground in the light of the improved results with prosthetic surgery.

Total elbow arthroplasty

Total elbow replacement is indicated for elbows with severe pain, limited range of motion, and pronounced loss of articular cartilage. The patient must agree to postoperative limitations of lifting no more than 2.5–5kg (5.5–11lb). The contraindications to total elbow arthroplasty are sepsis, the need for soft tissue coverage, severe muscle weakness or paralysis, and a non-compliant patient. There are two types that are commonly used: unlinked (Figure 5.4.4) and linked (Figure 5.4.5). In addition, more recently convertible implants have been designed which can be inserted as either unlinked or linked prostheses.

In an unlinked total elbow replacement, there is no linkage between the humeral and ulnar components, with a metal on polyethylene articulation. It relies on the ligaments and muscles for joint stability, with the theoretical advantage of decreased loading at the bone–cement interface. However, it carries a greater risk for instability. Significant pain relief has been reported in 79–94% with an 80%, 12-year survival for the Souter–Strathclyde implant with revision as the end point and a 90%, 16-year survival for the Kudo implant. An improved final arc of flexion has also been reported of 32 degrees to 136 degrees.

In a linked prosthesis, there is a sloppy hinge with a metal on polyethylene articulation that allows limited rotational varus/valgus motion between the humeral and ulnar components, to decrease the bone–cement interface loading. However, there is stress concentration at the hinge, which can lead to polyethylene wear, debris, osteolysis, and component loosening. The outcome of surgery in linked total elbow replacement is significant pain relief in 76–92%, with an improved final arc of flexion/extension of 29 degrees to 131 degrees. The 10–15-year survival of linked total elbow replacements with revision surgery as an end point is 92%.

A recent study compared three groups of consecutive patients who had undergone prosthetic elbow arthroplasty with the Souter–Strathclyde, Kudo, or Coonrad–Morrey implant for the treatment of RA. There were 33 elbows in each group. Clinical function was assessed on the basis of pain relief and the range of flexion. The study showed that this was similar in each group and that the component linkage with the Coonrad–Morrey implant prevented dislocation without an increased risk of loosening. Survivorship was assessed with use of a life-table method, with revision surgery and radiographic signs of loosening as the end points. Survival of the Coonrad–Morrey implant was better than that of the other two implants. The 5-year survival rates, with revision and radiographic signs of loosening as the end points, were 85% and 81% for the Souter–Strathclyde implant, 93% and 82% for the Kudo implant, and 90% and 86% for the Coonrad–Morrey implant. While radiographic evidence of loosening of the Coonrad–Morrey implants was less common, they noted focal osteolysis adjacent to 16% of the ulnar components and half of these cases progressed to frank loosening.

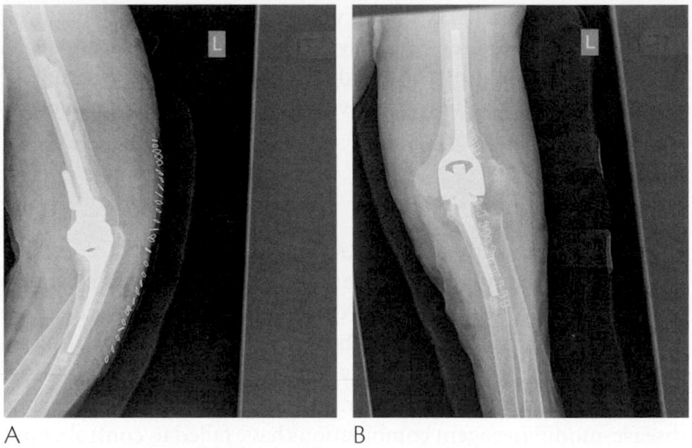

Fig.5.4.5 A linked total elbow replacement

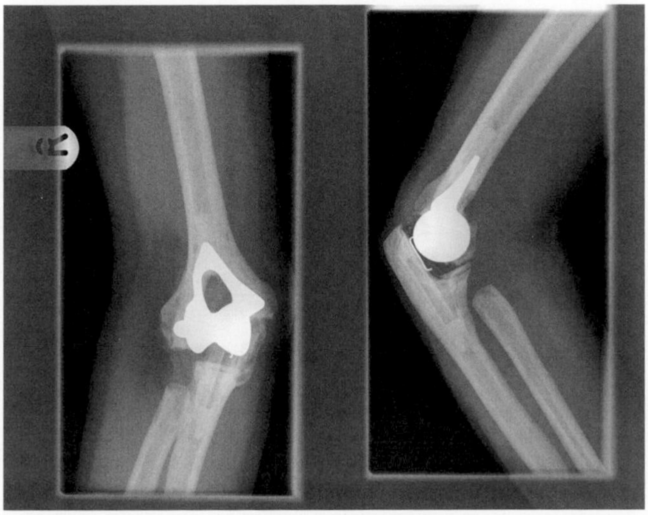

Fig.5.4.4 An unlinked Souter–Strathclyde elbow arthroplasty.

A discussion regarding the risks and benefits of elbow replacement should take place on several occasions prior to surgery. This should include the consequences of continued non-operative management together with discussion of the potential complications.

The complication rate following total elbow replacement is relatively high due to poor soft tissue coverage, the proximity of the ulnar nerve to the elbow joint, and the use of immunosuppressive drug therapy in patients with RA. The predominant complication is ulnar nerve damage, which, as a rule, is usually transient and reversible with permanent ulnar nerve damage uncommon. Deep infection is probably more common after elbow replacement compared to other joints and is reported to be from 2–11%. Wound healing has been a problem in 3–5% of patients, yet 75% of these required no additional surgical procedure.

Instability is a unique complication of the unlinked prosthesis and usually occurs soon after surgery. Inadequate soft tissue balance, either from the collateral ligaments or dynamically from the pull of the biceps, is the basic cause. The incidence of instability is less than 5%.

Intraoperative fracture has been reported in up to 5%, and if this occurs during an unlinked total elbow replacement, may require on-table revision to a linked prosthesis.

Aseptic loosening at 5 and 10 years requiring revision has been reported for the Souter–Strathclyde at 96% and 85% respectively. The longest follow-up of the Kudo implant gives a survivorship of 90% at 16 years. Twelve-year survivorship for the linked Coonrad–Morrey implant is 92%.

Summary

Fifty per cent of patients with RA have involvement of the elbow joint, usually bilaterally. Women are affected three times more commonly than men. There have been significant advances in the medical management of RA with the development of the disease-modifying agents. These are now used earlier in the disease, often in combination with each other. Anti-TNF drugs are used when disease-modifying agent combinations have failed to control symptoms. Intra-articular and intramuscular cortisone is an effective way of controlling flare-ups.

Synovectomy with or without excision of the radial head can be used earlier in the disease process when there is failure of medical management to control the symptoms of synovitis, particularly symptomatic radiocapitellar joint problems. The occasion for this procedure is diminishing with the advance of medical therapies.

Total elbow arthroplasty is indicated in severe RA where there is failure of medical management to control symptoms, particularly pain and loss of function. This gives good pain relief and restores a functional range of movement. When there is good bone stock a linked or an unlinked prosthesis can be used. When there is significant bone loss a linked prosthesis is used. However, there is a higher complication rate compared to lower limb arthroplasty, particularly ulnar nerve damage and wound healing problems. There are now published results of total elbow replacement beyond 10 years showing survival rates of between 80% (unlinked) and 92% (linked).

Further reading

Amis, A.A., Hughes, S.J., Miller, J.H., and Wright, V. (1982). A functional study of the rheumatoid elbow. *Rheumatology and Rehabilitation*, **21**, 151–7.

Gendi, N.S., Axon J.M., Carr A.J., *et al.* (1997). Synovectomy of the elbow and radial head excision in rheumatoid arthritis. Predictive factors and long-term outcome. *Journal of Bone and Joint Surgery*, **79-B,** 918–23.

Gill, D. and Morrey, B. (1998). The Coonrad-Morrey total elbow arthroplasty in patients who have rheumatoid arthritis: a ten to fifteen-year follow up study. *Journal of Bone and Joint Surgery*, **80-A**, 1327–35.

Ikävalko, M., Lehto, M.U., Repo, A., Kautiainen, H., and Hämäläinen, M. (2002). The Souter-Strathclyde elbow arthroplasty. A clinical and radiological study of 525 consecutive cases. *Journal of Bone and Joint Surgery*, **84**(1), 77–82.

Larsen, A.I., Dale, K., and Eek, M. (1977). Radiographic evaluation of rheumatoid arthritis and related conditions by standard reference films. *Acta Radiologica: Diagnosis*, **18**, 481–91.

Lee, B. and Morrey, B. (1997). Arthroscopic synovectomy of the elbow for rheumatoid arthritis. A prospective study. *Journal of Bone and Joint Surgery*, **79-B**, 770–2.

Little, C.P., Graham, A.J., Karatzas, G., Woods, D.A., and Carr, A.J. (2005). Outcomes of total elbow arthroplasty for rheumatoid arthritis: comparative study. *Journal of Bone and Joint Surgery*, **87-A**, 2439–48.

Mäenpää, H.M., Kuusela, P.P., Kaarela, K., *et al.* (2003). Re-operation rate after elbow synovectomy in RA. *Journal of Shoulder and Elbow Surgery*, **12**, 480–3.

Rymaszewski, L.A., Mackay, I., Amis, A.A., and Miller, J.H. (1984). Long-term effects of excision of the radial head in rheumatoid arthritis. *Journal of Bone and Joint Surgery*, **66-B,** 109–13.

5.5

Osteoarthritis of the elbow joint

Shantanu Shahane

Summary points

- Symptomatic, primary osteoarthritis of the elbow usually occurs in young men involved in heavy manual labour.
- Common causes of secondary osteoarthritis of the elbow are trauma, infection, bleeding disorders and neuropathic conditions.
- Clinically, the commonest presenting symptom is loss of motion. Patients can also complain of pain, locking and ulnar nerve symptoms.
- Plain X-rays are usually sufficient for diagnosis. They show reduction in joint space and osteophytes at the tip of olecranon and coronoid processes. Loose bodies are also frequently seen.
- Symptoms in early stages of arthritis are controlled by non-operative means. Steroids are rarely used in clinical practice.
- In advanced cases, numerous operative treatments including arthroscopic and open procedures are available.
- Total Elbow replacement (TER) for primary degenerative arthritis of the elbow is only to be considered as the last option and when stringent pre and post-operative requirements are followed.

Introduction

Osteoarthritis is defined as a 'non-inflammatory disorder of movable joints characterized by deterioration and abrasion of articular cartilage with formation of new bone at the joint surfaces'. Involvement of the elbow with this condition was once thought to be rare, although more recently its prevalence has been shown to be more common.

Prevalence and aetiology of primary osteoarthritis

The prevalence of symptomatic primary osteoarthritis of the elbow is around 2% and occurs most frequently in men involved in heavy manual labour. An increased incidence of osteoarthritis of the elbow in the dominant arms of middle-aged men in association with arthritis of the hip, knee, and metacarpophalangeal joints has been reported.

The use of pneumatic drills as an aetiological factor in the development of elbow osteoarthritis has been debated for a long time. However, a study has failed to show a direct relationship between the use of this type of equipment and the development of the condition.

Primary arthritis of the elbow has been shown to begin at the radiocapitellar joint as part of the normal ageing process with later involvement of the ulnohumeral articulation. It has been postulated that this may be due to the radiocapitellar joint performing a combined rotation and hinge movement as compared to the purely hinge motion in the ulnohumeral articulation. It is known that forces up to three times the body weight cross the elbow joint during strenuous lifting and up to six times during dynamic loading such as throwing or pounding.

Aetiology of secondary arthritis of the elbow (Box 5.5.1)

The most common cause of secondary osteoarthritis of the elbow is trauma. Intra-articular fractures of the distal humerus and radial head fractures can lead to the development of osteoarthritis. Management of this group of patients can be difficult due to loss of bone stock, presence of deformities, and previous surgeries.

Other causes of secondary arthritis of the elbow include: infection, bleeding disorders, and neuropathic pathologies.

Infection within the joint will result in destruction of the articular cartilage and should be treated with prompt washout and appropriate antibiotic therapy.

The commonest cause of haematologic arthritis is haemophilia. Recurrent bleeds with haemosiderin deposition and release of proteolytic enzymes results in destruction of the articular cartilage. Chronic arthropathy in the early stages can be managed well with a specifically designed regimen of exercises to maintain a functional range of elbow motion. In the later stages, synovectomy and total elbow replacement remains the mainstay of treatment.

Neuropathic arthritis predominantly occurs as a result of syringomyelia, tabes dorsalis, diabetes mellitus, congenital indifference to pain, and surgical denervation. The joint is subjected to repeated traumatic episodes not recognized by the patient due to loss of protective joint nociception and proprioception resulting in formation of a Charcot joint. As pain is rare, surgery is rarely considered and protective splinting remains the mainstay of treatment.

Box 5.5.1 Causes of osteoarthritis of the elbow

- Primary (begins at radiocapitellar joint):
  - Heavy manual work
- Secondary (can begin at any part of the joint):
  - Trauma
  - Infection
  - Bleeding disorders
  - Neuropathic pathologies.

Box 5.5.2 Clinical presentation

- Loss of motion
- Pain
- Locking
- Ulnar nerve symptoms.

Clinical presentation (Box 5.5.2)

Although secondary osteoarthritis can occur in either sex and at any age, primary osteoarthritis is predominantly seen in men rather than women by a ratio of 4:1. The disease usually presents in the fifth decade of life with the dominant extremity most commonly involved. The symptoms and signs include:

- *Loss of motion:* loss of extension is the commonest presenting feature and although flexion may also be restricted, the patients usually maintain a functional range of motion. Forearm rotation is less frequently affected
- *Pain:* the patient usually presents with aching discomfort which may be mild to moderate in nature. Acute pain is usually associated with episodes of locking. Pain is more evident in terminal extension (extension impingement) and less common in terminal flexion (flexion impingement). In advanced cases, the pain can be present throughout the arc of motion
- *Locking:* single or multiple loose bodies can be found in up to 50% of cases. Patients may present with an acutely painful elbow with a loose body interposed in the joint. The elbow may spontaneously unlock or can be unlocked by gentle manipulation
- *Ulnar nerve* entrapment*:* patients with arthritis of the elbow may also present with symptoms of ulnar nerve irritation. Osteophytes around the medial aspect of the joint cause compression of the ulnar nerve.

Investigations

Plain anteroposterior and lateral radiographs are usually sufficient to make the diagnosis and no other investigations are normally required. Radiographs typically show osteophytes at the tip of olecranon and coronoid processes. The olecranon and coronoid fossae also reveal ossification and osteophytes. There is reduction in the joint space and loose bodies are often present (Figure 5.5.1). Recently a radiographic classification system for primary osteoarthritis of the elbow has been proposed. Rettig and colleagues also propose that this classification system has validity in predicting postoperative outcomes.

Occasionally a computed tomography scan can be useful in locating loose bodies or delineating the extent of osteophytes prior to surgical planning.

Nerve conduction studies should be performed in cases of ulnar neuritis.

Treatment

Non-operative treatment

Symptoms in the early stages of arthritis can be controlled by lifestyle modifications, analgesics, and anti-inflammatory medication (Box 5.5.3). Although intra-articular steroids have been shown to be of some symptomatic relief, they are rarely used in practice due to their short-term benefits.

Splinting and physiotherapy are of use in post-traumatic elbows but are of little value once the degenerative process becomes established.

Viscosupplementation has been used to treat arthritic conditions around the knee and, more recently, the elbow. A study by Van Brakel and Eygendaal involved giving a series of three injections of

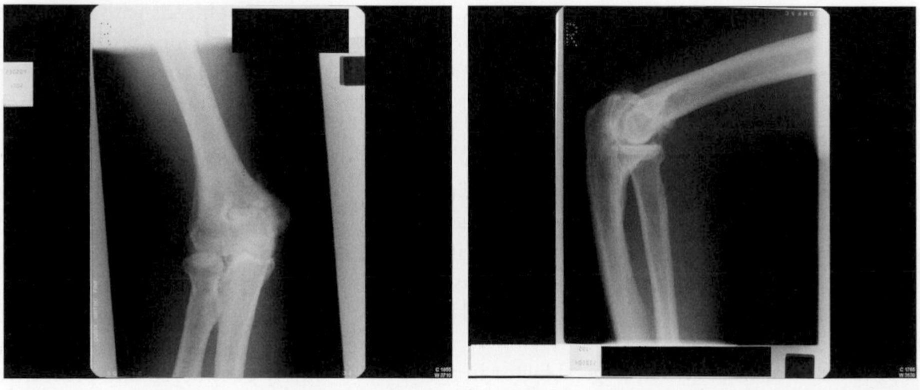

A B

Fig. 5.5.1 A) Anteroposterior radiograph of an osteoarthritic elbow: It shows reduced radiocapiteller joint space with ossification and loose bodies in the olecranon fossa.
B) Lateral radiograph of an osteoarthritic elbow: It shows osteophytes over the tip of olecranon and coronoid process with ossification and loose bodies in the anterior compartment.

Box 5.5.3 Non-operative treatment options

- Analgesics
- Non-steroidal anti-inflammatory drugs
- Intra-articular steroid injection
- Sodium hyaluronate injection.

sodium hyaluronate within a 4-week period for treatment of post-traumatic arthrosis of the elbow. It was seen to provide slight, short-term pain relief but no benefit was observed after 6 months. The authors did not recommend this treatment for post-traumatic arthritis of the elbow.

Operative treatment

A number of surgical options are available for the treatment of elbow arthritis (Box 5.5.4) which can broadly be divided into arthroscopic and open procedures. The exact choice of procedure depends upon the patient's symptoms, the radiological evaluation, and the surgical expertise.

Arthroscopy

The elbow is the most congruous joint in the body. Degenerative changes further reduce the intra-articular space making instrument manipulation more difficult. This in association with the close proximity of the major neurovascular structures makes elbow arthroscopy a technically demanding procedure with a steep learning curve. Surgeon experience and familiarity with elbow arthroscopy is essential in preventing complications during arthroscopic debridement.

Originally elbow arthroscopy was used for the removal of loose bodies but later it was also appreciated that osteophytes could also be excised. Recent studies have established elbow arthroscopy as an important tool in performing debridement, osteophyte and loose body removal, and capsular releases. Adams and colleagues described the results in 42 primary osteoarthritic elbows treated by arthroscopic osteophyte resection and capsulectomy with a minimum of 2 years' follow-up. They had 81% good to excellent results with minimal complications. However, like other studies, this review does not establish that an arthroscopic procedure is superior to open debridement, has improved outcomes, or results in earlier return to function. Additionally, radial head excisions can also be performed successfully arthroscopically, especially in post-traumatic arthrosis. Radial head excision is not often required in primary degenerative arthritis unless the patient experiences predominantly lateral-sided pain or has significant pain on forearm rotation.

Box 5.5.4 Operative treatment

- Arthroscopic debridement
- Outerbridge–Kashiwagi procedure/ulnohumeral arthroplasty
- Tsuge procedure
- Column procedure
- Interposition arthroplasty
- Total elbow arthroplasty.

Open procedures

Joint debridement procedures

These procedures are useful when conservative measures fail to provide adequate symptomatic relief.

Outerbridge–Kashiwagi procedure. Kashiwagi described a joint debridement procedure which he attributed to Outerbridge and called the Outerbridge–Kashiwagi or OK procedure. This is a simple technique allowing the removal of loose bodies and excision of osteophytes. It is performed using a posterior surgical approach. If indicated, the ulnar nerve can also be decompressed at the same time.

Technique of OK procedure: the procedure can be undertaken either in a supine position with a sandbag under the scapula or in a lateral decubitus position with the arm supported by a bolster. Under tourniquet control, a midline central incision is made over the posterior aspect of the elbow joint approximately 8cm above the tip of the olecranon. The triceps is split in the line of its fibres and the posterior capsule of the joint is exposed. The capsule is incised and any loose bodies in the posterior compartment removed. Osteophytes around the tip of the olecranon are excised. A bone burr is then used to fenestrate the floor of the olecranon fossa providing an opening into the anterior compartment of the elbow. Loose bodies from the anterior compartment are identified and removed at the fenestration by flexing and extending the elbow. The tip of the coronoid process is then brought into view by flexing the elbow and coronoid osteophytes removed using a fine osteotome. Osteophytes around the coronoid fossa can be removed using a Kerrison rongeur. This also partially releases the anterior capsule. The finger can then be passed through the fenestration to confirm the adequacy of resection (Figure 5.5.2). The joint is then thoroughly lavaged and closed in layers over a suction drain. The drain is removed at 24 hours and mobilization commenced with the help of therapists.

Ulnohumeral arthroplasty. The OK procedure was modified by Morrey (1992) and termed the ulnohumeral arthroplasty (UHA). Morrey elevates the medial half of the triceps rather than performing a triceps split. He believes this causes less blood loss and less swelling. He also uses a bone trephine to create the fenestration into the anterior compartment rather than a burr since he feels that this provides a more predictable and cleaner resection and creates less bone debris. The placement of the trephine is vital so as not to compromise the integrity of the trochlea, capitellum, or lateral and medial columns. Morrey also uses a more aggressive postoperative regimen. This involves the use of a brachial plexus block with a catheter for 2–3 days together with continuous passive motion and the use of splints to maximize the operative gain.

Results: Minami and Ishii (1986) presented their initial results showing good pain reduction and improvement in motion. Their subsequent study showed some deterioration of the results with time. Recurrence of symptoms was seen in 20% of cases at 10 years and recurrence of radiographic changes in up to 50% at 5 years. Morrey's study (1992) highlighted similar conclusions.

Several other studies have shown good mid- to long-term results of open UHA confirming its durability as a good procedure for this

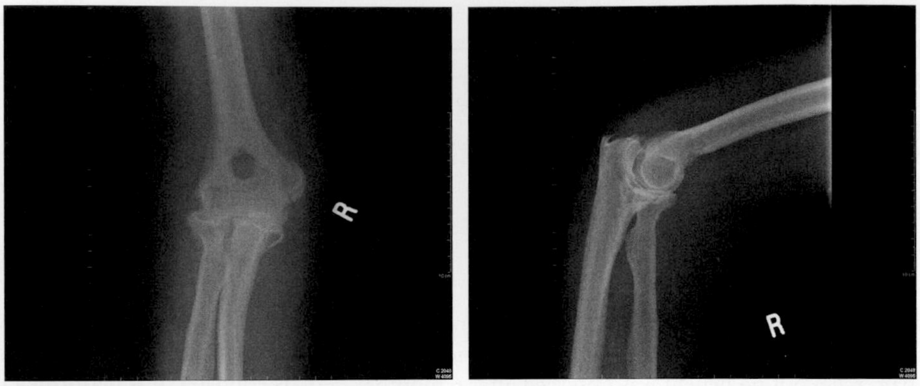

Fig. 5.5.2 Postoperative anteroposterior and lateral radiographs after ulnohumeral arthroplasty: fenestration in the olecranon fossa is visible. It also shows that loose bodies and ostephytes have been removed.

A B

condition. Antuna et al. (2002) reported good or excellent results in 34 of 46 patients at an average of 80 months after surgery. To avoid postoperative ulnar nerve complications, they recommended decompression or mobilization of the nerve in patients who had preoperative flexion of less than 100 degrees, where a flexion gain of more than 30–40 degrees was expected or in patients who had preoperative ulnar nerve symptoms. Wada et al. (2004) reported satisfactory results in 85% of patients at an average of 121 months after surgery. They also found that 76% of their patients returned to preoperative strenuous labour after surgery. None of the elbows in these discussed studies converted to total elbow replacement in spite of the follow-up being up to 13 years in some cases.

Tsuge debridement procedure. Tsuge and Mizuseki (1994) advocated a more extensive surgical procedure especially in young patients with more aggressive disease. The procedure involved isolation and protection of the ulnar nerve followed by reflection of the extensor mechanism medially. The radial collateral ligament together with the posterior portion of the medial collateral ligament was then divided and the joint dislocated. Loose bodies were removed, the capsule released, and all osteophytes around the olecranon and coronoid excised. The olecranon and coronoid fossa were then deepened and, if required, the radial head reshaped. Continuous passive motion was then continued for 7 days postoperatively. The authors reported reduced pain and improved motion in most of 29 of their cases at a mean of 64 months.

Column procedure

Some patients with osteoarthritis of the elbow present predominantly with symptoms of loss of motion. They develop progressive loss of extension with a reasonably pain-free mid arc of motion. This confirms a predominantly extrinsic contracture involving periarticular capsule ligamentous structures. The column procedure is useful in such patients in order to gain a functional range of motion especially if the extension deficit exceeds 20 degrees. The procedure involves a lateral Kocher incision with elevation of the brachioradialis and extensor carpi radialis brevis in order to gain exposure to the anterior aspect of the joint. The anterior capsule is then excised with removal of loose bodies and ostephytes. The triceps is then elevated to gain access to the posterior aspect of the joint and a similar procedure is repeated posteriorly. Continuous passive motion is instituted postoperatively to maintain the surgical gain. The Mayo clinic experience showed excellent pain relief and a substantial gain in range of motion following this procedure in spite of an heterogenous group of pathologies.

Interposition arthroplasty

This technique involves reshaping of the distal humerus and proximal ulna, interposition of a membrane between the elbow joint surfaces, and suturing it to the humeral side. Skin, fascia, and Achilles tendon allograft are most commonly used as interposition tissue. Collateral ligaments are either repaired primarily or reconstructed. A unilateral hinged fixator keeps the joint slightly distracted and allows early active range of motion. The procedure is suitable in young patients (under 60 years old) suffering from incapacitating pain due to traumatic or primary degenerative arthritis affecting the elbow and who have failed to respond to joint debridement procedures. Recent sepsis, an unfused epiphysis, and grossly unstable elbows are contraindications for this procedure. The technique also does not guarantee enough stability for heavy manual work. Larson and Morrey in 2008 updated the Mayo experience of 69 consecutive elbows that underwent interposition arthroplasties using achilles tendon allgraft and a hinged fixator. Three fourths of the patients suffered from post-traumatic arthritis. They concluded that this is a good salvage procedure for young active patients with severe inflammatory or post-traumatic arthritis, especially with limited elbow motion. They emphasized to exercise caution when using this procedure in patients with instability or severe pain.

Total elbow replacement

The indications for total elbow replacement are constantly evolving. It is an established and effective treatment in patients with inflammatory arthritis but its role in young patients suffering from primary degenerative arthritis is still limited. It is particularly unsuitable in patients planning to undertake manual work after replacement surgery. It is recommended that after total elbow replacements patients do not lift more than 4–5 kg with the operated arm as a single event or more than 1 kg repeatedly. Currently, total elbow arthroplasty is only indicated in patients with primary osteoarthritis of the elbow who are older than 65 years of age, are retired, have low activity levels, experience pain throughout the range of motion, or who have substantial deficits in motion in whom all other interventions have failed. In addition the patients must be happy to comply with postoperative restrictions which are essential after such a procedure.

Espag et al treated 10 patients with primary osteoarthritis of the elbow using an unlinked total elbow replacement. At a mean of 68 months after surgery, one had loosened and needed revising and a further two showed radiographic signs of loosening but 9 out of 10 were satisfied with the procedure.

Summary

Osteoarthritis of the elbow is a common condition. Patients present with symptoms of pain and stiffness and occasionally complain of locking due to the presence of loose bodies. Ulnar nerve symptoms may also coexist. X-rays are usually diagnostic and often no other investigations are required.

Conservative treatment is a good option in the early stages but surgical treatment may become necessary. Arthroscopic and open procedures are both effective in removal of loose bodies, capsulectomy, and osteophyte excision. The choice of procedure depends upon the patient symptoms, radiological appearances, and surgical expertise.

Interposition arthroplasty is only rarely performed. Total elbow replacement is also rarely indicated in this group of patients as they are often young and involved in manual work.

Further reading

Adams, J.E., Wolff, L.H., Merton, S.M., and Stienmann, S.P. (2008). Osteoarthritis of the elbow: results of arthroscopic osteophyte resection and capsulectomy. *Journal of Shoulder and Elbow Surgery*, **17**(1), 126–31.

Antuna, S.A., Morrey, B.F., Adams, R.A., and O'Driscoll, S.W. (2002). Ulnohumeral arthroplasty for primary degenerative arthritis of the elbow: long term outcomes and complications. *Journal of Bone and joint Surgery*, **84,** 2168–73.

Espag, M.P., Back, D.L., Clark, D.L., and Lunn, P.G. (2003). Early results of souter-strathclyde unlinked total elbow arthroplasty in patients with osteoarthritis. *Journal of Bone and Joint Surgery*, **85B**:3, 351–3.

Kashiwagi, D. (1978). Intraarticular changes of the ostearthritic elbow, especially about the fossa olecrani. *Journal of Japanese Orthopaedic Association*, **52**, 1367–82.

Krishnan, S.G., Harkins, D.C., Pennington, S.G., Harrison, D.K., and Burkhead, D.K. (2007). Arthroscopic ulnohumeral arthroplasty for degenerative arthritis of the elbow in patients under fifty years of age. *Journal of Shoulder and Elbow Surgery*, **16**(4), 443–8.

Larson, A.N. and Morrey, B.F. (2008). Interposition arthroplasty using achilles tendon allograft as a salvage procedure of the elbow. *Journal of Bone and Joint Surgery*, **90**:12, 2714–23.

Mansat, P. and Morrey, B.F. (1998). The "column procedure", a limited surgical approach for the treatment of stiff elbows. *Journal of Bone and Joint Surgery*, **80-A**, 1603.

Minami, N.M., and Ishii, S. (1986). Outerbridge Kashiwagi arthroplasty for osteoarthritis of the elbow joint. In Kashiwagi, D. (ed.) *Proceedings of the International Congress on the Elbow, Kobi, Japan*, pp. 189–96. Amsterdam: Excerpta medica.

Minami, M., Kato, S., and Kashiwagi, D. (1996). Outerbridge-Kashiwagi's method for arthroplasty of osteoarthritis of the elbow: 44 elbows followed for 8-16 years. *Journal of Orthopaedic Science*, **1,** 11.

Morrey, B.F. (1992). Primary arthritis of the elbow treated by ulnohumeral arthroplasty. *Journal of Bone and Joint Surgery*, **74-B**, 409–13.

Morrey, B.F. (ed.) (2000). *The Elbow and Its Disorders*. Philadelphia, PA: W.B. Saunders.

Rettig, L.A., Hastings, H., and Feinberg, J.R. (2008). Primary osteoarthritis of the elbow: lack of radiographic evidence for morphologic predisposition, results of operative debridement at intermediate follow up, and basis for a new radiographic classification system. *Journal of Shoulder and Elbow Surgery*, **17**(1), 97–105.

Tsuge, K. and Mizuseki, T. (1994). Debridement arthroplasty for advanced primary osteoarthritis of the elbow: Results of a new technique used for 29 elbows. *Journal of Bone and Joint Surgery*, **76-B**, 641–6.

Van Brakel,R.W. and Eygendaal, D. (2006). Intra-articular injection of hyaluronic acid is not effective for the treatment of post-traumatic osteoarthritis of the elbow. *Arthroscopy*, **22,** 1199–203.

Wada, T., Isogai, S., Ishii, S., and Yamashita, T. (2004). Debridement arthroplasty for primary osteoarthritis of the elbow. *Journal of Bone and Joint Surgery*, **86-A**, 233–41.

5.6

Elbow arthroscopy

Amir A. Qureshi and Stuart M. Hay

Summary points

- Indications relate to experience
- Neurovascular considerations are paramount
- Elbow Arthroscopy is an evolving technique.

Introduction

Burman reported a cadaveric study of elbow arthroscopy as early as 1932, but it was not until recent times that the technique became popular for treating elbow disorders. Advances in instrumentation as well as arthroscopic skills are the most probable reasons for the increase in use of the arthroscope in and around the elbow joint.

Elbow arthroscopy remains a technically challenging procedure. The reported complication rate is ten times higher than that of shoulder or knee surgery and careful attention to detail is required to help avoid iatrogenic neurovascular complications. The purpose of this chapter is to explore the current indications and contraindications for the procedure, give a description of preoperative planning, patient positioning, and the portals available, and review the results reported in the literature.

Indications

The original indications for elbow arthroscopy were for diagnosis and for removal of loose bodies. As surgeons became more proficient in this procedure, however, the range of pathology dealt with by arthroscopy has expanded. An example of its application is the osteoarthritic elbow where arthroscopy can be used after non-operative treatment has failed, as an intermediate step before arthroplasty. Indication is closely allied to experience and the indications have been related to five stages of surgical experience by Savoie as below:

- Stage I: beginning elbow arthroscopy:
  - Diagnostic arthroscopy before open surgery
- Stage II: limited experience with elbow arthroscopy/experienced arthroscopist with other joints:
  - Diagnostic arthroscopy
  - Confirmation of instability before open repair
  - Loose body removal
  - Spur debridement
  - Excision of posterolateral plica
  - Arthroscopic irrigation/debridement of contaminated joints
- Stage III: experienced elbow arthroscopist:
  - All stage II surgeries
  - Arthrofibrosis (open nerve protection)
  - Extensor carpi radialis brevis (ECRB) debridement for lateral epicondylitis
  - The arthritic elbow: synovectomy, spur excision, radial head excision, and ulnohumeral arthroplasty
  - Complete management of osteochondritis dissecans
  - Fractures: non-displaced or minimally displaced
  - Olecranon bursa removal
  - Synovectomy for rheumatoid arthritis, chronic infectious arthritis, or other arthritides
- Stage IV: advanced elbow arthroscopist:
  - ECRB repair
  - Varus/posterolateral rotatory instability reconstruction
  - Displaced intra-articular fractures
  - Triceps tendon repair
  - Ulnar nerve release
- Stage V: experimental—the future:
  - Allograft posterolateral reconstruction
  - Fascial interposition arthroplasty
  - Medial ulnar collateral ligament repair/reconstruction
  - Radial tunnel release
  - Distal biceps repair.

Debridement of the arthritic elbow and removal of loose bodies remain the most common indications for elbow arthroscopy, but simultaneous debridement of impinging osteophytes (Figure 5.6.1) and release of capsular contracture can also be performed. In fact, a three-dimensional computed tomography scan prior to the operation in order to identify all potential osteophytes needing debridement has been recommended.

Debridement of ECRB in the treatment of lateral epicondylitis (tennis elbow) can be effectively performed arthroscopically.

Instability, osteochondritis dissecans, and fractures are more recent additions to the indications of elbow arthroscopy.

If debridement/synovectomy is entertained in the deformed rheumatoid elbow, this should be performed by an experienced arthroscopist as the risk of neurovascular injury is particularly high.

With regards to the paediatric population, Micheli et al. (2001) have reported a series of 47 patients aged 3.5–17 years who underwent elbow arthroscopy for osteochondritis dissecans, arthrofibrosis and joint contracture, synovitis, acute trauma, and posterior olecranon impingement syndrome. Using a modified Andrews elbow scoring system (MAESS), 85% of these patients had a good to excellent result with 90% returning to sports free of any limitations. They concluded that elbow arthroscopy was both safe and effective in the paediatric and adolescent population as long as there was a careful selection process and the arthroscopist was experienced.

Contraindications

Disordered anatomy caused by trauma, arthritis (including rheumatoid disease), previous surgery (especially ulnar nerve transposition), or an overlying cellulitis may be regarded as contraindications. Congenital conditions may be a relative contraindication. Biceps tendon injury and isolated radial tunnel syndrome are also relative contraindications.

Preoperative preparation (authors' practice)

On the day of the operation the patient is seen on the ward and placed in the position for surgery. This is because the skin around the elbow is very mobile and will alter in position with changes in patient position. The medial and lateral epicondyles, radial head, subcutaneous olecranon tip, ulnar nerve, and area of interest are then marked with a permanent marker. Whilst identifying these structures the authors go through the procedure and the structures at risk, to reinforce informed consent.

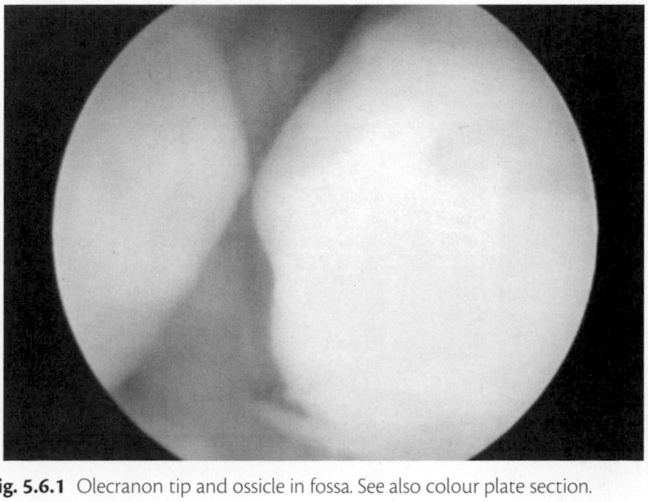

Fig. 5.6.1 Olecranon tip and ossicle in fossa. See also colour plate section.

Anaesthesia

General anaesthesia allows full muscle relaxation and enables the patient to be positioned as required without discomfort (especially if the patient is positioned in the lateral decubitus or prone position). We routinely use additional regional blocks for postoperative pain relief although these do not allow for immediate postoperative exclusion of nerve injury.

Patient positioning (Box 5.6.1)

Supine

Original description: Andrews and Carson (1985).

Positioning: the patient is positioned supine at the edge of the operating table. The affected limb is suspended by overhead traction of 5–10lb (2.25–4.5kg) (e.g. 'Chinese finger traps'). The shoulder is abducted to 90 degrees and the elbow flexed to 90 degrees.

Advantages: since the elbow is held in an anatomic position, orientation of the structures is made easier for the arthroscopist. Excellent visualization of the anterior joint can be achieved. This is particularly useful for fixation of anterior radial head or coronoid fractures. Importantly, it also allows for maximal airway exposure if there are any anaesthetic concerns.

Disadvantages: it is more difficult to access the posterior compartment. In addition, an assistant is required to prevent the arm from swinging when instrumented. This can be partly overcome by modifying the position—having the shoulder flexed to 90 degrees thereby suspending the forearm over the chest. A secondary advantage of this modification is that the anterior neurovascular structures are pulled away from the working area by the force of gravity.

Prone

Original description: Poehling et al. (1989).

Positioning: the patient is positioned prone with the shoulder abducted 90 degrees. The upper arm is placed in a holder allowing 90 degrees of elbow flexion.

Advantages: gravity pulls the neurovascular structures further anteriorly, away from the working area. Full extension to near full flexion of the arm can be produced. The entire elbow is readily accessible.

Disadvantages: patient needs intubation for airway protection.

Lateral decubitus (author's preference)

Original description: O'Driscoll and Morrey (1992).

Box 5.6.1 Patient positioning

- Supine
- Prone
- Lateral decubitus.

Positioning: the patient is placed in the lateral position with the affected side up. The upper arm rests on a padded support. The table is tilted 20 degrees towards the operating surgeon to avoid potential antecubital fossa compression and minimize patient roll-back (Figures 5.6.2).

Advantages: the position allows excellent access to the anterior and posterior aspects of the elbow without some of the disadvantages of the positions mentioned earlier, particularly regarding anaesthesia implications.

Disadvantages: access to the medial side is limited but can be improved by positioning the elbow higher than the shoulder.

Instrumentation

- A high arm tourniquet
- Fluid management system: the authors use pressure fluid distension for the procedure—we advise experimenting with this preoperatively
- 4-mm 30 degree scope with 2.7-mm arthroscope available: most cases can be performed with the 4-mm 30 degree scope. A 2.7-mm scope may be needed in the case of a tight lateral compartment or smaller elbows, for example, in the paediatric group.

Portal positioning

Of all the joints, arthroscopy of the elbow arguably carries the greatest risk of iatrogenic neurovascular damage. It is therefore essential to have a thorough knowledge of the anatomy of the available portals (Box 5.6.2) and their precise locations as margins for error are very small. The distance to the nerves from each portal has been elegantly documented by a number of cadaveric studies.

We regard it as essential to distend the elbow prior to making the entry portal. This is achieved by using 20–30mL of arthroscopic fluid (Figure 5.6.3A). Capsular distention pushes the neurovascular structures further away from the initial portal site and allows for easier entry into the joint. The site of injection is the centre of a triangle formed by the lateral epicondyle, subcutaneous olecranon tip, and radial head. This site is known as the 'soft spot' or infracondylar recess.

Box 5.6.2 Portal positions

- Anterolateral
- Proximal anterolateral
- Mid lateral
- Anteromedial
- Proximal anteromedial
- Posterolateral
- Direct posterior
- Posterior retractor portal
- Accessory lateral portal.

In establishing a portal, care must also be taken to minimize the risk of injury to the superficial cutaneous sensory nerves. Only the skin is incised, with a small blade and then a haemostat is used for blunt dissection in the pericapsular tissue. A blunt arthroscopic trochar and cannula are next inserted aiming towards the subcutaneous olecranon tip. Saline issuing from the cannula confirms intra-articular placement.

The authors begin by establishing the anterolateral portal followed by the anteromedial portal using a within-out technique. However, some prefer to begin with the anteromedial portal.

Steinmann (2003) has given an excellent account of the described portals in his review of elbow arthroscopy (Figures 5.6.3B,C).

Due to an unacceptably high risk of injury to the ulnar nerve, there are no posteromedial portals.

Anterolateral portal

Position: 3cm distal, 1cm anterior to lateral epicondyle. The trochar is aimed towards the centre of the elbow joint and passes through ECRB and supinator. Clearly the precise measurement will depend on body habitas and will need to be modified appropriately.

Structures at risk: radial nerve (1.4mm away on average) and posterior antebrachial nerve (7.6mm away on average).

Function: passing all instruments through this port minimizes the risk of injury to the radial nerve. Used to scope the anterior trochlea, coronoid fossa, coronoid process, proximal radioulnar joint, and radiocapitellar joint.

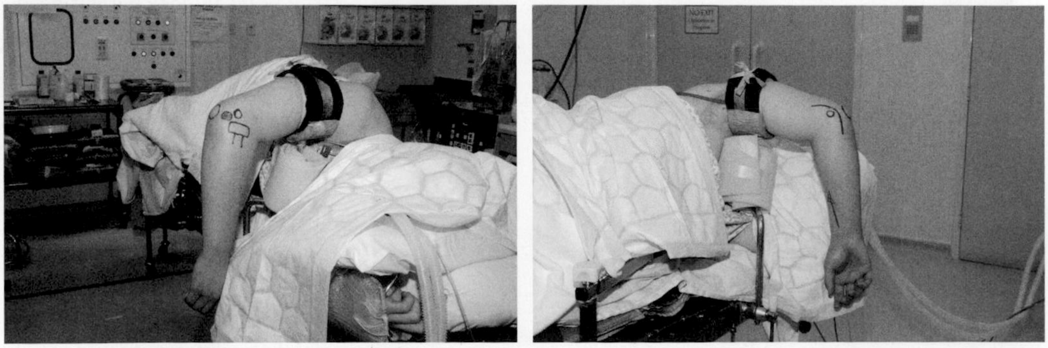

A B

Fig. 5.6.2 Lateral decubitus position.

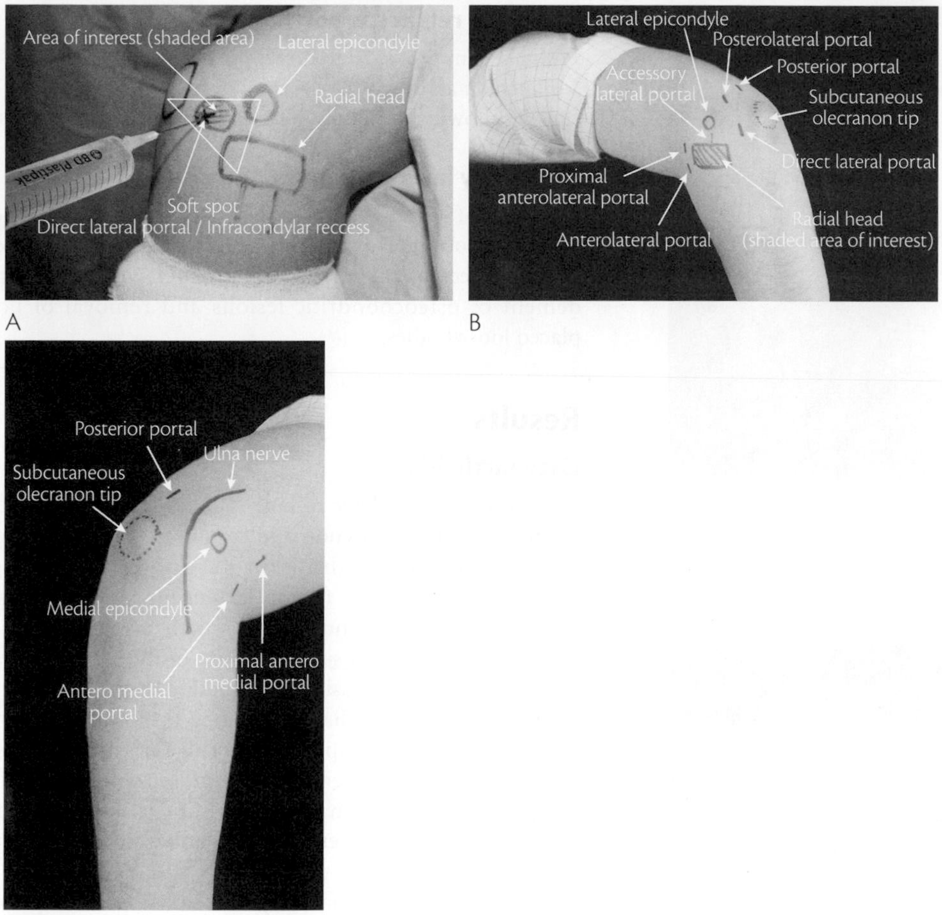

Fig. 5.6.3 A) Fluid distension of elbow prior to introducing scope. B) Portal sites, lateral view. C) Portal sites, medial view.

Proximal anterolateral portal

Position: 2cm proximal, 1cm anterior to lateral epicondyle.

Structures at risk: radial nerve (9.9mm) and posterior antebrachial nerve (6.1mm).

Function: preferred by some surgeons to the anterolateral portal due to its greater distance from the radial nerve. However, scoping the coronoid fossa or medial trochlea may be more difficult.

Mid or direct lateral portal

Position: the centre of a triangle formed by the lateral condyle, subcutaneous olecranon tip, and radial head (the soft spot).

Structures at risk: lateral antebrachial nerve (between 6–16mm in 90 degrees elbow flexion and mid pronation).

Function: scoping the intra-articular olecranon tip and fossa, posterior trochlea, olecranon articular surface, posterior capitellum, radial head, and radioulna articulation. May be of particular use in osteochondritis dissecans of the capitellum and for the removal of loose bodies.

Anteromedial portal

Position: 2cm distal, 2cm anterior to medial epicondyle. The trochar is aimed at the centre of the elbow joint and passes through the brachialis and common flexor origin.

Structures at risk: medial antebrachial cutaneous nerve (1mm away). Median nerve 7–14mm away with the elbow flexed at 90 degrees. The ulnar nerve is, on average, 20mm away in 90 degrees of flexion but it should be palpated prior to making the portal, checking for any possible subluxation from the cubital tunnel. Needless to say, particular caution is due in the case of a prior ulnar nerve transposition—in which case the surgeon would be advised to avoid this portal.

Function: good visualization of the anterolateral capsule, radiocapitellar, and ulnohumeral joints. Useful as an accessory portal when working in the medial gutter.

Proximal anteromedial portal

Position: 2cm proximal to the medial epicondyle, immediately anterior to the intermuscular septum. The trochar is aimed towards the radial head gliding across the anterior distal humerus.

Structures at risk: medial antebrachial cutaneous nerve (2.3mm average), ulnar nerve (12mm average), and median nerve (12.4mm average). The same considerations regarding the ulnar nerve apply with this portal as described earlier.

Function: good visualization of the radial head, lateral capsule, and coronoid (Figure 5.6.4) but poor visualization of the radiocapitellar joint and radial fossa. Useful as a retractor portal.

Posterolateral portal

Position: lateral joint line level with the tip of the olecranon with the elbow in 90 degrees elbow flexion. Trochar aimed at centre of olecranon fossa.

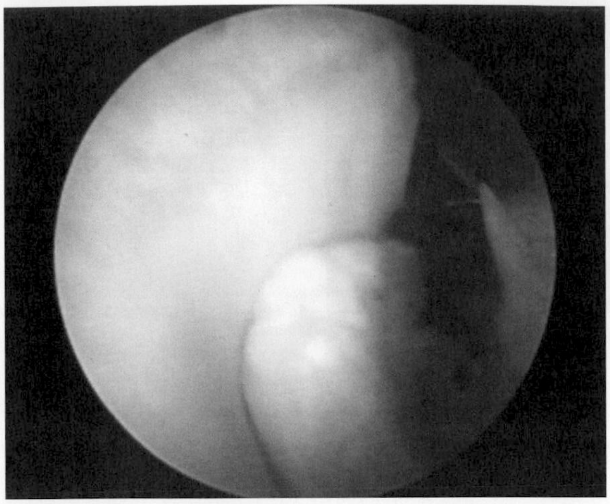

Fig. 5.6.4 View of coronoid tip from anteromedial portal. See also colour plate section.

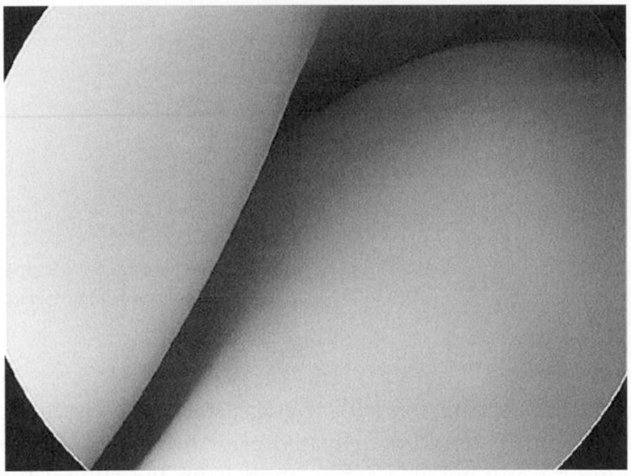

Fig. 5.6.5 View of radiocapitellar joint from posterolateral portal. See also colour plate section.

Structures at risk: average distances at 90 degrees of flexion—medial brachial cutaneous nerve 22mm, posterior antebrachial cutaneous nerve 22mm, and ulnar nerve 26mm. the ulnar nerve is palpated before portal placement.

Function: excellent visualization of the posterior elbow (Figure 5.6.5) including the olecranon fossa and tip, medial and lateral gutters, and the posterior radiocapitellar joint where loose bodies are frequently missed.

Direct posterior portal

Position: 3cm proximal to the tip of the olecranon. Sometimes a scalpel may be needed to penetrate the elbow joint due to the bulk of triceps. Trocar aimed at centre of olecranon fossa.

Structures at risk: average distances at 90 degrees flexion:—medial brachial cutaneous nerve 15mm, posterior antebrachial cutaneous nerve 30mm, and ulnar nerve 20mm. The ulnar nerve is palpated before portal placement.

Function: debridement of the posterior elbow joint. As an accessory portal to the posterolateral portal.

Posterior retractor portal

Position: 2cm proximal to direct posterior portal.

Function: a Howarth elevator can be passed to elevate the joint capsule allowing better visualization of the olecranon fossa.

Accessory lateral portal

The author (S.M.H.) also uses an accessory lateral portal positioned on the radiocapitellar joint line directly between the anterolateral and the direct lateral portals. It has proven very valuable for debridement of osteochondritic lesions and removal of posteriorly placed loose bodies.

Results

Osteoarthritis

Adams et al. (2008) have recently published their results of arthroscopic osteophyte resection and capsulectomy. Forty-one patients with primary osteoarthritis in 42 elbows showed significant improvements in mean flexion, extension, supination, and Mayo Elbow Performance Index scores with 81% good to excellent results. Pain decreased significantly. Complications were rare and included heterotopic ossification and ulnar dysesthesias.

Cohen et al. (2000) have compared the results of arthroscopic debridement with an open Outerbridge–Kashiwagi (OK) procedure (Figure 5.6.6). Overall they found no difference between the two procedures although arthroscopic intervention provided better pain relief, whereas open debridement resulted in an improved flexion range.

Savoie et al. (1999) have reported a series of 24 patients with osteoarthritis treated with arthroscopic debridement, partial resection of the coronoid and olecranon processes, and fenestration of the olecranon fossa. Eighteen of the 24 patients had arthroscopic radial head excision. They report significant pain reduction and an improvement of average arc of motion of 81 degrees. The paper records a complication rate comparable to open ulnohumeral arthroplasty.

Kelly et al. (2007) have reported a series of 24 patients with elbow joint osteoarthritis treated with arthroscopic ulnohumeral arthroplasty, leaving the radial head intact. Debridement of the radial head, anterior and posterior osteophytes, and capsular release

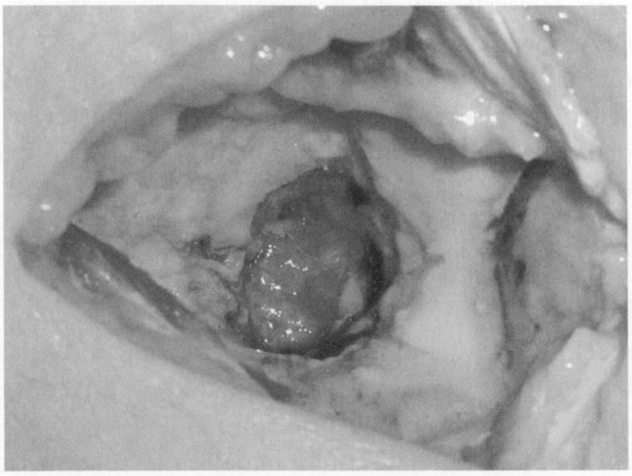

Fig. 5.6.6 OK procedure. See also colour plate section.

alone was performed. Their results showed 14 patients with an excellent result, seven good, three fair, and one poor. The average flexion–extension arc improved by 21 degrees. Twelve patients had no limitations in their daily activities, and 12 experienced occasional problems. No surgical complications were reported. They concluded that resecting an arthritic radial head was not essential.

Rheumatoid arthritis and synovectomy

The rheumatoid elbow presents a particular challenge to the elbow arthroscopist mainly caused by deformity, obscured vision, and synovial hypertrophy (Figure 5.6.7).

Lee et al. (1997) have reported a series of 14 elbows in 11 patients with good 3–4-year results (93% excellent/good) but with subsequent rapid deterioration.

Horiuchi et al. (2002) have reported results of arthroscopic synovectomy in 29 elbows (27 patients). They graded preoperative radiographs from 1–4 using the system of Larsen et al. (1977) forming three groups: 1/2, 3, and 4. They found only elbows with Larsen grade-1 or 2 arthritis had a favourable long-term result with regard to total function. The postoperative results were unsatisfactory for Larsen grade-4 elbows.

Arthrofibrosis

Nerve injury is the predominant concern when performing arthroscopic release of arthrofibrosis. Phillips et al. (1998) reported a series of 25 patients with elbow arthrofibrosis treated with arthroscopic debridement. At 18 months, all patients demonstrated increased motion and decreased pain, although one patient had a reoperation due to continued symptoms. They found that patients with post-traumatic arthritis tended to have greater contractures preoperatively, compared to those patients with degenerative arthritis, but had greater improvement postoperatively. This series reported no perioperative or postoperative complications and concluded that arthroscopic release and debridement of arthrofibrotic elbow joints achieved equal improvement to that of open techniques, with less morbidity and earlier rehabilitation.

Jones et al. (1993) have reported a series of 12 patients with good results, although one patient had residual posterior interosseous nerve palsy.

Radial head excision

Menth-Chiari et al. (2001) have reported a series of 12 patients who underwent arthroscopic excision of the radial head either due to post-traumatic arthritis after fracture of the radial head, or due to rheumatoid arthritis. All except one patient had significant pain relief and complete relief of mechanical symptoms. There were no infections or neurovascular injuries reported.

Lateral epicondylitis

Owens et al. (2001) have reported a series of 16 patients with recalcitrant tennis elbow who underwent arthroscopic surgical debridement of ECRB. There was only 75% follow-up data due to patients' military reassignment, but the group found that all patients had an improvement with an average return to unrestricted work at 6 days.

Peart et al. (2004) report a series of 87 patients, 54 treated with an open and 33 with an arthroscopic procedure. No significant difference in outcome was noted although an arthroscopic release led to an earlier return to work and required less postoperative therapy.

A systematic review of the literature found similar results in endoscopic, percutaneous, and open procedures.

Osteoarthritis dissecans

Rahusen et al. (2006) reported a series of 15 patients with osteoarthritis dissecans treated with arthroscopic debridement (Figure 5.6.8). Their results showed no significant improvement in range of motion, but use of the MAESS showed a significant improvement from 65.5% (poor) to 90.8% (excellent). There was a reduction in pain level and the average return to work occurred 3 months postoperatively.

The role of drilling or microfracture of the capitellum remains unproven.

Miscellaneous

There are a number of reports of novel use of the arthroscope in managing conditions of the elbow such as osteoid osteoma and treatment of posterolateral elbow impingement in professional boxers· The treatment of throwers' elbow/plica has also seen an increasing role of the arthroscope, and the author (S.M.H.) reports

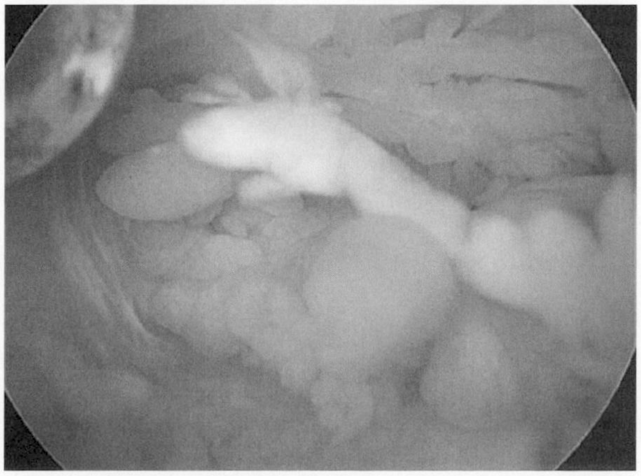

Fig. 5.6.7 Synovitis. See also colour plate section.

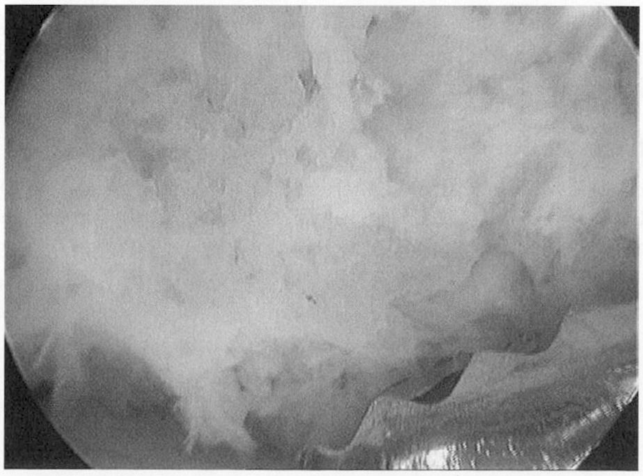

Fig. 5.6.8 Debridement of osteochondritic capitellum. See also colour plate section.

arthroscopic removal of a silastic radial head replacement. These are indications of the developing nature of the technique.

Complications

Kelly et al. (2001) have reported the complications of elbow arthroscopy in 473 patients. Four (0.8%) had a complication classified as major (septic arthritis). Minor complications occurred in 11%, which included prolonged drainage from, or superficial infection at, a portal site after 33 procedures, 12 transient nerve palsies (five ulnar, five superficial radial, one each of posterior interosseous, medial antebrachial cutaneous, and one anterior interosseous palsy). Rheumatoid arthritis followed by contracture was the most significant risk factor for temporary nerve palsy.

This study found no permanent nerve injuries. It also reports the findings of The Arthroscopy Association of North America who conducted two separate surveys. Of the 1648 elbow arthroscopies in both surveys, only one nerve injury was documented.

The authors of this comprehensive study of complications suggest that the use of retractors was the single most important technical step in preventing serious nerve injuries especially when performing synovectomy or capsulectomy. The second factor was arthroscopic/open identification of the nerve when performing a capsulectomy around nerves.

With regards to prolonged portal drainage, Kelly and colleagues found that all were from lateral portals and recommended the use of a locked horizontal mattress suture to minimize the risk of this complication.

Conclusion

As with many areas of arthroscopic surgery, the technique of elbow arthroscopy, its indications, and its success has evolved considerably in recent years. However, it is a technically demanding and a dangerous procedure for which a detailed working knowledge of the surrounding neurovascular anatomy is essential. It remains the preserve of the experienced arthroscopist and we strongly concur with Savoie (2007) that graduated progression where indication is titrated against experience remains the mandatory approach.

Acknowledgements

The authors are very grateful to Alun Jones and Andy Biggs at Robert Jones and Agnes Hunt Hospital, Oswestry, for their help in producing the illustrations.

Further reading

Adams, J.E., Wolff, L.H. 3rd Ed, Merten, S.M., and Steinmann, S.P. (2008). Osteoarthritis of the elbow: results of arthroscopic osteophyte resection and capsulectomy. *Journal of Shoulder and Elbow Surgery*, **17**(1), 126–31.

Andrews, J.R. and Carson, W.G. (1985). Arthroscopy of the elbow. *Arthroscopy*, **1**, 97–107.

Burman, M. (1932). Arthroscopy of the elbow joint: A cadaver study. *Journal of Bone and Joint Surgery*, **14**, 349–50.

Cohen, A.P., Redden, J.F., and Stanley, D. (2000). Treatment of osteoarthritis of the elbow: A comparison of open and arthroscopic debridement. *Arthroscopy*, **16**(7), 701–6.

Horiuchi, K., Momohara, S., Tomatsu, T., Inoue, K., and Toyama, Y. (2002). Arthroscopic synovectomy of the elbow in rheumatoid arthritis. *Journal of Bone and Joint Surgery*, **84-A**, 342–7.

Jones, G.S. and Savoie, F.H. 3rd. (1993). Arthroscopic capsular release of flexion contractures (arthrofibrosis) of the elbow. *Arthroscopy*, **9**, 277–83.

Kelly, E.W., Morrey, B.F., and O'Driscoll, S.W. (2001). Complications of elbow arthroscopy. *Journal of Bone and Joint Surgery*, **83-A**, 25–34.

Kelly, E.W., Bryce, R., Coghlan, J., and Bell, S. (2007). Arthroscopic debridement without radial head excision of the osteoarthritic elbow. *Arthroscopy*, **23**(2), 151–6.

Larsen, A., Dale, K., and Morten, E.E.K. (1977). Radiographic evaluation of rheumatoid arthritis and related conditions by standard reference films. *Acta Radiologica*, **18**, 481–91.

Lee, B.P. and Morrey, B.F. (1997). Arthroscopic synovectomy of the elbow for rheumatoid arthritis. A prospective study. *Journal of Bone and Joint Surgery*, **79-B**, 770–2.

Menth-Chiari, W.A., Ruch, D.S., and Poehling, G.G. (2001). Arthroscopic excision of the radial head: clinical outcome in 12 patients with post-traumatic arthritis after fracture of the radial head or rheumatoid arthritis. *Arthroscopy*, **17**(9), 918–23.

O'Driscoll, S.W. and Morrey, B.F. (1992). Arthroscopy of the elbow: diagnostic and therapeutic benefits and hazards. *Journal of Bone and Joint Surgery*, **74-A**, 84–94.

Owens, B.D., Murphy, K.P., and Kuklo, T.R. (2001). Arthroscopic release for lateral epicondylitis. *Arthroscopy*, **17**(6), 582–7.

Peart, R.E., Strickler, S.S., and Schweitzer, K.M. Jr. (2004). Lateral epicondylitis: a comparative study of open and arthroscopic lateral release. *American Journal of Orthopedics*, **33**(11), 565–7.

Phillips, B.B. and Strasburger, S. (1998). Arthroscopic treatment of arthrofibrosis of the elbow joint. *Arthroscopy*, **14**(1), 38–44.

Poehling, G.G., Whipple, T.L., Sisco, L., and Goldman, B. (1989). Elbow arthroscopy: A new technique. *Arthroscopy*, **5**, 222–4.

Rahusen, F.T., Brinkman, J.M., and Eygendaal, D. (2006). Results of osteochondritis dissecans for the elbow. *British Journal of Sports Medicine*, **40**(12), 966–9.

Savoie, F.H., Nunley, P.D., and Field, L.D. (1999). Arthroscopic management of the arthritic elbow: indications, technique, and results. *Journal of Shoulder and Elbow Surgery*, **8**, 214–19.

Savoie, F.H. (2007). Guidelines to becoming an expert elbow arthroscopist. *Arthroscopy*, **23**(11), 1237–40.

Steinmann, S.P. (2003). Elbow arthroscopy. *Journal of the American Society for Surgery of the Hand*, **3**(4), 199–207.

Steinmann, S.P. (2007). Elbow arthroscopy: where are we now? *Arthroscopy*, **23**(11), 1231–6.

5.7

Bursitis of the elbow

Andreas F. Hinsche

Summary points

- Inflammation of the bursa
- Non-Septic or Septic
- Repetitive Micro-traumata
- Bloods, XR, USS, MRI, Aspirate
- Splintage, NSAID, Antibiotics, I+D
- 85% Staph. aureus

Introduction

A bursa (Latin for purse or bag) is a small fluid-filled sac lined with synovial membrane providing a gliding plane and/or a cushioning effect between tendon, muscle, and bone. Several deep and superficial bursae around the elbow have been described; however, only a few are of clinical relevance.

Bursitis is the inflammation of a bursa through either mechanical irritation (non-septic bursitis) or infection (septic bursitis).

Inflammation of the lateral and medial epicondylar bursae are rare sequelae of tennis elbow or a subluxing ulnar nerve and respond to treatment of the underlying pathology. The *bicipital radial bursa* is often the cause for symptoms deep in the cubital fossa. Differentiation of this from tendinitis, a partial tear of the distal biceps tendon, and secondary compression of the posterior interosseous nerve can be difficult and requires magnetic resonance imaging for exact diagnosis and treatment. The clinically most significant elbow bursa is the superficial olecranon bursa (Box 5.7.1).

History and clinical examination

Olecranon bursitis has a male predominance with a mean age of 45 years, a prevalence of 3:1000, and an incidence of 1:1000 which is seasonal with the peak in summer. The olecranon bursa develops only after the age of 7 years and increases in size thereafter. In up to 54% the history includes a precipitating trauma but other risk factors need to be considered:

- Macrotrauma (occupational or recreational)
- Repetitive microtraumata (overuse, leaning on elbow)
- Immunosuppression (alcoholism, chronic obstructive pulmonary disease, systemic corticosteroid therapy, diabetes mellitus)
- Systemic inflammatory disease (gout, rheumatoid arthritis, psoriasis)
- Previous posterior elbow surgery
- Structural abnormalities (olecranon spur).

The clinical examination should begin with a routine elbow assessment including range of motion, nerve function, and pre-existing elbow pathologies (osteoarthritis, rheumatoid arthritis, and post-traumatic disorders). Localized clinical features of olecranon bursitis include: swelling, erythema, increased skin temperature, fluctuance, and tenderness

Attention should be given to scarring in the elbow region (previous surgery, healed sinuses, haemodialysis) and areas of possible skin breakage (open or healed).

It is important to differentiate between non-septic (more than 60%) and septic bursitis (Box 5.7.2) since early diagnosis is essential for appropriate treatment.

Septic arthritis of the elbow must be considered in the differential diagnosis and when present there is usually a painful reduction of joint movement. Aspiration of the elbow will normally confirm the diagnosis.

Box 5.7.1 Bursae around the elbow

- Lateral epicondylar bursa
- Medial epicondylar bursa
- Bicipital radial bursa
- Superficial olecranon bursa*

*Clinically most important.

Box 5.7.2 Regional and systemic signs of septic olecranon bursitis

- Induration
- Spreading cellulitis
- Lymphangitis
- Lymphadenitis
- Fever and shivering.

Investigations

If the bursa contains sufficient fluid, an aspiration is recommended in order to exclude or confirm infection. This can guide fast and efficient treatment. Aspiration also enables microscopic examination of the fluid for crystal formation. The extent of further investigations is dependent on the presenting symptoms and may require:

- Blood screening tests (inflammatory parameters including full blood count, erythrocyte sedimentation rate, and C-reactive protein)
- Radiographs of the elbow (pre-existing underlying bony pathology, effusion, osteomyelitis)
- Ultrasonography (soft tissue oedema, joint effusion)
- Magnetic resonance imaging (fluid collection, joint effusion, intra-articular pathology, reactive tissue changes).

Staphylococcus aureus is the most common organism found in septic olecranon bursitis (85%). Other organisms that may be present include Gram negatives, mycobacteria, as well as fungi. It has been suggested that the clinical spectrum of septic olecranon bursitis differs when it is caused by organisms other than *Stapylococcus aureus.*

Treatment options

Most cases of olecranon bursitis do not require hospitalization and can be treated ambulatory (Box 5.7.3).

Box 5.7.3 Treatment of olecranon bursitis

- Non-septic:
  - Splintage
  - NSAID
  - Intrabursal steroid injections
- Septic:
  - Splintage
  - Antibiotics—oral/intravenous
  - Surgical excision.

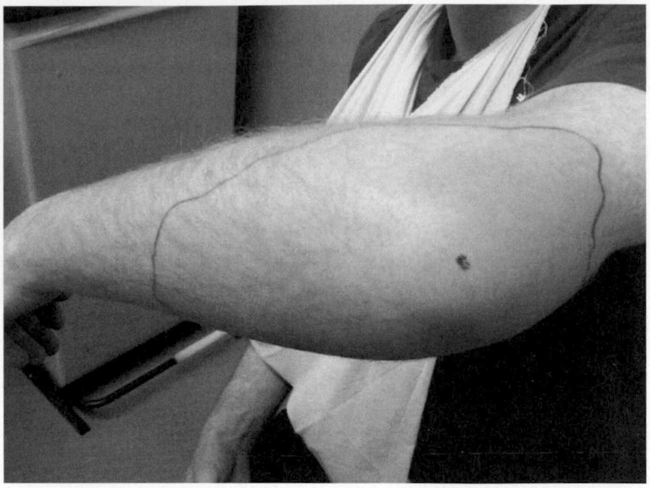

Fig. 5.7.1 The typical features of a traumatic, septic olecranon bursitis: scab over entry wound, swelling, induration, and spreading cellulitis.

Non-septic olecranon bursitis

This can be successfully treated with splintage, reducing elbow movements and thereby resting the overlying soft tissues. This should be combined with oral, non-steroidal anti-inflammatory drug (NSAID) treatment. Whilst intrabursal corticosteroid injections can be a very effective treatment option, the concern over local long-term effects remains. Any associated underlying systemic disease such as gout or rheumatoid arthritis must also be addressed if treatment is to be effective. The symptoms in patients with non-septic olecranon bursitis resolve more slowly when compared to septic bursitis.

Septic olecranon bursitis

Early treatment involves a combination of elbow splintage and oral antibiotic therapy. However, once the clinical picture shows advanced signs (Figure 5.7.1) such as local cellulitis, lymphangitis, and lymphadenitis or systemic effects with shivering and fever, the antibiotic therapy should be administered intravenously. The duration of therapy is guided by the response to treatment but prolonged treatment courses are not uncommon.

If the olecranon bursitis remains refractory to conservative treatment or a bursal collection with septicaemia develops, surgical excision of the bursa should be performed. Although normally the initial response to such treatment is good, the complication rate remains a concern for the treating clinician. Recurrence, a chronic discharging sinus, and wound breakdown are common (up to 25%) along with worrisome complications. In order to reduce such problems, several surgical techniques have been described:

- Skin incision skirting the tip of the olecranon
- Postoperative immobilization in 45 degrees of elbow flexion
- Application of a compression bandage postoperatively
- Wound drain.

If the extent of the bursa is difficult to determine, the use of methylene blue and hydrogen peroxide staining can be used. In an attempt to prevent wound healing problems following resection of the bursa, endoscopic techniques with excellent results have more recently been described.

A chronic discharging sinus can initially be treated non-operatively with regular changes of wound dressing in the outpatient department. If signs of infection develop, antibiotic therapy is required and is based on the culture and sensitivity report.

Should the sinus remain refractory to such treatment, revision surgery should be contemplated. The use of talcum powder in revision surgery has shown favourable results. For chronic and recurrent wound breakdown, more advanced reconstructive soft tissue techniques, such as local and free flap, may be required.

Further reading

Degreef, I. and De Smet, L. (2006). Complications following resection of the olecranon bursa. *Acta Orthopaedica Belgica* **72**(4), 400–3.

Ogilvie-Harris, D.J. and Gilbart, M. (2000). Endoscopic bursal resection: the olecranon bursa and prepatellar bursa. *Arthroscopy* **16**(3), 249–53.

Stewart, N.J., Manzanares, J.B., and Morrey, B.F. (1997). Surgical treatment of aseptic olecranon bursitis. *Journal of Shoulder and Elbow Surgery* **6**(1), 49–54.

SECTION 6

The Hand and Wrist

6.1

Assessment and investigation of chronic wrist pain

I.A. Trail, D. Temperley, and J.K. Stanley

Introduction

Advances in the understanding of the anatomy, biomechanics, and pathology of the wrist over the last few years have greatly increased the number of diagnoses that the upper limb surgeon must consider in the management of wrist disorders. At the same time, new methods of investigation are able to demonstrate wrist pathology with increasing accuracy. The aim of this chapter is to give an overview of the techniques of clinical assessment and diagnostic investigations that are useful in the management of chronic wrist pain.

Clinical assessment (Box 6.1.1)

Of paramount importance in the diagnosis of chronic wrist pain are a careful history and a thorough physical examination. Attention must be paid to the position of the wrist at the time of injury and the location of pain. Swelling and local tenderness are noted and the ranges of motion and grip strength of the injured and uninjured side are measured.

History

The mechanism of injury and the position of the wrist at the moment of impact can give useful information on likely injuries. Was the wrist flexed or extended? Was it the thenar or hypothenar eminence that struck first? The latter is particularly important when considering the possibility of intercarpal ligament damage. The magnitude of the force is also informative. Injuries that involve sudden transmission of body weight through the wrist are liable to cause fracture or intercarpal ligament damage. However, pain that follows a blow to the side of the wrist on a hard surface is unlikely to represent a serious injury.

The precise location of pain is most valuable. All too often, however, patients are unable to localize the pain and the best that can be achieved is localization to a specific area, for example, the radial or ulnar aspect of the radiocarpal joint or the distal radioulnar joint.

An indication of the severity, frequency, and duration of pain is useful in determining the management. Constant severe pain suggests infection or tumour. The activities that aggravate intermittent wrist pain should be ascertained. Persistent swelling would suggest an arthropathy. Mechanical symptoms (snapping, clicking, and so on) may be due to carpal instability.

Physical examination (Box 6.1.2)

The localization of swelling and local tenderness can be invaluable. Loss of motion can have a significant effect on the patient's function and the plane of principal loss can suggest potential diagnoses, for example, restricted or painful ulnar deviation in ulnar impaction or radial deviation with dorsiflexion in dorsal rim arthritis.

Osteoarthritis and other pathology of the first carpometacarpal joint can be detected by eliciting pain on the simple manoeuvre of applying traction to the thumb and pressing downwards over the base of the first metacarpal. More proximally, pathology of the scaphotrapeziotrapezoid joint can be reproduced by balloting the distal pole of the scaphoid. It should be remembered, however, that osteoarthritis of this joint can be associated with inflammation

Box 6.1.1 Clinical assessment

This is paramount in assessment. In particular:
- Position of wrist at injury
- Site of pain
- Swelling and local tenderness
- Specialist clinical tests
- Grip strength.

Box 6.1.2 Special clinical tests

- Distal radioulnar joint shear
- Watson's test
- Finkelstein's test
- Triquetrolunate ballotment
- Pisotriquetral shear
- Midcarpal shift
- Metacarpal rotation.

of the adjacent flexor carpi radialis tendon. As a consequence, resisted flexion and radial deviation will reproduce the pain.

Tenderness in the anatomical snuff box is said to be pathognomonic of fractures of the scaphoid bone. However, pressure in this area may be uncomfortable in the normal wrist, so the opposite side should be examined for comparison. Stability of the scapholunate joint can be demonstrated by two means. Firstly, the joint can be balloted using the thumb and index fingers of both hands. Secondly, Watson's manoeuvre is performed by applying pressure to the palmar aspect of the distal pole of the scaphoid as the wrist is moved from ulnar deviation into radial deviation (Figure 6.1.1). If an audible or palpable painful clunk is produced, the test is deemed positive. In the normal wrist, the scaphoid flexes along with the lunate as the wrist moves into radial deviation. If the scapholunate joint is unstable, pressure from the examiner's thumb prevents flexion of the scaphoid and allows dorsal displacement of the proximal pole as the wrist moves from ulnar to radial deviation.

In de Quervain's syndrome there is usually swelling and local tenderness over the tendons of the first dorsal compartment. Finkelstein's test is useful confirmatory evidence. The 'intersection syndrome' produces pain, swelling, and local tenderness over the radial wrist extensor muscles as they run under the muscles of the first dorsal compartment. Tendon disorders are characterized by a longitudinal distribution of tenderness and swelling, extending proximal and distal to underlying joints. In joint conditions, these signs are more typically orientated transversely and can be elicited on all surfaces of the joint.

On the dorsal surface, point tenderness may be seen in cases of 'occult' ganglion. Simple ballottement of the lunotriquetral joint will reproduce symptoms due to instability or other pathology at that site. The lunate is grasped between the index finger and thumb of one hand of the examiner. The examiner's opposite thumb and index grasp the triquetrum and pisiform. The examiner then attempts to displace the lunate and triquetrum in a palmar/dorsal direction, looking for pain and/or instability, and comparing the findings with the contralateral normal wrist. Midcarpal joint instability is often manifest by clicking or voluntary clunking of the wrist. The provocative manoeuvre used to confirm this diagnosis is performed by applying an axial load to a pronated and slightly flexed wrist, which is then brought into ulna deviation. This may reproduce the painful click.

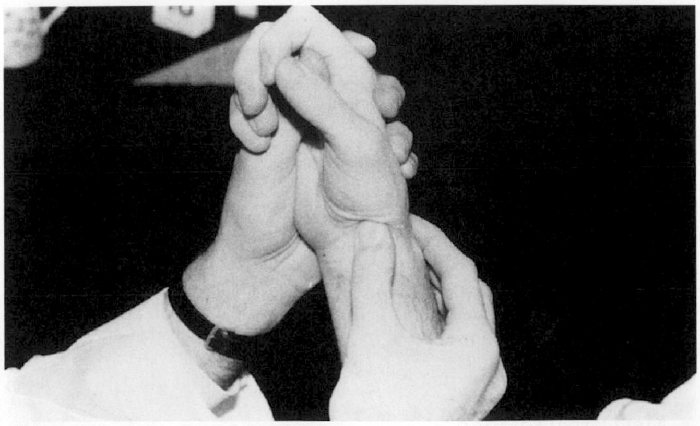

Fig. 6.1.1 Watson's manoeuvre (see text).

Volarly pisotriquetral pathology can be identified by compressing the pisiform onto the triquetrum both ulnarly and radially as well as from proximal to distal. This manoeuvre is helped by flexing the wrist. Firm ulnar deviation of the wrist may produce ulnar-sided wrist pain in the ulnocarpal impaction syndrome, which results from impingement between the lunate and triquetrum distally and the triangular fibrocartilage complex and ulnar head proximally. More distally, afflictions of the carpometacarpal joints such as a carpal boss have been demonstrated by direct ballottement of the each joint. A particularly effective manoeuvre is to flex the appropriate metacarpophalangeal joint to 90 degrees (thus tightening the collateral ligaments) and then to rotate the metacarpal by radial and ulnar deviation of the flexed finger. Reproduction of the pain at the carpometacarpal joint is highly suggestive of pathology at that site.

The distal radioulnar joint and ulnocarpal area are responsible for many cases of wrist pain. Pathology of the distal radioulnar joint, such as osteoarthritis and osteochondral defects, can be demonstrated by direct ballottement, which can be undertaken by compressing the articular surface or by producing a shear force in the anteroposterior plane (it appears clinically that the distal ulnar moves but this is fixed and in fact it is the distal radius that moves). The latter can also be used to demonstrate instability, but comparison with the contralateral wrist is essential. Finally, it is also important to be aware of the possibility of inflammation or tendonitis affecting the extensor carpi ulnaris and flexor carpi ulnaris tendons. Localized tenderness here is quite specific and pain is reproduced by resisted extension or flexion in the appropriate plane.

Limitation of the range of motion strongly suggests intra-articular pathology. The flexion/extension and radial/ulnar deviation ranges can be measured directly with the use of a goniometer and compared with the contralateral side. Pronation and supination are performed with the elbow flexed to 90 degrees so as to prevent rotation at the shoulder. Pain on active resisted motion suggests a disorder of tendon or tendon sheath.

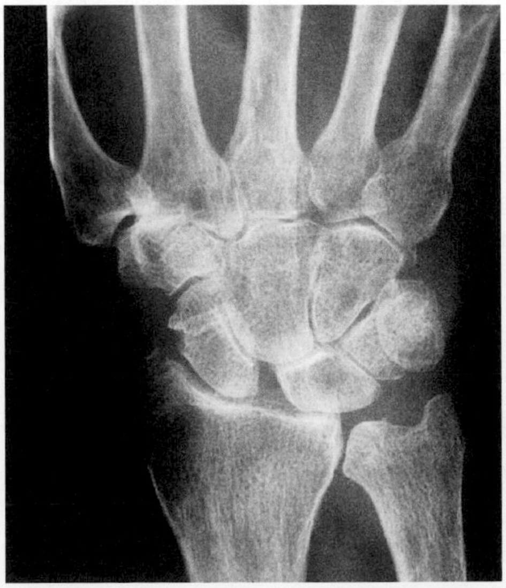

Fig. 6.1.2 Scapholunate dissociation due to scapholunate ligament rupture. The gap between the scaphoid and lunate is greater than the lunotriquetral joint space and exceeds the upper limit of normal.

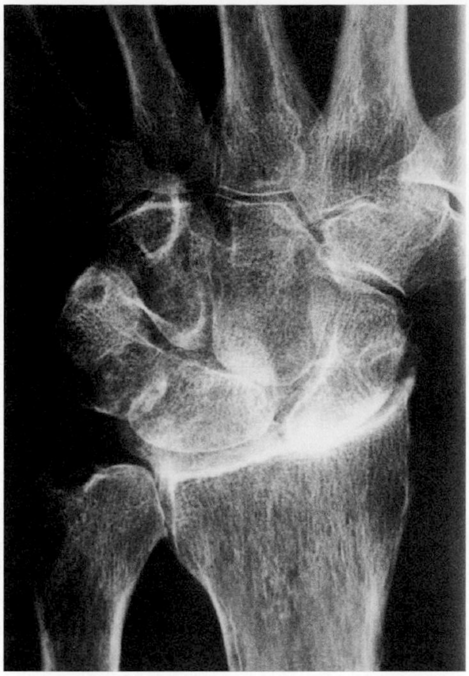

Fig. 6.1.3 Scapholunate advanced collapse (SLAC wrist). The scapholunate interval is widened. There is marked osteoarthritis in the radioscaphoid joint and early changes are seen in the scaphocapitate and capitolunate joints. The radiolunate surfaces are preserved.

Grip strength can help to evaluate the level of disability experienced by the patient. The measurements are made with a dynamometer with the elbow flexed and the forearm and wrist in neutral. Clinical estimation of grip strength is unreliable. Grip strength should diminish with fatigue on repeated testing. Rapid alternating tests between normal and abnormal hands may reveal an increase in strength (from an initial low level) on the abnormal side in patients whose symptoms are modified by psychological factors. The plot of grip strength against width of grip should show a bell-shaped curve with maximal strength at the middle position. A flat plot suggests that the voluntary effort is submaximal.

Imaging

Imaging of the wrist is often very helpful. The mainstay is plain radiography, with the addition of stress views when necessary. Specific clinical problems can be further examined with isotope bone scanning, ultrasound, arthrography, computed tomography (CT), or magnetic resonance imaging (MRI). The choice of imaging modality and the interpretation of the results depend upon knowledge of the clinical information derived from the history and physical examination.

Plain radiography

The standard radiographic assessment of the wrist comprises posteroanterior (PA) and lateral views of the wrist. The films are taken with the wrist in the neutral position with regard to flexion/extension and pronation/supination, so that measurements of intercarpal angles and relative radioulnar length are reproducible.

Special views may be required when particular diagnoses are suspected. An oblique view may show degenerative arthritis of the pisotriquetral joint. Fractures of the hook of the hamate may be seen on the carpal tunnel view.

Stress views are valuable in the assessment of carpal instability. All carpal instabilities are abnormal movements of the proximal row. The proximal row receives no tendon insertions and depends for its stability on the ligaments that bind the bones to each other, to the distal row and to the radius and ulna. Abnormal movement between two of the proximal row bones is termed carpal instability dissociative. Abnormal movement of the whole proximal row is termed carpal instability non-dissociative. Scapholunate dissociation is an example of dissociative carpal instability; midcarpal instability is non-dissociative.

PA radiographs in ulnar and radial deviation, and clenched fist views in PA and lateral projections, apply load to the proximal carpal row and may show displacement that is not evident on static films. Stress views increase the sensitivity in the diagnosis of ligamentous injury. On PA views the scapholunate gap should be no greater than the lunotriquetral gap, normally not more than 3mm. A larger gap suggests scapholunate dissociation or scapholunate ligament rupture (Figure 6.1.2), although there is considerable normal variation and comparison views of both wrists have been suggested. In the presence of scapholunate ligament disruption, forces acting on the wrist may cause flexion of the scaphoid, with an increase in the angle between the scaphoid and the lunate on the lateral radiograph. The normal angle is between 30–60 degrees. Angles of 80 degrees or greater indicate rotatory subluxation of the scaphoid. If, in addition, the lunate is dorsally angulated on the radius the appearances is termed dorsiflexion instability (dorsal intercalated segment injury) scapholunate angle of less than 30 degrees indicates volar intercalated segment injury, which usually results from disruption of the ulnotriquetral ligament complex.

Chronic scapholunate ligament rupture leads to flexion of the scaphoid decreasing the contact area and thus increasing the load in the radioscaphoid joint, leading to radioscaphoid osteoarthritis with proximal migration of the capitate and the subsequent involvement of the scaphocapitate and hamate/lunate joints. This degenerative pattern is known as the scapholunate advanced collapse

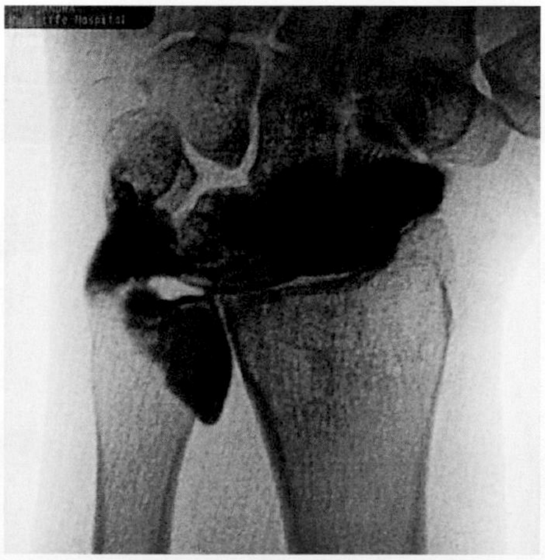

Fig. 6.1.4 Arthrography of the radiocarpal joint, performed with digital imaging. Contrast passes though a tear in the radial attachment of the triangular fibrocartilage into the distal radioulnar joint, where it coats the underside of the triangular fibrocartilage. (Courtesy of the Department of Radiology, Nuffield Orthopaedic Centre, Oxford.)

(SLAC) wrist and may occur naturally) as well as after trauma (Figure 6.1.3). Other common patterns of primary degenerative arthritis are of the scaphotrapeziotrapezoid joint and the first carpometacarpal joint. Less commonly, arthritis may involve the triquetrolunate, radiolunate, or pisotriquetral joints.

Fluoroscopy

Fluoroscopy enables wrist movement to be viewed dynamically and shows the abnormal movements occurring in instability. Recording the examination on videotape allows replay in slow motion. Fluoroscopy may show dynamic instabilities which cannot otherwise be demonstrated. It is especially useful in assessing the 'catch-up clunk' that can occur in scapholunate and midcarpal instabilities. In radial deviation, the proximal carpal row is normally flexed with respect to the distal row but moves smoothly into extension during ulnar deviation. In unstable wrists, the proximal row remains in flexion initially but makes a sudden movement or 'clunk' into extension as the joint is taken into ulnar deviation. The clunk may be painful and palpable, and may occur in reverse during radial deviation.

Wrist arthrography

Wrist arthrography was the principal means of diagnosing tears of the intrinsic ligaments of the wrist, the scapholunate and lunotriquetral ligaments, and the triangular fibrocartilage prior to the development of arthroscopy and MRI. The wrist comprises three anatomically separate compartments: the distal radioulnar joint, the radiocarpal joint, and the midcarpal joint. In wrist arthrography, radio-opaque contrast is injected into the radiocarpal joint. The contrast is usually mixed with local anaesthetic and is injected away from the site of expected abnormality to avoid obscuring the area with extravasated contrast material. The joint is distended. If there is a perforation of the scapholunate ligament or the lunotriquetral ligament, contrast may be seen to flow through the tear into the midcarpal compartment. A triangular fibrocartilage tear may be identified as contrast passes through it into the distal radioulnar joint (Figure 6.1.4). The injection of contrast should be visualized with fluoroscopy, as the route by which it reaches the midcarpal joint may not be apparent from postinjection radiographs. Standard radiographs after injection are PA (in neutral and with radial and ulnar deviation), lateral, and both obliques.

Unfortunately the demonstration of a communication between the wrist joint compartments does not necessarily imply a traumatic tear or that the abnormality is the cause of symptoms. Communications are common in asymptomatic wrists. Degenerative perforations of the triangular fibrocartilage are present in 40% of cadavers in the fifth decade. Abnormal arthrograms are found in the opposite asymptomatic wrist in most patients with wrist pain and abnormal arthrograms. Given this and the fact that arthrography has a relatively low accuracy when compared with arthroscopy the use of this investigation has declined.

Nuclear medicine

Three-phase isotope bone scanning using ^{99m}Tc-MDP is a useful technique in assessing chronic wrist pain, particularly where a cause is not initially evident. Bone infection and tumour, osteonecrosis, fracture, and arthritis usually appear as areas of increased uptake on bone scans. In chronic wrist pain, bone scanning is most likely to be helpful in the diagnosis of occult fractures and osteonecrosis of the carpal bones. Osteoid osteomas,

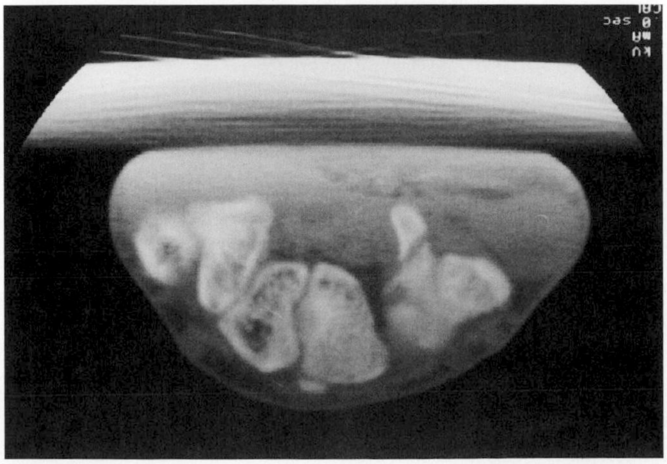

Fig. 6.1.5 Axial CT scan through the distal carpus, showing a fracture of the base of the hook of the hamate. Radiographs taken after a wrist injury appeared normal, but an isotope scan (not shown) showed increased uptake over the hamate.

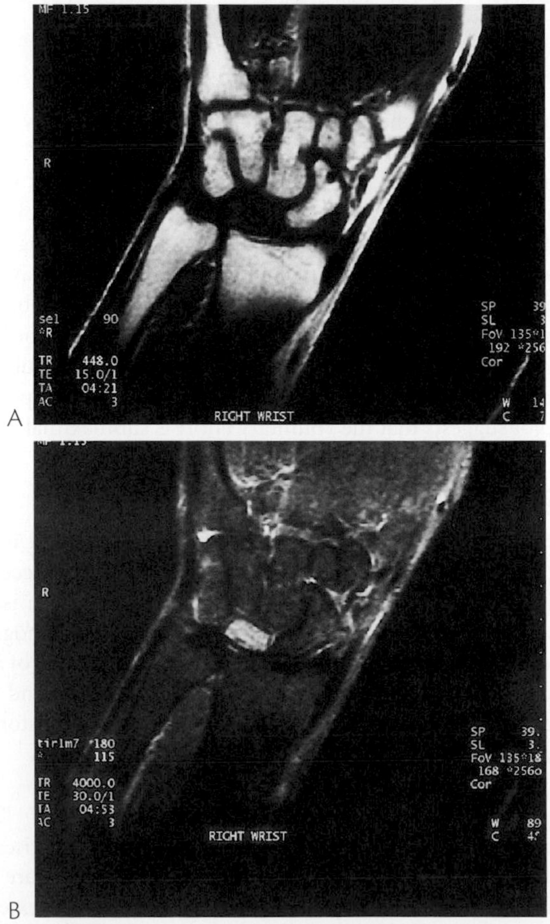

Fig. 6.1.6 A) *T1*-weighted coronal MRI scan shows loss of normal high signal in the lunate due to avascular necrosis (Kienböck's disease). B) *T2*-weighed images show high signal owing to oedema. (Courtesy of the Department of Radiology, Nuffield Orthopaedic Centre, Oxford.)

occasionally found in the wrist, show intensely increased uptake. Bone scanning is best used in patients with chronic wrist pain where there are no definite diagnostic signs on clinical or radiographic assessment. It is not useful in the diagnosis of carpal instability.

Tomography

Standard or trispiral tomography is useful in the diagnosis of occult fractures of carpal bones and in the assessment of fracture healing. Indications for tomography are broadly similar to those for CT, which has largely superseded it.

Computed tomography

CT shows excellent bony detail but is less useful in the investigation of soft tissue abnormalities. It is the technique of choice in the assessment of occult fractures, and in the assessment of position or healing of a known fracture when this cannot be achieved with plain radiographs (Figure 6.1.5). The examination must be tailored to the likely diagnosis e.g. thin slices (1–2mm) in the long axis of the scaphoid for assessment of union. CT scanning is also the preferred method for demonstrating healing of bone grafts and bone invasion by a soft tissue mass. Axial CT images of the symptomatic and opposite normal distal radioulnar joints in pronation and supination can be used to detect subluxation, which may be evident only in extremes of rotation.

Computed tomography arthrography

Arthrography is accurate in the detection of scapholunate ligament tears, but does not show the exact size and position of the tear. These can be accurately visualized used CT arthrography and, where this information will influence treatment, the technique is useful. CT arthrography is performed after standard arthrography; thin-section axial and coronal scans are taken through the wrist.

CT arthrography is more accurate than current MRI scanners in visualizing the scapholunate ligament. It is useful in demonstrating carpal fractures occurring in association with ligamentous injuries, but it is less likely to be helpful in triangular fibrocartilage or lunotriquetral ligament tears. The technique may also be helpful in detecting loose bodies in the wrist.

Ultrasound

Ultrasound is a quick, cheap, and simple method of imaging the wrist. It allows the examiner to assess the wrist clinically at the same time and does not involve the use of ionizing radiation. However, it is operator dependent. Ultrasound waves do not penetrate bone, precluding its use in bony and some deep soft tissue assessment. The major uses of ultrasound are in the assessment of tendon pathology and in the assessment of palpable swellings.

Tendon ruptures and other pathology, especially tenosynovitis, can readily be diagnosed with ultrasound. The advantage over MRI scanning is that the patient can be clinically assessed by the operator at the time of scanning.

Ultrasound is also useful in the assessing of lumps and masses around the hand. It is most useful in assessing ganglia; as in other areas of the body any mass that might signify aggressive or malignant pathology should be initially assessed with urgent MRI scanning where possible.

Ultrasound has also proved useful in the assessment of occult foreign bodies, and is increasingly used to help in the diagnosis of early inflammatory arthritis. It can also be used to ensure accurate placement of injections.

Magnetic resonance imaging

MRI has developed into an invaluable imaging tool in the diagnosis of chronic wrist pain. Its main advantages are the excellent contrast discrimination between different soft tissues and the ability to image in any plane. It is non-invasive and does not use ionizing radiation. Cortical bone does not return a signal but MRI is sensitive to bony abnormalities because of the signal returned by marrow fat. Fractures that are occult on plain radiographs can be seen on MRI, where on T_1-weighted images they show a low signal line through the normally high signal marrow fat with surrounding marrow oedema. MRI is the most sensitive technique in the diagnosis of early avascular necrosis On T_1-weighted MRI, avascular necrosis shows loss of the high signal of marrow fat (Figure 6.1.6). Later changes, including cyst formation, bone collapse, and osteosclerosis, are also well seen.

MRI has an accuracy of about 90% in the diagnosis of triangular fibrocartilage tears. Tears are characterized by a gap across the triangular fibrocartilage containing high signal; the normal triangular fibrocartilage shows as a low-signal disc (Figure 6.1.7). Degenerative perforations of the triangular fibrocartilage are common over the age of 40 years and thus a tear may not be the cause of a patient's symptoms. The scapholunate ligament and lunotriquetral ligament are not always visible, and so MRI is not entirely reliable in demonstrating tears. Tears may appear as absence of the ligament or high-signal fluid crossing the ligament. MRI is not as sensitive as arthrography in the detection of scapholunate ligament and lunotriquetral ligament perforations, and as with the triangular fibrocartilage the functional significance of a perforation may be uncertain.

MRI shows tendon pathology clearly. In tendinitis the tendon is enlarged. Tendon oedema and fluid within the tendon sheath return a high signal on T_2-weighted images. These conditions are most commonly seen in de Quervain's syndrome. Rupture of the tendon may be obvious. In arthritis, cartilage loss can be seen and erosions are said to be identifiable earlier than on radiograph. Joint fluid can be distinguished from pannus because the latter enhances after intravenous gadolinium.

MRI is valuable in the diagnosis of both cystic (Figure 6.1.8) and solid masses in the wrist and hand.

Increasingly MRI is performed with injection of contrast medium particularly to look for ligament/triangular fibrocartilage complex (TFCC) tears. As with standard arthrography, the presence of a tear does not of necessity mean it is traumatic nor that it is the cause of the patient's symptoms.

Arthroscopy

Arthroscopy has recently assumed the position of pre-eminence in the investigation of chronic wrist pain. Arthroscopy can provide information about the altered mechanics and pathology of the wrist, and can identify pathologies that would otherwise remain undetected. However, interpretation is sometimes difficult, not least because of the high prevalence of asymptomatic wrist lesions such as TFCC perforations.

In patients with symptoms suggestive of a scapholunate interosseous ligament tear but with normal radiographs, instability can be

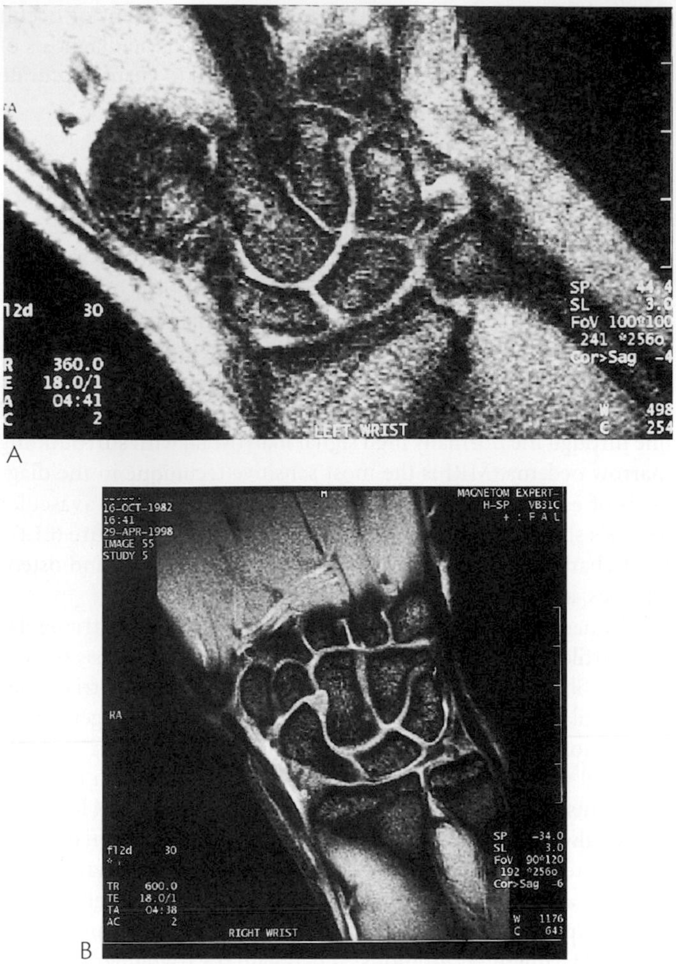

Fig. 6.1.7 A) Coronal *T1*-weighted MRI scan shows a high-signal defect in the normally low-signal triangular fibrocartilage, indicating perforation of the central portion of the triangular fibrocartilage, in a patient with abutment of the long ulna against the carpus. B) The normal triangular fibrocartilage of another patient is shown for comparison. (Courtesy of the Department of Radiology, Nuffield Orthopaedic Centre, Oxford.)

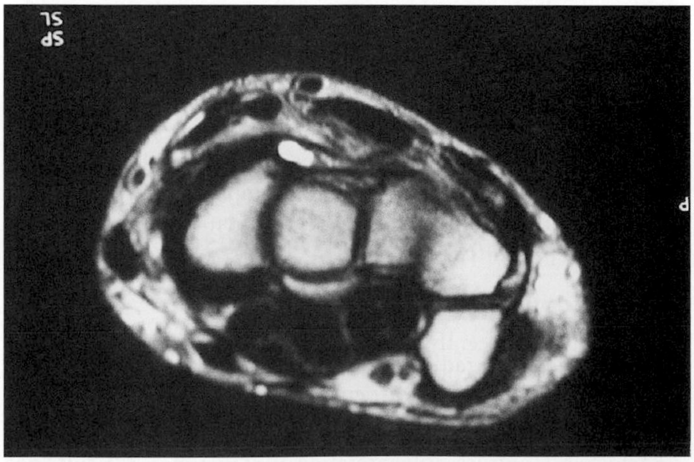

Fig. 6.1.8 Axial MRI image shows a small high-signal occult dorsal wrist ganglion. (Courtesy of the Department of Radiology, Nuffield Orthopaedic Centre, Oxford.)

Box 6.1.3 Investigations

- Plain radiography: the mainstay and usually diagnostic
- Fluoroscopy: for dynamic assessment
- Nuclear medicine: useful for non-specific localization
- CT scan: best for bone problems
- MRI: best for soft tissues
- Arthrography: best for ligament injuries/TFCC tears. Usually done with CT or MRI
- Arthroscopy: the gold standard assessment.

established by dynamic manoeuvres undertaken during radiocarpal and midcarpal arthroscopy.

Conclusion

There is no single clinical sign or investigation that can lead to an accurate diagnosis in cases of chronic wrist pain. The wide range of diagnostic investigations now available has revealed many pathological abnormalities in the painful wrist, although these changes are also seen in asymptomatic wrists. It is therefore essential to correlate the clinical information with the results of diagnostic studies before making decisions on management.

Further reading

Gilula, L.A. and Weeks, P.M. (1978). Post-traumatic ligamentous instabilities of the wrist. *Radiology*, **129**, 641–51. [The radiological basis for diagnosis of carpal instability is described. Line diagrams alongside radiographs aid the understanding of interpretation in this area.]

Gilula, L. and Yin, Y. (1996). *Imaging of the wrist and hand*. Philadelphia, PA: W.B. Saunders. [A comprehensive textbook of imaging of the wrist and hand. All imaging modalities are described. An initial section covers physical examination of the wrist. The description of plain radiography includes instability as well as normal variants.]

Oneson, S.R., Scales, L.M., Erickson, S.J., Timins, M.E. (1996). MR imaging of the painful wrist. *Radiographics*, **16**, 997–1008. [This paper gives a clear, easily understood, and well-illustrated account of the MRI findings in the major causes of chronic wrist pain.]

Watson, H.K. and Ballet, F.L. (1984). The SLAC wrist: scapholunate advanced collapse pattern of degenerative arthritis. *Journal of Hand Surgery*, 9A, 358–65. [The original description of the scapholunate advanced collapse wrist. The radiological features that are seen during progression from mild to severe disease are covered.]

6.2

Degenerative arthritis of the wrist

Peter Burge

Introduction

A strong, stable, mobile and painless wrist is the key to function of the hand. The multiple joint compartments of the wrist show very different susceptibility to degenerative arthritis. The frequency of involvement of joints of the wrist determined from study of 210 radiographs was radioscaphoid (RS) joint 55%, scaphoid-trapezoid-trapezium (STT) joint 26%, both RS and STT joints 14%, and other joints 5%. The fact that either the proximal or distal surface of the scaphoid was affected in 95% of cases emphasizes that bone's importance in the function of the wrist.

Radiocarpal osteoarthritis (Box 6.2.1)

Aetiology

Primary osteoarthritis of the radiocarpal joint is uncommon but may be associated with calcium pyrophosphate crystal deposition disease (CPDD) and with haemochromatosis. Most cases are secondary to conditions that damage articular cartilage or to injuries that increase surface pressure on articular cartilage by altering loading and joint contact areas. The causes of secondary degenerative arthritis are listed in Box 6.2.2.

Degenerative arthritis of the radioscaphoid joint is the final common pathway for several disorders that alter the mechanics of the wrist. The path of motion of the scaphoid in the elliptical radioscaphoid joint is controlled by ligamentous attachments to the radius and to the lunate. The scaphoid flexes during radial deviation and extends during ulnar deviation. The radiocarpal load is shared 60:40 between scaphoid and lunate. Injuries that destabilize the scaphoid, either by ligament disruption or by scaphoid fracture, affect the radioscaphoid joint in three ways: excessive scaphoid flexion; decreased articular surface contact; and increased radioscaphoid loading. The articular cartilage that is in contact with the unstable scaphoid (or, in the case of a scaphoid fracture, the unstable distal fragment) deteriorates rapidly in the face of this mechanical challenge, while the spherical and relatively unloaded radiolunate joint is preserved. Later, the capitolunate joint is

Box 6.2.1 Causes of secondary degenerative arthritis of the radiocarpal joint

- Intra-articular fractures of the distal radius
- Scaphoid non-union, malunion, and avascular necrosis
- Scapholunate instability
- Kienböck's disease
- Preiser's disease (idiopathic osteonecrosis of the scaphoid)
- Lunate fracture.

Box 6.2.2 Radiocarpal arthritis

- Cause:
  - Primary arthritis is uncommon
  - Mostly secondary, especially related to scaphoid problems (SLAC and SNAC wrist)
- History:
  - Pain
  - Stiffness
  - Reduced grip strength
  - Previous injury
- Examination:
  - Swelling
  - Tenderness
  - Reduced ROM (remember the functional range)
  - Reduced grip strength
- Investigations:
  - Radiology is characteristic
  - Other tests are infrequent.

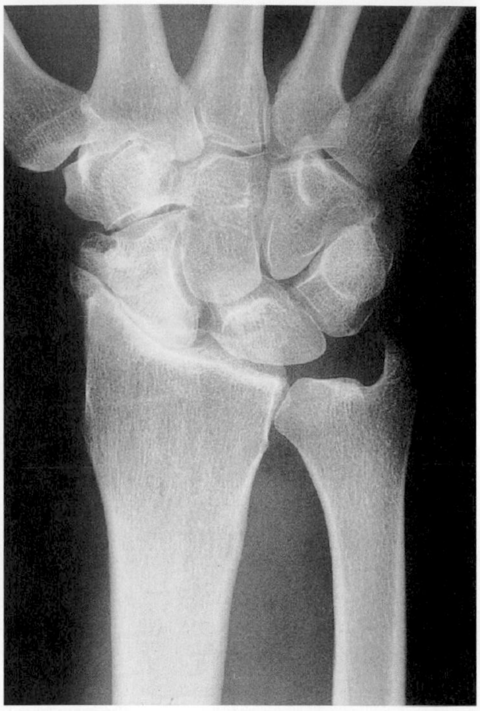

Fig 6.2.1 Radiograph of the scapholunate advanced collapse (SLAC) wrist, showing involvement of the radioscaphoid and midcarpal joints. The radiolunate joint is preserved.

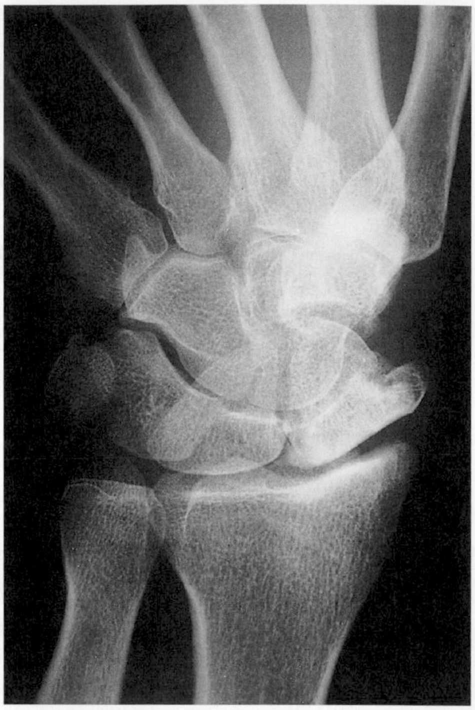

Fig 6.2.2 Early radioscaphoid osteoarthritis with beaking of the radial styloid and formation of osteophytes along the dorsal rim of the radius and the adjacent surface of the scaphoid.

affected. This characteristic pattern of degeneration is referred to as the ScaphoLunate Advanced Collapse (SLAC) wrist (Figure 6.2.1).

Clinical features

In the early stages, activity-related pain is experienced intermittently on the dorsoradial aspect of the wrist. As the process extends to the midcarpal joint, pain generally increases and is associated with loss of wrist motion and with loss of strength. In some cases, however, pain correlates poorly with the radiographic appearance and function remains good.

Radiography

The first sign of radioscaphoid osteoarthritis is beaking of the radial styloid. Loss of height of articular cartilage in the radioscaphoid joint and subchondral sclerosis follow. The changes are most marked along the dorsal rim of the radioscaphoid joint and may be associated with osteophytes that are best seen on oblique radiographs (Figure 6.2.2). Chondrocalcinosis may be seen in cases resulting from CPDD (Figure 6.2.3).

Non-operative management

Modification of activity, splintage, and analgesic medication are appropriate for modest symptoms. Steroid injection can give useful medium-term relief in patients who prefer to avoid operative treatment. Modest loss of wrist motion is consistent with good function. About 70% of normal daily activities can be accomplished within the range of 40° extension, 40° flexion, and 40-degree radial/ulnar deviation. Many patients adjust to their disability and do not require operative management.

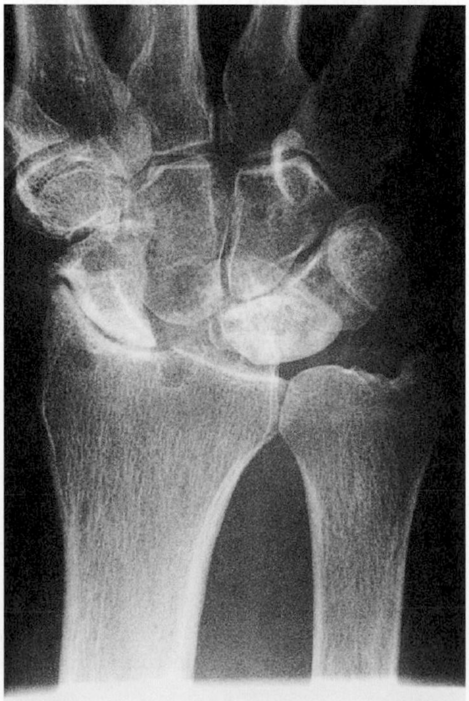

Fig 6.2.3 Severe SLAC wrist associated with CPPD. Note chondrocalcinosis in the triangular fibrocartilage.

Operative management

Wrist pain that persists despite non-operative management may require operative treatment (Box 6.2.3). The options are as follows:

Proximal row carpectomy

Excision of the proximal row of the carpus requires intact articular cartilage on the head of the capitate and the lunate fossa of the radius (Figure 6.2.4). The wrist is immobilized for 3–6 weeks. Strength and mobility improve over at least 12 months. A review of 22 cases after a minimum of 10 years found 14 patients very satisfied, four satisfied, and four failures requiring arthrodesis.

Scaphoid excision and midcarpal arthrodesis

The preservation of the spherical radiolunate joint in the late stages of the SLAC wrist allows it to be used as the sole articulating surface. Radioscaphoid impingement is relieved by excision of the scaphoid and the midcarpal joint is stabilized by arthrodesis (capitolunate or capitate-lunate-hamate-triquetrum) (Figure 6.2.5). Several studies have shown that proximal row carpectomy fares at least as well as scaphoid excision/midcarpal arthrodesis with regard to range of motion (ROM) and strength, and does not have the disadvantages of fixation-related complications, prolonged immobilization, and risk of non-union. However, scaphoid excision and midcarpal arthrodesis is the only alternative to total wrist arthrodesis when damage to the head of the capitate precludes proximal row carpectomy.

Radiocarpal arthrodesis

Arthrodesis of the radiocarpal joint is indicated for osteoarthritis confined to the radioscaphoid and/or radiolunate joints Intra-articular fracture of the distal radius is the most common cause.

Total wrist arthrodesis

Wrist arthrodesis is the definitive and durable solution for osteoarthritis of the wrist. The joint is fused in 15–25 degrees of extension and 0–15 degrees of ulnar deviation. Plate fixation has significantly a higher fusion rate than other techniques and is the method of choice for degenerative and post-traumatic arthritis (Figure 6.2.5).

Box 6.2.3 Treatment of radiocarpal osteoarthritis
◆ Non-operative (usually adequate): • Activity modification • Non-steroidal anti-inflammatories • Splint • Steroid injection ◆ Operative: • Denervation • Proximal row carpectomy • Partial fusion • Total fusion • Arthroplasty.

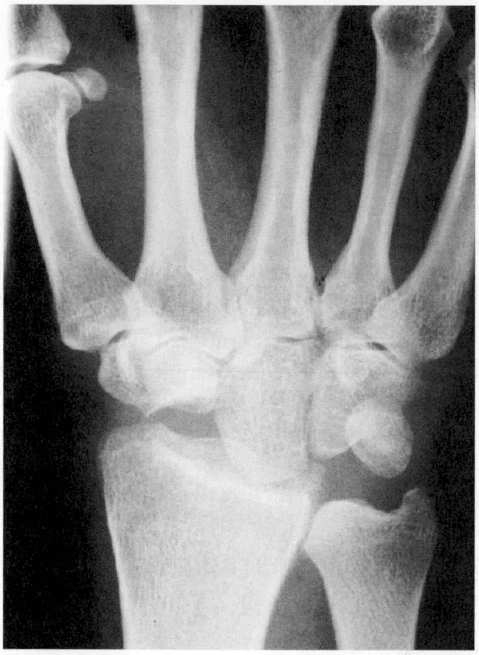

Fig 6.2.4 Proximal row carpectomy. The head of the capitate articulates with the lunate fossa of the radius. The tip of the radial styloid may require excision to prevent impingement against the trapezium.

The arthrodesis must include the radioscaphoid and midcarpal joints, but inclusion of the third carpometacarpal joint is controversial. In most cases, sufficient cancellous bone graft can be obtained from the distal radial metaphysis, obviating the need for iliac crest graft.

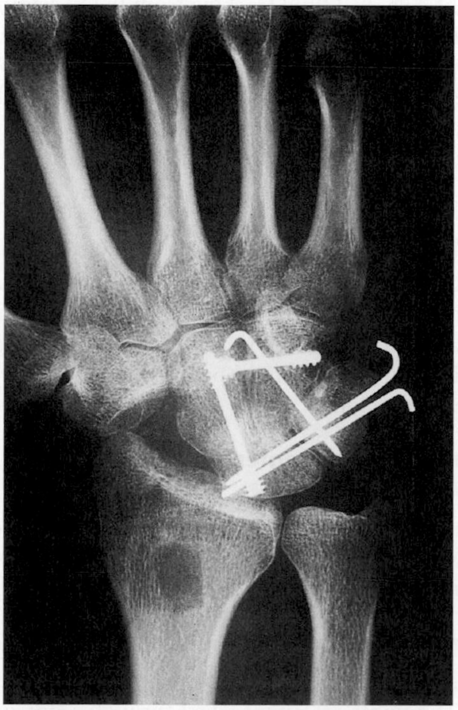

Fig 6.2.5 Scaphoid excision and midcarpal fusion for SLAC wrist.

Total wrist arthroplasty

Wrist arthroplasty is indicated mainly for severe rheumatoid arthritis. Patients who wish to maintain dexterity for low-demand activities of daily living may be suitable for wrist arthroplasty, but they must be willing to accept permanent restrictions in activity. Many patients with degenerative arthritis are young and active, and not suitable for wrist arthroplasty.

Wrist denervation

Division of multiple nerve branches that supply the wrist joint has been used to reduce pain from osteoarthritis and other painful disorders, either on its own or combined with other procedures. So-called total denervation requires multiple incisions around the wrist. Partial denervation, usually comprising the terminal branches of the posterior and anterior interosseous nerves through a dorsal approach, is also used. Preoperative diagnostic nerve blocks are believed to be helpful in predicting the effect of denervation.

Scaphoid-trapezoid-trapezium osteoarthritis (Box 6.2.4)

Aetiology

Osteoarthritis of the scaphoid-trapezoid-trapezium (STT joint) may be idiopathic, associated with CPDD, associated with trapeziometacarpal osteoarthritis, or secondary to trauma (intra-articular fractures and, possibly, ligament injury).

Clinical features

Pain on the dorsoradial aspect of the wrist is the characteristic symptom but the severity of pain is variable and asymptomatic. STT osteoarthritis is frequently seen on radiographs taken for another purpose. Local tenderness may be present over the dorsal and/or palmar surfaces of the STT joint. Loss of wrist motion is usually slight. Synovial fluid tracking from the STT joint along the flexor carpi radialis (FCR) tendon sheath may form a ganglion cyst just proximal to the wrist crease. STT osteoarthritis should be suspected when a ganglion cyst is seen at this site in an older individual. Rarely, osteophytes at the margins of the scaphotrapezial joint irritate the flexor carpi radialis tendon or flexor pollicis longus tendon, causing tendinitis or rupture.

Radiography

Loss of articular surface height in the scaphotrapezial and/or scaphotrapezoid joints is the earliest sign of STT osteoarthritis. Later, subchondral sclerosis, osteophytes and cysts appear (Figure 6.2.6). Oblique views are useful in showing the scaphotrapezial and trapeziometacarpal joints.

Non-operative management

Splintage and analgesic medication are the first line of treatment. Steroid injection may be given through dorsal or palmar approaches, and be guided by fluoroscopy if necessary. Non-operative treatment is sufficient for most cases.

Operative management

Arthrodesis of the STT joint is appropriate for isolated STT osteoarthritis. The joints are approached through a dorsoradial incision, avoiding branches of the superficial radial nerve. The alignment of the scaphoid and the spatial relationship of the three bones should be preserved, so as to avoid distortion of surrounding joints. Cancellous bone graft from the distal radius is packed between the decorticated surfaces and the bones are fixed together with pins, screws, or staples (Figure 6.2.7). If pins are used, their

Box 6.2.4 STT osteoarthritis

- Common
- Often asymptomatic or minimally symptomatic
- History:
  - Pain
  - Stiffness
  - Reduced strength
- Examination:
  - Tender over STT joint
  - Reduced ROM
- Treatment:
  - Non-operative (usually adequate):
    - Splints
    - Steroid injection
  - Operative:
    - STT fusion,
    - Excision of distal scaphoid
    - Trapezectomy for pantrapezial osteoarthritis

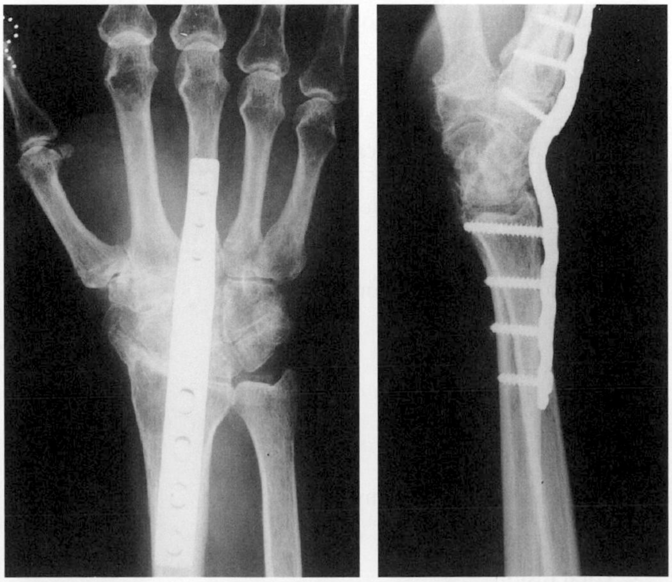

A B

Fig 6.2.6 Total wrist fusion for severe SLAC wrist, using a plate and distal radial bone graft (A, B).

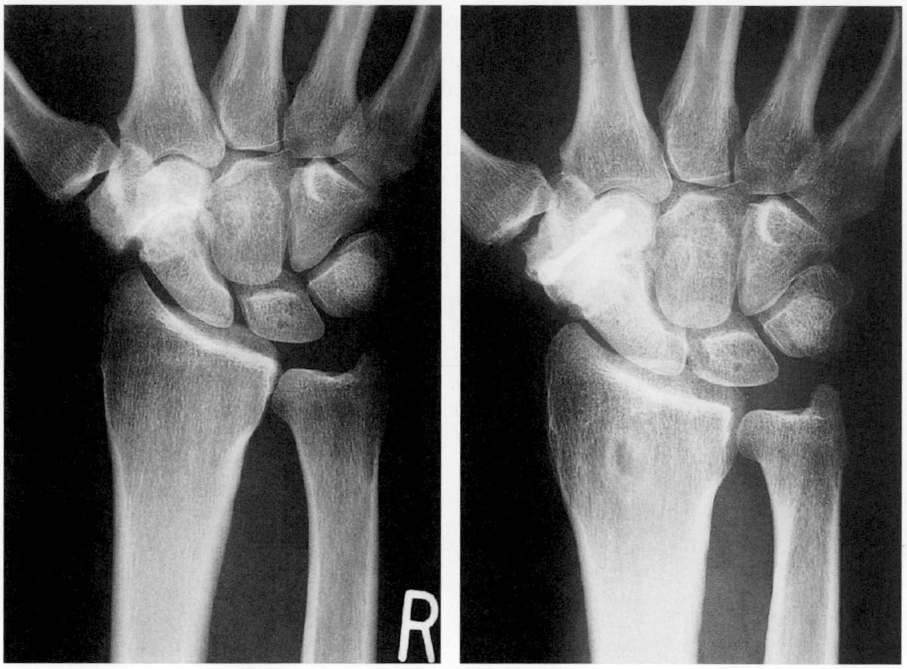

A B

Fig 6.2.7 A) Scaphoid-trapezoid-trapezium (STT) osteoarthritis. B) STT joint fusion.

ends should be left under the skin and removed later under local anaesthesia, to avoid the risk that pin-track infection will lead to septic arthritis. Good pain relief is usually achieved. However, complications are frequent (20–30%), including superficial radial neuroma, pin-track infection, and non-union. The postoperative range of wrist motion is approximately 75% of normal. Excision of the distal scaphoid is an alternative but the long-term results are unknown.

When both STT and trapeziometacarpal joints are involved, the trapezium should be excised. It may also be useful to undercut the scaphotrapezoid joint to minimize the risk of persistent pain from the scaphotrapezoid joint.

Pisotriquetral osteoarthritis (Box 6.2.5)

Aetiology

The pisiform is a sesamoid bone that lies within the flexor carpi ulnaris tendon and articulates with the triquetrum. Pisotriquetral osteoarthritis may be idiopathic or due to fractures of the pisotriquetral articular surfaces or instability of the pisotriquetral joint. It may also be associated with associated with loose bodies in the pisotriquetral joint and with entrapment or irritation of the ulnar nerve.

Clinical features

Pain over the palmar/ulnar surface of the wrist is the hallmark of pisotriquetral arthritis. Pain is frequently aggravated by flexion or ulnar deviation of the wrist. Local tenderness is present over the pisiform. Pain and crepitus may be elicited by compression and mediolateral movement of the pisiform against the triquetrum. Signs of ulnar nerve entrapment should be sought.

Radiography

Sclerosis of the pisiform may be apparent as an increase in density on the PA radiograph, but the joint is shown best on a 20-degree supinated oblique view or via computed tomography (CT). Osteophytes, sclerosis, and loss of articular cartilage height are seen on the underside of the pisiform and the adjacent surface of the triquetrum (Figure 6.2.8).

Non-operative management

Steroid injection through an ulnar approach can reduce pain substantially, though the effect may be short-lived.

Box 6.2.5 Pisotriquetral osteoarthritis

- Uncommon
- Often asymptomatic
- Examination:
  - Local tenderness
  - Positive shear stress test
- Treatment:
  - Non-operative: steroid injection
  - Operative: excision.

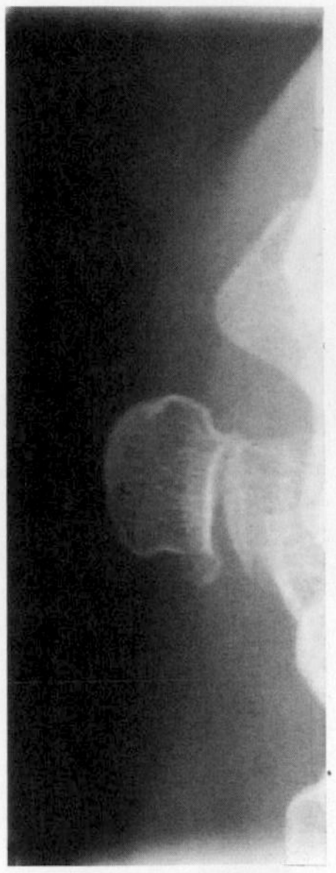

Fig 6.2.8 Oblique view showing osteoarthritis of the pisotriquetral joint.

Operative management

Excision of the pisiform is effective in relieving pain. It should be performed through a palmar or ulnar approach, protecting and, if necessary, decompressing the ulnar nerve and preserving the continuity of the flexor carpi ulnaris tendon. Excision does not appear to reduce wrist function significantly.

Further reading

Adams, B. D. (ed.) (2005). Wrist arthritis. *Hand Clinics*, **21**, 507–654. [Many aspects of degenerative arthritis discussed in this issue.]

Cooney, W.P., Linscheid, R.L., and Dobyns, J.H. (1997). *The Wrist. St Louis*, MO: C.V. Mosby. [A comprehensive and copiously illustrated textbook on the entire range of wrist disorders.]

Weiss, K. E. and Rodner, C. M. (2007). Osteoarthritis of the wrist. *Journal of Hand Surgery*, 32A, 725–46.

6.3

Kienböck's disease

Ilana Langdon and Grey Giddins

Summary points

- Uncommon but well recognised
- Cause – avascular necrosis
- Probably related to ulna positive variance
- History and examination may be suggestive but rarely diagnostic
- Radiographs or MRI are diagnostic
- Treatment is non-operative or operative
- Various operations are performed especially ulna shortening
- Most patients do well even with poor radiographs.

Introduction

Kienböck described avascular necrosis of the lunate in 1910. Over twice as many men than women are affected, with onset usually in the twenties or thirties. Kienbock's disease is usually unilateral. Although relatively uncommon, the pain, stiffness, and loss of strength may be devastating for otherwise healthy individuals, often in manual employment.

Anatomy

Vascular supply (Figure 6.3.1)

Kienböck's disease results from vascular compromise to the lunate. Like the scaphoid, most of the surface of the lunate is covered by hyaline cartilage. However, the dorsal and volar poles have small areas with ligamentous and capsular attachments including blood supply. Lee originally described the arterial anatomy in 1963. Gelberman elaborated on this using latex injection; most lunates have vessels entering from both the dorsal and volar sides with intraosseous anastomosis.

Biomechanics

The lunate has been described as the 'keystone' of the carpus. It transmits over 50% of the compressive load across the wrist joint. Approximately 80% of the load is transmitted through the radius and 20% through the ulna via the triangular fibrocartilage complex. The different compliance of the two interfaces may cause shear within the lunate.

The shape of the lunate may also affect force transmission; a triangular lunate may be more susceptible to microfracture than a square or rectangular lunate.

Aetiology (Box 6.3.1)

Vascular compromise is the common endpoint in Kienböck's disease; however, the relative contributions of intrinsic anatomical variants versus extrinsic trauma are contentious.

Intrinsic factors

Ulnar variance (Figure 6.3.2)

Ulnar variance as a risk factor for Kienböck's disease was first described in 1928 by Hultén, who compared the radiographs of 400 normal wrists with those of 23 patients with Kienböck's disease; 23% of normal wrists were ulnar negative, in comparison to 74% of the Kienböck's patients. Sixteen per cent of normal wrists were ulnar positive as opposed to none of the patients with Kienböck's disease.

Some other clinical studies have confirmed this association, others have not. Some studies have questionable validity, poor radiographic standardization, or controls. The consensus remains that Kienböck's disease is more common with an ulnar negative variance.

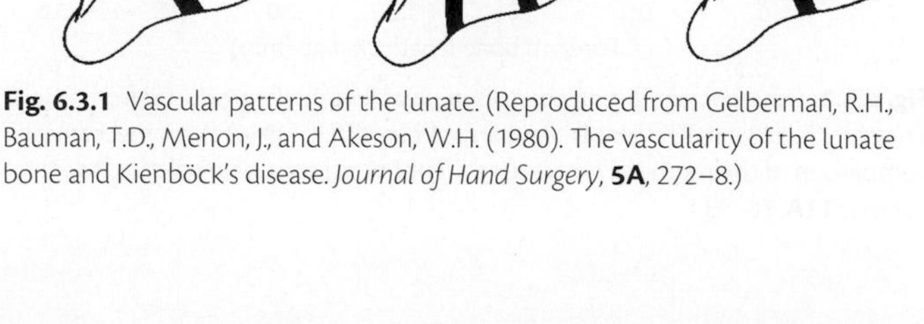

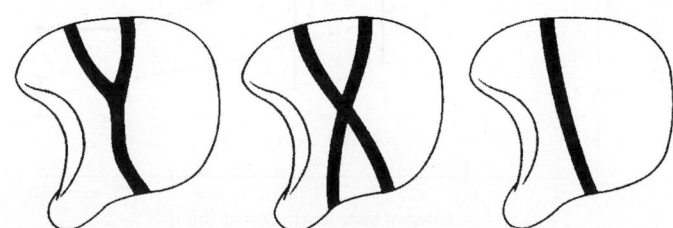

Fig. 6.3.1 Vascular patterns of the lunate. (Reproduced from Gelberman, R.H., Bauman, T.D., Menon, J., and Akeson, W.H. (1980). The vascularity of the lunate bone and Kienböck's disease. *Journal of Hand Surgery*, **5A**, 272–8.)

Box 6.3.1 Causation

- Idiopathic
- Probably related to:
  - Intrinsic factors—vascular insufficiency
  - Increased loading—ulna negative variance (controversial)
- Probably not due to direct trauma.

Biomechanical studies demonstrate the significant effect of changes in ulnar length on lunate strain; ulnar lengthening or radial shortening of 2mm more than halves lunate strain.

Vascular susceptibility

Kienböck speculated that injury may disrupt the lunate's blood supply. The rarity of Kienböck's disease following lunate and perilunate dislocations shows that the lunate can usually survive the loss of a major proportion of its vascular attachments.

Extrinsic factors

Fracture

External injury as an aetiological factor is suggested by increased frequency in manual labourers and in the dominant hand and by its infrequent bilateral occurrence. Clinical studies and cadaver models show susceptibility to fracture in hyperextension.

Vascular and traumatic susceptibility may be cofactors. The arterial supply has few or sometimes no anastomoses. Even a non-displaced stress fracture could disrupt this, causing devascularization. Conversely, a primary vascular injury would weaken the lunate, making it vulnerable to micro-shear fracture.

Clinical evaluation (Box 6.3.2)

Patients usually present with a gradual onset of wrist pain, but may describe a precipitating injury.

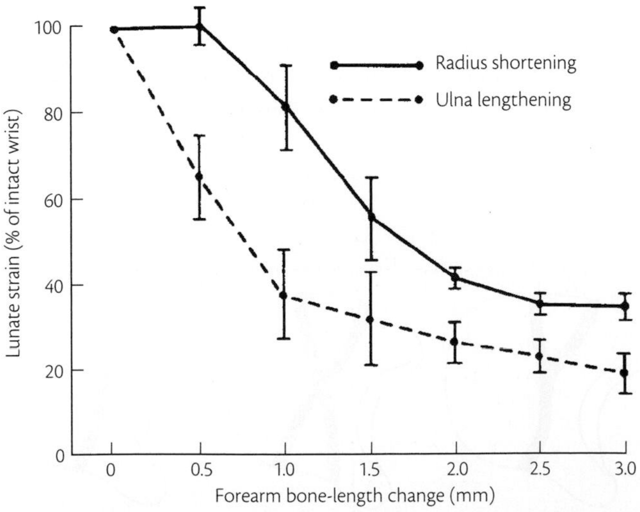

Fig. 6.3.2 Lunate strain during changes in ulnar length. (Reproduced from Trumble, T., Glisson, R.R., Seaber, A.V., and Urbaniak, J.R. (1986). A biomechanical comparison of the methods for treating Kienböck's disease. *Journal of Hand Surgery*, **11A**, 88–93.)

Box 6.3.2 Assessment

- History:
  - May be vague
  - There may be an minor injury starting the symptoms
- Examination:
  - May be local tenderness
  - Loss of range of movement esp extension

The physical findings are non-specific, but consistent. Inspection may reveal dorsal wrist swelling. Pain and tenderness is localized in the mid-dorsal area. Kienböck described exacerbation of pain on percussion of the third metacarpal head longitudinally. Wrist flexion and extension are decreased, as are radial and ulnar deviation to a lesser extent. Forearm rotation is usually normal. Grip strength is typically approximately halved.

Diagnostic tests (Box 6.3.3)

Confirmation of the diagnosis requires imaging; including plain radiography, radionuclide bone scan, computed tomography (CT) and/or magnetic resonance imaging (MRI).

Plain radiography

Plain radiographs including posteroanterior and lateral views are essential. The posteroanterior view must be taken with the forearm in neutral rotation, for true assessment of ulnar variance.

Changes on plain radiographs follow a consistent pattern, as described in the staging section. Initially, the lunate may appear normal or may have subtle horizontal lines suggesting compression fracture. Next the lunate appears more dense, consistent with avascularity. Lucency may be seen below the subchondral bone, similar to that seen in avascular necrosis of the femoral head. As the lunate collapses and fragments, the capitate begins to migrate proximally (Figure 6.3.3). The scaphoid falls into palmar flexion, similar to the pattern seen with scapholunate dissociation. In advanced cases, degenerative changes of the radiocarpal and intercarpal joints are seen.

Bone scans

Radionuclide imaging is useful in early disease, when history and examination are suggestive but radiographs are normal (Figure 6.3.4). Increased uptake ('hot spots') may be seen in all three phases: flow (angiogram), immediate (blood pool), and delayed (bone), suggesting hyperaemia of the soft tissues and bony reaction or repair.

Box 6.3.3 Investigations

- Radiology: usually diagnostic except in early (stage I) disease
- Nuclear medicine: can be used but superseded by MRI
- MRI: diagnostic.

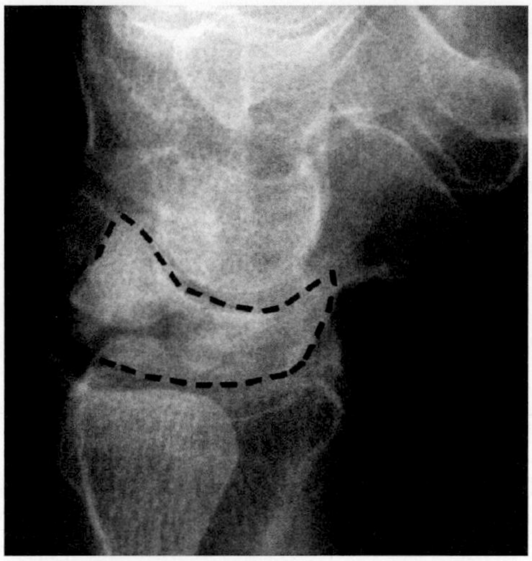

Fig. 6.3.3 Stage III lunate collapse.

Magnetic resonance imaging

MRI scanning in Kienböck's disease is now well established for early detection, assessment of bone viability, and evaluation of the response to treatment, rendering CT and bone scanning much less important (Figure 6.3.5).

Cancellous bone has adipose and haematopoietic tissue, and so high signal intensity on T_1-weighted images. Acute and chronic processes, including fracture, ischaemia, necrosis, and repair, alter marrow composition, decreasing signal intensity. MRI can identify lunate injury when plain films are still normal; the T_1 image abnormalities in Kienböck's disease are consistent. MRI cannot reliably distinguish between necrosis and reactive tissue; the zone of avascularity may be exaggerated.

MRI is also used for postoperative evaluation; return to normal signal intensity is observed in patients who undergo radial osteotomies for diseased lunates with normal shape.

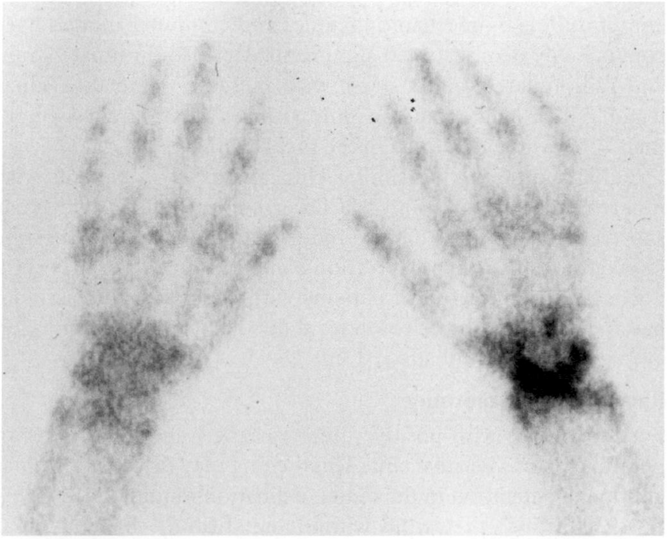

Fig. 6.3.4 Bone scan.

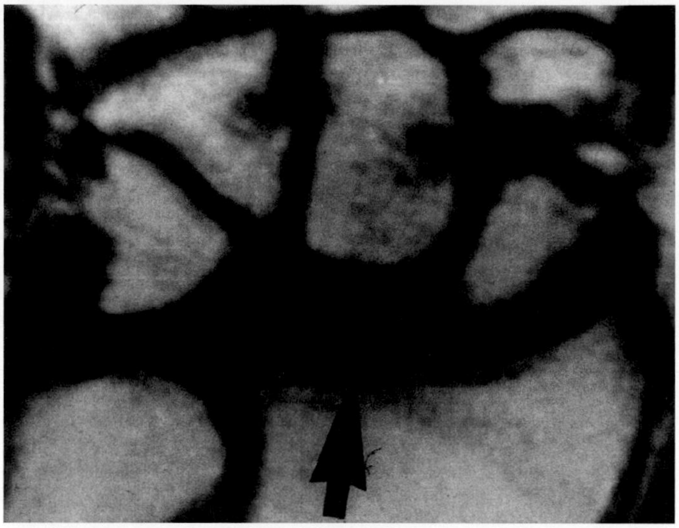

Fig. 6.3.5 MRI in complete avascular necrosis

Imaging algorithm

A diagnostic algorithm is shown in Figure 6.3.6. If history and examination suggest Kienböck's disease, plain radiographs are taken. If they show changes consistent with avascular necrosis

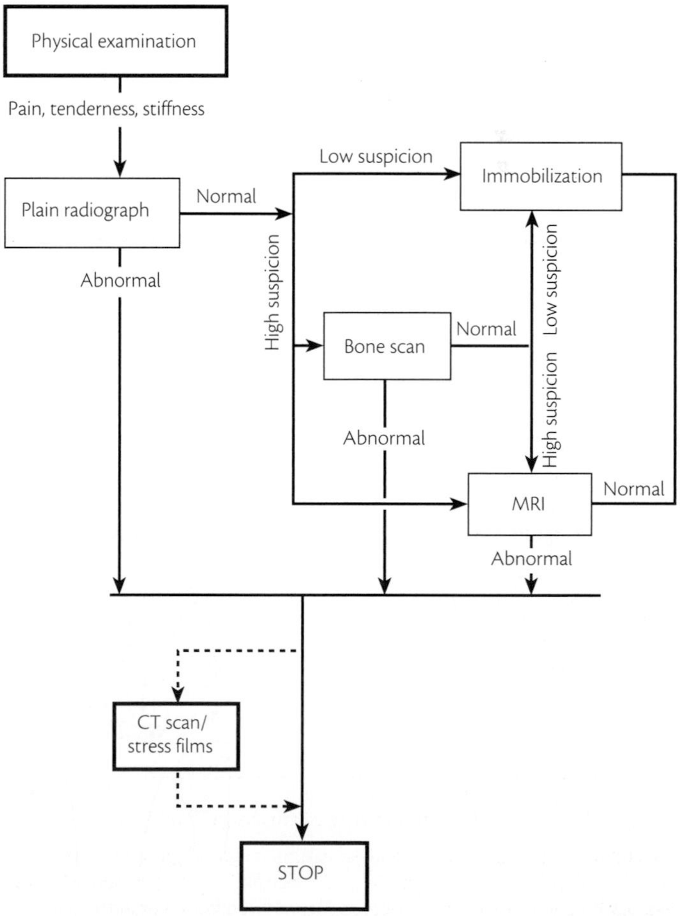

Fig. 6.3.6 Imaging algorithm.

(i.e. sclerosis, fragmentation, collapse), then no further tests are necessary.

With normal radiographs, a bone scan or MRI is indicated; either can show Kienböck's disease before plain radiographs. MRI is usually preferred to radionuclide imaging after normal plain films, as it can also show differential diagnoses and anatomical detail. Bone scanning remains useful for patients in whom MRI is contraindicated.

Staging

Staging is based on imaging and is divided into five distinct groups (Figure 6.3.7):

- Stage I: early disease with either normal radiographs or small linear compression/stress fractures
- Stage II: increased radiodensity, normal overall bony architecture
- Stage IIIA: collapse and fragmentation, typically with proximal capitate migration
- Stage IIIB: as stage IIIA, but with scapholunate dissociation and scaphoid flexion
- Stage IV: collapse with degenerative changes.

Management (Box 6.3.4)

Treatment options depend on staging, and include immobilization, revascularization, lunate unloading procedures, intercarpal

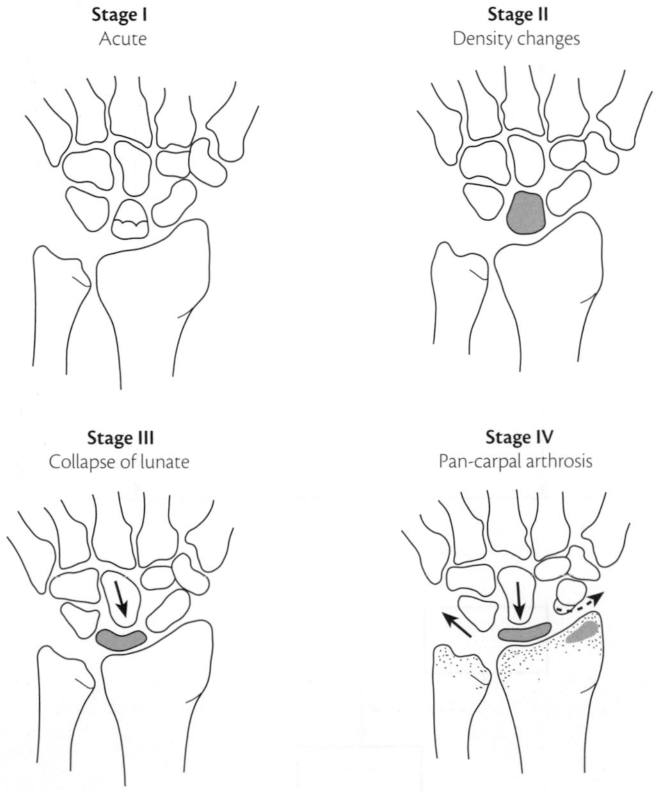

Fig. 6.3.7 Staging of Kienböck's disease. (Reproduced from Alexander *et al.* (1990).)

Box 6.3.4 Treatment

- Non-operative
- Immobilization
- Steroid injection.

fusions, and salvage procedures. Analysis of results is complicated by the poor correlation of clinical with radiographic findings, as with many wrist disorders.

Immobilization

Radiographic deterioration is common. Long-term studies show that no lunate ever returns to normal and that degenerative changes developed in half even when they are immobilized. However, radiographic changes did not correlate with clinical symptoms; despite these findings, most had either no pain or pain only with heavy work.

Revascularization

In a series of patients treated with dorsal metacarpal vascular bundle implantation (the majority of patients also underwent lunate core debridement and iliac crest grafting combined with either external fixation or scaphotrapeziotrapezoid fusion) after a mean of nearly 6 years, 50 of 51 patients had decreased pain and average improvement in grip strength of 13kg.

These techniques seem promising, especially combined with other techniques to protect or unload the lunate, during revascularization.

Unloading procedures

Other procedures designed to reduce stress through the lunate include ulnar lengthening, radial shortening, radial wedge osteotomy, capitate shortening, and intercarpal fusion.

Ulnar lengthening and radial shortening

'Joint-levelling' procedures were developed in response to the perceived relationship between ulnar minus variance and Kienböck's disease. Despite the controversy regarding the significance of variance, multiple biomechanical studies and computer models have convincingly demonstrated significant decreases in lunate strain and radiolunate contact stress with increases in relative ulnar length. Ulnar lengthening by 3mm reduces lunate strain by more than 70%, with 90% of that in the first 2mm.

Radial shortening has similar clinical success in patients with ulnar minus variance, and has fewer complications than ulnar shortening (Figure 6.3.8). The radius should be shortened to the level of the ulna, with compression plate fixation.

Long-term follow-up of patients with Kienböck's disease who had radial shortening osteotomies show that grip strength was, on average, 90% of the unaffected side.

Radial wedge osteotomy

For individuals with positive ulnar variance, and for some with neutral variance, relative ulnar lengthening may risk creating ulnar abutment. Alteration in the radial inclination modifies load transmission through the carpus without significantly changing ulnar variance.

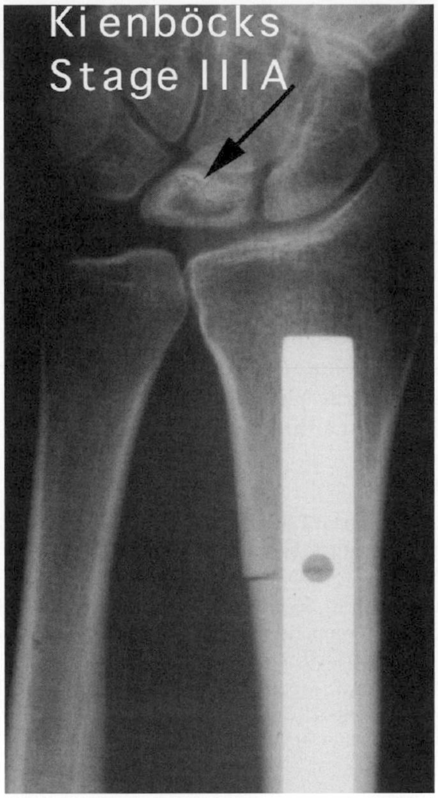

Fig. 6.3.8 Radial shortening.

Patients receiving osteotomies to *decrease inclination* are either pain free or have pain only with strenuous activity.

Intercarpal fusions

A variety of intercarpal fusions have been described that either directly (e.g. capitate shortening with capitate–hamate fusion) or indirectly (e.g. scaphotrapeziotrapezoid fusion) unload the lunate. They are particularly useful alternatives in ulnar positive variance or possibly when some lunate collapse has already occurred.

Capitate shortening

A 2- to 4-mm thick section of the capitate waist is removed with internal fixation of the remaining portions, generally combined with capitate–hamate fusion. Two-dimensional modelling of the procedure has predicted a 66% decrease in compressive load across the radiolunate articulation, with increases in scaphotrapezial load and triquetrohamate load.

Scaphotrapeziotrapezoid fusion

Scaphotrapeziotrapezoid fusion has been used in Kienböck's disease to unload the lunate indirectly (Figure 6.3.9); it also treats the rotation of the scaphoid seen in advanced cases. Biomechanical studies demonstrate that scaphotrapeziotrapezoid fusion with the scaphoid in neutral flexion reduces lunate strain by approximately 70%.

Patients treated by scaphotrapeziotrapezoid fusion had either no pain or mild pain with strenuous activity, but reduced range of motion (flexion 18%, extension 23%, radial deviation 69%); 13 of 15 returned to their original occupation. Some patients will require secondary excision of the lunate, and others will require late salvage procedures.

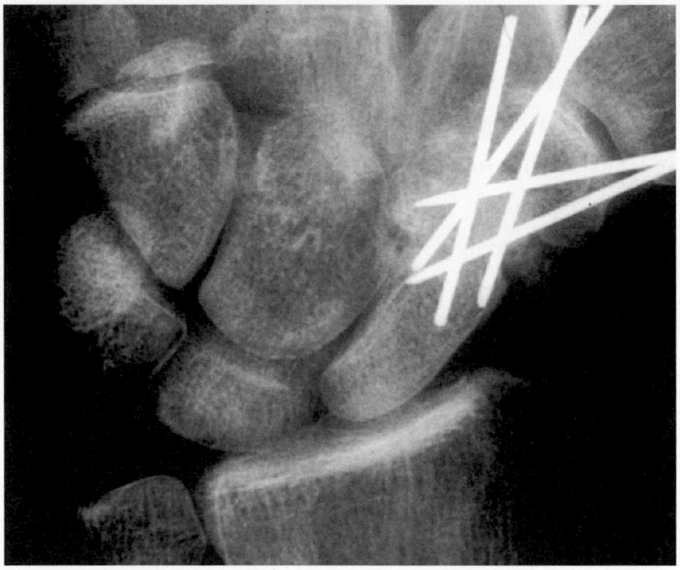

Fig. 6.3.9 Scaphotraziotrapezoid fusion.

Other intercarpal fusions

Scaphocapitate fusion can both unload the lunate and stabilize rotatory subluxation of the scaphoid. Cadaver and two-dimensional modelling studies predict significant unloading of both the capitolunate and radiolunate articulations. Clinically reports show wrist flexion and radial deviation are reduced by more than 60%, but there is good relief of pain and most patients returned to their original occupation. Although carpal height is maintained, some wrists show early radiocarpal degenerative change.

Isolated capitatohamate fusion has been used as a lunate unloading procedure. Although clinical success has been reported, cadaver studies and two-dimensional modelling do not demonstrate significant decreases in lunocapitate loading, radiolunate loading, or lunate strain.

Prosthetic arthroplasty

Silicone lunate replacement, which was introduced by Swanson (1970), gained popularity for treatment of stages II to IV of Kienböck's disease. It has also been used in combination with intercarpal fusions to limit the loading of the implant. The original implant, made of standard-grade elastomer, was later replaced by a high-grade elastomer with a deeper concavity to resist dislocation, and a titanium implant has also been designed, but not widely used. Despite early clinical successes, reports have continued linking silicone elastomer implants to particle debris synovitis. The long-term follow-up of patients with implants has shown radiographic and clinical deterioration.

Other treatment alternatives

Other primary treatments reported in the literature include sensory denervation of the wrist, forage of the distal radius, simple lunate excision, excision of the lunate with soft tissue interposition, and bone grafting of the lunate combined with external fixation.

Salvage

Total wrist arthrodesis is the procedure of choice following failed treatment, particularly when secondary osteoarthritis has

Box 6.3.5 Treatment

- Operative
- Revascularization for early (stage I and some stage II) disease
- Unloading the lunoradial joint
- Radial osteotomy
- Intercarpal fusion
- Wrist arthroplasty
- Salvage procedures especially proximal row carpectomy.

developed or if return to manual occupation is required. If the articular surfaces are relatively preserved and loss of motion is unacceptable, proximal row carpectomy is an alternative as both a primary or salvage procedure. Most patients will have either mild or no pain. Wrist motion is generally improved slightly while grip strength more than doubles.

As designs improve, third-generation total wrist arthroplasty is becoming an accepted alternative to arthrodesis in non-manual workers.

Conclusions

The diagnosis of Kienböck's disease is based on history, examination, and imaging. Staging is based on plain radiographs, with additional information primarily from MRI.

For stages I, II, and III, the aim of treatment is prevention of further collapse during healing and revascularization. Protection or unloading of the lunate is achieved by various techniques, depending on ulnar variance. In negative or neutral ulnar variance, radial shortening has established effectiveness. Capitate shortening, radial wedge osteotomy, proximal row carpectomy and intercarpal fusions are alternatives for patients with positive variance.

In stage IIIB, a scaphocapitate or scaphotrapeziotrapezoid fusion also corrects rotatory scaphoid subluxation.

For stage IV a wrist arthrodesis is generally indicated.

Further reading

Gelberman, R.H., Bauman, T.D., Menon, J., and Akeson, W.H. (1980). The vascularity of the lunate bone and Kienböck's disease. *Journal of Hand Surgery*, **5A**, 272–8.

Trumble, T., Glisson, R.R., Seaber, A.V., and Urbaniak, J.R. (1986). A biomechanical comparison of the methods for treating Kienböck's disease. *Journal of Hand Surgery*, **11A**, 88–93.

Weiss, A.P., Weiland, A.J., Moore, J.R., Wilgis, E.F. (1991). Radial shortening for Kienböck disease. *Journal of Bone and Joint Surgery*, **73A**, 384–91.

6.4

The distal radioulnar joint

Ruby Grewal, James H. Roth, and G.J.W. King

Summary points

DRUJ Stabilizers:

- Primary: TFCC
- Secondary: interosseous membrane, extensor retinaculum, dorsal carpal ligament complex, and the forearm muscles especially the pronator quadratus.

Investigations:

- Plain or stress radiography
- Arthrography
- CT: for bone alignment especially DRUJ arthritis and subluxation
- MRI: for soft tissue constraints
- Arthroscopy.

TFCC Pathology:

1. Traumatic
   - Central or peripheral
   - Treatment: Central — debridement, Peripheral — repair/decompression.
2. Degenerative
   - Mainly due to ulnocarpal impingement
   - Treatment: decompression by shortening or Feldon wafer.

DRUJ OA:

- Treatment: Steroid injection or Surgery
- Surgical Options
- Darrach's
- Partial resection
- Sauve-Kapandji
- Replacement.

Introduction

Derangements of the distal radioulnar joint (DRUJ) are common causes of acute and chronic ulnar wrist pain and dysfunction. This chapter will focus on triangular fibrocartilage complex (TFCC) disorders, ulnar impaction, instability, and degenerative arthroses. Fractures and dislocations, congenital and developmental disorders, and rheumatic diseases affecting the DRUJ are covered in other chapters.

Anatomy and biomechanics

The anatomy and biomechanics of the DRUJ are complex and interplay with the proximal radioulnar joint, interosseous membrane, and the ulnar carpus during forearm and wrist motion. Pathology at any one of these may affect their composite function.

The DRUJ is a trochoid articulation between the sigmoid notch of the radius and the ulnar head. The sigmoid notch has a 47–80-degree arc of curvature and a radius of approximately 15mm. The ulnar head is semicylindrical in cross-section. It has articular cartilage covering 90–135 degrees of its circumference and a radius of curvature of 10mm (Box 6.4.1 and Figure 6.4.1). Although 60–80 degrees of the ulnar articular surface engages the sigmoid notch in neutral rotation, the contact is less than 10 degrees at the extremes of rotation. Minimal bony constraint allows a wide arc of motion but at the expense of intrinsic instability that is limited primarily by soft-tissue restraints.

The primary soft tissue stabilizer of the DRUJ is the TFCC (Figure 6.4.2). It separates the DRUJ and the radiocarpal joint, and comprises the triangular fibrocartilage (TFC), the dorsal and palmar radioulnar ligaments, the ulnocarpal meniscus homologue, and the sheath of the tendon of the extensor carpi ulnaris (ECU). The palmar ulnocarpal ligaments are intimately related to the TFCC and contribute to ulnar wrist stability.

The TFC is triangular in shape and biconcave on its distal surface. It arises from the distal margin of the sigmoid notch and courses medially where its apex inserts into the fovea at the base of

Box 6.4.1 Anatomy of the DRUJ

- Sigmoid notch: arc of 47–80 degrees
- Ulna head: arc of articular cartilage 90–135 degrees
- Contact: mid part up to 80 degrees but <10 degrees at extremes.

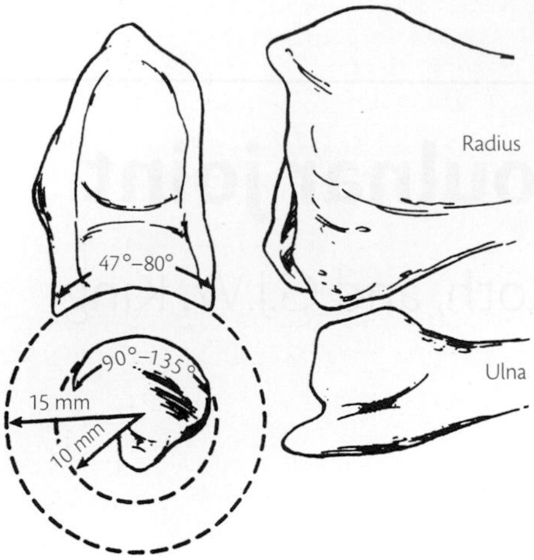

Fig. 6.4.1 Osseous anatomy and congruity of DRUJ. The articulation between the sigmoid notch of the radius and the ulnar head is viewed both end-on (left) and dorsally (right). The radius of curvature of the sigmoid notch is greater than that of the ulnar head, allowing sliding of the ulna relative to the radius with forearm rotation. The ulnar head has a greater arc covered with articular cartilage than the sigmoid notch. (Reproduced from Chidgey (1995).)

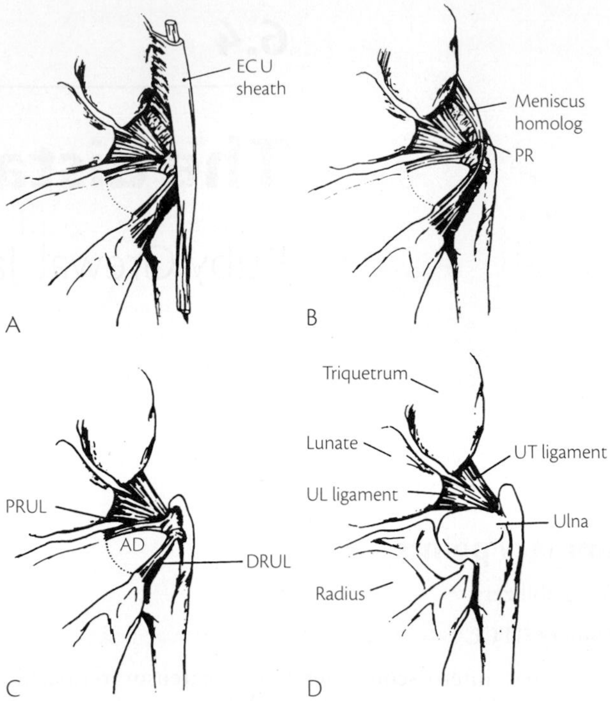

Fig. 6.4.2 Ligaments of the DRUJ and dorsal views of the TFCC. A) All components of the TFCC shown. The sheath of the ECU is an important stabilizer of the DRUJ; the infratendinous portion is sometimes referred to as the ulnar collateral ligament. B) The meniscus homologue attaches to the dorsal margin of the radius and the palmar/ulnar aspect of the triquetrum. As it passes the palmar radioulnar ligaments it forms the roof of the prestyloid recess, a synovial lined recess that may connect to the palmar aspect of the ulnar styloid. C) The meniscus homologue has been removed to show the TFC, also termed the articular disc (AD), and the dorsal and palmar radioulnar ligaments (DRUL, PRUL). D) The articular disc has been removed to expose the ulnolunate (UL) and ulnotriquetral (UT) ligaments, which extend form their respective carpal bones and lunotriquetral ligament to the foveal area and base of the ulnar styloid. (Reproduced from Chidgey (1995).)

the ulnar styloid. It is thickest (approximately 5mm) at its ulnar insertion, and thinnest centrally at its origin from the radius (approximately 2mm). The central portion, or articular disc, is avascular chondroid fibrocartilage with interwoven collagen fibres arising from the hyaline cartilage of the lunate fossa, and is adapted to compressive loading. The origin is reinforced by thick collagen bundles projecting 1–2mm from the radius creating a juncture that is a common site of TFC tears. In contrast, the TFC thickens dorsally and volarly to become the dorsal and volar radioulnar ligaments, comprising well-vascularized connective tissue with longitudinally oriented collagen fibres that arise from and insert into bone and are best suited to resisting tensile loads.

Perforations of the TFC are found with increasing prevalence with age over 30 years Excessive length of the ulna with respect to the radius (positive ulnar variance) is directly proportional to the age-related incidence of TFCC perforation, and inversely proportional to TFCC thickness.

Of the TFCC components, the palmar and dorsal radioulnar ligaments are the primary stabilizers of the DRUJ, and the joint is most stable when these are in tension at the extremes of rotation. The sheath of the ECU, the floor of which has been called the ulnar collateral ligament, extends from the ECU groove on the dorsal ulna to insert on the dorsal base of the fifth metacarpal. Its role in stabilizing the distal ulna is augmented by the dynamic effects of the ECU tendon.

The volar ulnolunate and ulnotriquetral ligaments arise at the base of the ulnar styloid, where the apex of the TFCs attaches. They course along its volar margin to diverge and insert independently into the lunate and triquetrum and into the lunotriquetral interosseous ligament. They act primarily in stabilizing the ulna and palmar carpus and resist dorsal displacement of the distal ulna.

The secondary stabilizers of the DRUJ include the bony conformation of the sigmoid notch, the interosseous membrane, the extensor retinaculum, the dorsal carpal ligament complex, and the forearm muscles that cross the pronation/supination axis, especially the pronator quadratus (Box 6.4.2). Watanabe and colleagues found that sectioning the joint capsule affected DRUJ stability in pronation and supination. They also demonstrated that dorsal capsular imbrication contributed to stability in pronation and volar capsular imbrication contributed to stability in supination. This effect was seen in positions of rotation greater than 60 degrees and was most evident in full pronation and supination.

The central 80–85% of the TFC is avascular and has no potential for healing. The peripheral 15–20% of the articular disc and the dorsal and palmar ligaments are well vascularized and are capable of healing (Figure 6.4.3).

The radiocarpal joint carries about 80% of the compressive load across the wrist; 20% is transmitted via the TFC and ulna in wrists

Box 6.4.2 Stabilizers of DRUJ

- Primary: TFCC
- Secondary: interosseous membrane, extensor retinaculum, dorsal carpal ligament complex, and the forearm muscles especially the pronator quadratus.

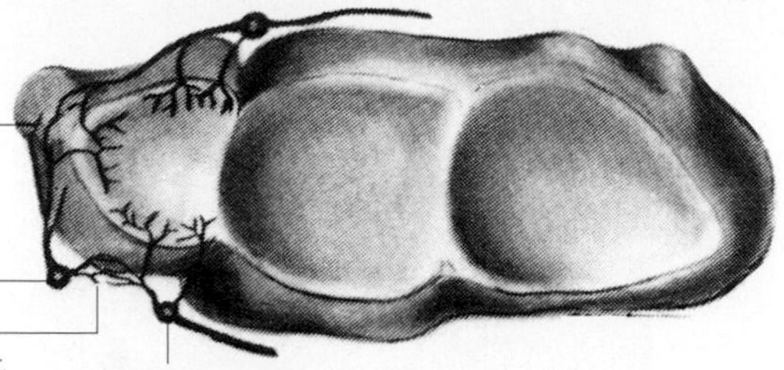

Fig. 6.4.3 Vascularity of TFCC. The TFC is viewed from its carpal side to demonstrate the sources of its arterial supply, and the poor vascularity of the centrum and its radial attachment. (Reproduced from Thiru-Pathi *et al.* (1986).)

with neutral ulnar variance. The load distribution between radius and ulna shows only a weak positive relationship to ulnar variance, probably because negative ulnar variants have thicker TFCs. However, surgical changes in ulnar variance alter force transmission dramatically: a 2.5-mm increase raises the ulnocarpal load to 42%; and a 2.5-mm decrease or excision of the disc lowers it to 4.3%. Up to two-thirds of the articular disc can be excised before changes in axial load transmission occur.

Evaluation

History and physical examination

The clinical assessment of patients with ulnar wrist pain includes the history of injury or onset of symptoms, the nature of the symptoms, and a provocative examination directed at localizing the pathological anatomy.

Provocative manoeuvres such as the 'ballottement', 'shuck', and 'shear' tests attempt to distinguish lunotriquetral abnormalities from the TFCC disorders. A positive 'ulnar fovea sign' identifies foveal disruption of the distal radioulnar ligaments and ulnotriquetral ligament injuries. The DRUJ is assessed by palpation, the 'grind test', attempting to elicit the 'piano key' sign and comparison with the opposite side, bearing in mind that signs may be dependent on the rotational position of the forearm (Table 6.4.1).

Imaging studies

Plain radiographs

Since the relative length of radius and ulna varies with rotation of the forearm, standardized positioning with the forearm in neutral rotation is critical for meaningful study and comparative measurements of the DRUJ (Figure 6.4.4).

Table 6.4.1 Provocative tests

Test	Evaluates	Technique	Finding
Lunotriquetral grind test	Lunotriquetral pathology	Examiner stabilizes hand and wrist with one hand and uses the other thumb to push the ulnar side of the radially toward the lunate	Pain
Shuck test	Lunotriquetral stability	Examiner's thumb on pisiform and fingers on dorsal lunate, deviation of wrist radially and ulnarly; or the pisiform and triquetrum are stabilized with one hand while the other shucks the medial carpus back and forth in a dorsoplamer direction.	Pain on dorsal aspect of the wrist at the lunate or lunotriquetral interval
Lunotriquetral ballottement or shear	Lunotriquetral stability and inflammation	As for scapholunate ballottement but with the lunate in one hand and the pisiform/triquetrum in the other; the bones are translated with respect to one another	Pain and/or instability at the lunotriquetral interval
Pisotriquetral shear test	Pisotriquetral stability	Examiner's thumb is hooked on radial aspect of pisiform and it is pulled toward the ulna	Pain or instability
Pisotriquetral grind	Pisotriquetral joint synovitis or arthritis	Examiner's thumb on pisiform and fingers of same hand on dorsal triquetrum, and joint is compressed	Pain or crepitus with compression
TFCC load and shear test	TFCC	Examiner grasps distal radius and ulna in one hand and metacarpals in the other; wrist is ulnarly deviated, then flexed and extended	Pain with ulnar deviation = positive load test
			Pain and snapping with flexion and extension = positive stress test
ECU instability	ECU instability	Examiner grasps distal radioulnar area and palpates the ECU in its groove on the dorsal ulna; forearm is then pronated and supinated; track of the ECU is palpated and a finger is used to hook it just distal to the ulnar head; ECU is then stressed in various angles of pronation and supination	Instability of ECU from the normal confines of the groove
Piano key test	TFCC instability with palmar sag of the carpus relative to the ulna	Patient's hand is placed palm down on table and attempts to force pisiform onto the table	Distal ulna shifts from slightly dorsal downward toward the table; must compare with contralateral for normal
DRUJ ballottement or shear test	DRUJ stability and arthritis	Examiner grasps distal ulna in one hand and the distal radius in the other; the forearm is then pronated and supinated and the radius and ulna are translated on each other in various positions	Instability, pain, and/or crepitus; must compare with contralateral side for normal
DRUJ grind test	DRUJ synovitis or arthritis	Examiner squeezes middle third of forearm to compress ulnar head into sigmoid notch and forearm is slightly rotated	Pain and crepitus

Adapted from Terrill (1994).

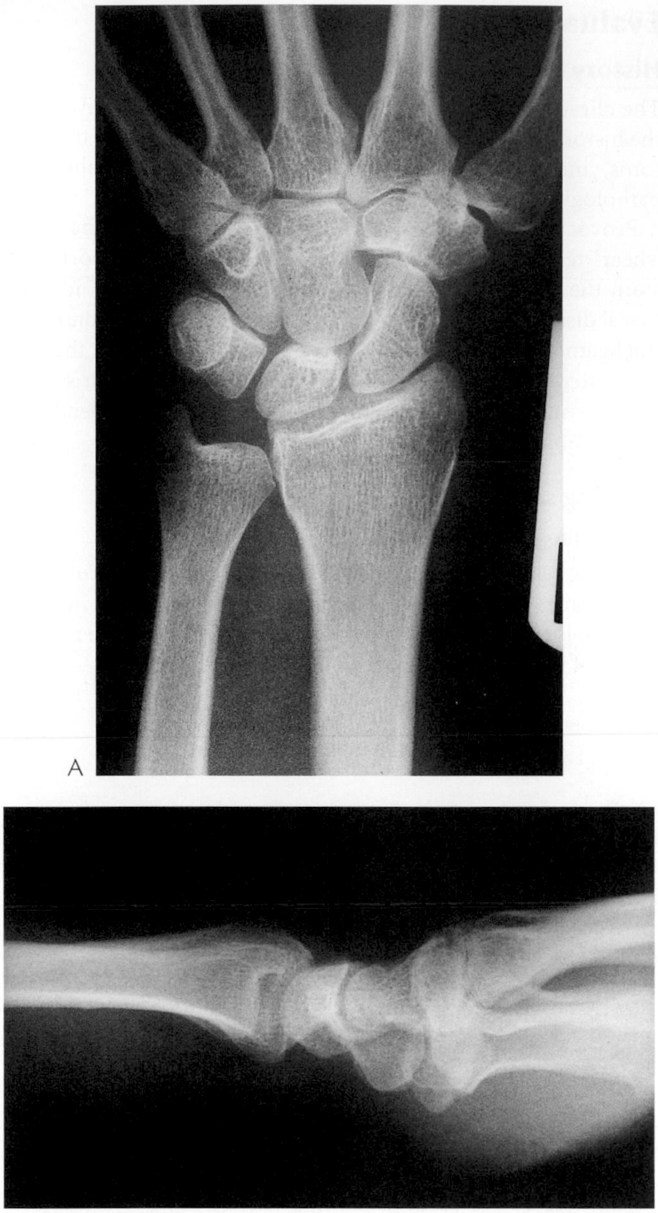

Fig. 6.4.4 Anteroposterior and lateral radiographs of the wrist. Normal radiographs of the wrist. The anteroposterior radiograph (A) demonstrates neutral ulnar variance and no evidence of degenerative changes of the DRUJ. The lateral radiograph (B) shows the normal overlap of the radius and ulna. The scaphoid proximal pole is central in the lunate, demonstrating a true lateral of the wrist and confirming that subluxation of the DRUJ is not present.

Stress or provocative views causing subluxation or ulnar impaction, such as full pronation while making a tight fist, may be useful in demonstrating instability patterns or impingement.

Arthrography

Arthrography can demonstrate the integrity of the soft tissue structures around the DRUJ (Figure 6.4.5).

While intercompartmental dye tracking may suggest an anatomical abnormality, the relation to symptoms is far from clear. Attritional abnormalities increase with age such that up to 50% of asymptomatic wrists will demonstrate 'lesions' by age 50. In a study of post-traumatic wrist pain, 74% of patients had 'abnormal' communications in the asymptomatic opposite wrist.

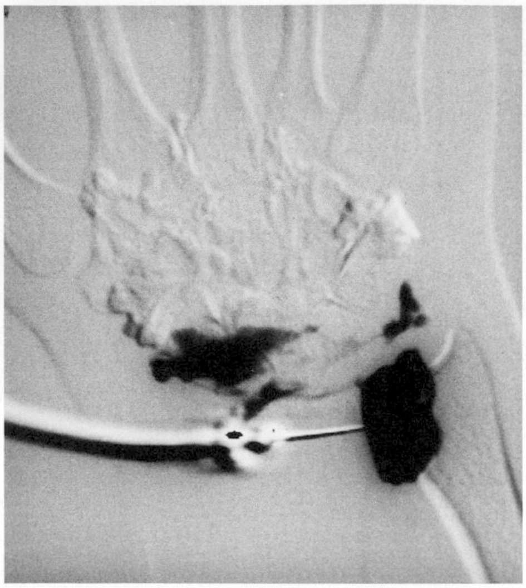

Fig. 6.4.5 Arthrogram with TFC tear of a 45-year-old woman with a history of chronic ulnar wrist pain and clicking. Injection of the DRUJ with contrast dye demonstrates a communication with the radiocarpal joint, confirming a TFC tear.

Computed tomography

Computed tomography (CT) is useful in diagnosing DRUJ subluxation and dislocation, as well for assessing the congruity of the articular surfaces in fractures and arthritic conditions of the sigmoid notch and ulnar head (Figure 6.4.6). To assess subluxation, CT scans of both wrists in neutral and both full supination and pronation are recommended and stress CT scans may be helpful.

Magnetic resonance imaging

While CT scanning best defines bony anatomy, magnetic resonance imaging (MRI) is the preferred method for non-invasive evaluation of the soft tissues, in particular the TFCC and associated ligaments. Using a wrist coil, T_2-weighted images best demonstrate traumatic tears, as synovial fluid has a high-intensity signal that provides contrast to fill defects (Figure 6.4.7). With T_1-weighted images, degenerative and traumatic tears are seen but difficult to distinguish. Radiocarpal joint injection of gadopentetate

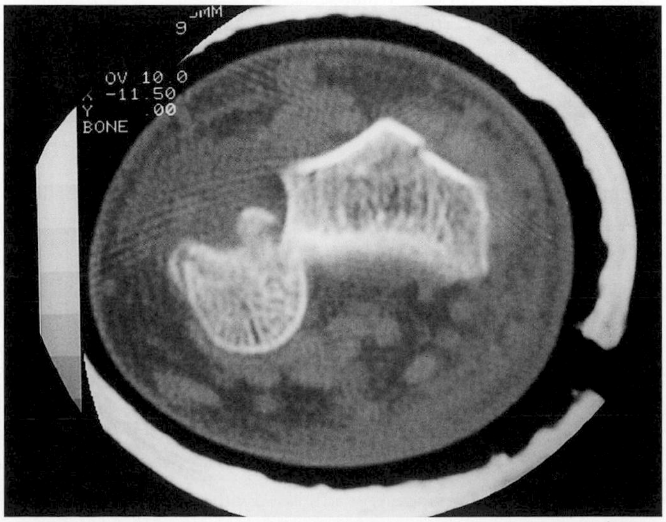

Fig. 6.4.6 CT scan of dislocated DRUJ of a 54-year-old man with an acute distal radial fracture. Plain radiographs suggestive of a DRUJ subluxation. A CT scan performed through plaster confirms a volar dislocation of the ulnar head.

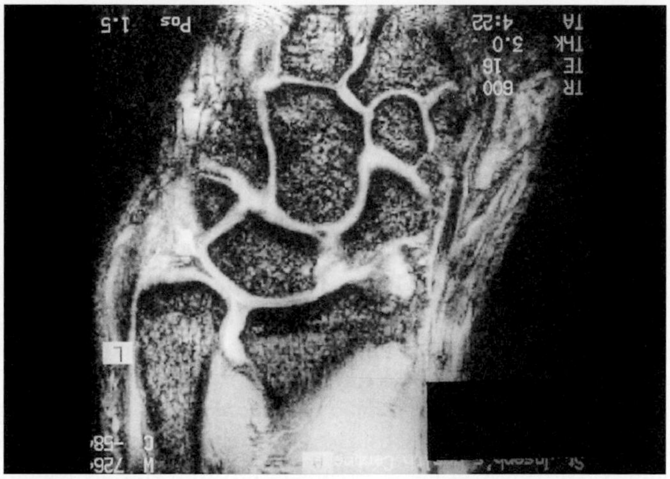

Fig. 6.4.7 MRI of TFC tear. MRI of a chronic TFC tear due to ulnar impaction from positive ulnar variance. The discontinuity in the TFC can be seen, as can the effusion in the DRUJ.

dimeglumine augments diagnostic accuracy for TFCC tears and has taken over from standard arthrography.

Arthroscopy

Arthroscopy is the 'gold standard' assessment of the wrist and TFCC but the DRUJ is difficult to visualize and so arthroscopy of the DRUJ is performed infrequently.

Distal radioulnar joint disorders

DRUJ disorders can be classified as acute, i.e. fractures and dislocations (see Chapter XX) or chronic. Chronic DRUJ disorders include TFCC tears, instability, arthritis, extensor carpi radialis subluxation, and contracture.

Triangular fibrocartilage complex

Palmer classified TFCC lesions as traumatic (type I) and degenerative (type II) (Table 6.4.2). Class II lesions are generally associated with ulnocarpal impaction syndrome. Traumatic and degenerative lesions may lead to DRUJ instability, which may be static or, more commonly, dynamic.

Type I: traumatic injuries

Type I injuries may result from various combinations of distal–proximal compression, shear, torsion, and radioulnar tension. Acute lesions are most frequently secondary to a fall on an outstretched hand in a patient who has ulnar neutral or positive variance.

Box 6.4.3 Investigations

- Plain radiography: look for variance and shape of DRUJ
- Stress radiography: for instability
- Arthrography: for TFCC tears
- CT: for bone alignment especially DRUJ arthritis and subluxation
- MRI: for soft tissue constraints
- Arthroscopy: difficult and limited role

Table 6.4.2 TFCC abnormalities

Class I: traumatic	
Type A	Central perforation
Type B	Ulnar avulsion
	With distal ulnar fracture
	Without distal ulnar fracture
Type C	Distal avulsion
Type D	Radial avulsion
	With sigmoid notch fracture
	Without sigmoid notch fracture
Class II: degenerative (ulnocarpal impaction syndrome)	
Stage A	TFCC wear
Stage B	TFCC wear + lunate and/or ulnar chondromalacia
Stage C	TFCC perforation + lunate and/or ulnar chondromalacia
Stage D	TFCC perforation + lunate and/or ulnar chondromalacia + lunotriquetral ligament perforation
Stage E	TFCC perforation + lunate and/or ulnar chondromalacia + lunotriquetral ligament perforation + ulnocarpal arthritis

Adapted from Palmer (1989).

Patients often present weeks or months after injury. Treatment is directed at relieving pain and restoring stability, with the specific approach being determined primarily by the vascularity of the injured TFCC component and its potential for healing. If positive ulnar variance or significant cartilage damage exists, consideration should be given to ulnar recession to avoid persistent ulnar impaction postoperatively.

Type I injuries are further subclassified.

Type IA lesions occur in the central articular disc and are not associated with DRUJ instability. As this avascular area has no ability to heal, arthroscopic debridement is the treatment of choice. Up to two-thirds of the central TFC can be excised without altering force transmission or DRUJ stability providing the peripheral 2mm of the disc, and the dorsal and volar radioulnar ligaments, are preserved.

Type IB lesions occur in the well-vascularized periphery of the TFC, at the base of the ulnar styloid. They may be associated with an ulnar styloid fracture and/or mild instability of the DRUJ. Significant displacement of the ulnar styloid fragment in unstable injuries requires reduction by closed means or by internal fixation. Type IB injuries may also be associated with acute ECU subluxation that will require reduction and possibly stabilization. Because these tears are located in the well-vascularized periphery of the TFC, they have potential to heal, therefore surgery is not required if the DRUJ is stable. If the DRUJ is unstable, the TFC should be repaired using either an open or arthroscopic technique. Each technique has its proponents.

Type IC injuries are least common and involve disruption of the ulnocarpal ligaments. Although readily diagnosed arthroscopically they may be repaired by open or arthroscopic methods.

Type ID lesions occur when the TFC detaches radially, from the sigmoid notch of the distal radius. Like IC tears, these injuries are also uncommon. They are frequently painful and destabilizing but are difficult to treat because of the avascularity of the radial margin

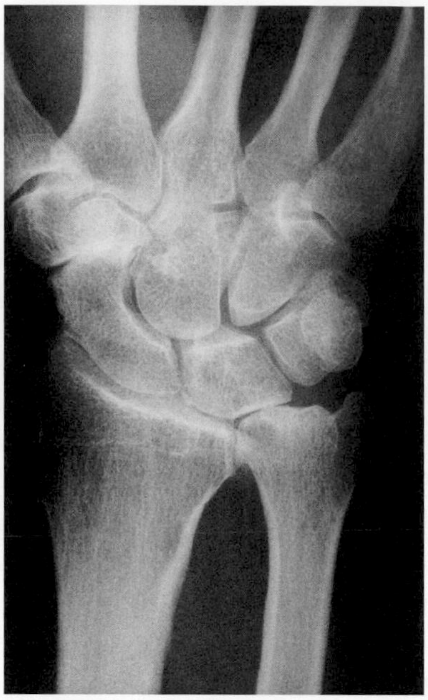

Fig. 6.4.8 Ulnar impaction syndrome in a 65-year-old man with a history of chronic ulnar wrist pain worsened by twisting and ulnar deviation of the wrist. Radiograph demonstrates ulnar positive variance with degenerative changes at the articulation between the ulnar head and the lunate.

of the articular disc. Management is controversial, but successful reattachment of the disc margin to the radius has been described both open and closed.

Type II: degenerative problems

These disorders comprise a spectrum of clinical and pathological sequelae resulting from recurrent compressive loading through the ulnar carpus, TFCC, and ulna, and have been variably referred to as ulnocarpal 'loading', 'abutment', 'impaction', or 'impingement' syndrome.

There are five stages, beginning with TFCC wear and progressing through perforation, lunate and/or ulnar chondromalacia, lunotriquetral ligament disruption, and finally ulnocarpal arthritis.

Clinical features may include: ulnar wrist pain accentuated by rotation (especially pronation), ulnar deviation, and clenched fist loading; tenderness and/or crepitation in the region of the TFCC; and a tendency to ulnar neutral or positive variance. Sclerosis and/or cystic changes in the ulnar head and/or lunate may be seen with plain radiography, joint narrowing, and/or chondromalacia on tomography, and TFC perforations and/or lunotriquetral tears on MRI/arthrography (Figure 6.4.8).

The onset of symptoms may vary from insidious to abrupt depending on any predisposing condition or injury, the pattern and repetitive use of hand, wrist, and forearm, and the loading applied. Positive ulnar variance may be a congenital variant of normal or may be acquired, e.g. post-traumatic radial shortening, premature physeal closure including Madelung deformity, and, most commonly, age-related relative radial shortening due to thinning of the radial head articular cartilage.

Non-operative treatment includes activity modification, anti-inflammatory medications, splints, and steroid injections.

A positive ulna variance can be corrected by shortening the ulna (Figure 6.4.9) (which is simpler) or lengthening the radius which is typically performed when there are other concomitant abnormalities such as dorsal tilt of the radius following fracture malunion.

If length discrepancy osteotomies will leave the DRUJ incongruous or if degenerative changes are already present then new or persistent symptoms are likely postoperatively and additional procedures as for DRUJ arthritis need to be considered (see later).

Alternatively, the 'wafer' procedure may be performed with minimal effect on radioulnar relations at the DRUJ. It involves resection of 2–3mm of the distal ulnar pole, leaving the styloid

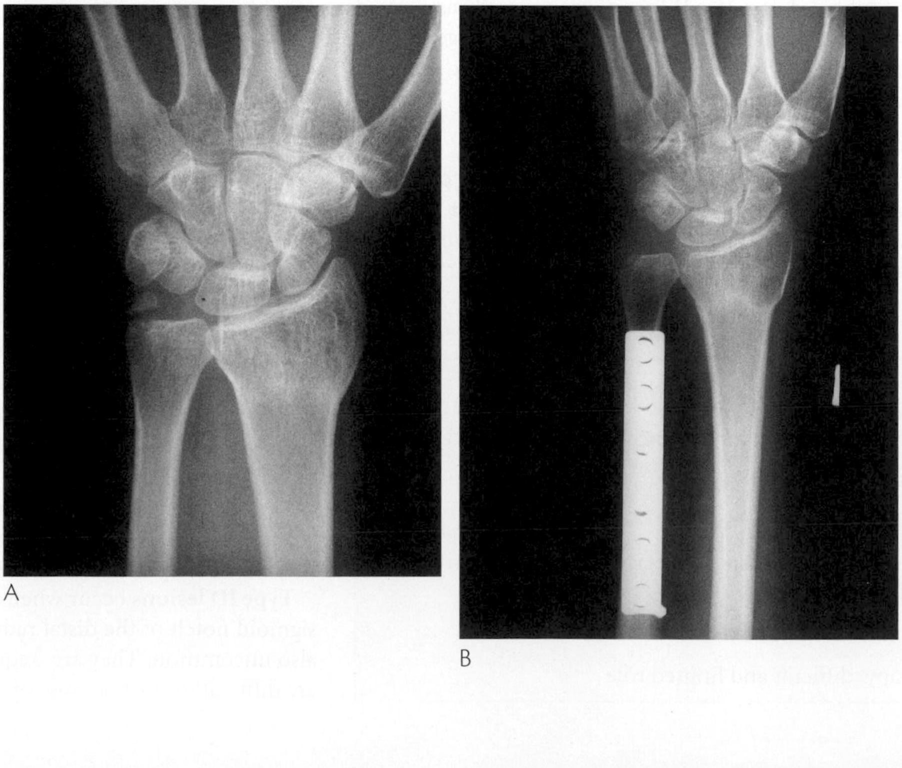

Fig. 6.4.9 Ulna shortening osteotomy for ulnar impaction syndrome in a 35-year-old woman with a history of chronic ulnar wrist pain and a documented TFC tear.
A) Anteroposterior radiograph demonstrates 2-mm ulnar positive variance. B) Radiographs following an ulnar shortening osteotomy demonstrate neutral ulnar variance. Her pain was relieved.

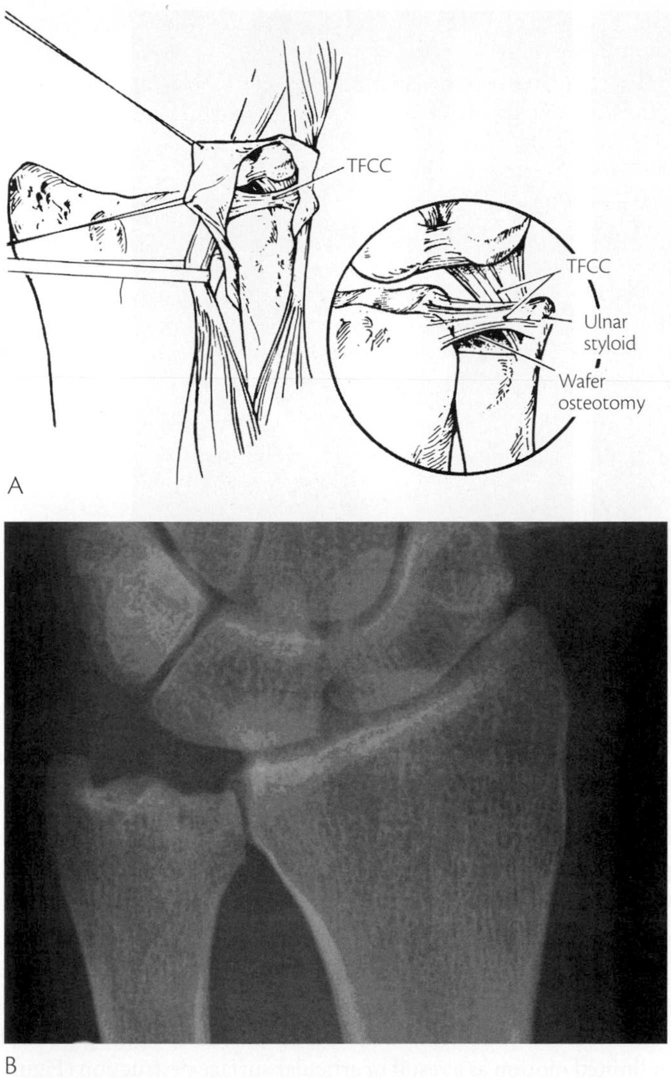

Fig. 6.4.10 Method of Feldon wafer resection. A) Diagram demonstrating the technique of wafer resection through a dorsal approach. The distal 2–4mm of distal ulna is resected while preserving the TFCC and ulnar styloid. (Reproduced from Feldon *et al.* (1992).) B) An anteroposterior radiograph demonstrating wafer resection of the distal ulna pre and postoperatively.

intact (Figure 6.4.10), via an open approach or arthroscopically through the perforated TFC.

The need to treat accompanying TFCC lesions is controversial. Some authors recommend arthroscopic or open debridement of central perforations and repair of any destabilizing peripheral lesions of the TFCC. Others believe that decompression of the ulnocarpal space by ulnar recession will suffice in most cases.

Distal radioulnar joint instability (Box 6.4.5)

By convention, instabilities, subluxations, and dislocations of the DRUJ have been described in terms of the direction of the ulnar head displacement relative to the radiocarpal unit. Strictly speaking though, it is the radiocarpal structures that move about the stationary ulna.

Although sometimes occurring in isolation, acute DRUJ instability or dislocation is seen in up to 60% of forearm fractures. It is especially common in complex distal radius fractures, where the TFCC and/or the sigmoid notch may be disrupted. Failure to recognize and manage these injuries adequately can result in chronic DRUJ dysfunction and instability.

Box 6.4.4 TFCC pathology

Traumatic

- Common
- Central or peripheral
- Treatment:
  - Central—debridement
  - Peripheral—repair/decompression.

Degenerative

- Common, may even be 'normal'
- Mainly due to ulnocarpal impingement
- Treatment: decompression by shortening or Feldon wafer.

Chronic DRUJ instability may result from disruption of any of the three major determinants of stability: the ulnar head/sigmoid notch articular congruence and alignment; the relative length, rotational, and angular relationship of the radius and ulna; and the integrity of the primary soft tissue stabilizers of the DRUJ (i.e. the TFCC). The adequacy of each must be ensured to restore stable DRUJ function. The presence and degree of instability and malunion is best evaluated clinically, and confirmed and quantified with plain radiography and a CT scan of both the involved and contralateral forearms and wrists.

Instability that results from malunion of forearm fractures may be improved by corrective osteotomy. Reattachment of the TFCC to the fovea has been described for minor degrees of instability, and if associated with an ulnar styloid fracture the bone fragment may be reduced and internally fixed if large or excised if small (Figure 6.4.11).

In the absence of a radial or ulnar malunion, soft tissue reconstruction alone can be undertaken. Many techniques for reconstruction of the distal radioulnar ligaments have been described. Each uses a tendon graft, which is weaved through drill holes in the distal radius and ulna and tied onto itself. The most anatomic, and the one most commonly used, is the technique described by Adams and Berger (Figure 6.4.12). It has been reported to restore clinical stability in 12 of 14 patients, and recovery of strength and range of motion averaged 85% of the unaffected wrist.

Chronic DRUJ instability may also be treated with hemiresection interposition arthroplasty. In a series of 23 patients, 17 had good to excellent results, and 21 had increased range of motion.

Box 6.4.5 DRUJ instability

- Common, often asymptomatic
- Treatment:
  - TFCC repair
  - Complex reconstruction with tendon graft.

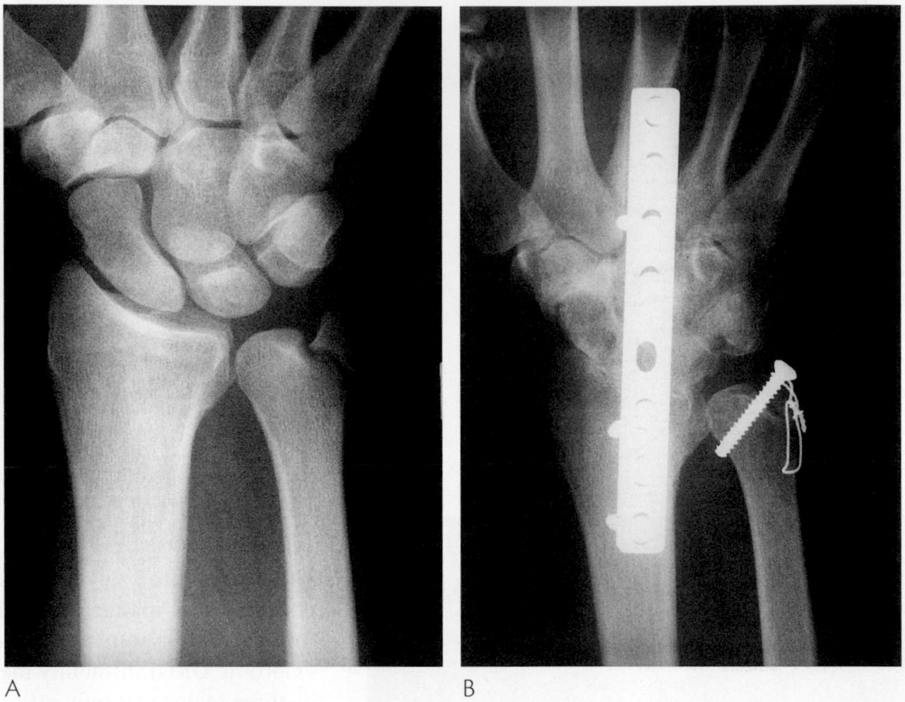

Fig. 6.4.11 Open reduction and internal fixation of ulnar styloid nonunion. A) Anteroposterior radiograph of a 25-year-old laborer with a painful wrist following a distal radial fracture. Arthroscopic examination demonstrated moderate degenerative changes in the radiocarpal and mid-carpal joints with intercarpal ligament injuries. B)He was successfully treated by a wrist arthrodesis and internal fixation of the symptomatic ulnar styloid nonunion.

Radioulnar fusion (a one-bone forearm) should be considered in patients doing heavy labour or who have failed soft tissue reconstructions (Figure 6.4.13).

Distal radioulnar joint arthritis (Box 6.4.6)

DRUJ arthritis may be primary or secondary to fracture malunion. The commonest cause is inflammatory arthropathy, e.g. rheumatoid arthritis (RA).

Non-operative management includes activity modification, anti-inflammatories, splinting, and steroid injections. Four types of DRUJ 'arthroplasty', with multiple variations, are in common use: excision of the distal end of the ulna (Darrach procedure); hemiresection interposition arthroplasty; DRUJ arthrodesis with creation of a proximal ulnar pseudarthrosis (Sauvé–Kapandji procedure); and ulna hemiarthroplasty.

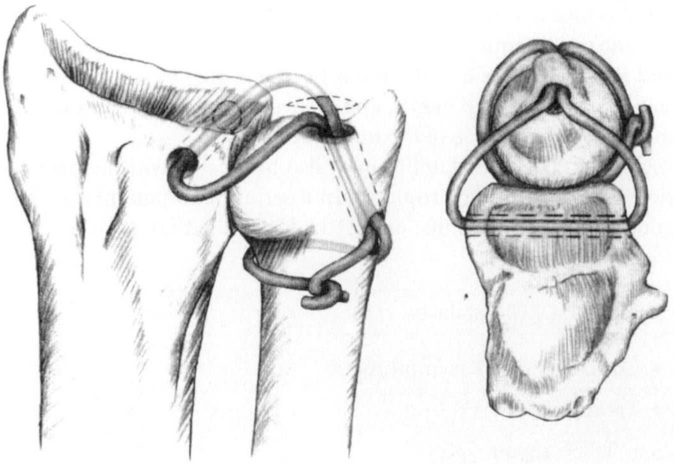

Fig. 6.4.12 Adams technique of distal radioulnar ligament reconstruction (dorsal and axial views).

Darrach procedure

The Darrach procedure is a subperiosteal excision of the ulnar head with or without the ulnar styloid. It may be considered in any condition that interferes with DRUJ function, causing painful or limited motion as a result of articular surface destruction (Figure 6.4.14). Because the 'DRUJ' is rendered unstable it is best performed with a minimal resection in low demand patients, typically patients with inflammatory arthropathy or elderly patients following a Colles' fracture.

Hemiresection interposition arthroplasty

Several variants of this procedure have been described. They attempt to minimize instability of the distal ulna by maintaining bony contact between the ulnar shaft and the TFCC attachments. In the hemiresection interposition arthroplasty of Bowers, only the articular portion of the ulnar head is removed, retaining the shaft/styloid relationship and interposing tendon, muscle, or joint capsule between the distal ulna and radius to limit contact. This procedure requires an intact or reconstructable TFCC to confer any advantage over a Darrach procedure.

Stylocarpal impingement may occur as the ulna migrates toward the radius. Concomitant ulnar shortening osteotomy should be performed in ulnar positive wrists, or if impingement can be anticipated preoperatively.

In the 'matched' distal ulna resection, the ulnar head is partially resected in an oblique fashion parallel to the inclination of the sigmoid notch. The ulnar styloid is removed and ulnar shortening distally is possible. Most are pain free and the remainder are significantly improved (Figure 6.4.15).

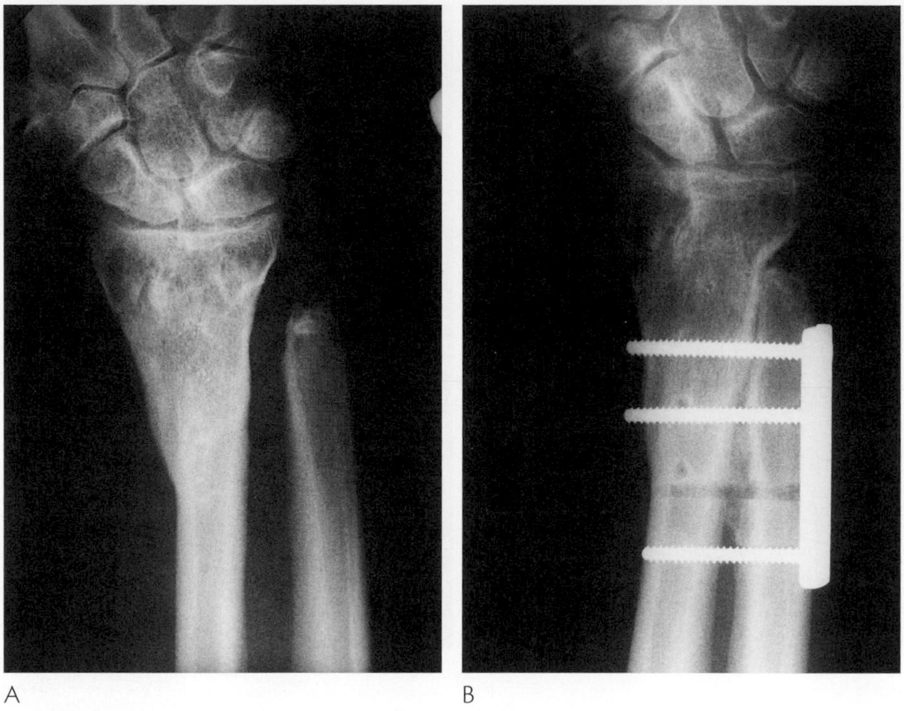

Fig. 6.4.13 Radioulnar arthrodesis in a 23-year-old labourer with unstable and painful ulnar stump following failed matched resection. A). Pain relieved by radioulnar arthrodesis using iliac crest bone graft (B).

Sauvé–Kapandji procedure

The arthritic DRUJ is fused and a mobile pseudarthrosis is created by excision of segment of distal ulnar shaft (Fig 6.4.16). While effective in relieving pain at the DRUJ, adequate bone must be resected at the proposed pseudarthrosis to allow full forearm rotation but prevent ossification between the segments of ulna.

The indications for this procedure remain unclear. Excellent results for relief of pain, range of motion, and patient satisfaction have been reported. Instability of the proximal ulna segment and radioulnar convergence are the commonest problems. Although infrequently symptomatic, when they are they can be difficult to treat although ulna hemiarthroplasty articulating with the underside of the fused ulna head is a recent salvage option.

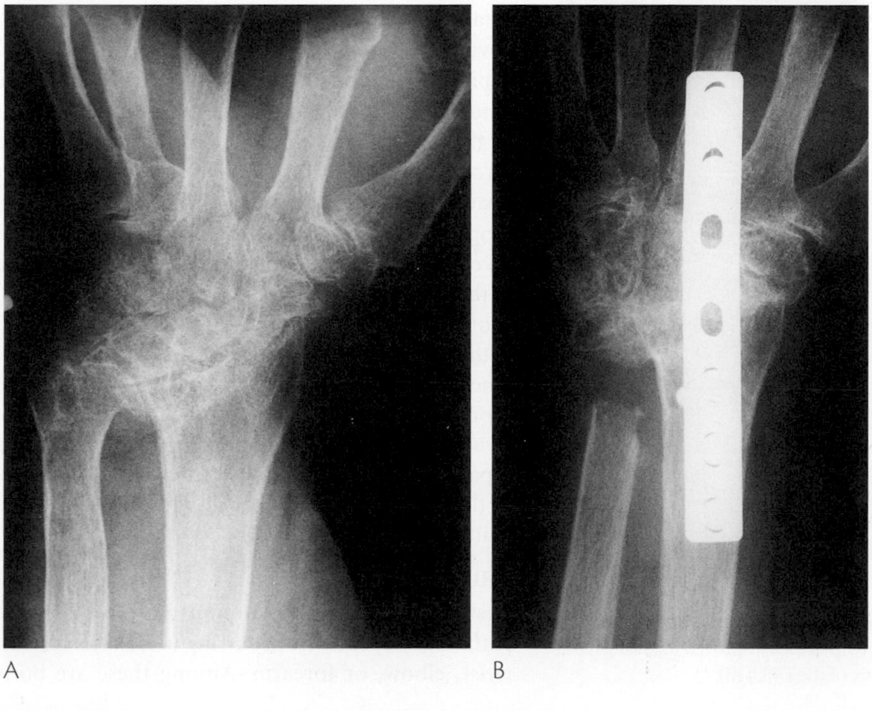

Fig. 6.4.14 Darrach procedure in a 54-year-old woman with long-standing rheumatoid arthritis and disabling wrist pain. (A) Pain and function improved following wrist arthrodesis and Darrach resection of the distal ulna (B)

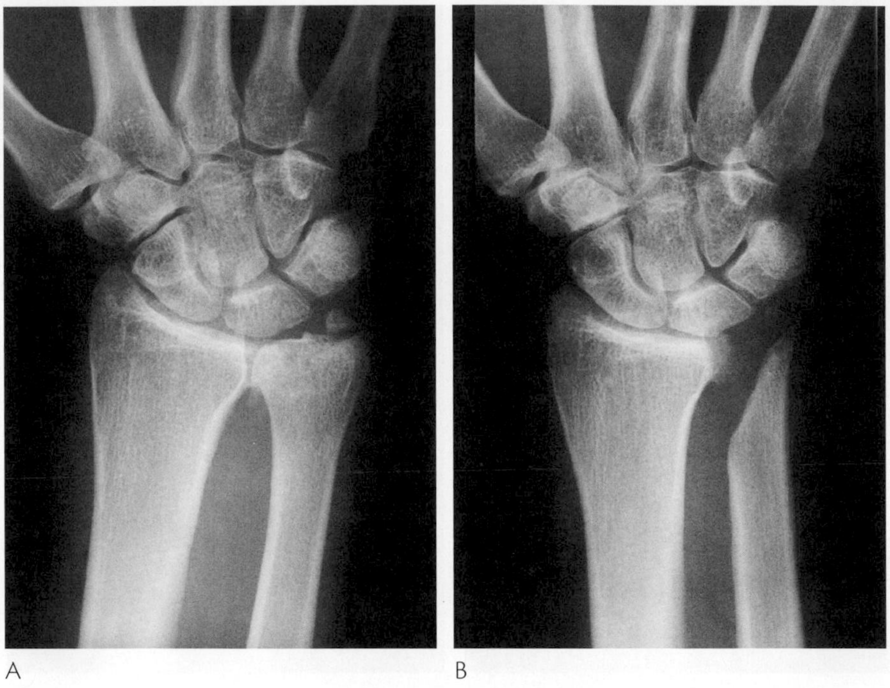

Fig. 6.4.15 Matched hemiresection interposition arthroplasty in a 48-year-old woman with chronic ulnar wrist pain and crepitus from DRUJ arthritis. B) Pain improved following matched resection of the distal ulna and interposition of a portion of the extensor retinaculum.

Arthroplasty

Replacement arthroplasty of the ulnar head is an emerging technology with promising early results. The primary indication for ulnar head arthroplasty is pain and stiffness secondary to rheumatoid, degenerative, or post-traumatic arthritis; failed excisional arthroplasty (Darrach or hemiresection interposition arthroplasty); bone tumour (Figure 6.4.17); and less commonly, an unreconstructable fracture of the ulnar head or neck due to comminution or poor bone stock. Ulnar stump instability or radioulnar impingement syndrome after excisional arthroplasty can also be successfully managed with this technique. There are various metal or pyrocarbon options. Silastic replacements have been abandoned because of implant failure. While the solid prostheses have shown favourable early results, long-term outcomes have not yet been reported.

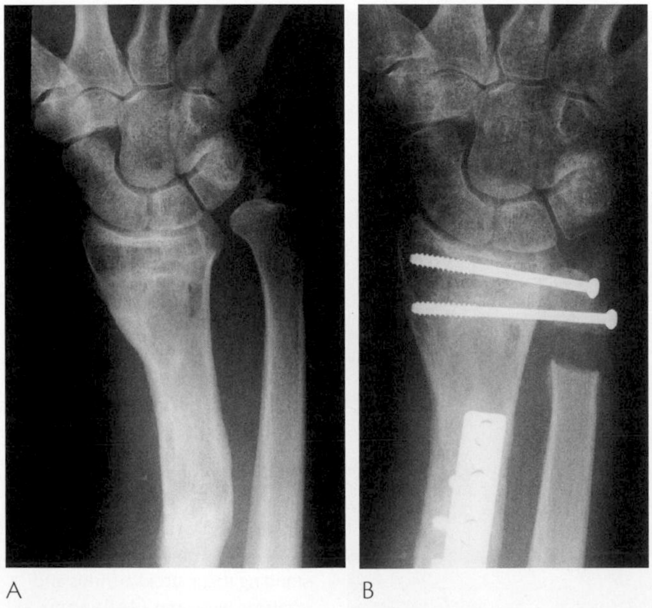

Fig. 6.4.16 Sauvé–Kapandji procedure in a 29-year-old man with a long-standing forearm malunion and dislocation of the DRUJ. A). Pain improved following radial osteotomy and a Sauvé–Kapandji arthrodesis of the DRUJ (B).

Other DRUJ-related disorders

Extensor carpi ulnaris subluxation

The course and action of the ECU tendon change with forearm rotation. In full pronation the ECU is linear and acts as an ulnar deviator while in supination it is an extensor of the wrist. In full supination, especially with ulnar deviation, the course of the ECU tendon is angular with the tunnel at its apex. Forcible contraction of the ECU in this position creates a strong ulnar translocating force that may disrupt the ECU sheath. This position and mechanism are often recalled by patients, in conjunction with a 'snapping' or 'popping' sensation. Examination in the acute setting will reveal local features of inflammation and painful ulnar subluxation of the ECU provoked by supination and ulnar deviation. Treatment acutely is with 6 weeks of forearm immobilization in pronation with the wrist slightly extended and radially deviated to reduce the tendon. Surgical repair may also be used acutely and is appropriate for chronic painful ECU snapping that has been untreated or failed non-operative immobilization. Operative treatment may consist of repair of the sheath lesion, reefing of local tissues, reconstruction of the tunnel using retinacular flaps or other tissues, and/or deepening of the ulnar groove.

DRUJ contractures

Restriction of forearm motion may result from a multitude of pathological processes occurring in isolation or combination at the wrist, elbow, or forearm. Among these are bony abnormalities

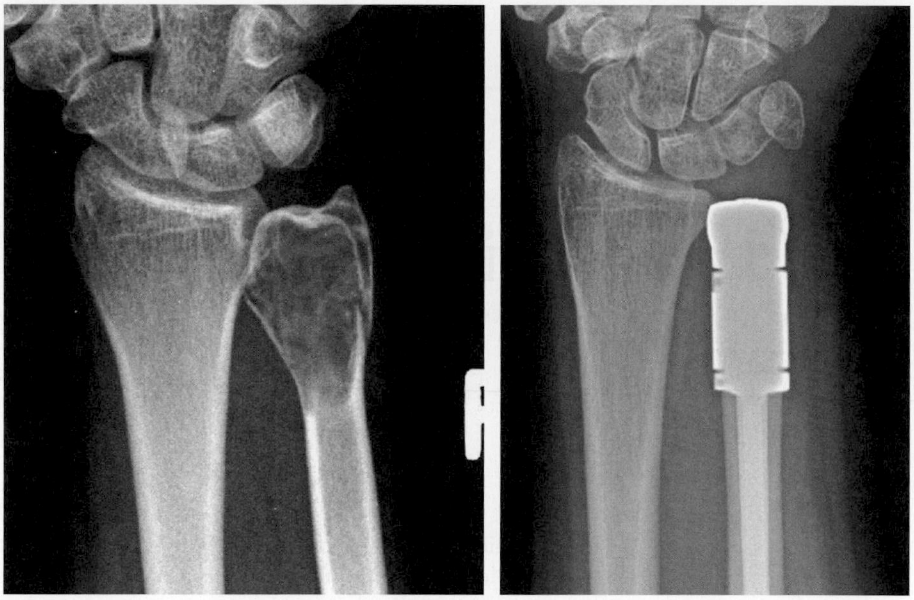

Fig. 6.4.17 Distal ulnar hemiarthroplasty (E-centrix) used to reconstruct a benign bony tumour. A) Preoperative radiographs. B) Postoperative radiographs with an E-centrix prosthesis incorporating an available spacer block to compensate for bone deficiency.

(congenital or acquired shaft or articular incongruence of the radius and ulna, synostoses), neuromuscular disorders (paralytic, spastic, or post-traumatic contractures), interosseous membrane insufficiency (instability, contracture), and proximal or distal radioulnar joint restrictions (articular deficiency, mechanical interference, soft tissue instability, or capsular contracture).

DRUJ capsular contracture is uncommon and generally post-traumatic. It may be associated with bony abnormalities. It may also result from prolonged forearm immobilization. Pathologically, the normally lax joint capsule becomes shortened and thickened with fibrosis, especially on the palmar side. Contracture of the palmar capsule restricts supination; contracture of the dorsal capsule limits pronation. Pronation contractures with restricted supination are most common. However, global limitation due to involvement of both the dorsal and volar capsule may occur.

Non-operative treatment with physiotherapy, dynamic splinting, and serial casting is often effective; if it fails, surgical release may be useful provided that there is no suggestion of joint incongruency. A volar capsulectomy is performed, proceeding dorsally as needed to restore motion. Care must be taken to preserve the radioulnar ligaments, TFCC, and articular surfaces. Intra-articular adhesions are lysed and the forearm is gently manipulated in rotation and translation under anaesthetic.

Box 6.4.6 DRUJ arthritis

- Common, especially in RA
- Treatment:
  - Steroid injection
  - Surgery:
    - Darrach's
    - Partial resection
    - Sauve-Kapandji
    - Replacement

Summary

Derangements of the DRUJ are a significant cause of ulnar wrist pain that have traditionally been poorly understood. Our improved understanding of the normal anatomy and biomechanics of this region has lead to a more successful approach to the diagnosis and treatment of DRUJ disorders.

Further reading

Adams, B.D. (2005). Distal radioulnar joint instability. In: Green, D.P., Hotchkiss, R.N., Pederson, W.C., and Wolfe, S.W. (eds) *Operative Hand Surgery*, fifth edition, pp. 605–44. New York: Churchill Livingstone. [A comprehensive, organized, and well-illustrated discussion of DRUJ anatomy, biomechanics, assessment, pathology, and treatments. Management options are reviewed with the experience of the author and major surgical techniques are well described.]

Chidgey, L.G. (1995). The distal radioulnar joint: problems and solutions. *Journal of the American Academy of Orthopaedic Surgeons*, **3**, 95–109. [An excellent overview of the current understanding and recent advances relating to the DRUJ, its derangements, and their management.]

Katolik, L.I. and Trumble, T. (2005). Distal radioulnar joint dysfunction. *Journal of the American Society for Surgery of the Hand*, **5**, 8–29. [The major clinical problems involving the distal radioulnar joint including injuries to the TFCC, instability, and degeneration, are discussed in detail.]

Kleinman, W.B. and Graham, T.J. (1996). Distal ulnar injury and dysfunction. In: Peimer, C.A. (ed) *Surgery of the Hand and Upper Extremity*, pp. 667–709. New York: McGraw-Hill. [A comprehensive discussion of distal ulna disorders. It includes a thorough review of DRUJ biomechanics, anatomy, and diagnostic evaluation. Derangements of the DRUJ are reviewed in an organized fashion with the perspective of the authors and operative techniques described in detail.]

6.5

Rheumatoid arthritis of the hand and wrist

J. Stothard

Summary points

- RA is common
- Medical treatment is the mainstay and newer anti-TNF drugs are reducing morbidity and thus referral for surgery
- Assessment is primarily clinical
- Investigations – Primarily radiographs
- Treatment
  - Non-operative
  - Steroid injections are often very useful
  - Operative
  - Site and condition specific
- In general
  - DRUJ – excision ulna head
  - Wrist – partial fusion, arthrodesis, arthroplasty
  - MP joints – synvestomy, arthroplasty
  - PIP joints – soft tissue rebalancing, arthrodesis
  - DIP joints – arthrodesis
  - Thumb MP and IP joints – arthrodesis

Introduction

The hands and wrists are frequently affected in rheumatoid disease. Function can be impaired by painful acute inflammation of joints or by their later destruction. Involvement of tendons can lead to rupture, bulky synovitis may cause secondary nerve compression syndromes, and painful subcutaneous nodules may interfere with use of the hands.

Disease-modifying drug therapy has reduced referrals to surgeons for treatment of persistent acute inflammation of joints and tendon sheaths. Early synovectomy of joints is effective in relieving pain but does not appear to protect them from destruction over the long term. However, the benefit of tenosynovectomy of flexor and extensor tendons is frequently long lasting.

Patients generally present to the surgeon in the late stage of rheumatoid disease. Requests for surgical advice may be for one or more of the following problems:

- Painful joints
- Loss of movement interfering with function
- Loss of strength interfering with function
- Cosmetic deformity.

Assessment (Box 6.5.1)

Assessment of the rheumatoid hand and wrist should involve not only 'look, feel, move, and radiograph' but also an assessment of function. A systematic approach is essential to avoid being distracted by obvious cosmetic deformities. Functional deficits may be due to joint disease, but the equally important effects of tendon

Box 6.5.1 Assessment

History

The prime symptoms are:

- Pain
- Stiffness
- Weakness
- Cosmesis.

Examination

The most important is pain, but remember:

- Instability
- Local versus combined stiffness
- Active and passive loss of movement
- Neuropathy
- Also remember to assess other local joints, e.g. shoulder/elbow.

rupture, nerve compression, and cervical radiculopathy should not be forgotten.

Patients should be asked how far they can reach with the hand—to the mouth, to the top of the head, to the natal cleft. These abilities are strongly influenced by disease at the elbow and shoulder. They should also be asked what they can do with the hand in these positions. Can they feed, dress, and attend to personal hygiene independently? Does disease of the lower limbs compel the patient to bear weight with the hands through a stick or crutch? Questions about common activities of daily living will identify specific functional problems and help to determine the surgical priorities.

Inspection of the hand should note the deformities, which frequently reflect zigzag compensatory phenomena such as flexion contracture of the proximal interphalangeal joint accompanied by fixed hyperextension of the distal joint (boutonnière deformity). Deformities may be in more than one plane (Figure 6.5.1). Ulnar deviation at the metacarpophalangeal joints is frequently associated with palmar subluxation and pronation (especially in the index finger). Palpation will detect residual synovitis and signs of active disease in joints and tendon sheaths. Sensory testing is useful in detecting peripheral nerve entrapment; motor testing is more difficult as weakness and wasting may be due to disease in adjacent joints.

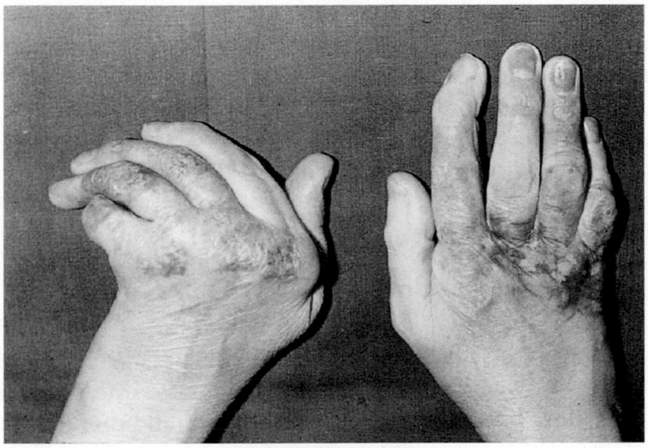

A

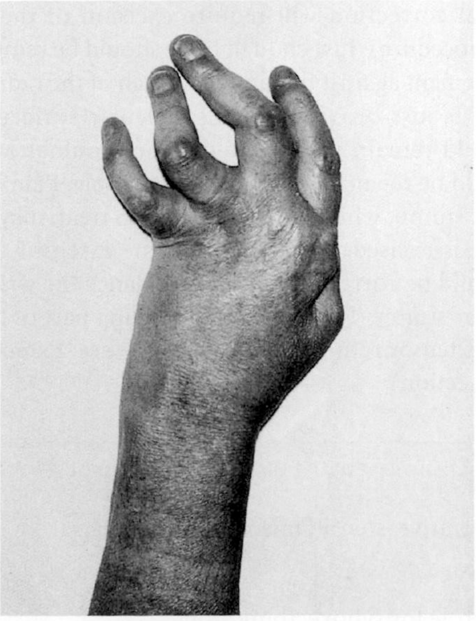

B

Fig. 6.5.1 A) Rheumatoid hands showing typical ulnar drift on left side. B) Radial deviation of wrist and ulnar deviation of metacarpophalangeal joints (one zigzag deformity) plus boutonnière deformity of the fingers (another zigzag deformity).

Movement is the most detailed part of the examination and must include the following:

- Detailed assessment of active movement of each joint
- Comparison with the passive range: a difference between active and passive range of movement indicates loss of tendon function (adhesion or rupture), or paralysis (nerve entrapment)
- Are deformities correctable passively?
- Assessment of overall movement, such as fingertip to palm distance (Boyes' index) and ability to touch the thumb to index and middle fingers for tripod pinch grip. The fingers may be able to grasp narrow objects such as the examiner's single finger. If movement is limited, grip may be restricted to larger objects. The patient may use the tip of the thumb for key pinch, or may be obliged to bypass an unstable terminal segment and use instead the head of the proximal phalanx.

Radiographs may show far greater bone and joint destruction than the functional assessment and examination had suggested. Radiographic abnormalities are not themselves an indication for surgery but are useful in determining the surgical options that are available (e.g. joint destruction precludes synovectomy).

Assessment by an occupational therapist experienced in rheumatoid disease can be most helpful, by observing the patient in a simulated home and kitchen environment, by selecting aids which may improve function, and by clarifying the need (or lack of need) for surgery.

Medical assessment includes degree of control of disease activity and monitoring of drug treatment, especially for 'new' drugs such as anti-tumour necrosis factor (TNF)-alpha agents for which temporary withholding of the drug is advised by manufacturers over the course of major surgical procedures.

Priorities for treatment (Box 6.5.2)

The priorities for treatment of the rheumatoid hand and wrist are pain relief and restoration of function. Cosmetic improvement would be regarded as a bonus but is seldom an indication for surgery on its own. The patient's expectations of outcome should be assessed carefully, bearing in mind that surgery often relieves pain but is much less effective at improving strength and movement. Unrealistic expectations should be corrected by counselling before surgery is undertaken. Not every patient with deformed hands needs surgery. Young patients whose lifestyle is affected by mild disease should be advised to modify their activities. Older patients

Box 6.5.2 Treatment priorities

- Pain
- Prevention of future problems, e.g. tendon ruptures
- Improved function
- Cosmesis
- Surgery should mostly be performed only once the systemic disease is under control.

who have minimal pain and satisfactory function despite deformity will not be improved by surgery.

Relief of pain is the most common indication for surgery at the wrist. A painful wrist will prevent good use of the hand, even if the fingers and thumb are in good condition. A painful thumb will affect many everyday actions, especially if it is also unstable. Souter emphasized that surgery of the rheumatoid hand and wrist should begin with simple and reliable procedures, so that the patient's confidence is gained, before moving on to less predictable operations. Provision of a pain-free wrist and stabilization of the thumb are top of Souter's list.

Assessment of the wrist should attempt to localize pain to the radiocarpal joint, to the distal radioulnar joint, or to both joints. The site of local tenderness and the provocation of pain by flexion/extension and forearm rotation are useful.

In the thumb, stability is more important than movement. When hand function is compromised, the thumb should be regarded as a stable 'post' against which the fingers can act. When finger movement is also limited, key pinch to the side of the index finger may be the only achievable type of pinch. It is acceptable to fuse the metacarpophalangeal joint and the interphalangeal joints of the thumb if its basal joint is mobile. An iliac crest graft may be needed to maintain length in cases of severe bone loss. Surgery of the painful subluxed basal joint will fail and basal subluxation will recur unless secondary web contractures and fixed deformities of more distal joints are corrected at the same time.

In the fingers, the priority is to maintain movement at the base of the digit. In severe cases, movement at the metacarpophalangeal joints and stability of the interphalangeal joints in a functional position may be all that can be achieved. In less severe cases, surgical correction at the metacarpophalangeal joints (e.g. by silastic interposition arthroplasty) may give good finger function, especially where the metacarpophalangeal joints are diseased but the interphalangeal joints are spared. Stiffness of the proximal interphalangeal joints in hyperextension (swan-neck deformity) can severely limit grip even if the metacarpophalangeal joints are mobile; surgical correction is often helpful. However, stiffness of the proximal interphalangeal joints in flexion is compatible with good power grip and seldom needs surgery.

Tendon rupture is a potentially preventable cause of functional loss in rheumatoid disease and merits careful assessment. Early clearance of persistent tenosynovitis and elimination of bony spicules will reduce the risk of rupture of additional tendons. The ruptured tendon should be regarded as diseased and not suitable for direct repair. Reconstruction is by transfer of a synergistic intact tendon, by side-to-side suture to an adjacent intact tendon, or, occasionally, by tendon graft. Fusion is sometimes simpler and more appropriate than tendon transfer (e.g. interphalangeal joint of thumb after flexor pollicis longus tendon rupture). The cause of rupture (e.g. ulnar head) should be treated to eliminate the risk to other tendons, even if tendon reconstruction is impracticable.

Loss of function caused by sensory deficiency secondary to nerve compression can often be improved by nerve decompression. For median nerve compression at the wrist, synovectomy of the flexor tendons should be added if there is obvious bulky synovitis.

Wrist and distal radioulnar joint

A stable pain-free wrist is essential for good function of the hand. Although the wrist is seldom the first joint affected by rheumatoid disease, it is ultimately affected in over 90% of patients with severe arthritis. Surgery is frequently required to deal with pain, weakness, and instability of the rheumatoid wrist and distal radioulnar joint.

Synovectomy

In the acute stage of pain and swelling, pain is frequently due to synovitis of the overlying flexor and extensor tendons rather than to disease in the wrist joint itself. In these cases, swelling and local tenderness will follow the synovial tendon compartments, which extend proximal and distal to the wrist joint. Tenosynovectomy (see later) may be useful. However, open synovectomy of the wrist joint is technically impracticable because of the many small joints and the difficulty in reaching their palmar recesses through a dorsal approach. Chemical synovectomy may be considered, or arthroscopic synovectomy may be performed.

In cases of continued pain with minimal destruction, wrist denervation has been used successfully and detailed descriptions of the techniques are available. Preoperative assessment by local anaesthetic blocks of all nerves supplying the wrist is mandatory. The author has found denervation useful in juvenile rheumatoid arthritis, where painful stiffness is a greater problem than joint destruction.

Two patterns of deformity are commonly seen in the stage of late destruction of the wrist and distal radioulnar joint. The carpus may supinate on the forearm, with translation of the extensor carpi ulnaris tendon over the axis of flexion/extension so that it ceases to act as an extensor of the wrist. The ulnar head becomes prominent dorsally. In other cases, destruction of the distal radius affects the palmar surface more than the dorsal surface, leading to palmar subluxation of the carpus.

Distal radioulnar joint (Box 6.5.3)

Distal radioulnar pain may arise from synovitis alone, from destruction of the joint surfaces, or from loss of radial length with impingement of the ulnar head on the carpus. Persistent synovitis with healthy joint surfaces is an occasional indication for distal radioulnar synovectomy. More often, joint damage will be obvious and surgical correction will require excision of the ulnar head (Darrach procedure). Just enough bone should be removed to clear any impingement against the sigmoid notch of the radius. The level of excision is just proximal to the articular surface. The ulnar stump should remain within the distal radioulnar joint capsule, which should be repaired as securely as possible. Painful instability of the ulnar stump, which is very difficult to treat, may occur if too much bone is excised. Subluxation of the extensor carpi ulnaris tendon should be corrected, so as to rebalance the wrist and stabilize the ulnar stump. This is performed using part of the proximal half of the extensor retinaculum as a 'sling' (see 'Extensor tenosynovectomy' section).

Box 6.5.3 Treatment of the distal radioulnar joint

- Non-operative: steroid injections often help
- Operative:
  - Little role for synovectomy alone
  - Darrach's procedure is very successful
  - Extensor tendons need to be checked

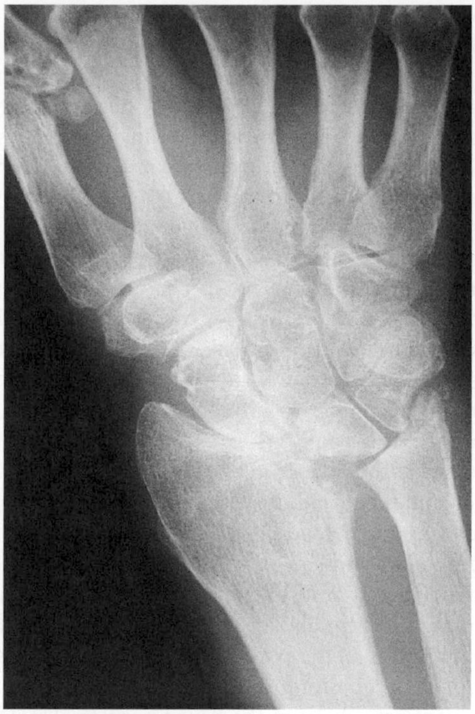

Fig. 6.5.2 Erosion of the lunate fossa of the radius with loss of support of the lunate and early ulnar translation of the carpus.

The results of ulnar head excision are much more satisfactory and predictable in rheumatoid arthritis than in post-traumatic disorders. Progressive ulnar translation of the carpus may occur after ulnar head excision. Although it is probably due more to softening of radiocarpal ligaments by disease (Figure 6.5.2) than to loss of support of the ulna, ulnar carpal translation is a contraindication to ulnar head excision. The presence of spontaneous radiolunate fusion, or a shelf of bone projecting toward the ulna from the lunate fossa of the radius, protect against ulnar carpal translation. Radiolunate fusion may be performed at the time of ulnar head excision in patients who are thought to be at risk of carpal translation because of limited radiolunate contact or excessive radial inclination.

An alternative to ulnar head excision is the Sauvé–Kapandji procedure, in which the ulnar head is fused to the sigmoid notch of the radius and a segment of distal ulnar shaft is excised to allow rotation through the resulting pseudoarthrosis. Although a stable radioulnar surface is provided, the procedure may not prevent ulnar carpal translation. Instability of the proximal ulnar stump may cause troublesome impingement against the shaft of the radius.

Wrist arthroplasty

Arthrodesis and arthroplasty are the surgical options for the severely damaged radiocarpal joint. Excision arthroplasty has been unsatisfactory in rheumatoid disease. Swanson silastic interposition arthroplasty has a high failure rate by fracture and bone resorption over the longer-term failures are seen particularly in patients who load the wrist heavily or who gain a large range of motion. Silastic arthroplasty remains a satisfactory procedure for patients with low demands and well-balanced wrists, aiming to achieve no more than 30 degrees each of flexion and extension, but is now rarely performed.

Cemented metal on polyethylene total wrist arthroplasties have been beset with problems of bone resorption, fracture, loosening, and infection. Cementless implants and improved methods of rebalancing wrist tendons may help to improve the results. Salvage of failed arthroplasties remains difficult because of the loss of bone stock. All wrist arthroplasties bridge the midcarpal joint but many do not 'line up' with the normal anatomical 20–24 degrees of radial inclination and 10-degree volar inclination of the radiocarpal joint so must have a propensity to fail because of shear stresses. Many designs have had to be withdrawn from the market because of unacceptable early and medium-term failure rates.

Wrist arthrodesis (Box 6.5.4)

Total arthrodesis provides excellent stability and relief of pain in the rheumatoid wrist in cases where arthroplasty is inappropriate or contraindicated (Figure 6.5.3) Arthrodesis is also indicated for salvage of failed arthroplasties. In the patient with severe bilateral wrist disease, a total arthrodesis will provide stability and freedom from pain on one side while a motion-preserving procedure (arthroplasty or limited wrist fusion) will retain some flexibility on the other side. However, many patients function very well with bilateral wrist fusions and are pleased with the stability and relief of pain. When considering the indication for bilateral fusion, the movement of the elbow, shoulder, and forearm rotation should be taken into account; a functional assessment by an occupational therapist may be invaluable. At least one wrist should be fused in neutral, rather than slight extension, so as to permit perineal hygiene.

Total wrist arthrodesis is achieved much more easily in rheumatoid disease than in post-traumatic arthritis. Simple fixation with a Steinmann pin from the third metacarpal into the radius will suffice. An additional wire or staple is sometimes needed to control rotation. The porotic bone and poor soft tissue envelope of most rheumatoid wrists do not lend themselves to fixation by plates. In wrists with marked palmar subluxation, the gain in length achieved by fusion may improve power in the finger tendons. Fusion in juvenile rheumatoid patients is occasionally needed for pain relief and correction of gross deformity but risks limiting growth of the distal radius. Splinting and wrist denervation should be attempted for pain relief before considering fusion.

Flexor and extensor tendons

Synovitis involving the flexor and extensor tendons is common in rheumatoid disease. It is more obvious on the extensor surface, particularly on the back of the hand where the tenosynovium

Box 6.5.4 Treatment of the wrist

- Non-operative:
  - Splints
  - Steroid injection
- Operative:
  - Almost no role for synovectomy
  - Partial fusion is increasingly used
  - Total fusion is reliable but overperformed
  - Arthroplasty is controversial.

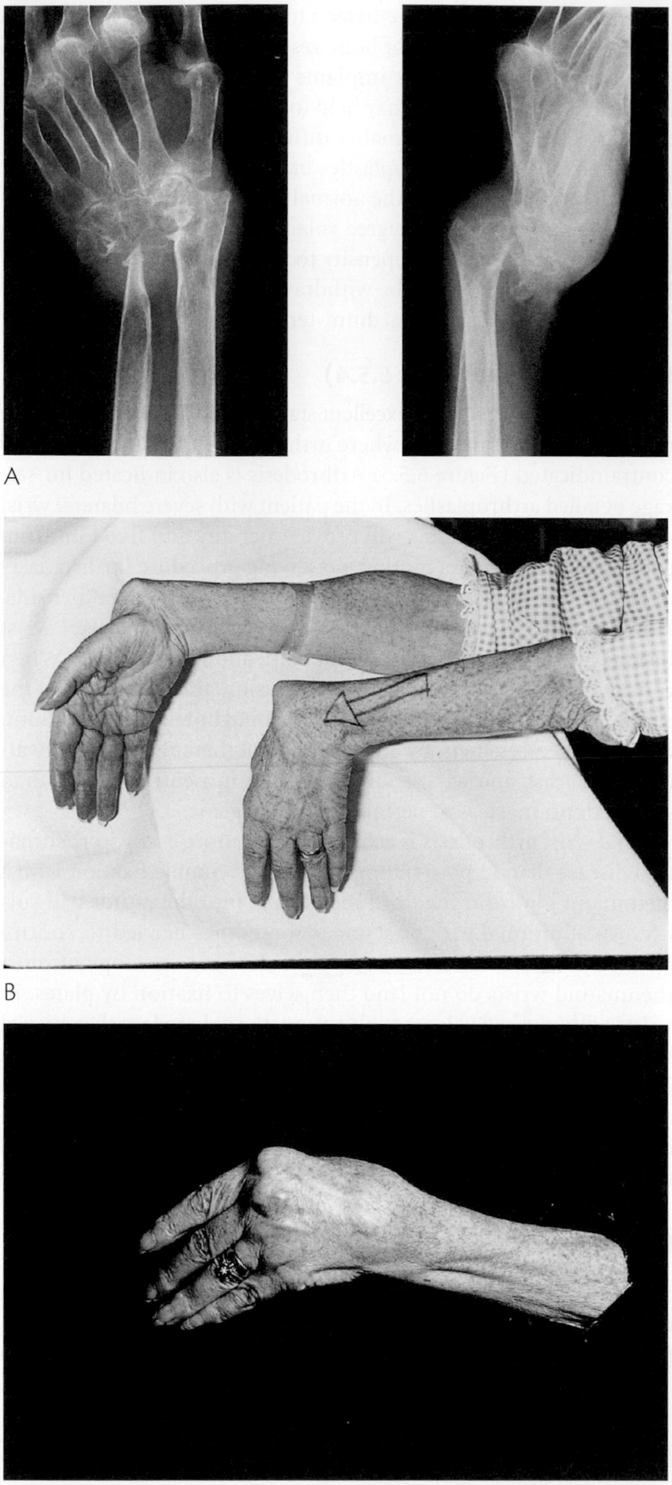
A B C

Fig. 6.5.3 A) Destructive arthritis of left wrist. B) Loss of function because of destruction. C) The same wrist after Steinmann pin fusion.

extends beyond the distal limit of the extensor retinaculum and may produce a sizeable swelling. The swelling extends proximally but is less evident beneath the unyielding extensor retinaculum.

Flexor tenosynovitis produces less obvious swellings, but restriction of active movement and crepitus as bulky tendons move beneath pulleys are common. The swelling is seldom visible or palpable beneath the flexor retinaculum, but appears in the palm, distal forearm, and digits. Restriction of active flexion, or persistent pain and stiffness in the presence of healthy joints, should always raise the suspicion of flexor tenosynovitis, even if swelling is minimal. Median nerve compression secondary to flexor tenosynovitis may cause pain without the sensory symptoms which characterize its presentation in the non-rheumatoid patient.

The consequences of tenosynovitis are pain, restricted active motion, and tendon rupture. Two mechanisms cause tendon rupture: destruction of tendon fibres by invading synovial tissue, and attrition on rough bony prominences. Typically, the extensors of the fingers are abraded sequentially by the ulnar head. A bony spicule protruding from the scaphotrapezial joint into the carpal canal may damage the flexor pollicis longus tendon, followed by the profundus tendon of the index finger, the superficialis tendon of the index finger, and the profundus tendon of the middle finger.

Rupture of extensor tendons causes drooping at the metacarpophalangeal joints and loss of active extension. Provided that the metacarpophalangeal joint is healthy, passive extension is normal. Two important differential diagnoses may mimic extensor tendon rupture. Subluxation of the extensor tendon to the ulnar side of the metacarpophalangeal joint diminishes its power so that it cannot extend the joint actively from the flexed position. However, if the joint is extended passively, the tendon returns to its normal position and can maintain the extended position. Rarely, loss of active metacarpophalangeal joint extension is due to compression of the posterior interosseous nerve by synovitis around the radial neck. A complete palsy is usually obvious, but partial lesions may affect only one or two extensor muscles. As the wrist is flexed, the viscoelasticity of the paralyzed muscles pulls the metacarpophalangeal joints into extension, whereas the metacarpophalangeal joints will remain drooped if the tendons have ruptured.

Unfortunately, the occurrence of tendon ruptures does not correlate well with pain or tenosynovial swelling. The patient with profuse extensor tenosynovitis is certainly at risk of rupture. Dorsal wrist pain on active resisted finger extension may signify impending rupture. However, ruptures which are due to attrition on bone frequently occur without warning or pain. Ruptures of the extensor digiti minimi and flexor digitorum superficialis tendons may pass unnoticed by patient or doctor, but their detection is vital because they indicate that other ruptures may be imminent.

Extensor tenosynovectomy (Box 6.5.5)

The indications for extensor tenosynovectomy are tenosynovitis which persists after appropriate medical management and incipient or actual tendon rupture. In common with other wrist operations in rheumatoid disease, a straight longitudinal dorsal wrist

Box 6.5.5 Extensor tendons

- Commonly rupture especially over the ulna head
- Sequential ruptures are common
- Reconstruction is very valuable and more reliable early
- The cause—typically distal ulna—needs to be excised
- The tendons are repaired with transfers or grafts

incision is preferred because it minimizes the risks of skin necrosis and dorsal sensory nerve damage. It can be reopened for subsequent wrist operations as necessary. The essential steps are removal of diseased tenosynovium, excision of bony spurs (e.g. ulnar head), and replacement of part or all of the extensor retinaculum beneath the tendons to protect them from later disease in the wrist joint. The third, fourth, and fifth compartments are frequently involved and should be opened routinely. Tenosynovectomy of the second and sixth compartments may also be necessary. The first compartment is seldom involved.

The frequency of rupture of the extensor tendons in a review of 202 cases was as follows: extensor pollicis longus, 20%; extensor digitorum (little), 17%; extensor digitorum (ring), 15%; extensor digitorum (middle), 7%; extensor digitorum (index), 2%; flexor pollicis longus, 12%; flexor digitorum profundus (index), 7%.

The ruptured tendons are not amenable to direct repair as their stumps are diseased and have retracted. Reconstruction is generally by transfer of an intact and expendable tendon into the ruptured tendon (Figure 6.5.4), but a tendon graft may be used if the original muscle is in good condition and no expendable tendon is available for transfer.

Commonly used transfers are shown in Table 6.5.1. The wrist extensor tendons can be used for transfer if the wrist is fused, but their excursion is limited and they may be too short to reach the distal tendon stumps.

Table 6.5.1 Commonly used transfers

Tendon(s) ruptured	Suitable tendon for transfer
EPL	EIP
EDM	EIP
EDC × 1	Suture to adjacent extensor tendon or EIP
EDC × 2	EIP or adjacent suture or both
EDC > 2	EIP or tendon graft or combination

EPL, extensor pollicis longus; EIP, extensor indicis proprius; EDM, extensor digiti minimi; EDC, extensor digitorum communis.

Flexor tenosynovectomy (Box 6.5.6)

The indications for flexor tenosynovectomy are persistent painful tenosynovitis, incipient or actual tendon rupture, median nerve compression in the carpal canal, and triggering. As in the extensor system, timely tenosynovectomy is vital in preventing tendon rupture and preserving function of the hand.

At the wrist, the tendons are exposed by dividing the flexor retinaculum and extending the incision proximally and distally as necessary. The diseased tenosynovium is removed from the musculotendinous junction to the lumbrical insertion, taking care to minimize retraction of the median nerve. The floor of the carpal tunnel is inspected for bone spicules, which most commonly arise from the scaphotrapezial joint. Spicules are excised and the capsule repaired by direct suture or local capsular flap.

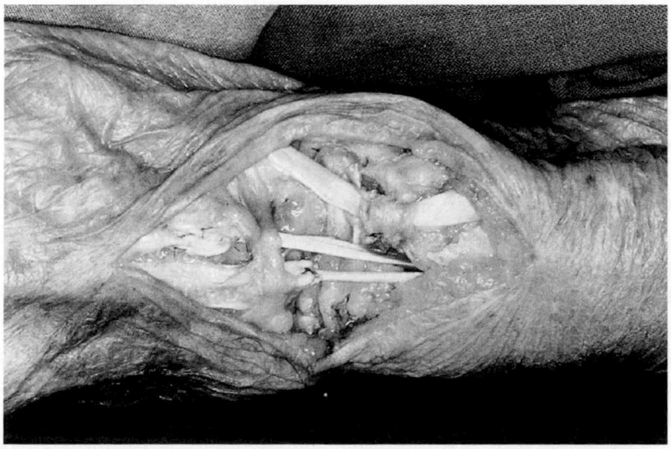

Fig. 6.5.4 Operative illustration of reconstruction of multiple extensor tendon ruptures. The only intact finger tendons are extensor indicis proprius and extensor digitorum communis to index finger. The former was transferred to extensor digitorum communis to ring and little fingers; the latter shared with extensor digitorum communis middle finger. The distal ulna has been excised. Note the stabilization of extensor carpi ulnaris using part of the extensor retinaculum as a sling (see text).

Segments of the digital flexor sheath can be exposed through transverse or zigzag incisions. Tenosynovitis is seen most often beneath the A1 pulley and just distal to the A2 pulley (Figure 6.5.5), but can affect the entire sheath. Diseased synovium and intratendinous nodules are excised. Release of the A1 pulley in rheumatoid disease is controversial, as it may allow ulnar migration of the flexor tendons and aggravate ulnar drift deformity of the metacarpophalangeal joints. Some surgeons prefer to decompress the digital sheath by excision of the ulnar slip of the superficialis tendon, a procedure that achieves decompression at the A2 as well as at the A1 pulley and which removes any possibility of entrapment of the flexor digitorum profundus tendon between the two slips of the superficialis tendon.

The management of flexor tendon rupture is also controversial. Rupture of flexor pollicis longus requires prompt exploration of the carpal canal and removal of the cause of rupture (osteophyte from the scaphotrapezial joint or invasive tenosynovitis), to prevent rupture of other tendons. Active flexion of the interphalangeal joint can be restored by transfer of a superficialis tendon, but the range of motion thus gained is usually small. Fusion of the interphalangeal joint in slight flexion is often preferred in the weak hand of the rheumatoid patient, as it gives a stable thumb with good power transmitted from the short muscles.

Loss of both tendons within the digital sheath is disabling but reconstruction is difficult. Transfer of the flexor digitorum superficialis tendon from another finger can be used if a healthy distal flexor digitorum profundus stump is present; otherwise tendon grafting may be necessary despite its unpredictable outcome.

Options for reconstruction of ruptured flexor tendons are shown in Table 6.5.2. The results of tendon reconstruction are dependent

Box 6.5.6 Flexor tendons

- Less often affected
- A CTR often suffices to settle symptoms
- Sequential rupture is much less common
- Reconstruction is with transfers or grafts

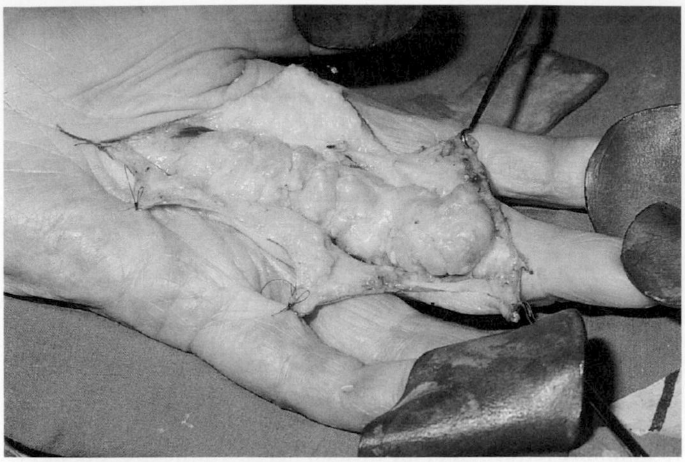

Fig. 6.5.5 Flexor tenosynovitis in the digital sheath.

on the number and level of the ruptures. Full active flexion is seldom regained.

Metacarpophalangeal joint

Many factors have been implicated in the production of ulnar deviation at the metacarpophalangeal joints. Synovitis at the metacarpophalangeal joint causes distension of the joint capsule and stretching of the collateral ligaments. The lax joints are then vulnerable to malalignment under the influence of muscle and other forces. The main factors appear to be the strong forces applied by the flexor tendons, which produce palmar subluxation, and by the thumb, which exerts pressure on the sides of the fingers during grip and pinch. If movement of the fingers is painful, the thumb may become the main source of functional grip and its use for key pinch against the sides of the fingers, rather than 'tripod' pinch to the tips, may deform the lax metacarpophalangeal joints. Subluxation of the extensor tendons and tightness of the ulnar intrinsic muscles are commonly seen in ulnar deviated fingers, but whether they are a contributory cause or a consequence of ulnar drift is uncertain (Box 6.5.7). Ulnar drift at the metacarpophalangeal joints is also associated with radial deviation deformity of the wrist, but again it is unclear if the wrist deformity is a cause or a consequence of ulnar drift. It is clear, however, that surgical correction of ulnar drift will fail if fixed radial wrist deviation is not also corrected.

Table 6.5.2 Commonly used transfers

Tendon(s) ruptured	Salvage procedure
FPL	IP joint fusion
FDS	None
FDP – wrist	Suture to adjacent FDP tendon or tendon graft
FDP – finger	DIP joint fusion
FDP + FDS – finger	Tendon graft or FDS transfer from another finger

FPL, flexor pollicis longus; IP, interphalangeal; FDS, flexor digitorum superficialis; FDP, flexor digitorum profundus; DIP, distal interphalangeal.

Box 6.5.7 Metacarpophalangeal (MP) joints

- Ulna drift is caused by:
  - Deforming forces of life, especially pinch and holding
  - Pull of tendons which worsen as the deformity progresses
  - Laxity of restraining structures especially ligaments
  - MP joint surgery
- Non-operative treatment:
  - Splintage is used but unproven
  - Steroid injections often help
- Operative treatment:
  - Synovectomy and soft tissue balancing has a role but recurrent deformity can occur early
  - Silastic MP joint replacement is well established and reliable
  - Silastic joints often break up but patients only infrequently need revision surgery.

The early stages of metacarpophalangeal joint synovitis are amenable to medical management. Synovectomy is effective in relieving pain and swelling that have persisted after appropriate medical treatment, but probably does not alter the course of the disease. Synovectomy may be performed in isolation or in combination with soft tissue reconstruction.

Synovectomy and soft-tissue reconstruction are indicated when synovitis is associated with passively correctable ulnar deviation and well-preserved joints without palmar subluxation. Subluxation of extensor tendons to the ulnar side of the metacarpophalangeal joint often occurs at this stage. The reconstruction may require release of tight intrinsic muscles, centralization of extensor tendons, reefing of lax radial collateral ligaments, and transfer of ulnar intrinsic tendons to the radial side of the adjacent digit (crossed intrinsic transfer). The intrinsic tendon may be attached to the radial aspect of the proximal phalanx, to the fibrous flexor sheath, or to the radial lateral band. Ulnar deviation of the index finger may be improved by reefing the tendon of the first dorsal interosseous muscle.

The extensor tendon is centralized by reefing of the radial sagittal bands and, if necessary, release of tight ulnar sagittal bands. Alternatively, a distally based strip of extensor tendon can be passed palmar to the deep transverse metacarpal ligament and sutured back to the remaining tendon. This type of reconstruction may cause some limitation of extension but it is effective in securing the alignment of the tendon (Figure 6.5.6). Persisting ulnar deviation may be improved by reefing of the radial collateral ligaments, but at the risk of some loss of metacarpophalangeal joint movement.

The essence of postoperative management is to allow early motion but protect against ulnar deviation forces until the soft tissues have healed. If the reconstruction is secure, protection in a static splint between exercise sessions for 6 weeks is sufficient. Alternatively, a dynamic extension outrigger splint supports the metacarpophalangeal joints in extension and radial deviation but allows flexion.

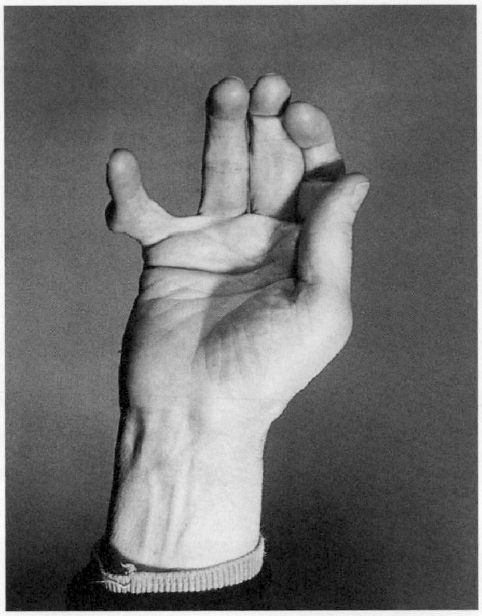

Fig. 6.5.6 Ulnar deviation of little finger suitable for extensor loop procedure. The patient is failing to control abduction with a thick rubber band around ring and little fingers.

Metacarpophalangeal arthroplasty is required for fixed ulnar deviation, palmar subluxation, and metacarpophalangeal destruction. Excision arthroplasty does not provide stability and may be followed by progressive loss of bone stock. Hinged and other total replacement arthroplasties have a high rate of early failure. The gold standard is the Swanson silastic flexible implant arthroplasty. A fibrous capsule forms around the implant, which pistons freely in the medullary cavities and acts as a spacer which maintains length and supports the soft-tissue reconstruction.

Not all patients with metacarpophalangeal joint destruction require metacarpophalangeal joint arthroplasty. The best indications are relief of pain and correction of deformity which is interfering with function. Moderate ulnar drift is compatible with satisfactory function, particularly if metacarpophalangeal joint pain is modest and interphalangeal movement is good.

Silastic metacarpophalangeal arthroplasty has given consistent and predictable relief of pain and improvement of ulnar deviation. The active flexion range at long-term review is 35–55 degrees. Mild recurrence of ulnar deviation may occur over several years, depending partly on the rate of progression of the disease. Particulate silicone synovitis is rare around metacarpophalangeal joint implants. Fracture of the implant occurs but does not necessarily cause symptoms or necessitate removal of the implant.

Metacarpophalangeal arthroplasty is performed through a single transverse or multiple longitudinal incisions. The metacarpal head is removed at a level just distal to the origin of the collateral ligaments. Release of the ulnar collateral ligament may be needed if ulnar deviation is severe. Release of the palmar plate may also be necessary. It is vital that sufficient space is created to accept the implant without buckling on flexion and extension. The medullary canals are reamed to accept the largest implant which will fit comfortably.

The implant provides a flexible and stable base for the soft-tissue reconstruction, which is vital to the success of the operation. The reconstruction may include intrinsic release, crossed intrinsic transfer, and extensor realignment. The radial collateral ligament may require reefing or, if it is deficient, reconstruction using the radial half of the palmar plate.

Postoperative management aims to encourage the formation of a soft tissue envelope which allows flexion/extension but is stable from side to side. Dynamic splintage, as described earlier for synovectomy and soft-tissue reconstruction, is widely used. However, crossed intrinsic transfer may remove the need for dynamic splintage.

Proximal interphalangeal joint (Box 6.5.8)

The proximal interphalangeal joint is a hinge joint which allows motion from 0–120 degrees. The stout collateral ligaments and palmar plate confer good lateral stability and resistance to hyperextension. Synovitis of the proximal interphalangeal joint produces a spindle-shaped swelling of the finger and rapidly limits movement. Synovectomy is indicated for persistent painful synovitis in the face of adequate medical therapy. Access is limited and may require incisions between the central slip and the lateral band on each side. The incisions are closed securely to prevent palmar migration of the lateral bands.

Deformity of the proximal interphalangeal joint is common in rheumatoid arthritis and is usually in the sagittal plane. It reflects disturbance of the delicately balanced muscle and tendon systems which act across the proximal interphalangeal joint.

Swan-neck deformity

Swan-neck deformity is hyperextension at the proximal interphalangeal joint and flexion of the distal interphalangeal joint. It results from imbalance in the tendon systems which cross the proximal interphalangeal joint and is generally due to weakening of a tendon insertion or static joint restraint by diseased synovium. Because the three joints are interdependent though their tendon

Box 6.5.8 Proximal interphalangeal (PIP) joints

- Instability is a particular problem.
- Early treatment is much more effective and can prevent later problems
- Swan neck deformity: can be caused by problems at the MP, PIP, or DIP joints
- Boutonniere deformity: caused by central slip failure
- Treatment:
  - Swan-neck deformity—should be treated early with soft tissue balancing
  - Boutonniere—rarely needs treatment
  - Joint destruction
  - Arthrodesis is simple and reliable but less good for the ring and little fingers
  - Arthroplasty works reasonably well in low-demand patients.

and ligament systems, swan-neck deformity can be caused by synovitis at any one of the three finger joints. Swan-neck deformity can occur only if hyperextension is possible at the proximal interphalangeal joint.

Proximal interphalangeal joint synovitis weakens the palmar plate and superficialis insertion, allowing hyperextension of the proximal interphalangeal joint. Later, the lateral bands migrate dorsally as the transverse retinacular ligaments elongate and a secondary extension lag appears at the distal interphalangeal joint.

Destruction of the terminal tendon of the dorsal aponeurosis by synovitis at the distal interphalangeal joint may also initiate swan-neck deformity. Without the attachment of the terminal tendon, the dorsal aponeurosis migrates proximally and pulls excessively on the central slip, resulting in hyperextension of the proximal interphalangeal joint.

Flexion deformity at the metacarpophalangeal joints is often associated with swan-neck deformity. Many factors may be involved, including intrinsic muscle contracture.

Swan-neck deformity has been graded into four types, depending on the mobility of the proximal interphalangeal joint and the condition of the joint surfaces.

- *Type I*: the proximal interphalangeal joint is mobile in all positions of the metacarpophalangeal joint. The zigzag posture is due to imbalance
- *Type II*: proximal interphalangeal joint flexion is full while the metacarpophalangeal joint is flexed but limited when the metacarpophalangeal joint is extended. Intrinsic tightness is present
- *Type III*: the proximal interphalangeal joint is stiff in all positions of the metacarpophalangeal joint but the joint surfaces are healthy
- *Type IV*: the proximal interphalangeal joint is stiff and the joint surfaces are damaged.

The disability of swan-neck deformity is due mainly to lack of flexion of the proximal interphalangeal joint. If the proximal interphalangeal joint is mobile, it may 'lock up' in hyperextension and flex with a snap as flexion effort is increased and the lateral bands slide from dorsal to palmar over the sides of the joint.

Type I swan-neck deformity may require no treatment. Locking of the proximal interphalangeal joint in extension (Figure 6.5.7) can be prevented by blocking hyperextension with a figure-of-eight splint. If a thermoplastic splint is effective, a more durable splint may be constructed from metal and worn like a ring. Hyperextension may also be corrected by tenodesis across the palmar aspect of the proximal interphalangeal joint, using one slip of the superficialis tendon which is detached proximally and sutured to the A2 pulley. Alternatively, the lumbrical tendon can be rebalanced as a flexor of the proximal interphalangeal joint. Fusion of the distal interphalangeal joint may also be useful, particularly when the swan-neck deformity is due to elongation of the terminal tendon.

Type II deformity is due to tightness of the intrinsic muscles. Proximal interphalangeal joint flexion is limited when the metacarpophalangeal joint is extended but normal when the metacarpophalangeal joint is flexed (the intrinsic tightness test). The restriction is often increased by deviation of the metacarpophalangeal joint to the radial side, showing that the tightness is greater on the ulnar side. A distal intrinsic release is performed, excising a triangle of the dorsal aponeurosis which includes the ulnar lateral band and adjacent oblique fibres. A tenodesis or tendon rebalancing may be required, as for type I.

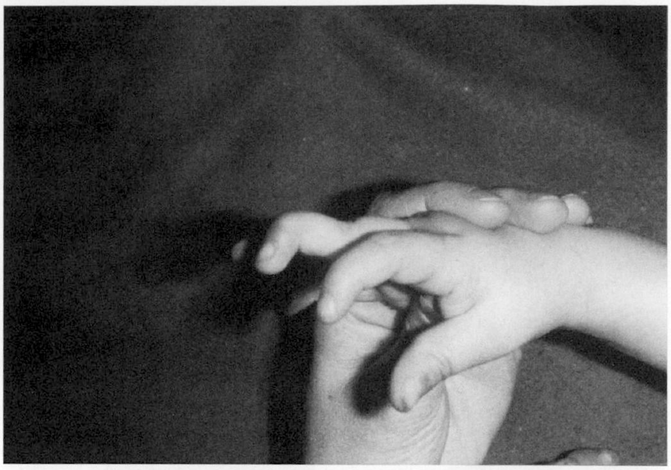

A

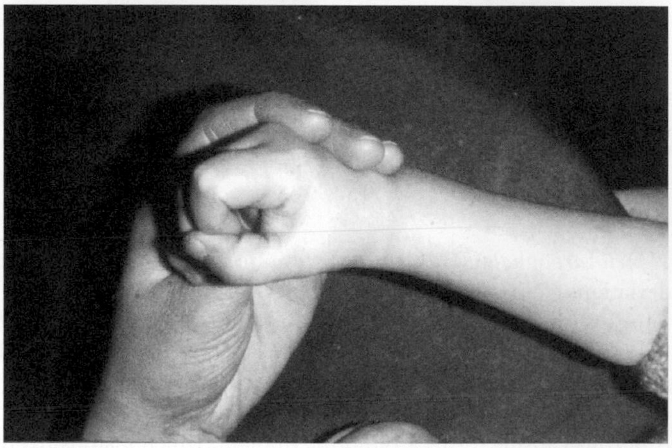

B

Fig. 6.5.7 A) Swan-neck deformity locking in extension and unable to grip examiner's thumb. B) The examiner's thumb has pushed the metacarpophalangeal joint into flexion, allowing full active flexion and grip (type II swan-neck deformity).

If the swan neck deformity was initiated at distal interphalangeal joint level as a 'mallet finger' fusion of the terminal joint in a position just short of full extension may need to be added.

Type III deformity prevents grasp because the proximal interphalangeal joints are fixed in extension. Passive flexion is prevented by soft tissue contracture which may involve the dorsal aponeurosis, the dorsal capsule of the proximal interphalangeal joint, and the skin. The lateral bands are fixed dorsally and cannot slide toward the palm to allow flexion. Manipulation of the proximal interphalangeal joint may restore flexion in less severe cases. An oblique skin release over the middle phalanx may be needed if the skin blanches on flexion. The joint can be stabilized temporarily with a pin across the joint. This procedure may be useful in psoriatic arthropathy, where the finger joints characteristically become stiff at an early stage without marked joint destruction. Mobilization of the lateral bands from the central slip may be needed in more severe cases. These procedures may be performed at the same time as metacarpophalangeal joint arthroplasty.

Type IV deformity is best managed by arthrodesis (see later). In selected patients, Swanson or pyrocarbon arthroplasty of the proximal interphalangeal joints can be considered, provided that tendon imbalance is corrected. Arthroplasty should be restricted to the proximal interphalangeal joints of the ring and little fingers, which require flexion for power grip. The index and middle fingers are also used for tripod pinch to the tip of the thumb; stability of pinch is more important than additional flexion in these digits. Aids such as large-handled cutlery can mitigate the effects of loss of flexion.

Arthrodesis of the proximal interphalangeal joint should be performed using a technique that gives stable fixation, allows early movement of other joints, and does not require plaster immobilization. Tension band wire fixation provides stable fixation without unduly prominent metalwork (Figure 6.5.8) and avoids protruding pins with their inconvenience, risk of infection, and need for removal before fusion is secure. Care must be taken to preserve the cancellous bone of the head of the proximal phalanx; excessive resection exposes the hard cortical bone of the neck and may delay union. The angle of fusion depends on the digit and the range of motion of other joints in the hand. The angles usually selected are: index 35 degrees; middle 45 degrees; ring 55 degrees; and little 65 degrees.

Arthrodesis of the distal joint is performed in a few degrees of flexion, though greater flexion may be required to accommodate to deformity of other joints or for specific functional needs. Tension band fixation is stable and avoids protruding pins, but an oblique K-wire and interosseous wiring technique is easier in these small joints. Fixation with a Herbert screw is also effective (Figure 6.5.9).

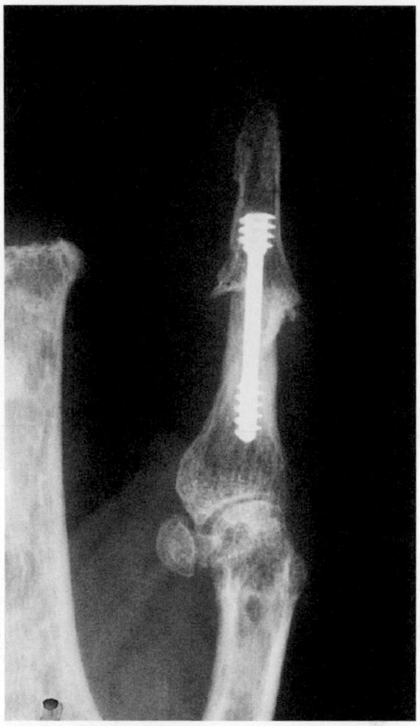

Fig. 6.5.9 Interphalangeal joint fusion using a Herbert screw.

Boutonnière deformity

Boutonnière deformity comprises flexion of the proximal interphalangeal joint and hyperextension of the distal joint. It is compatible with surprisingly good function in the rheumatoid hand, especially if some flexion is possible at the distal joint (Figure 6.5.10). Boutonnière deformity in the fingers always results from disease at the proximal interphalangeal joint, leading to destruction of the central slip. The lateral bands migrate in a palmar direction, where they become fixed by contracture of the transverse retinacular ligament. In this position, they no longer act to extend the proximal interphalangeal joint and their pull on the distal joint is excessive. Unfortunately, the results of soft tissue reconstruction of rheumatoid boutonnière deformity are unsatisfactory. If surgery is needed, it should be fusion of the proximal interphalangeal joint in a functional position. Tenotomy of the extensor tendon over the middle phalanx may improve the range of flexion of the terminal joint in less severe cases.

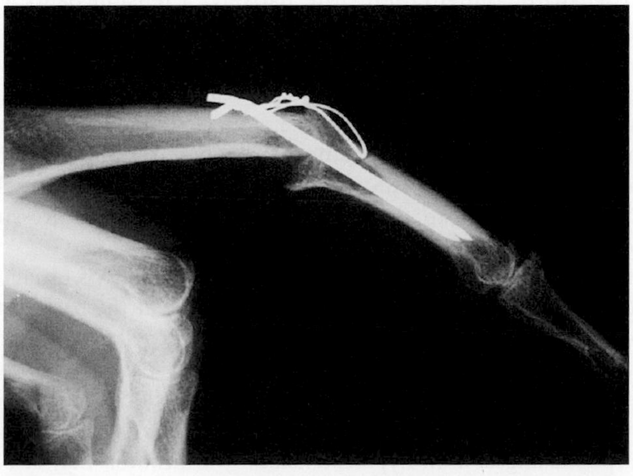

Fig. 6.5.8 Proximal interphalangeal joint fusion using tension band wire technique.

Lateral deformities and instability of the proximal interphalangeal joint are usually due to joint destruction; arthrodesis in a functional position is the only way to improve grip. In cases of mutilating arthritis with multiple joint destruction, loss of length, and instability, the principle is to provide stable fingers in the best functional position with movement concentrated at the base of the finger. It may be necessary to fuse both proximal and distal interphalangeal joints.

Thumb (Box 6.5.9)

The joints of the thumb are frequently affected by rheumatoid disease. Any of the three joints can be affected. The thumb is used in nearly all daily activities and the complaint is almost always of painful interference with function rather than of pain alone. The loss of pinch strength is frequently associated with instability of one or more joints. Repeated loading of the distended and inflamed joints leads to failure of the ligaments and to deformity. As in the fingers, the interdependence of the joint mechanisms results in a zigzag posture in which the failure of one joint leads to opposite deformity of adjacent joints.

Deformities of the thumb fall into three patterns.

1) *Boutonnière thumb* Flexion at the metacarpophalangeal joint with hyperextension at the interphalangeal joint. The basal joint is not affected. The primary deformity is usually at the

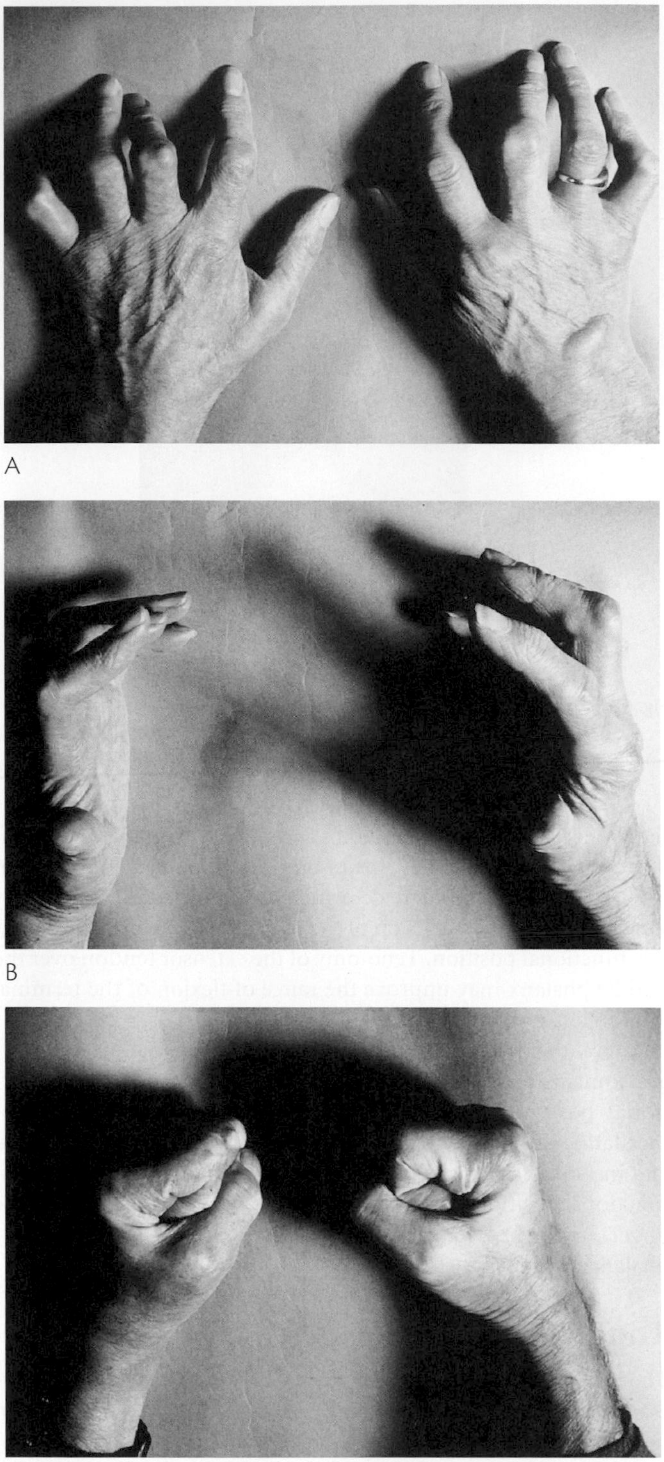

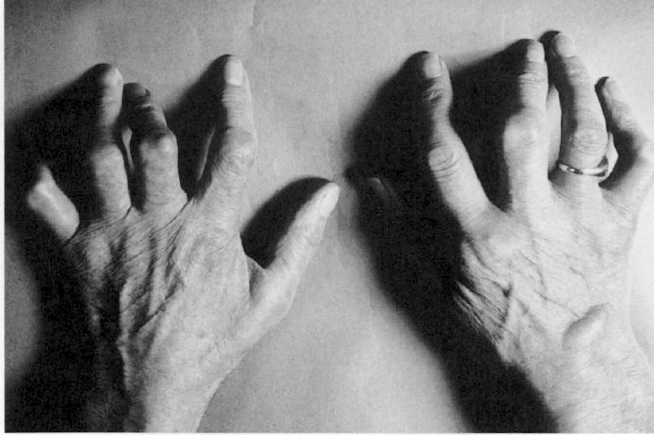

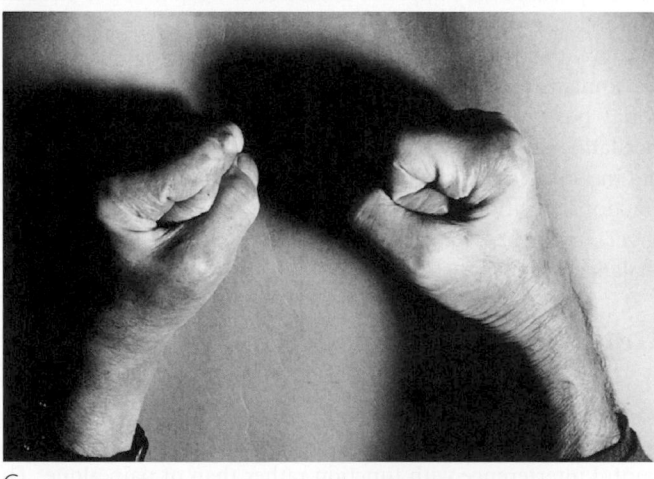

A

B

C

Fig. 6.5.10 A) Flexion contractures of multiple proximal interphalangeal joints. B) Lateral view, showing attempted extension. C) Full active flexion and good function.

Box 6.5.9 Thumb

The thumb is very important but relatively simple to treat

- Carpometacarpal joint:
  - It is often destroyed/subluxed but usually does not need treatment
  - Trapezectomy ± ligament reconstruction is reliable
- MP and IP joints:
  - Soft tissue procedures are unreliable
  - Fusion is reliable and well tolerated.

metacarpophalangeal joint, where synovitis weakens the dorsal hood and the resulting flexion posture leads to secondary hyperextension at the interphalangeal joint

2) *Swan-neck thumb* Damage of the basal joint causes dorsal subluxation with flexion and adduction of the first metacarpal, hyperextension of the metacarpophalangeal joint, and flexion of the interphalangeal joint

3) *Lateral instability* Lateral deformity is due to failure of the radial collateral ligament and/or destruction of the metacarpophalangeal or interphalangeal joints. Metacarpal adduction can occur secondarily.

A more complicated classification into six types has been proposed by Nalebuff and others, but the scheme listed here describes the great majority of thumb deformities.

In considering treatment, the thumb must be regarded as providing a stable post against which the fingers can work to provide pinch grip. Mobility is needed at the basal joint so that the thumb can be positioned appropriately. At the metacarpophalangeal and interphalangeal joints, stability is more important than movement. Therefore instability at these joints should be managed by arthrodesis in 0–20 degrees of flexion. In the author's opinion, silastic interposition arthroplasty has no place in the treatment of the rheumatoid thumb.

Arthrodesis of the interphalangeal joint of the thumb is performed by a tension band wiring technique through an S-shaped dorsal incision with care to protect the nail-bed. At the metacarpophalangeal joint, the bones are large enough to use a 'chevron' method in which a V-shaped notch is made in the head of the metacarpal and the base of the proximal phalanx is trimmed to fit it. The large surfaces of cancellous bone will fuse rapidly and can be held with K-wires at 90 degrees to each side of the V in a crossed-wire configuration. Alternatively, a tension band wire technique can be used, as in the proximal interphalangeal joint of the finger (Figure 6.5.11). In the case of marked bone loss in mutilating arthritis, it may be necessary to fuse both metacarpophalangeal and interphalangeal joints to maintain length or indeed to gain length by interposing corticocancellous grafts from the iliac crest. This apparently drastic surgery can improve function remarkably and help to maintain the patient's independence for dressing, cooking, and eating.

In the swan-neck thumb, the primary abnormality is usually at the basal joint. The aim of providing mobility at the base of the thumb precludes fusion. Trapezial excision arthroplasty with stabilization of the metacarpal base using a distally-based strip of the flexor carpi radialis tendon is effective and straightforward. Release of the contracted muscles of the thumb web and correction of metacarpophalangeal joint hyperextension by arthrodesis may also be necessary.

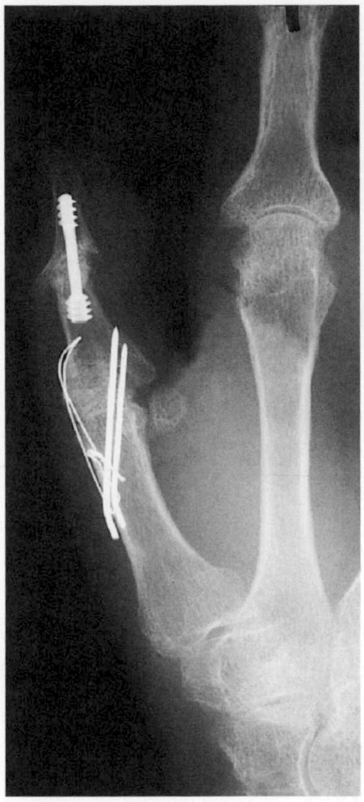

Fig. 6.5.11 Thumb metacarpophalangeal joint fusion using tension band wire technique. The interphalangeal joint has been fused with a Herbert screw passed from proximal to distal before fixation of the metacarpophalangeal joint.

Rheumatoid nodules

Nodules on the hand are more than a cosmetic problem. They occur commonly on the dorsum of the proximal interphalangeal joint, where they are easily knocked, and in the pulps of the digits, where they cause pain and interfere with grip. Many patients have relatively little joint destruction and their function can be improved by removal of painful nodules. Excision under local or regional anaesthesia may be very helpful, but patients should be aware that the tendency to form nodules can continue for many years and many operations may be needed.

Further reading

Feldon, P., Millender, L.H., and Nalebuff, E.A. (1993). Rheumatoid arthritis of the hand and wrist. In: Green, D.P. (ed) *Operative Hand Surgery*, third edition, pp. 1587–690. New York: Churchill Livingstone. [Detailed description of indications for surgery, operative procedures, and postoperative care.]

Flatt, A. (1995). *Care of the Arthritic Hand*, fifth edition. St Louis, MO: Quality Medical Publishing. [This book gives lucid descriptions of the pathology and mechanics of deformity in the rheumatoid hand and wrist, as well as covering assessment and operative treatment in detail.]

Lister, G.D. (1993). *The Hand: Diagnosis and Indications*, third edition. Edinburgh: Churchill Livingstone. [A concise and clear description of the pathology, clinical assessment, and indications for surgery.]

Ruby, L.K. and Cassidy, C. (eds) (1996). *Hand Clinics*, **12**(3). [This issue of Hand Clinics is devoted to rheumatoid disease and contains many good review articles.]

Souter, W.A. (1979). Planning treatment of the rheumatoid hand. *Hand*, **11**, 3–16.

6.6

Osteoarthritis of the hand

T.R.C. Davis and N.D. Downing

Summary points

- Prevalence of hand osteoarthritis increases with age
- Most hand osteoarthritis causes few symptoms
- Non-operative management is sufficient for the majority of cases
- Surgical treatment is sometimes required
- Total joint replacements have significant failure rates.

Prevalence and aetiology

Osteoarthritis of the hand is uncommon under the age of 50, but is very common, although usually painless, in older people. Some hand joints are more susceptible than others: over 50% of women aged 55–65 years have distal interphalangeal, about 40% have proximal interphalangeal, one-third trapeziometacarpal, and a fifth metacarpophalangeal joint osteoarthritis (Box 6.6.1).

The aetiology of hand osteoarthritis is poorly understood. 'Repetitive manual work' has been implicated as an aetiological factor with little, if any, supportive evidence. Most hand osteoarthritis is idiopathic (cause unknown) and this may either be localized to the hand or generalized. Idiopathic osteoarthritis is more common in women and has a hereditary predisposition.

Secondary hand osteoarthritis may occur as a complication of intra-articular fractures and infections. However, only a minority of properly treated intra-articular fractures develop symptomatic osteoarthritis and most joint infections are now treated promptly before the articular cartilage is destroyed.

Isolated osteoarthritis of the index and middle finger metacarpophalangeal joints is seen in haemochromatosis and may be the first clinical manifestation of the condition.

Clinical presentation

Hand osteoarthritis commonly causes joint stiffness, hand weakness, and deformity. It rarely causes disabling pain and only a few of those affected require treatment. For example, only 30% of women with radiological trapeziometacarpal joint osteoarthritis experience any pain. Thus when assessing patients with hand pain and radiological osteoarthritis, it is vital to confirm that the osteoarthritis is causing the pain and is not merely coincidental.

Finger interphalangeal joint osteoarthritis

History, examination, and radiographs (Box 6.6.2)

Osteoarthritis of these joints is usually painless. However, it commonly causes finger stiffness which may cause loss of dexterity and weakness. Osteophytes and soft tissue hypertrophy produce the characteristic Heberden's (distal) and Bouchard's (proximal) nodes (Figure 6.6.1).

Painful osteoarthritic interphalangeal joints are usually mildly tender and painful when stressed (rocked from side to side). Interphalangeal joint extension is usually preserved, but the range of flexion gradually reduces and may become painful at its extreme. Crepitus may be elicited and mucous cysts (ganglia arising from a joint) sometimes appear on the dorsum of the osteoarthritic distal interphalangeal joint. These may cause nail deformity.

Radiographs should include the metacarpophalangeal and both interphalangeal joints of the involved finger, not just the affected joint, in order to see the condition of the neighbouring joints. The standard views are posteroanterior and lateral for the interphalangeal joints, with an additional oblique view for the metacarpophalangeal joint.

Box 6.6.1 Incidence of osteoarthritis of the hand

- Common in those over 50
- In women aged 55–65 years:
  - 62% distal interphalangeal joint (DIPJ)
  - 40% proximal interphalangeal joint (PIPJ)
  - 33% thumb base
  - 20% metacarpophalangeal joint (MPJ)
- *But* often pain free.

Box 6.6.2 Finger interphalangeal joint osteoarthritis: assessment

- History: usually clear. May be a history of injury
- Examination:
  - Deformity
  - Tenderness
  - Stiffness
- Investigation:
  - Plain radiography—confirms diagnosis
  - X-ray features are *not* well correlated with symptoms.

Management (Box 6.6.3)

Painless osteoarthritis causing stiffness and hand weakness may improve with physiotherapy and is not an indication for surgical treatment. Interphalangeal joint osteoarthritic pain is commonly transient and may respond to conservative measures such as reassurance, rest, activity modification, analgesia, physiotherapy, and steroid injections. Surgery is reserved for patients with persistent joint pain which restricts activities and does not respond to conservative measures. The surgical options are arthroplasty and arthrodesis, and both have their drawbacks (Box 6.6.4).

Interphalangeal joint arthroplasty

Arthroplasty of the distal interphalangeal joint has been reported but is seldom performed as distal interphalangeal joint arthrodesis causes little disability.

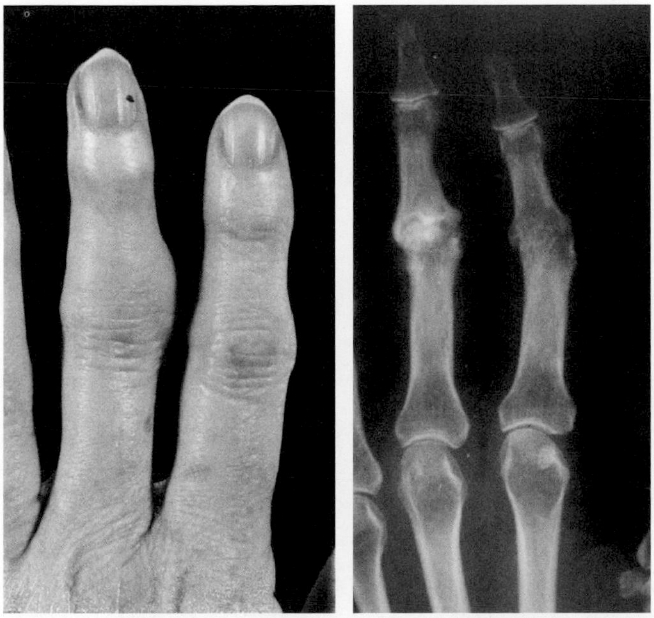

A B

Fig. 6.6.1 A) Osteoarthritic swelling of the distal interphalangeal (Heberden's nodes) and proximal interphalangeal (Bouchard's nodes) joints. B) Radiographs show advanced osteoarthritis. The index finger proximal interphalangeal joint has spontaneously fused.

Box 6.6.3 Finger interphalangeal joint osteoarthritis: non-operative treatment

- Activity modification
- Non-steroidal anti-inflammatories
- Splint
- Steroid injection.

Proximal interphalangeal joint arthrodesis causes considerable disability and elderly patients with osteoarthritis of this joint are usually satisfied with a silicone interposition arthroplasty (Figure 6.6.2). Pain relief is predictable in the majority of cases but as a general rule the range of movement remains the same as preoperatively. Silicone interposition arthroplasty should be used with caution in younger patients who place greater demands on their hands as these implants have a limited lifespan and may fracture or wear and cause silicone synovitis. Furthermore, they have little collateral stability and thus pinch strength is weak. Silicone synovitis may cause severe osteolysis which makes salvage surgery difficult. Silicone proximal interphalangeal joint arthroplasty may be performed through dorsal, palmar, or lateral approaches with equivalent results.

Dissatisfaction with the results of silicone interposition arthroplasty has lead to the development of two-piece proximal interphalangeal joint replacements. Initial designs were simple hinges

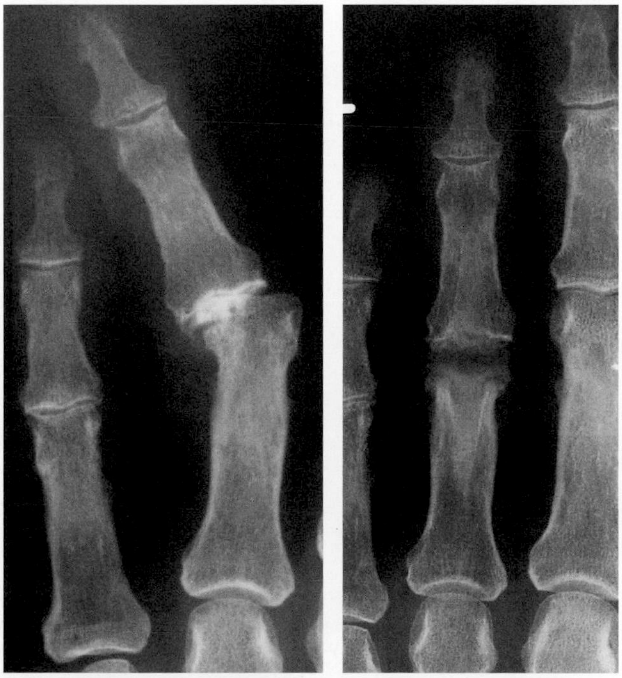

A B

Fig. 6.6.2. A) Advanced proximal interphalangeal joint osteoarthritis causing angular deformity. B) This was treated with a silicone interposition arthroplasty.

allowing single-plane motion and these rapidly loosened. Subsequent semiconstrained surface replacement designs preserve the collateral ligaments, seek to balance the flexor and extensor forces, and require minimal bone resection. The first surface replacement design was developed by Linscheid and Dobyns in 1979 and was modified in 1997. The results of 66 of these at a mean follow-up of 4.5 years revealed 32 good, 19 fair, and 25 poor results Significant complications, including instability, angular deviation, swan-neck deformity, subluxation, and flexion contracture, were seen in 19 cases, but there was no loosening.

Further development of surface replacement arthroplasty has concentrated on the bone–implant interface and on the material composition of the implant. There is currently much interest in pyrolytic carbon implants (Figure 6.6.3), which are known to have excellent wear properties. Short-term results are encouraging, with predictable pain relief and generally good patient satisfaction, though with high complication and reoperation rates. Metal and polyethylene implants have also been developed. Currently no clear advantage over silicone interpositional arthroplasty has been demonstrated.

Interphalangeal joint arthrodesis

This is the standard treatment for painful distal interphalangeal joint osteoarthritis. Although the best cosmetic result is achieved by fusing this joint in extension, fusion in slight flexion may produce better function.

Proximal interphalangeal joint arthrodesis is the best option for young manual workers who require strong resilient fingers, especially for the index finger. The position of fusion is debated: around 30–40 degrees for the index finger increasing to 45–60 degrees for the little finger. Arthrodesis of the index proximal interphalangeal joint is better tolerated as pinch is facilitated and power grip minimally compromised. Some patients with arthrodesis of a single proximal interphalangeal joint subsequently request amputation.

Arthrodesis techniques

Both interphalangeal joints are usually arthrodesed through a dorsal approach. The articular surfaces are either resected with appropriately angled saw cuts (difficult to judge accurately) or rongeured to create concentric cancellous surfaces. The latter technique allows some adjustment of the fusion angle and preserves more length. The arthrodesis can then be stabilized with K-wires, a tension band wire, a lag screw, or a headless bone screw (Figure 6.6.4). The critical point is that the bone ends are held in close approximation for the 8–10 weeks needed to achieve bone union.

Arthrodesis results

The reported non-union rates for distal interphalangeal joint arthrodesis range from 0–20%. Not all distal interphalangeal joint non-unions are painful and require revision surgery. The proximal interphalangeal joint is larger and more accessible than the distal joint and thus is easier to fuse and has a higher union rate.

Mucous cyst treatment

See Chapter 6.13.

Metacarpophalangeal joints of the fingers

Primary metacarpophalangeal joint osteoarthritis is usually asymptomatic but painful secondary osteoarthritis can occur following severe intra-articular fractures or infections (e.g. following a human bite sustained in a fight).

Occasionally, an otherwise painless osteoarthritic joint can lock in flexion as a result of the radial collateral ligament catching on an osteophyte on the metacarpal head (Figure 6.6.5) (best seen on the posteroanterior oblique radiograph). This locking usually affects the index or middle fingers. Joint distension with local anaesthetic and manipulation is the first-line treatment though the prominent osteophytes often need excision.

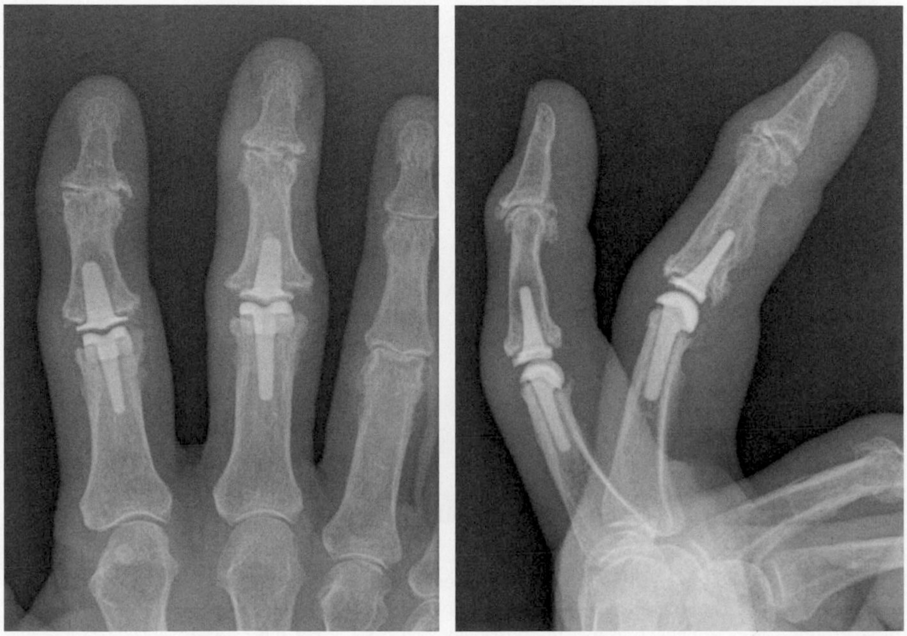

A B

Fig. 6.6.3 Pyrocarbon proximal interphalangeal joint implants.

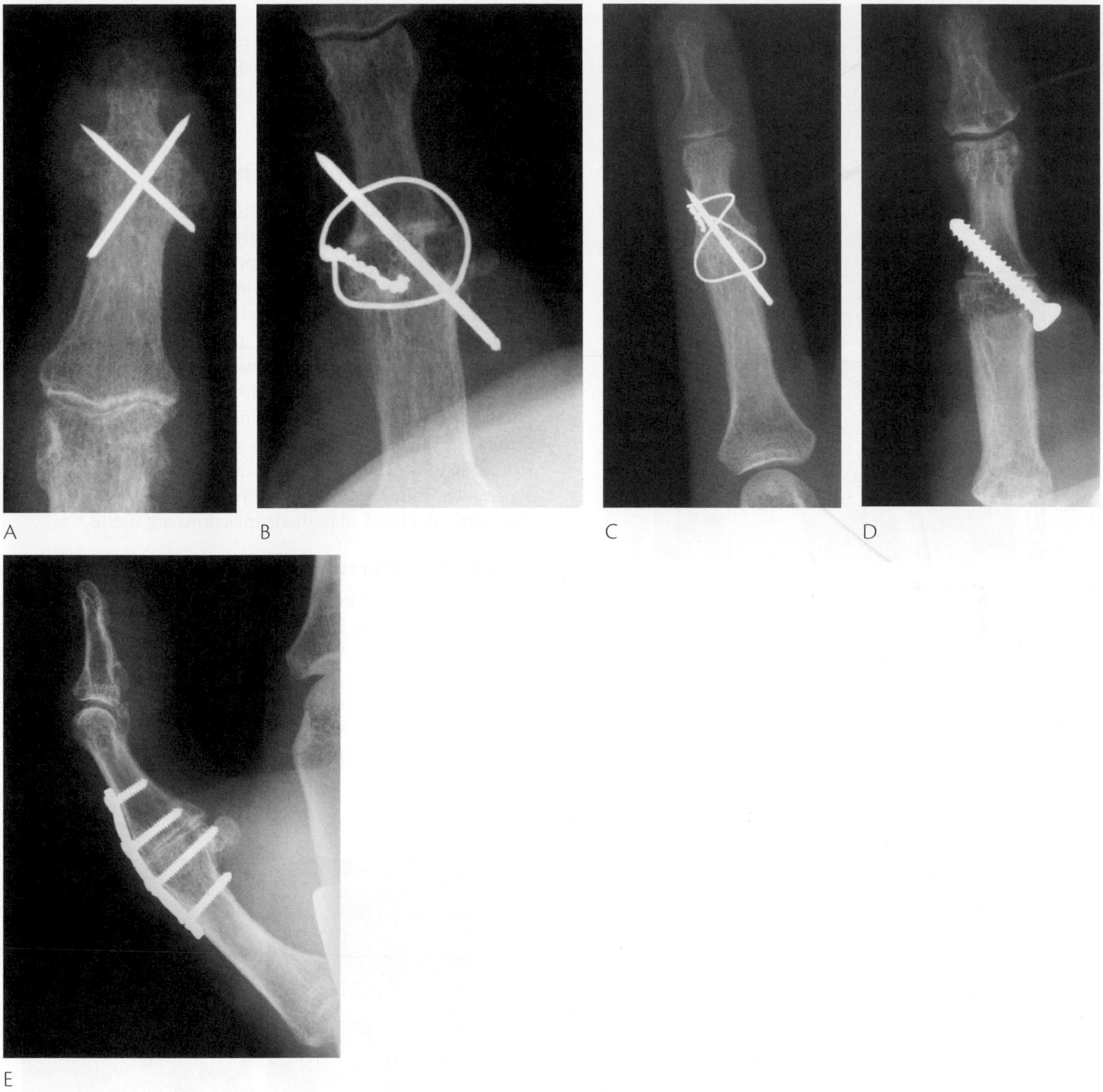

Fig. 6.6.4 Arthrodesis techniques for the metacarpophalangeal and interphalangeal joints of the hand. A) Crossed K-wires. B) K-wire and circlage wire. C) K-wire and tension band wire. D) Lag screw. E) Mini-fragment plate.

Box 6.6.4 Finger interphalangeal joint osteoarthritis: surgery

- Arthroplasty: unreliable either silastic or newer resurfacing implants
- Arthrodesis:
  - Reliable but awkward
  - Better in the DIPJs and index PIPJ
  - But less good for MPJs and ulnar PIPJs.

Management

Painful metacarpophalangeal joint osteoarthritis can be treated by arthrodesis or arthroplasty. Options for arthroplasty include excision, silicone interposition, or surface replacement.

Arthrodesis

Arthrodesis of the metacarpophalangeal joint is a disabling procedure though it is sometimes indicated in young manual workers, especially for the index finger. Fusion in 25 degrees of flexion is recommended though better function may be achieved by fusing

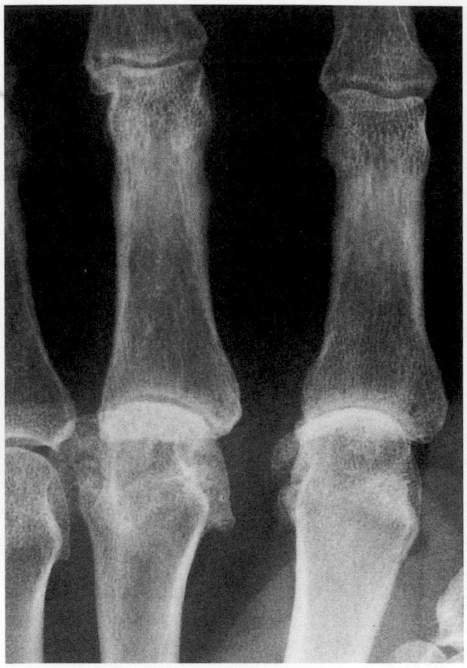

Fig. 6.6.5 Metacarpophalangeal joint osteoarthritis.

the ring and little fingers in 35–45 degrees of flexion. The bone ends can either be prepared as flat saw cuts or as a matching peg and socket and the arthrodesis can be stabilized with K-wires, a tension band wire, lag screws, or a dorsal mini-fragment plate. If the arthrodesis is stabilized with a plate, external splintage may not be required postoperatively. However, all the other fixation techniques require splint immobilization until bony union (6–8 weeks).

Excision arthroplasty

Excision arthroplasty is an option for young manual workers in whom silicone arthroplasty is contraindicated. In palmar plate arthroplasty, the metacarpal head is excised and the metacarpal attachment of the palmar plate is reattached to the dorsal surface of the metacarpal neck. Although this surgery inevitably results in a weak finger, typically a 50-degree arc of movement is preserved and pain relief in the short term is satisfactory. In the long-term, bone resorption and metacarpal shortening may occur, causing progressive instability and palmar subluxation. Because of a lack of collateral instability, excision arthroplasty is probably not indicated for the index finger metacarpophalangeal joint.

Silicone implant arthroplasty

Silicone implant arthroplasty is well established in rheumatoid surgery and is an option for the osteoarthritic metacarpophalangeal joint, particularly in the elderly, lower-demand patient.

Surface replacement arthroplasty

The potential for complications with silicone implant arthroplasty, such as implant fracture and silicone synovitis, has lead to the development of fixed fulcrum articulating designs. Failure of early hinged and ball and socket designs prompted progression to unconstrained and semiconstrained surface replacement arthroplasties which preserve soft tissue support and require minimal bone resection. Materials and designs continue to evolve. Short-term results of the latest design of pyrolytic carbon implant (Figure 6.6.6) are encouraging, with excellent pain relief, range of motion, and maintenance of pinch and grip strength, but its long-term outcome is unknown.

Osteoarthritis of the thumb

The treatment aim for thumb osteoarthritis is to create a painless stable thumb which is sufficiently strong to allow the patient to resume his or her normal daily and work activities. Arthrodesis is a successful treatment for single joint (trapeziometacarpal, metacarpophalangeal, or interphalangeal) thumb osteoarthritis. Indeed, reasonable thumb function is preserved following combined thumb metacarpophalangeal and interphalangeal joint arthrodeses, provided that the trapeziometacarpal joint is mobile and painless. If two or more thumb joints are osteoarthritic, it may be difficult to decide whether both are painful or all the pain arises from one joint. In this instance careful examination of each joint separately, while the others are carefully supported, is essential and intra-articular local anaesthetic injections are useful.

Incidence and prevalence (Box 6.6.5)

Trapeziometacarpal joint osteoarthritis is usually idiopathic and is particularly common in postmenopausal women (25%), although it is usually asymptomatic. It only rarely causes sufficient symptoms to warrant surgery. Symptomatic thumb metacarpophalangeal joint osteoarthritis is usually idiopathic but can complicate chronic ulnar collateral ligament laxity and severe intra-articular fractures. Interphalangeal joint osteoarthritis is common but usually only causes minor symptoms.

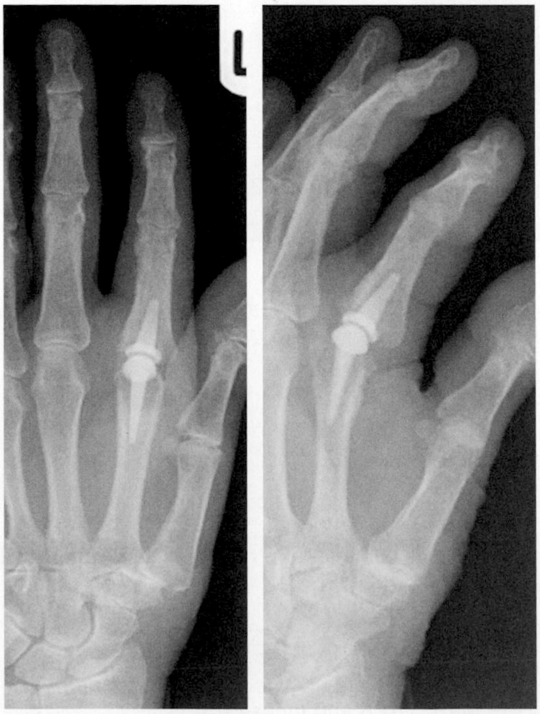

A B

Fig. 6.6.6 Pyrolytic carbon metacarpophalangeal joint replacement.

Box 6.6.5 Thumb base osteoarthritis

- Common, found in 25% of postmenopausal women
- Typically minimally symptomatic
- Probably due to beak ligament failure.

Anatomy

The thumb metacarpophalangeal and interphalangeal joints are similar to their finger counterparts but have different ranges of movement. The interphalangeal joint mean range of movement is −30 to 60 degrees; the metacarpophalangeal joint range of movement is variable and the normal range is determined by examining the contralateral normal thumb.

The basal thumb articulation consists of the trapeziometacarpal, the scaphotrapezial, scaphotrapezoid, trapeziotrapezoid, and trapezial–second metacarpal joints (Fig 6.6.7). The scaphotrapezial and scaphotrapezoid joints constitute part of the midcarpal joint though the former also allows some thumb abduction and adduction. Most basal thumb movement occurs at the trapeziometacarpal joint which has a saddle-shaped articulation allowing palmar abduction, radial abduction, adduction, and opposition. This joint is inherently unstable and its stability depends on the palmar ('beak') ligament. Trapeziometacarpal joint laxity is a common finding in young females and is usually asymptomatic. It may predispose to osteoarthritis in later life

Classification of basal thumb osteoarthritis

Basal thumb osteoarthritis may be classified according to which joints are degenerate and the radiological appearance of the trapeziometacarpal joint. The trapeziometacarpal joint alone is osteoarthritic in most cases but the scaphotrapezial and scaphotrapezoid joints are also osteoarthritic in 10% of cases. Trapeziometacarpal osteoarthritis is graded 1 to 4 according to its radiological appearances. In stage 1 the joint is painful when stressed and standard radiographs are normal though stress views show joint subluxation. In stage 2 there is minor osteoarthritic change and in stage 3, moderate change. In stage 4 there is subchondral sclerosis and joint space narrowing, with osteophytes and cysts. Although a higher proportion of patients with stage 4 osteoarthritis complain of symptoms, extreme radiological osteoarthritis may be asymptomatic and minor radiological osteoarthritis may be very painful: hence the distinction between stages 2–4 is of little clinical value.

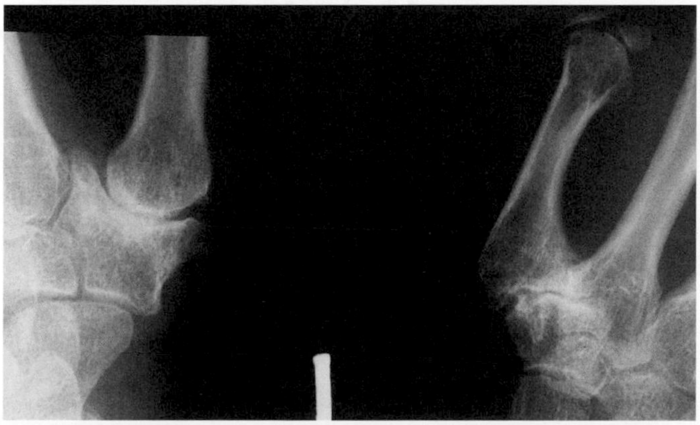

Fig. 6.6.7 Anteroposterior and lateral views of the base of the thumb showing trapeziometacarpal joint osteoarthritis. The anteroposterior view shows the four articular surfaces of the trapezium.

History and examination (Box 6.6.6)

Patients complain of pain around the involved joint that is typically use-related. The clinical findings are similar to those described for the finger joints.

The majority of patients with painful trapeziometacarpal osteoarthritis are middle-aged women who initially complain of gradually worsening basal thumb pain which occurs with or after use. This pain usually develops spontaneously though it is sometimes precipitated by a fall or other injury. Night pain is uncommon but patients may be woken at night by symptoms of carpal tunnel syndrome, which coexists in 32% of cases. Functional disability (e.g. undoing screw top jars, writing, and turning door keys) should be assessed.

In the early osteoarthritic stages, the trapeziometacarpal joint is tender and painful when stressed or moved under axial compression ('grind' test). In advanced disease, osteophytes are palpable and the thumb has the characteristic adduction deformity (Figure 6.6.8). This adduction deformity is usually accompanied by compensatory metacarpophalangeal joint hyperextension to maintain hand span.

Radiographs

The basal thumb articulations, as well as the thumb metacarpophalangeal and interphalangeal joints are clearly seen on anteroposterior and lateral views in the plane of the thumb (Gedda views). Trapeziometacarpal joint laxity and subluxation (stage 1) is assessed using stress views (Figure 6.6.9). However, painless joint laxity is exceedingly common in young females.

Management

Osteoarthritis causing minimal symptoms is treated by standard conservative techniques as described earlier. Surgery should be deferred until conservative methods have failed and thumb pain significantly restricts normal daily activities.

Metacarpophalangeal and interphalangeal joint osteoarthritis

Arthrodesis in about 15 degrees of flexion is the treatment of choice for painful thumb interphalangeal joint osteoarthritis. Isolated thumb metacarpophalangeal osteoarthritis is also best treated by arthrodesis in about 10–20 degrees of flexion. Both joints can be arthrodesed using any of the techniques described for the fingers.

Box 6.6.6 Thumb base osteoarthritis: history and examination

- Assessment: history and examination are often clear cut
- There may be subluxation
- Radiography is diagnostic
- Note subluxation and possible scaphotrapeziotrapezoid osteoarthritis.

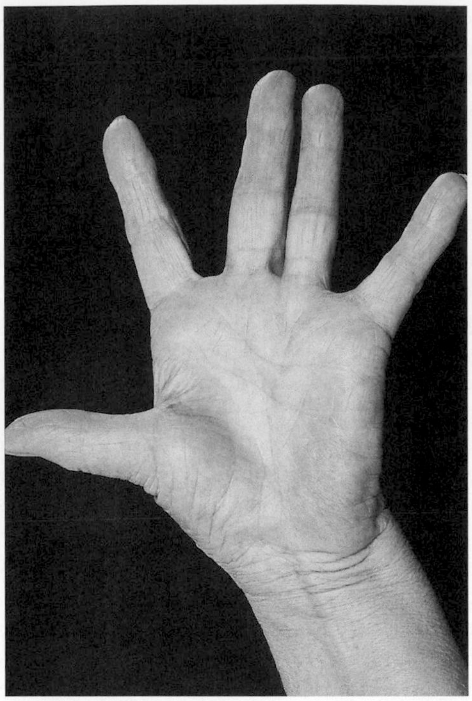

Fig. 6.6.8 The typical basal thumb adduction and metacarpophalangeal joint hyperextension deformities of advanced trapeziometacarpal joint osteoarthritis.

If thumb metacarpophalangeal and trapeziometacarpal osteoarthritis occur concurrently and the latter joint has an adduction deformity, a metacarpophalangeal arthrodesis or volar plate stabilization should only be performed if a trapeziometacarpal arthroplasty (excision or other) is also performed.

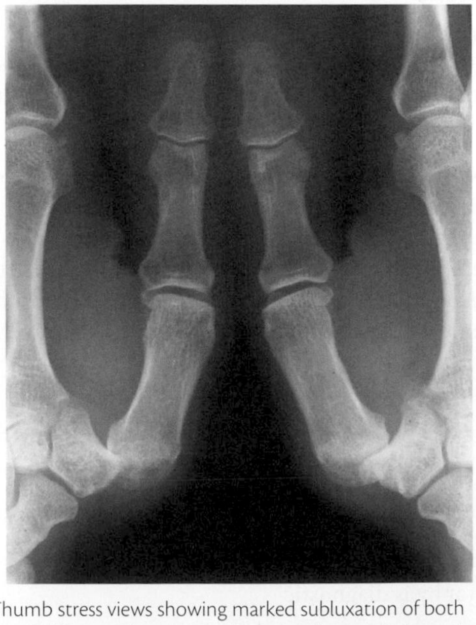

Fig. 6.6.9 Thumb stress views showing marked subluxation of both trapeziometacarpal joints. These stress views are taken with the patient pushing her thumb tips together as strongly as possible in order to provoke subluxation of the trapeziometacarpal joints.

Basal thumb osteoarthritis

Painless trapeziometacarpal joint adduction deformity is not usually an indication for surgery.

Conservative management

Thumb splints can provide useful pain relief but are poorly tolerated. Intra-articular steroid injections may produce significant pain relief for several months though rarely give lasting benefit. If trapeziometacarpal osteoarthritis is causing significant functional restriction and pain, then surgery should be contemplated.

Surgical management

The surgical treatment options can be divided into five general categories:

- Trapeziometacarpal joint capsular reinforcement
- Thumb metacarpal osteotomy
- Trapeziometacarpal joint arthrodesis
- Trapeziometacarpal arthroplasty with preservation of the trapezium and scaphotrapezial joint
- Excision of the trapezium with or without soft tissue or silicone interposition or ligament reconstruction.

The appropriate surgical procedure depends on the patient's age and activities, the severity (stage) of the osteoarthritis, and the condition of the scaphotrapezial joint (Box 6.6.7).

Trapeziometacarpal joint capsule reinforcement. For stage 1 disease (painful laxity with no radiological changes of osteoarthritis). The palmar ligament and joint capsule are reinforced, usually with a length of the flexor carpi radialis tendon (Figure 6.6.10) and the thumb is then immobilized in a plaster cast for 4–6 weeks.

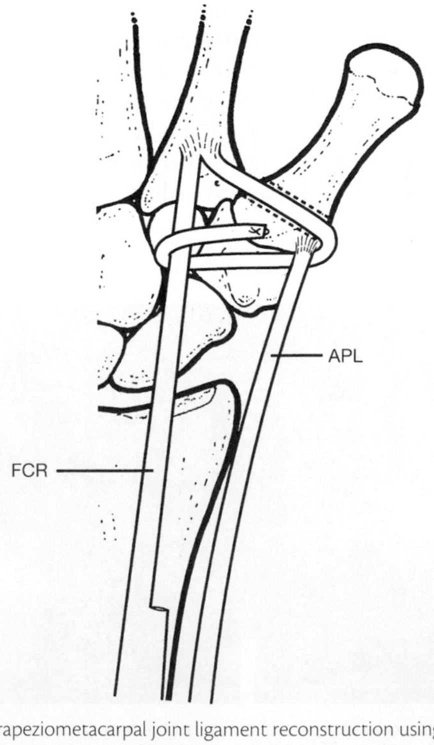

Fig. 6.6.10 Trapeziometacarpal joint ligament reconstruction using flexor carpi radialis tendon. A K-wire is used to stabilize the trapeziometacarpal joint for 6 weeks postoperatively. APL, abductor pollicis longus. FCR, flexor carpi radialis.

High success rates have been reported, although complete pain relief is not always obtained and trapeziometacarpal joint abduction and extension are often restricted.

Metacarpal osteotomy. A radial closing wedge osteotomy is performed at the base of the thumb metacarpal. Good patient satisfaction with the procedure has been reported with Stages 1, 2, and 3 osteoarthritis, but this procedure is unpredictable and has not gained widespread popularity.

Trapeziometacarpal joint arthrodesis. This is historically indicated for young manual workers who need to retain strong thumb pinch. It is contraindicated if both the trapeziometacarpal and scaphotrapezial joints are osteoarthritic as the latter joint may become more painful. The joint is best fused in the 'clenched fist position' (20–30 degrees of radial abduction and 20 degrees of palmar abduction) which preserves reasonable thumb span and allows opposition to the ring fingertip. The arthrodesis can be stabilized with K-wires, a tension band wire, or a small plate (Figure 6.6.11) and the thumb is immobilized until union occurs (6–8 weeks). Ten per cent non-union rates are typical though these are not always painful. A small amount of basal thumb movement remains due to the scaphotrapezial joint. Some patients have difficulty performing fine dextrous tasks, especially if the metacarpophalangeal joint has a restricted range of flexion. Arthrodesis does not restore normal thumb pinch strength and a 30% reduction is typical, such that it may not provide any better function than a trapeziectomy and ligament reconstruction in young manual workers.

Basal thumb arthroplasty. The majority of patients with painful basal thumb osteoarthritis are middle-aged or elderly women who do not place large force demands on their thumbs. In these patients it is best to preserve basal thumb mobility and some form of arthroplasty should be performed. Patients without scaphotrapezial joint osteoarthritis can be treated with a trapeziometacarpal arthroplasty which either preserves or excises the trapezium. If the scaphotrapezial joint is osteoarthritic then an arthroplasty which excises the trapezium should be performed.

Trapeziometacarpal total arthroplasty. Most trapeziometacarpal total arthroplasties are of a constrained or semiconstrained ball and socket design, with all metal or metal-on-polyethylene articulations. There are cemented and cementless designs (Figure 6.6.12). In the short term, these implants have a high success rate in terms of pain relief and restoration of function. Promising medium-term (up to 5 years) results have been published for some prostheses but others have been shown to have high loosening and dislocation rates.

Surface replacement prosthesis designs have been developed that require minimal bone excision. The lack of constraint inherent to these designs should reduce the risk of loosening, but their short-term results are disappointing.

Independent long-term follow-up studies are required as presently it is not known whether total arthroplasty produces better results than simpler and cheaper procedures such as trapeziectomy. The salvage procedure for failed total arthroplasty is trapeziectomy.

Trapezium excision arthroplasty. Trapeziectomy without additional soft tissue procedures was the standard treatment for trapeziometacarpal joint osteoarthritis for many years but fell out of favour because it was reputed to have a protracted rehabilitation time (6 months), cause thumb weakness, and be complicated by subluxation, dislocation, or painful degeneration of the scaphometacarpal pseudoarthrosis. Numerous modifications to 'simple' trapeziectomy have been devised to prevent these problems, including insertion of a silicone trapezial implant, interposition of

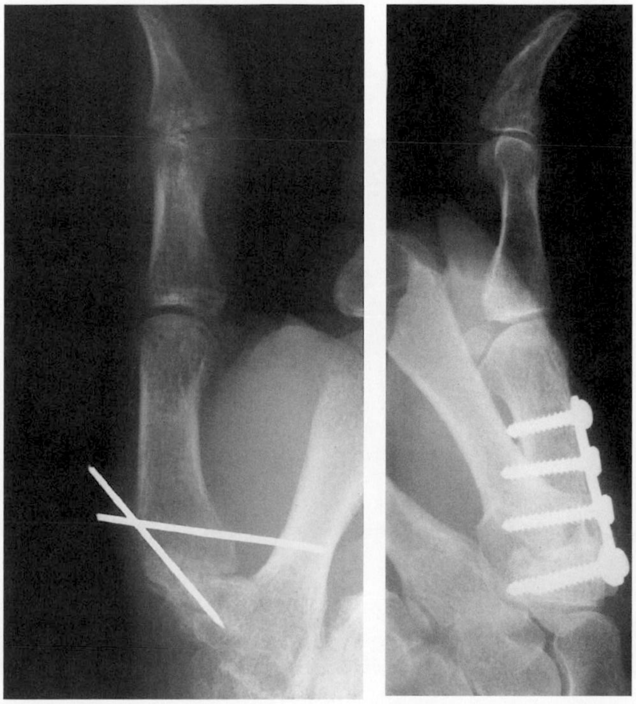

(a) (b)

Fig. 6.6.11 Trapeziometacarpal joint fusion using (A) K-wires and (B) a small-fragment T-plate.

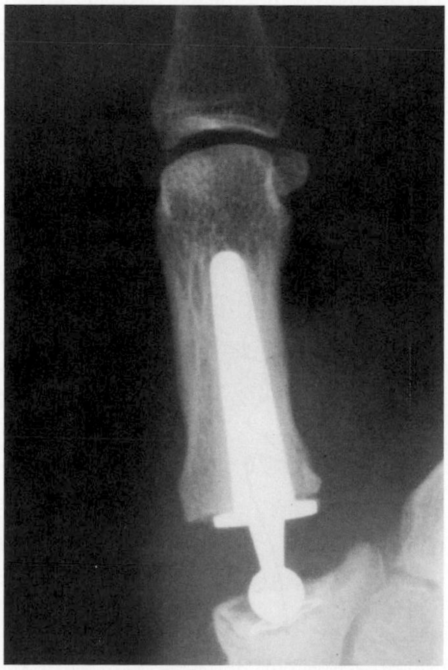

Fig. 6.6.12 Trapeziometacarpal total joint arthroplasty.

a rolled-up ball of tendon into the trapezium void (tendon interposition), and construction of a suspensory ligament between the bases of the thumb and index metacarpal bones (Figure 6.6.13). All these procedures aim to prevent the base of the first metacarpal articulating with the distal pole of the scaphoid and the suspensory ligament is also intended to prevent pseudarthrosis subluxation and dislocation.

Trapeziectomy with insertion of a silicone trapezium implant. This is no longer widely performed, predominantly because of the risk of silicone synovitis which occurs when silicone wear particles cause a painful foreign-tissue body reaction. This can cause severe bone loss though long-term studies suggest that this complication, as well as implant dislocation or subluxation, are uncommon

Trapeziectomy with tendon interposition. Trapeziectomy with tendon interposition is still widely used. Palmaris longus, flexor carpi radialis, and extensor carpi radialis longus have all been used with satisfactory results.

Trapeziectomy with ligament reconstruction. Many techniques of ligament reconstruction have been described. Most commonly the flexor carpi radialis, the abductor pollicis longus, or a combination of both tendons is used to suspend the thumb metacarpal base. Excess tendon may be interposed in the trapezial void, and a K-wire may be used to stabilize the construct during early healing.

Rehabilitation

Considerable swelling and pain can occur following trapeziectomy and strict postoperative elevation is essential.

After simple trapeziectomy, splintage in a plaster slab for 2 weeks followed by early motion, resting in a removable splint, is well tolerated. Formal physiotherapy is not usually required.

During trapeziectomy with ligament reconstruction, a K-wire may be passed across the scaphometacarpal pseudarthrosis to prevent proximal migration of the thumb metacarpal before the suspensory ligament becomes sound. The thumb is therefore immobilized in abduction in a plaster backslab until the K-wire is removed (4 weeks), after which some rest it in an abduction splint for a further 2 weeks. The thumb is generally immobilized for no more than 2 or 3 weeks following a total arthroplasty.

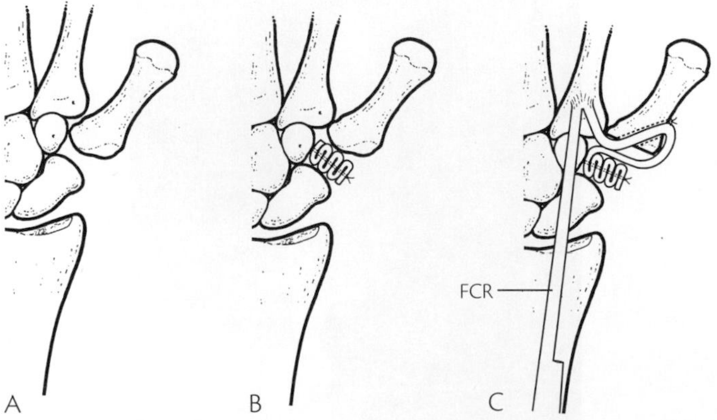

Fig. 6.6.13 A) Simple trapeziectomy. B) Trapeziectomy with tendon interposition. C) Trapeziectomy with ligament reconstruction and tendon interposition.

Box 6.6.7 Thumb base osteoarthritis: surgical treatment

- Soft tissue, i.e. ligament reconstruction for early disease
- Joint surgery for most
- Trapezectomy is simple and reliable
- Trapezectomy and soft tissue reconstruction is popular but not more reliable
- Arthrodesis best for manual labourers
- It can be technically difficult
- Joint replacement is as yet not established.

Results

There are good published results for all the surgical treatments of basal thumb osteoarthritis. Most patients regain good thumb function within 3 months. Typically 80–90% of patients achieve a painless thumb or only experience mild aching after use. All surgical procedures are reported to produce thumbs which have 70–80% of normal key and tip pinch strengths.

There is no good evidence that any procedure produces a better result than simple trapeziectomy in which the trapezium is excised, the trapezial void is left empty, and no ligament reconstruction is performed. Comparative studies have shown no advantage of adding suspension to simple trapeziectomy. Recurrence of pain and adduction deformity are uncommon following both simple trapeziectomy or trapeziectomy with ligament reconstruction.

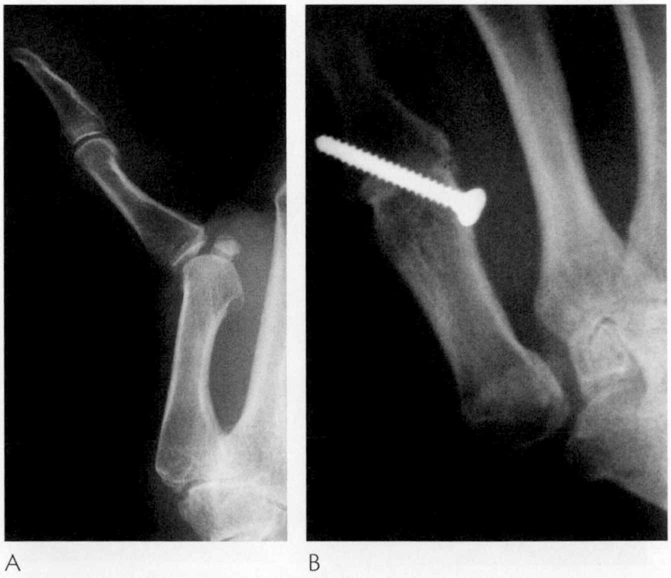

Fig. 6.6.14 A) Trapeziometacarpal joint osteoarthritis with adduction deformity and a compensatory metacarpophalangeal joint hyperextension deformity. B) This was treated with a trapeziectomy and metacarpophalangeal joint fusion.

Management of metacarpophalangeal hyperextension deformities

A compensatory metacarpophalangeal joint hyperextension deformity may occur in conjunction with the trapeziometacarpal joint adduction deformity found in severe osteoarthritis. Many would recommend that this is treated surgically to prevent recurrence of the basal thumb adduction deformity (which may cause implant/pseudarthrosis subluxation/dislocation) and improve thumb dexterity and strength. Hyperextension deformities of more than 30 degrees may be managed by metacarpophalangeal joint palmar plate advancement, sesamoid tenodesis, or fusion (Figure 6.6.14).

Complications

Complex regional pain syndrome, which may cause prolonged finger stiffness and hand disability may occur following procedures involving excision of the trapezium and should be treated urgently with intensive physiotherapy. Troublesome scar tenderness and paraesthesia may occur if superficial branches of the radial nerve or the palmar cutaneous branch of the median nerve are divided or stretched during surgery. Trapeziectomy is occasionally complicated by subluxation of the scaphometacarpal pseudarthrosis which may cause an adduction deformity and basal thumb pain, but the incidence of this problem is unknown.

Further reading

Bravo, C.J., Rizzo, M., Hormel, K.B., and Beckenbaugh, R.D. (2007). Pyrolytic carbon proximal interphalangeal joint arthroplasty: results with minimum two-year follow-up evaluation. *Journal of Hand Surgery*, **32**, 1–11.

Carroll, R.E. and Hill, N.A. (1969). Small joint arthrodesis in hand reconstruction. *Journal of Bone and Joint Surgery*, **51A**, 1219–21.

Davis, T.R., Brady, O. and Dias, J.J. (2004). Excision of the trapezium for osteoarthritis of the trapeziometacarpal joint: a study of the benefit of ligament reconstruction or tendon interposition. *Journal of Hand Surgery*, **29**, 1069–77.

Shin, A.Y. and Amadio, P.C. (2005). Stiff finger joints. In: Green, D.P., Hotchkiss, R.N., Pederson, W.C., and Wolfe, S.W. (eds) *Operative Hand Surgery*, fifth edition, pp. 417–59. New York: Churchill Livingstone.

Tomaino, M.M., King, J., and Leit, M. (2005). Thumb basal joint arthritis. In: Green, D.P., Hotchkiss, R.N., Pederson, W.C., and Wolfe, S.W. (eds) *Operative Hand Surgery*, fifth edition, pp. 461–85. New York: Churchill Livingstone.

6.7

Dupuytren's disease

Peter Burge

History

The first observation that contracture of a finger resulted from thickening and shortening of the palmar fascia was recorded in the notebook of Henry Cline Sr of St. Thomas' Hospital, London in 1777. Guillaume Dupuytren was born in the same year and published a detailed description of the condition that bears his name in 1831. Both Cline and Dupuytren performed palmar fasciotomy. It is remarkable that all of the operations in routine use today, except dermofasciectomy, were described before 1850.

Prevalence

Geographic variation

Dupuytren's disease shows a striking geographic variation in population prevalence, with high prevalence in Norway (30% of men over 60 years) and England (approximately 15% of men over 60 years), and much lower prevalence in the Mediterranean basin. It is very uncommon in Africa and rare in much of Asia.

Age and sex

The prevalence of Dupuytren's disease is strongly related to age. The onset is earlier in men and the disease is more common in men at every age (Figure 6.7.1).

Aetiology (Box 6.7.1)

Genetic predisposition

A genetic influence in Dupuytren's disease is supported by the geographic variation in prevalence and by clustering of cases in families. Many pedigrees show a pattern consistent with an autosomal dominant model of inheritance with variable penetrance but other cases appear to be sporadic. Investigation of the genetic influence is complicated by the high prevalence, late age of onset, incomplete penetrance, and the possibility that some cases have non-genetic causes. The search for a causative gene has not yet yielded conclusive results.

Smoking and alcohol

Smoking and alcohol independently increase the risk of Dupuytren's contracture.

Epilepsy

An association with epilepsy has been suggested by several studies, but a large case–control study has not confirmed it.

Diabetes

Dupuytren's disease has an increased prevalence in both type I and type II diabetes. The disease is more evenly distributed across the palm and the predilection for the ring and little fingers that is seen in idiopathic cases is less marked.

Trauma

In rare cases, there seems to be a clear link between a single episode of trauma and the subsequent appearance of Dupuytren's disease at the same site. However, causal relationships with repeated trauma or types of manual work have not been established, and there is no association with exposure to vibration.

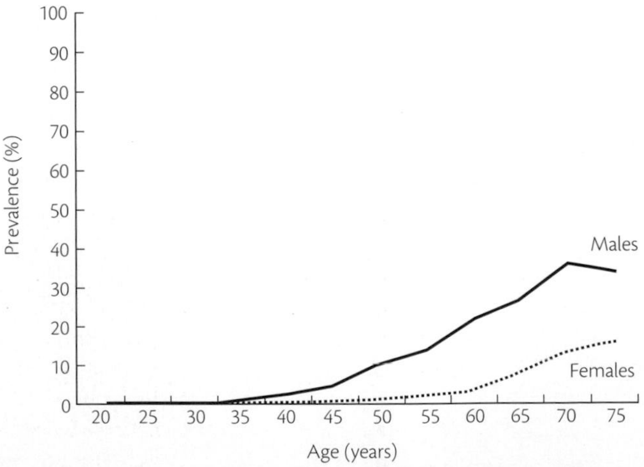

Fig. 6.7.1 Population prevalence in males and females in Norway. (Data from Mikkelson, O.A. (1990). Epidemiology in a Norwegian population. In: McFarlane, R.M., McGrouther, D.A., and Flint, M.H. (eds) *Dupuytren's Disease*, Volume 5, pp. 191–200. Edinburgh: Churchill Livingstone.)

Box 6.7.1 Causes

- Strong for genetics, diabetes, smoking
- Weaker for trauma and alcohol.

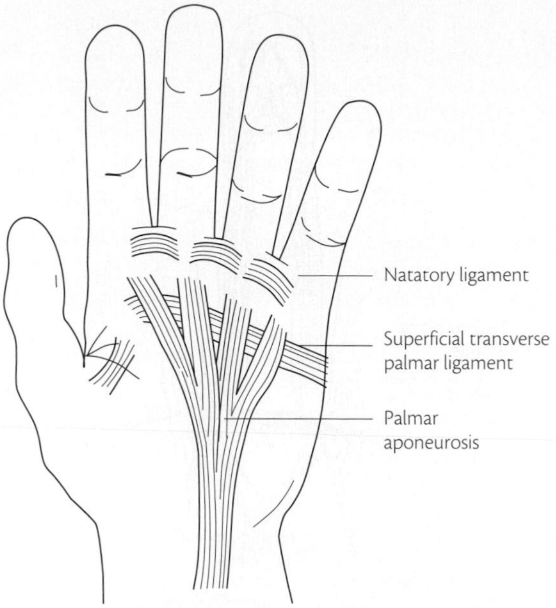

Fig. 6.7.2 Anatomy of the palmar fascia. (Reproduced from Strickland, J.W. and Leibovic, S.J. (1991). Anatomy and pathogenesis of the digital cords and nodules. *Hand Clinics*, **7**, 645–57.)

Pathogenesis

The pathogenesis of Dupuytren's disease remains elusive. Theories have centred on traumatic, neoplastic, and inflammatory processes. Histologically, the disease has many of the features of wound healing, including proliferation of fibroblasts, presence of myofibroblasts, and synthesis of collagen. The normal palmar and digital fascia is replaced by cords of collagen that are thicker and, in cases of contracture, shorter than the original bands. The collagen has a higher ratio of type III to type I collagen than normal fascia.

Myofibroblasts are a characteristic feature of Dupuytren's disease. They share the morphological characteristics of both fibroblasts and smooth muscles cells but are probably derived from fibroblasts. Myofibroblasts contain arrays of cytoplasmic actin filaments (stress fibres) that attach to specialized adhesion sites at the cell membrane, through which force could be transmitted to the extracellular matrix. The mechanical environment may influence the differentiation of myofibroblasts. The role of transforming growth factor (TGF)-β1 and other growth factors in this proliferative disorder remains unclear at present.

Clinical features

Anatomy of palmar fascia

The concept that Dupuytren's disease affects normal palmar and digital fascial structures and does not arise in a haphazard manner is fundamental to its safe and effective treatment and confirms the importance of thorough knowledge of the normal fascial anatomy.

The palmar and digital fascias form a three-dimensional array of ligaments that have transverse, longitudinal, and vertical components. The longitudinal fibres anchor the skin and resist shearing forces during gripping. They are connected to the skin and skeleton by vertical fibres and to each other by transverse fibres. The palmar fascial structures are called bands or ligaments in the normal state and cords when affected by Dupuytren's disease.

Each ray has a pretendinous band of fascia that runs longitudinally from the proximal palm to the base of the digit (Figure 6.7.2) and terminates in three ways: into the skin between distal palmar and proximal digital crease; into the spiral band; and deeply towards the metacarpal neck (the band of Legueu and Juvara) (Figure 6.7.3). The lateral digital sheet of fascia is continuous with transversely orientated layers termed Grayson's and Cleland's ligaments (respectively palmar and dorsal to the neurovascular bundle) (Figure 6.7.4).

The pretendinous cord may continue directly into the finger to run into the lateral digital sheet and/or Grayson's ligament. Alternatively, it may connect only with the spiral cord and thence into Grayson's ligament, to insert into the base of the middle phalanx or the overlying flexor tendon sheath. The spiral band passes deep to the neurovascular bundle; as it becomes contracted, the spiral cord pulls the bundle in a superficial direction so that it comes to lie immediately under the skin of the distal palm (Figure 6.7.5). The bundle is easily divided if the incision is carried directly down to the cord (Figure 6.7.6). A useful clue is that the skin is not adherent to the cord (since the cord lies deep to the bundle and its surrounding fat); a quantity of fat can be palpated between skin and spiral cord, whereas a pretendinous cord is more centrally placed in the ray and more likely to be adherent to the overlying skin.

Dupuytren's contracture is much more common in the ring and little fingers than in other digits (Figure 6.7.7).

Ectopic Dupuytren's disease

Knuckle pads are nodules of fibromatosis in the subcutaneous tissues over the dorsal surface of the proximal interphalangeal joints (PIPJs), described by Garrod in 1893 (Figure 6.7.8). *Plantar fibromatosis* (Lederhose disease) presents as nodules in the plantar

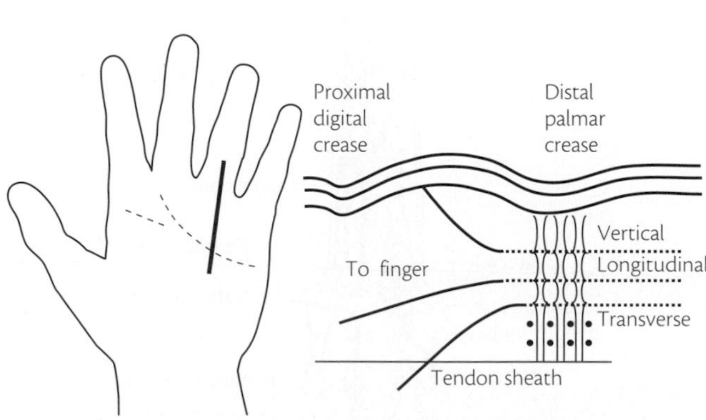

Fig. 6.7.3 Longitudinal section thought the distal palm, showing the three terminations of the pretendinous band into the distal palmar skin, into the spiral band and deeply towards the tendon sheath. (Reproduced from McGrouther, D.A. (1982). The microanatomy of Dupuytren's contracture. *Hand*, **14**, 215–36.)

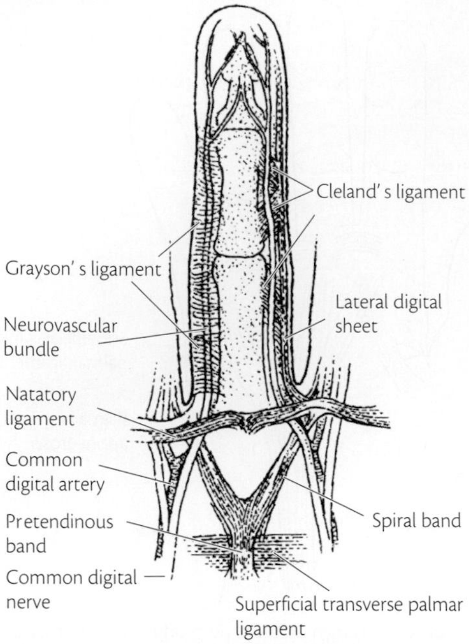

Fig. 6.7.4 The fascia of the distal palm and finger. The spiral band runs deep to the neurovascular bundle and links with the lateral digital sheet and Grayson's ligament. (Reproduced from Strickland, J.W. and Leibovic, S.J. (1991). Anatomy and pathogenesis of the digital cords and nodules. *Hand Clinics*, **7**, 645–57.)

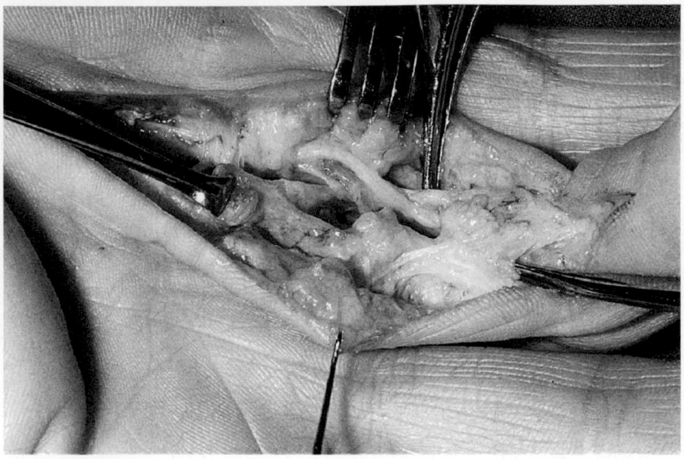

Fig. 6.7.6 Spiral cord displacing the radial digital nerve of the ring finger.

fascia that may cause discomfort or interfere with footwear (Figure 6.7.9). *Penile fibromatosis* (Peyronie's disease) is associated with Dupuytren's disease. Ectopic fibromatosis may be associated with severe or aggressive Dupuytren's disease.

Management

Non-operative treatment

Splintage

There is no good evidence that splintage prevents or retards the progression of contracture.

Steroid injection

Steroid injection of palmar nodules may reduce bulk and local tenderness. It has no reliable effect on contracture.

Collagenase injection

A randomized controlled trial of enzymatic fasciotomy by injection of collagenase has shown good correction of deformity but complications, recurrence rate and the cost–benefit relationship has not been defined.

Indications for operative treatment

The primary aim of operative treatment is to straighten bent digits and the secondary aim is to minimize the risk of recurrence. Surgery cannot cure the disease, which probably extends in a subclinical fashion throughout the hand. The choice of procedure

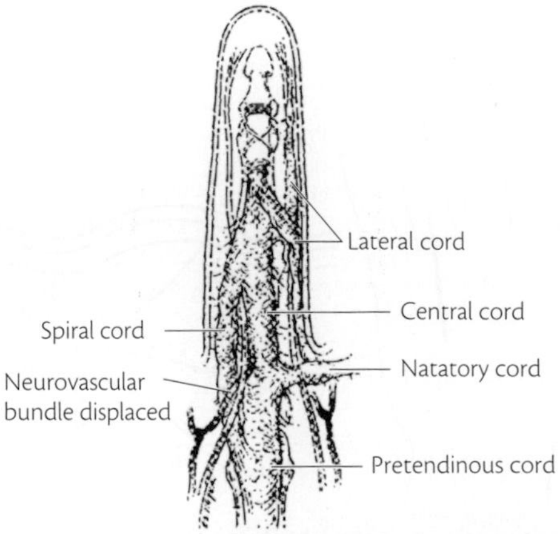

Fig. 6.7.5 Common patterns of involvement of fascia in the finger. (Reproduced from Strickland, J.W. and Leibovic, S.J. (1991). Anatomy and pathogenesis of the digital cords and nodules. *Hand Clinics*, **7**, 645–57.)

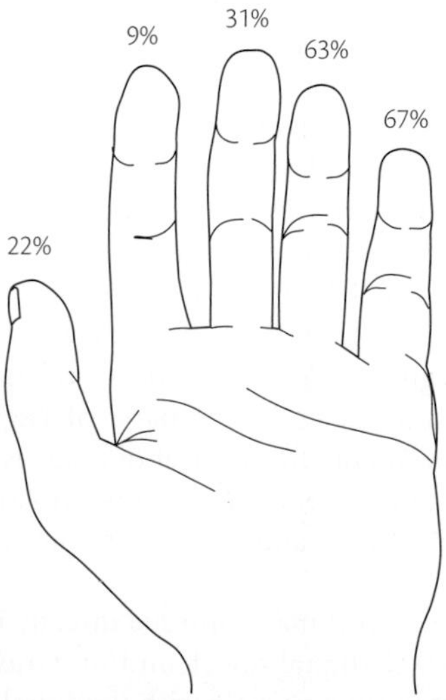

Fig. 6.7.7 Frequency of operation by digit in series of 670 Northern European patients. Many patients had operation on more than one digit. (Data from MacFarlane, R.M., Botz, J.S., and Cheung, I.I. (1990). Epidermiology of surgical patients. In: McFarlane, R.M., McGrouther, D.A. and Flint, M.H. (eds) *Dupuytren's Disease. Biology and Treatment*, pp. 201–8. Edinburgh: Churchill Livingstone.)

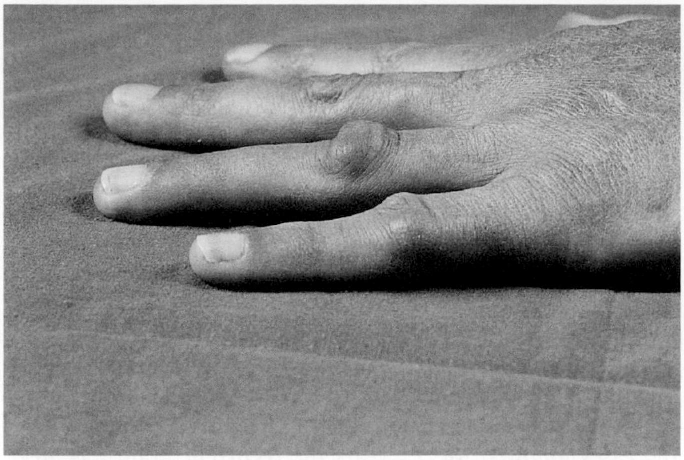

Fig. 6.7.8 Knuckle pads are areas of fibromatosis in the subcutaneous tissue over the dorsum of the PIPJs.

remains as controversial as in Dupuytren's day and good evidence to support one method of treatment over another is lacking.

Metacarpophalangeal joint

Metacarpophalangeal joint (MPJ) contracture is correctable almost regardless of its severity and secondary joint contracture is rare. The indication for surgery is a contracture that is interfering with function of the hand. Hueston's table-top test is a good guide; if the hand cannot be placed flat on the table *and* the patient reports limitation of hand function, operation may be considered.

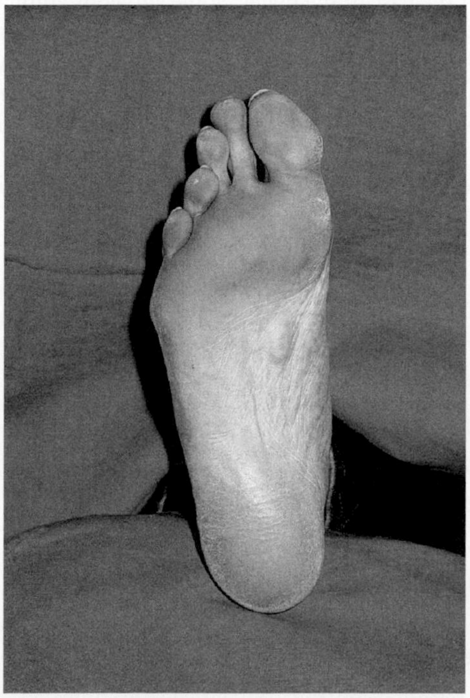

Fig. 6.7.9 Fibromatosis of the plantar fascia (Lederhose's disease).

Box 6.7.2

- Pathogenesis: overactivity of myofibroblasts
- Sites:
  - Commonly ring and little fingers
  - Ectopic sites suggest a stronger diathesis.

Proximal interphalangeal joint

Excision of contracted fascia often fails to restore full extension of the PIPJ because of secondary shortening of other structures that cross the palmar aspect of the joint, especially the check-rein ligaments of the palmar plate and the accessory collateral ligaments. Shortness of skin, involvement of the flexor tendon sheath, and shortening of the flexor muscles also limit extension in some cases.

The secondary contracture is variable and unpredictable, but generally the greater the severity and duration of contracture, the greater the risk of secondary joint contracture.

It might seem, therefore, that early operative treatment is appropriate. But the average residual PIPJ contracture after fasciectomy of the little finger is approximately 25 degrees and the patient is unlikely to feel that the operation was beneficial if the preoperative contracture was less than 30 degrees.

Serial measurements of the contracture with a goniometer at intervals of a few months can be most helpful. Progressive contracture is a good indication for surgery, as both patient and surgeon can see that deterioration is otherwise inevitable and a residual contracture after surgery will be more acceptable.

Distal interphalangeal joint

Involvement of the distal interphalangeal joint (DIPJ) is uncommon but often associated with a contracture of the PIPJ of the little finger by a band that spans both joints.

Information to patients

The risks of surgery should be explained and recorded. Risks specific to fasciectomy include delay in wound healing, incomplete PIPJ correction, temporary or permanent digital nerve impairment, limitation of flexion, recurrence and complex regional pain syndrome (CRPS) type 1.

Anaesthesia

Brachial plexus block by the axillary route gives excellent anaesthesia and postoperative analgesia. It is rare for patients to require any more than simple oral analgesia thereafter. Pain that requires strong analgesics usually signifies a complication such as tight bandage, haematoma, or infection, and requires inspection of the wound. General anaesthesia is sometimes needed for tourniquet discomfort or restlessness during a lengthy procedure. Intravenous regional anaesthesia gives a less satisfactory operative field and does not provide postoperative analgesia.

Operative methods

Understanding of the operative treatment of Dupuytren's disease is simplified by considering separately the *incision*, the *management of the diseased fascia*, and the *mode of closure*.

Box 6.7.3 Consent

- Crucial as the indications are relative
- Risks: especially incomplete correction, recurrence, nerve injury, CRPS.

Incision

A good incision should provide well-vascularized skin flaps, extensile exposure, and access for identification and preservation of the digital nerves and arteries. In the digit, a midline longitudinal incision gives excellent exposure and generally leaves the most heavily involved skin at the edge of the wound. Conversion to one or more Z-plasties breaks up the linear scar and provides some lengthening. Transfer of Z-plasty flaps is difficult in the stiff flat palmar skin; the author prefers a longitudinal incision in the digit that is extended in zigzag fashion in the palm, closing the digital component with a single large Z-plasty in the proximal segment (Figure 6.7.10).

The Bruner zigzag incision also provides good exposure. However, raising large flaps over a midline longitudinal cord of Dupuytren's disease may damage the subdermal plexus at the base of the flap, leaving its tip ischaemic. The modified Bruner incision, with shorter flaps, is less prone to this problem (Figure 6.7.10).

Multiple ray disease in the palm is more easily exposed through a transverse distal palmar crease incision that can be extended as necessary into each digit and proximally in the palm. The palmar skin in each web is supplied by perforating vessels and will survive provided that these vessels are preserved.

Management of diseased fascia

The contracted fascia may be divided or removed; removal may be segmental, regional, or total.

Fasciotomy

Percutaneous fasciotomy can be employed for well-defined bowstringing cords that cause contracture at the MPJ but recurrence is common. Under local anaesthesia, a knife is slid between skin and cord and used to separate skin from cord. The knife is then turned through 90 degrees and used to cut the cord from superficial to deep as the cord is held taut by pulling the finger firmly into extension. The wound is dressed and an extension splint is worn at night for a few weeks. Fasciotomy is relatively safe if performed at or proximal to the distal palmar crease, as the digital nerves lie beneath the superficial transverse ligament at that level. In the distal palm and finger, fasciotomy carries a risk of nerve injury because of the variability of the position of the neurovascular bundle.

Needle fasciotomy. French rheumatologists developed needle fasciotomy as an alternative to fasciectomy. As with percutaneous fasciotomy, the technique is more effective at the MPJ than at the PIPJ, and recurrences are more common than after fasciectomy. In 100 cases followed for 3.2 years the recurrence rate was 58%. Damage to digital nerves and flexor tendons appears to be less frequent than one might imagine.

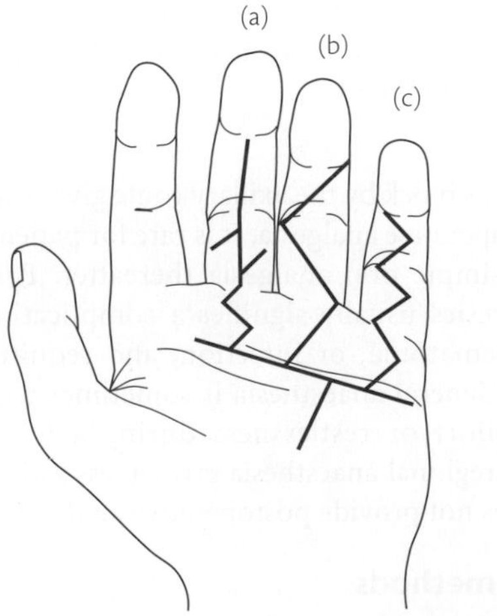

Fig. 6.7.10 Incisions for fasciectomy. A) Midline longitudinal incision converted to Z-plasty in the proximal segment of the finger. B) Bruner zigzag incision. C) Modified Bruner incision.

Segmental fasciectomy

Though several short C-shaped incisions, 1-cm segments of contracted fascia are excised. There is no attempt to remove all affected fascia from a digit. Postoperative extension splintage is continued for several months. The concept is that breaking up the longitudinal transmission of force in the fascia encourages the remaining fascia to remodel. Recurrence rates are reported to be similar to those of regional fasciectomy.

Regional fasciectomy

Regional fasciectomy is the most widely performed procedure for Dupuytren's contracture and has a low rate of recurrent MPJ contracture. The digital neurovascular bundles are identified proximally and traced distally (or vice versa), removing diseased fascia that is causing contracture from one or more rays. Safety dictates that the nerves are identified at points where their location is predictable—at the distal palmar crease, over the middle phalanx, and (usually) at the base of the finger. Some surgeons emphasize thorough clearance of diseased fascia from the fingers while others limit the excision to the cord causing contracture. It is not known if the former approach reduces the risk of recurrence. But the difficulty of any subsequent procedure is increased by extensive dissection. The more tissue is left undisturbed around the neurovascular bundle, the easier its dissection will be at the next operation.

Box 6.7.4 Treatment

- Non-operative: little role
- Surgery:
  - Indication—table top test
  - Fasciotomy—best for older patient, MPJ disease
  - Fasciectomy—the mainstay
  - Dermofasciectomy and full thickness skin graft—for recurrence or a bad primary disease with a marked diathesis
  - PIPJ release—controversial, largely not indicated.

Closure

The options for handling the wound after dealing with the fascia are:

Direct closure

Zigzag incisions are closed directly. A longitudinal midline incision is closed with one or more Z-plasties, which are cut after fasciectomy is completed as the orientation will depend on the location of thin skin. The author leaves the proximal limb of the palmar wound open, to minimize the risk of haematoma.

Open palm technique

In primary Dupuytren's disease, no skin is missing. The transverse distal palmar can be left open and allowed to heal spontaneously. Skin that has undergone shortening over the contracted fascia will return to its original length as the open wound heals. The open palm technique is not appropriate when there is a true shortage of skin; in this case, a graft is required.

The open palm method is associated with a low incidence of complications. Haematoma cannot occur and the risk of skin flap necrosis due to tension is avoided. The chief disadvantages are the need to wear a dressing for up to 4 weeks and a slight risk of infection of the open wound. The open method is less applicable in the fingers, where the wound interferes with rehabilitation.

Dermofasciectomy and skin grafting

Hueston's concept that recurrence of Dupuytren's disease is reduced substantially if the overlying skin is excised and replaced with a full-thickness skin graft is supported by many studies. An absolute indication for grafting is lack of viable skin flaps at the completion of fasciectomy. Relative indications include skin shortage, recurrent disease, aggressive primary disease, and primary disease in a young patient. The proximal digital segment is the area most often needing replacement (Figure 6.7.11). As grafting requires an intact flexor tendon sheath, a longitudinal or zigzag incision is used for exposure and the skin is excised only if the tendon sheath has remained intact after completion of the fasciectomy. The graft should extend to the midaxial line on each side, to avoid the risk of contracture of the scar along its edges. The graft may be obtained from the medial surface of the arm, from the antecubital fossa or from the groin crease. Graft take is very reliable if attention is given to precise operative technique and haemostasis.

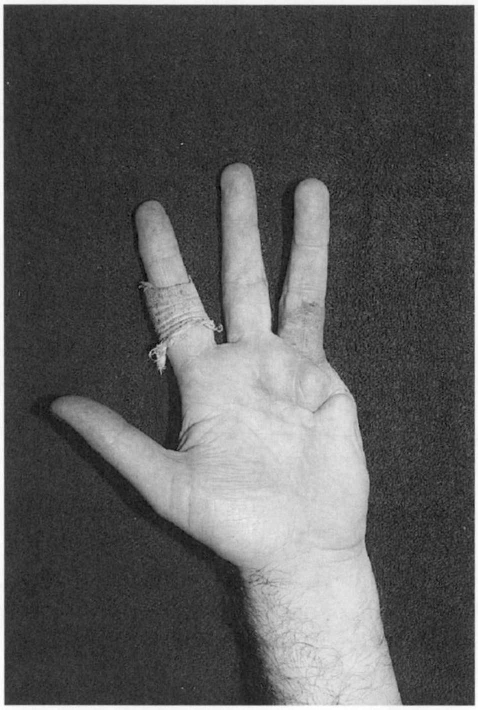

Fig. 6.7.11 Dermofasciectomy and full-thickness skin graft for recurrent disease at the base of the ring finger. The little finger had been amputated previously for recurrence after several fasciectomies.

Proximal interphalangeal joint release

Release of the secondary capsular contracture of the PIPJ is controversial and data on its effect are limited. Although release of the check-rein ligaments and accessory collateral ligaments can improve a contracture persisting after fasciectomy, the decision to proceed to joint release should balance the likely gain against the significant risk of losing flexion, which is more disabling than loss of extension. Tenotomy of the terminal tendon of the dorsal aponeurosis over the middle phalanx can improve flexion of the distal joint when Dupuytren's disease results in a boutonnière deformity.

Dupuytren's disease of the thumb web

The thumb web is affected in at least 25% of cases undergoing surgery on the ulnar side of the hand but in most older patients the contracture is minimal and does not require operative treatment. However, thumb web contracture may be severe and disabling, especially in individuals showing risk factors for aggressive disease (young age at onset, family history, and ectopic disease). A cord affecting the thenar fascia along the radial border of the thumb may cause contracture at the interphalangeal joint. Contracture of the thumb web may be due to fibres passing from the radial end of superficial transverse ligament of the palm to the thenar fascia, or to involvement of the fascia running in the crest of the web between the thenar fascia and the base of the index finger (Figure 6.7.12), with contracture of the index. Moderate contractures can be treated by regional fasciectomy but in severe cases restoration of the width of the thumb web requires dermofasciectomy and skin grafting.

Postoperative management

Dressings

Non-adherent dressings of paraffin gauze, dry gauze, and wool are held with a non-elastic bandage. Many surgeons feels that a palmar plaster slab from forearm to fingertips helps to control wrist position for the duration of the regional anaesthetic block, relieve pain, and prevent reactionary bleeding, which can occur if the hand is moved excessively in the first day or two. The fingers sit in midflexion; no attempt is made to hold them in extension, so as to avoid tension on skin flaps. Some surgeons inspect the wound the next day. The author leaves the dressings in place for 2–4 days unless a skin graft has been used, in which case the hand is immobilized for 7 days.

Hand therapy

Supervision by a hand therapist and diligent exercise by the patient are crucial to achieving consistent results after fasciectomy. The first priority is restoration of flexion by active exercise, with the

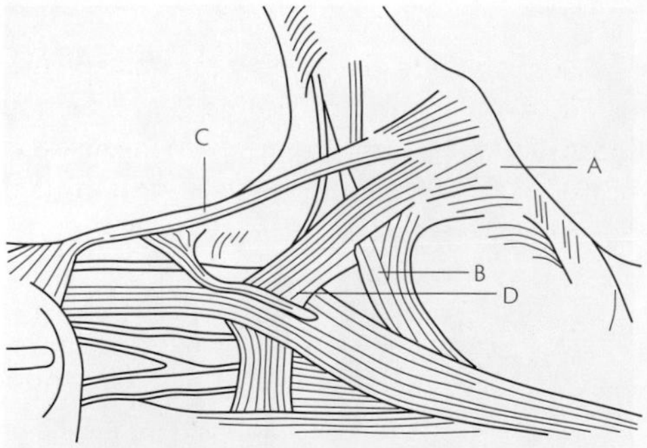

Fig. 6.7.12 Palmar fascia on the radial side of the hand. A) Thenar eminence fascia. B) Longitudinal fibres of the superficial palmar aponeurosis. C) Distal transverse commissural ligament. D) Proximal distal transverse commissural ligament. (Reproduced with permission from Tubiana, R. (1999). Dupuytren's disease of the radial side of the hand. *Hand Clinics*, **15**, 149–59.)

objective of flexion of the fingertip to the palm within 2 weeks of surgery. A palmar thermoplastic extension splint is worn at night until the scar is mature. Silicone inserts attached to the inner surface of the splint may assist scar remodelling.

Recurrent disease

Incidence

A new contracture after operative management can be due to *extension* (appearance of disease in previously unoperated areas), *recurrence* (new disease in the previous operation field), *scar contracture*, or some combination of these. Recurrence is common and exceeds 50% at 10 years, though not all recurrences require further surgery. The usual presentation of recurrence is a contracture of the PIPJ, most frequently in the little finger.

Assessment

Assessment of recurrent disease should include evaluation of the digital nerves (by two-point discrimination), digital arteries (by digital Allen's test), severity of contracture, and quality of skin (Box 6.7.5). Digits that lack a patent digital artery are surviving on collateral vessels and are at risk of ischaemia during extensive procedures; they are poor candidates for surgery. Digital nerves may be densely adherent to scarring from previous operations and their preservation may be difficult.

Management

Surgery for recurrent Dupuytren's disease is more difficult and more risky than primary operations. The indication for operation is a recurrent contracture that is interfering with function of the hand, but the decision is influenced by the condition of the finger. The state of the digital nerves, digital arteries, and skin will give an estimate of the risks of surgery and these can be balanced against the severity of contracture and degree of functional impairment. An additional factor is the pattern of recurrent disease. A well-defined cord lying beneath good skin is favourable. Diffuse thickening with adherence to skin is not.

Recurrent palmar disease is amenable to fasciectomy and is seldom problematic. The difficulties lie in the finger, where the mixture of scar tissue and recurrent disease may greatly hamper the safe dissection of nerves and arteries. It is also important to preserve the tendon sheath, as most cases of recurrence will require skin grafting. If the tendon sheath is deficient, closure with the original skin flaps or by a local flap will be needed.

> **Box 6.7.5** Recurrence
>
> - Common
> - Common finger more than pain
> - Especially little finger, strong diathesis
> - Treatment:
>   - Usually dermofasciectomy
>   - Increased complications.

Dermofasciectomy and full-thickness skin grafting is the procedure used most frequently for recurrent disease (see Figure 6.7.11). The rarity of recurrence beneath a skin graft, demonstrated by Hueston, probably reflects the importance of residual disease in skin flaps as a source of recurrence; when this skin is excised, recurrence is rare. Recurrence can occur, however, at the graft margins.

Skin grafting also corrects the skin shortage that is often evident at the base of the finger in recurrent disease and it allows removal of skin flaps of uncertain viability.

Salvage procedures (Box 6.7.6)

Flap cover

Local skin flaps have limited application in Dupuytren's disease and are used mainly in surgery for recurrent disease when the flexor tendons are exposed.

Proximal interphalangeal joint arthrodesis

Arthrodesis of the PIPJ in 30–40 degrees of flexion can overcome severe recurrent contractures that are not amenable to fasciectomy. Some skeletal shortening is necessary to overcome the flexion deformity. Arthrodesis is most applicable in the little finger, especially when some hyperextension at the MPJ compensates for the fixed PIPJ.

Proximal interphalangeal joint arthroplasty

Silicone rubber implant arthroplasty of the PIPJ has been used in combination with fasciectomy and dermofasciectomy. A good arc of motion cannot be expected and the possibility of recurrent deformity remains.

Amputation

Liberal use of skin grafts in recurrent disease has reduced the need for amputation. Patients who request amputation of the little finger should be warned of the adverse effect on power grip, reminded that a flexion contracture of 60 degrees at the PIPJ is compatible

> **Box 6.7.6** Salvage procedures
>
> - Flap cover
> - PIPJ arthrodesis
> - PIPJ arthroplasty
> - Amputation.

with good function if the MPJ will extend fully and advised about the risk of a painful neuroma. But amputation may be appropriate for a digit that is interfering with function because of persistent contracture after multiple operations. Its dorsal skin may be useful in resurfacing the adjacent digit or palm.

Complications

Operative complications

Digital nerve injury

Dissection of the digital neurovascular bundle is the essence of fasciectomy—once the bundle has been protected, excision of the diseased fascia is straightforward. Manipulation of the nerve may impair its function temporarily. Division of a digital nerve should be a very rare event during a primary fasciectomy if appropriate care and magnification are employed. The nerves are at much greater risk at second or subsequent operations because they may be heavily embedded in scar or recurrent disease. A divided digital nerve should probably be repaired, though most patients are at an age where useful recovery is unlikely.

Digital artery injury

The plentiful cross-connections between the two digital arteries will ensure survival of the finger if one artery is damaged. However, every effort should be made to preserve both arteries because of the likelihood that further operations will be needed. Loss of one artery will restrict the surgeon's room for manoeuvre at any subsequent procedure and will increase the risk of digital ischaemia. Injury of a single digital artery is not an indication for repair. Repair may be required if the other artery is also damaged. Spasm of the arteries may be caused by extensive dissection or by forcible stretching of the finger into extension. Positioning in flexion, patience, and application of warm saline will usually restore perfusion.

Postoperative complications

Dupuytren's contracture causes moderate functional impairment that is proportional to the loss of extension. Complications of surgery can lead to much more severe functional loss, particularly if the range of flexion is compromised. Prevention of complications is crucial to achieving consistently good results.

Skin necrosis

Small areas of skin loss (<5mm) create a risk of sepsis but will heal spontaneously. Larger areas may need excision and skin grafting. Spontaneous healing of larger areas is slow and likely to result in scar contracture, especially at the base of the finger.

Haematoma

Haematoma is a potentially disastrous complication that may lead to permanent loss of flexion, skin necrosis, or infection. The risk can be minimized by careful attention to haemostasis and by appropriate drainage, either by leaving a portion of the palmar wound open or by inserting a drain.

Infection

Maceration of skin in the folds and pits of a severely contracted digit increases the risks of infection. Prophylactic antibiotic therapy should probably be given if any pit or crease is macerated, but antibiotics are not needed routinely. A preliminary palmar fasciotomy under local anaesthesia may allow the skin to be brought into good condition for fasciectomy a short time later. Infection may develop in wounds that have been left open, in which case the response to appropriate antibiotic therapy is usually good.

Flare

The combination of diffuse swelling, stiffness and shiny redness of the hand has been termed 'flare'. Its cause is unknown but it may represent a minor variant of CRPS type 1. Treatment comprises elevation, control of pain and swelling, active exercise, and extension splintage at night. Early recognition and treatment are essential in preventing permanent loss of finger flexion.

Complex regional pain syndrome type 1

This serious complication is rare but can have devastating consequences for function of the hand. The cardinal features are excessive pain, swelling, stiffness and vasomotor instability. Early recognition and treatment are essential (see Chapter 1.11).

Conclusion

Dupuytren's disease affects at least 10% of older men of Northern European origin. Its cause and predilection for the ulnar side of the hand are unexplained. Operative treatment aims to straighten bent digits, not to cure the disease. Deeper understanding of the nature of the disease will be required to devise means of modifying its behaviour and, in particular, reducing the likelihood of recurrence after surgery.

Further reading

Rayan, G.M. (ed) (1999). Dupuytren's Disease. *Hand Clinics*, **15**(1).

Rayan, G.M. (2007). Dupuytren disease: Anatomy, pathology, presentation, and treatment. *Journal of Bone and Joint Surgery*, **89A**, 189–98.

Shaw, R.B., Jr., Chong, A.K., Zhang, A., Hentz, V.R., and Chang, J. (2007). Dupuytren's disease: history, diagnosis, and treatment. *Plastic and Reconstructive Surgery*, **120**, 44e–54e.

6.8

Tendon disorders

Will Mason and David Warwick*

Summary points

- The term tenosynovitis should be restricted to inflammatory disorders; De Quervain's syndrome and trigger finger do not show inflammatory changes histologically and are more appropriately termed tenovaginosis
- The cause of most tenovaginoses is unclear; they are occasionally secondary to trauma and rarely linked to overuse
- Rupture of individual tendons may not require surgical reconstruction but it is important to establish the underlying cause of rupture to prevent sequential rupture of adjacent tendons.

Congenital anomalies

Congenital anomalies of the tendons and tendon sheaths of the hand and wrist are common but rarely cause symptoms of pain or functional impairment. Asymptomatic anomalies are important as they may cause confusion in the interpretation of the physical examination.

Palmaris longus

Palmaris longus is absent in about 15% of hands and anomalous in 9%. It is implicated in the pathogenesis of carpal tunnel syndrome as it is absent in only 3% of patients with this condition. Its clinical significance is its use as a tendon transfer or free tendon graft.

Flexor pollicis longus

The Linburg–Comstock anomaly consists of a tendinous slip or tenosynovial adhesion connecting the flexor pollicis longus tendon to the flexor digitorum profundus tendon of the index finger. It is found in 25% of cadavers and can cause pain by restricting independent movement of the index and thumb. The pathognomonic sign is obligatory flexion of the index finger when the thumb is flexed actively. There is pain in the wrist if flexion of the index is blocked as the thumb is flexed. The anomaly is usually only problematic in musicians. Surgical division of the connection is usually curative.

Flexor digitorum superficialis

The flexor digitorum superficialis tendons of the index, middle, and ring fingers generally have individual muscle bellies and can act independently. Only 60% of little fingers have an independent flexor digitorum superficialis tendon. About 20% have no discernable function of the tendon though it may be present. This can lead to uncertainty when interpreting physical signs after lacerations of the little finger. In the remaining 20% the little finger superficialis tendon is linked to that of the ring finger. This can be demonstrated by the standard and modified flexor digitorum superficialis tests: the little finger cannot be flexed actively at the proximal interphalangeal joint whilst the other digits are held extended. When the ring finger is released, the ring and little finger proximal interphalangeal joints can be flexed together, but independently of the other digits.

Abductor pollicis longus

Abductor pollicis longus is subject to considerable variation in the number of tendon slips and their insertion. Slips may attach to the abductor or extensor pollicis brevis tendons, the trapezium, joint capsule, or thumb metacarpal.

Extensor pollicis brevis

The extensor pollicis brevis tendon is also rather variable. Its anomalies include absence, connection with abductor pollicis longus, and insertion into the distal phalanx or extensor hood in place of (or in addition to) the proximal phalanx. In 30–60% of wrists, the extensor pollicis brevis tendon runs in a subcompartment of the first extensor compartment. Symptoms of de Quervain's syndrome may persist if a subcompartment is overlooked at the time of release.

Extensor digitorum communis

Anatomical variations in the contribution of the extensor digitorum communis tendon to the little finger account for the variable deficit that results from rupture or laceration of the extensor digiti minimi. Rupture of extensor digitorum minimi, which may herald

* The authors acknowledge the contribution of Mr Peter Burge to this chapter in the first edition.

rupture of extensor digitorum communis in rheumatoid arthritis, may pass unnoticed unless independent extension of the little finger is tested.

Terminology of tendon disorders

The terminology of tendon disorders is unsatisfactory. The terms tendinitis and tenosynovitis mean inflammation of the tendon and tenosynovium respectively. These conditions have recognizable and reproducible physical signs (swelling, tenderness, and crepitus along the line of the tendon), as well as characteristic pathological changes on histology (e.g. rheumatoid arthritis). In the absence of these features, and especially in the context of pain in the workplace, it is inappropriate to assign these diagnoses. The term tendinosis, which makes no aetiological or pathological assumptions, is preferable, but its use is not widespread. In many cases, a recognized tendon disorder can be diagnosed (e.g. de Quervain's syndrome). If the clinical picture does not conform to a recognized disorder, but is clearly attributable to the action of a tendon, then a neutral term such as flexor carpi ulnaris tendon pain is appropriate. Terms such as forearm pain or non-specific arm pain can be used when the symptoms and signs are poorly localized.

Tenosynovitis

Pathology

Tenosynovitis is inflammation of the tenosynovium. Tenosynovitis is ultimately a pathological diagnosis, but a clinical diagnosis may be made in the presence of the characteristic features of tenderness, swelling, and crepitus along the line of the tendon sheath, along with restricted tendon excursion. Not all the signs are necessarily present simultaneously, but it would be difficult to justify the diagnosis of tenosynovitis in the absence of localized tenderness.

Tenosynovitis may be acute or chronic. Pyogenic tenosynovitis (see Chapter 6.14) is the commonest cause of acute tenosynovitis but rarely acute gout, calcium pyrophosphate deposition, and repetitive trauma may be responsible. Rheumatoid disease (see Chapter 6.5), mycobacterial infection, fungal infection, foreign body, sarcoidosis, gout, and amyloid may cause subacute or chronic tenosynovitis. Chronic flexor tenosynovitis can lead to median nerve compression.

Mycobacterial infection

Infection with atypical mycobacteria such as *Mycobacterium kansasii* and *Mycobacterium marinum* is now more common than tuberculous tenosynovitis (see Chapter 6.14). Mycobacterial infection should be considered whenever chronic tenosynovitis is not clearly associated with inflammatory arthritis and appropriate specimens sent for histology and mycobacterial culture.

The management is tenosynovectomy, which is both diagnostic and therapeutic, followed by appropriate antimycobacterial chemotherapy.

Retained foreign body

Foreign material within the tendon sheath may incite an inflammatory response in the absence of infection. The thorns of the blackthorn tree (*Prunus spinosa*) and *Pyrocantha* species are particularly liable to cause a subacute aseptic inflammation of joint or tendon sheath. The flexor tendon sheath of the finger is the most common site. Small foreign bodies may be identified by ultrasound examination. Tenosynovitis generally resolves once the foreign material is removed.

Painful disorders of tendons and tendon sheath (Box 6.8.1)

Pathology

There are several conditions, including de Quervain's syndrome and trigger finger, which have previously been attributed to inflammation of the tendon, sheath, or synovial lining, and which have been called 'tenosynovitis'. The clinical features of tenosynovitis may indeed be seen when the tendon sheath is affected by an inflammatory disorder such as rheumatoid arthritis. However, histological studies of the common idiopathic forms of these disorders seldom show inflammation of the tendon, tendon sheath, or tenosynovium.

The pathological changes of de Quervain's syndrome and trigger finger, which are the only conditions to have been studied in detail, are similar. The changes comprise an increase in extracellular matrix, thickening of the collagen fibrils, and areas of fibrocartilage metaplasia in the tendon sheath. Fibrillation or delamination of the tendon surface may be seen. Evidence of inflammation is notably absent. In the absence of clinical or pathological evidence of inflammation, it is illogical to refer to 'tendinitis' or 'tenosynovitis'.

Aetiology

The cause of these common disorders is unclear. The symptoms may be initiated by a single injury such as a direct blow or sudden strain. While damage by overuse is an intuitively plausible theory, the evidence that these disorders are initiated by excessive activity is scant, except in the case of intersection syndrome (peritendinitis crepitans) affecting the second extensor compartment. However, the symptoms that these conditions produce are often aggravated by activity.

Management

Rest, avoidance of aggravating activities, splintage, and analgesic medication constitute the first line of management. Injection of the

Box 6.8.1 Tenovaginosis and other tendon condition

Causes

- Mostly wear and tear of life. Congenital causes are rare. Work related causes are infrequent and contentious
- The pathology is often not primarily in the tendon:
  - De Quervain's and trigger finger—the sheath
  - Tendon ruptures—underlying pathology of bone or synovitis.

Presentation

- Pain
- Triggering
- Failure.

tendon sheath with corticosteroid, which can be dramatically effective, is the second line of treatment. Complications of steroid injection are uncommon. Infection is very rare but potentially disastrous. Tendon rupture is also very rare and is probably due to underlying pathology in the tendon or its surroundings (e.g. rheumatoid arthritis) rather than to the injection itself. Atrophy of dermis or subcutaneous fat results from inadvertent injection into the subcutaneous tissues, which should be avoided. Surgical decompression of the affected tendon may be needed in cases that fail to respond to non-operative treatment.

De Quervain's syndrome

The first dorsal compartment of the wrist, containing the tendons of abductor pollicis longus and extensor pollicis brevis, is the site of this painful disorder (Figure 6.8.1). The cause is unknown. It occurs spontaneously, more often in females than males, and may arise during or just after pregnancy. The chief symptom is pain during use of the thumb. Loss of ulnar deviation of the wrist and triggering of the abductor pollicis longus tendon are seen occasionally in severe cases. The physical signs are pain on resisted active extension of the thumb, swelling and tenderness over the compartment, and a positive Finkelstein's test. The test described by Finkelstein is reproduction of pain by 'grasping the patient's thumb and quickly abducting the hand ulnarward'. Another test, originally described by Eichhoff but often attributed erroneously to Finkelstein, deviates the wrist ulnarward while the thumb is held in the palm beneath the flexed fingers. The differential diagnosis includes the intersection syndrome and arthritis of the trapeziometacarpal, scaphotrapezial, or radioscaphoid joints.

Management comprises rest, analgesics, thumb splintage, and steroid injection. Injections are effective in the long term in at least 80% of cases but injection into the extensor pollicis brevis tenosynovium resulted in 100% success in one series. Care should be taken to avoid subcutaneous extravasation of long-acting steroid, which can produce an unsightly patch of atrophic skin and subcutaneous tissue.

Operative release is indicated if pain persists or recurs after injection. It requires a longitudinal division of the roof of the first dorsal compartment and of any subcompartments (30–60% of first dorsal compartments have a septum that separates the abductor pollicis longus tendon from the extensor pollicis brevis). A transverse skin incision gives good exposure and a better scar than a longitudinal incision. It is crucial to protect the superficial radial nerve; a neuroma can be very troublesome. Release of the retinaculum toward the dorsal edge of the compartment leaves a palmar ridge of retinacular tissue that may help to prevent the uncommon complication of palmar subluxation of the abductor pollicis longus tendon on wrist flexion.

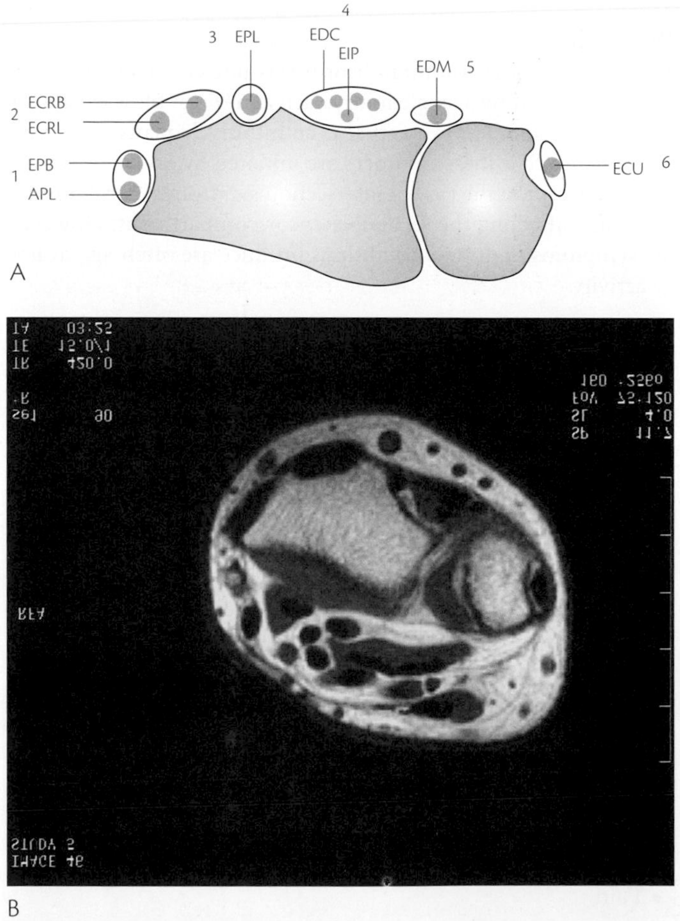

Fig. 6.8.1 The six extensor compartments at the wrist, shown (A) diagrammatically and (B) on axial MRI. (Courtesy of Dr E. McNally, Department of Radiology, Nuffield Orthopaedic Centre, Oxford.)

Intersection syndrome (peritendinitis crepitans)

This condition is probably the only tendon disorder for which a consistent association with overuse has been demonstrated. Repetitive gripping activities, such as weightlifting and rowing, are often implicated. It is characterized by pain, tenderness, swelling, and, in severe cases, crepitus where the abductor pollicis longus and extensor pollicis brevis muscle bellies run obliquely across the second dorsal compartment. This point lies about 5cm proximal to the radial styloid and is well above the site affected in de Quervain's syndrome. The pathology was previously thought to be due to friction between the first and second compartments causing tendinitis. However, Grundberg and Reagan (1985) found tenosynovitis in the second extensor compartment in each of 13 cases; in every case the symptoms were relieved by decompressing only the second compartment.

Conservative treatment of rest, splintage, and steroid injection is usually effective. Operative release of the second extensor compartment is rarely required.

Flexor carpi radialis

The flexor carpi radialis tendon passes over the wrist joint in a fibro-osseous tunnel lined with synovium, running past the ulnar side of the tubercle of the scaphoid and along a groove in the medial face of the trapezium before inserting onto the base of the second metacarpal.

Pain related to the flexor carpi radialis tendon may arise spontaneously, typically in females of late middle age (in whom it may be associated with scaphotrapezial osteoarthritis), but may occasionally be associated with activities requiring strenuous flexion of the wrist.

The patient complains of pain localized to the tendon at the wrist. There is tenderness and swelling of the tendon sheath. Pain is aggravated by resisted flexion of the wrist. The differential diagnosis includes de Quervain's syndrome, palmar wrist ganglion, and scaphotrapezial osteoarthritis. Treatment is by rest, splintage, analgesics, and steroid injection of the sheath. Operative release of the sheath is occasionally required.

Other tendons

Pain syndromes may be associated with several other tendons, including extensor pollicis longus, extensor indicis proprius, flexor carpi ulnaris, and extensor carpi ulnaris. The diagnosis is made from the findings of pain, swelling, local tenderness, and pain on active resisted tendon action. The management follows the lines described previously.

Trigger digits

Trigger digits in adults

Trigger digit in adults is caused by a nodular thickening of the flexor tendon that is accompanied by stenosis of the first annular (A1) pulley of the tendon sheath at the level of the metacarpophalangeal joint. It occurs most often in middle-aged females. The ring finger, middle finger, and thumb are the most frequently affected digits.

Trigger digit presents with clicking or locking of the finger during flexion and extension. The digit may lock in flexion, typically with the finger flexed into the palm (Figure 6.8.2). Locking is often most troublesome on waking, requiring forcible extension using the opposite hand. Although locking appears to affect the interphalangeal joints of the fingers or the interphalangeal joint of the thumb, pain and tenderness are felt over the tendon sheath at the level of the metacarpophalangeal joint. The thumb occasionally locks in extension. Persistent locking of the finger may lead to a fixed flexion contracture at the proximal interphalangeal joint, especially in diabetic patients. Triggering at the A3 pulley is a rare variant described in bowlers that affects the flexor digitorum profundus and therefore the distal interphalangeal joint only.

Most cases arise spontaneously in otherwise normal individuals. There is no relationship to occupation but repetitive gripping activities may cause acute transient triggering. Triggering may be due to intratendinous nodules or tenosynovitis in rheumatoid disease, or to a tendon flap caused by a partial tendon division. Trigger digit is common in diabetes and in association with amyloidosis and mucopolysaccharidoses. Several digits may be affected in these groups of patients.

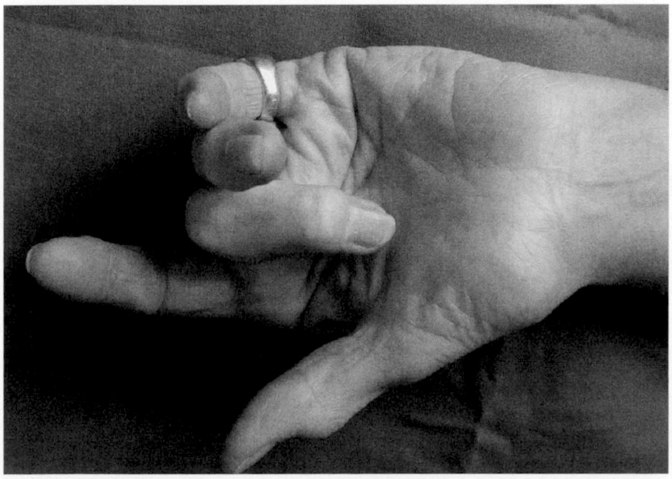

Fig. 6.8.2 Trigger middle finger locked in flexion.

Triggering may resolve spontaneously. Mild triggering may need no treatment apart from reassurance. Splintage of the interphalangeal joints in extension at night improves locking on waking and may suffice in mild cases. Taping of the proximal interphalangeal joint by day may prevent flexion to the point of locking. Steroid injection of the tendon sheath cures about 70% of cases but is less effective in diabetic patients.

In the non-rheumatoid patient, surgical release of the A1 pulley is indicated for persistent or severe triggering with almost 100% success for open release. Percutaneous release with a needle shortens recovery while being equally effective and safe. In longstanding cases with persistent proximal interphalangeal joint contracture and tendon thickening, division of the proximal part of the A2 pulley or resection of the ulnar slip of flexor digitorum superficialis may be required.

Release of the A1 pulley is contraindicated in rheumatoid as it may exacerbate a tendency to ulnar drift. Synovectomy and resection of the ulnar slip of flexor digitorum superficialis is preferred.

Trigger thumb in children

Trigger thumb is the most common hand condition requiring operative treatment in children. A young child, usually between the ages of 6 months and 3 years, presents with a painless fixed flexion contracture of the interphalangeal joint of the thumb. On rare occasions, there is a history of triggering. Thickening of the flexor tendon and its sheath is palpable at the level of the metacarpophalangeal joint. It is often termed 'congenital' although this seems inappropriate, as no cases were found during examination of 4719 newborn infants and children rarely present before the age of 6 months. The cause is unknown. The differential diagnosis is congenital clasped thumb, which is caused by absence or hypoplasia of the thumb extensors. Trigger thumb may resolve spontaneously; almost half of 53 patients recovered after observation for a mean of 7 months. Spontaneous improvement after age 3 is uncommon. If the thumb is reducible, splinting is more effective than observation alone in improving triggering. For persistent triggering, operative treatment involves division of the proximal pulley with care to avoid the digital nerves, which are close to the midline and lie immediately beneath the skin.

Trigger finger in children

Trigger finger is rare in children, accounting for about 14% of trigger digits. Unlike the thumb, locked trigger finger is uncommon. The middle finger is most commonly affected, followed by the ring and little fingers. Spontaneous recovery is common and splinting for trigger finger in children has had mixed success. Unlike adult trigger finger, release of the A1 pulley alone results in 44% recurrence In some cases, there is nodular thickening of the tendon and A1 pulley release alone suffices, while in others, there appears to be an abnormal relationship between the deep and superficial flexor tendons. In these patients, partial division of the A2 pulley or resection of one of the slips of flexor digitorum superficialis is effective.

Trigger wrist

Rarely, thickening of the tendon or synovium or may impede gliding at the wrist. This may cause triggering of the wrist (true trigger wrist) or fingers as well as median nerve compression. The cause is usually flexor tendon tenosynovitis for which tenosynovectomy and carpal tunnel release is usually curative. It is occasionally due to a discrete mass or extensor tendon pathology.

Tendon rupture (Box 6.8.2)

Tendon rupture is an important condition in the hand, not only because it impairs function but also because in some cases it can be prevented by timely intervention. The pathology of tendon rupture involves mechanical factors that increase tendon stress and pathological processes that weaken the tendon. Mechanical factors include abrasion on sharp surfaces (fractures, implants), change in direction, tendon anomalies (abnormal interconnections), and acute or chronic overloading. The tendon may be weakened by inflammation (rheumatoid disease, systemic lupus erythematosus, crystal deposition, osteoarthritis), ischaemia, or metabolic causes (chronic renal failure, systemic or local steroids).

Rupture of the extensor pollicis longus or flexor carpi radialis tendons is almost always an isolated lesion with a very low likelihood of other ruptures. Rupture of the finger extensors and of the tendons passing through the carpal tunnel is often sequential, so that detection of the first rupture and prompt intervention are crucial in preventing further loss of function.

Osteoarthritis

The classical lesion of attrition rupture of extensor tendons was described by Vaughan-Jackson in two cases of osteoarthritis of the distal radioulnar joint (Figure 6.8.3A). The roughened ulnar head erodes through the dorsal capsule and then lies in contact with tendons in the fifth and fourth compartments. Rupture is generally painless and sequential, beginning with the extensor digiti minimi tendon. Since extension of the little finger can, in many cases, be activated by a tendon slip from the extensor digitorum communis of the ring finger, rupture of extensor digitorum minimi may pass unnoticed until the ring and little finger drop together. Loss of independent extension of the little finger (Figure 6.8.3B) signifies rupture of extensor digitorum minimi and the need for appropriate surgery of the distal radioulnar joint.

Osteoarthritis of the radiocarpal, scaphotrapezial, and distal radioulnar joints can lead to tendon ruptures within the carpal tunnel. Osteoarthritis of the scaphotrapezial joint may cause rupture of the flexor carpi radialis tendon (Figure 6.8.4), the proximal stump of which may form a painful fusiform swelling in the distal forearm.

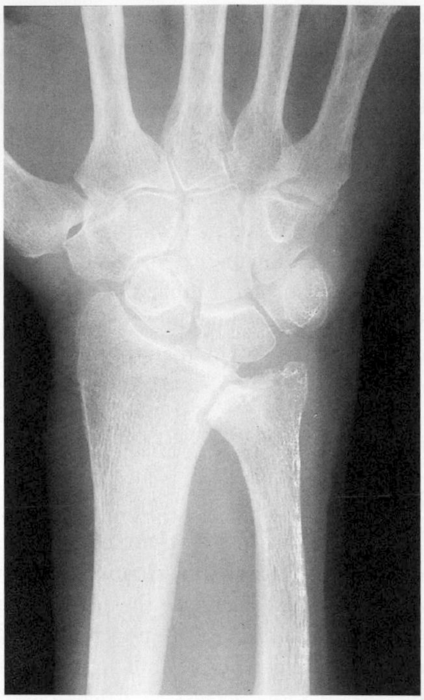

A

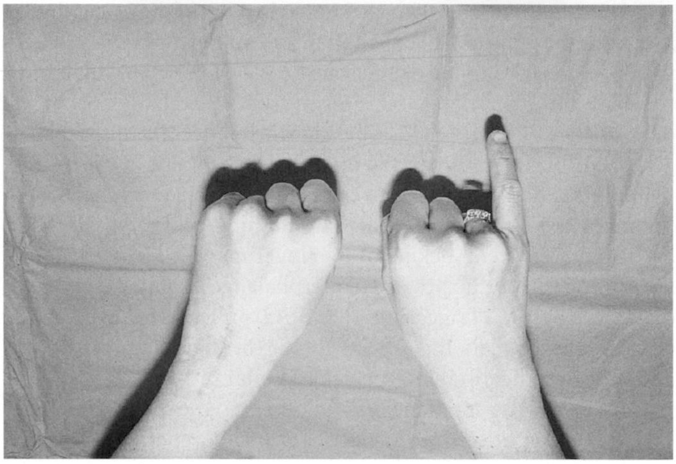

B

Fig. 6.8.3 A) Osteoarthritis of the distal radioulnar joint. B) Loss of independent extension of the little finger, owing to rupture of extensor digiti minimi.

Box 6.8.2 Treatment of tendon rupture

- Rest and waiting (many resolve spontaneously)
- Splintage for some conditions
- Steroid injections
- Release of tendons sheaths open or percutaneously
- Open reconstruction of tendon failure and removal of the cause, e.g. Darrach's procedure.

Distal radial fracture

The most common tendon rupture is of extensor pollicis longus, occurring a few weeks after fracture of the distal radius. The incidence is approximately 1% of all distal radial fractures. The rupture occurs typically in undisplaced fractures. The pathogenesis is uncertain but ischaemia probably plays a role. The tendon may be vulnerable to narrowing or irregularity of its sheath as it passes around the dorsal tubercle of the radius. At this point, it is subject to bending forces, has a poorly vascularized segment and lacks mesotenon. Nutrition at this point is from diffusion from the synovial fluid which may be hindered by haematoma contained in the

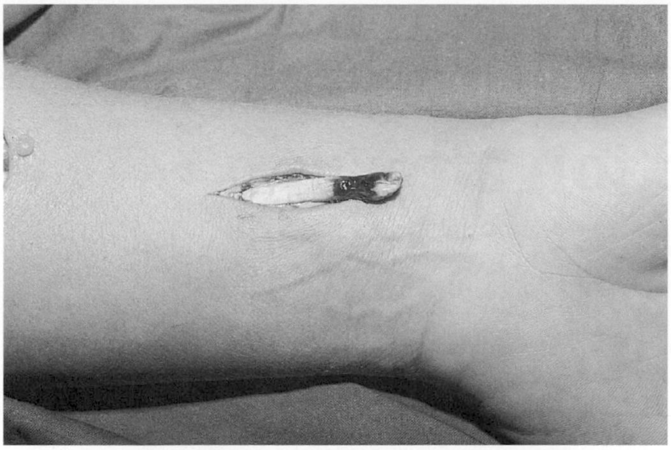

A

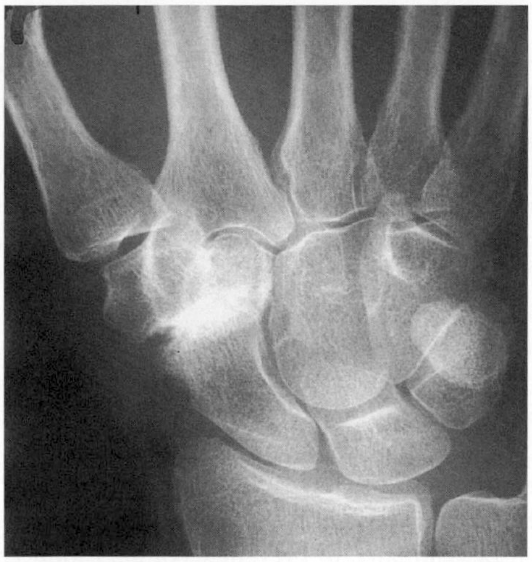

B

Fig. 6.8.4 A) Rupture of the flexor carpi radialis tendon associated with (B) scaphotrapezial osteoarthritis.

intact sheath. The intact retinaculum also holds the tendon down against the sharp fracture edge.

Pain and crepitus over the third compartment with thumb movement is an indication for release of the retinaculum. Generally, however, the rupture occurs without warning.

There may be an extension lag at the interphalangeal joint (Figure 6.8.5), but a more reliable sign is loss of retroposition wherein the patient cannot lift the thumb off the table when the hand is placed flat—a movement that only extensor pollicis longus can achieve. Reconstruction by tendon transfer (using extensor indicis proprius or a slip of abductor pollicis longus) is straightforward and effective.

With the increasing use of plate fixation of the distal radius, iatrogenic tendon rupture is encountered. The distal edge of a dorsal plate can abrade the long finger extensors; excessive length of screws securing a volar plate may do the same. Dorsally angulated malunion of the distal radius may also cause rupture of flexor

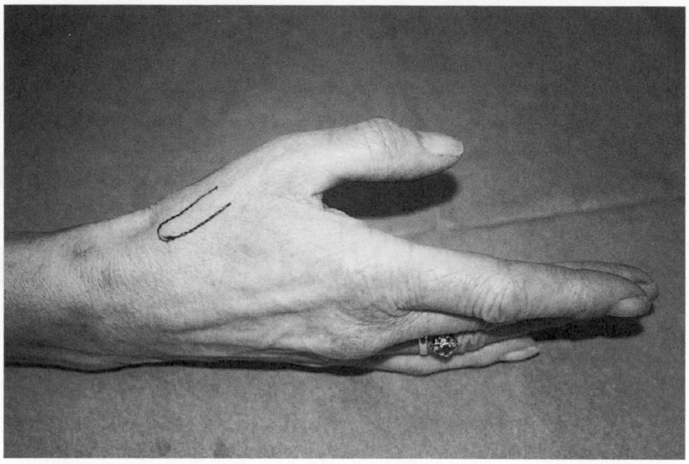

Fig. 6.8.5 Rupture of the extensor pollicis longus tendon after fracture of the distal radius. The palpable distal tendon stump is marked.

tendons in the distal forearm. Volar locking plates can cause flexor or extensor tendon ruptures.

Other causes of tendon rupture

Less common causes of tendon rupture include long-standing Kienböck's disease, scaphoid non-union, and scapholunate dissociation. The flexor digitorum profundus tendon of the little finger is particularly prone to rupture; this can be due to non-union of the hook of the hamate, calcium pyrophosphate deposition in the triangular fibrocartilage, pisiform–triquetral instability, and osteoarthritis.

When no definite cause can be found, the rupture is termed spontaneous. In flexor tendons these are rarer than avulsion from the distal phalanx. Typically they occur in zone III of the flexor digitorum profundus to the little finger. Although the aetiology is unclear, the likely predisposing factors include tendon anomalies, repetitive microtrauma, vascular alterations, and genetic influences.

Further reading

Clarke, M.T., Lyall, H.A., Grant, J.W., and Matthewson, (1990). The histopathology of de Quervain's disease. *Journal of Hand Surgery*, **22B**, 732–4.

Grundberg, A.B. and Reagan, D.S. (1985). Pathologic anatomy of the forearm: intersection syndrome. *Journal of Hand Surgery*, **10A**, 299–302.

Leslie, B.M., Ericson, W.B. Jr, and Morehead, J.R. (1990). Incidence of a septum within the first dorsal compartment of the wrist. *Journal of Hand Surgery*, **15A**, 88–91.

Trezies, A.J., Lyons, A.R., Fielding, K. and Davis, T.R. (1998). Is occupation an aetiological factor in the development of trigger finger? *Journal of Hand Surgery*, **23B**, 539–40.

Weiland, A.J. (1996). Repetitive strain injuries and cumulative trauma disorders. *Journal of Hand Surgery*, **21A**, 337.

6.9

Reconstruction after nerve injury

T.E.J. Hems

Summary points

- Late reconstructive procedures may improve function if there is persisting paralysis after nerve injury
- Transfer of a functioning musculotendinous unit to the tendon of the paralysed muscle is the most common type of procedure
- Passive mobility must be maintained in affected joints before tendon transfer can be performed
- The transferred muscle should be expendable, have normal power, and have properties appropriate to the function it is required to restore
- Tendon transfers can provide reliable improvement in function after isolated radial nerve palsy
- A number of procedures have been described for reconstruction of thumb opposition but impaired sensation after median nerve injury may limit gain in function
- Tendon transfers are possible to improve clawing of fingers and lateral pinch of the thumb after ulnar nerve palsy or other cases of intrinsic paralysis.

Introduction

Loss of function in a peripheral nerve is commonly caused by trauma but can also be caused by tumours, neuropathy, or infections such as polio or leprosy. Injury to a mixed peripheral nerve results in paralysis of the muscles that it innervates and loss of sensation in its cutaneous territory. Recovery may occur spontaneously in the case of neurapraxia or axonotmesis and may be possible after surgical repair of the nerve in cases of neurotmesis. Nerve regeneration is slow even under optimum conditions. Denervated muscles deteriorate rapidly and effective reinnervation is possible only if regenerating axons reach them within 1–2 years. Early repair of divided nerves is especially important where the injury is some distance from the muscles to be reinnervated, such as in the brachial plexus.

The results of a successful early nerve repair are often superior to those of late reconstructive procedures: nerve repair can increase muscle power in a paralysed limb; tendon transfer can only redistribute what remains. Partial nerve recovery may still be supplemented by other measures. However, tendon transfer potentially provides an earlier improvement in function than nerve repair and this option may better suit the patient's overall rehabilitation.

Reconstructive procedures must be considered when nerve repair has been unsuccessful, or was not performed. They may also be necessary where nerve or muscle function has been irretrievably damaged by other pathologies such as compression, tumour, and ischaemia.

The most commonly used reconstructive operation is transfer of a healthy tendon or muscle to replace the function of a paralysed muscle, but other options are occasionally indicated, including tenodesis, arthrodesis, and free muscle transfer. Reconstruction is usually delayed until the final result of nerve recovery is evident, but may be indicated much earlier if it is known that recovery is unlikely or, occasionally, to prevent secondary joint contractures. Reconstructive procedures to improve sensation are occasionally indicated.

Principles of tendon transfer

1) A *full range of passive movement* should ideally be available in all joints on which the transfer will act. Regular physiotherapy should be given from the outset in cases of nerve injury, as it is much easier to maintain movement than to restore it. In complex injuries, early skeletal fixation with repair of tendon injuries and provision of stable skin cover gives the best chance of providing appropriate conditions for subsequent tendon transfer
2) The transferred muscle should be *expendable*. Its use must not remove an important function. In cases of blunt trauma to a limb, it is common for more than one nerve territory to be affected. Therefore the full extent of nerve and muscle injury should be carefully evaluated to check which muscles are functioning
3) *Normal power* of the transferred muscle is desirable, as at least one grade on the Medical Research Council scale is generally lost by transfer. It is not always possible to satisfy this requirement, particularly after injuries to the brachial plexus; each case should be considered individually. It is rarely appropriate to transfer a muscle that has previously recovered after repair of its nerve

4) The *amplitude* and *power* of the transferred muscle should be appropriate to the function that is being restored (see later)
5) *Synergistic muscles* should be used for transfer where possible. For example, a wrist flexor which is synergistic in finger extension may be transferred to restore this movement. Experience has shown that synergistic muscles are more easily retrained to perform their new function
6) Some transferred muscles, such as brachioradialis, retain their *original function*, and their effectiveness therefore depends on the activity of the antagonist to that original function. If brachioradialis is transferred to flexor pollicis longus, for example, triceps must be strong enough to resist its normal elbow flexor action and allow its power to be transmitted distally to the thumb
7) The transferred tendon should have a *straight line of action*. Acute angulation should be avoided
8) The transfer is *attached to the tendon of the paralysed muscle* if this is available, thus achieving the most effective biomechanics at the insertion. In cases where some nerve recovery may occur later, the attachment is performed end-to-side.

Properties of muscles and tendons

There are three important mechanical properties of muscles:

1) The mass or volume of muscle fibres, which is proportional to work capacity
2) The average length of the constituent muscle fibres, which is proportional to excursion (the distance through which a muscle can contract). The excursion of a muscle is about one-third of the resting length of its fibres
3) The physiological cross-sectional area of a muscle, which is proportional to the maximum force of contraction.

The relationship between these properties depends on the architecture or arrangement of fibres within a muscle. The properties of forearm and hand muscles have been studied in cadavers and some of the results are shown in Table 6.9.1. The actual mass or volume of a given muscle varies considerably between individuals but the relative mass compared with other muscles in the same arm is quite consistent. Therefore mass is presented as the 'mass fraction', which is the percentage of the total weight of all the muscle in the forearm and hand. Physiological cross-sectional area was calculated by dividing volume of a muscle by the fibre length and is also presented as a percentage of the total called 'tension fraction'.

Muscles generate tension and create excursion, but tendons transmit the muscle work to the part of the skeleton that is to be moved. The amplitude of gliding of a tendon depends mostly on the excursion of its muscle but is also a function of the direction of the muscle fibres, amplitude being greater if the angle the fibres make with the tendon (pennation angle) is acute. The amplitude of tendon excursion is also influenced by other factors such as the freedom of gliding allowed by the paratenon, changes in direction around a pulley, and the crossing of articulations. The amplitude of gliding of the tendons of the extrinsic muscles of the hand also varies in the same tendon depending on the level at which it is measured. For example, the amplitude of gliding of the flexor digitorum profundus tendons is 5mm at the distal interphalangeal joint, 17mm at the proximal interphalangeal joint, 38mm at the carpal tunnel, and 85mm in the distal forearm. The maximal excursion for each tendon is shown in Table 6.9.2.

Table 6.9.1 Normal expected mean values for fibre length, mass fraction, and tension fraction for selected forearm and hand muscles in adult males and females (Brand et al., 1981), including abbreviated muscle names used in this chapter

Muscle	Resting fibre length (cm)	Mass fraction (%)	Tension fraction (%)
Adductor pollicis (AP)	3.6	2.1	3.0
Abductor pollicis brevis (APB)	3.7	0.8	1.1
Abductor pollicis longus (APL)	4.6	2.8	3.1
Brachioradialis (BR)	16.1	7.7	2.4
Extensor carpi radialis brevis (ECRB)	6.1	5.1	4.2
Extensor carpi radialis longus (ECRL)	9.3	6.5	3.5
Extensor carpi ulnaris (ECU)	4.5	4.0	4.5
Extensor digitorum communis (EDC)	5.8	6.3	5.5
Extensor digiti minimi (EDM)	5.9	1.2	1.0
Extensor indicis proprius (EIP)	5.5	1.1	1.0
Extensor pollicis brevis (EPB)	4.3	0.7	0.8
Extensor pollicis longus (EPL)	5.7	1.5	1.3
Flexor carpi radialis (FCR)	5.2	4.2	4.1
Flexor carpi ulnaris (FCU)	4.2	5.6	6.7
Flexor digitorum profundus (FDP):			
Index finger	6.6	3.5	2.7
Middle finger	6.6	4.4	3.4
Ring finger	6.8	1.1	3.0
Little finger	6.2	3.4	2.8
Flexor digitorum superficialis (FDS):			
Index finger	7.2	2.9	2.0
Middle finger	7.0	4.7	3.4
Ring finger	7.3	3.0	2.0
Little finger	7.0	1.3	0.9
Palmaris longus (PL)	5.0	1.2	1.2
Pronator quadratus (PQ)	3.0	1.8	3.0
Pronator teres (PT)	5.1	5.6	5.5
Supinator	2.7	3.8	7.1

Surgical techniques used in tendon transfer

Transferred tendons are passed through subcutaneous tunnels where possible, so as to allow gliding. Since the tendon is likely to adhere to the surrounding tissue to some degree, that tissue should be pliable; passage over unyielding surfaces such as bone and fascia should be avoided if possible. The transfer is usually attached to the tendon of the paralysed muscle by a tendon weave (Figure 6.9.1), which is considerably stronger than end-to-end suture. If there is sufficient overlap of the two tendons being joined, at least three passes through tendon should be made. Each pass is locked with non-absorbable sutures. Such a weave is very strong but is also

Table 6.9.2 Maximum excursion of the tendons in the adult hand

Muscle	Maximum excursion (mm)
Abductor pollicis longus (APL)	28
Extensor carpi radialis brevis (ECRB)	37
Extensor carpi radialis longus (ECRL)	37
Extensor carpi ulnaris (ECU)	18
Extensor digitorum communis (EDC)	50
Extensor pollicis brevis(EPB)	28
Extensor pollicis longus (EPL)	58
Flexor carpi radialis (FCR)	40
Flexor carpi ulnaris (FCU)	33
Flexor digitorum profundus (FDP)	70
Flexor digitorum superficialis (FDS)	64
Flexor pollicis longus (FPL)	52
Pronator teres (PT)	50

bulky, so there should be sufficient space to allow gliding. Where no tendon is available to receive the transfer, an attachment must be made directly to bone, using suture anchors or sutures passed through bone holes.

Tenodesis

Tenodesis is the automatic movement of a joint produced by motion of another, usually more proximal, joint. A tenodesis can be created surgically often by fixing a tendon to bone so that motion of a proximal joint causes a force on the tendon. For example, the EPL tendon can be anchored to the distal radius so that the thumb extends with wrist flexion.

Reconstruction for shoulder paralysis

The Glenohumeral joint

Paralysis of the important rotator cuff muscles and deltoid, which both stabilize the glenohumeral joint and produce abduction and external rotation, usually results from lesions to the C5 and C6 roots or the upper trunk of the brachial plexus. Although muscle transfer can sometimes help in cases of partial paralysis, shoulder arthrodesis is the only effective procedure for a completely flail shoulder.

Arthrodesis corrects subluxation of the glenohumeral joint and allows transfer of scapulothoracic motion to the arm, but at the expense of irreversible fusion of the glenohumeral joint. The active range of motion depends upon the function of the muscles controlling the shoulder girdle particularly serratus anterior. The usual position of fusion is around 30 degrees of glenohumeral abduction, 30 degrees of forward flexion, and 30 degrees of internal rotation. The technique involves exposure of the shoulder through an extensive posterior and lateral approach and decortication of the glenoid and humeral head. Internal fixation is provided by cancellous screws passed through the humeral head into the glenoid and a reconstruction plate placed from the spine of the scapula and acromium to the neck of the humerus (Figure 6.9.2). A spica cast is usually necessary for at least 6 weeks after operation. The mean range of active flexion and abduction was reported to be 75 degrees and 65 degrees respectively in a series of 11 patients (Figure 6.9.3).

Restoration of elbow flexion

Active elbow flexion is required for almost every activity of the upper limb. Because elbow extension is aided by gravity, triceps function is less vital. Elbow flexion may be lost as a result of supraclavicular injuries to the upper roots of the brachial plexus or infraclavicular injuries involving the musculocutaneous nerve. In cases where nerve reconstruction is unsuccessful, muscle transfer to restore elbow flexion may be worthwhile, particularly in patients who have satisfactory hand function. The possibilities for muscle transfer are greater in isolated musculocutaneous nerve damage than in supraclavicular brachial plexus injuries, where the donor muscles may also be completely or partially denervated. The following muscle transfers have been described:

- Pectoralis major
- Latissimus dorsi

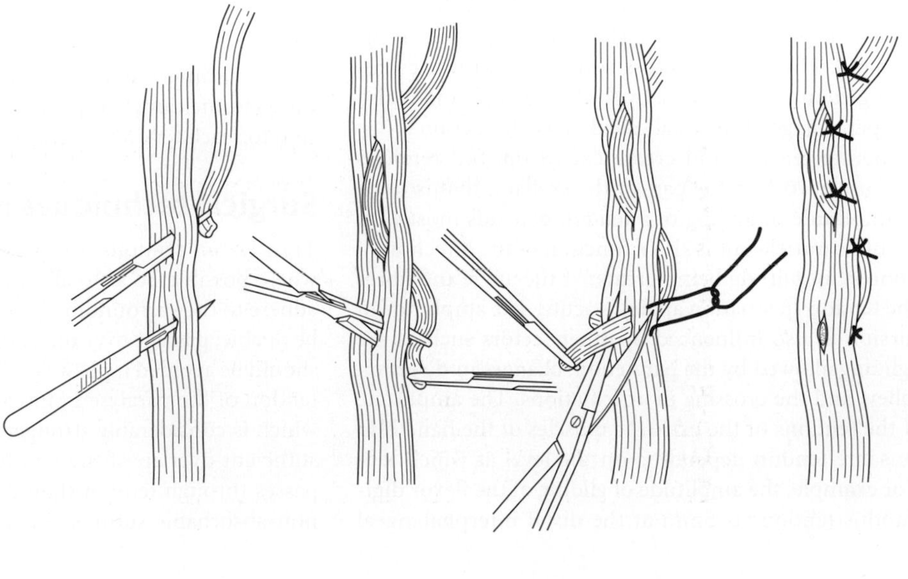

Fig. 6.9.1 Diagram illustrating a tendon weave. Where possible, the free ends of the tendons are buried to reduce adhesions.

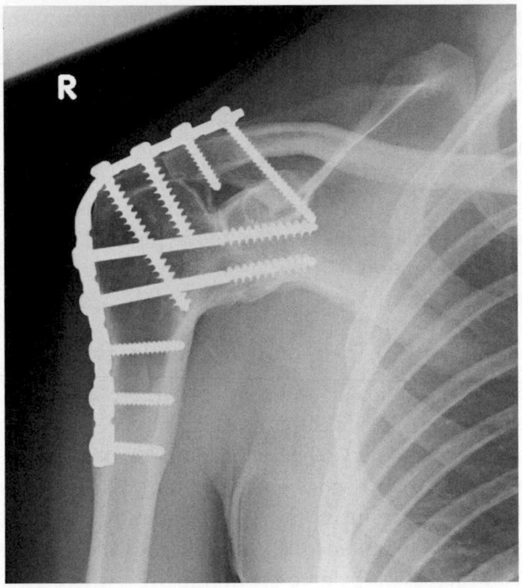

Fig. 6.9.2 Radiograph showing arthrodesis of the shoulder using a 4.5-mm pelvic reconstruction plate.

- Triceps
- Steindler transfer (transfer of the common flexor origin of the forearm to a more proximal position on the humerus)
- Functioning free muscle transfer (gracilis most commonly used).

Radial nerve palsy

The radial nerve is most commonly injured below its branches to the triceps, often in association with fractures of the humerus. Occasionally higher lesions occur which may be associated with more widespread damage to the brachial plexus. While triceps function can largely be replaced by gravity, it should be considered that, in the absence of supinator, the biceps can only supinate the forearm, if the triceps is stabilizing the elbow. Possible transfers to replace triceps include latissimus dorsi and deltoid lengthened with a tendon graft. It is not uncommon for the deficit to be confined to finger and thumb extension either as a result of injury to the posterior interosseous nerve or partial recovery of a more proximal lesion.

A patient with an irreparable radial nerve palsy needs tendon transfers to replace:

- Wrist extension
- Finger (metacarpophalangeal joint (**MPJ**) extension
- A combination of thumb extension and abduction.

Providing that the median and ulnar nerves are normal there are a number of possible combinations of tendon transfers for replacing these functions. Transfer of PT to ECRB for wrist extension appears to be universally accepted. Its use relies on the function being present in pronator quadratus. If PT is not available then the author has successfully used FDS to the middle finger. Wrist arthrodesis is rarely required and is generally undesirable since wrist movement enhances finger movement by the tenodesis effect.

Although the Jones (1916) transfer included the use of FCR and FCU for finger and thumb extension, it is now generally agreed that it is desirable to leave one wrist flexor intact. In making a choice between these donor tendons for transfer to EDC it is important to consider the balance of muscles that provide radial and ulnar deviation of the wrist. Those who prefer to use FCR argue that retention of a strong ulnar deviator of the wrist (FCU) is important for function of the hand. EPL function is restored with transfer of Palmaris longus.

Overall, the author has been slightly more impressed with the FCR set of transfers (Figure 6.9.4). The FCR has the advantage of having greater excursion than FCU. For posterior interosseous nerve palsy FCR should be used in order to balance radial and ulnar deviation. If PL is absent then EPL is usually included in the transfer for finger extension.

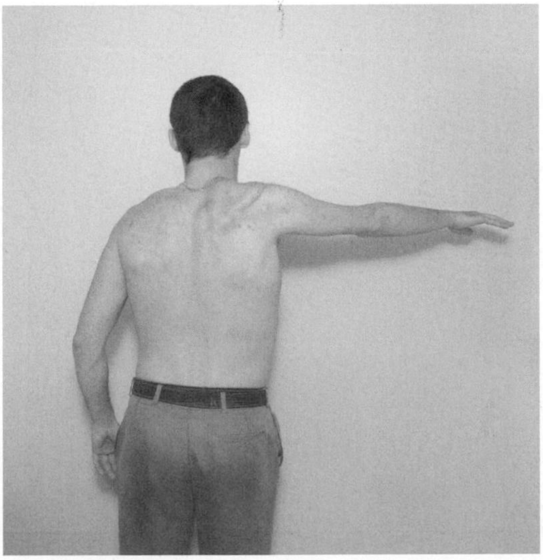

Fig. 6.9.3 Illustration of the range of abduction after shoulder arthrodesis.

Median nerve palsy

The median nerve is most often damaged either by trauma or by compression at the wrist or distal forearm. Hence the thenar muscles are denervated and opposition of the thumb is impaired. The degree of functional loss in isolated median nerve palsy is variable. Opposition is a combination of two movements: abduction or lifting of the thumb away from the palm of the hand; and rotation of the thumb into pronation so that the pulp surfaces of the thumb and index face each other. Before undertaking reconstruction it is important to overcome any contracture of the first web space. In the presence of severe sensory deficit in the median nerve distribution, patients are less likely to benefit from tendon transfer. A number of opposition transfers (opponensplasties) have been devised, and the circumstances of each case should be considered before making a choice.

Donor tendons include FDS to the ring finger, palmaris longus, extensor indicis, and abductor digiti minimi.

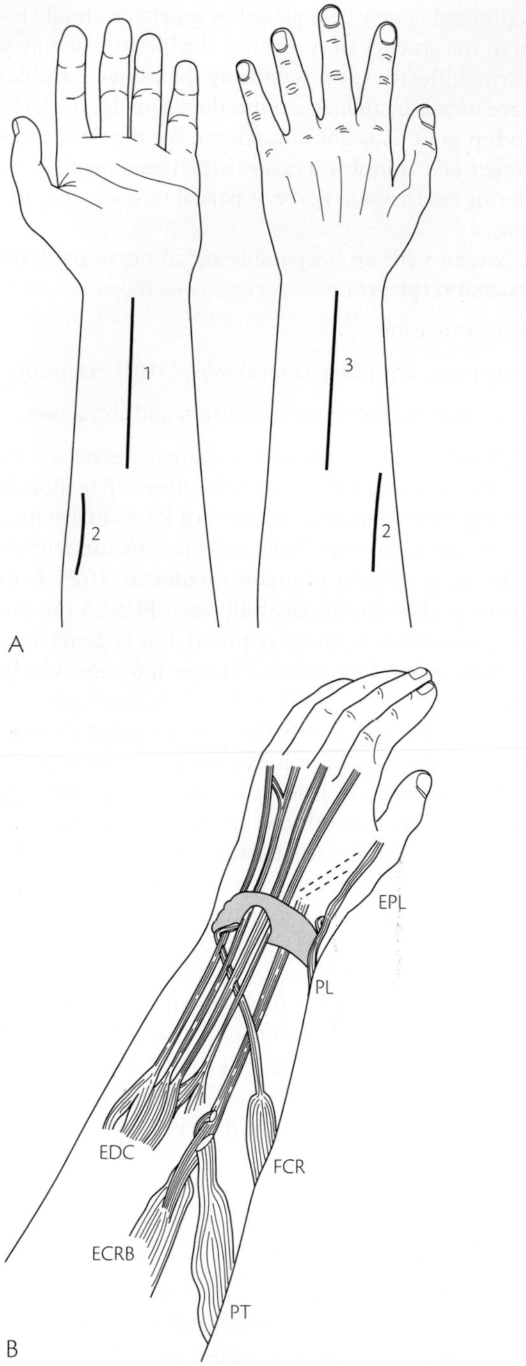

Fig. 6.9.4 Diagram illustrating the flexor carpi radialis set of transfers for low radial nerve palsy: A) Three incisions are required. B) The final positions of the transferred tendons.

Flexor digitorum superficialis opponensplasty

In this procedure the FDS tendon is divided at the base of the ring finger and delivered into an incision just proximal to the wrist crease. The tendon is passed through a subcutaneous tunnel round the ulnar side of the pisiform and then across the palm to the MPJ of the thumb. An attachment is then made to the tendon of APB or directly to the base of the proximal phalanx; there is some debate about the exact method of distal attachment.

Palmaris longus opponensplasty (Camitz transfer)

This is quite a simple procedure in which the PL tendon is mobilized in continuity with a strip of palmar fascia (Figure 6.9.5). The tendon is then passed through a subcutaneous tunnel from the forearm to the MPJ of the thumb, where it is sutured to the tendon of APB. This transfer has its greatest application in severe carpal tunnel syndrome where it can be carried out simultaneously with carpal tunnel release. However, the line of pull of PL tends to produce thumb abduction with little rotation and is therefore not a true opposition transfer.

Extensor indicis proprius opponensplasty

This transfer is particularly useful when there has been tendon damage at the wrist in addition to a median nerve injury or in high lesions of the median nerve. The extensor indicis tendon is removed at the index finger MPJ with a small portion of the extensor hood. It is delivered into an incision on the dorsum of the forearm and then passed, in a subcutaneous tunnel, round the ulnar aspect of the wrist and across the palm to the thumb MPJ, where it is attached to the tendon of APB (Figure 6.9.6). A similar opponensplasty can be preformed using EDM.

Hypothenar muscle opponensplasty (Huber transfer)

The abductor digiti minimi, which is an ulnar-innervated intrinsic muscle, can be transferred to restore opposition. The muscle is detached from its insertion and mobilized on its neurovascular pedicle which enters at the proximal end. It is then pulled through a subcutaneous tunnel and sutured to the APB. The Huber transfer is a good choice in children but involves quite an extensive dissection in adults. It has the advantage of using an intrinsic muscle which shortens throughout it length and therefore does not require tendon gliding.

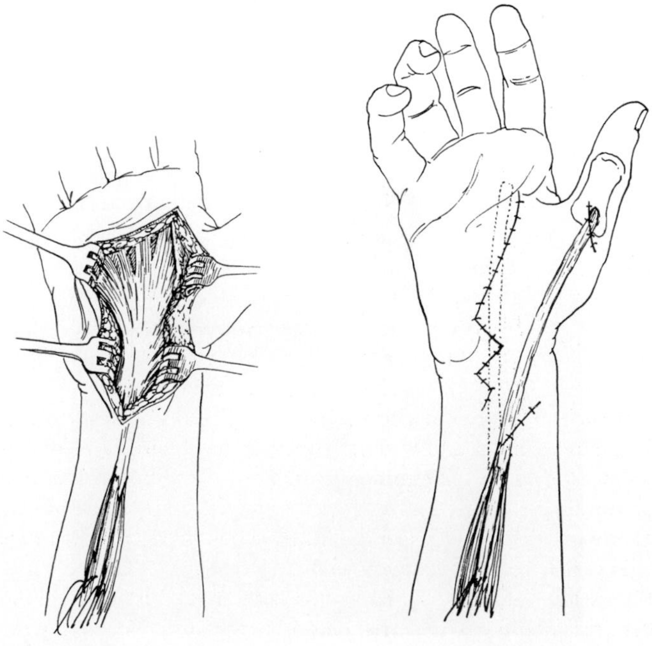

Fig. 6.9.5 Palmaris longus opponensplasty described by Camitz (1929).

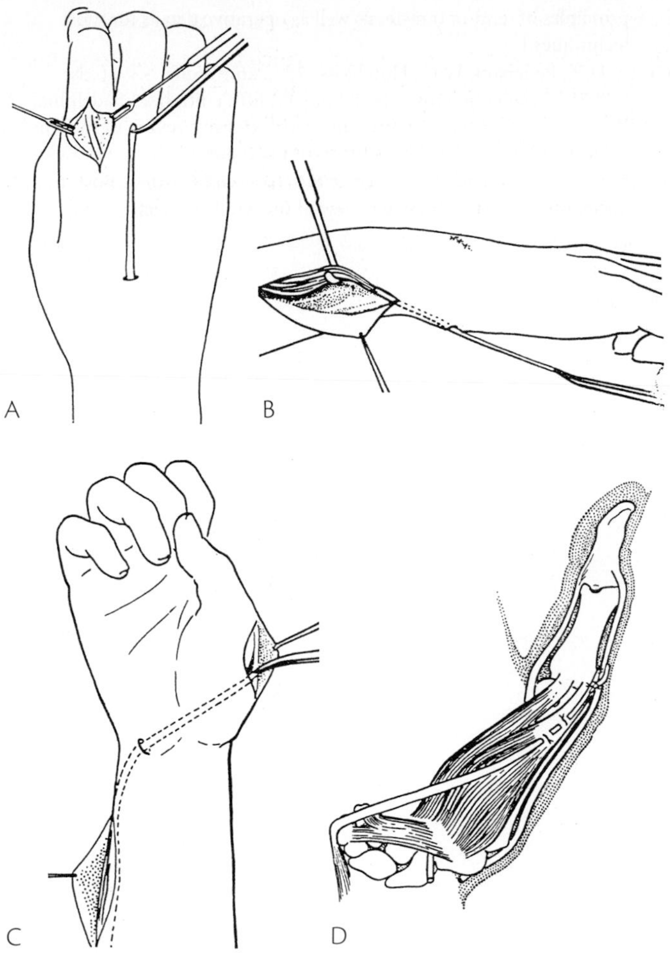

Fig. 6.9.6 Drawings illustrating the extensor indicis proprius opponensplasty (Burkhalter et al. 1973). A) The tendon is detached from the extensor hood on the index finger and the hood is carefully repaired. B) Through an incision on the dorsoulnar aspect of the forearm the muscle is transposed superficial to the extensor carpi ulnaris. C) The tendon of extensor indicis proprius is brought out in the area of the pisiform and then passed again subcutaneously across the palm to the thumb. D) Attachment is made to the abductor pollicis brevis tendon and extensor pollicis longus tendon.

High median nerve paralysis

In proximal injuries, such as those occurring in association with elbow injury, of the median nerve there is paralysis of FCR, FPL, FDS, and the radial half of FDP. In practical terms, transfers are usually performed to replace FPL and the FDP to the index and middle fingers. Tendons available for transfer include the brachioradialis and ECRL. The brachioradialis transfer to the FPL provides independent flexion of the thumb interphalangeal joint (IPJ). Flexion of the index and middle fingers can be obtained by side-to-side suturing of the FDP tendons so that the functioning ulnar half acts on all the digits. However, index finger flexion tends to be rather weak. Greater strength and independent flexion of the index finger can be restored by transfer of ECRL to FDP. The excursion of brachioradialis and ECRL is less than that of FDP and FPL. Therefore mobility of the wrist joint is important in enhancing the function of these transfers using the tenodesis effect.

Ulnar nerve palsy and other intrinsic deficiencies

The main motor deficit in ulnar nerve palsy is paralysis of the ulnar-innervated intrinsic muscles of the hand causing loss of flexion of the MPJs of the fingers, finger abduction and adduction, and thumb adduction. There is consequent clawing of the fingers and weakness of key pinch of the thumb. Paralysis of the ulnar half of the FDP and the FCU does not usually cause a functional problem. If necessary, the profundus tendons of the ring and little fingers can be attached to that of the middle finger in the forearm, so improving the strength of finger flexion. In addition to lesions of the ulnar nerve, damage to the lower roots of the brachial plexus can cause a similar deficiency of the intrinsic muscles of the hand.

Metacarpophalangeal joint flexion

The lumbricals and interossei, which insert into the extensor expansions of the fingers, normally act to flex the MPJs and extend the IPJs. If these muscles are paralysed and extrinsic muscle function is intact, the fingers will claw with hyperextension of the MPJs and flexion of the IPJs. In ulnar nerve palsy only the ring and little fingers are affected, but other causes of intrinsic paralysis (e.g. lesions of the lower roots of the brachial plexus) may affect all the fingers. If the MPJs are passively flexed then the EDC can extend the IPJs (Bouvier's manoeuvre). Normal finger flexion is initiated at the MPJ, so intrinsic paralysis also results in a loss of integration of MPJ and IPJ flexion. A number of procedures have been described to control the claw deformity.

Superficialis techniques

These techniques make use of the FDS tendons to replace intrinsic function. The FDS tendon to the middle or ring finger is divided and split into two or four slips. These slips may be passed through the lumbrical canals and inserted into the radial lateral band of the extensor mechanism of each finger. Alternatively, Zancolli (1979) recommended the 'lasso' procedure in which the tendon slip is looped through the annular pulley system at the base of the proximal phalanx and sutured to itself, so acting to flex the MPJs.

Transfer of extensor carpi radialis longus

Transfer of the FDS has the disadvantage that it does not add to overall grip strength. An alternative is transfer of ECRL. The tendon is lengthened using free tendon grafts to reach the lateral bands of the extensor mechanism of the fingers. In order to pass through the lumbrical canals on the volar aspect of the deep transverse metacarpal ligament, the tendons are routed either through the intermetacarpal spaces or through the carpal canal.

Thumb adduction

Paralysis of adductor pollicis and the first dorsal interosseous considerably weakens thumb–index pinch. Typically there is excessive flexion of the IPJ during pinch (Froment's sign). Tendons that can be transferred for thumb adduction include extensor indicis proprius, brachioradialis, and ECRL or ECRB. The choice depends to some extent on the power of abduction; weak abductors can be overpowered if a strong transfer such as ECRL is used. The tendon is passed through the second or third intermetacarpal space and then to the proximal phalanx of the thumb. If there is excessive flexion of the IPJ of the thumb (Froment's sign), this may be corrected by an FPL split transfer in which half the FPL tendon is transferred to EPL. The IPJ will then lie in a straight position.

Further reading

Brand, P.W. (1988). Biomechanics of tendon transfer. Hand Clinics, **4**, 137–54. [A classic review of the principles of tendon transfer including properties of forearm muscles. This issue is devoted to tendon transfer and contains many other useful reviews.]

Gelberman, R.H. (ed) (1991). *Operative Nerve Repair and Reconstruction*. Philadelphia, PA: Lippincott. [Includes a review of the history and principles of tendon transfer as well as operative details for most techniques.]

Green, D.P., Pederson, W.C., Hotchkiss, R.N., and Wolfe, S.W. (eds) (2005). *Green's* Operative Hand Surgery, fifth edition. Philadelphia, PA: Elsevier, Churchill Livingstone. [An extensive review of the whole subject with operative details for most procedures.]

Smith, R.J. (1987). *Tendon Transfers of the Hand and Forearm*. Boston, MA: Little, Brown. [An extensive review of the whole subject.]

6.10

Peripheral nerve entrapment

Krista E. Weiss and Arnold-Peter C. Weiss

Summary points

- Peripheral nerve compression syndromes are common when involving the median nerve at the wrist and the ulnar nerve at the elbow
- All patients are primarily diagnosed using a careful history and clinical examination
- Neurophysiological studies are very helpful especially in confusing presentations but do have a low false positive and false negative rate
- Conservative management should be tried in nearly all patients for 6-12 weeks
- Surgical treatment is generally very successful in relieving the symptoms of peripheral nerve compression
- Delayed treatment can result in permanent nerve damage which cannot be corrected by surgery.

General considerations

The term 'peripheral nerve entrapment' implies nerve compression based on impingement by adjacent soft tissue or bony structures, usually occurring in well-defined locations in the upper extremity. However, other factors frequently play a role in the onset of symptoms. Inflammation of the surrounding or adjacent structures can apply direct pressure to the nerve itself or increase pressure within a confined space. Systemic conditions, such as pregnancy, diabetes, and disorders of thyroid function, alter symptom manifestation and pressure applied to the nerve. Appropriate epineural blood supply also appears to be critical in the production of symptoms. Direct trauma to the nerve, although a relatively uncommon cause, can produce symptoms based on swelling, haematoma formation, or direct axonal injury. Similarly, abnormal tethering of the nerve can restrict its normal gliding motion leading to a traction phenomenon which impairs physiological function.

Peripheral nerve entrapment has several stages (Box 6.10.1):

- The first is intermittent impairment of the intraneural microcirculation. The raised pressure in the surrounding tissues intermittently exceeds the perfusion pressure in the epineurial vessels, which indirectly affects the resting membrane potential and propagated action potentials. Characteristically there are nocturnal and positional symptoms, for example, of early carpal tunnel syndrome, but otherwise normal function in the daytime; decompression provides immediate relief
- In the second stage, axonal transport is impaired and the myelin sheath may be lost from some fibres, leading to continuous symptoms and mild constant neural deficits such as muscle weakness and blunting of sensibility. Symptoms typically resolve within a few weeks of decompression
- In the third stage, axonal loss occurs through Wallerian degeneration. Recovery after decompression is slow (sometimes over a year) and may be incomplete.

Historically, peripheral nerve entrapment has been seen in the middle-aged and elderly population, more commonly in females than males, with a predictable and gradual progression of numbness and tingling. Patients with long-standing compression often presented with dense impairment of sensibility, with or without atrophic muscles, and with a poor prognosis for recovery after decompression. During the last 10–15 years, there have been increasing presentations from younger industrial or clerical workers undertaking repetitive hand tasks or using vibratory tools. The reasons remain unclear, although greater awareness of these conditions in the general population has contributed. The increase of workers' compensation claims for peripheral nerve entrapment has complicated the diagnosis and treatment of these conditions.

Clinical considerations (Box 6.10.2)

Nerve compression usually occurs gradually. Paraesthesia occurring at night or in response to specific activities is typical. Acute nerve compression is rare; patients note immediate symptoms of dense numbness and tingling in the appropriate distribution, often after a defined traumatic event. Bleeding and haematoma

Box 6.10.1 Stages of peripheral nerve entrapment

1. Intermittent impairment of the intraneural microcirculation
2. Impaired axonal transport and loss of some myelin sheath
3. Axonal loss occurs through Wallerian degeneration

The outcome is best with stage 1.

Box 6.10.2 Assessment and examination

- Assessment:
  - History—this is the mainstay
  - It should indicate the diagnosis and severity
- Examination:
  - Should confirm the diagnosis
  - Provocative tests include Tinel's sign
  - Fixed neurological changes indicate severity
  - Neurophysiology is often not required
  - Neurophysiology has false positive and false negative results.

formation secondary to the injury are the most common cause and patients with these findings are often best treated by immediate surgical decompression.

Since the clinical manifestations of impaired nerve function (sensory symptoms and muscle weakness or wasting) are projected to the distal terminations of the peripheral nerves, the site of the nerve lesion may, in theory, be deduced from the distribution of the symptoms. This is not always reliable. Assessment of the patient requires a careful interpretation of patient history and physical examination, as well as a thorough knowledge of the neural anatomy of the upper extremity. In most patients, clinical signs point to involvement of a single nerve. Once the affected nerve is identified, the site of compression can be localized by a combination of specific symptoms, physical signs, and electrodiagnostic testing. One should always be alert to unusual causes of peripheral nerve compression such as tumour surrounding the brachial plexus, radiation plexopathy, and the possibility of a double-crush phenomenon involving two sites of compression in the same nerve at different levels.

Sensibility testing can also provide valuable information although is rarely used in routine clinical practice. The Semmes–Weinstein monofilament test and vibration tests that examine the threshold for neural stimulation (a reflection of the function of single nerve fibres supplying one or more receptors) are more effective early since conventional sensory tests often show no abnormality in early and intermediate stages of neural entrapment. These are, in practice, only used in research. In contrast, static and moving two-point discrimination which test innervation density reflect the interpretation of signals from many overlapping receptor fields and require a considerable drop-out of fibres before performance is impaired. These tests are most frequently used to plot recovery after nerve repair.

Electrodiagnostic testing remains the most objective method available for investigating peripheral nerve compression (Table 6.10.1). The general assumption that electrodiagnostic testing is highly reproducible and completely accurate is incorrect. These tests are operator dependent, rely on the establishment of 'normal' values for each laboratory, and are affected by environmental conditions such as patient temperature, room temperature, and electromagnetic interference.

A summary of the physical signs and usefulness of electrodiagnostic testing in peripheral nerve compression

Carpal tunnel syndrome (Box 6.10.3)

Carpal tunnel syndrome is compression of the median nerve beneath the transverse carpal ligament in the wrist. It is the most common peripheral nerve entrapment syndrome, affecting about one in 1000 of the population per year, but its frequency of presentation may be increasing in parallel with greater community awareness.

Table 6.10.1 Common tests for peripheral nerve compression

Syndrome	Physical examination	Description	EMG/NCV usefulness
Carpal tunnel syndrome	Phalen's sign	Flex wrist for up to 60 s and look for numbness or tingling in fingers	+++
	Tinel's sign	Tap over median nerve at volar wrist and look for tingling radiation to radial fingers	
Pronator syndrome	Compression test	Compress median nerve at proximal forearm between pronator heads and look for numbness or tingling in fingers	+++
Guyon's canal compression syndrome	Tinel's sign	Tap over ulnar nerve at volar wrist and look for tingling radiating to ulnar fingers	+++
Cubital tunnel syndrome	Tinel's sign	Tap over ulnar nerve just behind medial epicondyle at the elbow and look for radiation of tingling to ring and small fingers	++
	Elbow flexion	Flex elbow fully and look for tingling in ring and small fingers	
Radial tunnel syndrome	Compression test	Compress or roll over radial nerve in the midportion of the proximal forearm (at mobile wad of Henry)	+
Wartenburg's syndrome	Tinel's sign	Tap over radial wrist and distal forearm and look for tingling in dorsum of thumb and index finger	+
Anterior interosseous syndrome	OK sign	Check for active flexion of thumb IP and index finger DIP joints (ability to make an OK sign with the fingers)	++

EMG, electromyography; IP, interphalangeal; DIP, distal interphalangeal.

Box 6.10.3 Carpal tunnel syndrome

- Median nerve compression at the wrist
- Very common
- Female incidence greater than male
- Typically bilateral
- Symptoms may be throughout the hand
- Provocative tests include Tinel's sign, pressure test, and Phalen's test
- Early disease may resolve non-operatively
- Splint, steroid injection
- Most patients require a carpal tunnel release
- The outcome is very reliable.

The classical clinical picture is of nocturnal paraesthesiae that wake the patient and are relieved by shaking the hands or hanging them in a dependent position. In severe cases, patients wake several times each night. In milder cases, patients will often note numbness and tingling upon waking in the morning, with fine motor activities of the hand, or when gripping the hand for extended periods of time (e.g. holding a steering wheel while driving a car). Numbness and tingling should be related to the median nerve distribution involving the thumb, index, and middle fingers, and the radial half of the ring fingers. Possible proximal causes of numbness and tingling, such as thoracic outlet syndrome, cervical radiculopathy, or pronator syndrome, should always be considered.

Physical examination includes tests of median nerve function (sensibility and thenar muscle power) and provocative tests. The two classic manoeuvres are Phalen's test and Tinel's test. In Phalen's test (generally performed on both hands simultaneously), the wrist is held fully flexed for up to 60s, noting the onset of paraesthesiae in the median nerve distribution. For Tinel's test, the examiner's finger or a rubber mallet is used to tap over the median nerve within and just proximal to the transverse carpal ligament, proving positive if the patient has distal radiation of 'electric shocks' or tingling in the median nerve distribution. Phalen's test is sensitive but sometimes renders false-positive results. Tinel's test is more specific but is less sensitive, so that a positive result is informative but a negative one is still consistent with carpal tunnel syndrome. Median nerve compression (the compression or pressure test) can also be used. The median nerve is compressed/pressed upon by the examiner's finger just proximal to the carpal canal. Like Phalen's test, if positive there is usually a response in 20s but it may be necessary to press for 60s.

Electrodiagnostic testing is the single best test in diagnosing carpal tunnel syndrome, and is especially invaluable when the clinical impression is inconsistent with the typical history and physical signs of the syndrome. Although this test provides the most objective examination of the median nerve, it should used in conjunction with the clinical signs and symptoms.

Conservative management includes use of a neutral-position wrist splint to be worn at night and during repetitive activities of the hands, and occasionally the use of oral anti-inflammatory medications. Steroid injections can offer two benefits in patients with a relatively short duration of symptoms: a cure (in less than half of patients) and diagnostic confirmation if there is a response even transiently.

Most patients eventually require surgical release of the transverse carpal ligament. Operative treatment is indicated in patients who have fixed neurological symptoms, i.e. thenar atrophy or constant sensory impairment (implying severe compression), although relief of symptoms may be incomplete. The carpal ligament can be divided open or with the newer techniques of endoscopic or mini-open ligament release. Open techniques are safer, with less chance of injury to the median nerve, common digital nerves, and flexor tendons, and a lower recurrence rate; however, increased palmar tenderness is a drawback (Figure 6.10.1). Though pillar pain is certainly not eliminated, endoscopic release provides the benefit of less palmar tenderness.

Postoperative splinting is not required routinely, and the outcome of splinting does not significantly differ from that of soft dressing. Concomitant internal or external neurolysis of the median nerve do not help and increase the risks, and so are not routinely performed.

Pronator syndrome (Box 6.10.4)

Entrapment of the median nerve in the proximal forearm is rare. Although called the pronator syndrome, compression may occur at various sites. Occasionally, patients will present with compression of the median nerve under a ligament of Struthers arising from a supracondylar process of the humerus. Alternative sites of compression as it passes through the proximal forearm and elbow region include the lacertus fibrosus, the origin of the pronator teres, and the arch of the flexor digitorum superficialis muscle distally. Patients classically complain of numbness in the radial three and a half digits and occasional thenar weakness. Unlike carpal tunnel syndrome, nocturnal paraesthesiae and tingling are generally absent with paraesthesiae chiefly occurring with forearm muscle contraction. Patients can complain of pain in the volar aspect of the proximal forearm. Phalen's test is generally negative. The pronator compression test, involving compression applied at the junction of the pronator heads with resulting dysaesthesiae and tingling in the median nerve distribution, may support this diagnosis. Flexing the elbow with the forearm in supination while simultaneously applying resistance can indicate compression at the lacertus fibrosus. If paraesthesiae occur while resisting forearm pronation with full elbow extension, the pronator site is indicated. The occurrence of median nerve tingling while the examiner resists isolated proximal interphalangeal joint flexion of the middle finger can indicate entrapment of the median nerve below the arch of the flexor digitorum superficialis muscle. Electrodiagnostic testing is essential.

Conservative treatment is to modify forearm and wrist musculature activity, possible through the use of a volar neutral position wrist splint. Occasionally heat and massage, as well as non-steroidal anti-inflammatory medications, can improve the condition. Surgical release of the median nerve in the proximal forearm may be required. Of the four sites which should all be checked during surgery after the median nerve is identified, the lacertus fibrosus and arch of the flexor digitorum superficialis appear to be most commonly associated with visual compression of the median nerve.

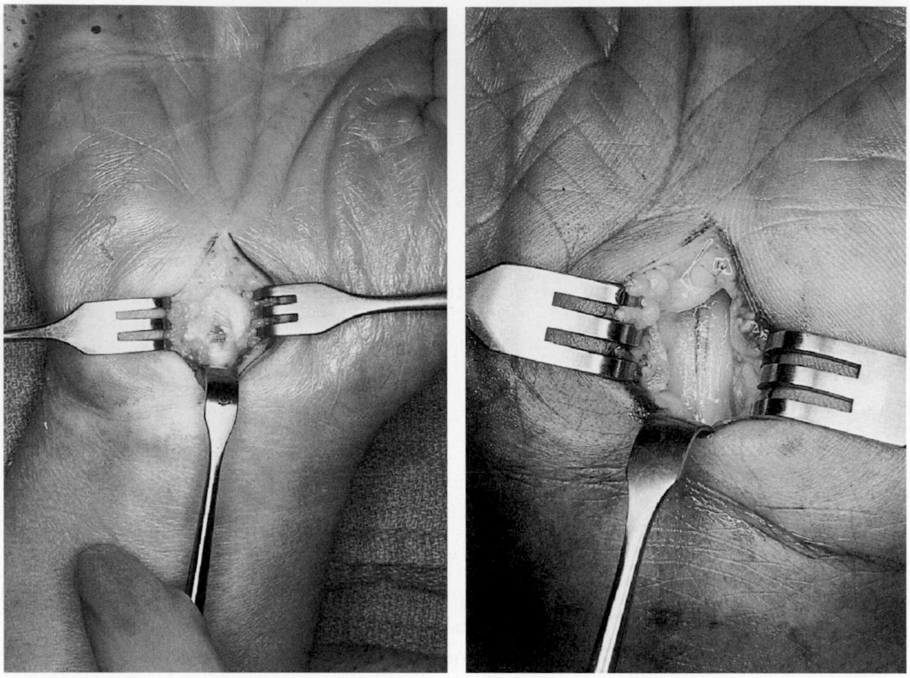

A B

Fig. 6.10.1 A) The palmar fascia has been divided through a 2.5-cm longitudinal incision at the proximal palm, allowing visualization of the transverse carpal ligament. Note a small amount of muscle tissue (the palmaris brevis) residing on top of the transverse carpal ligament. B) After transection of the transverse carpal ligament, excellent epineural blood flow returns to the median nerve.

The large blood vessels immediately adjacent to the median nerve should be protected during surgery (Figure 6.10.2). If a patient has had a previous carpal tunnel release without symptom relief, pronator syndrome should be considered but is still rare.

Anterior interosseous nerve syndrome (Box 6.10.5)

Isolated compression of the anterior interosseous nerve branch of the median nerve occurs but, again, rarely. The condition results in loss of motor function without sensory loss, usually seen with the loss of the ability actively to flex the distal interphalangeal joint of the index finger and the interphalangeal joint of the thumb (loss of the OK or ring sign). Patients may also experience non-specific aching and discomfort in the volar proximal forearm. Occasionally, the pronator quadratus can be deemed weak by testing resisted pronation with the elbow fully flexed to reduce the effect of the proximal pronator teres.

Anterior interosseous nerve syndrome is generally treated conservatively for 3–6 months, since most patients will recover spontaneously. If patients present with pain in both forearms or with symptoms extending proximally in the limb, transient brachial neuritis or Parsonage–Turner syndrome should be considered. The indication for surgical release of the anterior interosseous nerve is the lack of active flexion return in the distal interphalangeal joint of the index finger and that of the thumb, but the timing of surgery is controversial and almost always can be avoided. On rare

Box 6.10.4 Pronator syndrome

- Rare
- Due to proximal median nerve compression
- *Must* exclude carpal tunnel syndrome
- Diagnosis requires neurophyusiology.

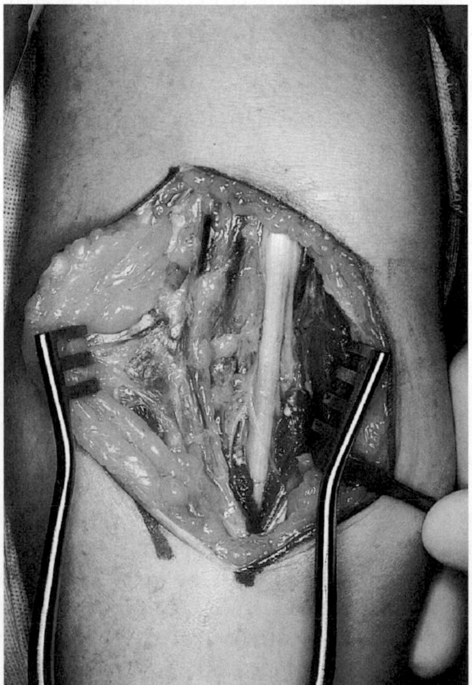

Fig. 6.10.2 After release of the lacertus fibrosus and pronator musculature, the relationship between the median nerve and adjacent vascular structures is easily seen.

Box 6.10.5 Anterior interosseous syndrome

- Uncommon
- Mostly viral
- Classically patients cannot make the 'O' sign
- Most patient recover spontaneously in approximately 6 months.

occasions, only one of the thumb or index finger is involved, generally indicating a more distal compression of the anterior interosseous nerve; one must be careful not to confuse this diagnosis with that of an isolated tendon rupture to either the flexor pollicis longus or the flexor digitorum profundus of the index finger especially in rheumatoid patients who can have isolated rupture of the flexor pollicis longus tendon. Flexion of the interphalangeal joint of the thumb when pressure is applied firmly to the flexor pollicis longus muscle belly in the forearm confirms that the tendon is intact.

Cubital tunnel syndrome (Box 6.10.6)

Cubital tunnel syndrome, or entrapment of the ulnar nerve at the medial elbow region, is the second most common peripheral nerve entrapment syndrome. The most common complaint is numbness and tingling in the little finger and ulnar half of the ring finger, commonly aggravated by repeated elbow flexion and extension, or by sleeping in a 'fetal position' with the elbows flexed. Weakness of the ulnar-innervated intrinsic muscles is a sign of severe or long-standing compression. Several other conditions may mimic cubital tunnel syndrome, though examination generally excludes cervical root entrapment, cervical rib or band, radiation plexopathy, and peripheral nerve tumours. If sensory symptoms involve the medial aspect of the forearm, the cause is probably proximal to the cubital tunnel.

Box 6.10.6 Ulnar nerve compression at the elbow

- Common (second only to carpal tunnel syndrome), almost always involves the little finger
- Typically presents later than carpal tunnel syndrome, i.e. with fixed neurological changes
- The diagnosis is often clear cut
- Examination:
  - Elbow—ROM, Tinel's sign, elbow flexion test
  - Hand—reduced sensibility especially little finger and dorsoulnar hand
  - Weakness of long (flexor carpi ulnaris < flexor digitorum profundus to RF(ring finger), LF(little finger)) and short (intrinsic) ulnar supplied muscles
  - Neurophysiology is generally requested
- Non-operative treatment: night splintage may work early
- Surgery: various techniques—the key is decompression
- Outcome: good but often incomplete recovery of fixed neurological changes.

Cubital tunnel syndrome can be distinguished from the much less common compression of the ulnar nerve at the wrist (Guyon's canal compression syndrome) by involvement of the dorsal sensory branch of the ulnar nerve, by weakness of the flexor digitorum profundus muscle of the small finger and flexor carpi ulnaris muscle, and by localization of Tinel's test to the cubital tunnel.

Conservative management includes a night elbow extension splint or, alternatively, wrapping a pillow with tape around the elbow in the fashion of a 'doughnut' to prevent elbow flexion during sleep. Steroid injection use at the cubital tunnel is best avoided due to a high incidence of fat necrosis, and non-steroidal anti-inflammatories are ineffective. Surgical decompression is indicated if conservative treatment fails or if muscle weakness or wasting is present.

The various operative procedures used for treatment of cubital tunnel syndrome all appear to provide 85–90 % improvement of symptoms. Surgical procedures include simple decompression of the cubital tunnel, decompression with partial medial epicondylectomy, and transposition of the ulnar nerve anteriorly. Simple decompression alone is generally indicated if Tinel's sign over the ulnar nerve at the elbow is localized to the cubital tunnel and the origin of the flexor carpi ulnaris. After simple decompression, the ulnar nerve must not sublux with elbow flexion and extension. If this does occur, partial medial epicondylectomy should be performed. Anterior transposition of the ulnar nerve is performed very variably depending upon surgeon preference. Indications include patients exhibiting significant involvement of the ulnar nerve with evidence of atrophy or weakness (Figure 6.10.3), especially in patients with fixed flexion deformities of the elbow. Since the nerve is being transposed anterior to the medial epicondyle, the medial intermuscular septum should be completely resected to avoid any 'tenting' of the ulnar nerve over this structure following transposition. The cubital tunnel release should be complete around the medial epicondyle, and the fascia, both deep and superficial overlying and within the flexor carpi ulnaris, needs to be completely released to prevent any further 'kinking' of the ulnar nerve distally. Transposition of the ulnar nerve can either be to the subcutaneous tissues above the fascia of the flexor pronator group, within the musculature of the flexor pronator group itself with the fascia repaired, or beneath the flexor pronator group with the origin repaired to the medial epicondyle. This is dictated by surgeon preference rather than scientific evidence.

Failure to achieve good results with these techniques may result from inadequate decompression, failure to ensure that the nerve is stable during elbow flexion/extension, or that it is free from compression in its new position.

Guyon's canal compression syndrome (Box 6.10.7)

Compression of the ulnar nerve at Guyon's canal (ulnar tunnel syndrome) is rare. Its numerous causes include space-occupying lesions (e.g., ganglion cysts), anomalous muscles, fractures of the hook of the hamate, thrombosis of the ulnar artery, repeated

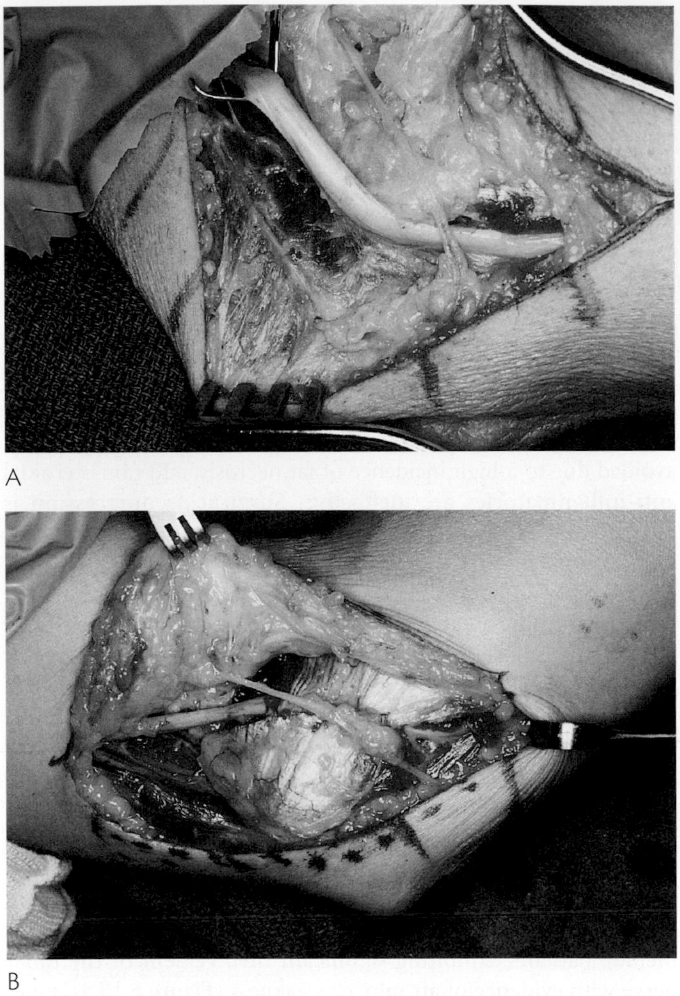

Fig. 6.10.3 A) During release of the ulnar nerve at the cubital tunnel prior to transposition, complete transection of the medial intermuscular septum and fascia of the flexor carpi ulnaris is required. Note the small branch of the medial antebrachiocutaneous nerve which should be preserved. B) After transposition of the ulnar nerve in an intermuscular fashion, superficial fascia is repaired forming an intermuscular tunnel.

trauma to the heel of the hand (hypothenar hammer syndrome), and long-distance cycling. Symptoms may be motor, sensory, or both, depending on the location of the compressive lesion relative to the ulnar nerve branches. It can be difficult to differentiate from more proximal compression, i.e. at the elbow. The signs of proximal compression as noted earlier should be looked for, as should local nerve irritability, i.e. a positive Tinel's sign over the ulnar nerve at the wrist.

Box 6.10.7 Ulnar nerve compression at the wrist

- Rare
- Often due to other local pathology
- Neurophysiology is essential
- Surgery should help.

The Allen test can often detect occlusion of the ulnar artery. Radiographic examination (e.g. computed tomography scanning) may identify a fracture of the hook of the hamate, while magnetic resonance imaging can define the nature and location of ganglia and other lesions.

Conservative management with rest and splintage is appropriate when compression arises from repeated local trauma or pressure. Since space-occupying lesions are so often the cause of compression within Guyon's canal, operative treatment is commonly needed. No matter the compression site, the ulnar nerve must be traced through the entire tunnel so as to ensure complete decompression, a process that generally yields good results.

Occasionally patients are seen who have carpal tunnel and Guyon's canal compression syndrome simultaneously. These patients can be treated by release of the carpal tunnel alone, since the procedure relaxes Guyon's canal. Alternatively, the vertical septa to Guyon's canal can be released through the same incision.

Radial tunnel syndrome (Box 6.10.8)

Entrapment of the posterior interosseous nerve produces two separate clinical pictures. In the first, a mass lesion around the neck of the radius may cause painless paralysis of the muscles supplied by the posterior interosseous nerve (see later). The second, termed radial tunnel syndrome, is a dynamic form of entrapment of the posterior interosseous nerve that cannot be unequivocally diagnosed following clinical and electrodiagnostic examinations.

Though a number of compressive sites have been described, the three most consistent are the fibrous edge of the extensor carpi radialis brevis muscle, the proximal edge of the supinator muscle (the arcade of Frohse), and the recurrent leash of radial vessels (the leash of Henry) that cross superficial to the posterior interosseous nerve (Figure 6.10.4). Patients complain of a deep-seated aching in the proximal forearm after strenuous muscle activity. Deep palpation where the posterior interosseous nerve enters the supinator muscle will produce marked tenderness, sometimes with radiation to the proximal forearm. Radial tunnel syndrome should be differentiated from lateral epicondylitis since these conditions can coexist. Pain with resisted wrist extension is generally directed towards the lateral epicondyle itself, and focal pain directly over the lateral epicondyle is typically indicative of lateral epicondylitis. Pain on resisted middle finger extension is occasionally seen in patients with radial tunnel syndrome. An injection of local anaesthetic that abolishes the pain and gives a temporary wrist drop provides further evidence to support the diagnosis. Electrodiagnostic studies,

Box 6.10.8 Radial tunnel syndrome/posterior interosseous nerve entrapment

- Rare
- Often overdiagnosed
- Signs and symptoms are often vague
- Local anaesthetic injection may help diagnosis
- Neurophysiology is often unhelpful
- Surgery is unreliable.

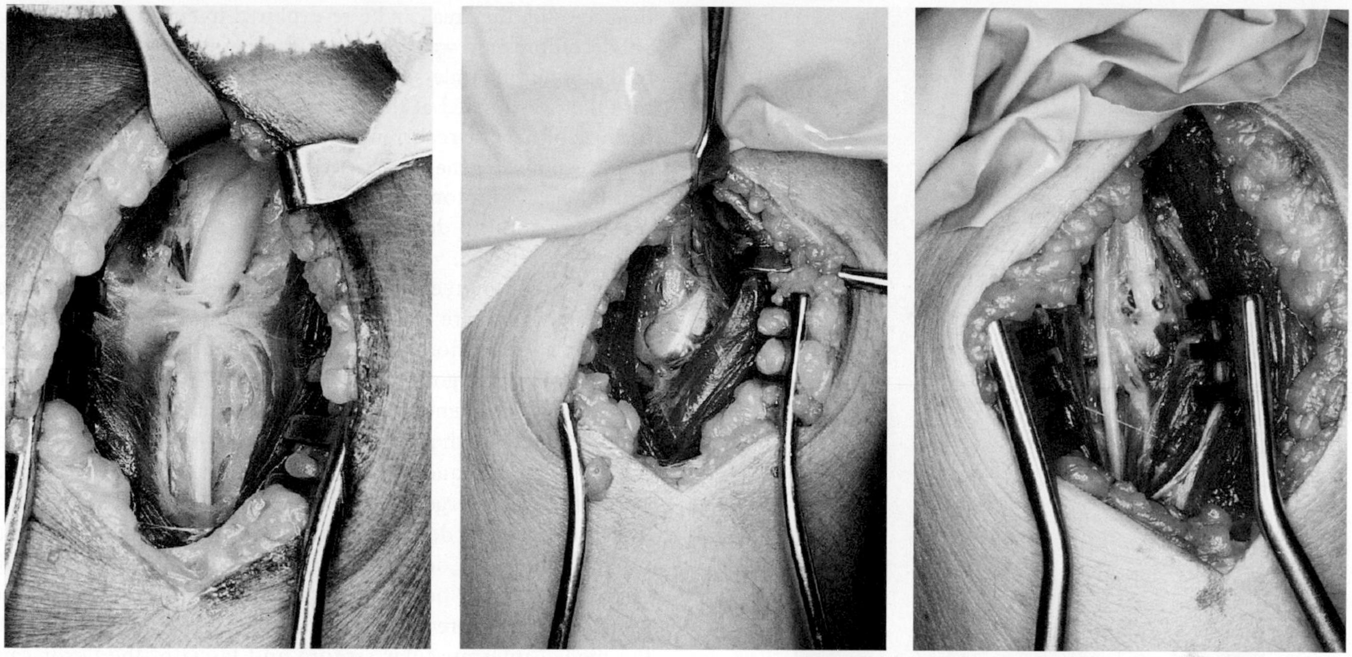

Fig. 6.10.4 A) Utilizing an exposure through the mobile wad of Henry musculature, the radial nerve is seen constricted by the recurrent radial artery (leash of Henry) vessels. B) Further distally, the posterior interosseous nerve dives underneath the arcade of Frohse. C) After complete release of the arcade of Frohse, the larger radial nerve is decompressed along with the smaller sensory branch of the radial nerve.

although extremely helpful if positive, are frequently normal in this dynamic compression syndrome.

Conservative management involves modification of upper-limb activity for 4–6 weeks and may be augmented by neutral wrist splinting. If conservative management fails, surgical decompression of the radial nerve, including the distal posterior interosseous nerve and sensory branch of the radial nerve, may be undertaken. Decompression should ensure release of the fascial tissues superficial to the radiocapitellar joint, coagulation and release of the recurrent radial artery known as the leash of Henry (ligating each vessel independently and sequentially), release of the fibrous edge of the extensor carpi radialis brevis, and, most importantly, release of the proximal edge of the supinator (the arcade of Frohse). In rare instances in which tenderness is also noted at the distal portion of the supinator preoperatively, release of the entire supinator or the distal edge may be required. Blunt finger probing along the radial nerve proximally and distally will exclude other areas of compression. The results of decompression of the radial tunnel have been quite variable. Coincidental undiagnosed lateral epicondylitis can lead to 'failure' of radial tunnel decompression so the lateral epicondyle should be addressed surgically if signs of lateral epicondylitis are present.

Posterior interosseous nerve palsy

Partial or complete loss of posterior interosseous nerve function may occur because of compression by a mass lesion within or at either end of the supinator muscle, most commonly caused by lipomas around the radial neck and rheumatoid synovial cysts. The diagnosis of a complete palsy is based on the loss of finger and thumb extension with weak and radial-directed extension of the wrist under the influence of extensor carpi radialis longus. Incomplete lesions, sometimes producing loss of extension of one or two digits, are easily confused with the much more common extensor tendon rupture. Operatively, the removal of the mass should be approached anterior to the proximal part of the supinator or posterior to the distal part.

Wartenberg's syndrome (Box 6.10.9)

Compression of the radial nerve sensory branch in the middle and distal forearm is very uncommon. The sensory branch of the radial nerve normally courses underneath the muscle belly of the brachioradialis and emerges from below its tendinous portion in the distal third of the forearm (Figure 6.10.5), where irritation, compression, or tethering may occur. Occasionally, a tingling or shocking sensation in the territory of the sensory branch can be provoked by forcefully pronating the forearm for up to 60s. The most useful sign is a positive Tinel's test directly over the sensory branch of the radial nerve as it enters under or exits from underneath the brachioradialis. Injection of a local anaesthetic can confirm

Box 6.10.9 Wartenberg's syndrome

- Uncommon
- Often clear from the clinical assessment
- Especially focal positive Tinel's sign
- Surgery usually helps.

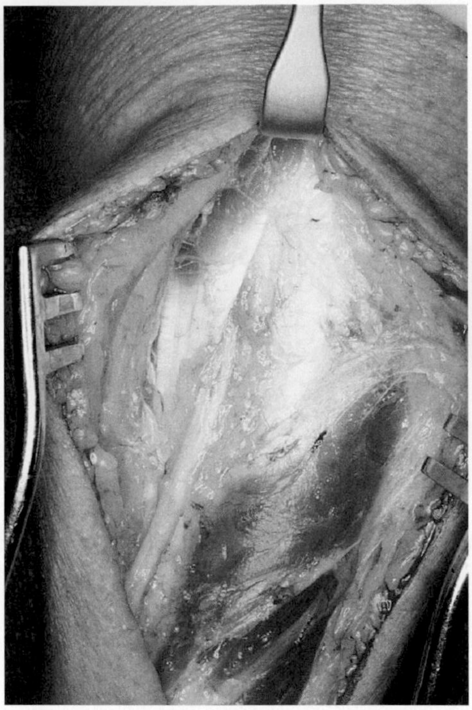

Fig. 6.10.5 In a patient with Wartenburg's syndrome, the sensory branch of the radial nerve exits underneath the edge of the brachioradialis tendon.

the diagnosis. This condition is found more proximal than de Quervain's stenosing tenovaginitis, which occurs at the radial styloid level.

Conservative management involves the use of a volar neutral position wrist splint to try to reduce inflammation. Surgical management generally involves release of any fascial and constricting fibres at the junction of the extensor carpi radialis longus and brachioradialis. Careful release of the sensory branch of the radial nerve through a 'no-touch' technique should be undertaken to ensure complete removal of compression. Occasionally, the edge of the brachioradialis pushes into the sensory branch of the radial nerve itself, requiring resection of half of the brachioradialis tendon to decompress the sensory branch of the radial nerve and provide a blunter edge with less overall constriction. Early mobilization is generally used in these patients to stop secondary adhesions. The results of surgery have been variable.

Recurrent peripheral nerve compression following failed decompression

On occasion, patients present with symptoms that have persisted or recurred after surgical decompression for three possible reasons: incorrect original diagnosis; incomplete previous decompression; or psychological concerns related to issues of compensation in the workplace. In this case, psychological factors as well as the peripheral nerves and musculoskeletal system (to exclude further causes of entrapment) must be examined. If these examinations are unsuccessful, the area can be re-explored to ensure that the original decompression was complete. The results of such surgery may be disappointing unless the surgeon is able to release a tight structure that was missed at the first operation. Symptoms may recur because of new or recurrent pathological changes in the areas of compression. In general, patients who have had a period of excellent relief of symptoms followed by recurrence fare better with a secondary surgical decompression than those whose symptoms were never relieved.

The two common examples of recurrent compression, although fortunately rare, are following carpal tunnel and cubital tunnel release. Patients who have undergone open carpal tunnel release will generally have good relief of symptoms but after several years can suffer a recurrence, especially if there are underlying pathological changes, such as amyloid deposition in chronic haemodialysis or diabetes. Frequently, these patients can be treated successfully by open revision surgery.

Failure following decompression of the ulnar nerve at the cubital tunnel region can occur after any procedure. Commonly, the release of the ulnar nerve was incomplete at the first operation or other structures were not dealt with adequately (most importantly the medial intermuscular septum and fascia of the flexor carpi ulnaris). Revision surgery is typically performed by transposing the ulnar nerve anteriorly.

Conclusion

Entrapment of the peripheral nerves is a common cause of symptoms in the upper extremity. Isolating the exact area of entrapment involves taking a careful history and a thorough physical examination to identify the nerve involved and to locate the site of compression. Conservative management can result in modest successes, especially if symptoms are of short duration and activities inciting the symptomatology can be curtailed for a period of time. Fortunately, surgical decompression also has met with a relatively high success rate if the diagnosis is accurate. Electrodiagnostic studies are an extremely helpful adjunct in establishing the diagnosis, but they can neither replace a careful history and physical examination nor make the diagnosis on their own. Isolated electrodiagnostic findings are not themselves an indication for surgery unless the diagnosis is supported by clinical evidence from the history and examination. With careful thought and planning, successful treatment of patients suffering from peripheral nerve entrapment is the rule rather than the exception.

Further reading

Barnum, M., Mastey, R.D., Weiss, A,P., and Akelman, E. (1996). Radial tunnel syndrome. *Hand Clinics*, 12(4), 679–89.

Bickel, K.D. (2010). Carpal tunnel syndrome. *Journal of Hand Surgery Am*, 35(1), 147–52.

Gellman, H. (2008). Compression of the ulnar nerve at the elbow: cubital tunnel syndrome. *Instr Course Lect*, 57, 187–97.

McCabe, S.J. (2010). Diagnosis of carpal tunnel syndrome. *Journal of Hand Surgery Am*, 35(4), 646–8.

Palmer, B.A. and Hughes, T.B. (2010). Cubital tunnel syndrome. *Journal of Hand Surgery Am*, 35(1), 153–63. Review.

6.11

Neurophysiological examination of the hand and wrist

Kerry R. Mills

Summary points

- Neurophysiological assessment includes:
  - Clinical assessment
  - Sensory testing
  - Motor testing
  - EMG
- Sensory testing (SAP) is generally the most useful
- Motor studies – there are 4 main measurements
- EMG – looks for (abnormal) spontaneous activity. It is operator dependent.

Introduction

The skilled manipulation of objects, often with both hands simultaneously, is a unique feature of human behaviour. This is achieved though complex neural circuits involving direct and indirect corticospinal connections, rich feedback networks from muscle, skin, and joint receptors, and multilevel integration in the cord, cerebellum, and cortex. Therefore it is not surprising that dysfunction of these networks, due to peripheral nerve lesions, leads to impairment of hand function and considerable disability.

The accurate diagnosis of conditions affecting the nerve supply to the hand is clearly important, and clinical neurophysiology is the discipline, par excellence, which can deliver this. Not only can nerve lesions be localized accurately, but it is also possible to assess the duration of the condition, the underlying pathology, and the prognosis.

Clinical neurophysiology begins by taking the history and examining the patient. Simple nerve lesions, such as carpal tunnel syndrome, may be the presenting feature of a more generalized disease, for example, diabetic neuropathy, thyroid disease, acromegaly, connective tissue disease, etc. The neurophysiological examination is planned to maximize the information that can be gained, but to minimize the number of shocks or needle insertions for the patient.

This chapter will describe the methods whereby neurophysiological investigations are conducted and the neurophysiological diagnosis and prognosis of lesions affecting the nerve supply of the hand. Normal values in nerve conduction studies depend critically on the precise technique used, including the type and positioning of electrodes and the temperature of the limb, and each laboratory will have its own normal ranges. For this reason, precise normal ranges are not quoted.

Methods (Box 6.11.1)

Nerve conduction studies involve exciting, usually percutaneously, a peripheral nerve by electrical stimulation and recording either from the same peripheral nerve at a distant site or from a muscle supplied by the nerve. The latency from the stimulus to the start of the response, the nerve conduction velocity, and the amplitude of the response are the most pertinent parameters to measure. Conduction measurements may be made from sensory, mixed motor and sensory, or from purely motor responses.

Conduction measurements depend on age (amplitudes become smaller and conduction velocities slower with age). Conduction parameters also depend on temperature. In routine practice, it is often not necessary to control temperature rigorously, but if the patient has cold hands and equivocal abnormalities are found, then the study should be repeated after warming the hands to above 32°C.

Box 6.11.1 Neurophysiological assessment

This includes:

- Clinical assessment
- Sensory testing (generally the more useful)
- Motor testing
- Electromyography (EMG).

Box 6.11.2 Sensory testing

- Stimulate the fingers and record proximally (SAP)
- SAP is dependent on:
  - Number of nerve fibres that are active
  - Synchrony with which individual action potentials arrive at the recording site.

Sensory studies (Box 6.11.2)

Ring electrodes placed around the fingers excite the digital branches of peripheral nerves which are, at this location, purely sensory. Recordings are made with surface electrodes from the skin overlying the relevant nerve. Because nerve responses are relatively small (in the microvolt range), electronic averaging may be required. The resulting nerve responses (Figure 6.11.1) are termed sensory action potentials (SAPs). The median SAP may be obtained by stimulating the thumb, index, middle, or ring fingers. The ring finger is usually split between median and ulnar innervation and hence the amplitude of response is smaller. The SAPs are usually obtained by stimulation of both digital nerves from each finger. They may also be obtained from stimulation of individual digital branches and even just recording in the finger but not the hand in order to localize any lesion. The radial sensory innervation of the hand and the dorsal branch of the ulnar nerve are tested by an antidromic technique.

The size of an SAP is principally dependent on two factors: the number of nerve fibres that are active and the synchrony with which individual action potentials arrive at the recording site. Thus patients with axonal degeneration-type peripheral neuropathies may have small or absent SAPs because of a reduced number of fibres; patients with demyelinating peripheral neuropathies may have small SAPs because of the dispersion of arrival times of action potentials at the recording electrodes.

In most nerve lesions likely to be encountered in the hand, sensory studies are more sensitive than motor studies.

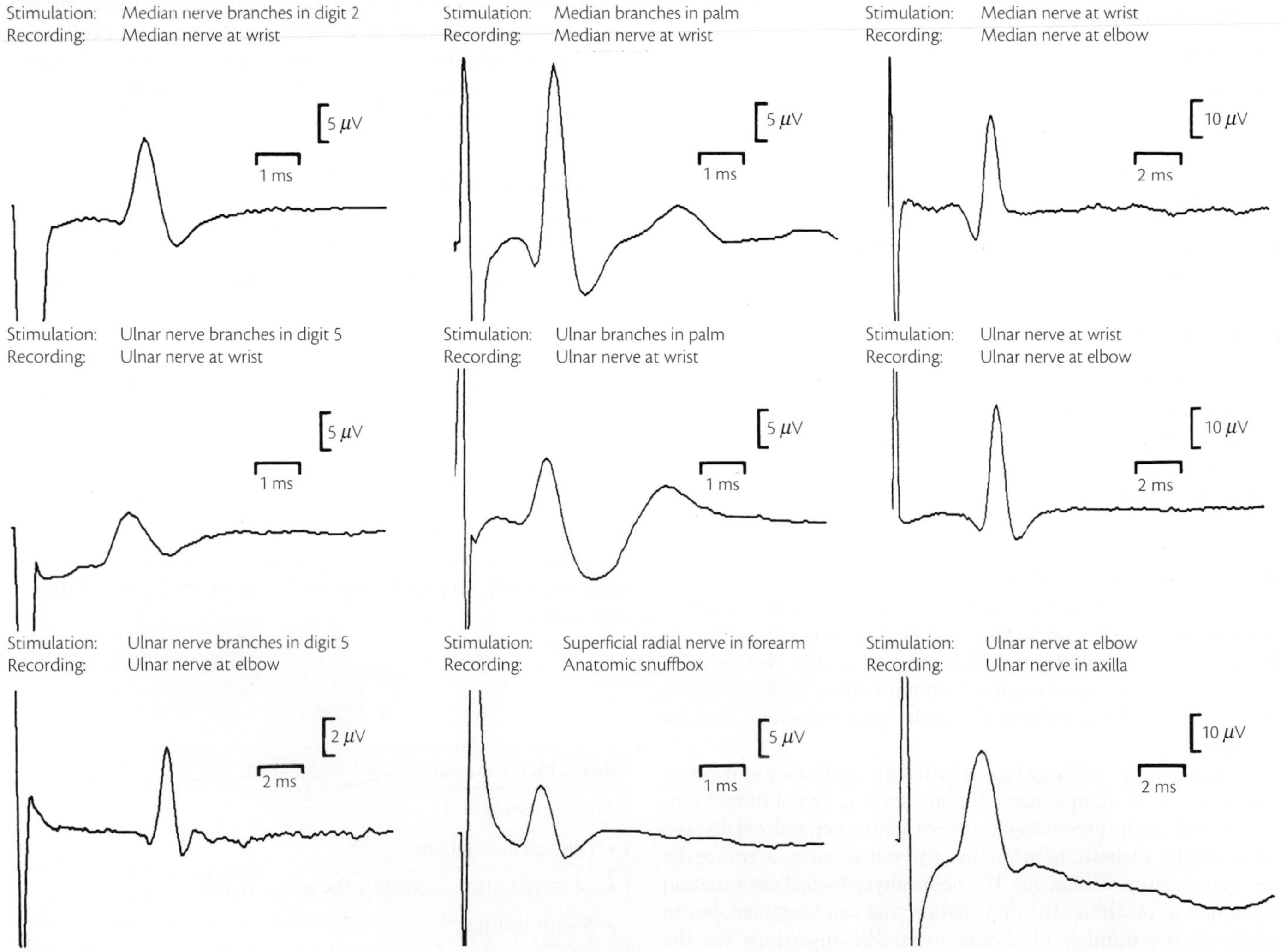

Fig. 6.11.1 Sensory action potentials (SAPs) and mixed-nerve action potentials (MNAPs) recorded over the median and ulnar nerves at various recording and stimulation points.

Mixed-nerve studies

When a mixed nerve, i.e. one containing both motor and sensory fibres, is stimulated, action potentials propagate in both directions in all nerve fibres. Measurements can be made both proximally and distally. This is useful in helping localize nerve lesions and is particularly valuable for assessment of the ulnar nerve.

Motor studies (Box 6.11.3)

In motor studies there are four main measurements: the latency from distal stimulation to the start of the muscle response (distal motor latency); the conduction velocity in motor nerve fibres; the amplitudes of compound muscle action potentials evoked by maximal nerve stimuli, taken to be roughly proportional to the volume of active tissue in the muscle; and the conduction in the proximal segments of each nerve. Surface electrodes are placed over the belly and tendon of the muscle of interest. For the median nerve, the abductor pollicis brevis (APB) muscle is used and for the ulnar nerve, either the abductor digiti minimi (ADM) or first dorsal interosseous (DIO) muscles. Electrical stimuli are applied to the relevant nerve at two or more locations and the latency of compound muscle action potentials is measured. By subtracting these latencies and measuring the distance between stimulation sites, the maximum conduction velocity can be calculated (Figure 6.11.2). It should be emphasized that this technique only assesses the fastest conducting (A) fibres in the nerve; these may be preserved in the face of quite severe motor nerve problems. The compound muscle action potentials (CMAPs) from proximal and distal stimulation sites are normally very similar in waveform and have amplitudes differing by no more than 20%. In the presence of conduction block (neurapraxia), the CMAP from a stimulation site proximal to the block is smaller than that obtained distal to the block (see Figure 6.11.3).

Late responses

When a motor nerve is stimulated, action potentials propagate in both directions: distally to the muscle where they evoke a CMAP, and proximally to the spinal motor neurons. Some motor neurons are re-excited by invasion of their soma and discharge again down the motor axons to produce responses in the muscle. These are termed F waves. Their importance lies in the fact that the latency of F waves assesses conduction over the whole length of the

Box 6.11.3 Motor studies

- The relevant nerve is stimulated and response measure with a surface electrode:
  - Median nerve—APB
  - Ulnar nerve—ADM or first DIO
- There are four main measurements:
  - The distal motor latency
  - The conduction velocity
  - The amplitudes
  - The conduction.

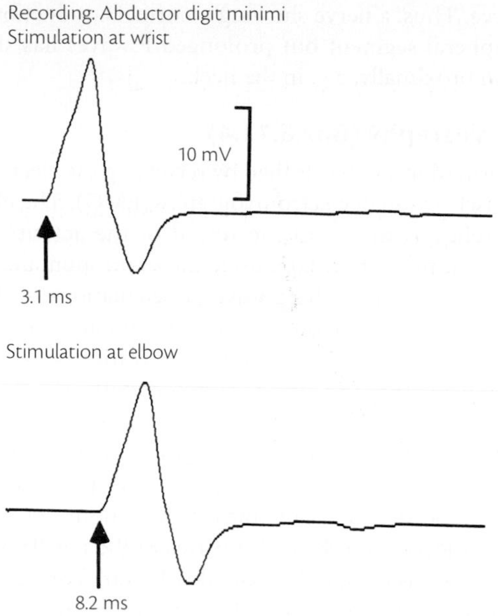

Fig. 6.11.2 Motor conduction velocity measurement. The ulnar nerve was maximally stimulated at the wrist and at the elbow. The latency of the response from the wrist was 3.1ms and from the elbow was 8.2ms. The difference between these two values (5.1ms) is the conduction time from elbow to wrist. The distance between the two stimulation sites was 270mm, giving a conduction velocity of 53m/s.

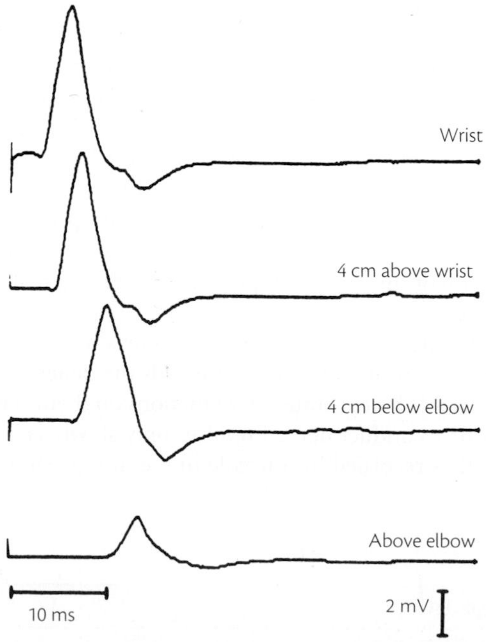

Fig. 6.11.3 Motor conduction study in a case of ulnar nerve entrapment at the elbow. Compound muscle action potentials (CMAPs) are recorded from the abductor digiti minimi muscle from supramaximal stimulation of the ulnar nerve at the sites indicated. There is a significant reduction in CMAP amplitude above the lesion indicating conduction block (neurapraxia). The conduction velocity from below elbow to wrist is 56m/s and across the elbow is 36m/s.

motor nerve. Thus, a nerve showing a normal conduction velocity in its peripheral segment but prolonged F waves has slowing of conduction proximally, e.g. in the neck.

Electromyography (Box 6.11.4)

Much information can be gleaned by recording the electrical activity in a muscle through electromyography (EMG). The electromyographer relies as much on the sound of the activity as on its appearance. At rest, a normal muscle shows no spontaneous activity. Fibrillations, positive sharp waves, fasciculations, and complex repetitive discharges may be encountered and are searched for in several muscle sites. During voluntary activation, muscle activity forms what is referred to as the recruitment pattern. The activity is recorded with a fine-needle electrode consisting of a concentric wire insulated from the shaft of the needle. Conventional concentric needle electrodes used in EMG record from a volume of muscle of radius of about 1mm. This means that about 200 individual muscle fibres are within the pick-up area of the needle. If all these fibres are active, as during a maximal voluntary contraction, then the signal recorded by the needle is complex. However, if the patient is requested to make a weak contraction then individual motor unit potentials can be discerned. These derive from a group of muscle fibres all innervated by the same spinal motor neuron and constitute part of a motor unit. The potential recorded is referred to as a motor unit potential. The waveforms, amplitudes, and firing frequencies of motor unit potentials give important clues to the pathogenesis of weakness (Figures 6.11.4A and 6.11.5).

Acute denervation of muscle is associated with spontaneous activity termed fibrillation, which is an electrical not a clinical sign. Traditionally this is described as sounding like rain on a tin roof. Fibrillations are potentials derived from single muscle fibres and are due to hyperexcitability of the muscle membrane. Acute denervation is associated with the proliferation of acetylcholine receptors on the muscle fibre membrane at sites outside the neuromuscular junction. Other forms of spontaneous activity having the same significance as fibrillations are positive sharp waves and complex repetitive discharges (Figure 6.11.4B). After an acute nerve lesion, fibrillations take 7–14 days to develop.

In complete nerve lesions, there is no possibility of reinnervation within the muscle and any recovery is by the process of nerve regeneration. This is a slow process and its success depends largely on the nature of the original injury and the distance of the lesion from the muscle.

In a partial nerve lesion, surviving motor axons in the muscle develop nerve sprouts which grow towards the denervated muscle fibres and establish neuromuscular junctions on them. These nerve sprouts at first conduct nerve impulses only slowly and so motor unit potentials recorded by a needle in the muscle show complex polyphasic waveforms of relatively low amplitude and may have satellite potentials. These potentials are sometimes referred to as 'nascent' and are a sign of early reinnervation (Figure 6.11.4C). As nerve sprouts mature, they conduct impulses faster and the satellite potentials now form part of the main motor unit potential. Thus, in chronic reinnervation, motor unit potentials are large in amplitude, and have relatively simple waveforms of longer than normal duration (Figures 6.11.4D and 6.11.6). The recruitment pattern in a chronically reinnervated muscle is incomplete due to the reduced numbers of motor units but the firing frequency of each motor unit is increased. This combination of reduced numbers of motor units with high amplitudes firing at high rates gives a characteristic sound on the EMG machine loud speaker which is easily recognized by the experienced electromyographer.

In muscle disease, a condition only infrequently encountered in hand muscles, motor unit potentials are small and spiky and the recruitment pattern is full (Figure 6.11.4E).

Box 6.11.4 EMG

- The electrode is placed in the muscle
- After acute denervation—fibrillations in 7–14 days
- Reinnervation—large motor unit potentials, and simple long waveforms.

Peripheral nerve lesions

Carpal tunnel syndrome

Sensory studies are usually more sensitive than motor studies. Diagnosis is achieved by demonstrating a slowing of conduction across the carpal tunnel. Orthodromic SAPs from the index finger to the median nerve at the wrist are compared with the ulnar SAPs from the little finger to the wrist (Figure 6.11.7). A median SAP peak latency more than 1.0ms greater than the ulnar value is taken as indicating significant median slowing. Occasionally, the middle finger is clinically more affected, and in this circumstance the SAP from the index finger may be normal but that from the middle finger delayed. Conduction velocity is calculated over the palm-to-wrist segment in the two nerves, and the ratio of ulnar to median conduction velocity is calculated; a ratio of greater than 1.25 indicates significant median slowing. Other protocols are in use but these are less reliable.

Motor studies measure the distal motor latency from the wrist to the abductor pollicis brevis muscle and the conduction velocity in the forearm segment. In moderate to severe cases of carpal tunnel syndrome, the distal motor latency is prolonged above the upper normal limit (Figure 6.11.8). Forearm conduction velocity is sometimes reduced in carpal tunnel syndrome, presumably due to retrograde demyelinating changes advancing proximally from the site of entrapment. If marked slowing of velocity is found, conduction velocity in another nerve should be measured in case there is a generalized demyelinating peripheral neuropathy.

EMG can occasionally be useful in carpal tunnel syndrome. It may document the degree of denervation, allowing prognostic statements to be made about the degree and speed of recovery. A weak abductor pollicis brevis that is not wasted, does not show acute denervation, and has a normal distal motor latency will recover to a greater extent and more quickly than a muscle that is wasted, shows active denervation, and has a prolonged latency.

A grading scale (Table 6.11.1) for the neurophysiological severity of carpal tunnel syndrome (from 0–6) has been developed and validated and may be useful as a guide to management. It has been shown that patients with very mild entrapment (grades 1–2) may respond better to steroid injection rather than surgery. Similarly, patients with very severe (grade 5) or extremely severe (grade 6)

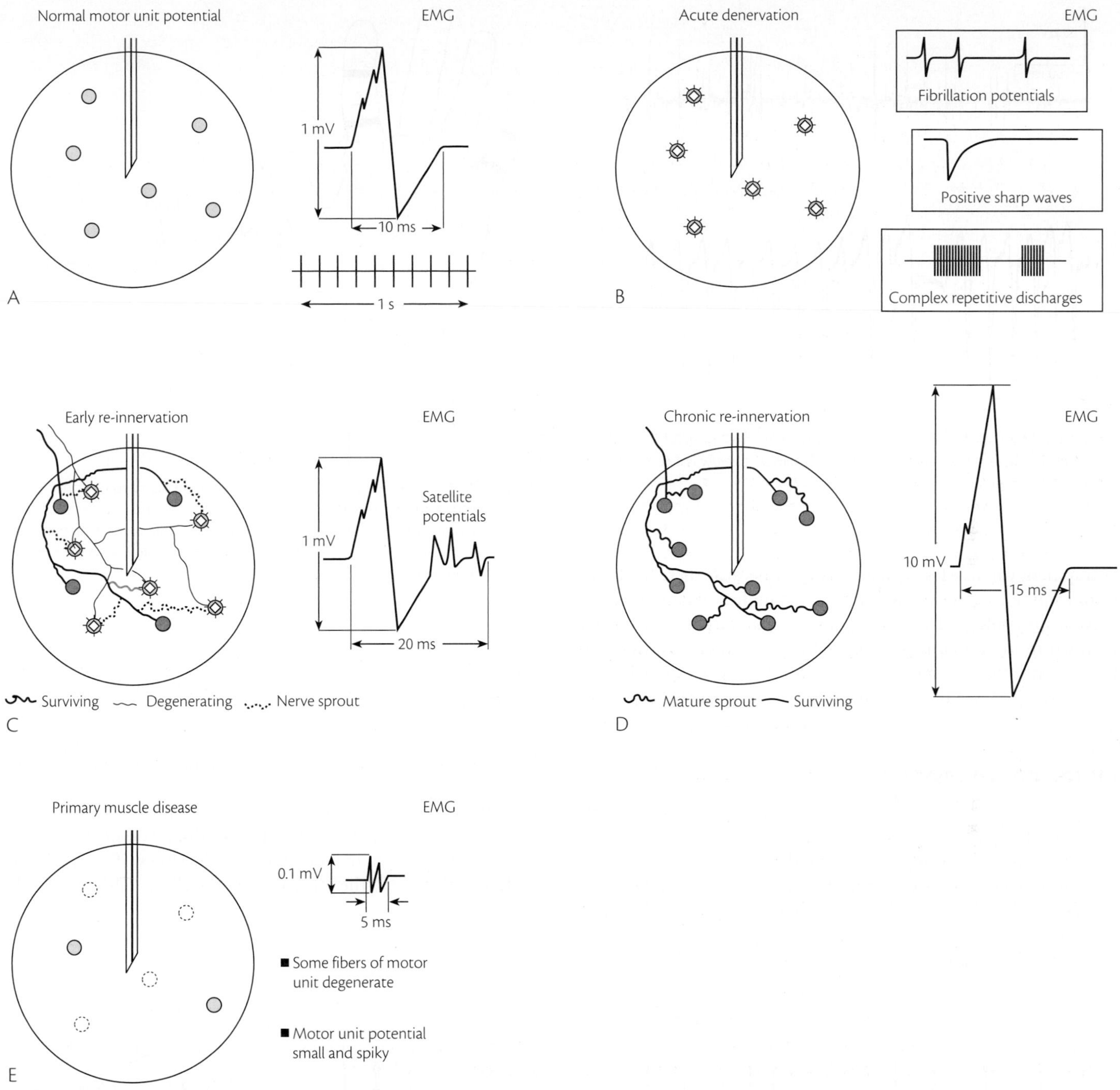

Fig. 6.11.4 A) The pick-up area of an electromyographic recording needle has a radius of about 1mm. Fibres belonging to one motor unit are indicated. The motor unit potential has an amplitude of about 1mV, a duration of about 10ms, and fires about 10 times per second when first recruited. B) In acute denervation, muscle fibres become supersensitive and produce spontaneous electrical activity in the form of fibrillations, positive sharp waves, or complex repetitive discharges. C) After a partial nerve lesion, degenerating axons (light line) are associated with fibrillating muscle fibres (open circles). Surviving axons (thick lines) are associated with normally functioning fibres (filled circles) produce nerve sprouts (dotted lines) to re-establish connection with the denervated fibres. The motor unit potential is complex, is of prolonged duration with satellite potentials, but is of normal amplitude. D) Nerve sprouts mature and the reinnervated fibres now assume the same fibre type as the parent fibres. The motor unit potential is now of long duration and high amplitude (say 10mV). E) In primary muscle disease, muscle fibres are lost and the motor unit potential is spiky in appearance and has a low amplitude (say 0.1mV).

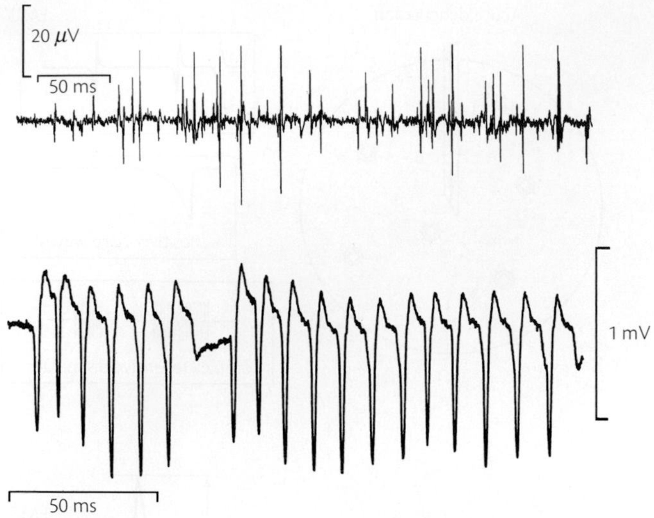

Fig. 6.11.5 Spontaneous activity recorded with an electromyographic needle in denervated muscle. Above are fibrillation potentials and below is a complex repetitive discharge.

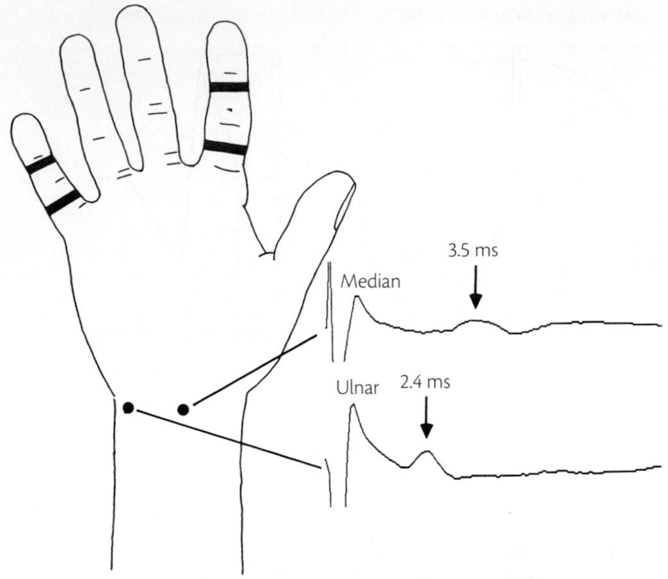

Fig. 6.11.7 Sensory action potentials recorded from median and ulnar nerves at the wrist from stimulation of the digital branches in index and little fingers, respectively, in a case of carpal tunnel syndrome. The median sensory action potential (peak latency 3.6ms) is significantly delayed compared with the ulnar sensory action potential (peak latency 2.4ms).

entrapment will fare less well after surgery because there has been a significant degree of axonal degeneration in the median nerve.

Neurophysiological assessment after 'failed' carpal tunnel release is much more difficult. It is best performed in comparison with preoperative measurements. Thus some clinicians, especially neurophysiologists, would recommend all patients have preoperative neurophysiology but this is not standard practice.

Ulnar nerve lesions

Symptoms in the hand may arise from ulnar nerve lesions in the palm, wrist, forearm, or cubital canal, and in general are more difficult to localize neurophysiologically than median lesions. By far the commonest site of entrapment is at or just proximal to the cubital canal at the elbow. Clinical examination is usually indicative: proximal lesions, i.e. at the elbow, may have weakness of the long ulnar supplied muscles, i.e. flexor carpi ulnaris and flexor digitorum profundus to the ring and little fingers and reduced sensation on the dorsum of the hand not present in lesions at the wrist or hand.

There are various steps in assessing ulnar nerve electrical function. The first is measurement of the ulnar SAP from the little finger to the wrist and a comparison with the median SAP from the index finger; a small or absent ulnar SAP confirms loss of sensory axon function but is no help in localization. The next measurement is the SAP from the little finger to the elbow; if this is absent, the lesion must be in the forearm or at the elbow. This may be the

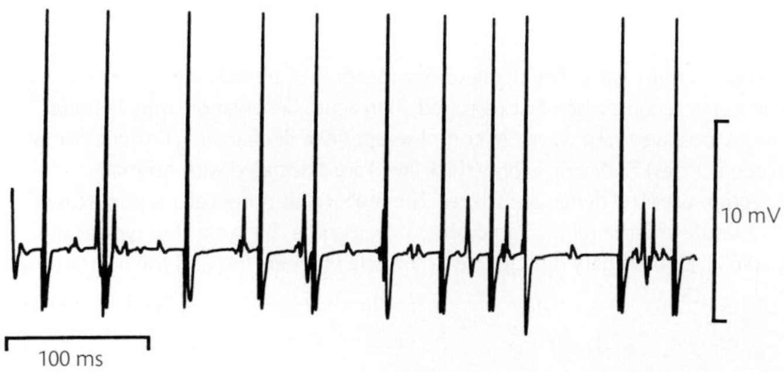

Fig. 6.11.6 Electromyogram recording from the first dorsal interosseous muscle from a patient with a severe ulnar nerve lesion. The patient is making a maximal voluntary abduction movement of the index finger. The electromyogram recruitment pattern is severely reduced, there being only a few motor units under voluntary control. The surviving motor units are of high amplitude and fire at high rates.

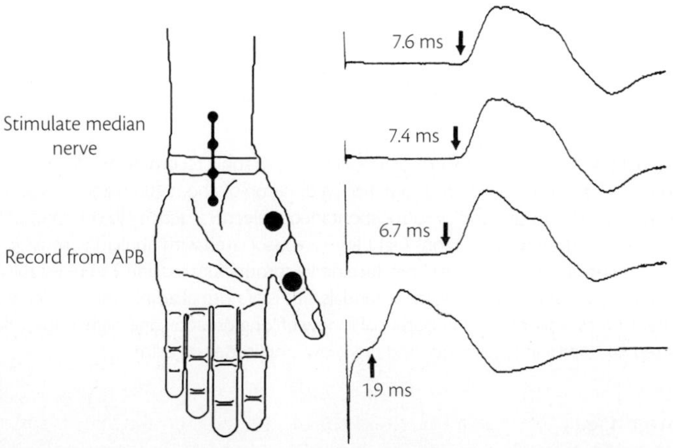

Fig. 6.11.8 Motor study in the carpal tunnel syndrome. The median nerve is stimulated at progressive steps across the wrist. Compound muscle action potentials recorded from the abductor pollicis brevis muscle (APB) have progressively shorter latencies but there is a discrete jump in latency as the site of slowing is crossed.

Table 6.11.1 Neurophysiological grading of carpal tunnel syndrome

Grade 0	Normal findings	No neurophysiological abnormality
Grade 1	Very mild	Two sensitive tests positive (e.g. ring-finger double peak, palm–wrist median/ulnar comparison)
Grade 2	Mild	Median sensory conduction velocity <40m/s Distal motor latency (APB) <4.5ms
Grade 3	Moderate	Median SAP present Distal motor latency >4.5ms
Grade 4	Severe	Median SAP absent Distal motor latency 4.5–6.5ms
Grade 5	Very severe	Distal motor latency >6.5ms
Grade 6	Extremely severe	CMAP (APB) <0.2mV

only neurophysiological abnormality in mild ulnar nerve lesions. The third comparison is of mixed-nerve action potentials by stimulating the ulnar and median nerves at the wrist and recording at the elbow. An absent ulnar mixed-nerve action potential with a preserved median mixed-nerve action potential from wrist to elbow again implies loss of fibres. The fourth step required for localization are mixed-nerve studies obtained by stimulating the ulnar nerve at the elbow and recording in the axilla. The ulnar elbow-to-axilla mixed-nerve action potential is normally at least twice the size of the ulnar potential from wrist to elbow, but in ulnar nerve lesions at the elbow, the mixed-nerve action potential from wrist to elbow will be small in comparison with the elbow-to-axilla potential, which will be normal.

Conduction block in motor fibres is an important feature to search for. It may explain weakness of hand muscles in the absence of wasting. Motor conduction is measured by recording from the abductor digiti minimi muscle whilst stimulating the ulnar nerve at various sites: the wrist; below the elbow; above the elbow, and in the axilla (see Figure 6.11.3). In young individuals, the CMAP obtained by stimulating the nerve at various sites is almost identical in amplitude. In older people (> 45 years), the CMAP amplitude from more proximal sites may be slightly smaller, but never less than 80%. If, in the absence of significant slowing of conduction, the CMAP drops between two stimulation sites by more than 50% then conduction block can be confidently diagnosed. This technique also allows conduction velocity to be measured in the various nerve segments; in ulnar nerve lesions the velocity often drops by more than 20m/s across the elbow. The abnormality may be accentuated by placing the arm in full flexion and repeating the study. Because of the difficulty of accurately measuring distance in the short segment across the elbow, a fall in velocity of less than 10m/s should be regarded as of doubtful significance.

Lesions of the deep palmar branch of the ulnar nerve (Figure 6.11.9A) are demonstrated by showing that the latency to the first dorsal interosseous muscle from ulnar stimulation at the wrist is prolonged but that to the abductor digiti minimi muscle is within normal limits The normal maximal latency difference between the two muscles is 4.0ms; differences greater than this suggest a lesion of the deep palmar branch, especially if there are also electromyographic signs of acute denervation in first dorsal interosseous muscle but not in the abductor digiti minimi muscle.

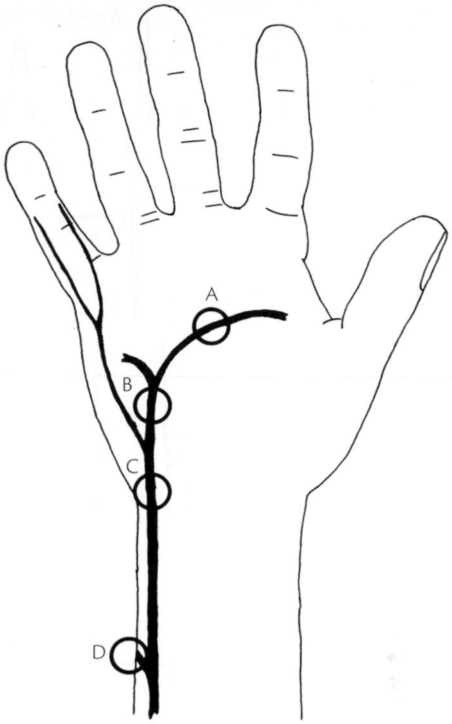

Fig. 6.11.9 Sites of ulnar nerve lesions in the palm and wrist: A) the deep palmar branch; B) in the palm distal to the origin of the sensory branch; C) in the wrist, proximal to the origin of the sensory branch; D) an isolated lesion of the dorsal branch.

Lesions of the dorsal branch of the ulnar nerve are also occasionally encountered (Figure 6.11.9D). These are usually produced by pressure from, for example, handcuffs around the wrist. In this case, the sensory potential from the fifth digit to the wrist is normal, but the SAP in the dorsal sensory branch is absent. It is essential in these cases to compare the SAPs from the two sides.

Rarer lesions of the ulnar nerve at the wrist include ulnar nerve entrapment as it passes into the hand through Guyon's canal at the base of the pisiform bone. In some cases, the lesion is distal in the palm in which case there will be denervation of abductor digiti minimi and first dorsal interosseous muscles but the ulnar SAP is normal (Figure 6.11.9B). Less frequently, the ulnar SAP is absent and there is denervation of the abductor digiti minimi muscle indicating a lesion proximal to the origin of the sensory branch in to the fourth and fifth digits (Figure 6.11.9C).

The differential diagnosis of ulnar and median nerve lesions always includes cervical radiculopathy, and differentiation of this common condition is vital to prevent unnecessary operations being undertaken. The crux of the issue is to demonstrate denervation in muscles not supplied by the nerve in question. Thus, in the differentiation of ulnar nerve lesions from C8–T1 radicular lesions, it is essential to show that ulnar nerve conduction is within normal limits, and that there is denervation in median supplied muscles that derive their nerve supply from the C8 and T1 roots.

A cervical rib or fibrous band compressing the lower cervical roots can also simulate median nerve lesions. There is often thenar atrophy. In this situation, the median SAPs from the index and middle fingers are normal but the potential from the fifth finger to the ulnar nerve is small or absent, due to degeneration of sensory

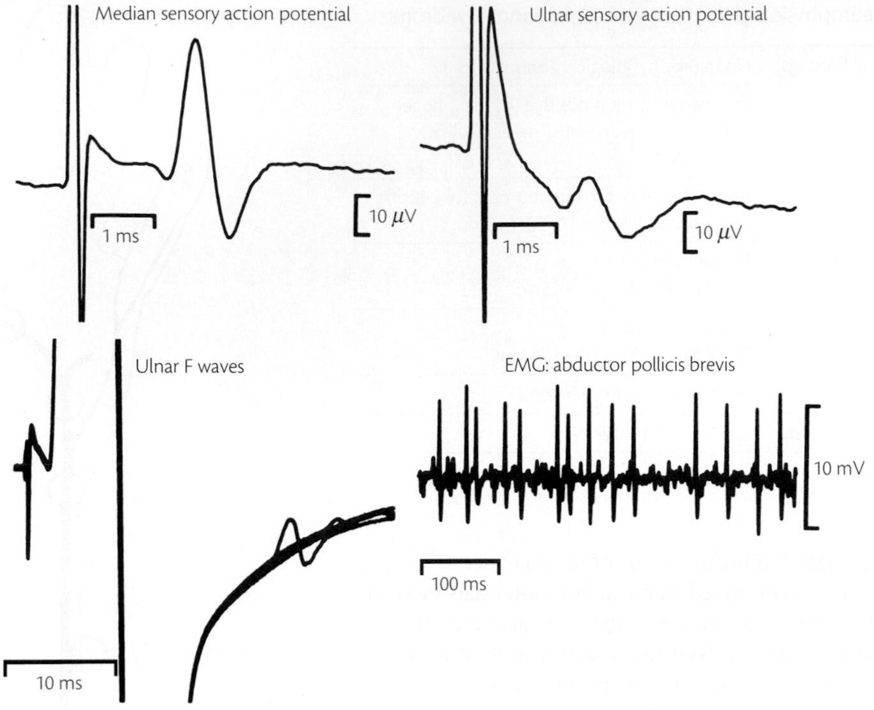

Fig. 6.11.10 Neurophysiological findings in a case of cervical rib syndrome. The ulnar sensory action potential is small, in comparison with the median sensory action potentials. The ulnar F waves are infrequent but are of normal latency, and there are chronic denervation and reinnervation changes in the abductor pollicis brevis.

fibres in the T1 root. The distal motor latency to abductor pollicis brevis is normal but electromyography will show it to be partially denervated (Figure 6.11.10). The F-wave latencies in the ulnar or median nerves may occasionally be helpful in demonstrating proximal slowing in the ulnar nerve fibres.

Other conditions that can simulate ulnar or median nerve entrapments and in which neurophysiology is useful in differentiation include generalized peripheral neuropathies, conditions causing mononeuropathy multiplex (polyarteritis nodosa, Churg–Strauss syndrome, systemic sclerosis, diabetes mellitus, rheumatoid arthritis, amyloidosis), amyotrophic lateral sclerosis, and spinal muscular atrophy, which often present as painless wasting of hand muscles, neuralgic amyotrophy which can cause focal muscle weakness, brachial plexus lesions (radiation plexopathy or neoplastic infiltration of the plexus), dystrophia myotonica in which EMG reveals characteristic myotonic discharges, and intrinsic cord lesions, especially syringomyelia. In this last case, because the lesion is central to the dorsal root ganglion cells, the SAPs from the fingers are preserved.

Radial nerve lesions

Lesions of the radial nerve are less common. In a complete radial palsy there will be wrist and finger drop and sensory disturbance over the dorsum of the hand. They may be traumatic, commonly due to fractures in the midshaft of the humerus or due to prolonged pressure as in 'Saturday night palsy'. EMG in these cases can be useful prognostically in differentiating between axonal loss where recovery is likely to be slow and incomplete, from conduction block (neurapraxia) where the prospects for complete recovery are much better. If, some 2–3 weeks after the injury, there are no signs of denervation in the paralysed muscles, there is a good chance of recovery. On the other hand, if the finger and wrist extensor muscles show marked acute denervation then a favourable prognosis is less certain, especially if there are no motor units in the muscle that can be activated by volition. These changes also apply in assessing other nerve injuries following open wounds both following injury and surgery. Thus there is little role for neurophysiology acutely but after 2–3 weeks denervation changes may indicate a poor prognosis.

The superficial branch of the radial nerve in the forearm may be externally compressed and gives rise to sensory loss and/or dysaesthesiae in the 'anatomic snuffbox'. Comparison of the radial SAPs from the two sides is useful in demonstrating this lesion.

Rarely, the posterior interosseous branch of the radial nerve may be entrapped as it enters the forearm. Clinically there may be pain in the elbow and forearm, and weakness of the wrist and finger extensors. Nerve conduction studies are usually unhelpful because it is difficult, even with needle electrodes, to stimulate selectively the deeply sited posterior interosseous nerve. However, EMG can be useful in demonstrating denervation in finger and wrist extensor muscles, but normality of the brachioradialis, the branch to which arises from the radial trunk before it enters the forearm.

Further reading

Bland, J.D.P. (2000). A neurophysiological grading scale for carpal tunnel syndrome. *Muscle and Nerve*, **23**, 1280-3.

Kimura, J. (1979). The carpal tunnel syndrome: localisation of conduction abnormalities within the distal segment of the median nerve. *Brain*, **102**, 619–35.

Liveson, J. and Ma, D. (1992). Laboratory reference for clinical neurophysiology. Philadelphia, PA: F.A.Davis.

Payan, J. (1969). Electrophysiological localization of ulnar nerve lesions. *Journal of Neurology, Neurosurgery and Psychiatry*, **32**, 208–20.

6.12

Tumours and hand reconstruction

D. Glynn Bolitho

Summary points

- Hand tumours are common
- The vast majority are benign
- Soft tissue – commonest Giant cell tumour of tendon sheath. Treatment marginal excision
- Bone – commonest – Enchondroma. Treatment – leave if incidental or currette +/− bone grafting
- Malignant – need full work up with detailed clinical examination, investigation, and planning in a multidisciplinary meeting
- Treatment is wide/radical excision often with partial amputation +/− plastic surgical reconstruction.

Introduction

A multidisciplinary approach which employs improvements in diagnosis, staging, adjuvant therapy, surgical resection, and particularly reconstruction has made limb salvage a viable option in the treatment of most upper-extremity malignancies. The adequacy of surgical resection should be paramount. However, reconstructive considerations should be contemplated during the phase of preoperative planning in order that the best possible functional and aesthetic outcome is achieved. Emphasis should be placed on a thorough evaluation by all members of the treatment team prior to the initiation of treatment. A broad range of techniques are available for both salvage and restoration of function.

In principle, the management of tumours of the bone and soft tissues in the hand and wrist differ little from those encountered elsewhere, except that vital neurovascular structures are more commonly juxtaposed and there is an inherent desire to preserve upper-extremity function. Certain tumours occur more frequently, e.g. ganglion cysts, epidermoid inclusion cysts, and giant cell tumours of the tendon sheath. Conversely, tumours common in other locations present rarely, e.g. metastatic carcinoma, lymphoma, and myeloma. The following guidelines may prove useful in the approach to the patient presenting with a mass in the hand:

- The majority of primary bone tumours of the hand are benign, but large deeply placed tumours in the soft tissues are frequently malignant
- The most common bone tumours in the hand are enchondromas and osteochondromas, except in the terminal phalanx where the most prevalent lesion is the epidermoid inclusion cyst
- The third most common site for giant cell tumours is the distal radius.

The approach to tumours of the hand and wrist incorporates the following principles:

- Clinical examination and investigations aimed at diagnosing and staging the tumour
- Biopsy
- Surgical resection
- Adjuvant treatment
- Reconstruction.

Principles of management (Box 6.12.1)

A multidisciplinary approach to management is mandatory for malignant tumours and some, typically larger, benign tumours. The initial goals of management include diagnosis and staging of

Box 6.12.1 Principles of management

The key steps are:

- Diagnosis:
  - Rarely from clinical examination or imaging
  - Tissue is required—incisional or excisional biopsy
- Staging: mainly through imaging, especially MRI
- Treatment:
  - Excision
  - Adjuvant therapy
  - Reconstruction
  - Always with an oncology team for malignancies.

the tumour prior to biopsy. The biopsy should be planned with the reconstruction in mind.

Patients presenting with a bony mass may be investigated by means of plain radiographs, computed tomography (CT), and magnetic resonance imaging (MRI). The usual criteria for the radiographic analysis of bone tumours include size, shape, location, gross architectural alterations, disturbance of the bony cortex, and the radiological appearance of the matrices of these tumours.

Staging of tumours of the hand and carpus involving bone or soft tissue

Most tumour surgeons employ the modified Enneking staging system for malignant neoplasms of bone (Table 6.12.1). This is generally also used for staging soft tissue tumours. This staging scheme depends on three primary determinants: the grade of the tumour (G), the anatomical location of the lesion (T), and the presence or absence of distant metastases (M). Benign tumours are usually designated G0, with low-grade malignant lesions classified as G1 and high-grade malignant lesions as G2.

The anatomical location is assessed by imaging studies including CT and MRI. The essential definition is whether there is preservation (T1) or violation (T2) of the involved compartment. For bony tumours, the involved bone fulfils the definition of a compartment, such that extraosseous extension is considered a T2 lesion. Soft tissue tumours that extend beyond the fascial compartment or involve the neurovascular bundle are considered to be T2 tumours.

For giant cell tumours of bone and chondrosarcoma, Campanacci (1976) has devised a grading system (Table 6.12.2). Giant cell tumours are graded into three radiographic types (calm, active, aggressive) and three histological types (typical, aggressive, sarcoma). Chondrosarcomas are also graded into three radiographic and three histological types (grades I, II, III). Cutaneous malignancies such as melanoma have their own unique staging scheme.

The American Joint Cancer Committee Staging System is usually employed in staging melanoma. This system is based primarily on tumour thickness and the presence of lymphatic metastasis. Tumour thickness and ulceration are the major determinants of prognosis. Subungual melanoma represents a specific clinical entity comprising 1–3% of all presenting melanomas. In these patients, tumour thickness is often difficult to determine due to fixation and biopsy techniques.

Staging workup

The approach to patients presenting with either bone or soft tissue tumours includes assessment of the grade of the tumour and the anatomical extent of the lesion, and determination of metastatic spread. The tumour is graded on the histopathology including special stains and even electron micrography. A working clinical diagnosis can usually be formulated on the basis of the physical examination, plain radiographs, and blood tests. This should enable the clinician to distinguish between benign tumours, primary malignant tumours, metastatic tumours, and lymphomatous deposits.

If the lesion is thought to be benign, an excisional biopsy without further workup is appropriate. Frozen section should be employed intraoperatively if there is any doubt. If the lesion is thought to be a primary malignant tumour, further imaging studies (CT or MRI) should be performed to stage the tumour accurately. MRI of the hand and wrist is accurate in the detection of mass lesions and can distinguish benign from malignant tumours in the most cases. In the case of suspected metastatic tumour, appropriate imaging of the probable primary source should be ordered. The focus of this search may be appropriately guided by the results of the biopsy.

Table 6.12.1 Enneking staging system for bone and soft tissue tumors

Stage	Grade (G)	Anatomic location (T)	Metastasis (M)
0	Benign(G0)	Any (T1 or T2)	None (M0)
IA	Low (G1)	Intracompartmental (T1)	None (M0)
IB	Low (G1)	Extracompartmental (T2)	None (M0)
IIA	High (G2)	Intracompartmental (T1)	None (M0)
IIB	High (G2)	Extracompartmental (T2)	None (M0)
III	Any grade	Any (T1 or T2)	Metastasis (MI)

Reproduced from Wolf and Enneking (1996).

Table 6.12.2 Grading of bone and soft-tissue tumors of the hand

Benign (GO)	Low-grade sarcomas (G1)	High-grade sarcomas (G2)
Bone		
Enchondroma	Giant cell tumor	Osteosarcoma
Osteochondroma	Desmoplastic fibroma	Ewing's sarcoma
Fibrous dysplasia	Chondrosarcoma	Lymphoma
Osteoid osteoma	Parosteal osteosarcoma	Chondrosarcoma
Bone cysts	Angiosarcoma	Hemangioma
Myeloma	Osteoblastoma	
Soft tissue		
Ganglion	Desmoid	Synovioma
Lipoma	Liposarcoma (LG)	Malignant fibrous histiocytoma
Neurolemmoma	Fibrosarcoma (LG)	Liposarcoma (HG)
Chondromatosis	Kaposi's sarcoma	Rhabdomyosarcoma
Glomus tumor	Epitheloid sarcoma	Malignant schwannoma
Giant cell tumor	Clear cell tumor	Hemangiopericytoma
	Angiosarcoma	

Reproduced from Mankin (1987).

Tumour resection (Box 6.12.2)

As a rule, neoplasms of the connective tissues spread locally by invasion of the adjacent vascular and connective tissues rather than by invasion of lymphatics. The adjacent normal tissues become compressed and may demonstrate a fibroproliferative response. This compressed fibroproliferative layer is known as the 'reactive zone'. Histological analysis of the reactive zone will frequently demonstrate microscopic tumour invasion. Discrete nodular metastases formed within the same compartment are known as skip lesions. These are more frequent with high-grade neoplasms such as osteosarcoma. Several studies have demonstrated the correlation of survival and local recurrence with the adequacy of

Box 6.12.2 Excision

- Intralesional: e.g. enchondroma
- Marginal: e.g. giant cell tumour of the tendon sheath
- Wide: e.g. ray amputation for subungual melanoma
- Radical: for the hand this would be and above-elbow amputation

local control. Based on the proximity of the surgical margin to the tumour and the pattern of tumour spread within the compartment, Wolf and Enneking have devised four types of surgical procedure:

- *Intralesional*: an amputation which exposes the primary lesion and thus leaves macroscopic disease. An example is the treatment of enchondroma by curettage
- *Marginal*: the surgical plane is in the reactive zone and there is a possibility of residual microscopic tumour or tumour satellite lesions. An example is the excision of a giant cell tumour of the tendon sheath
- *Wide*: a significant cuff of normal tissue is left surrounding the tumour, but not all the contents of the compartment are resected. The width of the margin should counter the possibility of local satellite lesions but a skip lesion may be left behind. A ray amputation falls into this category
- *Radical*: the entire compartment containing the tumour is excised en bloc. In theory, this entirely eliminates all local forms of recurrence, but is most costly in terms of loss of limb function. For tumours in the hand and wrist, this would constitute an above-elbow amputation.

There are no set guidelines for deciding when each of these four procedures should be applied. Table 6.12.3 gives a reasonable approach based on the tumour grade.

Factors that may affect this decision include the age and wishes of the patient, functional demands on the limb, and adjunctive chemotherapy or irradiation. At operation, it is vitally important to limit the dissection, and to observe meticulous haemostasis, to limit potential seeding of tumour cells. The biopsy and subcutaneous tract should be included in the specimen. A bone weakened by resection requires protection or definitive reconstruction. If the reconstructive procedure requires the harvest of autogenous tissue, the two surgical sites should be kept separated until such time as the specimen has been removed.

Finally, the entire ablative procedure should be performed only after careful planning and preoperative consultation with the oncologist and the pathologist. Only after an oncologically sound plan has been formulated should consideration be given to the restoration of limb function and form.

Table 6.12.3 Selection of appropriate surgical procedure

Stage	Procedure
0	Intralesional or marginal
IA	Marginal or wide
IB	Marginal or wide
IIA	Wide or radical
IIB	Wide or radical
III	Wide, or as necessary for local control

Reproduced from Mankin (1987).

Table 6.12.4 Primary bone tumors of the hand and wrist

	Total	Hand	Carpus
Netherlands Bone Tumour Registry (Sissons 1971)			
Benign	420	53 (12.6%)	3 (0.7%)
Malignant	626	8 (1.2%)	0
Total	1046	61 (6.1%)	3 (0.2%)
Mayo Clinic (Beard *et al.* 1988)			
Benign	1362	73 (5.3%)	5 (0.37%)
Malignant	2915	13 (0.44%)	1 (0.03%)
Total	4277	86 (2%)	6 (0.14%)

Reproduced from Feldman (1987).

Primary bone tumours of the hand and carpus

Primary bone tumours of the hand and wrist are uncommon. Of 1046 primary bone tumours in the Netherlands Bone Registry, only 64 (5.8%) occurred in the hand and 3 (0.2%) in the wrist (Table 6.12.4). Of the 420 benign lesions, 53 (12.6%) were in the hand and 3 (0.7%) were in the wrist. No malignancies involved the carpus, whilst eight (1.2%) were in the hand.

The classification of tumours is given in Table 6.12.5.

Adjuvant therapy (Box 6.12.3)

Postoperative adjuvant radiation therapy is usually employed in the management of malignant tumours when the surgical margin is narrow or for high-grade malignancy. Adjuvant radiation therapy

Table 6.12.5 Classification of bone tumors

Chondrogenic lesions
Chondroma
Enchondroma
Osteochondroma
Chondroblastoma
Chondromyxoid fibroma
Osteogenic lesions
Osteoid osteoma
Benign osteoblastoma
Osteosarcoma
Tumors of uncertain etiology
Giant cell reparative granuloma
Fibrosarcoma
Ewing's sarcoma

Box 6.12.3 Adjuvant therapy

- Radiotherapy is used but can give late stiffness
- Chemotherapy is used for specific malignancies.

should be considered in sarcomas larger than 6cm and where there is vascular invasion because of the poorer prognosis in these patients. Local recurrence of sarcoma with marginal resection and radiation is greater than with resection alone. The use of adjuvant radiation therapy diminishes local recurrence in extremity sarcomas. The use of preoperative adjuvant radiation therapy can be useful for diminishing tumour size prior to excision. In some patients presenting with sarcomas in the hand and forearm, adjuvant radiation therapy may facilitate limb-salvage surgery as an effective alternative to amputation.

Reconstruction (Box 6.12.4)

Soft-tissue reconstruction: a regional approach

More proximal lesions requiring division of branches of the brachial plexus should warrant a frank discussion with the patient as to the merits of amputation. Slow-growing soft tissue tumours seldom require additional skin coverage. The concomitant expansion of the adjacent tissues will usually ensure that skin closure can be achieved without difficulty. Reconstruction is more often required for rapidly growing tumours or where the provision of an adequate margin of resection dictates a greater need for skin coverage.

Digital coverage

Flap coverage following resection of small tumours in the digits is mandatory if such resection results in exposure of neurovascular structures or tendons. However, where the paratenon covering a particular tendon is intact, a full-thickness skin graft will often provide ideal coverage with minimal donor site morbidity. Where skin grafting is not an option, a local digital flap will provide good coverage of small defects. In principle, these are either harvested from the same finger (homodigital) or an adjacent finger (heterodigital).

Box 6.12.4 Reconstruction

- Thumb:
  - Very important for hand function
  - Length, stability, sensibility
  - Many options
- Dorsal hand: regional or free flaps
- Palm:
  - More specialist tissue
  - May need tissue from sole of foot
- Bone and joint: typically fusion for joint loss.

The use of heterodigital tissue for the reconstruction of a skin defect is only recommended following excision of benign tumours.

Thumb reconstruction

Amputation of the thumb constitutes a significant functional loss, rendering reconstruction a priority. The major goal of reconstruction is to provide a stable thumb of sufficient strength and length in the correct position. Lesser priorities for the reconstructed thumb are motion, sensibility, and appearance. Reconstructive alternatives following amputation of the thumb depend primarily on the length of the thumb remnant and the presence of the basal joint.

In subtotal amputations, metacarpal lengthening by distraction may provide adequate length. In total amputations, the options include osteoplastic reconstruction, pollicization, or toe-to-hand transfer. Which of these options is chosen depends on patient factors, such as compliance, suitability for microvascular surgery, and the level of the amputation, as well as surgical preference. Reconstruction of the thumb with tissue derived from the great toe gives the best results in patients suited to this procedure. This is by far the superior technique for thumb reconstruction. The tissue derived from the foot can be used in various ways. These include resurfacing of the skeletal thumb by the wrap-around technique, the trimmed great toe transfer, which minimizes the bulk of the great toe, and transfer of the second toe. Pollicization can yield excellent results, but in adults it is usually best reserved for the patient with pre-existent partial index finger amputation. Osteoplastic reconstruction, using a groin flap combined with bone grafting, is suitable for patients who are not candidates for microsurgery.

Dorsal hand coverage

In general the larger defects created by tumour ablation over the dorsum of the hand require flap coverage that cannot be satisfied by local tissue alone. One exception is where a fillet flap can be harvested from a digit to resurface a dorsal or palmar skin defect. The options include pedicled flaps from the groin or chest wall, regional flaps from the ipsilateral forearm, and free tissue transfers.

The groin flap

Based on the superficial circumflex iliac vessels, the groin flap has proved reliable for the resurfacing of dorsal hand defects. However, the use of the pedicled groin flap is limited to reconstruction following benign tumour resection. Although reliable, it commits the patient to a period of inactivity whilst the pedicle is attached, with the potential for stiffness in the small joints of the hand. Its use as a free flap obviates the need for a pedicle.

Forearm flaps

Flaps derived from the forearm include those based on fasciosepto-cutaneous perforating branches from the radial artery, the ulnar artery, and the posterior interosseous artery. They are referred to as the distally based radial forearm, ulnar forearm, and posterior interosseous flaps respectively, and are indicated for reconstruction following removal of benign tumours. Free tissue transfer is a better option for malignant tumours. Inherent in the use of local tissues for resurfacing skin defects is the concern about tumour seeding in the flap donor site. In the case of the radial and ulnar forearm flaps, there is the additional concern of deprivation of a major source of arterial inflow in the extremity. Donor site morbidity in the form of delayed healing is common, particularly where primary closure of the donor site is not possible. The posterior interosseous flap, although probably the least reliable of the group, has significantly less donor site morbidity.

Free tissue transfers

The ideal flap would provide durable coverage with the potential for a gliding environment without being too bulky. Broadly, the options include free muscle, skin, or fascial transfers. The success rate for free tissue transfer in large series now approaches, or equals, 100%. Cost analysis has demonstrated a significant saving with free tissue transfers compared with pedicled flaps.

There are many options with their own particular merits and limitations. They include: the gracilis and serratus anterior as small to medium free muscle flaps; the latissimus and rectus abdominis as large muscle flaps; the contralateral ulnar flap, the free groin flap, and the scapular flap as skin flaps; and the serratus anterior fascia, the superficial temporal fascia, the lateral arm fascia, and the scapular fascia as fascial flaps.

Coverage of the palm

The uniquely sensate glabrous skin of the palm is ideally suited to prehension. The particular aim of reconstruction in the palm should be sensate skin which is of similar volume, texture, and colour. For smaller defects, a large variety of local pedicled or island flaps can be applied. The reconstruction of large palmar defects of the hand remains a difficult problem because of the specificity of the anatomic structures and the highly sophisticated function of the palm. Free tissue transfer remains the preferred alternative for larger defects with exposed tendons, nerves, or other essential structures. The medial plantar flap provides the capability of transposing glabrous skin from the non-weight-bearing instep of the foot to the palm of the hand. Occasionally, owing to the relative abundance of subcutaneous tissue in the palm, vital structures may be protected such that a full-thickness or thick split-thickness skin graft from the sole of the foot will suffice.

Bone and joint reconstruction

The treatment of benign tumours of the phalanges is usually intralesional treatment involving curettage only or curettage and bone grafting. Amputation is usually indicated for benign tumours with extraperiosteal spread or for malignant tumours. The rate of metastasis of chondrosarcomas presenting in the phalanges is very low, unlike those occurring elsewhere in the body. Treatment of this locally aggressive lesion may be by curettage rather than amputation if the latter may result in significant functional loss.

Reconstruction is generally required for tumours of the metacarpals, the distal radius, and the distal ulna that fall into one of the following three categories:

- Recurrent benign tumour
- Benign tumour with extraperiosteal spread
- Malignant tumour.

This applies to tumours in stages 2 or 3 of the Enneking grading system, or grades 2 or 3 of the Campanacci radiological grade.

Reconstruction of the distal radius

The distal radius is a relatively common site for skeletal neoplasms and is the third most common site of giant cell tumours. Resection of the distal radius is indicated for malignant neoplasms, as well as for locally recurrent or invasive benign tumours. Many patients who fall into this category are relatively young and have high functional demands. The limited soft tissue coverage in this area and the proximity of neurovascular structures and tendons add to the difficulty in achieving clear marginal clearance of tumours of the distal radius. The pronator quadratus is a useful watershed on the volar aspect of the radius. Curettage remains the mainstay of management in cases where the tumour is confined within the radius. The resultant intramedullary bone defect can be filled with autogenous cancellous bone or methylmethacrylate cement, or it can be left unfilled. Cryosurgery or phenol instillation is used in an attempt to reduce the incidence of local recurrence. Giant cell tumours are particularly prone to recurrence after curettage, especially in the distal radius where recurrence rates of 50% have been reported. Malignant change in recurrent giant cell tumour may be associated with irradiation. For these reasons, en bloc resection and reconstruction of the distal radius may be necessary.

In the reconstruction of the distal radius, the surgeon needs first to decide whether or not to retain wrist motion. Factors contributing to this decision include the proximity of the tumour to the joint, the tumour grade, and patient preference. The reconstructive options that retain wrist motion include excision arthroplasty, prosthetic replacement, ulnar translocation of the carpus, allograft replacement, and the use of a non-vascularized fibular bone graft or a vascularized fibular bone graft. Depending on the nature of the bony defect, and if a decision has been made to sacrifice wrist motion, a vascularized or non-vascularized bone graft will usually be required at the time of the arthrodesis. However, recent reports have focused on the use of either osteoarticular allograft or vascularized bone grafts in the management of this difficult reconstructive problem.

The use of cadaveric osteoarticular allograft employs a size-matched fresh-frozen distal radial allograft. The advantages of this technique include the ability to provide an exact three-dimensional reconstruction and to reconstruct larger defects, including ligamentous reconstruction, and the absence of a donor site. Despite the encouraging results with this technique, non-vascularized autogenous bone grafts are predisposed to delayed union, stress fracture, resorption, and collapse.

The primary advantage of vascularized autogenous bone grafts is a lower fracture rate compared with large non-vascularized bone grafts or cadaveric bone grafts. Vascularized bone has a greater propensity to hypertrophy as well as a diminished tendency to non-union. Osteotomy sites heal in a fashion more akin to fracture healing than bone-graft incorporation. Furthermore, bony healing occurs irrespective of the dimensions of the vascularized bone segment. An additional advantage in the use of vascularized bone is the facility to provide skin as part of a composite skin–muscle reconstruction. In order to reduce the fracture rate further, the fibula can be double-barrelled for additional strength and bulk. When harvested correctly, the donor site morbidity should not be significant. When used for upper-extremity reconstruction, the vascularized fibula may not be capable of the hypertrophy seen in the lower extremity, particularly where the fixation is rigid.

Distal ulna

As for the distal radius, T1 lesions of the distal ulna may be treated by curettage and bone grafting. Tumours that are not amenable to curettage may be resected en bloc with good functional results.

Where the tumour extent allows subperiosteal resection, the ulnar collateral ligament and triangular fibrocartilage complex are amenable to reconstruction. This will significantly reduce the incidence of instability following resection. An ulna-stabilizing procedure may be necessary for the patient with demonstrable ulna instability following resection.

Outcome analysis

Standard systems have been derived for the evaluation of outcome following reconstructive procedures after tumour excision. It is recommended that these are used to facilitate comparison of reconstructive techniques.

Further reading

Bryan, P.S., Soule, E.H., Dobyns, J.H., Pritchard, D.J., Linscheid, R.L. (1974). Metastatic lesions of the hand, forearm. *Clinical Orthopaedics and Related Research*, **101**, 167–70.

Campanacci, M. (1976). Giant-cell tumor and chondrosarcomas: grading, treatment and results (studies of 209 and 131 cases). *Recent Results in Cancer Research*, **54**, 257–61.

Enneking, W.E., Eady, J.L., and Burchardt, H. (1980). Autogenous cortical bone grafts in the reconstruction of segmental skeletal defects. *Journal of Bone and Joint Surgery*, **62A**, 1039–58.

Enneking, W.E., Dunham, W., Gebhardt, M.C., Malawar, M., and Pritchard, D.J. (1993). A system for the functional evaluation of reconstructive procedures after surgical treatment of tumors of the musculoskeletal system. *Clinical Orthopaedics and Related Research*, **286**, 241–6.

Lister, G. (1985). The choice of procedure following thumb amputation. *Clinical Orthopaedics and Related Research*, **195**, 45–51.

Mankin, H.J. (1987). Principles of diagnosis and management of tumors of the hand. *Hand Clinics*, **3**, 185–95.

Wei, F.C., Chen, H.C., Chuang, C.C., and Chen, S.H. (1994). Microsurgical thumb reconstruction with toe transfer: selection of various techniques. *Plastic and Reconstructive Surgery*, **93**, 345–7.

Wolf, R.E. and Enneking, W.E. (1996). The staging and surgery of musculoskeletal neoplasms. *Orthopedic Clinics of North America*, **27**, 473–81.

6.13

Ganglia of the wrist and hand

Douglas A. Campbell and Peter Burge

Summary points

- Ganglia are common; typically age 20–40, in women more so than men
- Cause: unclear but associated with underlying ligament or tendon 'irritation' or joint osteoarthritis
- Diagnosis: usually obvious. Investigations are generally not needed
- Most recover spontaneously especially in children
- Good operative techniques are generally successful.

Incidence

Ganglia have featured in medical literature for over 250 years. They represent approximately two-thirds of all hand swellings and are most commonly seen between 20–40 years of age. However, they may be found in any age group. Annual incidence rates for ganglia of the wrist and hand are approximately 25 per 100 000 and 43 per 100 000 for males and females respectively

Pathology

Ganglia present as smooth round swellings which vary in consistency from soft to bony hard, depending on the pressure within them. They may be single or multiloculated but are seldom attached to skin.

Histologically, the ganglion wall consists of compressed collagen fibres lined by a few flat cells. There is no true epithelial or synovial lining membrane. The typical clear mucinous fluid within the cyst contains high concentrations of hyaluronic acid, together with glucosamine, globulin, and albumin.

Several lines of evidence indicate that the contents of ganglia originate from synovial cavities (i.e. joint or tendon sheath) nearby, but it is unclear if ganglion fluid is simply synovial fluid which has escaped from the joint or if it is formed by cells in the synovium at the origin of the ganglion. Ganglion fluid closely resembles synovial fluid in its composition. Ganglia are almost exclusively found near a joint or tendon sheath, with which a communication can often be demonstrated. Arthrographic and cystographic studies have shown that dye will frequently pass from joint to ganglion but, in the few cases studied, not in the reverse direction. The classical study of Angelides and Wallace (1976) examined the capsular attachments of 64 dorsal wrist ganglia under magnification *in situ*. In all cases, the ganglion arose from the dorsal surface of the scapholunate ligament. After dissection of the capsular portion of the ganglion from the scapholunate ligament, a small quantity of ganglion fluid seeped from the surface of the ligament in every case. Examination of this area under magnification showed that small gaps appear between the transverse ligament fibres in dorsiflexion and close in flexion. The capsular origin of the ganglion contained many small cystic spaces that were shown by serial sections to be parts of a tortuous continuous duct that connected the ganglion cyst with the joint. The hypothesis is that synovial fluid passes from the scapholunate joint along a continuous duct that acts as a one-way valve between the scapholunate ligament and the main ganglion cyst. Whether similar mechanisms operate at other sites of ganglia is unknown. The predilection for the four typical sites in the hand and wrist has not been explained. There is no good evidence to support traumatic or inflammatory aetiologies.

Clinical features

Patients present with swelling which may be accompanied by pain, stiffness, or weakness of the associated joint. Variation in size over time, especially a reduction in size, is virtually diagnostic of ganglion. Large ganglia may show the sign of fluctuance and may be transilluminated.

Obscure wrist pain is sometimes caused by an occult ganglion; there is local tenderness at one of the typical sites (usually the dorsum of the wrist) but the ganglion is too small to be visible or palpable. Occult ganglia can be identified by ultrasound or magnetic resonance imaging (MRI).

Ganglia resolve spontaneously in around 40% of cases. They may produce symptoms by extrinsic compression of adjacent structures such as the ulnar nerve in Guyon's canal and the median nerve in the carpal tunnel. Pressure on the terminal branch of the posterior interosseous nerve at the wrist may account for the pain caused by dorsal wrist ganglia.

Table 6.13.1 Classification of ganglia by site of origin

Ganglion	Site of origin
Dorsal wrist	Dorsum of scapholunate ligament
Palmar wrist	Radiocarpal or scaphotrapezial joints
Flexor tendon sheath	Flexor tendon sheath
Dorsal digital	Distal interphalangeal joint
Intraosseous	Bone adjacent to joint
Intraneural	Nerve adjacent to joint

Ganglia are most usually classified according to their site of origin (Table 6.13.1).

Dorsal wrist ganglion

The most common type of ganglion arises from the wrist capsule over the dorsal surface of the scapholunate ligament. The pedicle that connects the ganglion with its articular origin may pass some distance beneath the extensor tendons before coming to the surface, so the ganglion itself may present some distance from the scapholunate area (Figure 6.13.1). When planning the removal of a ganglion that is not located in the typical site, the possibility of a connection with the scapholunate ligament should be borne in mind, so that an incision can be designed to allow access for excision of the pedicle (the key to successful surgical treatment) without leaving an unsightly scar.

Palmar wrist ganglion

Palmar wrist ganglia typically present at the proximal wrist crease between the radial artery and the flexor carpi radialis tendon (Figure 6.13.2). Two-thirds originate from the radiocarpal joint at the scapholunate interval; the remainder arise from the scaphotrapezial joint. Ganglia arising from the scaphotrapezial joint may track along the tendon sheath of flexor carpi radialis and come to the surface some distance from their origin. Palmar wrist ganglia may occur in older patients in association with scaphotrapezial osteoarthritis. In these cases, the risk of recurrence is high unless the underlying arthritis is also treated by arthrodesis or excision arthroplasty. The symptoms seldom justify surgery of this magnitude.

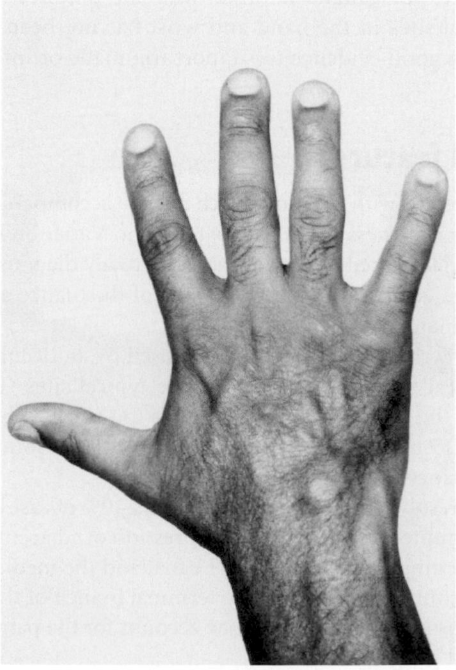

Fig. 6.13.1 Dorsal wrist ganglion presenting slightly to the ulnar side of the usual site of origin from the vicinity of the scapholunate ligament.

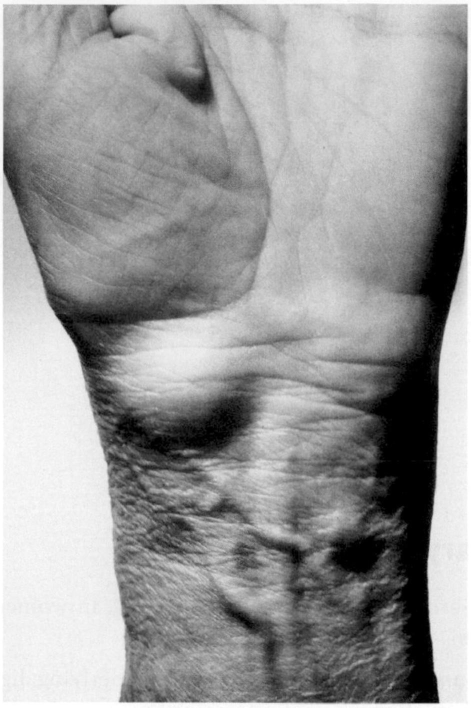

Fig. 6.13.2 Palmar wrist ganglion presenting between the flexor carpi radialis tendon and the radial artery.

These ganglia may be closely related to the radial artery and require careful dissection from it. A preoperative Allen test and tourniquet release before skin closure should be considered when excising palmar wrist ganglia.

Palmar wrist ganglia may be more extensive than clinical examination suggests. An extensile surgical approach is advisable, so as to deal with possible extensions under the thenar muscles, into the carpal tunnel, and along the sheath of flexor carpi radialis tendon. Excision of palmar wrist ganglia should be approached with caution. Small subcutaneous nerve branches are prone to produce painful neuromas if injured in this region. It is not always easy to identify the pedicle of the ganglion, the scar may be unattractive, and the recurrence rate is higher than for dorsal wrist ganglia (Table 6.13.2).

Flexor sheath ganglion

A 2- to 5-mm-diameter ganglion, also known as volar retinacular ganglion or seed ganglion, commonly arises from the A2 pulley of the flexor tendon sheath at the proximal digital crease.

Patients complain of accurately localized pain when gripping objects such as the steering wheel of a car or when carrying objects. The ganglion is small, hard, and tender. It sits on the external surface of the tendon sheath in the midline or just to one side it and

Table 6.13.2 Recurrence rates after surgical excision of wrist ganglia

Study	Ganglion type	Recurrences	Percentage recurrence
Angelides and Wallace (1976)	Dorsal wrist	3/346	0.9
Janzon and Niechajev (1981)	Wrist	21/165	13
Clay and Clement (1988)	Dorsal wrist	2/62	3
Wright et al. (1994)	Anterior wrist	14/72	19
Dias et al. (2007)	Dorsal wrist	40/103	39

does not move with the tendon. The ganglion may be punctured with a fine needle inserted in the midline of the digit, so as to avoid the digital nerves, and its contents dispersed by firm massage. If the ganglion persists or recurs, it may be excised together with a small disk of tendon sheath. Care should be taken to preserve the major part of the A2 pulley. Recurrence after excision is very uncommon.

Dorsal digital ganglion

Ganglia arising from the distal interphalangeal joint are sometimes known as mucous or myxoid cysts. They occur in older individuals and are often associated with early osteoarthritis of the distal interphalangeal joint. Pressure from the ganglion on the germinal matrix may produce a furrow in the fingernail; the furrow may appear before the ganglion is evident (Figure 6.13.3).

The ganglion arises from the joint capsule between the collateral ligament and the extensor tendon, presenting just to one side of the midline, typically between the distal joint crease and the eponychium but occasionally preoximal to the distal interphalangeal joint.

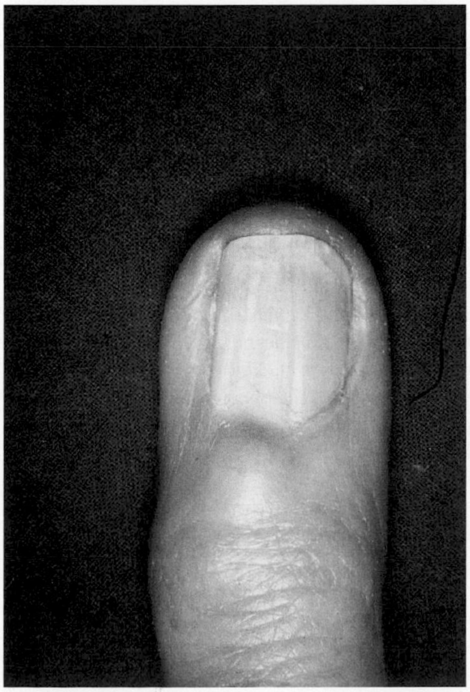

Fig. 6.13.3 Dorsal digital ganglion. Note the longitudinal furrow of the nail plate. (Courtesy of Dr R.P.R. Dawber.)

The overlying skin may become very thin, giving the ganglion a pearly appearance and leading to occasional discharge of clear viscous fluid.

Operative excision requires removal of the cyst in continuity with a block of joint capsule between the extensor tendon and collateral ligament. The nail matrix should be protected. A local synovectomy and removal of osteophytes may help to prevent recurrence. Small defects in the thin skin overlying the ganglion will heal spontaneously. In the rare case of a large defect, a full-thickness skin graft or dorsal advancement flap may be required. The risk of recurrence is probably less than 5%.

Intraosseous ganglion

Intraosseous ganglia are uncommon. The most frequent site is the radial border of the lunate (Figure 6.13.4), where a communication between the lesion and the scapholunate joint is usually found. Computed tomography (CT) examination and operative exploration often show a communication that is not evident on plain radiography. The predilection of intraosseous ganglion for bones on each side of the scapholunate joint suggests that intraosseous and soft tissue ganglia share a common, as yet unknown, pathogenesis.

Intraosseous ganglia may be found in patients with wrist pain but are not always the cause of it; other causes of pain should be excluded. Operative treatment is curettage and bone grafting, but relief of pain may be incomplete

Intraneural ganglion

Intraneural ganglia are rare. The ganglion is usually located within the nerve sheath and may extend for some distance above and below the point at which it is clinically obvious. The cause of intraneural ganglia is not clear. One theory is that synovial fluid gains access to the epineural sheath where an articular nerve branch enters the joint capsule and runs proximally into the main nerve trunk. Mucoid degeneration and fibrous tissue metaplasia have also been proposed. Although the most common site is within the

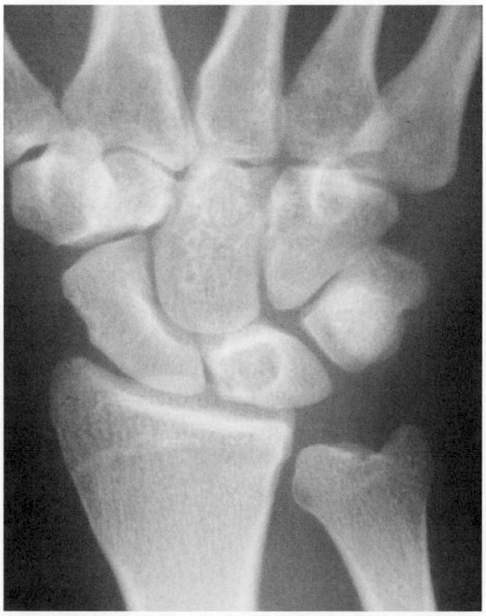

Fig. 6.13.4 Intraosseous ganglion cyst of the lunate.

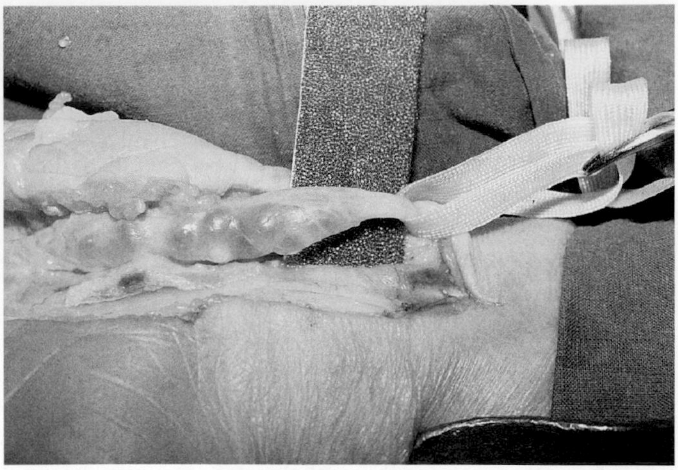

Fig. 6.13.5 Intraneural ganglion cyst of the ulnar nerve at the wrist

common peroneal nerve at the knee, intraneural ganglia have been reported in the radial, median, and ulnar nerves (Figure 6.13.5).

Investigation

A confident diagnosis of ganglion is usually possible on the clinical features alone. If necessary, the diagnosis can be confirmed by aspiration of the typical ganglion fluid. Ultrasound can demonstrate the cystic nature of the swelling. MRI is helpful in the diagnosis of occult wrist ganglia and in delineating the site and extent of ganglia that present in unusual locations.

Plain radiography is useful in excluding other causes of wrist pain and should be performed before a ganglion is treated operatively. CT imaging may be useful in diagnosis of intraosseous ganglion and identification of a communication with an adjacent joint.

Treatment

The management of ganglia is influenced by several facts: ganglia are harmless; some ganglia disappear spontaneously; recurrence is possible after aspiration or excision; and excision is not without complications.

The options for treatment of ganglia are reassurance, aspiration, and excision. Some patients are concerned about the development of a mass, but have few symptoms and are content with reassurance that the swelling is harmless.

Aspiration of ganglia requires a wide-bore needle, taking appropriate care of adjacent structures such as the radial artery. Studies of aspiration of ganglia have shown quite disparate rates of recurrence that may be explained by differences in case mix. Palmar wrist ganglia appear to have a significantly higher risk of recurrence after aspiration (Table 6.13.3). Aspiration may be accompanied by attempts to puncture the cyst wall with the needle or by instillation

Table 6.13.3 Recurrence rates after aspiration of wrist ganglia

Study	Ganglion type	Recurrences	Percentage recurrence
Nield and Evans (1986)	Wrist and hand	20/34	59
Zubowicz and Ishii (1987)	Wrist and hand	12/47	25
Richman et al. (1987)	Wrist and hand	56/87	64
Korman et al. (1992)	Wrist and hand	34/69	49
Wright et al. (1994)	Palmar wrist	20/24	83
Dias et al. (2007)	Dorsal wrist	45/78	58

of steroid, or followed by immobilization. It is uncertain if these manoeuvres reduce the risk of recurrence after aspiration Ganglia that recur after aspiration tend to do so within 3 months. Flexor sheath ganglia are too small for aspiration but can be dispersed by firm pressure after puncturing the cyst wall with a needle.

Successful excision of wrist ganglia depends upon the identification of the pedicle connecting cyst to joint. The pedicle should be excised together with a disc of surrounding joint capsule. Closure of the capsular defect is difficult, unnecessary, and may restrict movement of the wrist. Contrasting evidence exists regarding the use of immobilization after surgical excision. Most authors recommend that movement should begin as soon as possible postoperatively, since immobilization may lead to stiffness.

Arthroscopic excision of dorsal wrist ganglia is no more reliable at reducing recurrence rates than open excision.

Although recurrence is much less frequent after excision than after aspiration (Tables 6.13.2 and 6.13.3), the benefits of excision must be considered against the risks. The mere presence of a ganglion is not an indication for surgery. In addition to general risks of haematoma and infection, local complications such as tender or hypertrophic scars, injury to superficial sensory nerves, and loss of wrist motion occur in up to 8% of patients. These may mar the result. The small but real risk of complications should tilt the decision away from surgery unless the ganglion is persistent and the cause of significant symptoms.

Further reading

Andren, L. and Eiken, O. (1971). Arthrographic studies of wrist ganglions. *Journal of Bone and Joint Surgery*, **53A**, 299–302.

Clay, N. and Clement, D.A. (1988). The treatment of dorsal wrist ganglia by radical excision. *Journal of Hand Surgery*, **13B**, 187–91.

Dias, J.J., Dhukaram, V., and Kumar, P. (2007). The natural history of untreated dorsal wrist ganglia and patient reported outcome 6 years after intervention. *Journal of Hand Surgery*, **32E**, 502–8.

Greendyke, S.D., Wilson, M., and Shepler, T.R. (1992). Anterior wrist ganglia from the scaphotrapezial joint. *Journal of Hand Surgery*, **17A**, 487–90.

Zubowicz, V.N. and Ishii, C.H. (1987). Management of ganglion cysts of the hand by simple aspiration. *Journal of Hand Surgery*, **12A**, 618–20.

6.14

Hand infection

Lisa Leonard

Summary points

- Common
- Typically with common bacteria: *Staphylococcus* or *Streptococcus*
- Typically in common sites:
  - Fingertip
  - Tendon sheath
  - Deep palmar spaces
- Atypical infections such as MRSA becoming more frequent.

Introduction

Hand infections can result in severe disability, including stiffness, contracture, and amputation, particularly if treatment is inappropriate or delayed. Modern antimicrobial medication and prompt surgical intervention have made most infections in the hand treatable with the expectation that normal, or near normal, hand function will return. This expectation should not lead to complacency as infections in the hand can present in a myriad of ways and unusual organisms can sometimes evade definitive diagnosis by even the most astute clinician.

Incidence

This is difficult to determine and relates to the specific type of infection involved. One recent study of patients requiring admission to hospital in the United States found that human bites were the commonest infection (51%) followed by cellulitis (17%) and septic arthritis (11.8%). Paronychia was responsible for only 0.45% of admissions, although this is widely held to be the commonest hand infection overall.

Anatomy

The unique anatomy of the hand results in certain typical presentations of infection and dictates the principles necessary for subsequent surgical drainage. Dr Allen Kanavel, a Chicago general surgeon, treated hand infections in the preantibiotic era and undertook detailed studies of infection in the hand. The findings from these studies still underpin our understanding of how infections spread in the hand and how they may be effectively treated.

Fingertip

The fingertip is made up of multiple small compartments divided by connective tissue trabeculae. These trabeculae provide mechanical support to the fingertip pad and are filled with sweat glands that open in the skin and allow bacteria to enter. The nail complex consists of special tissues that are difficult to replace. The nail bed, below the nail plate, consists of the sterile and germinal matrix. Proximally the nail plate lies below the nail fold and to either side of the nail plate lies the eponychium.

Tendon sheaths

Tendon sheaths are double walled with a visceral layer closely adherent to the tendon (the epitenon) and a surrounding parietal layer adherent to the pulleys. These tubular structures are joined at their ends, forming a closed system that is a conduit for bacterial spread. The index, long, and ring finger tendon sheaths start at the distal interphalangeal joint (DIPJ), end at the A1 pulley in the palm, and drain into the midpalmar space. The thumb and little finger, however, have tendon sheaths that extend proximal to the transverse carpal ligament as the radial and ulnar bursae, respectively. These two bursae may communicate with each other, and enter the forearm, through Parona's space. The tendon sheaths are very close to the skin over the volar proximal interphalangeal joint (PIPJ) and DIPJ creases.

Deep palmar spaces

These were originally described by Kanavel. The spaces are bound by bones and soft tissues septae that dictate how infection spreads. The midpalmar space encompasses the area from the base of the palm to just below the web space and is bounded by the middle metacarpal bone radially and by the hypothenar eminence ulnarly. The thenar space is the area between the thenar eminence and middle metacarpal bone while the hypothenar space is over the hypothenar eminence.

Deep subfascial spaces

There are three more spaces in the hand that can become infected: the dorsal subcutaneous space (superficial to the extensors), the dorsal subaponeurotic space (between the extensors and the metacarpals), and the interdigital web space. These spaces are less well defined anatomically but infection here may present in a similar fashion to that of the deep spaces.

Box 6.14.1 Pathophysiology

- Systemic features e.g. immunocompromise, diabetes
- Local features e.g. repetitive insults, tissue damage
- Changing pathogens–MRSA becoming more common.

Pathophysiology (Box 6.14.1)

Systemic factors

Individuals who are immunocompromised for any reason are at greater risk of developing acute, chronic, atypical, and life-threatening hand infections. As a result they require more aggressive and prolonged therapy than other patients. Diabetics and drug abusers probably represent the commonest patients in this category but the very old and very young can also be affected.

Individuals with peripheral vascular disease resulting in poor blood flow to the extremities are also predisposed to infections, such as patients with scleroderma.

Local factors

The hand has natural barriers to infection, but local conditions can weaken these defences. Direct skin penetration from trauma or bites can introduce a variety of pathogens. Repetitive microtrauma or repeated environmental insults can also weaken defences and predispose to various chronic infections. Gross contamination, or crushing, results in devitalization of tissues that can allow opportunistic infections to occur. Surgical incisions and implants are other risk factors.

Changing pathogens

Staphylococcus aureus is the most common cause of skin and soft tissue infections in the hand, as elsewhere in the body. Methicillin-resistant strains have increasingly been identified (MRSA). In some institutions upwards of 50% of cases were caused by MRSA. It is important to recognize this changing pattern, modify antibiotic regimens appropriately, and obtain definitive microbial cultures whenever possible, even in apparently simple cases. Liaison with the microbiology team is advised. Human and animal bites are frequently infected by unusual, often more virulent, bacteria.

Clinical evaluation

History

A thorough history is essential, and suggests the likely organism(s) and best course of treatment. Careful enquiry must be made as to the mechanism of any precipitating injury, the environment in which the injury occurred, the time since injury, and any treatment that has been given. Risk factors for immune compromise, tetanus status, work activities, and hobbies should all be ascertained.

Examination

This should start with an assessment of any systemic signs of toxicity including temperature and vital signs. The regional lymph nodes should be palpated. The hand and forearm should then be inspected methodically, bearing in mind the anatomical considerations discussed earlier.

Box 6.14.2 Assessment

- History:
  - Typically diagnostic
  - Time from inoculation is critical
- Examination:
  - Classical features, e.g. red, swollen, tender, pus
  - Check for extension
  - Beware deep infections.

In an acute infection look for wounds and skin breaks, warmth, erythema, oedema, tenderness, and fluctuant collections. Differentiate uncomplicated cellulitis from that overlying an abscess or infected joint. All potential spaces should be palpated for tenderness, keeping in mind the possibility of spread along a defined space. For example, it is important to palpate the forearm in a little finger infection and palpate the midpalmar space in a middle finger laceration. It is sometimes useful to mark the extent of any erythema on the skin with a marker pen to allow subsequent comparative assessment.

In chronic infection the signs may be less florid with solid feeling, indurated tissues, sinuses, and ulcers.

Some infections have very characteristic appearances whilst other conditions can closely mimic infection. Some examples of this are discussed later in this chapter.

Common sites of infection (Box 6.14.3)

Fingertips

Paronychia

Paronychia affects the eponychial folds around the fingernail. Only refractory cases usually present to the hand surgeon.

Acute paronychia

Acute paronychia usually follows local trauma to the nail fold from biting nails, aggressive manicuring, or a hangnail. Pus below the nail plate can cause pressure on the germinal matrix and temporary or permanent arrest of nail growth.

Most acute paronychia are mixed infections. *Staphylococcus aureus* is the commonest bacterial isolate but other aerobic organisms such as *Streptococcus* spp. and *Eikenella corrodens* are also frequently present. Anaerobic species are also frequently isolated such as *Peptostreptococcus* spp. and *Bacteroides*.

Investigations are rarely needed.

Early acute cases can be treated with warm saline soaks, oral antibiotics (co-amoxiclav covers most of the common bacterial pathogens) and rest. Once an abscess develops it should be drained under ring block anaesthesia. If pus is found below the nail plate this should be removed to facilitate drainage.

Chronic paronychia

Chronic paronychia is a multifactorial inflammatory reaction to irritants and allergens often with superadded infection. The patient presents with a well-circumscribed, indurated, retracted, and rounded nail fold. The patient (92% female) often gives a history

Box 6.14.3 Common soft tissue sites for infection

- Paronychia—nail fold:
  - Acute and chronic
  - Typically *Staphylococcus*
- Felon—pulp infection
  - Typically *Staphylococcus*
  - Very quick onset of marked pain
  - Pus needs releasing
- Flexor sheath:
  - Usually follows puncture wound
  - *Staphylococcus* or *Streptococcus*
  - Surgical emergency to avoid tendon problems
- Deep palmar infections:
  - Uncommon and easily missed early
  - *Staphylococcus*
  - Requires surgical drainage.

of frequently soaking the hands in water. Housewives, bartenders, dishwashers, nurses, swimmers, and children who suck their fingers are often affected. Diabetics and patients with psoriasis can also develop this condition. Surgical exploration reveals no collection of pus.

In chronic paronychia, *Candida albicans* is implicated in up to 97% of cases. Subacute, superadded bacterial infection may also occur with normal nail fold colonizers such as *Pseudomonas aeruginosa.*

With a prolonged history, radiographs to exclude osteomyelitis and blood markers of inflammation (such as C-reactive protein) can be useful. If a fungal infection is suspected biopsy, Gram stain, or culture may be necessary.

Treatment includes activity modification and prolonged application of a topical antifungal. Oral antifungals are an alternative but neither approach consistently heals more than 40% of lesions. Eponychial marsupialization (excision of a crescent-shaped piece of skin proximal to the nail fold) should be considered if medical treatment fails.

Complications include stiffness, tenderness and hypersensitivity, nail growth disturbance, osteomyelitis, and recurrence. In chronic cases, nail discolouration may occur following secondary *Pseudomonas* colonization.

Felon

A felon is an infection of the palmar pad of the finger.

Often the patient gives a history of a minor injury to the fingertip such as a fingerstick test for glucose estimation. Due to the tight compartments in the pulp, pressure rises rapidly in this condition and results in severe pain, swelling, and throbbing of the digit. Tissue breakdown can occur with progressive ischaemia and osteomyelitis is a risk if the condition is not rapidly treated.

The commonest organism isolated is *Staphylococcus aureus* with methicillin-resistant strains being reported.

Investigations are similar to those for paronychia.

If the felon is treated very early, antibiotics and elevation may suffice when no collection of pus has formed, otherwise treatment involves incision and drainage under ring block anaesthesia with antibiotic coverage. The incision must be planned carefully to avoid a painful scar in an important functional area. A longitudinal, midaxial incision is usually best. Avoid the digital nerve, ensure that the incision enters all the affected compartments of the pulp, and leave the wound open after a thorough irrigation.

Complications are similar to paronychia but also include pulp necrosis and DIPJ septic arthritis.

Flexor sheath

Acute infections in the closed system of the flexor sheath can rapidly destroy the smooth gliding surfaces necessary for normal tendon function. Infection can also impair the blood supply to the tendon resulting in necrosis. This condition is a surgical emergency if devastating loss of function is to be avoided.

There is usually a history of a puncture wound on the volar side of the finger that can be very small. Animal and human bites can also be causative. Haematogenous spread rarely occurs and is most frequently gonococcal.

Kanavel described four cardinal signs of tenosynovitis:

1) Tenderness over the entire flexor tendon sheath
2) Swelling of the digit
3) Semiflexed position of the digit
4) Severe pain on passive extension of the digit.

Staphylococcus aureus and β-haemolytic streptococci are the most commonly isolated organisms. *Pasteurella multocida* is frequently found in association with animal bites. Other unusual organisms should be considered in the diabetic or immunocompromised patient.

This is primarily a clinical diagnosis, but blood tests and radiographs may be undertaken to monitor treatment and exclude foreign bodies, joint involvement, and unsuspected fracture.

Joint infection and inflammatory conditions, such as rheumatoid arthritis or gout, can mimic this condition.

Immediate drainage is almost always indicated for this condition. Ideally, microbiology specimens should be obtained prior to commencing antibiotics. Opening both ends of the flexor sheath via transverse skin incisions over the transverse palmar crease and the volar DIPJ crease and washing out using a paediatric feeding catheter is a useful technique. The catheter can be left in for sheath irrigation on the ward if necessary. Midaxial incisions are recommended if further exposure is required. Postoperative elevation and early motion are essential. Repeated washouts can be necessary.

Complications include stiffness and tendon necrosis.

Deep spaces of the hand

These infections present with swelling of the whole hand, particularly the dorsum where the fascial attachments are looser. There is often a history of penetrating injury. Local areas of exquisite tenderness may overlie a deep collection. The thenar space is the most commonly affected deep space and the interdigital webspace (collar button abscess) is the most commonly affected subfascial space. A characteristic of webspace infection is abduction of the adjacent digits caused by pus between the bases of the fingers.

Blood tests and radiographs should be obtained. Ultrasound can be helpful in localizing an abscess but should not delay treatment when there is sufficient clinical suspicion of a collection. Staphylococci are the commonest isolated organisms.

These infections are surgical emergencies. Various approaches have been described but in all cases adequate exposure is required whilst avoiding subsequent contracture and iatrogenic injury. A thenar space infection is best drained through volar (thenar crease) and dorsal (transverse parallel to the edge of the web space) approaches. A combined approach is also used for a collar button abscess. Postoperatively, the wounds are left open to drain with strict elevation, regular dressings, intravenous antibiotics, and early motion. Repeated washout can be necessary.

Complications include tendon adhesions, scarring, joint contracture, skin necrosis, and iatrogenic injury.

Joints (Box 6.14.4)

Septic arthritis is characterized by a purulent exudate within a joint caused by the introduction and proliferation of pyogenic bacteria. Rapid articular destruction can ensue frequently, making this condition a surgical emergency.

In the hand there is usually a history of penetrating trauma from a bite or foreign body. Joint arthroplasty infection can present acutely early after implantation. Many inflammatory conditions can mimic a septic arthritis and this should be borne in mind when taking a history. Common mimics include gout, pseudogout (particularly in the elderly wrist), rheumatoid arthritis, and reactive arthritis.

Symptoms of septic arthritis can include systemic sepsis, decreased range of motion, and severe pain on joint movement. With a longer history, in smaller joints, the findings can be less florid.

Staphylococcus aureus and *Streptococcus* spp. are the most commonly isolated organisms but Gram-negative and mixed infections can also occur.

Blood tests, including cultures, and x-rays should be obtained. A joint aspiration can be useful when the diagnosis is in doubt, particularly in the wrist. Visible organisms confirm the diagnosis.

Distal interphalangeal joint

This usually presents with an established infection where the articular cartilage is already destroyed. Surgical exploration is often not necessary as symptoms will settle on 6 weeks of oral antibiotics.

Box 6.14.4 Joint infection

- Common, especially DIPJ
- Usually a puncture wound
- Radiography is suggestive
- Aspiration is confirmative
- Typically *Staphylococcus*
- The more distal the less need for washout, especially DIPJ
- Antibiotics for 6 weeks.

Proximal interphalangeal joint

Arthrotomy is performed through a midaxial incision with excision of the accessory collateral ligament to gain access to the joint. Dorsal wounds or sinuses put the central slip at risk and this area should be explored if necessary to avoid a subsequent boutonnière deformity.

Metacarpophalangeal joint

Any wound on the dorsum of this joint should be assumed to be related to a punch injury and therefore be treated as a human bite and explored early. A dorsal longitudinal or curved incision is used, either splitting the tendon or opening the sagittal band to gain access to the joint. Look carefully for joint damage or retained fragments of tooth.

Wrist joint

A thorough arthroscopic washout can be used to treat this joint or an open arthrotomy between the third and fourth extensor compartments.

Wounds are left open postoperatively to heal by secondary intention. Strict elevation, regular dressings, and early motion (passive and active) are essential if good results are to be achieved. Repeated washouts can be necessary. The length of antibiotic treatment depends on patient factors and the organism identified. Intravenous antibiotics for 2 weeks followed by 4–6 weeks of oral therapy are usually suggested but consultation with the microbiology team is advised.

Results correlate with the durations of symptoms before treatment is started. Joint stiffness is very common as is joint arthrosis. Other complications include tendon adhesions and osteomyelitis. Salvage procedures include arthrodesis, resection arthroplasty, or amputation, depending on the site.

Bones (Box 6.14.5)

Osteomyelitis is rare in the hand because of the excellent normal blood supply. The commonest bone affected is the distal phalanx. A history of penetrating trauma or a contaminated open fracture is usually obtained but postoperative infection also occurs as does haematogenous spread, particularly in children. The presentation is with local signs of infection with or without a collection. Soft tissue signs may predominate and a high index of suspicion needs to be maintained, particularly with immunocompromised hosts. Systemic signs can be present.

The most common organism isolated is *Staphylococcus aureus*. Coagulase-negative staphylococci have been isolated in conjunction internal fixation devices and polymicrobial infection can occur with open fractures or in the immunocompromised.

Box 6.14.5 Bone infection

- Uncommon except with joint infection or following surgery
- Radiography may be diagnostic
- Aspiration is confirmative but often not needed
- Typically *Staphylococcus*
- Most settle with antibiotics for 6 weeks
- Surgical excision and reconstruction may be required.

Blood tests and baseline x-rays should be obtained. Soft tissue swelling is the earliest radiographic sign with osteopenia, osteosclerosis, and a periosteal reaction occurring at least 14 days after the onset of infection. Ultrasound, magnetic resonance imaging (MRI), and labelled white cell scans can be useful adjuncts but again this is primarily a clinical diagnosis.

Treatment classically requires thorough surgical debridement with the wounds left open and reinspected regularly until the infection is under control. Bone and soft tissue reconstruction may be required at a later stage but concerns over the ability to cover tissue defects should not be allowed to result in inadequate removal of infected tissues. Four to six weeks of intravenous antibiotics are commonly required but discussion with the microbiology team is essential.

Complications are common and include stiffness, deformity, loss of function, chronic pain, and cold intolerance. Amputation is sometimes necessary, depending on the site.

Subcutaneous tissues

Cellulitis

Cellulitis is a process of acute inflammation of the skin and subcutaneous tissue in which there is hyperaemia, oedema, and white cell infiltration. Successful bacterial proliferation has the potential for systemic spread in the blood or the lymphatic system and therefore requires adequate intravenous antibiotic therapy and high arm elevation.

The most commonly isolated organisms are Gram-positive streptococci and staphylococci but multiple pathogens can be causative, particularly in the immunocompromised, which should be treated aggressively.

Necrotizing fasciitis

This is a rapidly advancing infection of the skin, subcutaneous tissues, and fascia. It is associated with severe systemic sepsis and a high mortality rate. Risk factors include diabetes (particularly insulin dependent), HIV infection, and intravenous drug abuse but it can occur in previously well patients. A fulminant course is usually observed with severe pain and skin changes occurring progressively from hour to hour.

Two subgroups are identified. Type 1 infections are caused by mixed aerobic and anaerobic infections (80% of cases). Type 2 infections are caused by Group A streptococci alone or in combination with staphylococcal species.

Baseline blood tests including a clotting screen should be obtained, but aggressive surgical debridement and antibiotic therapy should not be delayed for any reason. Secondary thrombosis of the digital vessels can occur. A finger fasciotomy may help prevent loss of the digit in this circumstance. Supportive treatment is frequently necessary, often on the intensive care unit.

Complications include soft tissue reconstruction, difficulties with stiffness, and functional compromise. Mortality rates can approach 60% when chest wall involvement occurs.

Gas gangrene

This is fortunately rare. The history often includes trauma with a significant crush element. The clinical presentation is similar to that of necrotizing fasciitis but the formation of hydrogen sulphide and carbon dioxide in the soft tissues is characteristic. The gas can be visible on plain radiographs and results in palpable crepitus in the affected tissues. Muscle necrosis also occurs.

Various species of *Clostridium* have been implicated with *C. perfringens* being the most common.

Treatment is similar to necrotizing fasciitis but hyperbaric oxygen has a more established role.

Specific acute presentations

Animal bites

Dog bites

These are the most common animal bite, frequently affecting children under 12 years of age.

Infection manifests as erythema around the bite wound and malodorous discharge. Polymicrobial growth of aerobic and anaerobic bacteria is common. *Pasteurella* spp. were the most common isolates in one study with aerobes such as streptococci and staphylococci and anaerobes such as bacteroides also identified. The possibility of rabies and tetanus should be borne in mind.

Treatment includes irrigation of the wound, thorough debridement of any dead or infected tissues, and appropriate antibiotics.

Cat bites

Cats have needle sharp teeth which effectively inject any organisms deep into the tissues resulting in much higher subsequent infection rates.

Mixed flora are often encountered with *Pasturella multocida* commonly isolated. The possibility of cat-scratch fever, caused by *Bartonella henselae*, should be kept in mind.

Treatment is similar to that for dog bites.

Marine organisms

These are more commonly associated with chronic infection but acute infection with *Staphylococcus*, *Streptococcus*, *Pseudomonas*, *Aeromonas*, and *Enterobacter* have occurred following penetrating injury. Occasionally a venom is injected, resulting in immediate severe throbbing pain at the site of inoculation. In some cases severe local reactions can occur.

Leeches

Aeromonas hydrophila infection can be seen in association with the medicinal use of leeches to relieve venous congestion. This can result in cellulitis, myonecrosis, abscesses, endocarditis, and sepsis.

Human bites

Most of these injuries occur in relation to fighting. A puncture wound over the metacarpophalangeal joint following a punch to the mouth with a clenched fist is a particularly common presentation. The injury typically occurs with the fingers flexed fully but the patient presents with the fingers only partially flexed. The skin will therefore be in different relative position in relationship to the underlying joint and superficial exploration may not reveal the true depth of the injury. All such wounds should be thoroughly explored to actively exclude joint involvement.

The human mouth contains up to 190 species of aerobic and anaerobic organisms. *Staphylococcus, Streptococcus,* and *Eikenella corrodens* are the most common organisms isolated.

Transmission of viral disease, such as hepatitis B, C, and HIV, has been documented through human bites.

Prosthetic infections

Joint replacements in the hand are frequently carried out in the immunocompromised rheumatoid patient with infection rates up to 3%.

Organisms vary and tissue specimens should be obtained to guide antibiotic treatment.

Apart from very early infections, treatment almost always requires removal of the prosthesis and a thorough debridement of the affected tissues. Intravenous antibiotic therapy is required for a similar time period to osteomyelitis.

Late reconstruction or, rarely, amputation is considered when blood tests have normalized, all signs of infection have resolved, and the skin and soft tissues are supple. Late reconstruction may not be necessary if a reasonably stable, if stiff, scar joint develops.

Infections in intravenous drug abusers

The hand and forearm are common sites for attempted injection by drug abusers. They frequently present with infected abscesses, often at multiple sites. Many will present late with associated systemic sepsis. Underlying immunocompromise and concomitant infection with hepatitis B, C, and HIV should be borne in mind.

Polymicrobial infection is common. *Staphylococcus aureus* is the commonest isolate with methicillin-resistant strains rapidly becoming predominant. Microaerophilic streptococci and other anaerobes are also commonly found.

Ideal treatment includes aggressive surgical debridement, regular dressings, appropriate antibiotics, and early motion.

Complications are common in this group, who are often poorly compliant, and include osteomyelitis, necrotizing fasciitis, amputation, septicemia, and endocarditis

Infections in HIV patients

Upper-extremity infections in patients with HIV are more common in those patients with a concomitant history of intravenous drug abuse. The clinical presentation is similar to that of patients without HIV but the natural history of the infection is often more severe, particularly when AIDS has been diagnosed. AIDS patients may also have fingers that are red with painless erythema and periungual telangiectasia. Nails may be blue or show clubbing. Abscesses and spontaneous infection, such as with septic arthritis, are common. Necrotizing fasciitis is also more frequently encountered in this group.

Pyogenic organisms, including staphylococci and streptococci, respond well to standard aggressive surgical treatment.

Viral herpetic infections also occur and often do not run a self-limiting course but require oral or intravenous antiviral therapy to be resolved.

Unusual infections, including atypical mycobacteria and fungi, also occur in HIV patients and maybe helpful in indicating the onset of AIDS.

Herpetic whitlow

This is caused by herpes simplex virus (HSV) 1 and 2. The infection can occur in children and adults. HSV-1 infections usually occur following contact with infected saliva (finger sucking in children and occupational exposure in dentists, for instance). HSV-2 infections occur following genital contact. The incubation period is 2–14 days.

Early in the course of the disease there is intense throbbing and pain in the affected digit. Tingling can also occur. Erythema and mild swelling develop followed by the appearance of clear vesicles that gradually coalesce. The clear fluid may become turbid mimicking a purulent infection. The lesions gradually resolve over a 3-week period. Superadded bacterial infection can occur.

The Tzanck smear can be performed on vesicular fluid but is less sensitive than viral cultures at confirming the diagnosis. Immunofluorescent serum antibody titres can also be diagnostic.

No active treatment is usually indicated but attempts should be made to avoid autoinoculation and transmission. Deroofing the vesicles may provide some symptom relief and partial nail excision can be carried out for subungual pressure symptoms but this should be performed with care. Misdiagnosis and treatment as a bacterial felon can increase local complications and some authors have mentioned a risk of inducing viral encephalitis with this treatment. No recent studies have confirmed this. Recurrence can occur and can be severe in the immunocompromised.

Anthrax

This is caused by infection with *Bacillus anthracis*, a Gram-negative spore-forming bacterium. A history of direct contact with infected animals or animal products 2–7 days prior to symptoms and signs developing is characteristic.

Ninety-five per cent of cases present with the cutaneous form of the disease. Small, painless, red macules gradually progress to papules over 48–72h. These then become vesicular, rupture, ulcerate, and form a 1–5-cm diameter brown or black eschar which is painless. Tender regional lymphadenopathy, fever, and malaise with surrounding oedema may occur. Pulmonary and intestinal forms also occur.

Antibiotics do not affect the progress of the skin lesion but do sterilize the ulcer. Penicillin is the first-line choice, initially given intravenously. Surgical debridement is contraindicated because of the risk of spreading the infection.

Complications include malignant oedema, septicaemia, shock, renal failure, and death in 10–20% of untreated cases.

Mimics of acute infection

Many conditions can mimic acute infection in the hand.

Gout and pseudogout can present as a pyarthrosis or local soft tissue collection.

Acute calcific tendonitis presents as severe, acute pain over tendons or ligaments. This is often characteristic on plain x-ray.

Pyogenic granuloma presents as a raised, red friable lesion with a history of minor trauma. It is usually self-limiting but can be a significant nuisance. Silver nitrate applied to the surface may resolve the swelling but often takes several applications. For larger or persistent lesions curettage of the base under local anaesthetic is curative.

Pyoderma gangrenosum is a progressive, necrotizing, and ulcerative disease of the skin often, but not always, associated with inflammatory bowel disease or myelodysplastic syndrome. No organisms are grown on culture. Treatment is with oral steroids. Surgery risks precipitating a rapid deterioration of the condition. Complete healing should be expected.

Bony metastatic tumours can present acutely in the hand. The primary is most commonly the lung and the commonest affected bone is the distal phalanx. Soft tissue tumours also occur in the hand but usually present chronically. They include squamous cell carcinomas, basal cell carcinomas, melanomas, and keratoacanthomas.

Specific chronic presentations

Chronic infections in the hand occur infrequently and can present in numerous of ways. A high index of suspicion and a careful history are vital if an early diagnosis is to be made. Close liaison with the microbiology department is helpful if atypical infections are to be diagnosed and treated most effectively.

Mycobacteria species

Tuberculosis is still the commonest mycobacterium causing a chronic hand infection in less developed countries but *Mycobacterium marinum* is the commonest species in the developed world. *M. marinum* is commonly found in fish tanks or similar environments and such exposure should be sought in the history.

Mycobacterial infections present in an extremely varied fashion that can involve the skin, subcutaneous tissues, tenosynovium, bursae, joints, and bone. In the hand the commonest presentation is with chronic tenosynovitis, wrist joint infection, or dactylitis. *Mycobacterium leprae* presents very differently and is fortunately rare in the West.

Blood tests and x-rays should be obtained but inflammatory markers are frequently not raised. Microbiology specimens require specific handling and culture techniques for successful growth of organisms. Tissue specimens need to be cultured for aerobic and anaerobic bacteria, typical and atypical mycobacteria, and fungi. Polymerase chain reaction testing of tissue samples can sometimes be useful to confirm the diagnosis. Tissue should also be sent for histology as characteristic caseating or non-caseating granulomas can be diagnostic. If there is a history of travel to developing countries, protozoa and parasites may also need to be considered.

Treatment principles involve obtaining tissue to establish the diagnosis and prolonged antibiotic therapy, depending on sensitivities. Resistance is emerging so liaison with the microbiology team is important. Surgical debridement may be necessary if prolonged antibiotic treatment does not resolve the infection.

Cutaneous

This commonly presents as a nodular or pustular lesion or as a chronic paronychia.

Tenosynovitis

The flexor tendons are most commonly affected, presenting with a characteristic 'sausage digit' or carpal tunnel syndrome that can mimic rheumatoid tenosynovitis. Rice bodies may be palpable subcutaneously. Constitutional symptoms and inflammatory signs are usually absent. There may be a history of previous trauma, a surgical procedure, corticosteroid injections, or water contamination.

Complications include tendon infiltration and rupture, with bone involvement if the diagnosis is delayed for several years.

Arthritis

Pain is an early feature of this condition with swelling and a reduced range of motion. A monoarthritis is most frequent. Deformity and sinuses may occur over time.

Progressive x-ray changes occur with early soft tissue shadowing followed by subchondral cyst formation on either side of the joint and osteopenia. Later, joint destruction, subluxation, and ankylosis may occur.

Treatment consists of synovial biopsy for diagnosis followed by prolonged antibiotics (several months). More aggressive surgical debridement is restricted to cases that respond poorly to this regimen. Arthrodesis may be necessary in the long term.

Osteomyelitis

This typically occurs in the phalanges or metacarpals with local discomfort and pain and occasionally a pathological fracture. Fistulae may form.

Radiographic findings can resemble a tumour with bone destruction and honeycombing but preservation of articular cartilage. In a child the physis can be affected resulting in developmental deformity.

Hansen's disease (leprosy)

This is caused by *Mycobacterium leprae* and affects peripheral nerves and skin, particularly of the cooler peripheries. The highest incidence occurs in Asia and Africa with smaller numbers in South and Central America. Spread is probably from human to human via nasal droplet infection. In the upper limb the ulnar, median, and radial nerves are affected, usually in that order. The autonomic nervous system is also involved. Nerve damage is caused directly by infection, by immune reaction, and by compression of the thickened nerves. Cardinal signs are of an anaesthetic skin patch, nerve thickening, and a hypopigmented skin lesion. Without treatment, damage to anaesthetic digits may occur, deformity may arise from motor imbalance, and Charcot joints may develop.

Slit-skin smears (a cut in affected skin is scraped and smeared onto a glass slide) demonstrating acid-fast bacilli are diagnostic.

Treatment with multidrug therapy eradicates the bacteria. Later in the disease process, pain relief, nerve decompression, restoration of sensation, treatment of deformities, and rehabilitation may all be necessary.

Viral infections

Warts (human papilloma virus)

Human papilloma viruses (HPV) infect cutaneous and epithelia cells. In the hands 95% present as raised cauliflower-like lesions and 5% are flat. They are seen predominantly in children but adults, whose hands are frequently exposed to moisture, can also be affected. In the immunosuppressed, multiple lesions may develop and occasionally transform into squamous cell carcinoma (SCC). In addition, recent evidence points to infection with certain subtypes of HPV as being a cofactor with ultraviolet light exposure for developing SCC.

In children, 90% resolve spontaneously within 5 years. If therapy is indicated treatment with salicylic acid, as a keratolytic agent, has the best evidence of efficacy with a 73% clearance rate. Curettage and surgical excision are alternatives for recalcitrant lesions.

Complications include iatrogenic injury (e.g. to the nail germinal matrix) and recurrence.

Orf

Orf is caused by a pox virus that is endemic in sheep and goats. In animals it produces weeping lesions around the mouth and nose. It is transmitted to humans by direct contact, predominantly affecting farmers and slaughterhouse workers. Orf produces a red weeping nodule 1–2cm in diameter, 95% of which occur on the fingers, hand, wrist, or forearm. The lesions can be very large in the immunocompromised. A crust forms on the surface of the nodule. The lesion heals spontaneously after 4–6 weeks.

Diagnosis is confirmed (if necessary) by electron microscopy of suspensions from the lesions. Treatment is directed at preventing secondary bacterial infection, which may cause scarring, while the lesion heals. Giant lesions may require surgery.

Fungal infections

Fungal infections can be broken down into cutaneous, subcutaneous, and deep infections. Microscopically, fungi can be unicellular yeasts or moulds with multinucleated filamentous hyphae. Cutaneous and subcutaneous infections may occur in the general population but deeper infections occur most frequently in an immunocompromised host. These infections should be suspected in any patient who has an infection that does not respond to antibiotics, drainage, and debridement or with non-diagnostic cultures.

Cutaneous infections

These infections are caused by fungi that metabolize keratin. The nails or macerated skin, such as can occur between digits or in the clenched fist of patients with an upper motor neuron disease, are affected.

The diagnosis is confirmed by nail or skin scrapings with potassium hydroxide staining.

Candida albicans and trichophytosis (ring worm or tinea) are the commonest organisms encountered.

Treatment is with careful hygiene and topical antifungals.

Subcutaneous infections

This includes chronic paronychia (discussed earlier), sporotrichosis (rose thorn disease), and phaeomycotic cysts.

Sporotrichosis is caused by inoculation of *Sporothrix* (*Sporotrichum*) *schenckii* into the skin and subcutaneous tissues by a rose thorn or cat scratch. At the site of inoculation an erythematous nodule arises which becomes ulcerated with raised edges. Characteristic linear nodules appear subsequently along the course of the local lymphatics and lymphadenopathy ensues. A cycle of healing, ulceration, and discharge can continue for years if the diagnosis is not made. Biopsy and specific stains are required to confirm the diagnosis. Treatment is with oral antifungals.

Phaeomycotic cysts are rare and may arise following infection with fungi present on an implanted wood splinter. They usually require surgical removal.

Deep infections

These may affect the tenosynovium, joints, or bone, often with sinuses or ulcers, usually in an immunocompromised host. Organisms include *Aspergillus* spp., *Blastomyces dermatitidis*, *Candida* spp., *Coccidioides immitis*, *Cryptococcus neoformans*, *Histoplasma capsulatum*. *Sporothrix schenckii* may also present rarely in an extracutaneous form, often acquired through the lungs with a concomitant pneumonia. Aggressive therapy and close collaboration with the microbiology team are vital if treatment is to be successful.

Bacterial infections

Actinomycosis

This is caused by *Actinomyces israelii*, a normal inhabitant of the oral cavity. Only 2% of cases occur in the upper extremity. A closed fist injury is the commonest cause with the oral flora impacted into the metacarpal head. Persistent sinuses that drain yellow sulphur granules are characteristic. These granules are conglomerations of the microorganisms. Treatment is with penicillin. For late or recurrent infection with deformity, surgery might be required.

Mycetoma

Mycetoma is a chronic granulomatous infection caused by traumatic inoculation of a bacterium (actinomycetoma) or fungus (eumycetoma) present in the environment—as opposed to the endogenous human flora causing actinomycosis. The infection generally remains localized with swelling, nodule formation, and drainage through sinus tracts. Characteristic granules are discharged that can be black, white, yellow, pink, or red depending on the exact organism involved. Actinomycetes are advanced aerobic bacteria with some characteristics of fungi and are found in association with woody plants and soil. The commonest species are *Pseudallescheria* and *Nocardia*. Only 2–10% of mycetomas affect the hands, the majority occur in the feet. Males are five times more commonly affected than females and are usually not immunocompromised.

Treatment depends on definitive identification of the causal organism from the granules. Actinomycetoma should be treated with antibiotics. Eumycetomas should be widely excised initially with antifungal therapy to follow.

Brucellosis

Brucella spp. are widespread in animals and exposure to cattle, goats, or sheep is necessary for human infection to occur. The disease is endemic in the Mediterranean, Middle East, and South America. Presentation can be with osteomyelitis, septic arthritis, or dactylitis. Treatment is with a 4–6-week course of antibiotics.

Syphilis

Primary disease may present as an ulcer on the tip of the finger or as a paronychia with enlarged local lymph glands.

Secondary disease presents as dactylitis.

Tertiary disease presents with gummata that are chronic granulomatous swellings in any tissue from the skin to the bone.

Congenital syphilis may present as bilateral metacarpal and phalangeal dactylitis with sclerosis and bone destruction.

The causative organism is *Treponema pallidum*. Diagnosis is by serology and microscopy of the exudate from a lesion. Treatment is with antibiotics guided by local sensitivities.

Conclusion

Despite modern antibiotics, hand infections with a variety of organisms continue to be a source of morbidity and mortality. While *Staphylococcus aureus* continues to be the most common cause of infection, resistant strains and other organisms are increasingly being seen. Successful treatment requires identification of the infecting organism, appropriate antibiotic therapy, and proper surgical treatment, although aggressive surgery is less often required in the hand than the lower limb. The treating physician must have knowledge not only of the infecting organism, but also of the host factors contributing to infection. Microbiological advice should be sought for unusual organisms or organisms resistant to initial treatment.

Further reading

Hasham, S., Matteucci, P., Stanley, P.R.W., and Hart, N.B. (2005). Necrotising fasciitis. *British Medical Journal*, **330**, 830–3.

Kanavel, A.B. (1939). *Infections of the Hand.* London: Bailliere, Tindall & Cox.

LeBlanc, D.M., Reece, E.M., Horton, J.B., and Janis, J.E. (2007). Increasing incidence of methicillin-resistant Staphylococcus aureus in hand infections: a 3-year county hospital experience. *Plastic and Reconstructive Surgery*, **119**(3), 935–40.

Lew, D.P. and Waldvogel, F.A. (1997). Osteomyelitis. *New England Journal of Medicine*, **336**(4), 999–1007.

Swartz, M.N. (2004). Cellulitis. *New England Journal of Medicine*, 350, 904–12.

SECTION 7

The Hip

7.1

Indications for hip replacement

J. Miles and Timothy W.R. Briggs

Summary points

- Hip replacement is commonly performed as treatment of a multitude of degenerative hip disorders
- Pain, stiffness, and loss of function remain the primary indicators of the need for hip surgery
- As implant designs and surgical techniques have improved, the range of indications has expanded
- Contraindications and risks must always be counterbalanced with the potential benefits.

Introduction

Total hip replacement is one of the most successful of all elective operations in terms of symptomatic relief (Box 7.1.1). It provides long-term success: currently 90–95% implant survivorship is achieved to 10 years and 85% to 20 years. There are significant improvements in both joint-specific score measurements (such as the Oxford Hip Score) and more general measures of wellbeing (such as health-related qualify of life, HRQOL). Improvements in movement and pain relief translate to improved activity levels and well-being. Younger patients demonstrate the most marked improvement in joint-specific and general health scores postoperatively but all groups show a significant improvement in physical and social function.

Aetiology

Primary osteoarthritis remains the most common indication for hip arthroplasty (Table 7.1.1). Its use following fracture is becoming increasingly prevalent, either as an acute procedure at the time of a displaced subcapital fracture or as an elective procedure for secondary osteoarthritis. Inflammatory arthropathies and sequelae of childhood conditions expose a younger age group to hip replacement. Ankylosing spondylitis frequently presents with hip pain and should be considered in young male patients (Figure 7.1.1).

Box 7.1.1 Epidemiology of total hip replacement

- 1 million hip replacements worldwide in 2008
- 71 000 hip replacements in the UK in 2008
- 5% of individuals over 65 have hip osteoarthritis
- Women more commonly affected than men.

Table 7.1.1 Aetiology of primary hip arthroplasty

Indication	Percentage (Swedish Register)
Primary osteoarthritis	76.9%
Fracture	11.2%
Inflammatory arthritis	4.2%
Avascular necrosis	2.8%
Childhood disorder	1.8%
Other	3.1%

Indications for surgery

Johnstone and colleagues described the six most specific features of hip pathology which should be addressed by hip replacement; these are detailed in Box 7.1.2. The symptoms which are important to the patient are not always the same as the surgeon would imagine: leisure activities, sexual activities, and limb-length discrepancies are more important to the individual than surgeons recognizes (Box 7.1.3). See Box 7.1.4 for a summary of the indications for surgery.

Pain

This is usually the most prominent symptom of hip arthritis and the most significant indication for hip replacement. It begins with an intermittent ache which is related to activity and relieved by rest. The most common sites of pain are the groin, the anterior and lateral thigh, the buttock, and the knee. As the degeneration progresses, it tends to constancy, including pain at rest and pain waking the patient at night. Both surgeons and referring physicians agree that rest pain, night pain, and pain affecting activity are the most significant indicators that a hip should be replaced.

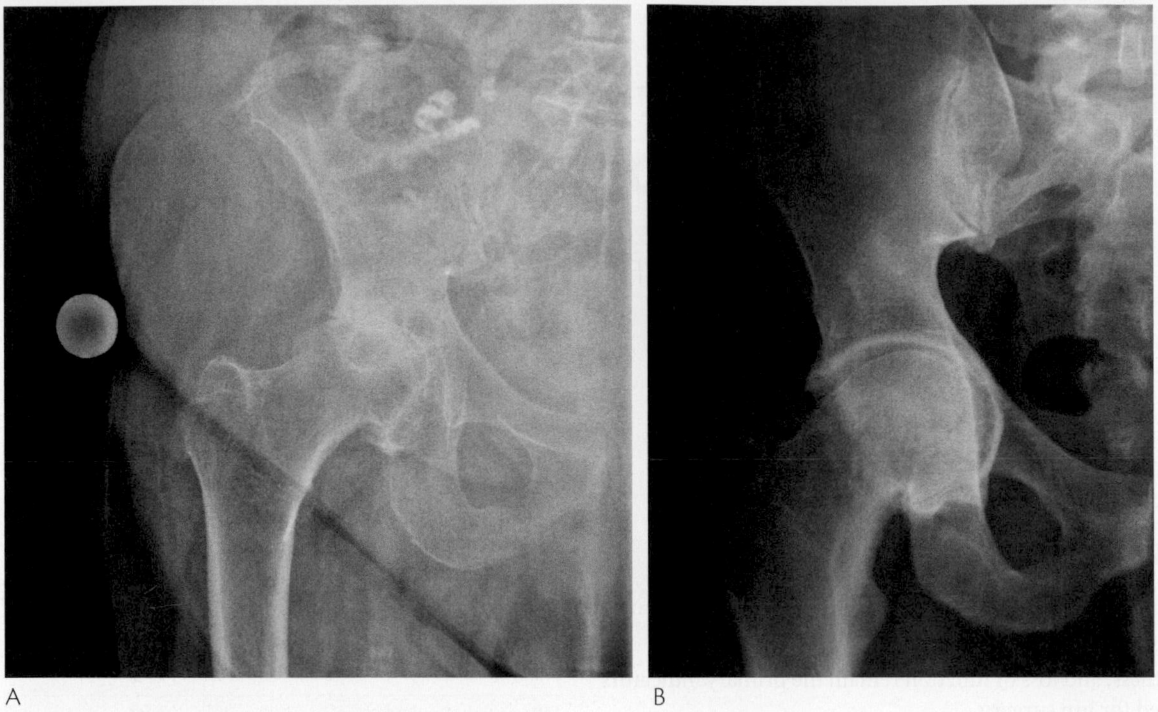

Fig. 7.1.1 A) Primary osteoarthritis of the hip.B) Protrusio hip as a presenting feature of ankylosing spondylitis.

Box 7.1.2 The important aims of hip replacement

- Pain relief
- Ability to work
- Increased level of activity
- Further walking capacity
- Satisfaction of the patient
- Physical examination parameters improved.

Box 7.1.3 Surgeons' rating of symptoms

- Rest pain
- Night pain
- Pain with activity
- Functional impairment
- Decreased range of motion
- Osteoarthritis x-ray changes
- Impaired social contact.

Examination of an early osteoarthritic hip reveals pain on flexion and internal rotation, with reduced range of motion and pain on abduction following with further degeneration.

There is no valid point at which pain can be defined as necessitating hip replacement: the balance of benefits against risks is determined, on an individual basis, between surgeon and patient.

Loss of function

Functional deterioration is usually closely linked to pain. Even moderate hip degeneration can lead to difficulties with pedicure and putting on footwear. Advanced arthropathy frequently affects the ability to climb stairs, access public transport, or rise from a chair. Loss of function can lead to loss of work, reduction in social well-being, and, eventually, dependence upon higher levels of support without intervention. Hip arthroplasty produces functional improvement in all areas, whatever the hip pathology.

Stiffness

The extreme rigidity associated with ankylosing spondylitis is frequently relatively pain-free, even in complete ankylosis. The typical flexion hip deformities are extremely disabling and significant improvement is offered by hip arthroplasty.

A previous hip fusion, even when successful, often produces low back pain, contralateral hip arthritis, and ipsilateral knee arthritis. Hip replacement is successful, whether the ankylosis is surgical or spontaneous (usually as a result of infection). Most patients achieve relief of pain in adjacent joints and an improvement in walking ability, although the latter is dependent on the persistence of gluteal function in the operated hip.

Gait abnormalities

Limp is a common symptom and can be due to limb-length discrepancy, capsular contractions, muscle weakness, and pain. The use of walking aids is usually well tolerated but the majority of patients walk unsupported after primary hip replacement.

Radiographic changes

Joint destruction and clinical deterioration of hip function tend to go hand in hand. X-ray appearances alone are not used as indication for arthroplasty without clinical need. It is also possible that severe symptoms can coexist with mild radiological signs of wear. In these cases, the injection of local anaesthetic into the hip joint can be used diagnostically; it is safe and reliable. Temporary relief of symptoms predicts successful hip replacement, but failure of relief suggests an alternative diagnosis should be sought.

Contraindications to surgery (Box 7.1.4)

Absolute contraindications

The presence of joint sepsis is an inescapable contraindication to surgery. Presence of distant infection with systemic upset (hyperthermia or raised inflammatory markers) or active cutaneous infection overlying the affected limb also precludes surgery. Chronic infective processes should be dampened as much as is possible before surgery.

Relative contraindications

Extremes of age are frequently cited as relative contraindications to surgery. Hip replacement has expanded to both ends of the age range as it has proven successful. It is now undertaken from teenagers to centurions with success. Its potential benefits in youth must be weighed up against the likelihood of multiple revisions. However, it is now the operation of choice in patients with arthritis above closed physes, having displaced fusion and excision due to their inferior results. Similarly, improved anaesthetic techniques have improved survivorship amongst the elderly. In a population of patients operated on at over 85 years of age, survivorship to 5 years after surgery is over 50% and to 10 years is over 35%.

Obesity is no longer an absolute contraindication to hip replacement as several papers have shown equivalent results in patients with a body mass index (BMI) above 30 to those with a BMI below 30. In morbid obesity, BMI above 40, the surgery is lengthy and more difficult but results remain satisfactory.

Neuropathic arthropathy, usually secondary to diabetes, syphilis, or syringomyelia, is a very rare cause of hip pathology and has previously been seen as an absolute contraindication to hip replacement. Although associated with high rates of complications, it is amenable to hip replacement in cases of severe joint destruction associated with significant symptoms. Similarly, sequelae of cerebral palsy can be treated with hip replacement but are associated with high rates of loosening or dislocation. It is best reserved for ambulatory patients with unilateral hip involvement; non-ambulatory patients may achieve pain relief with arthrodesis.

Manual labour in younger patients is now possible after hip replacement. Return to work has been shown to be mutifactorial, not just related to the type of work. Other factors include level of education, underlying illness, and the balance of social security benefits against work pay.

Significant medical comorbidity can be a relative contraindication: particularly poorly controlled diabetes, cardiac insufficiency, and respiratory failure. Cooperation between the patient, surgeon, physician, and anaesthetist is required to reach an informed decision. Similarly, local factors such as poor vascularity or soft tissue compromise can require input from vascular and plastic surgeons respectively in order to reach an informed decision as to whether hip replacement is advised.

Psychiatric disease, including dementia, should be evaluated to ascertain if the individual will be able to benefit from improved function and comply with basic postoperative requirements.

Box 7.1.4 Indications and contraindications for hip surgery

- Indications:
  - Pain
  - Loss of function
  - Stiffness
  - Gait abnormalities
- Contraindications:
  - Sepsis (local or distant)
  - Neuropathic hip
  - Systemic comorbidity
  - Inadequate vascularity
  - Psychiatric illness.

Further reading

Andrew, J.G., Palan, J., Kurup, H.V., Gibson, P., Murray, D.W., and Beard, D.J. (2008). Obesity in total hip replacement. *Journal of Bone and Joint Surgery*, **90B**, 424–9.

Crawford, R., Gie, G., Ling, R., and Murray, D. (1998). Diagnostic value of intra-articular anaesthetic in primary osteoarthritis of the hip. *Journal of Bone and Joint Surgery*, **80B**, 279–81.

Dreinhoefer, K., Dieppe, P., Til, S., *et al.* (2006). Indications for total hip replacement. *Annals of Rheumatic Diseases*, **65**, 1346–50.

Johnstone, R.C., Fitzgerald, R.H., Harris, W.H., Poss, R., Muller, M.E., and Sledge, C.B. (1990). Clinical and radiographic evaluation of total hip replacement. *Journal of Bone and Joint Surgery*, **72A**, 161–8.

Kärrholm, J., Garellick, G., and Herberts, P. (2008). *Swedish Hip Arthroplasty Register. Annual Report 2006.* Göteborg: Sahlgrenska University Hospital.

Ramiah, R.D., Ashmore, A.M., Whitley, E., and Bannister, G.C. (2007). Ten-year life expectancy after total hip replacement. *British Journal of Bone and Joint Surgery*, **89B**, 1299–302.

Suarez, J., Arguelles, J., Costales, M., *et al.* (2003). Factors influencing the return to work of patients after hip replacement and rehabilitation. *Archives of Physical Medicine and Rehabilitation*, **77**(3), 269–72.

Wright, J., Rudicel, S., and Feinstein, A. (1994). Ask patients what they want: evaluation of individual complaints before total hip replacement. *Journal of Bone and Joint Surgery*, **76B**, 229–34.

7.2

Approaches to the hip

J. Miles and Timothy W.R. Briggs

Summary points

- The development of safe and reliable approaches has allowed hip replacement surgery to be undertaken successfully
- There are four main approaches, each with their inherent advantages and disadvantages
- Awareness of the structures at risk with each approach reduces the risk of iatrogenic injury
- All of the approaches have been modified and improved upon to address specific weaknesses.

Introduction

Hip surgery has evolved from simple techniques, through excision arthroplasty and the development of modern total hip replacement surgery. As the operations have become more complex, visualization of the proximal femur and, in particular, the acetabulum has become increasingly important. An accurate and reliable approach is critical to the success of any primary or revision hip replacement. In order to achieve this, a variety of approaches have been pioneered and improved upon. Each has its own advantages and disadvantages and none can claim to be perfect (Table 7.2.1). There are a multitude of modifications but they can be grouped into four areas in order to simplify their comparison as listed in Box 7.2.1.

The anterior approach

The anterior approach uses the internervous interval between sartorius and tensor fascia lata, supplied by the femoral and superior gluteal nerves respectively. It was popularized by Smith-Peterson, who first described it in 1917, and further described its application in 'mold arthroplasty of the hip' in 1949. Subsequently, it has been adapted to allow for 'mini-open' femoro-acetabular impingement surgery and been incorporated into minimal invasive hip replacement surgery. It is performed supine, making bilateral surgery easier. It allows excellent views of the anterior femoral head and neck though is limited in acetabular exposure and visualization of the proximal femur can be difficult. In order to extend the approach, extensive dissection of the abductors from the ilium is required to expose the acetabulum in its entirety and division of the external rotators allows delivery of the proximal femur into view. In addition, the approach requires division of both origins of rectus femoris. The lateral femoral cutaneous nerve crosses the incision and should be preserved, as its division often produces a tender neuroma.

Less invasive surgery has modified the approach to include just the central portion of the incision and preserve the rectus femoris intact. Keggi and colleagues report excellent results with this minimally invasive surgical (MIS) approach. It does not require osteotomy or transection of any muscle belly or tendon so is proposed to allow quicker return to full function, reduced bleeding, and shorter hospital stay. It remains a matter of controversy with studies at other centres finding high complication rates, particularly with respect to component malposition, femoral fracture, and failure of femoral component fixation.

Box 7.2.1 Approaches to the hip for total hip replacement

- Anterior
- Anterolateral
- Direct lateral/transgluteal
- Posterior.

Position

Supine.

Landmarks

Anterior superior iliac spine (ASIS) and the iliac crest.

Incision

'J'-shaped incision, starting along the iliac crest and sweeping just below the ASIS and passing vertically along the anterior femur.

Procedure (Figures 7.2.1 and 7.2.2)

Identify and split the interval between sartorius and tensor fascia lata, erring towards tensor fascia lata to prevent damage to the lateral cutaneous nerve on the fascia of sartorius.

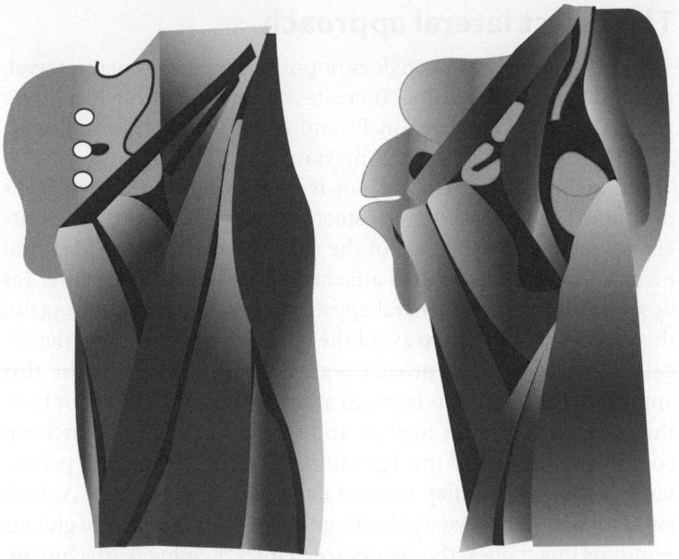

Fig. 7.2.1 The interval between sartorius and tensor fascia lata used in the anterior approach.

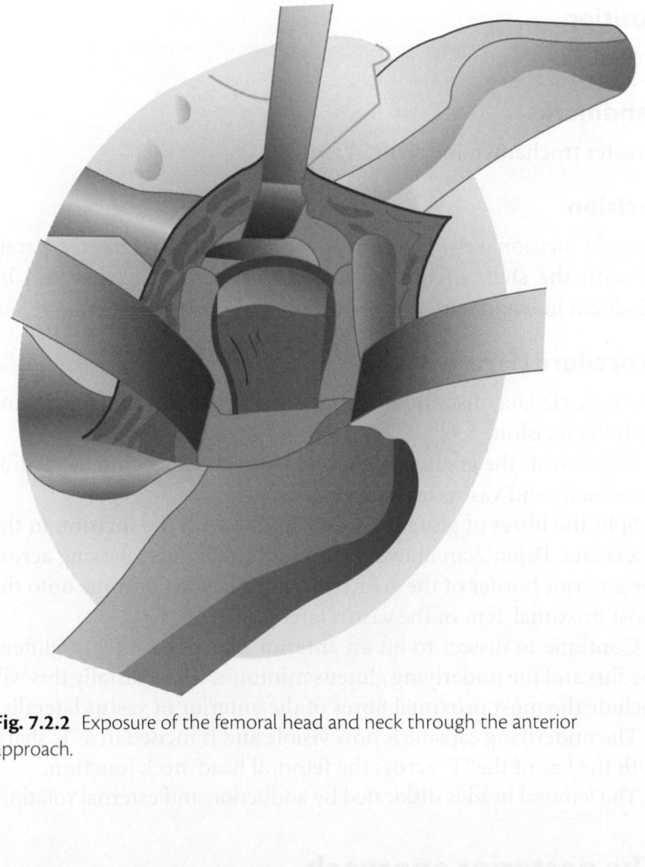

Fig. 7.2.2 Exposure of the femoral head and neck through the anterior approach.

This exposes the underlying muscles—gluteus medius and rectus femoris. Detach the direct head of rectus from the anterior inferior iliac spine and the reflected head of rectus from the superior margin of the acetabulum. The reflected head has fibres which blend with the anterior capsule—these should be carefully dissected.

Rectus femoris can now be retracted medially and gluteus medius retracted laterally. The capsule is now visible with iliopsoas passing medially to its insertion on the lesser trochanter.

Incise the capsule and the hip is exposed by adduction and external rotation of the leg.

The anterolateral approach

The anterolateral group of approaches all gain access through the interval between tensor facia lata and gluteus medius, utilizing a variety of methods of detachment of the hip abductors to expose both sides of the hip joint. It has its origins in the description by Watson-Jones in 1936 and was further advanced by McFarland and Osborne in 1954. It has been changed and applied to hip replacement by a multitude of famous hip surgeons, notably Charnley in the 1960s, Müller in the 1970s, and Hardinge in the 1980s. The patient can be positioned in either the supine or lateral decubitus position. The detachment of the abductors can be achieved in two ways: osteotomy of the trochanter (as popularized by Charnley) or transection of the anterior portion of distal gluteus medius and gluteus minimus tendon (as popularized by Müller). Both methods provide excellent access to both the acetabulum and the proximal femur and variations on the anterolateral approach remain very popular in total hip replacement and hemiarthroplasty of the hip.

As the posterior structures are maintained, the approaches allow inherently stable closure, reducing the rate of dislocation when compared with posterior exposures. Equally, both have disadvantages. Trochanteric osteotomy has an incidence of non-union, bursitis, and metalwork failure. The detachment of gluteus medius risks its denervation and the approach is associated with an incidence of Trendelenburg gait. Variations have been described in attempts to reduce the chance of a postoperative Trendelenburg gait; they propose avoidance of damage to the superior gluteal nerve (particularly the large and more significant superior branch). Learmonth's omega approach detaches the whole gluteus medius and minimus then splits vastus lateralis near its posterior border, avoiding denervation of most of it. Hanssen's approach involves a longitudinal split in the fibres of gluteus medius but much further posterior than that described by Müller. These approaches are described as modifications of the anterolateral approach but many, particularly that of Hardinge, fall into the direct lateral group.

Position

Lateral.

Landmarks

Greater trochanter and shaft of femur.

Incision

Slightly curved, apex posterior, incision centred over the greater trochanter passing parallel with the shaft of the femur, across the centre of the greater trochanter. Typically the incision will be 12–20cm in length for primary surgery.

Procedure (Figures 7.2.3 and 7.2.4)

Incise fascia lata, distally, and tensor fascia lata, proximally, in line with the incision.

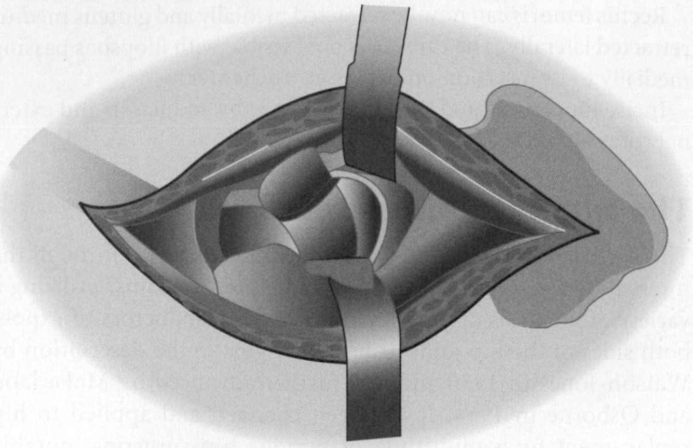

Fig. 7.2.3 The anterolateral approach.

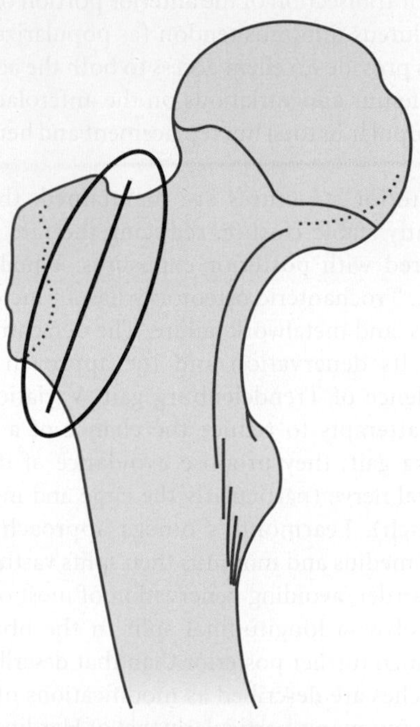

Fig. 7.2.4 The orientation of a trochanteric osteotomy.

This reveals the greater trochanter, with attached gluteus medius proximally and vastus lateralis distally.

If a trochanteric osteotomy is to be used, the greater trochanter is removed with a saw, starting 1cm below the vastus tubercle and aiming for the junction of the greater trochanter and the femoral neck. If an osteotomy is not used, the leg is externally rotated to stretch the gluteus medius and minimus. Dissect gluteus medius and the underlying gluteus minimus tendon off the anterior border of the greater trochanter. Use blunt dissection to reveal the anterior capsule of the hip, with the reflected head of rectus femoris. Dissect the reflected head off the anterior capsule.

To reveal the femoral head, the capsule is incised, typically in a 'T' shape centred on the femoral head and neck junction.

The hip is dislocated by adduction and external rotation.

The direct lateral approach

The direct lateral approach does not use an intermuscular interval, rather it is muscle splitting. It creates an interval through splitting gluteus medius fibres proximally and vastus lateralis fibres distally. The approach was pioneered by Harris, in 1967, again for use in 'mold arthroplasty'. The patient is held in the lateral decubitus position. The upper femur is osteotomized between the vastus lateralis tubercle and the base of the superior surface of the femoral neck, keeping the abductors attached to the greater trochanter (as described in the anterolateral approach—see Figure 7.2.4). Again, this has been modified to avoid the need for an osteotomy: the so-called transgluteal approach was described in 1979. In this approach, the incision is between anterior third and posterior two-thirds of both gluteus medius and vastus lateralis. The incision continues to bone and the dissection is carried out through periosteum, elevating each flap without damaging muscle fibres. A similar approach, described by Hardinge in 1982, leaves a cuff of gluteus minimus intact upon the greater trochanter, helping reattachment. The direct lateral approach has the ability to provide excellent exposure of the femur and is easily extended distally. However, proximal extension is not possible as splitting of the gluteus medius greater than 3–5cm above the tip of the greater trochanter risks damage to the superior gluteal nerve. This limits its application in cases of complex acetabular reconstruction.

Position

Lateral.

Landmarks

Greater trochanter and shaft of femur.

Incision

Straight incision passing directly over the greater trochanter, parallel with the shaft of the femur. Typically, the incision will be 12–20cm in length and centred on the greater trochanter.

Procedure (Figure 7.2.5)

Incise fascia lata, distally, and tensor fascia lata, proximally, in line with the incision.

This reveals the greater trochanter, with attached gluteus medius proximally and vastus lateralis distally.

Split the fibres of gluteus medius in line with the incision in the fascia lata. Begin 2cm above the greater trochanter, passing across the anterior border of the greater trochanter and continue onto the most proximal 2cm of the vastus lateralis.

Continue to dissect to lift an anterior flap, consisting of gluteus medius and the underlying gluteus minimus. More distally this will include the most proximal fibres of the anterior of vastus lateralis.

The underlying capsule is now visible and is incised in a 'T' shape with the bar of the 'T' across the femoral head-neck junction.

The femoral head is dislocated by adduction and external rotation.

The posterior approach

The posterior approach is another muscle splitting exposure: longitudinal split of the gluteus maximus fibres is used but there is no associated denervation as the muscle is innervated far medial from the split. The joint is exposed through division of the short external rotators of the hip. The lateral position is used. The exposure was

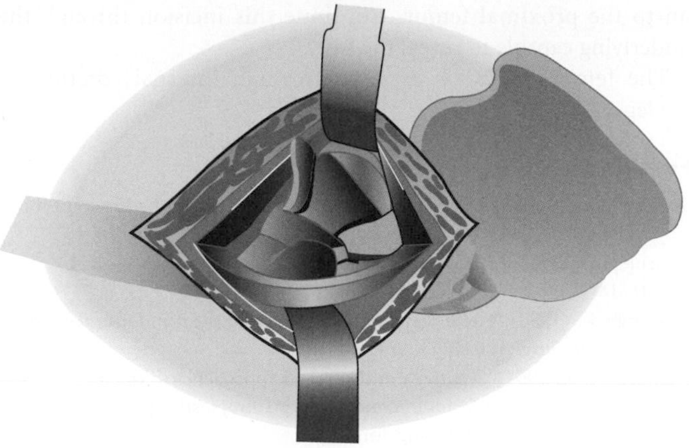

Fig. 7.2.5 The direct lateral approach to the hip.

introduced by Moore in 1957 and further detailed in his paper of 1959. The posterior approach does not encroach upon the hip abductors, far reducing the incidence of Trendelenburg gait after surgery. In addition it provides good visualization of both the pelvis and the femur, being easily extensile in both directions. The approach has also been condensed to only its central portion, as the mini-posterior approach, a form of minimally invasive approach. In this approach, the gluteus maximus tendon is not incised and pronator quadratus, the lowest short external rotator, is unviolated. Disadvantages of either posterior approach include the proximity to the sciatic nerve, which requires careful protection throughout and the division of posterior structures, which can result in an increased incidence of dislocation. The resistance to dislocation is dependent upon adequate repair of the short external rotators. A significant advance in the posterior approach has been the development of an enhanced posterior repair method, reducing dislocation rates from 5% to less than 1%. This method relies on direct fixation to bone: drilling through the proximal femur and passing sutures through the external rotators then through these

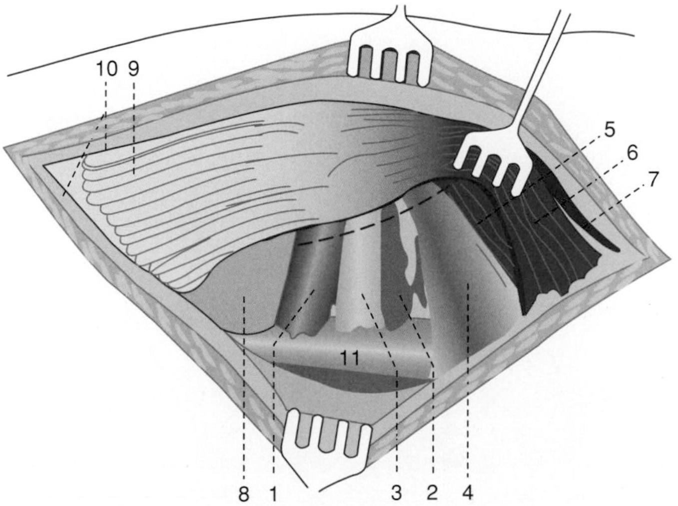

Fig. 7.2.6 Incision of the short external rotators in the posterior approach.

drill holes. When this technique is used, the rates of dislocation are comparable with those of the other approaches.

Position

Lateral.

Landmarks

Greater trochanter and shaft of femur.

Incision

Curvilinear incision centred on the posterior border of the greater trochanter. The proximal portion swings posteriorly, to lie parallel

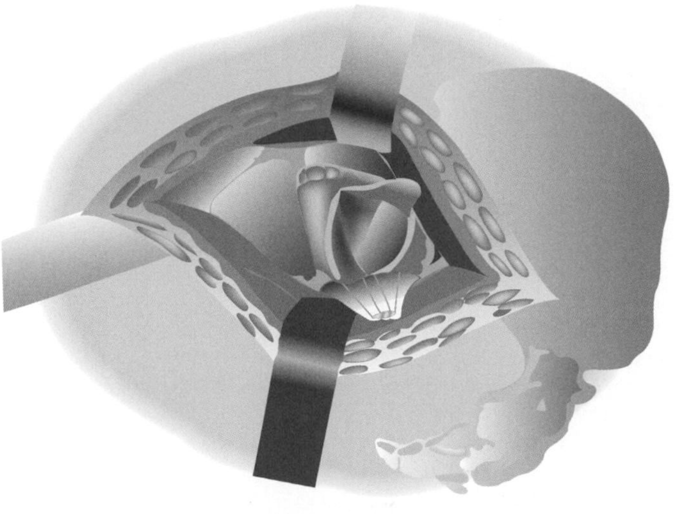

Fig. 7.2.7 The posterior approach to the hip.

Table 7.2.1 Approaches to the hip

Approach	Pioneer	Modifications	Advantages	Disadvantages
Anterior	Smith-Peterson (1917)	Keggi (MIS)	Excellent view of anterior structures, adaptable for MIS	Difficult to see acetabulum; lateral femoral cutaneous nerve
Antero-lateral	Watson-Jones (1936)	McFarland and Osborne; Charnley; Müller	Good visualization of pelvis and proximal femur, low dislocation rate	Metalwork problems (if osteotomy used), abductor denervation
Direct lateral	Harris (1967)	Transgluteal, Hardinge	Good proximal exposure, low dislocation rate	Superior gluteal nerve injury, poor exposure of superior acetabulum
Posterior	Moore (1957)	Pellicci repair	Excellent exposure of pelvis and femur, avoids abductor mechanism	Sciatic nerve injury, need for careful posterior repair to prevent dislocation

MIS, minimally invasive surgery.

to the fibres of gluteus maximus, passing posterosuperiorly towards the buttock. The distal portion lies along the posterior border of the shaft of the femur.

Procedure (Figures 7.2.6 and 7.2.7)

Incise fascia lata in line with the femur distally; more proximally the fibres of gluteus maximus are encountered and should be split bluntly in line with the skin incision, i.e. parallel with the muscle fibres.

This reveals gluteus medius, lying superficial and anterior to the short external rotators of the hip. By holding the hip in slight internal rotation and retracting under gluteus medius, the short external rotators are further exposed. Taking care not to damage the sciatic nerve, divide the external rotators close to their insertion on to the proximal femur. Continue this incision through the underlying capsule to reveal the hip.

The femoral head is exposed through internal rotation of the leg.

Further reading

Smith-Petersen, M. (1949). Approach to and exposure of the hip joint for mold arthroplasty. *Journal of Bone and Joint Surgery*, **31A**, 40–6.

Charnley, J. (1961). Arthroplasty of the hip: a new operation. *Lancet*, **1**(7187), 1129–32.

Hardinge, K. (1982). The direct lateral approach to the hip. *Journal of Bone and Joint Surgery*, **64B**(1), 17–19.

Hanssen, A.D. (1991). Anatomy and surgical approaches to the hip. In: Morrey, B.F. (ed) *Joint Replacement Arthroplasty*, pp. 516–20. New York: Churchill Livingstone.

7.3

Preoperative planning for total hip replacement, consent, and complications

R.W.J. Carrington and Rashid Khan

Summary points

- Preoperative planning is essential to achieve successful results after total hip replacement
- Obtaining informed consent is important for both surgeon and patient
- The surgeon must have a comprehensive knowledge of the aetiology and treatment of the common associated complications.

Introduction

Preoperative planning is of the utmost importance in performing total hip replacement successfully and obtaining reproducible results. For the surgeon, meticulous planning allows for efficient utilization of resources, the selection of appropriate implants, the need for any special equipment, and the anticipation of intraoperative difficulties. It shortens the learning curve when performing relatively new procedures, and achieves consistent results. Because total hip replacement is an operation aimed at improving quality of life, emphasis must be placed on prevention of complications rather than salvage afterwards.

Patients undergoing hip replacement are often elderly. The approach should be a multidisciplinary one. Patient education, attention to psychosocial needs, and early assessment of home circumstances will assure timely discharge home and increased satisfaction (Box 7.3.1).

Box 7.3.1 Preoperative planning: patient factors

- Patient education:
  - Details of operation
  - Rehabilitation, physiotherapy
  - Complications
- Discharge planning:
  - Assess home circumstances
  - Need for extra home care
- Assess patient expectations, set appropriate goals.

Clinical assessment

The process begins with the careful evaluation of the whole patient (Box 7.3.2). The indication for hip replacement must be well founded and appropriate. It is important to clarify that the signs and symptoms for which treatment is sought is attributable to the hip, and not the adjacent joint or overlying soft tissues. Childhood conditions such as developmental dysplasia of the hip, slipped upper femoral epiphysis, and Perthes' will have obvious consequences on the choice of implant due to altered anatomy, as will any previous surgery for these conditions.

Box 7.3.2 Preoperative assessment: history

- Pain
- Function
- Deformity
- Childhood orthopaedic disorders
- Previous limb trauma
- Past medical history
- Drug history
- Early referral to anaesthetist/physician to optimize any potential anaesthetic risks.

Box 7.3.3 Preoperative assessment: examination

- Gait
- Hip range of motion—active, passive
- Limb-length discrepancy
- Presence of scars
- Spine
- Knee
- Neurovascular status.

Box 7.3.4 Successful hip arthroplasty: restoration of biomechanics

- Restore centre of rotation
- Restore leg length
- Restore femoral offset.

Box 7.3.5 Radiographic assessment

- AP view of pelvis centred over pubic symphysis
- AP view of affected hip
- True lateral view of affected hip
- AP views taken with patient supine and hip in 10–15 degrees of internal rotation to counter the normal anteversion of the femoral neck.

The preoperative examination (Box 7.3.3) should include assessment of the patient's gait, as well as the spine and knee. Any conditions precluding the use of crutches or walking aids will have obvious consequences. Limb-length discrepancy, both true and apparent, should be established. The true limb length is measured from the anterior superior iliac spine to the medial malleolus; apparent length is from any midline structure, e.g. the umbilicus, to the medial malleolus. The commonest reason for apparent leg-length discrepancy is abduction or adduction contractures around the hip. When there is a difference between actual and apparent leg length, pelvic obliquity should be assessed with the patient sitting and standing. Pelvic obliquity due to causes above the pelvis, e.g. lumbar scoliosis, persists in the sitting position. Conversely, obliquity due to causes in or below the pelvis, e.g. gross arthritis, post-traumatic deformity of the pelvis, infection, or muscle contracture, resolves on sitting. In addition, leg-length discrepancy due to more distal causes, such as limb fracture, poliomyelitis, infection, and physeal trauma, should be excluded.

Correcting any leg-length discrepancy optimizes muscle function and provides the patient with improved gait and increased comfort, provided the stability of the hip replacement is not compromised, and sciatic nerve function not threatened.

Patients at high risk of postoperative dislocation, e.g. due to neuromuscular problems, should be identified. This may influence the choice of implant, e.g. the use of a larger femoral head to confer greater stability.

Radiographic review

The aim of implant positioning in hip arthroplasty is to restore the biomechanics (Box 7.3.4); templating helps to achieve this reliably and consistently. The traditional method of templating involves the use of transparent acetate templates held against hard-copy radiographs. The magnification of radiographs is generally in the region of 110–125%, and this needs to be known. Templates are usually supplied by the manufacturer.

Acetabular templating

Templating usually follows the steps of surgery, and attention is first turned to the acetabulum to determine the centre of rotation, and the cup position and size. A horizontal reference line can be drawn through the base of the teardrops, which represents the true floor of the acetabulum; it is also helpful to identify two further key anatomic landmarks—the ilioischial line and the superolateral margin of the acetabulum (Figure 7.3.1). Correct positioning and orientation of the cup is essential for the stability of the hip replacement. The cup should be sized so that it lies in 45 degrees of abduction, the medial border approximates the ilioischial line, and there is adequate lateral coverage. The inferior border of the cup is placed level with the teardrop line (Figure 7.3.2). In cemented cups there should be a 2–3-mm uniform cement mantle. The centre of rotation should be marked, and compared with the contralateral hip; templating the contralateral hip is useful in the presence of bone loss. Any osteophytes that need removal and cysts that require curettage and grafting are noted. Special care must be taken to seat the cup in the anatomically correct position in the presence of protrusio acetabuli, a lateralized acetabulum due to medial osteophytes and the dysplastic acetabulum; the use of bone graft may be required to augment any defects in these situations.

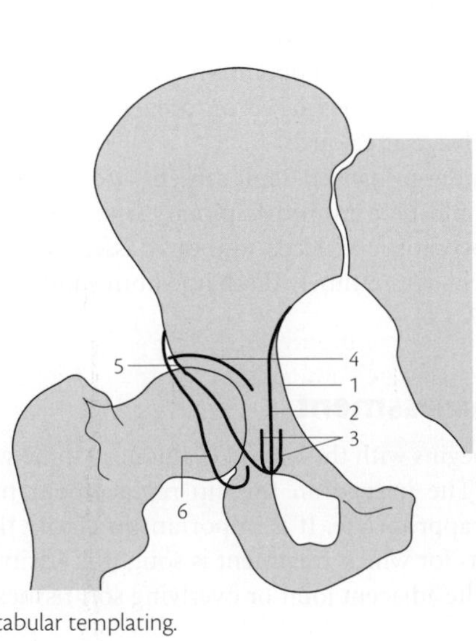

Fig. 7.3.1 Acetabular templating.

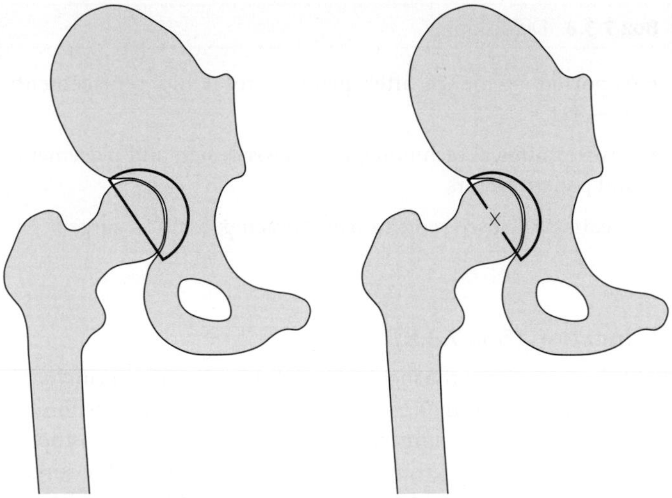

Fig. 7.3.2 Preoperative planning. The correct size and position of the acetabular component is chosen. The amount of acetabular bone that should be removed (left) and the hip center (×, right) are indicated.

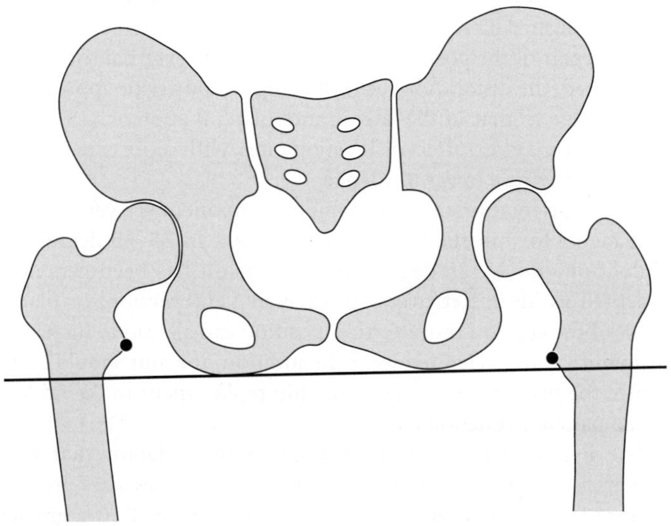

Fig. 7.3.3 Preoperative planning. Determination of leg length on the pelvic view by drawing a line, which hits the most distal part of the os ischii. The most medial part of the lesser trochanter has to be used as a femoral landmark.

Femoral templating

The aims of femoral templating are to restore femoral offset, optimize limb length and correctly size the stem. The anteroposterior (AP) view of the pelvis is useful to assess limb-length discrepancy. The teardrop line is used to orientate the pelvic axis; alternatively, a horizontal line drawn through the most distal part of the ischial tuberosities is also commonly used. The former is more accurate, as it lies nearer the centre of rotation of the hip joint. The vertical distance between this reference line and the most medial part of the lesser trochanters will enable measurement of any limb-length difference (Figure 7.3.3). The radiographic discrepancy should be compared with that measured clinically.

A line perpendicular to the femoral shaft at the level of the tip of the greater trochanter can be used to assess the desired level of the centre of rotation of the femoral head; caution must be exercised in the presence of coxa valga and coxa vara, as the true centre of rotation will then lie above and below the tip of the trochanter respectively. The stem size is chosen next, depending on the mode of fixation—for a cemented stem a 2–3mm cement mantle is desirable. For cementless fixation, adequate endosteal contact is required, either proximally or in the diaphysis, depending on prosthetic design. Finally, the femoral template is translated proximally or distally depending on the desired limb-length correction. The amount of limb-length change produced by surgery will be the vertical distance between the centre of rotation of the femoral component and the centre of rotation of the acetabular component.

The femoral offset should restore the offset of the normal hip; this can be judged from the contralateral hip if required. The offset is the horizontal distance between the centre of rotation of the hip joint and the longitudinal axis of the femur, and there is large anatomical variation (Figure 7.3.3). Failure to reproduce the correct offset will decrease the abductor moment arm, lead to a limp, increase joint reaction force and wear, and cause instability. Once again, the change in offset produced by surgery will be the horizontal distance between the centre of the femoral head and the centre of rotation of the cup on templating. Some stem designs allow for different offsets and neck-shaft angle. In addition, the angle and level of neck osteotomy can also be altered. In this way, it may be possible to adjust for anatomic variations in offset. Finally, when the surgeon is happy with the chosen size and position of the stem, the new centre of rotation and the position of the neck cut should be marked. Templating should usually aim for the middle range of neck lengths to allow for adjustment to a shorter or longer size of head intraoperatively if required.

The lateral view of the hip helps to plan the location of the femoral opening, and assess the femoral bow and the AP canal diameter. Any excessive femoral anteversion can be detected on a true lateral view. An inaccurate femoral entry point can lead to eccentric reaming and concomitant shaft perforation.

Digital radiographic technology is increasingly being introduced into hospitals in association with Picture Archiving and Communication Systems (PACS). This has changed the traditional templating process; the central issue here is of variable magnification in the digital images. An external scale marker of known dimension attached to the patient at the time of imaging is therefore needed to assess the magnification. On-screen templating requires specific digital software, and are now commercially available, although at considerable cost. The sequence of steps involved in templating is similar to those outlined earlier. The hope is that these will make the whole process faster and more accurate, and translate to improved patient outcomes.

Consent

Informed consent is a legal requirement before any surgical procedure. Effective communication is the key to enabling patients to make informed decisions. Successfully consenting a patient to treatment revolves around three key issues: the patient must have adequate mental capacity to make the decision; have sufficient information upon which to base their decision (Box 7.3.6); and reach that decision voluntarily without undue duress.

The surgeon should pass on that information which any reasonable patient would wish to know before giving consent. In the setting of hip replacement, this should include the common

Box 7.3.6 Consent: patient information

- Nature of patient's condition
- Nature and purpose of the procedure
- Probability of specific/general risks
- Other operative/non-operative alternatives
- Prognosis with no treatment.

risks and complications. If cardiopulmonary or systemic condition places the patient at high risk, the patient should be fully informed and guided with relatives in deciding whether to undergo surgery.

The doctor who consents should whenever possible be the one carrying out the procedure, or at least be appropriately qualified and familiar with all the details involved. The explanation given to the patient is of paramount importance and the signing of the consent form is of secondary significance. Due consideration should be given to language ability, appropriate setting, and adequate time.

A structured verbal discussion of the information has traditionally been the mode of imparting the information. Alternatively, a written information sheet may also be employed, and this may enhance patients' comprehension and recall of information.

The increasingly litiginous environment at present may endanger the surgeon's ability to practice. Good consenting practice is crucial both for the patient and for the surgeon. A recent review of malpractice claims of an insurance company that involved orthopaedic surgeons noted that all the claims involved elective surgery, and not a single emergency case. Poor communication was established as the critical factor linked to malpractice claims. Documentation in the surgeon's notes that informed consent took place was associated with a decreased risk of indemnity payment; dictating even a brief description of the informed consent processes—whether part of the clinic notes or the operative notes—is deemed as more legally substantive.

Complications of total hip replacement

Patients undergoing total hip replacement often have significant medical comorbidities, and the general risks of surgery must not be forgotten when obtaining informed consent. Cardiovascular, pulmonary, and renal complications can occur, and patients should be counselled as to these (Box 7.3.7).

Box 7.3.7 Complications of hip replacement

- Dislocation
- Infection
- Thromboembolism
- Limb-length inequality
- Neurovascular injury
- Fracture.

Box 7.3.8 Dislocation

- Reported incidence after primary total hip replacement: 0.2–7%
- Causes: surgical technique, prosthesis design and placement, and patient factors
- Treatment: closed reduction and bracing; revision surgery.

Dislocation (Box 7.3.8)

Published reports of the incidence of dislocation after primary hip arthroplasty vary from 0.2–7%, the majority occurring within the first few months after surgery. Variables that influence postoperative instability can be grouped into: factors related to the surgical technique; factors related to the prosthesis; and factors related to the patient.

The surgical approach has commonly been cited as a risk factor for dislocation, with the direct lateral and anterolateral approaches reporting lower rates than the posterior approach. A recent meta-analysis, however, concluded that there was insufficient evidence in the published literature to support this claim. Others have stated that if repair of the posterior capsule and short external rotators is performed, the dislocation rate following the posterior approach is comparable to that of the lateral/anterolateral approach. Surgical experience may also affect dislocation rates, with more experienced surgeons having a lower incidence.

Proper orientation of the acetabular component is a very important factor for hip stability. Cup placement in 35–45 degrees of abduction and 15–25 degrees of anteversion has been generally accepted as ideal. Retroversion, excessive anteversion, or placement of the cup in a more vertical position can all lead to increased instability and accelerated wear. In addition, the aim should be to centre the primary arc range of the hip replacement in the middle of the patient's functional range.

The use of larger femoral heads is another factor that may enhance postoperative stability. Larger femoral head sizes provide a more favourable head–neck ratio and therefore allow a greater arc of motion before impingement occurs. The use of constrained liners can also decrease instability rates; however, their use may be associated with increased polyethylene wear and loosening secondary to impingement.

Inadequate restoration of femoral offset results in decreased tension on the abductor musculature and subsequent instability. Preoperative templating should ensure that when the prosthetic stem is inserted, appropriate neck length and offset are restored. Restored hip mechanics confer stability via optimized abductor tension.

Finally, inherent neuromuscular disorders in the patient can affect hip stability by compromising soft tissue function. These can be grouped into central causes such as stroke, cerebellar dysfunction, Parkinson's disease, alcohol abuse, and peripheral causes such as peripheral neuropathy and lumbar stenosis.

Most cases of dislocation can be successfully treated with closed reduction and abduction bracing. Patients who experience multiple dislocations may require revision surgery; it is then crucial to identify the cause of dislocation, as this leads to optimal results. Surgical options include revision for malpositioned components, use of constrained acetabular components, larger femoral heads, and trochanteric advancement.

Infection (Boxes 7.3.9–7.3.11)

The reported rate of deep infection after total hip replacement is now around 0.3–2%. Infection arises either by contamination at the time of surgery or later by haematogenous spread; the airborne route is probably responsible for most cases. The commonest organisms are Gram-positive, with *Staphylococcus aureus* (50–65%) and *Staph. epidermidis* (25–30%) accounting for the majority. The remainder consist of other bacteria, fungi, and mycobacteria.

Also important is the suppression or elimination of infection at remote sites before surgery. Dental procedures produce a bacteraemia in nearly all patients, and should be covered with antibiotics, although this remains controversial. Any chronic skin ulcers should be treated prior to hip replacement. Patients should be screened to exclude concurrent urinary tract infections, and if identified, appropriate treatment instituted.

The use of ultraclean air and prophylactic antibiotics in combination has had a dramatic reduction in the rate of sepsis. The use of prophylactic antibiotics has been of paramount importance. Cephalosporins tend to be the antibiotic of choice because of their broad-spectrum activity. A preoperative dose at induction is always administered; the evidence for the recommended duration of prophylaxis thereafter is in favour of 24h, and not for longer periods.

Evaluation of a patient with suspected infection should include the use of blood inflammatory markers, plain radiographs, bone scans, and white cell scans. The goals of treatment are the eradication of infection and restoration of function; treatment itself is usually operative.

Box 7.3.9 Infection

- Reported incidence after primary THR: 0.3–2%
- Causes: primary contamination, secondary blood-borne
- *Staph. aureus* and *Staph. epidermidis* account for majority
- The use of ultraclean air and prophylactic antibiotics are the most important preventive measures.

Box 7.3.10 Patient factors predisposing to infection

- Immunosuppression
- Long-term steroid therapy
- Diabetes
- Morbid obesity
- Rheumatoid arthritis
- HIV.

Box 7.3.11 Infection: prophylaxis

- Ultraclean air in theatre
- Prophylactic antibiotics
- Identify and treat concurrent infections preoperatively (dental, urinary tract, cutaneous, etc.)
- Limit number of individuals in theatre
- Closed-air exhaust suits
- Avoid unnecessarily prolonging operating time.

Thromboembolism (Box 7.3.12)

Despite the use of thromboembolic prophylaxis for some time now, deep venous thrombosis continues to pose a significant risk after total hip replacement. In the absence of any prophylaxis, deep venous thrombosis rates are reported to be in the region of 40–60%, and the incidence of fatal pulmonary embolism about 0.5–2%; with prophylaxis, the corresponding rates are approximately 3–30% and 0.5 % respectively. Despite extensive research, the ideal agent for prophylaxis remains controversial; however there is agreement that some form of prophylaxis should be used. The results of randomized trials indicate that low-molecular-weight heparin, warfarin, and fondaparinux are the most effective agents, with or without the use of graduated compression stockings and/or intermittent pneumatic compression devices. Surgeons are concerned about bleeding associated with the use of prophylactic agents, as it can lead to haematoma formation, infection, and reoperation. Further controversy also surrounds the duration of prophylaxis; prophylaxis should, however, probably continue beyond discharge. The selection of a particular regimen depends on the experience of the surgeon and risk factors in individual patients.

Limb-length discrepancy (Box 7.3.13)

Limb-length discrepancy after total hip replacement may result in impairment of abductor function, pain, and a limp; it is one of the commoner reasons for significant patient dissatisfaction in an otherwise successful arthroplasty. The amount of disparity that causes

Box 7.3.12 Thromboembolism

- Reported incidences after primary total hip replacement: deep vein thrombosis 3–30%; fatal pulmonary embolism 0.5%
- Ideal agent for prophylaxis remains controversial
- Low-molecular-weight heparins widely used, but there are concerns regarding bleeding.

Box 7.3.13 Limb-length discrepancy

- Reported incidence in published literature variable
- Lengthening of more than 1cm may cause symptoms and patient dissatisfaction
- Preoperative templating and intraoperative assessment are both important to minimize incidence.

a clinically significant or functionally relevant shortening remains unclear, and published data are conflicting. This is probably due to variation in individual patients; the presence of concomitant spinal deformity, pelvic obliquity, and contractures of the contralateral limb all have an influence on the patient's functional leg length. Psychological issues and cosmesis are also important factors in the patient's perception of leg-length discrepancy.

Preoperative radiographic templating, as outlined previously, should be used to minimize the possibility of creating a significant leg-length discrepancy. A method of intraoperative assessment of leg length is also essential. A variety of methods are available: iliac fixation pins, intraoperative calipers, and computer-assisted navigation have all been described. Leg length can be compared by assessing the equivalence of knee joints and the malleoli. Measurement of distances from the tip of the greater trochanter to the centre of the femoral head, and the distance from the lesser trochanter to the centre of the femoral head should be compared to preoperative measurements. The toggle or 'shuck' test, in which the hip is distracted in the neutral position, also indicates length restoration; in general no more than 2mm of distraction should be possible.

Leg-length inequality may respond to the use of a shoe raise; persistent symptoms or significant patient dissatisfaction may necessitate revision surgery.

Neurological injury (Box 7.3.14)

The overall incidence of nerve injury associated with total hip replacement is 1–2%. Sciatic nerve injuries are by far the commonest, accounting for about 80%, followed by femoral, with obturator and superior gluteal nerve injuries accounting for a very small number. The posterior approach to the hip is traditionally associated with injury to the sciatic nerve, but the lateral approach may also be responsible. The aetiology of injury is usually unknown in a significant proportion of the cases. Out of the known causes, traction, compression, haematoma, constriction by suture, and heat from cement polymerization are generally responsible. Traction injury may be from intraoperative manoeuvres including dislocation and reduction, or from leg lengthening. Lengthening of greater than 4cm is generally accepted as a risk factor for nerve injury.

The majority of injury to the sciatic nerve affects the peroneal division; it is at increased risk of damage because it is tethered at both the sciatic notch and the head of the fibula, and is also located more laterally than the tibial division. For the femoral nerve, mechanisms of injury are similar to those that can lead to sciatic nerve palsy, and include direct injury from retractor placement, leg lengthening, and extruded cement. Obturator nerve injury is rare, and is usually due to cement extrusion, and anteroinferior quadrant screw placement. Injury to the superior gluteal nerve is a complication of the anterolateral or direct lateral approach to the hip.

If the postoperative clinical evidence points to injury of a nerve at the time of surgery, then that nerve must be explored. Loss of motor and sensory function, and in particular pain and numbness in the distribution of a nerve, should alert the surgeon to the possibility of its damage. Electromyography and nerve conduction studies are useful adjuncts in the diagnosis; however, they should not delay surgical exploration. Prompt diagnosis and early exploration is associated with a better outcome.

Vascular injury (Box 7.3.15)

Vascular complications after total hip replacement are rare—reported rates in the literature are in the order of 0.1–0.2%. They can either be perioperative, presenting with obvious haemorrhage, or late, causing pain or ischaemia due to a pseudoaneurysm. The commonly affected vessels are the common femoral, the external iliac, and the obturator. Vessels may be injured by direct mechanisms (scalpel, retractor, or reamer) or indirectly from a stretching injury, particularly in patients with atherosclerosis.

The use of screws to augment acetabular stability has also caused concern with regards to vascular injury. The quadrant system as described by Wasielewski and colleagues has become popular as a guide to safe screw placement (Figure 7.3.4). The acetabulum is divided into quadrants by two lines; the first from the anterior superior iliac spine extending distally through the centreof the acetabulum, and a second line perpendicular to, and bisecting, the first line. The anterosuperior quadrant risks external iliac injury, and the anteroinferior quadrant risks injury to the obturator vessels. The posterosuperior and posteroinferior quadrants are the safest for screw placement, and generally have the best bone quality.

Periprosthetic fracture (Box 7.3.16)

The reported incidence of periprosthetic fractures after total hip replacement varies, being in the region of 1–3% with cementless femoral stem implantation; the incidence is much lower using cemented stems. Fractures to the acetabulum occur much less frequently than occur in the femur. A recent report from the Swedish National Hip Arthroplasty Register found the accumulated incidence for primary hip replacements to be about 0.4%.

The surgeon must keep in mind patient factors that increase the chance of fracture, including age, female gender, and osteoporosis. Routine follow-up of patients after total hip replacement is critical in identifying those at high risk of fracture.

Box 7.3.14 Neurological injury

- Reported incidence: 1–2%
- Sciatic nerve injury commonest, followed by femoral, obturator, and superior gluteal nerve
- Causes include traction, compression, haematoma, constriction by suture, and heat from cement polymerization.

Box 7.3.15 Vascular injury

- Rare in primary total hip replacement; reported incidence: 0.1–0.2%
- Commonly affected vessels are the common femoral, external iliac, and obturator
- The use of screws to augment acetabular stability is a risk factor.

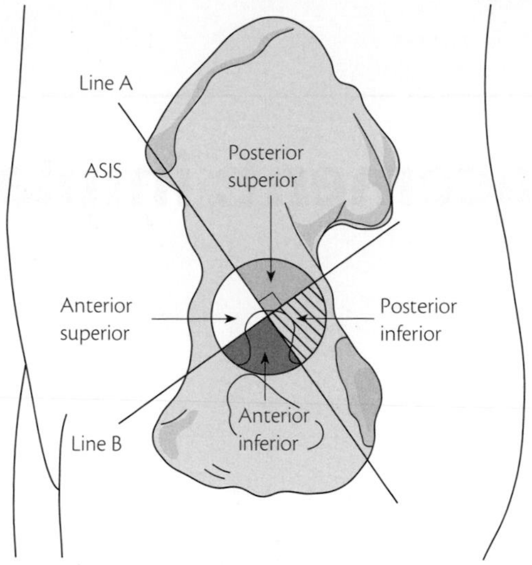

Fig. 7.3.4 Acetabular quadrant system. The quadrants are formed by the intersection of lines A and B. Line A extends from the anterior superior iliac spine (ASIS) through the center of the acetabulum to the posterior aspect of the fovea, dividing the acetabulum in half. Line B is drawn perpendicular to line A at the mid-point of the acetabulum, dividing it into four quandrants: the anterosuperior quadrant, the anteroinferior quadrant, the posterosuperior quadrant, and the posteroinferior quadrant. (Reproduced from Wasielewski *et al.* (1990).)

Box 7.3.16 Periprosthetic fracture

- Reported incidence in primary total hip replacement: approximately 0.4%
- Most cases involve femoral component
- Treatment options include: conservative management, fracture fixation, or revision arthroplasty.

Conclusions

In conclusion, careful preoperative planning ensures that the goals of total hip replacement are consistently and reliably achieved—the anatomical aims of restoring the centre of rotation, leg length and offset, as well as maximizing patient satisfaction. It ensures that the appropriate implants are available, shortens the learning curve for the surgeon, and minimizes the incidence of complications. Digital templating is gaining in popularity, and holds promise for the future.

The process of obtaining informed consent is an important component of the whole process, both for the surgeon and for the patient. Due attention must be given to the provision of adequate information to the patient, and appropriate documentation.

Finally, a comprehensive knowledge of the aetiology and treatment of complications associated with hip arthroplasty is necessary for safe practice. A hip replacement is an elective procedure that is very good at improving a patient's quality of life; the patient rightly has very high expectations. A meticulous approach will ensure the surgeon anticipates potential complications and minimizes them.

Further reading

Bhattacharyya, T., Yeon, H., and Harris, M.B. (2005). The medical-legal aspects of informed consent in orthopaedic surgery. *Journal of Bone and Joint Surgery. American Volume*, **87**, 2395–400.

Cuckler, J.M. (2005). Limb length and stability in total hip replacement. *Orthopedics*, **28** (9), 951–3.

Della Valle, C.J. and Di Cesare, P.E. (2002). Complications of total hip arthroplasty: neurovascular injury, leg-length discrepancy, and instability. *Bulletin of the Hospital for the Joint Diseases*, **60**(3–4), 134–42.

Della Valle, A.G., Padgett, D.E., and Salvati, E.A. (2005). Preoperative planning for primary total hip arthroplasty. *Journal of the American Academy of Orthopaedic Surgeons*, **13**(17), 455–62.

Jolles, B.M., and Bogoch, E.R. (2006). Posterior versus lateral surgical approach for total hip arthroplasty in adults with osteoarthritis. *Cochrane Database of Systematic Reviews*, **19**(3), CD003828

Kaltsas, D.S . (2004). Infection after total hip arthroplasty. *Annals of the Royal College of Surgeons of England*, **86**(4), 267–71.

Lidwell, O.M . (1986). Clean air at operation and subsequent sepsis in the joint. *Clinical orthopaedics and related research*, **211**, 91–102.

Lieberman, J.R., and Hsu, W.K. (2005). Prevention of venous thromboembolic disease after total hip and knee arthroplasty. *Journal of Bone and Joint Surgery. American Volume*, **87**(9), 2097–112.

Patel, P.D., Potts, A., and Froimson, M.I. (2007). The dislocating hip arthroplasty: prevention and treatment. *Journal of Arthroplasty*, **22**(4 Suppl 1), 86–90.

Van Flandern, G.J., (2005). Periprosthetic fractures in total hip arthroplasty. *Orthopedics*, **28**(9 Suppl), s1089–95.

Wasielewski, R.C., Cooperstein, L.A., Kruger, M.P., and Rubash, H.E. (1990). Acetabular anatomy and the transacetabular fixation of screws in total hip arthroplasty. *Journal of Bone and Joint Surgery. American Volume*, **72**(4), 501–8.

7.4

Total hip replacement: implant fixation

David H. Sochart

Summary points

- Cemented fixation in total hip replacement set the standard and has stood the test of time
- Improved generations of cementing technique have led to improved results
- The long term results of uncemented implants have improved with better designs and materials
- The most important determinant of the outcome and longevity of the implant is the quality and accuracy of the initial implantation

Introduction

Cemented fixation has been used successfully in total hip replacement for over 40 years, but uncemented implants were developed because of the higher rates of aseptic loosening noted in young, active patients. In 1987 Hungerford mistakenly attributed this mode of failure to the method of fixation and coined the term 'cement disease' but it was later realized that the cause was, in fact, osteolysis resulting from the generation of polyethylene wear debris.

There remains much debate over which type of fixation—cemented, uncemented, or hybrid—offers the most reliable and durable results. As technology and manufacturing processes have developed, the results for uncemented fixation have improved, but at the same time cementing techniques have advanced.

The basic arguments over fixation have been overtaken by tribological issues, but discrepancies remain with regard to the results published in the literature, usually of a single implant or technique from a single centre by the surgeon who designed it, and the findings of the national joint registries. Issues such as age, weight, activity, pathology, bone quality, canal morphology, experience, and cost, must always be considered and there are differences between the philosophies and performance of individual implants within the cemented and uncemented categories.

Wear, leading to the development of osteolysis, is the ultimate determinant of outcome in modern total hip arthroplasty, but neither implant can be studied in isolation, because it is the performance of the entire hip system (implants, bearing, and cement, if used) that will determine the function and longevity of the reconstructed hip.

Fixation with cement

Polymethylmethacrylate (PMMA) bone cement has been used in arthroplasty surgery for over 40 years, with many publications and registries confirming excellent long-term results, even in young patients. The constituents and properties of the successful cements have remained essentially unchanged, but the ways in which they are prepared and used have improved (Figure 7.4.1).

Cement consists of a powder and a liquid (Box 7.4.1), which, when mixed together, produce an exothermic reaction (40–46°C), with polymerization as the cement hardens. Modern cements contain radiopacifiers and may also contain chlorophyll to impart a green colour in order to differentiate cement from the bone.

The type of cement used is not simply an afterthought and the Swedish registry has confirmed that the specific cement used has a significant bearing on the risk of revision. Cements are available with a variety of setting times and viscosities, with the high viscosity cements having a lower reported revision rate. Most contain antibiotics, usually gentamicin, which has been shown to further reduce the risk of revision.

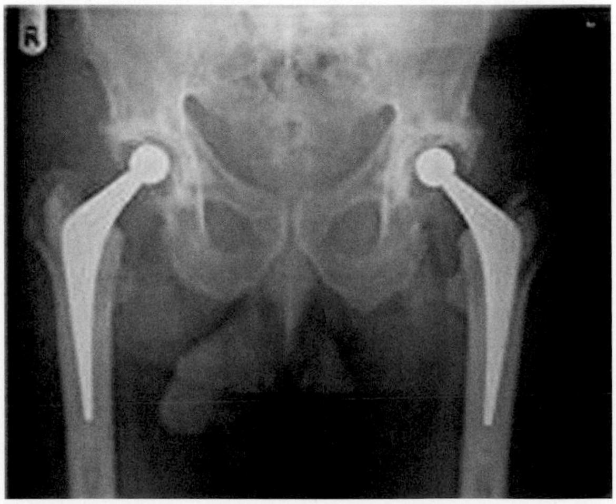

Fig. 7.4.1 Bilateral cemented total hip replacements.

Box 7.4.1 Constituents of a typical bone cement

- Powder:
  - Polymer: polymethylmethacrylate or copolymers of methylmethacrylate
  - Initiator: benzoyl peroxide
  - Radiopacifier: zirconium dioxide or barium sulphate
  - Antibiotic: gentamicin (optional)
  - Additives: dye—chlorophyll (optional)
  - Plasticizer: dicyclohexyl phthalate (optional)
- Liquid:
  - Monomer: methylmethacrylate
  - Activator: DMPT (N,N-dimethyl-p-toluidine)
  - Inhibitor: hydroquinone
  - Additive: dye—chlorophyll (optional)

If revising an infected arthroplasty the cement can be customized, based on the sensitivity of the infecting organism, by adding appropriate heat-stable antibiotics in powder form (less than 10% of the weight of the powder), and such cement can also be used to fashion a temporary spacer or beads for use in a two-stage procedure.

Bone cement has no adhesive properties and works as a grout, rather than a glue. During its insertion and working phase the cement is pressurized and interdigitates with the cancellous bone, hardening and creating a micro-interlock, forming a cement–bone construct, giving immediate stability. Meticulous preparation of the bony bed is essential and cancellous bone must be retained.

Pulse lavage removes debris or loose bone and the canal is dried to improve interdigitation and shear strength. Intramedullary bleeding is reduced by the local application of hydrogen peroxide, epinephrine, or chilled saline and by hypotensive anaesthesia.

The optimum cement mantle should be even and 2–4mm thick around the entire component, without any gaps, which would weaken it and allow wear debris to access the bony interface. Two interfaces are created (cement–bone and cement–implant), with cement being strongest in compression (93MPa) but weaker in shear (42.2MPa) or tension (35.3MPa).

The quality of the cement is important and the fatigue strength is increased by vacuum mixing or centrifuging which decrease the porosity. During cement insertion inclusions, voids, or laminations of fat, blood, or air should be avoided as this can reduce its strength by a factor of five.

A cement restrictor is placed 2cm beyond stem tip and a hollow centralizer should be used. Pressurization is maintained throughout to negate the effects of back bleeding, which forces the cement back out of the cancellous bone, and to take into account the initial cement expansion during the exothermic reaction and subsequent overall shrinkage (3–5%).

Cement must be stored at a constant temperature and should not be preheated or chilled because this makes its setting time unpredictable. Theatre temperature is important because a 1°C rise can reduce the setting time by up to 1min.

The type of cement, theatre, and storage environment and the quality of the cementing technique (Table 7.4.1) are crucial to the longevity of the arthroplasty, with the methods of bone preparation, cement insertion, and implantation differing between acetabulum and femur. Cemented fixation is demanding and time and care must be taken to ensure that all of the stages are performed as well as possible on each and every occasion (Box 7.4.2).

Uncemented fixation

The aim of uncemented fixation is to achieve initial press-fit stability with 'macro-fixation' of the component against the surface of the bone, which is prepared with a degree of under-reaming. Long-term stability is achieved by 'micro-fixation' with the subsequent ingrowth of the surrounding bone into the porous surface modifications of the implant. Hydroxyapatite (HA) can also be used to encourage this process, but initial stability is crucial, because excessive micromotion will prevent bony ingrowth.

Some early designs of femoral prosthesis were manufactured with gaps or surface irregularities to allow bone to grow through and anchor the prosthesis. One familiar example is the Austin Moore hemiarthroplasty, but in young or active patients this offered limited support and led to loosening. In others, HA was used to coat components, which had no other surface modifications, with the risk of the implants subsequently loosening if the coating separated from the implant or had been reabsorbed.

Modern uncemented implants feature coatings to part or all of their surfaces to encourage bony ingrowth, which will then provide long-term fixation. This process occurs within 6 weeks of implantation and some surgeons keep their patients partially weight bearing during this period. The initial fixation may be augmented by longitudinal flutes, spikes, fins, or screws (Figure 7.4.2).

The manufacturing of uncemented implants is more complex and time consuming than for cemented ones, as a result of which they are generally more expensive, but without significant improvements in prosthesis survival they will not be cost-effective.

The cemented acetabulum

Cemented high density polyethylene (HDP) acetabular components were popularized by Sir John Charnley as part of the low-frictional torque concept. The material of choice subsequently became ultra-high-molecular-weight polyethylene (UHMWP), with cementable highly cross-linked polyethylene (HXLP) implants

Box 7.4.2 Barrack classification of femoral cement mantles

- Type A: complete filling of the medullary cavity, a 'white-out'
- Type B: slight radiolucency (<50%) of the cement–bone interface
- Type C: 50–99% radiolucency, or a defective or incomplete mantle
- Type D: 100% radiolucency, or failure to fill the canal or cover the tip of the stem.

Table 7.4.1 Generations of femoral cementing technique

Generation	First	Second	Third	Fourth
Mixing	Bowl	Bowl	Vacuum	Vacuum
Restrictor	No	Yes	Yes	Yes
Gun	No	Yes	Yes	Yes
Pulse Lavage	No	No	Yes	Yes
Proximal Pressurizer	No	No	Yes	Yes
Centralizer	No	No	No	Yes
Improvements				
Mantle	NA	Yes	Yes	Yes
Cement quality	NA	NA	Yes	Yes
Stem position	NA	NA	NA	Yes

only recently being made widely available, despite the fact that this material has been used in modular uncemented cups for many years.

Modern components incorporate a long posterior wall to reduce the risk of dislocation and a flange to improve cement pressurization, implant positioning, and to act as a potential barrier to wear debris (Figure 7.4.3). PMMA spacers may be used on the back surface of some designs to avoid bottoming out, but may affect the integrity of the cement mantle. Metal backing, initially introduced for more even stress distribution, has been discontinued due to generally poorer results.

The process of bone preparation and cementing technique is crucial to long-term survival. The presence of a radiolucent line in zone 1 of the bone–cement interface on the 12-month radiograph is a predictor of early failure and represents suboptimal technique, rather than a fault in the philosophy of cemented fixation.

The bony bed is prepared by reaming to subchondral bone and the creation of multiple keyholes, increasing the surface area for cement interdigitation to provide fixation and rotational stability.

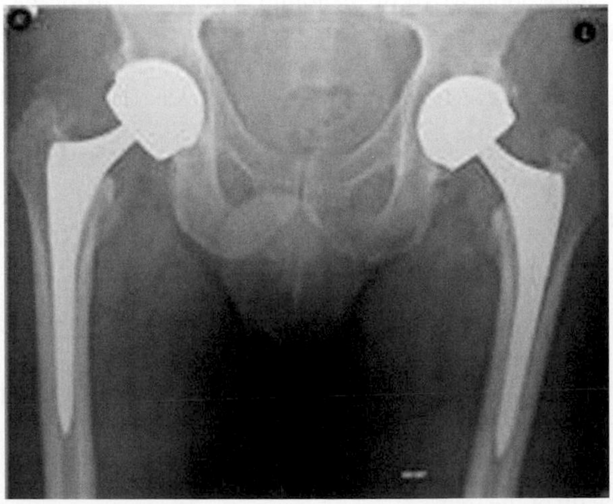

Fig. 7.4.2 Bilateral uncemented total hip replacements.

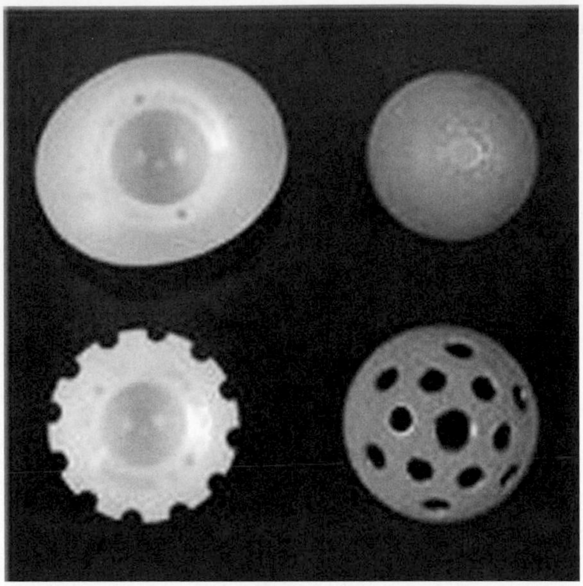

Fig. 7.4.3 Acetabular components: Top left clockwise: Flanged cemented, solid resurfacing , multi-hole uncemented, unflanged cemented.

The correct implant size is based on the size of the final reamer used and the preferred cement mantle thickness, following which the flange is trimmed, either by using a template or markings on the flange itself.

Charnley used three major keyholes (ilium, ischium, and pubis), with other cementing proponents advocating the use of multiple smaller ones, or a combination of both techniques.

The bone is washed and dried as thoroughly as possible and the use of a suction vent in the ilium, superior to the rim of the acetabulum, can assist with this. The cement is inserted and pressurized, avoiding laminations, with the cup being inserted at the appropriate time, then held and pressurization maintained until it sets. Any excess cement and osteophytes are removed to avoid impingement.

The uncemented acetabulum

Initial fixation can be achieved by press-fitting of a hemispherical component, or by the use of a threaded implant, screwed into the host bone.

The use of HA coatings without other surface modifications has now been abandoned, but HA continues to feature in modern designs. Threaded screw-in components were popular in mainland Europe, but have been superseded by the press-fit modular designs. These components may be either hemispherical or non-hemispherical and some have an expanded equator to enhance initial stability.

The press-fit cups are implanted by under-reaming of the acetabulum by 1–2mm, depending upon bone quality and prosthesis design, then the implant is impacted into place. The injudicious use of excessive impaction force must be avoided to reduce the risk of fracture.

If there are concerns regarding the quality of the initial fixation, augmentation can be achieved by additional screw fixation and components come in a variety of designs, some with no screw holes, and some with many (Figure 7.4.3). Screws must be accurately inserted to avoid tilting the prosthesis and distancing it from the surrounding bone. There will be one central hole in a modular cup for the insertion handle, and a cap is provided to occlude this prior to insertion of the liner. Some implants also feature spikes or fins to resist rotational forces, but solid resurfacing cups have no holes and a different design of insertion handle is required.

Modular cups were originally designed for use with polyethylene liners, but were associated with high rates of wear and osteolysis. This was more common with vertical implants (greater than 50 degrees) or when large heads articulated with thin liners. The phenomenon of backside wear was common, when a poor locking mechanism allowed motion to occur between the liners back surface and the inside of the metal shell. This is an example of type 4 wear between two surfaces which are not intended to articulate and the debris produced can access the bony interface via unplugged screw holes, leading to the development of pelvic osteolysis, in keeping with the concept of the effective joint space, as described by Schmalzreid and illustrated by computed tomography studies published by Engh.

Modern implants have improved locking mechanisms, polished inner surfaces, and caps to occlude the screw holes. The modular shells also permit the use of liners with different bearing materials such as highly cross-linked polyethylene, ceramic or metal, but long-term survivorship results of these implants are not yet available.

The cemented femur

The development of cemented femoral components has seen the divergence into two main categories, with the establishment of the composite beam (shape-closed) and taper-slip (force-closed) philosophies (Figure 7.4.4).

Composite beam implants have rough surfaces to promote bonding with the cement and may have a collar designed to load the calcar. Once inserted the stem should not move and any debonding or subsidence, at the implant–cement or bone–cement interface, represents loosening and failure.

Taper-slip components are polished, collarless, and taper in two or three planes. There is no bonding with the cement and the stems are designed to subside within the cement mantle, which must therefore be regular, complete, and of the highest quality. Stems are collarless to permit subsidence and polished to avoid abrasion of the inner surface of the cement mantle and the generation of debris, which led to high failure rates in matt finished collarless stems. A hollow centralizer is used to optimize stem positioning, avoid the creation of defects in the cement mantle, promote controlled subsidence, and to eradicate end-bearing, which would lead to distal load transmission.

Subsidence utilizes the viscoelastic properties of cement in a process called creep, which is non-recoverable deformation under load. As the femoral prosthesis is loaded, the cement deforms and the implant subsides within the mantle. The stem subsides and becomes more securely fixed within the mantle, generating hoop stresses within it. These stresses are then transmitted to the surrounding bone, which, because it is being loaded, will not undergo stress shielding, which could lead to the eventual loss of proximal support and loosening. This is in accordance with Woolf's law and the aim of polished tapered stems is to load the femur as proximally and 'physiologically' as possible.

Good long-term results have been achieved with both composite-beam and taper-slip stems, but when the importance of the philosophies or the bone cement are ignored, unacceptably high failure rates can occur as was seen with the Capital hip femoral prosthesis or the use of Boneloc cement.

Cementing technique is crucial and has progressed from the original 'first generation' bowl mixing and finger-packing, to vacuum mixing, pulsatile lavage, restrictors, retrograde filling with a gun, pressurization, and the use of centralizers (Table 7.4.1).

The cement mantle should be even, with a minimum thickness of 2–4mm, and the stem in neutral alignment, filling more than half of the femoral canal. Varus alignment of the stem leads to a higher failure rate, but probably reflects a global failure in the surgical technique and implantation rather than in the cemented philosophy.

Results from the Scandinavian joint registries have confirmed improved survivorship with the advent of each generation of cementing technique, confirming that the results of cemented arthroplasties are technique dependant.

The uncemented femur

There are two main categories of uncemented femoral components depending upon where in the femur the initial press-fit mechanical stability is achieved. The stems can be straight or curved, and feature a variety of porous coatings, beads or fibre-mesh (Figure 7.4.4). The implant may have a collar to prevent subsidence, whilst attempting to load the calcar.

The first category are the stems designed to provide metaphyseal fixation with fit and fill implants, which have porous coating only on the proximal part of the prosthesis. The distal stem may be polished or slotted to prevent distal loading and reduce the incidence of thigh pain.

The proximal coatings on early metaphyseal stems were often incomplete, leading to the development of osteolysis due to wear debris accessing the interface, but modern implants feature circumferential coatings to prevent this and aim to load the femur more 'physiologically' via the metaphyseal region.

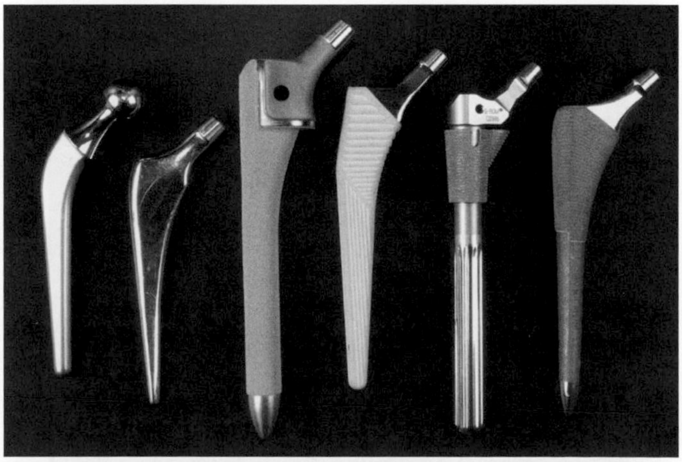

Fig. 7.4.4 Femoral components: (L>R) – Cemented Charnley (composite beam), Cemented Polished triple taper, Uncemented fully coated calcar replacing, Uncemented fully coated, Uncemented S-ROM with proximal sleeve, Uncemented proximally coated metaphyseal filling.

Because of the success of metaphyseal filling designs and the realization that the distal part of the stem may, in fact, be redundant, shorter or stemless implants, also designed to achieve metaphyseal fixation, have recently entered the marketplace. These stems are often identical to the proximal portion of a design that has been in use for a longer period, but there are no long-term results available, and claims that they will achieve the same results as the stems upon which they have been based can not be supported.

The implants designed to achieve distal diaphyseal fixation are extensively porous coated along all, or most, of the intramedullary surface and may feature longitudinal flutes to enhance rotational stability.

These extensively coated implants obtain the majority of their fixation distally and therefore risk the development of stress shielding, with subsequent proximal femoral bone loss. Because of the extensive coating these stems may also be harder to revise without causing significant additional loss of bone, as a result of which specialized instruments may be necessary for their safe extraction.

Uncemented implants are associated with a greater risk of intraoperative femoral fracture, which if undisplaced and unrecognized can progress to a complete fracture in the early postoperative period. If recognized at the time of surgery the fracture can be stabilized with cerclage wires or cables and the patient kept non-weight bearing for a period. Thigh pain is more commonly reported with uncemented implants, particularly the larger, stiffer, extensively coated ones.

Uncemented femoral components are not recommended for use in patients with a stove-pipe or Dorr type C femur, but such femoral anatomy is also associated with a higher failure rate of cemented implants.

Hybrid fixation

Conventional hybrid fixation consists of a cemented stem with an uncemented cup (Figure 7.4.5). The uncemented modular shells were originally used with a polyethylene liner, but with the growing popularity of alternative bearings, different articulations, and larger head sizes are becoming more popular.

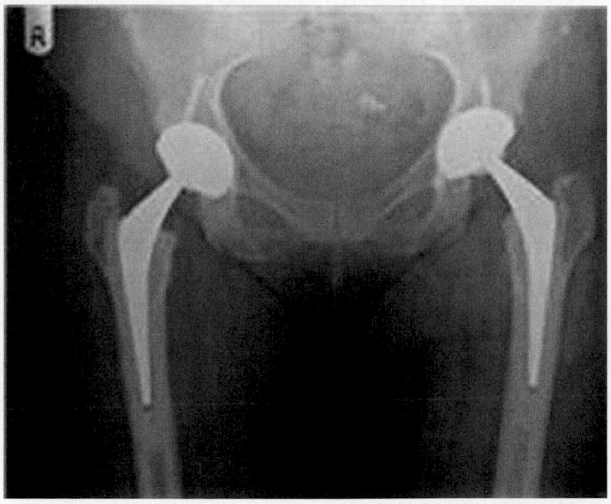

Fig. 7.4.5 Bilateral hybrid total hip replacements.

There has also been a recent trend towards the reverse hybrid (uncemented stem and cemented cup) with a metal or ceramic head articulating on a polyethylene bearing.

Good results of hybrid fixation using metal on polyethylene articulations have been demonstrated in the Scandinavian registries, but long-term results of reverse hybrid hips or alternative bearings have not been reported.

Conclusion

The use of a specific implant, whether cemented or uncemented, does not guarantee success. It is the process of implantation, with precise aseptic and surgical technique and the optimal use of the carefully selected components, which will reduce the risk of complications, improving the function and longevity of the arthroplasty.

The results of early uncemented designs were inferior to contemporaneous cemented implants, due to poor implant design and excessive wear of thin polyethylene liners, with many designs being withdrawn, replaced, or becoming obsolete long before any meaningful results could be established.

There is, however, a growing body of evidence from publications and registries that well-designed and well-performed uncemented implants can achieve equivalent results to well-designed and well-performed cemented ones, in most age groups.

The greatest influence on the outcome of any given design of total hip replacement remains the accuracy with which the surgeon implants the prostheses at the time of the operation and the technique of implantation will ultimately take precedence over the technology or specifics of the implant with respect to achieving the best long-term results.

Further reading

Barrack, B.L., Mulroy, R.D., Harris, W.H. (1992). Improved cementing techniques and femoral component loosening in young patients with hip arthroplasty. *Journal of Bone and Joint Surgery*, **74B**, 385–9.

Charnley, J. (1979). *Low Friction Arthroplasty of the Hip: Theory and Practice.* Berlin: Springer-Verlag.

Dorr, L.D., Mackel, A., and Faugere, M.C. (1988). Histologic validation of a new x-ray classification of hip changes in patients with osteoarthritis requiring total hip replacement. *Orthopaedic Transactions*, **12**, 464.

Engh, C.A., Massin, P., and Suthers, K.E. (1990). Roentographic assessment of biologic fixation of porous surfaced femoral implants, *Clinical Orthopaedics and Related Research*, **257**, 107–28.

Havelin, L.I., Engesaeter, L.B., Espehaug, B., Furnes, O., Lie, S.A., and Vollset, S.E. (2000). The Norwegian arthroplasty register: 11 years and 73,000 arthroplasties. *Acta Orthopaedica Scandinavica*, **71**, 337–53.

Makela, K.T., Eskelinen, A., Pulkinnen, P., Pavolainen, P., and Remes, V. (2008). Total hip arthroplasty for primary osteoarthritis in patients fifty-five years of age or older. *Journal of Bone and Joint Surgery*, **90A**, 2160–70.

Malchau, H., Herberts, P., Eisler, T., Garellick, G., and Soderman, P. (2002). The Swedish total hip replacement register. *Journal of Bone and Joint Surgery*, **84A**(Suppl 2), 2–20.

Sochart, D.H. (1999). Relationship of acetabular wear to osteolysis and loosening in total hip arthroplasty. *Clinical Orthopaedics and Related Research*, **363**, 135–50.

Sochart, D.H. and Porter, M.L. (1997). The long-term results of Charnley low-friction arthroplasty in young patients who have congenital dislocation, degenerative osteoarthrosis or rheumatoid arthritis, *Journal of Bone and Joint Surgery*, **79**, 1599–617.

7.5

Implant choice for primary total hip arthroplasty

Parminder J. Singh and Richard E. Field

Summary points

- Types of acetabular components available
- Types of femoral components available
- Types of bearings

Introduction

Until the mid twentieth century, degenerative disease of the hip joint could be treated by excision arthroplasty, arthrodesis, or interposition arthroplasty. Excision arthroplasty developed as a necessary strategy in the management of osteomyelitis and joint sepsis. Hip arthrodesis provided a painless and stable junction between trunk and lower limb, but created functional restrictions and increased the stresses and strains on the lumber spine, contralateral hip, and ipsilateral knee. Interposition arthroplasty started as a simple surgical strategy in which a patient's own muscle and fascia were interposed between the damaged articular surfaces. This was superseded by implantation of a shell over the reshaped femoral head (Smith– Peterson cup). Interposition cups were replaced by hemiarthroplasties secured into the proximal femoral bone with varying degrees of rigidity and stability. The hemiarthroplasties were superseded by articulating monobloc implants secured to both femur and acetabulum (Total Hip Replacement, THR). THR development has followed two fairly distinct paths. On one route, monobloc implants were adapted to minimize host bone resection. This has led to our current generation of metal-on-metal hip resurfacing and epiphyseal replacements. On the other route, monobloc implants have been modularized to provide devices that are optimized for fixation to host bone, and offer a variety of articular combinations with differing tribological advantages.

Half a century of THR development has created a cornucopia of hip replacement options to choose from. Today's surgeons are required to treat patients who may seek hip replacement while still relatively young and with many years of active life ahead of them. Hip surgeons face a spectrum of clinical conditions all of which are best treated by THR. However, equally strong arguments exist for different implant combinations in different clinical conditions. Surgeons ultimately choose particular implants because of their unique interpretation of available scientific and clinical literature, their clinical experience, their willingness or desire to embrace potential advances in implant design, and patient demand for benefits that have been promulgated though conventional media and the internet. This chapter considers the evolution, merits and shortcomings of the different component fixation and bearing options that are available to current orthopaedic surgeons.

The early hemiarthroplasties and first THRs were implanted without any defined strategy for fixation of the implant to host bone. In Norwich, cobalt chrome, metal-on-metal, uncemented hip replacements were implanted in the 1940s and in the 1950s. The need for better femoral component fixation to host bone was rapidly recognized, and in 1953, polymethylmethacrylate (PMMA), an acrylic material used by the dental profession, was introduced. Initial results were poor because the cement was used to secure the prosthesis rather than to provide a mantle that would stabilize the implant and facilitate even transfer of loading stresses on the surrounding bone. Once this concept was understood and its efficacy demonstrated, cement became widely used in the United Kingdom. Incremental improvements in cementing techniques have been introduced and PMMA cement can provide consistent and reliable, long-term fixation for cemented femoral stems.

Some authorities considered that the cement-stem interface would be a weak link. Indeed, in the USA, the Food and Drug Administration (FDA) were initially cautious about sanctioning bone cement for general use. As an alternative, cementless fixation strategies were developed to strengthen the mechanical bond between stem and the adjacent bone. Holes were drilled into femoral components such as the Austin Moore prosthesis. Besides making the implant less heavy and saving metal, it was hoped that this would create a mechanical lock between bone and implant. The strategy provided limited benefit and attention turned to creating microscopic irregularities on the surface of the prosthesis. Roughening of the prosthesis surface proved more effective and has led to the application of porous coatings to the component surface. More recently, accelerated osseous attachment has been demonstrated by application of hydroxyapatite, which is the crystalline component of natural bone.

In summary, excellent long-term results have been achieved using cement fixation of the femoral component, as shown by the Swedish hip registry and many other publications. Likewise long-term results of the uncemented stems have been published with excellent long-term survival.

The subject of the optimal bearing surface is widely debated. Experimental work has demonstrated that the coefficient of friction in an animal joint (μ = 0.02) is lower than that of a skate sliding on ice (μ = 0.03). This observation led to the search for a low friction bearing, and in 1956 a Teflon-on-Teflon (polytetrafluorethylene) bearing was tried. Early results demonstrated that Teflon-on-Teflon bearings lasted only 2 years and acted as an irritant. This led to the concept of resection of the femoral head and insertion of a metal femoral prosthesis. Metal-on-Teflon bearings fared no better with marked Teflon wear and osteolysis. In the same group of patients it was recognized that a larger femoral head caused higher volumetric wear. However, a small head (22.25 mm) caused linear penetration into the Teflon cup, compromising joint stability. The use of Teflon was therefore abandoned.

In 1962, a high molecular weight polyethylene acetabular cup was introduced. This was used in combination with a stemmed, cemented femoral component and 22.25 mm femoral head. Patients were thrilled with the outcomes of the cemented metal-on-polyethylene hip replacement, and enjoyed dramatic improvement in their quality of life. The combination proved effective, with low wear, and it was widely adopted as a result. The cemented metal-on-polyethylene hip replacement has provided the benchmark for subsequent developments and evolution of THR surgery. THR is one of the most successful advances in modern orthopaedic surgery, with over a 90% clinical success rate at 10 years.

Designs such as the Charnley, Exeter, Stanmore, and Lubinus femoral stems have excellent, long-term results published in the literature. However, minor modifications of these designs have provided significantly inferior outcomes. This finding led to the recognition that different designs of THR provide different mechanisms of fixation and load transfer. For example, the Capital hip prosthesis was promoted as a copy of the Charnley design. The device was provided in versions manufactured as both stainless steel and titanium. The latter option ignored the fact that most polished tapered stems with published long-term results had been made from stainless steel. The Capital stems manufactured from titanium performed significantly less well than the stainless steel variant. Another example was the use of the matt-finish Exeter stem, first used in 1976. The matt stem, revision rate for aseptic loosening was four times higher, at 10 years' follow-up. As a result of these poor results, a highly polished surface was reinstated to the Exeter stem, with excellent long-term results.

Many factors influence the longevity of a THR, including patient, surgical and implant factors. During the mid 1990s, there was growing awareness that the so called, advances in prosthesis design did not necessarily provide additional benefit to patients. It was identified that many prostheses are marketed with little or no scientific evidence to support the claims that are made regarding their potential advantages over existing designs. A directive on medical devices of the Council of the European Communities recommended that implant performance and side-effects should be assessed by clinical trials (Council Directive 93/42/EEC 1993) and some form of clinical investigation has become obligatory before a new implant can carry a CE mark. In 2000 the National Institute for Clinical Evidence (NICE) introduced benchmark performance criteria for implant use in the UK National Health service, and this strategy has been further developed by the Orthopaedic Data Evaluation Panel (ODEP) who have developed benchmarking of implant performance at 3, 5, 7, and 10 years. It is now widely recognized that the introduction of new implants must be supported by reliable pre-clinical testing, phased introduction, and diligent post-market surveillance.

Box 7.5.1 Summary Box

- Degenerative disease of the hip joint—treated by excision arthroplasty, arthrodesis or interposition arthroplasty
- Total hip replacement evolved
- Cemented fixation
- Uncemented fixation
- Optimal bearing surface debated
- New device must have reliable pre-clinical testing, phased introduction, and diligent post-market surveillance

Cemented stems

The optimal cement mantle thickness is not proven; optimal thickness may vary with different stem geometry. High strength stainless steel appears to be a satisfactory material in preference to titanium. Collars and flanges must be avoided in order to allow the taper to subside and function properly. Stem positioning within the femoral canal is improved with the use of centralizers and stem cannulation. The stem should be polished and tapered so that it can subside within the cement mantle and generate minimal cement debris. Whether the ultimate design should be single, double, or triple taper is not yet known, although both single and double tapers are associated with excellent results. No long-term results are yet available for triple tapered stems.

Cemented femoral stems probably remain gold standard for total hip arthroplasty. Long-term results for the Charnley (>80% survivorship from revision for aseptic loosening and/or radiographic loosening at 25 years) and Exeter stems (91% survivorship from revision for aseptic loosening at up to 33 years) are currently the gold standards in femoral fixation. They have an excellent track record in older patients (more than 65 years), but are also used in younger patients with comparable results to the uncemented stems.

The cemented stem is particularly useful with the stove pipe femur, previous femoral fracture, or previous osteotomy where one would not expect to achieve a tight fit for ingrowth with an uncemented stem. Cemented stems are also indicated in cases of poor bone quality such as Rheumtoid arthritis, osteoporosis, or Paget's disease.

Cement is used for fixation of the femoral stem in THR. The cement forms a seal around the femoral neck: this prevents the ingress of wear debris particles into the medullary canal of the femur. More importantly, cement allows stress transfer from stem to bone. In this respect, the femoral component can be viewed either as a composite beam or a load taper. To achieve optimal long-term results with a femoral component design, one must consider stem geometry, surface finish, and prosthesis cement interface.

Box 7.5.2 Summary Box

- Optimal cement mantle still debated
- Stainless steel
- Collar vs collarless
- Composite beam vs taper slip
- Centralizers and stem cannulation
- Bi-tapers and triple tapered
- Cement allows stress transfer from implant to bone

The cement/implant interface may rely primarily on the intrinsic stability of the implant within its cement mantle (i.e. the shape of the interface). Alternatively, fixation may depend heavily on adhesion at the cement/implant interface. In either situation, cement/implant displacement of 0.5 mm or less is characteristic of a well-fixed device.

Biomechanical theories of load transfer

Each cemented femoral stem design uses one of two mechanisms to transmit forces from stem to femur. A composite beam system requires strong stem/cement and cement/bone interfaces. In a loaded taper system, no bond between stem and cement is necessary. Both types of stem have performed equally well in the long term.

A composite beam requires all components to be rigidly bonded, with no movement between them. A tapered stem, however, must be capable of movement within its cement mantle. As a patient bears weight on a tapered, cemented femoral stem, the load is transmitted from the prosthetic femoral head and forces the taper to subside within the cement mantle. This subsidence generates radial compressive forces within the cement and subsequent hoop stresses within the bone. These forces are created throughout the length of the femoral stem, reducing proximal stress shielding.

Stem material

Cemented stems are fabricated from a variety of metals, including cobalt chromium, stainless steel, and titanium. Improved manufacturing techniques and the use of high strength stainless steel and cobalt chrome meant that stem fracture is now regarded as a thing of the past.

Stem length

Most conventional femoral stems extend to the isthmus of the medullary canal, to stabilize alignment and prevent varus migration. More recently, bone conserving joint replacements are emerging. Hip resurfacing, epiphyseal replacement, and mid head resection stems are being implanted and evaluated.

Stem offset

In a series of two hundred cadaveric femora, typical femoral offset was found to be 40–50 mm. Use of a short-necked femoral component can decrease offset in a reconstructed hip. This results in relatively medial abductor insertion, shortening the abductor lever arm, and reduced mechanical efficiency. Reduced offset increases the energy required for normal gait and may cause an abductor lurch, limit the range of motion, and decrease hip stability.

Increasing femoral offset lengthens the abductor lever arm, reducing the abductor muscle force required for normal gait. A lateral position of the femur also reduces impingement of the femur on the pelvis, and improves soft tissue tension. However, an increased offset may cause trochanteric bursitis due to increased pressure from the fascia lata. Also, an increased offset creates a larger bending moment on the prosthesis, which may increase strain in the medial cement mantle. This effect could contribute to early failure of the femoral component.

Stem shape

Before considering stem shape, it is helpful to consider the modes of loading, including axial forces, bending forces, and rotational forces. The mechanism of transfer of axial and bending forces is predominantly affected by the mid-frontal plane shape. The cross-sectional (horizontal plane) shape determines rotational stability of the stem and stress distribution within the cement mantle.

Collar or Collarless

Considerable debate has surrounded the need for a collar. A collar is a medial extension of the stem that projects at the level of the calcar cut. The collar of a cemented femoral component allows direct load transfer from the implant to the medial cement mantle and/or the bone of the medial femoral neck. The collar can decrease tensile stress in the stem and reduce migration. The second function of a collar is to control insertion when the stem is smaller than the broach, so that the implant reaches the same level as the broach. A collar should be considered only in composite-beam stems.

A collarless design should be considered in stems with a tapered design, which allows the stem to move distally and engage with the cement mantle. This increases compressive loading in the cement and reduces tensile and shear stresses and ultimately reduces calcar resorption.

Surface finish

Controversies exist with regard to the optimal stem surface finish for cement fixation. Polished stems with a roughness (Ra) of less than 1 micrometer create little abrasion with the cement mantle. Matt surface finish with a Ra of less than 2 micrometer will create abrasion with the cement mantle in the presence of excessive micromotion. In some cases, roughened stems have failed earlier than polished stems of the same design. Surface finish may be a critical factor in the durability of cement fixation with specific stem geometries. A Ra of greater than 2 micrometer is expected to cause excessive abrasion with the cemented mantle in tapered stems causing premature failure.

Stem alignment

Implant malposition can impair long-term survival of cemented THR, probably due to increased cement mantle stress.

There are two principal causes of malposition: implantation with the component in varus or valgus, and failure to centre the stem in the cement mantle. Implant positioning can be optimized with a stem centralizer or a cannulated stem.

Cement Mantle Stresses and optimal thickness

Control of mantle geometry is vital in controlling cement stresses. During normal weight bearing activities, cement stresses are highest in the proximal mantle and around the distal stem tip. When a stem subsides, it generates hoop stresses in the cement. Creep and stress relaxation dissipate hoop stresses, which are succeeded by radial compressive stress. In general, lower stem/cement friction results in increased cement loads in compression, and decreased shear forces. PMMA has greater compressive than tensile strength, so preferential loading in compression rather than shear is advantageous.

It has been demonstrated that stems with a 2–5 mm medial mantle have the best outcome, and that 3–4 mm cement mantles appear to have the best stress curves. However, this has challenged by others, and to a greater extent by the 'French paradox'. Two French-designed cemented femoral components both fill the medullary canal of the femur.

Stress risers

Stems with a square cross-section have more rotational stability than oval stems. However, sharp edges create peak stresses in the cement, which can lead to microfractures particular in areas where the cement mantle is thin.

Cement plug

Pressurization of acrylic cement is necessary for optimal fixation. Although this is most frequently achieved with a cement gun, it is possible to pressurize the implantation site by converting it into a closed space, with an intramedullary plug. Plug performance varies with canal diameter: in larger canals, plugs are more prone to migration. A successful plug should resist a cement pressure of 50 psi in clinical use. This can be more difficult in canals of >14 mm diameter.

Pre-Op Planning for THR

Pre-operative templating of the hip can be undertaken to determine a number of factors. On the acetabular side to determine the centre of rotation, identify any issues around coxa profunda or dysplasia. On the femoral side determine the centre of the femoral head, femoral offset, neck shaft angle, and an impression of the femoral canal shape. Also the relationship of the tip of the greater trochanter to the centre of the femoral head. Be clear where the piriform fossa is in order to avoid varus placement of the stem.

Factors that may lead to inaccuracy during templating include external rotation of the femur giving the appearance of coax valga and altered impression of femoral offset. Coxa vara may lead to thoughts around post operative lengthening and hip instability. Limb length can be assessed radiologically by drawing a line at level of, and parallel to, ischial tuberosities and intersecting the lesser trochanter on each side. A comparison of the two points of intersection measurement differences will determine any evidence of limb shortening.

Box 7.5.3

- Optimal Stem offset 40–50 mm
- Reduced offset leads to reduced mechanical efficiency
- Increased offset leads to larger bending moment on the prosthesis
- Collars for composite beam stems
- Collarless for taper slip stems
- Polished surface finish

Bearing surface

Improvements in femoral and acetabulum implant anchorage over the last 20 years have significantly extended THR implant lifespan; the formation of wear debris, however, leads to resorption and osteolysis, considerably shortening implant lifespan in active patients. Most wear related particulate debris originates from the bearing surfaces.

Wear remains is a significant problem. Alternative bearing surfaces are constantly being developed with improved tribological properties to reduce the amount of biologically active particle generation that can lead to osteolysis and aseptic loosening. The bearing surface include highly cross linked polyethylene, metal-on-metal articulations, ceramic on ceramic surfaces and composite bearing surfaces.

Highly cross linked polyethylene

In the past, polyethylene cups were manufactured from ultra-high molecular weight polyethylene (UHMWPE) by extrusion, bulk compression moulding, or net shape moulding followed by gamma sterilization in air with wear rates approximating 0.1 to 0.2 mm/year.

In order to reduce wear rates highly cross-linked UHMWPE was introduced in 1998. Gamma irradiation in the order of two to four times that used in traditional UHMWPE and electron beam radiation are used in conjunction with thermal treatment to induce cross linking of polyethylene particles and reduce free radicals that oxidize and weaken the polyethylene. The highly cross linked polyethylene has improved resistance to wear. However, too much radiation can lead to the material becoming prone to fatigue fracture. Very highly cross-linked polyethylene (PE) shows very significant improvement in terms of wear at five years' follow-up compared to conventional PE, but the behaviour of this new concept will need to be monitored in the long term.

Use of larger femoral head articulating with the cross linked UHMWPE provides the potential for increased range of movement, reduced frequency of dislocation and reduced risk of component impingement without volumetric wear.

The incidence of dislocation has been reported as 1–4% in primary THR and up to 16% in revision cases. Acetabular component with an elevated rim is thought to improve the postoperative stability. The presence of elevated liners can reduce the incidence of dislocation in primary THR from 3.8% to 2.2%. The largest benefit is gained in revision hip replacement surgery. The majority of dislocations are reported have been posterior caused by flexion, adduction, and internal rotation. Beware, that the elevated liners may increase the incidence of anterior dislocation due to impingement between the femoral neck and elevated lip of the liner during external rotation. In addition, they may also contribute to increased polyethylene wear.

If the femoral component is placed with adequate ante-version, excessive internal rotation is needed before the hip dislocates posteriorly. The abductors do not allow enough external rotation for the hip to dislocate anteriorly. Excessive anterversion of the femoral component reduces the chances of dislocation, but also limits external rotation. Excessive retroversion may predispose to posterior dislocation.

Metal-on-Metal Articulation

Metal-on-Metal articulations were first introduced with the McKee Farrar hip replacement. The main advantage are seen both in vitro on wear simulators and in vivo with retrieved implants in which the wear rates are low and increased range of motion to impingement secondary to the availability of larger diameter femoral heads. Retrievals analysed after 21 years of implantation revealed acetabular linear wear rates of 4.2 μm/year, which was 25 times lower than the wear rate of traditional UHMWPE. However, as a result of imperfect manufacturing, the implants were vulnerable to seize and subsequently loosen. More recently, improved manufacturing has led to better tolerances leading to lower wear rates. Wear rates of metal-on- metal bearings typically have 1 to 2 years run in period with wear rates of 20–25 ɥm/year; a steady state wear rate of only 5 ɥm/year is typically observed. Similarly, to the wear pattern, metal-on-metal bearings produce ion levels that are high initially during the 1 to 2 year run in phase and then decrease. However, the main concern around metal-on-metal articulations is the effects of the metal ions debris.

Concerns exist regarding the generation of metal ions seen in both the blood, serum, and urine of patients with metal-on-metal implants. As ion excretion is renal, use of a metal-on-metal bearings in significant renal impairment should be with caution. Metal particles (0.05 μm) are far smaller than polyethylene particles (~1μm) and can thus cross the placental barrier. Women of child-bearing age should be counselled accordingly.

Large ball metal-on-metal bearings are particularly susceptible to high levels of metal ion generation. Raised metal ion levels have been reported if the cups are implanted with high inclination angles (> 50 degrees). These metal ions have theoretical, although not proven, risks related to carcinogenic and biologic concerns. Additionally, concerns exist regarding hypersensitivity. In a few cases, a synovial reaction to Metal-on-metal articulations has been identified to cause ALVAL (Aseptic Lymphocyte dominated Vasculitis Associated Lesion,). This reaction has been reported to occur in approximately 1% of cases with a female preponderance. The patients may present with a pseudotumor or pain leading to muscle and neurological damage.

Although a metal-on-metal bearing may be considered a viable alternative to either polyethylene or ceramic implants, outstanding and unresolved issues continue to exist with this bearing, as they do with the alternatives.

Ceramic on Ceramic

Ceramic on ceramic bearing have been used since the 1970's. Alumina-alumina friction couples are hard, scratch resistant and provide a low friction coefficient, with wear particles that do not cause any osteolysis. Alumina bearings have shown low wear rates of 0.025 mm/year comparable to those of metal-on-metal articulations and up to 5000 times lower than metal-on-polyethylene. Ceramics are inert materials. The disadvantage of ceramic bearing is with their brittle nature. Improvements in manufacturing have reduced fracture rates down to 4 per 100,000 patients. Zirconia is a less brittle ceramic than alumina and fracture risk is theoretically lower. The current generation DELTA ceramic is a zirconia-alumina composite and is rapidly becoming the ceramic bearing of choice.

Box 7.5.4 Summary Box

- With Ultra High Molecular Weight Polyethylene Gamma irradiation and Cross linking can improve resistance to wear
- Metal-on-metal manufacturing has significantly improved
- Metal-on-metal concerns regarding metal ions, hypersensitivity, ALVAL, and pseudotumor
- New DELTA ceramic is a hard, scratch resistant bearing that provides a low friction coefficient

Acetabular Biomechanics

The surgeon should aim to restore the normal hip centre during acetabular reconstruction which helps restore normal biomechanics. Reaming down to the true floor of the acetabulum will medialize the hip centre and may improve the efficiency of the abductors. Implantation of the acetabular component laterally, reduces the abductor arm moment and increases joint reaction forces. The final position of the cup is critical to allow physiological movement without impingement. Cup placed in 30–40 degrees of abduction and 15–20 degrees of anteversion are regarded as a safe range. When cups are abducted less than 30 degrees, impingement occurs in flexion. When a cup is abducted more than 50 degrees, the femoral head is vulnerable to sublux out of the acetabulum. The bearing surfaces are also susceptible to higher rates of linear and volumetric wear.

Acetabular implant for hip replacement

Factors that influence the outcome of acetabular replacement are design materials, means of fixation, operative technique, and patient-related parameters. Threaded cups have failed to demonstrate any improvement in results and have been widely abandoned. The idea of metal backing has some theoretical advantages. However, metal backing has failed to provide any improvement when used for cemented cups. Presently, uncemented porous-coated or hydroxyapaptite acetabular components are the most popular option but it should be noted that advocates of fully cemented cups do provide equally strong data to support their preference.

Cementless cup

Uncemented acetabular components usually have a coated or textured surface to encourage bone growth into the surface for biological fixation. The components may also have screw holes via which screws can be implanted; or spikes, pegs, or fins to help hold the implant in place until the new bone forms. Sufficient initial fixation is required for osseo-integration and secondary stability of the press fit components. Ideally the component surface should lie with in 50 micrometers of the acetabulum to facilitate host bone attachment. Whilst screws provide additional fixation, there is a paucity of evidence to support that the screws act as sources of fretting, generating wear debris leading to osteolysis. By reducing the number of screws these mechanisms of wear debris are minimized. However, the unfilled screw holes also can act as conduits for wear debris generated from the liner to affect the attachment of the bone onto the cup surface.

Hemispherical and Rim Fitting cups

Cementless hemispherical cups are implanted in the acetabulum following 1–2 mm under reaming. Acetabuli should not be under reamed by more than 2 mm. Excessive under reaming of the acetabulum may lead to an acetabular fracture in. Cementless rim fitting (peripheral flare) cups are implanted in the acetabulum typically following size for size reaming. Either type of cementless cup usually has the option of supplementary fixation with screws. In addition, once the outer shell of the cup is implanted, the appropriate liner can be inserted.

Rim fitting cups may be more appropriate for protrusio or where the acetabulum has the potential to be over medialized. Failure to restore normal lateral offset in cases of protrusio may cause the greater trochanter to impinge off of the anterior edge of the acetabulum, potentially leading to posterior instability. Bone grafting the medial wall with cancellous autograft taken from the femoral head may be also required.

Cemented Acetabular Component

Whereas improved cementing techniques have produced a marked reduction in the rate of femoral component loosening, the incidence of acetabular loosening has been only slightly influenced by such improvements.

Cementless Femoral component

In the 1980s, new implant designs were introduced to attach directly to bone without the use of cement. The stem material tends to be manufactured from titanium which is less than 50% less stiff compared to cobalt chrome alloys which favours proximal load transfer. The proximal stem geometry in the majority can be either anatomical, trapezoid or rectangular. With respect to the distal stem geometry, cylindrical stems seat in the diaphysis and tapered stems allow metaphyseal seating.

Box 7.5.5 Summary Box

- Restore the normal hip centre
- Cup placed in 30–40 degrees of abduction
- Cup placed in 15–20 degrees of anteversion
- Uncemented porous-coated or hydroxyapaptite acetabular components available
- Biological fixation
- Hemispherical and rim fitting cups
- Cemented cups

The stems also have a surface that is conducive to attracting new bone growth. Most are textured or have a surface coating around much of the implant so that the new bone actually grows into the surface of the implant to provide secondary biological stability. The surface porosity is achieved via plasma-spray, grit-blasting, or bead sintering allowing bone ongrowth and fibre metal allowing bone ingrowth and hydroxyapaptite encouraging osseointegration.

Precise preparation the femoral channel must match the shape of the implant itself very closely. New bone growth cannot bridge gaps larger than 1 mm to 2 mm. Cementless femoral components tend to be much larger at the top, with more of a wedge shape. This design enables the strong cortex of the bone and the dense, hard spongy cancellous bone just below it to provide support. The prosthesis should have minimal stiffnes and maximum stablility.

Risk factors for intra-operative fracture include female gender, rheumatoid arthritis, increasing age, osteoporosis, and altered bone morphology/ deformity. Intra-operative fracture is more common in cementless than cemented stems.

Initially, it was hoped that cementless THR would eliminate the problem of bone resorption or stem loosening caused by cement failure. Although certain cementless stem designs have excellent long-term outcomes, cementless stems can loosen if a strong bond between bone and stem is not achieved.

Patients with large cementless stems may also experience a higher incidence of mild thigh pain. Causes of thigh pain include motion at the bone prosthesis interface, varus stem position in the presence of distal cortical hypertrophy, and excessive stress transfer from stem to host femur. Patients should be initially managed with time, since thigh pain may subside over the first 2 years.

Likewise, polyethylene wear, particulate debris, and the resulting osteolysis (dissolution of bone) remains problematic in both cemented and uncemented designs.

Cementless THR is most often recommended for younger, more active patients and patients with good bone quality where bone ingrowth into the components can be predictably achieved. Cementless stems are not the stem of choice for patients with stove pipe femurs, previous fracture, or previous osteotomy since these patients would not be expected to achieve a tight fit which is necessary for ingrowth. Poor quality bone stock is more likely to undergo plastic deformation and to allow subsidence of the femoral component.

Hybrid Total Hip Replacement

A hybrid THR has one component, usually the acetabular socket, inserted without cement, and the other component, usually the femoral stem, inserted with cement. This technique was introduced in the early 1980s, so long-term results are just now being measured. A hybrid hip takes advantage of the excellent track record of cementless hip sockets and cemented stems.

Box 7.5.6 Summary Box

- Uncemented stems with surface coatings
- Interference fit and biological fixation
- Implant should have minimum stiffness and maximum stability
- Not ideal with stove pipe femurs

Femoral head

The femoral head range in size from 22 mm up to 44 mm in THR. Larger femoral heads can be used in combination with resurfacing type acetabular components. The larger the femoral head, the larger the range of motion before impingement occurs against the acetabulum and therefore therefore has less dislocation risk.

Longevity and Outcomes

Hip replacement operations are highly successful in relieving pain and restoring movement. However, the ongoing problems with wear and particulate debris may eventually necessitate further surgery, including replacing the prosthesis (revision surgery) in damaged host bone.

Future

Improvements in the wear characteristics of newer polyethylene and the advent of hard bearings (metal-on-metal or ceramic) and bone conserving hip replacements may help resolve some of these problems in the future.

Further Reading

Alter, P., Lengsfeld, M., and Schmitt, J. (1999). Stress analysis of an anatomically-adapted femur shaft prosthesis (Lubinus SPII). *Zeitschrift fur Orthopadie und ihre Grenzgebiete*, **137**, 129–35.

Andriacchi, T.P., Galante, J.O., Belytschko, T.B., and Hampton, S. (1976). A stress analysis of the femoral stem in total hip prosthesis. *Journal of Bone and Joint Surgery [Am]*, **58-A**, 618–24.

Beckenbaugh, R.D. and Ilstrup, D.M. (1978). Total hip arthroplasty. A review of three hundred and thirty-three cases with long follow-up. *Journal of Bone and Joint Surgery [Br]*, **60-A**, 306–13.

Beim, G.M., Lavernia, C., and Convery, F.R. (1989). Intramedullary plugs in cemented hip arthroplasty. *Journal of Arthroplasty*, **4**, 139–41.

Callaghan, J.J., Salvati, E.A., Pellicci, P.M., Wilson, Jr. P.D., and Ramawat, C.S. (1985). Results of revision for mechanical failure after cemented total hip replacement, 1979 to 1982. *Journal of Bone and Joint Surgery [Am]*, **67A**, 1079–85.

Charnley, J. (1979). *Biomechanic in low friction arthroplasty of the hip.* Springer-Verlag, New York.

Charnley, J. (1982). Evolution of total hip replacement. *Faltin Lecture-Annales Chirugiae et Gynaecologiea*, **71**, 103–7.

Cobb, T.K., Morrey, B,F., and Ilstrup, D.M. (1996). The elevated-rim acetabular liner in total hip arthroplasty: relationship to postoperative dislocation. *Journal of Bone and Joint Surgery* [*Am*], **78**(1), 80–6.

Coudane, H., Fery, A., Sommelet, J., Lacoste, J., Leduc, P., and Gaucher, A. (1981). Aseptic loosening of cemented total arthroplasties of the hip in relation to positioning of the prosthesis. New utilization of the Tschuprow-Cramer statistical test. *Acta Orthopaedica Scandinavica*, **52**, 201–5.

Ebramzadeh, E., Sarmiento, A., McKellop, H.A., Llinas, A., and Gogan, W. (1994). The cement mantle in total hip arthroplasty: Analysis of long term radiolgraphic results. *Journal of Bone and Joint Surgery* [*Br*], **76A**, 77–87.

Ebramzadeh, E., Sangiorgio, S.N., Longjohn, D.B., Buhari, C.F., and Dorr, L.D. (2004). Initial stability of cemented femoral stems as a function of surface finish, collar and stem size. *Journal of Bone and Joint Surgery [Am]*, **86-A**, 106–15.

Haboush, E. J. (1953). Arthroplasty of the hip based on biomechanics, photoelasticity, fast-setting dental acrylic and other consideration. *Bull Hospital Joint Disease*, **14**, 242–77.

Hallan, G., Lie, S.A., Furnes, O., Engesaeter, L.B., Vollset, S.E., and Havelin, L.I. (2007). Medium- and long-term performance of 11 516 uncemented primary femoral stems from the Norwegian arthroplasty register. *Journal of Bone and Joint Surgery [Br]*, **89-B**, 1574–80.

Johnston, R.C., Brand, R.A., and Crowninshield, R.D. (1979). Reconstruction of the hip: a mathematical approach to determine optimum geometric relationship. *Journal of Bone and Joint Surgery [Am]*, **61A**, 639.

Johnston, J.A., Johnston, D., Hanaway, R., *et al.* (1995). Occlusion and stability of synthetic femoral canal plugs used in cemented hip arthroplasty. *Journal of Applied Biomater*, **6**, 213–8.

Kelikian, A.S., Tachdjian, M.O., Askew, M.J., and Jasty, M. (1983). Greater trochanteric advancement of the proximal femur:a clincal and biomechanical study. *Proceedings of the Eleventh Open Scientific Meeting of the Hip Society*, pp. 77. IN The Hip, CV Mosby, ST Louis.

Kerboull, M. (1987). The Charnley-Kerboull prosthesis. In: Postel M, Kerboull M, Evrard J, Courpeid J, eds. *Total hip replacement*, pp. 13–7. Berlin, etc: Spring-er Verlag.

Koster, G., Willert, H.G., Ernstberger, T., and Kohler, H.P. (1998). Centralization of the femoral component in cemented hip arthroplasty using guided stem insertion. *Archives of Orthopaedic and Traumatic Surgery (Germany)*, **117**(8), 425–9.

Kristiansen, B. and Jensen, J.S. (1985). Biomechanical factors in loosening of the Stanmore hip. *Acta Orthopaedica Scandinavica*, **56**, 21–24.

Kuiper, J.H. and Huiskes, R. (1996). Friction and stem stiffness affect dynamic interface motion in total hip replacement. *Journal of Orthopaedic Research*, **4**, 36–43.

Kwak, B.M., Lim, O.K., Kim, Y.Y., and Rim, K. (1979). An investigation of the effect of cement thickness on an implant by finite stress analysis. *Int Orthop*, 1–4.

Lee, A.J. and Wrighton, J.D. (1973). Some properties of polymethacrylate with reference to its use in orthopaedic surgery. *Clinical Orthopaedics.* 1973; 95:281–287.

Levy, R., Nobel, P., Scheller, Jr. A., Tullos, H., and Turner, R. (1988). The clinical reproducibility of precise asymmetric femoral cement mantle for total hip replacement. *Orthop Trans*, **12**, 591.

Malroy, T.H. (1981). A plastic intramedullary plug for total hip arthroplasty. *Clinical Orthopaedics*, **155**, 37–40.

Mann, K.A. and Kim, B.S. (2000). Influence of stem shape on fatigue fracture of the cement mantle in femoral hip components. *Procs Orthopaedic Research Society.*

Massoud, S.N., Hunter, J.B., Holdsworth, B.J., Wallace, W.A., and Juliusson, R. (1997). Early femoral loosening in one design of cemented hip replacement. *Journal of Bone and Joint Surgery [Br]*, **79**, 603–8.

Murray, D.W., Carr, A.J., and Bulstrode, C.J. (1995). Which primary total hip replacement? *Journal of Bone and Joint Surgery [Br]*, **77**(4), 520–7.

Neumann, L., Freund, K.G., and Sorenson, K.H. (1994). Long-term results of Charnley total hip replacement. Review of 92 patients at 15 to 20 years. *Journal of Bone and Joint Surgery [Br]*, **76-B**, 245–51.

Nizard, R.S., Sedel, L., and Christel, R. (1992). Ten year survivorship of cemented ce-ramic- ceramic total hip prostheses. *Clinical Orthopaedics*, **282**, 53–63.

Noble, P.C., Alexander, J.W., Lindahl, L.J., et al. (1988). Anatomical basis of femoral component design. *Clinical Orthopaedics*, **235**, 149–165.

Oh, I., Carlson, C.E., Tomford, W.W., *et al.* (1978). Improved fixation of the femoral component after total hip replacement using methacrylate intramedullary plug. *Journal of Bone and Joint Surgery [A]*, **60**A, 608–12.

Oh, I., Bourne, R.B., and Harris, W.H. (1983). The femoral cement compactor: an improvement in cementing technique in total hip replacement. *Journal of Bone and Joint Surgery [Am]*, **65A**, 1335.

Olsson, S.S., Jernberger. A., and Tryggo, D. (1981). Clinical and radiological long term results after Charnley-Muller total hip replacement. A 5 to 10 year follow-up study with special reference to aseptic loosening. *Acta orthopaedica Scandinavica*, **52**, 531–42.

Robertson, D., Lavalette, S., Morgan, and Angus, P.D. (2005). The hydroxyapatite-coated JRI-Furlong hip: OUTCOME IN PATIENTS

UNDER THE AGE OF 55 YEARS. *Journal of Bone and Joint Surgery [Br]*, **87-B**, 12–15.

Sarmiento, A., Turner, T.M., Latta, L.L., and Tarr, R.R. (1979). Factors contributing to lysis of the femoral neck in toatal hip arthroplasty. Clinical Orthopaedics, **145**, 208–12.

Savilahti, S., Myllyneva, I., Pajamaki, K.J., and Lindholm, T.S. (1997). Survival of Lubinus straight (IP) and curved (SP) total hip prosthesis in 543 patients after 4-13 years. *Archives of Orthopaedic and Traumatic Surgery*, **116**, 10–13.

Shetty, A., Slack, R., Tindall, A., James, K.D., and Rand, C. (2005). Results of a hydroxyapatite-coated (Furlong) total hip replacement: A 13-TO 15-YEAR FOLLOW-UP. *Journal of Bone and Joint Surgery [Br]*, **87-B**, 1050–54.

Singh, S., Trikha, S.P., and Edge, A.J. (2004). Hydroxyapatite ceramic-coated femoral stems in young patients: A PROSPECTIVE TEN-YEAR STUDY. *Journal of Bone and Joint Surgery [Br]*, **86-B**, 1118–23.

Skinner, J.A., Todo, S., Taylor, M., Wang, J.S., Pinskerova, V., and Scott, G. (2003). Should the cement mantle around the femoral component be thick or thin? *Journal of Bone and Joint Surgery [Br]*, **85**-B, 45–51.

Soballe, K. and Christensen, F. (1988). Calcar resorption after total hip arthroplasty. *Journal of Arthroplasty*, **3**, 103–7.

Suominen, S., Antti-Poika, I., Tallroth, K., *et al.* (1996). Femoral component fixation with and without intramedullary plug. A six year follow up. *Acta Orthopaedic and Traumatic Surgery*, **115**, 276–79.

Vaughan, P.D., Singh, P.J., Teare, R., Kucheria, R., and Singer, G.C. (2007). Femoral stem tip orientation and surgical approach in total hip arthroplasty. *Hip International*, **17**, *212 –7*.

Verdonshot, N. and Huiskes, R. (1997). Cement debonding process of total hip arthroplasty stems. *Clinical Orthopaedics*, **336**, 297–307.

Verdonschot, N. and Huskies, R. (1998). Surface roughness of debonded straight-tapered stems in cemented THA reduces subsidence but not cement damage. *Biomaterial*, **19**, 1973.

Williams, H.D.W., Browne, G., Gie, G.A. Ling, R.S.M., Timperley, A.J., and Wendover, N.A. (2002). The Exeter universal cemented femoral component at 8 to 12 years: A STUDY OF THE FIRST 325 HIPS. *Journal of Bone and Joint Surgery [Br]*, **84-B**, 324–34.

Wroblewski, B.M. (1986). 15-21 Year results of the Charnley low friction arthroplasty. *Clinical Orthopaedics*, **211**, 30.

Wroblewski, B.M., Taylor, G.W., and Siney, P. (1992). Charnley low friction arthroplasty:19–25 year results. *Clinical Orthopaedics*, **15**, 421.

Wroblewski, B.M., Siney, P.D., and Fleming, P.A. (2002). Charnley low-frictional torque arthroplasty in patients under the age of 51 years: follow-up to 33 years. *Journal of Bone and Joint Surgery [Br]*, **84-B**, 540–3.

Wroblewski, B.M., Siney, P.D., and Fleming P.A. (2007). Charnley low-friction arthroplasty: SURVIVAL PATTERNS TO 38 YEARS. *Journal of Bone and Joint Surgery [Br]*, **89-B**, 1015–18.

7.6

Bearing surfaces

Gordon Blunn

Summary points

- Traditionally bearings were made from polyethylene and cobalt chrome. These bearings are still most commonly used for knee replacements. In hip replacements due to osteolysis caused by polyethylene wear alternative material combinations at the bearing surface are used
- Highly cross linked plastics have been developed and have been shown to reduce wear. There are a number of different types available which differ in their performance
- Metal on metal bearings first used in the 1960s have also been developed and show very low wear rates. These bearings are more susceptible to edge loading and the resulting metal ion release can result in adverse biological reactions leading to failure
- Whilst ceramic on plastic surfaces have been used for a considerable amount of time the reduction in wear is not as great as with well functioning metal on metal bearings
- Ceramic on ceramic bearings have been used for a considerable time and show even lower wear rates than metal on metal bearings. In the past there has been an incidence of catastrophic fracture of these bearings but developments in materials technology have considerably reduced these events.

Introduction

Joint replacements of the hip and knee are among the most successful of surgical procedures. The changing demography of the population means that in future more total joint replacements are going to be performed. For example, in 2003, the number of primary total hip replacements performed in the United States was around 220 000 and this is expected to increase to over half a million in 2030. The number of primary total knee replacements is expected to rise exponentially with the ageing population. Patients today are also generally more active than those of three decades ago when hip and knee replacements were first being developed. The success of total joint replacements also means that younger patients are being treated with these procedures. Therefore extending implant longevity and improving function to meet the increased demands of today's patients are important. One of the limiting factors to increasing the longevity of total joint replacements, particularly hip replacements, has been the performance of the bearing surface. In the 1990s, alternative bearings to cobalt-chrome on ultra-high-molecular-weight polyethylene (UHMWPE), such as metal-on-metal and ceramic-on-ceramic, saw a resurgence in use due to aseptic osteolysis, which is associated with the release of UHMWPE wear debris. Development of the materials and design of alternative bearings has continued in an effort to reduce problems associated with wear at the articulation. Alternative bearing surfaces have been used predominantly for total hip replacement with total knee replacements still using conventional UHMWPE on cobalt chrome. This chapter will focus on the problems associated with wear of UHMWPE and then concentrate on the development of alternative bearing surfaces.

Problems associated with wear of UHMWPE (Box 7.6.1)

In the 1980s, endosteal lysis was thought to be associated with the breakup of the cement mantle and release of cement debris. The use of uncemented stems was introduced because it was believed that cement was detrimental to the long-term fixation of components, particularly in younger active patients. It was not until the late 1980s that wear particles released from polyethylene bearings were identified as being the main contributors to aseptic osteolysis

Box 7.6.1 Conventional UHMWPE

- Wear of the bearing surface leads to the release of small particles less than 1μm in size
- These particles are phagocytosed by macrophages, causing an inflammatory reaction which leads to activation of osteoclasts, aseptic osteolysis, and loosening of the implant
- The average wear rate for hip replacements with a 22-mm head (linear penetration) is around 0.1mm/year
- A threshold has been established of 0.05mm/year. Below this threshold, osteolysis rarely occurs
- Frictional torque and sliding distance increase with larger heads and for this reason, bearings of less than 30mm have to be used.

and long-term implant loosening. Small particles released from the plastic bearing surface are phagocytosed by macrophages, which then release a number of cytokines, the most important being tumour necrosis factor (TNF) alpha, interleukin-1 and -6, and prostaglandins. These cytokines recruit other macrophages and also promote osteoclastic bone resorption. Macrophages can only phagocytose particles less than 8µm in size and larger polyethylene particles are engulfed by foreign body giant cells (Figure 7.6.1). This may well be one of the reasons why aseptic osteolysis for knee joint replacements is not as common as that seen in hip replacements.

The main wear mechanism responsible for knee joint replacements is delamination which is a spalling of the plastic surface leading to the formation of large plastic shards which are engulfed by foreign body giant cells. In the hip joint, predominantly particles considerably less than 1 µm in size are released from the acetabular plastic bearing surface due to adhesive and abrasive wear mechanisms. Calculations have shown that millions of wear particles are released from the acetabular cup on a yearly basis. Examination of worn polyethylene hip and knee joints shows a contrasting appearance. The plastic articulating surface of worn tibial components due to delamination is characteristically rough and flaky. For UHMWPE acetabular components, the worn region is often finely polished and smooth (Figure 7.6.2). Clinically this leads to a linear decrease in the wall thickness of the acetabular cup which can be identified and measured on sequential clinical radiographs. The linear wear rate determined from a number of clinical studies using UHMWPE has been shown to be on average 0.05–0.1mm per year. For a 22-mm diameter cup this represents a volumetric loss of around 38mm^3. This wear rate is associated with successful cases where there is little evidence of osteolysis. In any clinical series there is a distribution around a mean where in some instances the wear rate may be considerably higher and osteolysis evident. The concept of a wear threshold has been introduced by Dumbelton and co-workers. They suggested that a wear rate below 0.05mm per year would not cause osteolysis and this was based on the observation that osteolysis was rarely seen in patients with wear rates of 0.1mm per year.

A wear rate threshold implies that wear particles released in low numbers do not have any effect and this may be associated with the clearance of macrophages containing the particles from the joint via the reticular endothelial system. UHMWPE wear particles have been identified in regional lymph nodes (inguinal) and aortic lymph nodes as well as in the spleen.

When Sir John Charnley introduced polyethylene as a bearing surface for total hip replacements in 1963 he did so in combination with a specific design. He referred to the design concept as 'low friction arthroplasty', indicating the benefits of having a relatively small, 22-mm diameter head which reduced frictional torque and a thick plastic acetabular component which dissipated the stresses. For UHMWPE bearings there are advantages of having a small femoral head which is associated with the sliding distance imposed on the bearing surface as it moves. Relative to the acetabular cup, for a given rage of movement a smaller head moves less than a larger head and

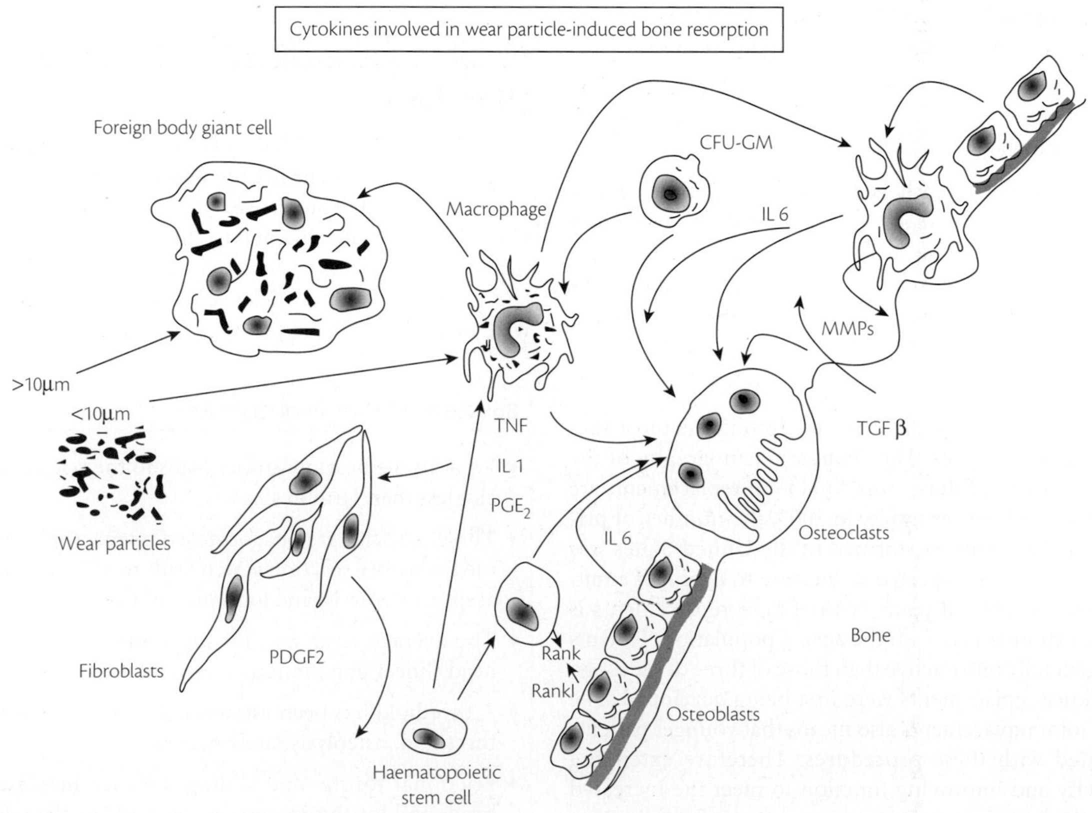

Fig. 7.6.1 Simplified diagram of part of the biological response to wear particles; wear particles under 10µm are phagocytosed by macrophages. The macrophages secrete cytokines including TNF alpha, which lead to further inflammation and induces bone resorption by osteoclasts.

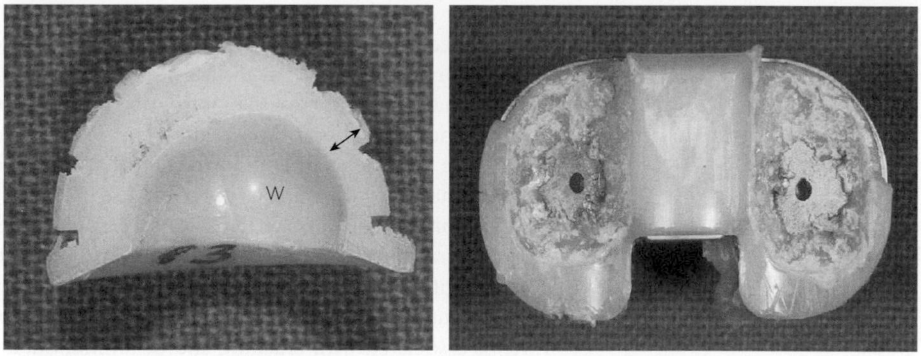

A B

Fig. 7.6.2 Photographs of worn acetabular cup (A) and worn tibial components (B). This shows the smooth worn region of the cup cause by abrasive and adhesive wear (w) and the thinner acetabular wall associated with the wear region (arrowed). The tibial plastic has worn down to the metal base plate and in contrast to the cup, the worn plastic has a flaky appearance caused by delamination wear.

consequently the sliding distance is less. This leads to reduced wear with smaller heads and is the reason why conventional UHMWPE bearings surface are restricted to below 30mm in diameter. The disadvantage with smaller head sizes when compared to larger heads, is that in theory there is a reduced range of movement due to earlier impingement of the femoral head on the rim of the cup. There is also a greater incidence of disarticulation due to the distance required for dislocation to occur, which is less with smaller heads.

Alternative bearings

Alternative bearing surfaces have been developed in response to the high wear rates of metal on conventional polyethylene and subsequent osteolysis caused by the generation of wear debris from these bearings.

These alternative bearings include:

- Cross-linked polyethylene
- Metal-on-metal bearings
- Ceramic-on-ceramic bearings
- Ceramic-on-polyethylene
- Metal-on-ceramic bearings.

Cross-linked polyethylene (Box 7.6.2)

In the 1990s it was recognized that sterilization using gamma irradiation in air led to a gradual increase in the oxidation of the plastic. Work from John Collier's laboratory (Dartford, United States) showed that plastic components sterilized by gamma irradiation and stored in air over several years gradually developed a characteristic subsurface zone of oxidation (Figure 7.6.3). This was a result of the irradiation process which caused chain scission and

Box 7.6.2 Cross-linked polyethylene

- Gamma irradiation causes the generation of free radicals which can cause both cross linking and oxidation
- XPEs are made using high doses of irradiation promoting cross-linking and by a heat treatment that drives off the free radicals
- There are a number of different XPEs available with different performances and material properties
- XPEs have been shown to substantially reduce the wear of the acetabular cup.

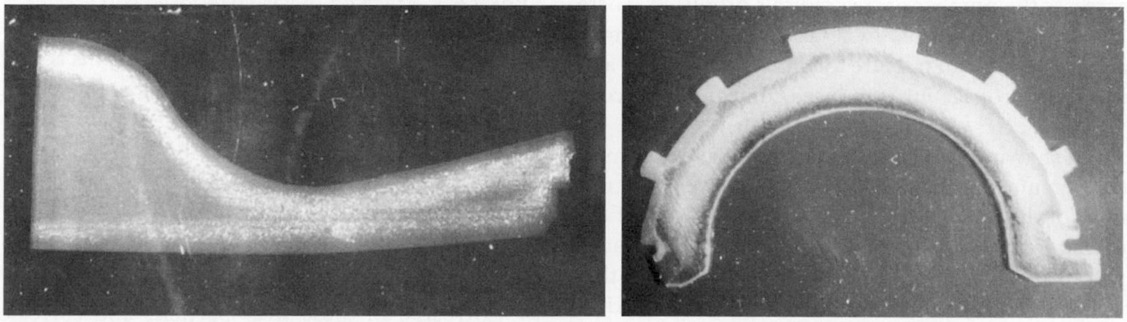

A B

Fig. 7.6.3 Sections through part of a plastic component from a knee joint component (A) and an acetabular cup (B) showing subsurface embrittled regions caused by plastic oxidation. The embrittled plastic has been stained with a strong acid discolouring the oxidized polyethylene.

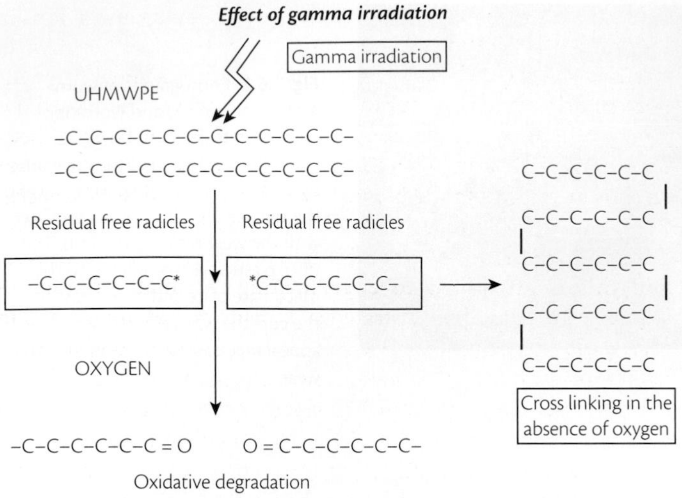

Fig. 7.6.4 The effects of gamma irradiation in air and in an inert environment.

free-radical generation (Figure 7.6.4). In air, these free radicals combined with oxygen resulting in embrittlement of the plastic. In retrieved components it was shown that this led to enhanced delamination and surface wear. Around this time it was also shown that irradiation in an inert environment had a beneficial effect. This was because the free radicals which were generated by irradiation cross-linked the polyethylene molecules, stabilizing the material. Hip simulator work showed that oxidation was detrimental and increased the surface wear rate, whilst cross-linking reduced wear. Largely driven by work from several groups in the United States, highly cross-linked polyethylenes (XLPs) have been produced. Generally these XLPs are made by irradiating UHMWPE with electron beam or gamma irradiation at relatively high doses (compared with those used for sterilization), followed by a heating step which eliminates the free radicals produced by irradiation, before machining the component and terminal sterilization. Elimination of the free radicals is an important step in reducing the long-term oxidative degradation and embrittlement of the XPEs. There are variations on this theme associated with the dose of irradiation, the temperature used to drive off the free radicals, and on the final sterilization step. Optimizing the amount of cross-linking has been a key consideration in the development of XPEs. A dose of up to 10kGy has been used clinically. This is around three times the amount of gamma irradiation used to achieve sterilization. However, high cross-linking promoted by increasing the dose of irradiation increases the number of free radicals produced. These free radicals have to be eliminated by a heating step which may reduce the fatigue strength and fracture toughness of the XPE, and the resistance to crack propagation is reduced compared with conventional UHMWPE.

XPEs have been shown in hip simulator tests to have extremely low wear rates, even under adverse conditions associated with rim loading, abrasion of the femoral head, and mal-positioning of the implants. Some laboratory hip simulator studies where the wear of XPEs was compared with conventional UHMWPE showed that XPEs reduced wear by over 90%. Other studies on different XPEs have shown less improvement. Due to the low wear rate of cross-linked plastics it has been proposed that these materials can be used in large diameter (>32-mm) acetabular cups. Hip simulator studies even under extreme conditions have shown that XPEs can potentially be used for large diameter plastic acetabular bearings.

Laboratory and short-term clinical studies have provided strong evidence that XPEs improve the longevity of total hip arthroplasty; however, the application of this material to total knee arthroplasty may not be so beneficial. Due to the fact that knee joint replacements are not as conforming as in the hip, high contact stresses are generated on the tibial plastic. This is one reason that delamination wear and cracking of the plastic is seen in knee replacements and less frequently in hip replacements unless there is rim contact. The cross-linking process reduces the resistance to crack propagation which is associated with cracking and delamination, and this may limit the role of XPEs in total knee arthroplasty. This reduction in the resistance to cracking is related to the heating process which is required to remove the free radicals. Retrieval of some components has shown oxidation, delamination, and cracking of XPE plastic and residual free radicals have been detected. This is associated with one particular XPE where it is claimed the free radicals were not eliminated because the heating step only annealed the plastic and the temperature was not high enough to melt the material which drives off more free radicals.

Recent advances in processing XPEs addresses the problems associated with the reduction in the resistance to crack propagation. One development utilizes vitamin E which is infused into the XPE after the irradiation step. Vitamin E is an antioxidant and works by scavenging free radicals in the plastic. In this way, although heated, the plastic is not re-melted during the infusion of vitamin E after the initial gamma irradiation step. It has been proposed that in this process the benefits of cross-linking can be achieved without the detrimental effects associated with remelting. Polyethylene manufactured using the technique is known as 'E-poly'. Another second-generation XPE utilize three relatively low-level irradiation steps, each separated by an annealing step to drive off the free radicals that are generated each time. In this way, a high level of cross linking can be achieved without reduction in the material properties. This material is known as X3 polyethylene.

Metal-on-metal (Box 7.6.3)

At the same time as XPEs were being developed, there was resurgence in the use of metal-on-metal bearings. The low wear rate associated with these bearings was another way of avoiding the

Box 7.6.3 Metal-on-metal hip replacements

- Wear on metal-on-metal hip replacements is characterized by a run-in period of relatively high wear and then a steady state period where the wear is lower
- Very low wear rate
- Wear rate increases when the cup is inserted at high inclination angles
- Wear particles are small in the nanometre size range
- Corrosion of these wear particles and corrosion from the bearing produces increased levels of metal ions in the bloodstream.

osteolysis associated with conventional plastic acetabular cups. Metal-on-metal bearings have a long track record of use. Relatively small numbers of these bearings were successfully used in the McKee–Farrar hip replacement which was developed in the early 1960s. Contemporary metal-on-metal designs are different from the bearings used in the McKee–Farrar hip replacement. Modern designs utilize better manufacturing techniques enabling the femoral head to contact the acetabular bearing at the pole of the cup whereas, for the McKee–Farrar design, clutching of the bearing due to peripheral contact sometimes occurred. Provided the geometry and surface finish of the bearing surface is well controlled, modern designs may be lubricated by a fluid film. This is important because it cuts down friction and reduces wear of the bearing. Fluid film lubrication is related to the movement of the femoral head which captures a film of fluid that is drawn into the bearing as it moves. The clearance of the head at the equator of the cup is critical and this is known as the diametral clearance. Too large a clearance and a fluid film does not form under physiological conditions. Movement is also key; for a given range of motion, the larger the head, the faster the movement and the greater the entraining velocity (Figure 7.6.4). It has been shown that fluid films form less readily in small metal-on-metal bearings. For metal-on-metal bearings the wear rate is more sensitive to macrogeometry and lubrication than a metal-on-UHMWPE bearing.

The wear rates of first-generation metal-on-metal bearings have been shown to be two orders of magnitude less than a conventional metal-on-UHMWPE bearing. For second generation, numerous metal-on-metal hip replacements hip simulator testing has shown that a metal-on metal has considerably less wear than a metal-on-UHMWPE couple. The volumetric wear in hip simulator tests of second-generation bearings has been shown to be less than $1mm^3$ per million cycles. Initially wear is relatively high but reduces to a steady state after about one million cycles. Metal-on-metal bearings are said to have a self-polishing capacity and bed-in over time. A million cycles represents about 0.5–1 year of use in patients. The wear rates measured from retrieved metal-on-metal bearings are higher than that seen in hips simulators but are still very low compared to metal on UHMWPE. *In vivo* wear of metal-on-metal bearings cannot be measured using radiographs because there is no distinction between the bearing surfaces and the wear rates are extremely low. Retrieval analysis of second-generation metal-on metal bearings has shown wear of $25mm^3$ for the first year, and as low as $5mm^3$ per year thereafter.

As with any other bearing articulations there are advantages and disadvantages with metal-on-metal. Wear particles released from metal bearings are between 20–100 nanometres and are an order of magnitude smaller than debris released from UHMWPE bearings. The smaller size metal debris *per se* is believed to be less aggressive than plastic wear particles. The macrophage is thought to take these small particles up into the cell by a different mechanism which does not lead to the release of cytokines associated with phagocytosis of plastic debris. However, wear of the metal-on-metal bearings is a major concern. In theory, under fluid film lubrication wear should be low but physiological conditions associated with movement and gait, as well as the surgical positioning of the cup, all lead to the release of metal debris and ions. The metal ions are generated either through direct corrosion of the bearing surface or by the corrosion of the metal wear debris.

In patients with metal-on-metal hip replacements, metal ions in serum have been shown to be three to five times higher than in controls (metal-on-UHMWPE). These ions are secreted from the body in urine; however, due to the continual release there is always a pool of ions in the blood. In line with the observation of bedding-in of the bearing seen in simulator studies, there is a higher level of metal ions in the bloodstream during the first postoperative year. Metal ion levels are higher in patients where the cup has an inclination (abduction) angle of greater than 50 degrees and this is attributed to edge loading. A small number of studies have also demonstrated a transitory rise in metal ion levels after patients have exercised. So, for example, a study from Oswestry, showed a significant increase in serum cobalt and chromium of over 10% immediately after the exercise. This is an important study because the rise in blood cobalt and chromium levels was immediate, indicating that metal ion levels may be a combination of direct corrosion and release of ions from the bearing surface and generation of wear particles that subsequently corrode. Current work is showing the importance of direct corrosion of the metal-on-metal bearing surface in contributing to ion levels in the blood stream.

The long-term biological consequences of the exposure to ions and wear particles remain largely unknown; however, adverse physiological effects have been identified in the follow-up of patients exposed to cobalt-chromium implants. It has been shown that implants generally have the potential to cause structural chromosome changes in marrow cells and in circulating lymphocytes but the incidence is greater in patients with metal-on-metal bearings. The clinical consequences of these chromosome changes, which include aneuploidy, deletions, translocations, and fragmentation, in a small number of cells are unknown. It is difficult to link these chromosome changes to any increase risk of developing cancer. However, the risk of developing haematopoietic cancers in patients with metal-on-metal hip replacements may be very slightly increased.

In a relatively small percentage of patients, wear debris and metal ion release from metal-on-metal bearing surfaces has been linked to newly recognized condition which is characterized by local necrosis, deposition of fibrin, and the agglomeration of lymphocytes around blood vessels, often deep within the synovial capsule. This condition has been termed aseptic lymphocyte-dominated vasculitis associated lesion (ALVAL). This is also linked with the formation of soft tissue masses within the capsule and surrounding soft tissue which is referred to as a pseudotumour. These masses may contain fluids or be more cellular and the main histological features of these masses are extensive necrosis and lymphocytic infiltration. Pseudotumours may also be linked to a hypersensitivity response. Metal ions can initiate a hypersensitivity response. A delayed cell-mediated hypersensitivity can occur, in which cytokines are released by T lymphocytes and an increased activation of macrophages is seen. Metal ions, such as nickel and chromium, can initiate a hypersensitivity response and in the normal population the incidence of sensitivity to metal ions is around 10%. This number is doubled in patients with well-functioning total hip replacements and increased further in patients with loose implants requiring revision. Whether the increased metal sensitivity is a cause or effect of the loosening is not known.

Ceramic bearing surfaces (Box 7.6.4)

Ceramic-bearing surfaces have been used over several decades and ceramic femoral heads have been implanted for more than 40 years. Just like other bearing surfaces there has been a general improvement in their wear characteristics and performance over time. The key to the wear resistance of ceramic surfaces is their hardness which prevents scratching (Table 7.6.1). These materials are also hydrophilic, more wettable than cobalt-chrome surfaces, and hold onto a fluid film which may be important for the lubrication of ceramic-on-ceramic bearing surfaces (Figure 7.6.5). Ceramic bearing surfaces can be used either as ceramic-on-ceramic coupling or as a ceramic femoral head articulating with a UHMWPE socket. In the past this was conventional polyethylene but XPEs are being increasingly used.

The perceived problem with ceramic heads is their history of catastrophic failure which is associated with their inherent low fracture toughness and ductility. Zirconia oxide ceramic femoral heads were introduced approximately 20 years ago to address the problems associated with alumina fracture. At that time, zirconia oxide femoral heads were three times stronger than their alumina oxide counterparts; however, zirconia oxide hardness is lower.

Several studies have shown the wear rate of UHMWPE total hip replacement is reduced when the femoral head is ceramic, although some studies have conversely shown a high penetration rate of UHMWPE liners by zirconia oxide heads. Overall, the penetration rate is between two to three times lower with ceramic-on-UHMWPE than with a metal-on-UHMWPE bearing. A small number of other studies have described higher wear with zirconia oxide heads with penetration rates equivalent to those seen with metal-on-UHMWE bearings. The reason why some zirconia oxide bearings demonstrate a contradictory behaviour may be associated with changes in the phase structure of the head. Paradoxically, zirconia oxide owes its strength to a material phase transformation from a tetragonal phase to the monoclinic phase. The natural state of pure zirconia oxide is the monoclinic phase but by a small addition of yttria during processing, a stabilized tetragonal phase is produced. A slight volumetric change occurs with this phase change which happens when there is a release of stress in the material. This is important for strength because the phase change compresses cracks in the material making them less able to propagate thus strengthening the ceramic. However, if this change happens on the surface, the monoclinic phase will increase the roughness of the femoral head increasing the polyethylene wear. This surface phase change can be accelerated by heating in an aqueous environment and this is one reason why zirconia oxide femoral heads should never be autoclaved. The phase change does not occur with alumina oxide femoral heads. Linear polyethylene wear against alumina heads is reported to be as much as a factor of five to ten times lower than metal versus polyethylene.

Although technology to prevent ceramic fractures is improving, an alloy has been developed composed of niobium and zirconium marketed as Oxinium. This alloy's surface can be transformed into a relatively thick (4–5μm) zirconium oxide (i.e., zirconia) ceramic-like material using a thermal process. This process combines the strength and toughness benefits of using a metal alloy head with the wear properties associated with zirconia oxide. The oxide layer

Box 7.6.4 Ceramic bearings

- Ceramic heads are either alumina oxide or zirconia oxide
- With a ceramic femoral head the wear rate against UHMWPE is reduced compared with a metal head. Well-functioning ceramic-on-ceramic bearings show the lowest wear rates on all bearing surfaces
- Low wear is associated with the hydrophilic surface and the hardness of the ceramic
- Incidence of catastrophic failure due to fracture of the ceramic components
- Fracture rate has been reduced due to the development of alumina-zirconia mixtures.
- As with metal-on-metal bearings, ceramic-on-ceramic bearings are susceptible to edge loading.

Table 7.6.1 The material properties of ceramic materials compared to wrought cobalt-chrome

	Strength Bending Mpa	Modulus GPa	Hardness HV	Toughness $mNm^{-3/2}$
Al2O3	400	380	2500	5-6
ZrO2	1200	200	1300	9-10
CoCr *w*	1500	230	450	

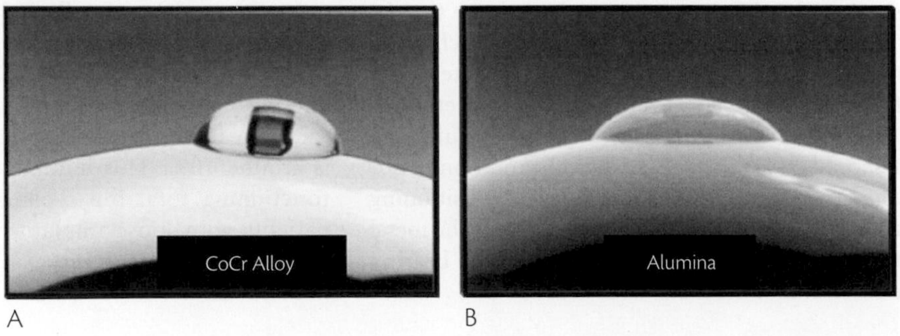

Fig. 7.6.5 Photographs showing drops of water on the surface of metal (A) and ceramic (B) bearing surface demonstrating reduced contact angle of the drop on alumina oxide surfaces.

is not a coating but rather the surface zone of the metal alloy. The oxide/metal interface is continuous, without pores or voids which might be detrimental to oxide adhesion. Laboratory studies have demonstrated the superior wear performance against UHMWPE with Oxinium heads generating significantly less volumetric wear compared with cobalt-chromium alloys. This technology can also be applied to the femoral component of knee joints. For knees, the femoral component does not contain nickel or chromium which may be beneficial in cases of metal sensitivity. Tests in a knee simulator comparing wear rates produced by Oxinium and cobalt-chrome femoral components against polyethylene revealed 42–85% less wear in the Oxinium group. Oxinium and cobalt-chrome femoral heads have also been compared under both smooth and roughened conditions in hip simulators; Oxinium heads exhibited lower wear rates.

Before discussing ceramic-on-ceramic articulations, it is important to understand how the advances made in manufacturing alumina oxide components have improved their fracture toughness and the strength. In the 1980s, femoral heads made from alumina oxide were produced using long sintering times which were necessary to produce alumina femoral heads with low porosity; however, this resulted in the growth of large grains in the material making it susceptible to fracture resulting in the catastrophic fracture of a small number of femoral heads. Thus in the 1970s a clinical fracture rate of one head per 2000 was reported or 0.05%.

Additions of CaO or MgO prevented grain growth reducing the grain size and reducing the fracture rate by an order of magnitude. Reports on the rate of fracture of the second generation ceramics are considerably lower than first generation with rates as low as four per 100 000 or 0.004%. The latest developments (third generation) produce ceramics which are even stronger. These ceramics are composed of alumina oxide matrix combined with zirconia oxide giving the components both wear resistance (associated with hardness of alumina oxide) and additional strength (associated with zirconia oxide component). Due to the development of pores during the sintering process, the size of femoral heads for second-generation ceramic was restricted to under 32-mm diameter but with the introduction of the newer ceramic mixtures the head size has increased to up to 40mm. The improvement in the manufacturing tolerances associated with the femoral spigot has also contributed to a decrease in the fracture rate.

If fracture of the femoral head does occur, the problems are substantial. Fragmentation of the ceramic usually means that it is difficult to clean out the joint during the revision procedure. The hard particles of ceramic that are left behind will increase the wear of the revision bearing. Often the tapers of the hip stem will be severely damaged, making it difficult to replace the head on the damaged taper, and in these situations the stem has to be revised.

Ceramic-on-ceramic wear rates are usually very low and in the range of 0.003mm per year; a factor of ten less than the lowest polyethylene wear rates. The wear particles that are released from ceramic bearings have been isolated and have been shown to be small, do not release ions, and are biologically well tolerated. There have, however, been reports that in series of successful ceramic-on-ceramic bearings there are often outliers where the wear is much larger. The reasons for this remain unclear but may be associated with the surgical technique in placing the acetabular cup, leading to edge loading. In these cases, wear is characteristically seen as a roughened region on the ceramic which is often linear at the periphery of the bearing area and in the form of a stripe, referred to as striped wear. Striped wear is caused by the ball slightly distracting from the socket and then impinging on the cup rim. Alumina acetabular components also have been susceptible to edge chipping and it has been recommended to place the acetabular component in the pelvis at 45 degrees to optimize the distribution of forces over the surfaces of the ball and cup, and to avoid neck-socket impingement.

Another concern regarding ceramic bearings which may be associated with striped wear, edge loading, and poor lubrication is the development of a 'squeaky' hip. Various studies have indicated that the incidence of squeaking is low, at well under 1% in most clinical series, and that apart from the annoying squeak there are no other symptoms. Simulator tests have shown that squeaky hips are usually associated with dry bearings and *in vitro* squeaking can be reduced by lubricating the hip joint, but unfortunately this is not possible clinically.

Metal-on-ceramic bearings

Unlike the metal-on-metal and ceramic-on-ceramic bearings used for hip replacements, bearings used in other engineering applications are often made of dissimilar materials with one material being harder than the other. In this sort of bearing combination, relatively greater wear occurs on the softer member of the bearing pairing. Hip simulator studies have shown that although not as low as ceramic-on-ceramic, metal-on-ceramic pairings were found to have wear rates approximately 30–100-fold lower than the metal-on-metal pairings. In these hip simulator studies, most of the wear was generated from the metal acetabular cup and relatively little from the ceramic head. In simulators, metal particles from the ceramic-on-metal bearings were also smaller than from metal-on-metal bearings. Friction of ceramic-on-metal combination bearings was less than for metal-on-metal combinations which indicated reduced wear and greater fluid film lubrication. Clinical trials conducted recently, have also shown a corresponding decrease in metal ion release in the bloodstream in patients from metal-on-ceramic hip replacements when compared to metal-on-metal bearings. The wear particles from the metal-on-metal articulation were similar in composition and shape to particles found in retrieved tissues from around metal-on-metal prostheses. The use of differential hardness ceramic-on-metal pairings reduced the wear rate compared to metal-on-metal hip prostheses.

Conclusions

Undoubtedly the use of alternative bearing surfaces has reduced wear at the hip joint. Table 7.6.2 shows the advantages and disadvantage of different bearing combinations. These new and developing technologies have been applied more to hip joint replacement than to knee joints. The reason for this may be that the incidence of osteolysis in the knees is relatively low compared to hip replacements. This may be associated with the kinematics of the replaced knee where the crossover motion characteristically seen in hip replacements is much less. Also, with the recognition of the effect that sterilization in air had on polyethylene in the 1990s and with the subsequent improvements in processing standard UHMWPE used for tibial components, delamination wear was significantly reduced.

Table 7.6.2 Advantages and disadvantages of bearing surfaces. Readings may vary according to the published study but these are representative. Note that for polyethylene articulations wear is expressed as linear penetration whereas for hard-on-hard bearings wear is expressed as a volumetric wear rate

Bearing	Advantages	Disadvantages	Clinical wear rate*
UHMWPE-on-metal	Long history of use Low cost	High wear Aseptic osteolysis Can only use small heads	0.05–0.2mm/year
Cross-linked polyethylene	Low wear Relatively low cost Larger head sizes can be used	Short history of use Variable wear seen depending on the exact process Decrease in the resistance for crack propagation.	0.003mm/year
Metal-on-metal	Very low wear, not as expensive as ceramic-on-ceramic Large heads can be used Self polishing Long history of use with first-generation bearings	Metal ion release Hypersensitivity's Susceptible to cup angle Wear in period	25mm^3 for run in wear, and 5mm^3 per year thereafter
Ceramic-on-UHMWPE	Generally lower wear than with metal-on-UHMWPE Long history of use Low cost	Wear rate is probably not low enough to prevent osteolysis	0.03mm–0.1mm/year**
Ceramic-on-ceramic	Very low wear Wear debris is not as biologically active as with other bearings. Long history of use	Small incidence of catastrophic fracture Susceptible to cup angle High cost	0.025–5μm^3/year
Metal-on-ceramic	Wear lower than with metal-on-metal bearings Large heads can be used	Debris released is metallic Short history of use	Clinical data not available

*Readings may vary according to the published study but these are representative. Note that for polyethylene articulations wear is expressed as linear penetration, whereas for hard-on-hard bearings wear is expressed as a volumetric wear rate

**This is an estimate based on a number of studies which show variable results.

For orthopaedic surgeons the number of different alternative bearing couples available for hip joint replacements and the body of scientific information backing up and rationalizing each one makes the choice overwhelming. It should be remembered that, to a certain extent, the range of alternative bearings developed by manufactures was a response to the considerable issues faced in the 1990s with aseptic osteolysis as a result of plastic wear, and these bearings have not yet stood the test of time. Although there is no substitute for clinical data, since the mid 1990s there has been considerable improvement in the way that these alternative bearings have been preclinically tested which provides safeguards to patients. The choices that surgeons make are often associated with the patients that they are treating, and in today's environment, having a choice of different bearing surfaces is advantageous for both economical and performance-related issues.

Further reading

D'Antonio, J.A. and Sutton, K. (2009). Ceramic materials as bearing surfaces for total hip arthroplasty. *Journal of the American Academy of Orthopaedic Surgeons*, **17**(2), 61–2.

Dumbleton, J.H., Manley, M.T., and Edidin, A.A. (2002). A literature review of the association between wear rate and osteolysis in total hip arthroplasty. *Journal of Arthroplasty*, **17**(5), 649–61.

Isaac, G.H., Thompson, J., Williams, S., and Fisher, J. (2006). Metal-on-metal bearings surfaces: materials, manufacture, design, optimization, and alternatives. *Proceedings of the Institute of Mechanical Engineers, Part H*. **220**(2), 119–33.

Jasty, M., Rubash, H.E., and Muratoglu O. (2005). Highly cross-linked polyethylene. The debate is over in the affirmative. *Journal of Arthroplasty*, **20**(4 Suppl 2), 55–8.

Revell, PA. (2008). The combined role of wear particles, macrophages and lymphocytes in the looseningof total joint prostheses. *Journal of the Royal Society Interface*, **5**(28), 1263–78.

Ries, M.D. (2005). Highly cross-linked polyethylene: the debate is over—in opposition. *Arthroplasty*, **20**(4 Suppl 2), 59–62.

7.7

The young arthritic hip

Ahmad K. Malik and Aresh Hashemi-Nejad

Summary points

- Impingement:
  - Primary femoroacetabular impingement:
    - Cam type
    - Pincer type
    - Combined cam and pincer
  - Secondary femoroacetabular impingement:
    - Slipped upper femoral epiphysis (cam type)
    - Protusio (pincer type)
    - Retroverted acetabulum (pincer type)
    - Malunited femoral head/neck fracture (cam type)
    - Acetabular fracture (pincer type)
    - Perthes disease (cam type)
- Instability:
  - Developmental dysplasia of the hip (treated/residual and untreated)
  - Dislocation
  - Subluxation
  - Dysplasia
- Inflammatory:
  - Juvenile idiopathic arthritis
  - Rheumatoid arthritis.

Aetiology of arthritis in the young adult hip

The cause of osteoarthritis of the hip can be viewed as a mechanical dysfunction resulting from either instability (hip dysplasia) or impingement, or a combination of both. Treatment is directed at the underlying disease process. Where there is no or minimal degenerative changes radiographically in a young patient who is normally fit and healthy, a reconstruction procedure is the preferred option (see Chapter 7.9). If there is evidence of severe osteoarthritis, an arthroplasty or salvage procedure should be considered.

History

Obtain the pertinent information: patient's age; occupation; and onset, nature, and duration of pain. Are there any limitations of work or sporting activities? Past medical history of childhood illness or pain affecting the hip along with any previous operation should be documented, along with any positive family history. History of trauma or any other associated illness should be gathered.

It should be ascertained whether the pain is present on weight bearing or at rest, such as sitting. History of locking is very suggestive of intra-articular pathology, such as labral tears, loose bodies, or chondral flap.

Examination

- Assessment of gait pattern and sitting posture
- Abductor strength, neurovascular status, and limb lengths
- Active and passive range of motion.

Patients with hip dysplasia typically have good hip flexion and, due to femoral anteversion, good internal rotation. In femoroacetabular impingement (FAI), passive flexion of the hip to 90 degrees with adduction and internal rotation will be restricted and will elicit pain in the groin similar to the pain they are complaining of. This is the basis of the impingement test. In Perthes disease, abduction in extension will be severely restricted in the presence of hinge abduction.

Imaging

Radiographic (Figures 7.7.1–7.7.4)

The anteroposterior (AP) pelvic radiograph illustrates the femoral head and its sphericity. The position of the joint centre and any subluxation can also be noted by integrity of Shenton's line. The acetabular coverage of the femoral head is depicted as is the acetabular inclination, also known as the sourcil (the weight-bearing superior dome of the acetabulum), which should measure 0–10 degrees and is between a line parallel to the weight-bearing dome (sourcil) and a line parallel to the inter-teardrop line. Loss of joint space and version of the acetabulum can also be seen. The vertical centre edge angle of Wiberg should be greater than 25 degrees.

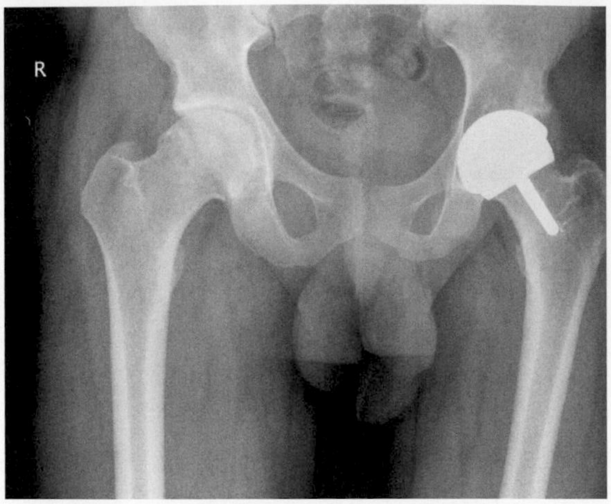

Fig. 7.7.1 Plain AP radiograph of pelvis. A 38-year-old male who had bilateral slipped upper femoral epiphysis as a child with 'pistol grip' deformity resulting in impingement. Left side successfully treated with hip resurfacing.

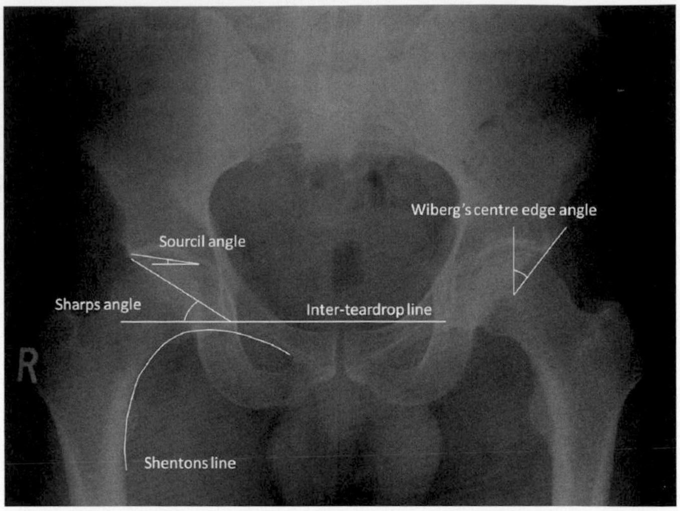

Fig. 7.7.3 Common radiographic angles. Acetabular angle (of Tonnis) or Sourcil angle normal value 0–10 degrees. Vertical centre edge angle (of Wiberg) normal value ≥25 degrees; note small cam lesion left hip.

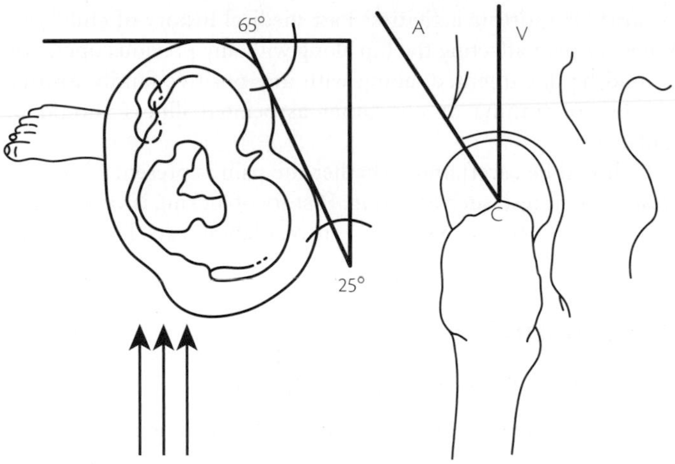

Fig. 7.7.2 Technique for false-profile lateral radiograph and measuring anterior centre edge angle. The anterior centre edge angle is calculated from a false-profile radiological view of the pelvis. The subject stands at an angle of 65 degrees oblique to the x-ray beam, with the foot on the affected side parallel to the x-ray cassette. The focal distance is 1m. The tip of the greater trochanter forms the horizontal centre, and the vertical centre is midway between the symphysis pubis and the anterior superior iliac spine. A vertical line through the centre of the femoral head subtends the anterior edge angle by connecting with a second line through the centre of the hip and the foremost aspect of the acetabulum.

The anterior or lateral centre edge angle quantifies the anterior cover of the femoral head, and angles of less than 20 degrees are considered abnormal. An AP projection may also show cyst formation at the superior lateral aspect of the acetabulum representing damage at the labrochondral junction.

A retroverted acetabulum can be identified through the 'cross-over' sign (Figure 7.7.4). The cross-over sign is seen when the anterior rim of the acetabulum 'crosses over' its posterior rim, as their outlines are traced from proximal to distal on the radiograph. Retroverted acetabulae have been correlated with radiological evidence of osteoarthritis of the hip. A comparison of six radiographic projections to assess femoral head/neck asphericity demonstrated that the Dunn view in 45-degree or 90-degree flexion or a cross-table projection in internal rotation best show femoral head/neck asphericity, whereas AP or externally rotated cross-table views are likely to miss asphericity.

Computed topography

Computed tomography (CT) is useful in assessing the congruency and coverage of the femoral head and as an aid to preoperative planning for osteotomy.

CT can provide detailed information on bony architecture and any subtle pathology such as cam lesions (Figures 7.7.5 and 7.7.6). It also can assess version and is extremely helpful in imaging grossly abnormal anatomy.

Magnetic resonance imaging

This is used valuation of painful hip and exclusion of other sources of hip pathology. It allows for assessment of concavity of head neck junction. The angle of Notzli (Figure 7.7.7) is used to confirm cam lesion. A normal alpha angle is approximately 40 degrees while patients with FAI have average alpha angles of 74 degrees. The gadolinium enhanced magnetic resonance imaging of cartilage has the potential of predicting outcome of Bernese pelvic acetabular osteotomy by assessing the integrity of the cartilage.

Treatment

Femoroacetabular impingement (Figure 7.7.8)

The concept of FAI started to become widely accepted at about the same time that enthusiasts of hip arthroscopy started to publish their experiences and results. One of the main indications and supposed benefits of hip arthroscopy was the diagnosis and *debridement* of labral tears. Unfortunately, results were disappointing due to the fact that the labral tear was not the underlying pathology but usually a result of FAI which itself went untreated. The study by Beck and colleagues has shown that cam impingement in particular leads to extensive damage to the acetabular cartilage and that

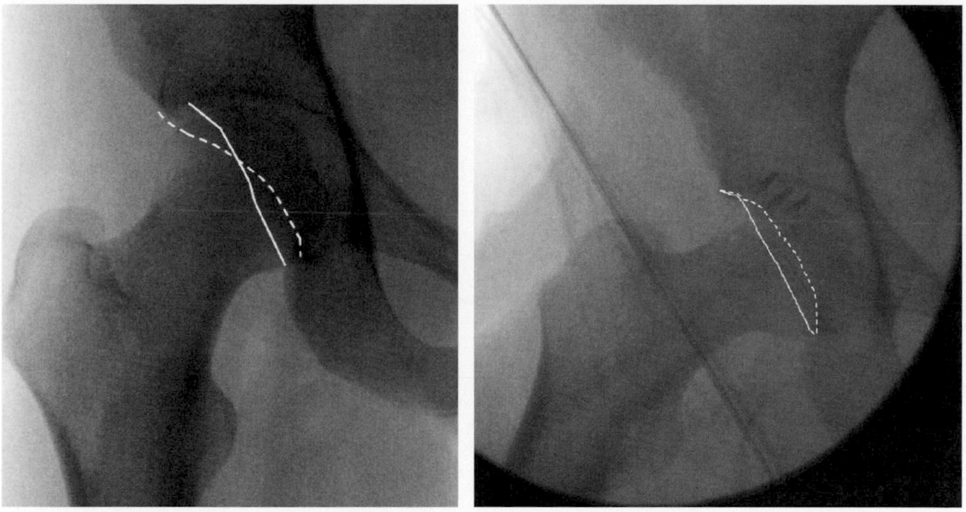

A B

Fig. 7.7.4 The cross-over sign in acetabular retroversion. A) Preoperative film shows cross-over sign, dotted line represents anterior rim of acetabulum. B) This patient was treated successfully for a pincer lesion with acetabular rim resection and labral refixation. The anterior dotted line and posterior solid line meet at the sourcil edge as they should in normal hips.

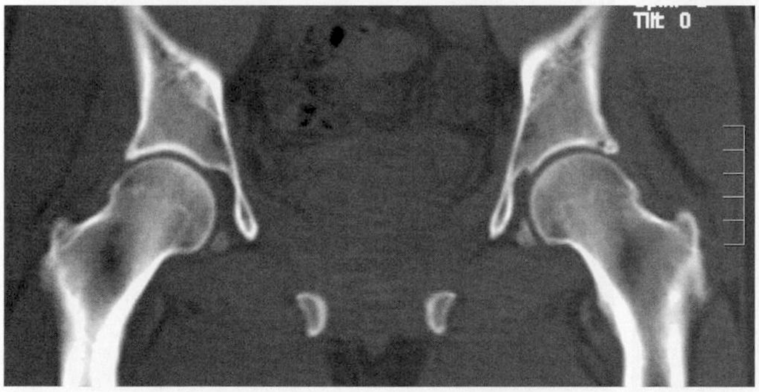

Fig. 7.7.5 Coronal CT image of pelvis. A cam lesion is evident in the left hip. Note the cyst at the superior lateral margin of the acetabulum, this almost certainly indicates underlying labral or chondral pathology.

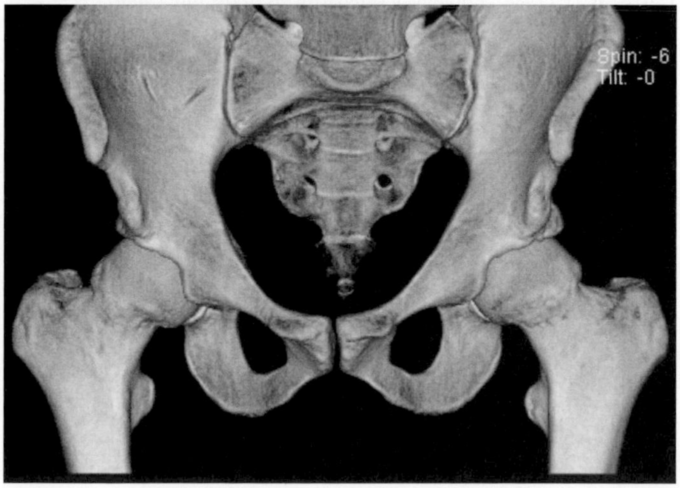

Fig. 7.7.6 Three-dimensional bilateral cam lesions in a 27-year-old triathlete.

separation between the labrum and the cartilage arises because the cartilage is ripped off the labrum. The tear of the labrum is only part of the pathology and is secondary to impingement.

The aim of surgical treatment for FAI is to improve the femoral head–neck offset thereby improving joint clearance and preventing abutment of the femoral neck against the acetabulum. The open surgical approach pioneered by Ganz and colleagues involves dislocation of the femoral head through a trochanteric flip osteotomy and allows full visualization of the femoral and acetabular articular surface. Excision osteoplasty is performed to regain a spherical femoral head and appropriate head–neck offset; acetabular rim excision is performed where there is a prominent anterolateral rim and any damage to the labrum can be addressed. Open dislocation of the femoral head involves technically challenging surgery with a long learning curve. Complications following open dislocation of the hip include heterotrophic ossification (37%), failure of trochanteric fixation, incomplete trochanteric union (27%), and sciatic nerve injury. The approach is extensile and requires sacrificing the ligamentum teres and 6–8 weeks of non-weight bearing with crutches until the trochanteric osteotomy unites.

Hip arthroscopy has recently become popular, but even in experienced hands cam lesions, and in particular acetabular rim trimming and labral refixation, can be technically very difficult. Complications following arthroscopic treatment include sciatic and femoral nerve palsy, perineal injury, and intra-articular breakage of instruments. Arthroscopic treatment of FAI is said to have results comparable to the open procedure although outcome measures were unclear and the methodology unclear.

Treating impingement of the hip through a direct open approach is not a novel idea. Even the authors behind the Bernese surgical dislocation of the hip routinely open the hip joint through a modified Smith–Petersen approach to assess for any impingement following periacetabular osteotomy, and, when necessary, undertake a resection osteoplasty of the femoral head–neck junction. A direct anterior approach allows for easy access to the site of impingement and correction of cam, pincer, and labral lesions. This can be performed after intra-articular assessment and treatment by hip arthroscopy or on its own. At the Royal National Orthopaedic hospital it is the senior surgeon's preference to use a mini-arthrotomy based on the Heuter approach.

Resection of the cam lesion by whatever technique should not exceed 30% of the femoral neck as the risk of femoral neck fracture becomes unacceptably high.

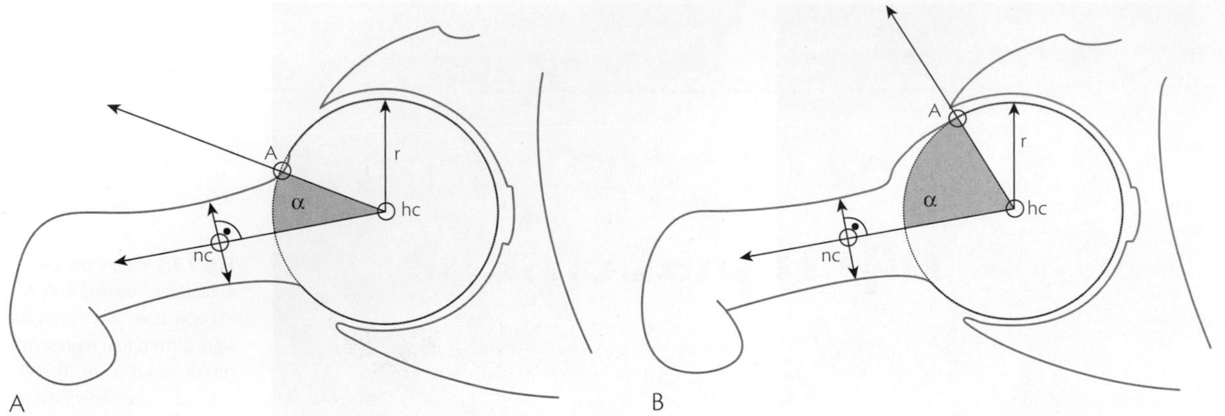

Fig. 7.7.7 Alpha angle (of Notzli). A is the anterior point where the distance from the centre of the head (hc) exceeds the radius (r) of the subchondral surface of the femoral head. Alpha angle is then measured as the angle between A–hc and hc–nc, nc being the centre of the neck at the narrowest point. A) shows a hip in a normal subject and B) a typical deformation resulting from a Cam lesion.

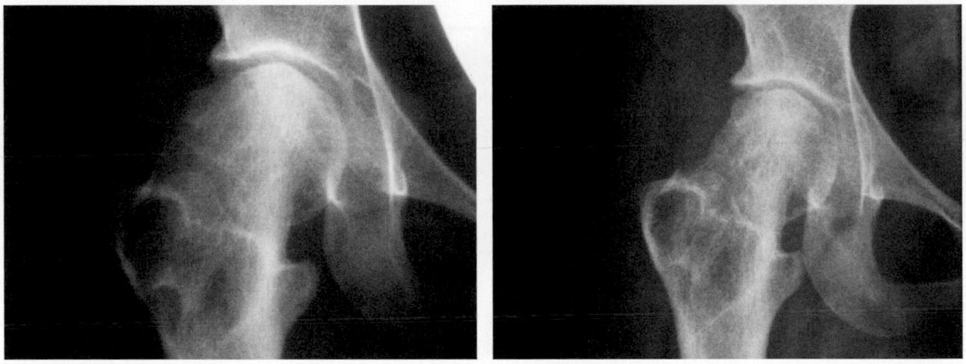

Fig. 7.7.8 Treatment of femoroacetabular impingement. A) A young female with history of slipped upper femoral epiphysis; B) treated successfully for femoroacetabular impingement with osteochondroplasty through a mini-arthrotomy.

Further reading

Buckwalter, J.A., Mankin, H.J., and Grodzinsky, A.J. (2005). Articular cartilage and osteoarthritis. *Instructional Course Lectures*, **54**, 465–80.

Cooperman, D.R., Wallensten, R., and Stulberg, S.D. (1983). Acetabular dysplasia in the adult. *Clinical Orthopaedics and Related Research*, **175**, 79–85.

Ganz, R., Leunig, M., Leunig-Ganz, K., and Harris, W.H. (2008). The etiology of osteoarthritis of the hip: an integrated mechanical concept. *Clinical Orthopaedics and Related Research*, **466**, 264–72.

Ganz, R., Parvizi, J., Beck, M., Leunig, M., Notzli, H., and Sienbrock, K.A. (2003). Femoroacetabular impingement: A cause for osteoarthritis of the hip. *Clinical Orthopaedics and Related Research*, **417**, 112–20.

Goodman, D.A., Feighan, J.E., Smith, A.D., Latimer, B., Buly, R.L., and Cooperman, D.R. (1997). Subclinical slipped capital femoral epiphysis. Relationship to osteoarthrosis of the hip. *Journal of Bone and Joint Surgery*, **79A**, 1489–97.

Harris, W.H. (1986). Etiology of osteoarthritis of the hip. *Clinical Orthopaedics and Related Research*, **213**, 20–33.

Ito, K., Minka 2nd, M.-A, Leunig, M., Werlen, S., and Ganz, R. (2001). Femoroacetabular impingement and the cam-effect. *Journal of Bone and Joint Surgery*, **83B**, 171–6.

Murphy, S.B., Ganz, R., and Muller, M.E. (1995). The prognosis in untreated dysplasia of the hip. A study of radiographic factors that predict the outcome. *Journal of Bone and Joint Surgery*, **77-A**, 985–9.

Myers, S.R., Eijr, H., and Ganz, R. (1999). Anterior femoroacetabular impingement after periacetabular osteotomy. *Clinical Orthopaedics and Related Research*, **363**, 93–9.

Notzli, H.P., Wyss, T.F., Stoecklin, C.H., Schmid, M.R., Treiber, K., Hodler, J. (2002). The contour of the femoral head-neck junction as a predictor for the risk of anterior impingement. *Journal of Bone and Joint Surgery*, **84-B**, 556–60.

7.8

The complex primary total hip replacement

James Donaldson and Richard Carrington

Summary points

- Hip Dysplasia
  - Despite screening programs, a large number of patients are affected by dysplastic hips and their sequelae
  - An understanding of anatomical abnormalities is crucial
  - Appropriate techniques and implants make arthroplasty feasible
  - Complications are significantly higher than standard primary hip replacements
- Protrusio Acetabuli
  - Technical difficulties include inadequate medial wall and restoring offset, hip centre and leg lengths
  - Neck may need to be cut in-situ; bone graft is usually necessary and ideally should be taken from the femoral head
  - Antiprotrusio cages or custom implants may be needed in cases with excessive bone loss
- Arthrodesed hip to total hip replacement
  - Careful evaluation of the gluteal muscles is mandatory and predicts final walking ability and patient satisfaction
  - Long-term effectiveness of total hip replacement in ankylosed hips is satisfactory but there is a higher complication rate

The dysplastic hip

Introduction

The severity of hip dysplasia varies widely and adults with dysplastic hips pose a number of technical challenges, ranging from the identification and preparation of the true acetabulum, preparation of the femoral canal, and stable reduction of the components.

Patients who have hip dysplasia are often young and active, and have had previous operations on their hip. Total hip replacement in such patients has been associated with high rates of complications and revision. It is therefore critical to understand the complexities of total hip replacement and to plan any intervention thoroughly.

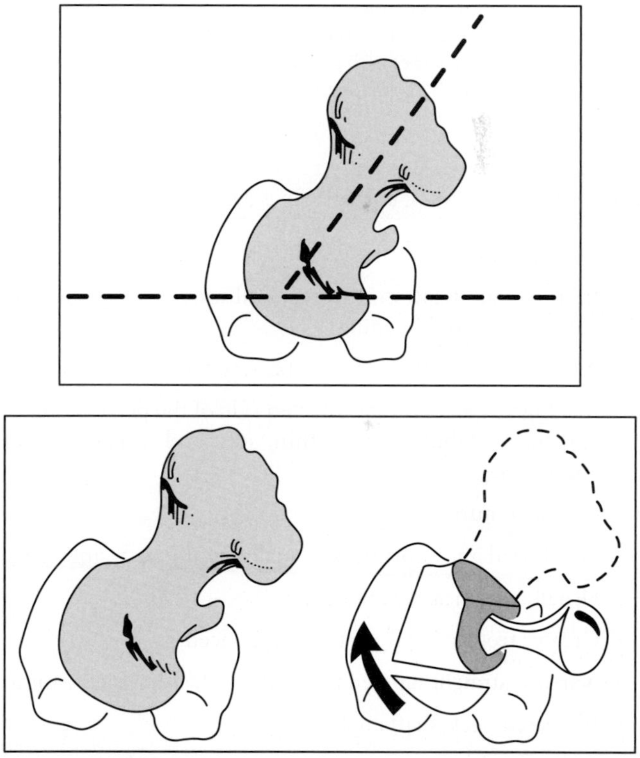

Fig. 7.8.1 The distorted anatomy of the proximal aspect of the femur, which includes excessive anteversion of the femoral neck and posterior displacement of the trochanter. (Reprinted with permission from Haddad, F., Masri, B., Garbuz, D., and Duncan, C. (1999). Primary total hip replacement of the dysplastic hip. *Journal of Bone and Joint Surgery*, **81A**, 1462–82.)

Anatomy

The anatomical abnormalities depend on the severity of dysplasia. Characteristic features are listed in Box 7.8.1(Figures 7.8.1 and 7.8.2).

Assessment

Common symptoms and signs include:

- Pain
- Limb-length discrepancy

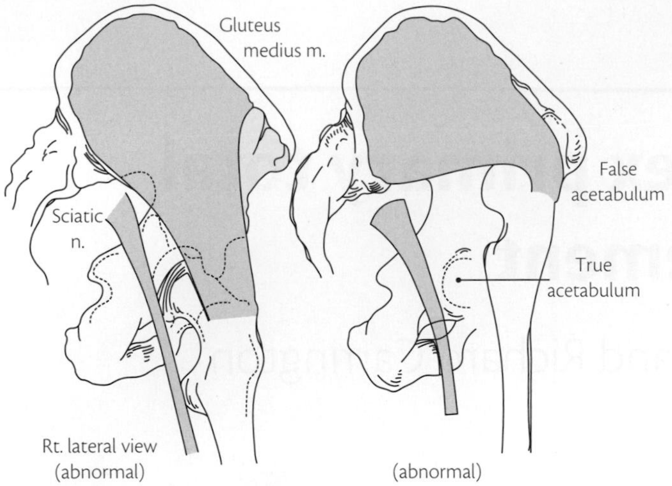

Fig. 7.8.2 Posterolateral view of a congenitally dislocated hip. The femur is riding high against the false acetabulum at a thin portion of the upper ilium; the femoral neck is markedly anteverted and smaller than usual. A true acetabulum is present but poorly developed. Reprinted with permission from Amstutz, H. (1991). *Hip Arthroplasty*. New York: Churchill Livingstone.

Box 7.8.1 Characteristic features of hip dysplasia

- Acetabulum:
  - In a low subluxation, the acetabulum is shallow but may have a wide, oval opening
  - Anteromedially, the wall may be very thin
  - In a high dislocation the affected side of the pelvis is smaller and the acetabular wall is thin, soft, and in some grossly anteverted
- Proximal femur:
  - Small head and short neck. Usually significantly anteverted
  - Usually significantly anteverted
  - Greater trochanter is posterior displaced
  - Narrow, straight tapered femoral canal with a tight isthmus
  - Increased neck-shaft angle
- Soft tissues:
  - Shortened hamstrings, adductors, and quadriceps
  - Horizontal orientation of the abductors from proximal migration of the femoral head
  - Thickened hip capsule
  - Shortened sciatic nerve, vulnerable to lengthening
  - Altered normal course of femoral nerve and profunda artery.

- Limp
- Referred knee pain
- Abductor lurch
- Compensatory lumbar lordosis
- Positive Trendelenburg sign.

Classification

Crowe and colleagues classified dysplastic hips radiographically into four categories depending on the extent of femoral head proximal migration. The Crowe classification system is the simplest and most widely used and allows comparison of operative techniques.

Crowe classification (Figures 7.8.3–7.8.5)

- Grade 1:
  - Proximal displacement less than0.1% of pelvic height or less than 50% subluxation of the height of the femoral head
- Grade 2:
  - Displacement of 0.10–0.15% or subluxation 50–75% of the height of the femoral head
  - Usually do not have leg-length inequality or loss of bone stock
  - With low dislocation, the femoral head articulates with the false acetabulum which partially covers the true acetabulum; on x-ray there may be two overlapping acetabula
  - Inferior part of the false acetabulum is an osteophyte which is located at the level of the superior rim of the true acetabulum; visible part of the true acetabulum can therefore be missed
- Grade 3:
  - Displacement of 0.15–0.20% or subluxation of 75–100% of the height of the femoral head
  - Complete loss of superior acetabular roof
  - May have thin medial wall; anterior and posterior columns are intact
- Grade 4:
  - Displacement greater than 0.20% or subluxation greater than 100% of the height of the femoral head
  - True acetabulum is deficient but remains recognizable

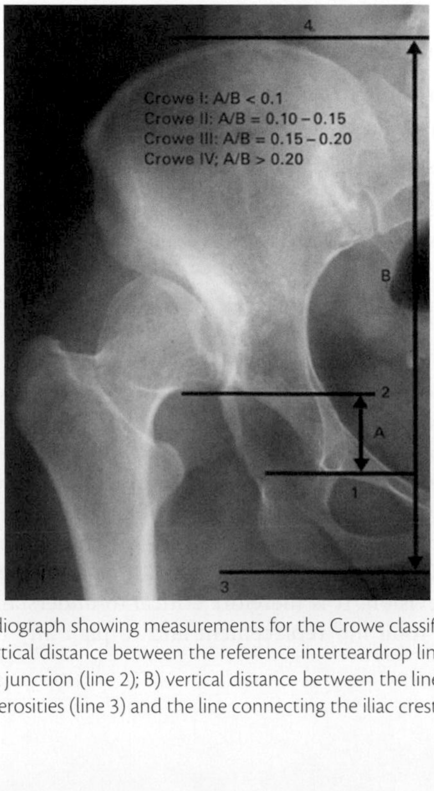

Fig. 7.8.3 Radiograph showing measurements for the Crowe classification system. A) Vertical distance between the reference interteardrop line (line 1) and the head-neck junction (line 2); B) vertical distance between the line connecting the ischial tuberosities (line 3) and the line connecting the iliac crests (line 4).

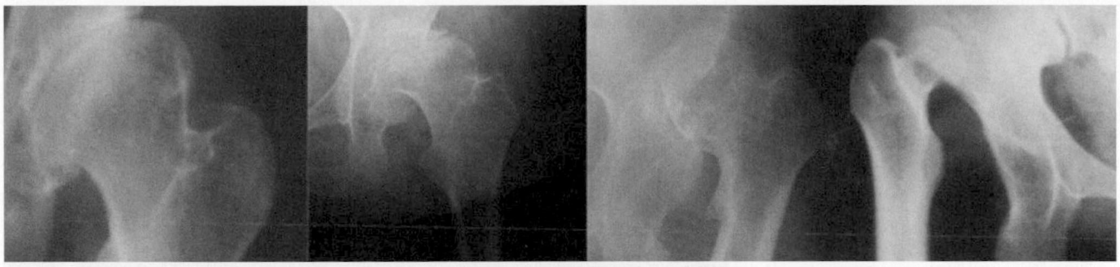

Fig. 7.8.4 Crowe 1–4 dysplastic hips.

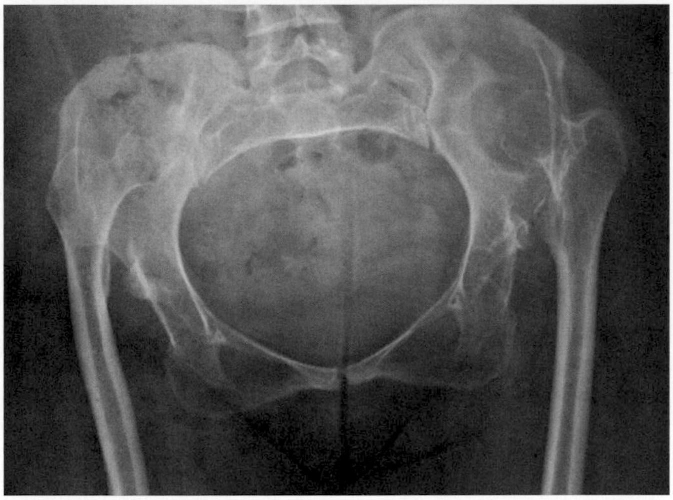

Fig. 7.8.5 Bilateral Crowe grade 4 hips.

Patients with Crowe grade 2 or 3 tend to develop degenerative changes earlier and proceed to total hip replacement at a younger age than grade 1 or 4.

Preoperative planning

Previous operations are common and add new surgical challenges. Previous femoral osteotomies make exposure more difficult and the procedure more technically demanding, but without significantly higher complication rates. Periacetabular and pelvic osteotomies may improve acetabular coverage but may alter available bone stock and careful assessment is necessary.

Retained metalwork and hardware can be problematic and its removal may be associated with significant morbidity. Some authors advocate the removal of hardware in the dysplastic hip setting routinely to avoid later difficulties with embedded or even intramedullary metalwork at a later date. *In situ* metal will need to be removed before a total hip replacement and specialized instruments and equipment may be needed. A staged procedure is sometimes necessary.

Preoperative planning is crucial in achieving a successful outcome. Useful investigations include:

- Radiographs
- Computed tomography (CT) scan can assess bone stock and degree of femoral anteversion
- A magnetic resonance image (MRI) scan can assess laxity of soft tissues around the hip.

Templating

- Acetabulum:
  - Position of true acetabulum should be identified
  - Need to decide whether to attempt to restore acetabulum to its original location or accept a non-anatomic (high hip centre) position
  - True acetabulum placement diminishes joint reaction force, facilitates limb lengthening, and improves abductor function
  - Assess degree of anteversion and adequacy of bone stock
- Femur:
  - Size of the femoral canal
  - Need for custom components
  - Need for rotational osteotomy. Consider if anteversion greater than 40 degrees
  - Need for relative equalization of leg lengths
  - Restoration of abductor function
- Components:
  - Estimate for size of components
  - Method of fixation
  - Need for bone graft
  - Special or custom made equipment.

Operative procedure (Figures 7.8.6–7.8.12)

The approach

Standard anterolateral or posterolateral approaches can be used with less severe degrees of dysplasia. Transtrochanteric or subtrochanteric

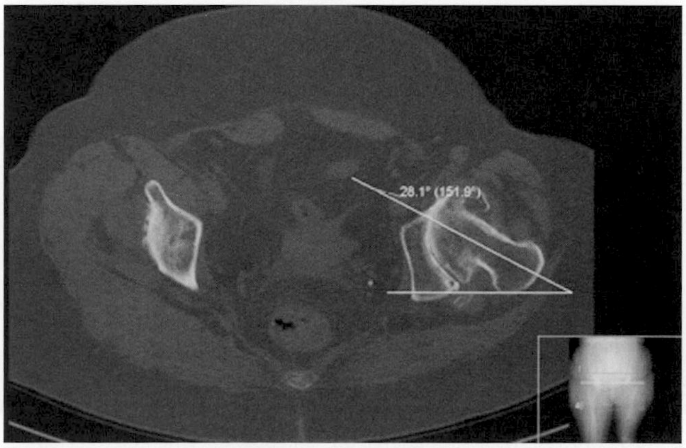

Fig. 7.8.6 CT scan assessing bone stock and femoral neck anteversion.

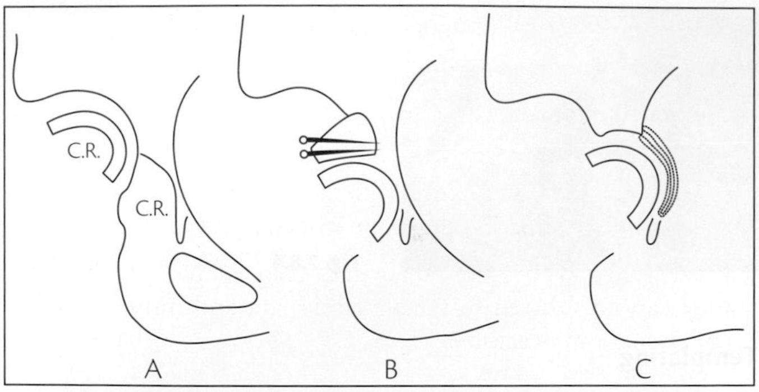

Fig. 7.8.7 Three alternative techniques that have been used for acetabular reconstruction during total hip arthroplasty in hips with a low dislocation. A) Superior placement of the cup. The cup is placed in the false acetabulum, and the superior location of the centre of rotation of the artificial joint is accepted. B) The superolateral augmentation technique with the use of a structural graft. C) The cotyloplasty technique. Complete coverage and anatomical placement of the cup are obtained with controlled medialization. (Reprinted with permission from Hartofilakidis, G. and Karachalios, T. (2004). Total hip arthroplasty for congenital hip disease. *Journal of Bone and Joint Surgery*, **86A**, 242–50.)

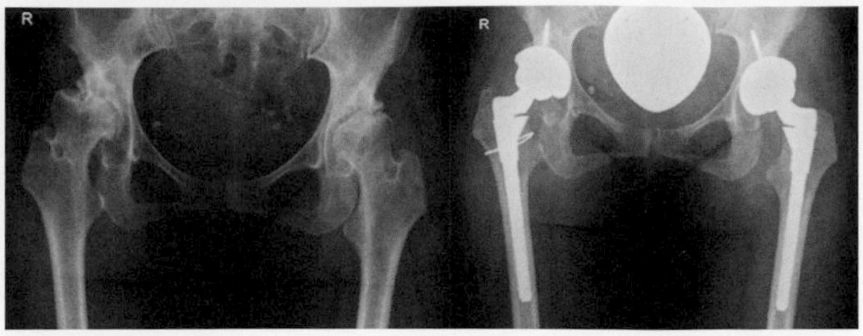

Fig. 7.8.10 Bilateral hip dysplasia pre- and post-bilateral hip replacements.

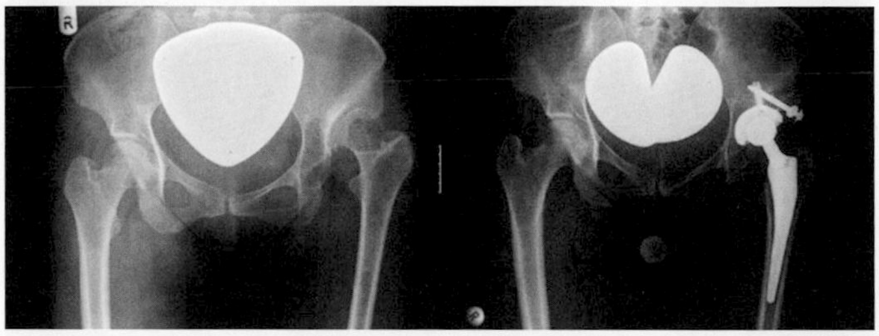

Fig. 7.8.11 Dysplastic left hip pre- and post-left total hip replacement with structural superolateral autograft augmentation.

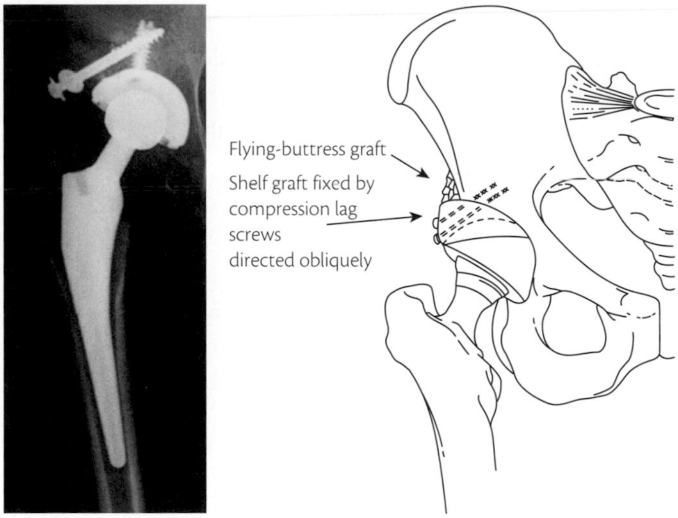

A B

Fig. 7.8.8 Crowe grade 1 dysplastic right hip pre- and post-uncemented total hip replacement.

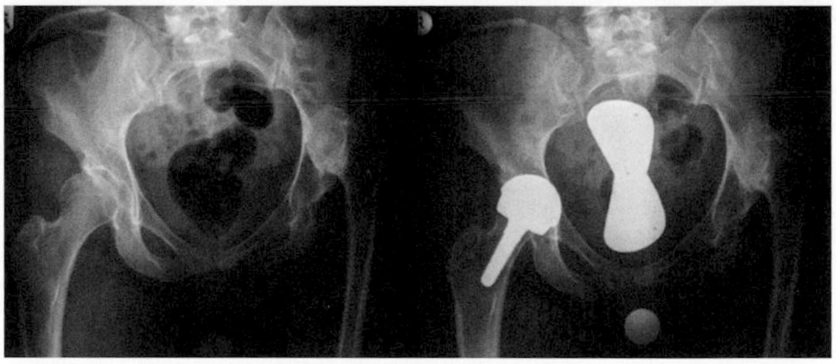

Fig. 7.8.12 Crowe grade 1 dysplasia right hip and grade 3 left hip. The right hip was more symptomatic and a Birmingham mid-head resection arthroplasty (Smith and Nephew) was performed..

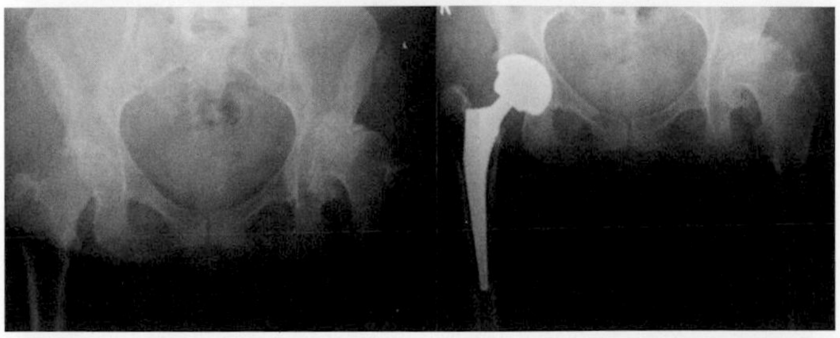

Fig. 7.8.9 Crowe 1 dysplastic right hip pre- and post-uncemented total hip replacement.

approach may be necessary for high dislocation or where abductor retensioning is required. This approach affords excellent exposure at the cost of the difficulties and complications of trochanteric reattachment.

The acetabulum

Obtaining satisfactory acetabular coverage is crucial. At least 70% contact should be with host bone. Either bone graft or cement can be used to fill superior defects.

When there is only a moderate reduction in bone stock, small acetabular components may be used. Sochart and Porter reported 97% 10-year survival and 58% 25-year survival of extra small Charnley acetabular components (38mm or less) usually with 22-mm heads.

Changes in the centre of hip rotation alter hip biomechanics. Acetabular placement can be non-anatomical or anatomical.

Anatomic (low hip centre)
◆ Better bone stock at site of true acetabulum ◆ May restore Shenton's line but acetabular coverage may be limited ◆ Use the transverse ligament as a landmark ◆ Loosening 13% at fifteen years (Linde and Jansen) ◆ May not be possible if hip is very stiff ◆ Large superior defect in superior wall can be filled with femoral head autograft and held with screws (Fig 7.8.7-B and 7.8.8) ◆ Uncemented fixation may be advantageous for implant survival but needs good coverage ◆ If acetabular component is small due to limited bone stock 22mm femoral heads can be used

Dunn and Hess recommended a deliberate fracture of the medial wall (cotyloplasty) to place the cup within the available iliac bone plus or minus augmentation with a mesh. The defect is then reinforced with autogenous bone graft and a small cup cemented in. This procedure advances the acetabulum medially and shifts the weight-bearing axis distal to the acetabulum, whilst gaining good anterior and posterior coverage (Figure 7.8.6C).

The femur

- Anteversion:
  - Significant anteversion (greater than 40 degrees) may necessitate a derotational osteotomy or the use of a custom or modular implant in which version of the femoral neck can be varied
- Femoral shortening:
  - The femur may need to be shortened to protect the sciatic nerve, especially if the acetabulum is brought down to its true level
  - Lengthening of 4cm or more is associated with increased risk of nerve damage. Leg lengthening of <4cm—no nerve palsy; lengthening >4cm—28% develop a nerve palsy
  - Shortening can be carried out at the level of the trochanter or in the subtrochanteric region
  - Subtrochanteric shortening is indicated when several centimetres of shortening is necessary or if derotation osteotomy required
  - Femoral neck shortening is combined with release of the psoas and external rotators
- Narrow femoral canal and short femoral neck often demands the use of a small, short, straight component. In Crowe grade 1, 2, or 3 a conventional implant can usually be used as long as the size of the femur is taken into account
- Distortion from previous osteotomies must be considered.

The abductors

- Osteonecrosis and trochanteric overgrowth in dysplastic hips may result in the greater trochanter lying superior to the centre of the femoral head
- May be resolved with:
  - Appropriate femoral component and increased offset
  - Extensive capsular release, psoas release, gluteus maximus tendon transposition
  - Abductor slide: stripping abductors off ilium and advancing them on the superior gluteal neurovascular bundle
- If the greater trochanter or the abductors cannot be reattached they can be sutured to tensor fascia lata and immobilized in abduction for 6 weeks.

Complications and outcomes

Complications are consistently higher in dysplastic total hip replacements compared with osteoarthritis hip replacements.

- Nerve palsy: 3–15% in published series. Maximum lengthening 4cm for dysplastic hips
- Dislocation: 5–11%
- Trochanteric non-union: 11–29%
- Fracture of the narrow femoral canal
- Impingement: increased if high hip centre used, particularly if the hip is placed medially. The femoral component impinges on the anterior acetabular column in flexion and internal rotation and impinges on the posterior column in extension and external rotation. Reduced with increased offset and release of rectus femoris
- Infection: higher rates reported may be due to longer operating times and more extensive soft tissue dissection and stripping.

Protrusio acetabuli

Introduction

Protrusio acetabuli was first described by Otto in 1824 as an intrapelvic protrusion of the femoral head occurring as 'an abnormal gouty manifestation' in adult women.

Protrusio may be primary or secondary and is thought to occur from the result of remodelling of the weak, medial acetabular bone after multiple recurring stress fractures. It is defined as displacement of the femoral head medial to the ilio-ischial line. In the early stages this heals with no apparent bone defect, in later stages the bone is severely fragmented. The deformity may progress until the femoral neck impinges on the side of the pelvis. Technical difficulties are, thus, normally encountered with the medial wall of the acetabulum in total hip arthroplasty.

Primary protrusion (Otto pelvis):

- Is characterized by progressive protrusion in middle-aged women
- Bilateral in one-third of patients and causes pain and limitation of movement at an early age
- Varus deformity of the femoral neck and degenerative changes are common.

Secondary protrusio may be bilateral or unilateral and due to:

- Paget's
- Marfan's

- Rheumatoid arthritis
- Ankylosing spondylitis
- Osteomalacia
- Septic arthritis
- Central fracture dislocation
- Total hip replacement and migration of the femoral head or cup.

Classification (Figures 7.8.13 and 7.8.14)

Sotelo-Garza and Charnley measured the distance between the medial wall of the acetabulum and the pelvic brim (ilio-pectineal line) radiographically. They recognized three grades:

1) 1–5mm (mild protrusion)
2) 6–15mm (moderate)
3) Over 15mm (severe).

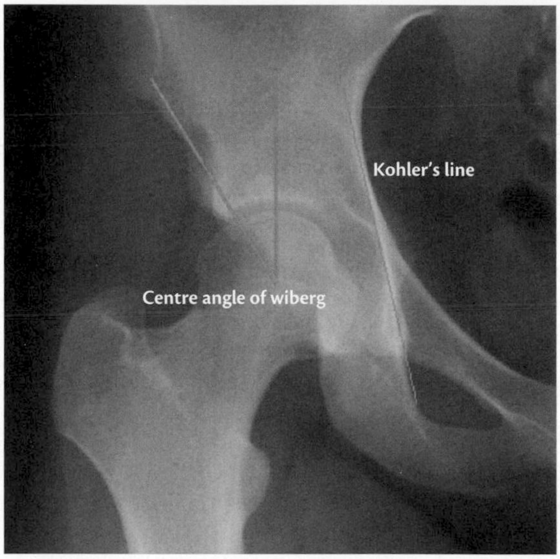

Fig. 7.8.13 Kohler's line and centre edge angle of Wiburg in a normal hip.

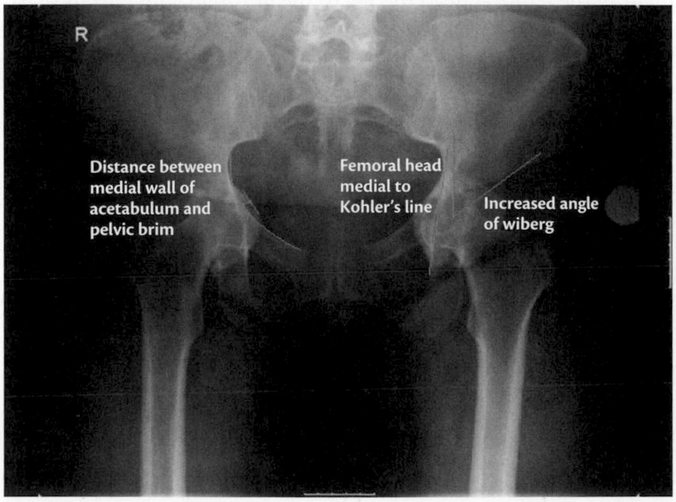

Fig. 7.8.14 Sotelo-Garza and Charnley method.

Radiographic diagnosis:

- If the medial wall of the acetabulum is 3mm or more medial to the ilio-ischial line in men and 6mm medial to it in women
- If femoral head is medial to Kohler's line (line from medial border of ilium to medial border of the ischium)
- If centre edge angle of Wiberg is greater than 40 degrees (normal = 35 degrees).

Preoperative planning

Successful total hip replacement depends upon restoring:

- The medial wall
- The 'hip centre' position
- The correct offset and abductor function
- Leg length inequality

and preventing recurrent protrusio.

Operative procedure (Figure 7.8.15)

Minor degrees of protrusio can be treated successfully with a standard total hip replacement. Moderate or severe degrees compromise the medial wall and an alternative should be considered. In some cases the neck cut will need to be made 'in situ' rather than risking a fracture whilst trying to dislocate the hip.

Bone graft

Bone grafting offers an elegant solution to managing the medial wall defect in protrusio. Various techniques have been described. It needs to be intimately opposed to the irregular host bed and compressible to allow sufficient incorporation and remodelling. Bone wafers meet these criteria better than a single massive graft as described by Heywood in 1980. Wherever possible, bone should be taken from the femoral head and supplemented by cancellous curettings from the femoral neck and greater trochanter. Morcelized bone graft is used for contained defects and can undergo revascularization and remodelling; it strengthens with time. Bone graft also allows cement to be inserted and offers resistance to compression. Using cement alone against the weak medial wall provides poor containment and fixation, which in turn leads to premature loosening.

Acetabulum

Uncemented components can be inserted over the bone graft in a more lateral and anatomic position and secured with acetabular screws. Ideally an acetabular component should contain a peripheral

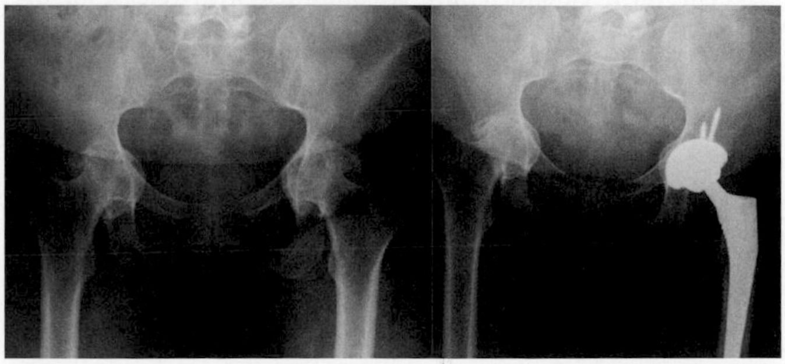

Fig. 7.8.15 Pre- and postoperative radiographs of primary total hip replacement in primary bilateral protrusio acetabuli.

flare, plus or minus peripherally placed screws, rather than a true hemisphere in order to prevent progressive medialization of the component. If a cementless cup is used, contact with host bone should be at least 50%. If contact cannot be made with at least 50% of host bone, then a cemented cup with a reinforcement ring or the technique of cementing into impacted bone should be used. In cases of extensive bone loss, antiprotrusio cages are necessary.

Reaming

It is essential not to deepen the acetabulum while reaming; the surgeon should ream to allow a good peripheral fit. The reamer can be used in reverse mode to mould and conform the graft to the acetabular floor.

Results

The adequacy of correction of the deformity and anatomical centre of rotation correlates with long-term prosthetic survivorship. Good results exist for grafted hips; cement or antiprotrusio cages alone may fail early and should be supplemented with bone graft to provide lasting support.

- Primary protrusio is uncommon and accounts for only a small percentage of cases
- Technical difficulties include inadequate medial wall and restoring offset, hip centre and leg lengths
- Neck may need to be cut in-situ; bone graft is usually necessary and ideally should be taken from the femoral head
- Antiprotrusio cages or custom implants may be needed in cases with excessive bone loss.

Conversion of arthrodesed hip to total hip replacement

Introduction

Hip arthrodesis can successfully provide long-term pain relief and will allow the resumption of manual labour and demanding physical activities. However, over time, it may be associated with a significant functional disability:

- Back pain:
  - Multilevel degenerate changes common
  - Leg-length inequality and fusion malposition exacerbate lower back pain
- Ipsilateral knee pain and instability:
  - More likely in an adducted fused position
  - Tendency for valgus deformity
- Contralateral hip pain: more likely if hip fused in an abducted position
- Painful pseudoarthosis.

Conversion to a total hip replacement may improve these symptoms as well as restoring leg-length inequality and improving hip mobility. Conversion of an ankylosed hip does, however, introduce a number of challenges:

- The effect of previous operations on both bone and soft tissues
- Atrophy of periarticular muscles
- The initial disease and indication for fusion.

Mid-term results have been satisfactory but complications, failures, restricted postoperative motion, and instability are more frequent than after primary hip replacement.

Preoperative planning

- Appropriate radiographs:
  - Anteroposterior and lateral
  - Judet views may identify anterior or posterior column deficiencies
- CT scan to assess bone stock
- MRI can be helpful in assessing the proximity of neurovascular structures and abductor muscle mass
- Position of fusion: patients with abnormal positions of fusion are more likely to have clinically significant soft tissue contractures and may require further soft tissue releases
- Further abductor muscle assessment:
  - EMG studies: routine use in assessing abductor function may be questionable
  - Some authors suggest palpation of abductor muscle contraction

Take care in offering conversion to total hip replacement when gluteal muscles are not continuous and the hip is fused in a good position.

Operative technique (Figure 7.8.16)

Numerous approaches have been described. The authors prefer a standard posterior approach although the direct lateral or a transtrochanteric approach is commonly used with success.

Gluteal muscles are assessed and any internal fixation devices will need to be removed. The femoral neck and the site of the fusion

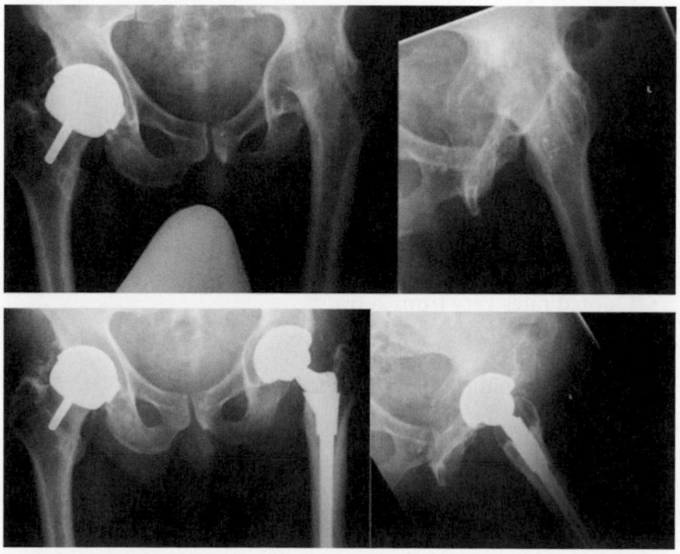

Fig. 7.8.16 Pre- and postoperative radiographs of conversion of an ankylosed left hip to total hip replacement; a previous right Birmingham resurfacing (Smith and Nephew) has been performed.

between the ilium and femoral head needs to be clearly visualized and preoperative planning is helpful in achieving this. If in doubt, an intraoperative radiograph can be obtained. Heterotopic bone is removed with an osteotome and the femoral neck is cut with an oscillating saw. Adequate exposure is necessary to identify the inferior margin of the acetabulum.

Technical considerations

- Acetabular component:
  - Consider constrained liner, especially if poor abductors
  - Structural grafting is sometimes required
- Femoral component: routinely prepared using modular implants to restore soft tissue stability, hip mechanics and a stable reduction
- Soft tissues releases are frequently required:
  - Percutaneous adductor tenotomy
  - Psoas release
  - If no abductors, the proximal femur can be sewn to the tensor fascia lata anteriorly and the gluteus maximus and iliotibial band posteriorly.

Postoperative rehabilitation

- Routine thromboprophylaxis and prophylactic antibiotics
- 'Slings and springs' until muscle control and then weight bearing depending on the type of implant fixation
- If any doubt about abductors, then an abduction brace for 6 weeks should be worn.

Results

The effectiveness of total hip replacement following hip fusion has been demonstrated in a number of series. Back pain is often relieved (70–90%) and leg lengths can be improved. Ipsilateral knee pain is less predictably relieved. Success is often more reliable in patients with spontaneous ankylosis.

Complications

More complications are generally reported than after conventional total hip replacement:

- Dislocation:
  - More common if early fusion (less than 15 years) due to underdevelopment of the abductor muscles
  - Quoted rates vary from 2–6%
- Infection: 2–6%
- Nerve palsy: sciatic and femoral 2–13%
- Heterotopic ossification:
  - Up to 13%
  - Some authors advocate the routine use of non-steroidal anti-inflammatory drugs

- Careful evaluation of the gluteal muscles is mandatory and predicts final walking ability and patient satisfaction
- Long-term effectiveness of total hip replacement in ankylosed hips is satisfactory
- Patients should be counseled about the higher rate of complications
- Trendelenburg gait will normally persist but abductor function may improve for up to 3 years.

Other difficult primary total hip replacements

Paget's disease (Figure 7.8.17)

- Characterized by increased bone resorption and secondary formation of abnormal new bone
- Deformed proximal femur and hypersclerotic bone are common
- Paget's disease may be incidental or a consequence of Paget's disease
- Degenerative changes in the hip joint are typically in the form of medial joint space narrowing compared to superior joint space narrowing in primary osteoarthritis
- If the acetabulum is involved, protrusio may occur in 25–50% of cases
- If the femur is involved coax vara and anterior or lateral bowing of the femoral shaft may occur
- As the disease progresses, the femur becomes sclerotic, and the intramedullary canal is sometimes obliterated
- Potential for serious bleeding perioperatively
- Consider cemented arthroplasty
- Increased incidence of early loosening and heterotopic ossification.

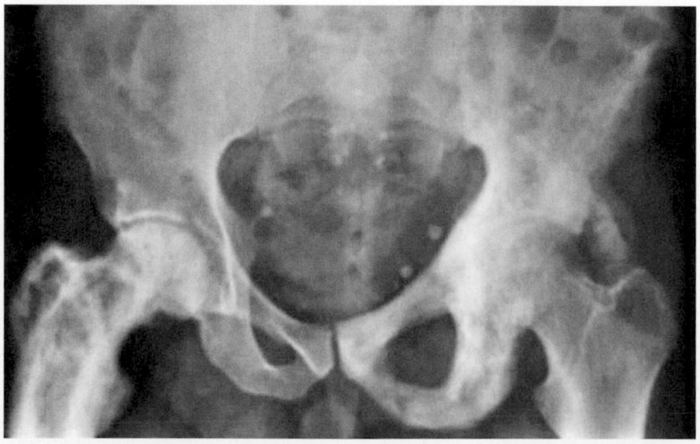

Fig. 7.8.17 Paget's disease in the right proximal femur and a degenerate left hip.

Postacetabular fracture

- Preoperatively:
  - Ensure no occult deep infection
  - CT scan to assess bone stock
  - Assess sciatic nerve carefully
- Extensile approach necessary to remove hardware
- May encounter altered anatomy
- May have large bony defects requiring bone graft and cages
- Higher postoperative complication rates because of scarring from previous surgery, retained hardware, and heterotopic bone
- Successful results but associated with earlier loosening than total hip replacements for primary osteoarthritis.

Slipped upper femoral epiphysis

- First described by Mueller in 1889
- The displacement of the femoral head usually results in a varus and external rotation orientation between the epiphysis and the metaphysis. When the deformity is severe or there are secondary complications such as chondrolysis or osteonecrosis, secondary osteoarthritis is an early complication
- Patients are often young and active and choice of implant is important; total hip replacement should only be considered when all other options have been exhausted.

Ankylosing spondylitis

- Preoperative respiratory and cardiac evaluation are necessary
- May be difficult to mobilize the hip joint if severe contractures or ankylosis; *in situ* neck osteotomy may be needed
- Uncemented femoral components only if bone is of good quality—often the femur has a 'stove pipe' deformity with straight lateral walls, making it unsuitable for press-fit or porous coated stems
- Heterotopic ossification only more likely if hip was completely ankylosed.

Osteonecrosis

- Osteonecrosis can be idiopathic or secondary to other pathology such as sickle cell disease, alcohol, or steroids
- Long-term studies show that patients with osteonecrosis who undergo total hip replacement are up to four times more likely to experience an overall failure from aseptic loosening or infection than those with osteoarthritis.

Further reading

Amstutz, H. (1991). *Hip Arthroplasty*. New York: Churchill Livingstone.

Cameron, H., Eren, O., and Solomon, M. (1998). Nerve injury in the prosthetic management of the dysplastic hip. *Orthopedics*, **21**, 980–1.

Crowe, J., Mani, V., and Ranawat, C. (1979). Total hip replacement in congenital dislocation and dysplasia of the hip. *Journal of Bone and Joint Surgery*, **61A**, 15–23.

Davlin, L., Amstutz, H., Tooke, S., Dorey, F., and Nasser, S. (1990). Treatment of osteoarthrosis secondary to congenital dislocation of the hip. Primary cemented surface replacement compared with conventional total hip replacement. *Journal of Bone and Joint Surgery*, **72A**, 1035–42.

Haddad, F., Masri, B., Garbuz, D., and Duncan, C. (1999). Primary total hip replacement of the dysplastic hip. *Journal of Bone and Joint Surgery*, **81A**, 1462–82.

Hamadouche, M., Kerboull, L., Meunier, A., Courpied, J., and Kerboull, M. (2001). Total hip arthroplasty for the treatment of ankylosed hips. *Journal of Bone and Joint Surgery*, **83A**, 992–8.

Hartofilakidis, G. and Karachalios, T. (2004). Total hip arthroplasty for congenital hip disease. *Journal of Bone and Joint Surgery*, **86A**, 242–50.

Merkow, R., Pellicci, P., Hely, D., and Salvati, E. (1984). Total hip replacement for Paget's disease of the hip. *Journal of Bone and Joint Surgery*, **66A**, 752–8.

Tachdjian, M. (1982). *Congenital Dislocation of the Hip*. New York: Churchill Livingstone.

7.9

Surgical options excluding total hip replacement for hip pain

Ahmad K. Malik and Aresh Hashemi-Nejad

Summary points

- Intra-articular steroid and local anaesthetic
- Soft tissue releases
- Synovectomy
  - Open
  - Arthroscopically
- Acetabular osteotomy
  - Bernese periacetabular osteotomy
  - Triple
  - Dial
  - Chiari
  - Shelf
- Femoral osteotomy
  - Varus
  - Valgus
- Hip arthroscopy
- Open surgical dislocation of the hip
- Hip arthrodesis

Introduction

This chapter outlines the main surgical options for hip pain excluding total hip replacement. The aim of surgery is to relieve pain and delay or halt further degenerative changes, negating the need for total hip replacement or delaying the age at which it needs to be implanted. The choice of treatment is dictated by the patient symptoms, underlying disease process, hip deformity, past treatment, and future patient expectations.

Due to the myriad of underlying causes of hip pain and arthritis in the young patient (see Chapter 7.7) not all, and likewise, perhaps more than one of the following surgical options may be employed during the course of management of the arthritic hip in the young adult.

Surgical options

Intra-articular steroid and local anaesthetic

For pain relief in patients with rheumatoid arthritis, juvenile idiopathic arthritis, and synovitis of the hip joint in the presence of minimal joint degeneration and absence of mechanical symptoms.

Used in conjunction with arthrogram and examination under anaesthesia to assess range of motion of hip joint and assessment for suitability of osteotomy (femoral, acetabular, or both) as well as verifying intra-articular nature of pain.

Surgical considerations

Should be performed under strict aseptic conditions with intraoperative fluoroscopy for correct placement of the needle. An anterolateral or direct lateral approach may be used. Injecting Omnipaque 300 dye confirms the needle is in the joint and helps outline the articular surface and aids in assessing joint congruency.

Intra-articular steroid and local anaesthetic do not alter disease progression radiographically and improvements in pain typically last for 12 weeks. Conflicting evidence in the literature exists regarding increased risk of infection in patients who have a subsequent total hip replacement shortly after their injection.

Soft tissue releases

Any condition leading to significant muscle imbalance and spasticity can result in soft tissue contractures. This in turn can result in substantial acetabular erosion, femoral head subluxation/dislocation, and in the skeletally immature increased femoral neck anteversion and coxa valga. Neuromuscular conditions such as cerebral palsy and myelomeningocele result in intrinsic muscle imbalance with resultant contractures.

Spastic hip subluxation and dislocation are common problems in patients with cerebral palsy often leading to a painful joint with difficulties in mobility (in previously ambulating patients), sitting, personal hygiene, and care. The adducted hip can also result in pelvic obliquity and subsequent scoliosis. The adductor longus and variably the iliopsoas are contracted in these patients. Release of adductor longus is performed by a medial open or percutaneous method. Release of iliopsoas at the level of the lesser trochanter or at the pelvic brim (to prevent loss of flexion power) is also performed. Soft tissue releases have proved to be beneficial in the prevention of spastic hip dislocation and progressive hip dysplasia.

In juvenile idiopathic arthritis, inflammatory synovitis leads to pain and muscle spasm with subsequent joint contractures. Effusion of the joint also leads to pain, the joint is then held in the position of maximal joint space, thereby reducing joint pressure, which in the hip joint is 45 degrees of flexion in neutral rotation. In the presence of fixed contractures, surgical release of psoas and the adductors relieves pain and increases mobility and function. More aggressive surgical release, including rectus femoris with or without open synovectomy, may also be indicated.

Hip dysplasia with marked subluxation or dislocation, adult acquired neurological diseases such as stroke or Parkinson's disease, and patients with longstanding hip pain can all develop muscle contractures around the hip joint. Patients undergoing a total hip replacement in the presence of tight adductors or iliopsoas may also benefit from surgical release to prevent deforming forces and improve range of motion and stability of the hip replacement.

Soft tissue releases have not shown to arrest or prevent degenerative changes in the hip joint radiographically or prevent the marked femoral neck anteversion seen in patients with juvenile idiopathic arthritis.

Synovectomy

Only a few conditions exist which solely affect the synovium around the hip joint, resulting in pain with or without mechanical symptoms. Juvenile idiopathic arthritis can lead to severe synovitis resulting in debilitating pain and decreased function. Open synovectomy results in significant improvements in pain, mobility, and walking ability.

Primary synovial osteochondromatosis of the hip is a rare benign condition characterised by multiple intra-articular osteochondral loose bodies and synovial hyperplasia, which may result in mechanical symptoms and degenerative arthritis if untreated. Open synovectomy can reliably remove the loose bodies and alleviate symptoms.

Pigmented villonodular synovitis of the hip is a rare disease. Synovectomy is generally accepted as the only surgical treatment for the disorder.

Synovectomy is traditionally performed through a Smith-Petersen approach or open dislocation of the hip. The latter has slightly better results in terms of recurrence of the primary disorder but is associated with increased morbidity. Synovectomy can also be performed arthroscopically.

Acetabular osteotomy

Reconstructive acetabular osteotomy is indicated in young active adults with symptomatic hip dysplasia and only mild arthritic changes as seen radiographically. Hip joint congruency is essential to the success of the operation and can be confirmed by preoperative imaging with either an anterior-posterior (AP) radiograph of the hip with the leg in abduction, on three-dimensional computed tomography (CT) reconstructed images. The false profile radiograph is a true lateral radiograph of the symptomatic acetabulum taken with the patient standing. The false profile radiograph is important as some patients who have dysplasia of the hip have nearly normal findings on AP radiographs and the lack of anterior coverage of the head is seen only on the false profile radiograph.

Examination under fluoroscopy with radio-opaque dye injected in the hip joint allows for a dynamic assessment of the joint congruency and can also help detect subtle labral pathology. The aim of the osteotomy is to return the hip joint to as near as normal anatomy and biomechanics, with improvements in pain and prevention of further degenerative changes. Reconstructive osteotomies include the Bernese periacetabular osteotomy, triple osteotomy and dial osteotomy. Where the hip joint is not congruent because of severely distorted anatomy, a salvage osteotomy is undertaken. These procedures rely on metaplasia of the capsule to fibrocartilage and therefore do not provide a long-lasting reconstruction. Common salvage procedures include the Chiari and shelf osteotomy.

Contraindications

Patients with inflammatory conditions; patients older than 50 years; the presence of arthritis or marked obesity. The presence of joint incongruence precludes any reconstructive osteotomy. Smokers should be cautioned of an increased risk of non-union.

Bernese periacetabular osteotomy (Figure 7.9.1)

The Bernese periacetabular osteotomy developed by Ganz and colleagues in the early 1980s is currently the most popular reconstructive pelvis osteotomy. The numerous advantages of this procedure include the need for only one incision, the use of three straight and reproducible bony cuts, the large range of correction possible with medialization of the hip joint centre, anterior and lateral rotation, version correction, preservation of a portion of the posterior column allowing for early partial weight bearing, and minimal internal fixation and no change in the diameter of the true pelvis therefore not interfering with child birth. The risk of non-union of the osteotomized fragment is negligible due to preservation of its blood supply. The procedure also allows for intra-articular assessment and repair if required of the labrum, as well as treatment of femoroacetabular impingement.

The longest follow-up to date by Ganz and colleagues at a mean 20 years, reports joint preservation of 60% at latest follow-up. Poor outcome was associated with pain and low functional scores preoperatively, severity of arthritis, positive anterior impingement test, limp, and age at surgery. Patient selection is therefore key to the success of this procedure. Previous Bernese periacetabular osteotomy does not compromise the results of subsequent total hip replacement.

Surgical considerations

The periacetabular osteotomy is performed through an abductor-sparing Smith-Petersen approach. Sequential soft tissue and bony steps as described by Ganz are performed which then allow for mobilization and correction of the acetabulum. The key aims in correction are:

1) Acetabular sourcil (weight-bearing surface) is repositioned to a more horizontal orientation
2) Lateral femoral head coverage improved with a goal of achieving 25–35 degrees centre edge angle
3) Translation of hip joint centre medially if required
4) Correct version (absence of cross-over sign)
5) Anterior femoral head coverage improved to 25–35 degrees on false profile view
6) The correction maintains or produces a congruent joint space and subluxation is corrected
7) Adequate head–neck offset is present or has been restored with osteochondroplasty

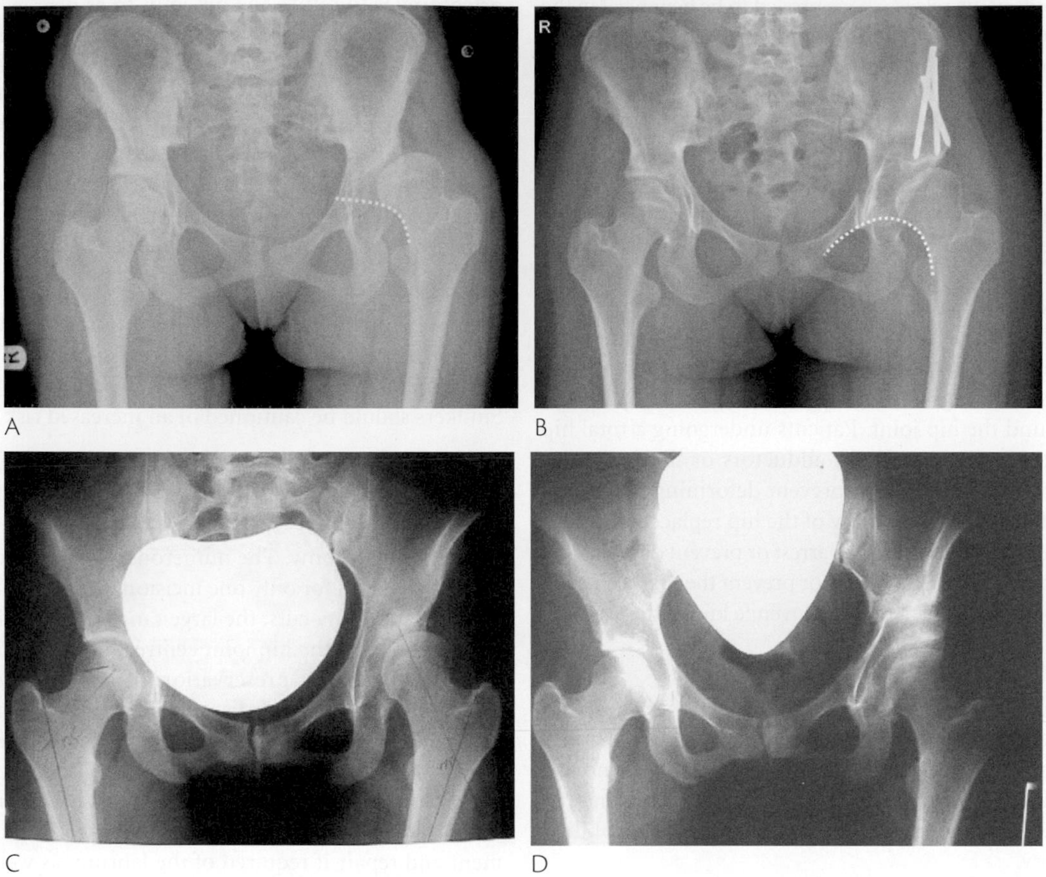

Fig. 7.9.1 Bernese periacetabular osteotomy and modfied Tonnis osteotomy. A) Hip dysplasia with subluxation, Shenton's line is clearly disrupted. B) Following Bernese periacetabular osteotomy, Shenton's line is restored and the sourcil is more horizontal. C) Preoperative film with decreased centre edge angle evident. D) Postmodified Tonnis osteotomy; the sourcil is horizontal and the centre edge angle is increased.

8) Adequate internal fixation with acceptable screw position

9) Hip flexion of ≥90 degrees and hip abduction ≥30 degrees.

Triple

The triple osteotomy includes cuts of the ilium, ischium, and pubis through three separate incisions. The acetabulum is then rotated to provide increased femoral head coverage. Although this is technically easier to perform than the dial or Ganz periacetabular osteotomy, the coverage it provides is less adequate (since the cuts are farther away from the acetabulum) and has the potential for non-union at the osteotomy sites because of inability to achieve adequate internal fixation. Steels osteotomy involves ischial cuts at a distance from the joint. The modified Tonnis osteotomy (see Figure 7.9.1) involves bony cuts closer to the joint. As the sacrotuberous and spinous ligaments are not violated, the mobility of the osteotomized fragment is limited. Large corrections with a triple osteotomy can result in pelvic deformity and as the posterior column is disrupted fixation of the osteotomized fragment can be compromised.

Dial

The dial osteotomy described by Eppright is one of a number of spherical osteotomies, mainly favoured in the Far East. It provides for excellent coverage with complete redirection of the acetabular articular surface. It is rarely used because it is extremely technically demanding and carries a high risk of penetration into the hip joint and resultant damage of the acetabular articular cartilage. Alternative surgical procedures, such as the Ganz periacetabular osteotomy, can achieve the same result with a less technically demanding and reproducible procedure.

Chiari

This procedure is reserved for non-congruent joints. The iliac bone is osteotomized just above the hip joint surface to the inferior part of the sciatic notch. The inferior segment of the pelvis is then displaced medially, resulting in increased femoral head coverage and medialization of the hip centre. Capsule is interposed between the femoral head and the proximal shelf of bone. This capsular tissue undergoes metaplasia into fibrocartilage. Long-term review of the Chiari pelvic osteotomy found that most patients had progressive degenerative changes and almost a third had severe pain at follow-up at 14 years. Outcome was enhanced when no preoperative arthritic changes were present, in younger patients, and a hip that was painless at the time of surgery.

Chiari osteotomy has no adverse effect clinically or radiographically on later hip replacement. It did, however, require less bone grafting and achieved better coverage by host bone when compared with hip replacements in dysplastic hips.

Box 7.9.1 Femoral osteotomy: indications

- Non-union of femoral neck fractures
- Osteoarthritis
- Correcting post-traumatic deformity, slipped upper femoral epiphysis deformity
- Legg–Calve–Perthes disease
- Avascular necrosis.

Shelf

This procedure involves using a corticocancellous graft to augment the anterolateral aspect of the acetabulum and to act as a buttress, increasing joint stability. The hip joint centre is unaffected as is the relationship of the femoral head with the acetabulum. This procedure is typically used in children with incongruent joints. Recent study in adults who underwent shelf osteotomy for symptomatic hip dysplasia revealed a survivorship with conversion to hip replacement as an end-point of 86% at 5 years and 46% at 10 years. In patients who had slight or no narrowing of the joint space preoperatively, the survival rose to 97% at 5 and 75% at 10 years.

Femoral osteotomy

Indications (Box 7.9.1)

One of the original and, to this day, main indications for proximal femoral osteotomy is the treatment of non-union of femoral neck fractures. A valgus osteotomy converts a shear force across the non-union site into a compressive force and this induces healing. In one study, 93% of hips went on to heal using this technique.

Pauwel is credited for introducing the concept of varus and valgus proximal femoral osteotomies as a method of increasing the weight-bearing surface across the femoral head. He believed that 'osteoarthritis results when abnormal forces act on normal tissue, or when normal forces act on damaged tissues' and treatment should therefore be directed at increasing joint congruency, which in turn results in a greater surface area and decreased load per unit area of the articular cartilage. Bombelli later added flexion and extension osteotomy in the sagittal plane to further optimize joint congruency.

Other indications for the use of proximal femoral osteotomy include correcting post-traumatic deformity, and treating healed slipped upper femoral epiphysis (SUFE) using a flexion with or without rotation osteotomy. Acquired varus deformity with hinge abduction following Legg–Calve–Perthes disease is corrected with a valgus extension osteotomy. The treatment of hip dysplasia with a varus (derotation) osteotomy is usually performed in conjunction with a pelvic osteotomy.

In the management of osteonecrosis a variety of osteotomies have been described, varus, valgus, flexion, extension, combined, or rotational all with the intention of moving the osteonecrotic area away from where it would transmit weight.

Surgical considerations (Figures 7.9.2–7.9.5)

Careful and meticulous preoperative planning is required to ensure a successful result. The position of 'best fit' and 'improved patient comfort' is key to achieving this. During preoperative examination it is important to assess the degree of passive movement, in particular

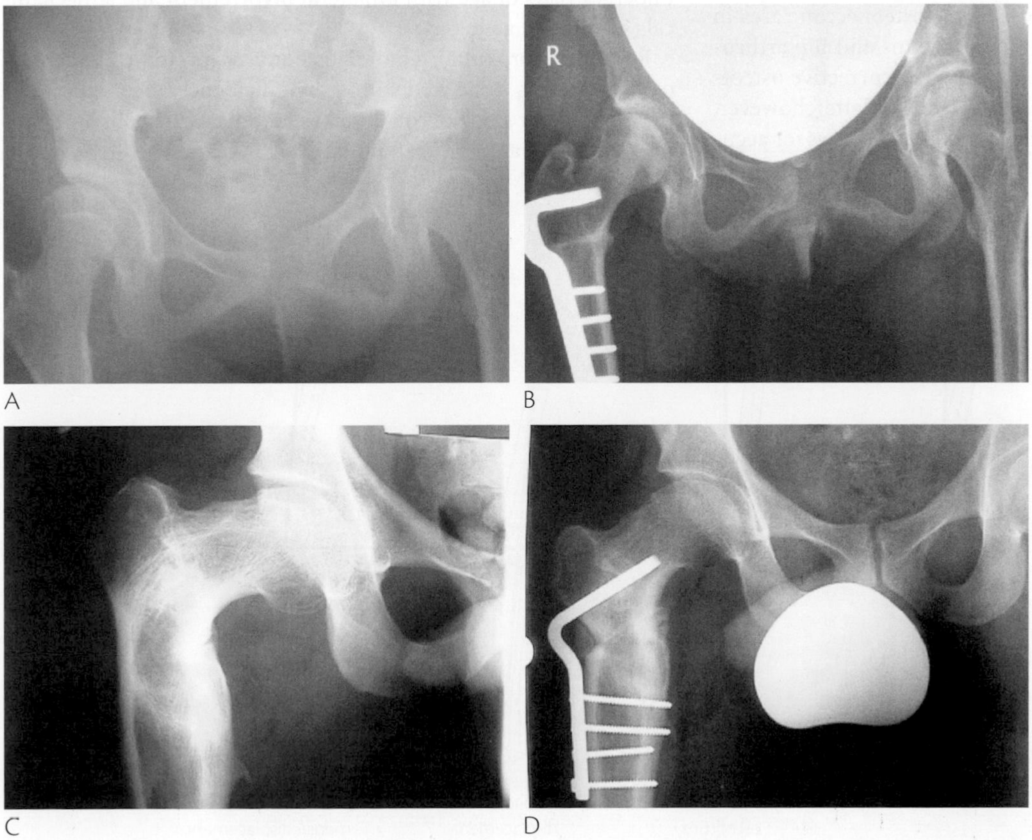

Fig. 7.9.2 Valgus and varus proximal femoral osteotomy. A) Marked bilateral valgus hips preoperatively B) Varus osteotomy with resulting increased head coverage C) Severe varus deformity right hip preoperatively D) Valgus osteotomy with normalised neck shaft angle.

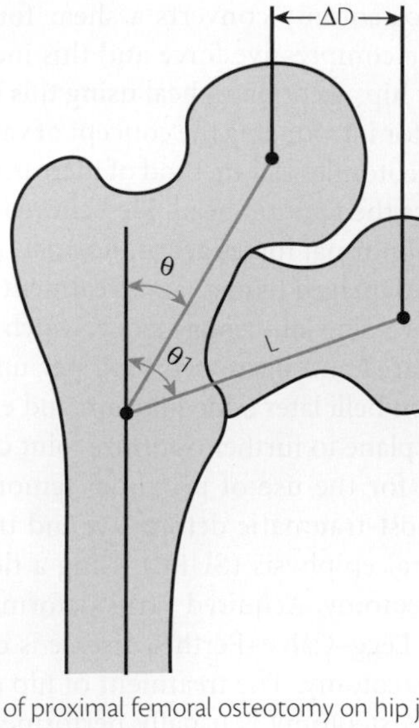

Fig. 7.9.3 Effect of proximal femoral osteotomy on hip joint centre. Valgus osteotomy causes lateralization and varus osteotomy results in medialization.

adduction and abduction across the hip. Following a varus osteotomy there will be loss of abduction, the minimum amount of abduction required prior to surgery is the amount of varus required plus 10 degrees, otherwise a fixed adduction contracture will ensue. Likewise, a valgus osteotomy will result in loss of adduction; therefore to avoid any abduction contracture postoperatively the patient should have at least the required angle in adduction.

Preoperative imaging with an AP of the hip taken in adduction/abduction is necessary. A false profile lateral view also reveals any anterior uncovering which may require correction. Magnetic resonance (MRI) scans are useful in isolating the osteonecrotic area in a patient with osteonecrosis of the hip. CT scans and hip arthrograms are also extremely useful in planning the corrective osteotomy and used according to surgeon preference. The latter, however, gives a dynamic understanding of the hip joint and allows for accurate assessment of position of 'best fit'.

Patients undergoing a varus osteotomy typically have lateral subluxation of the femoral head, associated with coxa valga. Following the osteotomy, the affected limb will be shortened and patients should be informed of this. Valgus osteotomy should result in reduced lateral impingement and an improvement in joint space on AP pelvis with the hip in adduction. It should also result in normalization of the relationship between the tip of the greater trochanter and the centre of the femoral head. In varus osteotomy the femoral shaft should be medialized, and in a valgus osteotomy the femoral shaft requires lateralization to avoid any alteration to the mechanical axis of the limb.

The affect on limb length and any resulting discrepancy following an osteotomy should be discussed in depth with patients preoperatively to ensure patient satisfaction.

Femoral osteotomy may distort the local anatomy which may jeopardize any future total hip replacement and this has to be taken into consideration by the operating surgeon. Best results are typically found in the young, non-obese patient with a good range of motion preoperatively.

Contraindications (Box 7.9.2)

Results of osteotomy

A study of 26 varus proximal femoral osteotomies for hip dysplasia in adults with a mean follow-up of 5 years reported no conversions to total hip replacement in the review period. There was significant improvement in symptoms and function with one case of non-union which was successfully revised. Best results were obtained in patients with long-leg dysplasia.

A review of intertrochanteric valgus-extension osteotomy performed for osteoarthritis reported 67% of the hips were good or excellent at final review. Better results were obtained in patients under 40 years of age with unilateral involvement and a mechanical (secondary) aetiology.

Rotational proximal femoral osteotomy for the treatment of osteonecrosis is associated with a high incidence of complications (55%). Another study of rotational osteotomy carried out in 18 hips in 17 patients at a mean follow-up of 5 years for osteonecrosis

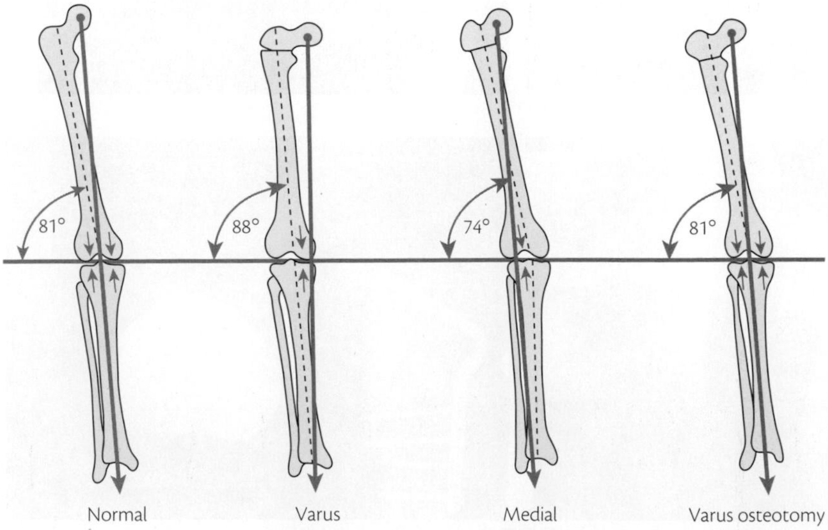

Fig. 7.9.4 Effect of osteotomy and displacement of shaft on mechanical axis.

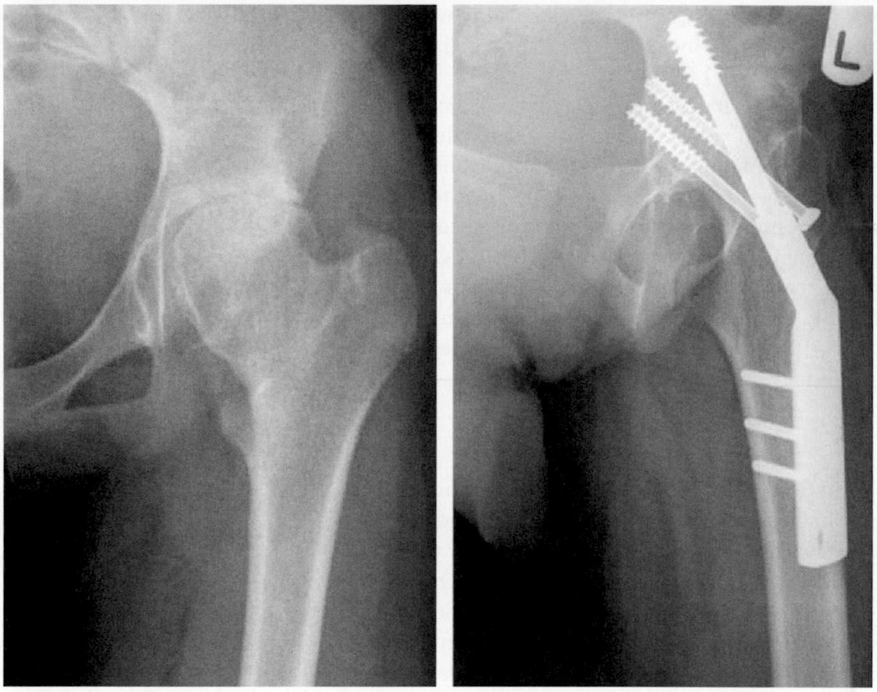

Fig. 7.9.5 Hip arthrodesis using compression hip screw technique. Twelve-year-old female with painful arthritis of the left hip who grew up in Africa. Arthrodesis achieved with use of compression screw. Union was achieved at 8 weeks postoperatively.

Box 7.9.2 Femoral osteotomy: contraindications

- Stiif painful hip
- Obesity
- Gross narrowing of joint space with sclerosis.

revealed satisfactory results in only three hips (17%) and 12 hips had been revised to total hip replacement; 83% of the patients had additional collapse. Varus and valgus osteotomies performed better with 74% and 85% good or excellent results respectively at medium-term review.

A previously osteotomized hip may be difficult to convert to a total hip replacement. Complicating factors include hardware removal, deformity of the proximal femur leading to inadequate prosthetic fit and fixation, or to intraoperative femoral fracture and risk of infection. In one large series of 305 total hip replacements in 290 patients who had a previous intertrochanteric osteotomy, it was noted that the operative time was longer and blood loss was somewhat greater than for primary total hip replacement. Technical difficulties were encountered in 23% of cases. The overall probability of failure at 10 years was 20.6%. The incidence of positive tissue cultures from the osteotomy site was 9%, and that of broken plates or screws 24.3% at the time of total hip replacement. Removing hardware as soon as bony union has been obtained as well as maintaining proximal femoral alignment with the femoral shaft on coronal and sagittal planes may facilitate and improve results of subsequent total hip replacement.

Hip arthrosopy

See Chapter 7.18.

Open surgical dislocation of the hip

See Chapter 7.7.

Hip arthrodesis

Once the preferred treatment of choice for end-stage osteoarthritis, the popularity of this procedure has faded as that of total hip replacement has risen since the early 1970s. The procedure is rarely performed today and most orthopaedic surgeons are inexperienced in its use, making it even less of an attractive option.

In adolescents and young adults with severe end-stage arthritis affecting a single joint, reconstructive and salvage procedures as discussed earlier may not be suitable. While total hip replacement offers the potential for immediate pain relief and good results in the short to medium term with regards to function, there remains considerable concern and reservation about the long-term outcome and durability of its use in the young active patient. Several long-term studies have shown that hip arthrodesis successfully relieves pain and allows patients to lead active lives.

The ideal patient is classically described as a young active male manual labourer who wants to return to work. In general, patients should be younger than 30 years of age and have end-stage monoarticular osteoarthritis. Ideal candidates are those with post-traumatic arthritis, osteonecrosis, and patients who have had sepsis such as tuberculosis. Patients should not have low back pain, ipsilateral knee pain, or contralateral hip pathology. MRI screening of the contralateral hip should be performed in patients with osteonecrosis to rule out early disease.

Surgical considerations

Hip arthrodesis can be achieved with the use of a Cobra plate applied to the lateral aspect of the femur and ilium. To gain access to the femoral head and acetabulum, a trochanteric osteotomy is performed which is then fixed over the plate. The Iowa technique involves performing a Chiari type osteotomy while the Vancouver technique avoids the need for this by medializing the socket.

Further techniques have been developed to avoid violation of the abductor mechanism which occurs using the earlier described techniques. Preservation of the abductors is important as the arthrodesed hip may be a stop-gap measure to delay a total hip replacement or a patient may choose to have a fused hip converted to a total hip replacement. Abductor-sparing techniques include the use of a dynamic compression screw and anterior plating (Figure 7.9.5). The hip should be arthrodesed in a position of 30 degrees of flexion, 5–10 degrees of adduction, and 10 degrees of external rotation. Abduction and internal rotation are associated with poor results.

Discussion

The functional limitations of hip arthrodesis relate to the loss of hip flexion, with difficulty in prolonged sitting in confined spaces, bending, putting on socks, and sexual activity. It is unclear whether patients today are willing to accept these limitations. The main long-term complication of hip arthrodesis is associated low back pain in up to two-thirds of patients, ipsilateral knee pain in half, and contralateral hip pain in a fifth of patients. Patients fatigue more easily due to the increased energy expenditure when walking. The main advantage is the relief of pain, return to active lifestyle, and preservation of bone stock.

Conversion of a fused hip to a total hip arthroplasty is generally associated with a favourable outcome. However, the technically demanding nature of the procedure should not be underestimated. Patients should be informed preoperatively of the possibility of a higher complication rate than that seen with primary total hip replacement.

Further reading

Ansari, A., Jones, S., Hashemi-Nejad, A., and Catterall, A. (2008). Varus proximal femoral osteotomy for hip dysplasia in adults. *Hip International*, **18**(3), 200–6.

Brand, R.A., Pedersen, D.R., and Callaghan, J.J. (1985). Hip arthrodesis. *Journal of Bone and Joint Surgery*, **67**A, 1328–35.

Chitre, A.R., Fehily, M.J., and Bamford, D.J. (2007). Total hip replacement after intra-articular injection of local anaesthetic and steroid. *Journal of Bone and Joint Surgery. British Volume*, **89**(2), 166–8.

Clohisy, J.C., Beaulé, P.E., O'Malley, A., Safran, M., and Schoenecker, P. (2008). AOA Symposium. Hip Disease in the Young Adult: Current Concepts of Etiology and Surgical Treatment. *Journal of Bone and Joint Surgery American Volume*, **90**, 2267–81.

De Roeck, N., and Hashemi-Nejad, A. (2002). The modified Tonnis triple pelvic osteotomy in the young adult - early results. *Hip International*, **13**, 215–19.

Ganz, R., Klaue, K., Vinh, T.S., and Mast, J.W. (1988). A new periacetabular osteotomy for the treatment of hip dysplasias. Technique and preliminary results. *Clinical Orthopaedics and Related Research*, **232**, 26–36.

Ganz, R., Gill, T.J., Gautier, E., Ganz, K., Krugel, N., and Berlemann, U. (2001) . Surgical dislocation of the adult hip: A technique with full access to the femoral head and acetabulum without the risk of avascular necrosis. *Journal of Bone and Joint Surgery (Br)*, **83**, 1119–24.

Kaspar, S., and de V de Beer, J. (2005). Infection in hip arthroplasty after previous injection of steroid. *Journal of Bone and Joint Surgery (Br)*, **87**-B, 454–7.

Miller, F., Cardoso Dias, R., Dabney, K.W., Lipton, G.E., and Triana, M. (1997). Soft-tissue release for spastic hip subluxation in cerebral palsy. *Journal of Pediatric Orthopedics*, **17**(5), 571–84.

Shannon, B.D. and Trousdale, R.T. (2004). Femoral Osteotomies for Avascular Necrosis of the Femoral Head. *Clinics in Orthopedic*, **418**, 34–40.

Steppacher, S.D., Tannast, M., Ganz, R., and Siebenrock, K.A. (2008). Mean 20-year followup of Bernese periacetabular osteotomy. *Clinical Orthopaedics and Related Research*, **466**(7), 1633-44.

Witt, J.D. and McCullough, C.J. (1994). Anterior soft-tissue release of the hip in juvenile chronic arthritis. *Journal of Bone and Joint Surgery (Br)*, **76**(2), 267–70.

7.10

Total hip replacement: modes of failure

Rob Pollock

Summary points

- Total hip replacements (THRs) may fail in various ways. They may become infected, they may be subject to aseptic loosening, they may dislocate, or a periprosthetic fracture may occur. The patient with a failed THR must be thoroughly assessed before treatment is contemplated
- Infection may be acute or chronic. Assessment involves clinical assessment, plain radiographs, blood tests (C-reactive protein and erythrocyte sedimentation rate), hip aspiration, and, sometimes, nuclear medicine. The acutely infected hip may be treated with one-stage revision. This involves thorough lavage, debridement, and exchange of all modular components as well as long-term antibiotic therapy. The gold standard of treatment for a chronically infected THR is a two-stage revision. Success rates of 80–90% can be expected
- Aseptic loosening typically occurs at the cement bone interface in hips where a metal-on-polyethylene bearing couple has been used. Bone resorption takes place as a result of an inflammatory response to small wear particles. After infection has been excluded the treatment of choice is a single-stage revision
- Dislocation may be the result of patient factors, implant factors, or poor surgical technique. It is imperative for the clinician to minimize the risk by selecting patients carefully, using the correct combination of implants and performing surgery accurately
- The management of periprosthetic fractures depends on how well the implants are fixed and quality of bone stock. Treatment ranges from simple fixation of the fracture through to revision augmented with strut allograft.

Introduction

THR is a successful treatment for osteoarthritis of the hip in the vast majority of patients. It reliably abolishes pain and restores function. Complications can and do arise, however, and the purpose of this chapter is to discuss the modes of failure of THR. Infection, loosening, implant failure, and periprosthetic fractures will be discussed.

Infection

Deep infection is a devastating complication of THR often requiring revision surgery. The incidence of deep infection after THR is 1–2%. Risk factors include diabetes, obesity, sickle cell disease, rheumatoid disease, HIV infection, cancer, and immunosuppressant therapy.

Aetiology and pathogenesis

The most common organisms include *Staphylococcus aureus*, *Staphylococcus epidermidis* and coliforms. These pathogens are usually commensal organisms living on the host but can be transmitted by medical staff. Methicillin resistant *Staphylococcus aureus* infections (MRSA) are rare and are usually seen in patients with associated comorbidity who have had prolonged antibiotic therapy and long hospital admissions. In patients with sickle cell disease, other organisms such as *Salmonella* are seen. In HIV, the infections can be atypical and include fungi as well as bacteria.

Some bacteria produce a glycocalyx that acts as a biofilm. This biofilm helps the bacteria to adhere to the implant, inhibits the action of macrophages, and protects the bacteria from antibiotics. Glycocalyx-producing bacteria are harder to eradicate than conventional bacteria and almost always require two-stage revision surgery.

Classification

Broadly speaking infection can be classified as acute, chronic, or delayed acute (see Table 7.10.1). Acute infections present within the first postoperative month. Chronic infections probably occur at the time of surgery but present some months or years later. There may be little to find clinically. Delayed acute infections are those that arise via haematogenous spread some months or years after implantation of the THR and are best treated as acute infections.

Prevention

Measures that can be taken to avoid infection are subdivided into patient factors and hospital factors. Patients should be optimized prior to surgery. Diabetes should be well controlled, sites of potential infection should be screened, e.g. urine, and any pending dental treatment or 'dirty' surgery, e.g. prostatectomy, should be

Table 7.10.1 Management of the infected THR based on the type of infection encountered

	Presentation	Cause	Treatment
Acute	< 28 days postoperative	Infection at time of surgery	Urgent debridement, lavage and exchange of modular components
Delayed	> 28 days postoperative	Infection at time of surgery	Two-stage revision
Delayed acute	Acute infection in a previously uninfected THR	Bacteraemia some months or years after THR	Urgent debridement, lavage and exchange of modular components

completed prior to THR. Hospital factors include using prophylactic antibiotics, laminar flow theatres, exhaust suits, minimizing the number of staff in theatre, careful soft tissue handling, antibiotic impregnated cement, wound lavage, and expert postoperative wound care.

Clinical features

Acute infections are normally associated with pyrexia, wound erythema, and purulent discharge. The presentation of chronic infections is more varied. Patients will often give a history of pain, particularly if the implants are loose. Clinically the picture ranges from a well healed, cool scar to a hot, erythematous thigh with draining sinuses.

Investigation

Standard investigations include plain radiographs, inflammatory markers (C-reactive protein (CRP) and erythrocyte sedimentation rate (ESR)) and hip aspiration. Characteristics of infection seen on plain radiographs include loosening, endosteal scalloping, and periostitis (Figure 7.10.1). Technetium-99 bone scans are hot in the majority of cases of infection but can also be positive in aseptic loosening. White cell scans using indium-111 have higher specificity for infection. Often it is difficult to distinguish aseptic from septic loosening. If a THR is deeply infected it is important to attempt to identify the offending organisms and their sensitivities prior to any revision surgery so an antibiotic regimen can be planned in advance. It is also essential to obtain tissue samples send at the time of revision surgery to confirm the suspected diagnosis of infection. These must be obtained prior to the administration of antibiotics perioperatively.

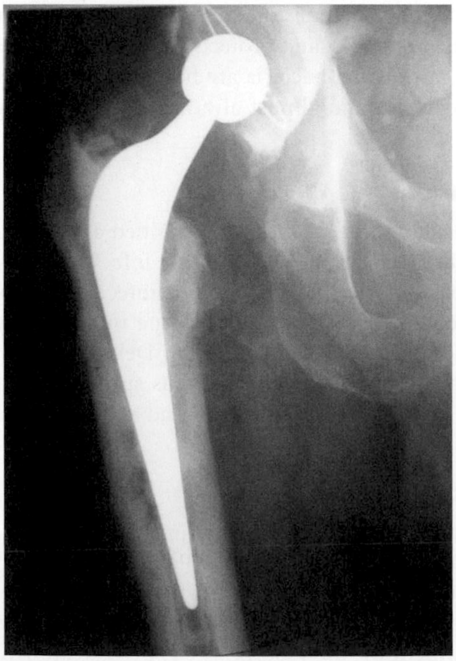

Fig. 7.10.1 Chronically infected THR with loosening of both components.

Treatment

The treatment strategy depends on the severity of symptoms, suitability of the patient for revision surgery and functional expectations of the patient. The goal in some patients is simply suppression of the infection and in others it is complete eradication of infection.

Patients who are not suitable for revision surgery, who have a solidly fixed prosthesis, and have a sensitive organism may simply be treated with long-term oral antibiotics.

Acutely infected THRs (including the acute delayed infections) can be salvaged with wound excision, aggressive debridement, extensive lavage, exchange of modular components, e.g. the head, acetabular liner, screws, hole eliminators, non-absorbable sutures, etc., and primary wound closure over a suction drain. Appropriate intravenous antibiotics should be started as soon as samples have been obtained for microbiology and continued until the inflammatory markers have returned to normal. The duration of treatment is usually 6–8 weeks. The reported success rate in eradicating infection using this treatment protocol is 80–90%.

Chronically infected THRs can be treated with either one- or two-stage revision. The gold standard in most hip revision centres is a two-stage revision. All of the implants and cement must be removed and a thorough 'membranectomy' performed. The femoral canal and acetabulum must be reamed until healthy bleeding bone is encountered and the whole surgical field subjected to extensive lavage. A temporary spacer is inserted and this is usually made from antibiotic impregnated cement. If the antibiotic sensitivities are known preoperatively, appropriate antibiotics can be incorporated into the spacer prior to insertion. The wound is closed over a suction drain and the patient mobilized. The same principles apply to the antibiotic regimen as for the acute infections discussed earlier. The reported success rate of two-stage revision in terms of eradicating infection is 90% in most series.

Aseptic loosening

Aseptic loosening is by far the commonest cause of failure of THR and the commonest indication for revision THR. Approximately 3000 revision THRs are carried out each year in the United Kingdom for aseptic loosening. This accounts for 55% of the revision burden for hips.

Aetiology and pathogenesis

When a cobalt chrome femoral head articulates with a polyethylene cup wear particles with a diameter of 0.3–10 microns are produced. These particles activate macrophages that, in turn, release cytokines (interleukin (IL)-1α, IL-1β, IL-6), prostaglandins (PGE-2) and tumour necrosis factor (TNFα). These factors not only cause osteolysis but also activate osteoclasts that resorb bone. The result is loosening at the cement–bone interface. Typically a polyethylene acetabular component wears at the rate of 0.1mm per year. Larger head sizes generate greater volumes of wear particles and thin polyethylene components are also more susceptible to wear. It is recommended that the minimum thickness of polyethylene should be 8mm in order to minimize generation of wear particles. Recently, highly cross-linked polyethylene and polyethylene containing vitamin E have been introduced with potential improvements in wear characteristics.

Cementless components can also be subject to aseptic loosening. They normally have a porous coating or are plasma sprayed with hydroxyapatite (HA). The intention is for the component to osseointegrate within the first few months of implantation. In order for osseointegration to occur, the implant must be stable at the time of implantation. Stability is achieved by 'press-fit' of the component. Surgical technique must be accurate and it is essential that the correct sized implants are used and inserted in the correct orientation. If primary stability does not occur, the component will move and fibrous ingrowth, rather than osseointegration, will occur, resulting in early loosening of the component. This phenomenon is more common with femoral components than acetabular components and the incidence is around 2% based on the early failure rates quoted in the National Joint Registry.

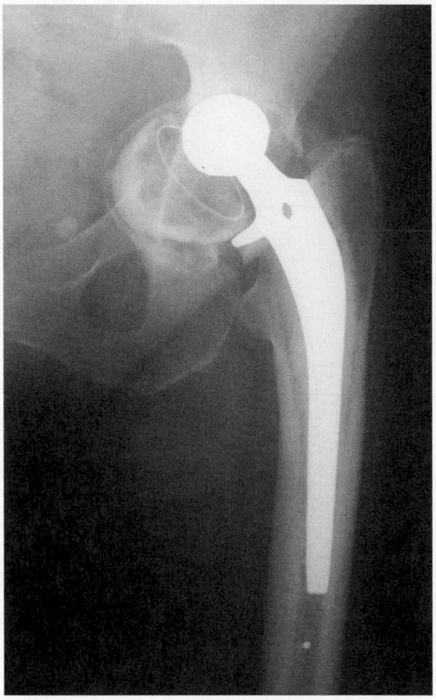

Fig. 7.10.2 Aseptic loosening of a THR. Using Harris criteria the cup is 'definitely' loose and the stem 'possibly' loose.

Clinical features

Loosening may be asymptomatic. Symptomatic patients usually complain of thigh pain. Classically this is 'start up' pain experienced first thing in the morning or when getting out of a chair after a period of rest.

Investigation

Diagnosis is made from the history and plain radiographs in the majority of patients (Figure 7.10.2). It is important to distinguish aseptic from septic loosening, as important management decisions need to be made. In aseptic loosening the CRP and ESR should be normal.

X-ray classification

Harris classified loosening into three groups; definitely loose, probably loose, and possibly loose, depending on the radiographic appearances (see Table 7.10.2). Furthermore, the zones of loosening around cemented femoral and acetabular components have been described by Gruen and DeLee (Figure 7.10.3).

Table 7.10.2 Harris classification of loosening after THR

Definitely loose	Migration of the prosthesis
	Cracks in the cement mantle
	Component breakage
Probably loose	Radiolucent lines around the whole prosthesis and cement mantle
Possible loose	Radiolucency affecting <50% of the prosthesis

Treatment

The treatment of choice for a non-infected, loose THR is a single-stage revision. The surgical procedure ranges from exchange of head and liner through to revision of both components. This is discussed in more detail in Chapter 7.11.

Dislocation (Figure 7.10.4)

The reported dislocation rate following THR is 1–3%. The causes of dislocation may be categorized as patient related, surgeon related and implant related. (See Table 7.10.3). The greatest risk of dislocation is within the first 3 months after surgery. Dislocations that occur after the first 6 weeks are more likely to become recurrent.

Aetiology and pathogenesis

Patient factors

It is reported that patients with hip dysplasia, rheumatoid arthritis, previous sepsis, those who have had previous hip surgery, and those who have previously suffered a fracture have higher dislocation rates after THR. Patients who lack full motor control of their hips are also at risk, e.g. alcoholics and those who have suffered a cerebrovascular accident. Poor compliance with postoperative rehabilitation and precautions may also result in dislocation.

Surgical factors

There are several factors that need to be considered including surgical approach, leg length, femoral offset, soft tissue tension, cup orientation, stem version, impingement, and soft tissue repair. Planning the THR in advance is mandatory. It is imperative that the choice of surgical approach and implants enables the restoration of normal anatomy and function. Traditionally the posterior approach had a higher dislocation rate than anterior or anterolateral approaches. With improvements in surgical technique and, in particular, repair of the posterior capsule the dislocation rates are now similar for all approaches.

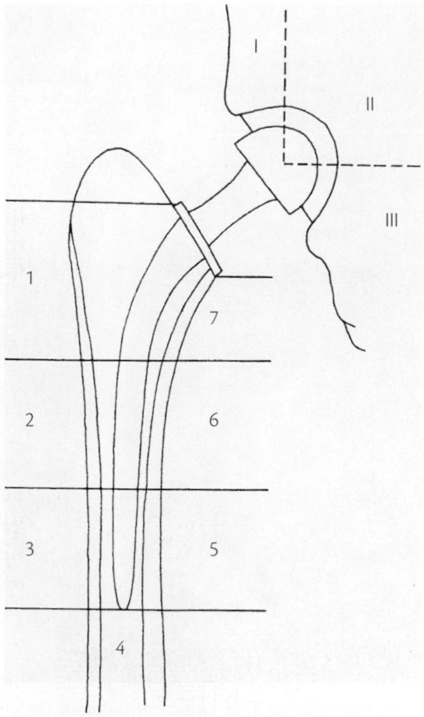

Fig. 7.10.3 Diagram showing the potential areas of lucency around the femoral and acetabular components of a THR according to Gruen (femur) and DeLee and Charnley (cup).

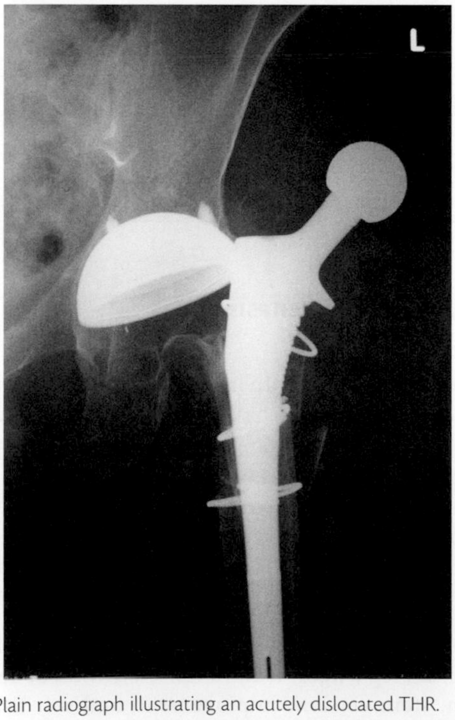

Fig. 7.10.4 Plain radiograph illustrating an acutely dislocated THR.

Lewinneck described a 'safe zone' for the position of the acetabular component. Cups inserted at an inclination of 45 ± 10 degrees and with 15 ± 10 degrees anteversion have greater stability than cups inserted in positions outside this range. Dislocation is more common when cups are inserted more vertically and with

Table 7.10.3 Potential causes of dislocation after THR

Patient factors	Implant factors	Surgeon factors
Developmental dysplasia	Head size	Posterior approach
Fracture	Head:neck ratio	Incorrect cup orientation (version + inclination)
Rheumatoid arthritis	Femoral offset	Incorrect version of femoral component
Alcohol abuse		Soft tissue tension
Epilepsy		Trochanteric avulsion
Age		Injury to hip abductors
Poor compliance		

incorrect version. When a trial reduction is performed with the definitive acetabular component correctly positioned, the femoral head should be congruently situated within the cup when the patient's leg is in a neutral position.

It is important to put the hip through a range of motion, particularly internal rotation in flexion and external rotation in extension, to identify potential impingement. Frequently, rim osteophytes need to be trimmed and hypertrophic capsule excised in order to prevent impingement. Finally, the soft tissue tension needs to be considered. If an anterolateral approach is used it is essential that the tendons of gluteus medius and minimus are repaired accurately.

Implant factors

For a hip to stay 'in joint' the implants need have a satisfactory head:neck ratio. The smaller the ratio the greater the risk of dislocation and the greater the ratio the less the risk (Figure 7.10.5). There has been a trend in recent years to use larger head sizes in order to prevent this complication. There is a trade off, however, between head size and production of wear particles. With

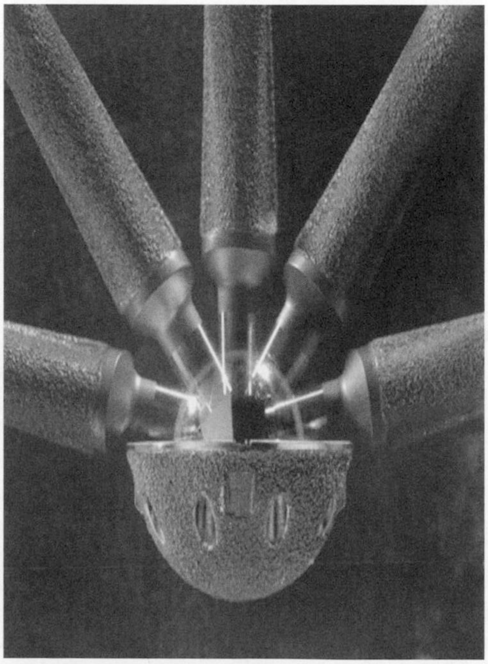

Fig. 7.10.5 Illustration showing that a THR with a large head: neck ration has a greater arc of motion before the point of dislocation.

metal-on-polyethylene combinations, larger head sizes, e.g. 32mm or 36mm produce a greater volume of particles, especially with acetabular components less than 8mm thick, and this may lead to early loosening. The wear properties of smaller heads, e.g. 22.225mm as used on the original Charley stem, are better but the dislocation rate is higher. To counteract this problem hard-on-hard bearings (metal-on-metal or ceramic-on-ceramic) are becoming more popular. These allow large head sizes (36mm and above) with a favourable head:neck ratio while avoiding the risk of aseptic loosening.

Prevention

Key points in preventing dislocation include careful patient selection, thorough preoperative planning, use of appropriate implants, accurate implant positioning, protection of the soft tissues, meticulous wound closure, and well-supervised postoperative rehabilitation.

Clinical features and investigation

The usual clinical picture is of a patient who performed a movement at the extreme of range of motion, who felt a 'clunk' and then experienced severe pain. The dislocated limb is always short. Posterior dislocations are normally associated with flexion and internal rotation whilst anterior dislocations are usually extended and externally rotated. Plain radiographs confirm the dislocation.

Treatment

The treatment of choice for a first dislocation is a closed reduction. Ideally the procedure should be carried out in the operating theatre under general anaesthetic. The hip should be screened with the image intensifier to check the orientation of the implants and for impingement.

For recurrent instability, the cause of dislocation needs to be identified. This can be with plain radiographs, screening under image intensification or with computed tomography (CT). The causes of dislocation should be corrected and this almost always requires revision surgery. Sometimes the modular components can simply be exchanged and soft tissue balance improved. Occasionally, extra measures such as constrained cups are required.

Periprosthetic fracture (Figure 7.10.6)

The incidence of periprosthetic fracture after THR is rising. Nowadays, in the United Kingdom, the average age of patients undergoing THR is 73 years. Approximately 8% of patients undergoing THR are over 85 years old and about 500 hip revisions are carried out each year for periprosthetic fractures.

Aetiology and pathogenesis

These fractures can occur intraoperatively or postoperatively. During surgery fractures are more common when using cementless components. The acetabulum is at risk when it has been deliberately under reamed and the shell is impacted with force in order to achieve 'press-fit'. The femur is at risk when inserting a 'press-fit', tapered implant. The type of fracture ranges from a simple, undisplaced crack in the calcar region to a grossly comminuted, displaced fracture. The femur is much more commonly fractured

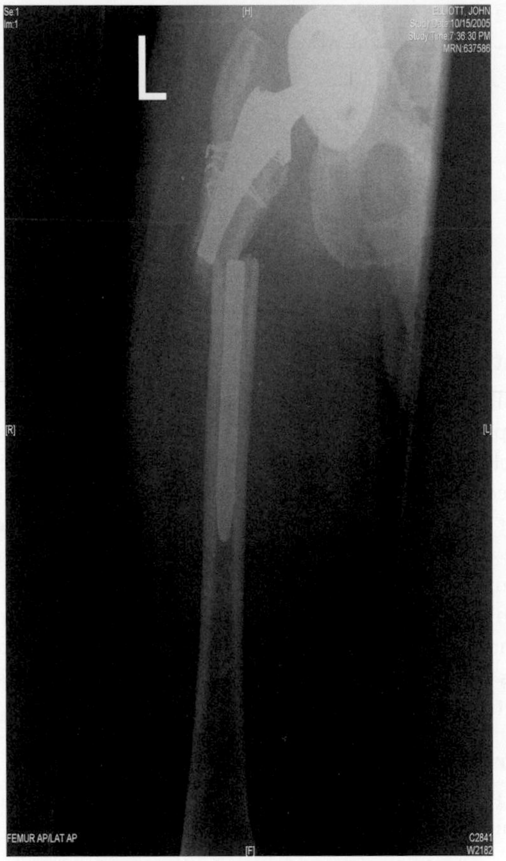

Fig. 7.10.6 Plain radiograph illustrating a fractured femoral component with associated periprosthetic fracture.

than the acetabulum and the calcar region should always be inspected after insertion of the femoral component.

Postoperatively, the fracture may follow significant trauma or may be a result of relatively minor trauma combined with a loose implant and/or osteoporosis.

Clinical features and investigation

The clinical features are those of an acute fracture of the proximal femur, namely, pain associated with shortening and external rotation of the leg. A thorough neurovascular assessment should be made with particular attention to the foot pulses and peripheral nerves. Plain radiographs should be obtained including an anteroposterior (AP) view of the pelvis and AP and lateral views of the whole femur.

Classification

Classification systems are described for intraoperative fractures but they are of limited use and do not guide patient management. The same can be said for postoperative acetabular fractures. In principle, acetabular fractures are classified as type 1 if the component is well fixed or type 2 if the component is unstable. As far as postoperative fractures of the femur are concerned, the Vancouver classification is the most widely used. This classification takes into consideration the location of the fracture, the stability of the implant and the quality of proximal femoral bone stock (see Table 7.10.4). Importantly, this classification system guides the management of the fracture.

Table 7.10.4 Vancouver classification of periprosthetic fracture

A	Fracture around the trochanteric region
B	Fracture around the stem
C	Fracture distal to the tip of the stem
1	Femoral component well fixed
2	Femoral component loose but bone stock good
3	Femoral component loose and bone stock poor

Prevention and treatment

Ideally all intraoperative fractures are identified during surgery and fixed appropriately. Stable acetabular fractures may be treated conservatively with a period of protected weight bearing. Unstable fractures need to be reduced and internally fixed. It may be necessary to augment the acetabulum with a cage or support rings to accommodate the cup. Intraoperative femoral fractures are best treated be temporary removal of the implant, reduction of the fracture, fixation with cerclage wires and then reinsertion of the implant.

The management of periprosthetic fractures in the postoperative period is guided by the Vancouver classification and is described in more detail in Chapter 7.12.

Further reading

Brady, O.H., Garbuz, D., Masri, B., and Duncan, C. (1999). Classification of the hip. *Orthopedic Clinics of North America*, **30**(2), 215–20.

DeLee, J. and Charnley, J. (1976). Radiologic demarcation of cemented sockets in total hip replacement. *Clinical Orthopaedics and Related Research*, **121**, 20–32.

Gristina, A.G., et al, The Glycocalyx, biofilm, microbes and resistant infection. Seminars in Arthroplasty. 1994 Oct; **5**(4): 160–70.

Gruen, T., McNeice, G., Amstutz, H. (1979). Modes of failure of cemented stem-type femoral components. *Clinical Orthopaedics and Related Research*, **141**, 17–27.

Johnston, R., Fitzgerald, R., and Harris, W. (1990). Clinical and radiographic evaluation of total hip replacement. *Journal of Bone and Joint Surgery*, **72A**, 161–8.

Kwon, M.S., Kuskowski, M., Mulhall, K.J., Macaulay, W., Brown, T.E., and Saleh, K.J. (2006). Does surgical approach affect total hip arthroplasty. dislocation rates? *Clinical Orthopaedics and Related Research*, **447**, 34–8.

Lewinneck, G.E., Lewis, J.L., Tarr, R., Compere, C.L., and Zimmerman, J.R. (1978). Dislocation after total hip-replacement arthroplasties. *Journal of Bone and Joint Surgery*, **60A**(2), 217–20.

Moyad, T., Thornhill, T., and Estok, D. (2008). Evaluation and management of the infected total hip and knee. *Orthopedics*, **31**(6), 581–8.

National Joint Registry for England and Wales. 6th Annual Report (2009). http://www.njrcentre.org.uk

Sanchez-Sotelo, J., Berry, D.J., Hanssen, A.D., and Cabanela, M.E. (2009). Mid-term to long-term follow up of staged reimplantation for infected hip arthroplasty. *Clinical Orthopaedics and Related Research*, **467**(1), 219–24.

7.11

Revision total hip replacement and complications in total hip replacement

J. Miles and R.W.J. Carrington

Summary points

- Revision hip replacement requires careful preoperative planning
- Accurate diagnosis is vital: particular attention must be paid to whether infection is present or not
- Extensile approaches are preferred
- Appropriate equipment is greatly helpful in explantation of the failed components
- Imaging, classification, and templating are useful in determining the best reconstruction techniques.

Introduction

Revision hip surgery is less commonly performed than primary procedures. The National Joint Register records that approaching 10% of operations are revisions or reoperations. However, this equates to 10 000 hip revisions in 2008 in England alone; the numbers are continuing to rise. In the United States, there were 43 000 revisions in 2002, accounting for 17.5% of hip replacements. Revision rates are 0.7% by 1 year and 1.3% at 3 years. Hip revision surgery accounts for disproportionately high costs to the health service: the operations are time consuming, require an extended hospital stay, and implant costs are higher. In addition, the rates of infection, dislocation, and mortality are all higher in revision surgery (Box 7.11.1).

The surgeon aims to answer a series of questions:

- *Is the pain coming from the hip?* Potential alternative diagnoses must be considered and may require further investigation to obtain an accurate diagnosis (Box 7.11.2).
- *Is the patient as well as possible?* Revision hip surgery is a major undertaking and the patient should be considered as a whole. In particular, the cardiovascular and respiratory systems should be assessed and any malfunction referred to a physician in case investigation and intervention are required. Common examples include lung function testing, cardiac angiography, and angioplasty

Box 7.11.1 Factors associated with failure

- Implant factors:
  - Press-fit non-coated stem
  - Polyethylene irradiated in air
  - Metal-backed cemented cup
  - Screw-in cup
- Patient factors:
  - Inflammatory arthritis
  - Hip fracture
  - Avascular necrosis
  - Paediatric hip disorder
- Surgical factors:
  - Low-volume surgeon
  - Poor cementing technique
  - Failure to restore offset

- *Is the hip replacement infected?* Differentiation between aseptic loosening and a septic hip is vital and discussed further later in this chapter. Decisions as to whether the procedure should be performed in two separate phases are also influenced by this information. If the hip is infected, identification of the causative organism is very useful
- *What is the degree of bone loss?* The magnitude and pattern of bone loss must be well understood for proper planning to take place. Consideration of modes of failure and sites of anatomical defect will determine whether one or other of the implants can be salvaged and determine the best reconstructive options available. The use of preoperative templating is then used to plan reconstruction of the bone loss.

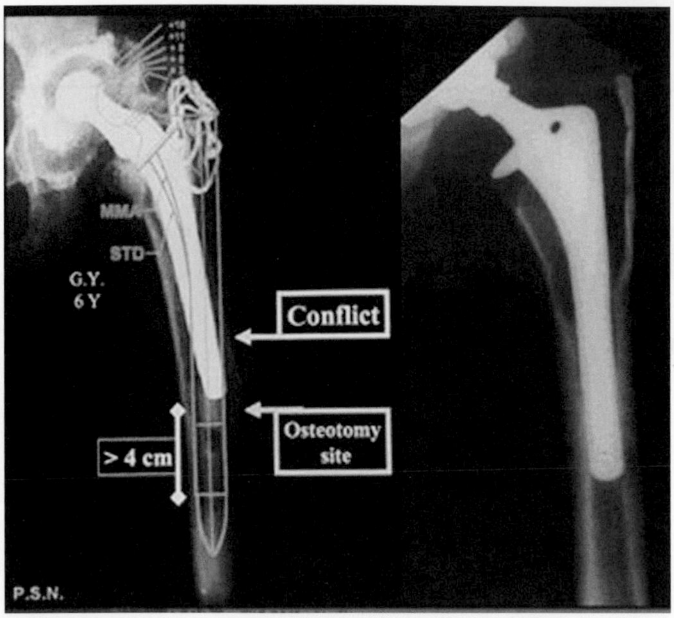

Fig. 7.11.1 Femoral templating and osteotomy planning.

Box 7.11.2 Differential diagnosis of a painful total hip replacement

- Degenerative arthritis of the lumbar spine
- Sciatica
- Spinal stenosis
- Peripheral vascular disease
- Stress fractures
- Malignancy
- Neuroma, particularly traumatic neuroma caused at time of surgery.

Box 7.11.3 Goals of surgery

- Restore centre of rotation
- Restore leg length
- Restore offset
- Restore anatomy and biomechanics
- Rigid fixation of implants.

- *Are there other problems with the hip replacement?* Common associated problems include leg-length discrepancy, recurrent dislocation, nerve injury and polyarthritis.

The key to successful revision hip surgery is preoperative planning. It can shorten the learning curve, anticipate intraoperative challenges, identify the correct approach, allow ordering of necessary equipment and identify appropriate investigations (Box 7.11.3).

Box 7.11.4 Preoperative investigations

- Blood tests:
  - Full blood count: baseline haemoglobin, white cell count rarely relevant
  - C-reactive protein: >20mg/L suggests infection
  - Erythrocyte sedimentation rate: >30mm/h suggests infection
- Microbiology and histopathology:
  - Hip aspiration or biopsy
  - Frozen section at time of revision
- Radiology:
  - Plain radiography-serial views can show migration as well as bone loss
  - Judet views—column integrity
  - CT scan
  - 3D CT reconstruction.

Investigations of a painful total hip replacement

Accurate investigation allows for proper planning of revision hip surgery (Box 7.11.4). All hips should have anteroposterior and lateral views of the pelvis and proximal two-thirds of the femur.

Judet views are used to assess the integrity of the anterior and posterior acetabular columns in particular. The iliac oblique view demonstrates the anterior wall and posterior column, whilst the obturator oblique view demonstrates the posterior wall and anterior column.

Computed tomography (CT) is useful for analysis of component orientation as well as existing bone stock. Three-dimensional (3D) reconstruction can provide further evidence of bone loss.

If there is intrapelvic cement or the acetabular component has migrated through the medial wall, angiography can be needed to demonstrate the vessels.

Approaches used in revision hip arthroplasty

Selection of the approach for revision surgery is even more critical than for primary surgery. There is no perfect solution through which all hips can be revised. Important considerations include the site of previous scars, the position and type of components to be removed, and the presence and extent of osseous defects. Adequate visualization is essential but must not be at the price of excessive damage to soft tissue or bone. Revision surgery is not always predictable and exposures should allow for flexibility when operative findings necessitate variance from the preoperative plan.

The posterior approach

The posterior approach is extensile and avoids damage to the abductor mechanism of the hip. It can be performed through extension of most previous lateral or posterior approach scars. More distal exposure of the femur can be achieved through release of the gluteus maximus and iliopsoas tendons. The exposure can continue with release of vastus lateralis, allowing exposure of the entire length of the femur if necessary. The acetabulum is also extremely well visualized. Reports vary as to whether this approach is associated with a higher rate of dislocation at revision surgery but more recent work suggests that the rate can be as low as with other approaches.

The anterolateral approach

This extensile exposure allows excellent visualization of the proximal femur and good exposure of the acetabulum. The vastus lateralis can be reflected anteriorly to allow access to the proximal femur. The risk of gluteal nerve injury is higher in revision surgery, with a corresponding increase in Trendelenburg gait pattern after the procedure.

Trochanteric osteotomy

Trochanteric osteotomy can be carried out to improve visualization of the acetabulum where complex reconstruction is anticipated. A variety of methods have evolved. A simple osteotomy can be carried out at the base of the greater trochanter, as described by Charnley. Whilst this provides excellent exposure of both sides of the hip, there can be problems with vascularity of the trochanter, reattachment, and metalwork failure. These can be compounded by proximal bone loss, weakening the greater trochanteric cortices and giving rise to trochanteric escape in 15–20% of patients in most revision series. The use of 'partial trochanteric osteotomy' can reduce these problems. The trochanteric flip begins its osteotomy posteriorly and stops to leave a 1-cm bone bridge supporting the incision of the gluteal tendons and the vastus lateralis, thus reducing the damage to the vascularity of the trochanter. Partial anterior trochanteric osteotomy removes a small sliver of anterior bone with the insertions of gluteus medius and vastus lateralis attached but leaves the insertion of gluteus minimus intact, making reattachment easier and subsequent escape less likely. A trochanteric slide also preserves the attachment of gluteus medius and vastus lateralis on one segment of bone, increasing vascularity, improving the biomechanics (the proximal pull of the fragment by gluteus medius is countered by the distal pull of vastus lateralis) of the reattachment, and reducing non-union rates to 4%.

The extended trochanteric osteotomy is useful in removal of femoral components with solid distal fixation, typically fully porous-coated cementless stems, and stems in significant varus. It has a high rate of union, typically less than 2% have non-union or malunion. The osteotomy begins with a 5–10 cm osteotomy posterior and medial to the greater trochanter, running down the linea aspera. A transverse arm passes anteriorly then the anterior osteotomy is completed anterior and medial to the greater trochanter. It involves elevation of vastus lateralis off the linea aspera and can be a cause of muscle necrosis if a previous anterolateral or lateral approach has been used, in which case the vastus lateralis fibres should be left inserting into the osteotomized fragment. Following extended trochanteric osteotomy, a longer femoral revision prosthesis will be required in order to achieve stable fixation.

The transfemoral approach allows excellent visualization of the femoral canal through exposure of the implant and any cement mantle across its entire length. This is achieved at the price of weakening the available bone stock, so it is used in combination with a very long prosthesis achieving distal fixation (such as the Wagner stem).

Component removal (Boxes 7.11.5 and 7.11.6)

The explantation phase requires planning and can be made significantly easier by the use of appropriate specialist instruments *but only if the surgeon has thought to have them available.*

Acetabular reconstruction

Hemispherical uncemented cups will work well in the majority of cases. They require a minimum of 50% host bone contact in order to osseointegrate (NB host bone is intact pelvis—allograft is not included). Care must be taken to remove any pseudocapsule or membrane which may reduce the percentage of implant to host bone contact. If host bone contact is anticipated to be below 50%, further techniques will be required.

Box 7.11.5 Removal of acetabular components

Cemented acetabular components

- Curved chisels to disrupt cement mantle
- Divide cup into quadrants
- Drill a pilot hole and screw slap hammer into polyethylene.

Uncemented acetabular components

- Simple liner exchange
- Curved chisels to the implant-bone interface
- Explant (Zimmer)
- Cement polyethylene liner into well-fixed metal shell.

Box 7.11.6 Removal of femoral components

Cemented femoral components

- Remove overhanging bone, cement, soft tissue
- Looped extractor
- System specific removal tools
- Cement removal instruments e.g. Moreland instruments or ultrasonic tools
- Bone window over thick columns of cement.

Uncemented femoral components

- Cortical windows or extended trochanteric osteotomy
- High speed carbide disk cutters to transect stem
- Specialized trephines and flexible osteotomes
- Bone window over pedestal at tip of prosthesis.

Table 7.11.1 American Academy of Orthopaedic Surgeons (AAOS) classification of acetabular deficiencies

Type	Lesion
I	Segmental deficiencies
a)	Peripheral
b)	Central—absence of medial wall
II	Cavitary deficiencies—an expanded and thin-walled socket
III	Combined deficiencies—I and II coexist
IV	Pelvic discontinuity—separation of the ilium from the ischiopubic portion of the pelvis
V	Hip arthrodesis

Type I defect (Table 7.11.1)

Segmental defects can be present in the anterior wall, posterior wall, medial wall, or superior margin of the acetabulum. Typically, these defects can be filled with augments or allograft. Augments can include the use of oblong cups or porous metal augments with screw fixation to bone. Impaction techniques of morcellized allograft work well in medial wall defects. Superior segmental defects can be treated with structural allograft and screw fixation to the ilium. Structural graft in particular is prone to resorption and collapse; thus one potential advantage of porous metal augments is avoidance of this complication.

Type II defect (Table 7.11.1 and Figure 7.11.2)

These cavitary defects have intact margins and floor of the acetabulum. They are often amenable to jumbo uncemented cup reconstruction, with or without morcellized allograft.

Type III defect (Table 7.11.1 and Figure 7.11.3)

These defects are a combination of segmental and cavitary bone loss. Their treatment, therefore, can require a combination of techniques. The use of antiprotrusio cages, with or without allograft, is more frequent. These gain superior fixation to the ilium via screws through a superior flange; inferior fixation is via an inferior hook in the obturator foramen.

Type IV defect (Table 7.11.1 and Figure 7.11.4)

In these cases, there is pelvic discontinuity and mechanical stability must be restored. Before the acetabulum is reconstructed, posterior reconstruction plating is performed to stop movement between the ilium and the ischium. Anterior plating is not necessary. Acetabular reconstruction cages are the mainstay of treatment; CAD/CAM components can be useful.

Femoral reconstruction (Box 7.11.7)

Cemented revision has advantages of immediate fixation, local delivery of antibiotics, and ability to flow into geometrically abnormal proximal femurs. It can, however, be difficult in severe bone loss and can be hard to re-revise. In addition, some series show high rates of early loosening because the internal femur is highly sclerotic, significantly reducing the microinterlock between cement and bone. If cement is used, meticulous cementing technique is vital. The use of impaction grafting is also successful in the femur, particularly in contained, proximal lesions.

Classification of femoral bone loss must be done after component removal to give an accurate evaluation of bone loss, as defects can be significantly larger after the explantation of the original stem.

If there is a cortical breach, the revision stem must bypass it by at least 5cm to reduce the chance of fracture.

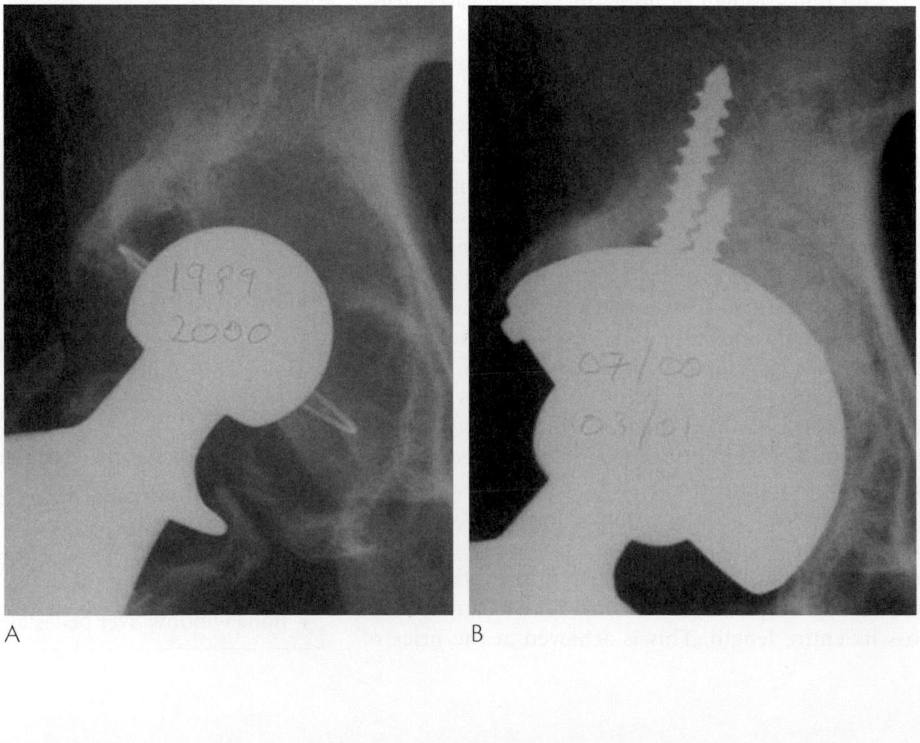

Fig. 7.11.2 Cavitary defect reconstructed with uncemented socket and morcellized allograft.

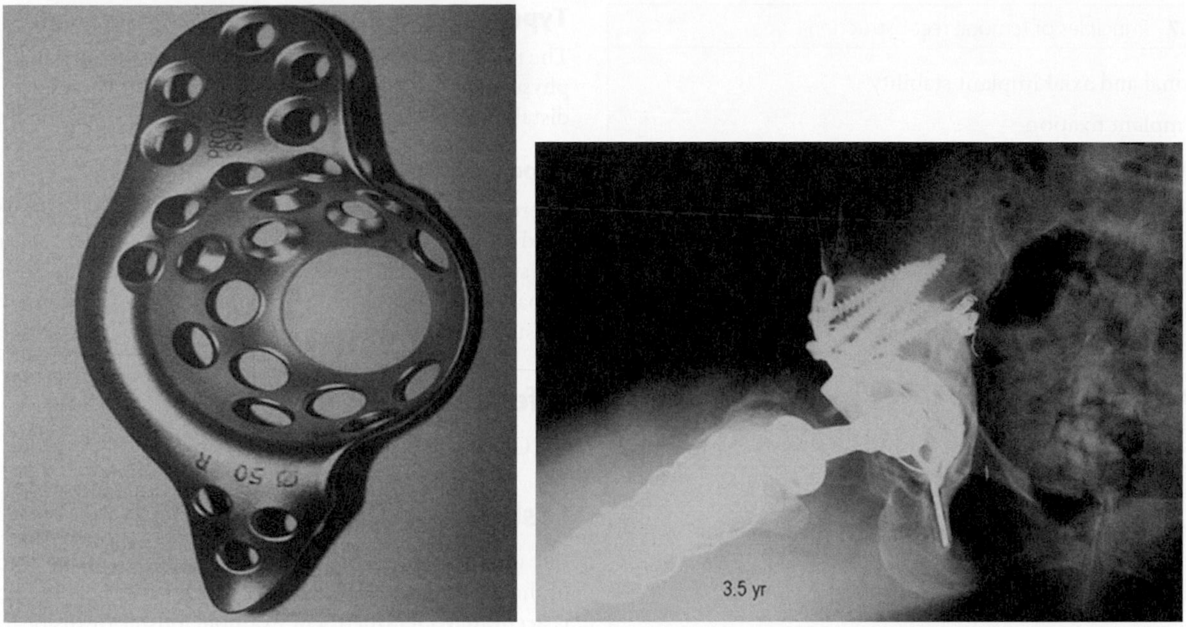

A B

Fig. 7.11.3 Antiprotrusio cage used to reconstruct combined defect.

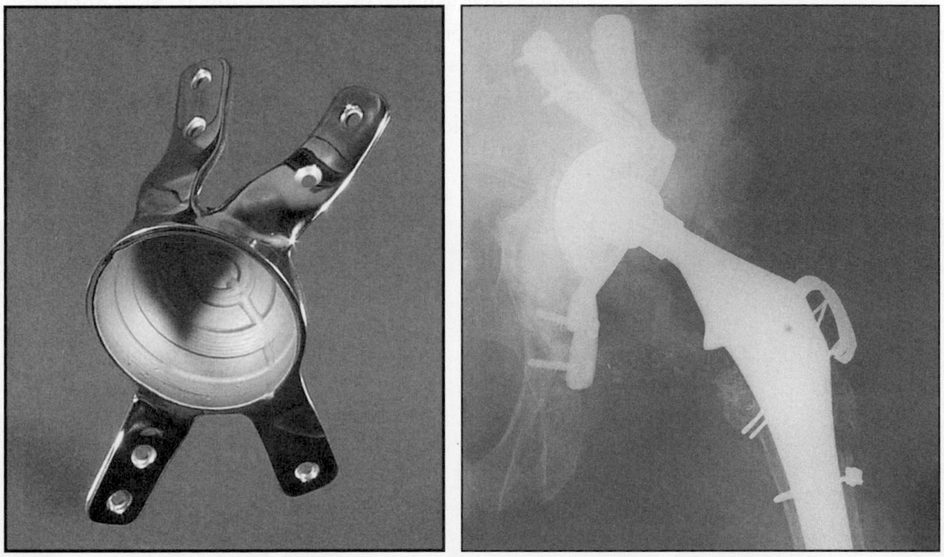

A B

Fig. 7.11.4 CAD CAM acetabular component.

If there is a completely intact cement mantle within healthy bone, a shorter stem can be cemented into the original cement mantle: a so-called cement-in-cement revision.

Type 1 defect

There is cancellous bone present, with minimal metaphyseal loss and an intact diaphysis. Proximal fixation is achieved with a porous coated, uncemented stem or use of a cemented prosthesis.

Type 2 defect

There is metaphyseal loss but the diaphysis is intact; this is a common finding at revision of cemented stems. An uncemented, proximally loaded, metaphyseal fitting stem can be used in less severe cases. If there is very poor proximal bone stock, an uncemented stem will require distal fixation and a fully porous coated stem is appropriate, with or without impaction bone grafting.

Box 7.11.7 Principles of femoral reconstruction

- Rotational and axial implant stability
- Rigid implant fixation
- Stability with range of movement
- Restore femoral integrity and continuity
- Prevent and/or augment bone loss
- Restore biomechanics.

Table 7.11.2 Paprosky classification of femoral abnormalities

Type	Lesion
1	Metaphysis and diaphysis intact
2	Metaphysis deficient, diaphysis intact, calcar non-supportive
3a	Metaphysis and diaphysis non-supportive; 4cm distal fixation near isthmus.
3b	Metaphysis non-supportive, diaphysis not intact due to severe bone loss; fixation available distal to isthmus
4	Extensive metadiaphyseal damage; cortical fixation at isthmus not reliable

Type 3a defect

The metaphysis is severely damaged and not supportive but there is at least 4cm of intact diaphyseal bone available for distal fixation. A fully porous coated stem can be used to achieve distal fixation, again with or without bone grafting.

Type 3b defect

The metaphysis is damaged and there is less than 4cm of intact diaphyseal bone distally. In this case a modular cementless stem with distal flutes is required in order to gain rotational stability.

Type 4 defect

There is extensive metaphyseal and diaphyseal bone loss, a widened femur and the isthmus is non supportive. A conical, cementless stem will not achieve stable fixation. Options include extensive impaction grafting (if the proximal cortices are intact), use of a prosthesis allograft composite, or proximal femoral replacement.

Infection

See Chapter 7.12.13.

Dislocation (Box 7.11.8)

The options for revision will depend upon the cause and direction of the dislocation. Success is more likely if the cause of dislocation is accurately identified. For example, posterior dislocation can be prevented by replacing the socket in a more anteverted position or removal of excessive anterior acetabular bone upon which the femoral neck may impinge. It is not always necessary to remove all components. In modular implants, a longer femoral head or lateralized acetabular liner may be an appropriate method of increasing offset. A larger diameter femoral head and bearing or use of a lipped liner will also increase stability. If this is not possible, the use of trochanteric advancement increases tension in the hip abductors. In cases with a significant soft tissue component to the dislocation (typically multidirectional instability with severe shortening or neurological disorder), the use of a constrained acetabular liner

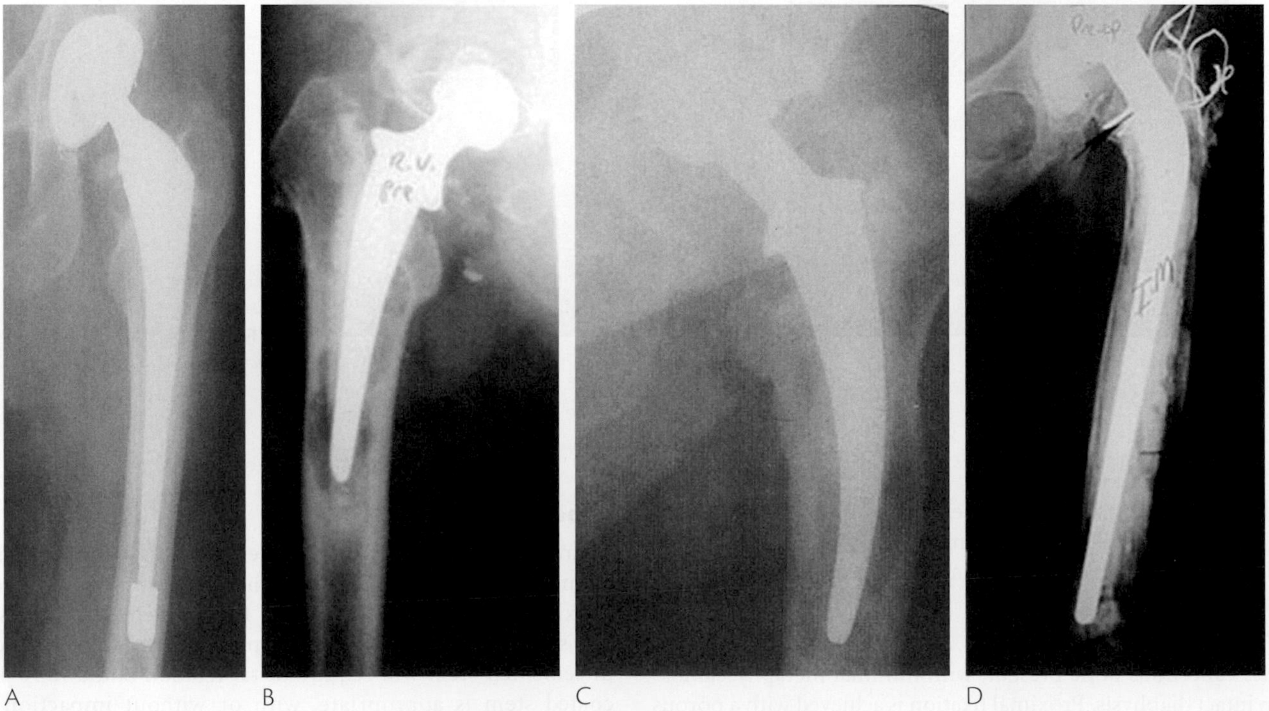

Fig. 7.11.5 Femoral defects by Paprosky classification: A)type 1; B) type2 C) type 3a D) type 4.

Box 7.11.8 Causes of dislocation

- Mechanical impingement of prosthesis components
- Impingement of prosthesis on bone/soft tissue
- Component malposition
- Trochanteric non-union
- Muscle weakness.

Box 7.11.9 Causes of neurological injury

- Retractor injury
- Lengthening
- Dislocation
- Direct trauma/haemorrhage
- Thermal injury from cement
- Acetabular screws.

can be necessary. This carries the disadvantage of reduced range of motion and higher rates of loosening. Revision to a bipolar femoral prosthesis alone can be used as a last resort in recurrent cases.

Periprosthetic fracture

See Chapter 7.12.12.

Nerve damage (Box 7.11.9)

The rate of nerve injury is 1–4% in primary hip replacement but rises to around 7% in revision surgery. Reconstruction of a dysplastic acetabulum also carries a higher risk of nerve injury.

The most commonly injured nerve is the posterior (peroneal) division of the sciatic nerve. The posterior division has a thinner perineurium than the anterior (tibial) branch and is more tethered at the fibula head, both of which are postulated to contribute to its increased rate of injury. Sciatic nerve injury is more common if the leg is lengthened at operation; lengthening less than 4cm tends to injure the posterior branch and lengthening over 4cm gives rise to complete sciatic palsy. Sciatic nerve injury is also caused by perineural haematoma, careless retractor positioning, and posterior capsular release, particularly in revision surgery. Dislocation can injure the sciatic nerve either perioperatively or postoperatively.

The femoral nerve is less commonly injured. It passes anterior to the hip, overlying the iliopsoas tendon, and can be injured in anterior capsular release or through careless placement of anterior retractors during acetabular preparation.

Injury to the superior gluteal nerve is rarely recognized after hip surgery; its inferior branch in particular is at risk in anterolateral and lateral approaches to the hip and its injury can lead to abductor weakness and Trendelenburg gait pattern.

Obturator nerve injury is rare and may be associated with extrapelvic extrusion of cement or antiprotrusio cages.

Vascular injury

Vascular injury is rarer than neurological compromise, occurring in well under 0.5% of hip replacement. Again, the incidence is far higher in revision surgery: if the acetabular component is significantly protruded into the pelvis, preoperative angiography is recommended.

The femoral vessels run parallel to the femoral nerve and are protected in a similar fashion, i.e. careful placement of an anterior acetabular retractor lateral to the iliopsoas muscle.

Medial wall penetration can injure the iliac vessels, though this is rare. Acetabular screw fixation also risks injury to the iliac vessels posteriorly or the obturator vessels anteriorly.

If bleeding is massive and uncontrolled, exposure and temporary clamping of the iliac vessels may be needed, followed by emergency intervention by a vascular surgeon.

Further reading

Alberton, G., High, W., and Morrey, B. (2002). Dislocation after revision total hip arthroplasty. An analysis of risk factors and treatment options. *Journal of Bone and Joint Surgery*, **84-A**, 1788–94.

Barrack, R. and Burnett, R. (2005). Preoperative planning for revision total hip arthroplasty. *Journal of Bone and Joint Surgery*, **87-A**, 2800–11.

D'Antonio, J., McCarthy, J.C., and Bargar, W.L. et al (1993). Classification of femoral abnormalities in total hip arthroplasty. *Clinics in Orthopedics*, **296**, 113–9.

D'Antonio, J., Capello, W., and Borden, L. (1989). Classification and management of acetabular abnormalities in total hip arthroplasty. *Clinical Orthopaedics and Related Research*, **243**, 126–37.

DeHart, M. and Riley, L. (1999). Nerve injuries in total hip arthroplasty. *Journal of the American Academy of Orthopaedic Surgeons*, **7**, 101–11.

Della Vale, C.J. and Paprosky, W.G. (2003). Classification and an algorithmic approach to the reconstruction of femoral deficiency in revision total hip arthroplasty. *Journal of Bone and Joint Surgery*, **85-A**(Suppl 4), 1–6.

Della Vale, C.J. and Paprosky, W.G. (2003). Classification and an algorithmic approach to the reconstruction of femoral deficiency in revision total hip arthroplasty. *JBJS*, **85-A**(Suppl 4), 1–6.

Dorr, L.D., and Wan, Z. (1998). Causes of and treatment protocol for instability of total hip replacement. *Clinical Orthopaedics and Related Research*, **355**,144–51.

Schmalzried, T.P., Amstutz, H.C., and Dorey., F.J. (1991). Nerve palsy associated with total hip replacement, risk factors and prognosis. *Journal of Bone and Joint Surgery (Am)*, **73**,1074–80.

7.12

Management of total hip replacement periprosthetic fractures

F.S. Haddad and F. Rayan

Summary points

- Periprosthetic fractures: intraoperative or postoperative femoral or acetabular fractures
- Third commonest reason for reoperation after THA
- Vancouver classification Type A, B, and C
- Three most important factors that determine treatment are:
  - Site of the fracture
  - Stability of the implant
  - Quality of the surrounding bone stock.

Introduction

Periprosthetic fracture of the femur after total hip arthroplasty (THA) surgery was first described in 1954 and the experience with periprosthetic femoral fractures was limited during this period.

Nowadays, the reconstructive orthopaedic surgeon deals with periprosthetic fractures quite frequently. Periprosthetic femoral fracture is a devastating complication after THA that can result in poor clinical outcome. They are challenging to treat, as they require the skills of both a revision surgeon and a trauma specialist. In this review we summarize the epidemiology, aetiology, classification, and various modalities of management.

Epidemiology and aetiology

The Swedish Hip Registry data have shown that periprosthetic femoral fractures were the third commonest reason for reoperation (9.5%) after total hip replacement, after aseptic loosening (60.1%), and recurrent dislocation (13.1%). Periprosthetic femoral fractures can be classified as intraoperative and postoperative. The cumulative prevalence of periprosthetic femoral fractures is 1.0% in primary total hip replacements and 4% in revision total hip replacements (Mayo Clinic Joint Registry). The incidence of intraoperative fractures is 0.3% in primary cemented and up to 5.4% in uncemented THAs whereas in revision surgeries the incidence is 3.6% in cemented and 20.9% in uncemented revision THAs. There is an increasing incidence of late postoperative periprosthetic femoral fractures that is attributable to many factors, including an increasing number of elderly patients at risk for falls, increasing numbers of young patients with total hip replacements at risk for high-energy trauma events, and the increasing numbers of revision procedures using cementless press-fit fixation or bone impaction allograft techniques. Periprosthetic femoral fractures usually occur with low-energy events, either after falls or spontaneously during activities of daily living. Patients may present with insidious pain and fracture with no history of fall or trauma. It should be borne in mind that osteolytic lesions often occur in asymptomatic hips.

Continuous surveillance of THR patients, especially younger ones with higher activity levels, may help in timely intervention and reduce the incidence of osteolytic-related fractures. In primary and revision hip arthroplasty, femoral fractures can occur after dislocation of the existing prosthetic stem, cement removal, during femoral canal preparation, and during insertion of the prosthesis.

Acetabular fractures occur during component insertion or removal. Postoperative acetabular fractures are associated with uncemented acetabular component insertion because of bone loss in a failed THA. The first description of acetabular fractures around THA was in 1972. The reported incidence of intraoperative acetabular periprosthetic fracture is less than 0.2%.The prevalence of such fractures has increased since the introduction of uncemented components. The prevalence of periacetabular fracture with pelvic discontinuity at acetabular revision is 0.9%.These fractures are attributed to trauma, osteolysis, under-reaming and oversizing of the components, osteopenia, and Paget's disease.

Classification

Various classification systems have been in and out of favour in the past based on site and pattern of fracture or implant instability. Some of the commonly used classification systems are given in Table 7.12.1.The Vancouver classification system for both intraoperative and postoperative femoral fractures has gained universal

Table 7.12.1 Classification systems for periprosthetic femoral fractures

Author (year)	Type					
Whitaker (1974)	Intertrochanteric	Around stem	Below stem			
Bethea (1982)	Below tip	Around stem	Comminuted			
Johansson (1981)	Proximal to tip	Around tip	Below tip			
Cooke (1988)	Comminuted	Around stem	Oblique below tip	Below tip		
Mont (1994)	Intertrochanteric	Around stem	Around tip		Comminuted	Supracondylar

Table 7.12.2 Vancouver classification of periprosthetic femoral fractures

A	A_L: lesser trochanter
	A_G: greater trochanter
B	B1: stable stem
	B2: unstable stem
	B3: unstable stem + poor bone quality
C	Fractures below the tip off the stem

acceptance (Table 7.12.2). This is the only periprosthetic classification system that has been subjected to psychometric testing for its reliability and validity. The factors that determine treatment are fracture location, stability of the implant and fracture, quality of host bone stock, patient physiology and age, and surgeon experience. This classification consolidated the three most important factors, i.e. the site of the fracture, the stability of the implant, and the quality of the surrounding bone stock.

Periprosthetic femoral fractures are classified into:

- Type A fractures: proximal metaphyseal, not extending into the diaphysis
- Type B fractures: diaphyseal, not extending into the distal diaphysis and, therefore, not precluding diaphyseal long-stem fixation
- Type C fractures: distal fractures extending beyond the longest extent of the longest revision stem.

Intraoperative fractures are subclassified into:

- Subtype 1, representing a simple cortical perforation
- Subtype 2, representing an undisplaced linear crack
- Subtype 3, representing a displaced, or unstable fracture.

The postoperative fracture type A is subdivided into A_L (involves lesser trochanter) and A_G (greater trochanter). Type B is subdivided into B1, B2, and B3 based on implant stability and bone stock quality. B1 fractures have a solidly fixed implant. B2 fractures describe those in which there is a unstable implant and B3 fractures have a unstable implant and a compromised bone stock.

Figures 7.12.1 and 7.12.2 shows comprehensive treatment algorithms for periprosthetic femoral and acetabular fractures which were described in 2004.

Management

The conservative treatment of periprosthetic fractures has become obsolete. These methods are fraught with complications. For example, revision rates as a result of prosthesis loosening have been reported in the range of 19–100%; reports of pseudoarthrosis rates range from 25–42%, and abnormal varus positioning of the femur occurs at an average rate of 45%. Subsequent revision is fraught with difficulties due to malunion. We no longer recommend the use of non-operative methods such as traction or cast immobilization as they increase the risk of thrombosis, embolism, pneumonia, pressure ulceration, and knee joint contractures. The goals of treatment are: to achieve early

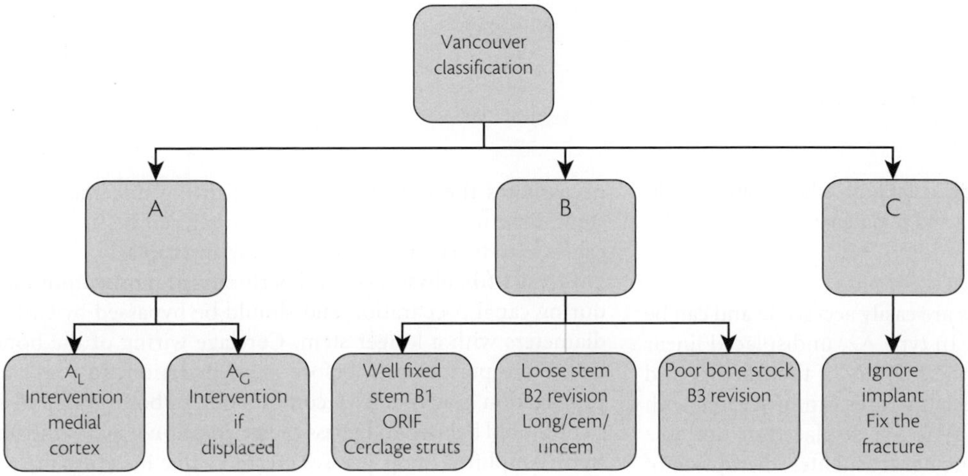

Fig. 7.12.1 Treatment algorithms for periprosthetic femoral fractures. ORIF, open reduction and internal fixation.

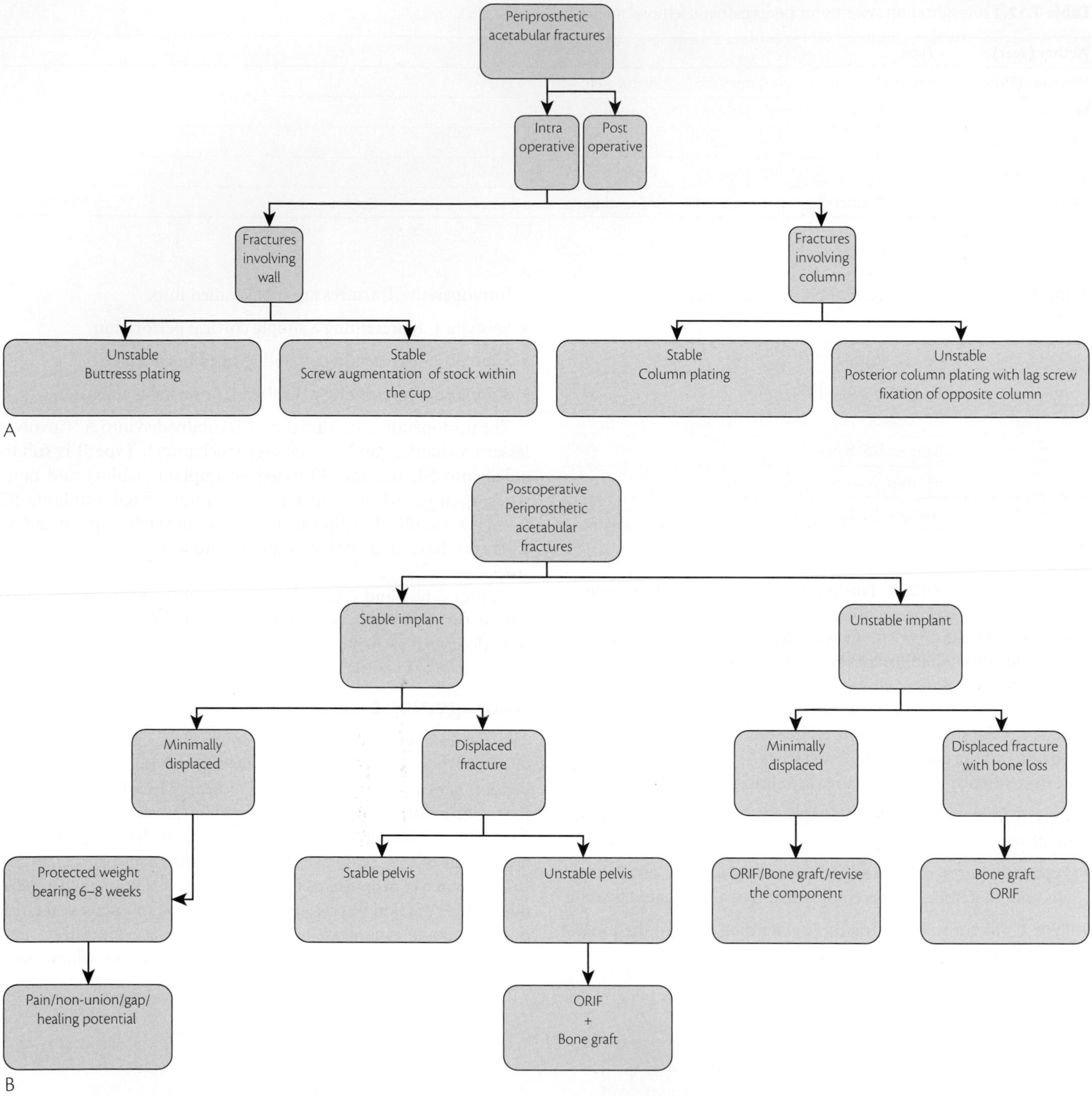

Fig. 7.12.2 Treatment algorithm for periprosthetic acetabular fractures.

union; anatomical alignment and length; a stable prosthesis; early mobilization; a return to premorbid function; and maintenance of bone stock.

Intraoperative fractures

In type A1, the cortical perforations are easily accessible and can be treated with simple bone grafting. In type A2, undisplaced linear cracks, the surgeon should assess the stability of the fracture and the stability of the implant and these fractures can be treated with cerclage wire or cable fixation. In type A3, displaced or unstable fracture of the proximal femur or greater trochanter, disruption of the integrity of the metaphyseal region of the proximal femur necessitates the use of a diaphyseal fitting uncemented femoral stem. Fracture of the greater trochanter can be fixed with wires, cables, or a trochanteric fixation claw and cables.

Type B1 (diaphyseal cortical perforation) most commonly occur during canal preparation and should be bypassed by two cortical diameters with a longer stem. Cerclage wiring of the bone at or below the perforation, before stem insertion, to prevent crack propagation is advisable. A combination of bone graft and cortical strut should be used to bypass the perforation if it is at the tip of the stem. Amplified hoop stresses created while inserting the prosthesis can cause undisplaced linear cracks (type B2). When recognized intraoperatively, they should be treated with cerclage wires or cables and the fracture should be bypassed. If unable to bypass the fracture with a longer stem, supplement with a cortical strut, or a plate and screws. Cortical onlay allograft struts increase cortical strength and are associated with good clinical results. Most of type B2 fractures are diagnosed only on the postoperative radiographs and they are treated with protected weight bearing for 6 weeks to 3 months until there are signs of healing. Type B3 (displaced fracture of the mid femur) occur during dislocation of the femur, broaching, femoral cement removal, canal preparation, and insertion of the prosthesis. The fracture should be adequately exposed, reduced, and fixed, with either cerclage wires or with one or two cortical struts. The continuity of femoral canal should be re-established and a femoral stem that bypasses the fracture by at least two cortical diameters should be inserted. For a stable implant, retain the stem augment with cables and cortical struts. Type C1 (cortical perforations) should be bone grafted and bypassed with a cortical strut. Type C2 (undisplaced linear crack extending just above the knee), if recognized intraoperatively and if fracture is potentially unstable, cerclage wires with or without an onlay cortical strut allograft should be used. Whereas in type C3 (displaced fracture of the distal femur that cannot be bypassed by a femoral stem) should be treated with open reduction and internal fixation. For intraopertive acetabular fracture, the surgeon needs to assess for component stability, augment fixation with screws, buttress plating, or graft, and if loosening present, revision is inevitable.

The main aim of treatment is provision of bony columns to support an acetabular component. If the fracture pattern is more extensive with a transverse component or if there is displacement, the surgeon should stabilize the posterior column and fix anteriorly with lag screws and graft if required.

Postoperative fractures (Box 7.12.2)

Type A_G are stable fractures treated with protected weight bearing up to 3 months and active abduction is avoided until union is achieved. Displacement greater than 2.5cm, trochanteric non-union, instability, or weakness of abduction are indications for internal fixation. When Type A_L fractures involve a large portion of the medial buttress, they may result in loss of implant stability and may warrant revision arthroplasty. These fractures are becoming more common with the increasing use of anatomical and tapered cementless stems.

The type B subgroup in the Vancouver system are probably the most crucial as they involve the bone in the vicinity of the femoral stem. They comprise more than 80% of late periprosthetic femoral fractures. There is a consensus that most fractures associated with a well-fixed stem (type B1 fractures) can be treated with open reduction and internal fixation whereas The mainstay of treatment for B2 type is revision of the femoral component using cemented or uncemented prostheses augmented with cerclage wires and strut grafts where indicated (Figures 7.12.3 and 7.12.4). Revision with a long-stem prosthesis permits stabilization of the fracture similar to that achieved when using an intramedullary nail, but the proximal femur may be a poor environment for recementing or proximal porous ongrowth if the index procedure was cemented. Uncemented prostheses help provide axial and rotational control in the diaphysis of the femur distal to the bone loss and comminution. In addition, they alleviate the potential concerns of cement inhibition or interposition on fracture healing. Fractures associated with a loose stem and extremely poor proximal bone quality (type B3 fractures), are treated with resection of the proximal femur and substitution with either a tumour prosthesis or an allograft prosthetic composite or a custom made implant (Figure 7.12.5). Every effort is made to preserve the abductor mechanism and reattach it to the implant or wrap the proximal femur around the implant.

Box 7.12.1 Goals of treatment

- Early union
- Anatomical alignment and length
- Maintenance of bone stock
- Stable prosthesis
- Bypass defects
- Adjuncts: cortical struts, circlage cables, plates
- Early mobilization.

Type C fractures are treated with open reduction and internal fixation.

The intramedullary blood supply is already compromised in periprosthetic fractures around THR. To add on to this the extra-osseous blood supply is interfered due to dissection involved with open reduction and internal fixation (ORIF) with or without wiring. Bone grafting of all periprosthetic femoral shaft fractures treated with ORIF is recommended. Percutaneous fixation of periprosthetic fractures with dynamic compression plating (DCP) is a good alternative. In locking plates the screw locks onto the plate, providing additional angular stability; the plates are designed for minimally invasive insertion, allowing extraperiosteal application, preserving the periosteal blood supply and reducing soft tissue damage. The plates allow unicortical screw placement which makes it useful when dealing with periprosthetic fractures, as screws may be placed without damaging the cement mantle. However, some fracture configurations may affect the outcome of internal fixation even when the stem is stable; for example, transverse fractures at the tip of the stem are very difficult to treat with plates alone, and in these cases revision of the stem may be preferred. The other common implant systems used are the cable plate fixation devices. The third-generation systems allow cable retightening which is particularly useful.

Cortical onlay strut grafting, first described for the treatment of femoral periprosthetic fractures, is an attractive option because it combines fixation with the potential to restore the bone stock and increase cortical strength. Excellent union rates with this technique have been reported. Through union with the host bone, the allograft also may enhance the host bone stock and strength.

Impaction grafting with long cemented femoral prostheses, bypassing the most distal fracture line, together with structural cortical grafts and/or plates, has also been attempted with encouraging results. An alternative of cement-in-cement revision to a longer stem is available for unfit patients providing the cement mantle is well preserved. This is particularly useful with tapered stems.

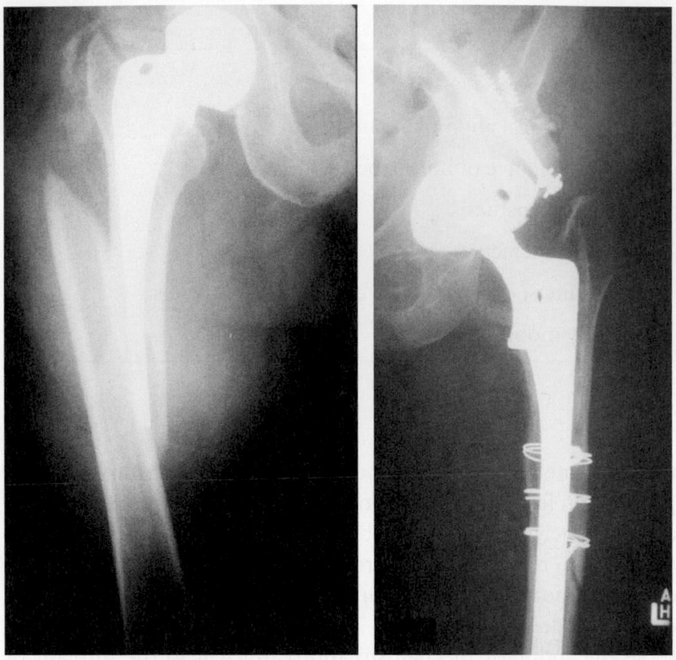

A B

Fig. 7.12.3 Type B2 fracture (A) and its revision with a long stem uncemented prosthesis augmented with cables (B).

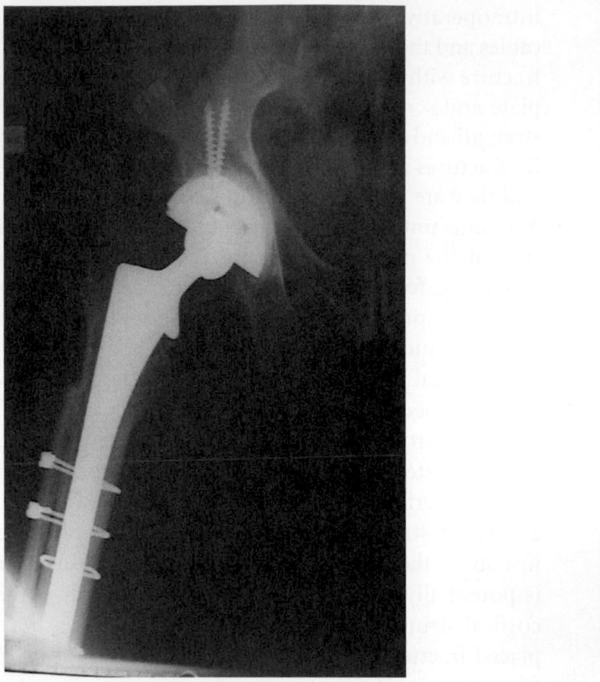

Fig. 7.12.4 Strut graft used to enhance the revision in Figure 7.12.3.

In acetabular fractures, the aim is to regain structural integrity of the columns and restoration of bone stock so that it allows stable fixation. All patients who are suspected of acetabular fractures after THAs should get standard and Judet views of the pelvis and a computed tomography scan to make an accurate diagnosis. These images are also used to define the anatomy. Patients with stable acetabular fractures are initially treated with 6–8 weeks of touch-toe weight bearing. In the presence of significant displacement revision surgery is necessary. Initial conservative treatment is justified to allow union and avoid stripping of the posterior column for late presenting fractures around cemented acetabular components with significant osteolysis and minimal displacement. If pelvic discontinuity is present at revision surgery they should be treated with tantalum sockets, cup cage constructs, or antiprotrusio cages (APC), with bone grafting and plating as necessary.

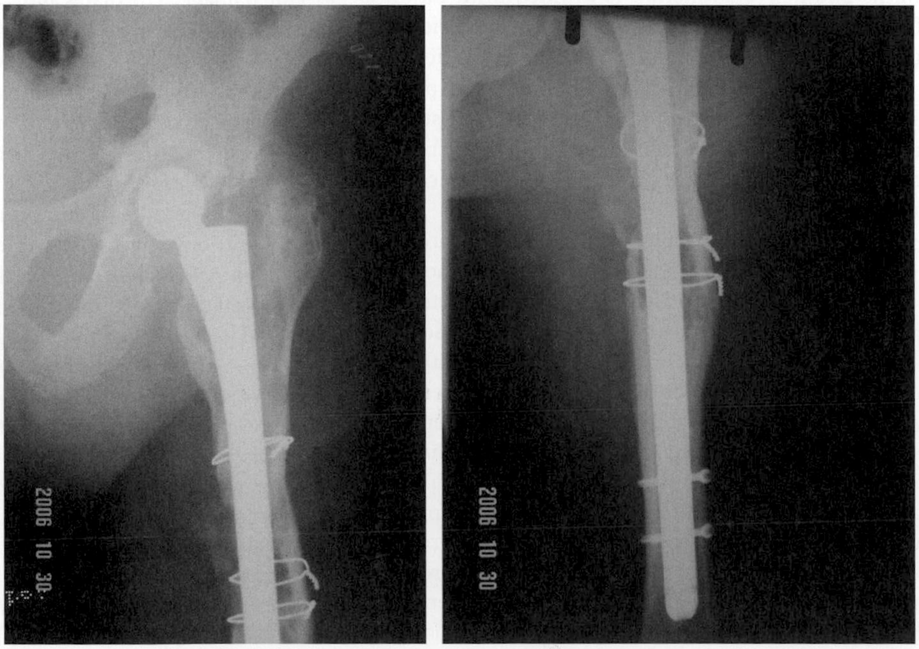

A B

Fig. 7.12.5 Vancouver type B3 fracture (A) fixed with distal locking revision stem (B).

Periprosthetic fractures around endoprostheses with epiphyseal or metaphyseal fixation

Further classification of periprosthetic fractures around endoprostheses with epiphyseal or metaphyseal fixation has been proposed into EM-B and EM-C. EM-B fractures are found with surface replacement endoprostheses, which occur at the boundary of the cup endoprosthesis and the neck of the femur, or which occur in the metaphysis in the case of metaphyseal-fixed prostheses. The implant should be exchanged for a stem endoprosthesis in cases of EM-B fractures. The EM-C1 fractures are infrequent fractures that occur at some distance away from a stable cup endoprosthesis or below stable metaphyseal anchored prostheses. Internal fixation is the ideal treatment for these cases.

The indication of osteosynthesis should depend on the location of the fracture, quality of the osteosynthesis, and on whether polyethylene wear is radiologically detectable or not. If wear is present, these fractures should be managed like EM-C2 fractures and treated primarily by complete exchange of the prosthesis. The EM-C2 fractures are fractures that occur at some distance below a loosened implant and are treated by prosthetic exchange.

Interprosthetic fractures

Interprosthetic fracture is also proposed as an extension of the classification of periprosthetic fractures. Type IA are the fractures that occur between a stemmed endoprosthesis of the hip and surface replacement prosthesis of the knee joint, and type IB are those that occur between two stem prostheses (hip and knee) The type IA fractures are subclassified according to the implant stability: fractures with stable implant as type IA1 and loose implants as type IA2. Type IA1 fractures are treated with internal fixation techniques. Type IA2 require exchange of the implant at the same time with a prosthesis that bridges the fracture by at least two diaphysis diameters. Type IB fractures usually require a total femur prosthesis, whereby a stable stem implant can be integrated into a special prosthesis in the form of a pin prosthesis.

Conclusions

Surgical decision-making in this complex group is influenced by various factors such as the patient's age, gender, femoral anatomy, bone stock quality, type and size of the prosthesis, surgical approaches, and techniques. The main strategies of management are: 1) identify the high-risk group, e.g. recurrent dislocation, loosening, subsidence and osteolysis; 2) perform revision arthroplasty before extensive bone loss results in periprosthetic femoral fracture; 3) in revision arthroplasties, it is prudent to obtain adequate surgical exposure, which may involve a trochanteric osteotomy, avoid eccentric or varus reaming, over-ream to avoid hoop stresses and fracture during the insertion of press fit stems, remove cement safely (by splitting it radially and at several levels or by ultrasound), and finally prevent propagation of fracture with the aid of prophylactic cerclage cables or wires.

Box 7.12.2 Management of postoperative periprosthetic femoral fractures

- Type A_G:
  - Protected weight bearing up to 3 months
  - Active abduction is avoided until union is achieved
- Type A_G with displacement greater than 2.5cm, trochanteric non-union, instability, or weakness of abduction
  - Internal fixation
- Type B1 fractures: ORIF
- B2 type fractures:
  - Revision of the femoral component using cemented or uncemented prostheses
  - Augmented with cerclage wires and strut grafts
- Type B3 fractures:
  - Resection of the proximal femur
  - Substitution with either a tumour prosthesis, or an allograft prosthetic composite, or a custom-made implant
- Type C fractures: open reduction and internal fixation.

Further reading

Duncan, C.P. and Masri, B.A. (1995). Fractures of the femur after hip replacement. *Instructional Course Lectures*, **44**, 293–304.

Franklin, J. and Malchau, H. (2007). Risk factors for periprosthetic femoral fracture. *Injury*, **38**(6), 655–60.

Fink, B., Fuerst, M., and Singer, J. (2005). Periprosthetic fractures of the femur associated with hip arthroplasty. *Archives of Orthopaedic and Traumatic Surgery*, **125**(7), 433–42.

Garbuz, D.S., Masri, B.A., and Duncan, C.P. (1998). Periprosthetic fractures of the femur: principles of prevention and management. *Instructional Course Lectures*, **47**, 237–42.

Haddad, F.S. and Duncan, C.P. (2003). Cortical onlay allograft struts in the treatment of periprosthetic femoral fractures. *Instructional Course Lectures*, **52**, 291–300.

Halliday, B.R., English, H.W., Timperley, A.J., Gie, G.A., and Ling, R.S. (2003). Femoral impaction grafting with cement in revision total hip replacement. Evolution of the technique and results. *Journal of Bone and Joint Surgery*, **85B**(6), 809–17.

Learmonth, I.D. (2004). The management of periprosthetic fractures around the femoral stem. *Journal of Bone and Joint Surgery*, **86B**(1), 13–19.

Lindahl, H., Garellick, G., Regner, H., Herberts, P., and Malchau, H. (2006). Three hundred and twenty-one periprosthetic femoral fractures. *Journal of Bone and Joint Surgery*, **88A**(6), 1215–22.

Lindahl, H., Malchau, H., Herberts, P., and Garellick, G. (2005). Periprosthetic femoral fractures classification and demographics of 1049 periprosthetic femoral fractures from the Swedish National Hip Arthroplasty Register. *Journal of Arthroplasty*, **20**(7), 857–65.

Masri, B.A., Meek, R.M., and Duncan, C.P. (2004). Periprosthetic fractures evaluation and treatment. *Clinical Orthopaedics and Related Research*, **420**, 80–95.

7.13

Management of the infected total hip replacement

I. Stockley

Summary points

- Diagnosis of infected hip arthroplasty requires a multidisciplinary team approach
- Aims of treatment are to eradicate infection, alleviate pain, and restore function
- Treatment should be conducted in specialist centers.

Introduction

Infection is a major complication of arthroplasty surgery with a reported incidence after primary operation of 0.2–1%. Its successful management depends on clear understanding of certain principles summarized in this chapter.

Pathogenesis

All surgical wounds are contaminated by bacteria and it is surprising that relatively so few become clinically infected. Over 95% of prosthetic infections that occur during the first year after implantation are due to perioperative contamination. Infection can also occur through the blood stream; such haematogenous infections tend to manifest later. Irrespective of the route, infection becomes established when the dose and virulence of bacteria overcome the host defences. The degree of virulence determines the speed of infection. In addition to surgical and environmental factors, patient factors play an important role, e.g. old age, chronic disease, immunosuppression, and a history of previous joint infection.

After implantation, body fluids immediately coat all surfaces of the prosthesis with a layer of serum proteins and platelets. Bacteria approach the surface of the prosthesis through an interaction of physical (van der Waals forces and hydrophobic interactions) and chemical forces (covalent and hydrogen ion bonds). There is then a race for colonization of the implant surface between the host's cells and the bacteria. If this race is won by bacteria, adhesion progresses to aggregation on the surface of the prosthesis. In doing so, bacteria change from being planktonic to sessile: they become encased in a matrix of polysaccharides and proteins to form a slimy layer known as the biofilm. This has the following properties:

- Enhancing nutrition to the bacteria
- Preventing detachment of the bacteria in adequate numbers thereby making diagnosis by aspiration difficult
- Acting as a protective barrier inhibiting phagocytosis and preventing penetration by antibiotics.

Gram-positive cocci dominate the list of pathogens identified accounting for over 50% of infections within several units. The majority are coagulase-negative *Staphylococcus* and *Staph. aureus*. Aerobic Gram-negative bacteria cause 10–20% of all deep infections and anaerobic bacteria are responsible for another 10–15%.

Classification

Infection can be superficial or deep.

- *Superficial*: superficial infections need to be treated with respect as they either represent a true superficial infection or an underlying deep infection presenting superficially.
- *Deep infection*: whilst several different classification systems have been described, that by Tsukayama and colleagues is most useful as it is a temporal classification with recommendations for treatment:
  - I: positive intraoperative cultures. Two or more specimens obtained intraoperatively have been cultured and found to be positive for the same organism
  - II: acute postoperative infection which is apparent within 1 month of implantation
  - III: chronic infection is of insidious onset occurring after the first month of implantation
  - IV: haematogenous infection occurs at any time after implantation from a distant source such as dental, urinary, or chest infection. The onset is often acute in a previously well-functioning hip.

As far as is known, haematogenous infection is relatively rare, many late infections being acquired from perioperative contamination.

Diagnosis of deep infection

Sometimes diagnosis is obvious, but not always: there is no single investigation which can conclusively confirm or refute its presence; no single test is 100% sensitive or specific and multiple tests are required.

Preoperative considerations

History

Most patients following hip arthroplasty have a very good clinical result. Any deviation from this, particularly in the first 12–18 months should raise suspicion of infection. The nature of the pain should be ascertained; is it mechanical in nature or present at rest, is it associated with fever or night sweats, in fact, has the hip ever felt right? Did the wound heal quickly or did it require antibiotics and district nurse input?

Examination

Pain and reduced range of movement may be present in acute infection otherwise the joint may be only mildly irritable. Frank pus, abscess, or sinuses may present or sometimes more subtle changes like skin discolouration and induration. In the majority of cases there will be nothing specific to find on examination.

Investigations

Blood tests

It is normal practice to measure the 'inflammatory markers' in the blood: the white cell count (WCC), the erythrocyte sedimentation rate (ESR), and the C-reactive protein (CRP). Full blood count often shows a normal WCC but patients with long-standing infection can develop anaemia of chronic disease and a raised platelet count.

The ESR takes up to 1 year from the index operation to return to normal levels but a raised level of 30mm/h or greater raises the clinical suspicion of infection. Other causes for a raised ESR must be taken into consideration.

The CRP is acutely raised after the index operation for 48–72h then falls rapidly over the next 2–3 weeks in the absence of infection. However, it may remain elevated in patients with rheumatoid arthritis for up to 8 weeks. After this time a level of 10mg/L or greater raises the clinical suspicion of infection.

Gaston has shown that serial measurements of CRP and ESR are more helpful than isolated results. A single elevated CRP and ESR was in his series, associated with a 50% chance of infection. This rose to 80% for persistently elevated test results. Normal levels—both isolated and in series—had a stronger predictive value in ruling out infection (90% and 94% respectively).

Imaging

Plain radiographs in isolation may show radiolucent lines, osteolysis, scalloping, and periosteal reaction but these can also be present in aseptic loosening. Serial radiographs are more useful for assessing changes over time as infective loosening tends to be more rapid in its progression.

With increasing use of uncemented prostheses, radiographic changes may be more difficult to interpret. Provided a prosthesis is not becoming loose overall, relatively marked signs somewhere at the bone–cement interface may be pain free.

Radioisotope scans although expensive and time consuming, may be useful. Indium-111 (^{111}In)-labelled white cell scans combined with technetium-99m (^{99}TC)-sulphur colloid marrow imaging have been found to be sensitive for loosening but not specific for infection. There is now interest in fluorodeoxyglucose positron emission tomography (PET scan) which may be more specific.

Aspiration and biopsy

Hip aspiration is regarded by many as the gold standard. In addition to diagnosing the bacteria responsible it also offers an antibiotic sensitivity profile. Bacteria spend most of their time in the sessile phase and so to optimize accuracy of the aspiration the following steps should be taken:

- Antibiotics should be stopped for a minimum of 2 weeks prior to aspiration
- Samples should be inoculated directly into enrichment media
- Prompt transfer to the laboratory should be ensured
- Prolonged culture for up to 14 days is necessary to ensure that slow-growing bacteria are identified
- Close liaison with a dedicated microbiologist is essential.

Numerous authors have found hip aspiration to be highly specific (see Table 7.13.1) and therefore making more invasive tissue biopsy unnecessary.

A simple WCC from the aspirate can be a useful adjunct. There is a reported sensitivity of 97% and specificity of 98% when there are 1.7×10^3 per microlitre white cells with a differential of 65% neutrophils.

Polymerase chain reaction

Polymerase chain reaction (PCR) allows detection of the bacteria in small numbers by amplification of microbial DNA but its usefulness is limited by a high rate of false positives.

Perioperative considerations

Frozen section

Although this investigation has been shown to be highly specific for the diagnosis of infection, it does not help with the preoperative diagnosis or yield antibiotic sensitivity profiles. It does, however, require an experienced pathologist. Whilst five polymorphs per

Table 7.13.1 Specificity and sensitivity of hip aspiration for infection

Author	Specificity (%)	Sensitivity (%)
Elson (1991)	87	84
Roberts (1992)	95	87
Lachiewicz (1996)	97	92
Spangehl (1999)	94	86
Williams (2004)	94	80
Farhan (2006)	91	82

high-power field is regarded as being consistent with a diagnosis of infection, the presence of ten polymorphs per high-power field gives an improved specificity of 99% without reducing sensitivity.

Gram stain

This simple test lacks any acceptable level of sensitivity and is not recommended for this purpose.

Intraoperative samples

Multiple intraoperative samples should be taken and sent for microbiological analysis. A fresh scalpel and forceps are used for each specimen and antibiotics withheld until the samples have been taken. It is imperative that these samples are sent directly to the laboratory. Three or more cultures growing a consistent micro-organism are thought to be diagnostic of infection.

The probability of diagnosing infection is increased with increasing number of positive results from all the investigations described here.

Management protocols

Eradication of the infection is the fundamental necessity taking precedence in the sequence of other curative measures, usually, but not always reimplantation. A stable implant will most usually be pain free.

The options are:

- Antibiotic therapy—rarely alone and usually accompanying surgery
- Surgical debridement with retention of prosthesis
- Single-stage revision
- Two-stage revision
- Excision arthroplasty
- Disarticulation.

Antibiotics

Surgery is not *always* the appropriate choice. In cases where the patient may not be fit for, or does not want surgery then long-term suppression with antibiotics can be an acceptable form of treatment. The prosthesis, however, must be soundly fixed and the infective organism sensitive to the antibiotic used. Nevertheless, it must be recognized that antibiotics alone will not eradicate the infection—only slow the infective process to some degree.

Surgical debridement with retention of prosthesis

Success rates of up to 84% have been reported with debridement and lavage with retention of the original prosthesis in cases of acute postoperative infection if performed within 2 weeks of the index procedure. After this time the chance of successful eradication of infection falls dramatically. A patient rarely presents during this time frame so making this treatment of later haematogenous infection much less successful.

Exchange arthroplasty

Exchange arthroplasty surgery offers the best way of eradicating infection along with restoration of function. This can be undertaken in a direct or staged manner. Results in the literature of each pathway are difficult to compare, but the key to success of both treatment modalities depends upon:

- Preoperative diagnosis of the infecting organism and its antibiotic sensitivity pattern
- Radical debridement
- Elution of antibiotic from bone cement.

Direct exchange

The major advantage of direct exchange surgery is that it is one operative procedure with benefits to both the patient and the healthcare system. It removes the morbidity of a temporary pseudarthrosis and lessens the cost of treatment.

The generally accepted criteria for performing direct exchange are:

- Cemented reconstruction
- Accurate preoperative bacteriological identification and an organism with an antibiogram appropriate to the antibiotics available
- Adequate bone stock and soft tissue support.

Direct exchange follows the principle that debridement removes all infected tissue and material, the dead space thus created is filled with the new implant which is fixed to the bone with cement acting as a depot for the release of local antibiotic. Recent published work has demonstrated the successful use of allograft bone as a delivery vehicle for antibiotics in single-stage surgery for infection using uncemented components. The combination of uncemented implants and an antibiotic bone compound used in a single-stage procedure has advantages and may improve long-term result.

It is generally accepted that direct exchange is less successful in eradicating infection than staged reconstruction. However, the difference is relatively small. The success of a one-stage procedure is highly dependent on the aggressiveness of the debridement, the experience of the surgeon, and close interaction with a microbiologist. Several European centres have reported excellent results treating all infections in this manner.

Although single-stage exchange has an obvious role we believe this should probably be restricted to the case of a single organism with known antibiotic sensitivities and reasonable bone stock.

Two-staged exchange

The only difference between direct and staged exchange is the interval phase. Radical debridement is essential to both. Antibiotics need to be administered either intravenously or to elute from bone cement (usually pellets or a spacer inserted during the interval phase as described later in this section) and after a period of weeks or even months the hip is reconstructed.

Following debridement, the extent of bone loss will be evident thereby allowing the surgeon to plan subsequent reconstruction. If bone graft is required, it can be safely used at the time of second stage without there being an increased risk of infection.

The interval phase allows for the administration of antibiotic. This can be given systemically or by elution from bone cement in the form of beads or a spacer. The advantage of cement elution is that it produces a much higher local concentration of antibiotic than could be safely given systemically. Local levels of gentamycin can be 10–100 times higher than the minimal inhibitory concentration of the causative bacteria whereas only 10% of the antibiotic available from the serum is found within bone when given systemically.

Any antibiotic can be added to the bone cement prior to polymerization as long as it is a sterile, dry powder which is heat stable and water soluble. It is usually mixed by hand in theatre at the time of surgery. The elution properties relate directly to the water uptake by the bone cement, antibiotic dissolves in the body fluid and elutes out. Generally no more than 4g of antibiotic should be added to each 40g packet of the polymethylmethacrylate (PMMA) polymer (10%) as above this level the biomechanical properties of the cement are affected.

Whilst the role of prophylactic antibiotics is established, is there a need for prolonged systemic therapy when the mainstay of treatment is surgical and such high concentrations can be delivered locally from the bone cement? Review of the literature is not particularly helpful when trying to evaluate the success of two-stage regimens. In Sheffield in the early nineties we took the decision to treat our infections in a two-stage manner on the principle of radical debridement, local elution of antibiotic without the need for prolonged adjunctive systemic therapy. Our results with respect to eradication of infection are comparable with other authors who have used prolonged courses of antibiotics, but have the advantage of reduced cost and no associated morbidity of prolonged therapy.

The timing of reimplantation is based upon the clinical progress of the patient as evidenced by the quality of soft tissues and falling ESR and CRP. The minimum period between stages is usually 6 weeks and there is no need for a prolonged interval before reimplantation according to the monitoring tests. If the soft tissues do not improve or inflammatory markers remain elevated it is preferable to explore and debride as opposed to delay.

The long-term results for successful eradication of infection with two-stage surgery range from 87–92% at 5- and 10-year follow-up.

The results for successful eradication of infection following one stage exchange range from 86–91% at 3- and 10-year follow-up.

Excision arthroplasty

If, following debridement, hip reconstruction is not possible or the patient declines further surgery, then excision arthroplasty remains a viable option. Whilst the results for eradication of infection are good, lower limb function, particularly in the younger more active and the elderly frail patients, is poor.

Disarticulation

Disarticulation is the final option available to the surgeon and should be reserved for life-threatening sepsis or irreparable neurovascular damage.

Summary

Diagnosis and treatment of infected hip arthroplasty requires a multidisciplinary team approach to eradicate infection, alleviate pain, and restore function. Each patient must be treated on an individual basis. The spectrum ranges from conservative suppressive therapy to radical ablation. Most cases that present will be chronically infected so the mainstay of treatment is surgical debridement, which must be radical and complete. Antibiotics obviously have an important but secondary role.

The surgery necessary for these infected cases does not involve any special techniques but it is extensive with respect to excision, becoming on occasion alarming unless the surgeon has at their disposal a comprehensive shelf of instruments and implants, adequate bone graft material, and time for long operative procedures. These are the main reasons why treatment of the infected arthroplasty should be conducted in specialist centres.

Further reading

Tsukayama, D.T., Estrada, R., and Gustilo, R.B. (1996). Infection after total hip arthroplasty. A study of one hundred and six infections. *Journal of Bone and Joint Surgery America*, **78**, 512–23.

7.14

Hip resurfacing

Deepak Kumar and Richard Carrington

Summary points

- Hip resurfacing has emerged as an alternative method of hip arthroplasty for younger patients
- It is technically more demanding than total hip replacement
- The reported early and mid-term results are good with revision rates below 5% at 7 years
- Long term effect of raised levels of metal ions remains a major concern
- Long term clinical follow up and further research must continue.

Box 7.14.1 Why hip resurfacing?

- Total hip replacement in younger patient has a higher failure rate
- Hip resurfacing has emerged as an alternative to total hip replacement in younger patients
- Bone preservation and better loading of proximal femur leading to less stress shielding
- Reduced risk of dislocation and leg-length discrepancy
- Low-wear bearing surface
- Hip resurfacing now accounts for 8–10% of all primary hip replacements.

Introduction

Hip resurfacing arthroplasty is an attractive concept, as it not only preserves proximal femoral bone stock at the time of surgery, but by optimizing stress transfer to the proximal femur it minimizes stress shielding in the medium to long term. The large diameter of the articulation offers inherent stability and optimal range of movement. Total hip replacement has a higher failure rate in younger patients, i.e. those under 55 years, compared to elderly patients. Hip resurfacing arthroplasty has emerged as an alternative to total hip replacement in younger patients (Box 7.14.1). In less than a decade, since its renaissance in the 1990s, resurfacing has become very popular with the number of implantations accounting for 8–10% of all primary hip replacements in countries such as the United Kingdom, Australia, and the Netherlands.

History

The first hip resurfacing arthroplasty was performed by Smith-Petersen in 1923. He temporarily interposed a thin hemispherical shell between the femoral head and acetabulum in patients with arthrosis and expected new cartilage to grow on the articular surfaces. Originally, the shells were made of glass, bakelite, or celluloid. In 1938, he first implanted metal shells made of vitallium (cobalt-chrome-molybdenum (Co-Cr-Mo) alloy). In the 1970s, the second generation of resurfacings were developed. They were total resurfacings with a metal-on-polyethylene bearing. The clinical results were disappointing. Their failures can be mainly attributed to osteolysis induced by wear particles from the thin-walled polyethylene acetabular component.

In the 1990s, recognizing this problem, the third generation of resurfacings with a metal-on-metal bearing was developed in Birmingham, United Kingdom, by McMinn and Treacy. After a few attempts of trial and error, they found that the best fixation was obtained with a cemented, stemmed femoral hemispherical Co-Cr-Mo cap and an uncemented hydroxyapatite (HA)-coated Co-Cr-Mo acetabular cup and in 1994, implantation of McMinn prosthesis was started. Now, at least 15 types of resurfacing prosthesis are available in the market. These prostheses differ in many details, such as shape, sizing, head coverage, clearance, metal alloy used, heat treatment, instrumentation, and so on. Just as with conventional hips, they exhibit differences in clinical outcome. The Swedish and Australian registries have listed a two- to threefold difference in revision rate between different makes.

Advantages and disadvantages

There are several theoretical advantages of hip resurfacing over conventional hip replacement but the lack of long-term data and emerging new modes of failure are the main disadvantages and cause for concern (Table 7.14.1).

Table 7.14.1 Advantages and disadvantages of hip resurfacing

Advantages	Disadvantages
Preservation of proximal femoral bone stock	No long-term outcome data
More normal loading of femur reducing proximal femoral stress shielding	Technically more demanding
Reduced risk of leg lengthening/shortening	Inability to adjust length and offset
Reduced risk of dislocation	New modes of failure—femoral neck fracture, femoral head collapse, local and systemic metal allergy
Improved function/activity level	Concern due to high levels of metal in blood and other tissues
Low wear bearing surface	
Easier revision of femoral component if required	

Table 7.14.2 Indications and contraindications

Indication	Primary osteoarthritis of hip in male >65 years
	Posttraumatic osteoarthritis
	Osteoarthritis of hip with proximal femoral deformity
	Osteoarthritis of hip with metal in proximal femur
	Osteoarthritis with mild developmental dysplasia of hip (mostly Crowe I)
Contraindication	**Absolute**
	Infection
	Loss of femoral head (severe bone loss)
	Large femoral neck cysts
	Osteoporosis (proven by DXA scan)
	Severe dysplasia of acetabulum (Crowe IV)
	Renal failure
	Relative
	Chronologic age >65 years
	Body mass index >35 years
	Varus neck-shaft angle
	Low head offset
	Moderate dysplasia of acetabulum (Crowe II and III)
	Osteonecrosis of the femoral head involving >30%
	Metal allergy
	With caution
	Femoral head cyst >1cm
	Female patient
	Patient with rheumatoid arthritis
	Tall and thin patient
	Leg-length inequality
	Child-bearing age group with incomplete family
	Use of glucocorticosteroids and endocrine disorders
	Malabsorption and alcohol abuse

DXA, dual energy X-ray absorptiometry.

Indications and contraindications

A man younger than 65 years with primary osteoarthritis with good bone quality and normal proximal femoral anatomy is the ideal candidate for hip resurfacing. Infection, osteoporosis, severe bone loss either of femoral head or acetabulum, and renal failure are the absolute contraindications for resurfacing. Patient selection for hip resurfacing is no less important than any other surgery. Important indications and contraindications are listed in Table 7.14.2.

Surgical technique (Box 7.14.2)

The National Institute of Health and Clinical Excellence (NICE) recommend metal-on-metal hip resurfacing arthroplasty to be performed only by surgeons who have received training specifically in this technique. Resurfacing can be carried out through a posterior or a direct lateral approach. The lateral approach to the hip has been advocated as a way of preserving the deep branch of the medial femoral circumflex artery thus preserving blood supply to the anterosuperior quadrant of the femoral head but with the lateral approach there is significant risk of abductor dysfunction. Abductor dysfunction is very poorly tolerated in young patients who wish to regain an active lifestyle. The posterior approach is currently favoured by most surgeons. The approach is more extensile than traditional posterior approach. Circumferential capsulotomy and gluteus maximus tenotomy is required for good exposure of femoral head and creation of a superior pocket is required to accommodate the femoral head and neck while acetabulum is prepared.

Easy resurfacing arthroplasties do not exist; with a steep learning curve, it remains a difficult procedure even in experienced hands. In particular, component positioning and cementing technique are critical factors—and the main causes of failure in retrieval studies. The main reason for early revision is fracture of the neck arising from the edge of the implant, which can be initiated by uncovered reamed bone and notching. Early revisions are more common in older patients and females, and bone quality seems to be a critical factor. Late revisions are without fracture and most of them show signs of wear and rim loading, which can be related to malpositioning. Varus placement of the femoral component leads to higher levels of stress and increases the probability of failure. It is recommended that a surgeon should strive to achieve a relative valgus placement of 5–10 degrees while avoid to notch the superolateral cortex of the femoral neck.

Computer-assisted navigation systems have been used with success to avoid malpositioning of components, especially in early phase of learning curve.

Results

Very good early and mid-term results have been reported from the centre of origin of Birmingham hip resurfacing prosthesis. They reported survival of 99.7% of 439 hips at a mean follow up of

Box 7.14.2 Surgical technique

- Hip resurfacing is a technically demanding procedure and needs specific training
- Lateral approach is advocated to preserve blood supply to femoral head but is associated with risk of abductor dysfunction
- Posterior approach currently favoured by most surgeons
- Circumferential capsulotomy and gluteus maximus tenotomy is required for good exposure
- Most failures can be attributed to technical errors, e.g. notching of superior neck, uncovering of reamed bone, varus femoral component, excessively open or anteverted acetabular component, or poor cementing technique.

3.3 years for patients under the age of 55 years, and 98% of 144 hips at a minimum follow up of 5 years for males under the age of 65 years and females under the age of 60 years. Their survival rates in multicentre studies have shown worse results. The National Joint Registry for England and Wales (2007) reported revision rates of 1.8% at 3 years; the Australian Orthopaedic Implant Register (2007) reported 3.7% at 5 years; and the Oswestry Hip Outcome Centre reported 4.6% at 7 years.

Complications

The main reasons for revision of a metal-on-metal hip resurfacing are femoral neck fracture, aseptic loosening, and pain (Box 7.14.2).

Femoral neck fracture (Figure 7.14.1)

Femoral neck fracture is a unique complication of resurfacing occurring in 0–7%. The causes of fracture can be related to the

Box 7.14.3 Complications of hip resurfacing

- Heterotopic ossification (28–68%)
- Neck narrowing (14–28%)
- Aseptic loosening (2%)
- Avascular necrosis (0.5–1%)
- ALVAL/pseudotumours (1%)
- Dislocation (<1%)
- Femoral neck fracture (0–7%)
- Osteolysis (rare)

patient, the surgical technique, or a combination of both. Patient-related factors include decreased bone mass, obesity, and inflammatory arthritis. Intraoperative characteristics that may lead to fracture if proceeding with resurfacing include cysts and/or exposed bone found in the femoral neck during preparation of femoral head. Surgical errors include notching of the femoral neck, preparing the femoral head and, therefore, tilting the prosthesis into excess varus (<130 degrees stem-shaft angle), and seating of the cup into retroversion.

Undisplaced fracture can be successfully treated with a few weeks of toe-touch weight bearing. Displaced fractures or undisplaced fractures failing to unite with conservative treatment can be treated by conversion to standard total hip replacement. If the cup is in a good position and well fixed, the hip can be revised using a standard stem with a large modular femoral head to articulate with the cup, otherwise both components can be revised.

Aseptic loosening

Aseptic loosening of the femoral component has been reported in some series, occurring in up to 2% of cases. Large areas of cystic

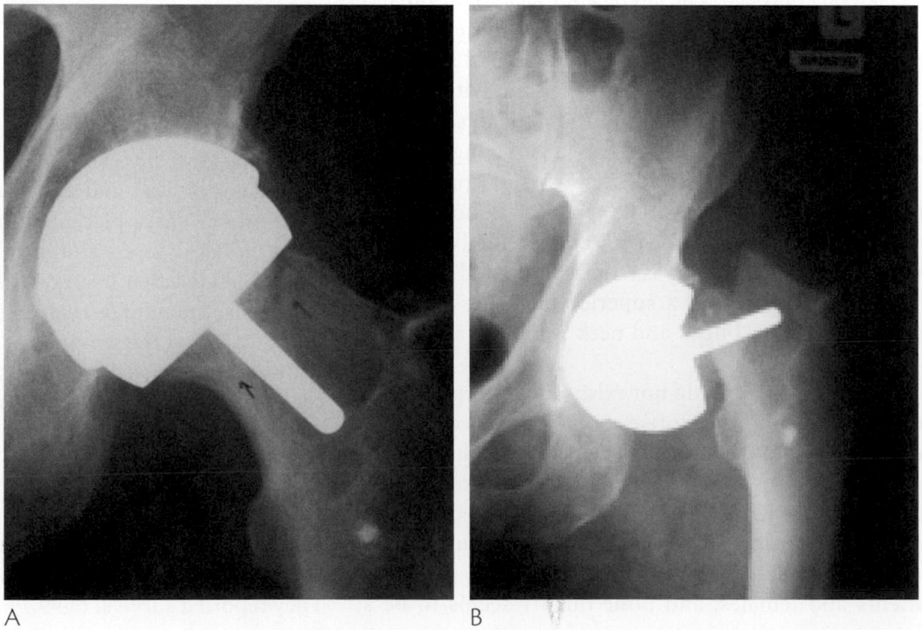

Fig. 7.14.1 A) Notching of the superior aspect of the femoral neck and a fracture line propagating from the superior implant-neck junction. B) Subsequent femoral neck fracture. (Reproduced from Shimmin, A., Beaulé, P.E., and Campbell, P. (2008). Metal-on-metal hip resurfacing arthroplasty. *Journal of Bone and Joint Surgery*, **90A**, 637–54.)

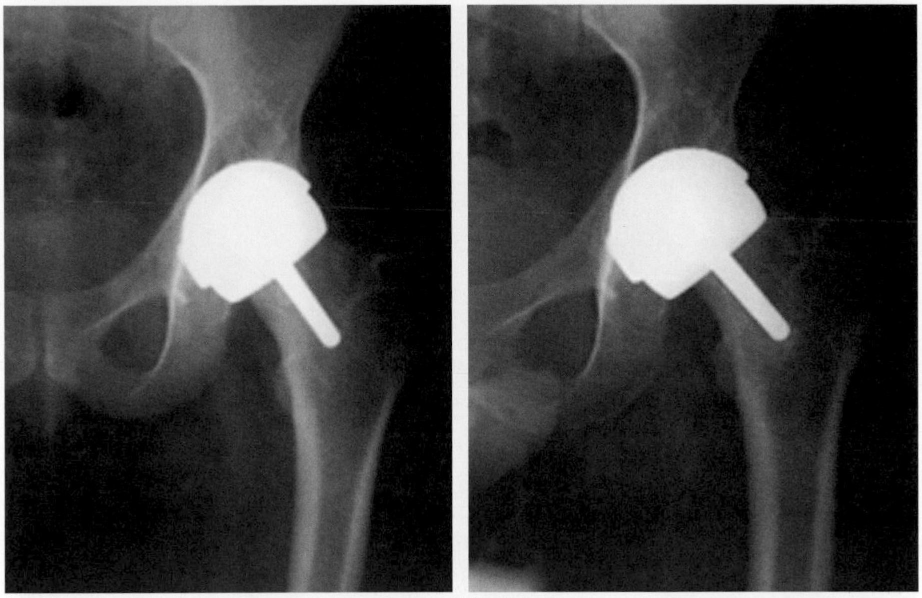

A B

Fig. 7.14.2 Anteroposterior radiographs of failing hip resurfacing due to histologically-confirmed avascular necrosis. A) Initial postoperative appearance and B) at 16 months showing collapse of the femoral head with migration of the femoral component. (Reproduced from Heilpern, G.N., Shah, N.N., and Fordyce, M.J. (2008). Birmingham hip resurfacing arthroplasty: a series of 110 consecutive hips with a minimum five-year clinical and radiological follow-up. *Journal of Bone and Joint Surgery*, **90B**, 1137–42.)

degeneration in the head leaving less surface area available for fixation and also a lower stem shaft angle are more frequently associated with aseptic loosening.

Avascular necrosis (Figure 7.14.2)

Hip resurfacing performed with a posterior approach has been shown to cause a 60% decrease in oxygen concentration in the femoral head and component insertion results in a further 20% decrease with no significant improvement occurring after wound closure. This raises concern regarding viability of femoral head after resurfacing, but excellent short-term results of resurfacing have been reported in patients with established osteonecrosis and it remains to be determined with longer follow-up whether femoral head viability has any significant effect on the outcome of resurfacing. True incidence of avascular necrosis is difficult to determine in asymptomatic patients due to overshadowing of metal on plain x-ray. Avascular necrosis of femoral heads accounting for revision have been reported in 0.5–1% of all resurfaced hips and may be held responsible for some of the neck fractures in the absence of other risk factors.

Heterotopic ossification

The approach for hip resurfacing is usually extensile and involves more tissue dissection and handling than conventional hip replacement. Heterotopic ossification has been seen in 28–60% of patients after hip resurfacing but only 7–8% develop Brooker grade 3 or 4. High-risk patients should have prophylactic treatment.

Dislocation

Hip resurfacing is inherently more stable than conventional hip replacement because of larger diametric clearance of femoral components. The reported incidence is less than 1% as opposed to 3–6% in conventional hip replacement.

Narrowing of the neck (Figure 7.14.3)

Some degree of narrowing of the femoral neck is seen in three-quarters of the patients who have had hip resurfacing but only 14–28% have more than 10% of narrowing. Female patients are 2.5 times more likely to develop neck narrowing and patients with higher (valgus) neck-shaft angle are also more at risk. Neck narrowing seems to stabilize with time with no adverse clinical or radiological features noted in cases followed-up for 6 years. No significant progression of narrowing was noted in these patients after 3 years.

Several other complications related to resurfacing arthroplasty have been reported including clicking, squeaking, soft tissue impingement, psoas tendinitis, nerve palsy, metallosis, osteolysis, raised metal ion levels, and aseptic lymphocytic vasculitis associated lesions (ALVAL) or pseudotumours (Figure 7.14.4).

The latter two have been investigated by many and remains focus of most research related to metal on metal bearing arthroplasty. The peak serum cobalt level and that of serum chromium level have been seen at 6 months and 9 months respectively. The serum levels of metal ions gradually decline as the bedding-in wear changes to steady-state wear but have remained higher than preoperative levels even at 2-year follow-up. Long-term impact of raised metal ion levels is unknown and remains a major concern against general acceptance of metal-on-metal hip resurfacing arthroplasty. The exact aetiology of aseptic periarticular soft tissue mass (pseudotumours) is unknown, but the two widely accepted explanations in the current period of time are T-lymphocyte-mediated delayed-type hypersensitivity reactions and/or direct toxic effect of a very high concentration of metal debris in the joint fluid. The individual biological response to the presence of wear debris seem to vary, and may be due to different toxic-effect threshold or immunological tolerance. They occur with an overall incidence of 1% in the first 5 years after implantation of metal-on-metal hip resurfacing and are commoner in females. Histological specimens harvested at the time of revision show inflammatory changes, vasculitis, and necrosis.

Periprosthetic osteolysis is a rare complication of metal-on-metal arthroplasty. The histological examination showing a perivascular accumulation of T lymphocytes and immunohistochemical analysis showing elevated levels of bone-resorbing

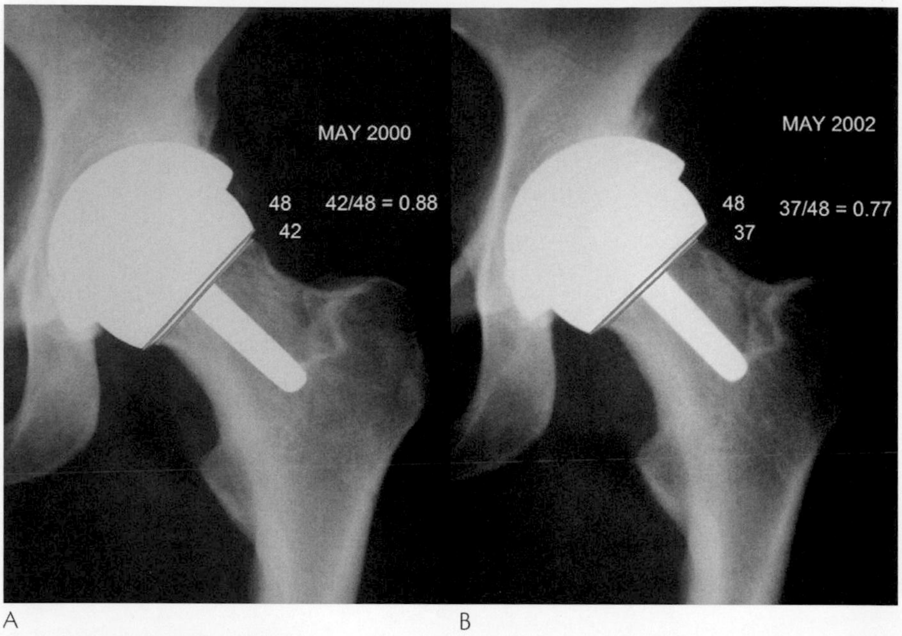

Fig. 7.14.3 Anteroposterior radiographs. A) A few weeks postoperatively, the neck prosthesis ratio was 0.88 and B) at 2 years, the component was radiologically stable but the neck prosthesis ratio dropped down to 0.77. Neck was narrowed by 12.5%. (Reproduced from Spencer, S., Carter, R., Murray, H., and Meek, R.M. (2008). Femoral neck narrowing after metal-on-metal hip resurfacing. *Journal of Arthroplasty*, **23**(8), 1105–9.)

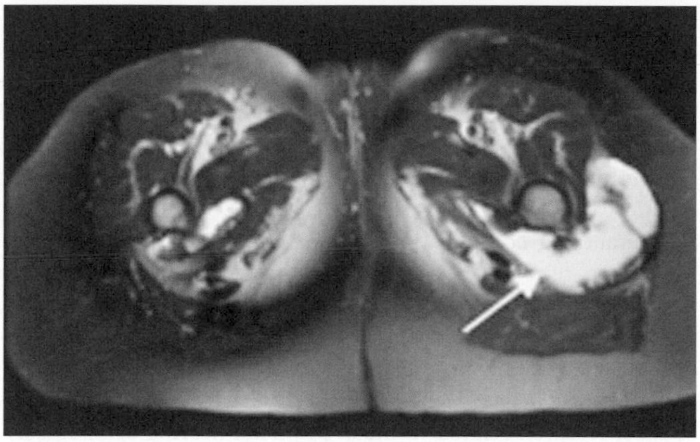

Fig. 7.14.4 Fat suppression T_2-weighted MRI scan showing a large posterolateral cyst arising from the posterior joint space (arrow). (Courtesy Pandit, H., Glyn-Jones, S., McLardy-Smith, P., et al. (2008). Pseudotumours associated with metal-on-metal hip resurfacings. *Journal of Bone and Joint Surgery*, **90-B**, 847–51.)

cytokines such as IL-1 and TNF-α produced by infiltrating lymphocytes and activated macrophages suggest that early osteolysis is associated with delayed-type hypersensitivity to metal.

Speculation of future association of metal-on-metal bearing arthroplasty with malignancy or genotoxicity is based on the findings of research related to intracellular metabolism of chromium and cobalt, which has been found to release free radicals (reactive oxygen and nitrogen species). Free radicals are known to be involved in protein oxidation, leading to their degradation, lipid peroxidation, and DNA damage.

Conclusions

Lessons from the failure of previous generations of hip resurfacing have helped to select better materials, improve implant design and manufacture, and also upgrade instrumentation. Cementless acetabular components and cemented femoral components fixation provide better and more reliable results compared to alternative methods of fixation. Orientation of implants and surgical time improve with experience as surgical technique has a steep learning curve. Patient selection is of paramount importance and not all patients with osteoarthritis of hip under the age of 65 years are candidates for hip resurfacing. Female patients tend to have a higher incidence of complications and they must be carefully warned before offering hip resurfacing at any age. Recent studies demonstrating excellent short-term results of metal-on-metal resurfacing in active patients younger than 60 years of age have established it as an alternative to conventional hip replacement.

The importance of long-term clinical follow-up of patients undergoing metal on metal hip resurfacing arthroplasty cannot be overstressed. The short-term success of resurfacing arthroplasty should not overwhelm and the research into the molecular and cellular mechanism involved in the pathogenesis of periprosthetic biological adverse reactions caused by metal wear particle must continue.

Box 7.14.4 Conclusions

- Survival rate above 95% at 7 years (reported from an independent centre)
- Female patients have higher incidence of complications at any age
- Long-term effect of raised levels of metal ions is unknown and remains a major concern against general acceptance
- Long-term clinical follow-up of patients and research into the pathogenesis of periprosthetic biological adverse reactions must continue.

Further reading

Amstutz, H.C., Beaulé, P.E., Dorey, F.J., *et al.* (2004). Metal-on-metal hybrid surface arthroplasty: two to six-year follow-up study. *Journal of Bone and Joint Surgery*, **86A**, 28–39.

Grigoris, P., Roberts, P., Panousis, K., and Bosch, H. (2005). The evolution of hip resurfacing arthroplasty. *Orthopedic Clinics of North America*, **36**(2), vii, 125–34.

Mabilleau, G., Kwon, Y.M., Pandit, H., Murray, D.W., and Sabokbar, A. (2008). Metal-on-metal hip resurfacing arthroplasty: A review of periprosthetic biological reactions. *Acta Orthopaedica*, **79**(6), 734–47.

Mont, M.A., Ragland, P.S., Etienne, G., Seyler, T.M., and Schmalzried, T.P. (2006). Hip resurfacing arthroplasty. *Journal of the American Academy of Orthopaedic* Surgeons, **14**(8), 454–63.

Treacy, R.B., McBryde, C.W., and Pynsent, P.B. (2005). Birmingham hip resurfacing arthroplasty: a minimum follow-up of five years. *Journal of Bone and Joint Surgery*, **87B**, 167–70.

7.15

Sports injuries in the pelvic region

Roger Wolman

Summary points

- The pelvis acts as a fulcrum for the forces transmitted between the lower limb and trunk especially on twisting and turning movements while running, and in the reverse direction when kicking. Sports injuries around the pelvis are therefore common in weight-bearing sports, such as running, football, rugby, and basketball
- Injury can occur to the various structures around the pelvis. Bone stress injuries affect the symphysis pubis, pubic rami, femoral neck, and sacrum. Stress fractures are more common in women and may occur as part of the female athlete triad (Box 7.15.1) where there is hypo-oestrogenaemia and low bone density
- Tendon injuries, including enthesopathies, most commonly affect the adductors, lower abdominals, glutei and hamstrings. Hip injuries can occur as a result of labral tears and femoroacetabular impingement. Sacroiliac joint instability may also cause symptoms especially in the buttock region. Synovitis of either joint may suggest an inflammatory arthritis
- Pain is the most common symptom. However it may be referred from elsewhere, especially the lumbar spine. Pain may also originate from other systems including the reproductive organs and the gastrointestinal and urinary tracts.

Introduction

Injuries around the pelvis usually cause pain, which tends to be in one of three regions:

- The anterior hip and groin
- The lateral hip
- The buttock.

There may be a degree of overlap of the site of the pain and sometimes, especially with primary hip joint pathology, the pain may be felt deeper within the pelvis. The diagnosis can usually be made following a detailed history and examination, which may include special tests. This can be confirmed by imaging, in particular magnetic resonance imaging (MRI) and ultrasound scanning.

Box 7.15.1 The female athlete triad

- Disordered eating—low energy intake
- Menstrual dysfunction—amenorrhoea
- Osteopenia—osteoporosis.

Anterior hip and groin pain

Groin pain may be caused by local pathology but several systems can cause referred pain into the groin. There is, therefore, a large differential diagnosis (Table 7.15.1).

Acute symptoms are usually due to strains and minor tears which can be managed expectantly with a good outcome. However, chronic groin pain is often complicated by the fact that multiple pathologies may coexist. Furthermore the aetiology of the so-called 'sports hernia', a diagnosis commonly made in athletes, is poorly understood. Therefore the assessment and treatment of chronic groin pain can be difficult.

Sports hernia and osteitis pubis (Box 7.15.2)

These two injuries often coexist and although the description of osteitis pubis is well established, the diagnosis of sports hernia is poorly understood. This injury has been described by many terms, such as sportsman's hernia, athletic pubalgia, and Gilmores groin. It is predominantly an injury of the male athlete. Both the aetiology and pathophysiology are controversial. The most common view is that it is due to a weakness or deficiency of the posterior inguinal wall. Findings at surgery include tears to the transversalis fascia or conjoint tendon and dilatation of the superficial inguinal ring.

The cause is thought to be the strong pull of overconditioned adductors against the relatively underconditioned lower abdominal muscles creating a shearing force across the front of the pelvis. This may also lead to instability of the symphysis, hence the association with osteitis pubis.

Symptoms and signs

The main symptom is a chronic, activity-related uni- (or bi-) lateral groin pain, which occurs in cutting and kicking sports, such as football, rugby and hockey. The onset is usually insidious

Table 7.15.1 Differential diagnosis of groin pain in athletes

Soft tissue	Bone	Joint	Referred pain
Sports hernia	Osteitis pubis	Femoroacetabular impingement	Lower back
Adductor strain or tendinopathy	Stress fracture—pubic ramus or femoral neck	Labral tears of hip	Sacroiliac joint
Rectus abdominis strain	Apophyseal disorder/avulsion fracture of rectus femoris	Synovitis/arthritis of the hip	Gynaecological:
Iliopsoas bursitis or tendinopathy			◆ Endometriosis
Obturator neuropathy			◆ Ovarian cyst
Inguinal hernia			Gastrointestinal tract
			Genitourinary system

Box 7.15.2 Features of 'sports hernia'/osteitis pubis

- Caused by a weakness of posterior inguinal wall
- May result in uni- or bilateral groin pain
- Often tenderness over pubic tubercle and superficial inguinal ring
- MRI may show:
  - Osteitis pubis
  - Tears at rectus and adductor insertion
- Treatment:
  - Conservative: rest, NSAIDs, physiotherapy
  - Surgery in non-responders.

initially with discomfort after a game. Gradually the pain comes on during a game, especially with cutting movements rather than running in a straight line. This then affects the ability of the athlete to train and perform. Examination findings are variable but can include tenderness over the pubic tubercle and around the superficial inguinal ring, which may be enlarged. There may be pain on testing the muscles groups attached around the symphysis, including the adductors and lower abdominals (tests include the adductor squeeze, double leg raise, and sit-up). Conventional hernia tests are negative.

Investigations

Imaging may show changes around the symphysis with changes on x-ray and bone oedema on MRI, both suggestive of osteitis pubis. MRI may also show tears and tendinosis of the rectus insertion and adductors. In experienced hands, changes can sometimes be identified on ultrasound.

Management

Treatment should initially be conservative. This should include a period of relative rest from the provoking activities. Non-steroidal anti-inflammatory drugs (NSAIDs) may help to control the pain while the symptoms of osteitis pubis may respond to an intravenous bisphosphonate. Physiotherapy should include conditioning exercises involving the muscle groups around the front of the pelvis with core stability/strength training involving the lower abdominals. A progressive training ladder gradually working back to full sporting activity should then be followed. This process to full recovery can take about 4 months.

In those who don't respond to this regimen or in those who want a quicker resolution of the injury (e.g. the professional athlete), surgery should be considered. The options are either an open or laparoscopic approach with exploration and repair of the abdominal wall, using a mesh or performing a modified Bassini repair. The success rate following surgery is extremely high with most studies reporting greater than 90% of the athletes back to full sporting activity within 4–8 weeks. Unfortunately there are no randomized, controlled trails comparing surgical with conservative interventions.

Adductor muscle strains and tendinopathy

These injuries are typically seen in footballers and ice hockey players. They usually occur acutely and can be graded from mild where minimal playing time is lost (grade I) to severe where there is almost complete loss of muscle function (grade III). The athlete complains of groin pain with tenderness over the adductor and/or at its insertion around the symphysis. There is pain on passive abduction and on active adduction. It is thought that without adequate rehabilitation there is a danger that an acute adductor strain may go on to a more chronic tendinopathy.

Rectus abdominis strains

These occur at the attachment to the superior pubic ramus as a result of excessive lifting or intensive 'sit-up' type exercises. There is usually tenderness around the site of attachment and pain on active contraction of the lower abdominals. The injury responds to relative rest and physical therapy.

Inguinal hernias

These occasionally cause groin pain in the athlete. There may be an obvious swelling with a positive cough impulse. They respond to surgical treatment.

Obturator neuropathy

The diagnosis of obturator neuropathy is controversial. It is due to fascial entrapment leading to exercise-induced pain together with weakness of the adductors and numbness in the distal medial thigh immediately post-exercise. Electromyography (EMG) may show denervation in the adductor muscle. It often responds to conservative therapy but may require surgical release.

Iliopsoas tendinopathy and bursitis

The iliopsoas arises from the lumbar vertebrae and anterior surface of the ilium and inserts into the lesser trochanter of the hip. It is a powerful hip flexor and recurrent kicking actions can lead to an overuse injury. This is seen typically in dance but may also occur in football. The athlete complains of groin pain while examination findings include pain on iliopsoas stretch and on resisted hip flexion. Treatment consists of rest from kicking movements and reconditioning of the iliopsoas.

A bursa lies adjacent to the tendon insertion into the lesser trochanter. This can sometimes get inflamed and swollen. Symptoms and signs are similar to iliopsoas tendinopathy. Treatment includes image-guided aspiration and injection of the bursa.

The 'snapping hip' syndrome

The snapping hip syndrome is a condition commonly seen in ballet dancers. It can be associated with pain and is most commonly due to the iliopsoas tendon as it passes over the anterior aspect of the hip (anterior snap). A less common cause in dancers is from the iliotibial band (ITB) as it passes over the lateral aspect of the hip (lateral snap). The anterior snapping hip can be confirmed on ultrasound assessment and usually responds to stretching exercises.

Femoroacetabular impingement/labral tear

See Chapter 7.16.

Synovitis of the hip

Sero-negative arthropathy typically occurs in the young adult population and may present as an isolated monoarthritis of the hip. Alternatively, hip involvement may be part of a more generalized arthropathy involving several large joints including the sacroiliac joints. The athlete will present with unilateral groin pain with limitation of movement of the hip. X-rays are usually normal but MRI may show evidence of both synovitis and bone marrow oedema. Treatment involves NSAIDs and possibly second-line agents. An image-guided steroid injection can be very effective especially in an isolated monoarthritis.

Stress fractures (Box 7.15.3)

Inferior pubic ramus

This occurs in distance runners, more commonly in females. The athlete will complain of groin pain and have localized tenderness. Early diagnosis can be made either by bone scan or MRI as changes occur within 48h whereas the plain x-ray may remain normal. Treatment involves rest from weight-bearing sport and correction of relevant biomechanical factors. The injury usually heals within 6–8 weeks.

Femoral neck

This injury is relatively uncommon, occurring in weight-bearing sports usually following a period of increased training. The diagnosis is often missed in the early stages as there is usually an insidious onset of exertional groin pain, a symptom that has a wide differential diagnosis. Furthermore, examination findings are often non-specific (with pain at end-of-range on hip examination) while plain x-ray is normal for several weeks. Diagnostic delay is therefore quite common and unfortunately this can lead to extension of the fracture with associated complications. Early diagnosis requires a high index of clinical suspicion supported by further imaging (either MRI or bone scan).

There are two types of fracture:

- Tension fractures occur on the superior surface and are prone to extend to a full fracture. These require urgent treatment with either early surgical fixation or strict bed rest
- Compression fractures occur on the inferior surface and are more stable. These usually respond to a period of non-weight bearing for 6–8 weeks, followed by a rehabilitation period gradually working back to full activity, which can take a further 6–8 weeks.

Apophyseal disorder/avulsion fracture of the rectus femoris

This injury occurs during adolescence, typically associated with sprinting and kicking. It occurs at the site of attachment of the rectus femoris to the anterior inferior iliac spine. It usually responds to conservative treatment but surgical re-attachment is occasionally necessary.

Lateral hip pain (Box 7.15.5)

Lateral hip pain typically occurs in long distance runners. It is commonly attributed to trochanteric bursitis. However, with improved availability of MRI and ultrasound scanning it is relatively uncommon to find a bursal swelling as the cause of lateral hip pain in an athlete. The trochanteric pain syndrome is a more useful description of this problem.

Trochanteric pain syndrome

The athlete complains of pain, which tends to radiate down the lateral aspect of the thigh. The aetiology is probably due to a tight

Box 7.15.3 Types of stress fractures

- Inferior pubic rami—common in female runners
- Neck of femur—pain on training, end-of-range discomfort, MRI to diagnose if x-rays normal:
  - Tension fracture, operative fixation
  - Compression fracture, non-weight bearing for 8 weeks.

Box 7.15.4 Causes of anterior hip pain

- Sports hernia/osteitis pubis
- Adductor muscle strain and tendinopathy
- Rectus abdominis strain
- Inguinal hernia
- Obturator neuropathy
- Iliopsoas bursitis/tendinopathy
- Femoroacetabular impingement
- Synovitis
- Stress fracture
- Apophyseal disorder and avulsion fracture of rectus femoris.

Box 7.15.5 Types of lateral hip pain

- Trochanteric pain syndrome:
  - Thought to be due to a tight ITB which then irritates the surrounding tissues
  - Non-surgical treatment is the mainstay; occasionally ITB lengthening needed
- Gluteus medius tendinopathy:
  - Tenderness around the greater trochanter
  - Treatment is non-surgical.

ITB as it passes around the greater trochanter. Occasionally this can cause a snapping hip. With time this leads to an irritation of the ITB, the adjacent soft tissues, or the bursa, which is then responsible for the pain. Treatment consists of ITB stretches, gluteal conditioning exercises, and sometimes a local cortisone injection. In recalcitrant cases, surgery involving lengthening of the ITB can help.

Gluteus medius tendinopathy

This is an increasingly recognized cause of lateral hip pain and tenderness around the greater trochanter. There may also be pain on stretching the gluteus medius. Diagnosis can be confirmed on either ultrasound or MRI. Treatment involves reconditioning exercises for the gluteus medius and, occasionally, image-guided injections.

Buttock pain (Box 7.15.6)

Referred pain from the lower back or sacroiliac joint is the most common cause of buttock pain.

Box 7.15.6 Types of buttock pain

- Sacroiliac joint pain
  - Can be due to instability or inflammation
  - Responds to physical therapy and addressing the cause
- Sacral stress fracture: uncommon, resolves in 8–12 weeks
- Piriformis syndrome:
  - Compression of sciatic nerve due to trauma or overuse
  - Responds to physical therapy and injections; rarely surgery needed
- Proximal hamstring tendinopathy/enthesopathy: usually insidious onset, responds to stretching and strengthening
- Apophyseal disorders of the ischial tuberosity:
  - Occurs in the adolescent athlete, treated with rest
  - Avulsion fracture of ischial tuberosity can occur and if widely separated may need surgical reattachment.

Sacroiliac joint pain

Sacroiliac joint pain can occur as a result of instability or due to inflammation. It causes unilateral buttock and possibly low back pain, which can radiate into the groin and the region of the symphysis pubis. It can also radiate into the thigh. Injury to the joint can occur as a result of intensive weight-bearing exercise especially in an athlete with a leg-length difference.

Treatment should consist of analgesia, correction of any biomechanical issues, and physical therapy techniques, including stability exercises. Therapeutic steroid injections may have a role to play. Surgical stabilization is rarely indicated.

Sacral stress fracture

This uncommon injury does occur in distance runners and has been reported in other sports including tennis and hockey. Risk factors include biomechanical abnormalities, such as leg-length difference. The athlete complains of low back and buttock pain sometimes radiating down the thigh. Diagnosis can be made on MRI. The injury usually resolves with rest within 8–12 weeks.

Piriformis syndrome

Piriformis muscle overuse or trauma can give rise to symptoms as a result of its close anatomical relationship with the sciatic nerve. The sciatic nerve may be compressed or otherwise irritated by the piriformis muscle causing pain, tingling, and numbness in the buttocks and along the path of the sciatic nerve. Treatment involves physical therapy, analgesia, and avoidance of contributory activities. Injections or surgical decompression are needed if symptoms do not resolve with conservative therapy.

Occasionally there may be a strain of the piriformis, which can cause buttock pain. Diagnosis can be made with clinical testing. The condition responds to conditioning exercises.

Proximal hamstring tendinopathy/enthesopathy

This injury typically occurs in sprinters as either a tendinopathy or as an enthesial injury at the attachment to the ischial tuberosity. It causes deep buttock and posterior thigh pain. Although it can come on acutely, it more commonly has an insidious onset. It can usually be diagnosed on physical examination and then confirmed on imaging. Most cases respond to physical therapy including mobilizations, stretching and strengthening exercises. Occasionally steroid injections or surgical release is required.

Apophyseal disorders of the ischial tuberosity

These occur in the adolescent athlete and present with proximal posterior thigh pain and tenderness with pain on testing the hamstring. Therefore they can often be mistaken for a proximal hamstring injury and treated inappropriately.

Apophysitis of the ischial tuberosity usually occurs as an overuse injury in early adolescence. Diagnosis can sometimes be made on x-ray but more obvious findings occur on MRI where bone oedema may be seen. Treatment consists of relative rest and gradual reconditioning of tight hamstrings.

Avulsion fracture of the ischial tuberosity

Usually occurs as an acute injury in late adolescence. The fragment of bone should be visible on x-ray. Usually this injury will respond to conservative treatment over a 6 – 12-week period. However, if there is a wide separation of a large fragment then surgical reattachment may be required.

Further reading

Cohen, S.P. (2005). Sacroiliac joint pain: a comprehensive review of anatomy, diagnosis, and treatment. *Anaesthesia Analgesia*, **101**, 1440–53.

Fredericson, M., Moore, W., Guillet, M., and Beaulieu, C. (2005). High hamstring tendinopathy in runners meeting the challenges of diagnosis, treatment and rehabilitation. *Physician Sports Medicine*, **33**, 32–43.

Hill, P.F., Chatlerjl, S., Chambers, D., and Keeling, J.D. (1996). Stress fracture of the pubic ramus in female recruits. *Journal Bone Joint Surgery*, **78B**, 383–6.

Johnston, C.A.M., Wiley, J.P., Lindsay, D.M., and Wiseman, D.A. (1998). Iliopsoas bursitis and tendinitis. A review. *Sports Medicine*, **25**, 271–83.

Swan, K.G. and Wolcott, M. (2007). The athletic hernia: a systematic review. *Clinical Orthopaedics Related Research*, **455**, 78–87.

7.16

Inflammatory and metabolic bone disorders of the pelvis

Richard W. Keen

Summary points

- Avascular Necrosis
- Paget's disease
- Transient Osteoporosis of the Hip.

Introduction

The pelvis and hip can be affected by a number of medical conditions, and it is important that orthopaedic surgeons are aware of these when considering a differential diagnosis in patients presenting with problems at these skeletal sites. This chapter will review and discuss the management of avascular necrosis and Paget's disease, which are two common conditions affecting the hip.

Avascular necrosis

Regional interruption of blood flow to the skeleton can cause ischaemic (aseptic or avascular) necrosis. Ischaemia, if sufficiently severe and prolonged, will kill osteoblasts and chondrocytes. Clinical problems arise if subsequent resorption of necrotic tissue during skeletal repair compromises bone strength enough to cause fracture with deformity of bone, and secondary damage to cartilage (Box 7.16.2).

Epidemiology

There is little accurate data on the incidence of osteonecrosis, although it is estimated there are approximately 15 000 new cases per year in the United States. The disease appears to occur more frequently in males than in females, with the overall male to female ratio being 8:1. The age of onset is variable, although the majority of cases are less than 50 years of age. The average age of female cases is, on average, 10 years older than male cases.

Pathogenesis

Osteonecrosis is often seen in association with a variety of different conditions (Box 7.16.1). Trauma with fracture of the femoral neck interrupts the major part of the blood supply to the head and may lead to osteonecrosis. Glucocorticoids and alcoholism are two important factors known to predispose to osteonecrosis.

The occurrence of disease in twins and a clustering of cases in families suggest a genetic basis to idiopathic osteonecrosis of the femoral head. Increased incidence of osteonecrosis in specific animal models also provides further evidence of the existence of susceptibility genes. In sporadic cases of osteonecrosis of the femoral neck, a number of genetic association studies have been conducted, linking specific genes to the pathogenesis of disease. The majority of the studies have, to date, focused on gene polymorphisms affecting the coagulation and fibrinolytic system. Genetic mutations have recently been identified in three families with osteonecrosis and dominant inheritance. Mutations in the type II collagen (COL2A2) gene (mapped on chromosome 12q13) proved to be the genetic cause of the disease. Type II collagen is the major structural protein in the extracellular matrix of cartilage.

Clinical features

The clinical presentation depends on many factors, including the age of the patient, anatomical site of involvement, and the extent and severity of this involvement. The femoral head is the most common location for the development of osteonecrosis, although it may also occur at other sites including distal femur, humeral head, wrist, and foot. Patients may develop pain that can persist for weeks to months before radiographs show any change, although patients can be asymptomatic. Avascular necrosis at the hip classically will present with pain in the groin, although this can be referred to the buttock, thigh, or knee. The pain is exacerbated by weight bearing but can also be present at rest. Gait may be affected and patients can present with a limp. Once the femoral head has begun to collapse, range of hip movement will be reduced and leg shortening may develop.

In osteonecrosis of the hip, involvement of the contralateral hip is present in 30–70% of cases at the time of first examination. Within 3 years of diagnosis, more than 50% of cases will have progressed in the contralateral hip to such a stage where surgical intervention is required.

Box 7.16.1 Causative factors associated with osteonecrosis

Traumatic
- Fracture of the femoral neck
- Dislocation or fracture-dislocation of the hip
- Minor fracture

Non-traumatic
- Alcohol
- Arteriosclerosis and other occlusive vascular disorders
- Bisphosphonates
- Carbon tetrachloride poisoning
- Connective tissue diseases
- Cushing's disease (OMIM #219090; OMIM #219080)
- Diabetes mellitus (OMIM #222100, OMIM #125853)
- Disordered lipid metabolism
- Dysplasia
- Fatty liver
- Gaucher's disease (OMIM #231000)
- Glucocorticoid treatment
- Human immunodeficiency virus
- Dysbaric conditions
- Hyperuricaemia and gout
- Legg–Calve–Perthe disease (OMIM #150600)
- Osteomalacia
- Pancreatitis
- Pregnancy
- Radiotherapy
- Sickle cell anaemia (OMIM #603903)
- Solid organ transplantation
- Systemic lupus erythematosus (OMIM #152700)
- Thrombophlebitis
- Tumours

OMIN, Online Mendelian Inheritance in Man database

Radiological features

In the earliest stages of the disease, plain radiographs will be normal. Magnetic resonance imaging (MRI) is useful to detect early pathological changes. The most characteristic image is a margin of low signal on T_1- and T_2-weighted images, and is observed in 60–80% of cases. Radionuclide isotope bone scans and computed tomography (CT) can also be used in cases where MRI is either contraindicated or has been inconclusive. Osteonecrosis can be staged according to the sequence of the radiological changes. These are detailed in Table 7.16.1 and shown in Figure 7.16.1.

Table 7.16.1 Staging of osteonecrosis

Stage	Findings	Techniques
0	All techniques normal or non-diagnostic Necrosis on biopsy	Biopsy and histology
1	Radiographs and CT normal Positive result from at least one of the additional investigations listed	Radionuclide scan MRI Biopsy and histology
2	Radiographic abnormalities without collapse (sclerosis, cysts, osteopenia)	Radionuclide scan MRI Biopsy and histology
3	Crescent sign	Radiographs CT
4	Flattening or evident collapse	Radiographs CT
5	As for stage 4, with narrowing of joint space	Radiographs
6	As for stage 5, with destruction of joint	Radiographs

Laboratory findings

In idiopathic osteonecrosis, laboratory investigations will generally be normal. Investigations may reveal potential contributory factors such as connective tissue disease, diabetes, hyperlipidaemia, and gout.

Histopathological examination of tissue from affected bone is consistent with the pathogenesis that is suggested from the radiographical examinations. It shows that these various processes of skeletal death and repair are focal, and may be occurring simultaneously.

Differential diagnosis

In stages 3 and 4 of the disease, the radiological features of the disease are specific. In the later stages 5 and 6, a differential diagnosis is not necessary as by this stage the bone and joint have been irreversibly damaged and the only treatment option would be joint replacement. In the earlier stages of the disease (1 and 2), other diseases of bone, cartilage, and synovial tissue should be considered in the differential diagnosis.

Treatment

Medical treatment includes non-weight bearing for osteonecrosis affecting load-bearing bones. This may be for 4–8 weeks. Vasoactive drugs such as prostacyclin may play a role in early stages of osteonecrosis. Bisphosphonates have also been shown to be effective in the treatment of osteonecrosis. Data has been observed for alendronate and more recently for zoledronate.

Surgical treatment for osteonecrosis involves core decompression. This reduces the intramedullary pressure within the ischaemic bone, and has been postulated to improve circulation. The outcome from core decompression at the femoral head, with regards to resolution of radiographic changes and improvement in symptoms, varies from 34–95% in the early stages of the disease. These results appear better than continuing with conservative measures such as non-weight bearing. In the later stages, joint

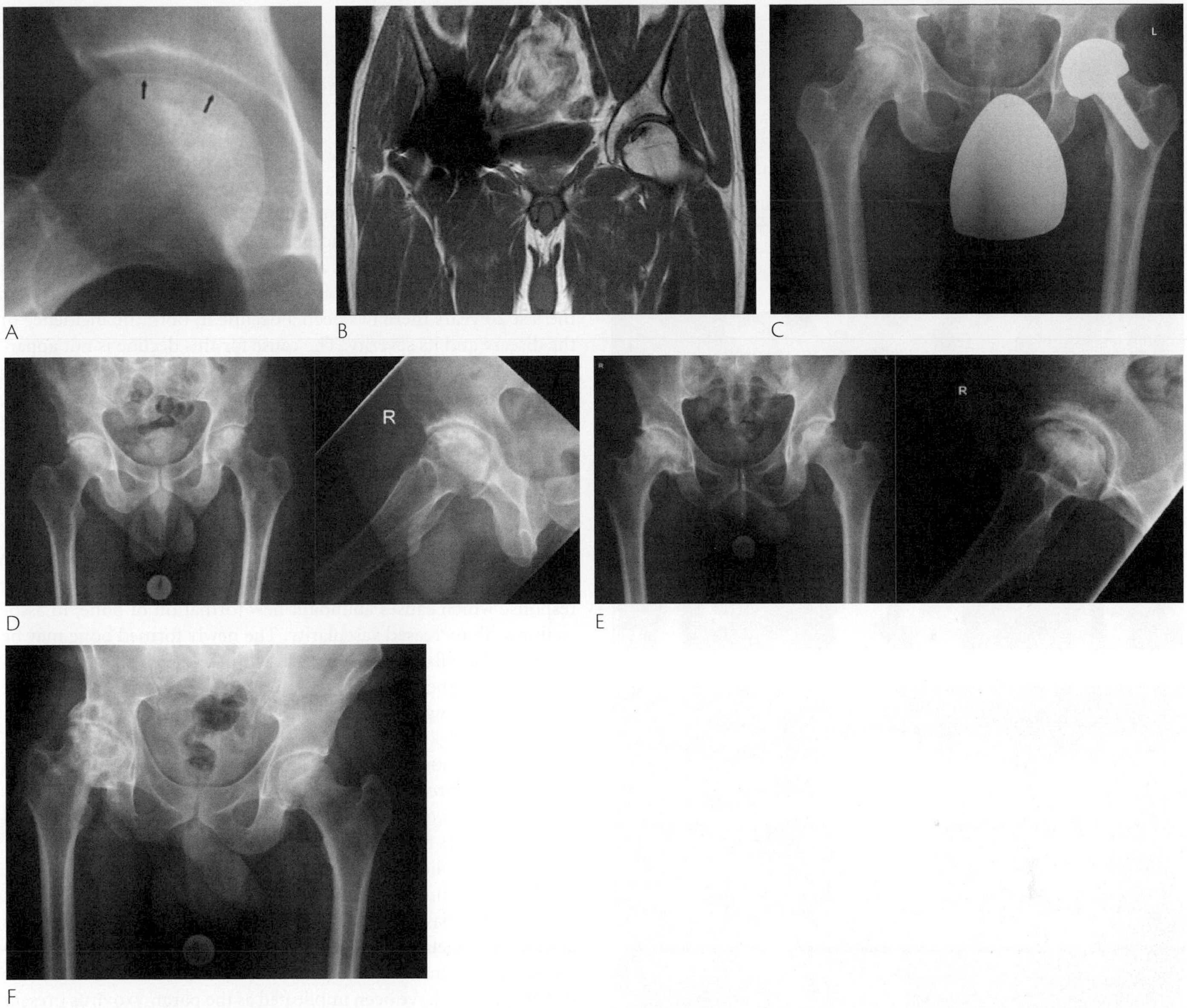

Fig. 7.16.1 Radiological changes in hip avascular necrosis. A) Area of subchondral hyperlucency (arrows)—the crescent sign. B) MRI showing an area of avascular necrosis present in the subarticular location of the left femoral head. There is artefact obscuring the right hemipelvis due to previous prosthetic replacement. C) AVN affecting the right hip with signs of previous decompression. A left Birmingham mid-head resurfacing arthroplasty has been performed for AVN on the left hip. D) Stage 4 AVN: radiolucent and sclerotic changes involve most of the femoral head, with flattening of the articular surface. E) Stage 5 AVN: sclerosis, lucency, flattening of the articular surface, and narrowing of the joint space right hip. F) Stage 6 AVN with joint destruction right hip.

Box 7.16.2 Avascular necrosis

- Often associated with other conditions, commonly secondary to trauma, steroids, and alcoholism
- Commonest site is the femoral head; presents with pain, exacerbated by weight bearing
- Graded from 0–6
- Treatment varies from non-weight bearing, prostacyclin, and bisphosphonates in the earlier stages to surgical decompression and joint replacement in later stages.

replacement is often necessary. Box 7.16.2 summarizes the key points relating to osteonecrosis.

Transient osteoporosis of the hip (Box 7.16.3)

This is a rare, self-limiting disorder. It can present idiopathically or may be seen in the third trimester of pregnancy. The cause is unknown, although it is thought to be related to local factors rather than a systemic cause.

Patients will present with unilateral or bilateral hip/groin pain. In some severe cases the condition can progress to hip fracture.

Box 7.16.3 Transient osteoporosis of the hip

- Rare, self-limiting. Can be idiopathic or associated with third trimester of pregnancy
- Presents with hip/groin pain and occasionally may fracture
- Diagnosed with plain radiographs, bone scan, or MRI
- Non-surgical treatment with non-weight bearing or bisphonates

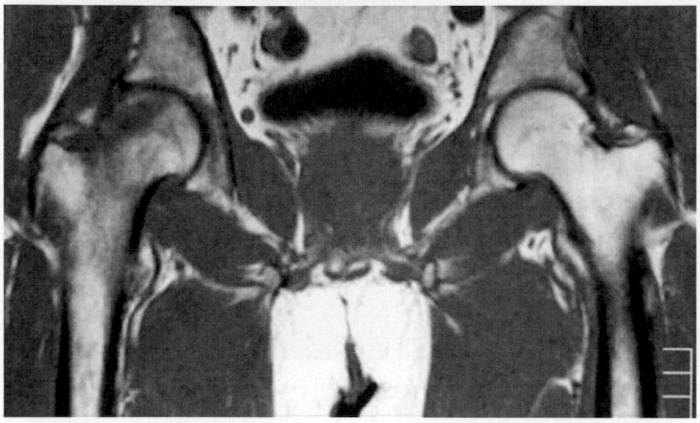
A

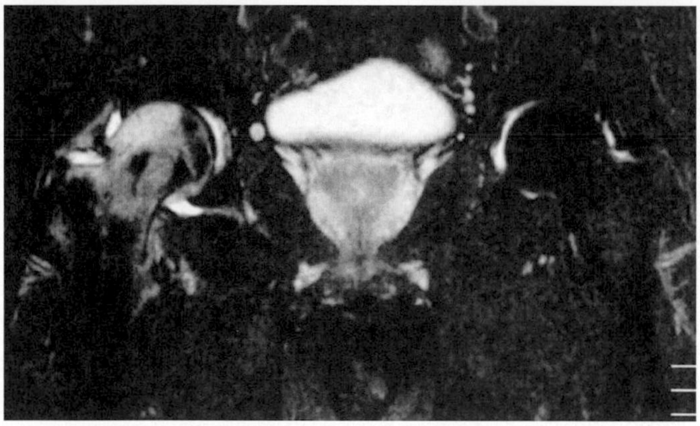
B

Fig. 7.16.2 A) Diffusely decreased signal intensity in the right femoral head and neck on T_1-weighted images and B) increased signal intensity in the same areas on T_2-weighted images. (Reproduced from Niimi, R., Sudo, A., Hasegawa, M., Fukuda, A., and Uchida, A. (2006). Changes in bone mineral density in transient osteoporosis of the hip. *Journal of Bone and Joint Surgery*, **88**B(11), 1438–40.)

In a small minority of cases the condition can migrate to affect either the contralateral hip or another skeletal site. There is evidence of radiological osteoporosis, assessed either with plain radiographs or dual energy x-ray absorptiometry (DXA). MRI demonstrates evidence of marrow oedema within the femoral head and/or neck (Figure 7.16.2). A joint effusion may also be present. The features may be similar to those for avascular necrosis.

The symptoms and the radiological features will generally resolve within 6–9 months. Patients may be managed with non-weight bearing if there is thought to be risk of hip fracture. Bisphosphonates have been shown to accelerate recovery in some patients.

Paget's disease

Paget's disease is the second most common metabolic bone disease in the United Kingdom. It was first described in 1877 by Sir James Paget (Box 7.16.4).

Epidemiology

The disease rarely becomes clinically evident before the age of 40 years, and shows an exponential increase in prevalence with age. Overall, the disease prevalence in the United Kingdom is estimated at 5% in those aged 55 years and over, rising to upwards of 10% in those aged 95 years. Recent epidemiological data suggest that over the last 20 years there has been a decline in both the incidence of the disease and its severity. The cause for this decline is not apparent, but suggests a possible environmental agent as an important activator in the disease process. Most studies have reported a slight sex bias, with men affected slightly more frequently than women, with ratios ranging from 7:6 to 2:1.

Pathogenesis

Paget's disease is a focal disorder of bone metabolism, primarily due to an increase in osteoclast-related bone resorption. The increased bone resorption is coupled with a vigorous osteoblastic response which causes abundant new formation of bone, in association with increased vascularity. The newly formed bone may be woven or lamellar in type (usually with abnormal spatial orientation), lacking the structural organization of the normal trabeculae and hence having greater flexibility and less resistance to deformation. Paget's disease is also usually associated with local enlargement of bone, suggesting that abnormal modelling is also involved in the disease process. The combination of structural and architectural bone abnormalities, in conjunction with biomechanical forces, accounts for the majority of the disease's clinical manifestations and complications.

The initial stimulus for increased bone turnover is unknown. Many studies have suggested a possible viral aetiology for Paget's disease, as pagetic osteoclasts have been found to contain paramyxoviral-like nuclear inclusions. The measles virus and the canine distemper virus have been implicated as the paramyxovirus present in pagetic osteoclasts and their precursors, although to date the viral material has not been isolated and their role in disease pathophysiology remains controversial.

Paget's disease has been demonstrated to have a familial tendency, suggesting a possible genetic cause for the disease. In patients with Paget's disease, 30–40% have been shown to have a first-degree relative similarly affected. In addition, several pedigrees have been identified where Paget's disease appears to be segregating as an autosomal dominant trait. To date, mutations or polymorphisms have been identified in four genes that cause classic Paget's disease or related syndromes. These genes include TNFRSF11A which encodes RANK, TNFRSF11B which encodes OPG, VCP which encodes p97, and SQSTM1 which encodes p62.

Clinical features

Paget's disease can have a wide spectrum of clinical presentations, ranging from asymptomatic to painful, disabling, and, very rarely, life threatening. In the majority of cases (greater than 80%), however, the disease is asymptomatic and is only diagnosed on the basis of an isolated increase in serum alkaline phosphatase or on

Table 7.16.2 Complications associated with Paget's disease

Focal	**Skeletal**	◆ Bone pain ◆ Bone enlargement ◆ Bone deformity ◆ Dental involvement
	Articular	◆ Secondary osteoarthritis
	Neurogical	◆ Deafness ◆ Hydrocephalus ◆ Nerve root compression ◆ Spinal cord compression ◆ Pagetic steal syndrome
Local	**Fractures**	◆ Fissure ◆ Pathological
	Malignancy	◆ Sarcoma ◆ Giant cell tumour
Systemic	**Cardiovascular**	◆ High output cardiac failure
	Metabolic	◆ Immobilization hypercalcaemia/hypercalciuria ◆ Secondary hyperparathyroidism
	Skeletal	◆ Increased vertebral fracture risk

classical radiological appearances following imaging. The clinical presentation of the disease is also dependent on the skeletal sites affected by pagetic lesions and their activity. Although any part of the skeleton may be affected, most commonly involved bones are the pelvis, femur, lumbar spine, skull, and tibia. The complications arising from Paget's disease can be attributable to local factors and to systemic factors. These are summarized in Table 7.16.2.

The most frequent symptom in patients with Paget's disease is bone pain. It has been suggested that this symptom is due both to increased vascular supply and to periosteal stretching caused by local bone growth. Pagetic pain is classically described as insidious and boring in nature, not usually aggravated by movement, and only progresses slowly. Sometimes, the pain also coexists with bone deformity and enlargement. In some cases it is difficult, however, to differentiate between pain due to Paget's disease and that due to secondary osteoarthritis and degenerative disease. Primary bone pain must also be differentiated from pain associated with certain complications of great clinical significance, i.e. fractures and sarcomatous change.

Painful fissure fracture (or pseudofracture) and complete pathological fracture occur in areas of high mechanical stress, particularly in the weight-bearing bones of the lower limbs. Fractures in pagetic bone usually follow very minimal trauma. The great majority of these are located in the subtrochanteric region or shaft of the femur and, less often, in the upper third of the tibia. Occasionally they are also seen at other sites such as the forearm, humerus or pelvic brim. Prolonged immobilization should be avoided following fractures in patients with Paget's disease as it can accelerate bone loss (leading to osteoporosis and an increased fracture risk) and can provoke hypercalciuria and hypercalcaemia.

Sarcoma arising in pagetic bone is the most serious complication of the disease, although is a rare event affecting fewer than 1% of Paget's patients. Sarcomatous change should be suspected when severe pain of sudden onset arises in bone known to have been previously affected by the disease. Such pain is usually unresponsive both to analgesics and medical therapy aimed to suppress pagetic disease activity. Other clues pointing towards a possible sarcoma include swelling at the site of the tumour, which may enlarge rapidly, and a significant rise in the serum total alkaline phosphatase. At present, the prognosis for patients with Paget's disease who develop sarcoma is poor with neither chemotherapy nor radical surgery having any significant effect on long-term survival.

Radiological features (Figure 7.16.3)

Plain radiographs are normally sufficient to make a diagnosis of Paget's disease. Additional investigations that may be required include isotope bone scan, CT, and MRI.

Laboratory findings

The main biochemical abnormality in Paget's disease is an increase in the serum total and bone-specific alkaline phosphatase (ALP). The extent of the increase in the ALP is proportionate to the number of skeletal sites involved, and in some patients with mild disease where there is little skeletal involvement the ALP may be normal.

In cases where the diagnosis is not clear, bone biopsy is indicated.

Differential diagnosis

The differential diagnosis includes osteomalacia, osteitis fibrosa, fibrous dysplasia, fibrogenesis imperfecta ossium, and metastatic bone disease.

Management

Historically medical treatment for Paget's disease has been reserved for the symptomatic management of pain in patients with active disease, or as an adjunct to surgery in those with serious complications (i.e. spinal cord compression). There are now a number of available therapies which have been successfully used to suppress abnormal osteoclast activity and control bone turnover. The treatment of choice would now be a bisphosphonate. With the advent of these agents, there is now a move to treat the disease earlier in either patients whose disease is only mildly active or in those who are asymptomatic. It remains unclear, however, whether this aggressive treatment of Paget's disease to normalize disease activity (as assessed by serum alkaline phosphatase or radionuclide imaging) will result in fewer long-term complications.

Surgical management

Surgery may be necessary for patients with severe complications, as highlighted earlier. The more common indication for surgery is in patients with secondary osteoarthritis who have pain that is not adequately controlled with conventional medical therapies. In these circumstances, total joint arthroplasty at both the hip and

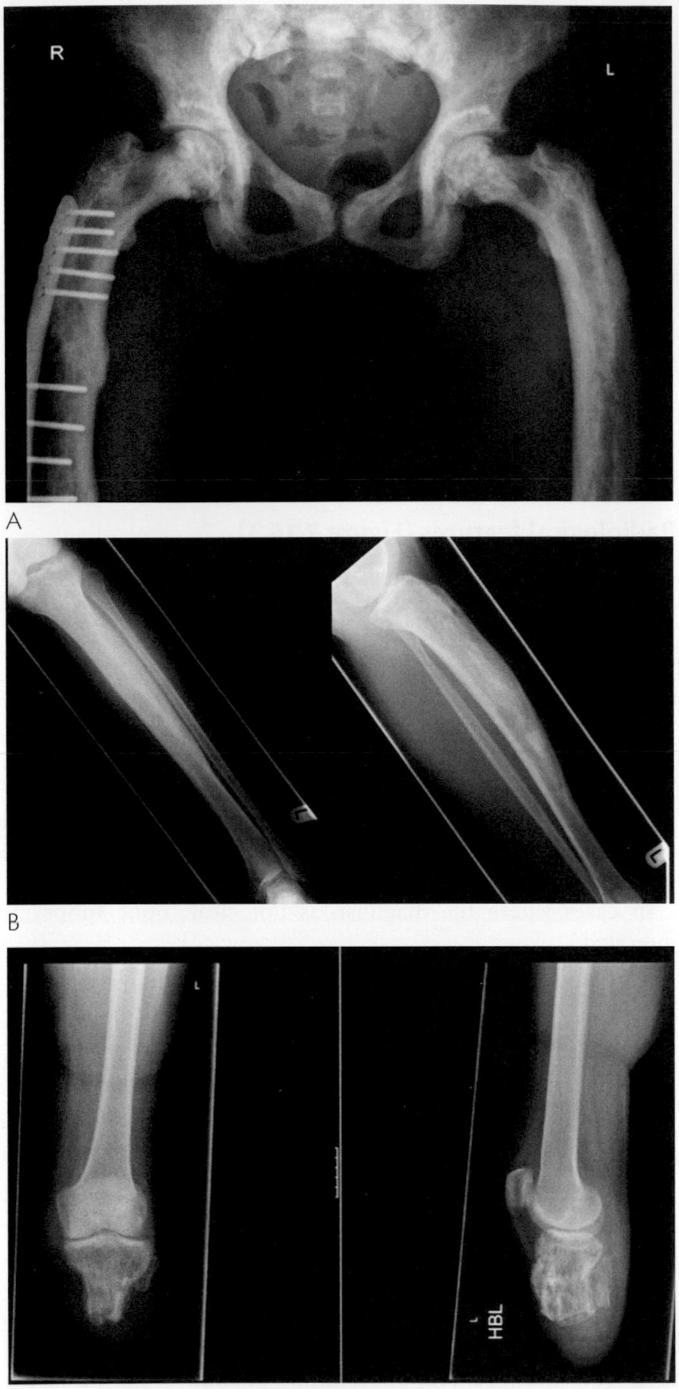

Fig. 7.16.3 Radiographic features of Paget's disease: sclerosis, coarse trabeculae, and remodelled cortices. A) Involving the pelvis and proximal femora; features of osteopetrosis also noted and pathological right femoral shaft fracture (internally fixed). B) Tibia with typical Paget's deformity. C) Tibia with residual Paget's proximally and below-knee amputation following sarcomatous change.

Box 7.16.4 Paget's disease

- Paget's is a focal disorder of bone metabolism
- Primarily due to an increase in osteoclast-related bone resorption, coupled with a vigorous osteoblastic response causing abundant new bone formation in association with increased vascularity. Abnormal remodelling is also involved, leading to a combination of structural and architectural bone abnormalities
- Often asymptomatic and found incidentally. Common sites are the pelvis, femur, lumbar spine, skull, and tibia. Commonest symptom is pain
- Diagnosed radiographically often, and with raised ALP
- Treated with bisphosphonates; surgery directed towards the complications of Paget's.

knee has been shown to be effective and safe in patients with Paget's disease. There has been concern that the operative procedures may be more difficult with surgery involving pagetic bone, and although not evidence based, many patients receive bisphosphonates treatment preoperatively in an attempt to suppress disease activity and reduce local complications. This area of practice requires further evaluation. In addition, although there has been long-term (between 5–10-year) follow-up of Paget's patients undergoing total hip arthroplasty, only limited data is available for those with total knee arthroplasty and again research is needed in this area. Most of the reported studies regarding surgical outcome have also focused on specialist centres, and it remains to be determined if outcomes are equivalent at other less specialized orthopaedic units.

Further reading

Disch, A.C., Matziolis, G., Perka, C. (2005). The management of necrosis-associated and idiopathic bone-marrow oedema of the proximal femur by intravenous iloprost. *Journal of Bone and Joint Surgery*, **87B**, 560–4.

Lai, K.A., Shen, W.J., Yang, C.Y., Shao, C.J., Hsu, J.T., and Lin, R.M. (2005). The use of alendronate to prevent early collapse of the femoral head in patients with nontraumatic osteonecrosis. A randomized clinical study. *Journal of Bone and Joint Surgery*, **87B**, 2155–9.

Liu, Y.F., Chen, W.M., Lin, Y.F., *et al.* (2005). Type II collagen gene variants and inherited osteonecrosis of the femoral head. *New England Journal of Medicine*, **352**, 2294–301.

Ralston, S.H., Langston, A.L., and Reid, I.R. (2008). Pathogenesis and management of Paget's disease of bone. *Lancet*, **372**, 155–63.

Steinberg, M.E. and Steinberg, D.R. (1991). Avascular necrosis of the femoral head. In: Steinberg, M.E. (ed) *The Hip and its Disorders*, pp. 623–47. Philadelphia, PA: W.B. Saunders.

7.17

Hip pain in the radiologically normal hip

Aresh Hashemi-Nejad

Summary points

- Patients who present with hip pain can have multiple origins of pathology—this may be intra- or extra-articular in origin
- In the majority, a definable diagnosis can be obtained through a detailed history, examination, and subsequent radiological evaluation
- However, there remains a group of patients who have intractable hip pain without a definitive diagnosis despite extensive non-invasive radiological investigation.

History

A detailed history is vital in the assessment of hip pain. Any history of trauma and the mechanism of injury should be noted. Overuse of the hip or an abrupt change in the level of activity may point towards a musculotendinous injury. Previous muscle strains or other injury should be documented.

The site, nature of the pain, location, duration, frequency, pattern, or radiation of pain should be recorded. The onset may be acute or insidious. There may be positions or activities which exacerbate the pain. There may be loss of function with inability to participate in certain activities or pain with sitting for prolonged periods.

The site of the pain can be an important indicator of its source. It aids in differentiating intra-articular pain from extra-articular pain (Table 7.17.1).

Table 7.17.1 Differential diagnosis of hip pain by site

Site of pain	Possible cause	
Anterior	Intra-articular	Arthritis Femoroacetabular impingement Labral pathology Loose bodies Chondral lesions Synovitis
	Extra-articular	Rectus femoris tendonitis Iliopsoas tendonitis Adductor tendonitis Ostetis pubis
	Referred pain	L2 nerve root compression Intra-abdominal/pelvic pathology
Lateral	Peritrochanteric space	Tensor fascia lata snapping Trochanteric bursitis Gluteus medius/minimus tendonitis/tears
Posterior	Local	Piriformis syndrome
	Referred pain	Lumbar spine radicular pain

Mechanical symptoms may be present. This also helps in not only differentiating intra-articular and extra-articular pathology but also inflammatory conditions which tend to have pain at rest and multiple joint involvement. The snapping hip is discussed in the 'Coxa saltans' section. Pinching or clicking may indicate a labral tear. A pop may be heard with an acute tendon injury. A change in sensibility or weakness in the leg may indicate pressure from an intervertebral disc. Relevant occupational and recreational history is important. Certain sports such as football, marathon running, gymnastics, and rugby have been associated with an increased incidence of degenerative hip disease.

A drug history should include amount of alcohol consumption and use of corticosteroids. Past medical history should enquire about the presence of any connective tissue and chronic inflammatory conditions as well as any history of carcinoma. Red flag symptoms include weight loss, fatigue, fever, or loss of appetite. Sepsis must be excluded. Abdominal and pelvic pathology such as appendicitis, prostatitis, and gynaecological conditions may masquerade as hip pain and should be considered.

Examination

Thorough examination of the hip should include examination of the lumbar spine and ipsilateral knee to rule out referred pain. Perform a full neurological examination of the lower extremities with assessment of sensation and motor power. Pain on resisted range of movement suggests a muscular or tendinous injury. Muscle weakness and altered sensation may be identified with nerve root compression. Straight leg raise and the sciatic stretch test may exclude referred radicular pain.

Investigation

Blood tests

Primary investigation of hip pain includes blood tests, including inflammatory markers.

Plain radiographs

A plain x-ray (anteroposterior and lateral) will exclude in the majority osteoarthritis, fracture, or avascular necrosis. The frog lateral radiograph is extremely useful in diagnosing and assessing the extent of avascular necrosis. Plain radiographs are unreliable in the diagnosis of un-mineralized loose bodies, labral tears, or chondral lesion. The signs of femoroacetabular impingement (FAI) are subtle and may also be missed.

Ultrasound

An ultrasound scan can be used to detect fluid within the joint, thickened or torn tendons, or fluid-filled bursae. Dynamic ultrasound can be used to find the source of a snapping hip, particularly a snapping iliopsoas tendon.

Magnetic resonance imaging

Magnetic resonance imaging (MRI) will demonstrate tendon thickening. Labral tears can be seen with the injection of contrast and are most reliably seen on the axial slices. In the presence of inflammation (iliopsoas and/or trochanteric bursitis or gluteus tendon tears) or fluid, there may be high signal intensity on T_2 scans. Both ultrasound and MRI can be used to help guide injections. MRI of the lumbar spine may exclude radicular causes of pain.

MRI and bone scans are indicated for suspicion of stress fractures in athletes and can aid the diagnosis of degenerative conditions and tumours.

Examination under anaesthesia

If still in doubt, examine under anaesthesia, assessing range of movement. A dynamic arthrogram is useful to assess congruency and stability. Intra-articular injection of local anaesthetic may help differentiate between intra-articular and extra-articular hip pain. Local anaesthetic and steroid injections into the trochanteric and iliopsas bursa are useful diagnostic tests and potentially therapeutic benefit.

Electromyogram studies may be useful in the assessment of extra pelvic compression of sciatic nerve.

Differential diagnosis

Labral tears

The diagnosis of a labral tear can be made on a clinical basis. Symptoms of a labral tear are analogous to those who present with meniscal tear.

The history may be of an acute traumatic event or related to overuse, especially in athletes. The pain may be positional or induced with activity that fails to relieve with rest. There may be an associated feeling of instability. Patients describe catching and painful clicking of the hip with restricted range of movement. Clicking can often be misdiagnosed as a snapping iliotibial or hypermobile psoas tendon.

FAI may predispose to labral tears. It is a common cause of hip pain in young adults. Morphological abnormalities of the hip result in abnormal loading and impingement. X-rays may appear normal at first, or there may be the presence of an acetabular subchondral cyst. The impingement test (flexion, adduction and internal rotation—FADIR test) is almost always positive. However, a negative FADIR test does not exclude a labral tear. A dynamic arthrogram will demonstrate impingement and labral tears in the majority. A magnetic resonance arthrogram (MRA) will also demonstrate a labral tear in the majority of cases.

Coxa saltans

Coxa saltans is described as external, internal, or intra-articular. The external type is the commonest. Outside of the hip joint a tight iliotibial band (or the anterior border of gluteus maximus) can cause an audible or palpable snap as it translates forward over the greater trochanter in flexion or adduction of the hip. A tight iliotibial band can also be demonstrated with the Ober test: with the patient lying on the unaffected side, passively abduct the upper leg and flex the knee to 90 degrees. Slightly extend the hip, and observe if the hip drops into the adducted position. Decreased adduction is a sign of tightness in the tensor fasciae latae and/or the iliotibial band.

Internal causes of coxa saltans are less common. The psoas tendon is felt to snap as it moves over structures located behind it. These include the iliopectineal eminence, a prominent inflamed iliopsoas bursa, the anterior inferior iliac spine, or, in some cases, the femoral head or prominent acetabular components following total hip replacement surgery.

Intra-articular causes of the snapping hip include loose bodies and labral tears or synovial chondromatosis.

The snapping hip can be voluntary and painless but may be painful especially with repetitive movement such as dancing or sport. There is an audible, palpable, and sometimes visible snap, usually as a muscle or tendon moves over a bony prominence. It is more common in the young athlete and women are more commonly affected than men. Athletes whose sport involves repetitive twisting about the hip have been identified as being particularly prone to develop a clicking hip

Bursitis

The bursae are fluid-filled sacs lined with a membrane similar to synovium. They may be normal, in areas where soft tissues are found to move over bony prominences, or they may develop as a result of repeated trauma. They serve to protect tissues from friction or pressure. Independently they are susceptible to acute or chronic inflammation and infection but may also commonly be involved in inflammatory conditions of an underlying joint.

Inflammation of the trochanteric bursae, separating the gluteal muscles from the greater trochanter, is a common cause of lateral hip pain. There may be visible swelling and tenderness over the prominent greater trochanter.

The iliopectineal bursa lies posterior to the iliopsoas muscle. It is the largest bursa of the hip. Inflammation may result in anterior hip pain with resistance to extension. There may be a palpable mass. Mild bursitis can cause a snapping hip syndrome (see earlier).

On T_2-weighted MRI scans, high signal may be seen in the presence of fluid within the trochanteric or iliopsoas bursae.

Tendonitis and muscle strains

Injuries to musculotendinous units usually occur with overuse (repetitive activity) or overload (sudden increase in activity). Symptoms can vary depending on the severity of strain or inflammation present.

Predisposing factors include abrupt change in level of activity, poor warm up, or a history of previous strains. These injuries can become chronic if not treated early and are significant causes of disability for athletic individuals.

A strain of the rectus muscle usually occurs in its middle third. There is pain and swelling over the anterior thigh with tenderness but little functional loss. Ecchymosis may be seen.

Gluteus medius syndrome is often seen in women who start vigorous walking or a new exercise programme. There will be tenderness over the insertion of gluteus medius and in severe cases a Trendelenburg gait. Gluteal tendonitis can be difficult to differentiate from a trochanteric bursitis. Resisted abduction will elicit pain in the gluteus medius tendon and, if still in doubt, an ultrasound or MRI scan can exclude fluid in the bursal sac.

Adductor strains are commonly seen in athletes. Following rapid deceleration or strong eccentric contractions of the muscle during activities such as kicking, a pop is heard and there is immediate pain and disability. Adductor longus is commonly affected. Pain is felt on palpation of muscle belly or over its insertion and on resisted contraction. Strains of the hamstring muscles occur with acceleration injuries, seen with sprinting or court sports.

Avulsion fractures around the pelvis occur in prepubertal athletes as a result of an actively contracting muscle encountering abrupt resistance such as a misstep, rapid acceleration, or eccentric movements.

Piriformis syndrome

Piriformis syndrome is usually a diagnosis of exclusion. It is a rare cause of posterior hip pain and it can be confused with sciatica. It often presents with intolerance to sitting and numbness and tenderness over the sciatic notch. Pain may be reproduced by bringing the hip into maximum flexion and internal rotation.

Blunt trauma is thought to result in haematoma formation and scarring between the muscle and the closely-related sciatic nerve. Branches of the nerve may in some cases pass through piriformis muscle resulting in further compression of the nerve on internal rotation.

There are six classical findings: trauma to the sacroiliac and gluteal region; pain in the region of the sacroiliac joint, greater sciatic notch, and piriformis that extends down the leg; exacerbation of pain with stooping or lifting; a palpable sausage-shape mass over piriformis muscle; positive straight leg raise; and gluteal atrophy depending on the duration of symptoms.

Management

Labral tears are increasingly managed by hip arthroscopy. The tears can either be debrided or repaired. Similarly, loose bodies can be removed arthroscopically in the majority. In the presence of FAI, debridement of either the acetabular rim and or the head-neck junction can be undertaken arthroscopically or, less commonly, via a mini open approach.

Snapping hip is usually painless and this can be managed by providing an explanation reassurance to the patient. In cases where the patient complains of pain, most respond to behaviour modification, physiotherapy with stretching exercises, and non-steroidal anti-inflammatory drugs (NSAIDs). In individuals who fail to respond to this treatment, a combination of local anaesthetic and steroid injection into the underlying trochanteric or iliopsoas bursa may be helpful. If symptoms are recurrent and painful, surgery can be undertaken either arthroscopically or via open surgery.

The management of bursitis includes rest, alteration in activity, and NSAIDs. There is often good response to aspiration and injection of steroids. In chronic cases, excision of the thickened bursa may be necessary. This can be undertaken either arthroscopically or via open surgery.

Tendonitis caused by overuse or overload injuries usually respond well to relative rest, ice, and anti-inflammatory medications. Use of orthotics may be beneficial where there are mechanical abnormalities, such as leg-length inequality or foot abnormalities. Muscle imbalance should be treated with appropriate flexibility and strengthening exercise programmes. Increasing joint flexibility and muscle strengthening exercises will prevent the risk of future injury.

The treatment of smaller avulsion fractures is similar to the treatment of strains of the muscle–tendon unit. Large avulsion fractures may need to be internally fixed.

Initial management of piriformis syndrome should again be conservative with stretching, physiotherapy, and NSAIDs. Some may respond to transrectal massage or electrical stimulation. Surgery in non-responsive cases involves release of the tendon and lysis of adhesions surrounding the nerve.

Further reading

Benson, E.R. and Schutzer, F. (1999). Posttraumatic piriformis syndrome: diagnosis and results of operative treatment. *Journal of Bone and Joint Surgery*, **81A**, 941–9.

McCarthy, J.C. (2002). *Early Hip Disorders. Advances in Detection and Minimally Invasive Treatment.* Boston, MA: Springer.

Meyers, W.C., Foley, D.P., Garrett, W.E., *et al.* (2000). Management of severe lower abdominal or inguinal pain in high performance athletes. *American Journal of Sports Medicine*, **28**, 2–8.

Peter, C.L. and Erickson, J. (2006). The etiology and treatment of hip pain in the young adult. *Journal of Bone and Joint Surgery*, **88A**, 20–6.

7.18

Hip arthroscopy: assessment, investigations, and interventions

Parminder J. Singh, John M. O'Donnell, and Richard E. Field

Summary points

- Learning objectives:
  - Understand hip arthroscopic anatomy
  - Awareness of indications and contraindications for hip arthroscopy
  - Understand what femoroacetabular impingement (FAI) is, and how to investigate and treat this condition
- Assessment: FADIR and FABER tests
- Investigations: plain x-ray, magnetic resonance imaging/arthroscopy, computed tomography scan in Pritchard O'Donnell (POD) position
- Interventions: central and peripheral compartments, periarticular space, lateral compartment, FAI correction—cam, pincer, or combined.

Introduction

The development of arthroscopic surgery to the hip joint has been slow for two reasons. Firstly, the hip is relatively difficult to access. Secondly, unlike the knee, shoulder, and abdomen, open procedures were not routinely undertaken on the hip so there was nothing to be superseded by arthroscopic techniques.

Arthroscopic examination of cadaveric hips was first described by Burman in 1931. Until 2003, hip arthroscopy was a procedure undertaken by enthusiasts to diagnose synovial pathologies, to remove intra-articular loose bodies, to resect damaged labral tissue, to debride damaged ligamentum teres ligaments, and to debride joints with early to moderate degenerative disease. Since the publication of Ganz's work on femoroacetabular impingement (FAI), orthopaedic surgeons have developed both open and arthroscopic strategies to address the damage caused by these mechanisms. With growing recognition of the efficacy and benefits of these interventions it has also become apparent that arthroscopic interventions achieve comparable outcomes, with less morbidity. In consequence, the orthopaedic community is gaining interest in learning and undertaking arthroscopic hip surgery.

As with all developing technologies, subdivision is inevitable. In the case of the hip, three distinct areas of intervention have evolved. These are:

1) The hip joint (central and peripheral compartments)
2) The periarticular space (ilio psoas tendon and periarticular structures)
3) The lateral compartment (trochanteric regions).

Arthroscopic anatomy

From the hip arthroscopist's perspective, the hip joint comprises central and peripheral compartments which are separated by the acetabular labrum (Figure 7.18.1). The central compartment can only be visualized when the bearing surfaces are separated through application of traction and fluid insufflation. While much of the peripheral compartment can be visualized while the hip is distracted, it is only after removal of traction and re-enlocation of the femoral head that joint movement can be visualized, FAI verified, and confirmation obtained that interventions have been effective.

The lateral compartment is deep to the tensor fascia lata. Arthroscopic access to this space allows visualization and interventions to the trochanteric bursa and gluteus medius and minimus tendons.

Indications, surgical techniques, and instrumentation for arthoscopic hip surgery are evolving and improving rapidly. To date, the majority of articles on hip arthroscopy provide anecdotal information, case reports, or results of short-term outcome studies. As yet, relatively few medium- and long-term outcome studies are available.

Indications for hip arthroscopy

Current indications for hip arthroscopy include: the presence of symptomatic acetabular labral tears; FAI; chondral lesions; osteochondritis dissecans; ligamentum teres injuries; snapping hip syndrome; iliopsoas bursitis; unexplained symptoms post-hip replacement; and removal of loose bodies.

Less common indications include: management of osteonecrosis of the femoral head; synovial abnormalities; crystalline hip

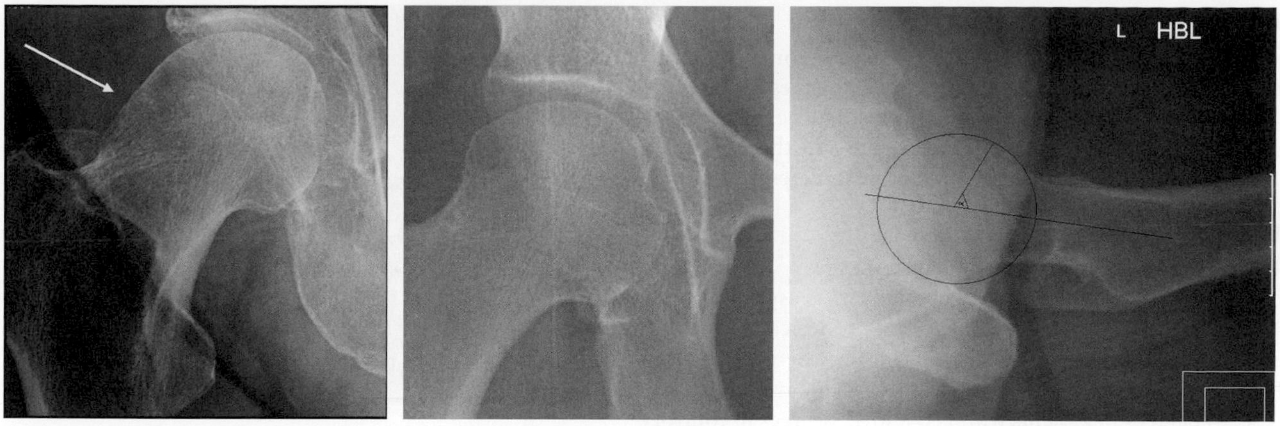

A B C

Fig. 7.18.1 A) Cam lesion. B) Coxa Profunda. C) Cross-table lateral.

arthropathy (gout and pseudogout); infection and post-traumatic haematomas; and intra-articular debris.

Some hip arthroscopists have noted that the symptoms of mild-to-moderate hip osteoarthritis can be temporized; particularly when peripheral osteophytes are causing mechanical symptoms. The benefit and duration of improvement are variable and these interventions require further evaluation.

Contraindications to hip arthroscopy

Conditions that limit the potential for hip distraction may preclude arthroscopy. These include: advanced osteoarthritis; osteonecrosis with femoral head collapse; significant protrusion; grade III or IV heterotopic bone; and joint ankylosis.

Types of impingement

Two distinctive types of FAI are recognized. 'Pincer impingement' occurs as a result of anterior overcoverage of the acetabulum or acetabular retroversion. 'Cam impingement' occurs when a non-spherical femoral head abuts against the anterior acetabulum, usually with the hip in flexion. In practice, it is common to see a mixed cam and pincer pathology, occurring along the anterior femoral neck and the anterior–superior acetabular rim.

Clinical presentation

Patients with hip impingement typically present with pain deep to the anterior portion of the tensor fascia lata muscle. In cases where cam impingement predominates, symptoms are often precipitated by prolonged upright sitting and internal rotation movement in flexion. Where pincer-type impingement predominates, abduction and external rotation movements may be more troublesome. A significant proportion of female patients with impingement will report exacerbation of their symptoms during sexual intercourse. Athletes, sportspeople, and dancers typically describe pain on training and early fatigue. These symptoms will improve with rest but always recur on resumption of exercise.

Clinical examination findings

A standard examination of the hip joint will often reveal asymmetric ranges of movement and evidence of irritability. Cases of cam impingement typically show reduced internal rotation of the hip in flexion. This may be bilateral. In cases of pincer-type impingement, ranges of movement may appear normal but with pain towards the extremes of movement.

Specific tests for impingement are:

- **FADIR test** With the hip in high flexion, adduction, and internal rotation (FADIR), abutment and impingement of the labrum and cartilage occurs. The reproducibility of this examination technique has been reported with a kappa value of 0.58 (95% CI: 0.29–0.87)
- **FABER test** With the hip in flexion, abduction, and external rotation (FABER), abutment of the abutment of the labrum and cartilage also can occur. The reproducibility of this examination technique has been reported with a kappa value of 0.63 (95% CI: 0.43–0.83).

Investigations

Plain radiographs

The first imaging study that should be requested is for plain x-rays of the hips. These should comprise an AP standing view of both hips, a standard lateral of the affected hip, and a cross-table true lateral of the affected hip. The AP view should be assessed both for degenerative changes and also evidence of the cam type deformity shown in Figure 7.18.1A and the profunda socket shown in Figure 7.18.1B, as well as the cross-over sign, indicating a prominent anterior acetabular wall, or acetabular retroversion.

The standard lateral view will reveal subchondral sclerosis and early subchondral cyst formation of the anterior acetabular rim and the cross-table true lateral will profile cam deformity or lack of concavity of the anterior head neck junction (Figure 7.18.1C).

Magnetic resonance arthrography

Where labral pathology is suspected, magnetic resonance (MR) arthrography is the preferred investigation. While these scans will show articular cartilage thinning, the contrast will seldom penetrate beneath delaminating articular cartilage and the extent of peripheral articular cartilage instability may be underestimated.

Alpha angles

Notzli and colleagues compared MR images obtained in 39 patients with FAI with MR images obtained in 35 asymptomatic control subjects. They measured the non-spherical shape of the femoral head–neck junction by measuring the alpha angle (see Figure 7.18.1C) at the anterior position. The average alpha angle was 74 degrees in patients with FAI and 42 degrees in control subjects (P=0.001). A cut-off angle of 55 degrees was proposed to diagnose FAI.

Pritchard and O'Donnell computed tomography scan

Where the shape of the femoral head–neck junction needs to be assessed for the presence of a cam deformity, computed tomography (CT) three-dimensional surface reconstructions allow the lesion to be visualized and surgical resection planned (Figure 7.18.2A).

A new CT view has been developed by Pritchard and O'Donnell (the POD view) to demonstrate FAI lesions. Figure 7.18.3A shows an axial CT scan through the hip of a patient with a typical cam deformity. A fibrocystic impingement lesion of the anterior head–neck junction is seen but no evidence of joint space compromise. In Figure 7.18.3B, the same hip has been scanned in the POD position (patient supine with the hip flexed, adducted, and internally rotated). The scan reveals the impingement lesions and also confirms articular cartilage loss at the point of impingement.

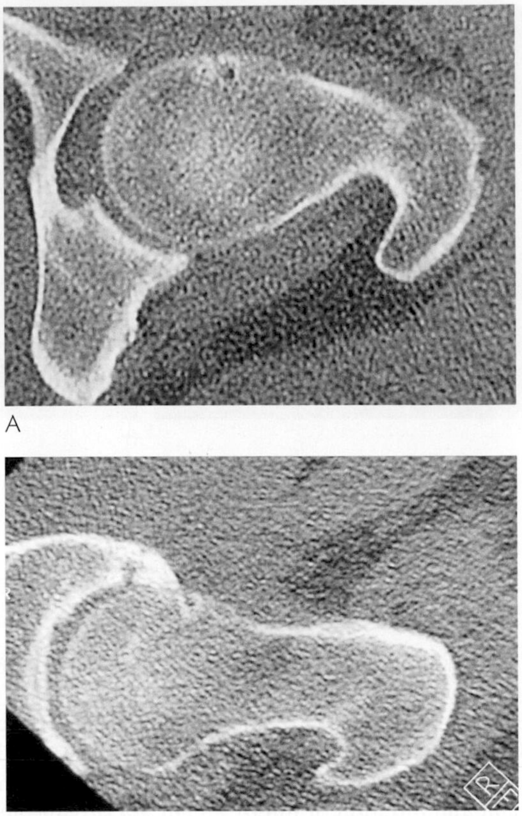

A

B

Fig. 7.18.3 A) Standard axial CT scan. B) Pritchard and O'Donnell (POD) protocol CT scan.

Treatment

Hip arthroscopy

Hip arthroscopy can be undertaken either in the supine or lateral decubitus position. Either the central or the peripheral compartment may be visualized first, and the use of an image intensifier may be used to facilitate portal placement.

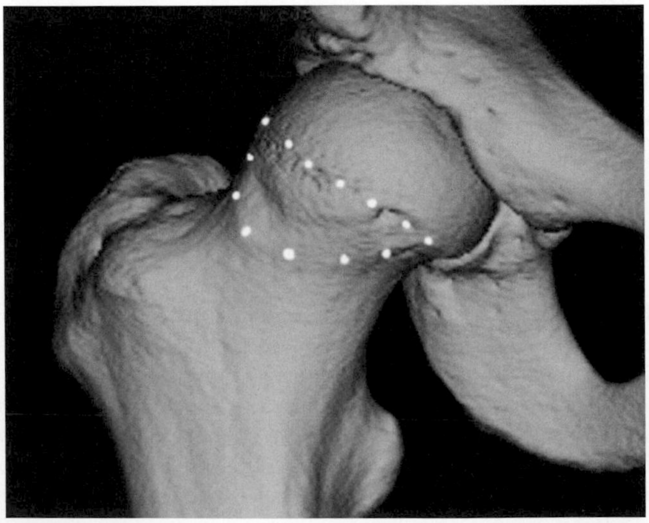

Fig. 7.18.2 A preoperative plan showing the marking out the bone for resection.

To enter the central compartment the limb is placed in traction with the leg in abduction and slight forward flexion. To achieve separation of the joint surface, traction must be applied in the direction of the femoral neck. This is achieved by combining a lateral force through the peroneal post in conjunction with a longitudinal force through the traction boot.

The force necessary for distraction is reduced by injection of saline into the joint. Most arthroscopy procedures can be completed via a viewing portal located just above the apex of the greater trochanter and an instrumentation portal 3–4cm more anteriorly. Additional portals can be created as required. An arthroscopic pump is used throughout to maintain constant distension of the joint with saline solution. A 70-degree arthroscope is used most commonly for central and peripheral compartment hip arthroscopy. A 30-degree arthroscope is useful for the lateral compartment and visualization of the distal iliospoas tendon.

Femoroacetabular impingement surgery

Arthroscopic recontouring of the non-spherical femoral heads seeks to eliminate trauma to the anterior acetabular margin and slow or prevent the development of osteoarthritis. Anterior acetabular wall overcoverage can be corrected by labral elevation, rim trimming, and labral repair. The arthroscopic approach minimizes postoperative morbidity and facilitates more rapid return to high-functioning lifestyles.

Labral surgery

Arthroscopic labral debridement has been reported as providing good or excellent results for two-thirds of patients with labral damage. Where reconstruction is viable, there is growing evidence that better outcomes are achieved with this treatment. However, if the underlying cause for labral damage is not addressed, any labral intervention will be followed by recurrence and progression of symptoms.

Arthroscopy of the soft tissues around the joint

Iliopsoas tendinopathy and anterior soft tissue fibrosis after total hip replacement

A minority of patients complain of persistent anterior hip pain after total hip replacement. Arthroscopic assessment and intracapsular release of the iliopsoas can be helpful in such cases.

Iliopsoas release at level of lesser trochanter if no periarticular tethering

Snapping iliopsoas tendon that is painful with no evidence of periarticular tethering can be treated by performing extra-articular arthroscopic psoas tenotomy at the level of the lesser trochanter.

Arthroscopy in the lateral compartment trochanteric regions

In the lateral compartment, tight or snapping iliotibial band, inflammed bursa, and gluteus medius and minimus tendinosis can all be treated arthroscopically. Gluteus medius sprains can be treated with coablation and tears can be repaired with anchor sutures.

Trochanteric bursitis can be treated with arthroscopic bursectomy combined with fascia lata releases.

Conclusion

Hip arthroscopy has become established over the past 10 years. Recognition of FAI has been the principal driver for the development of this field of hip surgery. While these interventions can provide excellent symptomatic relief of symptoms, it remains to be seen whether the natural history of premature hip degeneration will be modified.

Further reading

Biant, L. and Field, R.E. (in press). Hip arthroscopy after THR. *Arthroscopy*.

Ganz, R., Parvizi, J., Beck, M., *et al.* (2003). Femoroacetabular impingement: a cause for osteoarthritis of the hip. *Clinical Orthopaedics and Related Research*, **417**, 112–20.

Martin, R.L. and Sekiya, J.K. (2008). The inter-rater reliability of 4 clinical tests used to assess individuals with musculoskeletal hip pain. *Journal of Orthopaedic & Sports Physical Therapy*, **38**(2), 71–7.

Notzli, H.P., Wyss, T.F., Stoecklin, C.H., Schmid, M.R., Treiber, K., and Hodler, J. (2002). The contour of the femoral head-neck junction as a predictor for the risk of anterior impingement. *Journal of Bone and Joint Surgery*, **84B**, 556–60.

Sadri, H. and Hoffmeyer, P. (2008). Arthroscopic surgical treatment of coxofemoral conflic versus open surgery: comparison with at least 2 years follow-up. *Journal of Bone and Joint Surgery*, **90B**, 241.

SECTION 8

The Knee

8.1

History and examination of the knee

Tim Spalding

Summary points

- History and examination of the knee are linked and specific examination is determined by the likely diagnosis indicated by the history
- The 5 diagnostics groups are: Anterior knee pain; Traumatic injury to knee ligaments, meniscus, or other structures; Degenerative osteoarthritis; Inflammatory joint problem; and other problems
- General examination of the knee is still required with the patient, walking, standing, sitting, and lying supine
- Specific examination is targeted to 4 areas: The patello-femoral joint and extensor mechanism; Meniscal pathology; Ligament stability; and Arthritis. The pattern of signs elicited should lead to definitive diagnosis.

Introduction

Traditionally, examination of a joint involves the principle 'look, feel, move', but for the knee the order and sequence of examination changes, depending on the likely diagnosis suggested by the history. The history is key in detecting the characteristic patterns of symptoms that will direct examination. Specific direct questions may be needed to aid this process. This is not asking 'leading questions' but is rather 'direct questioning' and this helps focus the patient's mind onto the specific symptoms and the examiner onto specific possible diagnoses.

In addition, the level of disability caused by the symptoms as well as patient expectations need to to be carefully elicited as this will have a significant bearing on the management plan.

This chapter on history and examination of the knee breaks down the process into three parts: history, general knee examination, and targeted knee examination.

History

Clinical presentation

The three key features when addressing a patient with a knee problem are:

- *The main symptom or symptoms*: pain, swelling, locking, or giving way
- *Age of the patient*: younger age is more likely to be associated with a traumatic injury or anterior knee pain whereas older age usually indicates a degenerative arthritic process
- *Mechanism of onset of problem*: onset associated with trauma indicates specific injury to the anatomical structures in the knee whereas gradual onset over time indicates a degenerative process.

Main symptoms

Pain

In principle, the site, nature, character, and severity of pain are determined by specific questions.

General questions

- Location (vague widespread suggesting patellofemoral source or more localized to medial or lateral joint line)
- Nature (sharp, burning, dull ache, etc.)
- Exacerbating features (activity related or at rest)
- Pain radiation
- Progress over time (getting worse or better).

Specific scenarios

- Pain on medial aspect of knee on deep squatting: indicates a meniscal tear
- Joint pain radiating down leg: indicates arthritic aching process
- Pain at rest: usually indicates severe arthritis

Box 8.1.1 Principles of history taking

- Examination of knee directed by the history
- Accurate history taking will lead to five diagnostic groups:
  - Anterior knee pain
  - Traumatic injury to knee ligaments, meniscus, or other structures
  - Degenerative osteoarthritis
  - Inflammatory joint problem
  - Other problem.

- Pain at night: indicates inflammatory cause
- Pain worse on sitting for prolonged periods or on climbing/descending stairs: indicates patellofemoral problems
- Pain in multiple sites: indicates either a generalized problem or may indicate inappropriate pain response.

Swelling

Swelling usually indicates that there is a significant problem in the knee.

General questions
- Relation to onset of symptoms (early or late)
- Exacerbating features
- Relieving features.

Specific scenarios
- Swelling occurring within four hours from pivoting injury: usually indicates torn anterior cruciate ligament
- Swelling occurring greater than 4h after twisting injury: usually indicates a meniscal tear
- Swelling with activity: usually indicates a degenerative process
- Localized hard swelling on lateral joint line after activity: indicates lateral meniscal cyst from tear
- Extra-articular swelling: indicates a bursa
- Non-specific onset: indicates an inflammatory problem
- A very tense and painful swelling following injury: usually means haemarthrosis and a more significant injury.

Locking

This means the transient inability of the knee to go out straight rather than difficulty in flexing the knee. It is important to distinguish this from pseudo locking from the patellofemoral joint or following medial collateral injury where extension is limited by pain.

General questions
- Exacerbating factors (squatting, twisting, etc.)
- Relieving factors
- Exact description of locking (asking the patient what they mean by locking)
- Permanently blocked or intermittent
- True meniscal locking or false patella catching.

Specific scenarios
- Intermittent locking of the knee relieved by shaking the leg or a trick manoeuvre: indicates a loose body
- Inability to fully straighten the leg at any time following trauma: indicates a meniscal tear, osteochondral fragment, or anterior cruciate ligament (ACL) stump blocking full extension
- Transient locking on standing: may indicate catching of the worn arthritic surfaces.

Giving way

Giving way can also be described as buckling, not trusting the knee or giving out.

General questions
- Movements associated with the giving way (pivoting movements, straight line activities, or descending stairs)
- Description of giving way sensation (twisting knuckles sign or patella giving way)
- Relation to pain (pain before or after giving way).

Specific scenarios
- Rotational giving way mimicked by twisted knuckles: indicates ACL deficiency
- Knee giving way on pivoting to one side and feeling of patella jumping: indicates patella dislocation
- Knee giving way on squatting associated with medial pain: indicates meniscal tear
- Knee giving way on stairs with falling over: indicates patella dislocation. With ACL type giving way the patient is usually able to catch themselves
- Giving way after pain: usually due to quads inhibition associated with pain from the catching of worn surfaces.

Additional clinical features to elicit

Other specific detail is required to lead to an action plan and these include:

- Noises and sensations in the joint:
  - A feeling of something moving around indicates a loose body
  - A painful grating sensation indicates crepitus and possible damage to the joint surface
  - A thudding clunk usually indicates a meniscal tear catching in the joint.
- Severity of the symptoms in relation to lifestyle:
  - For the active individual this means sporting aims and desired activity levels
  - For the arthritic assessment this means walking distance, ability to climb stairs, pain at night, and interference with quality of life.

Conclusion of history (Box 8.1.1)

After taking the history then there should be a fairly good idea of the diagnosis or, if not likely diagnoses, then the main category of problem.

Essentially the patient will be in one of five categories:

- Anterior knee pain
- Traumatic injury to knee ligaments, meniscus, or other structures
- Degenerative osteoarthritis
- Inflammatory joint problem
- Other problem.

Examination

Examination starts with a general examination of the knee followed by specific examination to confirm a specific diagnosis that has been indicated by the history. The history and examination should lead to a management plan that may involve further targeted investigation or the initial stage of treatment.

General examination includes assessing the patient standing, walking, and lying supine, and includes active, passive, and provocative tests or movements. This should allow *specific* examination to concentrate on one of four areas (Box 8.1.2):

- The patellofemoral joint and extensor mechanism
- Meniscal pathology
- Ligament stability
- Arthritis.

General examination

Standing and walking

This includes general habitus, leg alignment, posture, change in alignment on walking, the presence of an antalgic hip gait, and muscle wasting. Looking at the leg starts as the patient walks in to the clinic and takes in to account their general demeanour, appearance, manner of walking, and mobility around the examination area. All these factors add information to the diagnostic equation.

Normal alignment, varus (bowlegged), or valgus (knock-kneed) alignment is noted and the presence of increasing deformity as a lateral or medial thrust on walking is also elicited (Figure 8.1.1).

Malalignment may also be rotational. Squinting patellae occur when the feet point forward but the knees squint towards each other representing abnormal femoral and tibial torsion. Isolated external tibial torsion may be noted if the patella points forward but the feet point outwards more than 10–15 degrees. There is clearly a wide range of what is normal and physiological varus or hyperextension, for example, may be a variant of normal.

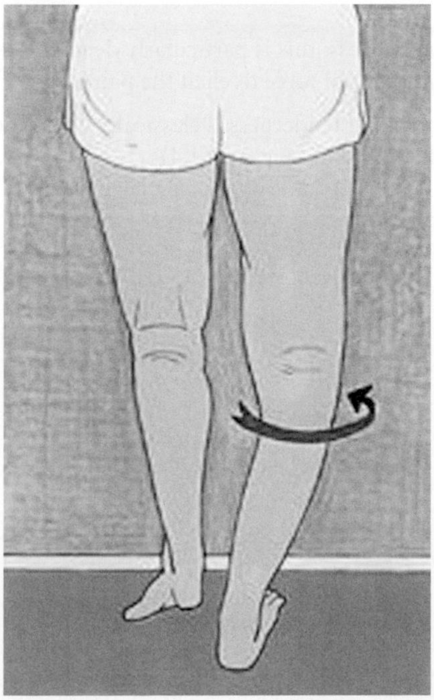

Fig. 8.1.1 Lateral thrust of the knee on walking, indicating malalignment.

Supine

Examination supine involves a combination of look, feel and move. In order to look properly we need to feel the knee aiming to detect and confirm specific appearances and problems.

- General inspection: this takes into account evaluating alignment, position of the knee, skin problems, scars, muscle wasting, bruising for site of trauma, and the manner in which the knee is held
- Presence of effusion: there may be obvious fullness of the knee or it is detected by the *bulge test* (milking fluid from the medial side via the suprapatella pouch into the lateral gutter and then stroking the lateral gutter with the back of the hand eliciting a bulge on the medial side) or the *patella tap sign* (squeezing the suprapatella pouch with one hand and balloting the patella [Figure 8.1.2])
- Fixed flexion deformity: the patient may hold the knee in a flexed posture indicating true locking or pseudo locking due to pain. The knee can be gently straightened to full hyperextension looking for any loss compared to the other side
- Range of movement (ROM): this will elicit how painful the knee is and therefore guide the remainder of the examination. In the obviously arthritic knee, ROM is the most important sign and palpation of tender points less so. By convention ROM is expressed by three numbers: passive hyperextension or recurvatum, active extension, and flexion, e.g. 5/0/135.

Specific examination

The patellofemoral joint and extensor mechanism

Inspection of the patellofemoral joint is initially best performed with the patient sitting with the leg flexed over the edge of the couch, noting the following features or signs:

- Position of the patellae: the patella normally faces forward and slightly up—higher indicates patella alta, lower indicates patella baja
- Position of the tibial tubercle: this should be directly inferior to the centre of the patella. Inspection gives a guide to the tibial tubercle trochlea groove (TT-TG) offset that is more formally

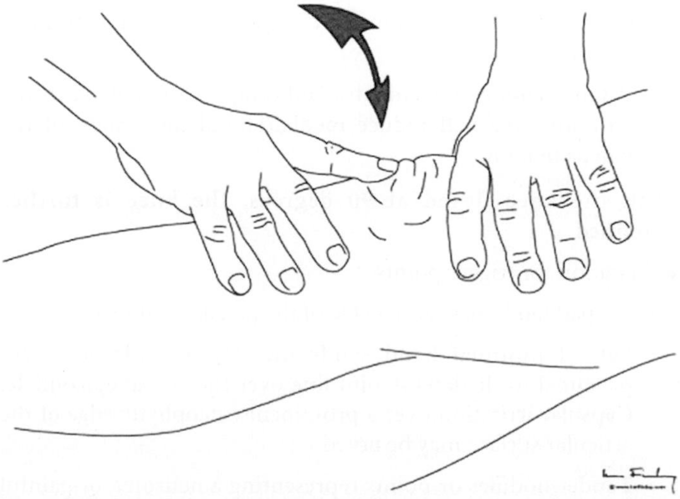

Fig. 8.1.2 Patella tap sign, bouncing the patella off the trochlea to demonstrate effusion.

quantified by computed tomography or magnetic resonance imaging scanning
- Patella tracking: on active extension the patella should track centrally toward the groin. Tracking laterally in extension as an inverted J-sign indicates lateral subluxation in extension and potential or real patellar instability
- Feeling the articulation: holding the hand gently over the patella detects crepitus.

With the patient lying *supine* the following tests can be performed:

- Detection of effusion: as previously described
- Palpation for tender points:
  - Tibial tubercle for Osgood–Schlatter's
  - Lower pole patella for patella tendinopathy (jumper's knee) or Sinding–Larsen Johansson syndrome in the adolescent. The patella is tilted from superior while pushing into the lower pole with the thumb
  - Superior pole of the patella for quads tendinopathy
  - Tenderness on the medial or lateral border of patella
  - Any specific trigger points looking for neuroma or tender nodules
  - Medial retinaculum for tenderness over the medial plica, felt as a chord on rolling the finger against the condyle (with the knee in extension)
  - Excessive patella tilt by holding the axis of the patella between finger and thumb
- Movements of the patella:
  - Patella glide is quantified as the proportion of patella width that it can move medially or laterally in either full extension or at 30 degrees of flexion (Figure 8.1.3)
  - Apprehension sign. Detected by gently trying to dislocate the patella laterally, eliciting an obvious sense of apprehension by the patient
  - Patellofemoral compression. Examined by compressing the patella into the groove and rocking the knee into flexion and extension, eliciting pain, catching, crepitus, or bare-bone grinding
  - Patella tendon movements. Tethering of the patella to the anterior tibia will reduce medial/lateral movement of the patella tendon.

With the knee flexed at 90 degrees, the knee is further examined

- Palpation for trigger points:
  - Fat pad tenderness either side of the patella tendon
  - Lateral iliotibial band syndrome. Deep tenderness 2cm proximal to the lateral joint line over the lateral epicondyle. Capsular irritation over a prominent osteophytic edge of the articular surface may be noted
  - Tender nodules or points representing a neuroma or painful scar.

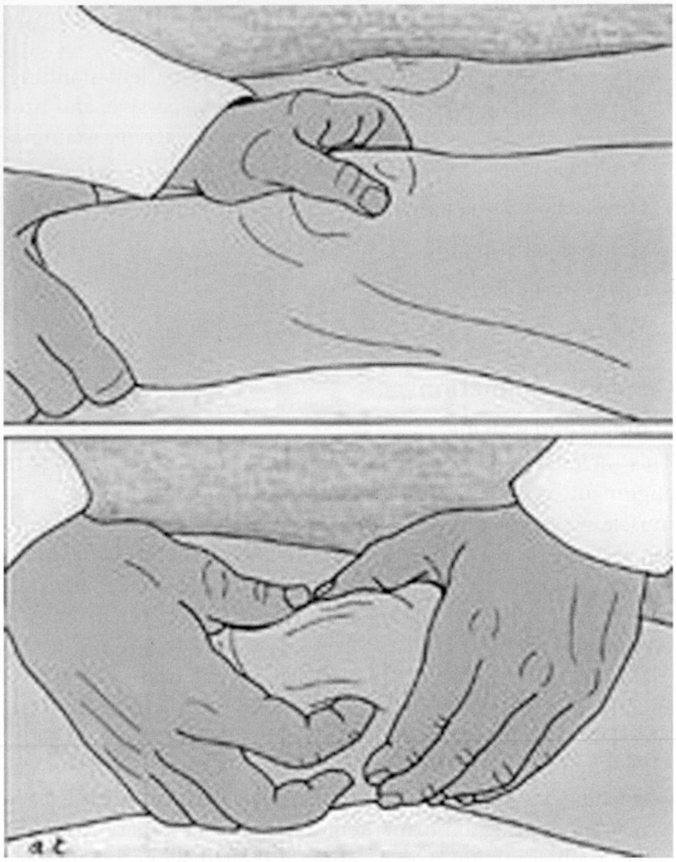

Fig. 8.1.3 Assessment of patella mobility by medial and lateral glide, expressed as a proportion of patella width that the patella moves.

Examination of the menisci

This is best performed with the knee flexed at 90 degrees.

Palpation

- Meniscal tenderness: this is particularly deep and therefore may take a fair amount of force to elicit the pain:
  - Medial meniscal tenderness is classically on the posteromedial part of the joint line (Figure 8.1.4)

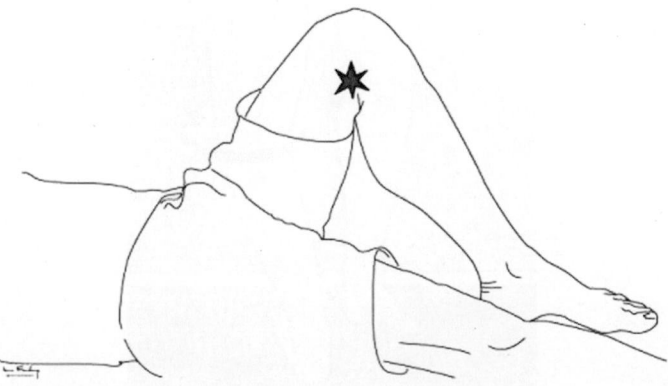

Fig. 8.1.4 Medial joint line tenderness is felt by deep palpation on the posteromedial part of the joint line between femur and tibia.

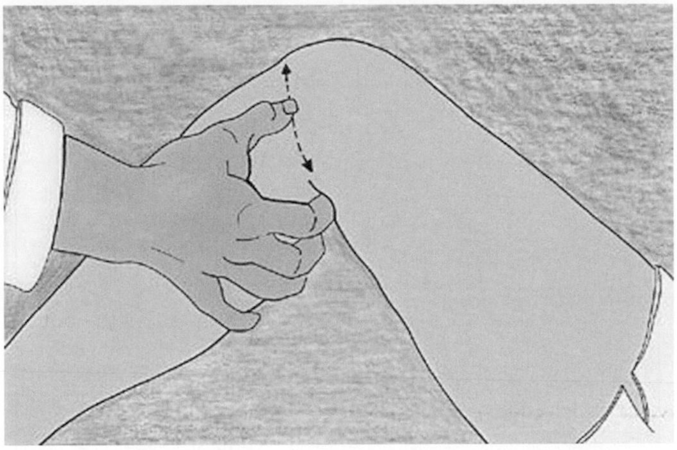

Fig. 8.1.5 Lateral joint line tenderness is felt in the mid lateral part of the joint, also by deep firm palpation.

- Lateral meniscal tear tenderness is on the midlateral aspect (Figure 8.1.5)
- Anterior joint line tenderness may indicate a bucket handle tear, especially if associated with a block to full extension

- Swelling: an associated fullness or obvious swelling may be sensed due to either an associated cyst (usually lateral) or sometimes the flap of a meniscus (typically medial).

Pain on movement

- Meniscal pain on full flexion: pressure on the meniscus is increased in full flexion and may be resisted by the patient
- McMurray's test: in this test rotation in forced flexion with compression over the medial joint line is positive if it elicits a clunk from a torn meniscus as the test was originally described. It is less reliable if used with simple detection of pain. (Figure 8.1.6)
- Squat or duck walking (mimics McMurray's manoeuvre): the patient is asked to squat and walk or waddle a few steps, eliciting their characteristic pain. This can be a very useful confirmatory test
- Apley's grind test: this is less commonly used but the patient is positioned prone, the knee flexed to 90 degrees and the tibia ground into the femur looking for pain from a meniscal tear.

Examination for ligament instability

The following ligaments or ligament complexes can be examined individually or in combination and the pattern of instability determined:

- Collateral ligaments
- Anterior cruciate ligament
- Posterior cruciate ligament
- Posterolateral corner
- Posteromedial corner.

Collateral ligament examination

Tenderness following acute injury is examined for with the knee at 90 degrees, applying deep palpation over the epicondyles and, for the medial collateral ligament, over the tibial attachment. Laxity and pain on stressing the collateral ligaments is detected at full hyperextension, 0 degrees extension and at 20–30 degrees with the purpose of detecting a difference with the other side. The patient should be asked whether the movement feels the same.

For detection of movement the knee is cupped by one hand using the fingers and the palm alternately as a fulcrum against the epicondyles, and the leg is levered to the side by firmly grasping the heel (Figure 8.1.7). Flexion beyond 20–30 degrees will result in rotation at the hip rather than opening of the knee.

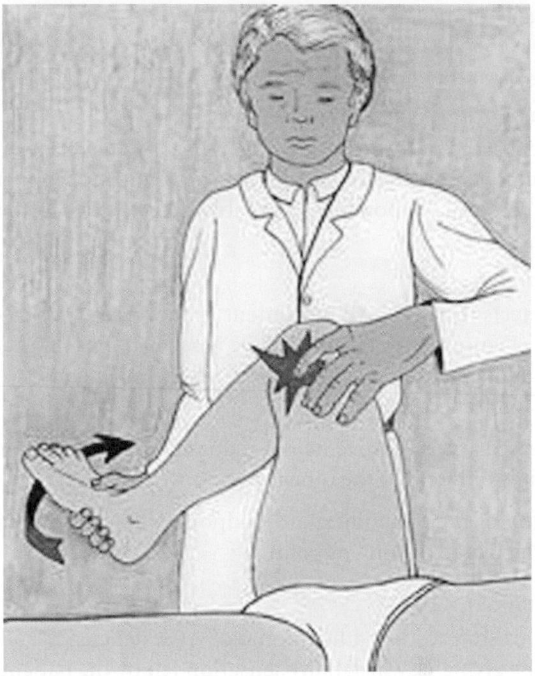

Fig. 8.1.6 McMurray test performed holding the knee to achieve full flexion and by applying rotational movements by grasping the heel.

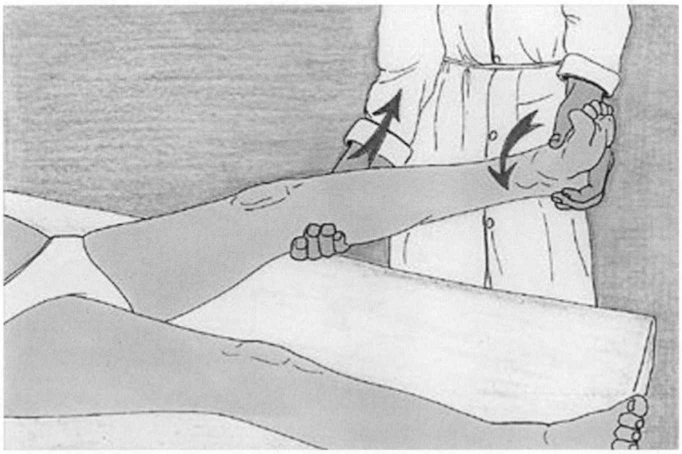

Fig. 8.1.7 Assessment of the collateral ligaments, achieved by cupping the knee and then applying medial and lateral movements of the leg by grasping the heel. The fingers and the palm are used as a fulcrum.

Integrity of the lateral collateral ligament can be checked by palpation in the 'figure four' position, feeling the chord-like structure running from fibula head to femur.

Anterior cruciate ligament examination

To detect laxity of the ACL the patient needs to be relaxed to avoid involuntary contraction of the hamstrings. With appropriate techniques it is usually possible to reliably detect laxity in the awake patient.

Lachman test

This detects increased AP movement in the knee at 10–15 degrees flexion (Figure 8.1.8). Firm AP force is applied, pushing back with the thigh hand and pulling forward with the tibial hand.

Two differences are sought:

- Increased anterior movement—it doesn't matter how much, just that it is different to the other knee
- Quality of the endpoint: hard endpoint, indicating some fibres may be intact, or soft endpoint.

Pivot shift test

The pivot shift test is pathogmonic of ACL deficiency and reproduces the giving way instability sensation felt by the patient.

The test has a reputation as painful and difficult to perform but with adequate support of the leg it is painless and easily reproducible. The principle is to detect a jumping, or familiar buckling sensation, as the lateral tibia slides from its normal position articulating with the lateral femoral condyle into an abnormal anterior subluxed position, and vice versa, at around 20 degrees flexion on bending and straightening the knee.

Figure 8.1.9 shows how the tibia is supported, between the examiner's side and over the examiner's forearm. The hand is then interlocked over the wrist of the other hand, which is applied against the lateral aspect of the proximal tibia and fibula. This is an active test involving participation of the patient. Initially their confidence is obtained by asking them to flex their knee from extension without the examiner applying any force on the leg.

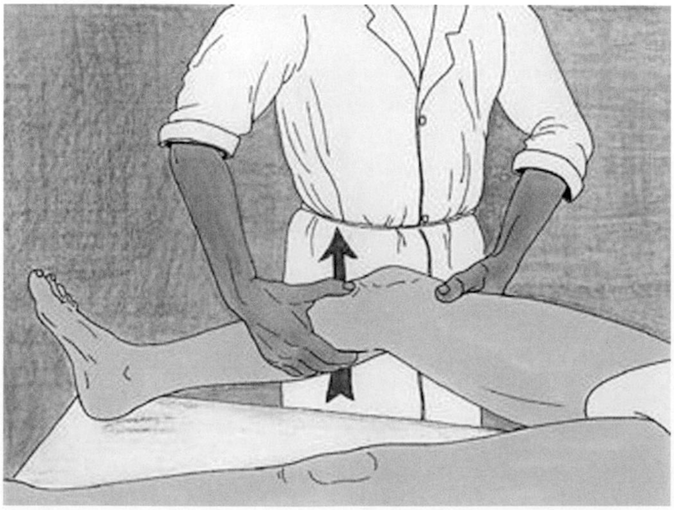

Fig. 8.1.8 Lachman test: the thumb and fingers of each hand, placed as near to the midline as possible—grip the leg in order to achieve direct anterior and posterior movement. A difference between the two sides in terms of endpoint or excursion is all that is required to indicate ACL injury.

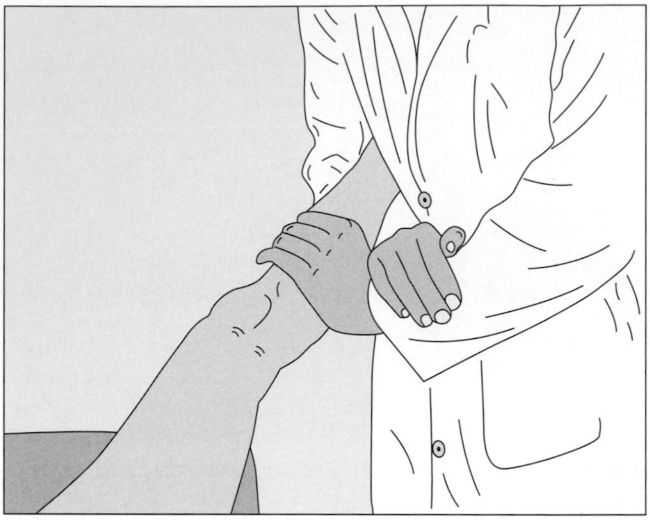

Fig. 8.1.9 Pivot shift test.

The examiner then flexes the knee passively by lifting from the patient's posterior calf, exerting an anterior force on the tibia. In a positive test the tibia is felt to slide or jump posteriorly back into place as the knee bends. Conversely as the knee is straightened the tibia is felt to sublux anteriorly. This can be an obvious clunk or a subtle glide. To emphasize the test, looking for reproduction of the patient's distrust of their knee, increasing load is applied, both in valgus and by inline compression, loading the lateral compartment to exaggerate the sliding of the femur over the dome of the lateral tibial plateau. When it is difficult for the patient to relax, the patient is asked to straighten their knee, thereby relaxing the hamstrings and allowing the pivot shift slide or clunk to be felt.

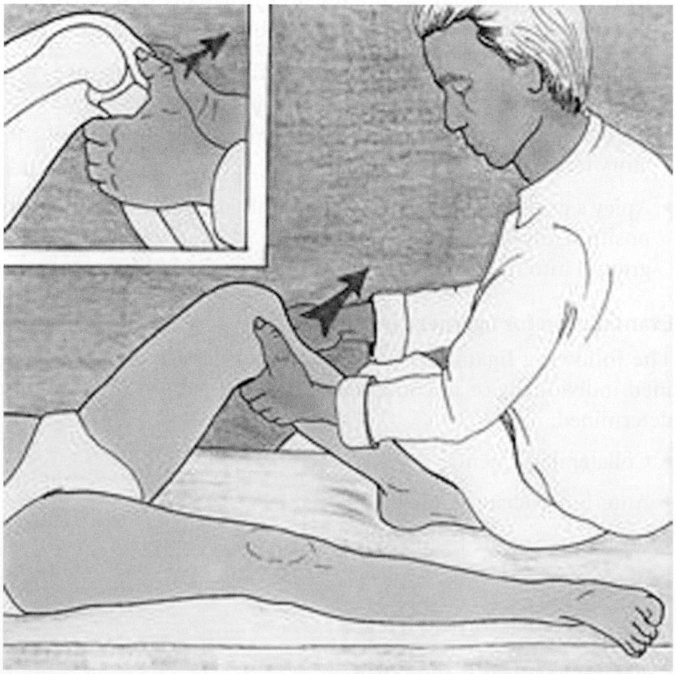

Fig. 8.1.10 Anterior draw test. The examiner sits just against the foot and exerts anterior pull on the tibia, holding the hamstrings out of the way with the index fingers while gripping the tibia with the palm of the hands.

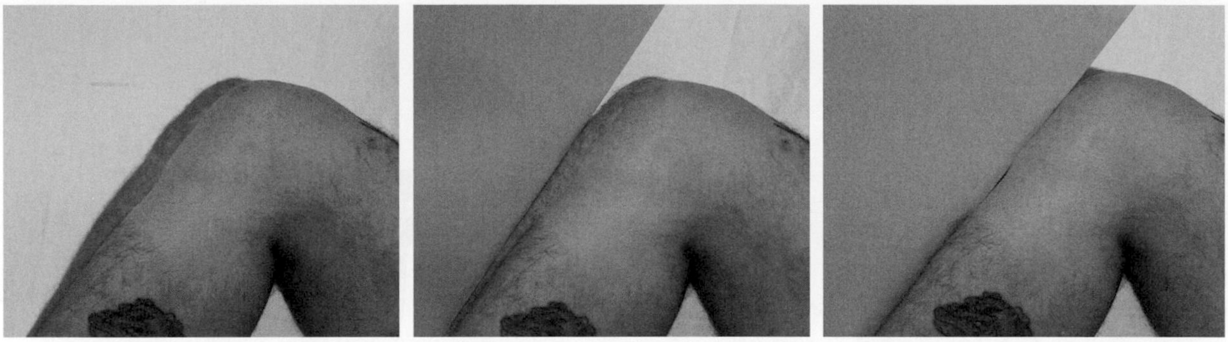

Fig. 8.1.11 X-ray packet sign showing normal gap between the edge and the patella (B) and the loss of gap (C) in posterior cruciate ligament insufficiency.

Anterior draw test

This test, in which the tibia is pulled anteriorly with the knee at 90 degrees (Figure 8.1.10), is much less reliable in the detection of ACL insufficiency. Paradoxically, it is very useful in detecting posterior sag and the step-off sign for posterior cruciate ligament insufficiency. The examiner sits against the foot and the palms grip the sides of the tibia exerting a strong anterior pull. The index fingers of both hands are used to 'knock out' posterior pull by the hamstrings.

Posterior cruciate ligament examination

The posterior cruciate ligament acts to resist posterior translation of the tibia. Laxity is best examined with the knee at 90 degrees.

Posterior sag

When both knees are viewed from the side, any sagging back of the tibial tubercle and upper tibia is noted as posterior sag. A straight edge such as an x-ray packet (if available) may be useful to demonstrate subtle sag (Figure 8.1.11).

Posterior draw test

With the knee at 80–90 degrees the tibia is pushed posteriorly to detect any increased posterior translation.

The step-off sign

This is perhaps the most useful sign in detecting posterior cruciate ligament laxity as it also helps to determine treatment. Figure 8.1.12 shows the three grades based on the stepping down from the tibia on to the femur. Grade II means the tibia is flush with the femur and when grade III is detected (tibia posterior to femur) there is likely to be injury to the posterolateral corner.

Posterior Lachman test

Increased posterior sag can also be detected at 15–20 degrees flexion when the tibia is pushed posteriorly in relation to the femur.

Posterolateral corner examination

Injuries to structures of the posterolateral corner result in increased external rotation of the tibia on the femur.

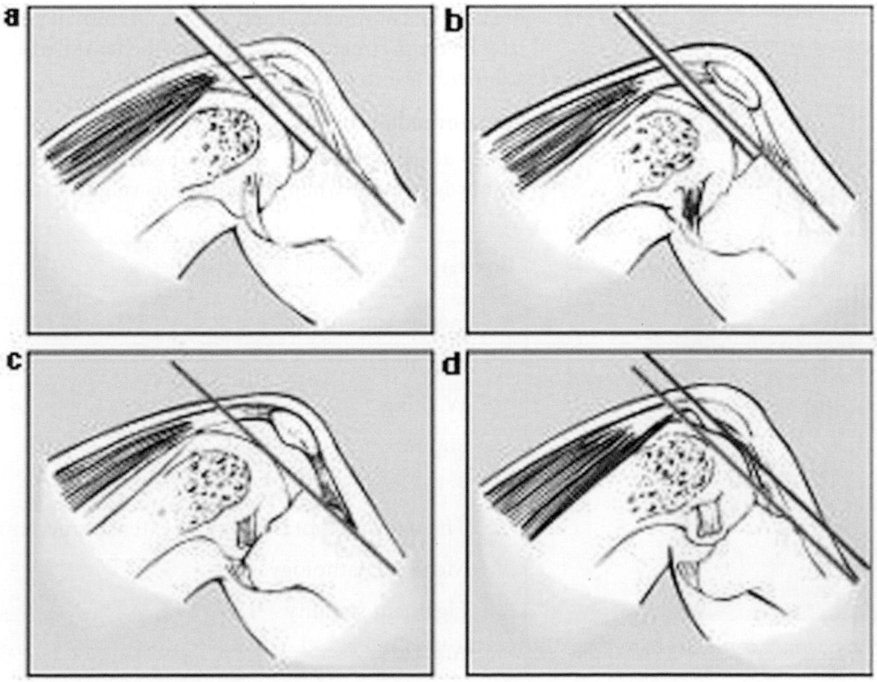

Fig. 8.1.12 The step-off sign classification in determining the amount of loss of the normal anterior position of the tibia in relation to the femur: a) Normal step-off, b) Grade 1: reduced step-off, c) Grade 2: tibia flush with femur, d) Grade 4: tibia posterior to femur.

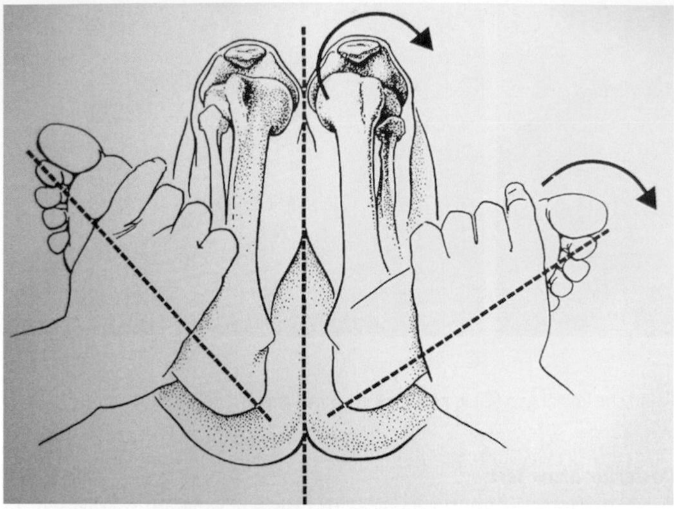

Fig. 8.1.13 Dial test demonstrating increased external rotation of the left tibia at the knee joint.

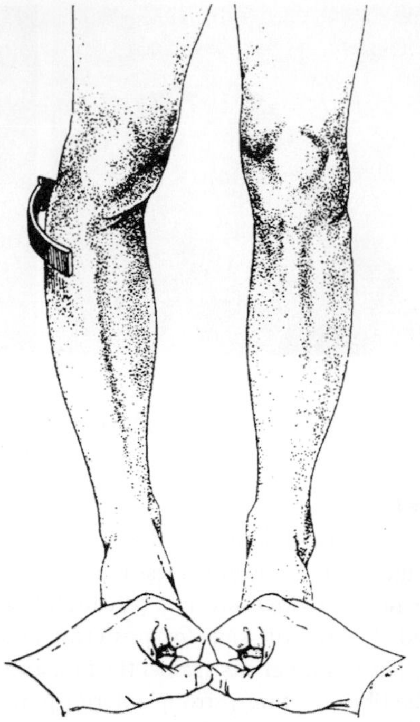

Fig. 8.1.15 External recurvatum test: the leg is picked up by holding just the big toe and the knee is seen to drop into varus, external rotation, and hyperextension, indicating injury to the posterolateral structures.

Dial test at 30 and 90 degrees

The patient can be supine or prone (Figure 8.1.13), but prone is probably more accurate. The examiner externally rotates the supported feet while an assistant keeps the knees together to eliminate femoral rotation. Greater than 15 degrees 'dialled' external rotation indicates injury.

Increased external rotation at 30 degrees suggests an isolated posterolateral corner injury whilst increased external rotation at 30 and 90 degrees suggests injuries to both the posterolateral corner and posterior cruciate ligament.

Lateral hypermobility at 90 degrees

With the knee at 90 degrees the knee is rotated by gripping the proximal tibiofibular joint and pushing it posteriorly in order to detect an increase in posterolateral mobility compared to the other side (Figure 8.1.14). Alternatively, with the patient sitting, the examiner spins out the tibia while the patient keeps their knees together (spin test). Increased posterolateral rotation can be noted by feeling and looking at the superior tibiofibular joint.

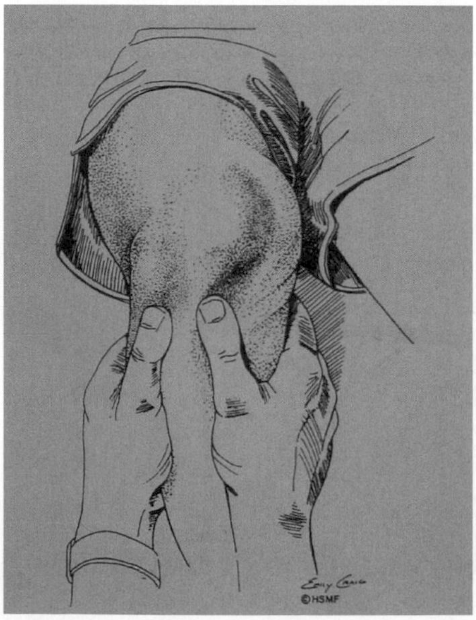

Fig. 8.1.14 Spin test: testing increased rotation externally of the tibia by rotating the tibia and noting the position of the tibial tubercle and the fibula head.

External rotation recurvatum test

When the legs are picked up by the big toe or forefoot then the knees fall into external rotation as the knee goes into hyperextension (Figure 8.1.15) when the posterolateral corner is stretched out.

Reverse pivot shift test

This test detects the opposite of the pivot shift phenomenon. The knee is supported in flexion with the foot externally rotated and the knee in compression and valgus. On moving into extension the lateral compartment reduces under the femur with a clunk. This is a difficult test to perform reliably.

Posteromedial corner

Injury to the posterior oblique ligament of the posteromedial corner is present when instability to valgus stress is present with

Box 8.1.2 Principles of knee examination

- General examination:
  - Standing
  - Walking
  - Supine.
- Specific examination:
  - The patellofemoral joint and extensor mechanism
  - Meniscal pathology
  - Ligament stability
  - Arthritis.

the knee in full extension. In this situation injury to one or both cruciate ligaments should be suspected.

Examination for arthritis or joint surface damage

The hallmark signs when examining for joint surface damage are signs associated with catching of worn articular cartilage surfaces. Fine crepitus on joint movement can be heard but it usually needs to be felt. Active movement loads the joint and the examiner places a hand over the moving part, either feeling with the fingers or the flat of the palm. Popping, snapping, or clunking may also be felt on movement under load and if painless are considered 'safe'.

Bare bone crepitus

When two bare bone surfaces are forcibly compressed together then there is very high friction and the surfaces momentarily stick together before sliding in a juddering fashion. This sign has been described as the *pepper mill sign* for obvious reasons and can be felt in the medial and lateral compartments by carefully forcing the knee into varus or valgus and slowly moving the joint under compressive load. With pausing, the thin synovial fluid is being compressed out of the articulation removing any lubrication benefit.

Range of movement

Loss of flexion and or extension is an early sign of joint degeneration. For consistency and accuracy, flexion is best measured with the patient reclined nearly supine, keeping the quadriceps at maximum length.

Palpation of articular surfaces

When the knee is at 90 degrees the distal articular surface of the medial femoral condyle is facing distally and is not covered by the patella. Deep tenderness on palpation of this surface is consistent with articular surface damage.

Popliteal cysts

Cysts and fullness in the popliteal fossa are best seen and palpated with the knee in extension and when standing.

Box 8.1.3 Specific knee diagnostic scenarios

Groups of symptoms and signs can predict likely diagnoses:

- History of non-contact rotational injury, and feeling of not trusting knee Rotational giving way mimicked by twisted knuckles: indicates ACL deficiency
- Description of knee 'dislocating' and persistent feeling of patella jumping out of joint on twisting movements: indicates patella dislocation
- History of twisting injury, knee effusion, and posteromedial joint line tenderness: indicates meniscal tear
- Knee giving way on stairs with falling over: indicates patella dislocation. With ACL type giving way the patient is usually able to catch themselves

Conclusion

History and examination are linked and specific examination is substantially determined by the likely diagnosis or group of diagnoses indicated by the history (Box 8.1.3). It is, however, important to undertake general examination of the knee with the patient, walking, standing, sitting and lying supine. Specific examination will then create a pattern of signs which should lead to definitive diagnosis (Table 8.1.1).

Table 8.1.1 Specific diagnostic signs

Diagnosis or disorder	Signs
ACL insufficiency	Lachman test +ve, Pivot shift +ve
Posterior instability	Reverse Lachman test +ve, posterior draw +ve, step-off sign (grading)
Posterolateral corner insufficiency	Prone dial test +ve, spin test +ve, reverse pivot shift test +/−ve, lateral knee thrust on walking
Knee arthritis (medial or lateral compartment)	Loss of ROM, bare bone crepitus. Varus/valgus malalignment
Patella instability	J-tracking patella, patella apprehension test +ve, increased patella glide
Medial meniscus tear	Effusion +ve, posteromedial joint line tenderness, McMurray test +ve, pain on squat walking
Lateral meniscus tear	Midlateral joint line tenderness
Patellofemoral arthritis	Effusion, pain on patellofemoral compression, crepitus felt on extending against gravity
Global anterior knee pain syndrome	Normal alignment tests, crepitus −ve, patella tendinopathy tests −ve

8.2

Cartilage repair in the young knee

Tim Spalding and Lars Peterson

Summary points

- Articular cartilage has a poor capacity to heal by itself
- Left alone, large areas are likely to progress into osteoarthritis
- The goal of cartilage repair is both short term improvement in function and long term durability
- There are several available strategies including non-surgical options, and these are formulated into an algorithm
- Cartilage repair is an advancing field and the future lies in bioengineering and high quality comparative clinical analysis.

Introduction

The treatment of articular cartilage injuries in the young knee poses a difficult management problem, because articular cartilage has a very poor capacity to heal. Repair occurs with poor quality fibrocartilage which does not have the endurance and function of normal hyaline articular cartilage and is unlikely to allow the patient to return to full function. Metal and plastic are final alternatives for the older more sedentary patient but the younger, more active patient poses a challenge.

This chapter outlines the structure of articular cartilage, explaining why it does not heal and outlines the treatment options available both now and in the near future with tissue engineering. The aim of articular cartilage repair techniques is the prevention or delay of later osteoarthritis, and so inevitably good evidence for the ideal treatment option is lacking due to the long follow-up periods required.

Cartilage injury—the beauty and the problem of hyaline cartilage

The behaviour of articular cartilage is determined very much by its biomechanical, biochemical, and morphological properties. Articular cartilage consists of distinct structural zones and the specific arrangement of the components and the fibres determines the characteristic properties of cartilage—namely to withstand high load with almost no friction. The coefficient of friction of the articular surface is less than that of ice on ice and, when damaged, friction increases so that much more effort is required to move the joint, resulting in acceleration of mechanical wear.

Articular cartilage has a very poor ability to regenerate itself following injury. This is because of its structure and lack of a neurovascular supply. Structure is important because the chondrocytes are trapped within the matrix and cannot migrate after injury to lay down new matrix of type II collagen and proteoglycans.

Full-thickness cartilage injuries that penetrate subchondral bone connect with the subchondral marrow elements resulting in migration of mesenchymal stem cells and fibroblasts which lay down repair tissue. This tissue is generally a fibrocartilage type of repair, heavy in type I collagen rather than the normal specialized type II collagen found in hyaline cartilage. Fibrocartilage does not have the same wear and endurance characteristics of type II collagen, hence the poor durability.

Natural history of articular cartilage injury (Box 8.2.1)

The natural history of chondral injury is unclear but it is generally accepted that a significant area of chondral damage is likely to lead to the development of degenerative change through enzymatic degradation and mechanical wear with the subsequent development of symptoms. Untreated lesions are likely to progress to osteoarthritis in the long term.

In degenerative joint disease, loss of articular cartilage is caused by a failure of the catabolic and anabolic ratio. This results in generalized destruction of the tissue under load and affects a large area of the chondral surface. This differs from traumatic cartilage

Box 8.2.1 Natural history of cartilage injury

- Articular cartilage has poor capacity to heal
- Any natural healing results in fibrocartilage repair with poor durability
- Current technologies aim to reproduce hyaline-like articular cartilage
- Future technologies aim to reduce healing time by development of scaffolds containing engineered tissue.

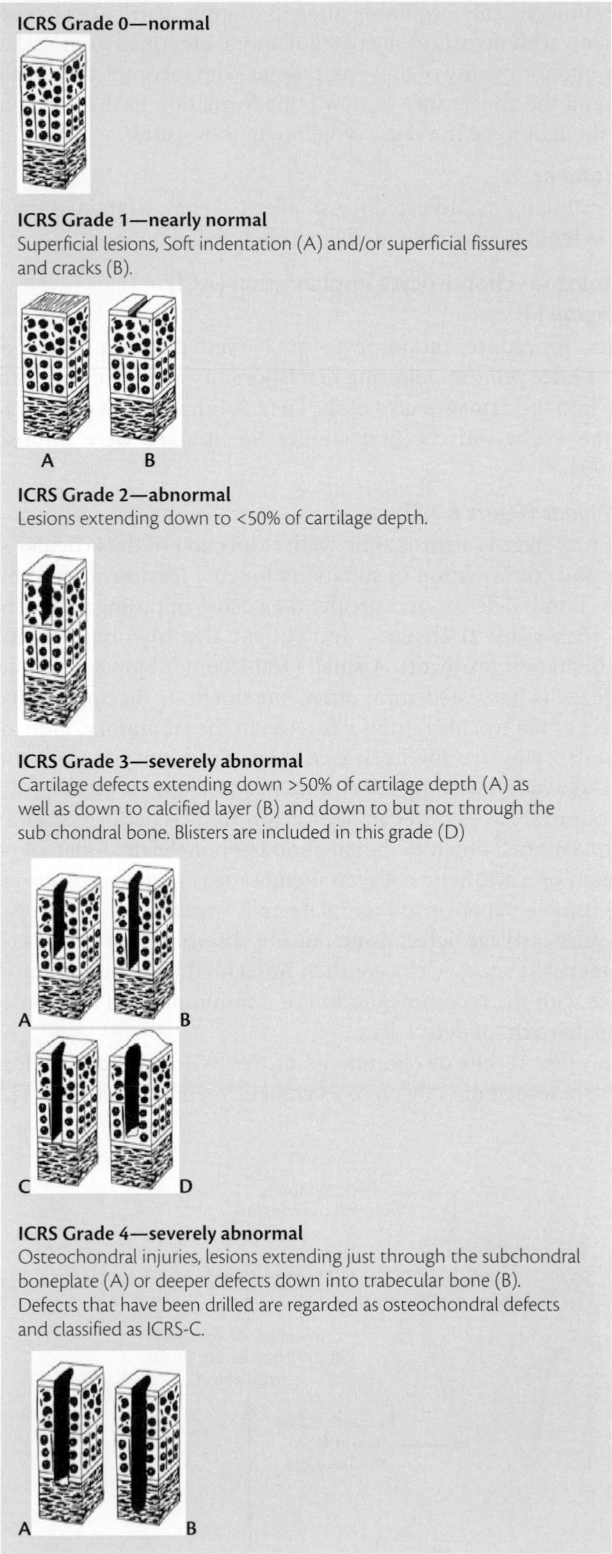

ICRS Grade 0—normal
ICRS Grade 1—nearly normal
Superficial lesions, Soft indentation (A) and/or superficial fissures and cracks (B).
A
B
ICRS Grade 2—abnormal
Lesions extending down to <50% of cartilage depth.
ICRS Grade 3—severely abnormal
Cartilage defects extending down >50% of cartilage depth (A) as well as down to calcified layer (B) and down to but not through the sub chondral bone. Blisters are included in this grade (D)
A
B
C
D
ICRS Grade 4—severely abnormal
Osteochondral injuries, lesions extending just through the subchondral boneplate (A) or deeper defects down into trabecular bone (B). Defects that have been drilled are regarded as osteochondral defects and classified as ICRS-C.
A
B

Fig. 8.2.1 International Cartilage Repair Society classification of chondral injury

lesions where a more isolated area of damage disrupts chondrocyte biosynthetic function, and this affects the structure and composition of the cartilage matrix. Cartilage defects are classified by the depth and size of the lesion (Figure 8.2.1).

Box 8.2.2 Articular cartilage repair

- Patient factors to consider for correction:
  - Alignment
  - Meniscus deficiency
  - Ligament insufficiency
- Lesion factors:
  - Size of lesion
  - Primary or secondary repair.

Articular cartilage repair (Box 8.2.2)

The goal of articular cartilage repair surgery is to improve patient symptoms and function and to achieve a durable surface which will alter the natural progression towards osteoarthritis. Repair with hyaline or hyaline-like cartilage instead of fibrocartilage has produced better clinical and mechanical results.

Treatment options (Box 8.2.3)

Non-surgical options

Non-surgical options for treating articular cartilage damage include reducing activity level, physiotherapy, taking simple analgesics, and non-steroidal anti-inflammatory drugs. Viscosupplementation injections and oral chondroprotective neutraceuticals such as glucosamine have also been tried but evidence for long-term benefit is lacking. Reducing load on the joint surface by changing activity level and by decreasing weight as appropriate may well decrease symptoms in the knee.

Arthroscopic debridement and thermal chondroplasty

Arthroscopic debridement techniques include mechanically smoothing (shaving) the roughened articular surface by removing unstable edges of articular surface and areas of fibrillation, washing out debris, and treating any torn menisci. In addition to mechanical shaving, energy can be applied using radiofrequency (RF) probes to produce ablate damaged tissue and seal fibrillation of articular cartilage. Heat applied to the proteoglycan protein results in shrinking and contraction of the surface producing a smooth and aesthetically appealing surface. Initial generations of RF probes,

Box 8.2.3 Options for surgical treatment

- Arthroscopic debridement provides short-term benefit relieving mechanical irritation to the joint
- Microfracture: stimulates repair from marrow cells and results in fibrocartilage repair tissue which may not have sufficient durability
- ACI techniques: expensive with long recovery time. Poorly assessed in comparative trials but hold the hope of long term durability
- Osteochondral grafting: transplanting healthy articular cartilage but limited by donor site morbidity.

however, produced significant heat damage to unpredictable depths and iatrogenic damage of surrounding articular cartilage with cell apoptosis and avascular necrosis of underlying bone were reported in early series. Current generations of RF probes, using plasma technology, produce a very controlled depth of heat penetration and careful use has resulted in few reported side effects.

Microfracture and marrow stimulation techniques

Background

Microfracture and other similar procedures are based on the principle that healing of articular cartilage is better if the bone marrow connects to the joint surface.

Surgical technique

Following cartilage debridement multiple small holes are made through the subchondral plate using specially designed sharp angled picks. The calcified layer of cartilage must be removed, usually by using a sharp curette, to provide a platform for the cells to attach to. Subchondral bone penetration occurs to a depth of 3–4mm and holes are spaced approximately 3–4mm apart. Ideally, a contained defect with sharp sided walls is prepared allowing the bone marrow blood in the defect to form a 'super clot'. Later differentiation into fibrocartilage then occurs.

Postoperative rehabilitation with a strict period of non-weight bearing is essential to allow the new tissue appropriate time to fill the lesion without being exposed to load. Rehabilitation, involving continuous passive motion therapy (CPM), is considered to be essential in postoperative management. Patients need to be aware of the requirement to use the CPM for 6h per day for 6 weeks or to perform at least 500 revolutions three times a day on a static bike without load.

Results of microfracture

Clinical results depend on the age of the patient, the size of the lesion, and the amount of fill that is achieved, as visualized on a magnetic resonance imaging scan. Younger (age <40 years) and active patients with smaller isolated traumatic lesions on the femoral condyles have the best long-term results. Results deteriorate with time, usually beginning after 18 months, particularly in older patients with defects in the patellofemoral and tibial joint surfaces. The inferior quality of the repair tissue, with incomplete defect filling and the appearance of new bone formation in the defect area are thought to be the cause of failure in these cases.

Indications

Microfracture is indicated for smaller (<2cm^2) contained lesions, not extending beyond underlying subchondral bone.

Autologous chondrocyte implantation (ACI)

Background

In this procedure, chondrocytes are harvested from a normal area in the knee prior to culturing in a laboratory and later reimplantation into the damaged area of the knee. Animal studies commenced in the 1960s and the first studies on humans were published in 1994.

Technique (Figure 8.2.2)

The first stage is arthroscopic, with inspection of the articular surface and confirmation of suitability for ACI treatment (full thickness chondral defect, area greater than 2cm^2, opposing surface with less than grade II changes, and patient able to comply with the rehabilitation protocol). A small (100–200mg) biopsy of articular cartilage is harvested from either the notch or the superomedial aspect of the trochlea using a curette. In the laboratory, individual chondrocytes are then released from the biopsy by enzymatic breakdown followed by cell culture in autologous serum.

Four to six weeks later an open arthrotomy is performed and the lesion curetted down to the subchondral bone plate. A flap of periosteum or a synthetic collagen membrane is prepared to the exact size using a paper or foil template and sutured over the prepared articular cartilage defect using fine 6/0 absorbable sutures to create a watertight space. Cells are then implanted by injection into the space with the recommendation of a minimum of 1 million cells per square cm of defect area.

In more recent developments of the ACI technique, cultured cells are seeded directly on to a synthetic membrane such as MACI

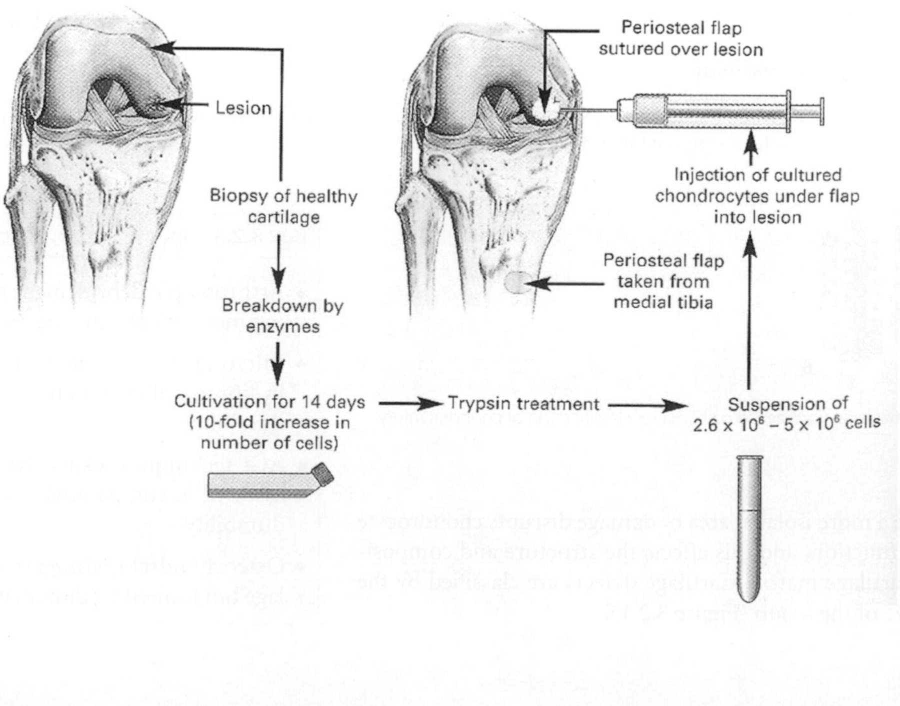

Fig. 8.2.2 Cartilage biopsy and preparation for autologous chondrocyte implantation.

(Genzyme UK) or into a three-dimensional matrix such as hyaluronic acid (Hyalograft-C, Fidia, Italy). Application of the patch in smaller contained defects arthroscopically has also been described.

Rehabilitation

Strict postoperative protocols are required, reducing load on the repaired area to allow healing. For tibiofemoral surface repairs 20kg of weight bearing is recommended whilst for patellofemoral surface repairs full weight bearing is allowed with limitations placed on stair climbing. Full rehabilitation is a lengthy process and tissue maturation continues for up to 3 years to create a resilient articular surface. Running or impact sports are not recommended for 9 months after surgery.

Histology and clinical results

Results are available with up to 16 years follow-up, and improvements have been demonstrated in more than 80% of the patients with relatively few complications. To date, six randomized trials have been published in addition to many case series. The short- to medium-term results from these early studies indicate no clear advantage of ACI over other surgical interventions but a more recent study comparing ACI with microfracture showed better histology and clinical results following ACI using characterized chondrocytes.

Returning to sports is an important goal of cartilage repair. In follow-up studies of ACI, clinical activity scores showed that return to sports including professional impact sports like football (soccer), ice hockey, and team handball, was possible in isolated femoral lesions and osteochondritis dissecans in eight to nine out of ten patients. In one study examining return to soccer in 45 patients, 92% had a good or excellent result on isolated femoral condyle lesions. Eighty-three per cent of high-skill level players returned to pre-injury level, with the highest chance in those who underwent surgery within 12 months of injury.

In another study of 35 young adolescent athletes undergoing ACI, 17 had previously had a failed microfracture procedure. All patients had a clinical improvement and returned to pre-injury level of sports. No failures were observed. The authors concluded that return to a high level of sports after ACI is possible, even if it takes 15 months to return to high-impact sports such as soccer.

Indications

ACI is primarily indicated for International Cartilage Repair Society (ICRS) grade III–IV contained lesions on one side of the joint or osteochondritis dissecans of the femoral condyle, trochlea, or patella. Salvage indications include uncontained lesions and those involving both sides of the joint (bipolar lesions).

Contraindications include rheumatoid arthritis and other systemic inflammatory joint diseases, as well as generalized osteoarthritis. Relative contraindications include obesity and smoking.

Osteochondral autograft transplantation

Background

This procedure involves transplanting healthy articular surface from one part of the knee to the damaged area as a functional osteochondral unit.

Technique

Healthy articular cartilage is normally harvested from the superolateral edge of the lateral trochlea or from around the intercondylar notch using harvesting coring devices of varying diameters. These cores of healthy tissue are then transplanted in to the damaged area as close to a perpendicular orientation as possible. The procedure can either be performed arthroscopically or using an open arthrotomy. Developments in instrumentation have allowed for this to become a reproducible, though demanding, arthroscopic procedure.

Results

Areas surrounding the grafted circles of tissue heal with fibrocartilage. It is recognized that harvesting itself damages the articular surface and approximately 25% of the grafted cartilage surface becomes non-viable after harvest. Initial outcome series reported good results for smaller lesions in 91% but there are few long-term studies or good comparative studies.

Indications

This technique is limited to full-thickness chondral and osteochondral defects in the knee with a maximum size up to 4cm^2 and less than 10mm in depth. For larger areas, donor site morbidity becomes unacceptable.

Realignment surgery

Any cartilage repair surgery will be compromised if the affected compartment is overloaded and it is essential to consider reducing the deforming force that may have initiated the damage process. A high tibial osteotomy can be performed to unload the medial compartment and a distal femoral osteotomy can be performed for lateral compartment overload. Anteromedialization of the tibial tubercle may be needed for trochlea or patella surface treatment with or without proximal soft tissue realignment.

Algorithm and factors for treatment

An algorithm for the treatment of articular cartilage defects affecting the femoral condyle or trochlea is given in Figure 8.2.3.

The natural history of a cartilage lesion is not fully understood, but lesions less than 1cm^2 usually do not progress. In addition, as some lesions do not cause symptoms it is important to tailor the treatment to various patient factors—it is not just one treatment for all patients. The three primary determining factors are the size of the lesion, patient demands or functional expectations, and whether treatment is primary or secondary with persistent symptoms following previous surgery. General patient factors include the age and gender of the patient, leg alignment, meniscal integrity, and ligament stability. However, overall factors including the financial cost of the procedure, experience of the surgeon, the implication of rehabilitation time for the patient, and the risk of complications also influence the decision.

Lesions up to 1cm diameter with unstable edges causing synovial irritation can be treated with simple mechanical debridement or radiofrequency treatment. For lesions 1–2cm^2 found at arthroscopy and considered to be causing symptoms, treatment depends on the patient's demands and simple debridement may be all that is necessary. Certainly procedures such as microfracture and grafting with synthetic or osteochondral plugs, which are indicated for the higher demand patient, should not be performed without ensuring the patient is aware of the commitment to rehabilitation.

For lesions over 2cm^2 the choice is more difficult. Up to 4cm^2 in the lower demand patient under age 40 then the fibrocartilage

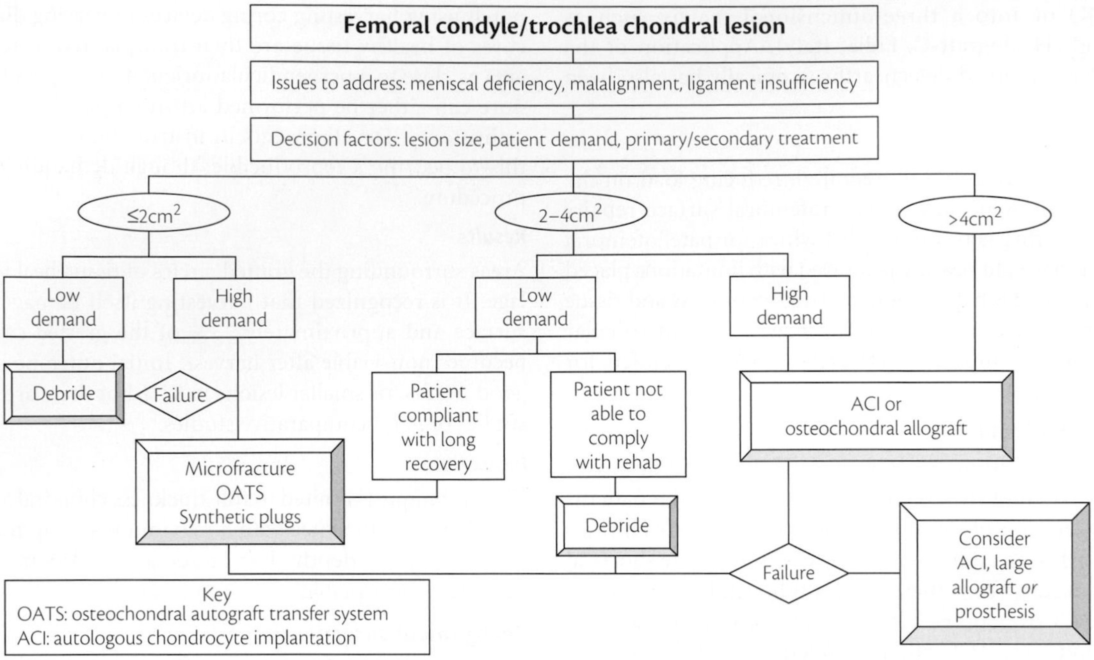

Fig. 8.2.3 Algorithm of treatment for chondral lesions.

repair induced by microfracture may be sufficient to protect the joint and relieve symptoms. In the higher demand patient, however, this is unlikely and ACI is indicated, taking into account the financial cost and the prolonged rehabilitation time.

Management of the larger lesions above 4cm^2 is more challenging and the prognosis is more guarded. Use of ACI in very large lesions is considered salvage surgery and alternatives such as massive allografts or prosthetic replacement need to be considered.

In revision cases, treatment is often determined by the first procedure and use of ACI is more likely to be indicated.

Future

The results of ongoing clinical studies are eagerly anticipated to answer remaining questions on the long-term results of articular cartilage repair surgery. Without treatment, articular cartilage injury is likely to result in post-traumatic osteoarthritis by degradation as the body lacks intrinsic repair capacity. Unfortunately, in the early stages of cartilage repair surgery, strict randomized trials were not performed and long-term data are therefore not available. Studies analysing the quality of the repaired surface indicates that only filling of the defect is required for early stage function but that the generation of hyaline articular cartilage is important for long-term durability.

It is clear that the goal of cartilage repair is to regenerate mature hyaline cartilage and to achieve this aim, regulation of chondrogenesis is required, involving either recruitment of host cells or differentiation of transplanted cells. In the advancing field of tissue bioengineering, scaffolds or matrices are being developed on which the cellular part of developing articular cartilage can grow. Much current research is focused on stimulation of this cellular growth with growth factors or genes.

It may be that development of *in situ* scaffolds that will capture the mesenchymal stem cells, such as the new bilayer scaffold made from poly(D,L-lactide-co-glycolide), PGA fibres, calcium sulphate, and surfactant (TruFit plugs, Smith and Nephew, USA) will provide a sufficient hyaline-like articular surface without the expense of culturing cells. Alternatively, the future may lie with cells held in synthetic scaffolds, including hyaluronic acid fleeces, collagen membranes, and hydrogels.

Demands for focal cartilage lesion treatment with cell therapy are likely to increase in the future and cartilage repair will continue to be one of the most rapidly advancing fields in knee surgery.

Further reading

Brittberg, M. (2008). Autologous chondrocyte implantation—technique and long-term follow-up. *Injury*, **39**(Suppl 1), S40–9.

Henderson, I., Lavigne, P., Valenzuela, H., and Oakes, B. (2006). Autologous chondrocyte implantation superior biologic properties of hyaline cartilage repairs. *Clinical Orthopaedics and Related Research*, **455**, 253–61.

Peterson L., Brittberg M., Kiviranta I., *et al.* (2002). Autologous chondrocyte transplantation: Biomechanics and long-term durability. *American Journal of Sports Medicine*, **30**(1), 2–12.

Rodrigo JJ., Steadman JR., Silliman JF., *et al.* (1994). Improvement in full thickness chondral defect healing in the human knee after debridement and microfracture using continuous passive motion. *American Journal of Knee Surgery*, **7**, 109–16.

Saris D., Vanlauwe J., Victor, J., *et al.* Characterized chondrocyte implantation results in better structural repair when treating symptomatic cartilage defects of the knee in a randomized controlled trial versus microfracture. *American Journal of Sports Medicine*, **36**(2), 235–46.

8.3

Magnetic resonance imaging of the knee

Ryan Shulman, Adrian Wilson, and Delia Peppercorn

Summary points

- ACL tear: abnormal fibres, tibial translation, PCL/patella tendon buckling, bone bruising
- Meniscal tear: signal change to free edge
- Bone bruising:
  - Reticular—not continuous subarticular bone
  - Geographic—extends to subarticular bone
- Posterolateral corner:
  - Oblique slices through fibular head
  - Consists of lateral collateral ligament, popliteus, popliteofibular ligament, and arcuate complex.

Magnetic resonance imaging (MRI) has revolutionized the investigation and treatment of the painful knee. It is non-invasive and avoids patient exposure to ionizing radiation. MRI has the advantage of establishing diagnoses in a painful knee without the morbidity of surgical intervention. It is now widely available and has moved from a simple diagnostic adjunct into a key planning tool. It offers improved management of theatre resources and it allows for more accurate planning of postoperative rehabilitation.

The role of MRI in management of the injured knee is determined by its cost-effectiveness and its ability to augment the diagnostic accuracy of clinical examination. Accuracy of clinical examination by specialist orthopaedic surgeons is comparable to MRI when interpreted by specialist radiologists (Table 8.3.1). Increasingly, MRI has been shown to be cost neutral. Whilst costs are high, diagnostic information reduces the need for unnecessary surgery.

Protocols

MRI protocols will differ slightly between units (Box 8.3.1). MRI T_1-weighted sequences are used to define local anatomy and can be used to identify trabecular microfracture. T_2-weighted sequences (with fat suppression) are most commonly employed to demonstrate oedema of both soft tissues and bone marrow. Proton density and T_2 gradient echo sequences are utilized to highlight meniscal pathology. Viewing images on a workstation is now preferred to hardcopy films with enhancement of brightness, contrast, and magnification with linking of orthogonal views. Comparison with plain radiographs complements interpretation of calcific lesions and assists identification of small avulsion injuries.

Bone bruising

Bone bruises are occult bony injuries and represent the local sequelae of chondral and microtrabecular trauma (Figure 8.3.1). Patterns of bone bruising can be pathognomonic for specific ligamentous injuries. Bone bruises have been described as reticular (oedema not extending to the subarticular cortical bone), or geographic (oedema which is continuous with the subarticular cortical bone). The long-term significance of these lesions has yet to be determined. However, histopathological studies of geographic bone bruises have demonstrated local chondrocyte and osteocyte death and have suggested that severe bone bruising may represent a precursor

Table 8.3.1 Diagnostic accuracy of MRI versus clinical examination in the acutely painful knee

	Medial meniscal tear		**Lateral meniscal tear**		**ACL (complete rupture)**		**PCL (complete rupture)**	
	Clinical[a]	MRI	Clinical[a]	MRI	Clinical[b]	MRI	Clinical	MRI[c]
Sensitivity	48/71	93	65/78	79	85/24	94	90	91
Specificity	94/87	88	86/90	96	94/98	94	99	99

[a] McMurray test/joint line tenderness
[b] Lachman test/pivot shift (without anaesthesia)
[c] MRI diagnosis of chronically PCL deficient knee has lower accuracy (57%)
ACL, anterior cruciate ligament; PCL, posterior cruciate ligament.

Box 8.3.1 MRI protocols

- T_1-weighted:
  - Local anatomy
  - Trabecular microfracture
- T_2-weighted:
  - Oedema in soft tissue and bone marrow
  - Meniscal pathology.

of early degenerative change. This could explain why degenerative changes develop despite successful anterior cruciate ligament (ACL) reconstruction and may provide justification for less aggressive rehabilitation programmes in patients with large subcortical lesions.

Cruciate ligament rupture

MRI is useful in the diagnosis of ACL rupture (Figure 8.3.1) and associated meniscal or chondral lesions. ACL rupture can be inferred from absence, discontinuity, or oedematous replacement of the normal ligamentous band that parallels Blumensaat's line. Less accurate indirect radiological signs such as buckling of either the posterior cruciate ligament (PCL) or patella tendons are evidence of anterior tibial translation (usually more than 5–7mm referenced from posterior margins of the tibia and femoral condyles). Difficulty arises from evaluation of partial tears, which should be correlated with clinical findings to determine appropriate management. Transient subluxation and impaction of the femur into the tibia at time of injury can lead to a 'kissing contusion' seen typically as bony oedema in the midportion of the lateral femoral condyle and posterior lip of the lateral tibial plateau. This 'traumatic pivot shift' is also responsible for the associated chondral, capsuloligamentous, and meniscal injuries.

Meniscal pathology

Clinical assessment of meniscal injuries (Table 8.3.1) is difficult and a combination of history and positive provocation tests are required for accurate diagnosis. In a systematic review of 32 papers, Ryzewicz and colleagues found that routine MRI was not indicated, as clinical assessment in experienced hands was of equal or higher reliability. However, MRI is able to assess the type of meniscal injury, aids surgical planning, and assists diagnosis with concomitant ligamentous injury where clinical examination becomes less reliable.

Detection of meniscal pathology involves identification of abnormal meniscal morphology and signal. Care should be taken as many asymptomatic individuals will have areas of high intrameniscal signal which is generally considered to be a normal consequence of aging. Abnormal signal, extending to the free edge of the meniscus, is accepted as representing a tear. However, a degenerative tear may not always represent the problematic pathology, and MRI review should not cease once a tear is identified. Meniscal fragments can become displaced into the intercondylar notch or settle into synovial recesses. It should also be noted that aberrant meniscal anatomy may mask injury. Remnants of a torn discoid meniscus can appear misleadingly normal.

Posterolateral corner injury

Posterolateral corner (PLC) injuries pose a difficult clinical problem. They often occur in conjunction with other ligamentous injuries and physical examination may be impossible in the acute setting. MRI allows evaluation of the PLC and can influence surgical management. Injuries to the PLC structures can be assessed with a variety of coronal, sagittal, and oblique views. Oblique coronal slices through the fibular head can more accurately demonstrate the popliteofibular ligament and inclusion of the fibular head in all sequences assists in diagnosis. Soft tissue oedema in the posterolateral aspect of the knee should always be viewed with suspicion. Osseous injuries such as occult arcuate fracture, Segond fracture, medial femoral condyle bone bruising, anterior rim tibial plateau fracture, and avulsion of Gerdy's tubercle should all be assessed. Each component should be reviewed and evidence of thickening, oedema, tear, disruption, or avulsion should be sought. However, the anatomical definition and individual variation of the PLC mean that defining all structures can be difficult. The popliteus, popliteofibular ligament, arcuate ligament, and lateral collateral ligament are primary structures considered for repair and thus their evaluation will provide the most useful information for surgical decision making.

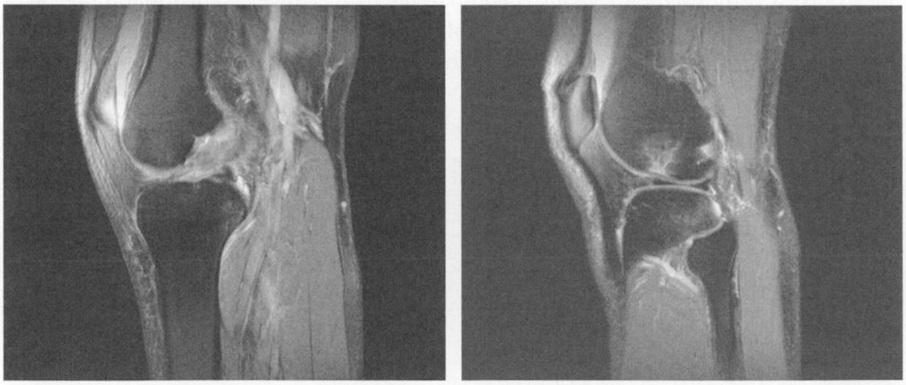
A B

Fig. 8.3.1 T_2-weighted (fat suppressed) images demonstrating A) ACL rupture–loss of fibre definition with oedema, and B) associated bone bruising of the lateral femoral condyle.

Postoperative imaging

Postoperative MRI is more difficult to interpret, although it is useful for the assessment of graft integrity, tunnel position, and tunnel widening following cruciate reconstruction, monitoring osteochondral defects or for missed meniscal pathology following arthroscopy. MR arthography using gadolinium has been employed to assess the postoperative meniscus and reconstructive grafts. Although this technique is invasive, it provides joint distension which facilitates imbibition of fluid into latent tears, potentially improving accuracy. However, at this time there are no convincing results to justify its routine use. Artefacts from modern metallic implants can now be minimized by various MRI techniques and do not preclude evaluation.

Miscellaneous pathology

MRI should be considered in the evaluation of other lesions in the knee joint. It can be used to provide prognostic data to patients with spontaneous osteonecrosis of the knee (SONK), examine the extent of spread of bony and soft tissue tumours (e.g. pigmented villonodular synovitis, PVNS), and evaluate postoperative cartilage repair after procedures such as chondrocyte implantation or marrow stimulating techniques.

Dramatic improvements in the quality of images produced by MRI over the past decade have provided clinicians with invaluable data that has undoubtedly saved patients from unnecessary surgery. It has also improved our understanding of pathology and the postoperative healing processes. As new technology improves resolution, and experimental techniques such as real-time MRI become more accessible, our understanding of individual patients' pathokinomatics will improve. The increasing quality of MRI will continue to augment clinical orthopaedic practice, and should ultimately result in improved outcomes for patients.

Further reading

Hayes, C.W. and Coggins, C.A. (2006). Sports-related injuries of the knee: an approach to MRI interpretation. *Clinics in Sports Medicine*, **25**(4), 659–79.

Nakamae, A., Engebretsen, L., Bahr, R., Krosshaug, T., and Ochi, M. (2006). Natural history of bone bruises after acute knee injury: clinical outcome and histopathological findings. *Knee Surgery, Sports Traumatology, Arthroscopy*, **14**, 1252–8.

Naraghi, A. and White, L. (2006). MRI evaluation of the postoperative knee: special considerations and pitfalls. *Clinics in Sports Medicine*, **25**(4), 703–25.

Oei, E.H.G., Nikken, J.J., Verstijnen, A.C.M., Ginai, A.Z., and Hunink, M.G.M. (2003). MR imaging of the menisci and cruciate ligaments: a systematic review. *Radiology*, **226**, 837–48.

Ryzewicz, M., Peterson, B., Siparsky, P.N., and Bartz, R.L. (2007). The diagnosis of meniscus tears: the role of MRI and clinical examination. *Clinical Orthopaedics and Related Research*, **455**, 123–33.

8.4

Osteotomies around the knee

Mui-Hong Lim and John Bartlett

Summary points

- Osteotomy about the knee can correct deformity and alter the alignment of the knee in different planes.
- Osteotomy of the knee is indicated for correction of alignment and offloading of affected compartment in osteoarthritis, instability, post cartilage repair and meniscectomy.
- Pre-operative planning for osteotomy of the knee involves patient selection, clinical and radiological assessment to achieve the desired knee alignment.
- Depending of the type of knee deformity, distal femoral or proximal osteotomy is indicated of the correction of the deformity.
- Osteotomy of the knee has been shown to provide pain relief and improve function in majority of patient.

Box 8.4.1 Aims of osteotomy

- Correct deformity
- Unload a damaged compartment
- Balance soft tissue.

Box 8.4.2 Principles of osteotomy

- As close to the site of deformity as possible
- Through cancellous bone
- In a mobile knee joint
- With stable internal fixation.

Introduction

Osteotomy of the proximal tibia or distal femur can alter the alignment of the knee in three planes—coronal, sagittal, or rotational axes.

The aim of the osteotomy might be to correct deformity due to fracture, growth plate arrest, or metabolic disease; to unload a compartment damaged by osteoarthritis or cartilage injury or to improve stability (Box 8.4.1).

The ideal patient will be active, young or middle aged, and have healthy bones and a mobile knee. The pathology will be either a unicompartmental problem or involve instability with deformity.

The principles of osteotomy involve creating the osteotomy as close to the site of the deformity as possible, preferably through cancellous bone with stable internal fixation (Box 8.4.2).

Principles of osteotomy

Osteotomy for osteoarthritis

The principle of osteotomy to unload a damaged compartment is based on the mechanical pathogenesis of osteoarthritis.

The mechanical axis (hip/knee/ankle alignment) of the leg is 0 degrees although the anatomical axis (femoro–tibial angle) is 5 degrees of valgus. This results from the distal femur being 8 degrees of valgus and the proximal tibia being 3 degrees of varus. With this alignment, 70% of the weight-bearing load passes through the medial compartment.

There are a number of factors which may increase this load, such as obesity. With an intact medial meniscus the surface contact area between medial femoral condyle and medial tibial condyle is $6cm^2$. Total meniscectomy reduces this to $2cm^2$ and hence a three times increase in load per unit area.

Articular cartilage is designed to withstand loads of $25kg/cm^2$—if the load exceeds $35kg/cm^2$ then matrix breakdown begins.

Cadaver studies have shown that in normal joints, very small changes in the relative alignment of the femur and the tibia produced marked changes in the amount of weight borne by the medial and lateral compartments of the knee. Osteotomy for osteoarthritis is based on this unloading effect on the damaged compartment.

Osteotomy for instability

Soft tissue surgery for correction of collateral instability is unlikely to be successful in the presence of malalignment with tension forces stretching the ligament repair or reconstruction. For example, lateral ligament instability will be aggravated in a varus knee. Corrective valgus osteotomy will relieve stress on the lateral soft tissues.

In a study relating gait analysis to results of valgus high tibial osteotomy (HTO), a low adduction moment gave uniformly good results whilst patients having a high adduction moment (varus thrust on walking) had only 64% good results.

With collateral ligament instabilities, balance of the knee is improved by osteotomy which moves the mechanical axis to the

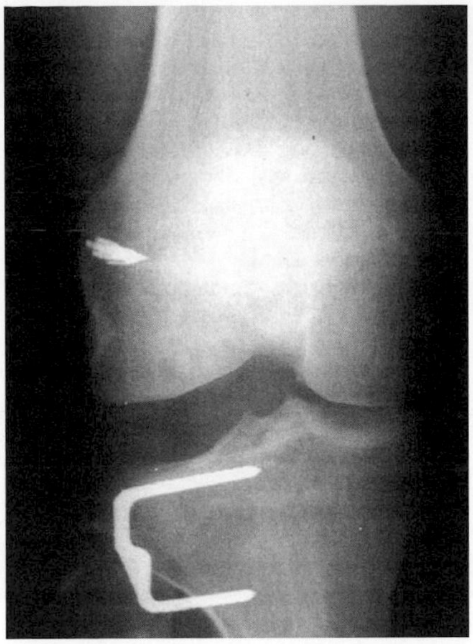

Fig. 8.4.1 Lateral collateral ligament laxity postosteotomy.

convex side. This relieves the tension stresses on the side of laxity although soft tissue repair or reconstruction is often also required to achieve stability (Figure 8.4.1).

The normal posterior slope of the medial tibial condyle is 6.7 degrees and the lateral tibial condyle 3 degrees. Any increase in slope will contribute to anterior translation of the tibia (and aggravate anterior cruciate ligament [ACL] instability) whilst a decrease slope will contribute to posterior translation (Figure 8.4.2). Any osteotomy that alters tibial slope may therefore influence cruciate stability.

Opening wedge HTO tends to result in increased tibial slope and thus increased anterior tibial translation. This is an advantage in posterior cruciate ligament instability resulting in symptomatic improvement. The converse is true of closing wedge HTO

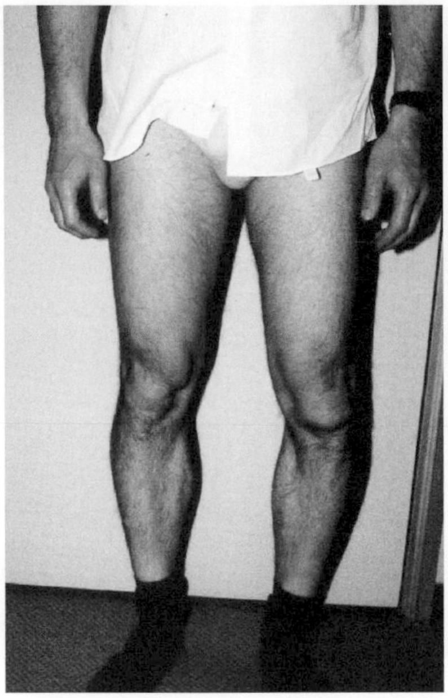

Fig. 8.4.3 ACL deficiency with genu varus.

where tibial slope tends to decrease, favouring its use in the ACL deficient knee.

Opening wedge HTO increasing the posterior tibial slope is also indicated in situations of hyperextension caused by premature closure of the anterior tibial growth plate or in some cases of soft tissue instability.

With varus plus ACL instability there is debate as to whether ACL reconstruction alone is sufficient to control symptoms or whether combined HTO and ACL reconstruction is more reliable. ACL graft forces are high in varus and internal rotation and most surgeons favour combined surgery (Figures 8.4.3–8.4.5).

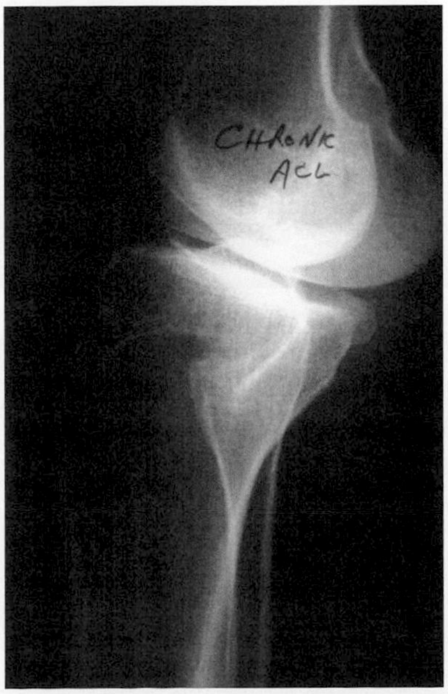

Fig. 8.4.2 Chronic ACL insufficiency with increased posterior tibial slope.

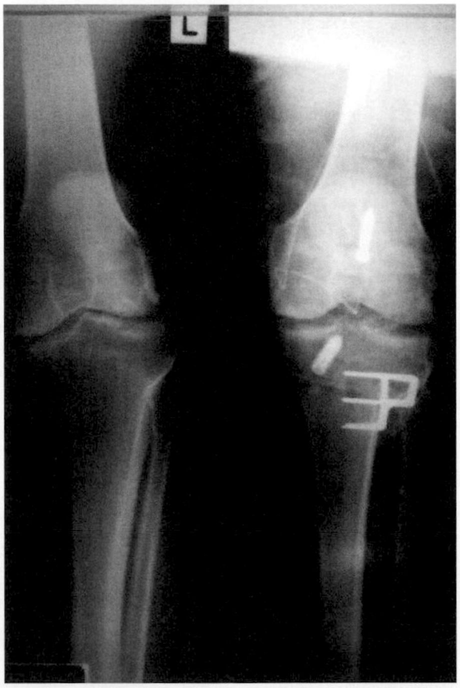

Fig. 8.4.4 Combined closing wedge HTO and ACL reconstruction.

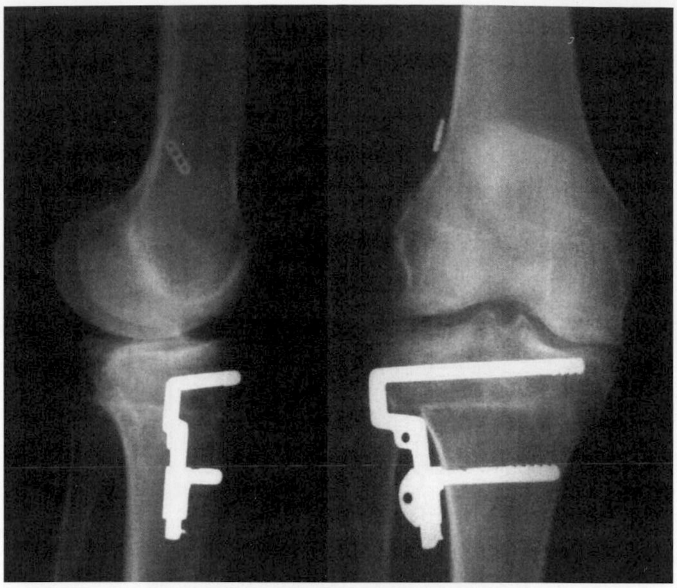

A B

Fig. 8.4.5 Combined closing wedge HTO and ACL reconstruction.

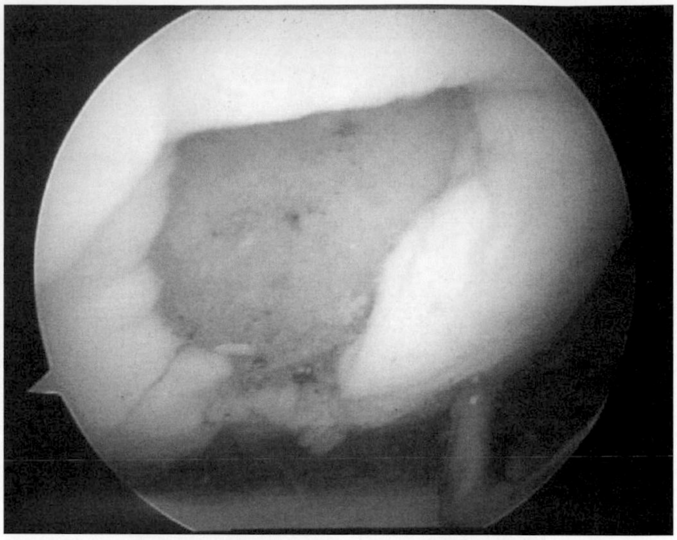

Fig. 8.4.6 Full thickness medial femoral condyle cartilage lesion.

Osteotomy for cartilage repair and postmeniscectomy

In the young patient with osteochondritis dissecans or post-traumatic full thickness articular cartilage loss on weight-bearing aspects of the femoral condyles consideration may be given to cartilage repair procedures such as microfracture, autologous chondrocyte implantation, or osteochondral grafting (Figure 8.4.6). Mechanical axis alignment becomes important as such procedures are unlikely to succeed if subject to excessive load. Hence osteotomy may be considered to unload a medial femoral condyle lesion in a varus knee or lateral lesion in a valgus knee. However, to reduce pressure on articular cartilage soft tissue release may also be required.

Meniscectomy

Meniscectomy predisposes to the premature onset of osteoarthritis, especially in association with malalignment (Figure 8.4.7). A long-term follow-up of arthroscopic lateral meniscectomy has shown a very high incidence of osteoarthritis.

When assessing the patient with postmeniscectomy pain, alignment is important. Magnetic resonance imaging or bone scan may confirm excessive stress in subchondral bone with thinning of

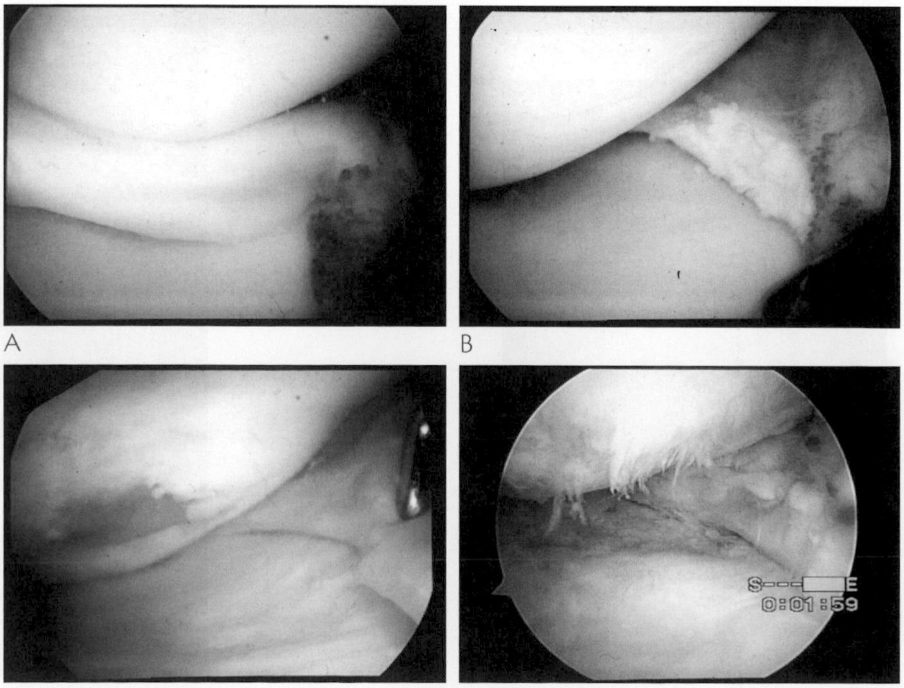

A B C D

Fig. 8.4.7 Development of secondary osteoarthritis postmeniscectomy.

articular cartilage and osteotomy may be appropriate to unload the damaged compartment.

Osteotomy versus replacement arthroplasty

Replacement arthroplasty of the knee involves a polished metal on ultra-high-molecular-weight polyethylene articulation. Polyethylene has a load to failure of 25MPa and this is exceeded in all high-impact activities which result in subsurface cracks, delamination, and fragmentation. Activities such as hiking and jogging also exceed polyethylene yield points.

As a result, the young, heavy, and active patient with osteoarthritis may be best managed with osteotomy whilst the older, lighter, and less active patient might be better managed with an arthroplasty. Comparative studies between tibial osteotomy and medial unicompartmental replacement have tended to favour arthroplasty, underlying the importance of patient selection for the appropriate procedure.

Preoperative planning

Osteotomy may be considered a four-dimensional procedure involving:

1) Positioning of the mechanical axis to a desired point
2) Manipulation of the tibial slope to influence anteroposterior stability
3) Consideration of rotation in cruciate, rotary, or patellar instability
4) Awareness of soft tissue balance with lax or contracted collateral and capsular ligaments.

Clinical examination

Active and passive range of movement is assessed noting fixed flexion or fixed angular deformity. The stability of the soft tissues and the mechanical axis alignment when weight bearing is recorded. The gait pattern is observed, especially noting any adduction moment or varus thrust.

X-ray evaluation

Standard anteroposterior, lateral, intercondylar, and skyline views are obtained for basic assessment.

A full-length standing hip/knee/ankle anteroposterior x-ray is required to assess the mechanical axis (Figure 8.4.8). Single leg standing x-rays will show greater deformity if a varus thrust is present on walking.

On occasion, varus valgus stress views are of value to assess soft tissue tension and determine whether soft tissue release is necessary for decompression or correction of alignment.

A bone scan may be helpful to demonstrate increased uptake in over loaded bones.

Determination of the desired position of the mechanical axis is critical to allow templating with measurement of the required angle of correction. In the varus osteoarthritic knee this is commonly at Fujisawa's point at 35% across the lateral tibial condyle. The degree of correction may also vary depending on the degree of joint damage with more correction required for greater degree of cartilage loss (Figure 8.4.9).

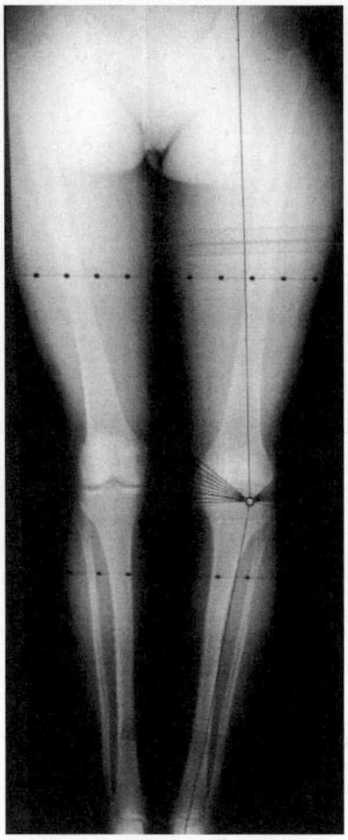

Fig. 8.4.8 Full-length standing hip/knee/ankle anteroposterior radiograph for assessment of the mechanical axis.

Operative technique

The amount of correction required to place the mechanical axis in the desired position and the tibial slope correction is measured using x-ray templates (Figure 8.4.10).

Intraoperative instrumented jigs allow measurement of the angular correction during surgery.

Computer assisted surgery

If the accuracy of computer navigation in osteotomy can be confirmed then it holds great promise for more accurate correction of deformity which should lead to improved results. The essential advantage of computer assisted surgery is accurate localization of the femoral head during surgery which should improve the accuracy of assessment of the mechanical axis.

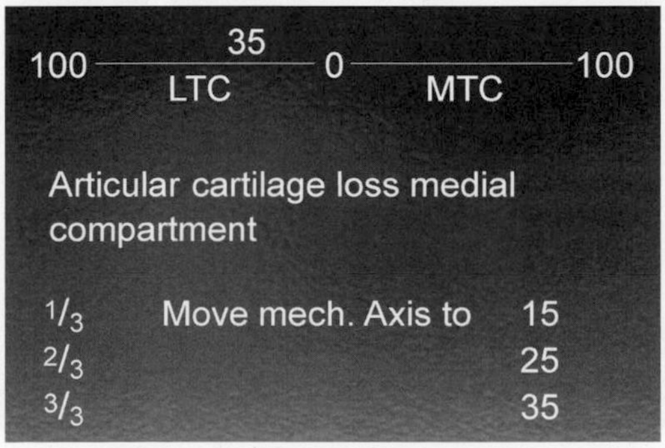

Fig. 8.4.9 Degree of correction based on Fujisawa's point and extent of joint space loss.

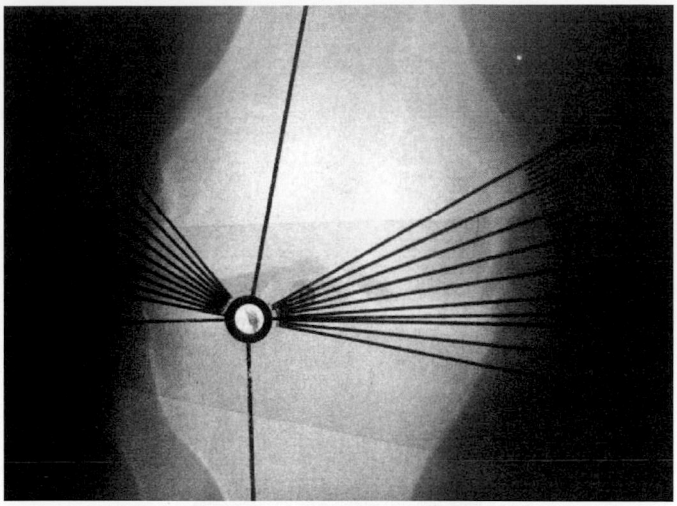

Fig. 8.4.10 X-ray template to guide the extent of correction.

Varus knee

Most commonly bone loss is on the tibial side and proximal tibial osteotomy is appropriate. This may be opening wedge from the medial side or closing wedge from the lateral side.

Closing wedge

A lateral approach involves reflection of tibialis anterior to expose the lateral surface of the tibia. A laterally-based wedge of bone immediately proximal to the tibial tubercle is excised. To allow closure of the osteotomy, release of the fibula is required and this may be performed at different levels. Release through the superior tibiofibular joint is safest and most popular; osteotomy of the fibular head or neck places the common peroneal nerve at risk; through the proximal third of the fibula threatens the nerve to extensor hallucis longus; and through the distal third of the fibula has a high incidence of non-union.

For stability of the osteotomy it is important to protect the medial tibial cortex and maintain correction with internal fixation.

The advantage of closing wedge HTO is bone-to-bone apposition which allows for early weight bearing and bone union. It is therefore favoured in older patients with osteoarthritis, large corrections of more than 12 degrees, and with associated ACL instability to reduce the posterior slope of the tibia.

Opening wedge

A medial approach releasing part of the superficial medial collateral ligament is performed and the osteotomy is directed proximal to the tibial tubercle towards the superior tibiofibular joint. Again the opposite cortex is preserved intact for stability. Gradual opening to the desired correction and stable fixation is required. For larger corrections bone graft is recommended—this can be autograft, allograft, or synthetic bone graft substitute. Major risks are fracture into the knee joint and non-union.

The advantages are that the fibula is not disturbed and there is less distortion of proximal tibial morphology which may be important should total knee replacement be required at a later date.

Opening wedge osteotomy is therefore recommended in younger patients, for corrections of less than 12 degrees or for posterior cruciate ligament instability or hyperextension because of the increased posterior slope of the tibia.

Valgus knees

In valgus knees the bone loss contributing to the deformity is most commonly on the femoral side (Figure 8.4.11). Hence a distal femoral osteotomy is recommended. As with the tibia this can be opening wedge or closing wedge but risk of non-union has led to closing

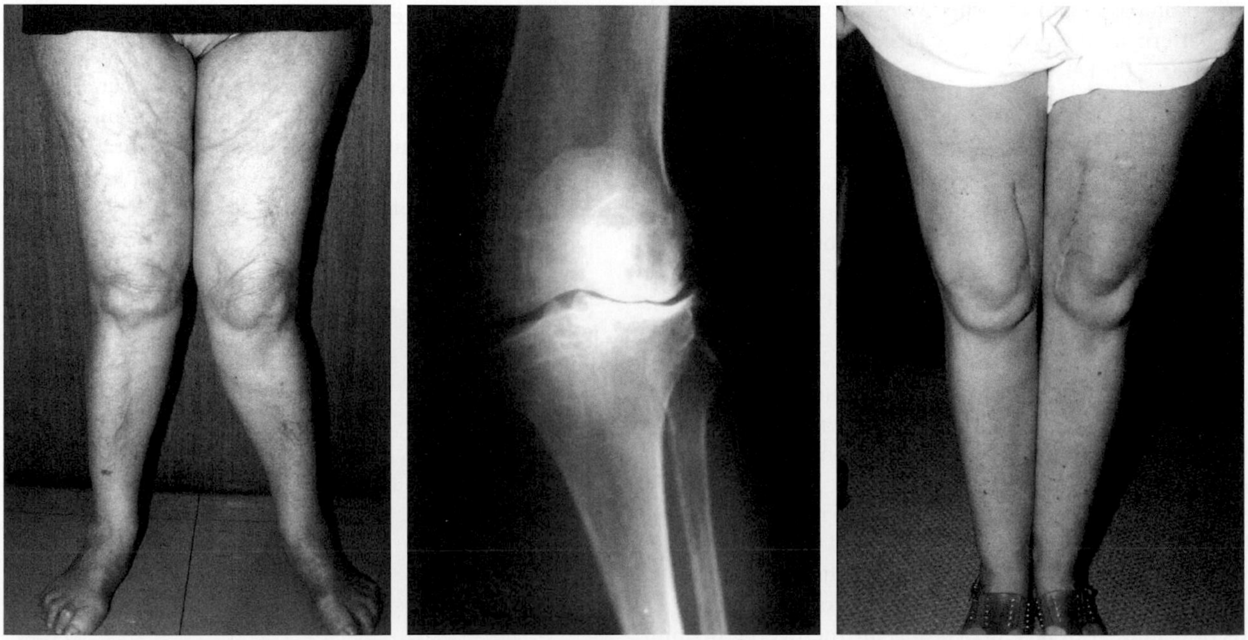

A B C

Fig. 8.4.11 A) Pre- and B) postoperative illustrations of a patient with genu valgum deformity.

wedge being more reliable. Again accurate intraoperative correction is required; protection of the opposite cortex and stable internal fixation to maintain correction, promote bone union, and allow early motion.

In some circumstances, e.g. previous lateral meniscectomy or fractured lateral tibial condyle, more minor valgus deformities may be corrected by a varus closing wedge HTO. However the correction should not exceed 8 degrees because of risks of creating an oblique joint line.

Recurvatum knee

Hyperextension or recurvatum deformity may follow premature closure of the anterior tibial growth plate, soft tissue instability, or fracture malunion (Figure 8.4.12).

Anterior opening wedge HTO and bone grafting will correct the deformity (Figure 8.4.13). If proximal to the tibial tubercle there is risk of increased patellofemoral pressure.

Opening wedge versus closing wedge

There is a place for both opening wedge and closing wedge HTO but on the femoral side closing wedge is favoured because of the high incidence of delayed union and non-union with opening wedge distal femoral osteotomy (Table 8.4.1, Figures 8.4.14 and 8.4.15).

Risks and complications

The risks of HTO are summarized in Box 8.4.3.

Evidence in favour of osteotomy

- Long-term survival correlates with maintenance of correction. The greater the valgus correction, the slower the progress of medial joint arthrosis

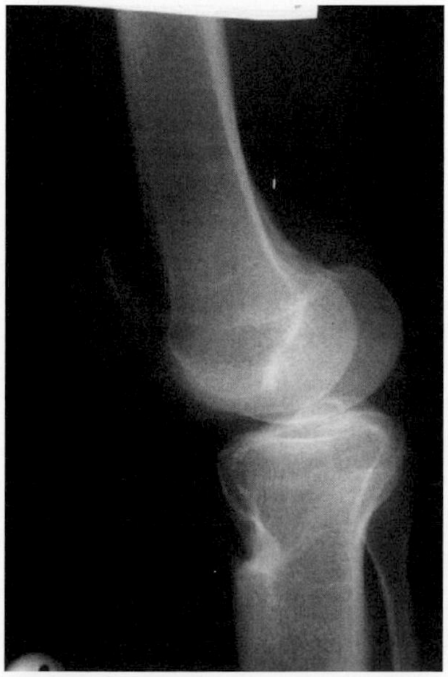

Fig. 8.4.12 Genu recurvatum deformity following premature closure of the anterior tibial growth plate.

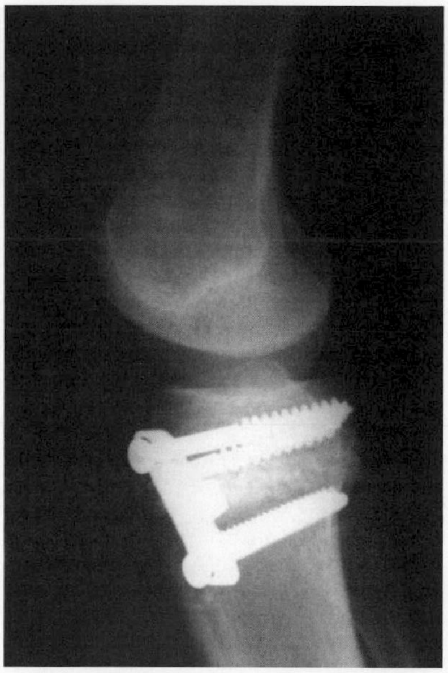

Fig. 8.4.13 Correction of deformity following an anterior opening wedge HTO.

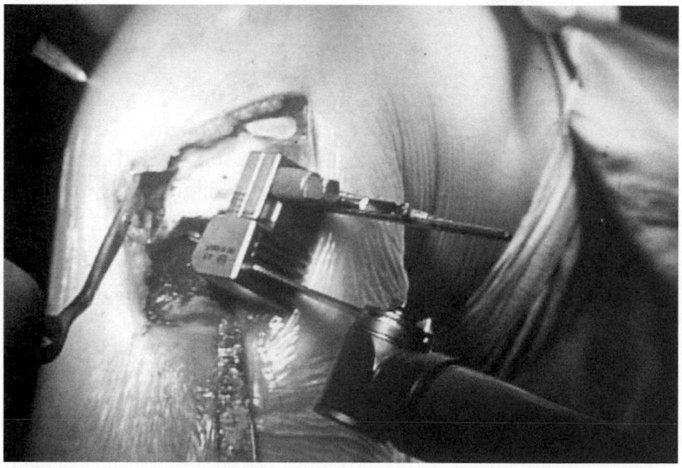

Fig. 8.4.14 Closing wedge osteotomy.

Table 8.4.1 Advantages and disadvantages of opening wedge versus closing wedge

	Advantages	Disadvantages
Closing wedge	No bone graft	Bone loss
	Early stability	Altered anatomy with offset tibial plateau and high fibula
	Early weight bearing	Patella infera
	Low non-union rate	Tendency to decrease tibial slope
Opening wedge	Less bone deformity	Bone graft
	Fibula not affected	Delayed union
	Common peroneal nerve not at risk	Fracture into joint on distraction
	Anterior compartment and tibialis anterior spared	Patella infera
		Tendency to increase tibial slope

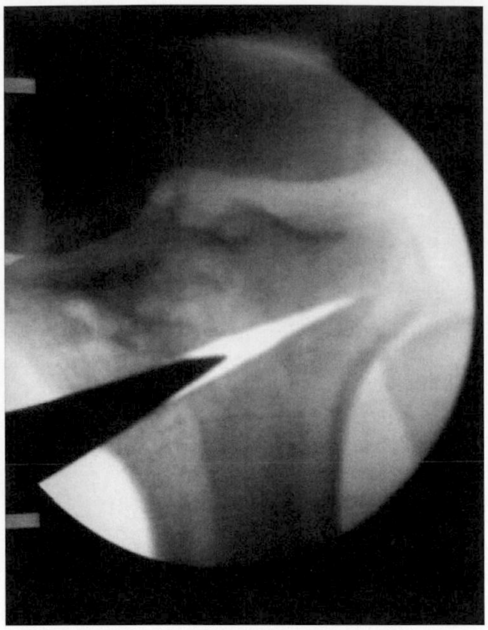

Fig. 8.4.15 Opening wedge osteotomy.

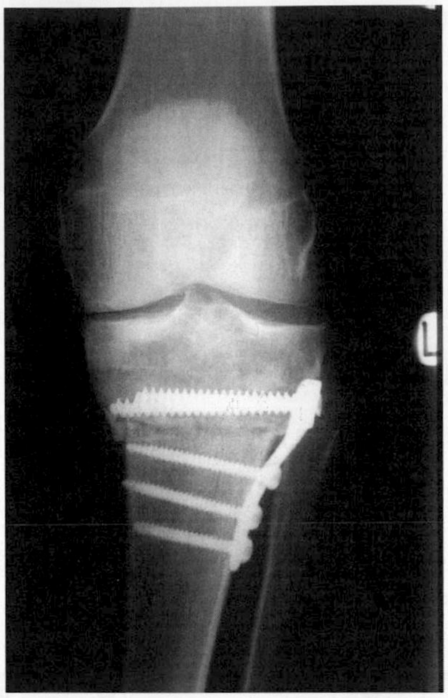

Fig. 8.4.16 Varus deformity after closing wedge osteotomy.

- If correction of deformity is maintained there is a lower incidence of subsequent revision to replacement arthroplasty. Using arthroplasty as the endpoint, it has been shown that survival at 10 years was 90% when the radiographic valgus angle at 1 year was between 8 and 16 degrees
- With bone scans performed before and after surgery there is a resolution of the preoperative increased uptake indicating unloading of the damaged compartment
- High articular cartilage and subchondral bone stresses are relieved by correction of malalignment
- High impact forces exceed the yield point of polyethylene and hence young, heavy, active patients are best considered for osteotomy
- Anteroposterior stability is altered by adjustments to the posterior tibial slope
- Fibrocartilage will heal across eburnated subchondral bone with restoration of joint space if adequate correction is obtained.

Box 8.4.3 Risks and complications of osteotomy

- Loss of correction
- Delayed union/non-union
- Common peroneal nerve injury
- Intra-articular fracture
- Vascular injury
- Compartment syndrome
- Patella infera.

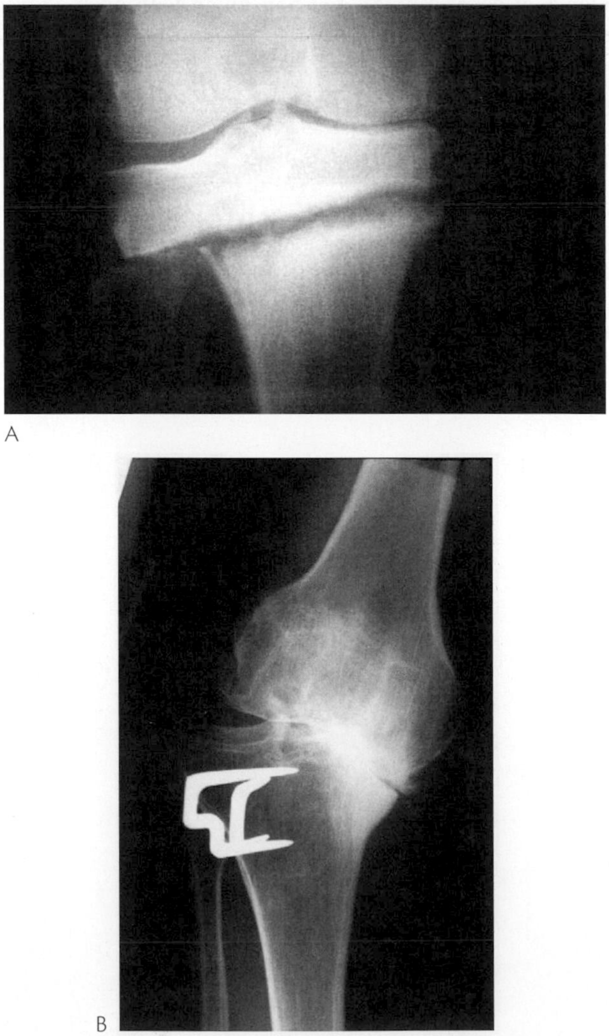

A

B

Fig. 8.4.17 Avascular necrosis of the A) proximal tibia and B) medial tibial condyle after osteotomy.

Long-term results of osteotomy

In general, osteotomy has been shown to improve function and provide pain relief for the majority of patients. A 10- to 21-year follow-up study on tibial osteotomy for varus osteoarthritis demonstrated that osteotomy allowed 10 to 15 years of pain relief, good range of motion and function in a large number of patients. However, results tend to deteriorate with time.

The 10-year survival rate of HTO varies from 51% to 90% in different studies.

In a Cochrane review (2007) based on 13 studies, most studies showed less pain and improvement in function scores after osteotomy, but no study compared osteotomy with conservative treatment.

Function can be improved with low-impact activities such as walking and stair climbing but improvement in true activity levels as measured on the Tegner scale has not been demonstrated.

Total knee arthroplasty after osteotomy

Inadequate symptomatic relief with persisting pain and limited function often associated with recurrent varus deformity or complications may require revision to total replacement arthroplasty.

A number of studies have reported poorer results in the osteotomy group with reduced flexion and higher reoperation rate with many concluding that total knee arthroplasty (TKA) after HTO is a technically more challenging procedure than primary TKA. The functional outcomes at a mean follow-up of 5 years after TKA in patients with a previous HTO tend to be inferior.

Others have reported a high rate of radiographic evidence of loosening with 8% of knees revised at 5.9 years postarthroplasty. Male gender, increased weight, young age at the time of TKA, coronal laxity, and preoperative limb malalignment have been identified as risk factors for early failure.

In contrast, a comparative study of patients who had bilateral total knee replacement following unilateral HTO reported that while patients with a previous HTO have important differences preoperatively, including valgus alignment, patella infera, and decreased bone stock in the proximal part of the tibia, results of arthroplasty in knees with and without a previous HTO are not substantially different.

Perceived difficulties are listed in Box 8.4.4.

The principles for revision of osteotomy to arthroplasty involve:

- A two-stage procedure with the first stage being removal of metal and arthroscopy in order to avoid added trauma and exposure
- Templating for the possible need of an offset fixation stem
- Choosing the exposure which least disturbs the extensor mechanism
- Resurfacing the patella because of altered height and tilt
- Dividing and substituting for the posterior cruciate ligament because it is contracted by changes in tibial slope
- Anticipating difficulty with soft tissue balance because of an oblique joint line and high fibula
- Cementing the tibial component because of abnormal proximal tibial bone.

Box 8.4.4

- Non-union or malunion
- Previous scarring with difficult access
- Extra exposure required
- Patella infera
- Soft tissue imbalance
- Oblique joint line
- Alterations to tibial slope
- Adherent neurovascular structures
- Removal of metal fixation devices.

In conclusion, most authors agree that it is technically more demanding to perform a total knee arthroplasty after an HTO.

Conclusion

Osteotomy about the knee is an effective method of unloading a damaged compartment and improving stability. Surgery for ligament reconstruction or cartilage repair will fail in the presence of malalignment. However, the aims and principles of osteotomy must be adhered to, together with careful preoperative preparation and surgical technique.

Maintenance of correction of the osteotomy correlates with long-term successful outcome.

Further reading

Fujisawa, Y., Masuhara, K., and Shiomi, S. (1979). The effect of high tibial osteotomy on osteoarthritis of the knee. An arthroscopic study of 54 knee joints. *Orthopedic Clinics of North America*, **10**, 585–608.

Hsu, R.W., Himeno, S., Coventry, M.B., and Chao, E.Y. (1990). Normal axial alignment of the lower extremity and load-bearing distribution at the knee. *Clinical Orthopaedics and Related Research*, **255**, 215–27.

Koshino, T., Wada, S., Ara, Y., and Saito, T. (2003). Regeneration of degenerated articular cartilage after high tibial valgus osteotomy for medial compartmental osteoarthritis of the knee. *Knee*, **10**, 229–36.

Sledge CB (1975). Structure, development, and function of joints. *Orthopedic Clinics of North America*, **6**, 619–28.

Walker, P.S. and Erkman, M.J. (1975). The role of the menisci in force transmission across the knee. *Clinical Orthopaedics and Related Research*, **109**, 184–92.

8.5

Arthrodesis of the knee

Andrew Floyd

Summary points

- Rare operation in developed countries
- Most often used for post infection damage in developing countries
- Still used as a last resort for failed knee replacements.

Introduction

Arthrodesis of the knee is a rare operation in the developed world—being largely a salvage procedure for a failed knee replacement—particularly following infection. In the developing world, it still has a place after primary joint infections, in particular tuberculosis and in post-traumatic osteoarthritis. Individual circumstances are paramount. A rigid straight knee might be a very disabling problem for a Western business man needing to travel by automobile or airplane. The same pain-free knee might be life saving in a subsistence farmer struggling to feed a family.

Indications

Arthrodesis of the knee should be considered in a painful and unstable knee joint which is not suitable for knee replacement. Stiffness of the joint would also favour arthrodesis. Suitability for knee replacement is addressed in a later chapter. Arthrodesis may be appropriate in paralytic conditions such as poliomyelitis but a locking caliper allowing the knee to flex for sitting is preferable in the majority of cases. The need to squat for toilet purposes is a relative but not complete contraindication for knee arthrodesis. Temporary preoperative immobilization of the knee in a cast is strongly recommended to allow the patient to assess the social and practical limitations of a permanently stiff knee. The ipsilateral hip and ankle joint should, ideally, be mobile and pain free. Bilateral knee arthrodeses make life extremely awkward and should be avoided if at all possible.

Without doubt the most common indication for a knee arthrodesis in the developed world is failure of a total knee replacement, particularly following infection. The presence of infection and lack of bone stock with poor blood supply makes this a particularly challenging problem best addressed by experienced knee surgeons with adequate facilities. Any infection should be treated energetically prior to an attempt at fusion. This should be by drainage and debridement supplemented with appropriate antibiotics. A two-stage procedure with initial implantation of antibiotic-impregnated beads may be necessary. In rare cases, where low-grade infection persists, arthrodesis may still be undertaken. Stabilization of the bone and soft tissues may, in some cases, enhance resolution of the infection.

Arthrodesis may also be appropriate following tumour resection around the knee where a knee replacement is not technically feasible.

Technique

While arthrodesis of a stable post-tubercular joint has a very high success rate and can be achieved with simple techniques, arthrodesis of an infected failed knee replacement with poor soft tissue cover and scanty residual bone is extremely challenging and will require very sophisticated techniques. The greatest advance in recent years has been the use of circular frames such as the Ilizarov system. Large blocks of well profused cancellous bone are straightforward to fuse—thinned out, devitalized cortical shells may be impossible.

Biological factors such as bone vitality, the state of the soft tissue envelope, and the virulence of the infection are paramount in decision making. Some form of rigid fixation is advocated in achieving knee arthrodesis. Techniques are summarized in Table 8.5.1.

Long intramedullary nails (Figure 8.5.1A) produce the highest success rate of all techniques. Intramedullary nails require accurate preoperative planning and measurement of both the medullary diameter and leg length. They are probably best supplied with a gentle anterior curve to simulate slight flexion at the arthrodesis. Although a curved nail may break more easily than a straight one, a curved nail is better at controlling rotation. Active infection, gross deformity, previous fractures causing obliteration of the medullary canal, as well as an ipsilateral hip replacement may be contraindications to the use of a long intramedullary nail. Shorter locking nails with a locking device at the knee are a possible alternative.

Double compression plating is an option (Figure 8.5.1B) but may have significant problems with skin closure if scarring, infection,

Table 8.5.1 Comparison of techniques

	Advantages	Disadvantages
Intramedullary nail	Early complete weight bearing High rate of union	Dissemination of infection Breakage of nail Rotation not always controlled Pre-existing femoral or tibial deformity
Double plating	Familiar technique Implants widely available. Rigid fixation with compression	Soft-tissue closure Second procedure to remove plate Stress riser at end of plates
External fixation	Useful in infected cases Achieves compression Can be fabricated in Third World situations	Unwieldy for patient Pin-tract problems: (a) infection (b) fractures (c) loosening

and other soft tissue problems exist. With intramedullary nailing, the femur and tibia will be in a straight line, whilst with plating the normal mechanical axis can be maintained. There is no evidence, however, that technical difference significantly affects the outcome. External fixators are particularly appropriate in infected cases. Two-plane fixation or double-ended pins provide superior fixation

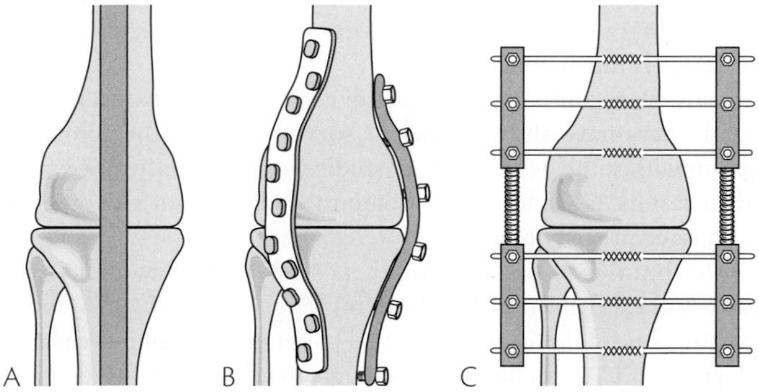

Fig. 8.5.1 Methods of mechanical fixation of arthrodesis of the knee: A) intramendullary nail; B) double-compression plating; C) external fixator.

to single-plane, one-sided fixators. Three to six pins above and below the knee confer a rigidity completely lacking in old-fashioned devices such as the Charnley clamp, aiding prompt union.

Ring fixators such as the Ilizarov device have achieved success where other techniques have failed at the expense of prolonged immobilization and a very awkward and bulky device for the patient's daily activities. The advantages of ring fixators are the ability to fully weight bear early, particularly in patients with poor bone quality.

Resection arthrodesis for tumour surgery may require the interposition of allografts or autografts—preferably vascularized autografts. In this situation, greater stress will be applied to the fixation device for a longer time. Such cases should be confined to surgeons and centres with sufficient experience and expertise.

Further reading

Arroyo, J.S., Garvin, K.L., and Neff, J.R. (1997). Arthrodesis of the knee with modular titanium intramedullary nail. *Journal of Bone and Joint Surgery*, **79A**, 26–35.

Damron, T.A and McBeath, A.A (1995). Arthrodesis following failed total knee arthroplasty. *Orthopaedics*, **18**, 361–8.

Garberina, M.J., Fitch, R.D., Hoffmann, E.D., *et al.* (2001). Knee arthrodesis with circular external fixation. *Clinical Orthopaedics and Related Research*, **382,** 168–178.

Fern, E.D, Stewart, H.D and Newton, G. (1989). Curved Kuntscher nail arthrodesis after failure of knee replacement. *Journal of Bone and Joint Surgery*, **71B**, 588–90.

Nichols, S.J, Landon, G.C., and Tullos, H.S. (1991). Arthrodesis with dual plates after failed total knee arthroplasty. *Journal of bone and Joint Surgery*, **73A**, 1020-4.

Wade, P.J.F. and Denham, R.A. (1984). Arthrodesis of the knee after failed knee replacement. *Journal of Bone and Joint Surgery*, **66B,** 362–6.

8.6

Total knee replacement

William J. Long and Giles R. Scuderi

Summary points

- Modern total knee replacement is a safe, effective, durable, and reproduceable solution to address symptomatic degenerative joint disease of the knee.

Introduction

The era of modern total knee arthroplasty (TKA) has undergone numerous design changes over the last three decades. It is an effective procedure that reduces pain and improves function. Despite multiple advances, surgical management and successful clinical outcomes continue to rely on the basic principles of accurate soft tissue balancing, well positioned components, and a neutrally aligned mechanical axis.

Indications

A complete history and physical examination are important in localizing pain and disability in the degenerative knee. Initial management may include non-steroidal anti-inflammatory drugs (NSAIDs), intra-articular injections, and possibly surgical arthroscopy. Other important modalities often overlooked in early management include an exercise programme and weight loss, both of which have been shown to be of benefit to patients with symptomatic arthritis.

Cemented TKA remains the gold standard for surgical management of symptomatic unicompartmental, bicompartmental, and tricompartmental arthritis of the knee that fails non-operative management. Predictable and durable results have been achieved in older and younger patient populations. Gender differences in preoperative functional decline and pre-existing quadriceps weakness suggest that a more aggressive approach and earlier intervention may be indicated when addressing females with progressive knee arthritis.

Athletic activity and high demand following TKA is a growing area of interest as little is known about the impact of these activities on long-term survivorship. Surgeon surveys have demonstrated that for the most part, moderate non-impact activities were recommended, although whether these guidelines are followed by younger, healthy, more active individuals is unknown. Implantable monitors may provide further insight into the forces in a total knee replacement following surgery, allowing surgeons to develop more scientific basis for these recommendations.

Design considerations

Fixation

Concern arose in total hip fixation when the well-designed cemented total hip system popularized by Charnley was applied to younger patients. Multiple centres reported higher rates of failures in this younger cohort which prompted the development of uncemented surfaces. Forces at the cement bone interface in the hip include a combination of shear, tension, and compression. This is distinctly different from the total knee setting, where the interface is primarily subjected to compressive forces, for which a cement interface is much better suited.

Long-term comparative studies of cemented versus uncemented total knees have shown superior survivorship in the cemented group with some designs. Other studies have demonstrated equivalent results. No studies have demonstrated superior survivorship with uncemented designs.

We continue to use a cemented, posterior stabilized design and have had excellent results in both our large outcome series, survivorship study, and in those selected patients less than 50 years old (Figure 8.6.1). A similar result, with greater than 95% survivorship at 10 years has also been noted elsewhere in younger patients.

Antibiotic cement

There are currently a number of commercially available, pre-mixed antibiotic cements for prophylactic use in total joint arthroplasty. Results from the Norwegian Arthroplasty Registry revealed at 1.8 times higher rate of infection when only systemic antibiotic therapy was used in cemented total hip arthroplasty. One randomized study in cemented primary total knees, demonstrated no infections with antibiotic cement, versus a 3.1% rate in total knees with standard cement. All infections occurred in patients with diabetes mellitus. These results provide evidence for the use of antibiotics in high-risk groups and have created debate as to the benefit of routine use of low-dose antibiotic cement in primary TKA.

Posterior cruciate ligament management

Excellent clinical results have been reported with both modern posterior cruciate ligament-retaining and posterior stabilized designs. A meta-analysis of eight randomized trials comparing the two techniques failed to demonstrate a difference in outcomes.

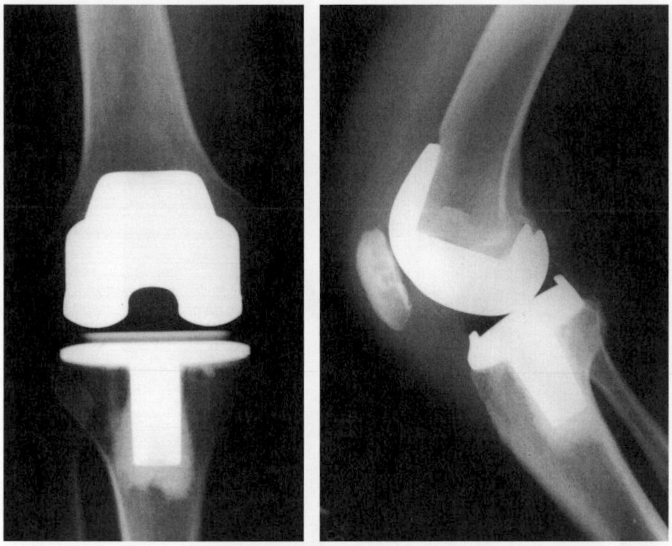

Fig. 8.6.1 A) Anteroposterior and B) lateral radiographs of a cemented IB II TKA functioning well at 15-year follow-up.

Some studies have shown superior outcomes with posterior stabilized components in specific subsets of patients. Rheumatoid knees have been shown to have a higher failure rate with one posterior cruciate-retaining design, though more recent studies have presented more favourable results with other posterior cruciate ligament-retaining designs. Patients with a planovalgus foot deformity are also at increased risk of failure when a posterior cruciate ligament-retaining component is used.

Fixed versus mobile bearing

Multiple studies have examined the clinical outcomes of mobile versus fixed bearing designs and have failed to demonstrate a benefit to the mobile bearing design. Bearing dislocation remains a risk with this design if the knee is not appropriately balanced. One of the strongest arguments for mobile bearings is that they are more forgiving of component malrotation, and thus decrease patellar based complications, but again this has not been shown clinically. A second theoretical benefit of mobile bearings is decreased wear. An early retrieval study has demonstrated increased polyethylene wear with this type of bearing, but this has not yet been confirmed in clinical outcome studies.

Articular conformity

We currently employ a conforming, high flexion design, with highly cross-linked polyethylene, for the vast majority of our primary TKAs. Our early outcome studies with this new design have been promising, as have *in vivo* biomechanical studies, but long-term follow-up does not yet exist.

Designs with flat-on-round articulations created point and edge loading resulting in increased failure rates. The current high flexion fixed bearing designs employed today involve a conforming articular tibial geometry. The tibial component allows a higher degree of flexion without posterior edge loading, and also has an anterior recess for the patellar component as the knee goes into deep flexion.

Patellar resurfacing

Improvements in implant design have resulted in a significant decrease in patellar component-related modes of failure in TKA. Modifications include more anatomical trochlear geometry, tibial polyethylene recession, and the redesign of metal-backed patellae. It must be emphasized that although metal backing has been associated with high rates of failure with some designs, this is not always the case and is likely to be design specific.

A number of randomized clinical trials exist comparing patellar resurfacing versus non-resurfacing in modern designs with no significant difference in outcomes shown. The two longest demonstrate no clinical difference at a minimum of 10-year follow-up.

Modularity

Tibial modularity was introduced for a number of reasons: biomechanical studies showed improved stress distribution with a metal-backed design; lower rates of loosening were observed in some early metal-backed designs versus a similar monoblock polyethylene component; and the option for isolated liner exchange existed if symmetric laxity or polyethylene wear occurred. However, recent long-term follow-up results have begun to question the benefit of modularity, as clinical results have demonstrated significant wear rates with some modular implants, although this is likely design, preparation (sterilization), and technique specific as other modular designs have not demonstrated increased wear.

Recent reconsideration of the monoblock design has been prompted by a number of long-term studies demonstrating excellent survivorship. A 98% survival at 14 years in patients over 75 years of age and no failures in a younger active population with monoblock designs were reported in recent studies. Other authors have not only noted excellent survival, but also a significant cost savings of over 700 USD per case.

A new design consisting of compression-moulded polyethylene on a porous tantalum base plate has introduced the possibility for long-term biological fixation into the porous metal surface. Basic science research involving porous metal has shown a number of benefits including its bone ingrowth qualities, the low modulus of elasticity, and initial friction fit. Early clinical results have been presented, but no long-term follow-up studies have been published.

Gender-specific designs

Review of the National Joint Registry for England and Wales demonstrated a lower level of satisfaction in females following TKA. Other authors have confirmed this observation with increased rates of pain and stiffness in radiographically well fixed and well aligned components. Anatomical studies as far back as 1996 have demonstrated important size and alignment discrepancies between male and female knees. The combined results of these anatomical and clinical studies have lead to gender-specific femoral component designs (Figure 8.6.2). Our early surgical results were reviewed, and demonstrated a statistically significant reduction in lateral patellar release rates in women with a modified femoral design. Clinical results following the introduction of these modifications are not yet available.

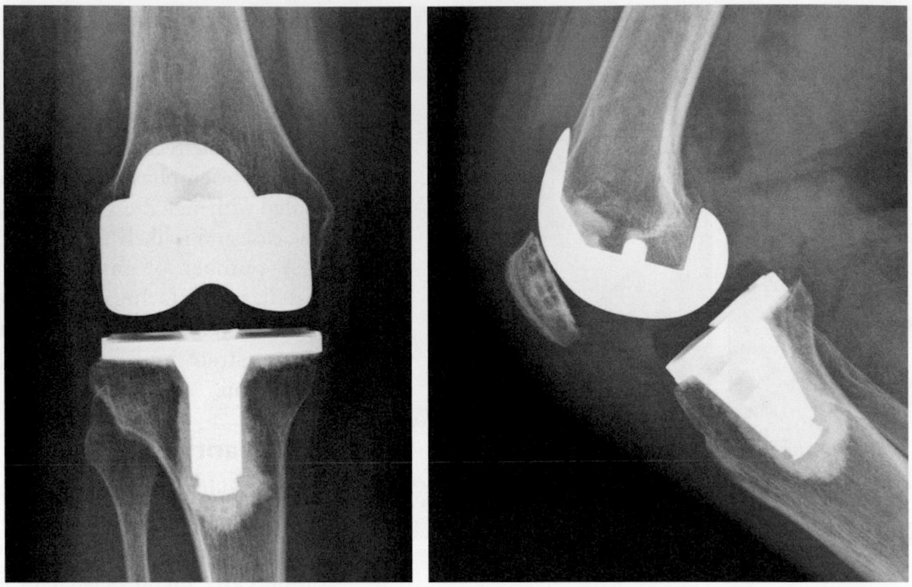

Fig. 8.6.2 A) Anteroposterior and B) lateral radiographs of a modern cemented Gender High Flex LPS TKA.

Surgical technique

Approach

A significant body of literature has recently been published regarding less invasive surgical techniques in TKA. Advances in perioperative management associated with these new protocols include preoperative education, multimodal pain management, rapid mobilization, and less invasive surgical techniques. Most studies have shown a steep learning curve, with limited early, or no benefits and more complications with mini-approaches. We favour a mini medial parapatellar approach as it is familiar to surgeons, can be gradually introduced, and can be extended to a formal medial parapatellar approach if necessary.

Ligament balancing

When alignment is not sufficiently corrected, due to poor bony cuts, or ligament imbalance, the components will be unequally loaded and subjected to excessive stress, resulting in eventual loosening of the prosthesis. Despite significant advances in component design and instrumentation, TKA remains a soft tissue balancing procedure. When a fixed angular deformity exists, the ligament on the concave side is contracted, and the other on the convex side is stretched. It is very rare for complete incompetence to exist. The principle of balancing of the collateral ligaments is to release the contracted side to the length of the stretched side.

Varus knees may require release of contracted medial structures including the superficial medial collateral ligament and the pes anserinus. Following standard bone cuts including a conservative tibial cut, a titrated subperiosteal release is preformed until gap balancing is achieved. When a varus–valgus imbalance exists, it is important to achieve soft tissue balancing prior to recutting bone.

Valgus knees are addressed by similarly releasing the contracted lateral structures. In this case our preferred technique is to 'pie crust' lateral structures, again in a titrated manner. Structures released include the arcuate ligament, lateral collateral ligament, and the iliotibial band. The popliteus tendon is preserved. Care must be taken when performing this procedure in the posterolateral region of the knee due to the proximity of the peroneal nerve. Good clinical success has been demonstrated with this technique in a number of studies.

In selected elderly patients with low physical demands, a constrained condylar knee prosthesis without ligamentous release is another option with no failures reported at an average 7.8-year follow-up.

Rotation

Rotational malalignment in TKA is associated with an increased rate of pain, wear, and patellar instability together resulting in mechanical failure. The most reliable reference for femoral component rotation is the epicondylar axis, which averages three degrees of external rotation with respect to the posterior condylar axis. Special consideration must be taken when simply referencing the posterior condylar axis when a hypoplastic lateral femoral condyle, or varus joint line obliquity exists.

On the tibial side, two popularly used techniques exist for establishing rotation. The first is to apply the tibial template and then flex and extend the knee allowing the tibial component to find the appropriate rotation, and then fix it in that position. The second method employs external landmarks including the medial third of the tubercle, the shaft of the tibia, and the second metatarsal. We employ the latter technique, and its superiority has been demonstrated in a recent comparison study.

Navigation

Significant advances have been achieved in surgical navigational tools. Studies have shown improvements in femoral component alignment alone; both tibial and femoral component alignment; and component rotation. Though this improved accuracy should be reflected in improved outcomes, this has not been demonstrated clinically. The benefit of computer-aided techniques in decreasing outliers (excess alignment errors) is particularly useful with unusual bony deformities; periarticular hardware precluding intramedullary femoral guidance; and in combination with minimally invasive techniques, where exposure and landmark recognition may be compromised.

In future, computer-aided guidance may also provide a benefit in surgical education and for the low-volume orthopaedic surgeon. Despite these benefits, the cost, increased surgical time, learning curve, and unfamiliar new technique, have been barriers to widespread adoption of computer navigation into total joint surgery.

Pain management

Current trends in pain management include a multimodal approach from the preoperative period through the outpatient rehabilitation phase. This includes NSAIDs, long acting narcotics, local infiltration, peripheral nerve blocks, and epidural pain management. In fact this may be the most important advance in patient care management as a result of the introduction of minimally invasive and rapid rehabilitation protocols. Early mobilization in turn, decreases associated postoperative morbidity including rates of deep vein thrombosis.

Outcomes

The success of cemented total knee replacement supports its continued use. Early posterior ligament-retaining designs, such as the Kinematic Total Knee Prosthesis (Howmedica, Rutherford, NJ) have had long-term success. In a 10–14-year follow-up study of this prosthetic design, the investigators reported a 6.5% revision rate. Results with a modular fixed-bearing posterior cruciate design at a minimum 15 years demonstrated a 92.6% survival rate. Of 139 patients there were five reoperations, four due to polyethylene wear, and one due to a loose cemented femoral component. Similarly, in the subset of patients under the age of 55, a 95% survivorship at 12 year follow-up has been published.

Results with the total condylar prosthesis, which sacrificed the posterior cruciate ligament, were excellent, supporting the belief that cemented knee replacement is a durable and predictable procedure. Despite this success, the posterior stabilized prosthesis was introduced. The intent was to design a prosthesis that improved stair-climbing ability, increased range of motion, and prevented tibial subluxation. The 9–12-year results with the posterior stabilized prosthesis and an all polyethylene tibial component demonstrated 87% good to excellent results. An analysis of failures revealed a 3% rate of tibial loosening. This prompted a modification to a metal-backed tibial component. In a subsequent 10–12-year follow-up study on this design, a 96% good to excellent result was reported. Despite the occurrence of two loose femoral components, there were no loose tibial components. Further modifications of patellar geometry, posterior femoral condylar offset, tibial shape, and conformity have resulted in the modern modular, cemented, third-generation posterior-stabilized prosthesis. Long-term studies do not yet exist for this design, but at a mean 48 months, no cases of aseptic loosening, no patellar complications, no evidence of osteolysis or wear, and an average Knee Society Knee Score of 96 were noted.

Speculating that the level of activity would influence the longevity of cemented TKA, the long-term results and functional outcome in patients who were 55 years or younger at the time of index procedure have been evaluated. All patients were rated good to excellent at an average follow-up of 8 years. The 18-year cumulative survivorship was 94%. This represented an active group of patients who regularly participated in exercises which placed high stresses on the cement interface. Although there was one case of polyethylene wear, there were no cases of component loosening.

Registry data

Registry data can provide some insight into both demographic as well as survivorship figures in large groups of patients followed over many years. Survivorship method analysis was performed on 2629 consecutive cemented primary TKAs performed by one surgeon (Dr J. Insall). The Total Condylar series had an average annual failure rate of 0.46% and a 21-year success rate of 90.77%. The Posterior Stabilized prosthesis with an all polyethylene tibia had an average annual rate of failure of 0.38% and a 16-year success rate of 94.10%, and this prosthesis with a metal-backed tibial component had an annual failure rate of 0.14% and a 14-year success rate of 98.10%. The Posterior Stabilized series with modular components had an average annual rate of failure of 0.59% and a 10-year success rate of 93.63%. The Constrained Condylar knee series had an average annual failure rate of 0.26% and a 7-year success rate of 98.12%.

Results from the Swedish knee registry of 41 223 primary arthroplasties, demonstrate decreased revision rates as the age at surgery increased. The overall cumulative revision rate (7.8% overall) decreased in the period 1976–1997 (7% decrease) primarily due to reductions in loosening (11%) and infection (7%). A 1.4 times increased risk of revision was noted with an uncemented tibial design. Overall loosening accounted for 44% of revisions. A satisfaction study in 27 372 patients operated on from 1981–1995 found that only 8% were dissatisfied at 2–17 years postarthroplasty, and that this was constant, regardless of when the procedure was performed over this 15-year period. A close review of population trends revealed a growing rate of total knee replacements, which is estimated to increase by at least one-third by 2030.

Review of the Norwegian Arthroplasty Registry demonstrated an 80.1% survival for unicompartmental knee replacements (n=2288), compared with 92% for total knee replacements (n=3032) and this value was lower in all age categories. Early failures in 7174 primary total knees implanted from 1994–2000 were examined. Five-year survival of tricompartmental total knees was 95–99% for different brands, and the differences were not statistically significant. When comparing bicompartmental to TKA, there was a higher rate of revision for patellar resurfacing following bicompartmental replacement, but a 2.5 times decrease in revision rates due to infection.

The Mayo Clinic Joint Registry, containing 11 606 primary TKAs, was analysed from 1978–2000. Higher survivorships in older patients, inflammatory arthritis, cruciate retention, and cemented all polyethylene tibial designs were noted. Survivorship was 91% at 10 years and 78% at 20 years.

An examination of 18 530 TKAs performed in Ontario, Canada from 1984–1991 was performed: 17,229 of these were primary total knees. Revision rates were estimated to be 4.3–8.0% at 7 years. Risk factors associated with significantly increased rates of revision included a younger age; an increased number of comorbid diagnoses; bilateral total knees; osteoarthritis; urban inhabitants; and having the primary knee surgery performed at a teaching hospital. The authors felt that the increased revision rate at teaching centres was likely due to the increased complexities of surgeries performed there, on patients with an increased number of comorbidities, but were not able to prove this.

Further reading

Diduch, D.R., Insall, J.N., Scott, W.N., Scuderi, G.R., and Font-Rodriguez, D. (1997). Total knee replacement in young, active patients. Long-term follow-up and functional outcome. *Journal of Bone and Joint Surgery*, **79A**, 575–82.

Font-Rodriguez, D.E., Scuderi, G.R., and Insall, J.N. (1997). Survivorship of cemented total knee arthroplasty. *Clinical Orthopaedics and Related Research*, **345**, 79–86.

Fuchs, R., Mills, E.L., Clarke, H.D., Scuderi, G.R., Scott, W.N., and Insall, J.N. (2006). A third-generation, posterior-stabilized knee prosthesis: early results after follow-up of 2 to 6 years. *Journal of Arthroplasty*, **21**(6), 821–5.

Long, W.J. and Scuderi, G.R. (2008). Fixed varus and valgus deformities. In: Lotke, P.A. and Lonner, J.H. (eds) *Master Techniques in Orthoaedic Surgery. Knee Arthroplasty*, 3rd edn, pp.111–126. Philadelphia, PA: Lippincott Williams & Wilkins.

Robertsson, O., Knutson, K., Lewold, S., Lidgren, L. (2001). The Swedish Knee Arthroplasty Register 1975-1997: an update with special emphasis on 41,223 knees operated on in 1988-1997. *Acta Orthopaedica Scandinavica*, **72**(5), 503–13.

8.7

Complications of total knee replacement

Bryn Jones

Summary points

- 81–89% overall patient satisfaction following total knee replacement
- 1 in 8 patients experience unexplained postoperative pain
- Obesity, increasing age, and medical comorbidities increase the risk of postoperative complications
- Prosthetic infection rate at 1 year is 1–2%
- Preoperative range of movement often determines postoperative range
- Low risk of acute vascular event and neurological and ligamentous injury
- Duration and method of venous thromboprophylaxis remains controversial
- Periprosthetic femoral and tibial fractures require stabilisation. Fixation of periprosthetic patella fractures is not recommended
- New surgical techniques and innovations require long term evaluation.

Introduction

The number of total knee replacements implanted continues to rise rapidly. In the United Kingdom between 1994 and 1995 there were a total of 25 000 total knee replacements implanted compared with 52 416 in England and Wales alone between 2006 and 2007 and for the first time the total number of knee replacements performed exceeded that of total hip replacement.

The increase in total knee replacements being performed has resulted from an increasingly elderly population, better implant design, improving medical care, and consumer pressure. Postoperative complications may therefore be expected to rise and the practising surgeon is likely to encounter such problems in their surgical career.

Outcomes of the total knee replacement

Total knee replacement has an estimated success rate in terms of patient satisfaction of 81–89% and most patients achieve a decrease in pain and an improved range of movement of the knee. However, approximately 22.6% of patients still report significant pain at 3 months after total knee replacement. Infection, instability, patellofemoral problems, and prosthetic loosening are the most common causes of pain; however, one in eight patients will continue to complain of pain postoperatively despite there being no obvious clinical or radiological abnormality. Patients with a poor range of movement preoperatively are less likely to have a satisfactory improvement in motion. In addition, young, female, and obese patient subgroups and those with severe arthritis may not see significant gains in postoperative functional outcome scores.

General postoperative complications (Box 8.7.1)

The 90-day mortality after total knee replacement is less than 1% with a reported incidence of less than 0.001% of intraoperative death. The peak time for an adverse event such as infection, death, or pulmonary embolus is within the first 30 days postoperatively. The 90-day rate of adverse events is 3.6% and is higher in older patients, male patients, and those with medical comorbidities. The presence of medical comorbidities also increases the need for extended rehabilitation. When compared to younger patients, patients over 80 years of age have an increased risk of death, myocardial infarction, pneumonia, postoperative confusion, and urinary tract infection. Patients in this age group, however, still have a mortality of almost half that of the general population.

Box 8.7.1 General postoperative complications

- <1% 90-day postoperative mortality
- 3.6% risk of suffering an adverse event at 90 days postoperatively
- Risk of adverse event increases with age
- Obesity increases risk of infection, implant malalignment, and early arthroplasty revision
- 1 in 8 patients will continue to have significant knee pain after arthroplasty.

Impaired cognitive function increases the general postoperative complication rate and some degree of cognitive impairment is still demonstrable in 18% of patients at 3 months postoperation. Intraoperative cerebral microemboli have not been shown to influence postoperative cognition.

Obesity and morbid obesity are increasing and are associated with an increased risk of wound leakage, superficial and deep infection, suboptimal alignment, increased early revision rate, avulsion of the medial collateral ligament, and increased length of stay and rehabilitation requirements. In addition, whilst such patients can gain significant improvement in their surgical outcome scores these scores are generally lower than those of non-obese patients. A higher incidence of radiolucent lines on postoperative x-rays may mean reduced long-term implant survival in patients who are significantly overweight.

Wound healing

Problems with wound healing can compromise a total knee replacement and prolonged wound drainage is associated with an increased risk of wound infection. Patients at risk of wound complications include those who are diabetic, obese, or immunocompromised through drug treatment or a systemic condition such as inflammatory arthritis (Figure 8.7.1). Eczematous skin lesions are heavily colonized with bacteria, incisions through psoriatic plaques are controversial, and, unless fully treated, incisions should avoid such areas.

A peripatellar anastomosis from the medial and lateral geniculates, anterior tibial recurrent, and supreme genicular arteries supplies the skin around the knee and midline or slightly lateral skin incisions are least likely to disrupt this supply. Small medial and lateral longitudinal scars can probably be ignored but if several longitudinal scars are present the most lateral should be incorporated into the incision. Transverse scars should be crossed as near to perpendicular as possible.

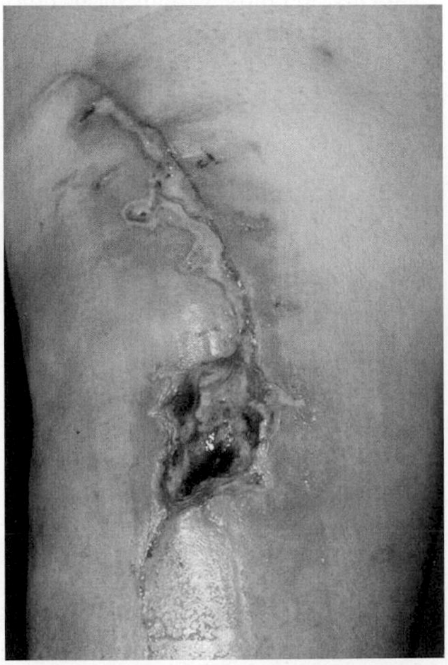

Fig. 8.7.1 Wound breakdown and infection after right total knee replacement.

Attention to surgical detail with careful haemostasis, avoiding excessive skin retraction or undermining of the skin and accurate tension-free wound closure promote satisfactory wound healing. Maintenance of adequate patient hydration, haemoglobin concentration, and saturation all improve oxygen delivery to the skin edges.

Partial thickness skin necrosis can be observed but may occasionally require debridement and skin grafting. Complete wound breakdown may require plastic surgical intervention to provide cover with a medial gastrocnemius or fasciocutaneous flap.

Infection (Box 8.7.2)

Approximately two-thirds of periprosthetic infections occur within 1 year of surgery with an infection rate of 1–2% at 1 year after total knee replacement. It is likely that such infections arise from bacterial contamination at the time of surgery.

Diagnosis is based on history, clinical examination, and further investigation. Not all infections appear as an erythematous, warm, swollen, painful knee with a discharging wound. No test is diagnostic for infection and a combination of investigations is often required. A rise in erythrocyte sedimentation rate (ESR) and C-reactive protein (CRP) level have a high specificity and sensitivity for infection *and* a raised serum interleukin-6 is very sensitive for infection.

A joint aspirate should be obtained for culture, white cell count and white cell differential count. Antibiotics should be stopped for at least 2 weeks prior to joint aspiration to increase successful identification of the infecting organism. Gram stain of a joint aspirate is not of proven value.

Bone scan sensitivity can be improved by the combination of a delayed white cell scan or monoclonal antibody white cell scan but all scanning techniques, including positron emission tomography scans, have a specificity for infection of approximately 80%. A negative bone scan virtually rules out infection.

Once an infection is confirmed, treatment is determined by the organism and the time since operation. If the infection occurs

Box 8.7.2 Prosthetic infection

- 1–2% prosthetic infection rate at 1 year after surgery
- Two-thirds of prosthetic infections occur within 1 year of surgery and are likely to be the result of surgical bacterial contamination
- Debridement and polyethylene exchange within 4 weeks of surgery may allow retention of the knee prosthesis
- In comparison with a single-stage revision a two-stage revision gives a higher chance of eradication of prosthetic infection (75% vs 90%)
- Sensitivity and specificity for infection increased by combination of investigations including:
  - Serological markers (CRP, ESR, and interleukin 1)
  - Knee aspirate for white cell count and differential ± arthroscopic biopsy
  - Triple phase bone scan + white cell labelled scan.

within the first 4 weeks of the total knee replacement then debridement of the knee and exchange of the polyethylene bearing can be considered otherwise complete revision of the implants in one or two stages is most likely to achieve eradication of the infection. In patients who are deemed not fit for surgery then suppressive antibiotic therapy plus knee aspiration may allow retention of the prosthesis. However this may lead to bacterial resistance causing further infective episodes. Identification of the causative organism is key to targeting any infection with appropriate antibiotics.

The stiff knee (Box 8.7.3)

Postoperative stiffness is often accompanied by pain and although definitions vary, its prevalence ranges from 1.3–12%.The definition of a range of movement less than 90 degrees at 6 weeks after the operation is often used.

Each patient with postoperative stiffness requires careful evaluation to assess the relevant contribution of patient factors, surgical errors, implant design, knee kinematics, perioperative complications, and postoperative rehabilitation.

Patient factors

Factors predictive of stiffness are confounding and vary between sexes but include high body mass index, previous knee surgery, patients on disability, diabetes, depression, and pulmonary disease. Stiffness is also more common in women, and women of a younger age with a low body mass index, high femoral flexion angle, and patella baja.

Preoperative range of motion influences postoperative range which is independent of prosthesis design. The presence of a preoperative flexion contracture contributes more to decreased range of movement postoperatively than reduced overall preoperative motion.

Intraoperative technical errors

A tight extension gap may result in a flexion contracture and a tight flexion gap or incorrect collateral ligament balancing may limit flexion. Oversizing or posterior placement of the femoral component can tighten the flexion gap whereas undersizing or anterior placement can increase the flexion gap and create mid-range flexion instability. Excessive femoral component flexion may impinge on and tighten the extensor mechanism in deep flexion.

Internal rotation of the femoral component can cause asymmetric tightening of the flexion gap and cause patellofemoral dysfunction.

Box 8.7.3 The stiff knee

- May be defined as ≤90 degrees range of movement at 6 weeks
- Aetiology variable and includes:
  - Patient factors
  - Intraoperative technical errors
  - Implant design
  - Postoperative complications
  - Postoperative rehabilitation.

Retention of significant posterior femoral osteophytes and/or failure to restore posterior condylar offset causes earlier impingement of the femur on the posterior aspect of the tibial component and this may limit flexion.

Patella resurfacing with excessive polyethylene thickness and implants with an increased trochlea height or similarly an anteriorly placed femoral implant can lead to overstuffing of the patellofemoral joint.

Elevation of the prosthetic joint line can cause patellar–tibial component impingement or midflexion instability.

Incorrect positioning of tibial implants which have a posterior slope can create a coronal malalignment and collateral ligament imbalance. Internal rotation of the tibial component can cause patellofemoral dysfunction. Excessive tibial polyethylene tightens both the extension and flexion gaps.

Implant design

The influence posterior tibial slope has on knee flexion is controversial. *In vivo* studies vary and a cadaveric study has demonstrated a 1.7-degree gain in flexion for every 1 degree increase in posterior slope; conversely an anterior sloping tibial component may reduce posterior femoral rollback and also limit flexion.

In vivo kinematics studies demonstrate a similar pattern of femoral rollback in total knee replacements as in native knees. Implants which do not allow sufficient posterior femoral rollback create early posterior impingement of the femoral component on the tibial component and this can cause paradoxical anterior femoral translation with tightening of the extensor mechanism.

Weight-bearing kinematics have demonstrated a reduced range of flexion in posterior cruciate ligament retaining designs when compared with posterior cruciate ligament substituting designs. The evidence for increased flexion with 'high-flexion' knee implant designs and mobile bearings remains unclear and may be design specific.

Perioperative complications

Infection, periprosthetic fracture, component failure, complex regional pain syndrome (types 1 and 2), heterotopic ossification, and postoperative medical complications may all influence postoperative range of movement.

Postoperative rehabilitation

Positive preoperative reinforcement, multimodal pain management, and physiotherapy can improve postoperative range of motion although the last of these remains controversial.

Treatment

Treatment should be aimed at identifying any remediable cause. A careful history of perioperative events, review of patient risk factors, and appropriate further investigations including interventional procedures such as joint aspiration and specialized imaging techniques are often required.

Improvement in a fixed flexion deformity of certain implants can improve up to 3 years after surgery. Non-operative treatment consists of intensive physiotherapy including passive stretching devices. Botulinum toxin injections can be effective where tight muscle groups can be identified.

Certain diagnoses such as infection usually require surgery; however, with minor implant malposition the risks of removing a well-fixed implant versus the perceived benefit of successful surgery have to be assessed. The results of revision knee surgery remain poorer than those for primary knee surgery and patients may still require manipulation under anaesthesia. Furthermore, less invasive procedures such as patella resurfacing and isolated tibial insert exchange have unpredictable results.

In cases where there is no discernable cause for stiffness following total knee replacement, manipulation under anaesthetic has been the traditional treatment of choice. Controversy remains as to the timing, degree of stiffness prior to, and outcome following manipulation. Recently, no difference has been shown between manipulation within 12 weeks of surgery and manipulation thereafter with the improved flexion maintained at 5-years follow-up.

As a result outcomes vary and perioperative complications such as patella or quadriceps tendon rupture, patella fracture, and haemarthrosis can occur.

Arthroscopy of a total knee replacement allows direct visualization of the implant and soft tissue/implant-related problems can be identified; however, it can be a technically challenging procedure. Arthroscopic debridement, including posterior cruciate release and manipulation, has been shown to improve range of flexion, at least in the short term, and is usually preferable to formal arthrotomy and debridement.

Patellofemoral dysfunction

There remains conflicting evidence from prospective studies regarding the functional value of patellar resurfacing in primary total knee replacement.

Concerns regarding persistent anterior knee pain without patellar resurfacing favour patellar resurfacing but historically complications related to patella replacement have ranged from 4–50%. Better understanding of knee kinematics, including implant rotation, has influenced modern surgical technique and the need to resurface the patella may be more influenced by implant design. However, secondary resurfacing of the patella is the most common reason for reoperation in primary total knee replacements despite unpredictable results in the short term and poor long-term outcomes.

Careful evaluation of the patient with apparent anterior knee symptoms is therefore required before committing to surgery and should include an assessment for infection and femoral and tibial implant stability, alignment, and rotation.

Peripheral nerve injury

The incidence of clinical peripheral neuropathy is approximately 1.3% with isolated common peroneal injuries being more common than combined common peroneal and tibial nerve injuries. Risk factors for nerve injury differ; however, include rheumatoid arthritis, preoperative deformity (valgus/flexion contractures), postoperative epidural anaesthesia, prolonged tourniquet time, and pre-existing peripheral neuropathy.

Individual experience in these injuries is low but expectant treatment is recommended with immediate local pressure relief and flexion of the affected knee to 20–30 degrees advised. Early neurophysiological investigations can be used to distinguish between nerve dysfunction and muscle dysfunction but are not prognostic of outcome. Immediate exploration of the nerve is not recommended unless a haematoma is suspected. Prevention of muscle contracture by early aggressive splintage and passive stretching is important regardless of the ultimate outcome.

Overall results are encouraging, in cases without nerve transection, with most patients showing some signs of recovery and up to two-thirds of patients with complete recovery occurring up to 18 months after initial injury.

Dysaesthesia in the common peroneal nerve distribution can be improved by decompression of the peroneal nerve.

Nerve injury can occur during any knee replacement surgery therefore attention to surgical detail such as careful retractor placement and avoidance of over releasing of soft tissue and excessive polyethylene insert thickness and care when applying dressings should be exercised at all times. Exploration, identification, and protection of the peroneal nerve intraoperatively have not been shown to reduce the risk of nerve injury.

Vascular injury (Box 8.7.4)

Acute occlusive vascular problems are rare (0.03–0.2%) after total knee replacement. Patients with a history of vascular disease, vascular calcification as seen on x-ray, previous vascular reconstruction, and possibly popliteal aneurysms are at risk of an acute vascular event.

Pedal pulses may be clinically impalpable in 36% of patients undergoing total knee replacement. The use of a tourniquet remains controversial as tourniquets may cause further vascular compromise and should be used with caution in high-risk patients.

Patients with an acute vascular injury typically present with a pale, cool, pulseless, and painful limb. Emergent vascular surgical intervention should be sought. The reported rates of amputation after these vascular complications range between 25–43% with most occurring in patients who have pre-existing atherosclerotic disease. An above-knee amputation is very rarely required and provides a very poor functional outcome.

Direct vascular damage can occur intraoperatively. The popliteal artery and vein, and tibial nerve, lie close to the posterior aspect of the knee and below the level of the joint the popliteal artery bifurcates and the anterior tibial artery becomes most at risk at this point. If an axial section of the proximal tibia is thought of as a clock face with 6 o'clock being anterior and 3 o'clock being lateral any penetration of the posterior tibial cortex between 3 o'clock and 11 o'clock can potentially damage neurovascular structures.

Significant bleeding problems may not be apparent until the tourniquet has been deflated. Any suspected vascular injuries require to be dealt with urgently and are easier to control before implantation of the prosthesis.

Ligament injury (Box 8.7.4)

Intraoperative collateral ligament disruption, as demonstrated by sudden ligament laxity, traditionally required conversion to a constrained type of knee prosthesis. However, repair and appropriate tensioning with postoperative bracing has been shown to offer a functional alternative in cases of medial collateral ligament damage.

The incidence of extensor mechanism disruption is said to be 0.17–2.5% and can be assessed with ultrasound or magnetic resonance imaging if there is clinical uncertainty as to its integrity. Treatment is determined by the level of disruption, degree of tear (partial/full), timing of disruption (acute/chronic), quality of host tissue, availability of autogenous or autologous tendon graft, and

Box 8.7.4 Neurovascular and ligament injury

- Acute vascular injury rare (<0.2%)
- 1.3% incidence of clinical peripheral neuropathy
- Common peroneal nerve injury most often injured
- Two-thirds of patients with nerve injury may recover nerve function (excluding nerve transection)
- Medial collateral ligament transection can be repaired acutely
- ≤2.5% incidence of acute extensor mechanism disruption.

the patient's functional demands. A reduced functional outcome can be expected.

Patellar tendon ruptures invariably require surgery and augmentation with either an autologous or allogenic tendon graft with protected rehabilitation.

Partial quadriceps tears can be treated satisfactorily operatively or non-operatively, whilst complete tears require operative treatment often with tendon grafting as rerupture rates can be as high as 40%.

Venous thromboembolism

Venous thromboembolism (VTE) is potentially fatal. Without thromboprophylaxis the risk of asymptomatic imaged deep vein thrombosis is 40–60% after total knee replacement but symptomatic VTE rates occur in only 2–5% of patients. Symptomatic pulmonary embolism and DVT occur at a mean of 12 and 20 days after total knee replacement. Thromboprophylaxis can be pharmaceutical or mechanical and most trials have shown that thromboprophylaxis reduces the incidence of all VTE events, including fatal pulmonary embolism. However, the duration and method of treatment remains controversial. Extended prophylaxis may be required for up to a month and mechanical prophylaxis is often poorly tolerated. TED stockings have not been shown to be of benefit in VTE reduction. Anticoagulants may require monitoring or parental administration and the perceived risk of clinically important bleeding remains a concern to many surgeons. New oral thromboprophylactic anticoagulants such as direct thrombin inhibitor or activated Factor Xa inhibitor demonstrate efficacy at least comparable to low-molecular-weight heparin without the requirement to monitor coagulation.

Knee joint dislocation

Knee joint dislocation occurs in about 0.2% of all total knee replacement types. It is increased in patients with a Charcot joint, revision surgery, and complex primary surgery. The mechanism of dislocation is usually a high flexion movement and not trauma. Diagnosis is based on history and clinical examination and confirmed with x-ray. Manipulation alone usually results in a poor outcome and revision with careful attention to ligament balancing and implant sizing and rotation is advised.

Periprosthetic femoral/tibial fracture (Box 8.7.5)

Intraoperative fractures of the femur or tibia are rare. Periprosthetic femoral fractures occur in approximately 2% of total knee replacements whilst whilst the incidence of tibial fractures is much less. Femoral fractures have been classified into types I(a/b)–III based on distal bone quality, implant stability, and fracture reducibility. Notching of the anterior femoral shaft at the time of implantation may be associated with periprosthetic fracture (Figure 8.7.2).

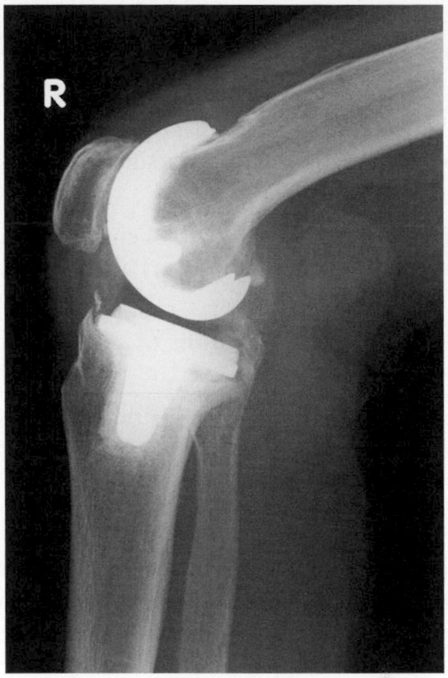

Fig. 8.7.2 Sagittal x-ray of right total knee replacement demonstrating excessive tibial slope and posterior placement of femoral component with resultant notching of femur.

Treatment should achieve a well-fixed and appropriately aligned knee replacement. Depending on the fracture configuration, quality of the bone, and the presence of an open femoral box, a retrograde intramedullary nail, a standard plate, or locking plate can be considered in cases where the femoral implant remains stable (type Ib). Early results with locking plates are encouraging particularly in cases where bone quality is poor however large clinical series and biomechanical data remain scarce. Type II fractures require a stemmed revision total knee replacement to achieve implant and fracture stability. In fractures which are not reconstructable and with poor bone (type III) a distal femoral replacement may be required.

Tibial fractures are treated on the basis of implant stability and may require a stemmed prosthesis with augments.

Periprosthetic patella fracture (Box 8.7.5)

The incidence of periprosthetic patellar fracture is 1.19% and occurs predominantly in resurfaced patellae though non-resurfaced patellae are also at risk. The majority of fractures are not associated with trauma and fracture classification is based on the integrity of the extensor mechanism, implant stability, and the state of the remaining patellar bone stock (Ortiguera and Berry types I–IIIa/b). The most common type of fracture involves an intact extensor mechanism with loosening of the patella implant (type III). Predisposing patient factors for fracture include osteoporosis, osteolysis, bone loss, high activity level, knee hyperflexion, and rheumatoid arthritis.

Surgically-related predisposing factors include central peg fixation and cementation, metal-backed uncemented patellae, patellar maltracking, and prosthesis malalignment.

Box 8.7.5 Periprosthetic fracture

- Femoral periprosthetic fractures most common (2%). Classification types I(a/b)– III
- Patella periprosthetic fracture classification: Ortiguera and Berry classification (I–IIIa/b)
- Patella fracture associated with central peg fixation, a metal-backed patella, prosthesis malalignment, and patella maltracking
- 92% failure of internal fixation of periprosthetic patella fractures
- 10–15mm minimum residual patella thickness recommended to avoid fracture.

A lateral release should be performed at a distance from the patella and removal of the prepatellar fat pad avoided to prevent disruption of the vascular anastomoses between the peripatellar and polar patella blood supplies. Patellar bone removal should be restricted as a patella with a residual thickness of less than 10–15mm is at risk of fracture.

A periprosthetic patellar fracture with disruption of the extensor mechanism presents with loss of active knee flexion; however, most cases present with no extensor mechanism disruption and require a radiological diagnosis.

Periprosthetic patellar fractures with a stable implant and intact extensor mechanism require a period of immobilization until radiological healing is demonstrated.

In the more complex cases with a disrupted extensor mechanism, open reduction and internal fixation has a very poor outcome with failure rates of 92%. In this situation excision of the avascular fragments and repair of the extensor tendon should be considered. If revision of the patella is not possible then partial/complete patellectomy should be considered.

Developments in total knee replacement surgery

Recent advances have seen the introduction of computer assisted and minimally invasive knee surgery and these have led to an increase in the complexity of surgical technique. Such innovations raise concerns about the risk of both traditional intra- and postoperative complications as well as some new to the individual technique. There is a significant learning curve for each innovation and longer operative times can increase infection rates, blood loss, or thromboembolic events.

Minimally invasive total knee replacement

Various minimally invasive surgical exposures exist and evidence from larger series, performed by technique enthusiasts, show comparable complication rates to traditional total knee replacement. A learning curve has been defined; one study demonstrated a 16% decrease in the major complication rate for each additional 50 procedures performed. Decreased intraoperative exposure can increase the risk of ligament damage, neurovascular injury, and intraoperative fracture. Inferior radiological outcomes secondary to compromised cementation and implant malposition have been observed.

Furthermore, the improved early functional recovery reported in minimally invasive surgery may, in part, be a result of the concurrent development of newer pain control modalities and changes in postoperative rehabilitation.

Computer-assisted knee surgery

Evidence of postoperative outcome in computer-assisted knee surgery is restricted to small series and short-term data; however, an improvement in mechanical axis alignment of the navigated total knee replacement has been demonstrated and a reduction in polyethylene wear and subsequent revision rate is predicted as a result. A reduction in total blood loss and postoperative confusion has been shown using computer-assisted surgery but controversy exists as to the extent of fat emboli reduction which may vary depending on how the femur is instrumented in conventional knee surgery.

Computer-assisted surgery relies on surgeon input of data and an understanding of the computer-generated information as well as a general understanding of total knee replacement surgery is key. Poor data entry or misinterpretation of data can result in surgical error and accurate assessment of tibial prosthesis rotation is difficult with the majority of currently available systems. Potential complications exclusive to computer-assisted knee surgery include distal femoral stress fracture and vascular damage associated with tracker pin insertion.

Conclusions

The number of total knee replacements continues to rise as a result of increasing indications for surgery and the ageing population. Patient demographics are changing and the average body mass index continues to increase. As a result, postoperative complications may be expected to increase. However, improvements in general medical care and an increased awareness and attention to surgical detail should enable surgeons to avoid certain complications and better treat others.

The future challenge will be to reduce complication rates in a more complex patient population, embracing those technologies and techniques shown to be of benefit and identifying early those which may not, in order to prevent both immediate and late complications.

Evidence supports a reduction in complication rates with an increased individual volume of knee surgery and a future trend may be for more individual knee specialist surgeons. However, controversy remains regarding the incidence, appropriate diagnostic intervention, and treatment of certain complications and evidence from numerically large and appropriate studies is often lacking. The increase in available arthroplasty registry data may provide some answers and allow observation of trends and monitoring of the effects of changes in surgical practice and implant design.

Further reading

Challdis B.E., Tsiridis E., Adamantios A.T., Stavrou Z., and Giannoudis P.V. (2007). Management of periprosthetic patellar fractures a systemic review of the literature. *Injury*, **8**, 714–24.

Denis, A.D., Komistek, R.D., Scuderi, R.G., and Zingde, S. (2007). Factors affecting flexion after total knee arthroplasty. *Clinical Orthopaedics and Related Research*, **464**, 53–60.

Kim, K.I., Elgol, K.A., Hozack, W.J., and Parvizi J. (2006). Periprosthetic fractures after total knee replacement. *Clinical Orthopaedics and Related Research*, **446**, 167–75.

Mandalia, V., Eyres, K., Schranz, P., and Toms, A.D. (2008). Evaluation of patients with a painful total knee replacement. *Journal of Bone and Joint Surgery*, **90B**, 265–71.

Parvizi, J., Tarity, T.D., Steinbeck, J.M., *et al.* (2006). Management of stiffness following total knee arthroplasty. *Journal of Bone and Joint Surgery*, **88A**, 303–14.

8.8

Revision total knee replacement

Kelly Vince and Jacob Munro

Introduction

No aspect of knee arthroplasty surgery has advanced more in the last decade than revision surgery—although the comparatively few revisions performed have left much of this information unappreciated in the literature. Repeat surgery was initially not considered feasible, and was then performed (and reported) identically to primary replacements. Eventually, special implant techniques and prosthetic systems emerged. A strong argument can be made that (with the exception of cases of infection and extensor mechanism allograft) the results of contemporary first revision arthroplasty, with the techniques described in this chapter will prove at least as, if not more, durable than current primary replacement. The same cannot be said for a second knee revision, emphasizing the importance of the initial opportunity. Given current population demographics and primary arthroplasty rates, a significant increase is expected in the need for revision knee arthroplasty.

A detailed understanding of how knee replacements fail is central to planning a successful revision. This means that a clear diagnosis and a deep appreciation of pathophysiology and biomechanics are essential. This information comes from a comprehensive literature, which cannot be quoted in depth in this format. However, the reader is directed to a few pertinent review articles which are a broad guide to the published data.

New appreciation of the rotational positioning of tibial and femoral components, quantifiable by computed tomography (CT), has implications for all patellar complications and not just tracking, instability, stiffness, and pain. Revision implant systems differ fundamentally from those that work well in primary surgery, with stem extensions, modularity, porous metals, and constrained articulations that enable surgeons equipped with the correct information, to help patients who were once consigned to pain clinics, or worse, arthrodesis and amputation.

The role of revision surgery is not simply to treat the older patient with a 'worn out' arthroplasty. Rather, it is the key piece in a strategy to ensure that the younger active patient, who may now be receiving a unicompartmental replacement, can be assured that a functional knee joint will be present through a long and active life.

Principles of revision total knee arthroplasty (Box 8.8.1)

Several principles underpin revision knee arthroplasty surgery:

1) Establish a diagnosis. This must emerge from a systematic, disciplined, and comprehensive approach to the problem knee replacement. The diagnosis should fit into a well-established 'differential diagnosis', and novel explanations for pain should be resisted. Infection must be considered in each case and a specific surgical plan should flow from the diagnosis. 'Revision knee arthroplasty' is not one, but several different operations depending on the cause of failure. A diagnostic algorithm may be established or a checklist consulted to ensure that nothing is overlooked (Figure 8.8.1)
2) 'Revise' the failed arthroplasty, do not simply perform a repeat operation. As such, revision describes a process of identifying what led to the initial failure and ensuring that an operation is conceived that will eliminate the causes of failure
3) Use revision implant systems. This does not mean a constrained or hinged implant every time. It does, however, mean a modular system that provides good options to ensure fixation with stem extensions, stability with a range of constraint options, and bone restitution with augments
4) The femur controls the soft tissues in the knee. That is to say, whatever we do with the tibial component will affect both the flexion and extension gaps of the knee equally. Furthermore, it is mainly the size (and to a lesser extent the position) of the femoral component that controls the flexion gap of the knee. By contrast it is the proximal–distal position of the femoral component that controls the extension gaps. This simple observation is the key to revision surgery technique (Figure 8.8.2)
5) Do a complete revision in virtually every case. Following from principle 4, if we do not revise the femur, we cannot control the soft tissues. If the tibia is exposed with the femoral component in place, collateral ligaments often stretch and sometimes fail. The resultant instability cannot be managed by revising the tibia alone, especially in the extreme case where constraint is required.

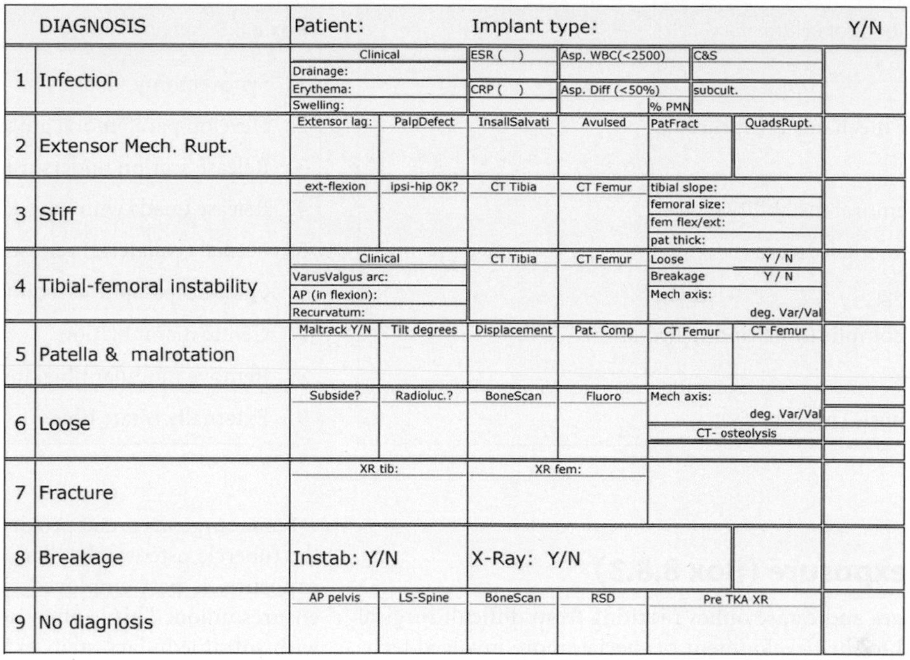

	DIAGNOSIS	Patient:		Implant type:				Y/N
1	Infection	Clinical Drainage: Erythema: Swelling:		ESR ( ) CRP ( )	Asp. WBC(<2500) Asp. Diff (<50%) % PMN	C&S subcult.		
2	Extensor Mech. Rupt.	Extensor lag:	PalpDefect	InsallSalvati	Avulsed	PatFract	QuadsRupt.	
3	Stiff	ext-flexion	ipsi-hip OK?	CT Tibia	CT Femur	tibial slope: femoral size: fem flex/ext: pat thick:		
4	Tibial-femoral instability	Clinical VarusValgus arc: AP (in flexion): Recurvatum:		CT Tibia	CT Femur	Loose Y / N Breakage Y / N Mech axis: deg. Var/Val		
5	Patella & malrotation	Maltrack Y/N	Tilt degrees	Displacement	Pat. Comp	CT Femur	CT Femur	
6	Loose	Subside?	Radioluc.?	BoneScan	Fluoro	Mech axis: deg. Var/Val CT- osteolysis		
7	Fracture	XR tib:		XR fem:				
8	Breakage	Instab: Y/N		X-Ray: Y/N				
9	No diagnosis	AP pelvis	LS-Spine	BoneScan	RSD	Pre TKA XR		

Fig. 8.8.1 Revision TKA worksheet.

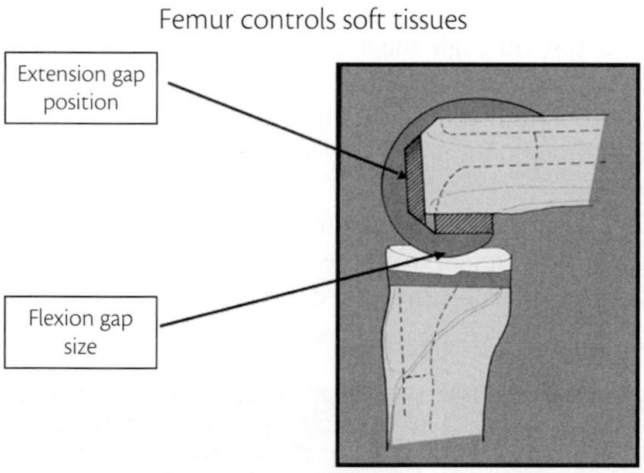

Fig. 8.8.2 Femoral component size and position. The key to revision TKA surgery.

Box 8.8.1 Principles of revision total knee arthroplasty (TKA)

- Establish a diagnosis
- 'Revise' the failed TKA—do not simply perform a repeat operation
- Use revision implant systems
- The femur controls the soft tissues and therefore the gap balance
- Do a complete revision
- Use a technique that 'couples' the tibia and femur through existing soft tissues.

Furthermore, the lateral condyle of a femoral component, with the knee flexed, impinges on the posterolateral corner of the tibial component threatening to rotate it internally.

Revision of the femur alone can be considered if the tibial component is ideally rotated (with a confirmatory CT scan) and there is clearly no need for constraint. Cases of loosening usually result from osteolysis, which affects the entire joint and is not restricted to one component. Revising one loose component today is often followed by loosening of the other component tomorrow. Complete revision, grafting of osteolytic defects, and elimination of an articulation that generates wear debris is more likely to succeed long term. Complete revision does not require finding compatible parts; it addresses the problem completely and is usually faster

6) Employ a surgical technique that couples the tibia to the femur, using the existing soft tissues. Accept that these tissues may have stretched or contracted and cannot be expected to resemble either what used to be or what is on the contralateral joint. Accordingly, do not choose component size as a function of the prerevision radiographs of either knee.

Failure modes and prerevision evaluation (Box 8.8.2)

There is a coherent argument for eight modes of failure (see Figure 8.8.1) that are amenable to revision arthroplasty and a ninth category (unexplained pain) that is an indication for further investigation and temporizing, but not surgery. All the cases within one diagnostic category will present with similar problems and respond to similar techniques. All can be managed with the '3-step technique' described in this chapter.

Box 8.8.2 Modes of failure

1. Sepsis
2. Extensor mechanism rupture
3. Stiffness
4. Tibial–femoral instability
5. Periprosthetic fracture
6. Loosening
7. Patellar complications and malrotation
8. Breakage
9. No diagnosis (no surgery).

Box 8.8.3 Surgical exposure

1. Synovectomy
2. Develop parafemoral gutters
3. Release scar on undersurface patellar tendon
4. Release quads with long scissors
5. Medial (collateral) release
6. Quadriceps 'split' if required
7. Gentle manipulation
8. Remove modular tibial insert
9. Externally rotate tibia.

Surgical exposure (Box 8.8.3)

Early challenges and catastrophes resulting from difficult surgical exposures led to the development of special, more involved techniques to avoid damage to the extensor mechanism and yet provide full access to the joint. Some of these divide the soft tissue of the extensor proximally and others detach the tuberosity distally. Initially, the very old 'Coonse–Adams' quadriceps tendon 'turndown' was adapted to knee arthroplasty surgery (Figure 8.8.3A). While sparing the patellar tendon attachment, it is aggressive and now largely obsolete, except for the most extraordinary circumstances. More limited manoeuvres, such as the 'quadriceps snip' or quadriceps 'split' often suffice (Figure 8.8.3B). An oblique (inferomedial to proximal lateral) arthrotomy of the quadriceps tendon has been described, but does not differ substantively from the 'snip'. Any transection of the quadriceps tendon close to the patella should be avoided.

Some surgeons prefer proximal soft tissue procedures and others the tubercle osteotomies. The osteotomy, while providing superb exposure, is best employed where adequate tibial bone quality ensures union. This is often not the case in the difficult revision, with intramedullary stem extensions and methacrylate cement (Figure 8.8.3C). Calamity may ensue when an osteotomy fails, as the extensor mechanism is in jeopardy.

The danger of forcing exposure is primarily to the extensor mechanism, where avulsion of the patellar tendon from either the tubercle or the patella is irreparable. The common practice of placing a pin through the tendon and into the tubercle does not reduce the force applied by an aggressive approach and risks tearing the tendon when enough force is applied. 'Peeling' of the insertion, though not universally accepted, is preferable to a transverse tear.

Collateral ligaments may suffer from forceful exposure where they are torn or ripped from the condyles. Though inelegant, this can be corrected with constrained implants and indeed a purpose-

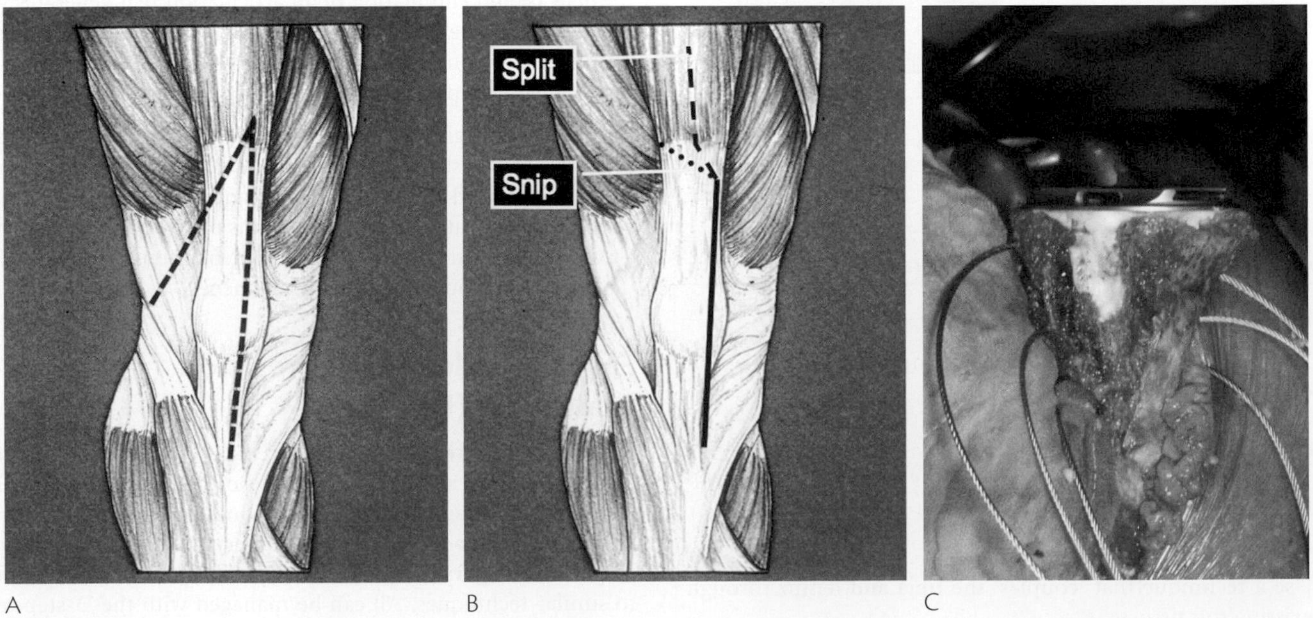

Fig. 8.8.3 Exposure—special manoeuvres. A) Coonse–Adams quadriceps turndown. B) Quadriceps split and snip. C) Tibial tubercle osteotomy with exposed proximal tibial cement.

ful removal of the collaterals from femoral condyles has been described for arthroplasty in the stiff knee, where it is referred to as a 'femoral peel'.

The best new information regarding surgical exposure in revision knee arthroplasty emphasizes the importance of patience and attention to detail. No aggressive manoeuvre should be invoked until there has been close attention to detail. The vast majority of cases, including stiff arthroplasties and reimplantations for infection can be exposed fully after:

1) Complete synovectomy
2) Resection of thick scar on the undersurface of the patellar tendon
3) Re-establishment of the parafemoral 'gutters'
4) Transection of scar between the anterior femur and the deep quadriceps with long-handled scissors
5) Release of the (deep) medial collateral ligament if indicated
6) External rotation of the tibia and
7) Gentle manipulation to stretch the quadriceps and
8) Removal of the modular polyethylene.

It may not be necessary to fully evert the patella for revision surgery (Figure 8.8.4).

Component removal (Box 8.8.4)

Numerous techniques and 'tricks' have been described for the removal of well-fixed arthroplasty components. A cautious approach that preserves bone is sound, but time must also be conserved as infection rates increase with longer surgery.

In general, the former sequence of component removal from cement followed by cement removal from bone can be expedited, in favour of sawing between the cement and bone. Simple techniques with a minimum of specialized equipment are useful. Very few components cannot be removed with standard reciprocating and oscillating saws, a narrow curved osteotome, half a dozen old flat osteotomes, mallet, punch, and perhaps one offset chisel.

The femoral component is immediately more accessible and once off makes it simpler to remove the tibia. A 'reciprocating saw' fits easily into the anterior, distal, and chamfered interfaces of both cemented and uncemented femoral components (Figure 8.8.5). A narrow curved osteotome reaches between the posterior condyle and bone, where the saw cannot go. A mallet blow via a 'punch' placed on the most superior edge of the femoral flange will easily dislodge the component once the interface is disrupted. Gigli saws, once favoured by some, may be difficult to control—excess bone is removed if the saw strays. 'Axial slap hammer extractors' once considered essential are not always available and will be difficult to attach to (right and left) asymmetric femoral components.

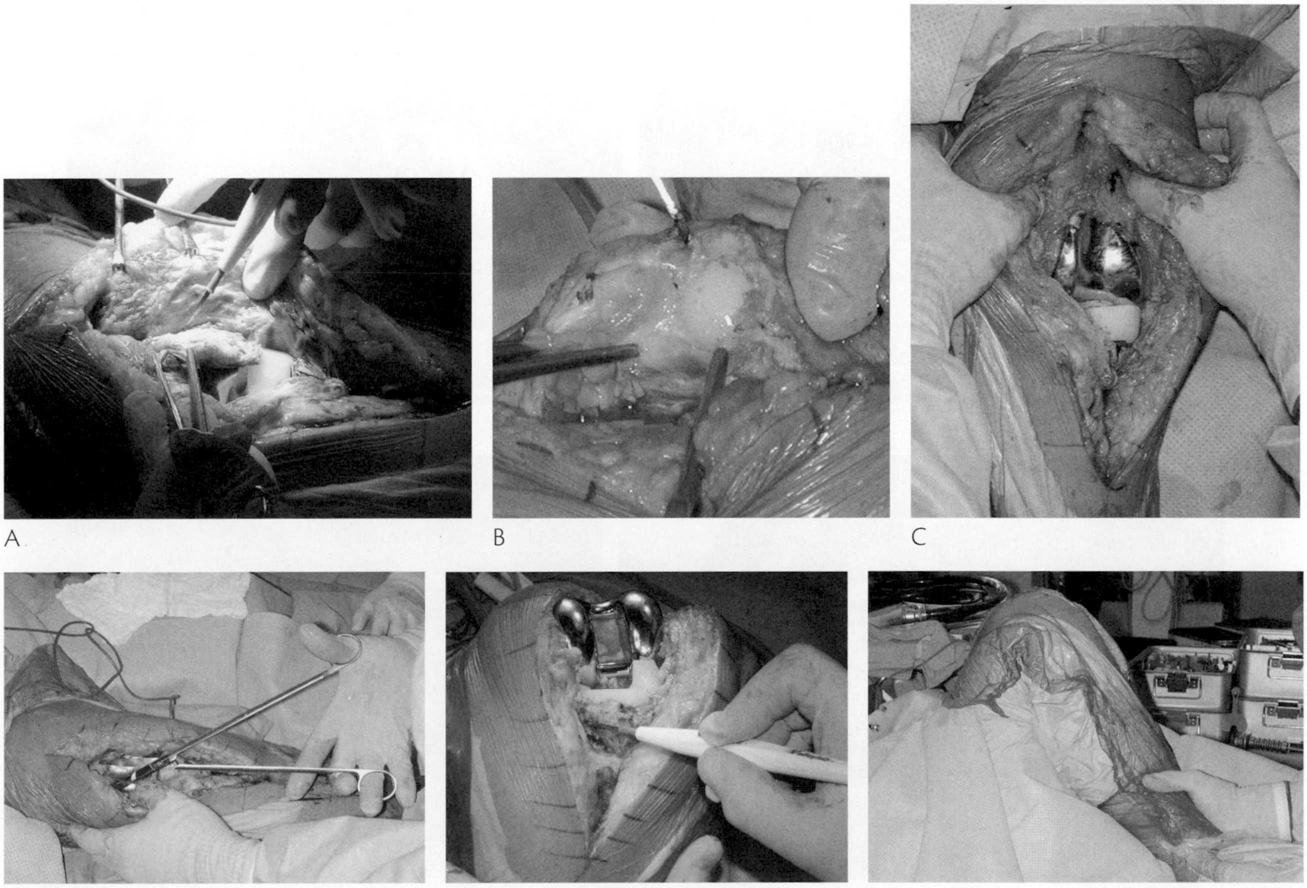

A B C D E F

Fig. 8.8.4 Exposure—the essentials. A) Synovectomy. B) Developing the parafemoral gutters. C) Releasing scar from the underside of the patellar tendon. D) Release of the deep quadriceps with long-handled scissors. E) Medial release. F) Manipulation to stretch the quadriceps.

Box 8.8.4 Component removal

Femur

- Reciprocating saw: anterior, anterior chamfer, and distal interfaces.
- Narrow, curved osteotome: posterior chamfer and posterior interfaces
- Punch and mallet to anterior femoral flange.

Tibia

- Oscillating saw between cement and bone: anterior and anteromedial
- Reciprocating saw between cement and bone: anterolateral and posteromedial
- Curved osteotome from posteromedial to posterolateral interface
- Stacked osteotomies.

They tempt the surgeon to remove the component (and consequently bone) with force before fixation has been disrupted.

Special situations arise where femoral components must be removed (revision of a revision) that are attached to stem extensions. In general, if the modular junction can be unlocked by the removal of locking screws, it will be advantageous to remove the component itself first. This exposes cement around the stem extension. Uncemented stems may come out with the component but if not, removal of the component enables the surgeon to work on the stem extension fixation directly. Once this has been done, the component may be reattached to the stem, providing an excellent grip. Alternately, only the axial screw may be reattached to the stem and a 'slap hammer extractor' applied to the screw and stem. Ultimately, a fully cemented long stem (which is not recommended for precisely this reason) may require an extensive anterior femoral window to remove cement and extricate the stem.

Tibial components may be approached with the large oscillating saw first, cutting between the bone and the cement to save time. Access will be limited by appurtenances (keels, pegs, spikes) on the underside. At that point the reciprocating saw, with its narrow

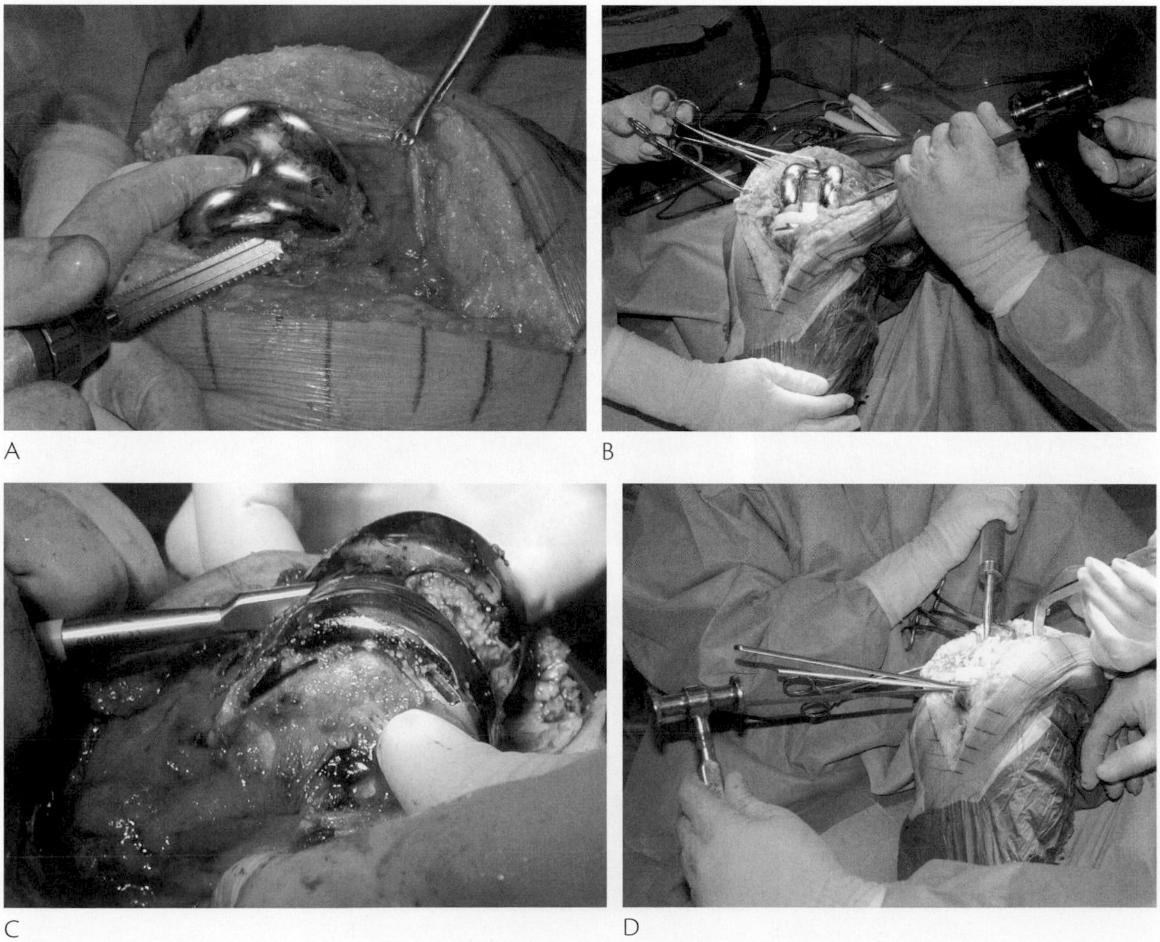

Fig. 8.8.5 Component removal. A) Reciprocating saw to anterior, distal, and chamfered interfaces. B) Narrow osteotome to posterior interface. C) Mallet and punch to anterior flange to remove femoral component. D) Stacked osteotomes to remove tibial component.

blade, helps but often cannot access the posterolateral corner, where an offset chisel works well, introduced from the medial side. The keel, though still fixed, will usually yield to 'stacked osteotomes' that gradually lift the component out of the residual cement mantle (Figure 8.8.5D). Special circumstances, such as extrication of the fully cemented porous-coated stem extension—now rarely encountered—may require creation of windows in the metal tibial surface to access the fixation interface.

Patellar components, if made exclusively of polyethylene are easily removed. An oscillating saw cuts between the cement and the bone, severing whatever posts penetrate into the patella. These are quickly dispatched with a burr, which can also be used to enlarge the diameter of the post hole and so remove all methacrylate, important in the treatment of the infected arthroplasty. Uncemented metal-backed patellar implants may be more problematic. It is worth hammering a narrow (¼-inch) osteotome into the interface. The thicker portion of the instrument will disrupt fibrous ingrowth. True bone ingrowth may require a 'diamond wheel' cutting device on a 'high speed, low torque' hand piece to disrupt the interface and sever the ingrown posts. These can then be removed with a 'pencil' tipped cutting head on the same burr.

Key to revision total knee arthroplasty technique (Box 8.8.5)

The key to revision knee arthroplasty surgery is simple: 'the femoral component controls the soft tissues'. This means that knee kinematics, the essential balance of stability and motion, can only be managed if the femoral component is revised. Furthermore, the flexion gap is controlled by the size and to a lesser extent, the position of the femoral component, while the extension gap is the product of the proximal distal position of the femoral component. Conventional soft tissue releases, integral to correction of deformity in primary arthroplasty, have a modest role in revision surgery—useful only when releases should have been performed in the primary, but were not.

Box 8.8.5 Femur controls soft tissues

- Flexion gap: function of femoral component *size*
- Extension gap: function of femoral component proximal distal *position.*

The '3-step technique' that follows is based on these principles. The technique is really only practicable if diaphyseal engaging stem extensions are used, preferably for the entire technique but certainly for the trial reduction. These stems establish and maintain trial component position independent of bone deficits. There are few primary instruments that work well in revision knee arthroplasty. It is almost dangerous to expect primary instruments to guide the reconstruction as the osseous landmarks that they reference from are no longer present. If the surgeon prefers fully cemented, shorter, narrower stems, they can be selected at the time of implantation—the longer tighter fitting trial components will have guided position and selection of augments.

Fixation (Boxes 8.8.6 and 8.8.7)

Cementless fixation has not supplanted methacrylate or the combination of methacrylate and 'press-fit' intramedullary stem extensions in general usage, as has been the case for revision total hip arthroplasty. A few committed practitioners have described techniques for revision knee arthroplasty without cement fixation.

Fully cemented stem extensions undoubtedly provide superb fixation (Figure 8.8.6A). They are, however, difficult to remove and by neither 'fitting' nor 'filling' the canal, they do not accurately guide position of the components. The arguments and literature against uncemented stem extensions (Figure 8.8.6B) is based on studies that have compared fully cemented stems with metaphyseal length uncemented stems. Clearly, the metaphyseal length stem is neither long enough to guide implant position nor improve

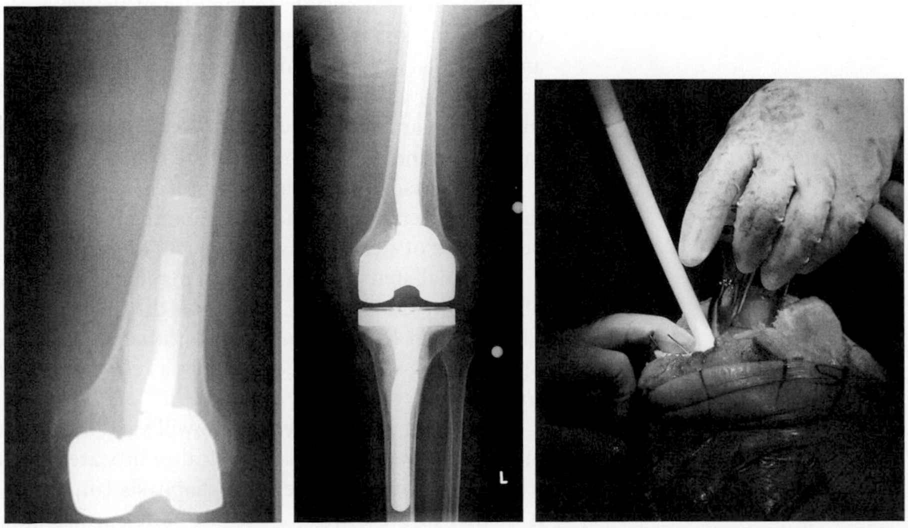

A B C

Fig. 8.8.6 Fixation options. A) Fully cemented stem. B) Uncemented stems. C) Cementing into the metaphysis.

Box 8.8.6 Viable fixation strategies

Fully cemented metaphyseal stems

- Advantages:
  - Solid fixation
  - Potential for antibiotic cement
- Disadvantages:
  - Does not guide position
  - Difficult removal.

Press-fit diaphyseal stems

- Advantages:
  - Guides position of components
  - Solid fixation
  - Easy removal
- Disadvantages:
  - Limited potential for antibiotic cement
  - Technique.

Box 8.8.8 Revision technique

1. Tibial platform
2. Knee in flexion
   - Femoral rotation
   - Femoral component size
   - Joint line
3. Knee in extension

fixation. Similarly, one would not expect the 'dangling' stem or one that does not contact the endosteum to aid fixation significantly.

If uncemented stem extensions are selected, cement that is limited strictly to the cut bone surface is probably inadequate as it does not provide fixation comparable to what is typically used in primary arthroplasty. The strategy that provides excellent fixation and alignment is the combination of asymmetric (to accommodate anatomy) diaphyseal length, modular stems with cement fixation extended a few centimetres, into the metaphysis (Figure 8.8.6C).

Three steps (Box 8.8.8)

Step 1: tibial platform

The tibial component, comprising one side of both flexion and extension gaps, is not useful for manipulating the dimensions of one gap relative to the other. It is, however, a 'platform' or 'foundation' from which the dimensions of both flexion and extension gaps can be established. Component position and fixation in the revision is not predicated on precise bone cuts as in the primary arthroplasty, but rather on a tight and accurate fit of an offset stem extension in the tibial canal, plus component contact with a majority of host bone. Small incongruities will be filled with cement. It will be the technique of inserting the stem extensions that determines component position. As a result, the sequence for preparing the tibial surface is:

1) A 'rough cut' to remove the component
2) Tibial reaming
3) An optional 'fine cut', based on an extramedullary guide attached to either the reamer or a trial tibial stem extension
4) Insertion of the trial tibial component.

Unless the primary knee has failed from varus alignment and loosening, most tibial components will, in this era of sound instrumentation, have been well aligned. As a result, the saw cut to remove the component should reproduce a reasonable alignment, including posterior slope, even without an instrument, by following the interface. Some surgeons will prefer a cut with minimal or no posterior slope for simplicity, but this is more likely to resect anterior bone and jeopardize the tibial tubercle. As is the case with much revision surgery, instruments that work well in primary surgery may not at revision. In the case of the tibia, extramedullary cutting guides cannot be pinned, between the existing tibial surface and the tibial tubercle and still enable resection of some bone. Pins hold poorly as the existing bone is deficient, soft, or sclerotic. Intramedullary guides are more promising in this situation, relating as they do, the position of the stem and that of the component.

The purpose of reaming is not to remove much tibial bone, but rather to measure the endosteal diameter as an indication of the best choice of stem extension. It paves the way for the insertion of a trial tibial stem and many systems may allow attachment of a tibial cutting guide to the reamer for the fine cut described earlier. The position of the reamer will ultimately be the position of a tightly fitting stem extension and as a result, the alignment of the component.

The correct reaming technique will vary with the design of the implant. However, two anatomical points are almost universally true: 1) the centre of the tibial diaphysis (on an AP radiograph) is medial to the centre of the cut bone surface and 2) the canal is anterior (on a lateral radiograph) to the centre of the cut tibial

Box 8.8.7 Non-viable fixation strategies

Fully cemented diaphyseal stems

- Disadvantages:
  - More fixation than necessary
  - Does not guide position
  - Destructive removal.

Press-fit metaphyseal stems

- Disadvantages:
  - Inadequate fixation
  - Does not guide position.

surface. For the reamer and stem extension to sit centrally in the diaphysis, the entry hole must be anterior and medial. The natural asymmetry of the tibia can be replicated expeditiously by placing an offset tibial stem extension in the canal medially, with the component oriented laterally on the cut bone surface above. When this trial component is inserted, the stem should fit nicely in the canal, the component will be centred on the cut bone surface, and neutral alignment preserved (Figure 8.8.7).

Applying the trial component upside down to the proximal tibia is a quick way to assess component sizing. Tibial templates that position punches and drill guides often do not fit on the irregular bone surface or cannot be held by pins in bad bone. They can be dispensed with in many cases, and the proximal tibia shaped with a rongeur or broach.

Maximizing tibial coverage is far less important than achieving correct rotational positioning and soft tissue coverage. Surgeons intent on maximizing tibial coverage will be tempted to rotate the component internally, to cover the larger posteromedial corner of bone. Revisions of the stiff knee may be complicated by an uncomfortably tight closure of the medial capsule—a situation that can be improved by undersizing the tibial component slightly and removing a small amount of medial tibial bone.

Step 2: knee in flexion

We can build the flexion gap, with the tibia as a foundation, and then match the extension gap to it. With the knee flexed to 90 degrees, we will: a) establish the rotational position of the femoral component; b) select the size of femoral component (anteroposterior dimension) to restore stability through the collateral ligaments when possible; and c) evaluate how this femoral component and a tibial insert affect the relationship between the patella and the joint line.

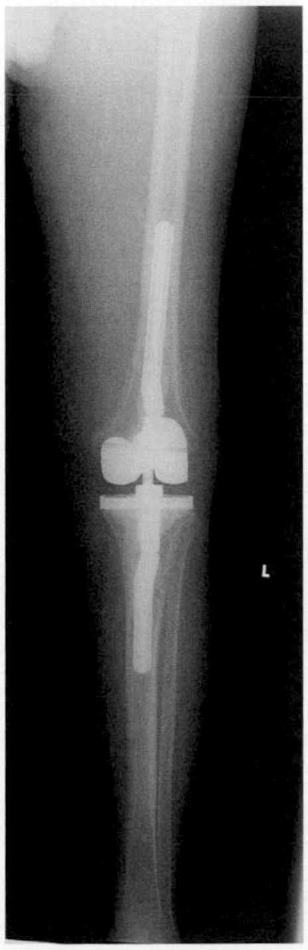

Fig. 8.8.7 Neutral alignment preserved with lateral offset of both tibial and femoral components.

Step 2a: rotational position of the femoral component.

Ideally, the medial to lateral axis of the distal femoral component will be placed parallel to the transepicondylar line. The epicondyles, obscure in ideal circumstances in the primary replacement, will be more difficult to locate in the revision. Nonetheless, they are the best indicators of correct rotational positioning, especially as there will be no posterior articulation and no trochlear groove or 'Whitesides line' to reference from. Preoperative CT will prove reassuring at revision surgery: the rotational position of the failed femoral component will have been quantified preoperatively and either replicated if acceptable or corrected if not.

Another, somewhat vague guide to rotation will be the residual posterior condylar bone, palpable in the back of the femur. Once the internally rotated component is removed and assuming symmetric bone loss, there will be more residual bone on the posteromedial side. This finding indicates a need for a posterolateral augmentation block to correct internal rotation. Finally, if rotation is off, the patella will track laterally; another indication for a corrective posterolateral femoral augment, assuming the tibial component has been oriented to the tibial tubercle.

An expedient way to visually and mentally commit to the desired rotational position for the femoral component is to create the intercondylar box cut at right angles to the epicondylar axis before reconstructing the flexion gap. Virtually every revision knee component will require some type of box cut and a minimum of instrumentation is required. The width of the box can be marked on the distal bone and a modest depth created. By the technique described here, we will not yet have decided where to seat the femoral component, proximally to distally until Step 3. The box bone, once removed, can be used as graft, whereas if the canal is drilled or reamed early, this bone will be destroyed. The notch, once created, is an unmistakable reminder of the desired rotation.

Step 2b: choose femoral component size to stabilize knee in flexion

The first of our 'keys to revision surgery' has not yet been implemented: the flexion gap will be 'controlled' by the (anteroposterior) size of the femoral component and to a lesser extent by its position. The largest component that can be sensibly implanted will be the one that extends from medial to lateral across the distal femur—any larger and it would overhang unacceptably. The maximum size might be necessary in the revision of a knee with flexion instability, where the flexion gap needs to be reduced. In most cases a size similar to the failed component will suffice. Sometimes (especially in revising the stiff knee with poor flexion) one or two sizes smaller may be appropriate. An easy way to assess the largest usable component is to place the trial component, articulation against distal bone, to compare medial lateral dimensions. It should be clear that the femoral component is never selected primarily for its medial–lateral fit, but rather for the effect that the anteroposterior dimension has on the collateral ligaments.

When the femoral canal is reamed, there is a tendency to enter the bone posteriorly and to lower the arm holding the reamer. As a direct result, the reamer assumes a 'flexed' angle relative to the medullary canal. This leads to impingement of the tip of a long

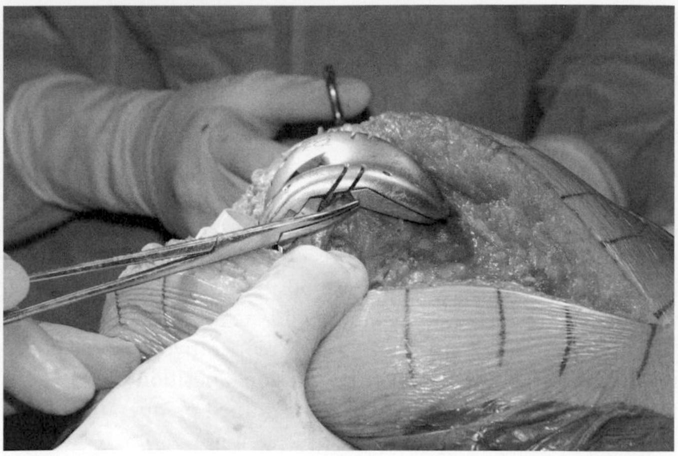

Fig. 8.8.8 Anterior entry point of femoral reamer often results in need for anterior augmentation.

press-fit stem on the anterior endosteum, which may give the impression of a tight press-fit, but which actually limits the diameter of the stem extension to something smaller than would be accomplished with parallel implantation. Most revision knees, if the femur is reamed parallel to the anterior cortex, will require some form of anterior augmentation on the femoral component (Figure 8.8.8).

Press-fit stem extensions ultimately become 'implantable instruments'. By lodging in the diaphysis, they ascertain alignment relative to the (distal half) of the femoral canal. Even if a surgeon prefers shorter, smaller diameter stems that will be fully cemented, using longer (i.e. 200mm for the femur) trial stems at this stage, as a means of determining alignment, position, and accordingly, the necessary augmentation, will help achieve the desired component position. The reaming technique can be manipulated (described later), to alter intramedullary stem position and arthroplasty alignment. If greater modification is required, then smaller diameter fully cemented stems will be required. At this point the stems in the femoral canal position the femoral trial reproducibly. A trial tibial articular polyethylene is required to stabilize the joint in flexion.

If the knee cannot be stabilized in flexion despite the use of the largest possible (extends from medial to lateral) femoral component, a very thick articular polyethylene and perhaps even block augments on the tibial baseplate, it is clear that the collateral ligaments are absent or have suffered plastic deformation. This is the first of two, specific indications for a constrained implant. If the extent of instability in flexion exceeds the 'jump distance' of a non-linked constrained articulation, this is an indication for a 'linked constrained' device or 'hinge'.

Step 2c: assess joint line relative to the patella

With the femoral component size and anteroposterior position established, the tibial articular surface that provides stability will also create a 'joint line' in flexion. There should be no confusion about the concept of joint line—it is not simply a two-dimensional 'line', but rather a three-dimensional 'shape' corresponding to where the tibia and femur articulate—from full extension to maximal flexion. For the purpose of revision knee arthroplasty and assuming a relatively 'normal' patellar tendon length, the joint line can be evaluated relative to the inferior pole of the patella.

A sound revision can be created from more than one size of femoral component, even if positioned identically in the anteroposterior plane (as viewed on a lateral radiograph). The flexion gap can be stabilized with a larger femoral component and a thinner articular polyethylene or alternately with a smaller femoral component and a thicker polyethylene. Both will be stable, but in the latter scenario, additional distal femoral bone would need to be resected to accommodate the thicker polyethylene in extension. The sequence of events becomes: smaller femoral component, more spacious flexion gap, thicker polyethylene, higher joint line in flexion, additional distal femur removed to accommodate thicker polyethylene, and so higher joint line in extension. The preferred combination of femoral and tibial components will be that with the best 'joint line'. Our recommendation is that this choice be made relative to patellar height and not a landmark on the femur or tibia (Figure 8.8.9).

Step 3: knee in extension

This final step is simple and invokes the second key to revision arthroplasty surgery: the extension gap is controlled by the proximal–distal position of the femoral component. At this point all the components have been selected and positioned on press-fit stems. The tibia cannot move, but by slowly and gently extending the knee, the femoral component will be pushed into the distal femur to precisely the point that it needs to be in order to make the extension gap equal to the flexion gap. If we push too far and place the knee in recurvatum, the femoral component will have migrated too far proximally into the femur. If we fail to eliminate a flexion deformity, the femur will be 'too proud' on the distal femur and the deformity will persist. Trial femoral components that include cutting slots facilitate this step. Small cuts on the residual, irregular bone once the knee is fully extended will create, millimetre for millimetre, the correct space to accommodate an augment that guarantees the position we require (Figure 8.8.10).

The correct femoral component proximal–distal position in this step is actually determined by the posterior soft tissues—capsule, hamstrings, and gastrocnemius. So, even if there has been collateral ligament failure, we may have the impression of full, stable extension because the fully extended knee is stabilized by the posterior structures. This is also the second point at which it may be

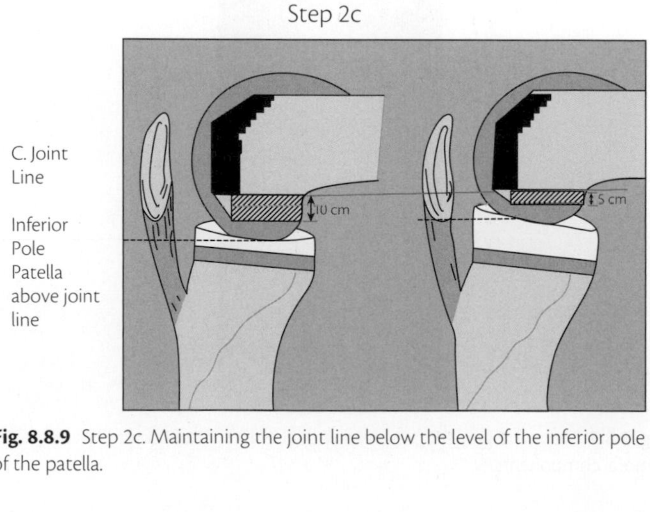

Fig. 8.8.9 Step 2c. Maintaining the joint line below the level of the inferior pole of the patella.

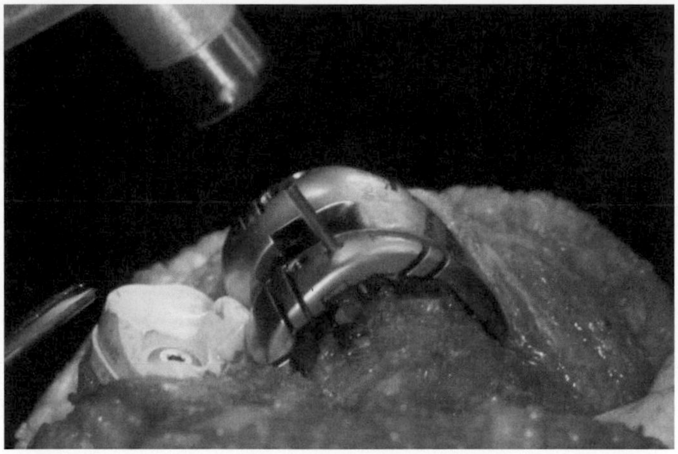

Fig. 8.8.10 Finishing the femur.

necessary to select a constrained prosthesis—if varus–valgus instability persists as a result of collateral ligament failure. It may be necessary to assess the knee in a few degrees of flexion to eliminate the confounding effect of the posterior structures.

How important is joint line height?

The earliest revision knee arthroplasties were performed with primary implants under challenging circumstances. With neither stem extensions nor augments in that era, surgeons were almost obligated to select the femoral component size that would fit the residual bone, once the failed implant had been removed. As we know from Step 2c of the revision technique described in this chapter, a smaller femoral component would necessitate a thicker polyethylene insert and inevitably an elevated joint line in flexion. To stabilize this knee, distal femoral bone loss either would have to be ignored to accommodate the tibial insert or, perhaps, distal femoral bone might be resected to achieve full extension. The results of early revisions were poor and the most glaring abnormality on postoperative anteroposterior radiographs was bizarrely thick polyethylene and an elevated joint line. The first efforts to remedy this situation led to a surgical technique that *began* by establishing the distal position of the femoral component, i.e. the (distal) joint line (or the joint line at full extension) as a preliminary reference point for the entire reconstruction. This was usually a calculated distance from an osseous landmark—often the fibular head. This strategy, though an improvement, did not address stability of the knee in flexion or recognize that there is a joint 'line' for every position of the knee from full extension to maximal flexion, because of the state of the soft tissues.

An illustration of the challenges of revision knee arthroplasty is to visualize a very badly failed knee replacement—perhaps a second revision or even a resection arthroplasty about to be reimplanted. The cruciate ligaments will have been long gone and the soft tissue balance is likely to have suffered plastic deformation or contracture. The hypothetical questions then become: if all normal bone and articular cartilage were restored in such a knee, and the compromised soft tissues left as they are, would this knee function well? Would it be both stable and mobile? After all, the original anatomical joint line would have been restored perfectly in all three dimensions. The reality is that the state of the soft tissues limits the ability of such an anatomical restoration of the joint line to work well in every case.

In contrast, a surgical technique that accepts that the envelope of soft tissue around the knee joint is likely to have changed, and that is based on the selection of femoral component (controlling as it does soft tissue tension) is much more likely to be succeed. Revision arthroplasty then becomes very much like pitching an unfamiliar circus tent, where poles are brought inside the collapsed structure and the outer fabric is erected.

Simply stated, the joint 'line' is not a line but rather a complex three-dimensional construct corresponding to the contact of the tibia with the femur through an entire arc of motion. It corresponds to the shape of the femoral component articular surface. There will be a joint line in flexion and extension and everywhere in between. Even restoration of a joint line that is normal in three dimensions may not produce a good joint. Pragmatism with respect to the state of the soft tissues is needed.

Step 4: the patella

The patella is best reserved for the end of the case because once the old patellar implant is removed the patella itself is more

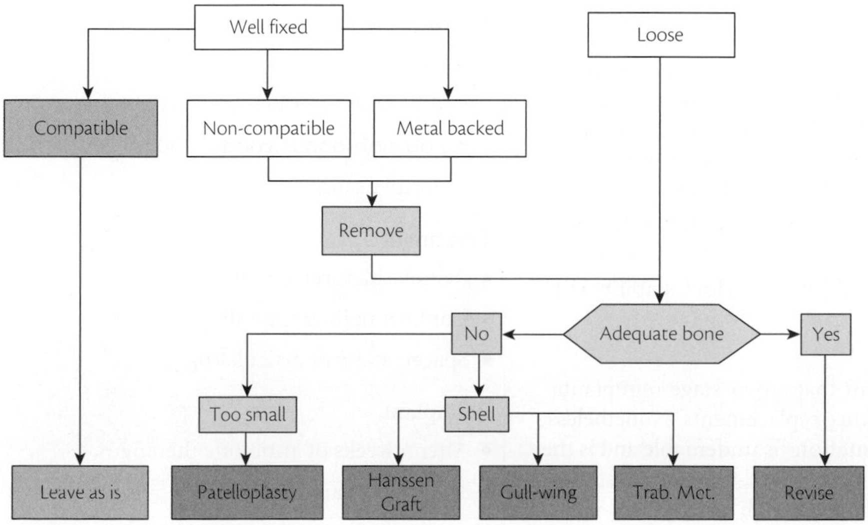

Fig. 8.8.11 Algorithm for treatment of the patella in revision TKA.

vulnerable to fracture. A treatment algorithm can be established (Figure 8.8.11) initially based on whether the implant is loose. A well-fixed patellar component that articulates compatibly with the revision femoral component should be left in place, unless the revision is being performed for stiffness and the entire construct is inordinately thick. Patellae with loose components may have adequate bone that would make revision feasible. If the residual bone is thin and perhaps scaphoid in shape (if only the anterior cortex is left) then reconstitution with particulate bone graft and a tensor fascia lata cover can restore thickness. Alternately the residual patella can be split from superior to inferior and both halves of the shell 'cracked up' to recreate a more conforming shape—the so-called gull-wing osteotomy. Newer porous metal implants, though more expensive and time consuming, produce excellent results and have largely supplanted the first two options. If the patella is too small, it may be left as is or reshaped slightly to enhance tracking. The patient with an extremely small or no patella, who suffers an extensor lag postoperatively, may benefit from an extensor mechanism allograft.

Specific techniques for specific causes of failure

Mode of failure 1: infection (Box 8.8.9)

Diagnosis of infection

Infection continues to be one of the most perplexing calamities to complicate knee arthroplasty surgery. The infection rate should be no greater than 2% and in most centres 0.5–1.0%. An aggressive and organized approach to the management of wound problems is essential to mitigate the risk of deep sepsis. The surgeon should also surrender early to the idea that the arthroplasty might be infected and act decisively so that a diagnosis will be established and not simply obscured by undisciplined use of antibiotics.

This means that all wound problems be taken seriously, as many cases of deep sepsis originate with superficial problems. Whilst many surgeons hesitate to aspirate an arthroplasty for fear of introducing infection, it is only by knowing what is inside the joint that therapy is likely to prevail. There is a strong rationale to aspirate any arthroplasty with late pain or an early wound problem before any antibiotic is administered. Introducing antibiotic without an aspirate compromises the prompt diagnosis of sepsis.

The knee presenting with pain months to years after the primary, whose history does not specifically arouse suspicion of infection and whose peripheral blood test for erythrocyte sedimentation rate (ESR) and C-reactive protein (CRP) is normal, may not require aspiration. When fluid is aspirated it should be sent not only for culture and sensitivity, but also for a cell count and differential. Solid evidence exists in the chronically painful knee, that white blood cell (WBC) counts in excess of 2500/mL, especially where there are more than 50% polymorphonucleocytes are consistent with deep sepsis. This may not pertain in the first few weeks after surgery.

Two stage versus one stage

There is almost universal agreement that a two-stage reimplantation protocol cures more infected knee replacements. Nonetheless, the appeal of 'single-stage' reimplantations is undeniable and is the practice of some surgeons. The debate lies in the relative success rates of both procedures. Common to both procedures is the importance of a precise bacteriological diagnosis and antibiotic sensitivity as well as an aggressive and complete debridement. It is good practice to obtain a radiograph (that images to the ankle) in the operating theatre with the patient still anaesthetized, once the surgeon feels that all foreign material has been removed. This often reveals more cement, frequently in the patella lug holes or the tibial metaphysis. Ultimately, and judicially, a radiograph that demonstrates 'no foreign material' is compelling evidence that the surgeon has understood and complied with a principle of treating infected arthroplasties: that all foreign material be removed. In addition, this radiograph will show bone deficiency in a way that is not feasible once a spacer has been implanted, and facilitates planning the reimplantation.

Two-stage reimplantation protocols represent the standard of care in most countries. Eradication of sepsis and acceptable knee function have been achieved with, in general, a 6-week period after the infected arthroplasty was removed during which the patient receives antibiotic therapy. Most surgeons use some type of antibiotic-impregnated methacrylate spacer and good results have been described with solid (non-articulating) spacers as well as those that resemble an arthroplasty and permit some motion. Some surgeons endorse autoclaving and reimplanting one or both of the implants that have been removed using limited fixation and antibiotic-impregnated cement. The rationale is to maintain motion and facilitate the reimplantation. To date, no compelling evidence exists that would suggest that any particular approach to 'spacers' has either better function or increased survival. While early reports on two-stage protocols included reimplantation at 6 weeks, immediately after antibiotic therapy was concluded, recent practice has included waiting, with the patient off of therapy for durations of weeks to months and reaspirating prior to reimplantation. No data demonstrate superiority of that concept to date.

Reimplantation surgery will challenge even the most experienced surgeon. Careful attention to detail in the surgical exposure (see earlier) will pay dividends. Tubercle osteotomies in this situation may be problematic—especially if performed for both the removal

Box 8.8.9 Mode of failure 1: infection

Diagnosis
- Suspicious history
- Aspiration:
  - WBC > 2000 WBC
  - Polymorphonucleocytes> 50%
  - Positive culture.

Treatment
- Remove all foreign material
- Confirm radiographically
- Spacer: static or articulating.

Reimplant
- After 6 weeks of antibiotic therapy
- ± Period off antibiotics.

and reimplantation. Bone quality is compromised and any hardware, even wires, left to hold the osteotomy runs against the principle of removal of all foreign material. The tubercle, ultimately implanted against stem extensions may not heal solidly, representing then a case of prior sepsis and extensor mechanism rupture.

The aggressive debridement, necessarily including curetting of the canal and wholesale removal of suspicious bone often leave the surgeon with challenges of bone defects and fixation. Porous metal augments advantageously address both issues and are very useful in reimplantation surgery. Fully cemented stem extensions have the advantage of excellent fixation and can include antibiotic, though less of a dose than can be used in spacers, because of the compromise to the mechanical properties of the cement. If the reimplantation suffers persistent or recurrent infection, removal of fully cemented stems may be a destructive prelude to amputation.

My preferred technique is a disciplined approach to establishing a bacteriological diagnosis, aggressive debridement on the removal, reimplantation at completion of the course of antibiotics without cessation of antibiotic therapy, long uncemented stem extensions and porous metal conical augments to enhance fixation whether large defects are present or not.

Mode of failure 2: extensor mechanism rupture (Box 8.8.10)

Acute or intraoperative ruptures of the extensor mechanism, often become chronic extensor ruptures until some tissue substitute, either an allograft (complete tibial tubercle, patellar tendon, patella, and quadriceps tendon construct) or autograft (semitendinosis) has been introduced. Ruptures anywhere from the tibial tubercle to the superior pole of the patella suffer similar results and this includes transverse, displaced patellar fractures with an extensor lag. This last entity should be removed conceptually from the category of fracture and treated as a chronic extensor rupture.

This is generally regarded as one of the most difficult problems to treat. The extensor rupture often occurs in an arthroplasty that is in some ways unstable. Then, when the extensor fails, global instability or posterior tibial dislocation (in flexion) often ensues. At other times, the patient with a chronically ruptured extensor will hyperextend the knee to prevent buckling. With time, this results in a recurvatum deformity. Maltracking is a common accompaniment to any patellar problem. Accordingly, revision knee arthroplasty is usually required when the extensor mechanism is reconstructed. Extensor mechanism allografts are used more frequently than other techniques and are generally successful in the short term if the graft is implanted under considerable tension. This is most likely due, not to stretching of the graft itself, but chronic retraction of the quadriceps up into the thigh during the period of rupture. If the graft is placed loosely, when the knee bends ands stretches the muscle, the lag recurs.

Mode of failure 3: stiffness (Box 8.8.11)

The stiff knee replacement is often accepted, with disappointment, by both surgeon and patient. Indeed, the patient who had very poor flexion prior to the arthroplasty probably has an extensor that is chronically scarred and tight. This cannot easily be completely overcome with revision surgery or therapy. In addition, the patient who truly has 'arthrofibrosis' and mounts an aggressive scar response to any surgery is unlikely to respond well to revision arthroplasty. Fortunately this is a very small minority of individuals. The majority of patients with good preoperative flexion who either bend less then 105 degrees or develop a flexion contracture exceeding 10 degrees will probably benefit from revision surgery, in particular if there is also pain. The scar that the surgeon confronts at surgery is then the result and not the cause of stiffness.

Revision is demanding for surgeon, patient, and the rehabilitation team. Once stiffness is chronic, very little will succeed short of a complete revision operation, with aggressive soft tissue release, and alteration of every feature of the knee away from stiffness towards mobility. For example, femoral components usually need to be reduced in size and implanted in neutral position (as viewed on the lateral radiograph), not flexed where they encroach on the flexion gap. Internal rotation of femoral and tibial components will be observed in the majority of stiff knees arthroplasties. The resultant tendency to patellar dislocation inhibits many patients from flexing past about 60 degrees. Those who succeed in regaining motion suffer patellar dislocations—those that don't become stiff. CT scanning, prior to revision, to quantify rotational position is urged. Patients who undergo expert and complete revision arthroplasty, with constructive alteration of component position and size may expect welcome pain relief, full extension and flexion on average to about 100 degrees.

Mode of failure 4: tibial–femoral instability (Box 8.8.12)

The unstable knee arthroplasty is at once the most intellectually challenging and, if approached successfully the most gratifying. Central to the problem of instability are four questions:

1) In what way is the knee unstable?
2) What forces have made it that way?

Box 8.8.10 Mode of failure 2: extensor mechanism rupture

- Preoperative evaluation:
  - Include transverse patellar fractures
  - Assess for instability
  - CT for malrotation
  - Probable complete revision
  - Extensor mechanism allograft.

Box 8.8.11 Mode of failure 3: stiffness

- Indications for revision:
  - Flexion <105 degrees
  - Flexion contracture >10 degrees
  - Pain
- Assess: CT scan for malrotation
- Complete revision required.

3) How can surgery mitigate those forces?
4) What means are available to stabilize the knee?

The frequent and unfortunate strategy to instability is often only: 'What constrained implant should I use?' If the deforming forces are not reduced, instability will recur, often with dire consequences.

The patient who reports 'that their knee arthroplasty is unstable is suffering from one or more of the following:

- Buckling from extensor mechanism failure, which either belongs in 'Mode of failure 2: extensor mechanism rupture' or 'Mode of failure 7: patellar complications and malrotation'
- Recurvatum which always raises the suspicion of extensor mechanism failure and compensatory 'back-kneeing'. If this originates from neurological compromise of the extensor, the prognosis is bleak and arthrodesis should be considered. Extensor rupture belongs in 'Mode of failure 2'. Structural recurvatum without neurological compromise, is generally from subsidence of a component, bone loss, and perhaps stretching of the posterior structures. This type of recurvatum will respond to revision arthroplasty
- Flexion instability: results from a flexion gap that is larger than the extension gap. Revision following the three steps described earlier will yield satisfying results, either by diminishing the flexion gap (larger femoral component) or by increasing the extension gap (posterior capsular release with or without resection of additional femoral bone)
- Varus–valgus instability from failure of one or both collateral ligaments usually requires a constrained revision prosthesis, along with realignment in the coronal plane (e.g. less valgus in the patient with medial collateral ligament failure) to reduce the deforming force. These cases may be further complicated by deformity at the hip, (developmental dysplasia or hip abductor weakness), the foot (tibialis posterior rupture and acquired flat foot deformity), and even in the spine where scoliosis can shift the centre of gravity, resulting in potent destructive forces at the deformed knee.

Some have postulated that a linked constrained device (hinge) will be necessary if the collateral ligaments have failed completely and that a non-linked device will suffice if some remnant of soft tissue envelope is present. While this may be a useful guide to some, it will fail if all the factors listed here are not taken considered.

Box 8.8.12 Mode of failure 4: tibial–femoral instability

- Varus–valgus: alignment and collateral ligaments
- Flexion instability: flexion > extension gap
- Recurvatum:
  - Structural: possible to revise
    —posterior laxity
    —component subsidence
  - Non-neurological quadriceps weakness:
    —i.e. patellectomy
    —correct at revision
  - Neurological quadriceps weakness:
    —i.e. polio
    —avoid revision
    —consider arthrodesis
- Buckling: correct patellar instability

Mode of failure 5: periprosthetic fracture (Box 8.8.13)

Fractures requiring surgery are more common in the supracondylar region of the femur than any part of the tibia. Patellar fractures, if transverse, represent a chronic rupture of the extensor mechanism and belong in 'Mode of failure 2'. Vertical patellar fractures can be treated non-surgically at first, to allow swelling and acute pain to subside. If a lag persists, or if the patellar component of a resurfaced knee is loose, surgery will be required. In most cases of vertical fracture, there will be a tendency to maltracking and these cases belong in 'Mode of failure 7'.

Supracondyar fractures usually occur in the patient with: a) osteoporosis; b) a stress riser (in the form of a supracondylar notch), and c) limited flexion so that during a fall the knee reaches its limit of motion and then the porotic bone yields. These fractures have been treated successfully in the past with both blade plates and plates with sliding screws. This was superseded by supracondylar locking nails and most recently have been replaced by locking plates with or without minimally invasive approaches.

Some low-demand patients with comminution and poor quality bone may require a revision arthroplasty either with a distal femoral allograft or more typically a tumour-style distal femoral replacement implant. Tibial fractures are generally the late sequel to extensive osteolysis and tibial component loosening. These require revision arthroplasty, not fracture fixation.

Mode of failure 6: loosening (Box 8.8.14)

Aseptic loosening was once thought to result from 'micromotion' at the interface that gradually increased in amplitude until the component came loose. Alternately, it has been attributed to bone overload and collapse. It has been correctly associated with varus alignment and the results of medial compartment overload since 1977. While some uncemented or partially cemented tibial components loosen early from failed ingrowth or inadequate fixation, and some femoral components loosen from gaps that are left between the posterior femoral bone and the femoral flange, virtually all late

Box 8.8.13 Mode of failure 5: periprosthetic fracture

- Open reduction and fixation when possible:
  - Favoured: locking plates
  - Feasible:
    —supracondylar nails
    —supracondylar plate.
- Revise with:
  - Tumour prosthesis
  - Distal femoral allograft.

Box 8.8.14 Mode of failure 6: loosening

- Early loosening:
  - Failed ingrowth
  - Cement technique
  - Alignment (varus)
- Late loosening:
  - Wear, particles, osteolysis
  - Revise with improved alignment
  - Eliminate prosthesis with poor interface
  - Full revision preferred
  - Polyethylene exchange possible in elderly

loosening will result from wear, particle generation, osteolysis, bone loss, and subsidence.

While partial revision with bone grafting may be appealing, the process of osteolysis is likely to progress through the joint and loosen the other components. Accordingly, complete revision is almost universally recommended. As with the unstable arthroplasty, causative factors must be identified and corrected specifically. Varus alignment is problematic, inducing inordinate forces on the medial component. A full-length radiograph showing hips, knees, and ankles is important; not only to appreciate the mechanical axis, but to plan how much valgus alignment can be tolerated to unload the medial compartment at the revision. Wear results not only from the articular surface, but the modular interface. A substandard modular locking mechanism and poor quality polyethylene may be implicated and should be replaced. CT scans depict the extent of osteolytic lesions with distressing accuracy.

Failures from osteolysis and loosening have constituted the majority of revision arthroplasties. Loosening of the revision is likely unless realignment reduces destructive forces, and fixation is supplemented by stem extensions that are either fully cemented or uncemented and fill the diaphyseal canal. The interface itself can be a problem—methacrylate cement against poor quality, sclerotic bone enjoys no interlock. By contrast, porous metal augments enhance fixation by providing a transition of interfaces from poor bone (that will yet grow into porous metal) and porous metal that on its other side accepts bone cement which provides an excellent bond to the implant. The porous implants can be impacted into the medullary canal of the tibia or femur without concern for rotational, flexion–extension or varus valgus position, so long as the augment does not impede the positioning of the component. Structural allografts, useful for massive bone defects are required less frequently as porous metal is commonly available.

Mode of failure 7: patella and malrotation (Box 8.8.15)

There is an ineluctable relationship between patellar maltracking and internal rotation positioning of the femoral and or tibial components. The relationship is additive, not compensatory. Furthermore, the effect of maltracking is responsible for virtually every patellar complication: as the patellar bone tries to slide off laterally and the polyethylene component stays in the trochlear groove, they may inevitably dissociate, yielding patellar fractures and component loosening or breakage. Maltracking invariably requires complete revision—the only way to correct rotational positioning of the components.

Box 8.8.15 Mode of failure 7: patellar complications and malrotation

- Consider malrotation in all patellar complications
  - Maltracking
  - Dislocation
  - Vertical patellar fracture
  - Component loosening
  - Patellar component breakage
- Evaluate with CT scan
- Complete revision required.

The tibial component will be correctly rotated when positioned directly behind the tibial tubercle. As the conforming articular polyethylene necessarily aligns itself under the femoral condyles, the only way that the tubercle and in turn the patellar tendon and patella itself can be positioned in the femoral trochlear groove, is to line the tibial component with the tubercle. Femoral components are most reliably aligned parallel to the transepicondylar axis—this being the only landmark available at revision surgery. A posterolateral augment will generally ensure more external rotation. These conclusions are not only logical but confirmed by the published data on CT scanning of knees with maltracking.

Mode of failure 8: breakage (Box 8.8.16)

Component breakage is far less common than previously. Some cases of tibial baseplate fracture were in fact cases of wear, osteolysis, and bone loss such that the component was unsupported and fractured. Posterior femoral condyles that have broken probably did so because of a gap between the posterior bone and an unsupported posterior condyle. Catastrophic polyethylene breakage is seen far less commonly as a result of better production methods, conforming articulations, and avoidance of thin modular inserts.

Box 8.8.16 Mode of failure 8: component breakage

- Relatively rare
- Do not include cases of wear and osteolysis- (loosening)
- Broken posterior stabilized spine invariably secondary to hyperextension
  - Subsidence after *loosening*
  - Recurvatum
  - Implantation with flexed femur and excess posterior tibial slope
- Poly wear and loss of conformity presents as late instability.

Complete revision to improve both is mandatory, except perhaps in one of the few indications for partial revision—late wear of a tibial polyethylene insert in an elderly, low-demand patient.

Fractures have been reported of posterior stabilized tibial spines. Closer evaluation confirms that the mechanism is generally hyperextension of the knee so that the anterior femoral flange strikes sharply against the base of the spine. In these cases the cause of recurvatum is usually (femoral) component subsidence. These cases require a complete revision with considerations appropriate to 'loosening' above.

Breakage of the more prominent (and vulnerable) tibial spine on non-linked constrained implants results either from alignment leading to potent varus or valgus forces, or malrotation that can 'twist' the spine off the baseplate. In each case complete, corrective revision is required.

Mode of failure 9: no diagnosis (no surgery) (Box 8.8.17)

The problem arthroplasty without a coherent diagnosis should not undergo revision surgery as the results are likely to be poor. This situation is a strong indication to evaluate the patient more thoroughly. Failure to identify a problem in the knee should be a strong reminder to revisit the hip and spine, perhaps even with a bone scan. Recent ESR and CRP, as well as an aspiration for cell count and differential are appropriate. A CT scan should be obtained to quantify tibial and femoral component position.

Radiographs that predate the primary, to answer whether the patient actually had sufficiently severe cartilage loss to expect that arthroplasty would be useful, are in order. Methodical palpation of anatomical landmarks on the knee may identify neuromas or tendinitis that will more likely respond to cryoablation or physical therapy. While always dangerous to attribute physical suffering to mental anguish, there is nonetheless a literature that correlates lower satisfaction with depression.

Box 8.8.17 Mode of failure 9: no diagnosis

- No surgery—results poor
- Methodical physical examination: spine and ipsilateral hip
- Consider:
  - Chronic regional pain syndrome
  - Tourniquet palsy
  - Limited arthritis prior to TKA
  - Occult infection
- Investigations:
  - AP pelvis radiograph
  - Technetium bone scan of spine, hip, and knee
  - CT scan component rotation
  - Reaspiration.

Conclusions

The conceptual appreciation of how knee arthroplasties fail, the surgical technique, and the implants themselves have improved dramatically over two decades. Any one surgeon performs relatively few revisions and so many of these advances have not been incorporated into their practice. The understandable, though at times misguided, desire to perform less surgery at revision has led to worse rather than better results. Diagnosis, and the coherent surgical plan that flows from it, is absolutely essential. Revision knee arthroplasty is not one procedure but rather about eight different operations depending on the cause of failure. The ideas, technique, and implants that work well for primary arthroplasty generally do not apply to revisions. New ideas and a methodical approach to surgical exposure, even for stiff arthroplasties has made the need for quadriceps snips infrequent and both patellar turn-downs and tibial tubercle osteotomies almost obsolete. While attention to the level of the joint line is appropriate, using it as the guiding principle in revision surgery complicates the technique unnecessarily and should be abandoned, remembering that this 'line' is actually a three-dimensional concept corresponding to the shape of the femoral articular surface.

The unsolved problems in revision knee arthroplasty are still infection and extensor mechanism ruptures. While strategies exist for these problems, the long-term results are less good.

By establishing a tibial platform, stabilizing the knee in 90 degrees of flexion and then selecting the proximal–distal position of the femoral component to balance the knee in extension, with a judicious use of constrained implants, the results of first-time revision knee arthroplasties may exceed those of primary knee replacement.

Further reading

Berger, R.A., Crossett, L.S., Jacobs, J.J., and Rubash, H.E. (1998). Malrotation causing patellofemoral complications after total knee arthroplasty. *Clinical Orthopaedics and Related Research*, **356**, 144–53.

Sharkey, P.F., Homesley, H., Shastri, S., Jacoby, S., Hozack, W., and Rothman, R. (2004). Results of revision total knee arthroplasty after exposure of the knee with extensor mechanism tenolysis. *Journal of Arthroplasty*, **19**(6), 751–6.

Vince, K., Chivas, D., and Droll, K.P. (2007). Wound complications after total knee arthroplasty. *Journal of Arthroplasty*, **22**(4 Suppl 1), 39–44.

Vince, K. (2006). Extensor mechanism rupture after total knee arthroplasty. In Scott, W.N. (ed) *Insall & Scott Surgery of the Knee*, 4th edn., pp. 1814–27. Philadelphia, PA: Churchill Livingstone.

Vince, K.G., Abdeen, A., and Sugimori, T. (2006). The unstable total knee arthroplasty: causes and cures. *Journal of Arthroplasty*, **21**(4 Suppl 1), 44–9.

8.9

Miscellaneous conditions around the knee

Paul Monk, Max Gibbons, and Tom Temple

Summary points

- Intra and extra-articular
- X-ray for bone or soft tissue origin
- Solid tumours consider malignancy
- MRI for diagnosis.

Introduction

The causes of knee pain are most often related to overuse or trauma. Other conditions can mimic common knee disorders and should be considered in the differential diagnosis in patients who present with a history and physical findings inconsistent with mechanical knee pain.

Synovial and bursal conditions

Synovial chondromatosis

Synovial chondromatosis is a monoarticular disease presenting more often in males, in the third and fourth decades of life. Clinically, patients present with knee effusions and episodes of locking and grinding. Radiographically, in the early stages of this disease, an effusion is present, but as the disease progresses, characteristic 'popcorn' calcifications are found in and around the joint (Figure 8.9.1).

Synovial chondromatosis is a metaplastic disease process whereby synovium modulates into cartilage. Hyaline cartilage coalesces on the fronds of synovium and becomes intra-articular loose bodies. When these cartilaginous loose bodies mineralize, this is called synovial osteochondromatosis.

If unrecognized, cartilage damage can occur from repetitive mechanical trauma resulting in joint arthrosis. Treatment involves either synovectomy (arthroscopic or open) and rarely in recalcitrant disease, chemical or radiation synovectomy. If intra-articular osteocartilaginous loose bodies are present, their removal in addition to synovectomy is necessary. Recurrences after synovectomy are relatively uncommon.

Rarely, malignant transformation occurs, usually marked by underlying osseous destruction and intra-articular nodular masses. Early diagnosis is important and either extra-articular resection or amputation is necessary to achieve local tumour control. Histologically, loss of the clustering growth pattern, myxoid stromal changes, necrosis, and spindling of cells in the periphery of the lobules are suggestive of malignant change. Pulmonary metastases may occur following malignant transformation.

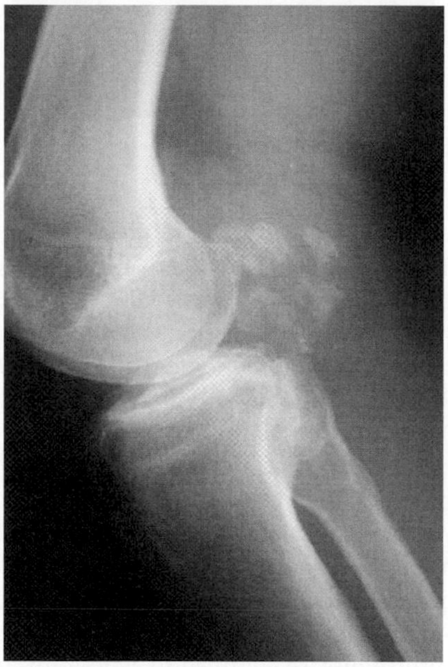

Fig. 8.9.1 Synovial chondromatosis—'popcorn' calcifications within the posterior knee joint.

Pigmented villonodular synovitis (Box 8.9.1)

Pigmented villonodular synovitis is a rare benign disorder affecting synovial joints and tendon sheaths. The knee is the most commonly involved large joint. It has been regarded as a reactive process, but recent cytogenetic evidence suggests a neoplastic aetiology. Two types of pigmented villonodular synovitis exist—a localized form is characterized by a solitary lesion, whilst the diffuse form is more aggressive in nature and usually involves the entire synovial membrane.

Local disease is usually heralded by mechanical symptoms such as locking and catching. Diffuse disease is characterized by pain,

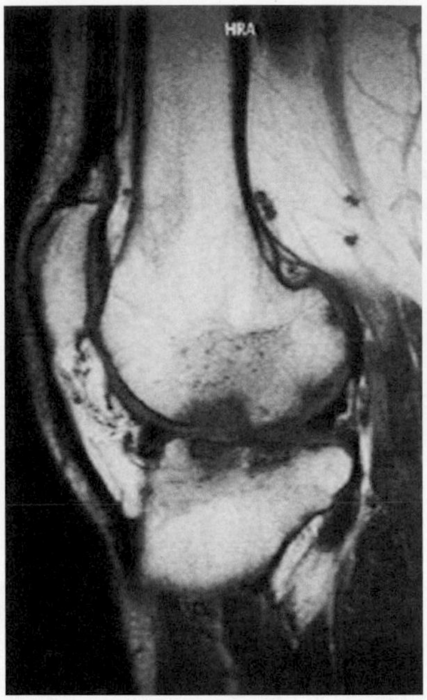

Fig. 8.9.2 MRI demonstrating multifocal pigmented villonodular synovitis with subarticular joint destruction.

swelling, stiffness, and eventually deformity. Diffuse pigmented villonodular synovitis can invade local structures extensively, including muscle, tendon, and bone, with periarticular cysts, erosions, and narrowing of the joint space. Magnetic resonance imaging (MRI) is useful in determining the nature of the disease (Figure 8.9.2). Multinodular intra-articular disease is characterized by patchy areas of fat and haemosiderin specific for pigmented villonodular synovitis.

With local disease, treatment is frequently successful with marginal complete arthroscopic or local excision, but with diffuse disease recurrence is greater than 45%. Arthroscopy and open total synovectomy alone may not relieve symptoms in these patients. With active diffuse disease confined to synovium, total synovectomy can give good short-term results. However, where the disease has extended out of the joint and into bone, local disease control is difficult. Arthrodesis and total joint replacement may be necessary for patients with diffuse and destructive disease.

Radiotherapy using intra-articular instillations of fibrosing agents is effective for refractory cases. External-beam radiotherapy has been used successfully as a salvage procedure for residual diffuse disease.

Even in patients with active disease, total synovectomy with total knee replacement will give good long-term results with recurrence of disease unlikely.

Box 8.9.1 Pigmented villonodular synovitis

- Reclassified as giant cell tumour of joint
- Benign metaplastic disease
- Nodular and diffuse forms
- MRI for diagnosis
- Open synovectomy and total knee replacement for recalcitrant disease.

Cystic lesions

Soft tissue ganglia arise from capsular, aponeurotic, bursal, and ligamentous structures as a result of myxoid degeneration of collagen fibres.

Extra-articular lesions

Extra-articular ganglia are usually painless or minimally symptomatic soft tissue masses located behind the knee in the popliteal fossa and originating from the posterior capsule. These masses do not communicate with the joint and insinuate around the semimembranosus tendon and the medial head of the gastrocnemius muscle. Popliteal or Baker's cysts are reported incidentally in 10–41% of MRI examinations of the knee. These masses can be found in children but are more commonly seen in adults, and the incidence increases with patient age. They are usually diagnosed incidentally and more commonly in adults with underlying mild to moderate arthritic changes in one or more compartments of the knee.

Synovial cysts can also arise in the tibiofibular joint and present as a painful effusion associated with restricted knee flexion and potentially compressive and invasive neuropathies of the common peroneal nerve.

Intra-articular lesions

These encapsulated fluid collections can also arise within the knee joint, most commonly the tibial insertion of the anterior cruciate ligament and can cause mechanical pain, restriction of motion, and locking of the knee.

Meniscal cysts arise from degenerative horizontal tears of the menisci. Lateral cysts are three to four times more common than medial cysts; however, medial cysts tend to be larger.

The best diagnostic study for evaluating cystic and cyst-like structures about the knee is MRI. These lesions appear uniformly hyperintense on T_2-weighted sequences and hypointense on corresponding T_1 images. Meniscal tears are also well visualized on MRI. It is important to establish a connection to the joint or aponeurotic structure because other lesions like myxoid sarcomas or synoviosarcomas can occur in the popliteal fossa and be mistaken for a common ganglion. Neurilemmomas arising from the nerve sheaths passing through the popliteal fossa can also mimic ganglia. However, these lesions are typically painful and are associated with dysaesthesias when compressed or percussed. On MRI they have an elongated appearance attenuated above and below (comet sign) and are in continuity with a nerve, often exhibiting a target sign (Figure 8.9.3). Moreover, on T_2-weighted sequences, they appear to be more heterogeneous with alternating bright and dark signals corresponding to intermixed cellular areas (Antoni A) and hypocellular areas (Antoni B) with superimposed haemorrhage and haemosiderin deposition in more long-standing lesions (ancient schwannomas).

Giant cell tumour of the tendon sheath is an occasional extra-articular mass occurring about the knee. Typically patients are in the fourth to sixth decade and present with pain and swelling that is mostly activity related. Giant cell tumour of the tendon sheath is a nodular form of pigmented villonodular synovitis and arises in tendons and aponeurotic structures. It is also heterogeneous on T_2-weighted sequences with varying degrees of dark signal depending on the degree of haemosiderin and collagen deposition within

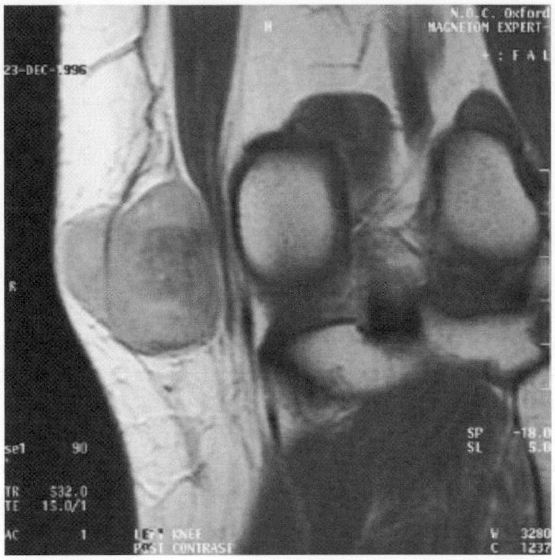

Fig. 8.9.3 Malignant schwannoma with a characteristic 'comet sign' on MRI. Peripheral nerve sheath tumour.

the tumour. Histologically, there are monomorphic round to spindled stromal cells and interspersed giant cells within a collagen matrix with moderate vascularity and haemosiderin-laden macrophages. The aetiology of this tumour is unknown. Local recurrences are uncommon after marginal or even intralesional excision.

Subchondral cysts

These fluid-filled voids are often adjacent to cruciate or meniscofemoral insertions. Most are asymptomatic but can, on occasion, be quite extensive and painful due to subchondral insufficiency.

Radiographs show a small well-defined radiolucent abnormality that is subchondral with sclerotic borders. MRI may show a fluid-filled abnormality that is bright on T_2 with little oedema in the adjacent dome. Subchondral cysts are reported in 1% of routine MRIs of the knee and treatment is not necessary.

Congenital conditions and osteochondromatosis (Box 8.9.2)

Congenital and developmental anomalies may result in morphological changes that clinically and radiographically can be confused with neoplasia.

Dwarfing conditions, such as achondroplasia, thanatophoric dysplasia, and spondyloepiphyseal dysplasia, because of abnormal physeal maturation, can cause peculiar changes in epiphyseal or metaphyseal development that may be mistaken as a tumour. Other conditions, such as chondroectodermal dysplasia or Ellis–von Crevald syndrome are associated with proximal diaphyseal exostoses. This is an autorecessive condition characterized by short stature, polydactyly, wide but dysplastic lateral tibial plateaux, and hypoplastic nails.

Chondrodysplasia punctata or Conradi–Hunermann syndrome is an autosomal dominant condition marked by asymmetric shortening with punctate mineralization of the epiphyses among other characteristic clinical features.

Metaphyseal destruction can be observed in patients with congenital syphilis, rubella, cytomegalovirus, and toxoplasmosis. Metastatic neuroblastoma and Wilms' tumour can also present as knee pain with corresponding destructive radiographic changes that require further clinical and radiographic staging followed by biopsy to diagnose and treat appropriately.

Multiple hereditary exostoses is also an autosomal dominant condition caused by a defect in the ossification groove of Ranvier or perichondral ring resulting in horizontal physeal growth and multiple periarticular osteocartilaginous excrescences that can be painful. These patients are of low to normal stature with abnormalities of the paired bones associated with valgus deformities of the elbows, wrists, knees, and ankles. Pain may result from tendonitis, bursitis, fracture through the exostosis, osteonecrosis of the cartilaginous cap, and malignant transformation which can occur in up to 5% of affected individuals. Malignant transformation is rare before skeletal maturity and is usually marked by increased growth of the mass associated with pain that is present with activity and rest. Other rare complications of osteochondral exostosis are compressive neuropathies, particularly around the knee, and vascular claudication, especially large lesions in the popliteal fossa.

Radiographically, osteochondral exostoses are metaphyseal or metadiaphyseal based at the ends of long bones. They typically grow away from the physis pointing away from the joint. On computed tomography (CT), a diagnostic feature is corticomedullary continuity between the tumour stalk and underlying medullary canal. The cartilage cap is usually thin, with a thickness of less than 1.5 cm; however, in a growing child and in proximal appendicular and axial sites, it can exceed 1.5cm and raise suspicion for malignant transformation. In patients with malignant change, apart from an excessively enlarged cap, there is underlying destruction of bone and mineralization within the cap appearing as arcs and rings, stipples, or flocculations. Dystrophic calcification can be seen in tumours undergoing osteonecrosis, and the clinical appearance of acute pain along with these radiographicchanges which evolve over several weeks or months can arouse suspicion for malignant transformation. Ultrasound scanning and MRI are useful in screening for malignant changes. Osteochondral exostoses can be prodigious in the proximal humerus and proximal femur, but most commonly occur as solitary masses about the knee.

Treatment is observation for asymptomatic lesions. For patients with pain, excision through the base of the stock to include the cartilage cap and overlying bursa is necessary. Axial imaging is important for preoperative assessment of the relationship of the mass to adjacent neurovascular structures. If malignant transformation is suspected, staging studies are necessary prior to biopsy and definitive surgical management.

Box 8.9.2 Osteochondromatosis

- Autosomal dominant
- Paired bones
- Metaphyseal
- CT demonstrates corticomedullary continuity
- <1% malignant transformation.

Dysplasia epiphysealis hemimelica (Trevor's disease)

This is a rare condition characterized by epiphyseal-based osteochondral proliferation of tissue that causes pain, joint incongruity, and early arthrosis if untreated. This condition may involve more than one joint.

Radiographically, there is intra-articular osteochondral tissue growth resulting in joint asymmetry and incongruity. Fluid sensitive Short Tau Inversion Recovery (STIR) MR images show hyperintense signal in the periphery reflecting the high fluid content in articular cartilage. Treatment involves resection and contouring of the joint surface to create a congruous joint. Early arthrosis is likely despite treatment and certain without.

Enchondromas are 'cartilaginous rests' arising from physeal cartilage (Box 8.9.3). The cells do not undergo scheduled apoptosis and calcification, but instead become entrapped in bone and migrate away from the physis with continued growth (Figure 8.9.4). The size varies from a few centimetres to involvement of nearly the entire shaft of a long bone. Most enchondromas are asymptomatic and recognized incidentally in the evaluation of more common traumatic and degenerative knee conditions. However, they may be biologically active following skeletal maturation and cause pain and discomfort, and thus are considered 'active enchondromas'.

Rarely, a solitary lesion can undergo malignant transformation over time, marked clinically by increased pain, occasional pathological fracture, and a soft tissue mass. Radiographically, deep endosteal scallops, greater than two-thirds of the cortex, cortical destruction, and the presence of a soft tissue mass strongly suggest malignant transformation.

Patients with multiple enchondromas (Ollier's disease) or multiple enchondromas associated with haemangiomas (Maffuci's disease) are at increased risk of developing chondrosarcoma; this risk is reported to be 25% in affected individuals.

Osteogenesis imperfecta, a disease of abnormal bone collagen, is manifest by frequent fractures and bowing deformities. In the tarda form of disease the clinical manifestations, and hence diagnosis, may not be as apparent, raising the possibility of child abuse in some children. Occasionally, fractures about the knee, particularly the distal femur, may heal with exuberant callus associated with massive swelling and be confused with an aggressive sarcoma. This diagnosis is particularly difficult for the unsuspecting pathologist, since large atypical osteoblasts with hyperchromatic nuclei coupled with mitotic activity arouses suspicion of osteosarcoma.

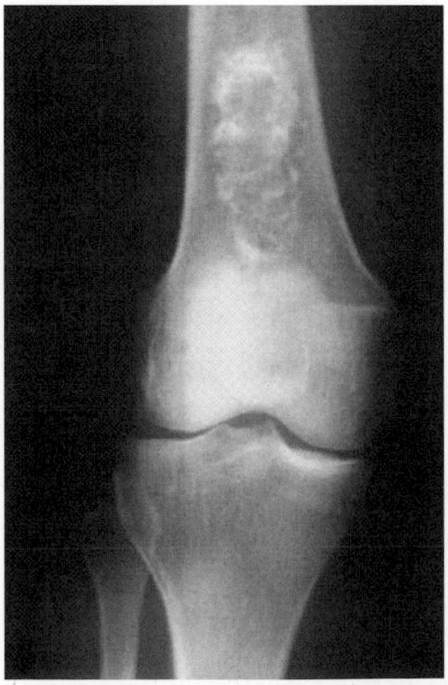

Fig. 8.9.4 Typical enchondroma with extensive mineralization.

Box 8.9.3 Enchondromas

- Common incidental finding on radiographs
- Multiple = Ollier's disease
- Immature cartilage islands
- <1% risk of chondrosarcoma
- Endosteal scalloping of >2/3 of cortex = active disease.

Enthesiopathies–osteochondroses

Cortical desmoid

This is a common variant found in adolescent patients at or near the insertion of the medial gastrocnemius muscle in the posterior medial aspect of the distal femur. Almost all are found incidentally. This abnormality is commonly mistaken for an aggressive neoplasm, specifically osteosarcoma. Radiographically, it is a cortically-based radiolucent abnormality without matrix production but with an internal sclerotic border. The well-delineated border is best seen on CT, while MRI shows a small soft tissue mass and surrounding oedema. They can be quite large and are often bilateral. Observation is the preferred treatment.

Osgood–Schlatter disease

This common condition occurs in young active adolescents, presenting with activity-related anterior knee pain and mild aching discomfort when sitting for periods of time. It is most common in males and is a traction apophysitis with occasional fragmentation and hypertrophic bone formation at the insertion of the patellar ligament.

Pain can be elicited by resisted quadriceps contraction and direct pressure over the tibial tubercle. Treatment consists of rest, activity modification, anti-inflammatory medicines, and isometric quadriceps exercises. Steroid injections should be avoided to prevent later patellar ligament rupture.

Pellegrini–Stieda disease

Avulsion injuries of the medial collateral ligament with subsequent repair may result in mineralization at or near the femoral insertion of the ligament, known as Pellegrini–Stieda disease. It is asymptomatic and found incidentally on trauma radiographs for other conditions. A remote history of injury is usually elicited, while physical examination may yield normal to mild valgus opening on stressing the knee. It should not be confused with a periarticular soft tissue mass such as synovial sarcoma or a periosteal osteosarcoma. The mineralization pattern is smooth regular and consistently located at the insertion of the medial collateral ligament in the distal femur.

Bipartite patellae

This is a common condition often confused with fracture and primary tumours. Unlike fracture, the edges of the bipartite patellar fragments are smooth, non-tender to palpation, and located in the superolateral aspect of the patella. This condition is best appreciated on oblique knee radiographs. There is no joint effusion unless there is an unrelated intra-articular injury or other knee pathology. In most cases, the lesion is bilateral.

Traumatic and vascular conditions

Myositis ossificans

Blunt and, less commonly, penetrating injuries of the soft tissue can result in haematoma, inflammation, and necrosis of muscle and fat, which, in the process of repair, can modulate into bone formation. Patients relate a history of fairly significant trauma, most often a deep contusion. Over several weeks to months, this indurated area becomes a firm, sometimes fixed, mass which becomes progressively less painful. Restricted joint motion is common immediately after an injury but improves with time. Late pain and discomfort is usually secondary to mechanical irritation, whereas night symptoms and rest pain are not present. Generalized soft tissue myositis with joint contractures and ankylosis can be seen in patients with acute pancreatitis and burns. Fibrodysplasia ossificans progressiva can present with generalized soft tissue periarticular masses as well as joint ankylosis. This disease is transmitted in an autosomal dominant fashion, though most cases are sporadic. It is generally manifested in early childhood as a large, rapidly progressive soft tissue mass that is often confused with sarcoma. The diagnosis can be made by inspecting the hands and feet, which reveal shortened first rays. In the foot, a common feature is brachymesodactyly with a portion of the proximal phalanx fused to the head of the first metatarsal giving the appearance of a hallux valgus deformity. It is important to recognize these constellations of physical and radiographical findings to avoid biopsy or attempted resection of the soft tissue mass which may worsen the condition.

Other radiographical findings include exostoses, hypoplastic posterior spine elements, a shortened anteroposterior diameter of the cervical spine, and a shortened femoral neck. Radiographical mineralization is observed in the axial and appendicular skeleton. Knee contractures and ankylosed joints occur later in the disease. Patients generally succumb to pneumonia and respiratory failure due to involvement of the intercostal muscles and marked spine and chest wall deformity. The heart and diaphragm are spared.

Isolated myositis around the knee must be distinguished from other mineralized soft tissue masses such as surface-osteosarcoma. Radiographically and histologically, myositis is characterized by a 'zonation phenomenon' whereby maturation progresses from the epicentre of the lesion to the periphery. For malignant tumours, maturation proceeds from peripheral to central, thus the periphery of the tumour is least differentiated. The mineralization pattern in soft tissue sarcomas is disorganized and the radiographical pattern is 'dystrophic'.

Like parosteal osteosarcoma, myositis ossificans can be separated or densely adherent to bone giving it a 'pasted on' appearance. Parosteal osteosarcoma invades the cortex of bone in over two-thirds of cases and involves the medullary canal in one-third. Both parosteal osteosarcoma and myositis ossificans can be differentiated from osteochondral exostoses by the absence of corticomedullary continuity.

Osteochondritis dissecans

Osteochondritis dissecans lesions are relatively common in young patients and adolescents. The typical manifestations of the disease are knee pain and an effusion; occasionally mechanical symptoms occur in patients with loose bodies or detached osteochondral fragments. The aetiology remains unclear. The majority of lesions are in the weight-bearing portion of the lateral aspect of the medial femoral condyle. Lateral femoral condylar lesions are less common and felt to be post-traumatic in nature resulting from patella subluxations and dislocations. Tibial osteochondral defects are rare.

These lesions are typically seen on radiographs as subchondral lucencies with internal sclerotic borders; occasional loose osteochondral bodies can be seen in the lateral or medial gutters or the suprapatellar pouch. Both CT and MRI are useful in discerning the exact size and location of the chondral defect. The appearance and location are characteristic and should not be confused with chondroblastoma, subchondral cysts, or Brodie abscess. Treatment depends on the size and degree of displacement of the osteochondral fragment.

Osteonecrosis (Box 8.9.4)

Spontaneous osteonecrosis of the knee (SONK) most commonly involves the medial femoral condyle and medial tibial plateau and is generally idiopathic. Secondary osteonecrosis is associated with systemic conditions such as rheumatoid disease, Caisson's disease, alcohol consumption, renal transplantation, steroid therapy, and systemic lupus erythematosus.

SONK is characterized by the presence of dead bone in the subchondral area of the weight-bearing portion of the femoral condyle. It is associated with subchondral fracture and collapse.

The aetiology remains uncertain but local trauma in a diseased joint causes ischaemia and disturbance of local circulation leading to increased subchondral pressure and ultimately necrosis.

Radiographs may appear normal in the early stages of osteonecrosis but with progression of the disease an area of radiolucency in the subchondral bone with a halo of sclerotic bone becomes evident (Figure 8.9.5). MRI detects early changes in the bone marrow, whilst technetium bone scans are less reliable. MRI findings include a well-defined area of low signal, best seen on T_1-weighted images. Patients with condylar lesions greater than 5cm^2 or a width of greater than 40% develop pain, deformity, and secondary destruction of the joint often requiring surgical intervention.

Non-operative treatment in the early stages of the disease includes pain relief and supportive physiotherapy exercises to

Box 8.9.4 Osteonecrosis

- Spontaneous osteonecrosis of knee and secondary osteonecrosis
- Medial femoral condyle
- Minor trauma
- Characteristic features on T_1 MRI
- Unicondylar knee replacement for end-stage disease.

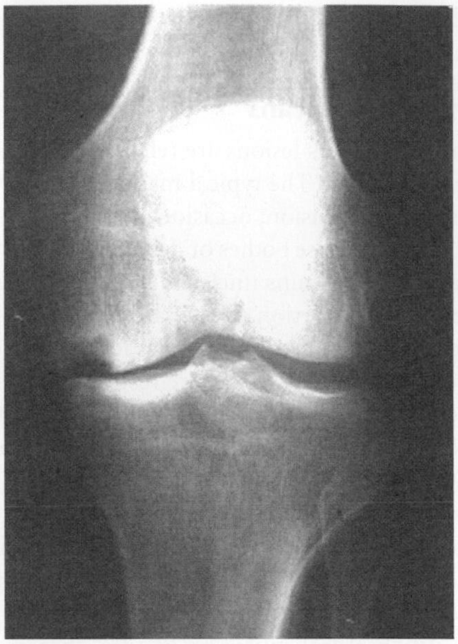

Fig. 8.9.5 Osteonecrosis of the medial femoral condyle.

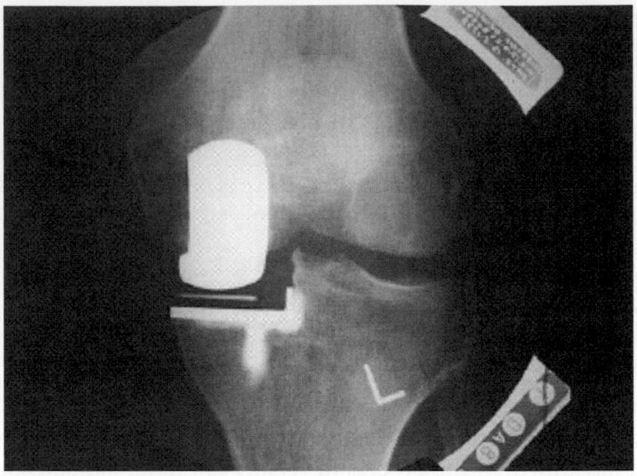

Fig. 8.9.6 Oxford unicompartmental knee replacement for refractory osteonecrosis of the medial femoral condyle.

improve quadriceps and hamstring strength, resulting in full resolution of symptoms in 80% of cases. Effective surgical options include arthroscopic debridement, drilling and bone grafting, and proximal tibial osteotomy. However, total or unicompartmental knee arthroplasty is indicated for lesions evolving into subchondral collapse and significant arthrosis. Success rates are 55% for arthroscopic procedures and up to 95% for arthroplasty (Figure 8.9.6).

Melorheostosis

A rare periosteal or cortically based hyperostosis involving the long bones of the lower extremity. It can be very extensive or more limited about the knee. In those lesions where it is more focal it can be confused with other bone-producing conditions such as juxtacortical osteosarcoma or myositis ossificans.

Radiographically, melorheostosis involves only one side of the cortex and only one lower extremity. It often crosses joints, especially the knee. It has been described as having the appearance of 'dripping candle wax'.

Pain is a constant feature of this disease. Often patients will present with a mass and knee effusion. With disease progression, ankylosis can supervene, and pain due to progressive hyperostosis may rarely require amputation for palliation.

Further reading

Ackerman, D., Lett, P., Galat, D.D. Jr., Parvizi, J., and Stuart, M.J. (2008). Results of total hip and total knee arthroplasties in patients with synovial chondromatosis. *Journal of Arthroplasty*, **23**(3), 395–400.

Adelani, M.A., Wupperman, R.M., and Holt, G.E. (2008). Benign synovial disorders. *Journal of the American Academy of Orthopaedic Surgeons*, **16**(5), 268–75.

Michael, J.W., Wurth, A., Eysel, P., and Konig, D.P. (2008). Long-term results after operative treatment of osteochondritis dissecans of the knee joint-30 year results. *International Orthopaedics*, **32**(2), 217–21.

Murphey, M.D., Rhee, J.H., Lewis, R.B., Fanburg-Smith, J.C., Flemming, D.J., and Walker EA. (2008). Pigmented villonodular synovitis: radiologic-pathologic correlation. *Radiographics*, **28**(5), 1493–518.

Narvaez, J., Narvaez, J.A. Rodriguez-Moreno, J., and Roig-Escofet, D. (2000). Osteonecrosis of the knee: differences among idiopathic and secondary types. *Rheumatology* (Oxford), **39**(9), 982–9.

8.10

The patellofemoral joint

Simon Donell

Summary points

- The symptomatic patellofemoral joint is difficult to manage.
- It is difficult to be certain that the pain felt by the patient is actually arising from the joint.
- The majority of symptomatic patients should be managed conservatively with exercises aimed at improving muscle control.
- Surgical treatment gives best results in patellofemoral instability when there are defined anatomical abnormalities that are then corrected.
- Surgical treatment of patellofemoral arthritis has uncertain outcomes.

Introduction

Disorders of the patellofemoral joint present in one of two ways:

1) Anterior knee pain and/or
2) Extensor mechanism instability.

Anterior knee pain may arise from the patellofemoral joint, or may arise remotely—typically the hip. Surgical management of anterior knee pain has uncertain outcomes. On the other hand instability may be mechanical or functional. If mechanical then successful surgical correction should be considered.

Around 40% of elective referrals to an orthopaedic department are for knee pain, of which about a third are for pain felt anteriorly. Accurate assessment and appropriate management is therefore essential. The algorithm for elucidating the likely problem starts with the age of the patient (see Figure 8.10.1).

Anatomy

The patellofemoral joint has evolved in man in response to bipedal gait. To effect hip abductor power the greater trochanter of the upper femur has become more lateral. This has resulted in the quadriceps line of action becoming more valgus with respect to the insertion of the patellar ligament into the tibial tubercle, creating an angle (the quadriceps or Q-angle). To overcome the resulting lateral pull to the patella, the lateral trochlear facet of the femoral sulcus has become more flared, to act as a buttress against lateral patella displacement.

The patellofemoral joint is made up of the quadriceps tendon, patella and patellar ligament, and tibial tubercle along with the medial and lateral retinaculum within which lie the medial patellofemoral ligament and lateral patelloiliotibial band ligament. Other condensations within the medial and lateral retinaculum (e.g. the medial and lateral patellotibial bands) are also described, but are of less clinical relevance. The soft tissue envelope (including the patella) is known collectively as the 'extensor mechanism of the knee'. Recently it was realized that the distal femoral sulcus may develop abnormally resulting in trochlear dysplasia.

The patella is a sesamoid bone that acts as a marker for the alignment of the extensor mechanism. The trochlear groove and an arch of articular cartilage around the intercondylar notch make up the femoral side of the joint. Except in deep flexion, the tibial articular surface comes into contact with a different part of the femur to the patella and the majority of intercondylar notch osteophytes result from patellofemoral disease. The femoral sulcus acts like a pulley for the extensor mechanism. The forces exerted through the normal patellofemoral joint depend on activity such that at level walking it is half body weight, on going upstairs is three to four times body weight, and on squatting it is seven to eight times body weight.

Kinematics

The movements of the patellofemoral joint are complex. In full extension only the distal part of the patella articular surface is in contact with the femoral groove. It mainly rests on the synovium overlying the supracondylar fat pad. As flexion increases, the contact area on the patella sweeps proximally as a broad strip until 90-degree flexion, when the proximal part is in contact with the distal groove. From 90-degree flexion the odd (or extreme medial) facet articulates with the lateral edge of the medial femoral condyle, and the lateral facet articulates with the medial edge of the lateral femoral condyle. The medial facet lies in contact with the synovium overlying the anterior cruciate ligament. In deep flexion the patella effectively bridges the intercondylar notch. At 135 degrees of flexion the patella articulates with parts of both

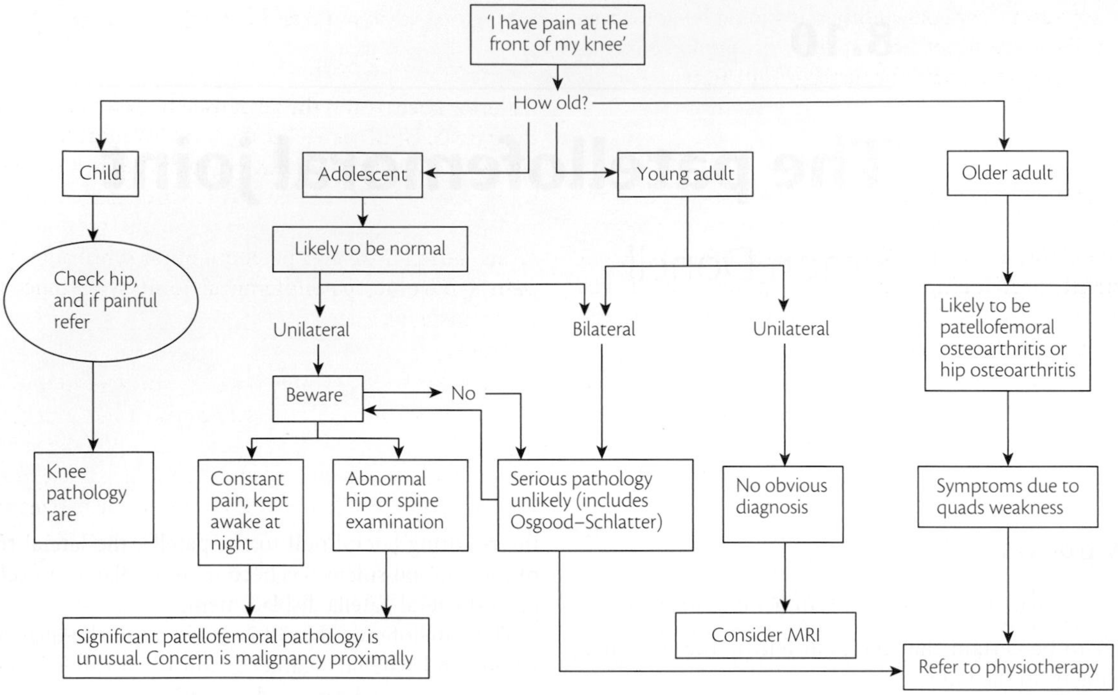

Fig. 8.10.1 An algorithm for initial management of anterior knee pain.

the medial and lateral femoral articular surfaces that also come into contact with the anterior meniscal horns (Figure 8.10.2).

Wherever there is uncovered articular cartilage, a synovial fold, usually enveloping fat, covers the articular surface. These folds include the peripatellar fringe of synovium, the supracondylar fat pad, and the infrapatellar fat pad with its alar folds. In extension, the supracondylar fat pad has a distal leading edge (abolished at arthroscopy by the introduction of fluid) which descends into the femoral sulcus as the knee flexes. It moves proximally as the knee extends, aided by the intra-articular negative pressure, and the action of the articularis genu muscle. As the patella articular surface contact sweeps superiorly during flexion, the synovium of the infrapatellar fat pad covers the exposed part. Specifically the alar folds point proximally in the midline. Beyond 90-degree flexion

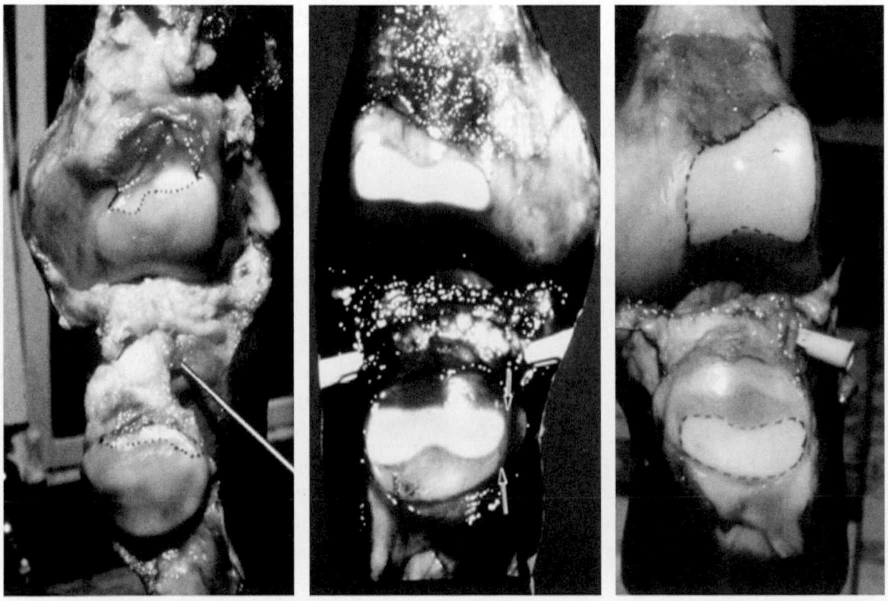

Fig. 8.10.2 The contact areas of the patellofemoral joint during flexion (kindly provided by John Goodfellow).

the alar folds move away from one another. It should be noted that the articular surfaces are swept by synovium during knee movement. This is probably important for cartilage nutrition.

Imaging

Standard plain radiographs are adequate as a screen for patellofemoral problems. The anteroposterior (AP) standing view gives the least information. The lateral view should have the posterior femoral condyles strictly overlapping. The trochlear groove can then be properly assessed. Figure 8.10.3 shows the normal groove. The skyline view (tangential patella) may be taken in various degrees of knee flexion. The sulcus angle is useful as a screening tool. If greater than 140 degrees, this is associated with patellar instability. The angle changes according to knee flexion (Figure 8.10.4) and therefore is not useful for research purposes, as this is difficult to control.

Computed tomography (CT) is helpful, and shows the shape of the subchondral bone. It can measure the rotational alignment of the lower limb as well as the patellar tilt angle, and tibial tubercle–trochlear groove (TTTG) distance (Figure 8.10.5). The TTTG is more useful than the Q-angle as it measures where the patella should be, rather than where it is. The normal TTTG is 10mm.

Magnetic resonance imaging (MRI) is very useful. It gives information on the chondral shape, as well as bony and soft tissue abnormalities, not only within the patellofemoral joint, but also the tibiofemoral joint.

Isotope bone scanning can be useful in unexplained anterior knee pain, and can confirm abnormal metabolism within the bone.

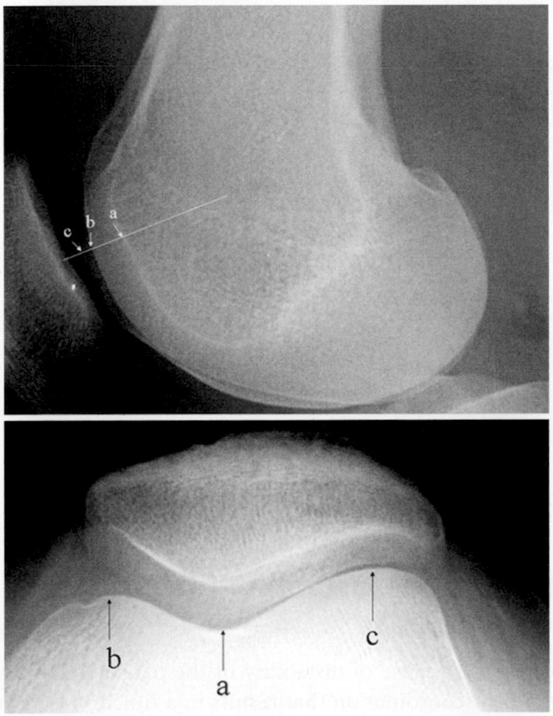

Fig. 8.10.3 The normal trochlear groove on lateral x-ray and skyline. Note the groove line (a) passes directly on to the line of the anterior distal femoral cortex.

Clinical presentation (Box 8.10.1)

Anterior knee pain

Anterior knee pain is the term used to describe pain in and around the patella. Until the 1970s, the term 'chondromalacia patellae' was synonymous with patellofemoral pain, because softening was noted on the undersurface of the patella. This term has now been replaced by 'anterior knee pain', which is a symptom and not a diagnosis. Other terms used are: patellofemoral syndrome, patellofemoral pain syndrome, patellofemoral joint syndrome, and extensor mechanism disorder.

Aetiology

There are two principal views as to the aetiology of anterior knee pain. The first is patellar malalignment with respect to the femoral sulcus. This causes localized peak loading of the articular cartilage which results in chondral damage and pain. Correction of the malalignment should therefore decrease the patient's symptoms by offloading the affected area. However, there is poor correlation between articular cartilage lesions and pain. Patellar malalignment may only explain some patellofemoral pain symptoms.

Until recently it has been suggested that anterior knee pain may be due to a wide range of physiopathological processes such as an increase in intraosseous pressure and increased bone remodelling. However, the most recent view is that the tissues of the patellofemoral joint are in balance at a molecular level (tissue homeostasis) and supraphysiological mechanical loading and chemical irritation of the nerve endings has a direct effect on unbalancing this. An inflammatory cascade then occurs resulting in peripatellar synovitis. The peripatellar synovium is richly innervated and has been shown to be extremely sensitive to light touch. Once the synovium is inflamed, it will be continually aggravated by activities of daily living, resulting in prolonged symptoms.

However deciding what causes the pain and which structure is involved is still controversial. Many patients with marked patellar malalignment never experience pain, whilst others, with apparently no malalignment, or changes to their activities, experience problems. Disorders that can present as anterior knee pain are outlined in Box 8.10.2.

Adolescent anterior knee pain (Box 8.10.3)

Pain felt at the front of the knee is common in adolescence, affecting both a third of boys and girls. Of these, a third of the girls and a tenth of the boys present to primary care physicians. Adolescent anterior knee pain should not be considered a disease. In this group it is important to confirm that there is no abnormality in the knee. Despite symptoms, examination of the knee is normal. Specifically there

Box 8.10.1 Presentation of patellofemoral disorders

- Anterior knee pain (exclude hip and spine disorders):
  - Extensor mechanism pathology
  - Hypermobility syndrome
  - Postural problems
  - Psychological
- Extensor mechanism instability.

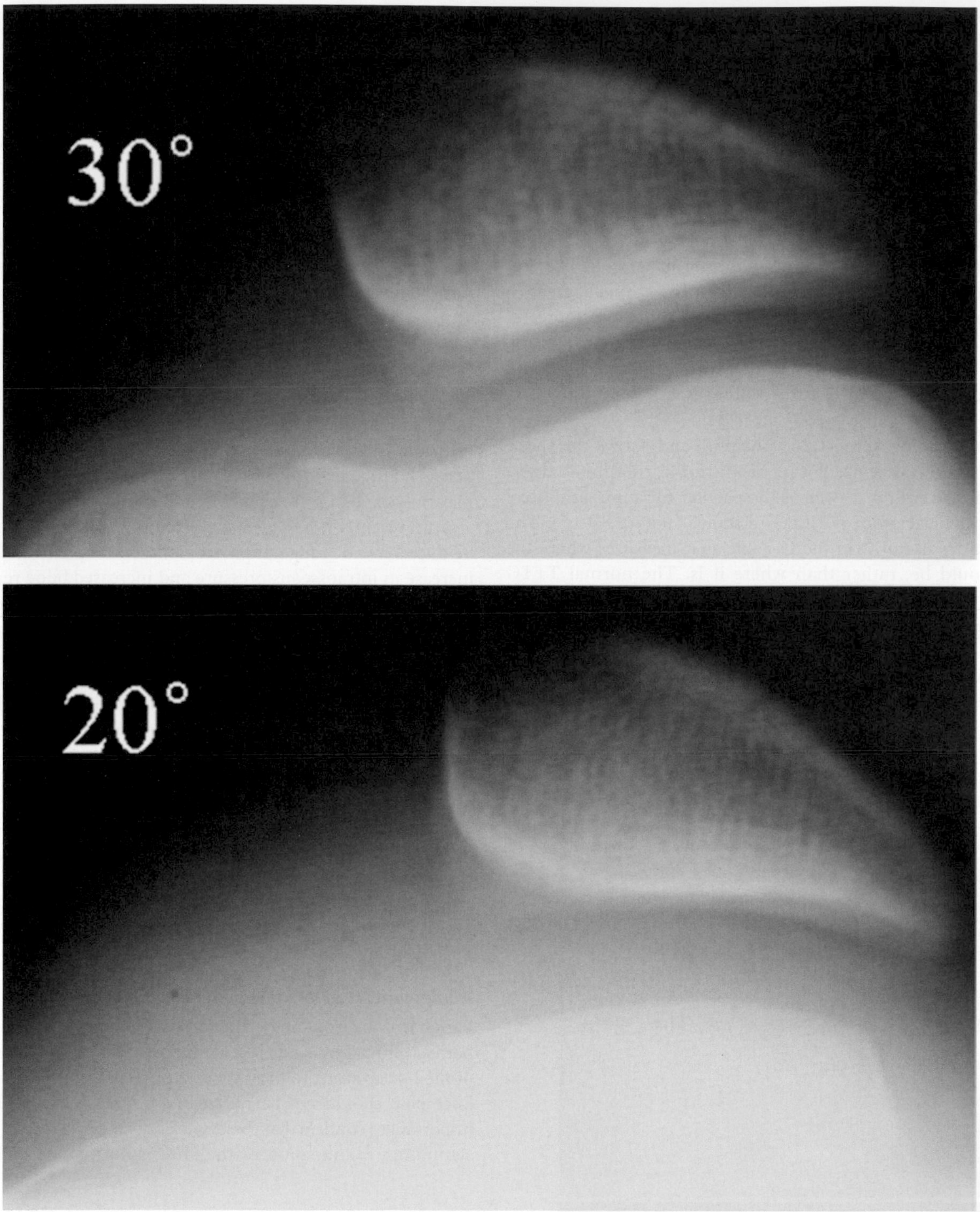

Fig. 8.10.4 Skyline x-ray of the patella in patellar instability showing the sulcus shape worsens as knee flexion is decreased.

is no effusion, the vastus medialis obliquus is present and functioning, there is no patellar apprehension, the patellar tracks normally, there is no evidence of meniscal pathology, the ligaments are intact, and the patient can squat. Variations and abnormalities that may be found are: hypermobility syndrome, spine or hip pathology, tight musculature, and rotational or postural abnormalities of the lower limb. The long-term prognosis is good.

Patellofemoral instability (mechanical and functional)

The commonest cause of instability of the patella is poor muscle power and/or coordination that results in a functional instability. Various anatomical abnormalities may be present that increase the risk of patellar dislocation, but if functional stability can be achieved,

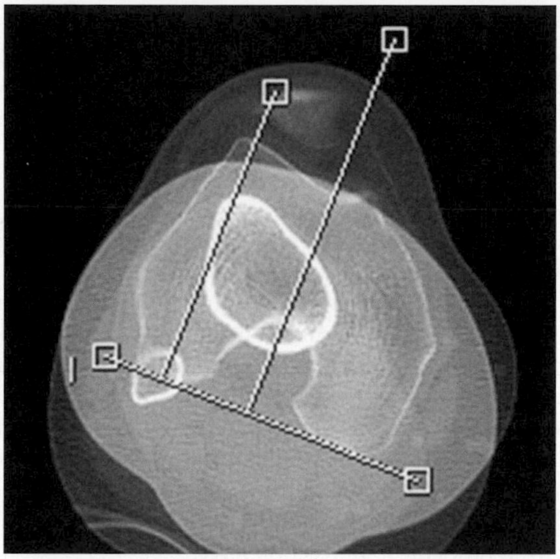

Fig. 8.10.5 CT scan in extension with the quadriceps lax showing superimposition of the femoral condylar cut with the tibial tubercle cut; showing the tibial tubercle–trochlear groove distance (TTTG).

Box 8.10.2 Disorders that can lead to anterior knee pain

- Adolescent anterior knee pain
- Patellar malalignment syndromes including dislocation
- Patellofemoral arthritis
- Patellofemoral pathology:
  - Infections
  - Tumours
  - Osteochondritis dissecans
- Extensor mechanism pathology:
  - Patellar tendonitis
  - Sinding–Larsen, Osgood–Schlatter syndromes
  - Quadriceps tendonitis
- Patellofemoral chondropathy
- Tibiofemoral pathology:
  - Meniscal tear
  - Pathological plicae
- Hip pathology
- Tumours:
  - Osteoid osteotoma
  - Osteosarcoma/Ewing's sarcoma
- Disorders of posture:
  - Tight quadriceps/hamstrings
  - Hyperlordotic lumbar spine
  - Pronated feet
- Complex regional pain syndromes
- Psychological problems.

Box 8.10.3 Adolescent anterior knee pain

- Exclude serious disease
- Exclude osteochondritis dissecans
- Anatomy of knee is normal
- Related to sports
- Settles with rest
- Expectant treatment.

the surgical correction of the abnormalities is unnecessary. This is similar to the situation found in anterior cruciate ligament rupture.

Patellar dislocation is the extreme of a continuum of malalignments of the extensor mechanism which include a tight lateral retinaculum with a lateral tilt of the patella, and subluxation of the patella. The displacement is laterally. Medial displacement of the patella is typically iatrogenic. It is important to note that although the patella may be subluxated or dislocated, the problem is not the kneecap. Various factors may lead to patellar instability:

- Extensor mechanism malalignment
- Trochlear dysplasia
- Hypermobility syndrome.

The single biggest risk factor for recurrent patellar dislocation is a positive family history.

Extensor mechanism malalignment

Epidemiology

The incidence of patellofemoral dislocation is reported to be 5–43 per 100 000. The factors associated with dislocation are listed in Box 8.10.4. Of those patients who present with a primary dislocation, about 17% will go on to have a recurrence. Of those who present with a dislocation, 50% have a history of previous dislocation or subluxation. However, in a recent randomized controlled trial the only factor that was associated significantly with recurrent dislocation was a positive family history.

Box 8.10.4 Risk factors associated with patellar dislocation

- Female adolescents
- Following primary dislocation
- History of subluxation or dislocation
- Younger
- More severe dislocation
- Family history
- Risk factors for developmental dysplasia of the hip:
  - First-born girl
  - High birthweight
  - Breech delivery
  - Caesarean section.

Classification

There are many ways to classify joint dislocation/subluxation. In the patellofemoral joint it is important to appreciate the difference between a dislocation in a joint with pre-existing normal anatomy, from one where the anatomy is abnormal. To dislocate a normal patellofemoral joint requires significant force to be applied to the medial side of the patella (typically in a tackle in football). Because the femoral sulcus is normal, the risk of an osteochondral fracture is high. If an osteochondral fracture occurs, prompt treatment is needed if long-term disability is to be avoided. These can be considered as a true 'traumatic' dislocation. Those with abnormal anatomy can be considered to sustain an 'atraumatic' dislocation. This is not to say that there has not been an injury, but usually there is no direct blow to the patella, or it has occurred with minimal force. Atraumatic dislocators have a low risk of osteochondral fractures. In the acute setting, examining the opposite knee will show whether there are anatomical abnormalities, as these are bilateral.

Extensor mechanism maltracking may also be classified according to whether the patella dislocates in extension or flexion. The former is more common. The latter is always due to a tight lateral retinaculum, and usually tight quadriceps. Both have to be addressed if surgical correction is anticipated. The terms 'habitual' and 'obligatory' are also used. They can be defined as voluntary dislocation in the former and involuntary in the latter although they are frequently used interchangeably.

Dejour classified extensor mechanism malalignment into major, objective, and potential patellar instability. Major is when dislocation has been documented and is associated with significant abnormalities, objective is when instability symptoms are associated with abnormalities, and potential is in the asymptomatic patient with anatomical abnormalities. He has a further group called 'painful patellar syndrome' where there is pain, but normal anatomy. This is the group where operative intervention is unlikely to be helpful. Abnormal anatomy can be stretched medial structures, especially the medial patellofemoral ligament (hypermobility syndrome), patella alta, or trochlear dysplasia. A combination of these is typical in major and objective patellar instability.

Trochlear dysplasia

In the last 10 years the importance of the shape of the femoral sulcus in patellofemoral pathology has been realized. Abnormalities in shape can lead to pain, and also increase the risk of an unstable extensor mechanism. The normal femoral sulcus has an angle of under 140 degrees, when measured from the subchondral bone. It is present at birth as cartilage, and continues into adulthood. Dysplasia may occur with overgrowth of the distal physes, which may abolish or, in extreme cases, reverse the angle. It is most important in the first 20 degrees of knee flexion, and may not be obvious on standard skyline films because they are taken at more than 30 degrees flexion. Dejour classified trochlear dysplasia on the plain lateral x-ray into types I, II, and III (Figure 8.10.6). The normal groove runs smoothly into the anterior cortical line of the femur. If it passes anterior to this, crossing the medial condylar line to reach the lateral condylar line anterior to the anterior condylar line, then this shows trochlear dysplasia. If the patella tracks normally, it raises the joint reaction force.

It should be noted that the groove in the dysplastic trochlea lies medial to the normal groove position. CT scans can also measure the patellar tilt angle, and the TTTG distance. If the TTTG distance is greater than 20mm then either the tibial tubercle may be moved medially 10mm or the trochlear groove laterally to correct it to normal. The former is achieved by a tibial tubercle osteotomy, and the latter by trochleoplasty. A trochlear boss of greater than 6mm and a Dejour type III dysplasia would indicate that a trochleoplasty may be beneficial.

Rarer is a lateral condylar hypoplasia. The groove line does not pass anterior to the anterior femoral cortical line, and neither does the lateral condylar line. There is therefore no lateral buttress to resist lateral translation of the patella secondary to the Q-angle. This can be corrected by the Albee trochleoplasty, which elevates the lateral femoral condyle. If performed for hyperplasia, it precipitates patellofemoral osteoarthritis (PFOA).

It can therefore be seen that patellar instability is associated with anatomical abnormalities. Figure 8.10.7 shows the differences in trochlear shape, patellar position, length and thickness of the medial structures, most notably the medial patellofemoral ligament (MPFL), and also indicates laxity or tightness in the

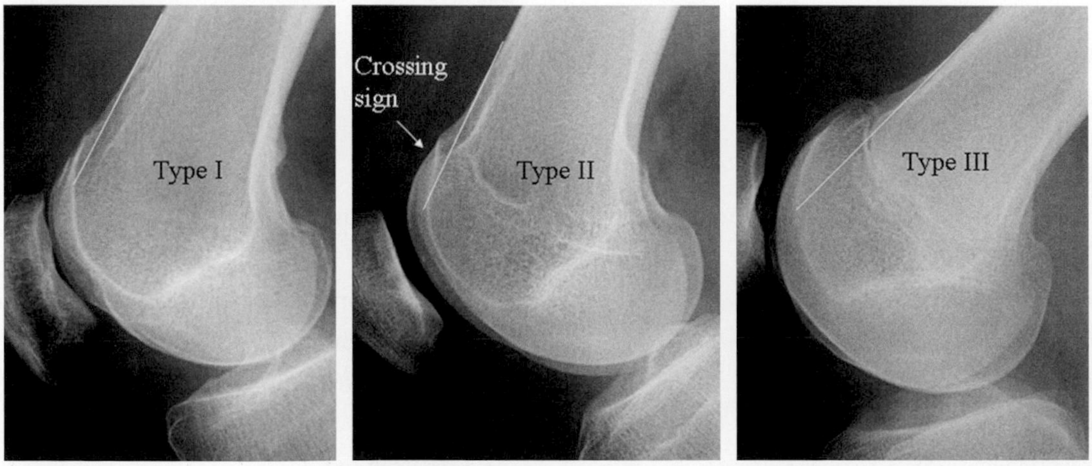

Fig. 8.10.6 Dejour's classification of trochlear dysplasia based on the lateral x-ray.

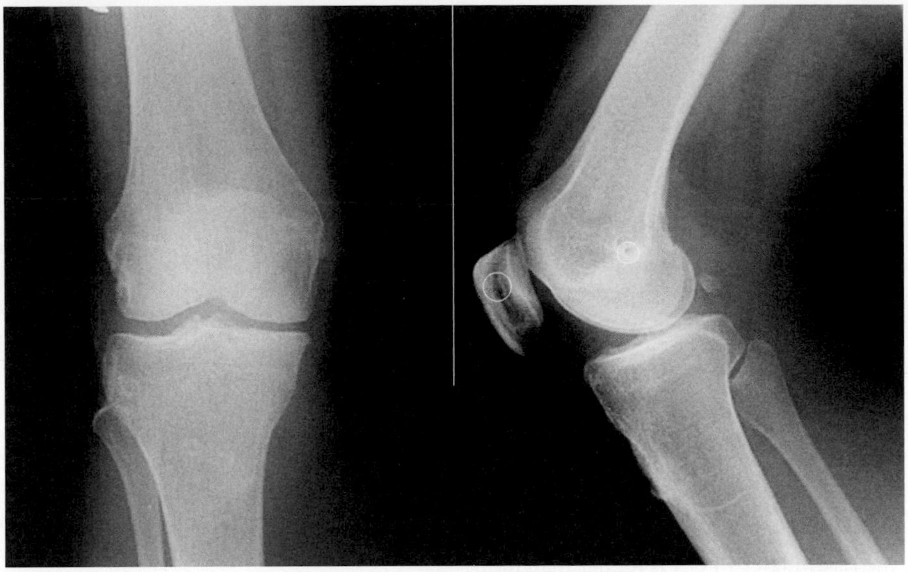

Fig. 8.10.7 Post-operative x-ray showing tunnel positions following MPFL reconstruction.

lateral retinaculum. Note that the lateral retinaculum is lax in the figure, and therefore lateral release is not appropriate.

Hypermobility syndrome

This is a genetically-based disorder of collagen covering a wide variety of genetic abnormalities from the extreme of Marfan's and Ehlers–Danlos syndromes to benign joint hypermobility syndrome. Screening involves assessing the Beighton score. This tests joint flexibility. True hypermobility syndrome is assessed using the Brighton criteria (Box 8.10.5).

Hypermobility syndrome is diagnosed in the presence of two major criteria/one major and two minor criteria/four minor criteria. Two minor criteria will suffice where there is an unequivocally an affected first-degree relative.

Patients who are hypermobile may experience pain that will not be improved by an operation. Given that they have very elastic tissues, the folly of performing a lateral release becomes evident in this group. Operations for instability have a poor outcome, mainly because the operative repair stretches over time. However a medial patellofemoral ligament reconstruction with a hamstring graft shortens the lever arm enough to stabilize the patella. Lateral release should not be performed. Because of the tissue elasticity, it is not usually necessary to perform a trochleoplasty for a shallow or flat dysplasia, since there does not seem to be a significant increase in the joint reaction force after stabilization.

Surgical procedures (traditional) (Box 8.10.6)

Surgical interventions to correct patellar maltracking are traditionally divided into proximal realignment (lateral release and medial reefing) and distal realignment (Roux–Goldthwait and tibial tubercle transfers). The traditional management is a lateral release, combined with a double-breasting medial reefing proximally, and Roux–Goldthwait or medialization of the tibial tubercle (Elmslie) distally. This works and normally controls the dislocation. However, in the presence of a significant trochlear dysplasia, where there is no groove for the patella to track in, then the risk is that either the patella redislocates, or the increase in the joint reaction force caused by the patella tracking over the trochlear boss leads to pain and later PFOA. Few patients partake in sports

Box 8.10.5 Brighton criteria for diagnosing hypermobility syndrome

- Major criteria:
  - Beighton score of 4 out of 9 or greater (currently or historically)
  - Joint pain for >3 months in 4 or more joints
- Minor criteria:
  - Beighton score of 1–3 out of 9
  - Joint pain (>3 months) in 1–3 joints or back pain (>3 months), spondylosis, spondylolysis/spondylolisthesis.
  - Dislocation/subluxation in >1 joint, or in 1 joint on >1 occasion
  - Soft tissue rheumatism >3 lesions (e.g. epicondylitis, tenosynovitis, bursitis)
  - Marfanoid habitus (tall, slim, span/height ratio >1.03, upper: lower segment ratio <0.89), arachnodactily
  - Abnormal skin, striae, hyperextensibility, thin skin, papyraceous scarring
  - Eye signs: drooping eyelids or myopia or antimongoloid slant
  - Varicose veins or hernia or uterine/rectal prolapse.

Box 8.10.6 Operations for instability

- Traditional:
  - Proximal re-alignment
    —Lateral release
    —Medial reefing
  - Distal re-alignment
    —Roux–Goldthwaite
    —Tibial tubercle osteotomy
- Current:
  - Medial patellofemoral ligament reconstruction
  - (Trochleoplasty)

after this treatment, and the risk of later PFOA is higher than non-operated patients. It should be noted that operated patients, however, have had more symptomatic knees.

More popular in the USA is proximal realignment with a Fulkerson osteotomy. This moves the tibial tubercle anteromedially and therefore reduces the joint reaction force. This helps if there is a trochlear dysplasia.

Surgical procedures (new)

Medial patellofemoral ligament reconstruction

Over the last 10 years newer surgical procedures have been introduced. The importance of the MPFL has led to a number of different variations to reconstruct or repair it. One method is a free hamstring graft anchored to the upper medial border of the patella, and inserted into the origin of the MPFL between the medial epicondyle of the femur and the adductor tubercle.

This is a proximal realignment and avoids the need to do other procedures, especially if the patient is hypermobile. MPFL reconstruction has the advantage over traditional proximal realignment procedures in that it can be performed as a day case, does not interfere with the quadriceps, and so allows earlier return to function, and does not need splintage.

Trochleoplasty

In the last decade there has been increasing interest in addressing hyperplastic trochlear dysplasia by deepening the trochlea. A number have been described, but the consistent feature is that the excess subchondral bone is removed and the 'boss' lowered. The articular surface is not removed, unlike some older described excision or abrasion procedures. The trochleoplasty can be subdivided into those that create a flexible osteochondral flap and those that create a thick one (Figures 8.10.8 and 8.10.9). In the former the articular surface has to be normal. The flap or flaps created are then anchored to the subchondral bone by a variety of methods. The aim of the trochleoplasty is to remove the boss, recreate the lateral buttress, and lateralize the trochlear groove. It is hoped that it will avoid later-onset PFOA.

Summary of patellar instability

Acute patellar instability is managed conservatively, where the aim is to achieve functional stability with strong coordinated muscles. Traditional treatment with plaster casting for acute dislocation is falling out of favour to temporary orthosis and early physiotherapy. There is no evidence that this is improves or worsens the outcome but patients prefer it. Recurrent instability may not need surgical treatment as patients may develop coping strategies. If operative treatment is decided upon, then patellar tracking can be controlled by MPFL reconstruction alone. It is now felt that lateral release should be avoided, especially in hypermobility syndromes. This also may be unnecessary when a deepening trochleoplasty is performed as this slackens the lateral structures.

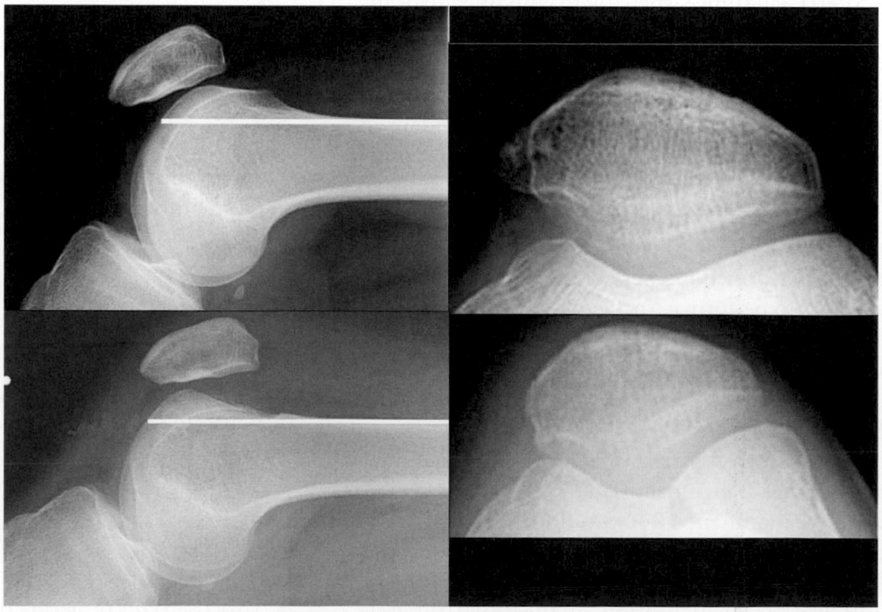

Fig. 8.10.8 Pre- and post-operative images of trochleoplasty.

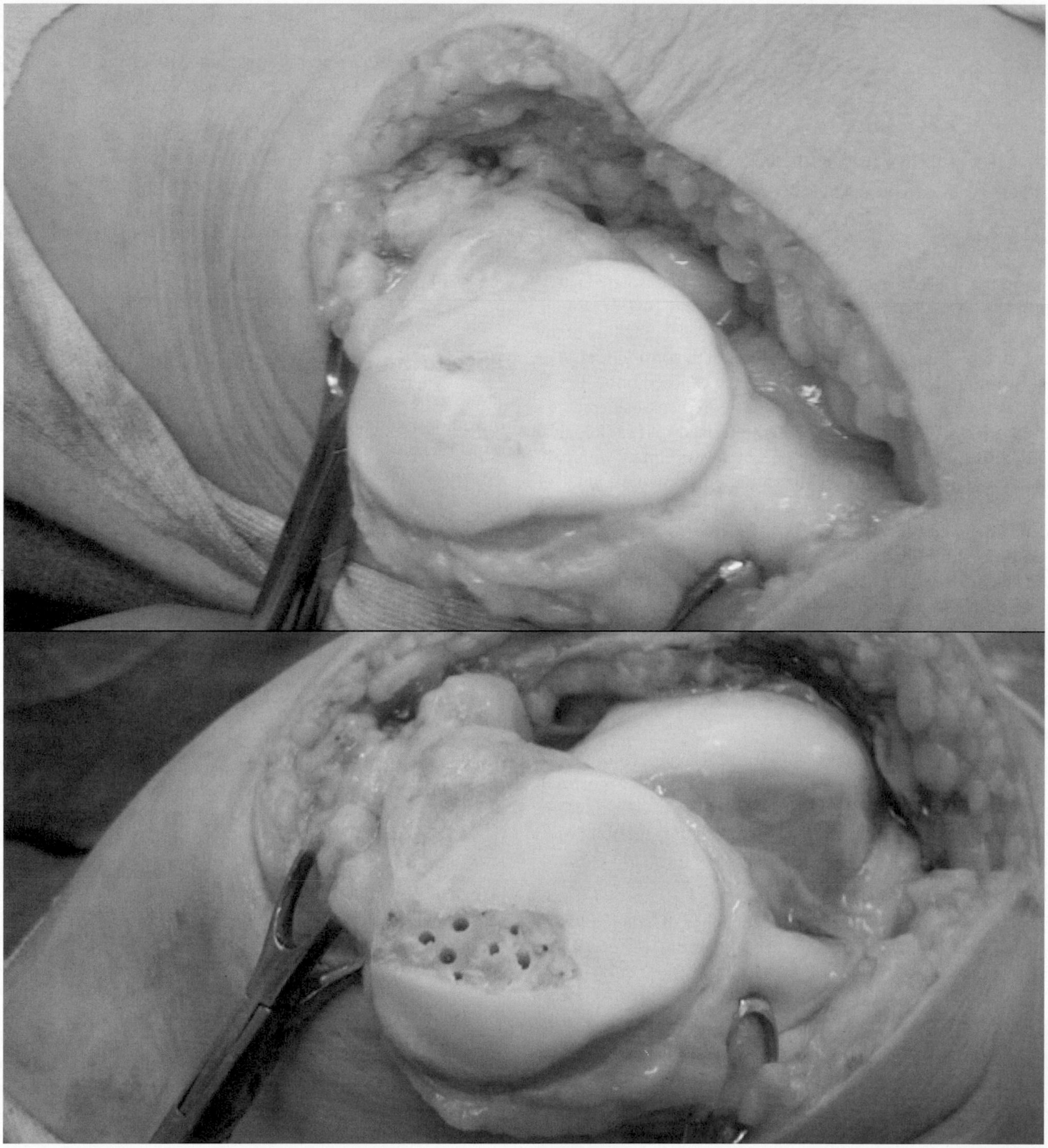

Fig. 8.10.9 Intra-operative photograph showing microfracture of the damaged patellar articular surface.

Dysplasia may need to be addressed if the patella tracks over a significant trochlear boss.

Patellofemoral osteoarthritis (Box 8.10.7)

PFOA affects an older age group than patellofemoral instability. Since the patellofemoral joint sustains the highest loads of any joint, it is no surprise that wear of the bearing surface is a common finding as age increases. However, symptomatic isolated PFOA is uncommon. It appears that about 5% of patients with radiographic changes of patellofemoral degeneration are actually symptomatic, which interestingly matches the anterior knee pain rate following unresurfaced patellae in total knee replacement. In a population of symptomatic osteoarthritic knees presenting over the age of 60 it

Box 8.10.7 Patellofemoral osteoarthritis

- Radiological changes are common over 50 years old
- Hip osteoarthritis must be excluded as source of anterior knee pain
- Selected patients may benefit from patellofemoral replacement
  - PFOA secondary to trochlear dysplasia has best outcome.

was found that 19% of men and 17% of women had isolated patellofemoral disease as compared to 5% of men and 10% of women between the ages of 40–60 years. This emphasizes that failure of the bearing surfaces increases with age. It is useful to consider PFOA as present when both surfaces of the joint have exposed bone. Lesser articular cartilage loss or damage can therefore be considered as a chondropathy. However, it must be emphasized that radiological changes in the patellofemoral joint do not always equate with pain or loss of function. This means that a patient may have anterior knee pain and marked radiological changes, but the pain may arise from elsewhere, notably the hip.

It would be anticipated that trochlear dysplasia would lead to PFOA. The evidence for this is increasing and it is interesting that patellofemoral arthroplasty is most successful in this group. Pre-existing trochlear dysplasia is difficult to assess in patients with PFOA and bone loss.

Management of patellofemoral osteoarthritis

Conservative

The majority of patients with radiographic changes of PFOA (Figure 8.10.10) have no symptoms. If symptomatic, most will improve by building up quadriceps strength and coordination. However there is no evidence that any particular rehabilitation regimen is beneficial.

Surgical

Clinical outcomes for the surgical management of isolated PFOA are sparse, and usually case series are not exclusive to isolated PFOA. Traditionally total patellectomy was the operative treatment of choice, but the outcomes were poor due to loss of extensor power, and continuing pain. More recently, excising any lateral osteophytes or part of the lateral facet (partial lateral facetectomy) with a lateral release has been reported with variable success (Figure 8.10.11). Tibial tubercle osteotomy moving the tubercle anteriorly (Maquet) has been done with generally poor results, and more recently the Fulkerson osteotomy has been used. However, as with osteotomies for tibiofemoral osteoarthritis, more certain outcomes seem to be had from joint arthroplasty. Recently figures for significant numbers of patients undergoing patellofemoral joint replacement with medium-term outcomes are encouraging (Figure 8.10.12).

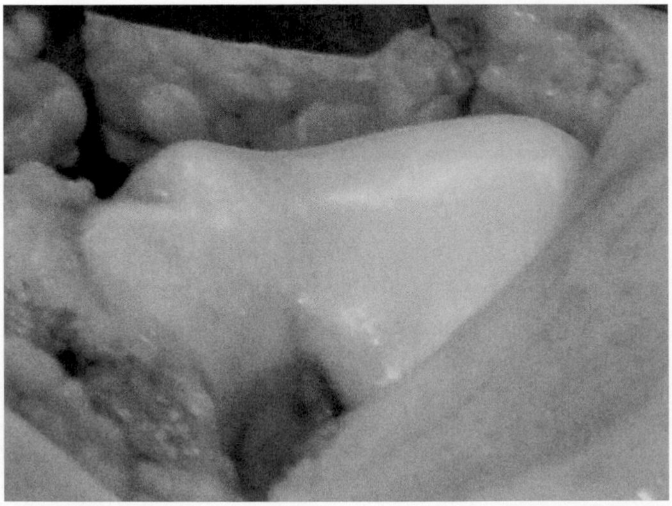

Fig. 8.10.10 Intra-operative photograph of a dysplastic distal femur.

Patellofemoral pathology

The patella may present with pathology in the bone. Infections including tuberculosis, Paget's disease, secondaries and primary bone tumours have been reported, but are rare. Management depends on the pathology and is not specific to the patella.

Osteochondritis dissecans

Osteochondritis dissecans (OCD) affecting the patellofemoral joint is described as 'anterior' OCD and is rare. It more commonly affects the patella than the trochlear groove. It is thought to occur secondary to trauma, and may lead to a loose body. Treatment is as for OCD in the tibiofemoral joint.

Patellofemoral chondropathy

Considerable efforts have been expended on repairing localized damage to articular cartilage. The standard method is microfracture. Other techniques have been described includeing carbon-fibre patches (matrix-support prosthesis), autologous periosteal transplantation, osteochondral plugs (mosaicplasty), and autologous chondrocyte implantation, ACI). Observational case series give good results, but as the quality of the scientific methodology improves the results look less good when compared to microfracture, although the latter may be worse in larger lesions. As stated earlier there is poor correlation between pain and the site of any lesion. Many of the lesions are traumatic in origin and secondary to trochlear dysplasia. Attempts at repairing the articular surface without addressing the dysplasia are therefore doomed to failure. The poor results of ACI in the patella probably reflect this. There is currently interest in the use of stem cells to repair damaged articular cartilage, but this is in its infancy.

Extensor mechanism pathology

Osgood–Schlatter/Sinding–Larsen syndromes

Pain arising from the soft tissue envelope is usually due to mechanical overload. In adolescence this may present as elongation of the tibial apophysis (Osgood–Schlatter syndrome) that may become symptomatic where the pathology is described as an osteochondrosis. The patients are usually sporty and in Osgood–Schlatter syndrome present with a prominent tibial tubercle that may be tender. Treatment is aimed at activity modification to reduce the symptoms to a level the patient can tolerate. Any pain should settle with rest and not keep the patient awake. If it does, and after excluding a

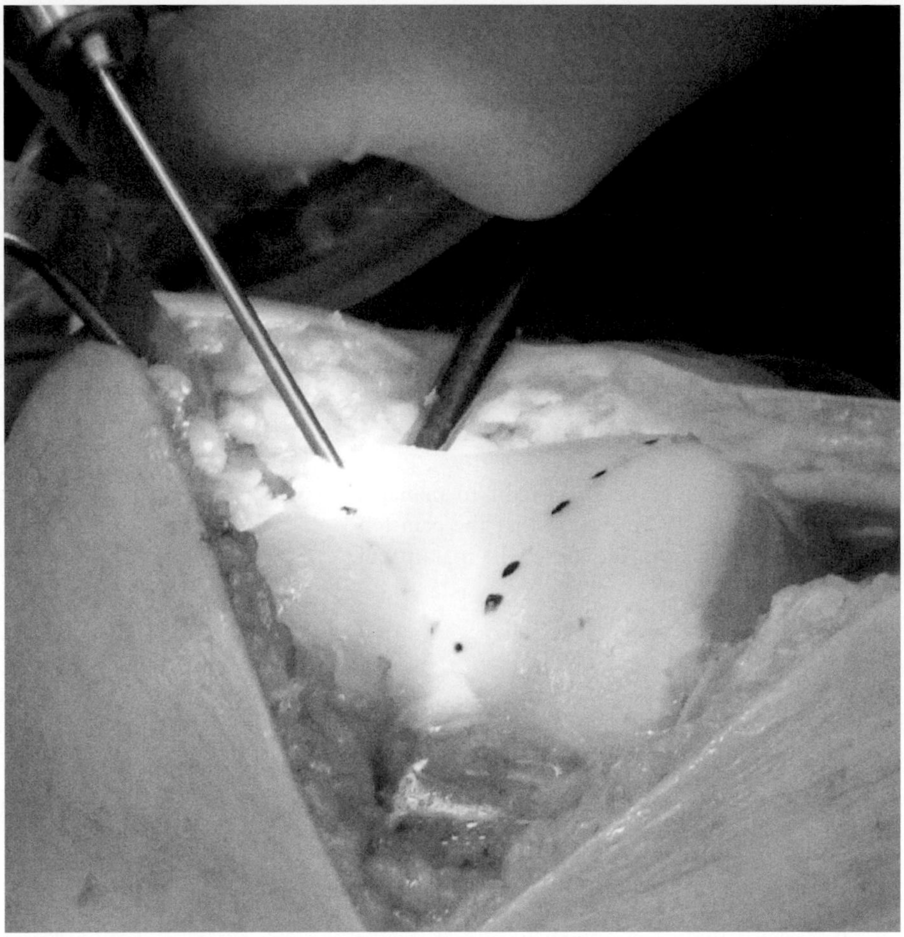

Fig. 8.10.11 Intra-operative photograph showing arthroscope light illuminating the articular surface during burring of the excess cancellous bone.

tumour, a period resting in a cylinder cast may be tried. This enforces rest and discourages teachers from over-exercising the pupil.

Osteochondrosis of the distal pole of the patella (Sinding–Larsen syndrome) is rarer but behaves similarly. In adult life the residual effect is an elongated distal pole, and implies an enthusiastic athlete in adolescence

Jumper's knee

Older patients, typically over 30 years old, may develop pain in the patellar ligament, or less commonly in the quadriceps ligament, when it is described as a tendinitis. It is also called jumper's knee and is similar to tennis elbow. The pathology is not inflammatory but a tendinosis. It is associated with tight musculature, typically the quadriceps. It reflects the loss of elasticity in the tissues with increasing age, thus causing stiffness. Typically it occurs in patients who are trying to maintain their athletic abilities and results in extensor mechanism overload. Treatment includes addressing the psychological aspects of the patient's desire to stay young.

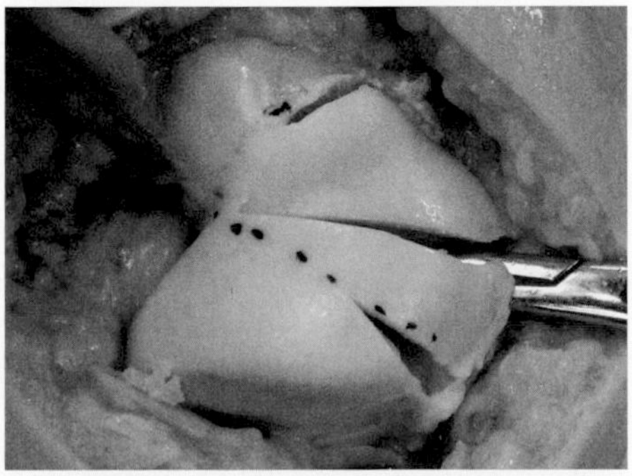

Fig. 8.10.12 Intra-operative photograph with knee viewed from lateral side showing rongeurs protecting the two osteochondral flaps, just after the new groove has been fashioned with an osteotome.

Infrapatellar fat pad pathology

Tumours such as ganglia and osteochondromata, arising within the infrapatellar fat pad are rare and present as anterior knee pain. Clinically there is fullness present either side of the patellar ligament, compared to the opposite side, which is tender. More difficult to diagnose is a haemangioma as this does not cause a swelling. Diagnosis is usually made on MRI scanning, which is the ideal way to investigate fat pad pathology.

All these lesions are easily investigated using MRI, especially when there is a doubt in the diagnosis, and concern about infection or tumour.

Stress fracture and bipartite patella

Stress fracture of the patella can occur in osteoporotic bone or more rarely in normal bone. Transverse fractures may need surgical intervention. The risk seems to occur if there is a tight lateral retinaculum (with a tilted patella on skyline x-ray) and a significant force is applied as in jumping, or tripping over a dog. The result is an autolateral release. Excision of the fragment is advised. A childhood variant is a sleeve fracture with loss of the articular surface. This needs early surgical repair.

It may be difficult to distinguish this fracture radiographically from a bipartite patella. The bipartite patella may have more than one fragment. Typically the fragment lies superolaterally, and occurs in 1% of knees. On skyline view it may be non-fused part of the patella, or a separate fragment that overhangs the lateral condyle. If symptomatic, an MRI scan may show oedema in the fragment, or reveal the cause of the anterior knee pain.

Summary

The symptomatic patellofemoral joint is difficult to manage, principally because it is difficult to be certain that the pain felt by the patient is actually arising from the joint. The majority of symptomatic patients should be managed conservatively. Surgical treatment gives best results in patellofemoral instability with defined anatomical abnormalities that are then corrected.

Further reading

Amis, A., Firer, P., Mountney, J., Senavongse, W., and Thomas, N.P. (2003). Anatomy and biomechanics of the medial patellofemoral ligament. *Knee*, **10**, 215–20.

Donell, S.T. (2006). Patellofemoral dysfunction – extensor mechanism malalignment. *Current Orthopaedics*, **20**, 103–11.

Dye, S.F. (1996). The knee as a biologic transmission with an envelope of function. *Clinical Orthopaedics*, **325**, 10–18.

Goodfellow, J., Hungerford, D.S., and Zindel, M. (1976). Patello-femoral joint mechanics and pathology. Functional anatomy of the patello-femoral joint. *Journal of Bone and Joint Surgery*, **58B**, 287–91.

Mihalko, W.M., Boachie-Adjei, Y., Spang, J.T., Fulkerson, J.P., Arendt, E.A., and Saleh, K.J. (2007). Controversies and techniques in the surgical management of patellofemoral arthritis. *Journal of Bone and Joint Surgery*, **89A**, 2788–802.

8.11

Surgical techniques of anterior cruciate ligament reconstruction

Julian Feller

Summary points

- The principal indication for ACL reconstruction is instability, either existent or predicted
- In general, it is crucial that the knee has settled and motion has been restored prior to surgery
- Accurate tunnel position is the most important aspect of surgery

Anatomy

The primary function of the anterior cruciate ligament (ACL) is to control anterior tibial translation relative to the femur. The ligament also plays a role, however, as a secondary restraint to internal rotation of the tibia on the femur, particularly towards extension. The axis of this internal rotation is within the medial compartment where the convex medial femoral condyle articulates with the concave medial tibial plateau. There is greater anteroposterior translation of the convex lateral femoral condyle on the somewhat convex tibial plateau during flexion and extension of the knee. This translation can increase with disruption of the ACL.

This can be clearly demonstrated by the typical pattern of 'bone bruising' seen on magnetic resonance imaging (MRI) following an ACL rupture (Figure 8.11.1). There is bruising on the posterior aspect of the lateral tibial plateau beneath the posterior horn of the lateral meniscus and corresponding bone bruising over the distal lateral femoral condyle where the posterior horn of the lateral meniscus and subjacent posterolateral tibia have impacted during subluxation of the knee. In ACL deficient knees it is this translation that occurs with twisting and turning, that can give rise to the patient's symptoms of giving way.

The translation can be reproduced by the pivot shift test. In this test the iliotibial band passes from anterior to the axis of knee flexion when the knee is extended, to posterior to this axis as the knee is flexed beyond about 30 degrees. As this occurs, the tibia, particularly its lateral half, reduces from its anteriorly subluxed position. The test is accentuated by a valgus stress being placed on the knee and therefore requires intact medial structures to resist this valgus force.

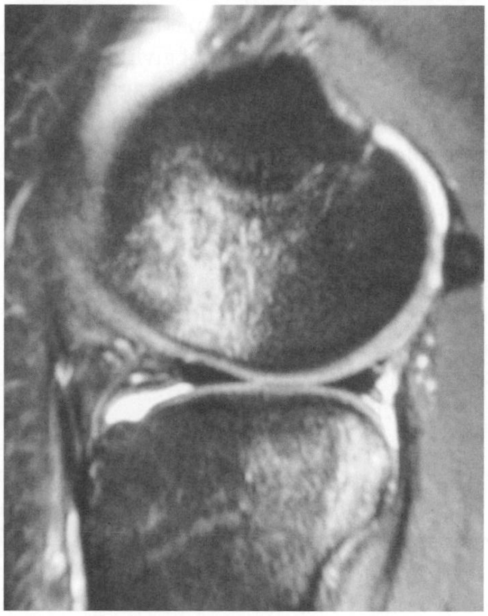

Fig. 8.11.1 Sagittal MRI showing typical lateral compartment bone bruising.

Two discrete bundles of the ligament have been described. They are the anteromedial and posterolateral bundles. Their attachment sites on the femur and tibia are such that the two bundles change their orientation to one another in varying degrees of flexion. Both bundles appear to contribute to both sagittal and axial plane stability but to varying degrees depending on the angle of knee flexion. There has been recent interest in trying to reconstruct both bundles separately to improve knee stability.

Natural history

The natural history of an untreated ACL rupture remains unclear, but there is clearly an increased risk of osteoarthritis (OA) that increases with the time from injury. There appear to be a number of factors that influence the outcome of an ACL rupture. These can be broadly classified as associated injuries, biochemical consequences, and biomechanical consequences (Box 8.11.1).

Associated injuries can include meniscal tears, chondral damage, injury to the subchondral bone, and other capsuloligamentous disruptions. Meniscal tears, particularly those of the medial meniscus, appear to increase the risk of subsequent OA. Given the poor capacity of articular cartilage to heal, any concomitant chondral injury will also increase this risk. The role of bone bruising seen on MRI is still somewhat uncertain but does appear to be associated with subsequent articular cartilage degeneration. Although some ACL ruptures may appear to be 'isolated', it seems doubtful that the ACL can in fact rupture without some concomitant damage, even though this may not be apparent at arthroscopy or on MRI.

A number of degradative enzymes, degradation products, and inflammatory markers have been found to be elevated following ACL rupture, and to remain elevated many months after the injury. Some of these biochemical changes may lower the threshold of the articular cartilage to injury, thereby making it more susceptible to the effects of trauma during episodes of giving way. There may also be some individuals who have a more aggressive biochemical response that increases their risk of developing OA.

If the individual goes on to have repeated episodes of giving way, the menisci and articular surfaces will be put at further risk of injury. Even if the individual is able to avoid episodes of instability, there are more subtle but persistent biomechanical changes in the knee following an ACL rupture. Abnormal kinematics and kinetics in day-to-day activities such as walking may impose abnormal loads on the articular cartilage that has already been compromised by injury or which has a lower threshold to injury because of associated biochemical changes.

It is unclear whether ACL reconstruction can reduce the subsequent development of OA. The evidence is limited and conflicting. Intuitively, one would imagine that by stabilizing the knee and preventing subsequent instability, further meniscal and chondral damage can be avoided, thereby protecting the knee. However, some studies have shown a somewhat alarming incidence of OA in football players who have suffered an ACL rupture. The incidence increases with time from injury and is not influenced by whether an individual has an ACL reconstruction or not.

One of the difficulties in interpreting the few studies available that do look at the longer-term outcome of ACL reconstruction, is that surgical techniques have evolved considerably over a relatively short time and indeed continue to change. One can always hope that new and apparently improved surgical techniques may be more effective in reducing the subsequent development of OA.

Nonetheless, the risk of OA will always be influenced by the presence of associated injuries as well as by more general predisposing factors such as young age at the time of injury, female gender, weight, and a familial tendency towards OA. In addition, a successful ACL reconstruction allows the individual to return to sporting activities that put the knee at risk of reinjury and also potentially allow the threshold for injury to the articular cartilage to be exceeded.

Indications for surgery (Box 8.11.2)

Given the uncertainty surrounding the natural history of ACL rupture and the effect of reconstructive surgery on it, the principal indication for ACL reconstruction at present is to eliminate instability symptoms.

In the chronic situation this is relatively straightforward as the individual presents with recurrent episodes of giving way.

In the acute setting the situation is much less clear. For active individuals who wish to continue in sports that involve twisting and turning, an initial trial of non-operative management may not be attractive or appropriate. In this situation the aim of an ACL reconstruction is to avoid predicted instability. The likelihood of instability will depend not only on the sports to which the patient wishes to return, but also the laxity of the knee on examination.

It should, however, be noted that the laxity of the knee does tend to change with time. In the first weeks or even months after injury there is often a general healing response of the knee and specifically the ruptured ACL. This can result in more subtle signs of ACL insufficiency than 3 or 6 months following the injury, when the examination findings are frequently much more obvious.

Some efforts have been made to assess the likelihood of an individual being able to cope without reconstructive surgery based on their response to an initial period of rehabilitation. The broader application of this research remains to be established.

At the present time, the literature does not support ACL reconstruction solely to protect the menisci and reduce the risk of OA. However, if a meniscal tear is repaired in the setting of an ACL rupture, the knee should probably be stabilized by ACL reconstruction in order to improve the chances of a successful meniscal repair.

Once the decision to perform an ACL reconstruction has been made, it is important that the chances for a successful outcome are optimized. This means that the knee needs to be in an appropriate state for surgery to be performed and that the patient is prepared for both the surgery and the subsequent rehabilitation. In the chronic situation, these considerations are less of an issue. In the acute situation, however, the knee is often stiff and swollen and the patient anxious about the diagnosis and outcome.

It is important to remember that ACL reconstruction is essentially an elective procedure. The main reasons for performing surgery on a relatively urgent basis are the presence of a locked knee or

Box 8.11.1 Factors leading to OA following ACL rupture

- Concomitant injuries
- Biochemical response
- Biomechanical consequences.

Box 8.11.2 Indications for ACL reconstruction

- Instability
  - Current
  - Predicted
- Protection of a meniscal repair.

significant associated capsuloligamentous injuries that are deemed to require primary repair.

Before embarking on surgery, it is preferable that knee swelling has largely resolved, or that the haemarthrosis or effusion is no longer tense, and that a good range of motion has been restored. Particular attention should be paid to extension. Patients who have not achieved near normal active extension preoperatively often find it difficult to actively achieve full extension after surgery. Difficulty regaining active extension preoperatively is usually a result of inhibition of quadriceps function secondary to pain and/or a haemarthrosis and swelling of tissues within the intercondylar notch. A true mechanical block to extension is relatively uncommon with the first injury and full extension can usually be restored by appropriate physiotherapy. This makes the subsequent restoration of extension after surgery much faster and easier for the patient.

Similarly, it is helpful to have good quadriceps function prior to surgery, even though there may be relative quadriceps weakness and reduction in bulk. It is much easier to restore quadriceps function following the trauma of surgery if it has been restored preoperatively.

Even in the professional athlete, a case can be made for letting the knee 'settle' prior to surgery as this may well result in a reduced rehabilitation time and a better overall outcome.

Anterior cruciate ligament rupture in the skeletally immature

ACL rupture can occur at all ages although the peak incidence is in the late teenage years and early twenties. ACL ruptures in the skeletally immature pose a number of additional considerations.

Children and adolescents often recover very quickly following a musculoskeletal injury. As such, the diagnosis of ACL rupture may go unrecognized as may the significance of subsequent giving-way episodes. As in adults, irreparable meniscal lesions in the young are associated with an increased risk of OA, but because of the young age at which the index injury occurs, the age at which the OA becomes symptomatic will also be early. Advanced OA in a young patient remains a problem with no easy solution.

Whether a child with an ACL rupture should be managed non-operatively is unclear. The success of non-operative management will depend on the laxity of the knee, adequate rehabilitation, the use of a brace, and the compliance of the child in avoiding situations that put the knee at risk of giving way. The latter is more difficult if a prolonged period of non-operative management is planned. The potential advantages and disadvantages of non-operative management need to be weighed against those of operative management. The main potential problem associated with early surgical reconstruction is damage to the growth plates.

For patients within 1 or perhaps 2 years of skeletal maturity, the risk of injury to the growth plates from ACL reconstruction using standard techniques is minimal. Although it may be prudent to use a soft tissue graft with no hardware crossing the growth plate, satisfactory results have been reported with patellar tendon grafts where either the bone block or the interference screw lies across the growth plate.

However, when there is considerable remaining growth, the potential for injury to the physis is more significant. As a result, alternative strategies have been suggested, such as extra-articular reconstruction or an intra-articular reconstruction in which the tunnels are entirely within the epiphyses. If the latter approach is taken, it must be recognized that the growth plate has a somewhat undulating morphology and any bone tunnels should be placed well clear of the growth plate.

Despite these concerns, however, there are surprisingly few complications reported from using a standard technique of soft tissue reconstruction with routine bone tunnels that pass through both the tibial and femoral growth plates. Although it has been

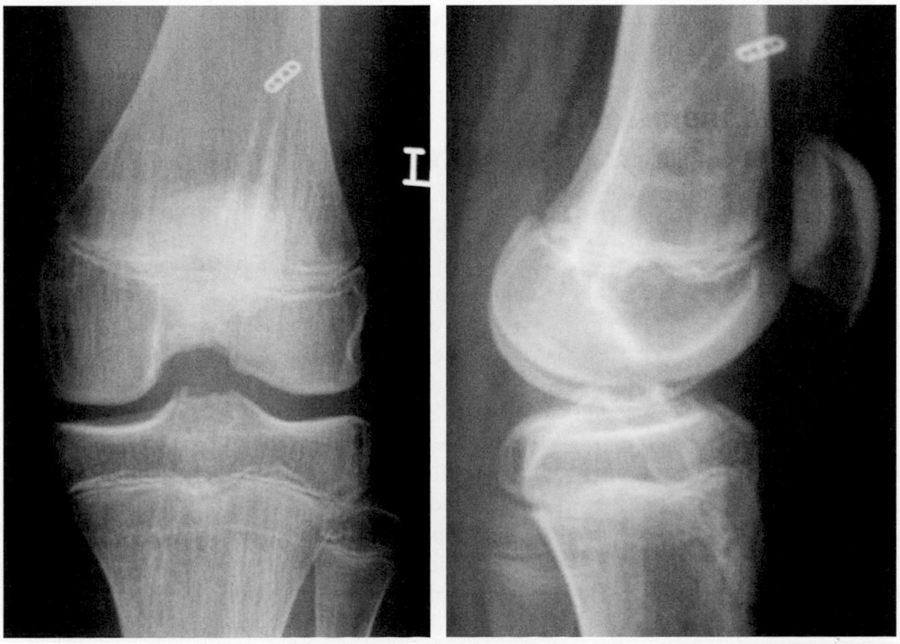

A B

Fig. 8.11.2 X-rays of an ACL reconstruction in a skeletally immature patient showing a relatively vertical orientation of the graft, particularly in the coronal plane.

suggested to make the tunnels slightly more vertical in orientation in order to reduce the cross sectional area of a tunnel at the level of the growth plate, the surgeon needs to be aware that such a strategy may also affect the positioning of the tunnels in both the tibia and femur. There is the potential to place the tibial tunnel too posterior and the femoral tunnel too high in the intercondylar notch (Figure 8.11.2).

Following ACL reconstruction in the adolescent or child, a number of studies have shown that there is probably an increased risk of graft rupture in teenagers compared to those in their twenties. Whether this increased instance of rerupture can be reduced by more conservative rehabilitation or the use of a brace has not been established at the current time.

Principles of anterior cruciate ligament reconstruction

The key principles of intra-articular ACL reconstruction are to take an adequate graft and insert the ends into appropriately placed bone tunnels in the femur and tibia using fixation that is able to withstand the forces applied during the first few months of rehabilitation, until integration occurs.

Errors in surgical technique probably constitute the commonest cause of early graft failures. Of the various errors in technique that are possible, poor placement of the bone tunnels is the most likely to lead to graft failure.

Intra-articular reconstructions can be combined with an extra-articular procedure, either involving the rerouting of the iliotibial tract or use of a free graft. However, there is little evidence to indicate that this provides a superior result compared to an intra-articular reconstruction alone.

The operative procedure should always be preceded by an examination under anaesthesia to not only document the degree of ACL insufficiency, but also to identify associated ligamentous pathology. If the preoperative examination has resulted in consideration of repair of a medial collateral ligament injury, it is worth re-examining the knee after performing the ACL reconstruction to determine whether the medial laxity has been reduced to a level where non-operative management is deemed appropriate. In the author's view, this means where there is no medial laxity at zero degrees of extension and laxity in flexion is less than 5mm greater than the normal side.

Similarly, arthroscopic inspection of the whole of the knee joint should be undertaken as part of the reconstructive procedure. If the medial meniscus is to be repaired using inside to out sutures, it is generally easier to harvest hamstring tendons prior to the passage of sutures.

Graft options

In selecting a graft, the strength and fixation options available for that graft need to be considered against the morbidity associated with graft harvest.

The range of available grafts varies from one country to another. Autograft tendons are the most commonly used, although in some centres allografts are readily available and therefore frequently used as a first choice.

Autograft tendons may be harvested from the same side as the injured knee (ipsilateral) or from the contralateral knee. Contralateral tendon harvest is more frequently used in revision surgery, but is an option for primary surgery and may be associated with a more rapid overall recovery of function.

The middle third of the patellar tendon with bone blocks from the adjacent patella and tibial tuberosity and the semitendinosus tendon either alone or in conjunction with the gracilis tendon make up the bulk of autografts. Usually four strands of hamstring tendon are used, either a quadrupled semitendinosus tendon or a doubled semitendinosus tendon and a doubled gracilis tendon. However, three- and five-strand grafts have also been used. Other autograft options include quadriceps tendon and fascia lata.

The choice between patellar tendon and hamstring tendons continues to be debated. Satisfactory results have been reported with both graft types and although meta-analyses have generally shown slightly less anterior knee laxity with patellar tendon grafts, this may not be the case if hamstring grafts of fewer than four strands are excluded. Both grafts can be associated with morbidity that can be significant to the patient. Patellar tendon grafts are associated with an increased incidence of pain on kneeling whereas hamstring grafts are associated with reduced hamstring strength.

A variety of allograft tendons can be used including Achilles tendon, patellar tendon, and tibialis anterior or posterior tendons. Allografts have the advantage of no harvest morbidity but have the disadvantage of cost, potential for disease transmission, and possibly greater knee laxity in the longer term. The results of allograft reconstructions appear to be less satisfactory in younger and more active patients.

Synthetic grafts have largely fallen out of favour due to long-term mechanical failure.

Graft strength

The relative strength of hamstring and patellar tendon grafts depends on the dimensions of the graft that is harvested and on how many strands of hamstring construct are used. It appears that a four-strand hamstring graft is generally stronger than a 10-mm wide patellar tendon graft, but it is unclear what impact this has on the long-term function of the graft and the risk of reinjury. All commonly used grafts, however, appear to be of sufficient strength to withstand the forces generated in the early rehabilitation period.

Graft harvest

There are many techniques described for harvesting of the middle third of the patellar tendon or the hamstring tendons.

Patellar tendon grafts can be harvested via traverse or longitudinal incisions which can be single or double. Transverse incisions or two separate longitudinal incisions are designed to reduce the risk of damage to the infrapatellar branches of the saphenous nerve and thereby preserve sensation on the anterior and anterolateral aspects of the knee and proximal leg. The bone plugs from the adjacent patella and tibial tuberosity are usually harvested with the aid of a small oscillating saw and osteotome. The blocks can then be shaped into cylinders or other shapes.

The hamstring tendons are generally harvested via an anteromedial incision over the distal attachment of the pes anserinus. The incision can be longitudinal, oblique, or transverse. The sartorius fascia needs to be incised to expose the underlying gracilis and semitendinosus tendons. These are harvested using a tendon stripper.

The fascial bands which attach the semitendinosus tendon to the medial gastrocnemius must be divided under direct vision. If a closed tendon stripper is used, the tendons need to be detached distally and secured with a whip stitch to allow passage of the stripper. If an open tendon stripper is used, this can be done with a distal attachment intact. When passing a tendon stripper, it is important to keep in mind the orientation of the tendons. When the gracilis tendon is being harvested, the tendon stripper should pass along the medial aspect of the thigh. When the semitendinosus tendon is harvested the orientation should be in a more lateral direction. The harvested tendons are then cleaned of extraneous tissue and attached muscle. Depending on the type of fixation being used they are then whip stitched at one or both ends

For hamstring grafts it has recently been suggested that harvesting some of the adjacent periosteum and incorporating this into one or both ends of the graft can improve subsequent healing of the tendon wall of the bone tunnel. Whether or not this translates into better long-term clinical results remains to be seen.

Intercondylar notch preparation

Intra-articular ACL reconstruction can be performed via an arthrotomy or using arthroscopy. In general, better visualization of the intercondylar notch can be obtained using arthroscopy but the surgeon should have the appropriate arthroscopic skills prior to embarking on arthroscopic ACL reconstructive surgery.

Surgeons vary in terms of their preference for preservation of native ACL tissues. The first principle should be to have adequate vision to ensure good tunnel placement. This may mean removing all of the remnants of the torn ACL. However, with experience the surgeon may well be able to leave much of the native tissue intact, but still remove any tissue that may impinge and result in so-called Cyclops lesion. Whether this has any functional benefit is difficult to determine but it may be associated with better revascularization of the graft, and possibly restoration of some proprioceptive function.

Although notchplasty was previously regarded as a routine component of ACL reconstruction, it has become apparent that a well-positioned graft is unlikely to impinge in the intercondylar notch in extension and therefore the role of notchplasty is limited to removing osteophytes or enlarging an intrinsically narrow or 'gothic notch', essentially to improve visualization to the posterolateral wall of the notch.

Bone tunnel preparation

Most commonly, the ACL is reconstructed using a single-bundle technique. Previously the ideal attachment sites on the femur and tibia were thought to be those which resulted in an isometric graft. However, it appears that relatively few fibres of the ligament are truly isometric and that different parts of the ligament are under tension at different angles of knee flexion. Because of this, emphasis has been placed on trying to reproduce the anatomy of the native ligament in order to more closely reproduce its biomechanical characteristics.

In recent years there has been increased interest in using a double-bundle or even a triple-bundle technique in an attempt to even better recreate the complex biomechanics of the intact ACL. Double-bundle techniques aim to reconstruct the anteromedial and posterolateral bundles of the ACL separately. Whilst cadaveric studies have indicated restoration of more normal biomechanics, clinical results to date do not demonstrate any clear functional outcome benefit compared to a well-performed single-bundle reconstruction. Further prospective randomized studies are required to clarify the role of double-bundle reconstruction. This chapter deals only with the technique of single-bundle reconstruction.

There are a variety of drill guides available for use in the preparation of the bone tunnels. However, it is important to remember that they are only used to improve the ability of the surgeon to place the tunnels in the positions which the surgeon believes to be correct. The guides do not in themselves indicate the correct position of the bone tunnels. The same applies to computer navigation of tunnel placement.

In general, the tibial tunnel is drilled from outside in over a guide wire, although retrograde drilling has been used. More options are available for the femoral tunnel. The tunnel can be drilled from inside to out or from outside to in. If drilling inside to out, the tunnel can be created by drilling through the anteromedial arthroscopic portal or by using a transtibial approach, drilling through the tibial tunnel. Retrograde drilling can also be used.

The essential principle is to align the graft in such a way that it controls both anterior tibial translation and internal tibial rotation without compromising terminal extension or full flexion of the knee (Figure 8.11.3).

In the coronal plane, a more vertically orientated graft (Figure 8.11.4) provides less chance of controlling rotation but may have a better chance of controlling anterior tibial translation, provided the sagittal plane alignment is satisfactory i.e. not too vertical (Figure 8.11.5). If too vertical, the graft may impinge on the posterior cruciate ligament and limit full flexion. A more horizontally placed graft (in the coronal plane) will be better able to resist rotation but less able to resist anterior tibial translation. Hence the interest in a double-bundle technique which allows for two bundles to be inserted in different alignments.

If a graft is too anterior on the femur or tibia, there will impingement of the graft on the anterior margin of the intercondylar notch in extension, resulting in either a restriction of extension, or amputation or failure of the graft (Figure 8.11.6).

The aperture of the tibial tunnel should lie in the footprint of the native ACL and should be as medial and anterior as possible without causing impingement of the graft on the roof of the intercondylar notch when the knee is extended. It should be noted that the anterior limit of the tibial footprint of the native ligament extends to the anterior attachment of the medial meniscus. The native ligament does not impinge in the intercondylar notch because of the shoe or foot shaped nature of its anterior extent. Grafts tend to be more cylindrical and therefore cannot extend as far anteriorly if impingement on the roof of the intercondylar notch in extension is to be avoided.

The aperture of the femoral tunnel should also be within the footprint of the native ACL and preferably towards its posterior margin as viewed arthroscopically. It is important to recognize that 'posterior' from an arthroscopic perspective is in fact superior from a strictly anatomical perspective. There has been a general trend to move the aperture of the femoral tunnel 'down' the lateral wall of intercondylar notch, once again when viewed arthroscopically with the knee flexed. Again, this results in an orientation of the graft that is better able to reproduce the function of the intact ACL. Using the analogy of a clock face, with the knee flexed to around 90 degrees, the aperture of the femoral tunnel of the left knee would be at the 2 o'clock position.

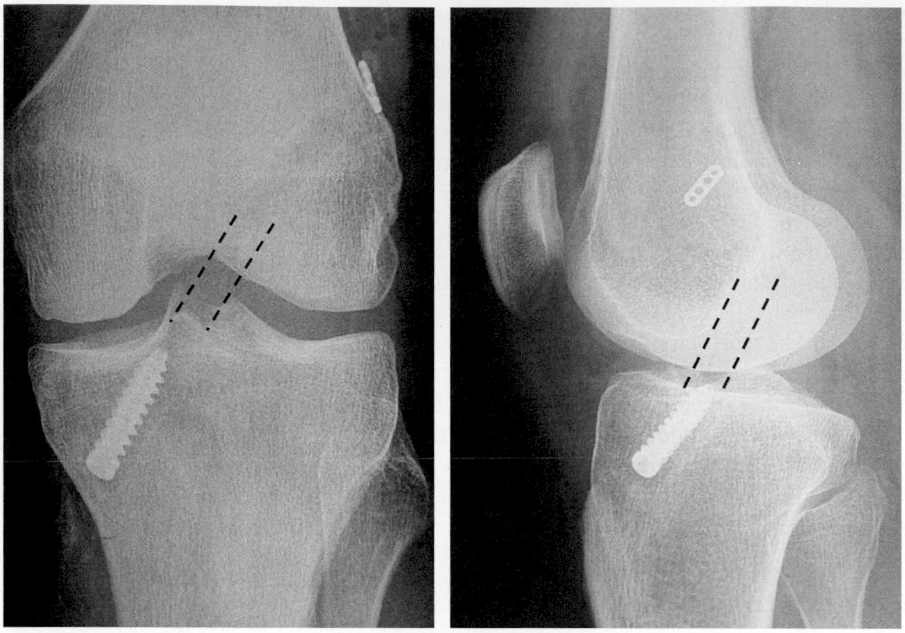

A B

Fig. 8.11.3 X-rays of a well-orientated graft in both the coronal and sagittal planes.

Although it is common practice, many experts feel that such a position cannot be achieved using a transtibial drilling technique and therefore recommend drilling via the anteromedial portal. In order to achieve a satisfactory femoral tunnel length to allow for an adequate length of graft to be placed in the tunnel, the knee needs to be flexed considerably, usually 110 degrees or more. This can make visualization of the back of intercondylar notch difficult. Drilling via the anteromedial tunnel also puts the articular surface of the medial femoral condyle at risk and care must be taken not to damage it with the drill tip.

If the femoral tunnel is drilled via the tibial tunnel careful attention needs to be paid to the angle of the knee flexion, the angle of the drill guide, and medialization of the starting point on the tibia during drilling of the tibial tunnel. In order to achieve a satisfactory position of the femoral tunnel, the tibial tunnel must start at the anterior margin of the superficial medial collateral ligament. Depending on the type of tibial drill guide that is used (tip aimer or elbow aimer), the guide needs to be set at a relatively shallow angle such as 45 degrees and the knee flexed to only 75–80 degrees to subsequently be able to obtain a satisfactory femoral tunnel position.

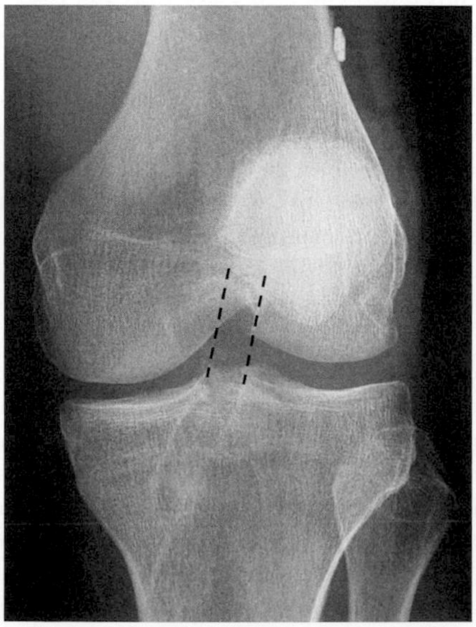

Fig. 8.11.4 X-ray of a graft that is vertically orientated in the coronal placement due to a 'high' femoral tunnel placement.

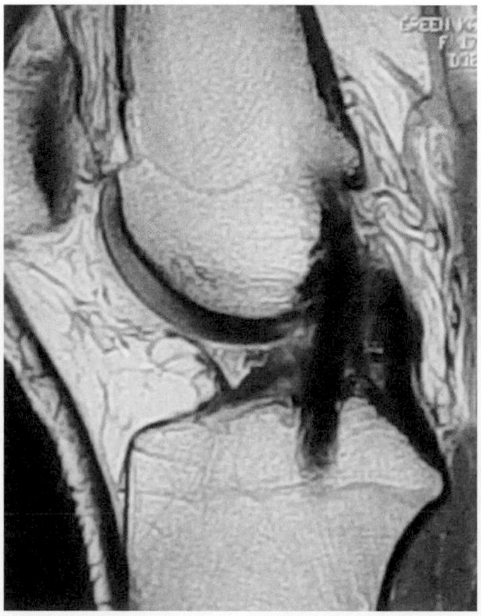

Fig. 8.11.5 Sagittal MRI of a graft that is vertically orientated due to the tibial tunnel being too posterior.

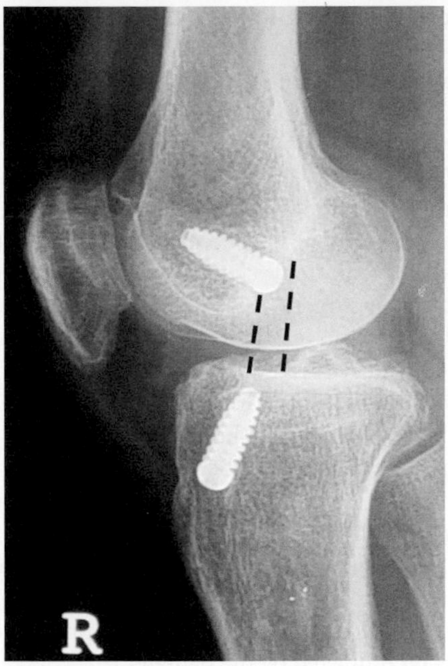

Fig. 8.11.6 X-ray of poorly positioned graft: the femoral tunnel is too anterior (distal) in the notch.

Generally cannulated drills are used to create the bone tunnels and are passed over a guide wire. Whichever technique is used for the femoral tunnel, it is helpful to mark the desired starting point on the lateral wall of the intercondylar notch with a curette or an awl, thereby creating a depression which helps to capture the tip of the guide wire.

Consideration should be given to the type of drills being used, whether these result in impaction or extraction of the bone and whether they have an 'acorn' or expanded type tip or are of a constant diameter. Impaction drilling may improve the strength of interference fixation devices. Using acorn-tipped drills can result in the tunnel walls not being parallel throughout their entirety if the guide wire loses fixation as the tip of the guide wire is approached.

Once the tunnels have been drilled and bone and articular cartilage debris removed from the joint, the graft is usually passed into the tibial tunnel, through the knee joint, and into the femoral tunnel by use of some kind of lead suture or tape exiting through the anterolateral cortex of the femur and distal and lateral aspect of the thigh. It is helpful to ensure that the external mouth of the tibial tunnel is clear of soft tissue to aid graft passage.

Graft fixation

Various forms of fixation are available. These can be broadly classified as aperture fixation or suspensory fixation. Aperture fixation typically involves the use of an interference screw or plug which is inserted longitudinally into the graft tunnel either between the graft and the wall of the tunnel or through the central portion of the graft, in either case pushing the remaining graft tissue hard against the wall of the tunnel. Suspensory fixation relies on a device being situated on the cortex of the femur or tibia and attached to the graft via some kind of loop. Suspensory fixation does have the advantage of being flexible and for use in most situations but it has been suggested that, being less rigid than aperture fixation, it might contribute to bone tunnel enlargement. This is more commonly seen with hamstring grafts than with patellar tendon grafts. Although most studies have not shown any deleterious effect of bone tunnel enlargement, more recent evidence does indicate it may be associated with increased graft laxity.

Transcondylar fixation is an alternative that can be used on the femoral side with a rod or pin passing through the proximal end of the graft. In the case of hamstring tendons, this is essentially a form of suspensory fixation with elimination of the loop between the fixation hardware and the graft itself, the aim of this being to reduce the effect of creep in the construct.

Many of the available fixation devices are offered in either metallic or bioabsorbable forms. Concern about metallic implants relates to their impact on subsequent MRI and the possible need for removal at the time of revision surgery, should this be required. Bioabsorbable devices do not interfere with MRI and it is possible for them to be ignored in a revision procedure depending on their position. There are various polymers that can be used in the manufacture of bioabsorbable implants and these can be combined with hydroxyapatite in attempt to improve bony incorporation. The rate of reabsorption varies considerably from one combination of polymers to another. In general, most bioabsorbable devices have been shown to provide initially similar biomechanical characteristics and clinical outcomes as metallic implants.

Whatever fixation type is used, pretensioning of the graft construct should be considered in an attempt to eliminate creep from the system. Pretensioning can be in the form of static pretensioning prior to graft insertion, or with cyclic loading of the graft following insertion and proximal fixation just prior to distal fixation.

The angle of knee flexion and the amount of tension applied to the graft at the time of distal fixation remains somewhat arbitrary. If the graft excursion in the tibial tunnel is minimal throughout extension and flexion, then there is probably little to indicate that one angle of knee flexion is preferable to another. It is unclear what the ideal tension within the graft should be at the time of distal fixation and it is also unclear whether this tension is maintained in the early postoperative period.

Perioperative management

Surgery can be undertaken on a day case or inpatient basis. It is usually performed under general anaesthesia, but can be undertaken with regional anaesthesia. Most patients can be discharged within 24h.

Initial postoperative analgesia can be aided by injection of local anaesthetic into the knee and graft donor site, femoral nerve, or iliacus block, or by single-shot epidural injection. Use of epidural anaesthesia may preclude management as a day case. Use of a femoral nerve block may require the use of a splint to compensate for quadriceps weakness.

Drain tubes, if used, can generally be removed within 6h postoperatively.

The use of splints and braces varies widely from one centre to another. Bracing may assist with analgesia and aid initial ambulation. Later in the rehabilitation period, bracing may protect the graft and reduce the incidence of bone tunnel enlargement following hamstring tendon grafts. There is little evidence to suggest that bracing results in an improved clinical outcome.

Rehabilitation

The principles of rehabilitation are to eliminate swelling, restore a full range of movement, restore adequate muscle strength, especially of the quadriceps and hamstring muscle groups, and to restore adequate neuromuscular control. Progression through the various stages should be based on the state of the knee, rather than just on the time since surgery.

Patients can weight bear as tolerated from immediately postoperatively but crutches are generally required for up to 3 weeks. Emphasis should be placed on restoration of full extension, equal to the normal opposite knee. Riding a stationary bicycle can usually be commenced by 4 weeks along with closed kinetic chain quadriceps strengthening exercises. The role of open kinetic chain quadriceps strengthening exercise is unclear. They may impose a potentially deleterious anterior strain on the graft and it probably safer to avoid such exercises in the first 12 postoperative weeks. Light jogging can be commenced by 12 weeks together with balance and landing drills. This is followed by the introduction of sport specific drills and a return to light training. A return to full training can start after 6 months.

The timing for a safe return to competitive sport is contentious. There are no proven criteria on which to base the decision. Although many surgeons recommend waiting until 12 months, many surgeons, including the author, feel 9–10 months is safe provided there is no effusion, an essentially full range of motion, no significant graft laxity, good strength, particularly of quadriceps, and good neuromuscular coordination.

Results of anterior cruciate ligament reconstruction

Overall satisfactory outcomes are achieved for the majority of patients, although *normal* static stability may only be achieved in as few as 50% patients depending on the type of graft and type of fixation used. Most studies do, however, report good or excellent results based on both a variety of outcome scales and also objective measures such as range of motion, anterior knee laxity, and muscle strength.

Rates of return to the same level of pre-injury sport are less than one would anticipate from the aforementioned results. Typical rates of successful return to the pre-injury level of sport are in the order of 60–70%, but may be as low as 50%. There are a number of reasons for this. Rotational stability is difficult to measure objectively and may be present despite other parameters being essentially normal. Patients may change their aspirations regarding return to sport after surgery. They may not want to face the risk of reinjury and further surgery and rehabilitation. Increasing age is also associated with reduced involvement in pivoting and contact sports. Patient confidence has also been shown to influence rates of return to sport, independent of knee function.

ACL reconstruction has yet to be shown to protect the knee from the development of OA, although protection of the menisci does seem to be achievable to some degree.

The results of surgery are best if both the patient and the knee are properly prepared prior to surgery, the surgery is done well (particularly tunnel placement), and appropriate postoperative rehabilitation is completed by the patient.

Further reading

Amis, A. A. and Dawkins, G. P. (1991). Functional anatomy of the anterior cruciate ligament. Fibre bundle actions related to ligament replacements and injuries. *Journal of Bone and Joint Surgery*, **73B**, 260–7.

Brand, J., JR., Weiler, A., Caborn, D. N., Brown, C. H., JR. and Johnson, D. L. (2000). Graft fixation in cruciate ligament reconstruction. *American Journal of Sports Medicine*, **28**, 761–74.

Goldblatt, J. P., Fitzsimmons, S. E., Balk, E., and Richmond, J. C. (2005). Reconstruction of the anterior cruciate ligament: meta-analysis of patellar tendon versus hamstring tendon autograft. *Arthroscopy*, **21**, 791–803.

Myklebust, G. and Bahr, R. (2005). Return to play guidelines after anterior cruciate ligament surgery. *British Journal of Sports Medicine*, **39**, 127–31.

West, R. V. and Harner, C. D. (2005). Graft selection in anterior cruciate ligament reconstruction. *Journal of the American Academy of Orthopaedic Surgeons*, **13**, 197–207.

8.12

Combined ligament injuries around the knee

Andy Williams and Ali Narvani

Summary points

- Any knee with major disruption of two ligaments is likely to have been dislocated at the time of injury
- Knee dislocations are associated with high risk of neurovascular injury. Angiography or vascular ultrasound is mandatory
- In knee dislocations, following immediate reduction and stabilization usually with a brace, acute repair of the ruptured soft tissue structure within 2–3 weeks of injury is likely to provide superior results compared to later reconstruction
- Management of most multiligament injuries is complex and requires surgical intervention therefore specialist centres are best to be involved early
- In cases with associated malalignment, osteotomy can improve the results of ligament reconstruction.

Introduction

These injuries include a spectrum of severities ranging from a cruciate ligament rupture plus a minor tear of a collateral ligament to frank dislocation of the tibiofemoral joint (Box 8.12.1). Since most dislocations spontaneously reduce, their incidence is considerably higher than was once thought. Any knee with ruptures of three or more ligaments or a major disruption of two ligaments has likely to have been dislocated at the time of injury. Awareness of this is important because of the risk of neurovascular injury associated with knee dislocation. Although the majority of these major injuries are associated with major trauma, in the morbidly obese, knee dislocation can occur with relatively minor injury.

Box 8.12.1 Knee dislocation

- Associated with ruptures of three or more ligaments or a major disruption of two ligaments
- High risk of neurovascular injury. Angiography/vascular ultrasound mandatory
- More common with major trauma, but associated minor trauma especially in the obese.

Acute management

This is dealt with in detail elsewhere in this book, but some important points need to be made. Firstly, awareness for the potential for a knee dislocation is important. Any knee that has multiple plane laxity may have dislocated, particularly one in which there is not a tense haemarthrosis from leakage of blood into the soft tissues through capsular tears.

Neurovascular injury should be ruled out. The authors' preference is that all such knees should have an angiogram as Doppler assessment cannot identify intimal flap tears of the artery that may need surgery.

If the knee is dislocated at presentation, it should be reduced immediately. Very rarely it is irreducible if the femoral condyle (usually medial) has protruded through a rent in the soft tissues. The initial management for the knee joint is then to maintain congruent reduction. If the posterior cruciate ligament (PCL) is ruptured, a fixed posterior subluxed contracture can develop. Regular x-rays to ensure maintenance of congruent reduction are important.

Usually an adequate brace will suffice, and allows early joint motion and icing to reduce swelling and avoid early contracture formation. Bridging external fixation should really only be used to protect arterial repairs or reconstructions. In other circumstances, an external fixator interferes with the ability to treat the soft tissues properly, runs the risk of pin tract infections, and frequently holds the joint in a subluxed position.

Magnetic resonance imaging (MRI) helps to establish the anatomy of the injury, but is no substitute for clinical assessment which gives greater detail about the severity of any instability.

Surgical management (Box 8.12.2)

There are few justifications for non-surgical management of a knee that has actually dislocated as this tends to lead to an unfortunate combination of stiffness, instability, and rapid deterioration with chondral damage. There is still considerable debate as to whether surgical repair or reconstruction of the injured ligaments should be undertaken within the first 2–3 weeks, or delayed 6–12 weeks following injury. Certain factors may determine the options available. If vascular reconstruction has been undertaken or there has been an open injury, then delayed treatment of the ligaments may well be necessary. Best results from treatment occur when surgery is undertaken around 2 weeks from injury. Any time after this

Box 8.12.2 Acute management

- Immediate reduction and stabilization usually with a brace
- Bridging external fixation if vascular repair/reconstruction
- Acute repair within 2–3 weeks of injury likely to provide superior results compared to later reconstructions, especially the posterolateral corner.

the repair of ruptured soft tissues is often impossible and only reconstructive procedures can be undertaken. Posterolateral corner injuries, in particular, are amenable to repair. The results of successful repair are always superior to reconstruction, presumably due to the restoration of normal anatomy with concomitant proprioception. In addition, where the cruciate ligaments are avulsed from bone, they too can be repaired with possible success. By reconstructing all injured ligaments simultaneously there is less risk of overload of the repair or reconstructions undertaken. The provision of congruent range of motion with stability allows the soft tissue envelope to heal at appropriate tension throughout the range of knee motion and is protective of the chondral tissues. Early mobilization also helps restoration of neuromuscular control of the limb.

Management of ligamentous injuries (Box 8.12.3)

These injuries are complex and specialist centres are best to be involved, particularly if early surgery is required.

Careful preoperative assessment is crucial in making the necessary surgical plans. Although most multiligament injuries associated with dislocation require early surgery, a number of injury patterns involving the medial collateral ligament (MCL) and more minor PCL injuries are best treated conservatively at first to allow these structures to heal with bracing. This greatly reduces the amount of surgery that is subsequently required.

Clinical evaluation of the knee includes observation of patterns of bruising and clinical tests of ligament laxity. Plain x-rays including long leg alignment films in chronic cases are essential. MRI scanning is helpful and also highlights significant osteochondral lesions or meniscal pathology.

Management of each component of the ligament injury

Anterior cruciate ligament

The management of anterior cruciate ligament (ACL) ruptures is covered elsewhere in this text (see Chapter 8.11). Even with an isolated ACL rupture, the majority of young active patients benefit from reconstructive surgery. In the context of a multiple ligament injury to the knee, however, ACL reconstruction is essential.

Posterior cruciate ligament

The extra-synovial nature of the PCL means that it does have some capacity to heal, particularly if the other ligament injured is the MCL which also has significant healing capacity. Bracing many of the combined PCL/MCL injuries for 6 weeks will restore normal stability and if any subsequent surgery is required it may be much more minor than if undertaken at the very early stage. Nevertheless, if it is clear that clinical assessment shows gross disruption of the PCL then early reconstruction is usually preferable. Clinical examination, which may require an anaesthetic in the acute situation, is best performed by the posterior drawer test. With the foot and therefore tibia in the neutral rotation position and the knee at 90 degrees of flexion, the tibia is pushed posteriorly. If a tibiofemoral 'step off' is present but less than the normal side, then this represents Grade 1 laxity. If the tibia is level with the front of the femur (i.e. there is no step off) then this is Grade 2 laxity. If the tibia has sagged behind the distal femur then this represents Grade 3 laxity. If Grade 3 laxity is present then there is virtual certainty of concomitant injury to one or both collateral ligament complexes.

Isolated Grade 1 injuries of the PCL need non-surgical treatment and invariably do well. Grade 3 ligament injuries have a poor prognosis and will require early reconstruction or repair (Figure 8.12.1). This will invariably involve treatment of at least one other ligament disruption. Controversy still reigns regarding the isolated Grade 2 lesions. Patients will often function well with this injury, but there is mounting evidence of significant arthritic damage in the longer term. There is as yet no evidence, however, that early stabilization in this way reduces the long-term risk of arthritis.

The PCL has two functional bundles of fibres, the anterolateral, which is more important, and the posteromedial bundle. Even in cases of complete rupture of both bundles of the PCL, *in vitro* 'bench' testing shows that the addition of a second posteromedial bundle to the reconstruction offers only modest benefit. In the context of acute reconstructions for knee dislocation, most surgeons would only undertake a single-bundle reconstruction. The question remains whether the addition of a posteromedial bundle in the reconstruction is of long-term advantage for more chronic cases.

In the case of a knee with multiligament injury, it is illogical to address all other ligaments apart from the PCL assuming that one will render the knee an isolated PCL-deficient one. Isolated PCL injuries do not involve extensive damage to the capsular structures

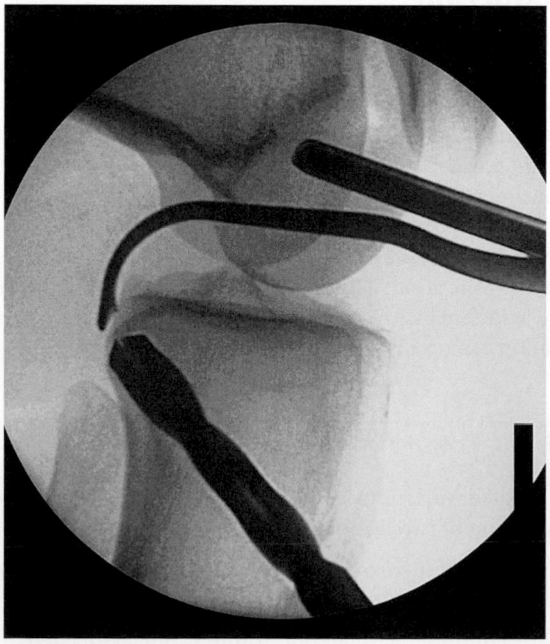

Fig. 8.12.1 Lateral intraoperative radiograph illustrating tibial tunnel placement for PCL reconstruction.

nor the proprioceptive deficit that occurs with a PCL rupture in the dislocated knee. If one was to reconstruct only one cruciate ligament the PCL should always take precedence. The ACL can always be dealt with at a later stage.

Medial collateral ligament complex

Most MCL injuries of all severities can be treated non-surgically. Those requiring early repair are those in which an MRI scan shows curling up of an avulsed MCL which clearly would not heal well, or cases in which the MCL is 'flipped' into the joint or where the meniscus has been extruded with the avulsed ligament. In addition, in cases where both cruciate ligaments are ruptured and require early surgery, failure to undertake early MCL repair is likely to overload the cruciate ligaments' repairs or reconstructions.

The MCL complex provides the primary restraint to valgus force, which needs to be assessed both in flexion and extension. Opening at all in extension indicates a failure of the posteromedial corner/posterior capsule. In addition, the deep MCL restrains external rotation. A secondary sign of MCL laxity in the presence of ACL laxity, is failure of tibial external rotation to abolish the anterior drawer sign. Knowledge of the anatomy of the medial ligament complex is critical to undertake an effective repair that does not render the knee joint stiff. This anatomy has been described by Warren and Marshall as being in three layers. The most superficial layer 1 can remain intact unless there is major disruption and only once this is incised is the magnitude of the MCL injury visible. The ligament can usually be repaired with suture and suture anchors.

In the chronic setting, most MCL laxity can be dealt with by opening layer 1 and undertaking plication of the loose deep MCL if the laxity is above the meniscus. If braced appropriately this double breasting of the tissue usually leads to good healing. If at arthroscopy it is clear that the laxity is inframeniscal, then layers 2 and 3 may need to be elevated from the tibia before reattachment in an appropriate position. The soft tissue quality may be poor and a simple plicating technique doomed. Although recent focus has been on the posterolateral corner, uncontrolled medial ligament laxity is far more challenging surgically. The superficial MCL and posteromedial corner can be stabilized using a four-strand hamstring tendon or patellar tendon allograft.

Posterolateral corner/lateral ligament complex

The structures involved include the lateral collateral ligament (LCL), the popliteus tendon and associated popliteofibular ligament, biceps tendon and gastrocnemius tendon, and the posterolateral capsule. The primary restraint to varus stress is the LCL. The popliteofibular ligament and attached popliteus tendon form the main restraint to external rotation. Significant injuries to the posterolateral corner are best evaluated by clinical assessment although with improved understanding of the structures comprising this region of the knee, MRI now is increasingly useful.

The LCL is tested by applying varus stress to the knee at 30 degrees but also in extension. Laxity in extension indicates disruption of the posterior structures/capsule. To assess the popliteofibular ligament there are a number of tests. Most knee specialists agree that the 'Dial test' is the most reliable. This can be undertaken in the clinic with the patient prone with external rotation of both legs applied simultaneously with the knee at 90 degrees and also, most specifically, at 30 degrees. An isolated posterolateral corner injury will reveal an excess of external rotation most clearly at 30 degrees. If the PCL is involved this increases the sign at 90 degrees. The test is said to be significant if there is more than 10 degrees side-to-side difference in excursion. Also with a PCL rupture, a so-called reverse pivot shift may be present. With the knee flexed and the leg externally rotated to cause posterior subluxation of the lateral tibia, the knee is then extended with concurrent applied valgus to compress the lateral articulation. A 'clunk' as the lateral tibial plateau comes forward into reduced position represents a positive result. It is essential to check the opposite knee since around 20% of normal knees have a similar finding. In the chronic case, assessment of gait is essential as significant posterolateral corner injury in the naturally varus aligned limb can lead to a dynamic varus thrust as a patient goes through the stance phase of gait. Particularly bad injuries also have hyperextension present. In these cases, lifting the limb with the great toe will lead to hyperextension, varus and external rotation (a positive Hughston test).

Determining the site of injury to the ligament complex can be helped by MRI scanning and also at arthroscopy where examination of the lateral compartment can show proximal avulsion of the popliteus from direct observation or identify whether opening up occurs above or below the lateral meniscus or indeed both.

Posterolateral corner injuries are best treated acutely since many of the structures can be repaired. This is particularly true in avulsion injuries of the fibular head (Figure 8.12.2). When the biceps, LCL, and popliteofibular ligament all come off as one, or the fibular head is fractured, simple reattachment restores normal laxity to the posterolateral corner. Fibular head fracture fixation is not easy. The common peroneal nerve should be identified and dissected free. The senior author has found that the tension band wiring technique is the most efficient way of fixing the fracture. In other cases in which there are midsubstance ruptures or proximal avulsion-type injuries the structures involved can be repaired directly. At the end of the repair stage of surgery it is essential to check the quality of repair as a reconstruction is usually also required to support the repaired tissues. There are a number of 'anatomical' reconstructive procedures described, but unfortunately none of them can provide the dynamic tensioning effect of the popliteus. It may be reasonable therefore to accept non-anatomical compromises such as the modified Larson procedure. This involves taking hamstring tendons from the lateral epicondyle of the femur through a tunnel in the fibular head (Figure 8.12.3). The advantage of this procedure is that it is more peripheral to the centre of the knee at which rotation occurs and therefore its lever arm for effectiveness against external rotation is maximal. If the lateral soft tissues are in reasonable condition then, in chronic cases, a useful option is to detach the lateral epicondyle which is then advanced to retension the posterolateral corner.

Posterolateral corner injuries have a significant rate of common peroneal nerve damage. In a series of 54 cases of posterolateral corner disruption the incidence of injury was 17% and in all but one case this occurred with distal injury to the ligament complex involving avulsion of the biceps' tendon with or without a fibular head fracture. If a common peroneal nerve injury does occur, then it is essential that an equinus contracture is not allowed to develop and that stretching and splintage are started early.

The role of osteotomy

The main use of osteotomy for multiple ligament injury to the knee is in chronic cases involving a posterolateral corner disruption and

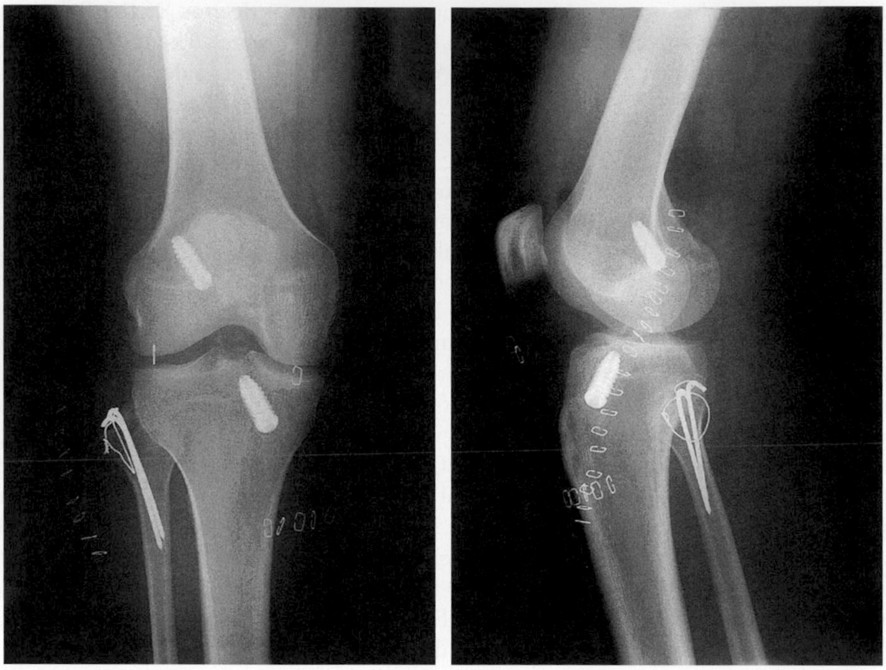

Fig. 8.12.2 A) Plain AP radiograph illustrating fibula fixation in combination with ACL reconstruction. B) Lateral view of radiograph if fibula fixation and ACL reconstruction.

natural varus alignment of the limb. In patients who naturally stand in varus, if the soft tissues are simply reconstructed alone then the dynamic stress applied to the reconstruction causes stretching out of the reconstruction or repair over time. In the normal varus knee, this stretching out does not occur since normal proprioception is present through the dynamic contraction of structures such as the biceps, popliteus, and lateral gastrocnemius and the lateral joint is kept closed down under limb loading. Unfortunately, after ligament injury this proprioceptive control is impaired and deliberate realignment of the limb in the coronal plane with osteotomy can be very useful. This is essentially a treatment for LCL laxity, although some authors have suggested that it may enhance restoration of rotational control.

The need for an osteotomy is determined by the presence of dynamic thrust seen on gait or excess varus alignment on long leg x-rays. In osteotomy for osteoarthritis a deliberate deformity is produced to shift the weight-bearing axis to the unaffected compartment of the tibiofemoral joint. When undertaking osteotomy for dynamic laxity for ligament problems, the correction needs to be much less aggressive. The aim is simply to bring the weight-bearing line through the centre of the joint. Calculation of the correct correction is, of course, important. A common error producing overcorrection occurs when there is a failure to recognize that part of the excess varus measured on long leg x-rays may be due to opening of the lateral joint compartment because of LCL laxity. As soon as the weight-bearing line comes across the midline, the lateral compartment will close down as it is loaded, so removing the lateral soft tissue laxity component of the deformity. It should therefore not be included in the calculation of the angle of correction required. A good working rule is that for every excess opening of 1mm, 1 degree of osteotomy correction should be subtracted. The addition of a valgus high tibial osteotomy in the treatment of posterolateral corner insufficiency can be dramatic. It can be undertaken as a preliminary procedure or at the same time as the ligament reconstruction.

The need for distal femoral osteotomy to produce varus in cases of chronic MCL laxity is much less common, but can also be very helpful.

It is easy to think simply in terms of the coronal plane, but the sagittal alignment of the tibial slope is also of great importance in treatment of multiple ligament injury to the knee. The steeper the tibial slope, the greater the tendency there is to anterior tibial translation under knee loading. Equally a flatter than usual or reversed tibial slope will lead to posterior subluxation. Deliberate control of tibial slope at the time of osteotomy can aid ACL or PCL laxity. In cases of ACL deficiency it is preferable to reduce the tibial slope and this is easily accomplished during lateral closing wedge upper tibial osteotomy. Since the approach to the tibia is lateral, the posterolateral corner is easily reconstructed at the same time. If as well as posterolateral corner insufficiency there is PCL deficiency present, then a medial opening wedge osteotomy is preferable. Since this osteotomy is anteromedial, increasing the tibial slope tends to occur when undertaking this procedure.

Realignment of the lower limb with an osteotomy can dramatically improve the quality of results from ligament reconstruction. It is a potent tool in the management of these complex problems.

Box 8.12.3 Chronic management

- Most chronic multiligament injuries require surgical reconstruction
- Grade 3 PCL injuries always associated with other ligament disruptions and usually require surgical repair/reconstruction
- Osteotomy can improve the results of ligament reconstruction in cases with associated malalignment.

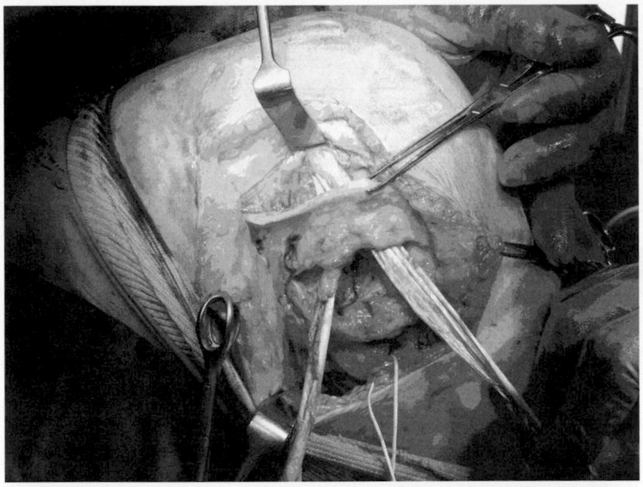

A

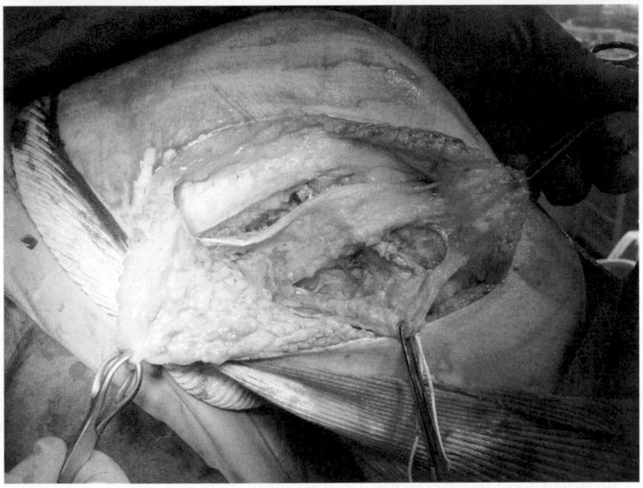

B

Fig. 8.12.3 Intra-operative photographs of posterolateral reconstruction. Following femoral fixation, hamstring graft is taken deep to the iliotibial tract (A), then through a fibula head tunnel (B).

Rehabilitation (Box 8.12.4)

This is complex and recovery will take place over 2 years following surgery for a knee dislocation. Most of the recovery occurs in the first 6 months, but patients should be counselled about the long process. Soft tissues should be dealt with early on with icing and patellar mobilizations to prevent fat pad contracture. Early motion is also important to reduce stiffness and help protect the joint surfaces. If a PCL reconstruction has been undertaken then flexion should be restricted to 60 degrees in the first few weeks as further flexion increase tension and may stretch the reconstruction. By 6 weeks from surgery, 90 degrees should be achieved in these cases with full flexion allowed by 12 weeks. To help protect the collateral ligaments, restricted extension can be helpful but tends to lead to a fixed flexion deformity which invariably results in a poor outcome. As a result many surgeons now insist on full extension (not hyperextension) as soon as possible after surgery.

Unlike ACL reconstruction, PCL reconstruction has a tendency to stretch and therefore the calf should always be supported when at rest for the first 3 months from surgery. In addition, when undertaking active flexion exercises, the therapist should apply an anterior tibial drawer to protect the PCL. The rehabilitation must progress much more slowly than that for ACL reconstruction.

Box 8.12.4 Rehabilitation

- Rehabilitation is complex and will take place over 2 years following surgery
- Most patients can manage activities of daily living and work following surgery
- Return to sport possible but carries significant risk of chondral damage.

Weight-bearing status is dependent upon the confidence in the reconstruction, but is generally encouraged as it helps restoration of normal lower limb muscle function.

A strengthening regimen should be started early but must avoid excess stress on the ligament. Proprioceptive drills start early on and become more challenging after 3 months.

Results

With an experienced surgeon the expectation is that at the end of surgical reconstruction in acute or chronic cases, normal laxity of all ligament groups should be obtained (and no more than grade I laxity by end of healing process). The long-term result is usually dependent on the presence or absence of significant chondral damage. In chronic cases, unfortunately most patients will have accumulated some chondral damage from the excess laxity in the ligament complexes, but even in acute cases chondral injury can mitigate against a good result. Although ligament laxity can be restored to near normal, the proprioceptive loss can never be fully addressed. Rehabilitation allows the patient to refine proprioception of the joint by enhanced feedback from structures around the joint. Unfortunately this is never normal and one must never forget what occurs in the situation of a Charcot joint. Some patients who are determined will certainly get back to sport, but particularly where long periods of running are involved, the risk that this will lead to chondral degeneration is high. Most patients are able to undertake activities of daily living and work without difficulty.

Further reading

Bottomley, N., Williams, A., Birch, R., Noorani, A., Lewis, A., and Lavelle, J. (2005). Displacement of the common peroneal nerve in posterolateral corner injuries of the knee. *Journal of Bone and Joint Surgery*, **87B**, 1225–6.

Harner, C.D., Waltrip, R.L., Bennett, C.H., Francis, K.A., Cole, B., and Irrgang, J.J. (2004). Surgical management of knee dislocations. *Journal of Bone and Joint Surgery*, **86A**, 262–73.

Liow, R.Y., McNicholas, M.J., Keating, J.F., and Nutton, R.W. (2003). Ligament repair and reconstruction in traumatic dislocation of the knee. *Journal of Bone and Joint Surgery*, **85B**, 845–51.

Recling, F.W. and Peltier, L.F. (2004). Acute knee dislocations and their complications. *Clinical Orthopaedics and Related Research*, **422**, 135–41.

Warren, L.F. and Marshall, J.L. (1979). The supporting structures and layers on the medial side of the knee. *Journal of Bone and Joint Surgery*, **61A**, 56–62.

8.13

Unicompartmental knee replacement

Hemant Pandit, Christopher Dodd, and David Murray

Summary points

- Ideal treatment option for end-stage osteoarthritis affecting a single compartment of the knee
- Unicompartmental knee replacement has many advantages over total knee replacement
  - Restores near normal kinematics
  - Usually gives a better range of movement
  - Patients require a shorter hospital stay
  - Fewer serious complications

Introduction

Primary osteoarthritis (OA) is common and predominantly presents after the fifth decade of life or later. In the USA, 12% of the adult population have signs and symptoms of the disease. It is a condition of the articular cartilage characterized by morphological, biochemical, molecular, and biomechanical changes to the cells and matrix which lead to softening, fibrillation, ulceration, and loss of cartilage. There is also sclerosis and eburnation of subchondral bone, with osteophyte and subchondral cyst formation. The aetiology is poorly understood and is believed to be multifactorial, with genetic and mechanical factors playing a major role. The characteristic manifestations of the disease are progressive pain, swelling, stiffness, and deformity which impede normal function and produce disability. The knee joint is one of the most commonly affected joints with an estimated incidence of 240/100 000 person-years. A number of characteristic patterns have been recognized in the knee: bilateral disease is more common than unilateral, tibiofemoral disease is more common than isolated patellofemoral disease, and finally with unicompartmental tibiofemoral disease, the medial side is more often affected than the lateral side.

Anteromedial OA of the knee was described as a pathological condition by White and colleagues in 1991. The cartilage erosion in the medial compartment is typically anterior or central in the tibial plateau, with preservation of cartilage posteriorly. There is a corresponding lesion on the distal femoral condyle. In extension, the femoral condyle sits within the tibial defect producing a varus deformity. The varus deformity corrects on flexing the knee as the preserved cartilage over the posterior part of the medial femoral condyle rides over the intact cartilage of the posterior tibial plateau. As a consequence, the medial collateral ligament is not shortened and the varus deformity remains correctible near extension. The anterior cruciate ligament (ACL) is usually preserved and it is postulated that retention of this structure prevents the OA from progressing to other compartments. This pattern of OA is believed to account for one in four osteoarthritic knees presenting for replacement in some centres. Knee replacement can be total or partial. In total knee replacement (TKR), both the medial and lateral tibiofemoral compartments are replaced with or without patella resurfacing. In partial or unicompartmental knee replacement (UKR), only the medial or the lateral (MCL) or the patellofemoral compartment is replaced.

The first UKRs used in clinical practice were the McIntosh (1954) and McKeever (1960) prostheses. More modern designs followed with the introduction of the Marmor (1972) and St Georg Sled (1976) implants. They have been widely used in both the medial and lateral compartments of the knee. Most UKR designs have a fixed polyethylene bearing (with or without a metal-backed tibia) and a polycentric femoral component. The medial Oxford UKR was designed by Goodfellow and O'Connor and was first used as a unicompartmental device in 1982. The design employs a spherical metal femoral component and a flat tibial base plate. Between the two an unconstrained polyethylene bearing is inserted. As the femur is spherical the bearing has fully congruent contact with both femur and tibia in all positions of flexion and extension. It therefore mimics the normal meniscus. The Oxford is the only UKR design which employs a fully congruous mobile bearing (Figure 8.13.1).

Surgical indications (Boxes 8.13.1 and 8.13.2)

In order to obtain good long-term results after UKR, the correct indications must be used. These are OA in the medial or lateral femorotibial compartment which may be primary OA or secondary due to osteonecrosis. In 1989, Kozinn and Scott suggested that

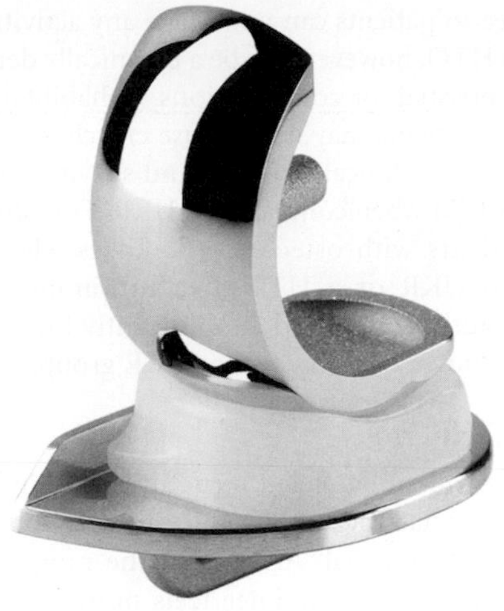

Fig. 8.13.1 Medial unicompartmental knee replacement.

the ideal candidate for a fixed bearing UKR is older than 60 years, not obese, and not extremely active with a preoperative range of motion of at least 5–90 degrees, a deformity of less than 15 degrees, and a clinically stable knee. According to Kozinn and Scott, contraindications for UKR are inflammatory arthropathy (e.g. rheumatoid arthritis), patello-femoral arthritis ligamentous instability, and tibial subluxation. The flexion deformity should be less than 15 degrees and the intra-articular angular deformity should be correctible suggesting that the collateral ligament is not shortened. The indications for the mobile bearing Oxford are different from those of fixed bearing UKR. There should be significant symptoms and anteromedial OA (or AVN). By this it is meant that there is full thickness medial OA with an intact ACL. There should also be full thickness lateral cartilage and a correctable varus deformity indicating that the MCL is functionally intact. These are best shown on a valgus stress x-ray. The Oxford group ignore the accepted contraindications as for the mobile bearing device they do not comprise the outcome. They therefore ignore age, obesity, chondrocalcinosis, activity, and patellofemoral joint damage. Previous high tibial osteotomy (HTO) is a relative contraindication as the failure rates of UKR with previous HTO are higher.

Surgical technique

Until 1997 UKR was usually performed through a surgical approach similar to TKR. In 1997, Repicci and Eberle showed that it was possible to resurface one compartment of the knee through a smaller incision extending from the proximal border of the patella to the proximal end of the tibia and that such an approach minimized the postoperative morbidity. This minimally invasive surgical (MIS) technique is now widely used to implant UKRs. Price and colleagues demonstrated that with a medial Oxford UKR, the average rate of recovery (as measured by time taken to achieve straight leg raise, 70 degrees of knee flexion, and independent stair climbing) was twice as fast as after an open incision UKR and three times faster than an open incision TKR. With MIS techniques, surgical damage to the soft tissues is reduced, injury to the quadriceps is minimal, patella is not dislocated, and the synovial reflections of the suprapatellar pouch remain intact.

Box 8.13.1 Prerequisites for UKR

- Isolated compartment arthritis (patellofemoral joint can be ignored)
- Intact ACL
- Correctible varus deformity
- Full thickness cartilage loss on both femur and tibia in the affected compartment.

Box 8.13.2 Contraindications for UKR

- Inflammatory arthropathy
- Previous HTO
- Ligamentous instability
- Tibial subluxation.

Results

The most commonly used unicompartmental prostheses, apart from the Oxford UKR have been fixed bearing devices. The early results of fixed bearing UKRs were not encouraging. Insall and Aglietti reported results of 32 fixed bearing UKRs. At 6 years postoperation only one was rated as excellent, seven knees as good, four as fair, and ten knees as poor. Seven knees (28%) had been revised. Similarly, Mallory and Danyi found a revision rate of 30% in a group of 42 procedures. More contemporary studies have also documented poor outcomes for some series of fixed bearing UKR—in particular the poor performance of the PCA fixed bearing UKR. This device has been shown to have poor survival and clinical outcomes, in association with catastrophic polyethylene wear.

Data from the Swedish Knee Arthroplasty Register illustrates that most commonly used contemporary fixed bearing devices in Sweden between 1990 and 1999 were the St Georg Sled, the Marmor, the Brigham, and the Miller–Galante prostheses. All four prostheses have a femoral component with polyradius geometry articulating with a flat polyethylene surface on the tibial side. Good clinical outcomes have been reported for each of these prostheses. The St Georg Sled is a fixed bearing device with an all polyethylene tibial tray. It was introduced into clinical use in 1985. Using the Bristol Knee Score system, Ansari and colleagues found that 92% of St Georg Sled prostheses reviewed had good or excellent outcome. More recently Ackroyd et al. reported the results of a series of 280 knees followed for a mean of 6 years, with excellent or good results were found in 77.9% of patients using the same knee scoring system. The designer of the Marmor implant has published the results of a series of 60 knees followed for 10–13 years. Using the HSS (Hospital for Special Surgery) rating system, 30 were excellent, eight good, four fair, and 18 poor. Seventy per cent of the patients had satisfactory results and pain relief was accomplished in 86.6% cases. Squire and colleagues published an independent series of Marmor prostheses that had been followed for a minimum of 15 years with a mean HSS score of 82. The Brigham prosthesis was introduced to clinical practice in 1981. Scott et al. reported 100 consecutive Brigham UKRs reviewed after 8–12 years, 64 knees (51 patients) being reviewed clinically at last follow-up. Of these, 87% had no significant pain. Argenson reported on the results of a series of 160 consecutive Miller–Galante prostheses with a mean preoperative HSS score of 59 improving to 97 at the final review (mean follow-up 5.5 years; range 3–10).

Various studies have been published demonstrating excellent results of the medial Oxford UKR with survival rates at 10 years of 94–100%. Svard and Price described a 95% survival of the implant at 15 years. Rajasekhar et al. reported on 135 Oxford UKRs implanted in a district general hospital by a single surgeon. The mean follow-up was 5.8 years (2–12 years). Five knees have been revised giving a cumulative rate of survival of the prosthesis at 10 years of 94% (95% confidence interval (CI) 84.0–97.8). Knee rating and patient function were assessed using the modified Knee Society scoring system. The mean knee score was 92.2 (95% CI 51–100) and the mean functional score 76.2 (95% CI 51–100). Although not all centres have achieved such good results, the Swedish Knee Arthroplasty Register has shown that those undertaking at least two replacements per month achieved a survival of about 93% at 9 years. These long-term results have also shown that with this device if the failures do occur, they tend to occur early. This is in part because of the fully congruous mobile bearing, which reduces the risk of long-term failure due to wear.

Table 8.13.1 summarizes the majority of the published 10-year survival results from series of 100 or more medial and/or lateral UKR.

UKR versus HTO

HTO is an accepted treatment for unicompartmental OA of the knee. A well done osteotomy should overcorrect the deformity of the mechanical axis of the limb to pass through the lateral side of the knee which unloads the medial compartment of the knee and reduces symptoms. This can overload the lateral compartment which in turn may fail. The advantage of HTO is that it maintains the native knee so patients can undertake any activities they want. Conventional HTO, however, can be a technically demanding procedure with potential for complications. Rehabilitation is usually prolonged and patients may have to use crutches for an extended period of time. The clinical outcome and survivorship after HTO tends to be inferior when compared to UKR. One study compared groups of patients with osteoarthritic knees who had either a St Georg Sled UKR or a HTO at a minimum follow up of 12 years. The authors reported a significantly lower revision rate and better functional outcome for the UKR group.

UKR versus TKR

UKR preserves all undamaged structures within the joint, in particular the cruciate ligaments, and can therefore restore knee function nearly to normal. After UKR the range of movement is better than after TKR, the knee feels more natural, and pain relief is as good or better. In terms of morbidity, infection is less common as is the requirement for postoperative blood transfusion. Recovery is more rapid and the postoperative gait is more physiological. Knee kinematics after UKR are restored to normal, unlike after TKR.

However, UKR has the disadvantage that the medium- and long-term revision rates are generally higher than for TKR. The primary reason for this is that UKRs are easier to revise than a TKR so they tend to be revised for less severe symptoms. Other reasons include:

- The high polyethylene wear rate of thin tibial components subjected to incongruous loading
- Imprecise (and inappropriate) patient selection
- Lack of instruments to accurately implant the device.

The issue of high polyethylene wear is dependent on the design of the implant. Fixed bearing devices tend to fail early because of wear in young active patients. The Oxford UKR maintains high contact area (about $6cm^2$) throughout the range of knee movement and therefore the contact pressure is low with this device. Measurement of retrieved bearings has shown a mean linear

Table 8.13.1 Published 10 year survival results for UKR (with 100 or more patients at start)

Year	Author	Compartment	Prosthesis	Number	10-year survival (95% CI)
1986	Knutson	Medial	Marmor	2354	92 (89–94)
1988	Marmor	Medial/lateral	Marmor	228	70 (?)
1986	Knutson	Medial	St Georg	1345	89 (82–92)
1991	Neider	Medial	St Georg	548	80 (?)
1997	Ansari	Medial	St Georg	461	87 (81–93)
1998	Murray	Medial	Oxford	144	98 (93–100)
2001	Svard	Medial	Oxford	124	(90.7–99.3)
2004	Rajasekhar	Medial	Oxford	135	94 (844–97)
1991	Scott	Medial/lateral	Brigham	100	85 (67–99)
1998	Bert	Medial	MBUKA	100	87 (?)
2002	Argenson	Medial	Miller–Galante	160	94 (91–97)

?: Confidence intervals not mentioned in the publication.

wear rate of 0.03mm/year and even less (0.01mm/year) if the knee had been functioning normally with no impingement.

Over the years, the surgical technique and instrumentation have been refined. Provided a good UKR device is implanted correctly in correct patients, the long-term survival can be similar to that of TKR.

Revision of UKR to TKR

Revision of a UKR to a TKR is technically less demanding than revision of a TKR. This is primarily due to preservation of native bone in the retained compartment. The use of constrained or stemmed TKR implants is rarely necessary and bone graft if needed can be obtained from the revision cuts, thereby allowing the surgeon to use patient's own bone. Martin et al. reported the outcome of 23 Oxford UKRs revised to TKRs with a mean follow-up of 4.1 years. Only one patient needed rerevision for infection. In addition, in all the cases except one routine implant could be used without the addition of any augments or constraints.

Lateral UKR

Isolated lateral compartment arthritis is less common than its medial counterpart. It can occur as a sequel to a previous lateral meniscectomy or significant trauma and is usually associated with femoral valgus. Therefore, lateral UKR only account for around 10% of all UKRs. In the lateral compartment of the knee during flexion and rotation there is a large amount of movement of the femoral condyle on the tibia. Many designs of UKR do not account for this increased translation and the kinematics can be suboptimal. The increasing movement offered by a mobile bearing would seem ideally suited to address this problem and a mobile bearing lateral UKR would be a sensible choice. However, in the past, results of a mobile bearing lateral UKR have been disappointing with a 5-year survival of 82% with commonest reason for failure being bearing dislocation. Dislocation is thought to be much more common in the lateral compartment because in flexion, the lateral collateral ligament is slack whereas on the medial side MCL remains tight. This allows the lateral compartment to be distracted on average 7mm, whereas the medial can only be distracted on average 2mm. Recently a new design of Oxford Knee has been introduced specifically for the lateral side (Figure 8.13.2). This has a domed tibial component and a biconcave mobile bearing. When used with a modified surgical technique this has significantly reduced the risk of bearing dislocation with an improvement in range of movement.

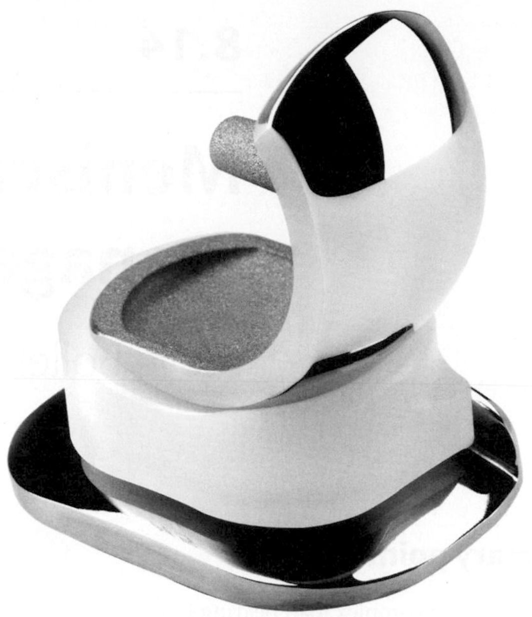

Fig. 8.13.2 Domed lateral unicompartmental knee replacement.

Summary

UKR has many advantages over TKR and is the preferred treatment option for arthritis limited to a single compartment of the knee. The procedure can be performed using minimally invasive surgical technique. Long-term failure rates can be reduced by proper patient selection, good surgical technique, and with the use of sophisticated instrumentation and optimal implant design.

Further reading

Kozinn, S.C. and Scott, R. (1989). Unicondylar knee arthroplasty. *Journal of Bone and Joint Surgery*, **71A**, 145–50.

Murray, D.W., Goodfellow, J.W., and O'Connor, J.J. (1998). The Oxford medial unicompartmental arthroplasty: a ten-year survival study. *Journal of Bone and Joint Surgery*, **80B**, 983–9.

Newman J.H., Ackroyd, C.E., and Shah, N.A. (1998). Unicompartmental or total knee replacement? Five-year results of a prospective, randomised trial of 102 osteoarthritic knees with unicompartmental arthritis. *Journal of Bone and Joint Surgery*, **50B**, 862–5.

Weale, A.E. and Newman, J.H. (1994). Unicompartmental arthroplasty and high tibial osteotomy for osteoarthrosis of the knee. A comparative study with a 12- to 17-year follow-up period. *Clinical Orthopaedics and Related Research*, **302**, 134–7.

White, S.H., Ludkowski, P.F., and Goodfellow, J.W. (1991). Anteromedial osteoarthritis of the knee. *Journal of Bone and Joint Surgery*, **73B**, 582–6.

8.14

Meniscal injury and management

Steve Bollen

Summary points

- Menisci have a complex load bearing function
- Loss leads to accelerated articular cartilage wear
- Injury is common but symptomatic relief straightforward with skilled arthroscopic surgery
- Peripheral tears have a blood supply and are potentially repairable.

Introduction

In the past, scant regard was paid to these collagenous structures, and almost any patient with a symptomatic knee, whatever their age, would have them totally removed through an arthrotomy with a Smillie knife.

Over time a more conservative surgical approach has evolved as surgeons have realized that menisci actually have an important role in knee function and that meniscectomized knees inevitably progress to accelerated osteoarthrosis. Arthroscopy has revolutionized the management of meniscal injury, allowing minimal resection or repair, with minimal morbidity and an extremely low complication rate.

Structure, function, and biomechanics

The menisci are semilunar in plan view, wedge-shaped in cross-section, and consist predominately of type 1 collagen, although types II, III, V, and VI are present in small amounts. Type II fibres are more prominent on the surface layers. They are attached circumferentially to the capsule and at either end to the tibial surface by strong ligaments (Figure 8.14.1). In addition, the posterior horn of the lateral meniscus has two ligaments (Wrisberg and Humphrey) which pass either side of the posterior cruciate ligament to the medial femoral condyle.

The predominant orientation of collagen bundles is circumferential, with a small number of radially orientated 'tie' fibres. When load is applied, the orientation of the fibres, with the meniscus fixed at either end, allows the generation of 'hoop stresses' and this in turn absorbs load across the joint. In the medial compartment the meniscus absorbs 40% of the load across the tibiofemoral joint and the lateral compartment 60% due to its higher relative surface area.

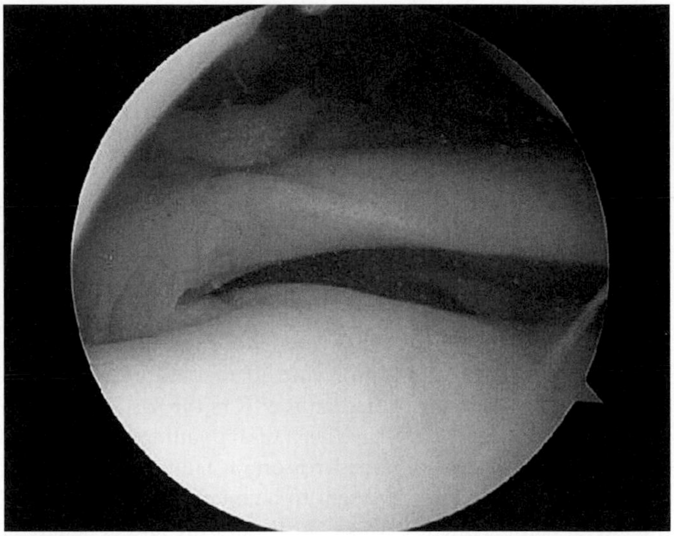

Fig. 8.14.1 A view of the posterior horn of the lateral meniscus showing its ligamentous attachment to the tibial plateau.

This becomes even more important when the anatomy of the tibial plateau on either side of the joint is taken into account. In the medial compartment the medial tibial plateau is concave and in the lateral compartment, convex. The consequences of loss of a meniscus are therefore much more severe on the lateral side of the joint, where without the meniscus there is almost point contact between the articular surfaces. The high contact stresses that this creates can lead to the rapid development of wear.

'Dynamic' magnetic resonance imaging (MRI) studies have shown that the medial meniscus is static during flexion and extension making the posterior horn vulnerable to tearing in extremes of flexion. The lateral meniscus, however, is extremely mobile during flexion and extension, virtually coming off the back of the lateral tibial plateau during full flexion.

The only common developmental variation is the discoid meniscus which almost exclusively occurs on the lateral side (Figure 8.14.2)

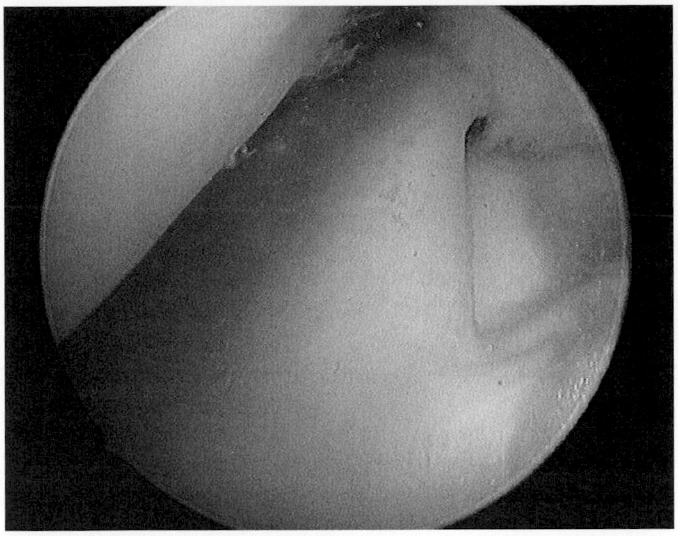

Fig. 8.14.2 A discoid lateral meniscus.

and has a prevalence of approximately 5%. This can produce symptoms at a very young age.

History

In the younger patient the typical history of injury is of a weight-bearing, twisting injury. Pain is localized to the affected joint line. Swelling usually occurs slowly overnight and often settles in a few days.

In non-sporting situations, patients with occupations that involve working with the knees in full flexion such as electricians, plumbers, etc., are prone to tearing the posterior horn of the medial meniscus.

In the more chronic situation, there is recurrent pain localized to the affected joint line and intermittent swelling.

Examination

Chronic meniscal injuries usually produce a degree of quadriceps wasting. There may be subtle losses of either terminal extension or flexion. It is important to look for a small effusion as this may confirm intra-articular pathology. There may be joint line tenderness and a positive McMurray's test.

Investigation

Plain x-rays (anteroposterior weight bearing, intercondylar and lateral) are useful, where early degenerative change may be identified and will exclude a number of other pathologies. Degenerative tears of the medial meniscus can produce narrowing of the posteromedial joint space on the intercondylar view.

MRI is only indicated where the diagnosis is in doubt after history, examination, and plain x-rays. MRI is neither 100% sensitive nor specific for either medial or lateral meniscal pathology and may completely miss a reduced peripheral bucket handle tear. It also has a false positive rate, especially in patients over the age of 40 where there is almost always a degenerate signal in the posterior horn of the medial meniscus which is difficult to distinguish from a degenerate tear.

MRI diagnosis should always be taken in conjunction with history and examination before subjecting the patient to surgery.

Differential diagnosis

Early compartment wear and small chondral lesions of the femoral or tibial surfaces can produce symptoms very similar to that of a meniscal tear and these may not be picked up on MRI scanning.

On the medial side of the joint, a medial plica and injury to the deep part of the medial collateral ligament (Figure 8.14.3) may also produce a clinical picture that is difficult to differentiate from a meniscal tear and these are also unlikely to be diagnosed on MRI.

Patterns of injury

Flap tears

Flap tears (Figure 8.14.4) tend to produce intermittent symptoms, with a feeling of catching and clicking. If in the middle third of the meniscus the patient may be able to feel something 'pop out' at the joint line. (If the lump always appears at the same site it will be a flap tear and not a loose body.)

Occasionally the flap will tuck itself underneath the rim of the meniscus—these tears often produce a fairly constant and quite significant pain. At arthroscopy there is a rounded appearance to the edge of the meniscus and the offending fragment can be retrieved into the joint with an arthroscopic probe, before resection.

Bucket handle tears

These tears may present with a locked knee or produce intermittent symptoms of true locking. A locked knee due to a torn meniscus presents with an inability to fully extend the knee with pain localized to the site of the pathology. Locking in full extension tends to be produced by patellofemoral pathology.

In the acute situation peripheral bucket handle tears may produce a haemarthrosis.

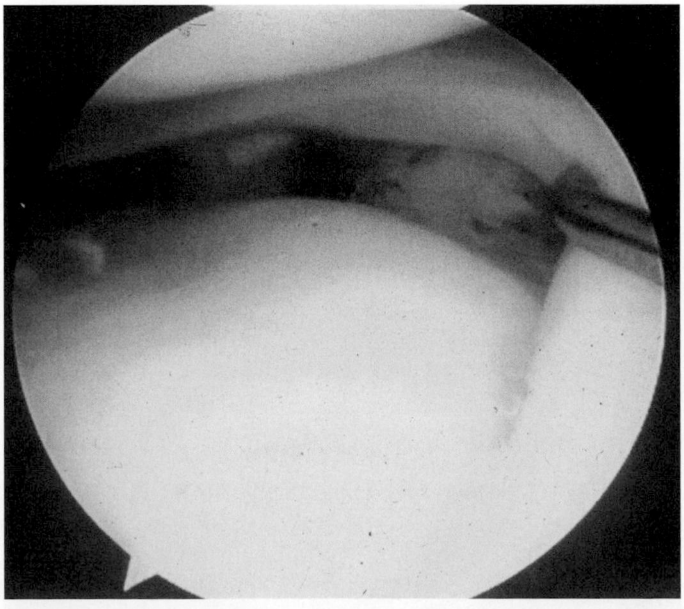

Fig. 8.14.3 An injury to the deep part of the medial collateral ligament.

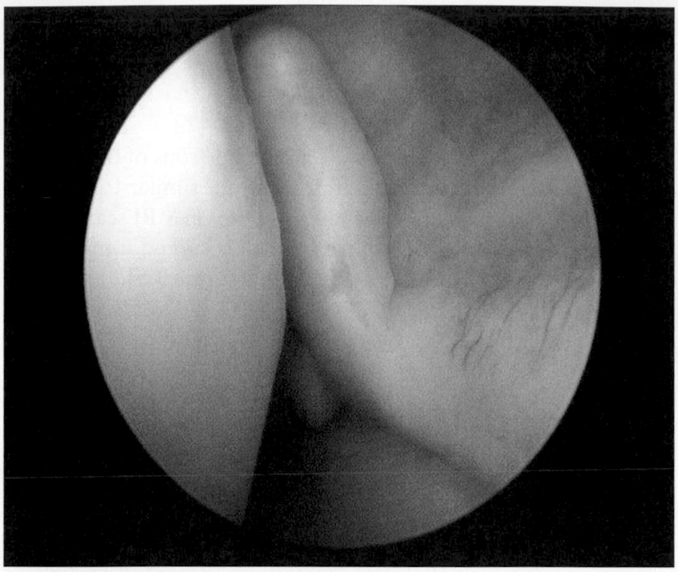

Fig. 8.14.4 A typical flap tear of the medial meniscus.

Once locked, the knee may spontaneously 'clunk' back into extension or, as patients learn how to unlock the knee, by hyperflexing and rotating the joint.

Horizontal cleavage tears

Horizontal cleavage tears (Figure 8.14.5) can act like flap valves allowing synovial fluid to be forced out of the joint during knee flexion and then not allowing it to return. This produces a meniscal cyst, classically seen on the lateral side. Meniscal cysts are not uncommon on the medial side but are less visible because of the broad medial collateral ligament.

Symptoms are of a chronic aching pain localized over the cyst, often worse at night. On the lateral side, a bony hard cyst may be found, localized to the joint line and, most pronounced at 45 degrees of flexion.

Almost invariably on the lateral side, there is a small radial tear at the junction of middle and anterior thirds with a horizontal cleavage behind it, leading into the cyst.

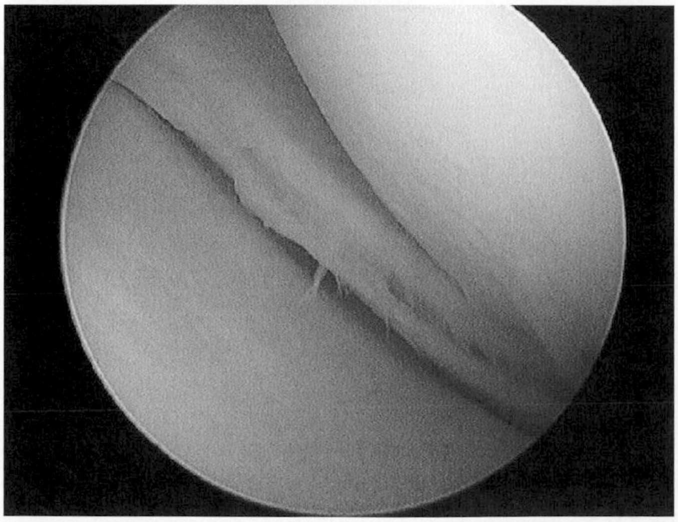

Fig. 8.14.5 A horizontal cleavage tear of the posterior horn.

Degenerate tears

Degenerate type tears are usually complex with a combination of flap and horizontal cleavage patterns. Sometimes initial inspection may appear relatively normal but there may be an inferior partial thickness tear which then leads in to a horizontal cleavage component.

On the medial side with degenerate posterior horn tears, there may be limitation of flexion and difficulty with squatting. Patients often also complain of pain at night when sleeping on their side with the knees placed together.

Treatment

There are some tears that do not require treatment. Partial thickness or short (less than 5mm) full thickness split tears that are stable and small radial tears can safely be left, particularly if they are asymptomatic.

The majority of symptomatic meniscal tears are treated by arthroscopic resection of the damaged portion of the meniscus leaving as much normal tissue as possible. This results in a speedy resolution of symptoms with minimal morbidity.

Portal placement is critical in making resection technically easier. For a lateral meniscal tear an anterolateral portal for the arthroscope and a medial portal in the middle of the 'soft spot', with the knee in the 'figure 4' position, for the instruments, allows ready access to most of the meniscus. Slightly extending the knee makes surgery to the anterior horn easier.

On the medial side, an anterolateral portal and a low medial portal just over the anterior horn allows access to the posteromedial aspect of the joint. This is aided by a side post at mid-thigh and a strong assistant (or a leg holder) to open out the joint which can sometimes be very tight. Surgery to the anterior third may be aided by swapping the arthroscope to the medial portal and arthroscopic tools to the lateral.

A variety of sharp specialist tools with upbiters, sidebiters, and arthroscopic shavers are essential to provide speedy, low-morbidity surgery, without damage to the surrounding articular cartilage.

In degenerate tears of the posterior horn of the medial meniscus, where there is virtually always a horizontal cleavage component, it is important to remove the inferior leaf of the horizontal cleavage to prevent recurrence of symptoms.

In the absence of associated pathology, recovery to full activity takes on average 4–6 weeks on the medial and 6–8 weeks on the lateral side following resection of a meniscal tear.

Meniscal repair

It was King who first observed that menisci have a limited and peripheral blood supply and that meniscal tears could heal, but only when they involved the peripheral third of the meniscus. This work was expanded by Arnoszky and Warren and their work led to the development of a variety of techniques for repairing appropriate meniscal tears rather than just excising them.

The current techniques of repair are either inside–outside (passing suture needles through the meniscus and out through a separate lateral or medial incision) if the tear involves the anterior two-thirds of the meniscus, or inside–inside with a 'stapling' device if the tear involves the posterior horn. Devices available include bioabsorbable darts, arrows, and screws as well as devices

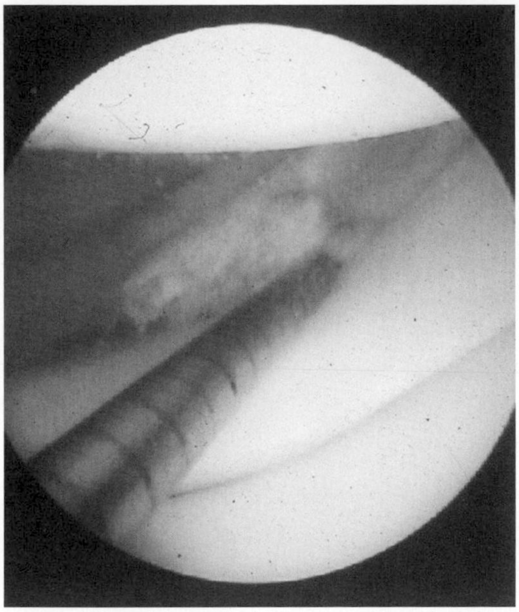

Fig. 8.14.6 A red on red lateral meniscal bucket handle tear—an ideal indication for repair.

that use preknotted sutures. It is important to mix superior and inferior surface sutures to prevent the meniscus rucking up.

In an intact knee, a bucket handle tear involving the periphery of the meniscus with bleeding on both sides of the repair ('red on red'), healing rates are in the region of 66% (Figure 8.14.6).

Rates of healing decrease if the tear is more than 4 weeks old, the peripheral rim width is greater than 4mm, or the patient is over 40 years of age. Rates of healing are better if the repair is done in conjunction with anterior cruciate ligament reconstruction.

Rehabilitation after repair is controversial with a range of protocols recommended from non-weight bearing and restricted range of motion, to full weight bearing with no restriction of range of movement or limitation of activity. Early full weight bearing and motion do not seem to be detrimental to healing rates, although limiting knee flexion to 90 degrees for 6 weeks and only returning to sport at 12 weeks seems a sensible approach.

The future

As the consequences of this common injury have become recognized, the challenge has been to find a solution that will prevent premature degenerative change occurring, lessen patients' symptoms (predominately pain), and improve function. This has largely been on two fronts.

Meniscal replacement

Clinical trials of the use of collagen scaffolds sutured into the meniscal defect with the aim of allowing healing to occur were carried out in the early 1990s. Despite promising initial and even medium-term results, this technique has not gained widespread acceptance.

Future developments may include implantation of patients' fibrocytes into the synthetic collagen matrix, the use of growth factors, and tissue manipulation with gene therapy.

Meniscal transplant

Another key development has been the development of meniscal transplantation, where a suitably sized meniscal allograft is either sutured to a meniscal rim, or is transplanted with a bone bock and ligaments at either end and fixed into a suitably prepared bed.

The experience in both Europe and the USA has been encouraging with satisfactory early to medium-term results in reducing patient symptoms. Long-term results still remain uncertain, however, as does the best technique for preservation, sizing, and implantation.

Further reading

McDermott, I.D. and Amis, A.A. (2006). The consequences of meniscectomy. *Journal of Bone and Joint Surgery*, **88B**, 1549–56.

Seedhom B.B., Hargreaves D.J. (1979). Transmission of the load in the knee joint with special reference to the role of the menisci. *Engineering in Medicine*, **8**, 220–8.

Tenuta J.J. and Arciero R.A. (1994). Arthroscopic evaluation of meniscal repairs – factors that affect healing. *American Journal of Sports Medicine*, **22**, 797–802.

Vedi, V., Williams, A.M., Tennant, S., Hunt, D., and Gedroyc, W. (1999). Meniscal motion – an in vivo study employing magnetic resonance imaging in near real-time in the weight-bearing and non-weight-bearing knee. *Journal of Bone and Joint Surgery*, **81B**, 37–41.

Verdonk, P.C.M., Verstraete, K.L., Almqvist, K.F, *et al.* (2006). Meniscal allograft transplantation: long-term clinical results with radiological and magnetic resonance imaging correlations. *Knee Surgery, Sports Traumatology, Arthroscopy*, **14**, 694–706.

SECTION 9

The Foot

9.1

Ankle and hindfoot arthritis

Paul H. Cooke and Andy Goldberg

Summary points

- Hind foot arthritis is usually treated orthotically but may need surgical fusion
- Severe ankle arthritis requiring surgical intervention is uncommon
- Arthroscopic debridement of early ankle arthritis is effective
- End stage ankle arthritis can be treated by fusion or arthroplasty
- Ankle replacement has a higher failure rate than hip or knee arthroplasty
- Correct alignment of the hind foot and forefoot are essential for good results.

Introduction

The ankle, hindfoot, and midfoot function as a mobile unit, which provides shock absorption in the early stance phase of gait, and changes to a rigid unit in the late stance phase allowing transmission of power necessary for push off.

Within this complex, the ankle moves principally in dorsiflexion and plantarflexion, the subtalar joint in inversion/eversion, and the midfoot in rotation.

In early stance phase, the plantar fascia and interosseous ligaments are relaxed, the arch is low, and the joints of the hind- and midfoot are mobile, allowing shock absorption by the foot without damaging impacts being transmitted that could cause injury to the foot, the leg, and the trunk.

In later stance phase, the plantar fascia tightens and the arch is restored (by the windlass mechanism, Figure 9.1.1), and all the interosseous ligaments tighten, making the foot rigid. This allows power to be transmitted through the foot, and the weight of the body to be transferred forward without the foot collapsing.

This rigidity is critical to function of the hind- and mid foot, and the patient's ability to stand and walk, so the mainstay of treating disorders of these regions is directed to relieving pain and stabilizing the foot—usually by orthotics or fusion—whereas in the ankle movement may be more important so joint replacement is sometimes performed.

The outcomes of all midfoot, hindfoot, and ankle procedures are often limited, achieving a 'second best' result of a stable pain-free foot, with the ability to walk and function domestically, but rarely restoring the levels of function required for running, and athletic or high demands.

The problems of the hind- and midfoot and the ankle will be considered separately for clarity, although deformity and pain often occur together in all.

Hindfoot and midfoot arthritis

Anatomy

The hindfoot comprises the talus, calcaneus, and navicular bones, as well as their articulations, which are responsible for most of the inversion/eversion of the foot (subtalar joint) and rotation (talonavicular and calcaneocuboid joints).

In the midfoot the cuboid and cuneiform bones articulate to increase rotation of the foot, but the movements in the midfoot are less than those of the hindfoot.

Dorsiflexion of the foot complex is really limited to the ankle and metatarsophalangeal level.

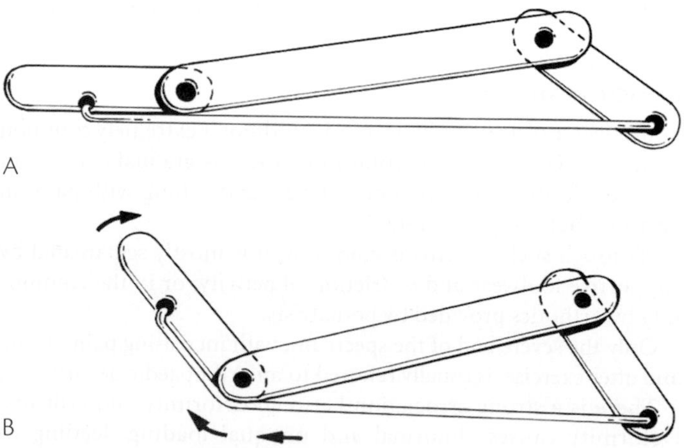

A

B

Fig. 9.1.1 A) In the flat foot position (early stance of gait) the toes are neutral to the metatarsals, the plantar fascia is relaxed, and the arch is low and mobile, because the interosseous ligaments are loose in this position. B) At end stance, the foot rolls forward, extending the metatarsophalangeal joint and winding up the windlass of the plantar fascia. This causes elevation of the arch and rigidity of the foot as the interosseous ligaments tighten.

Each of the joints of the hindfoot and midfoot allow some plantarflexion from their neutral position—contributing about 50% of the overall dorsiflexion/plantarflexion movement of the foot/ankle complex—but none of these joints allow any significant dorsiflexion.

The hindfoot and midfoot rely on a complex arrangement of ligaments between joints for stability, and on tendons which insert into or cross the region for movement.

The blood and nerve supplies of the region are rich, with abundant vessels and nerves which have to be respected by surgical approaches.

In contrast, the soft tissue envelope is thin, prone to injury, and gives little cover to underlying tissues or implanted metalwork.

Swelling of the soft tissues after surgery, especially with dependency during immobilization, makes the area prone to soft tissue break down. Furthermore, the bones of the hindfoot and midfoot generally (with the exception of the calcaneus) have few, if any, muscle attachments and therefore have relatively poor blood supplies. Hence the incidence of delayed or non-union after fusion is higher than in other areas of the body.

When arthritis and collapse occur, the pathological anatomy is changed, with complex deformities produced by unbalanced forces acting on bones and joints producing simultaneous subluxation, dislocation, and bone and joint deformity.

Correction of the deformities is difficult, and although it is tempting to plan simple angular corrections, careful consideration based on findings on clinical examination, biplanar radiographs, and, if necessary, scans often shows rotational and multilevel deformity. If function is to be restored, the deformities have to be corrected in all planes.

Thus, surgery in this area is fraught with potential problems due to geometric complexity and problems with healing. Surgeons undertaking this surgery need to understand these factors and also be able to manage the postoperative splintage, rehabilitation, and orthotic management of the patients.

For all these reasons, and at a time when experience of this type of surgery is waning—because of the virtual disappearance of polio and spina bifida within the United Kingdom— surgery to the mid- and hindfoot is now increasingly limited to specialist tertiary referral centres.

Presentation

Some degree of arthritis in the hind-/midfoot is extremely common with advancing age. Most commonly there is gradual collapse of the arch, leading to increasing stiffness and aching with pain on exertion, but rest pain is rare.

Although such arthritis is common, it is mostly self-treated by supportive footwear and restriction of activity, or in the community by orthotics provided by podiatrists.

Only the severe end of the spectrum, with increasing pain during and after exercise, is usually referred to an orthopaedic department.

There is a strong association between deformity and arthritis. Deformity causes abnormal and unequal loading, leading to arthritic wear and tear, and conversely arthritis often causes collapse of individual bones and abnormal alignment of joints affecting the stability of the longitudinal and transverse arches.

Aetiology

The causes fall into five groups (Box 9.1.1).

Box 9.1.1 Causes of hind- and midfoot arthritis

1) Post traumatic: especially major injuries and talar injuries
2) Systemic arthritis
3) Deformity
4) Coalition
5) Neuropathy.

Post-traumatic

A history of trauma is common in patients presenting to tertiary referral centres.

The hindfoot and midfoot are constantly exposed to low levels of trauma, being vulnerable with every trip and slip, and cumulative effects may account for the wear and tear changes commonly found with advancing age.

More major trauma has an association with arthritis, especially when joint integrity is affected.

Injuries to the talus are associated with avascular necrosis due to its poor blood supply, especially after fractures of the neck of the talus, and dislocations. Peritalar arthritis affecting ankle, subtalar and/or talonavicular arthritis then often occur.

Complex calcaneal fractures also often lead to subtalar arthritis. However, even badly destroyed joints sometimes lead to more stiffness than pain, and this may give relatively little restriction.

The risk of developing painful arthritis is linked to the severity of the original injury. The method of early treatment is less well associated with outcome. So open treatment of calcaneal fractures may not decrease the risk of later pain, but anatomical reduction makes any later reconstructive surgery easier and more effective.

In the midfoot, arthritis may follow fracture dislocations including Lisfranc injuries.

Good reduction of the fractures and dislocations is important, because with a well-shaped foot, orthotic management can often control symptoms without resorting to reconstructive surgery.

Systemic arthropathy (Figure 9.1.2A)

All forms of arthritis present in the hind- and midfoot.

Seronegative arthropathies present with heel pain due to enthesopathy.

Generalized osteoarthrithis presents with painful arch collapse, or localized arthritis - usually of the subtalar or talonavicular joints.

Rheumatoid arthritis commonly affects the region and may take one of two general forms. Proliferative synovitis can cause laxity, dislocation of the joints, and collapse of the arch, leading to planovalgus collapse with secondary arthritic changes.

In another group of patients—often with severely painful but less swollen joints—spontaneous ankylosis and eventually arthrodesis can occur. This is a common pattern in patients with rapidly progressive disease and in juvenile chronic arthritis.

Deformity

Deformity may occur due to weakness or imbalance. Two common patterns of deformity occur:

- Planovalgus deformity due to weakness of the tibialis posterior tendon (described in Chapter 9.5)

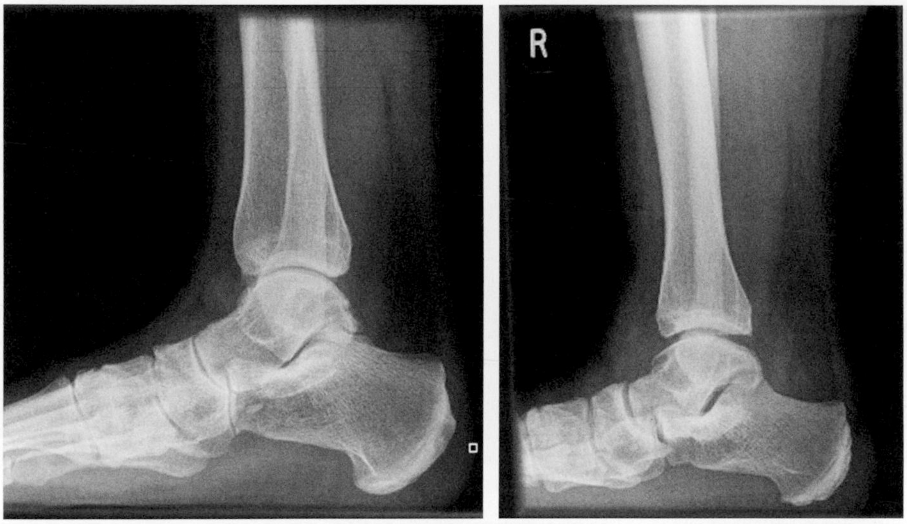

A B

Fig. 9.1.2 Degenerative changes occurring as a result of (A) generalized arthritis (rheumatoid arthritis) and (B) neuropathic degeneration (Charcot disease).

- Equinocavovarus occurs secondary to muscle imbalance between weak dorsiflexors and evertors and relatively stronger invertors and plantarflexors and is common in neurological disease and after other foot deformities, including congenital clubfoot.

Secondary to restricted movement

Congenital coalitions of the hind- and midfoot lead to pain and degeneration. The commonest coalitions—calcaneo navicular, and subtalar—lead to pain and degeneration in the talonavicular and subtalar joints respectively. These often present later as pain in adult life, and by this time degeneration is often established and take down of the joints is rarely indicated.

Stiffness, including surgically induced stiffness, may also lead to secondary degeneration.

Neuropathic (Figure 9.1.2B)

Charcot's joints are joints with severe degeneration—often with collapse and deformity—and occur in the presence of any sensory neuropathy. They are commonest in diabetes, usually in severe diabetes, and as such are dealt with in Chapter 9.3.

The careful clinician will always test for sensory loss when presented with a case of hind- and midfoot degeneration, using a tuning fork to test for vibration, and a Semmes–Weinstein filament to touch light sensation. A significant number of patients with early diabetes and other causes, including reversible neuropathies, will be diagnosed by these simple means—supplemented by blood screening for neuropathy when abnormalities are found.

Clinical presentation

Arthritis of the hind- and midfoot leads to stiffness, pain, or, more commonly, a combination of both.

Stiffness is not usually a great problem except when single joints are affected in younger people who still participate in sporting activities, or in patients where spontaneous ankylosis of the whole complex occurs (usually in rheumatoid arthritis). In these situations, stiffness may impose extra demands on other joints in the foot, ankle, or elsewhere.

Pain, whether in single or multiple joints, tends to be present on standing and walking, and absent when sitting, lying, or asleep.

Pain which wakens the patient from sleep can occur as an end stage of joint destruction, but should alert the clinician to the risks of infection or tumour.

Examination (Figure 9.1.3)

Examination of pulses, perfusion, and sensation are essential parts of examination of any foot condition.

Clinical examination also involves observing the foot standing (Figure 9.1.3A,B) and on tip-toe standing (Figure 9.1.3C), measuring dorsiflexion/plantarflexion (Figure 9.1.3D,E) of the foot (including ankle movement, Figure 9.1.3F), inversion and eversion (Figure 9.1.3G,H) and rotation (9.1.3I,J), as well as simple examination of power of the muscle groups (Figures 9.1.3K–N).

Simple investigation is usually more helpful than complex scanning, which is reserved for a minority of cases.

Investigations

Blood tests may be indicated to investigate arthritis and accompanying neuropathy.

Plain x-rays taken non-weight bearing will show structure, but weight-bearing films will show loss of joint space and deformity which may occur only on standing (Figure 9.1.3A). Oblique views may be useful to show coalition and Cobey (skiers) views will show the relative contributions of the ankle and the subtalar joints to deformity of the hindfoot in standing (Figure 9.1.3B).

Magnetic resonance imaging (MRI) scans can be useful to isolate a single inflamed joint, and computed tomography (CT) scans to demonstrate structure in complex situations, but when surgical intervention is considered, selective diagnostic injection of affected joints is the most useful supplementary investigation. The reason for this is that the joints are difficult or impossible to differentiate clinically—even by the most experienced clinician. The worst affected joint on x-ray is not always the most painful joint.

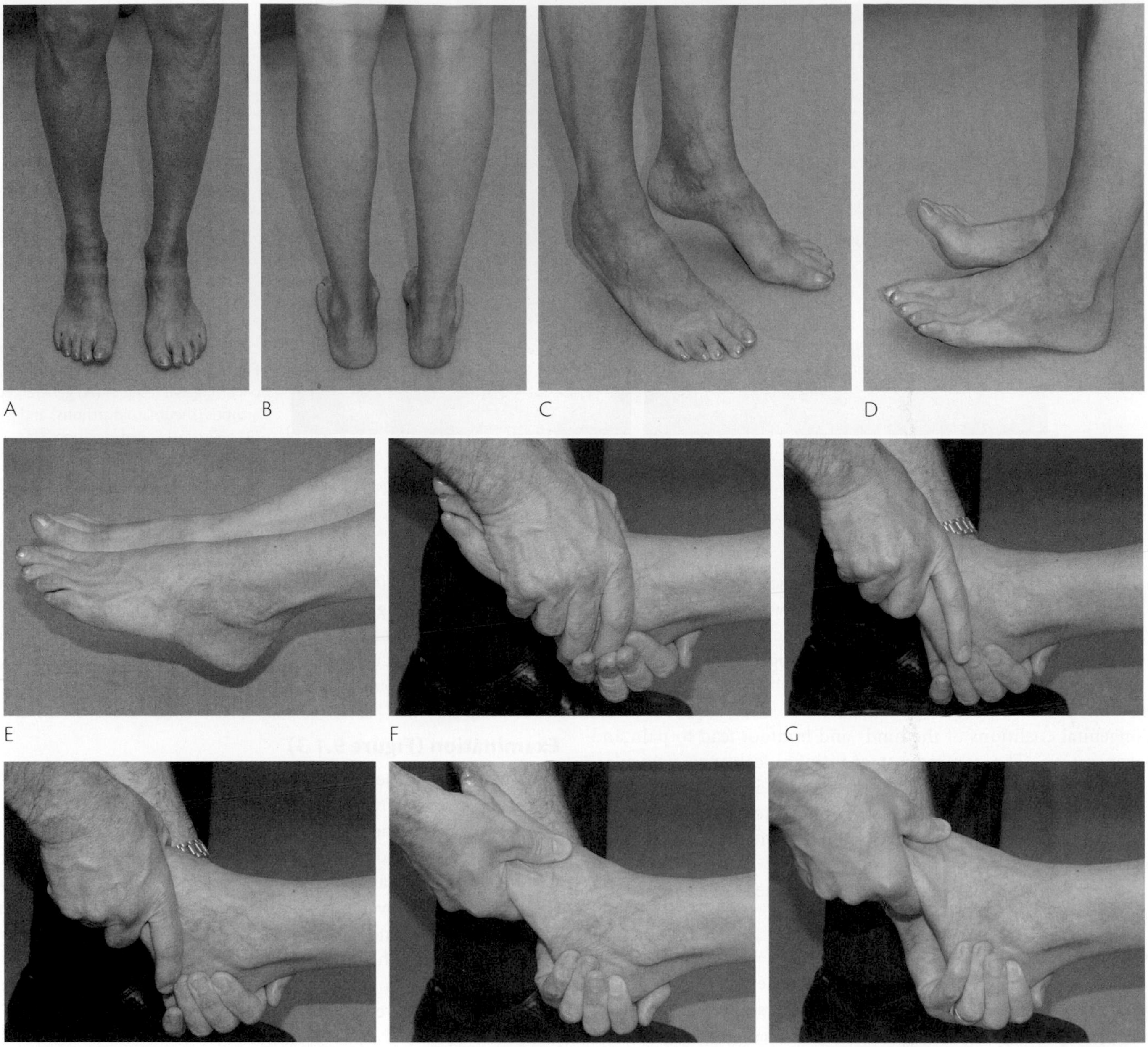

A B C D E F G H I J

Fig. 9.1.3 Examination of the ankle, hind-, and midfoot. A,B,C) The foot is observed from in front and behind in standing and on toe raising—note position and increased arch on tip-toe raise. D,E,F) Maximum foot and ankle dorsiflexion (D) and plantarflexion (E) are compared with the normal side (F) to measure isolated ankle dorsiflexion/plantarflexion, the subtalar and midtarsal joints are immobilized by the examiner's hand. G,H) Inversion and eversion are measured whilst immobilizing midtarsal rotation. This measures subtalar movement and any abnormal ankle movement present. I,J) The hindfoot is immobilized by the examiner's left hand while the forefoot is rotated to measure midfoot movement. K,L,M,N) (page 733) Pressure is exerted against the resistance of the examiner's hand to test power of dorsiflexion

Long-acting local anaesthesia is injected under image intensifier control along with x-ray contrast medium (Figure 9.1.4) to confirm that the correct joint has been injected, and that there are no connections into other joints (which occur commonly). The patient is instructed to undertake activity which would normally be painful and to complete a pain diary over the subsequent 12h to demonstrate whether the pain has been temporarily relieved. This can usually be performed by radiologists as an outpatient procedure, but when the joint is grossly destroyed this may require general anaesthesia. It may, on occasion, entail several injections to correctly identify which joint or combination of joints is symptomatic. This may seem tedious, but is preferable to the pain, inconvenience, frustration, and disability which arise if the wrong joints are fused.

Non-surgical management

Medical

Anti-inflammatories may be applied locally or administered systemically, and can be helpful as an adjunct to treatment by orthoses or surgery. They are rarely sufficient alone.

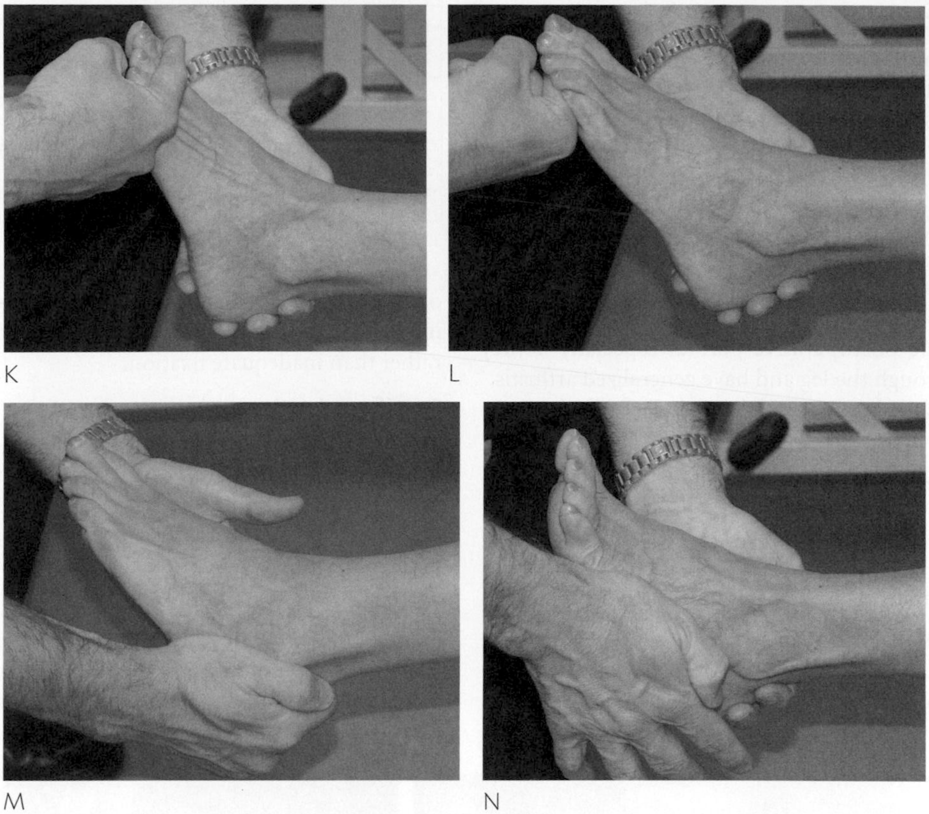

Fig. 9.1.3 (cont'd) (K), plantarflexion (L), inversion (M), and eversion (N).

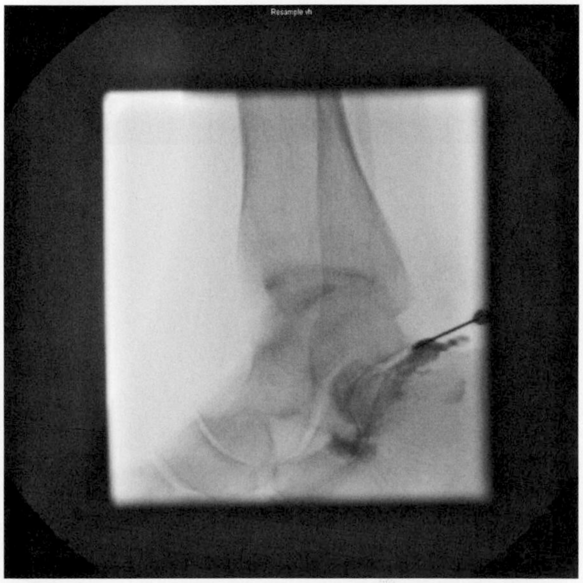

Fig. 9.1.4 Selective injection of joints is used to ensure which joint is the source of the pain prior to fusion. Contrast medium is always used to prevent false positive effects of local anaesthetic flowing between joints, as communications are common.

Blind or x-ray guided injections of depot steroids are more effective, but again are more usually combined with orthotic treatment, otherwise the pain inevitably recurs.

Orthotic management (Box 9.1.2)

Orthoses work by restoring anatomical alignment—reducing overload of affected joints by shock absorption and immobilization.

In general, orthoses will only be effective if deformity is corrected and deforming forces neutralized. Appropriate orthoses are described in Chapter 9.4 and may range from soft accommodative insoles, through to structural solutions such as ankle–foot orthoses (AFOs) or calipers.

Whatever type of orthotic appliance is used, it is important to remember to include adequate shock absorption in the system and consider footwear modification.

Box 9.1.2 Treatment of hind- and midfoot arthritis

- Diagnosis: x-ray, MRI scan, CT scan
- Orthotic treatment
- Localize symptomatic joints: selective injections
- Fusion
- Protect the foot from recurrence/transfer with orthotics.

Surgical treatment (Box 9.1.3)

Surgical treatment of hind- and midfoot arthritis is almost entirely limited to arthrodesis to relieve pain and correct deformity.

Arthroscopy of the subtalar joint is now performed in specialist centre but open surgery is still the norm.

It is important that deformity is reduced, and that muscle power is balanced to prevent recurrence.

Box 9.1.3 Principles of surgical and orthotic treatment of foot and ankle deformity and arthritis

- Place the foot directly beneath the leg
- Place the foot square on the ground in all planes
- Balance (or neutralize) the muscle power to avoid recurrence.

Arthrodesis

Arthrodesis can be difficult to achieve with the poor blood supply to the bones and fragile soft tissue envelope. The patient often has problems surviving the postoperative period, especially if they cannot bear weight through the leg and have generalized arthritis.

The principles of achieving successful arthrodesis are the same for all joints:

- Clearance of articular cartilage from the joint surface with minimal disruption to vascular supply
- Fixation of the arthrodesis (almost always by internal fixation)
- Protection of the limb from movement and/or weight bearing.

A bewildering range of screws of different metals and design, static and memory staples, and low profile and reconstruction plates are available to assist this surgery, but the commonest causes of failure remain poor tissue healing due to smoking or infection, inadequate surface preparation, or poor correction of deformity rather than inadequate fixation.

Specific arthrodeses

Although any joint in the hind- or midfoot may be fused in isolation, the commonest fusions performed are of the talonavicular joint or subtalar joint in isolation and triple fusion (of the talonavicular, subtalar, and calcaneocuboid joints).Technique is briefly described because standard textbooks and operative guides tend to describe outmoded techniques.

Talonavicular joint fusion (Figure 9.1.5A)

This is most commonly performed for isolated single joint arthritis to relieve pain. Although a limited degree of rotational correction

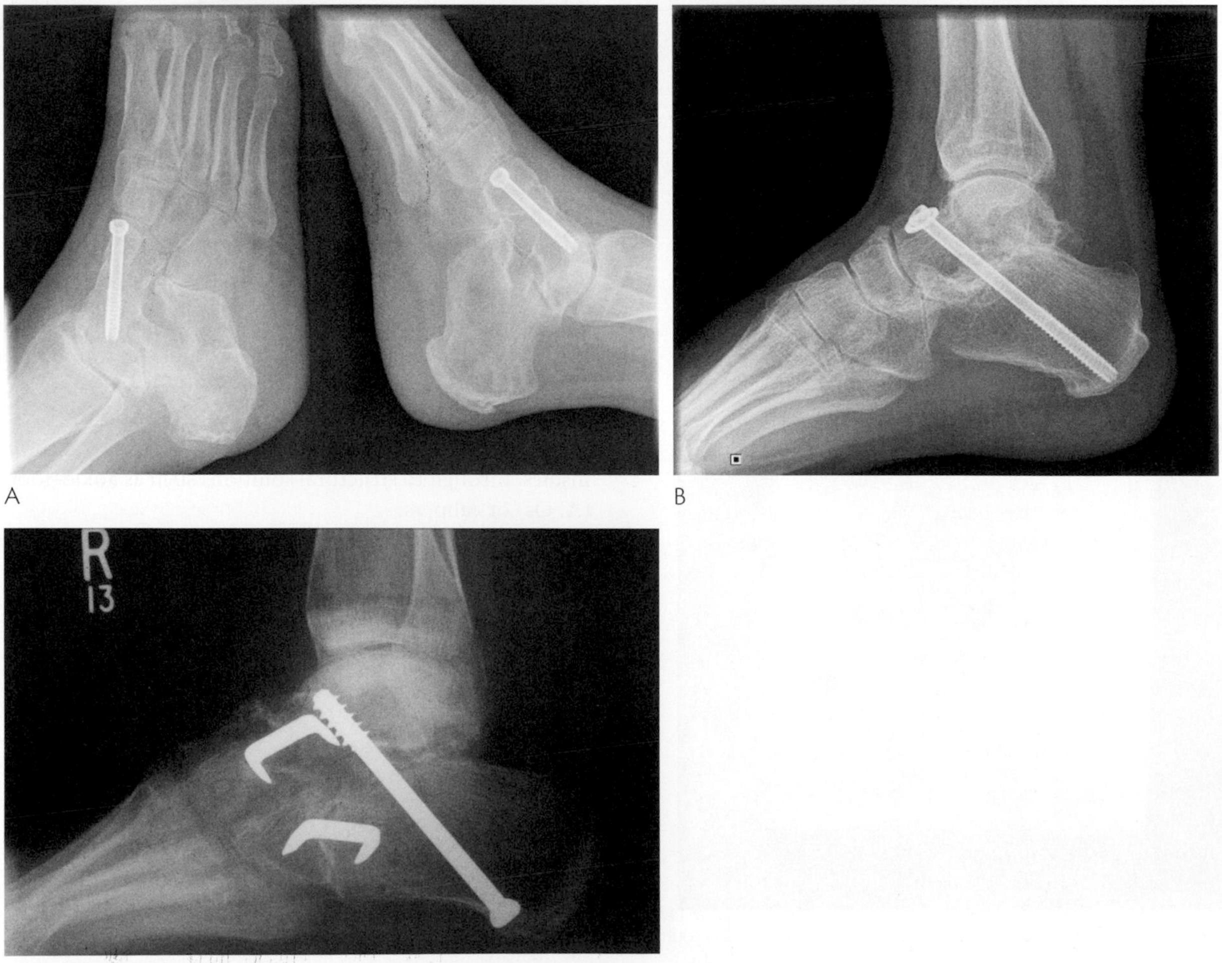

Fig. 9.1.5 A) Talonavicular fusion. B) Subtalar fusion. C) Triple fusion.

can be achieved when performed as part of a flat foot correction, it does not generally correct deformity well.

Preliminary examination and investigation is directed towards identifying predisposing factors, such as coalitions which may continue to generate pain if not addressed directly or by more extensive fusion.

In almost every case a preoperative, diagnostic injection arthrogram with local anaesthetic should be performed prior to surgery.

Procedure The joint is approached through a medial or dorsal approach. The articular cartilage is then removed from both joint surfaces.

The medial approach has the advantage of preserving cutaneous nerves, but in stiff joints it can be difficult to fully clear the lateral side of the joint. If it is not well cleared the remaining cartilage holds the joint open, and the risk of non-union is increased.

The dorsal approach gives easier clearance of the joint surfaces, but at the expense of producing numbness on the dorsum of the foot in about 50% of cases, after division of the medial branch of the superficial peroneal nerve.

Whichever approach is used, the arthrodesis should be rigidly fixed, usually by compression screws or staples.

Postoperative care The foot is elevated and protected in a cast or splint until the wound is healed, and then mobilization allowed—retaining the splint for at least 6 more weeks. Usually the patient will remain non-weight bearing during this time, unless a decision is made that because of general disease and/or excellent fixation this can be over-ridden.

After 8 weeks, radiographs are taken, and if union is seen to be proceeding, gradual weight bearing is allowed, usually in a lighter brace, followed by supportive insoles which are often retained in the long term.

The time to recovery is often prolonged, and we advise patients that it will take 6 months to return to the preoperative level of pain and function, and much longer to achieve their final result.

Results Although some papers describe a high rate of non-union in isolated talonavicular fusion, this need not be the case with thorough joint clearance and rigid fixation, and in non-smokers rates of union around 95% should be expected.

The theoretical advantages of isolated fusion are less than might be expected, and mechanical studies of isolated talonavicular fusion show that it creates considerable stiffness throughout the hindfoot complex.

Subtalar arthrodesis (Figure 9.1.5B)

Subtalar arthrodesis may be performed for pain relief, for correction of deformity, for stabilization, or a combination of these.

The principles of foot correction (discussed earlier) must be adhered to strictly to ensure good results.

Surgical techniques The standard approach to the subtalar joints (posterior, middle, and anterior facets) is via a lateral approach, starting at the tip of the fibula and directed towards the base of the fourth toe. Older transverse incisions such as the Ollier incision unnecessarily destroy nerves and vessels and are of historical interest only. Medial approaches are useful for correction of severe valgus.

The lateral incision exposes the sinus tarsi, which is cleared to show the three facets of the joint. These are cleared using osteotomes or burrs, using upward-cutting spinal bone cutters to clear the medial edges, to ensure safety of the posterior tibial nerve.

Once the surfaces are cleared and corrective cuts made, the joint is accurately reduced to place the hindfoot beneath the leg, checking that the midfoot and forefoot are well aligned. Bone graft may be inserted if large defects are present, but are not usually needed. Internal fixation is performed with compression screws, which may be inserted from above or below. Screws passed from below have the advantage of greater grip of the thread in the talus, and ease of passage, but may suffer sinkage into the calcaneum on compression, or cause screw prominence and damage to the heel pad.

Screws from above may give less reliable compression, and have a small increased risk of nerve damage, but are convenient when other surgery is performed at the same time as other procedures (such as ankle replacement). They minimize the risk of heel pad damage, and are easy to remove when needed if subsequent ankle arthroplasty is performed.

There are many modifications to technique and in some centres the procedure is performed arthroscopically.

Postoperative management Postoperative management mirrors that of talonavicular fusion, but the threshold for allowing weight bearing may be lower due to the essentially horizontal configuration of the joint.

Results Union is expected in over 90% of cases. Smoking, inflammatory arthritis, and infection predispose to non-union. Patients with longstanding pain and after calcaneal fractures may not achieve full pain relief.

Triple fusion (Figure 9.1.5C)

Triple fusion is performed to treat painful arthritis and correct deformity around the hind- and midfoot.

When correcting deformity, preoperative clinical assessment of the foot is critical to ensure that the necessary degree of correction is achieved, and also to ensure that any osteotomies, tendon transfers, etc. are performed at the same time. Triple fusion is often combined with other procedures such as heel osteotomy, dorsiflexion osteotomy of the first ray, and tendon lengthening, augmentation, or transfer.

Technique Triple fusion starts with the technique described earlier for subtalar fusion. The incision is extended distally to allow the extensor digitorum brevis muscle to be split, exposing the calcaneocuboid joint whose joint surfaces are prepared.

Talonavicular preparation is performed as for isolated talonavicular fusion, and then after corrective wedges etc. have been cut if needed, the joints are internally fixed—fixing the subtalar joint first, then the talonavicular and calcaneocuboid joints—carefully ensuring the exact position of the midfoot and forefoot, because the foot after triple fusion will be stiff to rotation and very intolerant of any overload, especially lateral overload of the midfoot.

Results Union occurs in more than 90% of cases. Non-union is 16 times more common in smokers. Recovery is often very prolonged, especially with regards to swelling and start-up pain.

The foot after triple fusion is stiff and often needs a total contact insole within the shoe. Walking should be possible without a limp, but the patient will often limp when running, and be unable to participate in active sports.

Ankle arthritis (Box 9.1.4)

Incidence and aetiology

Arthritis affecting the ankle is surprisingly uncommon when one considers the large number of injuries which are sustained at the ankle.

The number of operations performed for ankle arthritis is much less than the number performed for hip and knee arthritis. Although this may reflect the relatively successful outcomes of the latter procedures compared with procedures for ankle arthritis, the size of the discrepancy is such that it seems the ankle is relatively protected from arthritis and its effects.

In many cases of ankle arthritis a predisposing cause can be identified. The causes fall mainly into three groups:

1) Post-traumatic
2) Associated with systemic arthropathy
3) As a consequence of bleeding and bleeding diatheses.

Post-traumatic

Many patients give a history of previous fracture, often many years previously. There is an association between severe fractures, incompletely reduced fractures, fracture dislocations, malunited fractures, and arthritis.

Minor undisplaced, or well-reduced fractures do not appear to convey significant risk of later deterioration, but fractures (including tibial shaft fractures) which lead to angular deformity at the ankle may.

From a medicolegal standpoint, it appears that the fractures which have a significant chance of causing arthritis in the medium and long term will start to cause symptoms early, and certainly within 2 years of injury. It is uncommon for there to be a long completely symptom-free latent period before the onset of arthritis.

Less certain is the association between soft tissue injury and arthritis. Single soft tissue injuries rarely lead to ongoing problems, but recurrent instability of the ankle may do. Patients presenting with arthritic ankles frequently give a history of recurrent giving way and instability, and arthroscopic studies of ankles with chronic instability have shown universal chondral or osteochondral damage.

Secondary to systemic arthropathy

Of the inflammatory causes of ankle arthritis, rheumatoid arthritis is by far the commonest, although the ankle is also frequently affected in juvenile chronic arthritis (often in association with the other peritalar joints).

About half the patients admitted for inpatient treatment of rheumatoid arthritis have been noted to have significant affectation of the ankles. The ankle is also disproportionately involved in some other inflammatory arthritides.

Bleeding and bleeding disorders

Trauma to the ankle is a common occurrence for those with bleeding disorders, as in the general population. The ensuing haemorrhage causes arthritis. The number of patients affected is small, but the difficulties presented by their management and the requirement for resources can be great.

Damage due to repeated haemorrhage may also occur secondary to pigmented villonodular synovitis.

Box 9.1.4 Causes of ankle arthritis

- Trauma:
  - Recurrent dislocation
  - Severe fracture
- Generalized arthritis
- Bleeding disorders.

Anatomical considerations

For most purposes, the ankle may be considered as a simple, stable hinge joint, with stability provided by its bony shape and ligamentous restraints allowing controlled dorsiflexion and plantarflexion of the foot.

The tibial surface bears most of the load transmitted from the talus, and the curved surfaces of these two bones allows restricted dorsiflexion and plantarflexion to occur within the restraints of ligaments and capsule, with inherent lateral stability provided by the medial and lateral malleoli as well as the ligaments.

A deeper understanding of topographical and functional anatomy is necessary to understand pathological processes about the ankle, to plan surgical interventions, and to design prostheses for ankle replacement.

The ankle joint is in fact a composite joint, comprising the tibiotalar mortise joint and tibiofibular syndesmosis.

The fibula lies posteriorly as well as laterally. The fibula displaces and rotates during ankle movement. It also carries between 6–16% of the axial load during stance.

In the sagittal plane the talus is slightly saddle-shaped with a depressed centre and lateral condylar projections. This matches reciprocal shaping of the tibia, and thereby imparts lateral stability to the joint, which increases on weight bearing, and is additional to the restraint of the malleoli.

Both talus and tibia have curved surfaces when viewed from the side, but the radius of curvature of the talus is shorter than that of the tibial surface, so they are incongruent (Figure 9.1.6). The movement of this complex system is one of rotation about a moving instant centre aligned obliquely across the joint.

Anatomical changes in the arthritic ankle

During the development of ankle arthritis, the tibia usually first develops an anterior osteophyte. The changes have been described by Scranton and Mc Dermott as four stages of osteophyte formation:

- Stage 1: osteophyte on tibia only, less than 3mm
- Stage 2: osteophyte on tibia only, greater than 3mm
- Stage 3: tibial osteophyte greater than 3mm ± fragmentation, talar response
- Stage 4: tibia osteophyte greater than 3mm, talar osteophyte, degenerative changes.

At the same time other changes occur, with loss of joint space and flattening of the talus, which lead to restriction of movement.

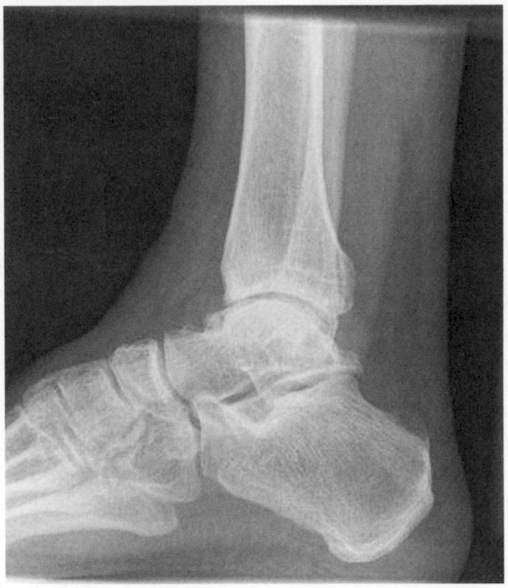

Fig. 9.1.6 Plain lateral radiograph in weight bearing shows that the talus and tibia are not exactly congruent. Incongruency increases with anterior arthritis.

Clinical presentation

Early arthritic changes present with symptoms and signs of inflammatory or mechanical arthritis, or with a combination of both.

Inflammatory changes cause swelling around the ankle, and stiffness after immobility. The ankle is painful to all movements, and the joint line is tender.

Mechanical symptoms and signs are more common. Early mechanical symptoms are typified by the symptoms of 'footballer's ankle'.

As osteophytes develop anteriorly, impingement occurs in dorsilexion (late stance phase). This progresses to pain during and after exercise, worse in dorsiflexion, such as ascending slopes and stairs. Patients may report relief of pain when wearing high heels. Later, posterior pain may develop due to 'hinge-opening'.

Later degeneration of the articular surface occurs. The gross changes observed arthroscopically usually affect the talus first. The region of the talus in contact with the osteophyte is often disproportionately affected, with longitudinal striations visible on the anterior surface of the talus.

Clinical signs

The anterior joint line should be palpated. Osteophytes are rarely palpable, but are often tender. Both feet should be examined and the range of dorsiflexion compared. Any restriction of dorsiflexion is significant. Osteophytes are always visible on radiographs, but oblique views may be needed to detect anteromedial or anterolateral osteophytes.

In moderate arthritis there will be pain on palpation of the joint line, and on joint movement, as well as swelling. The range of movement is restricted, often dramatically, with dorsiflexion lost first.

Deformity is not a constant feature in ankle arthritis, but may occur if degeneration occurs unequally across the joint. Once deformity begins, it increases abnormal loading and both the arthritis and the deformity often progress.

Non-surgical management

Medical

Oral non-steroidal anti-inflammatory drugs may be helpful in early arthritis. When symptoms occur during and after sport, they are most effective taken just prior to activity.

Injection of the joint may be useful for occasional overuse, for an exacerbation in a generalized arthropathy, for an isolated acute inflammatory episode, but has no place in the long-term management.

Orthotic management

In early arthritis, silicone heel inserts can impart relief by acting as shock absorbers. They also act to raise the heel slightly, reducing anterior impingement.

More often, an AFO is required. The orthosis should restore anatomical alignment, hold the joint rigidly, and provide shock absorption. Some mechanism should be incorporated to allow walk-through gait (for example, by adding a rocker to the shoe).

A well-tailored rigid AFO with a shock absorbing heel will be effective for many cases, but when major deformity needs to be corrected a caliper with strap may be more effective.

Surgical treatments (Box 9.1.5)

A wide range of surgical options are available to treat ankle arthritis:

Osteotomy

Takakura from Japan performed tibial osteotomy on 18 ankles (in 18 patients) with intermediate disease and tibial deformity and found improvements in pain, walking, and ability to perform activities of daily living over an average of nearly 7 years, although range of movement was not improved.

Osteotomy is reserved for cases occurring in young patients with deformity and preserved joints.

Distraction

Around the same time in Europe, Van Valburg described applying long-term joint distraction using an Ilizarov apparatus for 18–34 weeks. All showed an improvement in pain and range of movement with five gaining complete relief.

The length of treatment limits its use to cases in young patients.

Arthroscopy

Arthroscopy of the ankle can help in arthritis by synovectomy, anterior cheilectomy, surgery to chondral and osteochondral lesions, or by more extensive surgery such as distraction/debridement or arthroscopic arthrodesis (which is described later in the arthrodesis section).

Anterior spurs or osteophytes presenting as 'footballer's ankle' are dealt with as effectively arthroscopically as by open means, but with more rapid recovery—a return to preoperative activity is expected within 6–8 weeks.

Larger and more advanced (grade III/IV) osteophytes can also be removed arthroscopically, in isolation, or with general debridement of joint surfaces, although on occasions the increased range of movement is accompanied by increased pain.

Arthroscopic debridement can be combined with rigid intraoperative distraction (Figure 9.1.7). The method does not work for patients with significant deformity or instability, but may avoid or

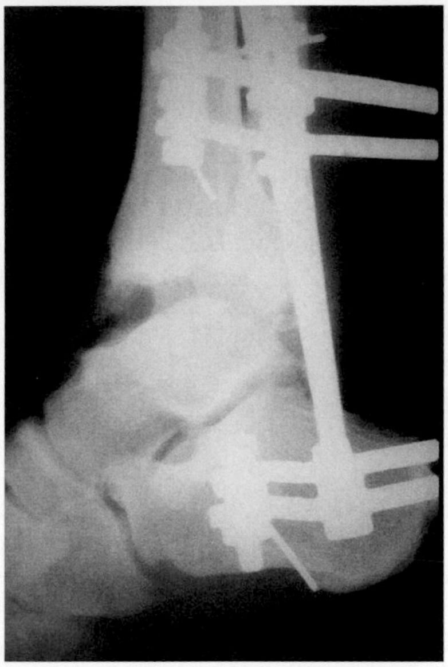

Fig. 9.1.7 A lateral radiograph of a degenerate ankle with distraction applied by an external fixator, showing that considerable distraction (and hence ligamentotaxis) is achieved during isolated distraction treatment or distraction arthroscopy.

delay arthrodesis in about half the cases, and can be useful for young patients wanting to avoid fusion.

Arthrodesis

Arthrodesis of the ankle has for many years been the mainstay of surgical treatment for ankle arthritis, but it remains difficult surgery. Sir John Charnley highlighted this and wrote that 'in the ankle it would appear that this joint does not possess the same natural potential for bony union as exists in the soft cancellous bone of the knee' and stated that the operation had 'a narrow latitude for technical error'.

Techniques

Almost every approach to the ankle has been described for arthrodesis. The methods of obtaining fusion are:

1) Open arthrodesis using internal fixation
2) Open arthrodesis using external fixation
3) Arthroscopic arthrodesis using internal fixation.

Compression arthrodesis is now favoured, using internal fixation when there is no infection and external fixation in the presence of infection.

Whichever method is used to obtain arthrodesis, the position of the foot after arthrodesis is important. The ankle should be held in neutral position with regard to both varus/valgus and plantar/dorsiflexion as well as in slight external rotation. The talus should be positioned directly beneath the tibia.

Gait analysis has shown that even small amounts of calcaneous (5 degrees) give a stiff gait with no push off (due to absence of third rocker) and equinus position imposes a vaulting gait.

Excessive varus is poorly tolerated by the subtalar joint and the foot, with painful callous forming on the outer side of the foot, and pain in the mid and forefoot occurring with only minor deformities. Excessive valgus may lead to painful fibula impingement or peroneal tendinitis, and both may lead to secondary pain in the knee.

If the foot is fused in neutral then the gross appearance of the gait is normal, but gait analysis shows that the walking speed is decreased, as are step length and single stance duration.

Preoperative conditions often dictate the risk of failure, with large deformities, previous ulceration or infection, and poor bone stock being bad prognostic factors. Rates of failure up to 20% occur in mixed series with large numbers of rheumatoid and elderly patients, and rates of 5% or less achieved in selected series with predominantly fit osteoarthritic patients. Cobb has shown that the rate of non-union is substantially increased by smoking.

Open arthrodesis using internal fixation Medial, lateral, posterior, anteromedial, anterolateral, anterior, and combination approaches are all used and in specific instances each will be indicated. The posterior approach may be appropriate when friable skin or skin graft lies anteriorly, medial approaches may be used to excise bone and correct valgus deformity, and conversely lateral approaches allow easy correction of varus.

The lateral approach (excising the fibula) and the anterior approach are currently the most popular open approaches. Whichever approach is adopted, it must allow full exposure of tibial and talar plafonds, and lateral aspects of the joint, with small accessory portals made if necessary to allow adequate internal fixation and correction of deformity. Lateral impingement of bone or peroneal tendons can be problematic after some approaches, but is avoided by partial fibula excision.

Postoperative regimens vary, but require 8–12 weeks minimum of cast immobilization to obtain union, with a similar period of protection in an orthosis or splint whilst consolidation occurs. A rocker bottom to the shoe is then frequently helpful.

Patients should be warned that they will get bony pain for up to 4 months after coming out of plaster, and this may continue to improve for a long time after surgery as full bony remodelling occurs.

Arthrodesis using external fixation Charnley popularized the use of external fixation for ankle arthrodesis. His method was originally mainly used for patients with polio and other neurological conditions and used a transverse incision (dividing extensor tendons as well as vessels and nerves), with through and through compression pins anteriorly through the tibia and calcaneum. It is no longer performed this way. Most surgeons now use triangulated frames or ring external fixators with fine wires reserving external fixation for the treatment of infected non-union, and for more complicated procedures performed with bone transport, skin transfer, etc.

Arthroscopic arthrodesis (Figure 9.1.8) In cases of painful articular arthritis with minimal (less than 10 degrees) varus or valgus tilt, arthroscopic arthrodesis may be performed. The degree of deformity which can be corrected increases with experience.

It has advantages in terms of postoperative pain (allowing early mobilization and short inpatient stay), and in speed and rate of union. It is particularly appropriate in patients with poor vascular supply, with bleeding disorders, or with skin grafts around the ankle.

A distractor is applied to the ankle, and after synovial clearance, anterior cheilectomy is performed to allow good visibility.

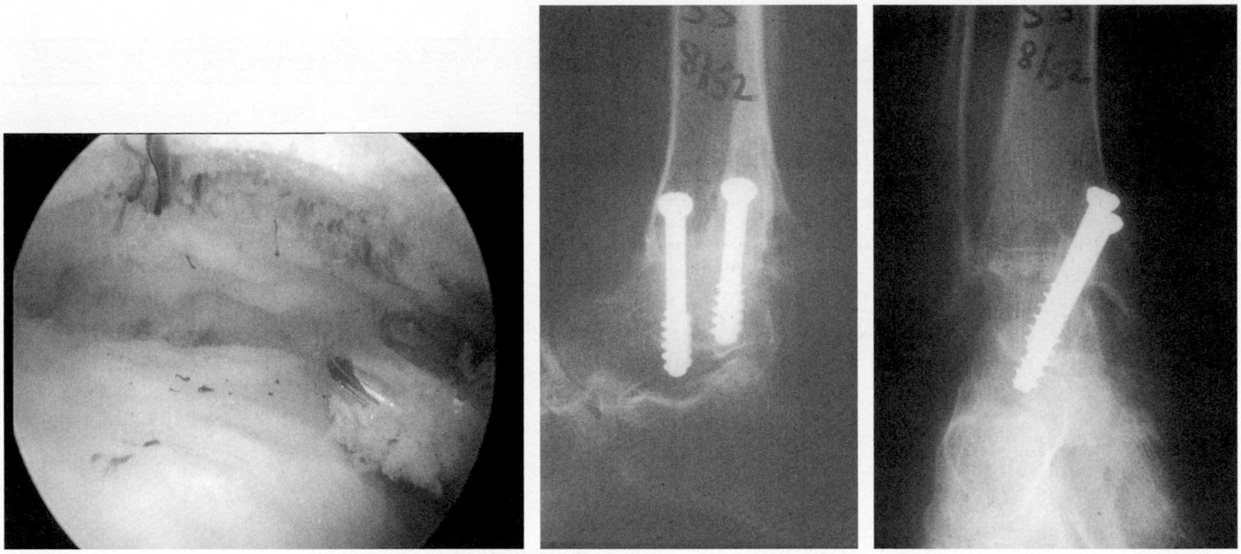

A B C

Fig. 9.1.8 Arthroscopic arthrodesis. (A) The cartilage removed down to cancellous bone at the end of surface preparation. (B) Radiograph at the end of surgery for implantation of internal fixation. (C) Radiograph at 8 weeks after surgery showing union.

The articular surfaces are then cleared down to cancellous bone using power burrs, and the lateral and medial gutters are similarly cleared of articular cartilage. Two cannulated screws are then passed (from the medial tibia down into the talus) under x-ray control.

A plaster is applied, and early weight bearing can be allowed within the bounds of pain.

The immediate postoperative radiographs almost always appear to have a substantial gap, but within a few weeks this fills in. Union may be observed as early as 4 weeks after surgery and is more rapid than after open surgery. External immobilization is usually maintained for 8 weeks, and then mobilization is encouraged from an appropriate brace. Although the initial and postoperative pain levels are much lower than after open surgery, it still often takes many months before all bone pain around the ankle subsides.

Ankle arthroplasty (Figure 9.1.9) Historically, ankle arthroplasty has been unsuccessful, with high rates of early and late failure, often of 10% or more per annum.

Clinical development has been slowed because of these failures, and because ankle arthrodesis is an effective treatment to relieve pain in many cases. However, arthrodesis has several drawbacks. The restriction of movement always imparts some disability and in patients with bilateral disease, and those with generalized disease, this may be severe. Both bilateral disease and multiple lower limb joint disease are common in patients with rheumatoid arthritis, and development of ankle prostheses has continued mainly because of the requirements of these patients.

In addition, long-term reviews of ankle arthrodesis have shown arthritic changes in adjacent joints with time.

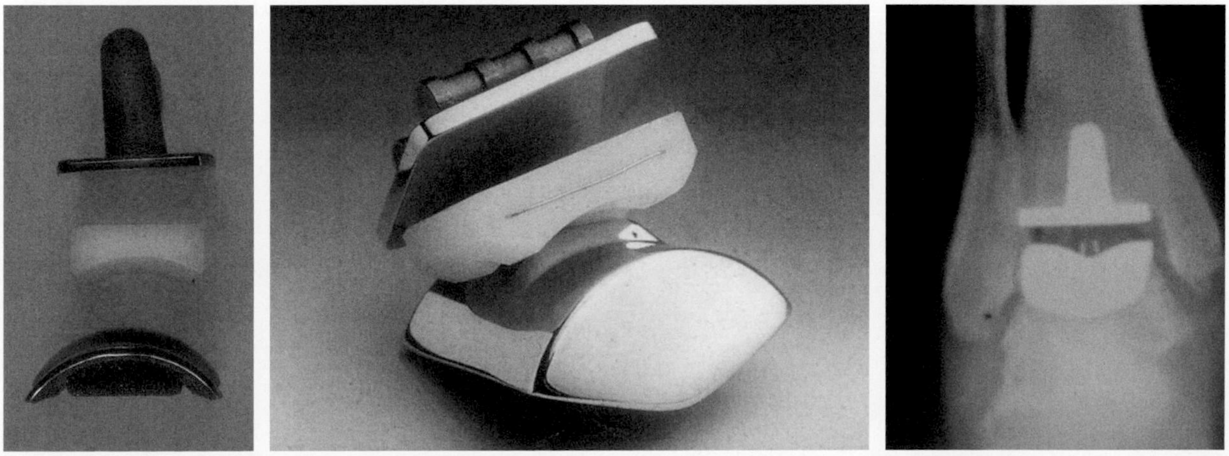

A (i) A (ii) B

Fig. 9.1.9 A) Two modern meniscal ankle replacements. B) Postoperative radiographs of a patient with a total ankle replacement.

Box 9.1.5 Surgical treatment of ankle arthritis

- Osteotomy: to correct deformity with minor degeneration
- Joint distraction: to avoid fusion in young patients
- Arthroscopy: for mild and moderate arthritis
- Distraction arthroscopy: a quicker way to simulate distraction
- Arthrodesis
- Arthroplasty.

Over more than 25 years a variety of designs have been tried, with hinge and non-constrained designs all described, but with high rates of failure.

The main causes of failure were sepsis and aseptic loosening. Constrained implants failed at a rate of around 10% per annum, with semiconstrained failing generally above 5% per annum.

The most popular designs of ankle replacements in Europe have a planar tibial surface, a curved talar surface, and a semiconstrained meniscal component. Early results suggest pain relief is good, functional restoration is reasonable, and the revision rate is around 1.5% per annum (although the confidence intervals are large due to small numbers).

There is a role for using a semiconstrained meniscal ankle replacement in bilateral disease, in rheumatoid disease, and in other circumstances where other joints are affected (Box 9.1.6).

Box 9.1.6 Which operation for who?

Fusion

- Young
- High demand
- Good compensatory joints
- Deformity
- Avascular necrosis, infection.

Arthroplasty

- Elderly
- Low demand
- Adjacent fusion
- No deformity
- ? Bilateral.

Conclusions

Hindfoot and midfoot arthritis cause pain and deformity or instability. Most cases can be helped by orthotic management. When orthotic management is inadequate, surgical treatment usually comprises of fusion in an anatomical position.

Ankle arthritis is rarer than arthritis of the hip or knee. The mainstay of surgical treatment is arthrodesis, which gives good results when union can be obtained in good position, but has a failure rate of 3–10 %. After arthrodesis, degeneration of surrounding joints may be accelerated.

As an alternative to arthrodesis, and for less severe cases, arthroscopic surgery may provide relief, and osteotomy may be considered to correct varus deformity.

Ankle arthroplasty has been unsuccessful in the past, but modern meniscal designs show better results, and may offer an alternative to arthrodesis in some circumstances such as bilateral disease, and multiple joint involvement.

Further reading

Cobb, T.K., Gabrielsen, T.A., Campbell, D.C. 2nd, Wallrichs, S.L., and Ilstrup, D.M. (1994). Cigarette smoking and non-union after ankle arthrodesis. *Foot & Ankle International*, **15**(2), 64–7.

Scranton, P.E. and McDermott, J.E. (1992). Anterior tibial spurs: a comparison of open versus arthroscopic debridement. *Foot & Ankle*, **13**, 125–9.

Takakura, Y., Takakura, Y., Hayashi, K., Taniguchi, A., Kumai, T., and Sugimoto, K. (1995). Low tibial osteotomy for osteoarthritis of the ankle. *Journal of Bone and Joint Surgery*, **77B**, 50–4.

Wood, P.L., Prem, H., and Sutton, C. (2008). Total ankle replacement: medium-term results in 200 Scandinavian total ankle replacements. *Journal of Bone and Joint Surgery*, **90B**, 605–9.

Wülker, N., Stukenborg, C., Savory, K.M., and Alfke, D. (2000). Hindfoot motion after isolated and combined arthrodeses: measurements in anatomic specimens. *Foot & Ankle International*, **21**, 921–7.

9.2

Disorders of the forefoot

Andrew H.N. Robinson and Maneesh Bhatia

Summary points

- The aim of modern forefoot surgery is to refunction the first ray, and balance the lesser rays around it
- The indications for surgery in hallux valgus are of pain over the bunion, or of pain with subluxation or dislocation of the lesser rays as a result of first ray insufficiency
- Hallux valgus surgery aims to reposition the metatarsal head over the sesamoids whilst maintaining length. The osteotomy should be stable to allow early mobilization
- The mainstays of the surgical treatment of hallux rigidus are dorsal cheilectomy and fusion of the first MTPJ
- 96% excellent and good results in reconstruction of the rheumatoid forefoot have been reported with fusion of the first MTPJ and resection of the lesser metatarsal heads.

Introduction

Over the last decade there has been a change from treatment of individual forefoot complaints in isolation to directing treatment at producing a balanced forefoot.

This chapter deals with the common forefoot problems of hallux valgus, hallux rigidus, sesamoiditis, and lesser toe deformity individually, and then summarizes the principles of reconstructing the whole forefoot.

Hallux valgus

Introduction

A bunion is a swelling of the first metatarsophalangeal joint (MTPJ) and is derived from the Latin for turnip (*bunio*). It is an imprecise term. Hallux valgus is a more precise term which describes the posture of the toe. Over 130 operations are described as no procedure addresses all cases.

Aetiology

Extrinsic factors include constricting and high heel shoes. Heredity is important with up to 84% of patients with juvenile hallux valgus showing a familial tendency—usually transmitted from mother to daughter.

Hypermobility and pes planus also contribute to onset and rate of deterioration.

The role of footwear is controversial, but high heels and tight pointed toe boxes increase the rate of progression of hallux valgus (Box 9.2.1).

Anatomy

The first MTPJ is prone to deformity as a result of its anatomy. The normal joint moves mainly in plantarflexion and dorsiflexion, but lateral movement is also possible.

Under the MTPJ are two plantar sesamoids. They lie in the two tendon slips of the flexor hallucis brevis, on either side of the flexor hallucis longus tendon and are thus radiological markers of the longitudinal axis of the first ray musculature.

The blood supply of the first metatarsal head comes from the plantar lateral part of the metatarsal neck, and should be preserved to prevent avascular necrosis of the first metatarsal head.

Pathogenesis

The pathogenesis of hallux valgus has been well described by Stephens. The proximal phalanx of the great toe moves into valgus and the first metatarsal splays, leading to metatarsus primus varus.

A groove develops on the medial side of the metatarsal head articular cartilage as it atrophies from the lack of normal pressure and defines the prominence of the medial exostosis—over which a bursa develops.

Erosion of the metatarsal crista between the medial and lateral sesamoids occurs early, and as the medial soft tissues become further attenuated, the metatarsal head moves medially from over the sesamoids. The medial sesamoid comes to lie under the eroded crista, and the lateral sesamoid on the lateral side of the metatarsal head in the first intermetatarsal space.

The extensor hallucis longus and flexor hallucis longus tendons remain in position while the MTPJ migrates medially and they come to act as bowstrings and exacerbate the deformity.

The adductor hallucis and the lateral head of flexor hallucis brevis also contribute to the development of the deformity. With time they become contracted, as does the lateral joint capsule.

The abductor hallucis and medial head of flexor hallucis brevis lose their abduction moment. The resultant imbalance causes dorsiflexion and pronation of the first toe.

These events combine to lead to first ray insufficiency and lesser ray overload. As a result, the second toe claws and eventually the second MTPJ dislocates.

Box 9.2.1 Hallux valgus: aetiopathology

- Aetiology: familial, high heels, hypermobility, pes planus
- Proximal phalanx moves into valgus resulting in metatarsus primus varus
- Hallux dorsiflexes and pronates
- The two sesamoids are the radiological markers of the longitudinal axis of the first ray
- Blood supply to first metatarsal head comes from plantar lateral aspect of metatarsal neck.

Presentation

Patients present with restriction in shoes (80%), pain over the bunion (70%), cosmetic concerns (60%), and pain underneath the second metatarsal head (40%). Lesser toe deformities, Morton's neuroma, corns, and calluses also occur as a result of first ray insufficiency and overcrowding.

Clinical assessment

The patient is examined standing to emphasize the hallux valgus and associated deformities.

Signs of generalized ligamentous laxity should be recorded.

It is important to assess the hindfoot, as planovalgus deformities and gastrocnemius-soleus tightness exacerbate loading and pain around the first MTPJ.

The degree of hallux valgus deformity and whether it is correctable is noted, as is pronation of the great toe. The range of motion of the first MTPJ is documented.

The lesser toes are examined for deformities and callosities, and the intermetatarsal spaces palpated for neuroma. The plantar surface of the foot should be checked for callosities.

Finally, first tarsometatarsal instability is assessed. The examiner immobilizes the lesser metatarsals with the thumb and fingers of one hand, with the ankle in neutral. The thumb and index finger of the other hand grasp the first metatarsal and move it from a plantar-lateral to dorsomedial direction.

Radiological assessment

Weight bearing anteroposterior and lateral radiographs of the foot are mandatory.

Box 9.2.2 Hallux valgus: clinical features

- Presentation: shoe restriction, pain, cosmesis, transfer lesions, lesser toe synovitis/deformity, callosities, Morton's neuroma
- Clinical examination should be weight bearing and includes:
    - Forefoot: degree of hallux valgus and pronation, correctibility of deformity, range of movements, lesser toe deformity, callosities
    - Hindfoot: planovalgus deformity, Achilles tightness
    - Ligamentous laxity: generalized and tarsometatarsal.

The hallux valgus angle (HVA) (normally less than 15 degrees) and intermetatarsal angle (IMA) (normally less than 9 degrees) are measured (Figure 9.2.1). The congruency of the joint is assessed. The relationship of the first metatarsal head to the sesamoids and presence of degeneration should also be recorded.

The distal metatarsal articular angle (DMAA) (normally less than 10 degrees) measures the angle between the articular surface of the first metatarsal head and the first metatarsal shaft (Figure 9.2.1)—this is sometimes called the proximal articular set angle (PASA). The DMAA is difficult to measure with high inter- and intraobserver variability.

The proximal phalangeal articular angle (PPAA) is the angle between the proximal phalanx and its proximal articular surface (normally less than10 degrees). Hallux valgus interphalangeus deformity is present if this value is increased, or if there is significant angulation between the proximal and distal phalanges.

The severity of the hallux valgus deformity is thus defined to help formulate surgical treatment.

Forefoot balance

Maestro and colleagues used anteroposterior standing radiographs to define the ideal forefoot morphotype and described a method of preoperative planning for forefoot osteotomies. According to their criteria a radiographically 'harmonious' forefoot displays a progression of the lengths of the lesser metatarsals, to give equal weight bearing across the forefoot (Figure 9.2.2).

Non-operative treatment

Hallux valgus can be treated with accommodative shoes made of soft leather with an extra wide and deep toe box. In the elderly and

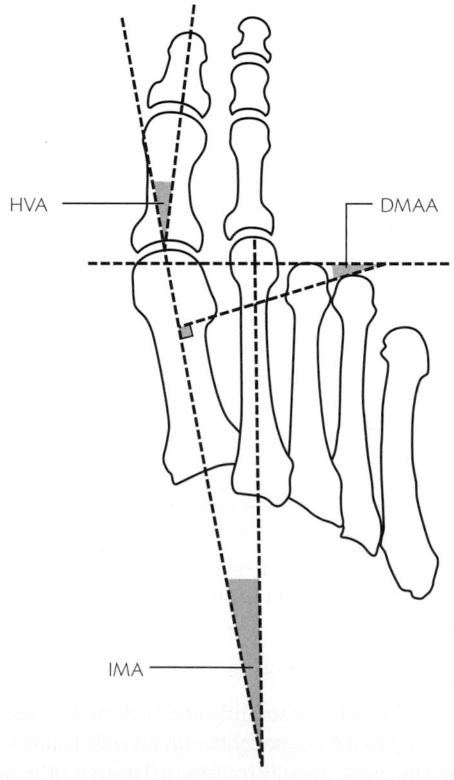

Fig. 9.2.1 Radiological assessment of hallux valgus. DMAA, distal metatarsal; HVA, hallux valgus angle; IMA, intermetatarsal angle.

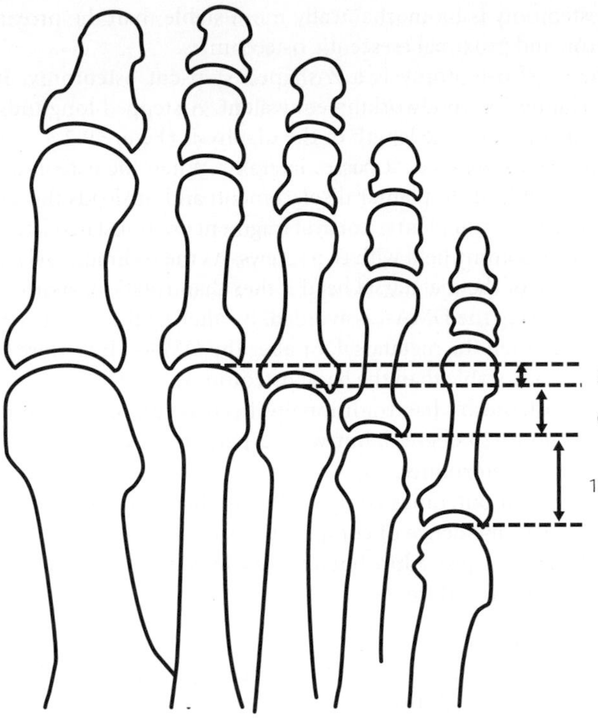

Fig. 9.2.2 The ideal metatarsal parabola, as described by Maestro. The first and second metatarsal heads lie at the same level.

those with neurological or vascular compromise this is the treatment of choice.

There is little evidence to substantiate the use of orthoses. A medial longitudinal arch support has been shown to reduce symptoms temporarily. There is no evidence that orthoses prevent the progression of hallux valgus.

Surgical treatment

The indication for surgery is pain over the bunion or in the second MTPJ as a result of first ray insufficiency.

The management of patient expectation is important. In the United Kingdom, 30% of orthopaedic litigation is as a result of foot surgery, of which 80% arises from forefoot surgery.

Only 60% of patients can expect to wear fashion shoes following surgery.

There are many surgical procedures; they can be broadly classified by the anatomical location of the procedure (Table 9.2.1).

Principles of surgery

- The technique should be technically easy and reproducible
- Osteotomies should be stable, with or without internal fixation
- The aim of surgery is to correct deformity and balance muscle power by repositioning the metatarsal head over the sesamoid apparatus
- The length and elevation of the firstmetatarsal should be maintained to prevent transfer lesions
- The metatarsal blood supply should be preserved to avoid avascular necrosis
- There should be a low hallux valgus recurrence rate.

Table 9.2.1 Eponymous osteotomies of the first metatarsal

Site of procedure	Eponymous or named examples
Medial cuneiform opening wedge	
First tarsometatarsal fusion	Lapidus
Proximal osteotomy	Crescentic (Mann); chevron (Stephens); opening wedge
Diaphyseal osteotomy	Scarf, Ludloff
Distal osteotomy	Chevron (Austin); Mitchell; Wilson
Distal soft tissue procedure	McBride
Bunionectomy and medial capsular reefing	Silver
First MTPJ excision	Keller
First MTPJ fusion	
Proximal phalangeal closing wedge	Akin

MTPJ, metatarsophalangeal joint.

Keller's procedure

This procedure involves resection of one-third of the proximal phalanx of the great toe. There is a high rate of recurrent deformity and the IMA is improved little. The procedure defunctions the first ray with loss of flexion power. Metatarsalgia from overload of the lesser metatarsal heads, cock-up deformity, and reduction of first MTPJ motion also commonly occur.

Salvage of failed Keller's procedure is technically demanding. Fusion of the first MTPJ is often needed, made more difficult by the shortening and bone loss necessitating structural interposition bone graft to re-establish length. This is associated with a high rate of non-union and other complications.

Keller's procedure should only be considered in an elderly household ambulator with low functional demands who would not tolerate a larger procedure or when infection is present.

Distal soft tissue procedures

Simple bunionectomy and medial capsular placation sounds attractive but does not address the pathology. At 5-year review the HVA and IMA are increased. Patients are dissatisfied in over 40% of cases.

McBride described lateral release and excision of the lateral sesamoid to correct hallux valgus, and a modified procedure, preserving the sesamoids, reduced the HVA by 14.8 degrees and the IMA by 5.2 degrees, but with an 11% incidence of hallux varus.

Modified McBride procedure is an important component of hallux valgus correction but is not sufficient in isolation in the majority of cases.

First metatarsal osteotomies

First metatarsal osteotomies are divided into proximal and distal. Proximal osteotomies allow a greater correction of IMA. Distal osteotomies are used for mild to moderate deformities, as they require less extensive exposure, with quicker recovery.

In recent years a new, intermediate group of diaphyseal osteotomies have become popular.

Distal metatarsal osteotomies

Wilson's osteotomy is an oblique metaphyseal osteotomy from distal medial to proximal lateral, which allows the metatarsal head to displace laterally and proximally. It corrects the IMA and HVA. Satisfactory results of bunion correction are described in 90% of patients but there is an average of 8.5mm shortening of the first metatarsal and 24% incidence of dorsal angulation. Metatarsalgia occurs in 35% of patients. Seventy-eight per cent of patients have callosities under the second metatarsal head. As a result of these shortcomings this osteotomy is not recommended.

Mitchell's osteotomy involves a double cut osteotomy through the first metatarsal neck, leaving a step which is used to 'hitch' the metatarsal head. The capital fragment is displaced laterally and plantarwards. Again, good clinical results have been reported with this procedure with a 91% patient satisfaction rate, but shortening of the first metatarsal can occur with an associated dorsal malunion. Thus transfer metatarsalgia occurs in 10–30% of cases, although the incidence of complications can be reduced by internal fixation.

The distal chevron osteotomy is a proximally based, V-shaped osteotomy of the metatarsal neck with lateral displacement of the capital fragment. It causes minimal shortening and is intrinsically stable. It is indicated for mild to moderate deformities. Excellent clinical results have been reported with little or no metatarsalgia and correction of the IMA by 4–8 degrees and the HVA by 11–18 degrees. Loss of correction and recurrence can occur, especially if used for more severe deformities. This risk can be minimized by cutting the osteotomy with a long dorsal or plantar arm and internally fixing the osteotomy. Variations include taking a medially-based closing wedge to correct the DMAA. Avascular necrosis of the first metatarsal head occurs in up 20% of patients. Thus many caution against undertaking a simultaneous chevron osteotomy and lateral release.

Diaphyseal osteotomies

Diaphyseal osteotomy has been recommended for IMAs between 14–20 degrees. After division of the diaphysis, either translation (Scarf) or rotation of the metatarsal (Ludloff) corrects the IMA (Figure 9.2.3). Lateral release and medial capsular plication are performed.

The Ludloff osteotomy is an oblique osteotomy, angled 30 degrees to the long axis of the metatarsal. The distal fragment is rotated and the metatarsal head turned plantarwards before internal fixation. Excellent clinical results are reported, with good correction and no metatarsalgia. There is minimal metatarsal shortening and

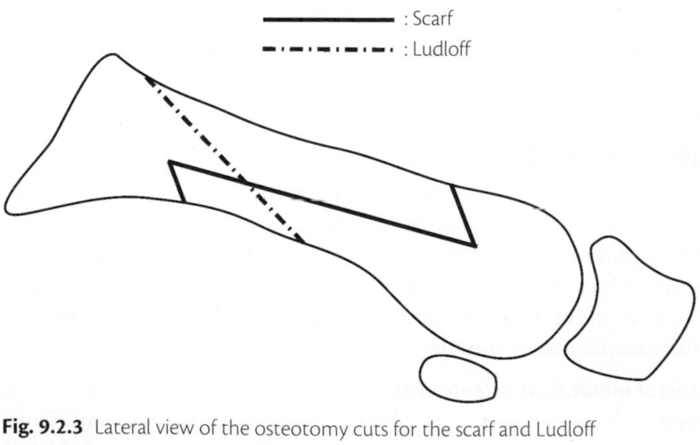

Fig. 9.2.3 Lateral view of the osteotomy cuts for the scarf and Ludloff osteotomies.

the osteotomy is biomechanically more stable than the proximal chevron and proximal crescentic osteotomies.

The scarf osteotomy is a Z-shaped step-cut osteotomy. It is named after its woodworking equivalent. A stepped longitudinal cut is made along the length of the diaphysis (Figure 9.2.3) and is sloped plantarwards as it passes laterally. When the osteotomy is displaced, it leads to plantar displacement, and off-loads the lesser rays. The head and plantar cortical fragment are translated laterally and the osteotomy held with two screws. As the technique relies on translation of the metatarsal head rather than rotation, shortening and increasing the DMAA is avoided. By altering the cuts it is possible to shorten the metatarsal, or alter the DMAA. It is more biomechanically stable than the basal osteotomies.

Scarf osteotomy has traditionally been recommended for an IMA of up to 20 degrees, but with experience it can be used for more severe deformities.

The clinical outcomes compare favourably with basal osteotomies with an incidence of complications of 4–11%. It is a technically demanding procedure but once mastered it is a highly effective and versatile procedure.

Basal osteotomies

Opening wedge, closing wedge, crescentic, and basal chevron osteotomies have all been described, normally combined with a distal soft tissue procedure, bunionectomy, and capsular reefing. They correct splay due to their proximal location, but increase the DMAA, and are used for moderate and severe deformities. An increased DMAA can be corrected by adding a distal biplanar chevron (the double osteotomy), and Akin osteotomy to correct hallux valgus interphalangeus (triple osteotomy). There is 81% patient satisfaction rate but a 19% incidence of major complications with an average 5mm of metatarsal shortening.

Opening wedge osteotomies cause elongation and stretching of the medial soft tissues and require bone graft. They have greater potential for stiffness and non-union. Distraction plates address some of these issues. A closing wedge osteotomy is easier but leads to shortening of the metatarsal, and rates of dorsal malunion of up to 38%.

Proximal crescentic osteotomy is formed with a crescentic saw blade (concavity directed proximally) through a dorsal approach, and held with a screw. It leads to minimal shortening of the first metatarsal and excellent results are described with patient satisfaction rates of more than 90% and good correction of the IMA and HVA even in severe cases. It is technically difficult and instability leads to dorsal malunion in up to 17% of cases. The proximal chevron osteotomy is technically easier and intrinsically more stable to dorsiflexion than the crescentic osteotomy, and causes fewer transfer lesions.

Arthrodeses

First metatarsophalangeal joint arthrodesis

Fusion is used to treat hallux valgus in patients with rheumatoid arthritis, severe metatarsophalangeal osteoarthritis, severe or recurrent deformity particularly in the older patient, neuromuscular disease and salvage following failed surgery. The success rate of fusion is 90% with high levels of patient satisfaction. A concomitant basal procedure is not needed, as the increased IMA corrects spontaneously.

First tarsometatarsal joint arthrodesis (Lapidus)

First tarsometatarsal arthrodesis with excision of a laterally-based wedge is performed in combination with a distal soft tissue procedure, in patients with hypermobility of the first tarsometatarsal joint, or for degenerative changes of the first or second tarsometatarsal joint. It is contraindicated in the adolescent with an open physis at the base of the first metatarsal, patients with a short first metatarsal or degenerative changes in the first MTPJ. The procedure is technically demanding and has higher rates of complication than metatarsal osteotomies. Satisfaction rates vary from 75–90% with fusion rates of 90%.

Conclusion

Hallux valgus surgery is technically demanding but has a high success rate in appropriately selected patients. The treatment protocol we recommend always uses internal fixation and is shown in Table 9.2.2.

Special situations

Juvenile hallux valgus

Bunions presenting in the preteen or teen years are classified as juvenile hallux valgus. Juvenile hallux valgus is more likely to recur than its adult counterpart. The patients have a higher DMAA and more hallux valgus interphalangeus than their adult counterparts. Care must be taken not to damage the physis, which is proximal in both the first metatarsal and proximal phalanx. In boys foot growth ceases around the age of 16 years, and in girls foot growth ceases around 14 years.

Hallux varus

The commonest cause of hallux varus is overcorrection at the time of hallux valgus surgery. Other causes are inflammatory arthritis and trauma.

Hallux varus presents with deformity, pain, stiffness, instability, clawing of the great toe, weakness, and difficulty with shoe fitting. Some varus is acceptable and when easily correctible does not require treatment. However, the treatment of symptomatic hallux varus is difficult—by soft tissue procedures or bony procedures including reverse scarf osteotomy and MTPJ arthrodesis. Arthrodesis remains the most reliable treatment.

Disorders of the sesamoids

The sesamoid bones of the hallux cause symptoms by intrinsic pathology (sesamoiditis) and by plantar prominence leading to plantar keratosis and pain.

Anatomy

The sesamoids lie within the tendons of the flexor hallucis brevis. Most patients have two sesamoids although in one-third of cases the sesamoid may be bipartite. Sesamoiditis, presenting with pain and tenderness of the sesamoids, may be due to fracture, degeneration of the joint between the sesamoid and metatarsal head, or avascular necrosis.

Treatment

Non-operative Both sesamoiditis and plantar keratosis are treated with pressure-relieving insoles. This is the commonest from of treatment.

Operative Surgery for sesamoid disease is of two types.

In those cases with increased pressure the first metatarsal is often plantarflexed, and in this situation a dorsally-based wedge osteotomy of the first metatarsal is used to correct plantarflexion. In cases with ulceration or with no plantarflexion, the prominent plantar surface of the sesamoid is excised.

In pure 'sesamoiditis' Brodsky reported good or excellent results in 23 cases treated by excision of the sesamoid. If a sesamoid is removed, it is important to repair the tendon of the flexor hallucis brevis, to avoid the development of hallux deformity postoperatively. Early orthotic management is started, otherwise transfer pain to the other sesamoid is common.

Hallux rigidus

Introduction

Hallux rigidus describes stiffness of the great toe, and is most commonly caused by osteoarthritis of the first MTPJ. It affects one in 45 people over 50 years of age. There is a decrease in motion, especially dorsiflexion. Other terms that have been used include hallux limitus or dorsal bunion to describe the dorsal osteophyte.

Aetiology

Hallux rigidus may be caused by trauma or osteochondritis dissecans. It is associated with a long first metatarsal, hypermobility of the first ray, pronation, hallux valgus interphalangeus, hallux valgus, metatarsus adductus, and inflammatory or metabolic conditions such as gout, rheumatoid arthritis, and seronegative arthropathy.

Table 9.2.2 An algorithm for treating hallux valgus

Mild hallux valgus (IMA up to 14°)	Normal DMAA	Short scarf osteotomy with a distal soft tissue procedure or long inferior limb chevron
	Increased DMAA	A short scarf osteotomy with a distal soft tissue procedure with added rotation of the metatarsal head
Moderate hallux valgus (IMA 14–20°)	Normal DMAA	Scarf osteotomy with a distal soft tissue procedure. Varus osteotomy (Akin procedure) added if needed to correct angular and rotator deformity
	Increased DMAA	As normal DMAA, but increased corrective rotation of the scarf osteotomy
Severe hallux valgus (IMA >20°)	Scarf osteotomy for most cases, but consider fusion instead	
Hallux valgus with first tarsometatarsal hypermobility	A first tarsometatarsal fusion with distal soft tissue procedure	
Hallux valgus with first MTPJ degeneration	First MTPJ arthrodesis	
Hallux valgus interphalangeus	Akin osteotomy	

IMA, intermetatarsal angle; MTPJ, metatarsophalangeal joint.

Presentation

Hallux rigidus presents with pain and stiffness of the first MTPJ.

In the early stages the pain is dorsal and worsened by walking or wearing high heels. Later the pain is deeper and may include sesamoid pain. The dorsal cheilus may cause pressure on the dorsal cutaneous nerve resulting in dysaesthesia and numbness along the medial border of the hallux.

Clinical assessment

The range of movement of the joint is restricted. Dorsiflexion is limited more than plantarflexion. Early in the disease, pain is only elicited at the extremes of dorsiflexion and plantar flexion, but in the later stages, crepitus and pain develops in the mid arc. The patient's gait becomes increasingly antalgic as the MTPJ stiffens and then progressive transfer of weight to the lateral border of the foot occurs. The interphalangeal joint often hyperextends in chronic cases, a callosity may also occur on the plantar aspect of this joint.

Radiological assessment

Standing anteroposterior and lateral radiographs reveal a dorsal osteophyte on the head of the metatarsal early on, with joint space narrowing, subchondral cyst formation, and sclerosis later.

Hattrup and Johnson classified the radiographic findings in 1988:

- Grade I: mild to moderate osteophyte formation with preservation of the joint space
- Grade II: moderate osteophytes narrowing of the joint space and subchondral sclerosis
- Grade III: marked formation of osteophytes with loss of the joint space, with or without subchondral cysts.

Non-operative treatment

Orthoses and shoe modification reduce motion, impingement, and mechanical stress on the joint. An extra-depth toe box avoids pressure on the dorsal osteophyte. A shoe with a low heel, stiffened sole, and a rocker bottom limits dorsiflexion.

Operative treatment

Injection or manipulation under anaesthetic and steroid injection may lead to reduced symptoms in patients with grade I changes.

Dorsal cheilectomy

Cheilectomy of the dorsal osteophyte and the degenerate portion of the articular surface on the head of the metatarsal preserves or increases motion, maintains joint stability, has low morbidity, and permits revision surgery. The osteophyte recurs in one-third of cases, although this does not correlate with clinical failure.

Following cheilectomy 97% of patients with minimal joint space loss have an excellent or good self-assessment score and a mean increase in dorsiflexion from 14.5 to 38.4 degrees. Poor results may ensue after cheilectomy in the patients with advanced degeneration. Thus cheilectomy is recommended in patients with grade I and II hallux rigidus.

It is sometimes performed with a dorsal closing wedge osteotomy of the proximal phalanx to increase the arc of MTPJ motion—a Moberg osteotomy.

Keller's resection arthroplasty

Keller's procedure is only rarely used and then only in low-demand and elderly patients. Some authors advocate capsular interposition arthroplasty in more active patients.

Metatarsophalangeal joint replacement

Hemiarthroplasty of the proximal phalanx and total joint replacement using Silastic® (Dow Corning), ceramic arthroplasty, and unconstrained metallic implants have been tried for hallux rigidus. There is a high failure rate of joint replacement in hallux rigidus. Given these unfavourable results in multiple studies with different implants, joint replacement is usually reserved for unusual circumstances such as rheumatoid arthritis with stiff midfeet in low-demand patients.

Arthrodesis

Arthrodesis of the first MTPJ is the mainstay of treatment for grade 3 hallux rigidus. It eliminates painful motion and maintains stability of the first ray. Complications include non-union, progressive arthritis of the interphalangeal joint, and lateral transfer metatarsalgia. The great toe is fused in 5–10 degrees of valgus to allow the great toe to lie alongside the second toe without impingement. The condyles of the proximal phalanx of the hallux are positioned 3–4mm off the ground at surgery. This is judged preoperatively with simulated weight bearing, comparing the toe to a flat surface.

Arthrodesis has been compared with Keller's procedure, hemiarthroplasty, and arthroplasty of the MTPJ. In all studies arthrodesis demonstrated superior results with fewer complications.

Lesser toes

Introduction

Deformities of the lesser toes should be considered in the context of the forefoot as a whole. For example, correcting a claw second toe with a dislocated MTPJ, without addressing an adjacent hallux valgus, usually fails. Firstly there is no space into which to reduce the toe, and secondly the deformity will recur if the underlying biomechanical cause of lesser toe overload is not addressed.

In this section the lesser toes will be addressed in isolation. The section on forefoot reconstruction addresses a more holistic approach which is often needed.

Box 9.2.3 Hallux rigidus

- Affects 1:45 people over 50 years of age
- Characterized by stiffness: hallux rigidus
- Aetiology: idiopathic, trauma, osteochondritis dissecans, inflammatory arthritis
- Hattrup and Johnson radiological classification
- Non-operative treatment: extra-depth toe box with stiffened, rocker bottom sole
- Dorsal cheilectomy indicated for early hallux rigidus
- Arthrodesis is the mainstay for advanced disease.

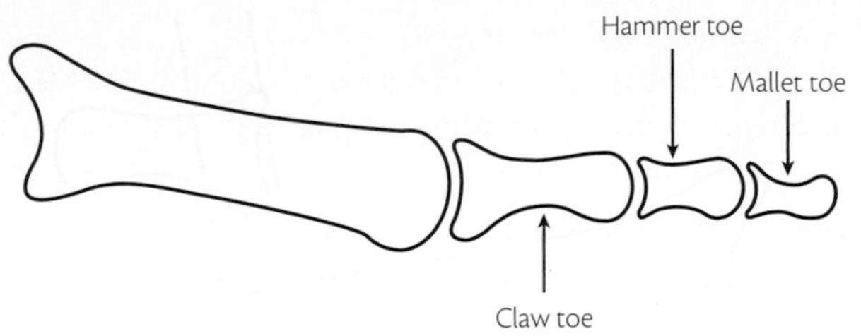

Fig. 9.2.4 Anatomy of the lesser toes.

Definitions

There are three principal deformities of the lesser toes. These are mallet, hammer, and claw (Figure 9.2.4). The deformities may be fixed or flexible.

Mallet toe

A mallet toe is flexed at the distal interphalangeal joint (DIPJ). Patients with mallet toes usually present with pain and callosities at the tip of the toe, where the sharp end of the distal phalanx impacts on the ground. Nail deformities are common.

Hammer toe

Hammer toes are flexed at the proximal interphalangeal joint (PIPJ), and usually at the DIPJ. Occasionally the DIPJ is extended—a boutonnière deformity.

Claw toe

Claw toes are the most complex and involve the same distal deformity as a hammer toe but with an extension deformity of the MTPJ. The most severe cases lead to subluxation or dislocation of the MTPJ.

Anatomy

The MTPJs are stabilized by two collateral ligaments and a plantar plate. The intrinsic and extrinsic musculature control movement of the toes (Figure 9.2.5). There are two extrinsic flexors and two extensors, none of which attach directly to the proximal phalanx. The short flexor inserts to the middle phalanx and the long flexor to the distal phalanx. The extensor mechanism is held centred over the MTPJ by the extensor hood. The extensor digitorum longus has a central slip that inserts into the middle phalanx but also has two slips connected to the distal phalanx—this is analogous with the anatomy seen in the hand.

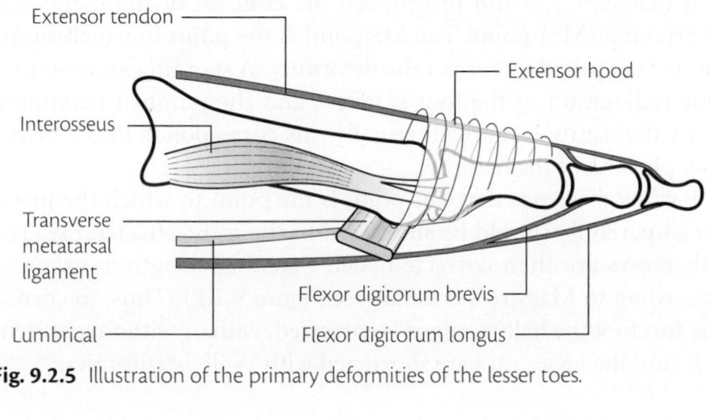

Fig. 9.2.5 Illustration of the primary deformities of the lesser toes.

The function of the extrinsic muscles is assisted by the intrinsic muscles. The interosseous and lumbrical muscles lie plantar to the MTPJ and act as flexors of this joint. They lie dorsal to the axis of the PIPJs and DIPJs and act as extensors of these.

Aetiology

Lesser toe deformities are common, occurring in 20% of individuals. Their incidence increases with age. They are commoner in women than men (4–5:1). The second toe is most commonly involved.

The most important aetiological factor in lesser toe deformity is probably shoes. Lesser toe deformity may also be a manifestation of neurological disease, compartment syndrome, and diabetes mellitus.

Presentation

Pressure produces callus, thus lesser toe deformity presents with deformity and painful callosities over the dorsal or plantar aspect of the foot.

The most severe and disabling symptoms are those in the MTPJ, where synovitis can progress on to subluxation and even dislocation of the joint.

Clinical assesment

The following points should be noted:

- The nature and type of the shoes worn
- Presence of systemic disease such as inflammatory arthropathy, diabetes mellitus, and peripheral vascular disease
- The exact location of pain
- Callosities
- Whether the deformity is correctable or uncorrectable.

Radiographic examination

Standing anteroposterior and lateral radiographs of the foot may help define subluxation or dislocation of the lesser MTPJs, Freiberg's disease, and hallux valgus and rigidus.

Non-operative treatment

In many patients, simple measures provide adequate treatment—a shoe with a toe box which is deep and wide enough to accommodate the deformed toes. Protection with padding or silicone toe sleeves can help, as can toe props. Calluses should be removed by a podiatrist, or the patient.

Patients with metatarsalgia may be helped by insoles with a metatarsal dome, or bar.

Operative treatment

The principles of surgery are:

- Treat the toe from proximal to distal: MTPJ, PIPJ, DIPJ
- Address correctable deformity with soft tissue procedures
- Address fixed deformity with bony procedures.

Mallet toes

A flexible mallet toe rarely needs correction. If necessary, treatment consists of a tenotomy of the long flexor tendon through a plantar approach. A fixed deformity is treated with excision arthroplasty or fusion of the DIPJ, each with simultaneous tenotomy of the long flexor tendon through the DIPJ. An alternative is terminalization of the toe.

Hammer toes

Correctable hammer toes rarely require surgery. When they do, a soft tissue procedure is performed, either a flexor to extensor tendon transfer (Girdlestone) or a long flexor tenotomy.

Fixed deformity is treated with a PIPJ fusion—usually with wire fixation—or excision arthroplasty where only the condyles of the middle phalanx are excised and a pseudoarthrosis is formed. This avoids the need for wires, but excessive resection can lead to a floppy toe. Excision arthroplasty is improved by interposition of retained redundant extensor tendon.

Claw toes

In claw toes there is an extension deformity of the MTPJ. Surgery to the MTPJ is incremental, until the deformity is corrected. A soft tissue release of the capsular structures including the collateral ligaments with tenotomy of the extensor digitorum brevis, and Z-lengthening of the extensor digitorum longus is performed.

If the MTPJ is subluxed or dislocated a bony procedure will be required which may be:

1) Du Vries arthroplasty: excising the distal 3–4mm of the metatarsal head, leading to arthrofibrosis (with about 50% reduced movement)

2) Weil osteotomy: the Weil osteotomy is an oblique osteotomy which translates the metatarsal head proximally, ideally without plantar displacement. This osteotomy is fixed with a small screw. The metatarsal head is translated sufficiently to allow the joint to reduce comfortably. The extensor tendons are left intact unless they remain tight at the end of the procedure, when they can be lengthened. It is difficult to cut the metatarsal parallel to the floor, especially in the second and third rays, with their steeper declination. Therefore a second cut excising a small segment is undertaken to prevent plantar displacement (Figure 9.2.6). Postoperatively the toe can be taped in 5–10 degrees of plantar flexion. Early mobilization is important to maintain mobility. The major complication of the Weil osteotomy is MTPJ stiffness as a result of impingement of the metalwork, prominent bone and arthrofibrosis

3) Proximal phalangectomy (Stainsby): in this procedure a generous proximal phalangectomy is undertaken, the plantar plate is mobilized and reduced, and the extensor tendon is interposed into the joint. The toe is stabilized with a longitudinal Kirschner wire. Ninety-three per cent of patients report excellent result or good results after this procedure. It leads to a weak toe.

Forefoot reconstruction

In some feet it is possible to address a single issue, for example, a hallux valgus or claw toe. In other feet the whole forefoot needs addressing. In this section the principles of forefoot reconstruction will be addressed.

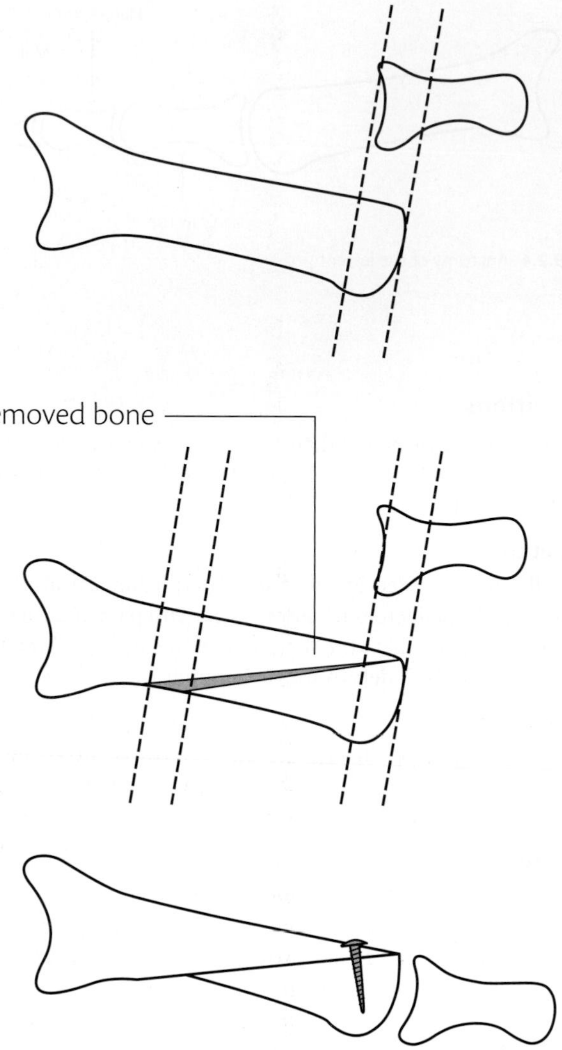

Fig. 9.2.6 Illustration of the Weil osteotomy.

First ray insufficiency

If there is hallux valgus this must be corrected to stabilize the first ray. This leads to resolution of the transfer lesions in some patients, but in patients with subluxed or dislocated lesser toes or those with secondary valgus drift of the lesser toes, the MTPJ needs to be reduced.

Barouk has outlined a number of principles for treating these feet (Table 9.2.3) and introduced the concept of the metatarsal shortening (MS) point. The MS point is the point to which shortening is required to correct the deformity. A standing anteroposterior radiograph of the foot is taken, and the point of maximum bony deformity is marked. Usually this corresponds to the proximal phalanx of the first ray.

Barouk proposes that this point is the point to which the metatarsal parabola should be shortened in the most affected ray. The other rays are then corrected such that their length is balanced according to Maestro's criteria (see Figure 9.2.2). Thus, to correct the forefoot the hallux valgus is corrected, with or without shortening, and the lesser rays are shortened with Weil osteotomies.

Table 9.2.3 Barouk's principles of forefoot reconstruction, with modifications

The hindfoot morphology must always be considered in addressing the forefoot
Internally fix osteotomies to allow early functional rehabilitation
Identify the point of maximum deformity, and plan your reconstruction around this 'MS' point
Balance the forefoot to establish a normal metatarsal parabola
If the surgery only affects a single ray, you only need to operate on this ray
A foot that fits a shoe, will function like a foot

MS, metatarsal shortening.

Box 9.2.4 Rheumatoid forefoot

- Typical deformities in the rheumatoid forefoot are hallux valgus and claw toes
- Non-operative treatment: pharmacological, total contact insoles, extra wide shoes with deep toe box
- Hallux MTPJ fusion
- Hoffman procedure (excision of lesser metatarsal heads) for the lesser toes
- Joint preservation can be considered in young patients with rheumatoid arthritis.

Rheumatoid forefoot

Pathophysiology

Ninety-four per cent of patients with rheumatoid arthritis (RA) have symptoms from the foot and ankle, with hallux valgus in the majority. The typical deformities in the rheumatoid forefoot are hallux valgus and claw toes. Overload and synovial inflammation of the lesser MTPJs leads to disruption of the collateral ligaments and capsule, and dorsal subluxation and dislocation of the MTPJ occurs. The dorsally dislocated phalanx forces the corresponding metatarsal head into plantar flexion. At the same time, the plantar fat pad also moves distally from beneath the metatarsal head. These factors increase plantar pressure. Consequently large plantar callosities and bursae develop.

Non-operative treatment

This comprises pharmacological treatment, shoe modification, orthoses, and steroid injections. Total contact insoles and rocker bottomed shoes can diminish peak pressures and shear stresses under the forefoot.

Operative treatment

Hallux

Excision arthroplasty Hallux valgus is the commonest deformity of the rheumatoid forefoot. Keller's procedure and excision of the first metatarsal head (Mayo's procedure) have both been used. Good initial patient satisfaction has been reported, but recurrent deformity, pain, and functional deterioration are common.

Arthrodesis Arthrodesis of the first MTPJ offers the advantages of good correction, relief of pain, and predictable outcomes, with union rates of around 90%. Several studies have compared arthrodesis with resection arthroplasty and have shown fusion to be superior for pain relief, cosmetic appearance, shoe-fitting, maintenance of alignment, and restoration of weight bearing under the hallux.

Hallux metatarsophalangeal joint arthroplasty Arthroplasty of the hallux MTPJ may be an alternative to resection arthroplasty or arthrodesis for the severely affected rheumatoid patient, usually with hinged double-stemmed silicone implants or ceramic or metallic arthroplasty. Moderate pain relief and patient satisfaction has been reported with the use of silicone implants but they may fracture or fragment, and cause synovitis in up to 29% of cases. Other complications include aseptic loosening of the implant, cock-up deformity, stiffness, and transfer metatarsalgia.

Lesser toe deformity

Excision procedures Hoffman described resection of the lesser metatarsal heads to allow deformity correction and relief of metatarsalgia. This procedure and its many variations have become the commonest treatment.

A transverse plantar incision, two longitudinal dorsal incisions, and a single transverse dorsal incision have been used to approach the lesser MTPJs, all with good reported outcomes. The plantar incision allows direct access to the dislocated MTPJs and excision of excess plantar fat pad and skin; alternatively, the dorsal incisions are felt to provide good MTPJ access while avoiding a scar on the plantar surface in patients who have impaired wound healing.

The Stainsby procedure, with generous proximal phalangectomy is also widely used.

Coughlin reported 96% good to excellent results with an arthrodesis of the first MTPJ and resection of the lesser toe metatarsal heads in 58 feet.

MTPJ preserving procedures Barouk and Barouk proposed joint-preserving surgery as an alternative approach to the rheumatoid forefoot. They reported excellent results using a scarf osteotomy for the first ray and Weil osteotomies of the lesser metatarsals. A recent study reported 88% excellent or good results following arthrodesis of the first MTPJ combined with multiple Weil metatarsal osteotomies of the lesser rays. Weil shortening can be difficult in dislocated MTPJs with joint destruction and soft bone.

Further reading

Barouk, L.S. (2000). Scarf osteotomy for hallux valgus correction. Local anatomy, surgical technique, and combination with other forefoot procedures. *Foot & Ankle Clinics*, **5**, 525–58.

Barouk, L.S. and Barouk, P. (2007). Joint-preserving surgery in rheumatoid forefoot: preliminary study with more-than-two-year follow-up. *Foot & Ankle Clinics*, **12**, 435–54.

Coughlin, M. (2000). Rheumatoid forefoot reconstruction: a long-term follow-up study. *Journal of Bone and Joint Surgery*, **82A**, 322–41.

Maestro, M., Besse, J.L., Ragusa, M., and Berthonnaud, E. (2003). Forefoot morphotype study and planning method for forefoot osteotomy. *Foot & Ankle Clinics*, **8**, 695–710.

Stephens, M.M. (1994). Pathogenesis of hallux valgus. *Foot and Ankle Surgery*, **1**, 7–10.

9.3

Diabetic foot

Andy Goldberg and Paul H. Cooke

Summary points

- Diabetic foot problems are of major socioeconomic importance
- Aetiology is multifactorial, with a neuropathic, vascular, and immune component
- A multidisciplinary approach must be adopted, with education and prevention being key aims
- If ulceration develops, restoration/preservation of an intact soft tissue envelope and the creation of a plantigrade foot that can bear weight are the key treatment goals.

Introduction

Diabetes affects 5% of the world's population. For diabetic patients, 30% of hospital admissions are for complications of the feet. With 20 million people worldwide suffering from Type 1 diabetes and up to twelve times that with Type 2 diabetes, their foot problems have a major social and economic importance.

Twenty per cent of diabetics develop clinically significant neuropathy after 10 years from diagnosis and 50% after 20 years. The longer the duration of the disease, the greater the risk of developing significant neuropathy.

Fifty per cent of diabetic foot problems and subsequent amputations can be eliminated by educating patients and physicians, and providing proper prevention and early treatment.

Aetiology

The aetiology of diabetic foot problems is multifactorial with a neuropathic, vascular, and immune component.

Neuropathic component

Neuropathy appears to be the most important factor in the aetiology of the diabetic foot and although not fully understood, involves the sensory, motor, and autonomic systems. Tight control of blood glucose levels reduces or prevents the development of neuropathy, but once developed it is irreversible.

Most patients complain of sensory changes in a glove and stocking distribution. Some have numbness and paraesthesia, others have hyperaesthesia or dysaesthesia, presenting as a burning sensation, usually nocturnal. It is this lack of sensation and, therefore, basic protective mechanisms, that makes problems of the diabetic foot severe and difficult for both patients and doctors.

Motor neuropathy leads to muscle weakness and intrinsic muscle atrophy. The plantar fat pad shifts and there is possibly rupture of some of the slips of the plantar fascia. The cumulative effect of these changes is less plantar protection of the bony prominences leading to callus formation, pressure necrosis, and ulceration. Patients with motor neuropathy may develop bunions, claw toes, and hammer toe deformities as a result of muscle imbalances.

Isolated mononeuropathy also occurs in diabetics, with the common peroneal nerve most typically being involved. This is characterized by unilateral foot drop, which must be differentiated from spontaneous rupture of the tibialis anterior tendon that is also seen in diabetics.

Autonomic neuropathy leads to loss of autonomic function and hence changes in blood flow and sweating, resulting in thick, dry, scaly skin and nail deformities.

Charcot neuroarthropathy is a non-infective destructive process that manifests as dislocation, periarticular fracture, or both, in patients with peripheral neuropathy. Although the incidence of

Box 9.3.1 Key facts on diabetic foot

- 3–4% of diabetics have foot ulcers or deep infections
- 15% of diabetics develop foot ulcers during their lifetime
- 30% of hospital admissions in diabetics are for pathologic conditions of the feet
- Severity of complications correlates with diabetic control
- Diabetic foot ulcers (DFUs) precede 70% of non-traumatic lower extremity amputations
- The risk of amputation increases eightfold once an ulcer develops
- 5 years after lower-extremity amputation, nearly two-thirds of these patients have died.

Charcot disease is very low (0.3% of diabetics), its impact on patients and treating surgeons is major and hence we have dedicated a section to Charcot disease at the end of this chapter.

Vascular component

Demonstrable peripheral vascular disease is present in 8% of adult diabetics at the time of diagnosis and increases to 45% after 20 years. The vascular deficiency in these patients is a mixture of large and small vessel disease and the presence of pulses does not necessarily mean the vascular supply is normal.

Immune component

Glycosylated immune proteins lose their efficiency in diabetics and granulocyte function is often impaired, especially if the patient is malnourished. These changes increase susceptibility to infection with organisms that would not normally affect a healthy host.

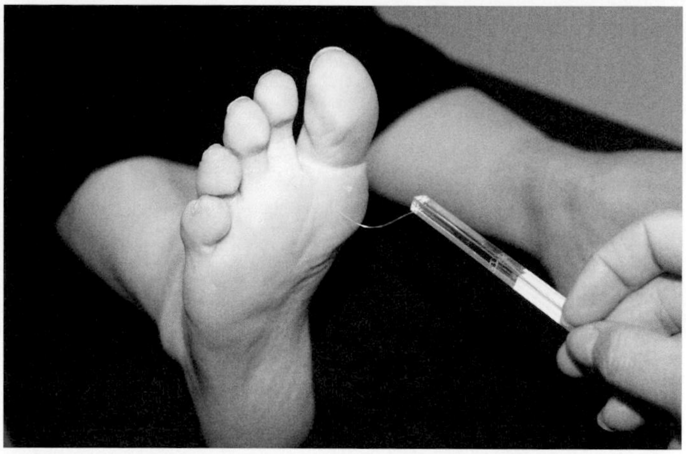

Fig. 9.3.1 A 5.07-calibre Semmes–Weinstein monofilament being used to test 10g of pressure, the threshold for loss of protective sensation. The patient is asked to note when they can feel pressure applied to each of the metatarsal heads and the tips of the toes.

Clinical presentation

Diabetic patients can present to the orthopaedic surgeon with four broad groups of problems:

- Ulcerations
- Infections
- Charcot's joints
- Skin and nail problems.

Clinical assessment

General assessment

In your history, establish the duration of the diabetes itself as well as any prior foot ulceration and whether or not any surgery has been performed. The duration of diabetes as well as the level of diabetic control correlates with the severity of vascular and neurologic change. It is also important to identify patients with ischaemic rest pain as opposed to those with dysaesthesia or insensitivity.

Foot assessment

Observe the patient's gait, both with and without shoes. In standing posture assess the hindfoot alignment as well as the arches of the foot.

During supine or sitting examination, document the general condition of the skin and toenails and in particular the presence of corns, calluses, and ulcerations. Note areas of bony prominence as well as those areas lacking normal fat-pad protection.

Examine light touch, pinprick, vibration sense, and deep tendon reflexes. The threshold for diagnosis of peripheral neuropathy is the inability to perceive 10g of pressure applied to the skin using the Semmes–Weinstein monofilament (Figure 9.3.1). The 5.07 monofilament is estimated to apply just over 10g of pressure and with this benchmark in population screening, plantar insensitivity is present in approximately 25% of adult diabetics.

Vascular examination

Feel the dorsalis pedis and posterior tibial pulses. If present and the capillary refill is brisk then further assessment is not usually helpful. If pedal pulses are absent, the ankle–brachial pressure index (ABPI) should be carried out using a handheld Doppler probe and a sphygmomanometer.

The ABPI in normal patients is usually around 1.1. An ABPI of less than 0.9 is regarded as abnormal. Critical ischaemia is indicated by an ABPI of less than 0.5 or one that is unrecordable. In diabetics, the ABPI may be spuriously high because of calcification in the distal vessels which prevents them from being compressed by the sphygmomanometer cuff around the calf, and so if the ABPI is over 1.3 then it is deemed an unreliable test.

If the patient has absent pulses or an abnormal ABPI then referral to a vascular surgeon is recommended. They will tend to carry out an arterial Doppler ultrasound (duplex scan) in the first instance as this is cheap and non-invasive. The wave pattern on the duplex provides important information. A triphasic waveform is consistent with normal vessel elasticity whereas a monophasic waveform indicates a calcified vessel. The measurement of toe pressures is also useful and an absolute toe pressure of 45mmHg is more predictive of healing than the ABPI.

If further information is required then magnetic resonance imaging (MRI) angiography is usual, although the use of contrast may be contraindicated in those with renal impairment.

Skin assessment

Skin breakdown is usually caused by shear forces. Plantar ulcers are due to weight-bearing pressure, whereas dorsal and side ulcers are, in the main, caused by shoe pressure.

The most widely used system to classify diabetic ulceration is the depth–ischaemia classification which looks at the size and depth of affected areas as well as the vascular status of the limb (see Table 9.3.1, Figure 9.3.2).

Investigations

Blood tests include a full blood count (FBC), renal function (urea and electrolytes, U&Es), liver function tests (LFTs to look at albumin levels for nutritional deficiency), and haemoglobin A1c (HbA1c) to look at longer-term diabetic compliance. If osteomyelitis is suspected you should request an erythrocyte sedimentation rate (ESR) and C-reactive protein (CRP).

Table 9.3.1 The depth–ischaemia classification of diabetic foot lesions*

	Definition	Treatment
Depth classification		
0	At-risk foot Previous ulcer or neuropathy and deformity.	Patient education. They should be taught to exam their feet regularly, wear appropriate footwear, etc.
1	Superficial ulceration No infection	Offload foot with a total contact cast, or walking brace
2	Deep ulceration exposing tendons or joints	Surgical debridement Culture-specific antibiotics
3	Extensive ulceration with exposed bone and/or deep infection (osteomyelitis) or abscess	
Ischaemia classification		
A	Not ischaemic	None
B	Ischaemia without gangrene	Vascular reconstruction as necessary (angioplasty or proximal and/or distal bypass using vein graft) or partial foot amputation
C	Partial (forefoot) gangrene	
D	Complete foot gangrene	Vascular intervention Major extremity amputation

*Adapted from Brodsky, J.W. (2007). Diabetic foot. In Coughlin, M.J. and Mann, R.A. (eds.) *Surgery of the Foot and Ankle. Vol II*, pp.1281–368. St. Louis, MO: Mosby.

Plain radiographs of the foot and ankle are standard. Permeative radiolucencies, destructive changes, periostatis, and new bone formation without reparative response suggests osteomyelitis, but plain film changes may lag 2 weeks or more behind the onset of osteomyelitis.

Bone scans (technetium-99m, ^{99m}Tc) and MRI are more sensitive than plain radiographs in detecting early bone changes of osteomyelitis and Charcot's joints. However, MRI is more sensitive and detects osteomyelitis earlier than a bone scan. Although MRI is useful in diagnosing occult abscess formation, especially if contrast is used, it is important to stress that no imaging techniques (plain radiographs, bone scans, or MRI) clearly distinguish neuroarthropathy from evolving deep bone infection and the diagnosis has to be made clinically.

Superficial swabs from ulcers will always grow mixed skin flora and are not helpful. If infection is suspected, deep biopsies should be obtained to direct antibiotic treatment.

Prevention

A multidisciplinary approach is used to manage the diabetic foot and the most important measures are education and prevention, in particular in stressing the importance of good accommodative footwear and diligent control of blood sugars (Box 9.3.2).

Box 9.3.2 Prevention

- Basic principles are education and prevention
- Good footwear
- Good glucose control.

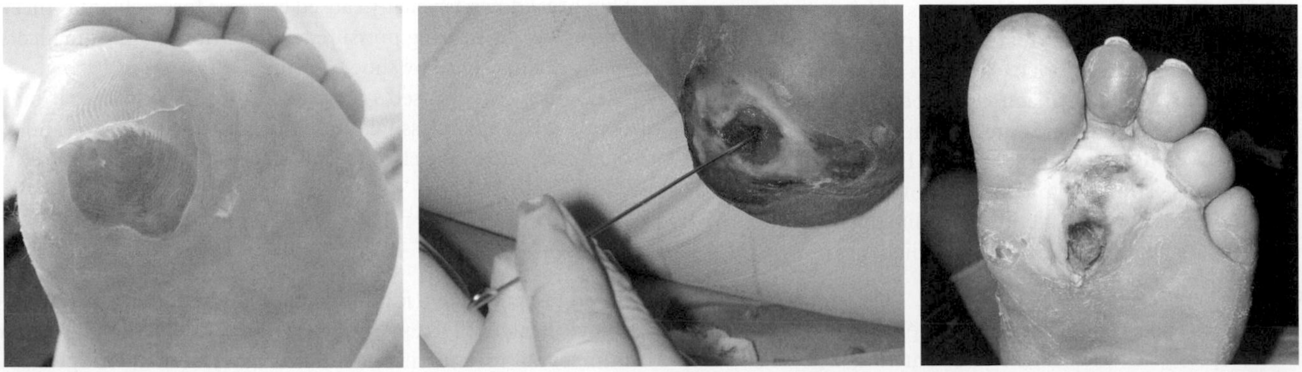

A B C

Fig. 9.3.2 Stages of the depth–ischaemia classification. A) Grade 1A, superficial ulceration. B) Grade 2A showing deep ulceration over the heel, which on probing reveals that it is down to bone. C) Grade 3C ulcer with osteomyelitis and a gangrenous second toe.

In patients with neuropathy it is important to stress that they need to examine their feet on a daily basis in front of a mirror, as they will not be alert to the same warning signs as those with sensate feet. It is also important to instruct diabetic patients in proper nutrition and the harmful effects of tobacco use.

Treatment

There is no set treatment for the diabetic foot and each treatment plan has to be individualized to the patient. There are, however, some broad goals for treatment, listed in Box 9.3.3.

Treatment protocols correlate with the specific grades found in the depth–ischaemia system (Table 9.3.1) which require full assessment of the ulcer and also the vascularity of the feet.

Most wounds treated in the outpatient setting are grade 1. The focus of treatment for grade 0 or grade 1 lesions is to relieve pressure. Options to modify weight-bearing pressure include specialized footwear, total contact casts, prefabricated walking braces, or custom ankle–foot orthoses (AFOs). The choice depends on the lesion and the specific problems of each patient.

Surgery on the diabetic foot

Surgery in the diabetic foot is frequently based on failure of non-operative management.

The goals of surgery include: relief or redistribution of pressure to ensure closure of the soft tissue envelope; to create a plantigrade foot that can weight bear; and one in which bracing, if appropriate, is a viable option.

Contraindications to surgery include significant underlying medical disease, severe malnutrition, and patients unable to comply with the postoperative course.

If there is vascular insufficiency then an opinion of a vascular surgeon should be sought with a goal of limiting the extent of amputation, potentially through revascularization methods such as angioplasty (including subintimal angioplasty to get distal revascularization) or femorocrural or femorodistal bypass.

If amputation is necessary, transcutaneous oxygen assessment is useful to assist in delineating the amputation level as attempts are made to maximize residual limb length to improve postoperative function. As prosthetic management will be necessary, preoperative evaluation by a prosthetist and rehabilitation specialist is recommended.

There are a large number of surgical treatment options available to treat the diabetic foot, full details of which are beyond the scope of this textbook; however, for simplicity Table 9.3.2 outlines a number of common problems and their treatments. Tendoachilles (TA) contracture commonly occurs in these patients and TA lengthening should always be considered as part of the treatment.

Box 9.3.3 Treatment goals

1) Restore or preserve an intact soft tissue envelope (get any ulceration to heal)
2) Create or preserve a plantigrade foot that can weight bear
3) Use bracing, orthotics, and appropriate footwear to maintain both of the above
4) Prevent amputation.

Table 9.3.2 Surgical options for treatment of the diabetic foot

Problem	Surgical treatment options
Hallux interphalangeal or metatarsophalangeal ulcer	Corrective osteotomy Excision of sesamoid through a medial approach Excision arthroplasty of 1st MTPJ (Keller's)
Lesser toe (metatarsophalangeal) ulcer	Elevation osteotomy at base of metatarsal Plantar condylectomy Metatarsal head excision
Hammer toe/claw toe deformities	Toe straightening procedure at the PIPJ (extensor tendon lengthening over MTPJ, MTPJ capsular release, division of IPJ collaterals, excision of distal third of proximal phalanx, interposition arthroplasty of extensor tendon to plantar capsule) PIPJ fusion
Mallet toe deformity	Flexor tenotomy Distal IPJ arthroplasty (see 'toe straightening') DIPJ fusion
Hallux valgus with lesser toe deformities or dislocation	Bunion correction (1st MT osteotomy and Akin varizing osteotomy for hallux interphalangeus) Keller's procedure Amputation of lesser toe 1st MTPJ fusion plus shortening/elevation of lesser toes (Weil osteotomies) 1st MTPJ fusion plus modified Hoffman procedure (resection arthroplasty of 2nd–5th MT heads
Midfoot ulceration overlying bony prominence (rocker-bottom foot)	Aggressive exostectomy Realignment arthrodesis (triple arthrodesis with or without wedge exostectomy. Note: tendoachilles lengthening is always required) Amputation
Ulceration secondary to ankle and hindfoot instability and deformity	Realignment arthrodesis (e.g.Tibiotalar-calcaneal arthrodesis) Amputation
Soft corns	Bony decompression via arthroplasty (excision or interposition)
Toenail disorders	Wedge excision of nail Zadik's procedure (great toe nail ablation) In osteomyelitis, consider terminal amputation

DIPJ, distal interphalangeal joint; IPJ, interphalangeal joint; MT, metatarsal; MTPJ, metatarsophalangeal joint; PIPJ, proximal interphalangeal joint.

Treatment of infections

Grade 2 lesions involve deeper soft tissues and require more aggressive wound management, in addition to pressure-relieving devices. If probing a wound demonstrates communication to bone then there is a high probability (more than 80%) of osteomyelitis.

Whilst available evidence does not support treating clinically uninfected ulcers with antibiotics, deeply infected ulcers should be admitted and started on appropriate intravenous antibiotics, empirically at first and then culture specific. Because infections in the diabetic foot tend to be polymicrobial, consultation with an infectious diseases expert is recommended to assist with selection and duration of antibiotics.

Aerobic Gram-positive cocci (especially *Staphylococcus aureus*) are the predominant pathogens in diabetic foot infections. Patients with chronic wounds or those who have received recent antibiotics may also be infected with Gram-negative aerobic rods (e.g. *Escherichia coli*) and those with foot ischaemia may have obligate anaerobic pathogens (e.g. bacteroides).

If the patient fails to improve clinically after appropriate wound care and antibiotics, an MRI is recommended to rule out occult abscess. Abscesses require drainage and if there is wet gangrene this must be carried out as an emergency.

Charcot disease

A complication of neuropathy in the diabetic population is Charcot disease. This neuropathic osteoarthropathy results in fragmentation, destruction, and dislocations of the bones of the foot and ankle. It was originally described by a French physician, Jean-Martin Charcot, in 1868 in a patient with tertiary syphilis. It was only described in diabetes in the 1930s although diabetes is now the commonest cause.

There are two theories of pathogenesis for the development of Charcot disease: neurotraumatic and neurovascular. The former involves repetitive trauma sustained by a joint unable to sense pain, whereas the latter refers to a sympathetic dysfunction with persistent hyperaemia and active bone resorption. The incidence of Charcot osteoarthropathy occurring in the diabetic population is 0.1–0.5%, despite up to 25% of diabetics having a clinically detectable peripheral neuropathy. The average time interval between the onset of diabetes and that of Charcot change is 16 years.

Despite it being a rare complication, it is one of the most severe of the problems encountered by the orthopaedic surgeon and therefore has a much greater impact on the treating surgeon's practice, than its frequency would suggest.

Charcot disease may be the first presentation of diabetes. In Charcot's disease the foot can assume significant deformity with a red, hot, swollen foot that mimics infection but without the clinical signs of overt sepsis such as fever, leucocytosis, and abnormal diabetic control. The muscle imbalance across a Charcot foot, with contracture of the Achilles tendon creates a static and dynamic equinus deformity of the ankle in which there is a pathological bending moment through the midfoot, leading to collapse of the arch and the development of a rocker-bottom deformity.

Contrary to common belief, 50% of Charcot feet have some pain, usually a deep pain.

Classification of Charcot

Eichenholtz characterized the natural history of Charcot neuroarthropathy into three stages as described in Table 9.3.3.

Anatomical classification of Charcot

Brodsky introduced an anatomical classification based on the regions of the foot most often affected by the Charcot process (Table 9.3.4). The most commonly affected areas are the midfoot, followed by the hindfoot, and lastly the ankle joint. The forefoot is involved only on rare occasions.

Table 9.3.3 Eichenholz stages of Charcot neuroarthropathy*

Eichenholz stage	Clinical	Radiography
I: fragmentation	Acute inflammatory phase: erythema, warmth, and swelling	Either normal; or debris, fragmentation of subchondral bone, subluxation, and/or dislocation
II: coalescence	Reparative phase: reduction in erythema, warmth, and swelling	New bone formation Coalescence of larger fragments Sclerosis of bone ends
III: consolidation	Healing phase: resolution of erythema and swelling; residual deformity	Remodelling, rounding of bone Decreased sclerosis

*Adapted from Eichenholtz, S.N. (1966). *Charcot Joints*. Springfield, Il: Charles C. Thomas.

Treatment of the Charcot foot (Figure 9.3.3)

The Eichenholtz stage I foot often presents with swelling and erythema and it is often very difficult to distinguish it from infection, although the patients lack the clinical signs of sepsis.

Admission and elevation of the limb to the level of the heart will often bring rapid (overnight) improvement in the appearance in Charcot, compared with infection where the signs will persist and may get worse.

Immobilization in a total contact cast is the mainstay of treatment for Eichenholtz stage I neuroarthropathy. Because one of the functions of the cast is to reduce swelling, it will tend to loosen quickly and so an initial cast should be changed after 5–10 days. Subsequent casts should be changed at intervals of 2–4 weeks.

The Charcot arthropathy process may take up to 2 years to run its course. The Eichenholtz stage I foot should be immobilized until it has progressed beyond the fragmentation stage, which can be 16 weeks or more.

Some surgeons have advocated the use of operative management of deformity during stage I neuroarthropathy, with arthrodesis *in situ* or realignment procedures. There is no data comparing this form of treatment with casting and it is not yet mainstream practice.

As increased osteoclastic activity is one of the processes leading to bony destruction, the administration of bisphosphonates have

Table 9.3.4 Anatomical classification of Charcot disease*

Type	Location	Typical joints affected
Type 1 (up to 60%)	Midfoot (Lisfranc)	Metatarsocuneiform and naviculocuneiform joints
Type 2 (30–35%)	Hindfoot (Chopart's) (any of the triple joints)	Subtalar-calcaneocuboid-talonavicular
Type 3 (<10%)	Ankle joint	Type 3A: ankle joint Type 3B: involves a pathologic fracture of tubercle of calcaneus (very uncommon)

*Brodsky, J.W. (2007). Diabetic foot. In Coughlin, M.J. and Mann, R.A. (eds.) *Surgery of the Foot and Ankle, Vol. II*, pp. 1281–368. St. Louis, MO: Mosby.

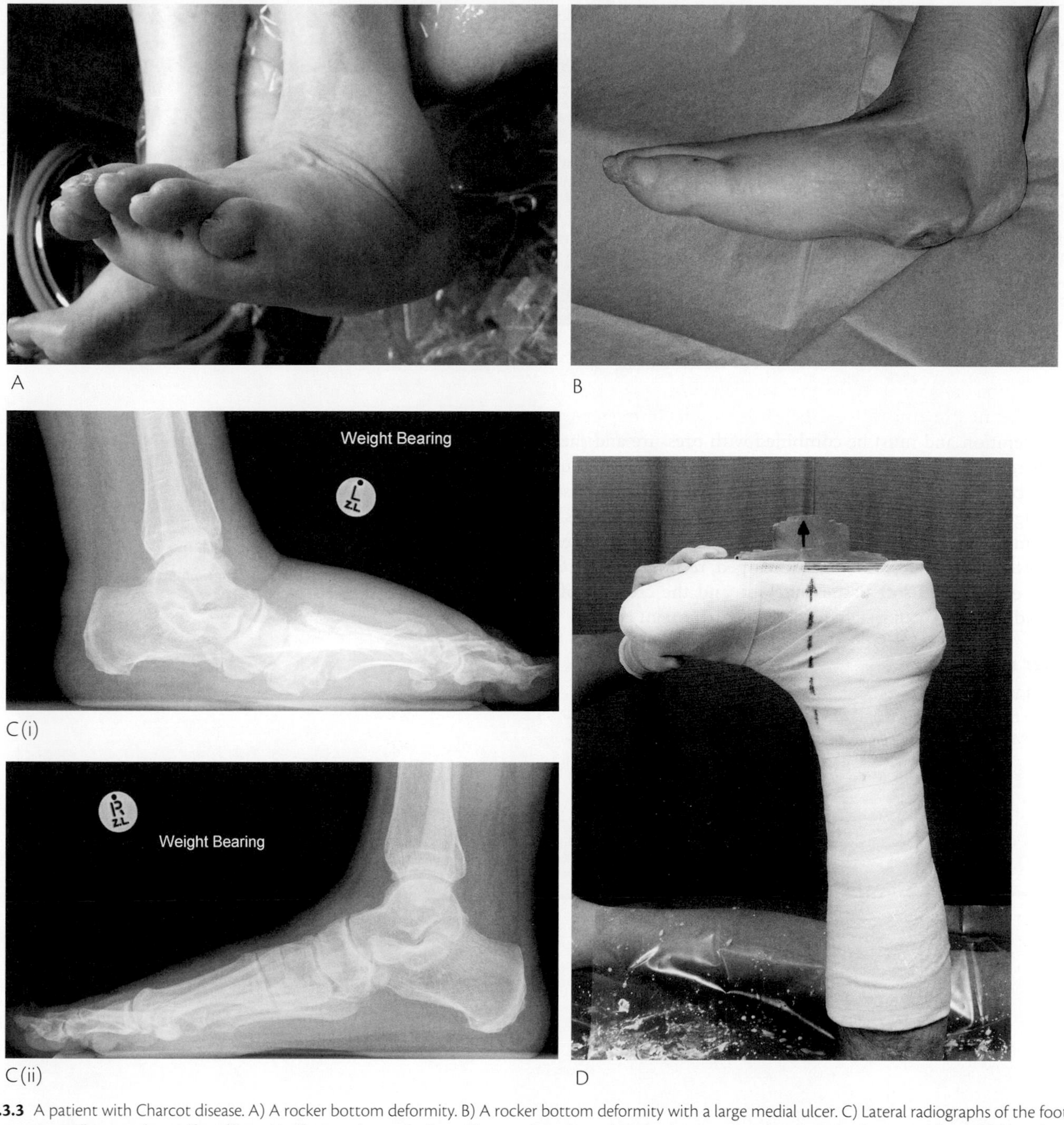

Fig. 9.3.3 A patient with Charcot disease. A) A rocker bottom deformity. B) A rocker bottom deformity with a large medial ulcer. C) Lateral radiographs of the foot demonstrating collapse at the midfoot (Note: hindfoot equinus as indicated by negative calcaneal pitch when compared to the opposite normal foot). D) A total contact cast with rocker-bottom sole (courtesy Mr N Geary).

been advocated in stage I neuroarthropathy. Randomized controlled trials have been carried out using parenteral pamidronate and alendronate demonstrating decreased markers of bone turnover, as well as reduced warmth in the limb over the period of the study. Whilst some groups are using bisphosphonates in the treatment of stage I neuroarthropathy, neither pamidronate nor alendronate are currently licensed for this use.

As the involved extremity passes through the Charcot stages, the focus of treatment turns to preventing limb-threatening complications. Surgery is used to correct deformity and reduce recurrent problems due to structural abnormalities (Figure 9.3.4). Accommodative orthoses should be prescribed to correct inequalities in pressure. Rocker-bottom shoes combined with an AFO or a Charcot restraint orthotic walker (CROW) may also be necessary to manage more severe deformities.

Conclusion

The diabetic foot is a major challenge. Neuropathy is the major factor leading to morbidity although neuropathy alone will not

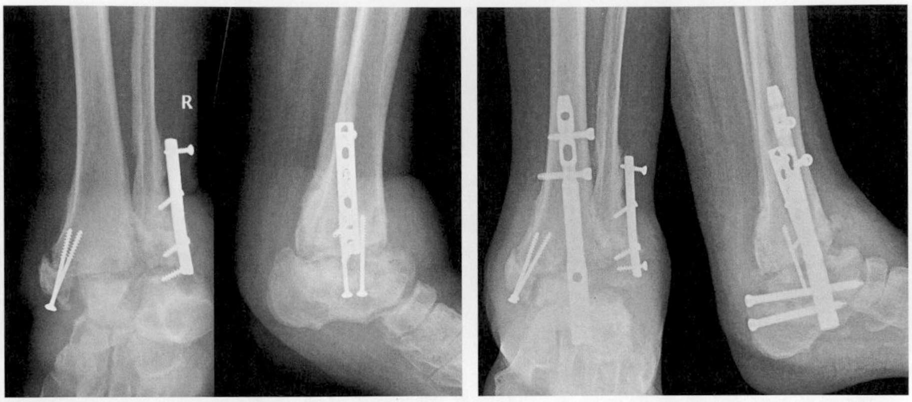

Fig. 9.3.4 Radiograph showing ankle and hindfoot destruction in Charcot disease after fracture and failed fixation. A) Preoperative anteroposterior and lateral. B) Postoperative after tibio-talar-calcaneal (TTC) fixation using an intramedullary nail.

cause ulceration and must be combined with pressure and shear forces across the soft tissues as well as underlying vascular and immune components. A multidisciplinary approach must be used in treating this important group of patients. The basic principles in the treatment of diabetic foot problems are education and prevention. However, once ulceration has developed, restoration or preservation of an intact soft tissue envelope and the creation of a plantigrade foot that can weight bear are key treatment goals.

Further reading

Brodsky, J.W. (2007). Diabetic foot. In: Coughlin, M.J. and Mann, R.A. (eds.) *Surgery of the Foot and Ankle, Vol. II*, pp. 1281–368. St. Louis, MO: Mosby.

Centers for Disease Control and Prevention. Diabetes Public Health Resource. Available at: http://www.cdc.gov/Diabetes.aspx

Lipsky, A.J., Berendt, A.R., Deery, H.G., *et al.* (2004). Diagnosis and treatment of diabetic foot infections. *Clinical Infectious Diseases*, **29**, 885–910.

Pinzur, M.S. (2008). Current concepts review: Charcot arthropathy of the foot and ankle. *Foot & Ankle International*, **28**, 952–9.

9.4

Orthoses of the foot and leg

Jo Mitchell and Paul H. Cooke

Summary points

- Orthoses may be corrective or accommodative
- Orthoses are described according to their anatomical application
- A knowledge of material properties, anatomy, and function is essential to prescribe
- Patients will only tolerate effective orthoses.

Introduction (Box 9.4.1)

Orthotic management of foot and ankle disorders is a little understood but important subject. Ortho- is derived from the Greek orthos, meaning straight.

Orthoses are externally applied devices used to modify the structural and functional characteristics of the neuromuscular or skeletal system through the application of forces.

Orthoses work in several ways:

- To correct malalignment and maintain correction
- To control motion (assist, resist, and/or stop)
- To augment weakened muscles
- To redistribute weight and generate a more natural loading pattern
- To accommodate fixed deformity.

A holistic approach is necessary when prescribing any type of orthosis. The cause of the problem and biomechanical deficit should be identified; then a device can be prescribed which effectively addresses the biomechanical problem.

Often, however, a compromise on the ideal form of orthotic treatment has to be made. This could be due to the fact that by controlling movement about a joint in one plane you may inadvertently affect movement in another plane which is unaffected. Other factors include the ability of the patient to put on and take off the orthosis independently and whether the item is cosmetically acceptable to the patient.

The correct terminology for describing an orthosis is generally accepted to be an indication of the joints that a device encompasses, for example, ankle–foot orthosis (AFO) and foot orthosis (FO). However, they can also be named after people or places (which should be avoided as it can be confusing) or by the function which they provide such as 'hallux valgus orthoses' (see next paragraph).

In this chapter we deal with orthoses in order from distal to proximal.

Toe splints

Hallux valgus orthoses to correct bunions will straighten the hallux when in place, but do not produce longstanding correction. They are most commonly used at night. Daytime splints are available but are difficult to wear within footwear. They can be useful as part of a postoperative regimen.

A variety of devices may be used on the lesser toes, usually decreasing pressure and friction rather than correcting deformity. Hammer toe 'crests' (banana splints) positioned in the sulcus raise the tip of the toe to relieve terminal corns. Silicon gel tubes reduce rubbing of the dorsum of clawed or hammer toes against the shoe; silicon polymer devices can be moulded in the clinic to protect and support lesser toe deformities.

Foot orthoses

Simple inlays (Figure 9.4.1A)

These are non-moulded and provide minimal support. They consist of a flat base made of card, leather, or closed-cell foam and can have valgus and/or metatarsal pads incorporated to support the arches of the foot. The base material may be full length or trimmed proximal to the metatarsal heads (three-quarter length). Off-the-shelf/prefabricated types are also available.

Box 9.4.1 Orthoses

- Orthoses correct deformity, maintain position, augment power, or accomodate
- Orthoses are off the shelf or made to measure (bespoke)
- Rigid materials correct and maintain position
- Soft materials cushion and accomodate
- Orthoses must fit the patient and their footwear.

Such an insole is often included within the shoe by the manufacturer, but the use of different materials, with increased cushioning by the use of foam or gel, allows improved shock absorption, and changes can be made to the surface of the insole to reduce shear forces.

Moulded inlays (functional foot orthoses, Figures 9.4.1B–D)

These are corrective, bespoke orthoses—manufactured by taking casts, impressions, or scanning the foot. They can be made of polypropylene/polyethylene, ethylene vinyl acetate (EVA) foam or composite materials and can be full, three-quarter length, or customized to suit the patient's needs (Table 9.4.1). Wedging or 'posting' can be added to the shell of the orthosis to correct or accommodate hindfoot and/or forefoot malalignment. Other additions can be incorporated, such as cushioning top layers and metatarsal pads.

EVA functional foot orthoses (FFOs) generally provide less control than polypropylene or carbonfibre foot orthoses and take up more room in the shoe. They are, however, more easily tolerated than rigid devices.

Heel cups (Figure 9.4.1E)

Where greater control of the subtalar and midtarsal joints is required the depth of the orthosis is increased to provide cupping around the heel. Heel cups are made of polypropylene and are generally three-quarter length so as not to interfere with forefoot function.

All these foot orthoses (and all ankle orthoses) are prescribed and fitted to address the patient's problem, but due regard must also be taken of the footwear needed to accommodate an orthosis.

Shoes may be open (slip on) or enclosed, and have laces, hook-and-loop fasteners (e.g. Velcro®), or elastic fitting. They can be made of soft or firm materials and have widely varying soles—both the materials (e.g. shock absorbing, rigid) used and their design (flexible, rocker profiles).

In general a lace-up or Velcro® fastened shoe is preferable to accommodate and optimally secure an orthosis. It is not normally possible to accommodate a FFO within a slip-on shoe or sandal. In these circumstances, patient compliance may necessitate compromise or, as they take up less space in the shoe, a simple inlay may be used.

So shoe choice is important; but equally important is the fit of the orthosis within the shoe. Inability to fit the orthosis inside the shoe is a common reason that foot orthoses are not used. Patients can be advised to find shoes with a removable insole (put there by the manufacturer) so that this can be removed and replaced with the foot orthosis, as in common sports shoes/trainers.

Orthopaedic footwear

Orthopaedic footwear may also be considered as an orthosis in that it is capable of applying forces to the foot in a controlled manner as well as performing an accommodative role.

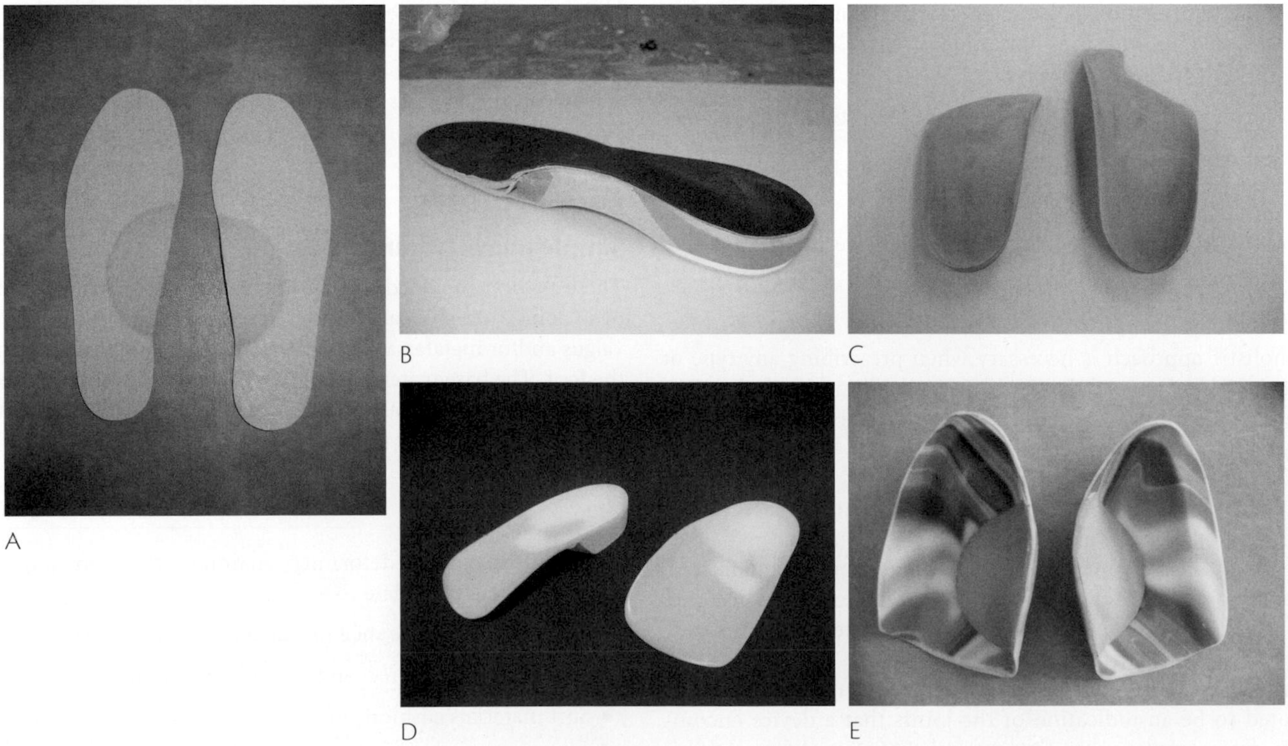

Fig. 9.4.1 Foot orthoses. A) A simple inlay with added medial arch cushion. B) A bespoke functional foot orthosis with medial posting. C) Functional foot orthoses may be of different lengths and materials. D) A rigid functional foot orthosis. E) A heel cup gives greater varus/valgus support.

Table 9.4.1 Materials commonly used in the production of moulded inlays

Rigid	Accommodative	Linings
Polypropylene	Ethylene vinyl acetate (EVA)—varying densities (open or closed cell)	Poron® PPT® Memory foam
Polyethylene		Leather
Carbonfibre composites		

Two types of footwear are commonly prescribed:

1) Made-to-measure (bespoke)
2) Off-the-shelf (stock).

Footwear adaptations

External adaptations such as raises (to accommodate leg length discrepancy), rocker soles (to enable heel rise in late stance with conditions such as hallux rigidus/limitus or ankle stiffness/fusion), floats (to increase the width of the heel, increasing stability), and wedges can be added to the patient's own footwear or to orthopaedic shoes.

Ankle orthoses (Figure 9.4.2A)

These are usually prefabricated braces used to stabilize the ankle (after injury or for chronic instability). They act solely on the ankle joint providing mediolateral control. These braces can also provide support in early arthritis or postoperatively.

Supramalleolar orthoses (Figures 9.4.2B)

Supramalleolar orthoses (SMOs) are custom-made devices which influence movements at the ankle joint and the foot.

They can be designed as a heel cup with high medial and lateral wings, anchored with Velcro® extending proximally over the malleoli, or with more extensive dorsal trim lines encapsulating the foot and ankle.

They are usually manufactured from flexible or rigid plastic and less commonly from blocked leather.

This design can control deformities in the transverse and coronal planes; however, it has no effect on saggital plane movements of dorsiflexion and plantar flexion.

Ankle–foot orthoses

The primary function of all ankle–foot orthoses (AFOs) is to control alignment and movements of the foot and ankle complex. A secondary effect may be to influence the hip and knee joints by influencing the ground reaction force.

Polypropylene AFOs are manufactured by taking a cast of the patient's leg in the corrected position. The polypropylene is moulded over the modified plaster model, thus producing a close fit and precise control of pressure distribution. After moulding, the device is trimmed to the required shape. Varying degrees of mediolateral stability can be achieved depending on the anterior trim lines and rigidity of the design.

Posterior leaf spring (Figure 9.4.3A)

A posterior leaf spring (PLS) AFO is used to aid or give passive dorsiflexion where flaccid foot drop occurs due to nerve damage (e.g. from a prolapsed disc) or in neurological disease.

The trim line is narrow between the calf and foot piece allowing dorsiflexion against resistance but returning the foot to a neutral alignment once plantar flexion power is removed, thus compensating for weak or absent dorsiflexors.

The addition of helical straps to reduce varus/valgus tendency increases mediolateral stability, and is used, for instance, in hereditary motor sensory neuropathy when inversion can be associated with foot drop.

Prefabricated AFOs are available and are useful assessment tools; however, custom-made designs are usually more comfortable and effective for long-term use.

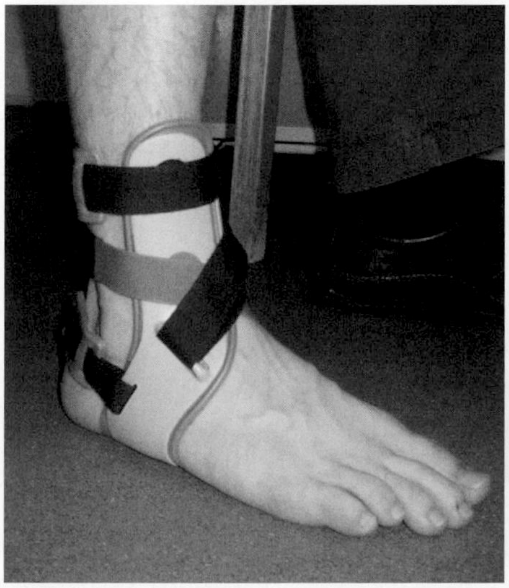

A

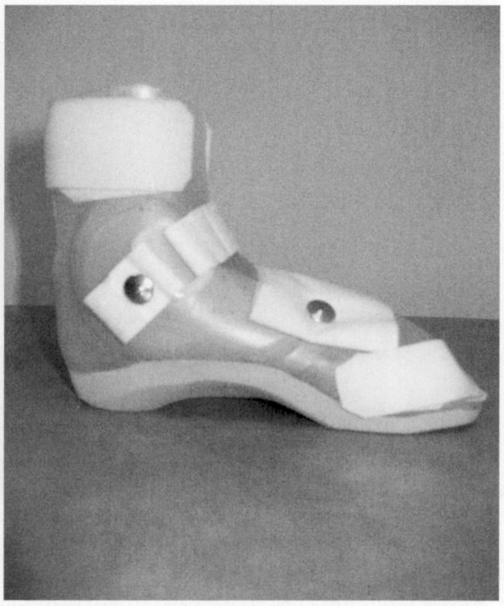

B

Fig. 9.4.2 Ankle orthoses. A) An ankle brace commonly used to treat or prevent lateral ankle ligament sprain. B) A bespoke supramalleolar orthosis (SMO).

Rigid ankle–foot orthoses (Figure 9.4.3B)

Rigid or solid ankle AFOs maintain the foot and ankle in a predetermined position. They prevent plantar flexion and dorsiflexion and offer good mediolateral control. Due to the rigidity of the design a rocker sole may be required to aid tibial advancement and walking.

Hinged ankle–foot orthoses (Figure 9.4.3C)

AFOS can be manufactured to incorporate hinges which can allow free motion, or restrict dorsiflexion and/or plantar flexion with the use of adjustable ankle locks, or aid dorsiflexion with the use of concealed springs. This can provide good control and allow movement, but is often at the expense of decreased cosmesis and increased bulk making footwear fitting difficult.

Anterior ground reaction ankle–foot orthoses (AGR-AFOs)

Anterior ground reaction ankle–foot orthoses (AGR-AFOs) can be a one-piece or two-piece design incorporating a rigid AFO with a removable front shell. They aim to bring the ground reaction force anterior to the knee and are used when there is excessive dorsiflexion and knee flexion as with crouch gait. A full range of knee extension must be present to allow them to work effectively.

Conventional ankle–foot orthoses (previously callipers), (Figure 9.4.3D)

These usually consist of one or two metal uprights attached to a metal, leather-covered calf band. They attach distally via a spur into a stirrup in the sole of the shoe.

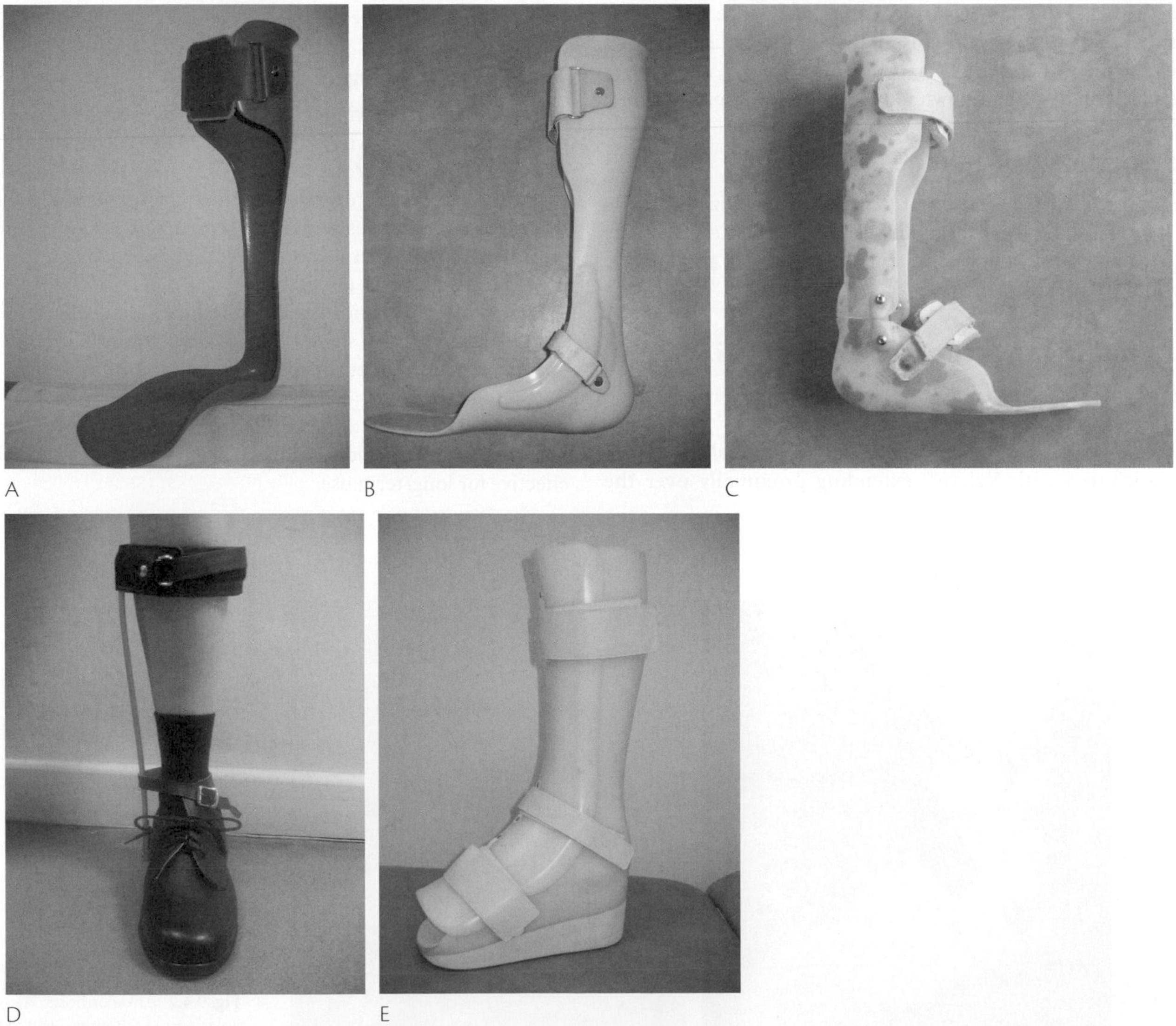

Fig. 9.4.3 Ankle–foot orthoses (AFOs). A) The posterior leaf spring orthosis has a narrow sprung segment at the ankle level. B) A rigid AFO. C) An AFO may incorporate hinges. D) A conventional AFO/caliper—here an inner iron with T strap to correct varus deformity. E) A Charcot restraint orthosis walker (CROW) is bivalve, total contact with liner.

The socket within the shoe can allow free motion or limit motion with the use of front (dorsiflexion) or back (plantar flexion) stops.

These can be used in conjunction with T/Y straps stitched to the shoe to aid valgus/varus instability.

Ankle joints can also be added to conventional calipers to:

- Stop/block motion
- Assist motion with the use of springs.

Conventional orthoses have largely been replaced by contemporary plastic designs. However, conventional orthoses offer an alternative when plastic orthoses are not tolerated.

Charcot restraint orthotic walker (Figure 9.4.3E)

The Charcot restraint orthotic walker (CROW) is a custom-moulded bivalved orthosis incorporating a total contact cradle inlay and a full EVA lining. It is used to immobilize the foot and ankle and to protect neuropathic feet during the early and intermediate stages of neuropathic Charcot disease, usually due to diabetes. On occasion it may be used long term as an alternative to amputation.

Conclusion

Orthoses are widely used in orthopaedic foot and ankle treatment either alone or as an adjuvant treatment and can help avoid, or delay, the need for surgery. Orthoses act to correct malalignment of body segments, control motion, accommodate deformity, and reduce pain and pressure. Patients rarely want to wear orthoses but patients who find that they can walk further, faster, or with less pain will often adapt their lifestyle and footwear to use these devices. It is often worth trying orthoses before proceeding to more invasive treatment.

Further reading

International Organization for standardization (1989). *ISO 8549-1: Prosthetics and Orthotics Vocabulary. Part 1: General terms for External limb Prosthetics ad External Orthoses.* Geneva: International Organization for Standardization.

International Organization for Standardization (1989). *ISO 8549-3: Prosthetics and Orthotics Vocabulary. Part 3: Terms relating to external Orthoses.* Geneva: International Organization for Standardization.

9.5

Tendon and ligament disorders of the foot and ankle

Matthew C. Solan and Mark S. Davies

Summary points

- Treatment of tendon and ligament disorders of the foot depends on accurate clinical diagnosis, supported by investigation
- The treatment of posterior tibial tendon dysfunction is guided by classification
- Ankle ligament injuries only need surgical treatment if very severe or chronic
- Achilles tendonitis is usually treated conservatively
- Rupture of the Achilles tendon may be treated operatively or conservatively.

Posterior tibial tendon dysfunction

Introduction

Tibialis posterior dysfunction is the most common cause of acquired flat-foot deformity in the adult.

Anatomy

The tibialis posterior muscle lies in the deep posterior compartment of the calf and is innervated by the tibial nerve (L4, L5). The musculotendinous junction is 4cm above the medial malleolus and the tendon passes behind the medial malleolus in its own sheath. It attaches mainly to the tuberosity of the navicula by three bands: anterior, middle, and posterior. The anterior is the largest (65%) attaching to the navicular tuberosity and inferior medial cuneiform. The middle band extends to the more lateral cuneiforms, cuboid, and metatarsal bases of the second, third, and fourth rays. The posterior band contributes to the soft tissue components of the acetabulum pedis.

Function

The posterior tibial tendon plays an important role in function of the foot and ankle. During gait the foot fulfils two purposes. As the foot contacts the ground it is flexible and acts as a shock absorber. By the end of the stance phase, the foot has changed into a rigid lever to maximize push-off strength. As a flexible shock-absorbing foot, the transverse tarsal (talonavicular and calcaneocuboid) joints are parallel and move in concert. With activity of tibialis posterior the heel inverts, the orientation of the transverse tarsal joints changes and flexibility is abolished.

Where tibialis posterior is dysfunctional the transition from flexible shock absorber into rigid lever does not occur. This places excess strain upon the medial column of the foot (the spring ligament in particular) and eventually leads to planovalgus deformity.

Clinical features

Posterior tibial tendon dysfunction (PTTD) is a progressive disorder. Johnson and Strom proposed a staging system that was later modified by Myerson (Table 9.5.1).

Most patients with early PTTD go unrecognized. It occurs mostly in people with pre-existing low arches. Posteromedial ankle pain and swelling occur first, but it is the 'collapse' of the medial longitudinal arch that usually prompts referral.

Once deformity becomes marked, fibular impingement develops.

Examination: standing

Walking aids, orthotics, and shoes are inspected for wear.

The medial longitudinal arch and the inclination of the heel are observed from behind. The 'too many toes' sign is a marker of forefoot abduction but not pathognomonic of PTTD (Figure 9.5.1).

The patient is asked to rise onto tiptoes. Normally both heels will invert. Failure of inversion indicates PTTD (Figure 9.5.2) but subtalar joint stiffness may cause the same appearance.

If double-stance heel rise is normal then single-stance heel rise is performed.

Table 9.5.1 Stages of tibialis posterior insufficiency. (I–III Johnson and Strom; IV added by Myerson)

Stage	Tendon	Deformity
I	Swollen	No deformity
II	Swollen and elongated	Mobile planovalgus
III	Swollen and elongated	Fixed planovalgus
IV	Swollen and elongated	Secondary ankle osteoarthritis

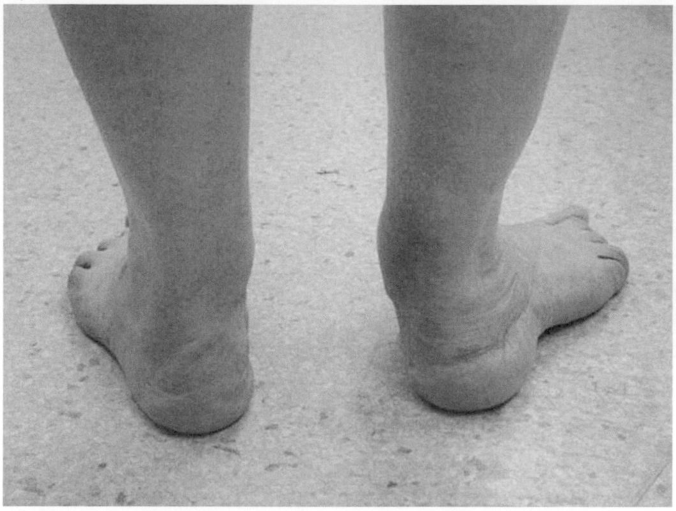

Fig. 9.5.1 Acquired flat foot—heel valgus, flat arch, and 'too many toes'.

This may be: impossible; more difficult than on the unaffected side; or fatigue easily with repetition—according to the severity of the PTTD.

It is important to consider the more proximal parts of the lower limb.

The leg must be exposed to allow knee alignment to be assessed as valgus deformity of the knee may be associated with an acquired flat-foot deformity.

To assess contracture of the gastrocnemius, the patient is asked to stand on their heels only, with the toes clear off the ground (forefoot ground clearance).

Examination: sitting

The pulses and sensation are checked.

Ankle and triple joint flexibility is assessed, and joint line tenderness noted. Silfverskiold's test demonstrates the severity of an associated gastrocnemius contracture by assessing the difference in ankle equinus observed when the knee is flexed compared to when the knee is extended fully (Figure 9.5.3).

The forefoot to hindfoot alignment is observed after reducing and holding the heel into neutral position beneath the tibia, then observing the relative position of the sole of the forefoot to the heel.

Where the first ray is elevated in relation to the fifth ray, the deformity is known as forefoot varus (Figure 9.5.4).

Differential diagnosis

Acquired flat foot in adulthood is most commonly caused by PTTD. Tarsometatarsal osteoarthritis, spring ligament injury, and subtalar joint inflammatory arthropathy are important differential diagnoses.

Clinical investigation

Plain weight-bearing anteroposterior (AP) radiographs show dorsolateral peritalar subluxation. Bilateral films allow comparison of the degree of uncovering of the talar head. A weight-bearing lateral film may demonstrate alignment of first tarsometatarsal and naviculocuneiform joints (Figure 9.5.5). These films and an oblique view should be studied for evidence of degenerative joint disease.

In advanced PTTD, an AP weight-bearing radiograph of the ankle may show ankle arthritis.

Ultrasound of the posterior tibial tendon is a useful means of confirming tenosynovitis, thickening, or rupture of the tendon but

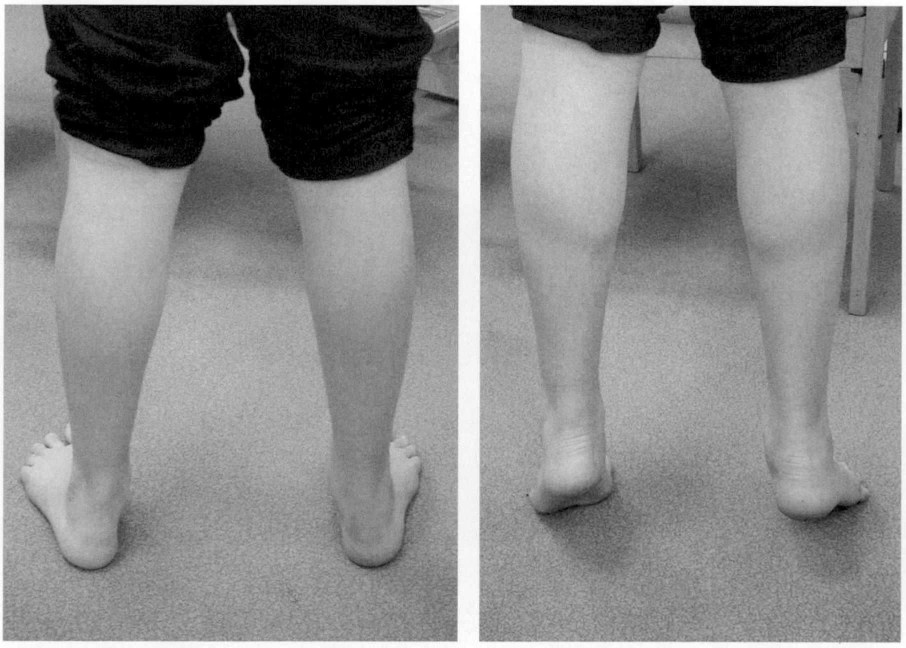

Fig. 9.5.2 Failure of (right) heel to invert on tiptoe raise.

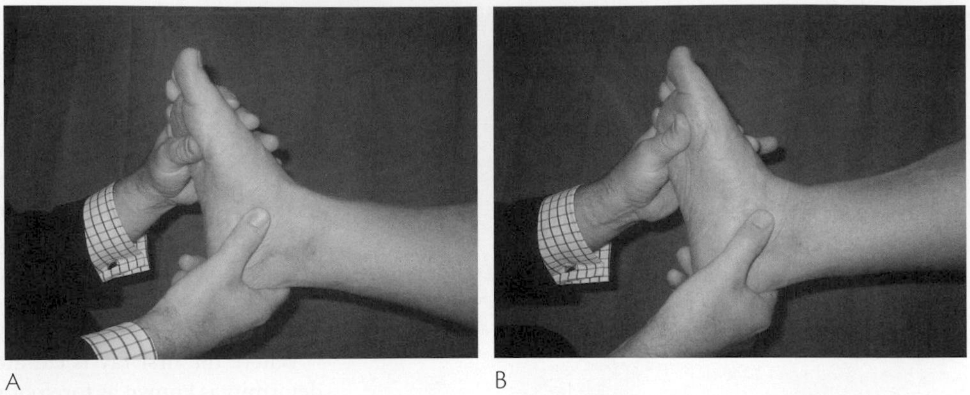

Fig. 9.5.3 Silfverskiold's test for isolated contracture of the gastrocnemius. A) Knee fully extended: limited dorsiflexion. B) Knee bent: dorsiflexion improves.

is operator dependent so may be less useful to the treating surgeon than a magnetic resonance imaging (MRI) scan (Figure 9.5.6).

Treatment

Non-operative

Physiotherapy and orthotic management are the mainstays of treatment. Physiotherapy addresses the gastrocnemius contracture and strengthens the tibialis posterior tendon and toe flexors.

Orthotic management

Orthotics may be corrective or accommodative. Functional foot orthoses (FFOs) extend only across the foot. More extensive devices (e.g. ankle–foot orthosis, AFO) are reserved for advanced stages of PTTD.

Details of specific orthotics are contained in Chapter 9.4.

Operative

Surgery for PTTD should achieve a stable, painless, and plantigrade foot.

Corrective knee surgery must be undertaken before the foot and ankle are addressed.

The stage of PTTD is a useful guide to treatment (Box 9.5.1).

If non-operative treatments for stage 1 PTTD do not work, tenosynovectomy may prevent progression of the tendinopathy and

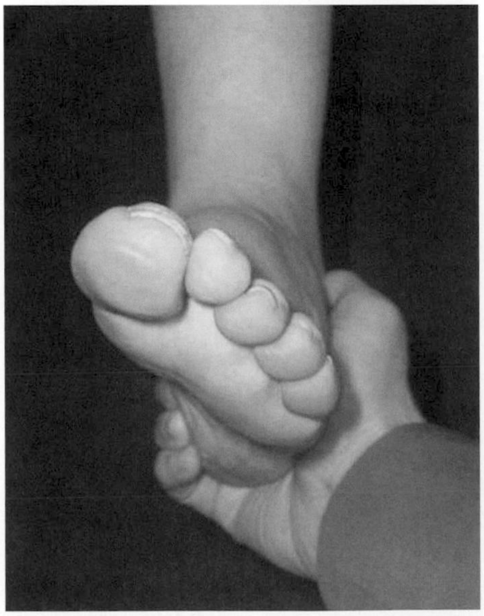

Fig. 9.5.4 Forefoot varus—assessed with heel corrected to neutral.

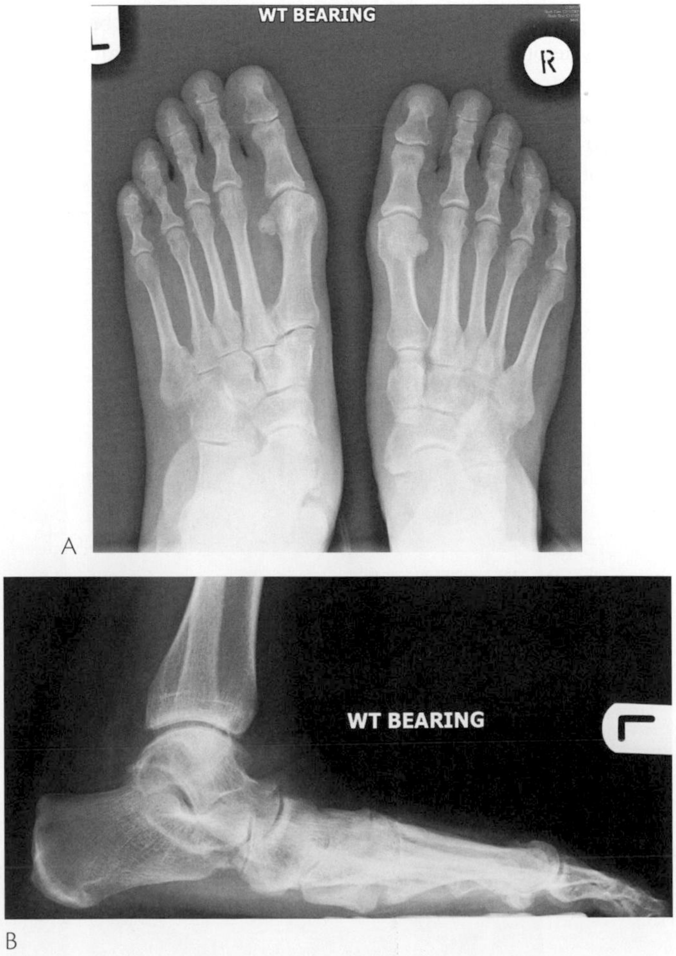

Fig. 9.5.5 A) Weight-bearing anteroposterior radiograph showing dorsolateral peritalar subluxation. B) Weightbearing radiograph with midfoot break.

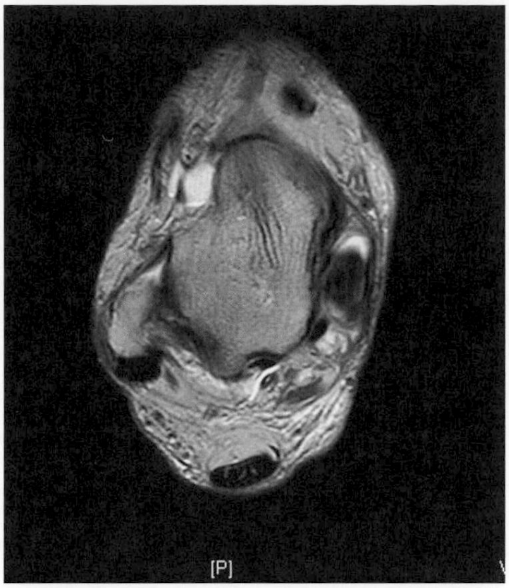

Fig. 9.5.6 Magnetic resonance image (axial) of posterior tibial tendon tendinopathy.

relieve the pain and swelling in about three-quarters of patients. In selected cases this may now be performed arthroscopically.

In stage 2, joint-preserving surgery with tendon transfer and osteotomy is preferable to arthrodesis. It is most successful where the forefoot varus is correctable.

The most widely used tendon is the flexor digitorum longus (FDL). This fails in isolation, so it is combined with medializing calcaneal osteotomy. The osteotomy protects the tendon transfer by correcting heel valgus and medializing the insertion of the Achilles tendon. Plication of the spring ligament and short plantar ligaments are also performed to restore static restraint.

In patients with medial column joint laxity, midfoot osteoarthritis, or hallux valgus, appropriate midfoot fusions and/or correction of the hallux valgus may be required to restore structure.

Surgical correction of associated gastrocnemius contracture should be performed if tight.

Alternative techniques to FDL transfer and calcaneal osteotomy include lateral column lengthening.

Where the hindfoot is stiff or there is significant degenerative joint disease (stage 3), corrective fusion is preferred. Traditionally, triple arthrodesis has been used, but produces considerable hindfoot stiffness.

Subtalar fusion may be used if there is no fixed midfoot deformity, with cuneiform osteotomy, midfoot fusion, or talonavicular fusion also sometimes required to correct the forefoot–hindfoot relationship.

Where the talonavicular joint is unstable, isolated talonavicular fusion may be considered.

In severe cases, where there is ankle degenerative joint disease, pantalar fusion or corrective triple arthrodesis followed by an ankle replacement are considered (Figure 9.5.7).

Prognosis

Surgical treatment of stage 2 PTTD gives satisfaction rates of 90% after 2 or 3 months' cast immobilization. It takes another 6–9 months for swelling to resolve and strength to improve.

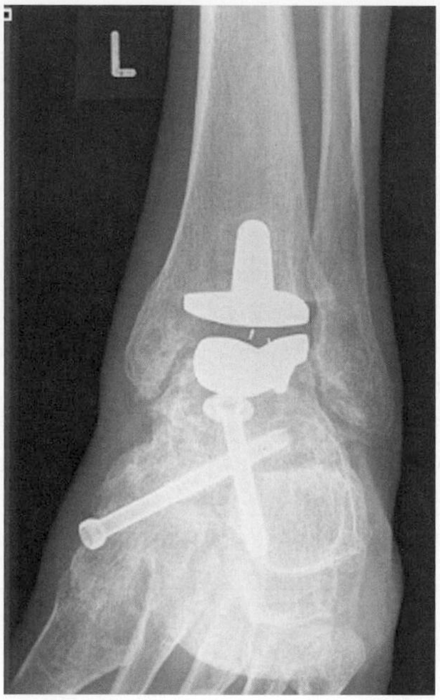

Fig. 9.5.7 Triple arthrodesis and total ankle replacement. Courtesy of Mr P. Cooke.

Selective or triple joint fusion for stage 3 PTTD also has good results, as long as plantigrade position is achieved.

Disorders of the ligaments of the ankle

Introduction

Ankle injuries make up 10% of attendances to Emergency Departments. The majority are inversion injuries resulting in localized pain, swelling, and bruising maximal over the anterolateral aspect of the ankle from damage to the anterior talofibular ligament (ATFL) and joint capsule.

Most are treated initially with rest, ice, compression, and elevation (RICE) followed by early weight bearing with an ankle brace. Physiotherapy concentrates on proprioceptive training and peroneal tendon strengthening.

Approximately 20–30% of patients suffer ongoing problems with their ankle. Table 9.5.2 shows the possible differential diagnoses.

Box 9.5.1 Tibialis posterior insufficiency

- The common cause of flat-foot deformity in adults
- Classified according to tendon involvement and flexibility
- Management plan: try orthotics first
- Flexible feet: corrective orthotics vs. tendon transfer/osteotomy
- Fixed deformity: accommodative orthotic vs. corrective arthrodesis.

Table 9.5.2 Differential diagnoses for the 'ankle sprain that does not get better'

Medial ankle pain	Lateral ankle pain	Anterior ankle pain	Posterior ankle pain
Deltoid ligament injury	Lateral ligament complex injury	Anterior impingement syndrome	Acute rupture of Achilles tendon
	Diastasis injury—inferior tibiofibular joint injury		
Chondral or osteochondral injuries	Chondral or osteochondral injuries		
Tendinopathy—tibialis posterior/flexor hallucius longus	Peroneal tendinopathy, recurrent dislocation of peroneal tendons	Tibialis anterior tendinopathy	Achilles tendinopathy
Stress fractures—calcaneus/navicular/talus/medial malleolus	Stress fractures—talus/distal fibula/cuboid		Stress fractures of posterolateral aspect of talus
Tarsal tunnel syndrome	Sinus tarsi syndrome		Os trigonum syndrome
Rare presentation of posterior impingement syndrome	Impingement syndrome Anterolateral Posterior		Posterior impingement syndrome
Referred pain from spine.Complex regional pain syndrome (CRPS)	Referred pain from spine. CRPS		

Predisposing factors

Varus ankle, tarsal coalition, cavovarus foot posture (e.g. Charcot–Marie–Tooth), and generalized joint laxity predispose to ankle sprain.

Anatomy

There are *three* groups of ligaments each of which has *three* elements (Table 9.5.3).

Acute lateral ligament sprain

Ankle sprains most commonly injure the ATFL. The calcaneofibular ligament (CFL) is involved in more severe cases.

Examination

Examination aims to define which ligaments are torn and to exclude fracture. Watson Jones described passive inversion of the ankle to test for ligament insufficiency. Test the ATFL by inversion with the foot plantarflexed and the CFL with the foot dorsiflexion).

Treatment

Early functional treatment is recommended initially for all grades of injury.

There is no evidence for surgery after an uncomplicated acute injury. RICE is supplemented by early weight bearing, physiotherapy, and bracing. Return to sport is gradual.

Syndesmosis injury

The syndesmosis is injured in 18% of ankle sprains. The mechanism of injury is external rotation with a dorsiflexion component. These injuries cause more disability than isolated injury to the lateral ligament complex.

Clinical evaluation

Tenderness is maximal at the distal tibiofibular articulation. The 'squeeze test' compresses the tibia and fibula together thereby stressing the syndesmosis. If this provokes pain then the test is positive. External rotation of the foot with the ankle dorsiflexed will also stress the inferior tibiofibular articulation. If the patient twists their body while standing on the affected leg only (sometimes called the Jive test) discomfort is produced in cases of subtle syndesmosis injury.

Radiographs

Plain radiographs and axial computed tomography (CT) of both ankles allows asymmetry of the tibiofibular joint to be detected. MRI can demonstrate injury to the component ligaments of the joint complex. Fluoroscopic examination under anaesthesia may show instability.

Treatment

Stable injuries are treated symptomatically.

A removable boot allows a graduated approach to rehabilitation. Recovery takes considerably longer for syndesmosis injuries than for sprain of the lateral ligament complex. There should be a low threshold for exposing the interior tibio-fibular joint through an anterolateral incision to ensure proper reduction.

An acute unstable syndesmosis injury should be treated surgically. The goals of surgery are anatomical reduction and stabilization.

When closed reduction is difficult, open or arthroscopic clearance of soft tissue from the medial side of the joint is performed.

Table 9.5.3 Ankle ligaments—rule of 3s

Group	3 components		
Lateral ligament	Anterior talofibular	Posterior talofibular	Calcaneofibular
Syndesmosis	Anterior inferior tibiofibular	Posterior inferior tibiofibular	Interosseous ligament
Deltoid	Superficial deltoid	Anterior deep	Posterior deep

Stabilization of the tibiofibular joint is then performed with a diastasis screw. The screw is used as a position screw, and *not* in lag mode. More recently, suture devices passed across fibula and tibia have become popular.

Screw removal should be scheduled for no earlier than 12 weeks from surgery. Weight bearing may be permitted prior to screw removal, but screw breakage is a possibility, especially where the screw engages the far medial cortex of the tibia (four-cortex technique).

In chronic cases the medial side of the ankle and the distal tibiofibular joint should always be explored. The syndesmosis is debrided and the ligament repaired or reconstructed.

Chronic lateral ligament insufficiency

Recurrent giving way of the ankle may be due to mechanical instability or functional insecurity.

Mechanical instability is where recurrent giving way of the ankle occurs in association with an abnormal displacement of the talus.

It is usually due to ligamentous disruption, osteochondral injuries or loose bodies, and peroneal tendon pathology can all contribute.

By contrast, functional insecurity is present when a patient complains of recurrent giving way, yet physical examination and radiological tests reveal a stable joint. Synovial impingement, peroneal muscle weakness, and poor proprioception are common causes of functional instability.

Synovial impingement

Synovial impingement may be caused by, or give rise to, recurrent painful episodes of giving way.

Synovial impingement may occur with or without joint laxity. The synovial impingement sign is a useful physical sign. It relies upon the examiner's thumb pushing inflamed hypertrophic synovium into the tibiotalar joint as the ankle is moved from plantar flexion into dorsiflexion, trapping the synovium and producing pain (Figure 9.5.8). The test is highly sensitive but not specific for isolated synovitis.

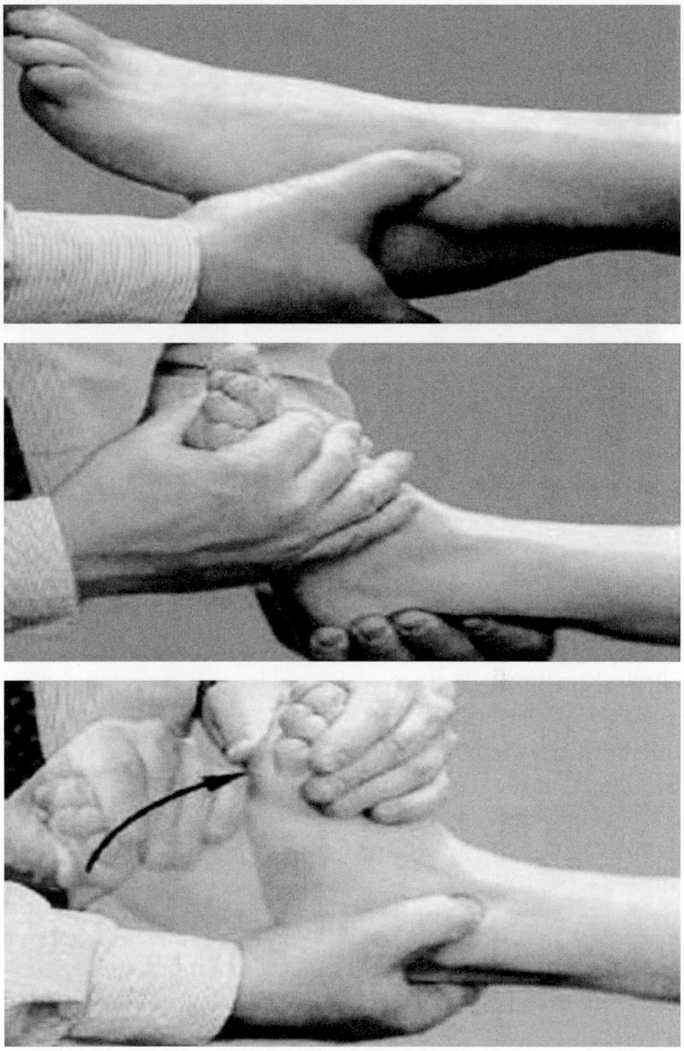

Fig. 9.5.8 Synovial impingement test. Reproduced with permission from Molloy, S., Solan, M.C., and Bendall, S.P. (2003). Synovial impingement in the ankle. A new physical sign. *J Bone Joint Surg Br.*, **85**(3), 330–3.

Patients with synovial impingement syndrome enjoy excellent results with examination under anaesthetic, arthroscopic assessment, and debridement of the joint.

Where clinical assessment reveals both synovitis and true ligamentous instability then the decision to simply debride the joint or to proceed to lateral ligament reconstruction at the same time is difficult.

Debridement of synovitis in isolation carries a quicker recovery time and requires no cast immobilization—advantages which must be weighed against the small chance of requiring a second procedure to reconstruct the ligament if addressing the synovial impingement alone provides insufficient improvement.

Osteochondral lesion of the talar dome (OLT)

Osteochondral lesion of the talar dome (OLT) is now the preferred term for this condition—although other terms such as osteochondral disease, osteochondral defect, and osteochondral fracture are also used.

A high index of suspicion is required for the diagnosis of OLT since symptoms may be vague and plain radiographs unrevealing. MRI scan is often required and will tend to underdiagnose the cartilage component and overdiagnose bony oedema.

Unstable cartilage on the dome of the talus may cause insecurity of the joint, an ill-defined 'deep' pain, acute pain, and clicking or just aching. OLT of the talus is treated by arthroscopic debridement of the unstable surface and underlying necrotic bone. In over 80% of patients the resultant fibrocartilagenous healing affords excellent symptom relief. For the 15 percent where debridement and microfracture fail repeating this procedure affords a further 80 percent success rate.

Occasionally, cases relapse and then treatment by cartilage graft, cartilage substitution, or, in the presence of major and/or increasing joint damage, even arthrodesis may be indicated.

Treatment of chronic instability

Non-surgical

Physiotherapy is important and focuses upon peroneal tendon strengthening and proprioception.

Activity modification, ankle support bracing, footwear modification, and orthotics are useful means of avoiding giving way.

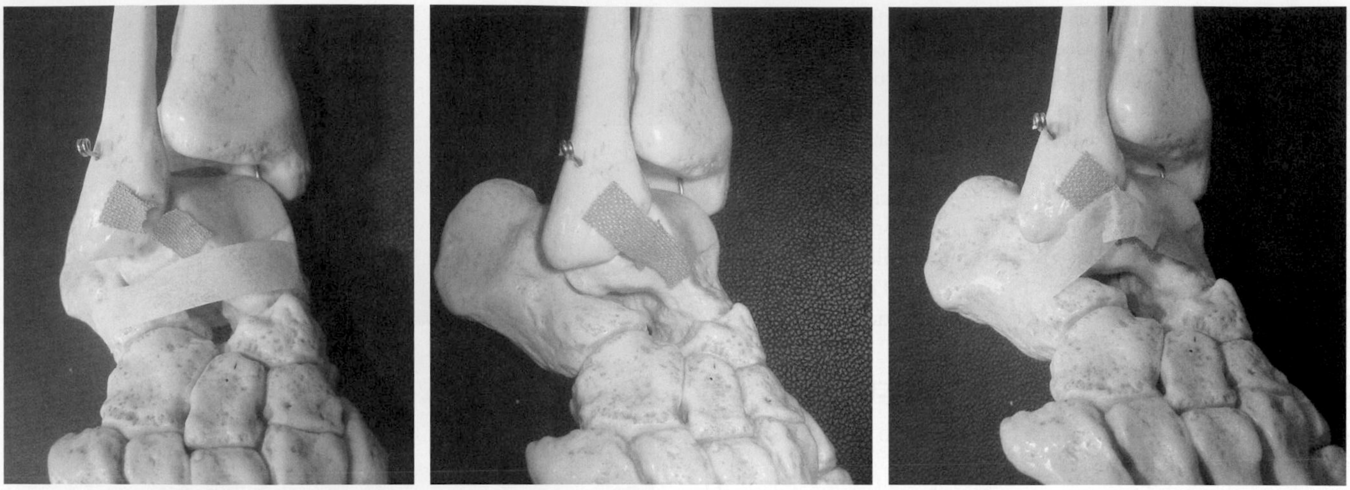

Fig. 9.5.9 A) Represents a torn anterior talofibular ligament. B) Represents a Brostrom repair. C) Brostrom–Gould operation: an anatomic lateral ligament procedure.

Surgery

Surgical treatment is reserved for ankles that have failed non-operative management.

Lateral ligament reconstruction

In cases requiring surgical stabilization, anatomical repair is preferred to non-anatomic reconstructions. This is because of the high incidence of degenerative change seen in follow-up after non-anatomic reconstruction (up to 60%), due to altered biomechanics. Non-anatomic reconstruction also has a high incidence of sural nerve damage and lengthy recovery time. It is therefore reserved for recurrent cases or very heavy patients, and robust sports.

Brostrom, in 1966, described anatomic repair of the attenuated ligaments. The most popular modification is that described by Gould who advocated advancing the extensor retinaculum across the repair (Figures 9.5.9). As well as reinforcing the repair, this increases subtalar stability.

Non-anatomic reconstructions use peroneus brevis to stabilize the joint.

Where lateral ligament insufficiency is consequent upon a cavus foot, consideration must be given to a dorsiflexion first metatarsal osteotomy and peroneus longus to brevis transfer.

Box 9.5.2 Ankle instability

- Ligamentous insufficiency is less common than synovial impingement
- Arthroscopic treatment for synovial impingement affords excellent results
- Conservative treatment with physiotherapy always precedes surgery
- Ligament reconstruction should usually be anatomic (modified Brostrom)
- Non-anatomic repair (e.g. Chrissman–Snook) for heavy people and revision surgery.

Aftercare for either requires 4–6 weeks' immobilization in cast or brace, followed by rehabilitation with an emphasis on proprioceptive re-education.

Lisfranc ligament injury

Introduction

Injury to the tarsometatarsal joint is frequently overlooked, especially as the patient often has multiple injures. It is a potent cause of late disability.

Purely ligamentous injuries to the tarsometatarsal joint complex result from more minor accidents and again often cause long-term symptoms.

Historical perspective

Lisfranc was one of Napoleon's surgeons who observed injuries in cavalry officers falling from their mounts while one foot remained in a stirrup.

Anatomy

The anatomy of the midfoot is complex. Stability depends upon bony and ligamentous anatomy, as well as dynamic (musculotendinous) stabilizers.

The wedge-shaped cuneiforms and metatarsal bases form a transverse arch. The second metatarsal base is considered to form the 'keystone' of the tarsometatarsal joint as it is the apex of the transverse arch and is recessed between the medial and the lateral cuneiforms providing lateral stability. In addition there are three groups of ligaments: dorsal, interosseous, and plantar (Figure 9.5.10). Without these ligaments the tarsometatarsal joint complex is inherently unstable.

Clinical features

Severe fracture or dislocation of the tarsometatarsal joint will be obvious, with gross swelling and deformity. The plantar ecchymosis sign, with a bruise under the foot at tarsometatarsal joint level, is seen. Tenderness is maximal over the second tarsometatarsal joint.

In contrast, a seemingly innocuous injury to the foot that presents late, once swelling and bruising have improved, is

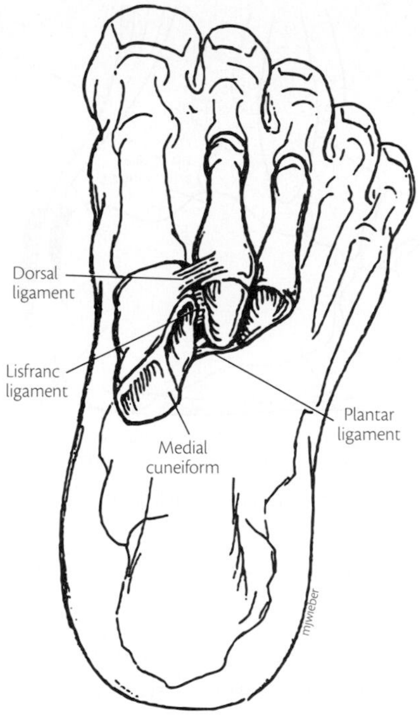

Fig. 9.5.10 Anatomy of the ligaments of the tarsometatarsal joint.

easily missed and requires careful examination and a high index of suspicion.

Differential diagnosis

Most cases of tarsometatarsal joint injury are presumed to be a 'sprained foot'. It is safer to assume that 'there is no such thing as a sprain of the midfoot'.

Investigation

In severe injuries, fracture and/or dislocation are usually obvious.

In contrast, in pure ligamentous injury, they may show no abnormality, particularly if taken non-weight bearing.

Positive radiographic features are the 'fleck sign' (a small avulsion of bone from the base of the second metatarsal) and an increase in the gap between the bases of the first and second metatarsal. The medial edge of the base of the second metatarsal should be aligned with the medial edge of the intermediate cuneiform. This is best assessed on an AP radiograph of both feet taken with the patient bearing weight (Figure 9.5.11A). Where plain radiographs are normal CT, MRI, or bone scan can be helpful (Figure 9.5.11B).

Targeted joint injection of local anaesthetic may be useful to confirm that pain is from the second tarsometatarsal articulation in chronic cases.

Treatment

Untreated, the ligamentous Lisfranc injury often results in a chronically painful foot with planovalgus deformity and tarsometatarsal joint arthrosis from which late salvage surgery in the form of corrective midfoot fusion gives unpredictable results.

Non-operative treatment

Non-operative treatment is only successful when no displacement is present, so a normal CT scan is a prerequisite.

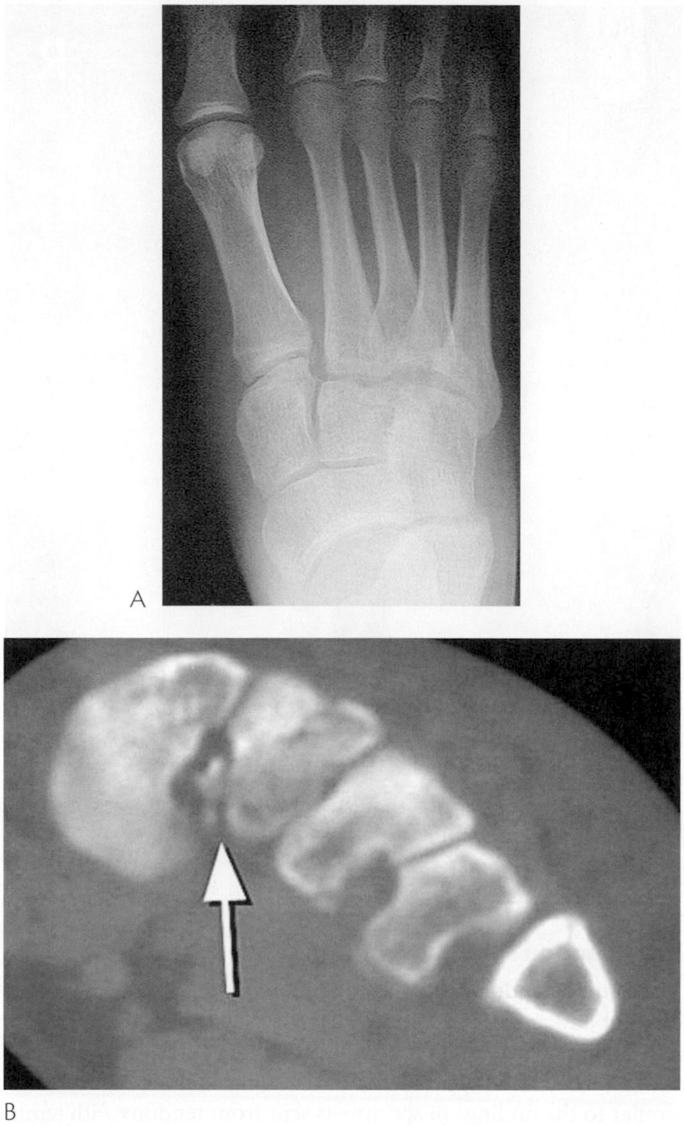

Fig. 9.5.11 A) An anteroposterior radiograph with increased space between base of M1 and M2. B) Computed tomography scan showing avusion fracture at base of M2.

Treatment comprises cast immobilization for 12 weeks with no weight bearing for the first half of this time period. Physiotherapy is required afterwards, as is prolonged support with a rigid FFO.

Operative treatment

When displacement is present, open reduction is preferred to give accurate reduction. Historically, K-wire stabilization was recommended. Screws across the tarsometatarsal articulation provide more stability but damage an already disrupted joint, so bridging plates are preferred by many surgeons.

In selected cases, primary fusion may be considered (Figure 9.5.12) to avoid repeated surgery and a protracted recovery.

Prognosis

Trauma to the Lisfranc joint is a potentially devastating injury. Even with good treatment, pain, stiffness and swelling lead to difficulty with sporting activities and shoe fitting in many patients.

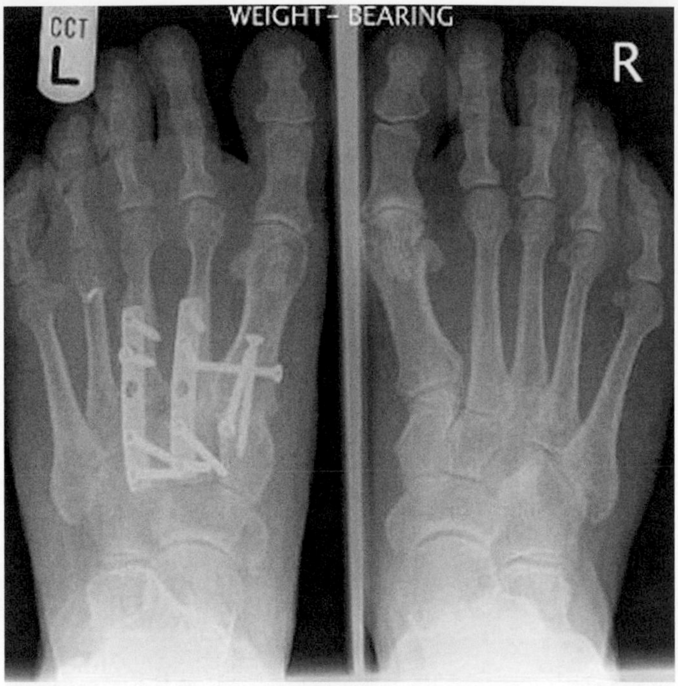

Fig. 9.5.12 Primary fusion for tarsometatarsal fracture dislocations.

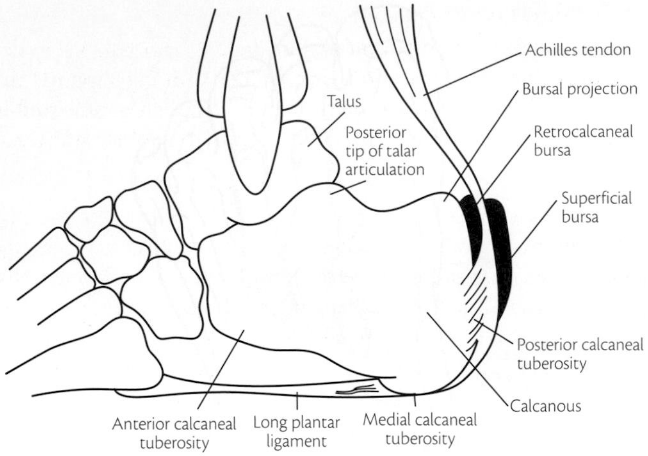

Fig. 9.5.13 Anatomy of the insertion af the achilles tendon. Courtesy of Prof. M.M. Stephens.

Patients should be warned that the foot is unlikely to return to full function, and may require long-term orthotic support.

Achilles tendon

Introduction

The Achilles tendon is the largest tendon in the body. In orthopaedic foot and ankle surgery, disorders of the Achilles relate to pain and swelling with resultant disability or to rupture.

The microscopic appearances of tendons that have ruptured are similar to the findings in specimens sent from tendons with tendinopathy without rupture, suggesting a pre-existing abnormality, prior to acute tearing.

However, many patients who sustain an acute rupture have never had symptoms while patients who endure chronic pain and swelling of the tendon rarely rupture.

Anatomy (Figure 9.5.13)

The Achilles tendon is the combined tendon of the three components of the triceps surae muscle. The gastrocnemii pass across both the knee joint and the ankle joint. Soleus does not extend above the knee. This distinction is important when stretching programmes are considered as part of a treatment programme, as the gastrocnemius cannot be properly stretched unless the knee is held in full extension.

The fibres of the Achilles tendon rotate through 90 degrees as they pass distally. The medial fibres proximally become the posterior fibres distally. Thus valgus collapse of the ankle tends to increase the twist and therefore tightness of the tendon.

The tendon inserts onto the middle one-third of the posterior surface of the tuberosity of the calcaneum. Structurally the insertion changes by way of transitional zone: fibrocartilage, mineralized fibrocartilage, and finally bone. This allows effective force dissipation.

The tendon immediately proximal to the site of insertion is related to the superior one-third of the posterior surface of the os calcis. This surface is covered by fibrocartilage and the tendon is protected by the retrocalcaneal bursa. Another bursa lies between the Achilles tendon and the skin.

Box 9.5.3 Lisfranc ligament injury

- Obvious fracture-dislocation or subtle ligament injury
- High index of suspicion—'no such thing as a midfoot sprain'
- Poor results but worse if missed
- Surgery open reduction and bridging plate fixation
- Consider primary fusion of tarsometatarsal 1–3.

Blood supply

The blood supply in the non-insertional region of the Achilles tendon is poor. This is important in the pathophysiology of tendinopathy and rupture.

Posterior heel pain

Posterior heel pain most commonly arises from the Achilles tendon. Pathology may arise from the insertion of the tendon or from the non-insertional region. This distinction is helpful.

Non-insertional Achilles tendon pathology is more common and is due to degenerative changes within the tendon, thickening of the paratenon, or a combination of the two.

Retrocalcaneal bursitis with insertional tendinopathy accounts for approximately 20% of all Achilles tendinopathies. Pure insertional tendinopathy makes up only 5%.

Terminology

Maffulli has clarified the nomenclature. The triad of pain, swelling, and impaired function should be referred to as Achilles tendinopathy.

Non-insertional tendinopathy

Achilles tendinopathy is common, but there are no reliable epidemiological data. An association with athletic training supports the theory that overuse is the principal cause, although it can trouble sedentary individuals as well. It is more common in older athletes.

Insertional tendinopathy

An enlarged posterosuperior border of the tuberosity of the os calcis is called the bursal projection (Haglund deformity), and may impinge against the tendon resulting in retrocalcaneal bursitis or degenerative change in the tendon. With retrocalcaneal bursitis the heel is swollen and maximally tender posteromedially or, more commonly, posterolaterally. It may also cause the heel counter of shoes to rub. This results in local swelling and tenderness.

Insertional heel pain may also be due to changes within the transitional zone of the tendon, to retrocalcaneal bursitis, or to both.

Patients with insertional tendinopathy complain of posterior heel pain that is maximal in the midline and inferiorly, at the insertion of the tendon.

Clinical assessment of posterior heel pain

A careful history determines the relationship of symptoms to: activity; new training regimens; poor warm-up technique; or to specific shoes. Atypical features in the history, such as night pain, should prompt investigations for enthesopathy or rare neoplastic causes.

Examination will reveal the site of maximal tenderness. The tendon is tender and swollen in non-insertional tendinopathy. Midline tenderness suggests insertional tendinopathy whereas maximal tenderness to the lateral (or less commonly medial) side of the tendon is due to bursitis.

Increased calcaneal pitch with heel varus makes the bursal projection of the calcaneum excessively prominent. Heel valgus with a low medial longitudinal arch and forefoot varus causes overpronation of the foot, tightening of the tendon, and secondary Achilles tendinopathy.

If a systemic inflammatory cause is suspected, general examination is performed and supplemented with blood tests.

Imaging

Plain radiographs may show deformity, bony lumps, and ectopic calcification (Figure 9.5.14A).

Ultrasound scan and MRI both provide useful information. MRI provides a permanent image (Figure 9.5.14B), but ultrasound allows dynamic assessment.

Treatment

Non-operative treatment

Patients must be informed of the natural history of non-insertional tendinopathy because the majority of patients improve and are only left with a palpable non-tender lump in the Achilles tendon in the long term.

Stretching regimens for non-insertional tendinopathy are effective, with 90% of patients responding. The patient and physiotherapist must understand that the knee has to be fully extended during the stretch for the gastrocnemius contracture to be improved. If the hamstrings are tight then stretches for this muscle group should be added to the regimen.

Steroid injection should be avoided except in proven cases of pure paratendinitis or bursitis, because of the risk of rupture.

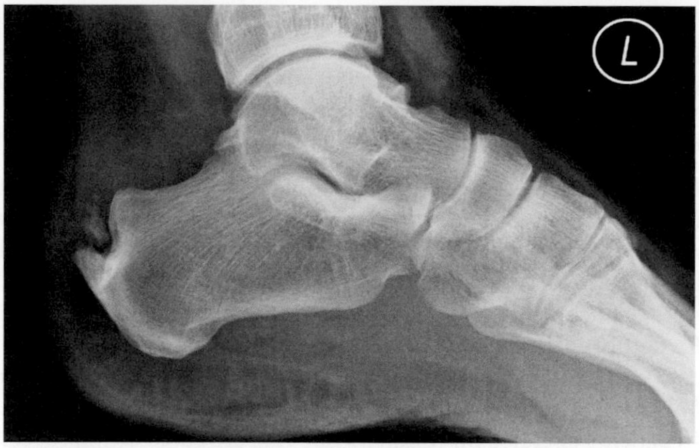

A

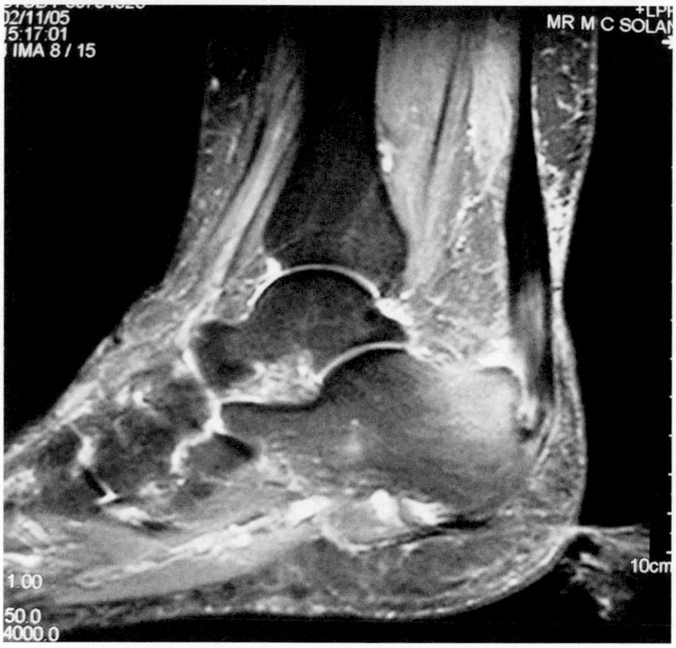

B

Fig. 9.5.14 A) Calcific tendinopathy. B) Insertional tendinopathy and bursitis.

Sclerosant injection therapy is successful in the treatment of non-insertional tendinopathy. Extracorporeal shock wave lithotripsy is under evaluation.

Patients with 'pump bumps' respond to education, modification of shoes, and occasionally an orthotic to lift the affected part, or a silicone lined sock. To avoid recurrence it is important that the patient understands that they must continue to be careful with shoes even after the symptoms resolve.

Retrocalcaneal bursitis can be managed in the same way. Corrective orthotics for planovalgus deformity can be helpful, but over correction is poorly tolerated, especially in running athletes. There may be some benefit from anti-inflammatory medication or gel, but steroid injection should only be considered if an MRI or ultrasound scan shows normal tendon.

Operative treatments

Open procedures Non-operative treatments are successful in about 90% of cases, so surgery is rarely required—especially as recovery times are often very long.

Non-insertional tendonitis Surgery is rarely required. Available procedures include decompression—performed open or percutaneously by multiple incisions and paratenon stripping. In severe cases, surgeons increasingly perform supplementary transfer of the flexor hallucis longus (FHL) tendon, to augment the Achilles tendon.

Haglund disease alone or in combination with retrocalcaneal bursitis Excision of the bursal projection is performed through a medial incision for osteotomy of the posteromedial and/or lateral bony prominence, minimizing risk to the sural nerve. At least 50% of the attachment of the tendon can be released without the need for suture anchor repair and without cast immobilization.

Combined excision of bursa and bony prominence results in 50% of patients being symptom free and a further 20% improved. In patients operated on within a year, 92% are cured or improved.

In rare cases where surgery is required for isolated insertional tendinitis, a posterior midline tendon splitting approach is used (Figure 9.5.15). The tendon is debrided, and may be completely detached and reattached. The success rates for pain relief are good, but the eventual outcome is often limited and not all patients improve sufficiently to resume sports.

The incidence of wound problems after surgery in the region of the Achilles tendon is small but troublesome. Minimally invasive surgical techniques for debridement to the retrocalcaneal bursa and bursal projection may offer reduced surgical morbidity.

Enthusiasts report no complications and a rapid return to normal function. The recovery time is equal in both methods, but the endoscopic group have fewer wound infections, fewer sensitive scars, and a lower incidence of altered sensation.

Acute rupture of the Achilles tendon

Overview

Management of the patient with rupture of the Achilles tendon is controversial. Operative repair offers advantages of predictability, but at the expense of surgical risk.

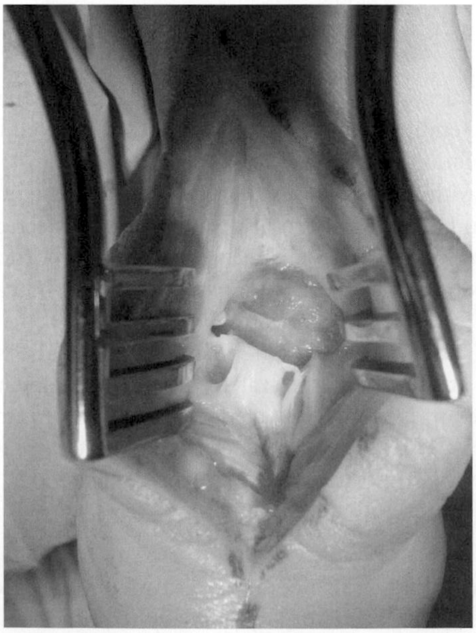

Fig. 9.5.15 Midline incision for tendon debridement and excision of spur.

Rehabilitation protocols have significantly changed with emphasis now on early weight bearing and movement.

Clinical features

Patients usually sustain a rupture of their Achilles tendon while engaged in athletic activity. The risk of rupture is greatest in unaccustomed activity.

Racquet sports (especially squash and badminton) have a reputation for injury, and anecdotally patients typically believe that their opponent has struck the back of their heel.

Sudden pain is a constant feature of the presentation, often with an audible tearing or snapping sound, though the pain may not last long.

Sadly even patients with classical presentations are misdiagnosed as having a sprained ankle, pulled calf muscle, or 'partial tear' of the Achilles tendon.

Clinicians may be deceived by the patient's ability to plantarflex using the muscles of the deep posterior compartment of the calf.

In the acute setting, soft tissue swelling and tenderness may mean that the gap between the tendon ends cannot be palpated. The only reliable way to diagnose rupture is to use the clinical test of Simmonds and Thompson. The patient lies on a couch or kneels on a chair with the feet and ankles hanging free. The examiner notes the resting posture of the ankles. The affected side will lie in a less plantar-flexed position, through loss of the pull of the gastrosoleus complex (Matle's test). The examiner then squeezes the normal calf and this action shortens the gastrosoleus muscle causing the foot to plantar-flex. When the manoeuvre is repeated on the affected limb there is no such movement at the ankle because there is no continuity of the tendon. To avoid confusion, the test should not be referred to as positive or negative—which is ambiguous—but as normal or abnormal.

Differential diagnosis

Sudden onset of posterior heel pain should be assumed to be due to a (complete) rupture of the Achilles tendon, until proven otherwise.

Investigation

Imaging is seldom required. Ultrasound or MRI (Figure 9.5.16) may be useful as an adjunct to clinical assessment where the presentation has been delayed or where there is a suspicion that the rupture is high, at the musculocutaneous junction—but may be misleading if clot or scar fills the gap.

Treatment

Achilles tendon rupture may be managed non-operatively or by surgical repair.

The benefits of surgical repair include a lower incidence of rerupture and the opportunity to achieve adequate tension in the tendon. Most surgeons specializing in foot and ankle surgery are proponents of repair. A review of the Cochrane database concluded that surgery is advantageous as long as complications can be avoided. Wound infection and/or breakdown, in an area with a thin soft tissue envelope, is the most important complication.

The decision to surgically repair a ruptured Achilles tendon is made after considering:

- Patient activity levels and expectation
- Timing of presentation after injury

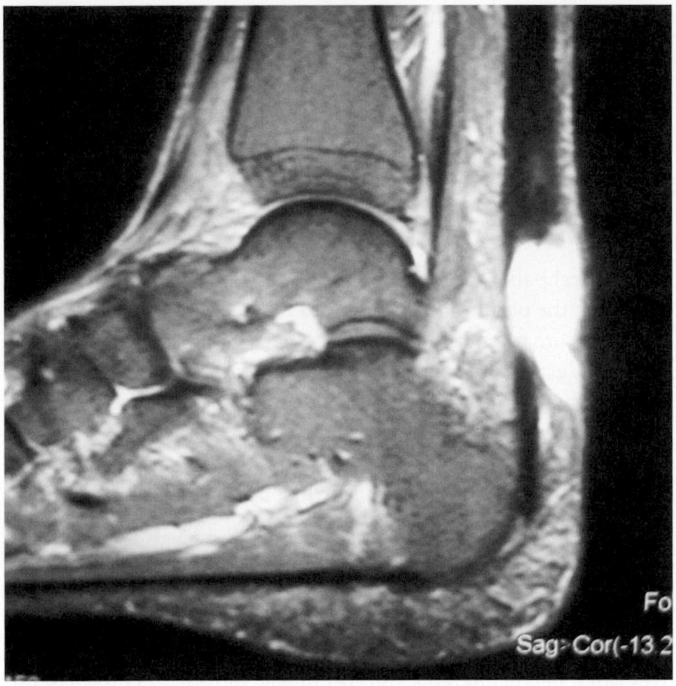

Fig. 9.5.16 Rupture after steroid injection.

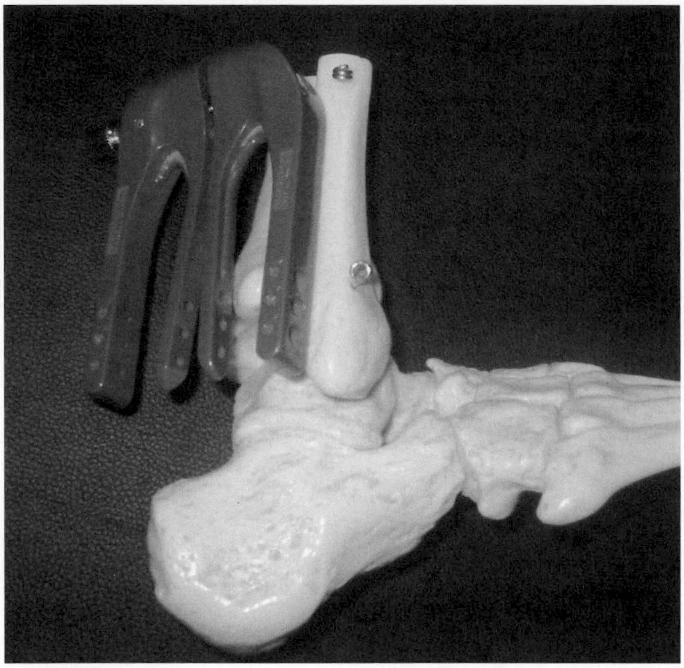

Fig. 9.5.17 Achillon® device.

- General health
- Local soft tissues.

At one extreme, the older patient who has poor skin, smokes, and presents immediately after an injury may be managed non-operatively—avoiding high risks of wound problems, but mindful of an increased rate of re-rupture.

A sportsman with a few days' delay in presentation should undergo surgical repair, as this allows the haematoma between the tendon ends to be evacuated and both length and tension of the tendon restored.

Conservative treatment

Conservative treatment should be active and is not 'treatment by neglect'. Equinus cast or functional immobilization should be monitored by ultrasound scans to confirm apposition of tendon ends at intervals during healing. After immobilization or functional treatment for 6 weeks, a heel raise allows the patient to gradually stretch out the repaired tendon during rehabilitation.

Open versus percutaneous repair

Open surgery allows direct visualization and robust repair but at the expense of possible wound complications. In an effort to avoid this, percutaneous repair has evolved. The incidence of painful sural nerve injury has been problematic.

The Achillon® device (Figure 9.5.17) facilitates percutaneous repair and has a very low incidence of nerve injury. Functional results after percutaneous repair are equal to those after open repair, but for those not familiar with its use, open procedures are more applicable.

Rehabilitation

Whether the tendon is repaired or treated conservatively, the rehabilitation protocol should allow the patient to bear weight from an early stage. This has been shown to improve collagen remodelling. With rapid rehabilitation it is often possible for the patient to be to bearing weight almost immediately and free from support by 6 weeks from the injury.

Delayed presentation of Achilles rupture

When a patient presents with a delayed Achilles tendon rupture a variety of terms may be used. Neglected may mean that the patient did not seek medical attention at the time of injury; Missed implies that the doctor, physiotherapist, or nurse failed to make the diagnosis.

When the rupture is not treated the natural history is for the tendon to heal, but at a length that prevents proper function of the triceps surae.

Clinical features

The patient may give a clear history of acute tendoachilles rupture that was not treated or of a minor exacerbation of chronic symptoms that was not appreciated to be a rupture. In either case, the presenting complaints are weakness, poor balance, difficulty with stairs, or inability to stand on tiptoes, with swelling of the ankle and pain.

On examination the ankle can be passively dorsiflexed further than the normal side; single-stance heel-rise is weak or impossible; the tendon is often thin at the site of rupture, if elongated healing has occurred; or deficient with a palpable gap.

Imaging

Plain films (lateral weight bearing of the foot and ankle) may show alterations of the normal soft tissue shadows, and may show features of insertional tendinopathy (calcification, Haglund deformity) which raises the possibility of distal rupture.

Ultrasound and MRI may confirm the diagnosis but also give information about the level of the rupture, the extent of retraction

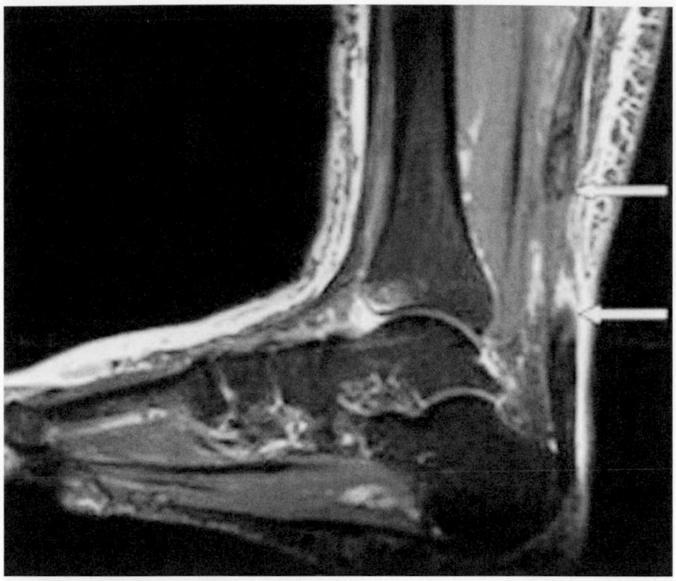

Fig. 9.5.18 Chronic Achilles rupture.

of the proximal stump, and the length of intervening scar tissue (Figure 9.5.18), but both may be deceptive and fail to differentiate between clot, scar, and tendon.

Treatment

Non-operative

This may be chosen when the patient reports minimal symptoms or if surgery is contraindicated. Physiotherapy strengthens the calf muscles and minimizes symptoms. Improvement may continue for more than 2 years.

Operative (Table 9.5.4)

Surgical treatment aims to restore plantar-flexion power to the ankle. There is a wide range of surgical techniques from which to choose. The choice is made according to the gap between the proximal and distal stump after debridement of scar tissue.

Available techniques include direct repair and indirect methods, and the more controversial autograft, synthetic graft, or allograft reconstructions.

End-to-end repair is unlikely to be successful if treatment is delayed for more than a few weeks. Advancement of the proximal stump can be achieved by means of V–Y-plasty or a 'turn-down' procedure. This produces a bulky repair with risk of wound problems and is less popular since the introduction of tendon transfer techniques.

Table 9.5.4 Repair of chronic Achilles tendon ruptures

Gap <1cm	End-to-end repair without augmentation
Gap 1–2cm	End-to-end repair with 'stress relaxation' of proximal portion
Gap 2–5cm	V–Y lengthening ± FHL transfer
Gap >5cm	FHL transfer ± V-Y lengthening

FHL, flexor hallucis longus. Adapted from Myerson, with permission.
Source: Foot and Ankle Disorders: Chapter 55 Disorders of the Achilles Tendon and Retrocalcaneal Region p1386–6.

Tendon transfer techniques may use peroneus brevis, FDL or (most commonly) FHL.

Reports of FHL transfer are good to excellent with negligible weakness of hallux flexion.

Synthetic graft should only be used in exceptional circumstances.

Plantar heel pain

Plantar heel pain is common, disabling, and usually due to plantar fasciitis at the point of insertion onto the heel.

Patients are often middle aged or elderly and present with severe heel pain, especially start-up pain that is most troublesome upon rising in the morning and improves, only to deteriorate again with prolonged standing or walking.

Atypical presentation in younger patients may be associated with stress fractures, enthesopathy, arthritis, tarsal tunnel syndrome, or lumbar radiculopathy.

Assessment

Patients should be examined for signs of a calcaneal stress fracture (calcaneal squeeze test) and for tarsal tunnel syndrome (Tinel sign over tibial nerve; altered sensation in sole of foot). Plantar fasciitis is classically maximally tender over the medial calcaneal tuberosity (Figure 9.5.19).

The majority of patients with plantar fasciitis have isolated shortening of the gastrocnemius, identified using Silfverskiold's test (Figure 9.5.3).

Treatment

Conservative treatment includes orthotics, physiotherapy (including ultrasound and stretching), night splints and lithotripsy. Patients who present early recover more quickly than those presenting late with established symptoms. The majority of cases respond, but in refractory cases, injection (preferably ultrasound guided) can be helpful. Rupture of the fascia is, however, a potential and serious complication (Figure 9.5.19B).

Open or endoscopic release of the plantar fascia insertion is sometimes performed, but the risk of provoking prolonged severe pain in association with acute flat foot and nerve damage means that it has not been adopted widely in the United Kingdom.

Peroneal tendons

Introduction

The peroneus longus and brevis tendons cause ankle symptoms either because of acute injury or because of chronic tendinopathy.

Box 9.5.4 Achilles tendon

- Rupture is complete (not partial) until proven otherwise
- Conservative treatment associated with higher re-rupture rate
- Surgical repair predictable but risk of wound problems
- Percutaneous techniques minimize wound
- Early weight bearing for both operative and non-operative cases.

Anatomy

Peroneus brevis lies anterior to longus as they course behind the lateral malleolus. Both are supplied by the superficial peroneal nerve (L5, S1 roots).

Proximal to the malleolus the tendons are invested in a synovial sheath. This extends beneath the peroneal retinaculum. After rounding the tip of the lateral malleolus, the tendons diverge, passing either side of the peroneal tubercle on the lateral wall of the os calcis. They pass beneath the inferior extensor retinaculum before following different courses. The brevis tendon passes to the styloid process of the fifth metatasal base. Peroneus longus passes beneath the cuboid and across the sole of the foot to insert on the plantar aspect of the base of the first metatarsal. At the point that the tendon changes direction it is strengthened by a sesamoid bone, the os perineum, which is often cartilaginous.

Clinical features

Injuries

Acute inflammation

Inversion injuries of the ankle may result in acute inflammation of the peroneal tendons leading to signs of: local tenderness; pain on passive stretch; and pain on active resisted movement. Swelling behind the fibula is characteristic.

Peroneal tendinopathy

The position of peroneus brevis, between the longus tendon and the fibula, makes it vulnerable to injury. It may also be trapped beneath the fibula when there is valgus deformity of the heel.

Imaging

Plain radiographs will not show the tendons but in the case of peroneus longus rupture may show proximal migration of a fracture through the os peroneum.

Ultrasound or MRI is more useful to show the structure of the tendons.

Box 9.5.5 Plantar heel pain

- Most commonly plantar fasciitis
- Atypical symptoms—young, night pain, malaise, or arthritis
- Treated with gastrocnemius and plantar fascia stretches
- Steroid injections may be effective
- Surgery usually avoided because of risk of complications.

Treatment

Non-operative treatments include activity modification and orthotic provision to address any cavovarus deformity or valgus collapse. Corticosteroid injection should usually be avoided.

Synovectomy can be performed arthroscopically. Open surgical exploration, with tenosynovectomy and repair or tendon debulking with tubularization of split/thickened tendons is indicated in severe cases with tendinosis/chronic rupture.

Peroneal tendon dislocation

The peroneal tendons dislocate from behind the fibula as a result of a twisting injury. In the normal ankle the peroneal retinaculum prevents this.

At the time of injury the tendons strip the retinaculum away from the bone of the fibula—a 'Bankart' lesion of the ankle.

Only occasionally does an avulsion fracture from the fibula make the injury apparent on plain radiographs. Neither MRI nor ultrasound is 100% sensitive.

A high index of suspicion is required to make the diagnosis in the acute setting.

After the acute symptoms have resolved, recurrent snapping of the tendons over the malleolus may be demonstrated by the patient.

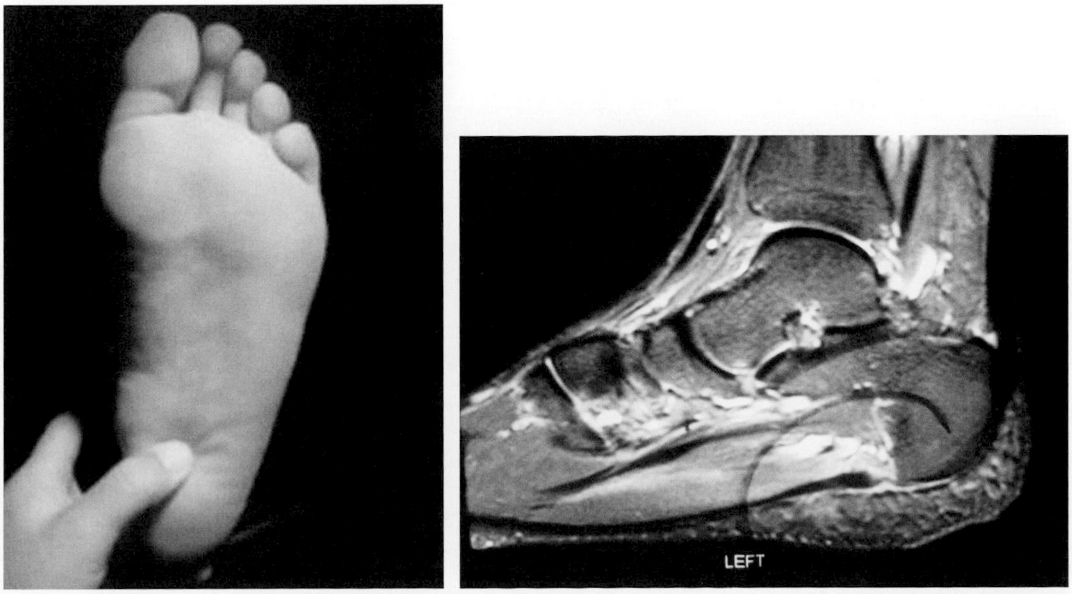

A B

Fig. 9.5.19 A) Site of tenderness in plantar fasciitis. B) Magnetic resonance image of plantar fascia rupture following injection.

Box 9.5.6 Peroneal tendons

- Vulnerable to inversion injury
- Peroneus longus may rupture through an os peroneum
- Dislocation due to retinaculum injury is often missed
- Anatomical repair advised.

Treatment of peroneal dislocation

After an acute injury cast immobilization may allow satisfactory healing. Surgery aims to repair the 'Bankart' lesion anatomically

In recurrent situations after failed surgery, various techniques have been described to augment the repair. The 'groove' behind the fibula can be deepened with an osteotomy or using a burr. A strip of tendon from the lateral portion of the Achilles tendon may be used to fashion a new retinaculum. Alternatively, the calcaneofibular ligament may be transposed into a position superficial to the tendons.

Results of repair are good, but 6–8 weeks of protection in a cast are required, and a lengthy rehabilitation period follows this.

Further reading

Khan, R.J., Fick, D., Brammar, T.J., Crawford, J., and Parker, M.J. (2004). Interventions for treating acute Achilles tendon ruptures. *Cochrane Database of Systematic Reviews*, **3**, CD003674.

Myerson, M. (1989). The diagnosis and treatment of injuries to the Lisfranc joint complex. *Orthopedic Clinics of North America*, **20**(4), 655–64.

Myerson, M.S. (1997). Adult acquired flatfoot deformity: treatment of dysfunction of the posterior tibial tendon. *Instructional Course Lectures*, **46**, 393–405.

Pijnenburg, A.C., Van Dijk, C.N., Bossuyt, P.M., and Marti, R.K. (2000). Treatment of ruptures of the lateral ankle ligaments: a meta-analysis. *Journal of Bone and Joint Surgery*, **82A**, 761–73.

Zengerink, M., Szerb, I., Hangody, L., Dopirak, R.M., Ferkel, R.D., and van Dijk, C.N. (2006). Current concepts: treatment of osteochondral ankle defects. *Foot and Ankle Clinics*, **11**(2), 331–59, vi.

SECTION 10

Medical Disorders of the Skeleton

10.1

Metabolic disease of skeleton and inherited disorders

Paul Wordsworth

Summary points

- Classic metabolic bone diseases include osteoporosis, osteomalacia, Paget's disease, and parathyroid bone disease
- Heritable disorders of the skeleton include numerous osteochrondrodysplasias, Marfan syndrome, and Ehlers-Danlos syndrome
- Investigation of short stature is indicated for those below 0.4 percentile, with skeletal disproportion and/or progressive shortness
- Genetic mutations for most of these conditions have been identified but clinical/radiographic features are usually diagnostic.

Introduction

The human skeleton serves both as a supporting frame and as an accessible mineral store. Bone is metabolically active throughout life and metabolic disturbances may have wide ranging consequences that are not restricted to altering its mechanics.

Structure

Bone consists of cells and an extracellular mineralized matrix (35% organic and 65% inorganic). About 90% of the organic component is type 1 collagen. The remainder includes many non-collagen products of the osteoblast (e.g. osteocalcin, osteonectin, and proteoglycans). The mineral is present mainly as calcium hydroxyapatite. There are two anatomical types of bone, trabecular (cancellous) and cortical, the proportions of which differ from one bone to another; vertebral bodies are predominantly trabecular, while the shafts of the long bones are cortical, reflecting their disparate functions. Trabecular bone contains more metabolically active surfaces in a given volume than cortical bone and is therefore more susceptible to conditions such as osteoporosis.

Bone cells

Three types of bone cell are clearly identifiable (Figure 10.1.1):

- Osteoblasts responsible for synthesis of the bone matrix
- Osteoclasts, which occupy areas of resorption and classically have a multinucleate appearance
- Osteocytes within lacunae in the mineralized bone, apparently in contact with other osteocytes through extensions in bone canaliculi.

Box 10.1.1 Bone

- Bone is a mineral store (1 kg. calcium)
- 90% is type 1 collagen
- In adults bone turnover is 25% cancellous but only 2–3% cortical bone/annum.
- Osteoblasts lay down bone after osteoclasts remove it.

In the adult, the annual turnover of old bone is approximately 25% in cancellous bone but only 2–3% in cortical bone. Imbalance between bone formation and resorption underlies many pathological states. Osteoblasts are pluripotent stromal cells which can also give rise to fibroblasts, chondrocytes, myocytes, and adipocytes. Osteoblasts respond to various systemic and local factors (cytokines) and also to mechanical stress. They synthesize the organic bone matrix (mainly collagen) and non-collagen proteins, and control bone mineralization. They also direct the activity of osteoclasts. Osteocytes, derived from osteoblasts, occupy lacunae within the mineralized bone, communicating with each other through gap junctions via their processes in the bone canaliculi. They probably have an important function in the detection of mechanical forces and the resultant response of bone to them. Osteoclasts have different cellular origins from osteoblasts, being derived from the haemopoietic system. They attach themselves to bone via integrins (vitronectin receptor) and produce a very acid environment within this sealed zone. Osteoclasts also have receptors to calcitonin, which suppresses their activity, but they are activated by prostaglandins.

Bone formation

Bone formation is largely dependent on osteoblasts. The stromal precursors of osteoblasts are found in the periosteum and the endosteal surfaces of bone. The local remodelling stimulus for new bone formation probably comes from product(s) of bone resorption which may include growth factors, cytokines, transforming

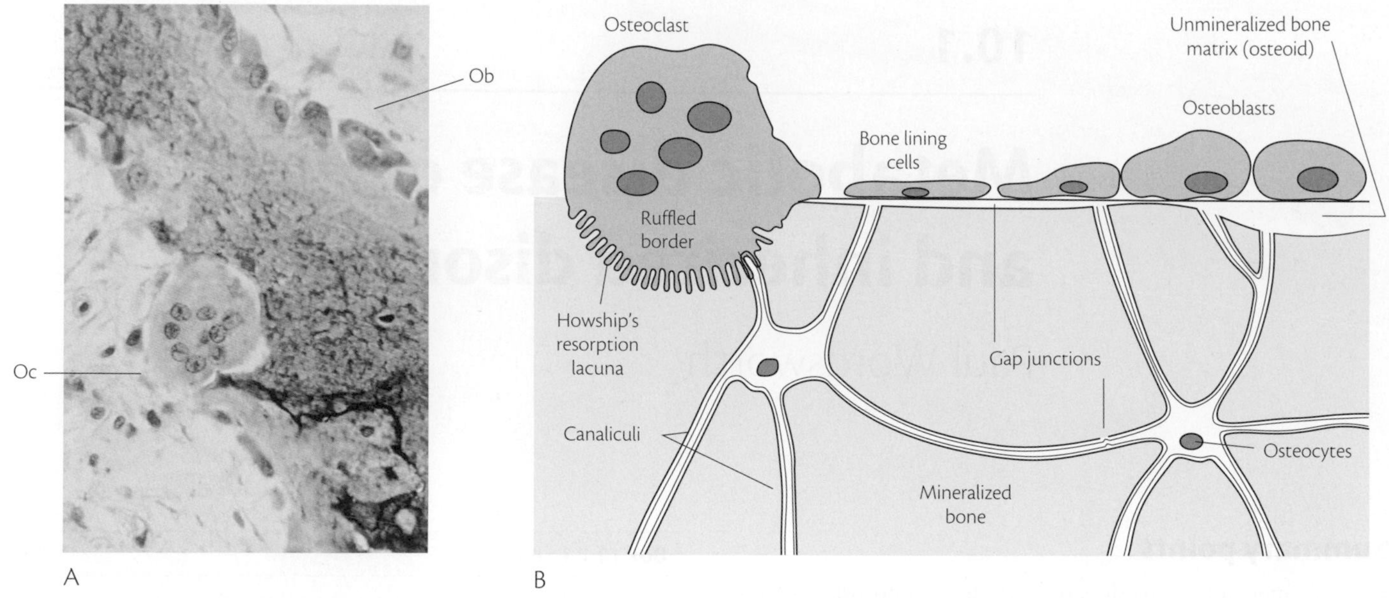

Fig. 10.1.1 A multinucleated osteoclast (Oc) in a resorption lacuna and a row of osteoblasts (Ob) on opposite surfaces of a bone trabecula (A) and the bone relationships of the osteocytes (B).

growth factor β (TGFβ), or bone morphogenetic proteins (BMPs) liberated from resorbed bone.

Bone resorption

Osteoclasts respond to systemic and local factors but not to mechanical stress. Calcitonin directly inhibits osteoclasts and also suppresses the generation of new osteoclasts, whereas bone resorption is increased by parathyroid hormone and $1,25(OH)_2D$. However, because osteoclasts actually lack receptors for either of these factors, their resorbing effects are mediated via the osteoblast. The number and activity of the osteoclasts are also increased by a variety of cytokines. Thus, in myeloma the malignant plasma cells release interleukin (IL)-1, IL-6, and TNF (tumour necrosis factor), all of which stimulate osteoclastic destruction of bone. The actions of the osteoclast are critically dependent on its ability to create an acidic resorption lacuna (Figure 10.1.2).

Bone mass

Peak bone mass is strongly genetically determined.In keeping with the mechanical functions of the skeleton, bone is laid down along its lines of stress. Osteoblasts respond to mechanical stress but the size and density of the skeleton is also related to nutritional intake, particularly of calcium, protein, and calories. The sex hormones (testosterone and oestrogen) encourage new bone formation. The complexity of these hormonal influences is emphasized in that oestrogen-deficient men get osteoporosis and the skeleton clearly depends on a full complement of sex steroids for its integrity. Growth hormone is an important anabolic skeletal agent during the early years of life, partly through the local production of somatomedins (insulin-like growth factors).

Collagen is the main product of the osteoblast, but there are also non-collagen proteins in bone. Osteonectin, the major non-collagen protein produced by human osteoblasts, binds strongly to calcium ions, hydroxyapatite, and native collagen.

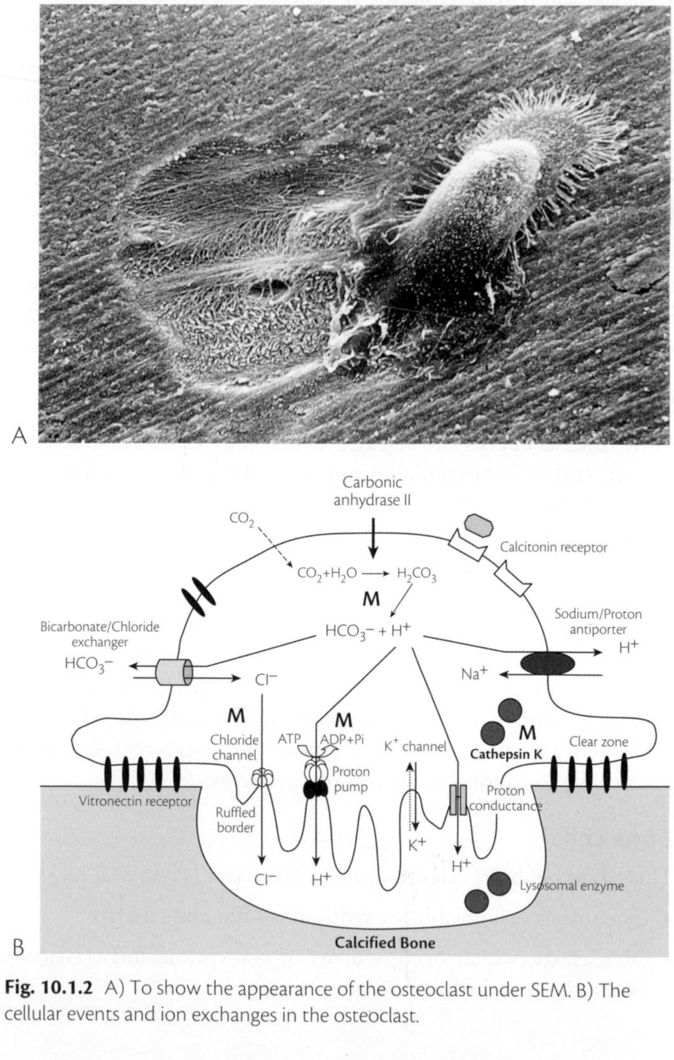

Fig. 10.1.2 A) To show the appearance of the osteoclast under SEM. B) The cellular events and ion exchanges in the osteoclast.

Box 10.1.2 Bone metabolism control

- Calcitonin inhibits osteoclasts
- PTH and 1,25$(OH)_2$D stimulate bone resorption
- Peak bone mass is strongly genetically controlled
- Sex hormones encourage bone deposition
- Demineralised bone matrix contains bone morphogenetic proteins
- Alkaline phosphatase is a good marker of bone turnover.

It has been known for many years that demineralized bone matrix contains substances capable of inducing ectopic bone formation. Because they are present in such small amounts these BMPs have only recently been isolated.

Bone mineral and mineralization

In most mineralized tissues, calcifying vesicles derived from chondrocytes or osteoblasts provide a focus for mineralization on bone matrix collagen. The precipitation of calcium within these vesicles is controlled by the action of alkaline phosphatase. In hypophosphatasia, deficient alkaline phosphatase activity results in defective mineralization and also accumulation of pyrophosphate in other tissues, where it results in ectopic calcification. Abnormal calcification or ossification may occur in many other pathological states and also as a consequence of ageing. Thus abnormal calcification of articular cartilage (chondrocalcinosis) may occur with increasing age.

Calcium and phosphorus balance (Box 10.1.3)

Total plasma calcium concentration is closely maintained at 2.25–2.60mmol/L. Nearly half of this calcium is in the ionized form. The skeleton contains approximately 1kg of calcium. Plasma calcium concentration is determined by a balance between intestinal absorption, renal excretion, and the exchange of mineral with the skeleton (Figure 10.1.3).

Parathyroid hormone and vitamin D (Figure 10.1.4)

Small changes in plasma calcium are detected in the parathyroid gland. Reduction in the plasma ionized-calcium concentration stimulates the release of parathyroid hormone (PTH), which increases calcium absorption through the gut, increases calcium reabsorption in the kidney, and increases bone resorption. The renal effect of PTH on calcium reabsorption is direct but, in contrast, the effect of PTH on increasing intestinal calcium absorption is indirect through its actions on vitamin D. 1,25$(OH)_2$D is the most important active metabolite of vitamin D. The action of PTH on increasing calcium absorption from the gut is therefore indirect through its effects on 1,25$(OH)_2$D production. PTH also encourages osteoclastic bone resorption indirectly by its effects on the osteoblast. Measurement of the plasma 25OHD concentration is a useful indicator of vitamin D status.

Calcitonin and other hormones

Calcitonin reduces bone resorption by the direct and reversible suppression of osteoclasts.

Excess corticosteroids (either therapeutic or in Cushing's syndrome) suppress new bone formation but can also be associated with exuberant callus formation after fractures. Androgens and oestrogens promote and maintain skeletal mass. Thyroxine increases bone turnover and resorption, thereby leading to bone loss. Excess growth hormone leads to gigantism/acromegaly (according to the age of onset). In contrast, growth hormone deficiency causes proportionate short stature and where there is general pituitary failure the reduction in gonadotrophins will also induce bone loss.

Biochemical measures of bone turnover

Total plasma alkaline phosphatase (largely derived from osteoblasts) provides a crude but readily accessible index of bone formation; it is increased during periods of rapid growth, following fractures and in conditions where bone turnover is greatly increased, such as Paget's disease.

The diagnosis of bone disease (Box 10.1.4)

Deformity, pain, and fracture are common features. To these may be added proximal myopathy (in osteomalacia and rickets) and the symptoms of any underlying systemic disease, such as renal failure, steatorrhoea, or myeloma. Other relevant factors are both family and menopausal history. Previous abdominal operations, including hysterectomy and oophorectomy, dietary history, and documentation of smoking, alcohol, and caffeine intake are all relevant to assessing the risk of osteoporosis.

Deformity and short stature

Short stature (defined as <0.4th centile) can be divided into proportionate and disproportionate forms, of which the most frequent is caused by short limbs. About three-quarters of children with short stature either have familial short stature or constitutional

Box 10.1.3 Calcium control

- PTH increases plasma calcium by:
  - Modifying gut absorbtion
  - Decreasing renal excretion
  - Reducing bone deposition
  - Increasing bone resorption
- Calcitonin—reduces bone resorption by suppressing osteoclasts.

Box 10.1.4 Diagnosis of bone disease

- Diet
- Family history
- Menstrual history
- Pain, and fractures
- Stature (proportionate vs disproportionate)
- Progressive deformity.

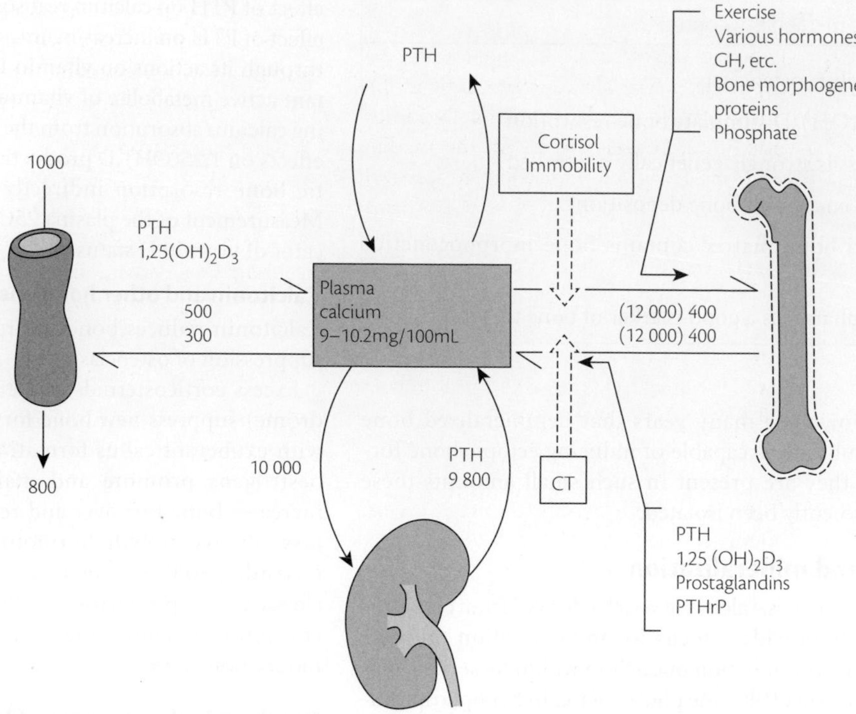

Fig. 10.1.3 Factors that control calcium balance. Units are in mg/day (to convert to mmol divide by 40) and refer to an adult. The figures in parentheses are an estimate of exchange through the cellular barrier of bone. CT, calcitonin; GH, growth hormone; PTH, parathyroid hormone; PTHrP, parathyroid hormone-related peptide.

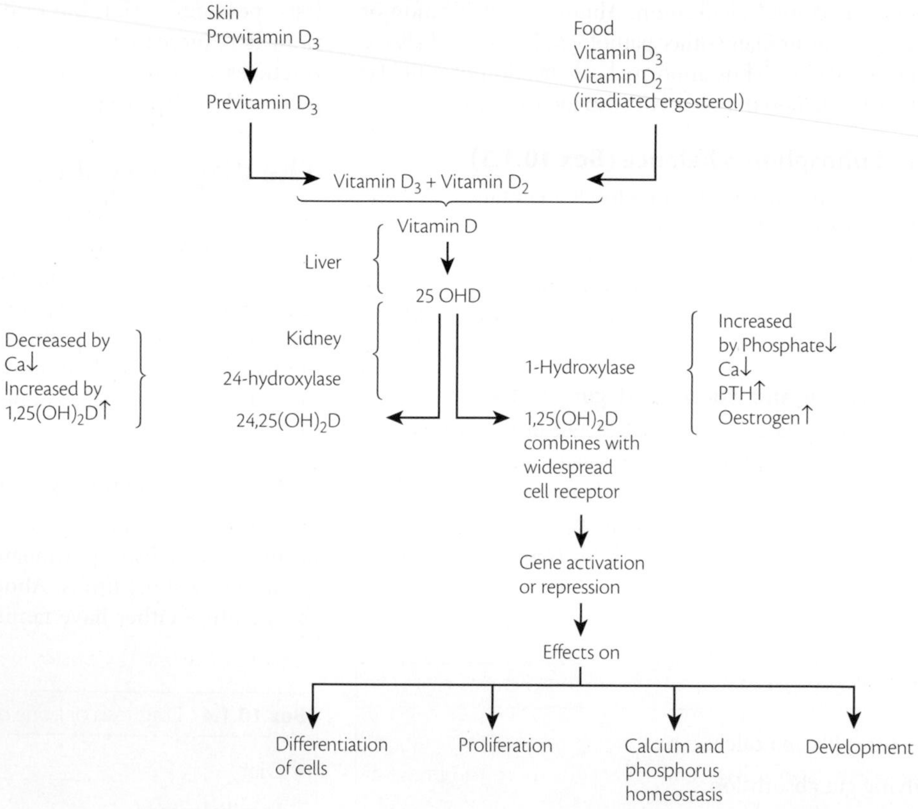

Fig. 10.1.4 The synthetic pathways and molecular and cellular effects of 1,25(OH)2D.

delay of growth and puberty; others have chronic disease (10%), syndromic short stature (6%), chromosomal abnormalities (5%), skeletal dysplasias (1%), or hormone deficiencies (1–2%).

Progressive kyphosis and loss of height is the commonest acquired deformity of adult life and is strongly associated with osteoporosis and osteomalacia. Other deformities include knock knees, bowed legs, enlarged epiphyses, and bossing of the skull in rickets; thick, bowed limb bones and an enlarged skull in Paget's disease; and very short, deformed limbs and trunk in severe osteogenesis imperfecta.

Bone pain and fracture

In osteomalacia, pain may be widespread and associated with tenderness on pressure. Osteoporosis is typically asymptomatic in the absence of fractures. Fissure fractures are characteristically found on the convexity of pagetic bone; Looser's zones on the medial borders of osteomalacic bones; and multiple vertebral compression fractures may be seen in osteoporosis. Degenerative joint disease is actually the most common cause of pain suffered by individuals with rare disorders of the skeleton.

Myopathy

Proximal muscle weakness is common in osteomalacia and rickets. The symptoms include a waddling gait and difficulty in climbing stairs. Limbs may be described as stiff rather than weak.

Physical signs

Abnormalities in physical signs may not be confined to the musculoskeletal system. Blue sclera (in osetogenesis imperfecta), lens dislocation in Marfan syndrome and tooth enamel defects (in hypoparathyroidism) are all examples.

Abnormal body proportions may give valuable clues to underlying conditions. The fingers may be abnormally long and thin (Marfan syndrome) or excessively short and mobile (pseudoachondroplasia). The spine is relatively short after vertebral collapse; scoliosis often dates from adolescence and is occasionally a clue to an inherited connective tissue disorder; a thoracolumbar gibbus is a particular (though not exclusive) feature of the mucopolysaccharidoses. Spinal deformity often produces secondary changes; thus a young patient with severe osteoporosis will develop a prominent sternum with ribs that impinge on the iliac crest and a transverse crease across the front of the abdomen.

Investigations

Biochemistry

Plasma

Fasting plasma calcium is normal in osteoporosis and also in Paget's disease unless the patient has been immobilized. Hypercalcaemia occurs in primary hyperparathyroidism, various neoplasms (including hypercalcaemia of malignancy), in sarcoidosis, vitamin-D overdosage and, rarely, in thyrotoxicosis. Hypocalcaemia is typical of parathyroid insufficiency and may be apparent in osteomalacia. However, hypophosphataemia is actually a more sensitive indicator of osteomalacia since calcium levels may be restored towards normal by secondary hyperparathyroidism. Plasma phosphate is reduced in primary hyperparathyroidism, in the humoral hypercalcaemia of malignancy and also in inherited hypophosphataemic rickets.

Plasma alkaline phosphatase is increased in primary hyperparathyroidism, but only where there is demonstrable bone disease. Plasma alkaline phosphatase is particularly elevated in young patients with active Paget's disease. It is variably increased in metastatic bone cancers and sometimes in active fibrous dysplasia of bone. Low levels are characteristic of hypophosphatasia.

Radiology

Magnetic resonance imaging (MRI) is very useful in the diagnosis and assessment of musculoskeletal disease because of the additional information it can provide about soft tissue and bone pathology. Bisphosphonate-labelled radioisotope scanning is useful in demonstrating the skeletal extent of Paget's disease, and the presence of bony metastases, Isotope scanning is preferable to multiple radiographs when assessing the distribution of abnormal bone but it is increasingly being supplanted by MRI.

Further investigations

Plasma PTH is useful when investigating hyper- and hypocalcaemia, PTHrP is useful for suspected hypercalcaemia of malignancy, and 25OHD and 1,25$(OH)_2$D levels are reduced in rickets and osteomalacia). Some guidance to the diagnosis can be gained from the age of the patient and frequency of the disorder (Table 10.1.1).

Osteomalacia and rickets (Box 10.1.5)

Osteomalacia usually results from a lack of vitamin D and in the growing skeleton it is referred to as rickets. Inherited hypophosphataemia and several other renal tubular disorders may also cause rickets.

Vitamin D synthesis in the skin is quantitatively more important than dietary intake. Asian immigrants and the elderly are most at risk from vitamin D deficiency.

Pathophysiology

Many patients have more than one cause for their osteomalacia; in the housebound elderly, vitamin D intake is often poor, exposure to sunlight limited, and renal glomerular failure progressive. Reduced exposure to sunlight is an indirect consequence of physical immobility and may contribute to osteomalacia in rheumatoid arthritis and other chronic diseases. Histology reveals an excess of unmineralized osteoid (Figure 10.1.5).

Clinical features

The main effects of osteomalacia are bone pain and tenderness, skeletal deformity, and proximal muscle weakness. In severe osteomalacia all the bones are painful and tender, sometimes sufficiently to disturb sleep and this may be accentuated over Looser's zones. In children growth rate is reduced, there is bowing of the long bones, enlargement of the costochondral junctions (rickety rosary), and bossing of the frontal and parietal bones. Later, osteomalacia may produce a triradiate pelvis, kyphosis, and chest deformities.

Investigations

Biochemistry

Classic vitamin D deficiency or malabsorption causes low plasma calcium and phosphate, low urine calcium and, eventually, an increase in the plasma alkaline phosphatase. The measurement of vitamin D metabolites is now routine; low plasma 25OHD level is a good indication of vitamin D deficiency.

Box 10.1.5 Osteomalacia

- Rickets in children leads to growth deformity
- On adults low 1,25$(OH)_2$D because of
  - Poor diet
  - Lack of sunlight
  - Inability to metabolize vitamin D.

Table 10.1.1 Diagnosis of disorders of the skeleton according to age

Age	Main presenting symptom	Most likely diagnosis	Frequency	Exclude
Over 50 years	Pain in the back; loss of height; fracture	Osteoporosis, most common in women	Common	Myeloma (especially in men); secondary deposits; coexistent osteomalacia
	Deformity of long bones; pain in hips; pathological fracture; deafness	Paget's disease of bone; most common in men	Common	Osteomalacia; hyperparathyroid bone disease; skeletal metastases;
	Bone pain; difficulty walking; unable to climb stairs; fractures	Osteomalacia	Uncommon, in adults	Carcinoma; polymyalgia rheumatica
	Bone pain and deformity; thirst; nocturia; depression; vomiting; constipation	Osteitis fibrosa cystica; most common in women	Rare	Carcinoma with hypercalcaemia; myeloma
20–50 years	Loss of height; unremitting bone pain; weight loss; systemic features	Probably secondary deposits; or myeloma	Rare	Osteomalacia; accelerated osteoporosis
	Muscle weakness; loss of height; bone pain	Osteomalacia	Rare	Late muscular dystrophy; neoplastic neuromyopathy; Cushing's syndrome
0–20 years	Bowing of bones; deformity; weakness	'Nutritional' rickets	Most common in Asian immigrants	Other causes of rickets; hypophosphatasia
	Multiple fractures; bruising at different times	Non-accidental injury	Not uncommon	Osteogenesis imperfecta
	Bone pain; ill health	Leukaemia	Uncommon	Osteomyelitis; rickets
	Pain in back; difficulty in walking; pain in ankles; less rapid growth	Juvenile osteoporosis	Rare	Leukaemia; osteogenesis imperfecta
	Failure to grow (short stature)	Many causes	Common	Particularly hypothyroidism; Turner's syndrome; and coeliac disease
	Excessive or disproportionate growth	Several causes, often familial	Less common than short stature	Marfan syndrome; pituitary tumour; homocystinuria; hypogonadism and chromosomal abnormalities
	Fracture and deformity at birth (often lethal)	Severe osteogenesis imperfecta	Uncommon	Hypophosphatasia; achondrogenesis; thanatophoric dwarfism

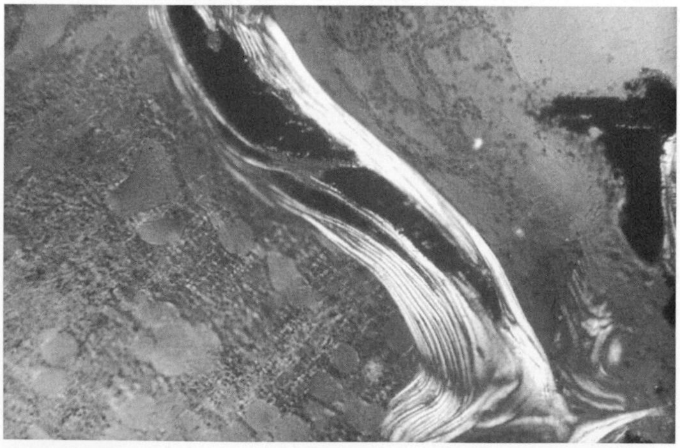

Fig. 10.1.5 Bone from a patient with osteomalacia. The birefringent osteoid is abnormally thick (up to 12 lamellae, arrows) and covers all bone surfaces. The bone preparation is undecalcified and viewed under polarized light (von Kossa stain; magnification ×300).

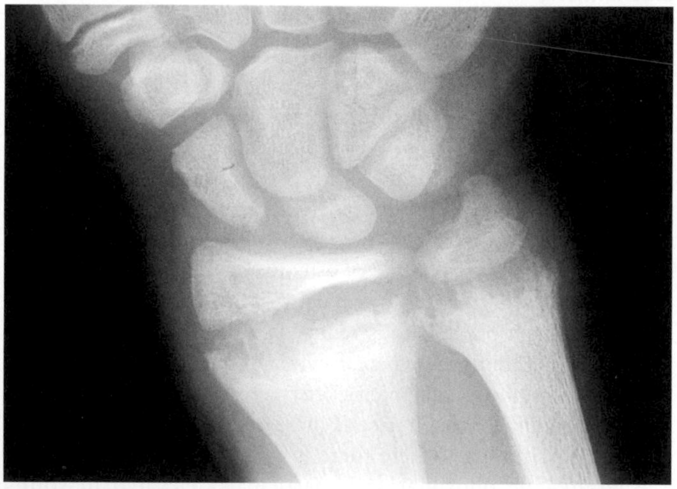

Fig. 10.1.6 The radiological appearance of rickets in a child with inherited hypophosphataemia. The growth plates are widened and the metaphyses cupped and ragged.

Radiology

In childhood rickets the main abnormalities are at the ends of the long bones, where the width of the growth plate is increased, and the metaphysis is widened, cupped, and ragged (Figure 10.1.6) but the radiological hallmark of active osteomalacia is the Looser's zone (Figure 10.1.7). This is a ribbon-like area of defective mineralization, which is seen particularly in the long bones, pelvis, ribs, and the scapulas. Looser's zones typically occur on the medial border of the femoral shaft or neck, contrasting with the multiple fissure fractures on the lateral convexity of the bone in

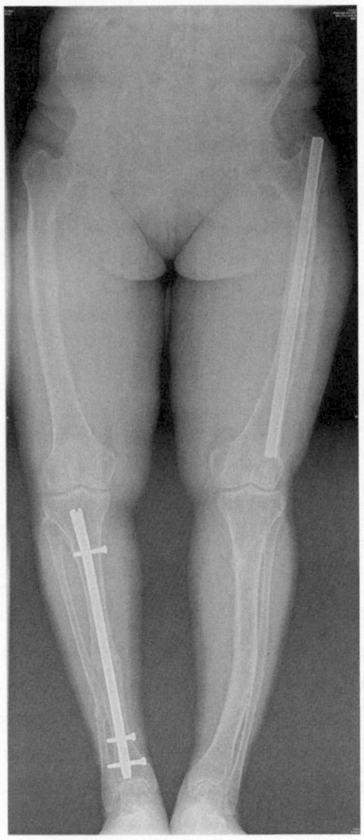

Fig. 10.1.7 X-linked hypophosphataemia Looser's zone, bowing and fissure fractures in the left tibia.

Paget's disease. The vertebral bodies are often biconcave ('codfish spine'). Additionally, in renal glomerular osteodystrophy, the end-plates may become relatively denser than the rest of the vertebral body, producing the so-called 'rugger jersey' spine.

Treatment

Rickets and osteomalacia should respond rapidly to vitamin D (or one of its metabolites). Increased mobility due to increased muscle strength is the first clinical response, despite a temporary increase in bone pain.

Paget's disease of bone (Box 10.1.6)

Paget's disease of bone is the most common metabolic bone disease after osteoporosis in the United Kingdom. It is characterized by excessive and disorganized resorption and formation of bone. The introduction of bisphosphonates, which act primarily on the abnormally active osteoclasts characteristic of the condition, has revolutionized the management of Paget's disease.

Box 10.1.6 Paget's disease

- Major genetic component
- Affects 750 000 in United Kingdom
- Rapid bone turnover with deposition of disordered bone
- Raised alkaline phosphatise
- Responds well to new aminobisphosphonates
- Premalignant in some cases.

Pathophysiology

There is now overwhelming evidence of a genetic contribution to a significant proportion of patients with Paget's disease.

Histology shows increased numbers of bone-resorbing multinucleate osteoclasts and active osteoblasts. The bone matrix is laid down in a haphazard fashion and loses its birefringence and strength; mineralization may be defective. Osteosarcoma, which occurs in Paget's disease, probably results from the excessive and prolonged activity of the bone cells. Pagetic bone is typically enlarged, vascular, deformed, and somewhat fragile. Fractures account for about 10% of all clinical presentations.

Incidence

Paget's disease affects about 750 000 people in Britain, of whom up to 40% may have an affected relative. It becomes more common with advancing years (approximately 3% of those over 40 years old) but only about 5% of affected individuals are symptomatic. In England there is a slightly increased prevalence in some northern regions and it is also more frequent in recent British migrants to Australia than in the indigenous population.

Clinical features

Most subjects with Paget's disease are asymptomatic but bone pain is the most common symptom in the rest. Pain may arise from the bone itself or from the neighbouring joints. In around 10%, pain due to fracture through pagetic bone may be the presenting complaint, while pain from fissure fractures (see Figure 10.1.8) or sarcomatous change are important but later complications.

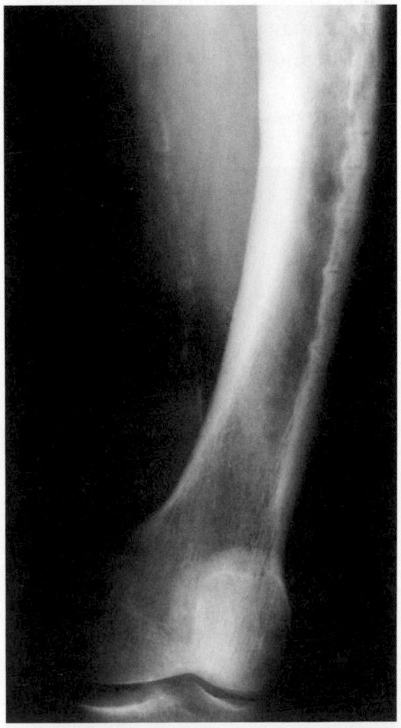

Fig. 10.1.8 Fissure fractures on the convexity of a femur affected by Paget's disease.

Clinically, the affected bones are enlarged, deformed, and warm. The enlargement is most clearly seen in bones such as the tibia and the skull: in the former the bone is typically bowed forwards; the latter shows a characteristic enlargement of the vault that is said to look like a 'tam-o'-shanter' hat, which appears to descend over the ears. Although any bone can be affected, including the maxilla and the phalanges, the most common sites for Paget's disease are the pelvis and the spine.

Deafness in Paget's disease is one of its most disabling symptoms; it has many causes, of which nerve compression is only one. Almost any nerve can be compressed by enlarging pagetic bone; the spinal cord is particularly at risk, due to the combined effects of increased bone size, vertebral collapse, and excessive vascularity. Paraplegia or cauda equina lesions may occur. Alterations in the shape of the skull may produce multiple cranial nerve palsies and brainstem lesions, with dysphagia, dysarthria, and ataxia.

Investigations

Biochemistry

There is variable elevation of plasma alkaline phosphatase that roughly correlates with the extent of clinical and radiological involvement with Paget's disease.

Radiology

The most characteristic appearance is an increase in size of the affected bones, which also appear sclerotic with abnormal trabecular architecture. Early in the disease a resorbing front may be seen in a long bone as a flame-shaped area (Figure 10.1.9). Excessive resorption is inevitably followed by disordered bone formation, causing thickening and deformity of the bone. Multiple partial fractures (microfractures, fissure fractures) are common on the deformed convex surface of long bones, particularly the femur and tibia (see Figure 10.1.8), contrasting with the Looser's zones of osteomalacia that predominantly affect the concavities.

Bone scintigraphy may be particularly informative in Paget's disease, demonstrating not only the extent and activity of the bone lesions but also the effects of treatment. MRI is particularly helpful in the demonstration of suspected fractures and in identifying sarcomatous change.

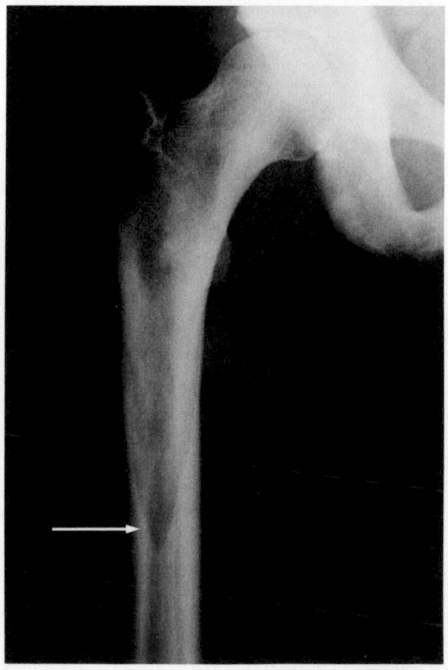

Fig. 10.1.9 A flame-shaped resorption front in a pagetic femur (arrowed).

Diagnosis

In prostate carcinoma with osteoblastic bone secondaries, the dense bones are not enlarged (in contrast to Paget's disease), and the prostate-specific antigen levels will be elevated in prostate disease but normal in Paget's disease.

Treatment

The newer aminobisphosphonates are particularly effective and many times more potent than the early bisphosphonates, such as etidronate. They may produce almost complete and permanent suppression of Paget's disease with few side effects. Calcitonin is useful to treat bone pain, for osteolytic Paget's disease and for preoperative treatment.

Surgical treatment

Fractures through pagetic bone require the usual surgical treatment but union may be delayed. When fracture occurs through a deformed bone the deformity should be corrected where possible. Elective osteotomy with intramedullary nailing or Ilizarov correction may be considered for a severe long-bone deformity. Spinal cord compression not responding to medical treatment requires surgery.

Hypercalcaemia

Malignancy is one of the most important causes of hypercalcaemia.

Where hypocalcaemia is prolonged, as in renal glomerular failure or coeliac disease, the parathyroid glands respond by increasing both in size and activity. Occasionally hypercalcaemia develops in such patients despite correction of the underlying disease due to one of the hyperplastic parathyroid glands becoming autonomous ('tertiary hyperparathyroidism').

Hypoparathyroidism

Parathyroid insufficiency most commonly occurs after surgical removal of the parathyroids but also in idiopathic hypoparathyroidism.

Osteogenesis imperfecta: the brittle bone syndrome

Osteogenesis imperfecta (OI) affects about 1 in 20 000 births and is a leading cause of lethal short-limbed dwarfism.

Pathophysiology

OI is a genetic disorder of type 1 collagen and affects those tissues which contain it. These include particularly bone and dentine but also the sclerae, joints, tendons, heart valves, and skin.

In the so-called 'mild' type I OI there is a reduction in the amount of bone (and hence in measured bone mineral density). In the extraskeletal tissues, the sclerae are thin (often blue or grey in colour), there is a varying degree of ligamentous laxity, hyperextensibility of the skin (sometimes with atrophic scars), and, uncommonly, incompetence of the heart valves.

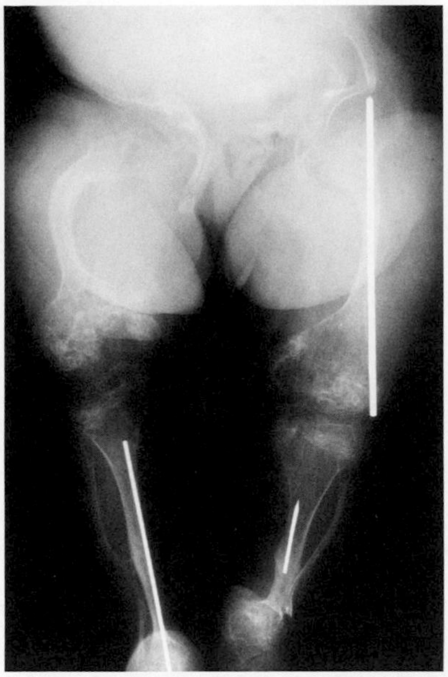

Fig. 10.1.10 Severe type III OI with intramedullary rods to treat and prevent fractures of the long bones. The bone of the metaphyses has a popcorn appearance.

Clinical features

Type I OI (60% of all patients) is the most frequent and least serious form. Fractures do not typically occur in the perinatal period and may even be delayed until the early menopause.

Type II OI is nearly always lethal, but not all infants with fractures at birth succumb immediately. A few survive the perinatal period to later merging with the type III (severe, progressively deforming) form.

Patients with type III OI are likely to survive but present major management problems because their disability is severe and progressive. Although intramedullary rods may be tried in some cases such patients rarely walk, even after multiple operations, and have a very short stature (>4 standard deviations below the mean) (Figure 10.1.10).

Diagnosis

In the first few years of life non-accidental injury is the main differential diagnosis. Although this may be suggested by multiple fractures at different sites and of different ages there are no pathognomonic signs. Some fractures, such as metaphyseal 'corner' fractures and posterior rib fractures are more often seen in non-accidental injury, but any type of fracture can also occur in OI. The distinction between OI and non-accidental injury is legally important and can be difficult. In adult life, mild OI may go unrecognized.

Marfan syndrome

In Marfan syndrome the fundamental genetic defect lies in fibrillin, one of the key microfibrillar components of elastic tissues.

Clinical features

Marfan syndrome is dominantly inherited. Its main effects are on the skeleton, cardiovascular, and ocular systems. In the typical patient with Marfan syndrome, overall height is increased and the limbs are long relative to the trunk. Long, thin fingers (arachnodactyly) are common. Scoliosis is common, may be severe, and worsens with the preadolescent growth spurt. Anterior chest wall deformity (pectus carinatum/pectus excavatum) is often associated with scoliosis (Figure 10.1.11).

Dislocation of the lens is the main ocular feature of Marfan syndrome, but the most severe complication is dilatation of the ascending aorta leading to aortic incompetence and/or dissection.

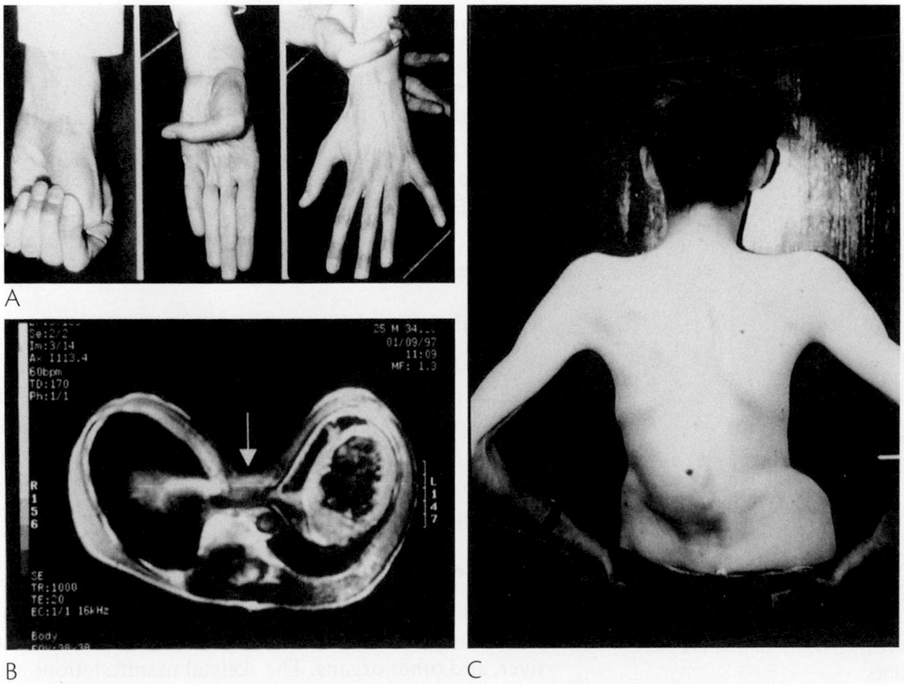

Fig. 10.1.11 Illustration of some of the clinical features of Marfan syndrome, including A) the positive wrist and thumb signs; B) severe pectus excavatum on axial MRI of the chest; and C) localized thoracolumbar scoliosis.

Treatment

There is no specific treatment yet for the underlying defect but many of the clinical manifestations require attention. Scoliosis may be progressive and severe. Bracing is largely ineffective and operative stabilization, ideally in adolescence, may be necessary. Epiphysiodesis may be considered in either sex where predicted height is in excess of that deemed to be socially acceptable.

Ehlers–Danlos syndrome

This heterogeneous syndrome includes individuals with the common clinical features of abnormal velvety hyperelastic skin, easy bruising, hyperextensible joints, and lax ligaments.

Alkaptonuria

The most important effects of this disease are on the spine (Figure 10.1.12) and later on the larger joints. The intervertebral discs lose height and later calcify. The spine becomes rigid and short and the lumbar lordosis is lost. In the large joints, such as the knees, shoulders, and hips, there are effusions and loose bodies. Ochronotic 'arthritis' is described with episodes of acute inflammation, reflecting the underlying pyrophosphate arthropathy. No effective medical treatment for the condition exists.

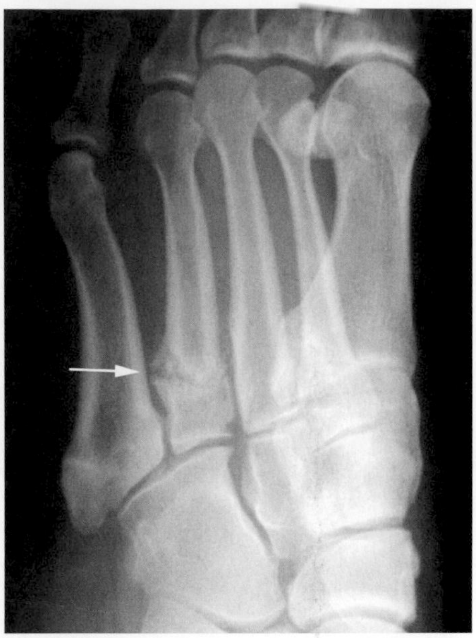

Fig. 10.1.13 Chronic fractures through base of the fourth metatarsal (arrowed) in a patient with the adult type of hypophosphatasia.

Hypophosphatasia

This rare disorder has similarities with rickets and osteomalacia. It is due to alkaline phosphatase deficiency which leads to defective mineralization of bone and varying degrees of fracture risk.

Clinical features

In the adult form, progressive stiffness, pain in the bones, and apparent 'stress' fractures can occur (Figure 10.1.13). Approximately 50% of such patients have a childhood history of bone disease or premature loss of deciduous teeth. Recurrent poorly healing metatarsal fractures occur. Partial fractures of the long bones characteristically occur on the convex outer surface (in contrast to Looser's zones in osteomalacia). Calcium pyrophosphate chondrocalcinosis is also common and may be associated with arthropathy (pseudogout).

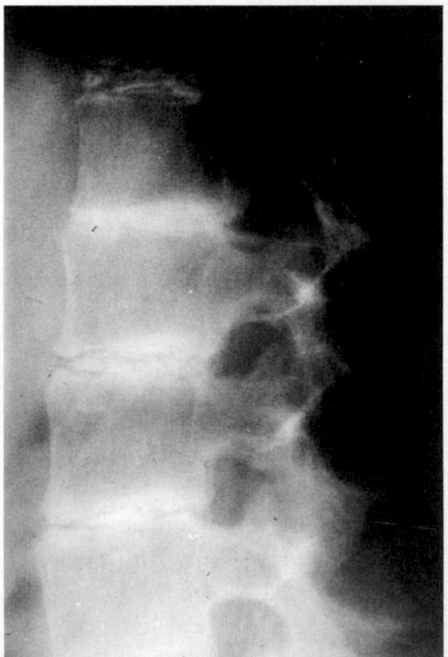

Fig. 10.1.12 The appearance of the spine in a man with alkaptonuria. There is universal calcification of the intervertebral discs.

Mucopolysaccharidoses

Failure of the normal lysosomal breakdown of complex carbohydrates or glycosaminoglycans leads to their accumulation in the tissues. Hurler's syndrome, the Hunter's syndrome, and Morquio's syndrome are such examples.

Hurler's syndrome

This is the most severe type of mucopolysaccharidosis and causes death at an early age.

The physical features include proportionate short stature, a typical facial appearance, a short neck with a lumbar gibbus and chest deformity, and a protuberant abdomen. Similar but less severe features are seen in the Hunter's syndrome.

Morquio's syndrome

In this disorder the orthopaedic manifestations are striking, but intelligence is normal. Characteristically the neck is short, the sternum is protuberant, and there may be a flexed stance with knock-knees. Importantly, the odontoid may be hypoplastic, leading to atlantoaxial instability, compression of the long spinal tracts, and paraplegia.

Gaucher's disease

This is a rare lysosomal storage disorder in which glucocerebroside-containing macrophages accumulate in the bone marrow, spleen, liver, and other organs. The skeletal manifestations are often severe and disabling. They vary from a characteristic but clinically insignificant failure of remodelling in the lower femora (Erlenmeyer-flask appearance) to diffuse and localized bone loss and osteosclerotic and osteonecrotic lesions, which cause pain and pathological fracture, often requiring precocious joint replacement surgery.

Skeletal dysplasias

Many of them are due to mutations in collagens

Most patients with skeletal dysplasias have restricted growth, and most are short-limbed. Achondroplasia is the most typical. Radiographs are essential to determine whether the metaphyses of the long bones or the epiphyses are primarily affected.

In achondroplasia, there are abnormalities in the epiphyseal growth cartilage. Radiological features include metaphyseal irregularity and flaring in the long bones, irregular and late-appearing epiphyses, a narrow pelvis in its anteroposterior diameter, with short iliac wings and deep sacroiliac notches. The spine shows progressive caudal narrowing of the interpedicular distance which is commonly associated with significant spinal stenosis. Spinal surgery for decompression of stenosis is commonly required and may be required at several levels. Eventual height can vary from about 80–150cm. Significant increase in height can be achieved by limb lengthening procedures.

Spondyloepiphyseal dysplasias

This heterogeneous group of disorders exhibits prominent spinal involvement and the short stature is partly due to shortness of the trunk. Hypermobility is marked and early osteoarthritis is quite typical, particularly in the hips. Joint replacement is often required in early adult life (Figure 10.1.14).

Proportionate dwarfism

The height of patients with epiphyseal dysplasias is variable but may be only slightly reduced.

Hereditary multiple exostoses

In patients with multiple hereditary exostoses (often referred to as diaphyseal aclasis) there is a juxtaepiphyseal disorder of bone growth, limited to bones developed in cartilage, which gives rise to cartilage-capped exostoses that point away from the joint. Stature is commonly normal. There may be mechanical interference with the normal functioning of affected joints. After skeletal maturity is reached there is a significant risk of malignant change in these exostoses that has been estimated at around 1% (lifetime risk). Any increase in size should raise the suspicion of malignant change which can be most effectively screened using ultrasonography to measure the thickness of the cartilage cap on the exostosis.

Cleidocranial dysplasia

In this rare condition the clavicles are hypoplastic or absent, the fontanelles remain open, there are supernumerary teeth and wormian bones may be apparent on skull radiographs.

Osteopetrosis

Patients with osteopetrosis (Albers–Schönberg disease) have increased bone density but pathological fractures are an important consequence of the abnormal architecture of the bone due to defective osteoclast function.

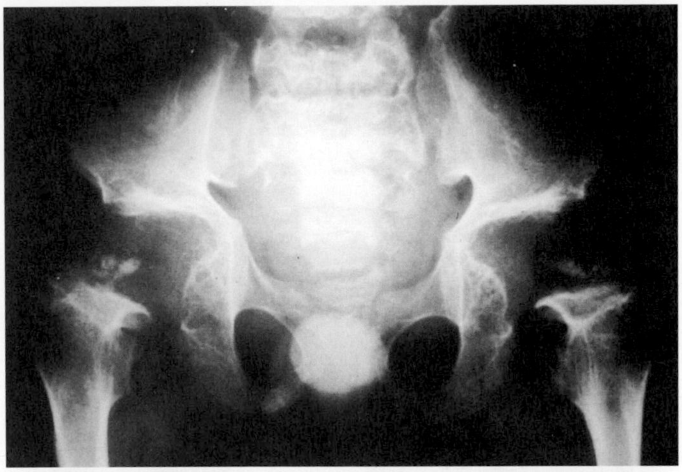

A

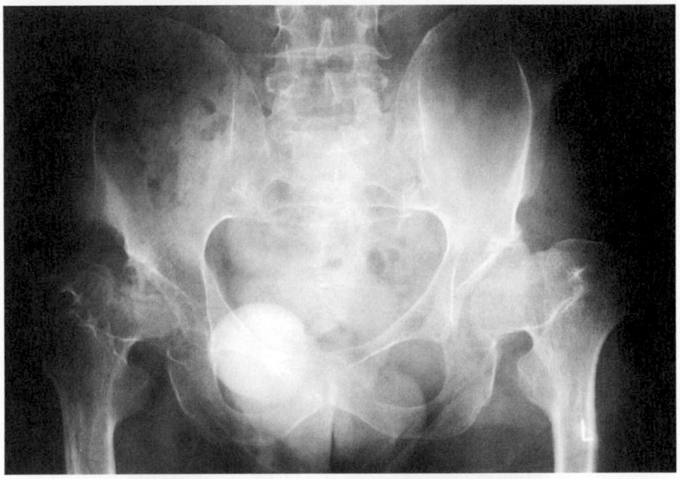

B

Fig. 10.1.14 Pseudochrondroplasia. A) Small proximal femoral epiphyses in a child with pseudoachondroplasia. B) Severe hip arthritis in a 26-year-old male with pseudoachondroplasia.

The mild forms vary widely in severity. The bones are relatively fragile despite being dense since they lack the normal capacity for remodelling along lines of maximum stress (Figure 10.1.15).

Fibrous dysplasia

Fibrous dysplasia of bone is a condition in which areas of immature fibrous tissue are found within the skeleton.

Monostotic fibrous dysplasia

This disorder is relatively common in orthopaedic practice. The lesions may occur in any bone and the most frequent presenting symptom at any age is a fracture, often of the upper end of the femur (Figure 10.1.16). There is a smooth-walled translucent area within the bone, often with thinning of the cortex and sometimes with associated deformity. The differential diagnosis is from other causes of bone cysts, including Paget's disease and hyperparathyroidism with osteitis fibrosa cystica. The large size of some of the defects in the shafts of the long bones may make conventional stabilization of fractures very difficult.

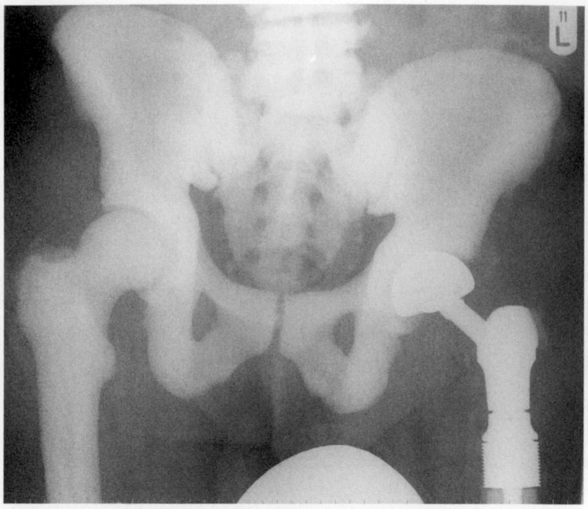

Fig. 10.1.15 The pelvic radiograph of a 72-year-old male with dominantly inherited mild osteopetrosis who sustained a fractured femoral neck late in life. The bones are uniformally dense and in this case show no 'endobones'.

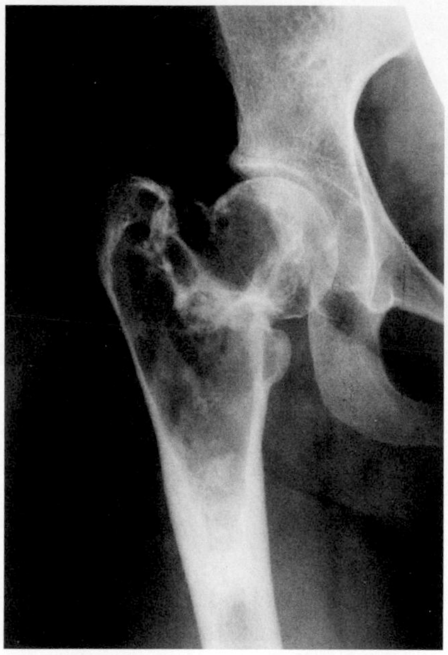

Fig. 10.1.16 Monoostotic fibrous dysplasia in a 23-year-old woman. A large cyst in the upper femur was the source of considerable pain, which settled for several years after treatment with intravenous pamidronate.

Polyostotic fibrous dysplasia

The bone lesions tend to increase in size and number but less rapidly after growth had ceased. The skeletal lesions may cause complications such as spinal cord compression, and may be associated with hypophosphataemic osteomalacia. Radiologically, the bones are deformed, the cortex may be difficult to detect, and the medullary bone takes on a 'ground glass' or 'smoky' appearance.

Ectopic mineralization

Deposition of calcium in the soft tissues (ectopic calcification) and on ectopic bone matrix (ossification) is often pathological, but the cause is frequently unknown.

Calcification can result from previous damage to soft tissues (dystrophic calcification) or from an increase in the circulating concentration of calcium or phosphate; (such metastatic calcification occurs in advanced renal osteodystrophy). Chondrocalcinosis is a particular example of ectopic mineralization which is common in the elderly but may also be pathological at a younger age. Dystrophic calcification occurs after infection, tumour, and trauma. In scleroderma, subcutaneous calcification in the fingers may be part of the CREST syndrome (calcinosis, Raynaud's phenomenon, oesophageal dysmotility, sclerodactyly, telangiectasia). The calcification can be very extensive but can also disappear rapidly. There is no specific treatment.

Calcific tendonitis

This is a particularly common form of soft tissue calcification to which many factors contribute. It may follow trauma but there is often no obvious injury. Calcific tendonitis may be associated with flares prompted by crystal shedding.

Chondrocalcinosis

In chondrocalcinosis, crystals of calcium pyrophosphate dihydrate (CPPD) are deposited in the fibrocartilage of the knees, the triangular cartilage of the wrists, the symphysis pubis, and elsewhere. CPPD may also form as linear deposits in the hyaline cartilage. It is most commonly age-related but may also reflect an underlying metabolic disturbance, such as haemochromatosis, hypophosphatasia, or hyperparathyroidism. One florid form of familial chondrocalcinosis causes early-onset polyarticular arthritis. It is useful to include examination of synovial fluid under polarized light microscopy in cases of acute monoarthritis to avoid missing pyrophosphate arthritis. However, the weakly positively birefringent crystals are smaller and less durable than the urate crystals causing gout. Intra-articular steroids help to settle acute episodes but there is no specific cure for the condition.

Ectopic ossification

Acquired ectopic ossification may occur at the site of local injury, such as after hip replacement or as a systemic response following paraplegia. It may occur in tumours and in a variety of other disorders, most notably infections, such as tuberculosis (Table 10.1.2).

Table 10.1.2 Some causes of ectopic ossification

Acquired	Local injury	
	Hip replacement	
	Traumatic paraplegia	
	Tumours	
	Others:	Diffuse idiopathic skeletal hyperostosis (DISH)
		Ossification of the posterior spinal ligament (OPLL)
		Ankylosing spondylitis
		Etretinate therapy
		Some metabolic enthesopathies (e.g. X-linked hypophospahataemia, Dent's disease)
Inherited	Pseudohypoparathyroidism	
	Fibrodysplasia (myositis) ossificans progressiva (FOP)	
	Progressive osseous heteroplasia (POH)	

Post-traumatic ossification

Local ossification can occur after total hip replacement but the incidence varies widely. It occurs more often in men than in women and is more likely to recur in certain individuals following surgery to the contralateral hip if ossification followed surgery to the first hip. The risk of such ossification may be significantly increased in patients with diffuse idiopathic skeletal hyperostosis (DISH, Forestier's disease). The bone mainly forms in the hip abductors. There is little evidence to justify routine use of prophylaxis for heterotopic ossification in hip surgery. However, in high-risk patients a single dose of radiotherapy perioperatively is more effective than anti-inflammatory agents.

Ossification after neurological injury

Extensive myositis ossificans may occur after injuries to the head or spinal cord in muscles distant from the injury after a significant delay. Affected muscles become swollen, red, and warm, and the differential diagnosis may include cellulitis, arthritis, and thrombophlebitis. Radiological calcification is initially absent (appearing at about 6 weeks or more after the injury), but an isotope bone scan or MRI will show changes well before that. Eventually organized bone appears. Because the bone affects the major periarticular muscles, it leads to joint fixation, particularly of the hips. Surgical removal of ectopic bone is technically difficult and usually ineffective. The ectopic bone recurs, especially if it is removed too early. The prevention of further ectopic bone formation after its removal may be delayed by non-steroidal anti-inflammatory drugs or radiotherapy, which should be commenced as soon as possible. Bisphosphonates are ineffective in the long term.

Myositis ossificans can also occur in neurological diseases, such as poliomyelitis and meningitis, and also after prolonged coma. It is not known why ectopic ossification occurs after head injury but interestingly head injury is associated with an increased rate of fracture healing and excessive callus formation. Ossification of the posterior longitudinal ligament of the spine (OPLL) is particularly described in Japan where it is a leading cause of myelopathy.

Fibrodysplasia ossificans progressiva

Fibrodysplasia ossificans progressiva (FOP) is rare, with an incidence of 1–2 per million. It is caused by activating mutations in ACVR1, a receptor for bone morphogenetic protein. Diagnosis depends on the combination of developmental abnormalities of the skeleton and progressive widespread myositis, leading to ossification in the major skeletal muscles.

Initially there is oedema and cellular infiltration throughout the muscle, with myofibrillar breakdown. Later endochondral ossification leads to mature bone, within which is haemopoietic marrow. The upper paraspinal trunk is typically first affected, and the peripheral skeleton and associated soft tissues are often spared. Typically, the affected muscle and/or associated fascia becomes swollen and hard, sometimes following injury; after a week or two these features subside, but the apparent improvement may be followed by ossification within the muscle and progressive joint fixation. Myositis usually begins in the upper paraspinal muscles in early childhood. By late childhood or adolescence, ossification will have usually occurred widely in the trunk but also within the muscles around the shoulders, hips, and less commonly knees, to fix these joints and to complete the disability (Figure 10.1.17). The large, striated muscles are affected; ossification does not involve the small muscles of the hands and feet, the diaphragm, the cardiac or the smooth muscles. Ossification in the muscles around the jaw may fix it almost completely.

The diagnostic skeletal abnormalities affect the big toes (Figure 10.1.18), to a lesser extent the thumbs and the cervical spine (Figure 10.1.19).

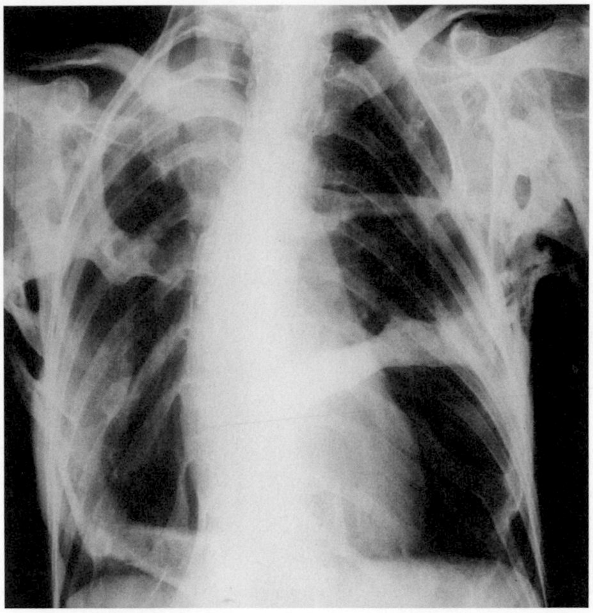

Fig. 10.1.17 Fibrodysplasia ossificans progressiva with widespread ossification of the muscles around the chest. The diaphragm is unaffected.

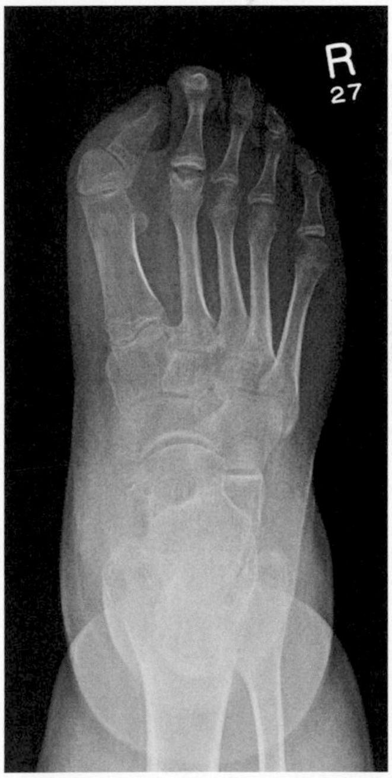

Fig. 10.1.18 Classic shortened monophalangic great toe in an adolescent with FOP.

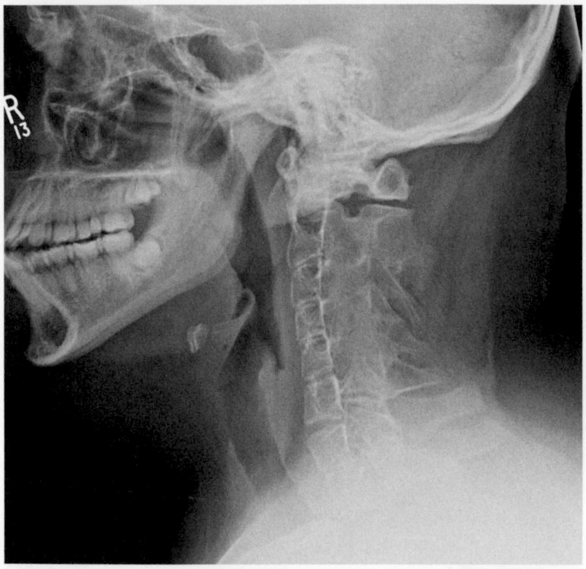

Fig. 10.1.19 The appearance of the cervical spine in FOP with failure to develop the normal zygoapophyseal joints giving the appearance of fusion.

Management

There is no effective treatment to prevent or reverse the abnormal ossification. Surgical removal of ectopic bone is technically difficult and may ultimately worsen the disability.

Miscellaneous bone disorders

Vitamin C (ascorbic acid) deficiency (scurvy) is reflected in weakness of collagen-containing tissues, notably causing haemorrhage and fractures. Extensive subperiosteal haemorrhage leads to pain and immobility; the legs are held in a 'frog-like' position. Radiographs in infancy show a widened zone of provisional calcification in the metaphyses and failure of new bone formation.

Prolonged parenteral nutrition can produce a form of bone disease similar to osteomalacia. The main symptom is periarticular bone pain, particularly in the ankles. The radiographic appearances suggest osteoporosis.

Deposition of excess fluoride in the skeleton can result from an excess in the diet (endemic fluorosis), from industrial exposure (during the manufacture of aluminium, steel, and glass, and from exposure to the dust of fluoride-containing rock), and from the administration of sodium fluoride in treatment. There is a generalized increase in bone density (with loss of the normal corticomedullary junction), and the tendons, ligaments, and sometimes muscles may be mineralized. Compression of the spinal cord and its roots, with progressive neurological disability has been described.

The prolonged use of vitamin A (retinoids) for the treatment of skin disease, such as psoriasis and ichthyosis, leads particularly to calcification of the spinal ligaments, causing stiffness and reduced mobility. There is a resemblance to Forestier's disease (diffuse idiopathic skeletal hyperostosis).

Chronic vitamin D overdosage leads to soft tissue calcification, especially in the arteries and kidneys. After several years, progressive stiffness in the spine, major joints, and feet lead to difficulty in walking. Radiographs show ligamentous calcification.

Lead poisoning in the growing skeleton produces a radiologically dense line near the growth plate.

Further reading

Firth, H.V. and Hurst, J.A. (2005). *Oxford Desk Reference: Clinical Genetics.* Oxford, Oxford University Press.

Online Mendelian Inheritance In Man, OMIM: http://www.ncbi.nlm.nih.gov/omim/

Royce, P.M. and Steinmann, B. (2002). *Connective Tissue and its Heritable Disorders,* second edition. New York, Wiley-Liss.

Smith, R. and Wordsworth, P. (2005). *Clinical and Biochemical Disorders of the Skeleton.* Oxford, Oxford University Press.

Spranger, J.W., Brill, P.W., and Poznanski, A. (2002). *Bone Dysplasias,* second edition. Oxford, Oxford University Press.

10.2

Rheumatoid arthritis

Sandeep Bawa and Paul Wordsworth

Summary points

- Rheumatoid arthritis (RA) is one of the most common disabling chronic diseases of the Western world.
- New biologic treatments have provided great benefit in the management of this condition, reducing morbidity and mortality.
- RA diagnosis requires careful clinical, biochemical, and radiological assessment
- Rheumatoid factor is not a reliable diagnostic test for rheumatoid arthritis (RA)
- The core of its management requires careful input from all members of the multidisciplinary team.

Introduction

RA is a chronic systemic inflammatory disorder predominately affecting synovial joints. It affects approximately 1% of the population in most developed countries. There is a female predominance but this is age dependent; at 30 years of age women are ten times more likely to develop RA than men but this diminishes to equality aged 60. There is a peak incidence between the ages of 35–55 years, although it can start at virtually any time of life. There is some evidence that RA is a relatively new disease in the West because historical writings and artistic depictions are uncommon until about 200 years ago in Europe. There is also some evidence that the incidence of RA may have diminished slightly in Europe in the past 20 years, which some authorities have attributed to protective effects of oral contraceptives. RA not only results in highly significant joint-related morbidity but also has a major effect on mortality; standardized mortality rates are increased two to threefold (mainly due to excess cardiovascular disease and infections). Its effects are not limited to the joints; extra-articular manifestations are common and systemic features, such as weight loss, malaise, and fever are prominent. There is no specific test for RA and its diagnosis depends on a combination of clinical, serological, and radiological findings.

Underlying causes

The cause of RA is unknown, but it is certainly associated with immunological abnormalities that place it in the realm of the 'autoimmune disorders'. Indeed it shares certain genetic susceptibility factors (human leukocyte antigen (HLA) genes, *CTLA4* and *PTPN22*) with other autoimmune diseases, such as systemic lupus erythematosus, autoimmune thyroiditis, and type 1 diabetes mellitus. These conditions also often cluster together in individuals affected by RA and their families, suggesting that there is an underlying autoimmune diathesis linking these diseases. The presence of autoantibodies to immunoglobulin (Ig) (rheumatoid factors) and cyclic citrullinated peptides (anti-CCP antibodies) is suggestive of disordered immune function. Likewise the chronic inflammatory infiltrate in the synovium and many other tissues; monocytes, macrophages, and T and B lymphocytes are all found in large numbers in the hypertrophied synovial pannus. The limited range of *HLA-DRB1* specificities associated with RA hints at a specific antigenic trigger for the disease but to date there is no convincing data as to its identity. Animal models, such as collagen-induced arthritis, have given some important insights into the underlying immunopathology despite their limitations. Basic research on the abnormal cytokine milieu in such animal studies was of fundamental importance to the introduction of anti-tumour necrosis factor (TNF) therapies for RA by Feldman and Maini that so revolutionized its management during the 1990s.

In contrast to the insights that have come from immunology, the contribution from epidemiology towards understanding the aetiology of RA has been relatively disappointing. Despite the widely held belief that infections may be involved in triggering RA, evidence for this is lacking. There is some evidence, particularly comparing indigenous South African populations in rural and urban communities, that increasing urbanization is associated with an increase in RA. Certainly the disease is uncommon in mush of rural sub-Saharan Africa. The risk of RA is increased by smoking and furthermore cessation from smoking is associated with improvements in disease activity.

Genetics

Identical co-twins of individuals with RA are three to four times more likely to be concordant for the disease than non-identical twins although overall concordance is still relatively low at around 15%. Non-twin siblings have a sixfold increased risk of RA compared to the general population and it has been estimated that heritability of RA is around 55%. Genetic susceptibility is complex and polygenic but major advances are now being made towards identifying the full component of genes involved by using genome-wide association scans. These are capable of identifying genes increasing the risk of RA by as little as 10–15%; good evidence exists for the *HLA-DRB1* locus, *PTPN22, CTLA4, STAT4, IL-2R,* and at least one gene on chromosome 6q.

Human leukocyte antigens

The human leukocyte antigen HLA-DR4, encoded by the immune response gene *HLA-DRB1*04*, is strongly associated with RA in the majority of populations that have been studied. In the United Kingdom, about 70% of patients with RA are HLA-DR4 positive compared with 35% of the normal population (odds ratio 4–5). In addition to HLA-DR4, other HLA molecules that share a high degree of structural homology with it, including HLA-DR1 and DR10 are also associated with RA. These molecules play a central role in the presentation of extrinsic antigens to the immune system and are implicated in numerous autoimmune diseases, suggesting involvement of specific components of the adaptive immune system in the aetiology of RA and related disorders. However, convincing evidence for this has yet to be presented in RA. The observation that individuals with RA, who do not carry HLA-DR4, are more likely to have mothers that possess HLA-DR4 as the non-inherited *HLA-DRB1* allele adds yet another intriguing layer of complexity to this ongoing immunogenetic mystery.

Pathophysiology

The most striking pathological finding is hypertrophy of the soft tissues around the synovial joints with evidence of chronic mononuclear cell infiltration. Histology of the synovium shows thickening of the synovial lining. The lining layer contains both fibroblast- and macrophage-like cells with evidence of *in situ* proliferation and migration into the lining layer. There is also a defect in apoptosis in the synovium that further increases the numbers of these cells. Many of the macrophages have a transformed appearance, neovascularization is prominent, and the synovial pannus is invasive with articular destruction beginning at the pannus/cartilage junction. T-helper cells (CD4+) are prominent, particularly in the perivenular space of the synovium. Cytotoxic (CD8+) T cells are present in smaller numbers but B cells and plasma cells locally synthesizing rheumatoid factors are also prominent. Within the joint macrophage-derived cytokines, such as TNF and interleukin (IL)-1 are found in high concentrations and appear to play a central role in mediating the chronic inflammation. There is currently much interest in the nature of the T-cell subsets involved in RA synovitis; in particular, the T_H17 subset of helper T cells that are thought to play a dominant role in establishing tissue non-specific inflammation. Insights into the pathology of RA have also come from the successful therapeutic targeting of disparate molecules on various cell types, including CD20 (B cells), TNF (macrophages), soluble IL-6 receptor, CD28 (T cells), and IL-1. RA is clearly the end result of several complex pathological pathways; while amelioration of the disease is possible by targeting specific components of these systems, the primary triggers for the aberrant immune mediated inflammation remain to be identified.

Clinical features

RA typically presents as a symmetric peripheral polyarthritis (Figure 10.2.1) although virtually any synovial joint in the body may be affected. The onset of the disease is usually insidious, with gradual recruitment of an increasing number of joints. Pain and stiffness, typically affecting the small peripheral joints, gradually increases in severity and spreads more centrally to involve the elbows, wrists, shoulders, ankles, knees, and hips. Systemic features such as malaise, weight loss, and low-grade fever are common and soft tissue problems such as carpal tunnel syndrome and flexor tenosynovitis may be prominent (Box 10.2.1).

Soft tissue swelling with tenderness, restricted movement, synovial effusion, redness, and warmth of the joints occurs with pronounced diurnal variation of symptoms, worse in the early morning and returning towards evening. The prolonged morning stiffness (>30min in duration) contrasts with the minor stiffness of osteoarthritis (rarely >5min in duration). The condition must be distinguished from other inflammatory arthropathies, such as systemic lupus erythematosus, seronegative spondyloarthropathies (see Chapter 10.4), crystal arthropathies (see Chapter 10.3), and viral arthropathies (rubella, parvovirus, hepatitis B and C). Several distinct patterns of onset are recognized: insidious onset with gradual recruitment of an increasing number of joints over weeks or months is common (approximately 60%); palindromic

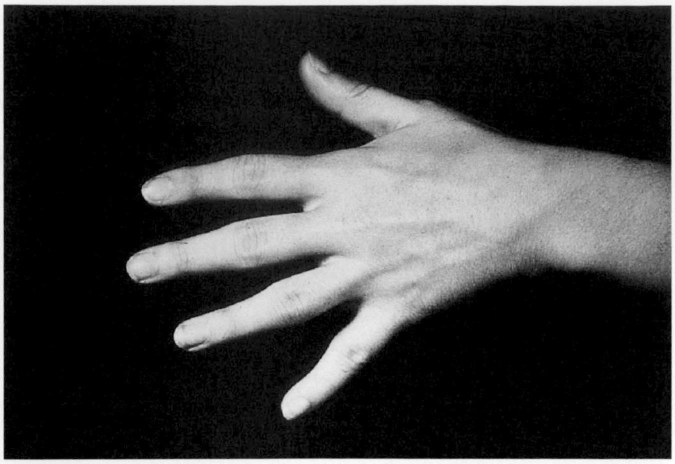

Fig. 10.2.1 Symmetrical synovitis affecting the proximal interphalangeal joints in early rheumatoid arthritis.

Box 10.2.1 American College of Rheumatology 1987 criteria for rheumatoid arthritis[a]

- Morning stiffness (>1h; >6 weeks)
- Arthritis in at least three areas (>6 weeks)
- Arthritis of hands or wrists (>6 weeks)
- Symmetrical arthritis (>6 weeks)
- Rheumatoid nodules
- Positive rheumatoid factor
- Radiographic changes in wrists/hands.

[a]Four criteria are required for the diagnosis.

rheumatism with short-lived episodes (<48h) of completely resolving synovitis (5%); episodic disease may relapse and remit in an unpredictable fashion but is quite uncommon; systemic onset disease particularly in middle-aged males may mimic malignancy or deep-seated infection; explosive onset disease (approximately 5%) is typically polyarticular but may resolve spontaneously after a variable time.

Physical signs

Synovial joint involvement usually predominates, typically in the periphery; soft tissue swelling, tenderness, stiffness, erythema, increased joint temperature; tenosynovitis, particularly in the flexor tendons of the fingers and the long flexors around the medial malleolus; carpal tunnel syndrome.

Synovial effusions may be present and a symmetric small-joint arthritis of the hands and feet with fusiform swelling of the fingers is common because of the prominent involvement of the proximal interphalangeal joints with sparing of the distal interphalangeal joints.

Swan-neck and boutonnière deformities of the fingers commonly develop and ulnar deviation together with volar and ulnar subluxation of the fingers at the metacarpophalangeal joints frequently occur (Figure 10.2.2). Deformities of the foot commonly lead to problems but are under-recognized; these include dorsal subluxation of the toes, spreading of the forefoot due to metatarsophalangeal joint synovitis, and collapse of the transverse arch of the forefoot (Figure 10.2.3).

Extra-articular features (Box 10.2.2)

These affect many patients with RA at some stage during the course of their disease but may be relatively mild and bear little temporal relationship to the joint activity. Many organs can be involved, and systemic disease contributes markedly to the adverse prognosis of RA. Men are particularly susceptible to rheumatoid vasculitis (lifetime incidence 1:9) which can be life threatening if it involves major organs. Cardiovascular disease is a major comorbidity in RA with chronic inflammation thought to be responsible for much of this. About half of the excess risk only can be attributed to traditional risk factors, such as hypertension, smoking, dyslipidaemia, etc. but these should be controlled aggressively along similar lines to the management of such risk factors in diabetes mellitus).

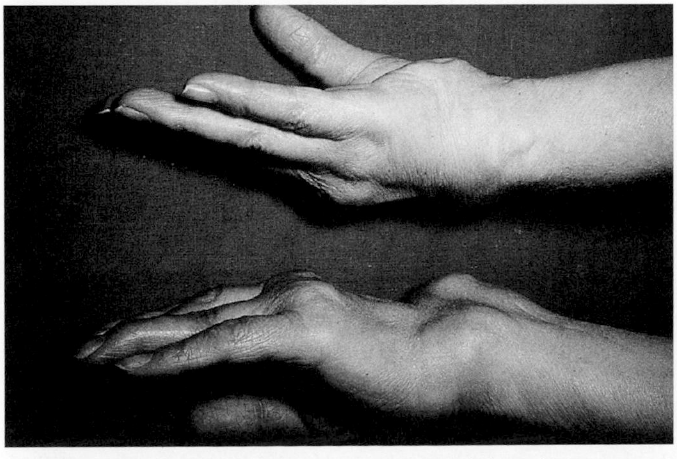

Fig. 10.2.2 Volar subluxation of the carpus, metacarpophalangeal joint involvement, and swan-neck deformity of the ring finger in established rheumatoid arthritis.

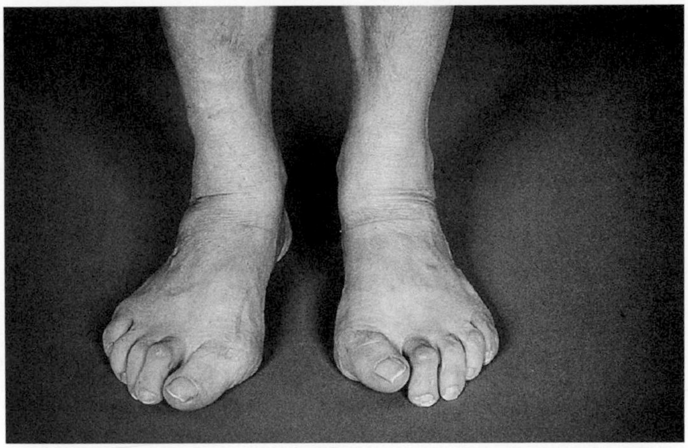

Fig. 10.2.3 Typical changes of the forefoot in rheumatoid arthritis with hallux valgus and dorsal subluxation of the toes.

Box 10.2.2 Extra-articular features of RA

- Haematology: normochromic normocytic anemia
- Respiratory:
  - Mild pulmonary fibrosis
  - Pneumonitis
  - Pulmonary nodulosis
  - Bronchiectasis
- Cardiovascular:
  - Pericardial effusion
  - Vasculitis
- Neurology:
  - Sensory peripheral neuropathy
  - Cervical myelopathy due to antlanto-axial or subaxial instability (Figure 10.2.4).
  - Entrapment neuropathies (carpal tunnel syndrome, ulnar neuropathy, tarsal tunnel syndrome)
- Bone: osteoporosis
- Eyes:
  - Superficial episcleritis
  - Scleritis
  - Sicca syndrome
- Felty's syndrome: neutropenia, splenomegaly, and lymphadenopathy
- Other: rheumatoid nodules, vasculitic ulcers

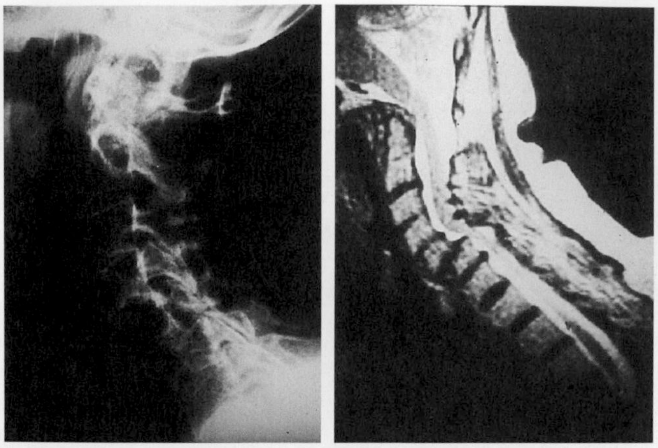

Fig. 10.2.4 A) Subaxial subluxation of the cervical spine in rheumatoid arthritis shown radiographically; B) MRI demonstrated significant cord compression.

Rheumatoid nodules

Intracutaneous or subcutaneous skin nodules occur in approximately one-quarter of patients and tend to be associated with more severe forms of RA and a positive rheumatoid factor. They are frequently found on extensor surfaces such as the elbow and forearm.

Investigation

The diagnosis of RA is mainly clinical (see Box 10.2.1). Pronounced elevation of inflammatory markers is usual but not invariably seen. A normal C-reactive protein in the presence of synovitis, particularly if rheumatoid factor is lacking, should raise the diagnostic suspicion of systemic lupus erythematosus. A normochromic, normocytic anemia is common and elevation of the platelet count is found in active disease. Anaemia may indicate anti-inflammatory drug-induced gastrointestinal blood loss, which may also induce thrombocythemia. Rheumatoid factor is found in around 80 per cent of patients but may be absent at the outset. There is increasing use of antibodies to cyclic citrullinated peptides (anti-CCP antibodies) in diagnosis since these are far more specific for RA than rheumatoid factor. Like rheumatoid factor they occur in around 80 per cent of patients and frequently predate the onset of symptoms. Most patients with RA develop erosions; these may be evident at presentation (Figure 10.2.5). And those patients destined to develop erosions will do so within the first 2 years of disease.

Rheumatoid factor

Rheumatoid factor is an antibody directed against the Fc portion of an IgG molecule (antigen). The antibody can be of various isotypes, IgM, IgG, IgA, IgE. Rheumatoid factor is present in about 75% of patients at initial diagnosis of RA, but can also be found in 10% of the normal population, those with chronic infections, and in patients with chronic inflammatory conditions—Sjögren's syndrome, systemic lupus erythematosus, hepatitis C.

Management

Curative treatment is not currently available and halting the progression of disease and maintaining function is therefore the cornerstone of medical management. The management of patients with persistent RA is best coordinated through a multidisciplinary team including medical, nursing, occupational therapy, physiotherapy, and surgical specialists amongst others.

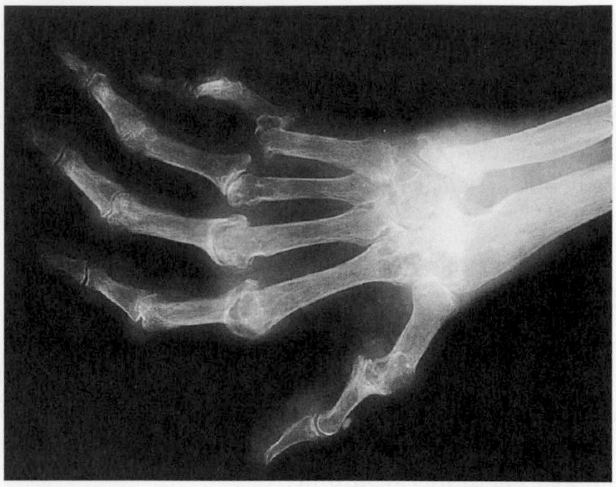

Fig. 10.2.5 Symmetrical erosive arthropathy in rheumatoid arthritis.

Drugs

At present no medication can be guaranteed to settle the inflammation and pain of RA. Drugs have traditionally been divided into those that afford rapid onset symptom relief (first-line drugs; non-steroidal anti-inflammatory drugs (NSAIDs)) and those which act more slowly to suppress inflammation (second-line; methotrexate). Anti-TNF biologic agents are now routinely used with good effect in those who fail to have an adequate response with second-line drugs.

Simple analgesics and NSAIDs

If symptom control is adequate these drugs should be used as first-line agents because of the low incidence of side effects. NSAIDs are effective in reducing inflammation, pain, and morning stiffness.

Second-line antirheumatic drugs

These include low-dose weekly methotrexate, sulfasalazine, and antimalarial drugs. Typically they reduce pain and inflammation over the course of several weeks or months and suppress erosive disease. The use of corticosteroids causes a rapid reduction in symptoms which can be very helpful while the second-line drugs begin to exert their influence.

Biological therapies

These include drugs such as anti-TNFα biologic agents, anti-CD20 monoclonal antibodies, (e.g. rituximab), and abatacept, a CTLA4/Ig fusion protein that interferes with T-cell signaling.

Physical treatments

The maintenance of muscle strength and joint mobility is crucial since both may be rapidly lost in the phase of active synovitis.

Advice from experienced physiotherapists and occupational therapists on a range of physical activities, footwear, and joint protection is essential, and simple orthoses may have a major impact on the patient's symptoms.

Surgery

Soft tissue surgery

It is unusual for nodules to require excision but this may be required if there is troublesome ulceration or pain over pressure points. Large skin ulcers may require plastic surgery to obtain adequate skin cover once underlying vasculitis has been controlled medically. Surgery for entrapment syndromes, flexor tenosynovitis, or rupture of the extensor tendon at the wrist are common indications.

Synovectomy

Considerable debate has arisen to the value of this procedure. Synovectomy of the knee is sometimes undertaken using radioactive yttrium.

Total joint replacement

Replacement of the hip and knee for end-stage RA is highly effective but operator dependent. Shoulder and elbow replacement is now commonly undertaken for pain relief and gives good results in carefully selected patients. At the shoulder it is probably appropriate to use hemiarthroplasty in those patients who have evidence of rotator cuff disruption. Pure ankle mortise joint disease is quite uncommon but may be an appropriate indication for joint replacement in carefully selected individuals. More commonly it occurs with widespread involvement of the hindfoot in which case arthrodesis may be more appropriate.

As a general principle, lower-limb problems should be tackled before those in the upper limb because of the requirement for walking aids which may place excessive demands on the replacement joints in the upper limbs. In the hand, more proximal joints should be dealt with first, thus stabilization of the wrist by arthrodesis should precede stabilization of the carpometacarpal and metacarpophalangeal joints of the thumb. Arthrodesis of the small joints of the fingers in a position of good function is often more effective than joint replacement. Silastic joint replacement of the metacarpophalangeal and posterior interphalangeal joints may be appropriate in certain circumstances but rarely maintains the range of movement and is best reserved for those who have significant pain at rest.

Neck

Patients with widespread erosive joint pathology may also exhibit neck pathology. This is important to recognize in the pre- and perioperative phase. Patients should be handled with care during anaesthesia. Patients with overt signs of cervical myelopathy with significant atlantoaxial or subaxial subluxation should be considered for spinal fusion with or without decompression as appropriate.

Further reading

Arnett, F.C., Edworthy, S.M., Bloch, D.A., *et al.* (1988). The American Rheumatism Association 1987 revised criteria for the classification of rheumatoid arthritis. *Arthritis and Rheumatism*, **31**, 315–24.

Elliott, M.J., Maini, R.N., Feldmann, M., *et al.* (1994). Repeated therapy with monoclonal antibody to tumour necrosis factor alpha (cA2) in patients with rheumatoid arthritis. *Lancet*, **344**, 1125–7.

Goldie, I. (1993). Is there any benefit in the surgery of rheumatoid arthritis? *Current Orthopaedics*, **7**, 120–6.

Kremer, J.M. and Phelps, C.T. (1992). Long-term prospective study of the use of methotrexate in the treatment of rheumatoid arthritis. Update after a mean of 90 months. *Arthritis and Rheumatism*, **35**, 138–45.

Rasker, J.J. and Cosh, J.A. (1989). Course and prognosis of early rheumatoid arthritis. *Scandinavian Journal of Rheumatology*, **79**(Suppl), 45–56.

Sewell, K.L. and Trentham, D.E. (1993). Pathogenesis of rheumatoid arthritis. *Lancet*, **341**, 283–6.

Sharp, J.T., Wolfe, F., Corbett, M., *et al.* (1993). Radiological progression in rheumatoid arthritis: how many patients are required in a treatment trial to test disease modification? *Annals of Rheumatic Disease*, **52**, 332–7.

Spector, T.D. and Scott, D.L. (1988). What happens to patients with rheumatoid arthritis? The long-term outcome of treatment. *Clinics in Rheumatology*, **7**, 315–30.

Symmons, D.P., Barrett, E.M., Bankhead, C.R., Scott, D.G., and Silman, A.J. (1994). The incidence of rheumatoid arthritis in the United Kingdom: results from the Norfolk Arthritis Register. *British Journal of Rheumatology*, **33**, 735–9.

Wordsworth, P. (1995). Genes and arthritis. *British Medical Bulletin*, **51**, 249–66.

10.3

Crystal arthropathies

Sandeep Bawa and Paul Wordsworth

Summary points

- Always exclude infection in acute hot joint
- Raised serum uric acid does not necessarily confirm a diagnosis of gout
- Aspiration and microscopy is essential for accurate diagnosis of crystal arthropathies
- Non-steroidal anti-inflammatory drugs and intra-articular steroids are the treatments of choice
- Wait 2 weeks for acute gout to settle before starting hypouricaemic therapy
- Aim for target urate of <300μmol/L.

Introduction

A number of crystals are associated with acute and chronic arthritis as well as periarticular syndromes and other soft tissue syndromes (Table 10.3.1). The most important of these are:

- Monosodium urate associated with gout
- Calcium pyrophosphate dihydrate associated with pyrophosphate arthropathies
- Calcium hydroxyapatite associated with calcific tendinitis.

Table 10.3.1 Crystals associated with joint disease

Crystal	Associated diseases
Monosodium urate	Acute and chronic arthritis Renal stones Gouty tophi
Calcium pyrophosphate dihydrate	Chondrocalcinosis Pseudogout Chronic destructive arthritis
Calcium phosphates (basic)	
Hydroxyapatite	Calcific periarthritis/peritendinitis
Octacalcium phosphate	Acute/chronic inflammatory arthritis
Tricalcium phosphate	Destructive arthropathy Soft-tissue calcinosis
Calcium oxalate, aluminium phosphate	Acute arthritis (renal dialysis) and in oxalosis
Xanthine	Asymptomatic deposition in muscles Acute arthritis (rare) Renal stones
Lipids	
Phospholipase (Charcot–Leyden)	Synovial fluid and tissues/eosinophilia
Cholesterol	Chronic synovial effusions

Gout

Gout is one of the oldest known forms of arthritis but the link with hyperuricaemia was only established in the nineteenth century. The fact that gout occurs exclusively in humans can be traced back to defunctioning mutations in the uricase gene. In other animals the accumulation of uric acid, a natural breakdown product of purine metabolism, is prevented by the action of this enzyme. The acute episodes of joint inflammation that characterize gout are said to be the most excruciating form of arthritis known. Acute gout is triggered by activation of the innate immune system through mechanisms that include the NALP3 inflammasome, activation of interleukin (IL)-1 and toll-like receptors. High levels of IL-1 provoke fever and neutrophilia; activated macrophages produce large amounts of tumour necrosis factor (TNF), and there is massive infiltration of the synovial compartment by neutrophils. As the attack continues and ultimately resolves there is a change in the cytokines produced by the macrophage population to a more anti-inflammatory profile with transforming growth factor (TGF)β and IL-10 supplanting TNF. The clinical features of gout are highly variable and include:

- Acute inflammatory arthritis (synovitis, bursitis), including the classic 'podagra' of the great toe
- Tophi with deposits of amorphous monosodium urate in the soft tissues
- Gouty nephropathy
- Uric acid stones.

Epidemiology

Gout is the most common inflammatory arthritis in adult men. Genetic, hormonal, and environmental factors are involved and the prevalence rises with increasing age and serum urate levels. The annual incidence of gout is approximately 0.3 per 1000, and its prevalence in males in the United Kingdom is 3–6 per 1000 adults. The male:female ratio is 8:1 and gout is rare in prepubertal boys and premenopausal women.

In addition to male gender, other risk factors include obesity, alcohol consumption, hypertension, renal failure, diuretics, social class, high protein intake, and a family history of gout. All these risk factors act through increasing serum urate concentrations. Hyperuricaemia is arbitrarily defined as a serum uric acid level two standard deviations above the mean (above 420μmol/L in adult males and 360μmol/L in adult females). Serum urate levels in boys rise at puberty while in women the pubertal rise is smaller and the level only approaches male values after the menopause. There are variations in serum urate levels between ethnic groups.

Several inherited enzyme defects can lead to the overproduction of uric acid. These are inherited as distinct Mendelian traits; X-linked (hypoxanthine-guanine phosphoribosyltransferase deficiency and phosphoribosylpyrophosphate synthetase overactivity), autosomal recessive (glucose-6-phosphatase deficiency), and autosomal dominant (familial urate nephropathy) patterns are recognized. Gout occurring before puberty, in premenopausal females, or where there is strong family history should prompt suspicion of an underlying enzyme defect.

Hyperuricaemia

Only 10–30% of hyperuricaemic subjects develop gout. Uric acid is derived from the purines of nucleoproteins through the intermediate metabolites xanthine, hypoxanthine, and guanine predominantly in the liver by the action of xanthine oxidase. Purines themselves are derived either from the diet or by de novo synthesis. Two-thirds of uric acid is renally excreted while the rest is degraded in the gut by bacteria. Lack of functional uricase which oxidizes uric acid to the more soluble allantoin is critical to the human predisposition to gout but other influences are also involved, notably diet and renal handling.

Hyperuricaemia results from overproduction or underexcretion of uric acid (Table 10.3.2). The majority of patients (90%) with primary gout are underexcretors of uric acid with an inability to increase uric acid excretion in response to a purine load. Fewer than 10% are overproducers of uric acid. A minority have underlying disorders of cell proliferation, including malignancy.

Clinical presentation

The first presentation of gout is usually acute monoarthritis although 10% of initial attacks are polyarticular. The first metatarsophalangeal joint is affected in 50% of initial attacks (podagra) and will be involved in 75% of goutees at some stage (Figure 10.3.1). Lower-limb joint involvement predominates (toes, ankle, knee, small joints of the hands and feet, wrist, elbow, and acromioclavicular joints in order of diminishing frequency). During the asymptomatic hyperuricaemic phase, up to 20% of patients have a history of renal colic from uric acid stones. Gouty arthritis and tophi have a predilection for cooler sites, such as the lower extremities and ears, because this reduces the solubility of monosodium urate.

Table 10.3.2 Causes of hyperuricaemia and gout

Impaired uric acid excretion
Idiopathic (primary)
Chronic renal disease
Increased tubular reabsorption (extracellular volume contraction) Dehydration, diuretics, diabetes insipidus
Decreased tubular secretion Starvation, diabetic ketoacidosis
Increased lactic acid production Alcohol, exercise, toxemia of pregnancy
Drug treatment Low-dose aspirin, ciclosporin, diuretics (especially thiazides and loop diuretics)
Hypothyroidism
Primary hyperparathyroidism
Glucose-6-phosphatase deficiency (von Gierke's disease)
Increased uric acid production
Idiopathic (primary)
Increased nucleic acid turnover Blood dyscrasias, e.g. leukemia, polycythaemia rubra vera Malignancies Severe psoriasis
Excessive purine intake
Increased purine synthesis (rare) HGPRT deficiency (Lesch–Nyhan) PRPP overactivity Glucose-6-phosphatase deficiency

HGPRT, hypoxanthine-guanine phosphoribosyltransferase; PRPP, phosphoribosylpyrophosphate synthetase

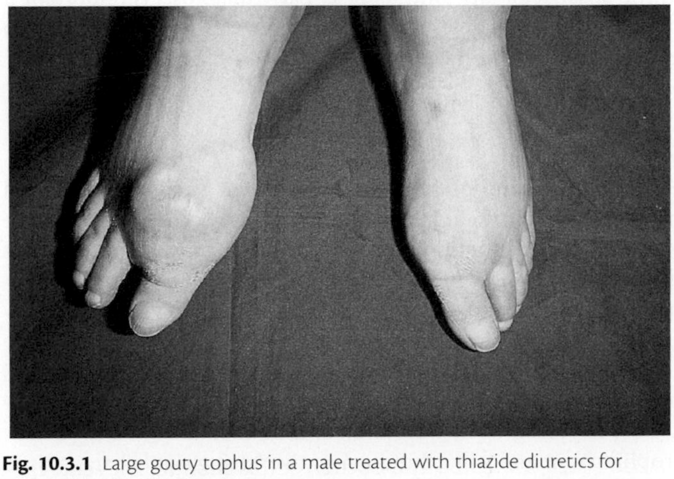

Fig. 10.3.1 Large gouty tophus in a male treated with thiazide diuretics for hypertension for 15 years.

Typical attacks have a rapid onset, often overnight, with the joint becoming swollen, hot, red, shiny, and extremely painful within a few hours (Figure 10.3.2). Inflammation is at a peak by 24h and can be associated with fever and malaise. Untreated attacks typically take 1–2 weeks to resolve spontaneously. Acute attacks may be

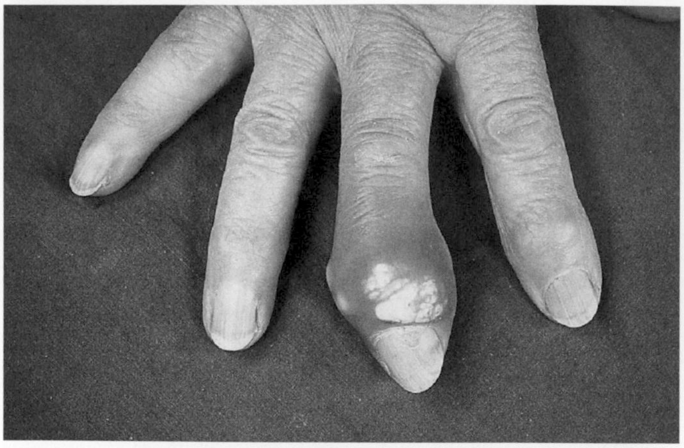

Fig. 10.3.2 Acute gout with tophus extruding through the skin.

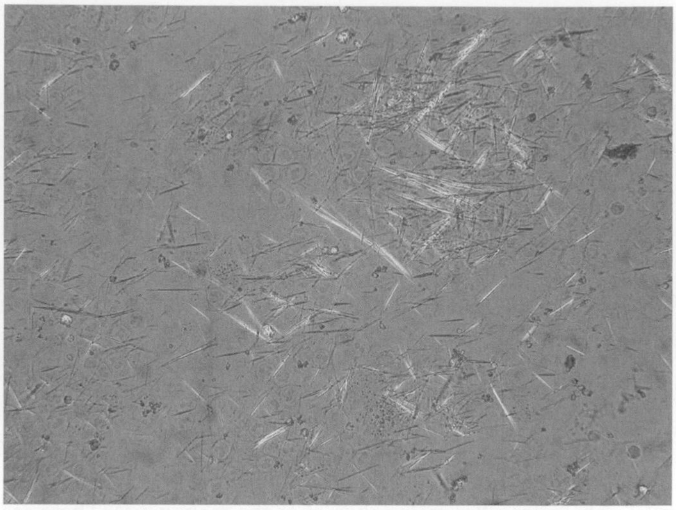

Fig. 10.3.3 Negatively birefringent under compensated polarized light.

triggered by dietary or alcohol excess, starvation, trauma (including surgery), haemorrhage, physical exercise, and severe systemic illness. Acute episodes may also be precipitated by sudden falls in serum urate after starting allopurinol or uricosuric drugs.

The course of gout is highly variable; some patients only ever have a single attack while others may rapidly develop polyarticular disease. A gradual evolution through several stages of disease is recognized (acute, episodic, interval, and chronic tophaceous gout). Joint involvement is usually asymmetric and monarticular initially; discrete episodes of inflammation with complete resolution occur in 'interval gout' while in the 'chronic gout' phase resolution is incomplete and there is always ongoing inflammation at one or more sites, causing progressive cartilage and bone erosion. Tophi may be present at any stage of the disease but are more typical of the late chronic phase. However, some individuals (particularly elderly women treated with thiazide diuretics) may develop massive tophi in the absence of any joint disease. Early diagnosis is important if one is to prevent potentially irreversible destructive arthritis in goutees destined for the more severe forms of the condition.

Investigations

Synovial fluid

Septic arthritis can present in a very similar fashion to gout and must be formally excluded. Ideally the diagnosis of gout should be established by aspiration of synovial fluid from the affected joint during an acute attack. It is confirmed by demonstrating intracellular 'needle-shaped' monosodium urate crystals that are negatively birefringent under compensated polarized light microscopy (Figure 10.3.3). Joint fluid for examination can be stored at 4°C overnight (or sometimes longer) since urate crystals are generally robust to storage. The fluid itself will be turbid from a high neutrophil count and will exhibit a negative 'string sign' characteristic of inflammatory synovitis due to the break down of high molecular weight aggrecan.

Laboratory tests

Hyperuricaemia (above 420µmol/L in adult males and 360µmol/L in adult females) is confirmed with serum uric acid levels, but raised levels alone do not confirm a diagnosis of gout. During acute attacks uric acid levels are often (approximately 15%) in the normal range, returning to the more typical steady state levels after 6 weeks or so. If the diagnosis of gout is seriously entertained it may be appropriate to obtain a series of measurements of morning (not fasting) serum urates once the acute episode has settled. During acute attacks there is often a neutrophil leucocytosis as high as $20–25 \times 10^9$/L. The sedimentation rate and C-reactive protein are typically markedly elevated.

Radiographs

Joint radiographs are rarely useful in establishing an early diagnosis of gout since they are usually normal until the disease becomes established. However, after repeated attacks erosions and secondary osteoarthritic changes may develop. Gouty erosions are classically seen as punched-out cortical lesions with sclerotic margins and overhanging hooks of bone, sometimes well away from the joint (Figure 10.3.4). Bone density is preserved. As uric acid crystals are radiolucent, tophi appear as eccentric soft tissue swellings with patchy calcification due to hydroxyapatite. Chondrocalcinosis may also occur.

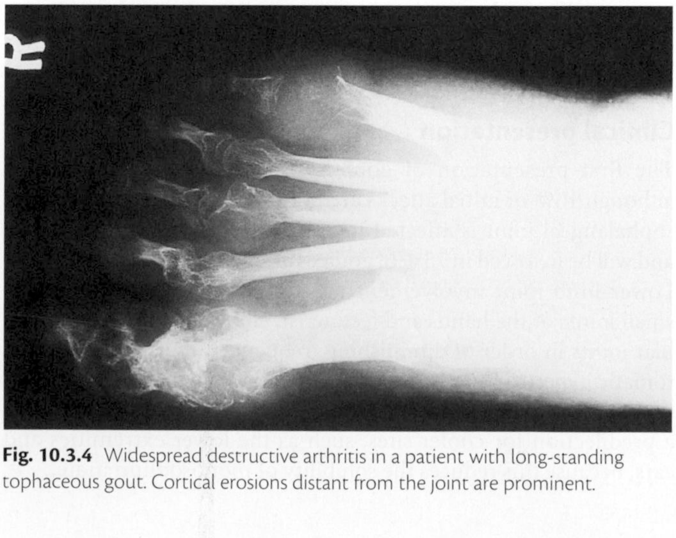

Fig. 10.3.4 Widespread destructive arthritis in a patient with long-standing tophaceous gout. Cortical erosions distant from the joint are prominent.

Treatment

Acute attack

The aim of treatment is to relieve pain and reduce inflammation. High doses of short-acting non-steroidal anti-inflammatory drugs (NSAIDs) given early in the attacks are usually effective but cannot be tolerated by some patients. They are contraindicated in renal failure because they decrease the glomerular filtration rate by one-third, cause fluid retention, and can be nephrotoxic.

Oral colchicine is a useful, rapidly effective alternative where NSAIDs cannot be used. The traditional dose schedules employed (1mg immediately followed by 0.5mg every 2h until symptoms improve) were associated for many with unacceptable side effects, such as abdominal cramps, nausea, and diarrhoea. It is now recognized that lower-dose schedules (500μg 2–4 times daily) are very effective while reducing the incidence of side effects very significantly.

Joint aspiration may relieve pain by reducing intra-articular tension and intra-articular corticosteroid injection is very effective in the acute stage. Oral or systemic corticosteroids may be useful in some patients for short periods, particularly in those with polyarticular problems. They may also be useful in some patients with ulcer disease because they are less gastrotoxic than NSAIDs.

Prevention

Gout is a potentially curable disease but treatment may require an alteration of lifestyle as well as long-term medication. It is sensible to make dietary alterations to achieve gradual weight of possible loss and a reduction in purine intake, to reduce alcohol intake, and if possible to avoid drugs that inhibit renal clearance of urate (e.g. diuretics). Aspirin in standard analgesic doses (600–2400mg/day reduces renal urate clearance but doses used in cardiovascular prophylaxis (75–150mg daily) have no significant effect on urate levels. Such measures may be enough to prevent further attacks but more commonly hypouricaemic agents will be required.

Hypouricaemic drugs are effective in lowering plasma urate levels, reducing the frequency of acute attacks, and decreasing the size of tophi. They are indicated in patients with the following:

- Recurrent troublesome attacks of acute arthritis
- Tophi or evidence of chronic gouty arthritis
- Associated renal disease including uric acid stones
- Very high uric acid levels (>550μmol/L), particularly with acute overproduction of uric acid, such as acute tumour lysis syndrome (in these individuals the prevalence of renal stones is 50%).

Allopurinol

Allopurinol lowers uric acid levels by inhibiting xanthine oxidase and hence the final conversion of xanthine and hypoxanthine to uric acid. It should only be started once the acute attack of gout has settled for 2 weeks. Maintenance treatment with low-dose NSDAIDs or colchicine (500mcg once or twice daily) should be used for the first 3 months of any hypouricaemic therapy because of increased risk of acute attacks of gout until lowered levels of urate are established. It should be used with care and in lower doses in the elderly, in patients with renal failure and those on azathioprine. Febuxostat is another xanthine oxidase inhibitor recently introduced for gout which may be useful in cases where allopurinol has been poorly tolerated.

Uricosuric drugs

These are useful particularly if allopurinol is not tolerated and in subjects who are under-excretors of urate. They prevent tubular resorption of uric acid, but are ineffective in renal failure (creatinine clearance <50mL/min). They are contraindicated if there is a history of renal stones. Sulfinpyrazone (50mg twice daily to 100mg four times daily) is commonly used. Benzbromarone (50–200mg daily) can be used in patients with moderate renal impairment when other uricosuric drugs are ineffective.

As with allopurinol, the aim of hypouricaemic drugs is to maintain the serum urate level below 300μmol/L. High fluid intake is recommended in the early weeks of treatment to prevent uric acid deposition within the kidney and the formation of uric acid stones.

Recombinant uricase

Human recombinant uricase is now available but has relatively limited applicability to the general treatment of gout. It is expensive, has a relatively short half-life, and requires weekly parenteral administration. It is occasionally used in the management of difficult cases or in the management of tumour lysis syndrome.

Calcium pyrophosphate arthropathy

The deposition of the calcium pyrophosphate dihydrate (CPPD) in cartilage is often an age-related phenomenon that does not necessarily imply any significant underlying joint problem. It may occur in normal cartilage or in cartilage already damaged by osteoarthritis. CPPD deposition within a joint can result in an acute arthritis.

Incidence

Chondrocalcinosis is uncommon in adults younger than 50 years old but occurs in up to 10% of the population over 65, increasing to 30% of those older than 85 years. Calcium pyrophosphate disease is more common in women and acute pyrophosphate arthropathy ('pseudogout') is the commonest cause of monoarthritis in the elderly (Box 10.3.1). An underlying metabolic abnormality is present in fewer than 10% of patients but should be sought in patients with younger onset disease.

Clinical features

The clinical features can mimic many different forms of arthritis; these include gout or septic arthritis, rheumatoid arthritis, osteoarthritis, Charcot joint, or even ankylosing spondylitis. Attacks of pseudogout often take longer to reach peak intensity than gout but may run a more protracted course. Larger joints, including the knees and wrists, are more frequently affected but virtually any joint may be affected. Chronic forms of pyrophosphate arthropathy have a variable pattern of joint involvement but should be particularly remembered in patients who have an unusual pattern of arthritis (e.g. ankle arthritis in the absence of injury, apparently degenerative arthritis of the metacarpophalangeal joints, or unexplained early onset arthritis).

Investigation

Synovial fluid

Acute pseudogout is diagnosed by microscopic examination of synovial fluid under polarized light. Calcium pyrophosphate crystals are rhomboid shaped and weakly positively birefringent.

Box 10.3.1 Classification of calcium pyrophosphate deposition disease

- Sporadic/idiopathic: associated with aging and joint disease
- Metabolic disease:
  - Hyperparathyroidism
  - Haemochromatosis
  - Gout
  - Hypophosphatasia
  - Hypomagnesaemia
  - Ochronosis
  - Wilson's disease
  - Amyloidosis
  - Haemodialysis
- Hereditary chondrocalcinosis: dominant inheritance described with loci on chromosome 8q and 5p loci (ANKH—a trans-membrane pyrophosphate transporter).

Both septic arthritis and gout can coexist with pseudogout, so the presence of crystals does not rule out these other conditions and fluid should also be sent for Gram stain and culture to rule out infection. Repeated joint aspiration and synovial fluid examination may be necessary to confirm the diagnosis since these crystals are harder to identify than urate crystals and are also less robust if left standing prior to examination.

Radiographs

Radiographs often show chondrocalcinosis as fine linear calcification parallel to the subchondral bone in articular hyaline cartilage (Figure 10.3.5). In fibrocartilage, ligaments, and joint capsules, calcifications appear as diffuse punctate linear densities. However, no more than 50% of individuals with pyrophosphate arthritis exhibit chondrocalcinosis so its absence does not exclude the diagnosis.

In pyrophosphate arthropathy, radiographs often show changes of arthritis at sites not normally seen in osteoarthritis, such as the radiocarpal joint of the wrist, metacarpophalangeal joints, the talonavicular or patellofemoral joint in isolation. Erosions of the femoral cortex superior to the patella and osteonecrosis of the medial femoral condyle also point towards a diagnosis of calcium pyrophosphate disease. In the axial skeleton, intervertebral disc calcification, sacroiliac erosions, and subchondral cysts in the facet joints can occur.

Blood tests

An atypical arthropathy may be the first clue to an underlying metabolic disease. In patients younger than 55 years a metabolic cause should be excluded. As a minimum screen the following tests are recommended: plasma calcium (hyperparathyroidism), ferritin and iron (haemochromatosis), magnesium (hypomagnesaemia) and alkaline phosphatase (hypophosphatasia).

Management

The principles of treatment are similar to gout; aspiration of the affected joint with injection of corticosteroids is the treatment of choice. NSAIDs at full dose, started at the onset of symptoms, are generally effective. Colchicine can also be tried but there is no effective long-term suppressive treatment known. Unfortunately, in cases where the pyrophosphate arthritis is secondary to another metabolic disorder, such as haemochromatosis, correction of the underlying metabolic disturbance (viz venesection to correct iron overload) will not prevent further progression of the arthropathy.

Basic calcium phosphate (hydroxyapatite) crystal deposition

Basic calcium phosphate, hydroxyapatite, is the calcium-containing mineral laid down in bone, dentine, and enamel. Hydroxyapatite and several other calcium-containing minerals may be found in soft tissues, tendon calcifications, and other forms of arthritis.

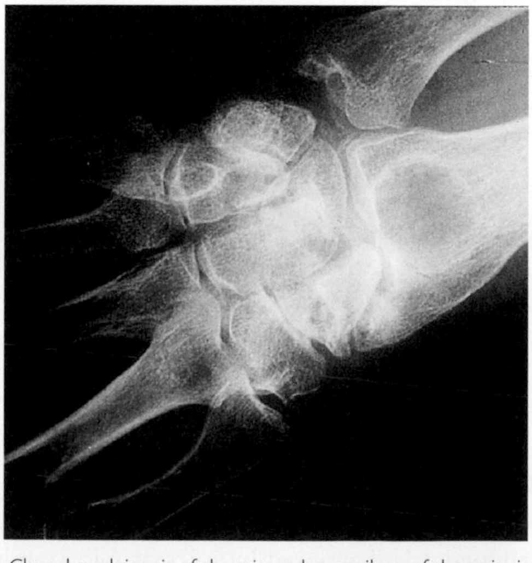

Fig. 10.3.5 Chondrocalcinosis of the triangular cartilage of the wrist in pyrophosphate arthropathy. A large cyst is also apparent in the distal radius.

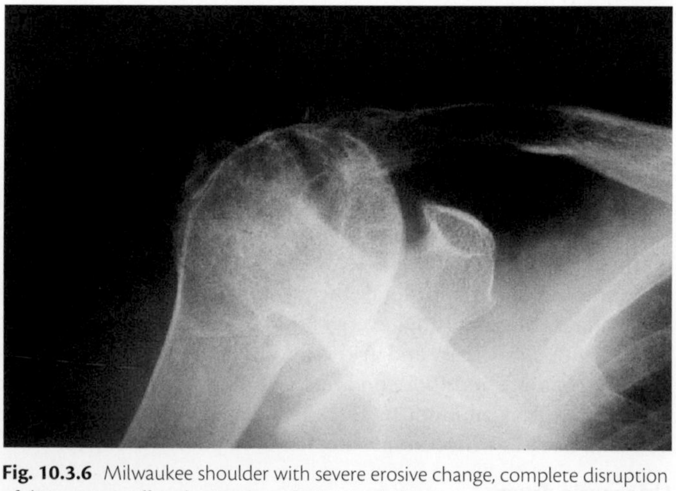

Fig. 10.3.6 Milwaukee shoulder with severe erosive change, complete disruption of the rotator cuff, and extensive soft-tissue calcification.

Collectively, these minerals are referred to as basic calcium phosphate which is associated with the following joint disorders: calcific tendinitis, acute calcific periarthritis, and apatite-associated destructive arthropathy (Figure 10.3.6).

Other crystals

Calcium oxalate crystals have a characteristic bipyramidal appearance and occur in effusions from patients with primary oxalosis, a rare recessive disorder, or end-stage renal failure.

Further reading

Beutler, A. and Schumacher, H.R., Jr (1994). Gout and 'pseudogout'. When are arthritic symptoms caused by crystal deposition? *Postgraduate Medicine*, **95**, 103–16.

Cohen, M.G., Emmerson, B.T., Doherty, M., Faure, G.C., Dieppe, P., and Schumacher, H.R., Jr (1998). Crystal arthropathies. In Klippel, J.H. and Dieppe, P.A. (eds) *Rheumatology*, pp. 8.14–9.2. London, C.V. Mosby.

Fam, A.G. (1992). Calcium pyrophosphate crystal deposition and other crystal deposition disease. *Current Opinion in Rheumatology*, **4**, 574–82.

Jones, A.C., Chuck, A.J., Arie, E.A., Green, D.J., and Doherty. M. (1992). Diseases associated with calcium pyrophosphate deposition disease. *Seminars in Arthritis and Rheumatism*, **22**, 188–202.

Jordan, K.M., Cameron, J.S., Snaith, M., *et al.* (2007). British Society for Rheumatology and British Health Professionals in Rheumatology guideline for the management of gout. *Rheumatology*, **46**, 1372–4.

Rosenthal, A.K. (1998). Crystal arthropathies. In Maddison, P., Isenberg, D., Woo, P., and Glass, D. (eds) *Oxford Textbook of Rheumatology*, pp. 1555–81. Oxford, Oxford University Press.

Terkeltaub, R.A. (1993). Gout and mechanisms of crystal-induced inflammation. *Current Opinion in Rheumatology*, **5**, 510–16.

10.4

Spondyloarthropathies

Inoshi Atukorala, Sandeep Bawa, and Paul Wordsworth

Summary points

- Spondyloarthropathies are related conditions typically associated with axial skeletal involvement, absence of rheumatoid factor, familial clustering, and a variable positive association with HLA-B27
- Ankylosing spondylitis is the prototype with sacroiliac joint involvement being a prerequisite for diagnosis
- Diagnosis is frequently delayed for several years but the use of magnetic resonance imaging to detect sacroiliitis greatly facilitates the establishment of an early diagnosis
- Psoriatic arthritis, reactive arthritis, and enteropathic arthritis have prominent peripheral joint involvement with variable degrees of spinal involvement
- Non-steroidal anti-inflammatory drugs and physical therapy are the cornerstones of management but slow-acting disease-modifying antirheumatic drugs only have a role in peripheral arthritis
- Anti-tumour necrosis factor biologic agents have revolutionized the treatment of the spondyloarthropathies.

Introduction

The spondyloarthropathies are a cluster of chronic inflammatory rheumatic diseases characterized by association with the genetic marker HLA-B27, and a variable predilection for spinal involvement. They include ankylosing spondylitis (AS), psoriatic arthritis, reactive arthritis (ReA), and arthropathies associated with inflammatory bowel disease. At the pathological level their major distinctive histological feature is extrasynovial inflammation at sites of mechanical stress known as entheses. These include the insertion of the joint capsule, tendon attachments, and chondro-osseous junctions. The cardinal features of the spondyloarthropathies are given in Box 10.4.1.

Box 10.4.1 Features of spondyloarthropathies

- Axial skeletal involvement
- Negative rheumatoid factor
- Variable association with HLA-B27
- Familial clustering
- Tendency to acute anterior uveitis.

Ankylosing spondylitis

AS is the prototypic spondyloarthropathy. It affects up to 5 per 1000 of the Caucasian population although only a minority of these (perhaps 20%) will develop severe symptoms. It is two to three times more common in men and has a peak onset around the third decade of life. Typical sites of enthesitis include fibrocartilaginous joints, such as the sacroiliac joints (pathognomonic of AS), costochondral junctions, and ligament and tendon attachments to bone (e.g. plantar fascia). The initial inflammatory phase is typically followed by fibrosis, ossification, and ankylosis. Synovitis of joints may also occur. Involvement of tendons by tenosynovitis is relatively common, particularly in the lower extremities. The net effects are persistent pain, stiffness, and cumulative deformity of the spine over the course of many years.

Axial skeletal disease predominates in AS and demonstrable sacroiliitis on imaging is mandatory for its diagnosis. The modified New York criteria for the diagnosis of AS are listed in Table 10.4.1. However, it should be noted that these rely on the presence of radiographic evidence of sacroiliitis, which may take many years to develop. Because of their lack of sensitivity, x-rays are now considered to be much less effective than magnetic resonance imaging (MRI) of the sacroiliac joints in the early diagnosis of AS but formal diagnostic criteria to take account of this are still in development.

AS is strongly familial (sibling recurrence risk is approximately 7%), reflecting the influence of several genes on susceptibility. The best known of these is the immune response gene, *HLA-B27*, found in more than 90% of patients with AS. More recently at least two other genes, *IL-23R* (interleukin 23 receptor) and *ERAP1* (endoplasmic reticulum aminopeptidase 1) have also been implicated. *IL-23R* is particularly interesting because it is also implicated in psoriasis and inflammatory bowel disease, two disorders that are commonly associated with AS. The *ERAP1* association is fascinating not only because of its potential role in the antigen presentation

Table 10.4.1 New York criteria for ankylosing spondylitis (1966)

1. Pain at dorsolumbar junction or lumbar spine	
2. Limitation of motion in anterior flexion, lateral flexion, and extension	
3. Chest expansion less than or equal to 2.5cm at fourth intercostal space	
Diagnostic requirements	
Either	grade 3 to 4 bilateral sacroiliitis with one or more clinical criteria
Or	grade 3 to 4 unilateral or grade 2 bilateral sacroiliitis with clinical criterion 2
Or	grade 3 to 4 unilateral or grade 2 bilateral sacroiliitis with criteria 1 and 3

pathway that involves HLA-B27 but also because it may also be involved in the shedding of cytokine receptors (including the tumour necrosis factor (TNF) and interleukin (IL)-1, and IL-6 receptors) that are heavily implicated in inflammation.

Clinical features

Most patients present with AS in early adult life; it is rare for the diagnosis to be made after the age of 40 years. Typical features include pain at the thoracolumbar junction, around the rib cage and alternating buttock pain. The inflammatory, rather than mechanical, nature of the pain is revealed by its response to moderate activity and anti-inflammatory analgesics, the presence of prolonged morning stiffness (>30min) and back pain during the second half of the night often waking the patient from sleep. The pain typically radiates into the buttock as far as the posterior midthigh but not below the knee, in contrast to the pain from lumbosacral nerve root entrapment.

Reduced lumbar spine movements in all planes occurs relatively early in the disease in contrast to the neck which typically occurs later. Rib-cage pain and loss of movement resulting from involvement of the costovertebral joints and/or the costochondral junctions may eventually cause a fixed chest with purely diaphragmatic breathing. The combination of loss of lumbar lordosis, progressive thoracic kyphosis, and the development of flexion contractures at the hips causes the classic question mark posture over a period of time (Figure 10.4.1). Osteoporosis may be present from an early stage but may be missed on bone density scans due to the spurious effects of new bone growth (syndesmophyte) around the vertebrae. Reduced bone density not only increases the risk of fractures but also exacerbates the tendency to thoracic kyphosis due to spinal wedging. Ankylosis of the cervical spine is also a major risk factor for cervical fracture in road traffic accidents.

The Achilles tendon and plantar fascia are commonly involved, often with pronounced local osteitis demonstrable on MRI. Peripheral joint involvement, particularly of the hips, knees, and shoulders, affects around 20% of patients. A coexistent history of inflammatory bowel disease and/or psoriasis occurs in about 15% of patients.

Around 40 % of patients sustain episodes of acute anterior uveitis which may be recurrent and sight-threatening; all patients with AS should be warned of this potential complication and advised to seek prompt specialist ophthalmic treatment with mydriatics and steroid eye-drops if they develop symptoms (typically a unilateral, painful red eye). Diaphragmatic breathing is clinically obvious in

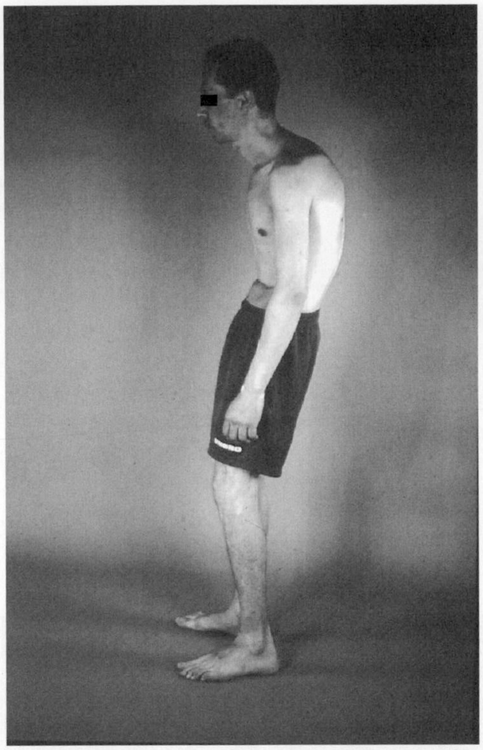

Fig. 10.4.1 Classic 'question mark' posture in ankylosing spondylitis with pronounced thoracolumbar kyphosis and flexion deformities of the hips.

those with a fixed rib cage due to costovertebral joint involvement and lung function may be somewhat restricted. Apical pulmonary fibrosis and cavitation mimicking tuberculosis radiographically is recognized but rare (in approximately 1%); colonization with bacteria, fungi, or *Aspergillus* species is an exceptional complication.

Aortitis causing incompetence of the aortic valve is an uncommon (approximately 1%) cardiovascular complication. Of far more clinical relevance in AS is the pronounced excess cardiovascular mortality from atheroma, similar to that for other chronic inflammatory diseases, such as rheumatoid arthritis and systemic lupus erythematosus. Accordingly any other cardiac risk factors, including hypertension, smoking, and hyperlipidaemia should be tackled aggressively.

Investigation

One of the most important challenges in AS for rheumatologists (and orthopaedic surgeons) lies in achieving early diagnosis. Too often the condition remains undiagnosed for several years or may be inappropriately treated with spinal immobilization or even surgery. Radiographic involvement of the sacroiliac joints is usually not evident early in the disease and a high index of suspicion is required in those with a history suggestive of inflammatory back pain. HLA-B27 testing, coupled with a careful assessment of the clinical history is useful in identifying those likely to be affected. However, because B27 is relatively common in the general population (approximately 10%) it is not a useful primary screening tool for back pain in the general community because of its lack of specificity. In contrast, when positive in an individual with inflammatory features (as outlined earlier) it is much more specific for AS. Further investigation of such B27-positive individuals by MRI can

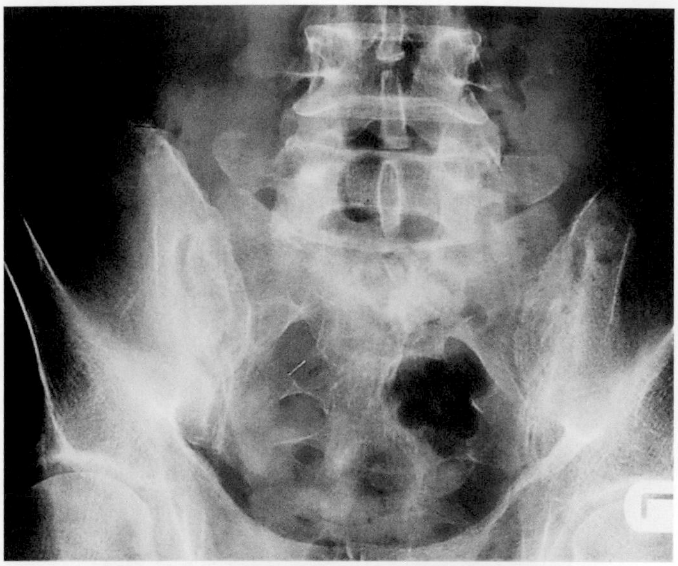

A

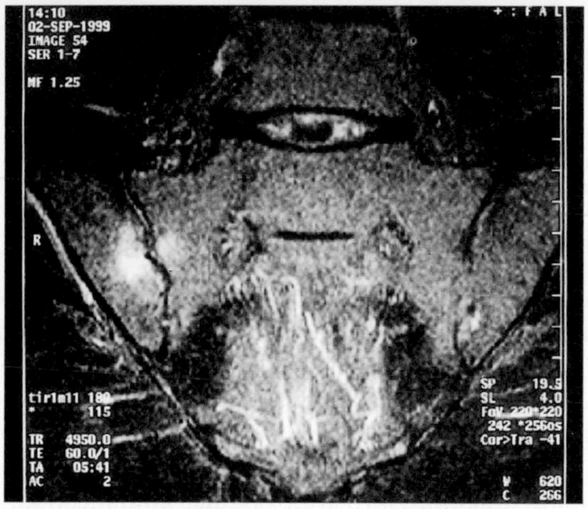

B

Fig. 10.4.2 A) Early radiographical evidence of sacroiliitis with slight marginal sclerosis and widening particularly evident in the right sacroiliac joint. B) High signal on fat-suppressed MRI sequences of the same patient indicating marrow oedema adjacent to the right sacroiliac joint confirming asymmetric sacroiliitis.

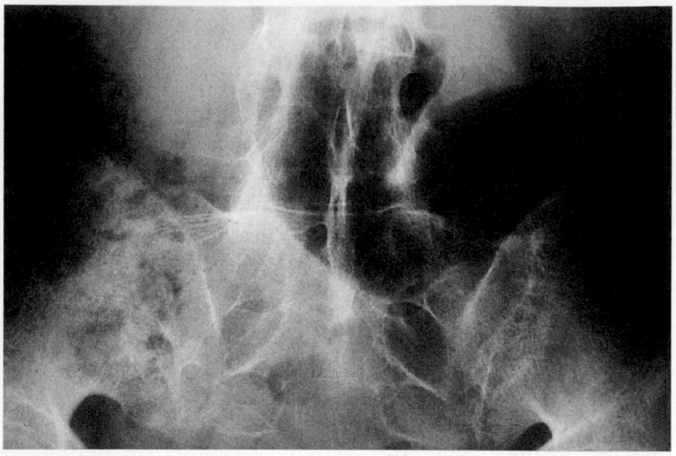

Fig. 10.4.3 Ankylosis of the sacroiliac joints and extensive ossification of the paraspinal ligaments in late-stage ankylosing spondylitis.

then be used to confirm the diagnosis beyond doubt. MRI of the sacroiliac joints using fat suppression techniques is highly sensitive at detecting early changes of osteitis. Although inflammatory changes may be seen widely in the axial skeleton, sacroiliitis is invariably present as the earliest sign of AS on MRI (Figure 10.4.2). Radiographic changes take longer to develop and are less useful in modern clinical practice. The earliest radiographic signs include sclerosis of both margins of the joint (often more pronounced on the iliac side) followed by erosion and widening of the joint. Ultimately ankylosis of the joint may occur (Figure 10.4.3).

Serum measures of inflammation, such as C-reactive protein, are frequently normal even in active AS although they can be markedly elevated in some individuals with pronounced systemic disease.

Management

Successful management is dependent on early accurate diagnosis and patient education. Physical treatment, combining postural and stretching exercises, is highly beneficial. Patient education and instruction in a regular domiciliary physical exercise programme is fundamental to a successful outcome. This can be supplemented as necessary by intensive courses of treatment (including hydrotherapy) during exacerbations of AS. The worst outcomes in AS are often associated with failure to recognize the condition, resulting in inappropriate immobilization or failure to implement an active physical mobilizing regimen. NSAIDs typically provide good relief from pain and stiffness in the majority of patients. However, conventional disease-modifying anti-rheumatic drugs (DMARDs), like sulphasalazine and methotrexate, are ineffective for axial skeletal disease. In contrast they may be helpful for the minority of patients with significant peripheral joint arthritis. Fatigue is a major problem for many patients with AS, particularly when sleep disturbance is prominent. Low doses of tricyclic antidepressants have a potential role in such patients in improving the quality of sleep and pain. However, the introduction of the anti-TNF biologic agents in recent years has revolutionized the treatment of AS and related disorders. For those who still have significant symptoms despite an adequate trial of non-steroidal anti-inflammatory drugs (NSAIDs) and physical therapy, anti-TNF drugs (monoclonal antibodies or recombinant soluble TNF receptor/IgG fusion protein) have the potential to suppress both axial and peripheral joint symptoms and improve the quality of life dramatically. However, the relatively high cost of these drugs and concerns about potential serious side effects (infection and malignancy) necessarily restricts their use to patients with more severe disease. Most patients treated with anti-TNF drugs show at least some improvement and around half demonstrate a 50% improvement. It remains to be seen whether these agents actually suppress the abnormal ossification of the spine that characterizes the condition in the long term.

The rigid fixed cervical spine and immobile chest may cause peri/postoperative difficulties when surgical intervention is required. Prolonged recumbency and postoperative chest infections are detrimental to the long term outcome of these patients. There is no convincing evidence that patients with AS are more prone to heterotopic ossification following joint replacement surgery than the general population.

Psoriatic arthritis

Approximately 10% of patients with skin psoriasis develop inflammatory arthritis but this is highly variable in its presentation. Skin involvement often predates the arthritis by many years but arthritis can be synchronous with or precede the skin disease. Nail involvement is evident in 70% of those who develop arthritis and the diagnosis can also be aided by a positive family history of psoriasis or psoriatic arthritis. The incidence of psoriatic arthritis is similar between the sexes.

Peripheral joint arthropathy (Figure 10.4.4) is more common than axial disease but is quite variable in extent (see later). Joint involvement in psoriasis is frequently coupled with nail changes, including nail pitting, discoloration, ridging, and onycholysis. Involvement of the distal and proximal interphalangeal joints of a single finger causes the appearance of a 'sausage finger'; such dactylitis is highly characteristic of psoriatic arthritis. Tenosynovitis contributes to dactylitis but overall this type of pathology can best be regarded as a particular form of enthesitis (see earlier) and is strongly correlated with destructive arthritis and a tendency to axial disease.

Psoriatic arthritis is associated with HLA-B27 but even in the presence of psoriatic spondylitis this association is somewhat less strong (approximately 60%) than in ankylosing spondylitis without psoriasis or inflammatory bowel disease. Asymmetric sacroiliitis or, vary rarely, spondylitis without sacroiliitis is more common in psoriatic spondyloarthropathy, which may also be associated with more florid syndesmophyte formation.

Box 10.4.2 lists the five classical patterns of psoriatic arthritis. These patterns may change over time in individual patients but with longer disease duration the overall trend is for the development of increasingly polyarticular disease.

Although many cases of psoriatic arthritis are relatively mild symptomatically and appear to have a relatively good prognosis, there is a strong tendency for increasingly polyarticular involvement over time. Early management of single swollen joints with intra-articular steroid injection and splintage should be effected and NSAIDs offered for symptomatic relief. Persistent synovitis, particularly polyarticular, erosive disease warrants DMARD therapy. Methotrexate, leflunomide, and sulfasalazine are all of some benefit but consideration should be given to biological therapies with anti-TNF drugs in patients who do not respond adequately.

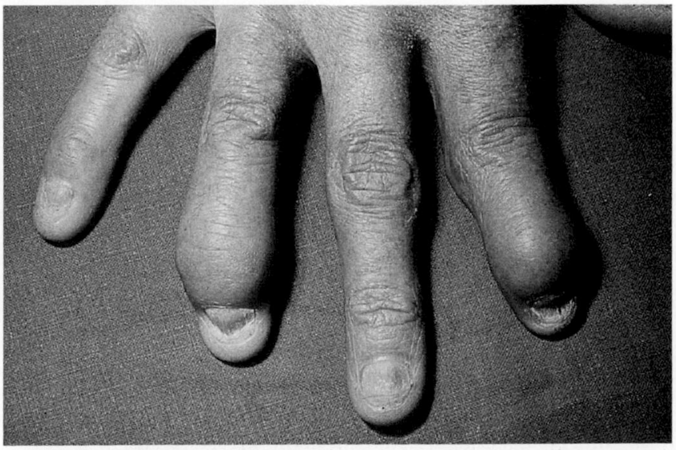

Fig. 10.4.4 Asymmetric peripheral arthropathy and nail dystrophy in psoriasis.

Box 10.4.2 The Moll and Wright classification of psoriatic arthritis

- Arthritis with distal interphalangeal joint involvement predominant
- Arthritis mutilans—a destructive erosive arthropathy
- Symmetrical polyarthritis—indistinguishable from rheumatoid arthritis (but rheumatoid factor and nodules absent)
- Asymmetric oligoarticular arthritis
- Predominant spondylitis.

Patients with psoriatic spondylitis should be managed in the same manner as AS. Anti-TNF drugs provide rapid symptomatic relief for most patients and prevent progressive peripheral joint destruction in psoriatic arthritis. These agents are also extremely effective for the cutaneous manifestations of psoriasis that are such a major source of distress for many patients with the disease.

Reactive arthritis

ReA refers to an episode of aseptic peripheral arthritis occurring within 1 month (typically 2–3 weeks) of a primary infection in another part of the body. The most common sites of infection are the gut or genital tract; *Shigella*, *Salmonella*, *Campylobacter*, or *Yersinia* species are implicated in postenteric ReA and *Chlamydia trachomatis* in the sexually acquired form. The precipitating infection is often not clinically apparent and a reasonably high index of suspicion may be required to make the diagnosis. The classic triad of urethritis, conjunctivitis, and arthritis was first described in association with endemic dysentery in the trenches during the First World War.

However, most cases of reactive arthritis currently present with joint symptoms alone. Between 60 and 80% of patients with typical ReA are HLA-B27 positive and this is associated with a more adverse prognosis. ReA is usually self-limiting but, particularly in the more severe HLA-B27 positive cases, persistent or recurrent joint symptoms occur (40% of patients at 15 year follow up). At prolonged follow up to 20% of patients with ReA may be found to have developed AS.

Clinical features

ReA typically presents as an acute asymmetric oligoarthropathy of the lower limb, with prominent knee and/or ankle synovitis. Rarely, it may present with more widespread synovitis including upper limb joints. An association with ocular inflammation (typically conjunctivitis and, rarely, anterior uveitis); enthesitis (Achilles tendonitis and plantar fascitis) and dactylitis is common (the classic 'sausage toe' or dactylitis is illustrated in Figure 10.4.5). A minority of individuals exhibit mucocutaneous features including keratoderma blennorrhagica, circinate balanitis, painless ulceration of the hard palate, and nail dystrophy resembling that seen in psoriasis.

Joint symptoms are typically self-limiting, varying in duration from a few days to several months. Spondylitis or isolated sacroiliitis is more likely to occur in the 15–40% of patients that develop chronic or recurrent arthritis: many of these patients have a family history of spondyloarthropathy or are HLA-B27 positive. Aortic regurgitation and cardiac conduction defects occasionally occur.

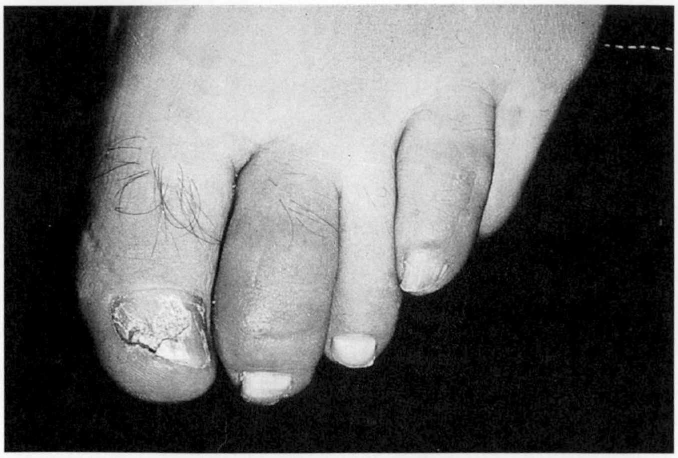

Fig. 10.4.5 Sausage toe in a patient with reactive arthritis. This appearance of dactylitis is common also in psoriatic arthritis.

Box 10.4.3 Diagnostic criteria for reactive arthritis

- Predominantly lower-limb asymmetric oligoarthritis
- Evidence of infection such as diarrhea or urethritis in the preceding month or laboratory confirmation of infection
- The presence of extraarticular manifestations (e.g. conjunctivitis, iritis, mucocutaneous manifestation).

Diagnosis

The diagnosis usually rests on the clinical history (Box 10.4.3). About half of those presenting with ReA have an obvious history of relevant infection although in the case of postenteric disease the causative organism is frequently not cultured because the infection has already cleared. ELISA (Enzyme-linked immunosorbent assay) for *C. trachomatis* will detect 50% of those with genital tract infection. Serology may demonstrate rising titres of antibodies to culprit organisms. Testing for rheumatoid factor or anti-CCP (cyclic citrullinated peptide) antibodies may help to exclude the alternative diagnosis of rheumatoid arthritis which has some prognostic value. HLA-B27 testing is not routinely required but may sometimes be useful when the diagnosis is unclear. Joint radiographs contribute little to diagnosis in the acute episode, but the presence of sacroiliitis may be of diagnostic and prognostic value. The sedimentation rate or C-reactive protein can be useful for monitoring disease activity during treatment.

Management

Rest, aspiration, injection of inflamed joints with corticosteroids, and regular use of NSAIDs will usually be sufficient to settle the synovitis and prevent irreversible joint damage. Most cases settle relatively quickly treated conservatively in this way but persistent synovitis may require DMARDs like sulphasalazine or methotrexate. Recurrent disease is not uncommon and is treated in the same way as acute disease. For resistant cases anti-TNF therapy is also effective. The role of antibiotic therapy in influencing ReA arthritis is controversial. However, it is standard practice to treat sexually acquired disease with tetracycline. It is also prudent to investigate for other possible venereal infections and to initiate contact tracing and treatment where appropriate.

Box 10.4.4 Classification of enteropathic peripheral arthropathy

- Type 1 (pauciarticular):
  - <5 joints
  - Acute self-limiting attacks (<10 weeks)
  - Often coincides with relapses of inflammatory bowel disease (IBD)
  - Strongly associated with extraintestinal manifestations of IBD
  - Associated with HLA-B*27 and HLA-DRB1*0103
- Type 2 (polyarticular):
  - 5 or more joints
  - Symptoms usually persist from months to years
  - Runs a course independent of IBD
  - Associated with uveitis but not with other extraintestinal manifestations
  - Associated with HLA-B*44 but not HLA–B*27.

Arthritis complicating inflammatory bowel disease

Seronegative arthropathy occurs in 5–10% of individuals with inflammatory bowel disease. It is twice as common in Crohn's disease as in ulcerative colitis. Spondylitis is well recognized, but the association with HLA-B27 is generally somewhat lower (60–80%) than in uncomplicated AS. Two forms of peripheral arthropathy are described, each with distinct clinical patterns and immunogenetic associations (Box 10.4.4). Neither form is erosive, although joint deformities may occur with type 2 disease.

Management focuses on good control of the inflammatory bowel disease. NSAIDs are effective in treatment of joint pains but can exacerbate bowel inflammation. Consequently, simple analgesics and intra-articular steroids should be used whenever possible. Sulfasalazine and methotrexate are both effective for the arthritis and bowel disease. When systemic corticosteroids are indicated for the bowel they will help the joint symptoms. Recent experience with anti-TNF drugs shows favourable results in resistant cases and is highly effective for the underlying bowel disease.

Further reading

Cuellar, M.L. and Espinoza, L. (2003). Psoriatic arthritis: management. In Hochberg, M.C., Silman, A.J., Smolen, J.S., Weinblatt, M.E., and Weisman, M.H. (eds) *Rheumatology*, pp.1259–66. St Louis, MO: Mosby Elsevier Limited.

Gladman, D.D., Antoni, C., Mease, P., Clegg, D.O., and Nash, P. (2005). Psoriatic arthritis: epidemiology, clinical features, course and outcome. *Annals of Rheumatic Disease*, **64**(Suppl II), ii14–17.

Khan, M.A. (2002). Update on spondyloarthropathies. *Annals of Internal Medicine*, **136**, 896–907.

Khan, M.A. (2003). Clinical features of ankylosing spondylitis. In Hochberg, M.C., Silman, A.J., Smolen, J.S., Weinblatt, M.E., and

Weisman, M.H. (eds) *Rheumatology*, pp.1161–81. St Louis, MO: Mosby Elsevier Limited.

Moll, J.M.H. and Wright, V. (1973). Psoriatic arthritis. *Seminars in Arthritis and Rheumatism*, **3**, 55–78.

Pradeep, D.J., Keat, A., and Gaffney, K. (2008). Predicting outcome in ankylosing spondylitis. *Rheumatology*, **47**, 942–5.

Toivanen, P. and Toivanen, A. (1999). Two forms of reactive arthritis? *Annals of Rheumatic Disease*, **58**, 737–41.

Wailoo, A., Bansback, N., and Chilcott, J. (2008). Infliximab, etanercept and adalimumab for treatment of ankylosing spondylitis: cost-effectiveness, evidence and NICE guidance. *Rheumatology*, **47**, 119–20.

10.5

Inflammatory connective tissue disease

Catherine Swales

Summary points

- Systemic lupus erythematosus (SLE) is the commonest multisystem connective tissue disease
- All patients with SLE are antinuclear antibody (ANA) positive, but not all ANA-positive patients have SLE
- Renal lupus carries a high mortality and requires aggressive immunosuppression
- Dermatomyositis may be associated with malignancy in the elderly
- The vasculitides are classified according to vessel size and ANCA (antineutrophil cytoplasmic antibody) profile
- Therapy for vasculitis includes corticosteroids, steroid-sparing agents, and cytotoxics.

Connective tissue disease

The inflammatory connective tissue diseases and systemic vasculitides are multisystem disorders which are often associated with abnormal immune responses towards self-antigens. The commonest connective tissue disease is systemic lupus erythematosus (SLE), which is characterized by antibodies directed against nuclear components.

Systemic lupus erythematosus

SLE is a multisystem disease with prominent involvement of small and medium vessels and serosal surfaces. Women are more commonly affected than men (~7:1) and the lifetime incidence in the United Kingdom is up to 1 in 1000.

Clinical features

SLE characteristically presents with vague constitutional symptoms, a photosensitive skin rash (Figure 10.5.1), arthralgia, oral ulcers, and Raynaud's phenomenon. Raynaud's phenomenon results from intermittent vasospasm of the digital vessels, usually in the cold. Digital pain is associated with the classic colour changes of pallor, cyanosis, and subsequently hyperaemia. Although involvement of virtually any organ system may occur in SLE, disease affecting the heart, lungs, kidneys, and nervous system is common.

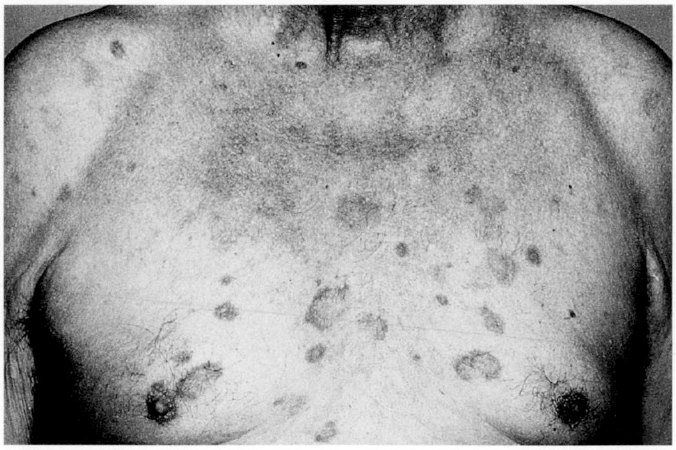

Fig. 10.5.1 Typical rash of subacute cutaneous lupus on the trunk.

Skin disease is frequently precipitated or exacerbated by exposure to sunlight and may be associated with an increase in the activity of systemic disease. Small-joint arthropathy affects up to 90% of patients, but clinically evident severe synovitis or joint effusions are relatively uncommon. Only 10–15% of patients develop progressive joint deformity (Jaccoud's arthropathy) and erosive disease is exceptionally rare. Serosal involvement is common, leading to development of pleurisy and pericarditis, occasionally causing significant effusions. Haematological abnormalities are common and an autoimmune thrombocytopenia, leucopenia, or haemolytic anaemia may be present. A normochromic normocytic anaemia is typical and lymphadenopathy is common. Renal involvement occurs in about half of those with SLE with the development of a glomerulonephritis. In many cases renal involvement may be entirely subclinical, manifesting only as asymptomatic proteinuria or microscopic haematuria, but progressive renal failure may develop. Neuropsychiatric features include headaches and mild depressive or behavioural problems. Seizures, strokes (particularly in the presence of the antiphospholipid syndrome, see later), and psychotic episodes may also occur.

Diagnosis

The diagnosis rests on a combination of laboratory and clinical criteria (see Table 10.5.1). Using current techniques, antinuclear

Table 10.5.1 The American College of Rheumatology revised criteria for diagnosis of systemic lupus erythematosus[a]

1	Malar rash
2	Discoid rash
3	Photosensitivity
4	Oral ulcers
5	Arthritis
6	Serositis (a) Pleuritis (b) Pericarditis
7	Renal disorder (a) Proteinuria above 0.5 g/24 h or 3+ on dipstix persistently (b) Cellular casts
8	Neurologic disorder (a) Seizures (b) Psychosis
9	Hematologic disorder (a) Hemolytic anemia (b) Leukopenia less than 4×10^9 (c) Lymphopenia of less than 1.5×10^9 on at least two occasions (d) Thrombocytopenia less than 100×10^9/l
10	Immunologic disorder (a) Positive lupus erythematosus cell (b) Raised antinative DNA antibody binding (c) Anti-Sm antibody (d) False-positive serologic test to syphilis present for at least 6 months
11	Raised titer of antinuclear antibody

[a]Four of the 11 criteria need to be met (serially or simultaneously) in order to make a diagnosis of systemic lupuse rythematosus.

antibodies are present in virtually all patients with SLE but are also detectable in about 30% of patients with rheumatoid arthritis and other connective tissue diseases. The presence of antibodies to double-stranded DNA (dsDNA) is much more specific for SLE (~90%). In addition antibodies to the 'extractable nuclear antigens' Ro, La, and Sm, and ribonucleoprotein (RNP) also occur in SLE.

Management

Raynaud's phenomenon is best managed by keeping the hands warm but calcium channel blockers, such as nifedipine, may be of additional benefit. Avoidance of direct sunlight and the use of high sun protection factor sunscreens may be all that is required to suppress the skin manifestations and arthralgia responds well to non-steroidal anti-inflammatory drugs and/or hydroxychloroquine.

Corticosteroids and steroid-sparing agents such as azathioprine should be reserved for patients who either do not respond to these measures or who have evidence of more severe systemic features. Treatment with high-dose corticosteroids and agents such as cyclophosphamide or mycophenolate mofetil is indicated in patients with serious major organ involvement. The 10-year survival rate for SLE exceeds 90%, although it is lower in those with major renal or neurological involvement.

The antiphospholipid syndrome

The antiphospholipid syndrome may occur in isolation or in association with other connective tissue diseases, particularly SLE. It is characterized by the tendency to thrombosis (both venous and arterial), recurrent early abortion, and thrombocytopenia. Diagnosis relies on the detection of either anticardiolipin antibodies or lupus anticoagulant and the treatment is based on life-long anticoagulation.

Scleroderma

Scleroderma is characterized by excessive deposition of collagen and small blood vessel obliteration, resulting in tissue ischaemia and atrophy.

Clinical features

Raynaud's phenomenon is an early feature of the disease and severe disease leads to finger pulp atrophy or even gangrene and osteolysis of the fingertips. Fibrotic changes lead to skin tightening, which may be accompanied by calcinosis. The fibrotic process commonly causes hypomotility of the gastrointestinal tract, causing dysphagia and reflux, malabsorption due to bacterial overgrowth in a hypomotile small bowel, and pseudo-obstructions. Respiratory failure due to interstitial lung disease or obliteration of the pulmonary vessels may occur and renal involvement causes severe hypertension and rapidly deteriorating renal function. Fibrosis of the capsules of joints sometimes leads to restricted movement and to the development of contractures.

Diagnosis

The diagnosis is largely based on clinical features although the erythrocyte sedimentation rate (ESR) may be raised and ANAs are demonstrable in over 50% of patients. The presence of anticentromere antibodies suggests more localized cutaneous disease, whereas antibodies directed against topoisomerase 1 (Scl 70) are most commonly found in those with progressive systemic disease.

Management

There is no specific treatment. Raynaud's phenomenon often responds to heated gloves, calcium-channel blockers, or sympathectomy but iloprost (a prostacyclin analogue) may be required for critically ischemic digits. Proton pump inhibitors and antibiotics may be used for oesophageal disease and bacterial overgrowth respectively. Angiotensin-converting enzyme inhibitors should be used in the management of hypertension associated with renal disease.

Dermatomyositis and polymyositis

These syndromes are characterized by inflammation of the muscles causing proximal muscle weakness and pain, with variable skin involvement. There is a clear association with underlying malignancy in the elderly.

Clinical features

The most common presentation is with progressive and symmetrical proximal muscle weakness. Progressive involvement of the pharyngeal and respiratory muscles may occur but involvement of myocardial muscle is rare. Skin involvement is very variable but includes heliotrope (lilac) discoloration of the eyelids and a scaly erythematous rash on the extensor surfaces of the fingers, elbows, and knees.

Diagnosis

The diagnosis is confirmed by the demonstration of markedly elevated muscle enzymes, e.g. creatine phosphokinase, and abnormal muscle biopsy and electromyography. If there is associated malignant disease it is usually clinically apparent and an exhaustive search for occult malignancy is not justified.

Management

Treatment is based on the use of corticosteroids and immunosuppressive agents such as methotrexate and azathioprine. The skin disease may respond to hydroxychloroquine. Although the prognosis is generally less good in the elderly, in whom an association with malignancy is more common, the overall 5-year survival rate is now nearly 90%.

Systemic vasculitis

The systemic vasculitides are characterized by an inflammation of blood vessel walls. Current classifications of the systemic vasculitides stratify the illnesses on the basis of the size of blood vessels involved and the detection of ANCAs (Table 10.5.2).

Polymyalgia rheumatica and giant cell arteritis

There is considerable overlap in both the clinical features and the pathology of these two syndromes. Both diseases affect the elderly and rarely present before the age of 55 years.

Polymyalgia rheumatica

This clinical syndrome is characterized by aching and stiffness of the shoulder and hip girdles. It is a common disorder in the elderly, affecting women more commonly than men. About one-third of cases are associated with coexistent giant cell arteritis. Characteristic symptoms are pain and stiffness in the muscles around the shoulder and hip girdles, in the absence of abnormal clinical signs. There is almost invariably elevation of the sedimentation rate and a mild normochromic normocytic anaemia is common. The condition is characterized by a dramatic response to low doses of oral prednisolone. Gradual withdrawal can commence once the patient is symptom-free and the acute phase has normalized.

Giant cell arteritis

Giant cell arteritis is a granulomatous vasculitis affecting large and medium-sized arteries, most typically in the territory of the external carotid. Typical features include severe unilateral headache with local tenderness of the inflamed artery (superficial temporal, facial, or occipital) and hypersensitivity of the scalp. Amaurosis fugax may occur with retinal artery involvement and this may presage complete occlusion of the vessel and blindness. There may also be claudication of the masseter muscle or tongue. The diagnosis is confirmed by biopsy findings of an affected vessel, but this should not delay the initiation of appropriate treatment in view of the potential threat to the patient's vision. Marked elevation of the ESR and a normochromic normocytic anaemia are typical. Treatment should be started immediately, to prevent blindness or other neurological consequences, with high-dose prednisolone. Steroid-sparing agents, such as methotrexate, may also be required.

Takayasu's arteritis

Takayasu's arteritis is a large-vessel vasculitis affecting the aorta and its major branches, causing vascular insufficiency. The clinical picture is associated with an elevated acute phase response and a normochromic normocytic anaemia. Arteriography is diagnostic. Treatment should be initiated with prednisolone and cytotoxic agents. When the inflammatory process has been controlled surgical intervention with angioplasty, arterial reconstruction, or arterial bypass grafting may be appropriate.

Behçet's disease

Behçet's disease is a systemic vasculitis of unknown aetiology with a particularly high prevalence around the Mediterranean, the Middle East, and the Far East. Characteristic clinical features include recurrent orogenital ulceration, uveitis, skin disease, and arthropathy, usually mono- or oligoarticular. Diagnosis is clinical, in association with an elevated inflammatory response. Treatment relies on corticosteroids and immunosuppression.

Polyarteritis nodosa

Polyarteritis nodosa is a necrotizing vasculitis affecting medium-sized arteries, leading to aneurysm formation. It may be associated with hepatitis B infection. Presenting features include constitutional upset, weight loss, abdominal pain due to mesenteric ischaemia, renal failure and hypertension, mononeuritis multiplex, and skin disease (purpura or livedo reticularis). Diagnosis relies on an elevated acute phase response, hepatitis serology, arteriography, and biopsy of an affected organ. Treatment involves corticosteroids and immunosuppression.

Table 10.5.2 A classification of systemic vasculitis based on size of involved vessels

	Aorta	Large artery	Medium arteries	Small arteries	Arteriole and venule
Takayasu's arteritis	<-------------------------------------->				
Giant cell arteritis		<-------------------------------------->			
Polyarteritis nodosa			<--------->		
Wegener's granulomatosis			<-------------------------------------->		
Churg–Strauss syndrome			<-------------------------------------->		
Microscopic polyarteritis				<-------------------------------------->	
Henoch–Schönlein purpura				<-------------------------------------->	
Vasculitides associated with the connective tissue disorders and rheumatoid arthritis				<-------------------------------------->	

Wegener's granulomatosis

Wegener's granulomatosis is a necrotizing granulomatous vasculitis of small and medium-sized vessels which predominantly affects the upper and lower respiratory tracts, kidneys, and eyes. There is evidence of a systemic inflammatory response and ANCAs (classically cytoplasmic) are present (cANCAs). Biopsy of an affected organ will also aid diagnosis. The systemic form of the disease is almost always fatal without treatment and immunosuppression should be started as soon as possible after presentation.

Churg–Strauss syndrome

Churg–Strauss syndrome is a granulomatous vasculitis affecting small and medium-sized vessels associated with a peripheral eosinophilia. It typically affects the lung (asthma, eosinophilic pneumonia), heart (myocarditis), peripheral nervous system (mononeuritis multiplex), and skin (vasculitic nodules). A peripheral eosinophilia and raised serum immunoglobulin E are typical. Treatment is with immunosuppression.

Microscopic polyangiitis

Microscopic polyangiitis is the commonest small-vessel vasculitis, leading to renal, skin, neurological, and pulmonary disease. Arthralgias, fevers, malaise, and weight loss may be prominent features. Diagnosis rests on demonstration of an elevated inflammatory response, renal biopsy, and antibodies against neutrophil cytoplasmic antigens (classically perinuclear, pANCA). Prompt treatment with prednisolone and a cytotoxic agent is crucial.

Henoch–Schönlein purpura

Henoch–Schönlein purpura is a small-vessel vasculitis characterized by immunoglobulin A deposition within vessel walls and glomeruli. The skin (especially the buttocks and lower limbs), joints, kidneys, and gastrointestinal systems are typically involved. The diagnosis again relies on biopsy of an affected organ. Children are usually affected and the disease in this age group is frequently self-limiting. Adult patients may require immunosuppression.

Further reading

Bertsias, G., Ioannidis, J.P., Boletis, J., *et al.* (2008). EULAR recommendations for the management of systemic lupus erythematosus. *Annals of Rheumatic Disease,* **67**, 195–205.

Lapraik, C., Watts, R., Bacon, P., *et al.* (2007). BSR and BHPR Guidelines for the management of adults with ANCA-associated vasculitis. *Rheumatology,* **46**, 1615–16.

Nataraja, A., Mukhtyar, C., Hellmich, B., *et al.* (2007). Outpatient assessment of systemic vasculitis. *Best Practice & Research. Clinical Rheumatology,* **21**(4), 713–32.

Rahman, A. and Isenberg, D.A. (2008). Systemic lupus erythematosus. *New England Journal of Medicine,* **358**(9), 929–39.

10.6

Osteoporosis

Malgorzata Magliano

Summary points

- Osteoporotic fractures affect one in two women and one in five men over the age of 50
- Previous fragility fracture increases future fracture risk and should prompt further assessment and treatment
- Clinical risk factors in combination with bone mineral density measurement allow identifying patients at risk
- Screening for secondary causes of osteoporosis is important, particularly in men and younger women
- Patients at high risk for future fracture should be offered appropriate treatment. Bisphosphonates together with adequate calcium and vitamin D supplementation constitute first-line therapy
- Compliance with treatment and clinical response need to be monitored.

Introduction

Osteoporosis is a skeletal disorder characterized by low bone mass and microarchitectural deterioration of bone tissue resulting in increased bone fragility and susceptibility to fracture (Figures 10.6.1 and 10.6.2).

Typically, osteoporotic fractures occur at the distal forearm, spine, and hip with increasing age. Globally, osteoporosis results in more than 8.9 million fractures annually with a lifetime fracture risk of between 30–40%. Fragility fractures are associated with high morbidity and mortality and result in significant costs to society. Given that number of osteoporotic fractures is likely to increase threefold over the next 50 years as a result of aging populations, identifying and treating individuals at risk is important. In 1994, the World Health Organization (WHO) produced diagnostic criteria for osteoporosis based on the measurement of bone mineral density (BMD). It defined osteoporosis as bone density value that is more then 2.5 standard deviations (SD) below the mean for young adults. Low BMD and factors such as older age, prior fracture, high rate of bone turnover, risk of falls, corticosteroid use, and family history allow the estimation of individual future fracture risk and guide therapeutic decisions. Effective therapies that can reduce the incidence of fracture are available but undoubtedly underused. The pathogenesis and epidemiology of osteoporosis, fragility fracture risk assessment, diagnostic tools, and current treatments are discussed in the rest of this chapter.

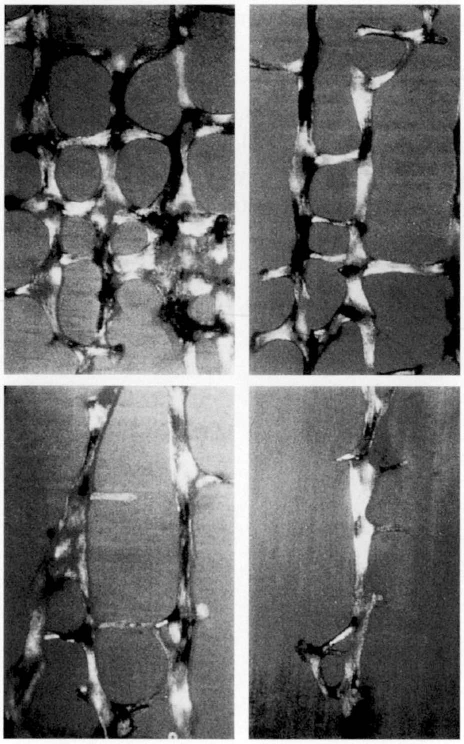

Fig. 10.6.1 The progressive loss of bone trabeculae with age.

Pathogenesis of osteoporosis

Bone undergoes constant remodelling which allows growth, repair, and adaptation to stress. The cycle of bone remodelling on endosteal surfaces starts with bone resorption initiated by osteoclasts. The resorptive cavity thus created is subsequently filled with new bone by osteoblasts. Mineralization of the newly laid down bone matrix (osteoid) completes the cycle which lasts 3–6 months.

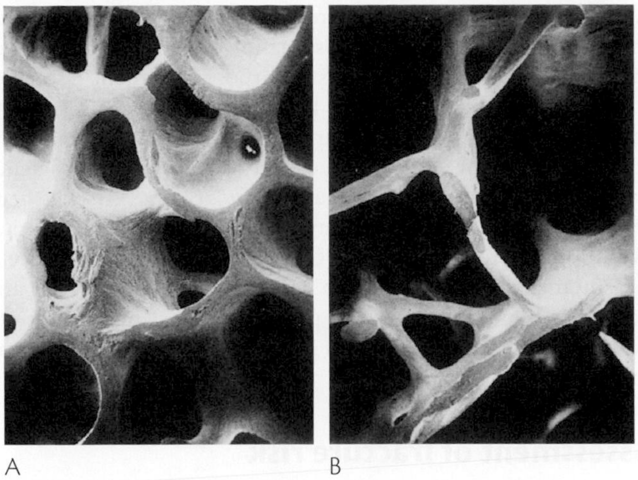

Fig. 10.6.2 Scanning electron microscopic appearance of normal and osteoporotic bone.

The balance between bone resorption and formation determines net bone acquisition or bone loss.

During skeletal growth, bone formation predominates, leading to gradual increase in bone size and density reaching peak BMD by about 25 years of age. About 50–85% of the variance in BMD is determined genetically. Low peak BMD can also result from prolonged childhood illness, low calcium intake, low body weight, or delayed puberty (Figure 10.6.3).

Reduction in BMD begins gradually, even in the early adult years in both men and women, and is thought to result from gradual reduction in new bone formation. In women, bone loss accelerates after menopause due to a significant fall in circulating oestrogen levels. This loss is particularly rapid in the first 5 years after menopause reaching up to 3% per year in the spine. Interestingly, low oestrogen levels in older men correlate positively with low BMD indicating that oestrogens are important regulators of bone formation in both genders. Bone loss in older people is influenced by a number of other factors including increased parathyroid hormone (PTH) levels, vitamin D deficiency, and low calcium intake. Other comorbidities, such as rheumatoid arthritis or medications (corticosteroids or aromatase inhibitors), contribute to accelerated bone loss and need to be considered as additional risk factors for fractures.

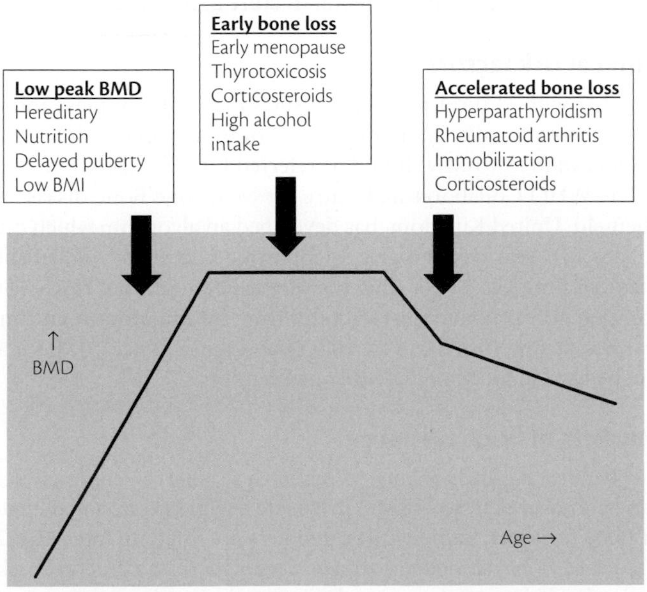

Fig. 10.6.3 Factors that can reduce bone mineral density throughout life.

Epidemiology of osteoporosis and osteoporotic fractures

As BMD decreases with age, prevalence of osteoporosis rises. Among people in their late 60s, 29% of women and 12% of men have osteoporosis at the hip. These numbers rise to 57% and 36%, respectively, by the age of 85. The incidence of fractures follows a similar trend, rising steeply after the age of 50. Osteoporotic fractures are twice as common overall in women. In the United Kingdom, the lifetime risk of any fracture at 50 years of age is 53% in women and 20% in men. The commonest non-vertebral fracture sites in over 55 years of age are the wrist, upper humerus, and hip.

Lifetime risk of a hip fracture in a white woman ranges from 11.4% in the UK up to 22.9% in Sweden. In men the risk is lower and ranges from 3.1% to 10.7%. Hip fractures affect mainly those over 70 years old and in 90% of cases result from a fall from standing height. Low BMD at the femoral neck is a strong predictor of future hip fracture risk but other factors are also important, including femoral neck length, angulation, and the distribution of cortical bone within the femoral neck. Thus it has been shown that cortical bone is well preserved inferiorly from 20 through to 90 years of age while there is a strong tendency for cortical thinning superiorly, with major implications for the integrity of the femoral neck in direct trauma as might happen in falls. The risk of falling itself is therefore also clearly an important risk for fracture. Hip fracture constitutes one of the commonest causes for acute admission to an orthopaedic ward and worldwide the cost of hospitalization for a hip fracture is estimated to be £10 300 per patient. Mortality after hip fracture is 10% at 30 days, rising to 30% at 1 year. Higher mortality is reported in older patients with multiple comorbidities and cognitive impairment and residual physical disability is common in this group. A year after hip fracture, 40% of survivors are unable to walk independently and 60% require assistance in at least one core activity of daily living.

Wrist fractures result from a fall on the outstretched hand and are commonest in perimenopausal women. Lifetime risk of a wrist fracture in a 50 year old white woman is between 16–20% worldwide. In men, the incidence remains low, rising slightly after the age of 85. Risk of wrist fractures correlates strongly with low BMD and these patients should undergo further screening for osteoporosis.

Lifetime risk of clinically diagnosed vertebral fracture varies from 3.1% to 15.1% in a white woman and from 1.2% to 8.3% in a white man worldwide. However, this represents the tip of the iceberg as only a third of vertebral fractures present on radiographs come to medical attention. The incidence of vertebral fractures rises after the age of 60. Most vertebral fractures result from bending or lifting light objects and less then 25% are due to falls. Vertebral fractures are associated with significant morbidity: chronic back pain, loss of height, kyphosis, and reduced mobility. Women with multiple vertebral fractures have increased mortality from cardiovascular and pulmonary causes.

Fractures of the proximal humerus, ribs, clavicle and pelvis are significantly increased in the elderly and if associated with low trauma should be treated as other fragility fractures.

Assessment of bone mineral density

Measurement of BMD using dual X-ray absorptiometry (DXA) is generally accepted for the diagnosis of osteoporosis. DXA measures the mineral content of the bone which is expressed as bone mass per projected area of the bone in g/m^2. BMD varies at different skeletal sites and measurements can be performed at the lumbar spine, proximal femur, the forearm, calcaneus, and the whole body. WHO diagnostic criteria for osteoporosis are based on BMD measured at the lumbar spine and the left hip. Individual BMD values are expressed in standard deviation units with reference to the mean peak bone mass of a young healthy adult, known as the T-score. Further comparison of BMD with the age and gender-matched range is expressed as the Z-score. Reduction in T-score and Z-score correlates with increased fracture risk. In postmenopausal osteoporosis it is generally accepted that fracture risk approximately doubles for each standard deviation in BMD below normal. Definitions of osteoporosis and osteopenia based on T-score values are described in Table 10.6.1.

Although DXA is widely used in everyday clinical practice, one has to be aware of its limitations. Bone densitometry allows two-dimensional measurement of bone density and is affected by bone depth. The presence of osteoarthritis with marginal osteophytosis, previous vertebral fractures, scoliosis, obesity, or aortic calcification can falsely elevate spinal BMD. Likewise, BMD measurement at the hip can be affected by anatomical variants, osteoarthritis, Paget's disease, or leg positioning. Peripheral DXA (PIXI) is used for measuring BMD at the forearm and calcaneus and can be used in fracture risk assessment if there is no access to axial DXA. DXA may also be useful to monitor patients on treatment, as the BMD is expected to rise. In younger patients, increase in BMD is most noticeable in the vertebrae where bone turnover is more rapid than in the hip. In older patients with degenerative changes in the lumbar spine, interpretation of BMD measurements may be difficult.

DXA provides an accurate and reproducible way of measuring BMD but does not provide information on bone microarchitecture. Other techniques are being developed to obtain a better understanding of factors that determine bone strength. Quantitative ultrasound measures attenuation of the ultrasound waves by the bone tissue and can be measured at the heel, tibia, radius, or phalanges. It can be helpful in estimation of the fracture risk but has not been accepted for diagnostic purposes. Magnetic resonance is increasingly utilized to assess trabecular structure of the bone and marrow fat content. In current clinical practice, magnetic resonance imaging (MRI) has use in identifying insufficiency fractures. In recent years computed tomography (CT) has been developed to assess bone microarchitecture. Volumetric quantitative computed tomography (vQCT) produces three-dimensional measurement of BMD and can separately analyse cortical and trabecular bone. It has proved precise in assessing response to treatment in clinical trials but its use is limited by higher radiation dose, cost, and availability.

Table 10.6.1 WHO classification based on axial BMD measurement

	Bone density
Normal	BMD value greater than 1 SD below the young adult reference mean (T-score ≥−1)
Osteopenia	BMD value that is between 1 and 2.5 SD below the young adult reference mean (T-score <−1 and >2.5)
Osteoporosis	BMD value that is 2.5 or more SD below the young adult reference mean (T-score ≤2.5)
Established osteoporosis	BMD value that is 2.5 or more SD below the young adult reference mean (T-score ≤2.5) and the presence of at least one fragility fracture

BMD, bone mineral density; SD, standard deviation

Assessment of fracture risk

Bone mineral density

The risk of non-vertebral fractures in people over 55 years old increases with reduction in femoral neck BMD. This association is the same for men and women. The strongest correlation between low BMD and fracture risk exists for wrist and hip fractures. However, only 44% of non-vertebral fractures in women and 12% in men occur in individuals with T-scores below −2.5, indicating that BMD alone is an imperfect tool for the assessment of fracture risk. The relationship between low BMD and fracture risk can be likened to the association between hypertension and stroke. Not all patients with elevated blood pressure will sustain a stroke but the risk of stroke is considerably increased in hypertensive subjects. Full evaluation of other risk factors is an essential part of fracture risk assessment that will guide a decision on treatment.

Previous fragility fracture

A previous fragility fracture constitutes a very important risk factor as it doubles the likelihood of any future fractures regardless of the site of the initial fracture. For example, a woman who has sustained a wrist fracture has a twofold increased risk of hip fracture. Prior vertebral fracture results in a fourfold increased risk of subsequent vertebral fracture and this risk increases further by two to four times for each additional vertebral fracture at baseline.

Clinical risk factors

Patients with clinical risk factors such as low body mass index (BMI), parental history of hip fracture, or other comorbidities that could lead to low BMD should be referred for DXA (Box 10.6.1).

The WHO Collaborating Centre for Metabolic Bone disease at Sheffield, United Kingdom, has developed an algorithm which calculates a 10-year risk of major osteoporotic fracture in women and men over the age of 50. This fracture assessment tool (FRAX®) computes the probability of fractures from information about clinical risk factors (listed in Box 10.6.2) and femoral neck BMD that can be used to guide therapeutic interventions.

Markers of bone turnover

Biochemical products of bone formation and bone resorption, which can be measured in serum and urine, are useful in assessing the rate of bone turnover. Some of these markers are listed in Table 10.6.2. Increased bone turnover correlates with increased fracture risk. Reduction in bone turnover markers on antiresorptive treatment can

Box 10.6.1 Indications for bone density scan

- X-ray osteopenia
- Fragility fracture (unless >75 years old)
- Untreated premature menopause (age <45)
- Amenorrhea (>1 year)
- Long-term steroids (>3 months at the dose of >5mg prednisolone/day)
- BMI <19kg/m^2
- Coeliac disease/malabsorption
- Primary hyperparathyroidism
- Chronic renal failure
- Post-transplant
- Cushing's syndrome
- Hyperthyroidism
- Hypogonadism.

Box 10.6.2 Risk factors for osteoporotic fractures incorporated in the FRAX® tool

- Age
- Female gender
- Previous fragility fracture
- Parental history of hip fracture
- BMI <19kg/m^2
- Long-term steroids
- Rheumatoid arthritis
- Presence of secondary causes for osteoporosis
- Cigarette smoking
- Excessive alcohol consumption (>3 units per day).

Table 10.6.2 Biochemical markers of bone turnover

Markers of bone formation	Markers of bone resorption
Bone alkaline phosphatase	Piridinoline (PYR)
Osteocalcin	Deoxypiridinoline (D-PYR)
C-terminal propepetide of type I collagen (P1CP)	N-terminal telopeptide (NT_X)
N- terminal propepetide of type I collagen (P1NP)	C-terminal telopeptide (CT_X)

be useful in assessing treatment compliance. Bone markers can be used in addition to BMD measurement in fracture risk assessment.

Clinical features of osteoporosis

Osteoporosis is an asymptomatic condition and is often detected only after a person has sustained a low trauma fracture. Clinical features of acute hip and distal radius fractures are described elsewhere. Vertebral fractures are often unrecognized and patients present late with an established thoracic kyphosis, loss of height, and variable back pain. Acute vertebral fracture should always be suspected in an elderly person with sudden onset of severe localized back pain. The commonest site for vertebral fractures is in the lower thoracic segment and at the thoracolumbar junction where localized tenderness over the relevant vertebrae is an important clinical indicator (Figures 10.6.4 and 10.6.5).

In most patients, the acute pain settles over 6–8 weeks but more diffuse low-grade discomfort may be prolonged. Patients with multiple fractures in the thoracic segment develop a deformity known as 'dowager's hump'. Spinal deformity results in secondary problems such as reduced chest expansion, early satiety, and abdominal pain. Acute rib fractures can follow episodes of coughing

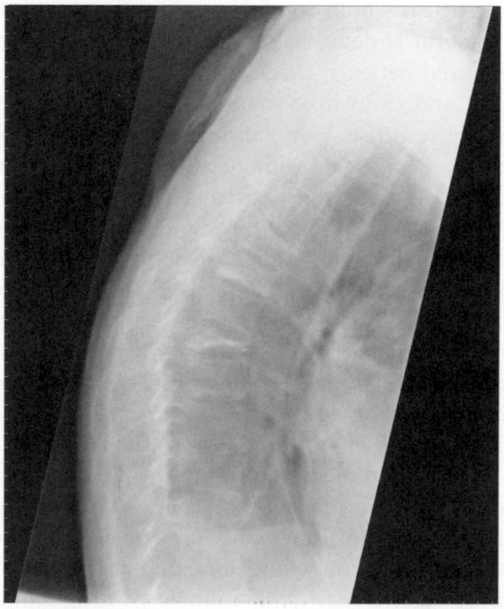

Fig. 10.6.4 Lateral x-ray of the thoracic spine in a 72-year-old man with rheumatoid arthritis who presented with acute midthoracic back pain. Vertebral fractures demonstrated at levels T5, T6, and T8.

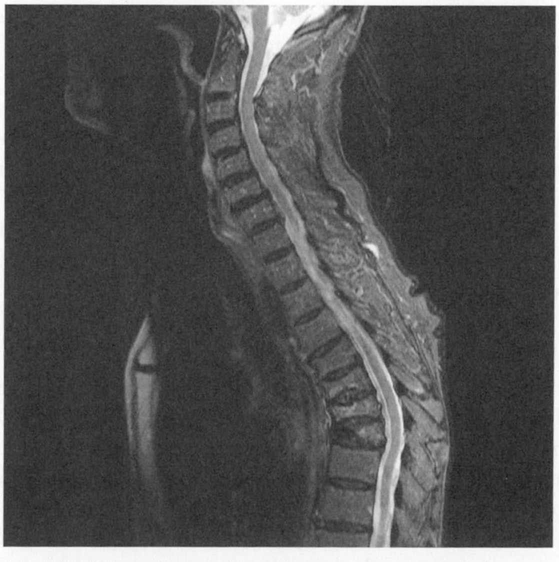

Fig. 10.6.5 MRI of the thoracic spine (STIR sagittal sequence) in the same patient as Fig 10.6.4 demonstrating wedge fractures at T5, T6, T7, and T8 with high signal in T6 and T7 vertebral bodies suggesting more recent fractures..

and produce pleuritic-type chest pain and localized rib tenderness. Pelvic insufficiency fractures should be suspected in a person following a fall if there is persisting buttock/hip pain on mobilization. Insufficiency fractures can be difficult to demonstrate on plain x-rays but can be well visualized on MRI (Figures 10.6.5 and 10.6.6).

Secondary osteoporosis

The majority of women who present with fragility fractures have postmenopausal osteoporosis but up to 30% of females and over 50% of males with osteoporosis have a secondary cause of bone loss (see Box 10.6.3). Patients with osteoporosis should therefore all have a set of simple blood tests to check for secondary causes (Box 10.6.4).

The commonest endocrine causes include hyperparathyroidism and thyrotoxicosis—both conditions are more common in older women. Vitamin D deficiency is common, particularly in older institutionalized patients; checking calcium, phosphate, alkaline phosphatase, and 25-hydroxyvitamin D levels is therefore recommended in those at risk. Eating disorders pose a particular therapeutic challenge and are an important cause of osteoporosis in young women. 'Female athlete' triad is increasingly recognized in women who sustain stress fractures and consists of disorder of eating, menstrual dysfunction, and osteoporosis. Secondary amenorrhoea is an important cause of low BMD in young women and may result from premature ovarian failure or pituitary insufficiency. Oestrogen replacement should be offered to young women with premature menopause. Gastrointestinal malabsorption should be suspected in patients with iron deficiency anaemia, low albumin levels, and hypocalcaemia. In elderly patients with an elevated erythrocyte sedimentation rate (ESR), serum protein and urine electrophoresis is mandatory to rule out multiple myeloma. Inflammatory conditions such as rheumatoid arthritis contribute to bone loss through production of inflammatory cytokines which stimulate osteoclastic activity. A number of drugs contribute to bone loss with systemic steroids being particularly important. Excessive alcohol intake is a common cause of male osteoporosis. Other causes of low bone density include heritable causes (e.g. osteogenesis imperfecta and hypophosphatasia), mastocytosis, and fibrogenesis imperfecta osseum. Mastocytosis is a rare disorder associated with osteoporosis that is caused by increased numbers of mast cells in the tissues. Clinical features include pruritus, flushing, nausea, diarrhoea, vascular instability, and a characteristic rash of urticaria pigmentosa. Fibrogenesis imperfecta osseum is an extremely rare acquired disorder in which the normal bone matrix is replaced by collagen-deficient tissue that is extremely fragile. Bone pain and multiple fractures occur and an association with paraprotein in the blood is well recognized. Some patients have responded to treatment with melphalan.

Glucocorticosteroid-induced osteoporosis

At some time in their lives, between 3–5% of the United Kingdom population receives corticosteroid treatment. Patients treated with systemic steroids have an increased fracture risk which increases within the first 3 months of corticosteroid treatment and declines towards baseline in the year following corticosteroid discontinuation. Fracture risk correlates positively with higher steroid dose and longer treatment duration but current steroid users have a twofold increased risk of fracture independent of BMD or previous

Box 10.6.3 Causes of secondary osteoporosis

- Endocrine:
  - Hyperparathyroidism
  - Thyrotoxicosis
  - Hypogonadism
  - Hyperprolactinaemia
  - Cushing's syndrome
  - Premature ovarian failure
  - Anorexia nervosa
  - Vitamin D deficiency
- Gastrointestinal:
  - Malabsorption: coeliac disease, inflammatory bowel disease
  - Liver cirrhosis
  - Primary biliary cirrhosis
- Inflammatory disorders:
  - Rheumatoid arthritis
  - Polymyalgia rheumatica
  - Ankylosing spondylitis
- Bone marrow disorders:
  - Multiple myeloma
  - Leukemia/lymphoma
  - Systemic mastocytosis
- Medications
  - Corticosteroids
  - Gonadotropin releasing hormone agonists
  - Anticonvulsants
  - Aromatase inhibitors
  - Long-term heparin
- Renal disease:
  - Chronic renal failure
  - Renal tubular acidosis
- Collagen disorders:
  - Osteogenesis imperfecta
  - Ehler–Danlos syndrome
- Others:
  - Post transplantation
  - Alcohol
  - Smoking
  - Prolonged immobility.

Box 10.6.4 Blood tests recommended in patients with osteoporosis

- Full blood count and ESR
- Urea, electrolytes, and creatinine
- Liver function tests
- Calcium, phosphate, and alkaline phosphatase
- Thyroid-stimulating hormone
- Serum and urine protein electrophoresis.

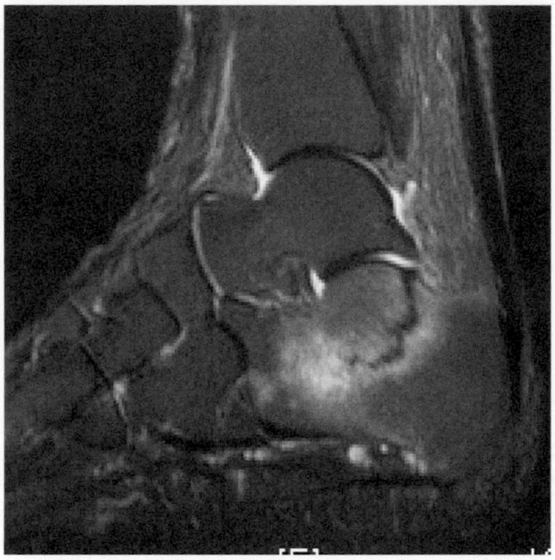

Fig. 10.6.6 STIR MRI of calcaneus showing insufficiency fracture and adjacent high signal.

steroid cumulative dose. Steroid-induced bone loss is greatest in the first 3 months of treatment and results from suppression of osteoblast function, increased bone resorption, and inhibition of intestinal calcium absorption. Fractures among steroid users occur at a higher threshold of BMD compared to steroid non-users, which needs to be considered when deciding on treatment. Starting prolonged steroid therapy at a dose greater than 5mg of prednisolone daily should trigger risk factor assessment and, if appropriate, the use of bone protective treatment. In younger patients, bone protection usually consists of maintaining adequate calcium and vitamin D intake. In patients over 65 years, treatment with bisphosphonates should be initiated, pending the result of DXA.

Osteoporosis of pregnancy

Pregnancy and lactation-associated osteoporosis presents with fragility fracture (usually vertebral) that typically occurs in late pregnancy or the early postpartum period. Although uncommon, osteoporosis of pregnancy can cause considerable pain and disability. The cause is unknown but pre-existing risk factors for low bone mass, such as low BMI, family history of fragility fractures, smoking, or vitamin D deficiency are often present. DXA shows reduction in BMD, particularly at the spine, which tends to improve with weaning and calcium and vitamin D supplementation. Bisphosphonates have been used successfully in some women postpartum. The condition only rarely recurs in future pregnancies.

Juvenile idiopathic osteoporosis

Osteoporosis should be suspected in children with low trauma fractures or radiographic osteopenia. Osteoporosis in a child usually results from other underlying causes such as low body mass, malnutrition, juvenile arthritis, endocrine abnormalities, or steroid therapy. Hereditable disorders of connective tissue such as osteogenesis imperfecta (OI) must also be considered.

Diagnosis of osteoporosis in childhood can be problematic. Standard DXA uses adult peak bone mass as a reference and will therefore produce misleading results. Paediatric normative data are available for the lumbar spine and total body and should be used if possible. Interpretation of bone density measurement must take into account pubertal onset and child's size. One of the most important measures is to ensure adequate intake of calcium, phosphate, proteins, and vitamin D and encourage physical activity. Bisphosphonates such as intravenous pamidronate are used in more severe cases, including the more severe forms of OI.

Management of osteoporosis

Elderly patients with prior fragility fracture should be commenced on treatment without the need for BMD measurement. In patients below 75 years of age, DXA can be helpful as it has additional value in treatment monitoring. For primary prevention, the intervention threshold will depend on the combination of BMD and clinical risk factor assessment as discussed earlier. A team approach is essential (Figure 10.6.7).

Lifestyle modifications

Lifestyle measures aimed at optimizing peak BMD are important from an early age. Adequate calcium intake of 1000–1500mg/day for an adult and vitamin D 400IU–800IU or 10–20mcg/day should be ensured. Vitamin K found in green leafy vegetables improves BMD while excessive caffeine and alcohol intake and smoking have detrimental effects on bone density. Weight bearing exercise such as walking, t'ai chi, and dancing improve balance, posture, and strength and are recommended.

Fall avoidance

Elderly patients with a history of falls require referral to fall services for further assessment and intervention. Hip protectors reduce the number of hip fractures but compliance is poor. They should be considered in institutionalized elderly patients.

Pharmacological interventions

There is an increasing number of therapies shown to improve BMD and reduce risk of fractures. They can be divided into: antiresorptive therapies, anabolic agents and those with dual mode of action (Table 10.6.3 and Figure 10.6.8).

Bisphosphonates are the most commonly used antiresorptive treatment. Bisphosphonate molecules contain P-C-P structure (two phosphonic acids bonded to a carbon), which binds to the hydroxyapatite on the bone surface, and two side chains which determine binding affinity and potency. Bisphosphonates inhibit osteoclast driven bone resorption and result in a modest increase in BMD in the first 2 years of treatment. In postmenopausal women, alendronate and risedronate reduce the risk of vertebral

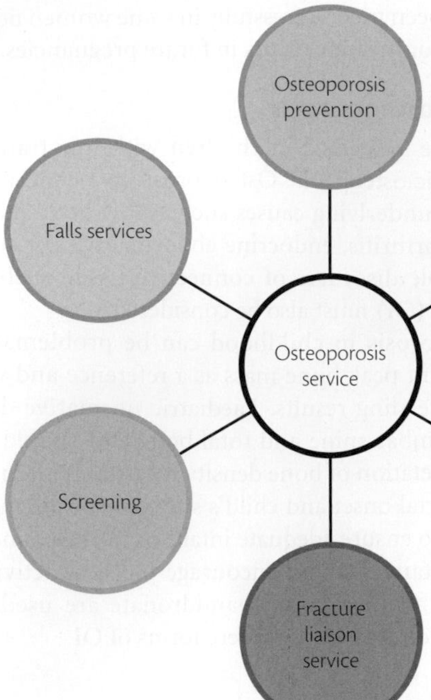

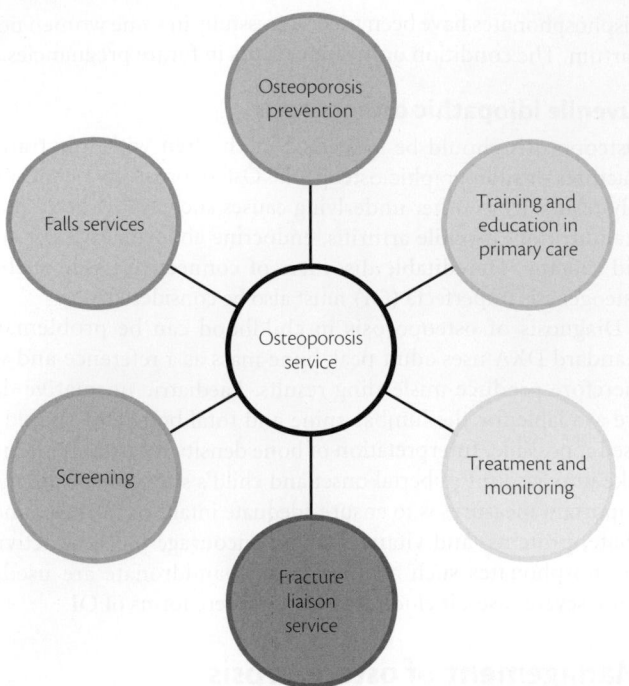

Fig. 10.6.7 A team approach to an effective osteoporosis service.

fractures by up to 50%, hip fractures by approximately 40% and other non-vertebral fractures by 20%. Ibandronate and etidronate have shown efficacy in preventing vertebral fractures only.

Oral bisphosphonates are poorly absorbed from the gut and must be taken on an empty stomach with copious water, remaining upright for the next 30–60min to avoid oesophageal side effects. Oral bisphosphonates should be avoided in patients with oesophageal stricture or recent peptic ulcer. For patients intolerant of oral bisphosphonates, intravenous forms, such as ibandronate or zoledronate, can be used effectively. Alendronate, risedronate, and etidronate are licensed for treatment of glucocorticosteroid-induced osteoporosis, while alendronate has an additional licence for treatment of osteoporosis in men. Bisphosphonates are renally excreted and are contraindicated in patients with renal failure.

Strontium ranelate has a dual mode of action with a modest inhibitory effect on bone resorption and stimulation of bone formation. In women with postmenopausal osteoporosis it has been shown to reduce vertebral fracture risk by over 40% and non-vertebral fracture risk by 16%. Strontium ranelate is particularly effective at reducing hip fractures in women over the age of 75 with low BMD (T-score <−3).

Raloxifene is a selective oestrogen receptor modulator (SERM). It has agonistic effects on oestrogen receptors in bone but acts as an oestrogen antagonist in the breast tissue and endometrium. Raloxifene is effective in the primary and secondary prevention of vertebral fractures in women with postmenopausal osteoporosis, demonstrating risk reduction of 30% and 50% respectively. It can be considered in younger women and has the additional advantages of improving lipid profile and reducing the risk of breast cancer. However, it does increase the risk of thromboembolism.

Hormone replacement therapy (HRT) improves BMD and reduces the risk of vertebral fractures in postmenopausal women although it has only weak action on the hip. In this age group the

Table 10.6.3 Pharmacological therapies for osteoporosis

Name	Administration	Vertebral fractures reduction	Non-vertebral fractures reduction
Alendronate	70mg/once a week or 10mg od PO	+	+
Etidronate	400mg od for 14 days every 3 months	+	
Ibadronate	150mg/once a month PO 3mg every 3 months IV	+	
Raloxifene	60mg od PO	+	
Risedronate	35mg/oew or 5mg od PO	+	+
Strontium ranelate	2g od PO	+	+
Teriparatide	20mcg SC daily for 18 months	+	+
Zoledronate	5mg every 12 months IV	+	+

IV, intravenous; od, once daily; PO, by mouth; SC, subcutaneous.

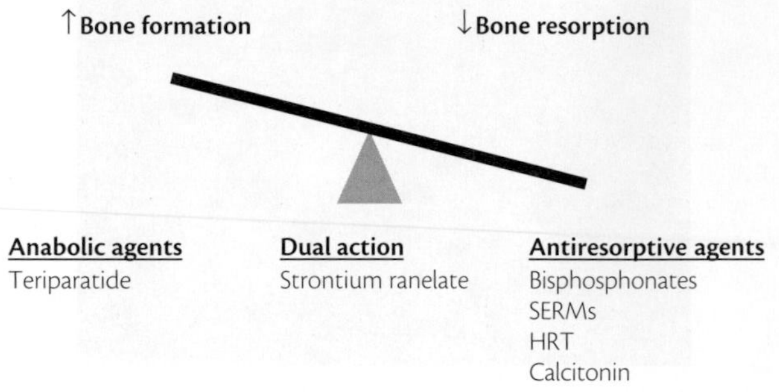

Fig. 10.6.8 Treatments for osteoporosis according to mechanism of action.

beneficial effect of the HRT on the bone tissue is rather offset by other undesirable effects, including increased risk of breast cancer, and cardiovascular and thrombotic events. In contrast, HRT is safe in young women in whom it should be considered when there is premature menopause in order to prevent early postmenopausal loss of bone.

Parathyroid hormone in intermittent doses has a potent effect on bone formation. Two recombinant forms of recombinant human PTH, 1-34 (teriparatide) and 1-84, have been developed. Teriparatide reduces the risk of vertebral fractures by 65% and non-vertebral fractures by over 50%. It is administered by daily subcutaneous injection for 18 months. In some countries its use is currently restricted to women with severe osteoporosis, with very low BMD and who fail to respond to other therapies.

Calcitonin, an endogenous peptide produced by thyroid C-cells, inhibits bone resorption. Salmon calcitonin administered intranasally produces a modest reduction in vertebral fractures. Both injectable and intranasal calcitonin has additional analgesic effects in patients with acute vertebral fracture, an effect which is most pronounced within the first week.

Vertebroplasty may be indicated for individuals where pain from acute fracture persists beyond 6 weeks and in whom there is evidence of persistent bone marrow oedema. Small volumes of methylmethacrylate cement injected into the vertebral body have a high success rate and low incidence of complication (Figure 10.6.9).

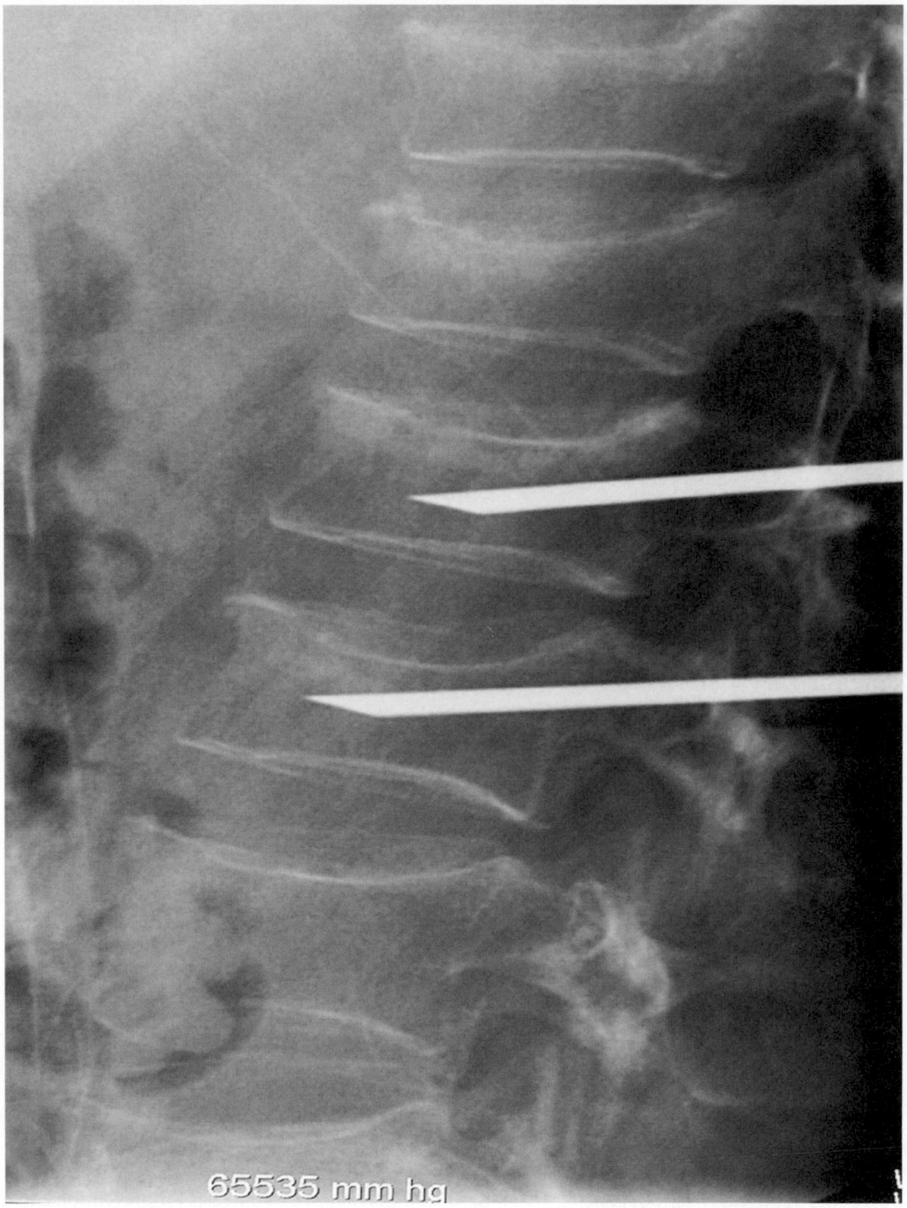

Fig. 10.6.9 Multilevel osteoporotic crush fractures of the thoracic spine with cannulae in situ in preparation for vertebroplasty..

Monitoring treatment response

Linear measurements of bone density in patients starting antiresorptive treatment demonstrated correlation between the increase in BMD and reduction in fracture risk (Figure 10.6.10). However, the magnitude of the fracture rate reduction cannot be explained by the often modest rise in BMD. In fact, a small reduction in fracture risk is observed in those patients whose BMD remains the same. Measurement of BMD at the spine and femoral neck every 2–5 years remains the internationally accepted strategy for monitoring treatment response or following BMD in untreated patients with risk factors. Additionally, in recent years, biochemical markers of bone turnover have been developed to assess responses to treatment and also patient compliance. They have the advantage of providing a more rapid indication of treatment response as they reach a nadir within 3–6 months of the initiation of treatment. No formal guidelines exist on their routine use in clinical practice but failure of suppression of bone turnover markers should at least raise the suspicion that bisphosphonate compliance might be poor. Although current therapies are effective in fracture prevention some patients will continue to fracture. In such cases treatment compliance should also be reassessed and a change of the therapeutic agent considered (e.g. switching from oral to intravenous bisphosphonate).

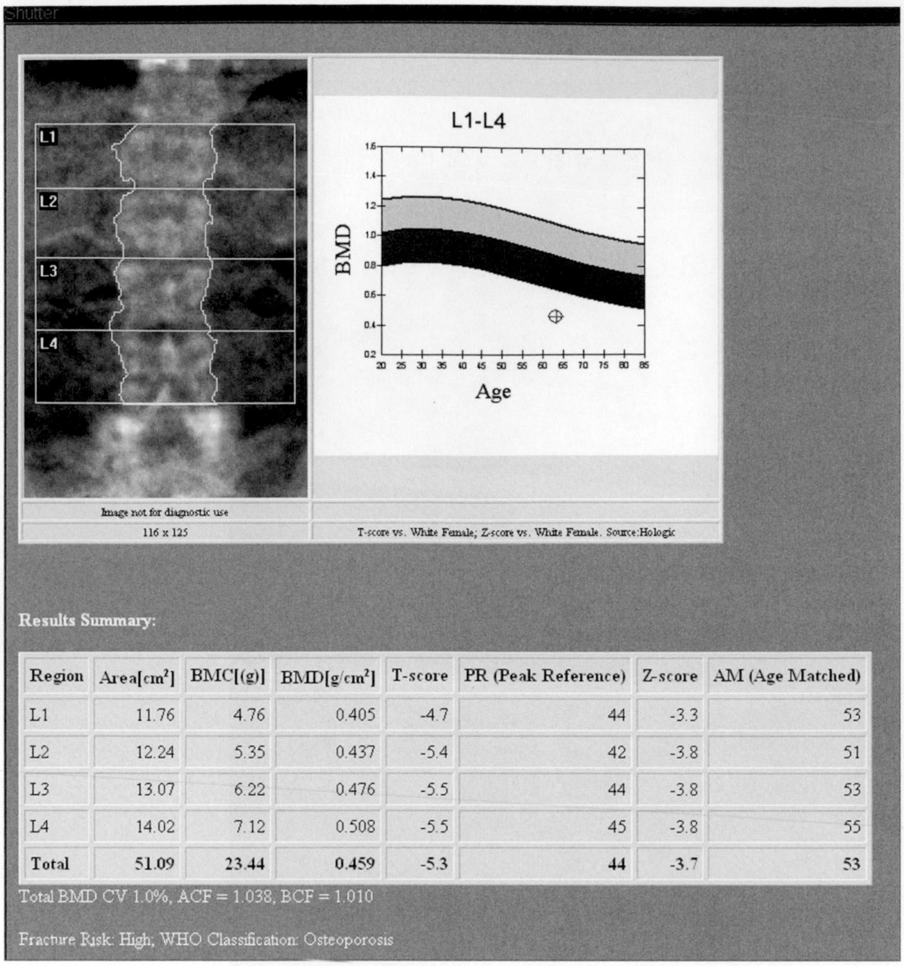

Region	Area[cm²]	BMC[(g)]	BMD[g/cm²]	T-score	PR (Peak Reference)	Z-score	AM (Age Matched)
L1	11.76	4.76	0.405	-4.7	44	-3.3	53
L2	12.24	5.35	0.437	-5.4	42	-3.8	51
L3	13.07	6.22	0.476	-5.5	44	-3.8	53
L4	14.02	7.12	0.508	-5.5	45	-3.8	55
Total	**51.09**	**23.44**	**0.459**	-5.3	**44**	-3.7	53

Fig. 10.6.10 Bone density measurement at the spine in a 51-year-old female with history of two renal transplants and long-term steroid therapy..

Summary

Osteoporotic fractures are an important cause of morbidity and mortality. Patients at risk should be recognized early as current therapies offer a significant fracture risk reduction. Having a fragility fracture is a major predictor of further fractures and orthopaedic surgeons can play an important role in identifying individuals who require further assessment and treatment.

Further reading

Cummings, S.R. and Melton, L.J. (2002). Epidemiology and outcomes of osteoporotic fractures. *Lancet*, **359**, 1761–7.

Kanis, J.A., Johnell, O., Oden, A., Johansson, H., and McCloskey, E. (2008). FRAX and the assessment of fracture probability in men and women from the UK. *Osteoporosis International*, **19**, 385–97.

Keen, R. (2007). Osteoporosis: strategies for prevention and management. *Best Practice & Research. Clinical Rheumatology*, **21**, 109–22.

Marsh, D., Simpson, H., and Wallace, A. (2003). *The Care of Fragility Fracture Patients*. London: British Orthopaedic Association.

Van Staa, T.P., Dennison, E.M., Leufkens, H.G.M., and Cooper, C. (2001). Epidemiology of fractures in England and Wales. *Bone*, **29**, 517–22.

WHO scientific group on the assessment of osteoporosis at primary health care level. Brussels, Belgium 2004. Available at: http://www.who.int/entity/chp/topics/Osteoporosis.pdf

10.7

Osteoarthritis

Kassim Javaid and Paul Wordsworth

Summary points

- Osteoarthritis is the outcome of many different disease processes
- Correlation between radiographic appearance and symptoms is poor
- Prevalence increases rapidly with age
- A multidimensional approach in treatment should include patient education, physical therapy, analgesia, and ergonomic assessment
- Surgical approaches to treatment should adopt a holistic approach.

Introduction

Osteoarthritis (OA) is the commonest joint disorder in the world and represents a heterogeneous disease process with the final outcome being joint failure. It can be defined pathologically, radiographically, or clinically. While in the past radiographic classification grades have been used to define OA, more recently OA is seen as a failed repair of damage that has been caused by excessive mechanical stress (defined as force/unit area) on joint tissues and combines both structural and symptomatic features to describe the failed joint. There are many causes of OA and the disease process affects not only the articular cartilage but also the subchondral bone, ligaments, joint capsule, synovial membrane, and periarticular muscles. Ultimately there is articular cartilage degeneration with fibrillation, fissures, ulceration, and full thickness loss at the joint surface with sclerosis and eburnation of the subchondral bone, osteophytes, and subchondral cysts. Clinical features are characterized by joint pain, tenderness, limitation of movement, crepitus, and occasional effusion without systemic effects. The failure of the joint to repair leads to pain and dysfunction. However, many people with severe radiographic changes are asymptomatic and progression, when it occurs, is usually slow and may halt intermittently.

Epidemiology

OA is the most common joint disorder in the world. It is more common in women and the prevalence increases rapidly with age, with 10% of the world's population aged over 60 years having symptoms attributed to OA. In 1990, OA was the tenth leading cause of non-fatal health burden in the world. In 2002, OA was the fourth leading cause of years lived with disability in the world. The global prevalence rates are shown in Figure 10.7.1. Using radiographic definitions, knee OA is present in 37% in those aged over 60 years and hip OA 27%. Symptomatic OA is much less common with rates of 4.9%. The lifetime risk of developing symptomatic knee OA is 45% (Figure 10.7.2).

Pathophysiology

OA is a dynamic process with a number of antecedents and represents a final common pathway for all insults to the joint. The typical initiating factor is a mechanical insult and the response of OA is a manifestation of the joint to repair and minimize the abnormal biomechanics. From community studies, at the knee OA may affect medial/lateral tibio-femoral joint (40%) and/or patellofemoral joint (60%).

Cartilage

The function of the chondrocytes in healthy cartilage is to maintain the matrix in terms of collagen, aggrecan, matrix metalloproteinases (MMPs), and cytokine constituents in response to loading. Risk factors for OA development divide into abnormal loading on normal cartilage or normal loading on abnormal cartilage. In OA, the abnormal loading experienced by the chondrocyte leads to promotion of matrix degradation and downregulating cartilage repair processes (Figure 10.7.3). The constituents of the articular cartilage change in OA with increased type II, IX, and XI collagen and aggrecan representing a matrix constitution similar to that seen in fetal development. The type of loading is critical, while repetitive loading promotes homeostasis of the articular cartilage, a single pathological compression of cartilage leads to an increase in catabolic MMP and aggrecanases in an attempt to resorb the damaged cartilage. Histologically, damage to the articular cartilage is evidenced by fibrillation, horizontal splits, partial and full thickness loss. Vascular invasion of the calcified cartilage leading to chondrocyte hypertrophy and replacement by bone further thins the articular cartilage.

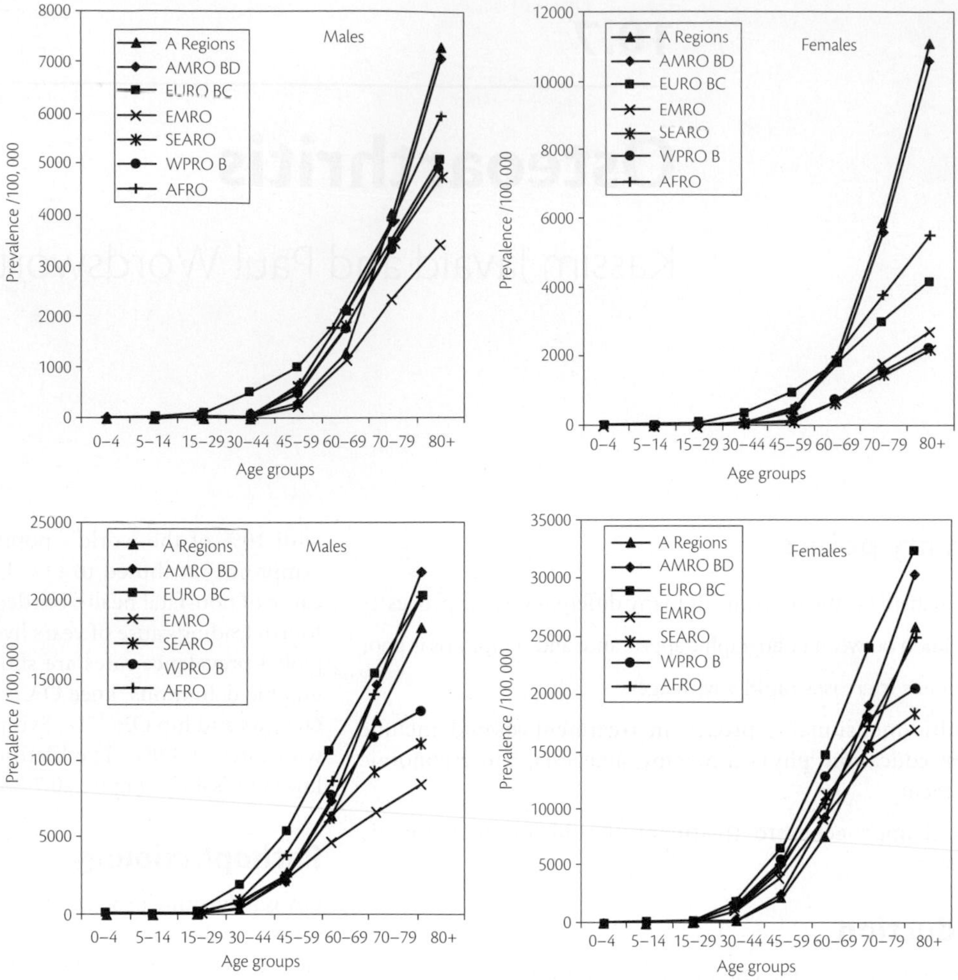

Fig 10.7.1 Global prevalence rates of OA of the hip (upper panel) and knee (lower panel) by age, gender and broad regions. A regions=; AMRO BD= USA Euro BC=European; SEARO= Pakistan; WPRO B= China/Japan; AFRO = African. Adapted from Symmons, D., Mathers, C., and Pfleger, B. (2006). *Global burden of osteoarthritis in the year 2000*. Geneva: World Health Organization.

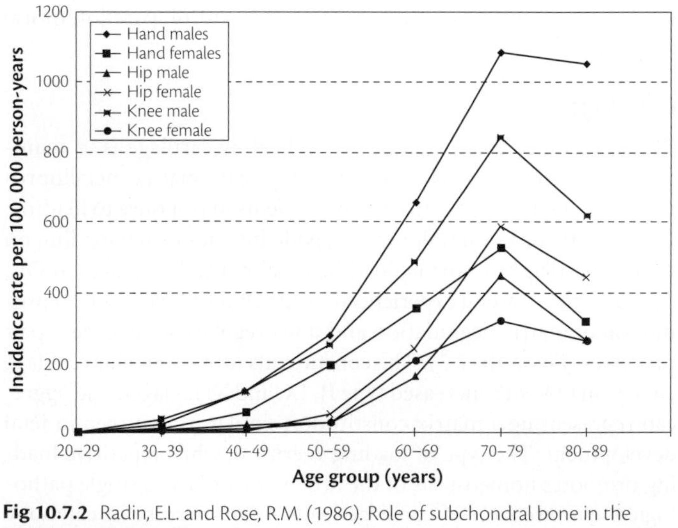

Fig 10.7.2 Radin, E.L. and Rose, R.M. (1986). Role of subchondral bone in the initiation and progression of cartilage damage. *Clinical Orthopaedics and Related Research*, **213**, 34–40.

Subchondral bone

There is a growing body of evidence demonstrating the role of bone as a key tissue involved in the pathogenesis of both structural and symptomatic features of OA. The principal role of the subchondral plate is mechanical with the cortical and trabecular bone compartments acting as shock absorbers, continually responding to loads applied to them by viscoelastic dampening. In the longer term, stress on the subchondral bone lead to remodelling, via the osteocyte network and Wnt signalling and alteration of the material properties. In OA, these changes in material properties reduce its capacity to absorb and dissipate the energy from loads through the joint. Perturbations in the trabecular structure result in increased load associated in interosseous pressure in the medullary area and this may be represented by bone marrow lesions as seen on magnetic resonance imaging (MRI), which have also been associated with arthritic pain and change in bone marrow lesions may correlate with change in symptoms.

In addition to structural changes, the subchondral plate of bone and underlying trabecular/cortical structures are innervated with nociceptive sensory nerves and there is now increasing evidence identifying bone as a source of pain in OA. From bone scintigraphy, extended bone uptake was strongly associated with knee pain in patients with knee OA (odds ratio 3.71 (2.26–6.12)). Of the neuropeptides, both calcitonin-related peptide and substance P are expressed in bone with the potential of mediating bone pain. These neuropeptides can function as both afferent nociception via substance P as well as efferent influences on bone remodelling via CGRP (calcitonin gene-related peptide), an inhibitor of osteoclast motility and stimulator of osteoblast proliferation.

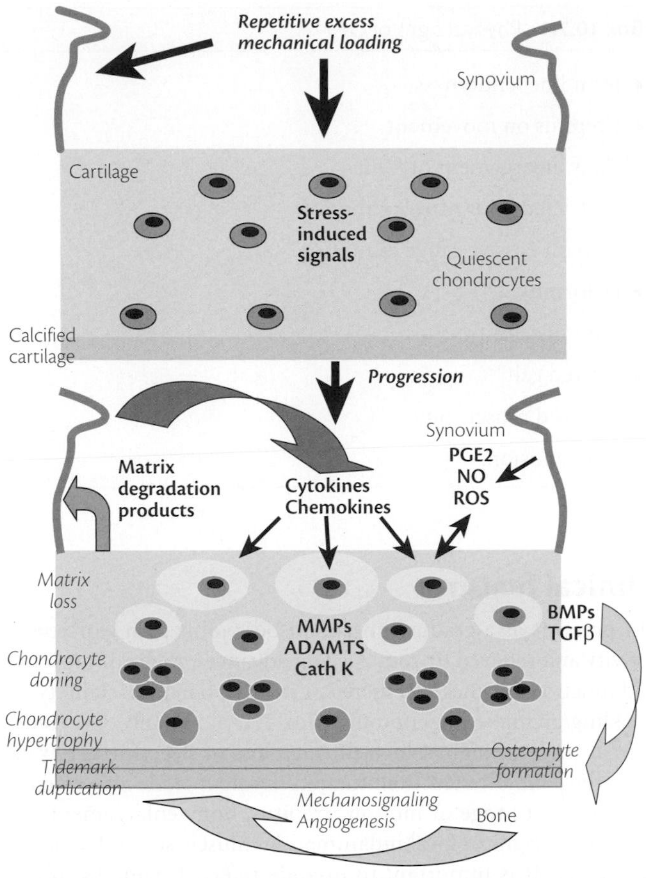

Fig 10.7.3 Matrix and cellular changes in OA. Adapted from Goldring M. (2007). Osteoarthritis. *Journal of Cellular Physiology*, **213**, 634.

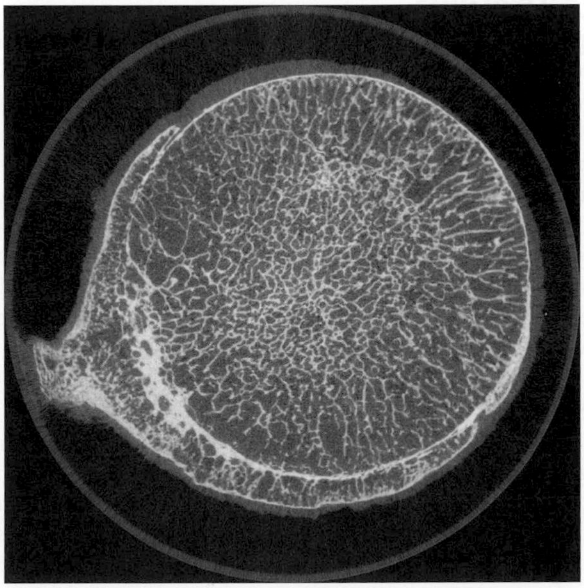

Fig 10.7.4 Bone changes in hip OA.

Osteophytes are fibrocartilaginous outgrowths localized to the joint margins that form through a process of endochondral ossification and are the radiographic hallmark of OA (Figure 10.7.4). Recent work has highlighted the role of the Wnt signalling system as critical in their formation. The significance of osteophytes as a marker of skeletal adaption versus a pathological feature of maladaptation remains unresolved.

Inflammation and synovitis

While OA has been traditionally been regarded as a degenerative disease, it is now clear that local synovitis is very common in OA—these inflammatory changes are likely to be the consequence of cartilage and bone catabolism and are associated with severity of knee pain. The ability to visualize the joint non-invasively using both contrast and non-contrast imaging has demonstrated the almost universal presence of synovitis in OA. From histological specimens, the synovial membrane in OA is hyperplastic and may contain lymphocytic infiltrates. The synovium not only is a source of catabolic inflammatory enzymes but also is richly innervated and represents another source of pain.

Meniscus

In the knee, the semicircular fibrocartilaginous menisci cover two-thirds of the articular surface and are responsible for load distribution and shock absorbing in addition to roles in proprioception, joint stability, and joint lubrication. Damage to the menisci can be the result of trauma or degeneration. Traumatic injury to the menisci is manifest as vertical or radial tears. Degeneration is associated with flaps, complex tears, or maceration. Damage to the menisci also commonly involves extrusion of the mensci. Meniscal damage is extremely common in OA as well as in those without joint pain and the contribution of meniscal damage as a cause versus consequence of OA is not yet clear.

Muscle and ligaments

Muscles not only provide movement but also provide stability for the joint and absorb reaction forces to loading. During normal walking a load of three to four times body weight is generated and at the knee, periarticular muscles are activated in specific patterns to actively absorb this energy and protect the other tissues of the joint. There is growing evidence for the role of the quadriceps weakness not only as a consequence of symptomatic knee OA but also as a determinant, through the potential role of muscle to absorb energy, facilitating patella tracking and acting as a sensory input for joint proprioception, together with mechanoreceptors in the ligaments, capsule, menisci, and skin. Damage to the cruciate ligaments is recognized as a key antecedent for knee OA, although the onset for symptomatic disease may be delayed for many years.

Obesity

OA is a common complication of obesity. Obesity through increased mechanical loading is strongly associated with incident and progression of OA especially at the knee and is a risk factor for total joint replacement. In addition, obesity is associated with a loss of muscle strength relative to weight and poor balance. To compensate for this, obese people have an altered gait exerting greater forces during walking. In addition to mechanical factors, obesity is associated with low-level inflammation which may further contribute to joint damage.

Genetics

Despite the mechanical aetiology to OA, the significant heritability of OA has been confirmed using familial studies, twin studies, linkage analysis, candidate gene, and genome-wide association studies. Genetic influences on bone density and geometry, obesity, synovitis, and chondrocyte function all potentially influence the natural history of OA. Polymorphisms in the Wnt signalling pathway as well as metalloproteinases and cartilage constituents, such as cartilage intermediate layer protein and oligemeric matrix protein, have been associated with knee OA. While the individual genetic traits carry a modest increase in OA risk, identifying the combination of traits in the form of gene–gene and gene–environment interactions have the potential to both inform our understanding of the pathogenesis of OA as well as identify high-risk groups and potential therapeutic targets.

Central pain processing

In addition to local nociceptive stimulus at the joint leading to pain in OA, there is a growing body of evidence that a mechanism involving the peripheral nerves through increased innervation density, spinal cord via gating and hyperexcitability, and altered cortical processing such as locus of control, anxiety, and depression leading to altered inhibitory descending tracts have major affects on symptoms and response to therapy. The characteristic feature of central sensitization leading to chronic pain is that previously non-noxious stimuli such as walking are perceived as painful.

Clinical risk factors

The purpose of clinical risk factors is to assess risk of disease, aid diagnosis and identify possible therapeutic methods. They can be divided into modifiable and non-modifiable risk factors (Table 10.7.1).

Of the risk factors, some are associated with incident disease (high bone mineral density), others with progression (malalignment) and some with both (obesity).

Table 10.7.1 Modifiable and non-modifiable risk factors for OA prevalence and incident disease

Modifiable	Non-modifiable
Smoking	Age
Vitamin D deficiency	Ethnicity
Obesity	Female gender (perimenopausal)
Dietary (possibly vitamin D, vitamin C, and selenium)	Family history of OA
	Diabetes mellitus
Malalignment (progression)	Previous inflammatory arthritis
Occupation exposure (require knee bends)	Previous trauma (ACL rupture)
	Fracture through joint
Heavy manual work	Osteonecrosis
	Meniscectomy
	Congenital hip dysplasia
	Legg–Calve–Perthes
	Slipped femoral epiphysis
	Epiphyseal dysplasia
	Blount's disease
	Acetabular dysplasia
	Acromegaly
	Haemochromatosis
	Ochronosis
	Calcium crystal diseases
	High bone density

Box 10.7.1 Physical signs of OA

- Joint line tenderness
- Crepitus on movement
- Bony enlargement of joint
- Restricted joint range of motion
- Pain on passive range of motion
- Deformity
- Joint instability
- Altered gait
- Reduced muscle bulk
- Joint effusion.

Clinical features

OA presents as a gradual onset, episodic joint pain worsened by activity and relieved by rest. As pain advances, range of movement and function declines and there is a reduction in joint stability with buckling/giving way symptoms (Box 10.7.1). Finally, OA leads to pain at rest and night which through loss of sleep further exacerbates the pain. Physical examination should include assessment for obesity, joint range of motion, crepitus, bony enlargement, focal tenderness, signs of local inflammation, muscle strength, and joint alignment. It is important to exclude referred pain, e.g. hip OA presenting as knee pain.

Investigations

Imaging is used to confirm clinical suspicion and rule out other diagnosis. While radiographs may have features of OA, the absence of radiographic features does not exclude a diagnosis of OA; in addition the presence of features does not exclude other causes for the patient's symptoms. MRI is used to exclude other diagnosis where appropriate. Blood tests can not confirm OA and a full blood count, and renal and liver function tests should be performed if there is a plan to start non-steroidal anti-inflammatory drugs (NSAIDs), especially in the elderly. While biomarkers have been developed for OA, their use is limited to research studies at present.

Imaging

The aim of imaging is to diagnose, follow-up, and elucidate underlying mechanisms of disease in OA. Standard imaging assessment of a joint affected with OA is the plain projectional radiograph which gives a two-dimensional representation of the bone (osteophytes, subchondral sclerosis, subchondral cysts, and attrition) and inferences regarding soft tissue such as joint space narrowing, which represent both cartilage thickness and meniscal extrusion. The Kellgren and Lawrence score is maintained as one of the key assessment of disease severity (Table 10.7.2). More recent atlases (OARSI) classify each compartment separately. The standard views are semiflexed anteroposterior (AP) to assess joint space width and tibiofemoral bone changes, and the skyline or lateral to examine the patellofemoral joint. In contrast, MRI offers a three-dimensional

Table 10.7.2 Radiographic grading system

Grade	Classification	Description
0	Normal	No features of OA
1	Equivocal	Minute osteophyte
2	Definite	Definite osteophyte
3	Moderate	Moderate joint space narrowing
4	Severe	Severe joint space narrowing with subchondral sclerosis

view in any given plane of all the anatomical structures within the joint including cartilage (as measured by defects or volume), osteophytes, ligaments, tendons, synovium, capsule, bone contours, and marrow signal. MRI can detect lesions at an earlier stage in more subregions of the knee. In addition to structural features, the use of specific MRI sequences such as T_2 mapping and T_1rho, allow indirect assessment of the cartilage composition

Ultrasound can easily detect cartilage thickness, meniscal integrity, synovitis, and effusion. Scintigraphy use is limited due to the radiation exposure and poor specificity. Newer computed tomography (CT) scanners are able to offer detailed imaging of the bone structures but have lower soft tissue contrast than that of MRI, for example. CT arthrography provides an indirect method to visualize the cartilage and structures within the knee.

Treatments

Overview

The treatment aims of knee and hip are to reduce clinical symptoms of pain and stiffness, improve or maintain function, reduce disability, improve quality of life and limit disease progression, both symptomatic and functional. A key aim is patient education not only in terms of OA causes and consequences but also in terms of expectations regarding treatment, a major predictor for willingness to accept arthroplasty. The recent OARSI guidance, by consensus produced a list of recommendations for the treatment of hip and knee OA (Table 10.7.3). From a mechanical perspective, therapies that reduce the abnormal joint loading are likely to result in better patient outcomes rather than tissue directed therapies.

Education

Patient education should address the contributions of biological, psychological, and social factors in OA pain. Hence the treatment should be individualized and education should be tailored to the patient's needs and capabilities. Further, in terms of willingness to accept more invasive interventions such as arthroplasty, information regarding postoperative pain and its management, expected time to recovery, and duration of benefit are all likely to influence patient expectations and reported satisfaction after surgery. While difficult to achieve, weight loss is a key management strategy for obese patients presenting with OA. A modest weight reduction of 10% is associated with clinically significant benefits. Strategies that combine incentives, raising outcome expectations and building on self-efficacy, are more likely to succeed. Further, combining weight loss with exercise leads to a preservation of muscle strength.

Exercise and physiotherapy

Exercise is an integral part of the management of the patient with OA, especially of the knee. However, failure of adherence to exercise regimens and underuse by practitioners to recommend the correct exercise or refer to physiotherapy remain key hurdles. At the knee, a key aim is to improve muscle strength. There is observational evidence that greater quadriceps strength increases disease progression in the presence of malalignment but not in those with neutral knees (±5 degrees); there is no robust interventional evidence for this. Through appropriately targeted exercise, proprioception can also be improved. An exercise prescription is now recommended for muscle rehabilitation for patients with OA (Box 10.7.2).

Devices

The principal aim of a walking device is to reduce the compressive load across the affected joint surface. This is maximally achieved by using the walking device in the contralateral side which not only shifts body weight from the symptomatic limb but also lessens the adduction moment. The optimal height of the cane is to the superior tip of the greater trochanter, with the arm at 20–30 degrees flexion.

A properly fitted unloader brace of the knee attempts to correct the relative alignment of tibia to femur and improve mediolateral instability. Care needs to be taken to ensure adequate adherence to using the brace and these braces are not appropriate in those with bicompartment disease. In those with symptomatic patellafemoral OA, medial taping of the patella reduces symptoms by increasing the patellafemoral contact area during weight-bearing exercise that

Box 10.7.2 Exercise prescription

1. Refer to health professional for appropriate exercise prescription
2. Recommend supervised group or individual treatments, which are superior to independent home exercise for pain reduction
3. Supplement home exercise with initial group exercise
4. Do not depend entirely on exercise handouts or audiovisual material, which alone are ineffective
5. Target quadriceps, hamstrings, and hip abductors for strengthening
6. Minimize compressive joint forces
7. Remember that the type of strengthening exercise does not influence clinical outcome
8. Use a combined program of strengthening, flexibility, and functional exercises
9. Employ strategies to maximize long-term patient compliance to exercise.

Table 10.7.3 OARSI non-surgical recommendations for the optimal management of hip and knee osteoarthritis[a]

General	A combination of non-pharmacological and pharmacological modalities is required
Non-pharmacological	Patients should be given access to information and education about the objectives of treatment and the importance of changes in lifestyle, exercise, pacing of activities, weight reduction, and other measures
	The initial focus should be on self-help and patient-driven treatments and on adherence to the regimens, including regular phone contact
	Patients may benefit from referral to a physical therapist for evaluation and instruction in appropriate exercises to reduce pain, improve functional capacity, and provision of walking aids
	Patients should be encouraged to undertake, and continue to undertake, regular aerobic, muscle strengthening, and range of motion exercises. For patients with symptomatic hip OA, exercises in water can be effective
	Patients with hip and knee OA, who are overweight, should be encouraged to lose weight and maintain their weight at a lower level
	Patients should be given instruction in the optimal use of a cane or crutch in the contralateral hand with frames or wheeled walkers for those with bilateral disease
	In patients with knee OA and mild/moderate varus or valgus instability, a knee brace can reduce pain, improve stability, and diminish the risk of falling
	Patients should receive advice concerning appropriate footwear and insoles
	Thermal modalities, TENS, and acupuncture may be effective for relieving symptoms
Pharmacological	Acetaminophen/paracetamol (up to 4g/day) can be an effective initial oral analgesic for treatment of mild to moderate pain
	NSAIDs should be used at the lowest effective dose and their long-term use should be avoided if possible. In patients with increased gastrointestinal risk, either a COX-2 selective agent or a non-selective NSAID with co-prescription of a proton pump inhibitor or misoprostol for gastroprotection may be considered, but NSAIDs, including both non-selective and COX-2 selective agents, should be used with caution in patients with cardio-vascular risk factors
	Topical NSAIDs and capsaicin can be effective as adjunctives and alternatives to oral analgesic/anti-inflammatory agents in knee OA
	IA injections with corticosteroids can be used in patients have moderate to severe pain not responding satisfactorily to oral agents or in patients with an effusion due to knee OA or other signs of local inflammation
	IA injections with hyaluronate may be useful in patients with knee or hip OA
	Treatment with glucosamine and/or chondroitin sulphate may provide symptomatic benefit in patients with knee OA. If no response is apparent within 6 months treatment should be discontinued. Diacerein may have structure-modifying effects in patients with symptomatic OA of the hip
	The use of weak opioids and narcotic analgesics can be considered for the treatment of refractory pain Non-pharmacological therapies should be continued in such patients and surgical treatments should be considered

[a]Adapted from Zhang, W., Moskowitz, R.W., Nuki, G., *et al.* (2008). OARSI recommendations for the management of hip and knee osteoarthritis, Part II: OARSI evidence-based, expert consensus guidelines. *Osteoarthritis Cartilage* **16**, 137–62.
IA, intra-articular.

involves knee flexion rather than maintaining the alignment of the patella.

At the initiation of the gait, the heel strike transient represents the ground reaction force at the point of initial ground contact and is attenuated by many factors including the heel fat pad. The use of viscoelastic insoles lead to a more gentle heel strike moment. The use of lateral or medial wedged insoles to counter degrees of malalignment has not been shown to produce meaningful symptomatic benefit.

Analgesics

The role of analgesics has been questioned by the observation that patients treated with a NSAID had reduced joint pain but an increase in the medial joint loading, with the potential of accelerating progression. NSAIDs and COXII inhibitors are also associated with significant side effects and careful use is advocated by national guidance. The use of topical agents represents an alternative route of administration for NSAIDs and they are better tolerated with fewer side effects and good short-term pain relief. Other topical agents such as capsacin work by initiating an intense local irritation that then depletes substance P. These agents need to be applied three to four times a day to maintain efficacy.

Intra-articular therapies

A number of intra-articular agents have been used in OA. Corticosteroids have a good short- to medium-term effect in reducing pain and improving function. The current guidance is to limit injections to four a year. Hyaluronic acid derivatives have been used to inject large joints and while they improve pain and function do not appear to have a disease-modifying role.

Nutritional supplements

Ongoing trials are evaluating the benefit of vitamin D supplementation. Vitamin K use has not been shown to be beneficial in the general population. Other micronutrients such as selenium, carotene, and vitamin E and C have not been clearly proven to improve clinical outcomes.

Complementary therapies

A large number of complementary therapies have been used in the treatment of OA pain including glucosamine, chondroitin, avocado-soybean; however none have been robustly shown to improve clinical outcomes.

Summary

Although OA is the commonest arthritis globally, we still have little understanding of why patients develop the disease, why symptoms occur in some not others, and how to predict those that will develop severe symptomatic disease. This limitation of understanding has restricted the development of clinically effective interventions to date. In contrast, there is an historical low level of utilization of non-pharmacological interventions which have been shown to improve symptoms. There is an urgent need to combine universal implementation of recent guidance together with translation research to improve patient outcomes in OA.

Further reading

Frost, H.M. (2001). From Wolff's law to the Utah paradigm: insights about bone physiology and its clinical applications. *Anatomical Record*, **262**, 398–419.

Hawker, G.A., Wright, J.G., Badley, E.M., and Coyte. P.C. (2004). Perceptions of, and willingness to consider, total joint arthroplasty in a population-based cohort of individuals with disabling hip and knee arthritis. *Arthritis and Rheumatism*, **51**, 635–41.

Hunter, D.J. (ed) (2009). Osteoarthritis. *Medical Clinics of North America*, **93**(1), 1–244.

Zhang, W., Moskowitz, R.W., Nuki, G., *et al.* (2008). OARSI recommendations for the management of hip and knee osteoarthritis, Part II: OARSI evidence-based, expert consensus guidelines. *Osteoarthritis Cartilage*, **16**, 137–62.

SECTION 11

Infection, Amputation, and Prostheses

11.1

Chronic long bone osteomyelitis

Peter Calder

Summary points

Pathological features of chronic osteomyelitis

- Necrotic bone
- Compromised soft tissues with reduction in vascularity
- Ineffective host response
- Sequestrum formation
- New bone formation from viable periosteum and endosteum
- Formation of involucrum:

Treatment principles in chronic osteomyelitis

- Surgical debridement – remove all devitalized necrotic tissue
- Dead space management:
  - Soft tissue defect – avoid healing by secondary intention. Consider local and free flaps
  - Bone defects – small structural with autologous bone graft, consider Papineau 'open bone grafting' where free tissue transfer is not an option, distraction osteogenesis with bifocal and bone transport for large defects including fibula transfer
- Bone stability – movement needs to be eliminated
- Antibiotic therapy – based on culture and sensitivity, local administration with PMMA beads or collagen sponge, Lautenbach procedure in resistant cases.

Introduction

Prolonged infection of bone differs from 'acute osteomyelitis' not simply by duration of symptoms but also because of pathognomonic pathological, clinical, and radiological features.

Pathology

Necrotic bone with compromised soft tissues produces the features of chronic osteomyelitis. Infection may arise either from haematogenous spread, direct inoculation (through trauma), or by contiguous spread.

The dead bone becomes isolated by fibrous tissue and chronic inflammatory cells forming inflammatory granulation tissue with a resultant decrease in vascularization. This prevents an effective inflammatory response, reduces delivery of antibiotics to the area of infection, and leads to a decrease in dead bone resorption. Thus non-viable tissue with an ineffective host response results in chronic disease. The persistent dead bone is known as the *sequestrum*. Due to the decreased blood supply and poor resorption it will appear sclerotic. Erosion can occur after time due to the invading granulation tissue.

New bone formation occurs from surviving periosteum and endosteum in response to the infection and increased vascularity. The periosteal bone produced may encase the dead bone, this is known as the *involucrum*. This is disorganized and irregular and may be punctuated by tracks through which pus may drain. The involucrum may enlarge both in size and thickness sufficiently to become a 'new' shaft of bone. Endosteal bone can result in obliteration of the medullary canal.

Clinical features

Systemic features of infection may or may not be present. Local infected foci can be painful with associated purulent discharge emanating from connecting sinuses. Soft tissue changes include thickening from scarring of muscle and subcutaneous tissue. There may be joint contracture and/or skin adherence to underlying bone. Pathological fracture may occur.

Following treatment the infection is stated to be 'arrested' rather than 'cured' as subsequent host suppression can lead to a further exacerbation of infection from residual dormant organisms.

Box 11.1.1 Pathological features of chronic osteomyelitis

- Necrotic bone
- Compromised soft tissues with reduction in vascularity
- Ineffective host response
- Sequestrum formation
- New bone formation from viable periosteum and endosteum
- Formation of involucrum.

Investigations

Laboratory studies

Non-specific inflammatory markers including white cell count, erythrocyte sedimentation rate, and C-reactive protein. These generally offer no indication of severity of infection. In an acute phase of osteomyelitis, blood cultures may yield a causative organism.

Imaging

- *Plain radiographs.* These can demonstrate bone destruction but changes lag behind the onset of infection by at least 2 weeks. Soft tissue swelling and periosteal elevation may be seen as an initial change. Lytic changes require up to 75% of the bone to be lost before becoming apparent on the radiograph. The necrotic bone will have characteristic sclerosis with isolated sequestra separate from surrounding bone
- *Technetium-99m isotope bone scan.* There will be increased uptake in areas of increased blood flow or osteoblastic activity. The scan is, however, non-specific for osteomyelitis—decreased uptake may highlight sequestra
- *Computed tomography.* Bone images enable dead bone and sequestra to be delineated (Figure 11.1.1)
- *Magnetic resonance imaging.* This provides more accurate limits of bone and soft tissue involvement by the visualization of oedema on T_2-weighted images. Sinus tracts will also appear as areas of increased intensity (Figure 11.1.2)
- *Sinogram.* Continuity between skin and underlying sequestra can be highlighted and aid in operative planning. At the time of surgery, injection of methylene blue into the sinus tracts allows clear boundaries of involved tissue during surgical debridement ensuring excision of all devitalized and scarred tissue (Figure 11.1.3)
- *Biopsy.* Removal of infected tissue with culture and sensitivity is important in both confirmation of diagnosis and ensuring correct antibiotic administration.

Classification

Cierny and Mader developed a classification which takes into account both the physiological condition of the host, the functional impairment caused by the disease, the site of involvement, and the extent of bony necrosis. All influence outcome and by association enable comparison of treatment protocols.

- Physiological class:
  - *A host*: normal, immunocompetent with good local vascularity
  - *B host*: compromised, local (L) or systemic (S) factors that compromise immunity or healing
  - *C host*: prohibitive, minimal disability with morbidity expected or poor prognosis for cure
- Anatomical type:
  - *I—medullary*: lesion is endosteal with splinter sequestra within the canal
  - *II—superficial*: a true contiguous focus lesion. Compromised soft tissue results in an exposure of the underlying bone
  - *III—localized*: full thickness, cortical sequestration, and/or cavitation. The discrete lesion is within a stable bony segment
  - *IV—diffuse*: the lesion is permeative and circumferential. Instability is present either before or after thorough debridement. Stabilisation therefore is an essential factor in the treatment and thus differentiates a diffuse lesion from the other types

By combination of the physiological class (A–C) and anatomical type (I–IV) one of 12 clinical stages may be defined (Figure 11.1.4).

Treatment

The principles of treatment include eradication of all infected dead bone and scarred devitalized soft tissue (including contaminated hardware removal). Antibiotic therapy is administered sensitive to

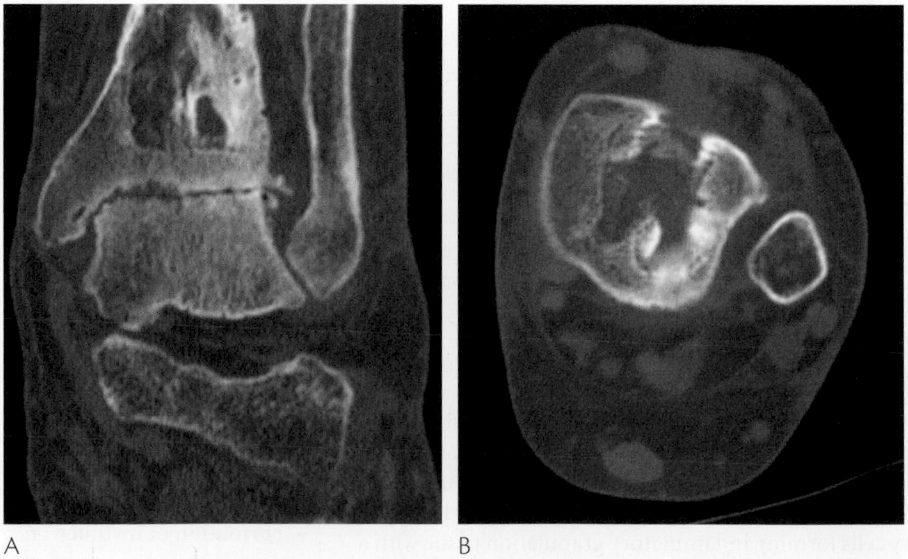

Fig. 11.1.1 Computed tomography scan demonstrating cortical destruction due to chronic osteomyelitis. Note also loss of articular cartilage due to spread to ankle joint.

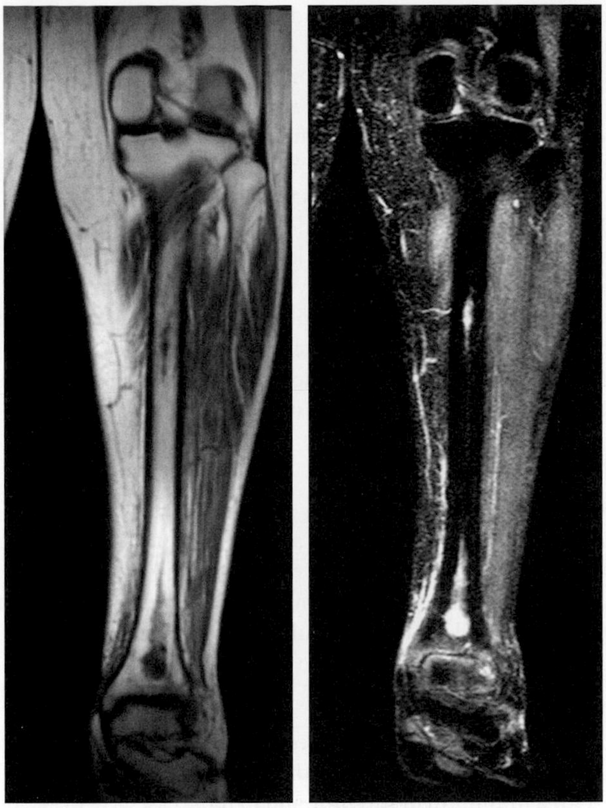

A B

Fig. 11.1.2 Magnetic resonance image showing oedema within the distal metaphysis. Note also involvement of the proximal tibia.

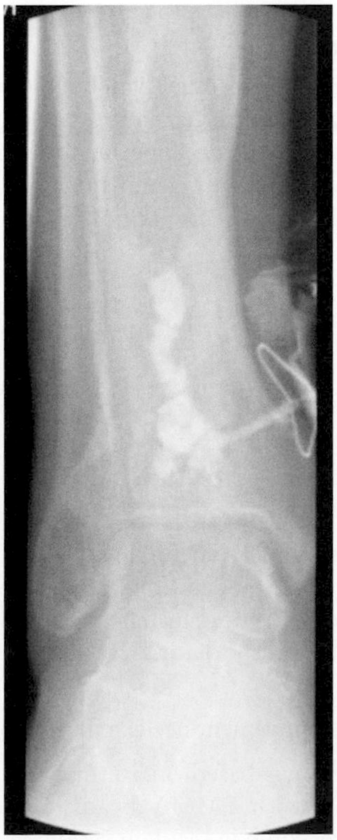

Fig. 11.1.3 Sinogram demonstrating continuity with metaphyseal infection.

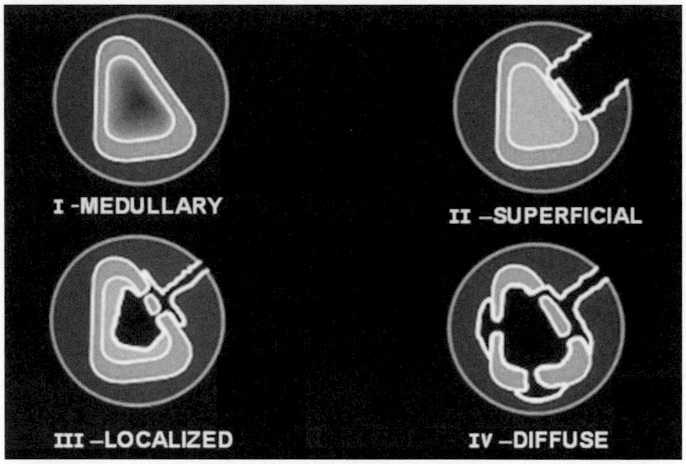

Fig. 11.1.4 Anatomical types of chronic osteomyelitis.

the causative organism; this can be either systemic or applied locally. Reconstruction of the limb requires achievement of a viable vascular environment and management of the resultant soft tissue and bone 'dead space' following debridement. Ideally a multidisciplinary approach best serves these complex problems, including a microbiologist interested in bone infection, plastic surgeon, and orthopaedic surgeon.

Surgical debridement

Skin incisions should allow direct exposure of the nidus avoiding devitalization of viable bone and soft tissues by raising unnecessary flaps. All sequestra, purulent material, and scarred and necrotic tissue is removed. Excise all sinus tracks. Sclerotic end caps over the intramedullary canal, from endosteal new bone formation, should be opened to encourage revascularization within the canal. Viable bone will demonstrate the 'paprika' sign with visible bleeding from the cut edges. This aids demarcation of healthy tissue and excision margins.

Inadequate debridement can lead to recurrence. Wide resection of greater than 5mm margins from devitalized bone have been shown to significantly reduce this risk.

Repeat debridement may be required prior to definitive soft tissue cover.

Dead space management

Soft tissue

Healing by secondary intention is to be avoided due to the resultant scar tissue which may be avascular and increase risk of recurrent infection.

Coverage of soft tissue defects may require local tissue flaps or, in larger deficits, microvascular free flaps. These can be combined with associated vascularized bone transfer such as fibula or rib (with attached intercostal muscle pedicle), to treat significant bone loss.

Bone defects

In the cases of small structural defects reconstruction may be achieved with autologous cancellous bone placed under viable soft tissue.

Where a free tissue transfer is *not* a treatment option and local flaps are inadequate 'open cancellous grafts' can be considered. After initial debridement, granulation tissue is allowed to form at the base of the defect. Grafting is then placed on top of this vascular bed with protection by antibiotic-soaked dressings. These are changed every 3–5 days until the graft has stabilized. Occasionally, spontaneous epithelialization occurs; otherwise formal skin grafting covers the area.

In large bone defects the Ilizarov method may be used. Distraction osteogenesis can reconstruct both bony continuity and restore limb length. Bifocal treatment involves acute closure of the bone defect following debridement with an osteotomy and gradual lengthening through normal healthy bone undertaken either proximally or distally to the infected area (Figure 11.1.5). When the defect is too large for an acute closure then bone transport can be undertaken. A segment of viable bone is transported through the tissues, either in an antegrade or retrograde direction, producing new bone in its wake. The transport doughnut then 'docks' with the opposing segment and heals. One main disadvantage using these methods is the time in frame waiting for sufficient stability to occur as the regenerate consolidates before the frame can be safely removed. An estimate can be made of 30–40 days in the frame per centimetre of new bone formed. An alternative is to transport the fibula en bloc to fill a massive tibial defect utilizing the ring external fixator. Distraction osteogenesis also stimulates neoangiogenesis and this increased vascularity induces an improved host response with accompanying improved delivery of antibiotics leading to the saying 'infection burns in the fire of regenerate'.

Bone stability is essential as movement may enhance infection and delay healing. Internal fixation can be used but bacteria can adhere to implants utilizing a glycocalyx which protects from the effects of local antibiotics. Due to an absence of blood supply, systemic antibiotics also fail. External fixators are therefore the method of choice in achieving adequate bone stability: either monolateral (especially in the femur) or ring fixators can be used.

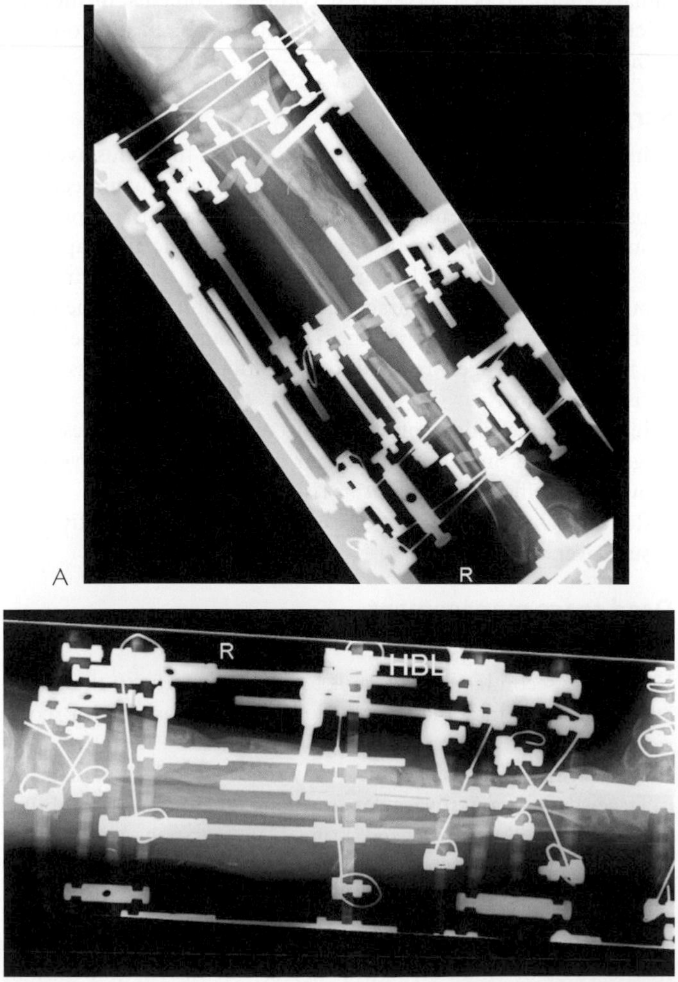

Fig. 11.1.5 Bifocal treatment of distal tibial osteomyelitis. The necrotic area is excised. The healthy bone ends acutely opposed. Lengthening proximally restores length.

Antibiotic therapy

When/which?

Ideally antibiotics should not be administered until bone bacterial culture and sensitivities are known. Broad spectrum antibiotics can be commenced immediately following debridement and harvesting of specimens until the biopsy results are known when the optimum antibiotic may be given on advice from the microbiologist.

Duration

Following debridement bone takes, in general, 3–4 weeks for revascularization to take place. Antibiotics should therefore be administered for a minimum of this time and in most cases a 6-week course is advised. Long-term parental use can be facilitated by insertion of a Hickman catheter or long line. Oral therapy can be considered, often after a 2-week course of intravenous antibiotics. Occasionally, combination therapy is advocated, for example, vancomycin and rifampicin in the treatment of methicillin resistant *Staphylococcus aureus.*

Local administration

This can be provided by using polymethylmethacrylate (PMMA) antibiotic bead chains or collagen-impregnated sponges. Antibiotic concentration has been shown to be 200 times higher at local sites than levels achieved with intravenous therapy. Aminoglycosides are most commonly employed, specifically gentamicin. The antibi-

Box 11.1.2 Treatment principles in chronic osteomyelitis

- Surgical debridement—remove all devitalized necrotic tissue
- Dead space management:
  - Soft tissue defect—avoid healing by secondary intention. Consider local and free flaps
  - Bone defects—small structural with autologous bone graft, consider Papineau 'open bone grafting' where free tissue transfer is not an option, distraction osteogenesis with bifocal and bone transport for large defects including fibula transfer
- Bone stability—movement needs to be eliminated
- Antibiotic therapy—based on culture and sensitivity, local administration with PMMA beads or collagen sponge, Lautenbach procedure in resistant cases.

otic levels diminish 2–4 weeks following placement and therefore ideally the PMMA beads should be removed. If infection persists then replacements can be placed following further debridement until the tissues are suitable for definitive reconstruction.

The Lautenbach procedure has been shown to be successful in treating long-standing infection when debridement and antibiotics have failed. Following intramedullary reaming, two double-lumen tubes are placed proximally and distally within the long bone traversing the whole canal. The outer tube is perforated at intervals and is used to drain the effluent. The inner tube is used to administer the antibiotics. The system provides a continuous circulation within the intramedullary cavity. Free drainage is performed for 30min every 4h. Irrigation fluid samples are taken twice weekly for culture and the tubes are removed after three negative cultures.

Miscellaneous

Brodie's abscess

This is a localized abscess that presents with pain but often the patients have no systemic signs. Typically there is a single lytic lesion located near the metaphysis of a long bone. *Staphylococcal aureus* is the commonest organism and simple debridement is often curative with appropriate antibiotics.

Sclerosing osteomyelitis of Garré

Radiographically there is thickening and distension but abscesses and sequestra are absent. The cause is thought to be due to a low-grade infection but cultures following biopsy are often negative. Patients present with pain and swelling but there is no accepted treatment; fenestration of the bone may be helpful.

Chronic recurrent multifocal osteomyelitis

Described as inflammation of the bone, this is similar to osteomyelitis but without infection present. It presents with insidious onset of pain at different sites. The natural history is for fluctuating symptomatic episodes resolving spontaneously after approximately 2 years. Treatment is aimed at pain control with non-steroidal anti-inflammatory medication. There is no use for antibiotics.

Further reading

Cierny, G., Mader, J.T., and Pennick, H. (1985). A clinical staging system of adult osteomyelitis. *Contemporary Orthopaedics*, **10**, 17–37.

Hashmi, M.A., Norman, P., and Saleh, M. (2004). The management of chronic osteomyelitis using the Lautenbach method. *Journal of Bone and Joint Surgery*, **86B**, 269–75.

Paley, D., Catagni M.A., Argnani F., *et al.* (1989). Ilizarov treatment of tibial nonunions with bone loss. *Clinical Orthopaedics and Related Research*, **241**, 146–65.

Shiha, A.E., Khalifa, A.R., Assaghir, Y.M., *et al.* (2008). Medial transport of the fibula using the Ilizarov device for reconstruction of a massive defect of the tibia in two children. *Journal of Bone and Joint Surgery*, **90B**, 1627–30.

Simpson, A.H.R.W., Deakin, M., and Latham, J.M. (2001). Chronic osteomyelitis: the effect of the extent of surgical resection on infection-free survival. *Journal of Bone and Joint Surgery*, **83B**, 403.

11.2

Miscellaneous orthopaedic infections

Sally Tennant and Peter Calder

Summary points

- Clinical features and treatment of: leprosy; brucellosis; syphilis of bone and joints; hydatid disease of the bone; mycetoma; salmonella infection; staphylococcus aureus infections associated with Panton-Valentine leucocidin; Poliomyelitis; Tuberculosis.

Leprosy

Leprosy is one of the oldest diseases known, and there are currently estimated to be 12–15 million cases worldwide.

Microbiology and pathology

The causative organism is *Mycobacterium leprae.* It is of very low virulence, and the incubation period varies from 3–5 years for tuberculoid leprosy and 9–11 years for lepromatous leprosy. Human beings are the only significant reservoir of the bacterium, and transmission is mainly by droplet spread and human contact via broken skin and nodules.

M. leprae selectively invades nerves. The extent of damage depends on the cell-mediated immunologic response of the patient. If immunity is high, bacterial multiplication is arrested early and a localized form of the disease results (tuberculoid type). An active granulomatous response occurs with destruction of axons and early neurological deficit results. If immunity is low, a severe and generalized form of the disease results (lepromatous type) with no immune response and no neural damage. These two types form the ends of the clinical spectrum of the disease, with intermediate types being described, and clinical presentation is varied.

Mixed nerve trunks are usually involved, at subcutaneous sites, often close to tight osteofascial canals or joints where the inflamed and swollen nerves are prone to further damage by joint motion and external trauma (Figure 11.2.1). The nerves involved are, in order of frequency, the ulnar nerve above the elbow (high ulnar type) or at the wrist (low ulnar type), the median nerve at the wrist, the common peroneal nerve at the fibular neck, the facial nerve, and the radial nerve.

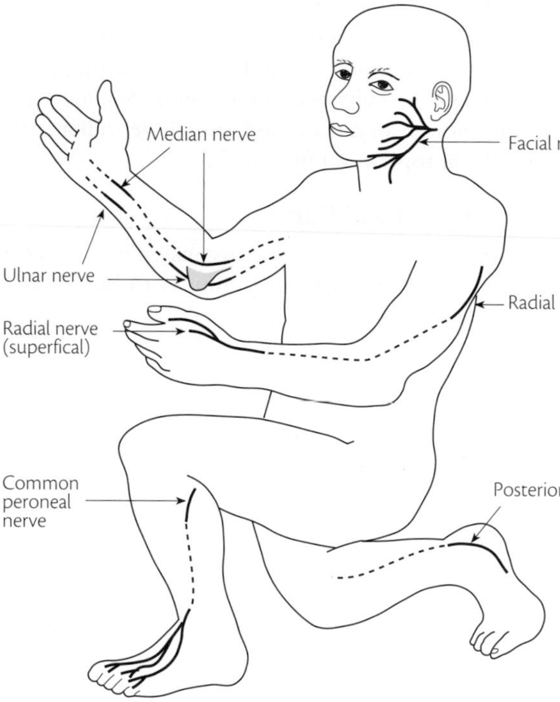

Fig. 11.2.1 The most common sites of affliction of the nerve trunks are all superficial and at osteofascial canals which are close to joints. This makes the inflamed nerves susceptible to repetitive trauma.

Clinical features and treatment

The hand

The neurological deficit in leprosy is often apparent as a claw hand. The commonest combination of deficit is a high ulnar and a low median nerve paralysis. Radial nerve involvement is less common and only occurs in combination with involvement of the other two nerves.

Corrective surgery may be performed after there is a good clinical response to leprosy treatment, with no tenderness over the nerve trunks and no history of neuritis during the preceding 6 months. Surgical procedures are designed to restore grasp and pinch.

The foot

Foot drop is the commonest deformity, resulting from involvement of the common peroneal nerve as it crosses the fibular neck. Rarely, tibial nerve involvement at the level of the ankle joint produces complete intrinsic muscle paralysis of the foot resulting in clawing of the toes. The development of a neuropathic foot leads to secondary deformities in untreated cases.

Ulcers are common in the anaesthetic foot, particularly in the presence of deformity, and occur particularly over pressure points. Skeletal deformities must be appropriately corrected so that high pressure zones are removed, and prevention depends on education in the importance of proper care of the foot.

Treatment in the acute situation may involve irrigation, drainage, and antibiotics. In the case of a chronic ulcer, thorough cleaning and debridement of all necrotic and infected tissues is performed, with elevation and daily dressings. The leg is then protected in a well-moulded below-knee walking cast.

Brucellosis

Various strains of *Brucella* can affect the joints and cause osteomyelitis. The lumbar spine or sacroiliac joints are commonly involved (Figure 11.2.2). Brucellosis may cause a monoarticular arthritis with isolation of the pathogen, or a polyarticular reactive arthritis where no organism is isolated. Differentiation from tuberculosis can be difficult, but characteristically brucellosis produces a combination of lytic and blastic lesions. X-rays show early bone repair with dense sclerosis and syndesmophytes. The characteristic radiological feature is erosion of the anterosuperior margin of the vertebral body (Pons sign) with rounding of the corner and decrease in the disc space. Doxycycline alone, or combined with streptomycin or gentamicin is usually effective.

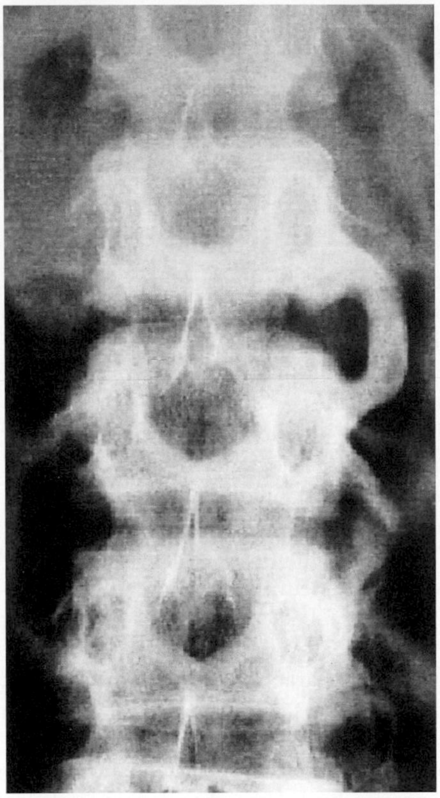

Fig. 11.2.2 Extensive brucellosis infection of the lumbar spine. There is less vertebral destruction than in tuberculosis infection, and there is prominent new bone formation with significant bridging spondylophytes (parrot beak appearance) even before complete cure of the disease.

Syphilis of bone and joints

Syphilis is caused by the spirochete *Treponema pallidum* and is sexually transmitted. The blood-borne organism lodges in the vascular metaphysis and produces a low-grade inflammatory response. In patients with inadequate host-defences, extensive necrosis of periosteum and bone occur with a yellowish gummatous sticky exudate (gumma). Beyond the central area of necrosis, an osteoblastic reaction is characteristic.

In the child, infection of the metaphysis interferes with endochondral ossification, with granulation tissue invading the zone of calcified cartilage. The long bones are particularly involved, especially the tibia, and the skull and nasal bones. The child with early congenital syphilis presents with a large tender swelling and reluctance to move the limb. Radiographs are typical, showing lucency of the metaphysis with sclerosis at the epiphyseal border. A fracture of the epiphysis may occur. Treatment usually produces rapid recovery with little subsequent interference with growth.

In late congenital syphilis, osteoblastic changes around the tibia, femur, and skull are seen. Asymmetric periosteal bone formation in the tibia produces bowing (saber shin). The phalanges and metacarpals appear spindle-shaped. Painless effusions of the knee may be seen in the second decade (Clutton's joints). Little residual damage is usually seen, and the child remains well.

In an adult, bone and joint lesions occur many decades after the primary stage, and are characterized by thickening of skull and

Box 11.2.1 Leprosy

- Caused by *Mycobacterium leprae*
- Low virulence, incubation period 3–5 years
- Selective invasion of nerves
- Upper limb—claw hand due to high ulnar lesion
- Lower limb—drop foot due to peroneal nerve involvement
- Tibial nerve involvement can result in neuropathic ulcers.

Box 11.2.2 Syphilis

- Caused by the spirochete *Treponema pallidum*
- Metaphyseal bone involvement, bone necrosis with a yellow gummatous exudates
- Lucency with surrounding sclerosis
- Asymmetrical periosteal bone formation in the tibia produces characteristic bowing (saber shin)
- Peripheral neuropathic changes can result in Charcot joints.

long bones without pain or inflammation. Extensive necrosis of bone occasionally leads to a draining sinus. Joints are involved only secondarily by direct extension. Peripheral neuropathic changes produce Charcot joints.

T. pallidum is highly sensitive to penicillin and the disease is completely curable.

Hydatid disease of the bone

Hydatid disease is caused by the parasitic tapeworm, *Echinococcus*, and is transmitted in the faeces of hosts such as dogs. Skeletal hydatidosis is rare (0.5–4%). There is a latent period of many years or decades before symptoms manifest, so that it is only seen in the second to fourth decades.

The vertebrae, long bones, the pelvis, skull, and ribs are affected in descending order of frequency. Extension of the cyst occurs along the medullary canal, but once the cortex is breached, the cyst expands into adjacent soft tissues. Cysts elsewhere are usual (liver and lung). Clinical presentation is usually with a pathological fracture or pressure over a neurovascular structure.

Radiographs show lucent areas with thinned out cortices and expansion of the bone. Resorption of bone without a periosteal or sclerotic reaction is characteristic (Figure 11.2.3). Calcification within soft tissue shadows is reported to be an important diagnostic sign of hydatid disease.

In the spine, the lower thoracic and lumbar vertebrae are most commonly involved. The trabeculae are eroded but the vertebrae maintain their shape until late, and the discs are relatively resistant. Large cysts form in paravertebral areas. Extension into the spinal canal often leads to neurological symptoms. Patients present with localized back pain with or without radicular pain, with paraparesis in more than 50% of cases. It is often confused with tuberculosis.

Treatment requires complete excision of the involved tissues and graft reconstruction, although this is rarely possible. Recurrence is therefore common. Drug treatment may occasionally be successful in eradicating the disease.

Mycetoma

Mycetoma is a fungal infection of the foot causing painless swelling, induration, and sinus formation with discharge of fungal grains (Figure 11.2.4). It is common in the tropics. Infection is usually via inoculation by a thorn prick; hence it is common in agricultural workers and barefoot walkers. It is caused by two main groups of organisms: the true fungi (infections termed eumycetoma) and actinomycetes (infections called actinomycetoma).

Radiographs show erosions of bone in eumycotic infections, and small cavities with sclerosis in actinomyctoic disease (Figure 11.2.5). Streptomycin or co-trimoxazole may be successful in the treatment of actinomycetoma, although eumycetomas are more resistant to chemotherapy. Surgical excision of the affected area (usually below-knee amputation) may be required in late or resistant cases.

Salmonella infection

Salmonella typhi and *S. paratyphi* can cause metastatic bone and joint infections by haematogenous spread. The long bones, chondrosternal junction, and the spine are common sites of involvement. Predisposing factors include sickle cell anaemia, young children, diabetes mellitus, and steroid therapy.

Osteomyelitis is the common mode of presentation, although septic arthritis can occur, either as direct extension from adjacent bone, or by haematogenous infection. Knee, shoulder, hip, and sacroiliac joints are commonly involved.

Salmonella gastroenteritis can also be accompanied by a reactive polyarthritis, presenting about 10 days following the gastrointestinal episode. Knees, ankles, and wrist joints are most commonly affected.

Radiographs show numerous punched out lytic lesions in the metaphysis extending into the diaphysis. Irregular sclerosis with subperiosteal bone formation is seen.

Salmonellae are highly sensitive to third-generation cephalosporins.

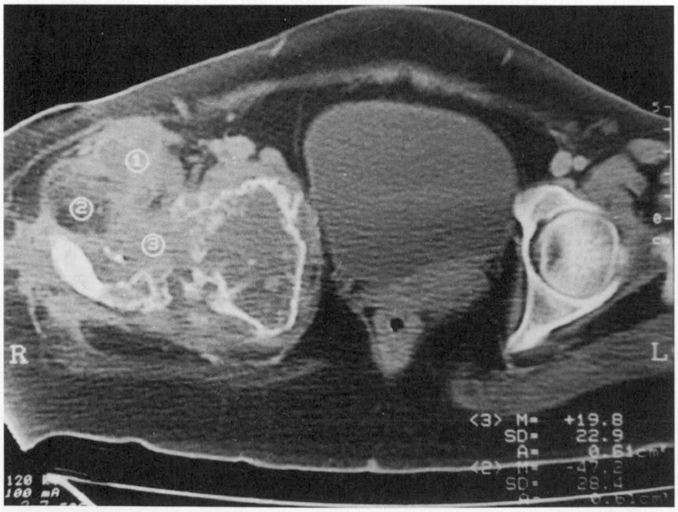

Fig. 11.2.3 Computed tomography scan of the pelvis demonstrating hydatid disease with destruction of the acetabulum.

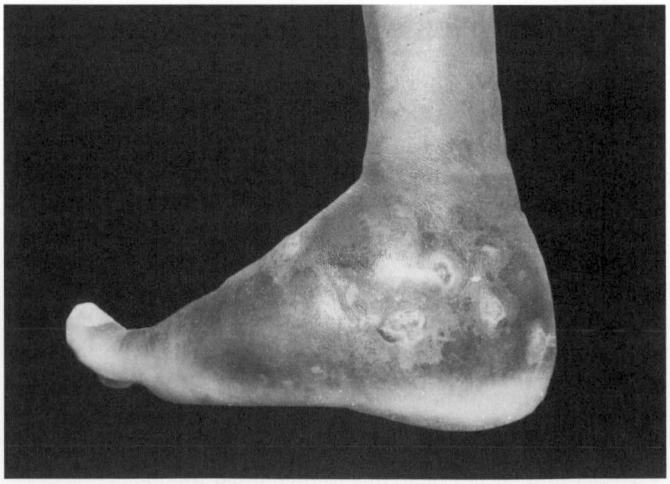

Fig. 11.2.4 Clinical picture of long-standing mycetoma showing 'tumefaction' with a swollen and misshapen foot. There are numerous closely placed sinuses extruding the characteristic granules which help in identification of the infecting organism.

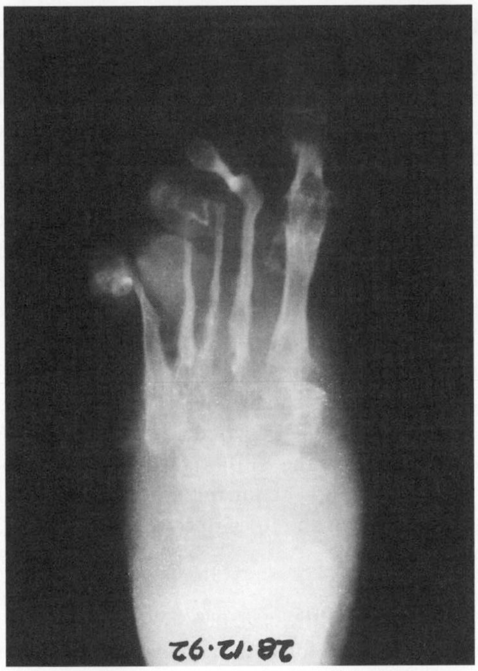

Fig. 11.2.5 In advanced mycetoma, although the foot is enormously enlarged, there is extensive destruction of the bones and the metatarsals appear thinned out. Muliple cavity formation in the tarsal bones and 'pencilling' of the metatarsals are characteristic. There is no sclerosis until super-added secondary infection occurs.

Staphylococcus aureus infections associated with Panton–Valentine leucocidin

Panton–Valentine leucocidin (PVL) is a bacterial exotoxin that is usually associated with skin and soft tissue infections and necrotizing pneumonia. However, in the last few years, an increasing number of musculoskeletal infections have been reported.

Microbiology and pathology

PVL can be secreted by methicillin-sensitive or methicillin-resistant strains of *Staphylococcus aureus*, and in Britain is secreted by 1–2% of *Staph. aureus* isolates. It produces a particularly virulent infection via leucocyte destruction, thereby impairing the immune response, and tissue necrosis. Deep venous thrombosis, septic emboli, and coagulopathy are common. In bones, intravascular coagulation means that pus rapidly becomes loculated, glutinous, and difficult to drain, and the true extent of bony and soft tissue involvement is often more extensive than suggested clinically.

Clinical presentation

Patients usually present with extremity pain with or without swelling, which may not be marked initially and may be misdiagnosed as minor trauma. If not treated appropriately and with a high index of suspicion, deterioration is rapid, with septic shock common. Full intensive care support with ventilation and inotropes may be required. Early magnetic resonance imaging (MRI) is vital to reveal the presence and extent of bone and joint involvement and guide appropriate surgery. Diagnosis requires identification of the PVL from the causative organism.

Treatment

A recent case series has emphasized the importance of early surgical intervention to debride poorly vascularized areas of infection. Joints must be aggressively and repeatedly washed out, with bones drilled and debrided thoroughly. Surgical eradication of all infected material is of paramount importance, and often requires repeated surgery. Clindamycin and rifampicin are usually advised as antistaphylococcal medication, and need to be continued for many months. Decolonization therapy in affected patients and close relatives may also be required.

The incidence of musculoskeletal complications following these severe infections is high. There should therefore be a high index of suspicion for all staphylococcal bone and joint infections, with routine requesting of the PVL status of every staphylococcal infection, early MRI scanning and aggressive surgery in positive cases.

Poliomyelitis

An acute viral infection causing neural damage to the anterior horn grey matter of the spinal cord resulting in an asymmetrical lower motor neuron palsy. The motor neuron cells are irreparably damaged or rendered temporarily functionless. Immunization has almost eradicated polio from many developed countries but it still remains prevalent in others—in India up to 150 000 new cases a year have been reported.

Stages of disease

- Acute: fever which lasts for a few days with rapid onset of flaccid paralysis. Muscles affected may be painful to passive stretch
- Recovery stage: lasts for 18 months to 2 years. Progressive recovery of muscle power, most recovery is within the first few weeks
- Permanent residual paralysis: adaptation to weakness and possible development of secondary skeletal deformity.

The lower limb is most frequently affected. Muscle imbalance results in deformity, the most common example is equinus due to paralysis of tibialis anterior with sparing of the triceps surae. Gait is affected with weakness in knee extension. Patients will walk with their hand on their affected knee preventing collapse in stance due to quadriceps weakness (Figure 11.2.6).

Progressive deformity will occur in the skeletally immature. Lack of stretch will produce a slower rate of growth of the affected muscle resulting in further contracture and possible bone deformity.

Common skeletal deformities

- Trunk: scoliosis
- Hip: flexion contracture associated with adduction/external rotation or adduction/internal rotation
- Knee: flexion, extension, valgus deformity
- Foot: equinus, calcaneus, midfoot varus and valgus
- Upper limb: pronation, supination, and/or intrinsic hand contractures.

Treatment principles

During the acute stage, appropriate splinting and limb posturing to avoid contractures. Passive range of motion exercises to minimize deformity due to muscle imbalance.

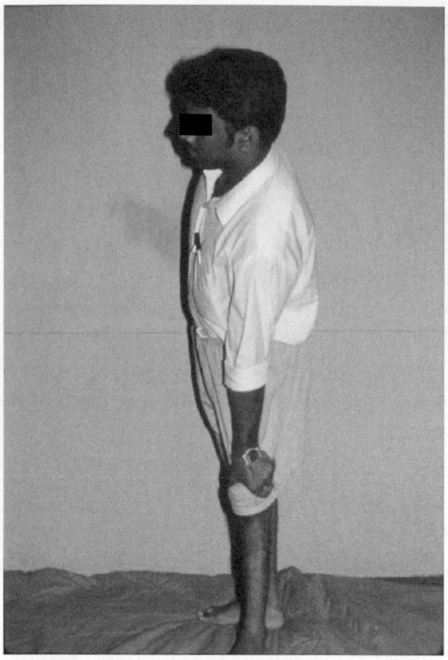

Fig. 11.2.6 A hand-on-thigh gait adopted for stabilizing the knee when the quadriceps is paralyzed.

Surgical principles

- Restoration of muscle imbalance with appropriate tendon transfers
- Joint deformity may respond to serial casting, moderate deformity corrected with tendon lengthening and capsule contracture release. Severe deformity may require corrective periarticular wedge osteotomies (e.g. supracondylar femoral extension osteotomy for knee flexion contracture)
- Joint stabilization by tendon transfer and/or orthotic support. Arthrodesis is a last resort
- Limb inequality can be achieved with shoe raises and by formal lengthening using distraction osteogenesis.

Box 11.2.3 Polio

- Viral infection
- Damage to anterior horn grey matter of spinal cord
- Stages of disease:
  - Acute fever lasts for a few days with rapid onset of flaccid paralysis
  - Recovery lasts up to 2 years, progressive recovery of muscle power
  - Permanent residual paralysis
- Immature skeleton can deform and fail to grow
- Treatment in acute phase to prevent contracture
- Surgery to restore function, tendon transfer, tendon lengthening, osteotomy, and lengthening procedures.

Tuberculosis

Tuberculosis (TB) continues to be a cause of death and disability in many parts of the world. Most commonly seen in underdeveloped countries, it is being increasingly seen in developed countries, attributed to global travel and immigration as well as increasing elderly populations and more people with suppressed immune systems—seen in patients taking immunosuppressive drugs and AIDS patients. The cause is mycobacterium, predominantly *Mycobacterium tuberculosis* (human type) although there are other types such as *M. bovis*, *M. africanum* (restricted to African countries), *M. canetti*, and *M. microti*.

Mycobacterium tuberculosis is an aerobic bacteria spread through air when affected patients cough, sneeze, or spit. It is a small rod-like bacillus and is classified as an acid-fast bacillus (AFB). The Ziehl–Neelsen stain dyes the AFB bright red. It does not grow on ordinary culture medium, requiring an enriched albumin base. There is a very slow growth rate with colonies only seen 2–4 weeks after inoculation.

Clinical manifestations

Pulmonary TB accounts for 75% of cases; skeletal tuberculosis is uncommon, involving 3–5% in total. Spinal involvement represents almost half of these cases (see Chapter 3.18). Haematogenous spread from a primary focus reaches the skeletal system by arterial vessels except the spine where spread via Batson's plexus of veins can also occur.

Systemic symptoms (Box 11.2.4) include fever, chills, night sweats, appetite loss, weight loss, and fatigue. Skeletal infection is usually mono-osseous or monoarticular. Localized symptoms characteristically involve pain and loss of function. With progression of disease, joints become deformed by destruction and assumption of a comfortable position. Joint involvement is seen to pass through characteristic stages—initial synovitis with soft tissue swelling, slight reduction in joint movement, and little pain. Early arthritis with decrease in joint space leads to advanced arthritic changes, significant restriction in movement, and increasing pain. Eventual joint destruction with minimal movement and severe pain on movement can lead to fibrous ankylosis.

Diagnosis is made with identification of the causative organism following biopsy. A high index of suspicion is often warranted in cases with minimal symptoms at presentation. A history of travel or recent immigration must be noted. The tuberculin skin test indicates exposure to the bacteria but does not indicate active disease and therefore may not be relied upon to make a diagnosis.

Treatment

Combination chemotherapy is mandatory, operative intervention is an adjunct to medical therapy. The choice of drug is dependant

Box 11.2.4 Systemic symptoms of tuberculosis

- Fever
- Night sweats
- Appetite and weight loss
- Fatigue and general malaise.

Box 11.2.5 Stages of tuberculosis arthritis

- Synovitis: minimal pain, doughy swelling, minimal loss of movement
- Early arthritis: painful movements, joint space narrowing, marginal joint erosions
- Advanced arthritis: fixed deformities seen, destruction of joint surfaces and adjoining bone
- Destruction: movements severely restricted and painful. Gross destruction of joint surfaces.

on sensitivity to the organism and must include one which is bactericidal. Multiple therapies are performed in an attempt to avoid bacterial resistance. Prolonged therapy, of several months, is necessary to eliminate small groups of 'persistent' bacilli. An initial intensive phase of three or four drugs is followed by a continuation phase of two drugs.

Surgical intervention due to the success of the chemotherapeutic drugs has a limited indication. Emergency decompression in tuberculosis paraplegia aside, abscess drainage may be conducted dependent on symptoms and functional loss and may not be required. Joint involvement requires drainage and potential debridement. Immobilization in a functional position can lead to a functional ankylosis. In the cases of joint instability, formal arthrodesis may be required. Joint arthroplasty can be considered but prolonged disease inactivity prior to surgery with 3 months of chemotherapy prior to joint replacement followed by several months of therapy postoperatively is advised.

Box 11.2.6 Primary antituberculosis chemotherapeutic drugs

- Isoniazid—bactericidal
- Rifampicin—bactericidal
- Ethambutol—bacteriostatic
- Pyrazinamide—bactericidal
- Streptomycin—bactericidal
- Para-aminosalicylic acid (PAS)—bacteriostatic.

Further reading

Antia, N.H., Enna, C.D., and Daver, B.M. (1992). *The Surgical Management of Deformities in Leprosy*. Bombay: Oxford University Press.

Arnold, S.R., Elias, D., Buckingham, S.C., *et al.* (2006). Changing patterns of acute haematogenous osteomyelitis and septic arthritis: emergence of community-associated methicillin-resistant *Staphylococcus aureus*. *Journal of Pediatric Orthopedics*, **26**, 703–8.

Fritshi, E.P and Fritschi, P. (1971). *Reconstructive Surgery in Leprosy*. Bristol: John Wright.

Gorbach, S.L., Blacklow, N.R., Zorab, R., and Bartlett, J.G. (1998). *Infectious Diseases*, second edition. Philadelphia, PA: W.B. Saunders.

Hastings, R.C. (1985). *Leprosy*. London: Churchill Livingstone.

Huckstep, R.L., (1975). *Poliomyelitis: A Guide for Developing Countries Including Appliances and Rehabilitation for the Disabled*. Edinburgh: Churchill Livingstone.

Lifeso, R.M. (1995). Current concepts review, tuberculosis of bone and joints. *Journal of Bone and Joint Surgery*, **78A**, 288–98.

Mitchell, P.D., Hunt, D.M., Lyall, H., *et al.* (2007). Panton-Valentine leukocidin-secreting *Staphylococcus aureus* causing severe musculoskeletal sepsis in children. *Journal of Bone and Joint Surgery*, **89B**, 123–42.

Moumile, K., Cadilhac, C., Lina, G., *et al.* (2006). Severe osteoarticular infection associated with Panton-Valentine leukocidin-producing *Staphylococcus aureus*. *Diagnostic Microbiology and Infectious Disease*, **56**, 95–7.

Srinivasan, H. (1993). *Prevention of Disabilities in Patients with Leprosy*. Geneva: World Health Organization.

Srinivasan, H. and Palande, D.D. (1997). *Essential Surgery in Leprosy: Techniques for the District Hospital*. Geneva: World Health Organization.

Warner, W.C. (2008). Paralytic disorders. In: Canale, S.T and Beaty, J.H. (eds) *Campbell's Operative Orthopaedics*, eleventh edition, pp. 1401–50. St Louis, MO: Mosby.

11.3

Amputations and prostheses

Rajiv S. Hanspal and Peter Calder

Summary points

- Amputation surgery should produce a new end-organ for locomotion with a prosthesis or interaction with the environment
- The choice of amputation level should be based on healing, functional expectations, and prosthetic use
- Success of rehabilitation depends on multi-disciplinary input and management of complications
- The prostheses prescribed should depend on functional need and expectation.

Introduction

Amputation, from the Latin amputare (to cut away), can be considered as one of earliest surgical procedures. Initially performed as a punishment, surgical techniques have been improved, mainly pioneered by military surgeons during the great wars, to produce functional stumps to support prosthetic wear and rehabilitation.

Indications for amputation

Amputation of a limb may be indicated to relieve symptoms (e.g. ischaemic rest pain), to remove a non-viable part of a limb (e.g. gangrene or a crushed limb), to preserve life (e.g. malignant tumour), or to improve function and quality of life (e.g. neuropathic foot or congenital limb deficiency). The commonest cause for amputation in the United Kingdom remains vascular disease (67%), including arteriosclerotic large vessel disease, and diabetic vascular disease. Only 9% of amputations are due to trauma, mainly being performed late after limb reconstruction has failed. Rarer causes include infection (7%), tumours (3%), neuropathic (1%) changes, and congenital limb deficiencies. Upper limb loss is much less frequent with a greater majority being secondary to trauma. The subject of congenital limb deficiency has been considered in Chapter 13.14.

The principles of amputation surgery

The purpose of amputation is not only to remove the diseased or damaged part of a limb to produce a healed stump, but equally to produce a new end-organ for locomotion (lower limb) or interaction with the environment (upper limb)(Box 11.3.1). Meticulous handling of the soft tissues is important to create a well healed functional stump. Tourniquet should be utilized in all cases except those with peripheral vascular disease.

Box 11.3.1 Indications for amputation

- Relieve symptoms—ischaemic pain
- Remove non-viable limb—gangrene
- Preserve life—malignancy
- Improve limb function—neuropathic foot, congenital limb deficiency.

- *Skin.* The stump should have healthy skin coverage which should be mobile and sensate. Avoidance of scar and skin adherence to the underlying bone is paramount
- *Muscle.* Conventionally the muscles are cut a few centimetres distal to the bone cut to allow retraction. The muscle can be debulked in order to reduce stump size (Figure 11.3.1). If myodesis is to be performed, as in a knee disarticulation or above-knee amputation, the muscles are cut approximately 5cm distal to the bone end to allow repair of the opposing muscles without tension
- *Nerves.* Gentle traction of the nerves before division with a sharp knife as proximal as possible to allow retraction and avoid the nerve end in the resulting scar tissue. Avoid over traction which can contribute to neuroma formation
- *Blood vessels.* Individual vessels should be ligated with either absorbable or non-absorbable sutures. Personal preference is for double ligation of major arteries. Meticulous haemostasis is required to avoid haematoma formation. Tourniquet should be released prior to muscle repair. A submuscular surgical drain should be placed
- *Bone.* Excessive periosteal stripping should be avoided. Optimum length is determined by amputation level, proximal joint function, and prosthetic requirement. For example, if no prosthesis is intended then an above-knee amputation may be made in the supracondylar region to maintain as much length as possible to aid balance.

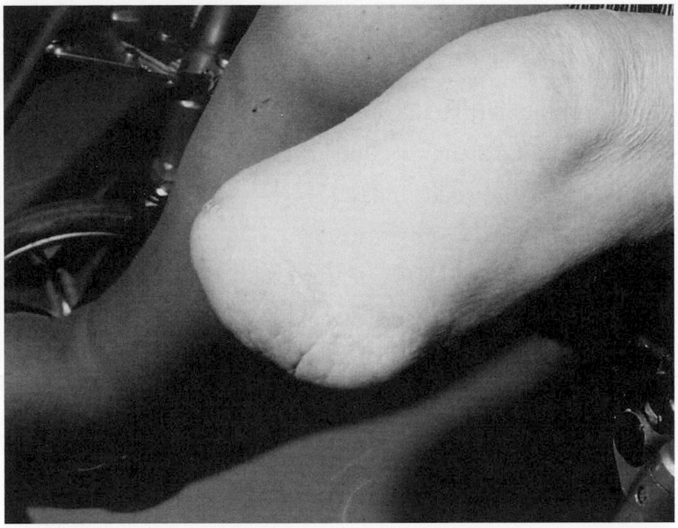

Fig. 11.3.1 Bulbous distal soft tissues in a transtibial stump will adversely affect limb fitting.

If gross contamination or major sepsis is present at the time of amputation, a delayed primary closure after 5–10 days is wise. Good perioperative pain control is essential. There is some evidence that epidural anaesthesia and analgesia in the perioperative period may reduce subsequent phantom limb pain.

Choice of amputation level

In general, amputations should be carried out at the most distal level at which healing can be achieved, though there are exceptions. An ideal stump for 'prosthetic' use of a lower limb should be of an appropriate length. In general, optimum femoral bone length is approximately 15cm proximal to knee joint level; for transtibial amputation residual bone length may be calculated as 8cm for every metre of height. Preservation of joints is important, though for prosthetic fitting adequate length and 'clearance distance', i.e. distance from the end of the amputation stump to the level of the contralateral joint line, is recommended. This is to ensure space to accommodate sophisticated prosthetic units and maintain level joints. Good end-bearing properties of through knee disarticulation, Gritti–Stokes amputation, or a Syme's amputation may be crucial to maximize function but may present problems of satisfactory appearance of the prostheses. Prostheses for Syme's amputation and knee disarticulation are cosmetically poor and these amputations should be avoided if 'cosmesis' is important.

Box 11.3.2 Principles of amputation surgery

- Skin: healthy, sensate, and repaired tension free
- Muscle: debulked to reduce stump size
- Nerves: gentle traction before division proximally with a sharp knife
- Blood vessels: double ligation
- Bone: avoid periosteal stripping with adequate length.

Fixed contractures in proximal joints compromise alignment and leads to unsatisfactory gait and weight bearing. Excessive contractures may preclude prosthetic use. For patients who are likely to walk or stand to transfer, an attempt should be made to preserve the knee joint. However, if a patient is likely to remain bed- or chair-bound, a through knee disarticulation or Gritti–Stokes amputation may be preferable to ensure satisfactory end bearing and bed mobility.

In the foot, a metatarsal amputation requires a minimum of prosthetic help and produces minimal disability. Hindfoot amputations like Chopart and Lisfranc procedures, tend to result in an equinovarus deformity, are prone to skin breakdown and are difficult to fit with a prostheses that can be worn with a normal shoe. Through hip and hindquarter amputations are fortunately rare, normally as a result of malignant disease or severe trauma. The prosthesis is required to embrace the whole pelvis and mobility remains poor.

In upper limb amputation, especially in the hand, no prostheses can adequately replace an injured hand, and so as much of the hand as possible should be preserved.

Rehabilitation

The rehabilitation programme should ideally start before the amputation. If the amputation was an elective amputation and an 'optional' treatment rather than a 'necessity', a pre-amputation consultation with the rehabilitation team is strongly recommended. Success in rehabilitation depends on the input of a multi-disciplinary team.

Physiotherapy should start early and include general mobility in bed, transfers, exercises of the stump and proximal joint, supervision of wound healing, and physical measures to control postoperative oedema. A rigid plaster of Paris dressing provides protection and reduces postoperative oedema, but there are risks of ischaemia and infection and is best avoided in dysvascular amputations, except in specialized units. Lightly elasticated tubular bandages are used followed by use of elasticated and graduated pressure stump shrinkers (e.g. Juzo™) once wound healing is ensured. Early walking aids (EWAs) allow the patients to stand and walk early with the physiotherapist and assist in control of stump oedema, improve standing and walking and morale. Commonly used types are the pneumatic post amputation mobilty (PPAM) aid (Figure 11.3.2) for the transtibial amputation with a maximum pressure of 40mmHg, or a Femurette™ for a transfemoral amputation (Figure 11.3.3).

Box 11.3.3 Amputation level

- Most distal level that healing can be achieved
- Preserve joints if possible (knee/elbow)
- Avoid amputation below joint contracture
- 'Clearance distance' to allow prosthetic joint placement
- In general:
  - 15cm proximal to knee joint for femoral stump
  - 8cm per metre of patient height for tibial stump
  - Syme's amputation gives better function than Boyd, Chopart, or Lisfranc.

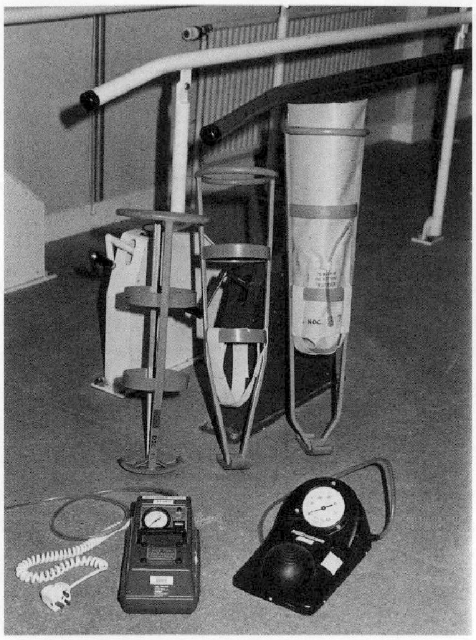

Fig. 11.3.2 The Pneumatic Post-Amputation Mobility Aid (PPAMAid) consists of an inflatable plastic sleeve within a metal frame, with rocker end.

Following provision of an appropriate prostheses, gait re-education is essential. It may be particularly complex if the prosthesis prescribed has complex components like hydraulic or microprocessor-controlled prosthetic joints. Rehabilitation should be planned with targeted goals to help the patient achieve maximum potential. Their general medical condition and presence of comorbidity are obvious influencing factors.

Commonly used outcome measures are listed in Box 11.3.4. Less commonly used outcome measures are the Trinity Amputee and Prosthetic Scales (TAPES) and the Prosthetic Profile of the Amputee Questionnaire (PPA).

Laboratory gait analysis is generally reserved for research or complex gait problems.

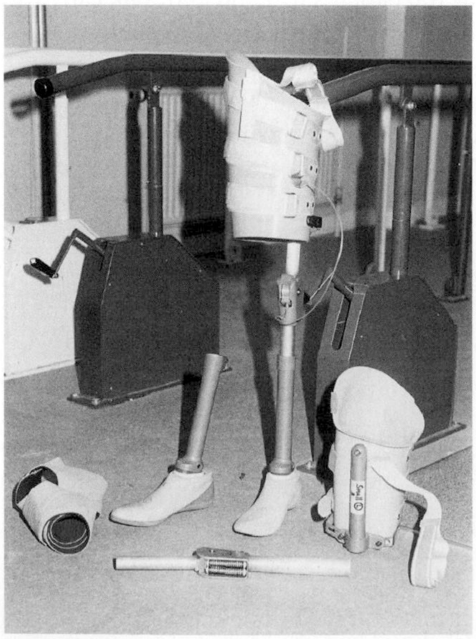

Fig. 11.3.3 Femurett early walking aid for transfemoral amputees; the length and alignment are readily adjusted using a single Allen key. Adjustable sockets in three different sizes can be interchanged quickly.

Box 11.3.4 Commonly used outcome measures in United Kingdom rehabilitation of the amputee with prostheses

- SIGAM Mobility Grade
- Harold Wood Stanmore Mobility Grade
- Locomotor Capability Index
- Timed Walking Test
- Socket Comfort Score
- Barthel Index for activities of daily living
- Hospital Anxiety & Depression Scale.

Problems following amputation

Surgical

Early

- Haematoma: avoid with meticulous haemostasis and avoidance of dead space
- Delayed healing due to ischaemia: appropriate level selection
- Infection: consider prophylactic antibiotics
- Skin necrosis: allow adequate skin flaps sutured without tension. Extensive necrosis in ischaemic limbs may indicate inadequate peripheral circulation and need to consider re-amputation at a higher level.

Late

- Soft tissue: contractures can occur if a limb is kept in a position of comfort, for example, hip flexion following above-knee amputation. Unopposed contracture of certain muscle groups can also result in joint deformity, for example, equinus deformity following Chopart amputation, hip adduction deformity following low transfemoral amputation, or hip flexion contracture following high transfemoral amputation. Muscle migration following fixation failure to bone can result in bony prominence and painful pressure points. Detachment of the myoplasty or myodesis may require revision surgery
- Epidermoid cysts, occasionally infected, may form as a result of skin movement and pressure of the brim of the socket, generally managed conservatively with socket adjustment, wound dressing, and antibiotic therapy, but if troublesome sinuses are formed, surgical intervention may be necessary
- Bursa formation over bony prominences: may need antibiotic therapy if infected or surgical excision if recurrent and refractory to conservative management
- Neuroma formation: always form at the end of the cut nerve. This is associated with excessive traction at time of division or if the end is within scar tissue
- Bone: bony spurs can occur which can produce painful pressure points. Widespread heterotopic bone formation is associated with excessive periosteal stripping. Recently heterotopic ossification (HO) has been found to be common in amputation following blast injuries.

General

- General problems include psychological problems and difficulty in accepting the limb loss. Counselling may be helpful and it is recognized that the need for psychological help is greater in traumatic amputees and in those who have had an upper limb loss and the time of this need is greatest at 12 months after the amputation
- Other problems include the increased energy requirement for walking with prostheses. This ranges from 10% over and above normal energy requirement for below-knee traumatic amputees, 60% for transfemoral amputees, to over 200% for bilateral transfemoral amputees
- Phantom sensation and phantom pain are recognized complications, though the incidence is decreasing with improved perioperative and multidisciplinary management in rehabilitation. Phantom pain may remain troublesome in 20–30% of amputees and may require various pharmacological or physical treatment modalities. Psychological therapies like distraction, relaxation, or cognitive behaviour therapy as part of a holistic pain management programme may be required in difficult cases. Rarely, nerve blocks or stimulator implants may be required.
- Increased incidence of degenerative changes in hip and knee joints and back pain due to mechanical factors from altered gait patterns are seen following long-term use of prosthesis.

Principles of prostheses

The most important part of any prosthesis is the socket, as this provides the interface between the residual limb and the prosthesis; if the socket is not comfortable, the most sophisticated prosthetic componentry will be of no benefit. Although leather and aluminium alloy are still used for some sockets, the vast majority are now made either of thermoplastic materials like polypropylene or of laminate plastic construction with glass- or carbon-fibre reinforced acrylic or polyester resin. Considerable forces have to be transmitted through the stump–socket interface of lower-limb amputees—several times body weight during vigorous activities. With the exception of amputations through or very close to joints, amputation stumps will only tolerate slight pressure directly under the distal bone end, so traditionally most sockets have been mainly proximally load-bearing, through the ischial tuberosity in the case of transfemoral, or the patellar tendon in the case of transtibial amputations. Most sockets now are of total-contact type, so that weight-bearing is spread more evenly, although the plaster cast of the stump from which the socket is made is first 'rectified', to increase loading in these tolerant areas and to reduce loading over areas such as the distal femur and head of fibula which are intolerant of pressure. Most sockets are worn over a cotton, wool, or polyurethane gel sock, but self-suspending suction sockets are worn next to the skin.

Most lower-limb prostheses used in the United Kingdom are now of endoskeletal construction, in which the socket is linked to the foot by an internal tubular structure of carbon fibre or aluminium, and this together with the joints, if applicable, and devices for adjusting the alignment of the socket and foot, are enclosed in a soft foam cosmetic cover with an outer woven, PVC, or silicone skin. Most, but not all, endoskeletal prostheses are of so-called modular construction, in which the component parts, apart from the socket, are prefabricated and clamped or bonded together, making assembly and subsequent adjustment or repair easier and quicker. In exoskeletal prostheses, the outer visible part of the prosthesis is the structural component.

The majority of upper-limb prostheses are of exoskeletal type. Even though they are much lighter than the natural limb which they replace, almost all prostheses feel heavy to the user, even more so for elderly amputees, so the aim is always to make the prosthesis as light as possible, compatible with strength. However, the extra comfort, stability, or function provided by more sophisticated componentry or socket materials often carries a weight penalty; this is the main disadvantage of electrically powered upper-limb prostheses. Summary of prostheses in Box 11.3.5.

Transtibial amputation

The two standard methods of fashioning a transtibial stump are the long posterior flap method (Figure 11.3.1), or the so-called 'skew-flap' technique (Figure 11.3.4). The difference is mainly in the skin flaps, as both employ a long posterior muscle flap, which is basically gastrocnemius, as most of the soleus should be removed distal to the level of bone section to avoid an excessively bulky distal stump. Both methods result in similar healing but the shape of the skew flap generally facilitates early limb fitting.

Most prosthesis for the transtibial amputation are endoskeletal construction and use a rigid plastic socket with cuff suspension and worn over a cotton sock. However, there is increasing use of silicone or gel liners which are worn next to the skin and also provide total contact and self-suspending properties (Figure 11.3.5). The figure describes this type of prostheses and not one with a cuff suspension.

The simplest type of prosthetic foot is the solid-ankle cushioned-heel (SACH) foot. More recently, various energy storage feet with different degrees of flexibility are available to suit different activity levels, including those for running.

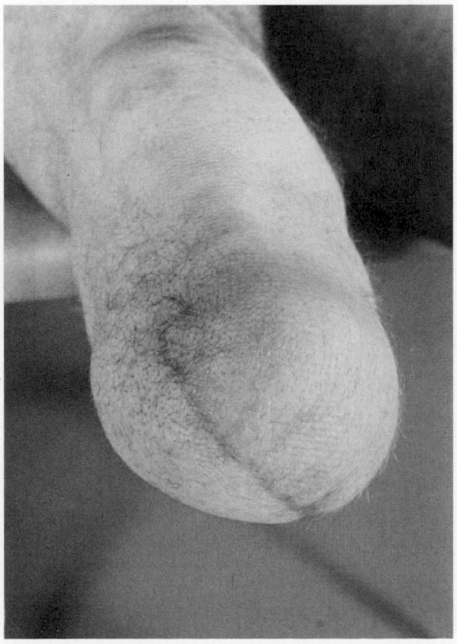

Fig. 11.3.4 Transtibial stump, fashioned by 'skewed' medial and lateral skin flaps.

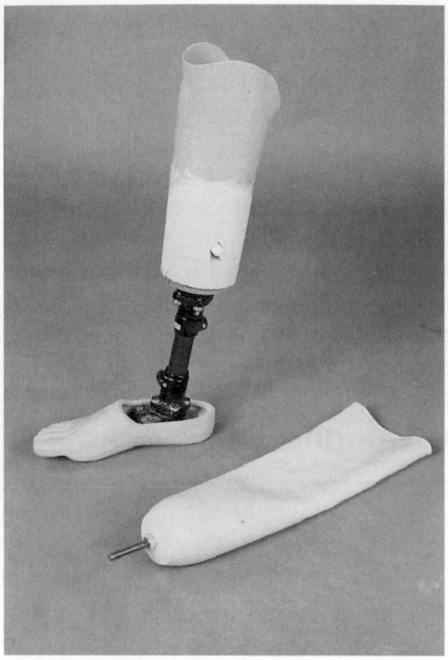

Fig. 11.3.5 Transtibial prosthesis with self suspending total contact socket with silicone liner. Note the button below the socket for releasing the spigot.

Transfemoral amputation

The choice of skin flaps is less critical than for transtibial amputation, but usually equal anterior and posterior flaps are used. The anterior and posterior muscle groups are stitched over the cut end of the bone and if vascularity is not impaired, a myodesis is performed by suturing the muscles to holes drilled into the distal femur.

Most sockets (Figure 11.3.6) are ischial bearing or ischial containment, and there is increasing use of total-contact sockets. Distal soft tissue support improves proximal comfort and avoids venous congestion and chronic oedema. The anterior wall of the socket needs to be high to avoid the ischial tuberosity slipping off the posterior seating area.

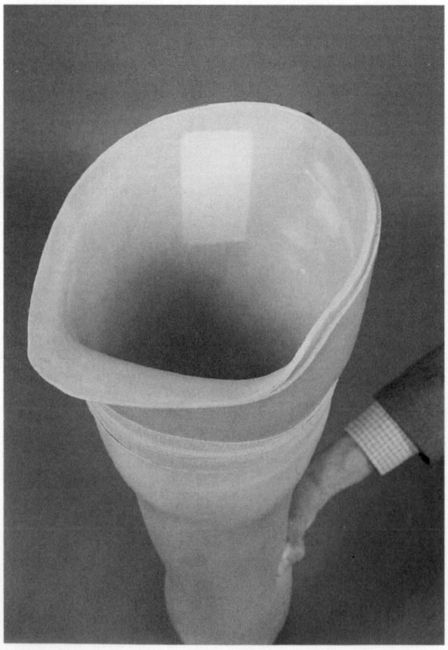

Fig. 11.3.6 Quadrilateral socket for transfemoral stump.

The prosthetic knee may be a semi-automatic locked knee which locks itself on extension and thus ensures safety in a stiff knee gait. It is unlocked for sitting. Alternatively, an optional lock may be incorporated thus giving the individual the 'option' to walk with a locked knee over difficult and uneven terrain. Fitter individuals who can control a free knee require both stance and swing phase control for optimal gait. Stance stability is largely a function of the correct alignment of the prosthesis (the weight line should be slightly in front of the knee axis when the knee is extended), but mechanical 'stabilized' knees provide enhanced stability by locking on weight-bearing even in slight flexion (up to about 25 degrees). Polycentric knees provide stance control by ensuring that the knee extends fully (usually into slight hyperextension) even if weight is placed on a slightly flexed (up to 10–15 degrees) knee. Swing-phase control can be in the form of an extension assist spring, by controlled friction, or by means of an adjustable pneumatic or hydraulic damper. An electronically-controlled pneumatic swing phase unit can be used; this measures the swing rate of the knee, and then selects the most appropriate of three preset positions (or an intermediate position) of a needle valve, to provide the optimal setting for different walking speeds. More recently, electronic knee units are available where microprocessor controls are available for both the swing and the stance phase of gait. Heavy-duty hydraulic knees, which provide both stance and swing-phase control in one unit, suit the most active users, but are heavier than other types and most require more effort to drive them. Recently introduced hydraulic knees require less effort and suit a wider range of individuals. Polycentric knees are more compact, and are indicated when clearance above the level of the sound knee is limited. The choice of prosthetic feet is similar to those described for transtibial amputations.

Upper limb amputations

Most upper-limb amputations are due to trauma, and in many cases this will determine the level of amputation and the site of the skin flaps; if there is sufficient healthy skin, equal length flaps on the flexor and extensor aspects are best.

Upper limb prostheses are generally of three types:

1) Cosmetic or passive function prostheses, where there are no moving parts and the limb is essentially for 'cosmetic appearances', though can be used in a 'passive manner'. If made of high-definition silicone, they look extremely realistic
2) Body-powered functioning prostheses with a range of different terminal appliances: many consider them cumbersome and cosmetically unacceptable but they remain most functional—the most versatile being the split hook. This type of prosthesis may be used for 'targeted function' at work or leisure
3) Myoelectric prostheses where surface electrodes are used within the socket which pick up electrical activity from the flexor and extensor muscles.

Hand

Even if the hand is severely injured, it is usually worth preserving as much of it as possible, although this may not apply if the remnant is devoid of sensation or if the wrist is immobile or flail. Even if only one digit remains, provided this has intact sensation, a simple

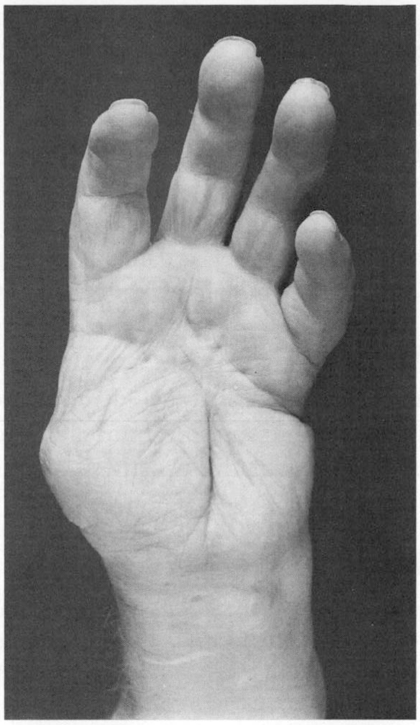

Fig. 11.3.7 Amputation of thumb.

opposition-type prosthesis can be fitted to give useful grip. Such a device would be needed if the thumb alone is lost (Figures 11.3.7 and 11.3.8), unless the index finger is to be pollicized. Loss of a single finger is not usually a great disability, except, for example, for a musician, but a minority do find this psychologically very disturbing and benefit from a silicone finger prosthesis, which can look very realistic. Recently, direct skeletal fixation of prosthetic fingers is being attempted. If all the digits are lost, a wrist-operated prosthesis can be fitted to provide useful grip.

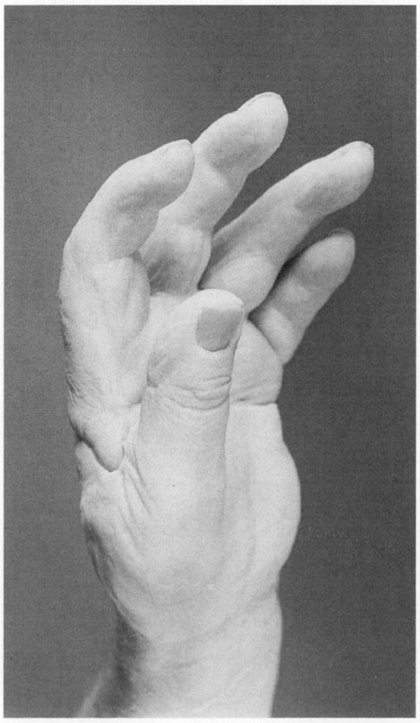

Fig. 11.3.8 Patient with amputation of thumb with silicone prosthesis.

Box 11.3.5 Summary of prostheses

- Socket:
  - Accommodates stump and interface between prosthesis and residual limb
  - Appropriate for load and pressure distribution, historically ischial tuberosity or patellar tendon bearing, now total surface bearing
  - Made of thermoplastic or composite, i.e. carbon fibre
- Suspension:
  - Rigid or soft belt
  - Self-suspension, e.g. bony contour (supracondylor supramalleolar)
  - Silicone or gel sleeves combine good skin protection and a suction concept of suspension
- Joints:
  - Knee: simple locked or free knee, single axis, four bar or multilink if space limited, hydraulic or pneumatic mechanisms more functional; these are typically weight or position activated
  - Microprocessor control of swing/stance current state of art
  - Ankle and foot: simple SACH to dynamic energy storage, or specific activity (running or water activity)
- Shaft/shank:
  - Carbon fibre, titanium, or aluminium
- Extras:
  - Torque rotator (to allow rotation of the prosthesis in vertical axis)
  - Telescopic devices for shock absorption
  - Cosmesis.

Wrist and forearm

Although a through-wrist amputation has the advantage over a transradial amputation of preserving pronation and supination, it is difficult to provide a prosthesis that is both functional and cosmetically acceptable, and the choice of prosthetic hands is much more limited. The lightest, easiest to operate, and most precise terminal appliance remains the split hook (Figure 11.3.9). This is connected by an operating cord to a loop around the opposite shoulder, and shoulder flexion or elbow extension will open the hook, which is usually closed by elastic bands (the number of bands determining the grip strength and the effort required to open the hook). These devices are described as 'voluntary opening'; voluntary closing hooks may also be used. Many, but not all, split-hook users also have a readily interchangeable cosmetic hand, which is covered in a PVC or silicone glove. Body-powered hands are heavier, provide less precise grip, and need more effort to open than split hooks, but look more natural. Electric hands provide similar function, with the option of powered wrist rotation, but many amputees reject them on account of their even greater weight. They may be operated by a switch in the prosthetic harness, or myoelectrically using

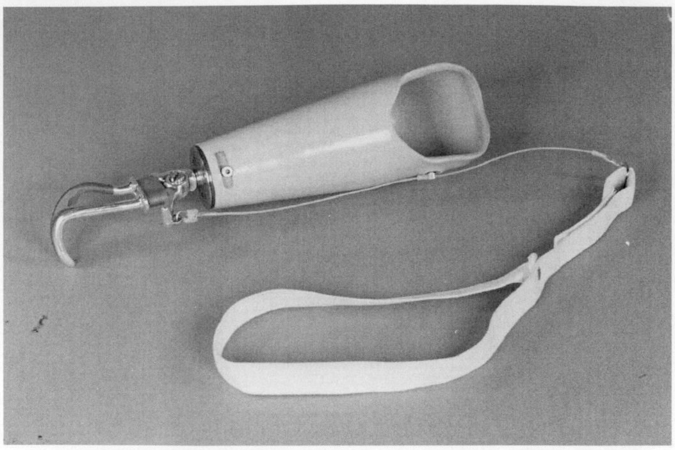

Fig. 11.3.9 Transradial prosthesis with split hook. Note operating cord and shoulder loop.

electrodes within the socket which pick up the electrical activity in the flexor and extensor muscles; this has the advantage, if a self-retaining supracondylar socket is used, of obviating the need for any harness or straps. A large variety of special attachments can be fitted to non-powered arms, such as tool holders, and appliances for driving, typing, or golf. Sockets are of rigid or flexible plastic, or leather, which is often favoured by those engaged in heavy work.

Elbow

Loss of the elbow joint results in a much greater disability, and a more cumbersome and less cosmetic prosthesis, which is more difficult to operate. Therefore the elbow joint should be preserved if at all possible, and it is worthwhile considering skin grafts and free flaps if these would make this possible. Although anaesthetic skin is a considerable disadvantage, because the loads on the skin are much less than with a lower-limb amputation, it presents fewer problems in the upper limb.

Shoulder

A functional prosthesis is not usually helpful for through-shoulder or forequarter amputations. A lightweight cosmetic arm is possible using a hollow, rigid PVC hand, and a foam shoulder cap (extending only just distal to the shoulder) is valuable for the very disfiguring forequarter amputation and allows clothes to hang normally.

Developments

Recent developments being trialled include direct skeletal fixation using osseointegration or intraosseous transcutaneous amputation prosthesis for attachment of the prosthesis to the amputation stump.

Further reading

BSRM, (2003). Amputee and Prosthetic Rehabilitation – Standards and Guidelines, 2nd Edition, Report of the Working Party (Chair: Hanspal, RS). British Society of Rehabilitation Medicine, London 2003.

Huang, C.T., Jackson, J.R., and Moore, N.B. (1979). Amputation: energy costs of ambulation. *Archives of Physical Medicine and Rehabiltation.* **60**, 18–24.

Jahangiri, M., Bradley, J.W.P., Jayatunga, A.P., and Dark, C.H. (1994). Prevention of phantom pain after major lower limb amputation by epidural infusion of diamorphine, clonidine and bupivacaine. *Annals of the Royal College of Surgeons of England,* **76,** 324–6.

Potter, B.K., Burns, T.C., Lacap, A.P., Granville, R.R., and Gajewski, D.A. (2007). Heterotopic ossification following traumatic and combat- related amputations: prevalance, risk factors and preliminary results of Excision. *Journal of Bone and Joint Surgery,* **89-A**, 476–86.

Robinson, K.P., Hoile, R., and Coddington, T. (1982). Skew flap myoplastic below knee amputation: a preliminary report. *British Journal of Surgery,* **69**, 554–7.

11.4

Acute osteomyelitis

Peter Calder

Summary points

- Bacteraemia resulting in bone deposition of bacteria
- Local bony tenderness, fever, and malaise may not be present initially
- WCC may be normal, ESR and CRP normally raised
- Plain radiographs normally take 10–12 days to occur
- Staphylococcus aureus remains the commonest organism
- Immediate antibiotics with surgical drainage of abscess formation.

Introduction

Osteomyelitis is inflammation of the bone caused by an infecting organism. It may be classified as acute, subacute, or chronic, determined by duration of symptoms.

Acute haematogenous osteomyelitis

Most commonly seen in children (see Chapter 13.1) it has a low incidence in adults following closure of the physis where capillary loops result in a predominance of metaphyseal childhood infection. In adults the immunocompromised host is most susceptible with infection seen most frequently in the elderly or adults with immune deficiency. The spine is the most common site (see Chapter 3.18) but any bone at any site may be involved. Bacteraemia results in deposition of bacteria at the sight of bone involvement but factors such as malnutrition or localized trauma may contribute to the resulting infection.

Clinical presentation

Pain with local bony tenderness but fever and malaise may not be present initially. Local swelling is associated with periosteal or soft tissue abscess formation. Associated erythema and warmth are cardinal signs of infection. There may be loss of local joint function and with extreme pain on swollen joint movement septic arthritis must be excluded, the infection extending through the bone to directly involve the joint. In long-standing cases, cortical bone destruction can lead to pathological fracture.

Investigations

- Blood tests: the white cell count may be normal. The erythrocyte sedimentation rate and C-reactive protein are usually raised
- Radiological: plain radiographs in the acute phase show no changes, Periosteal changes or cortical destruction normally take 10–12 days to occur
- Technetium-99m bone scans will demonstrate increased uptake
- Magnetic resonance imaging will show perisoteal reaction, soft tissue involvement, and bone marrow inflammation.

Microbiology

- The causative organism can be identified by blood cultures in approximately 50% of patients. Bone aspiration or pus specimens may be taken at surgical drainage
- *Staphylococcus aureus* remains the commonest causative organism in adult osteomyelitis
- *Pseudomonas* is often seen in intravenous drug abusers
- *Salmonella* osteomyelitis is reported in patients with sickle cell disease, most often affecting the diaphysis. This, however, is still less common than *Staphylococcus aureus.*

Treatment (Box 11.4.1)

- Systemic treatment should include limb splintage, analgesia, and fluid resuscitation
- Antibiotics: intravenous administration of broad spectrum antibiotics are commenced immediately after culture specimens taken (blood and/or direct bone aspiration). Change is then directed by sensitivity and specificity after culture. Continuation is generally for 6 weeks although this is controversial. Debate also is undecided over timing of change from intravenous to oral route
- Surgical drainage is indicated when significant subperiosteal or soft tissue abscesses are present. Drainage is usually via an incision centered over point of maximum tenderness. Bone drilling may be required both proximal and distal to the involved area to ensure complete drainage

Box 11.4.1 Treatment of acute haematogenous osteomyelitis

- An appropriate antibiotic, effective prior to pus formation
- Avascular tissues and abscesses require surgical removal
- After successful removal, antibiotics should prevent recurrence and primary wound closure can be undertaken
- Surgery should not damage further already ischaemic bone and soft tissue
- Antibiotics should be continued after surgery.

- Surgical exploration may also be indicated if a patient fails to improve symptomatically after 24–48h of antibiotic treatment
- Packing of the wound with a planned second look, further debridement, and wound closure may be considered. The use of antibiotic beads or collagen sponge is not usually required.

Outcome

Infection can recur several years following apparent successful primary treatment; most occur within 1 year, however. Therefore patients should be consented for recurrence and possible need for further treatment.

Subacute haematogenous osteomyelitis

This has a more insidious onset with few symptoms. Pain may be present for some weeks with minimal systemic symptoms or signs. Often no temperature or malaise is present.

Blood tests are usually normal; the erythrocyte sedimentation rate may be slightly raised in 50% of cases. Radiographs and bone scans are positive and a classification based on radiographic changes was proposed by Gledhill and modified further by Roberts and colleagues (Box 11.4.2).

Box 11.4.2 Classification of subacute osteomyelitis

- Gledhill (1973):
  - I: solitary localized zone of radiolucency surrounded by reactive new bone formation
  - II: metaphyseal radiolucencies with cortical erosion
  - III: cortical hyperostosis in diaphysis; no onion skinning
  - IV: subperiosteal new bone and onion skin layering
- Roberts et al. (1982):
  - V: central radiolucency in epiphysis
  - VI: destructive process involving vertebral body.

The lack of symptoms is thought to be due to increased host resistance. The differential diagnosis must include exclusion of a primary bone tumour and biopsy and curettage are advised. An organism is identified in only 60% of cases and those negative cases with a high index of diagnostic suspicion should be treated empirically with antibiotics for 6 weeks.

Further reading

Nade, S. (1983). Acute haematogenous osteomyelitis in infancy and childhood. *Journal of Bone and Joint Surgery*, **65B**, 109–19.

Peltola, H., Unkila-Kallio, L., and Kallio, M.J. (1997). Simplified treatment of acute staphylococcal osteomyelitis of childhood. *Pediatrics*, **99**, 846–50.

Gillespie, W.J., and Mayo, K.M., (1981). The management of acute haematogenous osteomyelitis in the antibiotic era. A study of the outcome. *Journal of Bone and Joint Surgery*, **63B**, 126–31.

Gledhill, R.B. (1973). Subacute osteomyelitis in children. *Clinical Orthopaedics and Related Research*, **96**, 57–69.

Roberts J.M., Drummond D.S., Breed A.L., *et al.* (1982). Subacute haematogenous osteomyelitis in children: a retrospective study. *Journal of Pediatric Orthopaedics*, **2**, 249–54.

11.5

Septic arthritis

Peter Calder

Summary points

- Painful swollen joint with significant limitation in movement
- Systemic symptoms, fever, and malaise
- Antibiotics following blood cultures, joint aspiration
- Wash out and joint splintage in position of function
- Low threshold to repeat washout if symptoms do not resolve.

Introduction

Septic arthritis indicates inflammation of the joint due to the invading organism. Bacteria within the joint space in adult septic arthritis may occur from haematogenous spread but most commonly occurs due to direct inoculation either from trauma or iatrogenic joint penetration, for example, intra-articular injection or arthroscopy. Contiguous osteomyelitis can also spread to local joints. Once again a high index of suspicion is required in the elderly or immunocompromised with a swollen joint as other symptoms may be reduced. Associated conditions including rheumatoid arthritis and other seronegative arthropathies predispose patients to septic arthritis, especially when joint aspiration and intra-articular steroid injections are undertaken.

Following infection, synovial infiltration with inflammatory cells, initially with polymorphonuclear leucocytes, are replaced with chronic mononuclear cells by 3 weeks. The inflammatory response results in an effusion which can become large enough to result in joint subluxation or even dislocation. This will also eventually result in articular cartilage destruction although the specific mechanism of this remains unknown—it is thought to be destructive enzymes within the exudate. This occurs as early as 4–6 days following initial infection, with total joint destruction by 4 weeks.

Clinical features

- Severe pain is present. This is significantly exacerbated with any attempted active or minimal passive motion. The patients generally lie very still and even movement of the examination couch can result in a terrible increase in pain
- Systemic symptoms are often present with fever and malaise (these may be absent in the immunocompromised patient)
- Local signs include a swollen joint with an effusion, warm to touch, with possible skin erythema
- Monoarticular involvement is typical with lower limb joints most often affected, the knee being the most common.

Investigations

- Blood tests will often show elevation of the white cell count, erythrocyte sedimentation count, and C reactive protein
- Radiology is usually unnecessary to make a diagnosis. Ultrasound, however, is particularly useful in demonstrating joint effusion, especially within the hip joint where it can aid in needle placement for aspiration
- Aspiration will confirm pus within the joint which can be sent for microbiology prior to antibiotic administration. A diagnosis is indicated with a synovial leucocyte count of greater than 50 000/mm^3 but this may be less in immunocompromised patients.

Organism

- *Staphylococcus aureus* remains the most common cause
- *Neisseria gonorrhoeae* is very common in young sexually active patients. This presents with polyarticular septic arthritis and a popular rash. Joint cultures are often negative but positive cultures may be obtained from the pharynx or urethra. In these cases appropriate antibiotics is usually sufficient treatment with surgical drainage unnecessary
- Adults with systemic lupus erythematosus have an increased risk of *Salmonella* infection and *Pseudomonas* and other Gram-negative organisms have a prevalence in intravenous drug abusers.

Treatment

The natural history of septic arthritis is known to result in eventual joint destruction and therefore this is an orthopaedic emergency which requires immediate treatment.

The principles of treatment include joint drainage and wash out. Systemic antibiotics are administered and the joint is splinted in a position of function. A drain can be placed to allow further drainage.

Drainage can involve formal joint arthrotomy and lavage or repeated joint aspiration. Arthroscopic lavage can also be considered in knee, ankle, shoulder, and elbow infection. My personal choice is open surgical drainage and wash out with saline.

If systemic and local symptoms do not resolve further, washout including formal open arthrotomy and debridement may be required within 24–48h following initial surgery.

The duration of antibiotics should continue for 4–6 weeks even if symptoms resolve quickly. After cessation of infection, treatment is concentrated on rehabilitation and restoration of joint function. Continual passive motion may inhibit adhesions and promote better nutrition to the cartilage. Residual joint deformity may respond to traction, serial casting, or dynamic splints. In the chronic ankylosed deformity, corrective osteotomy can place the limb in an optimal functional position.

Further reading

Dlabach, J.A. and Park, A.L. (2008) Infectious arthritis. In: Canale, S.T and Beaty, J.H. (eds) *Campbell's Operative Orthopaedics*, eleventh edition, pp. 723–52. St Louis, MO: Mosby.

Nade, S. (1983). Acute septic arthritis in infancy and childhood. *Journal of Bone and Joint Surgery*, **65B**, 234–41.

Smith, S.P., Thyoka, M., Lavy, C.B., and Pitani, A. (2002). Septic arthritis of the shoulder in children in Malawi. A randomised prosepective study of aspiration versus arthrotomy and washout. *Journal of Bone and Joint Surgery*, **84B**, 1167–72.

SECTION 12

Trauma

12.1

Fracture classification

Thomas A. DeCoster

Summary points

- The 2007 OTA Comprehensive Classification of Fractures and Dislocations is recommended as the standard for fracture classification
- Practitioners should be aware of the limited reliability and reproducibility of fracture classifications.

Introduction

The jargon of fracture description is learned early in orthopaedic training and helps to facilitate communication by identifying important parameter values in a qualitative way. The selection of adjectives such as 'a displaced comminuted closed tibia shaft fracture' identifies characteristics of an injury. Formal fracture classification is an extension of fracture terminology with specification of a number of groups with common and distinguishing factors (Box 12.1.1).

The benefits of classification include: 1) facilitates communication; 2) identifies prognosis and complication risks; 3) directs treatment; 4) enhances research.

Box 12.1.1 Qualities of a good classification system

- All inclusive
- Mutually exclusive
- Reliable
- Reproducible
- Clinically relevant
- Logical
- Facilitates communication.

All inclusive classification system

The classification should allow for all theoretical and practical patterns. A good example is the Neer classification of proximal humerus features which defines four anatomical parts to be considered. Since these four parts are present in every proximal humerus the classification is all inclusive.

Mutually exclusive classification system

The classification should allow for only one category for each pattern seen. A good example is extra-articular vs partial articular vs total articular. A poor example is the Gustilo and Anderson (1976) classification of open fractures. Type 1 open wound which is low energy, less than 1 cm long, and generally caused by bone piercing from the inside out while a type 2 wound is considered 1–5cm with a moderate amount of soft tissue damage. A given injury which is 0.9cm long with moderate soft tissue injury has qualities of both type 1 and type 2.

Reliability

Two different physicians should be able to identify the appropriate group or class to which each fracture should be assigned. Therefore it is necessary to select criteria which can themselves be reliably assessed and which physicians can learn, remember, and are willing and able to apply. Reliability can be measured by the kappa statistic which varies from −1 to 1 based upon agreement of two different reviewers: −1 indicates complete disagreement, 0 is random agreement, and 1 is complete agreement (Figure 12.1.2). It is a generally accepted consensus that values of 0–0.2 represent slight agreement, 0.21–0.4 fair agreement, 0.41–0.6 moderate agreement, and 0.61–0.8 substantial agreement (Figure 12.1.3). Other statistical measures of agreement reported in the literature which range between −1 and +1 include weighted kappa, Cronbach's alpha, and SAV of O'Connell. Weighted kappa gives partial credit for being close in contrast to kappa which is most applicable to a system where observations either agree or not. Alpha is particularly applicable to rank order analysis.

The reliability of this system decreases with increasing complexity and specificity at the group (fracture geometry) or subgroup (comminution pattern) level. The absence of a more reliable classification system is one measure of adequate reliability.

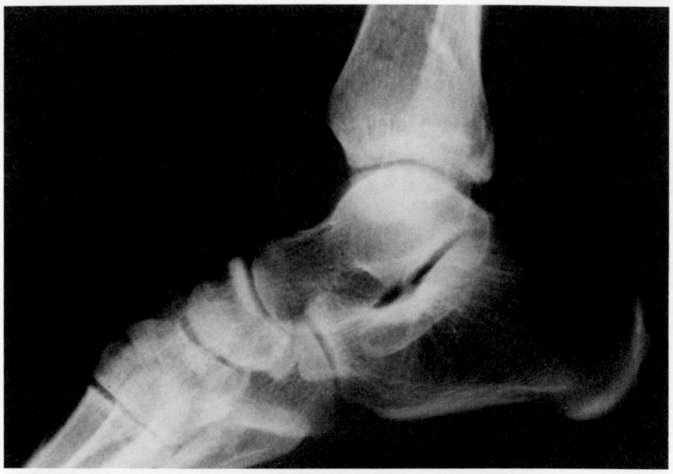

A

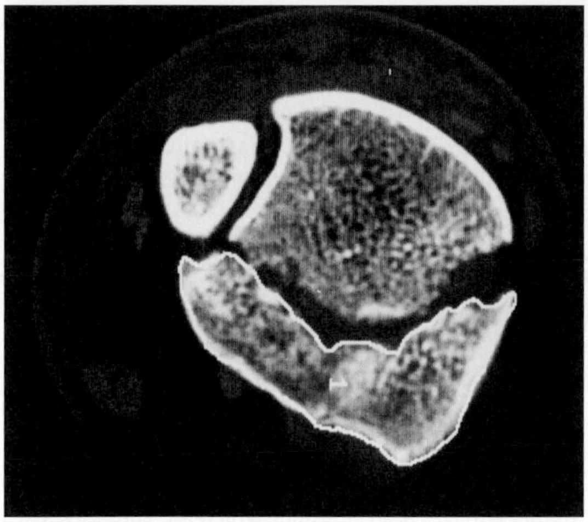

B

Fig. 12.1.1 Example of a poor fracture classification system. A) A lateral radiograph of a posterior lip distal tibia fracture where the fragment appears to be a small percentage of the distal articular surface (one-dimensional image of a two-dimensional concept). B) Demonstrates this fragment to be a large percentage of the distal tibial articular surface.

Box 12.1.2 Measuring reliability and reproducibility by definition

- +1 complete agreement
- 0 random agreement
- −1 complete disagreement.

Box 12.1.3 Qualitative descriptors of κ as a measure of reliability

- 0.81–1.00 excellent agreement
- 0.61–0.8 substantial agreement
- 0.41–0.6 moderate agreement
- 0.21–0.4 fair agreement
- 0.01–0.2 slight agreement.

Reproducibility

The appropriate classification should be consistent when one physician reviews the same case at different times. Reproducibility can also be measured by kappa or a similar statistic as previously described. The best classification is highly reproducible.

Clinical relevance

The classification should assist the physician in the care of the patient. Identifying prognosis, associated injuries, complication risks, and directing optimal treatment are the most common forms of clinical usefulness. Associated injuries may not be recognized without clues to their existence. The presence of associated injuries may make a dramatic difference in the significance of a fracture pattern. Recognizing a distal fibula fracture with talar shift as a Lauge–Hansen SER-4 helps identify by deduction the ligamentous injuries to the deltoid, anterior and posterior inferior tibiofibular ligaments which are not directly visualized on the radiographs.

Logical algorithm

The classification system is better if it is based on a logical algorithm. It should be possible to systematically answer a series of related questions about the fracture to arrive at the specific classification. The number of categories should be the fewest possible to effectively discriminate similarities and differences between groups. Allowance should be given for future developments in the field which may require subsequent revision of the classification system in a logical manner.

Facilitates communication

A classification system should facilitate verbal and written communication between clinicians. It should use standard terminology that is clearly defined and accepted and the definition should not change over time. Facilitation of communication could be considered a form of clinical relevance but is of sufficient importance to warrant specific inclusion as a desirable quality.

Problems with classification systems

The usefulness of a classification is usually time dependent. In the late 1970s intramedullary nailing of femoral shaft fractures was gaining clinical acceptance. The presence of comminution was associated with a significant incidence of complication of the technique, including poor rotational control and shortening. Winquist proposed a classification of femoral shaft fractures based upon increasing comminution and identified the percentage of circumference of the bone necessary to be in contact after nailing to reduce malunion to acceptable rates. At that time the classification was useful. Prior to intramedullary nailing there was no difference in outcome as a function of amount of circumference comminuted so the classification would not have been useful. Subsequent development of interlocking nails changed the usefulness of the classification from defining an indication for nailing to defining an indication for interlocking. Improvement in ease of interlocking made the technique useful without regard to amount of comminution so the Winquist classification of femoral shaft fractures was no longer of particular significance or usefulness. This illustrates that the Winquist classification of femur shaft fractures was clinically relevant during the time of difficult interlocking nails being prevalent.

The widespread tacit acceptance of most fracture classifications used clinically has been strongly challenged in recent publications. The reliability of applying various fracture classifications by different surgeons or reproducibility of a surgeon on two different occasions has been shown to be much lower than previously assumed. Current studies should and are focusing on the source of this variability. There is clearly a tendency for surgeons to adjust the classification based upon their own experience. In addition, clinicians have a limited and imperfect recall of definitions involved in classifications and this will result in some real error. Consensus classification has been proposed as a method to salvage classification schemes with poor reliability. Although this is appealing in theory, consensus classification has not yet been shown to be reproducible or reliable among different groups.

The radiographic interpretation of fracture lines is highly variable and dependent upon radiographic quality (contrast, completeness, obliquity). Reports of accuracy of radiographic measurements suggest more variability than commonly believed. For example, the imprecision in measuring Bohler's angle after a calcaneus fracture or the percentage of lost height in a lumbar spine fracture or the millimetres of displacement of a proximal tibia fracture all limit the usefulness of classifications which require those measurements. Another common problem is that the classification requires information not available from radiographs. Malleolar distal tibia fractures with large posterior tibial fragments have been considered for internal fixation based on the percentage of articular surface involved in the fragment. This is a two-dimensional concept, however this fragment is very poorly visualized on the anteroposterior or mortise radiograph and only one dimension can be measured on the lateral (see Figure 12.1.1). As more diagnostic information (computed tomography, magnetic resonance imaging, etc.), about a particular injury becomes available, the initial classification may not stand the test of time.

Not all of the problems are with the classifier. Classifications may give general typical scenarios without precise category definitions such as the Gustilo and Anderson open fracture classification. Open fractures caused by tornadoes are defined as type 3 without regard to their size. That may have helped explain the risk of infection in the patients treated in Minnesota but is not a generally good fracture classification scheme to be utilized worldwide.

A common mechanism of injury has often been applied to patterns of injury and fracture classification, such as the nightstick fracture (isolated ulna shaft) from fending off an attack by someone wielding a nightstick (truncheon); or boot-top fracture (midshaft tibia) from ski boot binding design in the 1970s. This technique is highly variable as the true mechanism of injury for a given patient is seldom known with certainty and hence speculation is usually required.

Eponyms have also been used to designate a certain fracture pattern by the person recognized as first publishing and being referenced on the significance of that particular injury. Thus distal radius fractures are commonly referred to as Colles fractures. Eponyms suffer from lack of precision and rarely mean the same thing to the speaker, the listener, or the original author. Fortunately these shortcomings have become recognized and the frequency of use of eponyms is rapidly fading in orthopaedic traumatology. There are probably better ways to pay tribute to our musculoskeletal forefathers than use of eponyms.

Current classification schemes and outcome measures suffer statistically from the tendency to clump rather than spread data across parameter values. For example, most clinical scores range from 0–100 but the range actually reported tends to be much more narrow, for example 50–89. In the extreme, if all patients score 70 then there can be no correlation of any variable to the outcome. When pain is scored as: no pain = 50 points; occasional mild pain with strenuous activity = 40 points; some pain with some activity = 30 points; severe pain with activity = 20 points; severe pain at rest = 10 points, then there will be a strong tendency toward 30 points. The more the results are clumped the less likely there is to be a correlation between variables and outcomes. Therefore a good fracture classification may poorly predict clinical outcome due to problems with measuring clinical outcome rather than deficiency in the classification system. Some authors have suggested rank order analysis to avoid the clumping problem of other outcome measures. Rank order forces the spreading of parameter values across the entire range. However, a drawback to this form of analysis is the lack of general applicability to patients outside the study.

AO/Orthopaedic Trauma Association classification system

The 2007 modification and republication of the Orthopaedic Trauma Association (OTA) fracture and dislocation classification compendium provides the current standard for the classification of fractures. This classification has now achieved widespread recognition, understanding, and acceptance in publications and orthopaedic practice. The 2007 version has reconciled differences that existed between the previous OTA and AO classifications by cooperation between the two groups and now the two are identical. This classification has been established as the standard by OTA, AO, SICOT, the *Journal of Orthopaedic Trauma*, and many other organizations and publications and can now be recommended as the standard fracture classification for general use.

The 2007 OTA fracture classification provides a complete system of fracture classification for all bones in the body that uses consistent methodology throughout the skeletal system. It is based on Muller's original principle of classification of long bone fractures with designation of a bone, then three bone segments/bone, three types/segment, three groups/type and three subgroups/group. This classification fulfils the criterion for a good classification system (Figure 12.1.2) and provides a wide spectrum of specificity. It can be used as a standard for terminology for very gross fracture types or extremely specific patterns for research purposes.

The OTA classification involves an alpha-numeric designation of the fracture which is particularly important with the current use of computerized search engines to look for information on a specific entity. The first number identifying the BONE (1–9), the second the bone SEGMENT (1–3), then a letter designating TYPE (A,B,C) followed by numbers (1–3) for GROUP and SUBGROUP separated by a decimal point. For example a comminuted fracture of the medial condyle of the distal femur would be coded 33.B2.3 (femur, distal, partial articular, medial, multifragmentary).

There are fundamental differences between various TYPEs of bone SEGMENT fractures. Proximal and distal segments of long bones are classified as extra-articular (A), partial articular (B), and

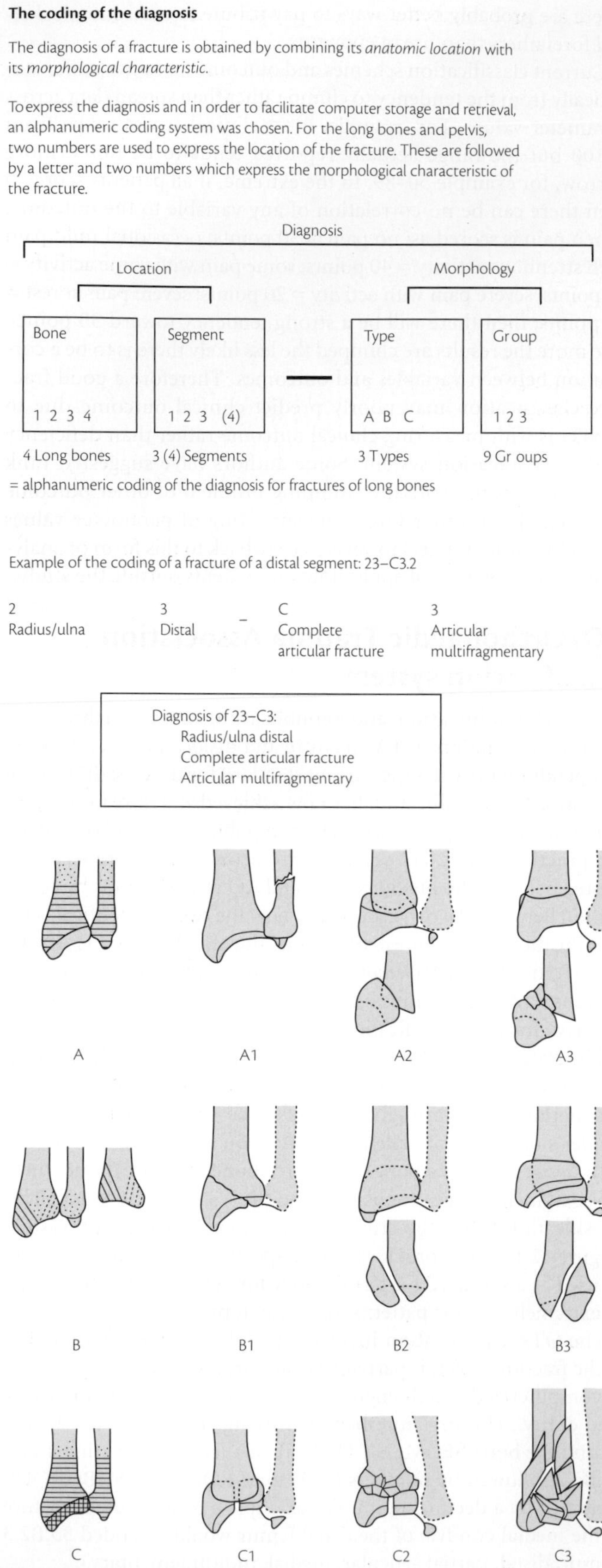

The coding of the diagnosis
The diagnosis of a fracture is obtained by combining its anatomic location with its morphological characteristic.
To express the diagnosis and in order to facilitate computer storage and retrieval, an alphanumeric coding system was chosen. For the long bones and pelvis, two numbers are used to express the location of the fracture. These are followed by a letter and two numbers which express the morphological characteristic of the fracture.
Diagnosis
Location
Morphology
Bone
Segment
Type
Group
1 2 3 4
1 2 3 (4)
A B C
1 2 3
4 Long bones
3 (4) Segments
3 Types
9 Gr oups
= alphanumeric coding of the diagnosis for fractures of long bones
Example of the coding of a fracture of a distal segment: 23–C3.2
2
Radius/ulna
3
Distal
C
Complete articular fracture
3
Articular multifragmentary
Diagnosis of 23–C3:
Radius/ulna distal
Complete articular fracture
Articular multifragmentary
A
A1
A2
A3
B
B1
B2
B3
C
C1
C2
C3

Fig. 12.1.2 The OTA/AO comprehensive classification of fractures method is based on the radiographic appearance of the fracture location and geometry.

total articular (C). Diaphyseal fractures are classified as simple (A), wedge (B), and complex (C). For the flat bones there are three types based on the same principle of increasing complexity. For example the types of talus (81) fracture are avulsion or process fractures (A), talar neck fracture (B), and talar body fracture (C).

The GROUP designation of fracture pattern typically involves anatomical specificity. For example, partial articular distal humerus (13B) fractures have three groups: lateral or capitellar (13B1), medial or trochlear (13B2), coronal plane (13B3). When anatomical specificity is not relevant, the groups are typically designated by degree and pattern of comminution. For example, total articular distal humerus fractures (13C) are grouped as articular simple, metaphysis simple (13C1), articular simple metaphysis multifragmentary (13C2), articular multifragmentary (13C3). This corresponds with the relative complexity of fracture, the treatment and the prognosis. There are a total of nine categories at the group level for each bone segment and this level of specificity would be more than adequate for the vast majority of clinical situations.

The SUBGROUP level of designation is useful when very detailed and specific categories are desirable as might be the case in research, database, or subspecialty discussions. It is more detail than would be necessary for most clinical situations. For example, distal humerus medial fractures (13B2) is sub grouped by the pattern of fracture as medial or Milch 1 (13B2.1), groove or Milch 2 (13B2.2), multifragmentary (13B2.3). There are three subgroups for each group (for example three subcategories of fractures of the trochlea of the distal humerus). There are a total of 27 categories at the subgroup level for each bone segment (all distal humerus fractures).

The OTA classification has been criticized as being overly complex. However, as illustrated earlier, the level of desired complexity can be chosen to match the needs of the user. If the information for the group or subgroup level is not known or needed, then designation at the level of type can be used. Furthermore, as illustrated by the example of trochlear fractures, the complexity at the level of subgroup is well within the skill set of the average orthopaedic surgeon with good quality plain radiographs, especially with easy accessibility to the standard reference.

The 2007 version of the OTA fracture classification is different from the 1996 version in several areas including hand, foot, flat bones dislocation, and the newly developed AO classification of fractures of bones with open growth plates (paediatric fractures).

Conclusion

A classification system may be imperfect; however it can still be useful. We should use the classifications which are the best available to help direct treatment and predict outcome. Directing treatment is one of the best forms and a classification which correctly partitions a family of related injuries into categories with unique treatments would be ideal. This correlation rarely survives more than a few years. We should continually strive to improve by testing and updating (perhaps once per decade) our classification systems to be logical, reliable, reproducible, and clinically relevant to direct treatment and identify risk.

Future directions

The 2007 OTA fracture classification is likely to continue to gain acceptance as the standard. New information about this classification in particular will be use to shape future modifications and improvements in the decades ahead. New information about fracture patterns and the predictors of treatment and outcome will also be forthcoming and this information will also result in modification of future versions (2017) of the classification.

Recognitipon of problems with current fracture classifications and the ongoing desire to optimize patient outcome will result in improved classifications in the future. Old and new classifications will be scientifically scrutinized and the reliable, reproducible, logical, clinically relevant ones will be selected for utilization. Ongoing efforts will focus on identifying and minimizing the sources of error or disagreement so as to optimize reliability and reproducibility. Factors will be scientifically and statistically analyzed for predictive value and important factors will be incorporated into fracture classifications.

There will be ongoing efforts to learn from our past and review clinical results as a function of existing fracture classifications. Treatments and outcomes as a function of fracture classification will continue to be reported with the potential for improvement as the tools we use (e.g. prospective fracture classification) are themselves improved.

New methods of classification will be further investigated. Consensus classification by a panel of experienced surgeons may be of benefit. Rank order and other non-parametric statistical analysis may also help solve the problems of poor agreement. The methodology by which we assess classification reliability will be standardized and improved.

There is considerable benefit and interest in generalized fracture classification systems (OTA, AO, SICOT). The ease of computerized and internet accessibility to fracture classification standards and educational tutorial tools will improve the accuracy and generalized utilization of the 2007 OTA fracture classification (e.g. OKO). Increased utilization and widespread acceptance will also depend upon the effectiveness of the classification and its ability to lump similar and distinguish dissimilar injuries in a comprehensible and usable manner.

Further reading

Dirschl, D.R. and Adams, G.L. (1997). A critical assessment of factors influencing reliability in the classification of fractures, using fractures of the tibial plafond as model. *Journal of Orthopedic Trauma*, **11**, 471–6.

Doornberg, J., Lindenhovius, A., Kloen, P., van Dijk, C.N., Zurakowski, D., and Ring, D. (2006). Two and three-dimensional computed tomography for the classification and management of distal humeral fractures. Evaluation of reliability and diagnostic accuracy. *Journal of Bone and Joint Surgery*, **88A**, 1795–801.

Marsh, J.L., Slongo, T.F., Agel, J., *et al.* (2007). Fracture and dislocation classification compendium – 2007: Orthopaedic Trauma Association classification, database and outcomes committee. *Journal of Orthopedic Trauma*, **21**(10 Suppl), S1–133.

Marsh JL. (2009). OTA fracture classification. *Journal of Orthopedic Trauma*, **23**(8), 551.

Martin, J., Marsh, J.L., Nepola, J.V., Dirschl, D.R., Hurwitz, S., and DeCoster, T.A. (2000). Radiographic fracture assessments: which ones can we reliably make? *Journal of Orthopedic Trauma*, **14**, 379–85.

Slongo, T., Audigé, L., Claver, J.M., Lutz, N., Frick, S., and Hunter, J. (2007). The AO comprehensive classification of pediatric long bone fractures: a web-based multicenter agreement study. *Journal of Pediatric Orthopedics*, **27**, 171–80.

12.2

Complications of fractures

James Wilson-MacDonald and Andrew James

Introduction

Complications of fractures include fat embolism and fat embolism syndrome, reflex sympathetic dystrophy, avascular necrosis, vascular injuries, crush injuries, gas gangrene, and tetanus. Vascular injuries are dealt with in Chapter 12.9. Avacular necrosis is discussed in the chapters on hip fractures and scaphoid fractures (Chapters 12.29, 12.50, and 12.51).

Fat embolism syndrome

Fat embolism syndrome is defined as the presence of globules of fat in the lungs and in other tissues. It occurs occasionally in long bone fractures (3.5%) and can rarely occur without trauma. It is commoner after multiple trauma (10%).

There is little correlation between the amount of fat in the lungs and the severity of the condition. Figure 12.2.1 summarizes the inflammatory cascade which occurs. Lipase is released by the lung which acts on the fat releasing free fatty acids and glycerol which are toxic to the lung.

The condition usually manifests itself 1–2 days after injury. Many features remain unexplained:

- It mainly affect the young
- It mainly occurs after lower limb fractures
- Most are closed fractures
- The elderly do not seem to be affected (e.g. hip fractures).

Table 12.2.1 summarizes the classical symptoms and signs (major and minor features). Tachypnoea, dyspnoea, and cyanosis are the earliest respiratory signs, but hypoxaemia may be detected earlier. Cerebral irritation can include headache and irritability to convulsions and coma. Embolization of fat into the dermis causes petechiae. They are transient but can be seen on the chest (Figure 12.2.2) neck, axillae, palate, eyelid (Figure 12.2.3), conjunctivae, and retina.

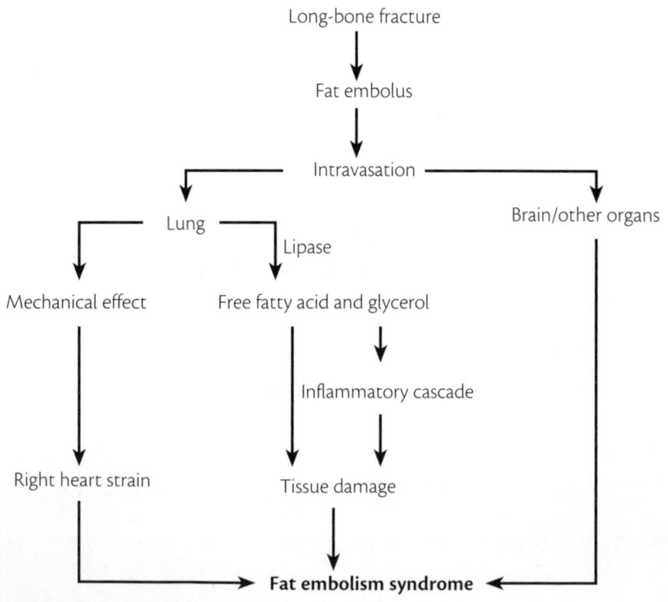

Fig. 12.2.1 Pathophysiology of fat embolism syndrome.

Table 12.2.1 Diagnosis of fat embolism (Gurd and Wilson 1974)

Major features (at least one)
Respiratory insufficiency
Cerebral involvement
Petechial rash
Minor features (at least four)
Pyrexia
Tachycardia
Retinal changes
Jaundice
Renal changes
Plus fat macroglobulinemia

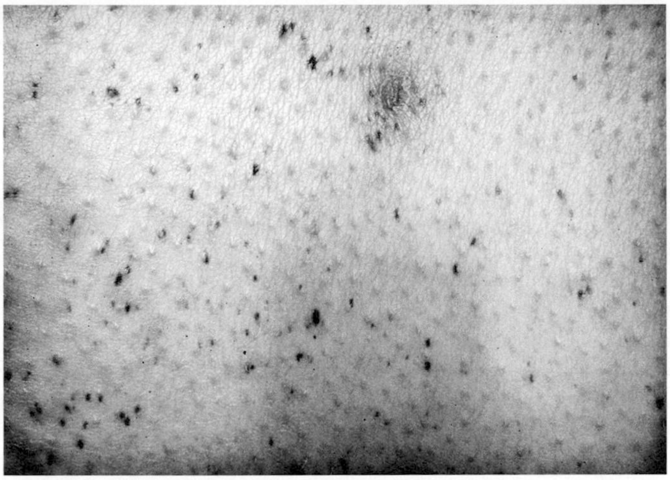

Fig. 12.2.2 Petechial hemorrhage on chest wall.

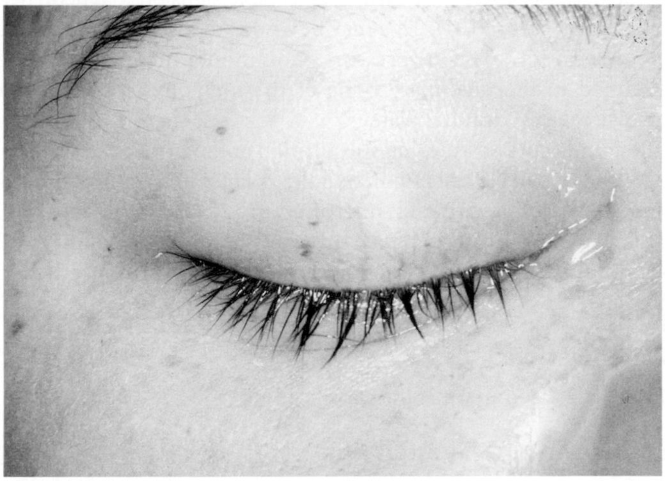

Fig. 12.2.3 Petechial hemorrhage on eyelid.

Diagnosis

The diagnosis is based on clinical and laboratory tests. These include:

- Low PO_2
- Macroglobulinaemia.

These should be combined with one major and four minor signs (see Table 12.2.1).

Pulmonary infiltrates on the chest radiograph, right heart strain, and ST segment changes on the electrocardiogram (ECG), together with anaemia, thrombocytopenia, and elevation of erythrocyte sedimentation rate, add support to the diagnosis but are not specific.

Management

The incidence of fat embolism syndrome can be reduced by appropriate early management of the trauma victim. Adequate fluid resuscitation and oxygen therapy with fracture splintage and careful transport are important first aid measures. There is no evidence that intramedullary reaming increases the incidence. The mainstay of treatment in the established case is respiratory support. Specific therapies have been proposed, including heparin, alcohol, and aspirin, but the findings were equivocal. Steroids have been studied in both prophylaxis and treatment. They are reported as effective in maintaining arterial oxygen levels and reducing serum free fatty acids, but the dose required is high and complications can be severe. At the present time they are not in routine use.

Results

The mortality rate approaches 15% mainly due to respiratory complications. Morbidity is mainly due to cerebral irritation.

A high index of suspicion and early treatment improves results.

Complex regional pain syndrome/reflex sympathetic dystrophy (Chapter 1.11)

Reflex sympathetic dystrophy is a syndrome characterized by intense or unduly prolonged pain, vasomotor disturbance, delayed functional recovery, and trophic changes. Many terms, including causalgia, Sudeck's atrophy, and algodystrophy, have been used to describe the condition. It can occur as a response to trauma. Up to 30% of patients with tibial fractures and distal radial fractures may be affected. The cause is not known. Livingstone's theory (Figure 12.2.4) is that there is a vicious circle initiated by capillary stasis, increased local pressure, and exudation, which is maintained by afferent fibre stimulation due to anoxia. The importance of inflammatory mediators and cytokines has been investigated but to date there is no reliable marker for reflex sympathetic dystrophy.

Clinical evaluation

The severity of reflex sympathetic dystrophy is not related to the magnitude of the initial traumatic insult. The condition commonly affects the periphery, although it is being increasingly recognized in the knee and shoulder. The elbow and hip are rarely

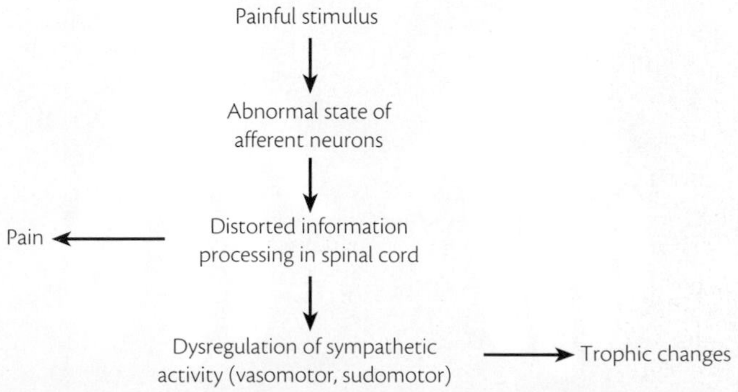

Fig. 12.2.4 Livingston's theory of the pathophysiology of reflex sympathetic dystrophy.

affected. It is more common in middle years but is recognized in children.

The clinical presentation is varied but three phases are commonly identified:

1) Acute or hyperaemic phase
2) Dystrophic or ischaemic phase
3) Atrophic phase.

The acute phase may occur soon after injury but may be delayed for several weeks. Pain and tenderness are the first signs. Hyperpathia (increased sensitivity to a noxious stimulus) and allodynia (pain caused by stimuli not usually noted to be painful) are common. In the acute phase the limb is swollen, dry, hot, and pink (Figure 12.2.5), with increased hair growth. In the second phase the limb often remains swollen but becomes blue, cool, and damp with sweat. It may be several months before the third stage is entered. This is characterized by atrophy and joint contractures.

Investigation

The diagnosis is primarily clinical. Several investigations are useful in assessing the severity and stage of the disease. Tenderness can be assessed using dolorimetry, joint stiffness can be recorded, and thermography can be used to assess vasomotor function. Bone scans are positive in the early stages, and when they return to normal there is visible demineralization on plain radiography.

Management

Early diagnosis is the key to successful management as the first two phases are reversible. The primary treatment of reflex sympathetic dystrophy involves reassurance, analgesia, and physiotherapy to maintain joint movement. In severe cases, treatment involves sympathetic interruption, for example, with intravenous guanethidine. Surgical sympathectomy is rarely indicated. A multidisciplinary team approach, including physiotherapists, pain specialists, and, in certain cases, psychologists, is helpful.

Results

Even in a mild form reflex sympathetic dystrophy gives rise to severe and permanent morbidity. There is little evidence in the literature for efficacy of the various treatments. It is essential to maintain movement to avoid long-term contractures after recovery.

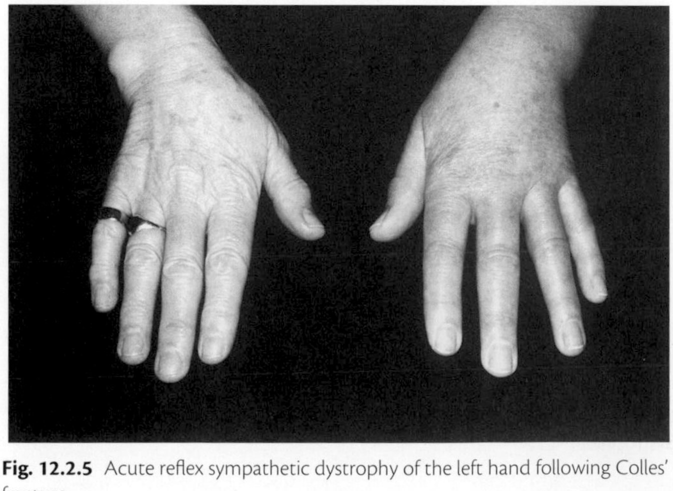

Fig. 12.2.5 Acute reflex sympathetic dystrophy of the left hand following Colles' fracture.

Avascular necrosis

This typically affects intra-articular bone after fracture (talus, hip, scaphoid, humeral head). In displaced talar neck fractures it may occur in up to 70% of cases.

Post-traumatic avascular necrosis may be due to any of these mechanisms. Avascular necrosis of the femoral head may occur as a result of tamponade due to intracapsular haemarthrosis or by vessel kinking or rupture. The degree of displacement and the interval between injury and reduction are important predictors of the likelihood of the occurrence of avascular necrosis.

The progression of the condition is independent of the initial mechanism. Within 2 weeks of injury, there may be histological signs of marrow necrosis with osteocyte death. Cell death leads to liposome release and tissue acidification. Saponification occurs in the presence of free fatty acids and calcium. Marrow oedema and tissue necrosis lead to the earliest detectable signs on magnetic resonance imaging (MRI). This may be associated with a quantifiable increase in intraosseous pressure. Commonly these changes are confined to the medullary bone of the metaphysis and do not involve the subchondral plate.

Repair occurs by creeping substitution and may take 2 years.

Without a viable cell population the normal process of remodelling does not occur and microfractures cannot be repaired. This can result in collapse of the subchondral bone and chondral flaps, both of which then lead to joint incongruity and arthritis.

Classification

Table 12.2.2 summarizes the classification.

Evaluation and investigation

Early diagnosis is important to limit transarticular load.

- MRI scan is the mainstay of investigation. Changes in marrow oedema can be identified
- Intraosseous pressure measurements may help with diagnosis
- Plain radiographs may show subchondral osteopenia (Hawkins sign seen in the body of the talus) which denotes continued vascularity in the absence of normal load. If there is no blood supply the bone is not resorbed
- Scintigraphy may show an area of reduced blood supply.

Management

Management is directed at preventing the complications of avascular necrosis, such as segmental collapse and osteoarthritis.

Clinical studies have shown clear evidence that the incidence of avascular necrosis in many injuries can be correlated with the severity of the initial injury and the delay to reduction. Therefore prompt accurate reduction with secure fixation can lessen the incidence of avascular necrosis, particularly in weight-bearing joints. This must be accompanied by evacuation of the associated haemarthrosis to reduce the effect of tamponade.

Table 12.2.2 Classification of avascular necrosis

Stage	Pain	Radiographic signs	Scintigram	MRI	Intraosseous pressure
Early	None	Normal	Normal	Normal	Increased
I	Minimal	Normal	Nondiagnostic	Early changes	Increased
II	Moderate	Porosis/sclerosis	Positive	Positive	Increased
Late			Positive	Positive	Increased
III	Advanced	Flat/crescent sign	Positive	Positive	Increased
IV	Severe	Acetabular changes	Positive	Positive	Increased

Early diagnosis allows preventive measures such as limiting weight bearing to be instituted to prevent propagation and segmental collapse.

Procedures to enhance revascularity have been advocated. Most commonly, these have been for the management of femoral head avascularity after intracapsular fractures of the proximal femur. Posterior muscle pedicle grafting has been used as an acute procedure and to enhance vascularity in established avascular necrosis. These techniques are infrequently used in modern practice, particularly with the increasing acceptance of hip arthroplasty.

Once segmental collapse has become established and symptomatic, reconstructive procedures such as arthroplasty and arthrodesis are indicated.

Vascular injuries

See Chapter 12.9.

Crush injuries

Major crush injuries of the limbs are mercifully rare. All structures can be injured by crush. Fractures may occur and prolonged crush can cause ischaemia. Muscle repair may be accompanied by fibrous tissue, and myositis ossificans can occur (20% of those with quadriceps haematoma).

In response to trauma, there is a tendency to hypovolaemia with expansion of the extracellular space. This results in an active antidiuresis with rapid renal tubular resorption. Excreted myoglobin and haemoglobin become concentrated in the renal tubules, causing tubular blockage, and may lead to acute renal failure. Sudden release and reperfusion of the affected limb may lead to metabolic acidosis and rapid rises in plasma potassium levels sufficient to cause cardiac arrest.

Investigation

On admission, a detailed assessment should include an ECG, relevant radiographs, measurement of electrolytes, arterial blood gases, and measurement of urinary output. Estimation of urinary myoglobin and haemoglobin are indicated if compromise of renal function is thought likely. Special investigations may include angiography if an associated vascular injury is suspected.

Management

General resuscitative measures should be instigated with administration of analgesia, intravenous fluids, and insertion of a urinary catheter. Electrolyte and acid–base derangement should be corrected. In the case of an open wound, precautions against infection should be taken with administration of broad-spectrum antibiotics and antitetanus prophylaxis.

Specific management of the injuries will be required. This will include fracture reduction and fixation, arterial exploration and reconstruction if indicated, and the limb deemed viable. The fracture pattern may demonstrate extreme comminution.

Decompressive fasciotomy of myofascial compartments surrounding and distal to the crush injury will be required. All non-viable tissue including muscle and bone should be excised. Wounds should be dressed without skin closure.

Complications

Complications can be local or general. General complications may include cardiac arrhythmias and acute renal failure. Cardiac manifestations of hyperkalaemia are reduction in P-wave amplitude and widening of the QRS interval into the ST segment. Sudden rises in serum potassium may result in cardiac arrest. Renal failure may occur as a result of myoglobinuria in the presence of hypovolaemia.

Deep venous thrombosis

The incidence of deep venous thrombosis (DVT) in trauma patients is high. A number of demographic studies have demonstrated an incidence approaching 60% after trauma. This may reach 80% in patients with femoral and tibial shaft fractures and in those with spinal cord injuries.

Pathology

The lower limb veins are most commonly affected due to local endothelial damage, venous stasis, and post-traumatic hypercoagulability and age. Direct trauma to the venous endothelium releases thromboplastic substances and exposes the basement membrane, initiating local thrombosis by the extrinsic coagulation mechanism. Trauma remote from the venous lining may also initiate these changes, explaining the widespread distribution of thrombi. Stasis, in association with immobilization and bed rest, may cause accumulation of platelets around valve cusps which promote the thrombotic process by the release of procoagulants. The frequency of deep venous thrombosis has been shown to rise with increasing periods of immobilization.

Pulmonary embolism may occur in up to 5% of patients.

Diagnosis

The clinical symptoms and signs of DVT are pain, tender swelling of the limb distal to the thrombus, and peripheral oedema. It is frequently associated with a low-grade pyrexia of less than 38°C. However, these signs are difficult to interpret, and clinical diagnosis may be difficult and will underestimate the number of cases seen.

Investigation

Impedance plethysmography and contrast venography are widely available to confirm the diagnosis of DVT. Contrast venography is the most specific test, but is invasive and requires transfer to the radiology department. Impedance plethysmography may be performed at the bedside, but is less specific for smaller distal DVT where proximal veins are patent.

Management

Prophylaxis

Prevention is best. Early mobilization and prophylaxis with low-molecular-weight heparin is widely used. The National Health Service in the United Kingdom has published NICE (National Institute for Health and Clinical Excellence) guidelines for prophylaxis. They recommend graduated DVT stockings for all adults, and 4 weeks of low-molecular-weight heparin for patients undergoing surgery for hip fracture. They also support the use of intermittent pneumatic compression where possible, and emphasize the importance of risk assessment for DVT.

Useful pharmacological agents include aspirin, heparin, fractionated heparin, and oral anticoagulants. The use of these agents in prophylaxis has to be balanced against the risk of haemorrhagic complication. For this reason, use of heparin in patients with acetabular, pelvic, or spinal fractures is not indicated in the first 48h after injury. Studies in patients with below-knee casts indicate that the incidence of DVT can be reduced by the use of fractionated heparin.

Treatment

Treatment of DVT depends on the anatomical site of the thrombus; asymptomatic below-knee thrombus may not require specific therapy. The standard treatment of symptomatic DVT is anticoagulation, initially with heparin, and commencement of warfarin therapy. Oral anticoagulants should be continued for 6–12 weeks, and clotting should be monitored to ensure that the dosage is within the therapeutic range.

In the event of a pulmonary embolus occurring during treatment of DVT, consideration can be given to insertion of inferior vena caval filters to prevent the formation of further emboli.

The complications of DVT include pulmonary embolism and postphlebitic limb.

Gas gangrene

Gas gangrene is a rapidly developing, spreading infection of devitalized tissue by toxin-producing clostridial species, especially *Clostridium perfringens* (formerly known as *Clostridium welchii*). It is a Gram- positive, anaerobic, capsulate, and non-motile bacillus. The most characteristic feature is the spore, which is produced whenever the organism faces adverse conditions. It is accompanied by profound toxaemia, massive tissue necrosis, and gas production, and is invariably fatal unless treated. Clostridial contamination is reported in up to 39% of wounds. The incidence is related to the interval between injury and treatment, as well as to the site and severity of injury.

Clostridial infection can be classified into three types.

1) Clostridial contamination occurs when the organisms are present without clinical disease
2) In clostridial cellulitis there is evidence of disease in the absence of dead muscle and little or no toxin production
3) Clostridial myonecrosis is the severe form known as 'gas gangrene'.

The exact processes by which clostridial contamination and cellulitis lead to gas gangrene are not clear, but a reduction in local oxygen potential is an important factor. The inoculum of *C. perfringens* required to produce fatal gas gangrene is reduced by a factor of 10^3 if the tissue is devitalized or contaminated with sterile dirt. The most important exotoxins are the α-toxins (lecithinase), although several others are well recognized (e.g. collagenase, hyaluronidase, and protease).

Muscle carbohydrate is fermented to lactic acid and 'gas' (mainly hydrogen and carbon dioxide). Putrefaction follows extensive necrosis. At this stage the characteristic smell is produced and the evolution of 'gas gangrene' is complete.

Clinical features

The original insult often involves a penetrating injury to muscle. The buttock and thigh are common sites. The incubation period can be as long as 4 days or as short as 6h. The progression of the disease can be rapid and devastating. Sudden onset of pain is the first symptom, followed by oedema and a thin serous ooze. The pain increases in severity and the skin becomes stretched, developing a 'bronzed' discoloration. Haemorrhagic vesicles may appear before areas of frank necrosis. Tachycardia out of proportion to temperature elevation and mental awareness marked by a 'terror of death' are characteristic. Profound shock follows in the untreated case, and death occurs within 48h. The mortality rate is about 30%.

Management

Emergency surgical debridement is required to save the patient's life, and compartment decompression. X-rays may show gas in the soft tissues, but its absence does not exclude the diagnosis.

A patient with suspected gas gangrene should receive intravenous penicillin. Consideration should be given to adding broad-spectrum antibiotics to cover other organisms. Hyperbaric oxygen is recognized to be of benefit in reducing toxin production and improving oxygen delivery to devitalized tissues.

Tetanus

Tetanus is a rare but often fatal disease caused by *Clostridium tetani*. All the clinical effects are caused by the effects of an exotoxin (tetanospasmin) on various receptor sites.

The incidence of tetanus is now rare in Western countries. In developing countries, where standards of hygiene and primary wound care are poor and the majority of the population are not immunized, it remains an important cause of mortality.

C. tetani is a Gram-positive, anaerobic, motile, and non-capsulate bacillus which forms a characteristic terminal 'drumstick' spore. The spore is very resistant and may remain dormant in wounds for long periods.

C. tetani is found in soil and faeces, but frequently contaminates the skin. A wound is identified as the portal of entry in only 60% of cases. Two factors favour progression of the infection: wounds with low oxygen potential or ischaemic tissue and wounds infected with other organisms. The initial traumatic lesion may appear innocuous compared with the outcome as clinically 'tetanus' is a disease of the central nervous system.

The incubation period varies from 3–21 days and is generally shorter in more severe cases. The period of onset is the time from first symptom to first spasm. This can vary from less than 24h to over 10 days; the shorter the period the more severe is the tetanus.

C. tetani produces two exotoxins. Tetanospasmin is a powerful neurotoxin which is carried slowly by peripheral nerves to the central nervous system, where it is avidly taken up by gangliosides. It is responsible for the characteristic clinical features of the disease. The toxin does not affect sensory nerves, the cerebral cortex, or the cerebellum. Tetanolysin is haemolytic and may contribute to the overall clinical picture.

The transit of the toxin in the peripheral nerves is slow; the first effect is produced in muscle groups with short motor neurons, i.e. the head and neck muscles. Severe trismus and dysphagia due to masseteric spasm ('lockjaw') are seen, and facial muscle spasm produces the characteristic risus sardonicus. The muscular spasm spreads to affect the neck, back, abdomen, and limbs. Opisthotonos—severe spasm such that the whole body is arched off the bed—may be seen.

Muscle spasm of increasing severity and duration may lead to crush fractures of the vertebrae and death from respiratory failure and exhaustion.

Diagnosis

The diagnosis is clinical. The organism is only cultured in one-third of cases, reflecting the specific anaerobic growth requirements of *C. tetani*.

Management

The treatment incorporates specific measures including wound care, passive immunization, and antibiotics. When a wound is identified it should be excised along with all devitalized tissue. *C. tetani* remains sensitive to penicillin, which should be given. Human tetanus immunoglobulin should also be given.

Supportive therapy may be needed depending on the severity of the case and sedation is often helpful. The most important factor is the maintenance of respiratory function and mechanical ventilation via a tracheostomy is required in severe cases.

Active immunization with absorbed tetanus toxoid is extremely safe and effective. If the wound is severe, passive immunization with tetanus immunoglobulin should be given. The American College of Surgeons Committee on Trauma (1986) has published a guide to prophylaxis against tetanus in wound management.

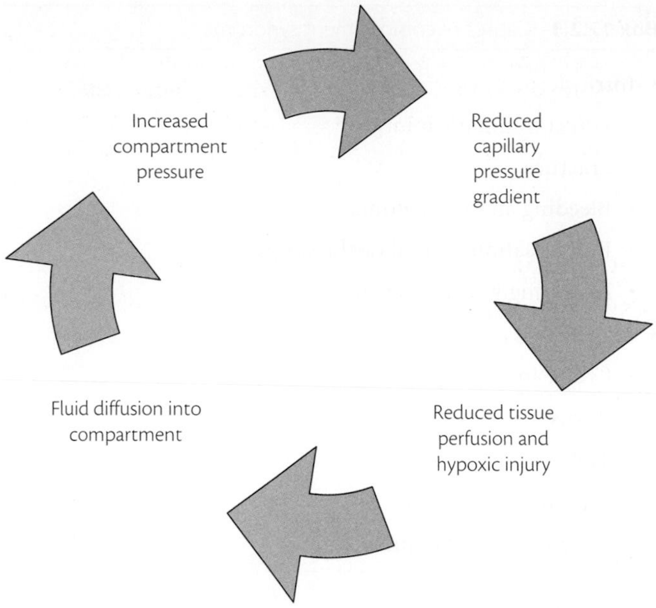

Fig. 12.2.6 Pathophysiology of compartment syndrome.

Compartment syndrome

Definition

Raised pressure within a closed compartment resulting in tissue ischaemia and if untreated, necrosis followed by fibrosis and muscle contracture.

Pathophysiology (Figure 12.2.6)

The capillary bed pressure is usually 20–30mmHg, and this is sufficient to create an adequate tissue perfusion, with an interstitial pressure of about 5mmHg. Compartment syndrome occurs when tissue pressure rises and tissue perfusion decreases or ceases. An increase in interstitial tissue pressure is possible in closed compartments, either by intrinsic or extrinsic causes. An increase in the volume in a contained compartment, giving rise to an intrinsic compression, may be caused by blood or other fluid shifts. Extrinsic compression similarly affects an increase in pressure.

If the pressure in the veins does not rise above the compartment pressure, the veins will remain collapsed, venous pressure rises and perfusion ends. Capillary pressure will then rise towards arterial pressure and there will be rapid diffusion of fluid out of the vascular compartment into the extracellular compartment of the muscle. The pressure in the compartment will continue to rise and the muscle becomes ischaemic. This hypoxic cellular injury causes a release of vasoactive substances, such as serotonin and histamine, which further increase endothelial permeability and extracellular fluid accumulation. Muscle necrosis will occur and myoglobin will be released.

It is important to note that arteries passing through this compartment are not squeezed shut during this process. This is because their intraluminal pressure is high (arterial blood pressure) and their walls are thicker and therefore resist compression. Therefore the presence of distal pulses does not exclude a compartment syndrome.

Box 12.2.1 Causes of compartment syndrome

- Intrinsic:
  - Direct traumatic injury
  - Fracture
  - Bleeding and haematoma
  - Extravasation of fluid (arthroscopy)
  - Following vascular repair
- Extrinsic:
  - Crush and entrapment
  - Burns
  - Tight cast or bandage
  - Prolonged tourniquet
  - Drug or alcohol induced stupor.

Prognosis

The prognosis is dependant on the speed of diagnosis and treatment. Acute compartment syndrome is a true surgical emergency.

Once a compartment syndrome is established, some measurable changes in the affected muscle may occur within 2h. Within 4–6h these changes will have significant long-term effects. After 12h there is likely to be severe irreversible damage.

Causes (Box 12.2.1)

Acute traumatic compartment syndromes can be divided into primary intrinsic, where swelling within the compartment is primarily responsible for the rise in pressure, and primary extrinsic, where there is a constricting cast or bandage. Intrinsic are much more common.

Intrinsic causes

Intrinsic compartment syndrome develops when the volume in an injured compartment rises following a traumatic injury. It is important to note that even open injuries may have intact fascial compartments. Bleeding or direct tissue injury may initiate the pressure increase. Manipulation and intramedullary nailing may precipitate compartment syndrome. This should not be used as a reason to delay these procedures but the surgeon must be aware of the possibility.

Extrinsic causes

Pure extrinsic causes are much less common and are unlikely to produce a compartment syndrome unless there is damage to tissues within the compartment leading to swelling. However, it is important to consider this when planning treatment, as removal of a cast alone can reduce compartment pressure by as much as 30%.

Non-traumatic

- *Chronic exertional compartment syndrome* is most commonly seen in high-level athletes. It is commonly bilateral and is frequently associated with small muscle hernias through the fascia. The differential diagnosis includes periostitis, tenosynovitis, tumours of bone or soft tissue, stress fracture, and nerve entrapment
- *Acute exertional syndrome* can present acutely in individuals who are not fit, but who are suddenly involved in strenuous exercise. The diagnosis here is given by the history which can only really be confused with acute tenosynovitis. If the symptoms do not rapidly resolve with rest, a fasciotomy is indicated
- *Following vascular reconstruction*: there may be acute swelling of muscles immediately after emergency embolectomy, especially if the limb has been critically ischaemic for some time.

History

There is a history of trauma, although this may have been quite minor, followed by a history of increasing pain over a period of hours. Pain as a clinical sign is unreliable if the patient's level of consciousness is altered. Most specifically, the patient will be extremely unwilling to move any part of the limb, especially the extremities. The patient may also complain that the limb feels numb or cold.

Examination

The cardinal sign is pain, especially when increasing or out of proportion. The patient has immediate and severe pain on passive stretching of the muscles of the involved compartment. It may be useful to distract children to ensure that it is not their fear of the injured limb being touched which produces the response.

Examination should then include a full release of any bandages down to skin and opening of any casts. This may produce some relief. The limb may also feel cold, have reduced sensation, and be pulseless; these are late signs and suggest a poorer prognosis.

However, it must be emphasized that the presence of normal sensation and pulses distal to a possible compartment syndrome does not exclude the diagnosis.

Investigation

The main diagnosis of compartment syndrome is based on clinical examination. A high index of suspicion is one key to making the diagnosis. Prompt decompression should not be delayed and if there is any doubt the surgeon should err on the side of caution and perform a fasciotomy. Intracompartmental pressure measurement can be performed and has a role in unconscious patients, and in those with unclear or unreliable clinical signs, such as children. Continuous monitoring may be needed in obtunded patients.

There are various methods available, most commonly a pressure transducer, is flushed, zeroed at the compartment level, and inserted into each compartment in turn to obtain a reading. Reproducibility and reliability of these measurements is poor. The pressure obtained can be used as an absolute value, or related to the diastolic or mean blood pressure.

Prevention

Circumferential bandages and casts should be avoided if at all possible in the first 12h after trauma or surgery. If they are used they should be split, and then closed or replaced when the swelling is no longer increasing.

All patients sent home with bandages or casts should be warned of the possibility of the development of a compartment syndrome.

Treatment

Casts, bandages, and padding need to be removed down to the skin. Soft cotton dressing soaked in blood can produce a tight constricting band. If removal of the cast compromises the reduction of the fracture, then this must be accepted. A compartment syndrome takes priority over fracture position. If there is not immediate and sustained improvement in pain and movement once the dressing has been released, an immediate surgical fasciotomy is required.

Fasciotomies should be performed open, as the skin itself can constrict compartments in severe swelling. Open fasciotomy allows the surgeon to avoid damaging nerves with a variable path through the fascia. The anatomy needs careful review before embarking on the fasciotomy. All compartments at risk need to be split along their whole length.

The fasciotomy should be left open, both to reduce pressure and to allow regular reinspection of the muscle. If any parts of the muscle fail to revascularize, they should be debrided. A second look should be performed at 48h and closure can be considered. Complete closure is often not possible and other methods of skin cover will be required. Mechanical closure devices are available but split-skin grafting, which can be later excised is the most commonly used technique. When compartment syndrome has occurred in the presence of an underlying fracture, the fasciotomy creates an open fracture, and should be managed with early coverage to avoid problems with hospital acquired infection.

Late fasciotomy

Delayed fasciotomy following a crush injury or failed revascularization can potentially do more harm than good. If there has been a full compartment syndrome for more than 12h, the chances of the muscle recovery is remote. Fasciotomy will result in extensive debridement of the compartments and expose large volumes of devitalized tissue to hospital-acquired organisms. Late fasciotomies have been associated with a high frequency of morbidity and mortality related to sepsis. Non-operative treatment will be associated with dangerous levels of muscle breakdown products and the risk of renal failure. Temporary dialysis or amputation will need to be considered.

Site

Compartment syndromes occur wherever muscles are bound within rigid fascia compartments. All muscles have an investing fascia, but some are more constrained than others, and it is these which seem to be most susceptible to compartment syndrome. Compartment syndromes of the hands and feet, and their treatments, are described in their relevant chapters.

The classic site is the flexor compartment of the forearm. In the lower leg it is the anterior tibial and the deep posterior compartments. However, compartment syndromes are well described in all of the five compartments of the lower leg (including the separate tibialis posterior compartment).

12.3

Orthopaedic approach to the multiply injured patient

Andrew C. Gray

Summary points

- Major trauma results in a systemic stress response proportional to both the degree of initial injury (1st hit) and the subsequent surgical treatment (2nd hit).
- The key physiological processes of hypoxia, hypovolaemia, metabolic acidosis, fat embolism, coagulation and inflammation operate in synergy during the days after injury / surgery and their effective management determines prognosis.
- The optimal timing and method of long bone fracture fixation after major trauma remains controversial. Two divergent views exist between definitive early intramedullary fixation and initial external fixation with delayed conversion to an intramedullary nail once the patient's condition has been better stabilised.
- There is agreement that the initial skeletal stabilisation should not be delayed and that the degree of initial injury has a more direct correlation with outcome and the development of subsequent systemic complications rather than the method of long bone fracture stabilisation.
- Trauma patients can be screened to identify those more 'at risk' of developing systemic complications such as respiratory insufficiency. Specific risk factors include: A high injury severity score; the presence of a femoral fracture; the combination of blunt abdominal or thoracic injury combined with an extremity fracture; physiological compromise on admission and uncorrected metabolic acidosis prior to surgery.
- The serum concentration of pro-inflammatory cytokine interleukin (IL) 6 may offer an accurate method of quantifying the degree of initial injury and the response to surgery.
- The effective management of the polytraumatised patient involves a team approach and effective communication with allied specialties and theatre staff. A proper hierarchy of the injuries sustained can then be compiled and an effective surgical strategy made.

Introduction

Injury is a leading cause of morbidity and premature death in the young. The initial treatment of seriously injured patients has improved with advances which include: minimizing the time at the accident scene; a more structured training for those involved in front-line trauma management; designated trauma centres with appropriate and adequate support from allied specialities. These improvements, combined with the early initiation of resuscitation protocols and early emergency interventions, have been attributed to improved patient survival after serious injury.

Orthopaedic trauma produces a systemic stress response, which is related to the degree of initial injury. Clinical outcome is determined by the magnitude of response both to the initial injury and its subsequent surgical management. The term 'second hit' has been applied to the process whereby an injured and physiologically vulnerable patient is exposed to further trauma as a result of the surgical management of his injuries. Therefore, the initial orthopaedic management of a seriously injured patient must balance between limited physiological tolerance and the optimal volume of fracture stabilization surgery initially required.

Pathophysiology (Box 12.3.1)

A number of physiological processes should be considered in managing the multiply injured patient. Hypoxia, hypovolaemia,

Box 12.3.1 Pathophysiology

- Impaired aerobic metabolism
- Interleukin-6 prognostic marker
- Acidosis may reflect inadequate resuscitation
- Fat embolism may complicate fractures
- Emboli may inhibit pulmonary function
- Proinflammatory cytokines may be prognostic.

electrolyte imbalance, pulmonary and systemic embolization, coagulopathy, and inflammation all evolve over the initial hours and days after injury. The processes overlap and can operate in synergy to produce indirect end-organ hypoxia and subsequent tissue damage. The pathophysiology is also affected by the injury severity with direct associated injuries (for example, blunt trauma to the chest), which can render the patient more vulnerable to the effects of initial fracture management. A patient's individual response to injury can also vary considerably, with acute respiratory distress and major organ dysfunction being the most serious sequelae.

Hypovolaemia

The stabilization of pelvic fractures which are causing haemodynamic instability is an obvious priority. Isolated adult femoral shaft fractures can also result in a range of blood loss from 300–1300mL and transfusion rates of up to 40% with a direct correlation to the degree of preoperative haemorrhage. Blood loss and transfusion requirements are higher after multiple lower extremity fractures and there is an increased frequency of acute respiratory distress.

The direct effects of hypovolaemia are to reduce end-organ tissue perfusion and oxygen delivery. This results in impaired aerobic metabolism and subsequent tissue damage. Indirect effects include the activation of platelets and the production of a hypercoagulable state. Proinflammatory cytokines are also upregulated during the early phase after injury as a direct result of hypovolaemia with overproduction being related to increased rates of acute respiratory distress, multiple organ failure, and mortality. Cytokines are acute-phase proteins implicated in the activation of the complement cascade and the expression of fibrinogen. Interleukin-6 (IL-6) is a predominantly proinflammatory cytokine secreted by macrophages and T lymphocytes. It has a relatively long half-life with a peak concentration that occurs 4–6h after injury and persists for several days. This makes it a potentially useful prognostic marker after injury where levels have been shown to correlate with mortality rate. In addition, excessive proinflammatory cytokine production stimulates the breakdown of muscle proteins and further contributes towards tissue damage after hypovolaemic shock.

Metabolic acidosis and base deficit

The correction of hypovolaemic shock is paramount to any trauma resuscitation protocol. However, standard measurements of heart rate and blood pressure do not always accurately indicate adequate tissue and end-organ perfusion. 'Oxygen debt' and 'occult hypoperfusion' are terms which have been applied to the haemodynamically stable patient, who has persistently elevated lactate levels and a deficit in tissue oxygenation after trauma. This type of patient is inadequately resuscitated and has uncorrected metabolic acidosis. A twofold increase has been demonstrated in postoperative complications in patients undergoing early (<24h) femoral fracture fixation with elevated lactate levels (i.e. >2.5 mmol/L) that were not corrected prior to surgery. The complications involve a range of systems including respiratory (acute respiratory distress syndrome, ARDS), as well as an increased incidence of infection. Higher rates of multiple organ failure and respiratory complications have been demonstrated after major trauma in patients with persistent (>24h) and uncorrected metabolic acidosis. Such patients are more susceptible to the 'second hit' phenomenon caused by emergency surgery. Adequate haemodynamic and acid–base resuscitation is essential prior to surgery in order to optimize outcome and improve mortality after serious injury.

Pulmonary and systemic fat embolism

Fat embolus is defined as fat within the circulation and can occur with or without clinical sequelae. Most long-bone fractures produce a mild, asymptomatic, and transient hypoxaemia detectable on pulse oximetry. The severity of hypoxaemia is correlated to pulmonary fat embolic load and tends to be greater after high-energy trauma or multiple long-bone fractures. Subsequent episodes of hypoxaemia can occur after manipulative or operative procedures on the fractured extremity.

The clinical manifestations of fat emboli are usually explained on the basis of mechanical effects. Fat globules are forced into the venous circulation as a consequence of pressure changes within the medullary canal. They are then transported in the venous system to the right side of the heart and thereafter enter the pulmonary circulation where they obstruct small arterioles and capillaries. Systemic fat embolization can occur due to arteriovenous shunting of emboli through the pulmonary circulation. In addition, a patent foramen ovale can also predispose to systemic effects by allowing emboli to enter the left atrium directly and bypass the pulmonary filtration process.

However, fat emboli also produce 'biochemical' effects after trauma. Lipase enzyme stimulation and catecholamine production stimulate the conversion of benign fat to toxic free fatty acids which can potentially damage end-organ endothelial lining. These toxic products contribute to the stimulation of coagulative and inflammatory processes (systemic inflammatory response syndrome, SIRS), which form part of a patient's systemic stress response after trauma.

Surgical procedures that instrument the medullary cavity are associated with increased intramedullary pressure and fat embolus production. Instrument design and surgical techniques have concentrated on reducing this fat embolic load. The use of unreamed nails, reamer aspiration irrigation systems, and intramedullary canal venting are all surgical techniques available to reduce the pulmonary and systemic fat embolic load during intramedullary long-bone fracture fixation.

Fat and bone emboli can enter the systemic circulation via a patent foramen ovale. Paradoxical embolization can also occur through arterial–venous shunts in the pulmonary circulation. Transcranial Doppler ultrasound has correlated shunt size to the volume of embolic material detected in the cerebral circulation. Chest injury is commonly associated; an altered pattern of pulmonary circulation caused by the chest injury may increase the degree of blood shunting within the pulmonary.

Coagulation

Trauma and subsequent surgery activates thrombogenic and fibrinolytic pathways within the pulmonary and systemic circulations. Increased perioperative levels of prothrombin fragments 1 and 2 and fibrin degradation products have been demonstrated in isolated femoral fractures treated with intramedullary fixation.

This activation and possible loss of coagulation control has been linked to the development of acute lung injury and other systemic complications after major trauma. Therefore a synergistic embolic and coagulative response can occur after trauma which can affect pulmonary function. The more severe clinical responses can produce a clinical picture similar to disseminated intravascular coagulation. Localized disseminated intravascular coagulation within the lung has been attributed to acute lung injury due to the production of microthrombi.

Inflammation

In the minutes that follow a traumatic event, the direct tissue damage and change in haemostasis produce an inflammatory response. This involves the activation of monocytes and granulocytes that produce pro- and anti-inflammatory mediators. The term systemic inflammatory response syndrome (SIRS) has been applied to the generalized inflammatory response to trauma. This initial proinflammatory response is produced predominantly from macrophages and is primarily involved in removing damaged tissue and beginning repair processes. This initial stress response is relatively short lived and the monocytes soon become deactivated and unable to respond to fresh stimuli. A compensatory anti-inflammatory response (CARS) is then activated with mediators directly linked to the development of immunosuppression after trauma.

Therefore this imbalance can result in a period of compromised immunity after serious injury. A more pronounced immunodepression is seen with increasing levels of haemorrhage and tissue damage. The clinical effects of this immune imbalance are an exacerbation of shock, increased fluid transudation into end-organ interstitial spaces, coagulative activation and a predisposition to infection. These processes are apparent in the days after injury and correspond to the scheduling time for many surgical procedures, which will involve further tissue trauma.

A recent development has been the use of pro- and anti-inflammatory markers in the prediction of patient outcome after serious injury. Elevated IL-6 levels have been demonstrated in the polytraumatized patient with further increases measured after intramedullary femoral fracture fixation.

Excessive release of proinflammatory cytokines appears to be central in the pathogenesis of complications such as acute respiratory distress. Amplified levels of proinflammatory cytokines IL-1β and IL-8 have been demonstrated from bronchoalveolar lavage samples in patients with high injury severity scores. However, there was no corresponding rise in systemic (serum) concentrations.

The accumulation of neutrophils and proinflammatory mediators has been demonstrated in the alveolar space during early acute respiratory distress. The alveolar space appears to be converted into an area of intense localized inflammation. Inflammatory cytokines can act as chemoattractants to draw neutrophils from the plasma into the interstitial space. This was demonstrated in a prospective clinical study, where neutrophils were isolated and examined from peripheral blood samples taken from healthy volunteers and from patients after major musculoskeletal trauma. The chemoattractant properties of IL-8 were demonstrated with enhanced neutrophil migration across porous tissue culture inserts in the injured group. The coupling of enhanced neutrophil migration with elevated IL-8 levels may be central to the development of pulmonary and other end-organ inflammation.

Intraoperative planning and strategy in the polytraumatized patient (Box 12.3.2)

General considerations

Care of patients who have sustained multiple injuries requires a team approach. During the initial phase in the Emergency Department this is usually coordinated by an accident and emergency consultant, with other specialties intervening in a coordinated and timely fashion, following ATLS protocol. The role of the orthopaedic team is to firstly assess for any musculoskeletal injuries that require urgent intervention. The haemodynamically unstable pelvis is an obvious example. Open fractures require antibiotic and tetanus prophylaxis with the application of a sterile dressing. Obvious skeletal deformity such as that caused by a dislocated ankle or long-bone fracture can also be reduced and temporarily splinted.

A careful secondary survey performed at this stage will often identify other orthopaedic injuries not identified during the initial Emergency Department assessment. Appropriate plain x-rays can be ordered to assess these areas, but in a timely fashion to minimize treatment delay. At this stage a list of injuries should be complied and effective communication with allied specialties will allow a hierarchy of injuries to be established. The most urgent life- or limb-threatening injuries should be dealt with first.

It is important to identify any logistical problems that may impede the surgical treatment plan. The optimal department for the patient's continued care should be established with intensive care specialists involved at an early stage if required. The availability of theatre and the relative orthopaedic trauma experience of the available theatre staff should be ascertained. Good communication with regards to the type and availability of the appropriate surgical hardware required will save time and allow adequate theatre preparation time. Inform the theatre staff of the likely sequence of surgical procedures and whether simultaneous management of different injuries is being considered. The availability of a radiolucent table greatly eases simultaneous fixation of long-bone and pelvic injuries. The intramedullary stabilization of long-bone fractures without the need for skeletal traction in the multiply injured can also reduce operative time, but requires adequate experience and good surgical assistance.

The physiological status of the patient throughout surgery should be monitored with the help of the anaesthetist. Appropriate invasive monitoring should be instigated with the insertion of a central venous and arterial lines and use of a Swan–Ganz catheter. These give vital information regarding the true haemodynamic and

Box 12.3.2 Intraoperative planning

- ATLS protocol with trauma team
- Radiolucent table best
- Prioritize procedures, e.g. pelvic fixation
- En bloc debridement and stabilization for open injuries
- Immediate/early reconstruction best.

metabolic status of the patient with pulmonary arterial pressure measurements being proportional to the degree of arterial hypoxaemia. The most urgent surgical procedures, such as the external fixation of an unstable pelvic fracture or the adequate tissue debridement of an open fracture, should be performed initially. Extremity injuries often require being redraped in order to ensure sterility. A few minutes of discussion before surgery in order to formulate a surgical plan can minimize the operative time. The management of contralateral upper and lower extremity injuries can be facilitated by a team approach with simultaneous fracture fixation, but requires adequate staff numbers. The floating knee can be stabilized with femoral and tibial intramedullary nails inserted through the same small incision in a retrograde and antegrade fashion respectively. Priority should also be given to injury types where bone, cartilage, and soft tissue damage is likely to progress with time. The dislocated shoulder or ankle may have been already reduced in the emergency department; however, a femoral head fracture/hip dislocation or displaced femoral neck or talar fracture are examples of injuries where a delay in treatment affects prognosis.

Open fractures

The Gustilo and Anderson classification system for open fractures is most commonly used and effectively describes the degree of soft tissue injury, periosteal stripping, and vascular injury. The vascularity and perfusion of damaged tissue should be assessed and allied specialties such as plastic surgery involved early. The wound should be minimally re-exposed and inspected as this may increase the contamination risk. Antibiotic prophylaxis reduces the incidence of infection and is usually prescribed for 3 days. The regimen can be altered depending upon the likely degree of contamination. Cephalosporins are most commonly administered with the addition of an aminoglycoside and penicillin (to cover *Clostridium*) in more contaminated wounds. Double antibiotic therapy is more effective specifically after type 3 open fractures.

A soft tissue debridement is only effective if it removes all necrotic and contaminated material. Serial debridement removes only tissue which is clearly necrotic on each operative visit. An immediate and more extensive 'en bloc' excision into viable tissue allows removal of all affected material and minimizes the infection risk of subsequent bone stabilization and reconstructive procedures.

An adequate excision of skin, subcutaneous fat, fascia, and muscle must be performed. Bone fragments contaminated or free from soft tissue attachments should also be removed. There is debate about the best type of lavage to use. Pulsatile lavage will not compensate for an inadequate tissue debridement and may obscure the tissue planes and cause secondary tissue damage. The use of normal saline or Ringer's lactate with low pressure lavage should suffice after an adequate debridement.

The initial soft tissue and bone excision should not be compromised by concerns about subsequent tissue defects and wounds should not be closed under tension. Skeletal stabilization should then be performed after the initial debridement. If the initial soft tissue debridement was considered inadequate then a second debridement should be considered within 48h. Early plastic surgery input with regards to soft tissue reconstruction is vital. The reconstructive ladder describes the available soft tissue options which range from primary closure or a simple split skin graft, to pedicled or free flap transfers. Immediate reconstruction is recommended and has been shown to reduce complication rates and speed patient rehabilitation. Delayed reconstruction (>72h) after extremity trauma increases the incidence of flap failure, delays bone healing, prolongs hospital stay, and increases the number of subsequent operative procedures required.

Pelvic injuries

The management of a haemodynamically unstable pelvis is a priority after serious injury. The mechanism of injury and accident details will often give an accurate guide to the most likely pattern of injury sustained. For example a rollover car vehicle accident is associated with a lateral compression (LC) pattern; a fall from a height would more likely produce a vertical shear (VS) fracture; forceful leg abduction and external rotation of the hemipelvis, (common after a motorcycle accident) can produce an anterior–posterior compression (APC) injury. Physical examination includes one gentle pelvic manipulation to assess stability and a careful secondary survey to exclude associated injuries with particular attention given to the spine and lower limbs. Urethral injuries occur in 15% of patients. The initial radiographs taken will include an anteroposterior radiograph of the pelvis which is useful in determining the type of pelvic injury. The pattern of fracture can predict the most likely associated injuries. APC patterns are associated with pelvic bleeding and damage to hollow viscera. LC injuries have a higher incidence of head and thoracic injury. Vertical shear fractures often damage the sacral plexus and have a higher incidence of neurological problems. A trauma computed tomography (CT) scan can be arranged in the haemodynamically stabile patient and gives useful additional information especially with regards to posterior ring integrity and the presence of blood in the pelvis. The primary ATLS survey establishes resuscitation and whether the patient is responding well, transiently or poorly to intravenous fluids. Haemorrhage into the thorax, abdomen, retroperitoneum, or from extremity injuries should be identified. An increased pelvic volume with the presence of hypovolaemia is an indication to apply a pelvic binder in the Emergency Department. External pelvic fixation should be applied prior to a laparotomy due to the tamponade effect provided by an intact abdominal wall. The open pelvic fracture should be assessed as to whether it involves the rectum and therefore risks faecal contamination. Haemorrhage from an open pelvic wound can be temporized by wound packing with skeletal stabilization of the pelvic injury. Wound management forms part of a secondary procedure with an adequate debridement and a temporary colostomy for faecal diversion.

If there is continued haemodynamic instability after pelvic skeletal stabilization then either pelvic angiography with embolization or pelvic packing is indicated. Controversy exists with regards to the optimal treatment method. Delayed embolization later than 3h after injury is associated with increased mortality rates. Good indications for arterial embolization in patients who have not responded to resuscitation and skeletal stabilization are: vascular 'blush' visualized on CT scan and an expanding retroperitoneal haematoma. Pelvic packing is a technique advocated for the exsanguinating and unresponsive patient and can form part of a damage control operative protocol.

Definitive pelvic fixation involves anterior symphyseal plating for displacements greater than 2cm. A vertically unstable posterior ring injury requires closed reduction and percutaneous screw fixation or direct open reduction with plates and screws.

Upper extremity injuries

The age, hand dominance, profession, previous injuries sustained, associated medial problems (e.g. diabetes), and drug history are all important factors to obtain once the life-threatening injuries have been stabilized. The time from injury allows an estimation of the ischaemic duration and likely tissue viability, whilst the mechanism and nature of the injury are indicators of the degree of tissue damage and contamination. Whilst circulation can be adequately assessed under an anaesthetic, motor and sensory function to the upper limb extremity should be assessed in the emergency department. This vital information should be obtained quickly and calmly with minimal distress or discomfort to the patient with adequate analgesia given prior to assessment. Plain radiographs should be obtained, with other useful diagnostic adjuvant being Doppler ultrasound and compartment pressure monitors. Preoperative planning should involve an estimation of the likely surgical time. This has implications with regard to the type of anaesthetic used (regional or general) and the application of a tourniquet.

After serious skeletal injury, limb revascularization is the first priority before soft tissue debridement and skeletal stabilization. Early intervention with vascular surgery aims to restore both arterial and venous blood supplies. Important considerations are:

- The use of an autologous reverse saphenous vein graft
- The hazardous systemic effects of restoring venous blood supply after prolonged tissue ischaemia and accumulation of toxic metabolites
- The use of temporary shunts to re-establish arterial blood flow quickly and minimize the tissue ischaemic time.

Reconstructive options include: primary closure (immediate or delayed); skin grafts; local, regional, pedicle, and free flaps. Amputation can be considered if functional reconstruction is not possible. This decision may be subjective, but is best made after the combined good judgement of the surgical team rather than any one individual. Scoring systems such as the mangled extremity severity score (MESS) are less applicable to the upper limb.

Early skeletal stabilization of upper limb injuries allows early rehabilitation, facilitates nursing, and reduces patient discomfort and morbidity. Open reduction and internal fixation of long-bone diaphyseal fractures after polytrauma with dynamic compression plates and screws is standard. External fixation or intramedullary long-bone stabilization is less successful than in the lower limb with higher iatrogenic and soft tissue complication rates. Concerns with regards to increased infection and non-union rates after open fractures or operations through contused soft tissues should not alter the method of fracture fixation. Acceptable (<15%) rates of non-union and infection after fixation of open forearm fractures with good functional results have been demonstrated in the majority of patients. Bone shortening is a useful technique which can achieve a stable construct following extensive bone and soft tissue loss. This is well tolerated in the upper limb. Intra-articular fractures of the shoulder, elbow, and wrist require reduction and stabilization. Options include: splint immobilization; open reduction and internal fixation; arthroplasty and arthrodesis.

Tendon and nerve injuries are best managed by early reconstruction. The location of the injury (e.g. zone 2 flexor tendons), the extent of the surrounding soft tissue damage, and the patient's associated injuries all influence outcome. Primary tendon repair restores anatomy with the ipsilateral palmaris longus tendon or long toe extensors being the most commonly used donor grafts if tendon substance has been lost. Although early reconstruction improves outcome, tendon transfer procedures are usually performed at a later stage once the patient has recovered and an accurate assessment of any functional deficits has been made. The key to successful rehabilitation is dynamic splinting whilst adequately protecting the tendon repair. Nerve reconstruction generally produces less satisfactory results even after direct repair in a clean and well vascularized environment. Nerves should be sutured without tension and if this cannot be achieved due to soft tissue damage, then nerve transposition or free non-vascularized grafts (e.g. sural nerve) for more extensive defects are commonly used options.

Lower extremity injuries

The initial patient assessment should determine patient age, pre-injury level of function, mechanism of injury, time from injury, and haemodynamic status. Associated injuries to the head, chest, abdomen, and pelvis should be documented. Peripheral nerve function and the vascular status of the lower limb are assessed, with specific injuries more likely to compromise neurovascular function. Examples include the dislocated hip which can affect sciatic nerve function and medial tibial plateau fractures which are associated with a higher incidence of popliteal vessel and common peroneal nerve injury. Sensation over the plantar aspect of the foot and the presence of pedal pulses (use Doppler ultrasound if required) should be determined in the severely traumatized lower limb as they affect likely limb prognosis. Open wounds are assessed with an estimation of tissue loss and contamination, with the application of sterile dressings and administration of antibiotic and tetanus prophylaxis. Obvious lower limb deformity can be corrected under adequate analgesia, prior to appropriate radiographs being obtained and splints or plaster being applied to ease patient discomfort.

There has been much recent debate with regard to the merits of limb salvage versus amputation. The MESS is one tool available to help assess the need for amputation. The measured parameters include: patient age, haemodynamic status, tissue ischaemic time, and the degree of soft tissue injury and contamination. Such scoring systems cannot substitute for sound clinical judgement, experience, and a team approach.

The main principles in the treatment of lower limb injuries are: adequate reduction and stabilization of long bone fractures; reduction and restoration of joint surfaces; and the maintenance of a viable soft tissue envelope. Reamed intramedullary stabilization of closed and open femoral and tibial diaphyseal fractures in the polytraumatized is standard with the main indications for external fixation being: severe soft tissue injury; poor patient physiological status; skeletally immature bone; and a narrow intramedullary canal. Intramedullary fixation is preferred for all other types of open fracture. Unreamed intramedullary nailing theoretically reduces the pulmonary fat embolic release from the fracture site. However, the stimulation of the periosteal blood supply and generation of autogenic bone grafting produced by reaming are thought to be reasons for the higher rates of non-union and implant failure associated with unreamed intramedullary fixation of both open and closed fractures.

The use of a radiolucent table can reduce operative time in the polytraumatized patient. It allows easier access to multiple injuries. Antegrade nailing is predominantly performed, with the main indications for retrograde femoral nailing being: the obese patient; distal femoral fractures; ipsilateral femoral and tibial shaft fractures (i.e. the 'floating knee'); ipsilateral femoral neck and shaft fractures; and the pregnant patient.

The joint disruption and associated soft tissue swelling that can accompany pilon or tibial plateau fractures can be initially treated with a spanning external fixator. This stabilizes the injury, restores limb length, and allows the soft tissues to recover, whilst ligamentaxis aids articular surface reduction. Definitive internal fixation using minimally invasive incisions can then be performed initially if the soft tissues and patient's physiological status allow. However, a staged procedure with initial external fixation and definitive stabilization performed 1–2 weeks after injury is a reasonable alternative with low risks of infection and complications. Displaced intracapsular hip fractures, hip dislocations, and acetabular fractures with radiological evidence of incarcerated bone fragments are the more common examples of proximal lower limb injuries that require urgent surgical intervention in order to reduce the incidence of bone necrosis and articular cartilage damage.

Risk factors for systemic complications after trauma surgery (Box 12.3.3)

Direct pulmonary injury can occur due to aspiration, pneumonia, pulmonary contusion, and toxic inhalation. Indirect end-organ damage can also occur as a result of sepsis, multiple transfusions, over-aggressive fluid management, and disseminated intravascular coagulation. Severe chest injury is relevant to orthopaedic trauma patients as there is much debate regarding the optimal method of long-bone fracture fixation in order to minimize secondary pulmonary damage. A higher Injury Severity Score (ISS) increases the likelihood of developing systemic complications after injury. This has been confirmed in a retrospective review of 1278 trauma patients. A correlation was established between: ISS, the systemic inflammatory response to trauma (SIRS), and the incidence of acute respiratory distress and multiple organ dysfunctions.

The screening of trauma patients to identify those 'at risk' of developing respiratory insufficiency and symptoms related to fat embolus is key to the early diagnosis and treatment of the condition. Following long-bone injury, males under the age of 30 years with significant and early hypoxaemia are considered to be at a higher risk of developing respiratory insufficiency. Age may be a key factor in the development of symptoms related to fat embolus. In a consecutive series of 274 patients with isolated femoral shaft fractures, a 4% incidence of fat embolism syndrome (FES) occurred. There were no cases in patients aged over 35 years. The risk of developing FES was also reduced by early intramedullary fracture stabilization within 10h of admission. All 11 cases of FES in this study occurred in patients aged under the age of 35 years who had delayed (>10h) femoral fracture stabilization. Elderly patients are also more susceptible to the systemic effects of trauma with a lower (50%) lethal ISS required in patients aged over 65 years. Prolonged bed-rest and poor mobility are associated with increased morbidity and mortality in this age group.

Predictors for respiratory distress in adults include youth, high ISS, the presence of a femoral fracture, the combination of abdominal and extremity injuries, and physiological compromise on admission.

Box 12.3.3 Risk factors

- High ISS
- Over or under transfusion
- Long bone/male/<30 years/hypoxaemia
- Elderly.

Damage control orthopaedics versus early total care following polytrauma

Background

Peripheral limb injuries that involve long-bone diaphyseal fractures constitute a leading cause of hospitalization related to non-fatal injury. The initial treatment of these injuries was often delayed in order to 'optimize' a patient's condition. Immediate surgical treatment to stabilize these injuries was thought to worsen prognosis owing to further tissue damage and haemorrhage. However, it became apparent that early skeletal stabilization actually reduced the incidence of complications and improved outcome. Early intramedullary long-bone fracture stabilization reduces mortality rate in seriously injured patients, with reduced respiratory complications, reduced mortality and length of stay.

A policy of early long-bone fracture stabilization has been recommended to improve and reduce the frequency of respiratory and systemic complications after injury. The term 'early total care' has been applied to the definitive and early (<24h from injury) reamed intramedullary fixation of long-bone fractures and is considered the optimal form of treatment and a surgical priority in the seriously injured.

However, concerns have been raised with regard to secondary pulmonary and systemic embolic events, possibly linked to reamed intramedullary surgical techniques in the seriously injured. Patients with a low injury severity benefited from early long-bone stabilization with fewer respiratory complications. However, this benefit was not seen in patients with an ISS of greater than 18.

The concerns regarding the physiological effects of early reamed intramedullary femoral stabilization have been extensively investigated by the Hanover group, and they concluded early reamed nailing in high ISS patients increased the risk of ARDS and multiple organ failure.

Conservative surgical techniques that reduce operative time and tissue insult were proposed in seriously injured patients to minimize the 'second hit' caused by surgery. The term 'damage control' was applied to these surgical techniques. The types of patients thought to benefit from 'damage control' were those who had sustained serious penetrating or blunt injury with persistent hypothermia, coagulopathy, and acidaemia despite resuscitation. In such patients, the risk of metabolic failure from surgery was considered greater than the risk of failing to complete the initial definitive procedure. The broad principles of 'damage control' surgery include: limited procedures to control haemorrhage and stabilize life-threatening injuries; physiological patient monitoring within

an intensive care environment; definitive surgery once the patient's condition has been optimized.

The anatomical areas where damage control surgery could be applied have expanded and now include trauma patients with pelvic and peripheral limb injuries. These alternative surgical strategies involve the use of temporary external femoral fracture fixation to minimize the 'second hit' of surgery in the physiologically vulnerable patient. Delayed conversion to definitive reamed intramedullary fixation is performed once the patient's condition has been optimized.

The use of external fixation is more common after pelvic fractures to reduce pelvic volume and limit blood loss. Initial external fixation is, however, a viable alternative to intramedullary stabilization of long-bone fractures. External fixation can provide adequate temporary stabilization in severely injured patients with a rapid operating time, reduced blood loss, and reduced pulmonary embolic load being potential benefits. Successful delayed conversion to definitive intramedullary fixation can be performed at an average of 5 days following initial treatment, but is reserved for the more seriously injured patients with a mean ISS of 29. This often includes associated injuries to the head, chest, and abdomen. Conversion to intramedullary fixation is performed at an average of 7 days after initial surgery with low infection rates (1.7%).

Advocates of this surgical strategy would indicate that following injury, the degree of initial trauma and the patient's subsequent biological response cannot be altered. Outcome can only be improved by minimizing the 'second hit' of surgery. Advocates of 'early total care' would argue that the degree of initial injury alone is the sole contributing factor to the development of subsequent systemic complications and that the method of fracture fixation is inconsequential given a background of severe injury.

There is agreement about certain principles;

- Initial skeletal stabilization should not be delayed
- The degree of initial trauma has a more direct correlation to the development of subsequent systemic complications than the method or timing of any peripheral extremity fracture stabilization.

A practical application of 'damage control orthopaedics' (Box 12.3.4)

There is no general agreement about which patients are suitable for 'damage control orthopaedics' (DCO) but it should be considered in multiple trauma patients with a significant chest injury or an ISS probably in excess of 30. Other patients can be treated by standard methods of long-bone fixation. Adequate haemodynamic and metabolic resuscitation are paramount prior to surgery. Uncorrected metabolic acidosis in the seriously injured appears to be a key feature with increased pulmonary and systemic complications after fracture fixation surgery. The clinical indicators used by the Hanover group, where DCO techniques have been most widely reported are: ISS higher than 20 with an associated chest injury; polytrauma with abdominal/pelvic trauma and shock (systolic blood pressure <90mmHg); ISS higher than 40 with no chest injury; x-ray evidence of bilateral lung contusions; mean pulmonary arterial pressure greater than 24mmHg; increase of more than 6mmHg in pulmonary arterial pressure after intramedullary reaming.

Box 12.3.4 Prevention of complications

- Urgent long bone stabilization
- May be best to ex-fix long bones initially
- Ex-fix pelvis
- Damage control
- Lung protective protocols.

They have also described certain clinical parameters associated with a poor outcome after serious injury. These include: inadequate resuscitation, coagulopathy, hypothermia, multiple blood transfusions (>25 units), multiple long-bone fractures, excessive surgical time (>6h), metabolic acidosis (pH <7.24), and an exaggerated inflammatory response judged to be an IL-6 measurement of >800pg/mL.

Damage control techniques have also been extended to include aspects of initial patient resuscitation. Aggressive fluid therapy has the potential to exacerbate lung interstitial oedema. Therefore, the concept of delayed fluid therapy may form part of a 'damage control' surgical protocol in order to avoid this complication. Invasive monitoring of central venous, arterial, and pulmonary arterial pressures allows a more accurate assessment of hypoxaemia and true haemodynamic status. The effects of surgery and other therapeutic interventions can then be closely monitored with regular blood sampling allowing oxygen, carbon dioxide, and lactate levels to be closely monitored.

Ventilatory strategies in polytraumatized patients have also altered. Conventional therapy is aimed to maximize oxygen delivery and obtain normal arterial blood gas measurements. This often involved the use of high tidal volumes and pressure ventilation techniques. These may have the potential to cause secondary pulmonary damage and could predispose to the development of acute respiratory distress after injury. Lung protective protocols are now often implemented in the seriously injured which involve less aggressive ventilatory intervention. The goals are to facilitate pulmonary recovery and to prevent any further alveolar damage. Low tidal volumes are used with pressure limited ventilatory techniques and non-toxic concentrations of inspired oxygen to achieve 'adequate' arterial blood gas concentrations.

With regards to surgery the 'DCO' concept can be extended out with the most recent debates with regard to femoral fracture fixation. A pelvic ring injury, where haemorrhage is poorly controlled and exsanguination imminent, can also be suitable for DCO. The role of angiography and arterial embolization has been debated. The time taken to perform this procedure has been shown to correlate with mortality rate. In order to avoid delay some trauma centres advocate minimally invasive pelvic fixation (with a pelvic binder or external fixator) followed by pelvic packing if this does not obtain haemodynamic control. Any haemodynamic, metabolic, or coagulative problems can then be corrected in an intensive care environment and definitive pelvic surgery arranged

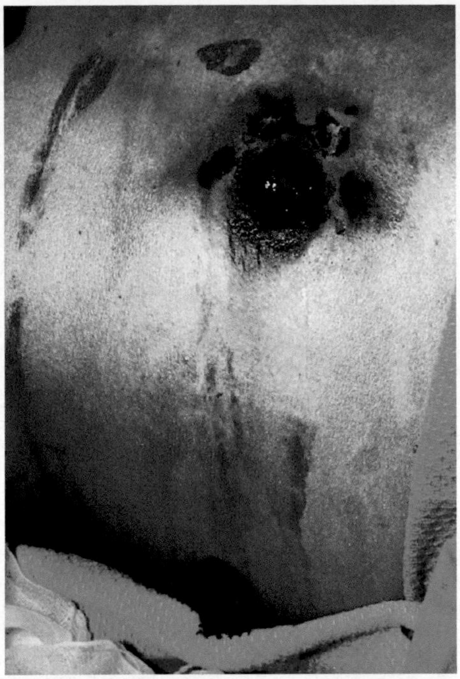

Plate 1 M16 gunshot wound to the side of the chest of a soldier. The entrance wound is larger than the exit wound, and is identified by powder burns.

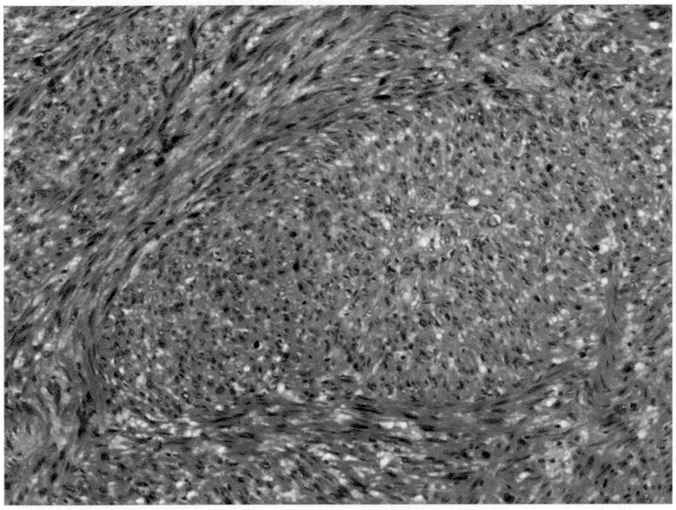

Plate 2 Typical microscopic features of high-grade leiomyosarcoma characterized by intersecting fascicles of eosinophilic spindle cells (10×; H&E stain).

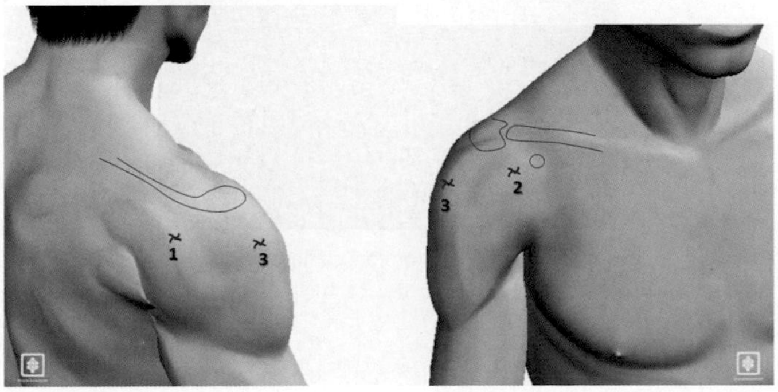

Plate 3 Portals for arthroscopic subacromial decompression.

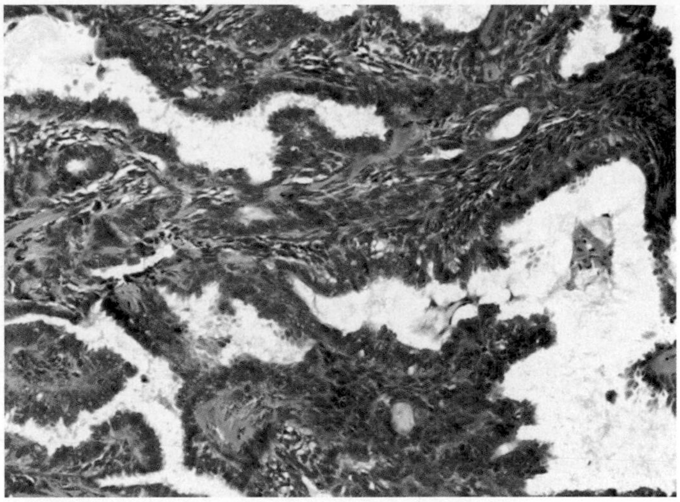

A

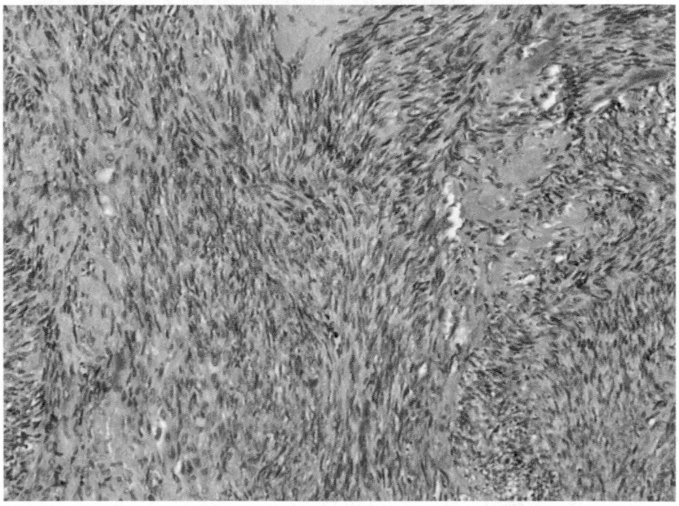

B

Plate 4 A) Biphasic synovial sarcoma showing glandular-like spaces with an intervening spindle cell component (10×; H&E stain). B) Monophasic synovial sarcoma is composed of fascicles of spindle cells with ill-defined basophilic cytoplasm (10×: H&E stain).

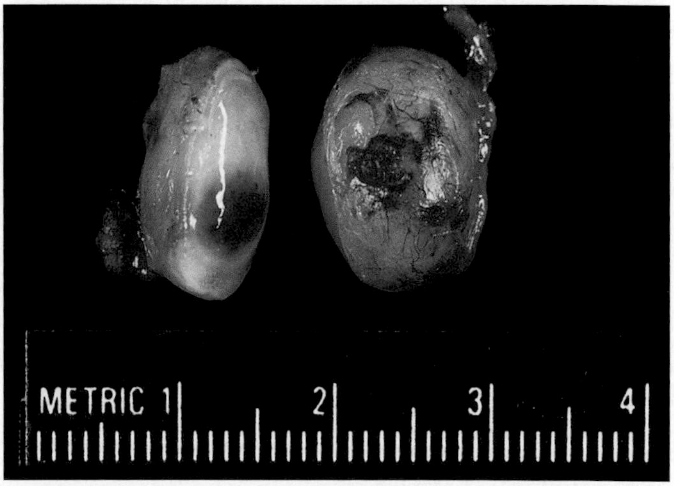

Plate 5 Characteristic macroscopic appearance of a schwannoma as an encapsulated eccentric growth of the associated nerve.

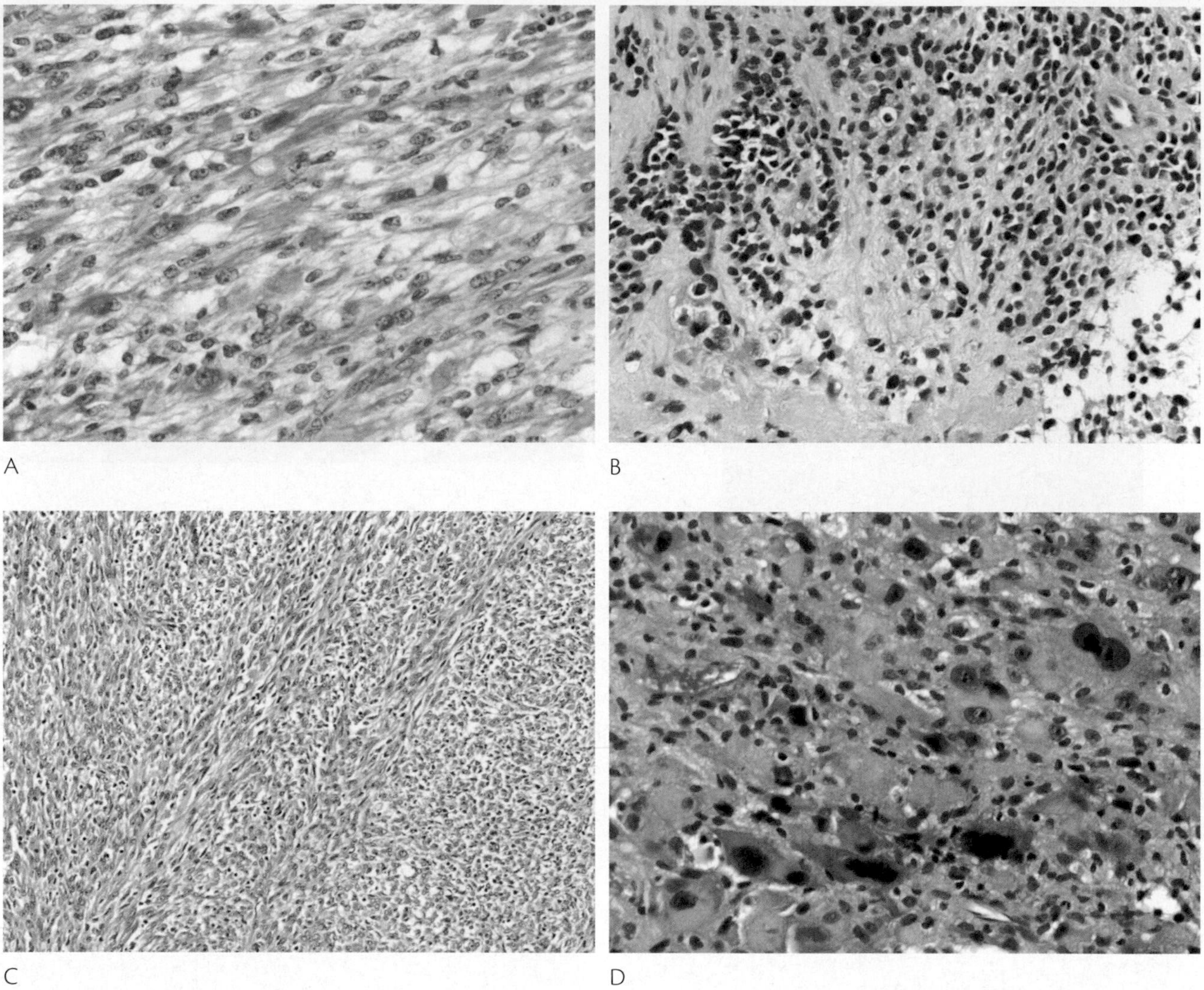

Plate 6 A) Typical embryonal rhabdomyosarcoma featuring fascicles of elongated spindle cells with striking rhabdomyoblastic differentiation (20×; H&E stain). B) Typical features of alveolar rhabdomyosarcoma showing small round blue cells with focal rhabdomyoblastic differentiation (20×; H&E stain). C) Intertwining long fascicles of spindle cells with eosinophilic cytoplasm and prominent nucleoli characterize the spindle cell variant of rhabdomyosarcoma (10×; H&E stain). D) Pleomorphic rhabdomyosarcoma is characterized by large cells with pleomorphic nuclei and eosinophilic cytoplasm (20×; H&E stain).

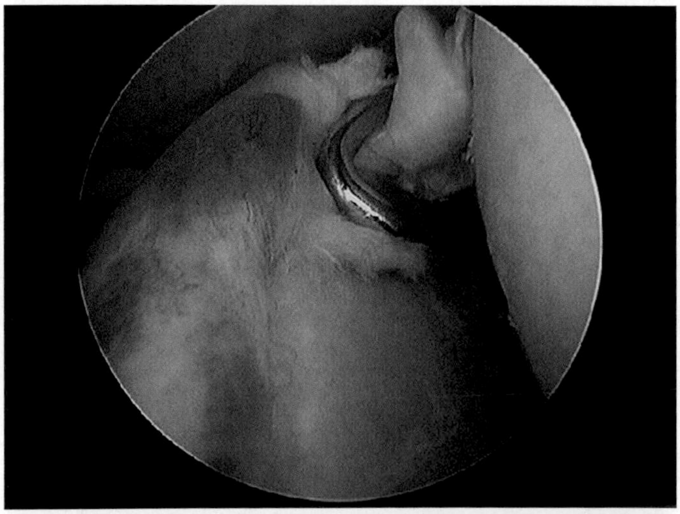

Plate 7 Posterior jerk test. Posterior instability is tested with the 'posterior jerk test'. This test is poorly described in standard textbooks. The arm is elevated in adduction and internal rotation, and the humeral head will gradually slip off the back of the glenoid; this is usually pain free. With the shoulder thus dislocated the arm is taken from adduction to abduction and the humeral head will suddenly relocate with a jerk; this is usually associated with pain.

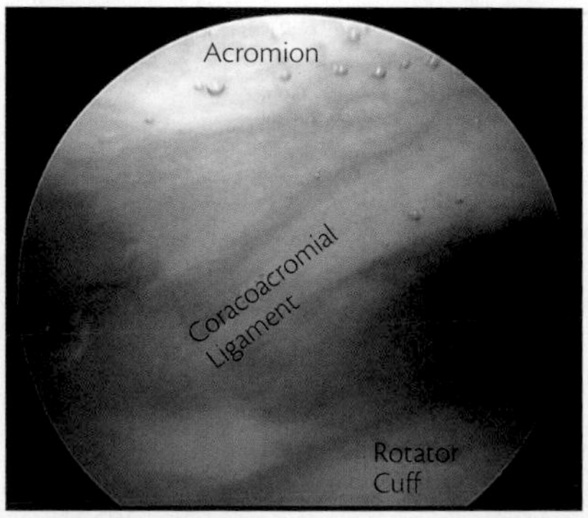

Plate 8 Bursoscopy view showing acromion, coracoacromial ligament, and bursal surface of rotator cuff.

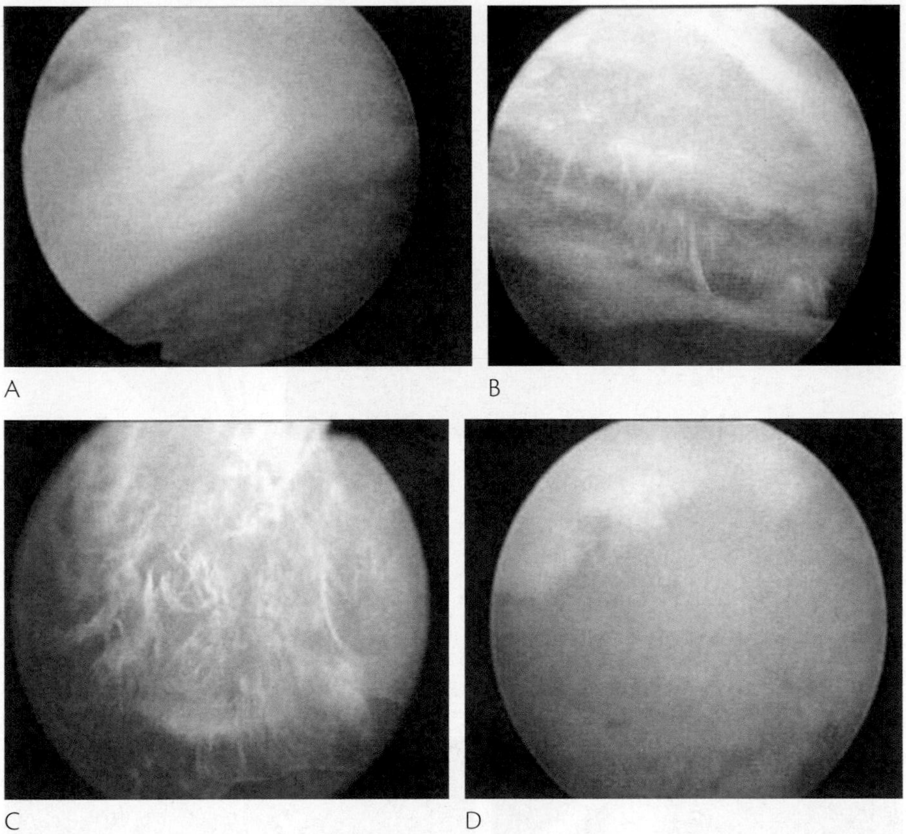

Plate 9

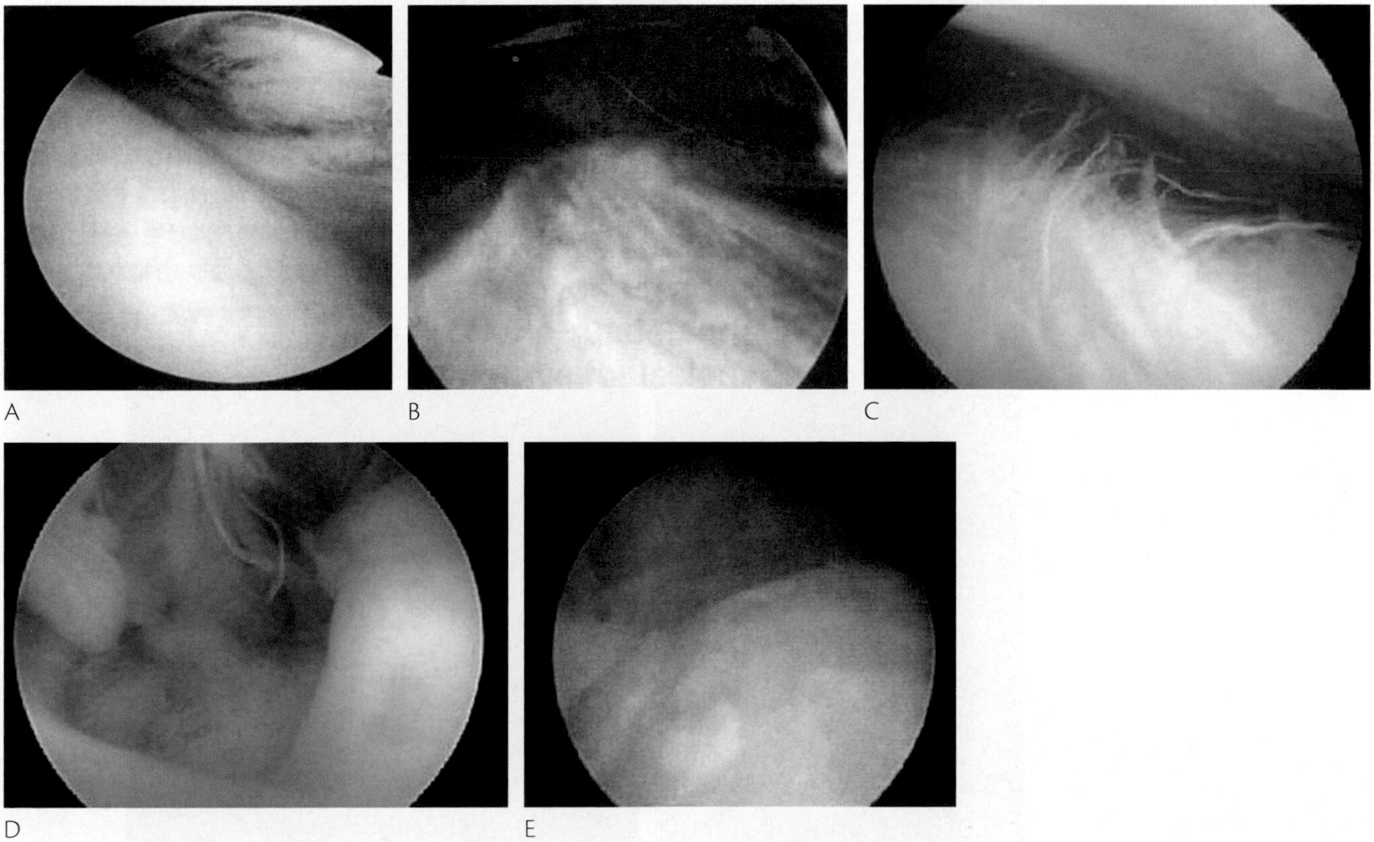

Plate 10

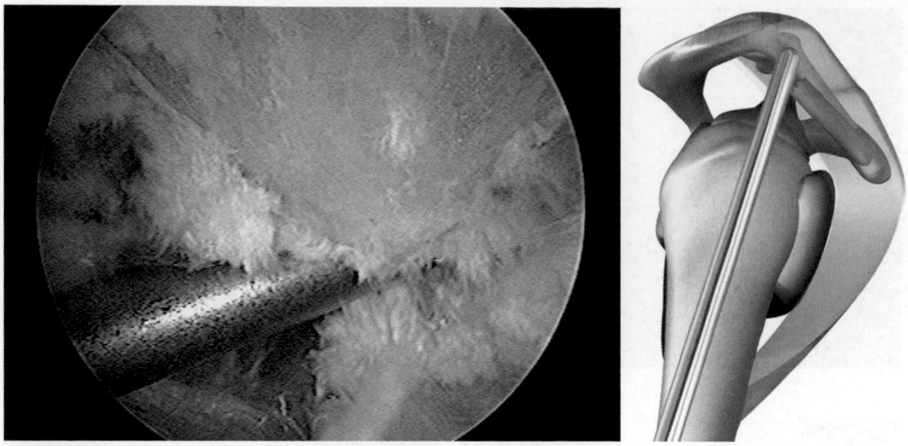

A B

Plate 11 Assessing resection level using shaver (scope and three-dimensional).

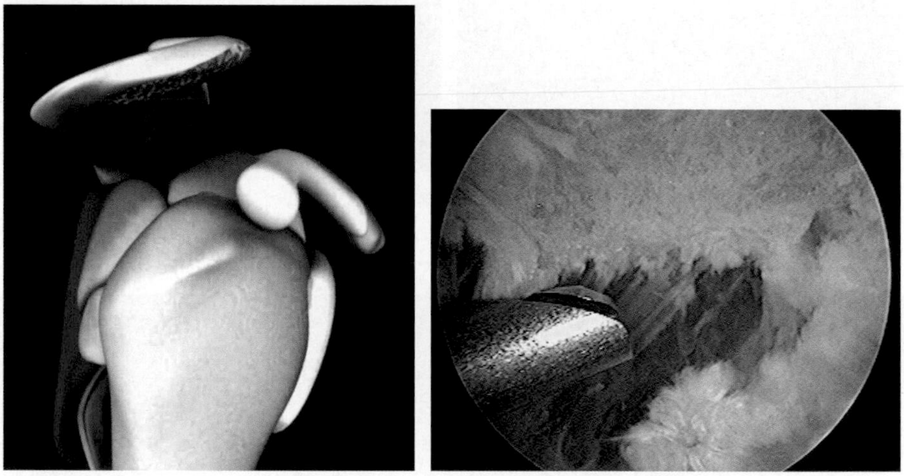

A B

Plate 12 Completed decompression images (scope and three-dimensional).

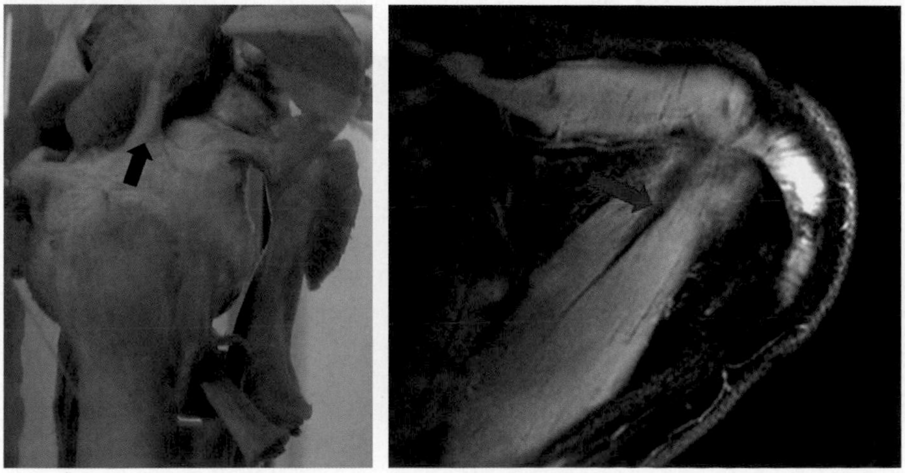

A B

Plate 13 Anterior oblique cord of supraspinatous (macroscopic, ultrasound, and arthroscopic views).

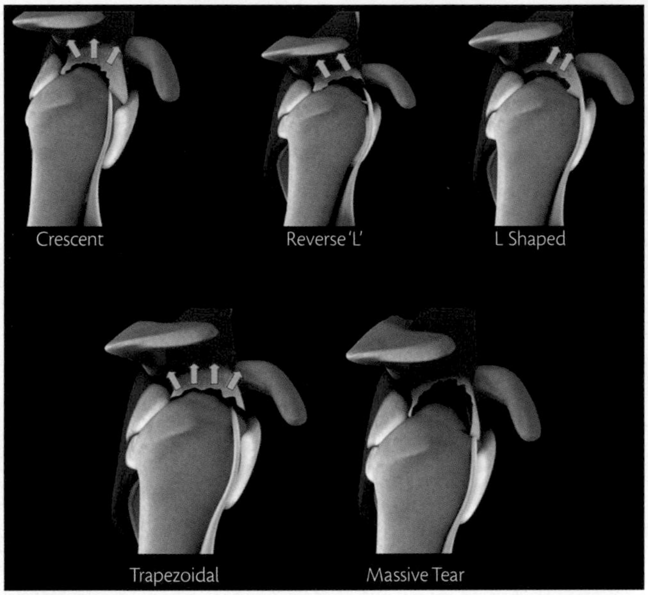

Plate 14 Tear patterns.

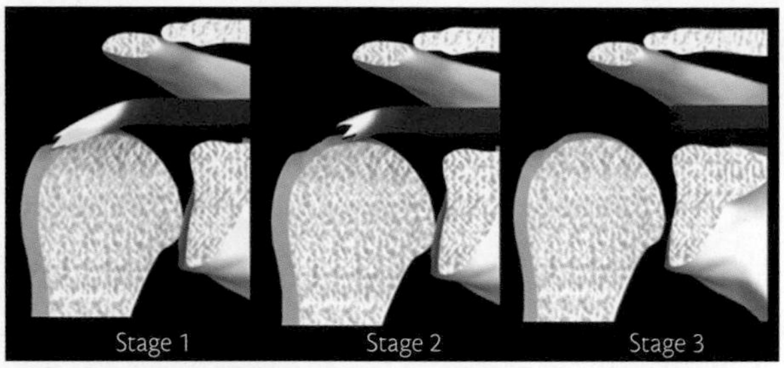

Plate 16 Patte classification.

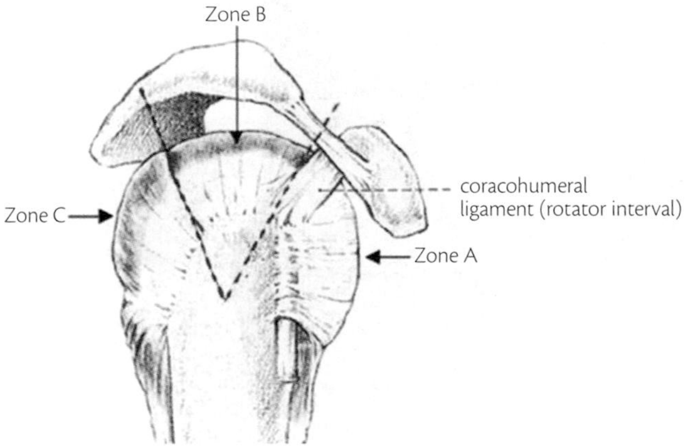

Plate 15 Habermeyer classification.

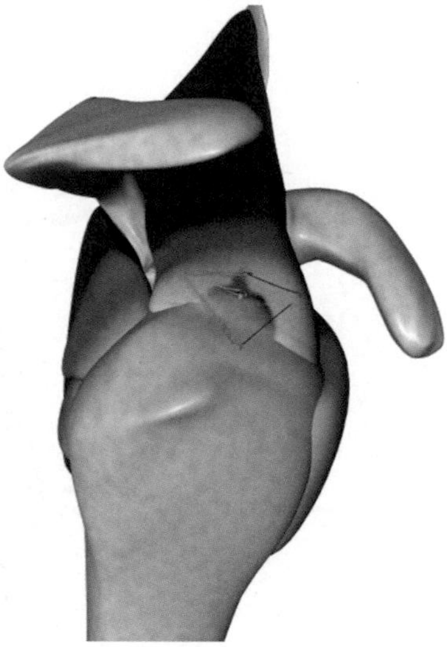

Plate 17 Simple and double row techniques for small tears.

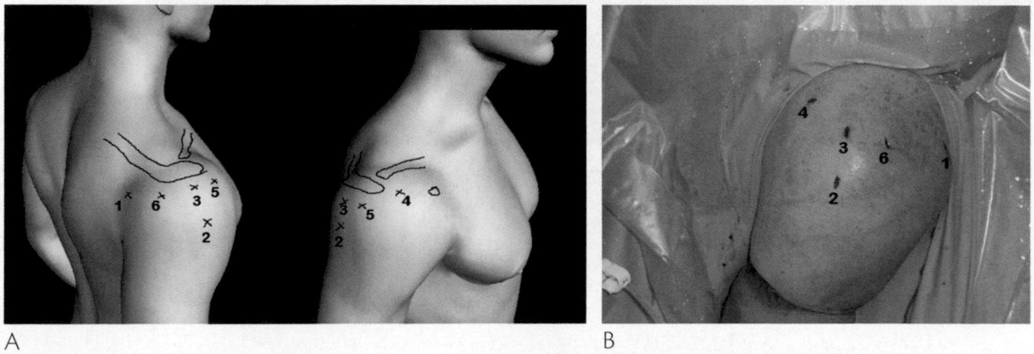

Plate 18 Portals for arthroscopic rotator cuff repair.

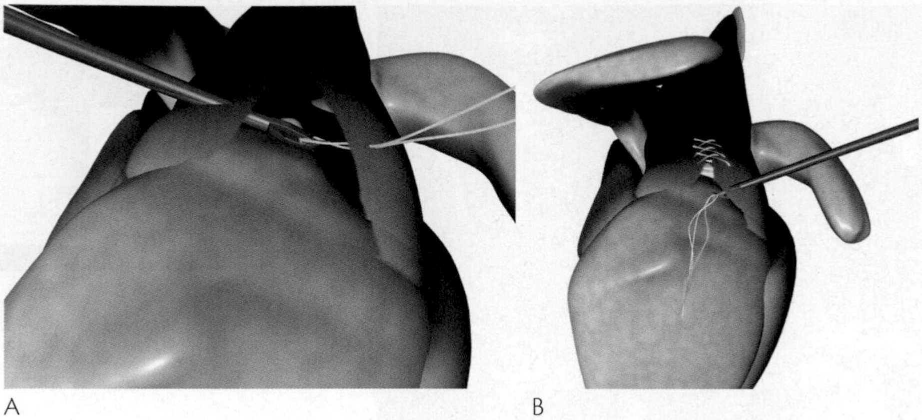

Plate 19 Margin convergence techniques.

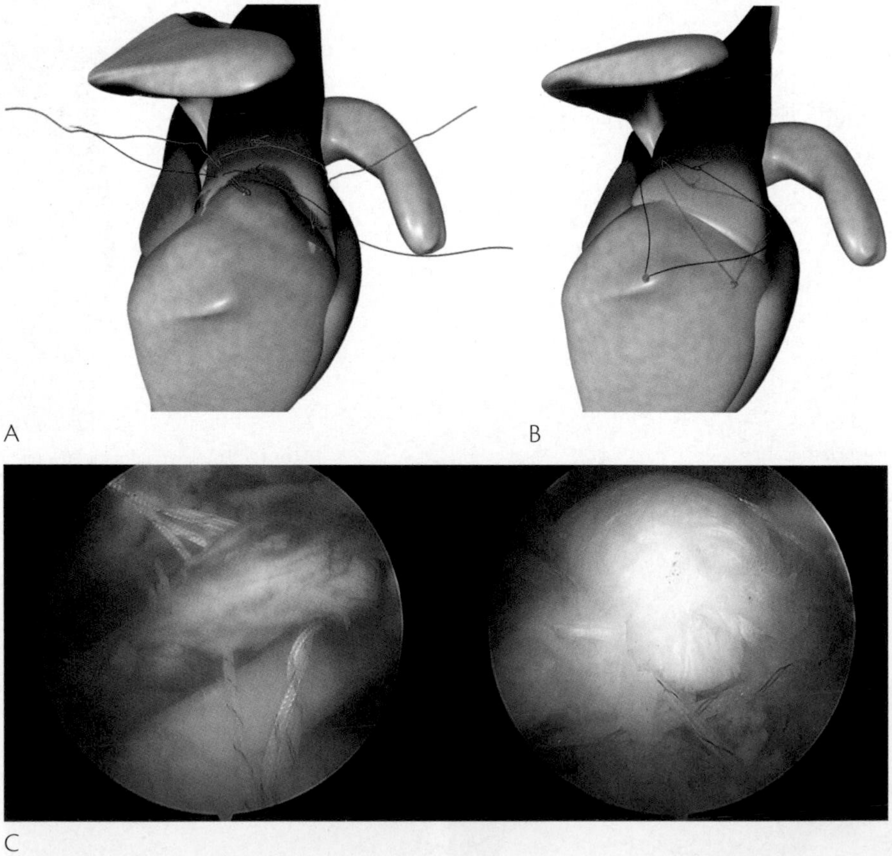

Plate 20 Double-row technique for large tears.

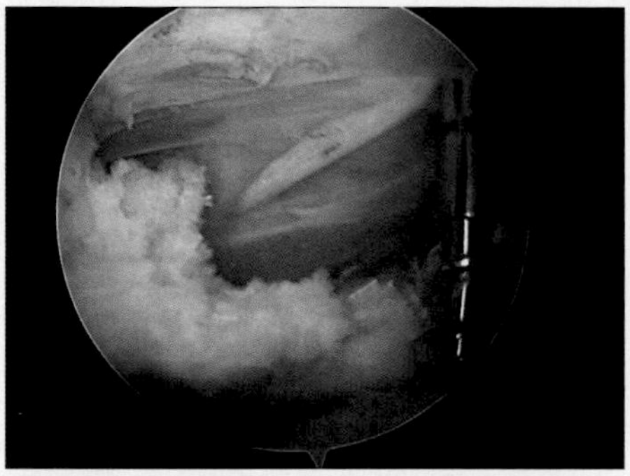

A

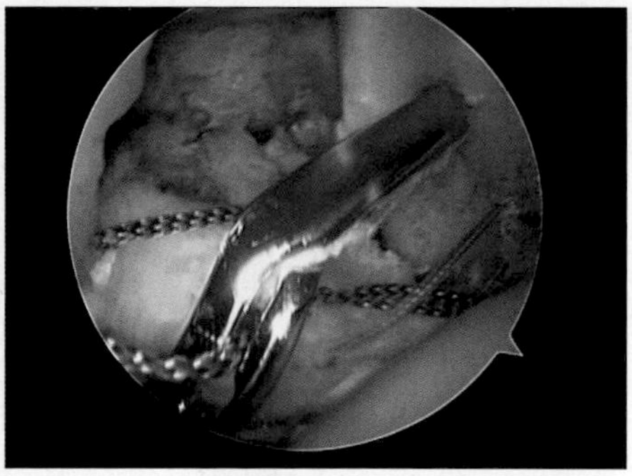

B

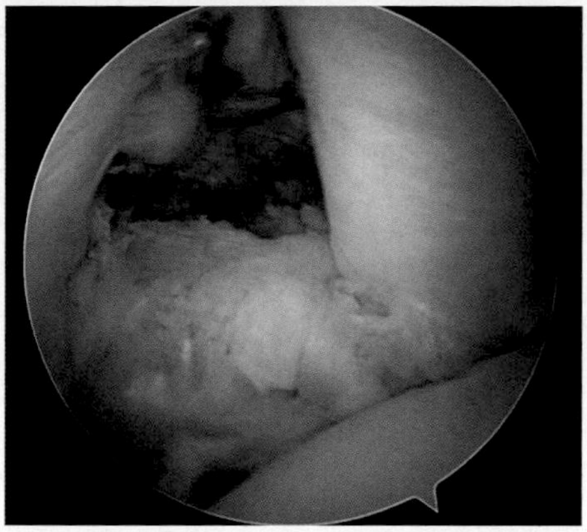

C

Plate 21 Arthroscopic subscapularis repair.

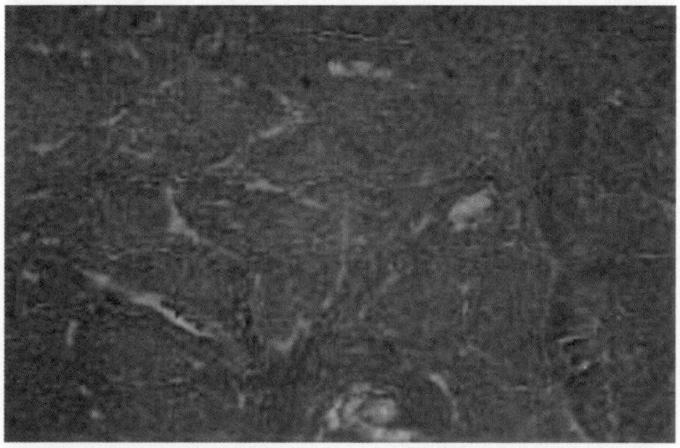

Plate 22 The histology of contracted (frozen) shoulder shows nodules and bands of type III collagen with fibroblasts and myofibroblasts.

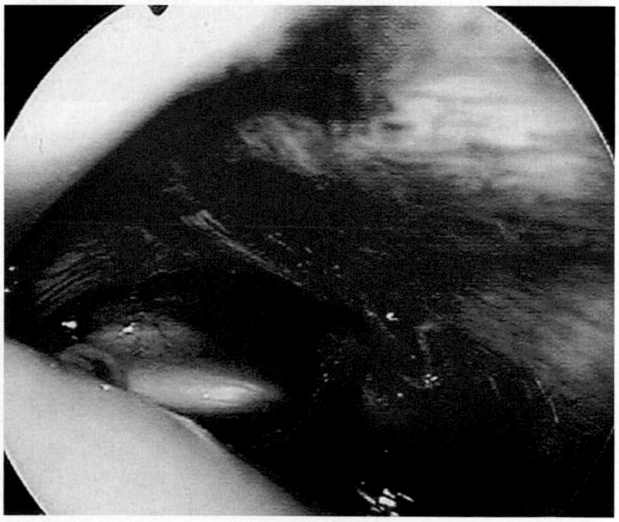

Plate 23 The main arthroscopic finding in contracted (frozen) shoulder is angiogenesis.

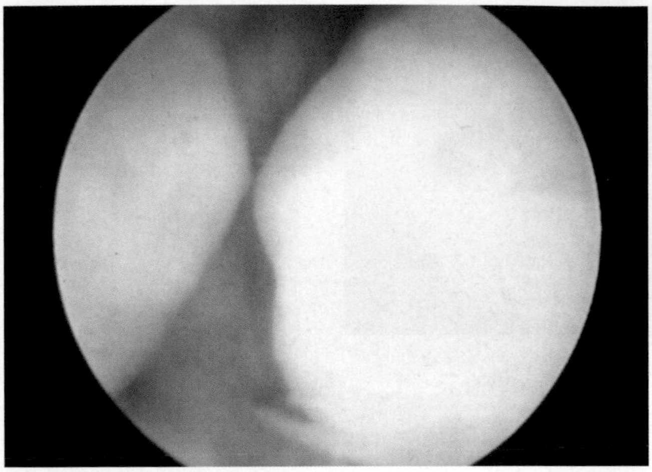

Plate 24 Olecranon tip and ossicle in fossa.

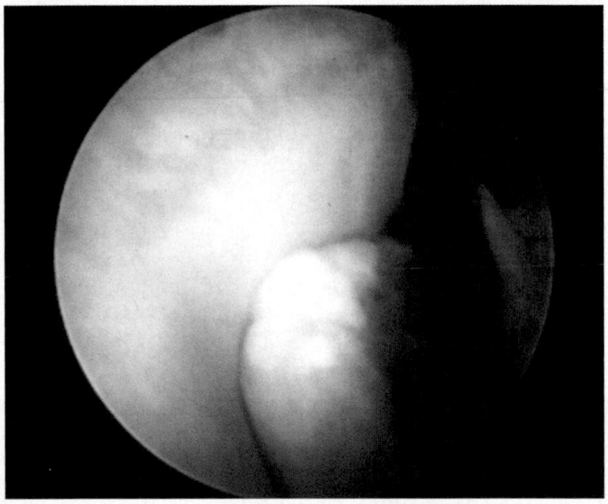

Plate 25 View of coronoid tip from anteromedial portal.

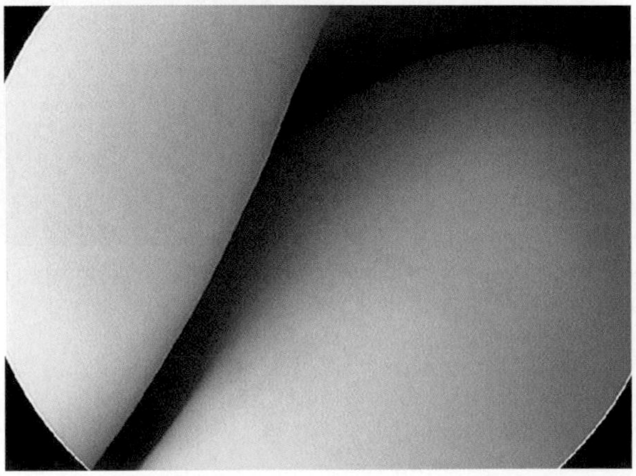

Plate 26 View of radiocapitellar joint from posterolateral portal.

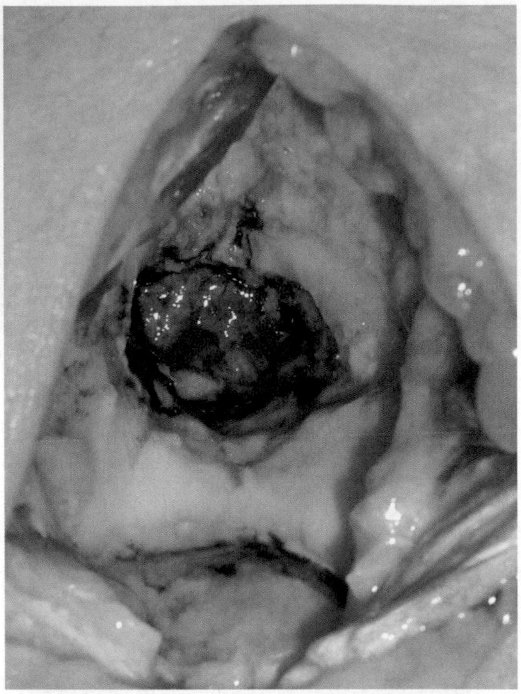

Plate 27 OK procedure.

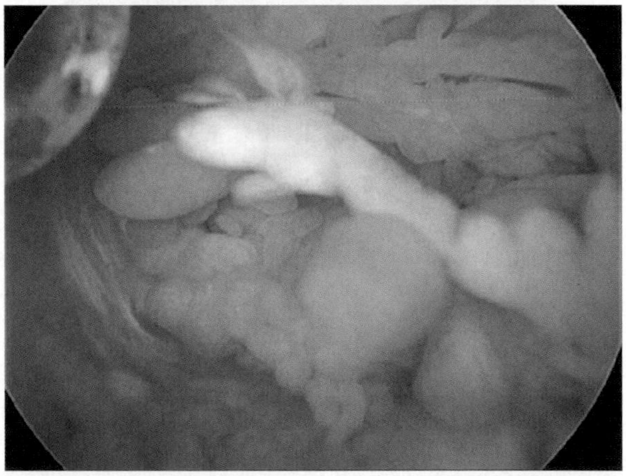

Plate 28 Synovitis.

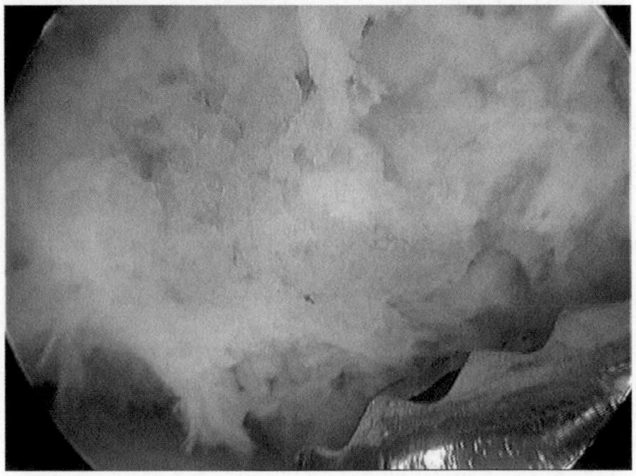

Plate 29 Debridement of osteochondritic capitellum.

12.4

Head, thoracic, and abdominal injury in the orthopaedic patient

K. Boffard

Summary points

- The orthopaedic trauma surgeon will be involved in the majority of poly trauma patients.
- It is essential that the associated non-orthopaedic injuries are identified and appropriately managed.

> It is my contention that failure to care for the surgical patient… is the most powerful disincentive to know the science of surgery. A surgical registrar who has not been exposed to the trauma patient and to intensive care is incompletely trained, unqualified, and unprepared for surgical practice or specialty training.
>
> Donald Trunkey, Address to the Association of Surgeons of Great Britain and Ireland, 1988

Head trauma

Extracranial injury

Scalp injuries

Laceration of the scalp may be associated with significant bleeding. Control with a compression dressing, and follow with deep sutures if necessary; debride and repair later. 'Haemostasis before cosmesis.' Haematomas under the galea can attain considerable size, and there is a significant danger of sepsis so these should be drained, rather than aspirated. Scalp infections may spread intracranially via the emissary veins.

Skull injuries

Skull fractures are described according to integrity of the overlying skin. A fracture can be diagnosed by digital exploration of the wound, or radiographically. Skull fractures can be divided into:

- External (skull vault)
- Simple
- Compound
- Fracture of base—diagnosis of basilar fractures is usually clinical:
  - Cerebrspinal fluid leaking from the nose or ear
  - Periorbital ecchymosis ('racoon eyes')
  - Ecchymosis behind the ear (Battle's sign)
  - Blood in the external canal is considered as a basilar fracture until proven otherwise by computed tomography (CT) scan.

Depressed skull fractures

Traditionally all depressed skull fractures (Figure 12.4.1) were elevated when the depth of the depression exceeded the thickness of the adjacent skull table, to alleviate compression of the underlying cortex. However, not all fractures need elevation in the absence of underlying focal injury.

Intracranial injury

Brain injuries

Severe brain injury accounts for almost half of all deaths from trauma and is a major cause of residual disability in trauma patients. Any other treatment (including orthopaedic or spinal fixation) should not prejudice the brain, or cause further damage. Any patients sustaining major injury should be suspected of having an associated cervical spine injury.

The availability of CT (Figure 12.4.2) scanning has been shown to reduce mortality, as the time taken to diagnose and evacuate an intracerebral haematoma is critical in determining outcome. However, the majority of patients with brain injury do not have a lesion suitable for neurosurgical intervention.

Brain damage is divided into:

Primary brain injury

This occurs at the time of injury and is irreversible, i.e. lacerations, contusions, axonal injuries of the white matter due to shearing forces. Only 35% of deaths due to brain injuries are due to primary brain injury.

Primary brain injury may be:

- Focal—focal injuries, which are usually caused by direct blows to the head, comprise contusions, brain lacerations, and intracerebral as a secondary procedure, once the patient's condition has been optimized.

There have also been concerns about intramedullary fracture fixation in the multiply injured patient with a head injury, but these have not been confirmed. Early fracture stabilization has the potential to reduce pain and minimize further soft tissue damage and fat embolism release, and should form part of the initial management of patients with a head injury along with adequate resuscitation. Improved neurological outcome does appear to be related to intracranial pressure monitoring and aggressive management if required. Optimal outcomes have been demonstrated by maintaining a cerebral perfusion pressure of above 70mmHg with intracranial pressures of below 20mmHg.

Further reading

Blow, O., Magliore, L., Claridge, J.A., Butler, K., and Young, J.S. (1999). The golden hour and the silver day: detection and correction of occult hypoperfusion within 24 hours improves outcome from major trauma. *Journal of Trauma*, **47**(5), 964–9.

Burgess, A.R., Eastridge, B.J., Young, J.W., *et al.* (1990). Pelvic ring disruptions: effective classification system and treatment protocols. *Journal of Trauma*, **30**(7), 848–56.

Fabian, T.C., Hoots, A.V., Stanford, D.S., Patterson, C.R., and Mangiante, E.C. (1990). Fat embolism syndrome: prospective evaluation in 92 fracture patients. *Critical Care Medicine*, **18**(1), 42–6.

Giannoudis, P.V. (2003). Current concepts of the inflammatory response after major trauma: an update. *Injury*, **34**(6), 397–404.

Gustilo, R.B. and Anderson, J.T. (1976). Prevention of infection in the treatment of one thousand and twenty-five open fractures of long bones: retrospective and prospective analyses. *Journal of Bone and Joint Surgery*, **58A**, 453–8.

Pape, H.C., Hildebrand, F., Pertschy, S., *et al.* (2002). Changes in the management of femoral shaft fractures in polytrauma patients: from early total care to damage control orthopedic surgery. *Journal of Trauma*, **53**(3), 452–61.

Schwab, C.W. (2004). Introduction: damage control at the start of 21st century. *Injury*, **35**(7), 639–41.

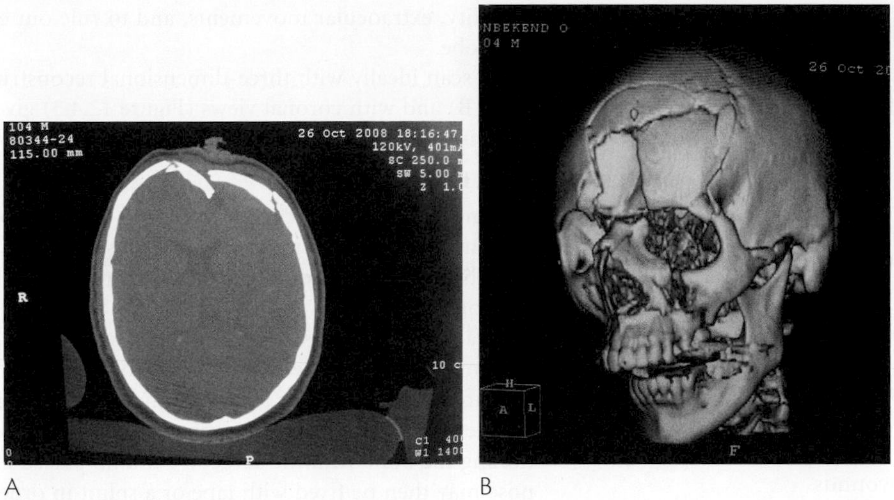

Fig. 12.4.1 A) CT scan of depressed fracture of skull. B) Three-dimensional reconstruction of same patient—45-degree view.

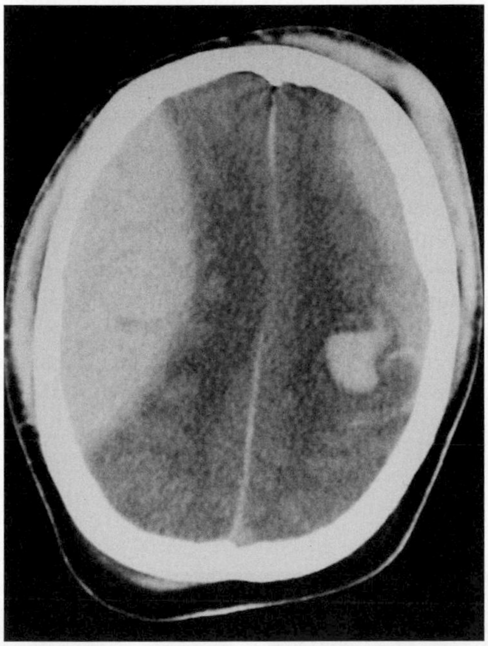

Fig. 12.4.2 CT scan showing combined extradural, subdural, and intracerebral bleed.

haemorrhage leading to the formation of a haematoma in the extradural, subarachnoid, subdural, or intracerebral compartments within the head

- Diffuse—diffuse brain injury causes diffuse damage to the axons. The distal segment of the axon undergoes degeneration. Profound deficits may result from this diffuse axonal injury.

Secondary brain injury

This occurs at a later stage, may be preventable, and to a significant extent, reversible, and is the cause of 65% of mortality due to brain injury. The injury is due to hypoxia, hypovolaemia causing hypoperfusion, and hypothermia. An understanding of these is fundamental, and the treatment of a head-injured patient should emphasize early control of the airway, adequate ventilation and oxygenation, correction of hypovolaemia, and limiting hypothermia. Hyperventilation is no longer routinely used. No surgery is possible and management is dependent on appropriate intensive care management of the patient.

Adjuncts to care

Antibiotics

Broad-spectrum antibiotic prophylaxis is recommended for both military and civilian penetrating craniocerebral injuries, including those due to sports or recreational injuries. Generally, a cephalosporin, or amoxicillin/clavulanate is recommended.

Prophylaxis is *not* recommended for fracture of the base of the skull.

Anticonvulsants

Seizure activity in the early post-traumatic period following head injury may cause secondary brain damage as a result of increased metabolic demands, raised intracranial pressure, and excess neurotransmitter release.

For patients who have had a seizure after a head injury, anticonvulsants are indicated and are usually continued for 6 months to 1 year.

Recent review of the available evidence has demonstrated that while prophylactic antiepileptics are effective in reducing early seizures, there is no evidence that treatment with prophylactic antiepileptics reduces the occurrence of late seizures, or has any effect on death and neurological disability.

Burr holes

Patients with closed head injury and expanding extradural or subdural haematomas require urgent craniotomy for decompression and control of haemorrhage.

In remote areas where neurosurgeons are not available, non-neurosurgeons (often orthopaedic surgeons) may occasionally need to intervene to avert progressive neurological injury and death. Surgeons in remote, rural hospitals in the United States of America have shown that emergency craniotomy can be undertaken with good results where clear indications exist.

Craniofacial injuries

Introduction

Face and neck injuries can be the most 'difficult-to-manage' wounds encountered.

Immediate management

Focusing on ABC priorities is vital: airway distress due to upper airway obstruction above the vocal cords is generally marked by inspiratory stridor.

- During airway control, maintain cervical spine immobilization. Up to 10% of patients with significant blunt facial injuries will also have a cervical spine (C-spine) injury. Obtunded patients with blunt facial trauma should be treated with C-spine immobilization. Unstable C-spine injury is very rare in neurologically intact penetrating face and neck wounds
- The airway may be partially or wholly obstructed from:
  - Blood or oedema resulting from the injury
  - The tongue may obstruct the airway in a patient with a mandible fracture
  - A fractured, free-floating maxilla can fall back obstructing the airway
  - Displaced tooth fragments may also become foreign bodies
  - Remove foreign bodies (strong suction, Magill forceps)
  - There is a real danger of airway obstruction due to haematoma. Early intubation is a key management requirement. Cricothyroidotomy or emergency tracheotomy may be necessary
- Injuries to the face are often accompanied by significant bleeding. Control of facial vascular injuries should progress from simple wound compression for mild bleeding to vessel ligation for significant bleeding. A Foley catheter inserted blindly into a wound and inflated, may rapidly staunch bleeding. Vessel ligation should only be performed under direct visualization after careful identification of the bleeding vessel. Blind clamping of bleeding areas should be avoided, because critical structures such as the facial nerve and parotid duct are susceptible to injury. Intraoral bleeding must be controlled to ensure a patent and safe airway. Do not pack the oropharynx in the awake, unintubated patient, due to the risk of airway compromise: first secure the airway with an endotracheal tube
- Complete assessment of remaining injuries (fractures, lacerations, oesophageal injury, ocular injuries)
- Penetrating injury may not follow classic Le Fort patterns but may have a significant soft tissue injury component (base of tongue, soft palate).

Evaluation

After initial stabilization, cleanse dried blood and foreign bodies gently from wound sites in order to evaluate the depth and extent of injury. Examination of the bony orbits, maxilla, forehead, and mandible and a complete intraoral examination of all mucosal surfaces for lacerations, ecchymosis, step-offs or mobile segments and malocclusion suggestive of a fracture, should be performed.

A cranial nerve examination must be performed, to assess vision, gross hearing, facial sensation, facial muscle movement, tongue mobility, extraocular movements, and to rule out entrapment of the globe.

CT scan ideally with three-dimensional reconstruction (Figure 12.4.1B) and with coronal views (Figure 12.4.3) gives an accurate assessment of the damage.

Nasal fractures

The most common fracture. Diagnosed clinically by the appearance and mobility of the nasal bones. Epistaxis must be controlled with direct pressure, anterior pack-gauze, or Foley catheter balloon tamponade.

Treatment is by closed reduction of the fractured bones and/or septum into their correct anatomical positions, up to 7 days after fracture. A blunt elevator is placed into the nasal cavity in order to elevate the depressed bony segment, while simultaneously repositioning the bone with the surgeon's thumb placed externally. The nose may then be fixed with tape or a splint in order to maintain the reduction.

Fractures of the mandible

The mandible is a 'ring structure' and in 50% of cases (like the pelvis) may be fractured in more than one site. The most common site is the subcondylar region.

Patients present with limited jaw mobility or malocclusion. Confirmation of the diagnosis is best by CT scan with coronal reconstruction. Dental Panorex is the single best plain film. PA mandible serves as a less reliable but satisfactory study (though subcondylar fractures are difficult to see).

Treatment is determined by the location and severity of the fracture and condition of existing dentition. Remove only teeth that are severely loose or fractured with exposed pulp. Even teeth in the line of a fracture, if stable, and not impeding the occlusion, should be maintained.

Immediate reduction of the mandibular fracture and improvement of occlusion can be accomplished with a bridle wire (24 or 25 gauge) placed around at least two teeth on either side of the

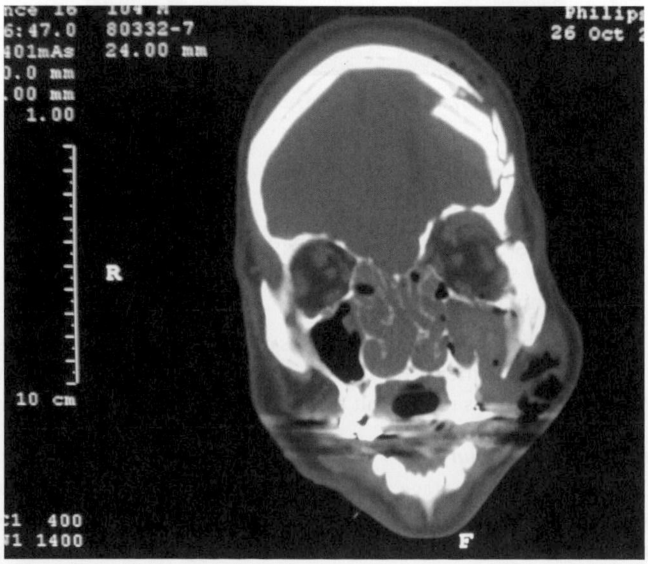

Fig. 12.4.3 CT scan in coronal plane.

fracture. More severe fractures with malocclusion will require immobilization with maxillary–mandibular fixation for ± 6 weeks.

Major midfacial fractures

These multibone injuries may be life threatening due to loss of airway, haemorrhage, or spinal injury. The haemorrhage is commonly from epistaxis, oral haemorrhage, or combination bleeding. Occasionally it can be catastrophic. Control is usually by a combination of pack tamponade and direct pressure. If uncontrolled, early sedation and intubation of the patient followed by appropriate packing may be life saving.

The fractures are associated with a significant amount of energy. They are particularly associated with central nervous system, cervical spine, and orbital injury.

Le Fort's classification of facial injuries

Facial bony injuries are classified into Le Fort type fractures (Figure 12.4.4 and Table 12.4.1), although not infrequently, the injuries may be a combination of several different components. Diagnosis is primarily by CT scan, with specific coronal views but clinical examination can be helpful and is performed by a gentle attempt to mobilize the hard palate and midface while stabilizing the skull.

Place the thumb and forefinger of one hand on the nasal bridge to stabilize, then with the other hand, determine mobility of maxilla by placing the thumb on alveolus and forefinger on the palate and attempting gentle distraction in an anterior–posterior direction.

Penetrating injury may not follow classic Le Fort patterns but may have a significant soft tissue injury component (base of tongue, soft palate). Normal principles of systemic palpation and inspection apply, looking for crepitus, tenderness, internal and external ecchymosis, and subconjunctival haemorrhage that might suggest fractures.

Management of facial fractures

The goals of fracture repair are realignment and fixation of fragments in correct anatomical position with dental wire (inferior, but technically easier), or plates and screws. With the exception of fractures that significantly alter normal dental occlusion or compromise the airway (e.g. mandible fractures), repair of facial fractures may be delayed for 2 weeks.

Wounds should be gently cleansed with saline and light scrub solutions; foreign bodies should be meticulously cleaned from wounds prior to closure. Devascularized wound edges require only minimal debridement. Facial lacerations should be closed in layers within 24h.

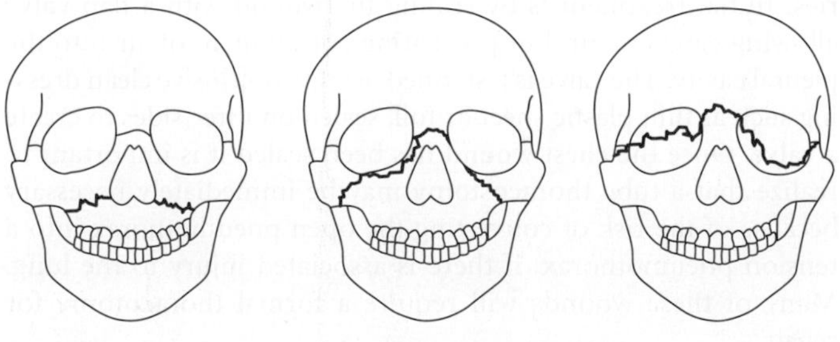

Fig. 12.4.4 Diagrammatic representation of Le Fort fractures.

Table 12.4.1 Anatomical and clinical presentation of facial fractures

Fracture	Anatomical	Clinical
I	Fracture separates the entire alveolar process from maxilla	Manipulation of the maxilla results in gross movement of the upper lip
II	Separation of midface, including the nasal bone, from the orbit (pyramidal).	Manipulation of the maxilla results in gross movement of the upper lip and nose
III	Detachment of the face from the skull (craniofacial disarticulation)	Manipulation of the maxilla results in gross movement of the whole face

If the patient's jaws are wired together, it is imperative that wire cutters be available next to the patient at all times.

The thorax

Introduction

Following major injury, 50% of fatalities are due to primary brain injury, 25% due to chest trauma, and in another 25% (including brain injury), thoracic injury contributes to the primary cause of mortality. Injury to the chest wall and thoracic viscera can directly impair oxygen transport mechanisms. Hypoxia and hypovolaemia resulting, may cause secondary injury to patients with brain injury, or may directly cause cerebral oedema. Conversely, shock and/or brain injury can secondarily aggravate thoracic injuries and hypoxaemia by disrupting normal ventilatory patterns or by causing loss of protective airway reflexes and aspiration.

A significant number of thoracic trauma-related deaths occur at the time of injury, for example, rapid exsanguination following traumatic rupture of the aorta in blunt injury or major vascular disruption after penetrating injury. Of those survivors with thoracic injury who reach hospital, a distressing proportion dies in hospital as the result of misassessment or delay in the initiation of treatment. These deaths occur *early* as a consequence of shock, or *late* as the result of adult respiratory distress syndrome (ARDS) and sepsis.

Most life-threatening thoracic injuries can be simply and promptly treated after identification by needle or tube placement for drainage. Only around 25% of injuries will require surgical intervention.

Thoracotomy performed in the Emergency Room (ERT) has specific indications, and is generally reserved for immediate control of haemorrhage following penetrating injury.

The spectrum of thoracic injury

Thoracic injuries are grouped into two types (Table 12.4.2):

- Immediate threat to life
- Potential threat to life.

The entity of the 'traversing mediastinal wound' in penetrating injury warrants specific mention. Injuries of this type frequently involve damage to a number of the mediastinal structures and are thus more complex in their evaluation and management.

Patients arrive in two general physiological states:

Table 12.4.2 Life-threatening thoracic injuries

Immediately life threatening	Potentially life threatening
Airway obstruction—tracheal injury	Simple pneumothorax
Tension pneumothorax	Simple haemothorax
Open pneumothorax	Pulmonary contusion
Flail chest/pulmonary contusion	Tracheobronchial tree disruption
Massive haemothorax	Blunt cardiac injury
Pericardial tamponade.	Traumatic rupture of the aorta (TRA)
Injury to the great vessels	Traumatic diaphragmatic herniation (TDH)
Air embolism	Oesophageal disruption

- Haemodynamically stable
- Haemodynamically unstable.

In patients with penetrating injury to the upper torso who are haemodynamically unstable, and the bleeding is into the chest cavity, it is important to insert a chest tube as soon as possible during the initial assessment and resuscitation. In the patient *in extremis* who has chest injuries or where there may be suspicion of a transmediastinal injury, bilateral chest tubes may be indicated. x-ray is *not* required to insert a chest tube, but *is* useful after the chest tubes have been inserted to confirm proper placement.

In patients who are haemodynamically stable, and those with blunt injury, x-ray remains the simplest initial screen for pneumothorax or haemothorax and to exclude pulmonary contusion. In these patients it is preferable to have the x-ray completed before placement of a chest tube—the decrease in air entry may not be due to primary lung pathology, and especially following blunt injury may be due to pulmonary contusion, or a ruptured diaphragm with bowel or stomach occupying the thoracic cavity.

Diagnosis

Diagnosis of thoracic injury is usually made, depending on the stability of the patient, using a combination of clinical examination, chest x-ray, CT scan, angiography, and magnetic resonance imaging (MRI) scan.

Clinical examination

The clinical examination of the chest will yield a significant amount of information. The trachea is checked for its position (central), the chest is examined in the standard fashion for pain, dullness to percussion, and alteration in breath sounds, and the heart is examined. It is essential to perform an examination of the chest posteriorly at an early stage, using a log-roll technique to protect the spine. The spine is examined for tenderness which may indicate vertebral injury. In penetrating injury, a search is made for additional wounds on the back.

Chest x-ray

A chest x-ray, initially taken supine will add valuable information to the clinical examination. Specific attention should be paid the 'ABCs' of the chest x-ray

- A: airway—including tracheal deviation, etc.
- B: breathing—lung fields, presence of contusion
- C: circulation—mediastinum and heart, particularly presence of a wide mediastinum
- D: diaphragm—the placement of a nasogastric tube may help clarify the position of the oesophagus, stomach, and left hemidiaphragm
- E: environment—rib fractures, associated fractures of scapula, etc.

CT scan of the chest

The chest CT scan is generally regarded as the 'gold standard' for diagnostic imaging. The scan should be performed with contrast, allowing CT angiography as required. The scan gives excellent information regarding the chest wall, lungs, mediastinum, great vessels, and bony structures.

CT scan should never be performed in the haemodynamically unstable patient.

Management of immediate threats to life

Tension pneumothorax

Tension pneumothorax is air under pressure in the pleural cavity due to a valve effect. It is associated with life-threatening cardiorespiratory compromise due to collapse of the affected lung, compression of the normal lung, and decreased venous return to the heart.

The presentation is dramatic, with a panicky patient who on examination has dyspnoea, cyanosis, tachypnoea, shock, distended neck veins. The symptoms are similar to those caused by cardiac tamponade. The trachea is shifted to the opposite side, best felt just above the sternal notch. Breath sounds are reduced or absent, and there is hyper-resonance on the affected side. The diagnosis is clinical. There is no time for x-rays! (Figure 12.4.5.)

Treatment is immediate decompression to relieve the pressure, by placement of a needle in the second interspace, midclavicular line, followed by a tube thoracostomy in the fifth interspace, anterior or midaxillary line.

Open pneumothorax

The incidence of open pneumothorax or significant chest wall injuries following civilian trauma is quite low, certainly less than 1% of all major thoracic injuries. True open pneumothorax is most often associated with close range shotgun blasts and major industrial injury. There is usually a large gaping wound commonly associated with frothy blood at its entrance. Respiratory sounds can be heard with to-and-fro movement of air. The patient often has air hunger and may be in shock from associated visceral injuries. Initial treatment is by sealing the wound with a flap valve allowing egress of air, but preventing entrainment of air into the pleural cavity. The valve is fashioned using an occlusive clean dressing such as thin plastic sheet or foil, sealed on three sides to create a valve. Once the chest wound has been sealed it is important to realize that a tube thoracostomy may be immediately necessary because of the risk of converting the open pneumothorax into a tension pneumothorax, if there is associated injury to the lung. Many of these wounds will require a formal thoracotomy for repair.

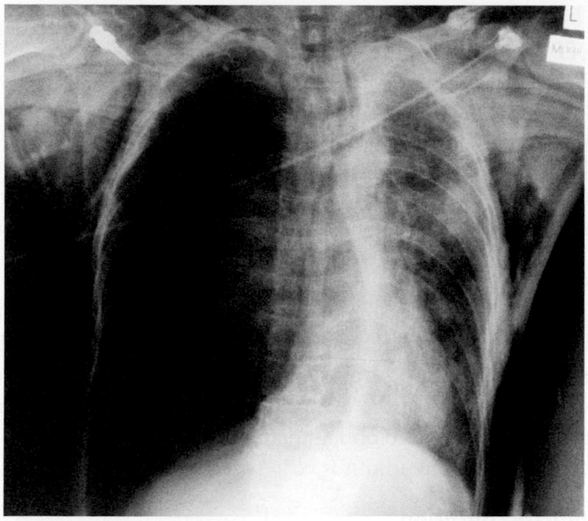

Fig. 12.4.5 Chest x-ray showing an untreated tension pneumothorax.

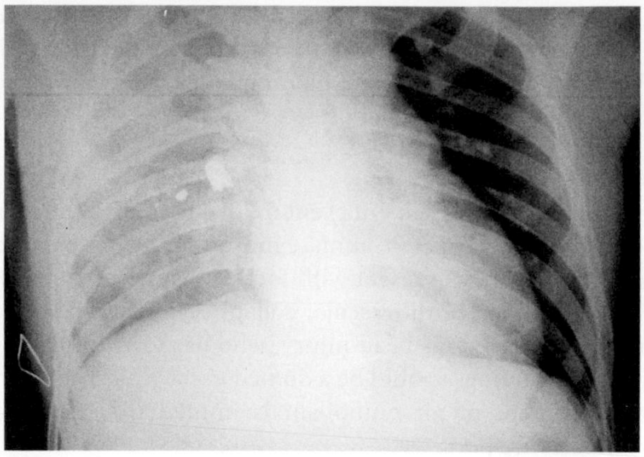

Fig. 12.4.6 Chest x-ray showing massive haemothorax.

Flail chest

Anterior or lateral fractures of three or more adjacent ribs in two or more places, causes a flail segment, which moves inwards during inspiration (paradoxical respiration). For flail chest the threat to life stems from the dual pathology of an underlying pulmonary contusion, and a decreased tidal volume (the chest wall moves inwards, rather than the lung expanding, on inspiration) causing a ventilation-perfusion defect, and thereby respiratory failure.

Diagnosis is initially based on the clinical examination and x-ray chest: Initial x-ray may not show pulmonary contusion. The initial blood gases may be normal—the first sign of respiratory failure is often a decreased arterial PCO_2 (due to hyperventilation), followed by a decrease in PO_2/FiO_2 ratio.

Traditionally, flail chest has been managed by adequate ventilation with humidified oxygen, symptomatic relief of pain (allowing more comfortable breathing), and, if necessary, internal splinting using artificial ventilation ('internal pneumatic stabilization'). While this undoubtedly is the method of choice in most instances, there has been increasing interest in open reduction and fixation of multiple rib fractures. In uncontrolled trials, there have been considerable benefits shown, with a shortening of hospital time, and improved mobility.

Massive haemothorax

Massive haemothorax is equally life threatening. Approximately 75% of patients with hilar, great vessel, or cardiac wounds expire shortly after injury, mostly due to a major injury of a great vessel. In about 15% of cases, the bleeding is from deep pulmonary lacerations. In blunt injury, with fractured ribs, this is most commonly an intercostal artery or the internal mammary artery. In a few patients, there may be injury to the hilum of the lung or the myocardium.

The diagnosis of massive haemothorax is invariably made by the presence of shock, ventilatory embarrassment, dullness to percussion, and shift in the mediastinum. Chest x-ray (Figure 12.4.6), will confirm the extent of blood loss but generally, tube thoracostomy is done immediately to relieve the threat of ventilatory embarrassment. Where possible, autotransfusion should be initiated. Note that clamping the drain does not tamponade the bleeding. The treatment of massive haemothorax is to stop the bleeding, and to restore blood volume. Essentially all such patients will require urgent thoracotomy.

Complications of haemothorax or massive haemothorax are almost invariably related to the visceral injuries. Occasionally there is a persistence of undrained blood which may result in empyema.

Injuries to the great vessels

Injuries to the great vessels from penetrating forces are infrequently reported, mainly due to the relative lack of survival prehospital. In those patients who present to the Emergency Department the injury has usually sealed. Diagnosis is usually made by CT scan with contrast, or using arteriography. The injuries can be treated by intravascular stenting or open surgery.

Penetrating cardiac injury and cardiac tamponade

In urban trauma centres, cardiac injuries are most common after penetrating trauma and constitute about 5% of all thoracic injuries. The diagnosis of cardiac injury is usually fairly obvious. The patient presents with a combination of exsanguination or cardiac tamponade. Patients with tamponade due to penetrating injuries usually have a wound in proximity, decreased cardiac output, increased central venous pressure, decreased blood pressure, decreased heart sounds, narrow pulse pressure, and, occasionally, paradoxical pulse.

Every stable patient with a potential cardiac injury and every patient with a penetrating precordial chest injury requires mandatory investigation. The diagnosis is made primarily by ultrasound, and every patient with a penetrating injury in the cardiac 'box' should have full echocardiography.

Pericardiocentesis has been suggested as a temporizing manoeuvre. However, it is technically unreliable, may exacerbate the injury, and may fail to diagnose a true tamponade. The treatment of all cardiac injuries is immediate thoracotomy, ideally in the Operating Room, but for the patient *in extremis*, thoracotomy in the emergency department can be life saving. The great majority of wounds can be closed with simple sutures or horizontal mattress sutures of a 3/0 or 4/0 monofilament suture. In an uncontrolled situation, a skin stapler is an excellent temporizing measure. A Foley catheter can be placed in the hole, the balloon inflated, and gentle traction applied until definitive surgery can take place.

Air embolism

Air embolism is an infrequent event following trauma. It occurs in 4% of all major thoracic traumas, mostly following penetrating injury. These patients present with focal or lateralizing neurological signs, or sudden cardiovascular collapse. Any patient with chest injury, without obvious head injury, who has focal or lateralizing neurological findings should be assumed to have air embolism.

The treatment of air embolism is immediate thoracotomy. Survival rates are poor.

Management of potential threats to life

Rib fractures

Fractures of first three ribs or three or more ribs have a mortality of more than 10% due to the energy required to cause such injury, and associated injury. It is essential to exclude associated injuries.

- Haemopneumothorax
- Ribs 1–3: aorta, subclavian vessels, trachea or major bronchi
- Ribs 4–8: lung contusion, cardiac contusion or rupture
- Ribs 9–12: diaphragmatic rupture, spleen, liver or kidney.

Diagnosis is primarily clinical. Anteroposterior compression of the chest elicits pain.

Fractures of ribs and fractures at the costochondral junction may not be seen on the chest x-ray.

Treatment is primarily symptomatic to allow adequate breathing:

- Pain control using a combination of narcotic and non-steroidal analgesia, e.g. ibuprofen 600mg three times a day orally, and morphine titrated intravenously (NB properly titrated, morphine will not cause respiratory depression)
- Intercostal nerve block
- Epidural analgesia
- Interpleural analgesia—very effective if a chest drain is already in place: 10mL of bupivicaine 0.5% and 10mL of lignocaine 1% are added to 30mL of sterile water and instilled into the pleural cavity via the chest tube, which is clamped for a short while
- Strapping the chest to splint the ribs is strongly contraindicated to avoid atelectasis.

Pneumothorax

The presence of free air in the pleural cavity, where the lung has been pierced by a fractured rib, or penetration of overlying chest wall has occurred.

Clinically, the presentation is often asymptomatic, although there may be associated dyspnoea, and the thorax may be resonant to percussion. Diagnosis is usually made on chest x-ray, although smaller ones may be missed, and may only be seen on a CT scan.

Significant pneumothoraces require a chest drain. There is usually an associated with a haemothorax. Small stable pneumothoraces (<2cm lung collapse on x-ray, normal blood gases, no dyspnoea) may be managed on oxygen, without drainage. This approach does not apply to patients scheduled for general anaesthesia or assisted ventilation, or interfacility transfer by air, because of the danger of developing a tension pneumothorax. In these instances, chest drainage is required. An adequate sized drain (36FG) is inserted through the fourth or fifth intercostal space, anterior axillary line. Chest physiotherapy immediately after insertion of the drain is of paramount importance. A single dose antibiotic prophylaxis is adequate.

Haemothorax

Defined as free blood in the pleural cavity, and are often asymptomatic (similar to a pneumothorax). A haemothorax is best diagnosed on erect chest x-ray. If a fluid meniscus is seen in the costophrenic angle on the erect film, this usually implies a minimum of 250mL of free blood, and an intercostal chest drain should be inserted as for pneumothorax.

Pulmonary contusion

Pulmonary contusion represents bruising of the lung, usually in association with direct chest trauma. In blunt injury, decreased air entry is most usually due to pulmonary contusion, and is often associated with multiple rib fractures. The pathophysiology is the result of ventilation–perfusion defects and shunts. This is treated symptomatically, and the patient may require early assisted ventilation and cardiovascular support.

Tracheobronchial injuries

Penetrating injuries to the tracheobronchial tree are uncommon and constitute less than 2% of all major thoracic injuries. Disruption of the tracheobronchial tree is suggested by haemoptysis, airway obstruction, subcutaneous emphysema, tension pneumothorax, and significant persistent air leak after placement of a chest tube. Diagnosis is usually by bronchoscopy. Most lesions are within 2cm of the carina. Initial management is a chest drain to treat the pneumothorax. Most distal lesions close spontaneously, but the remainder require surgical closure, or stenting.

Blunt cardiac injury

Blunt cardiac injury (previously known as myocardial contusion) is caused by direct blunt trauma over the precordium. It is commonly overdiagnosed. The most common presentation is suspicious mechanism of injury, and cardiac arrhythmia. Diagnosis is made on electrocardiogram and specifically on transoesophageal echo. Cardiac enzymes are not usually helpful, and are not part of the routine investigation of such injuries.

Contained rupture of the thoracic aorta

Aortic rupture is usually associated with acceleration/deceleration injury, either from road traffic crash, or from fall from a height. 80Eighty per cent are immediately fatal because of free rupture into the pleural cavity. The remaining 20% of ruptures are contained by the remaining adventitia, often with leakage into the (intact) pleura. There are often associated orthopaedic injuries.

Diagnosis is initially made on the basis of a high index of suspicion, and should be verified by:

- Chest x-ray (Figure 12.4.7A), which may show some or all of the following:
  - Widened upper mediastinum (>7cm)
  - Obliteration or loss of clarity of the aortic knuckle

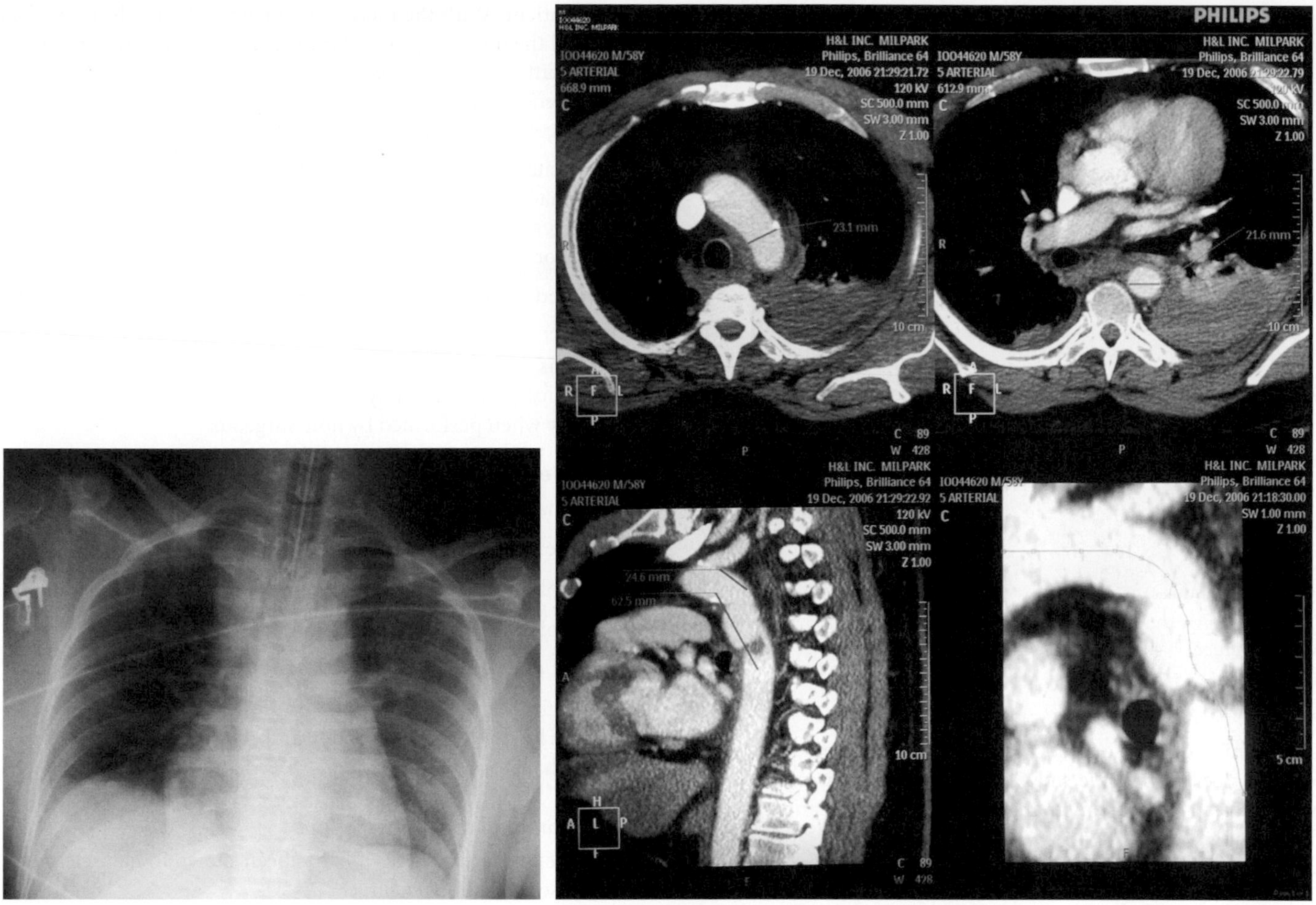

A B

Fig. 12.4.7 A) Chest X-ray showing widening of mediastinum and other signs suggestive of aortic rupture. B) CT scan showing traumatic dissection of thoracic aorta.

  - Deviation of the trachea
  - Depression of the left main bronchus
  - Deviation of the nasogastric tube to the right
  - Left haemothorax or left pleural apical cap
  - Fractures of the first and second rib—widened mediastinum is often present on supine x-ray. Once vertebral fractures have been excluded, an erect x-ray chest may be used to verify the 'widening' of the mediastinum. This manoeuvre is not entirely sensitive and specific to exclude ruptured aorta
- CT scan with contrast—the spiral CT scan (Figure 12.4.7B), with contrast is currently the 'gold standard' for diagnosis, since it will also help to differentiate the other causes of widened mediastinum, including prevertebral haematoma from a thoracic vertebral injury
- Transoesophageal echo—this is a useful, less invasive diagnostic tool in the stable patient and can be used to rule out associated blunt myocardial injury
- Aortic angiography—this is invasive, and is only suitable for the stable patient. The diagnostic procedure may, however, allow therapeutic stenting at the same procedure.

Keep the systolic blood pressure and pulse rate as low as possible (80–90mmHg) using beta-blockers to avoid converting a contained rupture into free (and fatal) rupture. Do not insert an intercostal drain, unless a free haemothorax is present.

Diaphragm injuries

Diaphragmatic injuries occur in approximately 6% of patients with midtorso injuries from penetrating trauma. The diaphragm normally rises to the fifth intercostal space during normal expiration. Any patient with injury to the chest wall below the fifth intercostal space is at risk of transdiaphragmatic penetration of the abdomen, and therefore intra-abdominal injury must be ruled out.

In blunt trauma, especially of the pelvis, there is a significant association with (particularly left-sided) diaphragmatic injury. Patients should have a nasogastric tube passed prior to chest x-ray (Figure 12.4.8), and visualization of the stomach in the chest is diagnostic.

The chest x-ray (preferably erect in the stable patient) may be helpful, and CT scan with contrast may assist. Laparoscopy is preferable to thoracoscopy, as it allows the diagnosis of intra-abdominal injury as well as the assessment of whether there has been breach of the diaphragm.

Optimally, all diaphragmatic injuries should be repaired, even small penetrating puncture wounds of no apparent importance.

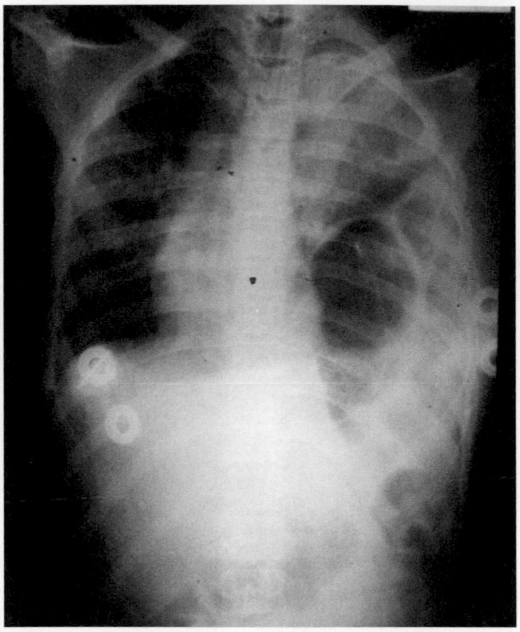

Fig. 12.4.8 Chest x-ray showing diaphragmatic rupture and stomach (with nasogastric tube) in chest.

Those injuries that are not repaired will present late, usually with incarceration of the small bowel, stomach, or colon, into the hernia defect. Subsequent strangulation may occur, and may be life threatening.

Oesophageal injuries

The incidence of oesophageal injury is very low. Occasionally, patients may present late with signs of posterior mediastinitis. Injuries to the thoracic oesophagus may present with pain, fever, pneumomediastinum, persistent pneumothorax in spite of tube thoracostomy, and pleural effusion with extravasation of contrast on gastrograffin swallow. Injuries to the cervical oesophagus are somewhat more frequent and are usually detected at the time of exploration of zone I and II injuries of the neck. In general, with penetrating injury of the neck, and penetration deep to the platysma, especially in inexperienced hands, the threshold for exploration should be very low.

Diagnosis is best using a combination of CT scan with contrast, or oesophagography. Once found, closure is performed, with drainage.

Complications following oesophageal injuries include wound infection, mediastinitis, and empyema, and if diagnosed late, the injury can be lethal.

Emergency Department thoracotomy

Improved emergency medical response times, and advances in prehospital care, have led to increased numbers of patients with cardiac and thoracic injury (who previously would have died in the prehospital environment), arriving in resuscitation *in extremis*. Salvage of these patients often demands immediate control of haemorrhage by thoracotomy and direct control. However, thoracotomy has often been attempted in hopeless situations, following both blunt and penetrating injury, and failure to understand the indications and sequelae will almost inevitably result in the death of the patient. With the increasing financial demands on medical care, and the increasing risk of transmission of communicable diseases, a differentiation must be made between the true emergency department thoracotomy, and futile care.

Thoracotomy may be divided into:

- Resuscitative thoracotomy which is an emergency procedure to treat haemorrhage in the chest. This can be performed in the Emergency Department (Emergency Department thoracotomy, EDT) or in the Operating Room
- Planned thoracotomy to repair damage in a relatively stable patient.

There is an extremely high mortality rate associated with all thoracotomies performed anywhere outside the Operating Room, especially when performed by non-surgeons.

Objective

The primary objectives of EDT in this set of circumstances are to:

- Release cardiac tamponade
- Control intrathoracic bleeding
- Control air embolism or bronchopleural fistula
- Permit open cardiac massage
- Allow for temporary occlusion of the descending aorta to redistribute blood to the upper body and possibly limit subdiaphragmatic haemorrhage.

Indications and contraindications

There are instances where EDT has been shown to have clear benefit. These indications include:

- Those patients with penetrating injury in whom there is a witnessed arrest and high likelihood of isolated intrathoracic injury, especially in penetrating cardiac injury ('salvageable' postinjury cardiac arrest)
- Those with severe postinjury hypotension (blood pressure <60mmHg) due to cardiac tamponade, air embolism, or thoracic haemorrhage
- Planned cross-clamping of the aorta in penetrating injury below the diaphragm, to allow circulation of the brain until local direct control has been achieved.

EDT is contraindicated when:

- In cases of blunt trauma
- There has been cardiopulmonary resuscitation in the absence of endotracheal tube intubation in excess of 5min or for more than 10min with endotracheal tube intubation.

Results

The results of EDT vary according to injury mechanism and location and the presence of vital and life signs. EDT has been shown to be beneficial in around 50% of patients presenting with signs of life after isolated penetrating cardiac injury and only rarely in those patients presenting without signs of life (<2%). In non-cardiac penetrating wounds, 25% benefit when signs of life and detectable vital signs are present, compared to 8% of those with signs of life only and 3% of those without signs of life.

Following blunt trauma, only 0.1% of patients requiring EDT are salvaged, regardless of their clinical status on admission.

When to stop Emergency Department thoracotomy?

EDT is a 'team event.' It should not be prolonged unduly but should have specific end points. If there is an injury repaired, and the patient responds, he/she should be moved to the Operating Room for definitive repair or closure.

EDT should be terminated if:

- Irreparable cardiac damage has occurred
- The patient is identified as having massive head injuries
- Pulseless electrical activity (PEA) is established
- Systolic blood pressure is less than 70mmHg after 20min
- Asystolic arrest has occurred.

The abdominal cavity

Introduction

Delay in the diagnosis and management of abdominal injuries is one of the most common causes of preventable death from trauma, with death usually resulting from major undiagnosed bleeding. Approximately 20% of abdominal injuries will require surgery. In the United Kingdom, Western Europe, and Australia, the trauma is predominantly blunt in nature, while in the military context, and in civilian trauma in the United States of America, South Africa, and South America, it is predominantly penetrating. There are significant differences between blunt and penetrating abdominal trauma, with regard to the assessment, investigations, and treatment.

Blunt intra-abdominal injuries may occur by means of three mechanisms:

1) Crushing of an organ against the spine or pelvis or the abdominal wall
2) Deceleration forces
3) Sudden increase of the intraluminal pressure and bursting of a hollow viscus.

Penetrating injury caused by stab wounds, (limited energy transfer) results in damage confined to the tract. Bullet or missile wounds have higher energy, resulting in energy transfer to the tissues surrounding the bullet tract, with direct damage from the missile, explosion of gas in hollow viscera, and degeneration or cell death beyond the confines of the tract itself.

It is important to appreciate the difference between surgical resuscitation and definitive treatment for abdominal trauma. Surgical resuscitation includes the technique of 'damage control', and implies only that surgery which is necessary to save life by stopping bleeding and preventing further contamination or physiological injury. It is part of the resuscitation process only, and the definitive surgery is initiated at a later stage when the patient is stable (see Chapter 12.3).

Resuscitation

Resuscitation of patients with suspected abdominal injuries should always take place within the ATLS® context. Attention is paid to adequate resuscitative measures, including pain control. Adequate analgesia (titrated intravenously) will never mask abdominal symptoms, and is much more likely to make abdominal pathology easier to assess, with clearer physical signs and a cooperative patient.

The diagnosis of injury following blunt trauma can be difficult. The knowledge of the mechanism can be helpful. Shoulder harnesses can cause blunt trauma to the liver and duodenum or pancreas, and rib fractures can cause direct damage to the liver or spleen. Lap belts can cause spinal injury, and shearing injury to intestine and mesentery, especially when incorrectly placed above the iliac crest. Pelvic facture are high-energy injuries and there is a significant association with intra-abdominal solid viscus injuries and rupture of the diaphragm.

Blood is not initially an irritant, and therefore it may be difficult to assess the presence or quantity of blood present in the abdomen.

Bowel sounds may remain present for several hours after abdominal injury, or may disappear following trivial trauma. This sign is therefore particularly unreliable.

Investigation and assessment of the abdomen can be based on three presenting groups:

1) The patient with the normal abdomen
2) An equivocal group requiring further investigation
3) The patient with an obvious injury to the abdomen.

Virtually all penetrating injury to the abdomen should be explored promptly, especially in the presence of hypotension.

Diagnosis

Diagnostic modalities depend on the nature of the injury.

- Physical examination
- Diagnostic peritoneal lavage (DPL)
- Ultrasound (FAST—focused abdominal sonography for trauma)
- CT scan.
- Diagnostic laparoscopy.

The haemodynamically normal patient

There is ample time for a full evaluation of the patient, and a decision can be made regarding surgery or non-operative management.

The haemodynamically stable patient

The stable patient, who is not haemodynamically normal, will benefit from investigations aimed at establishing:

- Has the patient bled into the abdomen?
- Has the bleeding stopped?

Thus, serial investigations of a quantitative nature will allow the best assessment of these patients. FAST also may be helpful in establishing the presence of free blood, though dependent on the operator. CT scan with contrast is currently the modality of choice (Figure 12.4.9).

The haemodynamically unstable patient

Efforts must be made to try to define the cavity where bleeding is taking place, e.g. pelvis or abdominal cavity, or even chest. Diagnostic modalities are of necessity limited, since it may not be possible to move an unstable patient to CT scan, even if it were to

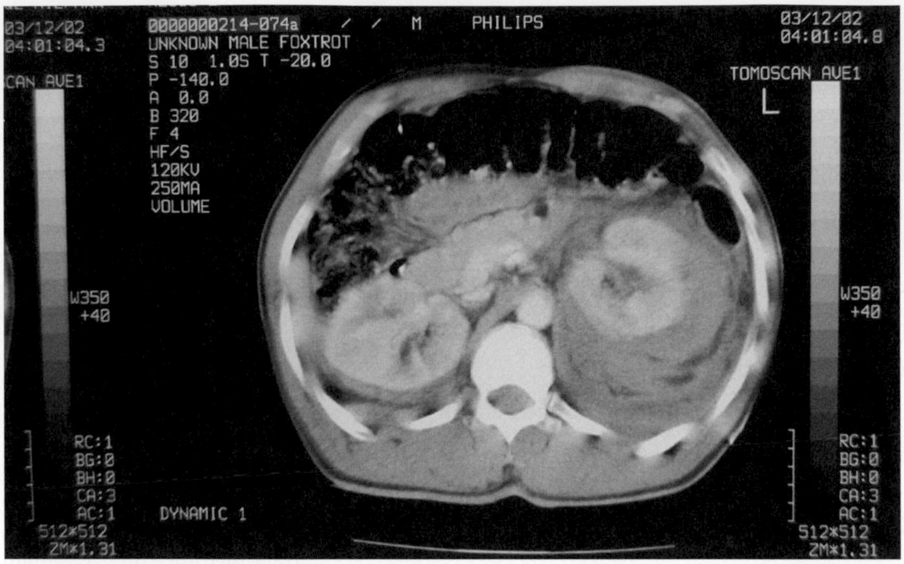

Fig. 12.4.9 CT scan of abdomen showing contained rupture of left kidney.

be readily available. FAST is the most useful, but is very operator dependent—important if the individual doing the scan is inexperienced in the trauma patient. DPL, although now rarely used in most European countries, remains one of the most common, most sensitive, cheapest, and most readily available and reproducible modalities to assess the presence of blood in the abdomen.

Treatment

The management of abdominal injury in association with orthopaedic injury should be contemplated as a 'Team' effort, with the goal being to treat threats to life first, using a combination of non-operative and operative methods.

Retroperitoneum

Injuries to retroperitoneal structures carry a high mortality and are often underestimated or missed. Rapid and efficient access techniques are required to deal with exsanguinating vascular injuries, where large retroperitoneal haematomas often obscure the exact position and extent of the injury. CT scan with contrast enhancement should be used wherever possible as the diagnostic tool of choice.

The retroperitoneum is explored when major abdominal vascular injury is suspected, or there is injury to the kidneys, ureters and renal vessels, pancreas, duodenum, and colon. Because of the high incidence of intraperitoneal and retroperitoneal injuries occurring simultaneously, the retroperitoneum is always approached via a transperitoneal incision. The decision to explore a retroperitoneal haematoma is based on its location and the mechanism of injury, and whether the haematoma is pulsating or rapidly enlarging.

Summary

Management of the patient with multiple truncal soft tissue and orthopaedic injuries presents a major challenge in the care of the trauma patient. It is critical in a successful outcome to:

- Appreciate which injuries are present
- Which injuries are major threats to life
- Prioritize and treat accordingly.

Further reading

Evidence based practice management guidelines on the management of trauma, can be found at the Eastern Association for the Surgery of Trauma web site: http://www.east.org/tpg.asp

Hirshberg, A. and Mattox, K.L. (2004). *Top Knife: the Art and Craft of Trauma Surgery*. Shropshire: TFM Publishing Ltd.

12.5

Massive transfusion

K. Boffard

Summary points

- Treatment of anaemia has changed substantially since the early 1990s
- Although massive transfusion may be necessary, trauma surgeons have modified their practice to provide aggressive control of haemorrhage, prevent hypothermia and acidosis, optimize haemodynamic management in intensive care units, and rationalize transfusion support in severely injured patients. The result has been an improvement in the outcomes of these patients
- Given the importance of early intervention in the care of the injured, understanding the physiology and true indications for early massive transfusion in trauma care has the potential to save many lives.

Definition

Massive transfusion is often defined as the transfusion of ten or more units of red blood cells in less than 24h, or more than 50% of the blood volume in 3h. A suitable massive transfusion protocol is suggested in Box 12.5.1.

The coagulopathy of massive trauma and haemorrhage

Among the most devastating of the complications of massive blood loss and fluid resuscitation is a bleeding diathesis. Paradoxically, although clotting is accelerated at the capillary level because of shock and tissue damage, the circulating blood becomes hypocoagulable. The coagulopathy of trauma is a syndrome of non-surgical bleeding from mucosal lesions, serosal surfaces, and wound and vascular access sites, the tissue oozing that continues after identifiable vascular bleeding has been controlled. It occurs in the presence of profoundly depressed concentrations of blood coagulation proteins and platelets, but also in the situation where normal clotting factors are present, but do not work. By the time that a trauma coagulopathy becomes obvious, the depletion of all clotting factors and platelets is already severe (Box 12.5.2). Even best case standard of care does not take into account the insensible losses of blood into tissue compartments, and the consumption of clotting factors at the site of injury.

In the initial phase of massive bleeding and massive transfusion, an important goal is to maintain reasonable concentrations of all the pro- and anticoagulant factors. Procoagulant factors and platelets help minimize surgical bleeding and prevent coagulopathic bleeding. Anticoagulant factors prevent clotting from spreading and causing further tissue injury. During massive transfusion, the major effort must be the maintenance of perfusion and oxygen transport. The early addition of plasma and platelets can help the coagulopathy of trauma. Stored blood is deficient in factors V and VIII and platelets but replete with fibrin split products and vasoactive substances. Timely administration of FFP and platelets will minimize the risk of coagulopathy after massive transfusion.

NB The use of starches is *contraindicated* in the actively bleeding patient, since all starches deplete the von Willebrand/Factor VIII complex, and may make the actively bleeding patient more coagulopathic, both from factor depletion and dilutional coagulopathy.

Also germane to the initial period of massive blood transfusion are the potential complications of acidosis, hypothermia, and hypocalcaemia. Hypothermia (<32°C) causes platelet sequestration and inhibits the release of platelet factors that are important in the intrinsic clotting pathway. In addition, it has consistently been associated with poor outcome in trauma patients. Core temperature often falls insidiously because of exposure at the scene and in the emergency department and because of administration of resuscitation fluids stored at ambient temperature.

The use of bicarbonate in the treatment of systemic acidosis remains controversial. Moderate acidosis (pH <7.2) impairs coagulation, myocardial contractility, and oxidative metabolism. Acidosis in the trauma patient is caused primarily by a rise in lactic acid production secondary to tissue hypoxia and hypothermia, and usually resolves when the volume deficit has been corrected and efficiency of circulation restored. Administration of sodium bicarbonate may cause a leftward shift of the oxyhaemoglobin dissociation curve, reducing tissue oxygen extraction, and it may worsen intracellular acidosis caused by carbon dioxide production. On the other hand, adrenergic receptors may become desensitized with protracted acidosis. Bicarbonate infusion, therefore, should be limited to persons with protracted shock.

Hypocalcaemia caused by citrate binding of ionized calcium does not occur until the blood transfusion rate exceeds 100mL/min (equivalent to 1 unit every 5min). Decreased serum levels of ionized calcium depress myocardial function before impairing coagulation.

Box 12.5.1 Guidelines for massive blood transfusion

Definition

Replacement of the whole blood volume within 24h, or 50% of the blood volume in 3h.

Activation

The protocol will be activated automatically by the Blood Bank after 2 units of packed red blood cells (PRBC) have been issued to a patient, *and* a request for a further 4 units of blood or more is subsequently requested within any 24-h period.

Blood specimens

- Group and crossmatch:
  - Leucodepleted blood should be used wherever it is available
  - Crossmatched blood if available
  - Uncrossmatched group O blood
- The following baseline blood specimens are required:
  - Full blood count including platelets
  - Prothrombin time (PT), activated partial thromboplastin time (aPTT), thrombin time, international normalized ratio (INR), fibrinogen, D-dimer
- Repeat after every 6 units PRBCs.

Avoid hypothermia

- Use an appropriate blood warmer
- Keep the patient warm using an appropriate patient warming device
- Maintain a warm environment.

Blood and blood products

- Blood Bank will issue the following products (as part of a 2- or 6-unit 'massive transfusion pack'). NB multiple 2-unit packs are preferable as they can be returned if the 'cold chain' is intact:
  - 2 units or 6 units of packed red cells using *freshest blood available*
  - 2 units or 6 units of FFP
  - 2 units or 6 units of platelets

or

- For every 6 units of blood issued:
  - 1 apheresis unit of platelets.

Administration

- Microaggregate filters are not advised.
- Once administration of the 'massive transfusion pack' blood is begun, administer all the above in a 1:1:1 ratio, (blood:FFP:platelets) or 6× 1:1 = 6:6: 1 apheresis platelet unit. After every 6 units of red cells, if ongoing bleeding or need for transfusion is present:
  - Give a further 4 units of FFP if PT or APTT are >1.5× mid normal
  - Give 10 units of cryoprecipitate if fibrinogen <1g/L
  - Give 10mL 10% calcium chloride *only* if the above additional doses are given
  - Give at least 1 unit of pooled platelets if platelet count <75000/mm^3.
- Return all unused 'massive transfusion packs' to Blood Bank as soon as possible

Endpoints of transfusion

- Any active surgical bleeding has been controlled
- No further need for red cells
- Temperature >35°C
- pH >7.3.

Box 12.5.2 Factors predictive of a severe coagulopathic state include:

- Massive rapid blood transfusion
- Persistent cellular shock:
  - Oxygen consumption index <110mL/min/m^2
  - Lactate concentration >5mmol/L
- Progressive metabolic acidosis:
  - pH <7.2
  - Base deficit >14mmol/L
  - Lactate >5mmol/L
- Refractory core hypothermia (<34°C).

Calcium gluconate or calcium chloride should be reserved for cases in which there is electrocardiographis evidence of QT interval prolongation or, in rare instances, for cases of unexplained hypotension during massive transfusion.

Fresh frozen plasma

Most trauma patients will need fresh frozen plasma (FFP) well before losing one blood volume. This is different from most recommendations which are based on more controlled circumstances, and is based on computer simulation of the amount of FFP required to avoid excessive plasma dilution compromising haemostasis. Most patients will require one unit of FFP for every unit of blood transfused. A unit of FFP also contains most of the citrate anticoagulant from the unit of blood from which it was originally derived. It contains about 0.5g fibrinogen, and normal levels of pro- and anti-coagulants. Solvent-detergent (SD) treated/freeze dried plasma (Bioplasma) carries about 20% less of these per unit given.

Cryoprecipitate

Cryoprecipitate contains fibrinogen, von Willebrand factor/Factor VIII complex, and fibrin stabilizing factor/Factor XIII. Cryoprecipitate may not be required in all cases of trauma. One unit of FFP (250mL) contains 0.5g of fibrinogen. One unit of cryoprecipitate contains 0.25g of fibrinogen, but in 10mL (rather than 250mL). Therefore in most cases, FFP will supply the needs required.

Platelets

A fall in platelet count occurs somewhat later than the loss of clotting factors. Unfortunately, a platelet count is not simple, since it gives no indication as to the function of the remaining platelets. Hypothermia affects platelet adhesion more than the enzymes, above 33°C, while hypothermia affects all aspects of coagulation below 33°C. There is some evidence in which there appears to be a survival advantage of receiving approximately 0.8 units of platelets per unit of red blood cells.

Recombinant factor VII

There is increasing use of activated recombinant factor VII (rFVIIa). Currently it is not approved for trauma patients.

Further reading

British Committee for Standards in Haematology, Blood Transfusion Task Force (2004). Guidelines for the use of fresh frozen plasma, cryoprecipitate, and cryosupernatant. *British Journal of Haematology*, **126**, 11–12.

Collins, J.A. (1974). Problems associated with the massive transfusion of stored blood. *Surgery*, **75**, 274–79.

Erber, W.N. (2002). Massive transfusion in the elective surgical setting. *Transfusion and Apheresis Science*, **27**, 83–92.

Hirshberg, A., Dugas, M., Banez, E.L., Scott, B.G., Wall, M.R. Jr, and Mattox, K.L. (2003). Minimising dilutional coagulopathy in exsanguinating haemorrhage: A computer simulation. *Journal of Trauma*, **54**, 454–63.

Holcomb, J.B. and Hess, J.R. (eds) (2006). Early massive trauma transfusion: State of the art. *Journal of Trauma*, **60**(6), S1–S96.

Miller, R.D., Robbins, T.O., Tong, M.J., and Barton, S.L. (1971). Coagulation defects associated with massive blood transfusions. *Annals of Surgery*, **174**, 794–801.

Philips, T.F., Soulier, G., and Wilson, R.F. (1987). Outcome of massive transfusion exceeding two blood volumes in trauma and emergency surgery. *Journal of Trauma*, **27**, 903–10.

Stulz, P.M., Scheidegger, D., Drop, L.J., Lowenstein, E., and Laver, M.B. (1979). Ventricular pump performance during hypocalcemia: clinical and experimental studies. *Journal of Thoracic and Cardiovascular Surgery*, **78**, 185–94.

12.6

Blast and ballistic injury

J. Clasper

Summary points

- Unlike civilian trauma most ballistic injuries are due to penetrating wounds
- Although weapons may change, the principles of treatment remain the same, prevent death by stopping bleeding, and prevent infection by removing dead and foreign material
- The severity of the injury is related to the energy transfer to the tissues as well as the specific structures injured
- Mass casualty situations may require Triage of the casualties.

Introduction

The principles of military surgery, to control bleeding and to prevent infection, are not new, and were documented during the Roman Empire by Celsus.

However, following the introduction of gunpowder in the Middle Ages, there have been major changes in the weapons of war, and this has lead to a different spectrum of injuries.

Conventional weapons can be divided into:

- *Small arms*: these include pistols, rifles, and machine guns and the injuries result from the interaction of the projectiles produced by the weapon and biological tissue the projectile strikes
- *Explosive munitions:* these include shells, bombs, and grenades, and in addition to the wounds caused by their projectiles, injury may also result from the effect of blast on the tissue.

Projectiles

In most wars, the majority of penetrating injuries are due to fragments rather than bullet wounds. During the First Gulf War, 90% of penetrating injuries seen in one British military hospital were due to fragments. These fragments may be from parts of a shell or grenade, or from objects such as nails or ball bearings packed around the explosive. In addition, any object in the vicinity of the blast, which is 'blown up' and accelerated away from the site of the explosion, can produce fragment wounds. Therefore it is appropriate to consider bullet and fragment injuries together as projectile (or missile) injuries.

Projectiles can cause tissue damage by either direct or indirect mechanisms. With low-energy injuries such as from handguns, tissue damage is confined to the wound tract, and is caused by cutting or crushing. Significant injury will only occur if a vital structure is directly damaged by the weapon.

However, with higher-energy missiles such as bullets, energy may be dissipated to the surrounding tissues, to produce indirect damage outside the wound tract, and a vital structure may be damaged without actually being involved in the wound tract. This is more likely to occur with high-energy wounds, especially, although not invariably, from high-velocity rifle bullets, and results in a cavitation effect, with the formation of a temporary cavity, behind the missile.

Cavitation

As the projectile passes through the tissue, energy is transferred to anything in contact with the projectile, and as a result of this energy, the tissue is accelerated away from the projectile. This results in the formation of a temporary cavity as the inertia of the tissue results in continued displacement even after the projectile has passed through the tissue. As well as the obvious injury caused by the compression and shear forces applied to the tissues, the negative intracavity pressure (with respect to atmospheric pressure), can result in increased contamination of the wound tract, by drawing material into the wound.

The effect of indirect damage is one of the factors in the increased mortality from high-velocity bullet wounds. In a report from Vietnam, bullets were responsible for 30% of penetrating wounds, but caused 45% of the deaths. It has been estimated that a casualty struck by a bullet, in a military conflict, has a 1 in 3 chance of dying. This compares to a 1 in 7 chance of dying if struck by fragments from a shell, and 1 in 20 if struck by a fragment from a grenade.

It is not, however, the energy transfer that determines the outcome, it is the specific tissue damage that occurs. Low-energy wounds to the heart or brain are more likely to be fatal than high-energy injuries to the limbs.

A number of factors affect the energy transfer from the projectile to the tissue (Figures 12.6.1–3).

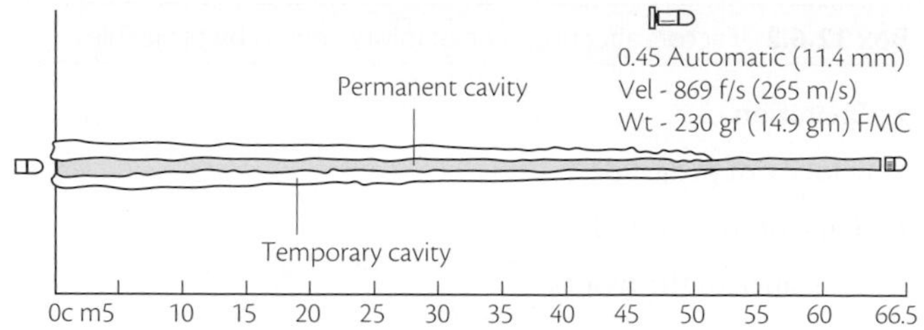

Fig. 12.6.1 Diagram representing the path of a low-velocity projectile (.45 caliber handgun bullet) in ballistics gelatin. The small size of the permanent and temporary cavity as well as the forward-facing (unchanged) orientation of the bullet should be noted. (Reproduced from Bowen and Bellamy (1988).)

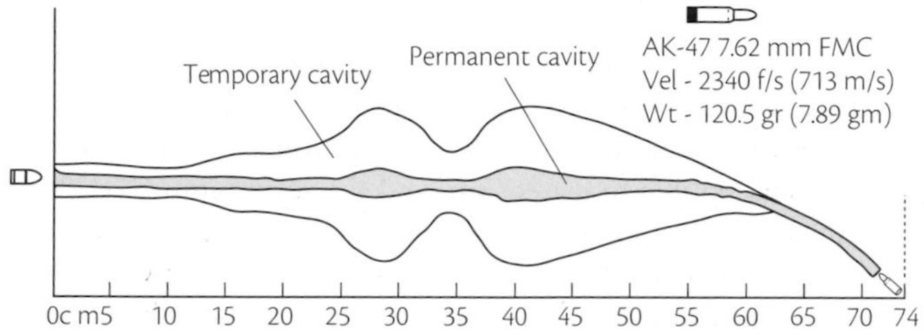

Fig. 12.6.2 Diagram representing the path of a high-velocity projectile (7.62-mm AK-47 rifle bullet) in ballistic gelatin. The increased velocity and yaw produce larger temporary and permanent cavities compared with the handgun bullet, but the projectile does not yaw significantly until almost 25 cm of penetration. Given the thickness of extremities and even the torso of an average individual, the projectile will have exited the target before it is able to release the majority of its kinetic energy. (Reproduced from Bowen and Bellamy (1988).)

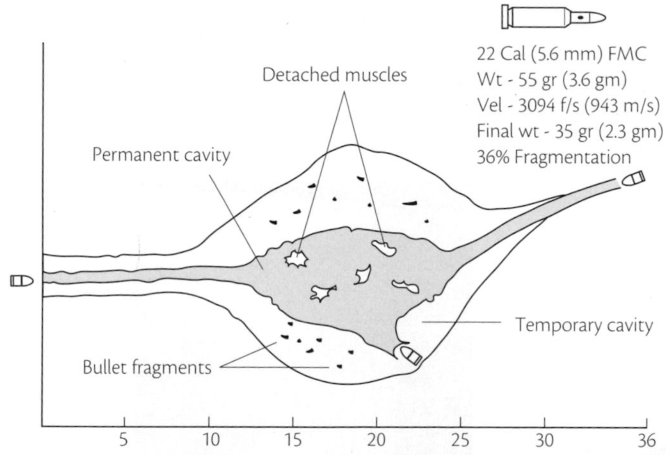

Fig. 12.6.3 Diagram representing the path of a high-velocity projectile (5.6-mm M-16 rifle bullet). The large temporary and permanent cavities are formed much earlier (approximately 10–25 cm) owing to the instability of the M-16 bullet and its correspondingly higher yaw rate. In addition, the M-16 bullet tends to fragment, which augments its kinetic energy release and tissue destruction. (Reproduced from Bowen and Bellamy (1988).)

Velocity of the projectile

As the kinetic energy possessed by a projectile is given by the formula:

Kinetic energy = ½ × mass × velocity^2

Box 12.6.1

Treat the wound *not* the weapon

changes in velocity have a significant effect on available kinetic energy, and the greater available energy accounts for the severe tissue damage seen after high-velocity missile injuries. However, high-velocity bullets do not invariably cause severe wounds, as the missile may pass through tissue without transferring significant energy. This occurs when the resistance of the tissues is low and the wound track is short, such that the bullet is not slowed, and therefore little energy is transferred.

For this reason it is incorrect to divide wounds into high or low *velocity*.

In addition, severe injury can occur from low-velocity projectiles, not only when a vital structure is directly injured, but also when the mass of the projectile is large. This is particularly true for close-range shotgun injuries, which can cause severe tissue injury.

Therefore it is the *energy transferred* to tissues that defines the work done in mechanical injury, and is the most appropriate index of physical injury.

Shape of the projectile

The smaller the area of the projectile presented to the tissue, the lower the resistance, and therefore the lower the energy transfer. Thus there is likely to be a lower energy transfer from a spherical object, such as a ball bearing, than a flattened irregular piece of shrapnel, for the same available energy.

With a bullet, the resistance afforded by the tissue is related to the orientation of the bullet. If the long axis of the bullet is aligned with the direction of travel, less energy is transferred than if the bullet yaws (or tumbles) and presents a greater surface area. Bullets are inherently unstable in tissues, and the resistance of the tissue may be sufficient to cause a bullet to tumble. This will result in greater energy transfer to the tissue and thus greater tissue damage. This is one reason why entry wounds are often small, and may be no larger than the diameter of the bullet, whereas exit wounds may be much larger, with torn skin, and a ragged star-like appearance.

In addition, any deformation, or breaking up, of a missile will result in greater energy transfer and more extensive wounding. This is the main reason for soft nose, or hollow nose bullets, or dum-dum bullets when the bullet was deliberately notched to encourage breaking up, producing more severe injuries. Such modifications were made illegal by the Hague Declaration of 1899. Even with standard bullets fragmentation can still occur, particularly if the bullet strikes bone, and this is accompanied by more severe wounding (Figure 12.6.4).

Resistance of the tissue

The energy transfer is also affected by the tissue involved in the wound tract, and is related to the resistance offered by the tissue. Muscle is denser than lung tissue, and greater energy transfer occurs when a projectile passes through muscle. More rigid tissue such as bone resists deformation, and offers a greater resistance, resulting in greater energy transfer.

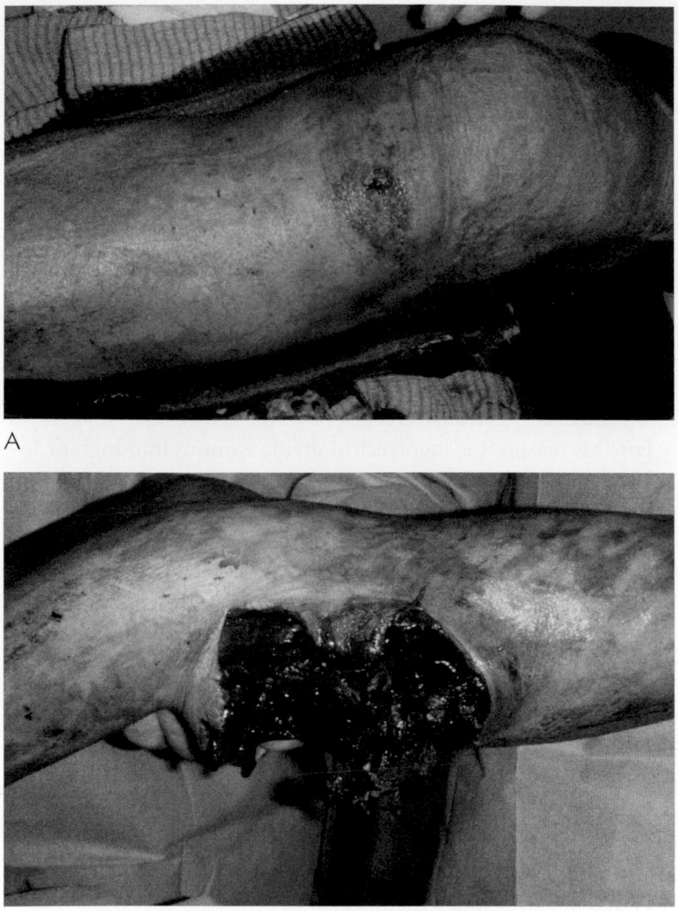

A

B

Fig. 12.6.4 Injury to leg from high velocity bullet with small entry wound (A), a large amount of energy was transferred as a result of contact with the proximal tibia resulting in significant fragmentation and a large exit wound (B).
Image courtesy of the Royal Centre for Defence Medicine.

Box 12.6.2 Factors affecting type of injury caused by projectiles

- Cavitation
- Velocity of projectile
- Shape of the projectile
- Resistance of the tissues.

The size of the cavity, although one determinant of the severity of an injury, is not the most significant factor; again it is the properties of the tissue injured which mainly determines the outcome. Muscle is able to withstand the distension produced by the temporary cavity, due to its elasticity, and although the tissue may be contused, recovery is possible (Figure 12.6.5). Less elastic tissue, particularly if enclosed by a fibrous capsule (e.g. liver), is unable to withstand the distension and severe disruption is possible. Brain is also very susceptible to distension, and the severe injury resulting from the compression and shearing is usually unrecoverable. This is one of the reasons that most high-energy transfer wounds in survivors are seen in the limbs, and are associated with extensive soft tissue injury, multifragmentary fractures, and highly contaminated wounds.

There are a number of factors that are important to appreciate at this stage (Box 12.6.2). Despite the division of wounds into high- and low-energy transfer, it is important to realize that these are merely two ends of a spectrum. It is, therefore, wrong to base treatment protocols, on the basis of a division of wounds into two types. The temporary cavity is not an all-or-none phenomenon, and the size of the cavity is related not only to the energy transfer, but also to the tissue involved. In addition, although the exit wound of a high-energy transfer wound is usually ragged and large, this is not always the case, and smaller entrance and exit wounds may be present despite high-energy transfer.

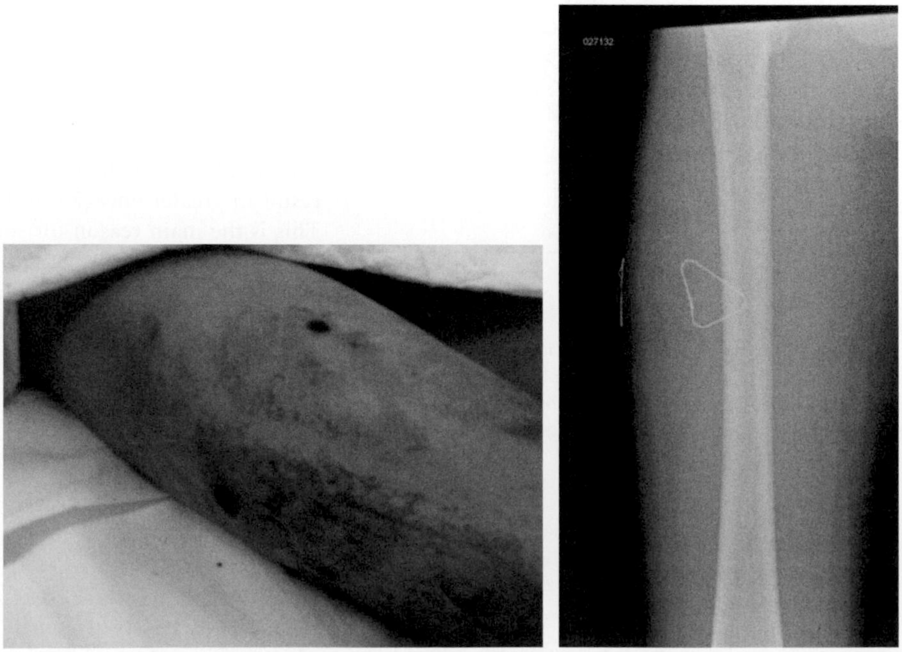

A

B

Fig. 12.6.5 Small entry and exit thigh wounds from a high velocity bullet (A). The short tangential missile tract resulted in relatively low energy transfer (B) and only minimal debridement was required. Image courtesy of the Royal Centre for Defence Medicine.

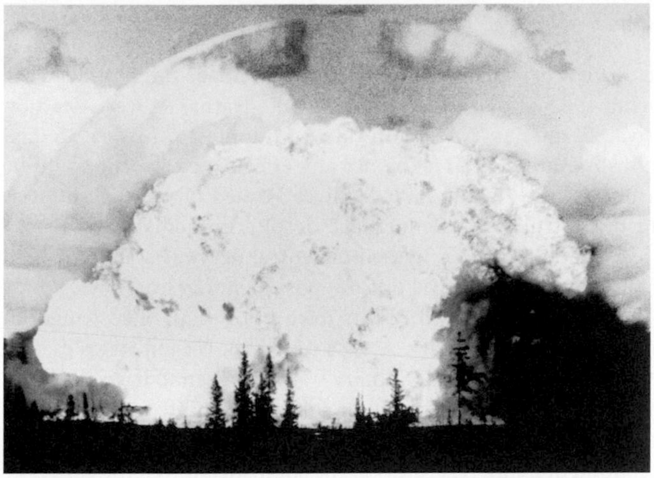

Fig. 12.6.6 This photograph of a large explosion illustrates several of the components responsible for blast injury. The thin line farthest from the blast center is caused by the difference in refraction between the compressed gas at the blast front and the surrounding air. In addition, debris can be seen being accelerated peripherally (perticularly at ground level) and the size of the fireball can also be appreciated. (Reproduced from from Zajtchuk *et al.* (1990).)

Explosive munitions

In addition to fragment wounds, explosive munitions can also cause injury from the blast and other mechanisms (Figure 12.6.6). Blast injuries can be considered as:

- Primary blast injury: including blast lung due to over pressure wave
- Secondary blast injury: including penetrating injuries from debris
- Tertiary blast injury: blunt injury due to blast wind throwing the casualty
- Quaternary blast injury: burns, fumes, building collapse, mental health, exacerbation of chronic disease.

Despite the different mechanisms, most injuries in survivors of explosions are due to penetrating trauma from fragments. Both the blast wave and blast wind are fatal close to the explosion, and this distance is dependent on the size of the explosive. However, the effects of the blast fall rapidly with increasing distance from the point of detonation, and therefore there is a very small zone where a casualty will survive the blast, but sustain significant injuries directly due to the blast wave or wind.

As a result, previous studies have demonstrated that 90% of fatalities occur before or very soon after arrival at hospital and most patients who survive are not severely injured, and have a relatively low Injury Severity Score (ISS <16, mean 8). Of the fatalities occurring after initial resuscitation, approximately 50% were due to severe head injuries, which would not have been amenable to treatment and would have been graded with an ISS of at least 16. In addition, burns may also be very severe if the casualty was close to the blast, but most of these patients will die from the other effects. In survivors, burns directly caused by an explosion are often superficial and confined to exposed areas. However, if the bomb was specifically designed as an incendiary device, or secondary fires result, then burns may be a significant problem.

Two other specific mechanisms should be considered—antipersonnel (landmines) and improvised explosive devices (IEDs) which are being used in current operations in Afghanistan and Iraq.

Landmine injuries

In general, landmines are designed as terror weapons, or to deny ground rather than to kill. The psychological effect of a survivor, with a traumatic amputation, is believed to be much greater than a death. A retrospective analysis from the International Committee of the Red Cross, of 757 victims of antipersonnel mines, has identified three patterns of injuries amongst survivors. Pattern 1 injuries occur when a buried mine is stepped on. Severe limb injuries including traumatic amputations of the lower injuries are common, as well as genital injuries. With pattern 2 injuries, the device explodes near the victim, this may be due to a buried mine activated by another individual, or due to a pull-action mine which is placed above ground level and is activated by pulling on a wire connected to the device. Lower limb injuries occur, but are less severe than in pattern 1, with traumatic amputations less likely. Injuries to the head, chest, and abdomen are common. Pattern 3 injuries occur when the device explodes whilst the victim is handling it. Severe facial and upper limb injuries are common in this group.

In addition other injury patterns can occur with specific devices. The M-16 series antipersonnel mines, which are designed to be propelled 1m into the air and explode 3s after the mine has been stood on. Most victims of properly functioning devices died, with severe injuries to the upper body and traumatic amputations of the upper limb being common.

Outcome of landmine injuries

Retrospective reviews of hospital admissions reports a low mortality rate after antipersonnel mine injury, 0–0.8%. When prehospital mortality is included a fatality rate of 1.7% has been reported.

Despite the low mortality rate, the morbidity after pattern 1 landmine injury is very high. As previously discussed, severe lower limb injuries, including traumatic amputations, can occur in approximately 90% of reported cases. In one study, patients required definitive surgical amputations. In addition, most of the patients sustained injuries to the other limb, and 13% of the patients sustained genital injuries. The majority of contralateral limb injuries were, however, salvageable.

Of the pattern 2 injuries, only 5% of the patients required amputation, but with pattern 3 injuries 80% of the victims sustained traumatic upper limb amputations, and many of the survivors required a definitive surgical amputation for non-salvageable injuries.

Multiple casualties and different injury patterns occur in victims of anti-tank mines, which contain far more explosive, and the outcome varies depending on the device and the type of vehicle involved. A 44% mortality rate has been demonstrated from injuries from the much larger anti-tank mines, due to severe central and head injuries. Many victims of anti-tank mines will die at the scene, and survival may be unlikely even if advanced medical care is available. Amongst survivors who reach medical care, the mortality appears to be relatively low. If significant delays are present, only patients with peripheral injuries will survive to reach hospital, resulting in an apparently low hospital mortality rate.

Improvised explosive devices

The United States Department of Defence defines these as devices placed or fabricated in an improvised manner incorporating destructive, lethal, noxious, pyrotechnic, or incendiary chemicals, designed to destroy, disfigure, distract, or harass and often incorporate military stores. In Iraq, they have been the leading cause of death amongst coalition troops, and during 2003–2008 resulted in 1690 fatalities.

The IEDs in Iraq are often camouflaged and are either laid under the road or by the roadside. Therefore targeted vehicles are in very close proximity to the device when it is detonated. The injury profile is related to the use of the explosive formed projectile (EFP). These are cylindrical charges, fabricated from commonly available metal pipe, with the forward end closed by a concave metal disc-shaped liner to create a shaped charge. Explosive is loaded behind the metal liner to fill the pipe. When the explosive is detonated, the conical metal plate (or lens) is deformed and reshaped into an aerodynamically efficient penetrator moving at high velocity (>1500m/s). The EFP then hits the target at high speed, delivering significantly high mechanical energy that could have only been previously provided with a large gun. Typically an EFP will perforate a thickness of armour equal to the diameter of its charge.

It appears that casualties caught in the trajectory of the EFP suffer catastrophic injuries whereas those sitting adjacent to the projectiles path suffered relatively less severe injuries. In addition, the types of injuries encountered were predominantly secondary blast injuries related to being hit by the large metallic EFP or large fragments of the EFP.

General principles in the management of military trauma

Golden hour

Much of civilian trauma planning has been based around the concept of the trimodal distribution of death, and in particular the golden hour (or first 2h after injury), when significant numbers of casualties can be saved by medical interventions.

There is now good evidence to demonstrate that there is no equivalent second peak military trauma, and that most deaths in conflict cannot be prevented.

A report on casualties of the 1982 war in the Lebanon, documented that 94% of deaths occurred within an hour, a further 2% over the next 3h and the remaining 4% over the next 75 days. This was with good initial treatment and evacuation. Moderately and severely injured casualties reached a physician within 30min in 80% of the time and within 60min for 95% of the casualties.

A report from Israel, during a period of low intensity conflict, reported 77% of deaths occurred within 30min, mostly from head and trunk injuries, and a further 6% died in next 30min, with 11% between 1–3h and 2% after 1 day.

This data suggests that there is a rapid, exponential drop in survival rate in those who ultimately die after military trauma, rather than the peaks seen with civilian trauma. To attempt to improve the survival rate after military trauma would, therefore, mean getting to the casualty very quickly after wounding.

However, even with very rapid evacuation to a medical team, survival is not possible for the majority of casualties who ultimately die. Review of outcome from a Lebanon refugee camp under siege during 1982, showed that amongst 160 deaths, 84 were dead on arrival, despite an evacuation time of minutes. A further 35 died within minutes of arrival before any effective treatment could be started. Of the 76 who arrived alive, 34 died of multiple injuries and uncontrollable haemorrhage despite immediate access to a surgeon, and a further 20 died of central nervous system or high spinal injuries. So survival was not possible for at least 86%.

This is consistent with results from both the United Kingdom and United States military. A 1984 report on United States casualties from Vietnam stated 'Military trauma is seen to have an all-or-none nature, sustaining a fatal or survivable and frequently minor wound. 80–90% of casualties evacuated from the field have little likelihood of dying regardless of the sophistication of the care'.

Triage

Triage, derived from the French *trier*, to sieve or sort, is the process of assessing the priorities of treatment and is usually applied when the injured (or injuries) exceed the available resources such not everything can be dealt with at the same time.

The principle is to identify the 'most needy' patients and prioritize their treatment to reduce overall mortality and morbidity. In times of high casualty flow (mass casualty situation) this may mean that the treatment of the most critically ill may be delayed to allow the most good to be done to the greatest number of casualties.

Triage is a military innovation but has been adopted widely in civilian settings for major incident and disaster medical management. Although the terminology will vary between systems the general principles are the same:

Priority 1

These are casualties with life-threatening injuries (for example, catastrophic haemorrhage, airway obstruction, or tension pneumothorax). Treatment can not be delayed.

Priority 2

These are casualties with serious injuries that require treatment within 2h. Most of these will result in significant, but not catastrophic, haemorrhage, or spillage of abdominal contents.

Priority 3

These are casualties whose injuries can safely wait for 4–6h or so before treatment. This will include fractures and open wounds, when there is no significant haemorrhage or ischaemia.

Priority 4

This priority is usually reserved for times of high casualty flow, when the demands exceed the available resources. It is usually reserved for those patients whose injuries are so severe that the prognosis is hopeless, e.g. open head injury with a Glasgow Coma Score of 3. Using resources to treat these patients at times of high demand may place other casualties at risk by delaying their treatment.

Management of military wounds

The initial management of injuries resulting from ballistic mechanisms should be exactly the same as that during peacetime.

Life-saving measures take priority; maintaining an airway, and ensuring adequate ventilation and circulation. Unless there is life-threatening haemorrhage from an open wound, it should not be dealt with until the secondary survey.

Surgical treatment

The aim of local surgery is reduce the risk of infection, one of the most important factors in the morbidity after ballistic injuries. All military bullet wounds should be formally explored to reduce the infection risk, although civilian trauma centres have reported the successful non-operative management of bullet wounds. These were, however, low-energy wounds, evacuated rapidly to a hospital and not associated with the factors discussed earlier.

When small shrapnel wounds, particularly multiple wounds, are present, not all need debridement. If wounds are small, there is no evidence of fracture or joint penetration and they appear to be superficial and low energy, then a conservative approach can be adopted provided regular review is possible.

Surgical technique

The principle of debridement is to remove all foreign and non-viable tissue. This must be methodical and thorough as inadequate surgery may be worse than no surgery.

Debridement starts with the skin, and often excision of the skin margins is all that is required; degloving injuries may require more extensive debridement of skin. Although minimal excision is required, the wound should be extended to allow its full extent to be visualized. For high-energy wounds considerable extension may be required. This should be in the long axis of the limb, with the exception of the flexor surface of a joint, when oblique incisions should be used.

Subcutaneous fat should be excised, but additional areas of degloving must not be created by overgenerous debridement.

The deep fascia should be incised along the complete length of the wound, including any extensions. Fasciotomies with complete longitudinal division of the deep fascia along the full length of the compartment should be carried out in most high-energy wounds.

Adequate debridement of muscle is essential, and often a large amount of necrotic muscle may have to be excised. The aim is to remove all non-viable tissue, with the aim of leaving only pink, healthy-looking, contractile muscle; however, it is not necessary to excise the wound track en bloc. Lack of capillary bleeding or contractility, colour and consistency (the 4 Cs) are guides to muscle viability, but experience is the best way of judging (Box 12.6.3). Debridement of muscle may result in considerable bleeding from the wound, and both the surgeon and anaesthetist should be prepared for this.

Box 12.6.3 Guide to assessing muscle viability

- Capillary bleeding
- Contractility
- Colour
- Consistency
- *Experience.*

Nerves and patent blood vessels should be left, as can tendons in continuity with muscles. Often, however, the tendons may be become desiccated and may have to be excised at a later date. Divided nerves ends can be marked with a non-absorbable monofilament suture; however, further damage to the nerve, by the marking sutures, must be avoided.

Difficulties can often occur in the debridement of bone, particularly the fate of the many small fragments. Bone fragments without any soft tissue attachments are avascular and should be removed. Often, however, periosteal and other soft tissue attachments are present and the viability of the fragment can be difficult to determine. Experience is probably the most important factor in deciding the viability of a bone fragment or muscle. Experimental work has suggested that there is limited spread of contamination beyond the fracture site and, therefore, exposure of intact bone beyond the fracture site is not necessary. However, the fracture site itself must be well visualized and washed out.

All wounds should be washed with copious amounts of fluid. It has been recommended that 9L are used for open fractures. In a military environment, it may be impossible to use this quantity of sterile fluids, but potable water can be used with a final washout of 1L of sterile saline. With high-energy transfer wounds, contamination can be spread along tissue planes, and these should be thoroughly irrigated.

Antibiotics

Although antibiotics are necessary in the treatment of open fractures, they must not be seen as an alternative to surgery. This is particularly true with the military wound that may be highly contaminated, and there may be a considerable time delay before appropriate management can be started. In a report on the United States of America's invasion of Panama, there was a wound infection rate of 22% in patients operated on in Panama. This compared with an infection rate of 66% when wound debridement was delayed until the patient was evacuated to the United States. The higher infection rate was despite the use of early broad-spectrum antibiotics, and delayed primary closure of the wounds.

Amputation

Primary amputation may be required as part of the initial debridement. Although the decision may be easy with a limb that is hanging off and obviously non-viable, the viability of less severe injuries can be difficult to determine.

Although scoring systems have been developed for civilian limb injuries, there is still no reliable predictor of the need for amputation. Even in the military environment, a second opinion should be obtained, if possible, prior to amputation. If the viability of the limb cannot be determined initially, it may be reassessed after 48h. However, with military casualties a return to the operating theatre cannot be guaranteed, as problems with evacuation or mass casualty situations may occur. The decision to perform bilateral or upper limb amputations injuries will often be delayed, but infection may threaten the life of the casualty and this must be considered.

Even with recent advances in medical treatment, amputation remains a commonly performed operation in the military environment with rates up to 19% reported among United States military personnel from recent conflicts, and 22.5% from the Balkans conflict.

In the military environment amputations should initially be carried out at the lowest level possible, rather than creating formal flaps at the time of the initial surgery. This allows for later revision to a definitive level at the time of wound closure. If a definitive stump is created at the initial operation, subsequent infection (of which there is a high risk) may require further shortening and compromise the ultimate result.

No attempt should be made to close the amputation site at the initial operation, despite the perceived advantages. This will lead to oedema, ischaemia, and infection requiring further debridement.

Closure of the wound

Delayed primary closure of ballistic wounds is the rule for military injuries; primary closure is associated with an increased risk of infection. Wounds are left open to allow for swelling, and to prevent raised tissue pressures, which will impair microcirculation and lead to further tissue death, predisposing to infection. Although certain injuries, such as wounds to the face or genitals, may need to be closed primarily, this should be the exception. High-energy transfer wounds, with comminution of the bone should never be closed primarily, and will often require plastic surgical techniques several days after the initial debridement. Delayed primary closure can be carried out between 2–14 days after initial surgery, depending on the nature of the wound, evacuation of the casualty, and available resources and casualty numbers. Heavily contaminated limbs that may require amputation can be reassessed at 48h, but for most wounds 4–5 days is the optimum period until the wound is closed.

Low-energy injuries are associated with small wounds and require minimal debridement. Often they can be left to close by secondary intention, but should not be closed primarily.

Exposed bone or tendon does not have to be covered at the initial operation, but consideration should be given to early closure of these wounds to prevent desiccation. Bone or tendon that is left exposed for long periods will usually require further debridement despite appearing viable at initial surgery.

Wounds can be dressed with plain gauze, which can be fluffed up, but the wound should not be packed. The purpose of the dressing is to allow absorption of fluid, and not to hold the wound open. Packing will increases wound pressure leading to further tissue death. Bandages and tape can be used to secure the dressing but must not be allowed to encircle and constrict the limb.

Delayed primary closure was originally a military practice developed due to of the risk of wound complications during casualty evacuation. Wounds were debrided at a forward surgical centre, and then delayed primary closure was carried out at a base hospital when the casualty could be observed more closely. Delayed suture of wounds at an interval of 2–4 days was recommended for the treatment of gunshot wounds during the First World War. The concept of delayed primary closure was defined in 1918 as closure of the wound before 'granulations' had formed; suture after this granulation tissue had formed was defined as secondary suture. One of the advantages of the technique was the ability to determine the microbiology of the wound prior to suturing. A high complication rate was noted following the suturing of wounds that were contaminated by haemolytic streptococci. The presence of other organisms was considered less problematic. At the end of the First World War this technique seems to have been neglected.

Box 12.6.4
Primary closure is associated with an increased risk of infection

In the Second World War, the technique of delayed primary closure of wounds from missile injuries was again described. The wounds were associated with fractures of the long bones, skull, and pelvis in servicemen. The treatment protocol involved careful debridement, lightly packing the wound with a Vaseline gauze dressing, and then encasing the limb in plaster. Delayed primary closure, was then performed, by direct suture or skin grafting at an average of 14 days following wounding. In a report of 2393 patients, complete success was achieved in 66.5%, and partial failure, with a small sinus or stitch abscess or partial loss of skin graft, in 26.8%. Overall, 93.3% of wounds had healed by the time the patient was discharged; complete failure with dehiscence or osteomyelitis occurred in only 6.7%. Unfortunately the healing rates for specific fractures, was not reported. The interval of 14 days was not planned, but was a result of the evacuation time to a base hospital.

Retained fragments

Many bullet wounds will be associated with an entrance and exit wound, and the issue of retained fragments will not arise. Most of the remaining fragments will be removed at the time of initial debridement, but some will be left behind, and are often diagnosed on later radiographs.

Retained fragments can usually be left, with only a small risk of subsequent infection. If the wound does develop an infection, secondary surgery will often be required, and the fragments can be removed at this stage. Consideration must be given, however, to the removal of retained bullets.

Civilian data suggests that intra-articular and intrabursal bullets should be removed due to the risk of lead arthropathy or systemic toxicity. This can, however, be left until the patient has been evacuated back to a base hospital, and arthroscopic techniques can be used. Bullets retained in soft tissues including muscle can be observed, and the current evidence would also suggest that bullets retained in bone can also be treated conservatively.

Further reading

Cleveland, M. and Grove, J.A. (1945). Delayed primary closure of wounds with compound fractures. *Journal of Bone and Joint Surgery*, **27**, 452–6.

Coupland, R.M. and Korver, A. (1991). Injuries from antipersonnel mines: the experience of the International Committee of the Red Cross. *British Medical Journal*, **303**, 1509–12.

Fraser, F. (1918). Primary and delayed primary suture of gunshot wounds. *British Journal of Surgery*, **6**, 92–121.

Helling T.S. and McNabney W.K. (2000). The role of amputation in the management of battlefield casualties: A history of two millennia. *Journal of Trauma*, **49**, 930–9.

Knapp, T.P., Patzakis, M.J., Lee, J., Seipel, P.R., Andollah, K. and Reisch, R.B. (1996). Comparison of intravenous and oral antibiotic therapy in the treatment of fractures caused by low-velocity gunshots. *Journal of Bone and Joint Surgery*, **78A**, 1167–71.

12.7

Management of open fractures

John McMaster

Summary points

- Restore soft tissue cover
- Prevent infection
- Achieve union
- Maintain function.

Introduction

A fracture is considered open when a wound causes a direct communication between the fracture and a contaminated environment.

Open fractures frequently occur in the high-energy polytrauma patient. Prioritized treatment is required to manage all injuries efficiently without detriment to non-life- or limb-threatening injury. Open fractures are frequently complex with significant soft tissue, neurological, and vascular damage.

Effective management of open fractures requires a multidisciplinary approach from the early management to the long-term follow-up. The management of open fractures continues to improve and evolve. Consensus documents, such as 'Standards for the management of open fractures of the lower limb' produced by the British Orthopaedic Association (BOA) and British Association of Plastic, Reconstructive and Aesthetic Surgeons (BAPRAS) are extremely important. They ensure continued improvement in clinical practice based on current literature and expert opinion.

Aetiology and epidemiology

The severity of soft tissue injury is proportional to the energy transferred to the limb and can be represented by the equation $E = mv^2/2$. The energy E dissipated is thus proportional to the mass m and the square of the velocity v. Energies involved in high velocity missile injury (900m/s) are significant due to the logarithmic influence of velocity. However, the energy transfer in relatively low velocity pedestrian road traffic accidents must not be underappreciated due to the significantly greater mass (1500kg, average car vs 3.6g, 5.56-calibre bullet). A 10mph collision with the bumper of a car will have ten times the energy of a high-velocity bullet.

The soft tissues will be damaged directly as result of both the impact and the fractured bone ends. This has the potential to produce a significant quantity of devitalized soft tissue. Subsequent damage can occur as a result of vascular compromise from arterial damage, pressure within the capillary beds, or reduced venous drainage.

Open fractures in the United Kingdom are estimated to occur with a frequency of 23 in 100 000 patients per year. They are more frequent in bones with less soft tissue coverage. Open phalangeal and open tibial fractures account for the majority (approximately 54%) of these fractures.

Classification of open fractures

In 1976, Gustilo and Anderson reviewed 1025 open fractures in long bones and described the first stage of their classification. They identified a prognostic classification system that took into account the energy involved and the degree of soft tissue disruption. The original classification was inadequate for the description of the more severely traumatized limbs. In 1984, Gustilo and colleagues modified their classification of type III injuries based on the degree of contamination, the extent of the periosteal stripping, and the requirement for vascular repair. This is the classification that is now most widely accepted and used (Table 12.7.1).

This classification system has been used to demonstrate the association between the severity of the soft tissue injury and infection: Grade I, 0–2%; Grade II, 2–5%; Grade IIIa, 5–10%; Grade IIIb, 10–50%; and Grade IIIc, 25–50%.

There are several limitations of this classification.

The classification is frequently misquoted in the published literature and with all classifications even relatively subtle changes to the wording can have significant impact.

It is currently accepted practice to classify the wound based on the findings after the initial debridement. Although this provides a more accurate assessment, it has not always been standard practice.

Overall the interobserver agreement for the Gustilo classification has been found to be moderate to poor, with agreement ranging from 42–94% for individual cases. One of the main areas of discrepancy is differentiating between Grade II and IIIa. The other criticism is the association of Grade IIIb fractures with the use of flaps. The classification should not be based on the perceived treatment. Not all Grade IIIb fractures will require a flap to achieve soft tissue coverage.

Table 12.7.1 Combination of original classification (1976) and modification of type III classification (1984) of open fractures

Type	Definition
I	An open fracture with a wound < 1cm long and clean[a]
II	An open fracture with a laceration > 1cm long without extensive soft tissue damage, flaps, or avulsions[a]
III	Either an open segmental fracture, an open fracture with extensive soft tissue damage, or a traumatic amputation[a]
IIIa	Adequate soft tissue coverage of a fractured bone despite extensive soft tissue lacerations or flaps, or high-energy trauma irrespective of the size of the wound[b]
IIIb	Extensive soft tissue injury loss with periosteal stripping and bone exposure. This is usually associated with massive contamination[b]
IIIc	Open fracture with associated with arterial injury requiring repair[b]

[a] Gustilo, R.B. and Anderson, J.T. (1976). Prevention of infection in the treatment of one thousand and twenty-five open fractures of long bones. *Journal of Bone and Joint Surgery*, **58A**, 453–8.

[b] Gustilo, R.B., Mendoza, R.M., and Williams, D.N. (1984). Problems in the management of type III (severe) open fractures: a new classification of type III open fractures. *Journal of Trauma*, **24**, 742–6.

A number of other classification systems have been developed to describe open fractures (e.g. AO classification, Ganga Hospital Score) and help in decision-making with mangled extremities (MESS, LSI, PSI, NISSSA, HFS-97). The AO classification and Ganga Hospital Score both acknowledge that the different components of the open fracture (bone, musculotendinous units, skin, nerves and blood vessels) will be injured in varying degrees. The GHS, Table 12.7.2, also attempts to take into account systemic components such as age, comorbidity, and polytrauma.

Table 12.7.2 Ganga hospital open injury severity score (GHS). A score for predicting salvage and outcome in Gustilo type IIIA and type IIIB open tibial fractures

	Score
Covering structures: skin and fascia	
Wounds without skin loss	
Not over the fracture	1
Exposing the fracture	2
Wounds with skin loss	
Not over the fracture	3
Over the fracture	4
Circumferential wound with skin loss	5
Skeletal structures: bone and joints	
Transverse/oblique fracture/butterfly fragment <50% circumference	1
Large butterfly fragment >50% circumference	2
Comminution/segmental fractures without bone loss	3
Bone loss <4cm	4
Bone loss >4cm	5
Functional tissues: musculotendinous (MT) and nerve units	
Partial injury to MT units	1
Complete but repairable injury to MT units	2
Irreparable injury to MT units/partial loss of a compartment/ complete injury to posterior tibial nerve	3
Loss of one compartment of MT units	4
Loss of two or more compartments/subtotal amputation	5
Co-morbid conditions: add 2 points for each condition present	
Injury - debridement interval >12h	2
Sewage or organic contamination/farmyard injuries	2
Age >65 years	2
Drug-dependent diabetes mellitus/cardiorespiratory diseases leading to increased anaesthetic risk	2
Polytrauma involving chest or abdomen with injury severity score >25/fat embolism	2
Hypotension with systolic blood pressure <90mmHg at presentation	2
Another major injury to the same limb/compartment syndrome	
Total score	

Rajasekaran, S., Naresh Babu, J., Dheenadayalan, J., *et al.* (2006). A score for predicting salvage and outcome in Gustilo type IIIA and type IIIB open tibial fractures. *Journal of Bone and Joint Surgery*, **88B**, 1351–60.

Rationale for the treatment of open fractures

The aim of the initial treatment is to limit the effect of the original injury. This is achieved by treating associated injury, preventing extension of the zone of injury, maximizing limb perfusion, and minimizing the bacterial load.

Antibiotics

Antibiotics should be administered as soon as possible and they have been shown to reduce infection risk by 59%. The choice of antibiotics should be based on the likely contaminants of the open wound, and the significant pathogens that need to be suppressed. It is important to appreciate that the bacterial flora within the wound changes and is influenced by antibiotics, surgical debridement, and bacteria acquired from the hospital environment. This influences the choice and timing of the antibiotics. Antibiotic requirements will also change with time and geographical location and this should be appreciated by individual hospital's antibiotic protocols.

Initial operative treatment

It is accepted that the biggest factor in the outcome of the injury is the quality of the initial debridement, and therefore this should be performed by an experienced surgeon. Wounds that require repeat debridement are associated with an increased risk of infection.

The aim of the initial operative intervention is to produce a clean healthy wound by removing devitalized tissue, maximizing tissue perfusion, and providing skeletal stability.

Remove devitalized tissue and foreign material

Healthy soft tissue can cope with a significant number of bacteria without developing evidence of infection. Civilian wounds with less than 10^5 per gram, at the time of closure, have been shown to heal uneventfully. The presence of nonviable material (devitalized tissue or foreign material) has been shown to reduce, by a factor of 1000, the number of bacteria required to cause infection. Ultimately the body's ability to deal with devitalized, contaminated tissue is dependent on local and systemic factors and the acceptable threshold is variable. It is important to appreciate that surgical devices (implants or sutures) should be considered foreign material and will become colonized and contribute to the risk of infection.

Several studies have looked at whether Grade I and II open fractures and low-energy gunshot wounds can be managed without operative debridement. These studies have reported acceptable results in both the paediatric and adult populations.

Assessing the characteristics of a wound by formal surgical exploration is superior to superficial inspection. Treating an open fracture wound non-operatively requires experienced surgical judgement and there should be a low threshold for surgical exploration and debridement.

In wounds that are heavily contaminated, associated with arterial injury requiring repair, or sustained as a result of crush it is often difficult to determine the adequacy of the debridement and these wounds should have a second look at 48h before planning definitive treatment (Figure 12.7.1).

Maximizing tissue perfusion

For the soft tissues to clear residual bacteria from the wound, they must be well oxygenated and this requires a good blood supply. Pressure within the soft tissues will compromise perfusion and increase the likelihood of infection. Wound debridement originates from the French word meaning to 'unbridle' or release. In modern parlance we use the word to describe the removal of devitalized tissue but forget at our peril the importance of decompressing the wound to maximize perfusion. Leaving the wound open not only prevents compressing the soft tissues with closure but also facilitates drainage, further decreasing wound pressure (Box 12.7.1).

Timing of debridement

Based on limited evidence it has been accepted practice to perform surgical debridement of open fractures within 6h. More recent studies have failed to identify any benefit from early debridement and an increase in deep infection rate has not been demonstrated with delays up to 48h. Based on the current evidence, BOA/BAPRAS guidelines for tibial fractures recommend that debridement is performed on a semielective basis within 24h of injury with senior orthopaedic and plastic surgery input. Emergency debridement should still be performed in grossly contaminated wounds (organic material, stagnant or sea water), compartment syndrome, multiply injured and devascularized limbs.

Skeletal stabilization

Skeletal stabilization has been shown to be advantageous in reducing infection rates in open fractures but the scientific basis is limited. However, it is accepted that skeletal stabilization provides stability to the injured soft tissue envelope. This prevents further

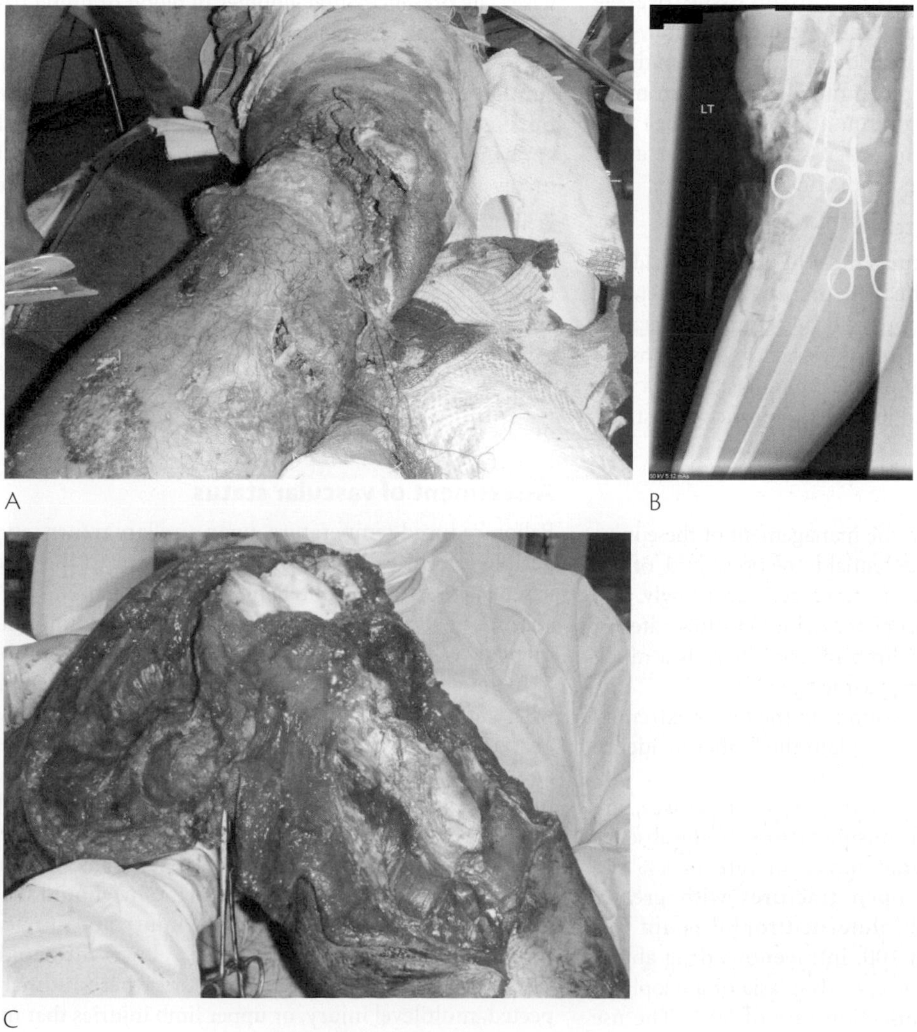

Fig. 12.7.1 Heavily contaminated open fracture requiring extensive soft tissue debridement. Images courtesy of the Royal Centre for Defence Medicine.

trauma, oedema, and reduced perfusion at the site of injury. The systemic and local benefits of skeletal stabilization are well established and facilitate early mobilization, nursing, and wound care.

Initial skeletal stabilization is temporary or definitive and the decision to use internal or external fixation will be dependent on the fracture, soft tissue cover, and local and systemic factors. An open wound devoid of devitalized tissue and foreign material will tolerate more contamination than a wound with an exposed implant. The timing of the planned soft tissue cover must be taken into consideration.

Timing of soft tissue coverage

Following successful debridement of open fracture wounds they remain at risk of infection while the wound remains open. The evidence would suggest that the vast majority of infections in open fractures are due to organisms that are not found in the wound at presentation. Early soft tissue coverage has repeatedly been shown to minimize the risk of infection from hospital-acquired organisms. The aim should be to achieve soft tissue coverage as soon as possible. The method of achieving coverage will be dependent on the soft tissues. Primary suture, delayed primary suture, and split skin grafting can be considered when the contamination is minimal and the soft tissue envelope is adequate to cover the implant. Primary suture has been shown to be safe when performed by experienced surgeons and will be discussed later in this chapter.

In those open fractures that have inadequate soft tissue coverage the best results (infection rate, flap failure, time to union, and function) have been achieved with debridement, fixation, and flap coverage within 72h. The current recommended optimum management involves debridement, fixation, and flap coverage as a single procedure. This technique has been shown to have a 3% deep infection rate in tibial fractures requiring flap coverage.

Involvement of multidisciplinary team

Any facility dealing with open fractures must be able to provide or access all of the relevant specialties. In the early management orthopaedic and plastic surgery input will be required. Vascular surgery will be required for Grade IIIc injuries. Complications are to be expected and the involvement of microbiologists with a specialist interest in bone infection and joint orthoplastic reconstruction clinics are beneficial.

Recognizing host factors

Host factors should be considered in the management of these injuries. Some of these factors have the potential to be optimized, others are indicative of high risk and should be managed accordingly.

Paediatric open fractures are associated with very low rates of infection in both upper and lower limb injury. There is a much higher rate of complications with increasing age.

A delay in neutrophil delivery to wounds in the lower extremity has been identified and this may help explain the higher incidence of infection in comparison to the upper limb.

Increased infection rates, in open long-bone fractures, are seen with systemic and local compromising factors. In the absence of compromising factors an overall infection rate of 4% has been reported. In comparison, open fractures with greater than three risk factors (or an absolute neutrophil count less than 1000; a CD4 count less than 100; intravenous drug abuse; chronic active infection of another site, or dysplasia or a neoplasm of the immune system) have an infection rate of 30%. The use of internal fixation in these high risk groups requires careful consideration.

In open tibial fractures, smoking has been demonstrated to increase the risk of infection (odds ratio 2.2), osteomyelitis (odds ratio 3.7), and non-union (37% less likely to be healed at 2 years). Cessation of smoking improves outcome but does not reduce the risks to non-smoking levels.

Initial management of open fractures (Box 12.7.2)

Open fractures are often high-energy injuries presenting as part of a polytrauma. The initial assessment and management should be carried out according to ATLS® principles. Ideally, prioritized activity can be concurrent rather than sequential. However during the primary survey attention may need to be directed at the open wound to address ongoing bleeding using pressure dressings or occasionally tourniquets.

Assessment of the wound

As a result of the significant deformation that can occur at the time of injury, open wounds may be some distance from the site of fracture. Any bleeding wound in proximity to a fracture should be treated with suspicion and assumed to be open until proven otherwise. The presence of fat globules in blood draining from a wound should be considered pathognomonic. In the case of pelvic fractures, open wounds may not be apparent on external inspection as communication may occur with the rectum or vagina. To avoid missing open fractures the entire limb must be visualized before applying dressings and splints. It is the responsibility of the person involved in this assessment to document clearly whether the injury is either open or closed. If an open injury is identified the characteristics of both the wound (size, location, and contamination) and surrounding soft tissues (degloving, abrasions and burns) also need to be recorded.

Microbiology swabs of the wound have not been found to be useful. In those cases that become infected the admission wound swabs are only representative of the organism involved in 8–18% of cases.

Assessment of vascular status

Pallor, reduced temperature, poor capillary return, and absence of peripheral pulses should alert the surgeon to the possibility of a vascular injury. To facilitate preoperative planning the presence or absence of all peripheral pulses in the affected limb must be documented. When pulses are not palpable it should not be attributed to hypotension. Doppler should be used to detect the presence and, where appropriate, the pressure of the distal pulses. Limbs which are grossly deformed should be manipulated into anatomical alignment with a vascular assessment both before and after manipulation. Positional ischaemia may resolve with a brisk hyperaemia following reduction. Failure to re-establish the circulation merits consultation with the vascular surgeons and further assessment of the vascular injury. Angiography should be considered, however in most cases the zone of injury and surgical target for reconstruction is clearly identifiable. A lower threshold for angiography should be used in blunt injury where intimal tear is suspected, multilevel injury, or upper limb injuries that may maintain peripheral pulses due to collateral circulation despite arterial injury (see Chapter 12.9).

Neurological assessment

Motor function is difficult to assess in the presence of a severe open fracture due to the pain and loss of muscle function. Light touch sensation is usually sufficient in the lower limb. Two-point discrimination is necessary to detect more subtle lesions, particularly in the upper limb.

Assessment of compartment syndrome

Despite significant soft tissue disruption it is still possible for open fractures to develop compartment syndrome. In the majority of cases this is a clinical diagnosis based on the patient's pain and evidence of muscle ischaemia on passive stretch. Neurological and vascular signs are late features. In the obtunded patient compartment pressure monitoring may be useful.

Wound cover

During this early phase the aim is to cover the wound as soon as possible and further exposure is to be avoided. The dressing should be sterile, moistened with normal saline, and occlusive. Antiseptic solutions are not recommended. The wound should be photographed and details documented. This should provide sufficient information prior to the next stage of treatment, and avoid the wound being repeatedly exposed. This simple measure has been shown to significantly reduce infection rates from 19% to 4%. Gross contamination should be removed from the wound. Exploration, debridement, and irrigation in the Emergency Department should be avoided as they are counterproductive.

Intravenous antibiotics

The first dose of antibiotics should be given as soon as possible. Current BOA/BAPRAS guidelines for lower limb open fractures recommend co-amoxiclav (1.2g 8-hourly in adults) or cefuroxime (1.5g 8-hourly in adults).

Clindamycin 600mg 6-hourly can be used instead of co-amoxiclav/cephalosporin when there is a history of penicillin-induced anaphylaxis should be administered within 3h and continued 8-hourly.

These antibiotics should be continued until the first debridement.

Tetanus prophylaxis

Tetanus prophylaxis must also be considered. Recommendations for prophylaxis are based on the condition of the wound and the patient's immunization history.

Splintage

Gross malalignment should be reduced, splintage applied, and the limb elevated. Splintage serves many purposes:

- Reduces bleeding by stabilizing the clot and reducing volume
- Pain relief
- Reduces local effect of displacement on skin, nerves, and blood vessels
- Temporary stabilization of soft tissue envelope reduces development of oedema
- Reduces complications relating to fat emboli.

Following application it is important to recheck distal neurological and vascular status and perform x-rays to check position.

Radiographic assessment

Prior to x-rays the limb should have already been assessed, the wound covered and the limb splinted. Good-quality anteroposterior (AP) and lateral radiographs of the fracture including the joint above and below is the minimum that is required. Significant bone displacement, bone loss and fragmentation indicate the presence of high-energy injury. Air in the soft tissue planes confirms that the fracture is open and indicates the zone of injury. Radio-opaque foreign material can be identified. Where possible, articular fractures should be investigated with computed tomography before the first operative intervention. This provides the surgeon with the best opportunity to reduce the articular surface with minimally invasive techniques.

Communication with other surgical teams

Ideally the wound assessment should be performed by the surgical team involved in the definitive care. Unfortunately this may not always be possible. Early communication will facilitate planning and avoid delays. Repeat assessment by the same team will allow evolving injuries (e.g. vascular and compartment syndrome) to be identified.

Primary operative intervention

Preoperative preparation

The surgery should be adequately planned. In cases where there may be soft tissue coverage problems it should be performed by the orthopaedic and plastic surgeons as a joint procedure.

Strategy

- The area should be given a 'social' wash with warm soapy water
- Further antibiotics should be given at induction. BOA/BAPRAS guidelines recommend co-amoxiclav (1.2g in adults) and gentamicin (7mg/kg, reduce if renal impairment)
- Following removal of the splint and dressings a further assessment of the limb can be performed
- Prep and drape for one- or two-stage procedure using alcoholic chlorhexidine solution, avoiding direct contact with the open wound
- Order of procedures, e.g. fasciotomies, vascular reconstruction, skeletal stabilization
- Skin incisions to allow adequate visualization. Where possible, fasciotomy incisions should be used to avoid perforator vessels. The surgeon should appreciate what secondary operations may be required to avoid compromising these procedures
- Consideration of the zone of injury will influence the necessary extent of the incisions, influence availability of local flaps, and the placement of fixation
- Debridement must be efficient and thorough. Random 'picking' at the wound should be avoided. Proceed in a sequential ordered fashion (superficial to deep, posterior to anterior, layer by layer).

Box 12.7.1 Debridement

- Adequate skin incisions:
  - Avoid compromising the next operation
  - Avoid further devascularization by using recommended fasciotomy incisions
- Adequate fascial release
- Excise all contaminated and devitalized tissue (unless articular bone):
  - 'Surgical steel is the best antibiotic'
- Irrigate
- Stabilize fracture and soft tissue envelope.

Make use of a second surgeon on the opposite side of the limb, operating alternately on each layer

- Standardized routine is helpful (especially in the middle of the night with non-specialist staff).

Equipment

- Ensure that all the required equipment is in the room and the theatre staff are aware of your plans. An appropriate quantity of irrigation fluid can be warmed in preparation
- Tourniquet—where possible a tourniquet should be fitted and can be used intermittently, which minimizes blood loss and allows the safe identification of nerves and vessels
- Image intensifier—fractures are most amenable to reduction at presentation. A short period of time spent maximizing alignment with external fixation will greatly facilitate minimally invasive definitive fixation techniques at the next sitting.

Potential problems

Complications will be avoided by preoperative consideration of potential problems. This will influence the choice of strategy and equipment.

- Patient's physiology—polytrauma patients may physiologically decompensate requiring the operation to be brought to a swift conclusion so that the patient can be optimized on the intensive care unit
- High-energy wounds will present with grossly distorted anatomy. A good knowledge of the anatomy will be required. Extending incisions to allow identification of nerves and blood vessels within normal anatomy is good practice, particularly if a limb is being perfused by a single vessel!
- Specific problems related to the different methods of stabilization
- Routine postoperative complications, e.g. compartment syndrome, infection, and deep vein thrombosis.

Intraoperative strategy

Vascular injury

Vascular injury that compromises the viability of the limb is a priority and reperfusion of the limb should be achieved within 4h, before irreversible ischaemic muscle damage occurs. The viability of the limb should be considered when the ischaemic time is greater than 4–6h.

Early reperfusion can be temporary or definitive (see Chapter 12.9). Adequate exposure and debridement should be performed rapidly to allow either definitive repair or temporary intraluminal shunting. A coordinated plan must be made with the vascular surgeons. If fasciotomy is likely to be needed it should be performed before the vascular repair. This will facilitate venous drainage and any perfusion provided by intact collateral vessels.

Skin

The size of the traumatic wound does not always reflect the degree of soft tissue damage. Skin wounds must be extended to allow an adequate estimation of the full soft tissue injury (Figure 12.7.2). The wound extensions should be made taking into consideration local fasciotomy incisions. In the tibia this will protect the fasciocutaneous perforator vessels. Consideration must also be given to access for internal fixation. Transverse incisions should be avoided when possible. The skin survives trauma well and routine excision is not appropriate, only non-viable or contaminated skin edges need excision. Usually excision of a few millimetres is the most that is required.

Degloving (Figure 12.7.3), occurs as a result of a shear force resulting in separation between the deep fascia and subcutaneous fat. This damages the perforator vessels that supply the skin and may devascularize large areas of skin.

Subcutaneous fat

Subcutaneous fat often has a poor blood supply and does not tolerate trauma as well as skin. This layer should be freely excised if there is any contamination or there is any question of viability.

Fascia

Any non-viable damaged or contaminated fascia should be removed. The fascia should be incised to decompress the underlying muscle and improve tissue perfusion. The surgeon should have a low threshold for performing complete fasciotomy of all compartments. Even if compartment syndrome is not present at the time of initial surgery it may subsequently develop.

Muscle and tendons

The identity and location of the muscle and tendon injuries need to be clearly documented to facilitate reconstruction at the time of definitive skin cover. It will also help establish if preoperative lack of function was due to a mechanical or neurological cause.

Necrotic muscle is the major medium for bacterial proliferation. All severely injured, ischaemic, and non-viable muscle must be removed. Assessing the viability of muscle may be difficult particularly in the presence of hypovolaemia, respiratory insufficiency, or temporary ischaemia (vascular injury or tourniquet). In general muscle viability can be assessed using the four Cs:

- Consistency
- Contractility—viable muscle will contract when gently pinched with forceps
- Colour—may be difficult to interpret due to blood under the myonesium

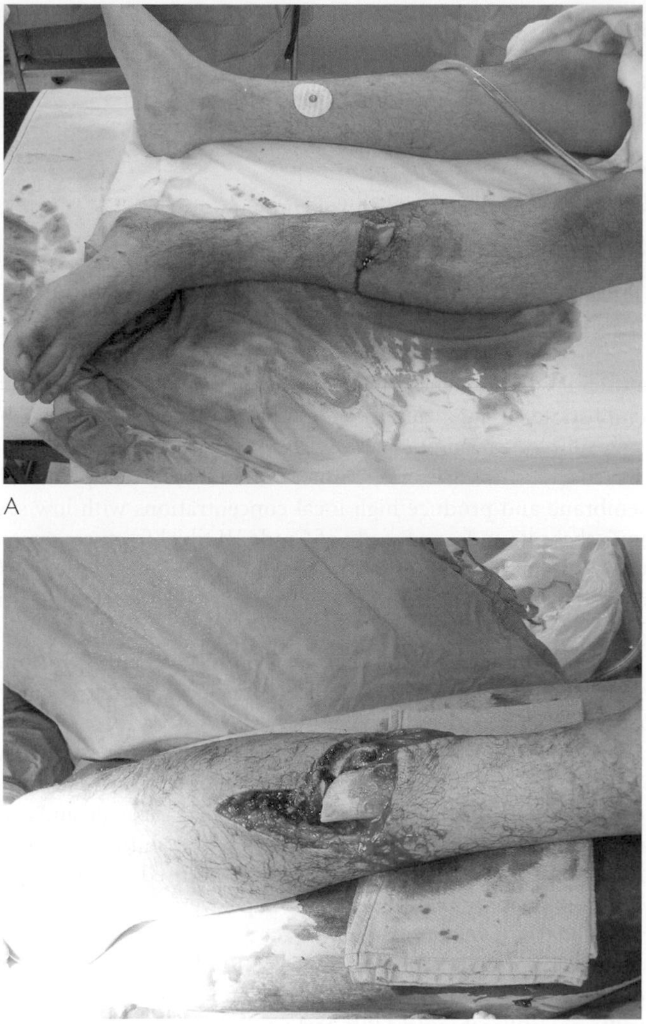

A

B

Fig. 12.7.2 Wound extensions should be performed to allow adequate visualisation and avoid unnecessary compromise to the residual blood supply.

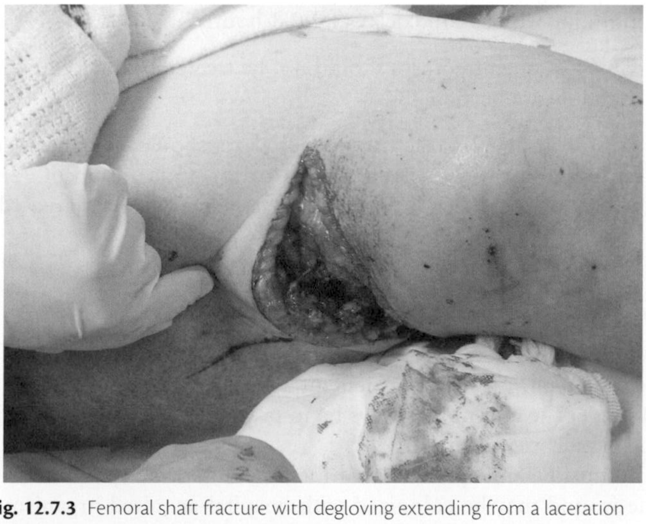

Fig. 12.7.3 Femoral shaft fracture with degloving extending from a laceration above the knee to the greater trochanters.

- Capacity to bleed—by the very nature of the procedure debridement of muscle must produce bleeding, to limit blood loss the majority of the debridement can be performed under tourniquet.

Nerves

Nerves in continuity should be maintained and cleaned. The epineurium of transected nerves can be tagged with a monofilament suture but care needs to be taken to avoid further damage. Identity and location of the nerve injury needs to be clearly documented.

Bone

Bacteria will colonize dead or ischaemic bone and produce a biofilm, making subsequent eradication very difficult. The tourniquet should be deflated to allow assessment of bleeding bone ends. Bone devoid of soft tissue attachment should be removed. These fragments should, however, be used to help judge fracture reduction before being discarded. An exception is made in the case of large articular fragments. These fragments need to be meticulously cleaned and reattached with absolute stability to facilitate union and revascularization. The viability of bone fragments that have some residual soft tissue attachments, in the absence of an available intraoperative assessment tool, continues to require surgical judgement. If the tissue is insufficient to resist the bone fragment detaching with a gentle pull it should be removed ('tug test'). The vascularity of a soft tissue bridge can be assessed using a hypodermic needle to elicit bleeding.

All fracture surfaces should be directly exposed and cleaned with a combination of nibblers, curettes, and scrubbing brushes.

Irrigation

The main purpose of irrigation is to wash away the loose particulate matter generated from the injury and the debridement. Tissue impregnated with foreign material and bacteria will not be effectively cleaned by washing alone. This should influence the volume of irrigation fluid used. There is no good evidence with regard to volumes required; however it is accepted practice to use large volumes (3–12L). Soap, antiseptics, and antibacterial agents have been investigated and demonstrated to have no additional benefit and in some circumstances are harmful.

Pulse lavage should not be used as this is associated with driving contaminants further into the tissues and increased bacterial seeding. It is also associated with trauma to the soft tissues. Although initially it is effective at reducing bacterial count there is a subsequent significant rebound.

Primary skeletal stabilization

At this stage the wound should be completely clean with all devitalized tissue and foreign material removed. The conditions should be sufficient to allow internal fixation to be considered. In addition to planning the method of fixation the wound should be classified and consideration should be given to how soft tissue coverage will be obtained. Where soft tissue cover is inadequate, involvement of the plastic surgeons is recommended. This is best performed at the time of the initial debridement as it will allow the fixation and soft tissue cover to be optimally planned.

Skeletal stabilization can either be temporary or definitive. Where debridement and soft tissue cover is considered adequate it is appropriate to proceed with definitive fixation. Despite adequate

Box 12.7.2 Preoperative management of open fractures

- Assess limb (if possible surgical team):
  - Wound
  - Surrounding soft tissue
  - Peripheral nerves
  - Pulses (± Doppler)
  - Compartment syndrome
- Photograph wound
- Sterile occlusive dressing ASAP
- Splintage
- Intravenous antibiotics ASAP
- Tetanus prophylaxis
- Diagnostic imaging:
  - X-rays
  - Consider angiography
- Consult other specialists where indicated (e.g. plastic surgeon)
- Consider transfer.

soft tissue coverage, if there is concern about the adequacy of debridement it is appropriate to use temporary stabilization and delay definitive fixation for 48h. Temporary stabilization with an external fixator should be considered when there is a soft tissue defect that would leave the implant exposed. The aim should be to perform definitive fixation at the same time as providing definitive soft tissue cover. Delays in covering exposed metal work are associated with increased infection rates (Box 12.7.3).

Placement of external fixators should avoid placing pins within the zone of injury or in areas of future internal fixation. Although conversion to internal fixation has been successfully reported up to 10–14 days following external fixation, colonization of the intramedullary canal from pin sites occurs rapidly. In general it is beneficial to convert from external to internal fixation as soon as possible.

Closure

There is good evidence to suggest that open fracture wounds can be closed primarily and early closure is associated with lower infection rates. This philosophy is based on the high prevalence of hospital-acquired organisms seen to cause infection in open fractures and the desiccation of exposed soft tissues. Dead space and drainage should be addressed as there will be a significant exudate as part of the inflammatory process. Failure to drain this fluid will further increase soft tissue tension and result in the accumulation of colonized fluid. Skin loss, heavily contaminated wounds, arterial injury, polytrauma, and compromising patient factors should be considered as contraindications to primary closure.

Primary closure requires experience, if in doubt leave the debrided wound and extensions open.

Dressings

The aim of the dressings, used following initial debridement, is to prevent external contamination and allow fluid drainage. The simplest dressing involves physiological saline soaked gauze.

Box 12.7.3 Temporary skeletal stabilization

- Pins should avoid zone of injury
- Pins should avoid position of future incisions
- Should not compromise soft tissue
- Should maintain length and alignment
- Casts are seldom indicated in long bone fractures.

Antiseptic solutions should not be used. Several large studies have demonstrated a significant reduction in infective complications by using antibiotic bead pouches. Beads are placed in the wound and covered with strips of non-circumferential adhesive semipermeable membrane and produce high local concentrations with low systemic absorption. In one study of Grade III tibial fractures treated with systemic both antibiotics, the addition of antibiotic beads reduced the rate of infection (39% vs 7.3%) and osteomyelitis (26% vs 6.3%).

Negative pressure wound therapy (NPWT) can also be recommended with a 1.9 times lower infection rate compared to standard dressings. These dressings have been shown to reduce oedema, increase local blood flow, encourage granulation, and reduce the size of the wound. The dressings can remain in situ for 48h and during this time the problems of dressing 'strike through' and contamination are avoided as the wound is sealed and continuously drained. Although NPWT dressings can be used to close open wounds and reduce requirements for flap coverage it is not recommended in the case of open fractures.

Current evidence demonstrates that NPWT and antibiotic bead pouches do not extend the 'window of opportunity' and the best results are still achieved with early soft tissue wound coverage (Figure 12.7.4).

Postoperative antibiotics

Antibiotics should be continued postoperatively, however there is no good evidence to guide clinicians on duration.

Current guidelines for open lower limb fractures recommend continuing with co-amoxiclav (1.2g) 8-hourly:

- Gustilo I open fractures should not be treated beyond 24h and certainly not beyond 48h
- Gustilo II and III fractures, prophylaxis should be continued until definitive soft tissue closure or for a maximum of 72h, whichever is shorter. This may have to be modified with regards to timing of debridement.

Secondary operative intervention

When there is uncertainty about the adequacy of primary debridement, further debridement at 24–48h can be considered. However the aim must always be to produce a clean wound with the first debridement.

It must be anticipated that at the time of secondary procedures the wound may be colonized with hospital-acquired organisms. Antibiotics with a different spectrum of activity are appropriate to cover these procedures involving the insertion and soft tissue

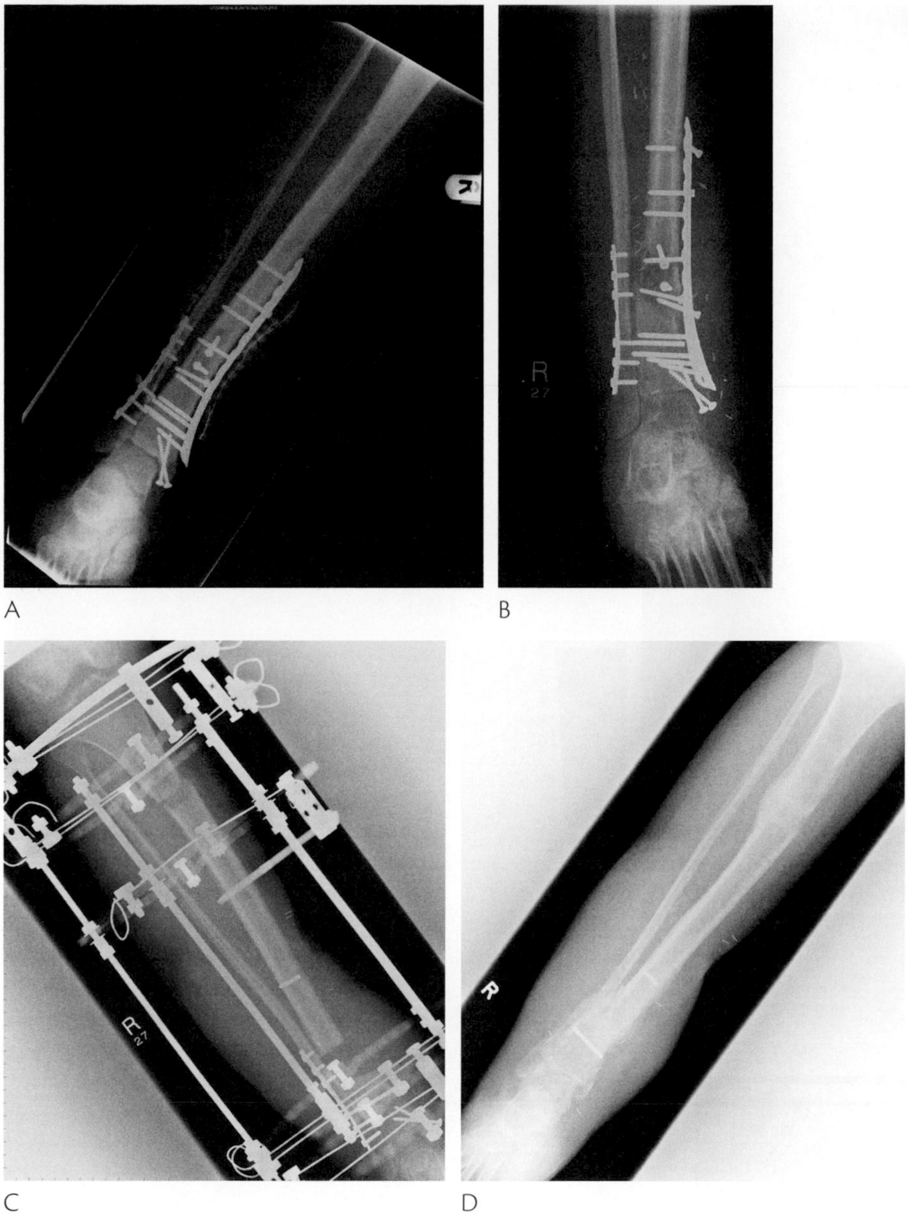

Fig. 12.7.4 A) Primary open reduction and internal fixation of Grade IIIb distal tibia fracture. Gentamicin bead pouch dressings. Definitive soft tissue coverage delayed, performed at day 7. B) Complicated by deep sepsis requiring debridement resulting in significant bone defect. C) Treated with circular frame and bone transport. Complicated by further soft tissue problems and re-fracture. D) Union and resolution of sepsis at 2 years postinjury.

coverage of internal fixation. Current BOA/BAPRAS guidelines for open lower limb fractures recommend:

When skeletal fixation and definitive soft tissue reconstruction is undertaken, gentamicin (7mg/kg, with appropriate adjustment in the elderly or those with renal impairment) and either vancomycin (1g) or teicoplanin (800mg). Vancomycin infusion will require to be started at least 90min before surgery.

Skeletal stabilization

The method chosen for definitive fixation of the fracture will depend on the fracture pattern. The method used should be optimal for bone healing and avoid further soft tissue trauma. Achieving early coverage of the implant is more important than the implant itself. Open fractures are associated with a higher incidence of non-union and early secondary surgery may be required to facilitate healing (11–58% in Grade III tibial fractures).

External fixation should be considered for definitive treatment of grossly contaminated wounds. Ring fixators provide additional benefit when there is bone loss, complex fracture patterns, and compromised soft tissues.

Intramedullary nailing has been demonstrated to be appropriate in the management of minimally contaminated open tibia and femur fractures. There are also significant benefits in terms of malalignment, subsequent procedures, function, and patient satisfaction. Reaming has not been shown to be detrimental. It has been recommended that if late conversion to intramedullary nailing from external fixation is considered there should be a delay of 7–14 days following removal of the external fixator to minimize the risk of infection.

Cast immobilization is generally not appropriate for either the temporary or definitive management of lower extremity long-bone open fractures in adults. In children Grade I and II open forearm

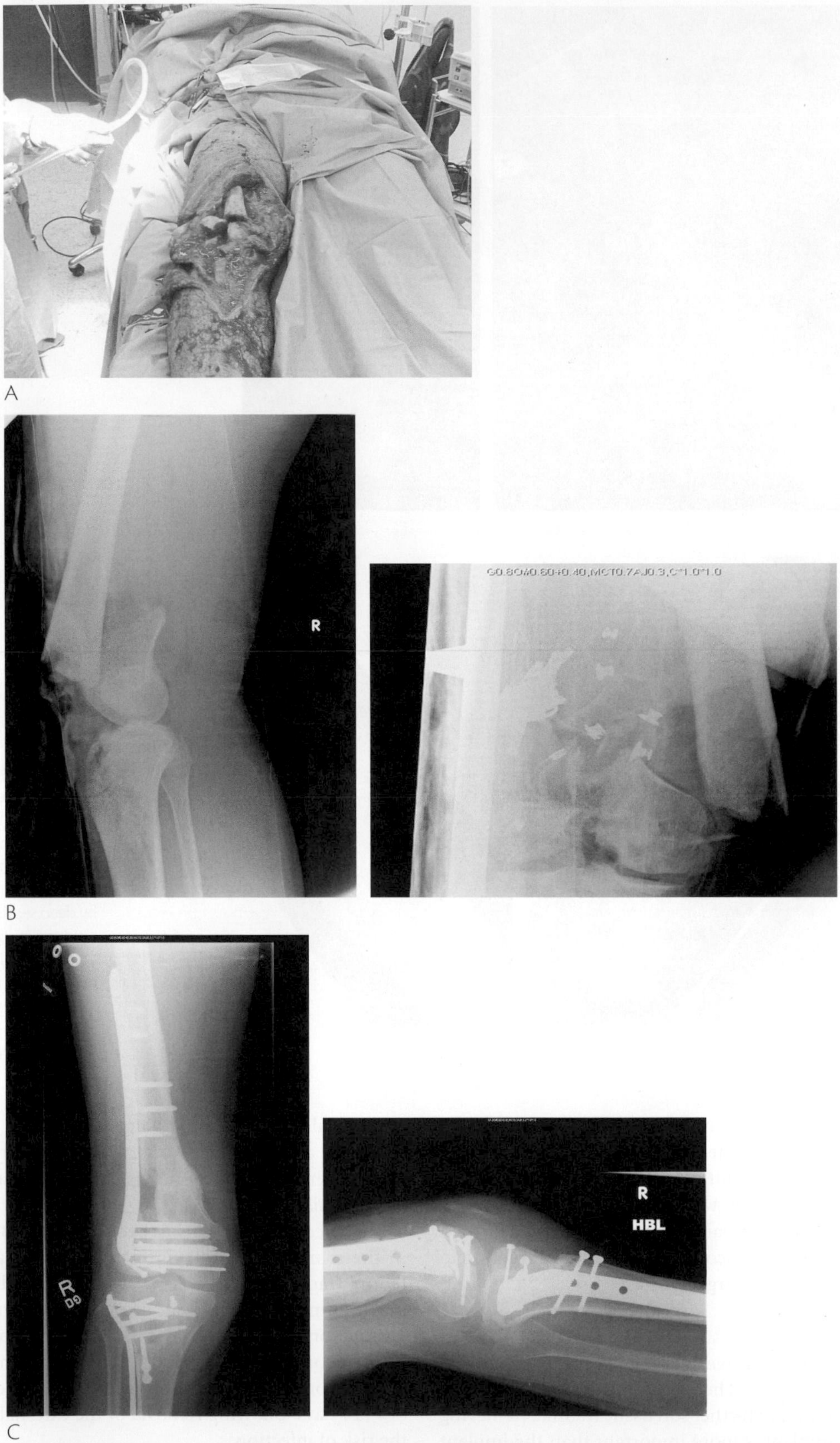

Fig. 12.7.5 A) A 21-year-old motorcyclist treated with debridement and external fixation as an emergency procedure. B) At 48h postinjury he was treated with internal fixation, reconstruction of extensor mechanism (hamstring tendon), gastrocnemius flap, and split skin graft. C) Multifragmentary distal femur and tibia.

fractures can be successfully treated with debridement and cast immobilization.

Soft tissue coverage

It should be considered best practice to achieve definitive skeletal stabilization and soft tissue coverage within 72h and certainly within 7 days (Figure 12.7.5).

In those wounds left open for a second look this should be performed at 48h and at this stage, soft tissue coverage can be achieved with direct skin closure, split skin graft, or flaps. Small residual defects, not involving exposed metal work can be left to heal by secondary intention. A 1cm^2 defect will take approximately 1 month to heal.

Definitive soft tissue coverage is covered in detail in Chapter 12.8.

Further reading

British Orthopaedic Association and British Association of Plastic, Reconstructive and Aesthetic Surgeons (2009). *The Management of Open Fractures of the Lower Limb.* http://www.boa.ac.uk

Gopal, S., Majumder, S., Batchelor, A., Knight, S., Boer, P.D., and Smith, R. (2000). Fix and flap: the radical orthopaedic and plastic treatment of severe open fractures of the tibia. *Journal of Bone and Joint Surgery*, **82B**, 959–66.

Naique, S.B., Pearse, M., and Nanchahal, J. (2006). Management of severe open tibial fractures: the need for combined orthopaedic and plastic surgical treatment in specialist centres. *Journal of Bone and Joint Surgery*, **88B**, 351–7.

Rajasekaran, S., Naresh Babu, J., Dheenadayalan, J., *et al.* (2006). A score for predicting salvage and outcome in Gustilo type IIIA and type IIIB open tibial fractures. *Journal of Bone and Joint Surgery*, **88B**, 1351–60.

Rajasekaran, S., Dheenadhayalan, J., Babu, J.N., Sundararajan, S.R. Venkatramani, H., and Sabapathy, S.R. (2009). Immediate primary skin closure in type-III A and B open fractures: results after a minimum of five years. *Journal of Bone and Joint Surgery*, **91B**, 217–24.

12.8

Soft tissue coverage

Christopher M. Caddy and Andrew N. Morritt

Summary points

- Soft tissue cover is a complex process
- Soft tissue cover requires specialist skills
- Soft tissue cover should ideally be performed in collaboration with a Plastic & Reconstructive Surgeon.

Box 12.8.1 Principles

- Replace like with like
- Minimal donor site morbidity
- Restore sensation if possible.

Box 12.8.2 Assessment

- Premorbid, e.g. smoking
- Soft tissue/vascular/neurological injury assessment
- Continues during surgery
- Avulsion/degloving will widen injury area.

Introduction

Soft tissue coverage of the extremities following trauma facilitates early wound healing and provides durable cover for exposed structures. Defects have traditionally been closed by using the simplest suitable technique from a reconstructive ladder, ranging from primary closure and skin grafting to flap cover. However, the expanded armamentarium available to the reconstructive surgeon permits the emphasis to shift from simply closing the wound to one providing an optimal functional and aesthetic result.

Outcomes are judged by the extent of restoration of form and function, and also by the donor site morbidity of the reconstruction. Losses should ideally be replaced with like tissue and cover should provide durable protection for underlying structures with minimal donor site morbidity. Attempts should be made to restore sensibility where possible as functional results will be enhanced. This chapter discusses options for soft tissue cover in the upper and lower extremities. Hand and wrist cover are discussed in a separate chapter.

General principles (Box 12.8.1)

Clinical evaluation (Box 12.8.2)

The approach to assessment and reconstruction of a surgical defect is similar in both extremities. The history should include an estimate of the forces causing the injury. The presence of peripheral vascular disease, diabetes mellitus, or a history of heavy smoking may influence the choice of reconstruction and are considered with age, sex, occupation, and pre-injury mobility status.

The limb assessment starts with the general trauma evaluation and continues in the operating theatre during initial debridement. High velocity, severe crush, or degloving injuries have extended zones of damage which are often unrecognized on initial inspection but should be suspected as soon as the details of the accident are known. The limb examination should pay particular attention to the vascular supply, skeletal integrity, and the presence or absence of nerve injury. The wound is examined to determine the extent of soft tissue loss, absence of other structures, and degree of exposure of vulnerable tissues (bone, tendon, nerve, cartilage, and vessels). The quality and availability of adjacent tissue is evaluated for possible use in local flap transfer. Avulsion or degloving mechanisms will further widen the affected area. Marginal tissues may not declare viability at the initial exploration and serial debridements are necessary until the wound is stable.

Investigations such as angiography should be requested if indicated, especially if free tissue transfer is being contemplated. Indications for preoperative angiography include patients with suspected vascular injury who may require acute vascular reconstruction (Gustilo 3C tibial fractures) and patients who have had previous regional surgery with possible alteration of recipient vessel anatomy.

A multidisciplinary approach is commonly necessary for the management of these patients, especially in the lower limb where complex fracture fixation procedures are undertaken prior to soft tissue coverage and early participation of all parties who will be involved in management should be encouraged.

Early management (Box 12.8.3)

The foremost principle in the management of any traumatic injury is early, meticulous surgical debridement and wound irrigation. In complex injuries, particularly with heavy contamination, serial debridement may be performed after 48–72h in order to determine more accurately the extent of tissue damage. Conservative

Box 12.8.3 Early management

- Meticulous debridement
- Serial debridement in complex injuries
- Intravenous antibiotics at outset and until wound closed
- Bacterial swabs from wound.

initial debridement in wounds with massive tissue loss allows for preservation of tissue which may otherwise be excised using a more radical approach. At the second debridement any obvious residual devitalized tissue can be excised. The wound should then be suitable for cover which can be undertaken at this stage. Alternatively, if free tissue transfer is proposed as a single-stage procedure, it is essential that all devitalized tissues are excised prior to coverage.

The bacterial count in the wound increases with time prior to surgery and intravenous antibiotic therapy is therefore commenced on admission and continued until soft tissue cover is achieved. Wound swabs should be taken intraoperatively and antibiotics adjusted according to bacterial sensitivities.

Indications for soft tissue cover (Box 12.8.4)

Where skin loss is minimal, wounds can be closed by primary suture following debridement and irrigation under appropriate antibiotic cover. During suturing the margins of the wound should be easily opposed without blanching and allowances made for postoperative swelling to avoid ischaemic skin necrosis (approximate—don't strangulate!). Wounds should not be closed primarily if under tension. If in doubt, sutures should be removed and another method of cover sought. In practice, most wounds can be closed either primarily or with a split skin graft.

Wounds that cannot be closed primarily can generally be closed by applying skin grafts or with flap cover. Skin grafts are also indicated in wounds where grafting would expedite healing in contrast to healing by secondary intention, and also where no advantage can be obtained by using a skin flap. The wound bed should be well vascularized and free from infection, which in practical terms means a wound bed consisting of healthy muscle, fascia, or granulation tissue. The presence of beta-haemolytic streptococci (Lancefield group A) is an absolute contraindication to grafting. Graft will not take on exposed bone, cartilage, or tendon unless the periosteum, perichondrium, or paratenon are intact. Absence of these well vascularized structures, or exposure of nerves or vessels, excludes the use of a skin graft and necessitates flap cover.

Flap cover may be from a local or regional source, or as a free tissue transfer. Flap transfer may be fascial, fasciocutaneous, muscle, or composites depending on the reconstructive requirements. Local random pattern flaps can be transposed, advanced, or rotated to cover small defects where the bed is unsuitable for a skin graft or where a flap would give a better cosmetic result.

Box 12.8.4 Soft tissue cover

- Do not oppose edges with tension
- Split skin graft needs vasularized bed
- Beta-haemolytic *Streptococcus* contraindication to grafting
- Low-energy injuries local flap.

The timing and choice of cover depends on the general condition of the patient including associated injuries, site, size, and depth of defect, extent of the zone of injury (macroscopic and microscopic), thickness of tissue required for reconstruction, donor site availability, and the need to perform secondary reconstructive procedures. In general, low-energy injuries unsuitable for primary closure or split skin grafting can be covered with local fasciocutaneous flaps, whereas extensive defects from high energy injuries often require free tissue transfer. Primary reconstruction of damaged tendons and nerves should only be performed if adequate cover can be provided simultaneously. Nerves and tendons that are not suitable for primary repair should be tagged following debridement and bony stabilization in order to facilitate easy identification during secondary reconstruction.

Technique of split skin grafting

Split skin grafts are most commonly harvested from the uninvolved thigh or buttock region under general or local anaesthesia with either an electrical or air-driven dermatome or a free hand knife. The donor site is prepared and draped in a sterile fashion. An epinephrine (adrenaline) containing local anaesthetic solution may be infiltrated subcutaneously preoperatively or applied topically following harvest to reduce blood loss and provide postoperative pain relief. The dermatome is set to the appropriate thickness, the donor site lubricated with liquid paraffin, and the graft cut by setting the dermatome flat on the skin, turning on the power and advancing it across the donor site using gentle downward pressure. The harvested skin may be meshed using a mechanical device or 'hand meshed' using a scalpel. Meshing allows egress of exudate which could otherwise accumulate under the graft lifting it from its bed. The donor site is dressed. A number of donor site dressings are available, including semiocclusive dressing such as calcium alginate (Kaltostat) or Lyofoam. The graft is spread, cut surface upwards, on a sheet of paraffin gauze. It is then placed on the wound and fixed with sutures or tissue glue (Histacryl), and a well-padded dressing is applied. The graft is typically inspected 5 days postoperatively and the donor site inspected 10–14 days postoperatively.

Principles of flap transfer

Careful planning and execution are of paramount importance for successful flap transfer. Flap design begins with projection of the recipient defect backwards (via a template) onto a suitable donor site. The flap should have a predictable circulation and be larger than the primary defect, allowing for safe single-stage transfer with tension free inset. Donor sites produce a secondary defect which may be closed directly or indirectly, using either skin graft or local flaps. Principles which improve the quality of the reconstruction include: elimination of dead space; atraumatic tissue handling; meticulous haemostasis; and the use of appropriate suture materials.

Fracture fixation methods and soft tissue cover

Complex injuries involving fractures with varying degrees of soft tissue loss require stabilization prior to coverage. The method of fixation used depends on the fracture site and type, size and characteristics of the wound and to a certain extent the preference of the orthopaedic surgeon. External fixation conveniently splints bone and soft tissues while providing access to the wound and can be applied rapidly with minimal risk of further devascularization of bone fragments and adjacent soft tissues. Internal fixation using plates and screws or intramedullary nails may be used primarily provided soft tissue cover can be achieved simultaneously. If the surgeon performing the external fixation is different from the surgeon providing cover, it is important that placement of fixation pins is discussed to avoid compromise of potential local donor tissues.

Timing of reconstruction

The timing of reconstruction depends on the mechanism of injury, wound status, condition of the patient and availability of appropriate surgical expertise. Early wound closure (defined by Byrd et al. as the first 6 days from injury and by Godina as the first 72h from injury) of complex lower extremity defects with vascularized muscle following radical debridement was associated with lower wound infection rates, a lower incidence of osteomyelitis and non-union, and lower anastomotic thrombosis rates, than delayed closure. In practice, initial evaluation, debridement, and bone stabilization are performed by the orthopaedic trauma team and the plastic/reconstructive surgeon is asked to provide soft tissue cover days later, thus missing the first 'window of opportunity' for reconstruction.

Ideally, all severe injuries are managed on a single site with dedicated orthopaedic and plastic/microsurgical surgeons with an interest in trauma. If the appropriate expertise is not available locally, it is essential that orthopaedic surgeons communicate with their local plastic surgery service or with appropriately trained and experienced orthopaedic colleagues before embarking on the first operative procedure. In cases where cover is delayed, it is important to avoid desiccation of the wound between operations.

Wound closure with vacuum-assisted devices

Topical negative pressure (TNP) wound care management systems have become increasingly popular over the last decade and their use in the management of limb trauma is continually evolving. Used in the appropriate wounds, TNP can reduce swelling and encourage the growth of granulation tissue allowing wound closure with split skin graft rather than a flap. However, used incorrectly it can delay appropriate radical debridement that may otherwise salvage early infected prostheses and metal work. In the military and acute trauma setting it can allow wound debridement and then sterile wound closure, so that appropriate transfer to a specialist centre can be achieved. Its usage should be regularly reviewed and restricted to those with appropriate training or when used in close collaboration with plastic surgery colleagues and it should not replace adequate surgical debridement.

Flaps available (Box 12.8.5)

Although numerous flaps have been described, the vast majority of defects can be covered adequately by using one of a limited number of 'workhorse' flaps.

Latissimus dorsi (Figure 12.8.1)

The latissimus dorsi muscle free flap is the workhorse of lower limb reconstruction, whereas the pedicled latissimus dorsi muscle or musculocutaneous flaps are useful in shoulder and arm reconstruction. The muscle is easily elevated, has a long pedicle enabling microvascular anastomosis outside the zone of injury, and can be folded which aids in dead-space obliteration. Dimensions averaging 25cm × 40cm in adults provide cover for defects extending from the proximal tibia to the ankle. The amount of muscle harvested can be tailored to the defect preserving innervation and function of the remaining muscle. Among the disadvantages of muscle transfer is weakness of upper extremity 'push-off', an activity of importance in some athletes and bell ringers!

Box 12.8.5 Flaps

- Multidisciplinary team essential
- Careful planning
- Stabilize skeleton first
- Early closure lower infection rate.

Serratus anterior

The serratus anterior muscle can be transferred as a free flap either alone or combined with the latissimus dorsi muscle for cover of medium to large defects in the distal third of the leg and foot. The upper slips of the muscle should be preserved during harvest in order to reduce winging of the scapula which would result from complete removal of the muscle. Although the donor site is closed directly, lack of an associated skin flap necessitates skin grafting for resurfacing.

Rectus abdominis

The rectus abdominis muscle can be used as a pedicled muscle or musculocutaneous flap for coverage of both groins or as a free muscle flap for coverage of lower limb defects. The blood supply is robust, considerable muscle bulk is available and the skin paddle can be carried anywhere along the muscle. If the skin island is placed at the level of the inframammary fold, a pedicled musculocutaneous flap can provide cover of the groin, trochanter, or anterior thigh as far as the knee. Disadvantages of flap harvest include abdominal weakness that results particularly in the inferior portion of the abdomen below the arcuate line, although hernias are rare and functional morbidity is minimal as the remaining rectus muscle compensates.

Gracilis

The arc of rotation of the pedicled gracilis flap allows for cover of ipsilateral groin defects or defects on the anterior and posterior thigh. The gracilis can also be transferred as a free muscle or musculocutaneous flap for coverage of limb defects. A neuromuscular flap can be used to provide motor input following muscle loss, e.g. for elbow flexion. Muscle harvest causes minimal functional morbidity and the donor site can always be closed primarily. However, long cutaneous skin paddles are unreliable distally and the flap may be difficult to raise in the obese.

Scapula flap

The scapula flap can be used to cover defects in the upper arm and axilla as a pedicled flap and defects in the forearm as a free flap. Composite flaps consisting of skin overlying the scapula, latissimus dorsi, and/or serratus anterior muscle are available for cover of large complex defects. Primary closure of the donor site is usual, although the scar over the scapula will almost always stretch leaving an unattractive donor site.

Groin flap

The groin flap has been popular for cover of hand and forearm defects. It is large enough for most upper extremity defects and can

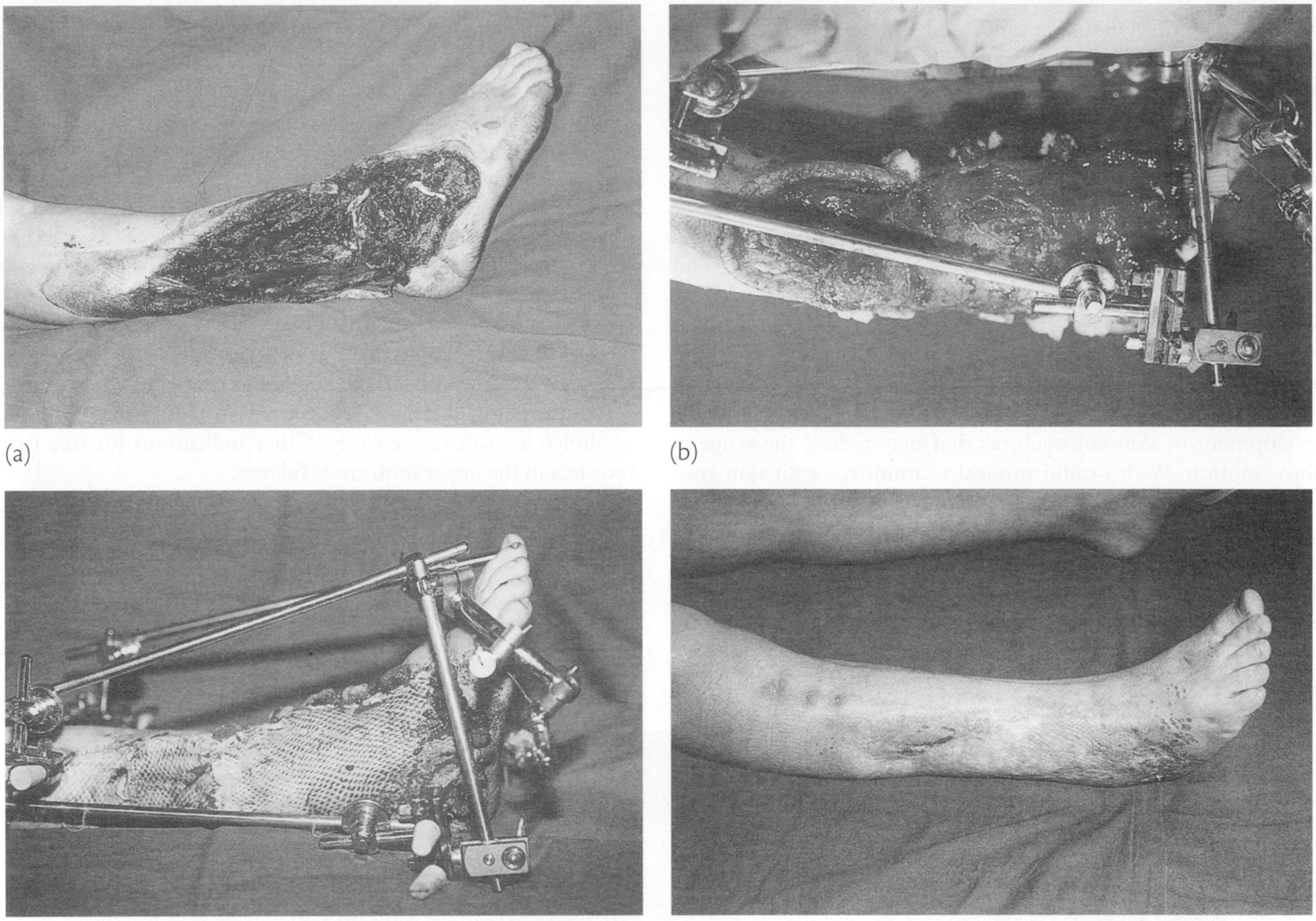

(a) (b) (c) (d)

Fig. 12.8.1 Latissimus dorsi flap cover of complex lower-limb injury in 12-year old male patient: A) initial presentation; B) following debridement, external fixation, and cover with a latissimus dorsi free flap; C) application of meshed split skin graft; D) late result showing stable soft-tissue cover.

be extended if necessary by delay procedures. The donor site can usually be closed primarily leaving an acceptable 'bikini-line' scar. The distal portion can be radically thinned to fit hand defects with a more acceptable contour although it may still be bulky in obese patients. As with all staged transfers the delay between stages may lead to stiffness which is compounded by the dependent position the arm is forced to adopt. Early aggressive hand therapy or use of this flap as a free tissue transfer can reduce this problem. Utilizing either method, groin flaps may require thinning procedures to improve contour.

Radial forearm flap

A large territory of forearm skin can be raised as an axial pedicle flap or as a free flap on the radial artery. Palmaris longus tendon and radial bone can be included for extensor or metacarpal reconstruction respectively if required. Composites of bone and skin can also be used for thumb reconstruction. The pedicled radial forearm flap is often used as a reversed flow distally based fasciocutaneous flap for cover of distal dorsal hand defects or degloved fingers in a mutilated hand. The vascular anatomy is constant and the excellent nerve supply allows its use as a neurovascular flap. The main disadvantages of this flap are the donor site morbidity and the sacrifice of the radial artery. The donor site may require a split skin graft for reconstruction which can be unsightly and should preferably not be used in female patients. Smaller donor sites that are still too wide for direct suture may close with a local sliding transposition flap. An Allen test should always be performed before raising this flap to confirm adequate ulnar artery vascular input to the whole hand.

Lateral arm flap

The lateral arm fasciocutaneous flap can be used as a pedicled flap to cover proximal forearm defects, or as a free flap to cover small to moderate size defects in the lower limb and distal forearm. Flaps with dimensions of 15 cm × 14 cm have been described but if the donor site is to be closed primarily the width should be limited to 6–8cm. The main advantage of the lateral arm flap over the radial forearm flap is that the nutrient artery is not essential to the vascularity of the distal upper extremity.

Adipofascial

For small to medium sized defects of the middle and distal third of the leg, turnover flaps of fat and fascia have been used as a bed for a split skin graft (Figure 12.8.2). They can be designed to incorporate a perforator in the base adjacent to the defect, and hence a more reliable blood supply. Donor sites that have been previously traumatized or degloved are unsuitable due to perforator damage and impaired vascularity. Success with these flaps requires some expertise and they should not be used for coverage of infected wounds. While muscle flaps are relatively resistant to bacterial contamination in contrast to fasciocutaneous flaps, adipofascial flaps have not been shown to have this property. Although donor site morbidity is minimal, the major disadvantage of this flap is the unpredictable take of skin grafts applied to the fascial surface.

Cover in specific anatomical regions

Upper limb (Box 12.8.6)

Where nerve, blood vessels, tendon, or bone are not injured or exposed, e.g. a deep friction burn or a skin avulsion injury, a split thickness skin graft can provide excellent cover. Where grafts cross the elbow joint, splinting and physiotherapy help to prevent the development of skin contractures that may reduce the range of elbow motion. With careful surgical technique, a split skin graft will heal sufficiently to allow mobilization within one week of the procedure. Pressure garments can be worn for 6–18 months to hasten graft maturation and improve the final appearance.

In some avulsion or degloving type injuries the skin flap can be used as a full thickness skin graft following defatting providing the surface of the skin flap is relatively undamaged. This has the advantage of providing skin with a good colour and texture match without donor site morbidity. Defects that are unsuitable for skin grafting require flap cover from local or regional sites or free tissue transfer.

Significant upper limb trauma is often associated with chest injuries and definitive cover may have to be delayed until the patient's condition is stable. Debridement with dressings or a split thickness skin graft, autogenous or autologous, can be used as a temporary biologic dressing. A pedicled latissimus dorsi flap may then be required to reconstruct defects in the shoulder and arm. Fasciocutaneous flaps such as the scapula or groin flaps may also be used to cover large forearm defects. For smaller defects, the lateral arm flap can cover defects above and below the elbow.

In more complex defects, free tissue transfer may be the method of choice for soft tissue cover. Other indications for free tissue transfers in the upper limb are as follows:

- Where simpler techniques are not suitable because of trauma to local donor sites or previous failures with use of adjacent tissues
- Where a one-stage procedure will allow for early mobilization and restoration of function

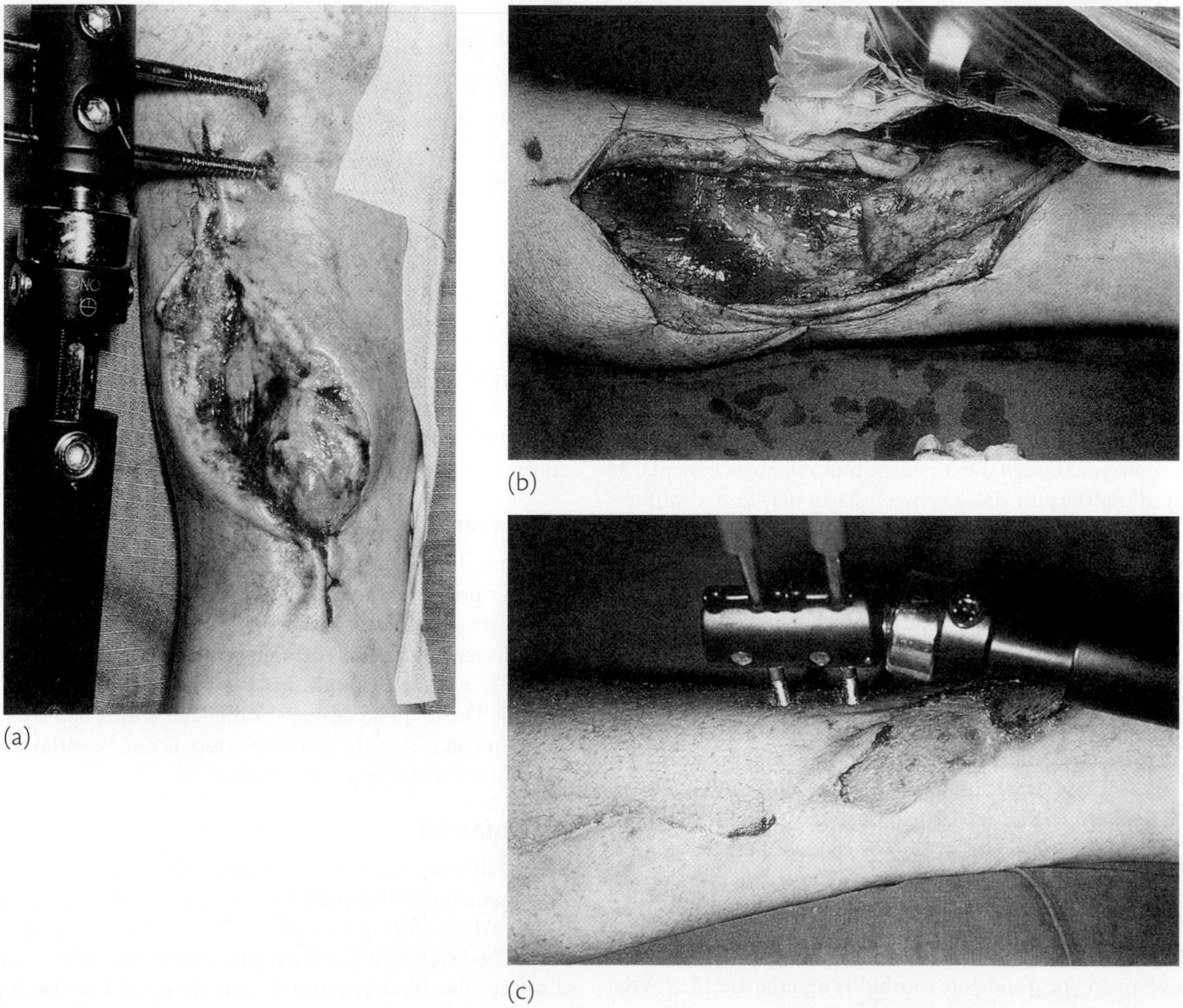

(a) (b) (c)

Fig. 12.8.2 Clinical example of adipofascial turnover flap. A) Delayed referral of patient with exposed tibia following trauma; B) adipofascial flap turned over and inset into defect; C) healed wound and donor site.

Box 12.8.6 Upper limb

- Early movement to avoid contractures
- Pressure garments useful
- Local flap may be used
- Latissimus dorsi or myocutaneous flaps may be required.

- Composite tissue transfers can be performed if required for reconstruction
- Staged pedicle transfers may be uncertain due to dubious vascularity of the recipient bed.

Lower limb (Box 12.8.7 and Figure 12.8.3)

Significant lower limb trauma is often associated with other injuries and while management of life-threatening conditions takes precedence over limb injuries, decisions regarding treatment of the injured limb need not be delayed. Prerequisites for reconstruction are vascular patency and tibial nerve integrity.

Groin and thigh

The circumferential muscle layer surrounding the femur in the proximal third of the thigh allows for most defects to be closed with split thickness skin grafts. When vessels or nerves are exposed following post-traumatic vascular reconstruction or occasionally with exposure of orthopaedic metalwork, a number of local pedicled flaps are available including: rectus abdominis, tensor fascia lata, gracilis, sartorius, vastus medialis, and vastus lateralis. When suitable local tissue is not available or composite tissue is needed, free tissue transfer should be considered.

Knee and proximal third of leg

Traumatic defects or exposure of orthopaedic metalwork following wound dehiscence in this region frequently require flap cover. Choices for coverage include proximally based fasciocutaneous flaps, local muscle flaps, and free tissue transfer. The gastrocnemius muscle is the most useful source of cover in this area. Based on proximal pedicles, the medial or lateral head of this muscle can be harvested for cover of medium sized defects from the proximal patella as far caudal as the junction of the upper and middle thirds of the tibia. Functional morbidity is minimal and split skin grafting of the muscle produces good surface contour.

Middle third of leg

Defects in the middle third of the leg can be covered with a soleus muscle flap. Based proximally, muscle vascularity is reliable to a point 5cm above its tendinous insertion. No functional deficit is noted following transfer although the long term effects on the

Box 12.8.7 Lower limb

- Need intact vascular supply and tibial nerve integrity
- Groin/upper thigh SSG or local flap
- Knee and upper leg—gastrocnemius local flap
- Middle third of lower leg soleus flap
- Distal lower leg and ankle fasciocutaneous flaps or free graft.

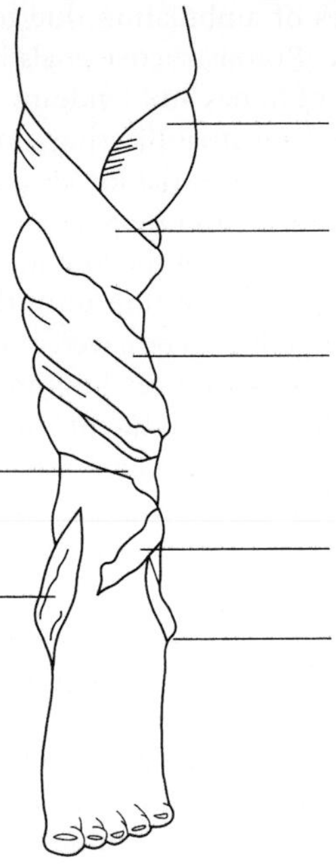

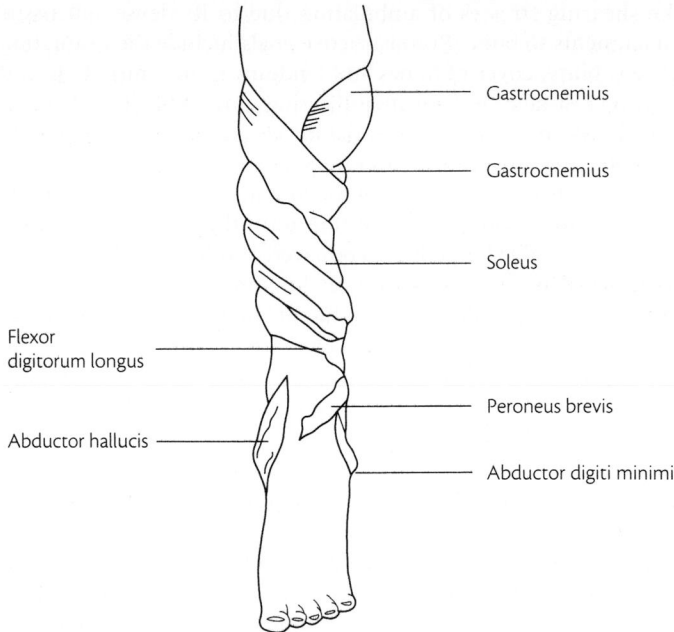

Fig. 12.8.3 Options for soft tissue cover in the lower limb.

venous pump mechanism have not been reported. High energy injuries with comminuted tibial fractures can result in soleus laceration and contusion excluding its use. In these cases, free tissue transfer of muscle from outside the zone of injury is indicated. For coverage of smaller defects the tibialis anterior muscle can be split longitudinally and flipped through 180 degrees to cover the tibial shaft. This technique preserves the innervation to the muscle and there is no functional deficit.

Distal third of leg and ankle

Defects in the distal third of the leg cannot easily be replaced with skin grafts as muscle cover is limited. Choices for cover include fasciocutaneous and free flaps. The axis of rotation of distally based fasciocutaneous flaps is designed with the base including one of two vascular perforators located 6cm and 12cm superior to the medial malleolus. These can be identified preoperatively using handheld Doppler. Fasciocutaneous flaps cannot be used when there has been extensive degloving as perforators will have been avulsed. Under such circumstances, in infected wounds, or where there is segmental bone loss, a free muscle transfer with a split skin graft is more appropriate.

Foot (Box 12.8.8)

Soft tissue cover in the foot can present a challenging prospect to the reconstructive surgeon with different requirements for dorsal and plantar surfaces. Dorsal skin is thin and pliable and provides a smooth undersurface to allow for tendon gliding whereas the weight bearing plantar skin is glabrous and able to withstand

Box 12.8.8 Foot

- Sensation important
- Dorsum—local or free fasciocutaneous flaps
- Plantar—local transposition or simple skin graft
- Free flap may be required in severe plantar injury.

the shearing stresses of ambulation due to its dense soft tissue attachments to bone. Reconstructive goals include the restoration of sensibility, cover of bones and tendons, to minimize bulk and provide resistance to tangential shearing movement. The ability to perceive deep pressure is essential for weight bearing, ambulation and long-term stability of coverage.

Skin grafts on the dorsum of the foot are susceptible to trauma from footwear and need protection until they are mature. Small defects unsuitable for grafts can be covered by local fasciocutaneous or muscle flaps (dorsalis pedis, lateral calcaneal, extensor digitorum brevis, abductor hallucis, or abductor digiti minimi). For more extensive defects, free fascial transfers (lateral arm, radial forearm, or temporalis) can be used with a skin graft. Free fascial flaps lack bulk and produce an excellent contour to the dorsum of the foot while permitting tendon gliding. Free fasciocutaneous or muscle flaps should be used for contaminated wounds or deeper defects.

The specialized plantar skin is best replaced with like tissue. Heel or forefoot defects with an adequate pad of subcutaneous tissue do well with a split or full thickness graft. Delayed application of skin grafts can reduce the severity of hyperkeratosis seen at the junction of plantar skin and skin graft. In wounds where the subcutaneous padding has been lost, the non-weight bearing skin of the medial instep can often be used for transposition to adjacent weight-bearing areas, i.e. lateral instep and heel. Axial flaps such as the medial plantar artery instep flap are useful for heel cover as they contain cutaneous nerves and are sensate. The toe fillet flap provides the best cover for forefoot defects with innervated skin, and minimal donor site morbidity. If the medial and lateral plantar nerves are intact, deep pressure sensation will be preserved offering protection from pressure necrosis to free flap cover. Muscle flaps, e.g. latissimus dorsi, provide bulk for padding of bony prominences and ambulation will be restored in most cases with appropriate rehabilitation. Rehabilitation of these patients is especially important with provision of custom-made shoes and instruction on foot care.

Chronic osteomyelitis (Box 12.8.9)

Chronic osteomyelitis has been defined as 'one or more foci in bone that contain pus, infected granulation tissue, sequestra, a draining sinus and resistant cellulites'. Treatment involves radical debridement of all devascularized bone, poorly vascularized soft tissue, and infected granulations. The wound is then left to heal by secondary intention, skin grafted, or covered with a flap. In cases where there is segmental bone loss skeletal reconstruction should be delayed and closure is best accomplished using free or pedicled muscle flaps. Reconstructive options once primary healing has occurred depend on the size of the defect and include: cancellous bone grafting; the use of vascularized iliac crest or fibula grafts; and the use of bone transport techniques.

Indications for amputation

The decision to amputate is made on a case by case basis, considering the injured extremity, the patient's age, associated injuries, and socioeconomic situation. While recovery and rehabilitation following complex lower limb reconstruction can often be a lengthy process, amputation often hastens recovery and return to work and with a suitable prosthesis can often provide a functional extremity. Disruption of the posterior tibial nerve is generally considered an indication for amputation because of the importance of plantar sensibility. Amputation should also be considered in massive degloving injuries of the foot as reconstruction will not recreate a normal foot.

Box 12.8.9 Osteomyelitis

- Radical debridement
- Then healing by secondary intention/SSG/free flap.

Results and complications

Valid comparisons of the results of soft tissue cover are difficult to make for the following reasons:

- There has been a lack of uniformity in the description of the soft tissue injuries
- Associated fractures have not been specified
- Criteria for wound closure have not been completely documented
- There has been variation in timing of cover in different published series.

Fasciocutaneous flaps provide reliable soft tissue cover in the extremities with a reported 97% success rate, as measured by wound healing and limb preservation. Free tissue transfer for cover of Gustillo grade III lower limb injuries has resulted in limb salvage rates of greater than 90%. In all series the highest success rate with the least complications occurred when patients were treated in the acute period. A major factor in obtaining better outcomes was the surgeon's learning curve with results improving with experience.

Long-term follow-up of 72 patients with Gustilo grade IIIB open fractures treated with free tissue transfer revealed a limb salvage rate of 93%, with 96% patient satisfaction. However, only 28% of these patients returned to long-term employment within 2 years in contrast to 68% of patients who underwent amputation for lower extremity trauma during the same period. This puts into perspective the fact that despite the technical ability to achieve salvage in a severely injured limb the surgeon must bear in mind the long-term goals of occupational rehabilitation before selecting patients for this treatment.

Further reading

Francel, T.J., Vander Kolk, C.A., Hoopes, J.E., Manson, P.N., and Yaremchuk, M.D. (1992). Microvascular soft tissue transplantation for reconstruction of acute open tibial fractures: timing of coverage and long- term functional results. *Plastic and Reconstructive Surgery*, **89**, 478–87.

Fix, R.J. and Vasconez, L.O. (1991). Fasciocutaneous flaps in the reconstruction of the lower extremity. *Clinics in Plastic Surgery*, **18**, 571–82.

Godina, M. (1986). Early microsurgical reconstruction of complex trauma of the extremities. *Clinics in Plastic Surgery*, **13**, 619–20.

Hallock, G.G. (1991). Complications of 100 consecutive local fasciocutaneous flaps. *Plastic and Reconstructive Surgery*, **88**, 264–8.

Moore, J.R. and Weiland, A.J. (1986). Vascularized tissue transfer in the treatment of osteomyelitis. *Clinics in Plastic Surgery*, **13**, 657–62.

Nanchahal, J., Nayagam, D., Khan, U., *et al.* (2009). Standards for the Management of Open Fractures of the Lower Limb. Royal Society of Medicine Press, London. http://www.bapras.org.uk/guide.asp?id=355#guide_278

12.9

Combined vascular and orthopaedic injuries

E. Chaloner

Summary points

- Early diagnosis of an arterial injury is critical in reducing the risk of limb loss
- Don't assume that missing pulses are due to arterial 'spasm'
- Don't assume that presence of distal pulses rules out a proximal vascular injury – arterial intimal tears can occlude the vessel many hours after the initial injury
- After an arterial repair has been completed there is still a risk of subsequent compartment syndrome from reperfusion
- Arterial shunts can procure some time for skeletal fixation prior to definitive arterial repair or grafting.

Introduction

Severe fractures and dislocations commonly cause injury to adjacent vascular structures. Certain patterns of injury such as femoral shaft fractures injuring the superficial femoral artery, popliteal artery injury after knee dislocation, and brachial artery injury after supracondylar fracture of the humerus are frequent because of the close anatomical relationship between certain blood vessels and bones or joints.

The major determinant of outcome following arterial injury is the early recognition of the possibility of vascular damage and its prompt investigation. This can be difficult as some arterial injuries can be caused to the intima of the artery alone with no obvious external bleeding or haematoma. Initially the perfusion of the limb can appear to be normal (even pulses can be intact) with thrombosis of the artery occurring several hours after presentation of the patient. Frequent reassessment of the distal vasculature in patients with fracture patterns that often injure blood vessels is necessary to prevent late diagnosis and the risk of limb loss or loss of function.

Major veins can also be damaged either in tandem with an arterial injury or as an isolated event. Venous injury rarely requires operative intervention but does raise the risk of later deep vein thrombosis (DVT) and subsequent ongoing morbidity from post-thrombotic limb syndrome.

Mechanisms of vascular injury (Box 12.9.1)

Penetrating trauma

Penetrating injuries causing both vascular and orthopaedic injuries usually result from gunshot wounds. A low-energy transfer missile ordinarily damages a vessel lying directly in its path and bony injury may be no more than the equivalent of a 'drill hole' (Figure 12.9.1). On the other hand, a high-energy transfer wound with a bullet striking bone will have an impact velocity which shatters bone into fragments producing secondary missiles which cause further injury (Figure 12.9.2). A cluster of pellets from a shotgun fired at close range will produce a concentrated 'spread' causing large defects in soft tissue and severe comminution of bone, as well as contamination from the wadding and clothing, features which are often underestimated on superficial inspection. The vascular and bony injuries caused by shrapnel and secondary missiles in bomb explosions may be further complicated by crush injury from falling masonry.

Blunt trauma

The severity of vascular injury resulting from blunt trauma—as observed following sudden deceleration in road traffic collisions, in falls, and in rail, air, and mining disasters—often exceeds that caused by penetrating agents. The shearing forces generated by violent angulation of fractures may cause sharp bony fragments to

Box 12.9.1 Mechanism of vascular injury

- Penetrating:
  - Low velocity—vessel directly in path
  - High velocity—injury may occur from secondary fragmentation or cavitation
- Blunt—shear forces resulting from:
  - Dislocations
  - Fractures.

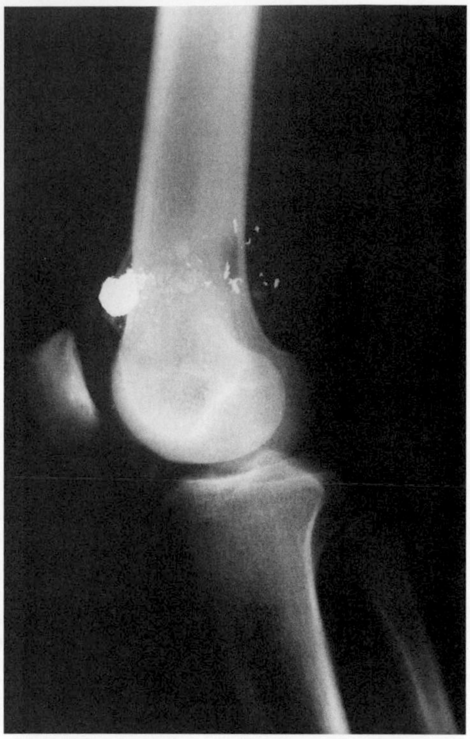

Fig. 12.9.1 Bullet created a 'drill hole' in lower femur, fracturing the anterior cortex, leaving the bone essentially intact, and transecting popliteal artery and veins. Reproduced from Barros D'Sa (1992).

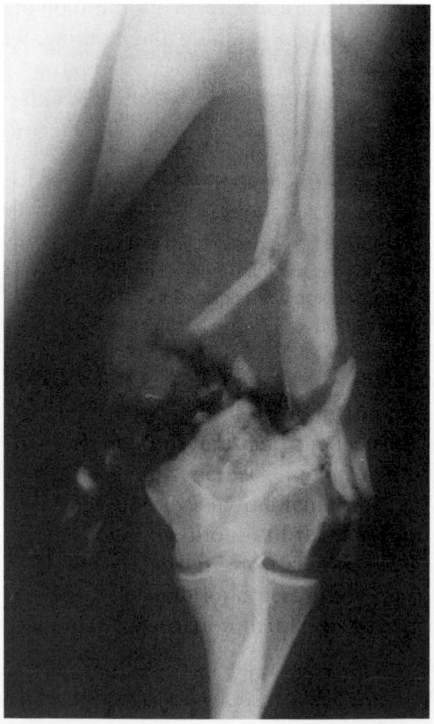

Fig. 12.9.2 High-velocity missile injury: gross comminution of humerus, transection of brachial artery and ulnar nerve. Reproduced from Barros D'Sa (1992).

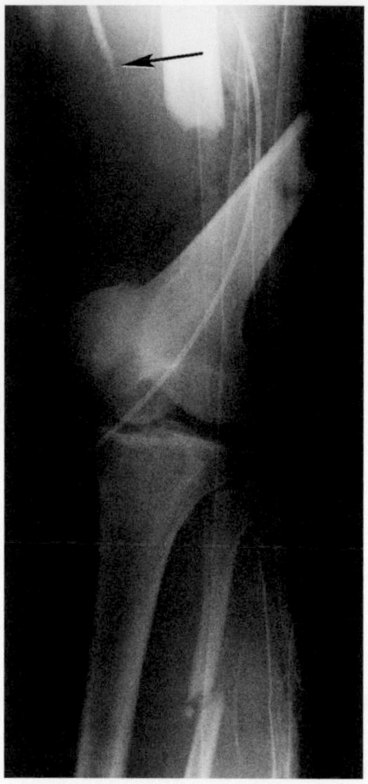

Fig. 12.9.3 Angiogram in a multiply fractured leg following a road accident showing injury at the femoropopliteal arterial segment.

lacerate or sever adjacent vessels (Figure 12.9.3) and indirectly stretch vessel segments at points of relative fixity, causing thrombosis. In posterior dislocations of the knee, the avulsive forces involved may result in tearing of tissues and in the process the layers of the popliteal artery, beginning with the intima, disrupt progressively. The dislocated knee has a tendency to reduce spontaneously, and notoriously the vascular injury may remain unsuspected and unrecognized on examination. In such cases, damage to the collateral system around the knee joint heightens the effects of ischaemia caused by popliteal artery injury. Fractures of the tibia associated with dislocation of the knee carry a vascular injury rate approaching 40% with a high risk of subsequent amputation if the injury is not recognized immediately.

In severe type IIIc open tibial fractures a constellation of factors inevitably combine to thwart success and are responsible for quite high amputation rates. In these cases, not only is there comminution of the fracture with bone defects and periosteal stripping but also severe muscle and skin loss, nerve trauma, and contamination compounded by injury to long segments of popliteal and crural vessels as well as collateral systems.

All these features may be found in blunt arterial trauma of the upper limb. In axillary vessel traction injuries the brachial plexus is also commonly affected.

Morphology of vascular injury (Box 12.9.2)

A variety of vascular injuries may occur in association with fractures and dislocations. These may be injuries in continuity, partial tears, or complete tears. True traumatic spasm is quite rare and ought not to be presumed, with at least some intimal damage present in most instances of 'spasm', in some cases permitting flow

Box 12.9.2 Injury morphology

- Partial lacerations more commonly result in exsanguination
- Complete division allows retraction and thrombosis
- Blunt venous injuries are difficult to repair
- Elderly arteriopaths are most vulnerable to complications.

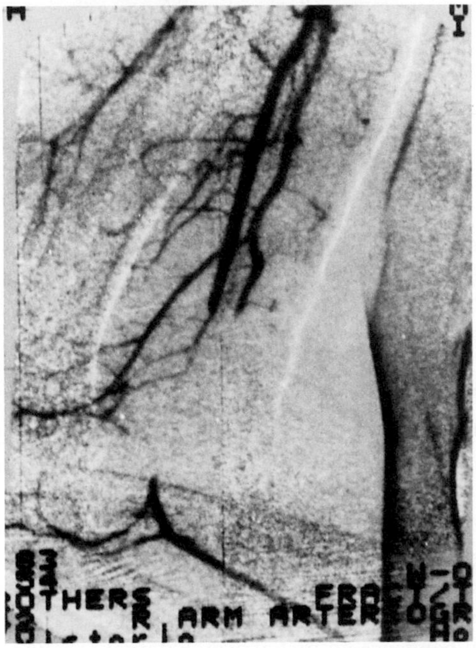

Fig. 12.9.4 Dislocation of left elbow, rupture of biceps and brachialis muscles, and traction injury and thrombosis of brachial artery causing severe ischaemia relieved by excision and vein graft replacement. Reproduced from Barros D'Sa (1992).

transiently before progressing to thrombotic occlusion (Figure 12.9.4). An intimal fracture may develop into an intimal flap, which in turn may lead to dissection and intramural bleeding, and in cases where the intimal tear is circumferential, thrombosis is common. The key message for the orthopaedic clinician is never to assume that loss of a pulse distal to a major fracture is due to 'arterial spasm', nor to assume that if a pulse is present on initial presentation that vascular damage is completely ruled out.

A lacerated artery, is usually unable to contract and in open injuries may cause rapid exsanguination. If it seals, a false aneurysm may develop which may present with later rupture (Figures 12.9.5 and 12.9.6). Concomitant injury to the adjacent artery and vein may produce an arteriovenous fistula (Figure 12.9.7), with or without an adjacent false aneurysm. On occasions fistulae can compromise flow to a limb; or in the long-term a proximal fistula may provoke a high-output cardiac state.

When a vessel is completely transected by a missile or a shard of metal, the free ends tend to constrict, retract, and become sealed by a plug of thrombus. This process is also seen in traction injuries, such as posterior dislocations of the knee, in which the avulsive forces stretch the intima until it fractures and curls back on itself, the media and adventitia disrupt, the ends constrict, and

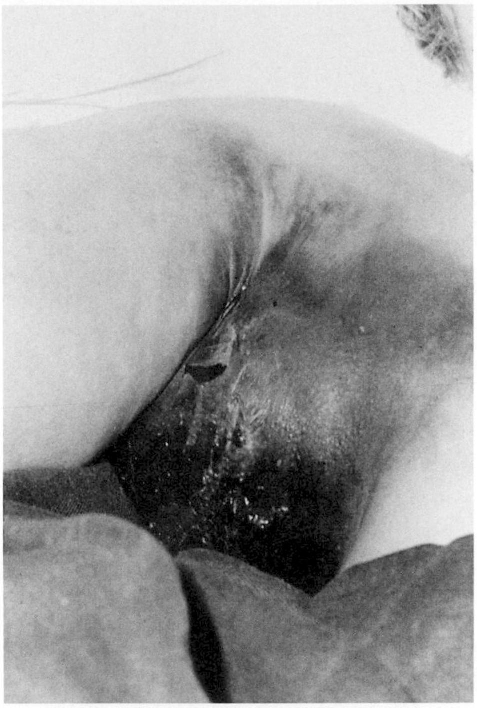

Fig. 12.9.5 Dislocated right shoulder: tear in the axillary artery resulting in a false aneurysm which ruptured producing massive axillary haematoma. Reproduced from Barros D'Sa (1992).

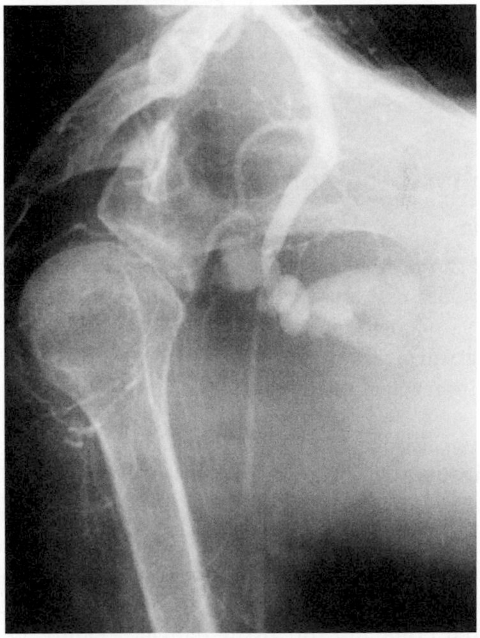

Fig. 12.9.6 Angiogram of the patient in Figure 12.8.5 showing the multiloculated cavity of a false aneurysm surrounded by clot. Distal vessel attenuated by both limited inflow and extrinsic pressure from haematoma. Reproduced from Barros D'Sa (1992).

thrombosis ensues. This does not occur in partial lacerations and can be associated with greater blood loss.

Venous injuries generally remain unrecognized until surgical exposure of an arterial injury. Those vein injuries sustained in blunt trauma do not easily lend themselves to repair.

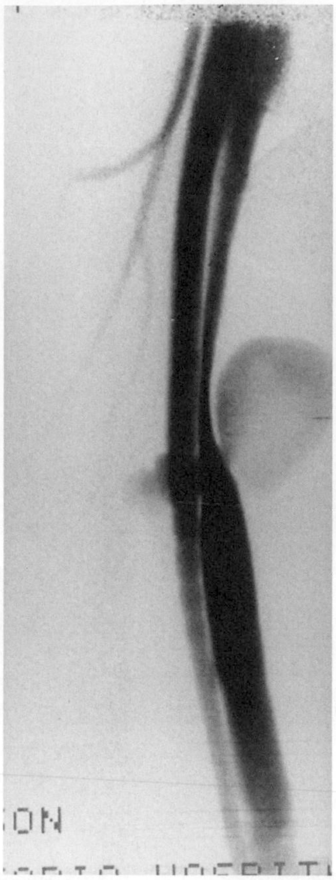

Fig. 12.9.7 Digital angiogram showing an arteriovenous fistula of the upper femoral vessels with associated false aneurysms. Reproduced from Barros D'Sa (1997).

Pathophysiology of vascular injury

Ischaemia

Arrest of arterial flow causes tissue hypoperfusion and hypoxia which, in some cases, is further compounded by hypovolaemic shock and vasoconstriction. Striated muscle has a low tolerance for continuing warm ischaemia and after 6–8h, depending on the degree of injury and availability of collateral flow, muscle death occurs.

Ischaemia–reperfusion

The restoration of blood flow after a period of ischaemia may cause the complex biochemical and cellular pathophysiological changes of ischaemia–reperfusion injury. Clamping or ligation of an adjacent injured main vein aggravates this process, as will the presence of associated bone and soft tissue damage (Figure 12.9.8). The extent of ischaemia–reperfusion injury is directly proportional to the severity and duration of striated muscle ischaemia. Ischaemia–reperfusion injury of a large mass of skeletal muscle has systemic implications, provoking multiple organ failure. An unrelieved rise in pressure may result in the development of compartment syndrome and ischaemic nerve damage. Again, the key point for the clinicians is not to assume that once the vascular reconstruction has been completed that everything will be fine—there is still the possibility of complications developing—particularly compartment syndrome and DVT.

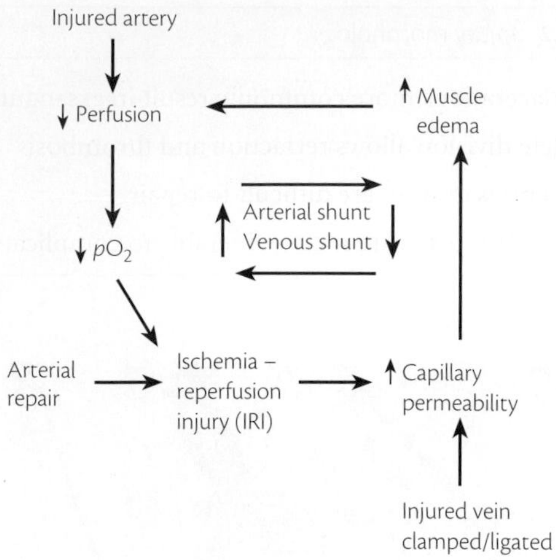

Fig. 12.9.8 Diagram showing the pathophysiological sequelae of arterial injury and repair, and the influence of ligating a concomitantly injured vein. The beneficial effect of adjuvant early arterial and venous shunting in countering that process is illustrated.

Management

Initial measures

In the multiply injured patient, resuscitative measures are taken to ensure an adequate airway, satisfactory ventilation, and correction of hypovolaemic shock. In many cases the orthopaedic team may be leading a resuscitation team and will therefore need to manage arterial or venous injuries in the acute phase until a vascular surgeon arrives. Many of these complex limb injuries are obscured by splints and bandages on first arrival. External bleeding should be controlled digitally and then by means of a pad and bandage. If arterial forceps or clamps are applied incorrectly they are likely to damage both vessels and nerves in the vicinity. Tourniquets tend to be poorly applied, often in a manner which accelerates the rate of bleeding, and if left unreleased will cause irreversible tissue and nerve damage. Information from bystanders as to the nature of the wounding agent, the amount of blood lost, and the time interval since injury will help in further decision making. Tetanus toxoid, prophylactic antibiotics, as well as appropriate analgesia, should be routinely administered.

Diagnosis and assessment (Box 12.9.3)

Clinical

A number of questions have to be answered in assessing the location, degree, and extent of vascular injury accompanying orthopaedic trauma:

- If bleeding is continuous, is it clearly arterial or venous, or of both types?
- If a haematoma is present, is it expanding or pulsatile?
- Is there evidence of a thrill or audible bruit indicative of arterial compression or arteriovenous fistula?
- Are there identifiable 'hard' signs of ischaemia, namely absent distal pulses, mottling, pallor, coolness, and numbness?
- If there are not, are 'soft' signs detectable, namely transient ischaemia, mild neurological deficit, or a small nonexpanding

Box 12.9.3 Diagnosis

- Clinical:
  - Bleeding, haematoma, bruits
  - Absent pulses, ischaemia, and failure to recover following reduction
- Investigation:
  - Ankle–brachial index (indicates need for angiography if <0.9)
  - Duplex scans
  - Angiography
  - Standard
  - One shot on table
  - Computed tomography (CT)/magnetic resonance imaging (MRI).

haematoma? The deficit caused by coincidental nerve injury cannot be evaluated with certainty in cases of profound ischaemia

- When signs of arterial injury are obscured in the shocked multiply injured patient, does circulatory recovery in the fractured limb lag behind its partner following resuscitation?
- Does reduction of the fracture or dislocation fail to restore distal flow?
- Even in the absence of signs of bleeding within the tissues around the knee, is there any evidence that a dislocated knee has reduced spontaneously and, if so, is there incontrovertible evidence that arterial injury is not present?

If the answers to these questions are neither clear nor unequivocal, further investigation is required.

Ultrasound

Doppler ultrasound pulse waveforms, segmental pressures, and ankle–brachial pressure indices may provide an early assessment of the presence of vascular injuries particularly in cases of blunt trauma, but should not be relied upon to definitively exclude injuries. In open injuries ultrasound is usually impractical.

Angiography

Angiography either delineates an arterial injury or excludes its presence (Figures 12.9.9 and 12.9.10). In the latter case it gives the surgeon the confidence not to intervene, preventing unnecessary exploration). When clinical signs are equivocal, angiography is advisable. The medico-legal consequences of missing an arterial injury leading to subsequent limb loss are obvious. Angiography is of particular importance in blunt injuries which cause instability or dislocation of the knee, sometimes in association with displacement of a fracture close to the knee. Even when distal pulses are palpable, the chance of an occult arterial injury going on to occlusion and loss of the limb remains, and therefore this condition demands a policy of routine angiography.

If angiography is likely to be delayed and an arterial injury is suspected clinically, it may be preferable to take the patient to the operating room and perform a one-shot single-plate on-table angiogram followed by urgent repair of the arterial injury. Timely angiography may also prevent disaster in cases of persistent ischaemia after reduction of a fracture, especially in the elderly atherosclerotic patient. Many hospitals now have facilities for CT or MRI angiography. The advantage of these modalities is that, particularly CT angiography, may be obtained quickly and allow for some visualization of the bone and surrounding soft tissue. If clinical doubt exists despite imaging that does not show an injury then meticulous and repeated clinical examination should be performed and, if necessary, surgical exploration to resolve any doubt of arterial injury.

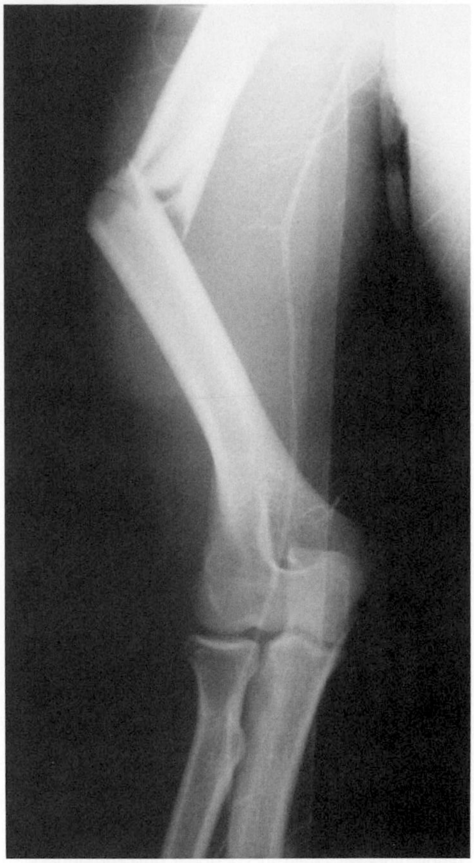

Fig. 12.9.9 Angiogram reveals some spasm in an otherwise intact brachial artery in relation to a midhumeral fracture.

The critical importance of time

In injuries involving fractures and vascular trauma it is important to abbreviate the period of ischaemia and minimize ischaemia–reperfusion injury following arterial repair. Control of bleeding, resuscitation, and surgical treatment should be overlapping rather than sequential stages of management. Life-threatening injuries of the head, chest, and abdomen naturally deserve priority, but delay in dealing with limb vessel trauma may result in a poor outcome. Even if the complex vascular injury is isolated to a leg, surgical intervention still requires adequate time for exposure, wound care, bone fixation, and repair of artery and vein.

Time pressure, should not progress to rushed surgical practice. Wound care and cleaning should be performed correctly and all

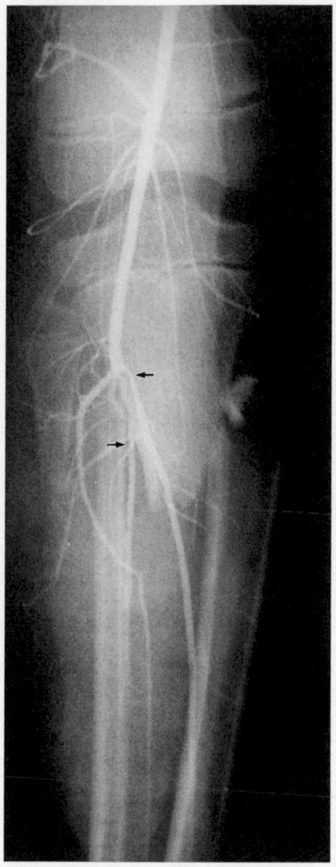

Fig. 12.9.10 Blunt injury with fractures of upper tibia and fibula with consequent distortion and spasm of the anterior tibial artery, high-grade stenosis of the tibioperoneal trunk (upper arrow), virtual occlusion of peroneal artery at its origin (lower arrow), and a patent posterior tibial artery. Reproduced from Barros D'Sa (1992).

repairs, be that of the vessels or damaged bones carried out meticulously. Stabilization of a fracture prior to repair of injured vessels deserves consideration. Some of the pain is relieved, movement of loose bone fragments ceases to injure the vessels and soft tissues, optimal lengths of graft are used to repair the vessels, and confidence is instilled by the knowledge that artery and vein repair will remain secure from disruption. However, this sequence of surgical action delays restoration of flow and correspondingly has an impact on the degree of ischaemia–reperfusion injury.

This time pressure may be relieved by using shunts for both artery and vein on exploration of the wound. The arterial shunt restores perfusion, minimizes ischaemia–reperfusion injury, and reduces compartment pressure. The venous shunt re-establishes drainage and further helps to prevent a rise in compartment pressure.

Initial operative steps

Standard longitudinal incisions are employed for access to vessels of the upper and lower limb. A posterior gentle S-shaped incisional approach to the midpopliteal artery is acceptable in some penetrating injuries. In the case of blunt trauma associated with instability of the knee, a medial approach, accepting some compromise to the integrity of the knee, is preferable. The injured vessel is controlled first by digital pressure and then by suitable vascular clamps applied to segments exposed on either side of an artery and vein injury. The damaged vessel must be adequately excised to leave pristine ends for suture. The proximal artery is released to flush out thrombus and a balloon catheter is used to retrieve clot from the distal vessel, a process which can be assisted by milking the limb upwards, especially when surgery is delayed. Heparinized saline (20IU/mL) is then perfused into the distal limb.

Operative discipline centred around shunting

Arterial and venous shunting

An indwelling shunt in a transected femoral or popliteal artery (Figure 2.9.11) immediately restores flow, buying valuable time for precise operative work. An outlying shunt should be considered for an extensive wound within which lengthy segments of vessel have been destroyed (Figure 2.9.12). An indwelling venous shunt in a severed adjacent vein (Figure 12.9.11) re-establishes venous drainage and will also discourage thrombosis. If the vein is simply clamped, an acute and unacceptable rise in compartment pressure will occur, invariably necessitating fasciotomy. In some multiply injured patients, the vascular surgeon, working alongside other

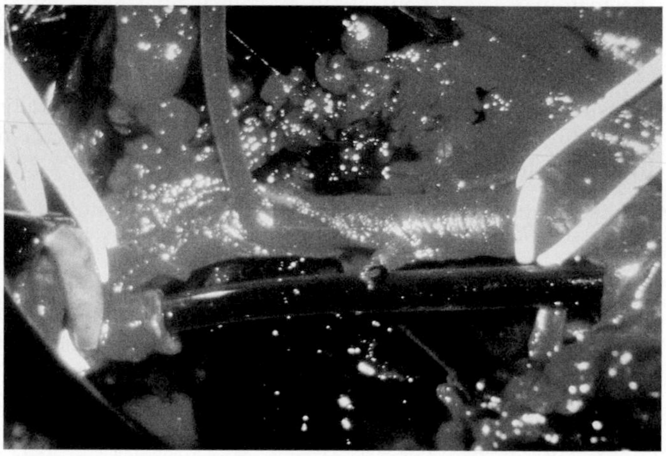

Fig. 12.9.11 Intravascular shunts: Brener shunt in torn popliteal artery (above) and Javid shunt in transected popliteal vein (below) preparatory to vein graft replacement of each vessel. (Reproduced from Barros D'sa (1988).)

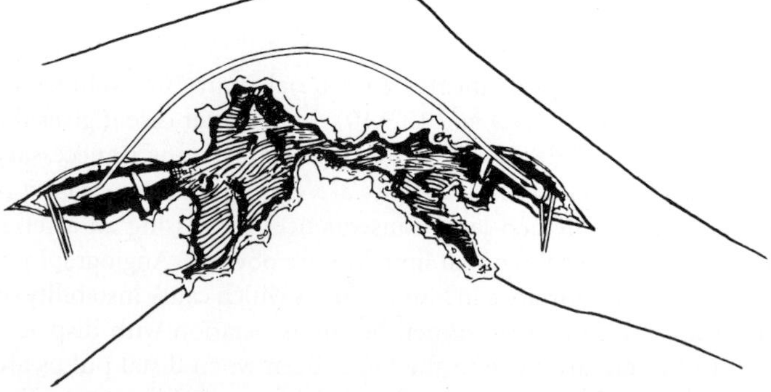

Fig. 12.9.12 In extensive injury an outlying shunt picks up flow proximal to the injured segment and revitalizes the limb distally. Reproduced from Barros D'Sa, A.A.B. and Moorehead, R.J. (1989). The rationale for arterial and venous shunting in the management of limb vascular injuries. *European Journal of Vascular Surgery*, **3**, 577–81.

specialists involved in life-saving surgery in the head or torso, may be able to place shunts in vessels in wounds of a lower limb, assuring its survival until definitive vascular repair some time later. A range of shunts are available and the surgeon should choose one which with they are familiar.

Wound care

The placement of shunts allows for ample time to survey the wound, identify nerve injury, remove debris, and irrigate the tissues. Restored arterial and venous flow provides sharper and more reliable demarcation between dead and viable tissue. Meticulous excision of nonviable tissues and debridement is especially essential in high-energy injuries. Free bone fragments and foreign bodies are removed, followed by copious irrigation, particularly in open contaminated wounds, a process which is of value in significantly lowering the concentration of the bacterial inoculum.

In the critically injured but neurologically intact limb (Figure 12.9.13A) restoration of flow by means of shunts (Figure 12.9.13B) will assist the surgeon in coming to a decision as to whether primary amputation may be more sensible than an attempt at major reconstruction.

Bone fixation

The use of long intravascular shunts in artery and vein (Figure 12.9.13B) will provide the necessary slack for the liberal manipulation of the bone fragments. At this stage the orthopaedic surgeon

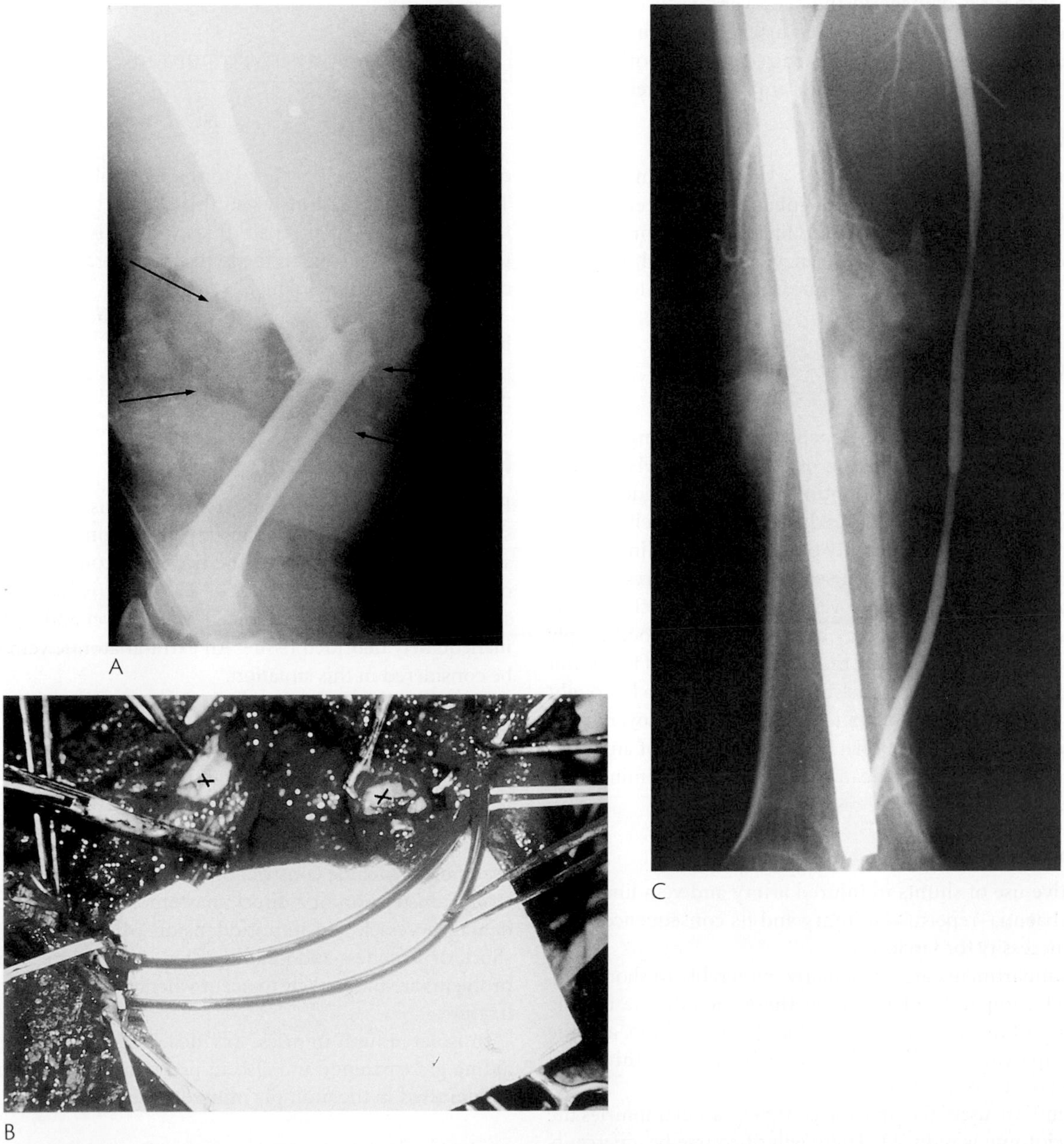

Fig. 12.9.13 A) Radiograph showing virtual dismemberment at mid-femoral level. Gap in soft tissues between arrows. B) Javid shunt bridging lengthy gap in femoral artery and perfusing distal limb; another shunt bridging adjoining femoral vein and draining the limb. Ends of a fractured femur (XX) being manipulated prior to fixation. (A) and (B) Reproduced from Barros D'Sa, A.A.B. and Moorehead, R.J. (1989). The rationale for arterial and venous shunting in the management of limb vascular injuries. *European Journal of Vascular Surgery*, **3**, 577–81. C) Angiogram many years later showing a healed fracture, an intramedullary nail, and a patent graft.

proceeds to restore skeletal integrity. He is under no pressure to compromise technique and will be guided solely by a desire to achieve the best possible orthopaedic outcome.

Arterial repair

Minor arterial injuries identified preoperatively may be amenable to treatment by endovascular means allowing the orthopaedic surgeons to proceed with bone stabilization in the presence of treated vascular injuries. Most injuries will not be suitable for endovascular repair in the trauma environment and will require open surgical repair. A variety of techniques may be employed by the vascular surgeon with the guiding principle of restoring both arterial and venous integrity in as many cases as possible. In lower limb injuries vein for repair should be harvested from the contralateral limb, particularly if there is damage to the deep venous system of the affected limb. If concomitantly injured artery and vein have not been shunted, the artery should be repaired first. If both vessels have been shunted, the order of repair is entirely immaterial.

Box 12.9.4 Treatment order

- Control bleeding
- Excise injured vessel
- Remove clot
- Heparinized saline
- Shunt
- Debride and washout wound
- Fracture stabilization/fixation
- Arterial repair
- Venous repair
- Soft tissue cover
- If fasciotomy necessary, perform early.

Vein repair

It is worth remembering that repair of a damaged vein not only renews free venous drainage but also enhances the patency of an adjacent arterial repair. Moreover, the likelihood of thrombosis, oedema, and chronic venous insufficiency is minimized. In a very small number of cases the development of limb-threatening venous gangrene is averted.

Wound closure

Vessel cover

The success of a vascular repair is dependent on achieving satisfactory vessel cover and the elimination of dead space by viable adjacent soft tissue and muscle. As shunting will have provided ample time for proper wound care at an earlier stage, some reliance can be placed on the quality and viability of tissue surrounding a completed vascular repair. If adequate soft tissue is not preserved to enable the repaired vessels to be covered then a superficial muscle such as the sartorius or gracilis may be freed with its blood supply intact and swung over to ensheath the repaired vessels. If that is not possible, then the skills of a plastic surgeon may have to be sought and free vascularized musculocutaneous flaps used to cover artery and vein repair and exposed bone. The construction of an extra-anatomic vein bypass through clean viable tissue may eliminate the need for these measures in some cases.

Fasciotomy

The adjunctive use of shunts in injured artery and vein limits the extent of ischaemia–reperfusion injury and its consequences, and reduces the necessity for fasciotomy.

Certain compartments are particularly vulnerable to short periods of raised compartment pressure; these include the muscle compartments of the forearm and hand in the upper limb, and the anterior compartment in the lower leg which lies within rigid osseous and fascial boundaries.

When shunts are used in managing complex vascular injuries the need for fasciotomy is reduced. There will of course be a percentage of patients who will require fasciotomy even when shunts have been used. If restoration of blood flow is delayed or fasciotomies are deemed necessary, then the procedure should be performed early as this will be beneficial to the residual collateral circulation. There may be occasions when this should be considered prior to the definitive vascular repair. If fasciotomy is delayed and tissue of tenuous viability (due to the ischaemia or trauma) is exposed, the chances of infection are high.

The clinician must repeatedly evaluate the need for fasciotomy before, during and after the vascular repair. Assessment should be based on clinical findings and, where necessary, compartment pressure monitoring.

Postoperative care

Early haemorrhage after surgery usually arises from debrided tissues or from a gap in vascular repair. Thrombotic occlusion and secondary haemorrhage are the two most common complications of vascular repair (Box 12.9.5). The latter is likely to occur as a sequel to a scenario of insufficient vessel cover and infection within inadequately debrided tissue. An extra-anatomic vein graft should be considered in this situation.

Close monitoring of pulses, Doppler ultrasound pulse waveforms, and pressures will provide warning of deterioration in arterial flow. Vigilance is required in anticipating complete thrombotic occlusion of a vessel repair. If flow is impaired and graft failure is suspected, angiography must be undertaken urgently and the vascular repair revised. The defects which can be expected to lead to graft failure include constriction at the site of lateral suture, purse-string constriction of a direct anastomosis, inadequate excision of damaged vessel, anastomotic tension when the vein graft is too short, or slackness and kinking when it is too long. These last two problems are more likely to occur when vessel repair precedes bone fixation.

In isolated limb injuries, low-dose heparin may be of value in aiding graft patency and also in preventing DVT. It may be contraindicated in the multiply injured patient.

Summary

The challenge of combined vascular and orthopaedic injury must be faced in the knowledge that a number of complications

Box 12.9.5 Postoperative problems

- Early haemorrhage
- Secondary haemorrhage
- Thrombotic occlusion:
  - Inadequate debridement of injured vessel
  - Stenosis:
    —Suture line
    —Graft too short
    —Graft kinked.

including amputation may occur, but these can be minimized by prompt intervention. Diverse factors play a role in achieving good results, namely early recognition of arterial injury, if necessary defined by angiography, a methodical approach to operative technique, often best formulated around the use of indwelling shunts in both injured artery and vein, diligent care of the wound, stabilization of bone before vascular repair, liberal use of interposition vein grafts including compound vein grafts of suitable calibre when necessary, timely and effective fasciotomy, and a willingness to revise repair in the event of failure.

Further reading

Ashwood, N. and Chaloner, E.J. (2003). Managing vascular impairment following orthopaedic injury. *Hospital Doctor*, **64**, 530–4.

Barros D'Sa, A.A.B. and Moorehead, R.J. (1989). The rationale for arterial and venous shunting in the management of limb vascular injuries. *European Journal of Vascular Surgery*, **3**, 577–81.

Huynh, T.T., Pham, M., Griffin, L.W., *et al.* (2006). Management of distal femoral and popliteal arterial injuries: an update. *American Journal of Surgery*, **192**(6), 773–8.

Korompilias, A.V., Beris, A.E., Lykissas, M.G., Vekris, M.D., Kontogeorgakos, V.A., and Soucacos, P.N. (2009). The mangled extremity and attempt for limb salvage. *Journal of Orthopedic Surgery and Research* , **4**, 4.

Fowler, J., Macintyre, N., Rehman, S., Gaughan, J.P., and Leslie, S. (2009). The importance of surgical sequence in the treatment of lower extremity injuries with concomitant vascular injury: A meta-analysis. *Injury*, **40**(1), 72–6.

Patterson, B.M., Agel, J., Swiontkowski, M.F., Mackenzie, E.J., Bosse, M.J.; LEAP Study Group. (2007). Knee dislocations with vascular injury: outcomes in the Lower Extremity Assessment Project (LEAP) Study. *Journal of Trauma*, **63**(4), 855–8.

12.10

Limb salvage versus amputation

Gregory M. Georgiadis

Summary points

- The decision to attempt limb salvage or amputate is difficult and depends on many factors
- Scoring systems provide guidelines only and not absolute treatment mandates
- Severe limb trauma results in a high degree of self reported disability regardless of treatment
- These injuries are best managed by a multidisciplinary approach.

Box 12.10.1 Leap project

- The Lower Extremity Assessment Project (LEAP) was a recent large prospective outcome study of patients with high-energy lower extremity trauma
- Patients were followed up to seven years
- Multiple published studies were generated.

Introduction

In the modern era there has been an increase in the incidence of severely traumatized extremities, often associated with open fracture and/or vascular injury. These injuries are now a leading cause of hospitalization among young adults. Most are due to motor vehicle related or industrial accidents or falls from heights. Military injuries are also increasing as well with recent conflicts in Iraq, Afghanistan, and other locations. With advances in surgical principles and techniques, many severely injured limbs that could previously be treated only by amputation can now be saved. However, these salvaged limbs are never normal. Almost all patients have some element of chronic pain. Others may have deformity, chronic infection, and many have a non-functional extremity or even require a late amputation. Financial, medical, social, and psychological problems due to prolonged and extensive treatments can also occur. Thus there is great interest in defining which injuries should have attempted limb salvage.

Recently the Lower Extremity Assessment Project (LEAP) completed a multicentre, prospective outcome study of 601 patients in the civilian population of the United States of America with high-energy lower extremity trauma (Box 12.10.1). This study group followed patients for as long as 7 years.

The severely damaged limb: defining the injury

The initial assessment of a severely injured extremity is based on a description and subsequent classification of the associated open wound. This is not an exact science, and clinical descriptions of open wounds may not always be accurate or reproducible. The Gustilo grading system is the most widely used method for describing open fractures in North America. However, studies have shown that the interobserver reliability of this system is only moderate, and that it alone may be inadequate for treatment decisions or comparison of published results.

The soft tissue injury is a key component of any high-energy extremity fractures (Box 12.10.2). However, the true nature and extent of the soft tissue injury after high-energy trauma is often not readily apparent from the outset. Frequently serial debridement over 2 or 3 days reveal the true extent of the injury (Figure 12.10.1). Despite the recognition that the nature and extent of the soft tissue injury has the greatest impact on the decision to attempt limb salvage or amputation, it still remains one of the most difficult aspects to reliably assess.

Surgeons can encounter lower extremities where the bone and soft tissues are so injured that the prognosis for salvage becomes questionable. The term 'mangled extremity' has been used to describe these limbs (Figure 12.10.2).

The mangled extremity is defined as one in which three of the four organ systems (skin, bone, vessels, muscle) have been severely injured. Further expansion of this definition is presented in Table 12.10.1.

The prototype for the mangled lower extremity is the Gustilo type III open tibia fracture. During treatment these injuries have numerous complications and problems. Rates of secondary amputation, deep infection, and non-union of 17%, 29%, and 43%, respectively, for grade IIIB open tibia fractures have been reported. For type IIIC injuries, these same figures increase to 78%, 57%, and 100%.

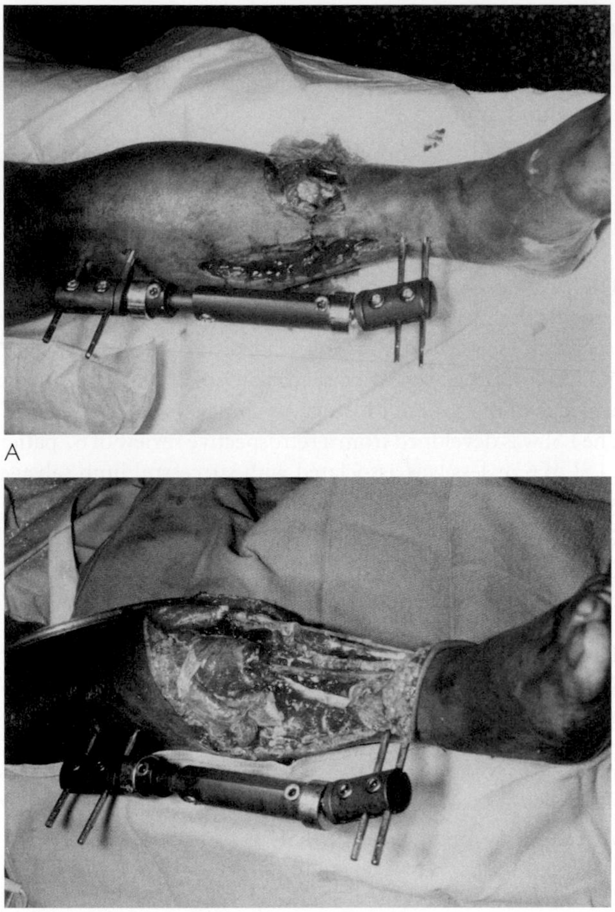

A

B

Fig. 12.10.1 A) Appearance of the open wounds after initial debridement and application of an external fixator. The leg was crushed between the bumpers of two cars. The true extent of the soft-tissue injury is not readily apparent. B) Appearance after serial debridements with removal of all devitalized tissue. The patient is left with large soft tissue and bone defects. The foot is viable, with intact pulses and plantar sensation. This patient chose below-knee amputation instead of attempts at limb salvage.

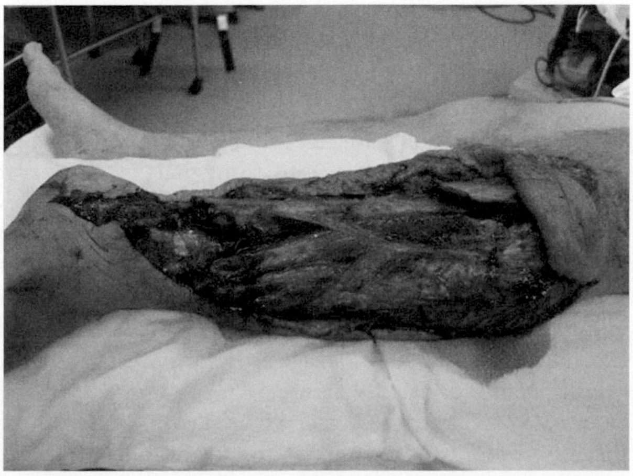

Fig. 12.10.2 Clinical appearance of a mangled extremity. This severe open, segmental open tibia and fibula fracture has extensive injury to skin, bone, vessels, and muscle.

Table 12.10.1 Definition of the mangled lower extremity

1	Severe injury to three of four major organ systems (skin, bone, nerve, vessel) in the same extremity
or	
2	Severe injury to two of four organ systems in an extremity, when the area of skin and muscle loss is greater than the circumference of the extremity and requires a free tissue transfer
or	
3	Severe injury to two, and minor injury to the other two, organ systems in an extremity, requiring surgical intervention
or	
4	Severe injury in two of four organ systems in an extremity, with greater than 5cm of bone loss and periosteal stripping

Reproduced from Bonanni *et al.* (1993). Journal of Trauma, **34**, 99–104.

Box 12.10.2 Soft tissue injury

- The soft tissue injury to the damaged extremity remains one of the most difficult aspects to reliably assess
- Gustilo grading system not reliable
- The true nature of the soft tissues may not be initially apparent.

Severe open tibia fracture with vascular injury requiring revascularization may be an indication for an early amputation. However, modern surgical techniques now allow many severely damaged limbs to be saved. For example a 93% salvage of type IIIC open fractures has been achieved in one study.

Indications for amputation after lower extremity fractures

In a patient with severe lower extremity trauma, the physician strives to restore the following:

- A painless leg
- Bony union
- No infection
- Equal limb lengths
- Protective sensation.

Frequently, however, in the mangled extremity all these goals cannot be attained. Prolonged warm ischaemia time, irreparable nerve injury resulting in an insensate limb, extensive crush injury, entrapment, limb avulsion or traumatic amputation, and multiple trauma with other life-threatening injuries are all indications for acute amputation (Box 12.10.3).

Extensive comminution and bone loss of more than 6–8cm, especially when combined with soft tissue loss, has also been considered an indication for amputation. Although a difficult and tedious procedure, local bone transport using distraction histogenesis is now being increasingly used to salvage these extremities. This technique not only restores bone loss, but helps unite non-unions, equalizes limb-length discrepancies, corrects angulatory deformities, and increases vascularity which is helpful in controlling osteomyelitis. Using these methods successful salvage of 11 of 12 patients with an average bone deficit of 12.5cm has been reported in one clinical study.

Precise indications for amputation or attempted salvage are difficult to define. Indications for primary amputation after open tibia fractures with vascular injury are as follows:

- Absolute indications: includes anatomical transection of the posterior tibial nerve and prolonged warm ischaemia time of over 6h
- Relative indications: include serious polytrauma, severe ipsilateral foot trauma, or an anticipated prolonged soft tissue or bony reconstruction.

Although these recommendations are generally accepted, there have been no follow-up studies to specifically verify them. The insensate foot was previously considered a major factor in considering whether to proceed with amputation or reconstruction. However, the LEAP study group have shown that initial plantar sensation is not prognostic of long-term outcomes. At 2-year follow-up after limb salvage, most patients initially reported as having insensate feet regained sensation (Box 12.10.4). The extent of the injury to the posterior tibial nerve can therefore not be reliably assessed at the time of injury. Nerve exploration is usually not indicated as it further damages the soft tissues.

Several clinical scoring systems have since been developed (Box 12.10.5). Their aim is to aid in the early decision-making on whether to proceed with attempts at limb salvage or to amputate the severely injured lower extremity.

Clinical scoring systems

A number of different scoring systems have been developed (Box 12.10.5). One of the first was the Mangled Extremity Syndrome Index (MESI). All these systems have resulted from retrospective reviews of relatively small numbers of patients. Others include the Predictive Salvage Index, the Mangled Extremity Severity Score (MESS), the Limb Salvage Index (LSI), and a modification of the MESS score, the NISSSA (for nerve injury, ischaemia, soft tissue injury, skeletal injury, shock, and age of patient). Recently, the Ganza Hospital Score (GHS) has been developed in India.

Each predictive scale attempts to quantitate the injury to the various organ systems of the extremity (skin, bone, nerve, vessel) by assigning a numerical score depending on the severity of the trauma. Some also include other factors like age, shock, and comorbid conditions.

Box 12.10.3 Amputation indications

- Long warm ischaemia time
- Irreparable nerve injury
- Extensive crush
- Limb avulsion or traumatic amputation
- Multiple traumas
- Severe ipsilateral limb trauma.

Box 12.10.4 The insensate foot

- An insensate foot on initial examination is not an indication for amputation
- Many patients without plantar sensation at presentation regain sensation and have satisfactory limb salvage.

The MESI was developed from a retrospective review of five patients with upper-extremity injuries and 12 patients with lower-extremity injuries. It was recommended that a score of below 20 should have limb salvage attempted. The MESI requires a thorough knowledge of the patient's history and injuries.

The LSI was developed from a retrospective review of 67 patients. An LSI of 6 or less was associated with successful limb salvage in 51 patients.

Both the PSI and the MESS scoring systems are less complicated then the MESI or LSI. In a retrospective review of 21 patients with pelvic and lower-extremity trauma, a PSI of less than 8 was compatible with a successful limb salvage.

The MESS score is perhaps one of the most referenced scoring systems. A MESS score of less than 7 was highly predictive of a successful limb salvage in a retrospective review of 26 patients.

The MESS score was used retrospectively to review 152 patients with 164 severely injured lower limbs. All cases with a MESS of 7 or more required amputation. A MESS of less than 7 was present for all salvaged limbs. However, many patients with a MESS of less than 7 also required amputation. Robertson felt the MESS was specific, but not sensitive, in predicting the need for a lower-extremity amputation after trauma.

In a retrospective study of 43 upper-extremity injuries, the MESS was found to have a 100% specificity, sensitivity, and positive and negative predictive value. This system was felt to be an early and accurate predictor of which upper extremity should be treated by amputation. The MESS was recently used in a combat setting and found to be useful.

The MESS score was modified to produce the NISSSA. In a retrospective review of 24 patients the NISSSA was more sensitive and specific in predicting amputation than the MESS.

The MESI, MESS, PSI, and LSI were analysed in a retrospective review of 58 limb salvage attempts over a 10-year period at a single institution. None of these four indices had the sensitivity or specificity required to predict limb salvage. The exact time to utilize a limb salvage index is unclear. The initial evaluation in the emergency department may be different from that in the operating room. Some information (patient age, comorbid conditions, exact time of injury, the true nature of the neurovascular injury, and many other pertinent factors) may only be available postoperatively. In addition, the degree of crush injury to the limb may be more apparent after several days than at the initial evaluation. It has been suggested that limb salvage scores may be most useful in early postoperative decision making.

The LEAP study group performed a prospective study to evaluate the use of clinical scoring systems to assist in the decision makeup process for limb salvage or amputation. The MESS, LSI, PSI, NISSA and Hannover Fracture Scale 97 (HFS 97) were studied in 556 lower extremity fractures. The study did not validate the

Box 12.10.5 Clinical scoring systems

- Both retrospective and prospective studies fail to support the validity of any scoring system as an absolute predictor of amputation or salvage
- Scoring system are best used as helpful guidelines, not a mandate.

Box 12.10.6 Limb reconstruction strategies

- Immediate internal or external fixation and early soft tissue coverage
- Increased use of local flaps, negative pressure therapy in addition to free flaps
- Staged procedures to achieve bony union likely.

utility of any of the lower extremity injury scores as absolute predictors of amputation.

In summary, despite persistent interest, scoring systems provide only helpful guidelines, not absolute mandates. The final decision for salvage versus amputation still rests with the clinical impression of the treating surgeon.

The timing of a traumatic extremity amputation

The initial decision to proceed with amputation or limb salvage is based on the surgeon's experience and available resources. The injured patient is often not able to make an informed decision and the extent of the injury may not be readily apparent.

Retaining an obviously necrotic or gangrenous limb can lead to higher morbidity and mortality. In one study forty-three patients with amputations after grade III open tibia fractures were reviewed; delayed amputations had increased incidence of sepsis, death, disability, operative procedures, and costs.

Earlier amputation and prosthetic fitting can be expected to result in shorter hospital stays, fewer surgical procedures, lower infection rates, and lower initial costs. Better rehabilitation and return to work occurs in patients who have amputations within 1 month of injury than those who had delayed procedures.

Emergency amputations have a higher incidence of anatomical stump problems than delayed amputations (57% versus 37%), and secondary amputation after limb salvage attempts probably does not compromise the final outcome.

If the initial decision to proceed with limb salvage is made, but the viability of the extremity remains questionable, the use of limb salvage scales has been useful for some authors. Rates of secondary amputation after initial attempts at limb salvage have been reported to be as low as 4% in series of 177 microsurgical free tissues transfers. Reported failure rates in other studies have ranged from 9–40%.

Timing of reconstructive procedures for limb salvage

Reconstruction begins after the initial debridement. The precise timing and type of procedures can vary widely. In general, early soft tissue coverage decreases infection rates. Subsequent staged procedures to achieve bony union are typically needed (Box 12.10.6).

Microsurgical free tissue transfers have lead to high rates of soft tissue coverage of open wounds. For the most severe injuries there may even be less wound complications using free flaps than rotational flaps. Nevertheless, these procedures are very labour intensive, and require close cooperation with microvascular surgeons.

There has been a renewed interest in local fasciocutaneous flaps for lower extremity trauma. In addition, negative pressure therapy (vacuum-assisted wound closure) has now begun to be used for high-energy soft tissue injuries. Both these developments have lead to a decreased need for microvascular free tissue transfer in some patients with large traumatic wounds.

In a polytrauma situation, provisional external fixation ('damage control') may be appropriate. Staged reconstruction can then follow once the patient's condition stabilizes. Prolonged used of external fixation, however, may be associated with increased complications.

The 'fix and flap' concept has been developed for treatment of severe open tibia fractures. This involves radical debridement followed by immediate internal fixation and soft tissue coverage. The final limb salvage rate in one series was 95%.

Outcome measures

In the past, outcomes were often measured by specific physician defined parameters: bony union, absence of infection, and final salvage of the extremity. Today patient perceived outcome parameters are just as important. This has lead to increased interest in health status and quality of life assessments.

Specific evaluation scales can either be disease specific or general measures of overall health. The SF–36 Health Status Profile takes about 10min to complete and is a popular health status questionnaire. The Musculoskeletal Functional Assessment (MFA) has been specifically developed for patients with musculoskeletal disorders. The Sickness Impact Profile (SIP) involves 136 statements about functional status in 12 categories. The SIP has been extensively used in outcome studies for lower extremity fractures, including all of the studies in the LEAP project.

Current challenges include selecting and evaluating outcome measures so that research and clinical studies can be adequately compared. There is no consensus on the best outcome studies to use; over 200 general orthopaedic musculoskeletal outcome measures are currently in use.

Outcomes of amputation versus limb salvage

Young adults after a traumatic amputation below the knee can be expected to be functional when fit with a prosthesis. Employment rates of 50% have been noted in several studies.

How do these patients compare long term with a severely damaged limb that has been salvaged? Some small, retrospective studies found no significant differences, and in fact noted that amputees seemed to fair slightly better. Other series reported opposite results.

Patients with foot and ankle injuries can be expected to have poorer salvage outcomes.

A major advance in our understanding of the outcomes of limb salvage or amputation has come from the LEAP study. This was a large, multicentre, prospective study of 569 patients in the United States of America. At 2 years there were no significant differences between the amputation and reconstruction groups. These results were maintained at 7 years. The SIP was the major outcome measure in this study. Outcomes did not improve over time. In fact physical and psychosocial function tended to deteriorate. Significantly poor outcomes were seen in patients who were older, female, non-white, as well as those who smoked cigarettes, had low self efficacy, lived in a poor household, had a lower education level, or were involved in litigation. Rehospitalization for major complications, foot amputation and severe soft tissue trauma were also poor prognostic factors.

Using different outcome measures for quality of life, similar results were noted in a group of patients from the Netherlands. Successful limb salvage patients in this series had more complications and required more operative intervention. Complications were most commonly related to problems with bone healing.

The LEAP study also provided information on outcomes after lower extremity amputations at different levels above the ankle. As expected, below the knee amputees had better timed walking speeds than above the knee amputees. However, there were no significant differences in the SIP scores between these two groups. Patients with an amputation through the knee however had significantly worse SIP scores.

In a meta-analysis of the recent literature, it was found that limb salvage and amputation patients had roughly similar lengths of initial hospital stay. However, limb salvage was associated with much longer rehabilitation and increased early cost. Limb salvage has higher rates of rehospitalization, more surgical procedures, and higher complication rates.

Lifetime costs of reconstructing a limb may be less than amputation. The long-term costs of an amputation in the Swiss healthcare system are nearly twice that of reconstruction if the financial impact of pensions and prostheses were considered. The costs of limb salvage using Ilizarov techniques were compared with amputation. The projected costs of a lifetime supply of prosthetic equipment exceeded the estimated cost of the Ilizarov reconstruction. The costs at 2 years between amputees and limb reconstruction are about equal, but lifetime cost for amputees are projected to be three times higher.

Reports of pain after limb salvage or amputation are difficult to interpret. Some studies show no significant differences between the groups. Others have noted more pain in limb salvage patients, while a number note more pain in amputees. So although many amputees can have chronic phantom and stump pain, limb reconstruction patients also appear to have a significant issues with chronic pain.

Employment rates appear to be similar in both groups. About half of the injured patients can be expected to return to work regardless of which treatment method was chosen. In the LEAP study, 53% of patients with an amputation and 49% with limb reconstruction return to work at 2 years.

Box 12.10.7 Outcomes

- Both amputees and limb salvage patients have a much higher incidence of self-reported disability than age matched controls
- Rates of pain, employment, and many outcome measures are similar in both groups.

Traumatic upper-extremity amputation and replantation

A patient's response to a unilateral upper-extremity amputation can be quite variable, and can depend on societal influences. However, the loss of a significant part of the upper extremity is generally considered more disabling than loss of a lower limb. A sensate salvaged upper extremity can be expected to function better than a prosthesis. Therefore the revascularization or replantation of an upper-extremity injury is usually desirable.

The best indications for replantation include sharp or guillotine amputations of the arm, forearm, or hand. Limb salvage rates of greater than 80% have consistently been reported in these situations. Mangled or crushed extremities can be expected to have much lower salvage rates. Single-digit replantation remains controversial, but thumb, multiple digit, or mid-palm amputations are indications for replantation.

The first successful replantations of digits, hands, and upper extremities were reported in the 1960s. Since then there has been an increasing realization that a viable but non-functioning limb may often be unsatisfactory to many patients. To date, however, there are no standardized methods to measure outcomes.

Functional recovery has been divided into one of four groups which included criteria on ability to work, range of motion, sensory recovery, and muscle power. An overall good to excellent functional recovery can be achieved in 69% of cases.

A very detailed 100-point grading system has been developed which includes range of motion, activities of daily living, sensory recovery, subjective symptoms, cosmesis, subjective satisfaction, and employment status. Good to excellent results were reported in 72% of the patients. Using a modified Tamai grading system, Ipsen *et al.* had a 47% rate of good to excellent results in long-term follow-up of their upper-extremity replantations and revascularizations.

Summary

The severely injured extremity cannot be expected to ever recover normal function. Modern techniques of vascular repair, local tissue transfers, negative pressure therapy, and free tissue transfer can provide reliable soft tissue coverage in many cases. Staged procedures to restore bony continuity are typically needed. Many severely damaged limbs can now be saved. Deciding which extremities should have attempted salvage remains extremely difficult. Predictive scoring scales can be very helpful in this area, but do not represent absolute mandates or replace the clinical judgement of the surgeon.

These injuries are best managed by a team approach. Close supervision of the entire treatment process, including surgery and subsequent rehabilitation, which can be expected to improve the final result. A salvaged extremity in and of itself does not necessarily yield a successful result. Much more emphasis is now being placed on final long-term function, patient satisfaction and quality of life, and return to useful employment.

In summary, patients with limb threatening lower extremity injuries have a high incidence of self reported disability no matter how they are treated. Long-term functional results of up to 7 years show no significant differences between lower extremity limb salvage and amputation. Reports of pain as well as rates of employment are similar. Certain clinical (rehospitalization for complications, associated foot and ankle trauma, severe soft tissue injury) and psychosocial factors (poor education, poverty, older age, female sex, lack of insurance, smoking, litigation, low self efficacy) can negatively effect outcomes.

Thus, amputation may remain the best solution for some mangled limbs despite modern reconstructive advances. It should not be considered a failure, but rather another treatment option.

Further reading

Bosse, M.J., MacKenzie, E.J., Kellam, J.F., *et al.* (2002). An analysis of outcomes of reconstruction or amputation of leg-threatening injuries. *New England Journal of Medicine*, **12**, 1924–31.

Gustilo, R.B. and Anderson, J.T. (1976). Prevention of infection in the treatment of one thousand and twenty-five open fractures of long bones. Retrospective and prospective analyses. *Journal of Bone and Joint Surgery, American Volume*, **58A**, 453–8.

McNamara, M.G., Heckman, J.D., and Corley, F.G. (1994). Severe open fractures of the lower extremity: a retrospective evaluation of the mangled extremity severity score (MESS). *Journal of Orthopaedic Trauma*, **8**, 81–7.

Melissinos, E.G., and Parks, D.H. (1989). Post-trauma reconstruction with free tissue transfer-analysis of 442 consecutive cases. *Journal of Trauma*, **29**, 1095–103.

Suedkamp, N.P., Barbey, N., Veuskens, A., *et al.* (*1993*). The incidence of osteitis in open fractures: an analysis of 948 open fractures (a review of the Hannover experience). *Journal of Orthopaedic Trauma*, **5**, 473–82.

Tamai, S. (1982). Twenty years' experience of limb replantation-review of 293 upper extremity replants. *Journal of Hand Surgery*, **7A**, 549–56.

12.11

Functional bracing

Augusto Sarmiento and Loren L. Latta

Summary points

- Inexpensive
- Avoids complications of internal fixation
- Allows mobilization of joints
- Weight bearing and movement as tolerated, guided by pain.

Introduction

During the past five decades, considerable progress has been made in the surgical treatment of a number of fractures, so much that many non-surgical modalities have been rendered obsolete and replaced by more effective surgical approaches. The most obvious examples are the fractures of the hip, and the femoral shaft. Rarely, are these fractures treated non-surgically.

Despite such progress, surgical treatments have their limitations and the potential for anatomical reduction is not necessarily synonymous with excellent clinical results. In some instances, complications such as infection are difficult to overcome. Plating and external fixators that rigidly immobilize fracture fragments can delay healing, because the osteogenic stimulus of interfragmentary motion is absent. In addition, the cost of surgical treatment is in many cases a great deal higher than that of conservative treatment.

It must be concluded that a rational balance between the two therapeutic approaches is essential for the best way to deal with specific clinical conditions.

Functional casting or bracing of certain long-bone fractures is a relatively new approach to care. It is a philosophy of management predicated on the premise that immobilization of fractured long bones and their adjacent joints is unphysiological and detrimental to healing, and that physiologically induced motion at the fracture site enhances osteogenesis. This premise does not fail to recognize that immobilization of fractures is often desirable, and in many instances the best means to achieve healing, while providing final acceptable cosmesis and limb function.

Our initial techniques for functional casting and bracing of fractures have undergone major change over the years, and have proven to be inappropriate in the care of many fractures such as metaphyseal and diaphyseal femoral fractures where internal fixation is more appropriate. Bracing of fractures of both bones of the forearm was practically abandoned because the implementation of the technique was difficult and the maintenance of reduction was often impossible. However, some profitable lessons were learned in the process, such as the realization that closed oblique or comminuted fractures of both bones if simply appropriately aligned, maintain the initial, usually acceptable, shortening without synostosis, while permitting unencumbered motion of the elbow and wrist. In addition it provided information regarding the ultimate limitation of motion that accompanies various degrees of angular deformity.

Bracing of diaphyseal tibial, humeral, and isolated ulnar fractures has been proven highly successful in most instances.

The diaphyseal tibial fracture (Box 12.11.1)

Functional casting and bracing offers good results in the vast majority of closed axially unstable diaphyseal tibial fractures that experience, at the time of the injury, an acceptable degree of shortening and an easily correctable angular deformity. Transverse fractures can also be managed in this way when a stable reduction can be manually obtained. These criteria were established upon recognition that the vast majority of closed fractures initially suffer less than 0.5cm of shortening. This degree of final shortening is inconsequential from the physiological, functional, and aesthetic point of view. Through clinical and laboratory investigations we have proven that the initial shortening does not increase with the introduction of graduated weight-bearing ambulation. Beyond those criteria, tibial fractures with intact fibula that demonstrate initial varus angulation should not be braced because of the likelihood of increased deformity.

Diaphyseal tibial fractures that are to be treated by non-surgical means are best stabilized initially with a well-padded above-the knee cast that extends from below the groin to the base of the toes. The knee joint is flexed to approximately 7–10 degrees. Further knee flexion to prevent weight bearing is not necessary as additional shortening does not increase in the case of closed tibias. If there is significant swelling at the time of the first evaluation of the patient, or additional swelling is anticipated because of the severity of the injury, a circular cast is not advisable. A posterior splint may be used or the posterior half of the bivalved above-the-knee cast. The ankle joint is best held at 90 degrees of flexion.

Forceful dorsiflexion should be avoided in order to prevent the development of recurvatum deformity at the fracture site. The limb should be elevated at rest and observed for compartment syndrome. The functional cast may be applied as soon as the acute symptoms subside, which in most instances occurs within the first 2 post-injury weeks. To apply it while the leg is still painful is an unwarranted and unnecessary experience. On the other hand, postponing its application until 'early callus' is seen on radiographs is also a misguided and erroneous practice. By the time callus is seen on the tibia, the faster healing fibula is likely to be solidly healed, creating a situation similar to that of an acute tibial fracture with an intact fibula, leading to the development of angular varus deformity.

If the cast is to be used in preference to the brace, it is best to postpone its application until the swelling has decreased to a greater degree, simply because the circular cast lacks the adjustable features to accommodate the reduction of swelling and limb atrophy that the brace possesses.

The application of the below-the-knee functional cast

The functional cast, mistakenly called a PTB (patellar tendon bearing) cast because it resembles the moulding of the PTB prosthesis worn by the amputee, is applied in three stages.

1) *First stage*: following the removal of the above-the-knee cast the patient must sit on a high table with the hip, knee, and ankle joints at 90 degrees. Both legs are exposed to facilitate reproduction of alignment. Stockinette and a thin layer of cotton wadding are applied. The cast can be applied without padding, but requires greater care during its removal. Plaster of Paris or synthetic material is used. The cast is moulded around the ankle which is held at 90 degrees of dorsiflexion. A recurvatum deformity at the fracture site can develop with excessive dorsiflexion (Figure 12.11.1A). It is not necessary at this time to pay attention to alignment or rotation of the fragments

2) *Second stage*: when the casting material begins to set it is firmly wrapped over the leg overlapping the portion of the cast over the ankle and extending to just below the tibial tuberosity. It is during this time that exposure of the normal leg is essential in order for the surgeon to duplicate the shape of the normal leg in the fractured one. The surgeon corrects any angulation or rotation seen during the above-the-knee cast stage. The soft tissues of the extremity are firmly moulded with particular attention being paid to the compression of the sub-popliteal space and the medial tibial condyle (Figure 12.11.1B)

3) *Third stage*: the cast is then extended over the femoral condyles with the knee at approximately 45 degrees of flexion and heel resting on the surgeons lap. This allows the quadriceps to relax in order that the patellar tendon can be firmly compressed as the material begins to set. The compression of the patellar tendon is not done in expectation that this soft tissue structure will become a weighty bearing area. The compression is performed only to facilitate posterior counter pressure of the subpopliteal calf (Figure 12.11.1C).

Box 12.11.1 Diaphyseal tibial functional casting/bracing

- Suitable for transverse fractures
- Suitable for axially stable fractures
- Suitable when there is an acceptable degree of shortening on the initial x-rays
- Not suitable when fibula is intact with varus angulation
- Convert to functional cast/brace when swelling and acute symptoms subside (usually within 2 weeks)
- Benefit of motion at the tibial fracture site before ulna unites.

The freedom of the knee joint is made possible by trimming the proximal cast (Figure 12.11.1D). Anteriorly, to just above the proximal pole of the patella; laterally, as far posteriorly as possible without impinging on the hamstring tendons; posteriorly, at a point opposite the tibial tubercle. The completed trimming should make possible full flexion and extension of the knee (Figure 12.11.1E, F).

Once the casting material has dried, ambulation with the aid of a walker or crutches may begin. Symptoms should dictate the degree of weight bearing. It is increased gradually.

Application of the below-the-knee functional brace

The surgeon might prefer to askew the functional cast, and go directly to the functional brace. The appropriate timing for its application is the same used for the application of the functional cast. That is, evidence of subsidence of acute pain and disappearance of significant swelling distally. If applied before these criteria are met, undesirable discomfort and persistence of distal oedema will result.

The brace can be custom-made or prefabricated. It extends from the level of the proximal pole of the patella and extends to just above the ankle. It must be held firmly in place against the soft tissue with Velcro straps (Figure 12.11.3A,B).

The brace is applied with the patient sitting on a high table, holding the hip and knee at 90 degrees of flexion. The functional brace is fitted over a layer of stockinette. The completed brace should allow full flexion and extension of the knee and ankle. If this is not possible because the brace is too long, the proximal or distal ends of the shells can be trimmed down with scissors (Figure 12.11.3C).

Instructions to the patient should consist of avoidance, during the first few days, of prolonged sitting with the knee flexed. Elevation of the leg and frequent active flexion and extension of the ankle expedite the subsidence of swelling and the restoration of motion. Ambulation can begin from the outset with the use of crutches. The degree of weight bearing is determined by the degrees of discomfort. There is nothing to be gained from forcing patients to bear weight if such an action is painful. The straps must be adjusted frequently several times during the first few days, and twice a day afterwards, in order to accommodate the new geometry of the limb created by the reduction of swelling. It is this firm compression that controls angular deformities.

The brace should not be removed for approximately 1 week, at which time the surgeon removes the brace and inspects the extremity. New x-rays are taken at this time. If clinically and radiographically there appear to be no problem, the patient is taught how to apply and remove the brace without assistance (Figure 12.11.4).

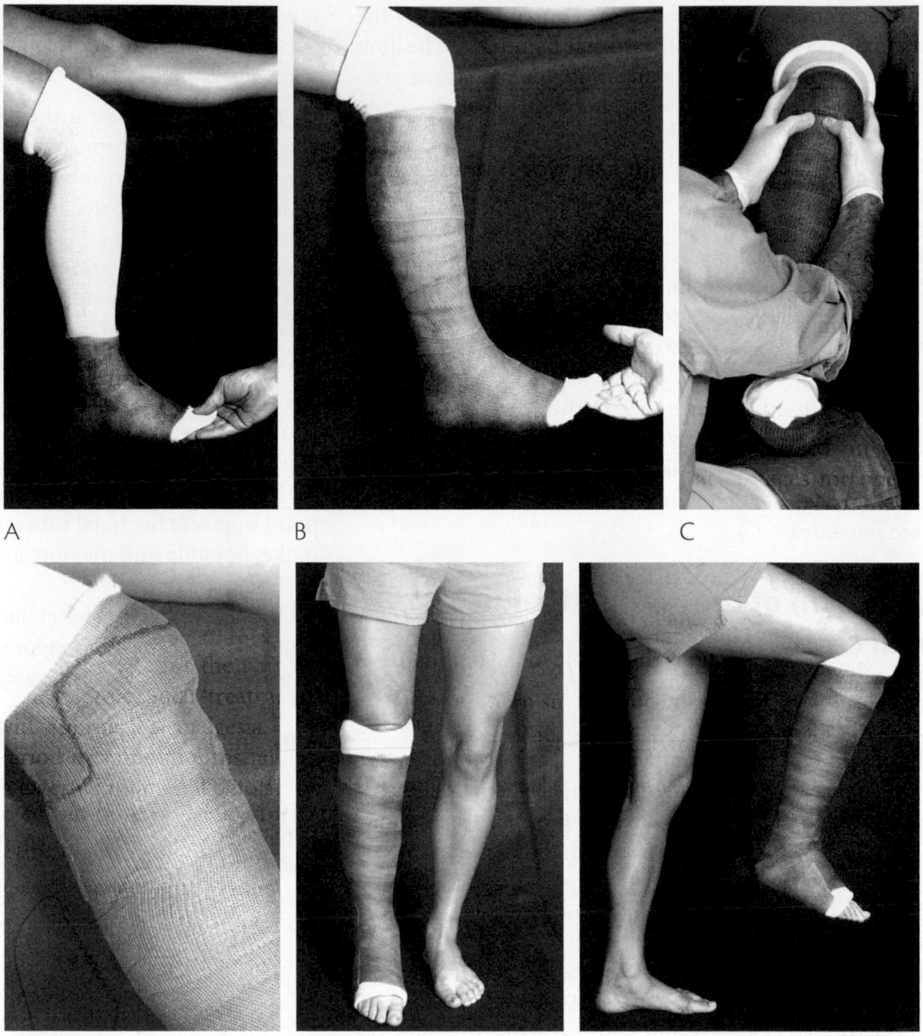

A B C D E F

Fig. 12.11.1 A) The ankle is held gingerly into dorsiflexion of 90 degrees. The casting material is wrapped from the toes to a couple inches above the malleolli. The arches of the foot are molded firmly. B) Once the casting material has dried over the foot and ankle, its application over the leg continues. C) The cast is then extended to include the femoral condyles. D) The cast is then cut to allow knee flexion. E) and F) Motion that should be possible upon its completion.

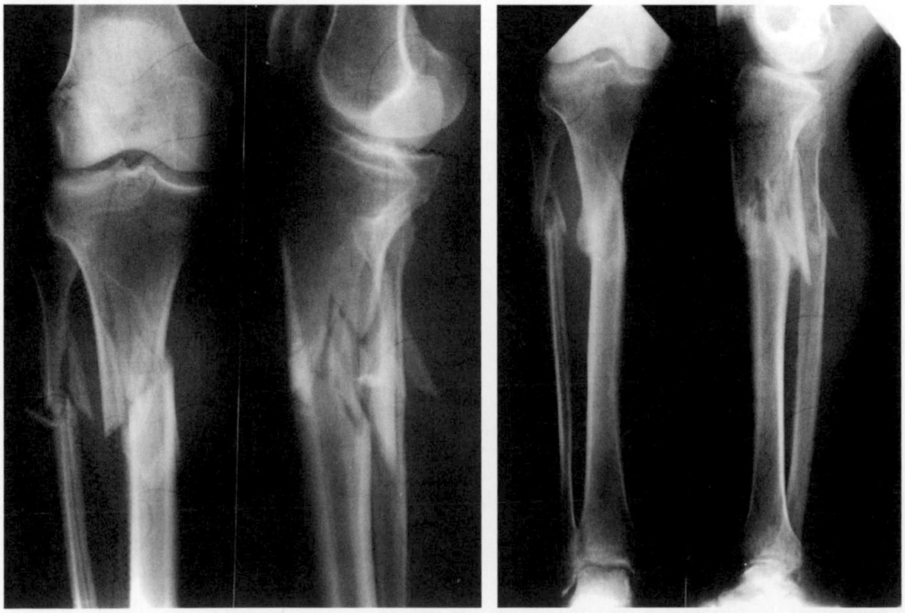

A B

Fig. 12.11.2 A) Radiograph of closed comminuted fracture of the proximal tibia and fibula. Notice the acceptable shortening seen at the time of the initial insult. B) Radiograph obtained after completion of healing. Notice that the initial shortening remained essentially unchanged.

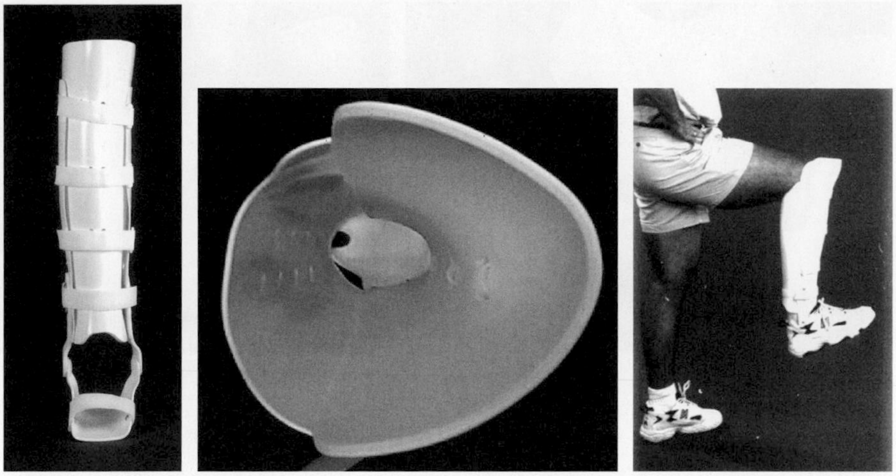

A B C

Fig. 12.11.3 A) The prefabricate brace illustrating the attached and removable distal ankle insert. B) The brace has two shells, which are held in place in order to permit their separation and to slide the components over the ankle without creating pain. C) Brace should allow full flexion and extension of the knee and ankle.

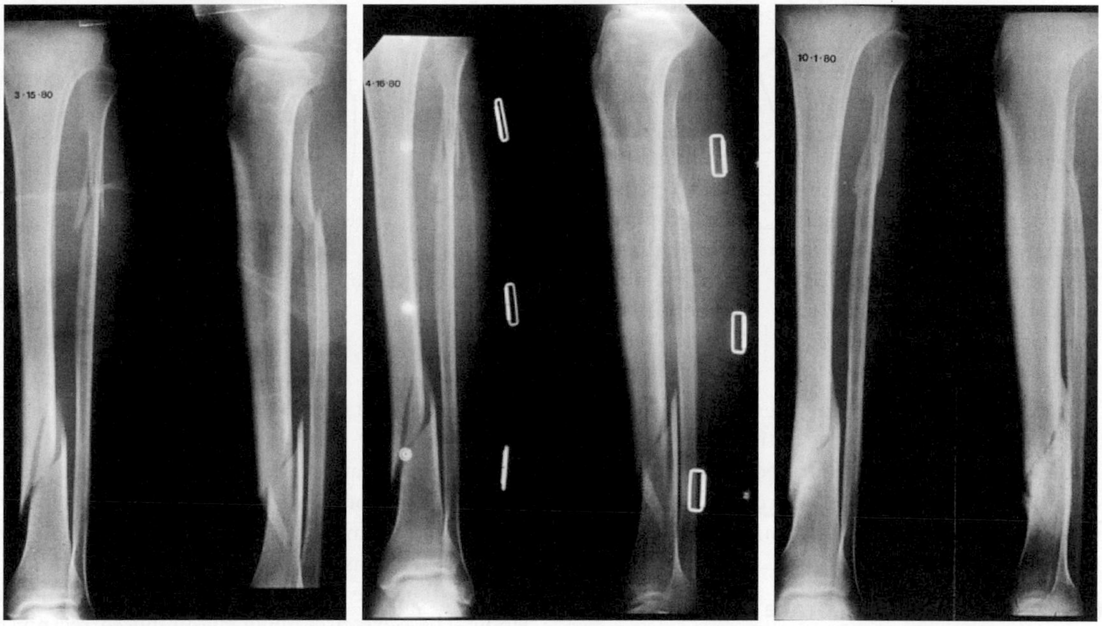

A B C

Fig. 12.11.4 A) Radiograph of closed oblique fracture of the distal third of the tibia and proximal fibula. Notice the acceptable initial shortening. B) Radiograph obtained after application of the brace. C) Radiograph taken after completion of healing. Notice that the initial shortening and alignment were maintained.

The humeral shaft fracture (Box 12.11.2)

Non-surgical functional treatment of diaphyseal humeral fractures has been highly successful, with a very low incidence of non-union and acceptable functional and cosmetic results.

Initial management

Patients with diaphyseal humeral fractures who are selected for non-surgical functional management are usually those with closed fractures that do not suggest extreme degrees of soft tissue damage, which is usually depicted by major axial separation between the major fragments. In order to provide comfort during the early acute stage of the process, an above the elbow cast or a coaptation splint is applied (Figure 12.11.5). The elbow should be held at approximately 90 degrees of flexion. A sling is essential, and must be attached while the shoulder is in a relaxed position; otherwise an angular deformity is likely to develop when the shrugged shoulder relaxes (Figure 12.11.6).

Box 12.11.2 Humeral shaft functional bracing

- Suitable for closed fractures without evidence of significant soft tissue damage (fracture gap)
- Initial treatment in cast or coaptation splint
- Apply brace from day 2, when pain and swelling settled
- Avoid applying sling with shoulder elevated, 'shrugged'.

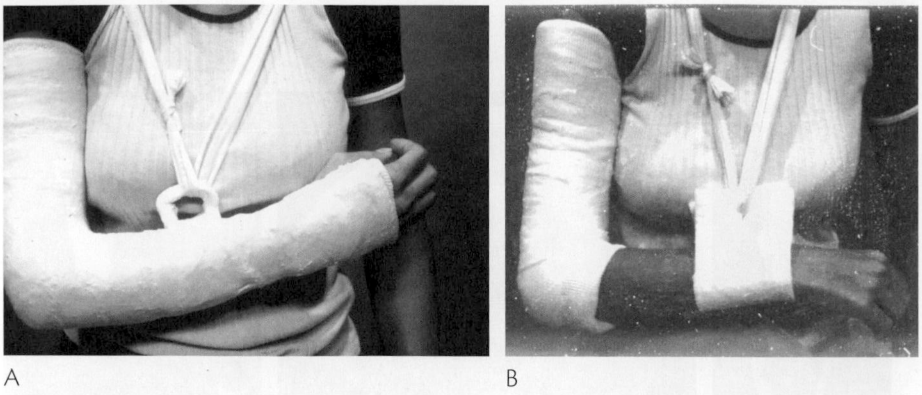

Fig. 12.11.5 A) Illustration of an above-the-elbow cast holding the elbow at 90 degrees of flexion. B) Illustration of a coaptation splint.

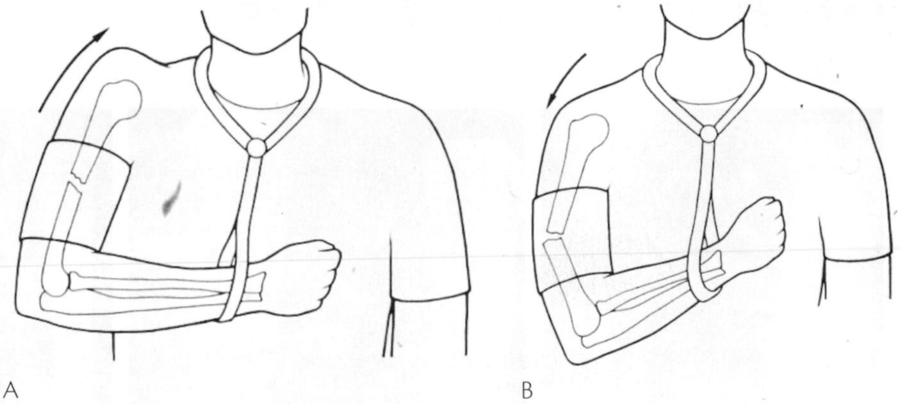

Fig. 12.11.6 A) A shrugged shoulder is a commonly seen problem at the time of application of the sling. B) As the shoulder relaxes a varus deformity readily occurs. It is important therefore to ascertain that when the sling is applied the shoulder is a relaxed position.

Circumduction (pendulum) exercises, in the sling, should begin within the first couple of days following the initial injury. Under no circumstances should the patient be encouraged to actively abduct or elevate the shoulder. These active exercises readily lead to angular deformity and increase the likelihood of non-union.

The application of the functional brace

In most patients with diaphyseal humeral fractures sustained from relatively low energy injuries, the functional brace may be applied within the first week of injury. However, if the extremity is still very painful and significant swelling is present at that time, it is best to postpone the application of the brace by a few more days.

The brace is applied while the patient is sitting in a high chair with the arm in a relaxed position. Since it is likely that the elbow will be limited in flexion because of the preceding days of immobilization, the arm should be supported by the patient's normal hand (Figure 12.11.7). A layer of stockinette is rolled over the upper arm, extending from the acromioclavicular level to below the elbow.

The prefabricated brace, which is made of two separate shelves, is slipped over the arm until it reaches a point below the axilla. Once this has been accomplished, the Velcro straps are firmly adjusted.

Braces that extend over the acromium do more harm than good. They have been allegedly designed to prevent their distal slippage. Although it is possible that in some stances this is accomplished, the necessary soft tissue compression is lost and pain or discomfort ensues.

Following the application of the brace, circumduction exercises, in sling, should be reinitiated. A few days later, in accordance with the degree of symptoms, the patient is instructed to start passive flexion and extension of the elbow. These exercises are then combined with active contractions of the flexors and extensors of the elbow. These exercises might favourably correct any rotary deformity that may have developed at the time of the injury. Once the elbow reaches full extension, and the acute symptoms have disappeared, circumduction exercises in extension may be started. These exercises must be conducted gingerly and without pain. During rest, the arm is best held in the sling until clinical evidence of early intrinsic healing has been demonstrated (Figure 12.11.8). Active flexion and abduction should be postponed until the fracture shows early callus formation in order to avoid angular deformities.

The isolated ulnar fracture (Box 12.11.3)

Plating of isolated ulnar fractures is a popular method of treatment. Postoperative infection is low and non-union and implant failure do not occur with great frequency. However, refracture following plate removal is not uncommon and the costs of surgical treatment remain high.

The popularity of surgical plating came as a result of observing that non-union was not infrequently encountered when the limb was immobilized in a cast that extended from the head of the

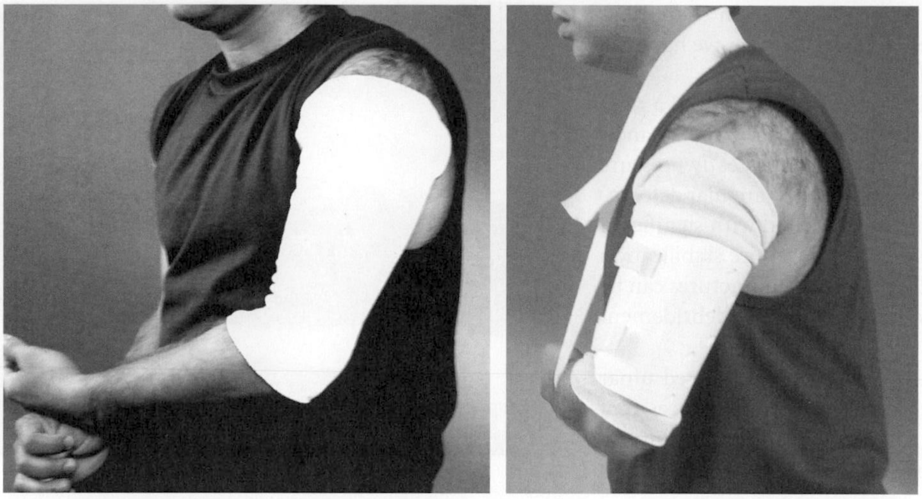

A B

Fig. 12.11.7 Illustrations of the sequential steps taken during the application of the functional brace. Notice that the brace is made of two shells that permit its application without the need for full extension of the elbow.

Box 12.11.3 Ulnar shaft functional bracing

- Usually the result of a direct blow
- Fracture is usually axially stable and supported by interosseous membrane
- Mild angular deformity correctable
- When the forearm is placed in a relaxed attitude of supination, the angular deformity usually improves
- Contraindicated in Monteggia fracture.

metacarpals to above the elbow. Such a cast had been used as it was believed that the joint above and below a fracture required immobilization. Today, the theory of rigid immobilization has been proven flawed, and replaced with evidence-supported data that freedom of motion of joints and physiologically induced motion at the fracture site are conducive to diaphyseal fracture healing. The high rate of success with functional bracing of isolated ulnar fractures makes it difficult to justify the routine plating of these fractures. There are, however, instances when open surgery is the treatment of choice, such as in the case of open fractures with severe soft tissue damage or major displacement of the fragments.

Since isolated ulnar fractures are usually the result of direct blows over the forearm, the most common displacement of the fragments is in a radial direction. Since the injury produces minimal to moderate damage to the interosseous membrane, its stabilizing role is rarely compromised. Shortening is not possible, since the intact radius prevents such a development. When the forearm is placed in a relaxed attitude of supination, the angular deformity usually improves. In any event, the common residual angulation does not result in a noticeable loss of prono-supination. It is our view that the surgical trauma produced at the time of plate fixation

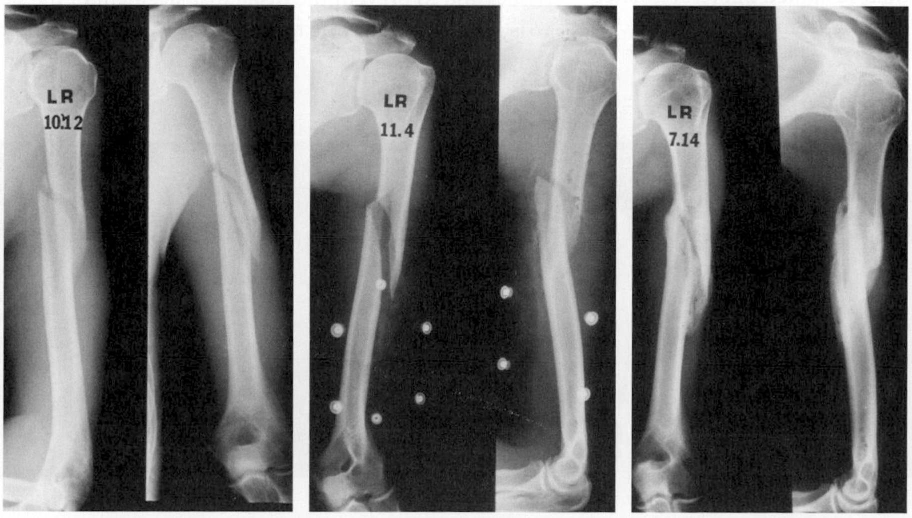

A B C

Fig. 12.11.8 A) Radiographs of a closed oblique fracture of the proximal humerus. B) Radiograph taken 2 weeks later, following the application of the functional brace. C) Radiograph obtained following completion of healing.

is more likely to create a greater degree of limitation of motion. A synostosis between the two bones is a complication we have not observed with the use of functional braces.

Initial angular deformity in a volar direction is usually of a mild degree and the clinical consequences are rarely of any significance. This type of angulation is easily correct by gently, steady pressure at the apex of the fracture for a few minutes. Major angular deformity may be seen in severe open fractures associated with significant amount of soft tissue damage. These fractures require stabilization with internal or external fixation. Low-grade open fractures can be treated with functional bracing following appropriate debridement of the injured soft tissues.

These observations suggest that the majority of isolated ulnar fractures can be successfully treated with functional braces that permit early use of the extremity without the need for complete prevention of prono-supination of the forearm and flexion and extension of the elbow and wrist.

We recognize that the functional brace does not immobilize the fractured fragments. This is a desirable feature, since immobilization retards healing. This is true for all other types of braces used in the care of tibial or humeral fractures. In the case of the ulna, the brace simply provides comfort and holds the forearm in the desirable relaxed attitude of supination, which assists in maintaining the two bones as far apart as possible.

Successful results have been achieved treating isolated ulnar fractures with the simply use of an elastic bandage. However, the brace provides a degree of comfort the bandage does not accomplish.

Instructions

Patients are encouraged to use the extremity to the maximum degree allowed by pain. In most instances the pain present at the time of application of the brace is only moderate. It is our opinion that the early introduction of function results in a more rapid disappearance of acute symptoms and faster healing. The brace should be short enough to make possible free motion of the wrist and elbow, regardless of the location of the fracture (Figure 12.11.9).

Flexion and extension of the elbow are rapidly regained. Pronation and supination required a longer period of time because such motions are more painful. In a few instances we have treated with functional braces patients who had sustained bilateral isolated ulnar fractures. Their recovery was rapid and uneventful.

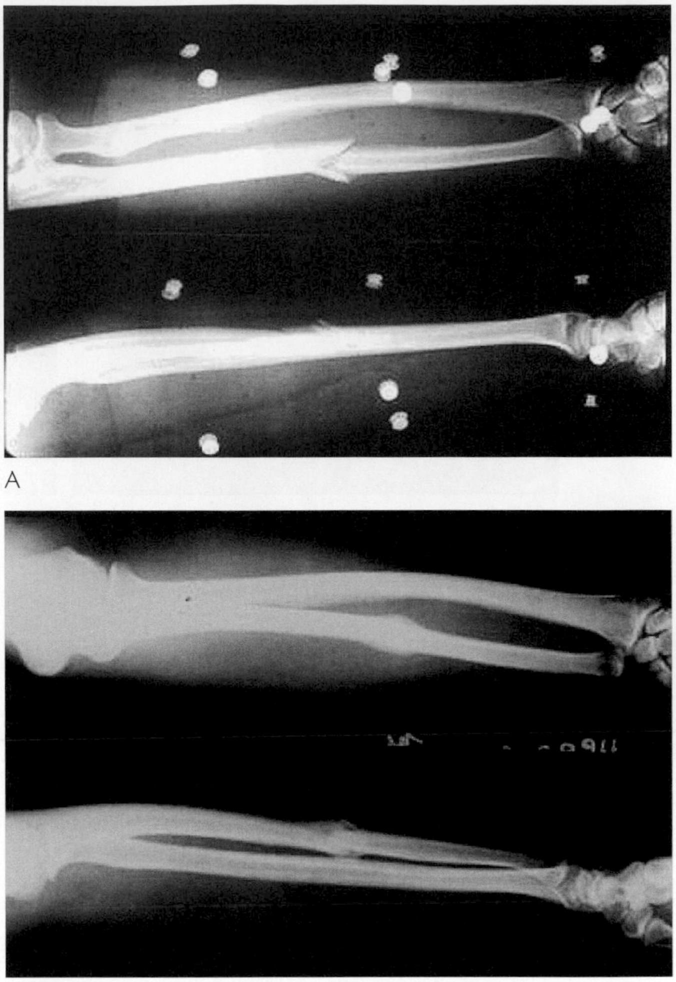

Fig. 12.11.10 A) Radiograph of non-displaced closed diaphyseal fracture of the ulna following the application of the functional brace. B) Radiograph obtained following completion of healing.

The brace should be adjusted on a frequent basis during the first few days in order to maintain the desirable compression of the soft tissues and to prevent the distal displacement of the sleeve over the wrist. The brace may be removed for hygienic purposes as often as

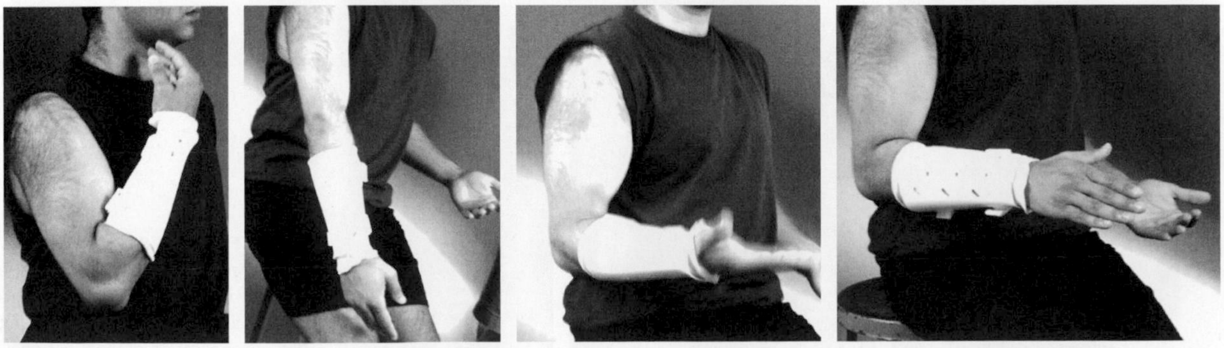

A B C D

Fig. 12.11.9 The brace should be short enough to make possible free motion of the wrist and elbow, regardless of the location of the fracture.

necessary and the collar-and-cuff permanently discontinued as soon as the symptoms subside.

Obviously, rigid immobilization of fragments is not necessary. All the brace accomplishes is probably nothing more than provision of comfort and protection to the arm from inadvertent forceful contact with hard objects (Figure 12.11.10).

Further reading

Martinez, A., Latta, L.L., and Sarmiento, A. (2003). Functional bracing of fractures of the proximal tibia. *Clinical Orthopaedics and Related Research*, **417**, 293–302.

Sarmiento, A. (2007). The functional bracing of fractures. *Journal of Bone and Joint Surgery*, **89A**, 157–69.

Sarmiento, A. and Latta, L.L. (2004). 450 closed fractures of the distal third of the tibia treated with a functional brace. *Clinical Orthopedics*, **428**, 261–71.

Sarmiento, A. and Latta, L.L (2006). On the evolution of fracture bracing. *Journal of Bone and Joint Surgery*, **88B**, 141–8.

Sarmiento, A., Latta, L.L. Zych, G., McKeever, P., and Zagorski, J. (1998). Functional bracing of ulnar fractures. *Journal of Orthopaedic Trauma*, **12**, 420–4.

Sarmiento, A., Latta, L.L., Zagorski, J., Capps, C., and Zych, G. (2000). Functional Bracing of Humeral Shaft Fractures. *Journal of Bone and Joint Surgery*, **82A**, 478–86.

12.12

Principles of plate and screw osteosynthesis

Glenn Clewer and John McMaster

Summary points

- Fixation using plates and screws requires an understanding of basic principles rather than simple pattern recognition
- Although plates and screws are simple mechanical devices their correct application requires good technique.

Screws—basic concepts (Box 12.12.1)

General principles of screw fixation

Screws have several components:

- *Head*
- *Shaft*—the shaft is comprised of a threaded section and in partially threaded screws there is also a non-threaded section. *Shaft diameter* is used to describe the diameter of any non-threaded sections. Threaded sections have both a *core diameter* and a *thread diameter*
- The screw thread has a *pitch* which defines the relationship between rotation and axial displacement of the screw (Figure 12.12.1). This is directly related to the inclination of the thread which determines the axial displacement that occurs with rotation
- *Tip.*

As a 'conventional' screw is tightened, a load is generated between the bottom of the screw head and the upper surface of the screw threads. As the axial load increases so does the fiction generated between the screw and bone. It is the friction that prevents the screw backing out, and this is dependent on the thread pitch. The steeper the pitch, the less friction and vice versa. Further tightening has the potential to generate load in excess of the ultimate strength of the bone. At this point, failure occurs at the interface between the screw and bone. The strength of this interface can be improved by using larger threads and washers, both of which reduce pressure on the bone.

Box 12.12.1
A *screw* is a mechanical device that converts a rotational movement (torque) into a linear movement (translation).

The corresponding drill for a screw accommodates the core diameter. In cortical bone, tapping is recommended to create a channel for the threads. In addition to cutting the threads the tap has flutes that allow the bone cuttings to be cleared. Conventional screw threads are not designed to 'cut' channels and there is a risk of the screw jamming, breaking, or stripping the threads.

Screw head

Head undersurface

Screw heads are required to interface with both bone and plates. Ideally this interface involves a large surface area and allows the screw to be angled. To accommodate these features a spherical undersurface is desirable (Figure 12.12.1). When screws are placed at an angle in cortical bone a counter sink can be used to increase the contact surface area and reduce pressure and the subsequent risk of failure of the underlying bone.

Head recesses

Recesses within the head accommodate the screwdriver. Different designs are available that aim to provide an effective coupling which is easy to use and resistant to damage on insertion and extraction. Hexagonal and 'star' recesses are the most frequently used in fracture fixation (Figure 12.12.2).

Threaded screw head

Many manufacturers of trauma implants have now utilized a threaded-head screw design, this allows the head of the screw to be 'locked' into the plate (Figure 12.12.3). The screw-plate construct acts as a fixed angle device and will be discussed later in the chapter.

Screw thread

Symmetrical threads

Thread symmetry refers to the profile of the thread. The upper and lower surfaces of symmetrical threads are the same. This design is

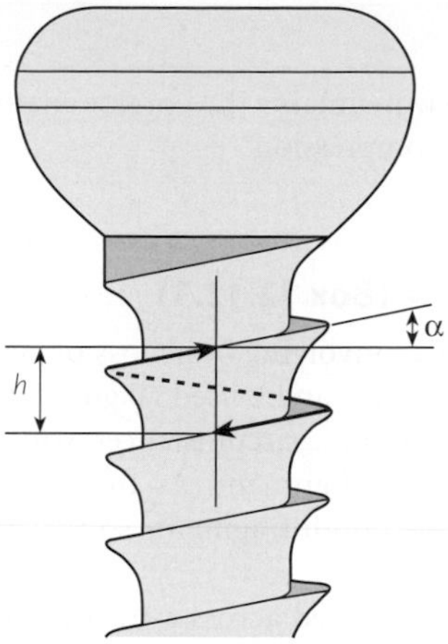

Fig. 12.12.1 Pitch of a screw: h, axial displacement with 360 degree rotation, α, inclination. The spherical under surface maximizes the contact surface area when placed at an angle and when used with plates.

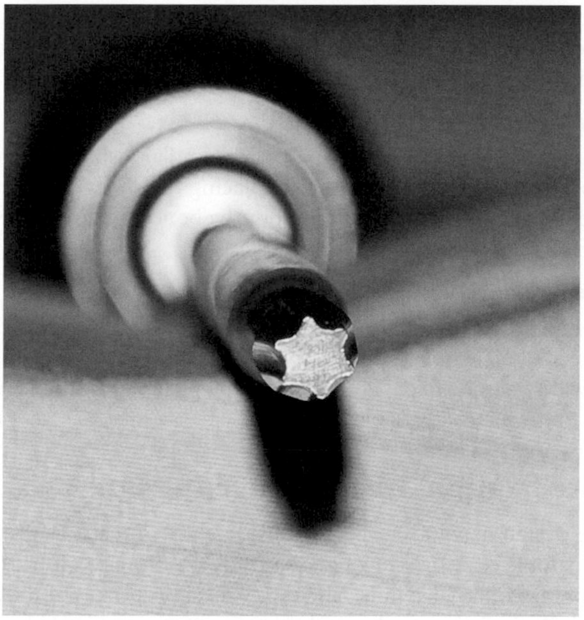

Fig. 12.12.2 Star drive screw driver.

easier to manufacture and is used in cancellous bone (Figure 12.12.4A).

Asymmetrical threads

This design is used for cortical bone screws (Figure 12.12.4B). The upper surface of the thread is flatter than the lower thread surface. The upper surface is more or less orthogonal to the axis of the screw increasing frictional resistance. The friction generated during insertion is minimized by the rounded undersurface.

Screw tips

Conventional cortical bone screws have a blunt tip and are designed to be used in a pre-drilled and pre-tapped hole. Self-tapping screws

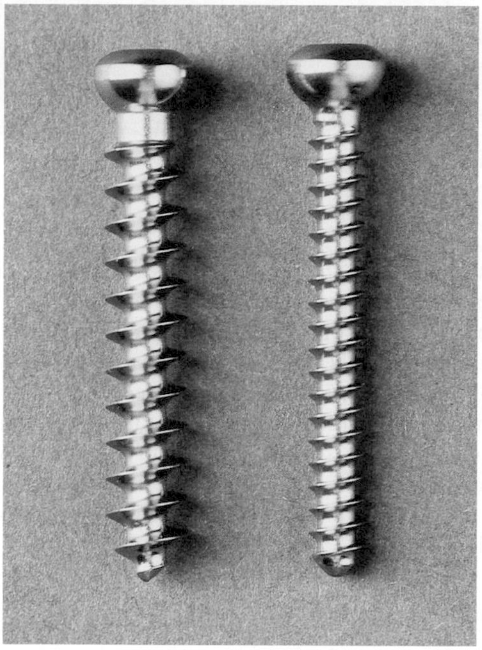

A B

Fig. 12.12.4 A) Symmetrical thread. This is the most common thread design used for screws in cancellous bone. The threads of cancellous screws are deeper, the pitch is greater and the outer diameter is larger than the corresponding cortical screw. B) Asymmetrical thread. This design is used for screws in cortical bone.

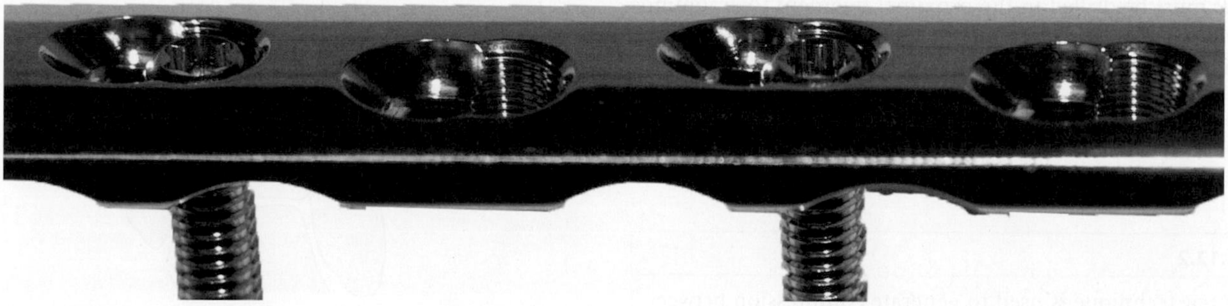

Fig. 12.12.3 Locking plate.

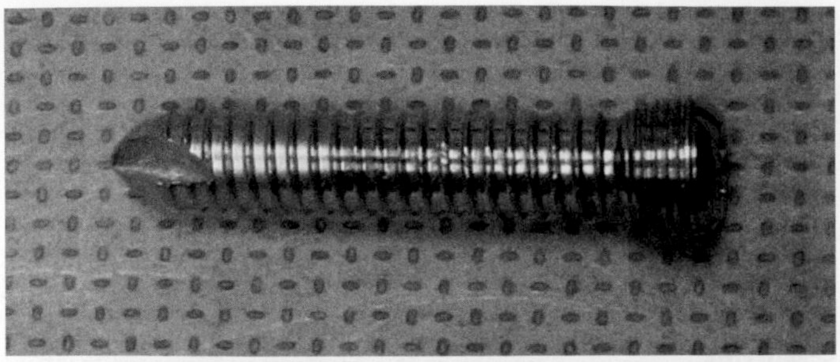

Fig. 12.12.5 Self-tapping screw tip.

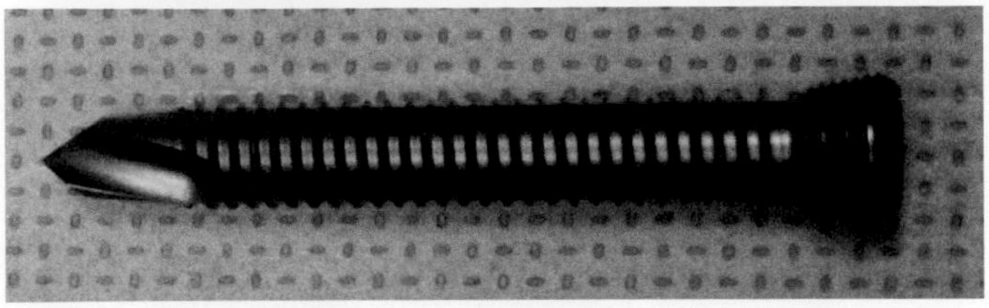

Fig. 12.12.6 Self-drilling/self-tapping locking screw.

have a cutting flute on the tip that allows the screw to cut its own thread through a pre-drilled hole (Figure 12.12.5). Self-drilling/self-tapping screws incorporate a drill tip and cut their own hole and thread (Figure 12.12.6). Self drilling screws should only be used for monocortical fixation. When used to achieve bicortical fixation there is a risk of stripping the thread in the proximal cortex. In strong cortical bone, the self-drilling tip will not advance at the rate dictated by the threads engaged in the proximal cortex. If bicortical fixation is required it is advisable to pre-drill and not use a self-drilling screw.

Methods of screw fixation

Lag screw (Box 12.12.2)

A lag screw generates displacement of one fracture fragment relative to another, generating compression at the fracture site. Interfragmentary compression helps create the stability that is required for direct bone healing. Lag screws should be placed at 90 degrees to the fracture site to maximize compression and avoid the risk of displacement.

Both partially and fully threaded screws can be used as lag screws. To generate compression at the fracture site the threads must only engage the distal fragment. When using a fully threaded screw a *glide hole* must be drilled in the proximal fragment to accommodate the outer diameter of the screw. A *threaded hole* is drilled in the distal fragment.

Box 12.12.2

A *lag screw* technique is used to generate compression between fracture fragments.

Box 12.12.3

A *positioning screw* maintains the correct anatomical alignment without exerting compression.

Positioning screw (Box 12.12.3)

Under circumstances involving bone loss or syndesmotic disruption, positioning screws can be used (Figure 12.12.7). Generation of compression under these circumstances would be undesirable as it would generate malalignment. As the screw is tightened the threads must engaged both fragments so that there is no relative displacement.

A positional screw placed across a fracture line can be used to maintain the compression generated by the prior application of reduction clamps or a compression device.

Plate screw

Plate fixing screw

The stability of a conventional plate screw construct is dependent on the friction generated at the bone–plate interface. For friction to be generated it relies on compression by the screws at the bone–plate interface and contact between the bone and plate.

Plate lag screw

The plate lag screw hole is prepared in a similar fashion to when a lag screw is placed in isolation. By placing the screw through the plate it achieves compression at both the bone plate interface and the fracture site (Figure 12.12.8).

Plate locking screw

The most common method involves a threaded screw head within a threaded plate hole (see Figure 12.12.3). With these implants the screw direction is fixed. Polyaxial locking plates allow the screw to lock to the plate at variable angles.

Plate fixation—basic concepts (Box 12.12.4)

Plate design may have evolved considerably from strips of metal, with simple circular screw holes, but they continue to function as temporary internal splints. The mechanical properties of the plate will influence the mechanical environment experienced at the fracture site and this will be dependent on the size and shape of the material used. Most orthopaedic trauma implants are made from

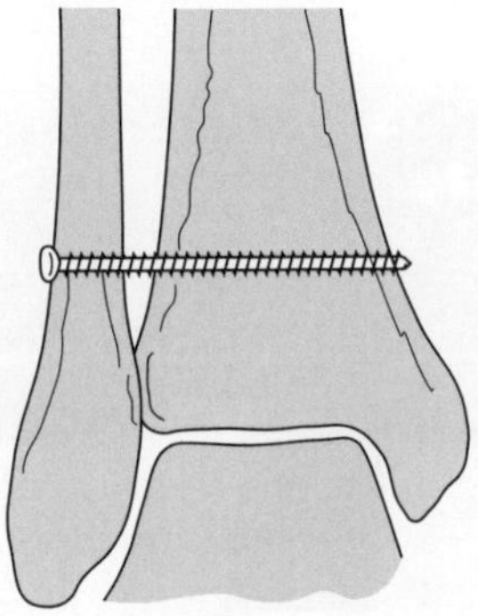

Fig. 12.12.7 Positional screw used to restore ankle joint alignment after disruption of ankle syndesmosis.

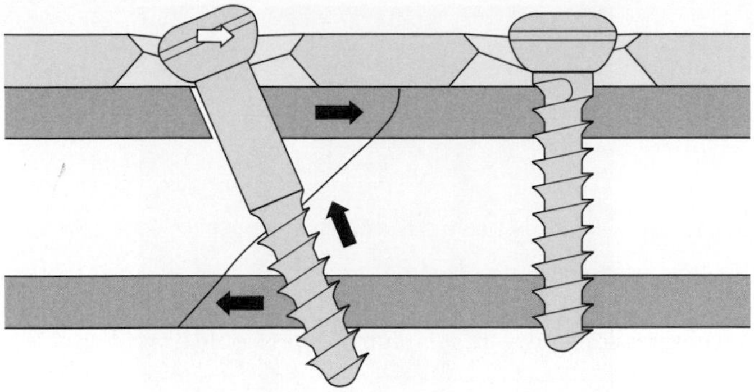

Fig. 12.12.8 Plate lag screw placed following plate fixing screw.

Box 12.12.4

A *plate* is a mechanical device that can temporarily take over the mechanical function of the bone to which it is applied.

stainless steel or titanium. Titanium has approximately 50% of the stiffness of stainless steel; however it is the dimensions rather than the elastic modulus that has the greatest effect on the mechanical properties of plates. Doubling the thickness of the plate has the potential to increase the stiffness by a factor of 16.

The strength of the fracture fixation construct is dependent on the mechanical interfaces between all the components. The strength of all plate-screw constructs is dependent on the bone–screw interface and this has been discussed in the previous section. The development of locking plates has resulted in improved biology and mechanics at the plate–screw and bone–plate interfaces.

Non-locking plate-screw fixation

In conventional non-locking plates, fixation strength is dependent on friction at the bone–plate and plate–screw interfaces. As the plate screw is tightened the plate is pulled against the bone increasing the friction between both of these interfaces. Loss of friction at the bone–plate interface will result in loosening of the construct. It can be expected that with the inevitable relaxation, of the relatively high application force generated by the screws, there will be loss of fixation. In screws that have been inserted with good technique this process will take months and this will be sufficient time to allow fracture healing. Screw tightening can cause high stresses at the interface between the undersurface of the screw head and the floor of the plate hole, causing incongruency as a result of the elastic and plastic deformation of the plate holes. Micromotion at this interface causes fretting corrosion and decreased friction between plate and bone. Any loosening will result in micromotion, bone resorption, and further loosening.

Another limitation of using high tensile force and friction is the detrimental effect to blood flow in the 'footprint' of the plate. This can result in necrosis and the potential for reduced bone healing, refracture with plate removal, and infection. Low contact plates have been developed to minimize this problem by reducing the surface area affected by bone necrosis without affecting friction. These plates allow soft tissue ingrowth and avoid creating large volumes of dead space.

Locking plate–screw fixation

Screw heads lock into the locking plate forming a construct with axial and angular stability. The plate does not need to be contoured precisely to the bone as it relies on the strength of the plate–screw interface rather than friction at the bone–plate interface for stability. It therefore functions as an internal fixator. This has a beneficial effect on the perfusion at the bone–plate interface. Relaxation is minimal at the plate–screw interface and the screws are subject to bending forces as opposed to the tensile loads experienced by non-locking screws. This allows the creation of stronger fracture fixation constructs in the presence of bone loss. For failure to occur at the bone–screw interface it must be accompanied by failure of all the screws on one side of the construct.

Methods of plate fixation

Plates can be considered load bearing when used to support the entire physiologic load in the absence of inherent fracture stability. When the reduced fracture contributes to stability the plate can be considered load sharing. The choice of plate will be dependent on the load to which it will be subjected and this is dependent on the anatomical position and the method of application.

The method used to apply a plate should be chosen according to the fracture pattern, soft tissues, and available reduction techniques. The methods of plate application are independent of whether a locked or non-locked plate is used (Box 12.12.5).

Neutralization

Simple fractures may be amenable to anatomical reduction and interfragmentary compression using lag screws. Fixation by this method alone is seldom sufficient as the fixation is likely to fail as a result of twisting and bending forces. The addition of a plate helps to neutralize these forces.

Compression

Plates can be used in compression mode by using the following methods:

- Dynamic compression plate holes
- Removable compression devices
- Pre-bending
- Plate lag screw.

Dynamic compression plates

Compression plates have oval holes that, viewed in longitudinal cross-section, have an inclined plane at one end (Figure 12.12.9). When a screw is inserted at this end of the plate the head slides

Box 12.12.5 Methods of plate application

- Neutralization
- Compression
- Buttress
- Antiglide
- Tension-band
- Bridge plate.

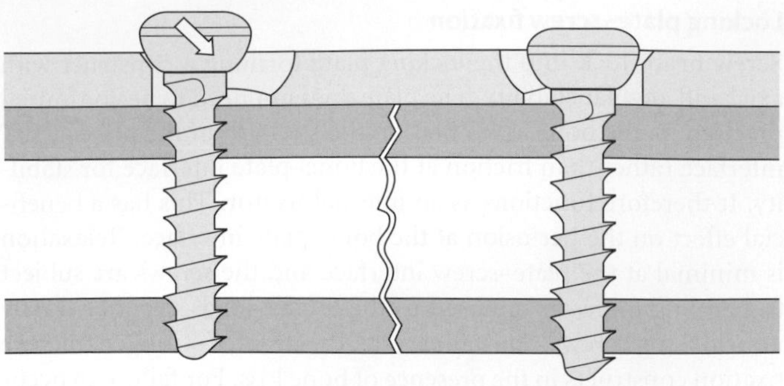

Fig. 12.12.9 Dynamic compression hole used to achieve interfragmentary compression.

down the incline resulting in axial translation of the plate and compression at the fracture site. This mode of usage relies on one end of the plate being rigidly fixed to the other fragment. The axial translation is small and the fracture needs to be anatomically reduced before application of the compression screw. The compression hole has been incorporated into plate designs that also accommodate locking screws (Figure 12.12.10).

Removable compression devices

These devices can generate compression once the plate has been firmly anchored to one side of the fracture (Figure 12.12.11). This technique requires a greater exposure but can generate more axial translation than can be achieved with dynamic compression holes. These devices can also be used in reverse to distract the fracture when performing indirect reduction techniques.

Pre-bending

When simple transverse fractures are fixed with compression applied through the plate there is a tendency for the fracture to gap on the opposite side. Placing a small bend in the plate with the apex

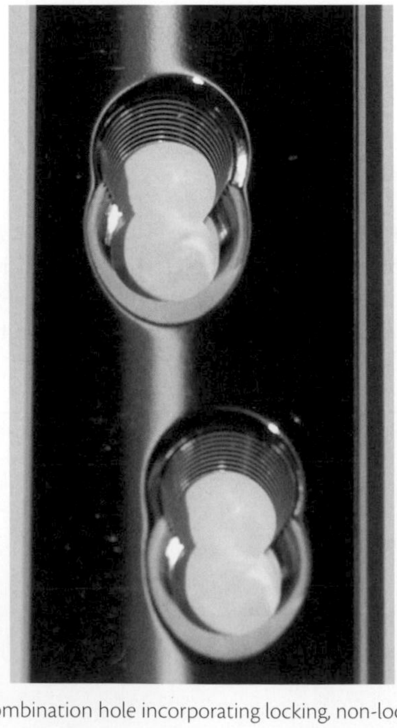

Fig. 12.12.10 Combination hole incorporating locking, non-locking, and compression options.

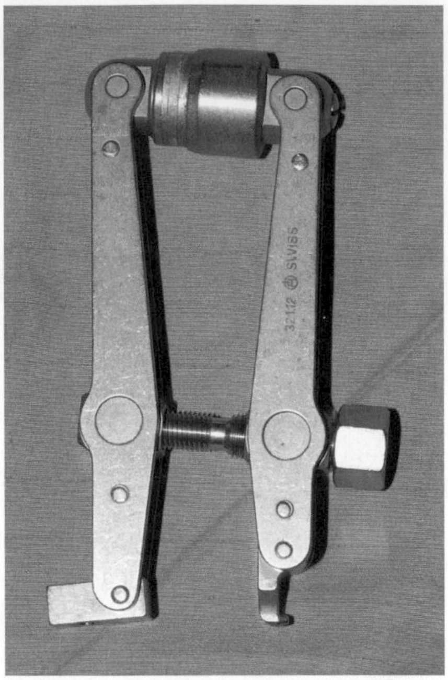

Fig. 12.12.11 Compression device.

at the level of the fracture causes the plate to sit off the bone. When the plate is then compressed down to the bone the elasticity of the plate results in compression of the bone on the opposite side.

Buttress and antiglide

Plates can be applied to resist specific deforming forces. Metaphyseal fracture fragments have characteristic fracture patterns and displacement can be prevented by using plates in a buttress or antiglide mode. Lag screw fixation alone is unlikely to provide sufficient stability to allow early range of motion. Buttress plates prevent displacement away from the axis of the limb in the same way as a buttress used in architecture prevents walls from falling outwards. Antiglide refers to plates used predominantly to prevent displacement in the axis of the limb. Antiglide plates can be used to hold the apex of the fracture as part of a minimally invasive technique that allows both reduction and stabilization using the plate (Figure 12.12.12).

Tension band

Plates can be applied in tension band mode and work in a similar manner to tension band wire constructs by converting tension within the construct into compression at the fracture site. For this method to be effective it requires bony continuity at the fracture site and a predominantly asymmetric load. This is best illustrated in the femur where the lateral cortex is in tension and the medial cortex is in compression. A plate applied to the lateral side will resist tension and facilitate compression of the fracture site.

Bridge plate

In complex multifragmentary fractures it may be impossible or undesirable to attempt to reconstruct the multifragmentary region of the fracture. Direct reduction, anatomical fixation, and absolute stability would necessitate further soft tissue stripping and runs the risk of de-vitalizing bone fragments and infection. An alternative method is to use indirect reduction techniques to restore length, axial alignment, and rotation without anatomical reduction at the

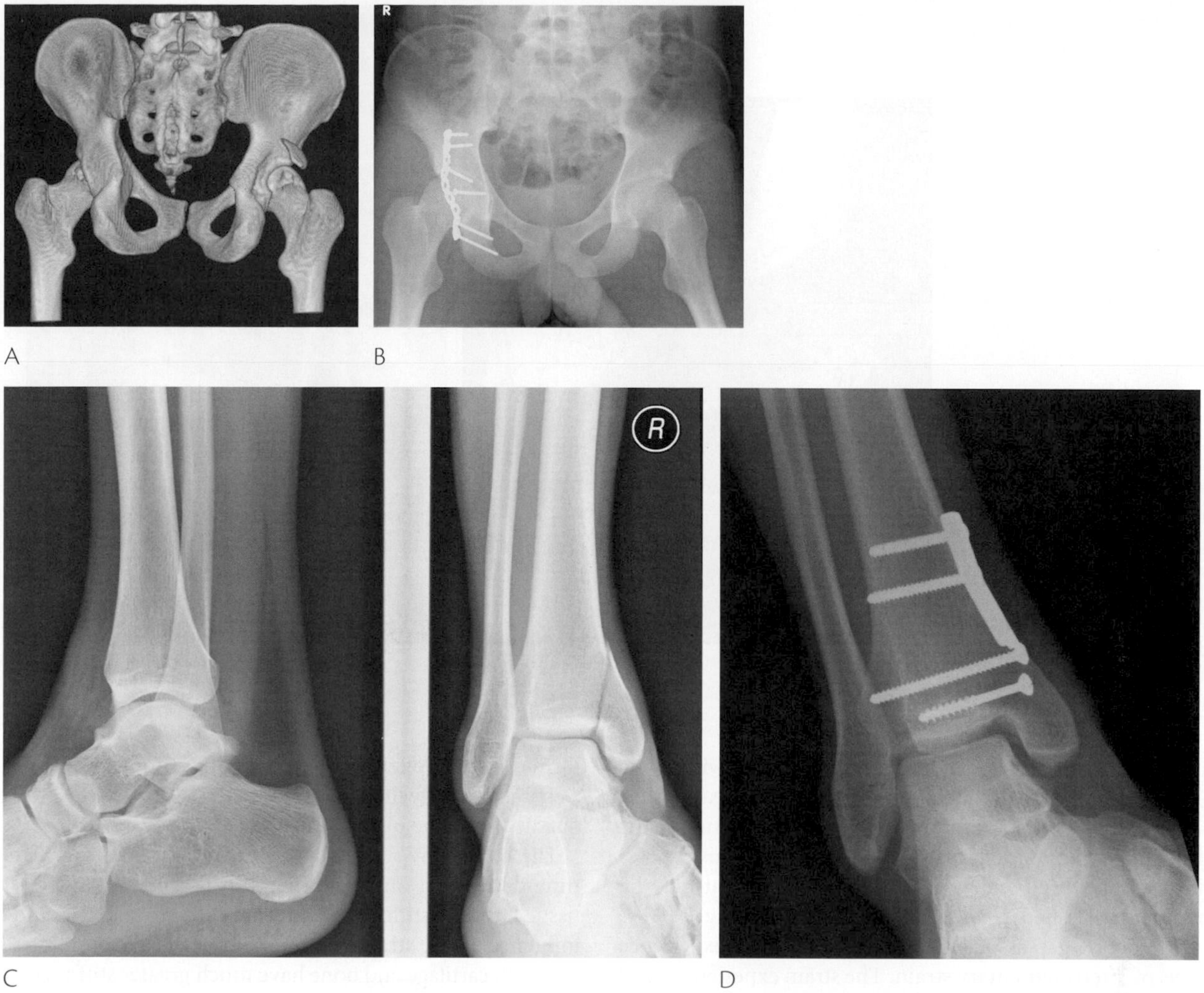

Fig. 12.12.12 A) Posterior acetabular wall fracture, B) stabilized with lag screws and buttress plate. C) Medial malleolus fracture, D) reduced and stabilized with percutaneous antiglide plate and lag screws.

fracture site. The plate functions as a load-bearing device until sufficient fracture healing has occurred.

Rationale of plate and screw fixation

When using a plate, consideration must be given to the mechanical environment that is being created at the fracture site. Bone healing is a complex process involving a multitude of biological and mechanical factors. Following the inflammatory phase, granulation tissue is formed within the fracture site, later this is then accompanied by the differentiation of cells into chondroblasts and osteoblasts producing hyaline cartilage and woven bone respectively. Lamellar bone eventually replaces hyaline cartilage by endochondral ossification and woven bone by bone substitution.

The tissue that forms within a fracture site is dependent on the mechanical environment, and in particular strain. Strain is a measurement of deformation and is reported as a percentage derived from the change in length divided by the original length (strain = $\Delta L/L$). Although not definitive, Perren's interfragmentary strain theory helps to explain the mechanics of fracture healing and how strain relates to plate fixation. Interfragmentary strain is influenced by both dynamic fracture displacement and fracture gap. The theory states that the strain experienced at the fracture gap determines the tissue that can form within the fracture gap. This is dependent on both the induction and tolerance of tissue within the fracture gap. The optimum strain range lies between that which is capable of inducing tissue formation, but below the threshold resulting in tissue disruption. Elongation strain below 2% is tolerated by lamellar bone and elongation strain below 10% is tolerated by cartilage and woven bone. Granulation tissue is more resilient and can tolerate elongation strains up to 100%. When strain is greater than 10% bone cannot form and resorption is the predominant process.

The strain experienced within an intact bone under physiological loading is very small (<1%). This is the optimum mechanical environment for the formation of lamellar bone and is seen to occur continuously as part of the remodelling process. Haversian osteones travel along the axis of the bone with osteoclast 'cutting cones' removing bone and osteoblasts laying down bone. The stability achieved by fixation using interfragmentary compression produces a strain environment, at the fracture site, which approximates bone. No resorption occurs and the 'cutting cones' are seen

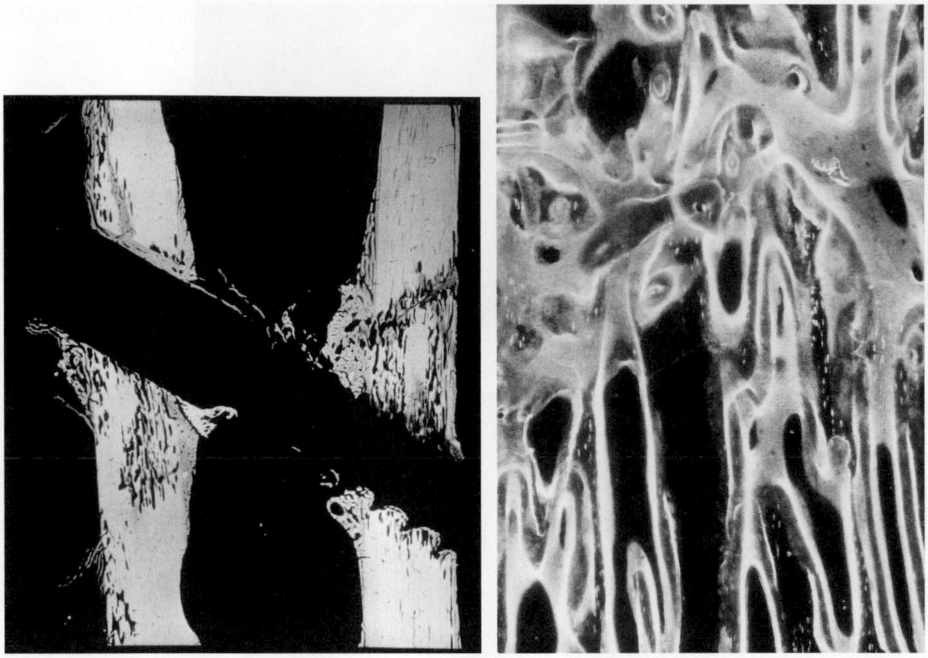

A B

Fig. 12.12.13 A) Microradiograph of a histological demonstrating an oblique osteotomy that was stabilized with a lag screw and neutralization plate. B) Magnified histological cut at the osteotomy site demonstrating Haversian remodelling.

to cross the fracture (Figure 12.12.13). Small defects within the fracture that are supported by neighbouring contact areas do not compromise stability and therefore will experience similar low interfragmentary strain allowing direct bone healing. This process is described as *primary bone healing* without callus but may be more accurately described as bone healing by remodelling.

A residual fracture gap associated with instability will experience higher levels of interfragmentary strain. The strain experienced will be dependent on many factors: physiological load, mechanical properties of fixation, fracture gap, and the position within the fracture relative to the fixation and fracture gap.

Small fracture gaps subjected to even small amounts of displacement will experience very high levels of strain preventing the formation of bone or cartilage and potentially resulting in bone resorption. This is the mechanism for resorption around loose implants. Poor technique will fail to provide a tight interface between the bone and screw, micromotion will create high strain environment within the interface resulting in resorption and further loosening. The proximal cortex is particularly important in non-locked constructs as movement perpendicular to the axis of the screw will cause the screw to 'toggle' around a fulcrum provided by the screw's fixation in the distal cortex. When the drill holes are being prepared care should be taken to avoid thermonecrosis as this will both compromise the bone–screw interface and increase the risk of infection. Thermal necrosis can be avoided by the use of a sharp, clean drill bit operating at the ideal speed and without undue pressure. The drill bit should be cleaned after drilling each hole.

Larger fracture gaps subjected to the same displacement will experience lower levels of strain and have the potential to facilitate the formation of hyaline cartilage and woven bone. Very low strain levels will not induce callus formation. Peripheral tissue will experience less strain as deformation is distributed over a greater volume of tissue. Fractures treated with non-rigid stabilization first form callus peripherally, in an area of optimum strain, resulting in a characteristic fusiform appearance. This is also seen to occur frequently in bridge plate constructs (Figure 12.12.14).

The strain environment within the fracture site changes with time depending on the stiffness of the new tissue. Granulation tissue has little stiffness, contributes little to stability, and has little influence on the strain environment of the surrounding tissues. In contrast, cartilage and bone have much greater stiffness and as they form they will reduce the strain experienced by the surrounding tissues. The reduction in strain has the potential to allow more cartilage and woven bone to form in a centripetal direction. Once the fracture is stabilized with mature callus it can then be replaced and remodelled by lamellar bone.

The orthopaedic trauma surgeon must harness these processes to successfully treat fractures with plates. Both the biology of the fracture and the strain environment must be optimized using a fixation technique that will maintain mechanical integrity until fracture healing is achieved. The technique will fail if the optimum strain lies outside the fracture haematoma, there is insufficient vascularity or the fixation fails prematurely.

The construct stiffness is one of the few factors that is directly controllable by the surgeon. Stiffer constructs can be created by fracture reduction, using larger implants and shorter working lengths. The physiologic loading can be controlled to a limited extent by the post operative regime.

Secondary bone healing with callus occurs with fixation that achieves *relative stability*. The effect of both the injury and open reduction on the soft tissues of complex diaphyseal fractures makes indirect restoration of mechanical alignment and fixation using relative stability techniques appealing. The strain is kept low as displacement is shared across multiple fracture lines with significant fracture gaps. It is not uncommon for these complex fractures to unite and consolidate resulting in a residual non-union of a simple fracture pattern. This problem can then be relatively easily resolved

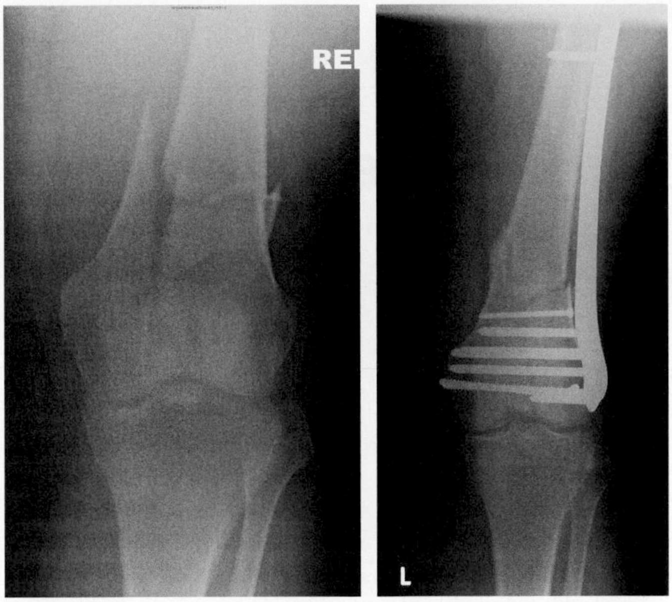

A B

Fig. 12.12.14 A) Intra-articular distal femur treated with reconstruction of the metaphyseal block and bridge fixation of the supracondylar fracture. The strain environment changes depending on the position relative to the plate and size of fracture gap. B) Fracture united with medial callus bridge, no significant bone healing adjacent to the plate.

by revising the plate construct to create absolute stability at this residual fracture site.

When a fracture is reduced and fixed anatomically with interfragmentary compression, the rigid construct created is mechanically similar to an intact bone and is described as having *absolute stability*. Absolute stability is desirable for treatment of both articular fragments and simple diaphyseal fracture configurations (Type A). In both cases restoration of alignment, to achieve a congruent joint surface or a mechanically aligned limb may result in a small fracture gap with the potential for high strain at the fracture site unless absolute stability is achieved. This is best accomplished with interfragmentary compression. Simple diaphyseal fractures can be managed with relative stability only if a sufficient fracture gap is maintained and elastic fixation techniques are used.

With early osteosynthesis techniques, emphasis was placed on anatomical reduction with open techniques, direct reduction, and absolute stability. This had the potential to adversely affect the biology by devascularizing bone fragments. Minimally invasive plate osteosynthesis (MIPO) techniques have been developed to minimize disruption of the soft tissues and fracture site. These techniques use image intensification and specific implants that allow restoration of alignment, relative stability, and bone healing through callus formation. These implants are designed to produce a more elastic fracture fixation construct that can be used for bridging and optimizes induction of callus. Consideration should be given to leaving a long enough working length between the screws on either side of the fracture to minimize the risk of plate breakage.

It is important to appreciate that, although technically more challenging, the advantages of MIPO techniques and implants can also be used to achieve anatomical reduction and absolute stability. Under these circumstances the plate can be used to utilize other modes of plate fixation (neutralization, compression, buttress, antiglide) in combination or isolation. It is the fracture configuration and soft tissues that determine the plate fixation technique, *not* the implant.

Complications specifically related to plate-screw fixation

- Infection:
  - Thermonecrosis
  - Necrosis under plate
  - Soft tissue stripping
- Screw failure:
  - Stripped threads—poor technique
  - Thermonecrosis
- Plate breakage:
  - Stress risers (e.g. short working length)
  - Poor choice of technique
  - Inadequate implant size
  - Non-union
- Non-union:
  - Mechanical—poor choice of technique
  - Biological—devascularization.

Further reading

Perren, S. (1979). Physical and biological aspects of fracture healing with special reference to internal fixation. *Clinical Orthopaedics and Related Research*, **138**, 175–96.

Perren, S. (2002). Evolution of the internal fixation of long bone fractures: The scientific basis of biological internal fixation. *Journal of Bone and Joint Surgery*, **84B**, 1093–110.

Rüedi, T.P., Buckley, R.E., and Moran, C.G. (eds) (2007). *AO Principles of Fracture Management*, Volumes 1 and 2. New York: Thieme.

12.13

Principles of intramedullary nailing

David Noyes and John McMaster

Summary points

- Intramedullary nailing provides the trauma surgeon with a biologic solution to the stabilization of both simple and complex long bone fractures
- An appreciation of the biomechanics and the technical difficulties is essential.

Introduction

The term intramedullary nail is used to describe a group of implants that are placed within the medullary canal of a long bone. Intramedullary nails form a construct with the bone and act to resist deformity. Nails may be used to prevent fractures, control fractures acutely, or in post-trauma reconstruction. Intramedullary nailing is the treatment of choice for many diaphyseal fractures and modern nail design has extended their application to include some metaphyseal fractures.

It is over a century since the first descriptions of intramedullary nailing. The technique was refined and popularized by the German surgeon Kuntscher who inserted his first femoral nail in 1939. He also introduced intramedullary reaming and, shortly before his death, described an implant that was the forerunner of the interlocking nail. It was Herzog who, in 1950, first introduced tibial nailing after bending the proximal part of a nail. Intramedullary nailing was further popularized through the 1970s and 1980s and has now become an indispensable tool for the orthopaedic surgeon.

Today, various flexible nailing systems are available with a wide range of applications, especially in the immature skeleton.

Definitions

Nails may be either solid or hollow. The latter are designed to be introduced over a guide wire. Hollow nails were traditionally open section (slotted) but are now more commonly closed section. Both solid and hollow nails have holes proximal and distal to allow the insertion of interlocking bolts. These bolts greatly increase construct stability by resisting torsional and axial forces. In the proximal femur, many nails provide an option to interlock by inserting a screw obliquely into the femoral head. These so-called 'cephalomedullary' nails are useful in the treatment of subtrochanteric fractures or ipsilateral neck and shaft fractures.

Interlocking may either be static or dynamic. Static locking provides a fixed relationship between the nail and the proximal and distal portions of the bone. Dynamic locking is produced via an elongated interlocking hole within the nail that allows axial compression while maintaining torsional stability.

Basic science

Biomechanics

The intramedullary nail and bone form a composite structure that is subject to load. The mechanical characteristics of this composite depend on the characteristics of the nail as well as the quality and integrity of the bone. The implant is central in the bone, close to the mechanical axis of the limb, which means it is optimally positioned to resist bending forces.

Intramedullary nails do not, nor are they intended to, abolish movement at the fracture site. This motion stimulates callus formation that bridges the fracture, gradually assuming more of the load and reducing stress upon the implant. The nail and interlocking bolts must be sufficiently durable to survive until fracture healing occurs. If, however, they are excessively rigid they will inhibit the stimuli required for fracture healing.

The strength of an intramedullary nail is a property of its cross-sectional geometry and the implant material. The rigidity of a cylindrical intramedullary nail in bending and torsion is proportional to the fourth power of the radius. Therefore, for a given amount of material, the further the material is distributed from the bending or torsional axis, the stiffer the structure becomes.

Producing a slot in a hollow nail reduces torsional strength by two-thirds, with little effect on the bending stiffness. The slot provides the nail with some radial flexibility, which decreases hoop stresses during insertion and increases contact area between the bone and implant after insertion.

Intramedullary nails are usually made of stainless steel or titanium alloys. The lower modulus of elasticity of titanium alloys has the theoretical advantage of less stress shielding of the bone, but no differences in healing or complication rates have been demonstrated. The geometry of the nail, specifically the diameter and wall thickness, are more significant factors for fracture healing.

The working length of a nail is the distance between the proximal and distal points of secure fixation to bone. With small-diameter interlocking nails without diaphyseal fit, this is usually the distance between the interlocking screws (Figure 12.13.1). The torsional rigidity of an implant is inversely proportional to the working length, and the bending rigidity is inversely proportional to the square of the working length.

Fatigue fracture is the usual mode of failure for intramedullary nails. Failure is usually associated with delayed or non-union, particularly in unstable fracture patterns where the bone contributes little to the overall construct. Nail design is an important factor that relates to the frequency of nail breakage. Defects in fabrication may also contribute to breakage. Smaller interlocking bolts used with smaller nails are more prone to fatigue failure. In studies examining interlocking intramedullary nailing in tibial fractures, smaller nails inserted without reaming had a higher rate of interlocking bolt failure. This problem is attributed to the size of locking bolt, and is not exclusive to unreamed tibial nails. Locking bolts used in 8- or 9-mm tibial nails are significantly weaker than the bolts used in femoral nails and larger tibial nails (≥10mm). Laboratory testing has shown that the number of cycles to fatigue failure of a 5-mm bolt would be expected to be more than 20 times greater than for a 4-mm bolt.

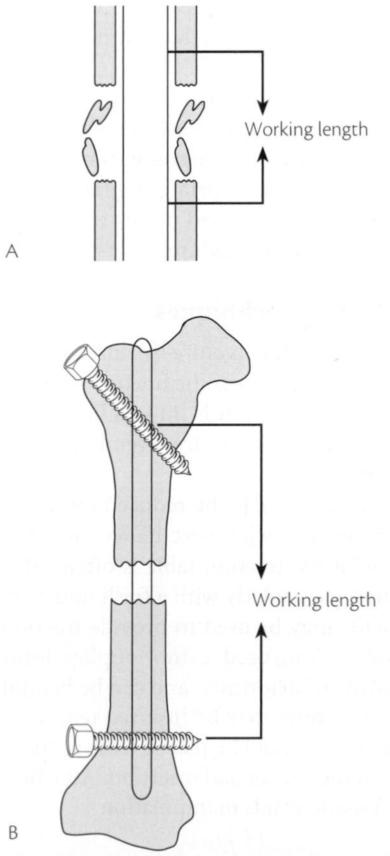

Fig. 12.13.1 (A) The working length of a tight-fitting nail is between points of secure cortical contact in the proximal and distal fragment. (B) In a small-diameter loose-fitting nail the working length is between the proximal and distal interlocking screws. Both the torsional and bending stiffness of the nail bone composite are inversely related to the working length.

Box 12.13.1 Positive influences upon nail–bone construct strength and durability

- Simple fracture pattern—reduced
- Implant close to mechanical axis of bone
- Larger diameter nail
- Short working length
- Non-slotted nail
- Larger locking bolts (5mm).

Reaming

Reaming of the medullary canal was first employed by Kuntscher to provide a better contact area between the nail and bone, thus improving the construct's stability. Interlocking bolts and smaller diameter nails can now provide much of this stability, but there are several other advantages to reaming. After reaming, a larger diameter nail can be passed with less chance of nail incarceration, fracture propagation, and implant failure. The morselized bone formed by reaming may also stimulate fracture healing.

Concerns about both the systemic and local effects of reaming have led some to advocate the use of unreamed nails. The pressure and abrasion from a reamer destroys medullary contents and acts as a piston, displacing medullary contents both locally and systemically. Reaming has, therefore, been implicated in fat embolism syndrome, respiratory distress syndrome, and multisystem organ failure. Recent studies have failed to confirm this link. Locally, reaming damages the endosteal blood supply, but, when compared to unreamed nailing, no ill effects have been demonstrated.

The arterial supply to the diaphyses of long bones is from the nutrient, metaphyseal, and periosteal arteries. The venous drainage of bone consists of thin-walled vessels running in the centre of the medullary cavity. The central two-thirds of the diaphyseal cortex receives its blood supply from the high-pressure endosteal circulation, and the outer third of the cortex is supplied by the low-pressure periosteal system. Cortical blood flow is, therefore, centrifugal. The direction of blood flow is reversed after a fracture, resulting from suppression of the intramedullary flow and increased vascularity of the periosteum.

Reaming damages the nutrient arterial circulation, but the clinical significance of this damage is uncertain. The periosteal circulation is only able to supply only the outer one-third of the cortex. Necrosis of the inner two-thirds of the cortex has been demonstrated in animals following reaming. A rapid regeneration of the nutrient system has been demonstrated with loose-fitting nails. Where the nail directly contacts the cortex, osteoclasts must remove necrotic bone to create a channel for vessels. At 12 weeks, the restoration of endosteal circulation is complete. The extent of revascularization varies and is influenced by the extent of original damage. Revascularization is facilitated by vessels, originating from the surrounding soft tissues, which traverse the external callus to reach the necrotic cortex. After reaming, there is an early periosteal vascular proliferation and hyperaemia, which is associated with periosteal new bone formation.

In an effort to reduce problems associated with reaming, some thought has gone into designing a new generation of reamer.

Box 12.13.2 Advantages and disadvantages of reaming

- Advantages:
  - Increased contact area between nail and bone:
    - —Shorter working length
    - —More rigid construct
  - Allows the use of larger diameter nails
  - Morselized bone acts as autograft
- Disadvantages:
  - Detrimental effects on endosteal blood supply
  - Concerns regarding systemic effects of displaced marrow contents.

The RIA (Reamer Irrigator Aspirator, Synthes) is a tool that irrigates while reaming, simultaneously aspirating the resulting mix of reamings and fluid. The RIA is a single-use instrument, with a steep cutting angle, designed to ream to the required diameter in a single pass, thus reducing operative time. The intramedullary pressures while reaming are significantly reduced, and throughout much of the process are negative. A reduction in local heat generation has also been demonstrated. Overall the RIA seeks to reduce the physiological impact of reaming both locally and systemically. The RIA is also useful for canal debridement after infected nail removal and harvesting bone graft from the femoral canal.

Indications

Intramedullary nailing is ideally suited to treating diaphyseal fractures, particularly in the femur and tibia. Nailing provides good stability via a minimally invasive technique, minimizing soft tissue disruption in the zone of injury. Avoiding further damage to the tissues surrounding the fracture site enhances revascularization and aids early bridging callus formation. The strength of the bone–nail construct will often allow for early weight bearing, accelerating rehabilitation.

Statically locked reamed intramedullary nailing is the treatment of choice for diaphyseal fractures of the femur. Reamed intramedullary nailing is the treatment of choice for displaced tibial shaft fractures and can safely be performed in all but the most severe open fractures. Locked intramedullary nailing of the humerus is indicated in patients with pathological fractures, otherwise open reduction and plate fixation is the preferable operative fracture treatment.

Other indications for intramedullary nailing include fixation of subtrochanteric, pertrochanteric, or supracondylar femur fractures, stabilization of arthrodeses, and as a guide for bone transport. Intramedullary nails are also indicated for fracture prophylaxis with metastatic bone tumours, and for tumour-like conditions, e.g. fibrous dysplasia.

Flexible nailing

Small diameter devices such as Ender's nails were traditionally used multiply to fill the medullary canal or were pre-bent to provide three-point fixation. These devices did not perform well in adult long bones, especially the femur and tibia, as they did not provide sufficient stability for healing.

Elastic or flexible nailing systems are now very much the preserve of paediatric long-bone fractures. These nails are bent prior to their insertion and are used in opposing pairs. When appropriately placed, the elastic recoil of these nails provides adequate internal splintage to permit fracture healing in the aforementioned bones.

This technique is further discussed in the Paediatric Trauma section (Section 14).

Operative technique

Patient positioning

In order to successfully place an intramedullary nail, patient positioning in the operating room is vitally important. Starting and interlocking points must be accessible, fractures reducible, and importantly all parts of the bone exposable to image intensifier.

The starting point is the where the nail first enters the bone and must be considered when positioning the patient. The point may be on-axis, such as the piriformis fossa for many anterograde femoral nails. Alternatively an off-axis starting point may be necessary, e.g. tibial nail, or desirable, e.g. trochanteric starting point femoral nail. Off-axis starting points increase forces required for insertion and may deform the fracture particularly if it is close to the starting point.

Limbs may be placed on traction or left free; both techniques have their pros and cons. The obese patient may provide difficulties; particularly with anterograde femoral nail insertion. Preoperative planning, appropriate implant selection and attention to the previously mentioned points will contribute greatly to the overall success of the procedure.

Fracture reduction techniques

It is desirable to reduce the fracture by closed means before passing a guide wire or solid nail across the fracture under image guidance. Sometimes fracture reduction is impossible by closed means and open nailing is indicated. There are several methods that may assist in closed reduction.

Tibial fractures can usually be reduced by closed manipulation and held, if necessary, with percutaneously applied reduction clamps. The use of the traction table is often sufficient to reduce femoral fractures, particularly with a fresh injury. Alternatively the femoral distractor may be used to provide traction and maintain reduction. The seldom-used F-tool applies indirect two-point forces, in the plane of deformity, and can be helpful in completing reduction. Shanz screws may be inserted temporarily to aid fracture reduction. They should be placed close to the fracture site and be unicortical on the side of nail insertion. Attachment of a universal chuck and T-handle aids manipulation.

Angulation control

Intramedullary nails are only well suited to reducing diaphyseal fractures. Diaphyseal-metaphyseal junction fractures are prone to predictable angular deformity with nailing. There is a tendency for oblique fractures to displace giving the appearance of the nail

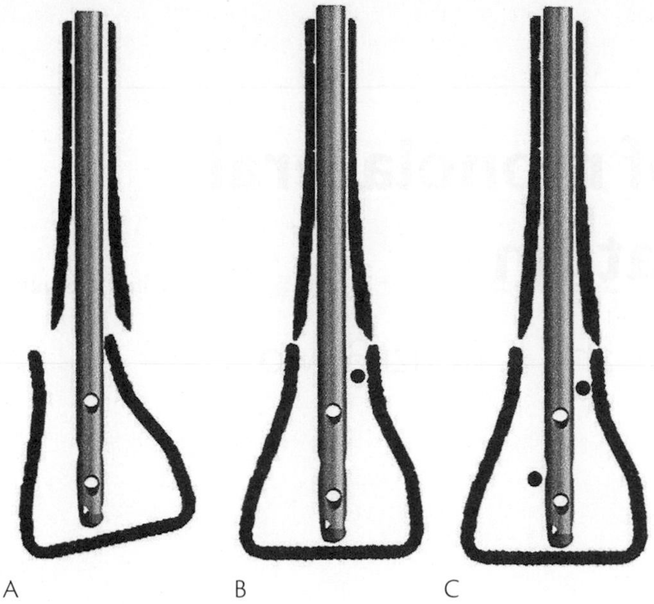

Fig. 12.13.2 The placement of a single blocking screw on the concave side of the deformity allows the nail to reduce the metaphyseal fragment (B). If the nail tip is not secure, a second contralateral blocking screw, in combination with diaphyseal fit, produces three-point fixation (C).

exiting the proximal fragment early and entering the distal fragment late. For successful fixation of these fractures the nail must be centralized within the short segment, using the correct entry point and ensuring appropriate nail tip position. Transmedullary blocking or 'Poller' screws may be used in conjunction with intramedullary nails to control this deformity. These screws can effectively extend the tight fit of the diaphysis and control the relationship between bone and nail. A single screw placed in the metaphyseal segment on the concave side of the deformity will allow the nail to reduce that deformity (Figure 12.13.2). The screw forms a third point of fixation together with the nail tip or entry point, and the point of diaphyseal contact. If there is insufficient anchorage of the nail tip then a second blocking screw is inserted contralaterally to the first.

Malreduction

Rotational malreduction is one of the most common problems to go undetected in the operating room. In one study 28% of patients who had undergone femoral nailing, in a high volume trauma unit, had a residual rotational deformity of greater than 15 degrees as determined by computed tomograhpy scan. These patients were also more likely to have ongoing functional problems.

Box 12.13.3 Adjuncts for fracture reduction when nailing

- Traction:
  - Whole limb—traction table or manual
  - Segmental, e.g. femoral distractor
- Externally applied pressure:
  - F-tool
  - Assistant
- Indirect invasive, e.g. Shanz pins
- Open reduction
- Image intensifier, e.g. avoiding rotational malreduction.

Clinical assessment or 'eyeballing' is not particularly sensitive and other techniques may need to be employed. Accurate assessment of rotation requires direct comparison with the normal limb. When performing intramedullary nailing without a traction table, it may be useful to prepare, and leave uncovered, the unaffected limb to allow this comparison. In the femur, radiological signs can be used to avoid malrotation. A comparison of lesser trochanter profiles with the patella facing anteriorly can be used before final locking. A less sensitive sign of malrotation is a sudden change of shaft diameter or cortical thickness on fluoroscopy. Changes may, however, be quite subtle, particularly in areas with a more rounded cross-section.

Further reading

Jaarsma, R.L., Pakvis, D.F., Verdonschot, N., Biert, J., and van Kampen, A. (2004). Rotational malalignment after intramedullary nailing of femoral fractures. *Journal of Orthopaedic Trauma*, **18**(7), 403–9.

Rüedi, T.P., Buckley, R.E., and Moran, C.G. (eds) (2007). *AO Principles of Fracture Management*, Volumes 1 and 2. New York: Thieme.

Stedtfeld, H.W., Mittmeier, T., Landgraf, P., and Ewert, A. (2004). The logic and clinical applications of blocking screws. *Journal of Bone and Joint Surgery*, **86A**(Suppl 2), 17–25.

The Study to Prospectively Evaluate Reamed Intramedullary Nails in Patients with Tibial Fractures (SPRINT) Investigators (2008). Randomized trial of reamed and unreamed intramedullary nailing of tibial shaft fractures. *Journal of Bone and Joint Surgery*, **90A**, 2567–78.

Wolinsky, P., Tejwani, N., Richmond, J.H., Koval, K.J., Egol, K., Stephen, D.J. (2001). Controversies in intramedullary nailing of femoral shaft fractures. *Journal of Bone and Joint Surgery*, **83A**, 1404–15.

12.14

Principles of monolateral external fixation

F. Lavini, C. Dall'Oca, and L. Renzi Brivio

Description

Monolateral external fixation is a system for the stabilization, reduction, and manipulation of bone segments by means of bone anchorage consisting of pins fastened to an external frame. Monolateral external fixators in their various forms have the advantage that they allow the use of half-pins (bicortical pins that do not penetrate both sides of the soft tissue envelope), thereby avoiding major damage to the neurovascular structures contralateral to the insertion point. The simple structure of monolateral systems permits rapid application and simplified preoperative planning, both of which are features particularly appreciated in traumatology.

The external construct may present different configurations according to the type of fixator used or the application for which it is designed (Box 12.14.1).

We can distinguish between two major types of monolateral fixators: *one-plane monolateral fixators* (Figure 12.14.1) in which clusters of pins are placed practically in the same plane, and *two-plane monolateral fixators* (Figure 12.14.2) in which pin clusters are placed in different planes and joined by the frame in two planes.

Monolateral fixators can also be differentiated on the basis of how the pins are connected to the frame. *Simple fixators* (Figure 12.14.3) have independent articulations which connect each pin with a rigid longitudinal rod, and *clamp fixators* (Figure 12.14.4) have pin clusters connected to a clamp which introduces the option of adjustments between the clamp and fixator body.

In addition, external fixators can be subdivided into *static fixators* and *dynamic fixators* on the basis of their intrinsic dynamization capability. This characteristic will be considered in the section on the biology of healing.

Box 12.14.1 Types of monolateral external fixation

- One plane versus two plane
- Simple versus clamp
- Static versus dynamic.

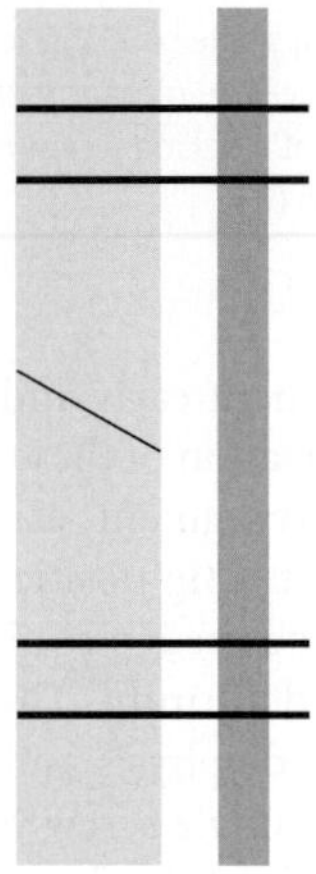

Fig. 12.14.1 Diagram of a one-plane monolateral fixator.

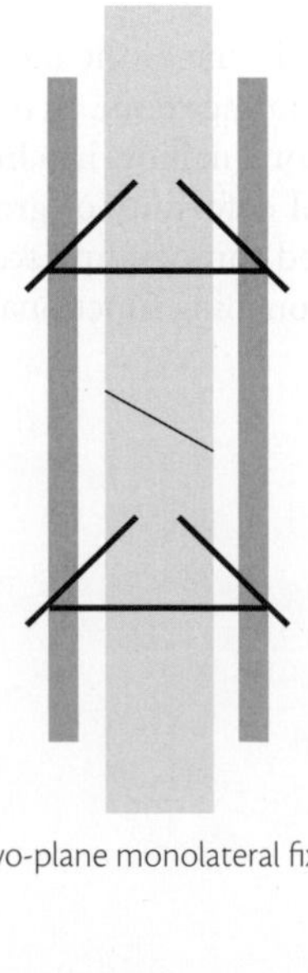

Fig. 12.14.2 Diagram of a two-plane monolateral fixator.

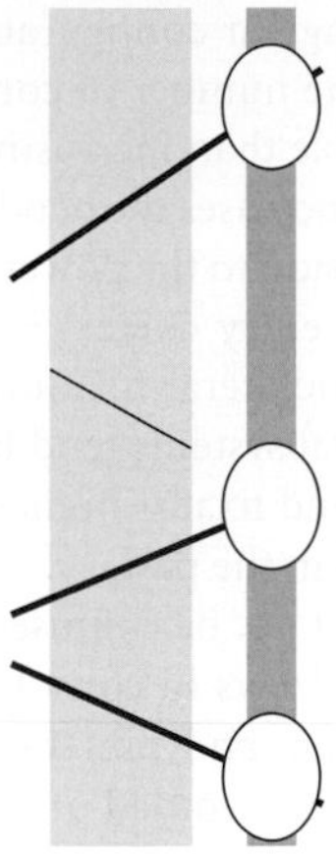

Fig. 12.14.3 Diagram of a simple fixator.

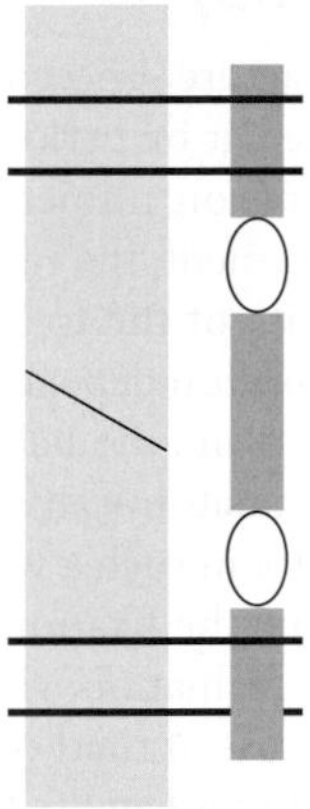

Fig. 12.14.4 Diagram of a clamp fixator.

Simple fixators have the distinct advantage that each pin can be placed at a different angle in relation to the fixator rod, and that the distance between two pins in a bony fragment can be freely chosen in relation to the soft tissue lesion and depending on the mechanical needs of the frame bone construct. A disadvantage is the need for reduction of the fracture prior to fixator application and the fact that external manipulation manoeuvres, particularly rotation, can only be performed by replacing one or more pins.

Advantages of clamp fixators are that they allow fracture reduction after the fixator has been applied and that subsequent adjustments can be performed fairly easily by loosening the universal articulations between the fixator body and the clamps. Disadvantages are the need to resort to supplementary external systems whenever gradual multiplanar adjustments are required; pin cluster placement and spread are strictly dictated by the clamp configuration.

Mechanics (Box 12.14.2)

The basic elements to be considered in the mechanics of a monolateral fixation system are as follows:

- Pins
- Wires
- Bone–fixator distance

Box 12.14.2 Mechanics of monolateral external fixation

- Screws:
  - Larger screws are stronger but weaken bone
  - Tapered conical screws gradually increase preload
  - Number of screws increases stability
  - Predrill screw holes to reduce thermal necrosis
  - Hydroxyapatite may enhance bone purchase
- Bone fixation distance—increased bone–fixator distance reduces stability
- Stability bone and fixator fastener—screw–body junction is weak point
- Geometry of frame—stability may enhance healing but too much rigidity may inhibit it.

- Stability of the bone–fixator fastening system
- Frame geometry. Nowadays, the barrier between monolateral and circular fixator is no more so rigid, due to the use of so called hybrid fixators that combine pins and transfixing wires joined by monolateral and circular frame. These are particularly useful in periarticular fractures in order to take advantage of the transfixing wires in the metaphysis and of the pins in the diaphysis
- Frame material. Radiolucent materials improves visualization of fracture reduction and healing. The mechanical properties have been tested mechanically and clinically and have shown stiffness characteristics comparable to the fixators currently employed.

The pins play the most important role in the stability of the entire system. When assessing the ideal type of pin, the following parameters must be considered:

- Pin diameter
- Number of pins
- Type of thread
- Pin insertion technique
- Pin material
- Pin coating.

The *pin diameter* must be such as to minimize the risk of breakage at the pin entry point. At the same time the pin must possess a sufficient degree of stiffness to ensure adequate implant stability. A pin hole greater than 30% of the diameter of the bone results in a 45% reduction in the torsional strength of the bone. The bending stiffness of the pin increases as a function of its radius by the power of four. If we know the diameter of the bone, the thickness of the cortex, the elastic modulus of the bone, the number of pins to be applied, the elastic modulus of the pin material, and the load applied, we can calculate the minimum pin diameter allowed in order to obtain a stable implant in relation to different bone–fixator distances.

In adult bone, a pin of diameter 6mm enables this requirement to be satisfied for bone–fixator distances up to 6cm, while maintaining the specific pressure at the entry cortex below one-third of the tensile strength of the bone tissue.

The load distribution in a monolateral implant is asymmetric, being greater at the entry cortex than at the exit cortex. For this reason a tapered conical pin can be employed and proves particularly useful. The taper ratio produces a gradual increase in radial preload. Pin–bone contact is optimized and the micromovements typical of a straight cylindrical pin inserted in a predrilled hole are avoided.

Increasing the *number of pins* leads to an increase in implant stability, as does spreading the pins across the bony segment. Maximal stability for a construct with two pins per segment occurs when one pin is close to the fracture site and one is as far away as possible. With a sufficiently rigid frame two or, at most, three pins per fracture segment will be enough to ensure adequate stability regardless of their spread.

The *type of pin thread* is determined by the shape, pitch, and pitch height. Various types of pins with different morphological characteristics are commercially available. The pin design must make allowance for the quality of the bone to which the pin is applied, with different designs being necessary for cancellous and cortical bone. The pitch vertex angle and the curvature radius at the base of the pin will have an effect on the insertion torque and thus on the temperature generated during pin insertion.

The *pin insertion technique* influences the bone–pin interface and thus the stability of the entire system over time. The use of self-drilling pins is associated with microfractures (particularly in cortical bone) and with the development of temperatures above 50°C which may cause thermal necrosis. Pre-drilling using very sharp drills minimizes thermal necrosis and bone damage, allowing the use of self-tapping conical pins which afford optimal bone purchase in that each thread cuts its own path as the pin advances. The advantage of such pins consists in their easy removal, often in the outpatient clinic, while the disadvantage is related to the fact that they cannot be backed out, even partially, without complete loss of bone purchase.

The pins must be made of biocompatible *material* and have substantial stiffness, making the use of stainless steel preferable. Titanium pins have been shown to be more elastic and this reduces pin loosening.

Pin coating with hydroxyapatite improves bone purchase by providing a better pin–bone interface. This reduces pin loosening and pin tract infection. They are recommended in implants applied for a long time and osteoporotic bone.

As the *bone–fixator distance* increases, implant stability decreases. This must always be borne in mind when deciding on the number of pins to be used and the initial weight-bearing load that the patient is to be allowed. In particular, in applications at the femoral level, the number of pins applied per fracture segment needs to be increased and the patient allowed to bear only a partial load for the first 2–4 weeks.

The weakest part of any system is the *junction* between the fixator body and the clamp, or directly between the fixator body and the pins. Here, one needs to know the mechanical yield characteristics of these elements through adequate information which should be provided by the manufacturers. In order to avoid secondary fracture displacements, the yield point of each system must be established in relation to the clinical bone–fixator distance, the load applied, and the fracture conditions.

The stability of simple and/or clamp fixators can be enhanced by increasing the number of pins or external rods. An example of this may be the delta or triangular configurations that can be created. In practice, increasing the number of components is less effective and clinically less desirable than increasing the size of the individual components, which increases the bending stiffness to the power of 4 and resistance to torsion to the power of 3. A greater pin diameter, particularly in the entry cortex, is also known to enhance implant stability in monolateral fixation. For these reasons, the latest types of monolateral systems tend have larger pin diameters and to use conical pins and fixator bodies of fairly large size compared with the rods used in the past.

However, stability must not be confused with rigidity, which is a condition which causes delays in consolidation, pseudoarthrosis, increased screw loosening, and pin-tract infections. Excessively rigid constructs should be avoided and the latest generation of stable fixators should incorporate fracture-stimulation systems such as dynamization.

Biology (Box 12.14.3)

The natural healing of a fracture proceeds through the well-known phases of inflammation, repair by periosteal callus formation, and remodelling, which depend on numerous variables such as the degree of soft tissue involvement, the reduction obtained, the type of fracture and the stability of the fixation. The type of healing obtainable with external fixation depends on the mechanical characteristics of the device used and the stability of the implant.

In a transverse fracture anatomically reduced and fixed with a rigid external fixation device in such a way that the weight-bearing forces are fully absorbed by the fixation system, healing is of the direct type, without callus formation, via a biological process akin to that associated with the use of rigid compression plates. Direct-type or contact healing requires lengthy time periods to restore the mechanical stability of the bony segment.

When an external fixator has been applied it is always necessary to consider the behaviour of the pin–bone interface, which deteriorates over time, in relation to the healing process. Thus the type of healing that should be achieved by external fixation must be of the periosteal type, as occurs without rigid fixation, which is quicker and stronger. It is only in this way that consolidation can be achieved in a relatively short period of time, which is essential for minimizing the most feared complications of external fixation such as pin loosening and pin-tract infection which in turn result in instability of the bone frame construct and may be a possible cause of pseudoarthrosis.

The conditions necessary for achieving periosteal healing with external fixation are as follows:

- Sparing of the soft tissues at the fracture site
- Adequate reduction
- Transmitting controlled micromovements to the fracture site.

Box 12.14.3 Biology of healing

Healing is enhanced by:

- Sparing fracture site
- Adequate reduction
- Micromotion at fracture site.

Sparing the fracture site can be achieved by placing the pins at an adequate distance from the fracture site (at least 1.5cm) and by seeking preferably a closed reduction solely by means of external manipulation of the segments. It has been demonstrated that the combination of external fixation with internal fixation with interfragmentary lag screws at diaphyseal levels to contain and reduce segmental fractures leads to an increased incidence of pseudoarthrosis. This is related to the different types of repair biology which the two systems create: interfragmentary—direct healing; external fixation—periosteal healing.

The reduction must be adequate and avoid large gaps which may indicate interposition of soft tissues, and axial alignment must be accurate. However, the reduction does not have to be anatomical where interfragmentary movements might be inhibited.

Micromovements are of fundamental importance for the development of the periosteal callus and distinctions need to be made in terms of quality, extent, and time of application. In this sense we can distinguish between static and dynamic fixators.

Lastly, from the biological standpoint, external fixation allows formation of new bone starting from an osteotomy or fracture site, when a gradual progressive distraction force of varying proportions depending to the bone response is applied. Distraction induces bone formation with an intramembranous-type ossification when the frame is stable; the newly formed bone eventually becomes mature and normally corticalized. This characteristic of bone repair under distraction can be exploited to remedy limb discrepancies and loss of bony substance as well as to perform gradual angular adjustments.

Dynamization (Box 12.14.4)

The term *dynamization* indicates converting a static fixation into a fixation which allows the passage of forces and/or the possibility of stimulating the fracture site with controlled micro movements. In a monolateral fixation, dynamization may be of three types:

- Passive
- Active
- Induced.

Passive dynamization is achieved when the fixator is placed in a static configuration and the patient applies a load to the limb in such a way as to exert a significant force (usually above 200N). In this case the micro movements are cyclic and are applied in an asymmetric manner on the fracture callus through the bending of the pins, which, in modern monolateral fixators, are the most elastic elements in the entire frame. In the long run, this type of dynamization will lead to asymmetric callus formation, thereby facilitating pseudoarthrosis (Figure 12.14.5).

Active dynamization is achieved by releasing the telescopic slides on the bodies of fixators possessing these features, hence the term

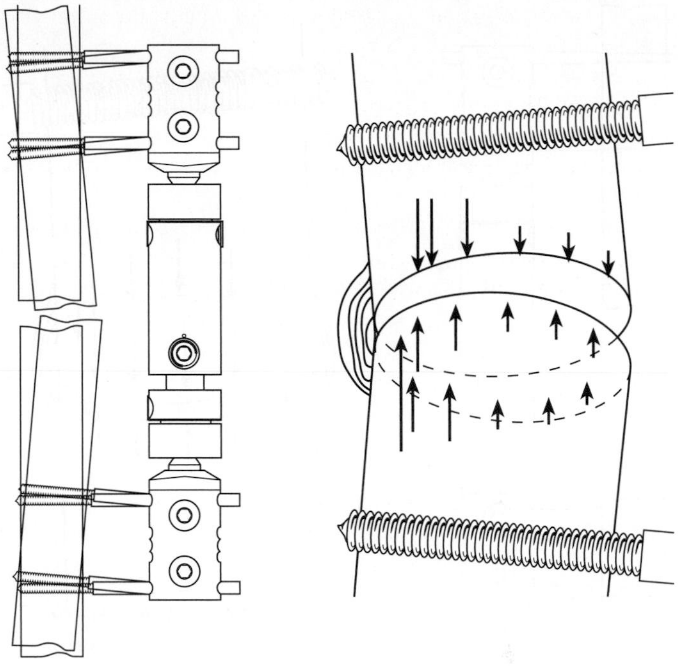

Fig. 12.14.5 Passive dynamization induces asymmetric stimulation of callus formation, thereby facilitating pseudarthrosis.

dynamic fixators (Figure 12.14.6). When bearing weight or applying a load, the patient brings about the progressive closure of the fracture gap; tissue stimulation is of the concentric type and is conducted mainly along the longitudinal axis of the telescopic element, which at the time of assembly must lie parallel to the main axis of the bony segment. This kind of dynamization may be of the free or controlled type. In the latter case, the fixator is equipped with systems which limit the excursion capability of the telesystem and at the same time provide for an elastic recoil after the loading phase.

It has been demonstrated that when all of the fixator joints were allowed to adjust simultaneously during dynamization, exact axial movement or uniform compression at a complicated fracture site was achievable. This study revealed that significant non-axial movements may occur during dynamization, and that such a deficiency can be corrected by relaxing certain fixator joints in addition to the sliding mechanism. The same modelling technique can also be applied in bone lengthening application to assure desirable limb alignment during the distraction process. These analysis results can aid the performance assessment of an external fixator and facilitate appropriate application of such a device to achieve either active or controlled axial movement.

Induced dynamization may be manual or mechanical and is applied according to known quantities and frequencies via external actuators. Kenwright *and colleagues* applied this type of controlled mechanical stimulation to tibial fractures, starting with a 1-mm movement at 0.5Hz for 30min daily a week after application of the fixator until a load of at least 200N was reached by ambulation. The patient group submitted to dynamization healed earlier than a control group treated with static fixation.

Induced dynamization can also be applied manually, with micromovements induced from the first week after surgery with the

Box 12.14.4 Dynamization of fixator

- Passive—asymmetrical by screw bending
- Active—telescopic slides
- Induced—manual or mechanical.

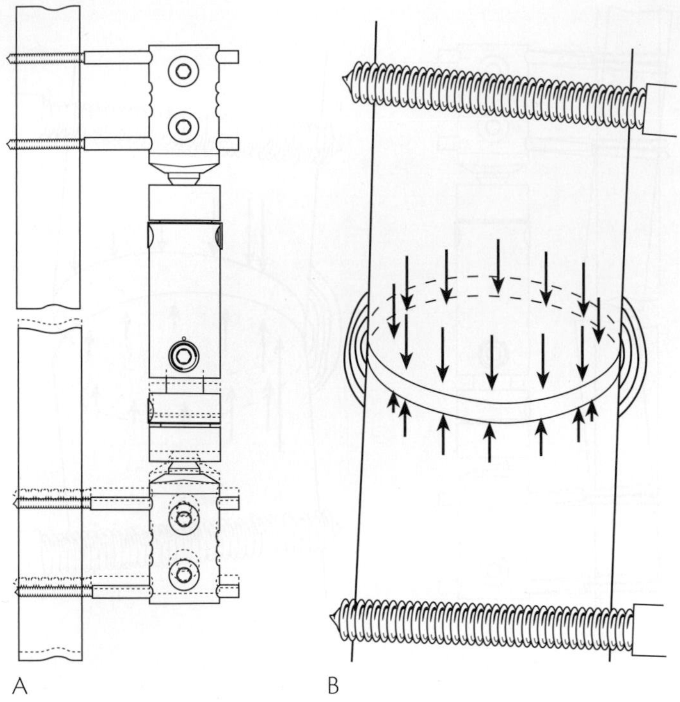

Fig. 12.14.6 Active dynamization allows symmetric stimulation of callus formation.

purpose of achieving early stimulation of callus formation even in bedbound patients or patients incapable of bearing weight on the limb.

The biological effects of dynamization have been demonstrated in a number of studies.

Indications and outcomes

From the anatomical standpoint monolateral fixation presents no limitations and as a result of the versatility and apparent simplicity of application it may be regarded as indicated for most traumatic or orthopaedic injuries.

In practice, however, it is necessary to define the limitations related to considerations of a mechanical nature, such as the stability of the fixation construct, the durability of the pin–bone interface, complications directly associated with external fixation, biological and clinical considerations, such as patient tolerance and the quality of the bone tissue or of the adjacent soft tissues, and the feasibility of adequate patient surveillance in the outpatient setting.

Therefore it is useful to define relative *contraindications* to external fixation (Box 12.14.5):

- Obesity
- Pronounced osteoporosis
- Psychological and emotional instability
- Impossibility of obtaining satisfactory patient compliance, particularly in terms of adequate scrupulous attention to loading rules, pin care, and regular attendance of scheduled ambulatory checkups.

There are also a number of relative contraindications related to the bony segment treated. Application of a fixator to the femur

Box 12.14.5 Contraindications to monolateral external fixation (relative)

- Obesity
- Osteoporosis
- Psychological or emotional instability
- Poor compliance.

entails crossing soft tissues of such thickness as to create a bone–fixator distance which makes the fixation construct comparatively less stable than in other segments and leads to more serious extension–flexion disorders of the knee.

The *indications* for external fixation in traumatology are as follows:

- Open fractures
- Complex closed fractures
- Fractures in multiply traumatized patients
- Pelvic fractures
- Complex joint fractures.

In orthopaedic surgery, monolateral fixation is used in the following cases:

- Lengthening
- Pseudoarthrosis
- Corrective osteotomies
- Reconstruction surgery for substance loss.

Open fractures (Box 12.14.6)

Monolateral fixation affords definitive treatment of open fractures. The systems currently employed achieve optimal stability, and frame stiffness can be adjusted over time to adapt to biological needs.

The prognosis of an open fracture depends mainly on the degree of soft tissue injury, the extent of the bone comminution, and the degree of bacterial contamination. Immediate stabilization of the bone lesion, administration of adequate broad-spectrum antibiotic prophylaxis (it is mandatory to perform a bacteriology specimen at the beginning of the debridement and at the end of the procedure in order to assess the pathogenic flora and adjust the antibiotic therapy), elimination of necrotic tissue with repeated debridements, and subsequent coverage of bone by replacing soft tissue substance losses as quickly as possible are necessary to optimize results.

Box 12.14.6 Open fractures

- Monolateral fixations allow stabilization, repeated debridement, and soft tissue coverage
- Healing rate >90%
- Malunion rate <5%
- 5% pseudoarthrosis.

These manoeuvres are facilitated by the use of monolateral external fixators. Stability is achieved without interference at the fracture site. In particular, it is of paramount importance that the fracture be adequately reduced. A partial load is permitted as soon as the patient's general condition allows and the soft tissue lesions are healing. Further fracture callus stimulation is subsequently applied by dynamization. A stable dynamizable monolateral external fixation should be generally regarded as a definitive form of treatment and not merely as a form of temporary stabilization.

Reports have demonstrated the possibility of achieving a healing rate of more than 90% with a malunion rate of less than 5% by the use of monolateral fixators. One study reported the outcomes of 101 open tibial fractures treated with axial dynamic fixators, including 63 grade III fractures, with pseudoarthrosis occurring in five cases and infection in six.

Recently there is a tendency to perform a temporary stabilization by external fixation in deep soft tissues lesions. After thorough care of the local damage, when there is evidence of recovery of the external mantle and absence of contamination, the external fixation, used for bony stabilization, can be substituted by internal synthesis as a definitive treatment. This is used following the principles of 'local damage orthopaedics' and it is intended to minimize the incidence of osteomyelitis and infected non-union. For this reason, the conversion must be performed only when the earlier mentioned conditions are contemporarily present, unless external fixation can be used as a definitive method of treatment.

Complex closed fractures

In diaphyseal open fractures of the lower extremity, an alternative treatment to monolateral external fixation is intramedullary nailing, which has a decreased rate of angular malunion. External fixation should be favoured when there is greater contamination or more severe soft tissue injury (Figure 12.14.7).

A monolateral external fixator allows rapid closed reduction which enables the surgeon to limit operative time and blood loss. This is useful in those patients with multiple trauma or at anaesthetic risk. Therefore this group of patients can be treated with external fixation even if the type of fracture would lend itself to other methods.

Femoral fractures in patients during growth, especially in multiple trauma, may be treated with external fixation. Other indications include unstable fractures, such as proximal-third fractures, and complex metaphyseal fractures, particularly those associated with a high-grade soft tissue injury.

Fractures in multiply traumatized patients (Box 12.14.7)

The multiply traumatized patient, particularly when simultaneously presenting with a thoracic or cranial trauma, requires early stabilization of the long bones in order to reduce the risk of acute respiratory distress syndrome (ARDS), to decrease time in the intensive care unit, and to decrease the period of ventilatory support.

If the stabilization is performed within 24h, the incidence of ARDS is 7%, compared with 39% if more than 24h has elapsed. However, certain injury combinations may preclude lengthy internal fixation procedures.

External fixation in its monolateral form allows early stabilization with closed reduction, minimal blood loss, and short operative times compatible with the severity of the associated lesions.

Box 12.14.7 The use of monolateral external fixation in multiple trauma

- Minimal blood loss and operating time
- Conversion to internal fixation only in first 2 weeks
- Early micromovement is essential.

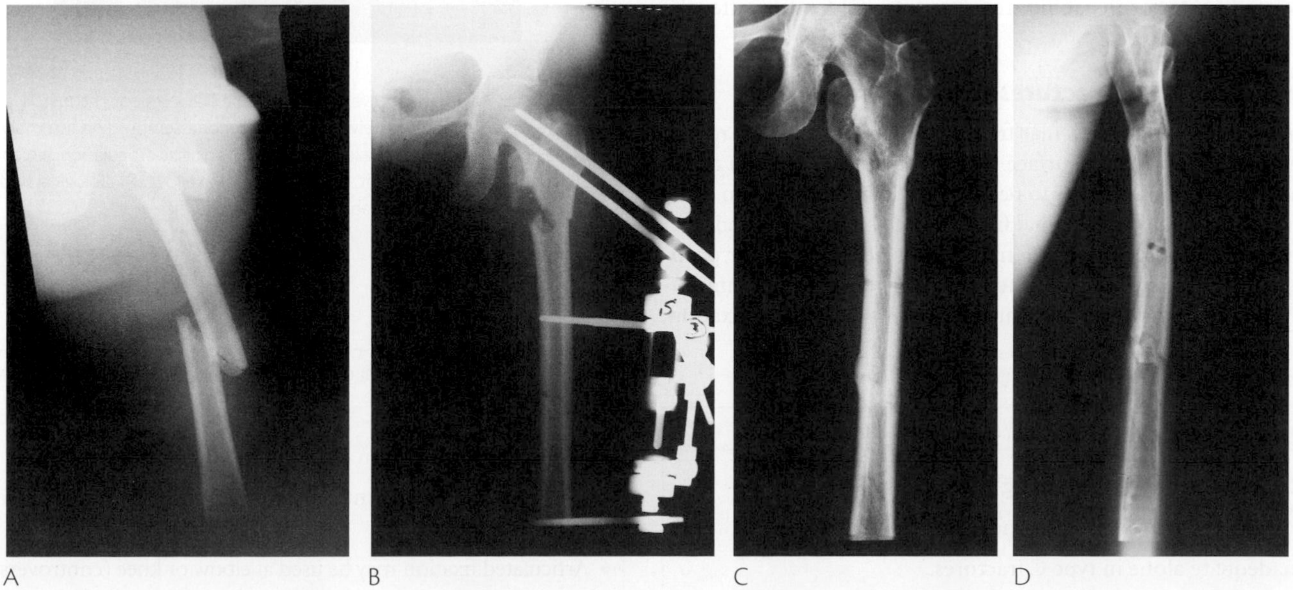

Fig. 12.14.7 Bifocal subtrochanteric metadiaphyseal fracture of the femur in a polytraumatized patient undergoing emergency treatment with open external synthesis. The clinical course was favourable with good callus formation and the possibility of removing the external fixator 18 months postoperatively.

The benefits of early stabilization are achieved with minimal surgical result.

If external fixation is chosen in the acute period for long-bone stabilization, it is necessary to decide whether the external fixation needs to be kept in place until healing is achieved or whether there is scope for replacement with intramedullary nailing so as to reduce pin-tract problems, increase fixation stability, and afford a better range of movement. Replacement operations must be decided on the basis of the type of fracture (periarticular fractures prove difficult to treat with intramedullary nailing) and the patient's general condition. Conversion from external to internal fixation should be done within 2 weeks of frame application to reduce the risk of osteomyelitis.

A definitive stable monolateral external fixator with a system for micromovement and subsequent dynamization is an alternative to internal fixation. Micromovement is necessary in the non-ambulant patient to ensure an adequate healing rate.

Pelvic fractures (Box 12.14.8)

The stabilization of unstable pelvic fractures in both the horizontal and vertical planes by external fixation is part of the surgeon's resuscitative armamentarium. Continuous blood loss and the resulting difficult haemodynamic compensation can be decreased by means of early stabilization with external fixation (Figure 12.14.8).

The retroperitoneal space can contain as much as 900–1000mL of blood which can collect in a very short period of time. External fixation can decrease pelvic volume and control motion which results in a reduction in mortality rates.

Pin insertion is possible either at the iliac crest level or below the anterior inferior iliac spine. In the former case, pin application is percutaneous, whereas in the latter it is open owing to the presence of the lateral femoral cutaneous nerve of the thigh. From the biomechanical point of view it is advisable to choose the anterior application in order to have a better grip of the pin–bone interface due to the thickness of the ileum in the area of insertion and a suitable mechanical performance of the frame in the horizontal plane. Associated posterior instability requires internal fixation after the patient stabilizes.

Complex articular fractures (Box 12.14.9)

The ideal treatment of articular fractures entails anatomical reconstruction of the articular surface and adequate stabilization of the meta-epiphyseal lesion so as to permit early rehabilitation. In complex articular fractures, external fixation may be used as an adjunct to obtaining these goals. These fractures present two major problems, namely articular incongruence and metaphyseal comminution. The metaphysis can be treated by means of external fixation,

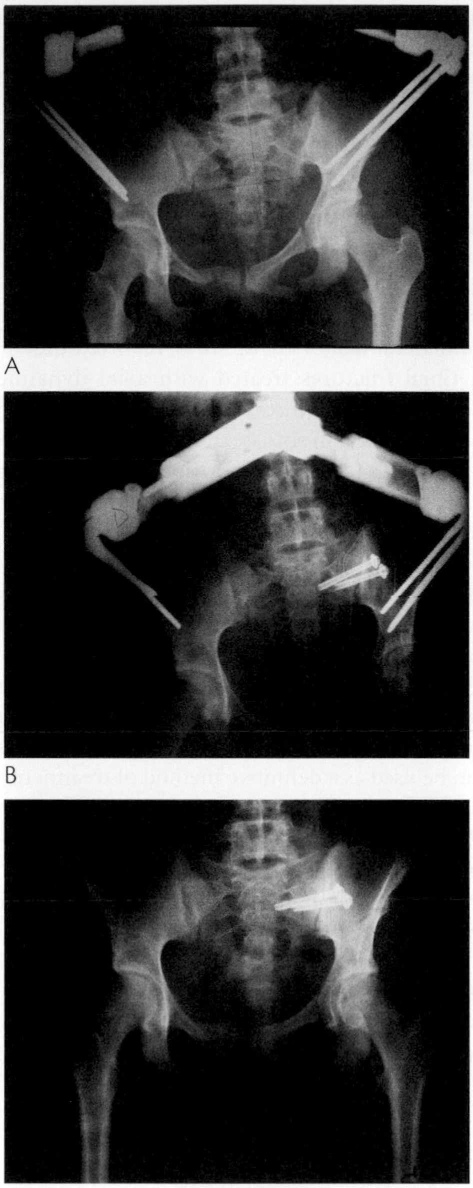

A

B

C

Fig. 12.14.8 Horizontally and vertically unstable pelvic lesion. The first manoeuvre is to stabilize the pelvis with an anterior assembly. This assembly is unable to ensure stability at the level of the left sacroiliac articulation, which is stabilized later when the patient's general condition allows. Radiological findings 3 months after surgery show stability of the pelvic girdle.

Box 12.14.8 Pelvic fractures and external fixation

- Reduced mortality if bleeding is severe
- May be used in isolation in most type B fractures
- Inadequate alone in type C fractures.

Box 12.14.9 Monolateral external fixation and complex articular fractures

- Monolateral frame can be used as temporary stabilizer
- Can reconstruct joint with percutaneous or minimally invasive fixation
- Articulated fixation may be used at elbow or knee (controversial).

which enables adequate alignment and good stability to be achieved. The treatment of articular incongruence is facilitated by the presence of the fixator distracting across the joint. The articular reconstruction is then obtained with an adjunctive percutaneous (closed reduction external fixation, CREF) or open minimal internal fixation (limited open external fixation, LOREF). In this case the open approach necessary for articular reduction is limited, stripping of periosteum is reduced, and the use of metallic elements is minimized, thus decreasing the risk of the serious complications, such as pseudarthrosis and infection, associated with wide open approach.

Most monolateral external fixators used for articular fractures are spanning fixators, i.e. they cross the involved joint. The external fixator is applied in distraction, utilizing ligamentotaxis with gripping elements placed at a considerable distance from the fracture site. Limited internal fixation of the articular surface is then applied secondarily. The external fixator may also serve as a tool for the definitive fixation of the articular lesion without additional internal fixation, when the reduction obtained is satisfactory, or when a 'biological' approach to the treatment of such lesions is adopted from the outset. Less commonly, the metaphyseal fracture may be treated by placing the monolateral fixator on the same side of the joint. This technique is useful in less comminuted cases, and has been utilized for the distal radius and proximal tibia (Figure 12.14.9).

These principles can be applied in various areas, such as the elbow, wrist, knee, or ankle. Experience with modern fixators spanning the elbow and fixing in the humerus and ulna, appears to be encouraging. A hinge articulated at the rotation axis of the elbow allows early mobilization of the joint, thus reducing the incidence of joint stiffness, which is a frequent and serious complication. This procedure appears to be particularly indicated for open or severely comminuted fractures. Furthermore it has been proved that a condition of fracture–dislocation is well addressed by the use of stable internal fixation to treat the bony lesions and an articulated fixator in order to achieve stability and to allow early motion while the ligaments are repairing. Ideally the fixator should be maintained for a period of 6 weeks.

Specific articular fractures

Numerically, the greatest indication for monolateral fixation in traumatology is for fractures of the distal radius using a spanning fixator with or without limited internal fixation. Occasional extra-articular distal radius fractures are amenable to fixation on the same side of the joint.

The following principles must be applied in external fixation of the wrist:

- Fixation of the second metacarpal only with half-pins
- Fixation of the radius, avoiding lesions to the superficial branch of the radial nerve (avoid percutaneous application)
- Reduction, avoiding excessive distraction and excessive ulnar deviation (a neutral position is preferable)
- Compare intraoperative trays with normal side for indication and length
- Bone graft or bone substitutes if there is comminution or shortening
- Reduction fixation is required with an intra-articular step-off
- If unstable, adjunctive fixation or reconstruction of the distal radioulnar joint
- Early mobilization of the fingers to facilitate rehabilitation.

The role of joint mobilization via articulated fixators for the wrist is still controversial. Prospective studies have demonstrated that with the Pennig dynamic external fixator there are no differences between the dynamized and the static group.

Similar principles apply to the treatment of intra-articular fractures of the knee. Complex fractures with meta-epiphyseal comminution or major involvement of soft tissues benefit most from external fixation. Knee stiffness is avoided by limiting transarticular external fixation to 40–50 days (Figure 12.14.10).

Twenty-one complex fractures of the tibial plateau were treated with closed reduction, application of a monolateral fixator, and fixation of the articular fragments. A range of movement of 115 degrees in 19 of the 21 fractures was reported, and the authors concluded that this procedure yields satisfactory outcomes. In this series most cases were treated with the external fixator on the tibia only, not spanning the knee joint.

High-energy fractures of the tibial plafond are a frequent indication for spanning external fixation. Pins can be applied across the ankle joint using an articulated clamp along the rotation axis of the tibiotalar joint. Release of this articulation at 3–4 weeks helps rehabilitation of the joint. The technique is safe and effective, and significantly decreases the treatment-related complications when compared with internal fixation with plates and screws.

Recent studies have demonstrated that the use of circular fixator for high-energy bicondylar tibial plateau fractures have marginal benefits over the use of plates and significant reduction of infections.

Lengthening (Box 12.14.10)

External fixation is a means not only of achieving stabilization and healing of fractures, but also of subjecting bony segments to gradual progressive distraction of an osteotomy area so as to obtain bone-segment lengthening.

The basic prerequisites for achieving such results are stability of the lengthening device and respect for the biological conditions which allow new bone formation, such as sparing of the periosteum, adequate waiting time prior to distraction, and customized distraction in relation to individual osteogenic capabilities.

Equally important is the preoperative patient assessment in order to minimize or prevent possible complications.

The joints adjacent to the segment to be lengthened must be stable and display normal functional capacity. Any muscular contracture must be evaluated in order to avoid aggravating it during lengthening. If necessary, tenotomies must be planned at the time of the first operation or to resolve unresponsive contractures during surgery. The amount of distraction possible must be assessed so as to plan a lengthening in one or more stages. In particular, congenital diseases are more prone to complications related to difficult muscle and tendon extension with the result that lengthenings often need to be done in several stages.

It is equally important to assess the coexistence of associated angular defects in order to be able to plan simultaneous angular

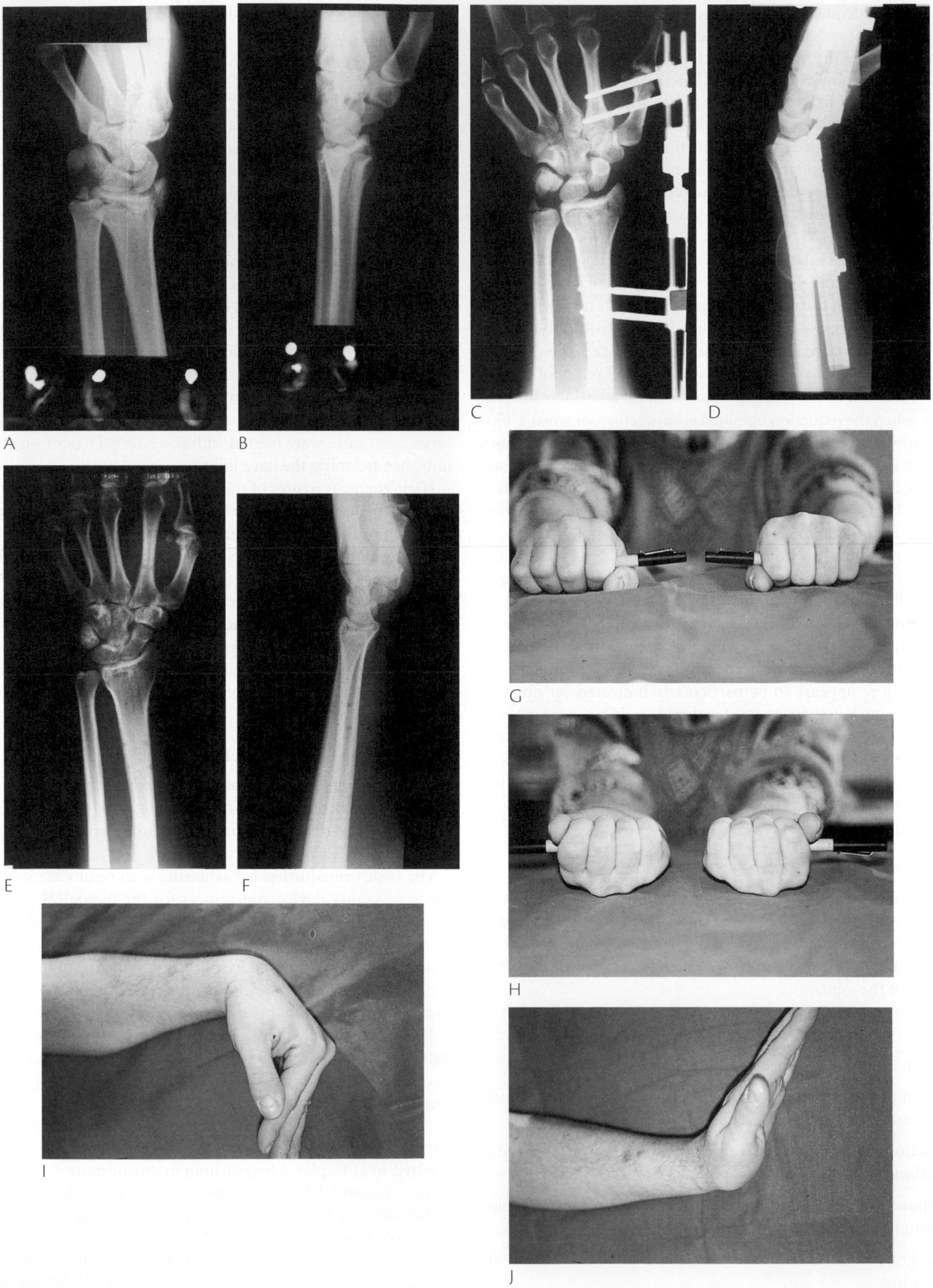

Fig. 12.14.9 Articular fracture of the wrist in a 37-year-old patient treated with an external fixator with ligamentotaxis. The reconstruction of the joint yields an excellent long-term clinical outcome.

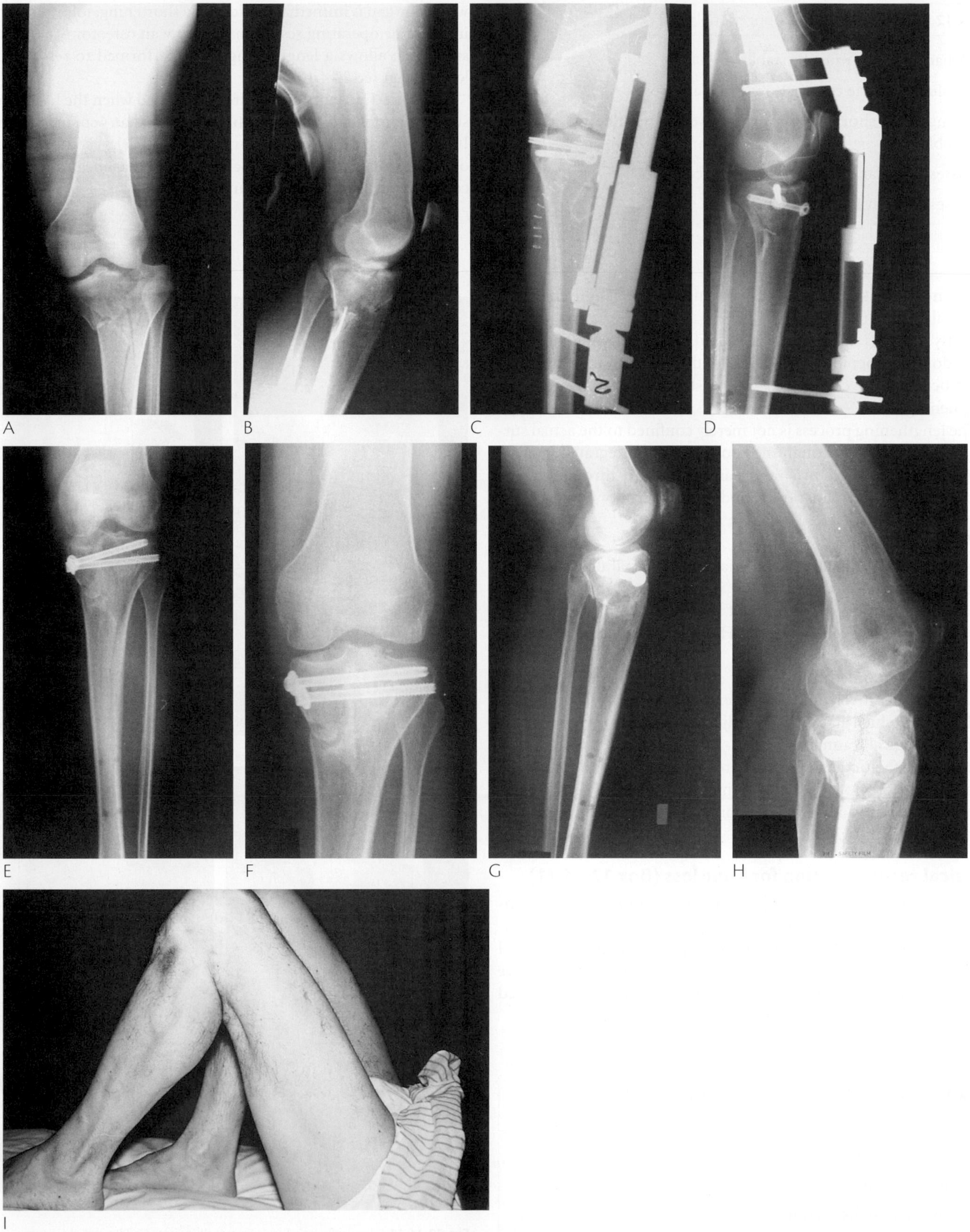

Fig. 12.14.10 High-energy episiodiaphyseal fracture of the proximal tibia. Owing to the epiphyseal comminution, the external stabilization is of the femorotibial bridge type. This is done in conjunction with minimal stabilization for the articular fracture. After 40 days, to allow articulation of the knee and definitive healing of the metaphyseal lesion, the bridge is removed and monosegmental stabilization is performed. Radiological and clinical picture 6 months after removal of the fixator.

Box 12.14.10 Lengthening using monolateral external fixator

- Adjacent joints must be stable
- Evaluate muscle contractures preoperatively
- Congenital shortening more prone to muscle and tendon problems
- Assess angular deformities and correct
- Assess neurovascular function.

adjustments or subsequent adjustments to the lengthening via manipulation of the callus.

Lastly, factors such as bone quality, the possible presence of endocrine–metabolic diseases, and neurovascular function must be carefully considered when establishing indications for lengthening.

The lengthening process is not merely confined to the actual surgery, but requires thorough monitoring by an integrated team of surgeons, physiotherapists, and paramedic staff throughout the distraction and consolidation period until the fixator is removed.

Osteotomy

Osteotomies for adjustment of axial or rotational defects can be stabilized in various ways. Often internal fixation is preferred because of the intrinsic stability of the method and the resulting possibility of early rehabilitation. However, the degree of adjustment has to be precise in order to obtain a good long-term outcome, and sometimes it is not simple to achieve the desired result intraoperatively. In this context, external fixation, especially with fixators which allow gradual adjustments, yields precise results with less surgical trauma.

In osteoarthritic genu varum, precision in realigning the load axis appears to be of fundamental importance for achieving clinically acceptable results in the medium to long term with less surgical trauma (Figure 12.14.11).

Surgical reconstruction for bone loss (Box 12.14.11)

Bone loss can be treated using the principles applied in lengthening. Bone transport may be used where a segment of bone previously osteotomized above or below the gap is gradually transported across the gap to 'dock' against the opposite segment (Figure 12.14.12). Alternatively, a compression–distraction can be used where the gap is immediately closed by shortening, followed, either in the same operating session or later, by an osteotomy at another site which allows a lengthening to be performed to restore limb length (Figure 12.14.13).

The bone-transport procedure is indicated when the loss of substance is more than 4cm in the tibia or more than 6cm in the femur. It is subject to the frequent complication of delayed consolidation or non-consolidation of the docking site, so that an additional procedure is needed to stimulate union.

Box 12.14.11 Surgical reconstruction using monolateral external fixator

For segmental loss (>4–6cm):

- Bone transport
- Compression distraction
- Treatment is lengthy
- Complications are common.

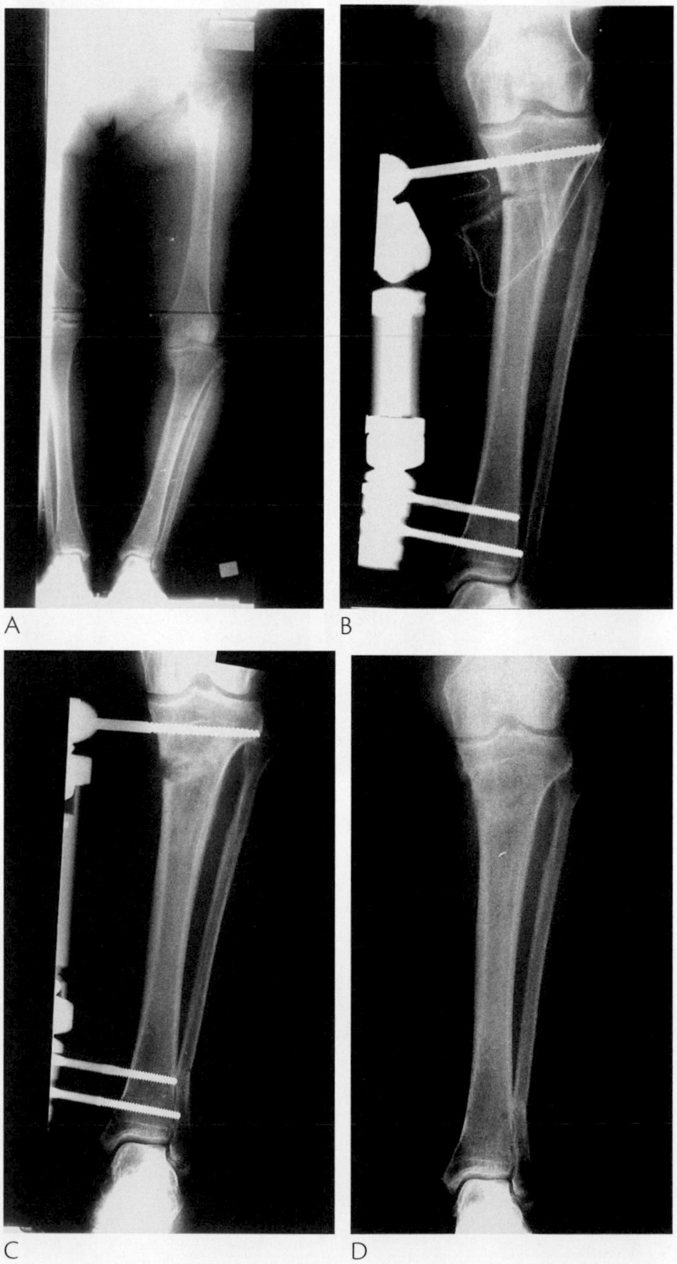

Fig. 12.14.11 Hemicallotasis for proximal tibia vara in a 58-year-old patient. Gradual correction enables adequate femorotibial alignment to be achieved, and the quality of the new bone formation allows lasting maintenance of the result, as demonstrated by follow-up findings 3 years after removal of the fixator.

Compression–distraction allows immediate contact between two viable contact surfaces. If the fracture site is clean and there is no risk of infection for the other sites of the same segment, a lengthening osteotomy can be performed concomitantly in a site which may be proximal or distal to the previously bridged gap. Shortening must not exceed 5cm to avoid vascular or soft tissue problems, although this depends on the characteristics of the injury. The fibula, if intact, should be resected 2cm more than the shortening distance.

The advantage of segment-shortening over bone transport is that it allows consolidation of the contact area without any additional intervention.

When assessing whether such surgical reconstruction is indicated, the surgeon must bear in mind the patient's age, the condition of the soft tissues, neurovascular function, and degree of patient compliance. The treatment is lengthy (on average 40 days per centimetre of gap to be bridged) and complications are common. For this reason, appropriate patient selection is mandatory and patients must be adequately informed and monitored.

The experience of the University of Verona Orthopedic Clinic is based on 38 cases, 15 treated with bone transport and 23 with compression–distraction for substance losses ranging from 3–11cm. All segments healed. The following complications have been reported: 11 (75%) pseudarthroses of the docking site, two axial deviations of 5–10 degrees (with compression–distraction), and seven (18.4%) pin loosening (with reinsertion).

Complications (Box 12.14.12)

The problems and complications relating to external fixation can be avoided or minimized by using scrupulous surgical technique and codified rules for patient follow-up, and having an adequate understanding of mechanics as applied to bone biology.

Problems are defined as mishaps which stand in the way of the realization of a given objective, without jeopardizing the final outcome.

Complications are defined as obstacles to the realization of a given objective which require treatment and may undermine or impair the final outcome.

Box 12.14.12 Complications of external fixation

- Screws:
  - Infection
  - Neurovascular damage
  - Osteolysis
  - Bending or breakage
  - Joint stiffness
- Fixator:
  - Jamming of dynamizable elements
  - Non-union
  - Malunion.

For this reason, we regard as problems only those deriving from minor pin-tract problems (grades 1 and 2 of the Checketts classification), which require improved nursing and closer cooperation between surgeon and patient.

Complications can be classified as follows:

- Complications related to monolateral external fixation
- Complications related to the conditions treated with external fixation.

The latter group are specifically related to the type of trauma or the type of orthopaedic condition treated and will therefore be addressed elsewhere in this book.

Complications due to monolateral external fixation can be further subdivided as follows:

- Complications due to bone-gripping elements
- Complications due to the fixator
- Complications due to contraindications to the use of monolateral external fixation.

Complications due to bone-gripping elements

Complications due to bone-gripping elements are as follows:

- Pin or wire tract infections
- Wire loosening
- Osteolysis
- Bone sequestrum
- Muscular stiffness
- Bending
- Breakage.

Vascular or neurological damage from a pin can be avoided by adequate care in placement. The monolateral system involves the use of pins whose entry point is well controlled and which penetrate only a few millimetres beyond the contralateral exit cortex.

The complications of pin-tract infection, osteolysis, and sequestrum are defined as major pin-tract complications and occur for the following reasons:

- Choice of the wrong type of pin
- Defective insertion technique
- Failure to comply with loading and dynamization indications
- Metal allergy
- Improper pin care.

Choice of pin type

Some systems require different types of pins for cortical bone and cancellous bone. Therefore it is necessary to choose the correct type of pin for the anatomic area to which it is to be applied. The total length of the pin must be based on the thickness of the soft tissues and on the size of the frame to which it is applied so as to allow adequate pin–fixator contact and at the same time care of the pin tracts. The length of the thread will depend on the diameter of the bone and must be selected so as to ensure adequate contact with both bone surfaces. The pin diameter must never exceed

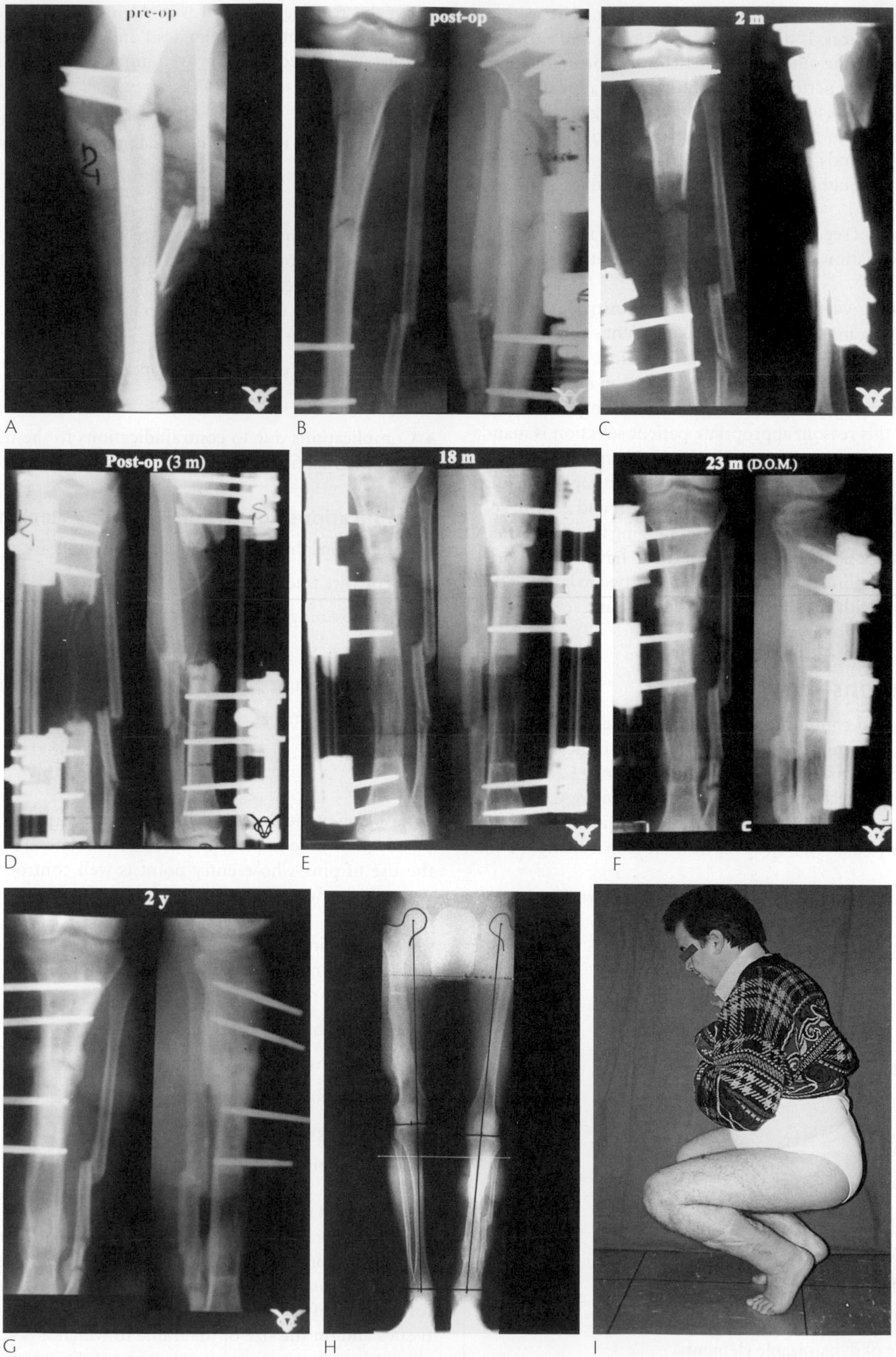

Fig. 12.14.12 Grade IIIB open fracture in a 36-year-old patient. Emergency fixation was followed 8 weeks later by necrosis of the intermediate fragment. For this reason, the necrotic segment was removed and an 11-cm bone transport procedure was commenced in a distal-to-proximal direction. After 18 months the transport was completed. After 23 months, the lengthening site was consolidated, but pseudoarthrosis of the docking site was found, requiring an additional osteomuscular decortication. Healing was achieved in this patient 2 years postoperatively. Follow-up 3 years after healing shows good function and an appropriate mechanical axis of the lower limbs.

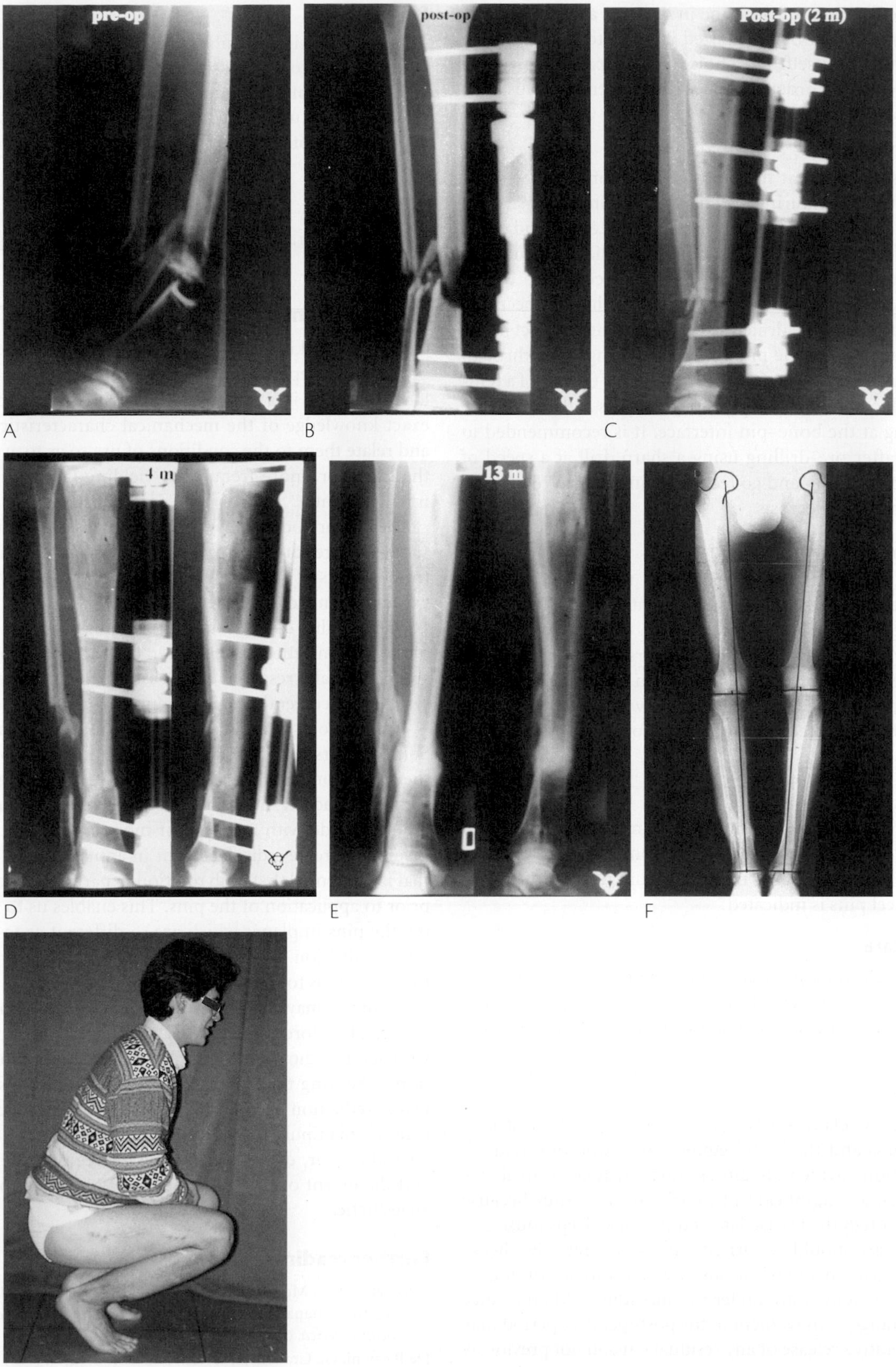

A B C D E F G

Fig. 12.14.13 Right tibia grade IIIA open fracture with 3.5-cm loss of substance in an 18-year-old patient. At 2 months after emergency fixation, reconstruction by compression–distraction was opted for. The acute shortening was 6cm, and lengthening was performed at the proximal submetaphyseal level. Lengthening procedure stopped at 4 months. Healing was achieved 13 months postoperatively. The follow-up 2 years after healing shows an excellent clinical and functional outcome.

one-third of the diameter of the bone in order to avoid secondary fractures, and must never be undersized in order to avoid bending or breakage of the pin itself. The choice of hydroxyapatite-coated pins is recommended in order to reduce the incidence of pins loosening and the rate of pin infections.

Insertion technique

The release of soft tissues at the point of insertion must be sufficient to prevent friction during articular excursion. In those cases where different types of pins are required for cancellous and cortical bone, care must be taken to ensure the drill diameter matches the type of pin used. The drill must always be equipped with a sharp bit in order to minimize damage due to thermal necrosis. Both bone surfaces must be drilled so as to guarantee correct insertion, avoiding any risk of the pin taking the wrong route through the bone. In those cases where it is recommended, the use of a template is essential to maintain parallelism of the pins and thus reduce preload bending at the bone–pin interface. It is recommended to apply the pins after pre-drilling using a sharp drill at a speed of 800rpm/min and the stop and go technique in order to reduce the thermal bone interface necrosis.

Loading and dynamization

The load must be graduated in relation to the type of fracture or condition treated, the type of bone segment to which the fixator is applied, the mechanical characteristics of the fixator, and the patient's weight. In dynamizable fixators, the dynamization must be implemented at the right time in order to limit pin stress and facilitate healing with a view to reducing total fixation time, which is directly proportional to the incidence of pin loosening.

Metal allergy

A preliminary investigation is necessary in order to establish whether the patient is allergic to any of the constituent materials of stainless steel. In such cases, the use of titanium pins or hydroxyapatite-coated steel pins is indicated.

Improper pin care

The methods of cleaning pin tracts must be properly explained to the patient. During the period in hospital after surgery, checks must be performed to make sure that the patient complies with the instructions given.

Muscle stiffness

There is a close correlation between the complications related to muscular stiffness and the bony segment and condition treated. Such complications, which are almost non-existent in tibial and humeral injuries, are significant in injuries of the femur because the pins pass through the fasciae lata and the quadriceps muscle.

Soft tissue release should be carried out intraoperatively, checking for any residual tension by means of extension–flexion movements while the patient is still under the anaesthetic. Maintenance of an adequate range of movement in the postoperative period may require postoperative release of any residual tension not previously identified.

Pin bending

This complication is unlikely to occur when using fixators with ball-joints, since the loads needed to bend pins are higher than the yield strength of the joint. However, pin bending is possible if the pin diameter is undersized and during lengthenings following early consolidation of the callus.

Pin breakage

This is possible if the pin diameter is undersized, particularly in cases of acute trauma when combined with breakage of the fixator body.

Complications due to the fixator

Generally speaking, there may be complications related to failure of the frame depending on the geometry of the fixator and on the loads to which it is subjected. For this reason we need to have an exact knowledge of the mechanical characteristics of the device and relate them to the conditions of use so as to avoid breakage of the frame or, more frequently, yielding failure with consequent misalignment.

The fixator body composed by anodized aluminium may also be subject to breakage due to tension–corrosion phenomena relating to the effects of certain disinfectants, the use of which should be expressly banned.

One possible complication of dynamizable fixators is jamming of the dynamization system when the fixator is subjected to excessive torsional stress. For this reason new jam-free dynamization systems are currently being produced.

The fixation system may be a contributory cause of malunion. Some fixators require reduction prior to application. However, all the latest monolateral fixators allow reduction adjustment with the fixator in place. It should be noted that whenever a rotatory adjustment is made with any type of monolateral fixation system, we invariably create a displacement in another plane, with the result that it is essential that limb rotation in particular should be reduced prior to application of the pins. This enables us to avoid positioning the pins in planes which are so different as to prevent subsequent reduction. If this should happen, the only way to overcome the problem is to reposition the pins.

Malunion may also be due to secondary loosening of the pins or frame. Therefore it is essential to monitor the patient over time with serial radiographs and give precise weight-bearing instructions, checking that the patient adheres to them scrupulously. If loss of reduction occurs, the fracture must be reduced by means of external manipulation of the segments, which can be done under anaesthetic or, depending on the degree of patient cooperation and the extent of the adjustment, may be performed without an anaesthetic.

Further reading

Checketts, R.G., Moran, C.G., and Jennings, A.G. (1995). 134 tibial shaft fractures managed with the Dynamic Axial Fixator. *Acta Orthopaedica Scandinavica*, **66**, 271–4.

De Bastiani, G., Graham Apley, A., and Goldberg, A. (eds) (2001). *Orthofix External Fixation in Trauma and Orthopaedics*. London: Springer.

Gruen, G.S., Leit, M.E., Gruer, R.J., and Petitzman, A.M. (1994). The acute management of hemodinamically unstable multiple trauma patients with pelvic ring fractures. *Journal of Trauma*, **36**, 711–13.

Kenwright, J., Richardson, J.B., Cunningham, J.L., *et al.* (1991). Axial movement and tibial fractures. A controlled randomized trial of treatment. *Journal of Bone and Joint Surgery, British Volume*, **73B**, 654–9.

Mohr, V.D., Eickhoff, U., Haake, R., and Klammer, H.L. (1995). External fixation of open femoral fractures. *Journal of Trauma*, **38**, 648–52.

Schandelmaier, P., Krettek, C., Rudolf, J., and Tscherne, H. (1995). Outcome of tibial shaft fractures with severe soft tissue injury treated by unreamed nailing versus external fixation. *Journal of Trauma*, **39**, 707–11.

Mahadeva, D., Costa, M.L., and Gaffey, A. (2008). Open reduction and internal fixation versus hybrid fixation for bicondylar/severe tibial plateau fractures: a systematic review of the literature. *Archives of Orthopaedic and Trauma Surgery*, **128**, 1169–75.

12.15

Principles of circular external fixation in trauma

Martin A. McNally and Maurizio A. Catagni

Introduction

The use of circular external fixators with fine tensioned wires has been extensively developed at the Scientific Centre of Reconstructive Orthopaedics and Traumatology in Kurgan, Russia and is now widely practised around the world.

Circular external fixation is not new. Dickson and Diveley presented their fixator of two arches connected by threaded rods and fixed by tensioned K-wires in 1932. Versatile tensioned-wire fixators were developed in Russia by Florensky, Rodin, and Gudushauri in the 1950s. Ilizarov explored the biomechanical and biologic effects of fine-wire fixation and designed a system of closed ring fixators which allowed dynamic, stable constructs in all planes. It is the ability to vary and control the mechanical properties of the construct which distinguishes circular external fixators from many other bone holding devices.

The 'ideal external fixation system' (Box 12.15.1) should allow:

- Varied frame design from simple interchangeable components
- Stable fixation of bone fragments, retaining mobility at neighbouring joints
- Maintenance of fracture stability under conditions of full weight bearing
- Controlled movement, in any direction, at any time during the treatment period, to enhance fracture healing, correct malalignment, or restore limb length
- Application with minimal soft tissue or osseus damage and without the need for open reduction of the fracture.

Box 12.15.1 The ideal external fixator

Circular frames allow control of the mechanical properties of fixation. The ideal frame should:

- Be versatile
- Be stable during load bearing
- Allow joint movement
- Allow correction of deformity
- Allow closed application.

These 'ideals' are difficult to achieve with a monolateral fixator but can be produced to varying degrees with even simple circular frame designs. With proper planning a circular frame can allow rehabilitation of the joints with full weight bearing and manipulation of the fracture fragments. Restoration of bone loss can progress within a stable limb segment with little effect on limb function.

Indications for circular external fixation in acute fractures (Box 12.15.2)

The Ilizarov method is established in the management of non-union, limb deformity, and leg lengthening. Primary circular fixation in acute fractures remains controversial. Outcomes of treatment are now clearer with recent studies comparing the Ilizarov method with other techniques.

It is helpful to divide indications into absolute and relative, separating those situations where circular external fixation has major advantages over other treatments and those where it may offer some additional benefits. The following indications are derived from the extensive experience in fracture care at our two institutions.

Absolute indications

- Fractures with bone loss (bone transport and bifocal compression-distraction)(see Chapter 00)

Box 12.15.2 Indications

- Articular fractures usually require ORIF
- External fixation best in non-articular fractures
- Combined approach reduces tissue injury around fracture
- Gradual reduction possible
- Apply Ilizarov Method, not just the fixator.

- Infected fractures (see Chapter 00)
- Non-articular metaphysodiaphyseal junction fractures
- Highly fragmented diaphyseal fractures
- Schatzker V bicondylar tibial fractures
- Fractures with pre-existing bony deformity or limb length discrepancy
- Delayed presentation with difficulty restoring alignment.

It should be remembered that articular fractures require accurate joint reduction and rigid fixation to allow healing, early movement, and functional recovery. Early weight bearing is rarely a prerequisite in treatment. External fixation works best when it can be applied without opening the fracture and where good limb alignment and early weight bearing is required. For these reasons, it is advisable to apply internal fixation to articular fractures and reserve the Ilizarov method for non-articular injuries. However, the two techniques can be used together, particularly in the proximal tibia with open reduction and limited internal fixation of the joint surface, combined with stabilization of the 'reconstructed joint fragments' on the tibial diaphysis using a circular fixator. This combination reduces soft tissue stripping around the fracture and allows adjustments to limb alignment after fixation.

A new fracture in a bone with a pre-existing deformity (especially shortening) gives an opportunity to treat the fracture with correction of the deformity. Ilizarov fixators allow placement of hinges at the CORA (centre of rotation of angulation) of the deformity with stabilization around the fracture. A corticotomy may be performed if the fracture is distant from the CORA.

When patients present late after fracture it may be difficult to reduce the fracture acutely to an acceptable position. Circular fixation can allow gradual reduction over several days. Similarly, some open injuries can have primary closure of the wound with the fracture shortened or angulated. The length and alignment can be restored gradually after wound healing with a circular frame.

The Taylor Spatial Frame (TSF) has been advocated in this mode. This computer-assisted frame allows multiplanar correction but must be used with all the principles of the Ilizarov method. The computer cannot compensate for poor planning, application, or understanding of the method.

Relative indications

- Schatzker VI articular fractures of proximal tibia
- Pilon fractures
- Fractures with severe joint destruction (allowing primary arthrodesis)
- Segmental fractures
- Articular fractures with instability of adjacent joints
- Midfoot and calcaneal injuries
- Open fractures in children.

There may be many more relative indications for circular external fixation. The following sections deal with fixation in specific fracture groups.

Upper limb fractures

Few acute upper limb injuries require circular fixators. In the humerus, severe bone loss, infected fractures, extensive highly fragmented fractures, and distal fractures with elbow instability may be relative indications. The Compass Hinge fixator allows protection of elbow ligament reconstructions and complex fracture fixations with a large range of motion. However, it should be noted that the application of a circular frame to the humerus is difficult, requiring extensive knowledge of cross-sectional anatomy.

In our experience there is almost no indication for ring frames in acute fracture of the clavicle, radius, or ulna. The principles of rigid internal fixation with early recovery of joint motion are perhaps best applied to these fractures.

Femoral fractures (Box 12.15.3)

Most diaphyseal femoral fractures can be treated by intramedullary nailing. External fixation has been advocated in those patients who have concomitant severe chest injury, contaminated open fractures, or multifragmentary fractures of the distal segment (knee bridging fixation). The hybrid advanced system of frame application allows stable fixation of the proximal femur without transosseous wires. This has extended the use of circular frames in this region.

Circular frames are useful in the upper femur in bone loss fractures of more than 2cm. We have applied frames to such fractures with extensive soft tissue injury, allowing stable bone fixation with full weight bearing within a few days. Compression–distraction or bone transport may progress in parallel with limb rehabilitation.

Circular fixation may also be employed where intramedullary nailing of a shaft fracture is technically impossible. Fractures occurring below an area of deformity in the proximal femur or adjacent to an implant may be well fixed with a ring frame.

In complete articular fractures of the distal femur, rigid fixation of the articular fragments will give the best joint surface for mobilization. In the elderly, osteoporotic bone stock and deficient soft tissues may make extensive open reduction and internal fixation (ORIF) inappropriate, risking high infection rates and fixation failure. Minimal internal fixation of the femoral condyles combined with circular fixation of complex metaphyseal fractures offers advantages of secure fixation of the joint surface with minimal disruption of the soft tissue envelope around the distal femur.

Box 12.15.3 Femoral fractures

- Indications:
  - Bone loss >2cm
  - Fractures which cannot be nailed
  - Fracture below deformity (e.g. old fracture)
  - Osteoporotic articular fractures
  - Primary arthrodesis after fracture
- Circular frames may have lower non-union and malunion rates than monolateral fixators.

Infrequently, destruction of the joint surface is such that it is impossible to reconstruct any useful joint. Circular external fixation is perhaps the method of choice for primary arthrodesis of the knee in this situation (Figure 12.15.1). If necessary this may be combined with restoration of limb length via a proximal corticotomy and distraction.

Tibial fractures (Box 12.15.4)

The tibia is unique in that it is easily accessible and has poor subcutaneous tissue cover over much of its length. Open operations may risk deep infection, wound breakdown, and non-union. Most closed and many open diaphyseal fractures are best treated with intramedullary nails but there remains a range of patients and fracture types in which these implants are suboptimal.

Circular fixators are best applied for non-articular fractures at the upper or lower metaphyso-diaphyseal junctions. These can be reduced closed with the fixator. They can be aligned easily and frames allow immediate weight bearing and short times to union. These fractures are often too proximal or distal to nail and plate fixation risks soft tissue complications, even with minimally invasive techniques.

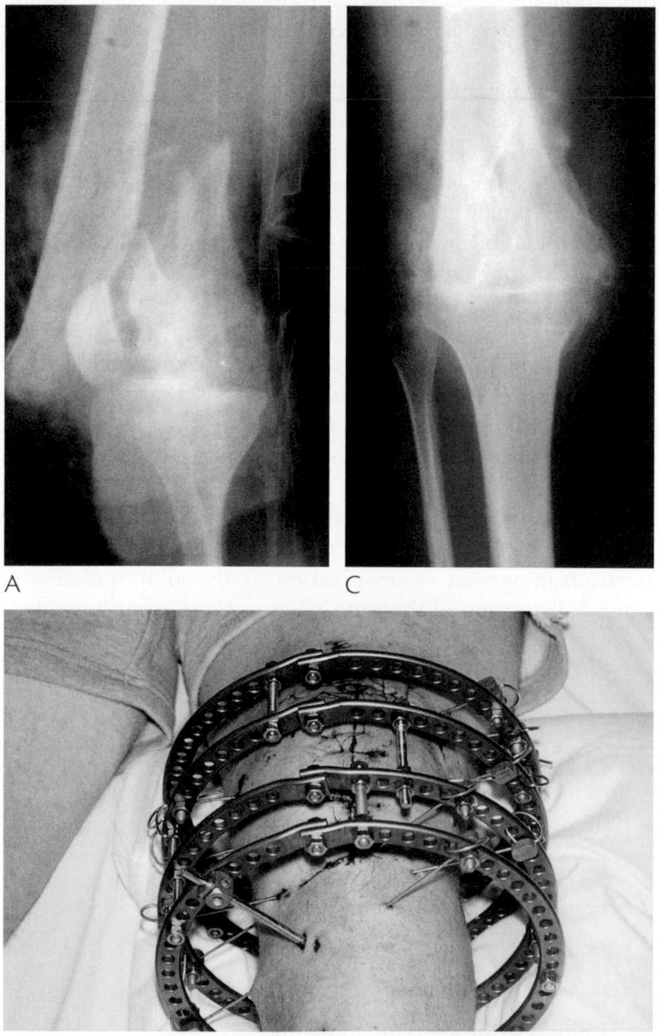

Fig. 12.15.1 A) A severe open fracture of the distal femur with loss of the joint surface and gross instability; B) a four-ring frame has been applied to allow primary fusion; C) complete fusion after frame removal.

Box 12.15.4 Indications in tibial fractures

- Significant bone loss
- Non-articular metaphyseal fractures
- Significant fracture comminution
- Associated soft tissue loss
- Combined with minimal ORIF in complex articular fractures
- Pilon fractures—fixator may cross the ankle joint for first few weeks.

In diaphyseal fractures with extensive fragmentation, circular frames allow excellent stabilization without further soft tissue injury around the tibia (Figure 12.15.2). In open fractures with soft tissue loss and a high-energy fracture pattern a circular frame may be applied with shortening of the limb to allow skin closure followed by gradual distraction after wound healing to restore limb length.

Segmental or complex open tibial fractures in children present fixation challenges. Intramedullary devices are contraindicated with active physes. Circular frame fixation may be used in these cases (Figure 12.15.3). Healing times are short in children, and frames can often be removed within a few weeks.

As stated previously, intra-articular fractures without dissociation from the tibial shaft (Schatzker I–IV) and similar ankle fractures (AO Muller Type B) require reduction and internal fixation. A few undisplaced articular fractures may benefit from circular fixation alone, particularly with poor skin cover.

Bicondylar fractures without joint surface damage (Schatzker V) can be well treated with circular frames applied in a closed manner. Careful reduction in the frontal and sagittal plane is needed. Schatzker VI injuries will usually need open reduction of the joint surface with internal fixation. The circular fixator provides excellent control of the shaft fracture.

Pilon fractures are characterized by comminution of the joint surface including coronal splitting of the plafond (Figure 12.15.4A, B). They require open reduction of the joint surface. Circular external fixation combined with minimal internal fixation provides adequate stabilization for sound bony union (Figure 12.15.4C). In many cases, the ankle joint is bridged with the fixator, distracting the joint, protecting the cartilage and preventing equinus contracture. Once the articular element of the fracture is uniting, the foot extension can be removed and ankle motion started (Figure 12.14.4D).

The components of circular external fixators (Box 12.15.5)

Circular fixators may look complex but they consist of simple parts which fall into four groups:

- *Rings* can be partial (1/2 or 5/8) or full. Carbon-fibre rings are lighter and radiolucent, allowing visualization of bone regenerate or fracture callus

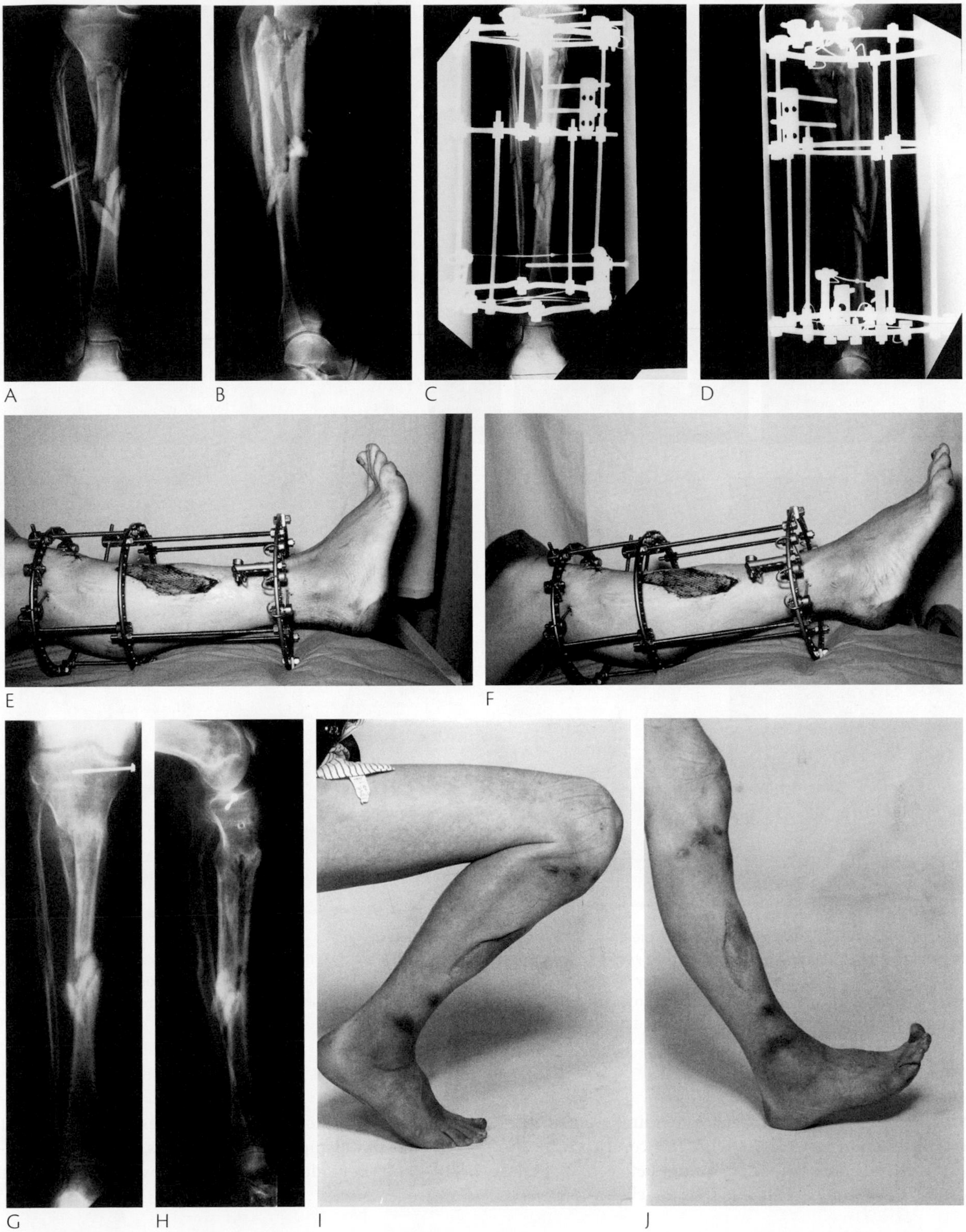

Fig. 12.15.2 A) Anteroposterior radiograph of a grade IIIb open tibial fracture with segmental fragmentation. B) Lateral radiograph demonstrates a coronal split of the diaphysis. C) A three-ring frame has been applied with smooth wires, olive wires, and half-pins for stabilization of each segment. D) The split diaphysis is held with two 'pushing' half-pins and compressed between the proximal and distal segments. E) and F) Ankle (and knee) motion is restored within 7 days of injury with a stable fracture and active mobilization. G) and H) Anteroposterior and lateral radiographs of the united fracture with good alignment and correct leg length. The proximal screw was used together with olive wires to secure an undisplaced fracture extending into the medial tibial condyle. I) and J) Functional outcome 7 weeks after frame removal.

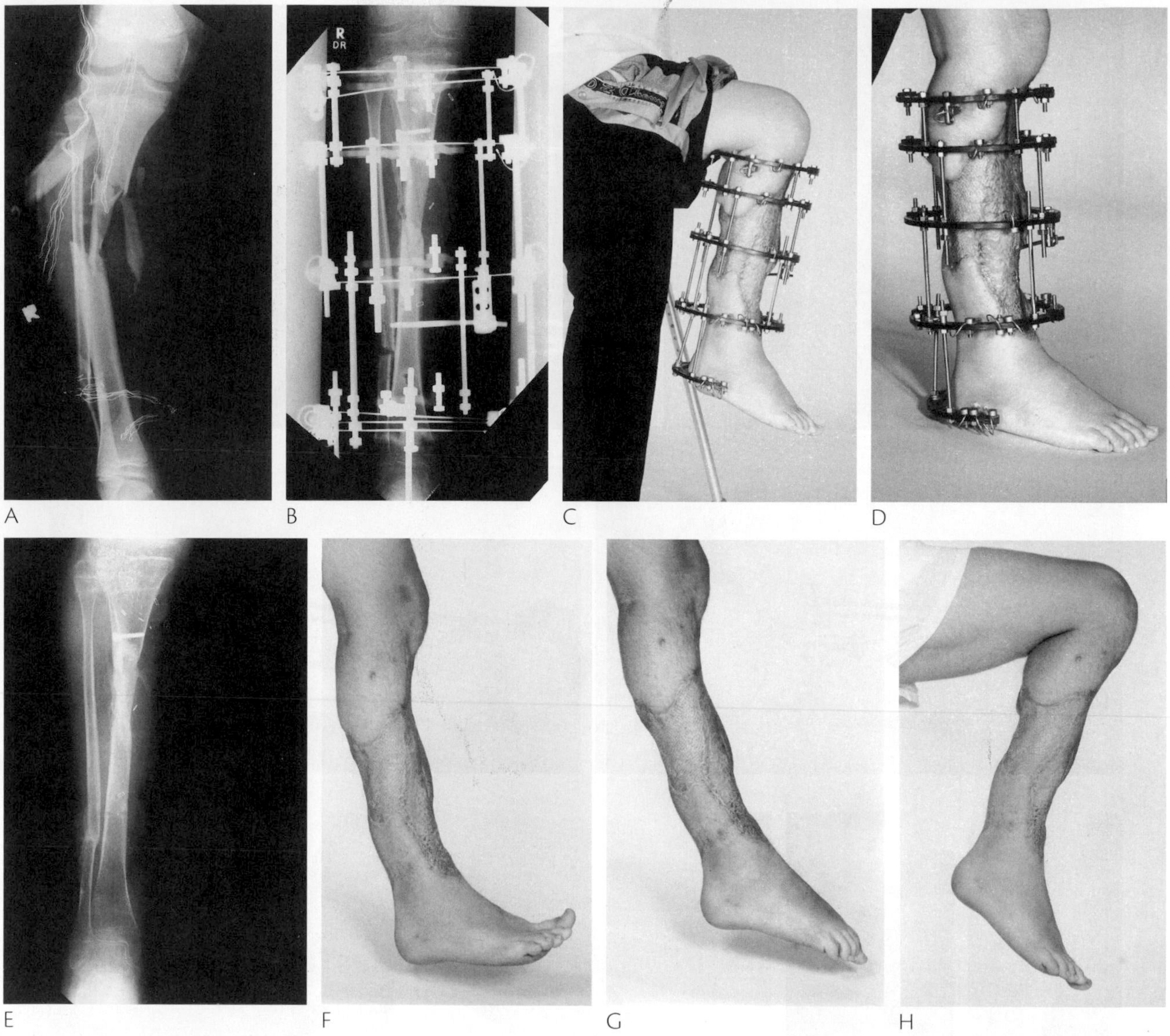

Fig. 12.15.3 A) Severe grade IIIb open fracture with circumferential soft tissue degloving and bone loss in a 14-year-old boy. B) A four-ring frame was applied with 5cm of acute shortening and skin grafting. The fracture was then gradually distracted to restore length. C) and D) The tibia is distracted over a 2-month period. The hindfoot has been included in the frame to prevent equinus deformity during distraction. The loss of the anterior muscles and soft tissue is demonstrated. e) Anteroposterior radiograph at frame removal with fracture union, good alignment, and correct leg length. The physes were unaffected by the injury or fixation. F), G), and H) Functional outcome 12 months after injury. Active ankle dorsiflexion remains reduced due to loss of muscle power.

- *Connecting rods* are usually threaded, providing gradual compression or distraction between rings but telescopic rods are also available. Four rods are normally required between each ring. The TSF uses six oblique extendable rods attached via universal joints
- *Fine wires:* flexible 1.5-mm and 1.8-mm wires provide transosseous fixation of the rings to bone. These are tensioned using a calibrated tensioning device. Olive or stopper wires are available with a bead one-third along the length of the wire to allow compression across oblique fracture lines or to move bone segments during treatment
  - Steel or titanium threaded half-pins may be used with fine wires, particularly in the humerus or proximal femur
- *Special parts* include plates, hinges, supports, slotted rods, arches, pin clamps, universal joints, and translation–rotation blocks. They allow fixators to move bone segments during osteogenesis.

General principles of circular fixator application (Box 12.15.6)

Meticulous preoperative planning with the patient and the radiographs is essential. Patients may spend many months in a frame and must fully understand the commitment that is required for a good outcome. If possible, patients should see a typical frame

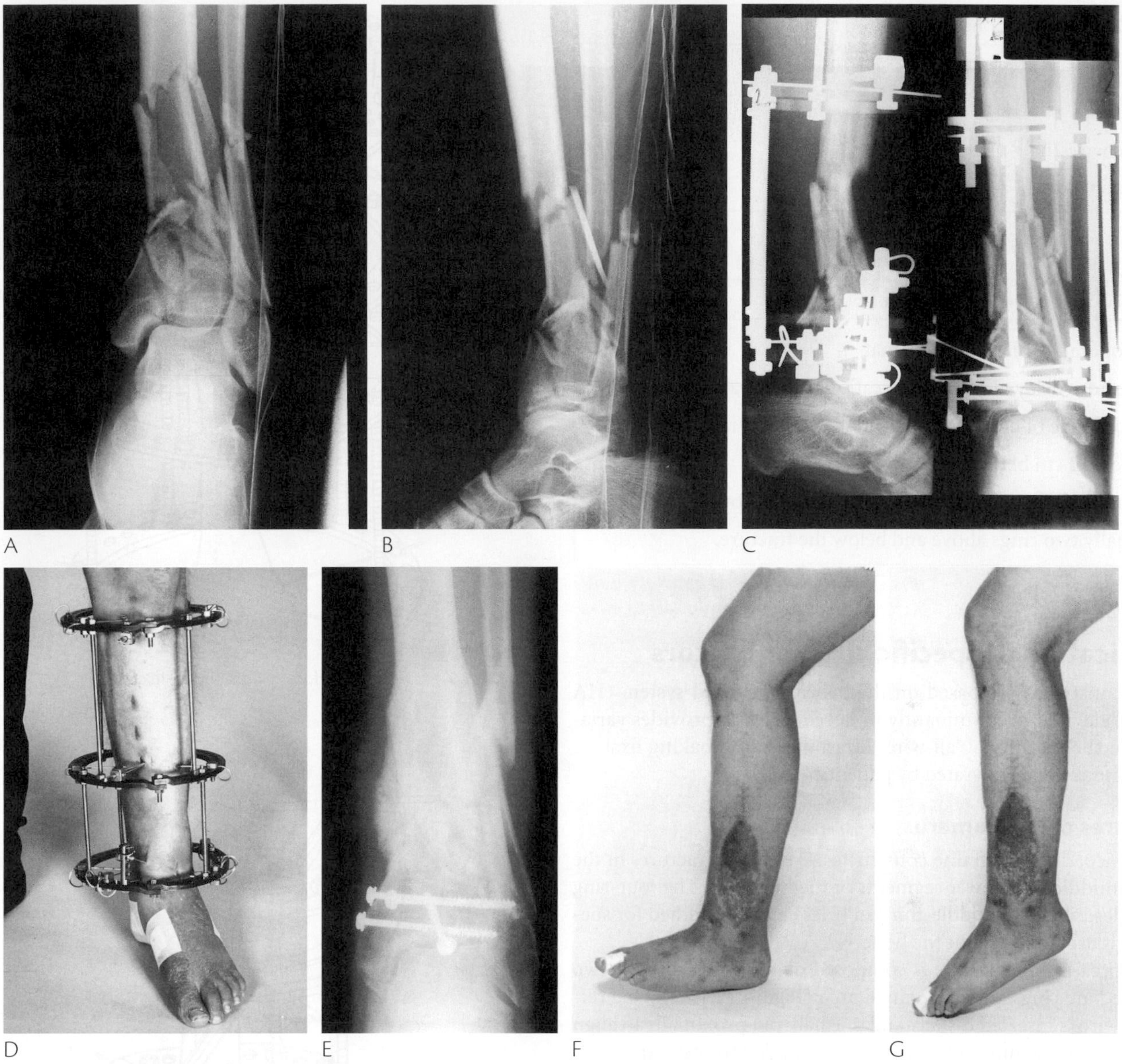

Fig. 12.15.4 A) Anteroposterior radiograph of an open Type C3 pilon fracture. B) Lateral radiograph demonstrates the metaphyseal destruction and coronal split of the joint surface. C) A three-ring frame is applied with minimal approach internal fixation to secure the joint surface. D) At 6 weeks the foot frame is removed and gentle ankle movement begins. Touch weight bearing is encouraged up to 10 weeks with increased weight bearing thereafter. E) Fracture union and frame removal at 19 weeks. The ankle mortise has been restored and alignment is good. F), G) Functional outcome at 28 weeks. The patient sustained a minor injury to a toe while jogging!

before surgery, appreciate the problems that may arise during treatment, and have access to information and help when problems occur.

It is usually inadvisable to apply a circular fixator for multiple lower-bone fractures or multisystem trauma during the initial surgery for open fractures and life-saving procedures. If a circular frame is indicated, the limb may be temporarily stabilized with a bridging monolateral fixator with later conversion.

A sound knowledge of the cross-sectional anatomy of the limbs is necessary for safe wire placement. Variations in neurovascular anatomy and displacement of structures by fracture must be sought to avoid nerve or vessel injury.

Frame application begins with the insertion of reference wires, usually at the ends of the long bones, under radiographic control. An understanding of the anatomical and biomechanical axes of the limbs allows correct frame orientation on these wires and prevents secondary deformities. Where possible, transosseous wires should be passed far enough away from joints to avoid an intra-articular passage, reducing the chance of septic arthritis.

Rings should be chosen that allow at least 2cm of clearance all around the limb. Very large rings are avoided as they reduce the stability of the frame and are inconvenient.

It is important to tension all fine wires around a circular frame. In general, tensions of 100–130kg are recommended to provide sufficient stability and axial loading.

Box 12.15.5 Components

- Rings
- Rods
- Fine wires/half-pins
- 'Special parts'.

Box 12.15.6 General principles

- Preoperative planning essential
- Consider delayed frame application in polytrauma patients
- Knowledge of cross-sectional anatomy essential
- At least 2 cm between ring and skin
- Avoid soft tissue tethering to protect joint motion
- Usually two rings above and below the fracture.

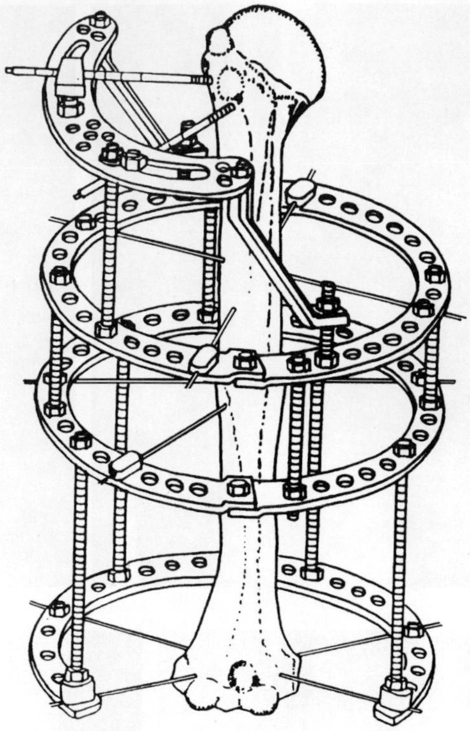
Fig. 12.15.5 Four-ring frame for a mid-diaphyseal fracture.

Application of specific circular fixators

These constructs are based on the hybrid advanced system (HA system) devised predominantly in Lecco, Italy. It provides variations on the traditional 'all-wire' Ilizarov designs, making fixation easier and is better tolerated by patients.

Fractures of the humerus

In practice, different frame constructs are used for fractures in the upper, middle, and lower segments of the humerus. The four-ring frame described for middle-third injuries can be modified for specific fractures throughout the bone.

The preassembled frame is composed of a 5/8 ring distally, two intermediate rings and a proximal arch (Figure 12.15.5). One reference wire is inserted distally and one half-pin proximally to align the frame to the humerus. The frame is applied to these and middle-third wires are added avoiding the neurovascular structures as shown. Additional distal wires and half-pins are placed. A modification of this frame may be used for bone segment transport in the treatment of humeral bone loss.

In some fracture patterns, or in obese patients, a variation of this system can be applied using two arches proximally, one intermediate ring, and the distal 5/8 ring (Figure 12.15.6). This frame, although less stable to angular motion, is tolerated better by patients.

Femoral fractures

The standard assembly incorporates a full ring distally, an arch proximally at the subtrochanteric level and one or two intermediate rings depending on the type and level of the fracture. Fixation distally includes a transverse reference wire and two half-pins. Proximal fixation is achieved by attaching two half-pins to the arch as shown. At the intermediate ring or rings, olive wires have traditionally been used to reduce and hold the fracture fragments in alignment. Transosseous wires in the mid-thigh are poorly tolerated by patients for the duration of treatment. Half-pins may be substituted, entering the thigh posterior to the iliotibial band.

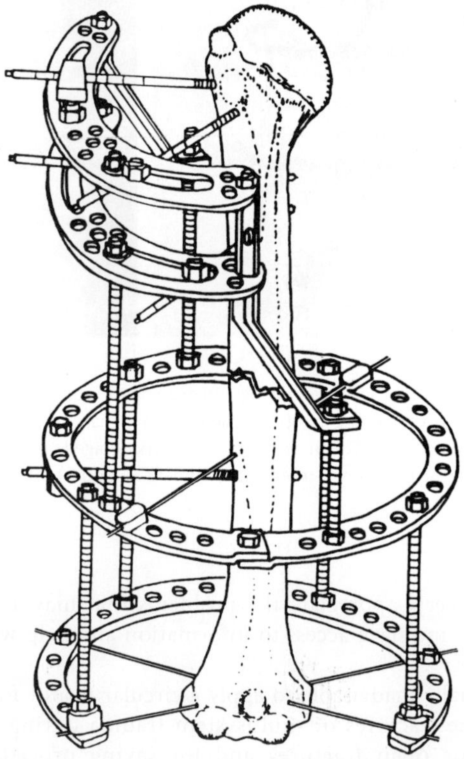
Fig. 12.15.6 Variant frame for diaphyseal injury in obese patients.

Proximal segment

The proximal section consists of one 90-degree and one 120-degree arch. It should be secured to the two-ring distal section by oblique support connectors. The proximal arch should be at the greater trochanter and the distal arch is at least 2.5cm proximal to the fracture. The distal ring is located at the base of the femoral condyles and the proximal ring is 2.5cm distal to the fracture (Figure 12.15.7).

The first reference wire is inserted at the base of the condyles in a transcondylar manner from lateral to medial and perpendicular to the anatomical axis of the femur. After placement of this wire, rotation must be checked. The proximal half-pin is inserted from posterolateral, at the level of the greater trochanter. During attachment of the half-pin to the arch, the frame must remain centred on the thigh. Wires and/or olive wires are then utilized to reduce the fracture. Reduction is confirmed with the aid of a C-arm image intensifier in both planes. After reduction, the remaining half-pins and wires are inserted as shown (Figure 12.15.7). Wires used for reduction, which are in a position which might cause irritation or pain, should now be removed.

Diaphyseal segment

This frame consists of four levels constructed to allow 5–6cm between the upper and lower sections, giving an unobstructed radiographic view of the fracture (Figure 12.15.8).

The frame is aligned as before. The proximal arch and distal ring are secured as before. The two central rings are fixed with lateral half-pins and tensioned wires passing from posterolateral to anteromedial, exiting anterior to the femoral artery.

Distal segment

A similar frame can be used for the distal segment, concentrating the three rings around the fracture (Figure 12.15.9). The two distal rings are connected with hexagonal sockets measuring 2, 3, or 4 cm, depending on the length of the distal fragment.

A variation is needed when the distal fragment is small and there is not enough space for two rings below the fracture. In this case a single distal ring is used, fixed as before but the frame is continued across the knee to include a ring at the proximal and distal tibial metaphysis. The femoral and tibial sections can be connected with hinges to allow some knee motion.

Tibial fractures

There are many variations in frame design for complex tibial fractures or intra-articular fractures but the following description provides a basic system for the commonest indications.

Complex proximal intra-articular fractures with dissociation of the tibial shaft (Schatzker types V and VI)

The preassembled frame consists of one ring above and below the metaphyseal fracture and a single ring on the distal tibia (Figure 12.15.10). The intra-articular component of the injury must be reduced anatomically. When there is no displacement, the frame can be applied without open reduction. Periarticular fragments may be secured with screws or olive wires.

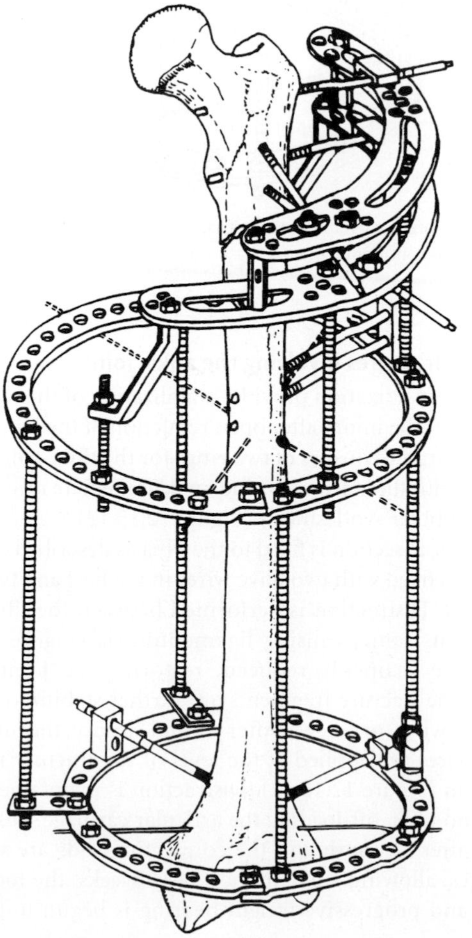

Fig. 12.15.7 Hybrid frame construct for proximal femoral fractures and non-unions.

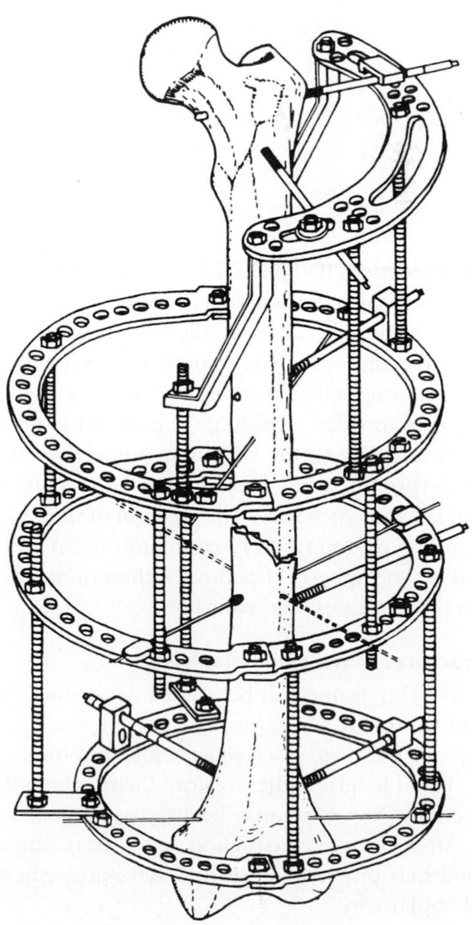

Fig. 12.15.8 Four-level frame for diaphyseal femoral fractures.

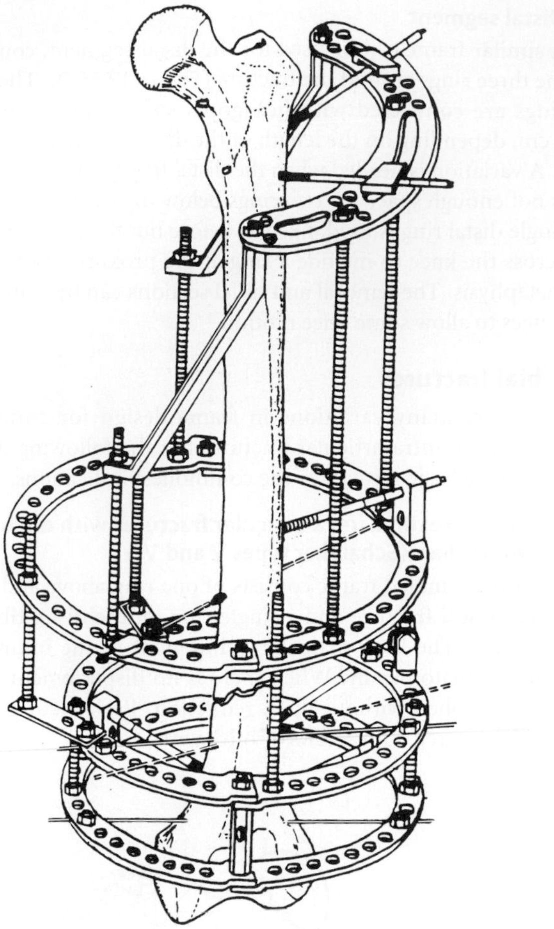

Fig. 12.15.9 Four-ring frame for distal femoral fractures. This frame can be used for intra-articular fractures with or without additional internal fixation.

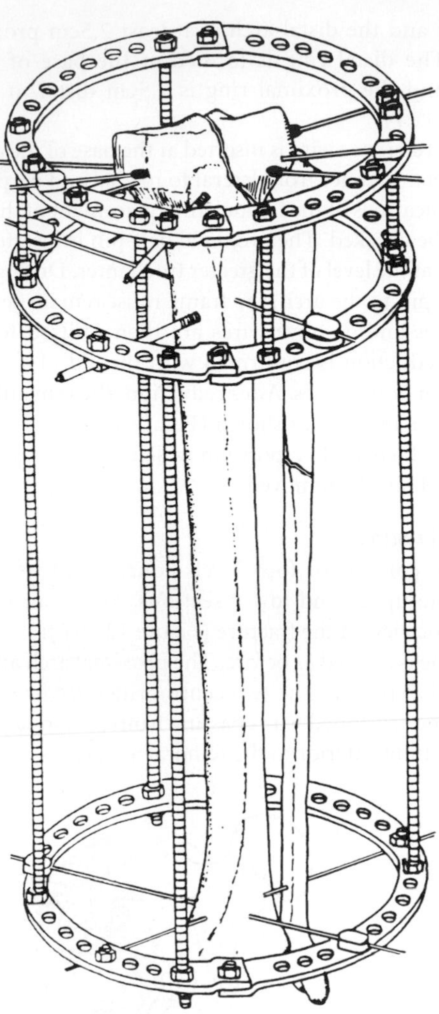

Fig. 12.15.10 Three-ring frame for proximal tibial articular fractures. Note the olive wires in the condylar fragments.

After joint reduction, two reference wires are passed transversely through the proximal and distal tibia perpendicular to the anatomical axis of the bone. The frame is aligned and further fixation is achieved with a second wire distally, passing through the fibula and tibia. The central ring is fixed with a single wire passing from anterolateral to posteromedial, avoiding the bulk of the muscles and a half-pin perpendicular to the subcutaneous surface of the tibia. Fixation on the proximal ring is completed with two olive wires on either side of the reference wire. The position of these wires can be varied depending on the fracture configuration. A similar frame may be used for metaphyseal fractures without joint involvement, especially in those with osteoporotic bone.

Complex fractures of the tibial diaphysis

A four- or five-ring frame will be needed depending on the fragmentation of the fracture (Figure 12.15.11).

Two reference wires are inserted as before and frame alignment is checked. Tibial length is then restored with gentle distraction, aiding reduction. Olive wires may be inserted to reduce the central fragments. After complete reduction, stability is improved with anteromedial half-pins and perpendicular wires where possible and a distal fibular wire.

Distal tibial fractures involving the ankle joint

Circular external fixation provides stabilization of the metaphyseal component of the injury after open reduction of the joint. The preconstructed frame consists of two rings for the tibia, connected to a foot frame with threaded rods, and an intermediate ring at the level of the tibiofibular syndesmosis (Figure 12.15.12).

The proximal section is fixed to the tibia as described earlier. The foot frame is fixed with two olive wires in the heel and two wires in the forefoot. Distraction is performed between the tibial section and the foot frame, causing ligamentotaxis (Figure 12.15.13). The fracture is openly reduced, restoring the joint anatomy perfectly. The fracture fragments are further stabilized with bone grafts, olive wires, or screws. After wound closure, the intermediate ring and wires are applied at the level of the fracture for further stabilization (Figure 12.15.12). Distraction is maintained between the foot and tibia, off-loading the articular cartilage. Distraction is removed after 1 month and the connecting rods are substituted with hinges, allowing ankle motion. At 6 weeks, the foot frame is removed and progressive weight bearing is begun until fracture union.

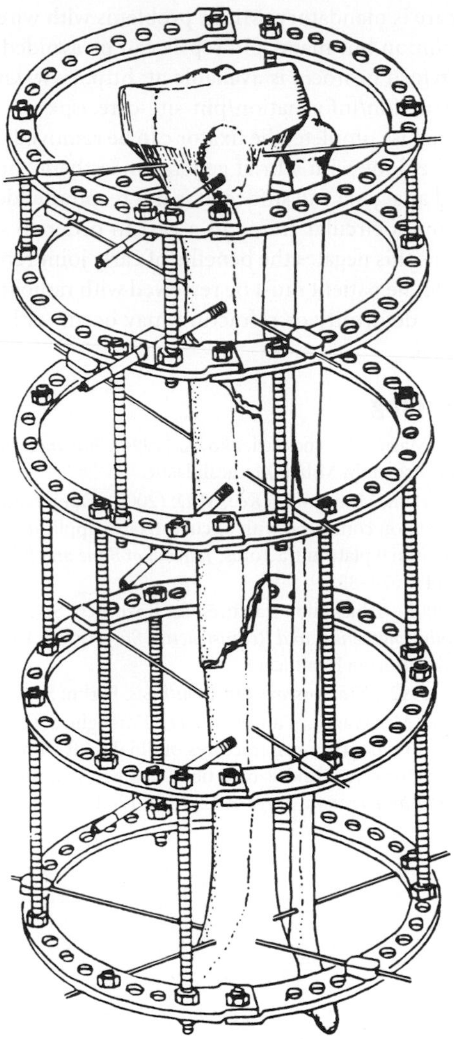

Fig. 12.15.11 Five-ring frame for stabilization of a segmental tibial fracture.

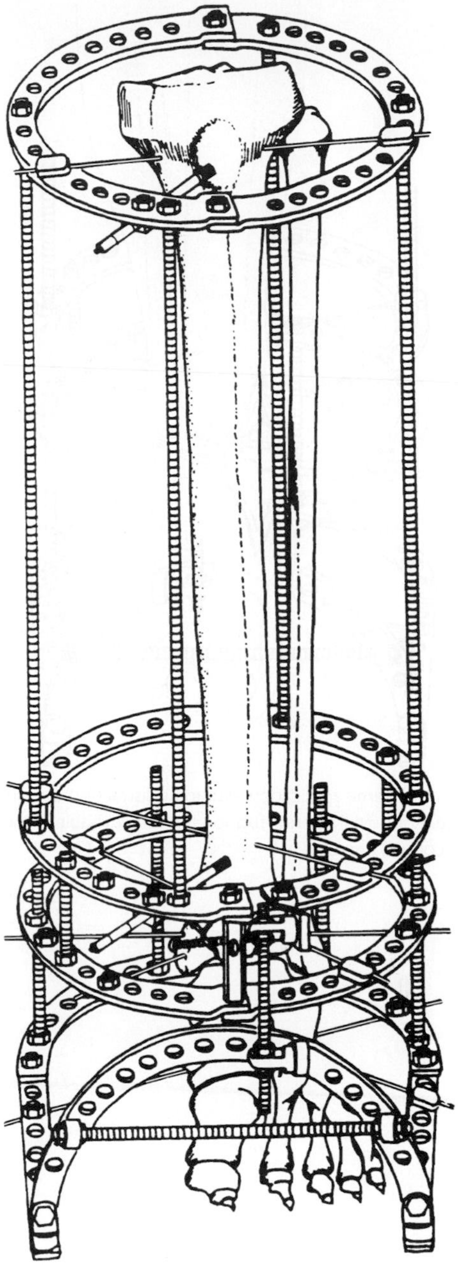

Fig. 12.15.12 Frame construct for distal tibial (pilon) fracture. The frame extends to the foot and the proximal tibia for improved stability.

Postoperative care of circular external fixators (Box 12.15.7)

Recovery of limb function is the primary goal of fracture care. The patient must be fully involved in the rehabilitation with education and encouragement. Passive and active joint motion begins on the day after surgery. This will require adequate analgesia and supervision with a physiotherapist. Resting splints for neighbouring joints (especially the ankle) will prevent contractures.

For intra-articular fractures, weight bearing may be delayed for several weeks but otherwise early loading will enhance fracture healing and reduce the time spent in the fixator.

The fixator must be regularly checked (initially weekly) to detect loss of wire tension or deformation of rods. Loose or broken wires will become painful and predispose to pin-site infection. If adjustments are being made for compression, lengthening, or angular corrections then patients should be encouraged to make the adjustments themselves. This promotes acceptance of the frame and integration into the normal activities of daily living.

Box 12.15.7 Postoperative care

- Engage the patient in all aspects of care
- Encourage early movement with physiotherapy
- Encourage early weight bearing in non-articular fractures
- Regular check for wire tension/fracture malalignment
- Pin-site care essential.

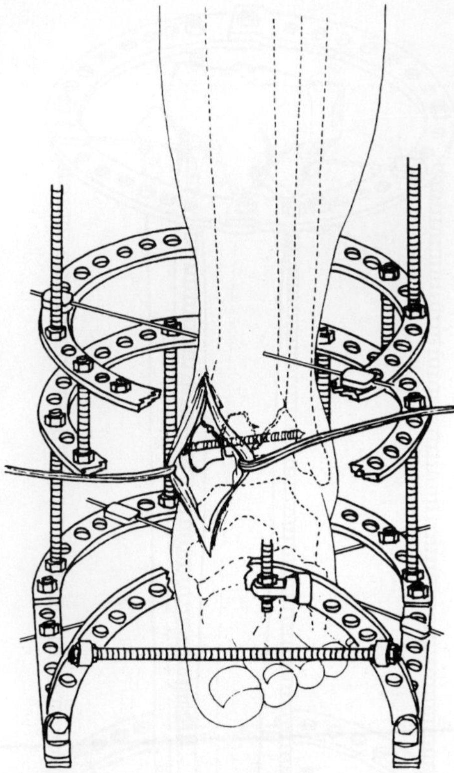

Fig. 12.15.13 Initial frame application with joint distraction can aid reduction of the joint surface. Additional internal fixation is often advisable in these fractures, particularly for coronal fractures.

Pin-site care is mandatory. Minor problems with wires and half-pins are common but major pin sepsis can be avoided with good care. The Oxford protocol is available at: http://www.noc.nhs.uk/limbreconstruction/information/pin-site-care.aspx

When union is complete, the fixator can be removed. In children this should be done with a brief general anaesthetic, but in adults sedation and analgesia will suffice. It is not recommended to transfer limbs from a circular frame to a cast in order to shorten the fixator time as this negates the benefits of early joint rehabilitation. After removal the patient must be reviewed with radiographs of the region as late deformity or refracture may occur with premature frame removal.

Further reading

Catagni, M.A., Malzev, V., and Kirienko, A. (1994). *Advances in Ilizarov Apparatus Assembly*. Milan: Medicalplastic.

Hall, J.A., Beuerlein, M.J., and McKee, M.D. (2009). Open reduction and internal fixation compared with circular fixator application for bicondylar tibial plateau fractures. *Journal of Bone and Joint Surgery*, **91A**(Suppl 2), 74–88.

Hutson, J.J. (2008). Tibial pilon fractures. In: Rozbruch, S.R. and Ilizarov, S. (eds) *Limb Lengthening and Reconstructive Surgery*, pp. 109–21. New York: Informa Healthcare.

Ilizarov, G.A. (1992). *Transosseous Osteosynthesis*. Berlin: Springer-Verlag.

Inan, M., Halici, M., Ayan, I., Tuncel, M., and Karaoglu, S. (2007). Treatment of type IIIA open fractures of tibial shaft with Ilizarov external fixator versus undreamed tibial nailing. *Archives of Orthopaedic and Trauma Surgery*, **127**(8), 617–23.

12.16

Absorbable implants for fracture fixation

O. M. Böstman

Summary points

- Use of absorbable fracture fixation devices eliminates hardware removal procedures
- Of the macromolecular biodegradable compounds, suited for the manufacturing of these implants, polylactide is the most widely used
- Small-fragment intra-articular fractures, especially at the elbow and at the ankle, are the most rewarding clinical applications
- Absorbable implants can be inserted through articular surfaces and, in children, also transphyseally
- Mechanical failures of the implants and redisplacements of fractures are rare, but local, transient inflammatory foreign-body reactions occurr
- In certain intra-articular applications the absorbable fixation devices are superior to metallic ones.

Introduction

When internal fixation is required for the treatment of a fracture, the implants used become unnecessary, and may even be harmful, as soon as there is secure union between the fragments. In contrast with metallic devices, absorbable implants leave no hardware in the tissues. Absorbable implants are radiolucent and do not interfere with magnetic resonance imaging (MRI). Metallic appliances sometimes require removal. In addition, they are associated with some other well-known minor disadvantages, such as excessive rigidity and corrosion. Hence efforts have been made during the past three decades to develop absorbable implants for fracture fixation. In this context, the terms absorbable, resorbable, and biodegradable are used interchangeably. A section on the use of calcium phosphate as bone void filler is also included.

Despite the obvious potential advantages of biodegradable internal fixation devices, such implants did not exist in clinical practice until the mid-1980s, when they were used first in maxillofacial surgery and then in orthopaedic fracture surgery. Once the physicochemical and technical problems associated with the construction and production of the implants were solved, development was rapid.

Description of implants

Chemical composition

Many organic macromolecular compounds are degradable and resorbable in living tissues, but few have the chemical and physical properties necessary for an internal fracture fixation device (Box 12.16.1). Most clinical experience to date has been with implants made from polyglycolic acid (PGA), polylactic acid (PLA), and polyparadioxanone, since these were the first materials used in clinical practice. More recently, other compounds, such as glycolide-trimethylene carbonate copolymer, have been used.

High-molecular-weight PGA and PLA are produced by ring-opening polymerization of the corresponding cyclic diester, glycolide, or lactide. Therefore the polymerization products are often called polyglycolide and polylactide respectively. These homopolymers, as well as copolymers of polyglycolide and polylactide in various ratios, have been used for manufacturing internal fixation devices. Because of the asymmetry of the lactic acid molecule, it occurs in two stereoisomeric forms. Consequently, PLA may be modified in stereoisomeric terms into polylevolactic acid (PLLA)

Box 12.16.1 Absorbable organic macromolecules suitable as materials for internal fixation devices

- Polyglycolide
- Polylactide in various stereoisomeric forms
- Glycolide–lactide copolymers
- Polyparadioxanone
- Glycolide–trimethylene carbonate copolymer
- Polyhydroxybutyrate/valerate
- Polycaprolactone
- Polyorthoesters
- Pseudopolyamino acids.

and a stereocopolymer of polydextro- and polylevolactic acids (PDLLA). Both PGA and PLA are α-hydroxy polyesters, but PGA is hydrophilic whereas PLA is hydrophobic because of its methyl groups. This difference influences the degradation rate of these polymers.

Physical appearance and geometry

Because of their thermal behaviour, several of the synthetic biodegradable polymers are difficult to shape into complex designs such as screws and plates. For example, PLLA is relatively brittle and rigid in room temperature. Also, the strict demands on the initial mechanical strength of the devices made by the clinical applications set limits on the geometric shaping of the implants.

Internal fixation implants which are now commercially available for orthopaedic applications include cylindrical pins, rods, screws, plugs, staples, anchors, tacks, arrows, and cords. The screw profiles are best suited for fixation of cancellous bone fragments. Staples, anchors, tacks, and cords are mainly intended to fix or reconstruct ligaments and joint capsules. Small PLLA plates are in clinical use principally in maxillofacial surgery but they are also suitable for certain small-fragment fractures of the extremities. Degradable cages have been developed for spinal surgery.

Biology and mechanics

Degradation

The degradation of absorbable polymers occurs principally by a simple hydrolytic reaction and, to a lesser extent, through non-specific enzymatic action (Figure 12.16.1), with the main route of final elimination being respiration. Despite these similarities in metabolism, the rates of degradation of different polymers vary greatly. As seen in experimental studies using light microscopy, PGA totally disappears from the tissues within 36 weeks, whereas PLLA still persists after 4.5 years. Also in clinical use, macroscopic remnants of PLLA devices have been found to be present in the ankle after 4 years and in the maxillofacial region after 5 years. The degradation rates of copolymers depend on the ratios of the constituent polymers.

In animal experiments, the polymer is seen to become gradually invaded by connective tissue as the degradation proceeds (Figure 12.16.2). The degree of final restoration of the original tissue

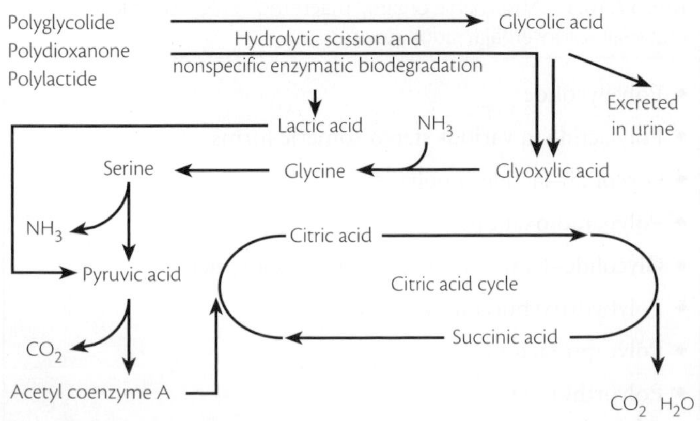

Fig. 12.16.1 Simplified scheme of the metabolic degradation of polyglycolide, polydioxanone, and polylactide.

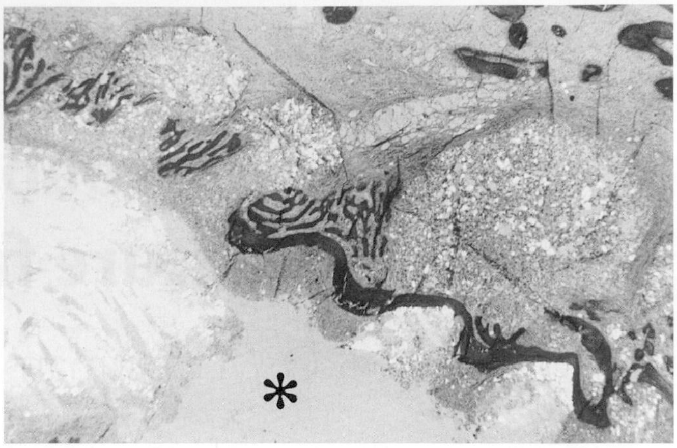

Fig. 12.16.2 A low-magnitude photomicrograph under polarized light illustrating the degradation of a polyglycolide screw 12 weeks after implantation in the cancellous bone of distal rabbit femur. Intense new bone formation is seen along the tissue–implant interface outlining the original screw profile. Remnants of the polymer have also migrated outside the implant cavity, which is filled with disintegrating polymer (asterisk).

architecture within the implant track varies greatly for reasons that are not yet fully understood.

Tissue response

Like any other medical implant, an absorbable fracture fixation implant must be free of infectious, toxic, immunological, teratogenic, and cancerogenic hazards. The results of biocompatibility studies in test animals cannot be directly extrapolated to humans. The only adverse reaction so far recorded for these implants in clinical use is a local transient inflammatory foreign-body reaction. Such a reaction has occurred in 2–25% of the patients depending on the type of implant used and the fracture site operated on. These reactions are discussed in detail later in this chapter.

Mechanical strength

The mechanical properties of absorbable implants must be discussed in terms of initial strength, strength retention during degradation, and elasticity. The initial strength is influenced more by the manufacturing technique of the implant than by the polymer utilized. Simple melt-moulding or extrusion of synthetic biodegradable polymers into pins results in weaker implants than when certain special manufacturing techniques are used. A reinforcing technique using high pressures and temperatures gives high-strength composite implants with fibres embedded within a matrix of the same biodegradable polymer. The initial flexural strength of a 4.5-mm diameter PLLA pin manufactured by a fibre-reinforcing technique is 245MPa. On the whole, the mechanical properties of absorbable materials are very different from those of stainless steel. Indeed, a direct comparison seems meaningless, since absorbable implants were not developed to mimic metallic ones.

The fixation properties of several types of absorbable implants have been tested under conditions simulating fractures in humans. In a study on the distal radius, satisfactory fixation was reported with PLA rods of diameter 2.7mm. A PLLA screw of diameter 6.3mm was found to be as good as a conventional metal screw for fixing a bone–patellar-tendon–bone graft for the anterior cruciate ligament in a bovine experimental model.

The strength retention of an absorbable implant is determined by its degradation rate. As already discussed earlier, the degradation rate is influenced by the micro- and macrostructural properties of the implant as well as by environmental factors. A rough estimate is that half of the initial bending and shear strengths is lost within 12 weeks when the implants are made of PLLA.

Some of the mechanical properties of biodegradable implants can be expressed in terms of Young's modulus of elasticity. The modulus of elasticity of absorbable polymers is much less than that of stainless steel. Rather, it is close to that of cortical bone and only slightly higher than that of cancellous bone. The ultimate mode of failure of an implant can be ductile or brittle.

Clinical applications

Upper extremity

In the upper extremity, absorbable implants have been used in the internal fixation of small-fragment fractures from the lateral clavicle to the phalanges. Other applications have been reported in addition to fractures (Box 12.16.2). Absorbable tacks, staples and anchors are used in reconstructive procedures on the ligaments around the shoulder joint.

The most common clinical applications for absorbable internal fixation devices in the upper extremity are displaced fractures of the humeral capitellum, the olecranon, the radial head, and the metacarpal bones. Exact reduction is necessary to secure the fixation when pins are used (Figures 12.16.3 and 12.16.4). The pins are inserted through the articular surfaces of the humeral capitellum (Figure 12.16.3) and the radial head (Figures 12.16.5 and 12.16.6).

Box 12.16.2 Clinical applications of absorbable implants in the upper extremity

- Displaced fractures
  - Lateral clavicle
  - Acromion
  - Glenoid rim
  - Greater tubercle of the humerus
  - Proximal metaphysis of the humerus (in children)
  - Supracondylar humerus (in children)
  - Lateral condyle of the humerus (in children)
  - Medial epicondyle of the humerus (in children)
  - Capitellum of the humerus
  - Radial head or neck (also in children)
  - Olecranon
  - Distal part of the radius (also in children)
  - Scaphoid
  - Metacarpal bones
  - Phalanges of the fingers
- Dislocations and ligamentous injuries
  - At the acromioclavicular joint
  - At the glenohumeral joint
  - At the first metacarpophalangeal joint
- Fixation of arthrodeses in the wrist and hand joints.

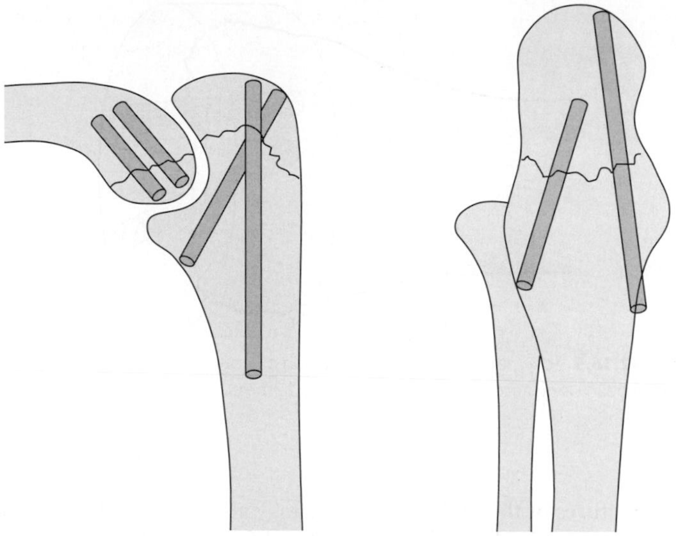

Fig. 12.16.3 Schematic drawing of the fixation of a fracture of the humeral capitellum and a fracture of the olecranon using absorbable pins. Pins with a diameter of 2.0mm or 3.2mm may be used.

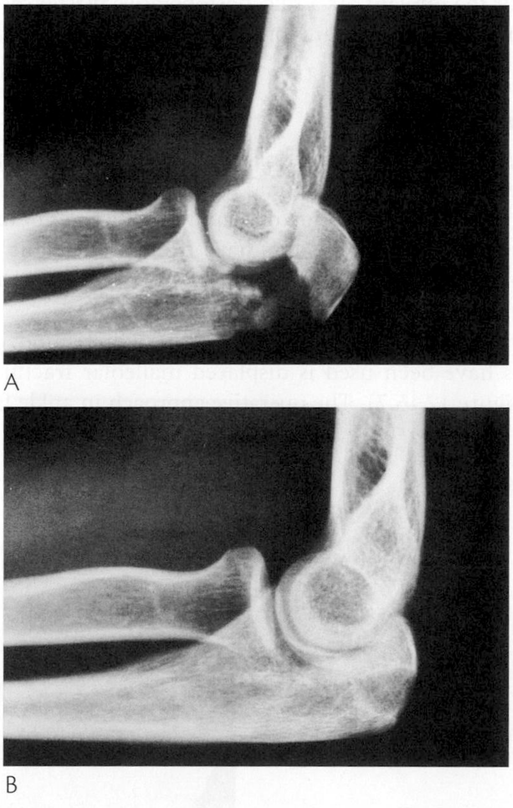

Fig. 12.16.4 Displaced fracture of the olecranon as seen (A) on admission and (B) 1 year after open reduction and internal fixation with two polyglycolide pins of diameter 3.2mm.

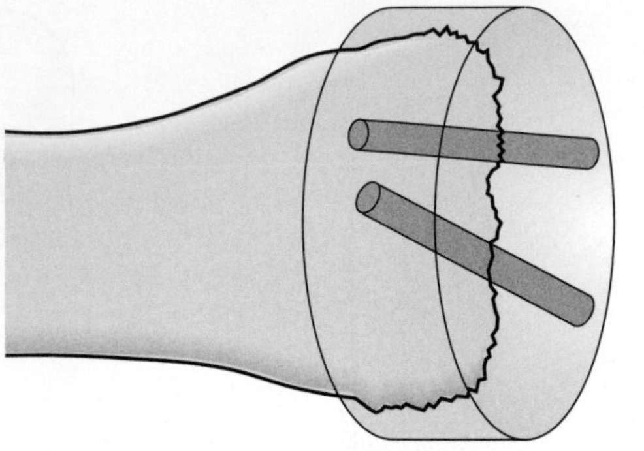

Fig. 12.16.5 Schematic drawing of the fixation of a displaced fracture of the radial head using absorbable pins of diameter 2.0mm.

In fractures of the olecranon screws may also be used. Absorbable pins are used in the fixation of displaced fractures of the distal part of the radius in countries where percutaneous pinning is a popular method of treatment of these fractures. Unlike K-wires, absorbable pins cannot be mounted on a chuck and be directly driven through bone fragments; a hole of the appropriate diameter must first be drilled for the implant. As a rule, postoperative plaster cast immobilization is used. In fractures of the metacarpal bones, small plates can be used.

Lower extremity

The spectrum of the clinical applications of absorbable implants in the lower extremity (Box 12.16.3) is as broad as that in the upper extremity. With the exception of diaphyseal fractures of the femur and tibia, absorbable implants have been used in the internal fixation of almost all kinds of fracture occurring in the lower extremity.

The most common fracture type for which biodegradable implants have been used is displaced malleolar fracture of the ankle (Figure 12.16.7). The operative approach in ankle fractures,

Box 12.16.3 Clinical applications of absorbable implants in the lower extremity

- Displaced fractures
  - Acetabular rim
  - Femoral head and neck
  - Supracondylar femur (in children)
  - Femoral condyles
  - Patella
  - Tibial condyles
  - Distal tibia (also in children)
  - Malleoli (also in children)
  - Talar body or neck
  - Calcaneus
  - Metatarsal bones (also in children)
- Refixation in osteochondritis dissecans
  - At the knee and ankle joints
- Fixation of osteotomies
  - Acetabulum
  - Tibial tubercle (Hauser's procedure)
  - First metatarsal for hallux valgus
- Fixation of acetabular cup in total hip replacement
- Fixation of bone–patellar-tendon–bone graft and meniscal tears
- Fixation of arthrodesis
- Ankle joint
  - Subtalar joint
  - First metatarsophalangeal joint.

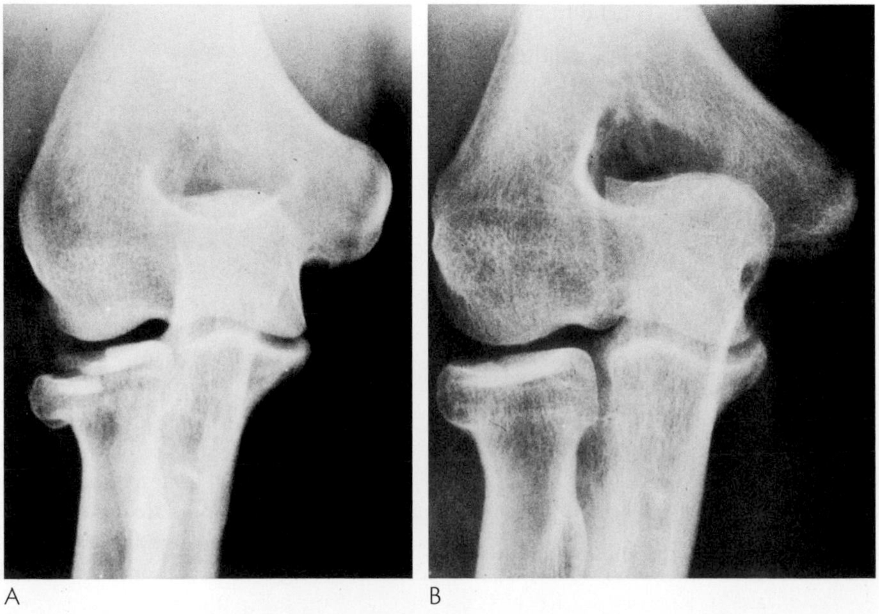

Fig. 12.16.6 Displaced fracture of the radial head as seen (A) on admission and (B) 1 year after open reduction and internal fixation with two polylactide pins of diameter 2.0mm.

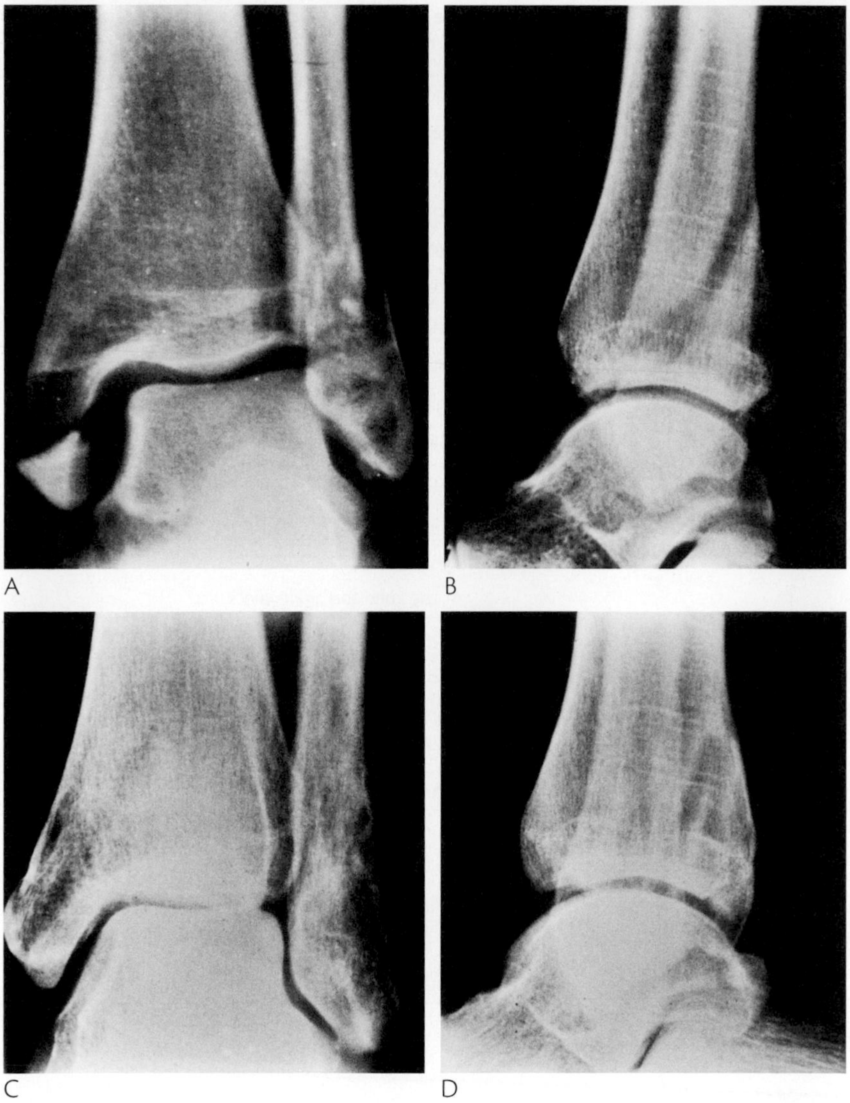

Fig. 12.16.7 A) Displaced anteroposterior and B) lateral views of a displaced bimalleolar fracture on admission and 2 years after open reduction and internal fixation using three 3.2-mm polylactide screws, one on the medial and two on the lateral side (C, D). The implant tracks are still discernible.

including disruptions of the syndesmosis, is similar to that used with metallic screws. However, a torque-limiting screwdriver is required to decrease the risk of screw breakage during insertion. After fixation, protruding screw heads can easily be cut off with an oscillating saw. Postoperative plaster cast immobilization has been used in the majority of the clinical studies reported.

Absorbable implants are used in many non-traumatic orthopaedic disorders in the lower extremity (Table 12.16.3). The two most common of these are the use of biodegradable interference screws to secure a tendon graft in reconstructive surgery of the anterior cruciate ligament, and the fixation of a torn meniscus by using a small absorbable arrow. Fixation of an osteotomy of the first metatarsal bone for hallux valgus (Figure 12.16.8) has been one of the more popular applications of absorbable implants.

Table 12.16.1 Absorbable organic macromolecules suitable as materials for internal fixation devices

Polyglycolide
Polylactide in various stereo-isomeric forms
Glycolide–lactide copolymers
Polyparadioxanone
Glycolide–trimethylene carbonate copolymer
Polyhydroxybutyrate/valerate
Polycaprolactone
Polyorthoesters
Pseudopolyamino acids

Fractures in children

The psychological advantages of avoiding implant removal procedures would seem to be of particular value in children. Indeed, absorbable pins have been used in the fixation of many kinds of displaced small-fragment fractures in children (Tables 12.16.2 and 12.16.3). Experimental studies have shown that as long as absorbable implants piercing the growth plate occupy 3% or less of the cross-section of the plate, no growth disturbance will occur. If this limit is observed, transphyseal insertion of absorbable pins through growth plates should be safe. A transphyseal fixation

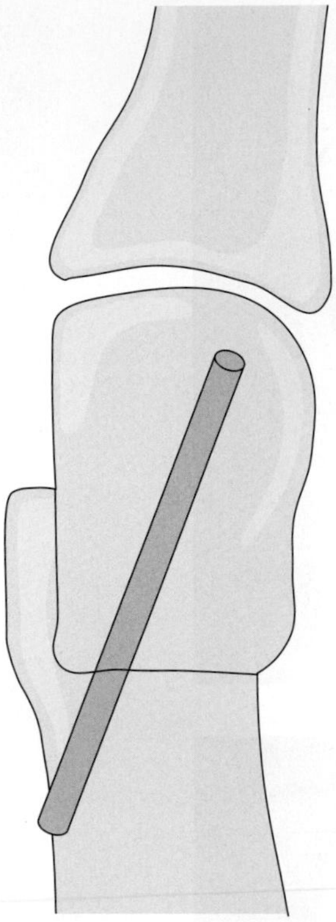

Fig. 12.16.8 Schematic drawing of the fixation of a chevron type of distal osteotomy of the first metatarsal bone for hallux valgus. A 2.0-mm polylactide pin is used.

Table 12.16.2 Clinical applications of absorbable implants in the upper extremity

Displaced fractures
Lateral clavicle
Acromion
Glenoid rim
Greater tubercle of the humerus
Proximal metaphysis of the humerus (in children)
Supracondylar humerus (in children)
Lateral condyle of the humerus (in children)
Medial epicondyle of the humerus (in children)
Capitellum of the humerus
Radial head or neck (also in children)
Olecranon
Distal part of the radius (also in children)
Scaphoid
Metacarpal bones
Phalanges of the fingers
Dislocations and ligamentous injuries
At the acromioclavicular joint
At the glenohumeral joint
At the first metacarpophalangeal joint
Fixation of arthrodeses in the wrist and hand joints

Table 12.16.3 Clinical applications of absorbable implants in the lower extremity

Displaced fractures
Acetabular rim
Femoral head and neck
Supracondylar femur (in children)
Femoral condyles
Patella
Tibial condyles
Distal tibia (also in children)
Malleoli (also in children)
Talar body or neck
Calcaneus
Metatarsal bones (also in children)
Refixation in osteochondritis dissecans
At the knee and ankle joints
Fixation of osteotomies
Acetabulum
Tibial tubercle (Hauser's procedure)
First metatarsal for hallux valgus
Fixation of acetabular cup in total hip replacement
Fixation of bone–patellar-tendon–bone graft
Fixation of arthrodesis
Ankle joint
Subtalar joint
First metatarsophalangeal joint

is not necessary in all fracture types in children that require internal fixation, since in many the fixation can be done proximally or distally to the growth plate. The most convenient way of inserting small polymeric pins of diameter 1.1–2.0mm is first to fix the fracture temporarily with one or two K-wires and then to replace the wires one after another with an absorbable pin (Figure 12.16.9). Of course, multiple tentative K-wire drillings through the physeal plates should be avoided. Transphyseal fixations should preferably be done using implants with a shorter degradation time than those made of PLLA. Pins made of PGA or polyparadioxanone are more suitable. The diameter must be chosen according to the size of the fragments and the estimated area of the growth plate.

Future applications

The future applications of biodegradable implants will be influenced by the development of the devices, the inventiveness of orthopaedic surgeons, and the accumulating experience of the advantages and disadvantages of the implants. An expanding field is the use of absorbable implants in many kinds of arthroscopic procedures of the shoulder and the knee. Degradable cages for fusion procedures of the spine are under development.

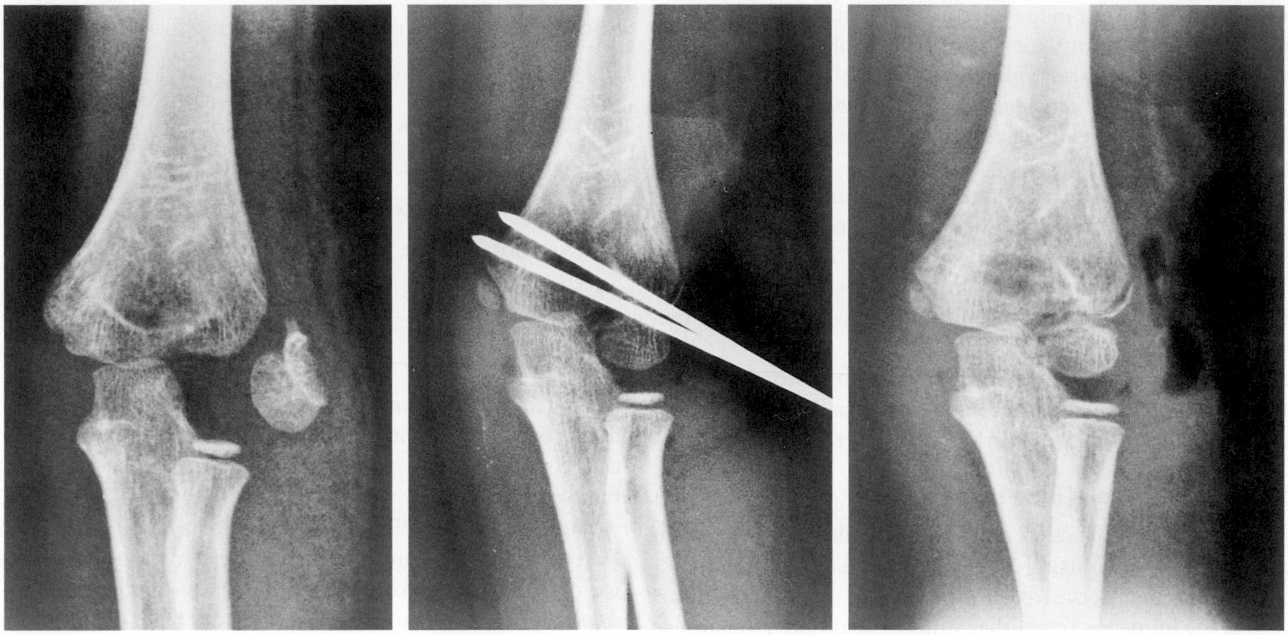

Fig. 12.16.9 A) A displaced fracture of the lateral condyle of the humerus in a 6-year-old child on admission. B) The fracture was reduced and temporarily fixed using two K-wires in an emergency operation. These were then replaced with transphyseally placed 1.5-mm polyglycolide pins. C) The fracture is shown 1 year later after uneventful union.

Advantages and disadvantages (Boxes 12.16.4 and 12.16.5)

The most obvious advantage of absorbable implants is that no removal procedure has to be considered after fracture union, osteotomy, or arthrodesis.

The fact that these implants are radiolucent and do not interfere with MRI is of particular value in applications at the shoulder and the knee joints. With regard to operative techniques, an advantage of absorbable pins is that they can be inserted through articular cartilage and left in place with less concern than when using metallic devices. However, because of their long degradation time, PLLA implants should not be left protruding in joint cavities.

A disadvantage of biodegradable implants is their loss of mechanical strength with time which makes the use of postoperative plaster immobilization advisable in many fracture types in order to minimize the risk of resdisplacement. Disadvantages that will probably resolve with time include the current limited assortment and the price of absorbable fracture fixation devices. At the time of writing, the cost of an absorbable screw is approximately five to eight times that of a metallic screw.

Box 12.16.4 Advantages of absorbable implants

- Removal not required
- No retained hardware
- Non-rigid
- Non-corrosive
- Can be inserted through articular cartilage and left in place
- Radiolucent and do not interfere with MRI.

Box 12.16.5 Disadvantages of absorbable implants

- Brittle
- Local foreign body reaction
- Loss of implant strength with time
- More expensive.

Results

Upper extremity

In labral and capsular stabilization procedures of the glenohumeral joint, the results of the use of absorbable tacks seem promising. Among the fractures in the upper extremity, a clear contraindication appears to be displaced fracture of the supracondylar humerus in adults, which is a fracture type with mechanical demands that are too high for the absorbable devices.

In contrast, displaced small-fragment fractures at the elbow joint seem to be a rewarding field for absorbable implants. Good results have been presented in fractures of the humeral capitellum and of the distal radius, the mechanical reliability of PGA rods was found to be good in a randomized study. Displaced fractures of the metacarpal bones can be successfully managed by small PLLA plates.

Lower extremity

Acetabular osteotomies performed for dysplasia have been successfully fixed using PLA screws in a series of 28 patients. The fixation of osteochondral flake fractures as well as fragments loosened by osteochondritis dissecans in the knee joint are established and generally accepted indications for absorbable implants. Absorbable interference screws are also widely used to fix the graft in reconstruction of the anterior cruciate ligament. However, the synovial tissues are at risk of developing aseptic inflammatory reactions to absorbable polymers.

The literature on displaced malleolar fractures of the ankle includes more patients than any other application. A fracture redisplacement requiring reoperation has occurred in approximately 1%. In two randomized studies comparing absorbable pins and screws with metallic implants no differences were found in the results of treatment.

Results have been satisfactory in fixation of osteotomies of the first metatarsal bone for hallux valgus as well as in fusion of the first metatarsophalangeal joint in rheumatoid arthritis.

Fractures in children (Box 12.16.6)

Among a variety of displaced fractures in 71 children with a mean age of 9.8 years treated using PGA pins, mechanical failure and severe redisplacement occurred in three out of 14 supracondylar fractures of the humerus. In another study of 50 different fractures, two cases with an osteolytic non-union of the radial head were observed. In a randomized study of 24 children with displaced fractures at the elbow joint, small-diameter PGA pins were found to be as effective as K-wires for fixation. This study did not include patients with supracondylar fractures of the humerus. Growth disturbances have not been reported.

Complications

Mechanical failures

Owing to the ductile mode of failure of fibre-reinforced absorbable implants, they lose their shear strength more slowly than their bending strength. Therefore angulation rather than lateral displacement between fixed fracture fragments is likely to occur when moderate overloading occurs.

Inflammatory reactions (Box 12.16.7)

An aseptic inflammatory reaction to biodegradable polymers occurs. The reaction presents clinically as a local painful fluctuant erythematous swelling approximately 0.5cm in diameter. Unless promptly aspirated or drained, it results in a discharging sinus. The bacterial cultures are negative but a secondary infection may ensue. The reactions occur in the final liquefaction phase of the degradation process of the polymer in question. Accordingly, they are seen on average 12 weeks postoperatively with implants made of PGA, but after 2–5 years with PLLA implants. The reactions usually subside within 4 weeks but occasionally show a protracted course. In biopsy specimens the lesions have the histopathological characteristics of a non-specific foreign-body reaction. Polymeric debris is seen lying intracellularly within abundant phagocytically active macrophages. Osteolytic changes may be seen on plain radiographs.

The incidence for PLA (<2%) seems to be lower than for PGA, at least as far as screws and ankle fractures are concerned. In contrast, use of PLA plates to fix mandibular fractures has resulted in a considerably higher rate of local inflammatory reactions (up to 40%).

Box 12.16.6 Use of absorbable implants in children

- Particular value of avoiding implant removal procedures
- Growth is not disturbed if the implant occupies <3% of the cross-section of the growth plate
- Transphyseal implants should have short degeneration time.

Box 12.16.7 Inflammatory reaction to absorbable implants

- Reported in 2–40% of cases
- Local swelling, fluctuant, erythematous
- Requires drainage to avoid sinus forming
- May have associated osteolytic reactions
- Does not interfere with fracture healing
- No difference in infection rate compared with metal.

Use of calcium phosphate as bone void filler

It is often difficult to achieve stable fixation and retention of a comminuted cancellous bone fracture associated with a significant metaphyseal defect. Augmentation by using calcium phosphate synthetic substitutes may then be helpful. Since these materials are resorbable, they are included in this chapter, although implants made of calcium phosphate actually are not fracture fixation devices. Calcium phosphate is available in a variety of different forms, including ceramic blocks, granules, powders and cements. Such devices provide an osteoconductive matrix for host osteogenic cells, but they are not osteoinductive unless specific osteoinductive substances are added. Calcium phosphate bone void filler appliances are relatively brittle and have little tensile strength. Their rate of integration depends on their crystalline size and stoichiometry.

One of the available resorbable ceramics is tricalcium phosphate. Another calcium phosphate-based bone substitute, synthetic coralline or cancellous hydroxyapatite is manufactured as a ceramic through a sintering process. Hydroxyapatite is not commonly used alone as an osteoconductive bone substitute because of its slow resorption and high brittleness. Tricalcium phosphate is less brittle and has a faster resorption. It has not yet been possible to exactly determine the resorption rate of calcium phosphate in humans. The resorption process occurs by dissolution and osteoclast activity.

Calcium phosphate can be manufactured as a cement by adding an aqueous solution to dissolve the calcium. An advantage of cements over blocks or granules is the ability to custom-fill the metaphyseal bone defects. Injectable cement can, however, be extruded beyond the boundaries of the defect, thus potentially disturbing or even damaging the surrounding tissues. If calcium phosphate migrates into a joint, it will not dissolve and become resorbed.

The ability of calcium phosphate bone substitutes to act as bone void filler in cancellous bone has been documented experimentally and clinically.

Conclusions

When judiciously used, absorbable implants provide a valuable extension of current internal fixation devices. In certain intra-articular fracture types they are already superior to metallic fixation devices. Avoiding hardware removals may provide economic benefits. So far, a methodical clinical use of absorbable implants has a history of only two decades. Although absorbable implants never will become universal for fracture fixation, these devices will undoubtedly be used in those specific clinical applications, in which they possess clear advantages over metallic devices.

Further reading

Böstman, O.M. (1991). Current concepts review. Absorbable implants for fracture fixation. *Journal of Bone and Joint Surgery*, **73A**, 148–53.

Böstman, O.M. and Pihlajamäki, H.K. (2000). Adverse tissue reactions to bioabsorbable fixation devices. *Clinical Orthopaedics and Related Research*, **371**, 216–27.

De Long, W.G., Einhorn, T.A., Koval, K., *et al.* (2007). Bone grafts and bone graft substitutes in orthopaedic trauma surgery. A critical analysis. *Journal of Bone and Joint Surgery*, **89A**, 649–58.

Svensson, P.J., Janarv, P.M., and Hirsch, G. (1994). Internal fixation with biodegradable rods in pediatric fractures: one-year follow-up of fifty patients. *Journal of Pediatric Orthopedics*, **14**, 220–4.

12.17

Stress fractures

M. Henry

Summary points

- Stress fractures are fractures occurring as the result of repetitive, submaximal loads, in the absence of a specific precipitating traumatic event.
- These fractures can be subdivided into two groups on the basis of aetiology. Whereas 'fatigue fractures' result from the excessive repetitive (i.e. abnormal) loading of normal bone, 'insufficiency fractures' are fractures resulting from normal forces acting on abnormal bone.
- Early diagnosis allows the initiation of effective treatment that can prevent prolonged pain and disability, as well as avoiding the progression to displacement or a non-union.
- While management decisions are generally focused on activity modification, protection of weight bearing, and immobilization, there is a subset of fractures at high risk for progression to complete fracture, non-union, or delayed union. These high-risk stress fractures, including tension-side femoral neck fractures and anterior tibial cortex fractures, require aggressive treatment to prevent the sequelae of poor healing.

Introduction (Box 12.17.1)

Stress fractures represent excessive loading of bone, resulting in repetitive microtrauma that exceeds the bone's ability to repair itself through osteoblastic remodelling. As the microtrauma continues, the rate of osteoclastic resorption of bone surpasses the reparative process, leading to failure of the bone. This process begins as a stress reaction, according to Wolff's law, then progresses to a stress fracture. The fractures are generally symptomatic well before any displacement occurs. A strong index of suspicion, thorough history, and appropriate use of imaging can lead to early diagnosis before progression to a complete, displaced fracture.

Box 12.17.1 Essentials

- Fatigue fractures—excessive use
- Insufficiency fractures—abnormal bone
- High risk fractures need active management.

Stress fractures have been reported in almost every bone. The relative frequency depends on the population studied, according to the age and the predominant activity in that population. The most commonly affected bones are the metatarsals, tarsals, tibia, femur, pelvis, and vertebrae. Although in the past there has been much emphasis on fatigue fractures in healthy individuals such as high-level competitive athletes or military recruits, insufficiency fractures are becoming more important as the population ages. Involvement in competitive youth sports is also increasing, resulting in the increased frequency of recognition of overuse injuries in the paediatric and adolescent populations. The female athlete has also been shown to be at increased risk of stress fractures compared to her male counterparts, which may be related to alterations in oestrogen levels and a resultant decreased bone mineral density.

Fatigue fractures

While early literature focused on fatigue fractures in military recruits, there has recently been increased recognition of stress fractures in all age groups and activity levels. Many reports show that these fractures are related to an abrupt increase in the duration, intensity, or frequency of activity. It is felt that the microtrauma sustained with repetitive loading, without adequate rest, leads to an increase in osteoclastic activity that exceeds the bones inherent adaptability and ability to remodel. Experimental work also shows that normal bone can sustain stress fractures under the repeated application of submaximal loads.

Insufficiency fractures

With an active, aging population there has been an increased recognition of stress fractures. While in many cases there is no description of a history of change in activity level, many of the patients sustaining stress fractures have been shown to have decreased bone density. Older patients with no apparent musculoskeletal disease have thus developed stress fractures. Similarly, there are reports of insufficiency fractures in patients with decreased bone density as a result of rheumatoid arthritis, lupus erythematosus, osteoarthritis, chronic renal disease, osteomalacia, and osteoporosis. Insufficiency fractures can also occur adjacent to joint replacements and arthrodeses.

Box 12.17.2 Epidemiology

- Incidence: 1%
- Commoner in females (oestrogen)
- Some runners incidence: 20%
- Common in tibia, metatarsals, and tarsals
- Spondylolysis in 6% of normal population.

Epidemiology (Box 12.17.2)

The reported incidence of stress fractures in the general athletic population is less then 1%. However, certain subgroups have much higher risk of developing stress fractures, such as runners with an incidence that may be as high as 20% (Table 12.17.1). One review of 370 athletes with stress fractures showed that the tibia was the most commonly affected bone (49.1% of fractures). Stress fractures of the tarsals (25.3%) and metatarsals (8.8%) were also commonly seen. This has been supported by subsequent studies, however one prospective study of 914 college athletes reported that the femoral shaft was involved in over 20% of stress fractures over a 2-year period. In this report, metatarsal fractures were shown to be more common in endurance runners, while tibial stress fractures were more common in sports with rapid decelerations such as tennis and basketball. Spondylolysis, a stress fracture of the pars interarticularis most frequently of L5, occurs in 3–6% of the general population, and is associated with activities such as weightlifting and gymnastics.

Many risk factors have been identified in the development of stress fractures. In competitive female track and field athletes, a history of menstrual disturbance, nutritional disturbance, and decreased bone mineral density have been identified as risk factors. In addition, anatomical variations such as leg length discrepancies, leg alignment, and bone geometry have also been shown to be related to stress fracture development. Insufficiency fractures in the elderly are clearly related to decreased bone mineral density.

Clinical features

Fatigue and insufficiency fractures can present with the clinical signs and symptoms of both benign and malignant skeletal disorders. There is commonly an insidious onset of pain over a variable period of time, from days to weeks. The pain is exacerbated by activity and relieved by rest, although some patients may continue to experience night pain. Although a careful history should elicit any recent trauma or changes in activity, the absence of such cannot rule out a stress fracture. The history should include general health, diet, occupation and activities, and a menstrual history in women, as well as more ominous features such as weight loss or constitutional symptoms.

Bone tenderness is the most obvious physical finding in superficial regions, while pain with a gentle range of motion or compression of the bone is also often useful. Stress fractures may cause local signs of inflammation such as local swelling or redness of overlying skin.

Table 12.17.1 Epidemiology of fractures—location and activity

Location of fracture	Activity associated
Metatarsals	Football, basketball, gymnastics, military training
Sesamoids of the great toe	Running, ballet, basketball, skating
Navicular	Basketball, football, running
Calcaneus	Military drills, running, aerobics
Tibia	Running sports, ballet
Patella	Running, hurdling
Femoral neck	Distance running
Pubic rami	Military drills, distance running
Pars interarticularis	Gymnastics, ballet, weightlifting, football

Differential diagnosis (Box 12.17.3)

The differential diagnosis of stress fractures is varied, and depends largely on the location, signs, and symptoms. A stress reaction, where the bone is weakened in an area of bone remodelling, has no physical disruption. Other pathological entities in the differential include avulsion injuries, infection, muscle strain, medial tibial stress syndrome (shin splints), exertional compartment syndrome, nerve entrapment, periostitis, and neoplasm.

Clinical investigation (Box 12.17.4)

A careful history and physical examination can usually be suggestive of a stress fracture; however, imaging studies are imperative to confirm the diagnosis. Plain radiographs are the first studies to order for suspected stress fractures. Although they are more likely to be normal within the first 2–3 weeks following the onset of

Box 12.17.3 Differential diagnosis of stress of insufficiency fractures

- Trauma (avulsion, muscle strain)
- Vascular (exertional compartment syndrome)
- Neurologic (nerve entrapment)
- Inflammatory (enthesitis, periostitis, tendonitis)
- Infection (chronic or acute osteomyelitis)
- Primary benign neoplasm (osteoid osteoma, eosinophilic granuloma)
- Primary malignant neoplasm (osteosarcoma)
- Metastatic neoplasm (carcinomas of breast, kidney, prostate).

Box 12.17.4 Investigation

- Pain commonest symptom
- X-rays abnormal at 2–3 weeks
- MRI scan most sensitive for diagnosis
- CT useful to assess healing.

symptoms, later films often show periosteal reaction, cortical lucency, or a fracture line.

Radionuclide imaging, using technetium-99 diphosphonate bone scans, is highly sensitive for stress fractures; however, it is not specific as increased uptake will be seen with any insult causing increased osteoblastic activity. Acute stress fractures will exhibit increased uptake in all three phases of the bone scan, whereas soft tissue injuries will only show increased uptake in phases 1 and 2.

Computed tomography (CT) can show fractures that are not demonstrated on plain radiographs, and can be used to evaluate and document fracture healing. The axial image acquisition of CT, however, can fail to delineate many stress fractures, as they are usually transversely oriented in the appendicular skeleton. Compared with magnetic resonance imaging (MRI), CT is better at delineating the osseous changes with stress fractures.

MRI is well documented to be superior for imaging and diagnosis of stress fractures. It is sensitive for detecting bone marrow oedema that occurs with stress reactions and stress fractures, and has the potential to demonstrate the presence of a fracture before changes are visible on plain radiographs or CT. However, oedema is somewhat non-specific and is also seen with both infection and neoplasm. The characteristic pattern of a stress fracture is a linear abnormal signal involving both the cortex and the medullary canal. Grading systems have been developed based on MRI or bone scan findings, with significant differences in time from diagnosis to return to sport according to the fracture grade (Table 12.17.2).

The majority of stress fractures are singular and oriented in the transverse plane, though multiple fractures in the same orientation may occur. Uncommonly a stress fracture may run in a longitudinal direction in long bones, typically in the anterior cortex of the distal tibia. These fractures have a confusing appearance on MRI, but have a characteristic pattern on several consecutive CT images, with a small cortical break and both endosteal and periosteal reaction.

Treatment (Box 12.17.5)

The key to the treatment of stress fractures is timely identification and diagnosis. Any intrinsic (hormonal, nutritional, etc.) or extrinsic (training regimen, activity level) factors must be assessed and corrected. Most fractures can usually be treated by analgesics, activity modification, and occasionally orthoses or casts. Stress fractures can broadly be divided into either low-risk or high-risk injuries. Low-risk stress fractures are often diagnosed on the basis of a thorough history, physical examination, and plain radiographs, without the need for advanced imaging modalities. A period of rest and restricted activities is usually adequate, with possible supplementation with bracing or cast immobilization. This period of relative inactivity is followed by a rehabilitation program with low-impact activities such as cycling or swimming, until the patient can perform without discomfort. The athlete can then gradually progress to higher impact activities and increase the intensity before returning to sport-specific exercises. In general, operative intervention for low-risk stress fractures is limited to those fractures that have failed non-operative management, non-unions, and malunions. Electromagnetic field therapy has been tried, but a recent prospective study failed to show a difference in time to healing between placebo and treatment groups.

Box 12.17.5 Treatment

- Timely diagnosis important
- Rest and immobilization for low risk fractures
- Surgery for failed treatment, non-union, and malunion
- Fix high-risk fractures.

High-risk fractures are those that have a tendency to progress to displaced complete fractures, and those with a propensity to go on to delayed union or non-union. Also of consideration is the morbidity of the development of a complete fracture. For this reason, stress fractures of the tension side of the femoral neck and fractures of the anterior cortex of the tibia are considered to be high risk. Other bones occasionally considered high risk include the patella, medial malleolus, talus, and fifth metatarsal. Because of the high complication rate, these fractures should be treated as acute fractures. Algorithms for the evaluation and treatment of suspected high-risk fractures have been developed.

Femoral neck stress fractures

Although uncommon, stress fractures of the proximal femur have a high rate of complications if the patient is not appropriately managed. Osteopenia and coxa vara may predispose the femoral neck to fracture. These fractures can occur on either the tension side, or more commonly, on the compression side of the neck. Compression side fractures of the inferior neck are stable injuries, and hence non-operative management is appropriate. In contrast, tension side fractures of the superior neck have a much higher risk of propagation across the neck, and are more likely to become complete and displaced. Complications of delayed or inadequate treatment include avascular necrosis, non-union, and delayed union. Given the significant morbidity of these outcomes, aggressive treatment including surgical intervention is indicated. Once a fracture has become displaced, many patients are unable to return to pre-injury activities,

Table 12.17.2 Grading of stress fractures*

Grade	Radiographic finding	Bone scan finding	MRI finding
1	Normal	Poorly defined area	Increased signal on STIR image
2	Normal	More intense	Poor definition on STIR and T_2 images
3	Discrete line	Area of sharp uptake	No focal cortical break on T_1 and T_2
4	Fracture or periosteal reaction	Intense localized transcortical uptake	Fracture line on T_1 and T_2

STIR, short T_1 inversion recovery.

despite appropriate surgical intervention. Percutaneous cannulated screw fixation will prevent completion of a tension side stress fracture and thus avoid the significant sequelae of a displaced fracture. As stress fractures take longer to heal than acute traumatic injuries, the patient with a displaced fracture needs to be kept non-weight bearing for 6 weeks, followed by 6 weeks of partial weight bearing.

Anterior tibial cortex fractures

The most common location of stress fractures in athletes is the tibial shaft. The incidence has been reported as 20–75% depending on the study group. Most frequently these fractures occur along the compression side of the tibia, the posteromedial cortex. These are seen more commonly in distance runners, and generally heal with activity modification alone. Less commonly, a stress fracture occurs on the tension side of the tibia at the anterior cortex of the mid-third. These fractures are more frequently seen in athletes with repetitive jumping activities Stress fractures in this area have the potential to progress to complete fracture. Initially rest and immobilization can be tried. The recalcitrant stress fracture of the anterior tibial cortex is best treated with reamed unlocked intramedullary nailing of the tibia.

Other high-risk stress fractures

Other fractures that the clinician must be aware of include those of the patellar, medial malleolus, talus, navicular, fifth metatarsal, and great toe sesamoids. Fractures at each of these sites have the tendency to progress delayed union or non-union, and must be treated appropriately to permit a return to sport and to avoid poor long-term outcomes. Frequently a high-risk stress fracture in one of these bones necessitates aggressive management and surgical intervention.

Stress fractures of the lumbar spine

Fractures of the pars interarticularis are the most frequent. Repetitive hyperextension places stress on the lumbar spine, predisposing certain athletes (ballerinas, gymnasts, and football lineman) to developing stress fractures of the lumbar spine, usually of the pars of L5. Spondylolysis, a stress fracture of the pars, is a result of mechanical failure. It is seen in 4–6% of the general population, but has been reported to be much higher (11%) in the previously-mentioned groups. Though there is a lack of consensus regarding the best management for spondylolysis, the most appropriate treatment plan starts with a removal from sports. Physical therapy to promote peripelvic flexibility and core strengthening to counter lordosis should then be undertaken. Stationary cycling and swimming are the only activities that should be allowed. Bracing may be indicated to decrease lumbar lordosis. After a 6-week period to allow healing, if the athlete is asymptomatic they may begin a return to sport programme. If symptomatic, ongoing physical therapy and bracing are indicated. For the athlete that fails non-operative management, surgical intervention such as a posterolateral transverse body fusion is indicated. Postoperative bracing is then continued for several months before sports are allowed.

Further reading

Beck, T.J., Ruff, C.B., and Shaffer, R.A. (2000). Stress fracture in military recruits: gender differences in muscle and bone susceptibility factors. *Bone*, **27**(3), 437–44.

Devas, M.B. (1965). Stress fractures of the femoral neck. *Journal of Bone and Joint Surgery*, **47B**, 728–38.

Giladi, M., Milgrom, C., and Simkin, A. (1991). Stress fractures. Identifiable risk factors. *American Journal of Sports Medicine*, **19**(6), 647–52.

Matheson, G.O., Clement, D.B., McKenzie, D.C., Taunton, J.E., Lloyd-Smith, D.R., and MacIntyre, J.G. (1987). Stress fractures in athletes: a study of 320 cases. *American Journal of Sports Medicine*, **15**, 46–58.

Nattiv, A., Puffer, J.C., Casper, J., *et al.* (2000). Stress fracture risk factors, incidence, and distribution: a 3-year prospective study in collegiate runners. *Medicine and Science in Sports and Exercise*, **32**(Suppl 5), S347.

Pepper, M., Akuthota, V., and McCarty, E.C. (2006). The pathophysiology of stress fractures. *Clinics in Sports Medicine*, **25**, 1–16.

12.18

Pathological fractures

D.E. Porter

Summary points

- Pathological fractures should be recognized before treatment, but often are not.
- If solitary and potentially malignant, pathological fractures should be investigated prior to treatment.
- Inappropriate management may compromise outcome.
- Maximize patient fitness for surgery.
- Preoperative assessment to look for other tumours e.g. CT scan of chest and abdomen.
- Biopsy if possible before definitive management.
- Aim to relive pain and restore function.

Introduction

In describing the mechanical effect of the environment on materials, cause and effect are related through stress and strain. A fracture occurs when the force applied to bone is greater than the ability of bone to dissipate the stress through its elastic properties as described by strain.

The skeleton which is constituted of bone of normal structure and physiology will require significant force to break at all ages. The patient's clinical history will register an impact of high energy and the radiographic appearance of the adjacent bone will appear normal. In contrast, bone may be weakened by a *pathological* process so that a fracture may occur with trivial force. Hence a pathological fracture is defined both by the application of trivial force, and, if sought, evidence of pre-existing weakened bone. It is important to elicit that minimal energy caused the fracture since bony fragments may obscure other evidence of localized bone loss. Consequently, inadvertent reaming of a primary malignant bone tumour or a hypervascular renal-cell cancer metastasis occurs with disappointing regularity and may compromise patient survival. Further evidence of localized bone disease is a subtle history of vague mechanical pain predating the fracture by days or weeks.

Types

Generalized

Bone may be weakened by:

- Generalized pathological processes:
  - Senile osteoporosis—the commonest
  - Osteogenesis imperfecta
  - Transient juvenile osteoporosis
  - Transient osteoporosis of pregnancy
  - Disuse osteporosis, e.g. cerebral palsy
  - Long-term steroids, chemotherapy and bisphosphonates
  - Osteopetrosis.
- Metabolic diseases (see Chapter 10.1):
  - Osteomalacia will cause incomplete stress fractures (Looser's lines) on the compression side of lower limb long bones
  - 10% of children with rickets are diagnosed as a result of an associated true fracture
  - Paget's disease causes both complete fractures and single cortex stress fractures on the distraction (anterolateral) side of the femur. Think of fracture through osteosarcoma although this disease is rare with bisphosphonate treatment.

Localized

Non-tumorous

- Osteonecrosis may result in dense mineral which is not immediately weak. Microfractures and crescentic collapse may occur during the revacularization phase. A specific type of osteonecrosis occurs following radiotherapy. Historically administered to the chest wall and shoulder-area in high dose in breast cancer, fractures of affected bone may occur up to 30 years following treatment. In such circumstances it is important to discriminate pure postradiation osteonecrosis from radiation-induced sarcoma by means of comparison with earlier radiographs and magnetic resonance imaging
- Bone infection rarely results in fracture
- The inherited defect of neurofibromatosis-associated pseudarthrosis is a special case which will not heal with conservative measures. Radical excision and reconstruction may be required with a risk of amputation in intractable non-union.

Tumorous

Although pain often drives a patient to seek the medical attention which results in the diagnosis of a tumorous lesion of bone, pathological fracture is perhaps the first presentation especially in benign lesions. Benign neoplastic lesions are most common in childhood and young adulthood. With increasing age, however, metastatic bone disease eventually becomes the most frequent cause of a localized pathological fracture.

Benign

All the benign intramedullary neoplasms of childhood can be associated with pathological fractures. Unicameral (simple) bone cysts are the most frequent but others include aneurysmal bone cyst, enchondroma, fibrous dysplasia, osteofibrous dysplasia, and eosinophilic granuloma.

In young adulthood, simple bone cysts seem to resolve and giant cell tumour can be added to the earlier list. Cortically based lesions such as fibrous cortical defect can result in a unicortical stress fracture. Even a pedunculated osteochondroma may fracture through its stalk and require excision.

Since the histology of new fracture callus includes plump active osteoblasts in a cellular osteoid matrix, it is important to inform the histopathologist of a fracture when sending material, otherwise a spurious diagnosis of osteosarcoma may be entertained.

Malignant

Primary malignant bone tumours infrequently present as a pathological fracture in childhood, although in osteosarcoma this complication may occur during biopsy or while undergoing neoadjuvant chemotherapy and awaiting surgery. Although univariate analyses suggest that pathological fracture is associated with poor survival, more recent multivariate studies point to other features of tumour aggression as more responsible for this. A chondroid tumour which fractures in one of the proximal long bones may hint of a chondrosarcoma, although in the hand or foot fractures tend to represent a benign enchondroma.

In the patient over 50 years old, a pathological fracture is usually due to metastatic disease. The usual suspect primary tumours are well recognized: breast, prostate, lung, thyroid, and kidney are all carcinomas. Added to this will be the myeloproliferative disorders of myeloma and lymphoma. Except for the special case of a late isolated renal cell carcinoma deposit, it may be impossible to cure the patient. However, an accurate diagnosis will provide the oncologist with the best chance of providing effective palliative treatment.

Investigation and diagnosis

The importance of identifying that a fracture is pathological cannot be emphasized too strongly. Among some doctors there may be a belief that cancers do not occur in children; others may believe that there can be no harm in promptly fixing all femoral long-bone fractures in the elderly.

Taking a comprehensive history and procuring good quality radiographs will go a long way to ensuring a minimum of mistaken diagnoses.

It is recognized that appropriate investigations may take several days to organize. In the interim it is important to reassure the patient and ensure that adequate analgesia is administered and fracture immobilization achieved. During this period, efforts can be made to maximize patient fitness for surgery—in particular hypercalcaemia of malignancy can be identified and corrected with fluid management and bisphosphonates. Clinical examination of lung fields, abdomen, prostate, and breast may be required. Further imaging may include magnetic resonance imaging of the local area, bone scintigraphy to assess for further skeletal lesions and computed tomography of the chest, abdomen, and pelvis where a primary adenocarcinoma is sought. Where the lesion proves to be solitary, a biopsy should be undertaken with the aim of discriminating a primary malignant bone tumour from a metastasis. This should be discussed with the local or regional bone tumour specialist service to ensure the biopsy method does not compromise further potential optimum management.

In the child and young adult, radiographs alone may be diagnostic, for example, in simple bone cysts of the proximal humerus and digital enchondromas. Age and site and tumour matrix may also be useful pointers in identifying fibrous dysplasia, giant cell tumour and chondroblastoma.

Where a skeletal metastasis is already identified, the risk of future fracture arises. If this risk is high, prophylactic fixation may be indicated. Where 50% of a single cortex is destroyed, pathological fracture may be regarded as inevitable. Furthermore, avulsion of the lesser trochanter points to an imminent hip fracture. It is recommended that each trauma unit has a named surgeon who has responsibility for liaison with colleagues and other specialists such as oncologists to allow early assessment and treatment of such impending fractures. Mirels has developed a scoring system which ranks radiographic and clinical features as shown in Table 12.18.1.

A score of 8 or above indicates a high likelihood of impending fracture and prophylactic fixation is recommended prior to radiotherapy.

Management

Generalized conditions

In most generalized conditions, bone will heal as rapidly or almost as rapidly as in normal bone. Choice of treatment depends upon the fracture configuration, comorbid factors, age, and mobility.

Localized conditions

In benign lesions, upper limb pathological fractures are perhaps more common than those in the lower limb. However, fractures in the lower limb are more difficult to manage with a higher malunion risk and so surgeons will be more likely to undertake prophylactic treatment of an impending femoral fracture. It is important to

Table 12.18.1 Mirel's scoring system for impending pathological fracture risk

	1	2	3
Site	Upper LIMB	Lower LIMB	Peritrochanteric
Pain	Mild	Moderate	Severe
Lesion	Blastic (sclerotic)	Mixed	Lytic
Size*	<1/3	1/3–2/3	>2/3

* As seen on plain x-ray, maximum destruction in any view.

advise use of crutches while awaiting surgery, or at least explain the risk of fracture to avoid accusations of neglect.

In many types of benign bone lesions, a fracture may stimulate osteogenesis within the lesion so that both fracture healing and lesional obliteration occur together. This is seen in simple and aneurysmal bone cysts, enchondromas, fibrous cortical defects, and fibrous dysplasia. It is recommended that the patient is followed-up until lesional obliteration. In the lower limb long bones, however, internal fixation may be necessary to achieve an accurate anatomical reduction. A giant cell tumour may represent a difficult reconstructive problem when an intra-articular fracture occurs around the knee. If there is sufficient bone to secure both medial and lateral cortices, then curettage, grafting, and plate fixation may be appropriate. Otherwise an extended tumour prosthesis might be required.

The British Orthopaedic Association has stated that the aim of surgery in a pathological fracture due to metastatic disease is to relieve pain and restore function. An over-riding principle is to provide immediate postoperative stability, allowing weight bearing, and to stabilize all lesions in the affected bone, where possible.

In long-bone biopsy-proven solitary metastases and in multiple bony metastases without biopsy a pathological fracture of the diaphysis or metaphysis is most reliably managed with a load-bearing implant—typically an intramedullary nail. The reason for this is that the fracture cannot be assumed to be capable of healing—at some point the tumour will grow again locally. The aim of surgery is therefore to stabilize the bone for the duration of the patient's life—typically this is 1–2 years in non-breast cancer, perhaps 2–5 years in breast cancer. Modern intramedullary fixation will not undergo fatigue-failure in cyclical loading within 2 years. It is probably worth stabilizing a long-bone fracture if life expectancy exceeds at least 6 weeks although each case is judged on its own merits with full involvement of patient and family in decision-making. Where surgery is too great a risk, then a portable epidural catheter may allow comfort and even some transfer-mobility. In renal cell metastasis, there is a risk of severe haemorrhage, so that preoperative angiography plus coil-embolization is warranted. In solitary renal cell metastases which have developed some years after nephrectomy, then treatment as for a primary malignant bone cancer might be undertaken with a high chance of cure.

Where a fracture is juxta-articular, then plate fixation together with bone–cement reconstruction is advisable. The exception to this, however, is a peritrochanteric fracture of the femur or proximal humerus fracture which may be treated by an intramedullary nail of reconstruction type, or a cemented joint prosthesis. The latter has a low failure rate. Occasionally, a tumour prosthesis may be required but the loss of some hip or shoulder abductor function will have to be accepted. A fracture through the ilium adjacent or proximal to the hip joint will require hip replacement with acetabular reconstruction. Harrington has described useful principles of surgical treatment depending on the anatomical site of the pathological pelvic fracture. Cement and metal pins will produce a 'reinforced concrete' effect proximal to the acetabulum into which a polyethylene cup can be cemented.

All reamings and curetted material should be submitted to histopathological examination to confirm the tumour diagnosis. Oncological postoperative treatment will be guided by the diagnosis and radiotherapy will frequently be directed to the tumour bed.

Certain cancers will not prevent fracture healing when treated with appropriate chemo-, endocrine, or radiation therapy. These include lymphoma, myeloma, thyroid, and breast and prostate cancer. New oncogene inhibitors in renal cell metastases now seem to provide a similar gratifying effect.

Further reading

British Orthopaedic Association (2001). *Metastatic Bone Disease: A Guide to Good Practice.* London: British Orthopaedic Association.

Harrington, K.D. (1995). Orthopaedic management of extremity and pelvic lesions. *Clinical Orthopaedics and Related Research*, **312**, 136–47.

Mirels, H. (1989). Metastatic disease in long bones. A proposed scoring system for diagnosing impending pathological fracture. *Clinical Orthopaedics and Related Research*, **249**, 256–64.

12.19

Management of segmental bone defects

Stuart J.E. Matthews

Summary points

- Segmental defects are a significant, but surmountable, problem for the Trauma surgeon
- The best results will only be achieved if all potential solutions are considered and used correctly in either: isolation; sequentially; or concurrently.
- Failure to correct a bone defect, during debridement of some open fractures, may be catastrophic. An appreciation of the techniques available to treat segmental defects is necessary to allow the surgeon to debride with confidence.

Introduction

A segmental defect may be defined in a number of ways. The simplest definition is wherever a segment of bone is missing and usually refers to the diaphysis of a long bone in colloquial orthopaedic parlance. Examples may include extrusion wedges debrided during surgery due to lack of soft tissue attachment or lost at the road side. Such situations refer to high-energy fractures of type B or type C pattern and the defect may be complete or incomplete, and so there may be bone-to-bone contact or a gap when the bone is restored to its original length.

A defect may also be defined by its size (Box 12.19.1). It thus may be referred to as a critical-sized defect or subcritical-sized defect. A critical-sized defect may be defined as one that cannot be successfully treated using standard techniques with cancellous autografts. Segmental defects are generally regarded as critical when in the region of 5cm or above.

Box 12.19.1 Definition
◆ Subcritical ◆ Critical.

Methods

Although cancellous bone grafting remains to this day the gold standard material for bridging and uniting complete or incomplete sized bone defects, there is a limit to the size of defect that may be treated using cancellous autografting. Other techniques and materials need to be considered:

- Bone graft:
  - Autograft[a]
  - Allograft[c]
- Demineralized bone matrix[c]
- Ceramics:
  - Calcium hydroxapatite[c]
  - Calcium phosphate[c]
- Free vascularized tissue transfers[b]
- Distraction histiogenesis[a, b]
- Bone morphogenic proteins)[a, b]
- LIPUS (pulsed ultrasound)[c]
- Tissue engineering.[b]

[a]Of use in subcritical-sized defects; [b]of use in critical sized defects; [c]no established role

Subcritical-sized bone defects

Autograft

Nature of autograft

Autograft may be cancellous bone from metaphyseal regions of a bone within the same patient or segments of cortical, usually corticocancellous bone, the latter providing structural support to the grafted area and often inserted as a pedicled or free microvascular tissue transfer although rib is used as a avascular graft in some circumstances such as the spine. Examples of pedicled flaps include the pronator quadratus to the scaphoid or a DCIA (deep circumflex iliac artery) to the neck of the femur. One of the most versatile of

Box 12.19.2 Cancellous autograft

- Osteoconductive, osteoinductive, and osteogenic
- Large quantities available in iliac crest and femur
- Associated donor site morbidity:
  - Bleeding
  - Infection
  - Nerve damage (lateral cutaneous nerve of thigh)
  - Iatrogenic fractures
  - Arterial injury
- Avoid in the presence of sepsis.

free flaps is a free fibular microvascular transfer. It has found applications in the treatment of segmental defects of the tibia, forearm bones, and the mandible. The needs of reconstruction surgeons have lead to applying free fibulas to other more inventive sites.

Properties of autograft

Cancellous bone graft consists of portions of spongy bone spicules with living bone cells.

Sources of autograft

The commonest source of autograft is cancellous bone and the commonest source harvested is between the two tables of the iliac crest, be it anterior or posterior. Methods consists of: trephine biopsies; lifting the superior cortex like a lid of a seaman's chest; peeling down ribbons of cortex from the outer table; scooping out the cancellous bone with either a gouge or using the acetabular (strawberry) reamer under power from a hip arthroplasty set.

Other sources include the femoral condyles or greater trochanteric regions at the hip. The distal radius is a ready source of cancellous graft when operating around the wrist and carpus where small volumes are required.

The main problem with cancellous autograft is the limited volume available to the surgeon which is much diminished in the elderly. Harvesting from all four iliac crests may be necessary to obtain a sufficient volume but even in fit young adult males all four crests are unlikely to yield more than 40–60mL with the average volume in a 75-kg man being 17g for the anterior crest and 40g from the posterior crest. The use of the reamer aspiration irrigator system passed through the intramedullary canal of the femur has yielded significantly greater volumes (20–90mL) of graft and there is evidence to show that even the irrigation fluid has osteogenic properties.

Morbidity of bone grafting

A variety of complications are associated with cancellous bone grafting. Not only is it common experience that the donor site is very painful and may indeed delay ambulation, but the technique has been associated with bleeding, infection, nerve damage (the commonest being lateral cutaneous nerve of thigh), and iatrogenic fractures and even arterial injury.

Indications for autografting

Autografting is the treatment of choice for non-critical bone defects and to encourage union in cases of delayed or non-union. Cancellous grafting comes sterile, is immunocompatible, and has no storage issues. Its availability is limited but may be increased by harvesting the femur with a Reamer Irrigator Aspirator (RIA) system.

The mechanical environment

Stability is essential (Figure 12.19.1). Too much micromovement may inhibit neovascularization of the graft. There may be a natural

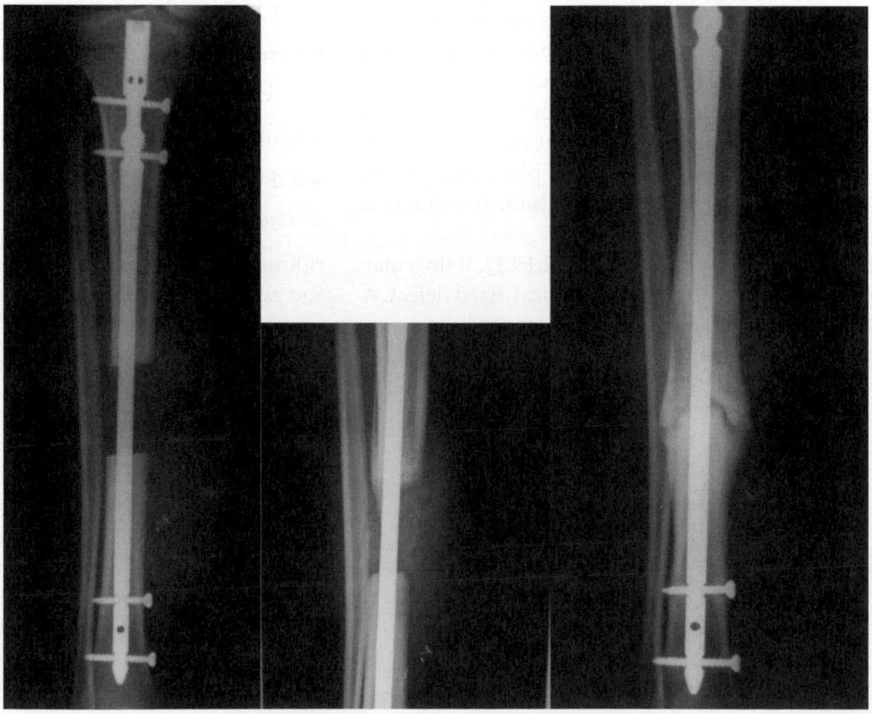

Fig. 12.19.1 Relative stability may result in non-union of the graft.

tendency to compare the defect to a segmental (type C) fracture and to apply relative stability, especially if the osteosynthesis uses a spanning plate.

The biological environment

Logically, as autograft is osteoconductive as well as osteoinductive, for successful neovascularization it is best if the graft is covered by a well-vascularized bed of healthy muscle and this may dictate the chosen surgical approach. Surgery is aided in instances where there is delayed management of segmental defects whilst the soft tissue bed matures following, for example, a free vascularized tissue transfer, by insertion of a spacer. A useful tool is a moulded piece of antibiotic-laden acrylic cement which leaves a cavity, following removal, that can accommodate an appropriate volume of graft as often the soft tissue envelope may be non-pliable and difficult to expand to accommodate sufficient graft to be of mechanical use.

There is a growing role for the mixture of autograft with human recombinant bone morphogenic proteins (BMPs) to enhance and extend autograft, especially in subcritical-sized defects. Its role in combination for critical-sized defects has yet to be established although the author has had anecdotal success using this technique.

Timing of grafting

Based on the premise that all osteosynthesis is a race between the bone uniting and load absorbing and implant failure, the surgeon is under pressure to graft as early as possible any segmental defects to prevent disastrous mechanical failure.

The options open to the surgeon are at initial closure in the open fracture scenario or delayed grafting. The majority of surgeons in the open fracture situation will opt for a delayed approach due to fear of sepsis complicating the graft which is regarded as a potential iatrogenic sequestrum. Sepsis will also cause graft lysis. Autograft, however, has the same propensity to become colonized as metal implants and the trend in recent years has been to internally fix open fractures at initium and thus grafting at the time of closure should not add significantly to the burden of implant related sepsis. Thus, if at the time of soft tissue closure, be it at the first sitting in a fix and flap setting (Figure 12.19.2), or delayed free flap, if the soft tissue bed is macroscopically healthy, then grafting may be performed with sepsis rates comparable to delayed grafting. This approach however is only appropriate in combined orthoplastic units when the zone of injury has undergone a sarcoma type excision from outside of the zone of injury, with immediate reconstruction.

In most situations, it may be considered appropriate to defer grafting to when any occult sepsis may have declared itself and any soft tissue reconstruction will have picked up a blood supply of its own and oedema has resolved, but before the soft tissues become scarred and woody. Appropriate timing is at 6–8 weeks after initial surgery when serum markers are normal (erythrocyte sedimentation rate (ESR), plasma viscosity (PV) levels, and C-reactive protein (CRP) levels) and the patient is no longer on antibiotics.

Small areas of unhealed skin graft at the edges should not delay surgery as long as the mentioned criteria are met. These areas may be excised as part of the incision and primarily closed. In all cases the surgeon should send five deep samples of tissue for microbiological evaluation and a sample for histology (to look for fungal hyphae). If three out of the five samples are positive for the same organism then infection, dormant or otherwise, can be assumed and a 6-week course of appropriate intravenous antibiotics given under the guidance of the microbiologist. Clinical control of sepsis is guided by regular charted ESR, PV, and CRP estimations.

Long-term effects

Autograft will incorporate and remodel but it is always of inferior mechanical strength compared to the original bone and morphologically it forms a solid but heterogeneous block. The cortex and medullary cavity are not reformed.

Ceramics and allograft-based materials

Ceramic implants such as calcium phosphate or calcium hydroxyapatite pastes have no place in the management of segmental defects. Their role is well established as metaphyseal void fillers and in this locus their use may be equal or indeed superior to autograft.

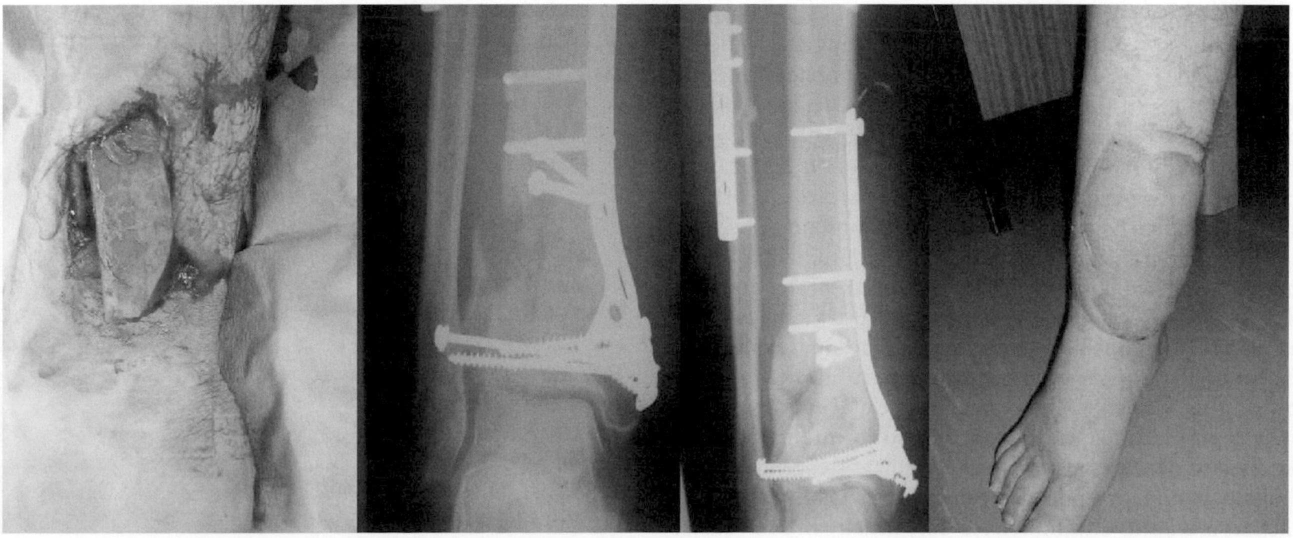

Fig. 12.19.2 Open pilon fracture primarily grafted at time of free flap coverage.

Box 12.19.3 Critical defects

- DH
- Acute shortening
- BMPs
- Free vascularized tissue transfer
- Tissue engineering.

Allograft has realistically only osteoconductive properties and little osteoinductive ones and cannot provide the rapid progress towards union to win the race against failure of osteosynthesis.

Demineralized bone matrix (DBX) has yet to establish a clear role but its protagonists refer to the BMP content. The use of BMPs is well established but evidence is that they are only effective in supraphysiological doses and the BMP content in DBX is of no proven clinical value.

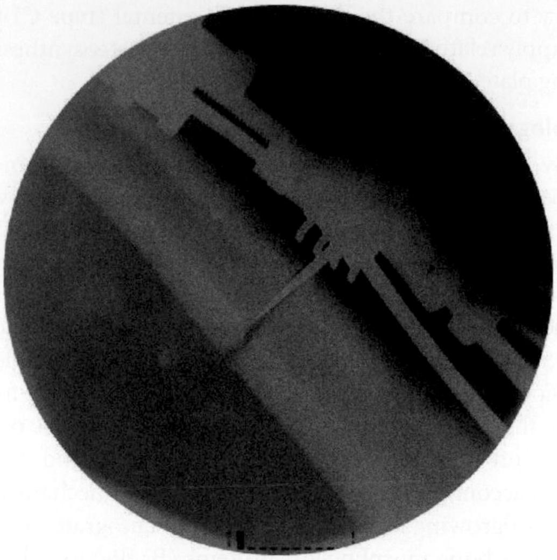

Fig. 12.19.3 Corticotomy with osteotome.

Critical-sized bone defects

The use of free osseous vascularized grafts such as DCMIA and free fibulas has been the mainstay of management of critical-sized defects and their role is well established. Their role in the management of diaphyseal long-bone defects has been superseded by distraction histiogenesis (DH) colloquially referred to as Ilizarov techniques, using circular frames and tensioned wires. The technique is now so mainstream that it will be described in some detail.

Distraction histiogenesis

DH has revolutionized the management of diaphyseal segmental defects of all sizes providing mechanical stability, the ability to modulate the new bone, and to simultaneously correct deformity, whilst at the same time creating new bone that has morphological features comparable to the original bone with similar mechanical properties once remodelling is complete. This technique, whilst powerful and at times spectacular, is not without its problems.

The theory behind the technique

An 'atraumatic' osteotomy is performed by lifting up the periosteum around the elected site for distraction. The bone is tensioned using the frame and the cortices are 'postage stamped' using a 2.5-mm drill. The postage stamping is connected with a sharp osteotomy (Figure 12.19.3), and slid along the axis of the cortex (without penetrating the medullary cavity). Particular care is paid to the posterior cortex and this may be broken by loosening the frame and rotating the bone ends around their longitudinal axis. The direction of rotation is chosen so as to slacken off major nerves. The frame is tightened down to compress the osteotomy which by this method is referred to as a corticotomy. The aim is to leave the periosteal and endosteal blood supply intact. Having said that, osteotomies performed with a Gigli saw appear as effective.

A latent period is required for callus to form and the frame is then used to distract the callus at a rate that osteogenesis occurs in a manner akin to endomembranous ossification. Rates of distraction are up to a millimetre a day, usually in four quarter millimetre increments during the day. For successful DH to occur the 'regenerate' bone requires mechanical stability avoiding shear and rotation. Axial compression is beneficial to regenerate bone and the beam loading biomechanics of circular frames lends itself to this as does a frame construct that is strong enough to allow weight bearing. Progress is monitored using radiographs that show a speculated area of regenerate bone of at least equal volume to the radiologically translucent fibrous interzone.

Ultrasound (Figure 12.19.4), is useful to look for cysts in the regenerate that are indicators that distraction is progressing faster than neovascularization and that distraction should be slowed down. Thus it is clear that the frame should hold onto each end of the bone as well as to the segment being transported. The technique of detaching a segment of bone to force it into the gap of missing bone is called bone transport and because there is a focus of distraction and a focus of compression at the other end, it is referred to as bifocal bone transport. The focus of compression is referred to as the docking site. When docking is complete, the docking site is compressed until union occurs by maintaining

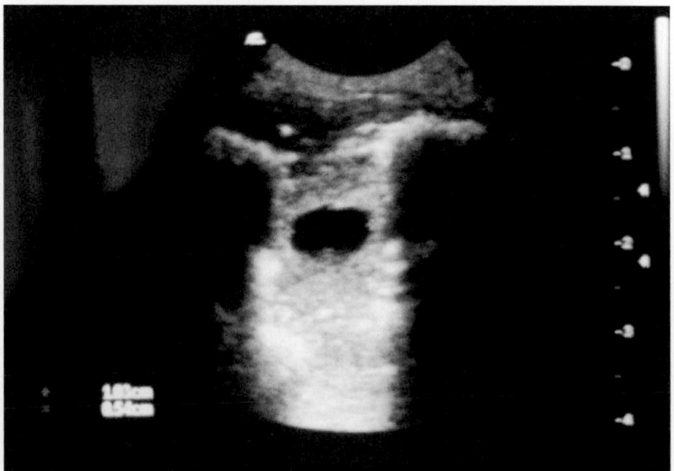

Fig. 12.19.4 Cyst on ultrasound in regenerate bone.

tension by compression for 1 day once a week or once a fortnight. It is not unusual to elect to autograft the docking site.

The docking site

Once docking is completed, the frame needs to stay on until the regenerate is strong enough. The rule of thumb is that the frame on time is 1 month for every centimetre of transport required. Frame removal time is determined by waiting until there is good cortical bone on all cortices radiologically and the patient can fully weight bear without pain. The frame may be progressively loosened over the next few weeks until it is effectively completely loose. The frame can be removed and the limb placed in a weight bearing cast for 6 weeks and early x-rays taken to ensure there is no catastrophic collapse of the regenerate bone. If this occurs a frame may need to be reapplied. This is a disastrous complication and must not be allowed to occur. The author would rather take the frame off a month too late than a day too early. Correction of a collapsed regenerate may be very difficult to achieve.

Frame-on times may be reduced by use of the monorail technique (Figure 12.19.5), and it is perfectly possible to transport a segment of bone over an interlocked intramedullary nail. Early fears about implant related sepsis have not proven to be a major problem. The advantage is that transport is very accurate, frame-on times are much reduced, and collapse of regenerate bone is avoided. Regenerate quality does not appear to be compromised.

Failure of regenerate bone may be dealt with a number of ways. One can go into reverse for a time and then go forwards more slowly. One can simply stop for another latent period and go forwards when radiology supports mineralization or autograft and anecdotally the author has used BMP7 with good results.

The two major issues with circular frames are pin/wire site sepsis and frame-on times. Other issues are failure of the technique to make new bone, neurovascular damage, and joint contractures and subluxations. Autografting may also be required to complete the treatment.

Wire site sepsis

In Ilizarov's unit in Kurgan in Russia, wire site sepsis (WSS) is not found to be a major problem. They have an aggressive outlook on wire site care regarding the wire site as a surgical wound with cleaning with alcohol, application of sterile dressings which are applied with the attendant being scrubbed, gowned, masked, and gloved. The dressings are left undisturbed until the next appointment is due unless there is a problem. In the United Kingdom, a laissez faire attitude has developed with wire sites with no dressings and patients being allowed to shower and go about their daily activities as if there was no issue. This has resulted in WSS rates of greater than 60%. A pragmatic approach more closely following the Russian method can reduce WSS rates to below 20%. One major factor in WSS is the technique of wire insertion.

The Oxford regimen for wire sites

At surgery each wire is dressed with an alcohol sponge that is half split and 'rides' on the wire site and is held close to the skin as a pressure dressing with the clips that slide up and down the wires. This forms a sterile sealed environment and prevents the formation of haematomas as well as movement of the skin edges against the skin which would otherwise break down the wire to skin symbiosis. The sponges are changed under sterile conditions at 48h with the skin pushed down from around the wire and 'descabbed' and cleaned with alcohol and redressed under sterile conditions with sterile dressings and the proprietary clips pushed down onto the dressings so as to supply enough pressure to prevent movement at the wire skin interface. Dressings are left undisturbed and changed once a fortnight unless a problem arises.

Surgical technique

Only sharp wires must be used. If a wire has failed during the process of insertion it must be discarded and a new one used. The wire is inserted under power. The wire insertion site, once chosen, is cleaned again with alcohol. The wire is pushed through the skin and the assistant stretches the muscle compartment that is to be traversed until the wire abuts the bone. The dominant hand of the surgeon holds the drill while the non-dominant hand holds the wire with an alcohol-soaked swab. Drilling occurs in short bursts so as to reduce the chances of thermal necrosis and the formation of a ring sequestrum. Once the wire enters the exiting muscle

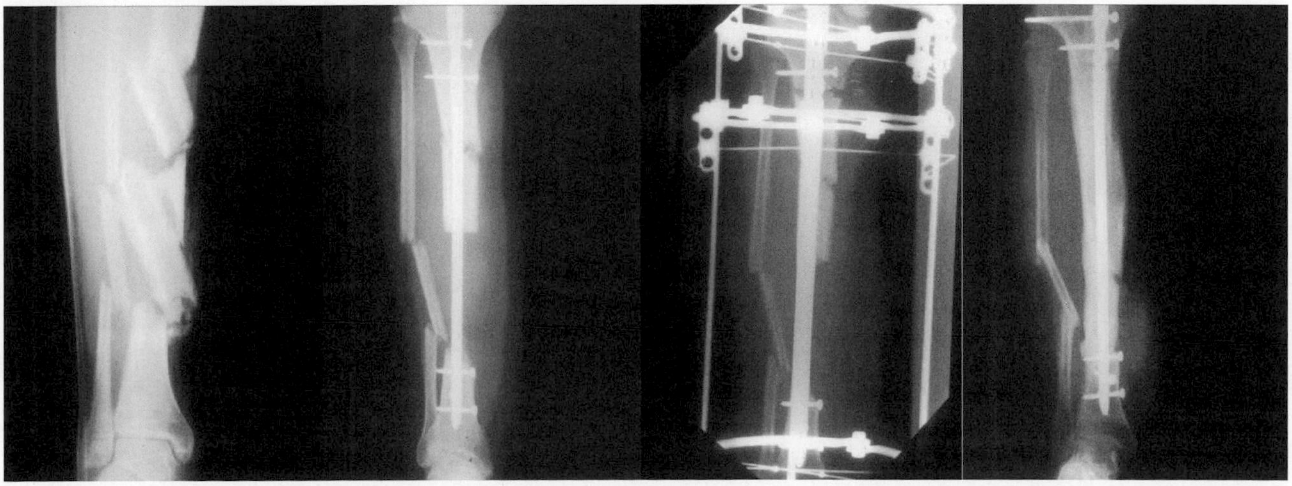

Fig. 12.19.5 The monorail technique minimises frame on time in large defects.

Box 12.19.4 Distraction histiogenesis
◆ 1mm/day (4 × ¼ mm increments) ◆ Consolidation phase (1 month/cm gained) ◆ Can be used in conjunction with intramedullary nail ◆ Complications: • Infection • Neurological damage • Vascular damage • Joint contracture • Non-union docking site • Failure of regenerate • Fracture.

compartment, the assistant passively stretches this too until the skin on the far side is breached. Power is not used when traversing muscle compartments and the wire is tapped with a mallet during this journey so as to reduce the risks of snagging neurovascular bundles.

Acute shortening

This procedure is a useful adjunct in fresh injuries in selected cases (Figure 12.19.6). It is only effective in acute cases when the soft tissue envelope is pliable. Once oedematous it is difficult to achieve. The bone ends may be squared off with a saw until healthy bone is reached and the fracture may be stabilized and even plated and compressed at the time of soft tissue cover, if needed. A deferred DH procedure may then restore the limb to its original length and the docking site has effectively already docked and has started to unite, aided by the limb hyperaemia which results from DH.

In transverse open wounds, shortening may allow primary closure and avoid the need for a free tissue transfer but it will cause longitudinal wounds to gape. It should always be done with the tourniquet released as arterial kinking of empty vessels can occur resulting in an ischaemic foot. If done without an inflated tourniquet, the bone ends can be gently apposed and the vascularity of the foot assessed.

The multidisciplinary team

No one should embark on Ilizarov surgery without adequate experience and ancillary support. The surgeon requires more than an industry produced course (although a useful introduction) and should ideally go on a Fellowship to learn and apply the technique under guidance and supervision. Also they should not perform

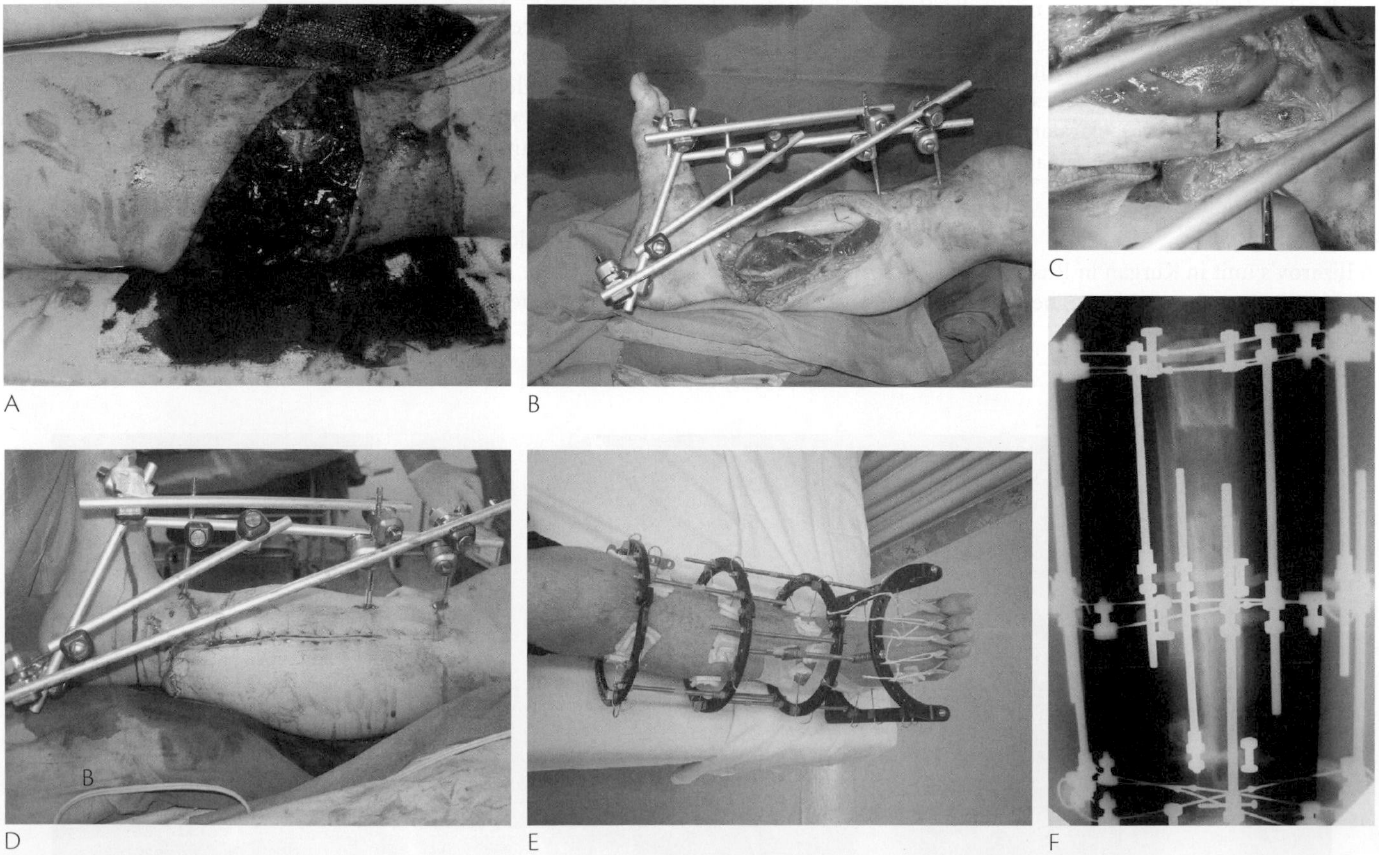

Fig. 12.19.6 A) Transverse wound in open fracture treated by acute shortening B) This acutely shortened limb was held with an external fixator. Note the dorsiflexed ankle. C) The bone ends have been squared off. D) Primary closure was achieved on day 1 by the plastic surgical team. E) An Ilizarov frame is used to relengthen the limb. Note inclusion of the foot. F) Secondary lengthening and compression of the fracture is performed once soft tissues are matured.

Ilizarov techniques on patients unless they have a similarly trained colleague or senior Fellow as part of the unit unless they are prepared never to go on holiday. The ultimate success of the procedure depends on a low complication rate with appropriate rehabilitation. The surgeon must work out of a unit with Ilizarov trained nurses and Ilizarov trained physiotherapists and clinical psychologists. A good x-ray in a septic leg with contractures is a failure.

Lastly, patient-related factors play a major role in the success or otherwise of this technique. Patients need to be fully cognitive of the principles that underlie this technique and be able to follow complex instructions, as well as understand the realistic objectives and how they are to be achieved.

Bone morphogenic proteins

BMPs are multifunctional cytokines of the transforming growth factor beta (TGF-β) superfamily. BMP2 and BMP7 are in commercial use. They work by inducing chemotaxis and mitogenesis and cause cellular differentiation and modulate vascularization and calcification. In the skeleton they orchestrate the pathway from mesenchymal stem cell to osteoblast and osteocyte. They work in supraphysiological doses and as such are as effective as autograft and are frequently used in combination for large defects. They are difficult to handle for the surgeon as come as granules like sand and so have poor handling characteristics and thus the use of drains is contraindicated. It is said that one ampoule has the same amount of BMP as contained in 10 000 human skeletons. Consequently expense has proved a barrier to their regular usage. They have a proven role in improving union rates in open fracture when used at the time of wound closure/coverage. The author has used BMP7 in combination with autograft when filling critical-sized defects with success (Figure 12.19.7). The response has been unpredictable but their role is well established in the treatment of critical and subcritical segmental defects and as usage is increased it is hoped that costs will decrease.

Free tissue transfers

These techniques require the involvement of an experienced plastic surgical team. They are a good 'one-stop shop' for massive defects and have certain attractions. Results have been very good long term but these techniques also have their problems.

There are difficulties with correcting and holding the mechanical axis of the bone. Non-union of one side or other in free fibulas is not uncommon. The graft takes a very long time (up to 4 years) to hypertrophy and may never completely do so. The quality and strength of successful cases is inferior to successful cases of DH. Donor site morbidity may be significant. Plastic surgical and orthopaedic objectives for the patient are not always entirely the same.

Tissue engineering

This is the exciting future with bespoke implants and mesenchymal stem cells harvested from the patient that are grown in culture onto a suitable anatomically formed implantable matrix with recombinant signalling molecules. Research is ongoing with regards to a suitable matrix on ceramics, starch-based materials, and nanomaterials. The aim is to provide normal living tissue at the site but stability is an issue as the tissue develops. This is presently experimental or used in specialist research units.

The unforeseeable future

Great hope is held for genetic manipulation following the mapping of the human genome but reality and hope have a temporal mismatch. Nevertheless it is clear that some individuals have an idiosyncratic response to injury and nature can work in tandem with the surgeon as exemplified in the case demonstrated in Figure 12.19.8. This patient sustained a segmental defect following trauma in which the bone was stabilized and the soft tissue defect made good with a free muscle flap. The patient was awaiting maturation of the soft tissues prior to embarking on a monorail bifocal bone transport but rapidly started weight bearing without pain.

Summary

Autograft is the gold standard for the treatment of subcritical segmental defects. Its volume is limited but may be enhanced by harvesting from the femoral canal using reaming aspiration irrigation systems.

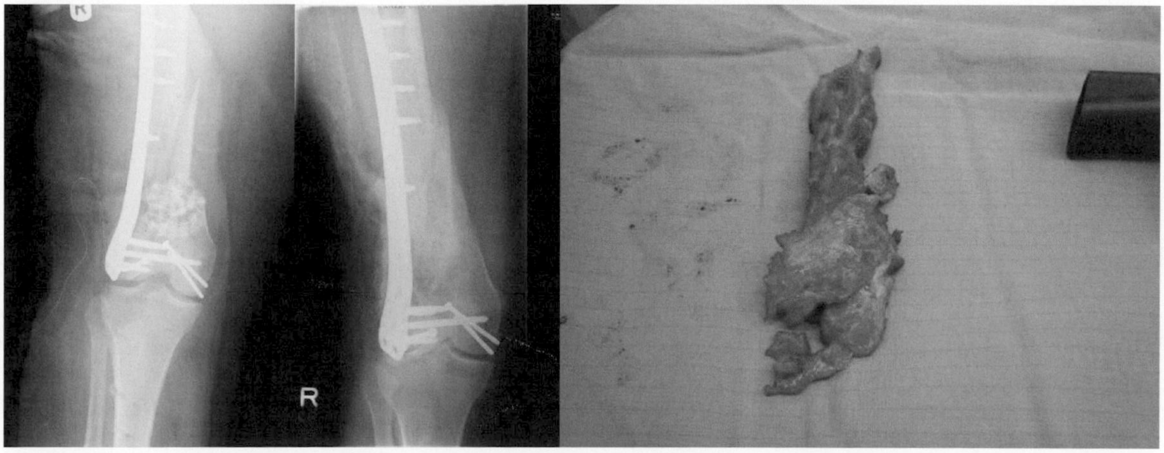

Fig. 12.19.7 BMP7 with autograft was used to treat this large defect which produced a large bone horn which required subsequent excision.

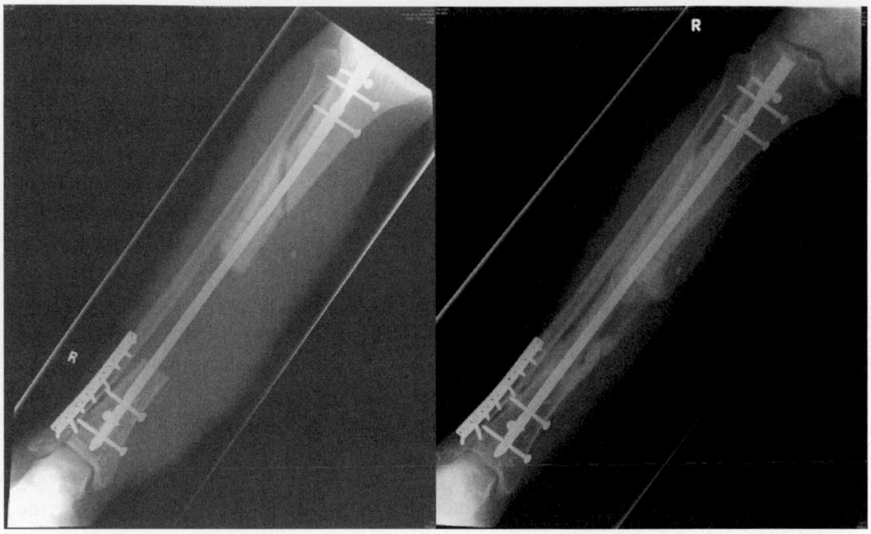

Fig. 12.19.8 Spontaneous filling in of a 10-cm defect after stabilization and free flap coverage.

Autograft mixed with BMPs have a role in the management of critical-sized segmental defects but DH and Ilizarov techniques are now the gold standard for managing critical-sized defects producing bone of near morphological normality.

The future lies with tissue engineering with signalling molecules and genetic manipulation with bespoke implants.

Further reading

Carrington, N.C., Smith, R.M., Knight, S.L., and Matthews, S.J.E. (2000). Ilizarov bone transport over A primary tibial nail and free flap: a new technique for treating Gustilo grade 3b fractures with large segmental defects. *Injury*, **31**(2), 112–15.

DeCoster, T.A., Gehlert, R.J., Mikola, E.A., Pirela-Cruz, M.A. (2004). Management of posttraumatic segmental bone defects. *Journal of the American Academy of Orthopaedic Surgeons*, **12**(1), 28–38.

Ilizarov, G.A. (1992). *Transosseous Osteosynthesis: Theoretical and Clinical Aspects of the Regeneration and Growth of Tissue.* Berlin: Springer Verlag.

Kadiyala, S., Jaiswal, N., and Bruder, S.P. (1997). Culture-expanded, bone marrow-derived mesenchymal stem cells can regenerate a critical-sized segmental bone defect. *Tissue Engineering*, **3**(2), 173–85.

12.20

Injuries to muscle–tendon units

S.D. Deo

Summary points

- Most injuries at junction of muscle and tendon
- Early gentle movement best for recovery
- Tendon heals more slowly than muscle
- Surgery may include direct repair or more complex procedures e.g. lengthening/augmentation
- Minimally invasive procedures often best e.g. Achilles tendon.

Introduction

Skeletal muscle is the human body's largest single tissue by weight, comprising 40–45% of total body weight. Muscle's main function is to generate power for movement and maintain posture. Other functions include storage of energy and blood volume and thermoregulation. Muscles have tendons at each end which insert into bone or fascia.

Muscle, the musculotendinous (or myotendinous) junctions, tendon, and bony insertion together form a *muscle–tendon unit.*

Acute injuries to muscle–tendon units are common and cause considerable morbidity due to the site of injury and the age of those affected. They can occasionally be life- or limb-threatening. Much clinical and research experience on these injuries is the result of work by sports medicine clinicians. Chronic injuries to muscle–tendon units are discussed in Chapters 4.6 and 8.9.

There are controversies and deficiencies regarding natural history, classification, and treatment of these injuries, particularly when one compares the literature on bony and articular surface injuries. An understanding of structure, pathology, and healing helps in understanding the basis of operative and surgical treatments.

Epidemiology (Box 12.20.1)

Epidemiologic data regarding the incidence and prevalence of muscle–tendon unit injuries in the general population are poor. Some estimate a point prevalence of muscle injury of 1–2% of the population in industrialized countries.

These injuries are uncommon in young children, but the incidence increases in the second decade to peak and plateau in the third and fourth decades. There is then a decline in acute injuries, and chronic or acute-on-chronic problems increase in frequency. They are more common in males.

The most common type is the indirect minimal or partial muscle rupture. These are the most commonly occurring sports injuries, but are also frequent in the workplace and therefore have a significant economic impact. The economic cost in the of acute non-articular soft-tissue problems in the United Kingdom has been estimated at over £1 billion per year

The incidence of muscle–tendon unit injuries seems to be increasing, due to increasing awareness and demand for treatment and increased adult participation in regular sport and exercise.

Current classifications are mainly based on the site, cause, and severity of injury. Unfortunately there is continuing confusion over nomenclature and terminology, and controversy over indications and optimal modes of treatment.

Anatomy

Skeletal muscle consists of multinucleate myocytes or fibres containing myofibrils which provide its contractile properties. Groups of muscle fibres form fasciculi. Groups of fasciculi form the whole muscle. There are other cells within muscle, such as stellate cells, which have important functions in healing and regeneration. Layers of connective tissue around muscle are the endomysium, which provides the extracellular space, the perimysium,

Box 12.20.1 Epidemiology

- Commonest third to fourth decades
- Commoner in males
- Incidence increasing
- Cost UK £1 billion per year.

which surrounds the fasciculi, and the epimysium, which surrounds the whole muscle (Figure 12.20.1A). A rich nerve and blood supply runs within these layers. The circulation within muscle is nutritive or non-nutritive; the latter are impedance and storage channels. The connective tissue sheaths fuse at the musculotendinous junction with tendon connective tissue.

Tendons are mainly composed of type I collagen (70% by dry weight) and are relatively acellular. Bands of collagen fibrils form fasciculi, and groups of fasciculi form bundles. Fasciculi are surrounded by the endotenon, containing nerves and small blood vessels. The outer connective tissue layer is the epitenon, which lies in loose areolar tissue (paratenon) or within a tendon sheath (Figure 12.20.1B). Tendon sheaths and bursae occur where moving structures are in tight apposition. The nerve supply is mainly efferent and the blood supply is poor, running in plexi between fasciculi. Watershed areas where the tendon blood supply is poorest have been identified and are linked to tendon pathology and rupture.

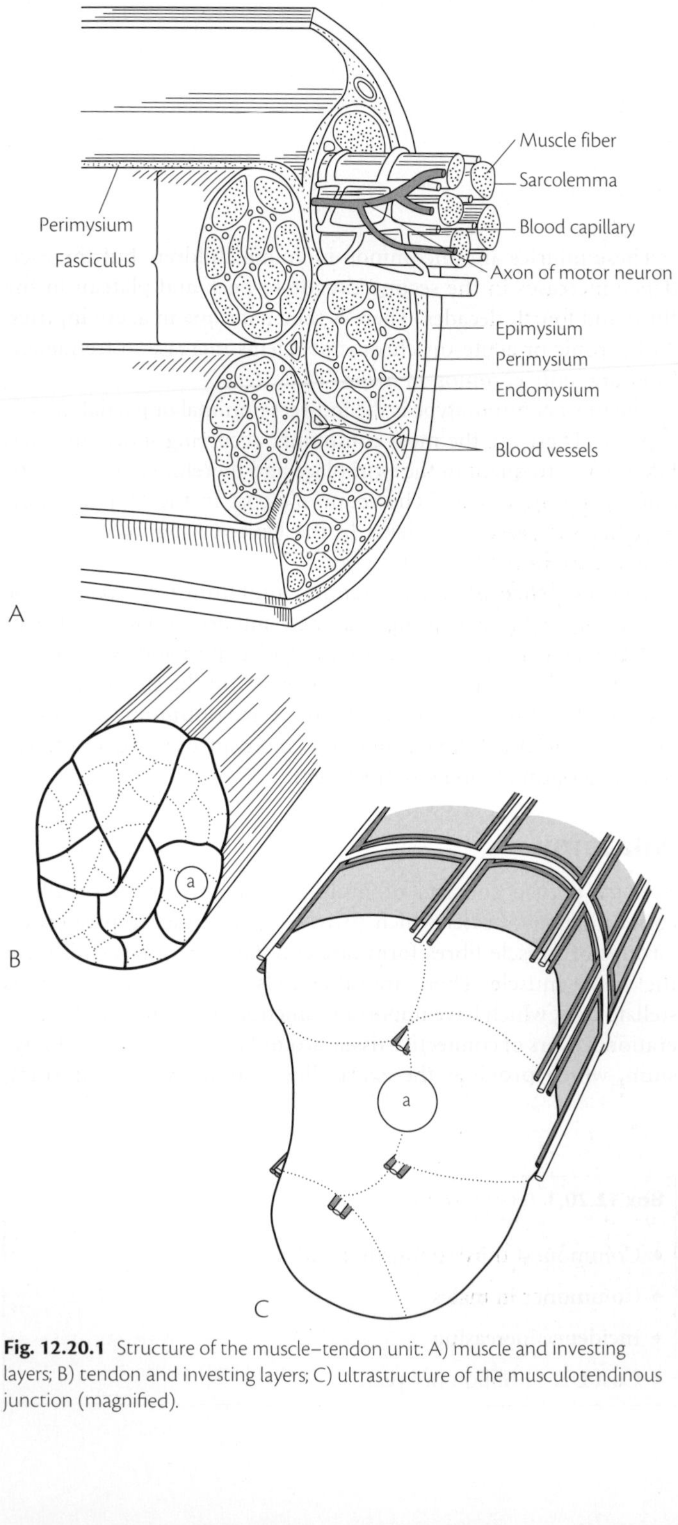

Fig. 12.20.1 Structure of the muscle–tendon unit: A) muscle and investing layers; B) tendon and investing layers; C) ultrastructure of the musculotendinous junction (magnified).

The *musculotendinous junction* is the interface between muscle and tendon. There is an intimate relationship between muscle fibres and collagen fibrils but no direct continuity (Figure 12.20.1C). The sarcolemma has multiple finger-like invaginations, known as terminal interdigitations, providing a large contact area to which collagen fibrils adhere. Adhesion is aided by glycoproteins and type III collagen. The junction is densely packed with sarcoplasmic organelles, mitochondria, and satellite cells, indicating potential for growth, repair, and regeneration. There is a portal blood supply and a rich efferent nerve supply.

The *osseotendinous junction* is also known as the *enthesis*. Tendons attach to bone at the periosteum and cortical bone, where they intermingle with perforating fibres of Sharpey, thus firmly anchoring them. If the attachment to bone is smooth, it implies the presence of a fibrocartilaginous plate which has anchoring properties.

Biomechanics (Box 12.20.2)

Muscle contraction, controlled by voluntary or reflex neural activity, produces a force depending on the number of muscle fibres available, muscle adaptation, muscle fibre type, muscle length, velocity of shortening, state of activation, and temperature.

Tendon properties vary depending on functional requirement, balancing tensile strength with elasticity. Tendons have high tensile strength, similar to bone, with 1cm^2 supporting 600–1000kg. Tendons display viscoelastic properties of stress relaxation, hysteresis, and creep. Overloading causes permanent lengthening damage—plastic deformation. Ultimate tensile strength is reached when all fibrils have failed—complete rupture.

The musculotendinous junction is important in force transmission, particularly during eccentric muscle contractions which occur in lengthening muscle; for example, landing from a jump causes eccentric contraction of the quadriceps, putting severe demands on the musculotendinous junction.

In vitro studies have shown that muscles tested to failure do so in the region of the musculotendinous junction on the muscle side of the junctional membrane. Muscle fatigue, prior injury, poorly conditioned muscle, and denervation all predispose strongly to. In human lower limbs, proximal rupture occurs in the proximal lower limb and distal rupture occurs in the distal lower limb. In the first and second decades the enthesis is the weakest part of the unit, and is thus more prone to injury.

Box 12.20.2 Biomechanics of tendons

- High tensile strength
- Overloading causes plastic deformation, then rupture
- Musculo-tendinous junction commonest site of injury.

Pathology and healing (Box 12.20.3)

General principles

The pathology of injury and healing are intimately connected. Injury incites an acute inflammatory response, of lag phase, lasting for 2–10 days, in proportion to and dependent on the degree of cellular injury and cell death. The inflammatory process will usually resolve and a cellular phase will commence. If there has been no tissue destruction, there is rapid resolution of the inflammatory exudate and return to normal, i.e. a grade I muscle injury. In the relatively avascular tendons, phases are prolonged. Sepsis or continuing injury will cause continuing inflammation. At 3–4 weeks postinjury the cellular regenerative phase will give way to a remodelling phase, which may go on for months.

Factors affecting healing

Local and systemic factors influencing muscle–tendon unit healing are shown in Box 12.20.5.

Pathological events following injury and healing in muscle

Traditionally it was thought that muscle mainly healed by scarring. However, the capacity for muscle to compensate and return to full function by regeneration and hypertrophy has been demonstrated.

Box 12.20.3 Healing

- Muscle:
  - Always some scarring
  - Mobilization is probably good
- Musculotendinous junction—healing is slower
- Tendon:
  - By week 4, 40% of strength has returned
  - Cyclical loading is probably good
- Osteotendinous healing—is rapid.

Box 12.20.4 Complications

- Early:
  - Crush
  - Compartment syndrome
  - Haematoma
- Intermediate:
  - Muscle pain and spasm
  - Sepsis
- Late:
  - Scarring
  - Wasting
  - Stiffness
  - Myositis ossificans.

Box 12.20.5 Factors influencing the type of muscle–tendon injuries

- Mechanism of injury (e.g. crush, cut, etc.)
- Severity (force applied etc.)
- Muscle involved
- Location of injury in the muscle tendon unit
- Pre-existing pathology (e.g. steroid therapy, degeneration)
- Other injuries (e.g. vascular, neurological)
- Acute/acute on chronic/chronic.

Soon after muscle fibre injury, the fibres at each end of the injury zone break into short cylinders back to the next intact Z-disc and hypercontract, restricting the injury, although there is fibre necrosis. Rupture of epimyseal vessels cause intermuscular haematomas with extensive ecchymosis and mild pain. Central ruptures cause intermuscular haematomas with more localized swelling, intense pain, muscle inhibition, and stiffness.

As well as necrosis and haemorrhage, there is acute inflammatory response with oedema and cellular infiltrate including macrophages which appear on days 1–2, ingesting debris but leaving the basal laminas. Muscle fibres from each end produce myotubes from their sarcolemmas, along which muscle fibres regrow. Satellite cells attach to the myotubes at day 3 and aid regeneration. Fibroblasts are also activated at this time. Regeneration occurs most rapidly and completely in clean muscle incisions, but has been noted after all muscle injuries. There is always some scar tissue formation proportional to the amount of muscle loss; thus healed muscle does not return to normal ultrastructurally. Remodelling follows. There is good evidence that mobilization may reduce the amount of scar tissue formation.

Musculotendinous junction healing

Events at the musculotendinous junction are similar to but slower than those in muscle, with a central core of necrosis and a zone of hypercontracted fibres. Myotube formation occurs at 7–14 days, new sarcoplasmic contents appear at 21–28 days, and the cellular phase continues for 5–7 weeks postinjury.

Tendon healing

In tendon the inflammatory response takes over 14 days to settle. The tendon ends fill with fibrinous clot and granulation.

Repair occurs by proliferation of fibroblasts, either tenocytes from the tendon or from surrounding connective tissue layers, which synthesize collagen commencing on day 7 and continuing for several weeks. Fibroblast numbers and metabolism peak at day 14 and then slowly decline. Tendon strength increases as collagen fibrils are formed and reorientate. By week 4 the tendon has regained 70% of its pre-rupture stiffness and 40% of its strength.

Remodelling commences at week 4. Eight weeks postinjury, peritendinous adhesions break down and the tendon strength continues to increase. The collagen fibres are realigned fully at 9 months and remodelling continues for a year postinjury. In sutured tendons the lowest breaking strength is at day 7. It is doubled at 2–3 weeks and again at 4–12 weeks postinjury.

Experimentally, cyclical loading and early mobilization improve collagen fibril realignment, capillary ingrowth, time to normal strength, and viscoelasticity, and reduce stiffness. Immobilization of muscle–tendon units reduces tensile strength at the musculotendinous junction, increases risk of strain injury, and causes a 30% reduction in vascular density following 3 weeks of immobilization.

Osseotendinous junction healing

Unlike other injuries, immobilization is a prerequisite for healing to occur. Given the age of the patients with disruptions at this level, healing is rapid and occurs by fracture-type healing of the bony avulsion.

Compartment and crush syndromes

In these two conditions, muscle injuries can cause limb- or life-threatening problems.

Compartment syndrome is caused by swelling confined by osseofascial compartments, causing interruption of the normal capillary arteriolar circulation which can result in a vicious cycle of cell death and further swelling, eventually causing infarction of muscle, nerves, and other structures within the compartment. Management of compartment syndromes is discussed in Chapter 12.2.

Crush syndrome may occur after any blunt trauma, classically entrapment or prolonged ischaemic revascularization injury where there has been extensive rhabdomyolysis causing release of muscle proteins and waste products. This leads to intravascular activation, circulatory collapse, and acute renal failure, which is also caused by intrinsic nephron damage by the free muscle products, frequently exacerbated by inadequate resuscitation.

Complications of muscle–tendon unit injuries

Complications can be classified by time of onset from injury or by cause—the injury itself or iatrogenic (see Box 12.20.4).

Classification

The type and severity of injury to muscle–tendon units is determined by a number of factors summarized in Box 12.20.5. There is no equivalent to the comprehensive classification system for fractures.

Muscle injury can be divided broadly into indirect and direct injury, in terms of the force transmission causing injury.

Indirect muscle injury

Indirect muscle injuries are most common and are also known as muscle strain injury, intrinsic muscle injury, pulled muscle, muscle sprain, or muscle tear. They occur when an abnormal force is applied to a muscle usually when it is activated and contracting, often eccentrically. Other factors associated with indirect injuries are muscle conditioning, fatigue, warm-up or muscle stretch, muscle temperature, anabolic steroid use, and previous injury.

Indirect muscle injury occurs most commonly at the musculotendinous junction in adults, the tendon in older patients, and the enthesis in young adults. In older patients there is often underlying degeneration within the tendon.

Muscles prone to indirect injury are those which cross two joints, contract eccentrically, and have a high proportion of type II fast-twitch fibres. Common sites of indirect injury are the medial head gastrocnemius (tennis leg), triceps surae, rectus femoris, adductor longus, semimembranosus, triceps brachii, and pectoralis major.

Indirect injuries form a spectrum from minor sprains to complete muscle ruptures, which have been graded as follows.

- *First-degree injury (grade 1)* is a strain with no significant muscle tissue disruption, but only with some disruptions of the connective tissue layers. There is minimal inflammation and no loss of strength or motion
- *Second-degree injury (grade 2)* implies damage to muscle fibres and connective tissue that compromises muscle function, i.e. a partial rupture. The partial rupture is associated with haemorrhage from ruptured blood vessels of the perimysium and, depending on its location, may cause a central haematoma
- *Third-degree (grade 3)* rupture implies complete disruption of some portion of the muscle–tendon unit, with concomitant loss of function and significant haemorrhage in the zone of injury.

Direct muscle injuries

Direct muscle injuries are divided into open and closed injuries. Closed injuries generally occur as a direct blow or crush as the result of sports injury (also known as extrinsic injury), blunt assault, industrial accidents, or road traffic collisions. Open injuries are associated with a sharp laceration or tissue loss such as those caused by glass, open fracture, gunshot injury, or burn. Direct injuries also form a spectrum from minimal to severe, and the O'Donoghue grading can be applied.

Other traumatic causes of muscle cell injury

Other causes of muscle cell injury are injuries to structures such as major blood vessels or nerves which result in muscle fibre death or dysfunction. Compartment syndromes can also cause muscle fibre death.

Management

Principles

Definitive management of patients with muscle–tendon unit injuries involves diagnosis treatment and rehabilitation of the patient. (This is summarized later in Box 12.20.9.) The terms emergency, initial treatment, and definitive treatment are not mutually exclusive; initial treatment of an indirect muscle injury is often definitive as well.

The first aim is to ensure the patient does not have a life- or limb-threatening condition; if this is the case the patient should be resuscitated and treated appropriately.

Clinical assessment

Clinical assessment involves history and examination, which is sufficient to diagnose most isolated injuries to muscle–tendon units. Compartment and crush syndromes, other injuries, and comorbidity should be identified, and this guides the need for further investigation and treatment. Initial clinical assessment is also a baseline for monitoring progress. Thorough note taking is advisable, particularly if treatment is going to be prolonged and multidisciplinary.

Differential diagnosis

A number of conditions can be mistaken for acute muscle–tendon unit injuries; some affect the muscle–tendon unit from within and some originate outside the unit, as summarized in Box 12.20.6.

History

The history should provide information regarding the injury and the patients to aid diagnosis and plan the extent of examination and investigation. Principle symptoms of muscle–tendon unit injuries are localized pain, swelling, and loss of function. Key points in the history are shown in Box 12.20.7.

Examination

The clinical examination should be sufficiently thorough to confirm or suggest one diagnosis and exclude others. The basic principles are to inspect, palpate, and move the affected limb passively and actively. The neurovascular status of the limb is examined and, where applicable, specific tests of muscle or tendon integrity should be performed. These are summarized in Box 12.20.8.

Joint movement is important in differentiating between intra- and extra-articular problems; for example, pain and reduced power on testing active external rotation of the shoulder implies an injury to the teres minor or infrapinatus components of the rotator cuff.

Thompson's calf squeeze test for the ruptured Achilles tendon is an example of a specific test of muscle tendon integrity.

Investigations

Investigations, summarized in Box 12.20.9, are not essential for all muscle–tendon unit injuries. There should be clear indications, which are to confirm a diagnosis prior to definitive treatment, to define which treatment option is optimal, to aid operative planning, to diagnose or exclude other pathologies, and/or to give prognostic information.

Box 12.20.6 Differential diagnosis

- Extrinsic:
  - Stress fractures
  - Ligamentous/capsular injury
  - Bursitis
  - Referred pain
  - Radicular pain
  - Peripheral nerve pain
  - Skeletal infection
  - Skeletal tumour
- Intrinsic:
  - Tendonitis
  - Myositis
  - Infection
  - Muscle hernia
  - Muscle tumour.

Box 12.20.7 History taking

- Evaluation of injury:
  - Circumstances
  - Timing
  - Ability to continue activity
- Evaluation of patient:
  - Age
  - Occupation
  - Location of symptoms
  - Onset of symptoms
  - Treatment to date
  - Past treatment
  - Social history
  - Level of sports performance.

Box 12.20.8 Examination

- Inspect
- Palpate
- Range of motion
- Neurovascular
- Specific tests.

Box 12.20.9 Investigations

- MRI
- Ultrasound
- CT
- Radiography
- Arthrography
- Bone scan
- Blood tests
- Urine tests
- Compartment pressure measurement
- EMG.

The investigation of choice for muscle–tendon unit injuries is magnetic resonance imaging (MRI), which gives excellent resolution of normal and pathological musculoskeletal and neurovascular structures shown in Figure 12.20.2. Ultrasound and computed tomography (CT) are also useful, particularly the former. Plain radiographs have a role, particularly in osseotendinous junction injuries and suspected fractures in conjunction with MRI are also useful.

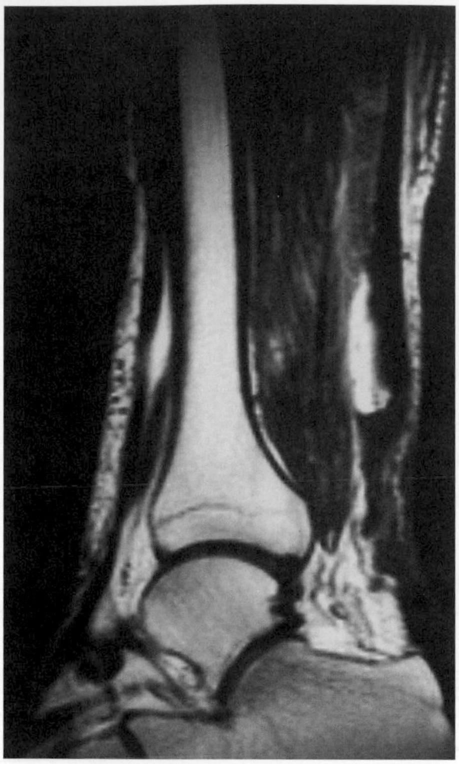

Fig. 12.20.2 Imaging of muscle–tendon unit injury: MRI scan showing rupture of the Achilles tendon.

Treatment

Principles of treatment

Most muscle–tendon unit injuries are treated non-operatively. The aims of treatment are to restore the muscle–tendon unit to normal function as quickly as possible and to prevent complications (see Box 12.20.4). Return to normal function can be improved by prompt adequate treatment and rehabilitation. A small proportion of patients will require specialized non-operative or surgical treatment, and in the latter a delayed operation or not operating may result in significant long-term morbidity.

Non-operative treatment

Emergency

Immobilization of the injured extremity, using a splint if necessary, is analgesic and avoids worsening the injury. Fluid resuscitation diuretics, dopamine, and dialysis are used for crush syndrome. Diagnosis, monitoring, and treatment are detailed elsewhere (Chapter 12.10).

Initial treatment

Painkillers, rest, ice, compression, and elevation (PRICE) form the initial treatment for a significant proportion of patients with muscle–tendon unit injuries. It is commonly used as a postoperative regimen as well. The regime minimizes the inflammatory process symptoms and therefore the formation of fibrous adhesions. It is adequate for most grade 1 and grade 2 acute muscle–tendon unit injuries. This type of treatment is usually indicated for the first 3 to 7 days post-injury.

Box 12.20.10 Treatment

- Pharmacological:
  - NSAIDs
  - Analgaesia
  - Sedation/muscle relaxants
  - Local anaesthetics
- Physical:
  - Initial 'PRICE'
  - Splinting
  - Movement/exercise
  - Therapeutic ultrasound
  - Short wave diathermy
  - Aspirate haematoma.

Definitive treatment (Box 12.20.10)

PRICE is frequently the definitive treatment. A smaller proportion of patients, particularly those seen in a hospital or clinic may require additional non-operative treatments.

Pharmacological treatments

Non-steroidal anti-inflammatory drugs (NSAIDs) are widely used for musculoskeletal problems and act by inhibiting arachidonic acid metabolism, reducing inflammation and platelet activation. They also have secondary analgesic properties. The exact mode of action of NSAIDs is unknown and qualitative proof of efficacy is poor. Inhibiting the cellular phase has theoretical risks of inhibition of healing.

Simple analgesics, such as paracetamol and opiate derivatives, have no direct effect on the injury, but are useful for symptom control. They can be used in conjunction with, or as an alternative to, NSAIDs.

Sedatives or *muscle relaxants* may be used to counter severe or painful muscle spasms, particularly in an anxious or agitated patient. They should be avoided in patients with head injury, if there is a specific contraindication, if there is a history of allergy or drug dependency, or if there is inadequate monitoring.

Local anaesthetics can be given proximal to a lesion as a regional block or epidural in lower-limb problems, for pain control, or for operative anaesthesia. In the acute situation there is a theoretical risk of masking a compartment syndrome, as blocks may cause sensory and motor deficits. *Hyperbaric oxygen* has been used in a few patients with muscle–tendon unit injuries.

There is no role for the use of corticosteroids in the acute phase of muscle–tendon unit injury.

Physical treatments

Rest, ice, compression, and *elevation* are most important in the first 72h postinjury.

Splinting, casting, or other forms of immobilization can be important in early management to help reduce pain and muscle spasm. They are also indicated for the definitive management of non-operatively treated tendon ruptures, most commonly of the Achilles tendon, as well as following surgical repairs. Various materials are available, including fibreglass and thermoplastics plaster of Paris. Splints can be removable, allowing for wound and skin care, and hinged to allow controlled joint motion.

Movement and exercise: understanding the normal healing process will guide the balance between immobilization to prevent rerupture or commencing mobilization to encourage faster return of normal blood supply and better remodelling. Ideally, exercise should be supervised, preferably by a physiotherapist.

Massage and *counter-irritation* have analgesic and potentially beneficial effects after the early inflammatory phase, similarly to other physical therapy treatment modalities (see later).

Ultrasound and *short-wave diathermy* are the most frequently used electrotherapy modalities in the treatment of muscle injuries. Others include electrical field stimulation and cryotherapy. Therapeutic ultrasound produces local thermal and non-thermal effects which reduces the duration of the inflammatory response by increasing macrophage and fibroblast activity, accelerates oedema and haematoma resorption, and improves the strength of scar tissue.

Needle aspiration of a persistent or worsening haematoma causing pain and muscle inhibition can be performed in the clinic or the radiology department. It must be carried out under aseptic conditions and a firm pressure dressing should be applied to the affected area to prevent recurrence.

Operative treatment

Rationale and timing

The decision to undertake operative treatment is based on a number of factors (Box 12.20.11). The potential benefits of surgery should outweigh the risks. The aims of surgery are as for treatment in general.

The timing of surgery is largely dependent on the pathology, although patient factors such as injury in top-class athletes are important. Acute compartment syndromes should be decompressed urgently as the warm ischaemic time to irreversible muscle damage is about 6h. After this period, and particularly after 10 days, there is marked adhesion formation and fibrosis, so that dissection and surgical trauma are more extensive, increasing the risks of complications and delayed healing.

Operative principles and technique

The principles of the surgery of soft tissues are summarized in Box 12.20.12.

Types of procedure

The main types of procedure are shown in Box 12.20.13. A combination of procedures may be needed.

Compartment decompression

The diagnosis of compartment syndrome and the surgical techniques used in its management are discussed elsewhere (Chapter 12.2).

Haematoma evacuation

Haematoma evacuation is only indicated as the sole procedure when a large intramuscular haematoma fails to resolve, increases in size, causes incipient skin and subcutaneous tissue necrosis, inhibits muscle activity or causes spasms, or is likely to progress to an ancient haematoma (commonly in thigh muscle groups). These types of haematomas are more common in patients with bleeding diatheses, and prompt correction of the clotting abnormality is the

Box 12.20.11 Factors affecting treatment

- Injury factors:
  - Compartment syndrome
  - Fracture
  - Complete rupture
  - Retraction of rupture
  - Open wound
  - Wound contamination
- Patient factors:
  - Age
  - Fitness for surgery
  - Comorbidity
  - Pre-injury level of function
  - Expectations of recovery
- Institution factors: e.g. personnel, expertise, etc.

Box 12.20.12 Surgical principles

- Asepsis
- Antibiotics if implants used
- Tourniquet is safe and indicated
- Adequate exposure
- Excise dead tissue
- Tension free apposition.

Box 12.20.13 Types of procedure

- Closed injuries:
  - Direct suture
  - V–Y lengthening
  - Reinsertion into bone and fixation
  - Augmentation, e.g. tendon, wire, graft.
  - Fasciotomy
  - Evacuation of haematoma
- Open injuries:
  - Wound excision
  - Delayed repair
  - Soft tissue cover procedures.

priority in such cases. Ultrasound guided biopsy is preferable in this group. Early haematoma evacuation may have a role in top-class athletes.

Direct suture

Direct suture or apposition is most readily used in fresh ruptures of the muscle–tendon unit at the mid-tendon, musculotendinous junction, or muscle belly. It can be a formally open technique or minimally invasive or percutaneous. Given the longitudinal alignment of the muscle fibres and tendon fibrils, simple suture techniques are not applicable and more complex sutures such as mattress, Kessler, or Strickland sutures are more applicable.

Lengthening with repair

Lengthening with repair is sometimes necessary to gain length to allow tension-free apposition of ruptured ends. Separation is caused by tissue loss at the time of trauma, fraying of tendon ends, retraction and shortening of the ruptured muscle, underlying muscle pathology, or a combination of these factors. An example of this type of repair is the V–Y lengthening of muscle, as used in quadriceps and Achilles tendon repairs (Figure 12.20.3B). Another method is to turn down flaps of the affected tendon as in rotator cuff or Achilles tendon repairs (Figure 12.20.3C).

Fixation to bone

Avulsed bone at the enthesis or avulsion of the tendon nearby may require direct fixation to bone. The former can be repaired using a small plate or toothed washer (Figure 12.20.3G), and the latter by using sutures with drill holes through bone or specially designed anchor sutures (Figure 12.20.3F, H).

Augmentation

A muscle–tendon unit repair can be augmented by using neighbouring muscle–tendon units as direct supports or brought into apposition as a flap, free fascia lata strips, implants such as Dacron or Marlex wrapped around the repair, or wires to protect the repair (Figure 12.20.3D, E).

Toilet and debridement

In the presence of an open contaminated wound, the priority is toilet and debridement to render the wound tidy, prior to definitive repair of the muscle–tendon unit and soft tissue cover.

Postoperative treatment

The initial priority is for early wound healing without infection. Early immobilization facilitates wound healing in the early phase. The immobilization time depends on the strength of the repair, the vascularity, the preoperative condition of the muscle–tendon unit and integument, and the treating physician's preference.

For the lower limb, a consensus period of immobilization would be 6 weeks, followed by increasing protected and supervised mobilization over the next 6–12 weeks, and a return to normal activity profile at 6–12 months depending on the injury, the strength of the repair, and the pre-injury level of function.

Rehabilitation

Principles

Rehabilitation is the third and final part of the management of a patient with a muscle–tendon unit injury, forming a continuum with diagnosis and treatment. It is frequently neglected by physicians.

Rehabilitation aims to restore to normal function, or as normal as pathology allows, the injured muscle–tendon unit, adjacent joints, the affected limb, and the whole patient. Additional aims are to reduce complications and prevent further injury both during the remodelling phase (reinjury) and in the longer term.

The rehabilitation phase should take into account the diagnoses, treatment, pre-injury level of activity, and expectations of recovery. Physical, social, ergonomic, and psychological factors should be considered in rehabilitation. Most rehabilitation is performed by the patient, guided by physiotherapists. Physicians commonly prescribe rehabilitation without supervising it. Less commonly, pain clinics, psychologists, and psychiatrists are involved.

Treatments in rehabilitation

The treatment options are similar to those used in the early treatment, although the emphasis is different. Mobilization and exercise, following splintage and immobilization, are the cornerstones of rehabilitation. Other treatment modalities include counselling and drugs.

Common muscle tendon injuries requiring repair

The most common closed muscle–tendon unit injuries requiring repair, excluding open direct injuries, are listed in Box 12.20.14. They are generally complete ruptures due to indirect trauma. Ruptures and subsequent repair of almost every muscle–tendon unit have been described. Further details are given in this section and in the relevant chapters.

Achilles tendon and distal musculotendinous injuries

Complete ruptures of the Achilles tendon are the most commonly operated tendon ruptures. They occur most frequently in the fourth and fifth decades, and are twice as common in males. This is the most commonly occurring tendon rupture in sport.

The location of ruptures (2–4cm from the calcaneal insertion) is the watershed area of hypovascularity most prone to microtrauma and degenerative change, strongly associated with tendon ruptures.

The usual cause is sudden dorsiflexion of a plantarflexed foot, although it can be caused by direct sharp or blunt trauma. The classic symptom is of a feeling of being kicked above the heel.

Box 12.20.14 Injuries often requiring repair

- Achilles tendon
- Rotator cuff
- Groin strain
- Quadriceps
- Patellar tendon
- Hamstring
- Biceps tendon
- Tibialis posterior
- Pectoralis major.

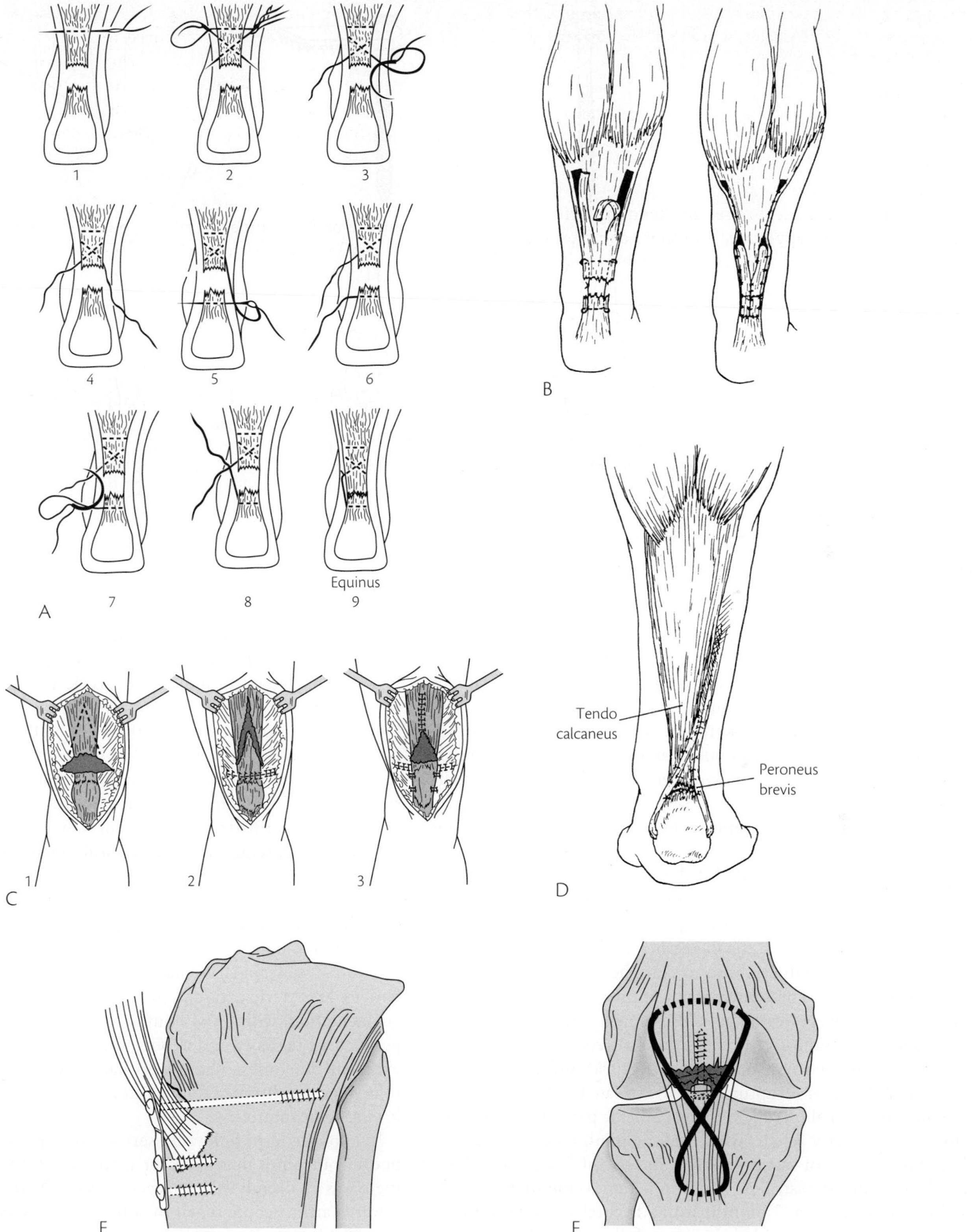

Fig. 12.20.3 Operative techniques of muscle–tendon unit repair: A) direct suture; B) V–Y tissue-advancement procedure; C) local flap advancement procedure; D) augmentation procedure with neighboring tendon; E) augmentation of repair with a tension band wire; F) fixation to bone with sutures through drill holes; G) fixation to bone with screw or plate, using a spiked washer or soft-tissue plate; H) fixation to bone with anchor suture.

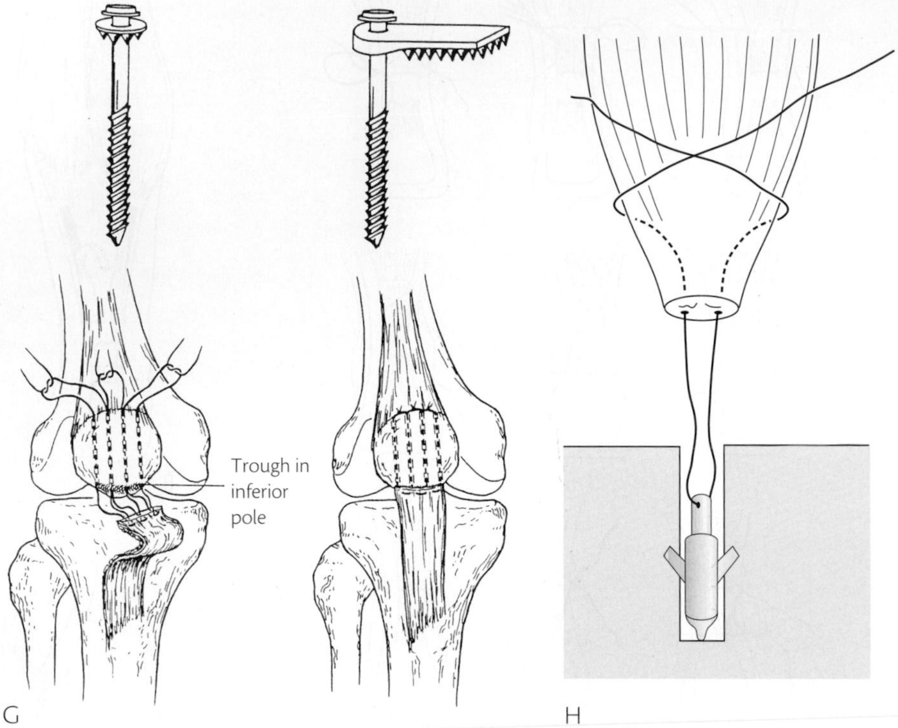

Fig. 12.20.3 (continued).

There is loss of active plantarflexion and no passive foot movement on squeezing the calf.

Partial ruptures do occur, but confirmation should be sought with ultrasound or MRI scanning, as the plantaris may continue to plantarflex the foot when the tendo-Achilles is ruptured. Musculotendinous junction injuries of the soleus or gastrocnemius are common, but rarely require surgery except in the case of high-class athletes.

Most authors agree that ruptures over a week old and reruptures should be treated operatively. More recently, non-operative treatment has been recommended if the gap that closes to less than 6mm in equines, as seen on ultrasound.

Developments in surgical technique include percutaneous repair (see Figure 12.20.3A) and the increasing use of a paramedian incision, which have reduced wound complication rates compared with earlier series. The immobilization time for both operatively and non-operatively treated patients is now 6–8 weeks.

In acute presentations the choice lies between the higher risk of rerupture if treated non-operatively (8–20%) and wound infection, breakdown, or rerupture (5–8%) if treated operatively.

Thus the optimal treatment for a fit athletic patient with an acute rupture is an early repair, which can be minimally invasive, followed by 4 weeks of cast immobilization or 'minimal immobilization' in a hinged cast, 2–4 weeks in a removable orthosis with passive ankle motion, 3 months with a heel raise and no running sports, and finally a graded return to full activity. Early weight bearing in an orthosis has not been found to be detrimental. Non-operative treatment would follow a similar course of immobilization, with a higher rerupture risk, and is a reasonable alternative.

Rotator cuff injury

Injuries to the rotator cuff cover the entire spectrum from minor strains to complete massive ruptures. There is a strong association with degenerative change within the cuff prior to injury in older adults. Acute-on-chronic ruptures in the middle-aged population make up the largest group of patients. Ruptures in young adults most commonly occur following a fall on the outstretched hand, injuring the supraspinatus. Full-thickness cuff tears are unusual in the younger age group (under 40), but the majority are acute and may be associated with fractures or dislocations. Definitive diagnosis may be difficult and is confirmed by arthrography, ultrasound, or MRI. Younger patients with ruptures make up a disproportionate group of those undergoing surgical repair. The epidemiology and specific management of rotator cuff injuries are discussed elsewhere (Chapter 4.3).

The majority of patients with full-thickness tears have fixation of the tendon to bone, possibly with intertendinous sutures, a transposition of subscapularis tendon, or a V–Y type repair. Other alternatives are Marlex, fascial autograft, or another tendon flap augmentation, with or without acromioplasty. Seventy to ninety per cent of patients undergoing surgery have reported good or excellent outcomes. Those who had surgery within 3 weeks of injury and no chronic radiological changes seemed to do best following acute injuries.

In a longer-term follow-up series younger women had slightly poorer outcomes than younger men, but at 4 years postsurgery there was an overall 94% satisfaction rate. There has been a move towards arthroscopic repair of some smaller acute tears over the past decade.

Aftercare of surgically repaired cuffs follows a regime of passive movements building slowly to active resisted motiown over 12 weeks.

Groin strain

Groin strain injury encompasses a number of muscle–tendon unit injuries around the inguinal and anterior hip area. The most common injury sites are the proximal adductor origin at the enthesis or tendon, the distal iliopsoas enthesis, the proximal insertion of the rectus femoris at the anterior superior iliac spine, or disruption of muscles inserting into or near the inguinal ligament. The last of these injuries, in the absence of a hernia, is sometimes termed 'the groin disruption syndrome' or 'sportsman's hernia'.

These injuries commonly occur acutely in athletes who sprint, and are commonly reported in the sports literature. MRI scanning, ultrasound, and herniography are valuable in confirming the diagnosis and the need for treatment.

Treatment for the majority of the injuries is non-operative. A large avulsion from the ischium or iliac spine can be fixed using a screw or small plate and screws. The groin disruption syndrome ('Gilmore groin') can be treated operatively with direct or augmented repair of disrupted parts with a reported 90% success rate, i.e. a return to sport.

Quadriceps tendon and muscle

Acute indirect injury commonly occurs in the rectus femoris muscle. The quadriceps muscles are also commonly affected by direct injury in sport, with the risk of a painful intramuscular haematoma, and in association with femur fractures. The most common cause of indirect injury is a fall or stumble against resistance, causing eccentric contraction.

The mean age of injury is about 45 years, more commonly in males. In patients over 40 the site of rupture is in the distal midtendon, while in patients under 40, rupture is more likely to occur near the distal enthesis. In middle-aged and elderly patients there is a strong association with chronic systemic diseases, such as gout, diabetes, or renal failure, or long-term steroid therapy.

Case reports and small series demonstrate good or excellent functional outcomes in over 90% of patients who receive early repair, followed by 6 weeks of immobilization in extension and rehabilitation for 3 months.

Injury to the muscle belly is more difficult to repair surgically and in most cases the treatment is non-operative, with splinting for 6 weeks followed by rehabilitation. A delayed presentation midbelly rupture may mimic a soft-tissue tumour, which should be excluded by investigations.

Patellar tendon rupture

Ruptures occur distally in the adolescent or proximally in the athlete aged over 20 years. There may be a history of a recent previous injury or chronic pain around the patellar tendon (jumper's knee). Compared with other muscle–tendon units, particularly the quadriceps, there is a lower association with chronic disease states or tendinopathy in older adults.

Repair often involves opposing the tendon to bone using drill holes and multiple sutures, or a tension band wire around the patellar tendon mechanism, or both. Bony avulsions can be fixed back using screws.

Hamstring ruptures

Partial injuries to the hamstrings are very common, particularly in activities involving sprinting. Complete ruptures are rarer, but occur most commonly in sprinting athletes. The most common site is the proximal enthesis and the rupture is often an avulsion injury, seen on radiography. The distal musculotendinous junction is the next most common site.

Isolated hamstring ruptures are being diagnosed with increased frequency using ultrasound and MRI.

Surgical repairs of bony avulsions and musculotendinous junctions with good results have been reported in a small series.

Biceps brachii

Most ruptures are due to sudden forced flexion of the arm against resistance. The most common site of rupture is the long head tendon proximally in the bicipital groove, followed by the proximal musculotendinous junction, the short head tendon, the muscle belly, and most rarely the distal enthesis. Rupture is generally well tolerated in terms of function and cosmesis.

Surgery may be indicated in athletes and heavy manual workers, if the symptoms persist, or if there is a cosmetic defect. Reattachment procedures using anchor sutures, drill holes, and sutures have been described, with good functional outcomes in up to 80%.

Tibialis posterior rupture

This rarely occurs as an acute event, and is usually an acute-on-chronic rupture in a middle-aged or elderly patient who notes pain posterior to the medial malleolus, followed by an acute correctable flat foot. In younger patients it occurs following a sharp laceration, usually due to glass.

Surgery involves exploration at the level of or proximal to the medial malleolus. Direct repair is not usually possible. A tenodesis to the flexor digitorum longus is used, followed by distal transfer of the latter into the navicular. Use of the flexor hallucis longus is a more complex procedure.

Pectoralis muscle rupture

This rupture occurs rarely in young adults lifting heavy weights. Considerable pain, bruising, and blood loss is associated with the injury. Scanning will differentiate partial from complete ruptures, and direct repairs have been reported with good or excellent functional outcomes.

Further reading

Cetti, R., Christensen, S.E., Ejsted, R., Jensen, N.M., and Jorgensen, U. (1993). Operative versus non-operative treatment of Achilles tendon rupture: a prospective randomized study and review of the literature. *American Journal of Sports Medicine*, **21**, 791–9.

Ciullo J.V. and Zarins, B. (1983). Biomechanics of the musculotendinous unit: relation to athletic performance and injury. *Clinics in Sports Medicine*, **2**, 71–86.

Gigante, A., Moschini, A., Verdenelli, A., Del Torto, M., Ulisse, S., and de Palma, L. (2008). Open versus percutaneous repair in the treatment of acute Achilles tendon rupture: a randomized prospective study. *Knee Surgery, Sports Traumatology, Arthroscopy*, **16**(2), 204–9.

Rees, J.D., Wilson, A.M., and Wolman, R.L. (2006). Current concepts in the management of tendon disorders. *Rheumatology (Oxford)*, **45**(5), 508–21.

Sharma, P. and Maffulli, N. (2005). Tendon injury and tendinopathy: healing and repair. *Journal of Bone and Joint Surgery*, **87A**, 187–202.

12.21

Dislocations and joint injuries in the hand

Peter Burge

Summary points

- Dislocation - X-ray first if possible, then early reduction
- Many injuries can be treated with splintage
- Many unstable injuries can be treated with percutaneous wire fixation
- Chronic instability most commonly affects the thumb
- CMC joint injuries often need wiring if unstable.

Function of joints

Joints have two functions: *movement* and *transmission of load*. The failure of these functions—leading respectively to *stiffness* and *instability*—may seriously reduce hand function. But the relative importance of movement and stability varies between joints; the metacarpophalangeal (MCP) joint of the thumb needs stability more than motion, whereas motion at the proximal interphalangeal (PIP) and MCP joints of the fingers is crucial for gripping.

The effect of stiffness depends on the distance between the stiff joint and the tip of the digit. The MCP and PIP joints contribute much more to the total arc of finger motion than the distal joint. Stiffness of the DIP joint is well tolerated if the other joints are supple, and, therefore, any treatment directed at the distal joint should not risk inducing stiffness at other joints. The index finger, which performs most of its functions in a semi-extended posture for pinch against the thumb, tolerates stiffness better than the ring and little fingers, which must flex fully to the palm during power grip.

The exposed position of the hand at work, at home and at sport places its joints at risk of excessive forces that may disrupt their capsules and ligaments. These injuries are very common and may cause prolonged disability, especially at the PIP joint.

Clinical assessment

Any joint that is bruised or swollen after injury may contain a fracture or ligamentous injury. It needs both clinical and radiological examination. Palpation of an injured joint can be guided by a mental picture of the underlying anatomy; tenderness is then localized to bone, ligament attachments and tendon insertions by gentle palpation with a fine blunt object such as a pen top. Radiographs of the injured joint should include anteroposterior and *true lateral* views, supplemented by oblique views if necessary. Computed tomography (CT) may be useful where superimposition of adjacent rays obscures the lateral view.

Dislocations should be reduced promptly (Box 12.21.1), in order to restore circulation and reduce pressure on the skin, but the state of the nerves and vessels must be determined and recorded before any manipulation is performed or local anaesthetic block is administered. If x-ray facilities are available without delay, a radiograph should be taken before reduction; it may provide valuable evidence of injury to articular surfaces, ligament attachments, and tendon insertions. The direction of the dislocation often influences subsequent management but may not be known if the reduction was performed prior to radiographs. Open dislocations should be reduced promptly in the operating room *after* the wound has been irrigated; otherwise contamination may be carried into the joint as a protruding bone is reduced.

Joint laxity may be demonstrated by stress examination and documented with a stress radiograph. Laxity may be masked by muscle spasm due to pain and it may be necessary to give a local anaesthetic block before a proper examination is possible.

Distal interphalangeal joint

Anatomy

The DIP joint is a hinge joint. The convex bicondylar head of the middle phalanx articulates with the base of the distal phalanx,

Box 12.21.1 Dislocations

- Reduce promptly
- X-ray before reduction if possible
- Open injuries should be reduced after wound debridement in the operating room.

which has matching biconcave surfaces separated by a vertical median ridge. The head of the middle phalanx is attached to the base of the distal phalanx by stout collateral ligaments and by the fibrocartilaginous palmar plate, which resists hyperextension. The terminal tendon of the dorsal aponeurosis attaches to the epiphysis of the terminal phalanx, while the profundus tendon inserts into the metaphysis. Dislocations are less frequent at the DIP joint than at the PIP joint, probably because of the short lever arm of the distal phalanx and the strength of the ligamentous supports.

Dorsal dislocation

Dorsal dislocation is the result of rupture of the palmar plate by a hyperextension force. Reduction is occasionally blocked by interposition of the palmar plate or the flexor tendon, in which case open reduction via a dorsolateral approach is needed. Lateral stability is seldom impaired. Active flexion may begin immediately and late instability is rare.

Dorsal fracture–dislocation

Dorsal dislocation may be accompanied by fracture of the palmar lip of the distal phalanx; stability after reduction depends on the size of the fragment and the joint may require pinning in the reduced position. If the insertion of the profundus tendon is detached, it should be reattached via a palmar approach.

Palmar fracture–dislocation

Avulsion fractures of the extensor tendon insertion ('mallet fracture') that involve more than 40% of the articular surface may be associated with palmar subluxation or dislocation of the DIP joint. The injury is usually the result of a blow that imparts flexion and axial compression force to the end of the finger. The subluxation is maintained by the unopposed action of the profundus tendon.

The indications for operative correction of the subluxation are controversial. Operative fixation is difficult unless there is a single large fragment. Surgical complications are common, and the results of non-operative treatment are generally good. Transarticular pinning of the reduced joint is the safest operative method.

Proximal interphalangeal joint

Anatomy

The PIP joint is a hinge joint and is stable to lateral stress at all angles of flexion. The head of the proximal phalanx has two convex condyles that articulate with matching surfaces of the middle phalanx.

The collateral and accessory collateral ligaments form, together with the palmar plate, a three-sided box that encloses the head of the proximal phalanx (Figure 12.21.1). The PIP joint cannot be displaced unless the box-like ligament array is disrupted in at least two planes. The collateral ligament arises from a depression just dorsal to the mid-axial line of the head of the proximal phalanx and inserts into the palmar lateral tubercle at the base of the middle phalanx. The accessory collateral ligament runs obliquely from the head of the proximal phalanx into the palmar plate. The palmar plate provides a static restraint to hyperextension; it is a tough fibrocartilaginous structure that has strong attachments to the palmar-lateral corners of the middle phalanx. The central portion of the palmar plate is rather loosely attached to the periosteum of the base of the middle phalanx. Proximally, the palmar plate has a long fibrous attachment ('check-rein ligament') to each side of the proximal phalanx at the distal margin of the A2 pulley.

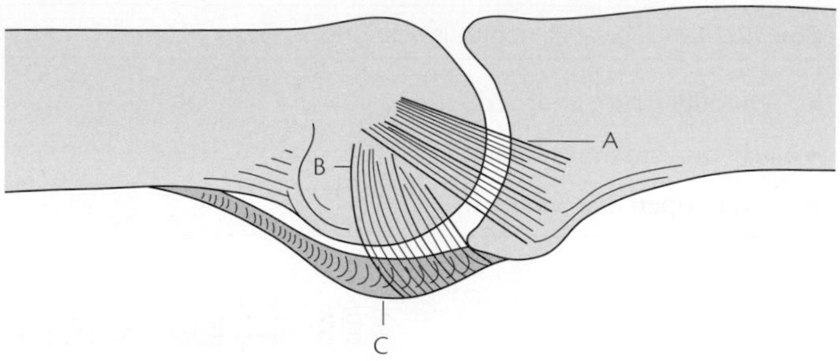

Fig. 12.21.1 Anatomy of the PIP joint. The proper collateral ligament (A), accessory collateral ligament (B), and palmar plate (C), form a three-sided box that encloses the head of the proximal phalanx.

PIP joint injuries

Ligament injuries to the PIP joint may be dorsal, lateral, palmar, or combined. The severity of injury varies from simple PIP joint sprains, which are common in athletes, to fracture–dislocation. Local tenderness may indicate the structures that are injured. Integrity of the extensor mechanism, collateral ligaments and palmar plate should be assessed and the joint should be observed for instability or deviation during active motion, under digital nerve block if necessary.

Dorsal PIP joint dislocation (Box 12.21.2)

Mechanism

Hyperextension force tears the distal insertion of the palmar plate or avulses a small bone fragment from its attachment at the base of the middle phalanx. The tear propagates longitudinally within the collateral ligament, or between the collateral and accessory collateral ligaments, allowing the base of the middle phalanx to dislocate dorsally (Figure 12.21.2). The dorsal component of the collateral ligament remains intact and the joint is stable to lateral stress after reduction.

Treatment

Dorsal dislocations are generally stable after reduction and require minimal treatment. The aim of treatment is early restoration of movement, but splintage in 10 degrees of flexion for 5–7 days may be useful for relief of pain. Swelling, discomfort and stiffness may persist for several months. The presence of a small avulsion fracture at the palmar lip of the base of the middle phalanx does not jeopardize stability or affect the management of this injury.

Open dorsal dislocation

Open dislocation of the PIP joint is usually associated with a transverse palmar wound at the level of the PIP joint; the skin splits as the joint is hyperextended. The serious risk of infection and stiffness may be underestimated if it is not appreciated that the wound communicates with the joint and with the flexor tendon sheath. Patients managed in the emergency room by closed reduction and suture are at risk of disastrous joint and tendon sheath infection. The wound should be debrided and the joint irrigated in the operating room.

Box 12.21.2 Dorsal PIP joint dislocations

- Generally stable after reduction
- Early movement as tolerated
- Beware open dislocations.

Box 12.21.3 Dorsal PIP joint fracture–dislocation

- True lateral x-ray necessary to assess joint reduction
- Treatment options:
  - Extension block splintage
  - Transarticular pin
  - Open reduction and internal fixation
  - External fixation-traction system
  - Palmar plate arthroplasty
  - Hemihamate arthroplasty.

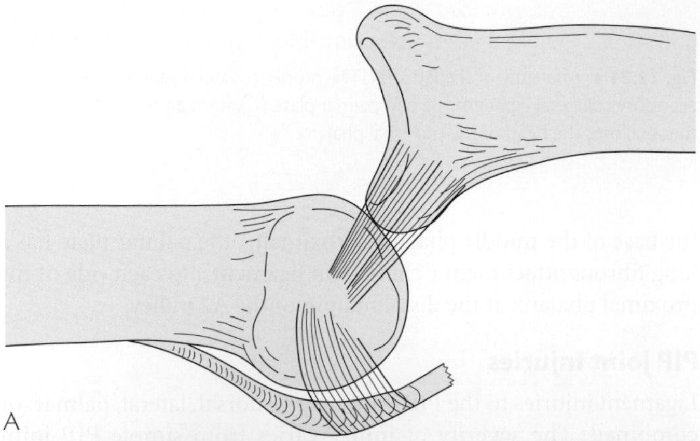

A

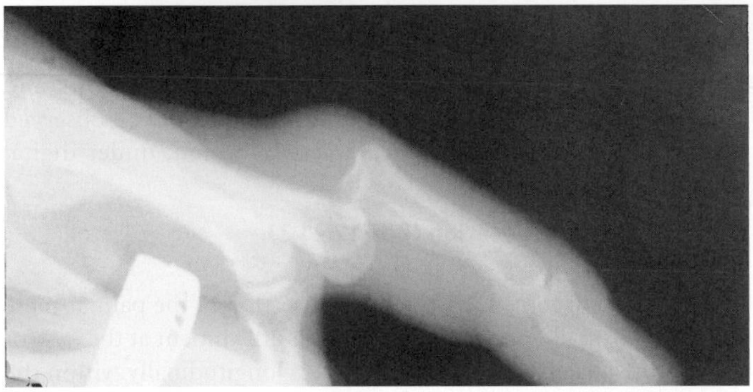

B

Fig. 12.21.2 Dorsal dislocation of the PIP joint. The line of injury passes though the distal insertion of the palmar plate and runs proximally along the fibres of the collateral ligament. The dorsal part of the collateral ligament remains intact (A, B).

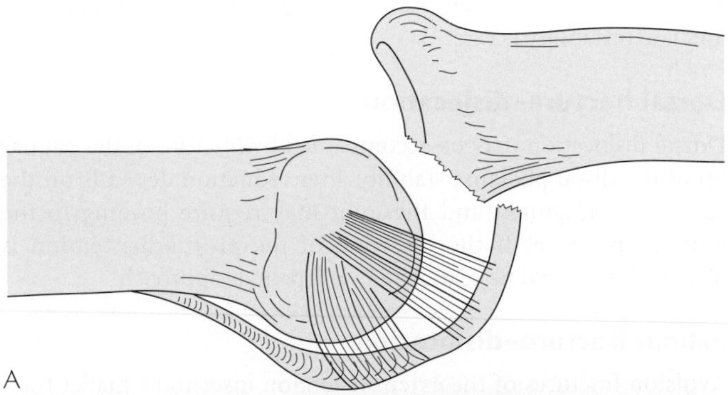

A

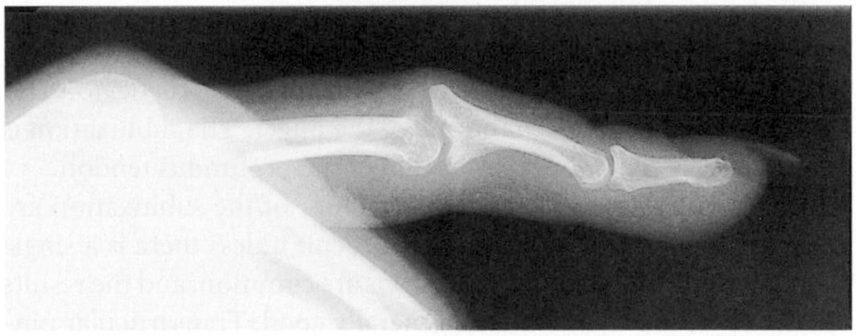

B

Fig. 12.21.3 A) Dorsal fracture–dislocation of the PIP joint. When the fragment comprises 40% or more of the base of the middle phalanx, it contains most or all of the insertion of the collateral ligament. B) Late result of untreated dorsal fracture–dislocation.

Complications

Flexion contracture is an unpredictable but common complication of PIP joint sprain or dislocation. The key to successful management is early recognition and treatment by static or dynamic splintage.

Dorsal PIP joint fracture–dislocation (Box 12.21.3)

Mechanism

The combination of hyperextension and axial loading produces a fracture of the palmar edge of the base of the middle phalanx and dorsal dislocation (Figure 12.21.3). Instability is directly related to the size of the fracture fragment. Since the collateral ligaments insert into the palmar aspect of the base of the middle phalanx, involvement of more than 40% of the articular surface effectively separates the ligaments from the middle phalanx and stability is lost. Stability is also impaired by loss of conformity of the articular surfaces, especially of the palmar lip of the middle phalanx.

Assessment

Swelling masks the deformity and the fracture–dislocation can be overlooked if a true lateral radiograph is not taken. Congruity of the joint surfaces is the aim of treatment; the relationship of the proximal phalanx to the middle phalanx is more important than the position of the palmar fragments. However, dorsal fracture–dislocation is a serious injury that may impair function of the PIP joint in the long term. Management is determined in part by the size and number of the fragments; however, the treatment of severe injuries remains controversial.

Extension block splintage

Fractures which comprise 10–30% of the joint surface may be stable in flexion, in which case the joint can be moved within a limited range in a splint which blocks extension. A dorsal padded aluminium splint is incorporated into a forearm cast and the splint is bent to block extension at the angle of flexion that is just sufficient to maintain a congruent reduction, usually about 50 degrees (Figure 12.21.4A). Active flexion is encouraged. The extension block is decreased by 10–15 degrees each week, provided that congruity is maintained on the lateral radiograph. The splint is worn for 4–6 weeks. Static or dynamic extension splintage may be needed to overcome a residual flexion contracture.

Operative treatment

Operative treatment is required when congruent reduction cannot be maintained in flexion, which is usually because the fracture comprises more than 30% of the articular surface, or because treatment was delayed. There is no consensus about the best means of operative stabilization.

Percutaneous pin fixation. The reduced joint is transfixed in about 25 degrees of flexion for 3–4 weeks by a pin inserted though the bare area of the middle phalanx, just distal to the central slip insertion (Figure 12.21.4B). The simplicity of this method, which concentrates on restoring the correct relationship between the proximal and middle phalanges rather than precise reduction of the fracture fragments, has much to commend it.

Open reduction and internal fixation. Open reduction may be performed through a palmar approach, opening the flexor sheath between A2 and A4 pulleys and retracting the tendons. A single large fragment that can be reduced and held with one or more small screws, but multifragmentary fractures are challenging and may require buttressing with a cage plate and bone grafting.

External fixation. Several ingenious techniques have been devised to exert traction on the middle phalanx whilst allowing movement of the PIP joint. The principle is sound but the technical aspects are demanding. The axis of motion of the device must coincide with the axis of the joint, and the device should permit joint motion without rotation of pins in the bone.

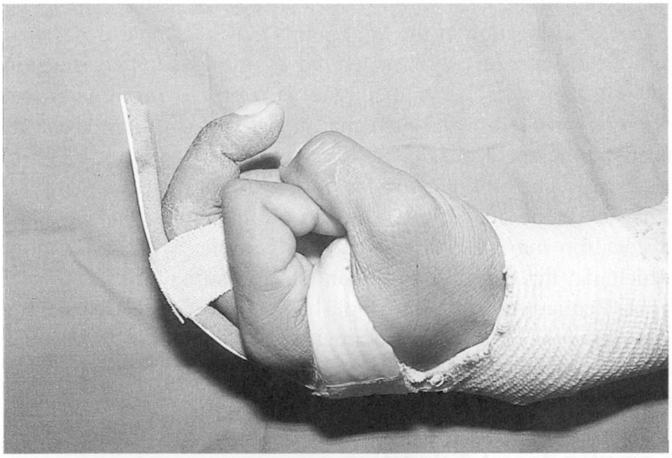

A

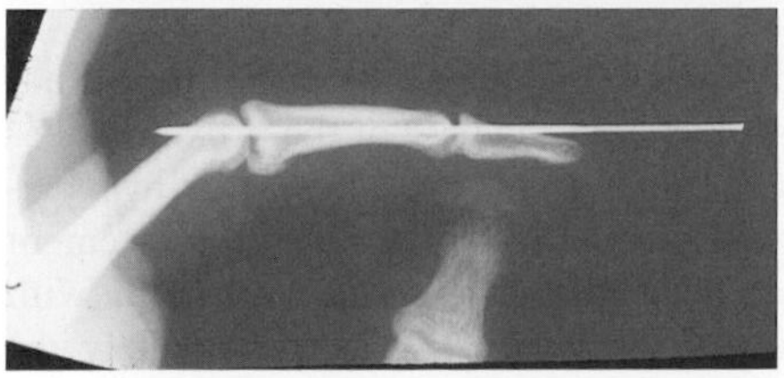

B

Fig. 12.21.4 Treatment of dorsal fracture dislocation of the proximal interphalangeal joint. (A) Extension block splintage. (B) Percutaneous pin fixation; note that the oblique pin does not cross the DIPJ.

Palmar plate arthroplasty. The palmar plate is used to reconstruct the articular surface of the palmar half of the middle phalanx. After excision of the bone fragments, the palmar plate is advanced into a transverse groove created in the defect in the base of the middle phalanx. The plate is held in place by a suture passed through drill holes in the middle phalanx and tied over a button on the dorsum of the finger or to a suture anchor. In late cases, it is usually necessary to excise the collateral ligaments in order to reduce the joint. The joint is immobilized for two weeks by a transarticular K– wire and then mobilized in an extension-block splint for a further two weeks. At 5 weeks, dynamic splintage may be needed to correct a flexion contracture.

Hemihamate arthroplasty. The damaged palmar lip of the middle phalanx is replaced with a size-matched portion of the hamate obtained from its distal dorsal articular surface between the ring and little metacarpals, thereby restoring joint stability and allowing early movement (Figure 12.21.5). This method is the best means of reconstruction of severe and late-presenting injuries.

Palmar PIP joint dislocation (Box 12.21.4)

Palmar dislocation of the PIP joint is more serious but much less common than dorsal dislocation. A rotational force tears one collateral ligament, the palmar plate and sometimes the central slip of the dorsal aponeurosis. The joint is unstable and liable to palmar subluxation, rotation and boutonnière deformity. If the central slip remains intact, reduction may be prevented by entrapment of the head of the proximal phalanx between the central slip and the lateral band. Early recognition and treatment of this serious injury is crucial in maintaining function of the finger, in contrast to dorsal dislocation which generally does well with minimal treatment.

Entrapment of the head of the proximal phalanx may be reduced by flexion of the MCP joint, which slackens the dorsal aponeurosis. If the central slip is intact, the joint can be immobilized in extension for two weeks and then mobilized with active flexion and dynamic and/or static splintage to prevent development of a flexion contracture. The joint should be reduced and held in full extension while the injured structures heal; this is most easily and reliably achieved with a transarticular pin. Open reduction and repair may be needed for displaced intra-articular fractures, irreducibility or fixed contracture.

Lateral PIP joint dislocation

Laterally directed force may rupture the collateral ligament and the ipsilateral half of the palmar plate, thus disrupting the box-like ligament array and allowing lateral dislocation. If the joint surfaces are congruous on x-ray after reduction and the joint is stable during flexion and extension, early protected motion is permitted. The finger can be supported during mobilization by taping to the adjacent digit on the side of the collateral ligament injury. Late instability is rare.

Box 12.21.4 Palmar PIP joint dislocation

- Open reduction occasionally required
- Splint in extension
- May need transarticular wire.

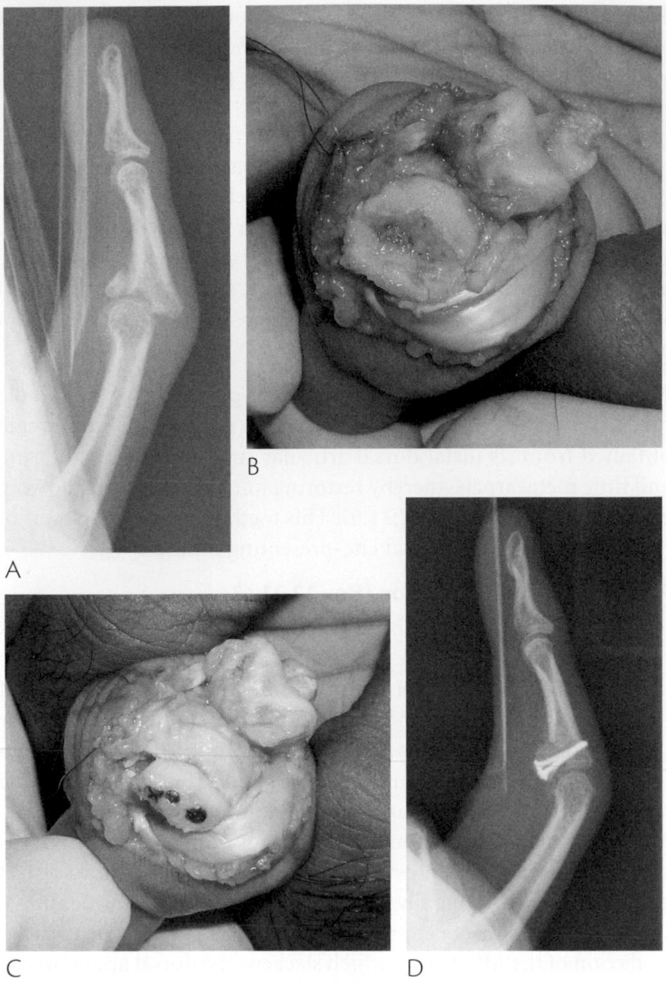

Fig. 12.21.5 Damaged palmar lip of middle phalanx (A, B) replaced by a size-matched graft from the distal surface of the hamate (C, D).

PIP strains

Lateral and hyperextension strains of the PIP joint are frequent in athletes. The primary restraint to lateral angulation stress at the PIP joint is the collateral ligament. Under load, the ligament fails at the proximal end and the tear then extends between the between the collateral and accessory collateral ligaments before running across the palmar plate. Protected active movement with buddy taping for 2–3 weeks is sufficient in most cases. Pain, swelling and stiffness often persist for several months after lateral ligament strains. Late instability is rare, but some joints develop troublesome flexion contractures that require static and/or dynamic splintage.

Hyperextension strains may be associated with avulsion of a small flake of bone at the distal insertion of the palmar plate. Flexion contracture is a common but unpredictable consequence of hyperextension injury and may require intensive splintage and exercise.

Hyperextension laxity is uncommon but may be aggravated by pre-existing ligament laxity or previous injuries. The finger adopts a 'swan–neck' posture with hyperextension at the PIP joint and flexion at the DIP joint, but mechanical difficulty in initiating PIP joint flexion is usually the presenting symptom. As the finger is flexed, the PIP joint 'hangs up' in hyperextension, snapping down into flexion as the voluntary effort is increased. Repair of the attenuated palmar plate, if possible, or construction of a new static restraint to hyperextension is required. Tenodesis using one slip of the superficialis tendon is a simple and reliable technique.

Metacarpophalangeal joints of the fingers

Anatomy

The strong collateral ligaments and palmar plate protect the MCP joints from dislocation. The palmar plate has stout attachments to the proximal phalanx but its proximal attachment is thinner and it lacks the fibrous 'check-reins' of its counterpart at the PIP joint. The MCP joint resembles the PIP joint in having a box-like arrangement of collateral and accessory collateral ligaments, which insert into the edges of the palmar plate. The MCP joint is linked to adjacent rays by the deep transverse metacarpal ligaments, which are continuous with the lateral edges of the palmar plate. The primary stabilising structures are the collateral ligaments. The palmar plate resists hyperextension and only contributes to lateral stability when it is taut in extension.

Dorsal dislocation (Box 12.21.5)

Dorsal dislocation of the MCP joint of the finger is uncommon (though it is the most common dislocation in children) and may affect the index and little fingers. The middle and ring fingers are protected by adjacent digits and are seldom dislocated unless the border digit is also injured. The thin proximal attachment of the palmar plate is torn by hyperextension force but the collateral ligaments remain intact.

Dorsal dislocation of the MCP joints may be *simple* or *complex*. Simple dislocation is characterized by marked hyperextension (60–80 degrees). The palmar plate is ruptured proximally and remains attached to the proximal phalanx; it is draped over the head of the metacarpal but does not block reduction (Figure 12.21.6A). The articular surface of the base of the proximal phalanx lies in contact with the dorsum of the metacarpal head. The dislocation may be converted to the complex type by traction, which may flip the palmar plate onto the dorsum of the metacarpal head. Reduction can be accomplished by direct pressure over the dorsum of the base of the proximal phalanx in a distal and palmar direction, pushing it back over the metacarpal head. Late instability does not occur and no splintage is needed.

Complex dorsal dislocation

Pathology

Complex dislocation of the MCP joint occurs when the palmar plate becomes interposed between the base of the proximal phalanx and the metacarpal head. The joint rests in modest hyperextension (20–40 degrees) (Figure 12.21.6B). Anterior displacement of the metacarpal head creates a prominence in the palm, with blanching of the palmar skin (Figure 12.21.6C), and a hollow just proximal to the base of the proximal phalanx dorsally. There may be an osteochondral fracture of the metacarpal head.

The primary block to reduction of a complex dislocation is the palmar plate, which remains attached distally to the base of the

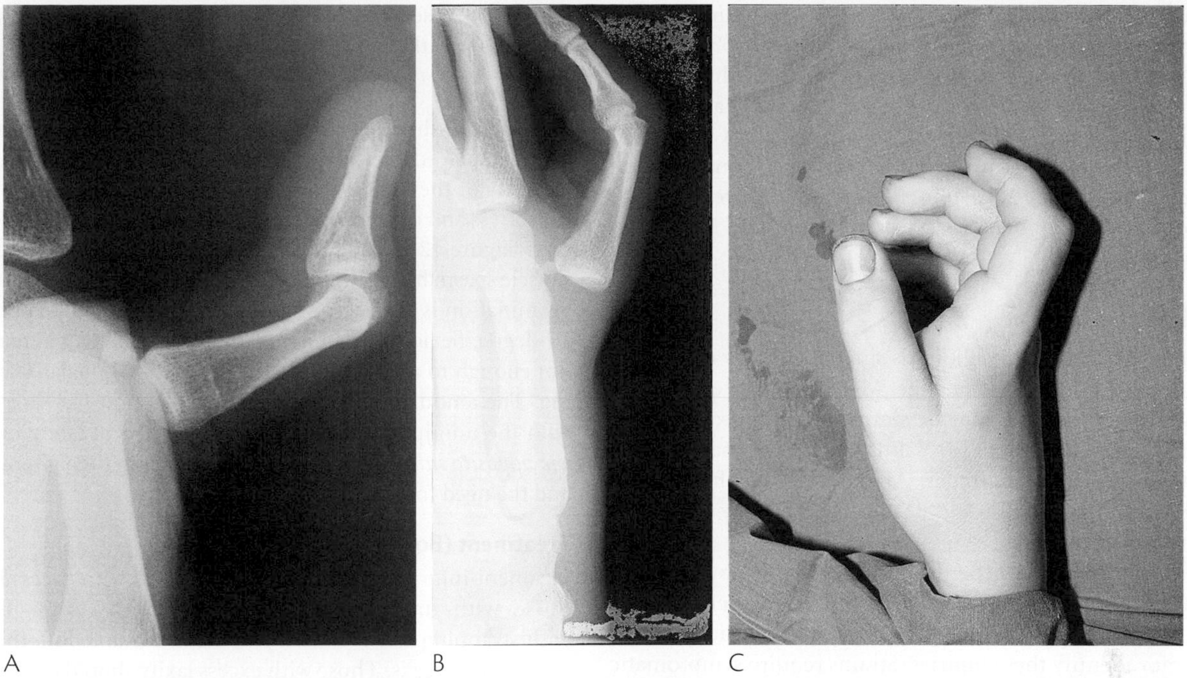

Fig. 12.21.6 Dorsal dislocation of the MP joint. A) Simple dislocation with marked hyperextension. B) and C) Complex dislocation of the index MP joint, with modest hyperextension and blanching of the palmar skin by the metacarpal head.

proximal phalanx and lies on the dorsal surface of the metacarpal head. Although closed manipulation is sometimes successful, open reduction is usually required.

Operative treatment

A dorsal approach to complex MCP joint dislocation avoids the risk of digital nerve injury in the palmar approach, allows access to osteochondral fractures and is both simpler and quicker than a palmar approach. The extensor tendon is split in the midline, exposing the base of the proximal phalanx and the palmar plate as it lies on the head of the metacarpal. Longitudinal incision of the palmar plate allows the two halves to slip back over the head of the metacarpal. The MCP joint is stable after reduction. Immobilization is unnecessary and may lead to stiffness. Recurrent dislocation and late instability do not seem to occur in the fingers, though injury to the palmar plate of the thumb MCP joint may contribute to hyperextension laxity.

Complex palmar dislocation of the MCP joint is rare but may require open reduction of the entrapped palmar plate or dorsal capsule.

Locked MCP joint (Box 12.21.6)

Locking of the MCP joint is characterized by the sudden onset of a flexion deformity that cannot be corrected passively. Locking may be acute, chronic or intermittent. Entrapment of the palmar plate on an osteophyte arising from the palmar/lateral corner of the metacarpal head is the usual cause of locking in older patients. Oblique views or CT may be needed to demonstrate the osteophyte; its removal will correct the deformity. Distension of the joint with local anaesthetic may lift the palmar plate off the osteophyte, but locking may recur. Other causes of locking include loose bodies, malunited articular fractures and entrapment of an interosseous tendon or collateral ligament on bony prominences of the metacarpal head.

Box 12.21.5 MCP joint dislocation

- Simple:
  - Presents with 60–80 degrees hyperextension
  - Reducible closed
- Complex:
  - Presents with 20–30 degrees hyperextension
  - Palmar plate entrapment
  - Open reduction required
  - Dorsal approach.

Box 12.21.6 Locked MCP joint

- Usually older patient
- Palmar plate caught on osteophyte palmar/lateral aspect metacarpal head
- Oblique x-rays or CT may be needed
- Closed and open reduction techniques.

Metacarpophalangeal joint of the thumb

Anatomy

The collateral ligaments and palmar plate are the primary stabilizers of the MCP joint of the thumb, but additional dynamic stability is provided by the insertion of the adductor pollicis muscle at the base of the proximal phalanx. The adductor aponeurosis lies directly over the ulnar collateral ligament and is formed from fibres that pass from the adductor muscle into the ulnar side of the dorsal aponeurosis. Stability is the most important attribute of the MCP joint of the thumb; movement is much less important provided that the basal joint is mobile. Indeed, some normal individuals have very little MCP joint flexion, but the average range is 75 degrees flexion, 20 degrees hyperextension, and 10 degrees abduction/adduction.

Dorsal dislocation

Dislocation of the thumb MCP joint is similar in many respects to dislocation of the index and little finger MCP joints. It results from forcible hyperextension and may be simple or complex, the latter resulting from interposition of the palmar plate. The management is the same as in the index finger. After reduction the stability of the collateral ligaments should be checked and any instability managed as described below.

Hyperextension injury of the thumb MCP joint may strain or rupture the palmar plate; comparing the range of hyperextension with the opposite thumb, using a local anaesthetic block if necessary, may identify these injuries. Strains require symptomatic treatment only. Complete ruptures should be immobilized with the MCP joint in 10–20 degrees flexion for 3–4 weeks to encourage healing of the palmar plate at its correct length. Hyperextension injuries occasionally lead to laxity and dynamic collapse of the thumb skeleton with hyperextension of the MCP joint and flexion at the IP and CMC joints. The collapse deformity can be corrected by capsulodesis or tenodesis of the MCP joint, if the joint surfaces are healthy, or by arthrodesis if the surfaces are degenerate.

Ulnar collateral ligament injury

Mechanism

Rupture of the ulnar collateral ligament is caused by forced abduction stress, with or without hyperextension. The degree of injury varies from a stable ligamentous strain to disruption of the collateral ligament, palmar plate and dorsal capsule. Motorcycle accidents, falls onto the outstretched thumb and ski-pole injuries are common causes of MCP joint ligament rupture. The ulnar collateral ligament resists laterally directed forces during pinch against the index finger; laxity of the ligament is associated with a weak painful pinch and predisposes to degenerative arthritis of the MCP joint.

Pathology

The ulnar collateral ligament is usually injured at its attachment to the proximal phalanx, where it may avulse a fragment of bone, but mid-substance ruptures are occasionally seen. An anatomical peculiarity of the ulnar side of the MCP joint may account for the poor results of non-operative management of complete collateral ligament ruptures. The ligament may slip around the proximal free edge of the adductor aponeurosis as the aponeurosis slides distally at the moment of injury—the Stener lesion. The aponeurosis then separates the torn end of the ligament and its site of attachment to the proximal phalanx (Figure 12.21.7A). The Stener lesion is present in the majority of complete ulnar collateral ligament ruptures. The ulnar collateral ligament may avulse a small fragment of bone at its insertion and the presence of a Stener lesion may be inferred from the position of the fragment on x-ray.

Assessment

Radiographs should be taken before stress testing is performed, lest an undisplaced fracture is displaced. If there is no fracture, the integrity of the ligament can be assessed by applying radial deviation stress and comparing the range of abduction with the opposite side (Figure 12.21.7B, C). It may be necessary to relieve pain and muscle spasm by infiltration of local anaesthetic before an adequate examination is possible. The examination should be performed in 15-degree flexion, which is sufficient to relax the palmar plate but not enough to allow rotation of the proximal phalanx during testing. The amount of laxity and the 'end-point feel' are compared with the uninjured side. A 30-degree excess of laxity *compared to the opposite side* indicates rupture of the ulnar collateral ligament and the need for operative repair.

Treatment (Box 12.21.7)

Ligament injuries which are not associated with excess laxity, and those with undisplaced avulsion fractures, may be treated with strapping but are often more comfortable in a thumb spica cast for 3–4 weeks. Those with excess laxity should be explored and repaired via a dorsoulnar incision, protecting the branch of the superficial radial nerve that lies here. Avulsion fractures which are displaced by more than 2mm should be reduced operatively and fixed with a K-wire, interosseous wire or small lag screw, depending on the size of the fragment. If a Stener lesion is present, the distal end of the collateral ligament is usually found turned back upon itself immediately proximal to the edge of the adductor aponeurosis. The ligament is usually torn at its attachment to the palmar and ulnar corner of the base of the proximal phalanx, and may be reattached by suture to local tissues or by a suture anchor. Protection of the repair with a transarticular pin is optional. The joint is mobilized after 4 weeks but protected from stress until the 8th week. Some limitation of MCP joint flexion is common but is not disabling in a joint where stability is more important than movement.

Chronic MCP joint instability

After 2 weeks from injury, the ruptured ligament shortens and it may be difficult to achieve a secure repair. The ligament may be reconstructed with a strip of palmaris longus tendon passed in a figure-of-eight fashion though vertical drill holes in the bone on each side of the joint. In the presence of degenerative arthritis, arthrodesis is an excellent procedure that provides stable pain-free pinch. Very little disability results from loss of MCP joint movement provided that there is good motion at the basal joint.

Radial collateral ligament injury

Tears of the radial collateral ligament account for about a quarter of MCP joint collateral ligament injuries. The ligament may tear at either end and there is no counterpart of the Stener lesion on the radial side of the joint. Pain occurs when pressure is placed on the radial side of the thumb, particularly when pushing against a surface with the hand flat. Excessive ulnar deviation occurs on adduction stress. Unstable radial collateral ligament injuries should be repaired.

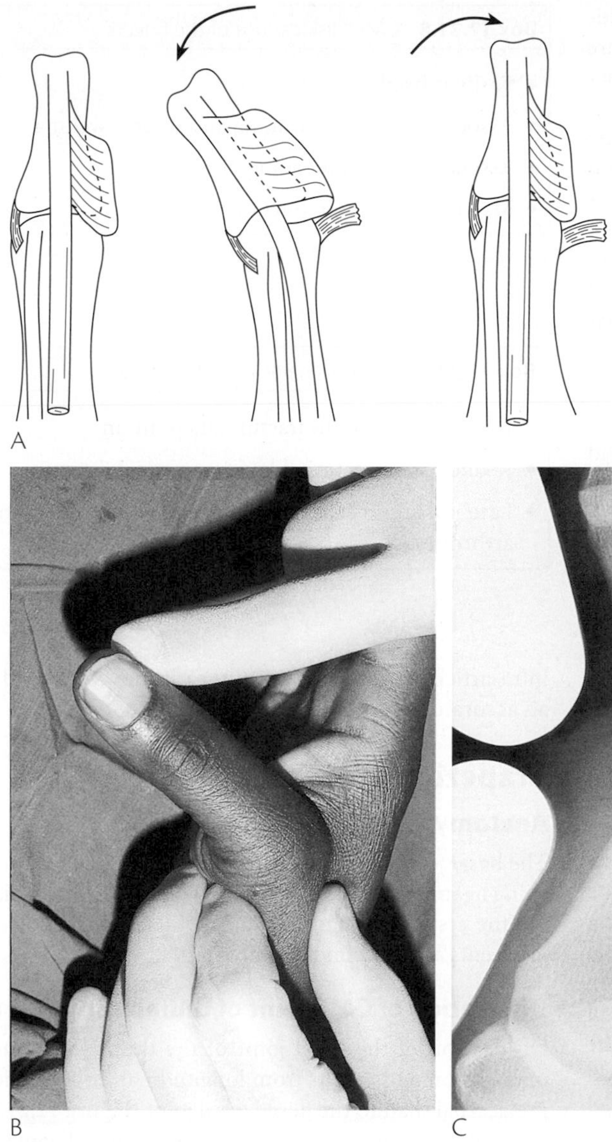

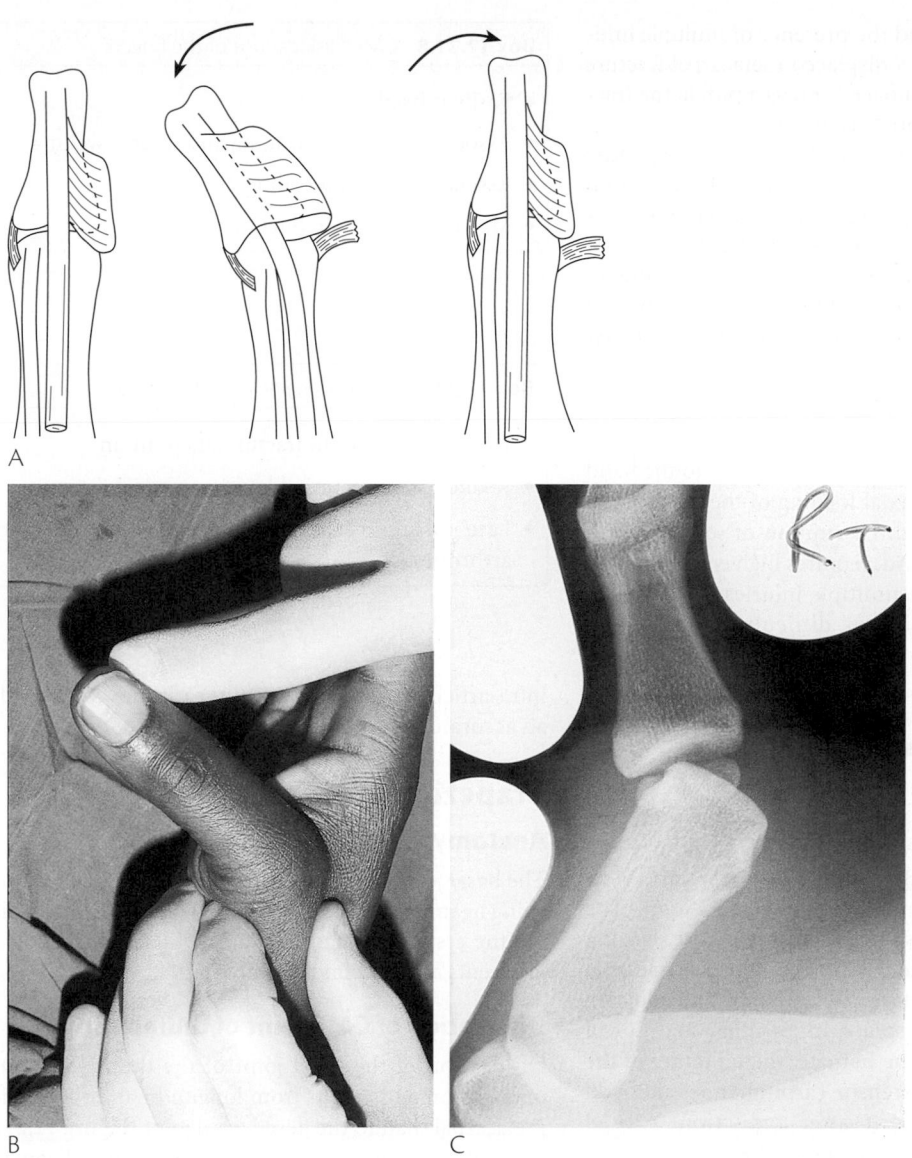

Fig. 12.21.7 Rupture of the ulnar collateral ligament of the MP joint of the thumb. A) The ruptured ligament flips out around the proximal edge of the adductor aponeurosis. B) and C) Laxity is shown on examination and on X-ray.

Carpometacarpal joints of the fingers

Anatomy

The CMC joints of the index and middle rays have interlocking articular surfaces and strong ligaments that allow very little movement. The base of the fourth metacarpal articulates with the radial facet of the hamate and has 10–15 degrees flexion-extension. The fifth CMC joint allows 15–20 degrees flexion as well as some rotation, aiding opposition of the thumb to the little finger and cupping of the palm. The deep branch of the ulnar nerve runs close to the palmar aspect of the fourth and fifth CMC joints, where it may suffer injury or operative damage.

Mechanism of injury

Dislocation of the CMC joints of the fingers may involve one or more joints, with or without fracture of the articular surfaces, and may be associated with fracture of adjacent metacarpal bones. The displacement is usually dorsal and the fifth ray is most frequently injured, though several types of multiple dislocation have been reported (Box 12.21.8).

Box 12.21.7 Thumb MCP joint ulnar collateral ligament injuries

- Radiograph before testing stability
- Relieve pain before testing stability
- Test in 15 degrees flexion
- Splint stable injuries
- Operative repair for most complete ruptures.

Assessment

Examination shortly after injury will often detect the dorsal displacement that may have been noticed by the patient. However, CMC joint dislocations are easily overlooked. Contributory factors are obliteration of deformity by swelling, inadequate radiographs or their incorrect interpretation and the presence of multiple injuries. The frequent combination of a displaced metacarpal fracture with CMC joint dislocation in an adjacent ray is a pitfall; the fracture catches the eye and the dislocation is missed.

Severe swelling of the wrist after a violent injury frequently conceals a serious carpometacarpal or carpal injury. The minimum radiographic examination comprises PA, true lateral view and oblique views in 30 degrees pronation and supination from the lateral position. CT examination may be very helpful in defining the injury and particularly in determining if comminution precludes operative reconstruction of the articular surfaces.

Dorsal CMC joint dislocation

Single CMC joint dislocations may result from blows to the hand or from falls, causing flexion and axial loading of the metacarpal. The fifth ray is most often affected. Disruption of several joints, especially the strong second and third, requires high energy trauma and these patients frequently have multiple injuries. The dislocations can usually be reduced without difficulty; stability can be assessed at the time of reduction and a K-wire inserted if necessary.

Dorsal CMC joint fracture dislocation

Undisplaced articular fractures of the CMC joints may be treated satisfactorily with external splintage of the wrist and protected motion of the fingers. Fracture–subluxation of the fifth CMC joint is sometimes called 'reverse Bennett's fracture' because of its similarity to fracture-subluxation of the first CMC joint. The fracture line runs obliquely across the metacarpal base, leaving the radial fragment attached to the base of the fourth metacarpal and hamate by the strong intermetacarpal ligaments and allowing the shaft of the metacarpal to displace in an ulnar and dorsal direction. The sloping surface of the hamate, the obliquity of the fracture line and the pull of the extensor carpi ulnaris tendon all contribute towards redisplacement after reduction. Closed reduction can usually be achieved without difficulty using a combination of traction and direct pressure but the injury is unstable and requires percutaneous pin fixation. The aim is restoration of the relationship between the metacarpal shaft and the hamate; slight displacement of the intra-articular fracture may be accepted. Open reduction is indicated for failed closed reduction, soft-tissue interposition or late presentation, and for open injuries.

Multiple CMC joint fracture dislocations are accompanied by severe swelling which precludes effective control by external splintage. Percutaneous pin fixation may be possible but it can be difficult to achieve in the presence of swelling and reduction is sometimes blocked by interposition of soft-tissues such as the extensor carpi radialis brevis tendon. Multiple pins are required and they tend to interfere with movement of the extensor tendons if the ends are left long. The potential for stiffness of the fingers in these severe injuries demands mobilization as soon as possible. Open reduction with fixation by buried K-wires, together with screw fixation of associated metacarpal fractures and large intra-articular fragments, permits early movement and also ensures an accurate reduction.

Box 12.21.8 CMC dislocations of the fingers

- Easily missed
- Associated with polytrauma and severe swelling
- Assess with oblique radiographs/CT scan
- May require open reduction.

Box 12.21.9 Trapeziometacarpal dislocation

- Dislocation without fracture uncommon
- Reduction often unstable—transarticular pin
- Late instability may require ligament reconstruction or arthrodesis.

Trapeziometacarpal joint

Anatomy

The basal joint of the thumb is saddle-shaped. The primary stabilizing ligaments are the anterior oblique and dorsoradial ligaments, but the first intermetacarpal, ulnar collateral and posterior oblique ligaments act as secondary stabilizers.

Dislocation of CMC joint of thumb (Box 12.21.9)

Dislocation of the basal joint of the thumb without fracture is uncommon and results from longitudinal force applied along the metacarpal shaft to the flexed basal joint (Figure 12.21.8). The dorsoradial ligament tears and the anterior oblique ligament is stripped subperiosteally from the base and proximal shaft of the metacarpal. Immediate closed reduction and maintenance of a stable reduction in a cast is associated with a good long-term outcome, but many joints are unstable and require percutaneous pin fixation. Painful instability is common in patients presenting late and may occur despite primary pin fixation.

Late instability of the basal joint predisposes to early degenerative arthritis. An anteroposterior stress radiograph with the radial surfaces of the thumbs pressed together may demonstrate instability. The treatment of painful instability or subluxation is determined by the state of the articular surfaces. Ligament reconstruction using a distally-based strip of the flexor carpi radialis tendon is appropriate if the articular surfaces are healthy. The tendon strip is passed through a drill-hole in the base of the metacarpal so as to replicate the function of the anterior oblique ligament. If painful instability is accompanied by degenerative change, the options are trapezial excision arthroplasty with ligament reconstruction and arthrodesis. The choice of procedure will be influenced

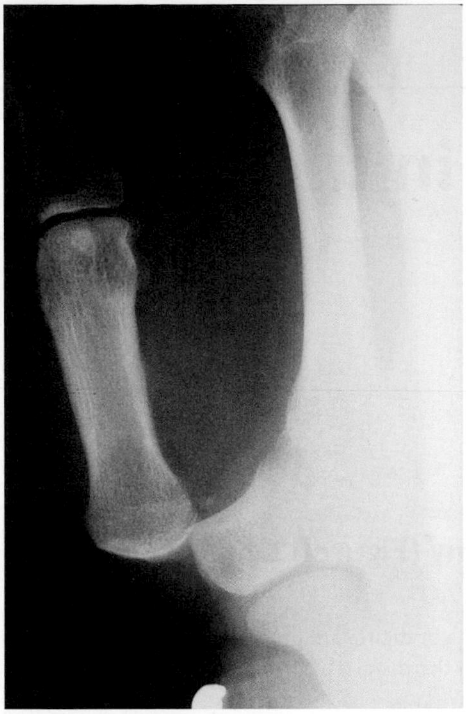

Fig. 12.21.8 Dislocation of the basal joint of the thumb.

by age, the state of other thumb joints and the requirements of the patient.

Further reading

Freiberg, A., Pollard, B.A., Macdonald, M.R., and Duncan, M.J. (2006). Management of proximal interphalangeal joint injuries. *Hand Clinics,* **22,** 235–42.

Glickel, S.Z., Barron, O.A., and Catalano, L. (2005). Dislocations and ligament injuries in the digits. In: Green, D.P., Hotchkiss, R.N., Pederson, W.C., and Wolfe, S.W. (eds) *Operative Hand Surgery,* pp. 772–808. New York: Churchill Livingstone.

Kiefhaber, T.R. and Stern, P.J. (1998). Fracture dislocations of the proximal interphalangeal joint. *Journal of Bone and Joint Surgery,* **23A**, 368–80.

Leibovic, S.J. and Bowers, W.H. (1994). Anatomy of the proximal interphalangeal joint. *Hand Clinics,* **10**, 169–78.

Waters, P.M. (2008). Surgical treatment of carpal and hand injuries in children. *Instructional Course Lectures,* **57**, 515–24.

12.22

Flexor tendon injuries

Robert Savage

Summary points

- Restoring continuity to the supple yet high tensile flexor tendon system presents a challenge unique in surgery. Although there is continuing debate about many details of technique, the central tenet of modern flexor tendon surgery is to repair and move the flexor tendons within a few days of injury
- Knowledge and experience count for everything at all points of patient care beginning with accurate and timely diagnosis. Emergency services should be arranged to relocate these injuries to appropriately trained surgeons and team-work with specialist hand therapists is an essential part of today's treatment
- While all flexor tendon surgery is complicated, it is simplest in the newly injured and unscarred digit, and the results of the correctly rehabilitated primary repair appear to be the best attainable
- However, occasions will arise when secondary surgery will be necessary and the appropriate skills must be learned.

History

In the early 1900s there were several reports of primary repair of divided flexor tendons using principles that were not so different to those we use today; however, Sterling Bunnell declared zone 2 of the finger 'no man's land' for primary surgery, on account of finger and tendon stiffness or repair failure. He advocated a delayed tendon graft, effectively removing the repair from the site of maximum adhesion in the flexor sheath and performing the two graft repairs at the finger end and in the palm. In Britain, Guy Pulvertaft became famous for his teaching on this technique in the 1950s and 1960s. Predominant suture materials were silk and wire.

The reversal of this policy back to early direct repair, pioneered by Kleinert and Verdan in the 1960s, and enhanced by improved postsurgery rehabilitation, showed that results can be better than after tendon grafting.

The last 30 years have seen progressive improvements following research into tendon healing, tendon suture mechanics, and protected mobilization after surgical repair; and the current trend is for multistranded repairs with early protected 'active' finger movement. We have returned full cycle, but mainly with good evidence of satisfactory outcomes.

Anatomy (Figure 12.22.1)

Tendons

The four flexor digitorum profundus (FDP) tendons pass from the forearm to the distal phalanges providing power grip. The ulnar

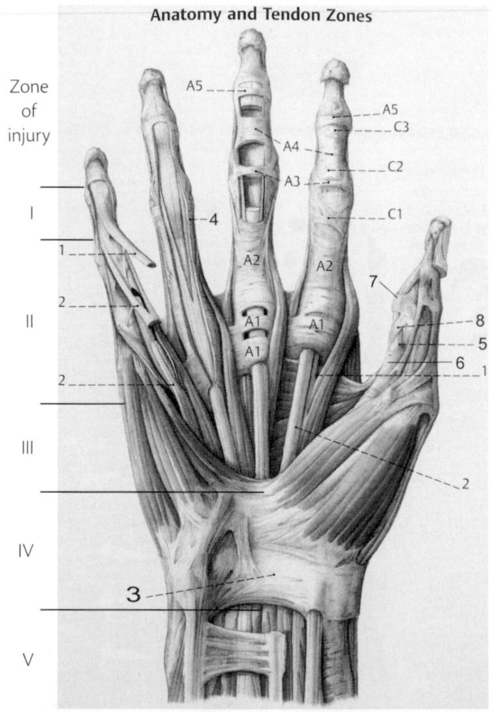

Fig. 12.22.1 Flexor tendons, fibrous sheath pulleys and zones of injury.
1 tendon of flexor digitorum profundus
2 tendon of flexor digitorum superficialis
3 flexor retinaculum
4 fibrous flexor sheath
A1–A5 annular parts of flexor sheath
C1–C3 cruciate parts of flexor sheath
5 tendon of flexor polllicis longus
6 A1 pulley of thumb
7 A2 pulley of thumb
8 oblique pulley of thumb
I–V zones of injury (relative to little finger).
Reproduced with permission.

three tendons are relatively conjoined, such that one cannot be flexed without the others flexing also.

Flexor digitorum superficialis (FDS) tendons insert to the middle phalanges and act individually. They contribute to power grip, and with the interossei, to dexterity, but are not necessary for full finger roll-up. In the finger, under the A2 pulley (see later) and at the decussation there is extra potential for tendon adhesion following repair.

Paratenon and vincula

Tendons are supported by paratenon via a thin mesentery within the palm, carpal tunnel, and distal forearm. In the finger there is no mesentery except where blood flow enters the tendon dorsally through two vascular pedicles, the long and short vincula; which give rise to a dorsal tendon artery and veins, that supply the tendon, branching into the tendon substance, becoming rarefied and absent towards the margins and volar aspect.

Fibrous flexor sheath—'the pulley system'

Within the finger the paratenon is supported by fibrous arches (pulleys) attached to the palmar lateral margins of the phalanges and volar plates.

The annular (A) pulleys prevent bowstringing of flexor tendons promoting mechanical efficiency during flexion. The toughest pulleys are:

- A1 at the metacarpophalangeal (MCP) volar plate,
- A2 at the proximal phalanx
- A4 at the middle phalanx.

Soft parts of sheath with cruciate fibres (C) allow the finger to bend:

- C1 and C2 at the proximal interphalangeal (PIP) joint
- C3 at the distal interphalangeal (DIP) joint.

The hard edges of the A2 and A4 pulleys may cause blockage of tendon movement against an irregular tendon repair or a partial division.

Zones of injury

- Zone 1 is distal to the insertion of FDS, where only FDP can be divided
- Zone 2 is where FDS and FDP coexist within the fibrous flexor sheath—the site for maximum adhesion potential
- Zone 3 is within the palm proximal to the flexor sheath but distal to the carpal tunnel. FDS is superficial to FDP and traumatic division may not be obvious
- Zone 4 is within the carpal tunnel
- Zone 5 is proximal to the carpal tunnel—from superficial to deep the structures are: palmaris longus, median nerve, FDS, FDP, with wrist flexors to each side.

Pathology of healing and repair

Following much controversy in which it was thought that tendons had little vitality and healing potential, dye injection studies in the rabbit flexor tendon model showed the vascular supply (see 'Paratenon and vincula' section).

Synovial nutrition

The fact that tendon is nourished by synovial fluid diffusion (in addition to blood flow) was shown when a segment of tendon was divided, devascularized, and allowed to retract within the fibrous flexor sheath. Sequential histological studies demonstrated cellular proliferation over the cut tendon ends and immature collagen fibrils.

Tendon healing without surgical repair

The rabbit flexor tendon was drawn proximal to the fibrous sheath, partly divided, and then allowed to retract within the sheath: the tendon was still in continuity, but nevertheless injured with a partial gap to observe. Sequential histology demonstrated gradual healing and maturation of the tendon gap, but notably without any adhesion to the tendon sheath.

Adhesion factors after surgical flexor tendon repair

The rabbit flexor tendon was partly divided (as earlier) and then subjected to three factors which occur during repair surgery: suture, sheath injury, and immobilization. Each single factor caused modest adhesion, paired factors caused moderate adhesion, and all three factors together caused dense restrictive adhesion.

Tendon and repair mechanics

Tendon strength

Laboratory testing showed breakage of human flexor tendons at 1200 Newtons (N) and tendon avulsion from bone at 600N. After injury significant weakening occurs for about 3 weeks.

Forces during activity

In patients having carpal tunnel surgery under local anaesthetic, light active unresisted finger and wrist movement induced tendon forces of 35N, and tip pinch, 120N

Friction

Tendon repair bunching, swelling, irregularities, knots, and gaps; and tissue adhesion, cause increased friction during movement.

Repair strength

The advantages of a multistrand repair are now established. Tendon repair strength is increased by:

- Suture strand number in a proportional relation. The approximate expected core strength, when combined with a simple peripheral suture is:
  - Two-stranded core repair, 20N
  - Four-stranded core repair, 40N (double Pennington/Kessler or modified four stranded Savage)
  - Six-stranded Savage core repair, 60 N

  60N approximately can also be obtained by a two-stranded core repair combined with either the very effective Halsted peripheral repair or the Silfverskiöld peripheral repair.
- Suture calibre—3/0 core suture is stronger than the usual 4/0 but can only be used if the finished repair is not too bulky

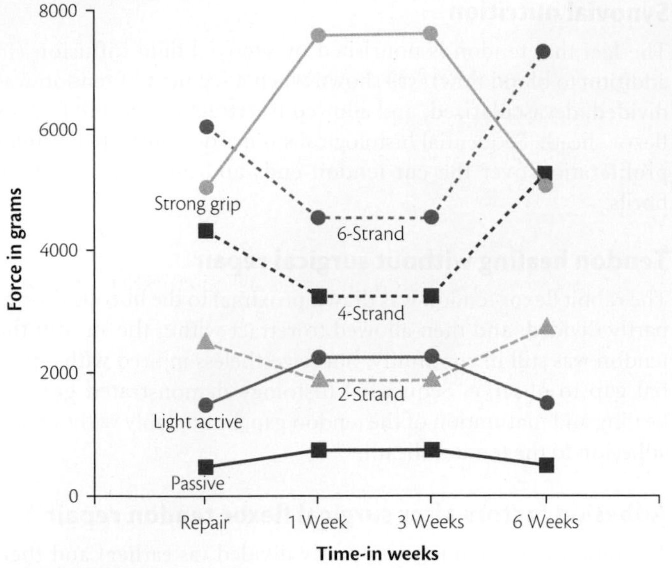

Fig. 12.22.2 Strength of two-, four-, and six-strand repairs plotted against passive movement, light active, and strong grip. Adjusted for friction, oedema, and stress. Reproduced with permission.

- Suture material—typically braided polyester and 'fibrewire' (Arthrex) is tougher (for the core suture) than polypropylene (for the peripheral suture)
- Effective 'anchor points' where the suture grips onto tendon fibres.

Core sutures 1cm from the cut tendon end and peripheral sutures up to 5mm from the cut tendon end share load to create a firm gap-resistant construct.

A summary diagram (Figure 12.22.2) shows that in theary a four-strand repair has a margin of safety during light active movement.

Clinical presentation

Complete division

Diagnosis is clear on finding a classic triad.

- A history of laceration by a sharp object, such as glass or a knife, over the palmar aspect of a finger, the palm, or wrist
- Finger resting posture is relatively extended compared to adjacent fingers
- Failure of the finger to flex on request.

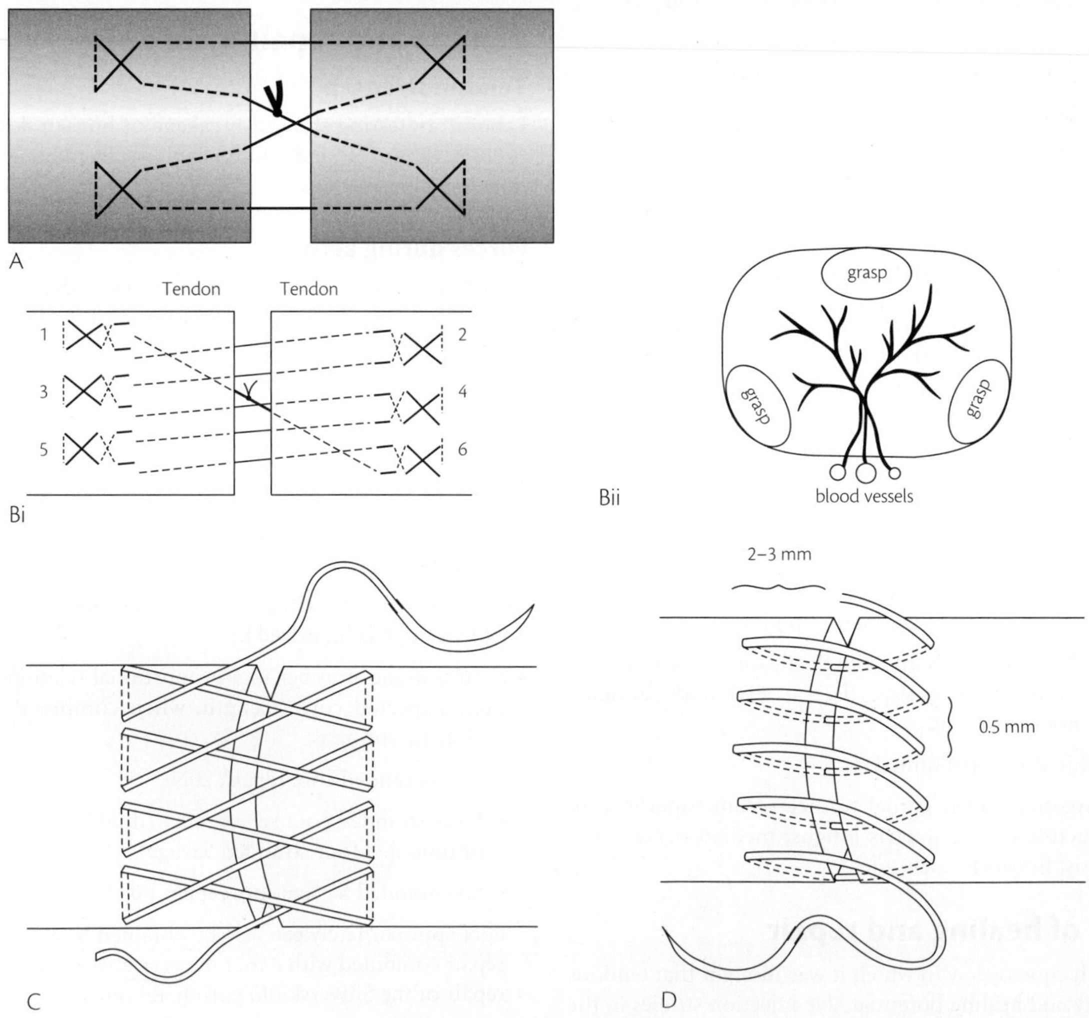

Fig. 12.22.3 Core and peripheral suture techniques. Reproduced with permission. A) Adelaide four strand suture; Bi) Savage six strand repair; Bii) Orientation of anchor points; C) Silfverskiöld cross-stitched peripheral suture; D) Simple peripheral suture.

Careful examination of all flexor tendons to the fingers, thumb, and wrist; and to all neurological and vascular structures relevant to the level of injury is essential. Special imaging is not required.

Partial tendon division

This injury can easily be overlooked because:

- The only sign is the skin laceration
- There is no loss of resting posture
- Nor inability to flex on request.

Suspicion of partial injury should be high, but particularly when considering a palmar laceration with the finger in a gripping action, when profuse bleeding suggests (neuro)vascular damage, and rarely when triggering, suggests the tendon is catching on a sheath edge.

Complex injuries

Association with crush or machine trauma and widespread tissue contusion, nerve injury, and/or fracture, will cause a poor outcome from resultant general scarring.

Closed rupture

In closed injury, rupture of the FDP insertion may result typically from a rugby tackle. The clinical signs are:

- No skin laceration
- Loss of resting posture
- Loss of active movement.

Non-traumatic causes of rupture include rheumatoid tendon disease and rarely, no particular cause at all.

Differential diagnosis

Rarely, anterior interosseous nerve palsy may cause loss of index FDP and flexor pollicis longus (FPL). Tendon blockage can result from trigger digit or rheumatoid nodules without tendon rupture.

Imaging

Magnetic resonance imaging (MRI) or ultrasound may be helpful in cases of repair rerupture and delayed partial tendon division.

Management (Box 12.22.1)

Partial tendon division

Diagnosis by local wound exploration is essential. The wound limit is sought to identify damage to tendon sheath, and the finger is moved to and fro to inspect the underlying tendon. It may not be possible to do this effectively under local anaesthetic, so doubtfully visualized and partial injuries must be explored fully under regional or general anaesthetic.

Complete tendon division

Complete injuries or unresolved suspected partial injuries must be treated by knowledgeable and practiced personnel, with referral and transfer to a centre of special expertise if the required skill is not available locally.

Non-operative treatment

Occasionally other factors will outweigh the importance of tendon injury, such as serious general ill health, age-related infirmity, or inability to comply with postsurgery rehabilitation through reasons of mental state, work, or domestic commitments.

Box 12.22.1 Primary repair of flexor tendons

- Immediate or up to 3 days is preferable
- Experienced surgeon and therapist
- Tourniquet and regional or general anaesthesia
- Zig-zag skin incisions
- Open windows in soft parts of flexor sheath
- A2 and A4 pulleys should not be disturbed unless essential
- Core and peripheral multi-strand repairs
- Sheath laid over tendon and not repaired.

Timing of surgery

Surgery within a few days of injury is ideal but delay up to about 5 days is acceptable. Beyond this time tendon adhesion and muscle retraction significantly reduce the possibility of a neat primary repair.

Consent for treatment should indicate reasonable chances of satisfactory outcome, dependant on compliance with rehabilitation: and moderate risk of infection, adhesion, repair rupture, and stiffness.

Surgery

An arm tourniquet is essential to obtain a bloodless field, so full regional or general anaesthetic is necessary. Surgery may take up to 1h and longer, particularly in cases of multiple tendon division, and microneural repair may be required.

Skin wound extensions (zig-zag) followed by carefully planned 'window' opening in the soft parts of tendon sheath (and sometimes partial opening of A2 and A4) relevant to the position of tendon division, will give access for the tendon repair. Proximal tendon retraction is likely unless prevented by an intact vinculum, where the cut end may be pushed distally by 'milking' the soft tissues, or flexing the finger joints. A separate proximal opening, such as in the palm for a finger injury, may be required to pass the tendon distally.

Careful handling of the divided tendon should minimize further surface and substance damage. Such damage is certainly increased with multi-stranded techniques and causes significant concern, but clinical outcomes suggest the advantages of increased strength outweigh the disadvantages of tissue damage.

Repair technique

There is mounting evidence that a minimum **four-stranded core** suture is required to obtain satisfactory results, e.g.:

- Double Pennington/Kessler: Adelaide (Figure 12.22.3A): Strickland and/or a complex peripheral repair, e.g.
- Silfverskiöld (Figure 12.22.3C): Halsted.

Six-strand repairs (Tang, Sandow, Savage) are equally or more effective.The techniques can be learnt in the laboratory, prior to attempting clinical work, aiming to achieve a robust smooth repair with no gaps.

Fibrous flexor sheath

The hard edge of annular pulleys may cause difficulty completing the repair or snagging of the completed repair, so minimal partial lateral release of a pulley is essential to obtain free movement of the repair. At completion of tendon repair the fibrous sheath is laid over the repair without suture closure.

Rehabilitation

Until healing is sufficiently advanced the finger cannot be used actively. During this time, and up to 6 weeks, a dorsal splint is applied to the wrist and fingers, preventing full finger extension and using a controlled movement programme. All resistance on the palm side, such as dressings, must be loosened from day 1 and removed later.

The repaired tendon must move within the flexor sheath to prevent one of the adhesion factors described by Matthews: immobilization. Force on moving the finger must be minimal so it does not exceed the repair strength.

A skilled hand therapist should direct the movement programme.

Controlled active motion

The currently named 'controlled active motion' regimen (CAM) is probably the most widely used rehabilitation programme in the United Kingdom and is the best suited for repairs of reasonable strength (Box 12.22.2). Originating in Belfast and also called by that name it described 'early active movement' but that was only a small part of the treatment.

- First, the fingers are mobilized passively to reduce joint and tissue stiffness
- Next, the fingers are exercised in a 'place and hold' manner: passive movement into flexion, and then the finger is held flexed actively, thus causing the tendon to move within its sheath
- All four fingers move together, remembering the conjoined action of FDP, and FDS is exercised individually
- Exercises are performed hourly
- As full a range of movement as can be achieved easily is satisfactory during the first few weeks, but preferable about three-quarters range, for the final one-quarter range requires most force. Provided the repair does not stick completely a full range can be regained later, as tissue swelling and adhesion subsides
- After 6 weeks the splint is discarded and light activity is permitted, but not gripping, pulling of can rings, and driving for a further 6 weeks during scar maturation
- An illustrated exercise and instruction chart helps with compliance to the tedious and restrictive regimen.

Box 12.22.2 CAM regimen

- Skilled hand therapist
- Early mobilization to prevent adhesions
- Dorsal blocking splint
- Passive and 'place and hold' exercises
- No active grasping for 6 weeks
- Gradual increase in activity over next 6 weeks
- No gripping for 12 weeks.

Splint position

In the CAM regimen the splint position should be

- Wrist 0-30 degrees extended
- MCP joints flexed 30–70 degrees
- IP joints 0 degrees.

There is least force on the flexor tendons during gentle active movement with the wrist in an extended position. The MCP flexed and IP extended position is the safe resting position to prevent joint contracture.

In the passive and elastic band regimen (below) the splint position is

- Wrist flexed 20 degrees
- MCP flexed 20 degrees
- IP joints 0 degrees.

Passive regimen

From the resting position (above) fingers are only moved by passive guidance from a therapist or the patient's other hand.

Kleinert elastic band traction

From the resting position (above) fingers are moved into a flexed position by elastic bands (attached to the finger nails and to the distal forearm), reducing force within the repaired flexor tendon. Finger extension is performed actively.

Complications

General swelling and stiffness are common and contribute to adhesion (see later) and poor function.

Infection

Pus formation and tissue necrosis is rare following adequate primary treatment, but leads to irrecoverable scarring and stiffness. Obvious infective cellulitis is also uncommon but minor degrees probably contribute to unwelcome tissue swelling.

Repair rupture

In partial repair rupture a scar bridges the tendon gap which sticks to the surrounding tissue, with resultant loss of movement and grip strength.

In typical complete tendon repair rupture the patient 'feels something go', and there is recurrence of the loss of resting posture and lack of active movement signs.

Adhesion

The repaired tendon sticks to neighbouring soft tissue, fibrous sheath, and bone, partly or completely, causing loss of finger movement and reduced hand function.

Results

Outcome is assessed by measurement of:

- Range of active movement
- Flexion and extension deficit
- Grip strength
- Quality of movement
- Rupture rate.

Good and excellent results

This implies near full movement and function. A combination of technical factors is required to achieve reliably good outcomes:

- High repair strength to give a margin of safety from repair dehiscence during mobilization
- Adequate sheath release to prevent repair impingement
- Highly skilled rehabilitation.

Mediocre to poor results

Stiffness, induced by varying degrees of adhesion or partial rupture, causes reduced flexor power with or without the quadriga effect (explanation under 'amputation'), flexion deformity with catching on tools and pockets, and reduced dexterity.

Rupture

Total failure of the treatment method is characterized by a floppy finger that fails to flex next to its neighbours. Published rupture rates of 2 strand core sutures, using the CAM regimen of 5–40 % in different hand centres in the United Kingdom using similar methods, have suggested that two-strand repairs are not adequate for all patients, and later studies strongly suggest that multistranded core and peripheral suture techniques, and improved therapy skill reduce the incidence of repair rupture to less than 5%.

Treatment of complications (Box 12.22.3)

General

For general swelling and stiffness prevention is the best treatment, by ensuring hand elevation and by maintaining movement. Modest infection is controlled by antibiotics but major infection may require tissue debridement.

Rerepair for repair rupture

Diagnosis and rerepair within several days may yield good results but the surgery is more complicated than the initial surgery. Excessive scarring in the tendon sheath and loss of tendon/muscle flexibility requires a two-stage tendon graft or salvage procedures.

Box 12.22.3 Options for repair rupture

- Presentation within several days—rerepair as for primary repair
- Later presentation:
  - 1- or 2-stage tendon graft
  - Leave alone
  - Tenodesis
  - Arthrodesis
  - Amputation.

Box 12.22.4 Flexor tendon grafting

- Imperfect results and frequent complications
- Donor tendon palmaris longus or fourth toe extensor
- Graft between FDS or FDP tendon proximally to distal phalanx
- Immobilize or CAM regimen
- Two-stage grafting using Hunter rod may reduce adhesions.

Tenolysis for adhesion

Where there is no separation of the initial tendon repair, adherent tendon is carefully dissected from surrounding paratenon in zones 3–5 and from the fibrous sheath in zones 1 and 2, retaining essential A2 and A4 pulleys. A continuous infusion local anaesthetic nerve block at wrist level is useful to ensure full active movement for a few days after surgery, and physiotherapy continues until all risk of recurrent stiffness has passed.

If the released tendon is ragged and weak, and where there is also gapping of the initial repair with a scar between the tendon ends, a two-stage tendon graft or salvage procedures may be necessary.

Tendon grafting (Box 12.22.4)

In one-stage tendon grafting the palmaris longus (or fourth toe extensor) donor is used, in an unscarred tendon sheath, for a severely damaged tendon or a segmental tendon loss.

Two-stage tendon graft

In the first stage, the damaged FDS and FDP tendons are excised and essential A2 and A4 pulleys are reconstructed if necessary. A flexible silicone (Hunter) rod (3- or 4-mm. diameter) is sutured to the FDP stump and passed within the flexor sheath to reach zone 5 where it is not connected to a tendon. A smooth synovial lining forms around the silicone rod, into which a tendon graft can be inserted 3–6 months later. Full passive mobilization is achieved following the first stage operation.

In the second stage tendon graft operation a palmaris longus tendon is drawn through the new synovial tube by the existing silicone rod, suturing the tendon graft to the distal FDP stump and to an appropriately flexible FDS or FDP tendon donor in zone 5.

Postsurgical rehabilitation is either by immobilization or by controlled active movement.

The potential for complications following tendon grafting is greater than following primary repair, with two repairs and the graft to fail or stick, and two periods of 3 months of physiotherapy; so great care is required in selecting a tolerant compliant patient.

Salvage procedures

Considering the difficulty in achieving success with a two-stage tendon graft these are common practical alternatives for treating failed tendon surgery. The principle is to focus on hand function overall, rather than to strive for one finger alone.

- *Leave it alone*: functional deficit may not be sufficient to merit intervention
- *Tenodesis*: FDP can be tenodesed across the DIP joint, thus transmitting FDS and intrinsic power to the finger tip
- *Arthrodesis*: arthrodesis can be done in either IP joint, though not usually both in one finger, and not for MCP joints which are flexed by intrinsic muscles
- *Amputation*: adhesion and reduced range of movement in one finger may reduce power in neighbouring fingers due to the conjoined nature of the FDP muscle and tendons (quadriga effect). Amputating the affected digit can free up the flexor system, restoring hand flexibility, power, and function.

Future directions

Future advances may come from simplified suture techniques, enhanced repair strength, and gadgets that achieve a strong repair reliably. Biological research may find methods that improve healing or reduce adhesion but currently none is available for clinical use.

Conclusion

Attention to all the important aspects of presentation, repair, and rehabilitation, in a team of knowledgeable experienced staff, should give near full movement and function following clean incised division of flexor tendons. However, many pitfalls and traps await the unwary occasional practitioner and the untrainable patient, so that poor results and complications are all too common.

Further reading

Elliot, D. (2002). Invited personal view. Primary flexor tendon repair – operative repair, pulley management and rehabilitation. *Journal of Hand Surgery*, **27B**, 507–13.

Matthew, J.P. (1989). Editorial. Early mobilisation after flexor tendon repair. *Journal of Hand Surgery*, **14B**, 363–7.

Strickland, J.W. (1989). Review Article. Flexor tendon surgery. Part 2: free tendon grafts and tenolysis. *Journal of Hand Surgery*, **14B**, 368–82.

Tang, J.B. (2007). Invited personal view. Indications, methods, postoperative motion and outcome evaluation of primary flexor tendon repairs in zone 2. *Journal of Hand Surgery*, **32E**, 118–29.

Viinikainen, A., Goransson, H., Huovinen, K., Kellomaki, M., and Rokkanen, P. (2004). A comparative analysis of the biomechanical behaviour of five flexor tendon core sutures. *Journal of Hand Surgery*, **29B**, 536–43.

12.23

Extensor tendon injuries in the hand and wrist

David M. Evans

Summary points

- Injuries common as tendons vulnerable
- 5 zones described
- Mallet finger usually treated in splint, but some fractures may require fixation
- Capener splint for boutonniere deformity, but sometimes surgery necessary
- Most open tendon injuries need direct repair
- Rehabilitation needs attention to detail.

Introduction

Extension of the wrist and fingers is vital to hand function. Although it is more obvious that flexion is required for pinch and grip, these functions can only be successfully accomplished if the extensor mechanism is intact. Extension allows the tactile surfaces of the hand and fingers to be exposed and brought into contact with objects being manipulated, and extension of the wrist both positions the fingers correctly for grasping and potentiates the long flexors of the fingers by passively increasing their tension, the tenodesis effect. Extension at the metacarpophalangeal (MCP) joints can only be produced by the long extensors of the fingers and thumb (the extrinsic system), but the interphalangeal (IP) joints are extended by both extrinsic and intrinsic systems, so that extensor tendon division proximal to the MCP joint does not eliminate all interphalangeal extension.

The extensor tendons transmit power from the muscle groups situated in the dorsal forearm compartments to the wrist, MCP, and IP joints, producing extension at four sequential joint levels across five rays. Contributions are received from the intrinsic muscles of the hand, entering the system distal to the MCP joints. This network of tendons can be injured at any point, by closed injury usually involving a traction force, or open penetrating, lacerating, or crushing injury. The consequences of such injury mainly affect joints directly controlled by the particular tendon(s) damaged, but effects may be seen at other joints, since the tendons in the system have to act across sequential joints which are inherently unstable without balanced control; they have complex interconnections, and the effects of unopposed antagonist muscles also have to be taken into account. The anatomy of the extensor tendons is shown in Figure 12.23.1.

Because of the exposed and vulnerable position of the extensor mechanism, injury to its tendons is common, occurring in all settings where the hand is at risk from injury, including the workplace, the home, especially the kitchen, and sports situations.

All tendons are vulnerable to sharp injury, and tendons weakened by age (as in mallet finger), trauma (as in extensor pollicis longus (EPL) rupture after distal radial fracture), and disease (as in rheumatoid arthritis) are more prone to closed rupture.

Figure 12.23.1 shows the zones into which the extensor tendons are divided for the purposes of classifying injuries and describing their treatment. In this chapter the zones of injury will be considered in sequence in all their aspects, starting with the most distal.

Injuries to the extensor mechanism

Zones 1 and T1

Mallet finger (Box 12.23.1)

Injuries resulting in loss of extension power at the distal interphalangeal (DIP) joint are most commonly closed injuries, but open laceration dividing the tendon close to its distal insertion has a similar effect.

Closed mallet finger

This common injury usually occurs in surprisingly innocuous circumstances, such as when the finger is stubbed or forced into sudden flexion while bed-making. Usually the patient is immediately aware of a flexion deformity but may not seek help straight away since the injury seems trivial. The injury either involves a stretching and softening disturbance of the tendon resulting in lengthening, or avulsion of a bone fragment at the tendon's insertion. The clinical effect is the same. Patients with normal joint ranges simply show a DIP flexion deformity allowing passive extension. If the proximal interphalangeal (PIP) joint allows some

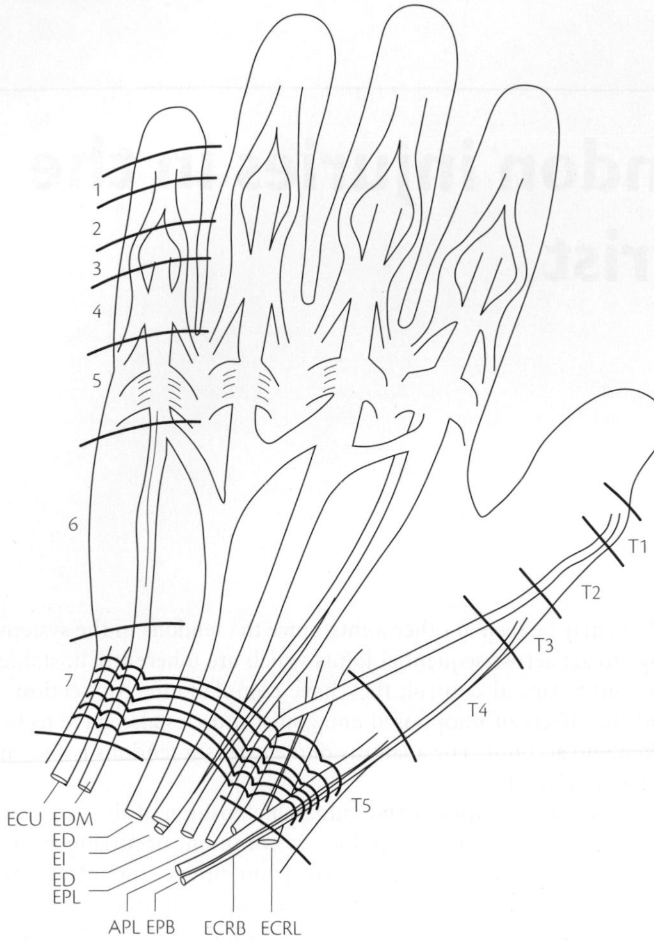

Fig. 12.23.1 The extensor tendons and their connections, and the zones by which injuries are classified. These are shown on the left for the fingers, and on the right for the thumb, with the prefix T.

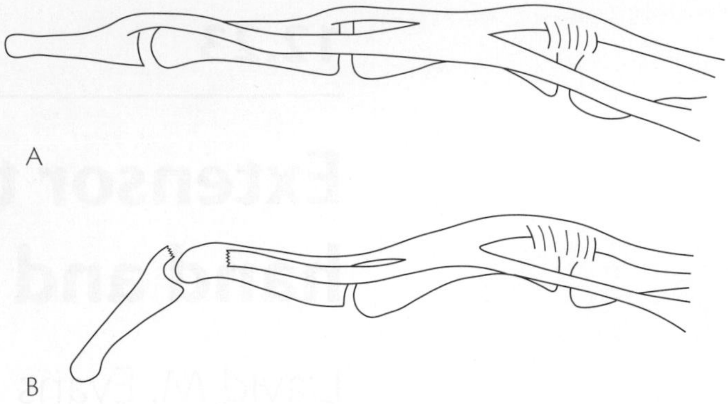

Fig. 12.23.2 A) The extensor mechanism of the finger. B) The change that results from division or rupture of the distal insertion. If volar plate laxity allows it, PIP hyperextension may occur, causing a swan-neck deformity.

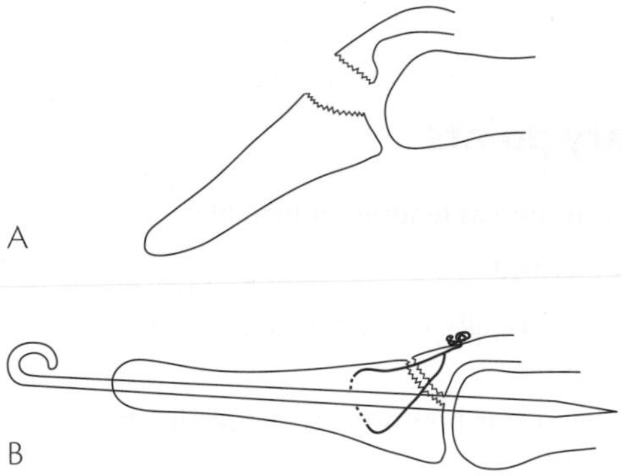

Fig. 12.23.3 A) and B) Mallet finger due to an avulsion fracture of the dorsal lip of the base of the proximal phalanx, showing the method of reattachment. A fine wire is used to hold the bone fragment in place through drill-holes in the distal phalanx. A K-wire maintains extension of the DIP joint.

Box 12.23.1 Mallet finger

- Splint 80% successful
- May have associated fracture
- Fix large bone fragments
- Can result in swan-neck deformity
- Fowler's release at 6 months for failed splintage
- DIP joint fusion if all else fails.

natural hyperextension, a swan-neck deformity may be observed within a few days. This results from the modification in force distribution of the extensor mechanism as it tries to migrate proximally following distal detachment. This proximal movement is restrained by the central slip attachment at the PIP joint (Figure 12.23.2), and the increased tension there can cause hyperextension, or restriction of full flexion where hyperextension is not possible. An understanding of this dynamic change is important.

Investigation includes radiography, with a lateral view to demonstrate an avulsion fracture (Figure 12.23.3).

Treatment of closed mallet finger without fracture is by splintage. Repair of the tendon gives poor results because it is stretched and denatured. Various splints have been described, although the simplest is a padded malleable metal splint placed dorsally across the DIP joint, strapped to the middle and distal sections of the finger to maintain DIP extension. The splint should not be bent dorsally with the intention of forcing the joint into hyperextension because the pressure exerted directly over the joint dorsally can result in skin damage or loss. Splintage should be continuous, and if the patient wishes to remove it to wash the finger, DIP extension should be maintained throughout, since any drop into flexion recreates the injury. This form of splintage needs to be maintained for at least 6 weeks, during which time the patient should be seen regularly and the condition of the dorsal skin checked for pressure. If after 6 weeks there is any tendency for persistent deformity, splintage should be continued, and often this is necessary for up to 10 or 12 weeks.

It is helpful if the patient can learn the habit of allowing the finger to sit in flexion at the PIP joint as this reduces the tension at the sit of distal tendon rupture.

Occasionally a red and slightly oedematous appearance develops over the middle phalanx, usually after splintage has been completed. This is not usually infection, though antibiotic treatment is wise, but it seems to represent inflammation or possibly avascular changes in the disrupted tendon. It settles slowly.

Correctly applied splintage for mallet finger is effective in approximately 80% of cases, although 10–20 degrees of extension lag may persist without functional disturbance. More than 30 degrees of lag can be corrected after a delay of 6 months by Fowler's release of the central slip at the PIP joint. This adjusts the imbalance between the tendon insertions at PIP and DIP levels, restoring tension distally, and can therefore only be done after complete healing of the disrupted tendon has occurred at its new length. Release can be performed under metacarpal block through a longitudinal incision on the side of the finger. The extensor mechanism is lifted intact by dissecting beneath the palmar edge of the lateral band, then the central slip is divided at its insertion without causing separation between lateral and central tendon components, or lateral migration of the lateral bands could cause a boutonnière deformity. This complication has to be protected against by splintage (see later) for 2–3 weeks after the operation. DIP extension is usually restored within days, the occasional failure being due to continued complete disruption of the distal extensor tendon. If the continued flexion deformity is severe enough, DIP fusion might be indicated.

A similar injury can affect the thumb, giving a flexion deformity of the IP joint, in contrast to loss of extension mainly at the MCP joint due to EPL rupture. Mallet thumb, like mallet finger, can be treated conservatively.

Avulsion fracture

A very small chip fracture can be treated by splintage, but large fragments include a significant proportion of the joint surface, which should be restored. The fragment is wired or sutured back in place through drill-holes in the distal phalanx (Figure 12.23.3), supporting the joint in extension with a percutaneous K-wire crossing the joint and kept in place for 3–4 weeks. A brief period of dorsal splintage may be needed after wire removal.

Zones 2 and 4, and T2

The extensor hood over the shafts of the proximal and middle phalanges is broad and flat, and because of its superficial position it is often divided by sharp lacerations. Because it is broad, division may be incomplete and therefore not obvious on clinical examination. The divided tendon can be approximated by simple interrupted sutures. Untidy injuries may involve loss of tendon, but it is usually possible to restore continuity unless tendon is actually missing, in which case a small graft may be needed. Skin cover needs to be secure. Adhesions form easily, and tenolysis may be needed later. This is particularly likely when tendon injury in this area is associated with an underlying fracture. Rigid internal fixation helps by allowing earlier mobilization, and separation of the tendon from bare bone should be attempted by periosteal repair (Box 12.23.2).

Box 12.23.2 Extensor tendon repair over phalanges

- Requires soft tissue cover
- Adhesion may require tenolysis.

Zone 3

Boutonnière deformity (Box 12.23.3)

This is caused by disruption of the central slip of the extensor mechanism at the PIP joint. It may be a closed injury due to forced flexion, or an open laceration at or proximal to the joint. Open laceration is not infrequently missed at the time of repair of a small laceration, because PIP extension can initially be produced by the lateral bands. However, propagation of the tear in the tendon between central and lateral components allows them to migrate palmar-wards round the joint, and they lose their extension force, becoming flexors. As they do so the pull at the DIP joint increases, causing hyperextension (Figure 12.23.4). The dysfunction is now obvious, and the patient seeks treatment, but delayed repair after this disturbance in the mechanism is often unsatisfactory.

When open tendon injury is identified primarily it should be repaired by direct suture with interrupted non-absorbable sutures (about 4/0), and the PIP joint supported in extension with a percutaneous K-wire for about 10 days. During this time, DIP flexion is encouraged, and after which active PIP movement is regained under the supervision of a physiotherapist. Some patients have difficulty in regaining movement.

Closed boutonnière deformity can also develop insidiously by the same mechanism, and patients frequently present 2–3 weeks later. Smith and Ross (1994) have described a test to detect the central slip rupture before it is clinically obvious. The wrist and MCP joint of the affected finger are passively flexed fully, and an intact central slip should produce full PIP extension. If it does not, there is laxity of the central slip, and early treatment is indicated.

The ability of dorsally placed lateral bands to extend the PIP joint is used in the method of closed treatment for this condition with a spring splint (the Capener splint) giving dynamic PIP extension while allowing active DIP flexion. This in turn helps to maintain the dorsal line of the lateral bands by tightening them. It is important that the splint selected is not tight, and the distal stems are short enough to allow DIP flexion (Figure 12.23.5). Splintage needs to be maintained for several weeks under the supervision of a therapist. Initially the joint is rested in extension in the splint, if necessary using a static volar splint until swelling has subsided to allow fitting of the dynamic splint. Then the patient is encouraged to start active flexion in the splint. Provided the treatment has been instituted early enough, migration of the lateral bands will be prevented and the torn tendon can heal without significant lengthening. If treatment is started too late, delayed reconstruction may become necessary. This is extremely difficult, and seldom gives entirely satisfactory results.

Various methods have been described, and involve either dorsal advancement and approximation of the lateral bands, use of a tendon graft, or a turnover procedure from the central extensor more proximally to secure reinsertion at the base of the

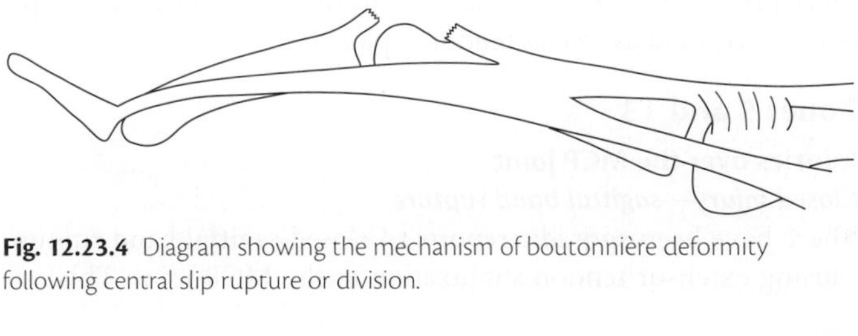

Fig. 12.23.4 Diagram showing the mechanism of boutonnière deformity following central slip rupture or division.

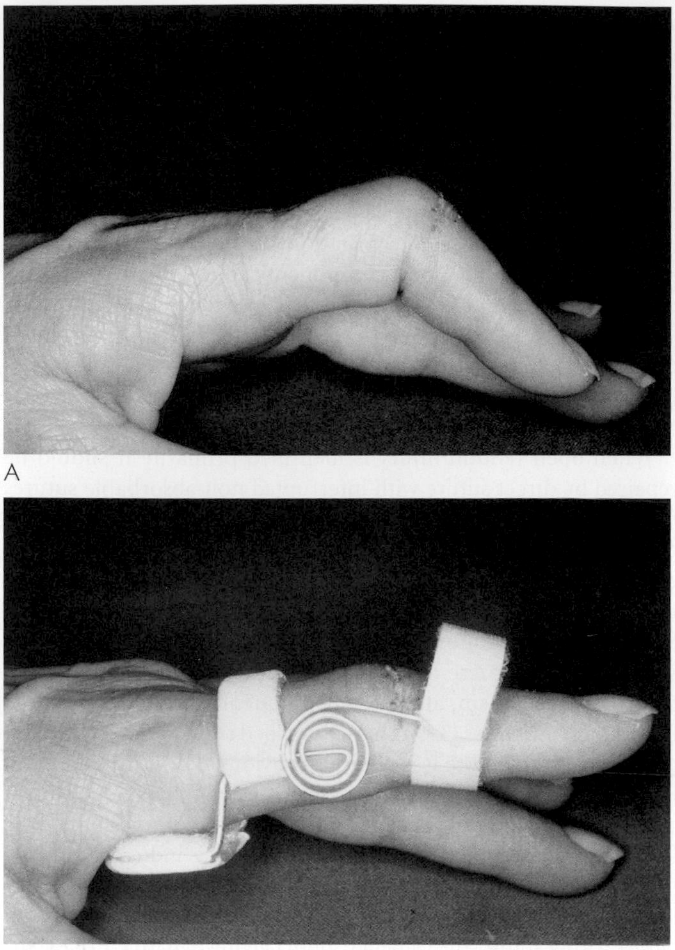

A

B

Fig. 12.23.5 The use of a Capener splint to correct boutonnière deformity.

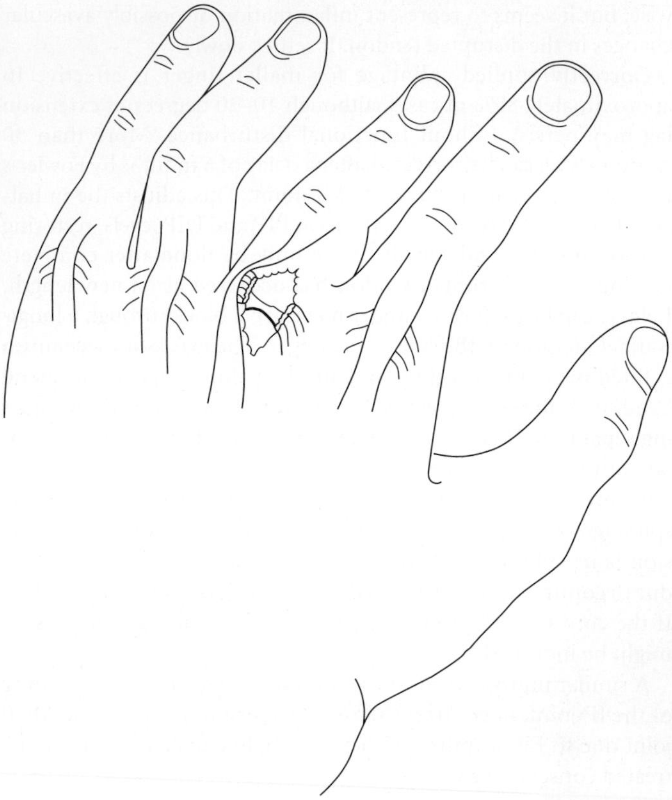

Fig. 12.23.6 Sagittal band rupture at the MP joint level, allowing the extensor tendon to slip off the prominence of the metacarpal head, weakening its ability to extend the finger, mainly at the MP joint. The rupture usually occurs on the radial side, allowing the tendon to slip in an ulnar direction, and the finger drops into some flexion and ulnar deviation, often with a little supination of the finger.

Box 12.23.3 Boutonniere deformity
◆ Early repair best ◆ Reinforce repair with splint ◆ Smith and Ross test to diagnose ◆ Capener splint several weeks.

middle phalanx. All methods should involve lengthening pf the extensor mechanism distal to the PIP joint. Support with a K-wire for 10 days is needed, and patients often experience stiffness, or recurrent deformity to some extent, or both. Physiotherapy and splintage may need to be continued for some time.

Skin loss associated with extensor tendon division presents a special problem, and soft-tissue repair, usually by local skin flaps, may be required as well as tendon repair.

Zones 5 and T3

Injuries over the MCP joint

Closed injury—sagittal band rupture

There have been sporadic reports of closed sagittal band rupture causing extensor tendon subluxation at the MCP joint. This can happen at any age, but requires more force in the young, and can occur with very little force when tendons are weakened, as, for example, in rheumatoid arthritis. The mechanism is usually a blow on the dorsum of the hand, particularly the base of the finger, with a clenched fist. The sagittal band, usually on the radial side, gives way, allowing the extensor tendon to move in an ulnar direction (Figure 12.23.6). From the beginning there is loss of full power of extension at the MCP joint, and this tends to increase as the tendon slides further across. It may reach a point of equilibrium, or deterioration may continue until there is full loss of extension.

If the injury is recognized immediately, splintage may be enough to allow healing without extensor tendon subluxation. Later referral usually leads to the need for direct repair of the tear of the sagittal band.

Extensor tendon division over the MCP joint (Box 12.23.4)

Open laceration at this level can occur as the result of a sharp injury such as a knife, or contact with a tooth during a fight. A limited sharp injury may not initially cause much loss of extension because intact sagittal bands on either side can splint the ends together. However, they easily split, allowing the tendon ends to separate with extensor lag at the MCP joint. Lacerations in this area should be carefully explored for unexpected tendon injury. The tendon is repaired using a core stitch and running marginal stitch.

Human bite injuries

It is common for a tooth to penetrate the stretched skin over an MCP joint, usually of the middle finger, during a fight. Because all

Box 12.23.4 Extensor tendon injury over MCP joint

- Early repair best
- Explore open injuries
- Bite injuries often present late
- Delay repair if active infection.

the tissues are stretched tight the tooth enters the joint, often causing delayed infection if appropriate action is not taken primarily. If the extensor tendon is in the path of the tooth it can also be divided. Because of the circumstances of the injury, the patient may not attend for treatment immediately. If he/she does, the wound should be explored, the joint irrigated and drained, and the central part of the tendon repaired if divided, under broad-spectrum antibiotic cover appropriate for oral flora. If treatment has been delayed and infection is developing, joint irrigation should be added to the regimen; tendon repair may be delayed if the infection is significant, and completed as a secondary procedure when infection has been eliminated.

Zones 6 and 7, and T4 and T5

Extensor tendon injury over the dorsum of the hand and wrist (Box 12.23.5)

The tendons are vulnerable to sharp injury throughout this area, but slightly less so at wrist joint level, being more deeply placed here, covered by the extensor retinaculum, and in the concavity of the joint in its neutral posture of slight extension. At the wrist, the tendons are more closely bunched together; therefore multiple tendon divisions are more likely than on the dorsum of the hand where they diverge.

The diagnosis is usually obvious from the posture of the fingers and the position of the laceration. Exploration usually requires extension of the original cut, and if that is oblique or transverse a zigzag design is best, taking into account the likely position of the divided tendon ends. When the injury is in the zone beneath the extensor retinaculum, it is necessary to reflect a section of the retinaculum to expose the appropriate compartment containing the injured tendons (see Figure 12.23.1). This is best done by lifting a flap based on one side or the other, rather than incising it longitudinally, which would allow bow-stringing. Extension is the usual posture of the wrist during contraction of the digital extensors, and so a pulley mechanism is needed.

When exploring multiple extensor tendon injuries it is important to identify and match individual tendons correctly, since slight differences of level of injury can create significant discrepancies in tension. Matching can be achieved by comparing the lengths of the tendons as they sit together, the direction and shape of each cut end, since they may vary in an identifiable way, and to some extent their position side by side, although this can be misleading as they can become transposed. Standard suture techniques are appropriate, such as the Kessler core stitch (4/0 non-absorbable braided polyester) and running 6/0 circumferential suture. Some extensor tendons are too flat to accommodate a three-dimensional suture such as this, and a simple mattress suture or continuous suture may be sufficient. Careful closure in layers of the surrounding gliding structures makes satisfactory excursion more likely. When treating more complex injuries, attention should be directed to the surface beneath the tendon as well as over it. Bone or fixation material must be separated from the repaired tendon, otherwise dense adhesion is very likely.

Wrist extensor tendons may be divided in deep lacerations in zone 7, always in association with division of more superficial tendons. Closed rupture occasionally occurs. Strong repair of the wrist extensors is essential for effective grip.

Box 12.23.5 Extensor tendon injury in the hand and wrist

- Multiple tendon injury common
- Repair may require division of retinaculum
- Strong repair necessary
- Must match tendon ends.

Postoperative rehabilitation (Box 12.23.6)

Following repair of a single extensor tendon, the hand and wrist are immobilized in extension. After 1 week the splint can be removed and the interphalangeal joints actively exercised under supervision. The splint is then replaced, but only extending to a point approximately 2.5cm distal to the MCP joint, so that some interphalangeal flexion is still possible. A further 3 weeks in this splint should allow tendon healing, and mobilization continues thereafter, under the care of a physiotherapist.

After primary repair of multiple extensor tendons, far superior results following early mobilization have been achieved with dynamic splintage (all excellent) as opposed to 40% excellent and 31% good following static splintage. Dynamic splintage can be started within days of repair.

Spontaneous rupture

It is not uncommon for EPL to rupture following Colles' fracture, usually with little displacement. The EPL at the level of the distal radius is poorly vascularized, and vulnerable to disruption of what blood supply it has, perhaps combined with interference in synovial nutrition through haematoma. Tendon transfer is usually required, and either extensor indicis or a slip of abductor pollicis can be used.

Injuries involving loss of soft tissue

Injuries to the dorsum of the hand involving extensive damage to or loss of soft tissue cover present additional problems. Usually when skin is lost, parts of the extensor tendons will be missing also,

Box 12.23.6 Rehabilitation

- Initial immobilization in extension
- Early dynamic splintage
- Fractures fixation must be kept separate (adhesions).

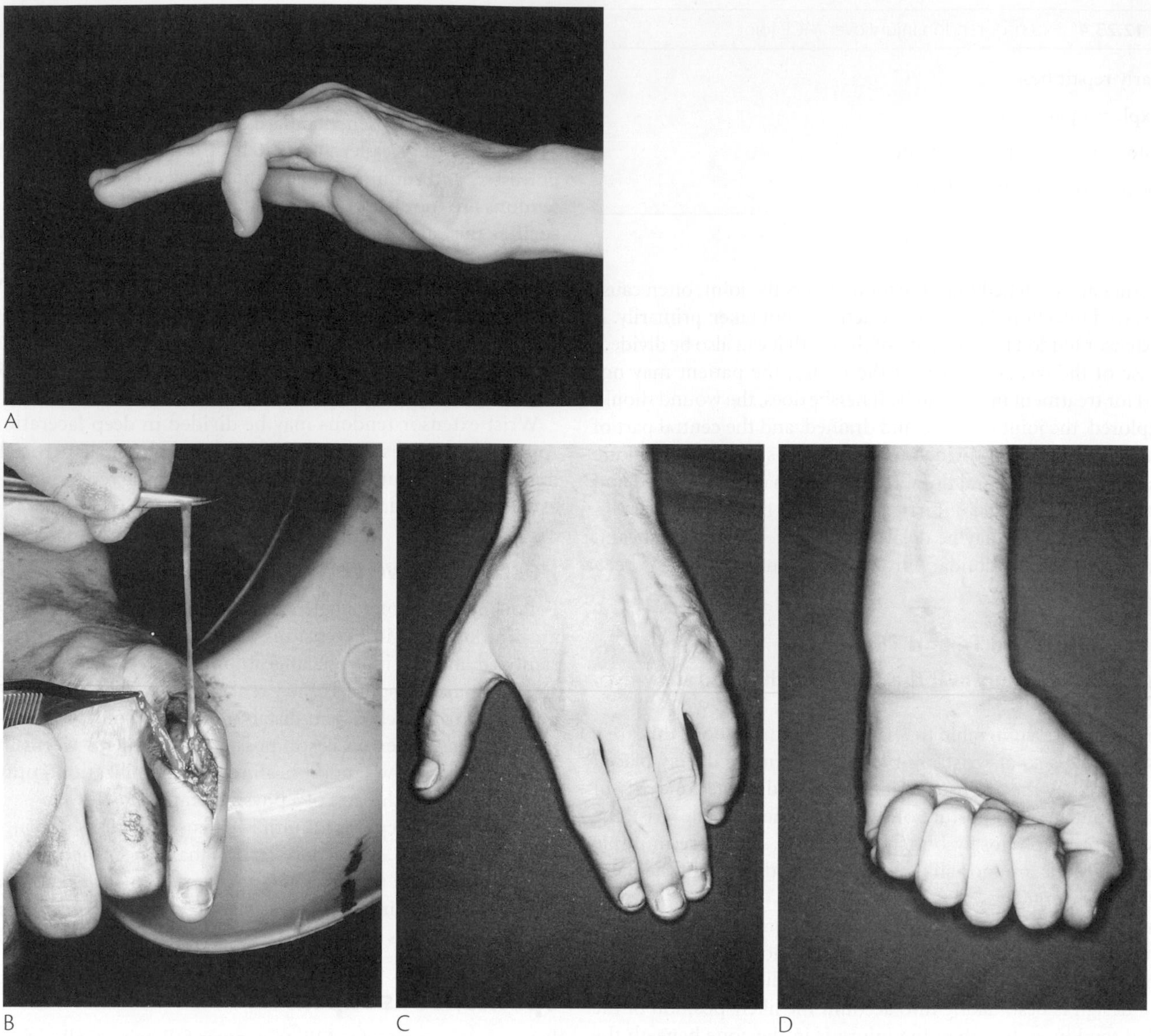

Fig. 12.23.7 A)–D) Loss of whole extensor mechanism of little finger due to infection following revascularization. Extension at the PIP joint was restored using a tendon graft attached to interosseous tendons on both sides of the finger, with the central part of the graft passed through bone at the base of the middle phalanx. DIP extension was produced by tenodesis from the distal insertion to the flexor sheath proximal to the PIP joint, reproducing the function of Landsmeer's oblique retinacular band.

and injuries involving crushing may be associated with metacarpal fractures or even bone loss. Primary reconstruction is always the goal, and if it is not possible immediately should be accomplished within 5 days. Reconstruction is geared to the precise details of the injury, and after thorough debridement may involve skeletal fixation, tendon repair or grafting, and skin replacement usually by flap cover. If there is doubt about the extent of tissue damage or viability, or the patient is not fit, it may be reasonable to bring the patient back to the operating room for a second look and definitive reconstruction after 48h. Under most circumstances, however, primary reconstruction is generally thought to be preferable.

Tendon grafting is less commonly indicated in the extensor mechanism than in the flexor tendons. Loss of an individual extensor tendon can often be effectively treated by suture of the distal end to the side of a neighbouring tendon, since independent extensor tendon function is less important. Loss of multiple tendons may require grafting, however, and multiple tendon grafting material may be needed. Long extensor tendons of the toes can be used, with slight donor morbidity, or strips of fascia lata, with none. These can be threaded through subcutaneous fat of a flap at the time of skin replacement. A composite free flap of skin containing tendons and their gliding mechanisms can be used, the donor site being on the dorsum of the foot. The composite dorsalis pedis flap gives an excellent reconstruction, but some feel that the morbidity of this donor site is unacceptable. If it is carefully resurfaced with full-thickness skin and 100% take is achieved, donor morbidity is minimal.

If a skin defect combined with extensor tendon loss has been healed by free skin grafting, it may be possible to reinsert a tendon graft by creating a tunnel beneath or around the grafted area with a silicone rod. The rod is subsequently replaced by a tendon graft.

Under some circumstances loss of skin and extensor tendons with replacement by free skin grafting alone can result in some restoration of finger extension. This presumably occurs by a tenodesis effect, with some force transmitted through inelastic scar tissue. It cannot always be relied on, but if it fails, a more elaborate reconstructive procedure is available.

Failed extensor tendon repair

Adhesions following extensor tendon repair can be effectively treated by tenolysis. Before doing this, time should be allowed for full resolution of post-traumatic scar tissue, and maximum joint ranges should be achieved by the physiotherapist. Good skin cover is a requirement. The technique requires careful dissection of the tendons from their surrounding bed with preservation of some extensor retinaculum if possible. Early protected mobilization is essential.

Rupture of repaired extensor tendons is unusual, and should be treated by tendon transfer or grafting, according to the availability of reconstructive material.

Further reading

Abouna, J.M. and Brown, H. (1968). The treatment of mallet finger. *British Journal of Surgery*, **55**, 653–67.

Chow, J.A., Dovelle, S., Thomas, L.J., Ho, P.K., and Saldana, J. (1989). A comparison of results of extensor tendon repair followed by early controlled mobilization versus static immobilization. *Journal of Hand Surgery*, **14B**, 18–20.

Fritschi, E., Hamilton, J., and James, J.H. (1976). Repair of the dorsal apparatus of the finger. *Hand*, **8**, 22–31.

Matev, I. (1969). The boutonnière deformity. *Hand*, **1**, 90–5.

Souter, W.A. (1967). The boutonnière deformity. *Journal of Bone and Joint Surgery, British Volume*, **49B**, 710–21.

12.24

Soft tissue hand injuries

Dominic Furniss and Anthony J. Heywood

Summary points

- Limit initial soft tissue damage
- Reconstruct key soft tissue elements
- Functional rehabilitation.

Introduction

Normal hand function is determined by a complex, delicate interaction of soft tissue and skeletal elements. Key soft tissue structures include musculotendinous units, neurovascular bundles, and skin. When the soft tissues are damaged by trauma, infection, or burns, function is compromised. Surgical and non-surgical management of soft tissue hand injuries is therefore aimed at limiting initial soft tissue damage, reconstructing key soft tissue elements, and functional rehabilitation of the hand and patient. Complex open hand injuries present a challenging problem to all reconstructive hand surgeons.

Compartments and spaces of the hand

The pattern of swelling after trauma and burns, the spread of infection and injected substances, and the susceptibility of tissues to raised intracompartmental pressure, are all influenced by anatomy. The complex arrangement of fascia and synovium in the hand forms a number of compartments and spaces, whose walls may contain the spread of infection, channel the spread of substances injected at high pressure, and prevent the dissipation of rising intracompartmental pressure. If neglected, infections may breach these anatomical boundaries and enter adjacent spaces and compartments.

A *compartment* is a volume of tissue partially or completely enclosed by anatomical structures. A *space* lies between anatomical structures, normally occupies a minimal volume, and contains only loose connective tissue and interstitial fluid or a small volume of synovial or other physiological fluid.

Compartments

Subcutaneous

Subcutaneous compartments contain fat, a variable amount of fibrous tissue, and nerves, blood vessels, and lymphatics. On the dorsum of the hand and fingers, the skin is not bound down, allowing massive swelling after injury, and the subcutaneous fat is a single compartment within which infection spreads easily. Along the sides of the digits, in the fingertip pulp, at the flexion creases, and in the palm, the skin is bound to the skeleton, via septa, cutaneous ligaments, and other fibrous structures which limit both distension and the spread of infection.

Muscle

There are ten muscle compartments in the hand containing intrinsic muscles (Figure 12.24.1). They comprise the thenar and hypothenar eminences, adductor pollicis, four dorsal interossei, and three palmar interossei. Their fascial envelopes allow very little distension and therefore their response to injury or inflammation is predominantly a rise in pressure.

Fibrous tunnels

In the hand the main tunnels are the carpal tunnel and Guyon's canal. Although the proximal and distal ends of these are not closed off by rigid structures, the structures within them are not capable of longitudinal displacement and so inflammation and oedema manifest themselves as raised intracompartmental pressure.

In the digits are the fibrous flexor sheaths (see Chapter 12.22). Within the fibrous sheaths are synovial spaces around the flexor tendons (a space within a compartment), where increased compartmental pressure may contribute to the damage caused by infection.

Spaces

Synovial spaces

- Joints: each joint and its synovial lining is a space where infection can develop and be contained.
- Tendon sheaths: the flexor tendons are surrounded by synovial sheaths in the fingers and at the wrist. Those of the thumb and little finger extend in continuity through the palm, known as the radial and ulnar bursae respectively, whereas those of the other fingers are absent in the palm.
- The extensor tendons at the wrist are enclosed in synovial sheaths but this is rarely a site of infection.

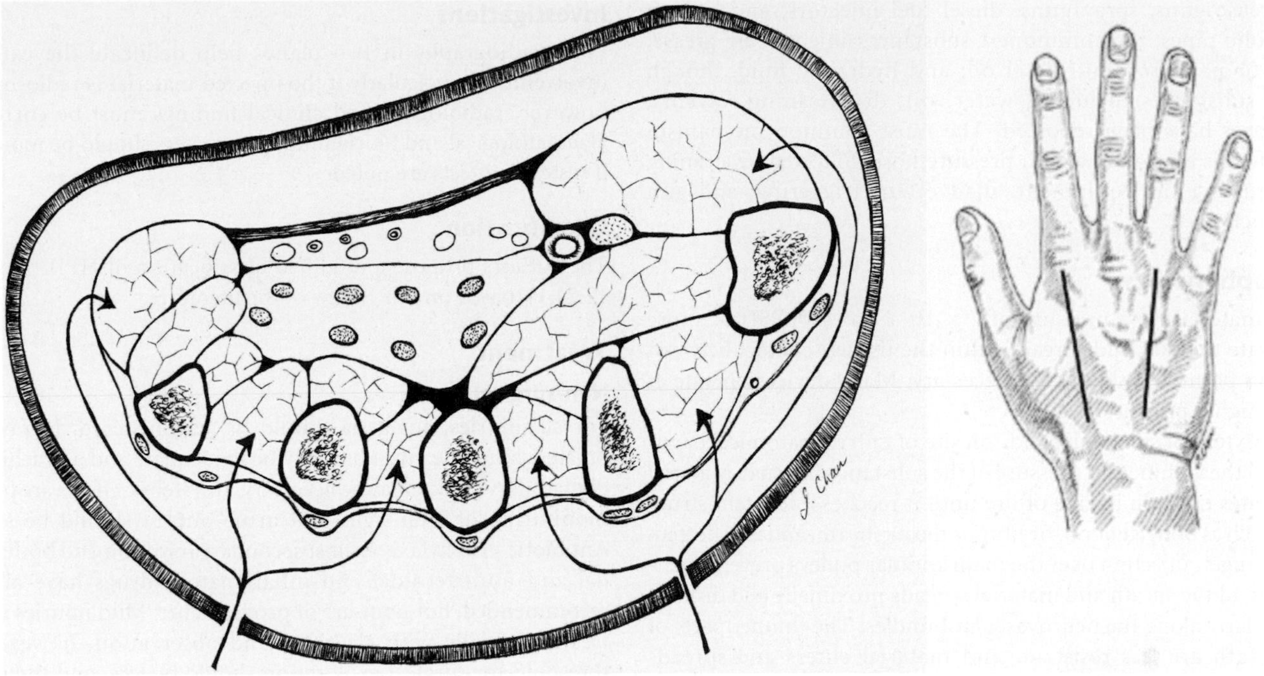

Fig. 12.24.1 Muscle compartments within hand and surgical access through 2 dorsal longitudinal incisions, overlying the second and fourth metacarpals (J Chan 2009).

Potential spaces

Web spaces

In the distal palm are the web spaces—strictly these are compartments—which contain fat, digital neurovascular bundles, and the tendons of the lumbricals and interossei. Their proximal limit is where these structures enter the fibrous tunnels between the palmar fascia and deep transverse metacarpal ligament. They are bounded medially and laterally by the fibrous flexor sheaths, and dorsally and palmarly by the skin of the web, with the natatory ligament on the palmar aspect.

Midpalmar and thenar spaces

Deep to the most superficial, longitudinally orientated layer of the palmar aponeurosis and the transverse palmar ligament a series of vertical fibres form septa on either side of each pair of flexor tendons, and attached to the metacarpals. The best developed of these pass from the radial and ulnar borders of the palmar aponeurosis to the third and fifth metacarpals respectively. Between these, the potential space deep to the long flexor tendons and superficial to the interossei is known as the palmar or midpalmar space (Figure 12.24.2). Radial to the third metacarpal, the potential space deep to the flexor pollicis longus tendon and superficial to the adductor pollicis muscle is the thenar space (Figure 12.24.2).

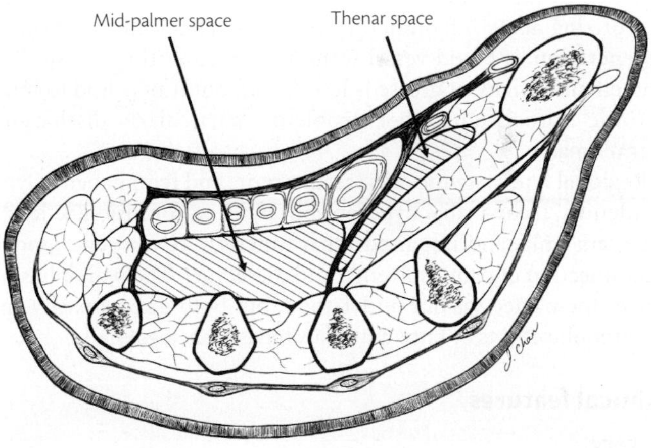

Fig. 12.24.2 Mid-palmar and Thenar deep spaces of the hand (J Chan 2009).

High pressure injection injuries

Background

High pressure injection injuries (HPII) are caused by devices used for injecting or spraying liquids or gases, and by leaks in pressurized pipes. They are uncommon, frequently underestimated, and even with the best treatment, both short- and long-term morbidity is often severe.

Importance

The exact incidence of HPII of the upper limb is unknown. Around two patients per year present to large hand surgery units in the United Kingdom and China.

Causes

Most HPII occur in young male manual workers, and the commonest injection sites are the index or middle fingers or the palm of the non-dominant hand. The commonest devices responsible are grease guns, spray guns, diesel fuel injectors, and leaking hydraulic pipes; the commonest substances injected are grease, paint or paint solvent, diesel oil, and hydraulic fluid, though other substances including water, oil, dry cleaning solvents, and gases have been reported. The most common mechanism identified is a break in a high pressure hose, followed by cleaning or adjusting the equipment, inadvertent triggering, and gun malfunction.

Pathophysiology

Fluid materials at a pressure of 7×10^5 Nm^2 (100PSI) or more penetrate the skin and spread within the tissues; contact between ejection point and skin is not necessary. Many devices operate at much higher pressures.

The extent of spread depends on site of entry, anatomical barriers, and the volume and pressure of the substance injected. Material penetrates tissue in its line of fire until it reaches a resistant structure, such as bone, tendon, or fibrous flexor sheath, and is deflected. In the finger, injection over the main annular pulleys prevents penetration of the sheath and material spreads proximally and distally, particularly along the neurovascular bundles. The thinner parts of the sheath are less resistant, and material enters and spreads throughout the synovial space. Joints are usually not penetrated. In the palm the palmar fascia and all deeper layers are penetrated through to the dorsum, with spread of material at all levels. Spread may be very extensive, and substances injected into the finger can reach the proximal forearm.

Early tissue damage is due both to direct physical and chemical effects, and to secondary ischaemia. Injections of paint rapidly dissolve in fat lobules, causing tissue necrosis and an intense necrotizing acute inflammatory reaction. This leads to fibrinoid degeneration of blood vessel walls and vascular thrombosis. The immediate toxicity of grease is less severe, but it may lead to more chronic fibrosis and other problems, particularly discharging granulomas.

Regional and systemic effects can occur, and lymphangitis, lymphadenitis, tachycardia, hypotension, pyrexia, confusion, leucocytosis, anaemia, and impaired renal function, have been reported after injection of paint, solvents, and diesel fuel. The pathophysiology of these effects is not understood, but both direct toxicity and the embolic effects of fatty materials have been suggested.

Clinical features

History

- Occupation
- Hand dominance
- Time of injury
- Site of injury
- Material injected
- Pressure of device.

Examination

- Puncture point usually trivial
- Circulation
- Sensation.

Investigations

Plain radiographs in two planes help delineate the extent of involvement, particularly if the injected material is radio-opaque; however, radiological and clinical findings must be correlated. Haematological and biochemical parameters should be monitored if systemic effects are noted.

Classification

The authors propose a modified classification of HPII (see Table 12.24.1), based on our review of the literature.

Treatment

Non-surgical

For all injuries, analgesia should be administered. Intravenous opiates should be given but may be inadequate and a brachial (*not* digital) nerve block may be necessary. If systemic effects are present, monitoring of vital signs and urine output should be started. Antibiotic prophylaxis against secondary infection and both steroidal and non-steroidal anti-inflammatory drugs have all been recommended, but none are of proven value. Mild injuries may be treated initially with elevation and observation, however, the threshold for surgical exploration should be low, and the patient prepared for surgery.

Surgical

Moderate and severe injuries, as well as patients with mild injuries who complain of increasing pain, require urgent exploration, decompression, and removal of as much of the injected material as possible. This is performed under tourniquet without forced exsanguination. Starting at the entrance wound the incision is extended proximally and distally until the full extent of spread is revealed—the smell of solvents can be a useful sign. Removal of all foreign material may be facilitated by use of the operating microscope and helps preserve vital structures. The skin should be left open, or at most partially and loosely closed. Inevitably some material is left, and repeat debridement at 48h should be performed.

Table 12.24.1 Classification of HPII[a]

Severity	Clinical features	Management
Mild	Air or water injected Grease confined to pulp only Low injection pressure No delay in treatment Circulation and sensation intact	Elevation Analgesia Close observation Ready for surgery if pain increases
Moderate	As for mild but with grease spread beyond pulp	Surgical decompression and debridement Leave wounds open Second look procedure after 48h Delayed primary closure
Severe	Paint or solvents injected Delay beyond 12h High injection pressure Extensive proximal spread Loss of sensation Poor circulation	Surgical decompression and debridement Leave wounds open Repeated debridement Late reconstruction Consider early amputation

[a]Modified from Wong et al. (2005).

Postoperative management

After operation the hand is elevated and splinted in the position of safe immobilization, and aggressive active and passive mobilization begun within a few days. Delayed primary amputation is necessary if the digit becomes clearly non-viable. Late reconstruction may include tenolysis, tendon grafting, neurolysis, nerve grafting, scar contracture release, and skin replacement.

Outcomes

Two factors have been shown to predict amputation in HPII: site of injection in the finger compared to the thumb or palm; and injection of an organic solvent (paint, paint thinner, diesel, or oil) compared to other substances. In addition, a delay to debridement of more than 6h lead to significantly more amputations when organic solvent injections were considered alone, but not when all HPIIs were analysed. Furthermore, there was a trend towards higher amputation rates with higher pressures of injection. The presence of infection and the use of steroids have not been shown to affect amputation rate significantly. In one series, all fingers which were noted to be poorly perfused at presentation were subsequently amputated.

Functional outcome of the hand is also poor. At an average 8.5 year follow-up a significantly decreased range of motion has been demonstrated at affected metacarpophalangeal (MCP), proximal interphalangeal (PIP), and distal interphalangeal (DIP) joints compared to the unaffected side. In addition, decreased grip and pinch strength, and increased two-point discrimination threshold has been recognized. Furthermore, 78% of patients complained of continuing cold intolerance, 61% of hypersensitivity, and 22% of constant pain in the affected digit. The average time to return to work was 7.5 months, and over half of patients had changed jobs or remained unemployed after the injury.

Compartment syndrome of the hand

Background

Compartment syndrome exists when the pressure within an anatomical compartment is increased to a level where the viability of the tissues within the compartment is compromised. The increase in pressure causes tissue ischaemia, especially of muscles and nerves within the compartment, and may lead to permanent loss of function. The fascial compartments of the hand are illustrated in Figure 12.24.1.

Importance

Incidence varies with aetiology and severity of the primary injury; in severe upper limb burns for example it is up to 70%.

Causes

The commonest causes are crush injuries and burns, but there are a large variety of potential causes, many of which can occur in patients who are unconscious and therefore do not display classical symptoms and signs (Box 12.24.1). Compartment syndrome is an important cause of iatrogenic morbidity as a complication of tight casts or dressings, intravenous drug administration, and arterial lines.

Box 12.24.1 Examples of causes of compartment syndrome in the hand

- Tight dressings or casts
- Crush injury—acute
- Crush injury—lying on hand
- Reperfusion injury—revascularization
- Burns
- Cold injury
- Snakebite
- Intra-arterial injection.

Clinical features

History

- Injury known to cause compartment syndrome
- High index of suspicion (especially in unconscious patients, or those with an insensate upper limb, for example, brachial plexus injuries)
- Pain out of proportion to injury
- Pain not controlled by immobilization and analgesics.

Examination

- Hand held in intrinsic minus position: MCP joints extended, PIP joints flexed
- Swelling and turgor of the compartment
- Pain on passive stretch
  - Interossei: MCP joint extended, PIP joint flexed, abduct and adduct digit
  - Adductor pollicis: palmer abduction of the thumb
  - Thenar: radial abduction and extension of the thumb
  - Hypothenar: extension and adduction of the little finger
- Paraesthesia in the distribution of nerves passing through the compartment
- Paresis of muscles supplied by nerves passing through the compartment
- Alteration of pulses and perfusion: late sign, muscle necrosis usually present.

Investigations

The diagnosis of compartment syndrome is clinical, and once made mandates immediate surgical intervention. Direct measurement of intracompartmental pressures can be achieved by a variety of methods, all of which involve the principle of placing a column of fluid between the compartment and a measuring device. Normal compartment pressure in an uninjured extremity is 0–8mmHg, and normal capillary perfusion pressure is 20–25mmHg. No consensus exists as to a threshold for compartment decompression, and indeed the threshold may vary depending on patient factors such as blood pressure, which affects capillary perfusion pressure. Furthermore, the multiple compartments in the hand make measurement a complex process even with the simplest techniques. We therefore recommend the measurement of intracompartmental pressures only where there is strong doubt about the presence of a compartment syndrome and a strong contraindication to surgical treatment, which is a rare situation.

Treatment

Non-surgical

The treatment of a suspected compartment syndrome is surgical decompression without delay. In the meantime, any external pressure, such as tight bandages or casts, should be removed. The hand should be placed level with the heart to maximize perfusion pressure whilst minimizing swelling and hypovolaemia should be corrected.

Surgical

The exact site of incisions is not critical, and all compartments can be reached through two dorsal incisions (see Figure 12.24.1). Should any doubt remain as to whether a particular compartment has been decompressed, a further incision over the compartment should be made. The carpal tunnel should also be released. Decompression of digits is not necessary unless the digit itself has been injured; the commonest indication is after burns (see later). The wounds should be left open and dressed.

In circumstances where the probability of a compartment syndrome is very high, such as after revascularization after a long ischaemia time, or following a severe crush injury, fasciotomies of the intrinsic muscles and carpal tunnel decompression should be performed prophylactically.

Postoperative care

After decompression, the hand should be elevated and splinted in the position of safe immobilization. After 3–5 days the patient should be returned to theatre and the skin closed if this can be done easily. If not, dorsal wounds should be covered with thin partial thickness skin grafts and the hand mobilized soon afterwards.

Outcomes

In a retrospective study of nineteen patients who had undergone hand and/or forearm fasciotomy for raised intracompartmental pressure, a good outcome in 13 patients and a poor result was recorded in four. In those four patients, the time from diagnosis to decompression was over 6h, and all four were obtunded or under general anaesthesia when the compartment syndrome developed. However, good results were achieved in three patients decompressed over 12h after diagnosis, so fasciotomy should still be performed when there is a late presentation.

Complications

Intrinsic tightness leading to intrinsic contracture is the characteristic complication of unrecognized or under treated compartment syndrome of the hand. This is caused by fibrosis of the affected lumbricals and interossei. Intrinsic tightness can be diagnosed clinically by increased resistance to flexion of the IP joints when the MCP joint is held extended compared to when the MCP joint is flexed. Symptomatically, patients with mild intrinsic contractures complain of persistent limited interphalangeal (IP) joint flexion months after injury. In more severe cases, flexion contractures of the MCP joints and extension contractures of the IP joints may develop. Severe complications of untreated compartment syndrome include digital necrosis, and persistent nerve dysfunction.

Burns

Background

Burns of the hands require specialist assessment and treatment. The British Burn Association recognizes that burns to the hands involving dermal or full thickness skin loss are more likely to follow a complex clinical course and therefore should be referred to a specialist burn care facility. Furthermore, the need for skin grafting of hand burns is independently correlated with reduced quality of life in burn survivors.

Importance

Hand burns are common, and occur out of proportion to their percentage body surface area. Many small injuries are treated as outpatients and the total incidence is unknown but high. In diverse countries such as the United Kingdom, United States of America, and Iran, two to three patients per 10 000 population per year are admitted to hospital with burns, and ten times this number may be treated without hospital admission; the arms and hands are involved in around 45% of cases. Both incidence and cause vary markedly with age, geography, and sex.

Table 12.24.2 Clinical features of burns

Feature	Depth			
	Epidermal	Superficial partial thickness	Deep partial thickness (deep dermal)	Full thickness
Colour	Pink or red	Pink	Pale, often punctuate red 'fixed staining'	White, black, brown
Texture	Normal	Normal	Normal	Leathery
Capillary refill	Brisk	Present	May be absent	Absent
Blisters	Absent	Present, may have burst	Usually absent	Absent
Exudate	Absent	Heavy	Light	Absent
Pain	Painful	Painful	Not very painful	Absent
Sensation	Present	Present	May be absent	Absent
Bleeding with pinprick	Present (not usually attempted)	Present	Present	Absent

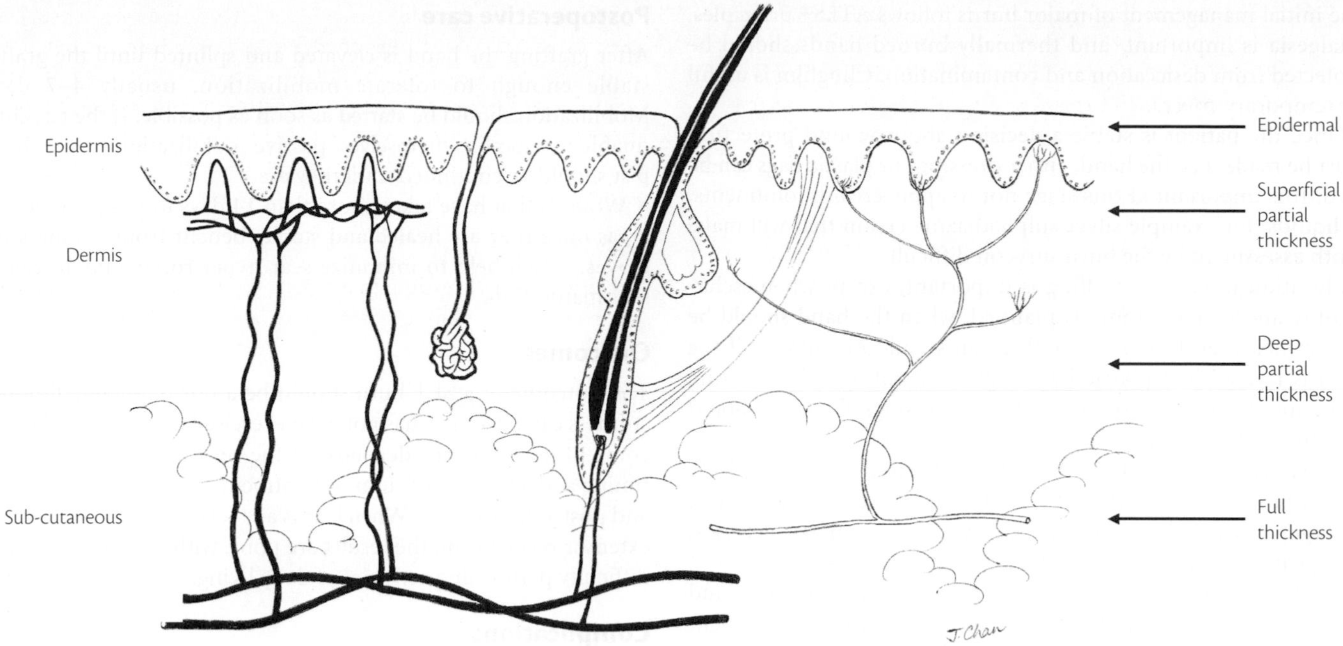

Fig. 12.24.3 Skin anatomy. A schematic diagram of skin anatomy with levels of injury corresponding to burn depth is shown. Epidermal and superficial partial thickness burns are more painful than deep partial thickness and full thickness owing to the preservation of more nerve endings. Superficial partial thickness and deep dermal burns heal without surgery because of epithelial cells lining adnexal structures such as hair follicles and sweat glands.

Causes and classification

The causes of burns are thermal, chemical, and electrical. The majority are thermal, caused by hot liquids, fire, and contact with hot objects. Chemical and electrical burns have their own special effects, and are not discussed further. The amount of damage in a thermal burn depends on the temperature and duration of burning.

Burns are classified clinically according to depth of skin necrosis (Table 12.24.2). Four grades of burn are clinically recognisable: epidermal, superficial partial thickness (SPT), deep partial thickness (DPT), and full thickness (FT) (Figure 12.24.3). Full thickness burns may also involve deeper tissues.

Burn depth forms the basis for decisions about management as it indicates whether the skin will heal and the likely degree of scarring. Epidermal burns, for example sunburn, heal spontaneously within 2–3 days and require treatment with moisturizer and mobilization. SPT burns heal in 7–14 days without scarring. DPT burns may heal in 14–21 days or more but often produce hypertrophic scars that contract and may interfere with function. FT burns heal by secondary intention, which is only acceptable if they are small. In the hand a distinction should also be made between palmar skin, which is thick, specialized, and more likely to heal well after apparently deeper burns, and dorsal skin, which is thinner, non-specialized, and less likely to heal well after anything more than SPT injury.

For all burns deeper than epidermal, oedema occurs in nearby tissues, and swelling reaches its maximum at 24–36h. A swollen, unsplinted hand takes up a position of wrist flexion, MCP joint extension, IP joint flexion, and thumb adduction, exactly the opposite of the position of safe immobilization, and if this is allowed to persist then secondary joint changes make mobilization difficult and can result in permanent joint contractures.

Coagulated protein contracts, and FT burns have lost their ability to stretch because of destruction of elastin within the dermis. Therefore, circumferential FT burns of the hand or digits, together with increased interstitial pressure due to oedema, may cut off the distal circulation and necessitate emergency release by escharotomy. With extensive FT burns a muscle compartment syndrome can also develop, especially if escharotomy is delayed.

Clinical features

History

- Obtain history from patient, witnesses, emergency personnel
- Identify likelihood of associated airway burn, inhalation injury, carbon monoxide or hydrogen cyanide poisoning–usually burns from a fire in an enclosed space
- Identify likelihood of associated escape injuries
- Estimate temperature and duration of contact, therefore depth of burn.

Examination

- ATLS® principles, assess hand as part of secondary survey
- Determine distribution and depth of burn (see Table 12.24.2).

Investigations

No special investigations are needed for hand burns. Various imaging techniques have been tried for measuring burn depth, but none has proved to be of practical clinical use.

Treatment

Non-surgical

Hand burns may occur as part of a larger burn, the systemic effects of which dominate the clinical picture at first, although the hands must be considered in the overall management plan from the start.

The initial management of major burns follows ATLS® principles. Analgesia is important, and thermally burned hands should be protected from desiccation and contamination. Clingfilm is useful for temporary cover.

Once the patient is stable a decision about wound protection must be made. For the hand, either dressings or plastic bags can be used. It is important at this stage not to apply creams, ointments, or liquids, for example silver sulphadiazine cream that will make depth assessment by the burn surgeon difficult.

Elevation to reduce swelling is important, except when escharotomy and/or fasciotomy is planned, when the hand should be kept at heart level. Active mobilization should be pursued if the burn is treated in a plastic bag or glove, combined with resting night-splints. If the burn is treated with dressings, the hand should be splinted in the position of safe immobilization.

Most chemical burns should be treated by immediate and copious lavage with water, although there are exceptions. Emergency workplace showers are available in many factories, along with specific antidotes for particular chemicals.

Domestic electrical injuries can cause cardiac arrhythmias and myocardial damage, and if evidence of either is found the patient should be monitored for at least 24h. High voltage electrical injury, often from industrial source, is a major emergency requiring immediate resuscitation and surgical exploration, fasciotomy, debridement, and vascular reconstruction, with amputation if the limb is irretrievably damaged.

Surgical

Escharotomy and fasciotomy, if indicated, are emergencies. Distal circulation in the burned hand may be difficult to assess, and the indication for escharotomy is a full thickness or possibly full-thickness burn that is circumferential or almost circumferential and might cause ischaemia. Both escharotomy and fasciotomy should be performed under general or regional anaesthesia, and if anything more than one hand requires escharotomy blood should be available for transfusion.

Apart from escharotomy and fasciotomy, the decision about operative or non-operative treatment and timing of surgery should be taken by a specialist burn surgeon. Decision making depends on the depth and distribution of the burn and on other injuries. SPT burns do not need surgery, but should be re-examined after 48h to make sure they are truly SPT and have not become deeper. Definite FT burns, dorsal or palmar, should be excised and grafted in a specialist unit. In large burns the hands are second only to the face and neck in order of priority for grafting.

The management of DPT burns is less clear cut. On the dorsum, the results of early tangential excision and skin grafting are so good that there is an argument for early surgery in all but definite SPT wounds, but this is controversial and good results can also be obtained by grafting only wounds that have not healed by 2–3 weeks. Grafts to the dorsum should be applied with the wrist and finger joints fully flexed in order to maximize the amount of skin applied and therefore prevent subsequent dorsal contracture. On the palmar surface depth is more difficult to assess and, because of the thickness of the skin, healing frequently occurs after burns that appear at first to be deeper than SPT. This is specialized skin and if it is capable of healing in 2–3 weeks or even longer without grafting, then this is likely to produce the best result.

Postoperative care

After grafting the hand is elevated and splinted until the graft is stable enough to tolerate mobilization, usually 4–7 days. Mobilization should be started as soon as possible. If the patient is unable to mobilize themselves, passive mobilization by the therapist should be continued until they are.

Wounds that have taken more than 14 days to heal, and grafted areas once they are healed and stable, benefit from compression gloves, which help to minimize scar hypertrophy and accelerate scar maturation.

Outcomes

The outcome of a SPT burn should be a normal hand, although stiffness can occur if it has not been exercised or splinted. The outcome of deeper burns depends on the severity of injury and the timing and adequacy of surgical treatment, splintage, mobilization and post-burn therapy. When burns are very deep, and involve the extensor mechanism, the results are poor, with loss of motion and difficulty performing activities of daily living.

Complications

Complications of hand burns are often a consequence of delayed healing with subsequent adverse scarring and contracture, or poor cooperation with therapy and splintage resulting in stiffness. Even with the best management, complications occur. Frequently seen problems include: first webspace adduction contracture, other webspace contractures, dorsal skin contractures, little finger abduction deformity, MCP joint hyperextension, PIP joint flexion contracture, extensor tendon adhesion, Boutonnière deformity, median and ulnar nerve compression neuropathy, amputation secondary to gangrene. Secondary surgery to release scars and reconstruct skin and soft tissues may be required. The growing hand is especially vulnerable and likely to need multiple secondary procedures.

Infection

Background

Hand infections are common, and the consequences of poor or delayed treatment can be severe. Infections may be acute or chronic, bacterial, viral, fungal, or protozoal. Most are acute, and most of these are bacterial. The following discussion applies to acute bacterial infections. The majority are due to trauma, including animal and human bites (usually the patient has punched someone in the mouth), but a few are haematogenous.

Importance

The total incidence is not known because many minor infections are treated by primary care physicians and accident departments, but large hand surgery units in the developed world may admit 40–100 patients per year with more serious infections. Accurate worldwide figures are not available.

Causes and classification

A large variety of bacteria have been cultured from hand infections. The most common organisms are flora of the mouth or skin, especially the gram-positive aerobes streptococci and staphylococci. However mixed infections are common and anaerobes are present not infrequently, particularly after human bites and in paronychia. Human bites have a high incidence of *Eikenella corrodens* and dog and cat bites of *Pasteurella multocida*. The majority of acute hand infections occur in immunocompetent hosts. However, a significant minority occur in patients with predisposing immunocompromise, caused by diabetes mellitus, HIV infection, or steroid treatment, for example. Immunocompromise may not be diagnosed prior to the onset of infection, and can predispose to infection with unusual organisms, including Gram-negative and mixed organisms, and mycobacteria. Clinicians must also be aware of the possibility of hand infection caused by community acquired meticillin resistant *Staphylococcus aureus* (MRSA). This may be particularly important as the delay before receiving appropriate antibiotics for patients with MRSA hand infections has been shown to be increased compared to those with non-MRSA hand infection.

Most infections are confined, at least initially, to a particular anatomical site, space, or compartment, and are classified accordingly. The classification and relative incidence of those infections requiring operative treatment are listed in Table 12.24.3. This is necessarily a biased estimate of the true frequency of different types of hand infection, as already it has been noted that many infections are treated successfully in a primary care or emergency department setting.

Clinical features

History

Most patients give a history of trauma, with a penetrating injury that may have been trivial, or a more severe injury that has been neglected. The history may suggest likely pathogens, but sometimes the history is unreliable, such as after a human 'bite'. A full general history should be taken, particularly regarding predisposing conditions and tetanus immunity. The duration of symptoms and severity of pain, particularly pain that has prevented sleep, indicate whether the infection is early or whether a localized collection of pus is likely.

Examination

Cellulitis

Cellulitis alone occurs most commonly on the dorsum of the fingers or hand, often following a minor wound, and is usually due to beta-haemolytic streptococcus. Erythema and swelling may spread rapidly, sometimes with associated lymphangitis and systemic illness, and there may be skin damage ranging from blistering to frank necrosis. Necrotizing fasciitis is uncommon but can affect the hand and upper limb as elsewhere.

Table 12.24.3 Hand infections: classification and relative incidence[a]

Infection	Incidence (%)
Human bite	51.4
Cellulitis	17.2
Septic arthritis	11.8
Subcutaneous abscess	9.9
Gangrene	2.7
Flexor sheath infection	2.5
Osteomyelitis	1.8
Dog bite	1.4
Web space infection	0.9
Paronychia	0.45
Cat bite	0.23

[a] Data from Weinzweig and Gonzalez (2002)

Nail-fold (paronychia/eponychia)

Mixed infections, particularly with *S. aureus* and anaerobes, are common. It starts with swelling, erythema, and tenderness around the nail-fold, usually on one side (paronychia), or at the base of the nail (eponychia). After 24h pus may be detectable, in the nail-fold and sometimes under the nail. In late cases the whole of the nail-fold, both sides and the base, may be involved.

Pulp-space (felon)

This is commonly due to a puncture wound and a foreign body may be present. Diabetics can get pulp infections caused by pricking their fingers for blood glucose monitoring. *S. aureus* and anaerobes are the commonest pathogens. Early on there may be localized cellulitis or a small collection of pus, but soon the whole pulp becomes swollen, tense, and very tender.

Other subcutaneous abscess

Localized subcutaneous infection may occur anywhere in the hand. In the palm the infection may extend via a narrow channel through the palmar fascia to form a subfascial abscess, which together with the subcutaneous component is known as a collar-stud abscess.

Tendon sheath infection (Box 12.24.2)

Infective tenosynovitis affects almost exclusively the flexor tendons. Most cases are caused by penetrating trauma, but some are haematogenous, and in these gonococcus is a likely pathogen. Kanavel's four cardinal signs are: digit held in slight flexion, fusiform swelling of whole digit, tenderness over the flexor sheath, and severe pain on passive extension. In early disease, the signs may be subtle. In tenosynovitis of the thumb and little fingers tenderness may extend proximally to the wrist and into the distal forearm via the radial and ulnar bursae.

Deep spaces

The potential spaces in the hand (Figure 12.24.2) can become actual spaces, occupied by pus, most often following a penetrating injury or extension of infection from a tenosynovial sheath or an adjacent deep space.

Web space

The fingers on either side of the web are abducted away from the web, and there is swelling and tenderness on dorsal and palmar aspects.

Thenar space

The thumb is held abducted, with tenderness and swelling over the thenar eminence, first web (palmar and dorsal), and index metacarpal, and pain on thumb extension or attempted opposition.

Box 12.24.2 Signs of tendon sheath infection

- Digit held in slight flexion
- Fusiform swelling of whole digit
- Tenderness over the flexor sheath
- Severe pain on passive extension.

Midpalmar space

The normal concavity of the palm is lost, there is dorsal swelling that may be more prominent than the palmar swelling, and finger movements, especially of the middle and ring fingers, are painful.

Joint

Septic arthritis may be caused by penetrating injury (when it may co-exist with tenosynovitis caused by the same injury), extension of another infection (most commonly tenosynovitis), or haematogenous spread from an infection elsewhere. In children *Haemophillus influenzae* is a likely pathogen, and in sexually active adults gonoccus should be considered. Bite wounds caused by punching someone in the teeth can result in septic arthritis of the MCP joints of the fingers if the joint is penetrated. An important anatomical point is that the wound occurs with the joints in maximum flexion, and if explored with the joints in extension the defects in the different layers (skin, extensor apparatus, joint capsule) will be out of line and the involvement of the joint missed if not looked for.

There is swelling and erythema around the joint, which is held in the position that maximizes its volume (MCP joint extension and IP joint partial flexion). The joint is tender, and any movement is painful.

Bone

Osteomyelitis of the hand is uncommon and affects almost exclusively the long bones. It may follow infections in adjacent tissues or compound fractures (including for example, a Seymour fracture) or may be due to haematogenous spread. *S. aureus* is the commonest pathogen, and *Haemophillus influenzae* is common in young children. There is local swelling, erythema, and tenderness over part of the affected bone.

Investigations

In acute infections the decision to operate is a clinical one. Plain radiographs in two planes may show foreign bodies, including broken teeth, but apart from these and soft tissue swelling most radiographs of infected hands are normal at the time of presentation. Microbiological specimens usually have to await surgical exploration, though in septic arthritis joint aspiration may confirm the diagnosis. Microbiology for osteomyelitis is best by bone biopsy. Blood cultures should be done in the presence of systemic illness.

Relevant biochemical and haematological tests should be done if an underlying cause such as diabetes or immune compromise is suspected.

Differential diagnosis

Many conditions can mimic acute hand infections, the more common differential diagnoses being acute arthritis, acute gout, herpetic whitlow, compartment syndrome, hand fracture, and rarely primary hand tumour.

Treatment

The principles of treatment are the same for all acute bacterial infections: surgical drainage of localized infections, elevation, splintage, antibiotics, and mobilization as infection is controlled and swelling subsides.

Non-surgical

Cellulitis and early osteomyelitis may be treated with elevation and intravenous antibiotics. Patients awaiting surgery for other acute hand infections are treated with elevation and analgesia. Antibiotic administration should be delayed until microbiological specimens have been obtained, unless there is a strong indication for starting them immediately, such as spreading infection or systemic illness.

Surgical

The decision to operate depends on history, examination, and suspected site of infection. Visible pus or fluctuation in nail-fold infections and subcutaneous abscesses may be obvious, but at other sites severe pain and/or loss of sleep strongly indicate localization and the need for drainage. Suspected septic arthritis and tenosynovitis require urgent drainage. Necrotizing fasciitis is a life-threatening emergency requiring immediate resuscitation and radical excision. Cellulitis needs surgery if an abscess develops or there is skin necrosis requiring excision. Haematogenous osteomyelitis is treated by operation if there is no improvement in 24h, and osteomyelitis due to compound fractures or extension of soft tissue infections is drained and debrided along with the primary lesion.

Surgical drainage should be performed in an operating theatre, under tourniquet control but without forced exsanguination. Incisions for localized infections at different sites should conform to general principles of hand incisions. Wounds should be left open or drained, and a planned wound inspection at 48h is recommended. If infection is severe, or the symptoms do not improve after initial treatment, earlier wound inspection and further exploration is indicated.

Postoperative care

Antibiotics should be started intravenously, the choice depending on likely pathogens, and local sensitivity patterns in consultation with microbiology colleagues. In most cases the choice should cover *Staphylococcus aureus*, beta haemolytic *Streptococcus*, and anaerobes. *Eikenella corrodens* and *Pasteurella multocida* are both usually sensitive to penicillins. Initial antibiotic treatment should be reviewed depending on clinical response and the results of microbiological investigation.

Hands should be splinted in the position of safe immobilization until acute inflammation is subsiding. Active mobilization should then be started, with resting splintage during the intervening periods and at night. As swelling diminishes, passive mobilization should be introduced with increasing active use and decreasing periods of splintage.

Outcomes

The outcome of a hand infection treated early and adequately should be a normal hand. Stiffness is the commonest complication (10–30%), and late or inadequate treatment can lead to irreversible damage to the tissues involved, spread to other tissues (including systemic and metastatic sepsis), and chronic infection both with the primarily infecting agent and other secondary organisms.

Complications

Cellulitis and pulp infections can cause skin and fat necrosis with exposure of deeper structures, especially extensor tendons, loss of pulp padding over distal phalanges, and osteomyelitis. Paronychia can lead to nail deformity, and sometimes chronic infection, often a secondary fungal infection. Tenosynovitis can cause scarring and adhesions between sheath and tendons, with loss of mobility, necrosis of the flexor tendons, extension into adjacent bone and joints, and more proximally into the deep spaces of the palm and wrist. Septic arthritis can result in secondary osteoarthritis or fusion. Septic PIP joint arthritis may lead to a septic boutonniere deformity caused by rupture of the dorsal capsule and destruction of the central extensor tendon slip. Osteomyelitis can lead to loss of bone and skeletal collapse.

Principles of management of open injuries

Background

Open hand injuries can present one of the most challenging problems to the reconstructive hand surgeon. Severe soft tissue injuries complicate the management of underlying fractures, and carry a worse functional prognosis. Adherence to the principles outlined in Box 12.24.3 will help to optimize long-term functional outcomes after these potentially devastating injuries.

Reconstructive techniques used for gaining soft tissue coverage have traditionally been conceptualized as a 'reconstructive ladder', whereby each rung of the ladder represents a more complex reconstruction, and the surgeon chooses the simplest possible reconstructive option. More recently, the concept of the 'reconstructive toolbox' has become more widely accepted, whereby not the simplest, but the *most appropriate* option from a toolbox of reconstructive techniques is applied to a particular clinical problem. This concept is particularly important in dealing with severe open hand injuries, where stable vascularized soft tissue coverage is vital to allow early mobilization and functional rehabilitation.

Importance

The incidence of all open hand, wrist and forearm injuries has been calculated as 966 per 100 000 person-years in a population-based study in Norway. Males were affected over twice as commonly as females, and this bias was more evident in more severe injuries. Furthermore, open fractures constituted 37.9% of hand fractures presenting to a hand surgery service in Hong Kong over a 10-year period.

Causes

The history indicates the type and degree of damage to both soft tissues and skeleton. Common injury mechanisms vary with geography, work and social factors. Industrial injuries commonly involve crushing and shearing forces, while domestic injuries are more frequently due to sharp cuts.

Box 12.24.3 Principles of management of open injuries

- Treat life-threatening injuries—ATLS®
- Aggressive early treatment allows functional rehabilitation
- Excise non-viable tissue
- Stabilize bony elements
- Early definitive soft tissue cover
- Total reconstruction may not be appropriate
- Soft tissue management takes precedence.

Clinical features

History

- Time, place, and mechanism of injury
- Determine functional needs and goals of patient—age, handedness, occupation, hobbies
- General medical history
- Smoking, and use of drugs.

Examination

- ATLS® principles, assess hand as part of secondary survey
- Vascularity
- Bony injury
- Musculotendinous integrity—examination may be compromised by bony injury
- Nerve injury—sensory, motor, autonomic.

Investigations

Plain radiographs in two planes, guided by the results of clinical examination, will demonstrate bony injuries. Occasionally, special views will be required in order to diagnose specific injuries. Laboratory studies as dictated by the clinical condition of the patient should be obtained.

Classification

We favour the classification described in Table 12.24.4, though other similar classifications have been described.

Treatment

Planning

The ultimate goals of reconstruction in relation to the individual patient should be determined in order to formulate a reconstructive surgical plan. For some patients, early amputation is the most appropriate reconstruction, allowing early functional rehabilitation, and early return to work.

Non-surgical

A rapid initial assessment and resuscitation following the principles of ATLS® should be undertaken. Wounds should be irrigated, and dressed with a non-adherent layer and saline-soaked gauze in order to prevent desiccation of the wound. If there is no suspicion of a vascular injury or compartment syndrome, the limb should be elevated. The open hand injury should receive the same tetanus and antibiotic coverage that any open fracture would receive.

Surgical

Wound excision

Wound excision is initiated at the skin surface and carried towards the depths of the wound. Any non-viable or grossly contaminated tissues should be excised. Marginally vascularized tissue, especially muscle, should be excised. Particular attention should be paid to

Table 12.24.4 Classification of open hand injuries[a]

Grade	Clinical features	Management
1	Clean wound <1cm	Excise and suture. Immediate bony fixation
2	Clean wound >1cm, no periosteal stripping, soft tissue envelope intact, low-velocity injury	Excise wound. Primary or delayed primary closure if possible. Early bony fixation
3	Contaminated wound, comminuted fracture, significant periosteal stripping, high-velocity gunshot wound, farm injury, blast injury	Excise wound (repeated if required). Stabilize skeleton. Vascularized soft tissue coverage (reconstructive toolbox). Early functional rehabilitation

[a]From Gonzalez et al. (1999)

the intrinsic muscles of the hand, as necrosis and subsequent fibrosis can lead to significant functional impairment. Critical structures, such as vessels, nerves and tendons should be retained. Any bone fragments which are maintained on a soft-tissue pedicle should be retained if not grossly contaminated. Any extensive wound in the palm should be extended to decompress the carpal tunnel. This extension not only prevents the development of acute carpal tunnel syndrome, but allows a reference to the planes of the palm.

Primary excision is undertaken under loupe magnification with the limb exsanguinated and tourniquet inflated. Secondary excision is carried out immediately afterwards with the tourniquet deflated to further trim any remaining devitalized tissue. Special attention should be paid to the soft tissue envelope after release of the tourniquet. Any parts which are to be amputated during the initial excision should be assessed for use as 'spare parts' in primary reconstruction, for example, a fillet flap may provide vascularized soft tissue coverage; a digit may provide bone graft.

After excision, the wound should be thoroughly irrigated with normal saline. If soft tissue reconstruction cannot be immediately performed, or if doubts remain as to the viability of some tissues, a 'second look' procedure at 24–48h should be undertaken. Subsequent skeletal stabilization and soft tissue reconstruction should be undertaken at the time of definitive soft tissue coverage.

Skeletal stabilization

The initial reconstructive step is skeletal stabilization. The most important consideration for skeletal reconstruction in the hand is obtaining stability. A stable bone base allows early rehabilitation, and a lack of rigid fixation is associated with a worse outcome. Anatomical length maintains the extrinsic and intrinsic relationships necessary for function. The particular form of stabilization undertaken depends on the precise fracture pattern. Segmental bone gaps can be primarily reconstructed with corticocancellous bone grafts.

Soft tissue reconstruction

Next, tendons should be trimmed and repaired using standard core and epitendinous suture techniques (Chapters 12.22 and 12.23). The A2 and A4 pulleys should also be repaired or reconstructed. If primary repair is not possible, silicone rods can be placed and a second stage reconstruction subsequently performed. The next procedure is vascular reconstruction, which is discussed in Chapter 12.27. Nerve reconstruction is undertaken next. Crushed nerve should be excised back to healthy fascicles, and the nerve repaired using an epineural technique under the operating microscope. If there is a nerve gap, conduits (reversed vein, muscle) or nerve graft—often harvested from amputated parts—can be utilized.

Definitive soft tissue coverage

Finally, vascularized soft tissue coverage should be obtained. The range of options available is large (Table 12.24.5), but some basic principles emerge:

- Skin grafts (full or partial thickness) can be used on vascularized beds, especially in non-critical areas
- Exposed tendon, nerve, bone, ligament, or joint requires flap coverage
- Flaps may be local, regional, or distant; pedicled or free. They may utilize an entire vascular pedicle, or be raised on a perforator.

Postoperative care

The hand should be elevated and splinted in the position of safe immobilization. A well-planned therapy regimen should be instituted in order to achieve maximal functional rehabilitation. The use of custom made thermoplastic splints from a few days postoperatively facilitates wound care and therapy. Skin grafts require immobilization for 5 days to prevent shear and allow adequate take, but otherwise skeletal fixation and soft tissue repair should be stable enough to allow early active motion. Desensitization therapy should also be started early following nerve repair.

Table 12.24.5 Commonly used flaps for soft tissue coverage of complex hand wounds

Area to be covered	Flap options
Digits	Step advancement, cross-finger, reversed cross-finger, flag flap, thenar, neurovascular island, groin
Thumb	Moberg, cross finger, Foucher, groin
Dorsum	Reverse radial forearm, ulnar forearm, Becker, posterior interosseous artery, groin, lateral arm
Palm	Reverse radial forearm, ulnar forearm, Becker, groin
Forearm	Groin, gracillis, latissimus dorsi, lateral arm, anterolateral thigh
Elbow	Lateral arm, brachioradialis, latissimus dorsi, radial forearm

Outcomes

The final outcome after treatment of open hand injuries depends on the extent of the injury, the surgical management, and the postoperative rehabilitation. This rehabilitation includes psychological and social support. Open fractures of the fingers and thumb have a significantly worse outcome than closed fractures. In the fingers, 46.6% of open fractures and 80.7% closed fractures have been reported as having a good or excellent outcome. For the thumb, the equivalent figures were 78.8% and 97.8%.

Complications

The complications of open injuries depend on the tissues injured. Failure to recognize the true zone of injury and perform adequate wound excision can lead to infection, sepsis, and even death. Skeletal fixation can result in non-union, malunion, or osteomyelitis. Joint contractures and stiffness can occur. Tendon repairs may rupture, or become adherent to scar tissue. Vascular repairs may thrombose. Nerve injury often leads to cold intolerance, hypersensitivity, and painful neuromas may form, in addition to incomplete sensory and motor recovery. Scars may become hypertrophic, and soft tissue ulceration may be problematic. Secondary procedures to address these complications include osteotomies, joint replacement, nerve grafting, sensory reconstruction, tendon transfers, tenolysis, arthrolysis, and contracture release.

Summary

Soft tissue hand injuries comprise a wide variety of pathologies. All share a common theme, in that optimization of outcome depends on early diagnosis and timely, adequate treatment. Non-surgical management, especially splintage and therapy, is a crucial component of a successful outcome, and a team approach is necessary. Even with optimal treatment, long-term results following some injuries are suboptimal, and mechanisms to rehabilitate the patient into society, work and leisure are important.

Further reading

Gunther, S.F. and Gunther, S.B. (1998). Diabetic hand infections. *Hand Clinics*, **14**, 647–56.

Luce, E.A. (2000). The acute and subacute management of the burned hand. *Clinics in Plastic Surgery*, **27**, 49–63.

Ortiz, J.A., Jr. and Berger, R.A. (1998). Compartment syndrome of the hand and wrist. *Hand Clinics*, **14**, 405–18.

Neumeister, M.W. and Brown, R.E. (2003). Mutilating hand injuries: principles and management. *Hand Clinics*, **19**, 1–15.

Wong, T.C., Ip, F.K., and Wu, W.C. (2005). High-pressure injection injuries of the hand in a Chinese population. *Journal of Hand Surgery*, **30B**, 588–92.

12.25

Nerve injuries

Grey Giddins

Summary points

- Nerve injuries are common
- The history is usually clear but the examination may be less so
- Neurophysiology is only useful after 3 weeks
- Imaging is of limited value as yet
- Treatment is removal of the cause/repair as appropriate
- Recovery is dependent upon many factors especially patient age, severity of the injury, how proximal the injury is and the type of nerve
- Post operative therapy is crucial
- Late reconstruction is primarily for motor function.

Introduction

Nerve injuries are common. They may occur simply such as a laceration of the finger, dividing a digital nerve, or may be part of a more complex picture such as a brachial plexus injury in a polytraumatized patient. The consequences of the injury are dictated by the likely recovery and the functional distribution of the nerve.

Incidence

The incidence of nerve injuries is not recorded. However, there are certain situations where there should be a very high suspicion that a nerve injury has occurred, such as dysfunction in the structures innervated by that nerve following an open injury, including a surgical wound. Certain orthopaedic injuries are commonly associated with nerve trauma, particularly shoulder dislocation, humeral shaft fractures, and supracondylar fracture of the humerus in the upper limb, and dislocations of the hip or knee and trauma around the fibula head in the lower limb.

Classification (Box 12.25.1)

The main classifications in use are those of Seddon (1942) and Sunderland (1978).

Seddon (1942) described three lesions: neurapraxia, axonotmesis, and neurotmesis.

Neurapraxia is a block to the conduction of electrical impulses without disruption of the nerve itself. It is essentially a physiological rather than an anatomic disruption, and thus secondary (Wallerian) degeneration does not occur. Typically, it is due to a blow, such as by bone fragments at the time of fracture, or short-term compression, such as by a tourniquet or plaster cast. The prognosis is excellent if the cause is removed. Typically, recovery is full, beginning within days and usually complete by 6 weeks.

Axonotmesis is a disruption of the axon itself but not of surrounding nerve tissue. It is usually caused by a more severe blow to the nerve, typically in a closed injury. Initially there is Wallerian degeneration proximally to the next proximal node of Ranvier and distally for the whole length of the distal axon. After about 10 days the distal end of the proximal axon starts to grow down its myelin sheath. Subsequently recovery occurs at a rate of about 1mm/day. Again, the prognosis is good if the cause is removed. However, recovery may not be full if there is fibrosis at the injury site, shrinkage of the nerve sheath distally, and/or end-organ degeneration. The further the distance from the site of injury to the site of recovery the less reliable the recovery.

Neurotmesis is a division of the axon and nerve sheath, typically following an open injury although it can occur with traction injuries such as to the brachial plexus. Any nerve palsy following an open wound must be assumed to be neurotmesis until proven otherwise. Wallerian degeneration will occur. Without surgery there is little hope of any nerve recovery. Even following expert surgical repair, recovery is rarely complete.

Sunderland (1978) classified nerve injuries into five subgroups on an anatomical basis. These are graded I–V: grade I is equivalent

Box 12.25.1 Nerve injuries

- Common
- Three types:
  - Neurapraxia (physiological disruption only)
  - Axonotmesis (disruption of axons)
  - Neurotmesis (disruption of nerves).

to neurapraxia, grade II is equivalent to axonotmesis, and grades III–V represent differing degrees of neurotmesis.

Each system has its advocates and neither is perfect.

Associated pathology

Various pathologies are associated with nerve injury and each has particular features depending on the site and type of injury, e.g. open digital nerve injuries are typically associated with injury to the contiguous digital artery. The main structures that can be injured in association are skin and soft tissue, blood vessels, bone, and spinal cord.

- *Skin and soft tissue:* contaminated wounds with soft tissue injury may lead to infection and a poor environment for nerve healing
- *Vascular injuries* the repair of a major blood vessel will be a priority
- *Bone* fractures can cause any grade of nerve injury from neurapraxia to neurotmesis. Stabilization of the fracture by a plaster cast or operatively by internal or external fixation is important to provide a stable environment for the nerve to recover
- *Spinal cord injuries* are associated with traction injuries, typically to the brachial plexus and rarely to the sacral plexus. As nerve roots are avulsed these become essentially an irreparable lesion, and there will be injury to the spinal cord with consequences in terms of both pain and dysfunction distally.

Clinical evaluation (Box 12.25.2)

The general features of clinical evaluation are described, with those specifically related to each nerve being referred to in detail subsequently.

History

The history is often clear cut. Important details to elicit are whether the wound is open or closed, the level of injury involved, and the time delay. A nerve injury associated with an open wound should always be assumed to be a neurotmesis until proven otherwise, typically at surgery. Low-energy closed injuries are associated with neurapraxia, and high-energy injuries are associated with axonotmesis and even nerve rupture. The time from injury is important, as this will also give guidance to the severity of the injury to the nerve and the appropriate treatment.

Box 12.25.2 Assessment of nerve injuries

- History:
  - Mechanism
  - Time from injury
- Examination:
  - Motor function
  - Sensory function
  - Autonomic function
- Investigation:
  - Neurophysiology (after 3 weeks)
  - MRI scan.

Examination

Examination for any nerve injury should look at motor function, sensory function, and autonomic function. With neurapraxia the dysfunction may be partial, but with axonotmesis or neurotmesis it will be complete. Autonomic dysfunction is the one truly objective sign in the early phases. Thus absence of sweating in the distribution of the nerve can only be associated with significant dysfunction, typically neurotmesis or axonotmesis. If there is doubt at initial clinical examination, the patient can be reviewed within 48h. Obviously, this presumes that there are no other major injuries dictating against this course of action.

The examination needs to be detailed and well documented. Pain can confuse the examination. Ideally, muscle function should be isolated and tested specifically. Sensory testing should be with light touch, pinprick, and two-point discrimination, if there is doubt.

Investigations

Investigation of the nerve injury

The main modalities for investigating nerve injuries are neurophysiology and magnetic resonance imaging (MRI) scanning.

Neurophysiology

Neurophysiology relies upon the secondary changes associated with Wallerian degeneration, particularly spontaneous muscular activity which shows as fibrillation potentials. This occurs from about 3 weeks after injury. Prior to this, neurophysiology has a limited role. Thus neurophysiology is mainly used about 6–8 weeks postinjury to assess nerves whose initial recovery was anticipated to be good but where this has not necessarily been the case. A typical example would be radial nerve dysfunction following a humeral shaft fracture which was believed to be either neurapraxia or axonotmesis from which a good recovery was anticipated, but at 6 weeks there had been little recovery. There seems to be no useful role for neurophysiology in assessment of acute injuries.

MRI scanning

In theory, MRI scanning will provide images of nerves and delineate their degree of disruption. At present this has not been achieved, although research is continuing.

Imaging of associated injuries

Bone

Plain radiographs usually suffice to delineate underlying fractures. If there is gross disruption of fracture fragments, this suggests a high-energy injury often associated with more severe nerve injuries.

Vascular injuries

If there is a doubt about vascular function, arteriography should be performed but not at risk of delaying exploration and repair of a major arterial injury.

Spinal cord injury

Spinal cord injuries can be imaged by MRI scanning, but the interpretation of these is difficult acutely.

Management (Box 12.25.3)

Management can be divided into initial management, conservative measures, operative repair, and secondary reconstruction.

Initial management

With closed injuries the limb should be rested, preventing further damage to the nerve. Associated fractures should be stabilized appropriately. With open injuries the wounds should be cleaned and dressed and preferably not reinspected too often as this leads to increased contamination. An alternative is to suture the wound under local anaesthetic without tension and await formal early surgical exploration as appropriate. With contaminated wounds debridement within 6h is considered essential with cover from appropriate antibiotics to minimize the risk of infection.

Conservative measures

Conservative measures are designed to provide an optimal environment for nerve recovery. This is also true following surgical repair. The two main modalities to address are motor and sensory dysfunction.

For motor dysfunction it is important to have a programme of physiotherapy and splintage to ensure that the muscle–tendon complexes continue to have good passive excursion and that joints also go through a full passive range of motion. This should ensure that whatever motor function does recover will work optimally. Splints such as those for radial nerve palsies may also allow continuing use of the arm.

The main concerns over sensory dysfunction are the risk of injury in anaesthetic areas and working on desensitization and retraining exercises as nerve function recovers. Thus patients are instructed in protection of anaesthetic areas and advised that, if injured, the wound should be covered as they often heal more slowly. Desensitization needs to be performed by the patient supervised by a hand therapist.

Nerve surgery

Surgery on nerves is best performed early, i.e. within 10 days of injury. Many series have shown that a delay in treatment causes a worsening of the prognosis, and in certain injuries, such as those to the brachial plexus, surgery becomes much more difficult once extensive local fibrosis has occurred. However, emergency nerve repair is not necessary; rather surgery is better performed by an experienced surgeon within several days rather than acutely by an inexperienced surgeon. At operation the nerve should be inspected: if it is found to be intact, it can simply be left, and the wound cleaned and closed; if the nerve is divided, and the environment is suitable, i.e. the skeletal structures are stabilized and the wounds are clean or cleanable, end-to-end repair should be performed using magnification. If there is doubt as to the cleanliness of the wounds, guided by the Rank–Wakefield classification, nerve repair should be delayed until asepsis can be guaranteed.

At nerve repair it is important to line up the nerves accurately either by inspecting the nerve bundles or by using external markings such as longitudinal blood vessels. Multiple sutures are applied, allowing good apposition without tension and preventing bulging of nerve fascicles. Typically 6.0 monofilament nylon sutures will be used for sciatic nerve injuries, 8.0 for median and ulnar nerve injuries in the forearm, and 10.0 for digital nerve injury. Any contiguous artery of size, i.e. any in the upper limb proximal to the wrist or in the lower limb proximal to the ankle, should be repaired even if the viability of the limb does not depend on this. It has been shown that the results of nerve injury are improved by repairing the neighbouring artery, presumably because of the increased blood supply locally but perhaps simply because of local splintage.

Where there has been extensive injury to the nerve or delay preventing a tension-free repair, nerve grafting should be performed. Classically, this is performed with nerve grafts from 'expendable peripheral nerves' such as the medial cutaneous nerve of the arm or the medial cutaneous nerve of the forearm in the upper limb, or the sural nerve in the lower limb. The nerve is cut to appropriate lengths, glued together with a fibrin glue, and sutured end-to-end to the nerve stumps after they have been trimmed back to healthy nerve ends. This provides a conduit down which the nerves can recover. Extensive work during the 1980s showed that freeze–thaw muscle grafts can also provide a suitable conduit over short distances (i.e. up to 5cm). This avoids sacrificing other peripheral nerves. However, they have largely fallen out of favour. Primary suture gives better results, and even with small gaps is preferable to grafting not least as the latter has to cross two anastomosis sites. Moreover, the results with long grafts (i.e. over 5–10cm) are not good, particularly if there is a poor vascular bed.

Recent laboratory and clinical studies have shown that bridging nerve gaps with a silicone tube, leaving a gap of 3–5mm between the nerve ends, gives comparable results to primary repair.

At the end of the operation, meticulous haemostasis must be achieved to prevent haematoma formation. The limb is splinted to prevent any tension on the nerve for 6 weeks whilst it is recovering except for digital nerve injuries where early mobilization gives better results. During this period and thereafter appropriate conservative measures must be instituted to optimize end-organ function.

Box 12.25.3 Management of nerve injuries

- Rest
- Debride contaminated wounds within 6h
- Physiotherapy to maintain range of motion
- Splints (e.g. for radial nerve palsy)
- Surgery:
  - Repair nerves within 10 days
  - Delayed repair for contaminated wounds
  - Line up nerve
  - Multiple small sutures
  - Repair contiguous major artery
  - Nerve graft for defect in nerve
  - Secondary surgery within 12–18 months.

Secondary surgery

Where a nerve repair has failed or recovery has been incomplete it may be appropriate to re-explore and graft the nerve. This can be of value for up to 6 months and sometimes up to 1 year following injury, but rarely thereafter. This is because of a combination of shrinkage and fibrosis in the distal nerve trunk, failure of the end-organs, particularly the motor endplates, progressive and irreversible changes in the central nervous system with loss of the parent motor neuron, changes within the receptor fields of sensory neurons, and, if therapy has not been adequate, distal secondary stiffness. At this point reconstructive surgery should be considered rather than further nerve surgery. This can address motor and sensory function.

It is difficult to improve *sensory function,* although for limited areas, such as the distribution of an important digital nerve (e.g. to the ulnar pulp of the thumb), innervated skin from another area can be transferred as in the Littler transfer or Foucher's modification. This will require some re-education, and although function will not return to normal it may be improved. This procedure is only infrequently performed and is very rarely indicated for more proximal lesions.

Motor function is the mainstay of secondary reconstructive surgery following nerve injury.

Pain

The treatment of pain following nerve injuries is difficult, particularly proximally involving the spinal cord, as with brachial plexus injuries (see later). For peripheral nerves it may occur with terminal sensory nerves such as digital nerves and the superficial branches of the radial nerve. The pain is typically localized to the distribution of the nerve, with burning pain and hypersensitivity. There is usually a neuroma at the site of nerve injury which is very sensitive. These can be extremely difficult to treat.

Prevention of pain by avoiding damage to nerves is best. If the nerve is damaged, primary repair should effect some restoration in nerve function which should prevent/minimize hypersensitivity and pain. Adequate postoperative analgesia and desensitization exercises also help. If pain is established, desensitization exercises and simple measures such as transcutaneous electrical nerve stimulation should be tried first. If these fail, nerve-suppressant medication such as amitryptyline, or gabapentin in increasing doses may help. If the pain is sympathetically mediated guanethidine or steroid and local anaesthetic blocks, may help but are becoming less common. Sometimes surgery is necessary, which aims at either burial of the neuroma in a less sensitive site, such as deep in a muscle or bone, or restoration of continuity in the nerve which appears to give better results. This can be performed with a nerve graft, although obviously the concern here is that one painful nerve site will be replaced by another. Cryotherapy to the injured nerve may help the pain and hypersensitivity but usually at the expense of some further loss of sensibility.

Results

The results of nerve surgery are very variable. However, grading is well classified according to the Medical Research Council (MRC) grading of 1954 and its 1975 modification (Table 12.25.1). It is important to note that, although this grading is quite sensitive when there is very little function, such as only a flicker of motor function, it gives only a crude indication of the loss of the first 50–70% of function. In the section on motor function a plus sign can be added to M4 to indicate some improved function, but this should not be used elsewhere in the grading.

Table 12.25.1 MRC grading of nerve surgery results

	Motor		Sensory
MO	No activity	SO	No sensation
M1	A flicker of muscle contraction	S1	Deep pain sensation only
M2	Muscle contraction enough to give movement without the effect of gravity	S2	Some superficial pain and touch felt
		S3	Superficial pain and touch felt throughout the nerve distribution with absence of hypersensitivity
M3	Muscle contraction enough to overcome gravity	S3+	As for S3 with some two-point discrimination
M4	Good but reduced strength	S4	Complete recovery
M5	Full strength		

Factors affecting nerve recovery (Box 12.25.4)

- *Age* The results of nerve repair decrease with age from as young as 10 years upwards
- *Nature of the injury* Recovery will be better in clean injuries than in extensive injuries such as closed traction injuries or where there is gross soft tissue loss. The results in gunshot wounds are particularly poor, with only 40% of patients having any return of function
- *Level of injury* The more proximal the injury, the less good is the recovery. This represents a number of factors including a decay in the quality of nerve recovery distally with time and particularly

Box 12.25.4 Results of nerve surgery

- Better prognosis:
  - Young patient
  - Clean injury
  - Distal
  - Large muscle group
  - No defect
  - Early repair
- Worse prognosis:
  - Older patient
  - Contaminated injury
  - Proximal
  - Small muscle group
  - Large defect
  - Delayed repair.

distal end-organ failure, as nerve recovery may take up to 2 years to reach end-organs such as the hand or foot. Recovery is rarely complete with distal injuries, however, and digital nerve repair in adults never gives normal sensibility

- *Type of nerve* Motor nerves to large muscle groups not requiring fine control have a good prognosis, whereas motor nerves supplying small muscles in the hand rarely have a good outcome. With pure sensory nerves, there is a significant risk of long-term chronic pain
- *Length of injured nerve* If a large segment of nerve has been injured or there has been a delay leading to nerve retraction and prevention of primary repair, the results of surgery will be less good as the results of nerve grafting are less good
- *Associated injuries* Associated skeletal injuries must be stabilized or the chances of a repair remaining intact are negligible. Significant vascular injuries should also be repaired even if this is not essential for limb viability, as nerve recovery is improved
- *Delay* It has been shown that primary nerve repair is much more successful than delayed repair. Ideally, nerve injuries should be repaired within a few days of injury (a maximum of 10 days), provided that local tissue conditions are favourable
- *Technical skills* It has not been proved that the skill of the surgeon results in improved outcomes. Nonetheless, it is widely believed that better results are achieved by experienced nerve surgeons using magnification than by occasional surgeons.

Complications (Box 12.25.5)

The main complications of nerve surgery are failure of recovery, pain, stiffness, and crossover sensation.

Failure of recovery

If sepsis is present, nerve recovery is very unlikely. It is also unlikely in the presence of ischaemic or hypovascular tissue where nerve repair and particularly nerve grafting are less successful. It can be difficult to decide when to re-examine a nerve following primary repair or grafting. It should normally be obvious within 3 months that there has been some progression of nerve recovery distal to the repair site. This will be indicated by return of function in the local motor or sensory supply and particularly by an advancing Tinel sign. This should be documented and is a very useful assessment of progressing nerve function. If there is a strongly advancing Tinel sign, the prognosis for nerve recovery is good. However, if there is also a Tinel sign at the repair site, this is less optimistic, and a strong Tinel sign at the repair site with none distally is a poor prognostic feature. Neurophysiological assessment may be able to indicate whether there has been nerve growth across the repair site. The main assessment of failure is clinical. If there is doubt, then re-exploration and revision nerve grafting should be undertaken. Nerve grafting is almost always required at revision surgery. It is unclear how many times nerve grafting can be undertaken following failure. However, if there is no recovery after two attempts, further success is unlikely. Again, the likelihood of successful nerve grafting after 12 months is minimal except in treating pain.

Box 12.25.5 Complications of nerve surgery

- Failure to recover
- Pain
- Stiffness
- Sensory crossover.

Pain

Pain is a significant problem as a complication of nerve injury and failure of recovery and was discussed earlier.

Stiffness

Stiffness is essentially a failure of therapy in the postinjury period although some stiffness will inevitably follow major nerve injuries. It is very debilitating as it will reduce the benefit from any motor recovery.

Crossover

Trophic nerve factors from the distal nerve stump will attract sensory and motor nerves from the proximal stump to the appropriate sensory and motor tubules distally. However, there will be crossover with motor nerves destined for one muscle going to another, and motor and sensory crossover. This reduces the efficacy of nerve recovery and can lead to problems of re-learning, particularly if there is sensory crossover. This can be reduced by retraining and is less of a problem in young patients who have greater cerebral plasticity.

Individual nerves

Upper-limb nerve injuries

Accessory nerve (Box 12.25.6)

The accessory nerve is particularly prone to injury by surgeons at biopsy of masses in the posterior triangle. The motor loss is to the trapezius with no significant sensory loss. However, there is often a significant problem with pain. The diagnosis should be obvious on the principle of nerve dysfunction in the line of an open wound although, sadly, referral and repair are often delayed especially following iatrogenic injuries.

Nerve grafting is almost always required. Good recovery in the nerves occurs in 80–90% of operations performed within 3 months, with no useful recovery after 1 year. If nerve repair has failed or not been attempted, pain may be a problem. Treatment of this is extremely difficult. If nerve repair fails, the scapula may be supported by a sling or transfer of levator scapulae and rhomboids. This may improve function but does not generally improve pain.

Box 12.25.6 Accessory nerve

- Posterior triangle surgery
- Usually requires nerve graft
- 80–90% success with surgery.

Box 12.25.7 Long thoracic nerve

- Iatrogenic/brachial plexus injury
- Nerve repair or muscle transfer.

Long thoracic nerve (Box 12.25.7)

The long thoracic nerve is typically injured in association with brachial plexus injuries (see later). The next most common cause is iatrogenic, at the time of axillary clearance. The motor dysfunction is paralysis of the serratus anterior causing loss of control of the scapula and disturbance of thoracoscapular movements. There is no sensory loss, but there is often a dull aching pain following injury. There are no reported series of repair of the long thoracic nerve, although sporadic cases show some value. If primary repair is not possible, local nerve transfer may be of value. If nerve surgery fails, muscle transfer of the pectoralis major or pectoralis minor to the lower part of the scapula improves thoracoscapular movement and diminishes pain.

Axillary nerve (Box 12.25.8)

The common causes of axillary nerve injuries are, again, brachial plexus injuries (see later), dislocations and fracture dislocations at the shoulder, and open wounds, particularly iatrogenic injuries. The motor loss is of deltoid paralysis. Patients with deltoid paralysis can often still achieve a full range of shoulder movement, particularly by using the rotator cuff muscles. Strength is reduced by about 50% in abduction and slightly less in flexion and extension. The area of sensory loss is the 'badge' area on the lateral aspect of the upper arm and is a minimal problem. Pain is not typically a problem.

Open injuries require exploration. Treatment of axillary nerve injuries following shoulder dislocation is less clear cut. Most surgeons wait for 6 weeks, anticipating a neurapraxic lesion and early recovery. If this does not occur, neurophysiological assessment should be performed together with a careful review to exclude a rotator cuff lesion which can present both similarly or in conjunction with an axillary nerve injury. If there is continuing doubt, the axillary nerve should be explored and, where possible, repaired using a nerve graft. This should be within 3 months of injury. The results of early surgery suggest that recovery to M4 or better should occur in about 80% of cases.

Radial nerve (Box 12.25.9)

Radial nerve palsy is one of the most frequent acute major nerve palsies in the upper limb. The most common cause is fracture of the shaft of the humerus with the nerve injured in the spiral groove. In most cases this is a neurapraxic lesion, or at worst an axonotmesis, and good recovery is anticipated. With high-energy injuries the nerve can suffer significant stretching and have an extensive lesion in continuity (see later) or even rupture.

Box 12.25.8 Axillary nerve

- Iatrogenic/brachial plexus injury/shoulder injuries
- Explore/repair open injuries
- Closed injury recovery usually by 6 weeks.

Box 12.25.9 Radial nerve

- Common
- Humeral fracture (80% recover within 6 weeks)
- Nerve repair success 80%
- Tendon transfers work well.

The motor loss is to the extensors of the wrist and hand, giving a classic wrist-drop posture. Sensory loss is in the dorsum of the first web space and is of little significance. Pain from these injuries is rare, in contrast with more distal radial nerve injuries.

The natural history of most radial nerve injuries following humeral fractures is recovery. Radial nerve palsy was reported in 57 of 765 fractures of the humerus (an incidence of 7.4%) of which 47 (82.5%) underwent full spontaneous recovery.

For low-energy injuries the wrist and hand should be mobilized with static or dynamic splintage. If there is no evidence of recovery at 6 weeks, neurophysiological assessment should be undertaken. If there is continuing doubt, open exploration should be performed. Whenever the fracture is opened primarily, the radial nerve should be inspected and repaired if ruptured. In all cases of high-energy injury there should be a high suspicion of a significant nerve injury and consideration should be given to early exploration.

A number of surgeons have reported on the results of radial nerve repair, particularly of military injuries which tend to be worse than civilian injuries. In civilian experience about 80% of repairs achieve M4 recovery or better distally. If nerve repair fails, tendon transfers give an excellent result. It is usual to wait for at least 18 months after nerve repair to see if there is any recovery in motor function, but such is the excellence of flexor–extensor transfers for radial nerve palsies that these may often be undertaken earlier.

Musculocutaneous nerve (Box 12.25.10)

This nerve is most commonly injured as a result of brachial plexus injuries (see later), and next most commonly via open wounds including iatrogenic injuries. The loss of motor function results in paralysis of the biceps, brachialis, and brachioradialis. The loss of sensation is to the lateral aspect of the proximal forearm and is of minimal consequence. This is primarily a motor nerve and as such does well with 90% of patients recovering at least M4 elbow flexion if repaired within 3 months.

If primary nerve repair fails, intercostal nerve transfer (neurotization) sometimes works well at providing some elbow flexion but the preferred transfer is the Oberlin transfer. A few of the motor fascicles from an intact ulnar nerve are transferred side-to-end to the musculocutaneous nerve. The nerve recovery is over a short distance and has minimal surgical morbidity. If neurotization is either not contemplated or fails, tendon transfer can be performed.

Box 12.25.10 Musculocutaneous nerve

- Brachial plexus injuries/iatrogenic
- Repair/nerve graft usually successful.

Box 12.25.11 Median nerve

- Self-inflicted/accidental lacerations
- Primary repair/nerve grafting better than delayed repair
- Tendon transfers can be used.

This is sometimes required for simple injuries, but is more common following brachial plexus injuries (see later).

Median nerve (Box 12.25.11)

The median nerve is commonly injured via self-inflicted lacerations at the wrist, accidental injury, or secondary to surgery. If the lesion is very proximal in the forearm, the median-supplied forearm flexors will be paralysed, namely the pronator teres, the flexor carpi radialis, all the flexor digitorum superficiales, and classically the profundus tendons to the index and middle fingers. Obviously this gives major dysfunction of the hand, particularly the radial side. More distal injuries would exclude the long flexors, but would include the median-supplied muscles of the thenar eminence which are primarily the abductor pollicis brevis and opponens pollicis, although there may be some ulnar supply to these. The loss of sensation is even more harmful, as it is in the radial three digits and includes the most important areas of the pulp of the thumb and the index and middle fingers. With distal injuries there is often only partial division of the nerve, in which case the loss is less and is variable.

The best results are with primary surgery, although very good results can be obtained from nerve grafting. Wrist injuries are often accompanied by injuries to the flexor tendons which also need to be repaired. If the injuries to the median nerve are within a few centimetres of the carpal canal, it is usual to release the carpal canal to avoid any local compartment problems.

The results of median nerve surgery very much reflect the factors discussed above. In a series of primary and delayed median nerve repairs, better results were achieved with primary repair (Table 12.25.2).

The results of nerve grafting are good; 100% of patients achieve good or fair sensory results and 80% good or fair motor results after median nerve repair. The most important factors for nerve grafting are age, closely followed by gap length, level of injury, and delay. Gap length and delay are of greater significance in sensory recovery than in motor recovery, whereas the level of injury has a greater effect on motor recovery than sensory recovery. This is also true for ulnar nerve grafts (Table 12.25.3).

Full recovery following median nerve injury will not be achieved in children over 10 years of age and adults. However, good functional recovery should be achievable. If there is very poor sensory recovery even after revision surgery, it is unlikely that complex nerve skin transfers would be performed to regain sensation, but this is always a possibility. Most secondary reconstructive procedures are aimed at tendon transfers.

Table 12.25.3 Results of median nerve grafting

					Overall recovery
Motor	M5	M4	M3	<M2	
100 cases	30	38	12	20	80% fair or good
Sensory	S4	S3+	S3	<S2	
104 cases	13	31	37	23	78% fair or good

Data from Frykman and Gramyk (1991).

Box 12.25.12 Ulnar nerve

- Self-inflicted/accidental lacerations
- Primary repair/nerve grafting better than secondary repair
- Tendon transfers/tenodeses sometimes useful.

Ulnar nerve (Box 12.25.12)

The ulnar nerve, like the median nerve, is commonly injured through open wounds, particularly at the wrist, which are either self-inflicted or due to a fall on glass. The sensory loss is less marked than the motor loss, particularly to the small muscles of the hand which tend to recover at best only incompletely, especially in adults.

Again, treatment is primary suture where possible and repair of the ulnar artery. The results of repairs of the ulnar nerve are similar to those of the median nerve and are shown in Table 12.25.4. If primary surgery fails, nerve grafting is worthwhile in most cases and usually gives some benefit (Table 12.25.5).

Clinical picture

Duchenne's sign is clawing of the hand in ulnar nerve injury. If the hyperextension is passively prevented by dorsal pressure over the metacarpophalangeal joints, the extensor tendons can extend the middle and distal phalanges. This is known as Bouvier's manoeuvre. In contrast, an attempt to extend the fingers further by flexing the wrist, in effect providing a tenodesing effect on the extensor tendons, increases rather than decreases the deformity. This is known as the André–Thomas sign. The inability to cross the middle and index fingers over each other due to loss of the interosseus function is known as the Pitres–Testut sign. An inability to

Table 12.25.2 Results of median nerve repair

Grade	Result of primary repair	Result of delayed primary repair
Good	19	5
Fair	7	8
Poor	0	2

Data from Birch and Raji (1991).

Table 12.25.4 Result of ulnar nerve repair

Grade	Results of primary repair	Results of delayed primary repair
Good	26	2
Fair	2	5
Poor	0	5

Data from Birch and Raji (1991).

Table 12.25.5 Results of ulnar nerve grafting

					Overall recovery
Motor	M5	M4	M3	<M2	
93 cases	12	26	23	32	65% good or fair
Sensory	S4	S3+	S3	<S2	
98 cases	13	20	43	22	78% good or fair

Data from Frykman and Gramyk (1991).

adduct the little finger to the ring finger, so that the little finger tends to stay in an abducted position, is known as Wartenberg's sign. Probably the best-known sign is Froment's sign, described in 1915, where an attempt to perform a key pinch between the pulp of the thumb and the side of the middle phalanx of the middle finger results in marked flexion at the thumb interphalangeal joint due to weakness or paralysis of the adductor pollicis and therefore the need to bring the flexor pollicis longus into action to provide strength. The descriptions of the clinical findings are based upon the classical innervation of the ulnar nerve. However, there is considerable variation, with a number of crossover patterns from the ulnar to the median nerve and vice versa. The most common is the Martin–Gruber communication, which occurs in about 17% of forearms (range 5–34%), where there is communication between the median and ulnar nerves in the proximal forearm. There are other rarer communications.

Reconstructive surgery

If nerve surgery has failed, the modalities to be addressed are sensation and motor function. It is rare to perform any surgery to improve sensation in the ulnar-supplied distribution to the hand. The main treatments are tendon transfers.

Digital nerves (Box 12.25.13)

In theory the repair of digital nerves should give excellent results, as these are pure sensory nerves often with only a short recovery distance. Unfortunately this is not the case.

Digital nerves are typically injured by lacerations, often in domestic situations but regrettably also iatrogenically. The concomitant digital artery is generally injured as well but does not normally require repair provided that the finger is viable. There is often associated injury to flexor tendons and even bone, and obviously these need appropriate primary treatment.

Repairs are performed using a microscope with fine sutures such as 10.0 nylon. Unlike for most repairs the results are better following early mobilization, primarily due to less stiffness. In children, full recovery can occur. In adults, even though normal two-point discrimination can be achieved, no patient achieves full recovery of sensation in the digit. Moreover, even if the nerve is not repaired there is often considerable recovery due to crossover sensation from the contralateral digital nerves. This does not indicate that digital nerve repair should not be performed, as a good recovery will improve function and reduce the risk of a painful neuroma at the injury site. Typically patients with injuries to the radial digital nerve to the index finger will bypass to the middle finger for fine sensibility.

Box 12.25.13 Digital nerves

- Lacerations (domestic and iatrogenic)
- Primary repair of nerve but not artery
- Mobilize early
- Crossover sensation common.

Lower-limb nerve injuries

Nerve injuries in the lower limb are less common than in the upper limb and have been less widely reported. The main reported nerve injuries are to the sciatic and common peroneal nerves. Less frequently nerves of the sacral plexus are injured particularly usually in association with pelvic fractures.

Sacral plexus injury (Box 12.25.14)

The sacral plexus is typically injured at the time of a pelvic fracture, often with fracture of the sacrum. Rarely, it will be injured by an open wound. Pelvic fracture is often associated with other life-threatening injuries, but it is important to try to delineate nerve injuries preoperatively as there is also a significant incidence of perioperative nerve injuries. Sciatic nerve injuries may also occur in these complex fractures and it is important to differentiate the two. The sensory loss following sacral injuries is over a much greater area proximally, and the motor loss will involve the hip flexor and knee extensors and there may be sphincter dysfunction.

Typically the sacral plexus suffers a traction injury like the brachial plexus and at present does not appear to be amenable to surgery, although with clean division successful repair has been performed. In the long term, recovery is at best incomplete and is often associated with pain.

Sciatic nerve (Box 12.25.15)

The sciatic nerve is mainly injured in association with pelvic fractures, and with fractures and dislocations of the hip. Regrettably, it can also be associated with hip replacement surgery. The injuries may be traction or division injuries and occasionally are due to compression. The incidence of pelvic injuries and fracture

Box 12.25.14 Sacral plexus

- Traction injuries usually with fracture
- Surgery rarely indicated
- Recovery often poor.

Box 12.25.15 Sciatic nerve

- Pelvic fractures/hip dislocations/hip replacement
- Severe in children
- Early reduction/stabilization improves results
- Fracture/surgical injuries should be explored early and repaired.

dislocations of the hip is reported at 8–12%, with the greatest risk in those involving injuries to the posterior column. Recovery appears to be improved by early reduction and stabilization of the fractures, with a good result expected in about 40–50% of patients, although the results are poor in at least one-third.

The incidence of nerve injury at hip arthroplasty appears to be about 1% (range 0.6–3.7%) after primary hip replacement, 2–3% after revision arthroplasty, and 6% in patients treated for congenital dislocation of the hip.

The treatment of nerve injuries in association with fractures or hip replacement is early exploration. Division of the nerve, compression of the nerve from a suture, or even a cement burn can occur. Appropriate treatment of these results in a much greater likelihood of good recovery.

The consequences of sciatic nerve injuries in children are particularly severe where there are limb-development problems as well as sensory and motor abnormalities. In particular, functionally significant leg-length discrepancy may occur. The lack of sensibility on a weight-bearing area leads to increased risk of skin breakdown, and the lack of muscle balance leads to risk of contractures.

Tibial and common peroneal nerve injuries (Box 12.25.16)

In the largest series reported on injuries of the sciatic nerve, the nerve was classified into the common peroneal and tibial divisions—345 injuries of the common peroneal nerve and 229 injuries of the tibial nerve were reported, and 145 nerve repairs were performed. One-third of the 72 cases of repair of the common peroneal nerve achieved functional dorsiflexion of the ankle. Eighty per cent of the 47 cases of repair of the tibial nerve regained functional plantar flexion of the foot. Recovery of sensation ranged from S2 to S4 and occurred in about two-thirds of cases. The main fixed deformities were equinus of the heel and clawing of the toes. Trophic ulcers were present in 14%, and pain and hypersensitivity of the foot were major problems in 50%. The discrepancy between function and neurological deficit is greater for the sciatic nerve than for any other nerve injury (Table 12.25.6).

The common peroneal nerve itself is typically injured around the knee, particularly as it winds around the fibula neck where it is both superficial and relatively immobile. It may be injured by local trauma to the knee, with knee surgery, and by open injuries. The most common injury is a rupture. Injury results in lack of anterior and peroneal compartment muscle function. The nerve has less supportive connective tissue and fewer autonomic fibres than the tibial nerve. Hence in traction injuries the motor and sensory nerves bear more of the injury. Open lesions should be repaired primarily and ruptures should be grafted. The results of surgery depend on both the severity of the injury to the nerve and the quality of local soft tissue. The results are generally good with clean simple wounds, but are less good with traction injuries. Delay is a significant problem following traction injuries, and a delay of over 6 months almost always leads to poor results. Early treatment can give significant recovery in about two-thirds of cases, but overall about 50% gain useful ankle dorsiflexion and a little over 50% gain protective sensation.

If there has been no adequate recovery after 1 year, further nerve surgery is probably not of value unless there was considerable doubt over the initial operation. Thereafter tendon transfer should be performed if static splintage is not adequate. The most useful is a tibialis posterior to tibialis anterior transfer which has been widely reported and in most cases gives a significant improvement in function.

Box 12.25.16 Common peroneal nerves

- Common peroneal:
  - Often traction injuries
  - Lacerations recover best with surgery
- 50% success with surgery
- Tendon surgery works well.

Table 12.25.6 Results of tibial and peroneal nerve repairs

	Cases	Surgical repair	Functional muscle action	S2–S4
Tibial	229	45	79% (Plantarflexion)	66%
Peroneal	345	72	35% (Dorsiflexion)	

Contractures present in 30%.
Trophic ulcers present in 14%.
Significant pain and hypersensitivity in 50%.
Data from Seddon (1975).

Iatrogenic nerve injures (Box 12.25.17)

There are four main types of iatrogenic nerve injury: surgical division, injection injuries, irradiation injuries, and compression neuropathy.

Direct surgical injuries are typically lacerations, although occasionally sutures will be placed around nerves or plates put upon nerves. If, following surgery, as for any open wound, there is dysfunction, particularly complete dysfunction in the line of the nerve, this should be explored as a matter of some urgency unless the surgeon identified and preserved the nerve right up to the end of the procedure. Even incomplete nerve dysfunction should be considered for early exploration, especially if there is a risk of partial compression such as around metalwork.

Box 12.25.17 Iatrogenic nerve injuries

- Surgical: explore early
- Injection: early decompression
- Irradiation: prognosis poor
- Tourniquet: usually recover
- Compression:
  - Usually recover
  - Up to 25% do not resolve
  - Consider decompression.

Fortunately, *injection injuries* are rare, and most commonly occur through injections near peripheral nerves in the upper limb now that the risk of sciatic nerve damage caused by buttock injections is well recognized. Any substance injected into a nerve causes an intense fibrotic reaction and early decompression is recommended. This can usually be avoided by checking whether the patient has tingling and pain in the distribution of the local nerve at the time of injection. If this is identified upon insertion of the needle, it can be withdrawn normally with no damage, but if injection continues then permanent damage will almost always occur.

There are two main risks from *irradiation injuries.* The most common is irradiation neuritis with intense fibrotic reaction which can occur many years after the irradiation. Symptoms occur typically 6–8 months after treatment, initially with pins-and-needles and sometimes with progression to severe and intractable pain. Operations rarely seem to improve function, particularly in the region of the brachial plexus where so many of these injuries occur following irradiation for breast carcinoma. There is a limited hope for free vascular grafting to bring in an increased blood supply on the basis that this is an ischaemic injury.

Most iatrogenic *compression neuropathies* are caused by tourniquets or pressure on nerves on the operating table.

Tourniquet neuropathies are infrequent. It is estimated that their incidence is between 1 in 5000 and 1 in 8000 cases. Although neurophysiological studies have shown that nerve abnormalities occur within as short a period as 20min, it appears that 2h is a safe upper limit for the use of a tourniquet in both upper and lower limbs. Although many surgeons have experience of using longer times without problem, this should be the exception and not the rule. Typically these lesions are neurapraxia or axonotmeses and recovery is full, but rare cases of permanent injury have been reported.

The most common perioperative injuries are to the common peroneal nerves in the lithotomy position, the brachial plexus in cardiac surgery, and the ulnar nerve whilst in the supine position. These have previously been felt to be benign lesions, which recover well, but this is not always so and a permanent deficit appears to occur in 5–25% of patients with brachial plexus lesions and 10–27% of patients with common peroneal lesions. Once these patients are identified, they should be assessed with early neurophysiology and if there appears to be a severe lesion consideration should be given to decompression of those sites where it may have occurred, most particularly the ulnar nerve at the elbow.

Further reading

Birch, R.B. and Giddins, G.E.B. (1996). Peripheral nerve injuries. In: Foy, M.A. (ed) *Medicolegal Reporting in Orthopaedic Trauma,* second edition. Edinburgh: Churchill Livingstone.

Frykman, G.K. and Gramyk, K. (1991). Results of nerve surgery. In: Gelberman, R.H. (ed) *Operative Nerve Repair and Reconstruction,* pp. 553–67. J.B. Philadelphia, PA: Lippincott.

Rank, B.K., Wakefield, A.R., and Hueston, J.T. (1973). *Surgery of Repair as Applied to Hand Injuries,* fourth edition. Edinburgh: Churchill Livingstone.

Seddon, H.J. (1942). A classification of nerve injuries. *British Medical Journal,* **ii**, 237–9.

Seddon, H.J. (1975). *Surgical Disorders of the Peripheral Nerves,* second edition. Edinburgh: Churchill Livingstone.

Sunderland, S. (1978). *Nerves and Nerve Injuries,* second edition. Edinburgh: Churchill Livingstone.

Sunderland, S. (1991). Factors influencing the quality of the recovery after nerve repair. In: *Nerve Injuries and their Repair: A Critical Appraisal,* pp. 395–411. Edinburgh: Churchill Livingstone.

12.26

Brachial plexus injuries

Grey Giddins

Summary points

- Serious injury, usually closed
- C5/C6 injuries commonest
- More proximal injuries have best results
- Early treatment leads to better results
- Direct repair if possible
- Arthrodesis or muscle transfer may be useful.

Introduction

Brachial plexus injuries are uncommon but very serious (Box 12.26.1). They may be closed or open, or occur as part of birth trauma. The treatment of these injuries has progressed but in most cases long-term disability persists due to the unpredictability of nerve regeneration. Secondary reconstruction is only of partial benefit. These injuries typically affect young males and they present a major challenge both to medicine and society as a whole.

Aetiology

The majority of brachial plexus injuries are closed, usually as a result of motorcycle accidents. This is demonstrated in Table 12.26.1 which shows experience from a tertiary referral centre in Switzerland. Open injuries occur more commonly in violent societies such as parts of South Africa and the United States of America. A significant percentage are iatrogenic lesions following removal of a lump from the posterior triangle of the neck.

Box 12.26.1 Brachial plexus injury

- Uncommon
- Serious effects
- Usually closed injury.

Table 12.26.1 Aetiology of brachial plexus injuries

	Percentage
Closed	
Road traffic accidents	
Motor cycle or bicycle	52
Cars	12–70
Pedestrians	6
Industrial accidents	7
Falls	10–24
Sports	5
Other	2
Open	
Lacerations	1
Gunshots	2–6
Iatrogenic	3

Data from Narakas (1987).

Incidence

The incidence of brachial plexus injuries is not known. There were estimated to be about 300–350 patients who suffer severe and permanent damage as a result of closed supraclavicular brachial plexus injuries each year in the United Kingdom. Recently the frequency appears to have diminished. There are many other milder lesions of the brachial plexus that recover well. The patients are typically inexperienced motorcyclists under 25 years old.

Anatomy

Normal

The brachial plexus is made up of five nerve roots from C5 to T1, but there is considerable variation and the plexus may be pre- or postfixed, i.e. coming from C4 or from as low as T2. The typical brachial plexus is shown in Figure 12.26.1.

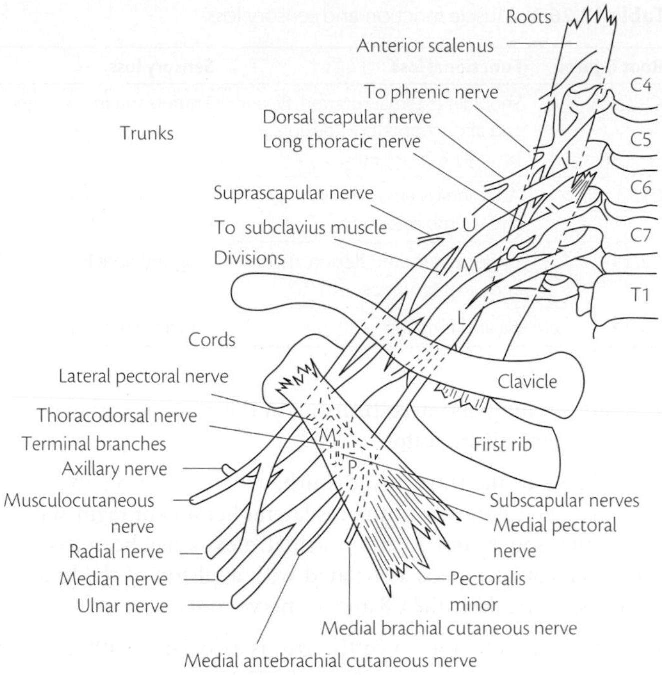

Fig. 12.26.1 The brachial plexus.

Box 12.26.2 Four types of injury

- Neurapraxia—good prognosis
- Rupture—postganglionic can recover
- Lesion in continuity—poor prognosis
- Avulsion:
  - Preganglionic
  - May be treatable surgically.

Pathological (Box 12.26.2)

Four types of injury can occur to the structures of the brachial plexus:

- Neurapraxia
- Rupture or division (neurotmesis)
- Lesion in continuity (a combination of anoxotmesis and neurotmesis)
- Nerve root avulsion.

Neurapraxia

Complete recovery should occur.

Rupture or division

This is a postganglionic lesion, i.e. one distal to the dorsal root ganglion. Therefore it represents a peripheral nerve injury with an opportunity for recovery provided macroscopic continuity is re-established, such as at surgery.

Lesion in continuity

This is also a postganglionic lesion. It represents stretching of a large segment of nerve but without rupture. This should, in theory, be a favourable lesion, but intense peri- and intraneural fibrosis leads to poor results.

Avulsion

This is a preganglionic lesion, i.e. a central lesion often associated with a direct spinal cord injury. Typically both dorsal and ventral roots are avulsed from the spinal cord but one or other alone may be avulsed. Historically this has been an irreparable lesion, but there are now some opportunities for surgical repair (see later). Preganglionic lesions are commonly associated with severe neuralgic pains.

Associated pathology

The main associated injuries are to bone and blood vessels.

Bone injuries

Typically there may be one or more fractures of the head or shaft of the humerus, fracture of the scapula, clavicle, or ribs, or a dislocation of the shoulder. There may also be other limb injuries associated with severe polytrauma.

Blood vessels

Major vascular injury, namely rupture of the subclavian artery, occurs in about 10% of supraclavicular and over 20% of infraclavicular lesions of the brachial plexus. The incidence is even higher in open wounds.

Other injuries

Head, spinal cord, and chest injuries occur in up to 10–15% of severe brachial plexus injuries.

Classification

The purpose of classification of brachial plexus injuries (Table 12.26.2) is to delineate the severity of the lesion. Two questions to be addressed are: Which nerve roots are involved? Are the injuries pre- or postganglionic? These are mainly addressed to closed injuries, as open injuries, typically with knives, are almost always postganglionic divisions of some or all of the brachial plexus.

Clinical evaluation (Box 12.26.3)

The diagnosis of a brachial plexus injury is usually obvious—typically a young traffic accident victim with a flail insensate arm. In some patients, however, the diagnosis may be less clear cut, for example patients after reduction of an anterior dislocation of the shoulder who cannot abduct their shoulder, which may be due to pain, a rotator cuff lesion, or an axillary nerve or infraclavicular plexus injury.

Table 12.26.2 The main patterns of closed supraclavicular injuries of the brachial plexus

Type	Pattern of injury	Incidence (%)
1	Rupture or avulsion of C5 and C6 (C7) with an intact (C7), C8, and T1	35
2	Rupture of C5 and C6 (C7) and avulsion of (C7), C8, and T1	30
3	Avulsion of the whole brachial plexus	20
4	Other—many other variations of injury may occur	15

Box 12.26.3 Clinical signs

- May not be immediately obvious (e.g. head injury)
- Assess motor/sensory function
- Tinel's sign (especially C6 root)
- Bruising along nerve trunks
- Swelling in posterior triangle (poor prognosis)
- Severe pain down arm (avulsion injuries).

Table 12.26.3 Muscle function and sensory loss

Root injured	Functional loss	Sensory loss
C5/C6	Shoulder external rotation, flexion and abduction, elbow flexion, possibly wrist extension	Thumb and index finger
C5/C6/C7	Additionally elbow, wrist, finger, and thumb extension	Additionally the middle finger
C8/T1	Finger and thumb flexion, median and ulnar intrinsics	Ring and little fingers
C5/T1	All arm function	All arm sensation

History

In severe brachial plexus injuries the history is often incomplete, especially from patients who have suffered a concomitant head injury. There will often be a history of high-energy trauma.

Examination

The initial examination will often show a completely flail insensate limb but is often not very specific and is complicated by associated pathology. There may be rapid return of function within 7–10 days after the initial neurapraxia has resolved. Nonetheless with the severe injuries that often require early surgical intervention the picture rapidly becomes clear. Specifically, sensory testing should be done as per the dermatome map (Figure 12.26.2).

Muscle testing should ideally be done for each muscle in the upper limb but there are general patterns which can be recognized (Table 12.26.3).

Certain clinical findings are of particular significance.

- A positive Tinel sign radiating to the hand is indicative of rupture. This is valid at 24h and is especially reliable for the C6 root
- Linear bruising along the course of the nerve trunks in the arm implies rupture of those trunks
- Severe swelling and deep bruising in the posterior triangle is a poor prognostic indicator
- Weakness of the trapezius, disturbance of sensation above the clavicle, and paralysis of the ipsilateral hemidiaphragm suggest that the upper root to the brachial plexus has been avulsed. Horner's syndrome is associated with avulsion of the brachial plexus, particularly the C8 and T1 nerve roots
- Severe pain radiating down the arm is associated with avulsion injuries.

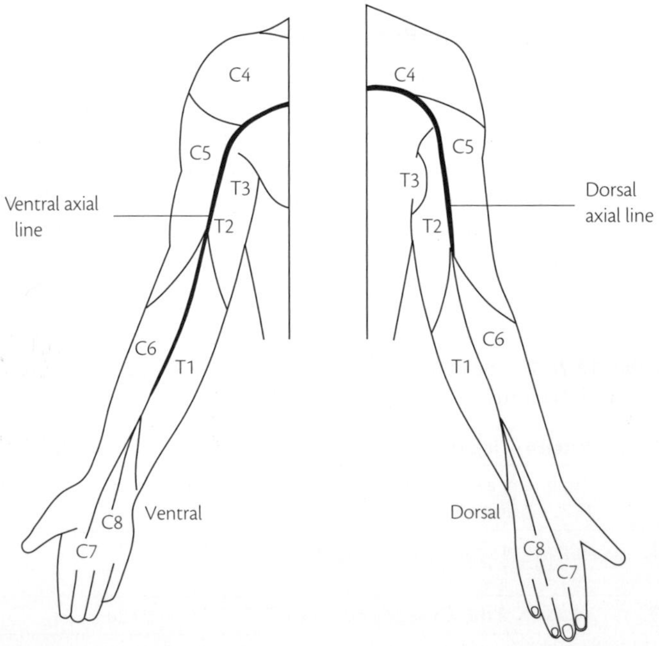

Fig. 12.26.2 Sensory dermatomes.

Investigation (Box 12.26.4)

Investigations can be subdivided into those for the neural injury and those for associated pathology. Obviously patients involved in severe polytrauma will require appropriate blood tests and other investigations.

Neural investigations

Plain radiographs

The key radiographs are those of the chest and cervical spine. Elevation of the ipsilateral hemidiaphragm on the chest radiograph suggests a phrenic nerve injury and possible C5 and C6 nerve root avulsion. Fracture or dislocation of the first rib or fracture of the transverse process of the seventh cervical vertebra are associated with C8 and T1 root avulsions. On the anteroposterior radiograph the cervical spine may be abducted away from the site of injury suggesting root avulsion.

Imaging of the cervical spinal cord

Myelography, computed tomography (CT) scanning with enhancement, and magnetic resonance imaging (MRI) scanning are all of

Box 12.26.4 Investigations

- Chest radiograph—diaphragmatic elevation/transverse process/rib fracture, neck abduction
- Neurophysiology has little acute role
- MRI scan may become valuable
- Consider:
  - Plain radiograph for skeletal injuries
  - Vascular studies
  - CT scan for head injury.

value but have significant false-positive and false-negative rates and so are not yet regularly used. Ultimately, however, MRI scanning to look at both the spinal cord and the brachial plexus may be of value.

Neurophysiological studies

These are of little value for 2–3 weeks until Wallerian degeneration has begun. Most severe brachial plexus injuries require surgery. This is recommended earlier than 2–3 weeks, hence neurophysiology has little role acutely.

Neurophysiology has been extended to use intraoperatively with scalp or cervical electrodes. These are of assistance in evaluation of the injured nerves at surgery. They are, however, not entirely reliable.

Investigation of associated injuries

Plain radiographs of skeletal injuries: these should be done as part of standard polytrauma assessment.

- Vascular studies: an arteriogram or digital subtraction arteriogram may be used for suspected subclavian artery or even aortic arch injuries
- CT scan for head injuries: where doubt persists as to the severity of the head injury this is an essential prerequisite to surgical intervention.

Management (Box 12.26.5)

The treatment of brachial plexus injuries can be divided into initial, non-operative and primary, and secondary operative treatments.

Initial management

The initial management of the brachial plexus injured patient is along advanced trauma life support guidelines. Vascular injuries are emergencies and require accurate diagnosis and urgent surgery. Surgical approach depends upon the site of injury. The vascular injuries specifically to the subclavian artery should be repaired with reversed vein grafts. Prosthetic grafts have a high incidence of thrombosis and lead to extensive local fibrosis. Skeletal injuries should be stabilized early, usually with rigid internal fixation. Humeral nails for humeral shaft fractures are easier and quicker to use but associated with higher non-union rates and do not permit examination of the radial nerve which can be ruptured in association with a brachial plexus injury.

Non-operative treatment

Neurapraxic lesions should be treated conservatively. It may be difficult to delineate these lesions absolutely. Indicators include mild lesions with a limited number of nerve roots involved. There is often patchy sparing of sensation or motor function and early recovery within the first 7–10 days. The treatment aims to prevent further damage to the brachial plexus by keeping the arm adducted to the chest for 4 weeks whilst preventing distal joint stiffness with physiotherapy.

A conservative approach should not be adopted for too long because of the much greater benefit of early over late operative repair. Thus, if the anticipated recovery is not occurring at 2–3 weeks, neurophysiological studies should be performed in conjunction with spinal cord imaging, and the decision for further treatment based upon these findings and the clinical progress.

Operative treatment

Primary operative treatment aims to restore nerve function whilst secondary operative treatment is that of muscle transfers and bone operations to overcome specific problems. There is only a very limited role for late nerve surgery.

Primary operative treatment

The standard surgical approaches are the transverse supraclavicular incision for proximal lesions and the deltopectoral approach for infraclavicular lesions (Box 12.26.6).

In the supraclavicular approach flaps of skin and platysma are raised, then after division of the omohyoid between stay sutures, whilst avoiding damage to the cervical plexus and vessels and the phrenic nerve, the brachial plexus is delineated posterior and lateral to the scalenus anterior muscle.

In the infraclavicular approach the deltoid and the pectoralis major are separated, the pectoralis minor is detached from the coracoid and reflected, and the plexus is then seen wrapped around the subclavian arteries.

Once the plexus has been displayed the lesions may be obvious. With increasing time from injury, however, this is less so and may be complicated by the degree of recovery that is shown. Diagnosis may be enhanced by intraoperative electrical testing both stimulating orthodromic across the lesion and antidromic recording from cervical or scalp electrodes. For neuromas and lesions in continuity, when there is a partial response to electrical stimulation across the lesion, the decision to resect and graft, or to leave is very difficult.

The following specific surgical treatments are available:

- Direct suture
- Conventional nerve grafts

Box 12.26.5 Management

- Treat vascular injuries
- Stabilize associated skeletal injuries
- Non-operative management for neurapraxia
- Surgery:
  - Direct suture for clean sharp injuries
  - Conventional nerve grafts
  - Nerve transfer for motor power or pain relief in preganglionic injuries.

Box 12.26.6 Results of primary surgery

- Best results with more proximal lesions
- Delay is detrimental
- 60% success for nerve grafts/transfers.

- Vascularized nerve grafts
- Nerve transfers.

Direct suture

Direct suture is rarely used and is only a possible option in early treatment of clean sharp injuries of the plexus. Even in such injuries, grafting is usually recommended. In clean injuries suitable for either direct suture or small grafts, the best results are achieved.

Conventional nerve grafts

The technique is as for standard nerve grafting (see earlier). The nerves used are typically one or more of the medial cutaneous nerve of the forearm, medial cutaneous nerve of the arm, and the sural nerve. It is essential that these are put in without tension. They are typically secured with fibrin glue and sutures. Postoperatively the arm is immobilized in a sling full time for 6 weeks to protect the repairs. Thereafter, physiotherapy is begun.

Vascular nerve grafts

Vascular grafts were first used in 1976 to provide a well-vascularized tube for nerve regeneration. It was hoped that this would overcome the problem of ischaemic scarred nerve beds. The reported results show that vascular grafts are only equivocally better than conventional grafting. The surgery is more complex and, therefore rarely used except in very scarring recipient sites.

Nerve transfers

These were first performed in the 1950s and are now well established. The most common are the accessory to suprascapular nerve transfers and transfers of intercostal nerves to median or musculocutaneous nerves. Their role is twofold. One is to provide further motor input to nerves distally to improve function. The accessory to suprascapular transfer can result in significant improved shoulder control and intercostal nerve transfer to the lateral cord can give grade III and even grade IV elbow flexion. They do require some relearning, but most patients manage this. The other role is to increase the sensory input to the distal nerves which can have a dramatic benefit in relief of pain especially with preganglionic injuries.

Results of nerve surgery

The results of nerve surgery are very variable and depend upon many factors, as with all peripheral nerve repair work (see Chapter 12.25). In essence, the recovery of the proximal muscles is best because there is the shortest distance from the nerve to recover and these muscles have a mass action so that fine innervation is not as important as in the finer actions of the small muscles of the hand. Furthermore, with nerve recovery to distal muscles there is often significant end-organ failure prior to the nerve reaching the muscle. Sensory recovery in the hand is at best protective.

The reported results are mainly with conventional nerve grafting and nerve transfers.

Nerve grafting

Of particular importance for the recovery after brachial plexus injury is the delay from treatment. Delays over 3 months are especially detrimental and after 6 months the chances of worthwhile regeneration are minimal. Repair of C5 and C6 by conventional nerve grafting gives functional flexion of the elbow and some control of the shoulder in 60% of cases.

Nerve transfer

Useful functional gain is achieved with the shoulder and elbow with significant relief of pain in over 60% of patients operated on within 3 months. Nerve transfers are particularly successful for preganglionic injuries of C5 and C6 and sometimes C7. They are much less effective for preganglionic injuries of C8 and T1.

Reconstructive surgery (Box 12.26.7)

There are various techniques of secondary operative reconstruction of brachial plexus injuries. The main ones are muscle transfers, arthrodesis, amputation, and surgery for the treatment of pain. These are always second best for 'good nerve regeneration will result in far better function than musculotendinous transfers'.

- Muscle transfers: the standard rules apply as for elsewhere (see Chapter 6.9). Muscle transfers are particularly useful for regaining elbow flexion and wrist and finger extension
- Arthrodesis is mainly used at the shoulder when there is good proximal shoulder girdle control so that the scapula muscles can support the weight of the arm and provide some movement. It can also help reduce the dragging on the brachial plexus from a very unstable shoulder, which can increase pain. Arthrodesis in the rest of the upper limb is rarely performed
- Amputations are now uncommon except in severe acute lesions with extensive vascular injuries. Later indications are for a flail and useless limb in a well-rehabilitated patient and occasionally for marked shoulder pain, particularly that associated with dragging on the plexus. Most of the amputations are proximal humeral amputations to maintain some shoulder contour.

The role of each reconstructive procedure is considered further in terms of the four main areas of use: the shoulder, elbow, forearm, and hand.

Shoulder

The complexity of surgery at the shoulder is often dictated by the level of function in the rest of the upper limb. Hence in injuries of C5 and C6 only, when nerve recovery has been poor, considerable efforts at improving the shoulder are worthwhile in order to use the very good hand and forearm function that the patient will have. For impaired shoulder function muscle transfer particularly of latissimus dorsi into the external rotators may be of value in regaining some active external rotation. If this is not possible, an external rotation osteotomy of the humerus may allow a more functional range for use of a good forearm and hand. For the flail or very weak shoulder arthrodesis is the most useful treatment. Gleno-humeral arthrodesis can be performed with internal or external fixation.

Box 12.26.7 Reconstructive surgery

- Muscle transfer for:
  - Elbow flexion
  - Wrist extension
- Arthrodesis for shoulder
- Amputation—occasionally for vascular injury or a painful useless limb.

Rarely, scapulothoracic fusion may be performed for poor thoracoscapular control.

Elbow

The lack of elbow flexion is a major disadvantage to patients who still have a good hand. Lack of elbow extension is less disabling as gravity can be used to achieve extension. The patients most troubled by lack of elbow extension are those who can abduct their shoulder above 90 degrees as the forearm then tends to fall, or those patients who need extension strength to get out of a chair or wheelchair.

Most elbow surgery is directed at regaining elbow flexion. The three main types of transfer are the triceps to biceps transfer, the pectoralis major to biceps transfer, and the Steindler flexorplasty, advancing the brachioradialis proximally up the arm. The triceps to biceps transfer gives the best results but with loss of elbow extension. The Steindler flexorplasty tends to give the worst results with weakness and risk of damage to the ulnar nerves.

Recently there have been cases of use of contralateral latissimus dorsi as a free muscle graft and in Japan in particular, surgeons are using gracilis as a free muscle transfer for both elbow and wrist and hand flexion. The latter typically gain M4 or M3 elbow flexion.

Forearm

The main problem is lack of forearm rotation. Active forearm rotation is very difficult to re-establish although re-establishing some pull on the distal tendon of the biceps may give some active supination. Surgery is mainly directed at improving the position of the rest of the forearm with a rotational osteotomy.

Hand

The most common problem that is treated is loss of finger and wrist extension. The extensors of the arm generally have more proximal root values than the flexors so for proximal brachial plexus injuries there may be retention of wrist and hand flexion but loss of extension. Tendon transfers are based upon the Robert Jones transfer (see Chapter 6.9) but obviously directed to which muscles are functioning well. Failure is more common that with peripheral nerve injuries as there is often partial involvement of the flexors. Retraining is also more difficult.

Pain (Box 12.26.8)

Pain can be the most severe consequence of a brachial plexus injury. It is more common with preganglionic injuries and with injuries of C8 and T1 than C5 and C6. It can lead to depression, opiate dependence, and suicide. It is typically crushing, burning, and vice-like often with superimposed shooting or lightening pains.

Box 12.26.8 Pain treatment

- Analgesics especially nerve irritant suppressants, e.g. amitriptyline
- Transcutaneous nerve stimulation (50% success)
- Nerve transfers (up to 80% success)
- Spinal cord surgery
- Rehabilitation.

These patients are difficult to treat and involvement in other activities such as work and the major role of successful rehabilitation back into the community. Specific treatments include analgesics, transcutaneous electrical nerve stimulation, nerve transfers, and spinal cord intervention.

Analgesics range from simple oral analgesics up to opiates. The latter, however, should be avoided if possible as they tend not be that effective and are associated with dependence. Neuralgical pains may respond in particular to carbamazepine, phenytoin, or amitriptyline.

Transcutaneous electrical nerve stimulation gives a significant reduction in pain in up to 50% of patients.

Nerve transfers, particularly intercostal nerve transfers, have been shown to be effective in reducing neuralgic pain. This was felt to be only with early surgery but even late surgery is of benefit in up to 80% of cases.

Attempts have been made at spinal cord intervention with interruption of spinal tracts and thermocoagulation of the dorsal root entry zone. Some patients have dramatic relief of symptoms and up to two-thirds are improved but there is a significant risk, of up to 10%, of lasting neural deficit, particularly affecting the lower limbs and possibly sexual function. Therefore spinal cord surgery is mainly used as a last resort.

Rehabilitation of patients following brachial plexus injuries is fundamental to their long-term function and integration back into their former lives. The key is a multidisciplinary approach with the surgeon or rehabilitation physician as the coordinator. Other team members include physiotherapists, occupational therapists, nurses, and retraining officers. The physiotherapists strengthen muscles, mobilize joints, and set up the transcutaneous electrical nerve stimulation. Occupational therapists make and fit splints and organize the retraining activities of daily living. The nurses provide ongoing support on the ward. The retraining officer is crucial in planning return to future work.

The future

Predictions about the future of brachial plexus injuries are difficult and unreliable. Adult brachial plexus injuries are becoming less common as motorcycle use appears less frequent especially in poor weather. Nonetheless as the evidence continues to accumulate of the efficacy of early intervention it is hoped that these patients will be referred earlier and will have more effective nerve surgery.

Recent work from Sweden has shown regrowth of implanted ventral rootlets into the spinal cord. This allows some regeneration of motor function into preganglionic injuries. Initial work in humans has shown some promise.

Nerve growth factors have recently been studied and shown to be present only in low levels in brachial plexus neuromas. In future, application of nerve growth factors at the time of operation may improve nerve recovery.

In reconstructive surgery the role of free muscle transfers has not been fully evaluated but is likely to broaden the scope of reconstruction.

Conclusion

Brachial plexus injuries sadly affect some of the youngest and most active members of the population and are a severe and debilitating drain on both patients and society. Too often they have been treated with a degree of therapeutic nihilism based on the belief that surgery has no role, as espoused at the SICOT Meeting in Paris in the 1960s. However, there is no doubt that early aggressive treatment of these patients can give significant benefit and even late attention to their problems can be very helpful.

When a man has nothing a little is a lot.
Sterling Bunnell

Further reading

Birch, R.B. (1992). Advances in diagnosis and treatment in closed traction lesions with a brachial plexus. In: Catterall, A. (ed) *Recent Advances in Orthopaedics*, No. 6, pp. 65–76. Edinburgh: Churchill Livingstone.

Birch, R.B. and Giddins, G.E.B. (1996). Peripheral nerve injuries. In *Medico-legal Reporting in Orthopaedic Trauma*, second edition. Edinburgh: Churchill Livingstone.

Breidenbach, W.C. and Graham, B. (1991). Vascularised nerve grafts. In: Gelberman, R.H. (ed) *Operative nerve repair and reconstruction*, pp. 569–86. Philadelphia, PA: J.B. Lippincott.

Carlstedt, T.P., Grane, P., Hallin, R.G., and Noren, G. (1995). Return of function after spinal cord implantation of avulsed spinal nerve roots. *Lancet*, **346**, 1323–5.

Narakas, A.O. (1987). Traumatic brachial plexus injuries. In: Lamb, D.W. (ed) *The Paralysed Hand*, pp. 110–15. Edinburgh: Churchill Livingstone.

Sedel, L. (1987). The management of supraclavicular lesions: clinical examination and surgical procedures. In: Terzis, J.K. (ed) *Microreconstruction of Nerve Injuries*, pp. 385–92. Philadelphia, PA: W.B. Saunders.

Wynn Parry, C.B., Frampton, V., and Monteith, A. (1987). Rehabilitation of patients following traction lesions of the brachial plexus. In *Microreconstruction of nerve injuries* (ed. J.K. Terzis), pp. 483–95. Philadelphia, PA: W.B. Saunders.

12.27

Replantation

D. Grinsell, D.R. Theile, and W.A. Morrison

Summary points

- Digital replantation is the best reconstruction available for the correct indications
- Amputated thumbs, multiple fingers, and paediatric replants are the strongest indications
- A functional result requires a mobile, stable, sensate digit of adequate length
- Replant survival and functional results are dependent on multiple factors including microsurgical expertise
- Spare part surgery is a unique opportunity to salvage tissue in an unreplantable limb.

Introduction

One of the guiding principles of reconstruction espoused by the father of modern plastic surgery Sir Harold Gillies was to replace like with like. In the successful replantation of an amputated part using microsurgery this principle is taken literally. Since the first reports of an arm replantation and the first thumb replantation, the reattachment of amputated parts has become common place and includes almost any extremity of the body.

Unfortunately successful replantation does not mandate satisfactory function, with the aim of survival alone being useless without a functional appendage. The potential adequacy of bone, tendon, and nerve repairs and joint flexibility must be predicted preoperatively before embarking on an attempt at replantation.

Mechanisms of amputation

The mechanism greatly influences the degree of damage caused to all anatomical structures and will have significant implications on survival and long-term function. It is prudent to give the patient a guarded outcome as occasionally even in ideal circumstances results can be disappointing.

The industrial machinery which cause amputations are many and varied and the injury can be further influenced by the reflex withdrawal response of the victim. A detailed description of the mechanism of injury combined with examination of the amputated part and radiographs will give clues to the extent of tissue damage but ultimately surgical exploration must determine the technical feasibility of replantation.

Box 12.27.1 Principles

- Replace like with like
- Give guarded outcome to patient
- Sharp injuries best
- Crush/avulsion worst.

Sharp or guillotine injuries

Sharp or guillotine injury is the most favourable mechanism of amputation although it is the rarest. Unfortunately it is seen most often at very distal levels where replantation is technically difficult.

Crush injury

Localized

Localized or moderate crush injuries caused by power saws and many industrial press-type machines are the most common form of injury. The tissue damage occurs over a wider area and often occurs at multiple levels. Following conservative trimming of damaged structures, this type of injury can usually be converted to the sharp type and whilst prognosis is worse than a sharp injury, in the absence of an avulsional component, a high survival rate can still be achieved.

Diffuse

Diffuse crush injuries caused by blunt squashing or high-velocity cutting machines reveal extensive contusion of skin and soft tissue as well as ragged tendon and nerve ends and often comminution of bones. There may be frank loss of tissue especially bone and skin and this may necessitate either local, regional, or free flap coverage.

Avulsion

Avulsion amputations result from a degloving or longitudinal force and are compounded by the natural withdrawal reflex of the victim. Typically, the vascular structures rupture and protrude from the proximal amputation stump while long tendon and nerve ends protrude from the distal part. Extensive damage occurs to the digital arteries over a variable length, often extending proximally to the next branch point and even into the palmar vessels, and may include skip lesions of thrombus. If the mechanism included a torsional component the arteries can look macroscopically normal in the absence of flow and this is due to intramural spiralling seen clearly with more proximal dissection under the microscope. In contrast, veins rupture rather than avulse. The veins are sheared at the same level of the skin and can be anastomosed primarily whereas the arteries nearly always require vein grafting.

Characteristic of avulsion is the extensive degloving of skin which remains with the amputated part, creating poorly vascularized distally based flaps following replantation. The ultimate fate of the skin depends on the extent of distal resection of the arteries in order to restore blood flow. It is possible to be left with an alive digit distally surrounded by a moat of necrotic skin requiring further reconstruction. In general the long-term functional prognosis is poor given the injury to nerves and tendons, especially if the latter have disrupted at their musculotendinous junction. One caveat to this is the classic isolated ring avulsion which often leaves the skeleton and flexor sheath intact and requires revascularization or replantation of the soft tissues alone thereby permitting early active mobilization and a more favourable outcome.

Confounding factors

Physical trauma may be combined with thermal or chemical burns which in the absence of blood supply to the amputated part can be impossible to assess. Incorrect storage can cause frostbite of the amputated part. Gross contamination requires widespread debridement of all tissues including bone and necessitates vein grafting of all vessels.

Indications for replantation (Box 12.27.2)

There are no absolute indications to replant. The decision whether or not to replant isn't always easy and demands experience both in replantation and hand surgery in order to maximize the chance of a successful functional outcome. The aim is to restore function, growth, and cosmesis. Stiff, cold, or painful fingers may be excluded from everyday use and also interfere with the function of the remaining undamaged hand. There remains a subgroup of patients who for religious or cultural reasons will categorically insist on replantation. Similarly some patients prefer to keep a non-functional digit as it affords a better cosmesis than a bothersome prosthesis. Thus whilst the delayed amputation of a finger at 12 months does not constitute a success, if there is any doubt, it is generally better to err on the side of replantation than primary amputation.

Box 12.27.2 Aims of replantation

- Aim to restore function, growth, cosmesis
- Within ischaemia time
- More distal injuries more favourable
- Thumb strongest indication in upper limb
- Multiple digits strong indication
- Better in younger patients.

Ischaemia time, level, mechanism of injury, number of digits amputated, associated hand injury, and age will all influence the potential for recovery.

Ischaemia time

The amount of muscle contained in the amputation is the critical determinant with respect to time to revascularization. Amputations containing minimal muscle generally present well before their maximum permissible ischaemia time has elapsed (warm 12–16h; cold <28h). More proximal amputations, particularly those in the forearm or the lower limb, contain significant portions of muscle and therefore have a much more limited warm ischaemia time than digits (6–8h). With viability unlikely and potentially life threatening consequences these replantations should probably not be attempted if the warm ischaemia time exceeds 8h.

Level of amputation

There are numerous classifications for the level of amputation but from a practical viewpoint there are five distinct types –

1) Type 0 (Distal) = distal to the distal interphalangeal (DIP) joint, or thumb interphalangeal (IP) joint
2) Type 1 = insertion of flexor digitorum superficialis (FDS) to DIP joint (Zone 1)
3) Type 2 = A1 pulley to insertion of FDS (Zone 2)
4) Type 3 = wrist to A1 pulley
5) Type 4 (major) = proximal to wrist or lower limb.

Although technically difficult, it has become obvious that distal replantations, only have to survive to be functional. They have the potential for the best results of any replant.

Only sharp type replantations in Type 1 have the potential to restore function, especially when they are multiple and to the ulnar side of the hand. Even with limited distal interphalangeal joint movement or sensation, the intact proximal interphalangeal joint will restore considerable palmar grip function and balance with the outstretched hand. Paradoxically, Type 2 amputations, with more to gain by replantation, are the poorest indication in a single digit because of the complexity of the structures involved. In practice very good function following a single digit non-guillotine injury in Types 1 and 2 levels is rare and replantation is generally contraindicated.

Replants in Types 0–2 have the relative advantage of not requiring any motor neural re-innervation. Amputations proximal to Type 2 in the hand are strong indications for replantation. Replantation of a clean-cut wrist-level amputation is the most rewarding. At the mid forearm level and above the prognosis worsens.

Whilst an amputation through a joint obviates the need for osteosynthesis and bony union and potentially allows for earlier mobilization, the range of motion resulting is universally disappointing. Repair of the unique stabilizing structures of the joint (usually the proximal interphalangeal joint) cannot hope to replicate the pre-injury status and therefore mobility.

Digit involved

The thumb contributes 40% of function to the hand and is the strongest indication for replantation at any level and at any age

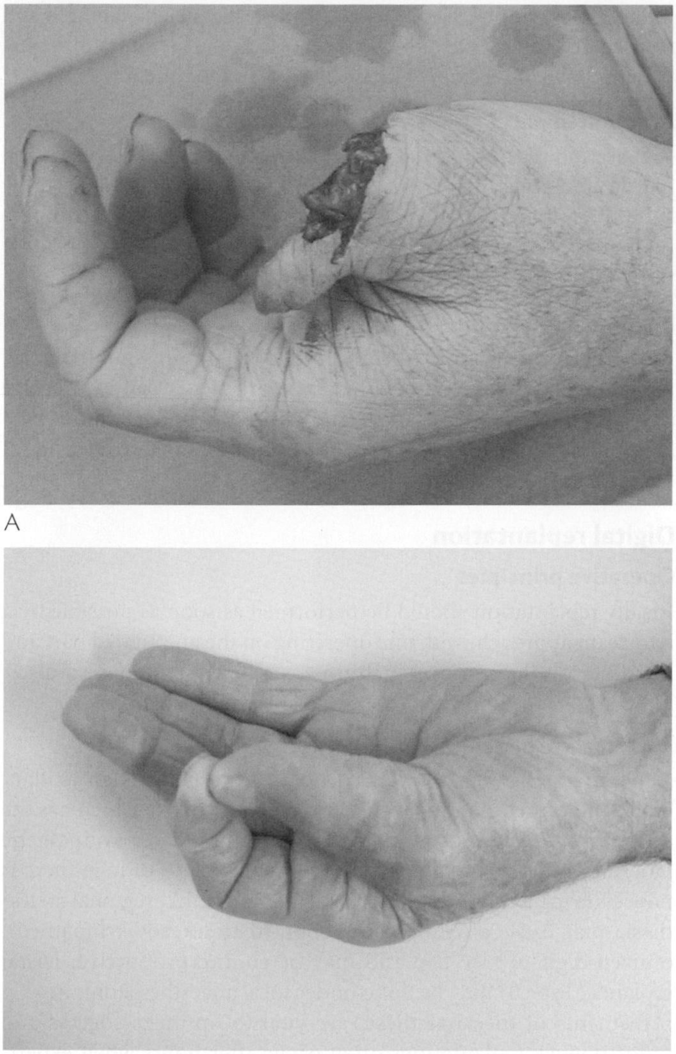

A

B

Fig. 12.27.1 (A) Total thumb amputation—a strong indication for replantation even in a 76 year old. B) Normal sensation and good function is attained.

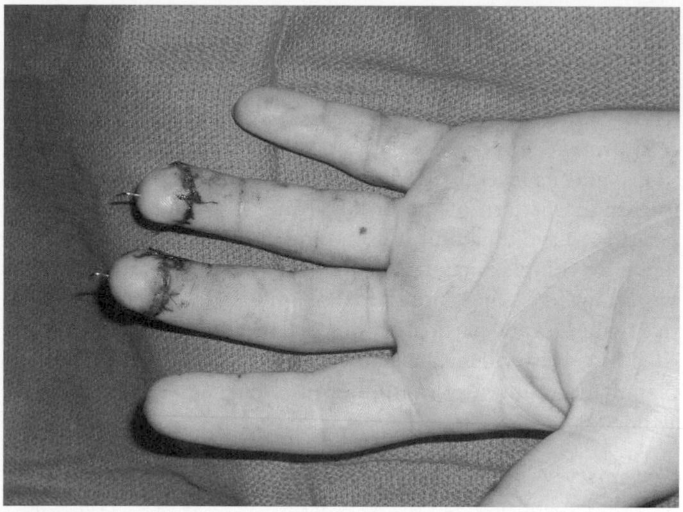

Fig. 12.27.2 Postoperative view of multiple distal replants of middle and ring fingers. These have the best functional and cosmetic results of all amputations.

(Figure 12.27.1). The mobility in three planes of the trapeziometacarpal joint also compensates for the stiffness postreplantation in the interphalangeal or metacarpophalangeal joints without a significant diminution in function. Replantation of a single finger should only be done in special circumstances, but single-digit amputations with a concomitant injury to another finger or part of the hand, magnify the disability and is a stronger indication (Figure 12.27.2).

Multiple-digit amputations are a strong indication for replantation. The barest use of the hand requires a stable, mobile thumb and a pillar against which it can oppose. The radial three digits are concerned with pulp pinch grip, and therefore sensory excellence is of greater importance than mobility. On the ulnar side of the hand however, power grip is the prime function and this requires digital length and mobility; sensation is relatively less important. The potential for joint movement, especially the proximal interphalangeal joint, is of prime importance. Amputations in Types 0 and 1 do not need sophisticated function as simple restoration of length will allow them to contribute to ulnar power grip.

Where multiple digits have been amputated and not all are suitable for replantation, the opportunity to select the least traumatized of them and transfer to the most appropriate stump should always be kept in mind. Most commonly this will involve the thumb.

Age

Young patients carry a better prognosis than the elderly. Due to the remarkable plasticity of the immature brain to create cortical reorientation, replantation of any digit at any level is strongly indicated in children. Beyond the age of 20, nerve regeneration occurs variably and unpredictably, and all but distal amputations should be expected to have significant limitations in their neurological function in terms of both motor and sensory modalities.

Clinical evaluation (Box 12.27.3)

History

The history should include the calculation of the ischaemic time, the nature and mechanism of the injury, and the presence of any contaminating agents. The patient's age, occupation, hobbies or sporting skills, and hand dominance should be noted. The status of the patient's tetanus prophylaxis should be checked. Any life-threatening medical comorbidities may make the decision to replant foolish.

Box 12.27.3 Clinical evaluation

- History/mechanism of injury/handedness
- Comorbidities
- Avoid unnecessary meddlesome examination of wound
- Hb/xmatch
- X-ray of amputated limb and injured limb.

Examination

The purpose of emergency examination is to evaluate the technical feasibility of restoring circulation and the potential for functional recovery so that an informed discussion with the patient can proceed prior to surgery. The amputated part will reveal the type of injury and its level. By deduction the proximal stump(s) should mirror the pattern of the distal segment, so that it is generally possible to avoid painful unwrapping of the proximal wound. In the more complex major limb and multiple-injury categories, it is important to exclude more proximal multiple-level injury, extensive tissue loss and particularly brachial plexus injury. Even in these situations it is evident that some form of surgery is inevitable, so that meddlesome explorations prior to anaesthesia should be avoided.

Consent

Problems often do not appear until intraoperatively and therefore preoperative consent should be as broad as possible and include grafts of veins, skin, nerve, and bone as well as local and free flaps.

Specific investigations

Most amputations have undergone some haemorrhage and therefore a haemoglobin/haematocrit and a blood group cross match should be performed routinely. Plain radiographs of both the injured limb and the amputated parts should be obtained and should demonstrate the joint proximal to the injury.

Management (Boxes 12.27.4 and 12.27.5)

Preoperative principles

Management of the patient

Although most amputations are isolated injuries the emergency management of the patient should be along trauma guidelines. As there are no absolute indications for replantation, other life-threatening injuries take priority. The patient should be adequately stabilized and resuscitated. There are numerous reports in the literature of digital replants being done hours or days later when the patient is stable.

Box 12.27.4 Management 1

- Stabilize and resuscitate
- Store amputated part cool and moist
- Haemorrhage control with compression
- Two-team approach to surgery
- General anaesthesia favoured.

Box 12.27.5 Management 2

- Debride
- Tag structures
- Bone shortening essential
- Repair extensor tendons
- Venous anastamoses first
- Then volar repair.

Amputated part

Preparation of the amputated part in a saline-soaked sterile gauze, placed in a sealed plastic bag, and packed in an ice-water slurry should be done immediately. Despite intensive research, no perfusate has been shown to be convincingly beneficial in cytoprotection of limb tissue.

Proximal limb stump

Haemorrhage can mostly be arrested by a compression bandage, with a tourniquet only used as a last resort. In cases of incomplete amputation with devascularization, the appendage should be splinted in an anatomical position to maximize any residual circulation.

Digital replantation

Operative principles

Ideally replantation should be performed as soon as possible by a two-team approach, with one operating on the amputated part and the other on the stump. Much time can be wasted unless a disciplined sequence of repair is followed shown in Table 12.27.1.

Anaesthetic requirements

General anaesthesia is favoured but if time permits an axillary block and catheter may be performed preoperatively which has the dual advantage of assisting with vasodilation due to a sympathetic blockade and providing postoperative analgesia. Although there is now evolving data in the anaesthetic literature that regional anaesthesia may cause a steal phenomenon to an already sympathectomized digit or free flap and may be counterproductive. Distal replants (Type 0) may be done under local anaesthesia only.

Elements of the anaesthesia are vital to optimize success and unfortunately replantations often occur after hours when experienced anaesthetists may not be available. It is incumbent upon the surgeon to ensure perfusion requirements to the digit are achieved. This includes a gentle induction and extubation, maintenance of a core body temperature of 37°C, a urine output of 1mL/kg/h, avoidance of vasopressors and diuretics, normovolaemia, and a haemoglobin of approximately 10. In our experience packed red blood cells followed by concentrated albumin are the best colloids to

Table 12.27.1 Repair sequence in digital replantation

Skeleton
Periosteum (dorsal)
Extensor tendon including lateral band/intrinsic
Veins
Dorsal skin
Periosteum (palmar)
Flexor tendon
Arteries
Nerves
Palmar skin

maintain intravascular volume, and with the use of depth of anaesthesia brainwave monitors, often volatile anaesthetic gases can be reduced with a subsequent improvement in systemic blood pressure.

Evaluation and exposure

Contaminating foreign material should be removed and conservative debridement of damaged tissue carried out. All vital structures should be systematically identified and tagged. Proximal damage and retraction of the digital artery and/or nerves will mandate a skin incision for exposure. A Bruner type incision is preferable, so that flap closure is possible over the microvascular anastomosis even if the incision itself cannot be fully closed because of swelling. The ends of the flexor tendons are located and a core suture is inserted into each.

Skeletal shortening and fixation

Bone shortening is an essential and frequently underrated initial step in replantation. Guillotine injuries and distal replants are the exception to the rule. The prime reasons for shortening are to allow good quality tension-free wound closure for primary healing, extensor tendon apposition, and nerve approximation. Although skeletal shortening does assist in vascular end to end repair, this is the least valid reason and in fact can lure the operator into inadequate resection of damaged vessels. In cases of disarticulation where shortening is not possible this may necessitate vein graft lengthening.

Rigid fixation to allow early movement is a vital operative step and the most difficult to achieve. Too often the functional benefit of successful revascularization is reduced by malunion although non-union is unusual. The dilemma resides in the balance between rigid low-profile plate fixation with its ensuing widespread periosteal stripping and the less invasive pin fixation favouring maximization of vascularity to the fracture but a consequent decrease in rigidity. Properly placed crossed K-wires carry a number of significant advantages as a method of skeletal fixation in replantation providing stable but not rigid fixation, minimal periosteal stripping and easy removal (Figure 12.27.3).

Dorsal repair

The extensor tendon, including the lateral bands and intrinsics, should be repaired with a continuous running technique. It is preferable to perform the venous anastomoses prior to the arteries to avoid unnecessary and prolonged bleeding if the reverse sequence is followed. In distal replants, some severe crush injuries and those with prolonged ischaemia where revascularization is doubtful then it is advisable to perform the arterial repair first. The dorsal digital veins are usually easily located in the subcutaneous tissue by the presence of small blood clots and the location of the veins on the distal amputation stump will mirror their position on the proximal stump. Occasionally adequate sized veins can be seen on the volar aspect. Radical resection is rarely necessary so direct anastomosis is common. The dorsal skin is closed cautiously over the venous anastomoses. Inadequate skin closure due to insufficient bone shortening or degloving risks venous exposure, desiccation, infection, secondary haemorrhage and late thrombosis after 4–5 days.

Volar repair

After periosteal repair the flexor tendons should be repaired by tying the core sutures previously placed and in so doing restoring the natural posture of the finger thus reducing tension on the

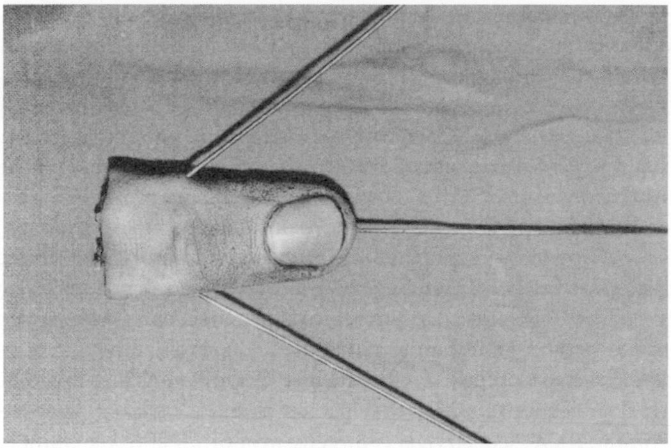

A

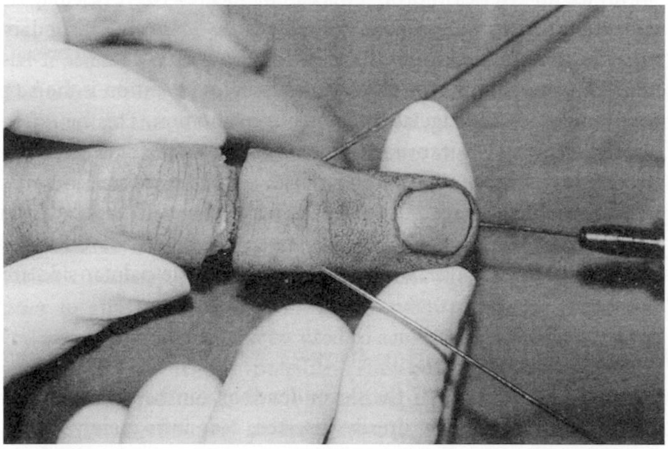

B

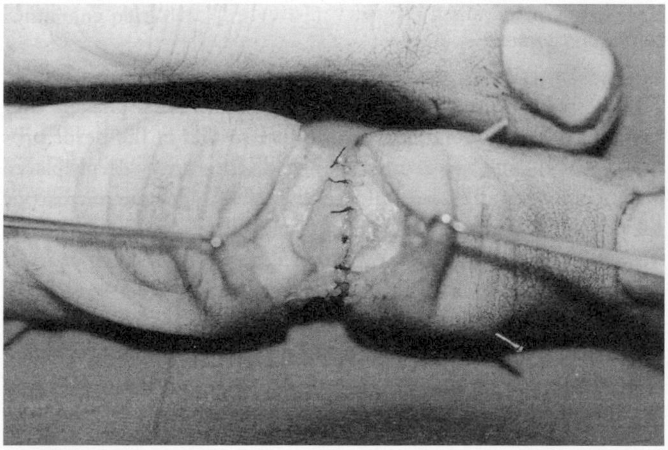

C

Fig. 12.27.3 Technique of K-wire fixation. (A) A longitudinal K-wire and two divergent wires are passed in a retrograde manner. (B) Correct alignment is maintained, as the longitudinal wire is driven proximally. Rotational alignment is corrected and the crossing K-wires are driven proximally, avoiding interphalangeal joints. The longitudinal wire is then removed. (C) Periosteal closure should be performed whenever possible.

neurovascular repairs. Digital arteries are identified by their constant dorsal relationship to the nerves in the fingers. Towards their termination in the distal phalanx they converge towards the midline to form an arcade with often a single midline artery deeply placed on the bone. The proximal vessels must be resected until pulsatile flow is encountered. If the vessel spasms, manoeuvres to restore flow include distraction of the vessel to its physiological length, a bolus of intravenous heparin, dependency of the limb, topical antispasmodics, and warm saline irrigation. Experience dictates an adequate distal artery seen under the microscope. Vein grafts should be harvested from the flexor aspect of the forearm and should be placed under mild tension in order to avoid redundancy. Where access is difficult, it is helpful to anastomose the distal end of the vein graft into the amputated part prior to skeletal fixation. Increased survival is directly proportional to the number of anastomosed vessels.

If no useful arteries and/or veins can be located for revascularization, afferent arteriovenous anastomosis may provide adequate perfusion or efferent arteriovenous anastomosis may provide outflow.

Both digital nerves should be repaired using an epineural suture technique. The medial cutaneous nerve of the forearm, the posterior interosseous nerve, or an interpositional vein graft are convenient donor sites if no rejected amputation segments are available. Skin closure should be tension free and designed so that vascular pedicles are covered. This may necessitate flap transpositions with skin grafts to the secondary defects (Figure 12.27.4). Circumferential dressings should be avoided when placing a volar plaster.

Major limb replantation (Box 12.27.6)

The capacity of replanted tissues to develop sensory reinnervation gives limb replantation a unique advantage over any contemporary prosthesis. The mixed nature of the proximal nerves involved, the large bulk of muscle, the local tissue destruction, and sometimes the avulsive mechanism of injury all weigh heavily against an ideal outcome. Larger vessels make vascular repair relatively simple, but permissible ischaemia times are severely reduced. The prognosis for significant recovery following repaired brachial plexus or proximal peripheral nerve injuries, even in ideal circumstances, is poor. In general, above-elbow replantations are contraindicated except in children. Double-level injuries, especially an associated brachial plexus avulsion are a contraindication.

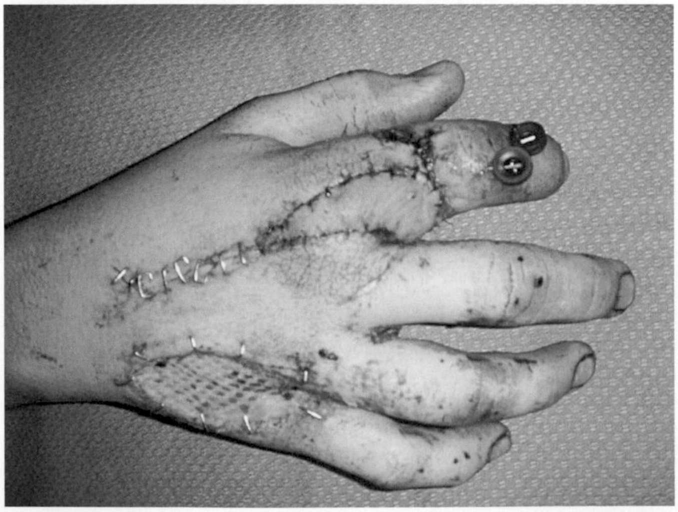

Fig. 12.27.4 Day 7 post index finger replantation and revascularization of ulnar 3 fingers. Venous flow through flaps as seen here can provide a simple and valuable source of soft tissue cover in multiply injured fingers when heterodigital flaps are unavailable.

Box 12.27.6 Major limb replantation in adults

- Shorter ischaemia time
- Easier reconstruction—structures larger
- Nerve recovery poor
- Above elbow/double level contraindicated
- Lower limb only if posterior tibial nerve intact.

In the lower limb the replanted foot or leg is likely to remain insensate and will cause difficulties for the patient during ambulation and with footwear. Patients tolerate below-knee prostheses well and rehabilitate rapidly. Therefore, except in children, replantation of lower limbs should be reserved for incomplete amputations where the posterior tibial nerve is in continuity.

Operative principles

There are several principles in major limb replantation that are not pertinent to the replantation of digits. Major limb replantation is a true surgical emergency. Contrary to traditional earlier credos, all major limb replantations should be revascularized *prior* to any bony fixation or other soft tissue repair. Temporary endarterectomy shunts can be used to rapidly restore arterial and venous continuity. Venous repair should always be delayed to allow toxins in the venous effluent to dissipate prior to reconnection into the circulation. Intraoperative cooling is also important in these large-muscle-containing parts.

Musculoskeletal repair

The objectives of bone shortening in major limb replantation are different from those in digital replantation. The priority is the permission of end-to-end nerve and musculotendinous repair and this may necessitate quite radical resections of 10cm or more. Fixation depends on level and site of the fracture and should be performed along AO guidelines. Despite the shortening, free flaps are frequently necessary to obtain wound closure.

Musculotendinous divisions are repaired in the same way as injuries in a non-replant situation. Side to side tenorrhaphies, secondary tendon transfers, or even secondary free muscle transplants may be indicated.

Neurovascular anastomoses

Adherence to microvascular technical principles is important. Only those vessels with demonstrable flow should be anastomosed. Grafts will almost always be necessary for arterial reconstruction. Because of high flow rates and high pressure demands over many years, the long-term fate of vein grafts in these sites is uncertain and consideration may be given to primary arterial grafts, for example from the thoracodorsal or opposite radial artery.

Reperfusion

If any doubt exists about the compartment pressures, prophylactic fasciotomies should be performed. These may include the interossei and a carpal tunnel release in the hand. Systemic reperfusion toxicity and myoglobinuria are theoretical grave risks after revascularization and are proportionate to the length of ischaemia of the part.

Postoperative principles (Box 12.27.7)

The patient should be kept warm, well hydrated, and comfortable with the limb elevated on pillows. Broad-spectrum systemic antibiotics are indicated for prophylaxis. Smoking is totally prohibited given its proven association with vascular spasm and increased risk of thrombosis. Visible access to the region of the amputation site is particularly important to detect early signs of local necrosis, sepsis, or vessel exposure. Given the propensity for myonecrosis in major replants it may be prudent to perform a 'second-look' operation after 24–48h in order to ascertain muscle viability.

Monitoring

Monitoring of capillary return, colour, and temperature should be hourly for the first 24h and every 2h for the next 24h. Healthy revascularized tissue should have a capillary return of 2s. Venous congestion is detected by a violet-blue colour and a rapid capillary return. When pricked the part will bleed briskly with dark blue blood. Absolute arterial obstruction is obvious. The digit is pale white and cold with no capillary return, the pulp is empty, and there is absence of bleeding on needle puncture. Partial arterial insufficiency is more difficult to recognize and may be misinterpreted as a venous problem. In this situation the finger may appear blue; however, the capillary return will be very slow or absent, and bleeding on needle puncture will be either absent or a delayed slow ooze of dark blue deoxygenated blood.

Anticoagulation

The paucity of human studies and conflicting animal studies make decisions regarding anticoagulation arbitrary. Anticoagulation regimens differ from centre to centre and range from no anticoagulation to full therapeutic heparinization varying on a case by case basis. We have experienced numerous cases of digital replantation that have clearly been salvaged by heparin. It is particularly valuable as a static dose intraoperatively in cases where reperfusion is protracted.

Mobilization

The goal of early active movement of replanted fingers, although theoretically tempting, is difficult in practice because of repairs on both extensor and flexor surfaces. Complete immobilization for approximately 3 weeks is the best option in most cases.

Box 12.27.7 Postoperative principles

- Keep patient warm
- Visible access
- Second look 24–48h
- Monitor vascularity
- Heparin may be used
- Immobilize for 3 weeks.

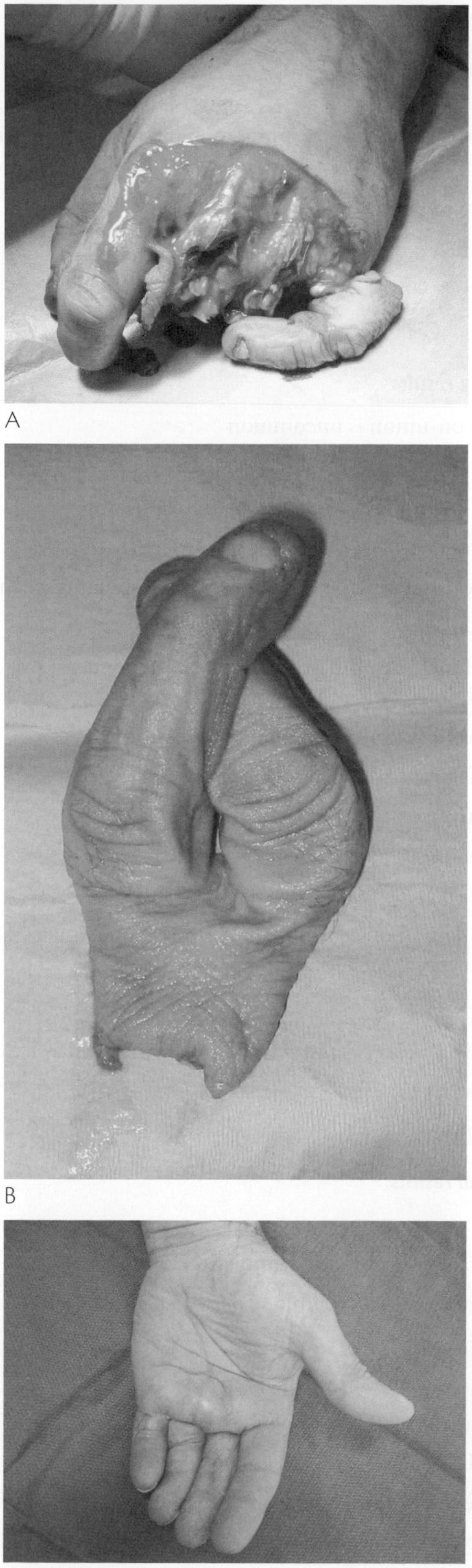

A

B

C

Fig. 12.27.5 (A) and (B) Attaining a good functional result in devastating hand injuries requires surgical skill and expertise, and a hint of luck. (C) Postoperative result of 3 finger replantation – even minimal function is beneficial to the patient.

Results

Digital replantation

Adults

Results in the literature are numerous and relatively consistent Based on a meta-analysis the following results can be expected.

Survival of replants

- Overall: 85%
- Guillotine: 90%
- Avulsion: 65%.

Functional results

- Bone: non-union is uncommon
- Nerves:
  - Two-point discrimination, 2mm to >20mm
  - Average, 9mm
  - More distal replants have superior two-point discrimination
- Vasomotor:
  - Incidence of cold intolerance is dependent on climatic conditions
  - Is due to the injury and not the replantation
  - Partial improvement occurs over years
- Subjective:
  - Overall 80% have subjective benefit
  - Older patients have lower satisfaction rates
- Rehabilitation: except for distal-tip replants, at least 4 months can be expected to elapse Before return to work.

Children

Results of digital replantations can be summarized as follows.

Survival

- Overall 70%.

Functional results

- Nerves:
  - Average two-point discrimination, 5mm
  - Normal sensation with one nerve repair only
- Motion:
  - 25% have a totally normal movement
  - The majority of the remainder have functionally useful digits
- Growth:
  - Depends on presence or absence of epiphyseal injury
  - Nearly all show growth commensurate with the child.

Major replantation

A number of reports of major replantation have been published. In an eloquent analysis the functional results of major replantation were superior to prosthetic reconstruction.

Complications (Box 12.27.8)

Arterial insufficiency

Arterial insufficiency requires prompt return to the operating room and results from inadequate shortening of damaged vessels thus revision is usually with vein grafts. If revision is unlikely to be successful, full systemic heparinization, warming, and placing the hand below heart level may be beneficial, but expectations should be guarded. Late vascular occlusion is rare but may occur in proximal amputation due to intimal hyperplasia.

Venous insufficiency

This is rapidly lethal and early detection is vital for salvage. Relative congestion may be relieved by elevation above heart level, but if this is not successful then exploration and revision should be undertaken. If this is not possible then either medicinal or 'chemical' leeching may be used.

Medicinal leech (*Hirudo medicinalis*)

Leech bleeding is due to release of hirudin which is a potent anticoagulant. Leeches should be applied as required when the digit takes on a bluish hue. Tetracycline or ceftriaxone should be administered to prevent *Aeromonas hydrophila* infection which is resident in the gut of *H. medicinalis*

Chemical leech

This technique involves making a chevron-shaped pulp incision and the injection of 500IU heparin into the subcutaneous tissue. Regular milking (every 30min) is required to ensure continued bleeding. Injections need to be repeated several times daily.

Infection

Despite the insalubrious manner in which many amputations occur, frank wound or bone infection is surprisingly rare. Haematoma and necrotic skin margins are the harbingers of infection which will threaten vascular patency. Thrombosis occurring after 4–5 days is ominously infective in origin and is generally unsalvageable, highlighting the essential need to obtain primary healing of skin. Early intervention with flap coverage is the only hope.

Late complications

Non-union, malunion, stiffness, and tendon rupture

It is very important to make detailed notes of any variation in neurovascular anatomy that has been created by the initial surgery to minimize risk during essential secondary surgery. Revision surgery on replanted parts is the most technically challenging of all hand surgery and may be threatening to the survival of the part.

Box 12.27.8 Complications

- Arterial insufficiency
- Leeching can be used for venous insufficiency
- Infection rare
- Arthrolysis tenolysis for stiffness
- Cold intolerance.

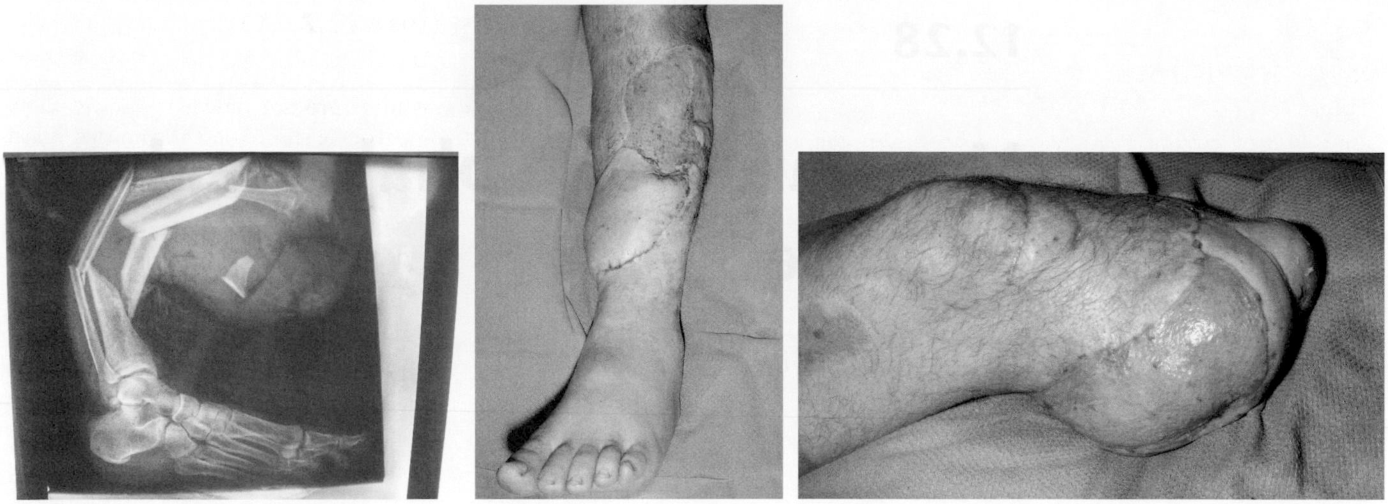

Fig. 12.27.6 (A) Multiple level injuries are a contraindication to replantation but can be a valuable source of "spare parts" in the form of free flaps. (B) Dorsalis pedis free flap used to cover contralateral compound tibia. (C) Free fillet of sole flap including calcaneum to salvage the knee joint and avoid a through knee amputation in the same patient. Residual bone length is augmented in order to fit a prosthesis and innervated durable skin cover is achieved.

Arthrolyses and tenolyses are frequently unrewarding. Therefore it is essential to perform optimal repairs at the time of the initial operation, even to the extent of primary nerve grafting if gaps are present. Silicone joints and tendon rods may also be considered to avoid reoperation through the replanted area, even though this risks infection.

Cold intolerance

The incidence of cold intolerance is initially high but improves with time. In our practice only a very small number of patients have sought reamputation although it has been a major problem in colder climates. It is highly likely to be due to the injury and not the amputation pre se.

Opportunism

In replantation opportunity strikes but once and it is of little use to realize later that some part of a non-replantable limb could have been used for an imaginative reconstruction. The durable sensate weight-bearing skin from the sole of the foot is ideal for resurfacing denuded upper tibial skeletal structures (Figure 12.27.6) and thereby avoiding above-knee amputations

Future developments

The ultimate dream for the replantationist is the transfer of human limb allografts. Surgical enthusiasm is currently in a state of flux following recent events. The first transplant was rapidly rejected. A more recent French attempt led to a second wave of hand transplants around the world.

There is precise documentation of the outcomes of at least 25 cases over several years. Most have had complications from the immunosuppression including transient rejection episodes, diabetes, and avascular necrosis of the hip; however, this has necessitated only two secondary amputations. The spectacular functional results from bilateral cases as well as a face transplant have tempered the chorus of objections from early hardliners. The achievement of lymphohaematopoietic chimerism is the Holy Grail as it will allow composite tissue transplantation without the inherent risks of immunosuppression.

In the longer term xenotransplantation of joints, muscles, tendons, and nerves from transgenic pigs may have a role in secondary reconstruction.

Further reading

Morrison, W.A., O'Brien, B., and MacLeod, A.M. (1977). Major limb replantation. *Orthopaedic Clinics of North America*, **8**, 343–8.

Morrison, W.A., O'Brien, B., and MacLeod, A.M. (1978). Digital replantation and revascularisation: a long term review of 100 cases. *Hand*, **10**, 125–34.

Tamai, S. (1982). Twenty years' experience of limb replantation—review of 293 upper extremity replants. *Journal of Hand Surgery*, **7**, 549–56.

Waikukul, S., Sakkarnkosol, S., and Vanadurongwan, V. (2000). Results of 1018 digital replantations in 552 patients. *Injury*, **31**(1), 33–40.

Wojciech, D. (2006). A met-analysis of success rates for digit replantation. *Techniques in Hand and Upper Extremity Surgery*, **10**(3), 124–9.

12.28

Metacarpal and phalangeal fractures

T.R.C. Davis and J.A. Oni

Summary points

- Proximal phalanx unicondylar and spiral fractures most unstable
- If axially stable can be considered for non-operative treatment
- Kirschner wires offer stability without excessive soft tissue dissection
- Ring and little finger metacarpal flexion deformity is well tolerated, but this is not the case for the radial metacarpals
- Displaced proximal and middle phalanx fractures are a common cause of stiffness
- Displaced condylar fractures are usually best reduced and fixed.

Incidence

Metacarpal and phalangeal fractures have a combined incidence of approximately 380 per 100 000 per year and are most common in 10- to 39-year-old males. They are frequently caused by sporting injuries or fights. Little finger metacarpal fractures account for 30% of all metacarpal and phalangeal fractures.

Classification

There are a variety of classifications systems which describe the site and pattern of the fracture, all of which have advantages and disadvantages. Whatever classification system is used it is important to classify fractures according to their stability.

Stable fractures are those which present in acceptable alignment and will not displace into unacceptable alignment if the hand is left free and mobilized. Thus most undisplaced fractures and most displaced little finger metacarpal neck fractures are stable. There are two subtypes of unstable fractures. The first includes fractures which present in acceptable alignment though are at risk of displacing into unacceptable alignment if mobilized. Undisplaced unicondylar and spiral fractures of the proximal phalanx are examples of this type. The second subtype includes all displaced fractures which present in unacceptable alignment and require reduction, after which they must be stabilized (splinted or internally fixed) in order to prevent redisplacement. Virtually all displaced fractures which need to be reduced are unstable, and for these it is also important to consider their likely axial stability after fracture reduction.

Axial stability describes a fracture's ability to oppose the constant tension in the digit's flexor and extensor tendons which attempt to shorten the fracture: transverse fractures have good axial stability while long oblique fractures have poor axial stability. The axial stability of a fracture, once reduced, is one factor which determines its suitability for non-operative treatment. Fracture stability should be viewed as a spectrum with absolute stability (undisplaced transverse third metacarpal fracture) at one extreme and absolute instability (severely comminuted open proximal phalangeal fracture with bone loss) at the other.

Clinical evaluation

History

The patient as well as the fracture must be assessed. Hand dominance, employment, and recreational activities, as well as ability to comply with the proposed treatment, must all be considered.

The mechanism and time of injury should always be ascertained. Twisting injuries are likely to cause fractures with rotational deformity and fifth metacarpal neck fractures are much more serious if there is a dorsal wound which was caused by a tooth (punching someone in the face). For open fractures it is important to determine the environment in which the injury was sustained (farmyard or clean environment).

Physical examination

The whole hand must be examined for swelling and bony tenderness so as not to miss multiple injuries (Figure 12.28.1), and skin sensation and perfusion distal to the fracture should also be examined, especially in crush injuries. Alignment should be carefully assessed though significant amounts of radial/ulnar and dorsal/palmar angulation can be masked by soft tissue swelling. It is of utmost importance to look for rotational deformities as these are poorly tolerated in the fingers and usually indiscernible on

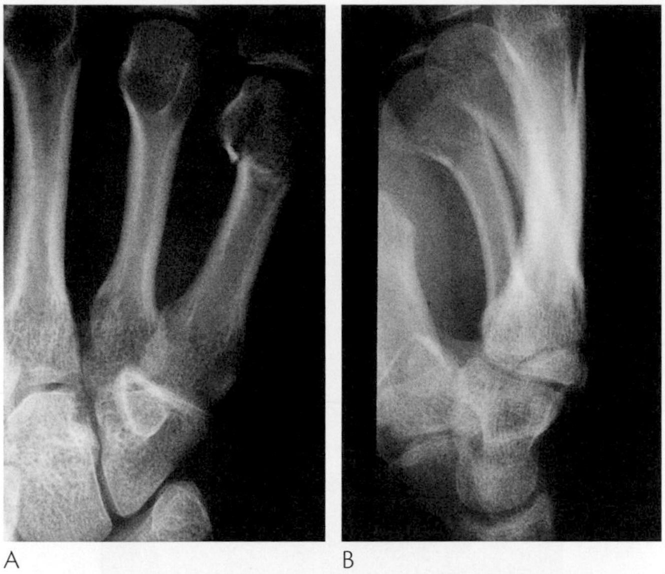

Fig. 12.28.1 This man punched a wall and sustained a little finger metacarpal neck fracture. Examination also revealed marked tenderness over the little finger carpometacarpal joint. There is no visible little finger carpometacarpal joint space on the posteroanterior radiograph, which suggests an injury, but this could easily have been missed but for the clinical findings. Further radiographs showed an impacted fracture–subluxation of the carpometacarpal joint.

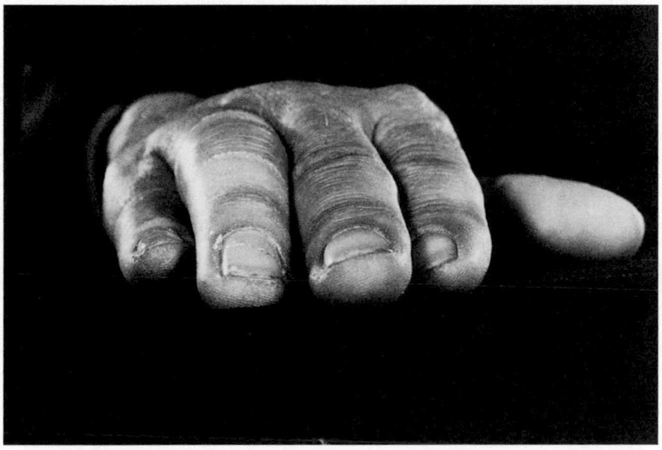

Fig. 12.28.2 The ring fingernail lies in a different plane to the other fingernails indicating a rotational deformity.

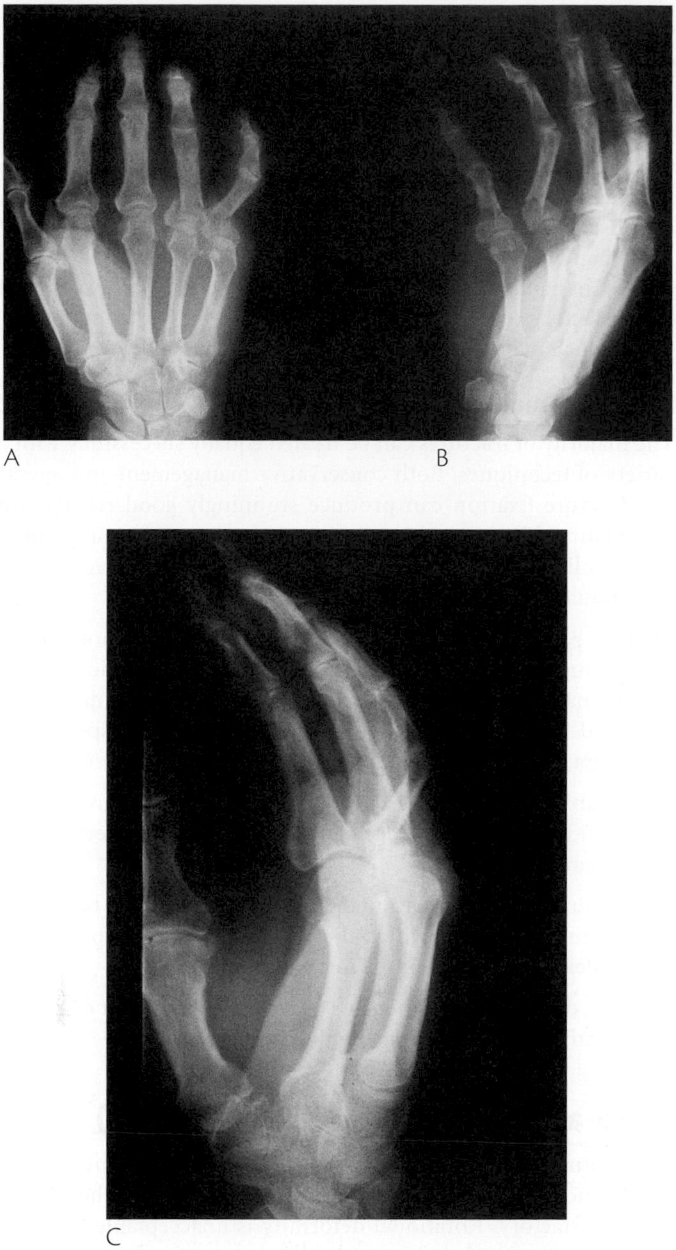

Fig. 12.28.3 A) Posteroanterior, B) oblique, and C) lateral views of fractures of the bases of the ring and little finger proximal phalanges. The fracture displacement is difficult to assess on the lateral view. The fingers are not superimposed on the oblique view which shows the dorsal angulation of the ring finger fracture.

radiographs. Although obvious if the patient can make a fist, most with fresh fractures cannot and rotational deformity is best assessed by examining the alignment of the fingernails with the fingers extended (Figure 12.28.2).

Investigations

Radiographs

Radiographs should be considered as a continuation of the clinical evaluation. Rather than simply requesting radiographs of the injured finger (or worse still the injured hand) one should request radiographs centred on the area of clinical tenderness where the fracture is suspected. The standard radiographic views for individual fingers are posteroanterior and lateral. Posteroanterior oblique views should also be obtained for finger metacarpal and proximal phalangeal fractures as dorsal angulation is frequently masked on the lateral view by the adjacent digits (Figure 12.28.3).

Anteroposterior and lateral views in the plane of the thumb (Gedda views) are usually sufficient for thumb fractures. Computed tomography (CT) scans, and other complex imaging techniques are rarely required.

Management

Initial management

If a closed fracture requires operative treatment or a manipulation and this cannot be performed immediately, the fracture should be temporarily splinted for pain relief. Patients with open fractures should always receive antibiotics and, if necessary, tetanus immunization.

All hand fractures should be screened by a surgeon with an interest in hand fractures. Such a policy reduces the prevalence of unsatisfactory results and prevents overtreatment of simple fractures, which in itself can cause stiffness and generate poor results.

Definitive management

The majority of fractures can be treated equally successfully with a variety of techniques. Both conservative management and operative fracture fixation can produce stunningly good results and humiliating failures. Although fracture factors such as alignment and stability are important determinants of treatment, consideration should also be given to the following.

1) The patient's expectations of treatment and motivation: although some patients cannot tolerate any cosmetic deformity, many are prepared to accept considerable malunion, provided that normal function is restored. This is especially if acceptance of malunion allows an earlier return to work
2) Rehabilitation resources: aggressive operative fracture fixation should only be performed if appropriate therapy services are available
3) Technical difficulty: trainees and assistants must be shown treatment methods which they will be able to perform independently and safely in the future
4) Cost: do the potential benefits of operative treatment over conservative management justify the extra costs?

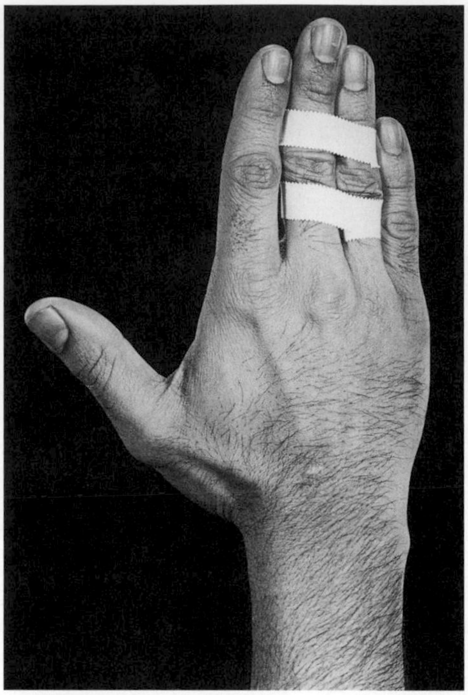

Fig. 12.28.4 Buddy strapping.

Extra-articular fractures (Box 12.28.1)

The treatment goal is union in an alignment which permits normal hand function and provides a cosmetic result which the patient finds satisfactory. Rotational deformity is unacceptable, particularly for metacarpal and proximal phalangeal fractures, and is a strong indication for operative fracture fixation. Metacarpal fractures can tolerate considerable shift and palmar angulation, and some radial/ulnar angulation without loss of function. Proximal phalangeal fractures are much less tolerant of malunion with acceptable limits of about 10 degrees of radial/ulnar angulation and 20 degrees of dorsal/palmar angulation.

Undisplaced and minimally displaced extra-articular fractures

The majority of undisplaced or minimally displaced fractures are stable and should be treated by early mobilization. For phalangeal fractures, this is usually achieved by buddy strapping (Figure 12.28.4) or a Bedford gaiter which holds the injured finger to an adjacent one so as to protect it from unexpected knocks. After 3 weeks most fractures are sufficiently sticky to discard all strapping. Alternatively, if the fracture is very painful or the hand is very swollen, stable fractures can be safely rested on a palmar slab in a comfortable position for 1 or 2 weeks and then mobilized once the pain and swelling have subsided. Stable fractures almost invariably achieve a good result.

However, minimally displaced spiral and long oblique fractures of the proximal and middle phalanges have little axial stability, are potentially unstable and may displace if mobilized (Figure 12.28.5). These fractures should be immobilized on a palmar slab or on an aluminum splint with the hand in the Edinburgh position for 3 weeks.

Displaced extra-articular fractures

The surgeon should assess the configuration of the fracture (transverse, oblique, etc.), so as to predict its axial stability following a closed reduction. If the reduced fracture has little or no axial stability (spiral and long oblique fractures) and accurate fracture alignment is vital, then the fracture should be treated operatively. If the fracture reduction has good axial stability (transverse and short oblique fractures) then the fracture may be treated non-operatively.

Conservative treatment methods

Unstable metacarpal fractures can be immobilized in plasters (Colles plaster, ulnar slab, or hand cast) which allow metacarpophalangeal and interphalangeal joint movement. Unstable proximal and middle phalangeal fractures require immobilization of the injured digit until the fracture becomes sticky (3 weeks). The position in which the injured hand is immobilized and the period of immobilization are of great importance. Fingers should be immobilized in the Edinburgh position (Figure 12.28.6), with the metacarpophalangeal joints flexed to at least 60 degrees and the interphalangeal joints virtually fully extended. In this position the collateral ligaments of these joints are taut and cannot shorten as a result of post-traumatic inflammation. Immobilization of

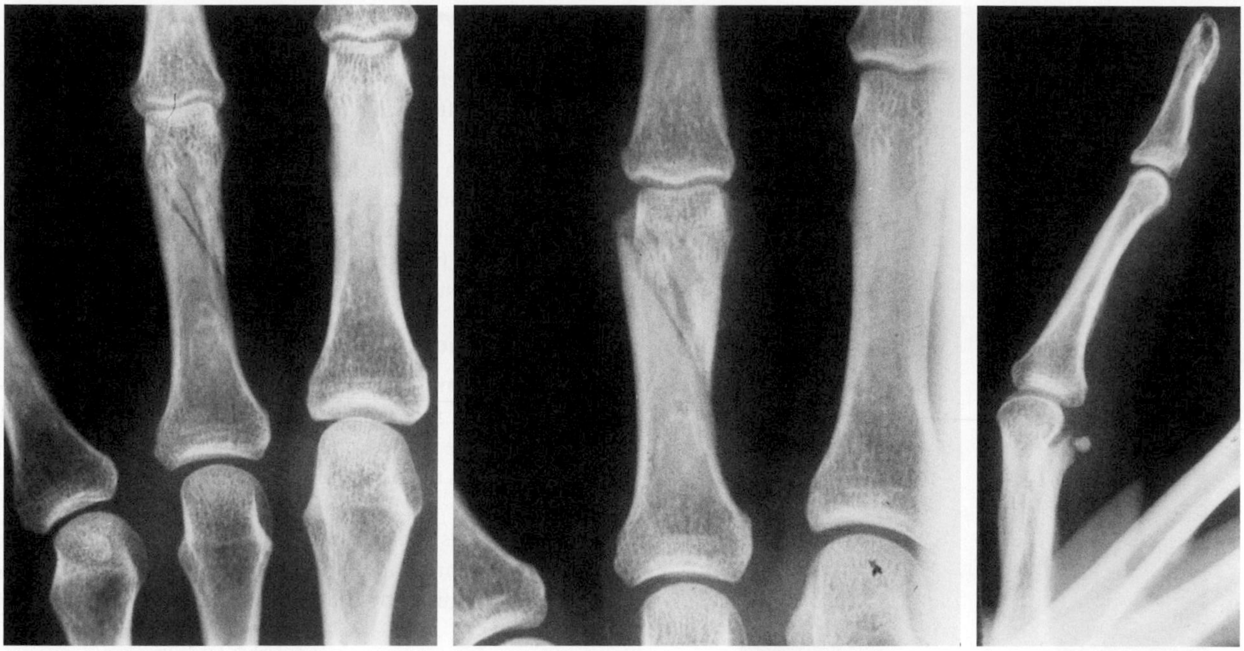

Fig. 12.28.5 A) Minimally displaced spiral fracture of the proximal phalanx which was treated with buddy strapping. B) The fracture displaced during treatment and the palmar bone spike (C) then blocked proximal interphalangeal joint flexion and had to be excised.

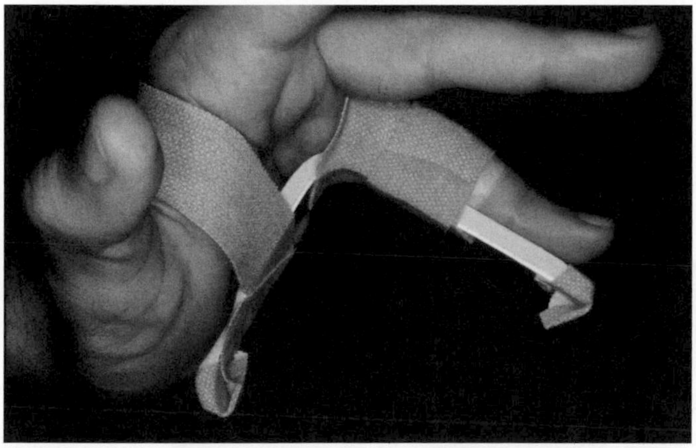

Fig. 12.28.6 The Edinburgh (intrinsic plus) position.

fingers with the metacarpophalangeal joints extended and the interphalangeal joints flexed is a potent cause of interphalangeal joint fixed flexion deformities and reduced metacarpophalangeal joint flexion. It is also a position in which most phalangeal fracture reductions are unstable and will redisplace.

Fractures treated conservatively should be followed up with weekly check radiographs to ensure that the splint does not slip and the fracture does not displace.

Although fracture union, as assessed by bridging callus on radiographs, takes many weeks to occur, firm clinical union is usually achieved after 3 weeks. It is thus rarely necessary to immobilize a finger fracture for longer than 4 weeks.

Operative treatment

Kirschner wires

These are widely used to stabilize fracture reductions and can be inserted following either a closed (percutaneous insertion) or open reduction. Two K-wires are usually used. Crossed K-wires can distract fractures and increase the risk of non-union (Figure 12.28.7).

The advantage of K-wires, especially if inserted percutaneously, is that they provide fracture stability without an extensive surgical exposure. However they may be difficult to insert and are provide relatively unstable fixation Thus, if an extensive surgical exposure with periosteal stripping is required to reduce a fracture, it is probably better to consider rigid internal fixation which allows early mobilization. Another disadvantage is that their tips inevitably protrude into the surrounding soft tissues and can cause irritation and pain, and interfere with rehabilitation. Furthermore, if their ends are left protruding through the skin, troublesome pin site infections can occur. Although these usually resolve once the K-wires have been removed, serious finger infections and osteomyelitis occasionally occur.

Rigid internal fixation

This is a demanding technique. Spiral and long oblique fractures can usually be fixed with lag screw fixation whereas transverse and short oblique fractures require plate fixation. The treatment aim of rigid internal fixation is to make an unstable fracture stable enough to allow early mobilization. Although the benefits of rigid internal fixation are obvious for some fracture types such as the unicondylar fracture of the proximal phalanx, it is uncertain for others whether internal fixation brings about an earlier return of useful function or a better end result than less invasive

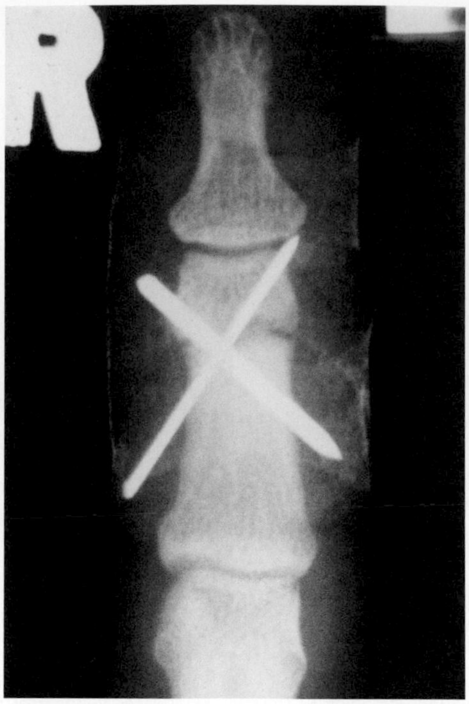

Fig. 12.28.7 Open fracture of the shaft of the proximal phalanx. This was treated with crossed K-wires which held the fracture in distraction and a non-union developed. The X-rays also show the track from another K-wire which was inserted and removed: this may also have contributed to the non-union by causing additional thermal injury.

treatment methods. Tendon adhesions and joint contractures readily develop and the surgeon, therapist, and patient must all be motivated to ensure that the finger is actively mobilized within 1 week in order to prevent these complications. Deep infections following rigid internal fixation are only rarely seen in the hand.

External fixation

External fixation is not widely used for closed hand fractures though is a useful technique for open fractures (Figure 12.28.8). It causes little soft tissue damage and usually provides sufficient stability to allow early fracture mobilization. There are numerous commercially available hand external fixators, and it is possible to manufacture one from Kirschner wires, the barrel of a syringe and bone cement. Pin site infections can cause troublesome deep infections. External fixators are usually removed after 3 or 4 weeks, once the fracture is sticky.

Dynamic traction

There are many dynamic traction devices, some of which are expensive and manufactured, while others are assembled out of K-wires by the surgeon during surgery. The principle aim of all these devices is to counteract the tension in the finger extensor and flexor tendons which will cause shortening of injuries without axial stability. This is achieved by applying a distraction force. Dynamic traction is commonly used for the treatment of complex intra-articular fractures of the base of the middle phalanx (Figure 12.28.9).

Specific extra-articular fractures

Extra-articular metacarpal fractures

Metacarpal base fractures of the thumb

Extra-articular fractures of the base of the thumb metacarpal displace into flexion. Provided that there is reasonable contact between the fracture surfaces, considerable deformity (up to a rather arbitrary 30 degrees) can be accepted without loss of thumb function. Most of these fractures are managed quite adequately in a scaphoid-type plaster for 3 weeks. However, if there is gross fracture displacement, comminution, or shortening, closed reduction and percutaneous K-wiring or open reduction and internal fixation (plate or K-wires) should be considered.

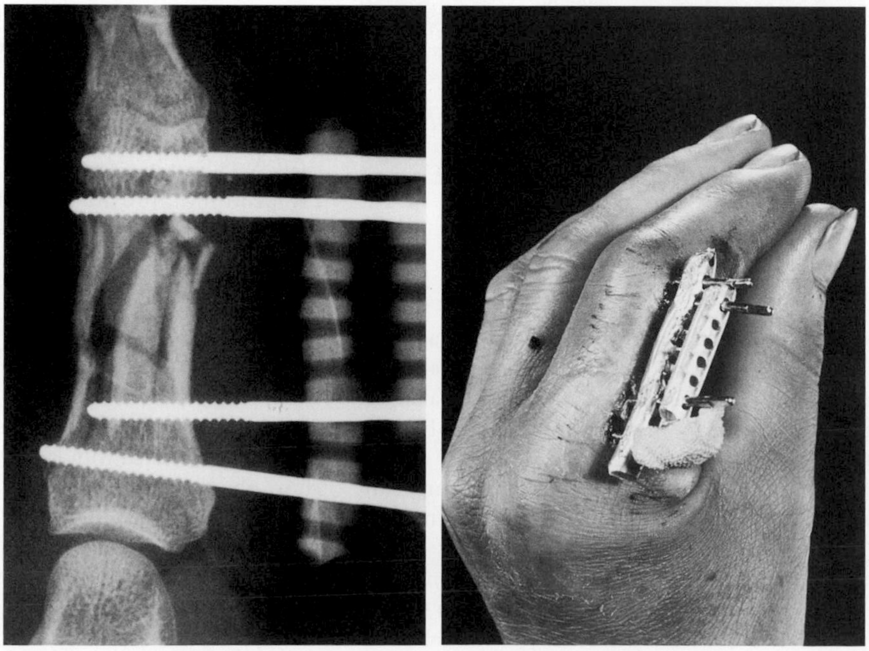

Fig. 12.28.8 Closed comminuted fracture of the index finger proximal phalanx which was been treated with a cheap though effective external fixator.

A B

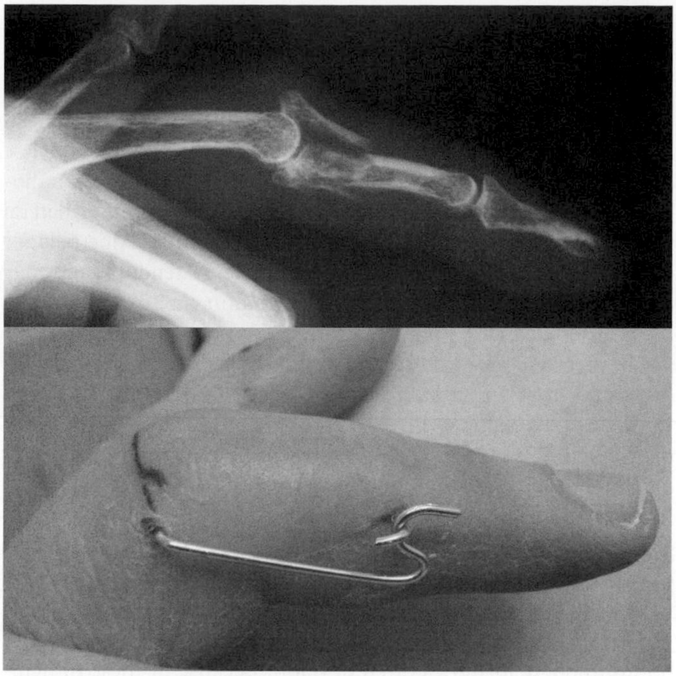

Fig. 12.28.9 Pilon fracture of the base of the middle phalanx. This was treated with dynamic traction using a device made from two K-wires. The proximal wire was inserted into the neck of the proximal phalanx and the distal one into the distal shaft of the middle phalanx. The two wires are linked under tension such that the devise distracts the fracture and proximal interphalangeal joint such that both heal 'out to length'. It will not restore perfect articular congruity.

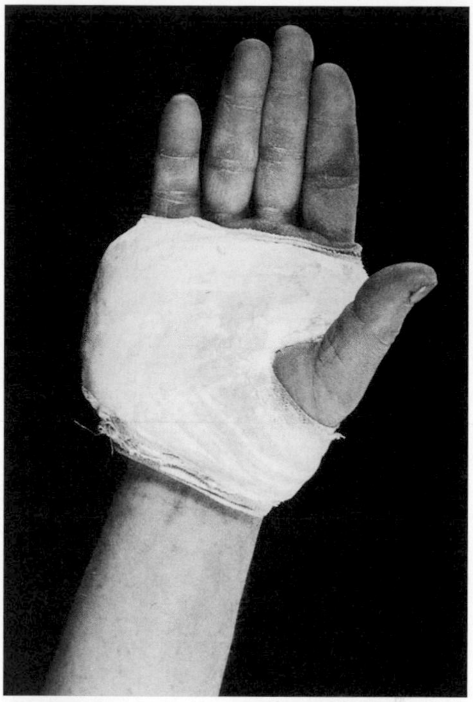

Fig. 12.28.10 A well-moulded hand plaster for metacarpal shaft fractures.

Finger metacarpal base and shaft fractures

These fractures, and all other metacarpal fractures, displace into palmar angulation and are most common in the ring and little finger rays. The intermetacarpal ligaments usually prevent rotational deformity though this can occur in all rays. It most commonly occurs with spiral fractures of the distal shaft of the little finger metacarpal.

Palmar angular malunion is well tolerated in the ring and little fingers which have mobile carpometacarpal joints and 'metacarpalgia' (synonymous with metatarsalgia) when gripping objects is most uncommon. However, it is more likely to occur following index and middle metacarpal fracture malunions as these rays do not have mobile carpometacarpal joints. Thus, although over 30 degrees of palmar angulation can be accepted in ring and little fingers without fear of significant functional disability, index and middle finger metacarpal shaft fractures with more than 30 degrees of angulation should be reduced. Although 30 degrees of palmar angular malunion of a ring or little finger metacarpal does not cause functional disability, it inevitably causes cosmetic deformity which is more prominent than that following metacarpal neck fracture malunion. For this reason the author usually offers to reduce and immobilize in plaster fractures with 30 degrees or more angular deformity. Fractures with less than 30 degrees of palmar angulation need not be reduced and should be treated conservatively, either by early mobilization or, if painful, by immobilization on a palmar slab for 3 weeks.

Treatment methods for fractures in unacceptable alignment include closed reduction and plaster immobilization (Figure 12.28.10) or percutaneous K-wiring, external fixation and open reduction and internal fixation with K-wires, screws, or plates. Although these fractures are easily reduced closed, it is difficult to maintain the reduction in plaster and redisplacement can occur, either during plaster immobilization or after the plaster has been removed at 3 or 4 weeks. For this reason, operative fixation should be considered for all fractures with rotational deformity and those which have completely 'stepped off' and telescoped (causing shortening). Operative fixation should also be considered when the cosmetic result is important, though one is trading in a bony bump and a sunken knuckle for a scar. Percutaneous K-wiring can be performed by reducing the fracture and passing three transverse K-wires, two distal and one proximal to the fracture, across from the fractured metacarpal into the adjacent metacarpal. Alternatively, these fractures can be stabilized by one to three intramedullary K-wires which are inserted through a small cortical window in the metacarpal base or neck. This technique is particularly suitable for the little finger metacarpal but is not as easy as it may appear (Figure 12.28.11). Most patients rapidly regain hand function and, if the K-wires are buried in the metacarpal shaft, they rarely migrate and require removal.

Lag screws can be used to fix spiral metacarpal shaft fractures but, if open reduction and internal fixation is the chosen treatment option, plate fixation is usually required. If plates are used, early postoperative mobilization is essential so as to prevent adhesion formation.

It is not unusual for patients with little finger metacarpal shaft fractures which have been reduced and stabilized in plaster to default from clinic and remove their plasters. Although such fractures may unite in gross palmar angulation (up to 60 degrees) and the cosmetic appearance may be unsightly, function is good.

Finger metacarpal neck fractures

Little finger metacarpal neck fractures are usually self-inflicted in a fight and displace into palmar angulation. Although this angular

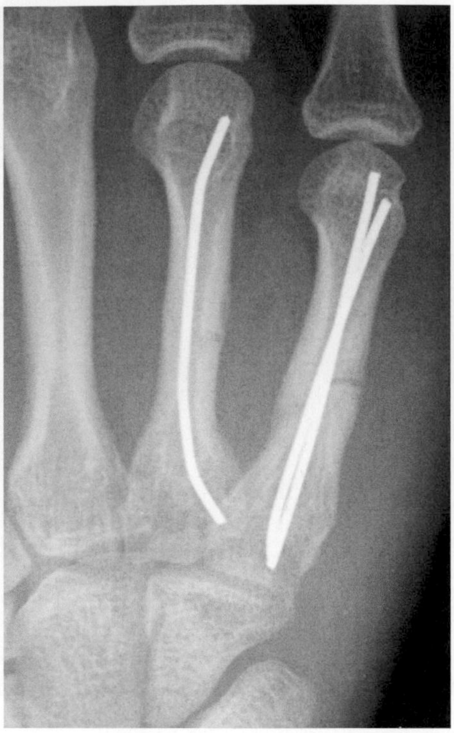

Fig. 12.28.11 These metacarpal shaft fractures, which were grossly displaced, were stabilized with intramedullary K-wires which were inserted through windows in the bases of the metacarpals and their ends were buried within the bones.

deformity is readily reduced, it is virtually impossible to maintain the reduction with closed methods. Excellent functional results can be achieved within 3 weeks by ignoring the fracture displacement and mobilizing even the most severely displaced fracture. The patient should be warned that he will be left with a bony bump and a sunken knuckle and initially may have a metacarpophalangeal and even a proximal interphalangeal joint extension lag. Operative fixation is reserved for fractures with complete step off or patients who cannot accept deformity. Metacarpophalangeal joint stiffness is not an infrequent complication of operative fixation, especially if blade plates are used.

Considerable palmar angulation can also be accepted in ring finger metacarpal neck fractures. However, index and middle finger metacarpal neck fractures must unite in reasonable alignment as these digits do not have mobile carpometacarpal joints which can extend and prevent the metacarpal head becoming prominent in the palm. Fortunately, metacarpal neck fractures in these rays are rare and they are usually only minimally displaced. Thus, most finger metacarpal neck fractures are treated conservatively.

Extra-articular phalangeal fractures

Extra-articular proximal and middle phalangeal fractures

Displaced fractures of the proximal and middle phalanges are a common cause of finger stiffness. This occurs either as a result of malunion or adhesion formation between the fracture and the flexor tendon or the extensor hood which enshrouds the dorsal and lateral surfaces of the proximal phalanx.

Proximal phalangeal fractures displace into dorsal angulation and are easily reduced by traction and flexion of the metacarpophalangeal joint. Fractures of the distal third of the middle phalanx also displace into dorsal angulation whereas proximal third fractures displace into palmar angulation. Middle phalanx fractures tolerate angular and rotational malunion better than fractures of the proximal phalanx.

Extra-articular fractures of the base of the proximal phalanx. These displace into dorsal angulation which is frequently missed on radiographs as the fracture is obscured by the other fingers on the lateral view. Malunion with dorsal angulation disrupts the fine balance between the extensor mechanism and the flexor tendons, and may result in a boutonnière deformity. In addition, an apparent loss of metacarpophalangeal joint flexion may occur. These fractures usually have a transverse configuration though there may be considerable dorsal comminution, especially in the elderly.

They readily reduce with metacarpophalangeal joint flexion and the reduction can then be maintained in a well-fitting plaster cast or Zimmer splint which holds the finger in the Edinburgh position. It is vital that the plaster/splint is checked and the fracture is radiographed weekly for 3 weeks, as the plaster/splint all too readily slips distally allowing metacarpophalangeal joint extension, fracture redisplacement, and proximal interphalangeal joint flexion (Figure 12.28.12). This is a potent combination for finger stiffness, and boutonnière deformities often develop. Because of these difficulties, some surgeons prefer to treat these fractures operatively, either with percutaneous K-wires, rigid internal or external fixation. A condylar blade plate provides good stability, but is uncompromising, very difficult to apply and may result in stiffness due to extensor tendon adhesions, especially if the patient is reluctant to move his or her finger postoperatively. It is not known whether any form of operative fixation produces better results than careful non-operative management.

Phalangeal shaft fractures. The majority of displaced transverse and short oblique fractures of the phalanges can be treated satisfactorily by closed reduction and immobilization in the Edinburgh position for 3 weeks. Spiral fractures have no axial stability after

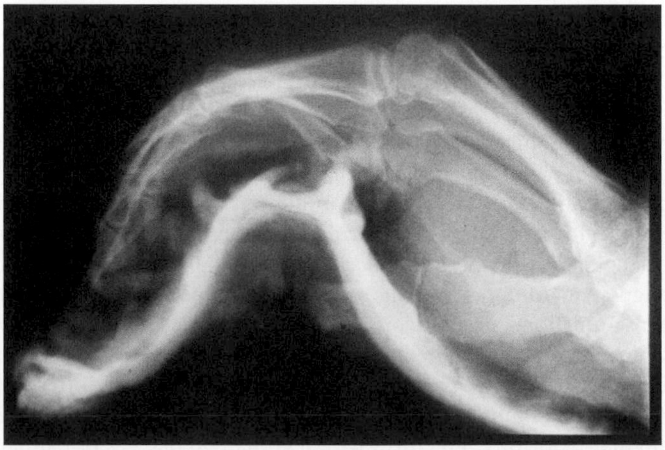

Fig. 12.28.12 These fractures of the bases of the ring and little finger proximal phalanges were treated by closed reduction and immobilization in a palmar slab. The immediate post-reduction radiographs (not shown) showed anatomical reductions with the fingers in the Edinburgh position. This radiograph was taken 1 week later and shows that the plaster has slipped distally allowing extension of the metacarpophalangeal joint, flexion of the proximal interphalangeal joint, and redisplacement of the ring finger fracture.

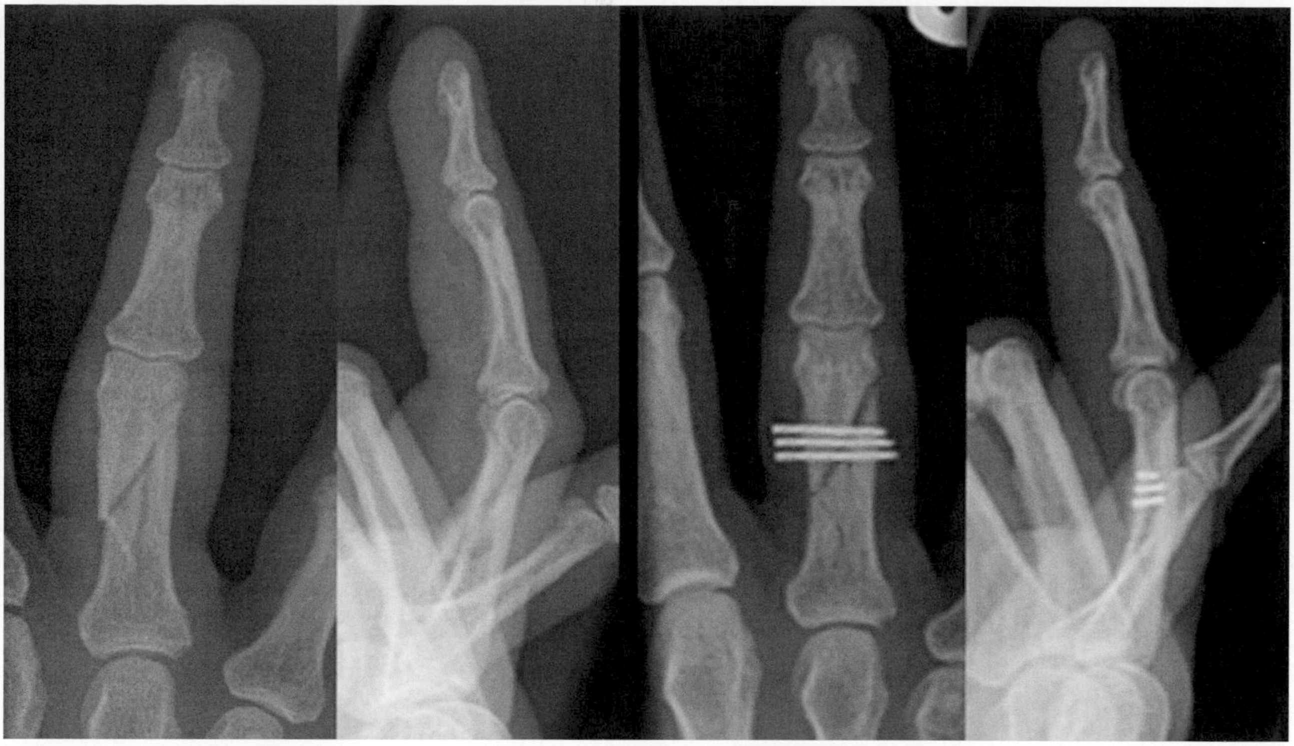

Fig. 12.28.13 Closed reduction and percutaneous K-wiring of a long oblique fracture of the proximal phalanx.

reduction, tend to redisplace and are a common cause of rotational malunion. Long oblique fractures may produce a bone spike which blocks proximal interphalangeal joint flexion (Figure 12.28.7). These fractures may be treated satisfactorily by closed reduction and K-wire fixation (Figure 12.28.13), or open reduction and lag screw fixation (Figure 12.28.14) with similar outcomes (Horton et al., 2003). Percutaneous K-wiring under radiographic control is not as easy as it may appear as the phalangeal shaft cortices are thick. Lag screw fixation is readily complicated by proximal interphalangeal joint fixed flexion deformities which can cause cosmetic deformity and loss of function, but are not usually severe if appropriate rehabilitation is provided.

Phalangeal neck fractures. Fractures of the neck of the proximal phalanx in adults are almost always transverse and can be treated non operatively by closed reduction and immobilization in the Edinburgh position which is modified slightly to incorporate slight flexion of the proximal interphalangeal joint (Figure 12.28.15). However these injuries often occur in young children who have caught the finger in the hinge-side of a door and these cannot be safely managed non-operatively due to poor compliance and chubby small fingers. These injuries will not remodel as they are away from the growth plate. Closed reduction and percutaneous K-wire fixation which transfixes the proximal interphalangeal joint is recommended in this situation. If the child presents late (more than 1 week, then it may be impossible to manipulate the fracture back into normal alignments, but an open reduction can usually be avoided by inserting a green hypodermic needle into the fracture (introduced dorsally) and using this to lever the distal fragment back into place: the fracture can then be K-wired (Figure 12.28.16).

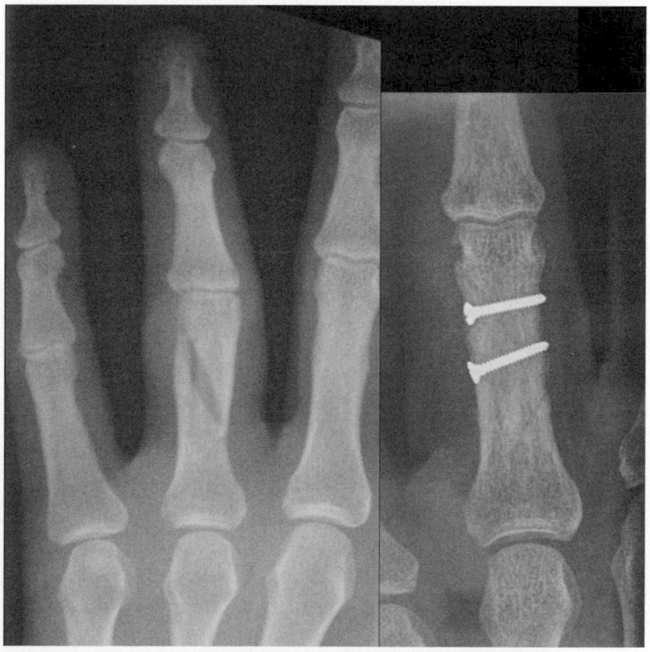

Fig. 12.28.14 Open reduction and lag screw fixation of a spiral fracture of the proximal phalanx.

Extra-articular distal phalangeal fractures

These can involve the tuft or the metaphysis. Tuft fractures are usually caused by crush injuries and often have associated painful subungual haematoma. These fractures should be treated conservatively though associated soft-tissue injuries (nailbed and skin lacerations) may require surgery and painful subungual haematoma should be

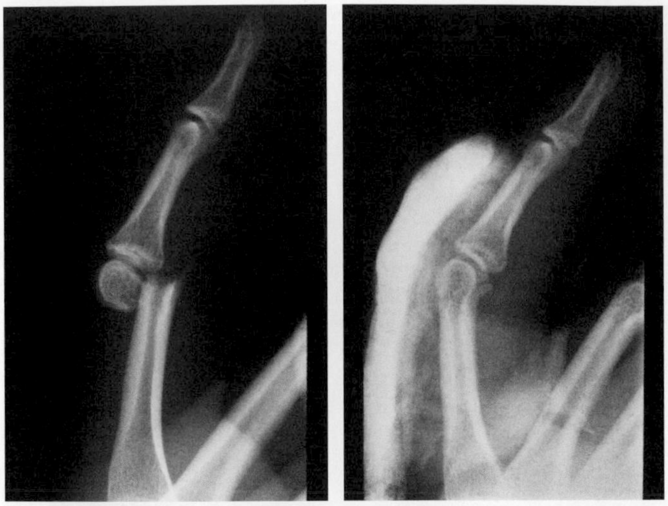
A B

Fig. 12.28.15 Fracture of the neck of the proximal phalanx. This was treated by closed reduction and placement in a dorsal splint which held the metacarpophalangeal joint flexed (60 degrees) and prevented full proximal interphalangeal joint extension. The interphalangeal joints could be flexed within this splint which was worn for 3 weeks.

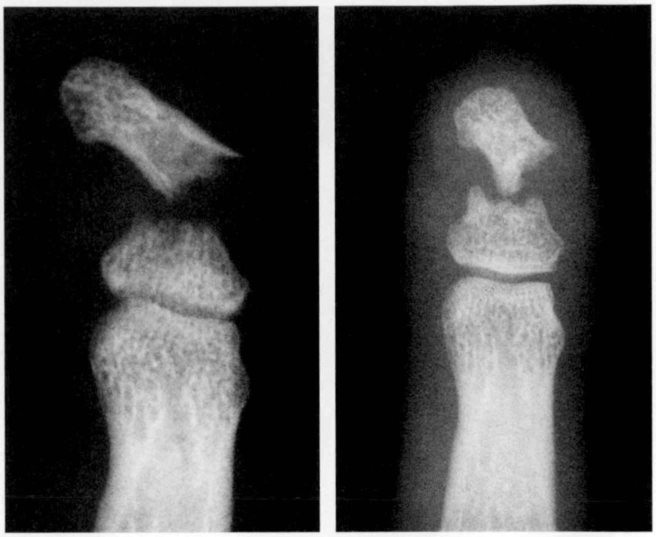
A B

Fig. 12.28.17 A) This fracture of the distal phalanx was not reduced and B) progressed to a painful non-union.

drained. They are best treated by early mobilization but can be splinted for 1 or 2 weeks if very painful.

Metaphyseal fractures also usually occur following crush injuries and again overlying nailbed injuries are common. If undisplaced, these fractures should be treated by early mobilization. If displaced, these fractures should be reduced in order to prevent cosmetic deformity and abnormal nail growth, and reduce the risk of non union (Figure 12.28.17). The reduction can usually be maintained by a dorsal or palmar splint though some prefer percutaneous K-wires.

Intra-articular fractures

Joint stiffness, joint instability, and post-traumatic osteoarthritis are specific complications of intra-articular fractures. These complications, as well as fracture alignment and stability, should always

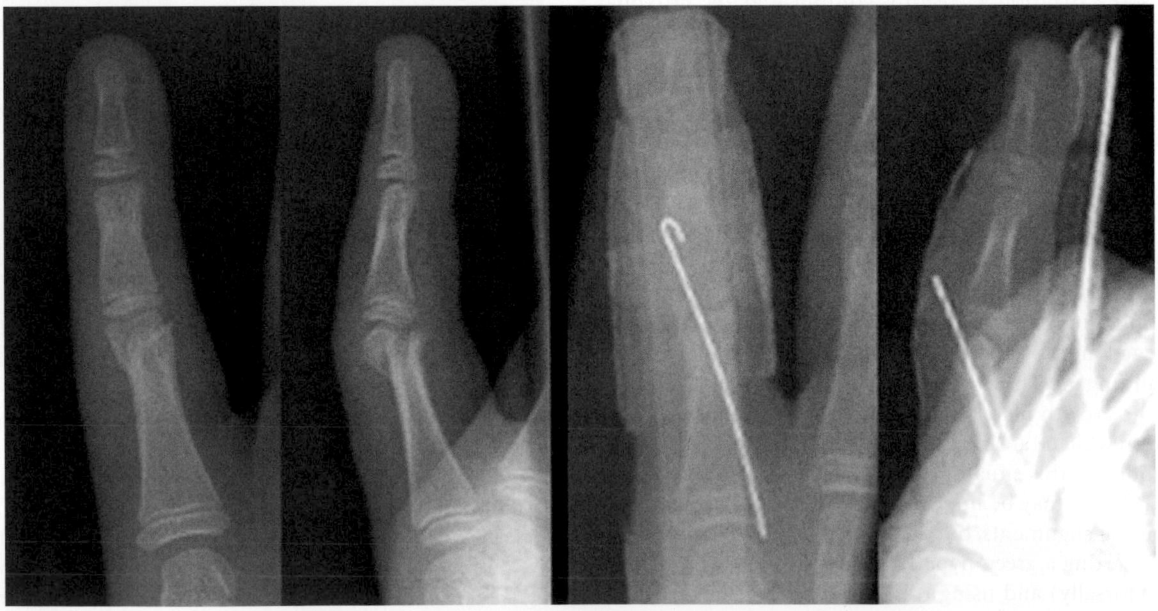

Fig. 12.28.16 Fracture of the neck of the proximal phalanx in a child who presented 1 week after injury. The fracture could still be levered back into position with a hypodermic needle which was inserted into the fracture.

Box 12.28.1 Non-articular fractures—general principles

- Beware of rotational deformity
- A malunion following conservative management is usually easier to treat than a stiff joint after operative fixation
- Metacarpals angulate palmarly; proximal phalanges angulate dorsally
- Metacarpals are more tolerant of deformity than phalanges
- The ring and little metacarpals are more tolerant of deformity than the index and middle metacarpals.

be considered when planning the treatment of intra-articular fractures. Furthermore, the likely outcomes of non-operative treatment (early mobilization or splintage) and operative fixation should be compared and the feasibility of worthwhile fracture fixation should be assessed.

As a general rule, the thumb and finger carpometacarpal, metacarpophalangeal, and distal interphalangeal joints tolerate articular incongruity reasonably well and rarely develop troublesome post-traumatic osteoarthritis or stiffness. In contrast, troublesome post-traumatic osteoarthritis and stiffness are well-recognized complications of some intra-articular fractures of the proximal interphalangeal joint.

Trapeziometacarpal joint fractures

Bennett's fracture of the thumb metacarpal is a two-part fracture–dislocation of the trapeziometacarpal joint without significant articular comminution (Figure 12.28.18). The palmar metacarpal fragment retains its attachment to the strong ulnar ligament of the thumb trapeziometacarpal joint and thus joint stability is restored following fracture union in anatomic alignment. Although Bennett's fractures are easily reduced thumb traction and abduction, the reduction is unstable and redisplacement often occurs if the fracture is treated conservatively in a Bennett's plaster. Such malunion causes persistent stiffness, weakness and pain and these fractures are more reliably treated by closed reduction and percutaneous K-wiring. The K-wire(s) may either pass between the bases of the thumb and the index finger or across the trapeziometacarpal joint. The thumb should then be immobilized in a scaphoid plaster for 4–6 weeks, thus allowing fracture union in good alignment. Of thumbs treated in this manner 80% are painless at 6-year follow-up and few of the remaining 20% experience significant pain or disability. However, 50% have radiological post-traumatic arthritis.

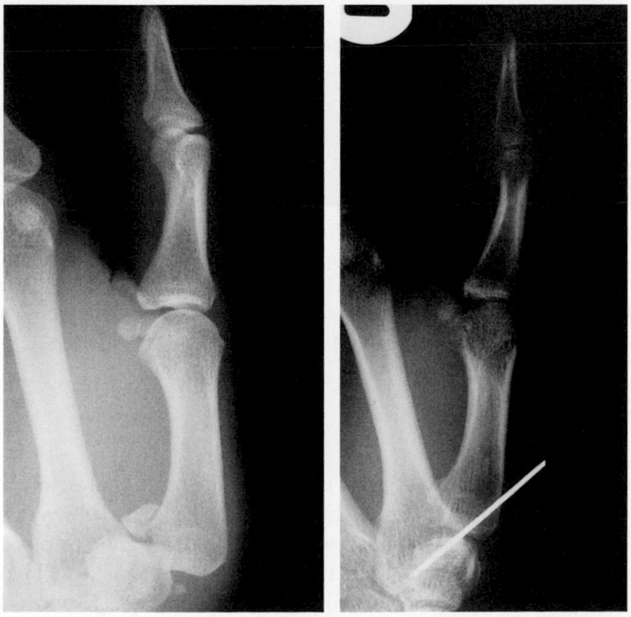

A B

Fig. 12.28.18 A) Bennett's fracture treated by B) closed reduction and percutaneous K-wiring.

For Bennett's fractures with large palmar fragments, open reduction and lag screw fixation is not inappropriate, though care must be taken not to damage sensory branches of the radial nerve or the palmar cutaneous branch of the median nerve.

Intra-articular fractures of the base of the thumb metacarpal with articular comminution are more difficult to treat. If the articular congruity and fracture alignment are reasonable, cast immobilization for 3 weeks may be the best option. Displaced fractures with two main articular fragments (Rolando's fracture) can be treated by open reduction and internal fixation with either K-wires or a T-plate. If there is a metaphyseal defect caused by cancellous bone impaction, this should be bone grafted. Operative fixation of these fractures is never simple and becomes technically much more demanding with increasing comminution. Ligamentotaxis using a small external fixator attached to the thumb and index metacarpal shafts is a worthwhile option for fractures with severe comminution.

Fractures of the base of the little finger metacarpal with carpometacarpal joint subluxation are similar to the Bennett's fractures. The small radial fragment retains the strong intermetacarpal ligament attachment and the little finger metacarpal base displaces ulnarly or, more usually, dorsally. Axial traction on the little finger readily reduces these fractures, which can then be stabilized with percutaneous K-wires which is passed through the base of the little finger metacarpal, either into the hamate bone or the ring metacarpal base.

Metacarpophalangeal joint fractures

Metacarpal head fractures

These usually occur as a result of an axial force (punch) and are most common in the index finger. Unless there is a large articular step (not gap), these fractures can be treated by active early mobilization with good results. If there is considerable articular incongruity and a single large fracture fragment (usually a palmar fragment), open reduction and internal fixation is indicated. However, many of these fractures are comminuted and difficult to fix as the bone is thin and friable. For such fractures conservative management with early mobilization is probably prudent.

Fractures of the base of the proximal phalanx

Collateral ligament avulsion fractures from the bases of finger proximal phalanges usually involve less than one-third of the articular surface. Such fractures should be mobilized in buddy strapping without fear of subsequent joint instability as persistent symptoms are unusual. Displaced avulsion fractures with larger

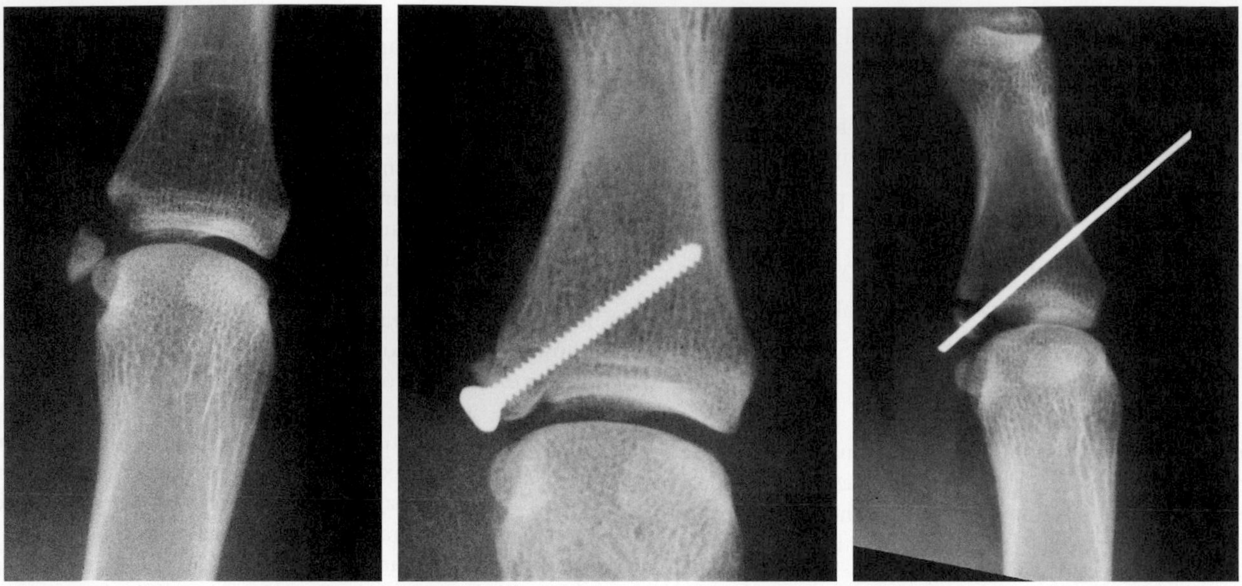

Fig. 12.28.19 Displaced avulsion fractures of the ulnar collateral ligament of the thumb metacarpophalangeal joint. These can be treated by open reduction and lag screw or by K-wire fixation.

articular fragments (more than 30% of the articular surface) should be treated by open reduction (palmar approach) and internal fixation, using either a K-wire or a lag screw.

Avulsion fractures of the thumb ulnar collateral ligament with less than 3mm of displacement can be satisfactorily treated by immobilization in a scaphoid-type plaster for 3 weeks. Avulsion fractures with greater displacement or marked rotation should be treated by open reduction and internal fixation, using a K-wire or a single lag screw if the fragment is sufficiently large (Figure 12.28.19). Avulsion fractures of the thumb radial collateral ligament are treated conservatively unless they involve a large portion of the articular surface. This rationale for treatment is based on the fact that ulnar collateral ligament stability is vital for pinch grip whereas radial collateral ligament stability is not critical to thumb function.

Proximal interphalangeal joint

Condylar fractures of the proximal phalanx

There is almost universal agreement that displaced unicondylar fractures of the proximal phalanx are best treated by open reduction and internal fixation. These fractures usually have no axial stability and, if treated conservatively, almost inevitably unite with shortening and palmar or dorsal displacement. This causes a radial/ulnar angulation when the finger is extended and a rotational deformity when it is flexed. The unicondylar fracture fragment is usually sufficiently large to permit open reduction and internal fixation with a 1.5-mm or smaller lag screw (Figure 12.28.20) which should be placed just proximal to the origin of the collateral ligament. Alternatively, these fractures may also be stabilized with one or two K-wires. Proximal interphalangeal joint movement is usually slightly diminished following unicondylar fracture fixation and a 10-degree fixed flexion deformity and an 80-degree arc of flexion are typical.

Bicondylar fractures of the proximal phalanx require careful assessment. If the general alignment of the proximal interphalangeal joint is reasonable and there is no angular or rotational deformity, the position of the fracture can be accepted. The finger is then rested in the Edinburgh position for 3 weeks. Surprisingly good results can be achieved with this method though most surgeons now favour open reduction and internal fixation using multiple K-wires, lag screws, or even a condylar blade plate. The best treatment method varies from fracture to fracture and some loss of proximal interphalangeal joint movement is to be expected.

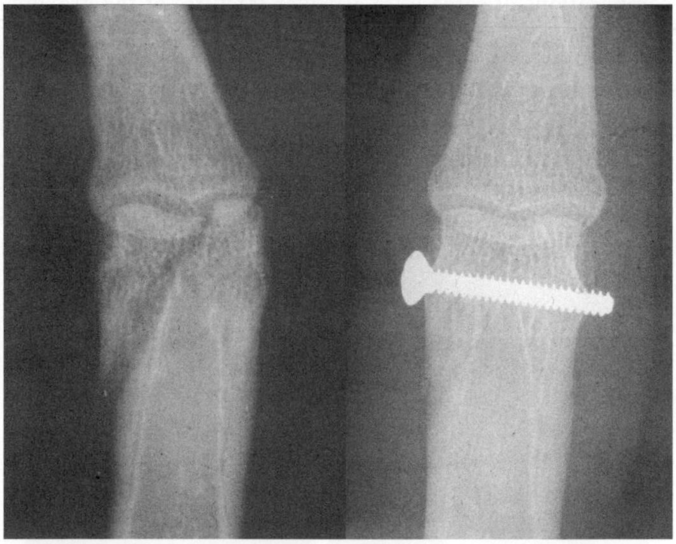

Fig. 12.28.20 Displaced unicondylar fracture of the proximal phalanx of a finger. If this is not stabilized the fracture fragment may displace further in a proximal direction as the fracture configuration has little axial stability. If allowed to unite with displacement it will cause an angular deformity and stiffness of the proximal interphalangeal joint. Lag screw fixation is demanding but permits early mobilization.

Intra-articular fractures of the base of the middle phalanx

These fractures can be classified as follows:

- Dorsal avulsion fractures of the central slip
- Palmar lip fractures with or without dorsal subluxation of the proximal interphalangeal joint
- Impaction fracture.

Dorsal avulsion fractures

These are avulsion fractures of the central slip of the extensor mechanism and they often allow palmar dislocation of the proximal interphalangeal joint. If the fracture fragment is sufficiently large, open reduction and internal fixation may be performed, especially if the proximal interphalangeal joint is dislocated and the reduction is unstable. A 1.5-mm or smaller lag screw or a K-wire can be used though care must be taken not to split the fracture fragment as the dorsal cortex is thin and the fragments are small (Figure 12.28.21). Smaller fracture fragments are treated with good results by splinting the proximal interphalangeal joint in extension for 3 weeks. However, radiographs should always be obtained with the finger in the splint in order to ensure that the fracture fragment lies in reasonable alignment and the joint, if previously dislocated, remains congruent.

Palmar lip fractures

Small palmar avulsion fractures without associated proximal interphalangeal joint subluxation or dislocation are caused by hyperextension injuries. These are treated by early mobilization but the patient should be warned that the proximal interphalangeal joint may remain swollen and tender for many months. Full finger flexion will only be regained once the swelling has settled, and there may be a permanent fixed-flexion deformity of the proximal interphalangeal joint.

Larger palmar lip fractures of the base of the middle phalanx cause dorsal subluxation of the proximal interphalangeal joint and are often comminuted with impacted central articular fragments (Figure 12.28.22). These injuries are caused by axial compression forces and are frequently inflicted by cricket or basket balls. Their prognosis depends on patient motivation, the degree of fracture comminution, and the percentage of the articular surface which is damaged. The proximal interphalangeal joint readily reduces with traction and flexion and the injury is then stable, provided that extension of the proximal interphalangeal joint is restricted. This can be achieved with extension block splintage, percutaneous K-wiring, dynamic traction or external fixation of the proximal interphalangeal joint. Some surgeons favour open reduction and internal fixation of these fractures, particularly those with more than 50% involvement of the articular surface, but this is complex surgery which is not always successful. Extension block splints are worn for 4–6 weeks and the results for fractures involving less than 30% of the articular surface are usually good This treatment method works well in motivated patients, but requires careful follow-up to ensure that the proximal interphalangeal joint does not resublux within the splint. Percutaneous K-wiring of the proximal interphalangeal joint in sufficient flexion to reduce the dorsal subluxation requires less patient cooperation. The K-wire is removed after 4 weeks and the finger is then actively mobilized, producing satisfactory outcomes. A few of these fracture–subluxations resublux after the K-wire, external fixator, or extension block splint is removed. All treatment methods usually produce a painless stable proximal interphalangeal joint which flexes to 90 degrees though has a 10–30 degrees fixed

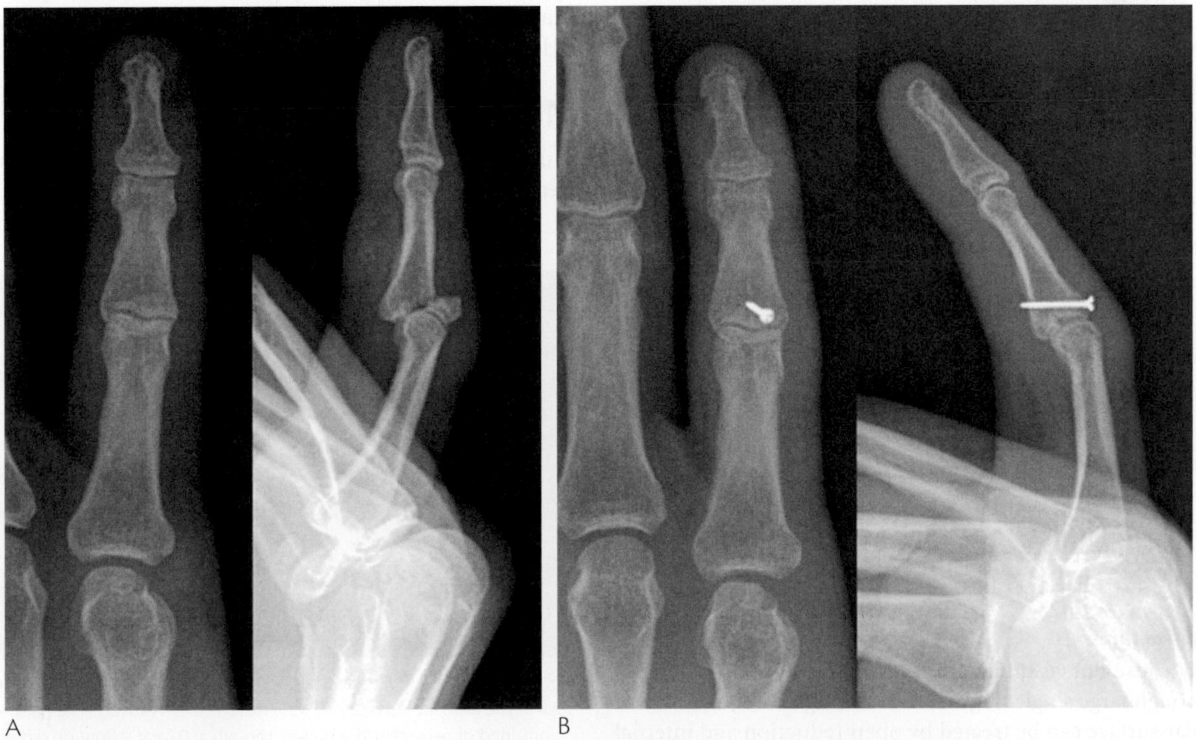

Fig. 12.28.21 A) Fracture of the base of the middle phalanx with displaced dorsal lip fragment. B) This was internally fixed and a good result was achieved.

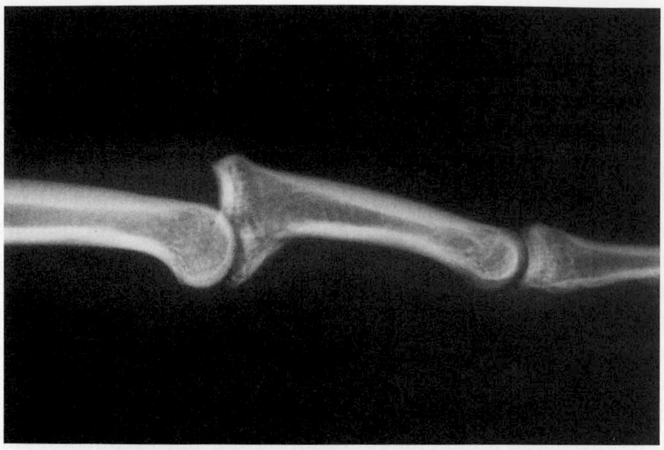

A

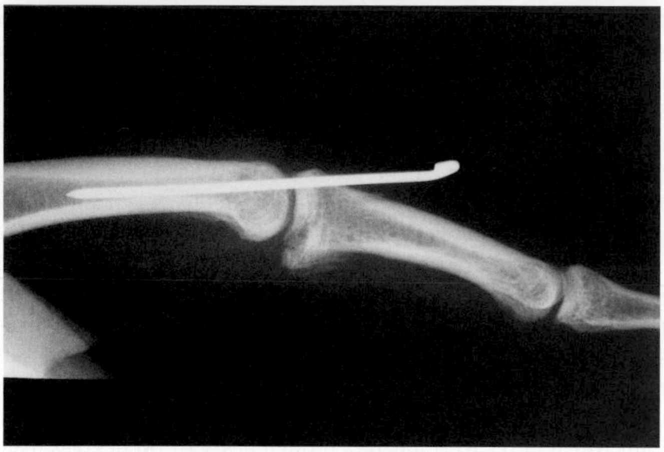

B

Fig. 12.28.22 A) Fracture of the base of the middle phalanx with dorsal subluxation of the proximal interphalangeal joint. B) This was treated by closed reduction and percutaneous K-wiring.

flexion deformity. The long-term results of non-operative treatment of these injuries are not as bad as may be anticipated and considerable joint remodelling can occur.

Distal interphalangeal joint fractures

Condylar fractures of the middle phalanx

These are treated in the same manner as those of the proximal phalanx.

Intra-articular fractures of the base of the distal phalanx

These can be classified as follows:

- Avulsion fractures of the flexor digitorum profundus insertion (covered in Chapter 12.22)
- Palmar lip fractures (avulsion fractures of the palmar plate)
- Avulsion fractures of the extensor expansion (mallet fractures)
- Other intra-articular fractures.

Palmar lip fractures

These may cause dorsal subluxation of the distal interphalangeal joint. Although large single fragments involving more than 30% of the articular surface can be treated by open reduction and internal fixation, the majority of these fractures have small fracture fragments and any associated joint subluxation can be reduced by splinting the distal interphalangeal joint in flexion for 4 weeks.

Mallet fractures

Mallet fractures can cause palmar subluxation of the distal interphalangeal joint (Figure 12.28.23). Their treatment is controversial but those with a fracture fragment which involves less than a third of the articular surface and no associated joint subluxation are reliably treated conservatively by splinting the distal interphalangeal joint in extension for 4–6 weeks. This is most easily achieved with a polyethylene Stack splint or thermoplastic which must be worn continuously. There is usually soreness at the fracture site for several months but this almost always resolves. Larger fracture fragments can also be successfully treated conservatively and some consider that this is also the treatment of choice for fractures with associated distal interphalangeal joint subluxation. Others consider that the presence of joint subluxation necessitates operative fixation, either with a lag screw or K-wires (Figure 12.28.24). Although there is a trend towards lag screw fixation of large fragment fractures, there is no evidence that this produces a better result than splintage, and the screw head is relatively bulky and the overlying skin is thin such that wound problems may occur. This is also discussed in Chapter 12.23.

Other intra-articular fractures

Most other intra-articular fractures of the distal phalanx are impacted and have small fragments. These should be treated conservatively with active mobilization as symptomatic post-traumatic osteoarthritis is unusual.

Open fractures

Open metacarpal and phalangeal fractures should be treated as other open fractures, with thorough soft tissue irrigation and debridement and fracture stabilization so that the damaged soft tissues can be inspected and gently mobilized. External fixation is particularly useful for these fractures.

Multiple hand fractures

Multiple fractures in unsatisfactory alignment are usually best treated by operative fixation, especially if there is more than one

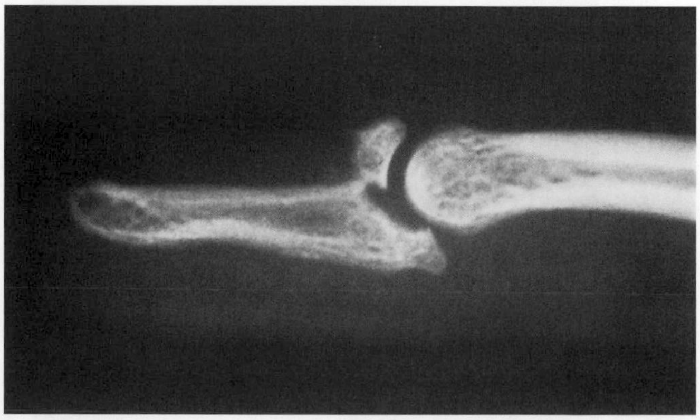

Fig. 12.28.23 This mallet fracture with palmar subluxation involved more than 50% of the articular surface but was treated conservatively. The patient complained of persistent discomfort though at 2-year follow-up did not consider this sufficiently severe to warrant surgery.

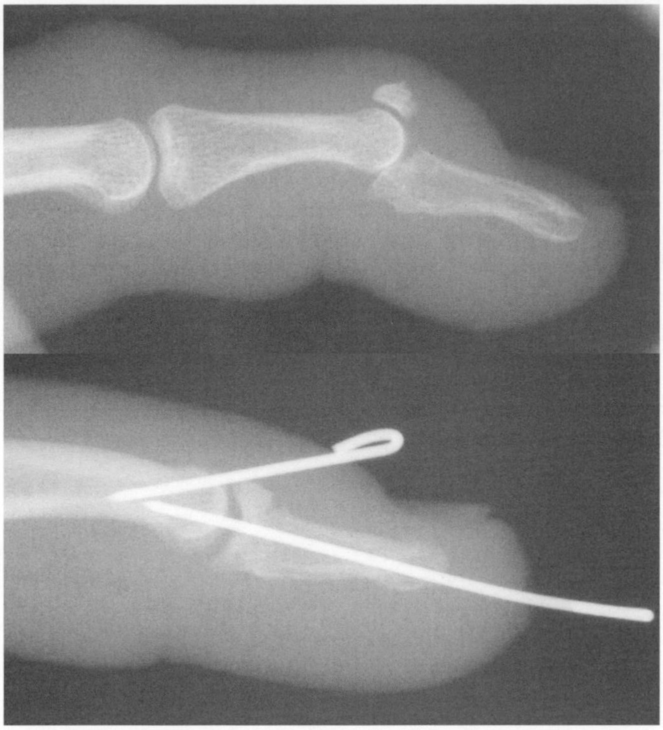

Fig. 12.28.24 Mallet fracture causing palmar subluxation of the distal interphalangeal joint. It was treated closed by flexion of the joint and placement of a K-wire in the head of the middle phalanx such that it passed dorsal to the avulsion fracture fragment and prevented it from extending and migrating dorsally. The main fracture fragment was then reduced onto the avulsion fragment and it and the distal interphalangeal joint were transfixed with another K-wire.

Box 12.28.2 Intra-articular fractures—general principles

- Troublesome post-traumatic osteoarthritis and stiffness are most common at proximal interphalangeal joint
- Carpometacarpal, metacarpophalangeal, and distal interphalangeal joints tolerate articular incongruity well
- Bennett's fractures and little finger carpometacarpal fracture-subluxations require reduction and pinning
- Unicondylar fractures of the proximal phalanx are treated with open reduction and internal fixation
- Beware of joint subluxation in palmar and dorsal lip fractures of the base of the middle phalanx.

fracture in each ray or each ray contains a different type of fracture. This is because it is difficult to manipulate and maintain multiple fracture reductions with conservative methods.

Metacarpal and phalangeal fractures in children

These fractures heal more rapidly than their adult counterparts. Although dorsal/palmar angular malunion may improve with remodelling during growth if the fracture is in the midshaft or at the end of the bone containing the growth plate, radial/ulnar and rotational malunion do not improve with growth.

In general, paediatric hand fractures should be treated in a similar manner to adult fractures. However, most extra-articular fractures which require operative fixation can be managed with K-wires and plate fixation is rarely indicated.

Complications

The major complications of metacarpal and phalangeal fractures are as follows:

- Malunion (rotational or angular) causing loss of hand function
- Finger stiffness
- Post-traumatic osteoarthritis
- Non-union.

Malunion

If a rotational deformity is detected within 8 weeks of injury, it is usually possible to take the fracture down and internally fix it in satisfactory alignment with K-wires or a plate. However, this is difficult surgery and the patient should be warned of the risks of osteotomy non-union and finger stiffness. A safer option, which should be used for rotational deformities detected after 8 weeks, is to regain full finger movement, allow the fracture to unite, and then perform a rotational osteotomy, either through the base of the fractured bone or through the base of the finger's metacarpal. The latter can be stabilized either with K-wires or a small plate, and is most unlikely to be complicated by finger stiffness.

Angular malunions which interfere with finger function are treated with a corrective osteotomy at the fracture site.

Finger stiffness

This can either be due to joint contracture or tendon adhesions and both can complicate either conservative treatment or operative fixation. Loss of finger extension, unless severe, usually causes little disability. Loss of finger flexion is much more disabling and can cause loss of dexterity and hand weakness, especially if it causes quadriga.

Stiffness due to joint contractures results in equal losses of active and passive movement. In stiffness due to tendon adhesions, the range of passive movement exceeds the range of active movement.

Joint contractures are difficult to treat but should initially be managed with physiotherapy and splintage. If this fails then surgical release of the contracted joint capsule and ligaments may be indicated, but the results of this surgery are unpredictable. In severe cases, the patient may be best managed with an amputation.

Tendon adhesions are also initially treated with vigorous physiotherapy. If they persist, a tenolysis should be performed once the fracture has firmly united. Postoperatively, the patient undergoes an intense course of physiotherapy.

Post-traumatic osteoarthritis

The treatment of this condition, if symptomatic, is no different from that of other types of osteoarthritis.

Fracture non-union

Fracture non-union is rare in metacarpal and phalangeal fractures, even though radiographic evidence of fracture union takes many weeks to develop. However, fractures which are treated operatively and fixed with distraction, frequently develop non-union. Non-union, if symptomatic, is treated by internal fixation and bone grafting.

Further reading

Aladin, A. and Davis, T.R. (2005). Dorsal fracture-dislocation of the proximal interphalangeal joint: a comparative study of percutaneous Kirschner wire fixation versus open reduction and internal fixation. *Journal of Hand Surg*ery, **30B**, 120–8.

Glickel, S.Z., Barron, O.A., and Catalano, III. L.W. (2005). Dislocations and ligament injuries in the digits: In: Green, D.P., Hotchkiss, R.N., Pederson, W.C., and Wolfe, S.C. (eds) *Green's Operative Hand Surgery*, fifth edition, pp. 342–88. Philadelphia, PA: Elsevier.

Hamer, D.W. and Quinton, D.N. (1992). Dorsal fracture subluxation of the proximal interphalangeal joints treated by extension block splintage. *Journal of Hand Surg*ery, **17B**, 586–90.

Stern, P.J. (2005). Fractures of the metacarpals and phalanges. In: Green, D.P., Hotchkiss, R.N., Pederson, W.C., and Wolfe, S.C. (eds) *Green's Operative Hand Surgery*, fifth edition, pp. 277–341. Philadelphia, PA: Elsevier.

Weiss, A.P. and Hastings, H. (1993). Distal unicondylar fractures of the proximal phalanx. *Journal of Hand Surgery*, **18A**, 594–9.

12.29

Scaphoid fractures

Simon Tan and Mike Craigen

Summary points

- Commonest fracture in the wrist
- Immobilization and serial X-ray is no longer the preferred method of management – use MRI scan
- Trend towards more frequent fixation especially displaced proximal fractures
- Untreated non-union leads to arthritis and pain
- Non-unions treated with bone grafting +/- fixation.

Essentials

The scaphoid is the most commonly fractured carpal bone. The typical patient is a young male. The bone is largely articular and has a tenuous vascular supply to its proximal pole. The scaphoid geometry and orientation make it difficult to interpret on radiographs and fractures can be occult on plain films. The practice of immobilization followed by delayed radiographic examination is ineffective and inconvenient to the patient. Magnetic resonance imaging (MRI) offers a cost effective, early diagnostic alternative. Non-displaced waist fractures are effectively treated non-operatively but there is a trend towards operative fixation. Displaced fractures and proximal pole fractures are unstable and operative fixation is preferable in such cases.

Scaphoid non-union is diagnosed if healing has not occurred 6 months from injury. Presentation may frequently be late. Proximal fractures are more prone to non-union. The eventual outcome of untreated non-union is osteoarthritis and pain, although these may not occur for some time. The success of surgical treatment is dependent on the site of the non-union, the age of the non-union, and the presence of avascular changes in the proximal fragment. Standard treatment involves bone grafting with or without internal fixation. Vascularized bone grafts are gaining in popularity, particularly when bone grafting has already failed once and when avascular necrosis (AVN) is present.

A predictable pattern of degenerative change is seen following established scaphoid non-union (scaphoid non-union advanced collapse or SNAC). Several different options for surgical salvage of advanced degeneration are described.

Introduction

Scaphoid fractures tend to occur in young and active patients, many of who are uniquely dependent on the integrity of upper limb function for work and sport. The trauma specialist managing these injuries should be confident in their diagnosis, initial management and management of medium- and long-term complications.

Incidence

Not everyone with a scaphoid fracture will seek medical opinion and the true incidence is impossible to ascertain. The diagnosis is commonly made speculatively in patients presenting with wrist pain following an injury and the actual number of patients with scaphoid fracture is probably less than one might expect. For the average district general hospital serving about 250 000 people, the incidence is about 35 per year or fewer than one per week.

This said, the scaphoid is still by far the most commonly fractured (Box 12.29.1) carpal bone accounting for 60% of carpal fractures. In Bergen, Norway, the annual incidence is 4.3/10 000 people; 82% of scaphoid fractures occur in males, with a mean age of 25 years. The incidence for men is highest between the ages of 20–30 years and decreases rapidly after this age. Incidence for men is significantly higher than the corresponding rates for women up to 50 years of age, whereas over the age of 60 the rates for men and women are similar.

In the United Kingdom, approximately 70% of scaphoid fractures occur at the waist, 20% at the distal pole, and 10% at the proximal pole. The fracture is rare in children and when present occurs most commonly in the distal pole.

Box 12.29.1 Scaphoid fracture

- Most commonly fractured carpal bone
- More common in males (82%)
- Most common between age 20–30 years
- 70% occur at the waist, 20% at the distal pole, and 10% at the proximal pole.

Anatomy

The term scaphoid derives from the Greek word skaphe meaning boat. It is the only bone that bridges the two carpal rows and creates a mechanical linkage between them (Box 12.29.2). Conventionally the bone is divided into three basic regions—proximal pole, waist and distal pole.

Three of the six surfaces of the scaphoid are articular. The distal surface articulates with the trapezoid and trapezium, its medial surface with both capitate and lunate, and its proximal convexity articulates with a corresponding concave fossa on the distal radial surface, the scaphoid fossa. The waist represents a non-articular strip, devoid of articular hyaline cartilage, and macroscopically is seen as a roughened ridge of bare bone. It forms a helix winding from the proximal end of the dorsal surface, around the lateral surface and terminating at the base of the tubercle volarly (Figure 12.29.1).

Blood supply

The scaphoid waist has consistently been shown to be the site of multiple vascular foraminae, which serve as entry portals for feeding arteries. Obletz and Halbstein's (1938) study of nearly 300 cadaveric specimens showed that the largest foraminae occur in the distal half of the bone. Thirteen per cent of scaphoids had no perforations in the proximal half of the bone and a further 20% had only a single foramen at or proximal to the waist (Figure 12.29.2).

The major blood supply to the scaphoid arises variably from the radial artery and its superficial palmar branch, although additional anastomosis from the anterior interosseous artery is described. The main feeding vessels enter the bone along the waist. The distal portion of the scaphoid has reliable direct arterial inflow, whereas the proximal pole is supplied by intra-osseous retrograde flow. Fractures of the scaphoid waist can disrupt the tenuous flow to the proximal pole.

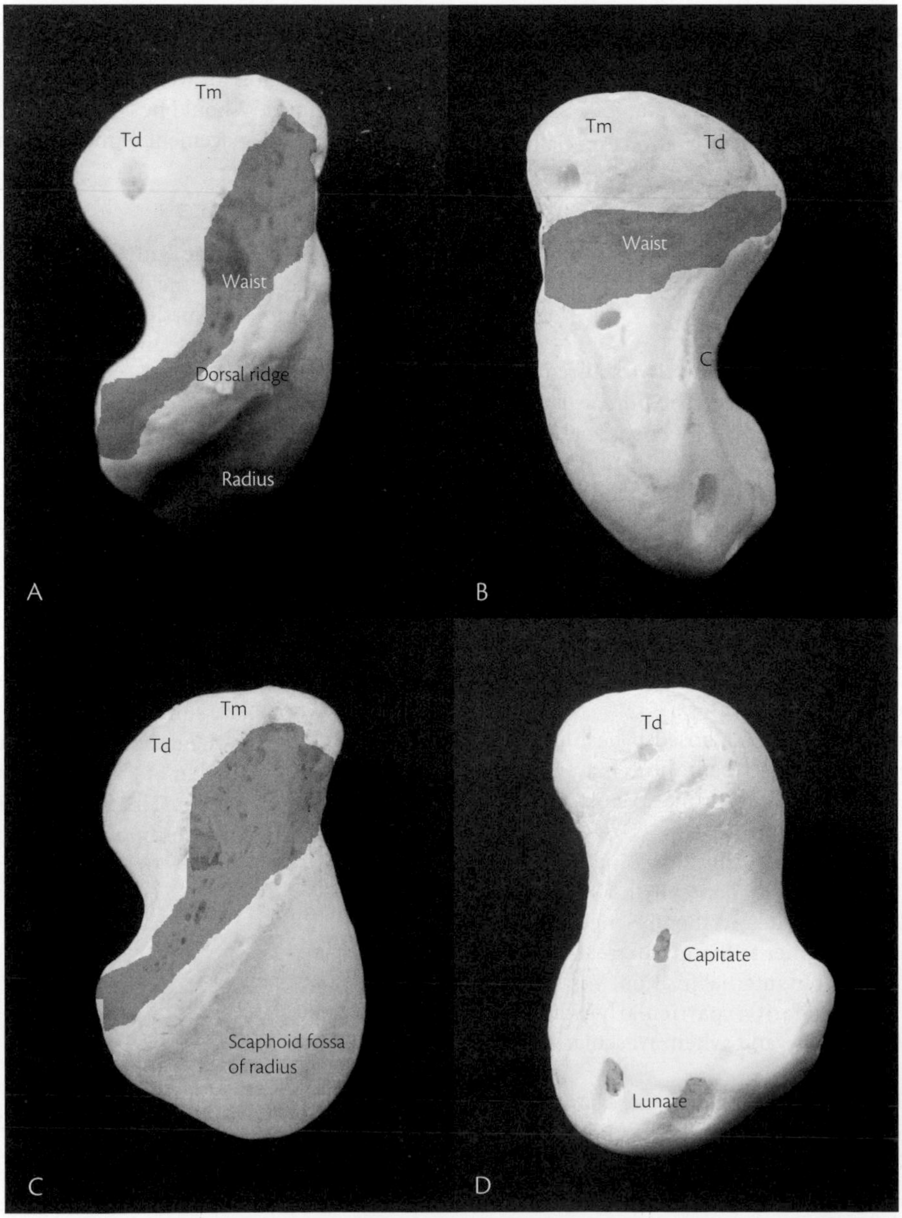

Fig. 12.29.1 Scaphoid anatomy. A left scaphoid as seen from: A) dorsal; B) volar; (c) lateral; and (d) medial. The articular surfaces are labelled: Tm, trapezium; Td, trapezoid and C, capitate. The waist (shaded area) represents a non-articular strip, which is devoid of articular hyaline cartilage and macroscopically can be seen as a roughened ridge of bare bone.

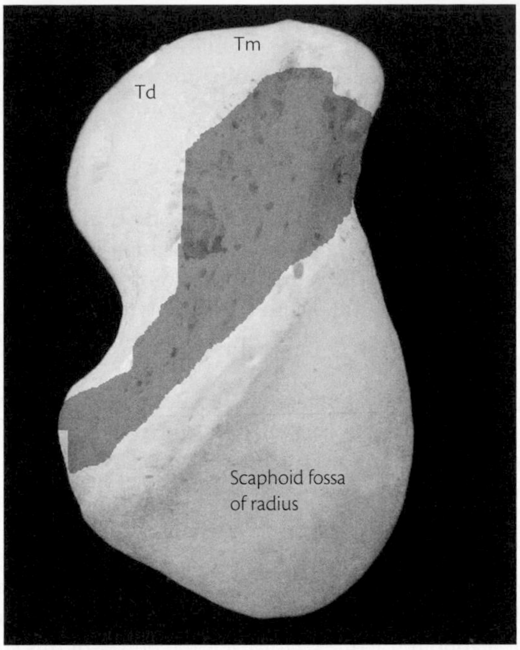

Fig. 12.29.2 The scaphoid waist is the site of multiple vascular foramina, which serve as entry portals for feeding arteries. Arterial foramina are seen here occurring at or distal to the scaphoid waist.

Ligaments

In bridging the proximal and distal carpal rows, the scaphoid spans both the lunate and capitate. Three important intrinsic ligaments secure it: the scapholunate ligament, the scaphotrapezial, and scaphocapitate ligaments. The most important of these is the scapholunate ligament connecting the proximal scaphoid pole to the adjacent lunate. The ligament prevents excessive scaphoid flexion and pronation, and lunate extension.

Wrist kinematics

The proximal carpal row (scaphoid, lunate, and triquetrum) has no direct musculotendinous insertion onto it. Its movement is determined by the shape of its articulations and ligamentous attachments.

The movement of the scaphoid is complex and varies between individuals. During normal wrist flexion–extension the scaphoid not only flexes and extends but also rotates around its longitudinal axis. In radioulnar deviation of the wrist the scaphoid moves in both the coronal and sagittal planes. With radial deviation, the scaphoid rotates in the coronal plane such that its proximal pole translates ulnarly, and in the sagittal plane it flexes. On ulnar deviation the scaphoid rotates in the coronal plane such that its proximal pole lies more radially, and in the sagittal plane it extends. The extent to which of these motions occurs in radioulnar deviation differs between individuals. In some the scaphoid predominantly flexes and extends, whereas in others the coronal rotation is the principal movement (Figure 12.29.3).

Fracture

In the presence of an unstable waist fracture, the scaphoid proximal pole will have a tendency to extend through its strong ligamentous attachment to the adjacent lunate and the distal pole will have a tendency to flex. The deforming forces on a scaphoid fractured at its waist are thus directed to cause intra-scaphoid flexion, the so-called 'humpback' deformity. With loss of the

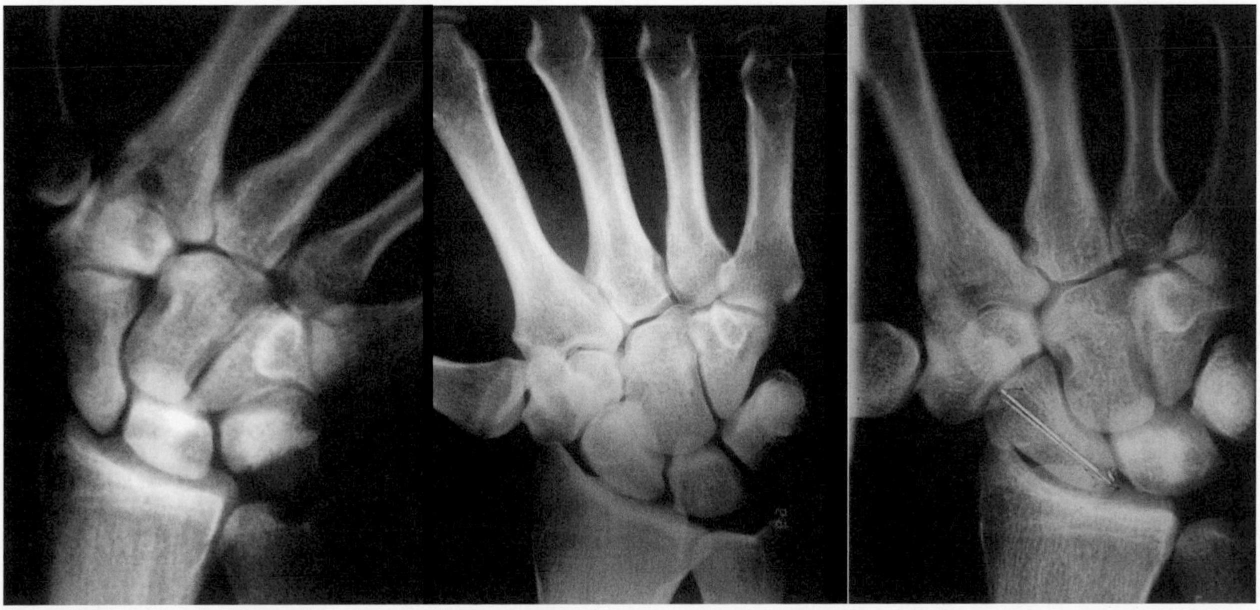

A B C

Fig. 12.29.3 PA radiographs of the wrist taken in (A) ulnar deviation and (B) radial deviation. On ulnar deviation the scaphoid 'extends' so that its long axis lies perpendicular to the x-ray beam, thus appearing longer. C) PA radiograph in a different individual demonstrating predominantly coronal rotation of the scaphoid with radial deviation.

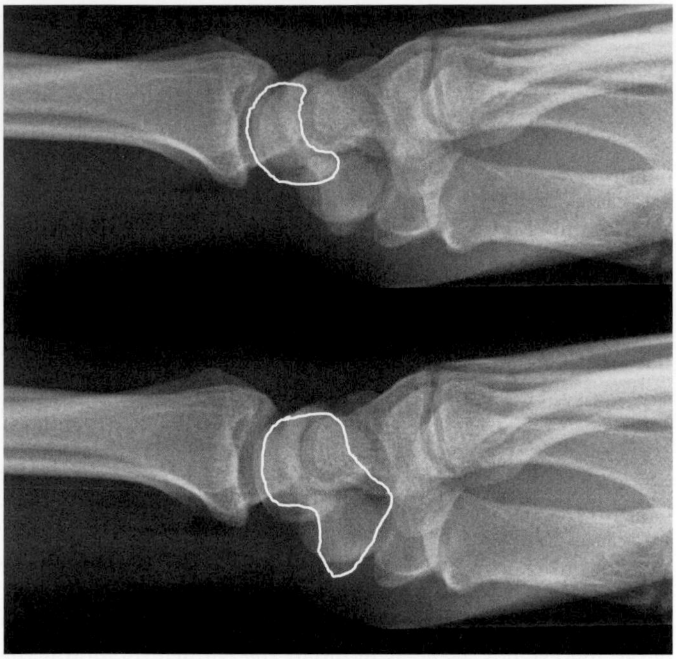

Fig. 12.29.4 DISI deformity. The lunate extends abnormally (top), and the scaphoid flexes abnormally (bottom).

Box 12.29.2 Anatomy

- Scaphoid largely covered with articular cartilage
- A helical, non-articular strip of bare bone forms the waist
- Feeding vessels enter the bone along the waist in the distal half
- Proximal pole blood supply is through intra-osseous retrograde flow
- Scaphoid bridges the proximal and distal carpal rows
- Scaphoid motion is complex.

linkage between proximal and distal carpal rows characteristic collapse of the midcarpal joint is seen (Figure 12.29.4).

In unstable fractures the distal pole of the scaphoid demonstrates relatively more movement than that seen in intact scaphoids whereas the proximal pole fragment becomes relatively fixed, and considerable motion can occur at the fracture site. This explains pseudarthrosis and cavitation seen with some non-unions and the pattern of secondary arthrosis seen with established non-unions, which is initially seen between the radial styloid and mobile distal scaphoid fragment.

Mechanism of fracture

The principle mechanism for scaphoid fracture is forceful wrist hyperextension, usually resulting from a fall onto the outstretched wrist. Less commonly a direct blow to the wrist may also cause fracture. In cadavers forceful dorsiflexion beyond 90 degrees results in carpal injuries and scaphoid fractures occur consistently if radial deviation is added. In this position the proximal scaphoid pole becomes locked between the distal radius and capitate, and the palmar ligaments supporting the proximal pole become taut adding further stabilization. The applied load at the distal pole thus generates bending forces within the scaphoid and failure occurs at the least supported portion, the waist.

Classification

Commonly, classification systems are based on the orientation of the fracture. Herbert and Fischer's classification incorporates fracture stability as well as delayed unions and non-unions. Acute injuries are divided into stable and unstable types and subgrouped according to fracture location and associated perilunate injury (Figure 12.29.5).

To date, no classification system has been shown to have satisfactory inter- and intraobserver reproducibility, and none have been able to reliably predict fracture union.

Fracture morphology is more accurately assessed with computed tomography (CT) and MRI than on plain radiographs. CT is more reliable and reproducible than plain radiographs at ruling out displacement. A correlation between displacement on MRI and fracture union has been found and a possible role for MRI in predicting union of scaphoid fractures. However, the power of this study was limited by the small number of non-unions seen, and further investigation is required.

Clinical features

The diagnosis of acute fracture of the scaphoid is suggested by the patient's age, mechanism of injury, and initial signs and symptoms. Clinical signs of scaphoid injury include: tenderness in the anatomical snuffbox, tenderness over the scaphoid tubercle, and pain on longitudinal compression of the thumb. All three signs are 100% sensitive but lack specificity. The use of these three tests in

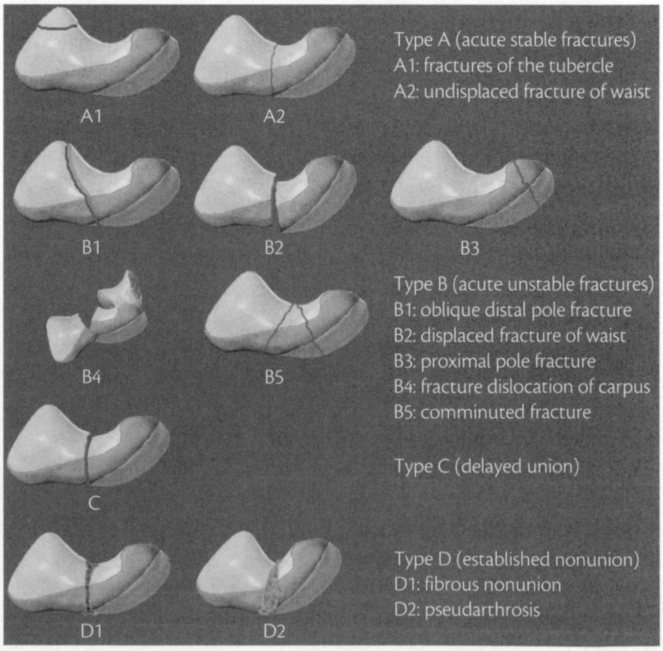

Fig. 12.29.5 Classification of scaphoid fractures described by Herbert and Fischer, 1984.

Box 12.29.3 Diagnosis

- Clinical signs lack specificity
- Up to 16% of fractures are occult on initial x-rays
- Repeat x-rays at 2 weeks are unreliable
- False positive results occur with bone scan
- MRI is sensitive and specific in fracture diagnosis
- MRI is cost effective in early definitive diagnosis following wrist injury.

combination improves specificity whilst still maintaining 100% sensitivity.

Clinical investigations

Due to its complex geometry and orientation, radiographs of the scaphoid are difficult to interpret (Box 12.29.3). A multitude of different radiographic views have been suggested for the scaphoid. Russe (1960) originally suggested four views (posteroanterior (PA), lateral and two oblique views taken in 15–20 degrees of supination and pronation respectively). Ziter (1973) popularized an ulna deviation view, which lengthens the scaphoid, and it is common to include this as a fifth view. The PA and pronation oblique are the most useful of the four Russe views in diagnosis of scaphoid fracture (Figure 12.29.6)

Although the majority of fractures are diagnosed with certainty on initial radiographs, 16% of fractures may be imperceptible on initial radiographs, the so-called occult fracture. When faced with clinical findings consistent with a scaphoid fracture but having normal-appearing x-rays, the classic teaching has been to immobilize the wrist and repeat x-rays at 10 days, and even at 3 weeks if tenderness persists. However, this practice does not improve diagnostic accuracy and is inefficient in terms of the economic impact of unnecessary immobilization, need for repeat clinical review, numerous repeat x-rays, and potential time of work.

Other imaging techniques have been proposed for detection of the occult fracture. Isotope scanning, CT, and MRI have all been shown to be useful.

The sensitivity of isotope bone scan is 100%, and a negative bone scan excludes fracture. However, bone scans are not totally specific. False positive results for fracture occur in up to 25% of scans. It is possible that 'bone bruising' is responsible for some positive bone scan results. Overtreatment of a significant proportion of patients occurs if based upon isotope bone scan results.

Diagnosis of fracture on CT relies on the presence of cortical or trabecula displacement at the site of injury and when no

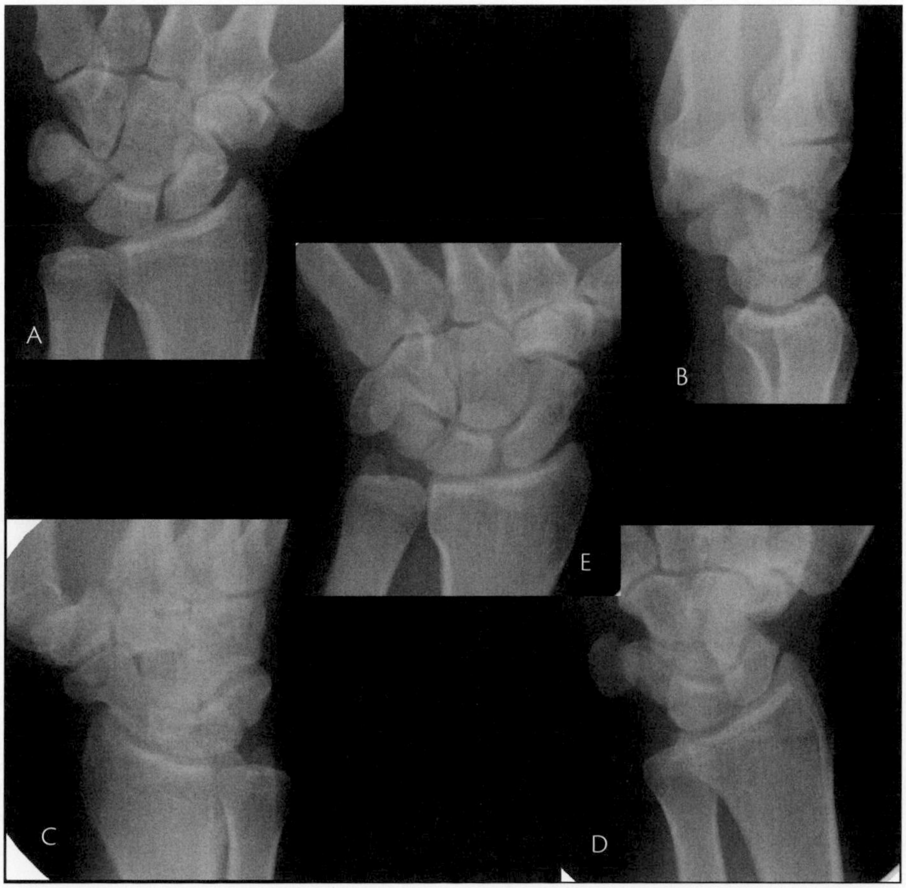

Fig. 12.29.6 Standard scaphoid views: A) PA; B) lateral; C) pronation oblique; D) supination oblique and E) ulnar deviated PA.

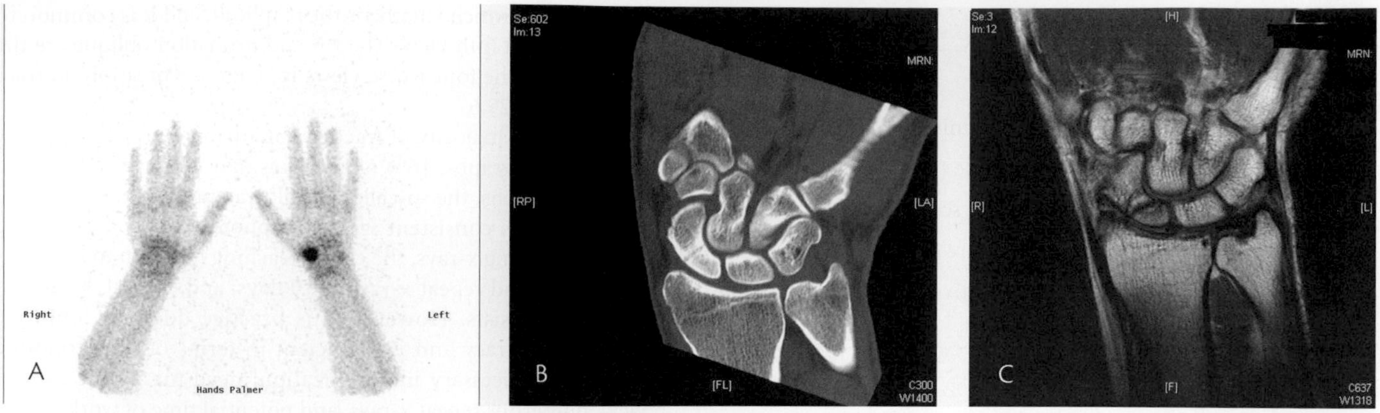

Fig. 12.29.7 Diagnosis: A) Isotope bone scan; B) coronal CT scan; and C) T_1-weighted MRI scan.

displacement is present CT can fail to identify injury which can be seen on MRI and bone scan (Figure 12.29.7).

MRI scanning is gaining in popularity as the investigation of choice when occult fracture of the scaphoid is suspected (Figure 12.29.7). Sensitivity has been reported at 100% and it is more specific than bone scan and has greater interobserver agreement in cases of fracture. MRI may highlight other bony and soft tissue pathologies that may be the underlying cause of symptoms in the patient with wrist pain following injury. Brydie has reported the largest series to date of MRI applied in routine clinical practice in suspected scaphoid injury. One hundred and ninety-five consecutive cases referred from the Accident and Emergency department with normal scaphoid series radiographs underwent MRI scanning. Scaphoid fracture was demonstrated in 19%, and in a further 19% a fracture of the distal radius or another carpal bone, not visible on plain radiographs, was demonstrated. MRI was estimated to have changed subsequent management in 92% of cases.

From a financial perspective, early MRI and conventional clinical surveillance with repeat x-rays have roughly comparable health-care costs. However, MRI is likely, overall, to be more cost effective when productivity and income loss are considered. Earlier definitive diagnosis in cases of suspected scaphoid fracture can prevent unnecessary plaster immobilization and prevent extended time off work and thus reduce on economic losses.

Treatment

Distal pole fractures (Box 12.29.4)

The distal pole is well vascularized and fractures in this area have a high rate of union.

Distal pole fractures can be extra or intra-articular. Extra-articular, distal transverse fractures are usually included with other waist of scaphoid fractures. Intra-articular fractures have been classified by Prosser and colleagues. Two predominant patterns of injury are seen: avulsions and intra-articular impaction fractures.

Avulsion injuries are the most common and represent detachment of the radioscaphoid ligament distal insertion on the radiovolar tip of the tuberosity. Treatment consists of splintage during healing, and most will heal uneventfully.

Impaction fractures are subclassified according to whether the radial side, ulnar side or both sides of the distal articular surface are involved. Radial sided fractures are the most common, unite readily and have a good prognosis. Immobilization of distal pole fractures in a short arm cast for 3–6 weeks is recommended. The long-term prognosis of distal articular fractures needs investigation, and the role of open reduction and internal fixation in preventing degenerative change when significant intra-articular incongruity exists is not known.

Box 12.29.4 Distal pole fractures

- Avulsion:
  - Most common
  - Heal with splintage
- Intra-articular:
  - Impaction fractures
  - Usually heal with cast
  - Ulnar sided fractures have poorer prognosis
- Extra-articular (transverse): treat as for waist fractures.

Scaphoid waist fractures (Box 12.29.5)

Stable, non-displaced fractures

Union rates in excess of 90% and as high as 95% are reported with cast immobilization. Currently, there is no way of predicting which fractures will unite. Although controversial, internal fixation of non-displaced fractures is gaining in popularity, and will be discussed in the 'Areas of uncertainty or controversy' section.

Unstable fractures

Fractures where there is displacement of more than 1mm in any direction are considered unstable and require more aggressive treatment than non-displaced fractures. Cast treatment in this situation does not reliably immobilize the fracture, and when more than 1mm displacement is present, up to a 55% rate of non-union is seen with cast treatment alone.

Scaphoid fracture can occur as part of a major carpal injury, the so-called transscaphoid perilunar dislocation. The pathomechanics of such injuries is described as a sequence of injuries around the lunate resulting in differing degrees of perilunar instability. When associated with perilunar instability, scaphoid fractures should be internally fixed as part of the procedure to restore stability to the carpus.

Box 12.29.5 Scaphoid waist fracture

- Stable, non-displaced:
  - 90% will heal in a cast
  - Fixation is controversial
  - Performed open or percutaneously
- Unstable fractures:
  - >1mm of displacement
  - Displacement more readily assessed on CT
  - Non-union common
  - Treat with internal fixation.

Proximal pole fractures (Box 12.29.6)

Fractures involving the proximal pole of the scaphoid have a poorer prognosis. The retrograde blood flow and consequent precarious vascularity increase the risk of AVN. Consequently, prolonged healing times of up to 6 months have been associated with cast treatment, and non-union occurs more commonly than with fractures at other sites. Healing rates following non-union surgery on proximal pole fractures are particularly poor and this adds further weight to the importance of achieving initial union in acute fractures.

The factors outlined constitute reasonable indication for internal fixation of all proximal pole fractures. Rettig and Raskin had favourable results from fixation with a Herbert screw using the dorsal approach in 17 proximal pole fractures. None failed to unite, average time to union averaged 10 weeks and there were no cases of AVN seen at an average follow up of 37 months.

Casting techniques

Theoretical advantages for immobilizing the wrist in differing positions have been postulated, but the position does not significantly affect union rate. An extended immobilization position, as opposed to a flexed one, leads to less restriction of extension at 6-month follow-up. The practice of immobilizing the thumb is commonplace and may add some comfort for patients. However, immobilization of the thumb confers no additional benefit over Colles type casts in terms of union. In cadavers, forearm rotation causes movement at a scaphoid fracture site, with average peak displacements of 2.1mm during forearm rotation in a short-arm cast. Clinically union rates of long-arm versus short-arm casts show no convincing difference.

Box 12.29.6 Proximal pole fractures

- Poorer prognosis
- 30% non-union with cast treatment
- Prolonged healing times with cast treatment
- AVN common
- Treat with internal fixation using dorsal approach.

Duration of immobilization and the assessment of union

It has long been accepted that scaphoid fractures should be immobilized until union has occurred even though prolonged immobilization may be necessary. Cases have been quoted where cast immobilization of up to 60 weeks, were used before union could be diagnosed! This situation is unacceptable in today's practice, but confidently diagnosing union continues to be a challenge.

Traditionally assessment of scaphoid union has relied upon clinical signs and serial plain radiographic examination. However, tenderness over the scaphoid disappears early, even in fractures, which have not united. The term '*clinically united*' has no meaning in the context of scaphoid fracture.

The scaphoid is mostly intra-articular, and no external callus is expected or seen with fracture healing on x-ray. Trabeculae crossing the fracture and sclerosis at the fracture line are said to indicate union. However, the shape, size and orientation of the scaphoid make it difficult to assess for these, and the appearance of trabeculae crossing the fracture may be artefactual. Radiographs taken 12 weeks after injury cannot be reliably and reproducibly used to assess union of a scaphoid fracture. Radiographs can only establish failure of union, and it is important that patients should be kept under review for a minimum of 6 months at which stage a non-union can confidently be ruled out on radiographs.

Prescribing the optimum duration of immobilization is a dilemma given that clinical and x-ray indicators of union, at or before 12 weeks, cannot be relied upon. Commonly, casting for an empirical 8 weeks is used for treating waist fractures. Extending immobilization to 12 weeks if union is doubtful at 8 weeks is acceptable, but casting should be dispensed with after 12 weeks.

CT scanning is increasingly being used to aid diagnosis of union in cases where doubt exists on plain radiographs. Continuity of trabeculae across the whole width of the bone constitutes union. One study described partial unions seen on CT scans performed at 12–18 weeks, where bridging trabeculae cross some areas of the fracture and gaps exist at other sites on coronal CT images. All 22 of the partially united fractures went on to fully unite without need of further immobilization (Box 12.29.7 and Figure 12.29.8).

Operative techniques

Method of fixation

Kirshner wires are a simple mode of fixation, but they provide less stable fixation than screws and protruding wires may cause damage to joint surfaces. Staples and plates have been described, but since fractures of the scaphoid are intra-articular, their application is limited. Standard screws have large heads, which cannot be buried and standard partially threaded screws may not be appropriately proportioned to allow compression.

Several different commercially available implants are now available, which have been specifically designed for scaphoid fixation. The original was the Herbert screw (1984), based on an original principle replacing the normal screw head with a second thread. The design allows for firm implant fixation in both proximal and distal fragments of the scaphoid and for the screw to be completely buried below the articular surface. The two threaded sections are proportioned specifically for the scaphoid, and by making the pitch of the thread at the tip of the screw greater than that of the thread

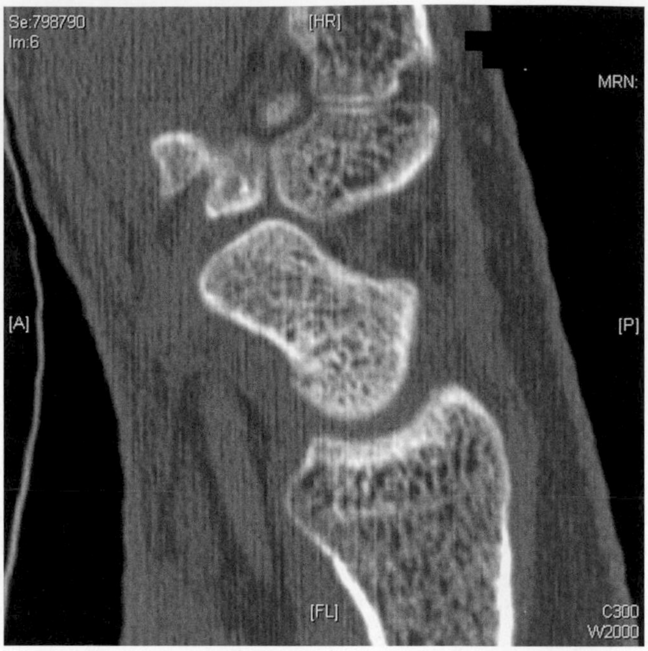

Fig. 12.29.8 Sagittal plane CT scan taken 8 weeks following injury demonstrating a partially united waist fracture. Bridging trabeculae can be seen crossing the dorsal half of the fracture.

Box 12.29.7 Assessment of union of scaphoid fracture
◆ Healing usually takes 8–12 weeks ◆ Clinical assessment unreliable ◆ X-rays not always reliable ◆ CT useful in doubtful cases.

Box 12.29.8 Outcome of scaphoid fracture
◆ 20% still have some pain 2.5 years after fracture united ◆ Malunion: • May cause pain • Humpback deformity may limit wrist extension • May result in osteoarthritis ◆ Secondary osteoarthritis seen in 5%, 7 years after fracture united.

replacing the head, compression is produced on screw insertion. (Figure 12.29.9).

Cannulated systems allow installation over a guide wire. They are easier to place and minimize exposure requirements. The Herbert-Whipple screw (Zimmer, Warsaw, IN) is a titanium device with variably pitched threads. The diameter of the non-threaded portion of the cannulated screw is larger than that of the original Herbert screw making it more resistant to bending loads.

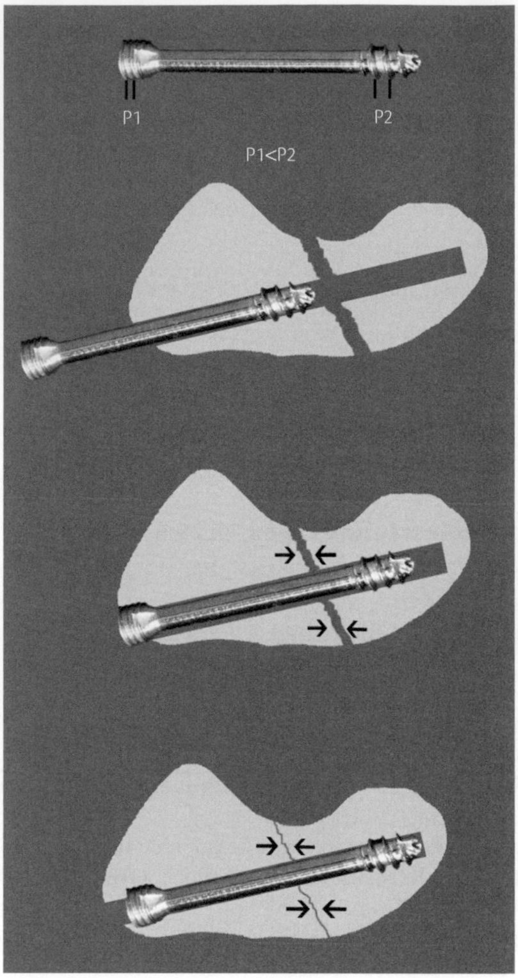

Fig. 12.29.9 Scaphoid compression screw with two threaded portions, each with a different pitch. The difference in pitch between the leading thread (P2) and the trailing thread (P1) governs the rate of drawing together of the two fragments to produce compression.

Prognosis (Box 12.29.8)

Union rates based on early radiographic evaluation of union at or before 12 weeks are unreliable. Studies, which have assessed for non-union at 6 months or a year, present more reliable estimates of union rate. For fractures of the waist of the scaphoid figures approaching 90% are realistic following cast treatment. For proximal pole fractures non-union occurs in up to a third of fractures treated non-operatively and for distal pole fractures this complication is rare.

Although, union is generally assumed to have a good outcome, injury to articular cartilage and altered carpal dynamics due to degrees of malunion, may result in persisting pain and secondary osteoarthritis following healing of a fracture. Persisting pain is reported by 20% of cases up to 2.5 years after fracture union. Radiographic evidence of secondary osteoarthritis is seen in 5% of wrists at a minimum follow-up of 7 years following healed fracture. The incidence of secondary degeneration is probably underestimated by plain x-rays and CT studies have suggested even greater frequencies (Box 12.29.9).

Box 12.29.9 Algorithm for suspected scaphoid fracture management

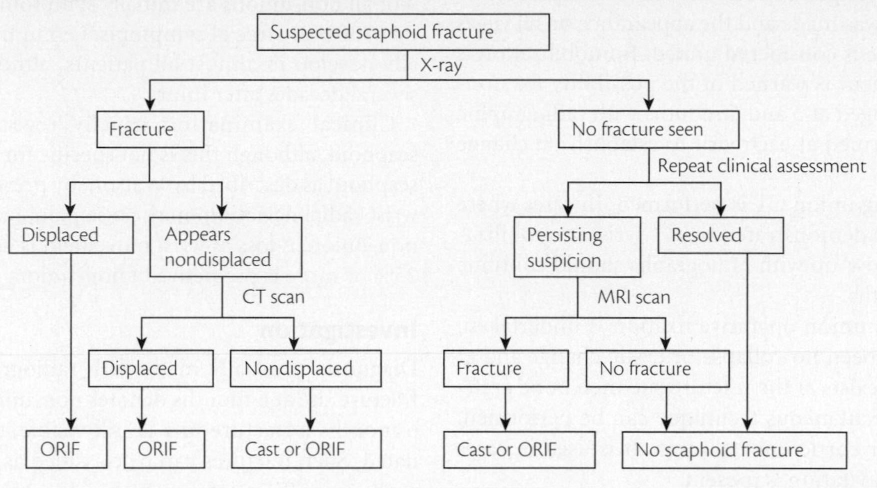

Areas of uncertainty or controversy

With the development of less invasive methods of fixation and a proliferation of new fixation devices, there has been an increasing trend towards internal fixation of acute, non-displaced scaphoid fractures. Proponents of fixation techniques suggest that more reliable union rates, quicker time to union, accelerated rehabilitation, and earlier functional recovery, are prime advantages over cast treatment. Five randomized controlled trials have compared internal fixation with cast immobilization for non-displaced scaphoid fractures, three using percutaneous screw insertion and two an open technique. In the largest trial, non-unions, diagnosed on CT scan at 16 weeks, were reported in 10 out of 44 fractures treated non-operatively and were subsequently fixed surgically. No non-unions occurred with operative treatment. The other four trials failed to demonstrate a significant difference in union rate between the two groups. Two trials reported significantly faster times to radiographic union in operatively treated fractures, one trial reported no difference and in the remaining two, time to union was not reported. None of the authors showed significant differences in range of movement and grip strength beyond 1 year, but three did show earlier return of these parameters in operatively treated fractures. Return to work was reported as being significantly earlier with operative treatment in three of the trials, but in one no difference was found.

Common complications following operative treatment appear to be largely related to the wound and include sensitive and hypertrophic scar, wound infection and cutaneous nerve dysaesthesia. The incidence of these may be less with percutaneous techniques. CRPS occurs rarely and can complicate non-operative treatment as well. Although postoperative complications are generally minor, the need for meticulous surgical technique remains paramount. Failure of surgical technique resulting in wire, instrument or screw breakage, implant protrusion into adjacent joints and intra-operative injury to joints, nerves or tendons can result in disastrous outcomes.

The case for fixation of non-displaced fractures remains controversial. Given that the majority of these cases will heal in a cast, a policy of fixation risks over-treating many patients and exposes them to avoidable surgical complications. Potential benefits from fixation are related to reliable healing and earlier functional recovery. The later advantage is transient and functional outcome, in the medium and long term, is equivalent following operative and non-operative treatments. For young and active patients, the population in which scaphoid fractures tend to occur, these benefits may seem attractive, but in providing informed choice, this needs to be balanced appropriately against any added risk.

Author's preferred treatment for non-displaced waist fractures

Where scaphoid fracture is suspected but not confirmed on initial good quality radiographs further clinical review is undertaken after 1–2 weeks, in which time most minor injuries will have settled. During this period the wrist need not be immobilized as long as the patient is told that the scaphoid may be fractured and they are given a clear explanation of the plan of action. The patient is asked to avoid undue wrist usage. If subsequent clinical examination still suggests fracture then MRI is performed so that a definitive diagnosis can be made.

When good quality radiographs (ideally scaphoid series consisting: PA; pronation and supination obliques; lateral and ulnar deviation views) show no evidence of displacement in all views the fracture can be treated accordingly as undisplaced. When doubt exists CT scan should be arranged.

In active patients with undisplaced waist fractures we offer operative fixation following the appropriate counselling on non-operative and operative interventions. If the patient chooses operative treatment percutaneous fixation is undertaken with a cannulated compression screw. We usually use a volar approach inserting the screw in a distal to proximal direction for waist fractures, and a dorsal approach inserting the screw from proximal to distal in more proximal fractures.

For patients with undisplaced waist fractures, who opt for non-operative treatment we adopt the '"aggressive" conservative' approach suggested by Dias. Patient are treated in a below elbow cast with the wrist in a functionally extended position and the thumb left free. The cast is removed after 6–8 weeks and scaphoid series radiographs repeated and compared to the initial series. If the fracture line can no longer be seen on views comparable to those in which diagnosis was made and the appearance on all views is satisfactory, the fracture is considered united. Immobilization is discontinued but the patient is warned of the possibility for non-union. Follow-up is arranged at 3 and 6 months with radiographic examination being performed at each visit to establish no change has occurred.

If doubt exists regarding union CT is performed. In cases where union or partial union is demonstrated by CT wrist immobilization is discontinued. Follow-up with radiographs should continue for a minimum of 6 months.

If CT demonstrates no union operative fixation is undertaken. In cases where there has been no collapse or cystic change and at operation no movement exists at the fracture site then bone grafting is not used and a percutaneous technique can be performed. Conversely, cancellous or corticocancellous graft is used in cases where collapse or cystic cavitation is present.

Non-union

A non-union exists when, given adequate time, the fracture has not united and healing activity has ceased, so that it will not unite without intervention. For the scaphoid, if non-union is defined as a persisting, clear gap at the fracture 1 year following injury, then the incidence of non-union following conservative treatment is 12.3% (Box 12.29.10).

Clinical presentation

The typical patient is male and in their twenties. Presentation may occur in four different ways:

1) Patients treated and followed up adequately in whom non-union occurs
2) Patients treated but followed up inadequately. The patient is discharged prematurely in the belief that the fracture has united, and represents with a non-union
3) Patients who were never treated because the diagnosis was not made following injury. They present later with symptomatic non-union, often after a further injury
4) Patients in whom scaphoid non-union is an incidental finding when examination is undertaken for another reason.

Box 12.29.10 Non-union

- Persisting fracture gap at 6 months
- Males in their 20s
- 30% symptom free at time of diagnosis
- Eventually symptoms will develop, although this may be decades later
- Secondary osteoarthritis rare before 4 years
- Secondary osteoarthritis inevitable in all patients.

Clinical features

Not all non-unions are initially symptomatic. At time of diagnosis up to 30% are free of symptoms. Left untreated, symptoms eventually develop in almost all patients, although this may not be for several decades after injury.

Clinical examination usually reveals tenderness over the scaphoid, although this is not specific for non-union. Stressing the scaphoid as described by Watson, by preventing the bone flexing in wrist radial deviation, may cause pain, but again is not specific for non-union. A loss of wrist movement is usually present, and loss of 25% or more is predictive of non-union.

Investigation

Diagnosis is usually made with radiographs. A clear gap at the fracture site at 6 months denotes non-union. Not uncommonly, at 6 months a fracture line is still visible, though partially consolidated. Such fractures can be classified as 'probably united' and in such cases CT is useful in confirming union (Figure 12.29.10).

Natural history

Osteoarthritis is the inevitable consequence of non-union. Although, radiographically arthritis is rarely seen before 4 years it is present in all patients with symptomatic non-union at an average of 8 years following injury. Even in the absence of symptoms from a non-union the natural history appears to be the same, and osteoarthritis will occur regardless of the patient being asymptomatic.

Treatment

The population that scaphoid non-union affects tends to be the young and active. If left untreated pain and osteoarthritis are the probable consequences. Therefore, non-union surgery is indicated in both symptomatic and non-symptomatic cases. A careful assessment for osteoarthritic change should be made, especially when the presentation is delayed. When significant arthritis is present, dealing with the non-union alone is no longer appropriate and salvage procedures are considered depending on symptoms.

The objectives of non-union surgery are:

- To achieve union of the fracture
- To decrease the incidence of osteoarthritis
- To abolish symptoms
- To improve function.

Surgery for non-union (Box 12.29.11)

Scaphoid non-union is treated by bone grafting with or without internal fixation. The standard exposure to the distal two-thirds of the scaphoid is through a volar approach. Dorsal approaches are utilized for proximal pole exposure and when utilizing certain vascularized bone grafting techniques.

Assessment of the non-union is made on direct inspection and with the aid of intraoperative radiographic examination. The following points are noted:

- The location and orientation of the non-union
- The deformity present. The scaphoid will demonstrate varying degrees of flexion deformity and loss of height
- The condition of the articular surfaces

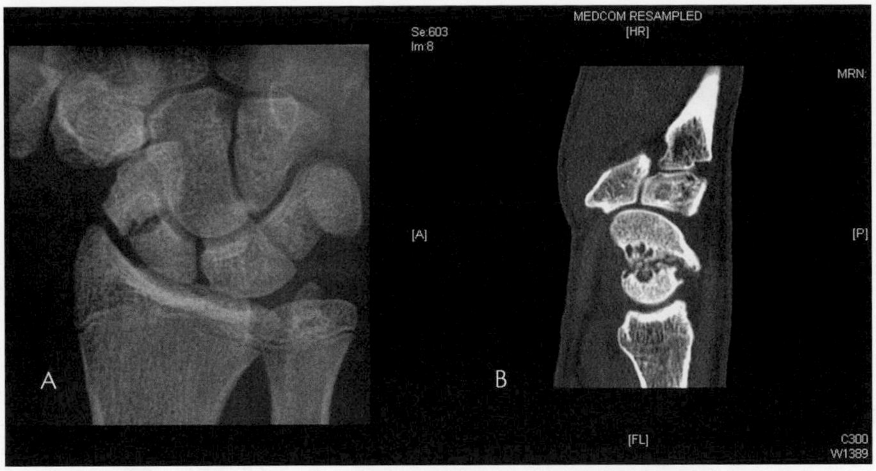

Fig. 12.29.10 Scaphoid non-union: A) PA radiograph demonstrating a clear fracture gap and cavitation; B) sagittal CT scan demonstrating collapse, cyst formation.

- The integrity of the scapholunate ligament complex. Coexisting scapholunate laxity can be present, although frank instability is rare
- The vascularity of the proximal scaphoid pole.

Following careful assessment the non-union is prepared to accept the desired graft. The edges of the fracture site are cut back to healthy bone using osteotomes. K-wires inserted as joysticks and laminar spreaders are useful in distracting the fracture to restore scaphoid dimensions so that the defect can be measured and the size and shape of the required graft ascertained.

Types of bone graft (Box 12.29.12)

Interposition grafts

Cancellous or corticocancellous graft can be harvested from the distal radius or the iliac crest. Harvesting from the distal radius can be performed from the volar aspect through a slightly extended volar approach, or through a separate dorsal exposure of Lister's tubercle. A trapezoid-shaped wedge is inserted with the broader surface volarly to correct the flexion deformity. The wedge shape causes a tendency to extrude, so some form of fixation is employed.

Inlay grafts

This technique involves excavating a cavity crossing the non-union site, from proximal to distal fragments, and inlaying strips of corticocancellous graft snugly across the non-union to immobilize it. Matti in 1937 originally described grafting done through a dorsal approach, Russe (1960) modified Matti's operation adopting a palmar approach (which he believed would be less likely to cause injury to the vascular supply of the scaphoid). The grafts can be harvested from iliac crest or distal radius and fixation may be reinforced with supplemental implant fixation.

Box 12.29.11 Surgery for non-union

- Usually volar approach
- Cut back dead bone
- Bone graft inserted in defect
- Fixation with cannulated compression device
- Postoperative cast for 6–8 weeks.

Box 12.29.12 Bone grafts

- Non-vascularized:
  - Distal radius or iliac crest
  - Interposition or inlay
- Vascularized, pedicled:
  - Volar radius (volar carpal artery or pronator quadratus)
  - Dorsal radius (1,2 ICSR artery)
  - Index metacarpal
  - Distal ulnar
- Vascularized, free: medial supracondylar femur.

Longitudinal pegs

Grafts are fashioned into a peg and positioned longitudinally in the same axis as a screw.

Vascularized bone grafts (Figure 12.29.11)

Vascularized grafts can be pedicled, based on local arterial branches feeding the transplanted bone, or free transfers. Grafts can be harvested from:

- The volar radius. A pedicle can be based on the volar carpal artery or on a strip of the distal margin of pronator quadratus. Graft harvest can be incorporated into an extended standard volar exposure of the scaphoid and flexion deformity secondary to the volar bone loss can be corrected
- The dorsal radius. The arteries supplying the dorsal radius are described by their relationship to the extensor retinaculum compartments. Vessels lie within compartments or in between (intercompartmental). The 1,2 intercompartmental supraretinacular vessel feeds the distal radius on its dorso-radial aspect and graft can be based on this pedicle
- The index metacarpal
- The distal ulnar based on the ulnar artery

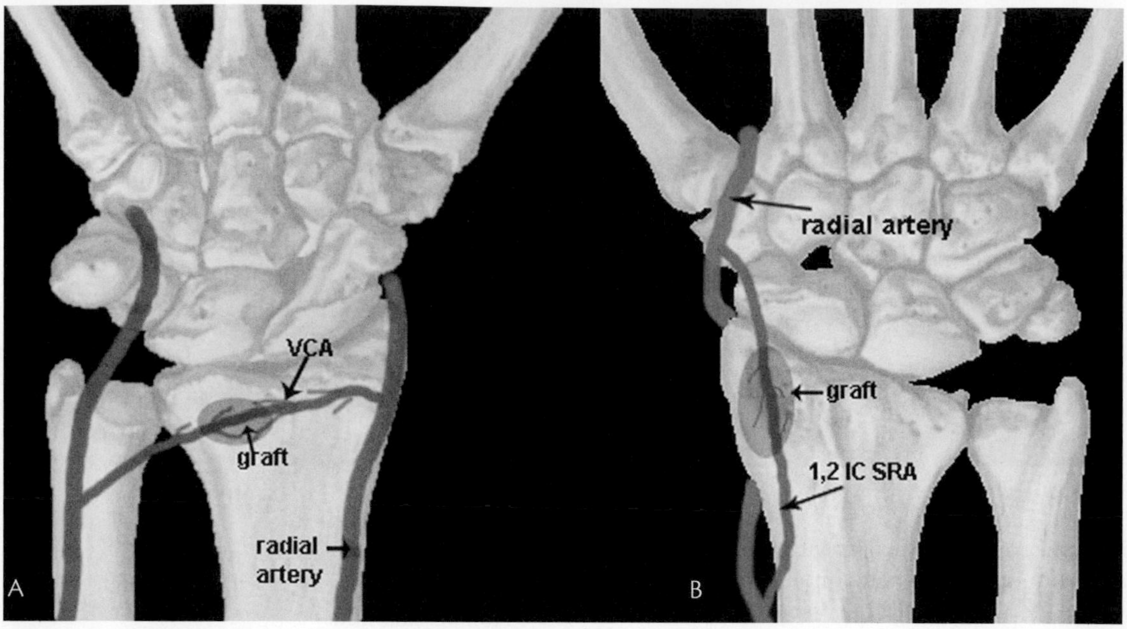

Fig. 12.29.11 Vascularized, pedicled bone grafts from the distal radius: A) volar. Based on the VCA (volar carpal artery) and B) dorsal. Based on a branch of the 1,2 IC SRA (1,2 intercompartmental supraretinacular artery).

- Free vascularized bone graft harvested from the medial supracondylar region of the femur and based on branches of the genicular arteries supplying the bone in this region. Anastomosis is performed onto the radial artery and its venae commitantes.

Prognosis (Box 12.29.13)

The following are important prognostic factors in bone healing following non-union surgery:

The site of the non-union

The convention to divide the scaphoid into proximal, middle (waist) and distal thirds is arbitrary and prone to intra- and inter-observer error. A more accurate method is to describe the non-union site as a ratio of the fracture fragments. Following non-vascularized bone grafting with internal fixation union rates vary from 27–100% depending on the site of non-union calculated using the fragment ratio method (Figure 12.29.12).

The time between injury and surgery

With delays of more than 5 years, mean union rates fall to around 60% following non-vascularized bone grafting with or without fixation. The effect that time from fracture has on union varies with the site of fracture, being weaker for more distal fractures.

Avascular necrosis of the proximal pole (Box 12.29.14)

Increased density of the proximal scaphoid on radiographs has traditionally been interpreted to denote avascularity. However, apparent increased radiographic density may not be due to avascularity and this method is unreliable. MRI and enhanced MRI with gadolinium offer more accurate assessment of blood flow. Intraoperative assessment remains the most reliable technique and absence of punctate bleeding from the bone is a poor prognostic indicator.

Although avascularity does not prevent union it is an important factor contributing to non-union. When the proximal scaphoid fragment is completely avascular it has no intrinsic repair capacity and must rely on repair from the distal fragment.

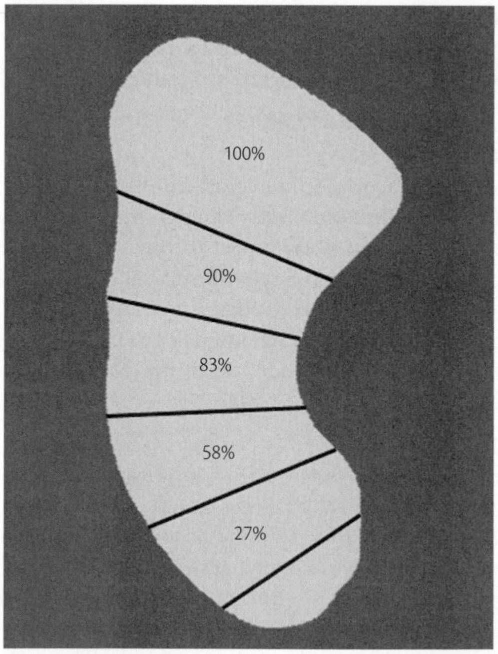

Fig. 12.29.12 Union rates following non-vascularized bone grafting and internal fixation for scaphoid non-union. Rates progressively worsen with more proximal site of non-union.

Smoking

Has a deleterious effect on bone healing, however, the effect it has on prognosis of scaphoid non-union is controversial. A greater than threefold risk of failure of non-vascularized bone grafting with screw fixation has been reported in smokers undergoing

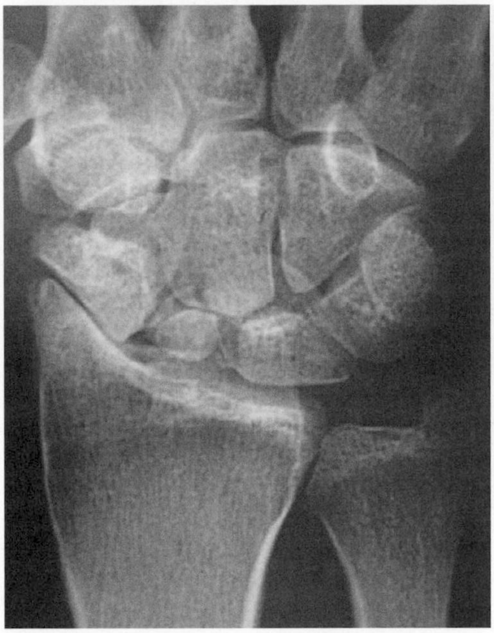

Fig. 12.29.13 Scaphoid non-union advanced collapse (SNAC). Degenerative changes start between the radial styloid and distal scaphoid fragment. The joint between radius and lunate is seldom affected.

Box 12.29.13 Outcome of non-union surgery

- 71% union with non-vascularized grafting and internal fixation
- Worse results with proximal fractures
- Worse results with increasing age of non-union
- Worse results with AVN of proximal pole.

non-union surgery, whilst others have shown smoking to have no influence on the rate of union following surgery.

Vascularized versus non-vascularized bone grafting

The union rates of non-vascularized bone grafting, with or without fixation, are reliably reported at 70–80%. Russe and subsequently Green contended that in the presence of complete AVN of the proximal fragment inlay grafting is highly likely to fail. Interposition grafts have been used in the presence of AVN with success in 53%.

Improving the vascularity of the proximal pole directly by implanting a vascular pedicle has not been successful, thrombosis of the implanted vessels and lengthy periods for bone revascularization to occur being cited as reasons. Vascularized pedicle bone grafts were introduced to overcome these problems.

There are currently no randomized series comparing vascularized versus non-vascularized grafting in the presence of AVN. Published series on pedicled distal radial vascularized grafting report union rates between 80–100%, but cohorts are heterogeneous for the presence of AVN. A recent meta-analysis shows that non-vascularized, interpositional grafts used in the presence of AVN have a union rate of only 47% compared to 88% when vascularized grafts are used. Recent publications on free medial

Box 12.29.14 Avascular necrosis

- Density on x-ray unreliable as a sign of AVN
- Assess with MRI
- Intraoperative assessment most reliable
- Consider vascularized graft.

femoral grafts used in the treatment of scaphoid waist non-unions, with an avascular proximal pole, report promising success rates.

The case for vascularized grafting remains inconclusively. For most waist fracture non-unions without other adverse features (AVN, failed previous surgery, long duration of non-union, proximal pole non-union) non-vascularized bone grafting is probably sufficient.

Secondary arthritis

The pattern of arthritis that develops in association with non-union is progressive and occurs in a predictable sequence (Figure 12.29.13). The term scaphoid non-union advanced collapse or 'SNAC' has been coined to describe this pattern, which closely parallels the pattern seen in chronic scapholunate ligament incompetence (scapholunate advanced collapse, SLAC wrist).

Non-union is usually associated with alteration in the shape of the scaphoid with flexion plus shortening leading to articular incongruity. With additional mobility of the fracture fragments and altered carpal motion, joint surfaces are exposed to excessive and abnormal forces, and the mechanisms for degeneration are established. The site of initial change is between the radius and mobile distal scaphoid fragment, stopping at the site of non-union. Osteophytes form at the tip of the styloid and subsequently the joint space is lost. The articulation between the radius and proximal pole fragment is preserved because both are spherical in nature, allowing congruency in all positions. Rotation of the distal scaphoid fragment and loss of the radius-distal fragment joint space allow the capitate to migrate. The capitate drives off the radial side of the lunate and destruction of the capitate-proximal fragment joint ensues followed by the capitate-lunate joint. The joint between radius and lunate is seldom affected (Figure 12.29.13).

Treatment (Box 12.29.15)

Radial styloidectomy

In the initial stages, where degeneration is isolated to the articulation between the radial styloid and distal scaphoid fragment, simple excision of the styloid can be performed. Excision is performed removing the degenerate styloid up to the junction of normal articular cartilage. Caution is needed to preserve the important extrinsic volar ligaments (radioscaphocapitate and radiolunate ligaments) as detaching theses may lead to instability.

Although some success for isolated styloidectomy is reported, pain relief is unpredictable as it is difficult to know whether pain is coming from the radioscaphoid arthritis or from the non-union. Combining grafting of the non-union with styloidectomy is a reasonable and logical alternative.

Excision of the scaphoid

A very small proximal fragment can be excised but resections of larger fragments of the proximal or distal poles, or the whole

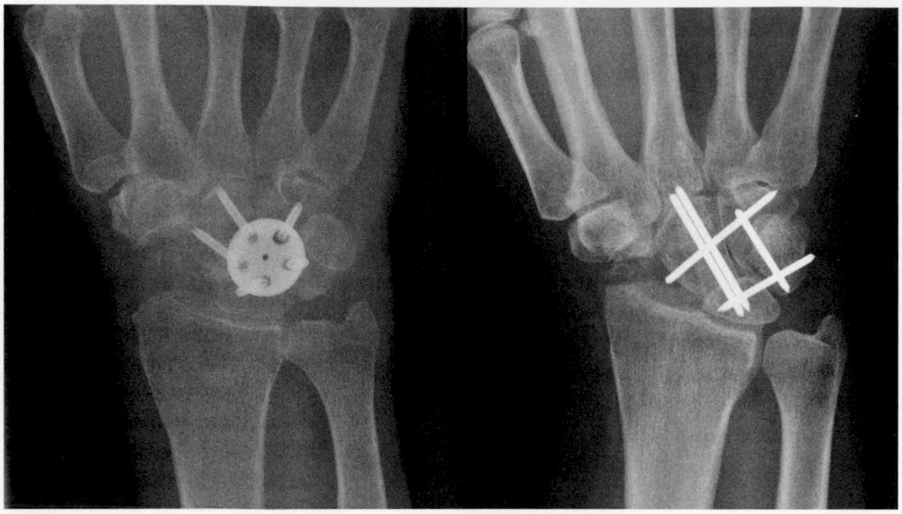

Fig. 12.29.14 Scaphoid excision and 'four-corner' fusion: A) 'hub-plate' and b) K-wires.

scaphoid, results in collapse of the carpus into a DISI deformity. Techniques to stabilize the carpus, following excision of part or all of the scaphoid, include some form of limited arthrodesis or some form of prosthetic replacement.

Limited carpal fusion

Watson popularized scaphoid excision with arthrodesis of the lunate, capitate, hamate and triquetrum ('four-corner fusion') for reconstruction of SLAC wrist. The procedure has successfully been applied to palliation for SNAC wrist. It can be used when degeneration has extended into the midcarpal articulation. The residual fusion mass articulates at the radiolunate articulation which is not usually affected until late in the arthritis process. In a series of 100 procedures performed by Kirk Watson and associates, the average range of motion was 53% and 59% of normal in flexion/extension and radioulnar deviation respectively. Grip strength reached 80% of normal (Figure 12.29.14).

Replacement of part or all of the scaphoid

Silastic implants have been widely used since their introduction including replacement of the proximal scaphoid pole and total scaphoid replacement. However, the problem of silicon synovitis causing cyst formation and progressive to total destruction of the carpus, has led to the abandonment of such arthroplasties. Alternative materials, including acrylics, metal alloy and cadaveric bones have failed to gain wide popularity. More recently the development of pyrocarbon implants has received some attention.

Excision of the proximal carpal row

Is an established treatment for SLAC and SNAC patterns of arthritis involving the articulation between the radius and scaphoid. Following proximal row carpectomy (PRC) the head of the capitate articulates with the lunate fossa of the radius, and these surfaces need to have good articular cartilage if this procedure is being performed. Evidence of degeneration at the lunate-capitate articulation should be sought on preoperative radiographs, but preservation of the articular surfaces can only be confirmed at time of operation. If articular damage exists then an arthrodesis procedure is preferable and patients are preoperatively counselled accordingly.

PRC is simpler to perform than limited fusion and lower rates of complication are reported. Good pain relief can be achieved with this procedure as well as improvements in grip strength. The range of motion in flexion-extension is 60–70% of normal. Progression of arthritis in the radius capitate articulation has been observed and this may be a concern, especially in younger patients, but the procedure has been shown to be durable at 10 years.

Denervation of the wrist

Denervation interrupts the sensory pathways from the pathological wrist. It is more conservative than other salvage procedures, with less potential for complication, and preserves wrist movement. However, the innervation of the different tissues making up the wrist joint is complex, and the exact sources of pain are not completely understood. Total denervation aims to interrupt all sensory nerves supplying the wrist. This is difficult as sensory afferents are numerous and variable. The technique requires the division of ten nerve branches through five separate incisions. Partial denervation selectively interrupts those regions most likely responsible for generating pain. The posterior and anterior interosseous nerves can be sectioned through a single dorsal incision, and high levels of patient satisfaction using this technique are reported. Other clinical reports suggest pain relief is somewhat inconsistent and only transient.

Complete arthrodesis of the wrist

In cases where advanced arthritis is causing marked pain, arthrodesis is reliable and predictable. The amount of movement that the patient has in the wrist when arthritis is advanced is usually, already, markedly limited. In such cases the further loss of movement is usually outweighed by the advantage of loss of pain.

Conclusion

The scaphoid fracture tends to occur in active, young males. Most fractures will heal with the appropriate treatment, but a few will go onto non-union. If left untreated a non-union, even when initially

Box 12.29.15 Surgery for secondary arthritis

- Radial styloidectomy
- Proximal row carpectomy:
  - Requires good proximal capitate
  - 60% range of flexion/extension
- Excision and 'four-corner' fusion:
  - Can be performed if midcarpal joint involved
  - 53% range of flexion/extension
  - 80% grip strength
- Denervation
- Total wrist fusion.

asymptomatic, will result in arthritis and eventually pain, although this may not be for several decades. The role of the surgeon is to make definitive early diagnosis and institute effective treatment. Unnecessarily long periods of immobilization should be avoided and early fixation may prove to be a more satisfactory strategy in the future. Despite newly developed techniques and implants for fixation non-union continues to occur. Our understanding of the factors involved in non-union has increased but the optimum treatment approach has yet to be defined.

Further reading

Barton, N.J. (1992). Twenty questions about scaphoid fractures. *Journal of Hand Surgery*, **17B**, 289–310.

Dias, J.J. (2001). Definition of union after acute fracture and Surgery for fracture non-union of the scaphoid. *Journal of Hand Surgery*, **26B**, 321–5.

Dias, J.J., Wildin, C.J., Bhowal, B., and Thompson, J.R. (2005). Should acute scaphoid fractures be fixed? *Journal of Bone and Joint Surgery*, **87A**, 2160–8.

Herbert. T.J. and Fisher, W.E. (1984). Management of the fractured scaphoid using a new bone screw. *Journal of Bone and Joint Surgery*, **66B**, 114–23.

Ramamurthy, C., Cutler, L., Nuttall, D., Simison, A.J., Trail, I.A., and Stanley, J.K. (2007). The factors affecting outcome after non-vascular bone grafting and internal fixation for non-union of the scaphoid. *Journal of Bone and Joint Surgery*, **89B**, 627–32.

12.30

Instabilities of the carpus

David Lawrie, Chris Little, and Ian McNab

Summary points

- Most injuries occur in hyperextension
- The force vector and size dictates the injury
- History and x-rays still prevail in diagnosis
- Classification has helped choose management
- Instability often associated with poor bone healing.

Introduction

Carpal instabilities can seem unduly complicated and unapproachable. With a better understanding of the anatomy and ligamentous support of the wrist, the instabilities seen become more logical, and the clinical assessments for instabilities makes more sense. Treatments of carpal instabilities, both acutely and established, are emerging with the growing appreciation of the kinematics and carpal kinetics of this complex of articulations.

Wrist anatomy (Figure 12.30.1)

The wrist represents a complex of articulations between the forearm bones, the carpal bones, which are arranged into two rows, and the bases of the metacarpals. The carpal bones are arranged into a proximal and a distal row This gives rise to a confluent joint between the radius/ulna (covered by the triangular fibrocartilage) and the proximal carpal row, called the radiocarpal joint (RCJ), and a second confluent joint between the proximal and distal carpal rows, called the midcarpal joint (MCJ). The bones of the distal carpal row articulate with the metacarpal bases.

The bones are connected by the intrinsic ligaments, and by ligaments within the capsule that pass from the forearm bones to the carpal bones, collectively called the extrinsic ligaments.

The bones of the distal carpal row are held tightly together by the intrinsic ligaments and so can be considered to act as a monoblock. The intrinsic ligaments of the proximal carpal row allow a greater degree of intercarpal motion. Both the scapholunate (SL) and the lunotriquetral (LTq) ligaments have weak membranous proximal portions (which can be seen arthroscopically from the radiocarpal joint) and stronger palmar and dorsal portions; the SL is stronger dorsally, and the LTq stronger on the palmar side. Fibres of the dorsal and palmar portions of these ligaments connect to form the scaphotriquetral ligaments at the MCJ. As long as the membranous portions of the ligaments are intact, there is no communication between the RCJ and the MCJ; communication through this portion of the ligaments occurs via traumatic or degenerate perforations, which are not necessarily clinically important. The MCJ is supported by intrinsic ligaments on the dorsum by the dorsal intercarpal ligament (DIC) which passes from the triquetrum to the scaphoid, trapezoid and trapezium, blending with the dorsal scaphotriquetral ligament, and on the palmar surface by the triquetrohamatecapitate ligament complex on the ulnar side, and by the scaphocapitate and scaphotrapezial ligaments on the radial side (the latter passing around to the dorsoradial aspect of the MCJ). These ligaments tend to fail by avulsion.

The extrinsic ligaments arise from the palmar and dorsal surfaces of the radius, and on the palmar side, the ligaments broadly form the shape of two inverted Vs running proximal to distal, one with its apex on the lunate (short and long radiolunate and ulnolunate ligaments) and the other with its apex on the capitate (the radioscaphocapitate ligament complex, and the ulnocapitate ligament). There is a sulcus between these two Vs on the radial side, connecting into the space of Poirier.

The palmar ulnocarpal ligaments and the palmar and dorsal radioulnar ligaments, along with the triangular fibrocartilage between them, form the triangular fibrocartilaginous complex, which is considered in more detail in Chapter 6.4. On the dorsum, the dorsal radiocarpal ligament forms the proximal limb of a radially-based V (the distal limb being the DIC intrinsic ligament) running transversely with its apex on the triquetrum. The extrinsic ligaments tend to fail by midsubstance rupture.

The carpal bones are connected by other ligaments outside the wrist capsule, notably the transverse carpal ligament (TCL) from the hook of the hamate and the pisiform to the distal scaphoid and the trapezium, forming the roof of the carpal tunnel, and the pisohamate ligament (which makes the floor of Guyon's canal). The TCL helps to maintain the convex-dorsal arch to the carpus in the transverse plane, and its division increases the width and volume of the carpal tunnel.

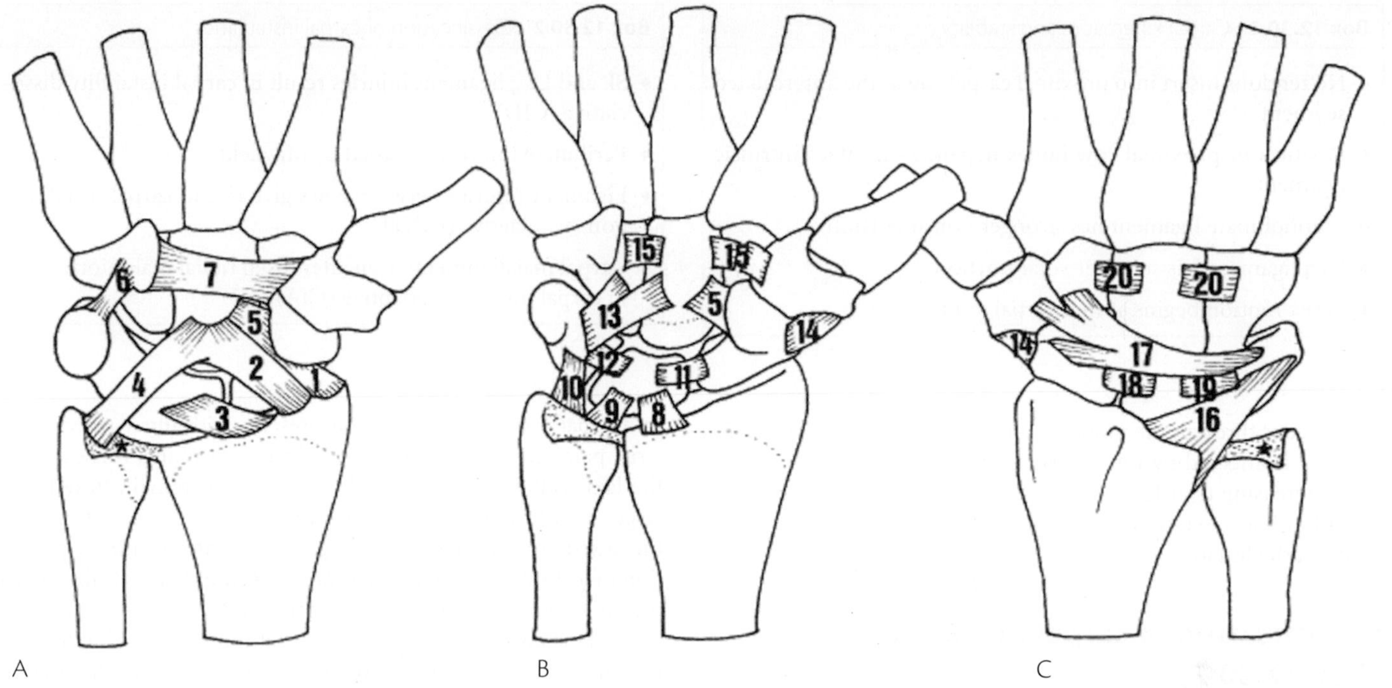

Fig. 12.30.1 Schematic representation of the most consistently present wrist ligaments. These drawings do not aim to replicate the exact shape and dimensions of the actual ligaments, nor their frequent anatomic variations. A) Palmar superficial ligaments: (1) radioscaphoid, (2) radioscapho-capitate, (3) long radiolunate, (4) ulnocapitate, (5) scaphocapitate, (6) pisohamate, and (7) flexor retinaculum or transverse carpal ligament. B) Palmar deep ligaments: (8) short radiolunate; (9) ulnolunate; (10) ulnotriquetral; (11) palmar scapholunate; (12) palmar lunotriquetral, (13) triquetral-hamate-capitate, also known as the ulnar limb of the arcuate ligament; (14) dorsolateral scaphotrapezial; and (15) palmar transverse interosseous ligaments of the distal row. C) Dorsal ligaments: (16) radiotriquetral; (17) triquetrum-scaphoid-trapezium-trapezoid, also known as the dorsal intercarpal ligament; (18) dorsal scapholunate; (19) dorsal lunotriquetral; and (20) dorsal transverse interosseous ligaments of the distal row.

Carpal kinematics and stability (Box 12.30.1)

As no tendons insert into the proximal row of carpal bones (excepting the sesamoid pisiform bone), the position of the bones is determined by the shape of the joint surfaces, the integrity of ligaments connecting the bones and the forces applied across the carpus by the tendons passing from the forearm to the hand and distal carpal row, making it act as an intercalated segment. There has been an evolution in thinking regarding how the wrist moves, from the 'row theory' (proximal and distal carpal rows acting as functional units) through the 'column theories' (with combinations of bones from the two rows acting as functional units for load transfer and positioning), to the 'oval ring theory' (with the distal carpal row, the scaphoid, the lunate and the triquetrum acting as linked elements in a ring, with failure of any element or the binding ligaments altering wrist motion and load transfer).

In summary, current thinking is that the helicoid shape of the triquetrohamate articulation and the alignment and ligament attachments of the triquetrum and scaphoid cause them to tend to extend and flex respectively. As long as the SL and LTq ligaments are intact, the lunate remains in a state of dynamic balance within the proximal carpal row; if the linkages within the proximal row fail, the lunate falls under the unopposed influence of the bone to which it remains attached, rotating into dorsi- or palmar flexion respectively.

Motion of the wrist starts with movement of the distal carpal row at the MCJ, with palmar flexion coupled to a degree of ulnar deviation and dorsiflexion to a degree of radial deviation. Palmar and dorsiflexion produces motion in the same direction of the proximal row bones, but with the scaphoid showing greater motion than the other proximal row bones, acting as the 'crank' in the three-bar linkage mechanism between the proximal and distal rows. When considering radial and ulnar deviation, wrists lie on a spectrum between 'row' wrists (where the proximal row slides towards the ulna during radial deviation, with rotation occurring in the coronal plane) and 'column' wrists, (where deviation in the proximal row is achieved by scaphoid flexion during radial deviation and by the triquetrum extending in ulnar deviation, the rotation occurring in the sagittal plane).

Normal range of wrist motion is 70 degrees each of palmar and dorsiflexion, 20 degrees radial and 40 degrees ulnar deviation and minimal intracarpal rotation (most occurring a the radioulnar joints); a range of 5 degrees palmar flexion, 30 degrees dorsiflexion, 10 degrees radial deviation, and 15 degrees ulnar deviation is said to be functional.

Carpal kinetics

While load distribution in the wrist is mainly dependent on hand and wrist positioning, most load transfer at the MCJ occurs through the capitoscapholunate articulation. In the main, about half the load will be transferred through the radioscaphoid articulation, about a third through the radiolunate articulation, and the

Box 12.30.1 Carpal kinematics and stability

- No tendons insert into proximal carpal row—the 'intercalated segment'
- Position of proximal row bones depends on intact intrinsic ligaments
- Scapholunate ligament has stronger dorsal portion
- LTq ligament has stronger volar portion
- Wrist motion begins at mid carpal joint.

Box 12.30.2 Classification of carpal instabilities

- SL and LTq ligament injuries result in carpal instability dissociative (CID)
- Perilunate injuries classified by Mayfield
- Ligament injuries between rows give rise to carpal instability non-dissociative (CIND)
- Carpal malalignments seen after distal radial malunions result in carpal instability adaptive (CIA).

remaineder through the ulnocarpal joint, although load transfer at the RCJ is affected by ulnar variance (relative lengthening of the ulna increasing transfer through the ulnocarpal articulation) and by radioulnar deviation (ulnar deviation increasing load transfer through the lunate).

Classification of carpal instabilities (Box 12.30.2)

The Mayo classification considers carpal instabilities (CI) to be dissociative (CID), non-dissociative (CIND), combined/complex (CIC) or adaptive (to forearm pathology, CIA); this is outlined in Table 12.30.1.

Most examples of CID reflect injuries to the intrinsic ligaments of the proximal carpal row, which can progress to perilunate dislocations with failure of other structures; as this happens, the instability moves into the CIC (complex) group.

The pathoanatomy of perilunate injuries was examined by Mayfield, who described a sequential failure of the structures around the lunate that gives rise to carpal instabilities and perilunate dislocations. In the usual pattern of soft tissue injury (so-called lesser arc injuries), the distal carpal row is subject to extreme extension and carpal supination from an indirect force, which is transmitted to the lunate via the scaphocapitate and scaphotrapezoid ligaments, the scaphoid and SL ligament; the extrinsic ligaments constrain lunate motion, causing tearing of the SL ligament (stage 1). If the force continues to be applied, the distal carpal row dislocates dorsally, tearing the capsule between the palmar extrinsic ligament Vs (stage 2). As the capitate translates dorsally, tension in the triquetrocapitate ligament pulls the triquetrum dorsally and into extension, tearing the LTq ligament (stage 3). At this point, the lunate remains attached to the radius by the short and long radiolunate ligaments and the dorsal capsule, the latter being vulnerable to rupture when the lunate is translated in a palmar direction by the displaced capitate, producing a palmar dislocation of the lunate (stage 4).

This normal Mayfield sequence may be associated with fractures of the radius or the carpal bones, in particular the scaphoid and the triquetrum. These injuries are termed greater arc injuries, and named by the pre-fix '*trans*- (name of fractured bone)', perilunate injuries. If force is applied to the ulnar side of the carpus, a so-called reverse Mayfield sequence of structural failure may uncommonly occur.

Damage to the ligaments crossing the MCJ can give rise to CIND instability patterns. This is most commonly seen in constitutionally lax individuals in whom a comparatively minor injury gives rise to on-going symptoms from the resultant manifest midcarpal instability. This often presents with ulnar-sided dorsal wrist pain and an associated sensation of clunking; this occurs as the laxity allows the proximal carpal row to remain flexed for a larger arc as the wrist moves from radial to ulnar deviation, with the flexed proximal row 'snapping' into extension with the perception of a clunk (often termed a catch-up clunk). This is the principle underlying the midcarpal pivot shift test.

CIND is also seen at the radiocarpal joint, either due to acute trauma (with extrinsic ligament avulsions), or in rheumatoid arthritis (with ulnar translation of the carpus).

CIA generally reflects carpal malalignments seen after distal radial malunions. Under these circumstances, abnormal inclination of the distal radial articular surface causes the proximal row to adopt an unusual position (e.g. dorsiflexed positioning following a dorsally-tilted malunion after a Colles pattern of fracture), with compensatory instability at the midcarpal joint (palmarflexed in the example given).

Clinical evaluation

Following an acute wrist injury, there should be a high index of suspicion for any underlying carpal bone fracture, ligament injury or dislocation. These injuries should be actively sought and excluded.

The mechanism of injury determines the magnitude of the forces that have been applied to the wrist and consequently the likely type of injury that must be excluded.

The injury can range from a high-energy road traffic collision (particularly involvig a motorcycle) to other high-velocity injuries such as a fall fronm a height, or during sport, that may cause perilunate dislocations and fracture–dislocations. Lower velocity falls on the outstretched hand/wrist may cause hyperextension and more isolated carpal fractures or ligament injuries. The patient often underestimates the injury severity, assuming that it is a trivial 'wrist sprain'. Other subtle or apparently trivial injuries that communicate significant extension, flexion or rotational forces to the wrist, such as when a power drill jams while drilling, should also raise suspicions.

Patients with perilunate dislocation injuries present with wrist deformity, limited motion, pain, and swelling. Single carpal bone dislocations may cause a subcutaneous prominence or a hollow over the dislocated bone. More subtle carpal instabilities will present with complaints of pain, swelling, and possibly clicking of the wrist.

Severe pain and swelling may make a careful complete wrist examination difficult in the early stages. However, the wrist should

Table 12.30.1 Classification of carpal instabilities

CID (DISI or VISI pattern)	
1	Scapholunate dissociation (early stages)
2	Lunotriquetral dissociation (early stages)
3	Axial dislocations of the carpus (if neither carpometacarpal joints distally nor proximal carpal row joints proximally are involved)
3A	Axial radial Peritrapezoid, peritrapezium, transtrapezium
3B	Axial ulnar Transhamate/peripisiform, perihamate/peripisiform, perihamate/transtriquetrum
CIND (DISI or VISI pattern or 'translatory' patterns)	
1	Radiocarpal Dorsal or volar Barton's fracture/dislocation Distal radius malunion (if extrinsic ligament damage is present or develops) Rupture of radiocarpal extrinsic ligaments (all ruptured equals radiocarpal dislocation; total or partial rupture can result in VISI, DISI, UT, DT, or VT) Radioscaphocapitate Short radiolunate Long radiolunate Ulnocapitate Ulnotriquetral Madelung's deformity (may occur with sufficient ulnar deformity) Ulnar translocation of the carpus Radiocarpal dislocation CLIP (if proximal instability present; the major instability in CLIP is the mid-carpal level instability) Proximal carpal row instability due to radiocarpal level damage only
2	Mid-carpal Proximal carpal row instability due to mid-carpal level damage only (the MCI of the literature)—a VISI deformity CLIP: the characteristic dorsal subluxation of the distal carpal row is due to damage at this level—a DISI deformity
CIC	
1	Any of the perilunate to lunate dislocation spectrum Dorsal and volar perilunate to lunate dislocations (ligamentous) Transosseous perilunate variants Trans-scaphoid dorsal perilunate and others
2	Any combination of two or more CID or CIND instabilities
3	CID which develops extrinsic ligament or additional intrinsic ligament insufficiency, i.e. stage 3 SLD with DISI
4	CIND which develops intrinsic ligament or additional extrinsic ligament insufficiency, i.e. proximal carpal row instability (either DISI or VISI) with extrinsic ligament damage at both radiocarpal and mid-carpal levels
CIA	
1	Any adaptive or apparent adaptive posture of the carpus not based on carpal injury, but reflecting changes in forearm or hand support structures Apparent CIND-DISI with a dorsiflexion malunion of a distal radius fracture (Colles type) Apparent CIND-VISI with a volar flexion malunion of a distal radius fracture (Smith type) Madelung's deformity with hypoplasia of the ulnar radius and displacement of the distal ulna

CIA, carpal instability adaptive; CIC, carpal instability combined; CID, carpal instability dissociative; CIND, carpal instability nondissociative; CLIP, capitolunate instability pattern; DISI, dorsal intercalated segmental instability; DT, dorsal translation; MCI, mid-carpal instability; SLD, scapholunate dissociation; UT, ulnar translation; VISI, volar intercalated segmental instability; VT, volar translation.

be inspected for haematoma, swelling, and altered shape. Subtle changes are best visualized by comparing the involved and uninvolved wrists.

Wrist palpation is performed following the bony anatomy, the distal wrist flexion crease is proximal to the carpus. There may be global wrist tenderness, but areas of maximum tenderness, and the structures that lie under them, should be identified and prioritized

The active and passive ranges of motion are assessed, noting any 'clicks' or 'clunks' indicating possible abnormal kinematics. A detailed neurovascular examination is performed.

Standard posteroanterior (PA) and lateral radiographs are obtained, with a radiographic wrist motion series, if wrist instability is suspected (see later).

Acute SL dissociation is generally suspected clinically but confirmed radiographically. However, most patients present with chronic SL dissociation (>6 months after injury). There may be an uncertain mechanism of injury, chronic dorsal or global wrist pain, swelling aggravated by lifting or gripping, and possibly wrist 'clunking'.

Physical examination may demonstrate, dorsal tenderness over the SL interval, a ballottable proximal scaphoid with pain and crepitus, and occasionally a 'click' demonstrable on ulnar to radial deviation, as the scaphoid subluxes or rotates out of the scaphoid fossa in radial deviation and relocates in ulnar deviation.

Watson's scaphoid shift test (Box 12.30.3) is performed as the examiner (seated opposite the patient) holds the patient's hand with the examiner's thumb overlying the distal pole of the scaphoid; the examiner's finger palpates the proximal pole of the scaphoid on the dorsum, and the patient's elbow is stabilized on the examination table. Starting with the patient's hand in ulnar deviation, the wrist is passively moved into radial deviation. Dorsally directed pressure, applied on the scaphoid tuberosity by the examining thumb, will cause the unstable scaphoid to 'back out' or sublux dorsally from the radial fossa. It is important to compare tenderness, pain, mobility, crepitus, and 'clicks' with the contralateral side. SL instability is likely when the test demonstrates an objective difference in stability of the two sides, or a palpable 'clunk' is elicited as the scaphoid proximal pole exits or returns to the scaphoid fossa.

LTq instability is a subtle clinical diagnosis. With an acute injury, there may be a history of a fall onto the ulnar side of the hand and ulnar sided wrist pain and swelling. LTq instability often presents as a chronic problem with ulnar-sided wrist pain and swelling aggravated by power grip, and popping or 'clunking' on radial/ulnar deviation. There is tenderness directly over the LTq interval, and increased pain, crepitus, and excessive motion compared with the other side, when performing a LTq ballottement test. During this test the examiner stabilizes the patient's triquetrum with their index finger volarly and the thumb dorsally. The patient's lunate is similarly stabilized with the examiner's other hand. The examiner attempts to 'shuck' the triquetrum back and forth on the stabilized lunate.

CIND conditions present following repeated stress or trauma with a history of underlying congenital ligamentous laxity in approximately 50% and poorly localized chronic wrist pain and tenderness (aggravated by activities). A 'catch-up clunk' of the proximal carpal row may be demonstrated (by either the patient or the examiner moving the wrist from radial to ulnar deviation or vice versa, or through a circumduction arc, possibly under axial compression).

Box 12.30.3 Investigations

- Watson's scaphoid shift test may demonstrated SL dissociation
- AP and lateral radiographs may not demonstrate acute ligament injury
- Clenched fist view may be helpful
- Gilula's lines is helpful in assessing for carpal dislocation
- Normal scapholunate angle is 30–60 degrees.

Normally the helicoid articulation between the triquetrum and the hamate, causes a tendency for the triquetrum to dorsiflex (with the tendency of entire proximal row to follow being balanced by the flexion moment from the scaphoid). In a traumatized or congenitally lax wrist, the laxity of the carpus permits exaggerated or prolonged flexion of the proximal carpal row in radial deviation. With ulnar deviation there is a delay before the proximal carpal row 'snaps' back into place and congruent articulation is restored.

Perilunate dislocations often occur in the context of high-energy trauma and a multiply injured patient and can cause characteristic wrist deformities. When the carpus is dislocated dorsally the radius is prominent in the carpal tunnel, on the palmar surface of the wrist as is the lunate in a pure lunate dislocation. Despite this up to 25% of these injuries are diagnosed late.

In dorsal perilunate dislocation the palmar skin and median nerve must be examined carefully. Median nerve damage is the most common associated injury and laceration of the palmar skin may indicate an open dislocation or fracture–dislocation. Palmar skin ischaemia may also be caused by pressure from the radius. Both arterial and compartment problems may occur and must be excluded. Bones or their fragments may be significantly displaced or even extruded.

Investigations

Imaging

Radiographic evaluation of wrist pain should include standard PA and lateral radiographs of the carpus. The PA film is centred over the radiocarpal articulation to assess accurately the SL interval, scaphoid position, LTq articulation, ulnar styloid, distal radius articular surface, and distal radioulnar joint.

The PA film is taken with the shoulder abducted 90 degrees, the elbow flexed at 90 degrees, neutral forearm rotation, an overhead x-ray beam, and the wrist placed flat on the x-ray plate, and 10 degrees x-ray beam radial angulation will enhance visualization of the SL interval. As discussed in Chapter 12.31, pronation causes relative shortening of the radius and will be apparent if the PA radiograph is incorrectly taken in this position.

Axial loading of the wrist, achieved with a 'clenched-fist' PA view, will accentuate any SL diastasis.

The lateral wrist film must also be taken in neutral forearm rotation, with the patient adjacent to a radiography table, the shoulder adducted, the thumb positioned toward the ceiling, and the wrist resting on the x-ray plate. A good lateral radiograph of the wrist should display: complete superimposition of the lunate, proximal scaphoid pole and triquetrum, the scaphoid tubercle overlies the pisiform, the radial styloid is in the 'centre' of the radius, and metacarpal shaft superimposition. If the lateral radiograph is incorrectly taken in ulnar deviation, then proximal carpal row dorsiflexion will produce an apparent DISI pattern.

Scaphoid views are obtained if there is tenderness in the anatomic snuffbox or if the PA and lateral radiographs suggest scaphoid pathology. The conned scaphoid waste view is obtained with the wrist in maximal ulnar deviation and 10-degree distal x-ray beam angulation. This produces an elongated, enlarged, detailed image of the scaphoid waste accentuating the trabecular pattern.

A wrist motion series includes flexion lateral, extension lateral, PA radial deviation, and PA ulnar deviation radiographs of both wrists. In ulnar deviation the scaphoid extends and appears elongated, while in radial deviation it should flex and appear shortened. SL diastasis usually accentuates in ulnar deviation and closes in radial deviation.

A so-called 'six shot' wrist series includes: PA, PA radial deviation, PA ulnar deviation, PA clenched fist, lateral, and lateral clenched fist views.

The normal SL interval on a PA radiograph measures 3mm or less. Diastasis beyond this indicates a possible SL dissociation. In SL dissociation, the scaphoid typically rotates out of the radial fossa into increased flexion. When viewed on the PA radiograph, this 'scaphoid rotatory subluxation' produces an 'end on' image of the scaphoid with overlapping cortical edges, known as the 'scaphoid cortical ring sign'.

Gilula described three smooth arcs, assessed on PA radiographs which can be traced along the proximal radiocarpal surface of the scaphoid, lunate, and triquetrum; the distal midcarpal surface of these same bones; and the proximal midcarpal surface of the capitate and hamate. An assessment of Gilula's lines provides a quick screen for fracture, dislocation, or instability of the carpus.

A PA distraction view (20–25-kg finger-trap traction) helps to define carpal fractures and dislocations in complex acute injuries such as perilunate dislocations. It can alert the physician to other injuries, e.g. palmar avulsion fracture of the triquetrum indicating a significant ulnar-sided ligament injury.

The normal lateral SL angle (formed by the intersection of the longitudinal axes of the lunate and the scaphoid) measures 30–60 degrees. An angle greater than 70 degrees is diagnostic for DISI pattern, while an angle less than 30 degrees represents a VISI pattern. A 'double check' for this diagnosis is the evaluation of the capitolunate angle (measured as the angle bisecting the longitudinal axis of the lunate and the capitate, normally 0 degrees) measuring greater than 15 degrees in a DISI deformity and less than 0 degrees in a VISI deformity. An apparently increased SL angle will appear with displaced scaphoid fractures and displaced/malunited Colles type distal radius fractures.

Arthrography

Standard arthrography has traditionally been used as an aid to the diagnosis of carpal ligament injuries. However as discussed in Chapter 12.31 (injuries to DURJ) false positive results can occur, particularly if, for example, there is a small perforation in an otherwise functionally competent SL ligament, which still allows contrast to pass from the radiocarpal to the MCJ. Arthroscopy remains the gold standard in the diagnosis of intraosseous ligament tears. Cadaveric studies have shown a high incidence of asymptomatic communications. Bilateral wrist arthrography has demonstrated similar communications in the contralateral asymptomatic wrists of patients evaluated for wrist pain.

Magnetic resonance imaging (MRI) or computed tomography (CT) scanning is now commonly performed as adjunct to plain arthrography, further improving its diagnostic accuracy, and providing extremely useful diagnostic information that helps to inform the patient and physician in the decision-making process prior to embarking on more invasive procedures.

Computed tomography scan

CT scanning is now widely available and is extremely useful, particularly in the context of acute injuries, for identifying suspected carpal bones fractures that remain 'occult' on plain radiographs, and for assessing preoperatively the true nature and full extent of complex wrist injuries. Unless it is combined with arthrography, it does not demonstrate wrist ligament injuries well.

Magnetic resonance imaging

Where high field strength magnets and dedicated wrist coils are employed, high-resolution MRI scans offer increasing accuracy in the diagnosis of carpal ligament injuries, particularly if combined with magnetic resonance arthrography (MRA).

MRI can demonstrate bone oedema, injury, and circulation, and intraosseous ligament damage, and increasingly also evidence of extrinsic or capsular ligament injuries. Gadolinium-enhanced MRI scans provide additional information about the vascularity and viability of carpal bones that is helpful in the context of scaphoid or lunate fractures, presenting with delayed or non-union.

Arthroscopy (Box 12.30.4)

Wrist arthroscopy remains the gold standard in the diagnosis of intra-articular wrist disorders and ligament injuries.

If non-invasive investigations have failed to identify a cause for a patient's wrist pain, particularly if follows a significant injury, then an examination under anaesthetic and diagnostic wrist arthroscopy should be considered.

Despite some limitations, which result from the necessity to place the wrist in traction, wrist arthroscopy provides a dynamic evaluation of the wrist including the status of: cartilage surfaces; synovium; most portions of the ligaments (intrinsic and extrinsic); the relative stability/motion between carpal bones; any anomalous structures, entrapped tissues, cartilage or bone debris, and tethering scar tissue.

Classifications of arthroscopic findings have been devised to facilitate accurate descriptions and to grade their significance as part of the decision-making process for treatment. For example, the classification of SL instability described by Geissler based on arthroscopic findings (Table 12.30.2).

Treatment

Carpal instability dissociative

CID is when instability arises due to injury between two bones in the same carpal row. Most commonly this occurs between the scaphoid and lunate or the lunate and triquetrum.

Table 12.30.2 The Geissler classification of SL ligament tears

Grade	Description
I	Attenuation or haemorrhage of an interosseous ligament is seen with the arthroscope placed in the radiocarpal space. There is no incongruency between the carpal bones with the arthroscope in the midcarpal space
II	Attenuation or haemorrhage of the interosseous ligament is again seen with the arthroscope in the radiocarpal space. There is an incongruency between the carpal bones when they are viewed from the midcarpal space
III	There is a separation between the carpal bones evident in the radiocarpal and the midcarpal space. A small joint probe passes through the gap between the carpal bones
IV	The gap between the carpal bones is wider, and a 2.7-mm arthroscope can be passed through this gap

Box 12.30.4 Anthroscopy

- Arthroscopy most sensitive technique for assessing intrinsic ligament injuries
- Geissler classified arthroscopic findings of SL injuries.

Scapholunate dissociation

Acute scapholunate dissociation (Box 12.30.5)

Following a ligament injury, the normal forces that act on the carpal bones can lead to the development of a progressive DISI carpal malalignment. This may be prevented if following an acute injury an anatomical reduction is achieved and maintained for long enough to allow the soft tissues to heal correctly.

Acute SL injuries without carpal malalignment may be treated with percutaneous K-wire fixation under image intensifier control. Temporary K-wires are inserted from the dorsum and used to 'joystick' the scaphoid and lunate to ensure anatomical reduction. Ideally two K-wires (mechanically more stable than one wire) are then passed from the scaphoid into the lunate to maintain position while the SL ligament heals. The wires are maintained for 8–10 weeks, so must be left buried under the skin to reduce the risk of infection. To reduce the risk of wire breakage, the wrist is immobilized in a below-elbow cast, until the wires are removed. Following which, intensive physiotherapy is commenced.

Some authors have reported good results with arthroscopically assisted K-wire fixation, allowing improved accuracy of reduction and wire placement. Arthroscopy also facilitates the debridement of any prominent ligament remains.

Complete disruption of the SL ligament may result in dynamic SL dissociation, where DISI malalignment of the carpal bones occurs only when forces are applied across the wrist. Following an acute injury of this magnitude, it is desirable to restore the anatomical position of the carpus and to formally repair the ligaments. The SL ligament can rupture through its midsubstance or be avulsed from (usually the scaphoid) with or without bone.

Although volar and dorsal approaches have been described, studies have suggested that a dorsal repair may be adequate. The wrist joint is approached between the third and fourth dorsal compartments. Anatomical reduction of the carpal alignment is achieved and maintained with buried K-wire fixation (as described earlier). A direct suture repair of midsubstance tears may be possible, but augmentation with bone anchors is often required. Small avulsion fractures are also reattached with bone anchors. The repair may also be augmented with a Blatt's dorsal capsulodesis, tightening the capsule between the radius and the distal scaphoid and preventing excessive scaphoid flexion. Postoperatively the patient is treated as previously described.

Static reducible scapholunate dissociation

If the presentation is delayed and the SL dissociation has not been treated in the acute phase, then the remains of the SL ligament retract and a primary repair is no longer possible. If the secondary restraint of the external ligaments fails progressively a permanent DISI carpal malalignment may develop. In symptomatic patients where carpal subluxation is still reducible and no degenerative changes have developed, a soft tissue reconstruction is possible.

Several ligament reconstruction techniques are described using tendon grafts, to maintain the normal carpal alignment. Perhaps the most popular tendon reconstruction currently is that described by Brunelli, who described using a distally based strip of FCR which is passed through a drill hole in the distal scaphoid. The remaining FCR tendon is then sutured across the SL interval to the remains of the SL ligament and attached to the distal radius. This was later modified to avoid crossing the radio carpal joint and instead the FCR tendon is (attached with a bone anchors to the dorsal lunate) and passed under the dorsal radiotriquetral ligament and then sutured back on its self. The long-term benefits of this procedure are not yet known.

Scapholunate advanced collapse wrist

Long standing SL dissociation may eventually lead to the characteristic progressive secondary degenerative changes described as a Scapholunate advanced collapse (SLAC) wrist. Many patients who reach this stage will respond to non-operative treatment. If this fails to control their symptoms then surgical intervention with one of the following salvage procedures may be considered.

The early stages of SLAC wrist involve the development of painful isolated radioscaphoid degenerative changes, which can be successfully treated with a radial styloidectomy. This pain relieving procedure does not correct the underlying pathological process, and degenerative changes may continue to progress across the midcarpal joint.

Proximal row carpectomy with excision of the scaphoid, lunate and triquetrum, creates a new articulation between the capitate

Box 12.30.5 Acute scapholunate dissociation

- In acute SL injures reduction, K-wire fixation ± SL repair should be performed
- In delayed presentation with no arthrosis, soft tissue reconstruction may be appropriate (e.g. modified Brunelli procedures)
- In long-standing injures with secondary arthrosis salvage procedures need to be considered (e.g. proximal row carpectomy or scaphoidectomy + four-corner fusion).

head and the lunate fossa of the radius. This procedure does not rely on successful bone healing at an arthrodesis site and so allows early mobilization. However, it requires healthy articular cartilage on both the capitate head and the lunate fossa, so is contraindicated when degenerative changes have already spread across the MCJ. Patients report good pain relief and a functional range of movement and grip strength. If symptomatic degenerative changes subsequently develop between the capitate head and radius a wrist arthrodesis can be performed.

Scaphoid excision and four-corner arthrodesis (capitate, lunate, triquetrum and hamate) is a successful procedure for an intermediate stage SLAC wrist. Various fixation techniques have been used to stabilize the arthrodesis site including K-wires, staples, screws, and more recently low profile circular plates. A supplementary circular bone graft can also be placed at the junction of the four bones. Healthy cartilage in the radiolunate joint is a prerequisite for this procedure, but it is successful at relieving pain even in the presence of degenerative change in the MCJ, between the capitate head and lunate.

In all the chronic wrist instabilities with associated degenerative change, pan-carpal wrist arthrodesis remains a salvage option. In order to obtain a successful outcome, solid fusion of the radioscaphoid, radiolunate, SL, capitolunate, scaphocapitate and capitate–third metacarpal joints needs to be achieved. Various fixation techniques have been described, including K-wires, interosseous pins, and dynamic compression plates. Dedicated AO wrist arthrodesis plates benefit from built in wrist extension, smaller 2.7-mm screws for the metacarpal shaft, 3.5-mm screws for the radius, and achieve high rates of successful fusion.

Lunotriquetral dissociation

Acute lunotriquetral dissociation

These injuries were previously treated non-operatively in a moulded cast. However this does not prevent the subsequent development of a chronic VISI deformity. The development of wrist arthroscopy has enabled the early diagnosis and treatment of LTq dissociation. It is desirable to reduce and fix these acute injuries with percutaneous K-wires, or to perform a repair by open or arthroscopically assisted means, in a manner similar to that for the treatment of acute SL dissociation.

Chronic dynamic lunotriquetral dissociation

As with the management of a delayed SL dissociation, the remains of the LTq ligament can be debrided arthroscopically. If the deformity is still reducible, tendon reconstruction may be attempted using a strip of ECU between the lunate and triquetrum, as described by Shin and Bishop. LTq arthrodesis has also been attempted, but with a relatively high rate of failure to achieve bony fusion.

Chronic static dissociation

Late ligament reconstruction is not possible, and if LTq arthrodesis does not adequately control the deformity, then a midcarpal or pancarpal arthrodesis should be considered.

Carpal instability non-dissociative

CIND occurs when the instability is due to dysfunction between the proximal and distal rows. The relationship between individual bones within a row however remains unaffected.

Radiocarpal dislocation

Pure dislocation of the radiocarpal joint is rare. It is more usually associated with an avulsion fracture of the radial styloid and urgent reduction is required. Neurovascular injury is commonly associated with these injuries. Following reduction, the radiocarpal joint is often unstable and open ligament reattachment may be required. Any associated radial styloid fracture is reduced and fixed restoring joint congruence and ligament stability.

Midcarpal instability

Acute midcarpal fracture dislocation is rare and should be treated in a similar manner to an acute perilunate dislocation. Chronic instability and malalignment of the MCJ represents a complex spectrum of conditions. When it presents as a dynamic problem, in the context of a congenital increase in ligamentous laxity, the initial treatment should be non-operative with splintage, activity modification and physiotherapy. Several soft tissue reconstructions and fusions have been described for patients with persistent symptoms, but these are all small studies.

Carpal instability complex

CIC covers a group of injuries in which there is disruption between bones of the same row and between separate rows.

Perilunate dislocation

Dislocation of the carpus around the lunate can be treated with an initial closed manipulation. If there are symptoms of median nerve compression then urgent carpal tunnel decompression is performed.

The extreme instability that results from these severe, often high-energy injuries, means that it is unusual for a true anatomical reduction to be achieved by closed manipulation alone. Therefore, early percutaneous K-wire fixation should be considered. Reduction of the lunate and scaphoid can be achieved using 'joystick' K-wires. Buried K-wires are then placed, in a similar manner to that described earlier for SL and LTq dissociations, to maintain the carpal alignment.

Severe injuries with gross instability, or those that are not fully reducible by percutaneous means, require open reduction via a dorsal approach which allows precise anatomical carpal alignment. The reduction is restored and maintained with the placement of transfixing K-wires. The dorsal approach facilitates the repair of the dorsal intrinsic and extrinsic ligaments. An additional palmar approach, via an extended carpal tunnel decompression, may also facilitate the reduction (especially of palmar dislocations) and a repair of the palmar wrist capsule.

Trans-scaphoid perilunate dislocation

The treatment of trans-scaphoid perilunate dislocations follows similar principles to pure perilunate dislocations. Urgent reduction and probable carpal tunnel decompression are required. It is important to achieve an anatomical reduction and stable fixation of the scaphoid fracture.

Open reduction and internal compression screw fixation of the scaphoid fracture and repair of the dorsal ligaments is best achieved via a dorsal approach. Arthroscopically assisted percutaneous scaphoid fixation may also be considered. The perilunate dislocation component of the injury is then stabilized with percutaneous K-wires as described earlier.

The wrist is initially immobilized for 8 weeks until the K-wires immobilizing the LT and MCJs are removed. Further immobilization may then be required if there is delayed healing of the scaphoid fracture. Ultimately, if a scaphoid fracture non-union develops it may require reconstruction with a bone graft and repeat fixation.

Patients should always be advised to avoid cigarette smoking to ensure the optimum bone-healing environment is maintained.

Greater-arc injuries

This variation of a perilunate dislocation involves fractures through the carpal bones adjacent to the lunate and is distinguished from the lesser arc injury in which there are purely ligamentous disruptions between the lunate and its neighbouring carpal bones. The classic injury involves fractures of the scaphoid, capitate, hamate, and triquetrum, but other fracture patterns or combinations of fractures and ligamentous injuries can occur. These severe injuries usually require open reduction via a dorsal approach, anatomical fracture reduction and internal compression screw fixation. Postoperative treatment is similar to that which is required following the lesser arc perilunate dislocation.

Scaphocapitate syndrome

This rare injury involves a scaphoid waist fracture and a transverse fracture of the capitate proximal pole, which then rotates through 180 degrees. The injury represents an incomplete greater-arc injury, propagated from the radial side of the carpus. Treatment includes open reduction and internal fixation and good results have been reported.

Results of treatment

Early reconstruction of SL dissociation has been show to have better outcomes compared with delayed treatment. In a study of 21 patients who underwent direct repair of the SL ligament with or with out capsulodesis, 19 patients had and improvement in their pain and grip strength. In addition a normal SL angle was maintained at 3-year follow-up.

There are few reports of the long-term results of delayed tendon reconstruction. Seventy-nine percent of patients undergoing a Brunelli reconstruction have satisfactory results. These results are promising, but the longer-term results are not yet known.

Radiocarpal arthrodesis is often avoided due to the potential for a reduced range of movement. However radiolunate fusion has been used with success in carpal instability. Pain relief was excellent and the preoperative range of motion was maintained. Radiocarpal fusion still allows movement at the MCJ, in particularly the functional 'dart throwing' movement (radial-extension toward ulnar-flexion).

Advanced degenerative changes (SLAC wrist) are best treated with either an excision of scaphoid and four-corner arthrodesis, or a proximal row carpectomy. A prospective study comparing these two procedures in 30 cases found no difference in pain or functional improvement. However, there were more complications in the four-corner arthrodesis group.

Proximal row carpectomy results in a high degree of patient satisfaction, a functional range of wrist motion and good pain relief but requires healthy articular cartilage on capitate head and lunate fossa.

If the degenerative SLAC wrist changes have extended to involve the capitate head then an excision of scaphoid and four-corner arthrodesis should give the best results. However, as with any midcarpal arthrodesis, it will result in the loss of approximately 50% flexion and extension and some radial deviation at the wrist.

In cases with advanced SLAC degenerative changes that require a pan carpal wrist arthrodesis as a salvage procedure, the AO wrist arthrodesis plate has been demonstrated as a reliable implant and technique.

Perilunate dislocations of the wrist are devastating injuries with poor results if left untreated. Despite treatment more than 50% of patients will go on to develop degenerative changes. However the incidence of carpal instability is reduced with open reduction and SL repair. If these injuries are treated appropriately at the time of injury, reasonable results can be achieved. In 14 patients with trans-scaphoid perilunate fracture dislocations whom underwent open reduction and internal fixation, all the scaphoid fractures healed and more than two thirds reported good functional recovery (Box 12.30.6).

The best reported results of radiocarpal dislocation have been with percutaneous K-wiring with or without open ligamentous repair.

Box 12.30.6 Treatment of perilunate dislocations

- Perilunate dislocations require urgent reduction and stabilization
- Urgent carpal tunnel decompression is often required
- If associated with a scaphoid fracture (trans-scaphoid perilunate dislocation) then scaphoid fixation is also required
- Care should be taken to exclude an associated capitate fracture.

Fractures of carpal bones other than the scaphoid

Evaluation and treatment

Lunate

Acute fractures of the lunate are relatively rare. They usually occur following a fall on a hyperextended wrist. Patients complain of pain and tenderness over the dorsum of the wrist. Standard poster anterior and lateral radiographs should be performed. If these appear normal, but a fracture is suspected, a CT scan should be obtained. Most small or undisplaced fractures can be treated non-operatively in a forearm cast. Displaced fractures require open reduction and internal fixation with cannulated screws (or K-wires). Wrist arthroscopy may be used to aid fracture reduction.

Perhaps the most common cause of lunate fractures is fragmentation secondary to the osteonecrosis seen in Kienböck's disease. The diagnosis of Kienböck's is usually based on the changes on plain radiographs. In the very early stages of the disease when radiographs remain normal, an MRI may be diagnostic. A more detailed discussion of Kienböck's disease is given in Chapter 6.3.

As with all carpal bone fractures, there may be a somewhat tenuous blood supply to the fracture site, and a harsh mechanical environment. Biological and mechanical factors should be addressed to ensure an optimal bone-healing environment is maintained and patients should always be advised to avoid cigarette smoke.

Triquetrum

Fractures of the triquetrum are the second most common carpal bone fracture. Tenderness over the ulnar side of the wrist raises the possibility of a triquetral fracture. Triquetral fractures may be associated with other carpal bone fractures or perilunate dislocations.

Small dorsal cortical triquetral fractures are common and may be due to impaction against the ulnar styloid or avulsion. These fractures can usually be treated with immobilization in a cast or splint. If they fail to unite and become symptomatic, then the fragment can be excised. Triquetral body fractures are usually identified on routine poster anterior radiographs of the wrist while dorsal chip fractures are generally identified on the lateral radiograph.

Triquetral body fractures can occur with perilunate injuries so these patients should be carefully examined for wrist instability. Open reduction and internal fixation should be considered for displaced triquetral body fractures.

Palmar ligamentous avulsion fractures are often not demonstrated on plain radiographs, but may be identified on CT scanning. These fractures may indicate a ligamentous injury with carpal instability. These injuries are managed as a LTq instability.

Trapezium

Fractures of the trapezium should be suspected in patients with pain at the base of the thumb after a direct blow. The fracture may be evident on plain radiographs or on a CT scan with sagittal reconstruction.

Trapezial ridge fractures may be identified on a carpal tunnel view. These usually represent an avulsion injury of the flexor retinaculum. These and nondisplaced trapezial body fractures may be treated by thumb spica cast immobilization for 4 weeks followed by mobilization if the fracture has healed clinically. Displaced trapezial body fractures with intra-articular extension require open reduction to restore the joint surface. Fixation is achieved with screws or K-wires. Subsequent symptomatic degenerative changes may later require arthrodesis or excision arthroplasty.

Trapezoid

Fractures of the trapezoid are extremely rare, most are detected on plain PA and lateral radiographs, but CT scanning will demonstrate fracture anatomy more precisely. Non-displaced fractures or small fragments should be treated conservatively in a short arm cast for 4 weeks followed by mobilization. Displaced fractures may require open reduction and pin or screw fixation.

Capitate

Capitate fractures can occur in isolation or in association with other carpal bone fractures and wrist ligament disruptions. Isolated non-displaced capitate fractures may be treated with cast and immobilization for 6 weeks followed by mobilization, provided clinical union is present. Isolated displaced capitate fractures require open (or arthroscopic assisted) reduction and internal fixation. Capitate fractures are prone to non-union and secondary post-traumatic osteoarthrosis. Capitate fracture non-unions should be treated with open reduction and internal fixation with bone grafting, possibly incorporating a partial arthrodesis.

Hamate

Hamate fractures either involve the body or more commonly the hook. Since hamate body fractures generally occur as a result of high-impact injury, a careful neurological examination is required. Standard PA, lateral, and oblique radiographs are obtained initially although a CT scan may be to determine the orientation of the fracture. Undisplaced, isolated body fractures can usually be treated conservatively with immobilization. If the fracture is displaced and involving the CMC joint, or if there is CMC joint instability, then reduction and fixation is required.

Fractures of the hook of the hamate typically present with hypothenar pain and tenderness. The diagnosis can often be difficult. A carpal tunnel view can be helpful, while CT scanning will usually confirm the diagnosis. Patients complain of pain in the hypothenar region which is worse on gripping. If diagnosed early, hamate hook fractures may be treated with a short arm cast for 4 weeks. However, painful hamate hook non-union is not unusual and can cause secondary flexor tendon attrition ruptures. Excision for hamate hook non-union through a carpal tunnel approach generally produces excellent results.

Pisiform

Pisiform fractures are uncommon, difficult to diagnose on radiographs, and are consequently often missed. As the Pisiform lies close to Guyon's canal, the ulnar nerve must be carefully examined. Pisiform fractures are treated with 4 weeks of short arm cast immobilization. If the fracture is comminuted, non-union occurs, or post-traumatic osteoarthrosis of the pisotriquetral joint develops, excision of the pisiform may be performed via a short longitudinal incision at the base of the hypothenar eminence (just distal to the distal wrist flexion crease). There is no significant loss of grip strength following pisiform excision.

Summary

Carpal instabilities represent a continuum of injuries, including subluxations, dislocations, unstable fractures, and fracture–dislocations, that are propagated from the radial or ulnar side of the wrist as a force is applied across a wrist (usually in hyperextension but occasionally in flexion). The force applied, site of application, force direction, and wrist position all determine the type of injury.

A detailed history and clinical examination with high-quality radiographs and if indicated a radiographic motion series remain the principle initial diagnostic tools. Additional imaging with standard arthrography, plain CT or MRI scans, or CT or MR arthrography are now providing increasingly accurate additional diagnostic information that can help the patient and physician to make informed decisions about treatment. Although more invasive, arthroscopy remains the gold standard investigation for diagnosing wrist ligament injuries.

The 'intercalated segment' concept helps to relate injuries to structure and function, to classify injuries, and to develop a logical approach to their diagnosis and treatment. Carpal instabilities can be classified as CID, CIND, or CIC, along with the simulated instabilities of 'CIA'. These injuries can then be further modified descriptively as DISI or VISI. Improved understanding of the complex anatomy and kinematics of the wrist is helping to further the development of rational surgical treatments for these problems, with earlier and more anatomic repair/reconstruction, and rehabilitation.

The carpal bones and their associated ligaments form an anatomically compact unit that functions by sharing forces throughout the carpus. Consequently, isolated carpal bone fractures are unusual but do occur. Because they are rare, they are often overlooked or passed off as insignificant.

Fractures of the proximal scaphoid, lunate, and capitate have a precarious interosseous blood supply and an increased risk for osteonecrosis. Symptomatic non-union of hamate hook fractures or pisiform fractures may be successfully treated with excision. Instability is often the 'common ingredient' in carpal injuries and its improved understanding and management remains central to the treatment of wrist injuries.

Further reading

Cooney W.P., Linscheid, R.L., and Dobyn, J.H. (eds) (1998). *The Wrist: Diagnosis and Operative Treatment.* St Louis, MO: Mosby/Mayo Foundation.

Garcia-Elias, M. (2008). The non-dissociative clunking wrist: a personal view. *Journal of Hand Surgery*, **33E**(6), 698–711.

Green, D.P., Hotchkiss, R.N., and Pederson, W.C. (eds) (2005). *Green's Operative Hand Surgery*, (Part III Wrist), fifth edition. Philadelphia, PA: Elsevier, Churchill Livingstone.

Lichtman, D.M. and Alexander, A.H. (1997). *The Wrist and Its Disorders*, second revised edition. Philadelphia, PA: W.B. Saunders.

Shin, A.Y, Battaglia, M.J. and Bishop, A.T. (2000). Lunotriquetral instability: diagnosis and treatment. *Journal of the American Academy of Orthopaedic Surgeons*, **8**(3), 170–9.

Stanley, J. (1995). *Safar Wrist Arthroscopy*. Philadelphia, PA: W.B. Saunders.

Walsh, J.J., Berger, R.A. and Cooney, W.P. (2002). Current status of scapholunate interosseous ligament injuries. *Journal of the American Academy of Orthopaedic Surgeons*, **10**(1), 32–42.

12.31

Injuries to the distal radioulnar joint

David Lawrie, Chris Little, and Ian McNab

Summary points

- Commonly missed injury
- Triangular fibro-cartilagenous complex integrity essential for DRUG stability
- Arthroscopy useful in assessing instability and the injury
- MRI increasingly accurate in diagnosis
- Ulnar shortening can be very useful in impingement.

Introduction

Once the acutely injured patient has been stabilized including a secondary survey, one must be vigilant regarding the potential for hand and wrist injury, which accounts for 17.6% of all missed fractures following blunt trauma. Injuries to the distal radioulnar joint (DRUJ) that are not detected or treated in the acute phase may present later with symptoms of ulna sided wrist pain or instability.

Relevant surgical anatomy and biomechanics (Box 12.31.1)

The ulna head articulates with the sigmoid notch of the distal radius (the DRUJ proper), and also with the ulnar side of the proximal carpal row (through the interposed triangular fibrocartilage—TFC). Injuries to the DRUJ can affect both articulations. The radius of curvature of the sigmoid notch is greater than that of the ulna head, reducing skeletal stability from bony congruence and allowing slide and glide motion in the DRUJ. The soft tissues around the ulna head are important for stability of the DRUJ and the proximal carpal row.

Load transfer from the hand is normally primarily radiocarpal (81.4%) but the proportion is dependent on the relative lengths of the ulna and radius (termed ulnar variance). When the ulna is lengthened by 2.5mm (positive ulnar variance), load transmission through the ulnocarpal articulation and TFC increases to 41.9% and reduces to 4.3% with 2.5mm ulnar shortening (Figure 12.31.1). The thickness of the TFC in a given individual varies depending on their ulnar variance. When assessing variance with post-traumatic

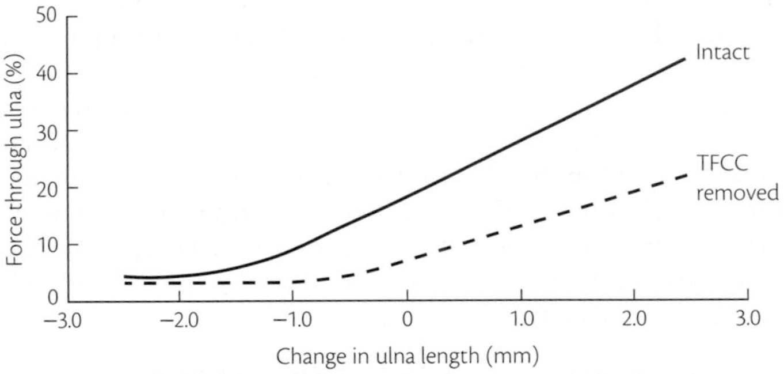

Fig. 12.31.1 Shortening of the ulna by 2.5mm results in a drop in ulnar load to 4.3%. Lengthening of the ulna by 2.5mm results in an increase in ulnar load to 41.9%.

ulnar wrist pain, comparison views of the uninjured side can be helpful. The TFC is also thinner in its central portion, where perforations are found with increasing prevalence with age.

Most people have a range of approximately 90 degrees of supination and approximately 80 degrees of pronation. Normal forearm rotation is important for many daily activities. The activities of daily living (ADL) require a 100-degree arc of forearm rotation. Supination is particularly important for ADLs and pronation very important for tasks such as use of a computer keyboard or mouse. While shoulder abduction can compensate for lost pronation, deltoid fatigues with prolonged abduction. Supination loses cannot be so easily overcome. With forearm rotation, the ulna remains essentially fixed and the radius rotates around the ulnar head. As the radius and ulna are joined proximally and distally, the relative lengths of the two bones (and so the ulnar variance) depends on the rotational position of the forearm; pronation is associated with relative shortening of the radius. This explains the ulnar-sided symptoms seen with forearm rotation in ulnocarpal impingement (see later).

The TFC is part of a complex soft tissue structure referred to as the triangular fibrocartilaginous complex (TFCC), the integrity of which is essential for DRUJ stability. The soft tissue can usefully be thought of as a complex of tissue whose form and function varies. The palmar and dorsal rims of the TFC form the palmar and dorsal radioulnar (RU) ligaments. The TFC and the deep portion of the ligaments insert into a fovea, the pre-styloid recess, which is found at the base of the ulnar styloid; this point marks the axis of rotation of the forearm. The superficial elements of the RU ligaments insert into the base of the ulna styloid. The insertion may be affected by basal ulnar styloid avulsion injuries, so explaining why DRUJ instability following trauma is much more common with basal styloid fractures than with tip fractures.

The blood supply to the TFC enters through its peripheral dorsal and palmar margins, giving these areas a rich blood supply and the best healing potential. The relatively avascular central portion has poor healing potential. Perforations of the TFC have been classified into acute and chronic lesions, and are described in Chapter 6.4.

During forearm rotation, the radius slides dorsally with supination (ulna head translates palmar) and palmar with pronation (ulna head translates dorsally). The tensions in the RU ligaments vary with forearm rotation, although studies have reached different conclusions regarding which become tense with pronation and which with supination. The apparently contradictory results were reconciled by an anatomical study that found that both the deep dorsal and superficial palmar ligaments tighten with supination (reciprocal changes seen with pronation).

The capsule of the DRUJ attaches to the proximal margin of the RU ligaments and the ulnocarpal ligaments (to the triquetrum and lunate) arise from the RU ligaments distally. On the dorsum, the capsule is thickened to form the floor of the fifth dorsal compartment and the floor of the sixth dorsal compartment explaining the crucial role of the extensor carpi ulnaris (ECU) and its subsheath in ulnar head stability.

Clinical evaluation: acute injury (Box 12.31.2)

Clinical examination of an acute wrist injury begins with examination of the forearm and elbow for fractures of the radius and ulna, elbow dislocation, fracture of the radial head, and dislocation of the proximal RU joint. Associated DRUJ and interosseous membrane injuries in this setting will have implications regarding treatment of the forearm and elbow injuries—the Essex-Lopresti injury (see Chapter 12.33).

Examination of the DRUJ itself begins by inspecting the location of the ulnar head. Dorsal prominence indicates dorsal DRUJ subluxation or dislocation, although swelling may partially obscure this. Palmar subluxation or dislocation may be less obvious clinically. The position, stability, and mobility of the distal ulna must be compared with that of the contralateral uninjured side.

By convention, DURJ instability causing a dorsal prominence of the ulna head is described as 'dorsal subluxation/dislocation' (usually accentuated in pronation). Palmar prominence of the ulna head is conventionally described as 'palmar subluxation/dislocation' (usually accentuated in supination). However, as stated earlier the ulna is actually the fixed bone in the forearm, around which the radius rotates. Thus, dorsal prominence of the ulna head actually represents palmar subluxation of the distal radius at the DURJ and vice versa.

Systematic palpation for deformity or tenderness in the region of the carpus, ulnar styloid, TFCC, and DRUJ must be performed. In the acute situation, it may not be possible to examine the full range of wrist motion, but it is important to establish that full forearm rotation is possible if a DRUJ injury is suspected.

DRUJ stability is assessed with the so-called 'piano key' test. The elbow is flexed and stabilized on the arm of the examining chair or couch. Attempts are made to translate the distal ulna out of the sigmoid notch of the radius in both palmar and dorsal directions, in positions of pronation, supination and neutral forearm rotation. Comparison is made with the contralateral uninjured side.

The neurovascular status of the hand must be evaluated, especially with palmar DRUJ dislocations, where the ulnar nerve and artery are at risk of injury.

Clinical evaluation: subacute or chronic injury

In the subacute setting, a careful history and physical examination are vital to establish whether ulnar-sided wrist pain is due to pathology in the DRUJ, TFCC, ulnar carpus, or other structures. If forearm rotation is reduced, it is important to establish whether it is due to incongruity of the DRUJ, proximal RU pathology, or malunion of a forearm fracture.

The patient should be asked to explain in detail the exact mechanism of injury, the specific movements that now provoke their symptoms, and, if possible, to indicate the precise anatomical origin of their pain, by pointing with a static finger. As with an acute injury, systematic direct palpation helps determine which of the ulnar-sided structures are involved in the injury.

It is important to establish the range of forearm rotation, especially the characteristic loss of supination in dorsal dislocations/subluxations, and pronation in volar dislocations/subluxations, and to compare this with the uninjured side to help determine the best method of treatment.

Ulnar-sided wrist pain may be due to increased contact forces between the ulnar head, the triangular disc, and the triquetrum or lunate. This ulnocarpal impingement is more common in the presence of positive ulnar variance and may be diagnosed clinically by

Box 12.31.1 Anatomy and biomechanics

- Ulna head articulates with the sigmoid notch of the distal radius
- Shallow sigmoid notch results in low skeletal stability
- Soft tissues key to stability:
  - TFCC
  - Ulnocarpal ligaments
  - ECU and sub sheath
- Central portion TFC prone to perforations (classified by Palmer).

Box 12.31.2 Acute injury

- Consider Essex-Lopresti injury when assessing injury
- Assess neurovascular status (especially ulnar nerve and artery)
- Ulna is fixed bone in the forearm around which the radius rotates
- DRUJ stability is assessed with the 'piano key' test
- Stability assessed in pronation and supination.

performing the following examination manoeuvre. The wrist is passively ulnar deviated, and a longitudinal axial load is applied to the wrist while it is then placed into supination and pronation. The test is positive if the patient's pain is reproduced. Logically the pain should be worst in pronation as this is the position where the radius is relatively shortened, but pain may also be provoked in supination.

The 'piano key' test (see earlier) can be further refined if it is also performed in wrist ulnar and radial deviation. If radial deviation increases the tension in the ulnocarpal ligaments sufficiently to reduce the amount of dorsal and palmar translation of the ulna head, then this indicates that following an ulna shortening osteotomy there may be some potential improvement in DURJ stability.

Tendonitis of the flexor carpi ulnaris (FCU) or ECU tendons may be diagnosed by tenderness or swelling along the tendon sheaths, pain on resisted flexion and ulnar deviation (FCU) or extension and ulnar deviation (ECU), and pain on passive stretch of these tendons (forced extension and radial deviation for FCU and forced flexion and radial deviation for ECU).

Investigations (Box 12.31.3)

Plain radiographs

A true posteroanterior (PA) radiograph of the wrist in neutral forearm rotation and a perfect lateral of the carpus and the distal radius are the key radiographs required to evaluate DRUJ congruity and reduction.

The true PA radiograph is taken with the shoulder in 90 degrees of abduction, the elbow in 90 degrees of flexion and an overhead x-ray beam. The hand and wrist are placed flat on the x-ray plate to achieve neutral forearm rotation. This view allows an accurate evaluation of the ulna variance. The styloid will appear directly in line with the ulnar cortex of the ulna in this view. If taken incorrectly in supination or pronation there will respectively be artificial lengthening or shortening of the radius apparent on the radiograph.

To determine if a true lateral projection of the wrist has been obtained, the alignment of the carpus should be assessed to ensure the scaphoid tubercle overlies the pisiform. With this projection, the true position of the ulna head relative to the radius will be shown.

To evaluate intra-articular fractures of the distal radius, ulna, and DRUJ, a computed tomography (CT) scan or two oblique views may be helpful.

Fluoroscopic examination

Live fluoroscopy of the DURJ is useful to assess its stability intraoperatively, or if subluxation or dislocation is suspected but plain radiographs cannot be obtained with the forearm appropriately positioned. A perfect lateral of the distal radius is obtained by live imaging, and the position of the ulna head is assessed. Dynamic stress fluoroscopy and clenched-fist views may be obtained to assess dynamic DRUJ and carpal instability. The ability to obtain and maintain reduction of the DRUJ can also be evaluated directly.

Computed tomography scan

CT scanning is the imaging modality of choice for suspected DRUJ subluxation or dislocation, distal radial fracture with DRUJ intra-articular extension, or DRUJ arthrosis (Figure 12.31.2).

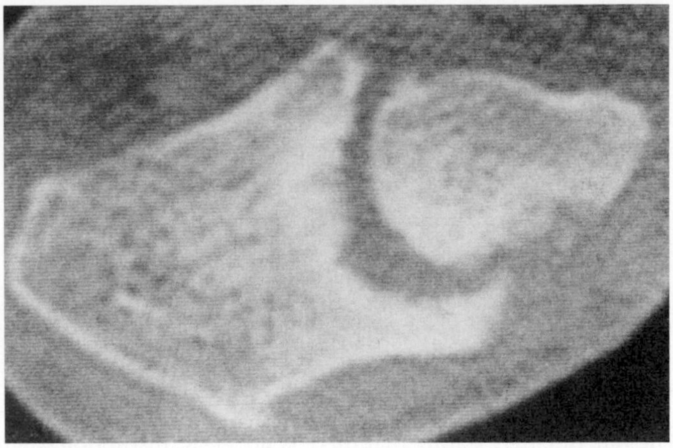

Fig. 12.31.2 CT scan through a grossly arthritic sigmoid notch.

Ulnar head stability within the sigmoid notch of the distal radius can be determined by CT evaluation of the position of the DRUJ in both pronation and supination, with simultaneous cuts of the opposite DRUJ with equivalent forearm rotation.

Arthrography

Arthrography or cine-arthrography may be performed if injury to the TFCC is suspected. Single or triple injection techniques may be employed. Magnetic resonance imaging (MRI) or CT scanning is now commonly performed as an adjunct to arthrography after obtaining plain arthrogram radiographs.

Flow of contrast from the DRUJ to the radiocarpal joint, or into the DRUJ after injection of contrast into the radiocarpal joint is diagnostic of a defect in the TFCC (Figure 12.31.3). Full-thickness central tears of the triangular disc are more commonly attritional and are seen in increasing frequency with increasing age. Peripheral tears that allow tracking of contrast around the triangular disc may result from trauma.

Studies have compared arthrographic findings to the 'gold standard' of arthroscopic findings. The rate of falsely identifying a TFCC lesion where none truly exists (a false-positive result) is low.

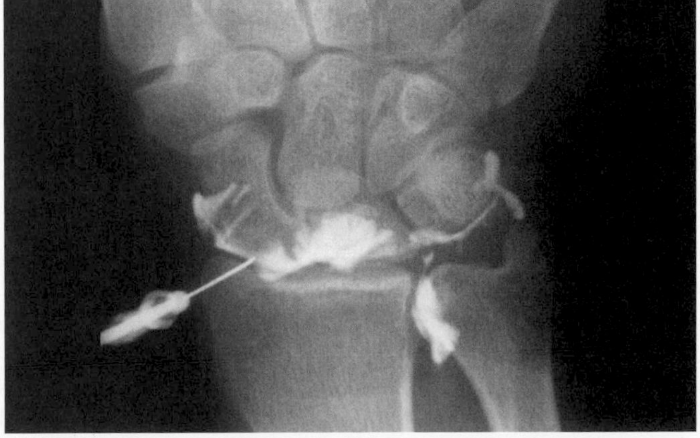

Fig. 12.31.3 An arthrogram, with dye being injected into the radiocarpal joint. A full-thickness tear of the TFCC from its origin on the sigmoid notch of the distal radius allows flow of dye into the DRUJ.

Box 12.31.3 Investigations

- Plain radiographs should include neutral rotation AP and lateral
- True lateral confirmed by scaphoid tubercle over lying pisiform
- Consider CT to confirm dislocation or subluxation
- Contrast flowing into DRUJ during arthrogram suggests TFC perforation
- Arthroscopy gold standard to assessing TFCC.

The rate of falsely stating that there is no TFCC disruption when one truly exists (a false-negative result) is substantially higher. In one study, of 32 patients with normal cine-arthrographic findings for TFCC tear, a subsequent wrist arthroscopy showed that 12 patients had full-thickness lesions of the triangular disc (location not specified). Imaging and clinical findings should always be correlated.

Magnetic resonance imaging

High field strength magnets and dedicated wrist coils are now producing high-resolution MRI scans that offer increasing accuracy in the diagnosis of acute ligamentous injuries of the carpus and TFCC, particularly when a combination of conventional and magnetic resonance (MR) arthrography is used. These investigations are now commonly performed to obtain additional diagnostic information, which helps to direct and inform the patient and physician, prior to embarking on more invasive procedures such as wrist arthroscopy, TFC debridement or repair, and RU ligament repair or reconstruction.

Arthroscopy

Arthroscopic examination of the wrist remains the gold standard for assessing the TFCC. It facilitates diagnosis of perforations (central, peripheral, partial or full-thickness), and chondral injuries of the distal radius, ulnar head, or proximal carpal row. Under surface partial thickness lesions can only be seen with DRUJ MR arthrography or arthroscopy.

Wrist arthroscopy is a useful diagnostic and therapeutic adjunct in the acute treatment of distal radius fractures. TFCC tears are present in as many as 66% of distal radial fractures.

Treatment (Box 12.31.4)

The treatment of DRUJ injuries is dependant of the time since injury, the type of injury, and any associated injuries.

Acute DRUJ instability

Acute isolated dislocations with no associated fracture are uncommon. By convention the direction of dislocation is defined by the displacement of the ulnar head in relation to the radius. Dorsal dislocation is more common than volar dislocation. If the injury is acute, reduction is usually easy. The stability of the DRUJ should then be assessed following the reduction. Dorsal dislocations tend to be more stable in supination and volar dislocations are more stable in pronation.

If there is only a moderate degree of DURJ instability then this can be treated in an above-elbow cast for 3–4 weeks followed by a forearm cast or splint. If the DRUJ is grossly unstable or requires extreme pronation or supination to maintain stability, then the addition of a percutaneous K-wire fixation across the distal radius and ulna should be considered. In these cases, the TFCC is disrupted and surgery to reattach the TFFC will also restore stability.

Distal radius fractures have an associated ulnar styloid fracture in 61% of cases. However, few of these result in DRUJ instability. Fractures of the tip of the styloid rarely lead to instability. If the fracture involves the base of the ulnar styloid (the site of TFCC attachment), and the DURJ is unstable clinically, then TFCC continuity and joint stability can be restored by internal fixation of the styloid fragment with either with a cannulated screw or 2 fine K-wires and a 'figure-of-eight' suture to act as a tension band (Figure 12.31.4).

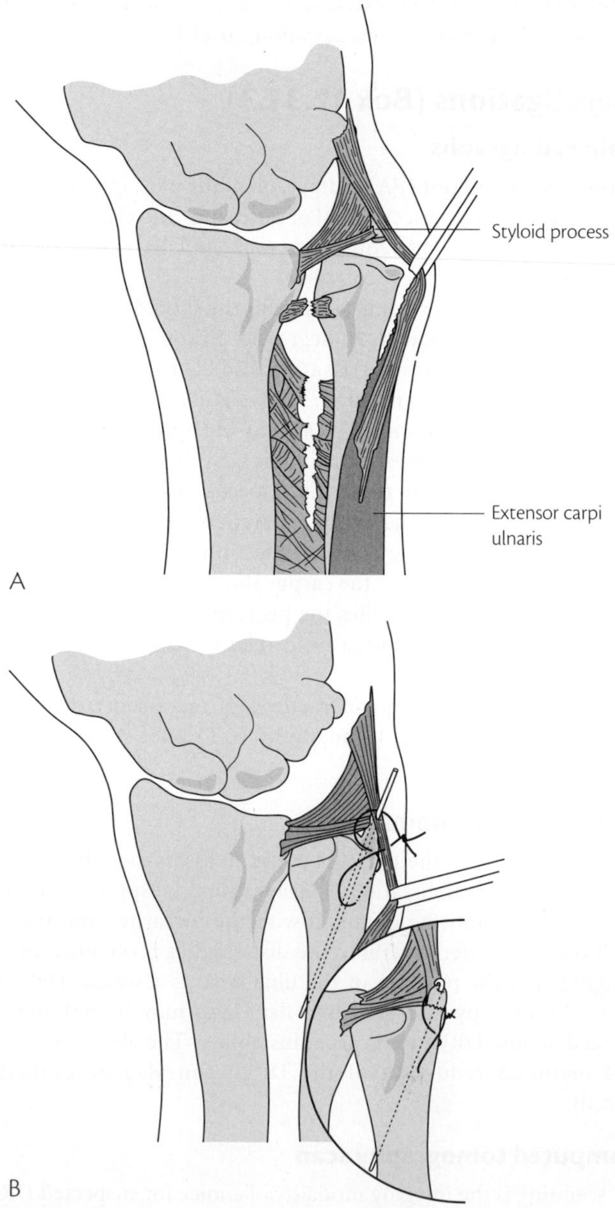

Fig. 12.31.4 The pathology and surgical technique of ulnar styloid process wiring.

Intra-articular distal radial fractures frequently involve the sigmoid notch and hence the DRUJ. The aim of treatment is to restore anatomical reduction of both the radiocarpal joint and the DRUJ, with stable fixation, to allow early mobilization of the joints.

If DRUJ subluxation or dislocation is associated with an extra articular forearm fracture (Galeazzi injuries and variants) or an elbow injury, then DRUJ stability is frequently restored by the reduction and stabilization of the forearm injury—particularly where the radial fracture is in the distal third. Having completed treatment of the proximal injury, assessment of the DRUJ reduction and stability should be made clinically and radiographically, and treated accordingly.

When closed reduction of the DRUJ is not possible, interposed soft tissue or bone fragments may be blocking reduction. Exploration is performed via a dorsal approach, through the floor of the fifth dorsal compartment, elevating an ulna-based capsular flap and repairing or reattaching the TFCC with transosseous sutures or suture anchors. Care has to be taken to avoid injury to the sensory branch of the ulnar nerve (Figure 12.31.5).

Chronic DRUJ instability

Symptomatic DRUJ instability is often associated with a malunited distal radial fractures. A trial of non-operative treatment should be undertaken initially with splintage and physiotherapy. If symptoms fail to improve and there is a malunion, then a corrective osteotomy will usually restore stability. If there is no bony deformity or secondary degenerative change, then soft tissue reconstructions may be attempted. Where possible the TFCC should be reattached. If the TFCC cannot be repaired, techniques have been described to reconstruct the volar ulnocarpal ligaments using a strip of FCU or both the volar and dorsal ulnocarpal ligaments.

DRUJ arthrosis

Degeneration of the DRUJ may arise due to intra-articular malunion or chronic instability. Symptoms may be controlled by intra-articular steroid injections. When injections fail to achieve adequate symptom relief, several salvage procedures have been described, but if they are performed in the presence of associated DURJ instability, this must also be addressed using appropriate soft tissue reconstructive procedures:

- Bowers hemiresection arthroplasty involves resection of the articular surface of the ulnar head but retains the ulnar attachments of the TFCC. If performed in isolation, this procedure may increase any existing instability
- The Sauvé–Kapandji procedure involves the creation of a distal RU fusion and a more proximal pseudarthrosis to allow forearm rotation. This procedure has the possible benefit of improved pain relief in arthritis; however, there is a risk of non-union, regeneration of the resected segment with loss of rotation, or significant symptomatic instability of the proximal ulnar stump (which is then difficult to address)
- The Darrach procedure involves resection of the distal ulna at the level of the ulnar neck and is best suited to patients with reduced functional demands
- DRUJ arthroplasty is possible, but requires restoration of stability. Part or all of the ulnar head can be replaced but the long-term results of these procedures are not yet known. Trials are also being undertaken on the new implants that replace both components of the DURJ.

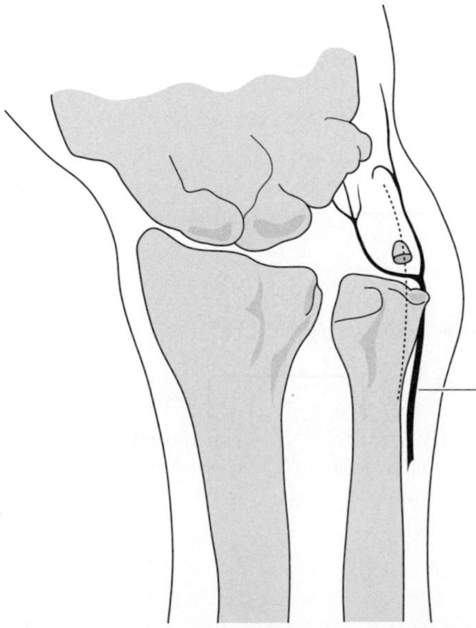

Fig. 12.31.5 The location of the dorsal sensory branch of the ulnar nerve, and its relation to the fractured ulnar styloid.

Box 12.31.4 Treatment

- Acute DRUJ instability may require re-attachment of TFCC ± K-wires across DRUJ
- If the TFCC is avulsed with a fracture at the base of the ulna styloid, it can be reattached with tension band wire
- If DRUJ dislocation is associated with a forearm fracture, anatomical fracture reduction usually reduces DRUJ
- Chronic DRUJ instability may require attempted TFCC reattachment, or a soft tissue reconstruction.

Ulnocarpal impingement (Box 12.31.5)

If a distal radial fracture heals in a shortened position, but with otherwise satisfactory alignment of the distal radial articular surface, then the sigmoid notch of the distal radial articular surface will lie proximal to the articular surface of the ulna head, which may cause DRUJ degeneration. The TFCC is tented over the ulna head, between the proximal ulnar aspect of the lunate and the ulna head, increasing load transmission in the ulnocarpal side of the wrist and progressive degenerative change between the ulna head, TFCC, and the ulnar carpus. Patients present with ulnar-sided wrist pain, especially during axial loading and ulnar deviation of the wrist and forearm rotation (Figure 12.31.6).

These distinctly different situations all require different surgical solutions:

- Occasionally, if the distal sigmoid notch joint surface is incongruent but the DRUJ articular surfaces are well preserved, a corrective distal radial osteotomy may be possible
- If the DRUJ joint surfaces are well aligned and preserved, and ulnocarpal impingement is the overriding problem, then an ulna

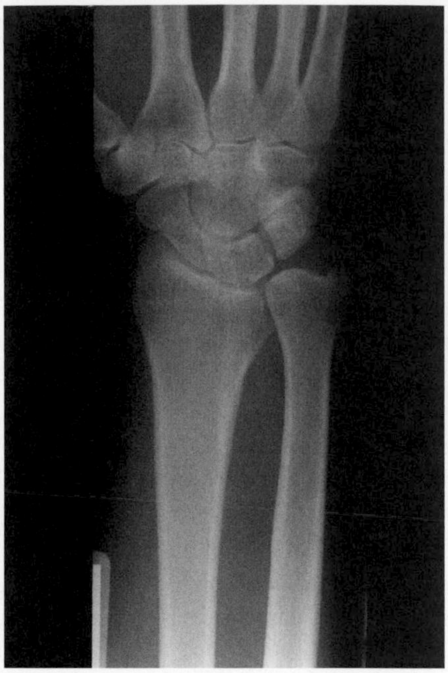

Fig. 12.31.6 The excessively long distal ulna, here a result of radial head resection prior to skeletal maturity, resulted in symptoms of ulnocarpal impingement.

shortening procedure is indicated. A minor degree of shortening (1–2mm) can be achieved by performing an intra-articular resection of the distal articular surface of the ulna head—a 'wafer' procedure (performed either open or arthroscopically)

- An ulna shortening osteotomy is indicated when a greater degree of shortening is required. This is reliably performed with an oblique osteotomy stabilized with a compression plate. The aim is to shorten the ulnar and to produce an ulnar neutral or mild ulnar minus variance and a congruent DRUJ

Box 12.31.5 Ulnocarpal impingement

- Ulnocarpal impingement occurs most commonly with positive ulnar variance
- Cystic change may be seen in ulnar corner of lunate
- Ulnar shortening by 2.5mm results in a drop in ulnar load to 4.3%
- Ulnar shortening performed using dynamic compression plate.

- If ulnocarpal impingement and DRUJ arthrosis are present, then one of the salvage procedures described earlier should be performed, whilst ensuring that adequate shortening of the ulna is also achieved.

Results of treatment

Early reduction of a dislocated DRUJ will ensure the best outcome. In one study, 25% of patients with dislocation of the DRUJ associated with a radial shaft fracture (Galeazzi), went on to lose more than 25 degrees of forearm rotation. In another study of 19 patients with DRUJ dislocation following Galeazzi fractures, it was shown that in patients in whom anatomical reduction of the DRUJ was achieved, there was minimal loss of function.

The results of soft tissue reconstruction for chronic instability have been variable. However, in one series of 14 patients who had a soft tissue reconstruction proceedure, stability was completely restored in 12.

One study using a Bowers procedure following malunion of distal radial fractures, all patients reported an improvement in their symptoms.

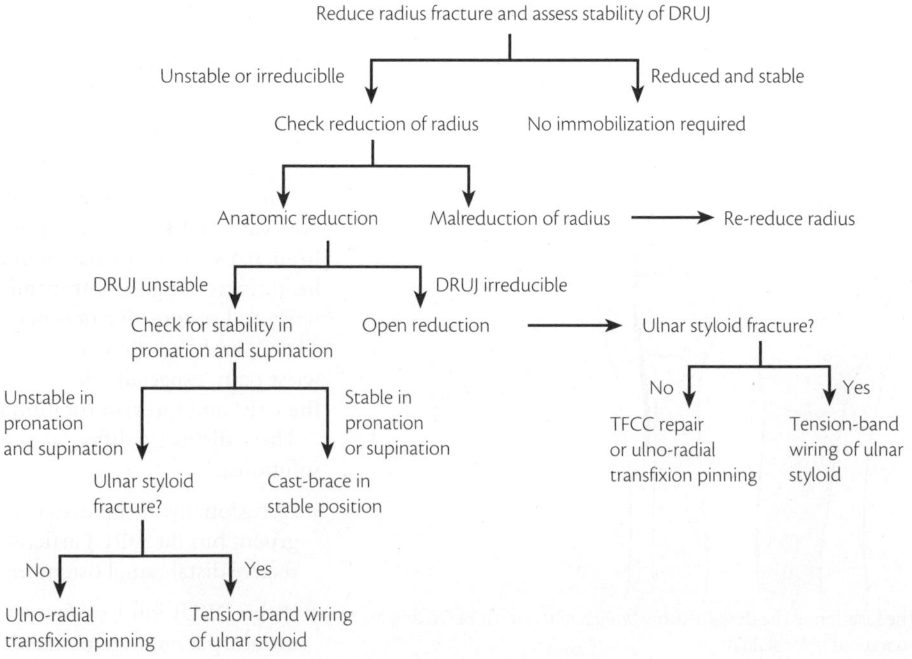

Fig. 12.31.7 Algorithm for decision-making in injuries of the DURJ and TFCC (courtesy of Dr S. Cheng).

Studies have reported that when using the Sauvé–Kapandji technique for post-traumatic instability, 11 of 17 patients were entirely pain-free with an additional five only complaining of minimal pain. Instability of the ulnar stump was a problem in two patients within the series.

The main complaint following a Darrach's procedure is instability of the distal ulna stump. Several studies have shown that the results are generally worse in patients with higher demands.

Several studies have shown high levels of success with the use of ulnar shortening for ulnocarpal impingement.

In a study of ulna head replacement in 13 patients, initial results (mean of 2 years) showed a reduction in pain scores of 50%. In one series, total DRUJ replacement was performed in 31 patients. Pain was greatly improved. Grip strength increased along with improved pronation and supination at a mean of 5.9 years follow-up.

Conclusion

The key to appropriate treatment of the DRUJ is early recognition of the injury. By defining the injury pattern acutely by history, clinical examination, and appropriate imaging, treatment of the upper extremity injury can proceed in an integrated fashion (Figure 12.31.7). Thus the goal of achieving full restoration of function to the injured extremity in as short a time period as possible may be realized.

Further reading

Büchler, U. (ed) (1996). *Wrist Instability.* New York: Informa Healthcare.

Cooney W.P., Linscheid, R.L., and Dobyn, J.H. (eds) (1998). *The Wrist: Diagnosis and Operative Treatment.* St Louis, MO: Mosby/Mayo Foundation.

Green, D.P., Hotchkiss, R.N., and Pederson, W.C. (eds) (2005). *Green's Operative Hand Surgery,* (Part III Wrist), fifth edition. Philadelphia, PA: Elsevier, Churchill Livingstone.

Lichtman, D.M. and Alexander, A.H. (1997). *The Wrist and Its Disorders,* second revised edition. Philadelphia, PA: W.B. Saunders.

Stanley, J. (1995). *Safar Wrist Arthroscopy.* Philadelphia, PA: W.B. Saunders.

Szabo, R.M. (2006). Distal radioulnar joint instability. *Journal of Bone and Joint Surgery,* **88A**, 884–94.

12.32

Distal radius fracture

Alastair Graham

Summary points

- Active treatment increasingly used
- It is important to recognize type B fractures
- CT useful to define complex fractures
- K wiring quick and simple but complex fractures often require plating
- Palmar locking plates useful for complex fractures
- Dorsal plates only used occasionally because of complications.

Introduction

Fractures of the distal radius were first recognized by Pouteau in 1783 and more widely recognized after Colles' description in 1814. Abraham Colles famously stated that 'one consolation only remains, that the limb will at some remote period again enjoy perfect freedom in all its motions and be completely exempt from pain: the deformity, however, will remain undiminished through life'.

This is one of the most common fractures in Western societies. With increasing longevity and activity in the middle-aged to elderly population the previous policies of 'benign neglect' may no longer be acceptable. Patients expect a strong and mobile hand. We should aim to achieve restore function quickly without exposing patients to additional risk.

Treatment of distal radial fractures is evolving rapidly. Published literature lags behind clinical practice by a year or two, textbooks even more so. Distal radial fracture management is remarkably diverse as surgeons apply traditional, contemporary, or innovative philosophies depending on factors such as published research, anecdotal belief, technical skill, availability of theatre time, and cost.

Classification

Fractures of the distal radius occur when a large loading force is applied between the proximal carpal row (particularly scaphoid and lunate) and the radial shaft. Various factors will determine the fracture pattern including the angulation of the wrist at the time of loading, the direction and magnitude of the force, the rate of loading, and the state of the underlying bone.

Eponyms are still commonly used but should probably be abandoned since they do not assist in management or prognosis. Many classification systems have been proposed. They should be simple to use, aid in decisions about management, allow an accurate prediction of prognosis, and also be used to define populations of patients in clinical research. In practice these ideals have not been achieved.

Deciding on stability is a useful aid to decision-making. Unstable fractures are those which will malunite if treated in plaster alone. This must be appreciated and treated to avoid long term deformity. Stability is judged from pre-reduction radiographs (Box 12.32.1).

Precise measurement of instability remains elusive. However, if any of these criteria are met then malunion could be expected with non-operative management. Many papers have shown that these factors correlate with final radiological outcome. However, they have not generally measured long-term clinical results using validated outcome measures. A key unanswered question is how malunion relates to long-term function.

The AO/OTA classification system is popular in current literature (Figure 12.32.1). This is a detailed classification with three main fracture groups and 27 fracture subtypes.

Recognizing type B fractures is important as the radiocarpal joint may sublux. These are fracture–dislocations of the wrist and patients can only regain useful function if the joint remains congruent.

Box 12.32.1 Factors associated with instability

- Age >65 years
- Osteoporosis
- Radial shortening >5mm
- Dorsal angulation >10 degrees
- Metaphyseal fragmentation
- Radial inclination >15 degrees
- Ulnar neck fracture.

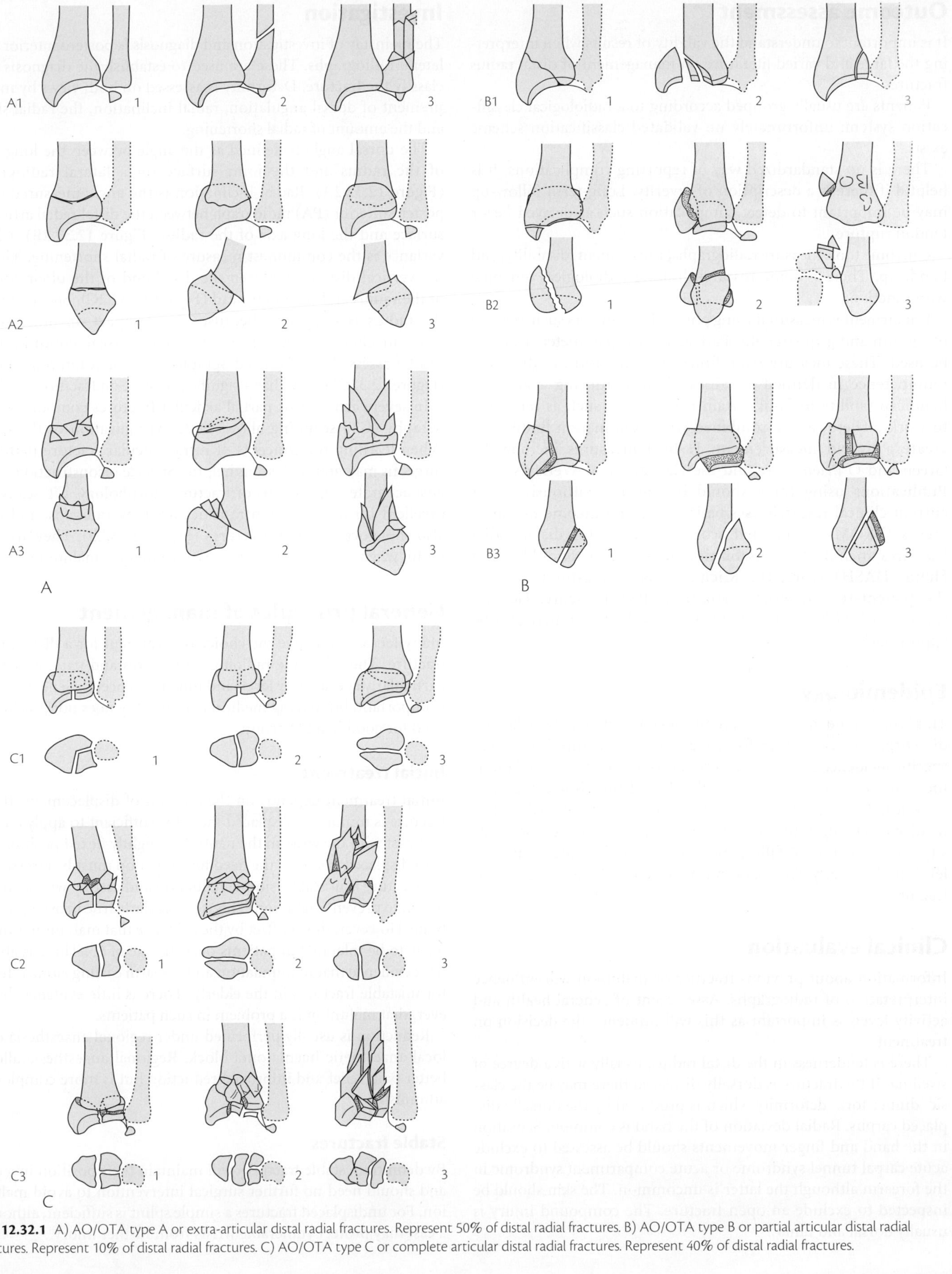

Fig. 12.32.1 A) AO/OTA type A or extra-articular distal radial fractures. Represent 50% of distal radial fractures. B) AO/OTA type B or partial articular distal radial fractures. Represent 10% of distal radial fractures. C) AO/OTA type C or complete articular distal radial fractures. Represent 40% of distal radial fractures.

Outcome assessment

It is important to understand the validity of results when interpreting the large and varied literature on management of distal radius fractures.

Patients are usually grouped according to a radiological classification system: unfortunately no validated classification scheme exists.

There is no standardized way of reporting complications. It is helpful if there is a description of severity. Long-term follow-up may be important to detect complication such as delayed flexor tendon rupture.

Outcome tools measure radiographs, impairment, disability, and handicap. There is some research linking radiological outcome with function.

Impairment is measured using physical parameters such as range of motion and grip strength. Patient-related parameters can also be used. These measure pain, function in the form of disability (competence in defined activities, such as turning a key), or handicap (ability to fulfil certain roles in life, such as returning to work). These can be combined with examination findings to create a hybrid measurement. Hybrid measures include the Green and O'Brien score and the Gartland and Werley scores. Publications using these should be viewed cautiously. Most current clinical research uses patient-related outcome measurements (PROMs). Validated scoring systems for distal radial fractures include the Disabilities of the Arm, Shoulder and Hand (DASH) score, the Michigan hand questionnaire and the patient-related wrist evaluation (PRWE) score. Generic functional health questionnaires such as the SF-36 may also be appropriate.

Epidemiology

This is one of the most common injuries encountered by orthopaedic surgeons accounting for 15–20%of all fractures. The age-specific incidence is consistent across various Western populations including Norway, Sweden, Scotland, and the United States of America. It affects four times more females than males. The incidence is rising as the population ages. Lower average bone density, increased rate of falling, poor vision, and increased activity levels in the elderly have all been implicated in the aetiology of this fracture.

Clinical evaluation

Information about previous fracture or malunion will influence interpretation of radiographs. Assessment of general health and activity levels is important as this will influence the decision on treatment.

There is tenderness in the distal radius, usually with a degree of swelling. If the fracture is dorsally displaced there may be the classic 'dinner fork' deformity which is produced by the dorsally displaced carpus. Radial deviation of the hand is common. Sensation in the hand and finger movements should be assessed to exclude acute carpal tunnel syndrome or acute compartment syndrome in the forearm although the latter is uncommon. The skin should be inspected to exclude an open fracture. The compound injury is usually dorsal and ulnar.

Investigation

The mainstay of investigation and diagnosis is posteroanterior and lateral radiographs. These are used to establish the diagnosis and classify the fracture. Deformity is assessed on both views by measurement of dorsal angulation, radial inclination, the radial shift, and the amount of radial shortening.

The dorsal angle is defined as the angle between the long axis of the radius and the joint surface on a lateral radiograph (Figure 12.32.2A). Radial inclination is the angle measured on a posteroanterior (PA) radiograph between the distal radial articular surface and the long axis of the radius (Figure 12.32.2B). Ulnar variance is the commonest measure of radial shortening. This is the vertical distance between the distal end of the ulnar corner of the radius and the ulnar head (Figure 12.32.2C). Shortening of the radius is important because of its impact on ulnar-sided wrist mechanics and symptoms. Metaphyseal comminution can be assessed on plain radiographs, is most commonly dorsal (Figure 12.32.2D), and has a significant effect on fracture stability.

In severe articular or partial articular fractures computed tomography (CT) scanning allows better visualization of the joint. When learning the concepts of intra-articular fracture patterns, surgeons may find such scans helpful. Surface reconstructions now give accurate impressions of fracture morphology. CT scans are excellent for measuring intra-articular steps and gaps, and may also show occult carpal fractures (Figure 12.32.3). They are also useful when planning corrective osteotomies for malunion.

General principles of management

Many factors influence the choice of treatment for a distal radial fracture. These include radiological features and patient factors, particularly age, activity level, and functional needs. General health is important, but having medical comorbidity does not preclude a need for good hand function.

Initial treatment

Initial treatment depends on the amount of displacement. If the fracture is minimally displaced then it is sufficient to apply a forearm cast with the wrist in the neutral or slightly flexed position.

In displaced fractures the need for reduction must be assessed. If the fracture is unstable, simple reduction and casting will be insufficient to prevent malunion. This is particularly true in osteoporotic bone. However, this is offset by the evidence that malunion is more likely to be tolerated in patients over the age of 65. There is abundant evidence that manipulation and forearm casting alone is futile for unstable fractures in the elderly. There is little evidence, however, that malunion is a problem in such patients.

Reduction is usually performed under regional anaesthesia or a local anaesthetic haematoma block. Regional anaesthesia allows better pain relief and improved reduction but is more complex to administer.

Stable fractures

By definition, stable fractures will maintain their position in a cast and should need no further surgical intervention to avoid malunion. For undisplaced fractures a simple splint is sufficient, although a cast may protect vulnerable wrists from further injury.

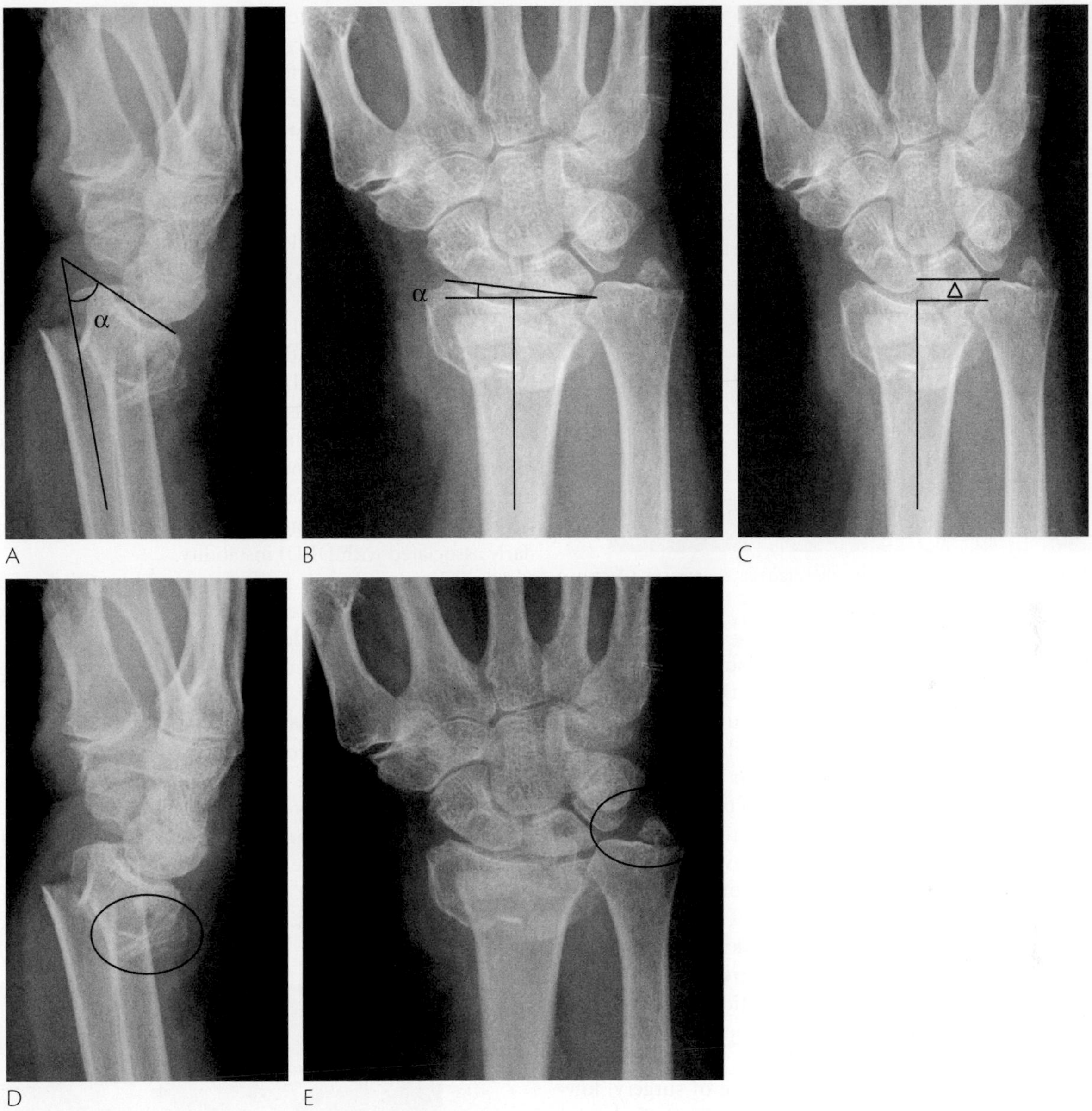

Fig. 12.32.2 A) Dorsal angulation. Normal is 11 degree palmar tilt. B) Radial inclination. Normal is 22 degrees. C) Radial length. Normally 0–2mm longer than ulna. D) Metaphyseal fragmentation. E) Associated ulnar styloid fracture.

Displaced fractures can be mobilized 3–4 weeks after reduction. Depending on whether the fracture is displaced in a dorsal or palmar direction it is customary to place the wrist in either palmar flexion or dorsiflexion although this may make little difference to the final outcome.

Unstable fractures

Management of unstable fractures of the distal radius is a contentious topic. Different methods of treatment are advocated. None has yet emerged as significantly superior. Management decisions should be based on the individual patient and the fracture type. Surgeons dealing with these injuries should ideally have a range of techniques at their disposal.

Many fractures deemed suitable for manipulation also fulfil the criteria for instability. This is particularly true in osteoporotic bone. Prediction of instability with any degree of certainty is difficult. While instability is defined radiologically there is only weak evidence that malunion affects function. Studies from London, Ontario found that in younger patients (under the age of 65), three unstable fractures needed surgery to prevent one patient from an unsatisfactory outcome, but that in older patients (over 65) eight unstable fractures needed surgery to prevent a single poor outcome. This work is supported by long-term retrospective studies showing that the majority of patients with malunited fractures still have excellent function. It is possible that early anatomical restoration and stable fixation will lead to a more rapid recovery but this is as yet unproven.

Displaced intra-articular fractures

Intra-articular fractures of the distal radius are common. Significant displacement at the metaphyseal fracture line is also common.

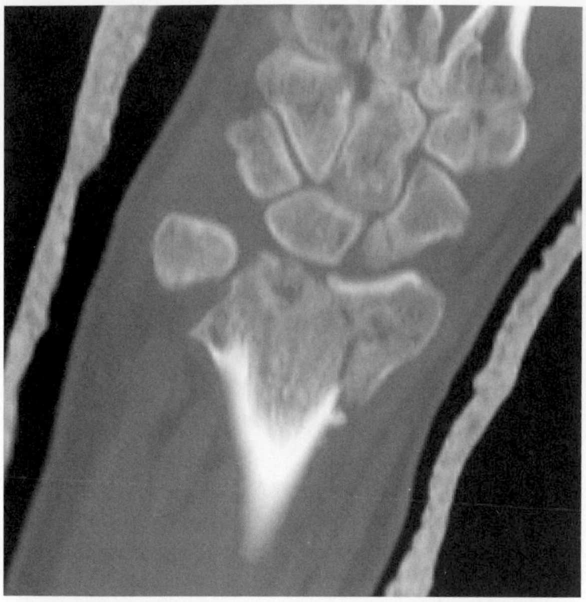

Fig. 12.32.3 Scaphoid proximal pole fracture detected on preoperative CT scan.

The distal radial articular surfaces, however, usually remain well-approximated: significant divergence between the articular fragments is rare. Accurate alignment of the joint surface may reduce the risk of post-traumatic osteoarthritis. In a widely-reported article, Knirk and Jupiter found that with articular malalignment of 2mm or more, radiographic osteoarthritis occurred in 100% of cases, 66% of which were symptomatic. However, patient numbers were small, associated metaphyseal malunion was not analysed separately, and non-validated classification and outcome measurements were used.

To minimize risk of malunion, surgical options include K-wiring, external fixation, palmar locking plates, and dorsal locking plates. Most interest at present is between closed reduction and K-wires or open reduction with palmar locking plate fixation. There is limited evidence comparing the results of these two.

Proposed benefits of K-wiring are speed, ease of surgery, low cost, and acceptable long-term results. Disadvantages include pin site infection, cutaneous nerve damage, prolonged immobilization, late loss of fixation, and tendon irritation.

Proposed benefits of plate fixation include more reliable anatomical restoration, stability for early mobilization, reduced rate of pain syndromes, and more rapid recovery. Disadvantages include high cost, operative time, the need for a more skilled surgeon, risk of deep infection, risk of late flexor or extensor tendon ruptures, and need to remove the plate if symptomatic.

In the displaced non-osteoporotic fracture with little metaphyseal comminution, manipulation with closed K-wiring of the fracture fragment is often adequate.

For displaced multifragmentary fractures many surgeons prefer a palmar locking plate. Some centres have used dorsal plates or combined palmar and dorsal plating for such cases. However, popularity for dorsal plates has waned because of the risk of extensor tendon irritation and frequent need for plate removal.

Some surgeons describe arthroscopic assistance to ensure that the articular fragments are perfectly reduced. There is slight evidence to support improved outcome.

If the radiocarpal articular surfaces are unreconstructable, one option is immediate salvage to a radioscapholunate arthrodesis. However, if the joint surfaces can be restored to approximate congruence and held with a plate or bridging fixator some patients obtain surprisingly good results, albeit with significant wrist stiffness.

Associated injuries

Patients commonly develop ulnar-sided wrist problems after distal radial fracture. Avulsion of the ulnar styloid is an indicator of disruption to the triangular fibrocartilage complex (TFCC), but stability of the distal radioulnar joint (DRUJ) depends on much more than this alone. If the radius is reduced anatomically the DRUJ is often stable. Patients with ulnar styloid fractures should be treated carefully. If the radius requires operative fixation, DRUJ stability can be assessed at the time of surgery. If, after radial reduction, there is marked instability on anteroposterior (AP) glide testing the ulnar styloid can be reattached by a variety of techniques including tension band wiring (Figure 12.32.4). Basal fractures are particularly associated with DRUJ instability.

Ulnar head and neck fractures should be fixed at the time of radial fixation if unstable. There are few published series of these injuries. Locking or blade plate fixation (Figure 12.32.5) is much more reliable than percutaneous K-wires which also prevent early mobilization.

High-energy injuries of the distal radius in younger patients are associated with injuries to the proximal carpal row. Scaphoid fractures are relatively rare in this situation; if the radial fracture requires operative fixation it is sensible to stabilize any scaphoid fracture at the same time using a compression screw. Injuries to intercarpal ligaments are surprisingly common when the joint is assessed arthroscopically. There is little evidence to support aggressive repair in such cases although the evidence is reasonable for

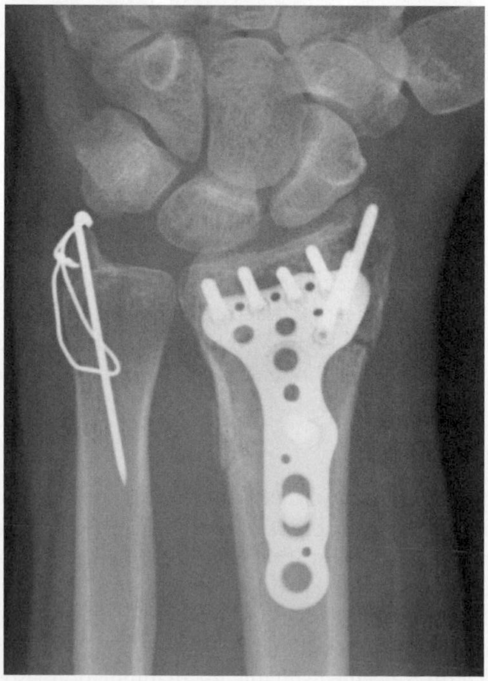

Fig. 12.32.4 After locking plate fixation of the distal radius, DRUJ instability was treated with a tension band wire to the basal ulnar styloid fracture.

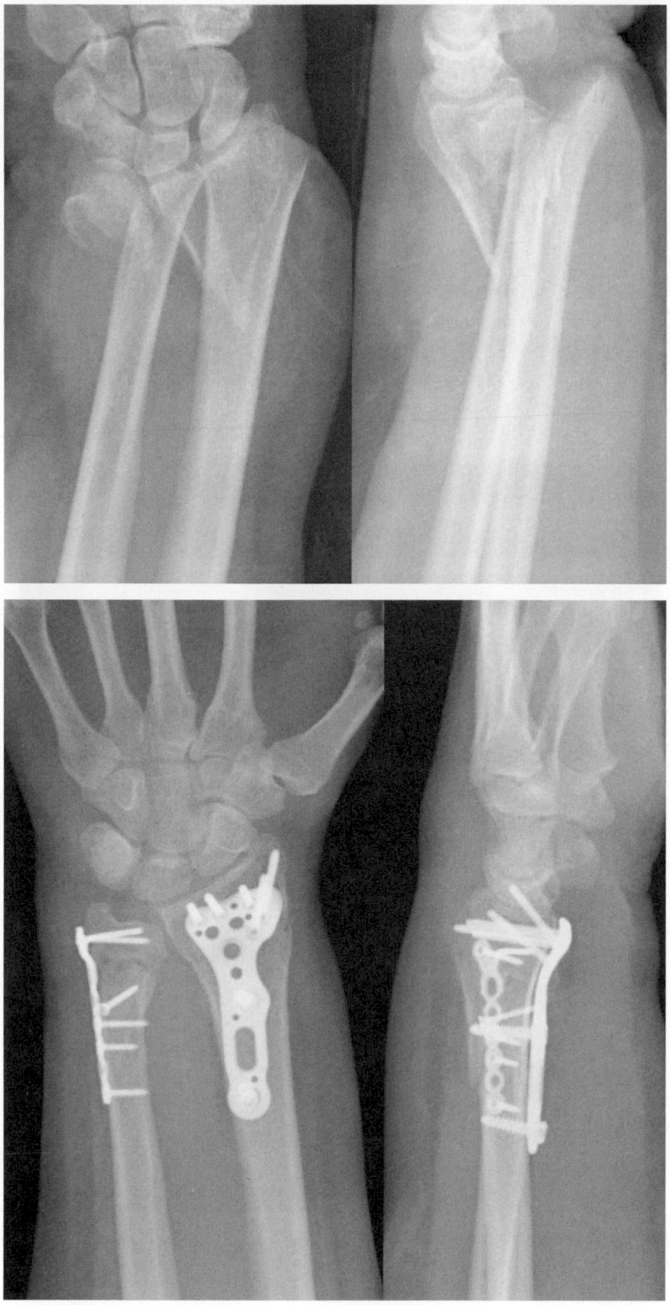

Fig. 12.32.5 Widely-displaced fractures treated with a locking plate to the radius and a 2-mm condylar blade plate to the ulna.

isolated ligament injuries in the absence of a radial fracture. Ligament repair often requires a period of protective immobilization which may delay mobilization of the radiocarpal joint, but this has not been studied. Conversely, occult intercarpal ligament injuries may heal spontaneously with traditional fracture immobilization, but remain unstable if the wrist is mobilized early after fixation of the radius.

Treatment options

Remanipulation and cast

Remanipulation of a distal radial fracture and application of a further cast has been the traditional method of treating unstable distal radial fractures. Lasting improvement following this method is rare, especially in the older age group. If maintained anatomical reduction is required other methods of treatment should be used.

Percutaneous wiring

Percutaneous pinning of distal radial fractures is usually performed with K-wires. Various methods of closed K-wiring have been advocated. In Kapandji's technique of intrafocal pinning the pins are introduced through the fracture to aid reduction as well as fixation (Figure 12.32.6). Plaster is usually used until fracture healing occurs.

Good results are reported using these techniques, although usually in younger patients. In the presence of osteoporosis or significant fragmentation, as is more commonly encountered in the older patient, it is more difficult to maintain a reduction: short and dorsal radial malunions are common. Specific risks include pin track infection, overcorrection of radial angulation, extensor tendon damage, and injury to cutaneous nerve branches.

Buttress plating

Buttress plating is generally used for palmar displaced fractures of the distal radius. The usual approach is through the bed of the flexor carpi radialis tendon sheath. Locking plates can be used to prevent the risk of dorsal malunion due to over-correction. Reports on the outcome of palmar buttress plating are sparse. Results are generally reported as good to excellent.

In palmar partial articular fractures (anterior marginal shearing fractures), the buttress effect of the plate may be adequate without screws in the distal fragment but redisplacement is common. A strong plate is required with good distal support (Figure 12.32.7).

In dorsal partial articular fractures there are various fixation options. One of these is to apply a dorsal buttress plate (Figure 12.32.8). Another is to reduce the fracture using percutaneous techniques, but then to hold the reduction with a palmar locking plate (Figure 12.32.9).

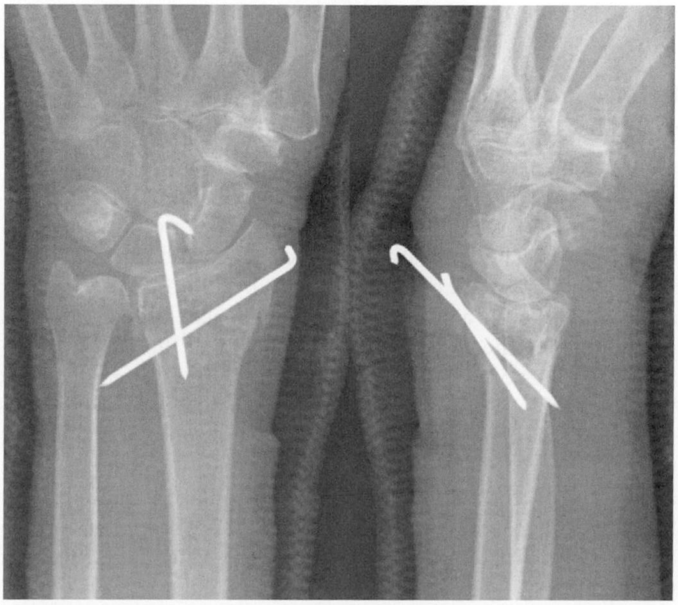

Fig. 12.32.6 A dorsal intrafocal Kapandji wire and a neutralization radial styloid wire used to stabilize an unstable osteoporotic fracture.

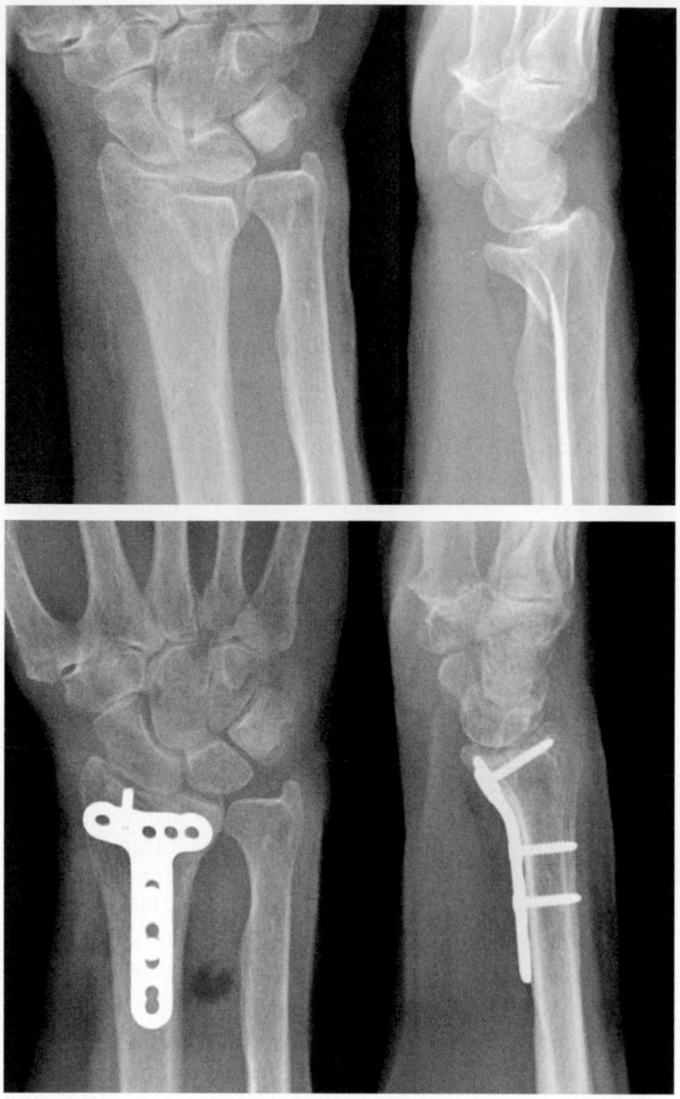

Fig. 12.32.7 A palmar-displaced partial articular fracture of the lunate facet held with buttress plate and additional locking screw for further stability.

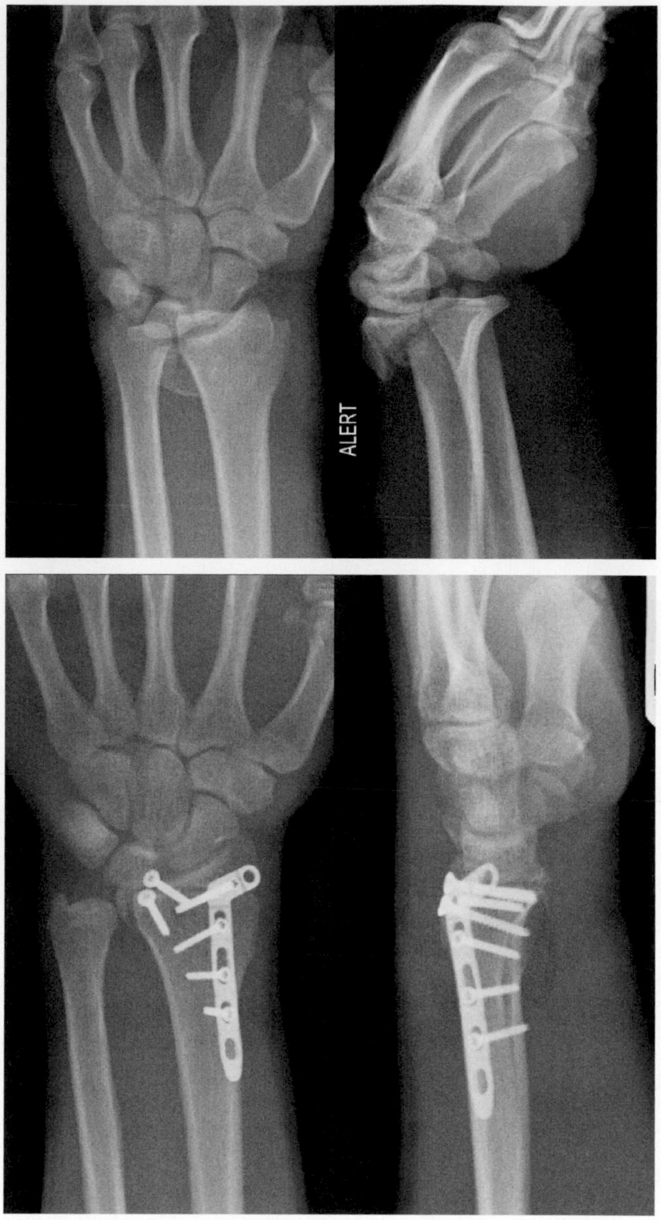

Fig. 12.32.8 Dorsally displaced partial articular fracture treated with dorsal buttress plating and lag screws.

Palmar locking plates

The philosophy of locking plate fixation is well-established. These plates allow reliable fixation of extremely unstable and multifragmentary fractures (Figure 12.32.10).

There are many techniques to achieve and then confirm anatomical reduction. The surgical approach can be modified to aid reduction. Reduction can be confirmed by eye, by fluoroscopy or with an arthroscope. With anatomically-designed plates some surgeons prefer to apply the plate to the radial shaft and then use this as a template to restore anatomical alignment. Others prefer to apply the plate to the distal fragments (after reduction of any interfragmentary displacement) and then reduce these to the shaft. A third method is to reduce and hold all fragments with temporary wires and then apply the plate, allowing for small adjustments in fixation for residual displacement. Different methods of reduction may be needed depending on the type of plate available and the nature of the fracture.

Locking plates come in a variety of shapes and materials. Generally larger lag screws are used for fixation to the radial diaphysis, while smaller locking screws or smooth locking pegs are used for distal fixation. Distal fixation should be into subchondral bone and may be parallel or divergent. Many plates allow fragment-specific fixation of both the lunate fossa and radial styloid. Some plates have fixed-angle locking while others allow polyaxial locking. Most plates are designed for the average distal radius but it is useful to have a variety of plate sizes and templates available. Finally, plates have a variety of devices for targeting the locking elements.

Open reduction and fixation of such fractures can be difficult. In the hands of an inexperienced surgeon the results may be significantly worse than with traditional treatment. Whichever plate is used, it is very important that both proximal and distal fixation is adequate for the type of fracture and any postoperative mobilization regime. It is important to ensure the metalwork does not irritate the

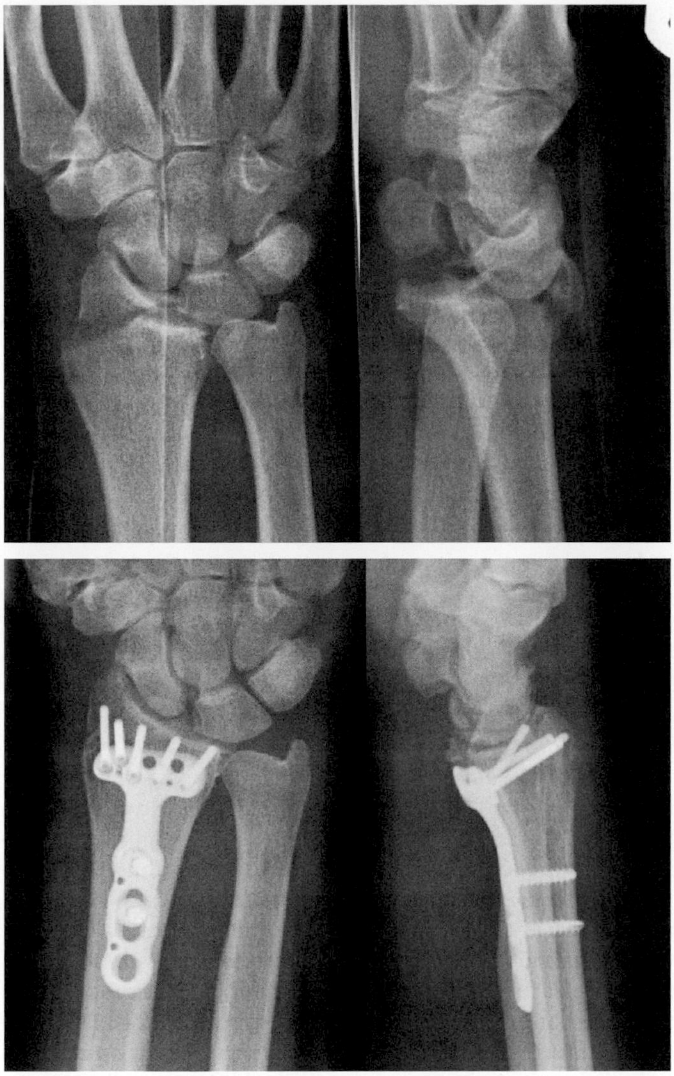

Fig. 12.32.9 Dorsally displaced partial articular fracture treated with arthroscopically-guided closed reduction, a palmar locking plate, and repair of the palmar radiocarpal ligaments. This method of treatment requires distally-angled locking pegs to resist recurrent migration of the dorsal articular fragments and associated carpus.

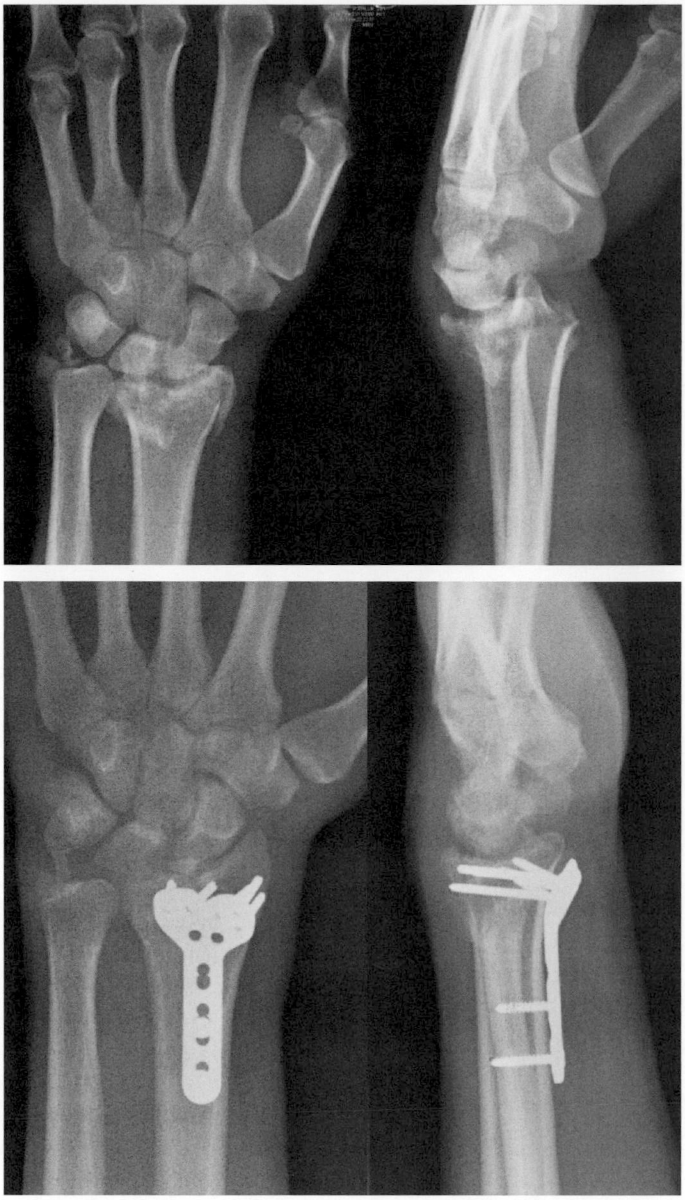

Fig. 12.32.10 Complex fracture with multiple articular fragments treated with palmar locking plate. The reduction is not perfect, but is adequate given the severity of injury. Locking plate fixation is surprisingly stable in such cases.

overlying flexor tendons at the end of the procedure: flexor tendon rupture is a more serious complication than radial malunion. There should be no penetration of distal screws or pegs into the extensor compartment (to avoid extensor tendon rupture). In this respect pegs may be safer than self-tapping screws. It is essential that no metalwork is inadvertently placed in the radiocarpal or distal radio-ulnar joints.

Dorsal locking plates

Palmar locking plates allow for fixation of dorsally unstable fractures with dorsal bone deficits. There is therefore less enthusiasm for dorsal plating. Dorsal plating can cause irritation and even rupture of extensor tendons. There may still be a role for combined palmar and dorsal plates in selected complex fractures. Dorsal partial articular fractures and those with central joint depression may also be held with dorsal plates (Figure 12.32.11).

External fixation

Traditional external fixation bridges the wrist joint using two threaded pins in the second metacarpal and two in the radial diaphysis proximal to the fracture. Successful reduction depends on ligamentotaxis.

Before the advent of locking plates, bridging fixators were popular for complex and unstable distal radial fractures. Non-bridging fixators between the radial diaphysis and articular fragment were an option for metaphyseal fractures. However, the use of fixators has dwindled as locking plates offer equally stable fixation but with the additional benefit of open anatomical fragment-specific reduction.

External fixation still has a role in open fractures and extremely distal multifragmentary fractures in which the joint surfaces are

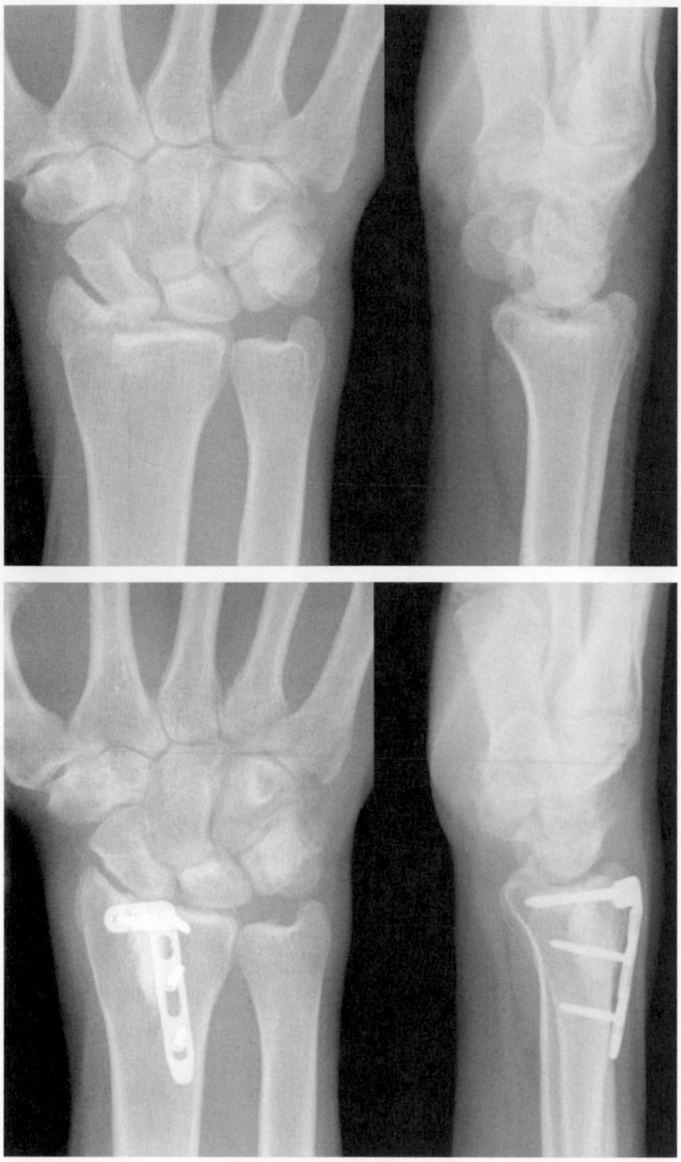

Fig. 12.32.11 A depressed central articular fragment elevated and stabilized with bone substitute and a dorsal locking plate.

not easily reconstructable but for patients in whom other options (such as radiocarpal fusion) are unattractive (Figure 12.32.12).

Bone grafting

Bone graft is traditionally used to augment fixation of unstable fractures. It can support the overall interfragmentary alignment when there is metaphyseal comminution. It can also be used to prevent subsidence after elevation of depressed articular fragments (Figure 12.32.11). The use of bone graft has waned with the advent of palmar locking plates as these rarely require augmentation.

Complications

Malunion

Malunion is probably the most common complication of distal radial fractures. Malunion, whether extra-articular or intra-articular, is associated with poor function. Intra-articular malunion is associated with radiocarpal arthritis on radiographs, although secondary radiocarpal salvage surgery (such as limited arthrodesis) remains uncommon for this indication.

Extra-articular malunion is common and involves loss of radial height, loss of radial inclination and dorsal angulation. In the short term this is commonly associated with ulnar-sided wrist pain and loss of rotation, particularly supination. In many patients the pain slowly improves. Long-term problems include ulnocarpal abutment syndrome (because of the shortened radius) and DRUJ instability (because of associated injury to the ulnar stabilizers as well as loss of soft tissue tension as a result of radial shortening).

If the radius is simply short but otherwise well-aligned, an ulnar-shortening osteotomy is a simple treatment. If there are significant translational and angular elements to the malunion, then a corrective radial osteotomy should generally be performed initially. For minor dorsal opening wedge osteotomies of 30 degrees or less a palmar approach can be used holding the osteotomy with a palmar locking plate. A variety of bone grafting methods have been described in association with this including bone autograft, bone substitutes and no bone graft at all. For larger corrections of 40 degrees or more, particularly in osteoporotic bone, a dorsal approach with structural autograft and plate or wire fixation may be more reliable and allows correction of more complex multiplanar malunions (Figure 12.32.13).

Excision of the ulnar head (a Darrach procedure) is not advisable in this situation and can have unpredictable consequences. Similarly the Sauvé–Kapandji procedure has an unpredictable satisfaction rate and is difficult to salvage later (An arthrodesis is performed between the ulnar head and sigmoid fossa of the distal radius along with creation of a soft tissue interposition pseudarthrosis just proximal to the arthrodesis site that preserves forearm rotation). An ulnar head replacement can be useful in cases of post-traumatic DRUJ impingement or to salvage unsuccessful earlier procedures. However, the long-term survival of these implants in active patients is not yet established. Occasionally patients develop DRUJ instability despite normal articular alignment. Such patients may require repair of elements of the TFCC or formal ligament reconstruction.

Occasionally patients present with severely limited wrist motion because of partial joint subluxation from underestimated partial articular injuries. The proximal carpal row is therefore unable to move in its normal axis, obstructing both radiocarpal and midcarpal motion. Such cases require an intra-articular osteotomy to restore normal mechanics.

Complications of casting

A tight cast can lead to swelling of the hand and fingers which if not relieved promptly leads to intrinsic contractures and finger stiffness. Overzealous wrist flexion prevents finger function and may create carpal tunnel symptoms. A common error is to extend the cast over the metacarpophalangeal joints which will also create stiffness. It is an avoidable tragedy if a patient recovers from a wrist fracture only to suffer iatrogenic finger stiffness as a result of poor plaster management.

Complex regional pain syndrome

The pathophysiology of complex regional pain syndrome (CRPS) remains obscure. The fault probably lies in cortical processing

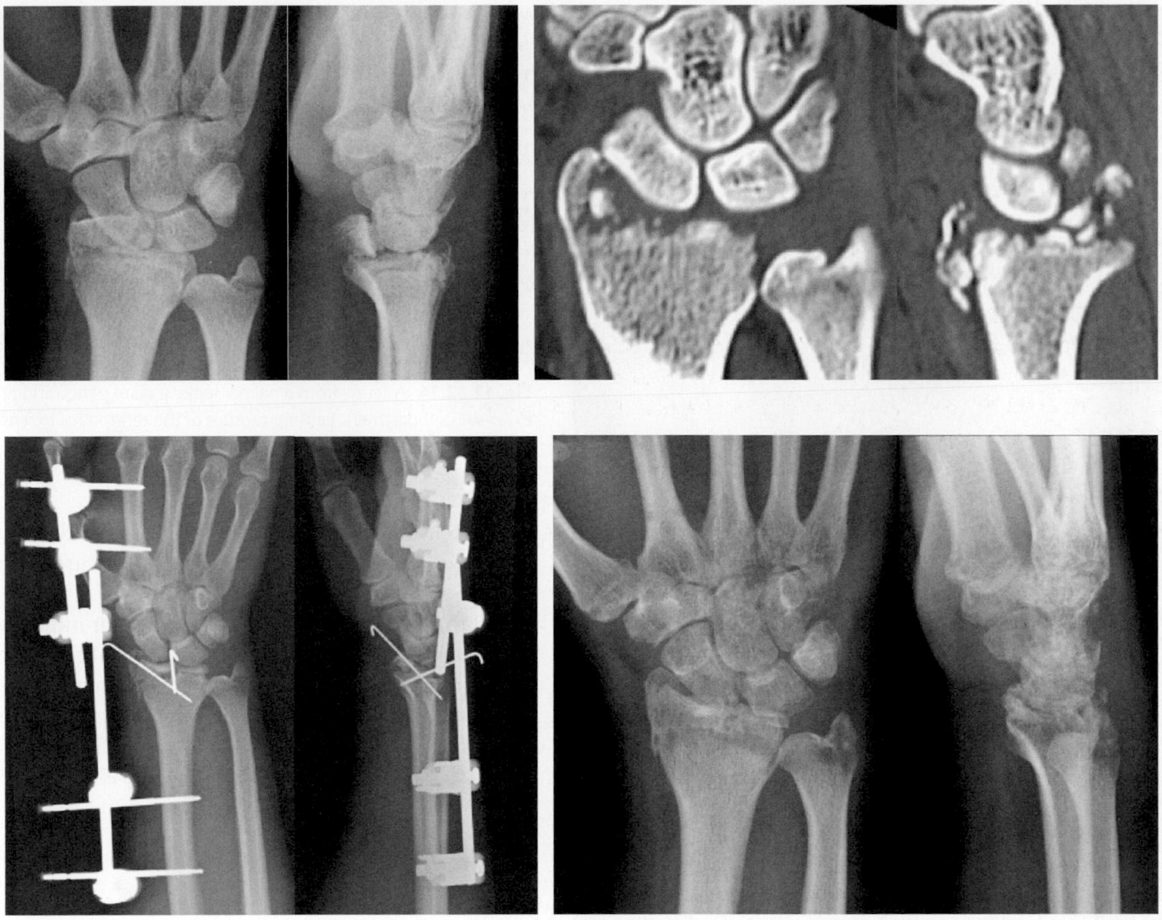

Fig. 12.32.12 A high-energy articular injury treated with open reduction and K-wire fixation of the largest fragments, but spanning external fixation to maintain overall alignment. Significant wrist stiffness is inevitable here, but this patient had surprisingly little long-term pain.

pathways rather than peripherally. It complicates as many as 25% of distal radial fractures treated in plaster.

Features include unexplained diffuse pain often extending beyond the zone of injury, altered skin colour and temperature, diffuse oedema, stiffness. Occasionally the pain is accompanied by fixed dystonic posturing. In later stages there are trophic changes in the skin, and osteopenia in underlying bones.

Most cases settle with activity, encouraged by physiotherapy and desensitization programmes. It should be treated intensively, and not allowed to fester. Protective splints should be avoided. Neuromodulation with low-dose amitriptyline or gabapentin is a useful adjunct in more severe cases. In patients with signs of sympathetic overdrive (marked colour changes and excessive sweating) guanethidine blocks can help. These patients have abnormalities in sensory cortical processing: sensory stimulation and retraining have also been used with devices such as the mirror box.

Infection

Infection can occur after operative fixation of any fracture. Pin site infection is common with K-wire and external fixation devices. It is easily diagnosed and usually settles with pin site care and oral antibiotics. Deep infection after internal fixation of the distal radius is rare. In general the treatment is to suppress the infecting organism with antibiotics until the fracture has united and then remove any metalwork. Early removal of metalwork risks creating an infected non-union which is then extremely difficult to manage.

Nerve compression

Nerve injury may occur after distal radial fracture as a result of the fracture or its treatment. Acute carpal tunnel symptoms may settle within hours of the injury, particularly if the fracture is provisionally reduced. Patients with persistent symptoms should have prompt carpal tunnel release. If the fracture is unstable it may be prudent to stabilize the fracture at the same time. There is some evidence that patients with acute carpal tunnel syndrome are more likely to develop a florid CRPS.

Ulnar nerve dysfunction is uncommon after distal radial fracture. Most cases are associated with displaced ulnar neck fractures and settle spontaneously. The terminal branch of the radial nerve may be damaged by percutaneous or open surgery along the dorsoradial surface of the wrist.

Tendon rupture

Extensor pollicis longus (EPL) tendon rupture is the most common tendon problem after closed injury. It is often associated with a minimally displaced or undisplaced fracture and may be due to a combination of trauma and poor blood supply. K-wire damage to extensor tendons can also occur, and surgeons should be particularly careful

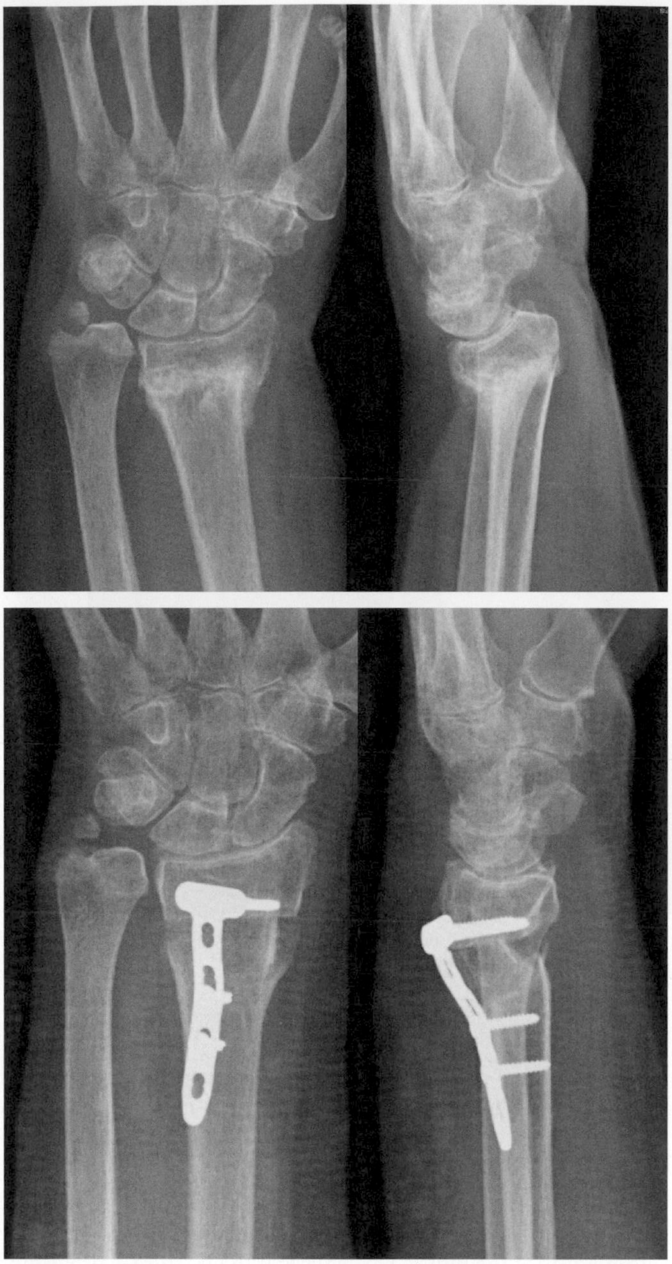

Fig. 12.32.13 Osteoporotic patient with intractable ulnar-sided wrist pain 18 months after fracture. Dorsal opening wedge iliac crest bone block held with dorsal plate.

when passing wires across the third and fourth extensor compartments, putting the EPL and extensor digitorum communis (EDC) tendons at risk.

Iatrogenic tendon rupture, however, has become much more common with the use of plate fixation (Figure 12.32.14). Dorsal plates have particularly high quoted rates of extensor tendon irritation and rupture. However, there are many reports of both flexor

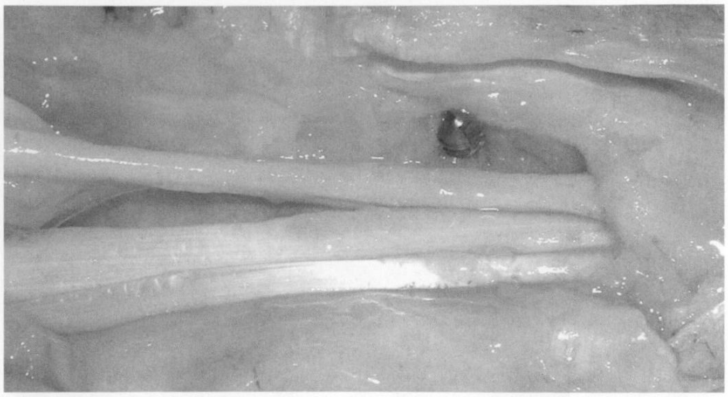

Fig. 12.32.14 A screw from a palmar locking plate penetrating the fourth dorsal extensor compartment causing rupture of the tendons of extensor indicis proprius and extensor digitorum to index and middle fingers.

and extensor tendon ruptures associated with the use of palmar locking plates. The majority of these ruptures relate to surgical technique.

EPL rupture is usually treated by extensor indicis proprius transfer: this is simple and reliable. Irritation of the EDC tendons and subsequent rupture is treated with urgent removal of the offending metalwork and then side-to-side transfers. Flexor tendon rupture (usually FPL or FDP tendons) is more difficult to treat. Urgent prophylactic removal of the metalwork is sensible, with bridging graft across any tendon defect.

Further reading

Chen, N.C. and Jupiter, J.B. (2007). Management of distal radial fractures. *Journal of Bone and Joint Surgery*, **89A**, 2051–62.

Downing, N.D. and Karantana, A. (2008). A revolution in the management of fractures of the distal radius? *Journal of Bone and Joint Surgery*, **90B**, 1271–5.

Fernandes, D.F. and Jupiter, J.B. (2002). *Fractures of the Distal Radius. A Practical Approach to Management*, second edition. New York: Springer-Verlag.

Grewal, R. and MacDermid, J.C. (2007). The risk of adverse outcomes in extra-articular distal radius fractures is increased with malalignment in patients of all ages but mitigated in older patients. *Journal of Hand Surgery*, **32A**, 962–70.

Jupiter, J.B. and Fernandez, D.L. (2001). Complications following distal radius fractures. *Journal of Bone and Joint Surgery*, **83A**, 1244–65.

12.33

Forearm fractures

Ben Ollivere and Matthew Porteous

Summary points

- Failure to restore anatomical alignment of the radius and ulna will result in significant functional limitations
- Plating techniques should be considered the gold standard in displaced fractures of the adult forearm.

Incidence, prevalence, and mechanisms

The function of the arm is to position the hand in space. Functional recovery after forearm fracture is dependent on the full return of forearm rotation, wrist and elbow function, and hand grip strength. The muscle envelope surrounding the forearm bones normally controls hand positioning but creates complex deforming forces in a fractured forearm. Complete recovery is reliant on the anatomical alignment and relationship of the radius and ulna. The intimate relationship between the radius and ulna and the articulation at each extremity makes management of these injuries challenging.

In the adult skeleton, forearm fractures are associated with high energy, and are consequentially seen more commonly in men. Open injuries are commoner in the forearm than any other bone excepting the tibia. Due to the high-energy nature of adult forearm injuries they not uncommonly present as multifragmentary fractures, often in the polytrauma patient.

In the elderly population diaphyseal forearm fractures are uncommon. A fall to the outstretched hand in the elderly usually presents with the more common distal radial or supracondylar fractures.

Anatomy (Box 12.33.1)

The forearm consists of the shorter radius laterally and the longer ulna medially (Figure 12.33.1). The relationship of the two bones is maintained by the distal radioulnar joint (DRUJ), interosseous membrane and proximally by the radial head and annular ligament. The interosseous membrane is the strongest of these elements and provides 75% of the stability.

Box 12.33.1 Anatomy

- Precise restoration of anatomy required for full function
- Interosseous membrane provides 75% stability
- Bowed radius rotates around straight ulna
- Proximal 1/3 fractures—proximal fragment supinated, distal fragment pronated
- Middle 1/3 fractures—proximal fragment neutral, distal fragment pronated
- Distal 1/3 fractures—distal fragment dorsiflexed and radially deviated.

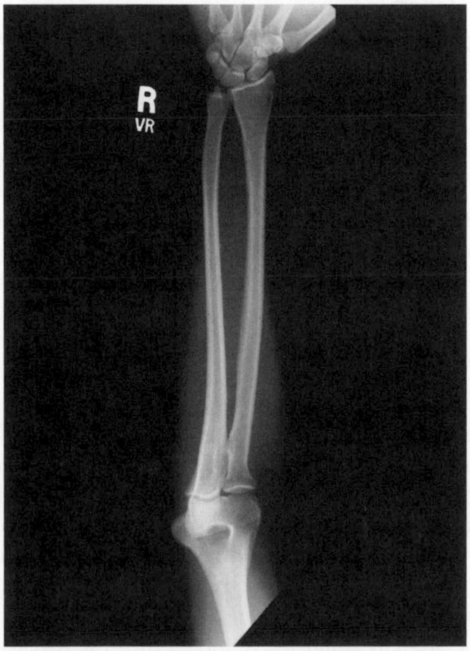

Fig. 12.33.1 Radiograph of the supinated radius and ulna demonstrating the normal radial bow and the forearm articulations at the radiocarpal, distal radioulnar, proximal radioulnar, and humeroulnar (elbow) joints.

The lateral bow of the radius allows the radius to cross the straight ulna mid-shaft in full pronation.

The radial tuberosity is found posteriomedially on the proximal radius allowing the biceps which inserts here to act as a forearm supinator as well as a flexor. Brachioradialis inserts into the styloid and acts as a pure flexor of the forearm. Distally the radius is grooved medially forming the sigmoid notch articulation with the DRUJ.

The olecranon process, of the proximal ulna, articulates with the trochlear groove of the humerus. The triceps tendon inserts into the olecranon posteriorly and brachialis into the coronoid anteriorly. Distally the head of the ulna articulates with a groove in the distal radius to form the DRUJ, the fulcrum for distal forearm rotation.

On the flexor surface three layers of muscles form the anterior compartment along with median, radial, and ulnar nerves. The first (superficial) layer is formed by brachioradialis with the muscles of the common flexor origin (pronator teres (PT), flexor carpi radialis (FCR), palmaris longus (PL) and flexor carpi ulnaris (FCU)). Flexor digitorum superficialis (FDS) lies deep to these and forms the second layer. The final third layer is formed radially by flexor pollicis longus (FPL), distally by pronator quadrates (PQ) and flexor digitorum profundus (FDP) lies on the ulna aspect.

The muscles of the common flexor origin arise from the medial humerus, proximal radius, and ulna. The flexor carpi radialis and ulnaris (FCU) cross the forearm without attachments to these bones. The deep flexors, unlike the superficial muscles, all originate from the forearm bones and interosseous membrane. The deep flexors arise more distally, FDP originates from the proximal two-thirds of the ulna, and the FPL originates from the middle third of the radius. Aside from the pronators, all forearm flexors insert into the bones of the hand.

The muscles on the radial side of the forearm include the extensor carpi radialis brevis and longus, and the brachioradialis. They all originate from the lateral humerus, and only the brachioradialis inserts on the forearm at the radial styloid. The common extensor origin is located on the lateral aspect of the forearm. It gives rise to extensor digitorum, extensor digiti minimi, and extensor carpi ulnaris. The deep extensors all originate on the dorsal surface of the forearm and interosseous membrane. From proximal to distal they are the abductor pollicis longus, extensor pollicis brevis, extensor pollicis longus, and extensor indicis.

The radial nerve divides into its two terminal branches, the superficial radial nerve and posterior interosseous nerve as it passes over the lateral epicondyle. The superficial branch passes over supinator and pronator teres before passing deep to brachioradialis and travelling down the forearm with the radial artery. The median nerve enters the forearm through the two heads of pronator teres. As it crosses the ulna artery it gives rise to the anterior interosseous nerve (supplying FPL, FDP and PQ). It passes between FDS and FDP before passing into the carpal tunnel medial to FCR. The ulnar nerve passes into the forearm through the cubital tunnel. It passes between the two heads of FCU and passes with the ulnar artery down the forearm. It enters the hand through Guyon's canal.

Anatomy of movement

The radius and ulna articulate proximally at the radial head and distally at the distal radial-ulna joint (DRUJ) while the interosseous membrane connects both bones along their length passing obliquely downwards from radius to ulna. The interosseous membrane functions to transmit load from the carpus through the radius to the ulna.

Pronation–supination functions around a complex series of movements. The axis of rotation is from the radial head through the distal ulna into the little finger. During pronation the radius rotates around the ulna at the DRUJ whilst the ulna is abducted (action of anconeus). The centre of rotation of the wrist stays static in space due to the ulna abduction. Conversely during supination, adduction of the ulna occurs (action of supinator) while the radius rotates about its axis. The articulation relies on a bowed radius rotating round a straight ulna to allow for 85 degrees of rotation in each direction.

As both bones work as an articulation with each other throughout their length any fracture within the shaft of either bone must be considered an intra-articular fracture, and this principle forms the cornerstone of management of these injuries.

Pathological anatomy

The deforming forces in forearm fractures have differing affects according to the level of the fracture. In proximal third fractures the proximal fragment is flexed and supinated by biceps and supinator whilst the distal fragment is pronated by pronator teres and quadratus. With middle third fractures the interosseous membrane holds the proximal fragment in neutral while the distal fragment is pronated. In distal third fractures brachioradialis dorsiflexes and radially deviates the distal fragment (Figure 12.33.2).

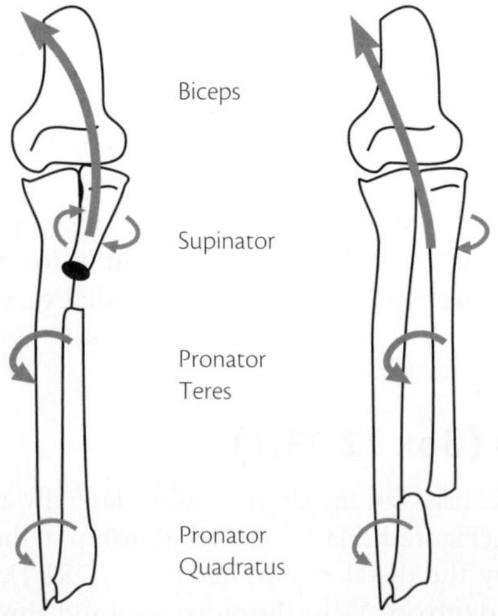

Fig. 12.33.2 The deforming forces in a forearm fracture. The displacement of the fragment depends on the level of the fracture. (adapted from Cruess RL (1973). The management of forearm injuries. *Orthop. Clin. North Am.*, **4**: pp. 969–982).

In indirect injuries the direction of angulation is determined by the rotation of the forearm. When pronated a flexion injury with dorsal angulation will occur while when supinated an extension injury with volar angulation will occur.

Associated injuries

The incidence of associated injuries is proportional to the severity and mechanism of the initial trauma. Open forearm fractures are associated with severe initial trauma consequentially the incidence of neurovascular injury is high. Neurological injury is reported to reach 9% in open both-bone forearm fractures. Careful neurovascular examination and documentation of findings is essential prior to any form of intervention, particularly after high energy trauma. It is prudent to take advice from a vascular surgeon prior to intervention in vascular injury as although reduction of the fracture will usually restore circulation there is an appreciable rate of associated intimal tears. The collateral circulation of the forearm and hand is usually excellent, and even in the presence of vascular injury the functional outcome is predominantly determined by associated musculoskeletal or neurologic injuries.

Compartment syndromes may occur in either closed or open forearm fractures but are usually the result of high-energy trauma. Compartment pressures may be elevated in any forearm injury, and are particularly common in the presence of a muscle crush injury. Compartment pressure monitoring should be considered an adjunct to careful clinical examination and is not the basis on which to make a diagnosis or treatment decisions. Complete open forearm fasciotomies of both flexor and extensor compartments should be undertaken immediately when a clinical diagnosis of compartment syndrome is reached or cannot be excluded.

Associated bony injuries have been reported to the scaphoid and floating elbows in adults. Complete examination of the upper limb and x-rays to include the joint above and below are essential to rule out these and other associated injuries.

Classification

Forearm fractures are usually described based on the location of the fracture (proximal, middle, and distal thirds) and involvement of the joints at either end. The location of the fracture can be used to determine the deforming forces and the most appropriate surgical approach.

Because the radius and ulna are joined by a proximal and distal joint, it is fundamental in the diagnosis and management forearm fractures that if there is a displaced fracture of one forearm bone, there must be a displaced fracture of the other or a dislocation of the proximal or DRUJ.

The Orthopaedic Trauma Association (OTA) and the AO–ASIF both developed more specific classification systems, which have now been merged. Although most commonly used in research it is simple to use. The classification is based around anatomical location (radius, ulna or both bones) and the increasing degrees of complexity in the fracture pattern (Figure 12.33.3).

The Bado classification is used to classify Monteggia fracture–dislocations based on the type of radial head dislocation, Figure 12.33.4.

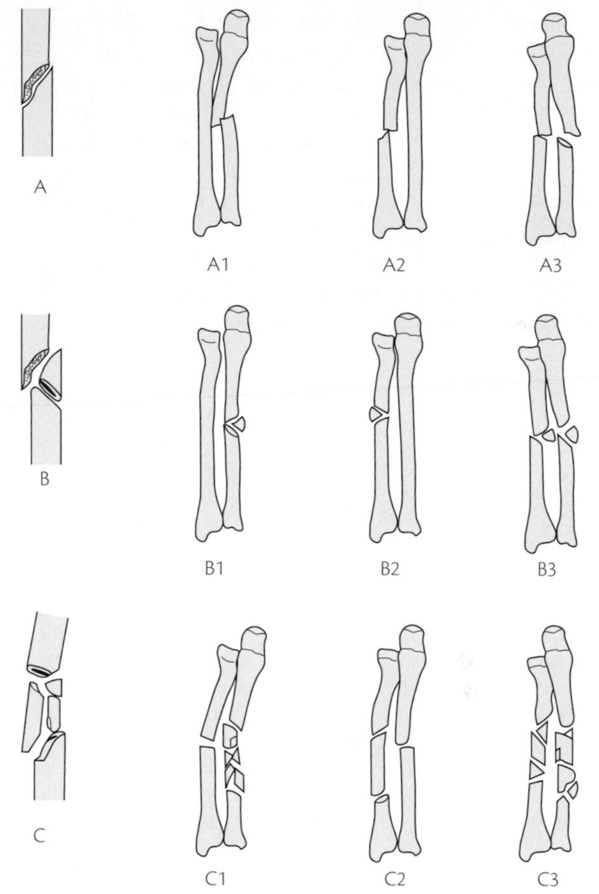

Fig. 12.33.3 The OTA/AO classification of forearm fractures is based on the fracture patterns designated in increasing complexity (types A, B, and C respectively). Subclassification of isolated ulna, isolated radius, and/or both-bone fractures are subclassified into 1, 2, and 3 respectively. http://www.ota.org/compendium/compendium.html

Physical examination

If the fracture involves complete cortical and periosteal disruption, displacement consisting of translation, shortening, angulation, and malrotation is not uncommon. Consequently, the clinical signs of a both-bone forearm fracture include obvious deformity, abnormal limb motion, prominent swelling, and severe pain.

The elbow and wrist should be palpated for tenderness, the skin inspected to rule out an open injury, and the forearm compartments evaluated. The competency of the ulnar and radial arteries should be established. A thorough neurologic examination of the radial, median, and ulnar nerves should be performed. All the relevant findings must be documented in the medical records.

Investigation

Plain anteroposterior and lateral radiographs centred on the forearm are required for diagnosis. The limb's malposition often prohibits true anteroposterior and lateral radiographs in this case two orthogonal radiographs will suffice. Plain films must include the wrist and elbow joint, but due to the divergence of the x-ray beams

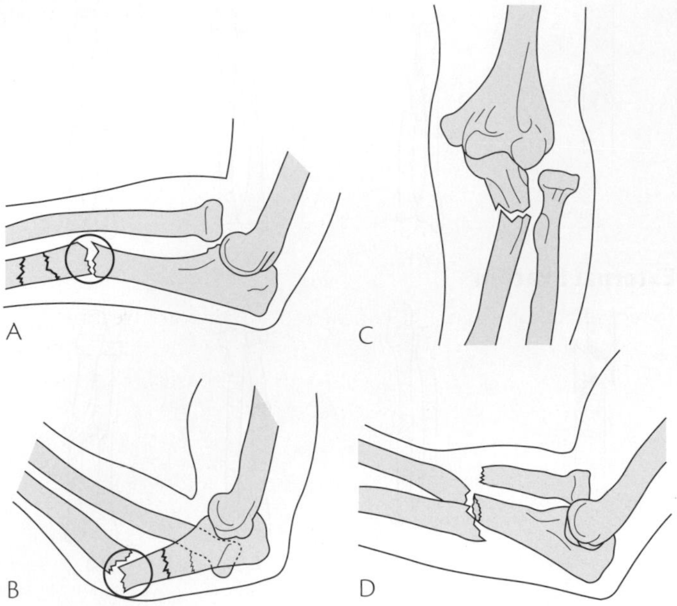

Fig. 12.33.4 The Bado classification of Monteggia fractures is based on the direction of radial head dislocation. (Type I is a fracture at the junction of the proximal and middle thirds of the ulnar with anterior angulation and anterior dislocation of the radial head. Type II is a fracture of the proximal ulna with posterior angulation and posterior dislocation of the radial head. Type III is a fracture of the proximal ulna with lateral dislocation of the radial head. Type IV is a fracture of the proximal ends of both bones with anterior dislocation of the radial head. (Bado JL (1967) The monteggia lesion. *Clin. Orthop. Relat. Res.*, **50**: pp. 71–86).

separate views should be obtained if there is any clinical suggestion of dislocation or bony injury at these joints. Careful assessment of the elbow is crucial to rule out radial head dislocation, and three views may be required in order to do so.

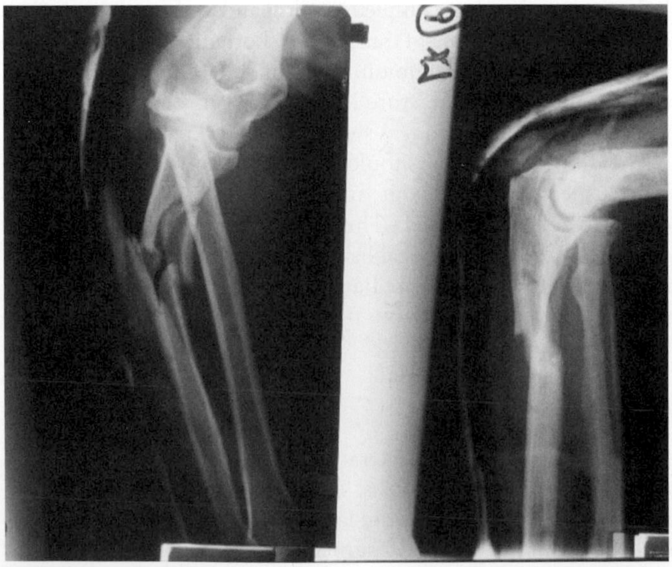

Fig. 12.33.5 A Monteggia fracture dislocation. The diagnosis is made by drawing a line down the long axis of the radius. It should bisect the radial head and capitellum in every view.

Management

External support consisting of a splint or rigid arm board should be secured to the traumatized limb to limit further soft tissue injury. If an open fracture exists, the wound must be swabbed, photographed, and a sterile dressing applied which should not be further disturbed until the patient is in the operating room. Although anatomically similar, forearm fractures represent a spectrum of injury mechanisms. Treatment of these injuries varies greatly in different populations and injury types.

The adult skeleton has no capacity to remodel and as whole forearm functions like a joint treatment should be aimed at anatomical reduction and fixation to minimize residual deformity and functional impairment. Open reduction and internal fixation is the treatment option of choice in all but totally undisplaced fractures of a single bone. If possible absolute stability and direct bone healing should be obtained by use of a lag screw and neutralization plate or by compression plating. In those circumstances where the state of the soft tissues or the fracture pattern make this undesirable, bridging plate fixation is an option. Temporary external fixation can be considered as a second line treatment, though this will often lead to some loss of function.

Treatment modalities (Box 12.33.2)

Manipulation and casting

Manipulation and casting has no place in the management of adult forearm injuries. As adults have a thin periosteum it is impossible to effectively manipulate and hold a both bone forearm fracture closed. Cast bracing can only be considered for select fractures that are non-displaced and minimally swollen in patients who can reliably tolerate the treatment. This group of patients will require frequent follow-up and may have to accept mild loss of motion and the risk of surgical intervention in the event of loss of position or non-union.

Plates

Plating is a type of fixation, not a mode of fixation or a type of healing. Plates can be used in the forearm in a variety of ways and it is important to decide on the aims of fixation prior to treatment.

Achieving absolutely stable fracture fixation is the conventional way of managing a displaced forearm fracture in the adult. In an oblique fracture patterns this is best achieved with a lag screw and

Box 12.33.2 Management of both-bone forearm fractures

- Very limited role for non-operative treatment
- Plate fixation (3.5mm) through separate approaches is the standard
- Assess stability proximal and DRUJs. NB Monteggia and Galeazzi fractures
- Early active range of motion should be encouraged when fractures fixed with absolute stability.

neutralization plate, while compression plating is required for transverse fractures. Preoperative planning is mandatory, and the surgeon should have decided the method and mode of use of the plate for each forearm bone before the operation starts. In normal adult forearm bone, conventional screws are normally adequate. Standard compression type plates should be used The lighter one-third tubular type plates have no place in the stable fixation of adult diaphyseal forearm fractures, although they can be used in small children. Compression plating in this manner has been shown to give a high union rate with a low rate of complications in children and adults (Figure 12.33.6).

Bridging plating in forearm fractures should be reserved for cases where there is extensive fracture comminution and/or soft tissue damage. This makes any attempt to achieve absolutely stable fixation likely to cause devascularization of bone fragments, which would lead to non-union. Although anatomical reduction of the fracture is not obtained, overall anatomical alignment of the radius and ulna is still necessary to prevent loss of pronation/supination. In using a bridging plate the surgeon is accepting some loss of function in an attempt to maintain blood supply to the fracture fragments and get them to heal.

Where the bone is of poor quality or the plate is used for bridging, then ideally a locking plate should be used. The advantage of the additional purchase provided by locking screws and no requirement to contour the plate accurately to the bone, may well justify their increased cost.

Intamedullary nailing

Elastic nailing in the adult is inappropriate as it does not provide stable anatomical fixation. Contoured interlocking intramedullary nailing systems are now available. Good early clinical results have been reported in small studies.

External fixation

External fixation should be considered a temporary treatment for open injuries with significant soft tissue damage. It is not common practice to use external fixation for these injuries. However, in some circumstances with extensive soft tissue trauma and bone loss, temporary external fixation may provide stability whilst awaiting definitive internal fixation.

Approaches to the radius

Henry approach

The anterior approach to the distal radius as described by Henry (Henry 1927), provides access to the distal two-thirds of the radius and may be extended proximally if required. The approach makes use of the plane between brachioradialis and FCR.

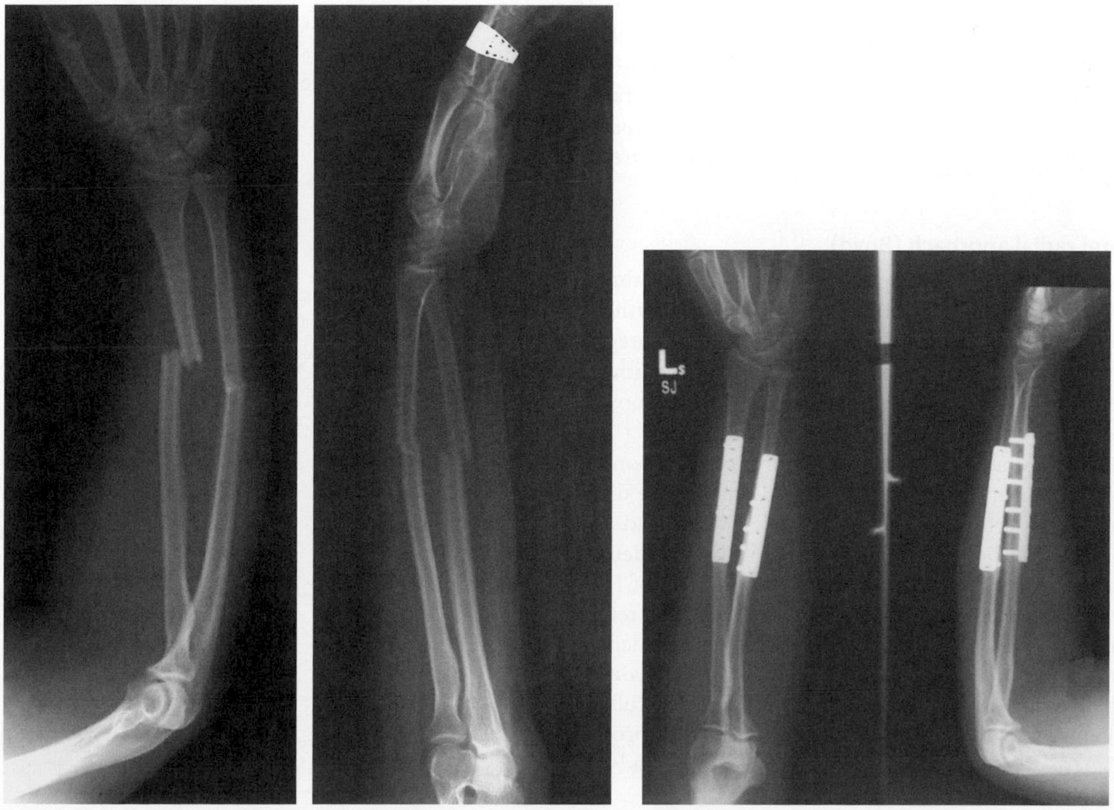

Fig. 12.33.6 Both-bone forearm fracture treated by open anatomic reduction and internal fixation of both bones with 3.5 mm dynamic compression plates. Absolute stability and primary bone healing has been achieved and the patient went on to uneventful union.

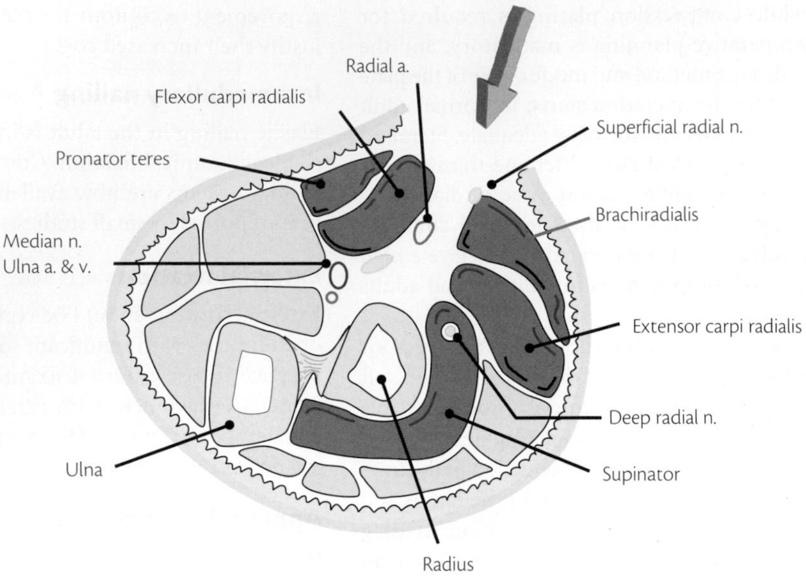

Fig. 12.33.7 The volar (Henry 1927) approach is an extensile approach to the forearm. The approach makes use of the plane between FCR and brachioradialis. Note the superficial radial nerve is taken radially and the radial artery deflected to the ulna aspect.

Position the patient supine with the arm supinated on an arm table. A curvilinear skin incision is made over the palpable border of FCR and extended proximally to within 5cm of the elbow crease. Identify the interval between brachioradialis and the flexor carpi radialis. The radial artery and the superior cutaneous branch of the radial nerve lie in this interval and must be identified before proceeding. Take the artery medially and the nerve laterally. Develop the plane with blunt dissection—a well-placed finger is often safest—to reflect the muscles. Pronation of the forearm will expose the radial boarder and FPL and PQ can be elevated on a subperiosteal flap, though in practice the fracture has often done this already (Figure 12.33.7).

Proximal lateral radial approach (Boyd)

Boyd describes a proximal approach to the radius which makes use of the plane between FDP and ECU. This is the authors' preferred proximal approach to the forearm for Monteggia and radial head fractures as it may be extended proximally into a Kocher's approach to the distal humerus and elbow if required.

The patient is positioned spine with the forearm pronated on the arm table. Make a skin incision from the lateral part of the distal 2cm of the triceps insertion, over the palpable radial head and along the subcutaneous border of the ulnar 6cm distally. Identify the radial boarder of the triceps tendon and the interval of ECU and FDP distally. Divide the ulnar insertion of anconeus and reflect the insertion remnant and FDP towards the flexor compartment as a subperiosteal flap (Figure 12.33.8). Lifting the belly of anconeus exposes the ulnar origin of supinator. Detach supinator carefully as a flap at its ulnar origin and reflect the muscle radially to protect the posterior interosseous nerve. This exposes the radial head and the proximal shaft of the radius.

Do not extend this incision distally beyond the proximal ¼ of the radius as both the dorsal interosseous artery and radial nerve are at risk. It may however be extended proximally to Kocher's lateral elbow approach.

Posterolateral approach (Thompson)

This approach provides access to the proximal two-thirds of the radial shaft, and makes use of the plane between ECRB and EDC. The patient lies supine with their abducted arm lying on an arm

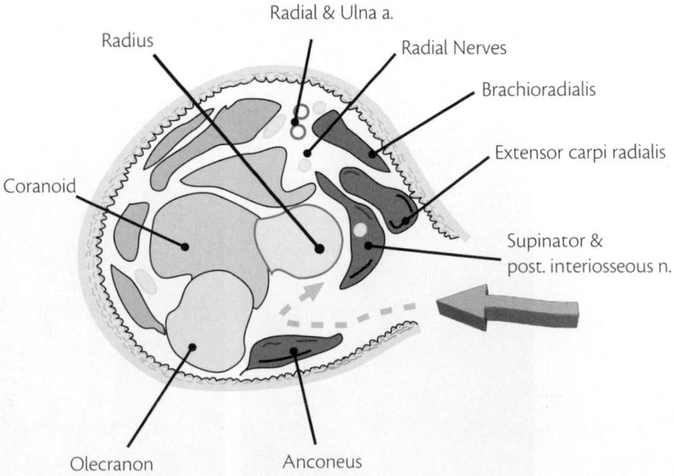

Fig. 12.33.8 The proximal lateral approach (Boyd) approach is a useful approach to the proximal forearm. The approach makes use of the plane between ECU and FDP. Note elevation of the supinator protects the posterior interosseous nerve. This approach may be extended proximally, but not distally.

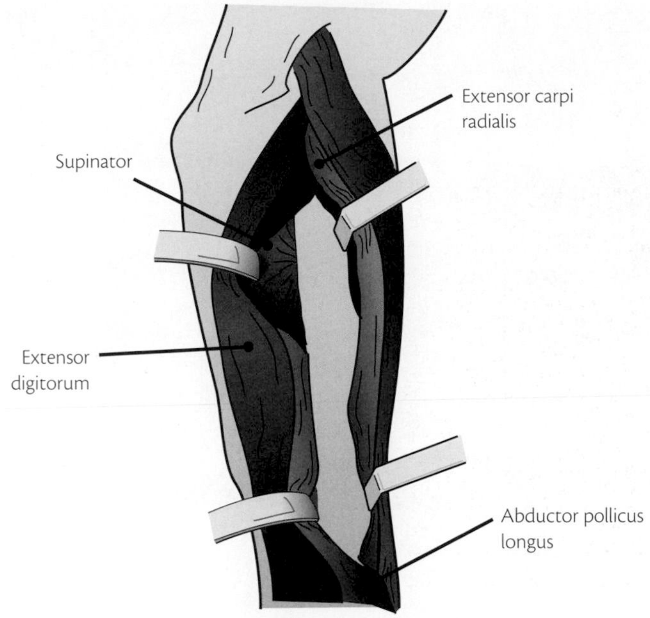

Fig. 12.33.9 The posteriolateral (Thompson's) approach is a useful approach to the whole posterior radius in the forearm. The approach makes use of the plane between ECRB and ECB. Note elevation of the supinator protects the posterior interosseous nerve. This approach may be extended distally, but not proximally.

table and the forearm pronated. The incision runs over the proximal two-thirds of a line from 1.5cm anterior to the lateral humeral epicondyle to the centre of the dorsum of the wrist.

Identify and split the interval between ECRB and EDC (Figure 12.33.9). This exposes the underlying supinator muscle. Supinator can be elevated off the radial shaft by subperiosteal dissection reflecting the muscle medially. It is important to start from distally and work proximally protecting the posterior interosseous nerve within the belly of the muscle. This may be helped by supinating the forearm. If required the nerve can be identified emerging from supinator inferiorly or within the muscle belly via a small muscle split.

Approaches to the ulna

The subcutaneous approach to the ulna is the only commonly used approach to the ulna shaft. Approach the ulna through an incision just volar to the subcutaneous border. Develop the incision through the deep fascia. Identify the plane between FCU and ECU and part the muscles using blunt dissection. The ulnar nerve lies deep to FCU should be protected throughout the dissection.

Post-treatment care

The postoperative regimen will vary from surgeon to surgeon and fracture to fracture. Early active mobilization to avoid stiffness is becoming more common after operative fixation, and this is the authors' practice. Fractures fixed with absolute stability should be aggressively mobilized although dangerous or heavy activities should be restricted until the fracture has united.

Complications

There is an appreciable risk of neurovascular damage in open procedures to the forearm, and these injuries represent the majority of interoperative complications. Reduced range of movement can be minimized with anatomical stable reduction that allows early rehabilitation. Other postoperative complica-tions include synostosis, refracture, infection, and loss of reduction.

Synostosis is a recognized complication of both bone forearm fractures. It is associated with high-energy injuries, malreduction, delayed surgery, single incision fixation of both bones, fractures at the same level in both bones, and excision of the radial head. After the ossification has matured (usually 1–2 years) the bone bridge can be excised and interposition performed.

It has been common practice in the past to remove forearm plates, and this is still common practice in children. However, the literature demonstrates a high refracture rate of up to 11% and a significant risk of wound complications and neurological damage particularly when removing plates from the radius. We do not advise or routinely remove plates unless crossing a growth plate or causing symptoms. Elective removal of plates should not be undertaken before 1 year and some authors have argued that the high refracture rate warrants a 2 year delay for plate removal.

Special cases

Monteggia fractures

It is important in any seemingly isolated ulna fracture to obtain good lateral and AP views of the elbow. Treatment is based around the nature of the ulna fracture, not the type of radial head dislocation. The same principles are used as for other forearm fractures. The radial head cannot be reduced closed in approximately 10% of cases due to soft tissue interposition, and open reduction is indicated. Annular ligament reconstruction is controversial. Bado type IV injuries with radial head fractur e dislocations require open reduction and internal fixation of large radial head fragments. If radiocapitellum stability is not compromised, small fragments of the radial head are best excised. Injuries with severe comminution of the radial head and significant ligamentous disruption, require radial head replacement to maintain stability.

Galeazzi fracture

A Galeazzi fracture is fracture of the distal third of the radius with an associated dislocation of the DRUJ. Also called the fracture of necessity by Campbell, the injury is often unrecognized and diagnosis relies on true lateral radiographs at the time of injury. Failure to anatomically reduce and hold this fracture pattern will result in almost universal poor outcomes. For this reason the authors advocate open reduction and internal fixation of the radius. This will usually reduce the DRUJ and if it is stable through a full range of pronation/supination then early functional rehabilitation can be considered. If the DRUJ remains unstable other treatment options are required (see Chapter 12.31) (Figure 12.33.10).

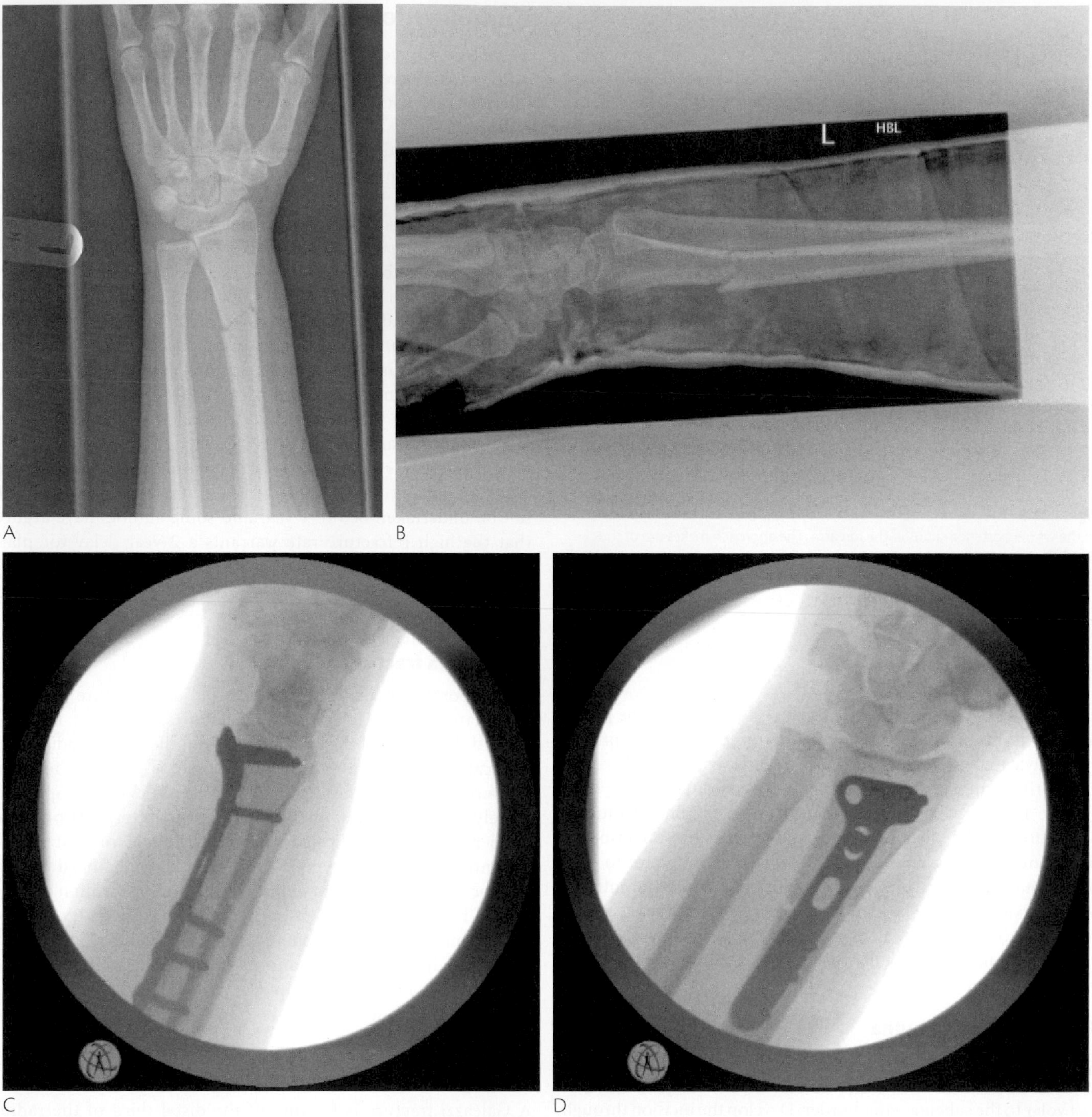

Fig. 12.33.10 Galeazzi fracture dislocation. Fixation of the radius often reduces the DRUJ.

Essex-Lopresti fracture

The Essex-Lopresti lesion is a fracture of the radial head in combination with a disruption of the interosseous membrane and disruption of the DRUJ. This is an unstable injury as the stabilizing function of the interosseous membrane is lost. Treatment should consist of reconstruction or replacement of the radial head to restore the radial length and stability.

Nightstick (single bone fractures)

The classic nightstick (truncheon) injury is described as a transverse fracture of the distal ulna. Typically caused by a blow to the ulna border of the forearm in an adult, who raises their arm over their head to ward off a blow, it may occasionally have a less violent aetiology and represent a fragility fracture. Radial fractures and displaced fractures of the ulna have been associated with a high incidence of non-union if managed conservatively. For this reason plate fixation is the treatment of choice.

Further reading

Bado, J.L. (1967). The monteggia lesion. *Clinical Orthopaedics and Related Research*, **50**, 71–86.

Charnley, J. (1950). *The Closed Treatment of Common Fractures* (fourth edition 2003). Cambridge: Cambridge University Press.

Rüedi, T.P., Buckley, R.E., and Moran, C.G. (eds) (2007). *AO Principles of Fracture Management*, pp. 627–79. New York: Thieme.

Hoppenfeld, S. and deBoer, P. (2003). *Surgical Exposures in Orthopaedics: The Anatomic Approach.* New York: Lippincott Williams & Wilkins.

Surgical technique and literature reviews: http://www.aofoundation.org/wps/portal/HomeFig. 12.33.6 Effective immobilization in plaster relies on use if the periosteal hinge to act as a third point for three-point fixation.

12.34

Elbow fractures and dislocations

John R. Williams and Brian J. Holdsworth

Summary points

- These are very complex fractures to treat; the elbow is intolerant of immobilization in the adult
- Posterior approach best for complex fractures
- AO classification widely used
- Most intra-articular fractures best internally fixed
- Most distal humeral fractures require two plates.

Introduction (Box 12.34.1)

Fractures of the elbow region are among some of the most difficult fractures to treat; they occur in three groups of patients: children, young adults typically following high-force injuries, and the elderly, where even low-energy trauma may cause severe fragmentation. This chapter deals only with adult fractures where the epidemic of osteoporotic elbow fractures is particularly challenging.

The adult elbow is intolerant of any immobilization. Hence there has been an increasing tendency over recent years to operatively manage elbow fractures.

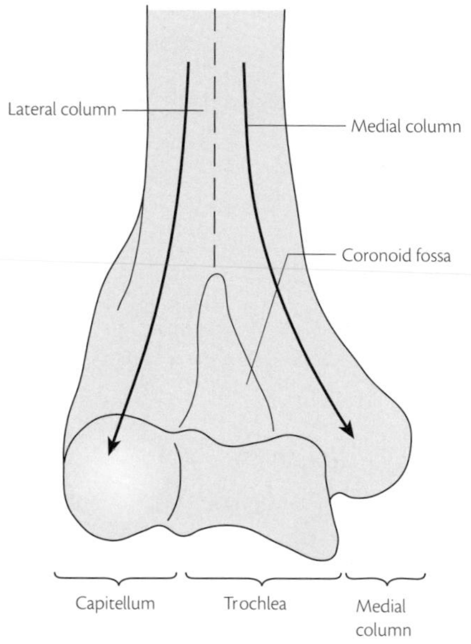

Fig. 12.34.1 Schematic representation of the trochlea, capitellum, and distal humeral columns (note the trochlea located between the columns while the capitellum forms part of the lateral column).

Distal humerus

Anatomy

The trochlea and capitellum make up the articular portion of the distal humerus and are held to the shaft of the humerus by the medial and lateral supracondylar ridges.

Medially, the trochlea sits like a cotton reel between the ends of the two supracondylar columns (Figure 12.34.1). The trochlear axis lies anteriorly, in internal rotation and in valgus relative to the humeral shaft. This creates the 'carrying angle' seen in the extended arm, and a perceived medial swing of the arm during flexion. The trochlea, with an arc of 270 degrees of articular cartilage, is supported by strong supracondylar columns that provide a valuable area for internal fixation. The proximal part of the medial column is entirely cortical bone and gives attachment to the common flexor origin while in the distal part, the true medial epicondyle, there is a little cancellous bone. This epicondyle gives origin to the medial collateral ligament, a crucial stabilizer of the elbow. As there is no articulation on the anterior surface of the medial column, screws can fully penetrate it. The inferior aspect of the epicondyle is also available for the insertion of screws passing proximally. Due care must be given both to the medial ligament and to the ulnar nerve passing behind and beneath the medial epicondyle. Avoid obstruction of the various fossae. The use of locking plates allows the plate not to be in compression contact with the bone preserving blood supply, but care must be taken to ensure that soft tissue compromise is not caused by overly prominent metalware.

Box 12.34.1 Principles

- The elbow is intolerant of immobilization
- Osteoporotic fractures can be difficult to manage
- Physiotherapy input essential.

On the lateral side the entire distal part of the column is available for screw fixation as the capitellar articular surface only occupies the anterior and distal aspects. The lateral column, flattened in its proximal part, is composed of cortical bone and readily accepts a plate. At a point approximately level with the middle of the posterior olecranon fossa, the lateral column sweeps anteriorly. In this region the anconeus muscle originates and on the anterior surface lies the radial fossa accommodating the radial head in full flexion. Particular care must be used when placing screws in this area otherwise the radial fossa or the articular surface of the capitellum will be penetrated leading to damage of the radial head.

Surgical approaches (Box 12.34.2)

The authors prefer the posterior approach to the elbow particularly for complex fractures. This gives optimal access to the distal humerus but requires an olecranon osteotomy.

The more limited medial or anterolateral approaches are rarely used and only for isolated fractures of the condyles without fragmentation.

The anterior approach of Henry should be limited exclusively to exploration of the anterior neurovascular structures.

The posterior approach

- Prone, arm on bar forearm hanging
- Extensile incision, medial to olecranon and locate nerve (minimizes flap over ulnar nerve)
- Olecranon osteotomy best (Figure 12.34.2). Chevron cut with power saw completed with osteotome. Repair with tension band
- Consider transposing ulnar nerve.

Classification

Many classification systems have been devised for distal humeral fractures. These have evolved in parallel with the change from non-operative methods to operative methods.

The AO group have defined an alphanumeric fracture classification system for the distal humerus (Figure 12.34.3). Jupiter and others have attempted to improve the AO system to reflect both fracture complexity and methods of reconstruction (Figure 12.34.4). The fractures are divided into three main groups.

- I. Intra-articular
  - A. Single column
  - B. Bicolumnar
  - C. Capitellar
  - D. Trochlear
- II. Extra-articular
- III. Extracapsular.

Box 12.34.2 Distal humerus—approaches

- Posterior approach with olecranon osteotomy most useful
- Lateral approach for isolated non-comminuted lateral condyle fractures
- Henry approach to explore vascular structures only.

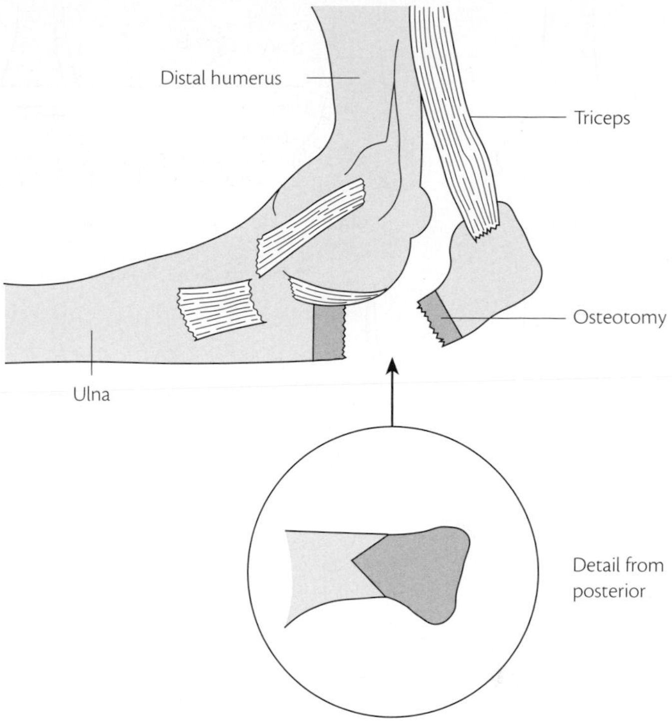

Fig. 12.34.2 Diagram of the technique of olecranon osteotomy to expose the distal humerus. The distally facing chevron cut is made into the mid-part of the greater sigmoid notch.

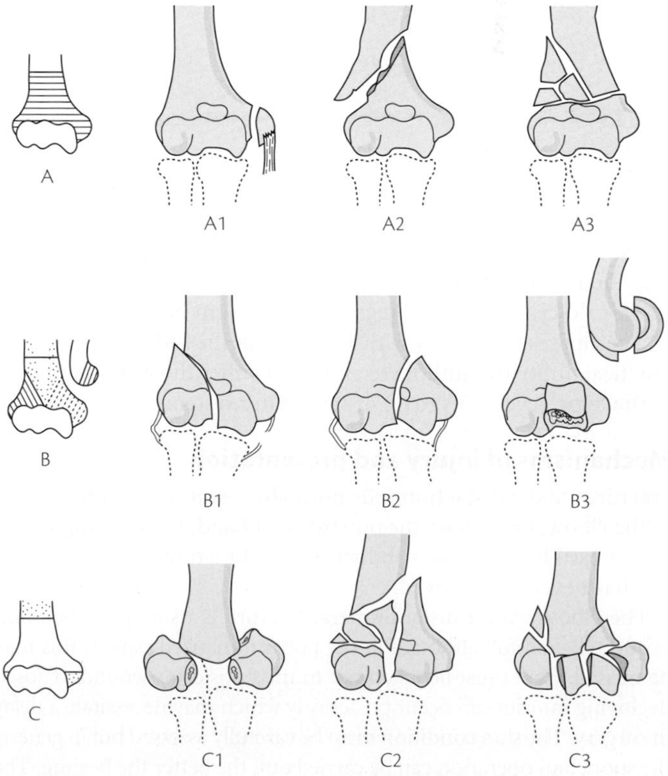

Fig. 12.34.3 The AO classification system for distal humeral fractures.

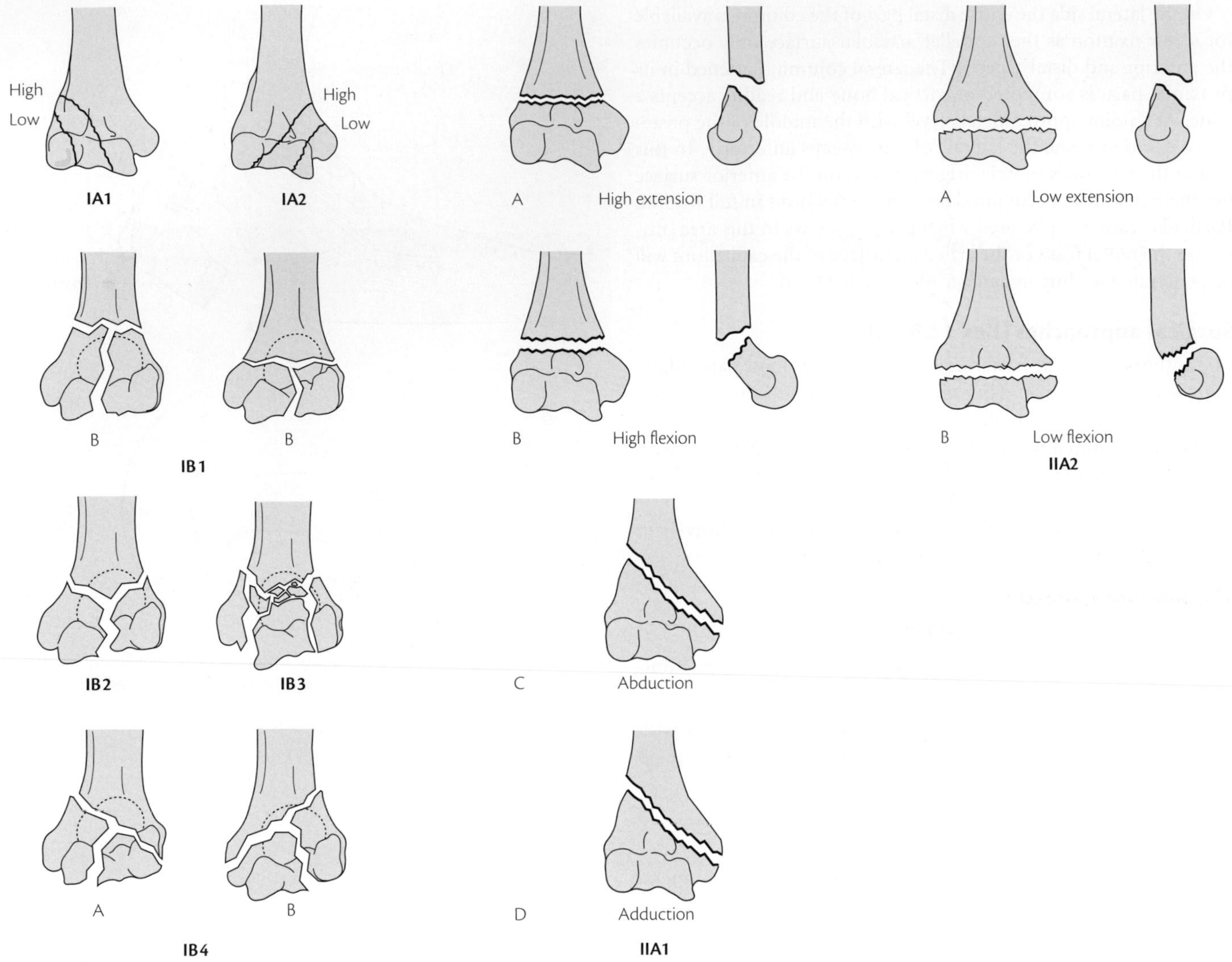

Fig. 12.34.4 The classification system for distal humeral fractures used by Jupiter and Mehne (1992).

The extra-articular fractures are either high fractures or low fractures. The extracapsular fractures are those of the epicondyles. They do not use the term condyle as they feel that it is neither helpful nor descriptive in this region. This system has only 19 classes and compares favourably with 61 classes in the full AO system. For practical utility the authors recommend either the AO system used to the 'type' level (13A to C) or the Jupiter system.

Mechanisms of injury and presentation

Fractures of the distal humerus normally result from a direct blow to the elbow, or a fall on the outstretched hand. Unicolumnar fractures possibly result from abduction or adduction forces, although this has never been proved.

The elbow with a distal humeral fracture is usually swollen and exquisitely painful; although in the polytraumatized patient this may be missed. Care must be taken not to miss posterior wounds. Closed degloving injuries can occur posteriorly which may necessitate a delay in surgery. The skin condition must be carefully assessed but in general the sooner an operation can be carried out, the better the healing. The distal neurovascular status of the limb requires careful examination.

Investigations (Box 12.34.3)

Standard anteroposterior and lateral radiographs of the distal humerus may be sufficient to appreciate the pattern of injury (Figure 12.34.5A, B). Traction radiographs obtained under anaesthesia at the start of the operation often allow a fuller understanding of the fracture pattern and facilitate surgical planning (Figure 12.34.5C, D).

Computed tomography (CT) scanning with three-dimensional reconstruction is increasingly helpful especially in elderly patients where elbow replacement is being considered.

Careful preoperative planning is essential for implant positioning and adequate reduction.

Box 12.34.3 Distal humerus—investigations

- Biplanar x-rays
- Traction film may be useful
- CT scan where total elbow replacement (TER) considered.

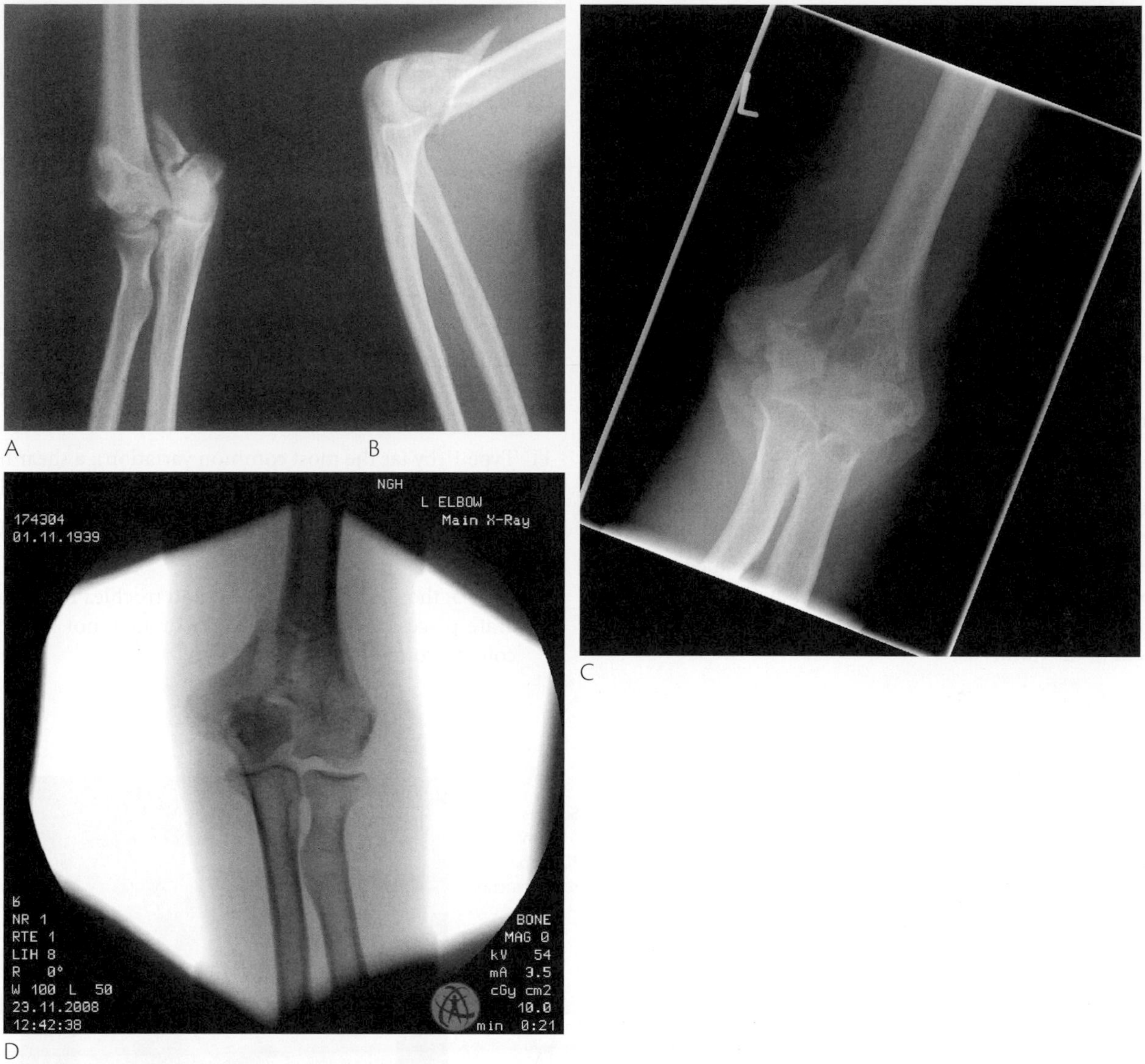

Fig. 12.34.5 A) and B) Radiographs of intercondylar AO 13C type distal humeral fracture. C) and D) Original antroposterior radiographs and in-theatre traction radiographs of AO 13C fracture.

Treatment (Box 12.34.4)

Intra-articular fractures

The authors recommend operative fixation for the majority of intra-articular elbow fractures, without any absolute contraindication. Closed methods usually require prolonged immobilization causing permanent stiffness in the adult elbow. The authors have not been impressed with the results of so-called 'bag-of-bones' treatment even in the frail elderly patient.

The goal of treatment must be an anatomically correct, congruent and mobile joint correctly aligned with the shaft. Fixation must be robust enough to resist the forces generated by early active motion of the joint particularly those directed posteriorly caused by tension in the forearm muscles with the elbow flexed. To this end humeral K-wires have no role other than temporary stabilization. Avoid 'one-third-tubular' plates which frequently break in this situation.

True single-column fractures are unusual but may be fixed using a transverse screw along the width of the trochlea with a supporting plate to maintain the strength and alignment of the distal humerus. The great majority of distal humeral fractures are safest fixed using two plates.

Box 12.34.4 Distal humerus—treatment

- Majority of intra-articular fractures should be fixed
- Capitellar fractures must be fixed
- Extra-articular intracapsular fractures either splint or fix or TER
- Extra-articular fractures usually need fixation.

Screws alone have often proved insufficient to resist the forces generated by early active movement leading to painful non-union. Supporting plates have proved much safer.

The bicolumnar fracture in any of its guises (T, Y, H, or Λ) poses the greatest difficulty in fixation. Improved techniques mean many of these fractures can be successfully stabilized using classical AO plating techniques (Figure 12.34.6A). The apparent advantages of fixed angle locking plates are yet to be proved in long term studies. The positioning of these plates in rotation is difficult if intra-articular penetration by locked screws is to be avoided.

These injuries should be operated on in the first 24–36h if swelling and any closed degloving injuries allow. All open injuries must be urgently stabilized. In exceptional circumstances temporary external fixation can have a role.

As the triangle formed by the epicondylar ridges and the trochlea is gradually reassembled it often proves necessary to make slight final adjustments. Because the distal humeral columns have a complex three-dimensional geometry, the 3.5-mm AO reconstruction plate (Synthes) which can be contoured in three dimensions is the 'workhorse' for the distal humerus especially on the medial side.

The posterolateral plate may be extended as far distally as the margin of the capitellar articular cartilage at the extreme inferolateral margin of the humerus.

On the medial side the plate may rarely be contoured through a right angle to cradle the medial epicondyle allowing a screw to pass upwards along the condyle. However, it is preferred to avoid risking damage to the medial ligament and to use a long transverse screw through the plate which can stop just above the tip of the condyle so avoiding later discomfort from prominent metalwork.

No screws must cross the anterior coronoid or posterior olecranon fossae (Figure 12.34.6B, C).

Bone graft from the iliac crest may, rarely, be needed to impart structural integrity to the fracture construct. Non-union is associated with inadequate implant stability.

Isolated capitellar fractures are rare. The pattern is usually of a coronal shear detaching the capitellum from the front of the lateral column of the distal humerus. Recent work has redefined coronal plane fractures of the distal humerus, into:

1) Type 1 (by far the most common variation): a shear fracture of the capitellum with/out part of the lateral trochlea ridge
2) Type2: those with the capitellum and whole trochlea as one piece
3) Type 3: those with the capitellar and trochlea fragments as separate pieces; these patterns may or may not have posterior column comminution.

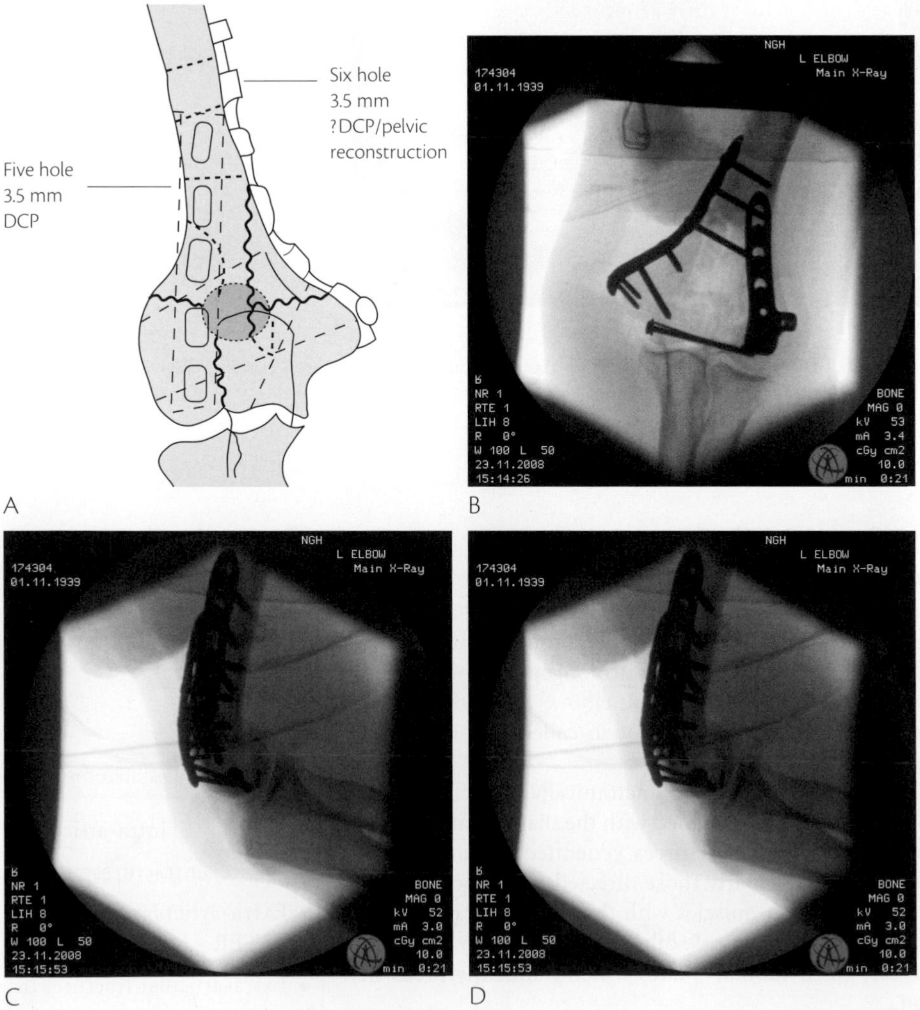

Fig. 12.34.6 A) Radiographs showing the internal fixation of the distal humeral fracture shown in Figure 12.34.5A,B using 'conventional plates'. B)–D) Radiographs showing the internal fixation of the distal humeral fracture shown in Figure 12.34.5A,B using 'locking plates'.

Operation is mandatory for these fractures. Small fragment screws from the back may be employed if there is sufficient cancellous bone attached to the fragment or buried head screws such as the Herbert screw or the Headless Compression Screw from Synthes (HCS) may be used from the front. If the articular cartilage is very damaged or the fragments comminuted, then excision of the capitellum alone may be the better option but beware of compromising the stability of the elbow by inadvertently also removing a substantial part of the trochlea. To achieve open reduction and internal fixation the authors use a lateral, posterolateral or full posterior approach (with olecranon osteotomy) depending on the level of access required. Beware on the initial radiographs a double outline to the displaced fragment as this is a clue to the fracture including a substantial part of the trochlea (Figure 12.34.7). Excision of such large pieces causes instability with subsequent arthritis.

Extra-articular intracapsular fractures

These fractures are all transcolumnar of varying sorts, either high and easy to fix or low and difficult. The low transcolumnar injuries usually occur in the osteoporotic bone of elderly female patients.

The higher extension fractures may be managed in some patients, as one would in a child, by closed reduction and splintage but at the expense of poor functional outcome. However, for the low fractures surgery is needed if painful non-union is to be avoided. In a few elderly patients, where the low transcolumnar fracture has scuffed off a thin shell of bone, the authors advise total elbow replacement as in displaced intracapsular fractures of the neck of the femur or anatomical neck of the humerus (Figure 12.34.8). Good medium-term results with the Coonrad–Morrey elbow have been reported either as a primary or as a secondary method for fractures in the elderly; most of the patients where secondary surgery was required had been treated with immobilization alone or with inadequate fixation often only K-wires.

Extra-articular extracapsular fractures

Extra-articular fractures include those of either the medial or lateral epicondyle. They are far less common in adults than children and normally require screw rather than K-wire fixation. As the fragments are often small, a 3.5-mm diameter cortical lag screw should be anchored into the opposite cortex. Particular importance should be attached to medial epicondylar fragments that may have all or a substantial part of the important anterior band of the medial collateral ligament attached to them. They may also carry with them the adjacent ulnar nerve, sometimes into the elbow joint.

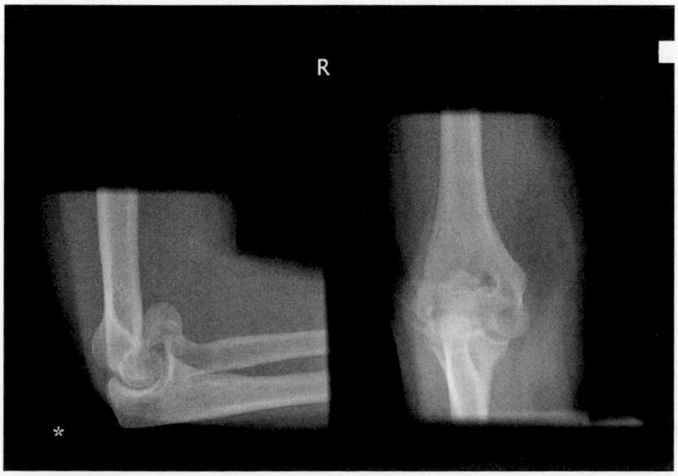

Fig. 12.34.7 Radiographs of a coronal plane fracture of the capitellum and trochlea showing the double shadow on the lateral view.

Postoperative management (Box 12.34.5)

Following operative fixation of distal humeral fractures early motion is of the essence. A successful outcome requires both pain-free motion of the elbow joint and union of the fracture. The use of a sling is allowed for pain relief on leaving the operating room. Plaster splints carry the risk of Volkmann's ischaemia and are best totally avoided as postoperative swelling is always considerable. However, the arm should be removed from the sling within 24h for active exercises to commence. Exercises include active or gentle active-assisted. The use of indwelling brachial catheters can be useful where pain control is difficult.

Complications and their management (Box 12.34.6)

Infection

Infection is an ever-present risk in either open fractures or those managed by open methods. The reported infection rates for distal humeral fractures range from 1–6%.

Vascular complications

Vascular complications are very rarely associated with adult distal humeral fractures. The clinician should be alert to the possibility of damage to anterior neurovascular structures, and may need to adjust the surgical approach should this be the case.

Neurological complications

Although the median nerve may be compromised anteriorly and rarely requires an anterior exploration, the most common neurological complication of distal humeral fractures involves the ulnar nerve. The incidence is around 5–7% of cases. It can be involved preoperatively, perioperatively, or later as 'tardy ulnar palsy'. In high-energy injuries the nerve may be lacerated by bone fragments, but more frequently it is damaged during the operation when it may be exposed to excessive traction or trapped between fragments. Because of disrupted anatomy, the nerve may be very displaced. Early identification proximal to the fracture and careful protection throughout the operation is mandatory. Late ulnar nerve palsy has sometimes been seen in relation to internal fixation devices impinging on the cubital tunnel behind the medial epicondyle.

Malunion and non-union

Malunion is a result of either failed surgery in the first instance or failed fixation which has united in a malreduced position.

Non-union may follow high-velocity injuries and is predictable if unstable fixation techniques have been used. Low transcolumnar fractures are more prone to non-union, perhaps as a result of their more precarious blood supply. Patients with non-union commonly complain of pain, instability about the elbow, and general weakness of the limb. Stable compression plating using two plates at right angles as described earlier, with or without bone graft, is normally effective in the management of such problems. O'Driscoll has shown success using parallel medial and lateral anatomical plates. In some circumstances, particularly low fractures in the elderly patient with non-union, salvage by a TER is the correct treatment. As the collateral stabilizing ligaments have then been lost, a semi-constrained hinge arthroplasty is needed.

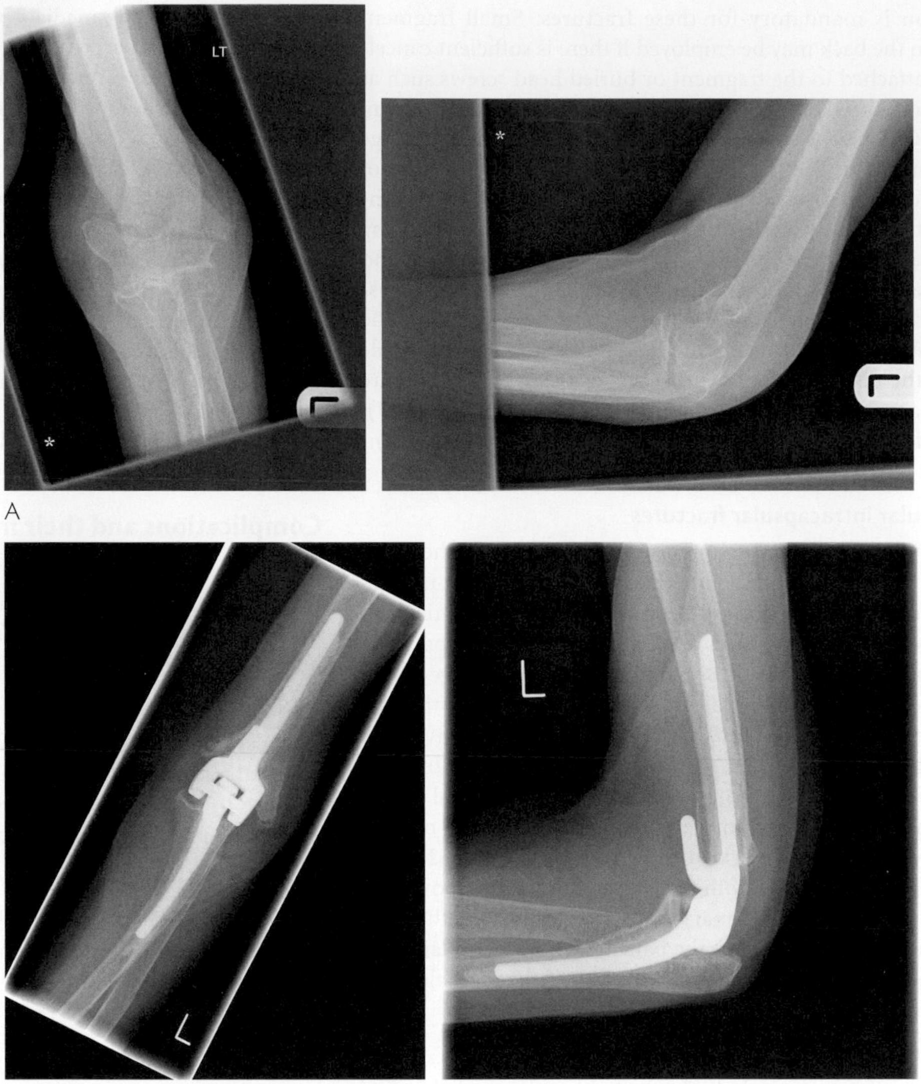

Fig. 12.34.8 Radiographs of A) a low extra-articular transcolumnar fracture treated with B) a Coonrad–Morrey 'sloppy-hinge' total elbow replacement.

Implant failure and non-union may also occur at the olecranon osteotomy. The incidence is in the range of 0–10% of cases. It is not often a clinical problem, though removal of tension band wiring is often needed for comfort. When symptomatic olecranon non-union occurs, refixation using a compression plate and a small bone graft is advised.

Stiffness and heterotopic ossification

Loss of range of elbow motion is very common following distal humeral fractures. Loss of extension is more prevalent and takes longer to resolve than restricted flexion. There is rarely any restriction of supination or pronation. The normal cause of the stiffness is contracture of the anterior joint capsule.

If stiffness below the normal functional range (30–120 degrees of flexion) persists beyond 6 months, intervention may be required. Most severely stiff cases referred for later treatment have been inadvisedly immobilized for several days or weeks immediately after operation. Early active motion is the best prevention.

Box 12.34.5 Distal humerus—postoperative management

- Movement is critical
- Physiotherapy important
- Flowtron may help
- Plaster splints best avoided.

Box 12.34.6 Distal humerus—complications

- Infection 1–6%
- Vascular complications unusual but must be vigilant
- Ulnar nerve may be compromised at injury or later (tardy)
- Non-union/malunion commonest with high velocity injuries
- Heterotopic calcification commoner with delayed fixation or immobilization
- Arthritis may follow intra-articular fractures.

Heterotopic ossification around the elbow appears to be mainly related to elbow dislocation, burns, or associated head injury. Massive new bone formation, also called myositis ossificans, only occurs in around 4% of cases. The incidence is much higher in cases where internal fixation has been delayed more than 7 days. Removing it by arthrolysis is very beneficial.

Osteoarthritis

Few papers discuss the incidence of osteoarthritis following fracture of the distal humerus, with or without internal fixation. Malreduction or malalignment of the articular surface predisposes the joint to osteoarthritis which occurs within 10 years in such cases. Jupiter's series followed-up at a mean of 5.8 years showed some narrowing of the joint space in 68% of cases, and extensive radiographic osteoarthritis in just over 20% of these. The changes correlated with fracture severity but not with the functional outcome.

In the authors' experience, patients with precisely anatomical reduction, even after severely comminuted intra-articular fractures, had little or no functional complaints even at 18 years and no radiological signs of deterioration in the joint. When instability remains after treatment, the joint very rapidly deteriorates and severe painful osteoarthritis ensues within very few years.

Outcomes from treatment

Results have improved and been maintained after stable anatomical internal fixation of distal humeral fractures in all age groups. Patients with severe comminution, major soft tissue damage, whether open or closed, such as follows high-velocity road traffic collisions, extensive falls, gunshot injuries, and side swipe injuries, tend to do worst.

Excellent long-term results, albeit with significant numbers lost to follow-up, have been reported with plate stabilization of distal humeral fractures using a number of validated upper limb outcome measures.

Olecranon and coronoid fractures

Introduction

The olecranon is the proximal articulating part of the ulna, proximal to the coronoid process but excluding the coronoid process itself. The subcutaneous position of the olecranon makes it vulnerable to trauma and various different fracture patterns are found with treatment options depending on the pattern. The majority of olecranon fractures are intra-articular except those of the very tip, although, some fractures in the centre of the trochlea notch may not involve articular cartilage.

Elbow instability after reduction of a dislocation is associated with some coronoid fractures.

Aetiology

Olecranon fractures are sustained as a result of direct trauma to the subcutaneous proximal ulna either in low-velocity falls or in high-velocity accidents which result in more complex injuries.

Classification of olecranon fractures

Colton's classification is a simple system that divides the fractures according to the anatomy and mechanism of the fracture (Figure 12.34.9). The fracture patterns are as follows:

- Group 1: avulsion injuries of the olecranon tip
- Group 2: oblique fractures
- Group 3: fracture–dislocations (Monteggia)
- Group 4: unclassified.

The AO classification attempts to classify all fractures of the proximal radius and ulna under one heading, namely segment 21. The classification system for the forearm bones differs from that for the other bones and this inconsistency makes it difficult to follow and of little clinical application.

Classification of coronoid fractures

Fractures of the coronoid process are classified as:

- Type I, fractures avulsing just the tip of the coronoid
- Type II, those that involve less than 50% of the coronoid, either as a single fragment or multiple fragments
- Type III, those involving more than 50% of the coronoid. These types are subdivided into type A (without elbow dislocation) and type B (with elbow dislocation), though transient dislocation may make the differentiation very difficult.

The isolated fracture of the anteromedial part of the coronoid with associated avulsion of the lateral ligament complex of the elbow has been recently recognized as the consequence of a varus injury to the elbow joint and frequently needs operative repair to stabilize the elbow and prevent the rapid onset of arthritis.

Symptoms and signs

Pain with proximal ulna fractures is localized to the posterior and medial aspects of the elbow. As the proximal ulna lies in a subcutaneous position, localized swelling from fracture bleeding is readily recognized and the fracture line may be palpated. A haemarthrosis may be observed by filling of the sulci on each side of the elbow. Open fractures usually present with wounds on the subcutaneous border. Isolated coronoid fractures are difficult to assess as the coronoid lies deep at the front of the elbow.

Investigations

Plain radiography remains the mainstay of radiological investigation of the elbow. Standard anteroposterior and lateral films can be augmented by the 'radial head, capitellar view' which can help visualize the coronoid. Where the elbow cannot be placed in extension, repeat radiography, with either sedation or 'on-table' traction views, can be valuable prior to any surgery. CT scans can be helpful in planning the operative strategy particularly with three-dimensional reconstruction images.

Treatment options

The goals of treatment of proximal ulna fractures are the restoration of triceps extension function with reconstruction of articular surface anatomy and alignment with joint stability.

For undisplaced fractures (Figure 12.34.10), where the triceps extension mechanism is intact, the elbow is immobilized for a minimum period of time, with clinical and radiographic assessment at 1 week in a sling followed by gentle active controlled movement under a physiotherapist's supervision. They rarely displace later and prolonged immobilization should be avoided.

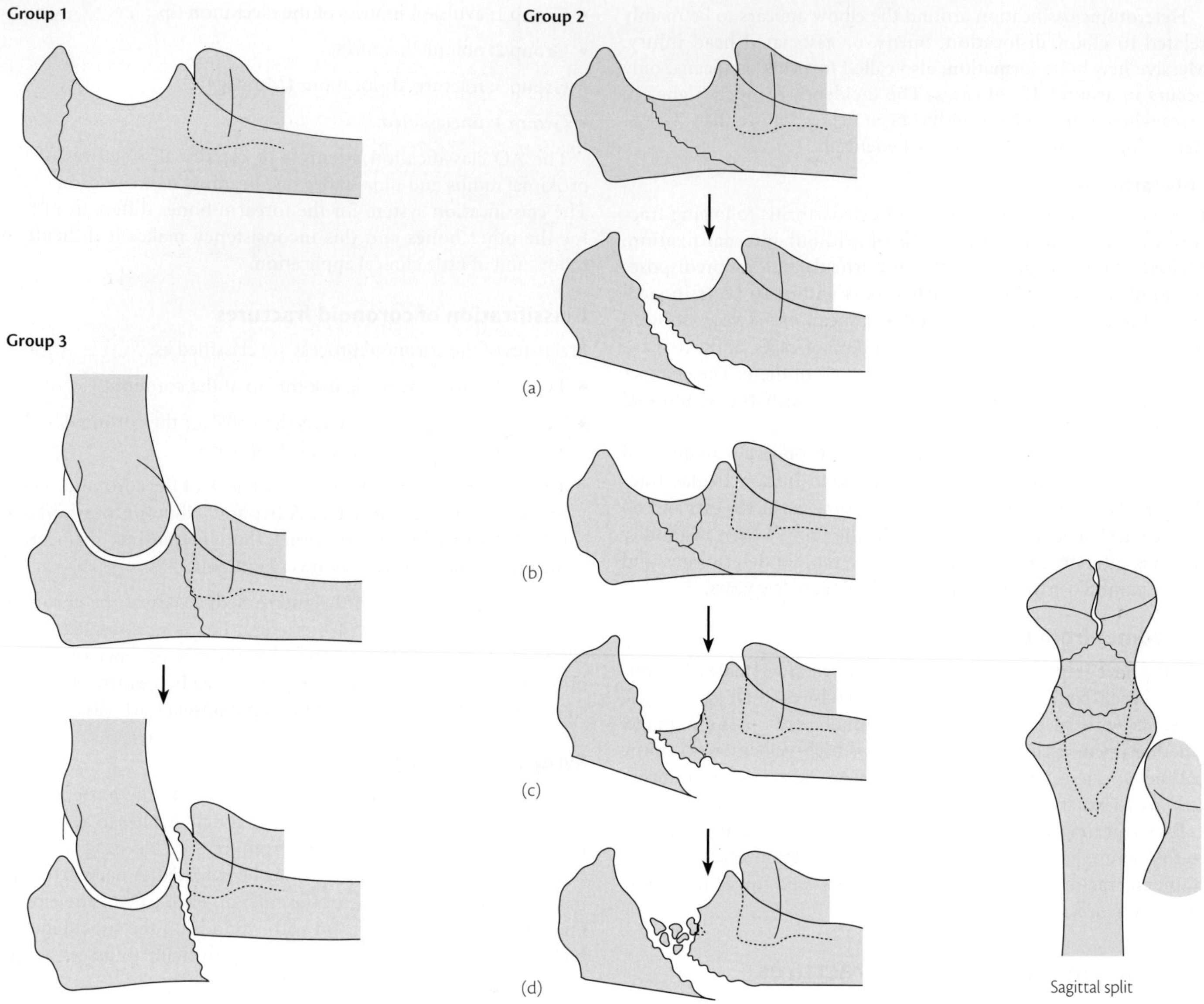

Fig. 12.34.9 Colton's classification system for fractures of the olecranon. (After Colton (1973).)

Extra-articular fractures

Extra-articular fractures of the tip of the olecranon are part of a spectrum of triceps avulsion injuries, most commonly seen in elderly patients presenting with loss of extension. If an appreciable gap (15mm or more) is noted then an ultrasound scan will demonstrate the state of the extensor apparatus. These injuries should be treated by triceps reattachment with strong non-absorbable sutures, with or without excision of the avulsion flake depending on its size. If missed, and presenting late the problem is compounded and a difficult repair with V–Y tendoplasty may be needed.

Transverse intra-articular fractures

These are the most common fractures of the proximal ulna and usually involve the mid-part of the greater sigmoid notch. Depending on the degree of confluence of the articular facets within the notch, transverse fractures affect varying amounts of articular cartilage. Simple, two-part fractures of this pattern are best internally fixed using the tension band principle (Figure 12.34.11).

The K-wires must be bent into a staple shape then driven through slots cut vertically in the triceps tendon and embedded deeply in the olecranon in order to avoid rapid loosening once triceps regains its power.

Some low-demand and surgically unfit elderly patients with intact triceps mechanism but some degree of fracture displacement do well without operation, simply allowing early motion but avoiding weight bearing through the arms for a few weeks.

Oblique intra-articular fractures

Displaced oblique fracture are not amenable to treatment by tension band wiring alone as the compression required by this technique is axial along the ulna and will displace an oblique fracture.

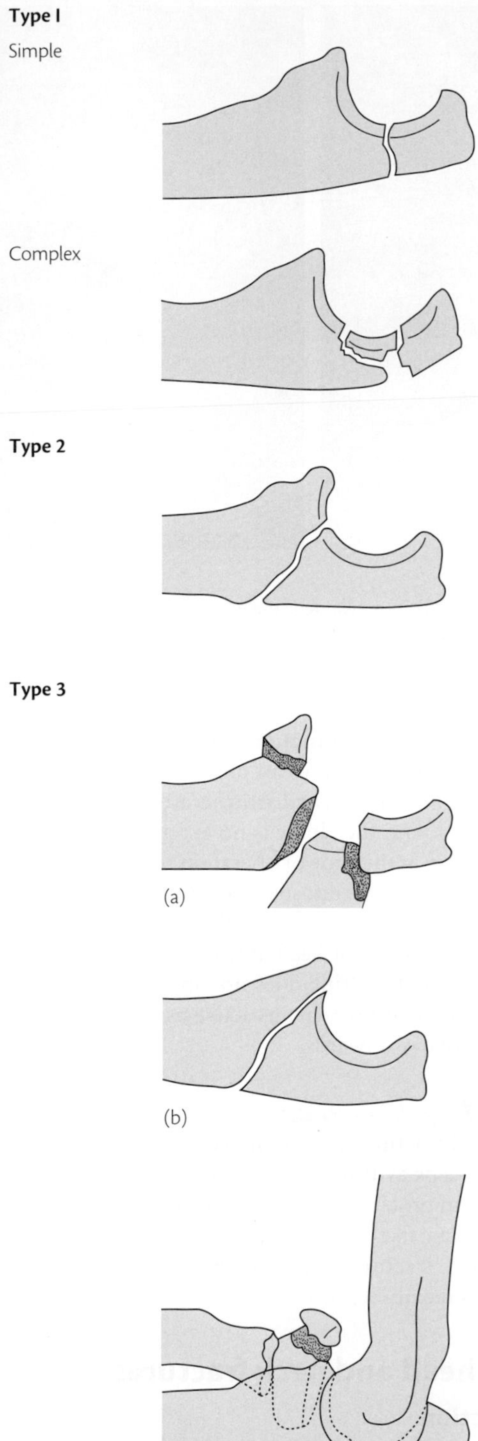

Fig. 12.34.10 A lateral radiograph of an undisplaced oblique fracture of the olecranon.

The fracture should be compressed with a lag screw and this should be 'neutralized' with a plate applied dorsally (Figure 12.34.12).

Comminuted intra-articular fractures

These fractures represent the greatest challenge in the management of proximal ulna fractures especially if associated with fractures of the radial head and/or distal ulna. There are frequently multiple planes of fragmentation. Reconstruction should try to achieve the objectives described previously. These are sinister injuries which risk total forearm ankylosis. Reconstruction may require a combination of techniques including 'bridge' plating, 'minimal' internal fixation, and the use of articulating external fixators. Although expensive and unforgiving anatomically-specific precontoured locking-plates (Figure 12.34.13) can be useful for very complex fractures of the proximal ulna.

In cases of limited stability due to either tenuous bony fixation or concomitant soft-tissue damage the use of skeletal fixators with wires or half pins is recommended (Figure 12.34.14).

The alternative to internal fixation of isolated fractures of the olecranon is the excision of the fragments and reattachment of the triceps to the remaining distal ulna. This is now rarely practised.

Coronoid fractures (Box 12.34.7)

Coronoid fractures occur either in combination with comminuted fractures of the proximal ulna or as part of an injury complex associated with elbow dislocation (15% of dislocations). They require internal fixation if they are type 3 injuries (whole coronoid) where the elbow is unstable as a result. Other coronoid fractures, if isolated injuries, can be mobilized within 3 weeks of injury.

Postoperative management

Rehabilitation is essentially as for distal humeral fractures. It is crucial to avoid immobilization—particularly in the very severe so called 'high Monteggia' injury with associated dislocation of the radial head.

Outcomes

A study of 52 patients reported 85% 'good' results with tension band wiring, for appropriate fractures, in terms of strength, range of motion, and function. This study reported a 25% incidence of problems with the K-wires backing out into the soft tissues; this problem was reduced if the wires were placed just through the anterior cortex of the ulna.

The results for comminuted proximal ulnar fractures and oblique two-part fractures stabilized using plates are good with minimal functional loss and good performance as measured by validated outcome measures.

Whatever method is used, due to the subcutaneous nature of the olecranon it is often necessary to remove the fixation sometime later.

Complications and their management

The main complication of olecranon fractures is the failure to achieve pre-injury ranges of motion, particularly extension. Poor ranges of motion are more common in complex multifragmentary

Box 12.34.7 Coronoid fractures—treatment

- Undiplaced briefly immobilize
- Extra-articular fractures repair
- Internal fixation.

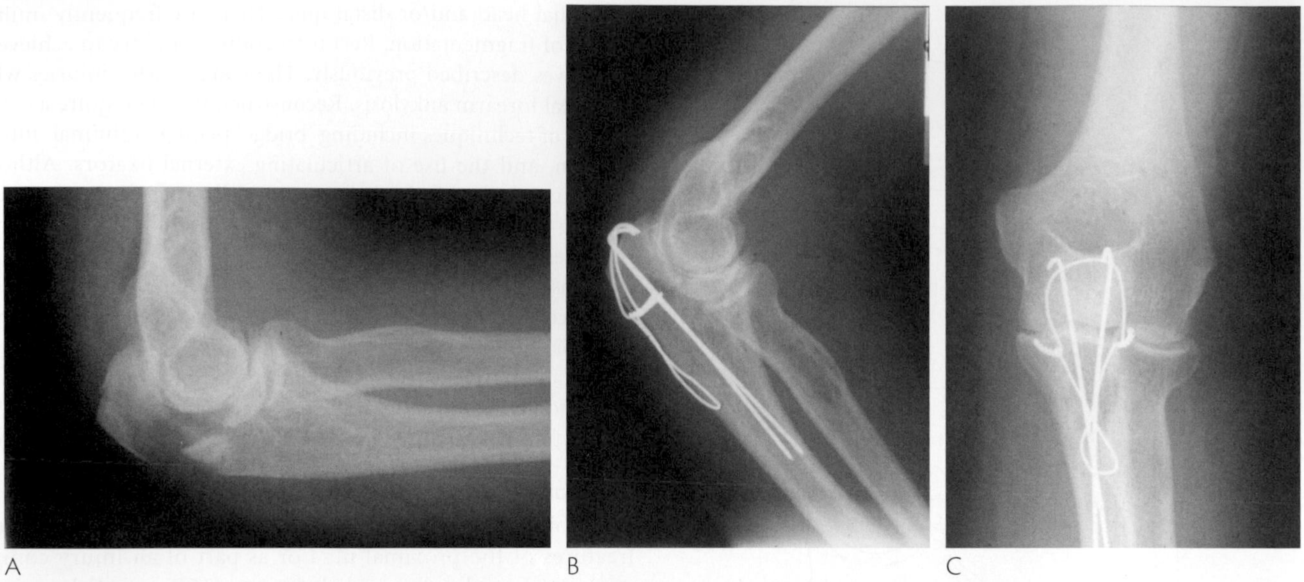

Fig. 12.34.11 A) A lateral radiograph of a displaced transverse fracture of the olecranon. B) and C) Tension band wiring of the fracture. (NB The longitudinal wires have not been passed through the anterior cortex in this case.)

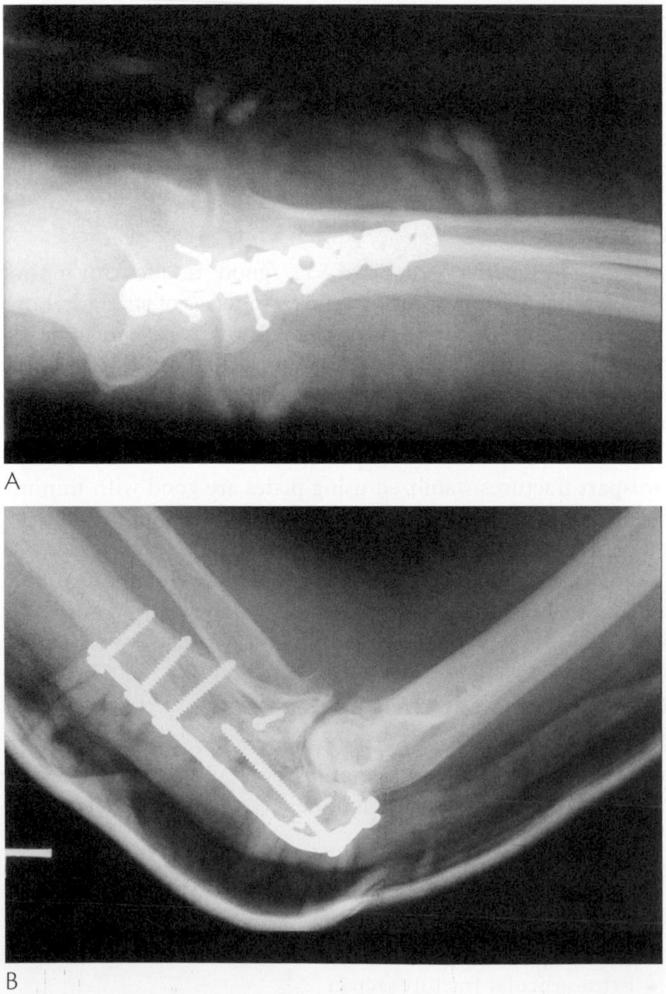

Fig. 12.34.12 An olecranon fracture stabilized with lag screws and a 3.5-mm AO reconstruction plate (anteroposterior and lateral views).

fractures. Early range of motion within a controlled environment helps to prevent loss of range of motion.

Malunion, non-union, and arthritis are complications of all fractures of joints, and the elbow is no exception. Surgical damage to the ulnar nerve at the time of operation should be guarded against, but this complication is unusual from the fracture itself. Heterotopic bone is of concern after severe elbow injury, particularly where associated with burns or head injury. Gentle passive elbow mobilization in the acute setting does not appear to lead to heterotopic bone, but the mainstay remains active use of the arm from the first postoperative day onwards.

Summary

Undisplaced fractures can be managed without operation. Extra-articular triceps avulsion injuries are best treated by triceps reattachment and protected motion. Displaced intra-articular fractures require internal fixation and early motion other than in a few unreconstructable fractures where fragment excision and triceps reattachment is recommended.

Radial head and neck fractures

Introduction

Radial head fractures are common, comprising 1.7–5.4% of all fractures. They involve about 20% of all elbow trauma. About 15–20% of proximal radial fractures are of the radial neck; but these are mainly in children. The management of simple radial head fractures is uncontroversial and successful, but controversial and less reliable for the more severe injury patterns. The majority of injuries fall into the simple group; however, care must be given to identify the small number of patients who fall into the complex injury group; particularly those with longitudinal injury patterns extending distally to the distal radioulnar joint (DRUJ)—the eponymous Essex-Lopresti injury.

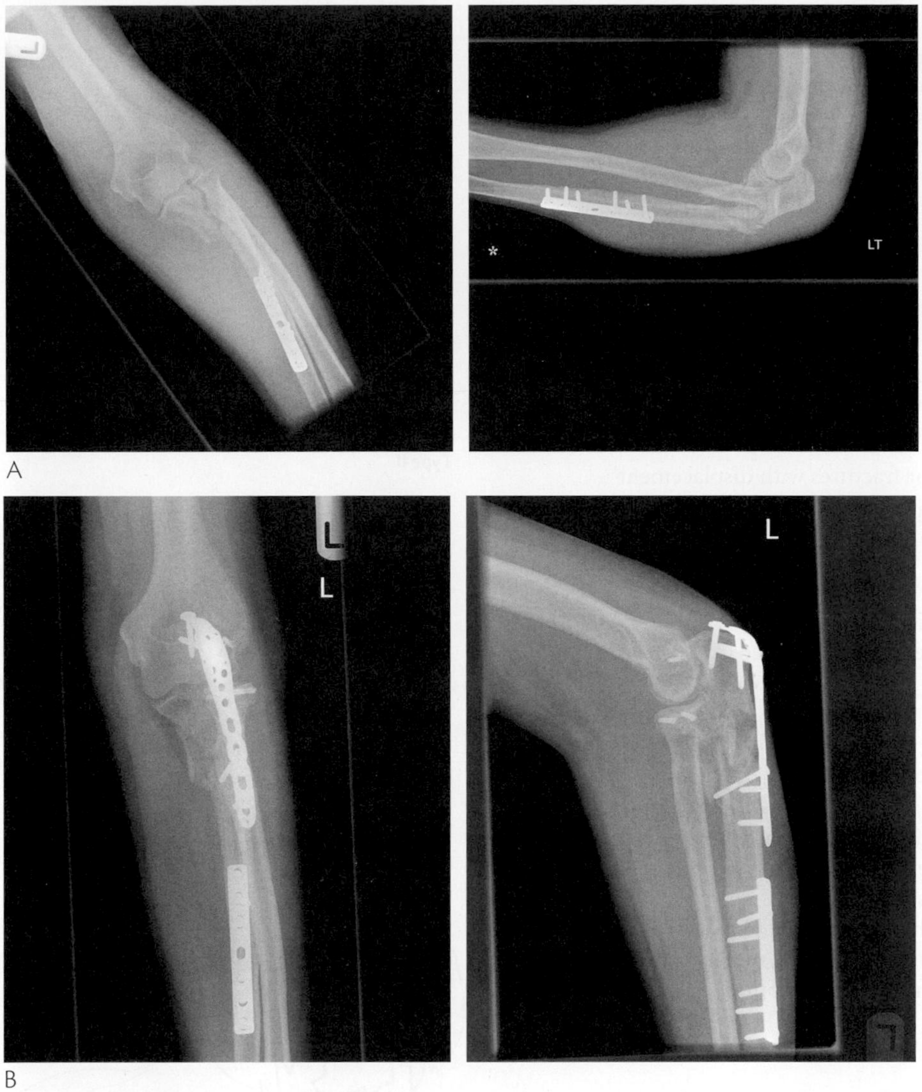

Fig. 12.34.13 A) A very comminuted olecranon fracture B) stabilized with a locking plate system (anteroposterior and lateral views).

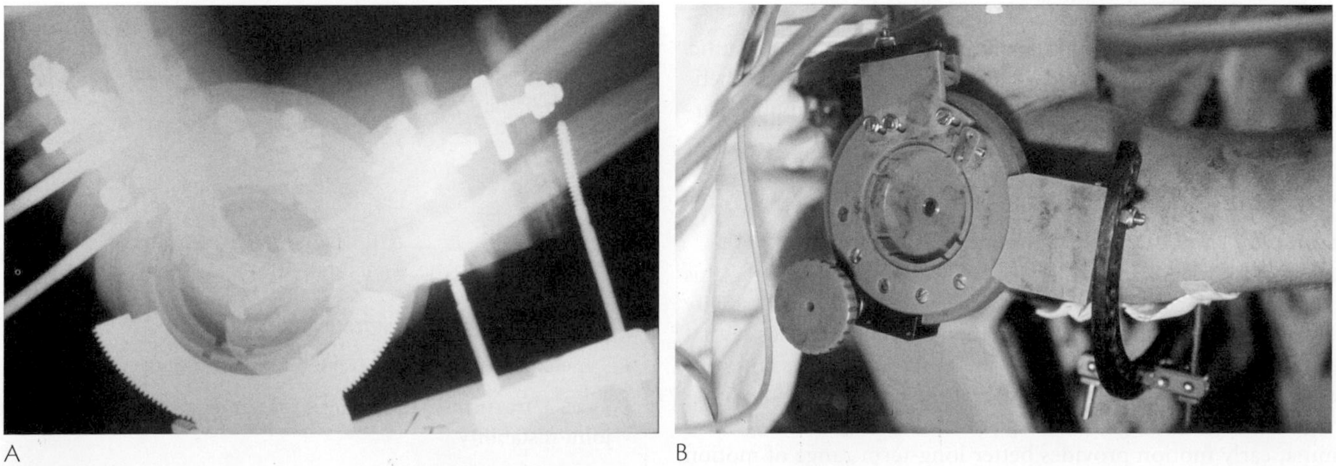

Fig. 12.34.14 A) A lateral radiograph and B) a photograph of a hinged external fixator applied to the elbow.

Aetiology

Radial head fractures are usually caused by a fall on the outstretched hand. The radial head is regarded as a secondary constraint to valgus instability. Displaced fracture fragments usually indicate damage to the very important anterior band of the medial collateral ligament with risk of lasting valgus instability. Disruption of the interosseous membrane between the radius and ulna which can extend into the wrist (DRUJ) is an important but rare injury associated with radial head fractures.

Classification

These fractures can be divided into three types

- Type 1 (62%) are 'fissure fractures or marginal sector fractures without displacement'
- Type 2 (20%) are 'marginal sector fractures with displacement'
- Type 3 (18%) are 'comminuted fractures involving the whole head'. No reference is made to the percentage of the articular surface that constitutes a 'marginal fracture'
- Type 4 fracture where there is a dislocation of the elbow (Figure 12.34.15) has subsequently been added to the basic classification.

Symptoms and signs

Fracture of the radial head, with or without associated damage to the anterior band of the medial collateral ligament, presents as pain and swelling on the lateral aspect of the elbow joint with a reduced range of motion, both to flexion–extension and forearm rotation. Examination will reveal tenderness over the radial head and occasional crepitus. The examination should include the medial aspect of the joint for bruising and tenderness suggesting medial collateral ligament damage and the wrist for DRUJ disruption. A haemarthrosis will be noted by loss of the normal medial and lateral sulci of the elbow.

Investigations

Radiological investigation of the radial head should include an anteroposterior and lateral view of the articulation. The lateral radiograph will demonstrate elevated anterior and posterior fat-pad signs due to the haemarthrosis. The oblique 'radial head, capitellar' view can be helpful. CT scanning is helpful only if reconstruction of complex fractures is being contemplated.

Aspiration of the elbow joint is both diagnostic and therapeutic. The direct lateral portal is used for aspiration and local anaesthetic can be introduced after aspiration of the 7–10mL of lipohaemarthrosis which accumulates.

Treatment options (Box 12.34.8)

Mason type 1 fractures: no or minimal displacement

Impacted non-angulated radial neck fractures are included in this group. Although early workers raised concern about the possibility of displacement of these fractures, the general consensus is that they should be mobilized early after joint aspiration. This improves the early results, particularly pain relief, but may have little long-term advantage for regained range of motion. As with all elbow trauma, early motion provides better long-term range of motion compared with immobilization. Mobilization can be aided by

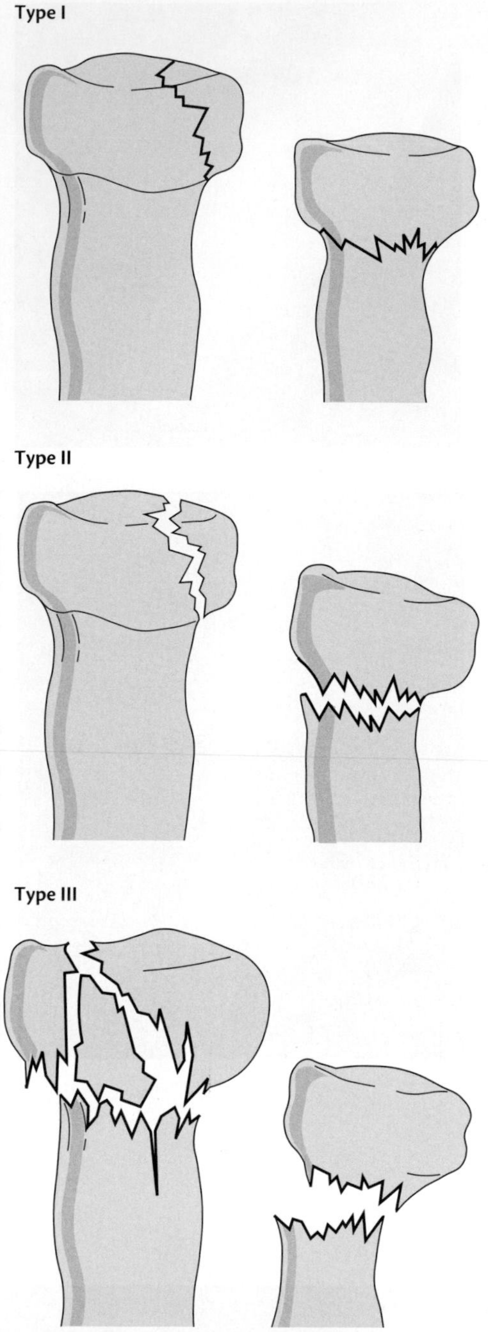

Fig. 12.34.15 The modified Mason classification of radial head fractures. (After McKee and Jupiter (2003).)

Box 12.34.8 Radial head fractures—treatment options

- Type 1: undisplaced aspirate and mobilize
- Type 2: fractures can be treated non-operatively sometimes
- Type 3: fractures—indications for surgery: block to motion or joint instability
- Type 4: radial head excision ± reconstruction.

application of ice to the anterior aspect of the joint to allow early full extension.

Mason type 2 fractures: displaced partial-articular fractures

If the radiocapitellar joint is stable and has no block to motion (as assessed after joint instillation with local anaesthetic), these fractures can be managed by initial splintage and then motion. Non-operative management can also be applied to radial neck fractures with less than 25 degrees of head/neck angulation. However some patients with a residual step of 2–3mm will complain for a very long time of clicking on rotation.

If there is a block to motion or joint instability, open reduction and internal fixation should be considered as radial head excision may lead to reduced grip strength and some proximal radial migration (of questionable significance in the absence of a true Essex-Lopresti injury).

Operative treatment is normally carried out through a standard lateral incision. Open reduction and internal fixation has been successfully achieved with standard raised head screws and a variety of sunken head devices including the traditional and cannulated Herbert (Figure 12.34.16) screws.

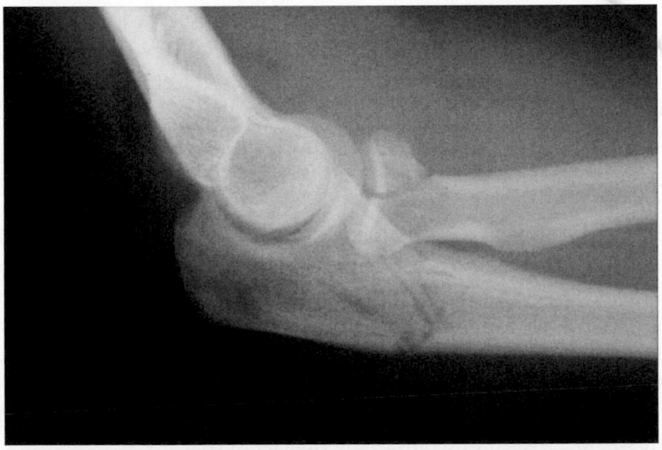

A

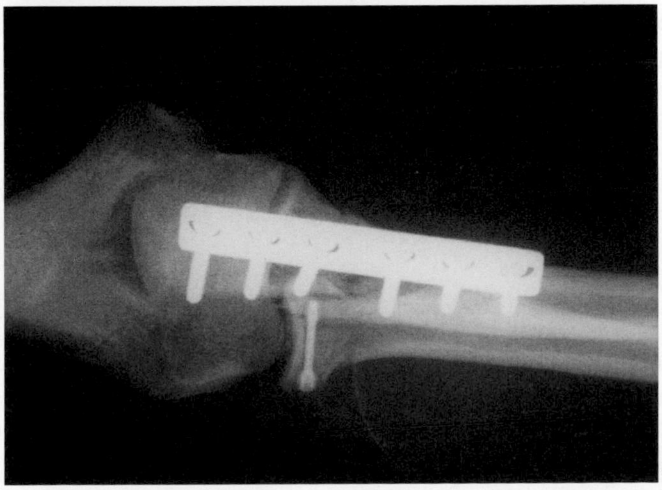

B

Fig. 12.34.16 A Herbert screw used for a radial head fracture. (NB Plate applied to oblique olecranon fracture.)

Where there is significant soft-tissue disruption either at the elbow or of the interosseous membrane, open reduction and internal fixation should be the treatment of choice of Mason type 2 fractures. If open reduction and internal fixation cannot be achieved for these fractures then radial head excision is carried out. If the fragment is small (less than one-third of the head) partial excision is an option. If the fragment is large then partial excision is less satisfactory than total excision. Where instability exists after radial head excision, treat by radial head replacement using a metal head (Figure 12.34.17).

Mason type 3 fractures: comminuted fractures

In these fractures open reduction and internal fixation is often not achievable. Consideration should be given to radial head replacement if there is valgus elbow instability or longitudinal forearm instability. In certain situations the elbow joint may be supported by a hinged external fixator or the DRUJ may be temporarily pinned.

Mason type 4 fractures: associated elbow dislocation

These fractures of the radial head are treated as their pattern would dictate were there no dislocation, noting the high incidence of ligamentous damage to the primary valgus constraints. Always screen the elbow after repair or replacement of the radial head as valgus instability may still be present. Direct repair of the anterior slip of the medial ligament should be considered and is not at that stage too difficult to achieve.

Outcomes

Non-operative treatment can produce good results in type 1 and 2 fracture, but is not reliable for all type 3 fractures. A retrospective review of 29 patients with Mason type 2 fractures showed significantly better results with open reduction and internal fixation than without. Overall results for type 4 fractures are poorer. Non-operative treatment with delayed excision if symptomatic has shown good result in a Swedish population for Mason 2 and 3 fractures.

Initial encouraging results, in small numbers of patients, using a metal replacement have been born out in the last decade. There are concerns regarding loosening of radial head replacements both monoblock and bipolar designs suggesting caution with their usage.

Complications and their management

Non-union and malunion occur with radial head fractures, and are more common with non-operative management. Instability of the elbow and the DRUJ are well-recognized complications. Heterotopic bone can occur at the elbow joint with radial head fracture particularly type 4 fractures and injuries associated with burns or head injury. Nerve injuries are uncommon, but the posterior interosseous nerve is at risk when exploring the radial head and neck. Grip strength is frequently decreased as is overall range of motion, particularly extension in the more severe grade of fracture.

Summary

Radial head fractures are common elbow injuries. They present with a haemarthrosis of the joint which should be aspirated. Undisplaced fractures are treated by early mobilization. Displaced

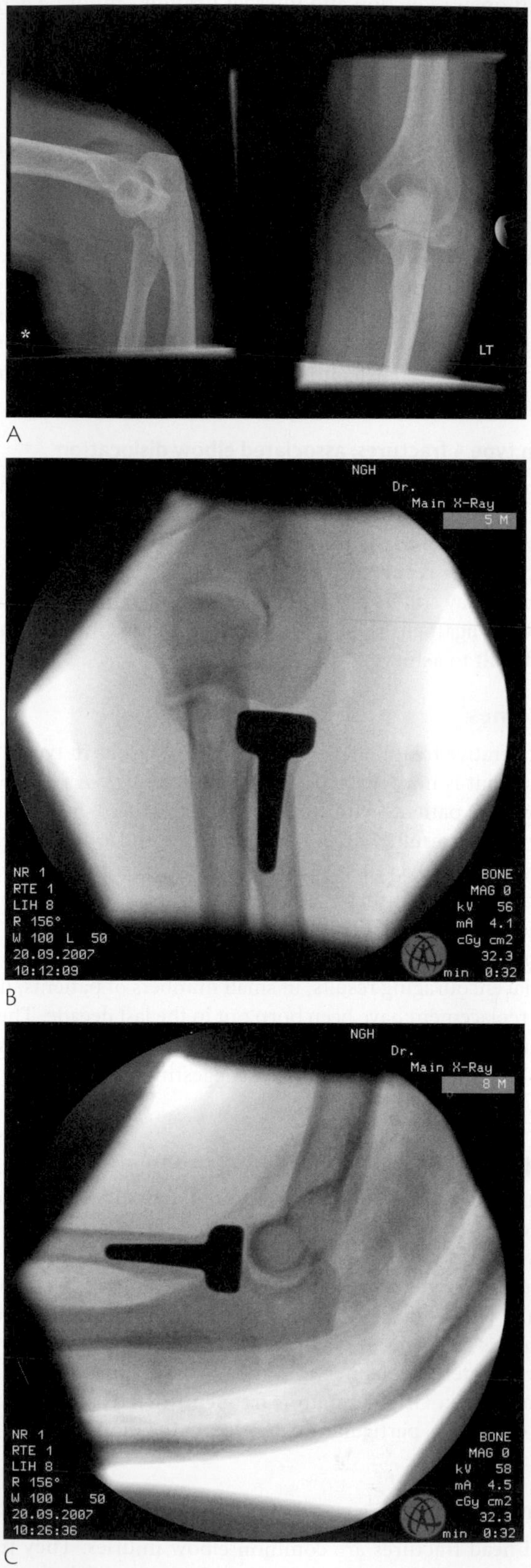

Fig. 12.34.17 Lateral radiographs of a comminuted radial head fracture treated with a metal radial head replacement.

fractures should be internally fixed where possible. Excision of the radial head is used where reconstruction is not possible. Radial head replacement should be carried out where there is marked valgus or any longitudinal instability. Radial head replacement, with a metal implant, can be helpful in complex fractures affecting the proximal radius and ulna to set the length prior to stabilizing the ulna. It is important to detect the Essex-Lopresti lesion. The so called 'terrible triad' injury of radial head fracture, coronoid fracture and collateral ligament injury (dislocation) require a comprehensive and aggressive surgical approach to regain elbow stability. They remain sinister injuries with a guarded prognosis.

Elbow dislocations and instability

Introduction

Acute elbow dislocation has an annual incidence of 6 per 100 000 population. The highest incidence is between the ages of 5–25 years; with the mode occurring in the late teens for both men and women.

Aetiology

The most common cause of elbow dislocation is a fall on the outstretched hand. In this position the olecranon tip impinges on the proximal edge of the olecranon fossa posteriorly and the ulna is levered out of joint by hyperextension.

An alternative mechanism for at least some elbow joint dislocations has been championed by workers at the Mayo Clinic. They suggest that rotatory forces associated with mild-elbow flexion and axial compression are the source of initially lateral ligament and capsule disruption.

Classification

Elbow dislocations are divided into simple (ligamentous injury only) and complex (those with significant associated fracture). Simple elbow dislocations are classified according to the direction of dislocation (Figure 12.34.18). Both lateral and medial collateral ligaments are torn in all elbow dislocations but lateral instability does not always result. Posterior dislocations are the most common (>80%). The other four possibilities—anterior, medial, lateral, and divergent—are all rare, especially the last of these.

Symptoms and signs

The patient presents with elbow pain and loss of motion. In the majority of elbows seen soon after dislocation, the abnormal anatomical appearance and malpositioning of the olecranon tip relative to the epicondyles is obvious. However, as the swelling increases this may become less apparent. It is important to document any prereduction deficit in distal neurological or vascular function.

Investigations

In many patients the diagnosis is evident without radiographs and reduction can be performed prior to taking radiographs. Where the diagnosis is unclear, standard anteroposterior and lateral radiographs are helpful. These radiographs should be repeated after reduction with the addition of the 'radial head, capitellar' views if further information about possible associated fractures is required.

Treatment options

Reduction can usually be carried out under analgesia and sedation in the accident and emergency department (Figure 12.34.19).

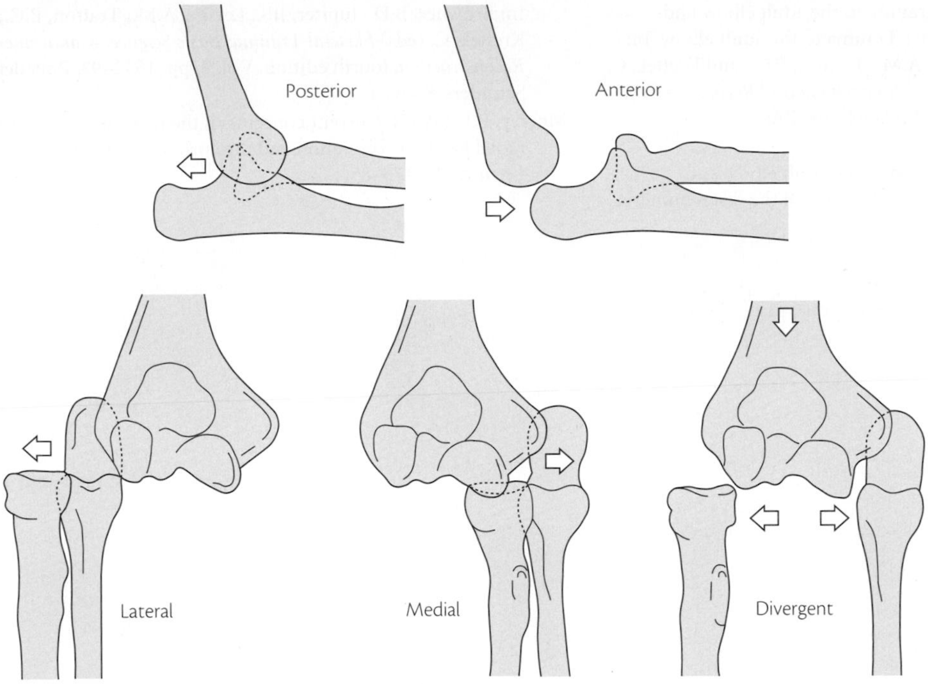

Fig. 12.34.18 The Classification system for elbow dislocations. (After McKee and Jupiter (2003).)

However, on some occasions or if diagnosis is delayed, general anaesthesia is required. Reduction is achieved by gentle traction on the forearm with counter-traction on the upper arm; medial or lateral displacement is corrected and the elbow is flexed to achieve the reduction. Relocation occurs with an audible or palpable 'clunk' and relief of the patient's symptoms. Following relocation an assessment of the range of stable motion is essential as well as checking post-reduction radiographs. Exact concentric reduction must be confirmed. In unusual circumstances—especially where diagnosis has been delayed or a redislocation missed open reduction is required.

Following reduction a short period (maximum 5 days) of immobilization in flexion is allowable (unless the joint is very unstable), but the aim should be early motion within the stable range of motion assessed at the time of reduction.

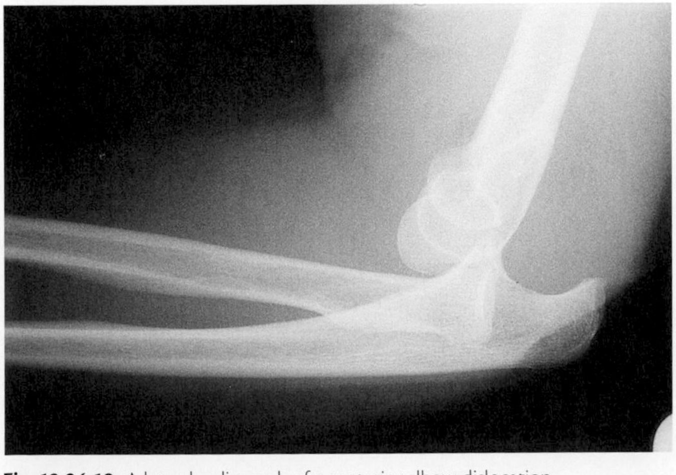

Fig. 12.34.19 A lateral radiograph of a posterior elbow dislocation.

Outcomes

The outcome following a simple dislocation is good. Those dislocations in which there is an associated fracture have a worse outcome.

Complications and their management

Complications of elbow dislocation include nerve and vascular impairment, chronic instability, stiffness, heterotopic bone formation, and myositis ossificans. Vascular complications need to be treated early with vascular exploration and fasciotomies. Nerve deficits can normally be treated expectantly unless open surgery has been performed in the vicinity of the nerve trunk. The management of other complications is discussed elsewhere.

Summary

Elbow dislocations are common injuries of adolescents and young adults. The majority occur posteriorly and may be associated with fractures of the coronoid or radial head. Dislocations associated with fractures have a worse outcome and may need surgery. Treatment is normally by closed reduction and early mobilization, aiming to prevent both chronic stiffness and chronic instability. Recurrent dislocation very rarely occurs in adults and the possibility should not prevent strongly advising patients to mobilize the elbow gently as soon as pain is tolerable.

Further reading

Jupiter, J.B. and Morrey, B.F. (2000). Fractures of the distal humerus in adults. In: Morrey, B.F. (ed) *The Elbow and its Disorders*, third edition, pp. 293–330. Philadelphia, PA: W.B. Saunders.

Linscheid, R.L. and O'Driscoll, S.W. (1993). Elbow dislocations. In: Morrey, B.F. (ed) *The Elbow and its Disorders*, third edition, pp. 441–52. Philadelphia, PA: W.B. Saunders.

McKee, M.D. and Jupiter, J.B. (2009). Trauma to the adult elbow and fractures of the distal humerus. Part 1 Trauma to the adult elbow. In: Browner, B.D., Jupiter, J.B., Levine, A.M., Trafton, P.G., and Krettek, C. (eds) *Skeletal Trauma: Basic Science, Management and Reconstruction*, fourth edition, Vol. 2, pp. 1503–41. Philadelphia, PA: Saunders-Elsevier.

McKee, M. and Jupiter, J.B. (2009). Trauma to the adult elbow and fractures of the distal humerus. Part II: Fractures of the distal humerus. In: Browner, B.D., Jupiter, J.B., Levine, A.M., Trafton, P.G., and Krettek, C. (eds) *Skeletal Trauma: Basic Science, Management and Reconstruction*, fourth edition, Vol. 2, pp. 1542–92. Philadelphia, PA: Saunders-Elsevier.

Morrey, B.F. (1995). Current concepts in the treatment of fractures of the radial head, the olecranon and the coronoid. *Instructional Course Lectures*, **44**, 175–85.

12.35

Humeral shaft fractures

Chris Little

Summary points

- Deformity is well tolerated
- Anterior approach for proximal shaft, but avoid damaging the axillary nerve
- Nerve lesions which do not recover within three weeks should be investigated with nerve conduction studies
- Most isolated fractures treated non-operatively
- Floating elbow, multiple injuries, open or pathological fractures consider fixation
- Open plating and nailing both give good results.

Introduction

Humeral shaft fractures are commonly closed injuries which will generally unite with non-operative treatment with good clinical function. A small proportion have an associated injury to the radial nerve, but this lesion is usually in continuity, and the role of early exploration of a nerve lesion present from the time of a closed fracture is controversial. The treatment options and their rationale are discussed.

Incidence and aetiology

In a Swedish study, humeral shaft fractures were seen to occur in 14.5 per 100 000, the incidence increasing with age. While in this study the majority were due to simple falls, high-energy trauma, penetrating trauma, and the indirect trauma of throwing and arm-wrestling, all caused non-pathological shaft fractures. Pathological fractures usually affect the proximal humerus but fractures through tumour deposits (particularly in multiple myeloma) and in patients with severe osteoporosis can be seen in the shaft.

Relevant regional and surgical anatomy

The humeral shaft connects the polyaxial shoulder joint with the elbow, which acts essentially as a hinge. The large range of motion in all planes at the shoulder joint means that malunion of shaft fractures are, for the most part, well tolerated. The humerus is well covered with muscle, minimizing the aesthetic impact of mild degrees of malunion.

The lateral aspect of the shoulder is covered by the deltoid muscle, innervated by the axillary nerve (a division of the posterior cord of the brachial plexus), which runs around the humeral surgical neck along with the circumflex humeral artery after passing through the quadrilateral space.

The anterior (or flexor) compartment of the arm contains the coracobrachialis, brachialis and biceps muscles. These are innervated by the musculocutaneous nerve, which runs in the plane between biceps and brachialis and has as its terminal division the lateral cutaneous nerve of the forearm. Brachialis receives an additional innervation from the radial nerve, the nerve that primarily supplies the posterior (or extensor) compartment muscle, triceps. The radial nerve arises from the posterior cord of the brachial plexus, runs along the posterior surface of the humerus in the spiral groove between the lateral and medial heads of triceps before passing through the lateral intermuscular septum to pass anterior the elbow joint, supplying the radial wrist extensors (extensor carpi radialis brevis from its posterior interosseous division) and brachioradialis.

The median (Figure 12.35.1) (from the lateral cord of the brachial plexus) and ulnar nerves (from the medial cord) traverse the arm without normally innervating any structures, the median nerve crossing anterior to the brachial artery from lateral to lie medial in the antecubital fossa, and the ulnar nerve passing from the anterior to the posterior compartment through the medial intermuscular septum, crossing the elbow behind the medial epicondyle within the cubital tunnel.

Approaches

The differential innervation of the compartments and sites of the neurovascular bundles dictates the common approaches to the humerus. The proximal shaft is usually approached through an anterolateral approach, which is extensile proximally into the deltopectoral approach to the shoulder and distally into the anterior approach to the elbow and forearm (Henry's approach). This uses the plane between the territories of the axillary and radial nerves posteriorly and the musculocuta-neous nerve anteriorly; brachialis is split to expose the anterior surface of the humerus, relying on its dual innervation, giving access to the whole length of the bone. The patient is positioned supine with the arm on a radiolucent hand table. The resultant scar is obvious.

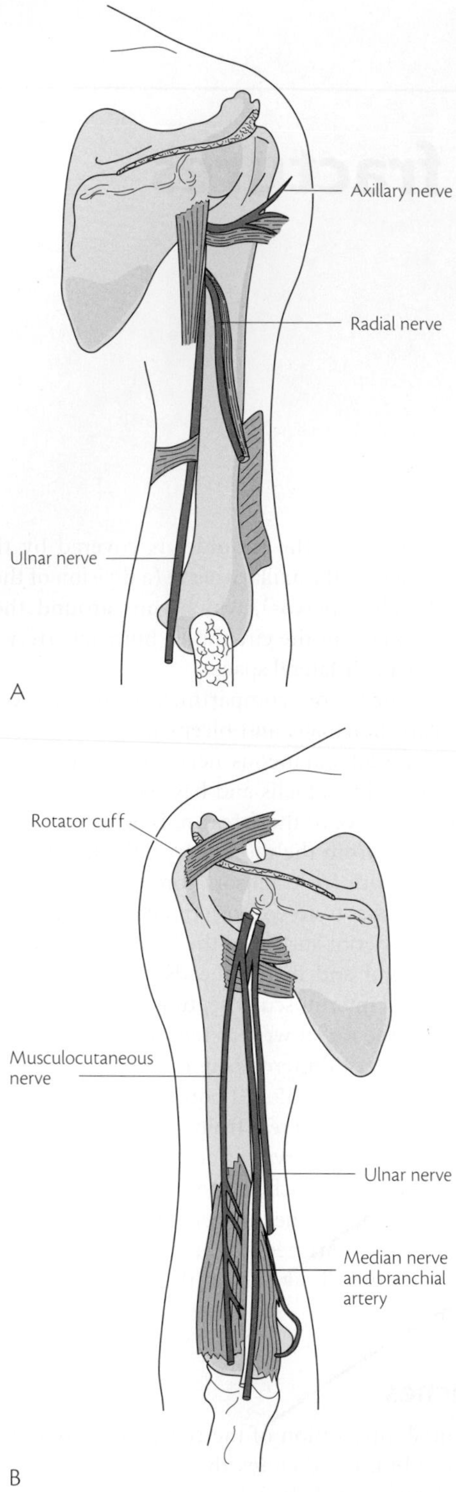

Fig. 12.35.1 A) Posterior and B) anterior drawings of the humeral shaft demonstrating the close relationship of critical neurovascular structures.

Distal shaft fractures, particularly with extensions into the distal metaphysis, are generally exposed through a posterior triceps-splitting or reflecting approach, which also allows exploration of the radial nerve in the spiral groove in the event of a radial nerve palsy. An early decision whether triceps continuity with the ulna, with its insertion into the olecranon, can be preserved (triceps reflection or splitting) or the extensor mechanism should be reflected in its entirety (olecranon osteotomy) needs to be made; this decision will largely be determined by the presence of a complex articular injury, requiring direct visualization of the distal humeral articular surface (and so requiring an olecranon osteotomy). Patient positioning is more difficult for posterior approaches, with the patient either lying prone or lateral with the arm in a gutter. Access for intraoperative imaging is also more challenging.

The medullary canal of the humerus runs from the head to just above the olecranon fossa distally. Access for intramedullary fixation techniques can be achieved antegrade through the humeral head (via a deltoid-splitting approach, but requiring violation the supraspinatus element of the rotator cuff). Care must be taken to avoid injury to the axillary nerve if the deltoid is split more than 4cm below the acromion. Retrograde insertion through top of the olecranon fossa is an alternative (via a posterior triceps-splitting approach) but risks creating a supracondylar fracture and makes locking in the proximal humerus more difficult.

History and clinical assessment

The energy of the injury is important to determine, to gauge the likelihood of associated injuries and of a pathological fracture, both of which may influence the chosen method of treatment. An assessment of the anticipated level of compliance with rehabilitation advice is similarly influential.

Examination of the patient should exclude associated injuries, treatment of which may well take clinical priority, and the patient's fitness for anaesthesia. Local examination focuses on the integrity of the soft tissue envelope and confirming the distal neurovascular function, in particular of the radial nerve (tested best by confirming finger extension at the metacarpophalangeal joint (MCP) joint, thumb retropulsion (an extensor pollicis longus function), and wrist dorsiflexion).

Investigations

Plain film imaging in two planes, without rotating the arm, will suffice in the majority of cases. Pathological fractures will usually be in patients with known metastatic disease, but staging investigations will be needed if the primary tumour is unknown. (see Chapter 12.18). Diaphyseal fractures with articular extensions may require cross-sectional imaging if the articular element cannot be accurately defined on the plain films.

Neurophysiological investigation of nerve lesions is appropriate at between 3–6 weeks if there is no evidence of clinical recovery. Leaving studies for a few weeks will allow denervation changes to be seen.

Treatment options

Non-operative (Box 12.35.1)

Given that mild malunions are accommodated with good function and that union with non-operative treatment is the norm, the overwhelming majority of humeral diaphyseal fractures can and are treated non-operatively. This should be an active process, with care directed to the type of brace used and to ensure that the risk of stiffness of the adjacent elbow and shoulder is minimized. Initial treatment with a plaster splint like a Bohler slab (to cover the

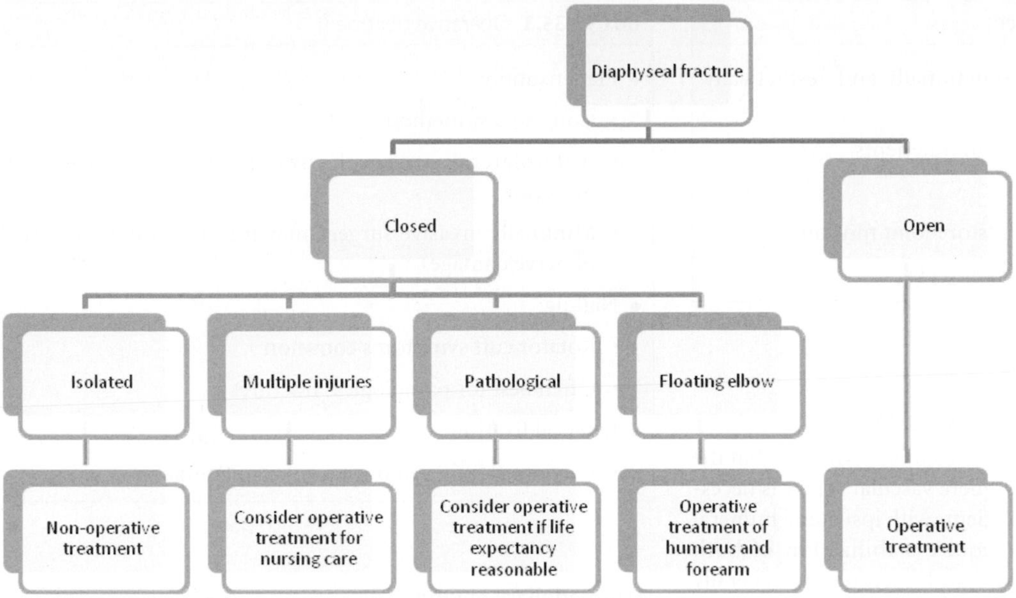

Fig. 12.35.2 Treatment algorithm for acute injuries.

shoulder like a cowl and splint the length of the humerus) to control pain is indicated, with collar and cuff support applied and instruction given to keep the elbow dependent so that gravity will assist reduction. If the humeral alignment is slow to achieve, reinforcement of the advice to keep the elbow dependent and application of a forearm cast to provide a little more gravity-assisted traction is appropriate. (Non-operative management is also dealt with in Chapter 12.11.)

Once the fracture swelling and discomfort has subsided, the protective slab can be replaced with a cooptation brace for the arm. This should be kept tight so that the hydrostatic tension within the muscle compartments will support the fracture, allowing micromotion to encourage union, but not too much motion so that union is prevented. Elbow motion should be encouraged.

Union should be expected by 8 weeks, and is achieved in over 90% of cases. Functional brace use may be associated with impaired shoulder function, but gives better elbow function than use of a U-slab throughout the treatment period.

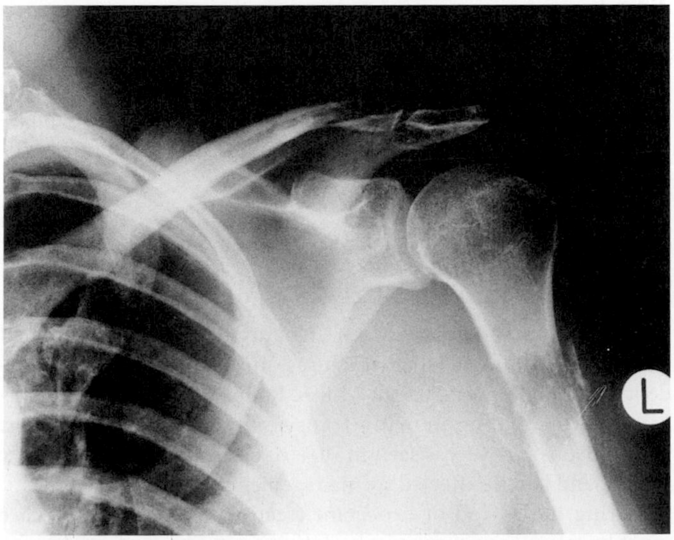

Fig. 12.35.3 Fracture through pathological bone in the proximal humeral shaft. Note the abnormal bone quality at the fracture site and the callus response. Whole length views of the humerus would be required to exclude multiple lesions, and additional imaging and investigation if the source of a primary tumour was not already known.

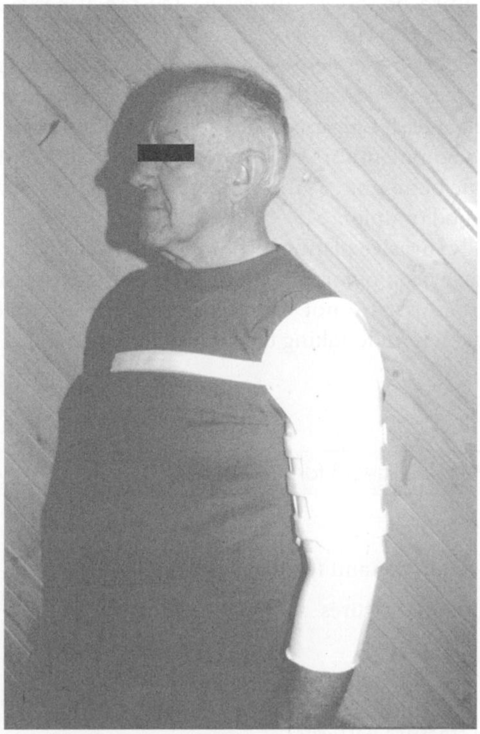

Fig. 12.35.4 A Sarmiento brace with strap.

Box 12.35.1 Non-operative treatment

- Mild degrees of malunion are functionally and aesthetically acceptable
- Gravity-assisted reduction to realign fragments
- Initial slab cowl for comfort
- Early functional cast-bracing to restore joint motion
- Union anticipated in over 90% by 8 weeks.

Operative

Indications for operative treatment (Box 12.35.2)

Open fractures require debridement and stabilization; in all but the most extreme soft tissue injuries, or where vascular repair is necessary, internal fixation is preferable. Patients with ipsilateral humeral shaft and forearm fractures also require stabilization of both skeletal injuries. Patients with pathological fractures are generally best treated operatively to give early pain control and return of function.

Other indications for acute fixation are relative, but include multiply injured patients (for ease of nursing care), patients where compliance with rehabilitation is likely to be poor, patients in whom a radial nerve palsy has developed during treatment (see later), and certain fracture configurations (relatively transverse fractures, especially in the proximal third, and certain distal shaft fractures when varus mal-union is less well tolerated).

Plate fixation

Open plate fixation of fractures when operative treatment is deemed necessary remains the most common treatment modality. The approach will usually be anterolateral, although fractures of the distal third or those with associated radial nerve lesions or extension into the elbow are better treated through a posterior approach. A large fragment plate (4.5mm) should be used due to the large forces applied to the implant during healing and rehabilitation, with at least four used holes in both the proximal and distal fragments. Some authors recommend the use of supplementary prophylactic bone-graft at the initial fixation to maximize the rate and likelihood of union.

Minimally invasive plating techniques, often using locking plate systems, have been reported with high union rates. As the neurovascular structures are not exposed during the approaches, care must be taken if undertaking this type of fixation.

Box 12.35.2 Indications for surgery

- Open fractures
- Ipsilateral upper and forearm fractures
- Pathological fractures
- Multiple injury
- Radial nerve palsy
- Special fracture patterns.

Box 12.35.3 Operative treatment

- Plate fixation:
  - Commonest method
  - Anterolateral approach unless distal fracture, then posterior
  - Minimally invasive surgery may improve union rates (risk of nerve damage)
- Nailing:
  - Rotator cuff symptoms common
  - Often best for pathological fractures
- External fixation:
  - Used for floating elbow/complex open fractures.

Intramedullary nailing

Initial enthusiasm for intramedullary techniques was dampened by reports of cuff impairment with antegrade insertion techniques, supracondylar humeral fracture with retrograde insertion techniques, comminution during nail insertion, fracture non-union (possibly related to poor rotational control), and problems with the instrumentation. Many of these problems have been reduced by improvements in the design and insertion techniques and instrumentation systems, and high union rates of close to 100% have been reported in series of both open and closed fractures. Similar union rates and function but more shoulder pain are reported in series that compared treatment by plate fixation or intramedullary nailing.

Intramedullary nailing has advantages in the treatment of pathological fractures (or impending fracture), where all but the most distal portion of the humerus can be stabilized, and potentially in obese patients, in whom access for open treatment may be difficult.

External fixation

While less commonly used than in other bones, external fixation is used for open injuries, to bridge a 'floating elbow' (associated ipsilateral humeral and forearm fractures) and in damage control situations with multiple injured patients.

Complications

Radial nerve palsy (Box 12.35.4)

While injuries to neurovascular structures have been described complicating humeral shaft fractures, most series report an incidence of radial nerve palsy of 11.8%. Radial nerve palsy is significantly more common with transverse and spiral fractures. Spontaneous recovery is seen in 71% of cases and overall recovery in 88% and is little affected by management.

During the period of expectant treatment and recovery, care must be taken to ensure wrist and digit contractures do not occur that will impair the ultimate function. Provision of a splint to hold the wrist dorsiflexed in a functional position and instruction in exercises to maintain passive motion of the wrist and digit joints is essential. Splints that provide a passive extension force to the MCP

Box 12.35.4 Complications—radial nerve palsy

- Seen acutely in 12%
- 71% recover spontaneously with expectant treatment
- Maintain passive elbow, wrist, and digit motion while recovery occurs
- Wrist extension splint safer than one with finger outriggers
- Neurophysiological evidence of nerve division mandates exploration at 6–8 weeks
- Tendon transfer better than late repair
- Expectant treatment may be reasonable for some lesions that arise during treatment.

joints while allowing active flexion can be used, but these splints risk creating a loss of flexion at the MCP joints if full flexion is not maintained (actively or passively) throughout the recovery period. If neurophysiological investigations suggest that the nerve has been divided, exploration and nerve grafting should be undertaken promptly to maximize the likelihood of the best possible outcome. If a long time has elapsed since the injury without evidence of recovery, tendon transfer will give a better functional outcome, although full passive motion of the wrist and digit joints is essential (see Chapter 12.25).

While most experts accept that initial expectant treatment of a radial nerve present from the time of injury is appropriate, the optimal treatment when nerve palsy arises during the treatment of a humeral shaft fracture is more controversial. Exploration of the radial nerve is advisable following palsy onset after intramedullary nailing or minimally-invasive plate fixation due to the potential for intraoperative nerve laceration. Nerve injury should be noted if a posterior approach has been used for open plating, but if an anterolateral approach has been used, exploration should be undertaken. Radial nerve palsy during non-operative treatment is the most controversial subject as in the majority of cases, exploration of the radial nerve in these circumstances showed an in-continuity lesion (as is the case with radial nerve palsy present from the moment of injury). As with radial nerve palsy from the injury, an initial period of expectant treatment and active monitoring with neurophysiological investigation at 4–6 weeks is reasonable, although early exploration can be justified.

Non-union (Box 12.35.5)

Rates of non-union with non-operative treatment range from 2–39%. Factors associated with failure to achieve union by non-operative means include the site of the fracture, with fractures of the proximal third being less likely to unite, and the pattern of the fracture, with transverse and short oblique fractures reported as being possibly less likely to unite.

Non-steroidal anti-inflammatory (NSAID) use has also been noted to be associated with non-union of humeral shaft fractures with a relative risk of non-union of 3.7 (95% confidence interval 2.4–5.6). However, in this retrospective study, NSAID use was only significantly associated with non-union at 61–90 days following injury (with opioid use in the same time window also showing a significant association with non-union), raising the possibility that the drugs were taken because of the pain of the impending non-union, and that the drug use may not be causal of the non-union.

Box 12.35.5 Complications—non-union

- Commoner in proximal fractures
- Transverse/short oblique fractures at risk of non-union
- NSAIDs may encourage
- Treat by onlay plating/grafting or reamed nailing.

Non-union may be treated by open plating with onlay bone grafting or by reamed intramedullary nailing.

Summary and conclusion

Humeral shaft fractures can occur at any age, although the incidence increases with age. The majority can and should be treated non-operatively as the outcome is generally good and the degree of malunion that commonly occurs is well tolerated with good function. Exceptions to the non-operative rule include open fractures, pathological fractures and humeral shaft fractures in multiply injured patients.

Non-union should occur in less than 10% of cases with non-operative treatment and can be treated with stabilization and bone grafting. While radial nerve palsy complicates over 10% of humeral shaft fractures, the overwhelming majority of lesions are in-continuity and can be treated expectantly with splintage and mobilization of the wrist and hand to maintain function, and clinical and neurophysiological monitoring to look for signs of early recovery. Prompt surgical treatment should be offered to patients in whom there is concern about radial nerve division.

When surgical stabilization is indicated, open plating and minimally invasive treatment with intramedullary nailing both give good results in terms of union and function, although there is a greater incidence of shoulder pain and dysfunction with antegrade intramedullary nailing. Minimally-invasive plate fixation has been reported, but the theoretical risk of iatrogenic nerve injury means caution should be observed. The role of external fixation in acute treatment is limited.

Further reading

Ekholm, R., Tidermark, J., Törnkvist, H., *et al.* (2006). Outcome after closed functional treatment of humeral shaft fractures. *Journal of Orthopaedic Trauma*, **20**, 591–6.

Hierholzer, C., Sama, D., and Toro, J.B. (2006). Plate fixation of ununited humeral shaft fractures: effect of type of bone graft on healing. *Journal of Bone and Joint Surgery*, **88A**, 1442–7.

Sarmiento, A., Zagorski, J.B., Zych, G.A., *et al.* (2000). *Journal of Bone and Joint Surgery*, **82A**, 478–86. Functional bracing for the treatment of fractures of the humeral diaphysis.

Sarmiento, A., Waddell, J.P., and Latta, L.L. (2001). Diaphyseal humeral fractures: treatment options. *Journal of Bone and Joint Surgery*, **83A**, 1566–79.

Shao, Y.C., Harwood, P., Grotz, M.R., *et al.* (2005). Radial nerve palsy associated with fractures of the shaft of the humerus: a systematic review. *Journal of Bone and Joint Surgery*, **87B**, 1647–52.

12.36

Fractures and dislocations of the shoulder girdle

Gregoris Kambouroglou

Summary points

- The function of the girdle is to position the hand in space
- The spectrum of injuries range from common and uneventful to rare and life threatening
- The functional outcome depends on individual demand, severity of the injury and the presence of complications.

Introduction

The shoulder girdle is a complex structure of three bones and five articulations that aims to position and support the function of the hand in space. As all joints, in order to serve the end-organ effectively the girdle requires range of motion, stability, and strength. Complex movement is shared amongst the five articulations resulting in a particular pattern of motion known as shoulder rhythm. In theory any pathology that affects these elements of girdle function may result in disability; however, as functional demands vary amongst patients and segmental disability may be compensated by the function of neighbouring joints, measurable deficits do not always correspond to functional disability. It is likely that in the average individual loss of 20% of girdle motion will not result in disability.

Acute glenohumeral dislocation

Anatomical considerations

The glenohumeral articulation is universal joint. In order to allow this range the joint depends less on osseous contact and stability relies more on the intra-articular and periarticular soft tissues. The structural and functional components of the glenohumeral joint (GHJ) stability have been extensively studied. The structures contributing to the joint stability are shown in Table 12.36.1.

The labrum provides a 50% increase in the congruency of the glenohumeral articulation whilst the middle and inferior glenohumeral ligaments are the primary ligamentous stabilizers of the joint.

Table 12.36.1 Glenohumeral joint stabilizers

Osseous	Static stabilizers	Dynamic stabilizers
Glenoid	Joint capsule	Rotator cuff
Humeral head	Labrum	Biceps tendon
Acromion	Glenohumeral ligaments	
	Coracoacromial ligament	

Pathological anatomy

A variety of traumatic lesions corresponding to the vector of the dislocation have been identified. The classic Bankart lesion associated with anterior dislocations represents the detachment of the capsulolabral complex from the anteroinferior portion of the glenoid. Correspondingly the Hill Sachs is an impaction fracture of the posterior part of the humeral head. Common fracture of the anteriorly dislocated shoulder is an impaction fraction of the glenoid with the great tuberosity fracture the next most common. Shearing fractures of the glenoid rim are discussed in the section on scapular fractures.

In posterior dislocations the impaction fracture is in the anterior part of the head (reverse Hill Sachs) and may be associated with avulsion of the lesser tuberosity or the subscapularis tendon.

Aging of musculoskeletal system results in inelastic tissues. Whilst fractures are more common in young adults, rotator cuff injuries have been identified in up to 85% of patients over 40 years of age. The presence of massive rotator cuff tears affects the outcome of shoulder dislocations.

Epidemiology

Anterior dislocation of the GHJ is the most common joint dislocation with a prevalence of 1.7%. It most commonly occurs as a sport related injury in young males and after a fall in elderly females. Posterior dislocation accounts for 2% of the GHJ dislocations. With the higher prevalence of high-energy injuries such as motorcycle crashes dislocations of the GHJ occur in conjunction with proximal humerus fractures (PHF). The obvious fracture and the difficulty of obtaining adequate imaging may result in a missed dislocation.

Clinical assessment, treatment principles, and outcomes

The history and clinical appearances are pathognomonic of the anterior dislocation of the GHJ. Caution is required in circumstances where the history is unclear or other clinical pathologies such epilepsy prevail. In contrast with the young adult the history of injury in the elderly can be vague, the complaints minor and the appearances subtle. Hence the diagnosis may be delayed or even missed.

Essential part of the clinical examination prior to any reduction manoeuvres is the neurological status of the arm. In anterior dislocation the axillary nerve is often involved although a recent study suggested a significant incidence of nerve involvement up to 48% when electromyographic (EMG) studies were used as a diagnostic tool. Multiple neural structures can be affected; however, the long-term prognosis is good with recovery evident 12–45 weeks following the injury.

Plain radiographs in two planes are the minimum standard of care regarding the imaging of the injury. Poor imaging may lead to error in diagnosis and management. The anteroposterior view must be in the plane of the GHJ. Axial views are difficult due to pain, however adequate analgesia and skilled radiography will produce adequate views in almost all circumstances. The direction and associated osseous injuries must be considered. The documentation of the dislocation is of importance in the long term in order to differentiate individuals with unidirectional traumatic dislocation from patients with multidirectional instability.

A multitude of reduction techniques have been describe for reduction of the anterior GHJ, the Hippocratic one being the oldest described. The principle of reduction, however, remains the same: adequate analgesia and monitored sedation followed by disimpaction, controlled traction, and reduction of the joint. Techniques that do not involve physicians in the process, such as the prone position and over the chair traction with weight application, are preferable. Contraindication to reduction in the emergency department is the dislocation with an undisplaced fracture of the humeral neck. Dislocations of the GHJ associated with humeral neck fractures are rarely successful in the Emergency Department and best avoided as the repeated trauma during the attempts may lead to a variety of complications and affect outcome.

Debate exists regarding the of postreduction after care. Multiple studies suggest no difference in the incidence of recurrent instability with or without immobilization in a sling and swathe or Velpeau bandage. An elegant study demonstrated that the avulsed capsuloligamentous flap (Bankart lesion) is best apposed to the glenoid neck with the arm in external rotation. However, the application of the finding in clinical practice has yet to be tested. Whilst the early surgical intervention has been lingering for some time, a recent well-structured study from Edinburgh suggested that early arthroscopic Bankart repair significantly decreases the risk of redislocation within the first 2 years in young individuals (15–27 years).

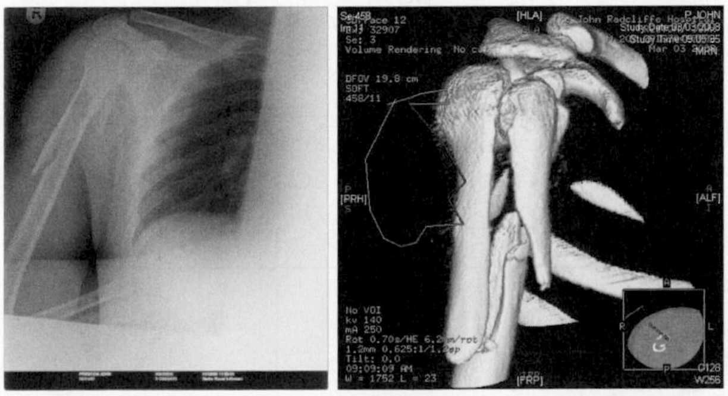

Fig. 12.36.1 Fracture of the proximal humerus with posterior dislocation of the humeral head.

Box 12.36.1 GHJ Dislocation: summary points

- Relies on osseous, static and dynamic stabilizers for stability
- Associated with:
  - Bankart lesion
  - Hill Sachs lesion
  - Tuberosity fractures
  - Rotator cuff tears
  - Glenoid rim fractures
- Prevalent in:
  - Young sportsman
  - Elderly females (often missed, occult associated injuries to the rotator cuff and plexus and early redislocation)
- AP and axial views
- Reduce with adequate analgesia and monitored sedation
- Consider arthroscopic Bankart repair in young (15–27 years).

It is hardly surprising that the redislocation is likely to occur in the 'sportingly active' group as the injury is sports related and they are unwilling to modify their activity. Multiple studies confirmed the fact and demonstrated a significant risk of up to 55% in the 2 years increasing to 66.8% at 5 years for the 15–27 age group.

Whilst recurrent dislocation is the most common injury-related complication in the young, the presence of rotator cuff damage and/or glenoid rim fracture predispose to redislocation of the GHJ in the elderly within the first 6 weeks. Pathognomonic of postreduction incongruence of the GHJ is painful rotation: in almost all non-fractured dislocations, rotation with the humerus in neutral position is comfortable and well tolerated. In the incongruent GHJ rotation is invariably limited and associated with pain and occasional crepitus.

Fracture dislocations can pose significant dilemmas and can be challenging to treat operatively. Reduction and fixation in young adults is preferable whilst in the elderly and low-demand patients with poor bone stock shoulder hemiarthroplasty may be the better option. Fractures of the greater tuberosity usually reduce once the GHJ is congruent. Displacement of the tuberosity fragment may occur, possibly suggesting associated rotator cuff tear. Early recognition will result in easier reconstruction and better outcome in terms of range of GHJ motion.

Fractures of the proximal humerus

Anatomical considerations

At the proximal end of the humerus the anatomical neck at 45 degrees to the shaft leads to the head that carries the head in

Box 12.36.2 Vascular supply to the humeral head

- Medial branch posterior circumflex artery—posteromedial capsule
- Ascending branch anterior circumflex artery—bicipital groove
- Thoracoacromial branches- insertion of the rotator cuff
- Intraosseous metaphyseal artery.

average of 20 degrees of retroversion. The rotator cuff attaches to the great tuberosity that is on average 8mm lower than the edge of the articular surface. The bicipital groove allows the uninterrupted and smooth function of the long heads of the biceps. Medial to the groove the subscapularis attaches to the lesser tuberosity. Studies have demonstrated that the vascular supply to the head is via four routes (Figure 12.36.2 and Box 12.36.2). Fractures through the anatomical neck of the humerus may have a significant risk of avascular necrosis (AVN) whilst fractures through the surgical neck will spare the blood supply to the head.

Epidemiology, mechanisms of injury, and classification

Proximal humeral fractures are common, compromising 5% of all fractures. It is a spectrum of injury ranging from physeal Salter–Harris II fracture in adolescents with excellent prognosis to high-energy fractures in young adults usually as the result of motor vehicle crashes. However, the majority of fractures occur in the seventh decade of life with a reported incidence of 63/100 000 population at an average age of 64.8 years. Fractures of the proximal humerus are now considered as 'fragility fractures'.

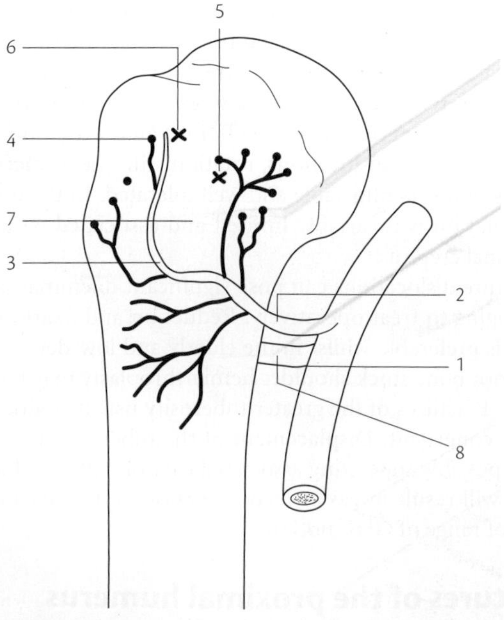

Fig. 12.36.2 (1) Axillary artery. (2) Anterior circumflex artery (ACA). (3) Ascending branch of the ACA. (4) Arcuate artery. (5) Lesser tuberosity. (6) Greater tuberosity. (7) Intertubercular groove. (8) Posterior circumflex artery (PCA).

The mechanism of injury is indirect force with fall on the arm or direct blow to the shoulder. The position of the arm, energy transfer upon impact and the bone stock will result in abduction, or abduction fracture patterns with or without dislocation of the GHJ.

Codman in 1934 described a distinct pattern of fracture of the proximal humerus and his observation remains valid to date: the proximal humerus fails in a predictable pattern due to the vector of force and the attachments of the musculotendinous units. The result is a fracture of the greater tuberosity, fracture of the lesser tuberosity and a fracture through the humeral neck. Neer's classification (Figure 12.36.3) is based on Codman's observations and despite criticism and individual interpretation it is still widely used providing a useful template for planning treatment. It classifies fractures according to the number of displaced fragments. Displacement was defined as 1cm and/or 45-degree angulation. This has led to fierce debate especially regarding the fractures involving the greater tuberosity (GT). Current thinking accepts displacement of no more of 5mm when referring to GT fractures. Evolution of knowledge resulted in recognition that valgus four-part fractures carry a different prognosis due to preservation of the head vascularity. Using Neer's criteria, 80% of PHF are undisplaced

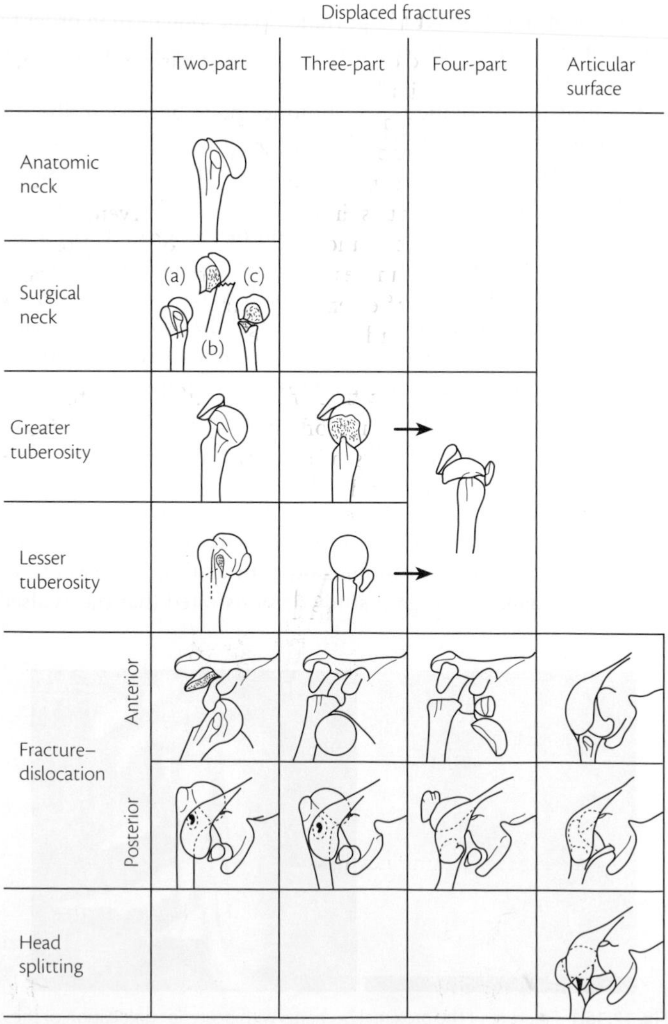

Fig. 12.36.3 Neer's classification system.

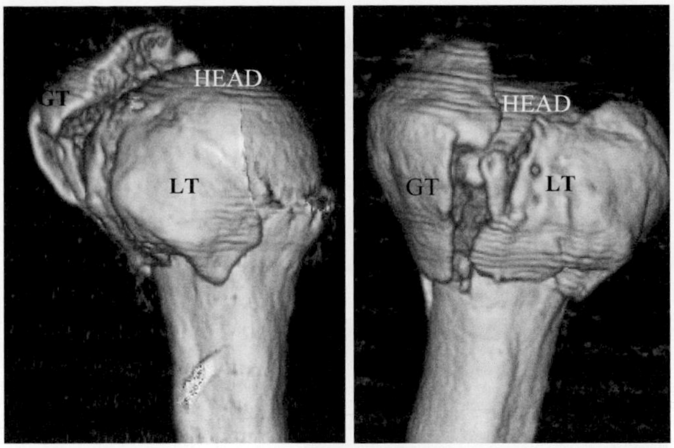

Fig. 12.36.4 Classic four-part valgus impaction fracture: GT great tuberosity, LT: lesser tuberosity,

and require symptomatic treatment followed by an intensive and structured rehabilitation programme.

The AO/OTA comprehensive classification is a useful system and distinguishes between extra articular, partial intracapsular, and intracapsular fractures.

Assessment and treatment principles

Clinical assessment should document the neurovascular status and the condition of the soft tissues.

Adequate imaging is essential to identify the extent of the fracture, the fracture pattern, and the state of the GHJ and neighbouring joints. Whilst most information can be obtained by adequate good quality plain radiographs, in patients were intervention may be appropriate, computed tomography (CT) of the proximal humerus with reformatted images has become the standard of care.

Patient particulars are of essence to complete the assessment prior to any decision regarding the treatment of the fracture (Box 12.36.3).

The most common complication of PHF is stiffness. As the GHJ heavily relies on the surrounding soft tissue structures for its function, early range of motion is of absolute essence in whatever method of treatment is followed.

Box 12.36.3 Patient factors affecting decision-making for PHF

- Injury-related complications:
  - Stiffness
  - Malunion
  - Non-union
  - AVN
- Treatment-related complications:
  - Stiffness
  - Infection
  - Construct stability
  - AVN.

GT fractures displaced more than 5mm are associated with rotator cuff tear and as such are potentially unstable fractures. Furthermore displacement may result in malunion and lead to impingement. However, the majority of the GT fractures displace superioposteriorly and as such result in an inefficient pulley mechanism resembling massive rotator cuff tear. Hence it is recommended that fractures of the GT displaced more than 10mm are best treated by reduction and fixation. Fractures displaced 5mm should be investigated for an associated tear at the interval. Repair is recommended if a tear is identified.

Displacement of the articular fragment (Figure 12.36.4) resulting in translation of the centre of GHJ rotation may affect the efficiency of the lever system. Correction of the head glenoid relationship restores the centre of rotation and minimizes the risk of pulley inefficiently.

High-energy fractures with or without dislocation in young adults is best treated with reconstruction of the proximal humerus and attachment of the tuberosities. It is postulated that replacement surgery of the humeral head with healed tuberosities is a more predictable procedure than primary replacement of a fracture dislocation that is associated with poor rotator cuff function and severe stiffness.

Fractures of the surgical neck and the metaphysis are usually undisplaced and the fracture configuration allows early mobilization. Widely displaced fractures are unstable; the distal fragment buttonholes through the muscles and may go on to a non-union (Figure 12.36.5). Fractures of the proximal humerus that require manipulative reduction are inherently unstable.

Displaced fractures of the proximal humeral third extending in the metaphyseal region are often unstable injuries associated with high incidence of delayed union/non-union. This appears to be especially true when patients report excessive clicking at the fracture site. Low energy fractures are associated with large soft tissue interposition whilst high-energy injuries result in medial and lateral fragmentation and subsequent gross displacement due deforming

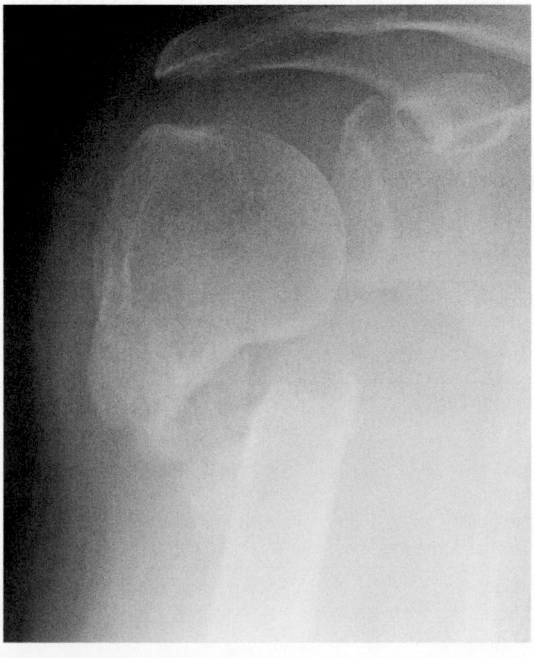

Fig. 12.36.5 Non-union of displaced PHF associated with functional disability.

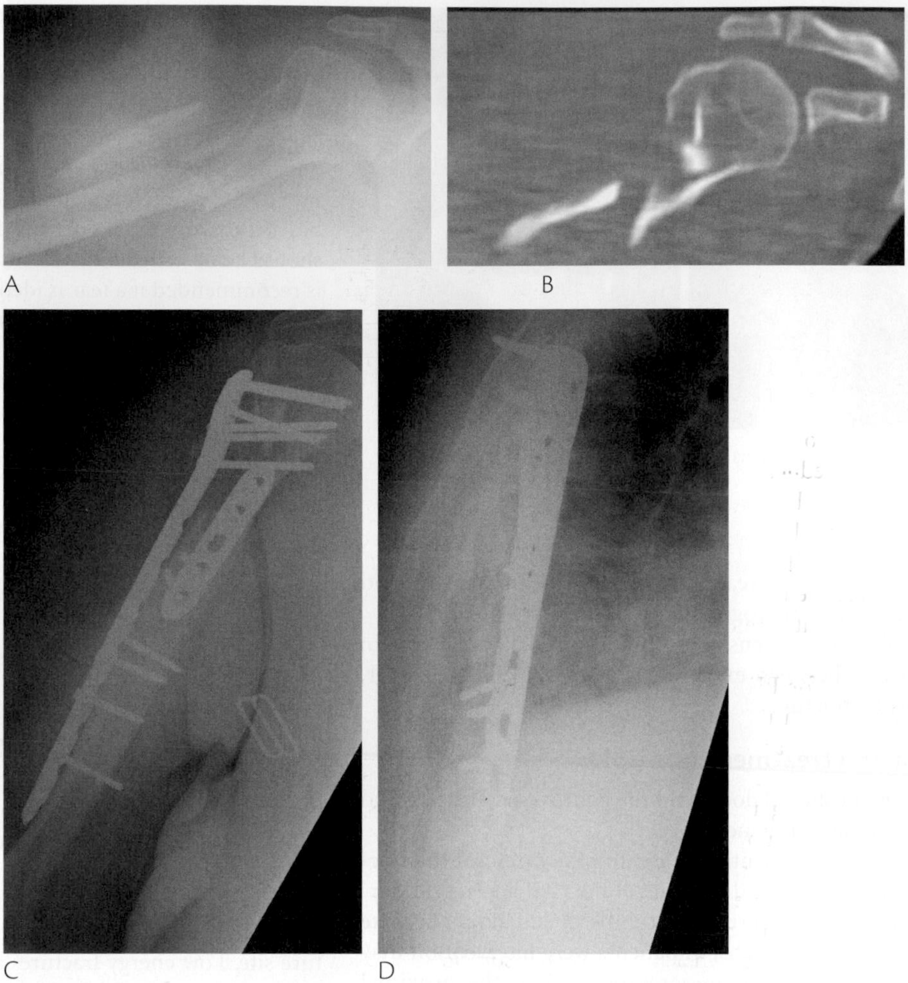

Fig. 12.36.6 A) and B) Highly unstable PHF extending to the GT and distally to the deltoid tuberosity. Highly unstable injury and patient factors led to the decision of primary reduction &fixation. C) and D) Postoperative radiographs.

forces from the muscle, weight of the arm, and body habitus. These are best treated operatively at the onset (Figure 12.36.6).

Sophistication of knowledge has led to less dogmatic approaches when it comes to fracture treatment. Most injuries can be treated non-operatively with acceptable results. Significant injuries will do badly whatever the intervention. It is the role of orthopaedists to identify the patients that appropriate operative treatment will affect the final outcome. Table 12.36.2 may act as an aid to decision-making.

Operative treatment

Historically, operative repair of PHF was associated with myriads of complications:

Complex fractures, poor imaging, poor understanding of the objectives of treatment, poor bone stock, unfamiliar territory, little experience, inadequate implants were some of the contributing factors that gave operative fixation of the PHF bad reputation. The good news is it could only get better: whilst operative treatment of

Table 12.36.2 Treatment matrix for PHF

Patient factors	Injury factors		
	Simple fracture undisplaced stable	**Significant injury: displaced # unstable**	**Devastating #: displaced fragmentation, dislocation**
Young/remodelling ability	Good outcome Symptomatic treatment and rehab	Allow for remodelling Good functional outcome	Surgery beneficial Variable functional outcome
Middle aged Type A/B host Good bone quality High functional demand	Good outcome Symptomatic treatment and intensive rehab	Surgery beneficial Good functional outcome	Surgery beneficial Variable functional outcome
Elderly fragility # Type B/C host Poor bone stock Low functional demand	Outcome depending on compliance	Unpredictable outcome Surgical intervention associated with increased risks	Very poor measurable outcome/ questionable functional outcome whatever the treatment modality

these injuries remains a challenge some of the factors mentioned are better understood. Due to small numbers of operative cases and variance of patient and injury characteristics it is difficult for the case series reported in the literature to be didactic and help the orthopaedic surgeon decide on the treatment modality.

Evolution of medical technology in imaging and multidisciplinary care of the frail patients has improved the patients' selection for operative treatment. The development of new plating systems to address the issues of osteopenic bone and fragmentation most often encountered in treatment of the PHF can only be seen as an advantage. However, the new technology is not a panacea and has not altered the indications for surgical treatment. In this context poor patient selection will result in relatively large treatment related complications.

The operative options are reduction and fixation and arthroplasty. The aim of reduction and fixation is to restore anatomy whilst preserving the blood supply to the bone and create a stable construct to allow early range of motion. Patients will need to follow a structured rehabilitation programme and the fracture will need to heal. There are technical issues relating to fragmentation and bone stock. Results are dependant on patient selection and surgeons' experience.

Hemiarthroplasty for PHF was recommended by Neer as the outcome following treatment of four part fractures was poor. Stableforth confirmed that the procedure was reliable, providing a pain-free shoulder at the expense of movement. Whilst there has been some understanding and improvement on technical aspects, length of the prosthesis appears still to be an issue with approximately 50% being too long or too short resulting in eccentric centre of rotation of the GHJ. More importantly it is now accepted that the poor functional status of a replaced fractured proximal humerus is directly related to migration, malunion and/or resorption of the tuberosities. Despite the evolution of design in shoulder prosthesis and the repair of the tuberosities this complication continues to date. Survivorship of the prosthesis does not appear to be a problem with a 94% survival rate at 10 years.

Complications

Complications of PHF are related to the injury and the treatment. In addition to immediate fracture related complications such as neurovascular compromise soft tissue disruption commonly experienced complications are listed in Box 12.36.4.

Post-traumatic stiffness is the most common complication of PHF as the shoulder girdle function is heavily dependent on the surrounding soft tissues in order to maintain a wide range of motion with efficiency. Injury severity and prolonged immobilization in internal rotation may result in recalcitrant stiffness and poor functional outcome. Fixed internal rotation or the lack of external rotation is probably the most disabling deformity. It cannot be overemphasized that the fracture pattern or final construct following intervention must allow early movement and in particular external rotation of the GHJ.

Most PHF will eventually heal with a degree of malunion. In the immature skeleton up to 45 degrees of angulation will remodel successfully. The true incidence of symptomatic malunion is unknown as it is poorly defined as to what constitutes malunion in PHF. In a retrospective review, of patients that underwent surgery for malunion, three types were identified (Table 12.36.3). They reported 69% successful reconstruction and 31% complication rate associated with poor outcome. In 79% of the patients there were associated soft tissue abnormalities with 80% being capsular contractures.

Box 12.36.4 Complications of PHF

- Injury
  - Stiffness
  - Malunion
  - Non-union
  - AVN
  - Osteoarthritis
- Treatment
  - Stiffness
  - Infection
  - Neurovascular damage
  - Hardware failure
  - AVN/Osteoarthritis.

The functional disability often is the result of additional global stiffness rather than structural alone. It appears that tuberosity malunion is the most responsive to treatment either with osteotomy or with acromioplasty, whilst replacement with prosthesis appears less successful and is associated with more technical problems as compared with primary hemiarthroplasty for acute fractures.

Non-union of the PHF is underreported. This may reflect the population characteristics and the practice of short follow-up without radiology. It is, not unreasonably, assumed that the clinical picture does not correlate with the imaging. Neer has described a distinct pattern of non-union and pseudarthrosis often seen in fractures of the surgical neck. Widely displaced two-part fractures of the proximal humerus are reported to have a 4.7% incidence of non-union. Mobile non-unions are symptomatic as patients often complain of painful clicking and lack of strength in the arm: they are unable to lift themselves off the chair or use their walking aid (Figure 12.36.7). This is a therapeutic challenge as reduction and fixation is challenged by poor bone stock. Hemiarthroplasty for non-union is technically demanding and often results in exchange of a flail arm with stiffness.

AVN is associated with fractures through the anatomical neck and historically with reduction and fixation of four-part fractures. It was initially thought that all four part fractures carried a significant risk of AVN; however the position changed once realized that

Table 12.36.3 Beredjiklian classification of proximal humerus malunion (1998)

Malunion of proximal humerus fractures	
Type 1	Tuberosity malunion >10mm
Type 2	GHJ incongruence
Type 3	Articular surface misalignment >45 degrees

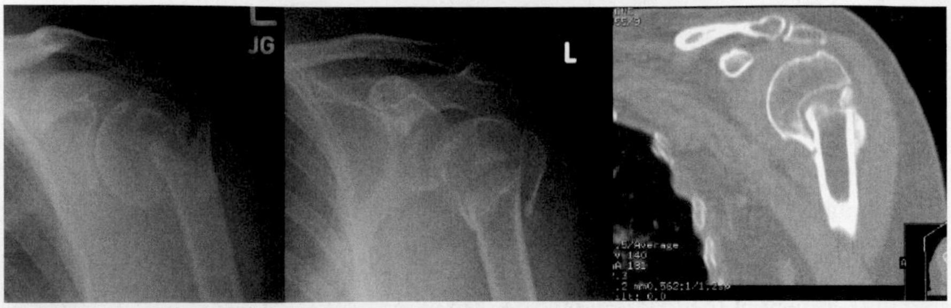

Fig. 12.36.7 Follow-up radiographs with classic appearance of PHF pseudoarthrosis.

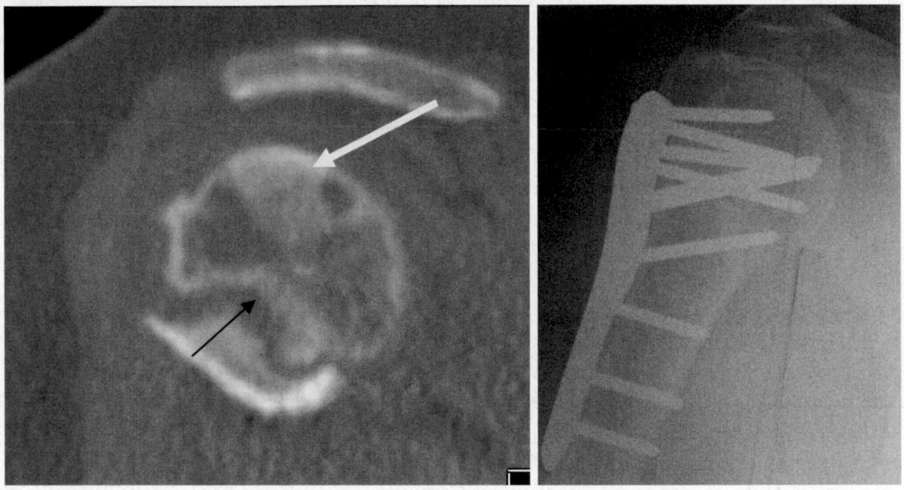

Fig. 12.36.8 Partial AVN (white arrow) in association with non-union (black arrow) following PHF; resolution following reduction grafting and fixation.

in valgus displaced fractures the vascular supply of the head fragment is preserved and the outcome is favourable. Appreciation of the vascular pattern of the humeral head and improved operative skills has led to a significant decrease of AVN following surgery. Recent report on the operative treatment of high-energy fractures suggested that the incidence of AVN is 35% with 20.6% partial (Figure 12.36.8) and 14.7% total. As expected patients with AVN did worse as assessed with outcome scoring tools.

Rehabilitation following proximal humeral fractures (Box 12.36.5)

Although stiffness in many circumstances is unavoidable, it is essential to commence physical therapy as soon as the fracture pattern or construct will allow. Results following early and late physiotherapy treatment show a significant difference in the outcomes at 1 year. The Neer regimen of four 3-weekly periods of passive range to resistance exercises with individual modifications to allow for patient characteristics seems to be universally accepted. Measurable improvement continues for approximately 6 months following injury, thereafter, functional improvement is most likely due to compensatory mechanisms and activity modification.

Box 12.36.5 Factors affecting outcome in PHF

- Injury pattern:
  - Displacement fragmentation and stability
  - Anatomical neck, head splitters
  - Dislocation
- Patient factors:
  - Age and bone quality
  - Pre-existing disease
  - Functional demands
  - Compliance and motivation
- Operative treatment:
  - No devascularization
  - Stable construct
  - Early mobilization.

Fractures of the clavicle

Introduction

As with all injuries, fractures of the clavicle it is a spectrum of injury with the majority of fractures resulting in an uncomplicated recovery and return to the pre-injury functional status.

Functional anatomy, epidemiology, and classification

The clavicle is an 'S' shaped bone with no medullary canal. The ossification starts in the 5th week of gestation, whilst the medial physis ossifies at the age of 25 years. It is the strut connection of the arm to the trunk via the sternoclavicular, acromioclavicular joints and the coracoclavicular ligaments and multiple muscle attachments. It is suspended like a crane via the trapezius, sternocleidomastoid and subclavius muscles and moves 30 degrees in the coronal plane, 35 degrees on the sagittal plane, and rotates 50 degrees to facilitate the version of the glenoid during GHJ movement clearing the arm of the trunk.

Fractures of the clavicle represent 10–12% of all fractures. The prevalence in the adult population is 30–64/100 000/year. It affects all ages with a peak in the young males during sporting activities. Motor-vehicle collision is the second most common mechanism of injury in males whilst the male to female ratio evens with advanced age. Direct impact is in most circumstances the mechanism of injury. Open fractures occur in 1.4% of the fractures treated in a level I trauma centre in the United States of America and are associated with head and torso injuries.

Altman in 1967 classified the fractures in medial, middle, and lateral thirds. Robinson identified subgroups within Altman's classification after collecting large number of data (Table 12.36.4).

Box 12.36.6 Clavicle fractures

- 89% of clavicle fractures heal uneventfully
- Displaced and fragmented fractures of the middle third may be prone to delayed/non-union and benefit form primary reduction and fixation.
- Operative management of middle third fractures is associated with faster recovery and significant complication rates
- Further work is required to identify the cause of symptoms in malunions
- Displaced/unstable fractures of the distal third are associated with high incidence of non-union (30%)
- Non-union of the distal clavicle is often asymptomatic and does not affect function.

Assessment and treatment principles

The clinical diagnosis is obvious in most fractures. Standard radiographs will include an anteroposterior and a 20-degree tilted view as displacement cannot be assessed on single view alone. In high-energy injuries associated girdle injuries or chest trauma may be present and these injuries may require immediate attention. This is especially true in the presence of open clavicle fractures. Widely distracted fractures of the clavicle should raise the suspicion of scapulothoracic dissociation, especially if accompanied by neurovascular compromise. In association with fractures of the scapula the disruption of the superior shoulder suspensory complex (SSSC) may lead to unacceptable displacement.

Eighty-nine per cent of all clavicle fractures go on to uneventful union with symptomatic treatment alone. Open fractures or fractures associated with vascular compromise are absolute indications for operative treatment in line with the general principles of orthopaedic trauma.

Reduction of the displaced fractures of the middle third was recommended using a figure-of-eight strapping. However, the reported results comparing simple sling and the figure-of-eight strapping did not show a difference in the final outcome. The figure-of-eight treatment has been abandoned in United Kingdom practice as it is associated with complications and does not affect outcome in terms of fracture healing.

The dogma that all clavicle fractures unite uneventfully has been challenged in the past with sporadic reports on case series of non-unions. Increasing number of reports identified subgroups of fracture patterns such as severe shortening and fragmentation to be associated with delayed/non-union. Furthermore, there has been some concern that malunion of the clavicle is associated with pressure phenomena and poor functional outcomes. Recent randomized studies suggest that certain fracture patterns may benefit from early intervention in terms of time to union. However the operative treatment was not without complications that were reported to be 37%.

Fractures of the lateral third of the clavicle are another subgroup that has attracted interest as the incidence of non-union is approaching 30% especially for the displaced Neer II/Robinson 3B type of fractures: it is accepted that these non-unions are mostly asymptomatic. In a 15-year follow-up, 95% of non-unions were asymptomatic. In a separate study only 14% of the non-unions required further surgery (Figure 12.36.9).

Operative repair of distal clavicle fractures is not without technical difficulties and complications mainly due to the inheritably unstable pattern of injury, poor bone purchase, and need of the fixation

Table 12.36.4 Epidemiology and classification of clavicle fractures

Type1: medial 1/5	Type 2: middle 3/5	Type 3: lateral 1/5
A1: undisplaced extra-articular 1.7%	**A1**: undisplaced 5.4%	**A1**: undisplaced extra-articular 16.2%
A2: undisplaced intra-articular 0.6%	**A2**: angulated with contact 13.5%	**A2**: undisplaced intra-articular 1.9%
B1: displaced extra-articular 0.2%	**B1**: simple wedge 37.5%	**B1**: displaced extra-articular 8.5%
B2: displaced intra-articular 0.3%	**B2**: segmental/ fragmented wedge 12.8%	**B2**: displaced intra-articular 1.4%
2.8%	**69.2%**	**28%**

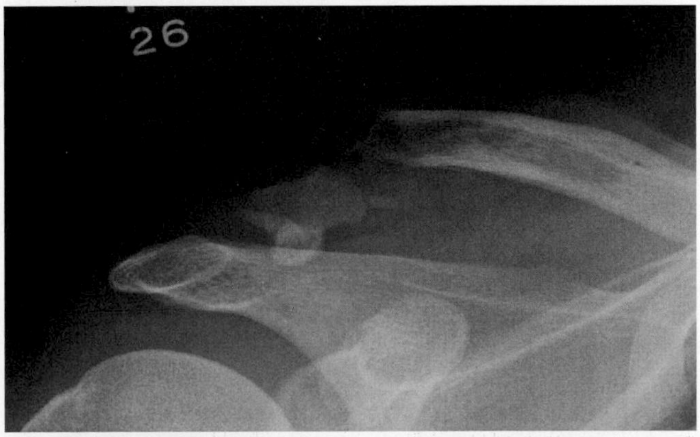

Fig. 12.36.9 Asymptomatic non-union diagnosed 3 years following injury in a 25-year-old sportingly active male.

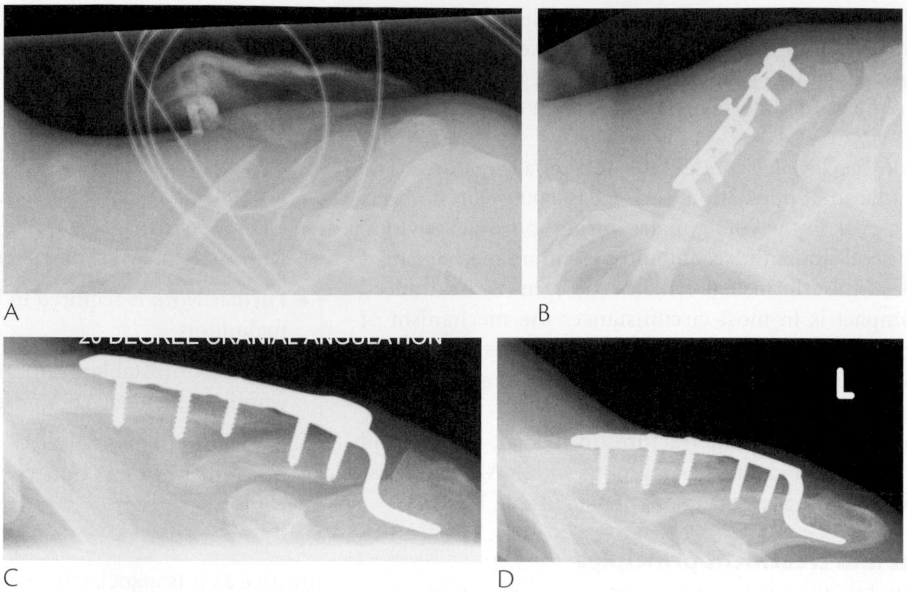

Fig. 12.36.10 Open fracture of the distal end of the clavicle in association with head injury: initial image (A) and early failure of fixation (B) due to patient's circumstances and poor distal screw purchase. Salvage using the hook plate (C, D).

crossing mobile areas around the shoulder. The variety of techniques illustrates the difficulty of the problem (Figure 12.36.10).

Box 12.36.7 lists the current thinking regarding indications for operative treatment of clavicle fractures.

Box 12.36.7 Operative treatment of clavicle fractures

- Absolute indications:
  - Neurovascular compromise (Figure 12.36.11)
  - Open fractures
- Relative indications:
  - Fragmentation middle third
  - Shortening >2cm
  - Threatened soft tissue envelope
  - Associated girdle/multiple injures

Acromioclavicular joint injuries

Anatomical considerations

The acromioclavicular joint (ACJ) is a diarthroldial joint with a meniscus and a strong capsule which in conjunction with the coracoclavicular ligaments suspends the scapula from the clavicle. The kinematics of the joint have been studied and a 20-degree arc of tilting, rotation and protraction has been identified.

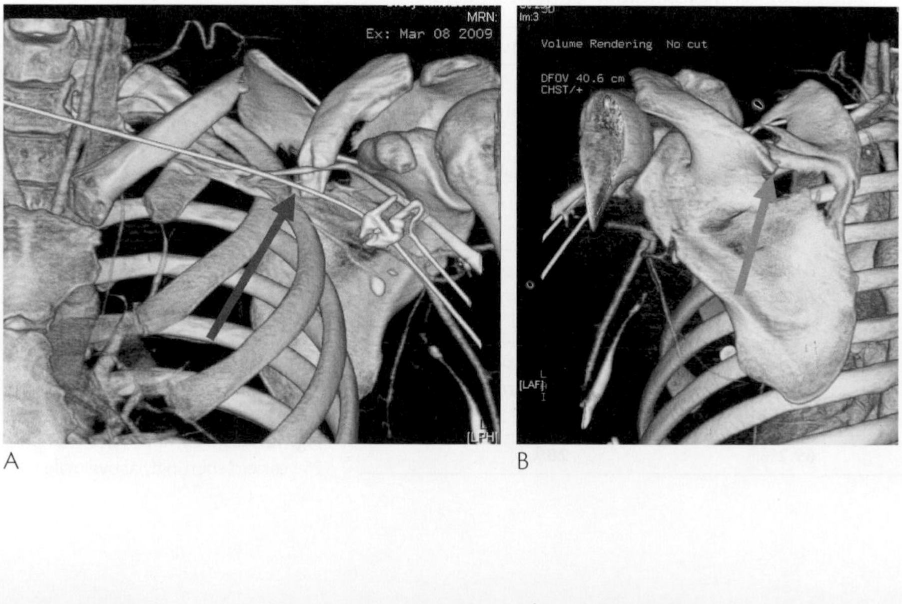

Fig. 12.36.11 A) Dramatic girdle injury with scapula fracture, clavicle fracture and associated neurovascular compromise: the distal clavicle hooked around the cord of the plexus (arrow). B) Arrow depicts scapula injury in keeping with suprascapular nerve injury.

Box 12.36.8 Rockwood classification of ACJ injuries

- Type 1: simple sprain of the joint no capsular/ligamentous damage
- Type 2: ACJ joint disruption/partial incongruence
- Type 3: ACJ dislocation with CC ligament disruption
- Type 4: posterior buttonhole through trapezius
- Type 5: deltoid detatchment gross displacement
- Type 6: inferior displacement subcoracoid space

Epidemiology, mechanism of injury, and classification

ACJ joint injuries are common in males as the result of sporting injuries with direct force on the shoulder. They represent 12% of the shoulder injuries and in their majority these are simple sprains.

The classification in Box 12.36.8 suggested by Tossy 1963 complemented by Rockwood appears to be universally accepted.

The mechanism of injury and corresponding clinical signs are pathognomonic of the injury. Radiographs exclude the presence of a fracture of the distal clavicle. Weight bearing comparative views are occasionally necessary to differentiate a type 2 from a type 3 injury.

Treatment principles, results, and complications

Universal agreement exists for type 1 and type 2 injuries: these are treated symptomatically (Box 12.36.9). Pain usually resolves within 3 weeks and function returns with simple physiotherapy exercises.

Whilst there is some debate regarding type 3 injuries, current evidence would support non-operative treatment. Patients are not easily convinced that the symptoms will soon settle and that the shoulder function will return despite the residual deformity. Follow-up consultation in 2–3 weeks allows more insight to the effects of the injury.

Evolving minimally invasive techniques in the acute setting has resulted in increased interest in early intervention as scarring in the region of the coracoclavicular ligaments may abolish the need for ligament transfer and reconstruction (Figure 12.36.12).

Symptomatic patients will respond to reconstructive surgery of distal clavicle excision, ligament reconstruction and augmentation. The Weaver–Dunn procedure with its many modifications remains the template for stabilization of the distal clavicle. Symptoms often relate to cosmesis, lack of strength, and/or painful clicking of the joint in order of frequency.

Early operative treatment is required for the more rare and severe disruptions that will impinge on shoulder movement such as the locked and widely displaced (Rockwood types IV and V) and subcoracoid (Rockwood VI) injuries.

Box 12.36.9 Treatment of ACJ injury

- Type I + II: non-operative
- Type IV, V, and VI: operative
- Type III: current evidence supports non-operative treatment
- Symptomatic patients benefit from distal clavicle excision, ligament reconstruction, and augmentation.

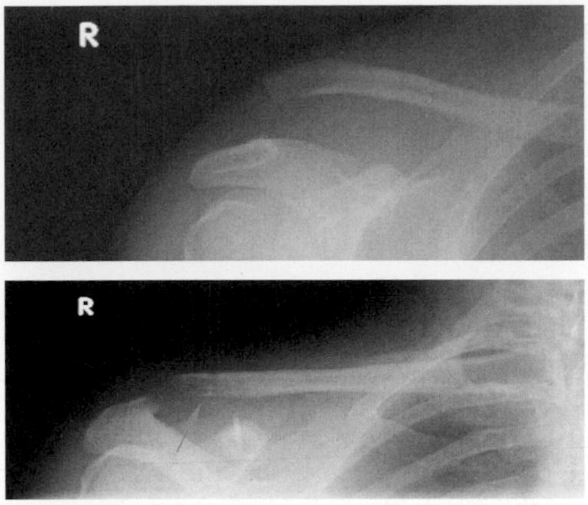

Fig. 12.36.12 Early operative treatment of Type III ACJ dislocation. Note calcification in the subclavicular region.

Numerous publications refer to the results of primary operative versus non-operative treatment and later reconstruction. The current practice varies depending the surgeon's experience and interpretation of the reported literature. It is reasonable to accept that the majority of these patients would do well either with or without operative treatment. With the exception of cosmesis, as a consistent indication for surgery, it is not obvious at presentation which subgroup of patients would benefit from early intervention.

Sternoclavicular injuries

Anatomy, epidemiology, and diagnosis

The sternoclavicular (SC) joint is a saddle joint connecting the clavicle to the axial skeleton. It has a range of motion of 35 degrees in the coronal plane and 70 degrees in the anteroposterior plane. For all practical purposes the articulation functions as a ball and socket joint. Stability relies partially in skeletal anatomy and more so in the strong and complex ligamentous structures (costoclavicular, interclavicular, anterosuperior, and posterior capsular reinforcement) and the subclavius muscle. The medial end of the clavicle physis ossifies by the age of 25, hence injuries to the region in young adults represent physeal fractures.

The mechanism of injury can be direct or indirect. As a result it can occur in a variety of injuries such as sport and motor vehicle accidents. The posterior dislocation may be associated with a dramatic clinical picture of airway obstruction whilst the sporting injuries can be easily overlooked.

The overall incidence of the injury to SC joint is reported as 1% of all dislocations and 3% of the dislocations of the upper limb. As with all injuries there is a spectrum of injury (Box 12.36.10).

Whilst the history of injury and clinical symptoms are significant often the deformity is mild (especially with posterior injuries) and the plain radiographs difficult to interpret. Special views and measurements have been recommended but CT is the investigation of choice (Figure 12.36.13).

Treatment, results, and complications

Immediate reduction of a posteriorly displaced medial clavicle is part of the ATLS protocol for emergency treatment of airway

Box 12.36.10 SCJ injury spectrum

- Sprain
- Subluxation
- Dislocation:
    - Anterior
    - Posterior
- Fracture dislocation.

Table 12.36.5 SCJ injury treatment matrix

Injury	Diagnosis	
	Early	Late
Sprain/ subluxation	Symptomatic treatment	
Anterior dislocation	Non-operative	Expectantly
Posterior dislocation	Closed reduction and evaluation under anaesthesia	Open reduction and ligament reconstruction
Chronic instability	Symptomatic treatment	Medial excision ± stabilization

compromise. In the less acute setting the treatment options vary according to the injury, the individual and the timing of the diagnosis (Table 12.36.5).

There are few relatively small case series in the literature reporting the results of operative techniques. Whilst there in no conclusive evidence regarding the treatment methods, it appears that open reduction with autologous tendon reconstruction without transfixation is associated with the best results (Figure 12.36.14) whilst medial clavicle excision and joint transfixion are associated with poorest results and highest incidence of complications respectively.

Complications relating to SCJ injuries are listed in Box 12.36.11.

Scapular fractures (Box 12.36.12)

Epidemiology and topographic classification

The scapula is a mobile platform suspended form the axial skeleton by the clavicular ligaments, the ACJ capsule and a variety of muscles. It provides the fulcrum (glenoid) for the arm movements and rotates to facilitate universal arm movement (scapulothoracic articulation) and is the site of origin for 17 muscles. Fractures of the

Box 12.36.11 SCJ complications

- Injury complications:
    - Associated mediastinal trauma (25%)
    - Pressure phenomena
    - Chronic instability
- Treatment complications:
    - Infection
    - Mediastinum injury
    - Loss of reduction, repair failure and implant failure, and migration

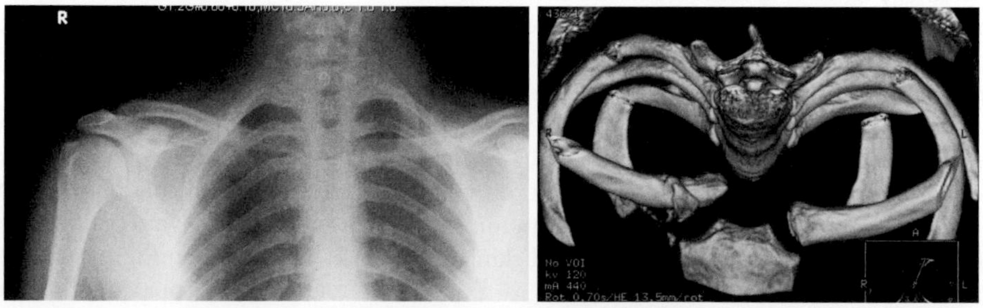

Fig. 12.36.13 Missed posterior fracture dislocation of the SCJ following rugby injury.

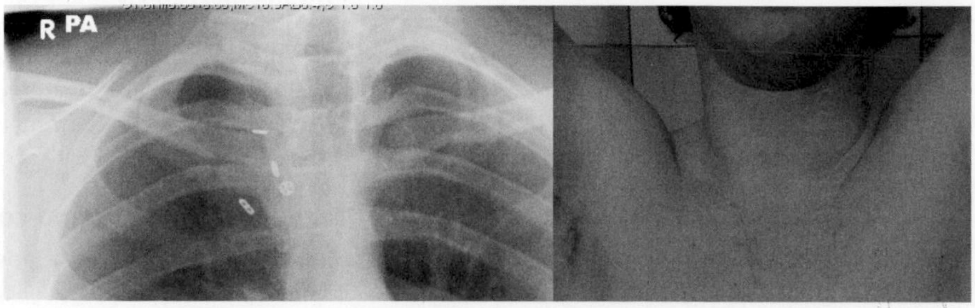

Fig. 12.36.14 Postoperative radiograph and clinical result following reconstruction.

Box 12.36.12 Scapula fracture

- Often associated with polytrauma and frequently missed
- 5–12% incidence of neurological and vascular complication
- Operative treatment rarely indicated
- Outcomes depend on injury severity and associated complications

scapula account for 1% of all fractures, 3–5% of fractures of the shoulder girdle, and occur in 3% of patients with multiple injuries.

Fractures of the scapula are subdivided according to anatomical topography. As considerable force is required for scapular fractures to occur, concomitant injuries are associated with particular fracture types (Table 12.36.6).

Assessment and treatment principles

Despite the history of significant trauma scapula fractures are missed at presentation in 43%. Likely reasons are the incidence of associated injuries (85–90%) mainly of the ipsilateral shoulder girdle or to the thorax and poor visualization on plain radiographs. It is expected that with the liberal use of CT to assess thoracic trauma the pick-up rate of scapula fractures will increase.

The incidence of associated neurological and vascular complications is reported to be 5–12%.

Glenoid and glenoid neck fractures

Glenoid fractures account for 10–15% of the scapula fractures. Approximately 10% are significantly displaced to pose a treatment dilemma. Hence the absolute incidence of displaced glenoid fractures to be considered for intervention is 1:10 000 fractures. Glenoid fractures are classified according to Ideberg based on the force vector of the humeral head on the glenoid fossa (Table 12.36.7).

Principles of treatment of articular fractures in terms of joint stability and congruence are valid and reproducible; however the true incidence of degenerative changes due to intra-articular malunion is unknown.

Glenoid neck fractures in association with a clavicle fracture were described as 'the floating shoulder'. The injury was considered highly unstable and thought to be associated with poor outcome. However, recent experience has questioned the dogma of instability of floating shoulders and clarified the indications regarding the need for intervention. Current thinking relates to the medial and caudal displacement of the glenoid fragment. It considered that caudal tilt greater than 40 degrees and medial displacement more than 1cm may affect GHJ motion and represent indication for operative intervention.

Table 12.36.6 Scapula fractures

Fracture type	Incidence	Potential complications
Glenoid fossa	10%	Joint instability
Glenoid neck	27%	Floating shoulder/displacement
Scapular body	35%	Significant chest trauma (50%)
Acromion and spine	23%	Fibrous union
Coracoid fractures	5%	Rare/diagnostic issues

Table 12.36.7 Ideberg classification of fractures of the glenoid

Type	Comments
I	Fracture dislocation
Ia	Anterior dislocation (Figure 12.36.15)
Ib	Posterior dislocation
II	Inferior displacement of the humeral head
	Operation indicated for articular anatomy and congruency of the GHJ
III	Superior displacement of the humeral head
	Operation suggested for articular step exceeding 5mm or disruption of the superior suspensory complex
	Outcome partly dependent on the associated injury of the acromion and acromioclavicular joint
IV	Operation suggested for articular step exceeding 5mm to avoid symptomatic post-traumatic arthritis, non-union, or instability of the GHJ
	Outcome depends on the complications
V	Combination of type II, III, and IV fractures
	Outcome depends on joint surface congruity and glenohumeral stability

Fracture of the scapula body

Fractures of the scapula body including the spine are the most common fractures of the scapula. In the absence of articular involvement the fractures are treated symptomatically with particular care to the associated chest injuries. Fractures that involve the supraclavicular notch may be associated with suprascapular nerve damage that in the context of loss of function due to pain may be difficult to diagnose early.

Acromion fractures

Fractures of the acromion are extremely rare as it is more likely that a direct force would result in injuries to the neighbouring anatomical structures mainly the acromioclavicular joint. Concerns and dilemmas with malunion and or symptomatic non-union are raised with significant displacement. Os acromiale may pose a diagnostic pitfall.

Coracoid fractures

Coracoid fractures compromise 2–5% of scapula fractures and have been related to a variety of mechanisms of injury. Fractures of the base are more common; despite the rarity of the injury six types have been recognized and operative treatment recommended for injuries associated with AC disruption.

Scapulothoracic dissociation

Scapulothoracic dissociation (SCTD) is a potentially life-threatening injury depicting a closed forequarter amputation with neural and vascular damage and essential disarticulation of the scapulothoracic joint. Since the original description in 1984 variations of

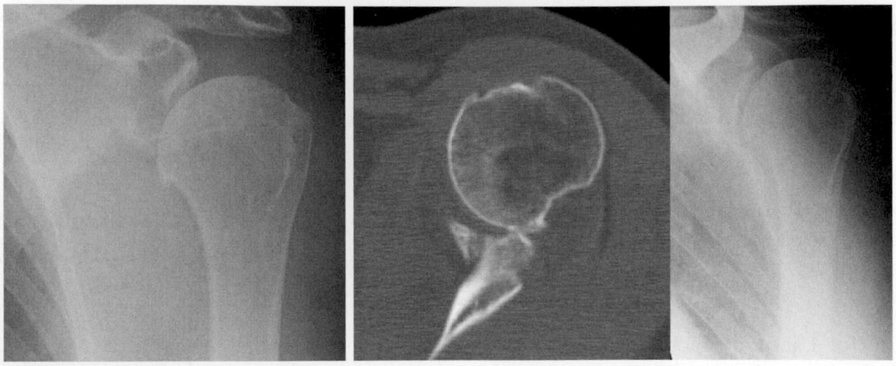

Fig. 12.36.15 Type Ia fracture of the glenoid treated non-operatively.

Table 12.36.8 Current classification of SCTD according to Zelle

Type	Clinical findings
1	Musculoskeletal injury (MS) alone
2A	Plus vascular disruption
2B	Plus neurological impairment of the upper extremity
3	MS and vascular and neural injury

the injury have been described and the spectrum of injury further classified (Table 12.36.8). Whilst immediate management relies on timely revascularization of the limb it appears that the long term outcome of injury heavily relies on the presence and extent of brachial plexus injury.

Management principles (Box 12.36.13)

Attention should initially address life and/or limb-threatening conditions.

Box 12.36.13 Indications for operative treatment of scapula fractures

- Glenoid involvement with step >5mm leading to joint incongruence
- Glenoid fossa fracture resulting in GHJ instability (>20% surface area)
- Caudal angulation glenoid >40 degrees
- Medial displacement of glenoid >1cm
- Displaced acromion/coracoid fractures
- Scapulothoracic dissociation.

Specific treatment for scapula fractures is based on small retrospective case series and knowledge boosts from their meta-analyses. Most scapula fractures are treated symptomatically. It has been estimated that, using current indications, an orthopaedic surgeon would operatively treat 1.5 fractures of the scapula during his/her career.

A recent meta-analysis of the literature identified 243 patients from 17 publications that had operative treatment for scapula fractures. Most of the fractures involved the glenoid (48%) and 20% involved the glenoid neck. Using a variety of scoring systems results were rated excellent and good in 84% and fair and poor in 16%. Operative treatment complications were infection 4.2% and nerve damage (suprascapular) 2.4%.

Further reading

Hardegger, F.H., Simpson, L.A., and Weber, B.G. (1984). The operative treatment of scapular fractures. *Journal of Bone and Joint Surgery*, **66B**(5), 725–31.

Altamimi, S.A. and McKee, M.D. Canadian Orthopaedic Trauma Society (2008). Nonoperative treatment compared with plate fixation of displaced midshaft clavicular fractures. Surgical technique. *Journal of Bone and Joint Surgery*, **90A**(Suppl 2, Pt 1), 1–8.

Fraser-Moodie, J.A., Shortt, N.L., and Robinson, C.M. (2008). Injuries to the acromioclavicular joint. *Journal of Bone and Joint Surgery*, **90B**(6), 697–707.

Robinson, C.M., Jenkins, P.J., Markham, P.E., and Beggs, I. (2008). Disorders of the sternoclavicular joint. *Journal of Bone and Joint Surgery*, **90B**(6), 685–96.

Neer, C.S. 2nd. (1970). Displaced proximal humeral fractures. I. Classification and evaluation. *Journal of Bone and Joint Surgery*, **52A**(6), 1077–89.

Nho, S.J., Brophy, R.H., Barker, J.U., Cornell, C.N., and MacGillivray, J.D. (2007). Management of proximal humeral fractures based on current literature. *Journal of Bone and Joint Surgery*, **89A**(Suppl 3), 44–58.

12.37

Imaging in spinal trauma

P. McNee, S. Gaba, and E. McNally

Summary points

- Clinical criteria and the nature of the injury determine who needs imaging
- Plain films are still commonly employed though CT finds more fractures
- Alignment, bony contour, cartilage (Disc and facets) and soft tissue are assessed in turn (ABC'S)
- CT is superior to MRI in assessing the bony configuration of fracture
- MRI is superior to CT in assessing the ligament tears and associated disc herniations
- Plain films have little role in the assessment of more chronic back pain and radiculopathy
- Sacral insufficiency fractures may be misdiagnosed as metastases on MRI.

Introduction

The aims of this chapter are to:

1) Describe how to clear the spine
2) Describe the common injury patterns and radiological findings.

The concept of risk of spinal injury is very important in helping to decide the appropriate imaging strategy. This is often difficult as a good history of mechanism and potential injury pattern is not always available.

The NEXUS study retrospectively applied the following clinical criteria in relation to potential cervical trauma: absence of midline tenderness, no focal neurological deficit, normal level of consciousness, no evidence of intoxication, and no evidence of distracting injury. If all of these criteria were negative then imaging was not considered necessary. The study included 34 000 patients and found that eight of 818 (1%) cervical spine fractures would have been missed; two of the eight were deemed serious. Their conclusion was that if the clinical criteria listed were all negative there was no need to perform any imaging.

The Canadian Cervical spine Rules (CCR) studies, through the application of clinical criteria, identified the following: persons of high risk who all required imaging, patients of low risk on whom it is safe to assess the active range of movement of the cervical spine, and finally patients with the ability to actively rotate their heads 45 degrees in both directions who required no imaging.

Prospective studies have been applied to both the NEXUS and CCR and found CCR to have a sensitivity of 99.4% for clinically important injuries, versus 90.7% for NEXUS.

In 2002 The British Trauma Society published a series of guidelines for the management and assessment of spinal injury that was, in essence, a hybrid of the conclusions of NEXUS and CCR, concluding that if a patient cannot be clinically cleared then imaging should be performed to exclude cervical spine injury.

Once the decision to image has been made, several imaging options need to be considered. Plain radiography is universally available. Traditionally the three view series (anteroposterior (AP), lateral, and peg views) has been employed. An essential requirement of the lateral view is that the cervicothoracic junction is demonstrated, as up to 20% of cervical injuries involve this segment. If traction on the arms fails to depress the shoulders sufficiently, a swimmer's view may be necessary. If clinical concern persists, computed tomography (CT) is indicated. The five-view series (the three-view series augmented by oblique views) is now largely redundant, as the obliques rarely add useful diagnostic information. CT scanning has largely replaced other x-ray techniques.

The plain film

The plain radiograph remains the essential first step in the assessment of the spinally injured patient. The majority of vertebral injuries can be accurately diagnosed and classified using AP and lateral views. Some fractures can be subtle and will only be detected by an ordered evaluation of the radiographs and by recognizing subtle changes in the normal anatomical relationships. Five per cent of cervical trauma radiographs are misinterpreted, resulting in delays in diagnosis with death or further neurological deterioration in up to 30% of the missed injuries. In half of these patients a complete three-series set of films had not been obtained.

Analysis in the cervical spine begins with the lateral view proceeding to the AP and peg views.

In turn, alignment, bony contour, cartilage, and soft tissue spaces (ABCs) are examined. Normal alignment on the lateral is confirmed by the integrity of three lines; the anterior vertebral line, the

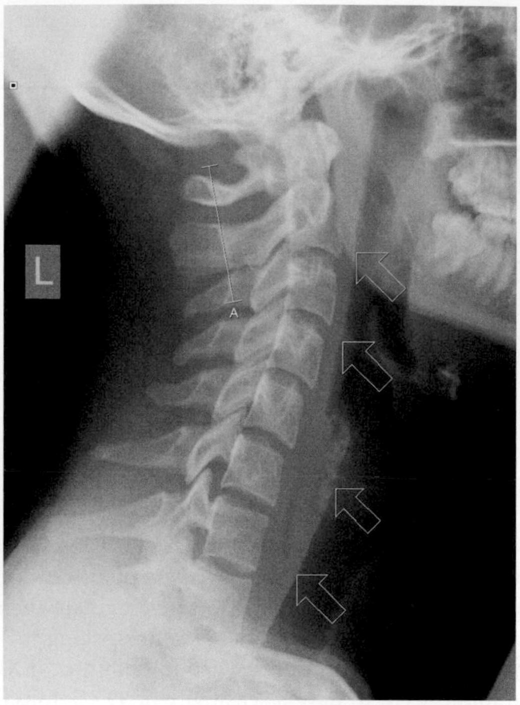

Fig. 12.37.1 The white line is drawn between the spinolaminar line of C1 and C3. The arrows delineate the precervical soft tissue space.

posterior vertebral line, and the spinolaminar line (Figure 12.37.1). Apparent subluxation of C2 on C3 is often identified in children and is physiological. This can persist up to the mid-teens. The most important portion of the spinolaminar line is between C1 and C3. A straight line joining the spinolaminar arcs of C1 and C3 should pass within 2mm of C2. This relationship is disturbed in patients with displaced fractures of C2 (Figure 12.37.2).

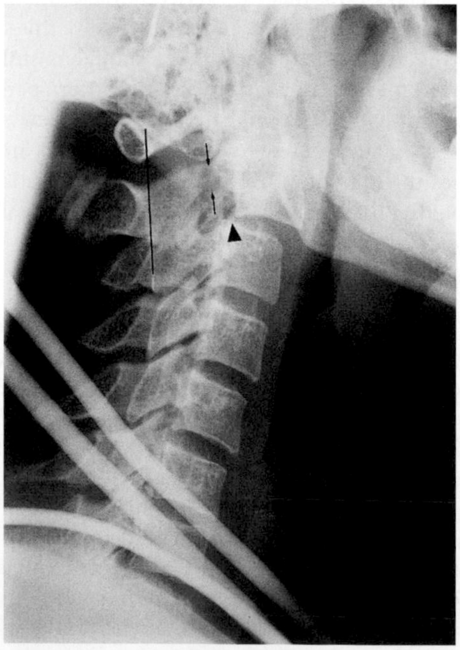

Fig. 12.37.2 Hangman's fracture. The posterior elements (black arrows). Note the minimal spondylolisthesis (arrowhead). An important clue is the disruption of the spinolaminar line. A line drawn between the spinolaminar lines of C1 (line) and C3 passes more than 2 mm anterior to the spinolaminar line of C2 (black line).

Assessment of 'cartilage' includes the disc spaces and facet joints. Loss of disc height is occasionally the only clue to a fracture through the disc, although this is most commonly a result of degenerative disc disease. The presence of traction spurs arising from the adjacent vertebral body margins is an associated sign in degenerative disease. The posterior facets should be superimposed one side upon the other if a true lateral has been obtained. Loss of parallelism is a feature of unifacet dislocation and should prompt a search for this injury.Even if alignment is normal, a careful assessment of bony contour is essential.

Soft tissue swelling can be a clue to underlying injury, but it is neither sensitive nor specific. Appreciable soft tissue shadowing does not develop until 6h after injury. At the level of the peg, the normal precervical space measures 5mm in adults and up to 7mm in children (Figure 12.37.1). Between C2 and C4, the normal precervical space depends on both age and weight according to the formula:

$$3.7\text{mm} - 0.02 \times \text{age (years)} + 0.01 \times \text{weight (pounds)}.$$

Less than 5mm is a useful guide. Below C4, an AP diameter of 22mm, or approximately the equivalent of vertebral AP diameter, is normal in adults. The normal atlantoaxial distance is less than 3mm in adults and less than 5mm in children. In some patients the precervical fat stripe can be seen as a black line within the precervical soft tissues. Anterior displacement of this line is a subtle sign of precervical haemorrhage or oedema. Posteriorly, the spaces between the spinous processes should be symmetric. Separation, which is often exaggerated on flexion, implies interosseus ligament rupture, which can be readily confirmed by magnetic resonance imaging (MRI). Widening of the interspinous distance also occurs with subluxed or perched facets.

The upper cervical spine

The distinctive anatomy of the upper cervical spine renders it prone to a different pattern of injury compared with the lower cervical spine. The upper cervical segments are also more commonly injured in children. A variety of measurements have been used to describe the normal relationships between the occiput and the atlas. Most of these are now superseded by sagittal CT reconstructions.

The atlantoaxial relationship can be examined using the ratio of the height of the atlantal spinolaminar line to the atlantoaxial interspinous distance. This ratio is normally 2. The distance between the spinolaminar line and the articular pillars can also be used to assess unifacetal dislocation. Abrupt alteration of this distance suggests spinal rotation and has a strong association with unifacetal dislocation following hyper flexion injury. Another common injury to C1–C2, rotary subluxation, will be discussed in relation to the peg view later in this chapter.

The posterior arch of C1 can be found anywhere between the occiput and the spinous process of C2. Angulation between the anterior arch and the dens is also commonly observed in normal individuals. The posterior arch of C1 is often not ossified and absence must not be misconstrued as a fracture. Abnormal widening may be seen (>10mm) between the spinous processes of C1 and C2 in patients with significant cord injury without other plain film findings.

The C2 vertebral body may show several fracture patterns, and careful review may be necessary to detect them. Small avulsions

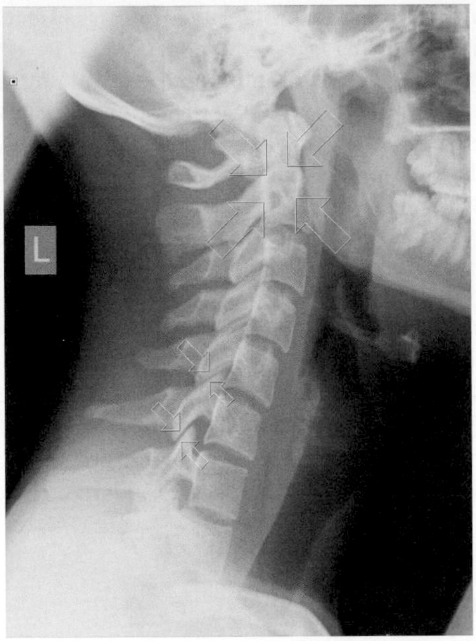

Fig. 12.37.3 Lateral cervical spine radiograph. The cervicothoracic junction is well seen. Note the white ring projected over the body of C2 (large arrows). If it is disrupted a careful search for a fracture is indicated. The smaller arrows indicate the posterior facets.

from the anteroinferior body of C2 may be the only clue. It is useful to look carefully at the apparent dense ring (Figure 12.37.3) projected over the C2 vertebral body, as disruption may be a clue to an underlying fracture, although in many cases this line is incomplete without injury. In a review of 165 injuries, 41% were dens fractures, 38% were traumatic spondylolistheses (hangman's fractures), 13% were extension teardrop fractures, and 6% were hyperextension dislocations. The remainder were fractures of the lamina and spinous processes. Consistent with other series, no type 1 dens fractures were reported, suggesting that a type 1 fracture, if it exists, is a rarity.

Dens fractures (Figure 12.37.4)

There are three types

- Type I: a fracture of the tip of the odontoid (rare)
- Type II: through the base of the odontoid
- Type III: through the body of the odontoid (commonest, 69%).

Hangman's fracture

Traumatic spondylolistheses (hangman's fractures) are divided into three types:

- Type 1 are undisplaced
- Type 2 are displaced
- Type 3 are associated with bilateral facet subluxation.

The lower cervical spine

The pattern of injury of the lower cervical spine differs from that of the upper two levels. Before diagnosing injury, a number of variations have to be recognized. The fourth and the fifth vertebral bodies can normally be slightly smaller than the adjacent third and sixth vertebral bodies without pathology being present. This can be particularly marked in children, possibly as a result of exaggerated hypermobility during ossification. In general, the difference between the anterior and posterior heights of a vertebral body should be no greater than 3mm. More than this implies an anterior wedge fracture.

The clay *shoveller' fracture* involves the spinous process of C6 or C7 (Figure 12.37.5). In hyperflexion sprain, it is a stable injury. The plain radiograph is often normal, and widening of the interspinous distance may be seen. The flexion teardrop is seen as a small anteroinferior fragment. It indicates an unstable injury and is often associated with abnormal neurology, particularly the anterior cord syndrome. The *hyperextension teardrop* is smaller and is more common in the upper cervical spine. Displacement is unusual and neurological abnormalities are less frequent. The plain film in *hyperextension sprain* is also normal unless views are obtained in extension.

The most obvious sign of *facet dislocation* on the lateral plain film is vertebral body subluxation. Half of these injuries are unilateral facet injuries and half are bilateral. In bifacetal dislocation, subluxation can reach 50% (Figure 12.37.6). In unifacet dislocation displacement is usually less than 25% and can often be difficult to detect, particularly if the film is rotated. Once suspected, a careful examination of the facets will reveal the

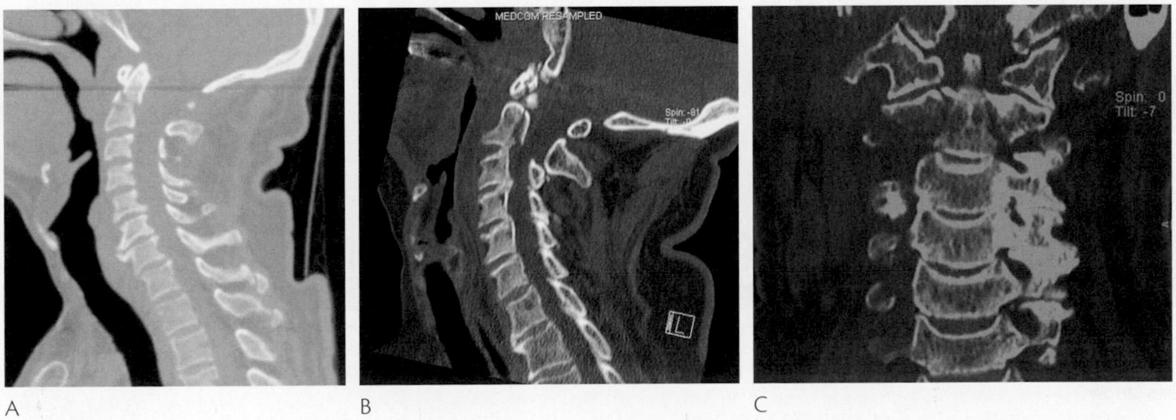

Fig. 12.37.4 CT upper cervical spine with sagittal and coronal reformats showing complex odontoid fracture extending into the body of C2.

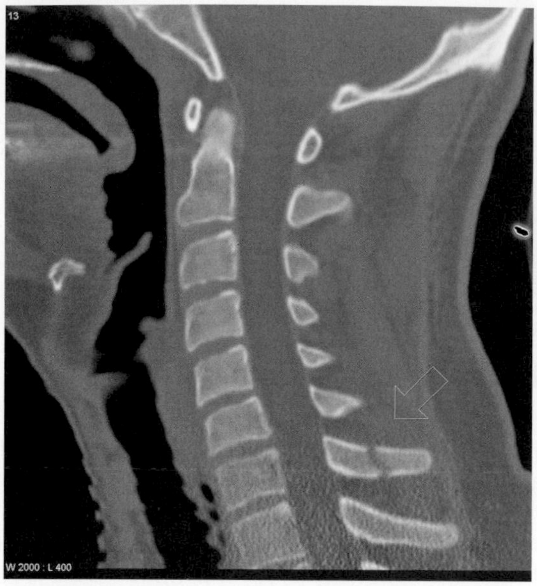

Fig. 12.37.5 Sagittal reformat showing Clay shovellers fracture through spinous process of C7 (arrow).

abnormality. Below a dislocation the facets are seen in the true lateral projection with the right facet overlapping the left. Above a unifacet dislocation, the facets on one side will lie more anterior to the other. The lateral mass is seen obliquely and resembles a bow tie. These injuries are frequently associated with fracture of the facet, best seen on CT. At the level of the injury, the superior articular process of the inferior vertebral body does not articulate with the corresponding inferior process of the vertebral body above. This is called the naked facet sign. Oblique views show loss of the normal 'tiled roof' appearance of the overhanging facets. Facet fracture–dislocation represents approximately 7% of cervical spine fractures. The incidence of neurological abnormality is high, up to 90% in some series, and is particularly common in bilateral injuries. MRI is necessary to exclude an associated disc prolapse which can cause neurological deterioration following facet reduction.

The diagnosis of a cervical injury may depend on the detection of abnormal alignment between vertebra. Immediately following injury, the presence of muscle spasm may cause the vertebra to maintain their normal relationships and obscure injury. Persistent pain following an injury is an indication of missed injury, and some centres employ flexion and extension views to exclude abnormal segmental motion. If flexion is adequate, the mandible should form an angle of at least 66 degrees with the horizontal. The film should be examined for angulation between the posterior border of the vertebral bodies and for fanning of the spinous processes. The latter is present when the interspinous distance is more than 2mm greater than the spaces above and below. Angulation of more than 3 degrees between vertebral bodies is considered abnormal. If the angle reaches 11 degrees the injury is considered unstable.

The anteroposterior view

The standard cervical AP view should be scrutinized for alignment along both lateral borders and the spinous processes. Abrupt loss of alignment of the spinous processes is seen in unifacet dislocation and may be the most obvious sign of this injury.

Subtle fractures of the lateral pillars may only be appreciated on the AP view. Sagittal oriented fractures appear normal on the lateral view in up to a third of cases and the majority are unstable. Fractures of the upper ribs imply a high-velocity injury which may be associated with lower cervical vertebral fractures and rupture of the great vessels.

The pedicles are also best seen in the AP projection. Absence of a pedicle may be due to destruction by tumour or congenital absence, although this is more common in the thoracic or lumbar spine. The AP view can be obtained with caudal tilt to show the posterior arch, or cranial tilt to give better delineation of the vertebral bodies. In cases where better definition is required, CT is usually employed to better effect.

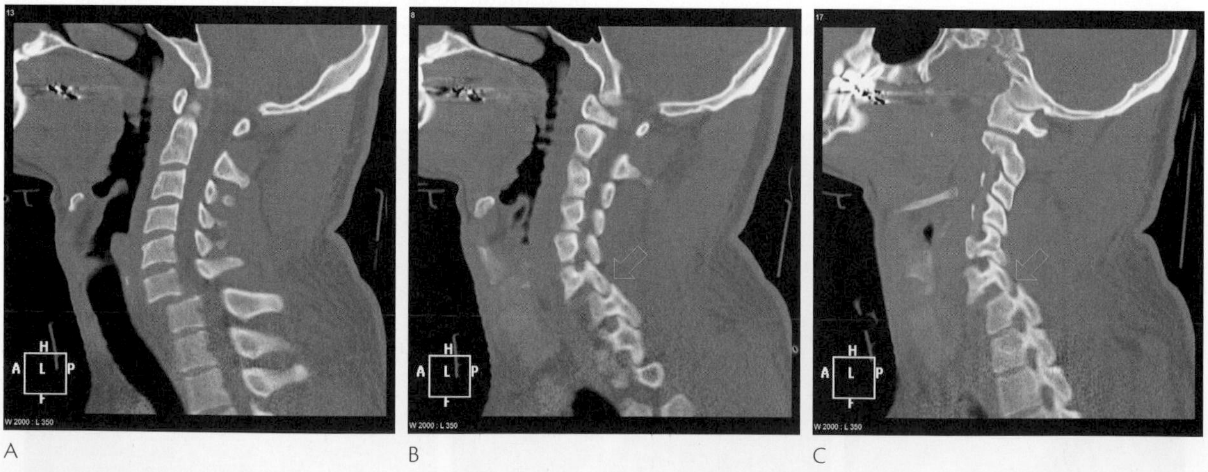

Fig. 12.37.6 Bilateral dislocated facets, sagittal and left and right parasagittal CT reconstructions showing marked anterior spondylolisthesis of C6 on C7 with bilateral dislocated facets (arrows).

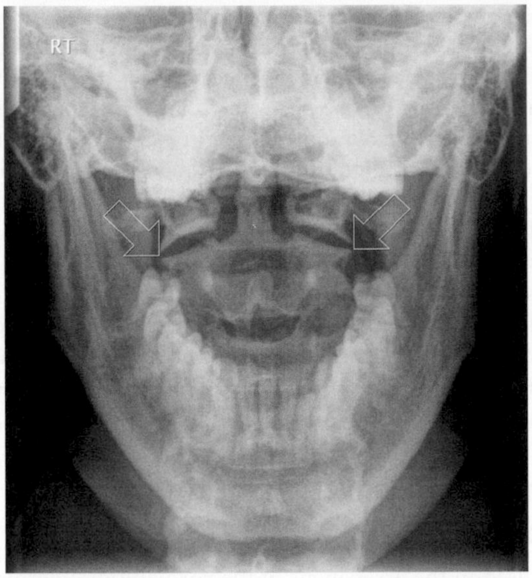

Fig. 12.37.7 Normal Peg view. Note the symmetry of the distances between the peg and the lateral masses of C1 and the normal lateral alignment (arrows).

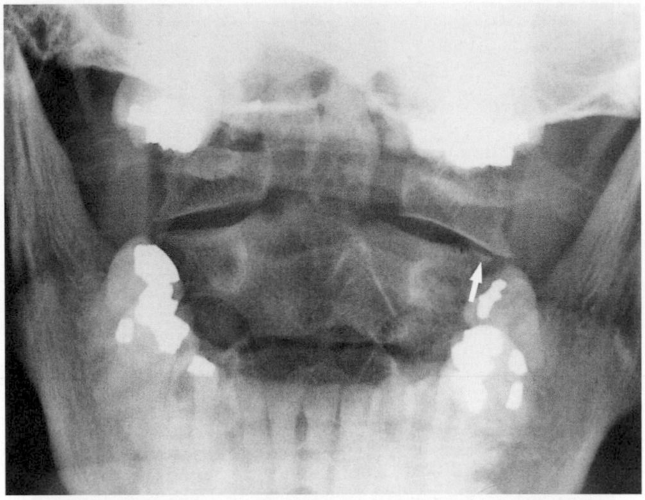

Fig. 12.37.8 Displaced lateral mass of C1 with associated fractures of the ipsilateral facet of C2 (white arrow).

The peg view

The AP projection of the peg shows its relationship to the lateral masses of C1 and C2. The combined distance between the peg and the lateral masses should be no more than 7mm (Figure 12.37.7). Displaced fractures of the arch of C1 (Jefferson fractures) are recognized by an increase in this measurement and by lateral displacement of the lateral mass of C1 with respect to C2 (Figure 12.37.8).

The classical Jefferson fracture involves four breaks in the arch of C1, two anterior and two posterior, although fewer are frequently seen (Figure 12.37.9).

The injury can also be unstable if there are fewer breaks but the posterior longitudinal ligament is torn. Many injuries of this type are not obviously displaced on initial plain films.

Asymmetry between the right and left spaces without an absolute increase in the total measurement occurs when there is rotation of C1 on C2. Abnormal rotation can occur following trauma, viral infection, or torticollis, particularly in children. Asymmetry may be seen in normal individuals even with correct positioning of the head. Failure to correct with 15 degrees of rotation to either side has been termed *fixed* atlantoaxial rotatory subluxation (ARS), and is said to distinguish traumatic rotation from other causes, but only if combined with positive clinical signs. Rotation also causes an apparent increase in the size of one lateral mass (that furthest from the film) and a decrease in the size of the other. In true fixed ARS, axial CT sections may show an associated fracture of the facet. In the absence of a fracture, haemorrhage, or synovial entrapment within the facet may account for the fixed rotation. CT is also used to classify fixed ARS based on the peg–anterior arch distance. A distance greater than 5mm implies an unstable lesion which requires surgery.

Undisplaced peg fractures can be difficult to diagnose in the early stages on standard plain films. Fractures are usually oriented in the axial plane and therefore can be overlooked on standard axial CT sections. Coronal CT reconstructions will show the fracture line; however, thin sections have to be acquired to provide sufficient resolution to avoid reformatting artefact. These problems can be overcome with multislice CT and orthogonal voxel acquisition (Figure 12.37.4).

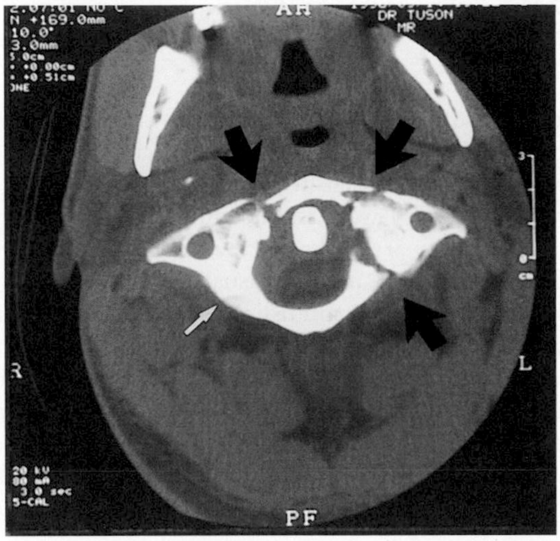

Fig. 12.37.9 Axial CT through C1, the ring is disrupted in three locations (black arrows) with slight lateral displacement of the left lateral mass. A faint line is seen in the intact arch (white arrow) this represents a vascular groove and not a fracture.

Plain film vs computed tomography

Plain film radiography has been the mainstay of spinal imaging for decades, but there is no doubt that even with excellent radiographic technique and accurate interpretation, a significant number of bony injuries are not detected. The percentage of missed injuries is age dependent and may be as much as 10–20%. With this high miss rate there is a strong argument for bypassing plain film radiography in favour of multislice CT in all apart from the low-risk groups, particularly as the multiply traumatized patient often requires CT imaging of the brain, chest, and

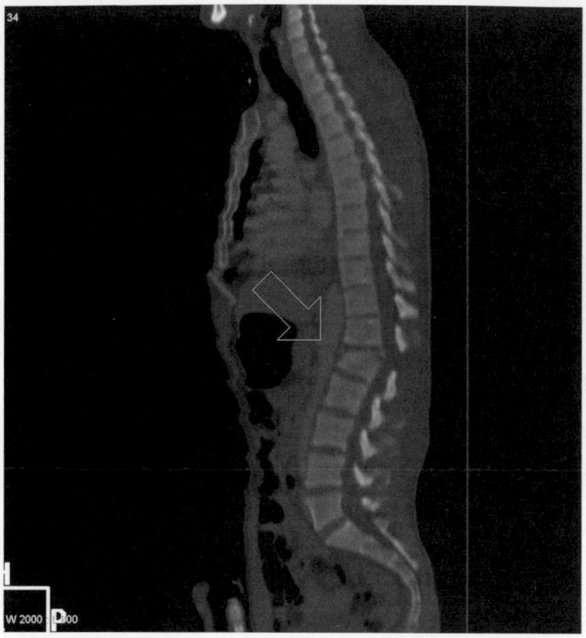

Fig. 12.37.10 Sagittal reformat of the whole spine from a polytrauma CT showing a wedge compression fracture of L1 with a small retropulsed fragment.

abdomen and other injuries. The main counterargument to screening with CT is radiation burden, particularly to the thyroid gland, which is very radiosensitive.

When single slice CT was first introduced it was used as a problem solving tool for areas like the craniocervical or cervicothoracic junctions that were not well visualized on plain film. Helical slice CT and subsequently multislice CT followed with the latter permitting 1-mm slice thickness and isotropic voxels enabling multiplanar image reformatting, have tended to be used to image the entire cervical spine between the foramen magnum and T4. This aids in the perception of difficult subtle fractures and dislocations particularly fractures through the pedicles, pillars and posterior arches. Sensitivities of 95% and specificities of 93% are quoted.

Improvements in CT technology and computing power have facilitated the development of isotropic voxel imaging using multislice CT. This means that slice thickness is now so thin that multiplanar reformatting can be performed on the original voxel data set (Figure 12.37.10). Not only are sagittal and coronal reformats used routinely, but oblique and three-dimensional modelling now become possible. The three main imaging plains axial, sagittal, and coronal are all complementary and useful in the detection and analysis of different fractures (Figure 12.37.11). Plain film radiography has no equivalent to the axial plane in which the CT data set is acquired and here lies the greatest advantage of CT over plain film and this is that the bony canal can be clearly demonstrated and the relationship of bony fragments to the canal can be directly delineated (Figure 12.37.12).

Magnetic resonance imaging vs computed tomography

MRI is used in the assessment of the cord and disc herniation in patients with neurological deficit and the assessment of ligamentous structures.

The four main indications for MRI are suspected spinal cord injury are, suspected ligamentous injury, radiculopathy, and progressive neurological deficit, which is an indication for *emergency MRI*. Sequence optimisation is particularly important in maximizing diagnostic yield. However, the basic examination of the cervical spine should include a T_1-weighted sagittal sequence, a T_2 or more preferably a fat saturated T_2 sagittal sequence and axial images with either T_1, T_2, or GRE T_2* images, or a combination of these. Further sequences can be obtained depending on the clinical scenario and bespoke investigation can be tailored as appropriate. For example if nerve root avulsion is suspected, specific axial oblique T_2 or T_2*-weighted images are obtained through the exiting nerve roots.

The T_1 images are particularly useful for displaying anatomy, for example the sagittal T_1 sequence beautifully demonstrates the anterior longitudinal ligament. Likewise the STIR (short-tau inversion recovery) or T_2 fat sat images are crucial for detecting

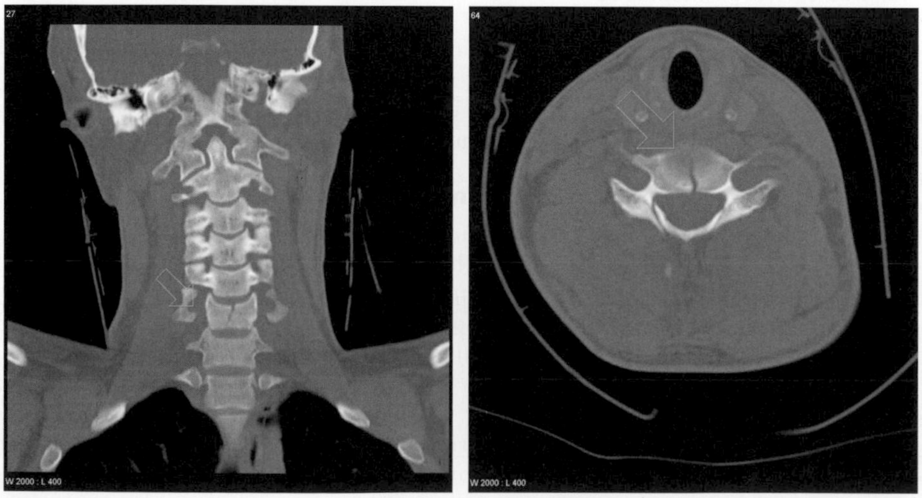

A B

Fig. 12.37.11 Coronal and axial CT showing sagittally orientated fractures through the vertebral body of C6 which was not visible on the plain film.

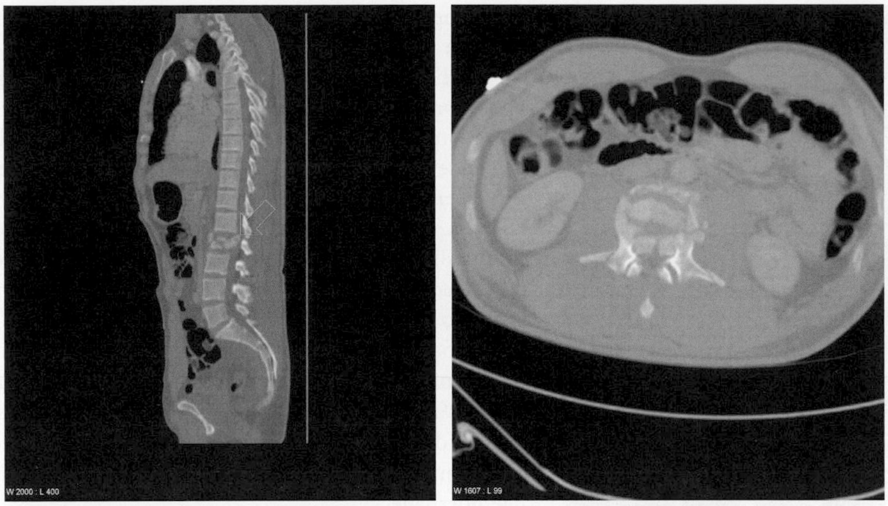

A B

Fig. 12.37.12 Sagittal and axial images showing burst L2 fracture, note the axial image clearly defines the relationship of the bony fragments and the canal.

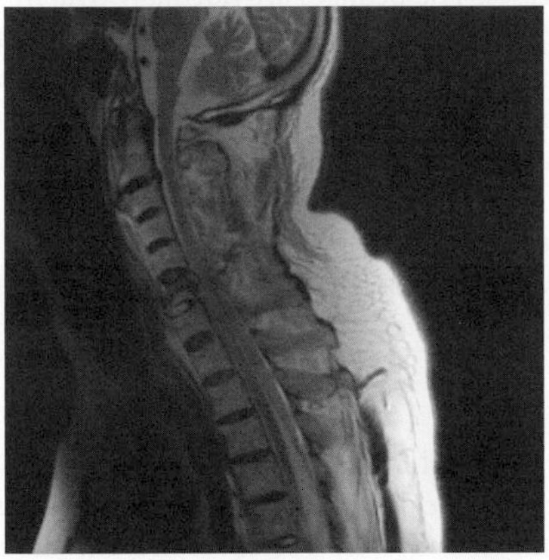

Fig. 12.37.13 Sagittal T2 image of the cervical spine showing a fracture through the sixth cervical vertebra, with a posteriorly displaced fragment causing spinal compression, note the abnormally high signal in the compressed cervical cord, also note the abnormally high signal in the C6/7 disc which indicates the fracture involves the disc.

bone marrow oedema and microfracture. CT and plain films miss 0.5% of significant injuries in the obtended patient.

Other indications for MRI in trauma include:

- Diffuse idiopathic skeletal hyperostosis (DISH) and ankylosing spondylitis
- SCIWORA (spinal cord injury without 'radiological' abnormality)
- Vertebral artery trauma, traumatic meningocoeles, CSF leaks after nerve root avulsions, post-traumatic syrinx, syringohydromyelia, and myelomalacia.

Posteriorly the interspinous ligaments lie between the spinous processes and lamina, they are not as conspicuous as the ALL and PLL on sagittal images but abnormal signal or haematoma in their location infers disruption and potential instability when taken into context with the other injuries seen. As well as assessing alignment of the longitudinal and interspinous ligaments, the paravertebral soft tissues and cord (Figure 12.37.13) should be examined, as vertebral fractures may be associated with paravertebral haematomas. The MRI signal characteristics of blood are complicated and evolve with time, as the oxygenated haemoglobin released from the red blood cells undergoes degradation via deoxyhaemoglobin and methaemoglobin to haemosiderin, all of which have different and definable signal characteristics.

Thoracolumbar spine

Injuries to the thoracolumbar spine account for approximately 60% of all spinal injuries. In adults, 90% are between T11 and L4, and the majority of these occur between T12 and L2. In children T4 and T5 also figure prominently. The standard projections are AP and lateral views, which can be supplemented by cone lateral views of the injured area.

On MRI, the axial images are best suited for assessing the paravertebral areas, canal and spinal cord. Haematoma is not uncommonly seen within the spinal canal, usually in the epidural space. Epidural haematomas may be compressive and reactive cord oedema is identified as high signal on the fluid sensitive sequences within the cord itself. Differentiation from cord haemorrhage can be achieved by considering the different signal characteristics of oedema and haemorrhage. Finally, the osseous structures should be considered, as previously stated it is well known that MRI is relatively insensitive to detecting fractures, even if STIR sequences are employed. The classic signal characteristics of a fracture are low signal lines on T_1 imaging (Figure 12.37.14) and associated high signal on T_2 (Figure 12.37.15) and other fluid sensitive sequences. If fat saturation techniques are employed, the fatty signal of the marrow can be negated to exaggerate the fluid signal associated with fracture and micro fracture, improving the pickup.

Anteroposterior projection

On the AP projection, the margins of the vertebral bodies can be difficult to distinguish owing to overlap with the posterior elements. A careful scrutiny of the superior and inferior margins will demonstrate wedging; however, this is much easier to assess on the lateral view. The upper thoracic vertebra can be difficult to assess on the lateral view; therefore particular attention must be paid to these on the AP view. Signs of vertebral injury on the AP view also include paravertebral haematoma, apical capping, and mediastinal

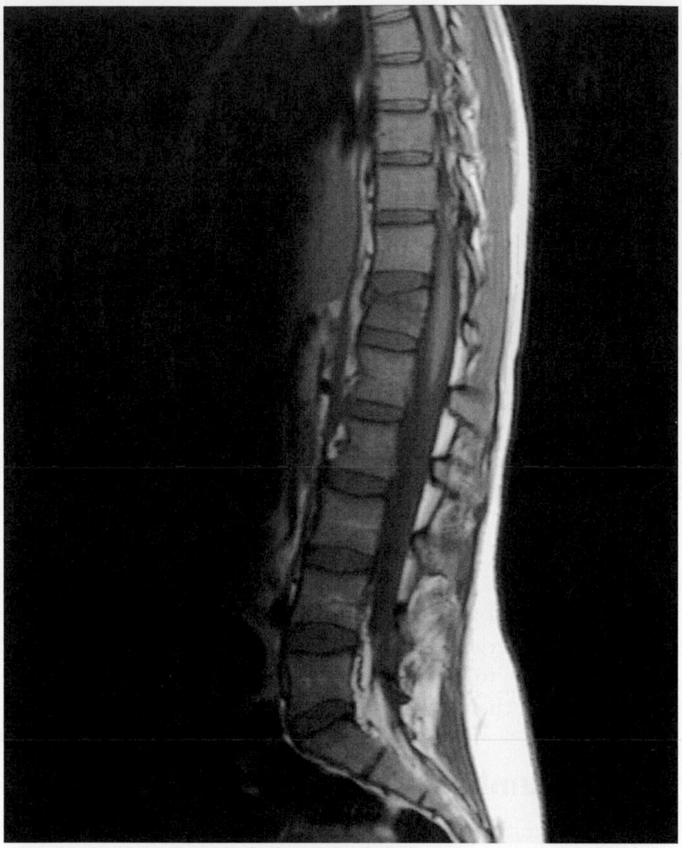

Fig. 12.37.14 Sagittal T1 image of the lumbar spine showing the characteristic low signal line through the T12 vertebral body representing the fracture line.

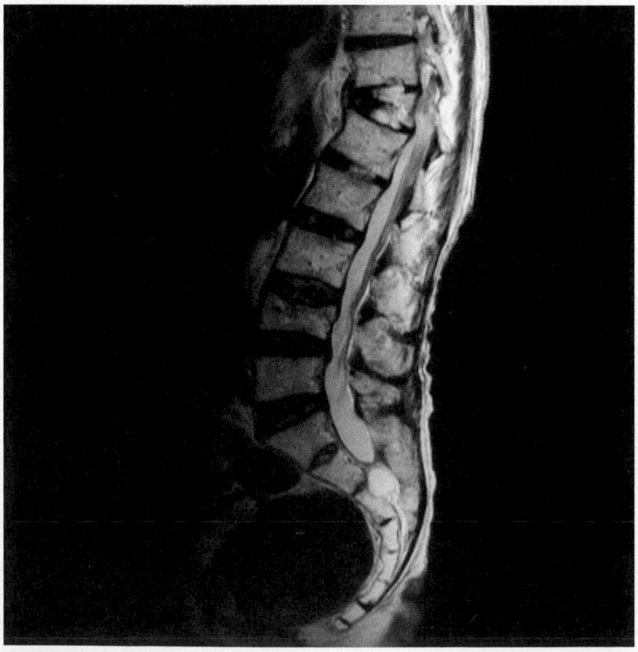

Fig. 12.37.15 Sagittal T2 image showing collapse of T12 with associated high signal, also note the loss of vertebral body height of L4, both fractures were osteoporotic in aetiology.

widening. These are also features of vascular injury. Aortic rupture causes a variety of plain radiograph changes, but the most reliable are tracheal or oesophageal deviation to the right, apical capping, and depression of the left mainstem bronchus. The right paravertebral line lies in close proximity to the vertebral column throughout its length; the left is slightly more laterally placed as a result of displacement by the aorta and can be up to 1cm from the vertebral column. A focal increase in these distances can occur with a paravertebral collection of blood or pus. Displacement due to an ectatic aorta or large osteophytes is the more common cause and tends to be diffuse rather than focal. Below the diaphragm, the psoas shadows may assist in the diagnosis of a paravertebral mass or haematoma. The left psoas shadow can be identified in more than 70% of individuals. The right is more variable in its appearance and is not seen in up to 60% of normal subject. Blurring or enlargement of the psoas shadow may be a sign of retroperitoneal haemorrhage.

Evaluation of the AP view should also include an assessment of the costovertebral joints, the pedicles, and the transverse and spinous processes. The pedicles are normally oval in shape and the spinous processes are teardrop shaped. The cortical margins of both structures should be carefully scrutinized for fracture. There is a gradual increase in the interpediculate distance between T1 and L5. An increase in this distance, following trauma, to more than 4mm greater than adjacent levels indicates involvement of the posterior column and a burst fracture. The presence of a fracture of the transverse process should prompt a search for associated renal injury.

The lateral view

The anterior and posterior margins of the vertebral body should be compared on the lateral view. Minor anterior wedging is acceptable, but the anterior vertebral margin should not differ from the posterior vertebral height by more than 3mm (Figure 12.37.16). More significant wedging causes retropulsion of the posterior vertebral margin into the spinal canal. The most common site of retropulsion is from the posterosuperior margin of the vertebral body. Signs of fragment retropulsion include a convex configuration of the posterior vertebral margin which may be associated with loss of the normal cortex and an increase in the posterior vertebral bony angle to more than 100 degrees. Fragments from both superior and inferior margins are next in frequency. CT will assess the precise nature of the retropulsed fragment and the degree of spinal canal compression; however, the latter does not necessarily correlate with the degree of neurological deficit. A limbus vertebra may mimic a compression fracture. It can be differentiated by its more rounded contour and the corticated fragment of bone isolated by herniated nuclear material (Figure 12.37.17).

When the fulcrum of force is anterior to the vertebral body, a 'lap-belt' or Chance fracture ensues (Figure 12.37.18). Distraction forces may result in tearing of the interspinous ligament, facet subluxation, or horizontal fractures through the vertebral body, pedicles, or laminas. Vertebral body height is characteristically increased.

The most common cause of pathological thoracic vertebral fracture is osteoporosis. The most common cause is postmenopausal

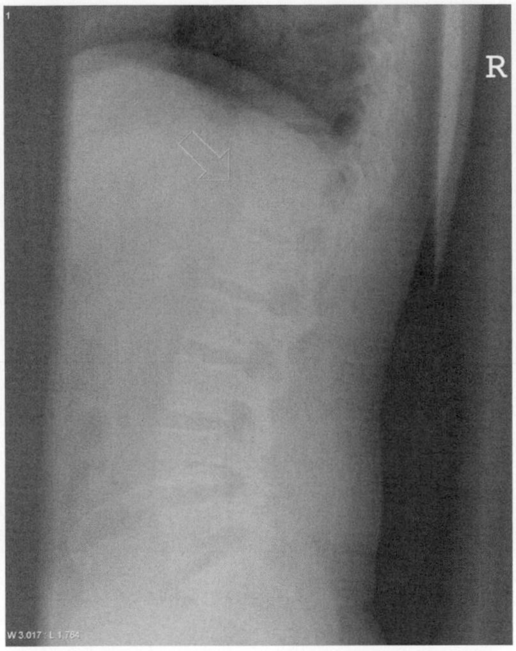

Fig. 12.37.16 Plain lateral radiograph showing loss of anterior height of T12 greater than 3mm indicating fracture.

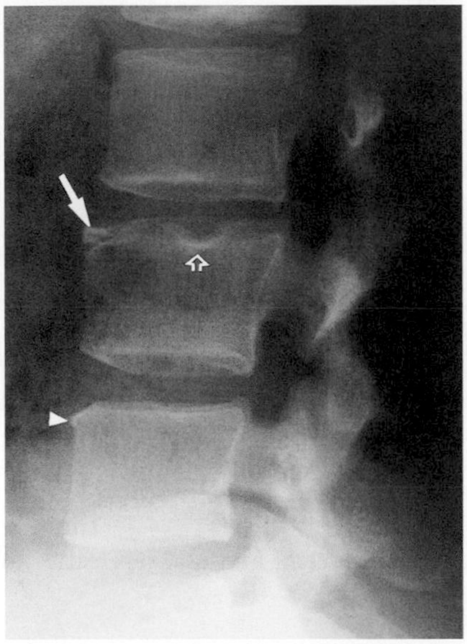

Fig. 12.37.17 Limbus vertebra. A residual ring apophysis (white arrow). Separated from the underlying vertebral body by prolapsed disc material. An incidental Schmorl node (open arrow) and traction spur (arrowhead) are noted.

osteoporosis, but myeloma as a cause of osteoporosis should be considered and excluded. Multiple osteoporotic fractures are more likely to be contiguous. Plain film changes suggestive of malignancy include involvement of the pedicles (usually spared in multiple myeloma), cortical destruction and a soft tissue mass. MRI is the investigation of choice in distinguishing benign from malignant

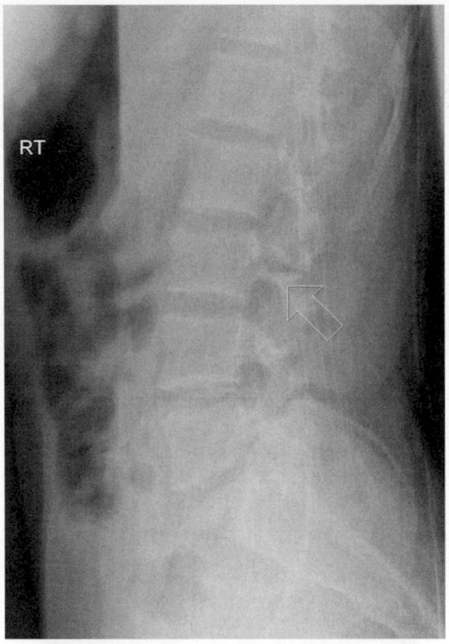

Fig. 12.37.18 Lateral lumbar spine showing Chance fracture of L3 with a horizontal fracture through the vertebral body which has propagated out through the posterior elements (arrow).

causes and in determining whether osteoporotic fractures are acute or chronic.

Displaced fractures of the pars interarticularis are readily identified on plain films. Undisplaced fractures may be identified on the lateral view, or, more easily, on the 45-degree oblique projections. This technique has been replaced by CT (Figure 12.37.19) and MRI. The authors consider MRI to be the more justifiable imaging technique, as it is more sensitive and does not involve ionizing radiation. These patients are often young, and a negative plain film in suspected pars defects often does little more to progress the differential diagnosis. Sagittal T_1-weighted MRI shows the defect as a focus of the intermediate signal within the pars and is the method of choice for the initial evaluation of the pars. In the majority of cases, an interruption to the normal bright marrow signal within the pars is seen on the sagittal T_1-weighted images. MRI also has the advantage of demonstrating the adjacent exit foramen in patients with associated root compression secondary to spondylolisthesis (Figure 12.37.20). Degenerative disc changes at the level above the pars defect can also be diagnosed. Traumatic spondylolisthesis can be distinguished from the degenerative type by a relative increase in the AP canal diameter. Sagittal STIR or fat-suppressed images may demonstrate oedema in the adjacent marrow secondary to attempts at repair; however, these changes are uncommon. In some cases, high signal is demonstrated within the pars in the absence of an established fracture and this is termed stress response. Differentiation of injury at this occult stage may be important in the training athlete, as modification of the training programme may prevent progression to established fracture. In patients with known pars fracture, CT is superior to MRI in determining healing. Skeletal scintigraphy, preferably with single-photon emission CT (SPECT), shows increased

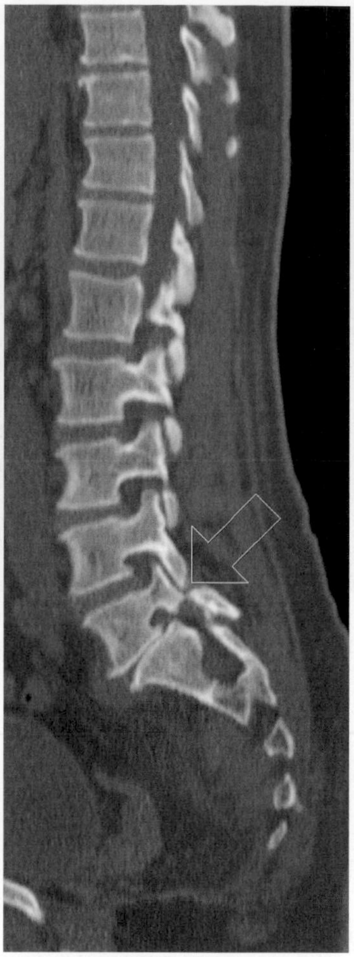

Fig. 12.37.19 CT sagittal reformat of lumbosacral spine, arrow indicates pars defect, also note minor anterior spondylolisthesis of L5 on S1 .

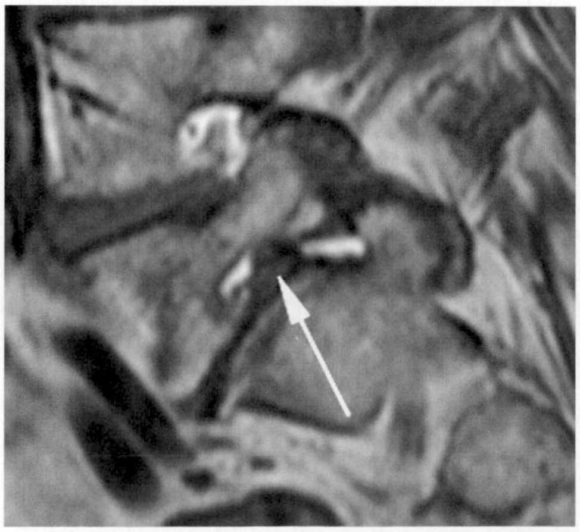

Fig. 12.37.20 Displaced pars defect with root compression. The arrow indicates a swollen distorted nerve root within a distorted exit foramen.

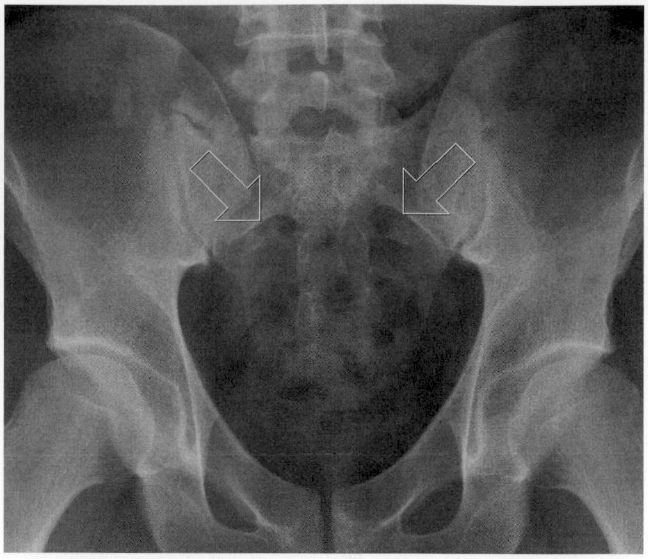

Fig. 12.37.21 Anteroposterior view of the pelvis showing the sacrum and arcuate lines (arrows).

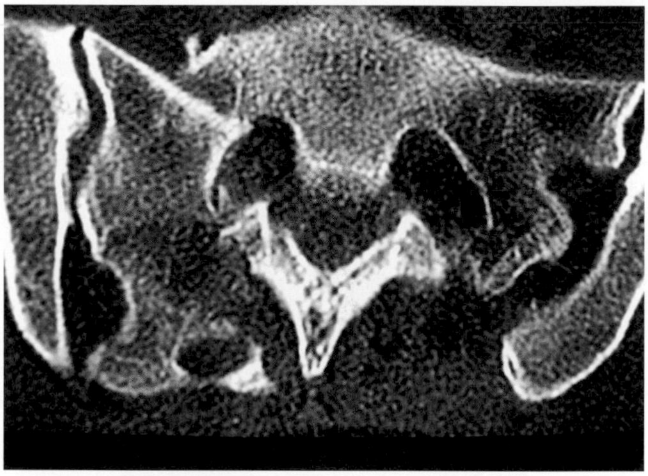

Fig. 12.37.22 Axial CT showing disruption of the arcuate lines secondary to sacral fracture.

uptake at these sites of repair and is also sensitive to the prefracture stage.

The sacrum, sacroiliac joints, and coccyx

The sacrum can be difficult to assess on plain radiographs, as anatomical detail can be obscured by overlying soft tissue. Particular attention should be paid to the lateral margin of the bone and the integrity of the arcuate lines (Figure 12.37.21). If either of these landmarks are blurred or interrupted, cross-sectional imaging with CT (Figure 12.37.22) or MRI may be necessary.

Fractures of the sacrum are frequent in the osteoporotic patient. One or both ala may be involved and a linking fracture may cross at the S2 level giving the classical H or Honda sign configuration. The fractures are easier to see on MRI than plain films. Fractures of the pubic rami are frequently present in these patients.

Coccydynia is a common problem in the general population, usually following trauma, particularly parturition. In these cases imaging is of little help. If sinister pathology is suspected by the clinical history and rectal examination, MRI or CT is the investigation of choice.

Further reading

Bohrer, S.P., Chen, Y.M., and Sayers, D.G. (1990). Cervical spine flexion patterns. *Skeletal Radiology*, **19**, 521–5.

De Smet, A.A., Robinson, R.G., Johnson, B.E., and Lukert, B.P. (1988). Spinal compression fractures in osteoporotic women: patterns and relationship to hyperkyphosis. *Radiology*, **166**, 497–500.

Gisbert, V., Hollerman, J., Ney, A. (1989). Incidence and diagnosis of C7-T1 fractures and subluxations in multiple trauma patients: evaluation of the Advanced Trauma Life Support guidelines. *Surgery*, **106**, 702–9.

Griffen, M.M., Frykberg, E.R., Kerwin, et al. (2003). Radiographic clearance of blunt cervical spine injury: plain radiograph or computed tomography scan? *Journal of Trauma-Injury Infection and Critical care*, **55**(2), 222–7.

Sliker, C.W., Mirvis, S.E., Shanamuganathan, K. (2005). Assessing cervical spine stability in obtunded blunt trauma patients: review of the medical literature. *Radiology*, **234**(3), 733–9.

12.38

Emergency management of the traumatized cervical spine

Jens R. Chapman and Richard J. Bransford

Summary points

- Unconscious patients should have CT scan of neck
- Emergency MRI if possible in spinal cord injury
- Avoid flexion/extension views if possible
- In spinal shock avoid over transfusion and consider epinephrine; high dose steroids probably not indicated
- Reduce dislocation acutely (MRI before in intact patients if possible)
- Do not put distraction injury into traction
- Urgent surgery for traumatic disc hernaition, expanding epidural haematoma, depressed lamina fracture or complex facet fractures with dislocation.

Prehospital care (Box 12.38.1)

A patient with spinal cord injury and neck deformity would usually benefit from a general realignment effort and subsequent protective immobilization prior to transport.

In children, placement on a conventional backboard can lead to undesirable cervical kyphosis as paediatric heads are disproportionately larger than those of adults. Using a specialized backboard with a cutout for the head or placing a folded blanket under the victim's torso helps to avoid this.

Exceptions to the principle of supine positioning of trauma patients on a hard board for retrieval purposes are rare. Neurologically intact patients who present with significant painful neck deformity, such as patients with ankylosing spondylitis, are preferably immobilized *in situ* with sandbags and folded towels in a semi-upright position to accommodate their deformity, provided that their vital signs are stable. It may also be helpful to ask the patient about their pre-injury posture and neck alignment as well as position of comfort, since patients with pre-existent neck deformity may be subject to further cord impingement and subsequent neurological deterioration attempts from ill-advised manipulation.

Box 12.38.1 Prehospital care

- On site management:
  - High degree of suspicion for cervical spine injury
  - Attention to ATLS guidelines for extrication
- Patient transport on spine board
  - For children use occipital cutout to avoid excessive flexion
- Use rigid neck collar ± sandbags and tape for patient transport
- Establish/document basic four-extremity neurological status prior to transport.

Emergency diagnostic measures (Box 12.38.2)

Clinical evaluation

Unconscious patients should receive an emergency head computed tomography (CT) scan as soon as possible to exclude intracranial lesions and caudal extension of this scan to include the cervical spine. This allows visualization of the entire cervical spine and the cervicothoracic junction.

Log-rolling is performed with proper spine precautions maintained by a team approach. The cervical collar is released during palpation of the neck. Strict spine precautions should be maintained in all trauma victims until appropriate radiographic and clinical clearance have been completed; however, positioning on a rigid board for more than 4h increases the risk of developing sacral or occipital decubiti.

Neurological assessment starts with determination of mental status and cranial nerve function and is followed by systematic spinal cord functional evaluation following the principles established by the ASIA system (American Spinal Injury Association 1992) (Figure 12.38.1). The effects of sedatives, muscle-relaxing medications, and limb injuries on rating motor strength should be considered during this evaluation. Formal neurological status evaluation for trauma patients routinely includes evaluation of the anal sphincter region for perianal sensation, spontaneous sphincter tone, quality of voluntary contraction, and presence or absence of bulbocavernosus reflex. For patients with neurological deficits, an attempt is made to establish the level of sensory and motor injury. Further differentiation of complete and incomplete neurological injuries is of importance with regard to timing of treatment and patient prognosis. Repeat neurological evaluations should be obtained and recorded to exclude neurological deterioration which may occur, for instance, in the event of a developing epidural haematoma or

STANDARD NEUROLOGICAL CLASSIFICATION OF SPINAL CORD INJURY

MOTOR

KEY MUSCLES

	R	L	
C2			
C3			
C4			
C5			Elbow flexors
C6			Wrist extensors
C7			Elbow extensors
C8			Finger flexors (distal phalanx of middle finger)
T1			Finger abductors (little finger)
T2			
T3			
T4			
T5			
T6			
T7			
T8			
T9			
T10			
T11			
T12			
L1			
L2			Hip flexors
L3			Knee extensors
L4			Ankle extensors
L5			Long toe extensors
S1			Ankle plantar flexors
S2			
S3			
S4–5			Voluntary anal contraction (Yes/No)
TOTALS	+	=	**MOTOR SCORE**
(MAXIMUM)	(50)	(100)	(100)

0 = total paralysis
1 = palpable or visible contraction
2 = active movement, gravity eliminated
3 = active movement, against gravity
4 = active movement, against some resistance
5 = active movement, against full resistance
NT = not testable

SENSORY

KEY SENSORY POINTS

	LIGHT TOUCH R	LIGHT TOUCH L	PIN PRICK R	PIN PRICK L
C2				
C3				
C4				
C5				
C6				
C7				
C8				
T1				
T2				
T3				
T4				
T5				
T6				
T7				
T8				
T9				
T10				
T11				
T12				
L1				
L2				
L3				
L4				
L5				
S1				
S2				
S3				
S4–5				
	(56)	(56)	(56)	(56)

0 = absent
1 = impaired
2 = normal
NT = not testable

Any anal sensation (Yes/No)

TOTALS: + = **PIN PRICK SCORE** (max: 112)

TOTALS: + = **LIGHT TOUCH SCORE** (max: 112)

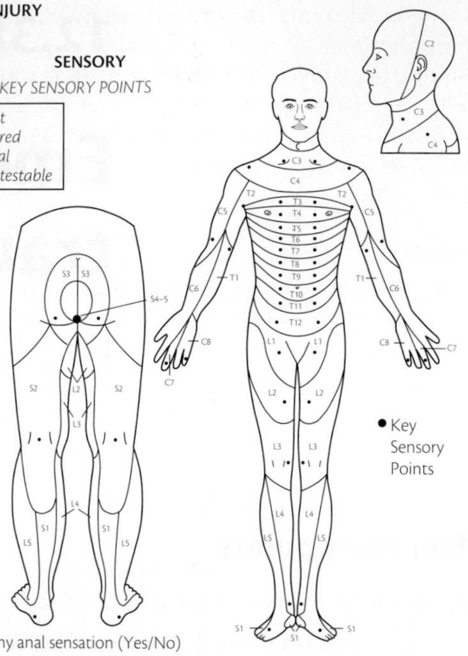

NEUROLOGICAL LEVEL *The most caudal segment with normal function*		R	L	**COMPLETE OR INCOMPLETE?** *Incomplete = presence of any sensory or motor function in lowest sacral segment*	**ZONE OF PARTIAL PRESERVATION** *Partially innervated segments*		R	L
	SENSORY					SENSORY		
	MOTOR					MOTOR		

A

This form may be copied freely but should not be altered without permission from the American Spinal Injury Association

ASIA IMPAIRMENT SCALE

☐ **A = Complete:** No motor or sensory function is preserved in the sacral segments S4–S5.

☐ **B = Incomplete:** Sensory but not motor function is preserved below the neurological level and extends through the sacral segments S4–S5.

☐ **C = Incomplete:** Motor function is preserved below the neurological level, and the majority of key muscles below the neurological level have a muscle grade less than 3.

☐ **D = Incomplete:** Motor function is preserved below the neurological level, and the majority of key muscles below the neurological level have a muscle grade greater than or equal to 3.

☐ **E = Normal:** Motor and sensory function is normal.

CLINICAL SYNDROMES

☐ Central cord
☐ Brown–Sequard
☐ Anterior cord
☐ Conus medullaris
☐ Cauda equina

B

Fig. 12.38.1 A) Motor and sensory checklist for post-trauma neurological examination. B) Neurological impairment scale.

malreduced spine. The presence of a bulbocavernosus reflex has been described as implying absence or resolution of spinal shock. Similar to neurological deficits secondary to spinal shock, patients with incomplete spinal cord injuries may recover some neurological function. Sacral sparing can present with signs of preserved voluntary anal sphincter contractility, perianal sensation, and voluntary long toe flexor function.

Imaging

The ABC principles as formulated in the Advanced Trauma Life support algorithm had recommended three initial trauma radiographs, consisting of anteroposterior (AP) chest, AP pelvis, and lateral cervical spine views for several decades. The more ready availability of rapid image acquisition CT-scan technology, such as offered with helical CT, allows for comprehensive imaging of head, cervical spine, and torso with pelvis regions and has largely replaced conventional imaging in the emergency department setting. Despite this technological advance, a lateral cervical spine radiograph still remains the single most relevant diagnostic entity for trauma in most centres (Figure 12.38.2).

Significant injuries to these transition zones of the cervical spine (occipitocervical and cervicothoracic spine) are among the most common regions of missed cervical spine injuries due to limitations placed on conventional radiographic imaging. Helical CT has been consistently shown to be more sensitive, less time consuming, and more cost effective compared to the traditional work-up, with increased patient radiation exposure the only major downfall. Practitioners need to remember that certain cervical spine injuries are not readily seen on axial CT images, such as type II odontoid fractures and distractive injuries. Reformatted views in sagittal and coronal planes are integral to establishing CT as the sole imaging modality of trauma patients. Specific fine cut CT-scans in defined regions may be helpful to detect specific injuries such as craniocervical dissociations.

Emergency magnetic resonance imaging (MRI) scanning is indicated in patients with cervical spinal cord injury, unexplained neurological deficit, discordant skeletal and neurological levels of injury, and worsening neurological status (Figure 12.38.3). Barring contraindication to MRI, such as presence of stimulators, pacemakers or ferromagnetic clips and other foreign bodies, urgent indications for scanning present predominantly in patients with non-osseous encroachment of the spinal cord. Emergency CT myelography should be considered if there are contraindications to MRI, or if MRI is not readily available. Although sagittal MRI sequences such as T_2-weighted images can be helpful in depicting discoligamentous injuries, this imaging study can usually be obtained on a non-emergency basis.

Dynamic radiographs, such as flexion–extension lateral radiographs of the cervical spine, are effective in assessing stability. However, in order to obtain flexion–extension radiographs, the patient must present without cognitive impairment and have a normal, entirely non-focal neurological examination with normal plain radiographs. Recent studies have suggested that follow-up flexion–extension radiographs are not efficacious when a negative CT has been performed in blunt trauma without neurological findings. Recent evidence has also suggested that initial CT imaging identified all unstable cervical spine injuries in obtunded trauma patients. Subsequent upright radiographs did not identify any additional injuries but significantly delayed spine clearance.

In the setting of a hectic Emergency Department we recommend against routine acute flexion–extension radiographs because of the risk of incurring neurological deterioration by failure to satisfy all the criteria mentioned earlier. Furthermore, a patient with an acutely sprained neck is unlikely to provide a useful neck motion effort in the acute postinjury phase, thus rendering the study less meaningful. We recommend putting the patient into a neck brace and then performing flexion–extension radiographs at 1 to 2 weeks.

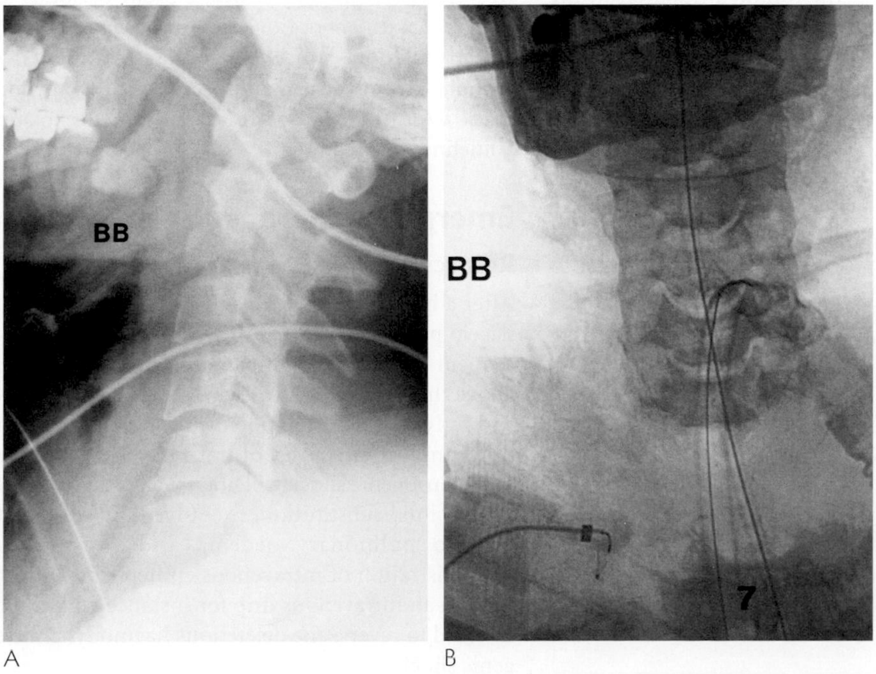

Fig. 12.38.2 A) This lateral cervical spine trauma radiograph of a 38-year-old male injured in a dump truck loading accident fails to visualize the C7 segment. It would be erroneous to 'clear' the cervical spine based on this radiograph. B) The anteroposterior radiograph of the cerviothoracic junction in the same patient reveals a displaced distractive injury to the C6–7 segment.

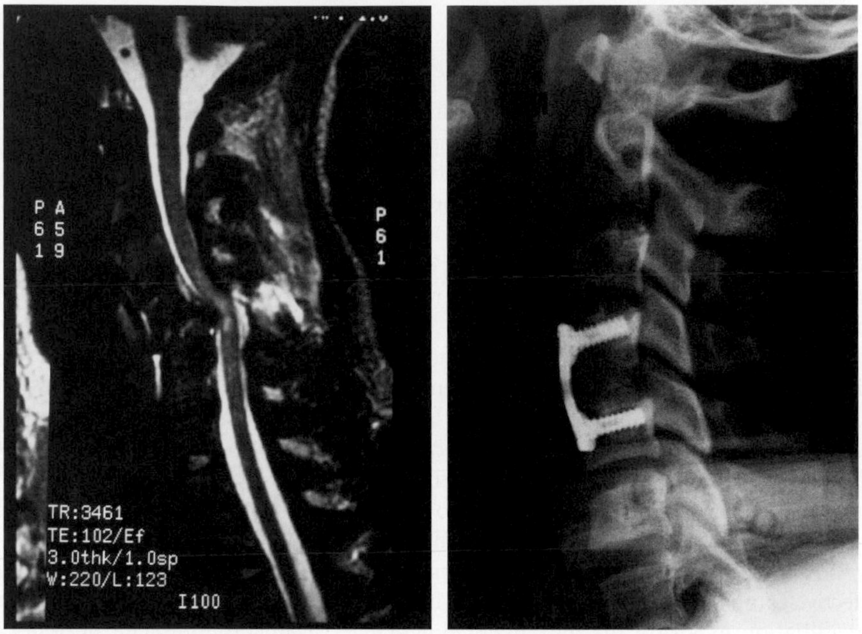

A B

Fig. 12.38.3 A) This 42-year-old female presented with neck pain and hyper-reflexia but no extremity motor or sensory deficits following a motor vehicle accident. An emergency MRI scan was obtained prior to attempting closed reduction of the bilateral facet dislocation in order to exclude a traumatic disc herniation. This sagittal MRI shows a C4–5 dislocation with cord impingement caused by the displacement of the spinal column and a retropulsed C4–5 disc. In patients with displaced cervical spine dislocations without significant neurologic compromise, an emergency neural imaging study, such as an MRI, can influence further management considerably. In this patient closed reduction would probably lead to retropulsion of the C4–5 intervertebral disc into the spinal canal with possible additional neural compromise. B) Treatment consisted of emergency anterior C4–5 discectomy with interbody fusion and plate fixation. The patient continued to demonstrate signs of myelopathy postoperatively, but maintained normal extremity motor and sensory function.

Injuries to the vertebral arteries (VAI) should be suspected in any patient with cervical spine trauma presenting with altered mental status. Injuries with significant vertebral displacement and displaced fractures involving the transverse processes should also alert the clinician to evaluate the patient for possible vertebral artery injuries. Any fracture extending into the foramen transversarium or with significant displacement, as in the setting of jumped facets, may be associated with overt or occult vertebral artery injury. Catheter angiography has been the gold standard for the diagnosis of VAIs; however, new 16-slice CT angiography seems to have sensitivity and specificity which is as good. Vertebral angiography can also be performed at the same time as aortic angiography (Figure 12.38.4). Magnetic resonance angiography and Doppler evaluation are non-invasive techniques for assessing cranial flow abnormalities with as yet unclear clinical implications. In those patients with identified vertebral artery injury, serial monitoring with transcranial Doppler over a 3-day period is used to assess for emboli. Treatment options include observation, antiplatelet agents, anticoagulation, and endovascular treatments. Although some authors have advocated antithrombotic therapy for most asymptomatic VAIs, there is a lack of class I evidence to support any strong guidelines for treatment.

Box 12.38.2 Emergency Department management principles

- Early recognition and treatment of cervical spine injury
- Serial neurological examination and documentation
- Radiological assessment:
  - Initial lateral x-ray (optional)
  - Spiral CT scan head and cervical spine through T1/2 disc space (preferred)
  - Beware non-contiguous injury (40%)
- Prevent further harm:
  - Immobilize with collar, sandbags or traction, move patient off backboard.

Emergency therapeutic intervention

Resuscitation

After a brief initial period of hypertension, spinal shock results in flaccid paralysis, decrease of systemic vascular resistance, and subsequent hypotension. In patients with thoracic spinal cord injury above the T6 level, loss of sympathetic input to the heart can lead to bradycardia and hypotension. Neurogenic shock may mask other important causes of trauma-related hypotension. Patients with neurogenic shock will not usually respond to continued intravenous fluid substitution. Excessive fluid resuscitation efforts may lead to pulmonary oedema and congestive heart failure. Administration of intravenous epinephrine (adrenaline) by bolus or with an intravenous drip for instance with dopamine is recommended to reverse the deleterious haemodynamic effects of neurogenic shock.

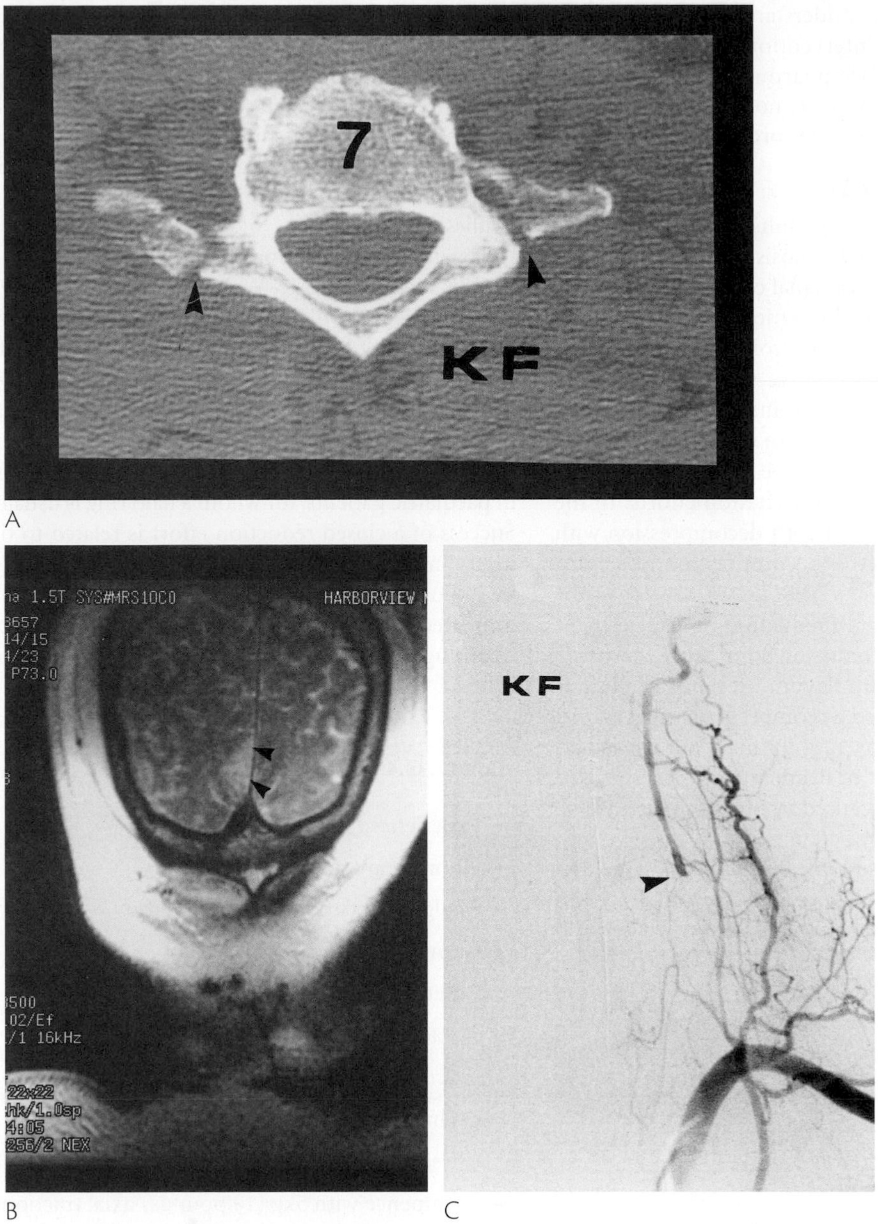

Fig. 12.38.4 A) This 52-year-old male presented with neck pain and confusion 24h after a fall from a height. A CT scan revealed a minimally displaced C6–7 fracture–dislocation. This axial image demonstrates bilateral C7 transverse process fractures. B) A cranial MRI scan showed unilateral cerebellar signal changes consistent with stroke (arrows). C) Vertebral angiography demonstrated bilateral traumatic vertebral artery injuries with complete flow disruption (arrow). The patient was treated with anticoagulants after urgent surgical stabilization of the cervical spine fracture.

Emergency pharmacological treatment

Some units give glucocorticoids to patients with spinal injuries. The rationale is based on animal experiments which show stabilization of neural membranes, prevention of uncontrolled intracellular calcium influx, decrease of lysozymal enzyme effects, and decrease of swelling and inflammation, thus limiting the effects of the secondary injury to the spinal cord.

Two multicentre studies have shown that high doses of methylprednisolone, using a loading dose of 30mg/kg over 1h, followed by 5.4mg/kg/h over 23h, is beneficial for adult patients presenting within 8h of spinal cord injury. However, there has been mounting concerns about the methodology of data analysis of these studies and the occurrence of side effects such as gastric bleeding and infections. This has led to the use of intravenous steroids for the treatment of spinal cord injury to be considered a 'treatment option'. There is near universal agreement, however, that methylprednisolone has no influence on recovery of neurological deficits for patients with spinal nerve root injuries or ballistic trauma.

New promising drug-based therapeutic approaches include regenerative strategies to neutralize myelin-mediated neurite outgrowth inhibition, neuroprotective strategies to reduce apoptotic triggers, the targeting of cationic/glutamatergic toxicity, anti-inflammatory strategies, and the use of approaches to stabilize disrupted cell membranes. All of these substances, however, are experimental in nature and far from routine clinical administration.

Of a number of other measures, hypothermia has received a great deal of more recent attention due to its purported benefits in the treatment of some high-profile individuals, despite previous studies failing to show benefits. Formal repeat review through larger spine societies led to rejection of the stated benefits of hypothermia as treatment for acute spinal cord injury. Although there is some hope for advancements in our understanding of modulating acute spinal cord injury, current intervention results have been modest or unclear at best. Therefore pharmacological measures currently remain focused on blood pressure normalization, correction of anaemia, and hypoxia to maximize cord perfusion.

Primary treatment (Box 12.38.3)

Hyperextension of the cervical spine in adults should be avoided due to its risk of increasing spinal canal stenosis. In adults, infolding of the ligamentum flavum may increase canal occlusion by 19%.

In spinal cord injuries, timing of the removal of any ongoing mass effect acting upon the spinal cord may contribute to potential neurological recovery. Animal studies have shown a brief time window of 6–8h during which removal of spinal cord compression can lead to reversal of spinal cord injury. In clinical reality such time frames are highly unrealistic to achieve and commonly are incompatible with other vital patient resuscitation efforts. In the cervical spine, however, indirect spinal cord decompression with cervical traction can facilitate effective decompression of a compromised spinal cord.

Application of cervical traction with reduction of displacement can decompress the spinal cord by reducing bony canal encroachment and flattening the ligamentum flavum. Reversal of physiological cervical canal occlusion caused by compression using cranial traction improves canal clearance by 12% in intact human cadaveric specimens. Similarly, the effect of ligamentotaxis can be used to reduce spinal canal compromise caused by burst fractures of the cervical spine and facet dislocations.

Skeletal cervical traction is unsuitable for patients with distractive injury patterns or specific conditions such as fractures in ankylosing spondylitis. Relative contraindications to cervical traction also present in patients with skull fractures, in distractive cervical spine injuries such as occipitocervical dissociations, and in combative patients who cannot be pharmacologically sedated. Reduction of a dislocated cervical spine in unconscious or anesthetized patients without spinal cord injury may endanger the spinal cord, and should preferably be performed with spinal cord monitoring or after a disc herniation is excluded with neural imaging studies.

Skeletal cranial traction should be applied by means of suitable devices such as Gardner–Wells tongs or a halo ring (Figure 12.38.5). These devices should be MRI compatible in order not to impair neural imaging in spinal cord injury patients. In trauma patients use of cranial sling setups such as a head halter device is not desirable due to the risk of airway encroachment, aspiration, and limitations of weight that can be safely applied (Box 12.38.4).

Conventional Gardner–Wells tongs are usually not appropriate in paediatric patients, for whom a halo ring is usually more suitable. Success of a closed reduction effort is related to timing following injury, monitored muscle relaxation and analgesia and by providing a controlled setup with shoulder pulldown and fluoroscopy unit. Reduction by manipulation is generally discouraged. Serial neurological re-evaluations are strongly encouraged to minimize

Box 12.38.3 Management of cervical dislocation

- Acute closed reduction:
  - Indications:
    - —facet subluxations/dislocations
    - —burst fractures with canal compression
  - Contraindications:
    - —skull fracture or distractive trauma
    - —ankylosing spinal disorder (relative)
- Timing
  - After initial resuscitation completed
  - Reduction prior to MRI scan in the awake, cooperative patient
- Note:
  - Urgent reduction in emergency department with fluoroscopy safe and effective
  - Preferred treatment for patients with cervical spine spinal cord injury
  - Disc disruption (22–50%) commonly associated with such injuries.

Box 12.38.4 Technique of closed reduction with skull traction

- Experienced personnel
- Fluoroscopy suite
- Analgesia/sedation/pulse oximetry
- Garner–Wells tongs
  - Betadine wash
  - 1% lignocaine
  - 1cm posterior to external auditory meatus
  - Finger breadth above ear
  - Use new stainless steel tongs if high weights anticipated
- Commence with 5kg (10 pounds) axial traction:
  - Increase in 5-kg (10-pound) increments every 5–10min with head in flexion trajectory
  - Neurological and radiological assessment at each step
  - Weights up to 65kg (140 pounds) may be required
- Cease if:
  - Neurological deficit—transfer to MRI/operating room
  - Mechanical block
  - >1cm distraction at injury level
- Reduction obtained
  - Decrease skeletal traction weight to <10kg (20 pounds)
  - Lower traction trajectory to horizontal angle
  - Place towel in interscapular region to maintain neck in extension
  - Patient placement in Rotorest-type bed (preferred).

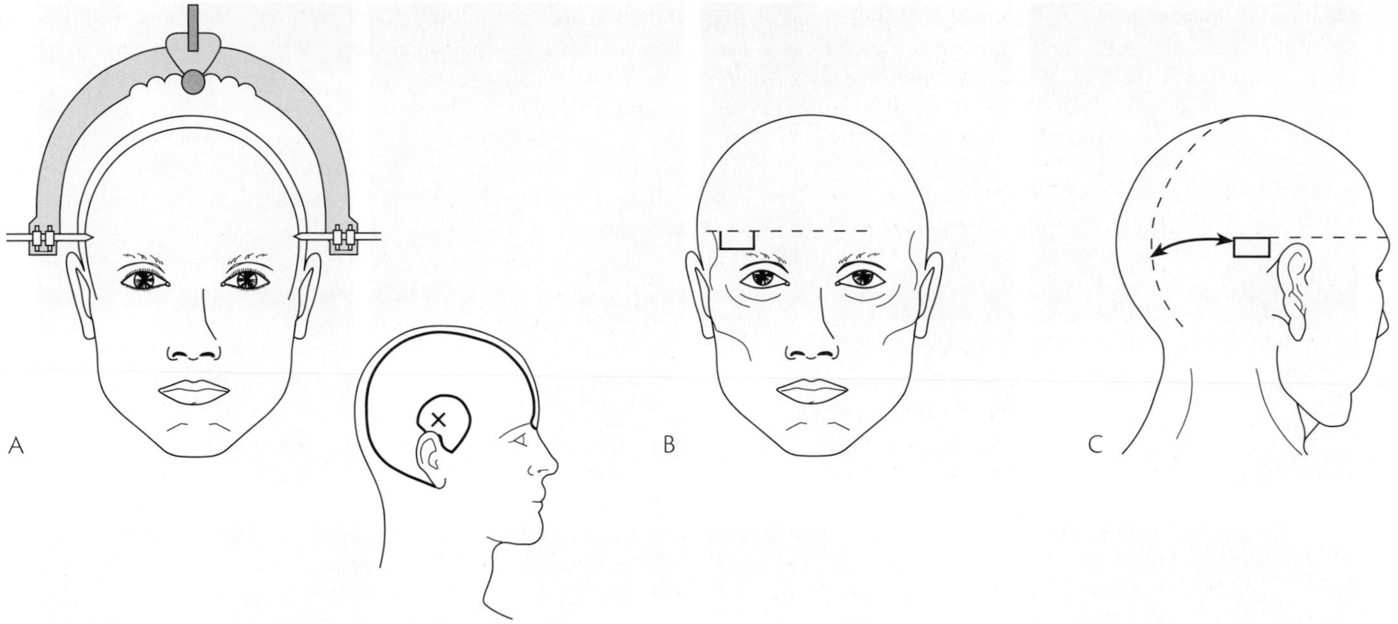

Fig. 12.38.5 A) This illustration depicts the preferred placement site for skeletal cranial traction devices such as Gardner–Wells tongs. Ideally the pins are secured to the outer table of the cranium by pins placed in line upwards to the external auditory meatus at a distance of 1cm from the outer earlobe, but below the equator of the skull. B), C) The pins of a halo-ring are preferably placed in the shaded areas depicted in the two diagrams. Anterior pins should avoid the supraorbital nerve and the frontal sinus medially and the temporal fossa laterally. The posterior pins should be placed in superior and posterior location relative to the mastoid process. The halo-ring should be located below the equator of the skull in order to minimize pin avulsion.

the risk of a secondary traction-induced neural deterioration being missed.

Halo-ring placement is more complicated than tong placement and requires at least one assistant or a dedicated halo positioning board (ACE-Fisher). Open-back halo rings have become increasingly popular due to greater ease of application and some improvement in patient comfort. Closed reduction of cervical dislocations is performed with the patient supine on a hard cushioned stretcher with both upper extremities pulled caudally by straps or surgical tape attached to the shoulders. We recommend intravenous analgesics, muscle relaxants, and nasal oxygen in responsive patients. Monitoring of vital signs such as automated blood pressure, pulse rate, and oxygen saturation is very helpful in titrating sedatives adequately. It is important that the patient remain awake in order to provide neurological feedback during the closed reduction.

Over-distraction should be avoided during cervical traction. We recommend starting with low initial weights of 2–5 kg (5–10 pounds), and checking a lateral radiograph for focal widening beyond 1.5mm between each cervical segment. Particular attention must be directed toward the occipital–cervical junction to assess for an undiagnosed craniocervical dissociation. If there is no over-distraction, traction weight is increased in 2- to 5-kg increments accompanied by clinical and radiological assessment (Figure 12.38.6). Older patients and patients with injuries of the upper cervical spine usually require lower weights to achieve the desired reduction results. Skeletal cervical traction weights usually should not exceed half to two-thirds body weight or approximately 45kg. Changes in the pull-angle that place the neck in a more flexed position can help in disengaging locked facets. Flexion is generally needed to reduce flexion type injuries in order to unlock the facets and allow them to translate back to their native position; in-line traction cannot accomplish this. Possible causes of unsuccessful closed-reduction efforts are inadequate muscle relaxation, presence of a fracture dislocation with comminuted lateral masses, or dislocations of the cervicothoracic junction.

Continued controversy surrounds the timing and technique of reduction of cervical spine dislocations. Reduction carries with it a theoretical risk of the intervertebral disc displacing into the spinal canal with potential for subsequent secondary neurological deterioration. Neural imaging, preferably in form of a MRI scan, has been suggested to rule out presence of a potentially cord compromising mass prior to embarking on closed reduction efforts (see Figure 12.38.3). However, the time taken for such imaging studies introduces a potentially critical delay in realigning and thereby indirectly decompressing the spinal cord. There is also a certain degree of risk in transferring a patient with an unstable dislocated spine from a trauma stretcher onto an imaging table.

The overwhelming majority of studies addressing this controversy of timing with a defined patient cohort have found immediate closed reduction to be a safe and effective intervention with successful reduction achieved in over 80% of patients and few, if any, cases of secondary neurological deterioration. While the incidence of visualized disc herniation on postreduction MRI has been described to range from 10–25% of patients, the vast majority of these lesions did not compromise the cord. Not surprisingly, the incidence of these disc herniations appears to be somewhat higher in patients with unilateral compared with bilateral facet dislocations. Based on these experiences the following protocol has become widely accepted: patients with neurological injury preferably receive emergent reduction using a formal skeletal traction sequence prior to receiving an MRI scan. In contrast, patients who are neurologically intact can be considered for prereduction MRI as long as this imaging modality is readily available. For cognitively impaired patients a best faith judgement call as to likelihood of

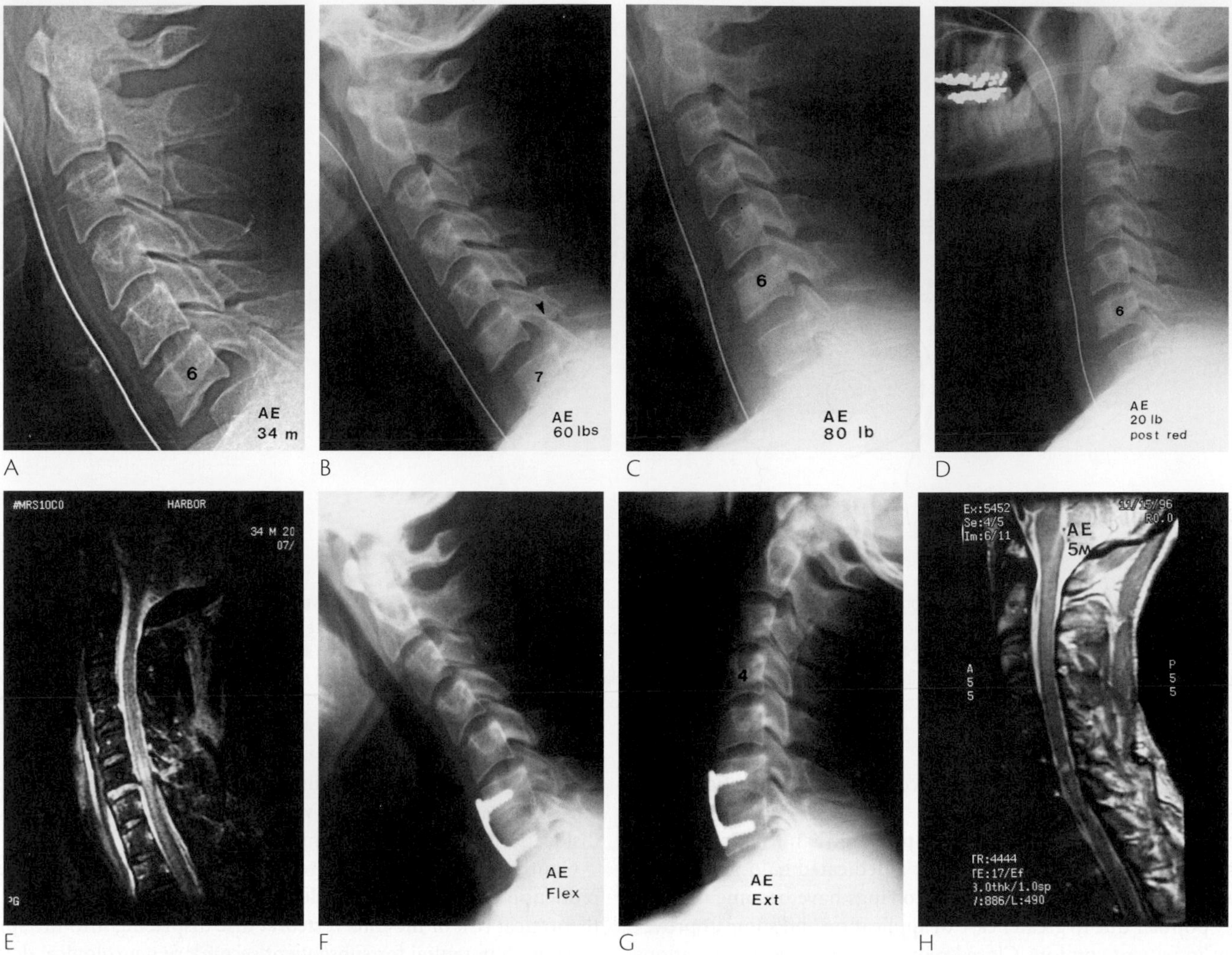

Fig. 12.38.6 This 34-year-old male presented within 4h of a barefoot waterskiing accident with a neurologically complete C6 tetraplegia. There was no sacral sparing present; the patient also had an absent bulbocavernosus reflex. Lateral plain cervical radiographs demonstrated a bilateral C6–7 facet dislocation. Along with intravenous methylprednisolone administration the patient underwent immediate closed reduction with cranial tong traction, without undergoing an MRI first. B) Following sequentially increasing cranial skeletal traction, the facets were found to be perched on lateral radiographs at 60 pounds traction. The patient noticed immediate recovery of trunk and leg sensation. C) The facet dislocation reduced with 80 pounds traction. No manipulation was used for the reduction sequence. Notice the overdistraction at the C6–7 interspace. D) Following reduction, the traction weight was reduced to 20 pounds in order to avoid potential damage from persistent overdistraction. The entire duration from initial presentation to complete reduction lasted for 45min. The patient was kept in a rotating bed. E) A postreduction MRI scan was obtained to exclude a persistent space-occupying lesion affecting the spinal cord. This T_2-weighted MRI scan demonstrates anterior and posterior discoligamentous injuries to the C6–7 segment and confirms absence of any residual cord compression. Increased signal within the cord substance is reflective of cord haemorrhage. F) and G) The patient received anterior cervical discectomy and fusion at C6–7 48h after injury. Apart from unilateral C7 root pain the patient made a full neurologic recovery within 5 days of his injury. These lateral cervical flexion–extension radiographs demonstrate solid fusion in anatomic alignment. H) At 5 months postinjury the patient received an MRI scan to assess his unilateral C7 radiculopathy. A focal area of spinal cord injury probably representing gliosis was noted at the C6–7 interspace. There was no evidence of any residual cord or nerve root compromise.

presence of concurrent spinal cord injury can be used to guide the decision of emergent traction reduction. In general, however, the risks of leaving a patient with a dislocated spine appear to outweigh the risks associated with expediently performed closed skeletal reduction. Should a traumatic disc herniation with cord compression be identified on neuroimaging, anterior surgical decompression and fusion are recommended instead of pursuing closed reduction. Similarly, patients with failed attempts at closed reduction should be considered for emergent surgical reduction and stabilization.

For patients with unstable cervical spine injuries unsuitable for early surgical stabilization traction may be considered as a temporizing alternative. In order to minimize the risk of thromboembolic disease, decubital ulcers, and pulmonary deterioration during prolonged recumbence spinal injury patients who are unsuitable for early surgical stabilization are preferably placed in dedicated hospital beds, which maintain spinal alignment while allowing for some horizontal mobilization such as afforded by rotating trauma beds (ROTOREST).

Of several contraindications to the application of cranial traction, patients with distractive injuries to the cervical spine are particularly concerning due to their propensity for further displacement and subsequent neurological deterioration (see Figure 12.38.1). Temporary reduction under gentle compression can be attempted by application of a halo ring and halo vest or placement of sandbags around the patient's head and securing it with tape placed across the head. For craniocervical dissociative injuries or similar upper cervical spine distraction injuries a reverse Trendelenburg position will likely cause further distraction. Postural reduction with a reverse Trendelenburg position can be achieved with the head protected by circumferential sand sacks; however, this positioning is unsustainable over a longer period due to increase in intracranial pressure and progressive cardiopulmonary compromise.

Emergency surgical intervention (Box 12.38.5)

Early surgical intervention is now felt to be generally safe and effective. It has consistently shown decreased pulmonary decompensation, and shortened intensive care and overall hospital stays.

Surgical intervention for patients with cervical spine injuries serves the purpose of decompressing the spinal cord, minimizing further trauma to the injured segment, realigning and stabilizing the spinal column, and mobilizing the patient expediently in order to maximize spinal cord recovery. Unlike cord injuries in the thoracic region, cervical spinal cord injuries offer a greater hope for recovery not only due to the propensity for root area functional return but also in terms of cord level recovery. Results of animal experiments and evolving clinical data support the concept of emergent surgical decompression and stabilization with current instrumentation techniques for cervical spine injuries with spinal cord compromise that are not reducible by closed means. A recent ongoing multicentre study also supported the hypothesis that patients with early surgical management have improved outcomes over those treated in a delayed fashion. There is also emerging evidence that surgery within 24h may reduce length of intensive care unit stay and reduce postinjury medical complications.

The role of routine emergent surgical intervention in spinal cord injury remains controversial. Fortunately, most displaced cervical spine injuries can be reduced with closed means using the protocol described earlier. Surgical intervention may be beneficial if indirect decompression of the spinal cord is unsuccessful. Patients with worsening neurological status in the presence of an unstable spine may also be considered for expedient surgical decompression and stabilization. Patients with conditions not amenable to indirect closed decompression, such as traumatic disc herniation, expanding epidural haematoma, depressed lamina fracture, or complex facet fracture dislocations, may similarly benefit from surgical decompression and stabilization (Figure 12.38.7). Patients with unusual distractive injuries, such as occipitocervical dissociations, or patients with acute injuries superimposed on pre-existent spine

Box 12.38.5 Consideration of urgent surgery

- Increasing neurological deficit
- Displaced fracture in ankylosing spinal disorder
- Unsuccessful closed reduction
- Uncooperative, unconscious patient
- Residual compression seen on MRI in patient with neurological deficit.

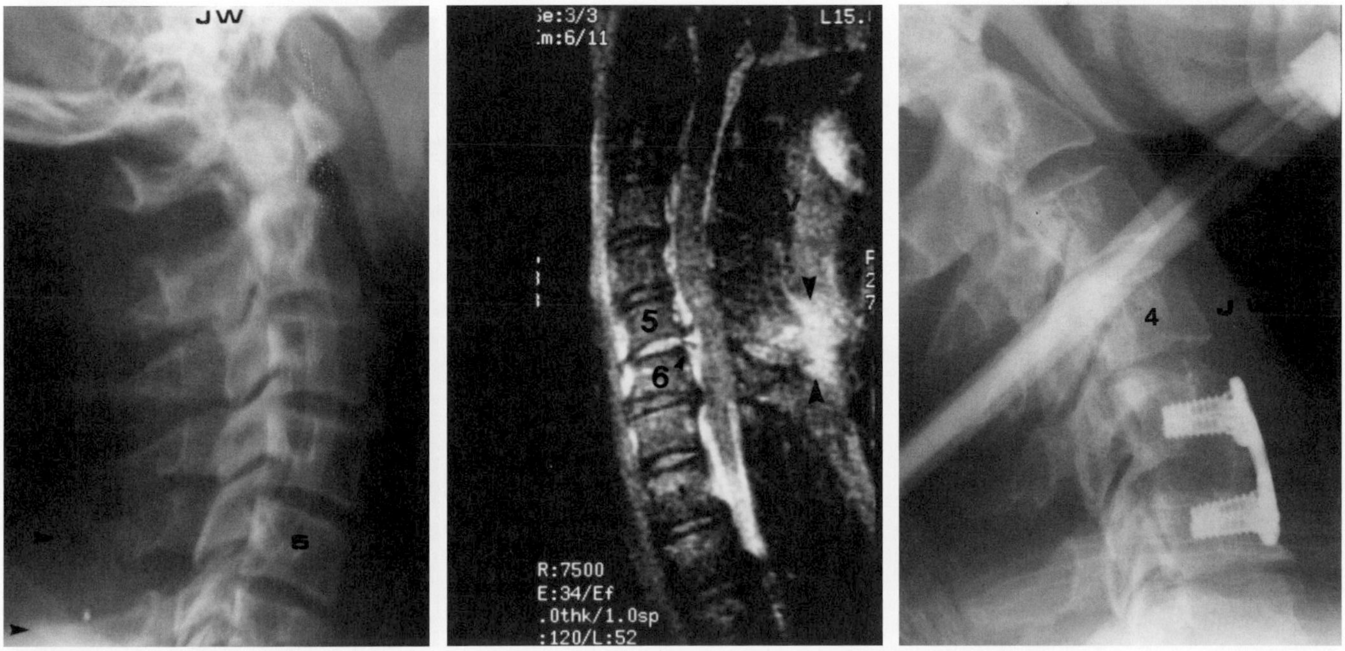

A B C

Fig. 12.38.7 A) This 36-year-old male presented with a complete C5-level tetraplegia and high-grade open fractures of three of his extremities following a high-speed rollover accident. Lateral cervical trauma radiographs demonstrated interspinous C5–6 widening and loss of facet parallelism. The patient received intravenous methylprednisolone and aggressive volume resuscitation. B) An emergency MRI scan demonstrates a large traumatic disc herniation at the C5–6 interspace and disruption of the posterior ligamentous structures of the same level. C) Concomitant with surgical care of the open extremity fractures, an emergency anterior C5–6 discectomy with bone graft and instrumentation was carried out. The time from injury to surgical decompression was calculated to be 6h. The patient improved to an ASIA D level of function within 5 months of injury and currently is a household ambulator living independently.

deformities, such as ankylosing spondylitis or diffuse idiopathic hyperostosis are also candidates for early surgical stabilization due to inability to maintain closed reduction in these patients.

From an anaesthetic point of view, atraumatic intubation and maintenance of normotension is desirable. In any emergent surgical undertaking, the potentially deleterious effects of a 'second hit' in form of hypotension on neural cell survival following initial resuscitation should be considered in preoperative planning. Spine instrumentation should be used with the goal to facilitate early mobilization and the minimum necessary bracing. In considering the various factors previously mentioned, there has been an international trend favouring anterior procedures with rigid locking instrumentation over posterior or combined surgeries for a majority of cervical spine injuries. Exceptions to this observation present in patients with ankylosing spinal disorders or patients with depressed lamina fractures.

Patients with VAI pose a different set of problems in management due to continued bleeding or intimal damage leading to thromboembolic events. Interventional angiography can allow for embolization or stenting of the lesion site as needed. Usually a period anticoagulant therapy is recommended for patients with emboli emanating from intimal vertebral artery injuries as long as spinal cord or unstable column injury has been excluded (Figure 12.38.4). Should the cervical spine injury require surgical care, it is desirable to expedite such surgery so that a suitable anticoagulant therapy for the concurrent VAI can be started as soon as deemed safe. Delay of spine surgery in a patient who has already been started on anticoagulant treatment is usually far more complicated.

Conclusions

From the perspective of spinal cord pathophysiology most primary cellular damage has occurred by 6h or 8h, with cord necrosis present at 24h post-trauma. Current treatment mainly aims to reduce secondary zone spinal cord injury by minimizing cord swelling and maximizing cord perfusion. To date, the most meaningful emergency intervention for cord-injured patients consists of the earliest possible closed reduction of cervical spine dislocations or burst fractures by controlled skeletal traction. While there are few indications for emergency surgical decompression and fusion, the preponderance of recent publications favour early intervention over delayed surgery in patients who have been adequately resuscitated.

Current literature has redefined the role of high-dose methylprednisolone in the management of spinal cord injuries as optional. Novel neuroprotective therapies, including rho antagonists, minocycline, and sodium/glutamate blockers are the main pharmacological agents undergoing investigation.

Preferably, care of patients with spinal cord injury should be concentrated at specifically designated centres at the earliest possible time to allow for comprehensive treatment and to enhance our understanding of these measures by using standardized intervention measures.

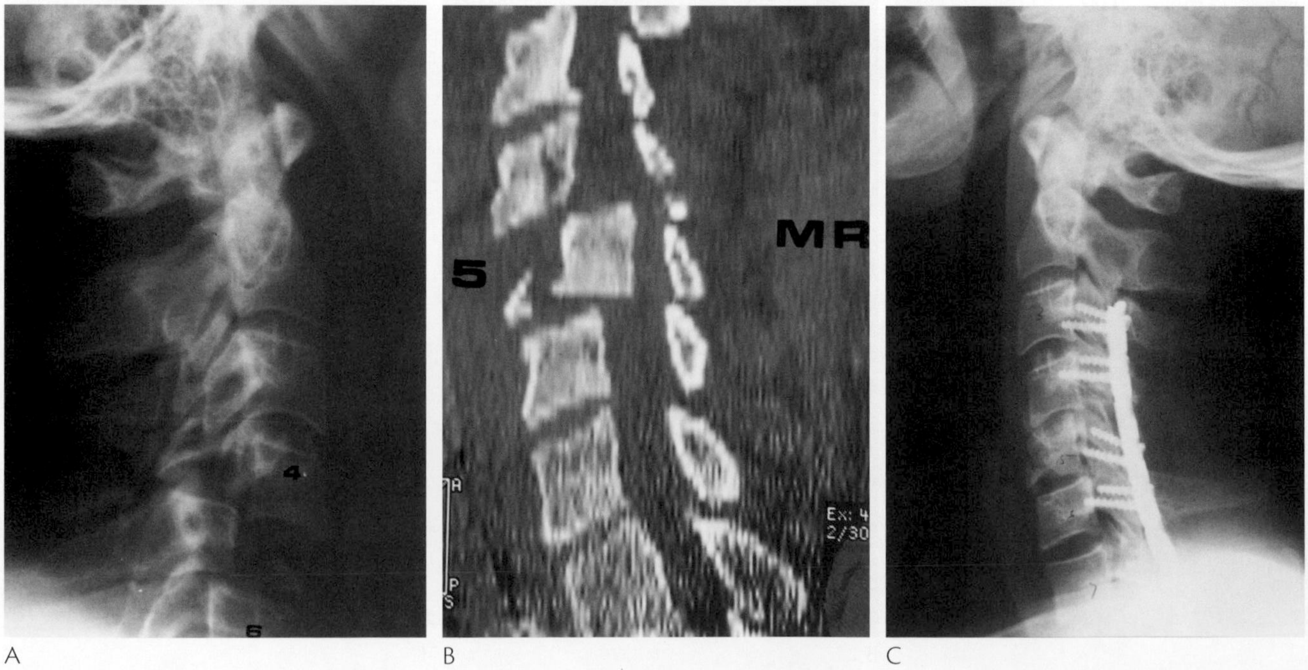

Fig. 12.38.8 A) This lateral cervical spine radiograph demonstrates a C5 burst fracture in a 38-year-old male following a headfirst fall. The patient presented with a complete C4 level tetraplegia. B) Closed reduction attempts up to 60 pounds failed to achieve a reduction. CT demonstrated severe canal impingement through the retropulsed vertebral body and multilevel lamina fractures. C) Owing to failed attempts at achieving realignment of the spinal canal with cranial traction, an indication for early surgical decompression and fusion was given. In light of the multilevel posterior element injuries, which were depressed upon the cord at the C5 level, a posterior approach with two-level laminectomy and posterior plate fixation C3–7 was chosen. This postoperative lateral cervical radiograph demonstrates healing of the injured cervical segments in satisfactory alignment. The patient's neurological function improved to a C6 ASIA A level.

Further reading

Blackmore, C.C. (2003). Evidence-based imaging evaluation of the cervical spine in trauma. *Neuroimaging Clinics of North America*, **13**(2), 283–91.

Brodke, W.P., Chapman, J.R., Andersen, P.A., *et al.* (1997). Anterior posterior stabilization of cervical spine fractures in spinal cord injury. *Orthopaedic Transactions*, **21**, 260.

Fassett, D.R., Dailey, A.T., and Vaccaro, A.R. (2008). Vertebral artery injuries associated with cervical spine injuries: a review of the literature. *Journal of Spinal Disorders and Techniques*, **21**(4), 252–8.

Fehlings, M.G. and Baptiste, D.C. (2005). Current status of clinical trials for acute spinal cord injury. *Injury*, **36**(suppl 2), B113–22.

Fehlings, M.G. and Perrin, R.G. (2006). The timing of surgical intervention in the treatment of spinal cord injury: a systematic review of recent clinical evidence. *Spine*, **31**(11 Suppl), S28–35.

12.39

Upper cervical injuries

Paul A. Anderson

Summary points

- Upper cervical spine injuries should be considered in all blunt trauma patients.
- Critical review of plain radiographs or CT should carefully examine the alignment of the articulations between the occiput-C1 and C1-2 to determine if ligamentous injury is present.
- The initial stabilization of unstable upper cervical injuries usually should avoid the use of traction in favour of the halovest.
- Definitive stabilization is based on fracture type and the status of the cranio-cervical ligaments.

Introduction

The upper cervical spine is a transitional zone between the skull and the mobile cervical spine. It protects the medulla oblongata, spinal cord, and vertebral arteries. Despite this important function, the upper cervical spine has a large range of motion with over 50% of rotational motion and 20% of anterior, posterior, and lateral bending, respectively. The anatomy is complex and has many anomalies that may be associated with important disease processes and surgical procedures.

This chapter will examine injuries of the occipital condyles, craniocervical articulation, the atlas, the atlantoaxial articulation, and finally the axis. Because these five different areas of injury are anatomically and kinematically related, injury to more than one of these locations occurs commonly.

Occipital condyle fractures

Occipital condyle fractures are increasingly being diagnosed with prevalent use of computed tomography (CT) for evaluation of blunt trauma patients following injury. The common mechanisms of injuries are from cranial trauma (impaction of the skull base on the cervical spine) or rapid head deceleration. Occipital condyle fractures should be suspected in all patients with high-energy closed head trauma, altered consciousness, lower cranial nerves paresis, upper cervical spine tenderness, retropharyngeal haematoma or swelling, and in those patients with atlantoaxial instability.

The occipital condyles are concave projections from the caudal surface of the occiput that lie in corresponding concavities of the lateral masses of the atlas. This creates a shallow articulation that is congruous along its entire extent. Normally, separation is less than 2mm between the occipital condyle and the atlantal lateral mass. The paired alar ligaments are primary stabilizers of the occipitoatlantal articulation and extend from the dens tip to tubercles on the inner surface of the occipital condyles. The other important stabilizer is the tectorial membrane which is the continuation of the posterior longitudinal ligament spanning from the posterior aspect of the dens to the basion at the anterior margin of foramen magnum.

Patient presentation

Occipital condyle fractures occur in 1–4% of patients with traumatic brain injury, and have an associated loss of consciousness in up to 65% of cases. In an awake patient, pain and tenderness can be elicited but this may not always be present. Range of motion may be reduced, although it is not recommended that this be checked until stability of the cervical spine is confirmed. Various neurological syndromes may occur, including the XII cranial nerve (hypoglossal) which exits on the anterior lateral aspect of the occipital.

Plain radiographs rarely visualize occipital condyle fractures although retropharyngeal swelling is commonly present. The diagnosis of occipital condyle fractures is usually by CT. The stability of these fractures is related to the status of the alar ligaments and therefore displacement between the occipital condyles and atlantal lateral masses should be carefully analyzed on sagittal and coronal CT reformations (Table 12.39.1). MRI has been shown to evaluate these structures in some instances but requires coronal and fat suppression techniques.

Classification (Figure 12.39.1)

There are three fracture types:

1) Type I fractures are comminuted fractures secondary to impactions of the occipital condyle on the lateral masses of C1. These are stable
2) Type II are skull-base fractures where the fracture line involves a large amount of the occipital condyle
3) Type III are traumatic avulsions from tensile forces of the alar ligament. These may be unstable.

Table 12.39.1 Occipital condyle fractures

Fracture type	Description	Proposed mechanism	Stability	Occ–C1 displacement	C1–2 displacement	Alar ligaments	Recommended treatment
I	Comminuted	Impaction from C1	Stable	None	None	Incompetent (temporarily)	**Collar**
II	Skull base fracture	Impaction from C1	Stable	None	None	Intact	**Collar**
	Separation	Impaction from C1	Unstable	Yes	None	Incompetent	**Halo vest** Occ–C2 fusion
III	Avulsion fracture No displacement	Alar ligament avulsion	Stable	No	None	Incompetent (temporarily)	**Collar**
	Avulsion fracture Minimal displacement	Alar ligament avulsion	Unstable	Yes	–	Incompetent (temporarily)	**Halo vest**
	Avulsion fracture AOD	Alar ligament avulsion	Unstable	Yes	+/–	Incompetent	**Occ–C2 fusion**

Author's recommendations are in bold face.

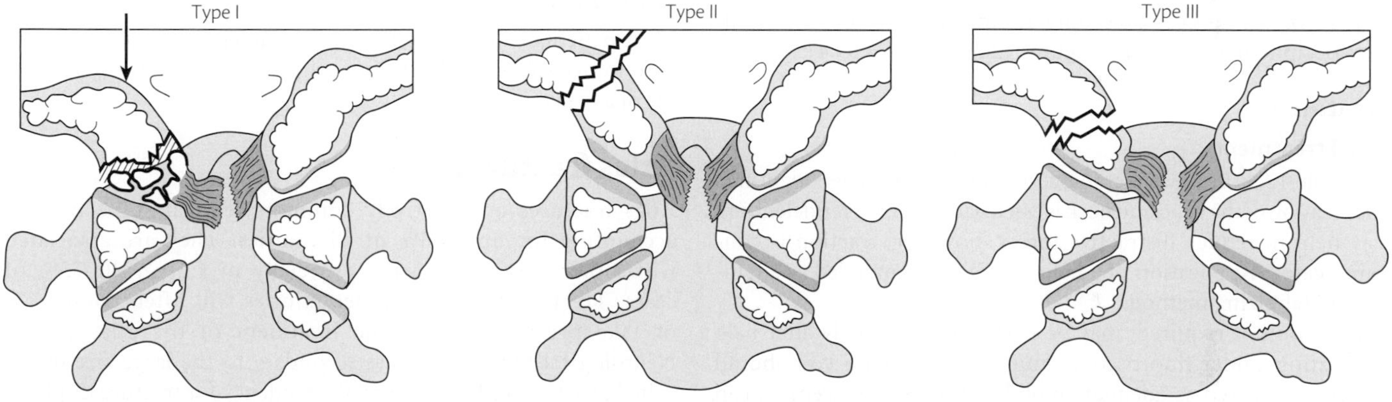

Fig. 12.39.1 Classification of occipital condyle fractures. Type I are stable impacted fractures secondary to axial loading. Type II are basilar skull fractures that involve the occipital condyle. They may be associated with complete separation of the occipital condyle from the skull base. Type III are avulsion fractures of the alar ligaments. They may be associated with occipitocervical instability.

Treatment

See Table 12.39.1.

Craniocervical instability

Craniocervical instability refers to injuries resulting in displacement or potential displacement between the occipital condyles and atlantal facet articulations, or injuries to the ligaments that stabilize these joints. Craniocervical instability is life threatening and until recently, survivors of dislocations were only reported in small case series. Most injuries are highly unstable. Spine clearance protocols using modern imaging including CT and, in some cases, magnetic resonance imaging (MRI) have led to an increasing recognition of these injuries. Neurological deficits occur in up to 40% of cases. Associated injuries are common.

Classification of craniocervical instability (Figure 12.39.2)

1) Grade I normal CT but increased MRI signal in craniocervical ligamentous structures or occipitoatlantal joints
2) Grade II, abnormal displacement of the occipitoatlantal articulation and abnormalities on MRI suggesting injury to AO joint, alar ligament or tectorial membrane.

A simple classification system is based on direction of displacement, Figure 12.39.2. Other systems take into account that there is a spectrum of injury severity as described below:

Diagnosis

Craniocervical injuries are often overlooked and have a delayed diagnosis in up to 40% of cases despite modern imaging. Also there is a strong association with delayed diagnosis and neurological

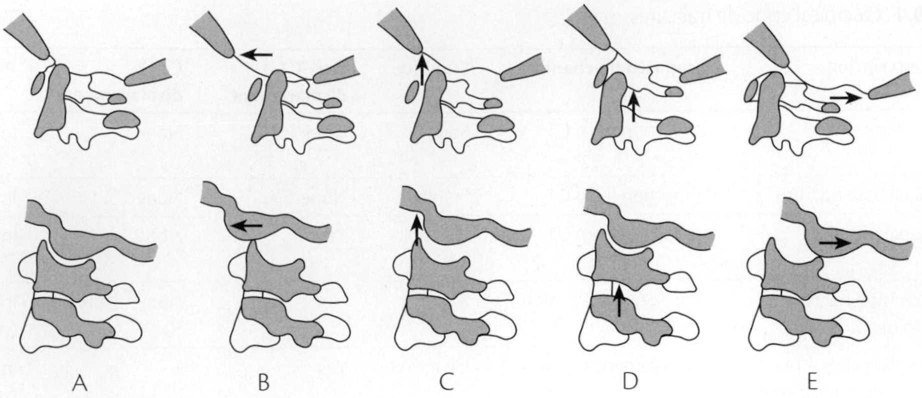

Fig. 12.39.2 Classification of craniocervical instability. A) Normal. B) Anterior occipitoatlantal dislocation. C) Vertical occipitoatlantal dislocation. D) Vertical occipitoatlantal dislocation with C1–2 diastasis. E) Posterior occipitoatlantal dislocation.

deterioration. Joint asymmetry is abnormal and gapping of more 2mm indicates disruption of the craniocervical ligaments. Another sensitive measurement based on two plain radiographic findings is the Harris rule of 12. First the basilar dens interval (BDI) is less than 12mm. Secondly the distance from the basion to a line drawn along the posterior aspect of the axis (posterior axillary line) is less than 12mm. Distances exceeding 12mm on either of these indicates occipitoatlantal injury (Figures 12.39.3 and 12.39.4).

Treatment

Initial treatment

See Table 12.39.2. Once a craniocervical injury has been identified stabilization of the head and neck is essential. Reverse Trendelenburg may help to reduce distractive forces, however, traction is contraindicated. Application of a halo vest is recommended as a temporary stabilizing method.

Reduction, if required, may be performed manually after halo application under fluoroscopic guidance. The halo vest should not be considered as adequate mobilization as displacement can occur and, in particular, distraction may be created at the craniocervical junction. Verification of alignment should be repeatedly performed while awaiting definitive treatment, especially after upright immobilization.

Definitive treatment

See Table 12.39.2

Outcomes

Most patients will achieve fusion, and unless there is a complete cord injury spinal cord function usually improves. Many patients die of associated injuries.

Atlas fractures

Atlas fractures are relatively common cervical spine injuries accounting for up to 8% of all injuries. They are associated with other cervical injuries, especially of C2, in 30–75% of cases. Treatment of these other injuries will often complicate or take precedence over the treatment of the atlas injury. Neurological injuries are rare secondary to the large size of the spinal canal at this location and the tendency for fracture displacement to occur radially with resultant increase in the size of the spinal canal.

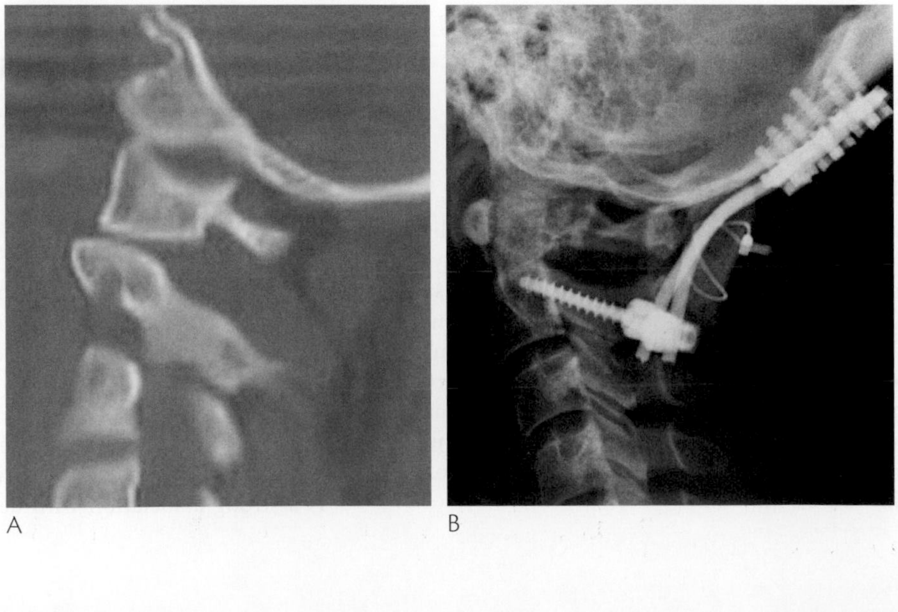

Fig. 12.39.3 Thirty-nine-year-old female involved in car crash sustained abdominal injury and open ulna fracture. She initially had laparotomy and debridement of forearm fracture. A) Sagittal CT shows subluxation of right occipitoatlantal articulation. This was present bilaterally. B) Reduction was achieved with a halo vest and a posterior occipitocervical fusion was performed.

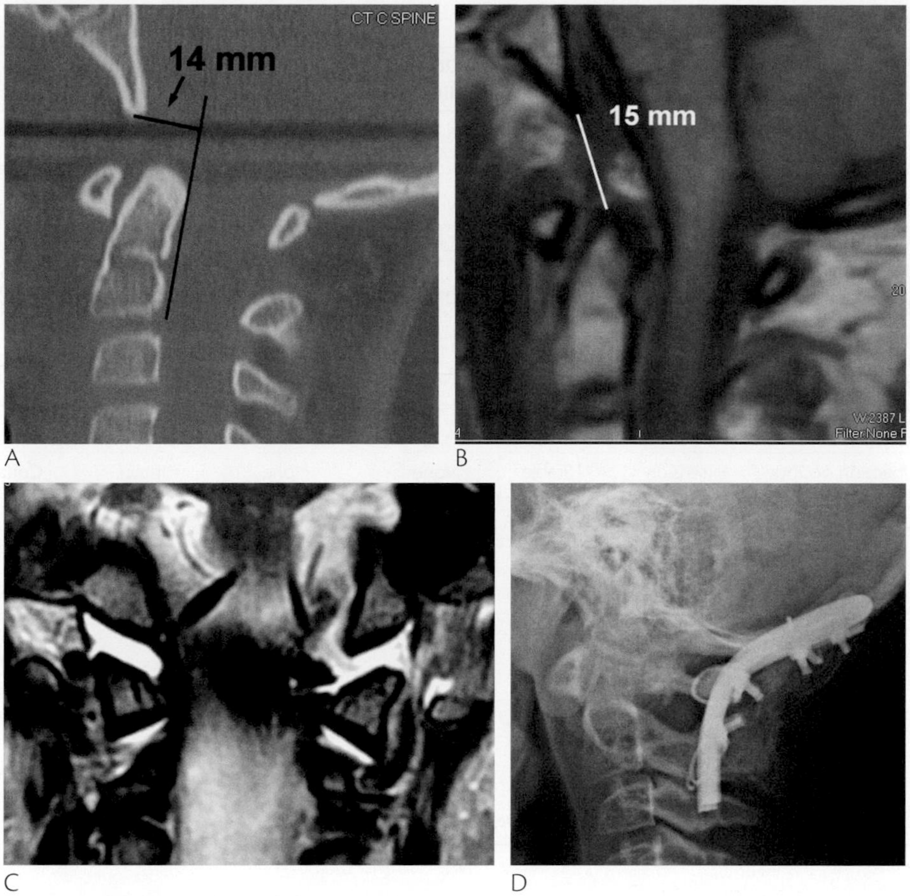

Fig. 12.39.4 Ten-year-old boy who sustained facial injuries and was noted to have XII nerve palsy. A) CT showing unrecognized increased interval between dens posterior dental line and basion suggestive of craniocervical instability. B) MRI 2 days later shows increased basion-dens interval now exceeding Harris rule of 12. C) Coronal MRI shows distraction at both occipitoatlantal and atlantoaxial facets. D) Postoperative occipitocervical fusion with cable-rod construct and rib bone graft.

Table 12.39.2 Patterns of craniocervical instability

Fracture type	Description	Stable	Occ–C1 displacement	C1–2 displacement	Alar ligaments	Recommended treatment
I	Normal CT alignment Positive MRI	Yes	No	No	Intact	**Collar**
II	Normal alignment Positive traction test	Unstable	+/–	+/–	Ruptured	Halo vest **Occ–C2 fusion**
III	Displacement >2mm	Unstable	Yes	+/–	Ruptured	Halo vest **Occ–C2 fusion**

Author's recommendations are in bold face.

The anatomical characteristics of the atlas lead to unique fracture patterns (Table 12.39.3). Displacement of the ring structure of the atlas usually requires a minimum of two fractures, especially when injury results from axial loading secondary to abnormal hoop stresses. The only structurally important musculoligamentous structures attached to the atlas are the transverse ligament and longus coli muscles making avulsion injuries rare. The large thick lateral masses favour injury patterns which involve the smaller arches. From an anterior projection, lateral masses are wedge-shaped. Therefore axially directed forces are transferred laterally and tend to laterally displace the lateral masses. This is resisted at first by the anterior and posterior arches, then by the transverse ligament and finally by the alar ligaments.

The mechanisms of injury are usually due to axial loading forces from blows to the cranium and hyperextension. Lateral displacement of greater than 6.9mm of the C1 relative to C2 lateral masses on plain radiographs is consistent with complete transverse ligament disruption. As the lateral masses displace, the cranium settles downward on the cervical spine with concomitant rostral migration of the dens with possibility of brain stem compression (Figure 12.39.5).

Table 12.39.3 Classification and treatment of atlas fractures

	Fracture type	Proposed mechanism	Forces	Stable	Occ–C1 displacement	C1–2 displacement	Transverse ligament	Recommended treatment
Anterior	Transverse avulsion	Avulsion longis coli	Extension	Stable	None	None	Intact	**Collar**
	Isolated arch	Shear from dens	Extension	Stable	None	None	Intact	**Collar**
	Plough fracture	Shear from dens	Extension	Unstable	None	Posterior	Intact	**Collar**
Lateral mass	Extraspinal	Impaction occipital condyle	Lateral compression	Stable or unstable	Caudal	Cranial	Intact	**Collar** **Halo vest**
	Separation	Impaction occipital condyle	Lateral compression	Stable or unstable	Caudal	Cranial	Ruptured	**Halo vest**
	Coronal with posterior AOD	Impaction occipital condyle	Lateral compression and extension	Unstable	Posterior	None	Intact	**Reduction and Occ–C2 fusion**
Posterior	Isolated arch	Impaction occiput and C2 lamina/ spinous process	Extension	Stable	None	None	Intact	**Collar**
Comminuted injuries	Comminuted Without TL injury	Impaction occipital condyle	Axial loading	Stable	None	None	Intact	Collar **Halo vest**
	Comminuted With TL injury	Impaction occipital condyle	Axial loading	Unstable	Caudal	Lateral and cranial	Ruptured	Collar **Halo vest** Posterior C1–2 fusion Posterior Osteosynthesis Anterior Osteosynthesis

The author's preferred treatment is in bold.

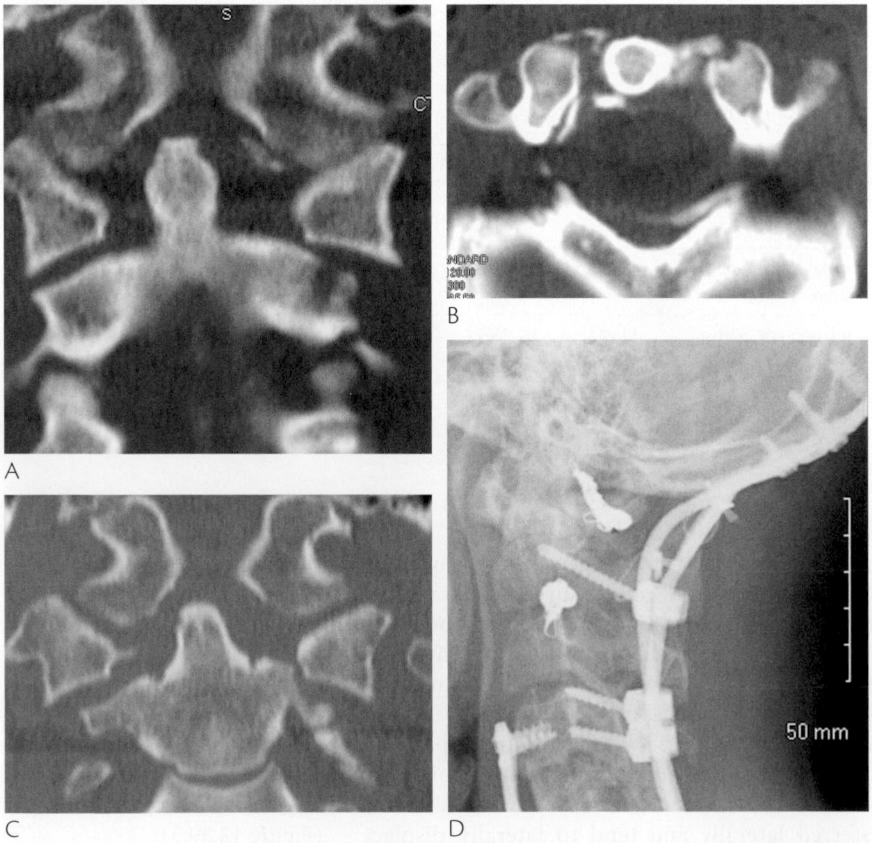

Fig. 12.39.5 Thirty-two-year-old motorcyclist sustained C5 and C6 burst fracture with complete C5 quadriplegia. A comminuted atlas fracture was treated with a collar. Two months later he developed brain stem compression from cranial settling and medullary compression from the dens. Traction improved alignment and posterior occipitocervical fusion was performed complicated by vertebral artery injury of a traumatic pseudoaneurysm. A) Fracture of the left lateral mass of C2 and 5mm displacement of C1 over C2 is seen on coronal CT. B) Bilateral anterior arch fracture and fracture posterior to right lateral mass of atlas. This creates potential for separation of the two lateral masses. C) Significantly more displacement of the C1 lateral masses over C2 is present. This indicates rupture of the transverse ligament. D) Postoperative lateral radiograph following laminectomy of C1 and occipitocervical fusion.

Classification

See Figure 12.39.6.

Stable fractures

Type 1 isolated arch fractures are stable, as are many Type 2 and Type 3 fractures when the transverse ligament is intact. This includes bursting-type fractures with less than 6.9mm displacement and lateral mass fractures without significant lateral displacement.

Unstable fractures

Type 2 bursting fractures with greater than 6.9mm displacement are unstable and may have progressive displacement despite treatment. The transverse ligament injury may be either an avulsion facture or midsubstance tear; the former having a better healing potential. The plough fracture with posterior C1–2 dislocation and the lateral mass fracture with occipitocervical dislocation are highly unstable.

Treatment of isolated atlas fractures

Stable injuries

Stable injuries can be immobilized in a collar for 6–12 weeks. Controversy exists regarding the stable bursting fractures as some authors recommend use of a halo vest. Serial upright radiographs including open mouth views should be critically analyzed for displacement during immobilization.

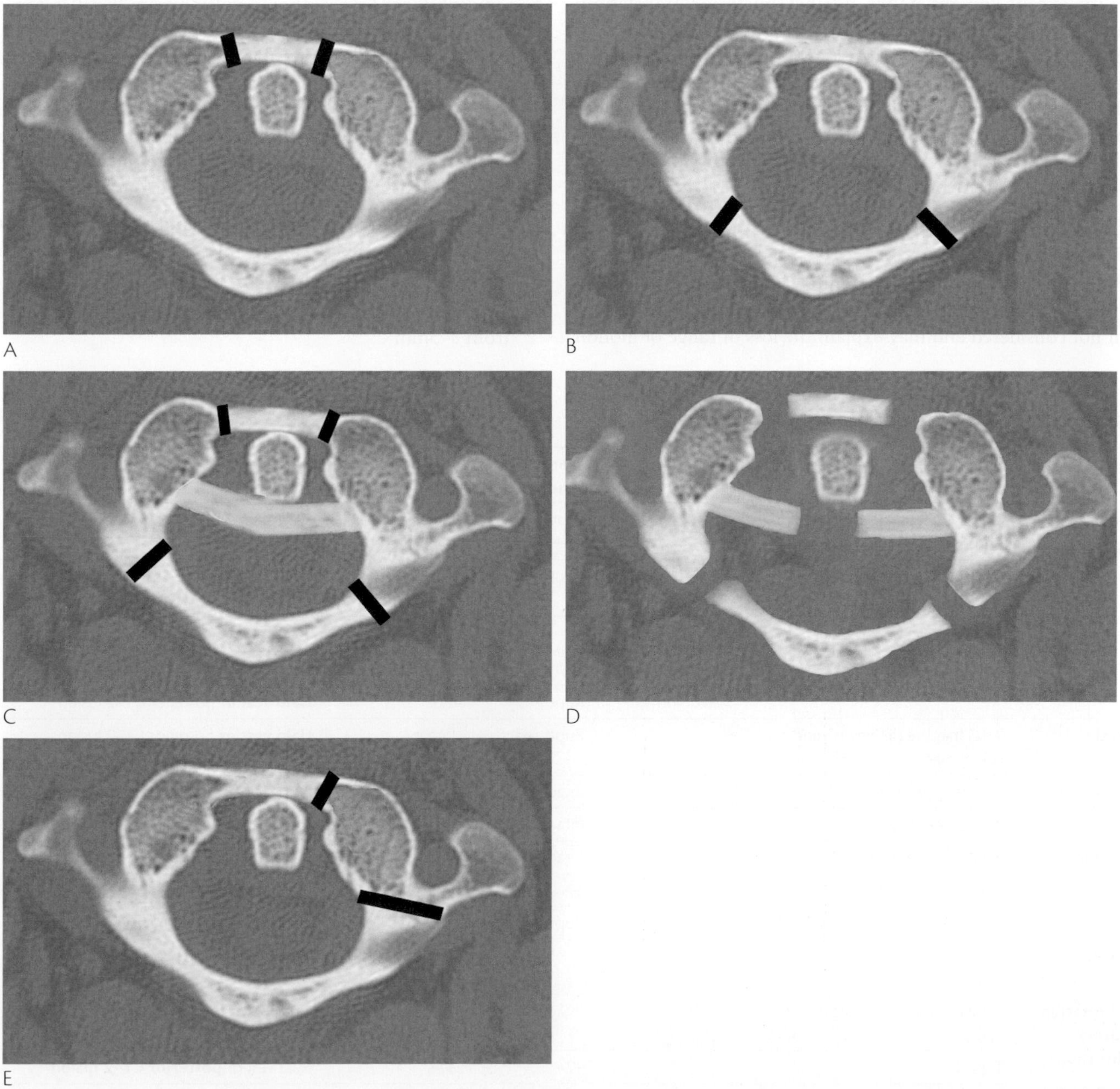

Fig. 12.39.6 Classification of atlas fractures. A) Type I: stable anterior arch. B) Type I: stable posterior arch. C) Type II: bursting fracture without TL ligament rupture. D) Type II: bursting fracture with TL ligament rupture. E) Type III: lateral mass fracture.

Unstable injuries

No consensus is available regarding the best treatment of the unstable burst-type fractures. Osteosynthesis is appealing, as reduction is theoretically obtained and no fusion is performed. Occipitocervical fusion is indicated for displaced fractures, excessive comminution, subluxation of the occipitocervical articulation, or when brain stem compression is present. In many of these cases, a C1 laminectomy is also performed (see Figure 12.39.5).

See Table 12.39.3 for details

Atlantoaxial instability

Atlantoaxial instability is rarely considered as a separate entity as it is frequently a component of other more obvious injuries (Table 12.39.4). The atlantoaxial articulation lacks inherent bony stability except for resistance against posterior translation. Ligamentous stability is provided by the transverse and alar ligaments. The C1–2 facet articulations are biconcave and have a wide range of motion and if imaged with the head turned (even minimally) may appear subluxated. The facet capsules are redundant to allow motion and, therefore, have little inherent strength. Injury to the alar and transverse ligaments or their bony attachments can result in displacement in anteroposterior, lateral, or axial (rotation) directions.

Aetiology

The most common aetiology of atlantoaxial instability is displaced odontoid and atlas fractures. Subluxation of the C1–2 facets is often not considered and may explain the loss of range of motion after healing. More specific injuries, generally considered as atlantoaxial instability, are transverse ligament rupture and rotatory subluxation. Transverse ligament rupture occurs from tensile failure of the ligament or bony attachment to the atlas associated with anterior shear so that anterior subluxation occurs.

Classification

Radiographically, atlantoaxial instability from transverse ligament rupture is present when the anterior atlantodens interval (ADI) exceeds 3mm in adults and 5mm in children. When the ADI exceeds 7–8mm then the secondary restraints, the alar ligaments, have been injured. Because of injury to the alar ligaments this condition may be associated with occipitoatlantal instability. Rarely, vertical atlantoaxial instability occurs as evidenced by diastasis greater than 2mm between the facets. The ligamentous injury may be a midsubstance tear or a bony avulsion from the atlas, the latter having a better prognosis for healing.

Rotatory subluxation occurs almost exclusively in children usually from low energy trauma or following infection (Grisel's syndrome). The child presents with a 'cock robin' head position: the head rotated to one side and tilted to the other. Radiographs are difficult to assess due to the head rotation. The injuries are best evaluated with CT and three-dimensional reconstructions. There are four types:

1) Type I is rotatory subluxation around the dens with intact transverse ligament. This is difficult to differentiate from normal physiological motion
2) Type II is associated with transverse ligament injury with ADI from 3–5mm

Table 12.39.4 Patterns of atlantoaxial instability

Direction	Injury type		Transverse ligament	Alar ligament	Treatment
Anterior	Odontoid fracture without transverse ligament rupture		Intact	Intact except Type 1	See Table 13.39.5
	Odontoid fracture with transverse ligament rupture		Ruptured	Intact except Type 1	**Posterior C1–2 fusion**
	Transverse ligament injury				
		Midsubstance	Ruptured	+/–	Halo vest
		Avulsion	Ruptured	+/–	**Halo vest or** posterior C1–2 fusion
Lateral	Atlas fracture (Jefferson's and lateral mass)		Ruptured	Intact	**Halo vest or** posterior C1–2 fusion
	Odontoid fracture		Intact	Intact	Odontoid screw or **posterior C1–2 fusion**
	Axis lateral mass fracture		Intact	Intact	**Halo vest or** cervicothoracic brace
Posterior	Atlas fracture (Plough)		Intact	Intact	**Posterior C1–2 fusion**
	Odontoid fracture		+/–	Intact	See Table 12.39.5
	Dislocation (Fielding Type IV)		Ruptured	Ruptured	**Posterior C1–2 or occipitocervical fusion**
Vertical	Alar ligament (atlanto-occipital instability)				**Posterior occipitocervico fusion**
Axial rotation (rotatory subluxation)	Type I (no transverse ligament injury		Intact	Intact	**Halter traction and collar**
	Type II		+/–	+/–	Halo vest or **posterior C1–2 fusion**
	Type III		Ruptured	+/–	**Posterior C1–2 fusion**

The author's preferred treatment is in bold type.

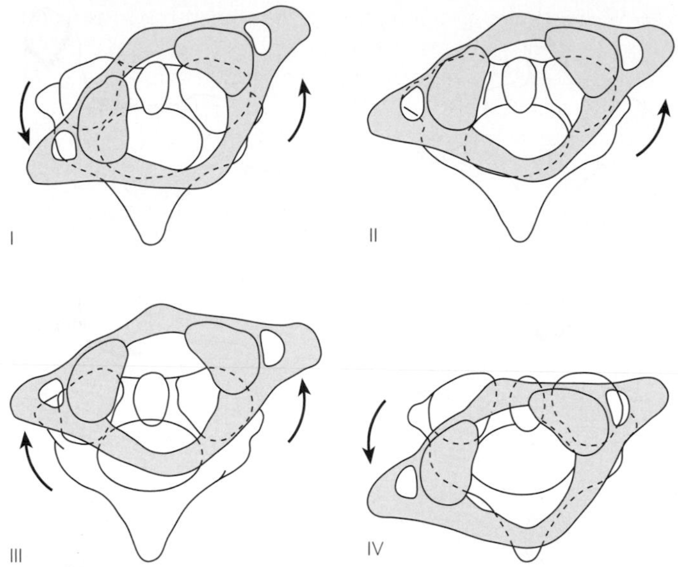

Fig. 12.39.7 Fielding classification of rotatory subluxation of the atlas. (After Wilson and McWhorter.)

3) Type III is similar to Type II with greater than 5mm ADI
4) Type IV is the rare posterior dislocation where the atlantal arch is posterior to the dens (Figure 12.39.7).

Treatment

The treatment of patients having other associated injuries such as atlas and odontoid fractures will be described elsewhere in this chapter. Isolated injuries resulting in atlantoaxial instability are discussed as to follows.

Transverse ligament rupture

The healing of isolated transverse ligament injury is dependent on the type of tear (midsubstance or bony avulsion), the severity of subluxation, and the patient age. Young children with smaller amounts of subluxation or patients who can be maintained in a reduced position and who have bony avulsion may be treated in a halo vest for 12 weeks. They are the assessed by flexion-extension radiographs at the end of treatment for atlantoaxial stability. Adults and patients without bony avulsions are best treated by posterior C1–2 fusion with screw fixation.

Rotatory subluxation

Traumatic Type I rotatory subluxations do not have a significant ligament injury and are treated by reduction and immobilization. Usually the reduction can be achieved by muscle relaxation and analgesia or halter traction. Resistant cases may require tong traction. After reduction immobilization for a short time in a collar is prudent. If redisplacement occurs, an injury to the transverse ligament should be considered.

Types II and III are characterized by presumptive injury to the transverse ligament. Initial treatment is aimed at reduction which can be accomplished by halter, tong traction, or halo. In acute injuries, the best treatment remains unknown given the rarity of these conditions. Options include halo vest immobilization or C1–2 posterior fusion. In younger patients, halo vest immobilization can be attempted. In the author's experience, recurrent deformity is common (Figure 12.39.10). Posterior C1–2 fusion with rigid fixation is indicated for adult patients or those who fail halo vest immobilization. Type IV injuries are associated with ligamentous injury to the alar ligaments and therefore an occipitocervical fusion should be preformed.

Vertical distraction injuries

Diastasis greater than 2mm between the atlantoaxial articulations indicates injury to the alar ligament and tectorial ligament creating an unstable craniocervical segment. These injuries should be treated with posterior occipitocervical fusion.

Odontoid fractures

Odontoid fractures are the most common fracture occurring in the axis and account for up to 25% of cervical injuries.

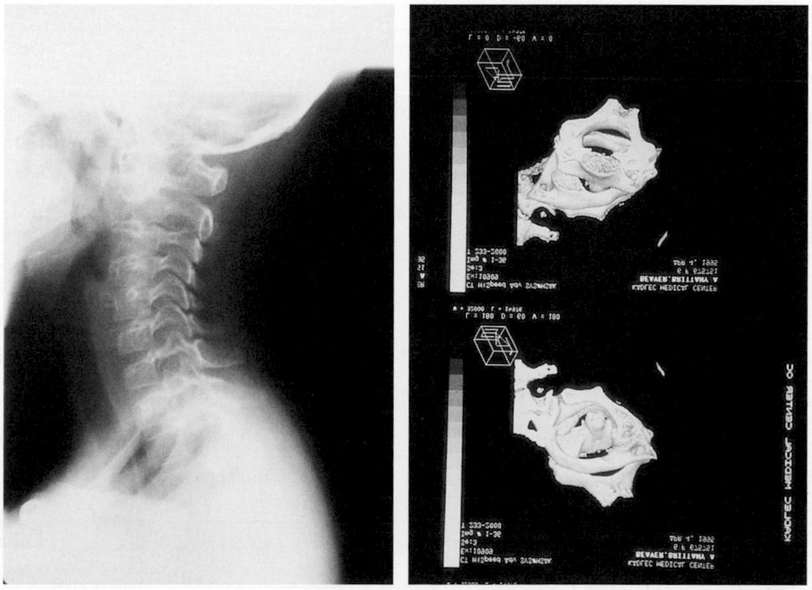

A B

Fig. 12.39.8 A 6-year-girl fell from a tree sustaining humerus fracture. Over the next 3 days she developed torticollis. A) One month later her lateral radiograph shows possible rotatory subluxation of the atlas. B) Three-dimensional CT reconstructions demonstrate Type II rotatory subluxation with an increased atlantodens interval. She was initially treated by reduction and halo vest but had recurrent subluxation 3 months later. Definitive treatment was a posterior C1–2 fusion.

Biomechanically, the odontoid process functions as an axis around which the atlas rotates. The relationship between C1 and C2 is maintained by the odontoid process, the atlas, and the transverse ligament. These combined structures prevent shear in the antero-posterior and lateral directions. Loss of stability from odontoid fractures places the spinal cord at risk and is a frequent cause of fatality especially in the elderly.

Classification (Figure 12.39.9)

Type I

Type I injuries are an avulsion fracture at the dens tip from the attachment of the alar ligaments. Because the alar ligaments are primarily responsible for craniocervical stability, Type I fractures may be associated with atlanto-occipital instability. This is assessed by critical analysis of the occiput–C1 and C1–2 articulations and the Harris rule of 12.

Type II

Type II injures occur through the waist of the odontoid and do not have fracture lines that involve the C1–2 articulations. Grauer has further classified Type II fractures to aid in determining treatment. Type IIA are non-displaced. Types IIB are displaced transverse or those with oblique fracture lines that are oriented anterior-superior to posterior-inferior. Type IIC are comminuted or have fracture lines that are oriented posterior-superior to anterior-inferior. Type IIB injuries are amenable to anterior screw fixation whereas Type IIC would be significantly more difficult to fixate as the fracture line runs parallel to the screw.

Type III

Type III are C2 vertebral body fractures at the odontoid base which extend into the atlantoaxial articulations. These involve cancellous bone and therefore have a good potential for osseous healing.

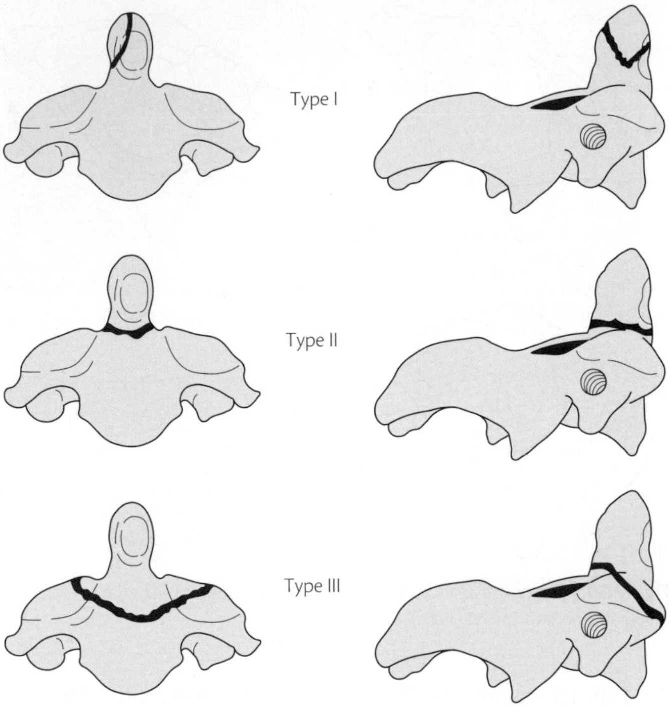

Fig. 12.39.9 Classification of odontoid fractures. (After Rechtine and Landsman.)

In addition to the fracture location, the status of the atlantoaxial articulations should be considered. Displacement may occur unilaterally or bilaterally in either anterior, lateral, or posterior direction. Rarely vertical distraction may be present. The presence of initial odontoid displacement and therefore accompanied by atlantoaxial subluxation is a major predictor of poor outcome and continued instability.

Table 12.39.5 Odontoid fracture

Fracture type	Description	Subtype	Stable	Atlantoaxial displacement	Transverse ligament	Recommended treatment
I	Dens tip fracture	Non displaced (occiput–C1)	Stable	None	Intact	**Collar**
		Displaced (occiput–C1)	Unstable	+/–	+/–	**Occ–C2 fusion**
II	Transverse fracture waist	Low risk	Unstable	<5mm	Intact	Collar **Halo vest** Odontoid screw Posterior C1–2 fusion
	Transverse fracture waist	High risk	Unstable	>5mm	+/–	Collar Halo vest **Odontoid screw** **Posterior C1–2 fusion**
	Transverse fracture waist	Elderly	Unstable	Cranial	Intact	**Collar** Halo vest Odontoid screw **Posterior C1–2 fusion**
	Transverse fracture synchondrosis	Paediatric	Unstable	Cranial	Ruptured	**Halo vest** Minerva cast
III	Body fracture		Unstable	+/–	Intact	**Collar** Halo vest

The author's preferred treatment is in bold.

Treatment

The choice of treatment should be based on a synthesis of the best available evidence, patient factors and patient preference (Table 12.39.5). Two recent systematic reviews provide evidence based data that can guide treatment although they are limited by the poor quality nature of the studies included in their analysis.

Type I

Type I injuries without atlanto-occipital instability are stable and can be treated with either simple immobilization or halo vest. Although only a few case reports are available satisfactory outcomes have been achieved with either treatment. Given the lower risk of brace management, the author recommends non-halo vest management. Type I fractures associated with occipitoatlantal instability are treated by posterior occipitocervical fusion.

Type II

Type II fractures have a poorer prognosis secondary to associated instability, and small fracture surfaces involving mainly cortical bone. Up to 50% develop non-union. Risk factors include

- Initial fracture displacement and angulation
- Displacement and angulation at the time of discharge
- Fracture gap greater than 1mm at discharge
- Patient age greater than 65.

Many treatments of Type II fractures are advocated but no consensus exists for the exact indications for non-operative treatment versus surgery or the best surgical approach. Overall healing rates using non-rigid braces, halo vests, odontoid screws and posterior fusion are 51.3%, 68.4%, 84%, and, 93.4% respectively. Based on this information in younger patients, the best treatment is defined by the relative risk of healing as well as the shared decision making with the patients.

In patients who are at low risk of non-union, halo vest immobilization for 12 weeks is recommended. Healing in all Type II patients treated by halo vests is 68% but in this selected group would be expected to occur in up to 80% of patients. Younger patients who are at risk for non-union are surgical candidates. Surgical indications include displacement greater than 5mm, or angulation greater than 20 degrees, inability to control fracture site displacement in a halo vest, or persistent fracture gapping.

Both anterior and posterior techniques can be used to treat Type II dens fractures. Posterior C1–2 fixation with rigid fixation has a high fusion rate with low rate of adverse events (Figure 12.39.10). The disadvantage of this technique is the loss of atlantoaxial rotation. Anterior odontoid screw fixation is an alternative for fractures with favourable patterns (Grauer IIB) that can be reduced (Figure 12.39.11). Odontoid screw is an osteosynthesis technique where no fusion is performed thereby theoretically maintaining atlantoaxial motion. Only about 50% of normal atlantoaxial rotation is preserved after odontoid screw fixation. Complications such as implant failure, loss of reduction, and non-union are significantly higher with odontoid screws compared to posterior fusion.

Type II fractures in the elderly (Figure 12.39.10)

Odontoid fractures occur in a bimodal distribution with peaks in the third and eighth decade, these latter are usually the result of low-energy trauma and initially may appear minimally displaced. However, these fractures are associated with a high mortality similar to that seen following hip fractures. Causes of death include respiratory failure, cardiac arrest, and thromboembolic disease. Other complications include decreased respiratory function, dysphagia, fracture displacement despite rigid immobilization, multiple medical comorbidities, and fixation failure. Much of the morbidity may be related to the treatment. The halo vest is poorly tolerated in this age group with high rates of complications and death reported. Surgery in the elderly patient with an odontoid

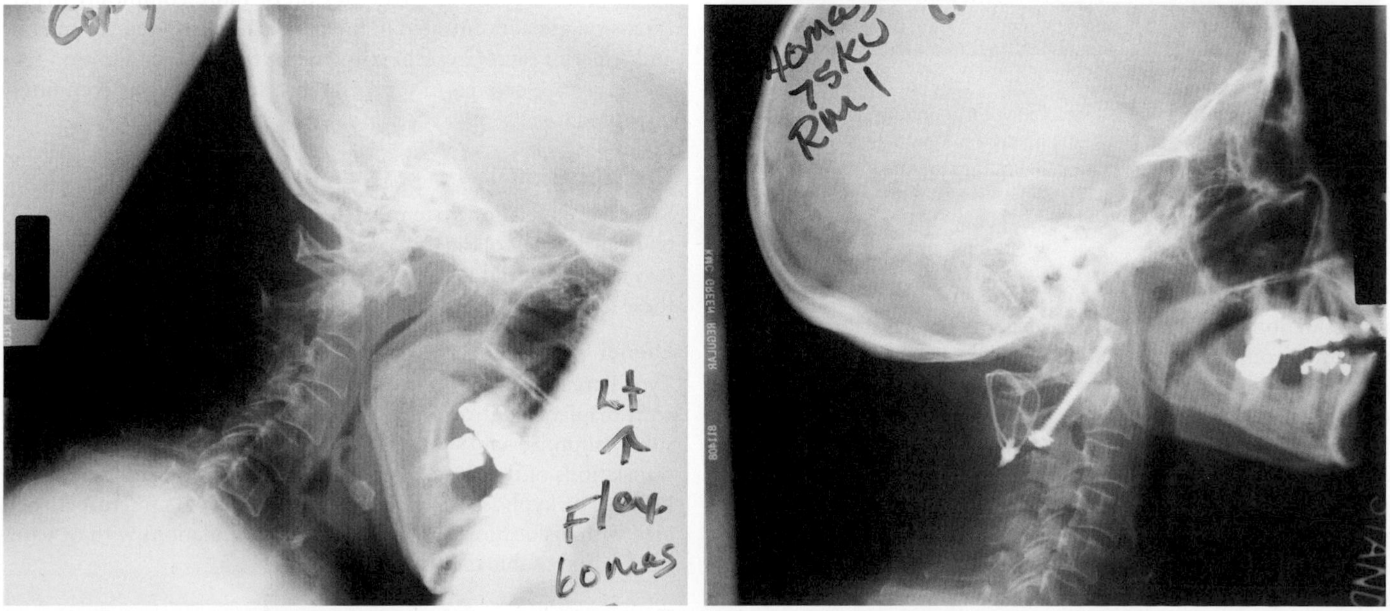

A B

Fig. 12.39.10 Posterior fusion of elderly patient with Type II odontoid fracture. A) Lateral radiograph of 80-year-old lady showing displaced Type II odontoid fracture. Non-operative treatment failed secondary to displacement and she was treated with posterior transarticular C1–2 screw fixation. B) Postoperative lateral radiograph.

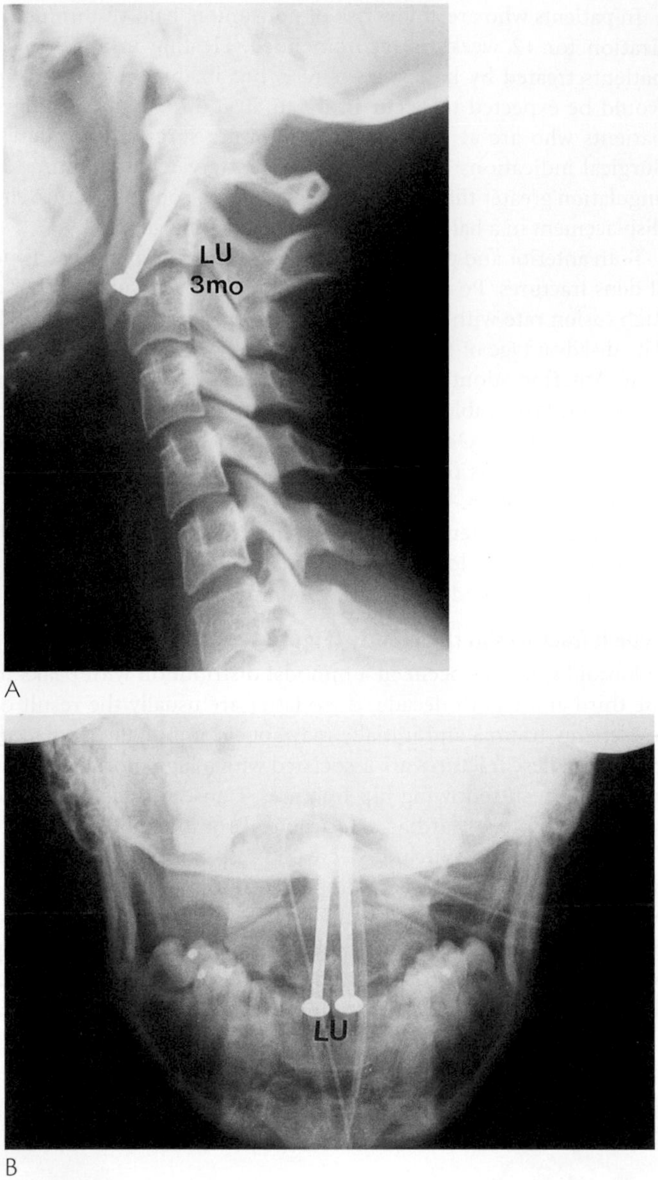

Fig. 12.39.11 Odontoid screw fixation of a Type II odontoid fracture.
A) A 32-year-old struck on head sustaining a Type II odontoid fracture. Lateral radiograph after odontoid screw fixation. B) Postoperative open mouth view. Note two screws were used but equal results have been published using a single screw.

fracture is challenging due to poor bone stock, difficulty in achieving reduction, loss of fixation, pre-existing deformity making screw placement difficult, and medical comorbidities. The choice of an anterior or posterior technique remains controversial. Higher rates of implant failure secondary to screw cut out from the C2 body and higher mortality have been reported after odontoid screw fixation compared with posterior C1–2 fusion with screw fixation. However the mortality rate is probably lower with surgery than without surgery (10% versus 20%).

The author's recommendation is that odontoid fractures in elderly patients are treated similarly to hip fractures. In healthy active patients with normal mentation, early surgery is indicated. In most cases this is achieved by a posterior C1–2 fusion with screw-based technique. Alternatively odontoid screw fixation can be performed in cases having adequate C2 bone stock and favourable fracture patterns. In patients with significant comorbidities, who are inactive, or have dementia, non-operative treatment in a collar is warranted. The goal is immediate immobilization and avoidance of complications. Such patients are not expected to heal their fracture but rarely will have long-term sequelae.

Type III

Type III fractures rarely require surgery. Surgical indications include instability despite non-operative treatment, and failure of fusion. Healing success with non-rigid immobilization and the halo vest are 92% and 94% respectively (see Table 12.39.5). Therefore this author recommends an attempt at immobilization in a cervicothoracic brace for Type III fractures. For failure of bracing, a posterior fusion is recommended.

Traumatic spondylolisthesis of the axis

Acute traumatic spondylolisthesis of the axis, also called hangman's fracture, is caused by a fracture in the area of the pars interarticularis creating separation of the anterior and posterior aspects of the C2 vertebrae. Displacement increases the size of the spinal canal, accounting for the rare association of spinal cord injury expected in cases of severe displacement. Despite the injury's ominous name, its overall prognosis is good with few patients requiring surgical treatment or having long-term disability.

The unique anatomy predisposes the axis to this injury. The axis is characterized by the dens or odontoid process which projects cranially from the C2 body around which the atlas rotates. The C2 body is connected to strong lateral masses by broad pedicles. The superior articular facet, which articulates with C1, is located on the cranial surface of the lateral mass. In all other vertebrae, the inferior facet is located directly under the superior facet but in the axis it is located posteriorly connected by a relatively small isthmus or pars interarticularis. This pars is a short tubular structure bounded by the C2 nerve root cranially and the vertebral artery caudally. Bending moments from hyperflexion or more commonly hyperextension are concentrated in the pars region between the inferior and superior facets, resulting in tensile fractures. In addition tensile forces are created in the C2–3 disc space which is commonly disrupted.

Classification

Several classification systems have been developed and all are based on displacement of the C2–3 disc and facet (Figure 12.39.12). These two factors should be considered when classifying and managing these injuries.

Effendi

Type I are non-displaced pars fractures. Type II have pars fractures with displacement or angulation of the C2–3 disc without facet subluxation. Several subtypes have been identified: those with only translations of the C2–3 disc and others with angulation, either in lordosis or kyphosis. Type III fractures are a pars fracture associated with dislocations of the C2–3 facet articulations with or without C2 body subluxations.

Treatment

Many treatment methods have been recommended for traumatic spondylolisthesis of the axis and they include collar immobilization,

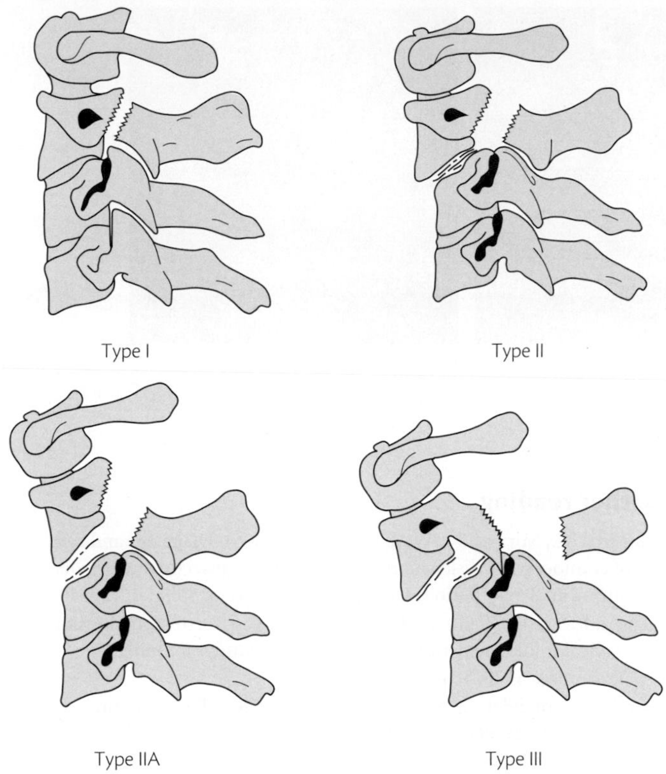

Fig. 12.39.12 Classification of traumatic spondylolisthesis of the axis. (After Rechtine and Landsman.)

rigid immobilization with a halo vest, anterior plate fixation of C2–3, pars interarticularis screw repair, and posterior C1–C2–C3 or C2–3 fusion (Table 12.39.6). The choice of treatment is most commonly recommended based on the degree of stability of the fracture. Unfortunately no consensus exists to define stability.

Almost all Type I and most Type II injuries heal with non-operative treatment although healing is often in a displaced position without clinical sequelae.

Type I

Immobilization of Type I fractures with a collar appears sufficient and healing is likely to occur in greater than 95% of cases.

Type II

There is no consensus regarding the treatment of Type II hangman's fractures. Successful non-rigid and rigid (halo vest) immobilization of Type II injuries have been reported. Multiple studies report greater than 95% healing with the halo vest. Anterior C2–3 interbody fusion with plate fixation and posterior fixation using either C2 pedicle screws or posterior C1–3, C2–3 instrumentation and fusion are also recommended. In the author's opinion, Type II hangman's fractures have an excellent prognosis and are best managed initially with a cervicothoracic brace. If this treatment option fails, a halo vest can be utilized. Surgical indications include failure to obtain or maintain fracture reduction, multiple injuries, and pseudoarthrosis. Either direct osteosynthesis with a C2 pedicle screw or anterior C2–3 fusion with plates and screws can be performed.

Type III

Type III injuries are unlikely to be reduced with traction and therefore open reduction and posterior C2–3 fusions is recommended. Stabilization of the pars fracture component can either be by transarticular C1–2 screws or by C2 pedicle screws.

C2 body fractures

Fractures of the C2 body exclusive of Type III odontoid fracture are heterogeneous in pattern although in general these injuries have a good prognosis. Fujimura classified these into four groups: extension avulsion from anterior-inferior corner of C2; low transverse fracture; comminuted body fracture; and sagittal plane fracture extending into the lateral mass.

Treatment

The majority of these injuries are stable, therefore non-operative treatment is appropriate. Non-rigid bracing is sufficient for

Table 12.39.6 Classification and treatment of traumatic spondylolisthesis of the axis (hangman's fracture)

Type	Description	Stability	C2–3 disc displacement	C2–3 facet joint	Recommended treatment
I	Non-displaced	Stable	None	Intact	**Collar** Halo vest
II	Displaced	Unstable	>3mm	Intact	**Cervicothoracic brace** Halo vest Osteosynthesis Anterior C2–3 fusion
	Angulated	Unstable	Kyphotic angulation	Intact	**Cervicothoracic brace** Halo vest Osteosynthesis Anterior C2–3 fusion
III	Associated C2–3 facet dislocation	Unstable	+/–	Intact	Open reduction and posterior C2–3 fusion with halo vest or collar **Open reduction and posterior C2–3 fusion with C2 pedicle screw**

The author's preferred treatment is in bold.

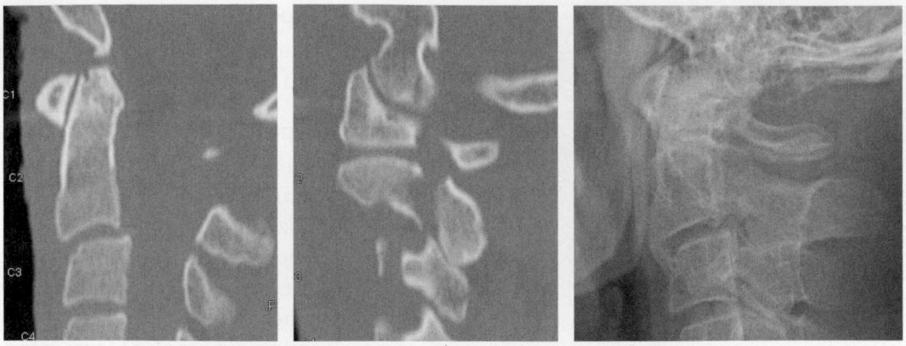

A B C

Fig. 12.39.13 A) Mid sagittal CT of 35-year-old male with Type II hangman's fracture. He was treated with a cervicothoracic brace. B) Sagittal CT demonstrating displacement of the pars interarticularis fracture. C) An anterior fusion of the C2–3 disc is seen on 3-month follow-up lateral radiographs.

non-displaced injuries (Figure 12.39.13). In displaced fractures, a halo vest should be considered. Surgery is indicated for failure of non-operative treatment, significant misalignment, and in spinal cord injured patients.

Conclusion

The stability of the upper cervical spine relies upon strong ligaments and unique osseous anatomy. Improved imaging with CT and MRI has enabled early diagnosis and an improved understanding of the pathophysiology of these complex injuries. Displacement of the occipitocervical or atlantoaxial articulations indicates disruption of key stabilizing structures and, in general, is an indication for surgery. More recent studies and systematic reviews have provided stronger medical evidence from which to base treatment decisions.

Further reading

Bellabarba, C., Mirza, S.K., West, G.A., *et al.* (2006). Diagnosis and treatment of craniocervical dislocation in a series of 17 consecutive survivors during an 8-year period. *Journal of Neurosurgery: Spine*, **4**, 429–40.

Bucholz, R.D. and Cheung, K.C. (1989). Halo vest versus spinal fusion for cervical injury: evidence from an outcome study. *Journal of Neurosurgery*, **70**, 884–92.

Dvorak, J., Schneider, E., Saldinger, P., *et al.* (1988). Biomechanics of the craniocervical region: the alar and transverse ligaments. *Journal of Orthopedic Research*, **6**, 452–61.

Hanson, J.A., Deliganis, A.V., Baxter, A.B., *et al.* (2002). Radiologic and clinical spectrum of occipital condyle fractures: retrospective review of 107 consecutive fractures in 95 patients. *American Journal of Roentgenology*, **178**, 1261–8.

Subach, B.R., McLaughlin, M.R., Albright, A.L., *et al.* (1998). Current management of pediatric atlantoaxial rotatory subluxation. *Spine*, **2**, 2174–9.

12.40

Subaxial cervical spine injuries

Sergio Mendoza-Lattes and Charles R. Clark

Summary points

- The spine study group classification describes three families of fractures
- Clinical examination can exclude a cervical spine injury in a non-distracted conscious patient without pain and neurological deficit
- CT scan is the investigation of choice where fracture is suspected
- Pure ligamentous injuries are rare
- Priorities are immobilization and assessment, reduction of dislocations and then surgical decompression and stabilization.

Introduction

Approximately 150 000 spinal injuries present to the Emergency Rooms of the United States of America every year, and roughly, 7.5% of these present with a neurological injury. Improvements in on-site resuscitation and in the delivery of emergency medical care have significantly improved the survival of patients with spinal cord injuries. Multiple classification systems have been proposed to describe the different injury patterns, and the principles laid out by Allen and Ferguson, where injuries are classified according to the mechanism of failure, continue to be valid and widely accepted.

The interpretation of clinical findings and imaging studies to identify different injury patterns constitutes the first part of a successful treatment plan. Injury patterns reflect the biomechanics, the direction and severity of trauma, and the degree of instability of the cervical spine. The classification system adopted by the Spine Trauma Study Group describes three families of injuries according to the relationship of the vertebral bodies with one another: compression, distraction, and translation/rotation. Additionally, the presence of neurological injury and the integrity of the discoligamentous structures (intervertebral disc, anterior and posterior longitudinal ligaments, supra- and interspinous ligaments, facet joint capsules, and ligamentum flavum) constitute important indicators of the severity of the injury.

Initial evaluation and management (Box 12.40.1)

Management of cervical spine injuries starts at the site of the accident, following initial resuscitation guidelines described by the American College of Surgeons and includes protection of the spine and spinal cord during the primary survey. From the initial extrication and on-site management, it should be assumed that all trauma patients have a cervical spine injury until otherwise proven.

Patients with altered mental status or those presenting with distracting injuries are at a particular risk. Some authors have estimated that 3–25% of spinal cord injuries occur during extrication, acute resuscitation, and transport. For this reason, a rigid cervical orthosis must be used at all times, until the cervical spine has been formally cleared, which requires a reasonable certainty that the patient's cervical spine is stable and free of significant injury. On the other hand, excessive use of a cervical orthosis can be associated with complications, including aspiration pneumonia, mandibular and occipital ulcers, limitations of respiratory function, and even possible increases in intra-cranial pressure. The protocol used in our institution for clearance of the cervical spine is described in Figure 12.40.1, and is further detailed as follows:

An awake and alert patient is better able to cooperate with the clinical examination than an obtunded or unconscious patient. Also, the presence of other injuries, such as chest or abdominal trauma, or other musculoskeletal conditions, can distract from the symptoms of a cervical spine injury.

Clinical examination is sufficient to rule out a traumatic injury to the cervical spine in patients that present alert and awake, and have no complaints of neck pain or neurological deficit. The patient should be able to rotate the neck at least 45 degrees in each direction and have a normal neurological examination. This practice guideline is supported by Class I data, and has been extensively adopted in many institutions.

If the patient is awake and alert, and presents with neck pain or tenderness, there is a 2–6% chance of a significant cervical spine injury that will require specific treatment. In this scenario, clinical examination alone has a negative predictive value of 96.7%, but a sensitivity of only 66.7%. For this reason, radiographic examination is mandatory. Similarly, imaging studies are also mandatory for all patients who present with altered mental status, neurological injury, or other distracting injuries.

The basic trauma cervical spine series includes anterioposterior (AP) and lateral radiographic views, as well as an open-mouth odontoid view. Cervical spine radiographic series alone are associated

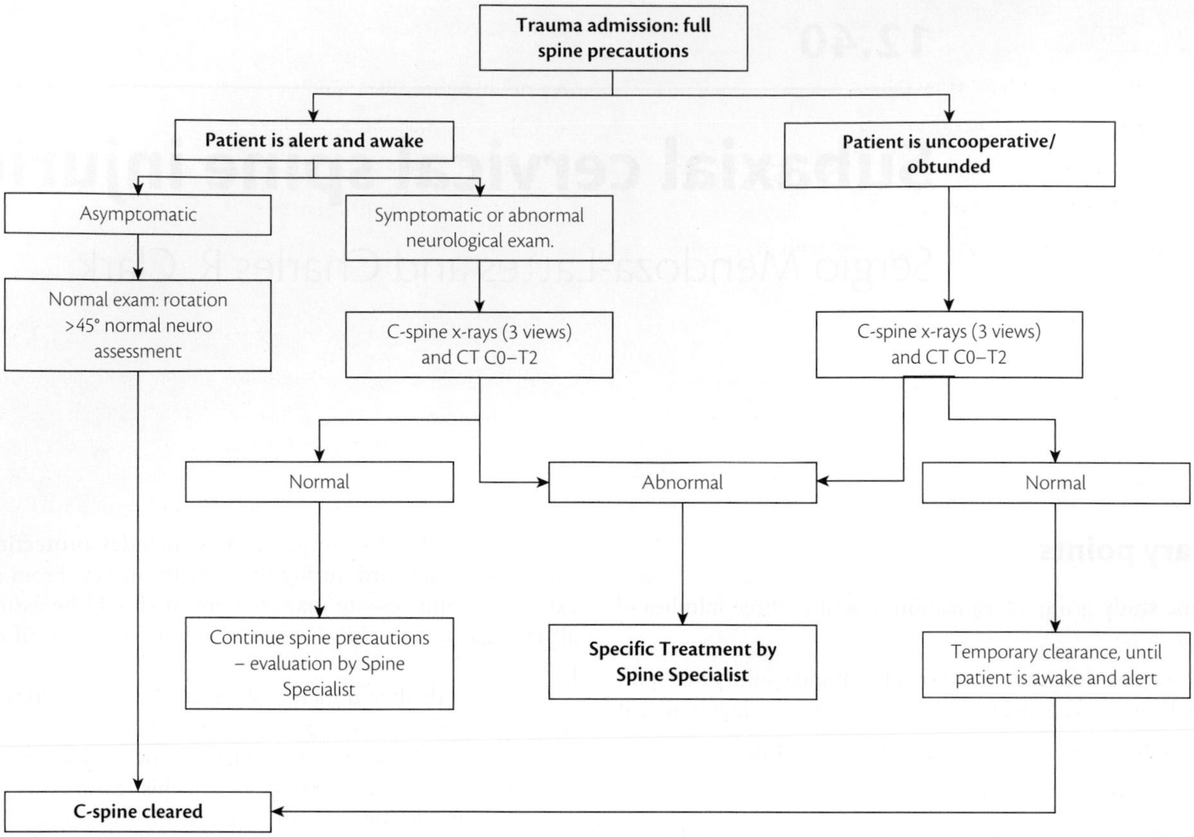

Fig. 12.40.1 University of Iowa Hospital cervical spine clearance algorithm.

1. Alert and cooperative patients are cleared based on their symptoms and physical examination.
2. If the patient is symptomatic, imaging studies are requested.
3. If the patient is obtunded and uncooperative, temporary clearance is awarded, following review of cervical spine trauma series and CT.
4. In patients with high-risk criteria (motor vehicle collision >35mph (56km), fall from heights >10 feet (3m), closed head injury, neurological deficits referable to the cervical spine, and pelvis/extremity fractures) cervical spine precautions including the permanent use of a cervical orthosis are maintained until the patient is awake and cooperative.

with 15–17% false negatives. Because most of the misdiagnosed injuries are located in the occipitocervical or in the cervicothoracic junction, the addition of computed tomography (CT) scan increases the negative predictive value to 99.7% by improving the visualization of these areas. Despite the absence of osseous injury, instability can exist as a consequence of disruption of the spinal ligaments and other soft tissue components of the motion segment. These purely ligamentous injuries are of rare occurrence (0.1–0.7%). Flexion–extension radiographs can be safely used to rule out instability when the basic trauma cervical spine series is normal, only if the patient is awake and cooperative. Nevertheless, fluoroscopy and passive flexion–extension radiographs present risk of iatrogenic spinal cord injuries in obtunded and non-cooperative patients. Dynamic fluoroscopic examination is only able to detect surgically relevant injuries in 0.56% of patients not detected by CT scan. Finally, magnetic resonance imaging (MRI) is not recommended as a screening tool, but may provide important information when planning treatment. In a recent study, MRI showed abnormalities in 21.1% of patients with normal CT scan and normal neurological examination, nevertheless, any of these injuries required additional treatment.

Obtunded and uncooperative patients are temporarily radiographically cleared following review of cervical spine trauma series and CT. Particularly if the patient presents with high risk criteria (motor vehicle collision >35mph (56km), fall from heights >10 feet (3m), closed head injury, neurological deficits referable to the cervical spine, and pelvis/extremity fractures) cervical spine precautions must include the permanent use of a cervical orthosis, until the patient is awake and cooperative and can than be clinically cleared (Figure 12.40.1).

Following diagnosis, specific treatment priorities are as follows:

1) Medical stabilization with immobilization of the cervical spine
2) Reduction of dislocations
3) Operative decompression, and spinal stabilization.

Initial airway management and fluid resuscitation have a positive impact on spinal cord perfusion. Reduction with skeletal traction should be initiated as soon as possible, and if reduction cannot be achieved, or if there are other compressing elements on the spinal cord, surgical decompression and stabilization is recommended as soon as the patient's condition has been optimized. The timing of surgery must be decided considering the characteristics of the injury, but also the general condition of the patient, and the local institutional and personnel. This continues to be a matter of

Box 12.40.1 Diagnosis

- Must identify injury to treat correctly
- Allen and Ferguson classification
- Assume all trauma patients have a cervical injury initially
- CT scan negative predictive value 99.7%
- May require other modalities to diagnose soft tissue injury.

controversy and significant research efforts. Animal models support acute decompression of the spinal cord, and there is an increasing body of clinical data to support this as well. Nevertheless, there is a lack of prospective trials to support early or acute intervention. Finally, the role of high-dose steroids is controversial and will not be discussed in this chapter.

Skeletal traction and closed reduction

If the spine is dislocated, or if there is significant impingement of the spinal cord by bone fragments, reduction with traction should be initiated on an emergent basis (Box 12.40.2). This procedure is safe if the patient is awake and cooperative. If neurological assessment is not reliable, as is the case of an obtunded or uncooperative patient, MRI is suggested prior to the onset of skeletal traction. The purpose is two-fold:

1) To identify any disc or endplate material that could potentially be retropulsed into the spinal cord during reduction
2) To identify signal changes in the spinal cord suggestive of contusion or disruption.

Reduction is achieved by applying direct axial skeletal traction with skull tongs or a halo-ring. After an initial application of 5–10kg (10–20 pounds), incremental additions of 5kg (10 pounds) are applied until reduction is confirmed. The patient should be awake but lightly sedated so as to reduce muscle contractures and facilitate reduction. The head can also be positioned so as to facilitate the reduction, usually with some flexion of the neck. After 20–30min in traction, the neurological status of the patient is monitored, and a lateral cross-table radiograph is obtained. If the spine is not reduced, additional weights are added, a neurological examination is performed, and a lateral cervical radiograph is obtained, as previously described. Our typical protocol includes adding weights up to approximately one-third of the body weight, if needed. At higher weights, tongs may displace, and a halo ring is preferable. Another advantage of a halo ring is that it may facilitate better control of the position of the head and neck relative to the axis of traction. Traction is contraindicated in ankylosed spines, such as those suffering from ankylosing spondylitis and diffuse idiopathic skeletal hyperostosis (DISH).

Non-contiguous cervical spine injuries occur in up to 15% of the cases and must be assessed before traction is initiated. Monitoring of plain films during reduction should also include evaluation for overdistraction at the level of injury. MRI is indicated to rule out the presence of disc material occupying the spinal canal if new or progressive neurological symptoms develop during the procedure.

Box 12.40.2 Traction

- Safe in conscious patient
- Otherwise need imaging first
- Increasing weights can be applied
- X-ray when weight increased.

Definitive management (Box 12.40.3)

Indications for surgery will depend on stability of the spine and the need for neural decompression. Understanding the principles and definitions of stability is fundamental for adequate management decisions. White and Panjabi have defined stability as the 'ability of the spine under physiologic loads to maintain its pattern of displacement so that there is no initial or additional neurological deficit, no major deformity and no incapacitating pain'. In the event of a traumatic injury, it must be recognized if these properties have been lost. For this purpose, these authors have also provided a checklist to guide the clinician in the determination of spinal instability, which is based on both clinical and radiological parameters. Unfortunately, there are no means to accurately determine instability. Injuries of the cervical spine represent a continuum, and in some cases, there may only be a very tenuous difference between indicating unnecessary surgery and avoiding a disastrous omission. Careful review of the points in this checklist will help guide clinical decisions. If the criteria provide for a particular injury to be considered unstable, surgery is indicated for the purpose of recovering stability. This is usually designed to counteract the disruptive forces that have acted upon the spine.

Radiolographic criteria are based on static and flexion-extension films (Figure 12.40.2). These criteria are based on biomechanical data obtained from serial sectioning of the ligamentous components of the spinal motion segment. These experiments showed that catastrophic failure could occur at physiological loads following sectioning of all posterior ligaments and one anterior ligament, or all anterior ligaments and one posterior structure. Furthermore, measurements made of intact motion segments showed a maximum displacement (measured between the posterior walls of adjacent vertebral bodies) of approximately 2.7mm and maximum angulation (measured between the inferior endplates of adjacent vertebrae) of 10.7mm. Only modest increases in displacement and angulation were observed before catastrophic failure occurred at physiological loads. The authors further suggested that to allow for variability in radiographic and measurement technique, measurements on a plain film lateral radiograph greater than 3.5mm of AP displacement or 11 degrees of angulation between adjacent vertebrae in excess of the angulation present in the levels above or below, imply potential instability in the clinical setting.

The number of cervical spine injuries without neurological impairment, or with incomplete spinal cord injuries arriving in emergency rooms, appears to be steadily increasing due to improved extrication and immobilization methods, on-site resuscitation, and improved trauma networks. The second most common reason for urgent surgery is in those patients with incomplete spinal cord injury with radiographic findings of ongoing spinal cord compression.

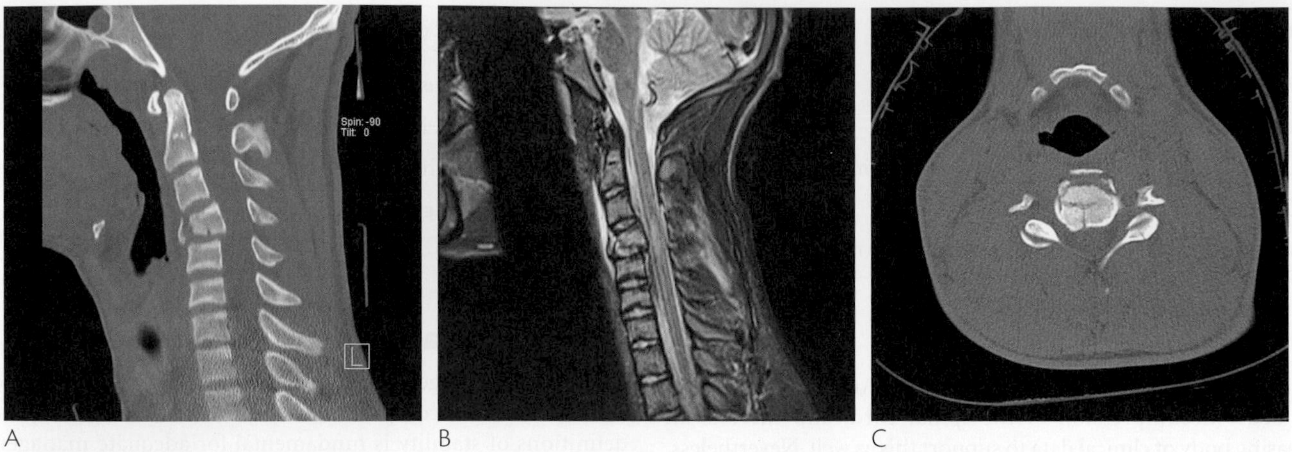

Fig. 12.40.2 Teardrop fracture of C4. Mid-saggital CT reconstruction (A), mid-sagittal T2-weighed MRI (B), and axial CT section through C4 (C) of an 18 year-old male who suffered an incomplete spinal cord injury following an accident while diving into shallow waters. An extensive signal change is observed in the spinal cord (B), as well as posterior soft-tissue disruption, reflecting damage through the posterior tension band. Characteristically, the posterior wall of the vertebral body of C4 is retropulsed, relative to C5 and C7. Also characteristic, in the axial CT image (C), are the coronal and saggittal fracture lines forming a 'T'.

Box 12.40.3 Definitive management
◆ Establish whether spine is stable or unstable.

Common injury patterns (Box 12.40.4)

Three distinct categories of injury patterns are recognized based on the primary mechanism of injury: compression injuries, distraction injuries, and translation or rotation injuries.

Compression injuries

Simple compression injuries are defined by failure of the anterior column (anterior half of the vertebral body), with sparing of the posterior cortex of the vertebral body. They are usually not related to any form of neurological injury, and may be treated by the use of a cervical orthosis for 8–12 weeks. Early in the course of treatment, and as soon as the patient has developed reasonable comfort, flexion and extension films are taken to asses for patterns of instability. Additionally, serial radiographs are recommended to monitor for the potential development of progressive deformity (kyphosis).

Burst fractures are those where the structure of the vertebral body has failed under compressive loads, extending through the posterior cortex. As the energy dissipates into the vertebral body, bony fragments are ejected in all directions, including retropulsion of bone fragments into the spinal canal, frequently involving the spinal cord. Surgical decompression is indicated for ongoing spinal cord compression and is achieved by means of a corpectomy. Stability is achieved by the interposition of a strut graft and anterior locking plate.

Distraction injuries

Distraction injuries may occur with an extension or with a flexion moment. Hyperextension injuries are most likely to occur in a rigid, spondylotic spine. The energy is dissipated through anterior osteophytes, vertebral body, and into the posterior ligaments and facet joints. Hyperflexion injuries damage the posterior tension band, including the supra- and interspinous ligament complex, ligamentum flavum, and facet joint capsules, resulting in facet subluxation or perched facets. Varying degrees of damage to the posterior longitudinal ligament and posterior annulus also occur.

Ideally, reduction of uni- or bilateral perched facets should be obtained by skeletal traction with an awake and cooperative patient. If this fails, then surgical reduction and stabilization is considered. This can be achieved from either anterior or posterior approaches. We recommend a preoperative MRI in these cases. If there is evidence of extruded disc material, posterior to the body of the inferior vertebra, an anterior approach is recommended. This will allow for anterior decompression of the spinal canal, reduction of the dislocated facet joints and stabilization by means of an interbody graft and an anterior locking plate. If there is no evidence of disc extrusion, a posterior approach is preferred, as it provides for easier reduction of the dislocated facet joints. Although posterior fusion with lateral mass screw fixation provides superior biomechanical characteristics, progressive kyphosis is likely to develop, particularly in cases where the inter-vertebral disc has been disrupted.

Hyperextension injuries commonly occur in previously spondylotic spines with varying degrees of ankylosis (see Figure 12.40.2). These injuries are increasingly common in our increasingly active aging population. The spinal canal is commonly stenotic (Torg's ratio <0.8), and the mechanism of hyperextension results in a pincer phenomenon, compressing on the spinal cord, between the posteroinferior margin of the superior vertebra, and the anterosuperior border of the lamina from the inferior vertebra. This will result in spinal cord ischemia, frequently manifest as central cord syndrome. Furthermore, if the spine is extensively ankylosed, a significant lever arm is formed over the fracture site, resulting in a highly unstable injury pattern. An increased retropharyngeal soft tissue shadow, a widened disc space with high-signal intensity on T_2-weighed MRI (otherwise degenerative disc spaces present with low-signal on T_2), anterior osteophyte avulsion or avulsion injury of the anteroinferior vertebral body should be warning signs of this highly unstable injury.

These patients commonly present with persistent cord compression, which may or may not be accompanied by bone or disc-ligament injury. If the spine is stable and the neurological status is static or improving, initial non-surgical treatment with close follow-up is recommended. Delayed or late decompression may be required if symptom improvement is stagnant. Alternatively, some authors advocate early surgical decompression.

If surgery is indicated for spinal cord decompression and the spine is considered stable, then the approach will be determined by the alignment of the cervical spine, and the number of affected levels. A posterior approach with a laminoplasty is recommended for a lordotic spine with multiple levels of compression. If the spine is neutrally aligned or slightly kyphotic, and if lordosis is obtainable on extension films, the same approach is accompanied by laminectomy and fusion with lateral mass screw fixation. Conversely, if the spine is focally kyphotic, and if the main compressive element is an anterior disc-osteophyte complex, then anterior surgical decompression and fusion is recommended.

Fractures through a previously ankylosed cervical spine require special attention. This may occur in ankylosing spondylitis, DISH (or Forestier's disease), or in extensive multilevel cervical spondylosis. The injured motion segment is extensively ossified, including most, if not all of the spinal ligaments, facet joint capsules, and even the inter-vertebral disc (ankylosing spondylitis). As a consequence of this, the fracture through the ankylosed motion segment will compromise all of the stabilizing structures, rendering significant instability, similar to a long-bone fracture, with long lever arms acting on the injury and the spinal cord.

These injuries frequently occur in elderly, osteoporotic patients, and result from low-energy trauma. They are frequently missed, and initial diagnosis is based on a high level of clinical suspicion. Once recognized, these injuries must be immediately immobilized, and treated as highly unstable. The patient depicted in Figure 12.40.3A presented with neck pain after a fall at home, and the lateral film shows a fracture line through an extensively ankylosed spine secondary to DISH. He was immediately placed on cervical orthosis, and taken to MRI for further evaluation (Figure 12.40.3B), where the injury was recognized to be displaced. The patient was indicated for emergent surgical fixation. Skeletal traction must be avoided, as it only contributes to further displacement. Surgical treatment, in the form of a multisegment posterior instrumentation is recommended to provide stability to the long lever-arms and poor bone quality. Postoperative immobilization is mandatory, and should be maintained until the injury and fusion have completely healed.

Box 12.40.4 Patterns of injury

- Compression fractures: brace
- Burst fractures: anterior fixation
- Facet subluxation/dislocation: traction and/or stabilization
- Ankylosis: very unstable fracture—may require decompression and/or stabilization
- Teardrop fracture: usually requires anterior/posterior fixation.

Translation or rotation injuries

These injuries are recognized by the presence of translation of one vertebra relative to the adjacent one. Translation can occur in the sagittal plane, coronal plane, rotational plane, or combined. In bilateral facet dislocation, the mechanism is of pure anterior translation, whereas in unilateral facet fracture or dislocation, the mechanism is that of rotational translation with a fulcrum around the intact facet joint. Translation can occur as a product of disruption of disc-ligament structures or fracture of the articular process. There is a wide spectrum of injuries ranging from unilateral or bilateral dislocated facets, to the fracture-separation of the articular process, where the dissociation of the articular process (Figure 12.40.4) from the vertebral body and lamina affects the relationship to both the superior as well as to the inferior motion segments. In general, the more elements that are compromised with the injury, the easier it is to obtain closed reduction. Unilateral facet dislocation, are the most difficult injuries to reduce.

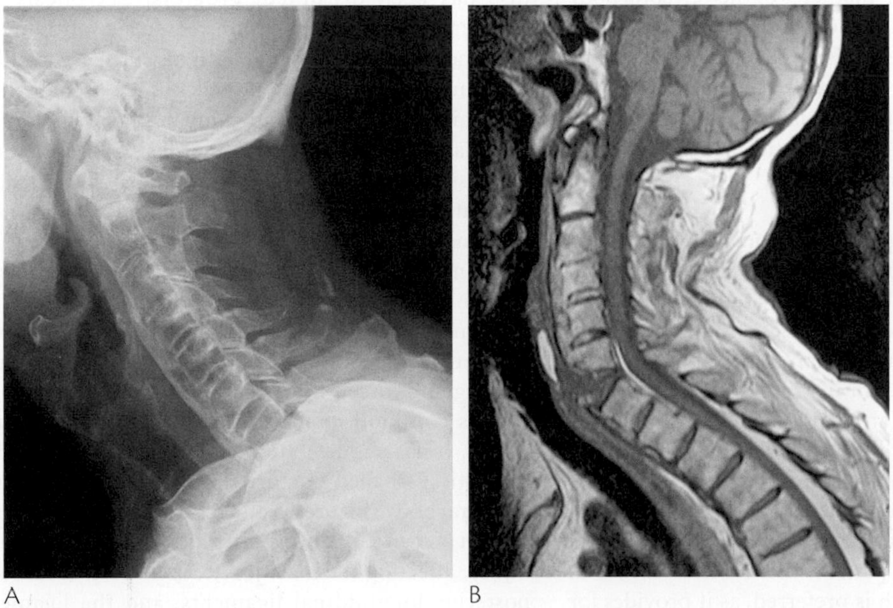
A B

Fig. 12.40.3 Lateral radiograph (A) and sagittal T1-weighed MRI (b) of a 70-year-old male who consulted in the emergency room with complaints of neck pain after a fall in his patio. In (A), a non-displaced fracture line through an extensive area of ossification of the anterior longitudinal ligament is observed. Once the patient arrived to the MRI suite, the injury has displaced into extension (B).

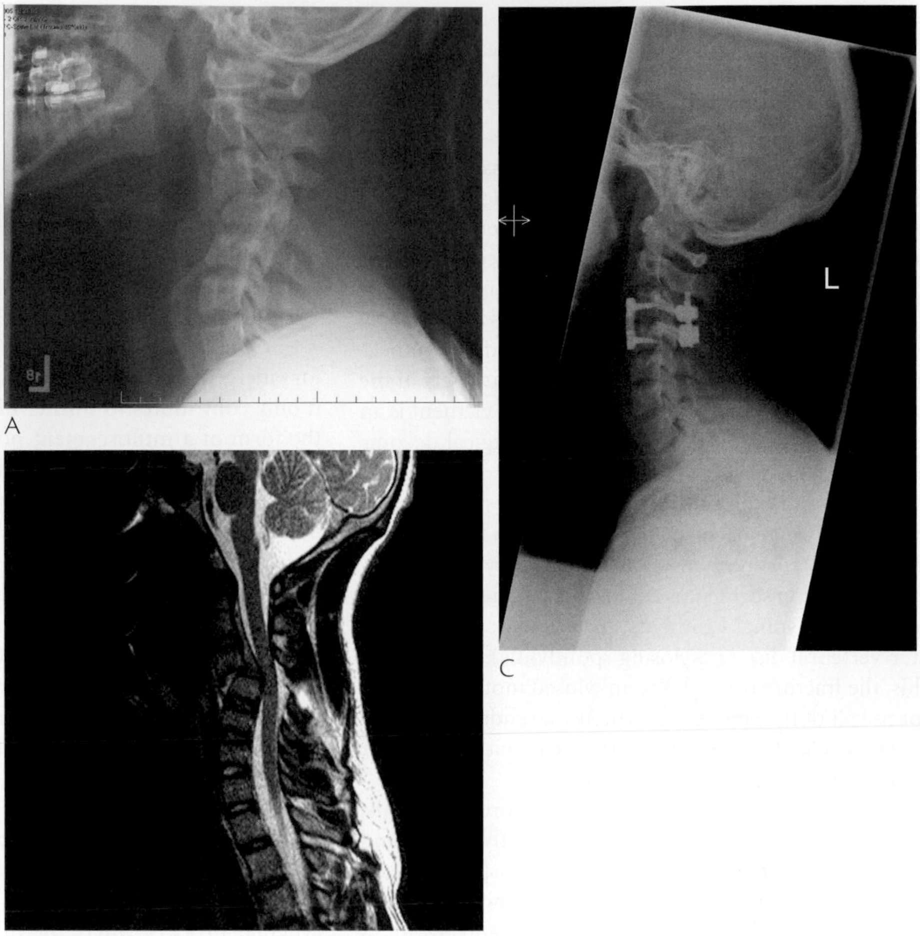

Fig. 12.40.4 Lateral radiograph (A) and sagittal T_2-weighed MRI (B) of a 16-year-old boy who suffered an incomplete spinal cord injury after an accident diving into a pond. Notice bilateral facet dislocations, as well as severe injury to the posterior tension band. After closed reduction had failed, anterior discectomy and decompression was followed reduction and reconstruction with an autologous tricortical interbody graft and anterior and posterior instrumentation (C).

Facet fractures and dislocations are easily recognized on plain films. In unilateral dislocation, the AP film will reveal a loss of colinearity of the spinous processes at the level of the injury. The lateral films will add varying degrees of vertebral body translation. If this listhesis is 25% of the AP diameter of the vertebral body or less, unilateral facet joint fracture or dislocation is the rule (Figure 12.40.5), whereas with a listhesis of 50% or more is commonly associated with bilateral dislocations (Figure 12.40.4). Unilateral facet fractures or dislocations usually present with radiculopathy secondary to foraminal stenosis, whereas bilateral facet fractures or dislocations frequently present with spinal cord injury.

Management consists of emergent reduction with the use of skeletal traction, following the previously described protocol. Approximately 25–50% of patients will fail close reduction and will require open reduction under general anesthesia. Once reduction is achieved, surgical stabilization is mandatory, and may be obtained by either anterior or posterior instrumented fusion. Prior to open reduction, we recommend an MRI to identify the presence of extruded disc material posterior to the body of the inferior vertebra. In such a case, an anterior approach is recommended. This will allow for anterior decompression of the spinal canal, reduction of the dislocated facet joints, and stabilization by means of an interbody graft and an anterior locking plate. If there is no evidence of disc extrusion, a posterior approach is preferred, as it provides for easier reduction of the dislocated facet joints. Posterior instrumentation with lateral mass screw fixation provides superior biomechanical characteristics when compared to anterior plate fixation and interbody graft. Nevertheless, in cases where the intervertebral disc has been disrupted, progressive kyphosis may develop. Furthermore, posterior fusion requires a more traumatic dissection and prone positioning, both of which are avoided in anterior fixation. Anterior fixation provides direct decompression, has similarly high fusion rates, and compares favorably in the restoration and maintenance of segmental lordosis. Nevertheless, if a fracture of the superior endplate of the vertebral body is associated with the translational deformity, anterior fixation alone is insufficient with early mechanical failure in two-thirds of the cases. In this situation, combined anterior and posterior fixation is recommended, similarly to injuries with significant posterior ligament complex disruption, such as the case of teardrop fracture-dislocations.

The teardrop fracture is an injury pattern that results from axial loading and forced flexion of the cervical spine (Figure 12.40.2). This is common in injuries occurring when diving in shallow waters. It has also been termed burst fracture dislocation. A characteristic T-shaped fracture through the superior endplate of the vertebral body (Figure 12.40.2A) is associated with varying degrees of facet and articular process fracture as well as severe disc-ligament injury, affecting the facet joints, intervertebral disc, anterior and posterior longitudinal ligaments, and the ligamentum flavum

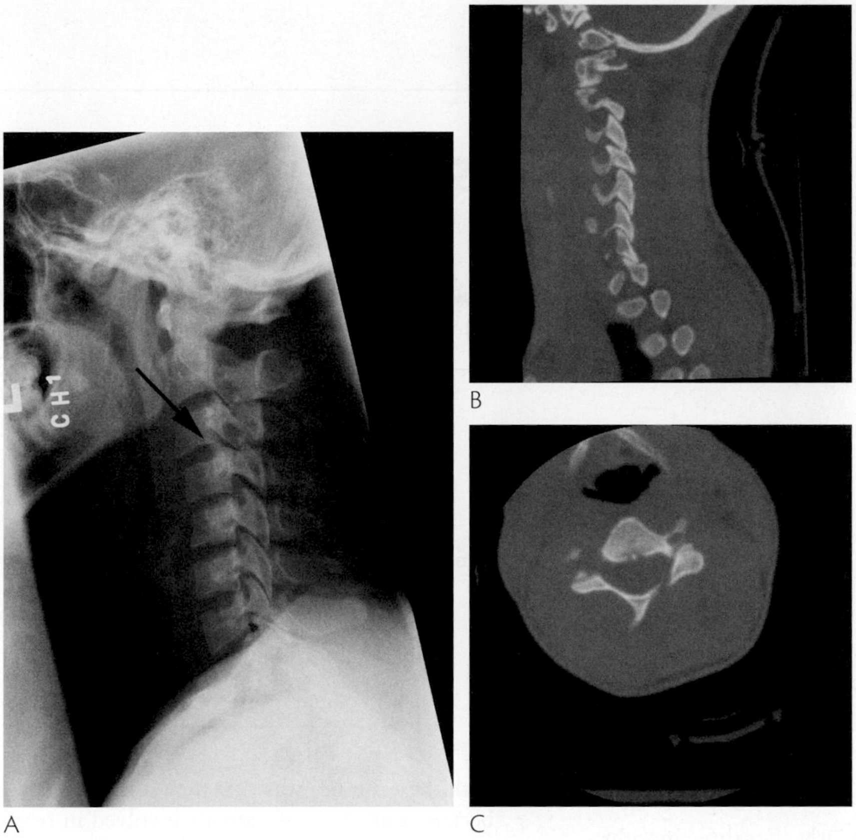

Fig. 12.40.5 Fracture-separation of the articular process of C4: Lateral radiograph (A), parasagittal CT reconstruction (B) and axial CT at the level of C4 (C) of a 24-year-old female who presented with left- sided neck and arm pain following a motor-vehicle collision. Notice in (A) and (B) that the articular process of C4 is horizontalized, dissociating from the inferior articular process of C3, as well as from the superior articular process of C5. Fracture through the pedicle and ipsilateral lamina can be seen in (C).

(Figure 12.40.2B). The superior vertebra is not only is axially loaded against the inferior vertebra, but also rotates over its axis, thus indenting its anteroinferior margin into the superior endplate of the inferior vertebra. This further displaces the posterior aspect of the vertebral body into the spinal canal, through a sagittal fracture line. The key feature is the displacement of the posterior vertebral body fragments into the spinal canal, both relative to the superior, as well as the inferior adjacent vertebral bodies. This finding must be recognized because it reflects a severe degree of discoligamentous complex injury, which results in continuous cord compression, as well as severe instability. Complete spinal cord injury is frequently present, and the recommended treatment includes decompression of the spinal canal through a corpectomy, and reconstruction with combined anterior and posterior instrumentation. Reduction by traction is rarely indicated, as the degree of disruption of the discoligamentous complex easily leads to over-distraction of the spinal canal and spinal cord.

Further reading

Allen, B.L. Jr, Ferguson, R.L., Lehmann, T.R., and O'Brien, R.P. (1982). A mechanistic classification of closed, indirect fractures and dislocations of the lower cervical spine. *Spine*, **7**, 1–27.

Anderson, P.A., Moore, T., Davis, K.W., *et al.* (2007). Cervical Spine Injury Severity Score – assessment of reliability. *Journal of Bone and Joint Surgery*, **89A**, 1057–65.

Bracken, M.B. (2001). Methylprednisolone and acute spinal cord injury: an update of the randomized evidence. *Spine*, **26**(24S), S47–S54.

Dvorak, M.F., Fisher, C.G., Fehlings, M.G., *et al.* (2007). The surgical approach to subaxial cervical spine injuries: An evidence-based algorithm based on the SLIC classification system. *Spine*, **32**(23), 2620–9.

Hadley, M.N., Walters, B.C., Grabb, P.A., *et al.* (2002). Guidelines for the management of acute cervical spine and spinal cord injuries. *Clinical Neurosurgery*, **49**, 407–98.

McKinley W., Meade M.A., Kirshblum S. (2004). Outcomes of early surgical management versus late or no surgical intervention after acute spinal cord injury. *Archives of Physical Medicine and Rehabilitation*, **85**, 1818–25.

12.41

Whiplash-associated disorders

Rouin Amirfeyz, Simon Kelley,
Martin Gargan, and Gordon Bannister

Summary points

- Whiplash costs UK economy approximately £3.64 billion per year
- Most occur after rear end vehicle collision
- Patients present with neck pain and stiffness, occipital headache, thoracolumbar back pain and upper limb pain and parasthesia
- Over 66% make a full recovery but 2% will be permanently disabled
- The outcome can be predicted in 70% after three months.

Definition

'Whiplash' is a collective diagnosis of the symptoms that follow indirect injury to the neck, spine, and adjacent structures. The term derives from one of a number of mechanisms of injury. The Quebec Task Force (QTF) on Whiplash-Associated Disorders (WAD) defined it as 'an acceleration–deceleration mechanism of energy transfer to the neck. The impact may result in bony or soft tissue injuries (whiplash injury), which in turn may lead to a variety of clinical manifestations (WAD)'.

Incidence (Box 12.41.1)

Since the introduction of compulsory seatbelts for the occupants of motor vehicles, the incidence of WAD has risen from 7.7% to 55%. Five per cent of the United Kingdom population have been involved in a rear-end collision. It is estimated that there are 300 000 claims for whiplash in the United Kingdom every year, losing 110 million man days at a cost of £3 billion to the United Kingdom economy, which includes NHS costs, social security costs, damage to property, and lost productivity. Of all personal injury claims, whiplash now accounts for 90% of the volume and 70% of the cost.

The incidence of acute whiplash injury is not known in many other countries, but a group of Norwegian neurologists reported that its incidence was much lower in Lithuania than in the United Kingdom or United States of America and attributed this to cultural differences. They demonstrated little difference in neck pain in car occupants involved in motor vehicle collisions than age- and gender-matched control subjects. Similar results were observed when controls were members of the same family. The difficulty with these studies was that they recorded rear-end collisions and because only 15% of patients involved in rear-end collision ever develop neck pain they were statistically underpowered. This was further compounded by the high prevalence of constitutional neck pain in Lithuania. This is 20% compared with 5% in Bristol and 7% in Belfast.

Box 12.41.1 Incidence

- 5% of the population have experienced WAD
- Annual cost £3 billion
- 90% of personal injury claims.

Biomechanics

The mechanism most commonly associated with whiplash injury is that of a stationary vehicle impacted from the rear, often with little or no vehicular damage. The speed of impact is important. Whiplash injury is unlikely to occur below 8–10km/h (5–7mph). The direction of impact also has an influence. In vehicles of a similar mass, front or side impacts require a higher velocity for tissue damage to occur compared with a rear impact.

Chronologically there are five stages during the transmission of force:

- Ramping: T1 vertebra moves superoanteriorly immediately on the impact, producing an extension moment
- S-phase: the extension moment results in hyperextension of the lower cervical spine with compensatory flexion of the upper cervical spine
- Transition: where the upper cervical spine starts to extend
- Hyperextension: the whole cervical spine goes to hyperextension
- Flexion: forward acceleration of the head pushes the cervical spine into flexion.

The lower cervical spine exceeds the physiological limits of hyperextension at lower acceleration than upper cervical spine. Peak cervical spine flexion has not been shown to exceed physiological limits suggesting that the lower, and to a lesser degree, the upper cervical spine are at risk for extension injury during rear impact probably in the s-phase, whereas pure flexion is a more unlikely mechanism of injury.

Pathology (Box 12.41.2)

The anatomical structures at risk are: intervertebral discs, paraspinal muscles, ligaments, and zygapophyseal joints.

Intervertebral disc: the high prevalence of disc disease in the asymptomatic population makes it difficult to ascertain the incidence of new disc injury in patients with WAD by magnetic resonance imaging (MRI) scan. A cadaveric study showed that shear forces of as little as 3.5g demonstrate excessive strain of the fibres of the annulus fibrosus, specifically at C5/6 level. Symptomatic cervical degenerative disc disease in patients suffering from WAD is both more common and occurs at a younger age compared to control population.

Paraspinal muscles: on MRI scans, the neck muscles of patients with WAD have significantly larger amounts of fatty infiltrate in all the cervical extensors than healthy control subjects particularly in the rectus capitis minor, rectus capitis major, and multifidi at the level of C3. These findings are independent of age, compensation status, body mass index (BMI), and duration of symptoms. It is, however, unclear whether the patterns of fatty infiltration are the result of local structural damage, nerve injury, or generalized disuse.

Ligaments and membranes: the findings of cadaveric studies are not truly applicable to underlying ligamentous involvement of WAD, as the latter has a different mechanism of injury with less energy transfer involved. High signal intensity is observed in alar ligament, transverse ligament and posterior atlanto-occipital membrane in individuals with chronic symptoms of WAD.

Zygapophyseal joints: if the whiplash mechanism is severe enough to injure the joint capsule, overstretching of the capsule of the facet is a potential cause of persistent neck pain. These data are reinforced by the therapeutic response of the zygapophyseal joints to intra-articular local anaesthetic blocks and radiofrequency neurotomy.

Classification

There are many published scoring systems for whiplash. Classifications commonly in use are the Gargan and Bannister which grades severity of symptoms (Table 12.41.1) and the QTF classification that also includes physical signs (Table 12.41.2).

The Gargan and Bannister grade is significantly associated with physical and psychological outcome measures and can be used as a self-administered questionnaire as it does not require physical assessment. It is a useful instrument for the evaluation of patients and an accurate method of classifying outcome and has a perfect inter-observer (Cohen's kappa coefficient = 0.82) and significant intra-observer reliability (intraclass correlation coefficient = 0.79).

The authors of the QTF classification concede it that was a consensus that required further work and it has neither been validated nor found particularly useful.

Box 12.41.2 Pathology

- Speed of impact important
- 5 stages of transmission
- Injury can occur to disc, muscles, ligaments, and zygapophyseal joints.

Table 12.41.1 Gargan and Bannister grading (1990)

Grade A	No symptoms
Grade B	Nuisance symptoms but which do not interfere with occupation or leisure
Grade C	Intrusive symptoms requiring intermittent analgesia, orthotics, or physical therapy
Grade D	Disabling symptoms requiring time off work and regular analgesia, orthotics, and repeated medical consultation

Table 12.41.2 Quebec classification (1995)

Grade 0	No symptoms or signs
Grade I	Symptoms of neck pain or stiffness but no signs
Grade II	Neck symptoms and objective stiffness and point tenderness
Grade III	Neck symptoms and neurologic deficit
Grade IV	Neck symptoms and fracture/dislocation

Clinical evaluation

History

Most patients will suffer their symptoms within 2 days, but they may be delayed by 12h or so. In up to 35% of patients the symptoms can be significantly delayed. The symptoms of whiplash are varied in their distribution and incidence (Table 12.41.3). In a prospective study of 504 patients from the south west of England who suffered a rear-end collision, 78% described neck pain lasting more than 1 week; 52% were still suffering neck pain at 1 year.

Table 12.41.3 Symptoms associated with whiplash injury

Symptom	Incidence
Neck pain	88–100%
Headache	54–66%
Neck stiffness	69%
Depressive symptoms	43%
Shoulder pain	40%
Low back pain	35%
Interscapular pain	20%
Dizziness	17–25%
Dysphagia	16%
Temporomandibular joint pain	15%
Arm and hand pain	14%
Auditory problems	4–18%
Visual problems	1%

The incidence of depressive symptoms after whiplash injury is common. In Saskatchewan, 42% of patients with normal mental health before whiplash injury who had ongoing compensation claims or medical treatment demonstrated depressive symptoms within 6 weeks of their accident. The symptoms of depression occurred early in the disorder suggesting that depression is significant component of whiplash injury.

Although headaches are a generally accepted symptom of whiplash, the origin is less clear. The strongest predictor of headache following whiplash injury is pre-existing headache. Acute headaches after rear-end collisions may be stress related. There is a strong association between occipital headache and pain in the neck and trapezii with continuing symptoms 15 years after whiplash.

Physical examination

The symptoms of whiplash are usually disproportionate to the physical signs. The most common sign is a reduced range of movement in a tender neck. The most common neurological deficit is decreased sensation. Significant irritation of the brachial plexus can be manifested by paraesthesia, coldness, discoloration, and hyperhidrosis of the upper limb. A positive Tinel's sign over the scalene muscles, supraclavicular fossa, cubital tunnel or carpal tunnel may be found. These signs were associated with an unfavourable prognosis exactly as were the distribution of symptoms described by Squires et al. (1996).

As some 40% of patients with irritation of the brachial plexus had a positive Tinel's sign in distal peripheral nerves, this suggests that proximal stretching may render the distal nerves more susceptible to subsequent compression. Alpar et al. demonstrated that carpal tunnel release in such cases relieved pain over the entire upper limb and reduced levels of substance P further reinforcing the concept of double-crush after whiplash. Paraesthesia occurs in 13–62% of cases and weakness in 18% (Table 12.41.4).

Investigations (Box 12.41.3)

There is no objective diagnostic test for WAD. Vertebral fractures are very rare. Therefore in the absence of high-energy impact, the need for a radiograph is questionable; however, the association of more severe symptoms after whiplash in those with radiological changes in the neck has been recognized for decades.

There is no correlation between electromyography (EMG) and patients' symptomatology, computed tomography (CT), and MRI findings.

Table 12.41.4 Signs associated with whiplash injury

Sign	Incidence
Reduced range of neck movements	87%
Neck tenderness	64%
Paraesthesia	13–62%
Discolouration	18%
Hyperhidrosis	39%
Weakness	12–18%
Coldness	10%
Postural abnormality	12%
Tinel's sign	20–42%

Box 12.41.3 Investigations

Imaging and nerve studies of little use.

The role for MRI is in patients with upper limb symptoms and signs. The difficulty with indiscriminate use of MRI is the high proportion of abnormalities unrelated to symptoms even in younger patients. Some clinicians have used MRI scans and clinical signs to target surgery. The fatty infiltrate in the cervical extensor muscles is specific in its presence and location in WAD patients and is independent of age, compensation status, BMI, and duration of symptoms.

As we understand more about the organic pathology of WAD, imaging studies may become increasingly useful.

Treatment (Box 12.41.4)

A variety of methods are advocated for the treatment of WAD, many of them controversial or not supported by the literature. The following text summarizes the available level 1 evidence.

- *Collar and immobilization:* soft collar is widely used in the immediate phase, but there is little evidence to support it. In fact its use should be discouraged as it slows down the recovery rate. Physiotherapy and mobilization is probably the best management. This reduces the pain and increases the range of movement 4 and 8 weeks after commencement of the treatment when compared with soft collar immobilization
- *Education:* educational pamphlets do not help patients both in short (2 weeks) or long term (3 months). However, once it is delivered in the form of a video the reduction in pain and the increase in the cervical range of movement are significantly better in 1, 3, and 6 months' follow-up
- *Self-mobilization exercises:* active cervical exercises in the range limited by pain decrease whiplash symptoms 6 weeks following injury and maintain the improvement for a year. It is best commenced within 4 days
- *Physiotherapy:* ice, active, passive, strengthening, and isometric exercises reduce the pain 6 weeks and 3 months postinjury. Maitland's manipulation protocol and McKenzie's principles are helpful if commenced within 4 days of injury. Magnetic field applied twice a day for 2 weeks combined with non-steroidal anti-inflammatory drugs (NSAIDs) is more effective than medications alone

Box 12.41.4 Treatment

- Little evidence for collar
- Education
- Exercises useful
- Physiotherapy useful
- Early steroids reduce symptoms
- Botulinum little evidence
- Radiofrequency neurotomy may help.

- *Self-mobilization exercises vs. physiotherapy:* there is controversy which is best
- *Chiropractic manipulation:* manipulation (a combination of high-velocity-low-amplitude thrust, muscle energy, and soft tissue techniques) in the acute phase is more effective than a single 30-mg intramuscular dose of ketorolac (NSAID) for immediate (1h) pain relief. Phasic exercises added to chiropractic manipulation increases the effectiveness of the delivered treatment on chronic WAD
- *Laser acupuncture:* laser acupuncture fails to improve the range of movement or reduce the pain when used in acute phase
- *NSAIDs:* 20mg of tenoxicam (a non-steroidal with a long duration of action) per day administered for 2 weeks, when started in the first 72h after accident effectively reduces the pain and increases the cervical range of motion at day 15. The observed difference in cervical range of motion was large enough to justify a clinically significant difference
- *Melatonin:* oral melatonin 5mg per day 5h prior to dim light melatonin onset does not reduce the pain, improve the sleep pattern or the quality of life (based on SF-36) in the chronic phase
- *Steroids:* intravenous methylprednisolone (30mg/kg in the first hour and 5.4mg/kg/h for 23h) started in the first 8h of the injury increases the short-term pain relief and reduces the long term sick leave
  - Injection of 1mL (5.7mg) of betamethasone into the zygapophyseal joints is not more beneficial than 1mL of bupivacaine 0.5% (local anaesthetic). The anatomical location of the painful joint should be confirmed on two separate occasions by pain relief following local anaesthetic injection. One should be aware that more than half of the patients report recurrence of pain after a week
- *Botulinum A toxin:* two different doses of botulinum toxin A has been tried in chronic WAD: 100 units. The injection sites are four to five 'most tender' spots in splenius capitis, rectus capitis, semispinalis capitis, and trapezius. In all three of these randomized controlled trials an improvement was observed in both the intervention and the control groups. None of these studies showed a significant difference between the two groups at the end of the trial (at 4–24 weeks). This might be due to the low number of patients in each arm
- *Percutaneous radiofrequency neurotomy:* percutaneous radiofrequency neurotomy of C3/4 to C6/7 facet joint capsule gives medium-term pain relief. The most commonly involved joint is usually the C5/6 facet joint. The median time for 50% of the pain to return is almost nine months
- *Cervical fusion:* there is no evidence to support surgical intervention for axial neck pain following suspected upper cervical ligamentous injury in WAD. In the case of radiculopathy, the evidence is not different from what is available for spondylosis and radiculopathy in general.

The following treatments are ineffective:

- Halter traction
- Kinaesthetic sensibility and coordination
- Cognitive behavioural treatment
- Pulsed electromagnetic therapy and transcutaneous electrical nerve stimulation
- Ultra-reiz current.

Prevention

The biomechanical principles to reduce whiplash injury are as follows:

- Decrease occupant acceleration
- Minimize relative spine movement
- Minimize forward rebound.

In the 1970s Saab introduced the fixed head restraint followed shortly after by Volvo. However, most head restraints are adjustable and 93% are poorly positioned.

Head restraints have been required by law since the1970s, but to be effective they must be positioned behind and as close to the occupant's head as possible. The major problem is that adjustable head restraints are less effective than a fixed version because they are often left in the down position, thus improperly positioned for many people.

Head restraints can and do reduce the incidence of whiplash injuries, especially among females.

Outcome (Box 12.41.5)

The established injury outcome of WAD is confounded by a diffuse literature that varies in its point of recruitment of patients. Only 54% of patients presenting in neurosurgical practice in Tennessee recovered, compared to 73% attending accident and emergency departments in the United Kingdom in the 1980, and 88% of patients filling insurance claims in Quebec, Canada.

Applying the Gargan and Bannister classification to series recruited from Accident and Emergency Departments in the United Kingdom and Sweden, 55% made a complete recovery, 22% recorded nuisance levels of discomfort, 16% had intrusive symptoms, and 7% were disabled.

Rate of recovery

The most comprehensive cohort study is a 4-year prospective review carried out for the Transport Research Laboratory in which symptoms reached a plateau at 2–3 years from injury. However the majority of patients reach their final state within 3 months.

Factors associated with outcome

Using univariate analysis, the literature identifies worse outcomes with the pre-accident variables of female gender, advancing age, known cervical spondylosis, previous whiplash injury, pre-existing

Box 12.41.5 Recovery

- 50–75% recover
- Most of recovery within 3 months
- Many factors affect outcome, e.g. cervical spondylosis
- Psychological effects important.

neck pain, pre-existing back pain, excessive use of primary care services, and a history of anxiety/depression. Accident variables associated with worse outcome include rear end impact, lack of awareness of the impending impact, and position in the front of the vehicle. Response variables associated with worse outcome include onset of symptoms in less than 12h, pain radiating from the neck to other sites, and abnormal neurological signs.

Behavioural response to whiplash injury

From the mid-twentieth century, a psychoneurotic response was observed in patients presenting with whiplash injuries (52–85%). The behavioural response to whiplash is often disproportionate to the trauma sustained and the physical signs demonstrated. As whiplash injuries present more frequently in the medicolegal than clinical context there are inevitable suspicions that symptoms may be exaggerated for gain.

There are two conflicting theories about this psychological response to WAD.

The somatopsychic response

Cognitive deficits have been found in patients after whiplash injury that could not be explained by their psychological history before the accident. Distress is at similar levels in all patients at a week but significantly higher after 2 years in those who have developed chronic symptoms. The pain caused by the whiplash injury probably precipitates the syndrome that follows.

The biopsychosocial model

Cultural influence

An Australian occupational health physician, reported on patients with 'late whiplash' syndrome reviewed in the course of his professional duties. He compared 300 patients from South Australia with 20 from Singapore. Whilst the former reported high levels of disability, the only ones to complain in Singapore were emigrant Australians. The data were anecdotal but supported by further work from New Zealand. Another study in 1986 compared the incidence of whiplash injuries in Victoria, Australia and New Zealand. The population sizes and numbers of cars were comparable but in Victoria there were 3.5 times the number of rear-end collisions, ten times as many claims for compensation, and five times as many took more than 2 months off work. In 1987, legislation required that all whiplash injuries be reported to the police and that victims pay the first 317 Australian dollars of medical expenses. Although this is highly suggestive of social manipulation, 10% of Australians reported continuing symptoms after the 1987 legislation.

The effect of previous psychological problems

A biosocial model has been proposed based on symptom expectation, amplification and attribution, and prior knowledge of expected symptoms. Adverse social circumstances and a vulnerable personality count as risk factors for poor psychological outcome but not the physical outcome. Patients who were frequent attenders with their general practitioners before the injury have a worse outcome.

The effect of WAD on the patient's psychological state

The initial reaction to RTA can be of anger, emotional shock, and frightened behaviour. These are usually temporary and settle with time. However, 1 year after the accident almost a third of the patients still show a form of psychological disorder, if looked for carefully by the employment of standard mental health diagnostic criteria, such as the diagnostic and statistical manual of mental disorders–fourth edition (DSM–IV).

The most common are as follows:

- *Travel phobia:* kinesiophobia, or fear of travel and movement, is more common in the victims of WAD (6% of patients) when compared to the patients with minor head injury. This phobia is associated with longer duration of neck symptoms
- *Post-traumatic stress disorder (PTSD):* this includes avoidance, re-experiencing, and hyperarousal. Buitenhuis et al. showed that hyperarousal symptoms at 3 weeks following the accident was related to more severe WAD symptoms both at 6 and 12 months. Therefore this can be a helpful outcome assessment tool at the time of initial evaluation
- *General anxiety:* there is a strong correlation in between chronic pain and anxiety. This is even more severe in males following WAD even though the coping strategies to counteract the effect of pain are virtually the same in both genders
- *Depression:* more than 40% of patients with no history of previous mental health problems develop depression in the first 6 weeks from the injury and another 18% develop depression at between 6 weeks to a year following the accident. Of these 60% usually settle, but 40% become recurrent or persistent. Early depressive symptoms are also a risk factor for developing widespread pain and, therefore, anxiety.

Physical and psychological aspects of WAD are not separate. They interact and therefore sometimes make it difficult to attribute the proportion of disability following relatively mild injury. 'Apparently disproportionate disability' has been coined as a term for those patients with exaggerated symptoms and unexpectedly slow recovery. This is a subconscious psychosocial process. It is a useful term as it combines different physical, psychological, and social aspects of the injury.

Risk factors for poor psychosocial outcome can be divided to five distinct groups:

1) Pre-accident characteristics such as poor social circumstances and previous psychological problems
2) Accident trauma causing disproportionate distress and phobia
3) Patients erroneous beliefs on the chronicity and severity of the problem
4) Further postaccident factors such as a second accident, bereavement and frustrating legal proceedings
5) Quality of care. Inconsistent and ambiguous medical advice.

On the basis of these, appropriate medical care involves attention on psychiatric as well as chronic pain management. Patient education plays an important role. Prerecorded audiovisual material reduces the amount of pain and therefore anxiety 1, 3, and 6 months after injury.

Further reading

Carragee, E.J. Hurwitz, E.L. Cheng, I., *et al.* (2008). Treatment of neck pain: injections and surgical interventions: results of the Bone and Joint

Decade 2000–2010 Task Force on Neck Pain and Its Associated Disorders. *Spine,* **33**, S153–69.

McClune, T. Burton, A.K. and Waddell, G. (2002). Whiplash associated disorder. A review of the literature to guide patient information and advice. *Emergency Medicine Journal,* **19**, 499–506.

Spitzer, W.O. Skovron, M.L. Salmi, L.R., *et al.* (1995). Scientific monograph of the Quebec task force on whiplash-associated disorders. Redefining whiplash and its management. *Spine,* **20**, 1–73s.

Squires, B. Gargan, M.F. and Bannister, G.C. (1996). Soft-tissue injuries of the cervical spine. 15-year follow-up. *Journal of Bone and Joint Surgery,* **78**B, 955–7.

Teasell, R.W. and Shapiro, A.P. (1998). Whiplash injuries: An update. *Pain Research & Management,* **3**, 81–90.

Watkinson, A. Gargan, M.F., and Bannister, G.C. (1991). Prognostic factors in soft tissue injuries of the cervical spine. *Injury,* **22**, 307–9.

12.42

Thoracic fractures

Christopher J. Dare and Evan M. Davies

Summary points

- Thoracic fractures are associated with severe trauma in young patients
- Multiple injuries are common
- Early fixation of unstable injuries is recommended to prevent neurological deterioration
- Almost all surgery best carried out posteriorly
- Long implants can be used
- Anterior reconstruction may be required where the anterior column is deficient.

Incidence (Box 12.42.1)

Thoracic spine fractures (T1–T10) are relatively less common than thoracolumbar and lumbar fractures (T11–S1) and very little is published specifically on the subject.

There are two peaks of incidence. Firstly in young men associated with high-energy injuries with a second peak in elderly women with low-energy fragility fractures.

The annual incidence of thoracic spine fracture is approximately 21 per 100 000 population. In approximately 40% of cases there are other associated injuries with an overall mortality rate of about 4%. The reason for the high rate of associated injuries is because the thoracic spine is splinted by the ribs, and hence much greater forces are required to cause a fracture in the younger age group. In about 16% of cases a spinal cord injury will also be present.

Mechanism of injury

Most thoracic fractures are simple wedge fractures. They are particularly common in elderly women and are associated with osteoporosis. These fractures are generally caused by low-energy or minimal trauma and are stable.

Other patterns of fracture are generally caused by high-velocity or high-energy injuries, and these are more common in young males. However, pre-existing pathology such as ankylosing spondylitis may predispose to other patterns of fracture without severe trauma.

Axial compression is the most common mechanism of injury. Facet dislocation is rare in the mid-thoracic spine. This is probably because of the orientation of the facet joints and the relative stiffness of the thoracic spine compared with the spine at the thoracolumbar junction. Many of these fractures are the result of seatbelt injuries. Thoracic spine injuries are often associated with a lower cervical spine fracture. Injuries in the lower cervical spine are often overlooked, and a high index of suspicion is required.

Box 12.42.1 Incidence

- Less common than other spine fractures
- 40% associated injuries
- Mortality 4%.

Aetiology of fracture

Motor vehicle accidents are the most common cause of fracture by either direct injury, such as ejection from a vehicle, or indirect injury, such as a major deceleration injury. In the United States of America gunshot injury is a common cause of thoracic spine fracture and spinal cord injury, but this is much less common in Europe (Table 12.42.1).

Spinal cord injury

For a number of reasons the spinal cord is relatively sensitive to injury in the thoracic spine:

1) The blood supply to the thoracic spinal cord is relatively poor
2) The thoracic spinal canal is relatively small compared with the size of the spinal cord—this is most marked in the mid-thoracic spine

Table 12.42.1 Etiology of thoracic spinal fractures in the United States

Motor vehicle accidents	33%
Gunshot	28%
Fall	24%
Other trauma	9%
Medical	6%

3) When fracture of the thoracic spine occurs, it is often due to very high forces. Translation or torsional injuries are more common, and these injuries are most commonly associated with spinal cord injury. Chest injury is also common after these fractures and occurs in about 24% of these patients. Chest injuries are not always apparent immediately after the injury, and in some cases a high index of suspicion is required to make the diagnosis.

In those with a spinal cord injury approximately 13% will not have a fracture of the bony elements. These fractures may be caused by stretching of the spinal cord, or vascular injury to the cord itself, so-called SCIWORA (spinal cord injury without radiological abnormality).

Not surprisingly, the more severe the fracture pattern the more likely it is to be associated with a neurological injury. In injuries involving the anterior and posterior elements three-quarters are associated with a neurological deficit and in those in whom a neurological injury is present all would have a dural laceration. The significance of a dural laceration is that the neural elements may become incarcerated in the lamina fracture itself and may benefit from decompression at the time of stabilization.

Surgical stabilization of patients with complete spinal cord injury probably reduces hospital stay, although the incidence of complications may be doubled in patients undergoing internal fixation.

Following a thoracic spine fracture the neural elements may be at risk particularly if the spine is unstable. Neurological deterioration has been well documented during hospital stay with the risk increasing the longer the spinal cord remains vulnerable.

Therefore it would appear that the optimum management of patients with unstable thoracic fractures and neurological damage is to protect the spine while resuscitating the patient and then to fix the fracture internally at the earliest opportunity to prevent the risk of neurological deterioration. In this respect, thoracic fractures are probably different from lumbar fractures, where no benefit has been found in urgent decompression and stabilization of unstable fractures in the absence of deteriorating neurology.

Diagnosis

Diagnosis of thoracic fractures is not always easy. In the majority of patients a clear history will be given and local tenderness will be found with radiological evidence of a fracture. However, in some circumstances distracting injuries make the diagnosis less straightforward:

- Proximal fractures (above T5)
- Fractures associated with head injury
- Fractures associated with patients who are intoxicated or on drugs
- Patients with multiple injuries
- Patients with associated pathology (e.g. ankylosing spondylitis)
- Confused elderly.

Risk factors for high energy thoracic fracture include back pain, a fall of 3m (10 feet) or more, a vehicle crash at 80km/h (50mph), Glasgow Coma Scale score less than 8, and neurological deficit. All these patients should be sent for radiography.

There should also be a high index of suspicion in elderly patients with low-energy falls or sudden-onset back pain in the absence of an obvious precipitant. Wedge compression fractures are common in the elderly with osteoporotic bone. Historically, if a fracture was aidentified, these patients would be treated expectantly with the vast majority going on to make a full recovery. However, other treatment options now exist for those who remain symptomatic.

All patients with suspected high-energy thoracic spinal injuries should be considered unstable until proved otherwise, and the patient should be protected from spinal cord injury by log-rolling and immobilizing the spine.

Unstable fractures are more commonly associated with the following:

- High-velocity injury
- Chest injury
- Multiple injuries
- Head injury
- Other pathology (e.g. ankylosing spondylitis).

Imaging (Box 12.42.3)

In most patients anteroposterior and lateral radiographs will demonstrate the fracture, but further investigation with thin slice computed tomography (CT) scanning may be necessary to establish whether or not the fracture is stable.

CT scanning is the most widely used investigation for assessing the stability of fractures. It gives the best definition of the bone structure, and allows assessment of the anterior and posterior structures. It will also demonstrate the amount of canal compromise caused by displacement of the fracture or by intrusion of bone fragments into the canal. If fine cuts are used, reconstruction of the CT scan can be very helpful in assessing the injury, the amount of displacement, and the amount of canal compromise.

The usefulness of magnetic resonance imaging (MRI) in high-energy thoracic fractures is limited. It may be useful to establish the presence or absence of a posterior soft tissue injury associated with an anterior injury, or to establish the type of spinal cord injury in those with paraparesis or paraplegia. In late injuries, deteriorating

Box 12.42.2

- Hyperflexion most common mechanism of injury
- Commonest in elderly females (osteoporotic)
- Ankylosing spondylitis predisposes
- Spinal cord injury common
- Chest injuries common
- Unstable fractures are best stabilized acutely if possible.

Box 12.42.3 Imaging

- Most fractures shown on x-ray
- Thin slice CT helpful in management
- MRI to assess cord injury.

neurological function should be assessed with MRI to examine the cord and to determine the presence or absence of a syrinx.

Ninety per cent of these fractures are stable.

MRI is of particular benefit in assessing fractures, particularly fragility fractures that remain persistently painful at a time when most would have settled or a least be symptomatically much improved (approximately 6 weeks).

Ongoing pain and high signal on STIR (short tau inversion recovery) sequence MRI are indicative of non-union of the fracture and such fractures are amenable to operative intervention.

Associated injuries

Associated injuries are relatively common after thoracic fractures, particularly displaced fractures. This is because they are mainly caused by high-velocity or high-violence forces (Table 12.42.2).

Head injuries are more common in fractures of the thoracic spine than in fractures elsewhere in the spine. This may be because of the high violence involved with so many of these injuries, and it is also possible that many of those with cervical injuries die before they can be transferred to hospital. It has been demonstrated that up to 40% of patients may have no tenderness at the site of a spinal fracture, and one of the risk factors for this is head injury. It is best to assume that those with a significant head injury have an unstable thoracic fracture until radiographs have excluded this.

Associated injuries are more common in thoracic fractures compared to thoracolumbar and cervical fractures.

A classic combination of injury in those with thoracic fracture is the association between sternal fracture, thoracic fracture, and rupture of the arch of the aorta. The sternal fracture is usually self-evident, but it is easy to miss one of the other two injuries because they can both cause serious back pain. The injury commonly occurs following high-velocity trauma in a road accident where the patient has been wearing a seatbelt. About 40% of those with thoracic fractures have associated chest injury, usually in the form of rib fractures. Haemopneumothorax is common and usually requires drainage with a chest drain. A chest radiograph and radiographs of the thoracic spine are mandatory in these patients, and an arch aortogram is required if there is suspicion of an aortic injury.

Other injuries associated with thoracic fractures include scapular fractures (2%), clavicle fractures (5%), rupture of the bronchus, subclavian injury, brachial plexus injuries, cardiac tamponade, rupture of the diaphragm, and intra-abdominal injury.

Multiple-level injuries occur in 10–15% of those with spinal fractures, and are common in those who fall from a height and in those subjected to high-violence injuries.

Non-operative management (Box 12.42.5)

Virtually all stable thoracic fractures can be treated non-operatively. Significant late deformity is very unusual, and most of these fractures can be treated with pain relief and bed rest initially, followed by mobilization and physiotherapy. Depending on the severity of their symptoms, many patients will not even require a period of bed rest. There is no evidence that bracing controls or limits the amount of kyphosis seen after simple wedge fractures, but the patient may be more comfortable in a three-point brace until the pain has settled down. The elderly do not tolerate brace-wear well, but it may be in these patients that the brace is best able to prevent progression of kyphosis after fracture. The standard orthosis is of little use in thoracic fractures above T6, and in these patients a thoracolumbar spinal orthosis with a cervical extension may be used. Below T6 a standard thoracolumbar spinal orthosis can be used.

Table 12.42.2 Incidence of associated injury

Site	Incidence
Head	26%
Chest	24%
Long bones	23%

Box 12.42.4 Caveats

- Head injury
- Sternal fracture, thoracic fracture, and aortic injury.

Box 12.42.5 Management

- Little evidence for bracing
- Brace ineffective in high fractures
- Some unstable fractures best treated non-operatively.

Box 12.42.6 Insufficiency fractures

- Usually treated with pain relief and/or bracing initially
- Must exclude underlying pathology, e.g. malignancy
- Consider vertebroplasty/kyphoplasty where symptoms >6 weeks.

Some unstable fractures may be managed non-operatively. For example, patients with complete spinal cord injury and without wide displacement of their fracture may be managed with bed rest followed by orthotic treatment for up to 3 months. The treatment used will depend on the preference of the treating physician.

Axial load or extension injuries over multiple levels are best treated non-operatively. Initial bed rest followed by immobilization in a brace for 6 weeks is best. However, if there is a neurological injury, the spine is probably unstable and surgical management is recommended in most cases.

Surgical management

Low-energy fractures

Treatment options now exist for the management of fragility fractures of the thoracic spine that remain symptomatic. Whole spine MRI is mandatory in this group of patients to exclude malignancy as the underlying cause of fracture or pain. If doubt exists, then vertebral body biopsy should be undertaken. Investigations should demonstrate concordance with pain, changes in plain radiology, and high signal on STIR sequence MRI at the same vertebral level.

It is not uncommon to find multiple vertebral compression fractures on plain x-ray in this patient group but not all may be

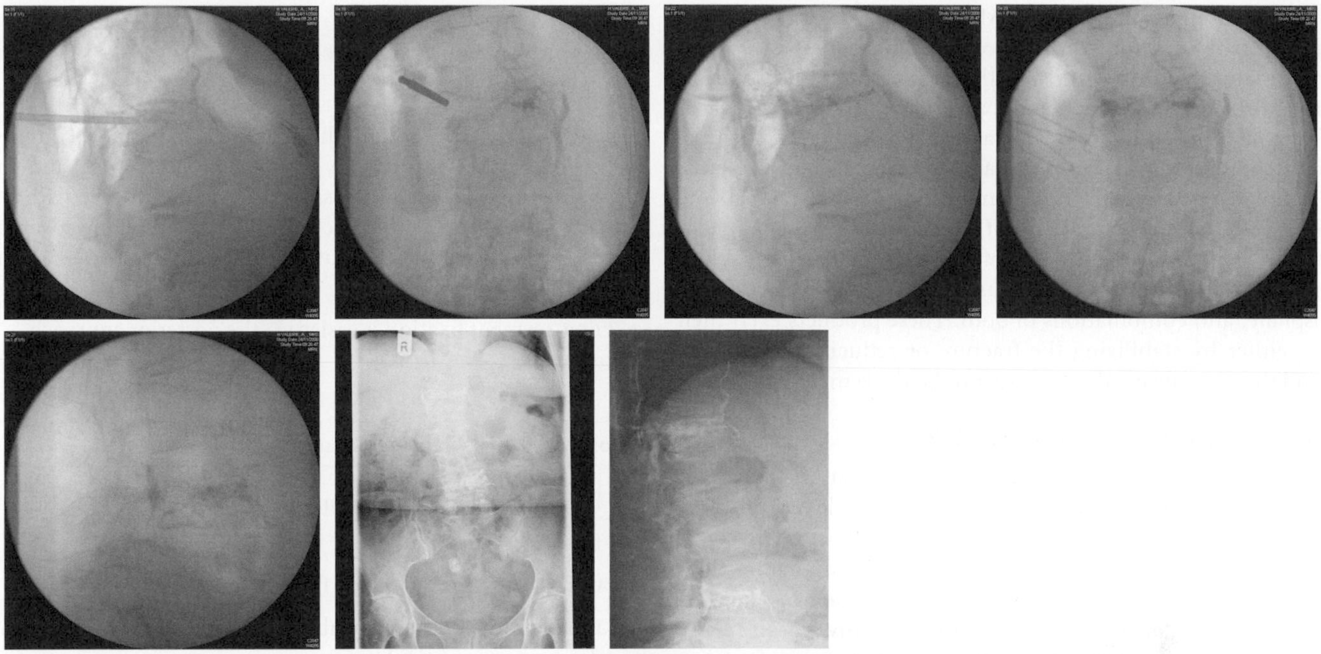

Fig. 12.42.1 Vertebroplasty demonstrating one of the complications, extravasation of cement, into the venous system which on rare occasions may result in cement embolus.

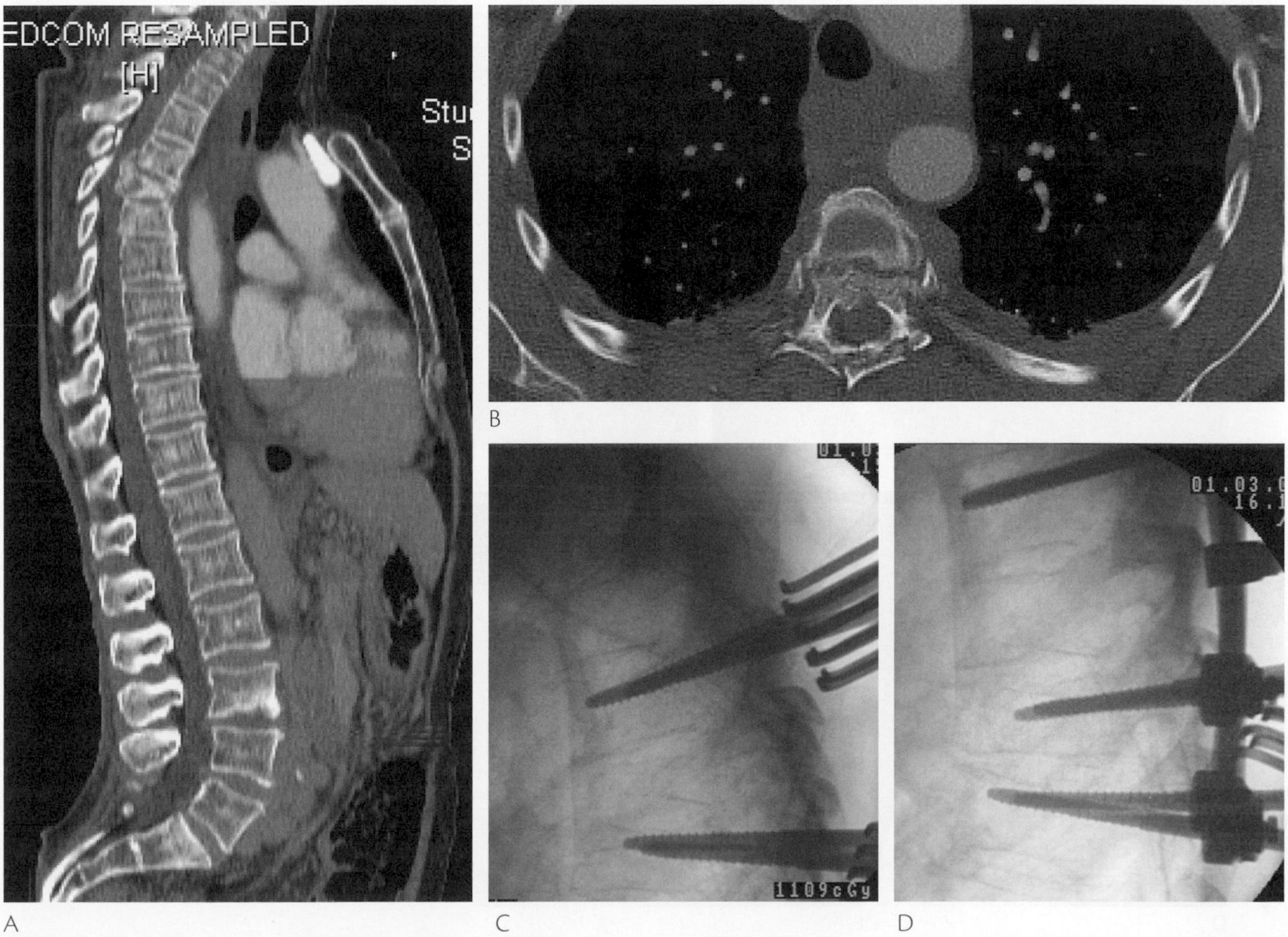

Fig. 12.42.2 High thoracic fracture at T5 associated with fractures of C6 and C7. A) and B) Sagittal and axial CT demonstrating acute kyphosis at level of the fracture with retropulsion of the posterior wall into the canal. C) and D) Demonstrates intraoperative images following pedicle screw placement before and after ligamentotaxis to reduce the fracture.

symptomatic hence the need for MRI (Figure 12.42.1). The vast majority of these fractures heal without ongoing sequelae. However, symptomatic fractures of greater than 6 weeks' duration can be treated with cement augmentation. A variety of systems are available ranging from products that are aimed at restoring the height of the vertebral body either using a balloon or metal stent to elevate the endplates with a delivery system to then fill the residual void with bone cement (kyphoplasty). If height restoration is not considered feasible than simple filling of the vertebral body may suffice (vertebroplasty). Bone cements used include PMMA, calcium phosphate, and combinations of both. These products exert their effect either by stabilizing the fracture or reducing nociceptive stimuli through the exothermic reaction of the cement.

High-energy fractures (Box 12.42.7)

Since the advent of the Harrington instrumentation there have been great advances both in the type and complexity of spinal instrumentation and in the surgical expertise of the modern spinal surgeon. Instrumentation and techniques now mean that fractures may be stabilized anteriorly, posteriorly or both and in some circumstances percutaneously or by minimally invasive means.

The approach to surgical stabilization of thoracic fractures depends on a range of factors:

- Fracture pattern
- Presence or absence of neurological injury
- Associated injuries.

The posterior approach to the thoracic spine is most commonly used. This is the traditional approach to the spine and most surgeons carrying out spinal surgery feel comfortable with it. In surgery to stabilize the thoracic spine after fracture, the advantages of the posterior approach outweigh the disadvantages in most cases:

- Long-segment fixation is easier via the posterior approach

Box 12.42.7 High-energy fractures

- Posterior surgery most common
- Long constructs
- Can reconstruct anteriorly from behind
- Deteriorating neurology absolute indication for emergency decompression/stabilization.

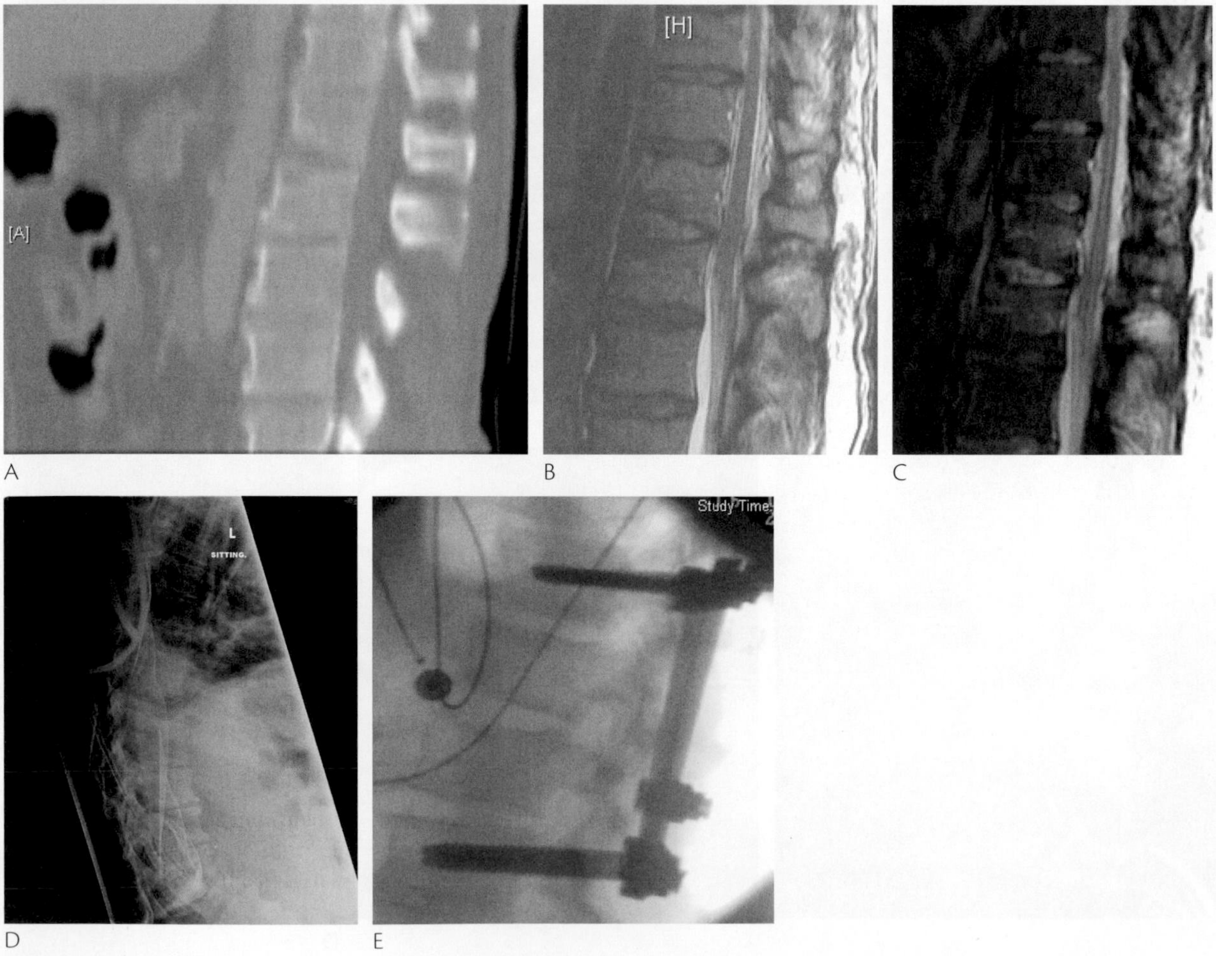

Fig. 12.42.3 Patient pedestrian versus cars, admitted with head injury and soft tissue Chance fracture of the thoracic spine. A) Sagittal CT demonstrating minor endplate fractures of adjacent vertebral bodies. B) Sagittal T2-weighted MRI demonstrating the fracture and increased signal in the intervertebral disc with increased signal in the posterior elements. C) STIR sequence demonstrating vertebral body oedema. D) Dynamic plain x-ray (sitting lateral) demonstrating gross ligamentous instability. E) Reconstruction of the posterior tension band utilizing a pedicle-based instrumentation system.

- The posterior approach does not compromise lung function which may already be impaired after injury
- Most fixation devices for thoracic fractures are designed for posterior use
- Fracture reduction, where necessary, is easier.

The importance of short instrumentation and fusion in the lumbar spine, in order to maintain its motion, has been emphasized. In the thoracic spine longer-segment instrumentation or fusion does not compromise the spine in the same way (Figure 12.42.2). The thoracic spine is relatively immobile compared with the lumbar spine, with most motion being in rotation. Patients tolerate a stiff thoracic spine much better than a stiff lumbar spine. Careful biomechanical consideration needs to be given to the type of construct required for fixation. There is no consensus on the optimal fixation technique. Constructs range from long to short and employ fixation methods from screws, hooks and wires although the trend is increasingly toward a pedicle screw based system. Most of the short-segment fusion devices depend on pedicle screw fixation for their stability. With this type of construct mobile segments may be preserved (Figure 12.42.3). At best a single mobile segment may be spanned and fused (ultra short segment fixation), if the injured vertebra is intact enough to support a screw. Alternatively two mobile segments may be spanned with fusion of the injured segment. This leaves the option of removing the metalwork with restoration of movement of the non-injured segment.

Non-pedicle screw constructs require a longer area of instrumentation (usually two segments above and two segments below the fracture) in order to achieve adequate stability.

Fracture patterns resulting in complete loss of anterior column support biomechanically would benefit form restoration of this support. This can be achieved from the posterior approach with a corporectomy via a costotransversectomy approach with or without sacrificing a thoracic nerve root. A reconstruction cage can then be sited to replace the fractured vertebral body. This combined with posterior column reconstruction gives a biomechanically robust construct, minimizing the risk of late kyphotic deformity or implant failure. A recent evolution in this construct, minimizing the surgical insult is to support the anterior column with bone cement through an open transpedicular approach using a hydraulically inflated balloon to reduce the fracture fragments and create a void to fill with bone cement, a technique known as balloon kyphoplasty.

In the neurologically compromised patient or the patient with deteriorating neurology it may be necessary to decompress the neural elements. Although this can be achieved with modern posterior instrumentation and ligamentotaxis, a more thorough decompression is achieved with an anterior approach. Following decompression anterior instrumentation is used to reconstruct and stabilize the anterior column. With associated major posterior ligamentous disruption this may also need to be augmented with additional posterior instrumentation.

The absolute indication for surgery is the patient with an unstable thoracic fracture with deteriorating neurology. Failure to stabilize these patients early on is likely to result in further deterioration and possibly paralysis. As discussed earlier, there is a high incidence of neurological deterioration in patients with unstable thoracic fractures, and they should undergo early stabilization to prevent neurological damage. This applies whether the patient is neurologically intact or has a partial neurological injury at presentation. In those with a complete and irreversible spinal injury there is not the same urgency for treatment. However, stabilization of a grossly unstable fracture in the presence of multiple injuries will help in the management of the patient; for example, it will allow the patient to be sat up and moved without danger.

Further reading

Hu, R., Mustard, C.A., and Burns, C. (1996). Epidemiology of incident spine fracture in a complete population. *Spine*, **21**, 492–9.

Keerlan, J.J., Diekerhoff, C.H., Buskens, E., *et al.* (2004). Surgical treatment of traumatic fractures of the thoracic and lumbar spine. A systematic review of the literature on techniques, complications and outcome. *Spine*, **29**(7), 803–14.

McLain, R.F. (2006). The Biomechanics of long versus short fixation for thoracolumbar spine fractures. *Spine*, **31**(11) Suppl, S70–S79.

Sesani, M. and Ozer, A.F. (2008). Single stage corpectomy and expandable cage placement for treatment of thoracic or lumbar burst fractures. *Spine*, **34**(1), 33–40.

Wardlaw, D., Cummings, SR., Meirhaeghe, J.V., *et al.* (2009). Efficacy and safety of balloon kyphoplasty compared with non-surgical care for vertebral compression fracture (FREE): a randomised controlled trial. *Lancet*, **373**(9668), 1016–24.

12.43

Thoracolumbar, lumbar, and sacral fractures

Philip Sell

Summary points

- High-energy trauma often results in serious spinal fractures. The junctional zone between the relatively stiff thoracic spine and the more mobile lumbar spine is particularly susceptible to injury
- The role of decompression in spinal cord injury remains uncertain at level three or four evidence
- Unstable fractures may be stabilized using modern fracture fixation methods enabling easier nursing care in polytrauma and earlier mobilization than non-surgical treatment
- There is level two evidence that stable thoracolumbar fractures have similar outcomes with surgical and non-surgical treatment
- There are many fracture classification systems that are not validated or have poor inter- and intraobserver error. Recent modern validated systems may in the future assist in the rational planning of interventions for spinal injury.

Introduction

A spectrum of injury can occur from the trivial to the devastating. The mobile junctional zones of the cervicothoracic and thoracolumbar junctions are more susceptible to injury than the deeply set lumbosacral junction. The relatively stiff thoracic spine is supported by the thoracic cage, the ribs and sternum.

In terms of nomenclature a fracture of the thoracolumbar spine involves any combination of the T11, T12, and L1 vertebral bodies.

At the thoracolumbar junction the spinal cord segments control lower limb and bowel and bladder sphincter function. Neurological dysfunction at this level can have devastating consequences for the patient.

A lumbar fracture is of the L2, L3, L4, and L5 vertebral bodies.

A sacral fracture is to any part of the sacrum between the superior endplate of S1 and the sacro-coccygeal junction and laterally to the sacroiliac joints.

Historical perspective

The development in care of spinal cord-injured patients owes much to the tragedies of the world wars. The reduction in morbidity and mortality of cord injured patients came about as a result of the political embarrassment of crippled soldiers dying from avoidable complications and poor nursing care. Centralization into specialized spinal injury units resulted in dramatic improvements for these patients. Powerful single personalities such as that of Guttmann at Stoke Mandeville in the United Kingdom influenced the whole of spinal rehabilitation for many generations.

The early mining industry with tunnel collapses produced spinal column injuries with regularity. The original Holdsworth classification of stability of spinal fractures into anterior complex and posterior complex was generated with the injuries sustained in the Nottingham coal mines.

Early surgical fixation devices such as the Harrington rod have no place in modern fracture management and are of historical interest only.

Aetiology and epidemiology

Motor vehicles in the form of cars and motorbikes are world wide the most common causative agent for thoracolumbar injury. Sports injuries from horse riding, mountain biking, climbing, and some extreme sports also contribute.

Earthquakes, particularly at night, are major natural disasters that can paralyse many thousands in a matter of minutes. The tremor wakes the population, they sit up in bed, flexed at the moment of ceiling collapse. In Oct 2005 in Northern Pakistan, 194 paraplegics were observed from a population of 600; 62% had lumbar level injuries, 25% thoracic, 9% thoracolumbar, and 4% were cervical or sacral.

A significant challenge is the patient group of 'jumpers'. They fall into two psychiatric categories: the psychotic that jumps under impulse or because of delusional voices. They have a high rate of recidivism; the depressed or those with a situational crisis rarely repeat after the cathartic injury. Significant lower limb injuries contribute to the complexity of management.

The ageing population increases the pool of those vulnerable to fragility fractures secondary to osteoporosis. The incidence of vertebral osteoporotic fracture is high worldwide. In the United States of America there are an estimated 700 000 osteoporotic vertebral body compression fractures each year. The natural history is one of resolution of pain. Modern treatment strategies aim at preventing future fractures with treatment after assessing bone mineral density.

Vertebroplasty and kyphoplasty involve the injection of the vertebral body with bone cement. This can be an effective treatment for pain. There are no published randomized controlled trials comparing this technique to natural history. There is level two, three, and four evidence to support this treatment.

Stability (Box 12.43.1 and Box 12.43.2)

This term is commonly used but poorly defined.

An injury to the spine must be assumed 'unstable' until clinical data from examination and imaging enables an evaluation of stability.

There is a spectrum of stability and the two main questions relate to immediate stability and long term stability. Neurological features and mechanical or structural features need consideration in this assessment.

- Question 1: Is this spine so 'unstable' that there is immediate risk to neurological structures?
- Question 2: Is this spine 'unstable' such that over the expected time frame of healing of the injury the spine will deform or displace to an extent that may impair function or structure of the spine?

In simple terms, neurological involvement, no matter how trivial, implies that at the moment of injury there was sufficient displacement of the fracture to produce damage to neurological tissue. Immediate stability is likely to be jeopardized, and long-term displacement has a high probability.

In the absence of neurological symptoms or signs immediate stability must be assessed in terms of probability of displacement in the short term producing neurological deficit and long-term increasing displacement producing pain, deformity, or embarrassment of neural function.

A simple fracture of a transverse process is an obviously stable injury. A burst fracture with rotation at the thoracolumbar junction with partial neurological involvement is obviously unstable.

Fracture classification systems assist in the assessment of stability.

There are insufficient series or tested protocols to recommend a classification system for children.

Clinical features

The spinal injury should be assessed as a part of the routine Advanced Trauma Life Support (ATLS) protocol: Primary and secondary surveys should occur. Modern imaging systems combined with clinical skills enable accurate assessment of stability at an early stage.

In the same way that repeated neurological assessment of patients with head injury is mandatory, so it is with patients who have a spinal column injury. An obtunded or consciousness-impaired patient must be assumed to have an unstable injured spine until evidence is available to 'clear' the spine.

Assessment should be context specific for polytrauma or isolated an injury.

Inspection and palpation

It is not possible to properly examine the spine of a supine patient. A 'log-roll' or spinal lift are the only two ways to move a patient before 'stability' has been established. A gibbus is a kyphotic deformity at the site of the fracture. It can only be seen on log rolling the patient. At this 'look, feel, move' moment, interspinous point tenderness and haematoma can be detected.

Neurological examination

The use of the ASIA (American Spinal Injury Association) chart (Figure 12.43.1) reduces observer error and makes recording of sensory and motor deficits easy. The chart itself has helpful reminders regarding the Medical Research Council (MRC) grading of muscle strength. It enables diagrammatic recording of the dermatome and myotome of neurological deficit.

Differential diagnosis

The diagnosis of a spinal fracture is confirmed with imaging. The energy transferred during acceleration or deceleration causes a structural failure of the components of the spinal column. The greater the energy the greater the injury. Whenever there is disproportionate tissue destruction or damage, suspect a secondary pathology. Pathological fractures secondary to metastatic or even primary tumour can occur with low-energy trauma.

Osteoporosis and osteomalacia have many causes. In older patients suspect fragility fractures as the cause of spontaneous spinal pain.

Osteoporosis produces decreased trabeculae thickness and strength. In the older spine the posterior elements are often osteoarthritic and so have sclerosis and falsely high bone mineral density. Loading of the osteoporotic vertebra results in fracture of the anterior superior aspect of the body, where there is greatest bone loss.

Pathological fractures occur as a result of metastatic spinal disease. Screening for metabolic bone disease to include plasma electrophoresis must occur in all patients with a pre trauma history of new back pain.

Clinical imaging

Consider:

Box 12.43.1 Key points in assessment and documentation

- Immediate mechanical stability
- Long-term stability
- Neurological stability.

Box 12.43.2 Stability

- Compression fractures and stable burst fractures are treated non-surgically
- Unstable injury patterns are treated surgically. Flexion distraction, fracture dislocation, and unstable burst
- The separation of stable and unstable burst fractures remains problematic.

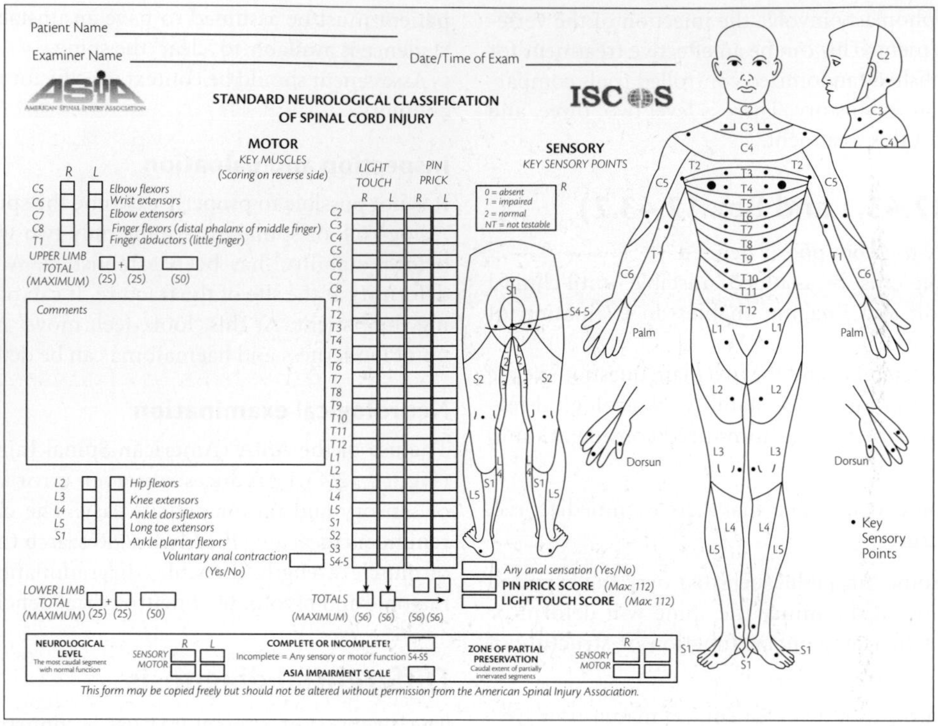

MUSCLE GRADING

0 total paralysis

1 palpable or visible contraction

2 active movement, full range of motion, gravity eliminated

3 active movement, full range of motion, against gravity

4 active movement, full range of motion, against gravity and provides some resistance

5 active movement, full range of motion, against gravity and provides normal resistance

5* muscle able to exert, in examiner's judgement, sufficient resistance to be considered normal if identifiable inhibiting factors were not present

NT not testable. Patient unable to reliably exert effort or muscle unavailable for testing due to factors such as immobilization, pain on effort or contracture.

ASIA IMPAIRMENT SCALE

☐ A =**Complete**: No motor or sensory function is preserved in the sacral segments S4-S5

☐ B =**Incomplete**: Sensory but not motor function is preserved below the neurological level and includes the sacral segments S4-S5

☐ C =**Incomplete**: Motor function is preserved below the neurological level, and more than half of key muscles below the neurological level have a muscle grade less than 3

☐ D =**Incomplete**: Motor function is preserved below the neurological level, and at least half of key muscles below the neurological level have a muscle grade of 3 or more

☐ E =**Normal**: Motor and sensory function are normal

CLINICAL SYNDROMES (OPTIONAL)

☐ Central cord
☐ Brown-sequard
☐ Anterior Cord
☐ Conus Medullaris
☐ Cauda Equina

STEPS IN CLASSIFICATION

The following order is recommended in determining the classification of individuals with SCI.

1. Determine sensory levels for right and left sides
2. Determine motor levels for right and left sides.
   Note: in regions where there is no myotome to test, the motor level is presumed to be the same as the sensory level.
3. Determine the single neurological level.
   This is the lowest segment where motor and sensory function is normal on both sides, and is the most cephalad of the sensory and motor levels determines in steps 1 and 2.
4. Determine whether the injury is Complete or Incomplete (sacral sparing).
   If voluntary anal contraction = No AND all S4-5 sensory scores = 0 AND any anal sensation = No, then injury is COMPLETE. Otherwise injury is incomplete
5. Determine ASIA Impairment Scale (AIS) Grade:
   Is injury complete? If YES, AIS=A Record ZPP
   NO ↓ (For ZPP record lowest dermatome or myotome on each side with some (non-zero score) preservation)
   Is injury motor incomplete? If NO, AIS=B
   YES ↓ (Yes=voluntary anal contraction OR motor function more than three levels below the motor level on a given side.)
   Are atleast half of the key muscles below the (single) neurological level graded 3 or better?
   NO ↓ AIS=C
   YES ↓ AIS=D

If sensation and motor function is normal in all segments, AIS=E

Note: AIS E is used in follow up testing when on individual with a documented SCI has recovered normal function. If at initial testing no deficits are found, the individual is neurologically intact; the ASIA Impairment Scale does not apply.

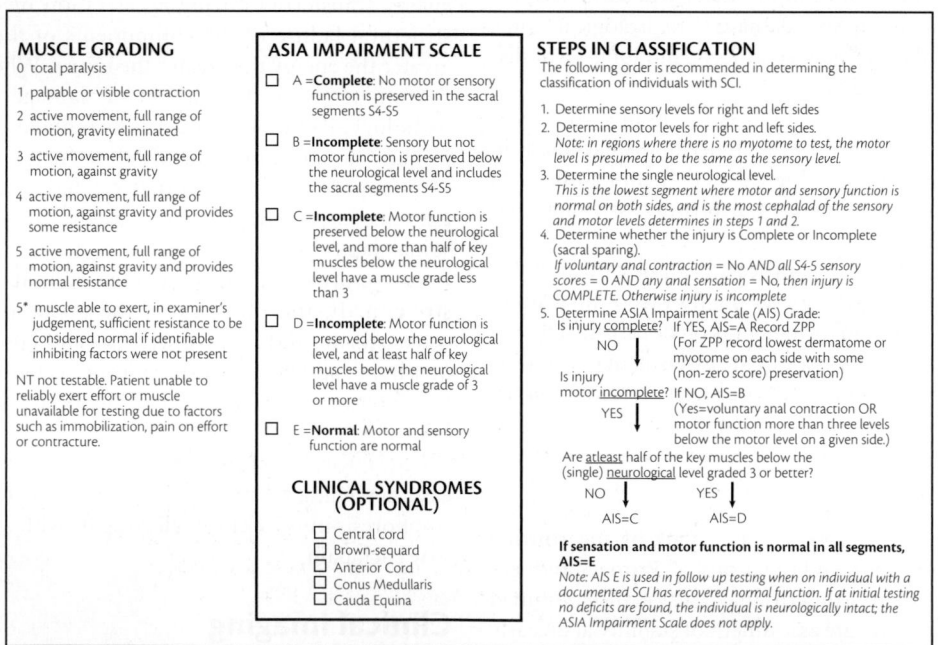

Fig. 12.43.1 ASIA chart.

- X-ray, coned view:
  - Plain AP and lateral
  - Sometimes enables greater definition of detail, redundant with computed tomography (CT) scanning
- Standing weight bearing x-ray: useful to determine stability in less severe injuries
- Flexion extension x-rays: used to detect abnormal dynamic movement
- CT scan: 5mm or thin slice 2–3mm give clear definition of bone, Abdominal scans for trauma should be viewed for fracture
- Magnetic resonance imaging (MRI) scan: used to assess posterior ligament and disc. Predictive role not yet clear and a high false positive rate

- Bone mineral density scan: use for assessment of osteoporotic fractures and consider prior to fracture fixation particularly in alcoholic or other at-risk groups.

Classification systems

The ideal classification system for thoracolumbar fractures awaits development. A classification system essentially compartmentalizes an analogue spectrum of injuries into discrete packages and creates arbitrary boundaries. This makes comparison, pattern recognition and treatment algorithms easier for those involved in the analysis of treatment options.

The ideal classification system provides the following functions:

- Language for communication
- Decisions about treatment
- Evaluate prognosis
- Compare results.

It should also be reliable, reproducible, all-inclusive, mutually exclusive, logical, and clinically useful.

As imaging technology has advanced so has the complexity of commonly used classification systems.

The early 'two complex' concept was superseded by the three columns. These were based on pain x-rays and subsequently CT scans.

The load sharing concept is a classification system that describes the loss of structural integrity of the anterior spinal structures and implies a need in certain circumstances to reconstruct the anterior complex of the spine. The system has good reliability but remains unproven in prediction of mechanical failure. The study is a retrospective evaluation of imaging and patient outcomes.

Denis three-column concept (Figure 12.43.2 and Box 12.43.3)

The three-column concept is in common use and has a practical value. It was developed from a retrospective review of 412 plain x-rays, 53 CT scans, and 120 patient records.

The fractures fall into four main categories, which have an interobserver agreement with a kappa of 0.606, which is moderate:

- Burst
- Seat belt type
- Compression
- Fracture dislocation.

The 16 subcategories have a poor interobserver error with a kappa value of 0.173.

The AO system has a comprehensive classification. The type A, Type B and Type C fractures are subdivided into three sub groups and each of these into a further three subgroups, a total of 27 types. The kappa scores of 0.475 for the main three groups of A, B, and C suggest fair reproducibility.

A specific study looking at reproducibility of the two most common classification systems used 33 sets of imaging and 19 observers. The Denis and the AO system for the classification of spine fractures have only moderate reliability and repeatability. The tendency for well-trained spine surgeons to classify the same fracture differently on repeat testing is a matter of some concern.

Fracture pattern is frequently the dominant or only factor forming the basis of spinal injury classification.

Box 12.43.3 The three anatomical columns

- SLL, supraspinatus ligament
- PLL, posterior longitudinal ligament
- ALL, anterior longitudinal ligament.

The Thoracolumbar Injury Classification and Severity Score

The Thoracolumbar Injury Classification and Severity Score (TLICS) is a system in evolution being validated and improved by the American Spine trauma study group. The three components held by a consensus of clinicians to be important in fracture management decision processes are included. They are

- Fracture morphology determined by radiographic appearance
- Integrity of the posterior ligamentous complex
- The neurological status of the patient.

The three main categories are similar to the AO system, that is, A) compression or burst B) translation or rotation C) distraction. The integrity of the posterior ligament complex is assessed and scored, and medical uncertainty is permitted as the ligament may be intact, suspected or indeterminate, or injured. A spectrum of neurological status is recognized and graded. There is clinical utility to the research by this active group.

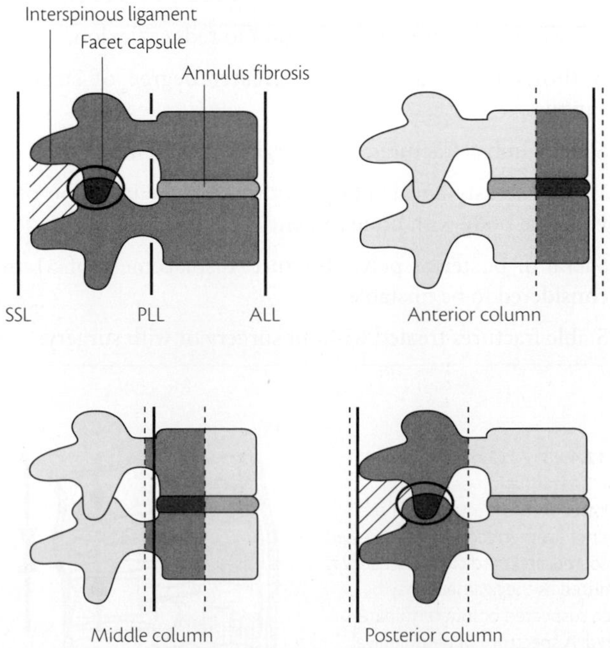

Fig. 12.43.2 The three anatomical columns: SLL, supraspinatus ligament; PLL, posterior longitudinal ligament; ALL, anterior longitudinal ligament.

Treatment (Box 12.43.4 and Box 12.43.5)

There is prehospital care, in-hospital care, and rehabilitation. In-hospital care must involve consideration of the risks of venous thromboembolic disease. Early mobilization improves outcomes. Rehabilitation and avoiding long-term disability is an important treatment goal.

Simple measures such as an early graded medical return to the workplace have significantly reduced the social morbidity of long-term impaired function. Reassurance by the physician is an important tool in this process. 'Mixed messages' and negative messages from health care professionals confuse patients and can act as obstacles to recovery. Most fractures have a favourable prognosis and spinal fractures are no exception. The outcome of many spinal disorders can be influenced by positive messages.

Non-surgical treatment can require greater supervision with serial assessments. If the fracture is deemed stable then early mobilization and return to activity as pain allows is the treatment of choice. Early aggressive pain control with appropriate support and early discharge is the most common treatment for stable injuries.

'Trunk' stability is when the patient can sit comfortably without support. A proportion of patients find bracing beneficial as a means of pain reduction. A Jewitt brace is small and lightweight. It has three-point fixation to reduce flexion. A custom moulded thoracolumbar orthosis provides a greater degree of structural support.

Early surgery may have advantages in trauma over delayed surgery with reduced morbidity.

Stable fractures can be treated without surgery or with surgery. The principles of fracture stabilization are

- Short segment fixation to preserve motion segments (Figure 12.43.4)
- Consideration of anterior reconstruction as well as posterior fixation if there is loss of anterior column support
- Posterior fixation two levels above and two levels below fracture if fitness for anterior reconstruction doubtful.

Box 12.43.4 Treatment options

- A Jewitt brace: three-point fixation to reduce flexion.
- A thoraco lumbar orthosis: greater degree of structural support
- Stable lumbar fractures: non-surgical treatment
- Vertebroplasty and kyphoplasty involve the injection of the vertebral body with bone cement
- Sacral or posterior pelvic fracture: displacement of >1cm is considered to be unstable
- Stable fractures treated without surgery or with surgery.

Box 12.43.5 Principles of fracture stabilization

- Short segment fixation to preserve motion segments
- Anterior reconstruction and posterior fixation if loss of anterior column support
- Posterior fixation two levels above and two levels below fracture if fitness for anterior reconstruction doubtful.

A randomized controlled trial (level two <80% FU) compared surgery to non-operative care in stable thoracolumbar burst fractures without neurology. There was no difference in outcome. The surgical group had an average Oswestry disability index of 20 points, the non-operative only 10 points, suggesting a better outcome for non surgical treatment in this group.

Medical uncertainty

The role of early decompression of spinal fractures that have a stable neurological deficit has not been confirmed.

The assessment of neurological status before 'spinal shock' has resolved is not absolute.

Clinical outcomes of anterior decompression and stabilization compared to posterior decompression and stabilization in the presence of an unstable injury and neurological deficit has insufficient evidence, but there is a trend for better results with anterior decompression and stabilization where there is evidence of anterior compression of the spinal cord or nerve roots.

Likely developments over the next 5–10 years

Current research centres on establishing predictive value to treatment algorithms that are based on classification systems. Biological means of improving the outcome of neurological deficit with stem cells or olfactory glial cells are in development.

Sacral fractures

Sacral fractures are often identified late. Local crepitus, deformity, or sacral de-gloving may be found. Rectal examination and assessment of sphincters and perineal dermatomes is essential. Five principals of assessment have been described

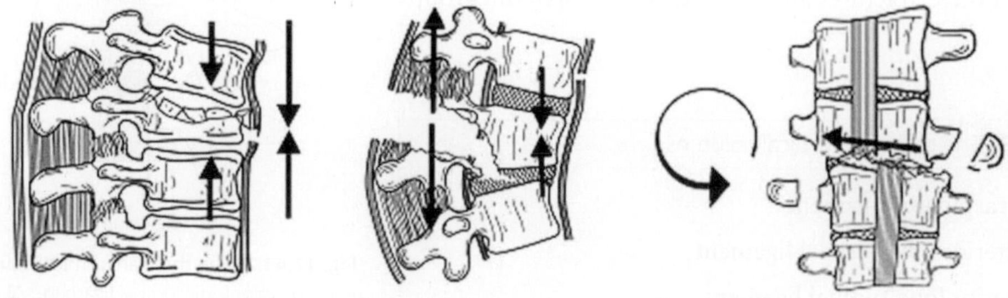

A B C

Fig. 12.43.3 A) Compression or burst. B) Translation or rotation. C) Distraction. The integrity of the posterior ligament complex is assessed and scored, and medical uncertainty is permitted as the ligament may be intact, suspected or indeterminate, or injured. A spectrum of neurological status is recognized and graded. There is clinical utility to the research by this active group.

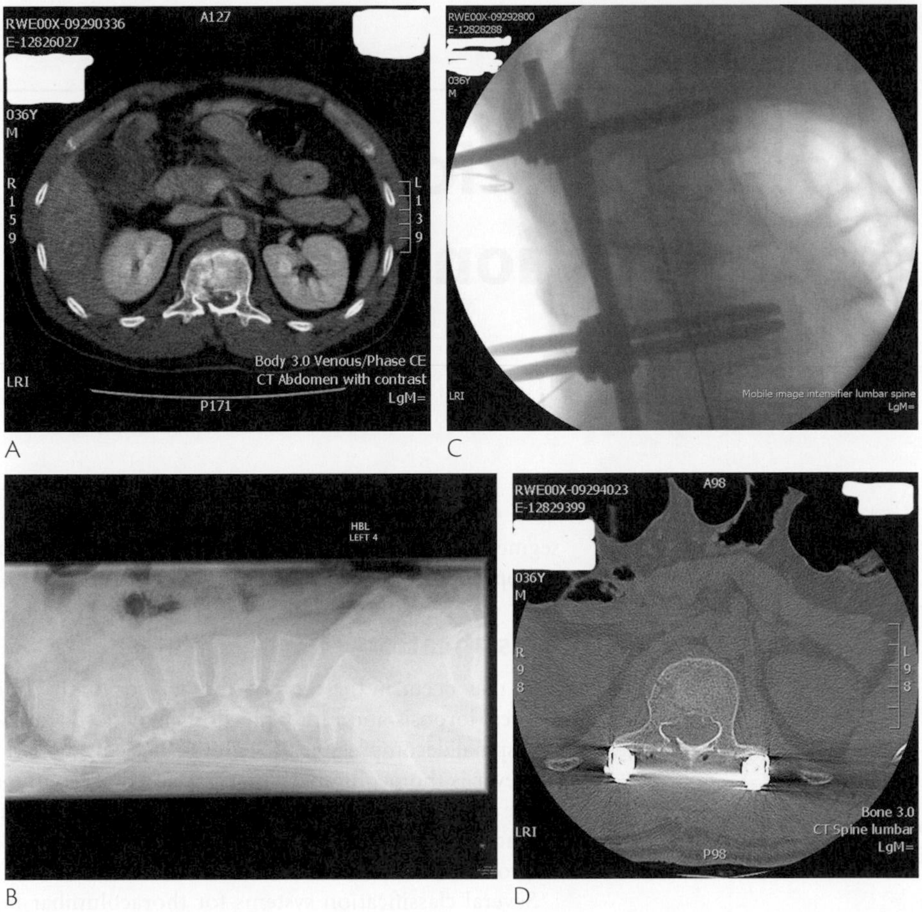

Fig. 12.43.4 Complete motor an sensory deficit in an isolated fracture L1, closed reduction and short fixation. A) Pre-operative CT; B) Lateral plain Xray; C) Intraoperative radiculogram was undertaken to confirm closed reduction of canal intrusion; D) Post-operative CT scan.

1) The presence of active bleeding
2) The presence of an open fracture
3) Neurological injury
4) The pattern and stability of the injury
5) The systemic injury load.

The fracture may be difficult to image with plain x-rays. CT scan is the imaging modality of choice. Radiological features such a fracture of the L5 transverse process may be associated with sacral fracture.

There are a number of classification systems, the most widely used is that of Denis. The three zones described in his retrospective series have an ease of use simplicity.

- Zone 1: completely lateral to the neural foramina
- Zone 2: involves the neural foramina but not the spinal canal
- Zone 3: extend into the spinal canal and may have associated fracture lines.

Any sacral or posterior pelvic fracture-displacement of greater than 1cm is considered to be unstable. Fracture fixation can be considered if the fracture configuration and patient fitness permits. Insufficiency fractures in metabolic bone disease may not be amenable to fixation.

Further reading

Bracken, M.B., Shepherd, M.J., Collins, W.F., *et al.* (1990). A randomised controlled trial of methoprednisolone in the treatment of acute spinal cord injuries. *New England Journal of Medicine*, **322**, 1406–11.

Denis, F. (1983). The three column spine and its significance in the classification of acute thoracolumbar injuries. *Spine*, **8**, 817–31.

Holdsworth, F.W. (1963). Fractures, dislocations and fracture dislocations of the spine. *Journal of Bone and Joint Surgery*, **45B**, 6–20.

Vaccaro, A R., Lehman, R.A., Hurlbert, R.J., *et al.* (2005). A new classification of thoracolumbar injuries: the importance of injury morphology, the integrity of the posterior ligamentous complex, and neurologic status. *Spine*, **30**, 2325–33.

Wood, K., Butterman, G., Mehbod, A., Garvey, T., Jhanjee, R., and Sechriest, V. (2003). Operative compared with non operative treatment of a thoracolumbar burst fracture without a neurological deficit: A prospective randomized study. *Journal of Bone and Joint Surgery*, **85A**, 773–81.

12.44

Post-traumatic spinal reconstruction

Brian J.C. Freeman

Summary points

- The commonest site for post-traumatic kyphosis (PTK) is the thoraco-lumbar junction
- Symptoms of PTK may include pain, progressive deformity, neurological deficit and unacceptable cosmesis
- Localized kyphotic deformity greater than 30 degrees increases the risk of chronic pain
- Surgical options for the correction of PTK depend on the magnitude and location of the deformity and whether the deformity is fixed or mobile.

Incidence

In the United States of America approximately 50 000 fractures of the spine occur each year. Between 7000 and 10 000 of these are associated with neurological deficit. The thoracolumbar junction (T10–L2) is the commonest site for such injury. This predilection may be explained by virtue of its unprotected position between two rigid lever arms formed by the upper thoracic and lower lumbar spine.

Post-traumatic kyphosis (PTK) is a common sequel to fractures in this region, particularly following neglected flexion–compression, flexion–distraction, and burst fractures. The resultant late deformity may result in pain, neurological deficit, or unacceptable cosmesis requiring complex reconstruction of the spine.

Anatomy

The spine has a characteristic alignment in the coronal and sagittal planes. In the coronal plane the spine is straight. In the sagittal plane, the spine is lordotic in the cervical and lumbar regions and kyphotic in the thoracic region. The normal cervical lordosis is 30–50 degrees, with the majority occurring at the C1–C2 level. The normal thoracic kyphosis is 10-40 degrees. The normal lumbar lordosis is 40–60 degrees with up to 75% occurring between L4 and S1. The thoracolumbar junction measured between the superior endplate of T10 and the inferior endplate of L2 usually measures 0 degrees.

In stance, the C7 plumb line should pass within a few millimetres of the posterosuperior corner of S1. The lordotic and kyphotic segments of the spine must ultimately *balance* the occiput over the sacropelvic axis for posture to be energy-efficient.

Classification

PTK may occur in the cervical, thoracic, or lumbar spine. Loss of cervical lordosis and lumbar lordosis may occur following posterior spinal decompressive procedures. The commonest site of PTK however is thoracolumbar junction. The thoracolumbar junction is the biomechanical transition zone between the relatively rigid thoracic spine and the highly flexible lumbar spine and is relatively unprotected.

Several classification systems for thoracolumbar injuries have been described. However, these often lack validity and reproducibility, serving only as descriptors of injury and not necessarily as predictors of outcome. The thoracolumbar injury classification severity score (TLICS) attempts to address this by assessing the fracture morphology, the integrity of the posterior ligamentous complex, and the neurological status of the patient. Careful use of this classification may improve the diagnostic accuracy of such injuries, resulting in more aggressive early treatment, potentially minimizing the risk of PTK.

Assessment

History (Box 12.44.1)

The present site and severity of pain should be ascertained. Pain may be localized to the original fracture site. It may result from a pseudarthrosis or failure of the fracture to heal, or it may be secondary to adjacent level intervertebral disc degeneration or facet joint degeneration. Alternatively, the pain may be remote from the fracture site. Malcolm et al. highlighted the problem of low back pain resulting from *muscle fatigue* as the posterior spinal muscles attempt to correct the sagittal imbalance produced by a more cranial PTK.

Patients may complain of loss of height or progressive deformity. Others will complain of discomfort when sitting in hard-backed chairs when the gibbus makes contact with the back of the chair. Others still will complain of unacceptable cosmesis. Neurological dysfunction may be evident with radicular-type symptoms suggestive of individual nerve root compromise or in more severe cases there may be spinal cord involvement with lower limb weakness, bladder, bowel, or sexual dysfunction.

Box 12.44.1 Presenting symptoms of PTK

- Pain
- Progressive kyphosis
- Instability
- Increasing neurological deficit
- Unacceptable cosmesis.

Examination

The patient should be examined in the standing position with attention paid both to frontal and sagittal alignment. The spinal balance should be formally assessed with a plumb line in both posterior and lateral views. The site and size of the gibbus should be noted. This will become more obvious if the patient is asked to bend forward. The range of motion in the spine should be assessed. An attempt should be made to ascertain whether the deformity is *fixed* or *flexible*. This may be done, for example, by asking the patient to lie on a flat couch to see if the deformity corrects. A complete neurological examination including abdominal reflexes and rectal examination should be carried out.

Investigations (Box 12.44.2)

Box 12.44.2 Investigations

- Plain radiography:
  - Standing lateral views
  - Flexion/extension films
- Computed tomography: sagittal/coronal reconstructions
- MRI to assess:
  - Posterior ligamentous complex
  - Adjacent intervertebral discs
  - Degree of neural compromise
- Provocative discography: to assess pain source
- Baseline SSEP: to allow spinal cord monitoring

Plain radiographs

Standing anteroposterior and lateral radiographs of the whole spine will allow assessment of the focal kyphosis by measurement of the Cobb angle. This is the angle subtended by a line drawn over the superior endplate and a line drawn over the inferior endplate of the vertebral body above and below the level of injury. These standing radiographs will also allow for an assessment of the global sagittal balance. The C7 sagittal plumb line should pass on average 40mm anterior to the posterosuperior margin of the S1 endplate. A hyperextension film over a bolster placed at the apex of the deformity will allow for an accurate assessment of the flexibility of the deformity (important in planning the surgical strategy). Serial lateral standing radiographs will allow assessment of progression of the deformity over time.

Computed tomography

Computed tomography with fine cuts (1–3mm) will allow a detailed evaluation of the bony architecture and fracture geometry. Sagittal and coronal reconstructions may confirm the presence of a pseudarthrosis at the site of the original fracture and also allow for detailed planning including the need for spinal osteotomy.

Magnetic resonance imaging

Magnetic resonance imaging is invaluable for assessing the integrity of the posterior ligamentous complex, the surrounding intervertebral discs, and subtle neural compression and changes within the spinal cord, such as myelomalacia or the presence of a post-traumatic syrinx.

Provocative discography

This is useful to confirm the source of pain. Under conscious sedation, the intervertebral discs adjacent to the injured vertebra are cannulated using a two-needle technique, followed by injection of radiographic contrast. If such an injection produced concordant pain reproduction, there would be a strong argument for inclusion of this level in the proposed fusion.

Somatosensory evoked potentials

Baseline somatosensory evoked potentials (SSEPs) are important to assess before surgery. If reproducible, they will allow the use of continuous intraoperative spinal cord monitoring to detect intraoperative spinal cord dysfunction before it becomes irreversible.

Management (Box 12.44.3 and 12.44.4)

The treatment of PTK depends primarily on the location and magnitude of the deformity, its stiffness on hyperextension films, and the anatomical source of pain. Conservative measures including non-steroidal anti-inflammatory medication and physiotherapy (aimed at optimizing the spinal extensor muscle activity and postural readjustment) should be given a fair trial before surgery is considered.

Indications for surgery include pain, progressive neurological deficit, progressive spinal deformity, and unacceptable cosmesis. Patients who have a localized kyphotic deformity of greater than or equal to 30 degrees have been noted to have an increased risk of chronic pain at the site of the kyphosis.

Goals of surgery include correction of the deformity, restoration of sagittal balance, provision of immediate stability, improvement of neurological function, and reduction in pain. In so doing, it is important to recreate a load-sharing and tension band system and to fuse only the damaged segments.

The basic principles used in the treatment of fractures still apply, however the surgical technique differs. This is because the kyphosis is often fixed, correction is more difficult to achieve than is the case for acute fractures because of the presence of osseous deformity, soft tissue retraction, and elongation. Also there is a higher risk of neurological impairment because of dural adhesions. Very rarely is only one segment damaged, in the majority of cases two segments are involved.

In any surgical correction it is important to use spinal cord monitoring during the procedure. The combination of SSEPs and transcortical magnetic stimulation motor-evoked potentials (MEPs) are extremely useful in detecting spinal cord lesions *before* they become irreversible. Prompt intervention during loss of spinal cord monitoring can lead to a return of normal spinal cord monitoring, thereby preventing a permanent neurological deficit.

A number of different surgical procedures have been described, depending on the magnitude and location of the deformity and whether the deformity is fixed or mobile.

Posterior-only instrumented fusion

This is particularly useful for flexible multisegmental deformities which lack focal angular kyphosis. Multiple extension (Chevron) osteotomies with segmental fixation may allow return of a normal sagittal contour. In this type of surgery, the importance of a comprehensive resection of the facet joints or fusion mass cannot be overemphasized.

Anterior-only instrumented fusion ± decompression

This technique requires either a thoracotomy or a thoracoabdominal approach, depending on the level of the PTK. For fixed kyphotic deformity, the anterior-only approach provides a less reliable and sometimes incomplete correction.

Benli et al. (2007) treated 40 patients with PTK with a mean age of 44.7 years (range 18–65 years) with anterior vertebrectomy, decompression and anterior fusion with costal or iliac crest bone graft. The preoperative kyphosis measured 51.4 degrees ± 13.8 degrees compared to a postoperative kyphosis of 7.0 degrees ± 7.6 degrees. At a minimum of 5-year follow-up, the mean loss of correction was 1.4 degrees ± 1.8 degrees. These authors reported complete resolution of pain in 36 patients with partial resolution of pain in the remainder. For those patients with neurological deficit before surgery (24 patients), all noted an improvement following surgery. Improvements in pain and functional assessment were noted, as well as total SRS-22 scores and each individual domain score (pain, function, mental status, self-image, and satisfaction).

Gertzbein (1992) in a study of 1019 *acute* spinal fractures noted that anterior surgery was *more* beneficial in improving complete

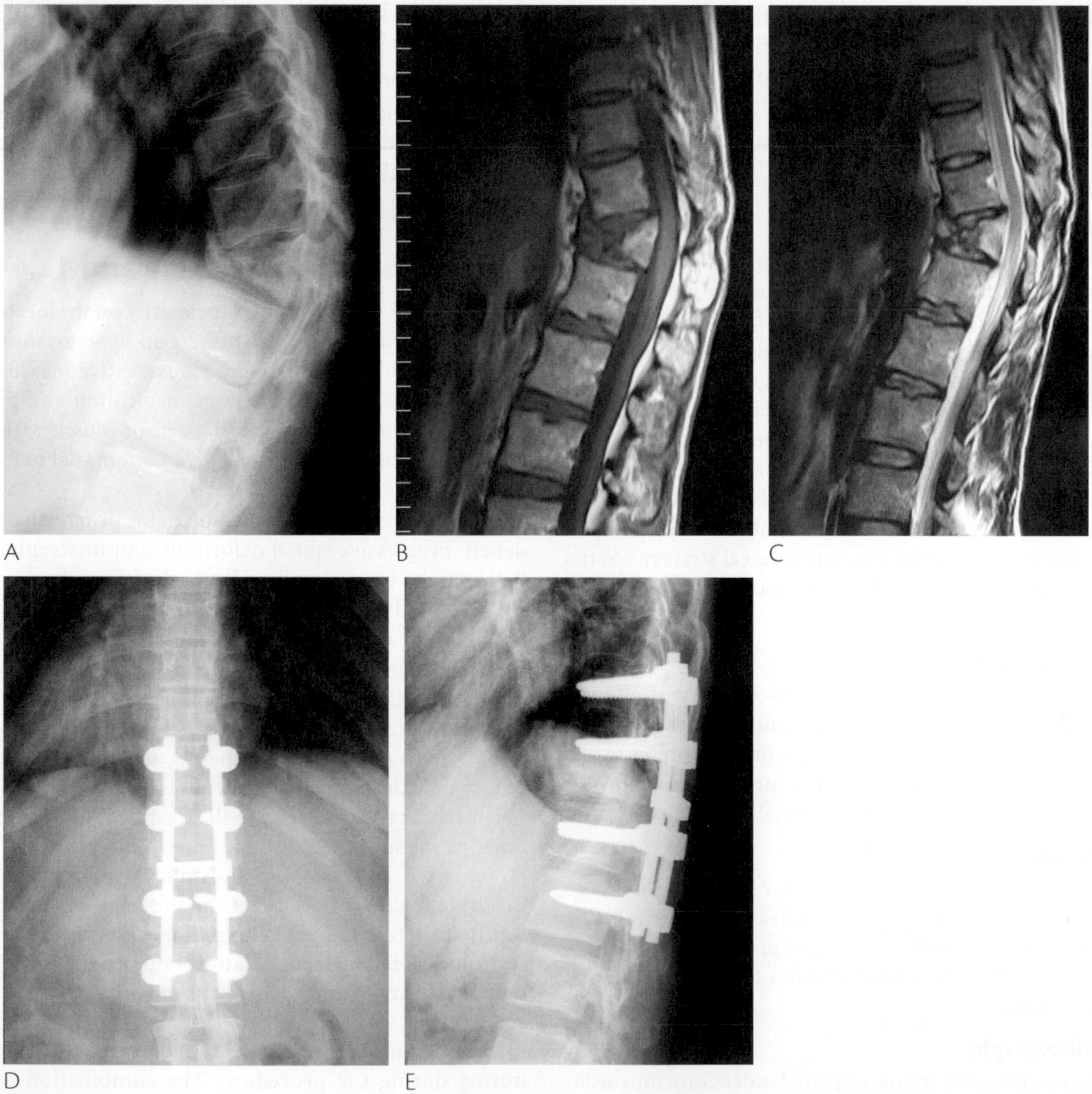

Fig. 12.44.1 Thirty-nine-year-old female sustained a burst fracture of T12. Initial treatment was conservative. A) Standing lateral plane radiograph. Kyphosis measures 50 degrees. B) Mid-sagittal T_1-weighted MRI scan. C) Mid-sagittal T_2-weighted MRI scan. D) Standing AP radiograph following pedicle subtraction osteotomy at T12 with posterior instrumentation from T10 to L2. E) Lateral postoperative radiograph. Kyphosis corrected to 10 degrees.

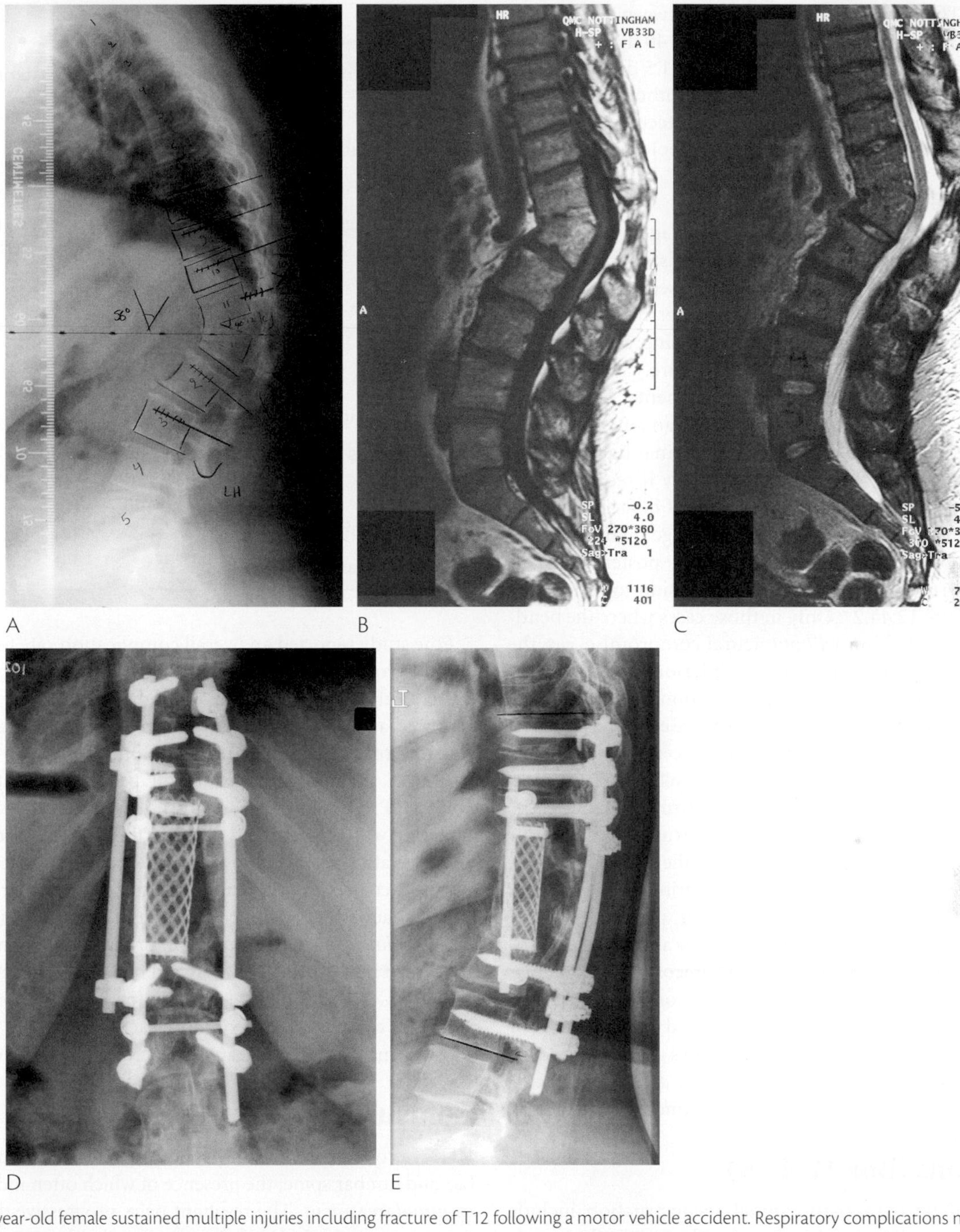

Fig. 12.44.2 46-year-old female sustained multiple injuries including fracture of T12 following a motor vehicle accident. Respiratory complications necessitated upright sitting posture in intensive care. Post-traumatic kyphosis developed with pain and progressive deformity. A) Standing lateral radiograph whole spine. Kyphosis angle 56 degrees. B) Mid-sagittal T_1-weighted MRI scan. C) Mid-sagittal T_2-weighted MRI scan. Note small remnant of T12 with spontaneous fusion between T11 and L1. No significant neural compromise evident. D) Following three-stage correction. Posterior pedicular fixation with anterior column reconstruction. Standing AP postoperative radiograph. E) Standing lateral postoperative radiograph. Kyphosis corrected to 15 degrees.

bladder impairment to partial impairment when compared to posterior surgery. For those patients with an incomplete neurological deficit, several authors have reported significant neurological recovery after anterior decompressive procedures even as late as two years after injury.

Pedicle subtraction osteotomy

This is an excellent posterior technique ideally suited for localized kyphosis requiring a large magnitude correction. Surgery below the conus medullaris (circa L1) is generally regarded as safer than that above the conus.

The technique involves removal of a posteriorly-based wedge involving the spinous process, pedicles and vertebral body followed by segmental fixation (Figure 12.44.1). This is a *closing*-wedge osteotomy thereby shortening the neuraxis. For this reason arguably it is safer than an *opening*-wedge osteotomy, which is now rarely performed.

Wu (1996) treated 13 patients with rigid PTK by pedicle subtraction osteotomy. All patients were male between the ages of

20 and 45 years. The initial fractures were all between T12 and L4. The mean kyphosis before correction measured 40 degrees (range 30–60 degrees), reducing to a mean kyphosis of 1.5 degrees (range −5 degrees to +5 degrees) postoperatively. The authors reported no neurological deficit, no implant failures, no infections and bony union was said to occur in all 13 cases at the osteotomy site.

Three-stage surgery (back–front–back)

Harms describes surgery consisting of three stages, usually performed in one operation. The first stage consists of a posterior release via a transversotomy. This consists of resection of the ligamentum flavum and undermining of the upper neural arch (to avoid posterior compression of the cord during and after the reduction), resection of the facet joints. Only rarely is a complete laminectomy required. Pedicle screws for segmental fixation are inserted at this stage. The second stage involves an anterior release consisting of excision of the anterior longitudinal ligament and intervertebral discs, along with a vertebrectomy if required. The anterior release is then followed by reduction of deformity, grafting and anterior instrumentation. The third stage involves return to the posterior approach for completion of the posterior instrumentation. The structure is loaded in compression to restore the tension band (Figure 12.44.2). Only in those cases where the bending films show *full* reduction *without* neural compromise, can the surgery be performed in two approaches (anterior and posterior).

This technique provides exceptional correction of sagittal plane deformity through segmental and progressive release/excision. The initial posterior approach allows an aggressive facetectomy ± osteotomy followed by anterior decompression/release allowing for a comprehensive correction of the kyphotic deformity. Finally the posterotension band is restored through an instrumented posterior arthrodesis. Disadvantages of this procedure are the prolonged anaesthesia, significant blood loss, and it may well be tiring for the surgeon.

Been et al. (2004) compared an anterior procedure alone (10 patients) with a one-stage combined anterior and posterior procedure (13 patients) for post-traumatic thoracolumbar kyphosis after simple type A fractures. The main indication for this surgery was *pain*. No significant difference was observed in the clinical or radiological outcome between the two techniques. The authors concluded that monosegmental correction with an *anterior procedure alone* was preferable to the more complex combined procedures.

Complications (Box 12.44.5)

Complications of post-traumatic spinal reconstruction include approach-related complications (e.g. pneumothorax, diaphragmatic hernia, paralytic ileus, chylothorax, retrograde ejaculation, dural laceration), neurological deficit (spinal cord, cauda equina, individual nerve roots), bleeding, infection, pseudarthrosis, and implant failure.

Box 12.44.3 Surgical considerations when correcting PTK

- Kyphosis often fixed
- Often multisegmental damage
- Correction difficult because of osseous deformity and soft tissue retraction
- Higher risk of neurological impairment.

Box 12.44.4 Surgical options for PTK

- Posterior only instrumentation ± Chevron osteotomy
- Anterior only instrumentation ± decompression
- Pedicle subtraction osteotomy—single stage
- Anteroposterior surgery for fully flexible PTK
- Three-stage surgery (back–front–back) for rigid PTK.

Box 12.44.5 Complications of surgery

- Approach-related complications
- Neurological deficit
- Blood loss
- Infection
- Pseudarthrosis
- Implant failure.

One study reported an overall complication rate for PTK surgery at 48%. Postoperative neurological deficit was observed in 8.3% of patients and 12.5% suffered a pseudarthrosis. Forty-two per cent reported a loss of correction of more than 10 degrees and 2% had further problems with instrumentation.

In PTK, the spinal cord is often draped over the anterior vertebral column. Pre-existing spinal cord injury, neural scarring, and cord tethering will all potentially increase the risk of neurological injury. Intraoperative neural injury to the spinal cord may occur as a result of traction, correction, mechanical damage or vascular events. Nerve roots or cauda equina may be injured as a result of a misplaced pedicle screw or *inadequate* decompression prior to reduction. Dural laceration is not infrequently reported and may relate to previous scarring. Major vessel injury has been reported involving the aorta and inferior vena cava caused by too vigorous retraction. Posterior screws that are too long may perforate the anterior cortex and cause vessel injury.

Conclusions

PTK is a common occurrence following fractures of the thoracolumbar and lumbar spine, the presence of which often indicates a failure of *initial* treatment. The resultant pain, progressive deformity, progressive neurological deficit or unacceptable cosmesis may offer compelling indications for surgical intervention. With careful planning and meticulous technique these symptoms can be treated with a degree of success, justifying such invasive and complex surgery.

Further reading

Harms, J. (1999). Post-traumatic kyphoses. In J. Harms and G. Tabasso (ed). *Instrumented spinal surgery. Principles and technique.* pp 72–94. Stuttgart, Germany: Georg Thieme Verlag.

Vaccaro, A.R., Lehman, R.A., Hurlbert, J., Anderson, P.A., Harris, M., Hedlund, R., *et al.* (2005). A new classification of thoraco-lumbar injuries: The importance of injury morphology, the integrity of the posterior ligamentous complex and neurologic status. *Spine*, **30**, 2325–33.

Wu, S.S., Hwa, S.Y., Lin, L.C., Pai, W.M., Chen, P.Q., and Au, M.K, (1996). Management of rigid post-traumatic kyphosis. *Spine*, **21**,2260–66.

12.45

Rehabilitation of spinal cord injuries

B. Gardner

Summary points

- Fragmentation of care is the greatest threat to the treatment of patients with spinal cord injury
- Level of injury defines disability
- Early care critical to prevent late complications
- Tertiary spinal cord injury may occur (e.g. syrinx of the spinal cord)
- Complications affect almost all body systems directly or indirectly.

Introduction

Prior to the Second World War most spinal cord-injured patients died soon after injury. The establishment of systems of comprehensive care, pioneered by the National Spinal Injuries Centre in Stoke Mandeville Hospital, changed this situation.

Spinal cord injury affects every system of the body. Successful rehabilitation depends on the effective management of all aspects. Failure of care in any area results in unnecessary morbidity and mortality. A multidisciplinary approach is essential if the optimum rehabilitation outcome is to be achieved.

The greatest threat to the successful rehabilitation of the patient is fragmentation of care. To avoid this, systems of care were initially developed in the United Kingdom, and later in Australia, New Zealand, the United States of America, and Canada, where all aspects of treatment could be addressed by those with the required training. Those systems where all facets of medical care following the accident and emergency department phase are dealt with in one centre have fewer complications than those that involve acute care in one hospital followed by subacute and chronic care elsewhere.

Definitions

A spinal cord injury is complete if there is no somatic motor or sensory function below the level of injury. If the arms are spared the patient has paraplegia. If they are involved the patient has tetraplegia. The level of injury is the lowest intact spinal cord segment. If there is residual function several segments below this then the injury is incomplete and the patient has either paraparesis or tetraparesis.

Box 12.45.1 Spinal cord injury

- 0–50/million/year
- Road accidents commonest cause
- Diving, rugby, and horse riding commonest sports.

Epidemiology (Box 12.45.1)

The incidence of traumatic spinal cord injury is between 10 and 50 per million in the population each year. The figure in the United Kingdom is towards the lower end of this range.

Prevention (Box 12.45.2)

The two components relevant to rehabilitation are prevention of the injury, and avoidance of the secondary deleterious effects that are the consequence of poor care.

Spinal cord injury is most commonly caused by motor vehicle accidents. Seat belts, both front and rear, side impact support systems, and inflation bags reduce the incidence and severity of injury.

Sports-related injuries are uncommon. In the United Kingdom the most common are, in order of frequency, diving, rugby, and horse riding.

Diving-related injuries can be partly prevented by good education, appropriate pool design, adequate poolside signs, and appropriate supervision by attendants trained in safe methods of retrieval.

Rugby injuries can be reduced by adherence to the rules of the game, the avoidance of participants playing out of position, and ensuring that players are suitably fit. Where complete tetraplegia is

Box 12.45.2 Prevention

- Vehicle design and road safety measures
- Sports training
- Stabilization of acute injuries.

caused by cervical dislocation, relocation within 4h of injury can produce full recovery in two-thirds of cases.

Avoidance of the secondary deleterious effects that are a consequence of poor care is dependent firstly on the recognition that a spinal injury may have occurred, and secondly on knowledge of, and expertise in the correct actions to take. Ten per cent of unstable spinal injuries in the United Kingdom are missed. Of these, circa 50% deteriorate neurologically due predominantly to inappropriate movement at the injury site, compared with less than 5% of those managed appropriately. Common sites where fractures are overlooked include the cervicodorsal junction and spinal fractures below the major fracture. If there are reasonable grounds for believing that there is an unstable spinal injury, appropriate steps must be taken to immobilize the spine until the diagnosis has been confirmed or refuted. The more the spinal cord is damaged the less complete its recovery and the worse the rehabilitation outcome.

Clinical management

Optimum rehabilitation outcome depends on good management of all facets that affect the spinal cord-injured person.

Management of associated injuries (Box 12.45.3)

Associated injuries must be well treated to ensure optimum rehabilitation outcome. Amongst the more important are the following.

Brain

Successful rehabilitation following spinal cord injury is dependent on the total involvement of the disabled person. Good executive function enables the spinal cord-injured person to lead a safe and well-integrated life. Relatively minor impairments of personality, memory, concentration, and intellect can interact with the other problems associated with spinal cord injury to make safe independent living and successful employment more difficult.

Limb joints and bones

People with spinal cord damage are more dependent on their arms than prior to injury. Joint damage, and to a lesser extent long-bone fractures, can severely impair transfers and wheelchair skills. Contractures are frequently very disabling.

Problems in arm joints commence at an earlier age after spinal cord injury because they are put under stress by the routine activities of wheelchair life. The onset of these difficulties is accelerated by damage sustained at the time of injury.

Peripheral nerve injuries, especially brachial plexus

Peripheral nerve and brachial plexus injuries occasionally occur in association with the spinal cord damage. Paraplegics require both arms for most activities. The affected arm cannot cope so well with transfers and wheelchair control.

Chest and abdomen

Chest and abdominal injuries, though life-threatening at the time of injury, are seldom important in rehabilitation terms.

Box 12.45.3 Associated injuries

- Treat brain injury
- Avoid contractures especially upper limb.

Neurology

The level, degree of completeness, and pattern of the spinal cord injury are of central importance in determining rehabilitation outcome and prognosis. There is no level of neurological disability, including ventilator dependency, that is incompatible with life in the community.

Methylprednisolone is seldom given in the United Kingdom as the harmful effects of the very high doses of steroids required outweigh the relatively small rehabilitation benefits.

Preserved sensation below the injury makes the paralysed person aware of complications such as pressure sores, fractures, and intra-abdominal events, thereby improving life expectancy through earlier diagnosis.

Neurological level (Box 12.45.4)

The neurological level of injury is the most important determinant of rehabilitation outcome. Each segmental level in the cervical region in particular is of vital importance.

Complete C3 and above patients usually require a greater or lesser degree of ventilatory support.

C4 level patients can almost always breathe independently but are otherwise almost totally dependent. Electric wheelchair mobility and high-technology control of the environment is achievable using retained head and neck control.

C5 level patients have good shoulder control as well as elbow flexion. With aids, such as feeding straps, limited function is possible. Assistance is required with every activity.

C6 level patients have good wrist dorsiflexion. Elbow extension can be achieved by means of trick movements. By locking the elbow, transfers are sometimes possible. Wrist dorsiflexion is associated with passive tenodesis of the fingers and the thumb. Upper-limb reconstructive procedures can be of great benefit at this level of injury. Active elbow extension can be achieved by the Moberg posterior deltoid to triceps transfer operation. Stronger hand key and grasp grips can be achieved by tendon transfers around the wrist, such as insertion of extensor carpi radialis longus into flexor digitorum profundus and brachioradialis into flexor pollucis longus. These procedures do not usually increase transfer capability. They improve upper-limb control and lead to improved quality of life.

C7 and C8 level patients lack fine intrinsic hand muscle control but have sufficient upper-limb function to achieve partial independence in transfers and activities of daily living.

Box 12.45.4 Neurological level

- C3 and above ventilator dependent
- C4 breathe spontaneously but otherwise totally dependent
- C5 limited function, assistance with every activity
- C6 can sometimes transfer
- C7/8 can transfer, some independence of activities
- T2–6 poor trunk control, difficulty transferring, poor trunk control
- L1 very limited ambulation sometimes
- Mid-lumbar younger patients can ambulate.

Upper-thoracic (T2–T6) level patients lack the abdominal and lower paraspinal muscle control required for good truncal balance. Wheelchair control and transfers are impaired as a result. Spontaneous spasms can cause problems in transfers. Ambulation is difficult and requires both long-leg orthoses and truncal braces.

Lower-thoracic (T7–T12) patients have greater abdominal and paraspinal muscle control and hence better truncal balance. Higher kerbs can be negotiated because of better wheelchair control.

L1-level patients frequently achieve ambulation using long-leg orthoses though this is seldom of functional benefit.

Mid-lumbar level patients have good quadriceps control. This usually allows functional ambulation in younger patients through using below knee orthoses.

Longer-term neurological consequences (Box 12.45.5 and Box 12.45.6)

The incidence of tertiary spinal cord change is commoner than had previously been recognized. These changes continue to develop throughout the life of the spinal cord-injured person. The most important is the spinal cord syrinx. The previously quoted incidence of syrinx formation of 2–4% was largely based on clinical diagnosis. It is now clear that the incidence of syrinx is much greater because the majority do not have clinical features. The incidence of syrinx at 5 years postinjury is 9%. In those injured over 20 years it is 20%.

The presence of a syrinx has important consequences for rehabilitation. Lifestyle should be altered to avoid those abrupt stresses, strains, and other events that could cause serious spinal cord deterioration. Falling from the wheelchair in a poorly executed transfer, for example, can be associated with loss of the use of a hand. The aetiology and management of syrinxes remains controversial. Surgery is not usually required. Continued review is essential.

A neurosurgeon with a specialist interest in the spinal cord-injured patient is an essential member of the multidisciplinary team.

Spine

Following the acute event, spinal problems are not usually an issue. Degeneration may occur at an earlier stage in the mobile motion segments above and below the injured one. This can give rise to increased spinal pain, stiffness, and altered neurological function. This contributes to the greater dependence that arises with aging. Deformities such as gibbus are seldom functionally important.

Long spinal fixations can be very disabling. A young person with paraplegia and a long fixation is usually totally independent in their younger years but when they are older their loss of truncal mobility cannot be so readily compensated by increased movement in his hips. This brings forward the stage at which dependence increases. Long fixations in the cervical region prevent the tetraplegic person from looking around, making driving a car more difficult.

Around 10% of spinal injured patients have fractures at multiple levels. Those below the level of the main injury are important if they cause neurological damage or deformity. For example, a complete cervical spinal cord-injured person with an L1 fracture must have the latter carefully treated if reflex bladder, bowel, and sexual functions are to be retained.

Progressive skeletal deformity is a particular problem in children. Regular careful review of their spinal position is required until skeletal maturity. Whereas gibbus does not significantly increase disability, scoliosis can be a significant problem. Sitting posture, the pattern of pressure on the ischial areas, cardiorespiratory function and transfers are impaired by scoliosis.

An orthopaedic spinal surgeon with a specialist interest in the spinal cord-injured person is an essential member of the multidisciplinary team.

Pain

Musculoskeletal and neurogenic pains are common following spinal cord injury. They can be intractably disabling. Treatment is frequently difficult.

Sometimes the pain makes it necessary for patients to shift from one position to another or to lie down at intervals during the day. Employment can be difficult for this reason and also because of the effect on concentration of the pain itself and its associated medication.

Neurosurgical intervention is rarely required. Behavioural approaches usually offer the best prospect for the patient learning to cope with the pain. An anaesthetist with a specialist interest in the spinal cord-injured person is an essential member of the multidisciplinary team.

Bladder

Lower urinary tract

Bladder sensation and control are impaired by spinal cord injury. All methods of bladder care are associated with events that can be distressing and inconvenient. With intermittent self-catheterization there is incontinence. Toilets are frequently inaccessible. With automatic drainage the urinary sheath occasionally disconnects causing soaking. Penile problems can prevent application of the sheath forcing bed-rest or an indwelling catheter. High voiding pressures can compromise renal function.

When partial bladder control remains there is often urgency and frequency that seriously impairs quality of life. Journeys depend on accessible toilets. Anticholinergics or intravesical botulinum toxin may help.

Bladder management in females is particularly difficult. There are no satisfactory external collecting appliances. The risk of incontinence and the smell of urine impair self-confidence and femininity.

A variety of urological procedures exist that benefit certain groups of patients. The more commonly used include augmentation cystoplasty, surgical or botulinum toxin distal urethral sphincterotomy, the artificial urinary sphincter, and sacral root stimulators. Many patients elect to have indwelling suprapubic or urethral catheters because their improved quality of life outweighs the increased risks of infection, bladder stones, intravesical bladder change, urethral discharge, catheter blockage and autonomic dysreflexia.

Upper urinary tract

Continued vigilance of the upper urinary tract is required throughout the life of the paralysed person. Asymptomatic upper tract problems such as calculi and dilatation can occur. An annual evaluation will usually suffice to ensure early diagnosis and treatment. Improved urologic techniques, such as lithotripsy, have reduced the morbidity of upper tract stones.

Experienced nurses are important sources of advice and help with incontinence aids and appliances.

A urological surgeon with a specialist interest in the spinal cord-injured person is an essential member of the multidisciplinary team.

Box 12.45.5 Consequences 1

- Up to 20% syrinx
- Long fusion can be very disabling
- Progressive deformity common in children
- Pain common
- Bladder and bowel function seldom normal.

Bowels

Upper gastrointestinal problems are seldom significant.

Faecal evacuation is usually a major problem. Most patients require suppositories or digital stimulation. Some require aperients. A disciplined pattern of bowel control is essential.

Episodes of incontinence can be very distressing. They are minimized by discipline and avoidance of precipitating factors such as hot curries.

Most paraplegics are able to manage their bowels independently by transferring onto the toilet followed by suppository insertion or digital evacuation. The rectum needs to be checked after bowel emptying to ensure that no faeces remain.

Most tetraplegics need assistance. Bowel evacuation whilst seated on a shower chair over the toilet and followed by a shower is usually effective.

Bowel problems are common in chronic spinal cord injury. Faecal evacuation may take a progressively longer time. Aperients become less effective. The life of the paralysed person can be greatly disrupted. Colonic irrigation or colostomy is sometimes required.

Nurses are the key team members advising on bowel care following spinal cord injury.

Joints

Wear and tear of upper-limb joints is increased. As paraplegic patients get older, episodes of upper-limb joint pain and stiffness occur with increasing frequency, especially in the shoulder girdle.

Heterotopic ossification can occur in the early stage following injury. Hip mobility can be severely impaired. Transfers and activities of daily living become more difficult. The ossification process eventually becomes quiescent. Surgery is rarely required. It should only be undertaken after ascertaining that there is no residual heterotopic activity. There is a small place for radiotherapy immediately following excision of abnormal tissue.

Contractures interfere with independent living, mobility, and transfers. They give rise to pain and disability. In tetraplegics, contractures of the shoulders, elbows, and wrists are a particular problem. In paraplegics, lower-limb contractures prevent ambulation and interfere with transfers.

Therapy to joints is essential at all stages following spinal cord injury, and especially in the acute phase. Splinting of hands and correct positioning of shoulders and elbows can prevent unnecessary upper-limb joint morbidity. Therapists should establish the treatments that should be continued by the patient, carers, and family.

In the chronic spinal cord-injured person long-bone fractures occur following relatively minor trauma. Internal fixation often fails because of the osteoporotic bones, infection, and the development of pressure sores. Immobilization in casts must be carefully supervised to avoid pressure sores.

Spasms

Spasms and spasticity usually occur in spinal cord injury. They are sometimes helpful but more usually a problem. They can cause embarrassment, hinder transfers and driving, impair sleep of both paralysed person and partner, and throw the legs and trunk out of position.

Treatment of spasms includes eradication of any precipitating cause, in particular intravesical and bowel-related pathology, good physiotherapy including standing, systemic drugs such as baclofen, tizanidine, and dantrolene, local injections such as botulinum toxin, and, occasionally, operative intervention such as insertion of an intrathecal baclofen infusion system.

Systemic medication for spasticity has adverse effects. Baclofen causes drowsiness and interferes with concentration, affecting both quality of life and employment. The intrathecal drug delivery systems can have complications such as tube dislodgement and kinking.

For the management of spasticity to be effective there must be expertise in the spinal cord injury centre in all relevant physiotherapeutic, medical, and surgical techniques. Intrathecal pump insertions should only be carried out by those with experience.

Respiratory system

Permanent ventilator-dependent patients can live safely in the community provided that they have sufficient care. A trained carer must at all times be 'in-line-of-eye' of the ventilated person. This carer must be able to carry out tracheal suctioning, tracheostomy replacement, ventilator reconnection, and bagging. Alarms to summon help immediately are required. With a portable ventilator and other suitable devices, good mobility including aircraft travel can be achieved. High tetraplegic ventilated patients value their lives even though these are impoverished in physical terms

Mid- and low-cervical patients have good diaphragmatic control but no intercostal or abdominal muscle function. Their cough is weak.

Respiratory impairment is the most important increased risk to life in tetraplegics. Carers need to be carefully instructed in the relief of choking, the assisted cough, postural drainage of the chest, the cough assist machine, and clearance of secretions.

Mid-thoracic paraplegics lack a good cough because their abdominal muscle control is absent. They require help with chest infections in their older years.

For the management of respiratory problems to be fully effective there must be a chest specialist available who has a special interest

Box 12.45.6 Consequences 2

- Upper-limb arthritis problem in older patients
- Heterotopic bone
- Contractures may occur
- Spasms common
- Ventilatory problems highest risk for life
- Autonomic dysreflexic episodes can be very troublesome.

in the respiratory problems of the spinal cord-injured. Expert anaesthetic support is required to make domiciliary ventilation as safe as possible.

Cardiovascular system

Postural hypotension is a common problem in the early stage following spinal cord injury. It is seldom disabling thereafter. It can cause muscle neck and shoulder girdle ischaemic muscle pain that is mistaken for spinal column pathology.

Autonomic dysreflexia is a serious potential problem in all patients with injuries at T6 and above. It can be precipitated by any stimulus arising below the level of injury. The most common are those from the bladder and the bowels. Some events, such as rectal electrostimulated semen emission and vibrator-induced ejaculation, are particularly potent stimuli.

During autonomic dysreflexic episodes the arterial blood pressure can rise to dangerously high levels. Cardiac dysrhythmia may occur. Patients may describe their heads bursting open with pain. Sweating may be so profuse that a change of clothes or bedding is necessary.

Because tetraplegics cannot deal with the factors that precipitate autonomic dysreflexia, care must be available to ensure that when such attacks occur they are dealt with promptly and safely. It is essential that staff, patients, family, and carers are fully conversant with the diagnosis and treatment of this unpleasant and dangerous complication.

Despite immobility and leg dependency, deep venous thromboses and pulmonary emboli are uncommon except in the early stage following injury. Anticoagulation is rarely required following the acute stage. In contrast, cardiac and arterial problems are common. Cardiovascular exercise through FES (functional electrical stimulation) cycling or rowing, treatment of dyslipidaemias, cessation of smoking, and attaining an ideal weight are essential.

Peripheral oedema and superficial vascular skin changes are common. Careful attention must be paid to the feet so that cellulitis and other complications are avoided. Chiropody is sometimes helpful. Cardiovascular risk factors need to be regularly reviewed.

Skin (Box 12.45.7)

Immobility and loss of sensation contribute to the risk of pressure sores. Careful discipline and good care will largely prevent their development. The insensitive skin must be inspected morning and evening. The minor red marks and skin abrasions that occur during transfers are best treated by rest in bed until the skin has returned to normal.

With aging, the skin and its underlying tissues become less resilient and the risk of pressure sores increases. Patients may go many years without a pressure sore and then develop a serious one.

During the acute stage following injury turning every 2h in bed is necessary. In the later stages such frequent turning is rarely required. Prone lying is an excellent way of maintaining the hips, minimizing spasticity, and preventing pressure sores.

Paraplegics are usually able to turn in bed independently in their younger years. They require increasing help as they get older. Various aids such as monkey poles are helpful. Tetraplegics usually require assistance with turns. The required time between turns in bed at night depends on the individual. A risk assessment will indicate if one or two people are required for turns.

Variable height beds make transfers easier. The ability to elevate the head of the bed aids independence. Rotating beds are seldom popular. Most patients prefer double beds that they can share with their partners. Beds that appear normal are preferred to beds with a hospital appearance.

Specialist mattresses increase the time between turns and reduce the burden on carers. They can make turns more difficult.

Different types of cushions are available. The appropriate one for the individual must be selected. A spare cushion is required in case the main one is damaged. Good posture is as important as cushions in the prevention of pressure sores. A Jay Back may be required to correct posture. The Jay Protector enables patients to go up and down steps on their bottoms and to travel more safely in vehicles when other methods for buttock support are not available.

The nursing staff of the centre must be conversant with teaching techniques for lifting and turning to patients, families, and carers. A posture and seating clinic is essential to ensure that the optimum seating system for the patient is defined.

Sexual function

Sexuality is severely impaired following spinal cord injury. Men sometimes feel incomplete because not only is normal sexual intercourse impossible but also they feel they cannot be full husbands, fathers, and breadwinners, or be involved in 'masculine' activities.

Women can lose their self-respect. Wearing attractive clothes such as skirts is limited by the leg-bag and the wheelchair. Urinary incontinence reduces self-confidence and produces a smell of urine.

Although many approaches are available to achieve erections, including oral medications, implants, intracavernosal injections, and external aids, the spontaneity, sensation, and orgasm of normal intercourse are lost. Oral phosphodiesterase inhibitors such as sildenafil produce effective erections in approximately 70% of impotent males.

Fertility in spinal cord-injured men is usually severely impaired. Obtaining semen is the first problem. Methods for achieving this include the penile vibrator, rectal electrostimulated semen emission, and microepididymal sperm aspiration. The second and more important problem is oligoasthenospermia.

Fertility centres are usually required for parenthood to be achieved. Their contribution includes preparation of the semen and treatments of the female partner to increase her fertility. Of the current techniques, intracytoplasmic sperm injection has the highest success rate. Men without any motile sperm, such as those who were prepubertal at the time of injury, can now become fathers.

Female intercourse is possible but passive. Orgasm does not occur except in women with lower levels of injury. Fertility is usually unimpaired

Box 12.45.7 Consequences 3

- Pressure sores prevented acutely by 2-hourly turns
- Specialist pressure relieving equipment may be needed
- Sexual function severely affected in men
- Affects male fertility
- Causes stresses in family life.

Both male and female spinal cord-injured people face limitations in their parental roles. Relationships and marriages are under greater stress following spinal cord injury. The prospects for maintaining and developing lasting relationships are reduced, particularly in young women.

The spinal cord injury service must have doctors, nurses, and therapists who are knowledgeable in the sexual problems that follow spinal cord injury. Sexuality and fertility clinics are important. A gynaecologist with a special interest in the particular problems of the spinal cord paralysed woman is essential. Close liaison with a fertility clinic is mandatory if optimum live birth rates are to be achieved for couples where the male partner is spinal cord-injured.

Mobility (Box 12.45.8)

Wheelchair selection requires expert therapist assessment. Different wheelchairs are necessary for different purposes. A sports wheelchair, a lightweight wheelchair, and an outdoor electric wheelchair may be required by the same person for use at different times.

The pattern of wheelchair requirement varies with the individual. It also changes with age. A young tetraplegic can cope with a lightweight manual wheelchair on level surfaces and up shallow slopes. In their older years they will require an electric wheelchair instead.

The range and type of wheelchairs that are available is enormous and constantly changing. Before the appropriate wheelchair for an individual is selected it must be evaluated in a practical setting. The most sophisticated wheelchairs allow control of the environment through systems built into the wheelchair. These chairs can also take portable ventilators. They can provide stand-up or reclining facilities.

The wheelchair must be integrated with an appropriate car for satisfactory mobility out of doors. The selection of the appropriate vehicle and its controls requires careful assessment in a specialized centre. The individual characteristics of the patient must be considered. Tall tetraplegics are restricted in the vehicle that they can use whilst seated in their electric wheelchair. Swivel seats aid transfers.

In general, tetraplegics at the level of C5 and below are able to drive. Those at C5 usually require a joystick control. Some at C6 and most at C7 and below can cope with vehicles with hand controls, automatic transmission, servo-assisted brakes and power-assisted steering.

Ambulation is seldom a functional form of mobility for paraplegics or tetraplegics but it can be useful as a form of exercise. For those with poor truncal balance, such as low tetraplegics and higher-thoracic paraplegics, orthoses that provide truncal support are necessary. With lower thoracic and upper-lumbar levels of injury, knee–ankle–foot orthoses usually suffice. Those with good quadriceps control usually ambulate with ankle–foot orthoses alone. The majority of spinal cord-injured patients who learn to ambulate soon cease to do so. Few regret having mastered the technique.

Public transport, such as buses and trains, is difficult. Air travel is usually feasible.

Recreational mobility equipment, such as the quadbike for mobility over rough ground, can be helpful.

A portable ramp is useful when visiting places where ramped access is not available.

Transfers

This refers to the way in which a paralysed person gets from one position to another.

Nearly all paraplegics become independent in level transfers. Most achieve the more difficult split-level transfers such as from easy chair to wheelchair and out of the bath. The most difficult transfers, such as getting from the floor into the wheelchair, are achieved by only the most able.

There is great individual variation between paraplegics in their capability with transfers. Factors associated with reduced ability include increasing age, poor truncal balance, spasticity, spasms, obesity, joint contractures and upper-limb problems such as muscle strains and nerve injury. Those with a low arm to trunk length ratio, for example, achondroplastics, seldom achieve independent transfers.

A few low-level tetraplegics become totally independent in transfers, usually with the aid of a sliding board. Most require help.

The minimum pattern of help required by each individual is best determined by a risk assessment after a course of rehabilitation in a spinal cord injury unit. Hoists are important transfer aids. Portable hoists are versatile but ceiling mounted ones take up less room.

Activities of daily living (Box 12.45.9)

This refers to the normal activities of daily life that the able-bodied take for granted. The occupational therapy department is vital in this area.

Paraplegics are usually independent. Tetraplegics are usually partially dependent, especially in lower-half activities such as washing, dressing, and personal hygiene. Obesity, poor truncal balance, increasing age, upper-limb musculoskeletal problems, spasms, spasticity, and short arms reduce the ability to carry out activities of daily life.

Higher-level tetraplegics benefit substantially from environmental control systems. . Provided that a single muscle can be voluntarily moved in an accurate and predictable manner then the environment can be controlled, such as closing curtains and using the telephone. An expert is required to advise which system is appropriate to an individual's needs.

Most paraplegics and tetraplegics benefit from remote control door-openers.

Box 12.45.8 Transport

- Public transport difficult
- Air travel possible
- Many can drive.

Box 12.45.9 Activities of daily living

- Paraplegics are usually independent.
- Tetraplegics are usually partially dependent
- Multiple adjustments to home usually required
- Recreational activities limited.

Paraplegics are usually able to manage wall-mounted shower seats. Higher-level paraplegics and low-level tetraplegics find the shower chair system more helpful.

Most paraplegics can manage a normal bath whilst they are young. This becomes more difficult with aging. A bath-board may then help. Eventually a specialized bath is required.

Psychology

The effects of sudden paralysis, potential double incontinence, impotence, infertility, loss of personal relationships, and all the other manifestations of spinal cord damage insinuate into every facet of life. The impact can be devastating. Despite this, depression is not a major consequence of spinal cord injury. Most paraplegic and tetraplegic people who have experienced a spinal cord injury unit have learned to minimize the effect of their disability. They seldom concentrate on what they cannot do. Children in particular adapt well. Counselling may be helpful at various stages though it is usually resisted.

The psychologist in the multidisciplinary team has an important role not only in diagnosing and treating patients but also in assisting family and staff in dealing with the psychological and emotional strains that surround spinal cord injury. A psychiatrist with a special interest is essential because first the risk of suicide is increased and second psychiatric conditions such as depression and schizophrenia can result in traumatic spinal cord injury.

Family

The enormous impact of paralysis on the family including parents, siblings, spouses, and children must be considered. Relationships can be destroyed. The old age of parents can be shattered by paralysis in their children. The ability of the spinal cord-injured person to be a complete father, mother, husband, or wife is severely impaired. The adverse effects on the family rebound on the patient who sometimes feels guilty for the suffering caused.

It is no longer widely accepted that family members should look after their spinal cord-injured relative. It is better for normal relationships to be retained. A wife should remain wife, mother, and lover, rather than become nurse and carer.

Family teaching days are essential. Chronic spinal cord-injured patients and their families provide invaluable insights based on experience to the families of those who have recently been injured.

Home

The accommodation in which most spinal cord-injured people live at the time of their injury is seldom suitable for life in a wheelchair. Early housing assessment is required.

Incomplete paraplegics who can ambulate and cope with stairs in their younger years find this increasingly difficult as they grow older. Many eventually become wheelchair dependent. Crutch and rollator walking take up more space that normal ambulation. Doorways and corridors need to be wider to take account of this.

Tetraplegics and complete paraplegics are safer in ground-floor wheelchair accessible accommodation. This is seldom achieved in the United Kingdom because most houses are two-storey, and most spinal cord-injured people like to remain in their own area. Accordingly, through-floor lifts and stair-lifts are usually required.

The precise housing requirements following spinal cord injury depend on the person concerned and the pattern of disability. It is seldom possible in the United Kingdom for all needs to be met by statutory authorities so compromise is almost always required.

There should be a covered way for the car and from the car to the front door together with adequate space for the patient to get in and out of the vehicle under cover. There should be appropriate, usually ramped, access to the house. Doorways and corridors should be of sufficient width to accommodate the wheelchair base and turning circle. Adequate storage space should be available to avoid equipment cluttering up corridors and living space. The main bedroom should be of sufficient size for ready wheelchair mobility and with adequate storage space for catheters, urinary sheaths, and other personal equipment. There should be an en suite toilet and bathroom to the main bedroom. For tetraplegics, and paraplegics in the later years of their lives, carer accommodation is required.

Paraplegic and tetraplegic people are less able to maintain their body temperature. Adequate heating is required. The temperature control of tetraplegics is compromised by their altered sympathetic nervous system, so air conditioning is required.

Recreation

Recreations possible before injury are seldom practicable afterwards. A home computer system is often helpful. High tetraplegics benefit from page-turners. Although some paraplegics and tetraplegics enjoy wheelchair sports, the majority are no more sporting that the rest of the population. Access to places of public enjoyment such as theatres and cinemas is often difficult.

Regular holidays help to maintain morale and family relationships. They are usually more expensive. Extra help is required.

Occupational therapists, and specialist clubs and societies can provide information. Many recreations such as skiing, scuba diving, piloting aeroplanes, sailing, abseiling, and various sports are possible.

Employment

This most important rehabilitation goal is often not achieved. The opportunities for employment following spinal cord injury are greatly reduced.

Many universities have facilities where spinal cord-injured people can study. Most succeed in obtaining good degrees. However, there is a great difference between obtaining a qualification and achieving employment. In general, the wheelchair dependent are disadvantaged when there is competition.

Those who had physical outdoor manual employment prior to injury, and in particular those with poor academic backgrounds, usually remain unemployed.

Academically capable patients and those who succeed in retraining in clerical skills still face many problems. It takes longer for them to get up and get going in the morning. At work the car must be under cover and with access from it to the place of work. The latter must be wheelchair accessible. Getting from one floor to another and from one building to another is usually difficult and sometimes impossible. There must be facilities at work to allow for episodes of incontinence. Employers have to accept that complications such as red marks and urinary tract infections will result in time off work. Drugs such as baclofen interfere with concentration and mental agility.

Although many paraplegics and some tetraplegics achieve some form of employment, it is more likely to be part-time than full-time, and intermittent rather than continuous, and involve early retirement.

Continuing medical care

In the chronic stage following spinal cord injury, complications such as pressure sores and urinary tract infections can arise. Some can be successfully treated at home. When hospital admission is required, this should be into a spinal cord injury centre. Annual comprehensive review in a spinal cord injury unit is required.

Aging

It is essential that the effects of ageing are taken into account when planning a spinal cord injury service. There is no stereotypical pattern for aging. Some people are intrinsically more able than others. Others have the effects of aging brought forward by problems such as contractures.

Community care

Low-level paraplegics are usually independent when young apart from domestic activities, shopping, certain obstacles out of doors, gardening, and home maintenance.

Mid-level paraplegics may require assistance with the standing frame, bath and car transfers, and lifting the wheelchair in and out of the car. Spasticity, spasms, intrinsic ability, obesity, truncal balance, and age are important.

Most low-level tetraplegics require some assistance. For example, they can feed themselves but not cut meat. They can drive a car but not transfer into it or lift in the wheelchair. Someone should be on hand to deal with an emergency such as autonomic dysreflexia or choking on food.

Whilst in general it is not appropriate for family members to be involved in the care of their relations, they frequently choose to do so and provide extremely good care.

In general, carers can carry out straightforward physiotherapy activities provided that they are initially trained and subsequently monitored by specialist physiotherapists.

Conclusion

The successful rehabilitation of a spinal cord-injured person is dependent on a full understanding of the particular individual including past history, current situation, and future aspirations. Treatment should be in a spinal cord injury centre that can manage all acute, subacute and chronic aspects.

The clinical service specifications of a modern United Kingdom spinal cord centre have been laid out. They include cooperation in the efficient retrieval and early admission of acute spinal cord-injured patients for specialized care, the provision of all necessary treatment in the acute, subacute, and chronic phases, life-long surveillance, readmission when required, and outreach services at all stages.

Further reading

Bedbrook, G. (ed) (1981). *The Care and Management of Spinal Cord Injuries.* New York: Springer-Verlag.

Bromley, I. (1991). *Tetraplegia and Paraplegia: A Guide for Physiotherapists,* fourth edition. Edinburgh: Churchill Livingstone.

Grundy, D. and Swain, A. (eds) (1993). *ABC of Spinal Cord Injury.* London: BMJ Publishing.

Parsons, K.F. and Fitzpatrick, J.M. (eds) (1991). *Practical Urology in Spinal Cord Injury.* Berlin: Springer-Verlag.

12.46

Pelvic ring fractures: assessment, associated injuries, and acute management

John McMaster

Summary points

- The contribution of the soft tissue and bone in each fracture pattern must be understood
- A large proportion of pelvic fractures will have significant associated injuries
- Successful management of haemodynamically unstable pelvic fractures requires advance planning.

Introduction

Pelvic ring fractures within the developed world are reported as having a yearly incidence of 23 per 100 000 population. Of 23 patients there will be three prehospital deaths, ten high-energy injuries, and ten low-energy injuries. Only high-energy injuries are discussed here. These are potentially life-threatening injuries and their outcome is very dependent on the early management.

Anatomy

The pelvic ring is formed by the sacrum and two innominate bones. The innominate bones are formed from the ilium, ischium, and the pubis. These bones are connected by the triradiate cartilage of the acetabulum which is fused by approximately 16 years of age.

Axial load is transmitted between the inominate bones and the sacrum via the sacroiliac (SI) joints. The SI joint has an irregular surface and a relatively small synovial cavity. There are small rotatory movements during gait. Posteriorly the joint is spanned by the interosseous and posterior SI ligaments that originate from the posterior iliac crests and insert across the entire sacrum. The sacrum effectively hangs between the innominate bones supported by the very strong posterior ligament complex; this is analogous to a suspension bridge (Figure 12.46.1B). The orientation of the SI joints contributes little to the mechanical stability. The majority of stability comes from the posterior SI ligaments. The anterior SI joint ligaments are weak in comparison.

The anterior part of the pelvis is formed by the pubic rami and a symphysis that is composed of hyaline cartilage, fibrocartilage, and ligament.

The pelvic floor is spanned by the sacrotuberous and sacrospinous ligaments (Figure 12.46.1A) and in combination they resist external rotation and shearing forces. The sacrotuberous ligament also resists flexion (sagittal plane rotation) (Figure 12.46.1C). To understand the contribution of these structures it is important to appreciate the orientation of the pelvis in the anatomical position. The muscles of the pelvic floor contribute little to the stability of the pelvic ring.

In single-leg stance the anterior part of the pelvic ring acts as a strut resisting compression. In double-leg stance the anterior part of the pelvic ring and pelvic floor ligaments are under tension.

The L5/S1 disc provides the connection between the pelvic ring and the lumbar spine this is augmented by the iliolumbar and lateral lumbosacral ligaments that connect the transverse process of L5 to the iliac crest and sacral ala, respectively.

When the pelvic ring is disrupted, the abdominal wall helps to limit pelvic volume; this is breached during a laparotomy.

Pelvic stability

Stability is defined as the ability of the pelvic ring to withstand physiological forces without abnormal deformation. This is a key concept in the management of pelvic injury.

When a force is applied to the pelvis, both the bone and ligaments fail sequentially in a predictable order. As the pelvis functions mechanically as a ring, disruption of one part necessitates disruption elsewhere. However, that disruption is not always complete and mechanical continuity can be maintained by the ligaments. The transition from stable to unstable patterns is dependent on the integrity of both the bone and ligamentous structures that make up the posterior part of the pelvic ring (Box 12.46.1).

A pelvic injury is described as *completely unstable* when a hemipelvis is unable to resist deformation in any plane. For this to occur

Box 12.46.1 Pelvic ring injuries

- Stable
- Partially or rotationally unstable
- Completely unstable.

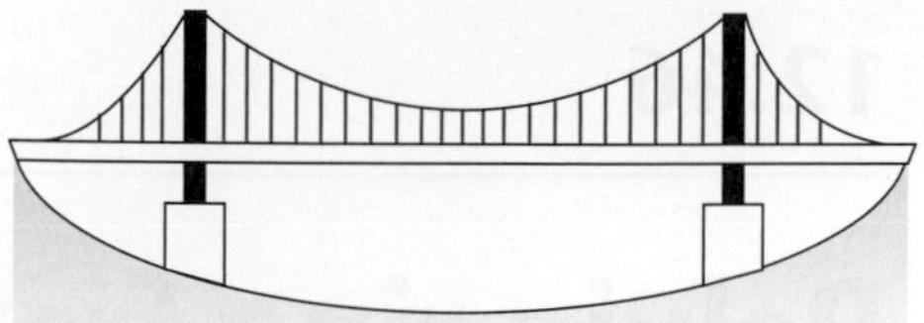

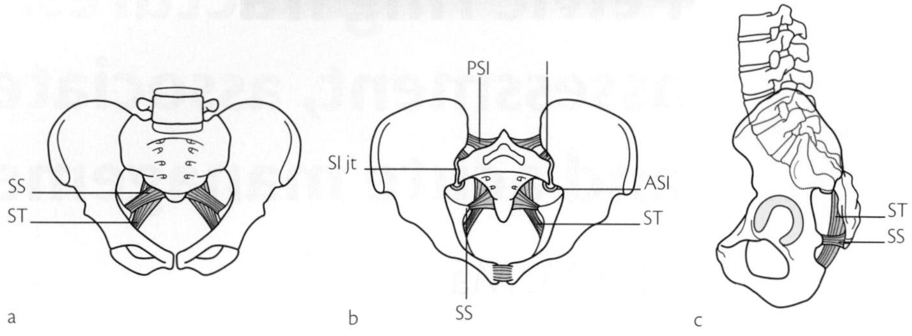

Fig. 12.46.1 A) AP view pelvis, B) Inlet view pelvis, C) Lateral view pelvis. ST, sacrotuberous ligament; SS, sacrospinous ligament; ASI, anterior sacroiliac ligament; I, interosseous ligament; SI jt, sacroiliac joint; PSI, posterior sacroiliac ligament.

there must be a complete disruption of the anterior and posterior pelvis (bone, joint, or ligament) resulting in a mechanical disconnection of the lower limb from the axial skeleton.

Pelvic injuries can also be considered *partially* or *rotationally unstable* when there is incomplete disruption of the posterior complex and pelvic floor ligaments. Vertical stability may be maintained, however there is loss of stability in the horizontal plane, e.g. internal or external rotation.

There are a group of *stable* pelvic ring fracture patterns that do not compromise the mechanical integrity of the pelvic ring. This group also includes avulsions (e.g. avulsion of rectus femoris with anterior inferior iliac crest) or direct blows (e.g. transverse sacral fractures below the sacrogluteal arch and iliac crest fractures). The management of these injuries will be dealt with in the next chapter (Chapter 12.47).

How the pelvis fails during loading is dependent on many factors such as bone density, rate of loading, contact surfaces, etc. The direction of force, however, is the key factor in determining injury pattern and allows us to understand the residual stability.

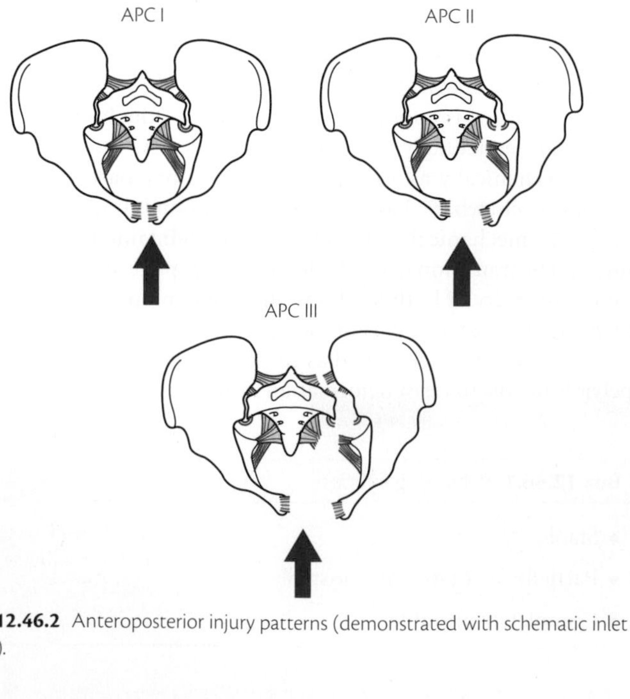

Fig. 12.46.2 Anteroposterior injury patterns (demonstrated with schematic inlet view).

Classification (Box 12.46.2)

Many classifications have been proposed; however, the two dominant concepts are stability and direction of force. The evolution of a classification based on direction of force has culminated in the Young and Burgess classification. The degree of residual stability has been used in the comprehensive classification system. The most recent version has been produced after collaboration between the AO group and the Orthopaedic Trauma Association (OTA) in 2007.

In addition, the Denis classification is commonly used to describe the sacral component of the pelvic fracture.

Young and Burgess pelvic ring fracture classification

The Young and Burgess classification system groups injuries according to the direction of force; anteroposterior compression (APC), lateral compression (LC), vertical shear (VS), and combined mechanism (CMI). APC and LC injuries are further subdivided according to severity. This classification has been used to correlate injury patterns with blood loss and associated injury.

Anteroposterior compression

The force is applied directly to the pelvis or through the flexed hip, along the femoral axis, in an anteroposterior (AP) plane. Failure occurs initially at the anterior ring through the symphysis or through vertically orientated fractures of the pubic rami. Direct AP blows may result in fracture of all four pubic rami. This can be seen in 'straddle' type of injuries where the rest of the pelvic ring and floor remains intact. More commonly with AP loading the hemipelvis externally rotates resulting in diastasis of the pubic symphysis.

An APC I injury occurs when the pelvic floor ligaments are stretched but maintain their mechanical integrity. With further external rotation the ligaments of the pelvic floor and SI joint start to stretch and then fail from anterior to posterior. With displacement of the symphysis in excess of 2.5cm it can be expected that the anterior SI and ligaments of the pelvic floor will have ruptured, resulting in an APC II injury. The integrity of the posterior SI ligament in isolation will prevent vertical displacement and therefore retain stability in this plane. With further external rotation the last structure to fail in this mechanism is the posterior pelvic ligament complex (interosseous followed by posterior SI), resulting in an APC III injury. Although vertical displacement may not be apparent

Box 12.46.2 Classification systems

Young and Burgess

- APC:
  - I—stable
  - II—rotationally unstable
  - III—completely unstable
- LC:
  - I—stable
  - II—rotationally unstable
  - III—LC ipsilateral and APC contralateral, 'roll over'
- VS: completely unstable
- CM: combined mechanism

AO/OTA classification

- A: stable
- B: rotationally unstable
- C: completely unstable

Denis

- Zone I: lateral to foramen
- Zone II: involving foramen
- Zone III: extends into spinal canal.

on the diagnostic imaging this injury is unstable in both the horizontal and vertical plane. Pure AP compression injuries may result in external rotation bilaterally.

Lateral compression

Lateral compression is the most frequent mechanism (up to 80%) and is seen with side impacts and crush. Failure of the anterior ring tends to occur through transverse orientated fractures of the pubic rami (ipsilateral, contralateral, or bilateral) (Figure 12.46.3). The most frequent method of failure posteriorly in a lateral compression fracture involves an impacted crush of the sacrum. Due to the impaction, intact posterior pelvic ligament complex (that spans the fracture posteriorly) and pelvic floor ligaments LC I injuries retain both vertical and horizontal stability.

In the case of LC II injuries there may be complete disruption of the posterior pelvis either through the SI joint, posterior ilium, or both. SI disruption occurs when the anterior sacrum acts as a pivot and the lateral compressive force produces a complete disruption of the posterior ligament complex. The 'crescent' fracture pattern is a fracture/dislocation through the anterior part of the SI joint and the posterior ilium. The 'crescent' refers to the posterior superior iliac crest that remains attached to the superior part of the posterior ligament complex. There is no impaction and therefore these injuries are rotationally unstable, the integrity of the pelvic floor ligaments provides 'relative' vertical stability. With significant internal rotation of the hemipelvis there is also the potential for superior rotation and subsequent leg length discrepancy.

LC III injuries are associated with more extreme internal rotation with associated external rotation of the contralateral hemipelvis and increased instability. This injury often results from a roll-over type mechanism rather than falls and lateral impact motor vehicle collisions that are seen commonly in LC I and II injuries. The pattern of associated injuries is also different with less head, chest, and upper abdominal injury.

Lateral compression can also cause isolated extra-articular fractures of the ilium (Duverney fractures).

Vertical shear

Axial loading, directly or through an extended leg, results in superior displacement of the hemipelvis and indicates complete disruption of both the anterior (pubic symphysis or vertically orientated pubic rami fractures) and posterior pelvic ring (sacrum, SI joint, or ilium) with rupture of the (pelvic floor) sacrospinous and sacrotuberous ligaments, (Figure 12.46.4). This injury mechanism is usually due to a fall from height or motor vehicle collisions and results in complete instability of the hemipelvis. Vertical displacement is usually apparent on the original x-rays.

Combined mechanism

The direction of force may not be readily apparent in some circumstances either due to a combination of sequential forces (e.g.

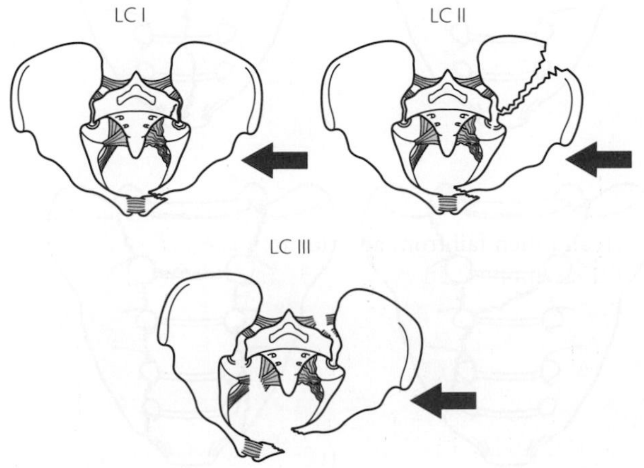

A

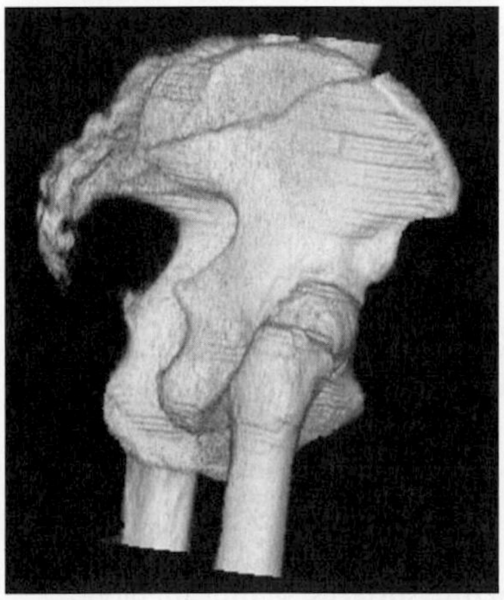

B

Fig. 12.46.3 A) Lateral compression injury patterns (demonstrated with schematic inlet view). B) Three-dimensional view demonstrating 'crescent fracture'.

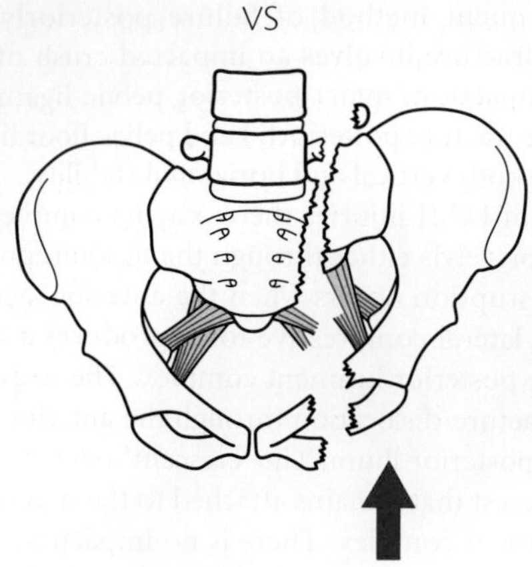

Fig. 12.46.4 Vertical shear injury pattern (demonstrate with schematic AP view).

ejection from vehicle followed by landing) or resultant force acting in a different plane. Common patterns include lateral compression/vertical shear and AP/vertical shear.

Comprehensive pelvic ring classification (OTA/AO)

The comprehensive classification is an alpha-numerical code used for coding throughout the body. In relation to pelvic injuries they are categorized according to residual stability of the pelvic ring. The code for pelvic ring is 61 and subdivided into A, B, and C. Group A represents stable pelvic ring injuries. Group B represents partially unstable injuries and Group C represents complete instability. Subclassification further describes the injury.

Details of the classification can be found at: http://www.ota.org/compendium/compendium.html

Denis fracture classification

The Denis classification describes the relationship of the sacral fracture to the sacral foramen and has been correlated with neurologic injury (Figure 12.46.5). Zone 1 injuries are defined as fractures restricted to the sacral ala lateral to the sacral foramina. Zone II injuries involve the sacral foramina but do not extend medially into the sacral canal. Zone II injuries may also result in instability at the lumbosacral junction. This is dependent on the relationship of the vertical fracture line with the L5/S1 facet joint. Fractures running lateral to the joint are not associated with instability, however fractures running into or medial to the facet joint have the potential for instability at L5/S1 as the facet joint is either defunctioned or separated from the axial skeleton.

Any fracture that extends into the sacral canal is defined as Zone III. Zone III fractures also include pure transverse fractures and complex fractures with a transverse component (e.g. 'U', 'Y', 'H' and 'Λ' patterns) (Figure 12.46.6). These complex fractures result in complete discontinuity between the spine and pelvis.

Associated injuries

Pelvic fracture should be considered a marker for high-energy injuries and associated injuries are very common. All of these associated injuries can have a significant impact on morbidity and mortality.

Vascular injury

In addition to the bleeding from fracture surfaces, significant blood loss may arise from venous and arterial vascular injury.

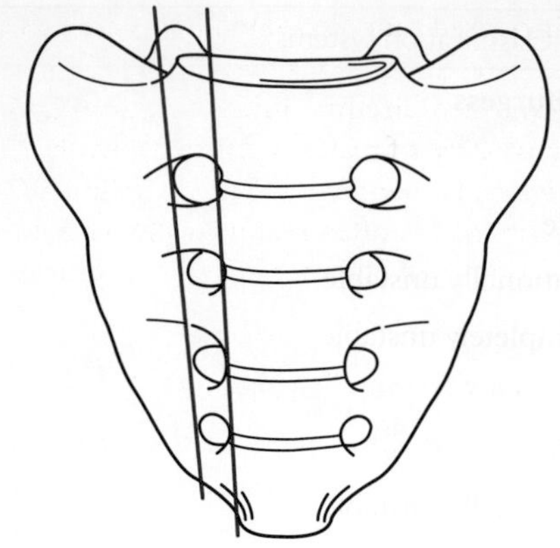

Fig. 12.46.5 Denis zones I, II, and III.

Venous bleeding is much commoner than arterial bleeding. Significant arterial bleeding source is identifiable in 4–15% of cases, and is commoner with more severe injuries of the pelvis. The superior gluteal is the most frequently injured in unstable posterior injuries and the pudendal and obturator vessels are the most commonly injured vessels as a result of the anterior ring injuries.

Genitourinary lesions

The frequency of associated injury to the bladder and urethra is reported at 7–25%. Injuries to the urinary tract are frequently multifocal and the overall frequency and anatomic distribution of urinary tract injury is similar in both APC and LC injuries. Although the fracture pattern is not predictive of urinary tract injury, the type of injury is related to the pelvic fracture pattern.

Bladder injury has been reported with a frequency of 9–16%, of these 60% are extra-peritoneal, 30% intraperitoneal, and the remainder are a combination of both. Extraperitoneal injuries result from a shearing force and commonly involve the anterolateral and base of bladder. Intraperitoneal ruptures tend to occur at the dome as the result of blunt injury to a distended bladder. Due to the high energy involved, pelvic fractures associated with bladder

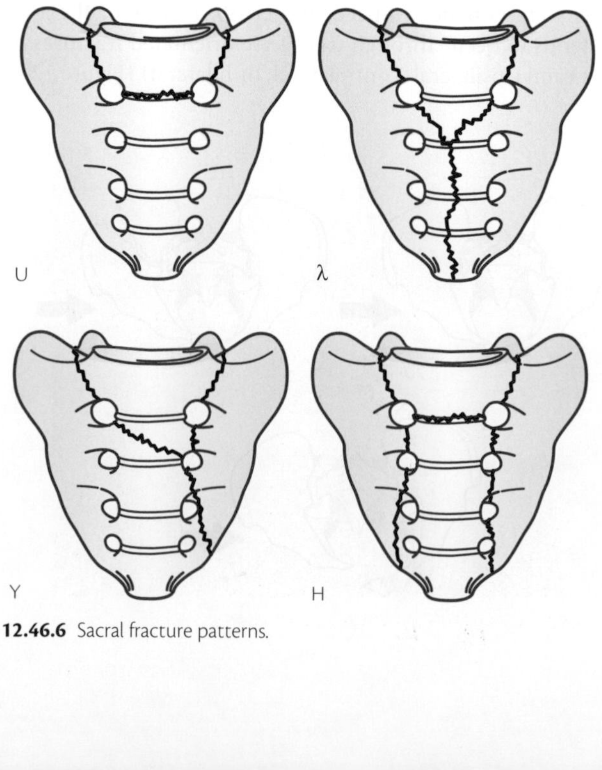

Fig. 12.46.6 Sacral fracture patterns.

rupture have increased mortality rates. Perforations can also occur directly from the fractured bone ends.

Partial and complete urethral injury (Figure 12.46.7) is seen in approximately 10–22% of males and usually involves the posterior part of the urethra, below the level of the sphincter. Female urethral injury is rare and is often secondary to laceration from fracture fragments. Injury involving the bladder sphincter can result in incontinence.

Abdominal and thoracic injury

The frequency of associated abdominal injury is 15–26%, and in unstable pelvic fractures the frequency of abdominal injury is up to 55%. Although the incidence of abdominal injury is high, only a proportion will require laparotomy, this can create difficulty in identifying, prioritizing and managing ongoing blood loss. Pelvic fracture with a liver injury requiring packing has been associated with a 60% mortality rate.

The rectum is held within the muscular pelvic floor, and when the pelvic floor is torn it is at risk of injury.

Abdominal compartment syndrome should be considered in patients with pelvic and abdominal injury, this may be secondary to visceral oedema or ongoing bleeding resulting in a tense abdomen, respiratory compromise and renal dysfunction.

Approximately 20% of pelvic fractures will have a thoracic injury greater than AIS (Abbreviated Injury Scale) 2.

Neurological injury

Pelvic fractures are frequently associated with central and peripheral neurological injury. In the United Kingdom, AIS scores higher than 2 for head injuries have been identified in 17% of cases. Head injury is particularly common in lateral compression injuries. This has been related to frequently occurring motor vehicle side impacts. Head injury has a significant influence on mortality and outcome.

Up to 25% of high-energy pelvic fractures will have an associated spinal injury.

Peripheral nerves are also susceptible to injury. The anterior lumbar, sacral, and coccygeal rami form nerves which traverse the pelvis providing motor and sensory function to the pelvic viscera, perineum, and lower limbs. Neurological deficit may be subtle and has been reported in up to 21%. The sacral nerve roots and lumbosacral trunk are at risk from posterior pelvic ring disruption either as a result of being crushed within sacrum or stretched due to pelvic or sacral displacement. The location of the sacral injury influences the risk of neurologic deficit: zone I, 5.9%; zone II, 28%; and zone III, 57% (within this group, bowel, bladder, and sexual dysfunction occurs in 76%). In transverse sacral fractures there is a higher incidence of bladder dysfunction at the S1–3 level compared with S4 and below.

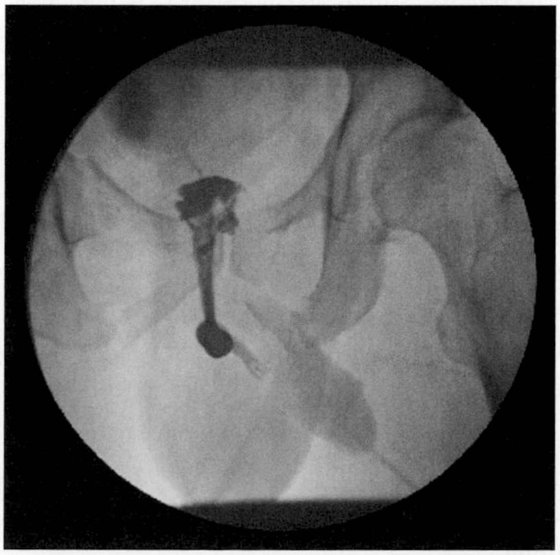

Fig. 12.46.7 Urethral rupture identified on retrograde urethrogram.

Initial assessment

Assessment of a pelvic injury should be conducted along ATLS® principles. With appropriately trained personnel many of the steps can be performed simultaneously rather than s equentially.

The following elements of the assessment are particularly pertinent to pelvic trauma:

- Haemodynamic assessment and response to resuscitation
- Evidence of other sources of bleeding
- Full blood count, clotting, acid–base, lactate, and cross-match
- AP pelvic x-ray as part of the primary series. Pubic symphysis diastasis greater than 2.5cm is suggestive of horizontal plane instability and more than 1cm distraction of the SI joint is suggestive of complete posterior instability. Pubic rami fractures displaced more than 1.5cm are suggestive of complete disruption of the obturator membrane and inguinal ligament. Occasionally unstable pelvic fractures may look relatively normal on the AP x-ray when a pelvic binder has been applied in the prehospital setting. Radiographic findings such as posterior fracture gap (rather than impaction), avulsion of L5 transverse process, lateral border of sacrum (sacrotuberous ligament), or ischial spine (sacrospinous ligament) or SI displacement of 5mm in any plane should alert the clinician of the potential for instability
- Temperature
- Rectal examination to identify abnormal rectal tone or sensation, high-riding prostate, or fresh blood suggestive of a rectal tear. Rectal examination can be performed with the patient supine
- Vaginal examination to assess for tears
- Evidence of genitourinary bleeding. Blood at the meatus (98% sensitive for urethral injury). If positive a retrograde urethrogram and cystogram (with pre- and postdrainage films) should be considered
- Evidence of significant soft tissue injury:
  - Degloving (Morel—Lavallée lesion)
  - Open fractures
- Evidence of abnormal leg position and limb length discrepancy
- Tenderness, palpable gaps, and crepitus both anteriorly and posteriorly. Posterior tenderness over the SI joint is suggestive of injury to the posterior ligament complex

- Evidence of neurological deficit in the lower limbs. Particular attention to entire motor and sensory distribution of the lumbosacral plexus including anorectal/bladder and gluteal muscle dysfunction
- Lower extremity pulses
- Log roll and physical assessments of stability should *not* be performed in the haemodynamically unstable patient. Radiographic findings are usually sufficient and the primary clot should not be jeopardized.

Further assessment and management

The appropriateness and urgency of further assessment and management is dependent on the haemodynamic stability.

Haemodynamically unstable pelvic fracture

There is controversy regarding optimum management. However, there is evidence and consensus that the outcome is improved if the treatment plan is protocol driven. Optimum management will be dependent on the institution and is best considered as a series of standard steps:

- Identify the patient at risk (Box 12.46.3)
- Resuscitate (Box 12.46.4)
- Identify source of bleeding (Box 12.46.5)
- Haemostasis (Boxes 12.46.6 and 12.46.7).

Quick, minor interventions can be life saving during the early phase as the majority of pelvic fractures will be amenable to simple interventions performed efficiently. Ongoing bleeding that does not stop with splintage and resuscitation will require surgical or angiographic control and this will take time to organize.

An early decision should be made with regard to transfer. This a contentious issue which requires senior input and a common sense approach. Transfer to an appropriate facility has been demonstrated to increase the probability of survival by 30%.

Identify the patient at risk

This should start in the prehospital environment and should influence the choice of appropriate receiving facility, avoiding medical 'speed bumps'. Many haemodynamically compromised patients will have achieved haemostasis by the time of presentation and will respond appropriately to resuscitation. The group that requires early identification are those patients who are haemodynamically unstable due to ongoing active bleeding. They will present as transient or non-responders to fluid resuscitation and are more likely to require early intervention. Identification of the 'sick patient' is the priority as this sets the tempo, direction and location of further aggressive management. 60% of deaths with pelvic fractures occur in the prehospital environment.

A post injury median survival time of 55min has been reported in pelvic fracture fatalities (54% <1h; 11% 1–2h; 16% 2–6th h). In general the primary survey (including diagnostic peritoneal lavage (DPL) or focused assessment with sonography for trauma (FAST)), and temporary stabilization of the pelvis should be achieved within 15min and the decision with regard to requirements for haemostasis within 20–30min.

Using physiological signs and readily available investigation will allow the correct management decisions to be made in a timely fashion. Pulse, blood pressure (BP), and respiratory rate allow an estimation of blood loss. The response to fluid resuscitation is also useful to determine adequacy of resuscitation and ongoing losses.

Box 12.46.3 Identifying patient at risk

- Haemodynamically unstable patient with suspected pelvic fracture should be transferred to an appropriate facility:
  - 30% increased incidence of survival
- Pregnant
- Elderly
- Systolic BP <90mmHg
- Response to resuscitation
  - BP <90mmHg after 2 units packed red blood cells (73% positive predictive value for arterial bleeding)
  - Haemodynamic instability associated with >40–60% mortality
- Base deficit:
  - >5mmol/L associated with significant bleed
  - 9mmol/L = average in non survivor group
  - >12mmol/L associated with 50% mortality rate
- Abnormal clotting
- Blood transfusion:
  - ≥6 units of blood in 12h associated with >40% mortality rates
- Triage Revised Trauma Score (T-RTS—based on Glasgow Coma Scale, systolic BP, and respiratory rate).
  - T-RTS ≤8 associated with a mortality rate of 65%.

Box 12.46.4 Resuscitation

- Activate trauma team (preferably prior to patient arrival) and early involvement of all additional involved specialities (blood bank, theatres, neurosurgery, urology, obstetrics, etc.), this will facilitate decision-making and avoid time wasting
- ATLS ® to deal with associated immediately life-threatening injury
- Pelvic binder/sheet—to reduce pelvic volume and stabilize clot
- Pack open pelvic wounds—to help formation of clot
- Avoid disturbing the clot with unnecessary movements
- 'Permissive hypotensive'/'balanced' resuscitation, until evidence of haemostasis (unless head or spinal cord injury)
- Aggressive correction and prevention of coagulopathy
- Maintain core temperature
- In the event of an early transfer ensure that resuscitation can continue.

Box 12.46.5 Identify source of bleeding

- ATLS® primary survey
- FAST + DPL to be considered (confidence in result?)
- Can the patient survive CT with contrast in your institution?

Lactate, Ph, and base deficit (BD) are useful indicators of hypovolaemic shock and when monitored will also reflect the response to treatment. Retrospective clinical review has identified BD as a better prognostic indicator than pH and is a sensitive marker for injury severity, blood transfusion requirements within the first 24h, incidence of multiorgan failure (MOF) and death. Patients with a BD higher than 5mmol/L should be considered at risk of having a significant bleed. Lactate levels are also reliable indicators of morbidity and mortality in pelvic trauma. One study demonstrated that survivors had significantly lower initial lactate levels (4.2 ± 1.8mmol/L) in comparison to those early deaths within a few hours (8.6 ± 2.5mmol/L).

The presence of coagulopathy early in the presentation of a trauma patient is a poor prognostic sign. Prothrombin time (PT) and partial thromboplastin time (PTT) are independent predictors of mortality. Initial abnormal PT increases the adjusted odds of death by 35% and an initial abnormal PTT by 326%.

Resuscitation

'Permissive hypotensive' or 'balanced' resuscitation, maintaining a systolic BP of 80–100mmHg and haemoglobin of 7–9g/dL, is appropriate in the initial management to minimize blood loss and the risk of rebleeding. This must only be used as a temporizing measure until the source of bleeding is controlled. This is not appropriate in patients with *head injury or spinal cord injury and care should be used in the elderly patient.* Under these circumstances it is important to maintain perfusion pressure.

To help control bleeding, a pelvic binder/sheet should be considered and open pelvic wounds should be packed.

The choice of resuscitation fluid is still an area of ongoing development; however, there is increasing evidence to suggest that early resuscitation with blood products is associated with improved outcome. The use of packed red cells (PRC) and fresh frozen plasma (FFP) in a 1:1 ratio is favoured by many trauma centres and the military.

Consideration must also be given to prevention and correction of coagulopathy. Platelets should be administered to maintain a platelet count in excess of 100 000/µL. Clotting can be further promoted with tranexamic acid and Factor VIIa. Factor VIIa is most beneficial when used before the patient becomes acidotic. Fibrinogen levels should be maintained >1g/L with cryoprecipitate.

Box 12.46.6 Indirect haemostatic techniques: decision making

- No useful comparative clinical trials available
- Any stabilization applied quickly is likely to be better than none
- How quickly can embolization be performed in your institution?
- Is the fracture pattern amenable to stabilization with a binder/sheet and will an external fixator provide improved reduction and stability in the short term?

Box 12.46.7 Direct haemostatic techniques: decision-making

- Mortality is related to the rate of bleeding and the speed at which it is stopped
- Is there evidence of ongoing haemodynamic instability despite adequate resuscitation and indirect methods? If yes, proceed with direct haemostatic technique ASAP:
  - Patients who respond to initial resuscitation with ongoing manageable resuscitation requirements are good candidates for AE—can the patient survive the time required to set-up, transfer, and perform AE in your institution?
  - If the patient has failed to respond to 2L of crystalloid and 2 units of packed red blood cells it is recommended that EPP is considered
  - In the patient with multiple potential sources of bleeding the operating theatre is the best environment to prioritize, treat, and reassess
  - If laparotomy is required, perform external fixation ± packing ± minimal internal fixation
  - If EPP is to be performed notify interventional radiology team, they will have time to set up during the operative procedure in the event that EPP fails
  - If evidence of ongoing haemodynamic instability despite skeletal stabilization and EPP assess and treat with AE
  - Repeat AE may be required.

In addition, it is also important to address hypothermia. A 1° decrease in core temperature is associated with a 10% decrease in coagulation function. All intravenous fluid must be warmed.

Identify source of bleeding

In polytrauma, having identified a patient at risk, it may not be clear what contribution the pelvic fracture has made to the haemodynamic status. Accurate assessment is essential as it avoids unnecessary time wasting procedures. Significant bleeding from limb fractures is easily identified through clinical and radiological examination; blood loss volumes can be estimated. Bleeding from open injuries is less easily quantified. The majority of thoracic bleeding can be excluded with the presence of a normal chest x-ray. One of the biggest dilemmas is differentiating between ongoing pelvic and abdominal bleeding. DPL, FAST, and computed tomography (CT) can help to determine the source of bleeding but they all have limitations.

The recorded sensitivity of DPL, FAST, and CT for detecting intra-abdominal injury is 1.0, 0.92, and 0.97 respectively. However, it is the lack of specificity that results in negative laparotomies, reported in one-third of cases. This has the potential to delay treatment of a pelvic bleed.

CT has high sensitivity and specificity but requires the patient to be transported to the CT scan. Emergency CT is extremely valuable in all high-energy pelvic injuries as in addition to information on the fracture pattern it allows the identification of visceral and spinal injury. In addition, CT can identify pelvic haematomas and contrast extravasation. Pelvic haematoma volumes higher than 500mL are associated with a 0.45 probability of ongoing pelvic arterial bleed. Contrast extravasation can indicate ongoing arterial bleeding demonstrable at angiography (positive predictive values 45–80% and negative predictive values of 85–99.6%). Although the negative predictive value is extremely high, a small number of these cases will require embolization and therefore the clinical situation must be monitored.

Although there is no reason for anything other than brief interruptions to resuscitation and monitoring, CT scanning may delay the necessary time critical intervention to stop the bleeding, and this must be balanced against the patient's physiology. If the patient's haemodynamic situation requires early intervention and does not permit CT, then DPL and FAST can be used to help in the decision-making and treatment priorities. However, they have greater limitations with regard to specificity.

FAST depends on availability and technical expertise and in general it has a reported sensitivity of 0.92 for detecting intraperitoneal fluid. However, in the context of a patient who is hypotensive (<90mmHg) from abdominal bleeding the sensitivity has been reported as 1.0. In practical terms if a patient is hypotensive, secondary to bleeding in the abdomen, and the FAST scan is negative an extra-abdominal source of bleeding should be sought.

If neither FAST nor CT are available then DPL can be considered, it has been reported as having a sensitivity of 1.0 with poor specificity (false positive rates for DPL have been reported as high as 29%). The accuracy can be improved with supraumbilical placement and good technique. In a hypotensive patient unless gross bleeding is identified on the DPL, bleeding is likely to be originating from an extra-abdominal source.

Haemostasis

Treatment should be directed at promoting and maintaining clot formation. The quicker a haemostatic technique is adopted the more likely it is to work. All interventions directed towards controlling pelvic bleeding will fail unless coagulopathy is aggressively corrected.

Indirect

In addition to the correction of coagulopathy clot formation is enhanced by reducing the pelvis. Reducing the pelvis reduces pelvic volume, increases stability, and apposes pro-thrombotic surfaces. This can be achieved by using non-invasive *or* invasive external compression devices. Stabilization of the pelvis has been proven to be clinically effective in reducing mortality rates and transfusion requirements. Once stabilization has been achieved the patient should be moved with caution to avoid clot disruption.

Non-invasive external pelvic compression This includes pelvic binders, bean bags, and sheets that can be applied to generate non-invasive circumferential pressure (Figure 12.46.8). The principal aim is to minimize movement and clot disruption at the fracture site. To further supplement stability the lower extremities can be held together with padded bandages applied to the thighs and ankles. These devices need to be used correctly (centred on the greater trochanters), with care to avoid neurological, vascular, visceral, and skin injury through over-reduction. They are quick to apply in the prehospital or resuscitation setting and avoid the problems of pin sepsis. It is not advisable to maintain them for long periods of time due to concerns about skin breakdown. The benefit of this technique has yet to be fully quantified and the limited studies available are not conclusive.

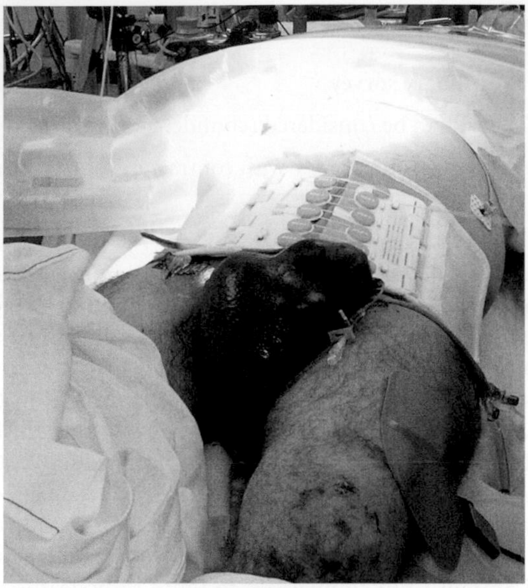

Fig. 12.46.8 Pelvic binder.

Anterior external fixation External fixation pins can be placed in the ilium through both the iliac crest, (Figure 12.46.9) and supra-acetabular region. The latter has biomechanical advantages but is technically more challenging to apply in the emergent situation. Application through the iliac crests is a familiar technique that can be performed quickly (in the emergency department, operating theatre or angiogram suite) without image intensification. Anterior

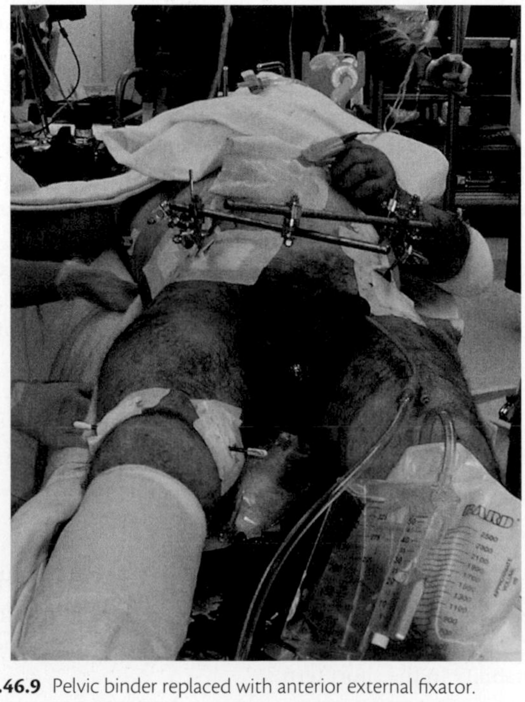

Fig. 12.46.9 Pelvic binder replaced with anterior external fixator.

external fixation has been associated with poor reduction and stability of the posterior ring. Any form of external fixation can be complicated by pin site colonization and sepsis. Ideally pin placement should avoid areas of degloving and if possible the position of future surgical incisions; however, these are secondary considerations in the emergency setting (discussed further in Chapter 12.47).

Posterior external fixation A pelvic c-clamp can be used for emergency treatment of posterior ring disruption. Pins are applied against the outer table of the posterior ilium, overlying the SI joints. The entry point for these pins is at the intersection of the femoral axis and a vertical line running through the anterior superior iliac spine. Posterior external fixation has the potential to reduce and stabilize the posterior ring more effectively than anterior fixation. The c-clamp must be applied with care to avoid placement of the pins in the sciatic notch and is contraindicated in iliac fractures. Over compression or pin perforation risks vascular, visceral, and neurological injury.

Internal fixation Certain fracture patterns and situations may warrant consideration of early internal fixation. In the presence of an open book injury undergoing a laparotomy it would be appropriate to consider plating the pubic symphysis. Posterior injuries could be considered for percutaneous SI screw placement; however, this is technically demanding and should not be undertaken if there is a risk of incurring an unacceptable time delay. Both of these options need to be considered before draping.

Direct intervention

Despite resuscitation, correction of coagulopathy and pelvic stabilization a small proportion of pelvic fractures will have persistent hypotension due to ongoing arterial and venous bleeding. They will require rapid direct haemostatic intervention for survival. In extremis, temporary occlusion of the aorta can be considered by clamping the aorta or insertion of a balloon catheter. Ligation of the internal iliac is of limited benefit due to the retroperitoneal haematoma and considerable anastomoses linking the right and left sides of the arterial and venous circulation.

Extraperitoneal packing (EPP) This procedure involves tamponade of the pre-sacral and paravesical vessels by placing packs into the extraperitoneal space of the true pelvis. This is achieved through a low midline incision. Once the extraperitoneal space is accessed little additional dissection is required due to the injury and the expanding haematoma. Large swabs are placed, from posterior to anterior, either side of the pelvic viscera. For maximum benefit it has been recommended that EPP should be performed within 30min. In those amenable fracture patterns, external fixation is added in conjunction with EPP. The packs are usually removed at second look surgery within 48h.

Routine post-EPP angiography has demonstrated an 80% incidence of ongoing arterial bleed. However, in another study, angiography was only performed in 17% when it was clinically indicated.

Packing has been shown to have a significant effect on haemodynamic status, reduced postpacking blood transfusion, and is suggestive of improved survival rates. It also allows other sources of bleeding to be dealt with by surgical intervention in the same location. It can be performed quickly during the time required to set up for angiography.

This technique requires the immediate availability of an operating theatre and necessitates an open procedure that has implications with regard to infection and abdominal compartment syndrome. It is likely to be less effective with bleeding from larger arteries and under these circumstances may only function as a temporizing measure to limit blood loss. Packing is associated with a 25–29% mortality rate.

Angiographic embolization (AE Figure 12.46.10) AE is an attractive technique for controlling pelvic arterial bleeding with an 85–100% success rate. However, it does not limit venous bleeding. The angiography suite should be equipped and staffed to allow optimum continuation of all the components of resuscitation. In extremis a balloon catheter can be rapidly inserted and used to occlude the aorta. A catheter is passed through the femoral artery at the groin or the left axillary artery if the groin is not accessible. Angiography can

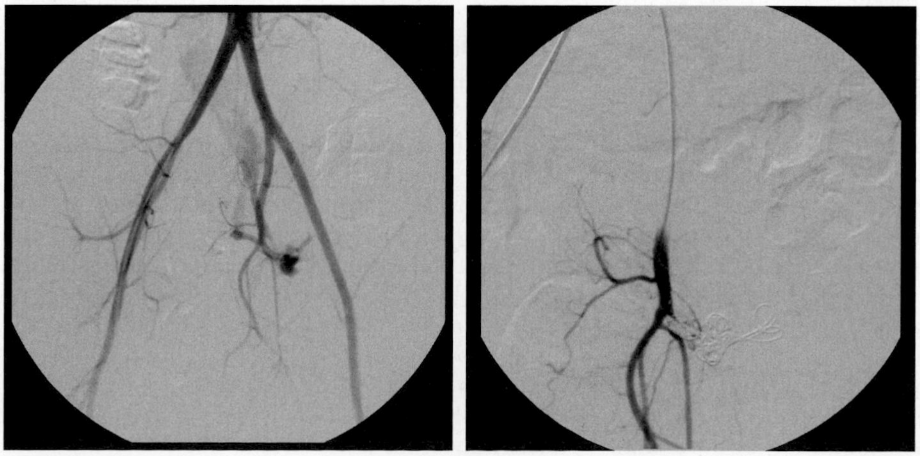
A B

Fig. 12.46.10 Angiographic embolization; A) traumatic AV fistula superior gluteal vessels, B) embolized with coils.

also look for sources in the chest and abdomen. Large vessel injury including the thoracic aorta is present in approximately 6% of those requiring embolization of pelvic arteries. Selective embolization techniques can be performed, however non-selective bilateral embolization procedures, including embolization of the internal iliacs, has been reported with good outcome. In some hospitals it is feasible to perform angiography in the operating room.

Review of the literature would suggest only 5% of all pelvic fractures are likely to benefit from embolization. However, there are subgroups that have been identified with an increased incidence of ongoing arterial bleeding: contrast extravasation and large haematoma volumes on CT; hypotensive patients (<90mmHg) who are transient or non-responders to resuscitation have a 44–76% incidence; BD of more than 6mmol/L (when used as a trigger it identified arterial bleeding in 100% of cases); over 60 years of age (over two-thirds of this group of patients will present with normal vital signs). Venography has been recommended if there is no improvement following AE as significant venous injuries have been identified. It is also appropriate to consider placement of an inferior vena cava filter (discussed further in Chapter 12.47).

If hypotension or a BD persists following any intervention, repeat angiography should be considered. Re-embolization has been required in 6–7.5% of reported cases.

The technique is both resource and time consuming, even in expert hands it requires time. It should be expected that AE will take an average of 90min, in addition to the transport and set-up time; however, this is very dependent on the institution. Successful embolization has not been seen to always result in an immediate improvement in haemodynamic status and reduced requirements for blood products. Not all identifiable small arterial bleeds (seen on CT and angiography) will require embolization. These factors have yet to be fully quantified. The extent of ischaemic complications related to AE is believed to be less with selective embolization techniques. However it is difficult to separate the effect of AE from the injury. Risks include:

- Gluteal muscle necrosis (<5%)
- Skin necrosis (may be sign of gluteal muscle necrosis)
- Visceral necrosis
- Lower limb paresis
- Urogenital dysfunction (has not been clearly demonstrated)
- Nephrotoxicity from the contrast agent.

The cumulative reported mortality rate is 43%.

Haemodynamically stable pelvic fracture

When the patient is haemodynamically stable, with or without intervention, further assessment is required prior to definitive management. Further imaging is required to define the injury. First-line investigation in most centres still involves inlet and outlet views. The inlet view is taken with the patient supine; with a 40-degree cranial tilt of the beam so that it is perpendicular to the pelvic brim. The beam is then rotated to a 45-degree tilt towards the feet to achieve the outlet view (Figure 12.46.11). In some circumstances obturator and iliac oblique films are useful to define the fracture pattern and exclude acetabular involvement. CT (1–2-mm cuts) is a more sensitive tool for identifying occult injury and with improving technology (e.g. three-dimensional reconstruction) and access, the requirement for inlet and outlet views will become more dependent on surgeon preference.

Under some circumstances, to determine stability, examination under anaesthesia and stress views can be used. Dynamic assessment is contraindicated in haemodynamic instability (wait 3–5 days), lumbosacral plexus injury, ipsilateral vessel injury, and lower limb fractures that prevent axial loading of the hemipelvis.

Provisional reduction and stability is important for pain relief and to facilitate definitive surgery. This can be achieved using the methods previously discussed with or without skeletal traction (skin traction is inadequate) to reduce vertical displacement. If external fixators are considered, application should be discussed with the surgeons performing the definitive fixation.

Management of associated injuries

Genitourinary lesions

A history of inability to void, blood at the urethral meatus, haematuria, high riding prostate, and inability to catheterize are suggestive of genitourinary injury. In the presence of these findings urethral catheterization is contraindicated and requires further investigation. Retrograde urethrogram can be performed through a Foley catheter with the balloon sited in the urethral meatus. The presence of a urethral injury demands a urological opinion and may necessitate a suprapubic catheter. Potential bladder ruptures are diagnosed with a retrograde cystogram. The bladder is then emptied and the x-rays are repeated if necessary. Small extraperitoneal bladder ruptures are treated with suprapubic catheter drainage alone, to prevent the accumulation of urine and the risk of sepsis. The majority of tears will be healed by 10 days, the remainder within 4 weeks. Large tears and intraperitoneal tears require surgical repair.

Male urethral tears can be managed with early realignment with a urethral catheter maintained for 4–6 weeks or urinary diversion using a suprapubic catheter for 3–6 months followed by reconstruction. Urethral tears are frequently complicated by stricture formation. In females with proximal urethral tears, early urethral realignment or reconstruction is recommended.

Surgical correction of impotence should be delayed 12–18 months due to delayed return in function.

A vaginal laceration in association with a pelvic fracture should be considered an open fracture. All vaginal injuries should be explored and debrided under a general anaesthetic.

Abdominal injury

In addition to the associated visceral injury seen with polytrauma involving pelvic fractures it is important to identify rectal injuries that may be in continuity with the pelvic fracture. These fractures should be considered as open due to the contamination of the fracture site by faecal organisms. The only evidence of this injury may be fresh rectal blood identified at PR. Rectal tears may not always be identifiable using standard investigations (proctoscopy, sigmoidoscopy, and contrast studies). However, the consequences of a missed rectal injury are serious. Therefore when there is a high index of suspicion, the general surgeons should be encouraged to perform a complete defunctioning colostomy with distal washout. A double barrelled colostomy is not acceptable as it does not completely divert the faecal stream. The colostomy should be placed sufficiently high on the abdominal wall to avoid

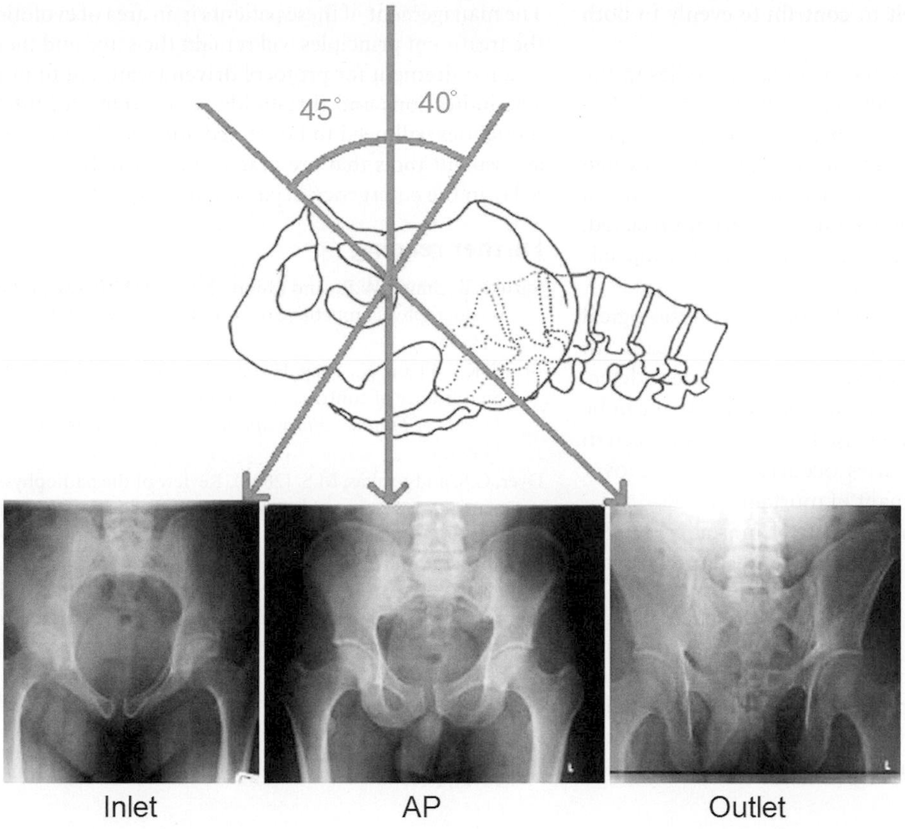

Fig. 12.46.11 AP, inlet, and outlet views. Axial and three-dimensional pelvic views.

interference/contamination of future pelvic surgery. This can be reversed at a later date.

In the haemodynamic unstable patient with pelvic and abdominal bleeding, damage control principles may be appropriate with minimal surgical intervention, packing of the abdomen and pelvis and application of an external fixator. These patients should be monitored for abdominal compartment syndrome. Further pelvic or intra abdominal bleeding may be amenable to AE.

Soft tissue injury (Figure 12.46.12)

Open fractures including those involving the rectum and vagina constitute 2–4% of all pelvic fractures. The mortality rate for open pelvic fractures is greater than 50%. In an open fracture there is less potential for tamponade and blood loss is limitless. In addition there are the problems with deep sepsis. Early studies (pre-1992) report infection rates of approximately 30%, compared with a 15% incidence in the modern literature. Although the reported incidence of infection has improved the mortality rate of open fractures remains high, 67%.

This problem should be managed, at presentation, according to the guidelines of all open fractures with early antibiotics, tetanus, and wound dressing followed by debridement, stabilization, and early soft tissue coverage. Defunctioning colostomy is required in those patients with an open injury involving the rectum or significant perineal wounds that are at risk of contamination.

Closed degloving injuries (Morel-Lavallée lesions) are associated with necrotic fat, fluid collection and bacterial colonization. These injuries may involve the planned surgical field and must be treated before fixation. Open and percutaneous techniques have been used successfully at both the same operation and as a separate procedure.

Mortality

Pelvic fracture should be considered a marker of severity and as demonstrated earlier in the chapter there are significant associated injuries. Many of these associated injuries will be fatal. The incidence of pelvic fracture as the sole cause of death (based on post-mortem studies) is very low, 3.7%, and approximately 50% of pelvic fracture deaths will have other potential causes of haemorrhage.

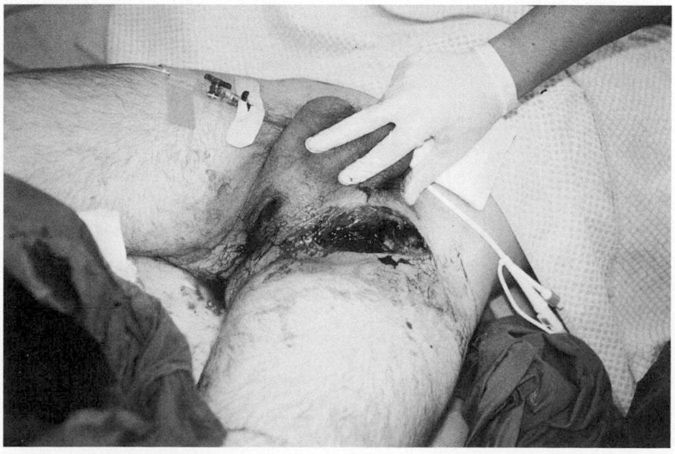

Fig. 12.46.12 Open pelvic fracture with communication of the wound in the left inguinal region to the ruptured symphysis pubis.

In general the pelvic fracture is felt to contribute evenly to both early and late deaths.

Generalized inpatient mortality rates, from large studies in the modern literature, are quoted at 3–20% (cumulative data 12.4%). These figures are dependent on the cohort, usually reflecting the referral pattern for the institution, and care should be taken when comparing figures. These figures are of little value in the clinical setting as the true lethality of this injury can be under appreciated. Haemodynamically unstable fractures have a much higher mortality rate, 40–60%.

In the polytrauma patient it is the cumulative physiological burden of the multiple injuries that often contributes to death. An ISS higher than 25 has been determined as an independent determinant of mortality. The level of physiological burden that can be survived is dependent on age with increased mortality rates seen in the over 40 age group. Pelvic injuries occurring in those over 65 years is an independent determinant of mortality.

Pelvic fracture in pregnancy is rare but fetal mortality rates of 35–80% have been reported; many of these deaths occur prehospital.

Summary

An understanding of the pathoanatomy of pelvic fractures will allow accurate classification and appropriate treatment. A significant proportion of pelvic fractures will be at additional risk of morbidity and mortality from extravasation and associated injuries. The management of these patients is an area of evolution. However, the treatment principles will remain the same and there will always be a requirement for protocol driven treatment to minimize delay. The indications and thresholds for current and future treatment modalities will need to be refined and ideally this will be based on assessment tools that are practical and can be used with minimal delay in the emergency department.

Further reading

Suzuki, T., Smith, W.R., and Moore, E.E. (2009). Pelvic packing or angiography: competitive or complementary? *Injury*, **40**(4), 343–53.

Brasel, K.J., Pham, K., Yang, H., Christensen, R., and Weigelt, J.A. (2007). Significance of contrast extravasation in patients with pelvic fracture. *Journal of Trauma-Injury Infection & Critical Care*, **62**(5), 1149–52.

Dyer, G.S. and Vrahas, M.S. (2006). Review of the pathophysiology and acute management of haemorrhage in pelvic fracture. *Injury*, **37**(7), 602–13.

Miller, P.R., Moore, P.S., Mansell, E., Meredith, J.W., and Chang, M.C. (2003). External fixation or arteriogram in bleeding pelvic fracture: initial therapy guided by markers of arterial hemorrhage. *Journal of Trauma-Injury Infection & Critical Care*, **54**(3), 437-43.

Spahn, D.R., Cerny, V., Coats, T.J., *et al.* (2007). Management of bleeding following major trauma: a European guideline [erratum appears in *Critical Care*, 2007, **11**(2), 414]. *Critical Care*, **11**(1), R17.

12.47

Pelvic fracture: definitive management

John McMaster

Summary points

- Pelvic fractures must be actively managed to avoid peri-operative complications
- Understanding stability is the key to pelvic fracture management. Fixation is used to compensate for instability until healing occurs
- Long term disability can occur despite optimum fixation.

Introduction

The aim during definitive management is to produce a stable, pain-free pelvis with minimal functional limitations and avoidance of complications.

Ideally optimal treatment in the acute and definitive phases of treatment should be complementary but can, however, conflict. This can be problematic if definitive treatment is to be performed in another facility. Even if the admitting facility is not involved with definitive management it is important that definitive treatment options are understood.

Interim management (Box 12.47.1)

During the period between early and definitive management the patient must be actively managed and steps should be taken to avoid complications.

Timing of definitive fixation needs to consider the disadvantages of early and late surgery. In the physiologically unstable patient, definitive fixation can be associated with higher levels of blood transfusion, organ failure, multiple organ failure, and death. Long operations have a greater physiological impact and are associated with a worse outcome. It is therefore appropriate to postpone definitive fixation until the patient is fit for surgery. Problems associated with the 'second hit' are believed to be minimized if surgery is delayed until after day 4. Fracture stability is part of the optimal treatment of open fractures and this will influence timing and method of fixation. Prolonged delay to surgery increases the risks associated with immobilization. It also increases the technical difficulty of achieving anatomical results and this has been associated with worse outcome. The technical difficulties of delay can be mitigated to a degree by holding the pelvis in a reduced position with external fixation and skeletal traction in the case of vertical displacement.

Venous thromboembolism (VTE) is a significant problem in pelvic fracture patients as they frequently have many of the well established risk factors:

1) Injury severity score higher than 15
2) Age greater than 40 years
3) Lower extremity fracture
4) Severe head injury
5) Vertebral fracture
6) Spinal cord injury
7) Delay to surgery.

The presence of any of these risk factors in association with pelvic fracture results in a significantly higher incidence of VTE. In addition, these patients may not have received appropriate thromboprophylaxis due to haemodynamic instability. Deep venous thrombosis (DVT) has been reported with an incidence as high as

Box 12.47.1 Interim management

- Active medical management
- Maintain temporary pelvic stabilization
- Thromboprophylaxis:
  - Mechanical
  - Chemical
  - IVC filter
- Avoid sepsis
- Pressure area care
- Laxatives.

61% in pelvic fractures that have not received DVT prophylaxis. With DVT prophylaxis the incidence is reported as 2–33%. Pulmonary embolus (PE) is reported as occurring in 2–13%. Fatal PE is reported with an approximate incidence of 1%. Early thromboprophylaxis is important as 6% of PEs occur within the first 24h.

Strategies to minimize the problems associated with VTE include early mobilization, screening, mechanical and chemical prophylaxis, and inferior vena cava (IVC) filters.

Although the majority of DVTs originate in the legs, in pelvic fractures approximately half involve the pelvic veins. Ultrasound and venography are poor investigations for deep pelvic vein thrombosis and magnetic resonance (MR) venography has been reported as the gold standard. There is no consensus at present with regard to screening.

Where possible, chemical thromboprophylaxis with low-molecular-weight heparin should be used; however, this can be problematic in this patient group due to both the acute haemorrhage and the need for operative intervention. Pulsatile compression devices are an alternative in those patients in which chemical thromboprophylaxis is contraindicated. Their use is limited in the presence of lower extremity injury and the benefit, on their own, has not been conclusively proven.

IVC filters can be used in high risk patients, those with established DVT and as an alternative to chemical prophylaxis (Figure 12.47.1). A review of studies (1983–2005) reporting on IVC filter use reports a 13% complication rate. Complications include malposition, migration, insertion site thrombosis, difficulty removing the device, and occlusion. Occlusion has been reported as 15%, but can be reduced to 8% with anticoagulation.

Pressure areas must be protected particularly in the unconscious patient and those on traction. Wound care will minimize the risk of sepsis from wounds and pin sites prior to definitive surgical treatment. Constipation should also be avoided as faecal loading causes discomfort and can greatly limit intraoperative image intensifier visualization.

Rationale for treatment (Box 12.47.2)

Treatment strategies need to consider residual pelvic stability, strength of fixation, deformity, pain and neurologic deficit.

Stability is the key to managing pelvic fractures. Stability can usually be interpreted from the clinical assessment, x-rays and CT (see Chapter 12.46). Where stability, in the vertical and horizontal planes, has been maintained, non-operative treatment can be considered with immediate full weight bearing as tolerated.

Where stability is deficient, fixation can be used to compensate until sufficient healing has occurred (pubic rami 4–6 weeks, sacroiliac (SI) joint 12 weeks). It is important therefore that the fixation used is capable of performing the task. Bone quality and the condition of the soft tissues will have a significant impact on the choice of fixation technique.

In displaced rotationally unstable fractures where vertical stability is maintained, as a result of the intact posterior ligament complex, anterior fixation alone is adequate. Posterior fixation is usually required in pelvic injuries with complete instability of the posterior pelvic ring.

Deformity also influences the treatment strategy. In lateral compression (LC) injuries significant internal rotation of the hemipelvis is also associated with rotation in the sagittal plane and subsequent relative leg length discrepancy (Figure 12.47.2). Significant leg-length discrepancy and internal rotation are indications for operative intervention. Thresholds for acceptable displacement will be dependent on the patient and it has been recommended that operative intervention should be considered for rotation greater than 10 degrees and leg-length discrepancy of more than 0.5cm. When the rotation deformity is sufficient to prevent external rotation it will prevent normal gait. Prominence and asymmetry of the pelvic bony prominences can also cause problems. Fractures involving the relative height of the ischial tuberosities will affect sitting stability.

Pain is a factor in both short- and long-term goals. Stabilization of fractures reduces pain and allows for easier and earlier mobilization. There are occasions in patients with minimally displaced stable pelvic ring injuries where a short period of temporary stabilization, provided by an anterior external fixation, for pain relief

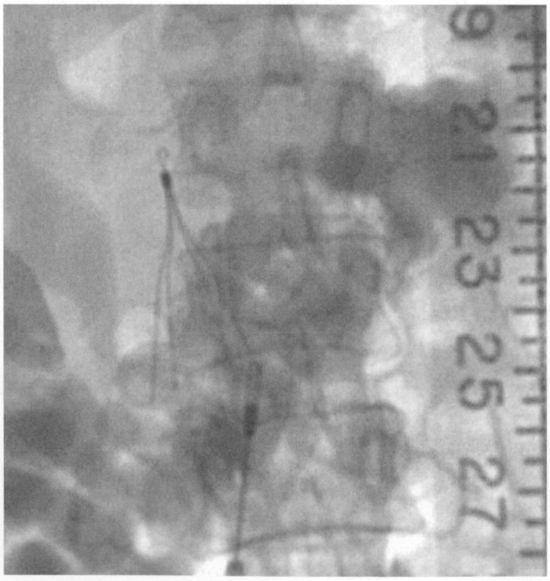

Fig. 12.47.1 IVC filter.

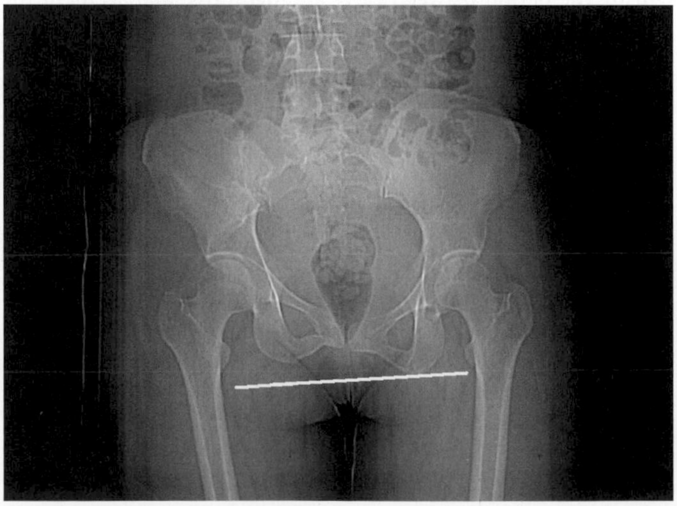

Fig. 12.47.2 LC II fracture with 2cm leg length discrepancy.

Box 12.47.2 Rationale for treatment

- Early mobilization
- Restore stability
- Avoid complications of displacement and consider intervention if:
  - Leg-length discrepancy >0.5cm
  - Reduced hip rotation >10 degrees
  - Sitting stability
  - Bony prominence
- Reduce early and late pain:
  - Dyspareunia >5mm pubic rami displacement in females
  - SI joint displacement >5mm associated with increased pain
- Decompression of sacral nerve roots.

will be of benefit. Pubic rami fractures can heal quickly and allow the frame to be removed.

In the long term, pain significantly affects outcome. Pubic rami fractures may cause dyspareunia and displacement of more than 5mm has been demonstrated to be problematic in females. Pain is particularly problematic in pelvic fractures involving disruption of the SI joint. Anatomical reduction of the posterior ring (<5mm displacement) is believed to correspond to a better outcome. However, this appears to be more significant in injuries involving the SI joint.

Treatment must avoid causing neurological deficit and there are certain circumstances and techniques that may place neurological structures at risk. Percutaneous techniques in particular SI screws require experience and adequate intraoperative imaging. Sacral fractures may result in neurological compromise as a result of compression at the time of injury or treatment.

The indications and outcomes of sacral nerve root decompression have not been fully established. Denis zone II and III fractures with identifiable compression may benefit from open reduction and decompression; delays of 2–3 days are believed to be acceptable. It is reported that there will be an overall improvement in at least 30% of cases regardless of treatment. Higher rates of recovery have been reported following decompression.

Treatment options

The categorization provided by classification systems helps to establish the residual stability of the pelvic ring. It is this understanding which allows the correct treatment decisions to be made.

Stable pelvic ring injury

These fractures do not compromise the stability of the pelvic ring and the vast majority can be treated non-operatively.

Avulsion fractures

Fractures of the anterior superior and anterior inferior iliac spines occurs as a result of avulsion of the sartorius and rectus femoris muscles, respectively. This most frequently occurs in adolescents. Treatment is symptomatic.

Transverse sacral fractures

Transverse fractures of the sacrum, below the level of the sciatic buttress, occur as the result of a direct blow. Operative treatment is considered when there is significant angulation particularly in association with a neurological deficit, but this is rare.

Iliac wing fractures

These fractures also occur as a result of a direct blow and may be associated with significant overlying soft tissue injury. Treatment is usually non-operative. When there is gross displacement that is likely to result in unacceptable cosmesis or gluteal muscle dysfunction, operative intervention can be considered (Figure 12.47.3). These injuries can be very painful.

Anterior posterior compression Type I

When displacement of the symphysis pubis is less than 2.5cm the ligaments of the pelvic floor and the integrity of the posterior ring is likely to be intact. Non-operative treatment is appropriate with weight bearing as tolerated.

A
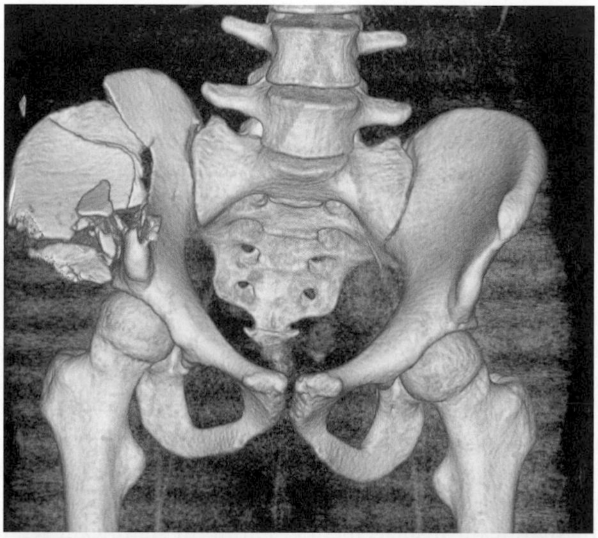

B
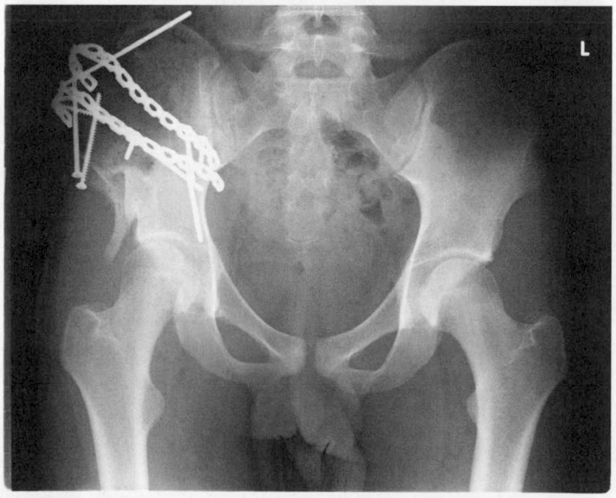

Fig. 12.47.3 This fracture was treated with open reduction and internal fixation to avoid problems with bony prominence and gluteal dysfunction. Full range of pain free movement and weight bearing was achieved at 6 weeks.

Lateral compression Type I

These fractures are associated with horizontally orientated pubic rami fractures and an impaction fracture of the sacrum. The pelvic floor and posterior ligaments remain intact. This is a stable fracture pattern that can usually be treated non-operatively. The patient can weight bear as tolerated.

Bifocal fracture of anterior arch

These fractures can occur without disruption of the posterior pelvic ring and are associated with straddle injuries, e.g. fuel tank of motorcycle. As pelvic ring stability has not been compromised the injury can be managed non-operatively; however, operative fixation should be considered with significant displacement.

Rotationally unstable, vertically stable pelvic ring injury

Anterior posterior compression Type II (Figure 12.47.4)

This fracture pattern is seen in APC injuries with disruption of the pelvic floor ligaments and displacement greater than 2.5 cm. The hemipelvis externally rotates on a hinge (intact posterior SI ligaments) and maintains vertical stability. Plating the symphysis restores stability of the pelvic ring in the horizontal plane and facilitates healing of the soft tissues in an anatomical position. Late plate failure as a result of fatigue is frequently seen, however at this stage stability has usually been achieved by the healed soft tissues. An external fixator can be considered instead of a plate if the soft tissues are not appropriate. The anterior fixation will be under tension in double leg stance and compression in single leg stance. Following operative fixation weight bearing is protected for 6–8 weeks although some authors have advocated weight bearing as tolerated.

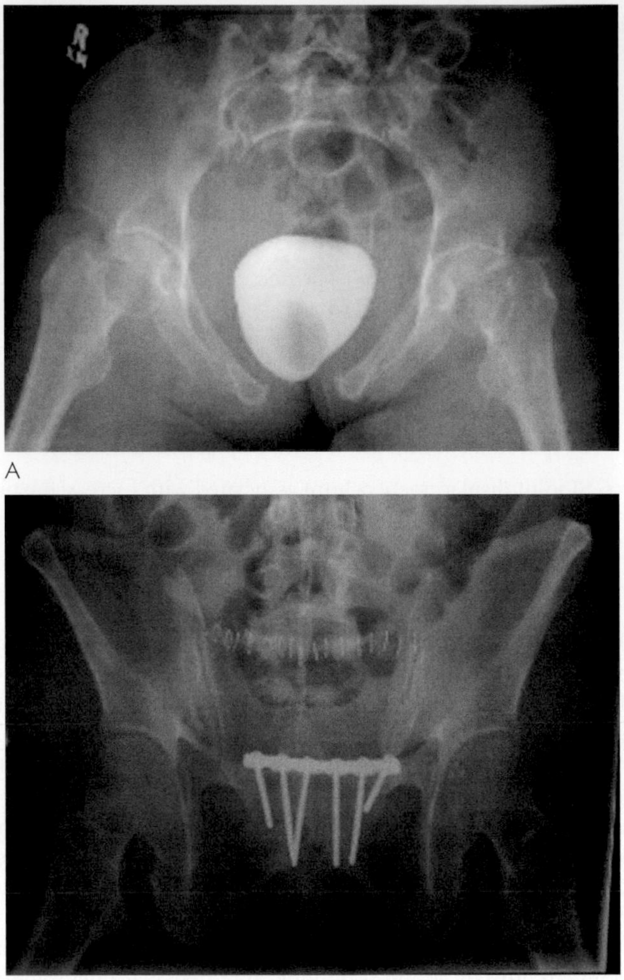

A

B

Fig. 12.47.4 APC II injury treated with symphyseal plate.

Lateral compression Type II

This fracture pattern is seen with *lateral compression associated with complete disruption of the posterior ring.* Horizontally orientated pubic rami fractures are associated with a fracture line that runs through the posterior ilium and often involves the SI joint. In both circumstances it is only the pelvic floor ligaments that remain intact, providing 'relative' vertical stability. Fractures of the ilium with significant displacement resulting in significant leg-length discrepancy or internal rotation should be considered for operative intervention. When a fracture/subluxation involves the SI joint, it is described as a 'crescent fracture' (Figure 12.47.5). This refers to the posterior ilium that remains attached to the posterior SI ligaments. These fractures are more unstable than lateral compression with anterior sacral crush and are usually treated operatively.

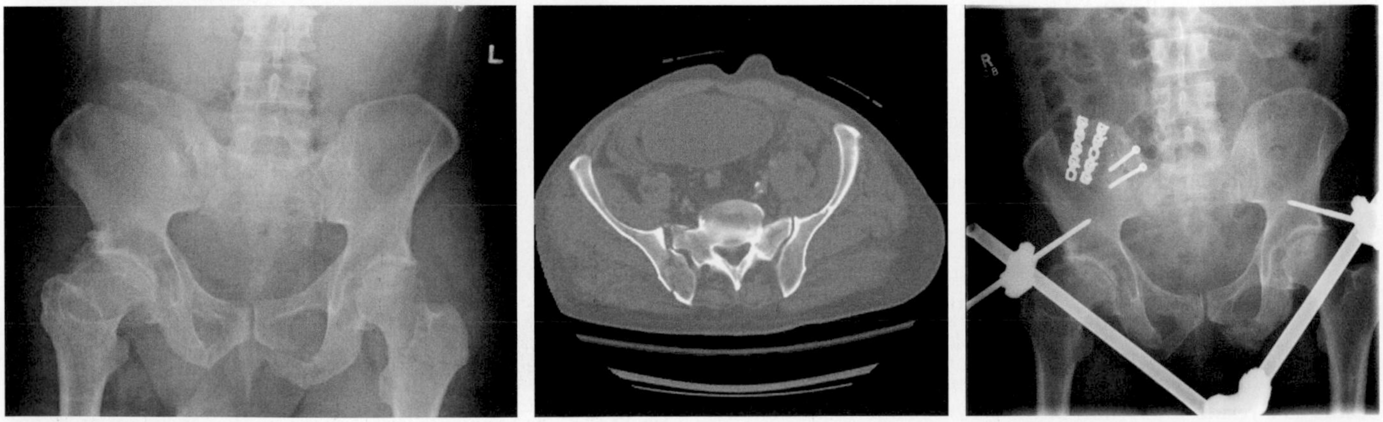

A B C

Fig. 12.47.5 LC II 'crescent fracture' treated with posterior open reduction and internal fixation and anterior supra-acetabular external fixator.

Anterior fixation is usually achieved by plating, external fixation or percutaneous screw fixation of the superior pubic rami. Posterior fixation is required to anatomically reduce the SI joint and this can be achieved using closed or open techniques.

Completely unstable pelvic ring injury

These fractures are vertically and rotationally unstable as a result of complete disruption of the anterior and posterior parts of the pelvic ring. Posterior disruption occurs through the ilium, SI joint, or sacrum. These fractures require both anterior and posterior fixation to restore stability.

In SI joint disruption, treated with open reduction, some surgeons will routinely fuse the SI joint.

Bilateral pelvic ring injury

Consideration and treatment is directed towards the individual components, as described earlier. However as the contralateral side cannot be relied upon to 'anchor' the fixation additional posterior fixation may be required to restore stability e.g. LC III or CMI (Figure 12.47.6).

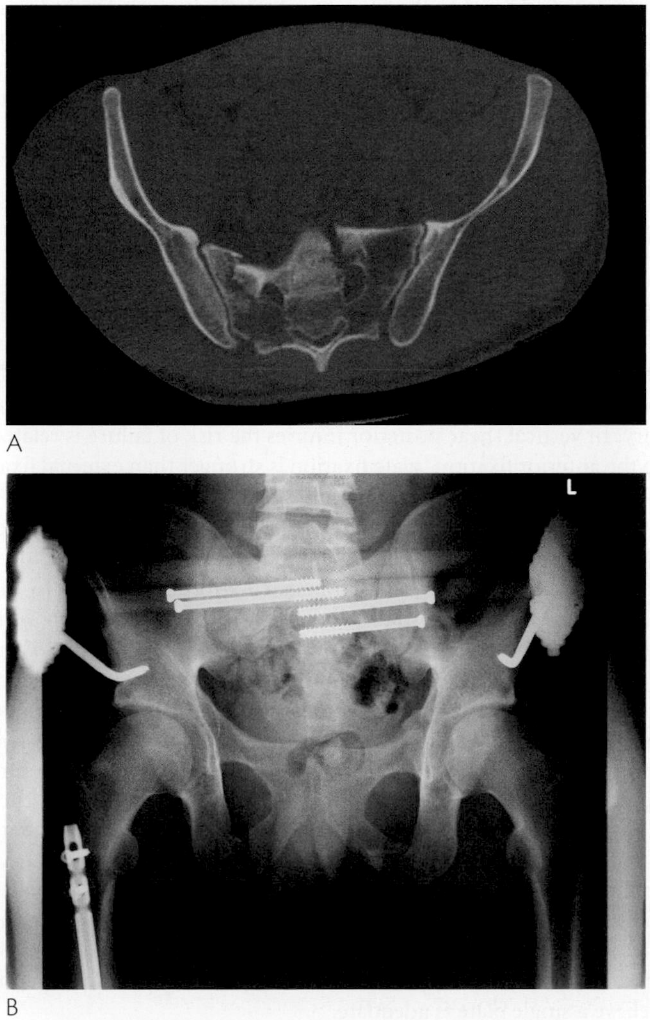

Fig. 12.47.6 LC III fracture treated with bilateral SI screws and anterior supra-acetabular external fixators.

Lumbosacral injuries

Complex fractures through the sacrum, with vertical and transverse components, or traumatic spondylolisthesis from bilateral L5/S1 fracture dislocations may result in complete mechanical discontinuity between the lumbar spine and pelvis. These are rare high energy injuries that are frequently fatal. More frequently, vertical sacral fractures running through or medial to the L5/S1 facet joint may cause instability between L5 and S1. Sacral fixation in isolation may be inadequate and lumbo-pelvic fixation should be considered (Figure 12.47.7).

Non-operative treatment

In the majority of pelvic fractures the optimal treatment will be non-operative. There will also be a small group of patients who will have indications for operative management but due to other circumstances are managed non-operatively. The aim is to mobilize early. The main limitations are pain and sufficient upper body strength to mobilize partial weight bearing. The patient will require adequate analgesia, a short period of bed rest followed by progressive mobilization with walking aids. Pain is a good indicator of healing and should be used as a guide to determine the progression from bed rest to mobilization with weight bearing as tolerated.

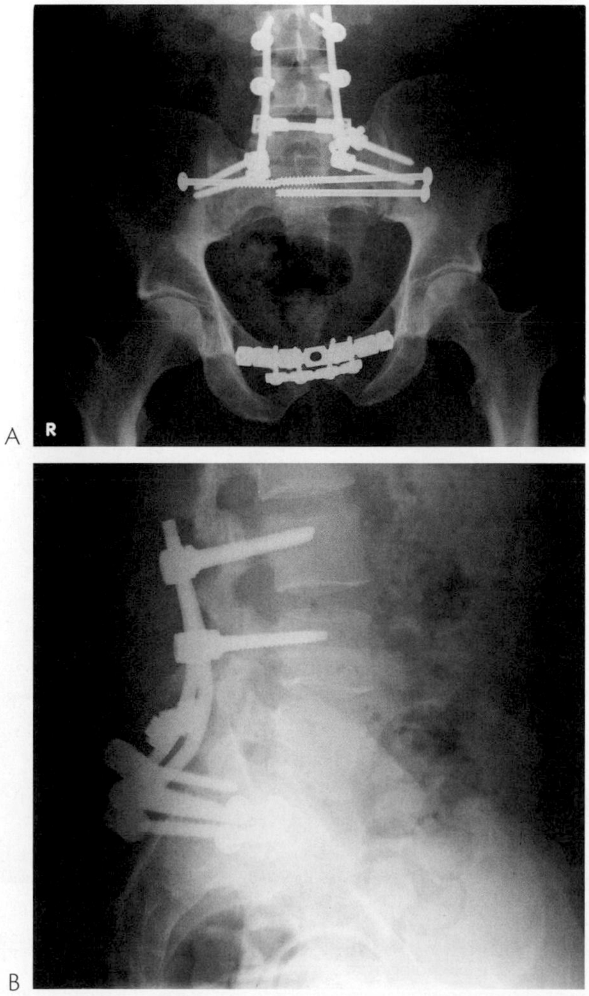

Fig. 12.47.7 Lumbopelvic fixation used to treat complex sacral fracture.

Operative treatment (Box 12.47.3)

External fixation

Anterior external fixation can be used in isolation or in conjunction with posterior internal fixation. Anterior external fixation is insufficient to maintain posterior reduction. Pins are placed into the iliac crest (Fig 12.47.8A) or supra-acetabular bone (Fig 12.47.8B). During the course of treatment external fixator pin sepsis may be problematic and both sites may be used consecutively.

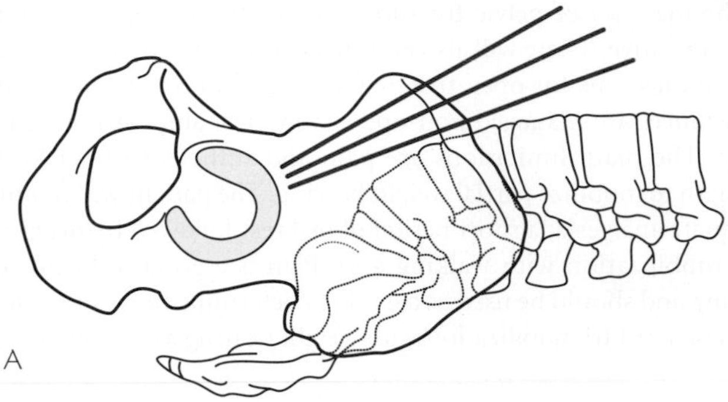
A

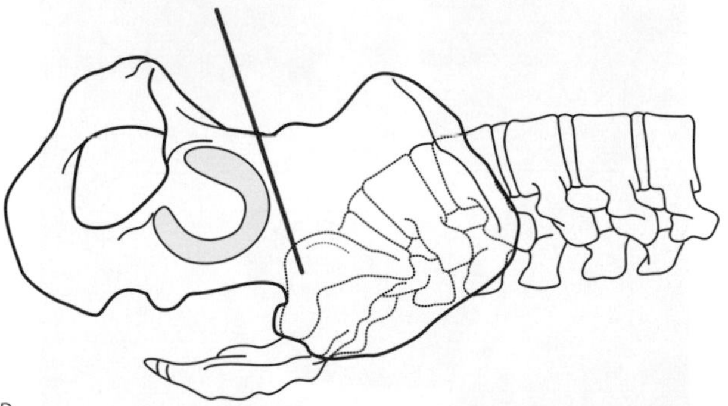
B

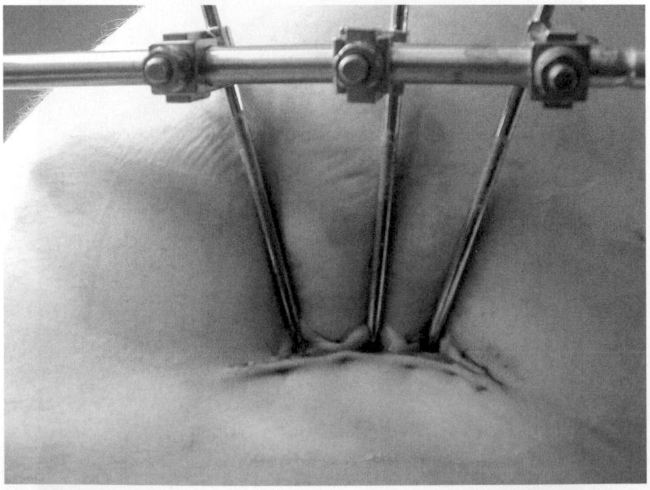
C

Fig. 12.47.8 A) Optimum placement of pins in iliac crest takes advantage of the thick strut of bone extending from the crest to the hip joint. B) Optimum placement of supra-acetabular pin is similar to that of the LC II screw. C) Poor placement of pins and obesity pre-dispose to skin necrosis and sepsis.

External fixation using convergent pins placed in the thick strut of bone running from the anterior iliac crest to the acetabulum is relatively quick and familiar to most orthopaedic surgeons. Three pins are placed between the inner and outer table of the iliac crest. It is preferable to only drill the outer cortex and use 5-mm pins. The use of self-drilling pins increases the risk of breaking out of the inner or outer table. An appreciation of the anatomy of the iliac crest is important to ensure correct pin placement, pins are commonly placed too vertical in both the sagittal and coronal planes. As the iliac crest overhangs the outer table there is also a tendency for the entry point to be too lateral. A K-wire placed on the inside of the inner table can provide a useful guide. Considerations must be given to the surrounding soft tissues. When an external fixator is used to reduce an open book fracture the position of the optimum skin incisions will change. To accommodate the change in position it is often helpful to place the skin incisions perpendicular to the iliac crest directed towards the umbilicus. It is very common for the abdomen to swell following pelvic fracture and if this is not anticipated, problems with skin necrosis and infection arise (Figure 12.47.8C).

The main purpose of anterior external fixators used in isolation is to restore horizontal stability in a rotationally unstable pelvis. Biomechanically this reduction is best achieved with supra-acetabular pins placed adjacent to the anterior inferior iliac spine directed posteriorly into the thick bone of the sciatic buttress. One or two pins can be linked with a simple frame to achieve this goal. Placement of these pins requires the image intensifier and therefore is rarely suitable in the acute management of haemodynamic instability.

External fixation, either used temporarily or definitively, is associated with a significant incidence of sepsis and aseptic loosening

Internal fixation

Anterior

Fixation of the pubic rami or symphysis pubis can restore the anterior pelvic ring. Not all pubic rami fractures will require fixation and those fractures with up to 1.5cm of displacement will have sufficient retained soft tissue stability that fixation may not be necessary. In vertical shear posterior injuries the risk of failure is related to the anterior fixation, plate fixation is stronger than external fixation and has been associated with less late displacement.

The approach used will depend on the position of the fracture. Disruption of the symphysis pubis and medial pubic rami fractures can be obtained through a Pfannensteil approach. Access to the superior aspect of the pubic symphysis is achieved by a split between the distal rectus abdomini. This allows access to the extraperitoneal space. Often the recti are torn and some of the dissection will have already been accomplished by the injury. A limited amount of sharp dissection of the rectus abdominis insertion will improve exposure. Reduction can be achieved with reduction forceps. In rotationally unstable injuries a single 3.5-mm reconstruction plate is usually sufficient when the bone quality is adequate (see Figure 12.47.4). Specialized plates are available that avoid leaving a stress riser (unfilled screw hole or thin part of the plate) directly over the symphysis. In completely unstable injuries double plating, with an additional plate applied anteriorly, can be considered in addition to the posterior fixation; however, some surgeons believe a single plate is adequate.

An alternative to plating the pubic rami fractures involves using pubic rami screws that can be inserted percutaneously in an antegrade or retrograde direction. Their trajectory is similar to that described for anterior column screws (see Chapter 12.49).

Posterior

Many methods and combinations have been described. The technique used will depend on the fracture position, configuration, and displacement. In addition the surgeon must also take into account the soft tissues, neurological deficit, patient positioning, available equipment, and experience.

Open or closed reduction techniques have been described. Open reduction techniques have the benefit of reducing under direct visualization but incur the risk of the open approach. Posterior approaches use either a midline incision or a longitudinal incision 2.5cm lateral to the posterior superior spine. The gluteus maximus and multifidus muscles can then be mobilized. Posterior open approaches have been associated with a high incidence of wound problems and infection (3–27%).

Mechanical differences have been identified between the fixation techniques. In general, two points of fixation are preferable and none of the techniques are sufficiently strong to allow unrestricted weight-bearing. Two SI screws or one SI screw and anterior SI plating have been shown to be the strongest constructs most commonly used. A lumbopelvic triangular construct can also be considered, however this is overtreatment for many fractures.

SI screws

SI screws are commonly placed through the posterior aspect of the ilium into the body of S1. If space permits, two screws can be placed in S1 or alternatively a second screw can be placed in S2 (Figure 12.47.9). The screws can be placed with the patient supine or prone. The percutaneous technique is very dependent on operator experience and good image intensification. The technique requires using the image intensifier to obtain good quality inlet, outlet and lateral views. Inaccurate placement is associated with the risk of injury to L5, sacral nerve roots (within the foramen and canal), iliac vessels, superior gluteal nerve and vessels. The risk has been shown to increase significantly when the sacral fracture is incompletely reduced or there is sacral dysmorphism. Nerve injury has been reported as less than 1%; however, it must be appreciated that this complication rate is not transferable.

Transforaminal vertical sacral fractures stabilized posteriorly with SI screws should be closely observed over the first 3 weeks as loss of fixation has been reported in 13%.

Sacroiliac plates (Figure 12.47.10)

Anterior SI plating can be performed through the lateral window of the ilioinguinal approach (see Chapter 12.49) using two orthogonal plates passing from the sacral ala to the anterior aspect of the posterior ilium. It has the advantage of being performed with the

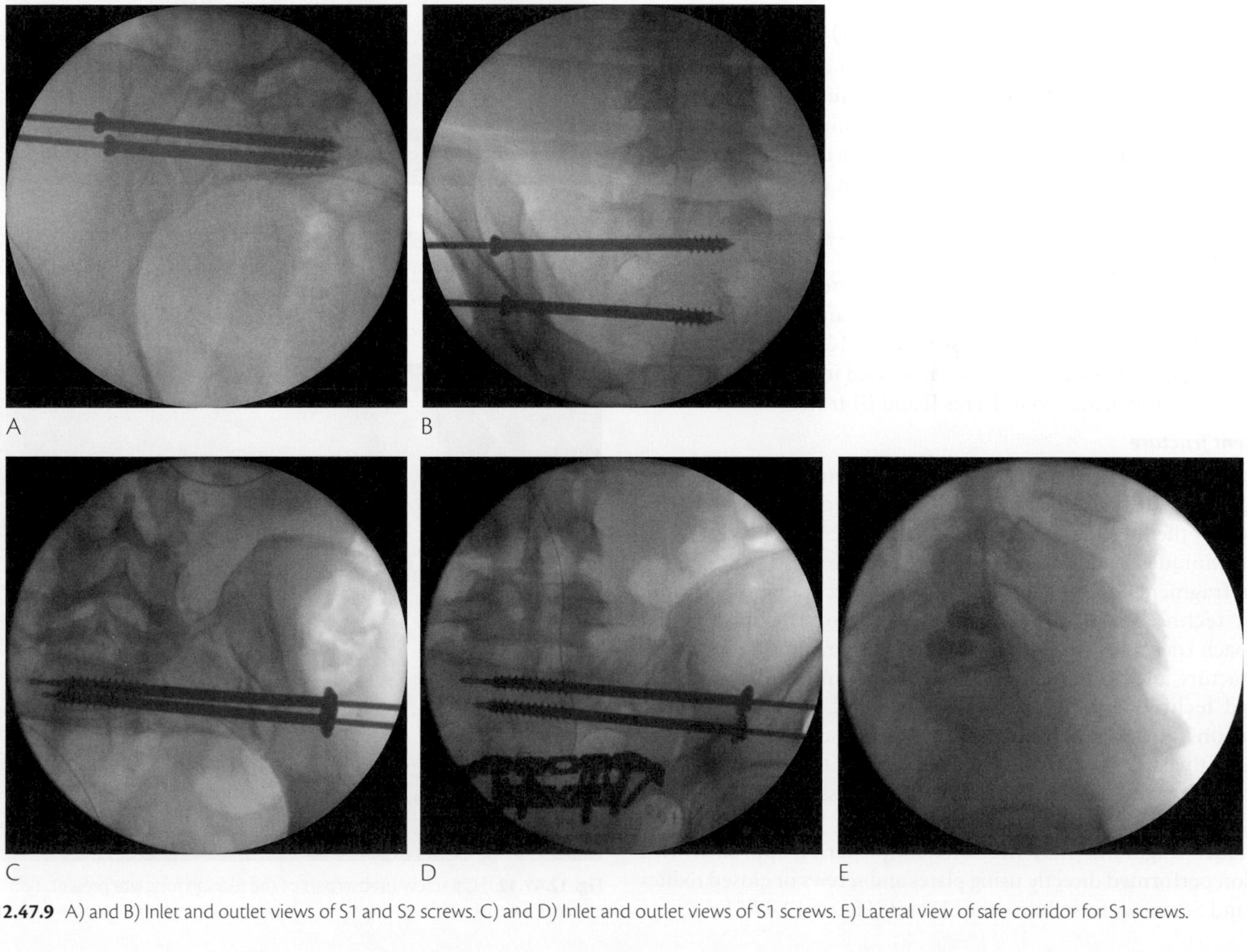

Fig. 12.47.9 A) and B) Inlet and outlet views of S1 and S2 screws. C) and D) Inlet and outlet views of S1 screws. E) Lateral view of safe corridor for S1 screws.

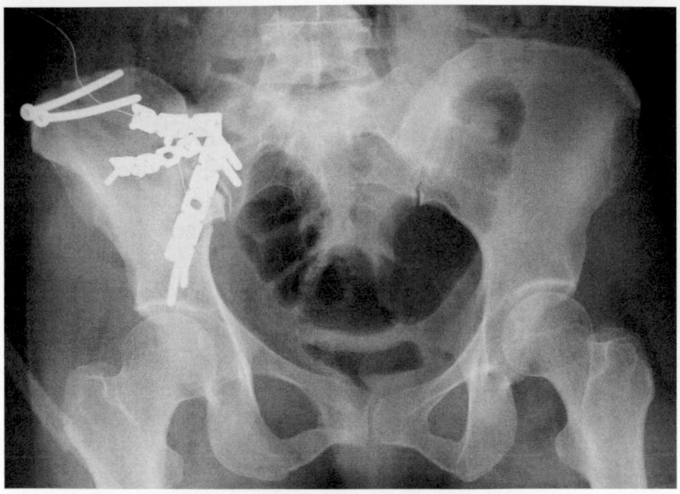

Fig. 12.47.10 Anterior SI plates (courtesy of R Keys).

patient supine using an incision with low morbidity. In addition it facilitates direct visualization of the reduction, direct placement of fixation and allows the SI joint to be debrided to facilitate fusion if required. However, it is restricted as it can only be used in a pure SI joint injury with an intact sacral ala. Only one screw in each plate can be inserted into the sacral ala due to the close proximity of the L5 nerve root which runs over the sacral ala approximately 1cm from the anterior aspect of the SI joint.

SI bars plus tension band plate (Figure 12.47.11)

These devices require posterior incisions that are associated with problems of wound breakdown; however, minimally invasive techniques have been described. Metal work prominence can be problematic in thin patients. Posterior plating can be used in conjunction with neural decompression and can maintain distraction in fracture patterns associated with compression.

Spinopelvic fixation

This is considered to provide the highest mechanical stability. Pedicle screws can be placed into L4 and L5 and linked to screws placed into the posterior ilium (see Figure 12.47.7). Cross links create a triangular construct. This can be used in lumbosacral injuries and can be considered in Denis II and III fractures.

Crescent fracture

The posterior ilium retains attachment to the posterior SI ligament complex. Anatomical reduction and fixation of this fragment to the rest of the ilium restores posterior stability. The choice of fixation techniques is dependent on the size of the crescent fragment. Large fragments are suitable for open or percutaneous fixation. Open techniques use the lateral window of the ilioinguinal approach (described in Chapter 12.46) with direct visualization of the fracture and SI joint. Anterior plating techniques can be used. Closed techniques have also been described. Following closed reduction one or two partially threaded 'LC II' screws can be passed through the supra acetabular corridor (similar to supra acetabular external fixator pin) across the sciatic buttress into the crescent fracture (Figure 12.47.12).

Smaller fragments may necessitate a posterior approach with fixation performed directly using plates and screws or closed reduction and SI screws to stabilize the SI joint (Figure 12.47.5).

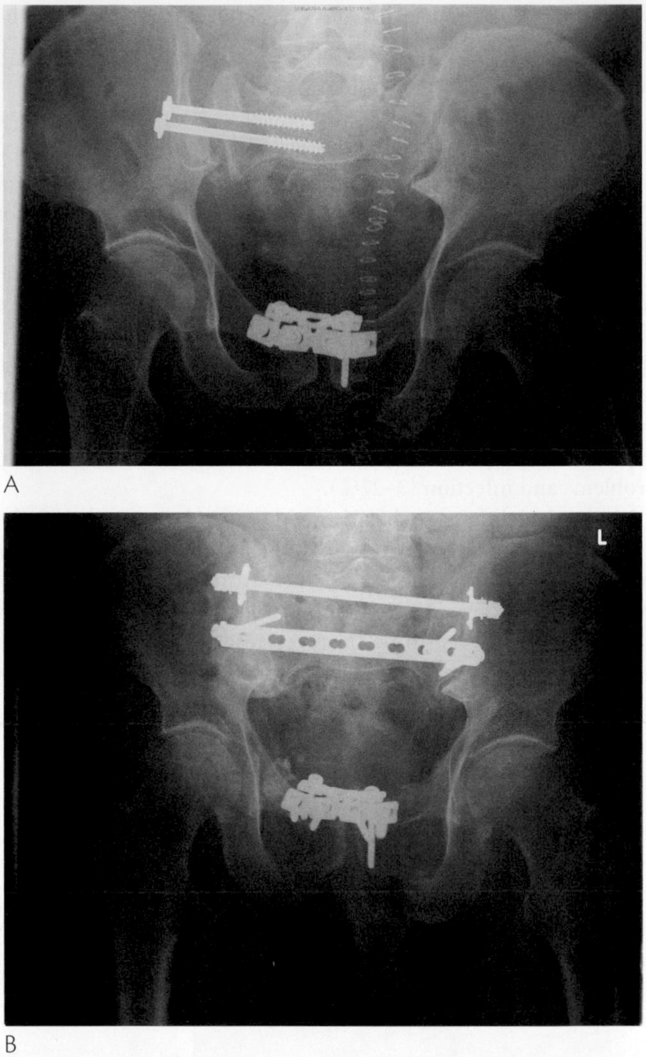

Fig. 12.47.11 A) Complete instability through SI joint treated with SI screws resulting in screw cut out and early failure. B) Salvage with posterior approach, SI fusion, and SI bar and plate.

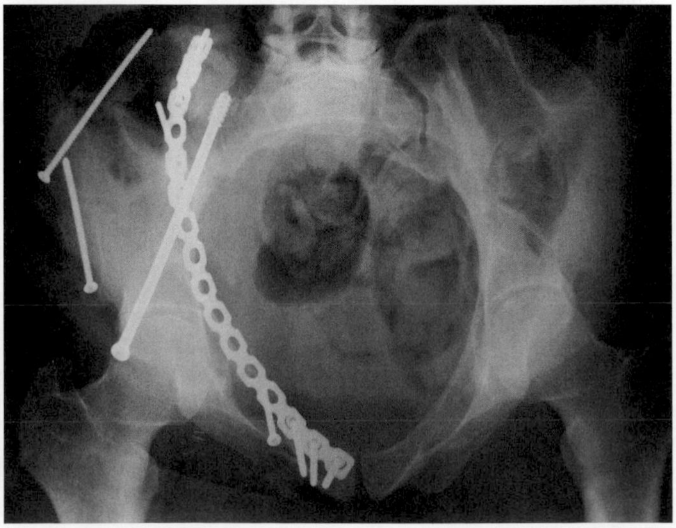

Fig. 12.47.12 LC II screw used as part of the fixation for a late presentation crescent fracture.

Box 12.47.3 Fixation techniques

- External fixation
- Internal fixation—anterior:
  - Plate
  - Rami screws
- Internal fixation—posterior
  - SI screws
  - SI plates
  - SI bars
  - Tension band plate
  - Iliac plates and screw fixation
  - LC II screws
  - Lumbopelvic fixation.

Postoperative management

Open reduction and internal fixation can be painful and this is often best managed during and after the operation with epidural analgesia. The epidural catheter is usually removed over the following 3 days so that the patient can start to mobilize.

Weight bearing as tolerated can be considered for fractures that retain horizontal and vertical stability. Fractures that require posterior fixation require protective weight bearing until sufficient healing has been achieved (8–12 weeks). The patient should be instructed by the physiotherapists to only touch weight bear (equivalent of the weight of their leg). Bilateral injuries will necessitate wheelchair mobilization until full weight bearing on one limb can be tolerated.

X-rays (AP, inlet, and outlet) should be performed postoperatively and if there are concerns about hardware placement a CT scan may be required. Further x-rays should be performed frequently if there are concerns about stability, otherwise routine follow-up at 6-weekly intervals until the fracture is united.

In addition to mobilization, physiotherapy should help with breathing exercises, hip range of motion exercises, and general conditioning.

Outcomes

Complications related to specific problems and techniques have already been discussed. General problems are discussed below.

Infection

Infection rate is very dependent on the technique used. Posterior approaches are the most problematic (3–27%). Percutaneous approaches have generally very low rates of infection; however it has been considerable in some studies and is believed to be secondary to soft tissue injury. Large series generally report infection rate at less than 5%.

Non-union

The overall incidence of this complication is unknown but appears to be very small. The risk of non-union increases with displacement and instability.

Function

There are no controlled trials to allow direct comparison of the outcomes of non-operative and operative treatment options. Much of the evolution has been based on comparison with historical studies and expert opinion. Many studies have attempted to correlate features related to pelvic fracture and outcome. The results of these studies are not conclusive. This has been attributed to significant confounding variables, in particular the measurement methods and associated injury.

In general there is acceptance that the outcome is worse with increased severity of pelvic injury. However, severe pelvic injury is more likely to be associated with a higher incidence of significant associated injuries and neurological deficit. In addition it can also make reduction harder. Pure SI joint injury appears to have worse outcome than fractures and fracture dislocations of the posterior ring, especially when associated with non-anatomical reduction. However anatomical reduction of any pelvic ring injury pattern does not guarantee a good outcome. The opposite is also demonstrated with some displaced unstable injuries reporting relatively good outcomes. Correction of leg length discrepancy has been correlated with better outcome scores in some studies.

Outcome measurement varies amongst studies and the methods used influence the ability to identify good and bad outcome groups. Health survey questionnaires such as SF-36 and Sickness Impact Profile are useful measures of general health but are influenced by the cumulative severity of all injuries. Some authors have used more pelvic specific scoring systems, e.g. Iowa Pelvic Score, Majeed, etc.

Many studies have inconsistently correlated outcome with classification systems that amalgamate very different osteoligamentous injuries into groups based on stability. Outcome based on injury types has demonstrated clear differences within these groups. APC injuries in general have worse outcome than lateral compression injuries however both are classified as rotationally unstable. In a large study comparing functional outcome rotationally unstable lateral compression patterns (LC II + III) had a good or excellent outcome in 92% compared with 74% in rotationally unstable APC injury (APC II); despite a difference in anatomical reduction 75% vs 94%. In the same study completely unstable fracture patterns had an anatomical reduction in 63% and a good or excellent outcome in 71%. It is also apparent that within the completely unstable fracture group there are different outcomes depending on the type of posterior injury.

A significant proportion of pelvic fractures are not associated with multisystem trauma and are satisfactorily managed non-operatively or with minor surgical intervention. As a result they will not need transfer to a specialist centre for treatment. Due to the relative rarity of the injury only the specialist centres are in a position to publish on the subject, resulting in a bias in the study population presented.

One of the most frequently used outcome measures is return to work. Although not directly comparable it does allow for the physical impact of the injury to be appreciated. Not all patients who return to work will return to the same job, however in most studies the majority do. Overall approximately 75% of pelvic fractures return to their original employment. In studies looking at rotationally unstable injuries, 85% return to work has been reported in contrast to 33–69% of completely unstable injuries. Difficulty in sitting has been reported as high as 60% in rotationally and completely unstable injuries.

Pelvic pain is a significant feature in the outcome of pelvic fractures. Low back pain is common in sacral and sacroiliac injury and the overall incidence has been reported at 17–90%.

In rotationally unstable injuries, pain of some degree is reported in 11–45%. In a study reviewing patients treated with external fixation they were functionally normal if the pelvis remained reduced but 80% required analgesia for posterior pain if reduction was not maintained. A German multicentre study identified persistent pain in 32% of rotationally unstable APC type injuries in contrast to 18% in those rotationally unstable fracture patterns that result from lateral compression.

In vertically unstable fracture patterns significant pain is reported in 30–90% and has been correlated with residual displacement. In these fractures the average patient has been reported as having an average visual analogue score (VAS) at rest of 2.8 and 4.1 when ambulating. This was noted to be higher in those patients with an unresolved lumbosacral injury or extremity injury.

The outcome of pelvic fractures is very dependent on the contribution of the frequently occurring significant associated injuries.

A significant proportion of severe pelvic injury have an associated neurological deficit. It is the presence of a neurological injury that has been a consistent determinant of poor outcome. In addition to neurological deficit the neurological injury is believed to contribute to pain. Nerve injuries have been reported in 5–17% of rotationally unstable (more common in APC type injuries) and 25–40% of completely unstable fractures. Nerve injuries seen in rotationally unstable fractures have been noted to be more likely to recover than in completely unstable injuries, 70 vs 29% respectively. In sacral fractures displaced more than 10mm, 87% were identified as having a sensory deficit, 45% motor dysfunction of the lower extremities, 52% voiding dysfunction, 36% bowel dysfunction, 39% altered sexual function, and 65% gait impairment. In this group only 33% returned to work.

In completely unstable pelvic fractures the frequency of long-term urinary dysfunction (frequency, incontinence, retention, urethral stricture and urgency) is 37%.

The psychological impact of being involved in an accident and sustaining serious injuries is becoming increasingly understood. Treatment of the physical problems in isolation may be inadequate in optimizing a patient's outcome.

Sexual function is an important aspect of pelvic fracture outcome as a result of residual pain, urological, neurological, vascular, and psychological injury. Overall approximately 75% of pelvic fracture patients return to normal sexual function. Unstable pelvic injury patterns are associated with a 29–40% incidence of sexual dysfunction. Male sexual dysfunction has a reported incidence of 30% within the general pelvic fracture population. Although the cause may be multifactorial, a vascular rather than neurological cause is most frequently reported. An important relationship has been identified between mental and sexual health. Within the group returning to their original work without sexual dysfunction, the psychosomatic and affective status is near normal, unlike those with sexual dysfunction who demonstrate depressive affectation.

Summary

Pelvic fractures and the associated injuries represent complex problems with variable outcomes. Many of the factors that determine outcome are predetermined by the injury. It is therefore important to optimize those factors that are amenable to treatment.

Further reading

Krappinger, D., Larndorfer, R., Struve, P., Rosenberger, R., Arora, R., and Blauth, M. (2007). Minimally invasive transiliac plate osteosynthesis for type C injuries of the pelvic ring: a clinical and radiological follow-up. *Journal of Orthopaedic Trauma*, **21**(9), 595–602.

Smith, W.R., Ziran, B.H., and Morgan, S.J. (2007). *Fractures of the Pelvis and Acetabulum.* Boca Raton, FL: CRC Press.

Yinger, K., Scalise, J., Olson, S.A., Bay, B.K., and Finkemeier, C.G. (2003). Biomechanical comparison of posterior pelvic ring fixation. *Journal of Orthopaedic Trauma*, **17**(7), 481–7.

Yinger, K., Scalise, J., Olson, S.A., Bay, B.K., and Finkemeier, C.G. (2003). Staged reconstruction of pelvic ring disruption: differences in morbidity, mortality, radiological results, and functional outcomes between B1, B2/B3, and C-type lesions. *Journal of Orthopaedic Trauma*, **16**(2), 92–8.

Ziran, B.H., Wasan, A.D., Marks, D.M., Olson, S.A., and Chapman, M.W. (2007). Fluoroscopic imaging guides of the posterior pelvis pertaining to iliosacral screw placement. *Journal of Trauma*, **62**(2), 347–56; discussion 356.

12.48

Fractures of the acetabulum: radiographic assessment and classification

John A. Boudreau and Berton R. Moed

Summary points

- This injury is relatively uncommon at 3 per 100,000 patients annually
- Understanding the complex anatomy of the innominate bone is key
- Assessment is based on interpretation of three basic plain radiographs supplemented by computed tomography
- Fractures are classified into five elementary and five associated types
- A systematic approach to the radiographic interpretation facilitates diagnosis and treatment.

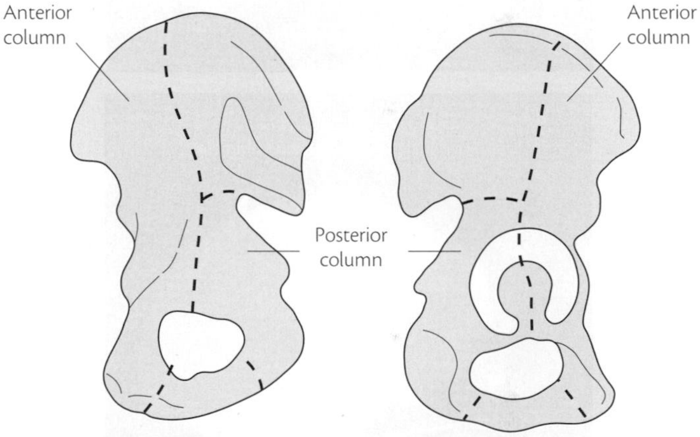

Fig. 12.48.1 Illustration of the surgical divisions of the innominate bone into the anterior and posterior columns. Letournel described the acetabulum as contained between the arms of an inverted Y formed by these two columns.

Incidence and mechanism of injury

Acetabular fractures represent a serious injury with disruption of the articular surface of the hip joint. Fortunately, these injuries are relatively uncommon with an incidence of about three per 100 000 patients annually in the United Kingdom. In 1998, there were 12 000 fractures of the acetabulum reported in the United States of America. This compares with 323 000 fractures of the femoral neck that occurred in the same time period. The majority of patients sustaining fractures of the acetabulum are injured in a motor vehicle or motorcycle collision, as a pedestrian struck by a motor vehicle, or in a fall from a height. For more than a decade, the reported annual incidence in the United Kingdom has remained stable. However, over time, there has been a change in demographics, with an increase in acetabular fractures caused by simple falls and an increase in the proportion of women with acetabular fractures.

Bony anatomy

The classification and treatment of acetabular fractures is based on a thorough understanding of the anatomy of the innominate bone. The innominate bone is formed as a condensation of pubis, ischium, and ilium at the triradiate cartilage which fuse at the time of skeletal maturity. The articular surface of the acetabulum can be visualized as being supported between limbs of an inverted Y of bone. Letournel was the first to describe the surgical anatomy of the innominate bone, identifying these two limbs as the anterior column or iliopectineal segment and posterior column or ilioischial segment (Figure 12.48.1). The anterior column refers to the anterior half of the iliac wing that is contiguous with the pelvic brim to the superior pubic ramus, as well as the anterior half of the acetabular articular surface. The posterior column begins at the superior aspect of the greater sciatic notch, and is contiguous with the greater and lesser sciatic notches inferiorly and includes the ischial tuberosity. The posterior column also contains the cortical surface of bone posterior to the acetabulum, known as the 'retroacetabular surface'. The coalescence of the pelvic brim and greater sciatic notch is referred to as the sciatic buttress and links the anterior and posterior columns (inverted Y of bone) to the axial skeleton (Figure 12.48.2).

Radiography of acetabular fractures

Three radiographic projections of the pelvis are used to evaluate fractures of the acetabulum (Figure 12.48.3): the anteroposterior (AP) view of the pelvis, the obturator (or 45-degree internal, Judet)

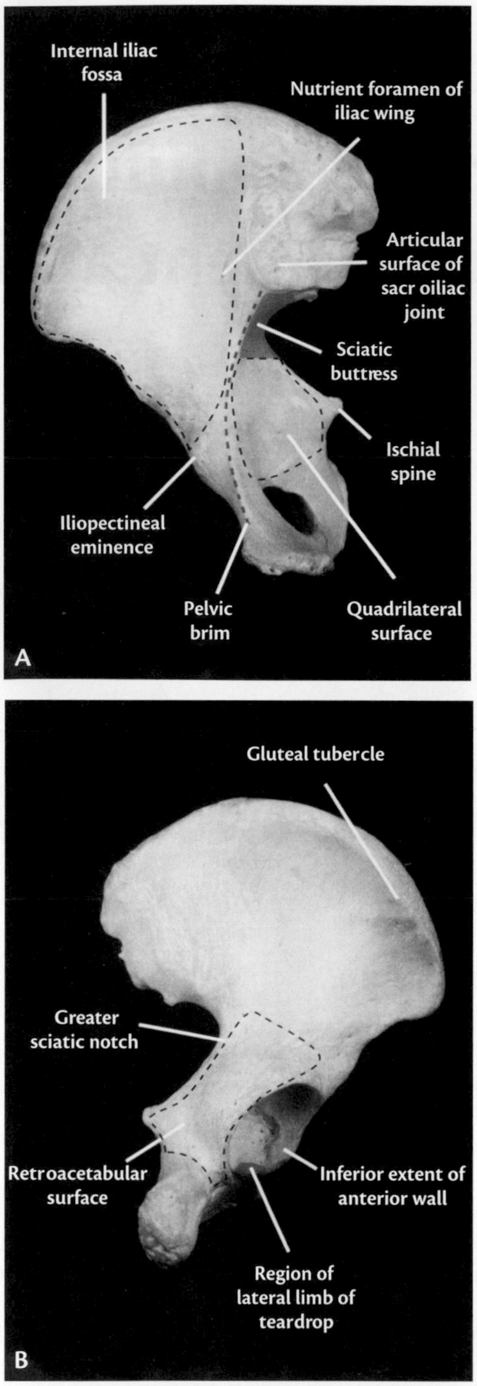

Fig. 12.48.2 A) Anatomical regions of the internal aspect of the innominate bone are illustrated. The quadrilateral surface is bound by the pelvic brim anteriorly, the greater and lesser sciatic notches posteriorly, the obturator foramen inferiorly, and the sciatic buttress superiorly. The iliopectineal eminence lies directly over the anterior wall of the acetabulum. The nutrient foramen of the iliac wing is a consistent landmark found adjacent to the sacroiliac joint. B) The external aspect of the innominate bone is shown. The retroacetabular surface is outlined.

oblique view, and the iliac (or 45-degree external, Judet) oblique view. Interpretation of plain films is based on the understanding of normal radiographic landmarks of the acetabulum and disruption of these landmarks represents a fracture involving that portion of the bone. Computed tomography (CT) and three-dimensional reconstructions are helpful to further define fracture patterns and assess for associated injuries (Box 12.48.1). However, it does not replace the standard radiographic evaluation.

Anteroposterior view

On the AP view, there are six basic landmarks (Figure 12.48.3A and Box 12.48.2). The iliopectineal line is the major landmark of the anterior column. The inferior three-quarters of the iliopectineal line represents the pelvic brim. The superior quarter of this line is formed by the tangency of the x-ray beam to the superior quadrilateral surface and the greater sciatic notch. The ilioischial line is formed by the tangency of the x-ray beam to the posterior portion of the quadrilateral surface, and is considered a radiographic landmark of the posterior column. The radiographic U or teardrop consists of a medial and lateral limb and represents a radiographic finding and not a true anatomical structure. The lateral limb represents the middle third of the cotyloid fossa in the acetabulum, and the medial limb is formed by the obturator canal and the anteroinferior portion of the quadrilateral surface. Because the teardrop and the ilioischial line both result, in part, from the tangency of the x-ray beam to a portion of the quadrilateral surface, they are always superimposed on the AP pelvis view of the normal acetabulum. Dissociation of the teardrop and the ilioischial line indicates either rotation of the hemipelvis, or a fracture of the quadrilateral surface. The roof of the acetabulum is a radiographic landmark resulting from the tangency of the x-ray beam to a narrow portion of the subchondral bone of the superior acetabulum. Interruption of the radiographic line of the roof indicates a fracture involving the superior acetabulum. The anterior rim represents the lateral margin in the anterior wall of the acetabulum and is contiguous with the inferior margin of the superior pubic ramus. The anterior rim is typically medial to the posterior rim, and has a characteristic undulation in its mid-contour in the AP pelvis view. The posterior rim represents the lateral margin of the posterior wall of the acetabulum. Inferiorly, the posterior rim is contiguous with the thickened condensation of the posterior horn of the acetabulum.

Obturator oblique view

The obturator oblique view (also known as the internal oblique view) is taken with the patient rotated so that the injured hemipelvis is rotated 45 degrees toward the x-ray beam (Figure 12.48.3B and Box 12.48.3). This view shows the obturator foramen in its largest dimension and profiles the anterior column. The iliopectineal line has the same relationship with the pelvic brim as on the AP view. The posterior rim of the acetabulum is best seen in the obturator oblique view. Comparison of the relationship of the femoral head with the posterior wall on the normal hip and the injured hip on the obturator oblique view will allow the surgeon to detect subtle amounts of posterior subluxation.

Iliac oblique view

The iliac oblique view (also known as the external oblique view) is taken with the patient rotated so that the injured hemipelvis is tilted at 45 degrees away from the x-ray beam (Figure 12.48.3C and Box 12.48.4). This view shows the iliac wing in its largest dimension, and profiles the greater and lesser sciatic notches, as well as the anterior rim of the acetabulum. Involvement of the posterior column is often best seen on this view. Fractures of the anterior column traversing the iliac wing can also be detected.

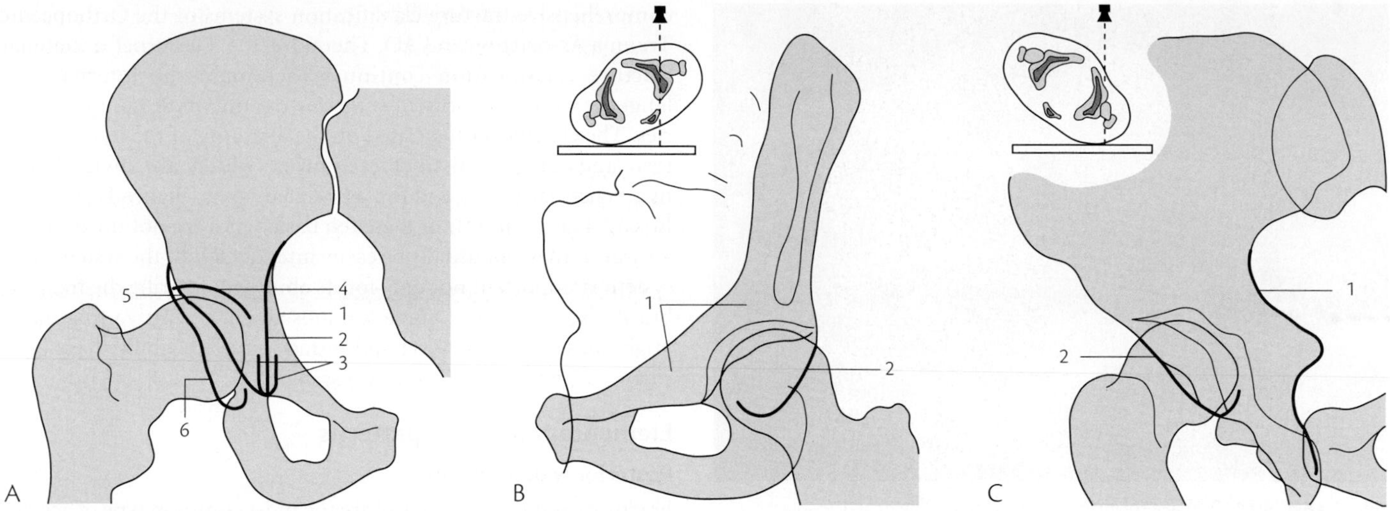

Fig. 12.48.3 A) Radiographic landmarks of the acetabulum on the anteroposterior view of the pelvis. 1, iliopectineal line; 2, ilioischial line; 3, teardrop; 4, roof; 5, anterior rim of the acetabulum; 6, posterior rim of the acetabulum. The iliopectineal line, the anterior rim, and teardrop are landmarks of the anterior column; the ilioischial line and posterior rim are landmarks of the posterior columns. (b) Obturator oblique view of the hemipelvis, obtained by turning the injured side 45° toward the X-ray beam. The obturator ring is seen en face, and the iliopectineal line is also present. 1, Area of the anterior column; 2, posterior rim of the acetabulum. Posterior wall fractures are best seen on this view. (c) Iliac oblique view, obtained by rotating the injured side away from the X-ray beam. The iliac wing is seen en face, and fracture lines extending into the iliac wing are often best seen on this view: 1, the greater sciatic notch is seen on this view, and represents the posterior column; 2, the anterior rim of the acetabulum is best seen on this view. Reproduced with permission from *Orthopaedic Knowledge Update 2*. Rosemont, IL, American Academy of Orthopaedic Surgeons, 1987.

Box 12.48.1 Investigations

- AP view of pelvis
- 45-degree iliac oblique view
- 45-degree obturator oblique view
- Axial two-dimensional CT scan ± three-dimensional reconstructions.

Computed tomography scan

Two-dimensional (axial) and three-dimensional CT scans are used as an adjunct to the analysis of the AP and oblique plain radiographic projections. After studying the plain films, the surgeon should use the two-dimensional CT to answer specific questions about the fracture that remain unanswered (Box 12.48.5). In addition, two-dimensional CT has been shown to be superior to plain radiographs in the detection of fracture step and fracture gap deformities. In order to obtain reliable and useful information, the

Box 12.48.2 AP x-ray—six basic landmarks

- Iliopectineal line (anterior column)
- Ilioischial line (posterior column)
- Radiographic U or teardrop
- Roof of the acetabulum
- Rim of the anterior wall
- Rim of the posterior wall.

Box 12.48.3 Obturator oblique x-ray—four landmarks

- Obturator foramen
- Posterior rim of acetabulum
- Anterior column.

Box 12.48.4 Iliac oblique x-ray—three landmarks

- Iliac wing (fractures of anterior column)
- Anterior rim of acetabulum
- Posterior column.

Box 12.48.5 Aspects of injury associated with acetabular fractures which can be recognized using axial CT

- Identification and orientation of additional fracture lines
- Injuries to the posterior pelvic ring
- Intra-articular osteochondral fragments
- Fractures of the femoral head
- Marginal impaction of the articular surface
- Size and location of anterior and posterior wall fractures
- Rotation of the fracture fragments
- Fractures of the quadrilateral plate not seen on radiographs
- Involvement of the superior acetabular articular surface.

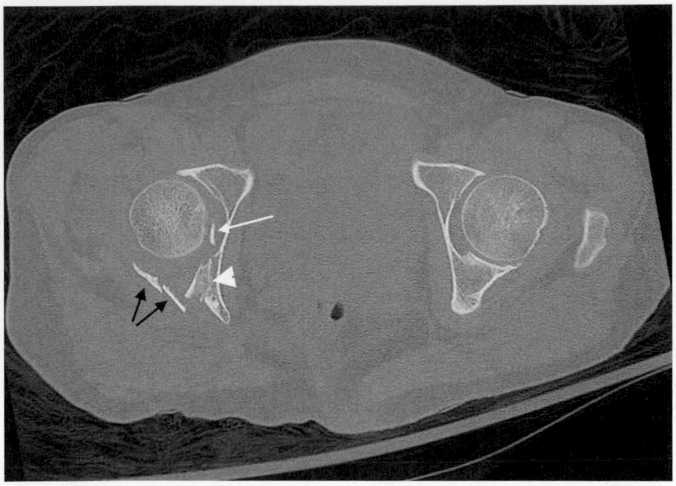

Fig. 12.48.4 Axial CT image through the acetabulum. The right acetabular posterior wall is fractured (black arrows). There is an intra-articular loose body between the femoral head and acetabulum (white arrow). The asymmetry of the contour of the posterior wall from side to side is secondary to marginal impaction (white arrowhead), which occurs when a segment of the articular surface and underlying cancellous bone adjacent to a major fracture line is impacted or depressed away from the normal contour of the joint. (Copyright Dr. Berton R. Moed.)

CT scan should consist of contiguous sections of no more than 3mm in thickness. Although the two-dimensional CT has also been advocated as a means to determine hip joint stability, this has proven unreliable. Furthermore, CT analysis may overestimate the extent of fracture comminution.

Three-dimensional CT scan technology has improved to the point that it is helpful in further defining the fracture pattern and thereby assisting in preoperative planning. However, it does not provide the diagnostic detail of the two-dimensional CT scan.

Fracture classification

The basic acetabular fracture classification developed by Judet and Letournel has been incorporated into the alphanumeric comprehensive fracture classification systems of the Orthopaedic Trauma Association and AO. Therefore, the 'Letournel' acetabular fracture classification continues to remain the international language of the majority of surgeons treating these complex injuries. The classification is based on the anatomy of the fracture pattern and has ten distinct categories, which are divided into five elementary types and five associated types (Figure 12.48.5 and Box 12.48.6). Variants of these ten basic types are not uncommon. However, they can usually be easily integrated into the system. This system is important not only for its ability to describe the fracture, but it also serves as a guide for subsequent operative treatment. High rates of interobserver and intraobserver reliability have been reported using this classification system.

Elementary fracture patterns

Posterior wall fractures

Fractures of the posterior wall are the most common type of acetabular fractures. The posterior wall fracture involves disruption of the

Box 12.48.6 Classification of acetabular fractures

- Elementary fracture patterns:
  - Posterior wall
  - Posterior column
  - Anterior wall
  - Anterior column
  - Transverse
- Associated fracture patterns:
  - Posterior column and posterior wall
  - Transverse and posterior wall
  - T-shaped
  - Anterior column (or wall) and posterior hemitransverse
  - Both-column.

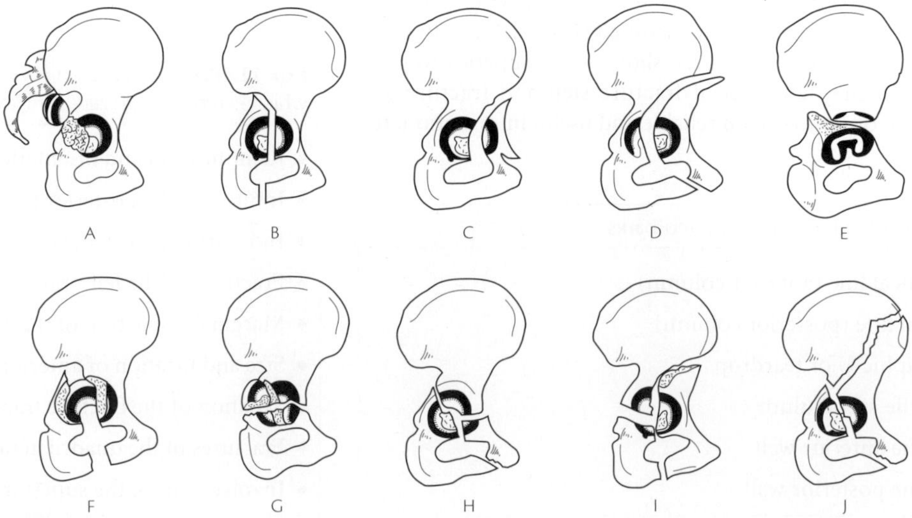

Fig. 12.48.5 Letournel classification of acetabular fractures is based on anatomic description of fracture patterns. There are 10 fracture types, divided into five elementary patterns and five associated patterns. The elementary patterns are: A, posterior wall; B, posterior column; C, anterior wall; D, anterior column; E, transverse. The associated patterns are as follows: F, posterior column and posterior wall; G, transverse and posterior wall; H, T-shaped; I, anterior column (or wall) with associated posterior hemitransverse; J, both-column. Reproduced with permission from *Orthopaedic Knowledge Update 2*. Rosemont, IL, American Academy of Orthopaedic Surgeons, 1987.

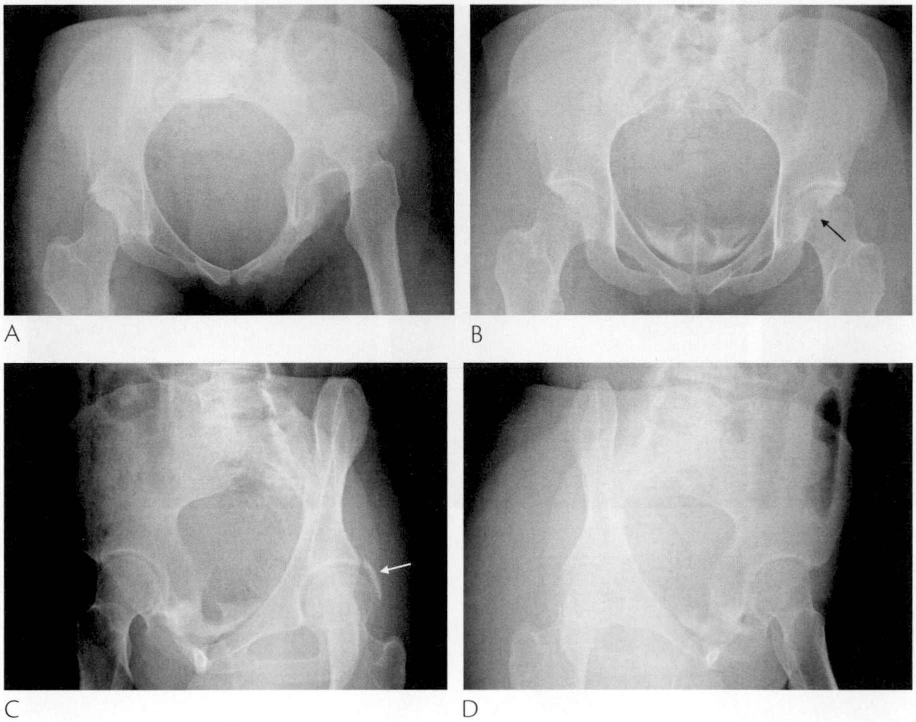

Fig. 12.48.6 Posterior wall fracture: A) initial attempted anteroposterior view of the pelvis shows the left femoral head dislocated without apparent bony injury. After closed reduction of the dislocation (B) repeat anteroposterior view shows all radiographic landmarks to be intact except the posterior rim (arrow). The obturator oblique (C) demonstrates the displaced posterior wall fracture (arrow). The iliac oblique view (D) shows an intact posterior column. (Copyright Dr. Berton R. Moed.)

posterior rim of the acetabulum, along with a portion of the articular surface and retroacetabular surface. Fractures can vary in size from a very small portion of articular surface to nearly the entire posterior wall, and can vary in location from the posteroinferior to the posterosuperior aspect of the acetabular articular surface. On the AP and obturator oblique x-rays, posterior wall fractures disrupt the posterior rim, but no other radiographic landmarks (Figure 12.48.6). Impaction of the articular surface (marginal impaction) (Figure 12.48.4) is a common associated finding. The typical posterior wall fracture does not disrupt the greater and lesser sciatic notches or extend into the quadrilateral surface. Extended posterior wall fractures represent a more severe injury that involve a disruption of the greater or lesser sciatic notches, and a portion of the quadrilateral surface. These fractures do not extend into the obturator foramen.

Posterior column fractures

Posterior column fractures (Figure 12.48.7) disrupt the posterior or ischial portion of the acetabulum and are best seen on the iliac oblique view. The majority of the retroacetabular surface is displaced with the posterior column. A vertical or oblique fracture line starting near the apex of the greater sciatic notch and crossing in the acetabular fossa, separates the anterior and posterior columns, and commonly enters the obturator foramen. There is usually an associated fracture of the inferior pubic ramus. The femoral head usually follows the posterior column posteriorly and medially. The ilioischial line is typically displaced relative to the teardrop. However, when a large portion of the quadrilateral surface remains intact with the posterior column, the teardrop will displace with the ilioischial line.

Anterior wall fractures

Anterior wall fractures disrupt the central portion of the anterior column (Figure 12.48.5C) and are rare fractures (1–2%). The inferior pubic ramus is typically intact. The iliopectineal line commonly has displacement in its mid-portion on the AP and obturator oblique views and the ilioischial line is intact. An anterior wall fracture variant has been described (Figure 12.48.8), which does not involve the pelvic brim and is a morphological equivalent to the posterior wall fracture.

Anterior column fractures

Anterior column fractures can occur at a variety of levels. The fracture is named based on where it exits the bone anteriorly. High fractures exit the iliac crest, intermediate fractures exit at the anterior superior iliac spine (ASIS), low fractures exit below the anterior inferior iliac spine (AIIS), and very low fractures exit at the iliopectineal eminence. The fracture typically involves disruption of the superior acetabular articular surface in the coronal plane. The iliopectineal line and anterior rim are typically displaced. Displacement of the superior articular surface is often best seen on the obturator oblique view. Inferiorly, the fracture disrupts the obturator ring through the ischiopubic ramus. Many variants have been described (Figure 12.48.9).

Transverse fractures

Transverse fractures divide the innominate bone into two portions, with a horizontally displaced fracture line, an intact superior acetabular fragment, and an inferior ischiopubic segment. The fracture begins at the pelvic brim, superomedially, and extends obliquely laterally and distally. The fracture line can cross the acetabulum at various levels and have been subdivided into three groups: transtectal fractures—the fracture line crosses the superior acetabular articular surface; juxtatectal fractures—the fracture line crosses at the junction of the superior acetabular articular surface and superior cotyloid fossa; and infratectal fractures—the fracture line crosses through the cotyloid fossa. Disruption of the vertical landmarks on the AP view (i.e. iliopectineal line, ilioischial line, anterior,

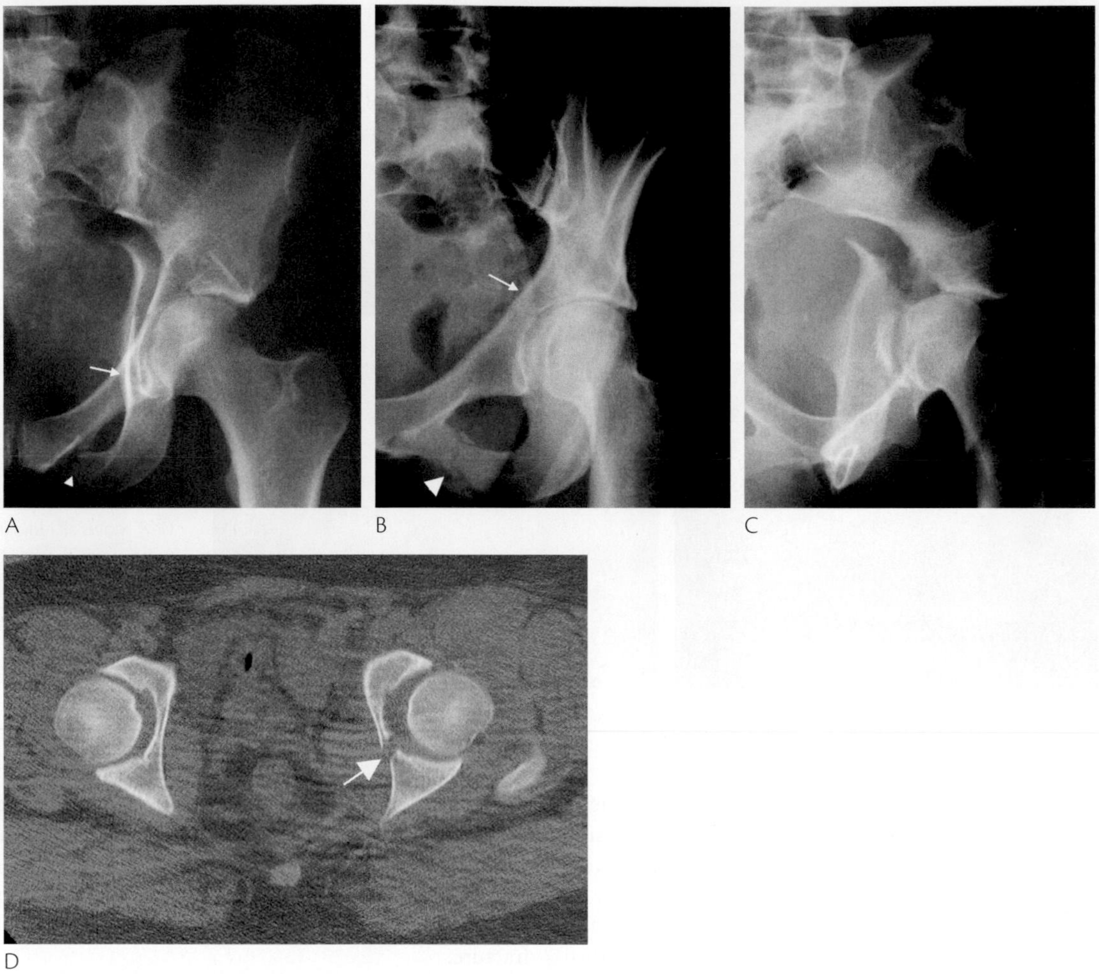

Fig. 12.48.7 Posterior column fracture: A) anteroposterior; B) obturator oblique; C) iliac oblique views and selected CT section. The anteroposterior view shows disruption of the ilioischial line displaced medial to the teardrop (arrow) and the fracture through the inferior pubic ramus (arrowhead). The obturator oblique view shows the intact iliopectineal line (arrow) and the fracture through the inferior pubic ramus (arrowhead). On the iliac oblique view, the fracture propagates through the greater sciatic notch. The CT shows the separation between the anterior and posterior columns (arrow). (Courtesy of Mr. Martin D. Bircher.)

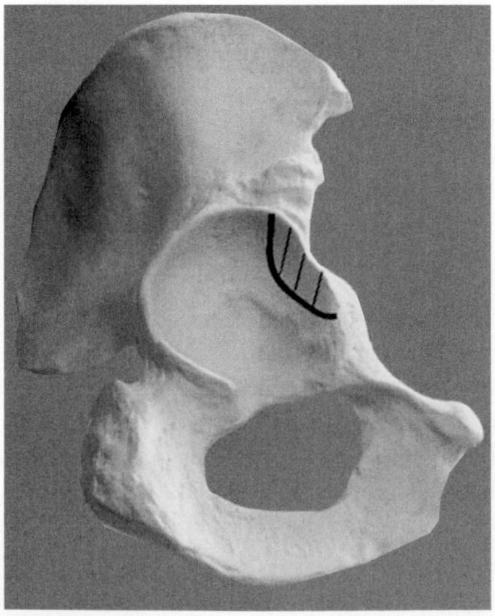

Fig. 12.48.8 Plastic bone model showing external aspect of the innominate bone. The anterior wall fracture variant drawn on the external surface of the innominate bone. (Copyright Dr. Berton R. Moed.)

and posterior rims) are noted. On CT scan, the fracture line is oriented in an AP direction in the axial section (see Figure 12.48.10D).

Associated patterns

Posterior column and posterior wall fractures

The association of a posterior column and posterior wall fracture represents a typical posterior column fracture, complicated by injury to the posterior wall. The femoral head usually dislocates with the wall component. Radiographic signs of a posterior column fracture with a dissociation of the ilioischial line and teardrop are commonly noted. Posterior wall fractures will be best seen on the obturator oblique view.

Transverse and posterior wall fractures

Associated transverse and posterior wall fractures are an extremely common type of acetabular fracture, approximately 20% of all acetabular fractures. The femoral head is often dislocated. This fracture combines a normal transverse configuration with a posterior wall fracture component. When the posterior wall fragment is minimally displaced, it may be missed on the AP pelvis, but is commonly seen on the obturator oblique view, as well as the CT.

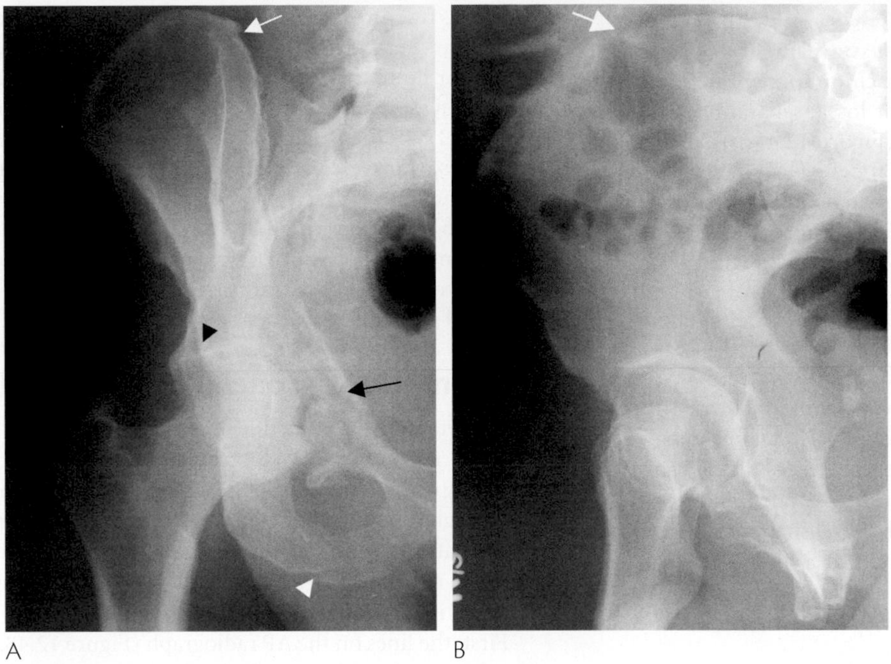

Fig. 12.48.9 High anterior column variant fracture: A) the obturator oblique view shows the typical high fracture through the iliac crest (white arrow), the displacement of the superior articular surface (black arrowhead), and fracture dividing the ischiopubic ramus (white arrowhead). A secondary fracture line extends through the anterior wall (black arrow). On the iliac oblique view (B), the posterior column is intact with the fracture again shown through the iliac crest (white arrow). (Copyright Dr. Berton R. Moed.)

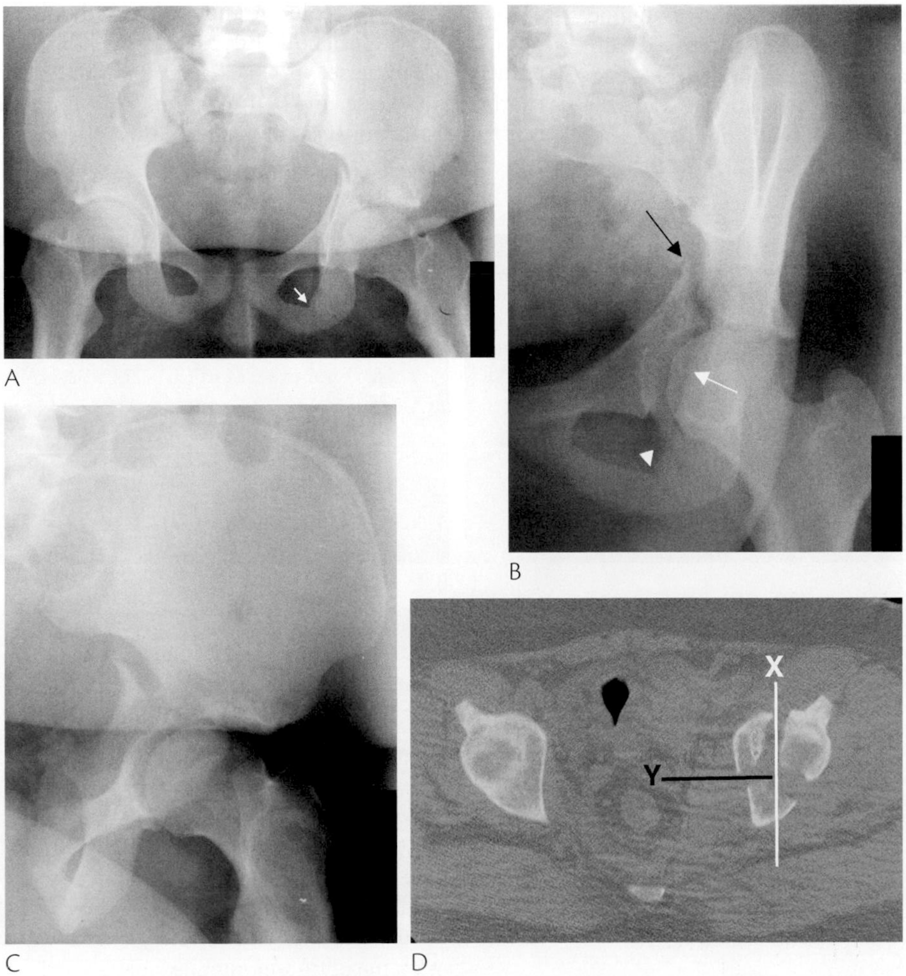

Fig. 12.48.10 T-shaped fracture: A) anteroposterior; B) obturator oblique; C) iliac oblique views; and D) selected CT section of a displaced juxtatectal T-shaped fracture. The anteroposterior view shows fractures through the iliopectineal and ilioischial lines and the ischiopubic ramus (arrow) with medial subluxation of the femoral head. The obturator oblique view illustrates displacement of the anterior column (black arrow), stem of the T through the acetabular fossa (white arrow), and fracture through the ischiopubic ramus (white arrowhead). The iliac oblique view shows disruption and displacement of the posterior column at the greater sciatic notch. The axial CT section (D) shows the juxtatectal position of the transverse fracture line (white line X) and the stem of the fracture (black line Y) separating the anterior and posterior columns. (Copyright Dr. Berton R. Moed.)

T-shaped fractures

T-shaped fractures are similar to transverse fractures with the addition of a vertical fracture in the ischiopubic segment along the quadrilateral surface and acetabular fossa, separating the anterior and posterior columns inferiorly (Figure 12.48.10). This inferior fracture is known as the stem of the T. The stem will typically extend through the obturator foramen, exiting through the ischiopubic ramus; however, it may also extend posteriorly (exiting through the ischium) or anteriorly (exiting near the pubic body). Medial or posterior subluxation of the femoral head can occur.

Anterior column and posterior hemitransverse fractures

Anterior column with associated posterior hemitransverse fracture combines an anterior wall or anterior column fracture with a transverse component posteriorly. The posterior component of this fracture pattern is identical to the posterior half of a transverse fracture. The distinction between the associated anterior column and posterior hemitransverse and the T-shape patterns is often subtle. The anterior injury is typically at a higher level and more displaced than the posterior hemitransverse component. Anterior subluxation of the femoral head is typical with an anterior column and posterior hemitransverse injury.

Both-column fractures

Both-column fractures by definition have the anterior and posterior columns separated from each other, and all articular segments of the acetabulum are detached from the intact portion of the posterior ilium (Figure 12.48.11). The both-column fracture is unique, in that it represents an acetabulum completely disconnected from the axial skeleton. If the femoral head medializes, the articular fragments can rotate around the head because the labrum is usually intact. This is called 'secondary congruence' and is unique to both column fractures. Both-column fractures are associated with the 'spur' sign. This represents the fracture edge of the intact posterior ilium that is seen prominently on the obturator oblique view. This spur sign is pathognomonic of a both-column fracture (Figure 12.48.11B). The surgeon should recognize that transverse fractures, transverse and posterior wall fractures, T-shaped fractures, and anterior column and posterior hemitransverse fractures all *involve* the anterior and posterior columns of the acetabulum, but are not 'both-column' fractures. In these four fracture types, a portion of the articular surface remains intact with the ilium and the axial skeleton.

Systematic approach to interpretation

The acetabulum is a complex three-dimensional structure and effort is required to develop the required interpretive skills. The majority of fractures can be classified from the information gleaned from high-quality plain radiographs. An organized approach to the examination of the three radiographs (AP and obliques) and the CT scan of a patient with an acetabular fracture must be used. One method is as follows.

First, the lines on the AP radiograph (Figure 12.48.3A) should be carefully analysed in turn. Is the iliopectineal line disrupted? If so, the fracture possibilities include the anterior wall, anterior column, transverse types, T-shaped, anterior column and posterior hemitransverse, and both-column. If the ilioischial line is disrupted, possibilities include the posterior column types, transverse types, T-shaped, anterior column and posterior hemitransverse, and both-column. With both lines disrupted, the possibilities are reduced to transverse types, T-shaped, anterior column and posterior hemitransverse, and both-column. Is the line along the posterior rim disrupted? If so, this will add the possibility of a posterior

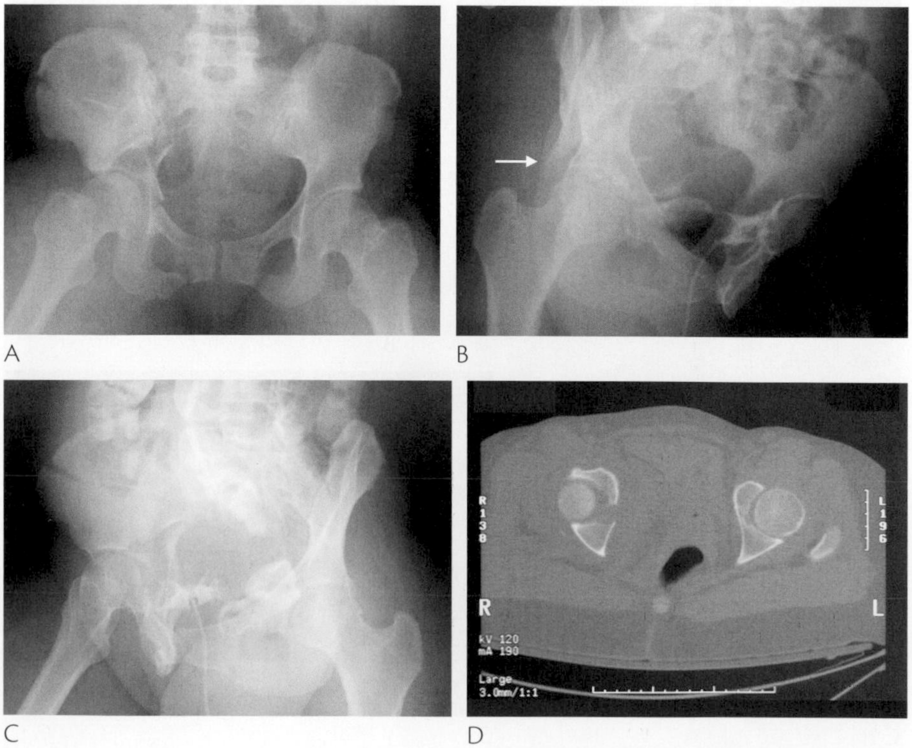

Fig. 12.48.11 Both-column fracture: A) anteroposterior; B) obturator oblique; and C) external oblique radiographs, and D) CT scan section through the hip joint demonstrating a both-column fracture of the acetabulum with secondary congruence. Although there are gaps between the intra-articular fracture fragments and the entire hip joint is medially displaced, a symmetric joint space is maintained. The spur sign is evident on the (B) obturator oblique view.

wall fracture. Is the ilioischial line displaced from its normal relationship to the teardrop? If so, this would indicate, in general, that the two columns are separated from each other.

Next the obturator oblique is examined. This view will refine the diagnosis made from the AP view. A suspected posterior wall component will become obvious, as well as disruption involving the anterior wall or column. Is the obturator ring fractured? If so, this, again, would suggest that the two columns are separated from each other. The presence of a spur sign (Figure 12.48.11B) is pathognomonic for a both-column fracture. The iliac oblique is viewed next. Injury to the posterior column is further defined, as well as the presence and location of fractures involving the iliac wing (for example; anterior column, anterior column and posterior hemitransverse, and both-column fractures).

Finally, the CT scan is studied to reveal the additional information described previously (Box 12.48.5). After this analysis, the plain films should be revisited to refine the diagnosis for fracture subtypes (for example, the level of transverse fracture or the path of the stem of the T-shaped fracture). If the diagnosis continues to be unclear, the three-dimensional CT scan can prove helpful. However, as noted previously, the three-dimensional CT scan has its limitations.

In some clinical situations, high-quality plain radiographs, especially the Judet oblique views, may be difficult to obtain. Investigators have reported on the advantages of equivalents to the plain oblique radiographs, which are reconstructed from CT scan data using three-dimensional CT modelling software. However, the use of this approach and an overall increased role for the three-dimensional CT scan, awaits further study, as well as technological improvements.

Summary

Acetabular fracture patterns can be complex; however, classification can be achieved with the use of appropriate imaging and a systematic approach. Classification is not only important for communication but is essential in allowing the surgeon to understand the fracture pattern and select the most appropriate surgical strategy.

Further reading

Beaule, P.E., Dorey, F.J., and Matta, J.M. (2003). Letournel classification for acetabular fractures: Assessment of interobserver and intraobserver reliability. *Journal of Bone and Joint Surgery*, **85A**, 1704–9.

Judet, R., Judet, J., and Letournel, E. (1964). Fractures of the acetabulum. Classification and surgical approaches for open reduction. *Journal of Bone and Joint Surgery*, **46A**, 1615–38.

Lenarz, C.J. and Moed, B.R. (2007). Atypical anterior wall fracture of the acetabulum: case series of anterior acetabular rim fracture without involvement of the pelvic brim. *Journal of Orthopaedic Trauma*, **21**, 515–22.

Letournel, E. and Judet, R. (1993). *Fractures of the Acetabulum*, second edition. New York: Springer-Verlag.

Patel, V., Day, A., Dinah, F., Kelly, M., and Bircher, M. (2007). The value of specific radiological features in the classification of acetabular fractures. *Journal of Bone and Joint Surgery*, **89**, 72–6.

12.49

Management of acetabular fractures

Berton R. Moed

Summary points

- Acetabular fracture patients often have associated injuries
- Restoration of hip joint congruity and stability are the treatment goals
- Stable concentrically reduced fractures can be considered for non-operative management
- Operative treatment is indicated for fractures with hip joint instability or incongruity
- Choosing the proper surgical approach is one of the most important treatment aspects
- Although the surgery is demanding, an experienced surgeon can obtain excellent results.

Introduction

Restoration of hip joint congruity and stability are the goals of acetabular fracture treatment. The achievement of these goals should minimize pain, prevent post-traumatic osteoarthritis, and thereby improve long-term functional outcome. Although certain fracture patterns may not require surgery to have a satisfactory outcome, in general, a patient with a displaced fracture in the superior weight-bearing area of the acetabulum should be managed with open reduction and internal fixation. However, the surgery is complex and demanding, even for the experienced surgeon, and has the potential for many serious complications. Therefore, many factors, including the patient's age, general medical condition, and associated injuries, must be considered prior to making definitive management decisions.

Patients with severe associated injuries should be treated non-operatively until their general condition improves. Continued poor general medical status and a long delay (>3 weeks) from injury to possible operative intervention may dictate a non-operative management course. Elderly, debilitated patients and others with pre-existing osteopenia require special consideration since the ability to achieve and maintain an anatomical reduction may be more difficult due to poor bone stock and extensive comminution. Furthermore, these patients often have sustained low-energy trauma resulting in a fracture pattern more amenable to non-operative care. Total hip arthroplasty may be a reasonable option either acutely or as a delayed reconstruction.

Initial management (Box 12.49.1)

In most cases, the patient with a fracture of the acetabulum has sustained high-energy trauma. Therefore, these patients often will have an associated injury that must be identified during the initial work-up. Consequently, the initial evaluation, even in those patients with an apparent isolated injury, should be part of a well-organized overall approach. Associated injuries can be life- or limb-threatening. In contradistinction to the unstable pelvic ring injury, a closed fracture of the acetabulum, occurring alone or in combination with other extremity fractures, should not be considered as the primary cause of hypotensive shock. An alternative source of haemorrhage should always be sought. However, laceration of the superior gluteal artery with severe bleeding can be caused by fractures of the acetabulum having wide posterior column displacement. One must be alert to this possibility, which is treatable by therapeutic embolization.

A detailed physical examination is a necessity. The soft tissues should be carefully evaluated, as soft-tissue injury has important implications for subsequent surgery. Acetabular fracture surgery through a compromised soft-tissue envelope is ill advised due to the increased risk of infection. Closed de-gloving soft-tissue injuries over the trochanteric region associated with underlying haematoma formation and fat necrosis (the Morel-Lavallé lesion) or open wounds may require debridement followed by delayed wound closure. More recently, a percutaneous method has been reported

Box 12.49.1 Initial management

- Assess and treat according to ATLS ® protocols
- Evaluate soft tissue, e.g. Morel-Lavallé lesion
- Evaluate neurology
- Reduce hip dislocation ± dynamic assessment of stability
- Skeletal traction
- Diagnostic imaging (see Chapter 12.48)
    - AP and oblique x-rays
    - CT.

in a small number of patients, using a plastic brush to debride the injured fatty tissue, which is then washed from the wound with pulsed lavage. A medium closed-suction drain is placed within the lesion and removed when drainage is less than 30mL over 24h. Fracture fixation is deferred until at least 24h after drain removal. The prevalence of post-traumatic sciatic nerve injury has been reported as being as high as 29%. Other peripheral nerves, such as the femoral nerve and obturator nerve, may also be injured. A complete and clearly documented neurological examination is extremely important both for patient prognosis and for medicolegal concerns.

Initial acetabular fracture management depends on the specific fracture pattern, the amount of fracture displacement, and the relative stability and congruency of the hip joint. The initial anteroposterior (AP) radiograph of the pelvis (which is often an adjunct to the ATLS® primary survey) can provide substantial diagnostic information and indicate the need for emergency treatment. This radiograph must be supplemented by further studies (oblique plain films and computed tomography (CT)—see Chapter 12.48) in order to define the injury completely.

Dislocation of the femoral head, which can be diagnosed on the initial AP radiograph, requires prompt reduction as the rate of osteonecrosis increases significantly if reduction is not performed within 12h of the injury. The reduction manoeuvre can often be performed in the emergency room setting. However, adequate sedation and pain medication are necessary. Subsequent failed closed reduction, pre-existing contraindications to conscious sedation, or doctor preference constitute indications for closed reduction using general anaesthesia. Immediately following reduction, confirmatory radiographs should be obtained. There is no need to stress an obviously unstable hip and redislocation may be injurious. Only when the fracture pattern suggests that the hip joint should be stable or stability is equivocal (such as with a small posterior wall fracture) should the hip be taken through a full range of motion to evaluate postreduction stability. As a diagnostic procedure, this examination is best performed using fluoroscopic visualization of the hip joint with the patient under general anaesthesia.

Patients with an acetabular fracture may not require skeletal traction. However, there are notable situations in which skeletal traction (preferably using a distal femoral, rather than a proximal tibial, traction pin) is either mandatory or desirable. Unstable fracture–dislocations require skeletal traction following reduction to prevent recurrent dislocation. When hip stability is in doubt, it is also prudent to use traction, pending further evaluation. Preoperative skeletal traction is also important to prevent further femoral head articular surface damage from abrasion by the raw acetabular bony fracture surfaces and may occasionally improve fracture position (Figure 12.49.1). Skin traction is ineffective and should not be used. Skeletal traction using a trochanteric pin is contraindicated due to its associated high infection risk and ineffectiveness in fracture reduction. In general, fractures with minimal or no displacement, both-column fractures in which the hip joint remains congruent and in acceptable position (so-called secondary congruence), and other displaced fractures not meeting operative criteria initially require only bed rest with symptomatic treatment. However, these patients, as well as those with fractures meeting operative criteria who do not require skeletal traction for fracture management, may benefit from skeletal traction for pain relief.

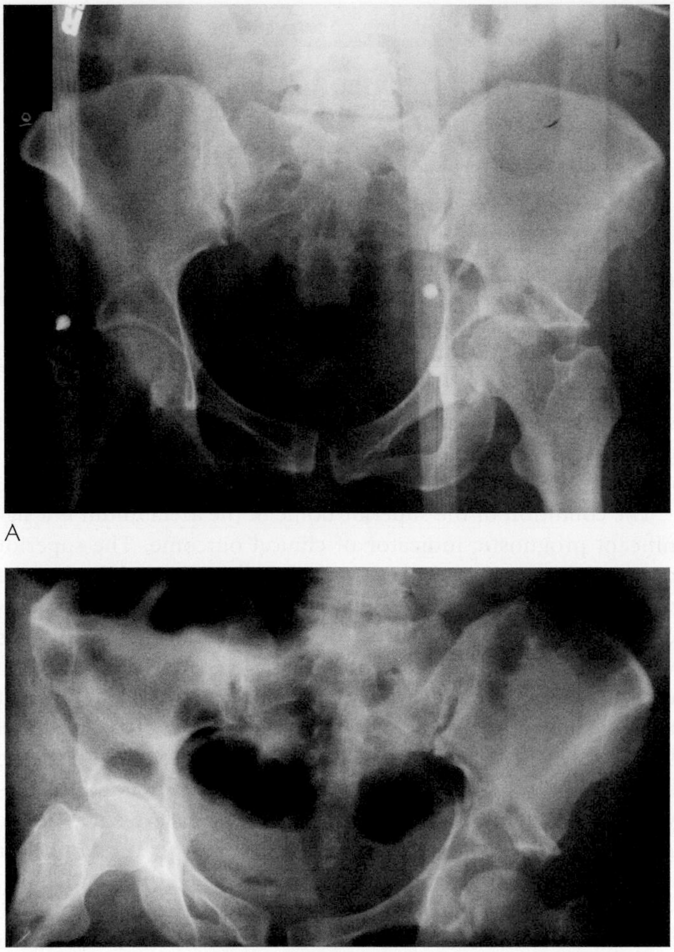

Fig. 12.49.1 Anteroposterior hip radiographs (A) before and (B) after the application of traction. Without traction the femoral head is medially subluxed, rubbing against the sharp corner of the superior acetabular fracture surface in this displaced transtectal fracture (A). The hip joint is distracted with the application of traction pulling the articular cartilage of the femoral head a safe distance away from the acetabular fracture surface (B).

Operative treatment of acetabular fractures is not an emergency and is generally delayed 3–5 days to allow for stabilization of the patient's general status and for preoperative planning. However, the time to surgery has been shown to be a significant predictor of radiological and clinical outcome. In one study, a good-to-excellent clinical outcome was more likely when surgery was performed within 15 days for elementary fractures and 10 days for associated types. The indications for emergency fracture fixation are uncommon (see later).

Non-operative management

Indications (Box 12.49.2)

In general, all stable concentrically reduced acetabular fractures not involving the superior acetabular dome can be considered for non-operative management. This group of fractures includes non-displaced and minimally displaced fractures, fractures in which the intact part of the acetabulum is large enough to maintain stability and congruity, and those with secondary congruence (Box 12.49.3). Non-operative management may also be selected for patients with

Box 12.49.2 Radiological criterion for non-operative treatment

- Displacement <2mm
- Stability
  - Roof arc angles
    - —medial 45 degrees
    - —anterior 25 degrees
    - —posterior 70 degrees
  - Dynamic fluoroscopy.

severe osteoporosis or severe underlying medical problems that preclude surgical intervention. This is a relatively small group, consisting mainly of elderly patients.

The condition of the superior dome of the acetabulum is a significant prognostic indicator of clinical outcome. The superior dome of the acetabulum is described as the superior third of the weight-bearing area of the acetabulum. Roof arc measurements can be used to decide whether or not an acetabular fracture has violated the weight bearing dome. This measurement has been used to determine if the remaining intact acetabulum is sufficient to maintain a stable and congruous relationship with the femoral head. In this way, operative verses non-operative treatment can be selected. The roof arc is measured on all three radiographic views with the leg out of traction. The medial roof arc is measured on the AP view. The anterior roof arc is measured on the obturator oblique, and the posterior roof arc is measured on the iliac oblique. To obtain these measurements, the first line is a vertical line through the centre of the femoral head and the second line is drawn from the centre of the femoral head to the fracture location at the articular surface (Figure 12.49.2). Roof arc measurements are not applicable to both-column fractures or those with a fracture of the posterior wall. The previous recommendations were that roof arc measurements greater than 45 degrees on the AP (medial roof arc), iliac oblique (posterior roof arc), and obturator oblique radiographs (anterior roof arc) indicate preservation of the weight-bearing dome, and these patients should be considered for non-operative management. More recently, however, biomechanical analysis has produced different criteria. Non-operative fracture management is considered with a medial roof arc angle of greater than 45 degrees, an anterior roof arc angle of greater than 25 degrees, and a posterior roof arc angle of greater than 70 degrees (Figure 12.49.3).

CT cuts of the superior 10mm of the acetabular articular surface are equivalent to the weight-bearing dome region, and can also be useful in determining if acetabular fracture lines involve this region. Although controversy exists regarding the exact amount of displacement that is considered acceptable when the superior dome of the acetabulum is involved, most authors recommend surgical intervention if displacement exceeds 2mm.

Displaced low anterior column, low transverse and low T-shaped acetabular fractures are amenable to non-operative treatment, provided the fracture position is stable and the joint remains congruent.

Displaced both-column fractures of the acetabulum may be considered for non-operative management in the presence of secondary congruence (see Chapter 12.48, Figure 12.48.11), defined as congruency between the femoral head and the displaced acetabular articular fragments without skeletal traction being applied. Parallelism between the femoral head and acetabular articular surface must be maintained in all three radiographic views, especially in a young patient. In addition, articular fragment displacement and medial joint displacement should not be so excessive as to limit motion. However, it must be recognized that fractures with secondary congruence do not have as good a prognosis as those reduced in anatomical position.

Fractures involving the acetabular walls should be treated non-operatively only if the hip joint remains completely stable. Recurrent dislocation and subluxation have disastrous

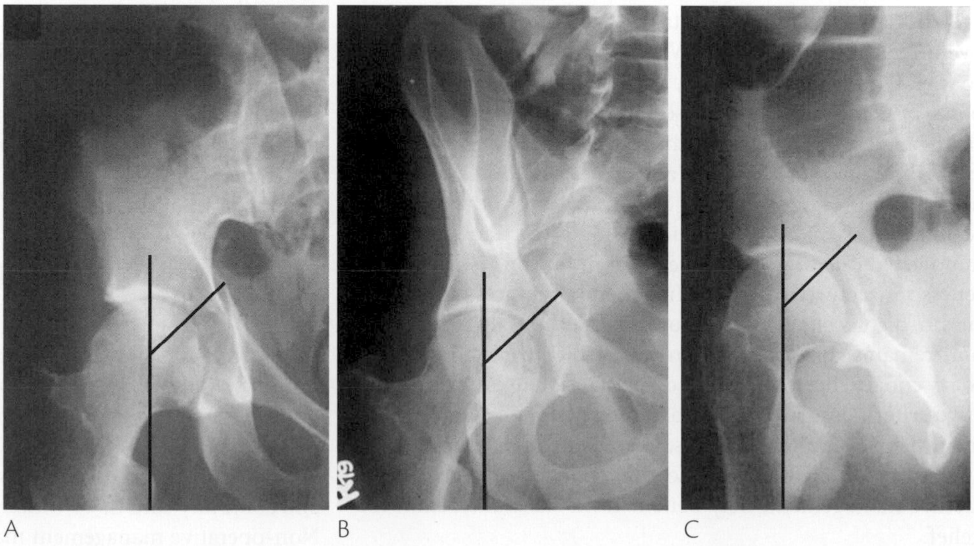

Fig. 12.49.2 A) Anteroposterior; B) internal oblique; and C) external oblique radiographs of a transverse fracture of the acetabulum of a 35-year-old man treated in 1992 showing roof arcs all approximately 50 degrees in measurement, indicative of a stable hip joint by the initial recommendations. (Copyright Dr. Berton R. Moed.)

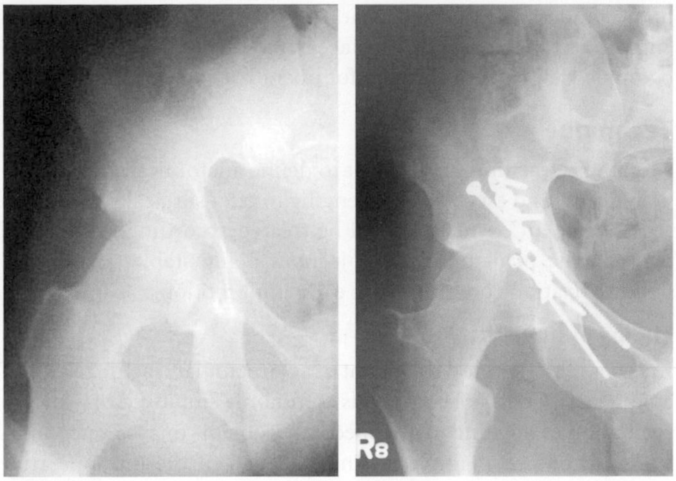

Fig. 12.49.3 Anteroposterior radiograph (A) of the patient from figure 12.49.2 obtained 3 weeks later showing gross medial subluxation of the hip, which would have been expected using the criteria of Vrahas et al. (1999). Subsequently, the patient underwent operative treatment, shown 3 years later (B) with an excellent clinical result. (Copyright Dr. Berton R. Moed.)

consequences. Although hip instability is much more common with fractures of the posterior wall, anterior wall fractures are also potentially unstable. CT studies of posterior wall fractures indicate that those involving greater than 40–50% are usually unstable, whereas fractures less than 20–25% are usually stable. However, there is evidence that these radiographic measurements are not reliable. When in doubt, it is safest to assume that all of these fractures are unstable until proven otherwise. Therefore, clinical evaluation of stability is mandatory if non-operative treatment is being considered. As noted previously, this examination is best performed using fluoroscopic visualization of the hip joint with the patient under general anaesthesia. With this method, the patient is placed supine with the hip in neutral rotation and full extension. The hip is then gradually flexed past 90 degrees while progressive manual force is applied through the hip along the longitudinal axis of the femur; simultaneously, fluoroscopic imaging of the hip is performed, first using the AP projection and then using the obturator oblique projection. If the hip appears stable (remains congruent) on this assessment, the exam is repeated with the addition of slight adduction and internal rotation (approximately 20 degrees). Frank redislocation is neither required nor clinically desirable. Therefore, posterior subluxation demonstrated in either view (as evidenced by a widening medial clear space or loss of joint parallelism) is indicative of dynamic hip instability. This technique has been proven to predict long-term stability and outcome. Acetabular wall fracture presenting in the absence of known hip dislocation is no guarantee of hip stability (Figure 12.49.4).

It seems obvious that all non-displaced and minimally displaced acetabular fractures should be considered for non-operative management. However, there have been advocates for percutaneous fracture fixation in this group of patients. The concern centres on the questionable stability of these fractures with the contention that a certain percentage will displace. Therefore early percutaneous fixation would avoid a subsequent more extensive open procedure or prevent the disaster of early traumatic arthritis in those (for whatever reason) not having the benefit of further treatment. However, only a very small number (less than 7%) of these non-displaced and minimally displaced fractures are potentially unstable and will significantly displace without traction. Rather than unnecessarily operating on a large number of fractures to prevent problems in these few or subject all of these patients to prolonged bed rest in traction, it makes more sense to try to identify those at risk for fracture displacement. Dynamic fluoroscopic stress examination with the patient under general anaesthesia, as noted earlier, is one proposed method of identifying these fractures at risk. However, the exact technique for performing this examination is ill defined for fractures other than the posterior wall. Another method is to closely observe all patients presenting with non-operative parameters via weekly radiographic follow-up, being prepared to shift immediately to operative management (percutaneous or otherwise) should joint instability or incongruency be detected.

Technique

The non-operative management of patients with acetabular fractures mainly consists of bed rest with joint mobilization and eventual progression to full weight-bearing activity. Bed rest is necessary in the acute injury phase only for symptomatic relief. Mobilization of the patient and the hip joint should follow as soon as symptoms allow. Patients should begin with touch-down partial weight

A

B

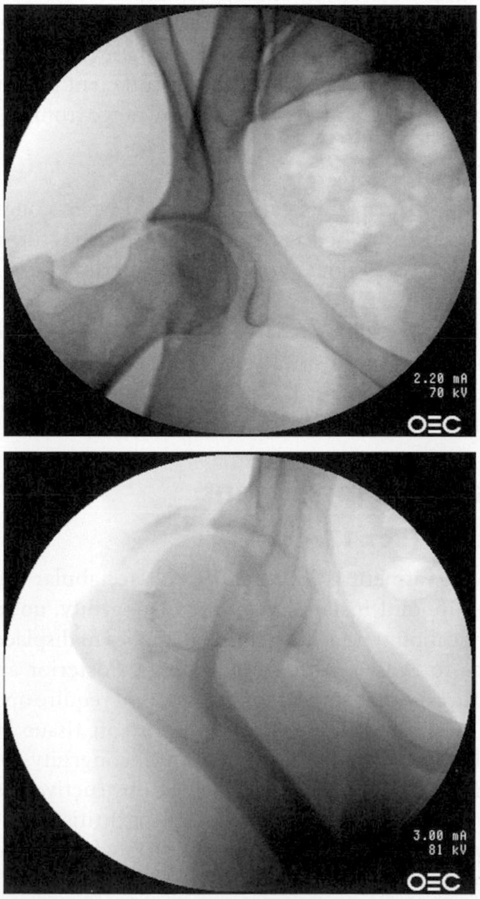

Fig. 12.49.4 Fluoroscopic internal oblique views of a fracture of the posterior wall of the acetabulum without history of hip dislocation and involving less than 20% of the articular surface and presumed stable. A) The hip is in neutral position and the joint is congruent. B) The femoral head is subluxed posteriorly with 70 degrees of hip flexion indicating occult instability.

Box 12.49.3 Fractures amenable to non-operative treatment

- Stable non-displaced and minimally displaced fractures
- Selected displaced fractures:
  - Remaining intact acetabulum maintains stability and congruency
    - —low anterior column fractures
    - —low transverse fractures
    - —low T-shaped fractures
  - Both-column fractures with secondary congruence
  - Wall fracture not compromising hip stability.

bearing of the affected extremity (<10kg). AP and oblique radiographs should be obtained at frequent intervals (weekly for the first 4 weeks) to confirm maintenance of satisfactory position. When there is adequate fracture healing, usually by 6–12 weeks, the patient should gradually progress to full weight bearing. Joint mobilization should be continued throughout the rehabilitation period. The use of formal physiotherapy or continuous passive motion modalities should be tailored to the individual.

Prolonged traction treatment should be reserved for those patients with operative indications related to fracture displacement, but having medical contraindications. In these cases, traction should be maintained until fracture healing is sufficient to allow progressive weight-bearing ambulation and may range from 4–12 weeks.

Results

Good or excellent results can be achieved when congruency and stability are maintained with non-displaced fractures and some displaced fractures not involving the superior dome. Displaced fractures of the superior acetabular dome and posterior acetabular fractures are generally associated with poor clinical results. Delayed reduction of the hip dislocation, injury to the femoral head, and continued instability are all factors contributing to a poor outcome in patients with acetabular fractures.

Operative management

Indications (Box 12.49.4)

Operative treatment is indicated for all acetabular fractures that result in hip joint instability and/or incongruity, no matter what the classification type. This statement applies to displaced fractures as well as to those with occult findings. Posterior and anterior wall fractures with instability of the hip joint require operative fixation. In addition, fragments of bone or soft tissue incarcerated within the hip joint may result in joint incongruity. Open reduction and removal of the loose body or obstructive tissue is indicated to prevent early onset of traumatic arthritis. Internal fixation should be performed in this setting as dictated by hip joint stability parameters.

Fracture displacement in the weight-bearing dome results in joint incongruity and constitutes one of the main indications for open reduction and internal fixation. As described previously, plain radiographs and CT can be effectively used to determine whether an acetabular fracture violates the weight-bearing dome. For the both-column fracture, loss of parallelism between the femoral head and the acetabular articular surface noted on any of the three radiographic views is an indication for operative management.

Technique

Acetabular fractures are difficult to define anatomically and radiographically, and especially challenging to treat surgically. However, these articular fractures should be treated according to standard orthopaedic principles: the objectives being stable, anatomical fracture fixation combined with early joint motion.

Timing of surgery

In general, the surgical treatment of an acetabular fracture is not an emergency. A delay of 3–5 days is commonly employed to allow for evaluation of any underlying medical problems or associated injuries and for preoperative planning. Much of the intraoperative manoeuvring for acetabular fracture reduction is performed indirectly, without direct exposure or complete visualization of the fracture fragments. These techniques rely on the presence of relatively mobile fracture fragments. Ten days following injury, early fracture healing begins to limit this type of fracture mobilization. Two weeks following injury, healing has often progressed to the point that this fracture mobility has been lost and a more extensive surgical approach is required for certain fracture types, such as the transverse, T-shaped, anterior column with posterior hemitransverse, and both-column patterns. After 3 weeks, callus formation is extensive to the point that the fracture is no longer considered to be an acute injury. It has been shown that a good-to-excellent clinical outcome is more likely when surgery was performed within 10–15 days. This compromised outcome is probably related to many factors beyond the more extensive surgical exposure with its attendant higher complication rate, such as acetabular cartilage damage and femoral head erosion. Therefore prolonged delay in operative treatment should be avoided if possible.

Indications for emergency open reduction and internal fixation are uncommon (Box 12.49.5). Treatment of open fractures of the acetabulum should follow the standard principles of open fracture management, which include emergency irrigation, debridement, and fracture stabilization. Fracture stabilization options include acute open reduction and internal fixation or traction followed by delayed open reduction and internal fixation. When an acetabular fracture is directly related to a vascular injury and fixation is an important adjunct to the vessel repair (i.e. femoral artery laceration with anterior column fracture), concomitant open reduction and internal fixation is indicated.

Planning and facilities

Plain radiographs and CT imaging should allow the surgeon to classify the fracture type and to achieve a precise understanding of the 'personality' of the fracture. The three-dimensional CT reconstruction may obscure some fracture lines. However, this study can

Box 12.49.4 Operative indications

- Documented or suspected hip instability
- Incarcerated bone or soft tissue leading to incongruity
- Fracture displacement in the weight-bearing dome.

be very helpful in visualizing the overall fracture pattern in the mind's eye (Figure 12.49.5). Drawing the fracture on paper or on a whole bone specimen is also very instructive. In this way the appropriate surgical approach, reduction technique, and hardware configuration can be planned with confidence that the required anatomical reduction and stable fixation will be accomplished.

Intraoperative traction is very important in obtaining fracture reduction. Therefore, purpose-specific traction tables, such as the Judet fracture table or the Jackson table, are recommended. The operating table should be radiolucent. Intraoperative C-arm fluoroscopy can then be used to assess fracture reduction and hardware location. Therefore fluoroscopy equipment and trained radiology personnel are needed. An extensive array of instruments and implants is also required (Figure 12.49.6). An oscillating drill is helpful for placing screws deep within the wound.

Reduction techniques and aids

Anatomical reduction of the intra-articular fracture fragments is the objective of acetabular fracture surgery. While correction of fracture displacement is very important, failure to appreciate and correct malrotation (which is considerable in many of the fracture types) is probably the most common cause of fracture malreduction. Developing an understanding of the deformity (gleaned from the preoperative imaging studies) is critically important. This will facilitate planning of intraoperative reduction manoeuvres. Various tools and techniques developed specifically for acetabular fracture reduction are essential. Long pointed reduction clamps, ball spike pushers, and Farabeuf clamps are extremely helpful in obtaining satisfactory reduction (Figure 12.49.7). Intraoperative traction, to unload the fracture fragments from the considerable deforming forces across the hip, is instrumental in assisting fracture reduction. Traction may be applied manually by a surgical assistant, either pulling on the leg or on a traction pin placed in the greater trochanter or distal femur. However, traction by this means is often difficult to maintain effectively. As noted earlier, operating room tables with traction capability are preferable. On board traction using a Universal Distractor is one possible alternative. A Schanz screw with T-handle attachment is helpful for traction and for direct fracture manipulation. K-wires and cerclage wires can be used to secure provisional fixation, and the reduction should be carefully evaluated using fluoroscopy or plain radiographs prior to permanent hardware placement. Fluoroscopy or intraoperative radiographs should be used throughout the procedure to confirm maintenance of reduction and appropriate placement of hardware (Figures 12.49.8 and 12.49.9).

Box 12.49.5 Timing of acetabular fracture surgery

- Emergency:
  - Recurrent dislocation despite traction
  - Irreducible hip dislocation
  - Progressive sciatic nerve deficit following closed reduction
  - Associated vascular injury requiring repair
  - Open fractures
  - Ipsilateral femoral neck fracture
- 3–5 days after planning is ideal
- Results deteriorate after 10 days to 2 weeks.

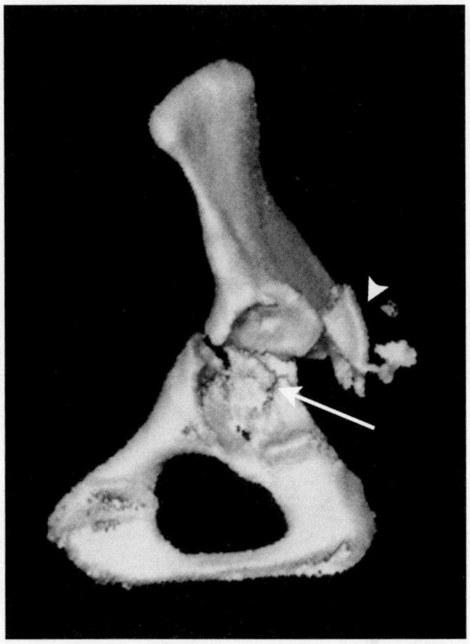

Fig. 12.49.5 Three-dimensional CT scan showing the main transverse fracture line, posterior wall fragments (white arrowhead) and intra-articular free fragment (white arrow), which are well visualized. (Copyright Dr. Berton R. Moed.)

Implants

After an anatomical reduction has been obtained, stable fracture fixation is best accomplished using interfragmentary screws augmented by plates. Cortical screws of 3.5mm and 4.5mm diameter are ideal for this purpose and should be available in lengths up to 110mm. Longer or smaller diameter (2.7mm or 2.0mm) screws may be required depending on the fracture configuration or comminution (Figure 12.49.8). These sizes may not be readily available in standard instrument sets. Therefore, preoperative planning is invaluable in these instances. Reconstruction-type plates of 3.5mm (Synthes

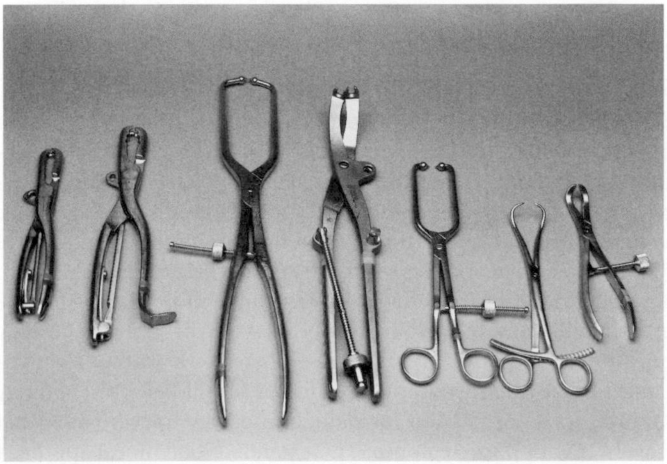

Fig. 12.49.6 Example of some of the instruments often needed for fracture reduction (Synthes, Philadelphia, PA).

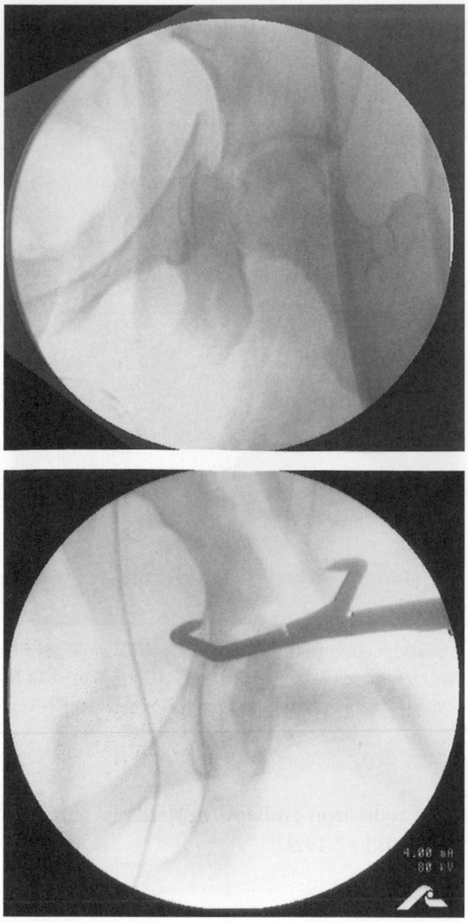

Fig. 12.49.7 Intraoperative fluoroscopic views of a transverse type fracture before (top) and after (bottom) reduction using a pointed reduction clamp. The clamp has been placed through the greater sciatic notch, correcting the displacement and malrotation. (Reproduced from Moed, B.R. (2006). Acetabular fractures: the Kocher-Langenbeck approach. In *Master techniques in orthopaedic surgery: fractures* (ed. D.A. Wiss), pp. 685–709, Lippincott Williams & Wilkins, Philadelphia, PA.)

or Stryker), which can be contoured to the curved, irregular surface of the pelvis and acetabulum, are appropriate for stable fracture fixation (Figure 12.49.9). Implant sites should be carefully selected to obtain satisfactory bony purchase while avoiding neurovascular injury and intra-articular hardware placement. Experience dictates the quantity of hardware required to achieve a stable fixation construct.

Surgical approach (Box 12.49.6)

Selection of the appropriate surgical approach is one of the most important aspects of the preoperative planning for acetabular fracture surgery. The main determinants in the decision-making process are the fracture type, the elapsed time from injury to operative intervention, and the magnitude and location of maximal fracture displacement. The mainstay surgical approaches to the acetabulum are the Kocher–Langenbeck, ilioinguinal, iliofemoral and the extended iliofemoral. The first three provide direct access to only one column of the acetabulum (posterior for the Kocher–Langenbeck; anterior for the ilioinguinal and iliofemoral) and rely on indirect manipulation for reduction of any fracture lines that traverse the opposite column. The extended iliofemoral approach affords the opportunity for almost complete direct access to all aspects of the acetabulum.

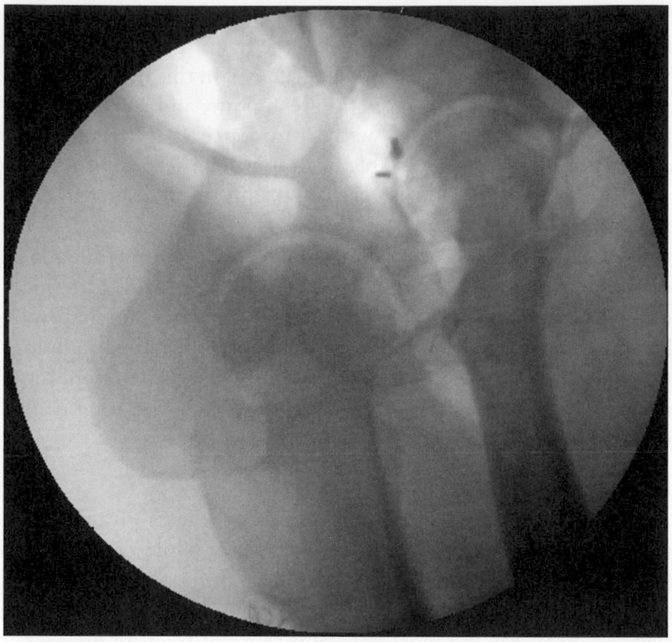

Fig. 12.49.8 Intraoperative fluoroscopic image of fracture showing the use of small interfragmentary lag screws (2.7mm and 2.0mm) to fix a small posterior wall fragment and documenting extra-articular screw placement.

Variations of the Kocher–Langenbeck include the addition of an osteotomy of the greater trochanteric or moving the proximal limb of the incision slightly more anterior (modified Gibson approach). These variations increase somewhat the anterior extent of the surgical exposure (see later). The modified Stoppa surgical approach, an extension of the standard Pfannensteil incision, is an anterior intrapelvic approach and can be considered as a variation of the

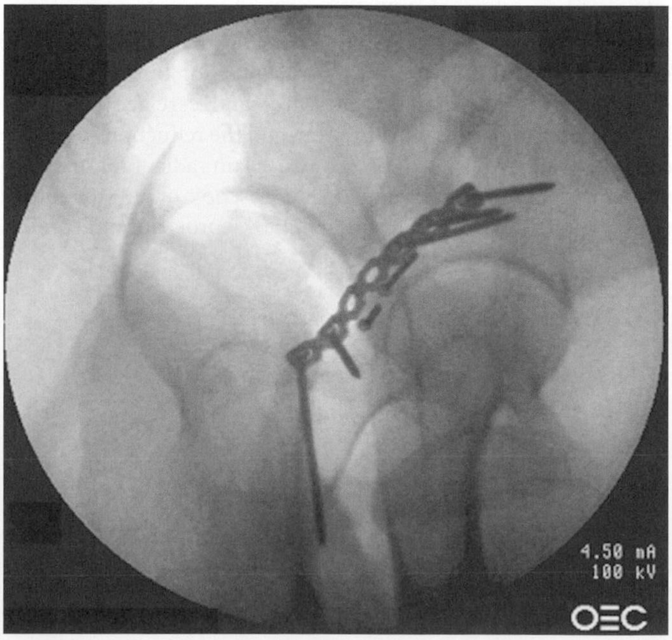

Fig. 12.49.9 Intraoperative fluoroscopic image of fracture from Figure 12.48.6 showing the use of a 3.5-mm reconstruction plate contoured to buttress the screw fixation.

ilioinguinal approach. This approach may provide improved visualization of the quadrilateral plate, while avoiding dissection of the femoral nerve and vessels. However, a secondary posterior incision (Kocher–Langenbeck) or one paralleling the iliac crest is often required. In addition, if the surgeon shifts his/her position to the opposite side of the operating room table from the ilioinguinal incision, all of the potential advantages of the modified Stoppa approach can be attained.

Modifications of the extended iliofemoral approach have been developed by others, such as the triradiate approach and the T-shaped variant. Each of these extended approaches has its distinguishing aspects. However, they are all variations on the same theme. The price to be paid for the greater surgical access is a greater risk of surgical complications.

As common sense would dictate, posterior fracture types require a posterior approach and anterior fracture types require an anterior approach. Fractures involving both columns demand some decision-making. In general, acute fractures without displacement through the weight-bearing dome can be reduced through a single surgical approach to that column of the acetabulum having the greatest fracture displacement, as long as the fracture lines traversing the opposite column can be accessed and manipulated by indirect reduction manoeuvres. Fracture mobility is gradually lost over time. Therefore, an extended approach (with its attendant higher complication rate) may be needed for delayed surgery of fractures that were otherwise amenable to a less extensive surgical exposure (see earlier). Other indications for the extended approaches include transverse and T-shaped fractures with displacement through the anatomical roof (weight-bearing area) of the acetabulum (i.e. transtectal fractures), T-shaped fractures having wide displacement of the vertical limb, and both-column fractures with sacroiliac joint involvement or segmental fracturing of the posterior column.

The full extent of an anterior approach is obtainable only with the patient in the supine position. Similarly, the posterior Kocher–Langenbeck approach is fully utilized with the patient prone. A simultaneous anterior and posterior surgical approach with the patient in the lateral position limits the access from either. Lateral patient positioning for other than posterior wall fracture fixation creates a tendency to use a more extensive surgical approach (i.e. extending a Kocher–Langenbeck to a triradiate or using simultaneous anterior and posterior incisions) when, with proper positioning and planning, less may have sufficed (Figure 12.49.10).

Box 12.49.6 Surgical approaches

- Posterior—Kocher–Langenbeck:
  - Modified Gibson
  - Trigastric trochanteric osteotomy
- Anterior—ilioinguinal:
  - Iliofemoral
  - Modified Stoppa
- Extended iliofemoral:
  - T-shape modification
  - Triradiate
- Combined anterior and posterior

Kocher–Langenbeck approach

The Kocher–Langenbeck approach is ideal for posterior wall fractures and posterior column fractures with or without an associated posterior wall fracture. Transverse and T-type fractures without displacement in the anatomical roof, treated within 15 days of injury, are also amenable to this surgical approach. In addition, for T-shaped fractures, the major displacement should be posterior, with only minor displacement occurring anteriorly at the pelvic brim.

The patient can be placed in the lateral or prone position. However, as noted previously, the prone position is preferred for the more complex fracture types. The knee must remain flexed throughout the procedure to reduce the risk of injury to the sciatic nerve. The incision begins approximately 6cm lateral to the posterior superior iliac spine, courses distally in a curvilinear fashion over the greater trochanter and extends in a mid-lateral position to the midpoint of the thigh. The fascia lata is sharply incised and the gluteus maximus muscle is bluntly divided toward the posterior superior iliac spine. The innervation of the gluteus maximus muscle comes from the inferior gluteal nerve, which runs from posterior to anterior in the muscle. Therefore the splitting of this muscle should stop as soon as the first nerve trunk is met, approximately at the midpoint between the greater trochanter and the posterior superior iliac spine. Next, the insertion of the gluteus maximus muscle into the femur is released. This allows posteromedial retraction of the muscle without excessive stretch on the inferior gluteal nerve. The sciatic nerve is then located along the posterior surface of the quadratus femoris muscle and traced proximally to the piriformis muscle. The short external rotators and piriformis tendon are divided and tagged with sutures to assist with retraction. These tendons should be incised approximately 1.5cm from their trochanteric insertion to avoid injury to the blood supply of the femoral head. Gentle retraction of the short external rotators allows visualization of the posterior column and retroacetabular space but provides only limited protection of the sciatic nerve.

The Kocher–Langenbeck approach provides direct visualization of the entire lateral aspect of the posterior column of the acetabulum (Figure 12.49.11). Visualization may be extended anterosuperiorly by dividing a portion of the gluteus medius insertion or performing a transtrochanteric osteotomy (Figure 12.49.12). Indirect access to the quadrilateral surface can be attained by the palpating finger or the use of special instruments placed through the greater sciatic notch. A posterior capsulotomy allows limited access to the posterior aspect of the joint surface. This access is increased in the presence of a fractured posterior wall. This approach has a relatively high risk for sciatic nerve injury and an intermediate risk for heterotopic ossification.

Modifications of the Kocher–Langenbeck approach

The modified Gibson approach differs from the Kocher–Langenbeck approach in its proximal dissection such that the interval between the gluteus maximus and tensor fasciae latae muscles is divided rather than splitting of the gluteus maximus muscle (Figure 12.49.13). In this way, the neurovascular supply to the anterior portion of the gluteus maximus muscle is not at risk. In

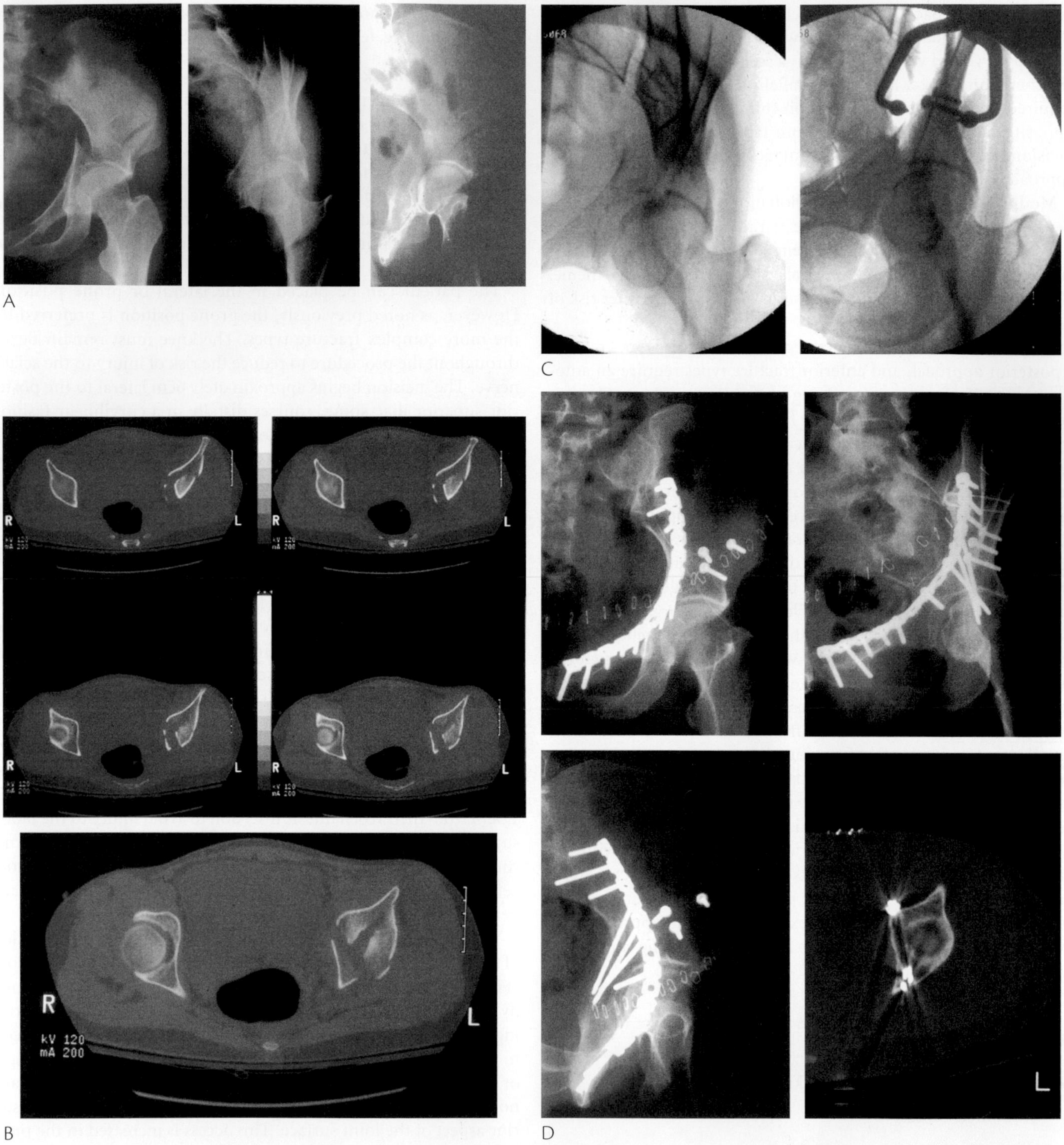

Fig. 12.49.10 A 30-year-old woman struck a tree while skiing, sustaining a both-column fracture. Evaluation of (A) the plain radiographs and (B) the CT scan revealed a posterior superior wall fragment in a fracture otherwise readily amenable to the ilioinguinal surgical approach. The addition of a second surgical approach might be considered. However, in this case the wall fragment was addressed through (C) the ilioinguinal approach by placing one tine of the reduction forceps along the external surface of the ilium accessed via limited elevation of the muscles along the iliac crest. (D). Postoperative radiographs and CT scan demonstrated an anatomical reduction.

addition, anterosuperior visualization and access are extended (Figure 12.49.12). Having a straight, rather than angled skin incision, may make the modified Gibson more cosmetically appealing, especially in obese female patients. Either the Kocher–Langenbeck or modified Gibson approaches can be combined with a trigastric trochanteric osteotomy, maintaining the gluteus medius, vastas lateralis and gluteus minimus muscle attachments to the mobile trochanteric fragment. In this way, intraoperative dislocation of the femoral head for inspection of the joint is facilitated.

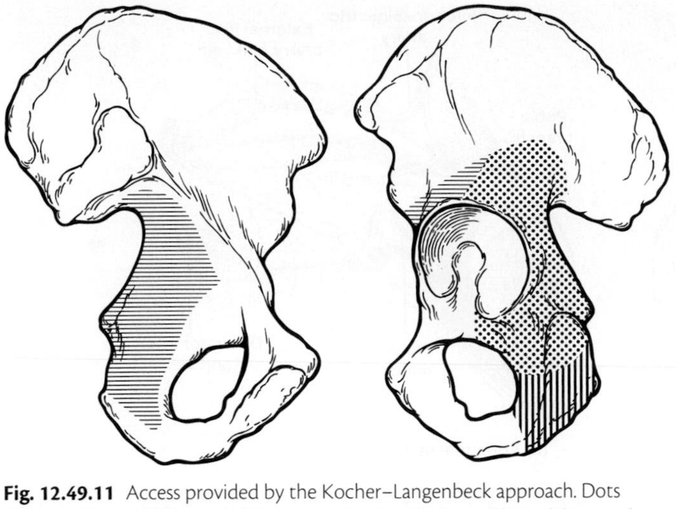

Fig. 12.49.11 Access provided by the Kocher–Langenbeck approach. Dots delineate the available area of direct visualization. Horizontal lines delineate the area of indirect access. Vertical lines delineate the area of visualization and access extended by release of the quadratus femoris muscle origin. (Copyright Dr. Berton R. Moed.)

Ilioinguinal approach

The ilioinguinal approach is indicated for fractures involving the anterior wall and anterior column. Transverse and T-type fractures in which the major displacement is anterior with minimal posterior displacement and both-column fractures having a non-comminuted posterior column fragment can also be managed using this approach. Again, these complex fracture types must not have displacement in the anatomical roof and must be treated within 15 days of injury.

The patient is placed supine on the operating room table. The incision extends from just posterior to the gluteus medius tubercle, paralleling the iliac crest to the anterior superior iliac spine and then coursing medially to the midline ending two finger-breaths above the pubic symphysis. The iliacus muscle is elevated from the internal iliac fossa. The aponeurosis of the external oblique muscle (along with the anterior aspect of the sheath of the rectus abdominis) is then incised from the anterior superior iliac spine to the midline, passing at least 1cm superior to the superficial inguinal ring. The aponeurosis is reflected distally revealing the spermatic cord in the male and the round ligament in the female. This structure is bluntly isolated along with the ilioinguinal nerve and retracted using a rubber sling. The now exposed inguinal ligament is split through its entire length revealing the laterally placed lacuna musculorum contents (lateral femoral cutaneous nerve, the iliopsoas muscle mass and femoral nerve) and the medially placed lacuna vasorum containing the external iliac vessels and lymphatics. The iliopectineal fascia, which separates these lacunae, must be incised to allow access to the quadrilateral plate and true pelvis. Separate rubber slings are placed around the lacuna musculorum contents and the external iliac vessels. In this way medial, middle and lateral surgical access 'windows' are created.

The internal iliac fossa, anterior aspect of the sacroiliac joint, and lateral portion of the anterior column can be visualized by retracting the iliopsoas medially. The quadrilateral plate can be accessed by retracting the iliopsoas laterally and the external iliac sheath medially. The superior pubic ramus is visualized by retracting the external iliac sheath laterally and spermatic cord medially. Lateral retraction of the spermatic cord (aided by release of the insertion of the rectus abdominis muscle) allows visualization of the symphysis pubis and access to the retropubic space. Prior to retraction of the vessels, care must be taken to look for an anomalous origin of the obturator artery, known as the corona mortis or other anastomoses between the obturator and the external iliac systems (Figure 12.49.14).

The ilioinguinal approach allows direct access to the entire pelvic brim and the internal iliac fossa (Figure 12.49.15). Indirect access

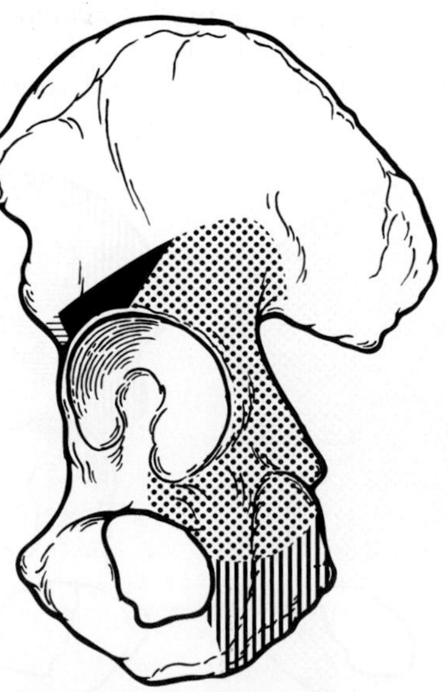

Fig. 12.49.12 Access provided by extension of Kocher–Langenbeck approach or use of the modified Gibson approach. Dots delineate the available area of direct visualization. Horizontal lines delineate the area of indirect access. Vertical lines delineate the area of visualization and access extended by release of the quadratus femoris muscle origin. Solid black area shows area of extended visualization and access.(Copyright Dr. Berton R. Moed.)

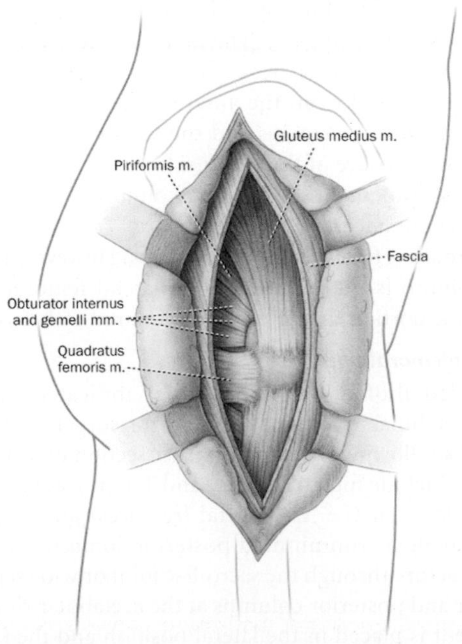

Fig. 12.49.13 The modified Gibson approach. (Reproduced from Moed, B.R. and McMichael, J.C. (2008). Outcomes of Posterior Wall Fractures of the Acetabulum: Surgical Technique. *Journal of Bone and Joint Surgery, American Volume,* 90A (supplement 2, part 1), 87–107.)

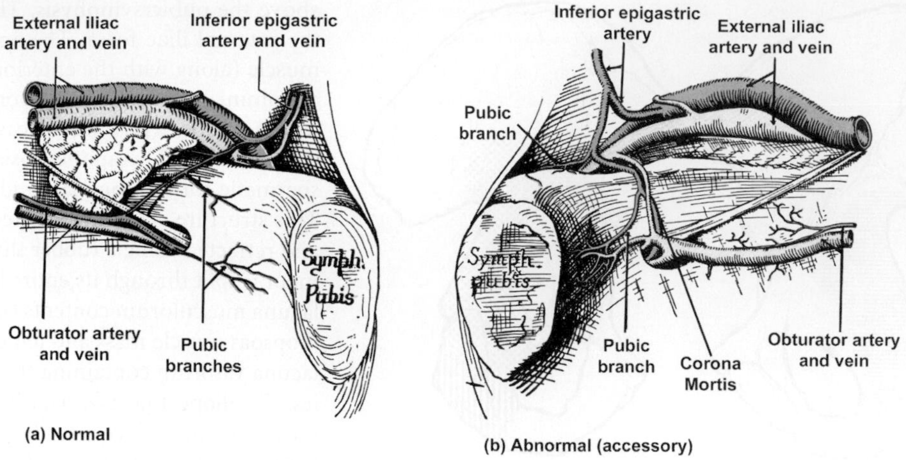

Fig. 12.49.14 Illustration of the commonly occurring small calibre anastomoses between the obturator and external iliac systems (A). Illustration of the true 'corona mortis', aberrant origin of the obturator artery from the external iliac system (B). (Reproduced from Grant, J.C.B. (1972). *Grant's atlas of anatomy* (6th edn). Williams & Wilkins, Baltimore, MD.)

to the quadrilateral surface can be attained by the palpating finger or the use of special instruments. This approach has the lowest rate of heterotopic ossification. The lateral femoral cutaneous nerve, the femoral nerve, the external iliac vessels, and the inguinal canal contents are all at risk for injury.

Iliofemoral approach

The iliofemoral approach has limited application. It is the approach of choice for anterior wall fracture variants (see Chapter 12.48, Figure 12.48.8). Although the ilioinguinal is usually the better choice, the iliofemoral approach may be used for high anterior column fractures.

The patient is placed supine on the operating room table. The incision extends from just posterior to the gluteus medius tubercle, paralleling the iliac crest to the anterior superior iliac spine and then coursing distally for approximately 15cm along the lateral aspect of the sartorius muscle. The iliopsoas muscle is elevated off the inner aspect of the iliac crest. The sartorius origin and inguinal ligament are released from the anterior superior iliac spine. The interval between the sartorius and the tensor fascia lata is developed to allow exposure of the anterior hip joint capsule, the anteroinferior iliac spine, and the anterior column as far medial as the iliopectineal eminence.

This approach is fairly simple and low risk. However, access to the anterior column is quite limited. The lateral femoral cutaneous nerve or some portion thereof is usually injured with this approach.

Extended iliofemoral approach

The extended iliofemoral approach is indicated for selected complex acetabular fracture types and for surgery delayed more than 2 weeks following injury (see earlier section on timing of surgery). These include high transverse and T-type fractures involving the acetabular roof (i.e. transtectal fractures) and both-column fractures having a comminuted posterior column component, a displaced fracture through the sacroiliac joint or wide separation of the anterior and posterior columns at the acetabular rim.

The patient is placed in the lateral position and the knee maintained in a flexed position to relax the sciatic nerve. An inverted J incision is used, extending from the posterior superior iliac spine along the iliac crest to the anterior superior iliac spine and then continued distally to the midpoint of the thigh angling toward a point 2cm lateral to the lateral aspect of the patella. The gluteal and tensor fascia lata muscles are elevated from the external surface of the ilium and are hinged on the superior gluteal neurovascular bundle. The hip abductors and the short external rotators are released from their insertion into the greater trochanter to complete the exposure of almost the entire external surface of the bone. Release of the reflected head of the rectus femoris combined with a circumferential capsulotomy at the acetabular rim provides direct visualization of the hip joint. The exposure can be extended medially by release of the sartorius and rectus femoris origins and elevation of the iliacus from the internal iliac fossa. However, this additional muscle stripping creates added risk of iliac wing and acetabular dome devascularization and increased risk of infection.

The extended iliofemoral approach allows exposure of the entire outer surface of the ilium, posterior column, posterior wall, and anterior column to the level of the iliopectineal eminence (Figure 12.49.16). The articular surface is exposed following

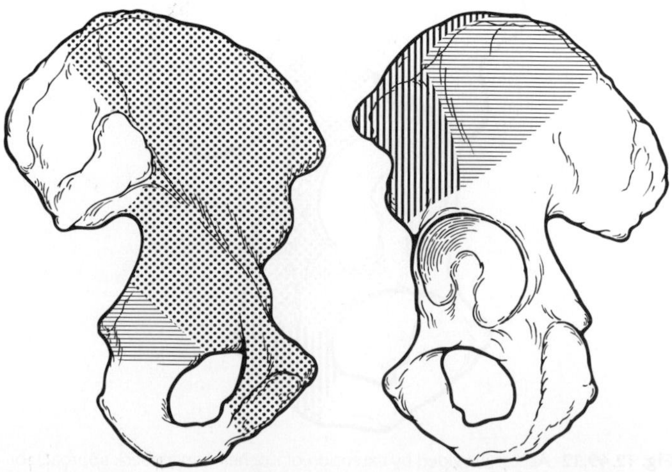

Fig. 12.49.15 Access provided by the ilioinguinal approach. Dots delineate the available area of direct visualization. Horizontal lines delineate the area of indirect access. Vertical lines delineate the area of visualization and access extended by release of the tensor fasciae latae muscle. (Copyright Dr. Berton R. Moed.)

capsulotomy, and access to the iliac fossa is also possible, as noted earlier. This approach has a high rate of heterotopic bone formation. The risk of infection is significant, over 8% in one series. There is also a risk of injury to the sciatic nerve and the superior gluteal neurovascular bundle. At one time it was postulated that severe abductor muscle necrosis would result from injury to the superior gluteal artery. However, extensive clinical experience and animal studies indicate that this is not a clinically significant problem.

Triradiate approach

The triradiate approach has indications similar to those for the extended iliofemoral. However, the exposure is more limited, lacking complete visualization of the iliac crest. The skin incision is Y-shaped, with the posterior limb being nearly identical to the Kocher–Langenbeck incision. The anterior limb of the incision extends from the greater trochanter to the anterior superior iliac spine. The skin incision is deepened through the fascia. Posteriorly, the approach is as for the Kocher–Langenbeck. A trochanteric osteotomy is performed to release the abductor insertion, and the glutei and tensor muscles are elevated from the external surface of the ilium. The triradiate approach can be performed when the surgeon cannot address the fracture through an initial Kocher–Langenbeck approach.

Combined anterior and posterior approaches

Combined anterior and posterior approaches were originally used in sequential fashion when one approach was planned, but proved inadequate for fracture fixation. One example of this is the inability to reduce or fix the posterior column of a both-column fracture initially approached using the ilioinguinal. Use of simultaneous anterior (iliofemoral or ilioinguinal) and posterior (Kocher–Langenbeck) approaches has been advocated for complex fracture patterns. The patient is first positioned supine and then turned 45 degrees toward the side opposite the fracture and secured in this position. The initial incision is used to approach the column with the greatest displacement.

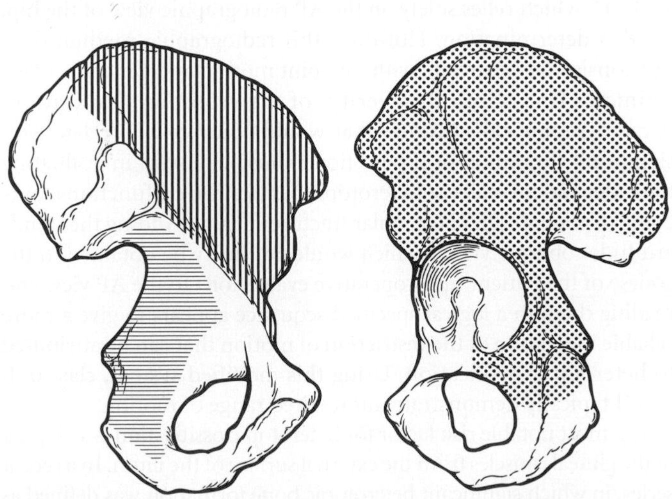

Fig. 12.49.16 Access provided by the extended iliofemoral approach. Dots delineate the available area of direct visualization. Horizontal lines delineate the area of indirect access. Vertical lines delineate the area of visualization and access extended elevation of the iliacus from the internal iliac fossa. (Copyright Dr. Berton R. Moed.)

Postsurgical care

Patients should receive prophylactic intravenous antibiotics, administered preoperatively and continued at least 24h postoperatively. Prophylaxis for thromboembolic disease (mechanical or chemical) should be routinely used during the perioperative period and continued up to 12 weeks postoperatively, until the patient regains mobility. Heterotopic ossification is associated with all approaches that involve stripping of muscle from the external surface of the ilium and is a particular risk of extended surgical approaches. Therefore, prophylaxis should be considered in these cases.

AP and oblique postoperative radiographs should be obtained, and repeat radiographs should be evaluated at routine 4- to 6-week intervals during the early postoperative period to check maintenance of reduction and fracture healing. A postoperative CT scan should be considered if there is concern for intra-articular hardware or inadequate reduction.

Postoperatively, the patient is mobilized as quickly as the associated injuries will allow. Sitting up on the first postoperative day, is followed by formal physical therapy for muscle strengthening and active range of motion exercises on subsequent postoperative days. Total hip arthroplasty precautions should not be needed, as internal fixation has rendered the hip joint stable. Partial toe-touch weight bearing of 10–15kg with crutches or a walker is required for 10–12 weeks. However, progression to full weight bearing must be tailored to the individual. Physical therapy should continue until muscle strength and range of motion are regained or a plateau is reached.

Results

Clinical outcome and the subsequent development of post-traumatic osteoarthritis strongly correlate with the adequacy of fracture reduction. Early studies considered residual displacement of up to 2–3mm as 'satisfactory' and demonstrated good, very good, or excellent results in approximately three-quarters of the study group.

A more recent study used less than 2mm of residual displacement as an anatomical reduction and at an average follow-up of 10.9 years demonstrated 81% good or excellent clinical result, whereas only 64% of patients with non-anatomical reduction achieved a good or excellent clinical result. The rate of anatomical reduction was found to decrease with increased fracture complexity, patient age, and time delay to fracture fixation. Many studies have demonstrated the detrimental effect of delay to surgery. This affects the ability to achieve anatomical reduction and clinical outcome. It has been demonstrated that anatomical reduction is more likely if performed within 15 days for elemental and 5 days for associated fracture patterns.

Certain fracture patterns appear to have better outcomes after surgical treatment than others. Both-column fractures are complex injuries and technically demanding. However, they have a generally better outcome than many fracture types, despite a higher rate of non-anatomical reduction. Despite anatomical reduction in only 57% of cases, good to excellent result were achieved in 77% of one study group. Posterior wall fractures present as a straightforward treatment problem with excellent anatomical reduction rates reported as high as 100%. However, despite the anatomical reduction obtained, clinical failure rates as high as 32% have been reported. Other studies have reported better results and this disparity has been shown to be in large part, to the inadequacy of radiographs in assessing the quality of the postoperative posterior wall reduction.

Complications

The common major early complications consist of infection, iatrogenic nerve injury, intra-articular screw placement, and thromboembolism. Late complications include heterotopic ossification, post-traumatic arthritis, and osteonecrosis of the femoral head.

Infection

The rate of infection is approximately 5% in most series of acetabular fractures treated operatively. The risk of infection is increased in patients with open fractures and local soft tissue injuries such as Morel-Lavallé lesions. Gastrointestinal or urological injuries are also associated with increased infection rates. Appropriate antibiotics, less extensive surgical approaches, and aggressive debridement of open wounds can help to decrease the rate of infection. The adverse affect of a deep postoperative intra-articular wound infection cannot be minimized. Complete joint destruction can be expected in 50% of these cases.

Iatrogenic nerve injury

Although the superior gluteal, obturator, or femoral nerves (among others) may be injured during acetabular surgery, the prevalence of these injuries is low. However, iatrogenic damage to the sciatic nerve is one of the major complications encountered in acetabular fracture management. These injuries are most commonly associated with the posterior and extended surgical approaches which involve direct exposure and retraction of the sciatic nerve. However, injury at the time of indirect reduction of posterior column displacement through an anterior surgical approach can also occur.

Iatrogenic nerve injury rates have been reported ranging from 2–9%. Intraoperative sciatic nerve monitoring has been advocated by some authors as a method to decrease the incidence of sciatic nerve injury. However, the rate of nerve injury appears to decrease as surgeon experience increases. A 2% incidence has been reported without nerve monitoring when performed by experienced surgeons in a large centre. At present, there is no clear data indicating that intraoperative somatosensory evoked potential nerve monitoring actually reduces the overall rate of iatrogenic sciatic nerve injury. Spontaneous motor potential monitoring is another option and preliminary results indicate that this method may prove to be more effective. At present, there is no substitute for attention to detail in the operating room with careful patient positioning and good surgical technique.

Intra-articular hardware

Although specific rates are not available, intra-articular placement of screws is a documented and often destructive complication of acetabular fracture surgery. Intraoperative fluoroscopy is the best method of preventing this complication and avoiding post-traumatic arthritis.

Thromboembolism

Post-traumatic and postoperative thromboembolism is a significant problem in acetabular fracture patients. Proximal deep vein thrombosis has been identified using magnetic resonance venography in 34% of acetabular fracture patients. Therefore, some form of mechanical or chemical prophylaxis is recommended to decrease the risk of thromboembolic complications. One study indicated that early (at the time of hospital admission) mechanical prophylaxis with foot pumps and the addition of enoxaparin on a delayed basis (5 days after admission) is a very successful strategy for prophylaxis against venous thromboembolic disease following serious musculoskeletal injury. For any patient who was required to return to the operating room, the enoxaparin was discontinued on the night prior to surgery and was resumed within 12h of surgery. Despite the use of prophylactic treatment, the prevalence of post-traumatic and postoperative thromboembolism approximates 11% and the value of screening, using Doppler ultrasound or magnetic resonance venography remains controversial. The placement of prophylactic vena caval filters is controversial but may be indicated in selected high-risk patients.

Currently, no prophylactic treatment consensus exists. Our approach consists of mechanical sequential compressive devices applied on hospital admission to both lower extremities, low-molecular-weight heparin for chemical prophylaxis as soon as the patient is haemodynamically stable and screening using duplex colour Doppler ultrasound. For patients who require operative intervention, the low-molecular-weight heparin is discontinued on the night prior to surgery and resumed within 36h after surgery. After discharge from the hospital, the patients are maintained on chemical prophylaxis until they have regained mobility, usually 6–12 weeks postoperatively. Vena caval filters are reserved for those high-risk patients having contraindications to chemical prophylaxis.

Heterotopic ossification

Heterotopic ossification has been reported as occurring in as many as 90% of patients after acetabular fracture surgery (range 18–90%) with severe involvement as high as 50% in some patient groups. The terminology 'severe heterotopic ossification' is often used to describe the amount of heterotopic ossification necessary to impair function. Greater than 20% loss of total hip motion is thought to be the best clinical definition for severe heterotopic ossification. Many reports have used the Brooker classification (Table 12.49.1), which relies solely on the AP radiographic view of the hip, for this determination. However, this radiographic method does not consistently correlate with hip joint motion and generally overestimates the clinical severity of heterotopic ossification. A radiographic classification that would accurately correlate with significant limitation of hip motion should be useful in evaluating the independent effect of heterotopic ossification on functional outcome in patients after acetabular fracture surgery. Adding the standard Judet oblique views (which would routinely be obtained in the course of the patient's postoperative evaluation) to the AP view and reading them in a logical specified sequence appears to give a more reliable indication of the restriction of motion that can be attributed to heterotopic ossification. Using this modified system, class 0, I, and II typically demonstrate unimpaired range of motion.

The most notable risk factor for heterotopic ossification is stripping of the gluteal muscles from the external surface of the ilium. In a recent series, in which significant heterotopic bone formation was defined as motion limited by greater than 20% and patients were not given prophylactic treatment, the following prevalence figures were reported: Kocher–Langenbeck 8%; extended iliofemoral 20%; ilioinguinal, 2%.

It appears that the rate of heterotopic ossification can be significantly reduced with the use of indomethacin and radiation therapy.

Table 12.49.1 Brooker classification

Class 0	No heterotopic ossification
Class I	Islands of bone in the soft tissues
Class II	Bone spurs from the pelvis or proximal femur leaving at least 1cm between opposing bone surfaces
Class III	Bone spurs from the pelvis or proximal femur leaving <1cm between opposing bone surfaces
Class IV	Apparent bony ankylosis of the hip

A recent prospective randomized study comparing indomethacin and radiation therapy demonstrated both to be safe and effective prophylactic agents. Non-compliance was the problem with indomethacin; radiation was strikingly more expensive. Use of a combination of irradiation and indomethacin essentially eliminated postoperative heterotopic ossification in one series as no progression of heterotopic ossification was noted, even when early ossification was seen on preoperative radiographs.

Heterotopic ossification is a significant potential postoperative complication of acetabular fracture surgery and prophylactic therapy is desirable. However, one must weigh the risk of prophylaxis and its potential for failure against the actual risk of occurrence in each particular clinical situation. A recent study in acetabular fracture patients has shown that the use of indomethacin increases the risk of long-bone non-union. Although genetic alterations in offspring may also be at issue, the possibility of induced malignant disease is the main concern with low-dose radiation therapy. However, for the radiation dosage and methods used for the prophylaxis of heterotopic ossification about the hip, the likelihood of induced malignancy is very low. Based on a review of the current evidence available in the literature, recommendations have been made regarding the use of heterotopic ossification prophylactic treatment (Box 12.49.7). Indomethacin is inexpensive, simple, safe, and probably works. As with other non-steroidal anti-inflammatory drugs, gastric and duodenal mucosal lesions may occur. In addition, gastrointestinal prophylaxis (such as misoprostol) should be considered to decrease the risk of these drug-induced lesions. However, the use of this drug, or that of any other gastroduodenal mucosal protective agent, in acetabular fracture patients receiving indomethacin for heterotopic ossification prophylaxis has not been studied. Irradiation should be considered in high-risk cases (e.g. head injured) and for adult patients (women beyond child-bearing age) requiring an extended surgical approach.

Box 12.49.7 Recommendations for heterotopic ossification prophylaxis

- Prophylaxis after acetabular fracture fixation using the ilioinguinal surgical approach or similar surgical approaches is not recommended
- Prophylaxis after acetabular fracture fixation using the extended iliofemoral surgical approach or similar surgical approaches is recommended
- Despite conflicting evidence, prophylaxis with indomethacin after acetabular fracture fixation through the Kocher–Langenbeck surgical approach or similar posterolateral surgical approaches is recommended
- Prophylaxis with irradiation after acetabular fracture fixation through the Kocher–Langenbeck surgical approach or similar posterolateral surgical approaches is not recommended.

Post-traumatic arthritis and osteonecrosis of the femoral head

Post-traumatic arthritis is a well-documented complication of patients sustaining a fracture of the acetabulum. The quality of the fracture reduction appears to be the main determinant for clinical outcome and for the risk of late traumatic arthritis. Damage to the femoral head at the time of initial injury is another important factor. Osteonecrosis of the femoral head is known to result from acetabular fracture associated with hip dislocation and can also result in post-traumatic arthritis. However, post-traumatic arthritis is more commonly due to wear of the femoral head against a malreduced fracture and often may be incorrectly attributed to osteonecrosis. Total hip arthroplasty or arthrodesis is indicated for patients with post-traumatic arthritis and disabling pain.

Special circumstances

Elderly patients

Displaced acetabular fractures in elderly patients may be effectively treated with open reduction and internal fixation. Good or excellent results at 2-year minimum follow-up have been reported, in 16 of 17 elderly (over 60 years old) patients treated surgically. However, elderly patients often have low-energy fracture patterns (anterior column or both-column) that have a relatively good prognosis with conservative treatment. The decision to perform open reduction and internal fixation should be based on the fracture pattern, the medical status of the patient, and the degree of osteoporosis. Extended surgical approaches are to be avoided. The alternative is non-operative treatment followed by total hip arthroplasty, as the symptoms dictate, with the knowledge that the prognosis for conservative treatment is poor. Unfortunately, studies indicate that, overall, the late outcome of total hip arthroplasty after acetabular fracture is inferior to that of arthroplasty performed because of degenerative arthritis. Therefore, open reduction and internal fixation combined with primary total hip arthroplasty, as a single operative procedure, has been advocated for a highly selected group of especially severe acetabular fractures, particularly those in elderly patients.

Associated femoral shaft fractures

Fractures of the ipsilateral femoral shaft are common, and should be acutely fixed. Acute fixation of both the femoral and acetabular fracture may be undertaken, but this is often not desirable or logistically possible. If the two procedures are staged, the antegrade operative approach for femoral nailing may compromise a subsequent acetabular approach. Therefore, retrograde nailing of the femoral fracture should be considered.

Total hip arthroplasty after failed acetabular fracture surgery

As noted earlier, the results of total hip arthroplasty after failed acetabular fracture surgery are inferior to those of primary total hip arthroplasty for degenerative hip disease. There is a significantly higher rate of acetabular loosening (53%) and revision (14%) compared with patients who did not previously sustain an acetabular fracture. Factors contributing to these poorer results include the young age of the patients, the predominance of males, and the residual osseous deficiencies. The surgery itself is also technically more demanding. Therefore the performance of acetabular fracture surgery should not be approached as a satisfactory staging procedure prior to a definitive total joint replacement.

Summary

Since the initial publications of Judet and Letournel in the early 1960s significant strides have been made in the treatment of acetabular fractures. There is no doubt that excellent results can be obtained by experienced surgeons and the expansion of educational activities specific to acetabular fracture care has increased the number of experienced surgeons. However, acetabular fracture fixation remains extensive surgery with a significant potential complication rate. Not all patients achieve a good or excellent result, related mainly to residual fracture displacement, infection, nerve injury, thromboembolic disease and heterotopic ossification. Efforts continue toward the refinement in operative techniques and improved prophylactic measures. However, the results of Letournel and Judet (1993) remain as the 'gold standard'. It is yet to be determined whether the advent of intraoperative, fluoroscopically-based three-dimensional image navigation systems, along with improved instrumentation for fracture reduction and fixation through limited-incisions, can better these results.

Further reading

Brooker, A.F., Bowerman, J.W., Robinson, R.A., and Riley, L.H. Jr (1973). Ectopic ossification following total hip replacement: incidence and a method of classification. *Journal of Bone and Joint Surgery,* **55A**, 1629–32.

Judet, R., Judet, J., and Letournel, E. (1964). Fractures of the acetabulum: classification and surgical approaches for open reduction. *Journal of Bone and Joint Surgery,* **46A**, 1615–46.

Letournel, E. and Judet, R. (1993). *Fractures of the acetabulum* (2nd edn). New York: Springer-Verlag.

Matta, J.M. (1996). Fractures of the acetabulum: accuracy of reduction and clinical results in patients managed operatively within three weeks of injury. *Journal of Bone and Joint Surgery,* **78A**, 1632–45.

Moed, B.R., Carr, S.E.W., Gruson, K., Watson, J.T. and Craig, J.G. (2003). Computed tomography assessment of fractures o f the posterior wall of the acetabulum after operative treatment. *Journal of Bone and Joint Surgery,* **85A**, 512–22.

Moed, B.R., Ajibade, D.A., and Israel, H. (2009). Computed tomography as a predictor of hip stability status in posterior wall fractures of the acetabulum. *Journal of Orthopedic Trauma,* **23**, 7–15.

12.50

Dislocations of the hip and femoral head fractures

A. Pohl

Summary points

- Most injuries are high violence, so look for associated injuries
- Immediate closed reduction usually best under general anaesthetic
- Do not proceed to open reduction without appropriate imaging studies
- Surgical approach depends on injury pattern
- Some long term complications can be minimized/avoided by appropriate early treatment (e.g. avascular necrosis).

Background

Hip dislocations are commonly associated with other local and regional fractures and injuries resulting in a high risk of chronic disability and early or accelerated degenerative joint disease.

Importance

Avascular necrosis of the femoral head is a common complication of hip dislocation and a knowledge of the blood supply to the femoral head is therefore essential.

The main source of intraosseous blood supply of the weight-bearing portion of the femoral head is the deep branch of the medial femoral circumflex artery (MFCA) which gives rise to several 'terminal' superior retinaculum vessels. The deep branch of the MCFA passes between the psoas tendon laterally and pectineus medially, and runs laterally on the inferior border of obturator externus, which it crosses posteriorly, coming to lie between quadratus femoris and the inferior gemellus. It courses anterior to the inferior and superior gemellus muscles and the interposed obturator internus tendon (i.e. deep to these structures as seen from a posterior surgical approach) and enters the hip capsule just above the superior gemellus muscle, and distal to the piriformis tendon. The terminal retinacular vessels course towards the femoral head, bound to the femoral neck by the reflected fibres of the hip capsule.

The inferior gluteal artery may often anastomose with the MFCA through a branch that runs along the piriformis tendon, but the lateral femoral circumflex artery provides little contribution to the vascularity of the femoral head. A portion of the femoral head around the attachment of the ligamentum teres to the fovea is supplied by the medial epiphyseal branch of the acetabular branch of the obturator artery in the young.

Underlying causes

The underlying cause of dislocations and fracture–dislocations of the hip is high-energy force dissipation. The relationship of the pelvis to the vector of force through the femur will determine whether an anterior dislocation, posterior dislocation, or fracture–dislocation will occur.

Clinical features (Box 12.50.1)

History

Most patients presenting with dislocations and fracture–dislocations of the hip have a history of severe trauma with a high force dissipation, such as:

- Industrial accidents
- Falls from a height
- Road traffic collisions.

Because of high force dissipation, victims in motor vehicle collisions may suffer multiple injuries and other occupants of the same vehicle may suffer the same fate.

An accurate history is invaluable and must be sought from the ambulance officers or those delivering the patient to hospital:

- Patients with head injuries may be unable to provide a reliable history
- Patients with multiple injuries may have difficulty localizing their pain, especially after treatment with narcotic analgesics
- Regional injuries to the legs, pelvis, abdomen, and spine may obscure a hip dislocations

Physical examination

The high force dissipation involved in hip dislocation requires that medical staff should follow the principles of the early management of these injuries recommended by the Advanced Trauma Life Support method. Patients should undergo a thorough secondary examination initially to look for injuries to other organ systems and should be reviewed clinically over the next few days to exclude missed diagnoses.

Patients with a hip dislocation commonly present with:

- Pain
- Classical deformity
- Restricted and painful hip movement.

The positional deformity of a posterior hip dislocation is one of flexion, adduction, and internal rotation. In the presence of an anterior dislocation, the hip typically assumes a position of external rotation abduction and some extension. When ipsilateral fractures of the femoral shaft or neck occur, however, the leg may assume a near-normal position and the diagnosis of hip dislocation may be missed.

Knowledge of the mechanism of injury should alert medical staff to possible associated injuries for which a careful search must be made. Opposing forces of an impact to the knee at one end of the leg and the momentum of the body at the other can result in injury anywhere between those two points. Abrasions and lacerations over the patella or proximal anterior tibia may indicate the site of force application. Injuries about the knee include proximal tibial fractures, patellar fractures, osteochondral fractures of the patellar and distal femoral articular surfaces, and distal femoral fractures. Patellar and knee ligament injuries may lead to instability of the knee which must be carefully assessed. The pelvis and spine must be examined thoroughly to exclude pelvic fractures, pelvic ring disruption, and spinal injuries.

A detailed assessment must be made for neurological injuries and if these are present they must be documented before and after reduction of the hip. Sciatic nerve injuries, particularly of the peroneal component, occur commonly in hip dislocations. Injuries to the lumbosacral trunk may accompany disruptions of the pelvic ring and spinal nerve root injuries may be present in patients with vertebral fractures.

Investigations

Imaging

Plain films

All patients subject to severe trauma should have radiographs of the cervical spine and chest, and an anteroposterior view of the pelvis, as recommended in the Advanced Trauma Life Support method.

The anteroposterior radiograph of the pelvis must be scrutinized systematically for evidence of hip dislocation. Check for:

- Any difference in size of the femoral heads (femoral head measurably larger in anterior dislocation; smaller in posterior dislocation)
- Symmetry of the hip joint space (asymmetrical with dislocation/subluxation or when fragments of bone, cartilage or soft tissues incarcerated in the joint)
- Integrity of Shenton's line (Shenton's line broken with dislocation/subluxation)
- Position of femoral shaft (adduction, internal rotation and flexion with posterior dislocation; abduction, external rotation and extension with anterior dislocation)
- Note: the lesser trochanter lies posterolaterally on the femur. It normally presents a small image that becomes more prominent with external rotation of the femur
- Associated fractures of the acetabulum (the presence, size and location of acetabular fractures determines the classification and treatment of hip dislocation)
- Associated fractures of the femoral head (large impaction fractures limit the stable range of hip rotation and influence prognosis. Undisplaced fractures must be recognized prior to attempting closed reduction of the hip. Displaced fractures may lead to an irreducible hip dislocation).

A series of pelvic radiographs, as described by Letournel and Judet, should be obtained when a hip dislocations is recognized, to improve the accuracy of diagnosis of associated fractures and the presence of incarcerated fragments in the hip joint. These additional views include an anteroposterior view of the hemipelvis and two 45-degree oblique views (Judet views), all centred on the femoral head. The pelvic series of radiographs allows an assessment to be made of the anterior and posterior walls and columns of the acetabulum. The three radiographs provide a profile of the anterior, middle, and posterior portion of the hip joint, which can be used to assess the integrity of the femoral head and acetabular surfaces. The three views can also be used to diagnose incarcerated fragments in the hip joint, as shown by incongruity of the joint, but only when the fragments are larger than 2mm. The Judet views are commonly omitted because of pain. Appropriate analgesia, however, is an integral part of resuscitation and the assistance of an anaesthetist may be sought when analgesia is inadequate. If the patient still cannot be positioned correctly for the Judet views, despite these measures, then the views should be taken under anaesthesia before a reduction is performed.

Repeat radiographs must be obtained immediately after reduction to determine the following:

- Adequacy of reduction
- The presence or absence of fragments of bone, cartilage, or soft tissue incarcerated in the joint space
- The number, size, location, and adequacy of reduction of fracture fragments of the femoral head and acetabulum
- The presence of associated fractures of the acetabulum and the femoral head and neck that may have been caused by the reduction or missed by the pre-reduction radiographs.

Box 12.50.1 General features of hip dislocations

- Hip dislocations often associated with local and regional fractures
- Leg position with a posterior hip dislocation—flexion, adduction, and internal rotation
- Leg position with an anterior dislocation—external rotation abduction and extension
- Sciatic nerve injuries, particularly the peroneal component
- Medial femoral circumflex artery—main branch to the femoral head
- Risk of avascular necrosis.

It is imperative for the plain radiographs to be interpreted precisely to diagnose all associated fractures and any incarcerated fragments in the hip joint. This information is essential for an accurate classification of the hip dislocation, and hence the choice of appropriate treatment and operative approach when surgery is indicated.

Computed tomography

The benefits of computed tomography (CT) compared with plain radiography include

- Greater resolution than plain radiography
- Visualization of the anteroposterior relationship of structures
- Visualization of the integrity of the articular surfaces of the femoral head and acetabulum in multiple axial slices
- Improved assessment of congruence
- Increased accuracy of diagnosis of impaction fractures of the femoral head or acetabulum (Figure 12.50.1).

The additional information provided by CT therefore improves the assessment of the size and displacement of fractures of the femoral head and the acetabular wall and hence the stability of the hip joint. Measurement of the percentage of remaining posterior acetabulum on axial CT scans after posterior dislocation of the hip provides a useful determinant of the stability of the joint (Figure 12.50.2). The incidence of instability is high when the remaining posterior articular surface is less than 34%. Hips with greater than 55% of the remaining posterior acetabulum will be stable.

Routine CT scanning has been recommended after successful closed reduction of hip dislocations and prior to planned open reduction, when closed reduction is unsuccessful. However, CT scanning may not be necessary after concentric reduction of simple (type I) posterior hip dislocations assessed on plain radiography. Nevertheless, the usefulness of CT scanning remains undisputed following dislocations of the hip associated with fractures or in the presence of an irreducible hip dislocation.

Magnetic resonance imaging

Magnetic resonance imaging (MRI) offers improved imaging of soft tissues compared with CT scanning. MRI scanning may be useful in the following:

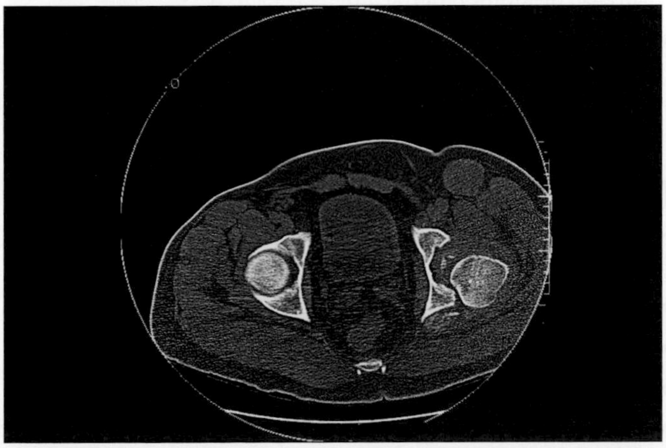

Fig. 12.50.1 Axial CT scan of a posterior hip dislocation demonstrates multiple intra-articular bony fragments, an impaction fracture of the femoral head, and a displaced fracture of the left posterior acetabular wall.

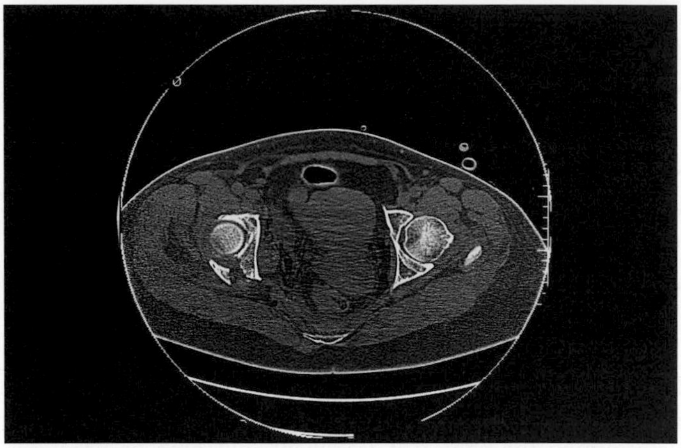

Fig. 12.50.2 A post-reduction CT scan of a posterior hip dislocation demonstrates a displaced posterior wall fragment (Levin type IV). Hips with greater than 55% of remaining posterior articular surface will be stable.

- Detection of fragments of cartilage or labrum incarcerated in the articular space after a hip dislocation
- Assessment of integrity of the articular surfaces and the labrum
- Evaluation of the blood supply of the femoral head.

From a practical perspective, MRI has limited usefulness in the initial evaluation of the multiply injured patient, because the procedure severely restricts access to the patient. MRI, however, may become a useful option after the patient is clinically stable.

Classification in relation to pathogenesis and treatment

Hip dislocations are classified as posterior or anterior, according to the position of the femoral head. The previously recognized term of 'central' dislocation has been superseded by a more comprehensive classification of acetabular fractures (AO Comprehensive Classification of Fractures of the Pelvis and Acetabulum). This subset of dislocations is discussed separately under acetabular fractures.

Thompson and Epstein subclassified posterior dislocations of the hip into five types. More recently described an improved subclassification of posterior hip dislocations that combined clinical and radiological findings, thereby providing a basic indication of treatment (Table 12.50.1).

Table 12.50.1 Levin classification of anterior and posterior hip dislocations

Type I	Pure dislocation or no significant associated fracture, congruent reduction, clinically stable postreduction
Type II	Irreducible reduction even under general anaesthesia, no significant associated fractures
Type III	Clinically unstable postreduction or incarcerated fragments of bone, cartilage, or soft tissue
Type IV	Associated acetabular fracture requiring reconstruction to restore joint congruity or hip stability
Type V	Associated femoral head or neck fracture (including impaction fractures)

The clinical findings included:

- Irreducibility
- Assessment of stability after reduction of the hip.

Radiological findings included:

- Joint incongruity
- Incarceration of fragments of bone, cartilage, or soft tissue between the articulate surfaces
- Associated fractures of the femoral head and acetabulum, based on findings on CT, MRI, and plain radiographs

Epstein subclassified anterior hip dislocations (Figure 12.50.3) into five types, but the subclassification took no consideration of the postproduction radiological findings and provided no benefit in determining the choice of treatment, outcome or prognosis. Consequently, a preferred subclassification is that of which follows the same pattern used for posterior dislocations (see Table 12.50.1).

Discussion on treatment

Early diagnosis and treatment is essential for the patient with a hip dislocation. Avascular necrosis of the femoral head correlates strongly with the duration of an unreduced hip dislocation. Prompt reduction of a dislocated hip is therefore mandatory. Epstein reported markedly improved long-term results with immediate open reduction compared with closed treatment. However, those improved results may have resulted from a visual clearance of loose bodies, from the hip joint, which could not be radiologically demonstrated at that time. The advent of CT scanning for postproduction assessment after hip reduction nullifies the advantage of visual assessment of loose bodies during open reduction. Most authors now favour an immediate attempt at closed reduction.

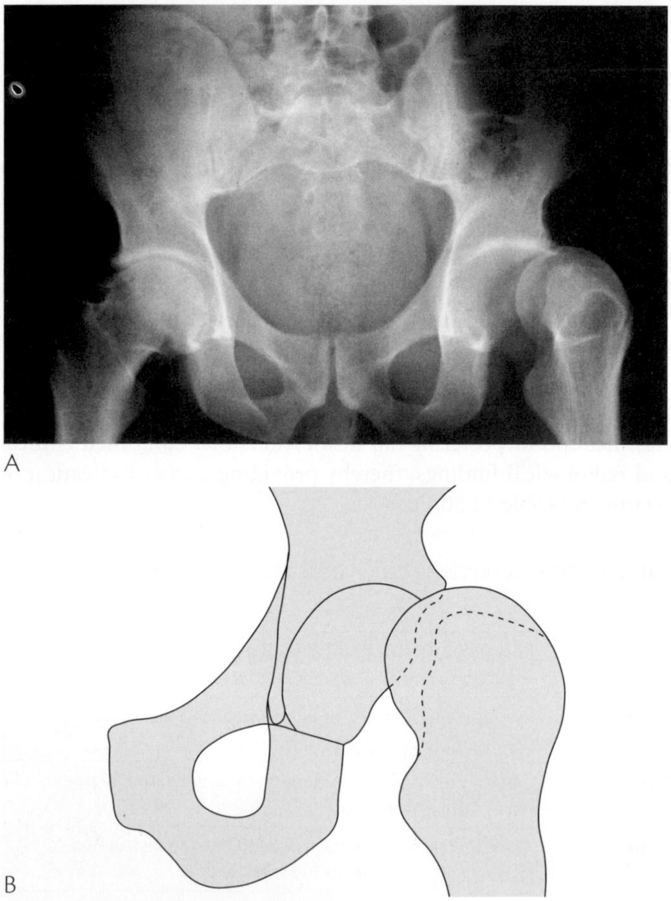

Fig. 12.50.3 Type 1 anterior dislocation, with classic position of abduction and external rotation. The dislocated femoral head is radiographically larger.

Ideally, a closed reduction should be performed under general anaesthesia if an anaesthetist is readily available. The reduction can be performed under intravenous analgesia and sedation just as easily in a well-equipped emergency department as in an operating room. Patients already intubated for the treatment of closed head injuries can have an immediate closed reduction of the hip. Patients undergoing a general anaesthetic for treatment of multiple injuries should have a closed reduction of the hip performed first.

If it is not possible for a patient to undergo an immediate general anaesthetic, then a closed reduction can be attempted in the emergency department. Only one attempt at closed reduction should be made, and only once the patient is adequately sedated. Forceful attempts at closed reduction should be avoided when the patient is inadequately sedated as further damage to articular cartilage can result. If the attempt at closed reduction is unsuccessful, the patient should undergo a closed reduction in the operating room under general anaesthesia and complete muscle paralysis. If a closed reduction is still unsuccessful, an immediate open reduction must be performed.

Before progressing to open reduction, the full pelvic series of radiographs must be available. Irreducible hip dislocations may be associated with the following:

- Fractures of the acetabulum or femoral head
- Buttonholing of the femoral head through the capsule
- Displacement of the piriformis muscle across the acetabulum
- Intra-articular loose bodies.

An accurate diagnosis of associated pathology is essential for preoperative planning of surgical approaches. For example:

- Fractures of the posterior acetabular wall should be approached through a posterior exposure of the hip joint
- Anterior wall fractures will require an anterior exposure
- Fractures of the femoral head are best approached through a surgical dislocation of the hip
- Intra-articular loose bodies may not be recognized in plain radiography and should be evaluated by CT scanning, but surgery should not be delayed if the CT scan cannot be performed immediately.

Methods of closed reduction

Standard principles of reduction of a dislocated joint should be followed:

- Apply traction in line with the deformity
- Then gently increase the deformity while maintaining traction
- Gentle rotatory movements of the hip may aid reduction
- Avoid forceful manipulative techniques (may cause increased risk of damage to the articular surface of the femoral head, a iatrogenic fracture of the femoral neck, or displacement of an unrecognized fracture).

Successful reduction is usually evidenced by an audible or palpable 'clunk', return of a leg to a normal position, and immediate relief of pain when the patient is awake.

Stimson described a gravity reduction technique in which the affected leg is left hanging off the end of the barouche or operating table, with the hip and knee in a position of 90 degrees of flexion. With one hand on the front of the ankle and the other on the calf of the affected leg, the surgeon can easily control the position of the leg, while directing an anterior reduction forced to the hip. In this technique the surgeon has the advantage of working in line with gravity.

An alternative method of production was described by Allis. In this technique, which is the author's preferred choice, the patient is left supine. The surgeon stands over the patient and pulls on the affected leg, against gravity, in the line of the deformity. When necessary, an assistant can apply countertraction to the pelvis. In large patients, when a lot of force is required, the assistant can gain a better hold by placing a towel over the skin first, before applying counter traction. The surgeon places one hand behind the calf and the other hand over the front of the ankle of the affected leg. By this means the position of the leg can be controlled, while an anterior reduction force is applied through the hip. When the surgeon has to apply greater force, various techniques can be used to gain a mechanical advantage. Bending forward at the waist, the surgeon can strut one elbow on an ipsilateral knee, placing the volar aspect of the forearm under the calf of the patient's affected leg. An anterior reduction force can then be applied by the surgeon flexing that elbow (Figure 12.50.4). When even greater force is required, the surgeon can use this same technique bilaterally. The ankle of the patient's affected leg is propped between the surgeon's knee and forearm. The patient's calf is supported in the surgeon's hands. An anterior reduction force can then be applied by the surgeon clasping both hands together and flexing both elbows (Figure 12.50.5). These techniques allow the surgeon to use safe back practices by applying traction through a technique of elbow flexion and not through back extension.

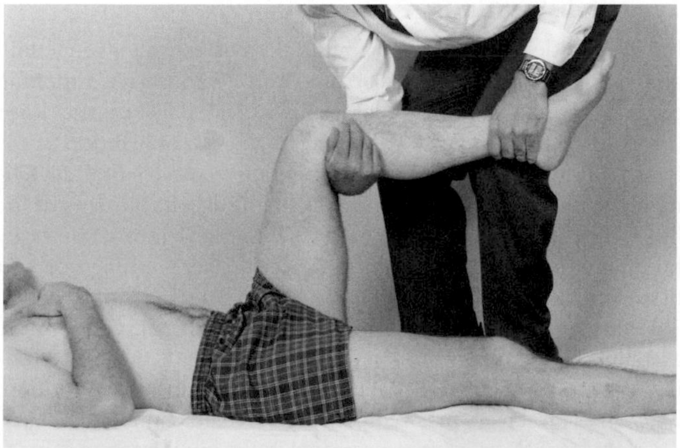

Fig. 12.50.4 Closed reduction of a posterior hip dislocation using the Allis technique. The surgeon stands over the patient, pulling on the affected leg. Bending forward at the waist, with an elbow propped on the knee of the same side, the surgeon places that forearm under the patient's calf, holding the ankle with the other hand. By flexing the elbow, the surgeon exerts an anterior reduction force on the patient's hip.

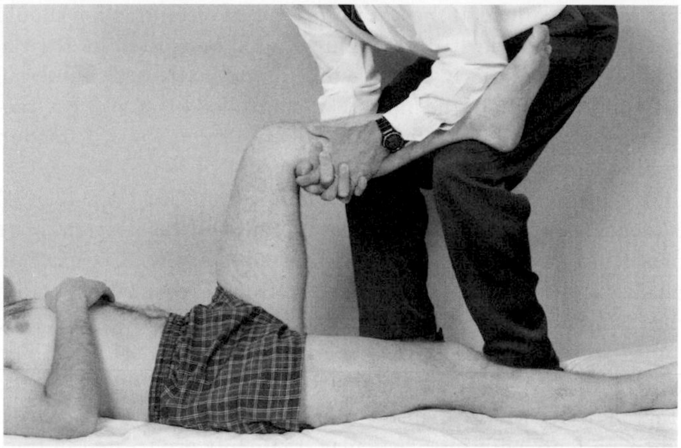

Fig. 12.50.5 Closed reduction of a posterior hip dislocation using the Allis technique. The surgeon can apply a greater reduction force by propping each elbow on a knee, using bilateral elbow flexion, rather than back extension, to reduce the dislocated hip.

Management of the reduction (Box 12.50.2)

After reduction of the hip has been verified radiographically, the stability of the hip must be assessed clinically, under continued sedation or anaesthesia (Box 12.50.3). This assessment is contraindicated in the presence of radiographic evidence of instability, including large displaced fractures of the posterior or posterosuperior acetabular wall, displaced fractures of the acetabular columns, or in the presence of a femoral neck fracture. The assessment of stability is made by applying a strong posteriorly directed force through the knee, with the hip flexed to 90 degrees in a neutral position of rotation and abduction/abduction. If any evidence of subluxation is detected, a CT scan is required.

Successful reduction of a dislocated hip and grading of the dislocation should be immediately confirmed with plain radiographs, including an anteroposterior and lateral view of the hip and an anteroposterior view of the pelvis. The radiographs should be carefully reviewed for evidence of incongruence or fractures of the acetabulum, femoral head, or femoral neck. If a previously unrecognized fracture of the acetabulum is diagnosed, additional Judet views should be obtained. A CT scan of the involved hip should be obtained for all dislocations of the hip associated with fractures (Levin types II–V) or when the presence of an intra-articular loose body is suspected.

Following closed reduction and assessment of hip stability, the affected leg is placed in traction. If the hip is stable, simple skin

Box 12.50.2 Investigations and management

- Anteroposterior view of the hemipelvis and two 45-degree oblique views—Judet views
- CT scans
- Hips with >55% of the remaining posterior acetabulum will be stable.
- If closed reduction is unsuccessful, an open reduction must be performed.

traction will suffice. If the hip is unstable, skeletal traction should be used. A posteriorly unstable hip should be treated in external rotation. An anteriorly unstable hip should be treated in internal rotation. Rotation of the hip can be controlled by applying a traction cord to one end of the traction pin. Placement of a traction pin must be correctly inclined to achieve this.

Widening of the hip joint is not radiographically (Box 12.50.4) evident on plain radiographs when fragments measuring 2mm are present in the hip joint. Therefore widening of the joint space on plain radiographs is a poor indicator of small loose bodies within the traumatized hip joint. Furthermore, although widening of the joint space is demonstrable when 4-mm fragments are interposed with in the hip joint, the widening does not equal the size of the fragment. There is a high risk of developing traumatic arthritis when patients with intra-articular fragments are treated in traction. Consequently it is imperative that the diagnosis of small loose bodies in the hip joint is not missed. Small loose bodies can be diagnosed by a CT scan taken with fine slices through the entire acetabulum. The scan should be processed for bone and soft tissue windows. When non-osseous loose bodies are present, MRI may be a useful alternative.

Once the radiographic imaging and clinical assessment of stability has been performed, the Levine grading of the dislocation can be completed. Management of the dislocation is largely determined by the Levine grading.

Type I dislocations

Type I injuries are pure dislocations or dislocations in which there is no significant associated fracture (Figure 12.50.6). A congruent reduction is obtained and the dislocation is stable after reduction. No surgical intervention is required. The patient is treated in gentle skin traction such as Hamilton–Russell traction. Active and passive range of motion exercises are permitted, but flexion beyond 90 degrees and internal rotation beyond 10 degrees are avoided for 6 weeks. Patients are mobilized weight-bearing as tolerated, once hip irritability resolves and leg control is regained.

Type II dislocations

In type II dislocations there is an irreducible hip dislocation (Figure 12.50.7). No significant associated fractures are present. The irreducibility is therefore due to the interposition of soft tissues, such as largely cartilaginous osteochondral loose bodies, the labrum, tendons, or muscle. An open reduction is required, with exposure of the hip joint on the side of the dislocation. If the hip remains unstable after reduction, further surgical exploration is required. If large tears of the capsule and labrum are present, these must be repaired. Concentric reduction of the hip joint must be confirmed radiologically in the operating room before surgical closure is performed.

Box 12.50.3 Indications for traction

- If the hip is stable, simple skin traction will suffice
- If the hip is unstable, skeletal traction should be used
- A posteriorly unstable hip should be treated in external rotation
- An anteriorly unstable hip should be treated in internal rotation.

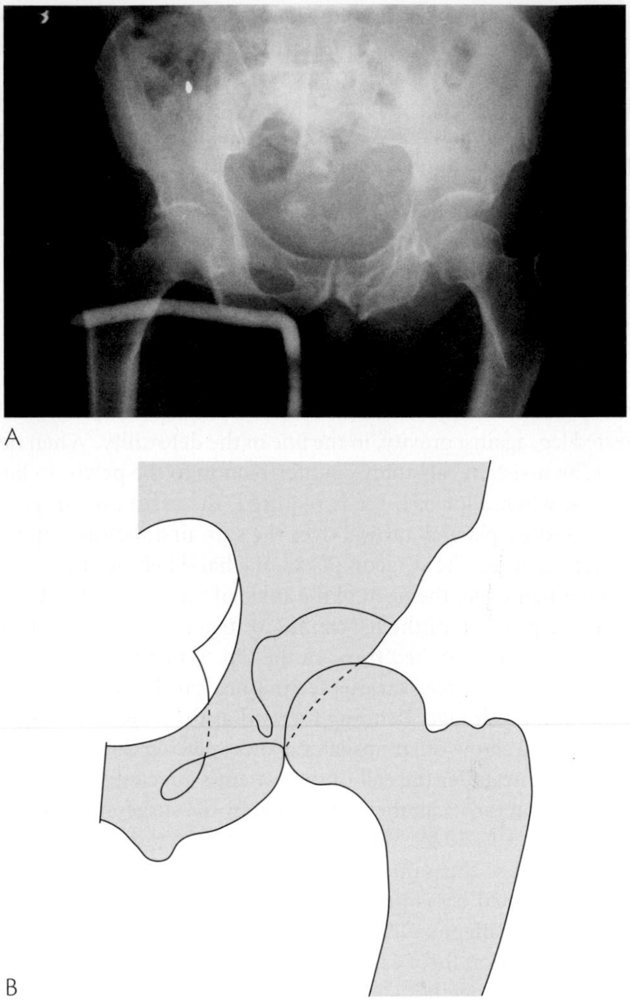

Fig. 12.50.6 Posterior hip dislocation with classic position of adduction, internal rotation, and flexion (Levin type 1). The dislocated femoral head is radiographically smaller while the femoral shaft of the flexed leg is radiographically larger.

Type III dislocations

In type II dislocations the hip is clinically unstable after reduction, or postproduction imaging demonstrates joint space widening or incarcerated fragments of bone or cartilage in the joint (Figure 12.50.8). The instability may be due to subluxation of the femoral head by incarcerated fragments, extensive labral detachment, or disruption of the capsuloligamentous attachments of the hip joint. Plain radiographs or CT scanning demonstrate bony fragments incarcerated in the articular space. Cartilage or soft tissue fragments are demonstrated best in MRI studies.

Minor capsuloligamentous disruptions or detachments of the acetabular labrum may be managed by non-surgical means, including bed rest or bracing of the hip within its stable arc of motion. Extensive labral tears may require surgical reattachment.

Fragments of tissue left incarcerated in the hip joint may damage the articular cartilage of the apposing femoral head and acetabulum. These fragments must be surgically cleared from the hip joint. Large fragments may be replaced where this is surgically possible. Smaller fragments must be removed, either arthroscopically or

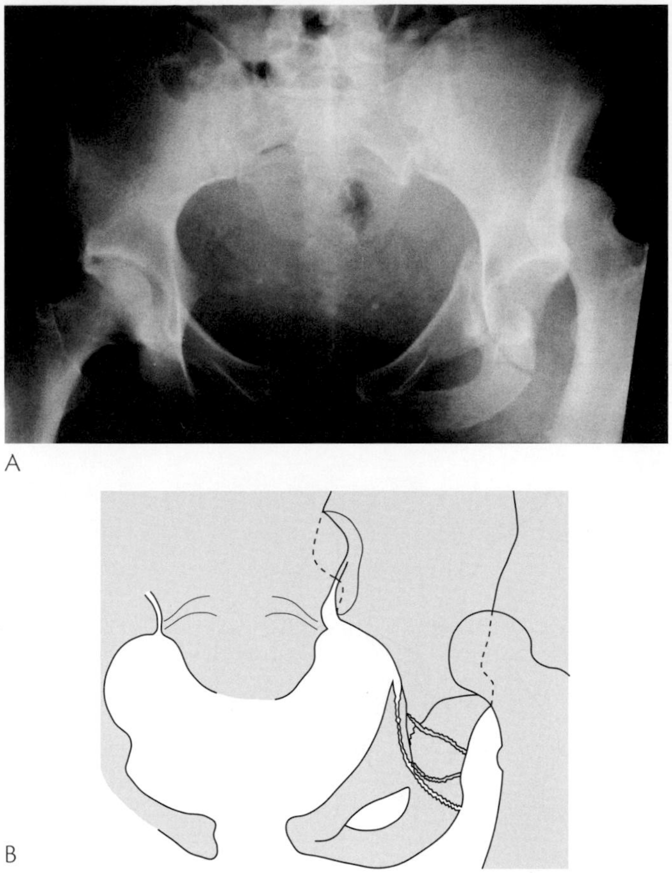

Fig. 12.50.7 Irreducible hip dislocation, due to psoas muscle interposition (Levin type II). This patient had also suffered an undisplaced transverse acetabular fracture and a type C pelvic ring disruption and minimally displaced ipsilateral superior and inferior pubic rami fractures.

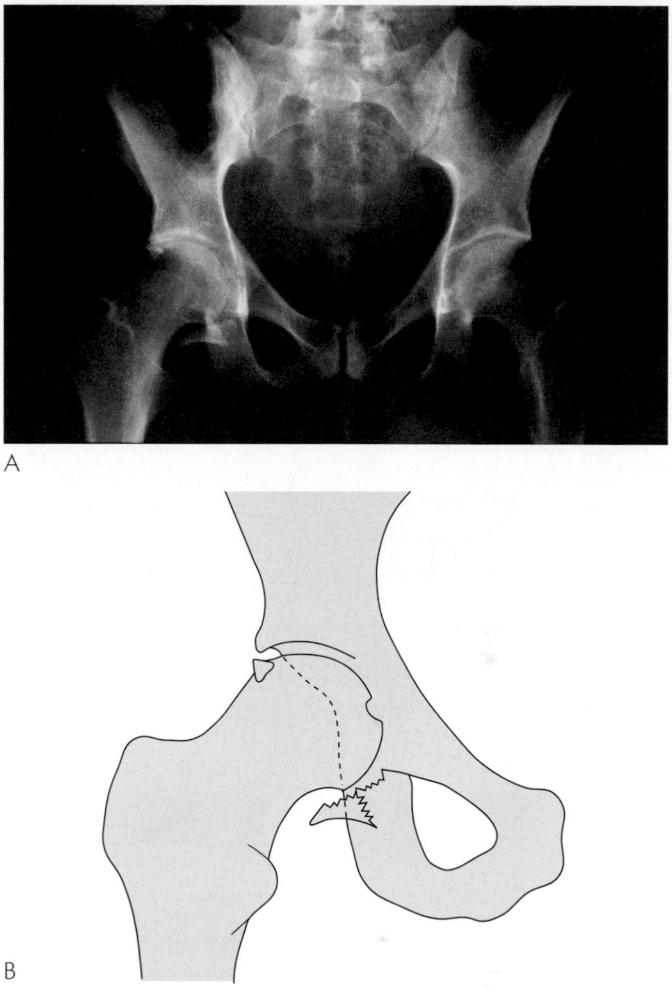

Fig. 12.50.8 Postreduction radiograph of a posterior hip dislocation demonstrates an incarcerated bony fragment superolaterally and a displaced fragment lying inferiorly (Levin type III).

by an open procedure. When an open procedure is performed, the surgeon should choose the surgical exposure which offers the most direct approach to the offending fragment. Concentric reduction of the hip must be demonstrated radiographically before wound closure. The stable range of hip motion must be determined by stability examination before the patient leaves the operating room. Postoperatively the patient is placed in Hamilton–Russell traction. Active and passive range of motion exercises are permitted within the clinically determined stable range of hip motion. Once hip irritability resolves and leg control is regained patients are mobilized weight-bearing as tolerated. A hip brace may be used when the stable range of hip motion would leave the patient vulnerable to redislocation when walking.

Type IV dislocations

Type IV dislocations are associated with fractures of the acetabulum requiring reconstruction to restore joint congruity or hip stability (Figure 12.50.9). Prolonged dislocation of the hip joint should be prevented whenever possible. The author initially places the patient in skeletal traction and performs a gentle closed reduction at the time of insertion of the traction pin. Definitive surgical management should be dictated by the acetabular fracture and not the hip dislocation.

Type V dislocations

Type V dislocations are associated with fractures of the femoral neck (Figure 12.50.10) or femoral head (Figure 12.50.11). The mechanism of injury in femoral head fractures is the same as that of hip dislocations. Typically the injury occurs with the femur in a neutral position with reference to abduction and relatively less flexion than in pure dislocations of the hip.

The majority of hip dislocations are posterior. The incidence of femoral head fractures associated with posterior dislocations has been reported at 7–13%. Femoral head fractures have been reported in up to 68% of anterior hip dislocations, but the number of reported cases is small. Femoral head fractures may result from indentation (Figure 12.50.12) or cleavage (Figures 12.50.11 and 12.50.13) of the femoral head by the acetabular lip at the time of dislocation, or from avulsion by the teres ligament.

Pipkin classified cleavage fractures of a femoral head into four types according to the position of the fracture and the presence of a femoral neck or acetabular fracture (Table 12.50.2). In a type I injury the fracture of the femoral head is caudad to the fovea (Figure 12.50.14 and 15A). In type II injuries the fracture of the

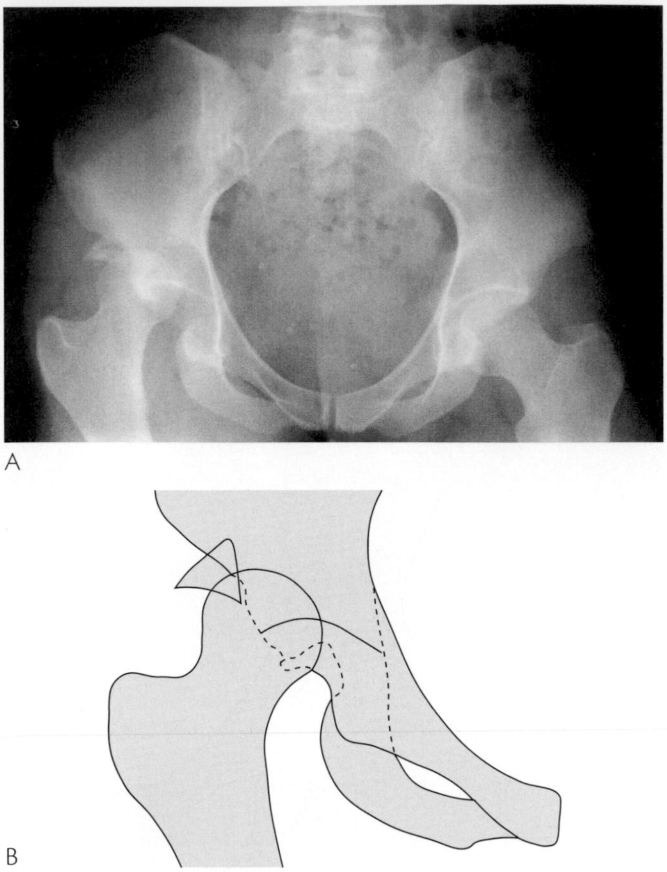

Fig. 12.50.9 Type IV dislocation with acetabular fracture.

femoral head is cephalad to the fovea (Figures 12.50.11 and 12.50.15B). A type III injury is a type I or a type II fracture with an associated fracture of the femoral neck that results in a segmental fracture of the femoral head (Figure 12.50.15C). A type IV injury has an associated fracture of the acetabular rim (Figures 12.50.13 and 12.50.15D).

Type 1 Pipkin fractures have been treated by closed reduction and traction. If postproduction radiographs demonstrate incongruence of the hip or the presence of intra-articular fragments, operative excision was previously recommended. Following experience gained in surgical hip dislocation the preferred treatment is open reduction and internal fixation for non-comminuted fractures sufficiently large to provide purchase for screw fixation.

Type II Pipkin fractures have been treated by closed reduction and traction, closed reduction and excision of the fragments, or open reduction and internal fixation. Following reduction the patient is treated in traction and early range of motion exercises are commenced.

Type III Pipkin fractures have been treated by closed reduction and traction, closed reduction and excision of the fragment, open reduction and internal fixation, and primary arthroplasty. Any attempt at closed reduction must be performed gently to avoid displacement of a femoral neck fracture, or the production of an iatrogenic fracture. If the attempt at reduction is unsuccessful, the surgeon should proceed to open reduction rather than resort to an excessively forceful closed reduction.

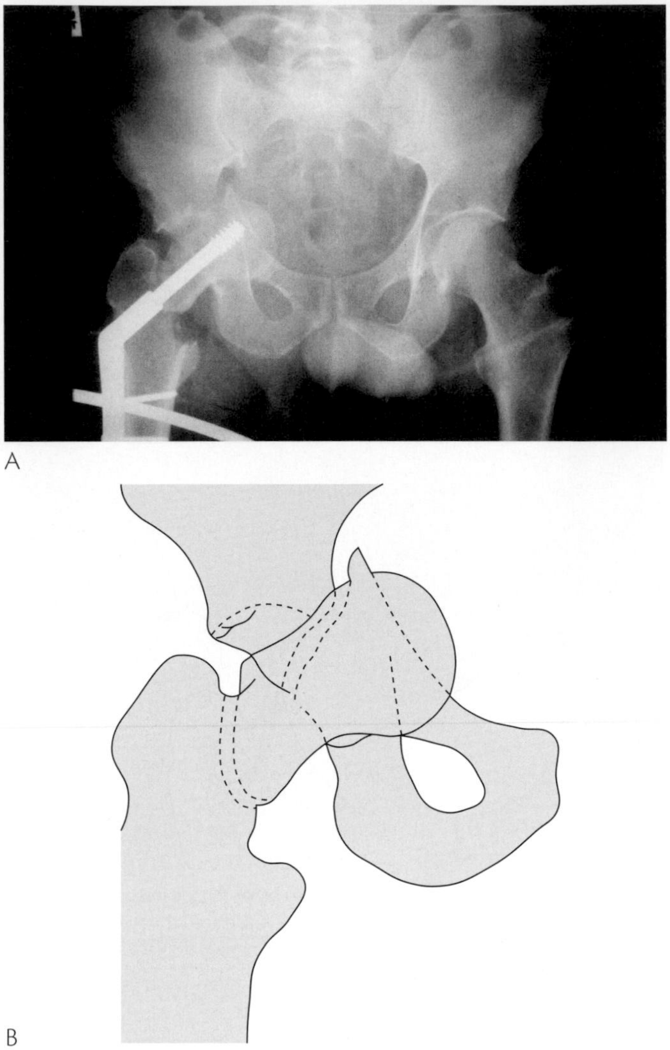

Fig. 12.50.10 Posterior hip dislocation with associated acetabular and femoral neck fractures (Levin type V). The classification assumes the grading of the most severe (femoral neck) injury.

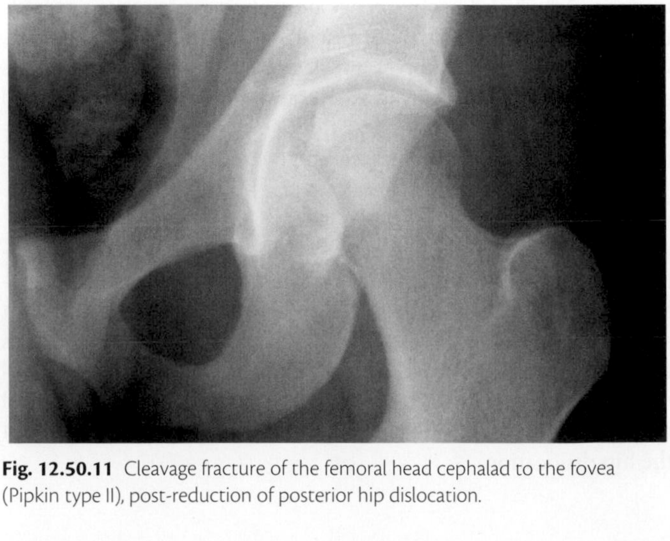

Fig. 12.50.11 Cleavage fracture of the femoral head cephalad to the fovea (Pipkin type II), post-reduction of posterior hip dislocation.

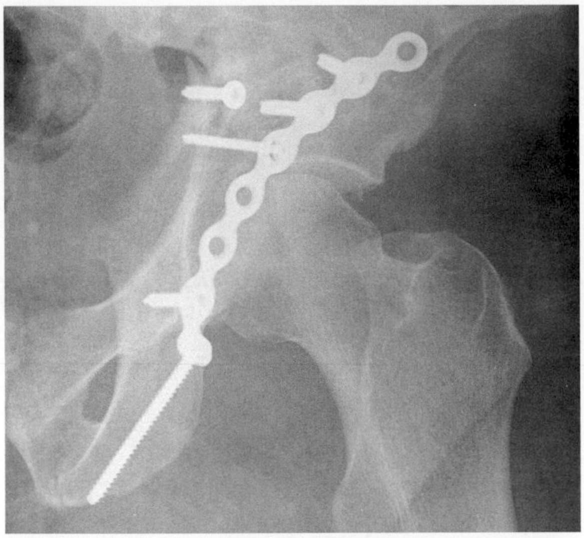

Fig. 12.50.12 Fracture dislocation left hip treated by closed reduction of hip dislocation and open reduction and internal fixation of transverse acetabular fracture. Note indentation on lateral portion of femoral head.

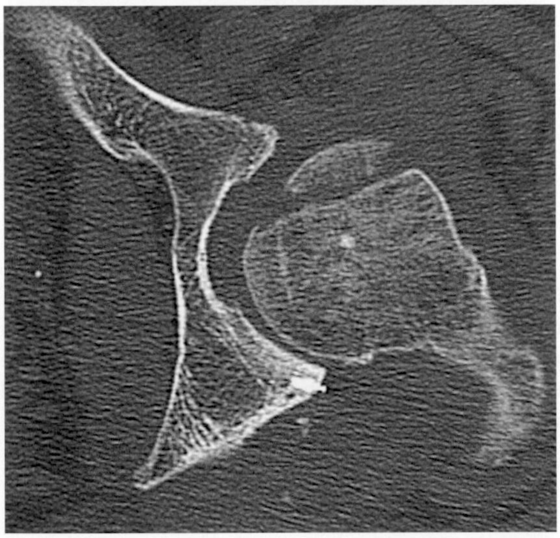

Fig. 12.50.13 CT scan: axial slice shows cleavage fracture anterior portion of femoral head.

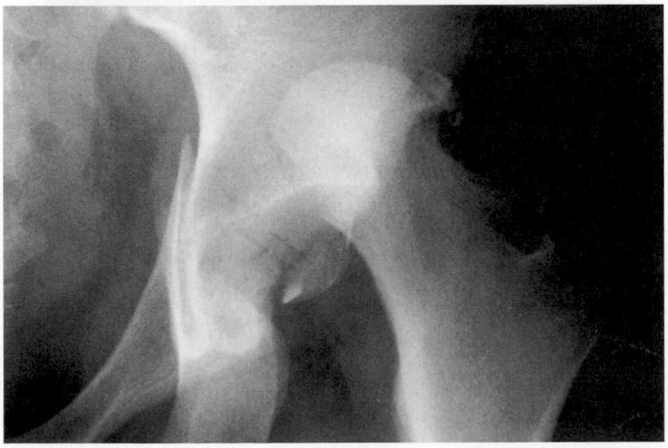

Fig. 12.50.14 Type 1 fracture of the femoral head, caudad to the fovea, with associated acetabular fractures (Pipkin type IV).

Table 12.50.2 Pipkin classification of femoral head fractures

Type I	(Hip) dislocation with fracture of the femoral head caudad to the fovea capitis femoris (Figure 12.50.14A)
Type II	(Hip) dislocation with fracture of the femoral head cephalad to the fovea capitis femoris (Figures 12.50.12 and 12.50.14B)
Type III	Type I or II injury associated with fracture of the femoral neck (Figure 12.50.14C)
Type IV	Type I or II injury associated with fracture of the acetabular rim (Figures 12.50.13 and 12.50.14D)

Type IV Pipkin fractures have been treated by closed reduction and traction, closed reduction and excision of the fragment, and open reduction and internal fixation. The acetabular fractures should dictate the treatment protocol. Undisplaced acetabular fractures may be treated non-operatively. When the indications for open reduction and internal fixation of the acetabulum are present, the fracture should be treated operatively and the femoral fracture can then be treated along the lines of type I and II fractures. Postoperative management is determined by the acetabular fracture.

Posterior hip dislocations may result in impaction (Figure 12.50.12) or cleavage fractures (Figures 12.50.13 and 12.50.14) of the femoral head that lie anteriorly. A surgical hip dislocation is ideal for operative reduction and internal fixation of these fractures and provides ready ease of access to the whole femoral head (Figure 12.50.16). Ganz and Beck have modified the technique by incorporating a step-cut of the greater trochanter. Placing the distal half of the trochanteric osteotomy deeper than the proximal portion, the intervening step between the two provides a mechanical block to proximal migration of the osteotomized trochanter after internal fixation. The patient's ipsilateral knee is flexed and the tibial shaft used as a reference to the plane of the osteotomy. In contrast, anterior hip dislocations are characterized by cleavage or impaction fractures on the posterosuperior and lateral portion of the femoral head.

Outcomes and complications (Box 12.50.4)

Treatment goals of anatomical reduction, restoration of hip joint stability, and removal of all interposed bone fragments have resulted in an improved prognosis of femoral head fractures. In general, the outcomes of Pipkin type I and II fractures are similar and are better than those of Pipkin type III and IV fractures.

Sciatic nerve injury

The sciatic nerve is frequently injured in hip dislocations. The peroneal component is most commonly affected. The reported incidence varies from 8–19% of patients with hip dislocation. Damage to the nerve may be secondary to pressure ischaemia or directly from laceration or impalement by bone fragments. Nerve tissue has little tolerance to ischaemia. Posterior hip dislocations with neurological deficit of the sciatic nerve should therefore be reduced as a surgical emergency. Increasing sciatic nerve dysfunction in the presence of displaced posterior wall or transverse acetabular fractures should be treated emergently by acute open reduction and internal fixation of the fracture. Paresis may develop acutely after reduction of a hip dislocation and warrants surgical exploration. Causes include:

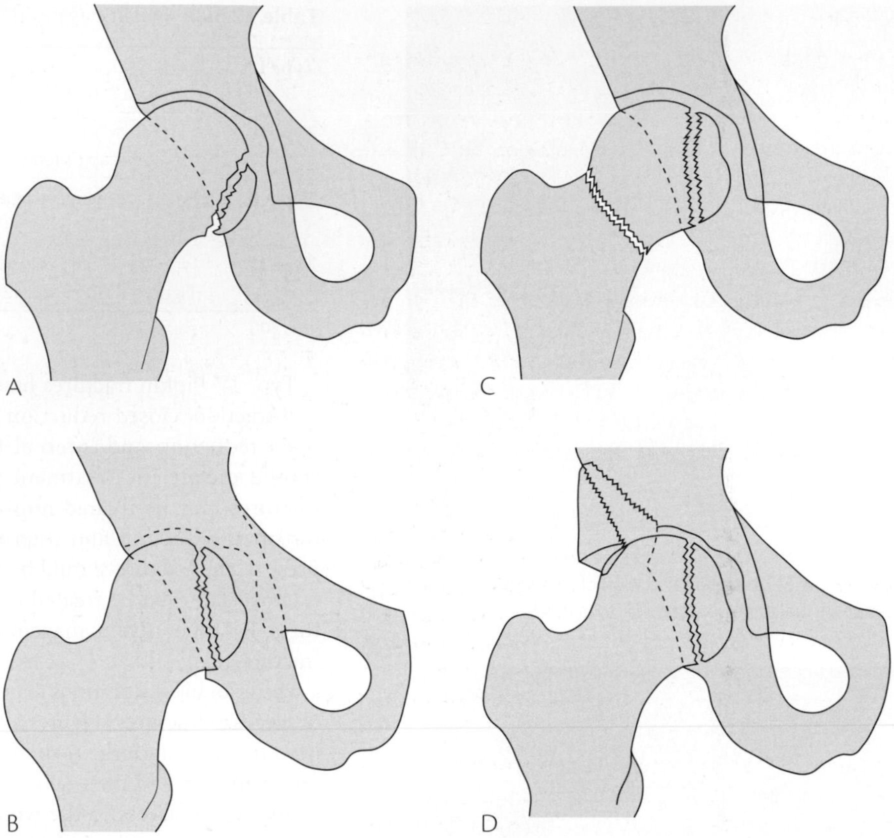

Fig. 12.50.15 Pipkin's classification of femoral head fractures. A) Pipkin type 1. The femoral head fracture lies caudad to the fovea. B) Pipkin type II. The femoral head fracture lies cephalad to the fovea. C) Pipkin type III fractures have a fracture of the femoral neck associated with a type 1 or type II fracture of the femoral head. D) Pipkin type IV fractures have a fracture of the acetabulum associated with a type 1 or type II fracture of the femoral head.

- Entrapment of the nerve in the joint
- Redislocation of an unstable hip
- Redisplacement of associated fractures
- Haemorrhage, especially with anticoagulation prophylaxis to thromboembolic disease.

Missed knee injuries

Posterior hip dislocations commonly results from a forceful blow to the front of the knee. Concomitant injuries may therefore occur to the patella, the femoral or tibial condyles, or to the knee ligaments. Posterior cruciate ligament injuries and posterolateral rotatory instability are the most common ligamentous injuries associated with posterior hip dislocation. Associated collateral knee ligament injury may occur when the causative force is applied to the tibia and not directly to the knee.

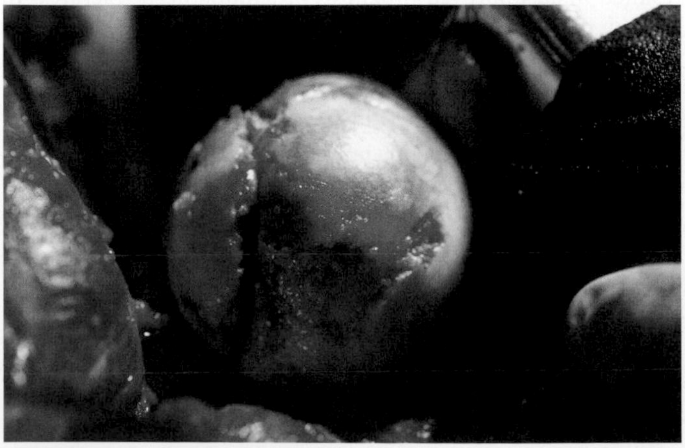

Fig. 12.50.16 Ganz surgical dislocation of hip showing full exposure of femoral head. Note anterior cleavage fracture and impaction fracture of superior aspect of femoral head.

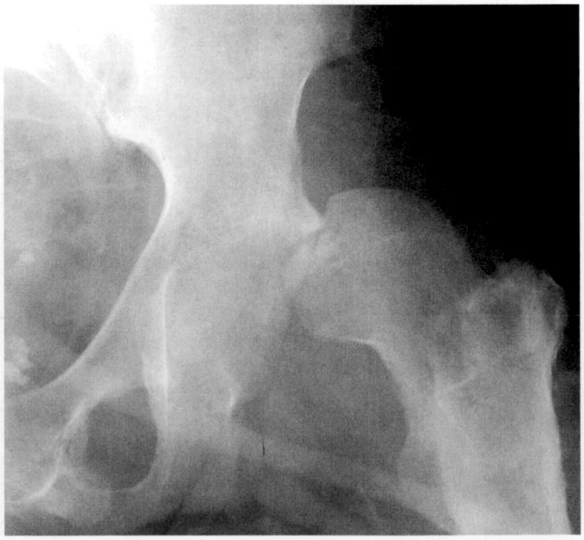

Fig. 12.50.17 Posterior hip dislocation with impaction fracture of femoral head on posterior acetabular wall.

Avascular necrosis of the femoral head

Avascular necrosis of the femoral head occurs more commonly after posterior hip dislocations than after anterior dislocation. The reported incidence after posterior hip dislocation varies from 3–50%. Changes occur in the extraosseous blood flow of the common femoral and circumflex vessels to dislocated hips. Internal rotation of the femur, posterior dislocation of the hip, and lateral displacement of the femur produces traction to the deep branch of the medial circumflex femoral artery, which have shown to be the major blood supply to the weight bearing portion of the femoral head. Delay in reduction may lead to avascular necrosis by prolonging ischaemia and by causing progressive arterial damage in the common femoral and circumflex vessels. The commencement of early weight bearing does not increase the incidence of avascular necrosis but may modify the severity of this complaint.

Recurrent dislocation

Recurrent hip dislocation may result from a deficiency of the bony and capsuloligamentous restraints of the hip joint, or an alteration of local muscle forces. Impaction fractures of the femoral head may also lead to recurrent dislocation in a manner similar to dislocation of the humeral head resulting from a Hill–Sachs lesion.

Heterotopic bone formation

The reported incidence of heterotopic bone formation associated with hip dislocation is 2%. The incidence increases after open reduction of dislocations, open reduction and internal fixation of associated fractures, delayed surgery, and in patients with a hip injury. Surgical excision may be warranted when heterotopic bone formation is disabling, but should be delayed until the process is quiescent. A bone scan may be helpful to confirm this.

Post-traumatic arthritis

The reported incidence of post-traumatic arthritis following uncomplicated hip dislocation varies around 11–16%. When hip dislocation is associated with acetabular fractures the incidence of post-traumatic arthritis rises markedly and has reached 88% in severe acetabular fractures. The incidence of post-traumatic arthritis decreased to 10% or less with accurate open reduction and internal fixation of acetabular fractures, but increased with age.

Box 12.50.4 Principles of treatment

- Treatment goals: anatomical reduction, restoration of hip joint stability, and removal of all interposed bone fragments
- Posterior hip dislocations with neurological deficit should be reduced as a surgical emergency
- Concomitant injuries may occur to the patella, femoral, or tibial condyles, or knee ligaments.

Box 12.50.4(b) Long term complications

- Avascular necrosis of the femoral head more common after posterior hip dislocations
- Recurrent hip dislocation
- Heterotopic bone formation
- Post-traumatic arthritis.

Conclusion

Appropriate management of hip dislocation requires a clear understanding of the mechanisms of injury, early recognition of systemic injuries, accurate diagnosis and grading of dislocations, and prompt effective treatment. Problems and complications must be anticipated to prevent their occurrence or to allow early and effective treatment when they occur. A comprehensive approach to the injury complexes associated with hip dislocation is mandatory for an effective outcome of treatment.

Further reading

Epstein, H.C. (1973). Traumatic dislocations of the hip. *Clinical Orthopaedics and Related Research*, **92**, 116–42.

Letournel, E. and Judet, R. (1992). Mechanics of acetabular fractures. In: Elson, R.A. (ed) *Fractures of the Acetabulum*, second edition, pp. 23–28. Berlin: Springer Verlag.

Letournel, E., and Judet, R. (1992). Radiology of the acetabulum. In: Elson, R.A. (ed) *Fractures of the Acetabulum*, second edition, pp. 29–43. Berlin: Springer Verlag.

Letournel, E. and Judet, R. (1993). Late complications of operative treatment within three weeks of injury: post-traumatic osteoarthritis. In: Elson, R.A. (ed) *Fractures of the Acetabulum*, second edition, pp. 551–8. Berlin: Springer Verlag.

Levin, P. (1992). Hip dislocations. In: Browner, B.D., Jupiter, J.B., Levine, A.M. and Trafton, P.G. (eds), *Skeletal Trauma*, pp. 1329–67. Philadelphia, PA: W.B. Saunders.

Matta, J. (1986). Planning definitive care: Indications for nonoperative and operative treatment of acetabular fractures. In: Mears D.C. and Rubash H.E. (eds) *Pelvic and Acetabular Fractures*, pp. 196–204. Thorofare, NJ: Slack.

12.51

Femoral neck fractures

Martyn J. Parker

Summary points

- Intracapsular fractures are classified by division into those fractures that are essentially undisplaced and those that are displaced
- Undisplaced fractures are generally treated by reduction and internal fixation
- Displaced fractures may be treated by reduction and internal fixation but this incurs the potential complications of re-displacement of the fracture, non-union, and avascular necrosis
- Displaced fractures in the elderly are generally treated with a replacement arthroplasty.

Epidemiology (Box 12.51.1)

Fractures in the elderly, particularly hip fractures, constitute one of the major current orthopaedic problems. The expected increase in the number of elderly persons, as well as an increasing age-specific incidence of hip fractures, make this already large problem even more important. Worldwide, an estimated 1.3 million hip fractures occurred in 1990. As more of the world's population reach their eighties, global numbers of hip fractures will increase to between 7 and 21 million by 2050. Much of this increase will occur in South America, India, and the Far East. Europe and North America can still expect an increase in numbers, but not by such dramatic amounts.

Having sustained a hip fracture there is an increased risk of later sustaining a similar type of fracture of the contralateral hip. The most plausible cause for this is the differences in femoral neck lengths, with a long femoral neck predisposing to an intracapsular fracture. Other causes may be the different degrees of osteoporosis in the femoral neck (cortical bone) and trochanteric area (cancellous bone), or the mechanism of the fall. Arthritis of the hip reduces the risk of an intracapsular fracture occurring but not an extracapsular fracture.

Box 12.51.1 Epidemiology of femoral neck fractures

- Average age is about 80 years, 75% female
- Major and increasing problem
- Risk increases exponentially with age
- Increasing incidence as more of the population live to their 80s
- The age-specific incidence is increasing particularly in developing countries.

Aetiology

Three principle factors are responsible for the occurrence of hip fractures in the elderly. These are a tendency to have falls with ageing, a diminution of protective mechanisms in falling (such as using their hands to cushion the impact of the fall), and weakling of the bone with ageing (Figure 12.51.1). Those who sustain a hip

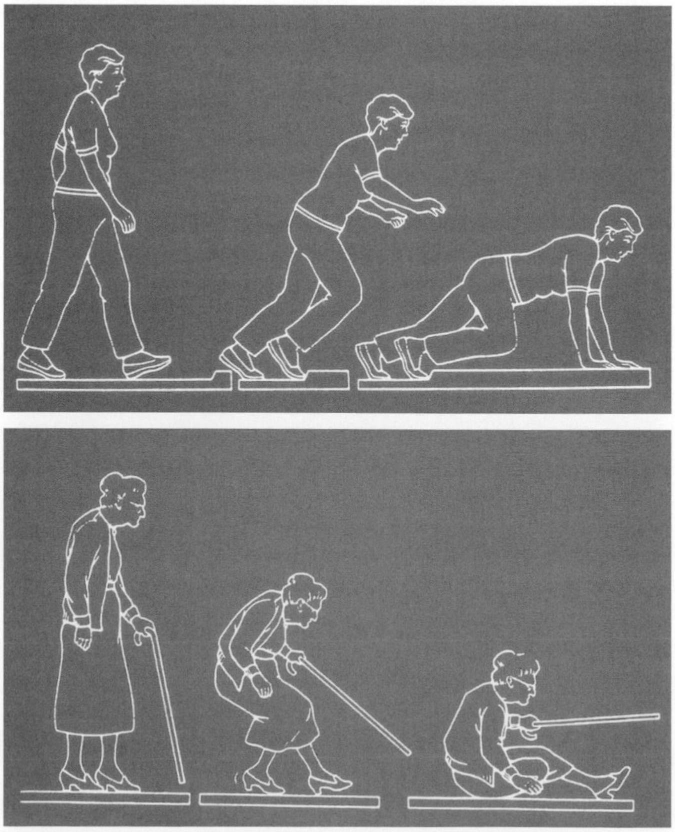

Fig. 12.51.1 Differences in the fall characteristics for a wrist and hip fracture. The more elderly who sustain a hip fracture do not have the forward momentum and lack the protective mechanism from the upper limb to cushion the impact of the fall. The fall is directly onto the hip.

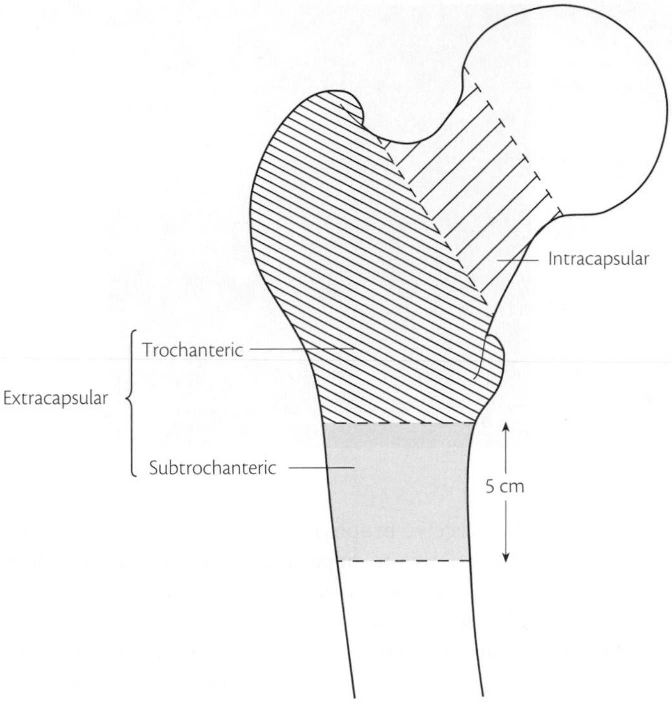

Fig. 12.51.2 Basic classification of proximal femoral fractures.

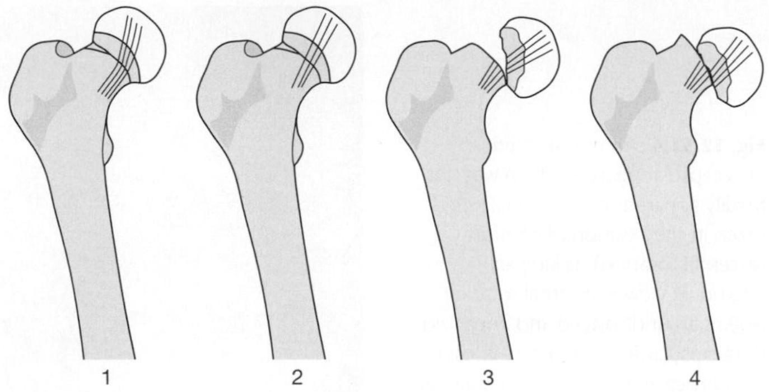

Fig. 12.51.3 Garden's classification of femoral neck fractures. Grades 1 and 2 are undisplaced fractures; grades 3 and 4 are displaced fractures.

fracture tend to be frailer with more associated medical conditions than their age-matched peers.

Classification

Proximal femoral fractures or 'hip fractures' can be primarily divided into two groups. Fractures proximal to the femoral attachment of the joint capsule are termed intracapsular (femoral neck, cervical) fractures, whilst those between the hip joint capsule insertion to a line 5cm distal to the distal part of the lesser trochanter are termed extracapsular fractures (Figure 12.51.2). Even this primary classification may cause confusion because fracture lines may cross these anatomical boundaries. In these circumstances the area in which the fracture line crossing the femur is predominately found should be taken. Where the fracture is situated running along the intertrochanteric line at the base of the femoral neck it is termed a basal fracture. These fractures are usually treated as trochanteric fractures (Box 12.51.2).

Ideally any classification of intracapsular fractures should be able to predict fracture healing complications, namely non-union and avascular necrosis. Unfortunately no system where radiographs are evaluated can reliably predict this outcome. In addition, most of the current classifications fail to reach acceptable degrees of intra- and interobserver variation. Garden classified cervical fractures into four groups depending on degree of dislocation evaluated on an anteroposterior (AP) radiograph (Figure 12.51.3). Whilst this is the most frequently quoted classification, in clinical practice there is poor interobserver agreement. Furthermore grade 2 fractures are rare and difficult to distinguish from the impacted grade 1 fractures. In addition the difference between the displaced fractures of grade 3 and 4 is of questionable value. Therefore the classification is only of value in differentiating between those fractures that are essentially undisplaced (Garden grades 1 and 2) and those that are displaced (Garden grade 3 and 4).

The Pauwels classification of femoral neck fractures is based on the angle of the fracture line with the horizontal. Whilst biomechanical studies indicate that those fractures with the more vertical angle (type 3) have greater shearing forces across the fracture. Garden grade 1 impacted fractures are included in the classification and will invariable be type 1, whilst displaced fractures are type 2 or 3. Clinical studies have failed to find and difference in fracture healing complications between types 2 and 3. Essentially the classifications system is again dividing fractures into displaced and undisplaced fractures.

The more recent AO classification has nine subdivisions. These subdivisions have not been shown to be of value in predicting fracture healing complications and the system has been shown to have unacceptable intra- and interobserver variation. In summary, it is recommended to simply classify intracapsular fractures into those that are essentially undisplaced and those that are displaced.

Box 12.51.2 The approximate incidence of the different fracture types

- Undisplaced intracapsular fractures: 14%
- Displaced intracapsular fractures: 42%
- Basal fractures: 3%
- Trochanteric two part: 12%
- Trochanteric multifragment: 25%
- Subtrochanteric fractures: 4%.

Diagnosis

After falling, the patient, who is usually an elderly woman, lies on the floor unable to get up by themselves. The leg is usually shortened and the limb externally rotated with all movements causing pain. The fracture is diagnosed by an AP and lateral radiograph of the hip. Occasionally, for an undisplaced fracture the radiographic signs may be minimal causing a delay in diagnosis, during which time the fracture becomes displaced. A third radiograph with the hip in 10 degrees of internal rotation and the film centred on the hip may be useful to make the diagnosis (Figure 12.51.4).

For those patients in which a hip fracture is suspected but there is no apparent abnormality on the plain radiographs additional

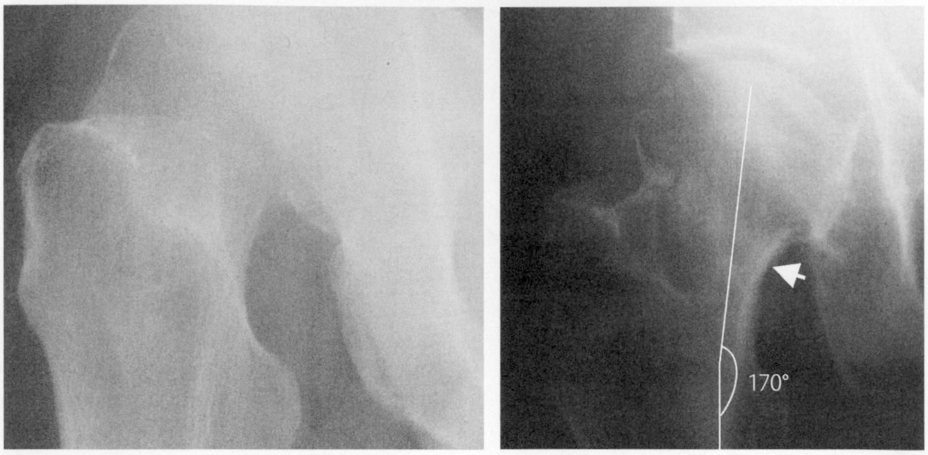

A B

Fig. 12.51.4 An undisplaced intracapsular fracture which was not readily apparent on the initial x-rays taken in the position of comfort (external rotation). Taking an additional view in internal rotation reveals an undisplaced and impacted intracapsular fracture. There is loss of the cortical continuity laterally and an area of impacted bone (arrow). The trabeculae of the femoral head now have an angle of 170 degrees (normal 160 degrees) as the femoral head has tilted.

investigations are required. A magnetic resonance imaging (MRI) scan of the hip is now the investigation of choice (Figure 12.51.5). In addition to revealing a hip fracture, this investigation will reveal alternative diagnoses such as a bone haematoma, pubic rami fracture, or soft tissue injuries.

Alternative investigations that may be used are an isotope bone scan or computed tomography (CT) scan of the hip (Box 12.51.3). If bone scintimetry is used, this should ideally be undertaken at least 2 days after the injury to reduce the risk of a false negative result.

Management (Box 12.51.4)

Thromboembolic prophylaxis for hip fracture patients remains a controversial topic. The progressive improvements in hip fracture management, with an increasing proportion of patients having early surgery and mobilization, has markedly reduced the incidence of thromboembolic complications. Furthermore the frail elderly patients who sustain a hip fracture are at increased risk of adverse bleeding complications (intestinal, intracerebral, and wound) from pharmacological prophylaxis. This means that there will be a fine balance between the adverse effects of prophylaxis and the benefits. The Cochrane review of randomized trial of heparins, demonstrated a reduction in thromboembolic complications with heparin but a tendency to an increased mortality to those allocated to receive prophylaxis. Aspirin has been recommended as an alternative to heparin by one clinical guideline. The largest clinical study on this indicated a reduced incidence of thromboembolic complications (2.5 to 1.5%), but an increased risk of wound haematomas (2.4 to 3.0%) and a tendency to a reduced mortality with aspirin. Mechanical prophylaxis appears to be effective but is costly and time consuming. Antiembolism stocking have not been proven to be effective for hip fracture patients.

Traditionally, traction was applied to the limb with the aim of decreasing pain while waiting for surgery and to reduce the facture and thereby improve the femoral head circulation. Randomized trials have since demonstrated that traction has no effect on the degree of discomfort encountered. No clinical studies have evaluated the effect of traction on femoral head blood flow.

If the fracture is to be managed surgically, then if possible this should be undertaken within 48h of the injury. Delaying surgery further will increase the complications of recumbencey (pressure sores, thromboembolic complications, pneumonia), prolong the pain, and increase hospital stay. There will be a small group of patients (5–10%) in whom surgery needs to be delayed to improve their fitness for surgery (Box 12.51.5). Anaesthesia for hip fracture is invariable by means of general anaesthesia or a regional block with spinal anaesthesia. Spinal anaesthesia may have marginal benefits over general anaesthesia but the evidence base for this is limited.

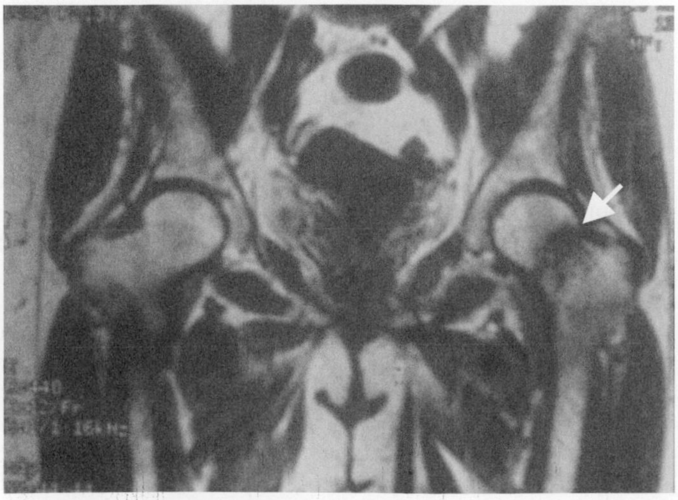

Fig. 12.51.5 MRI scan of an intracapsular hip fracture.

Pathophysiology

Fracture healing for a femoral neck fracture is dependent on a stable fracture position and good circulation. The femoral head receives it blood supply from three sources:

- Through the marrow vessels. This is disrupted for all fractures

Box 12.51.3 Investigations of femoral neck fractures

- Radiographs are indicated in any patient complaining of hip or groin pain after a fall who is unable to weight bear
- If initial pelvis and lateral views are normal, a third film with internal rotation can be taken
- MRI is the investigation of choice to detect fractures not evident on plain films
- Alternative investigations are isotope bone scan or CT scan.

Box 12.51.4 Key aspects of initial management

Assessment

- Diagnosis established
- Examination of the patient for associated injuries
- Review for medical conditions that may require treatment or influence management
- Consideration for possible aetiological factors for the fall
- Assessment of the patient's prefracture mobility and mental state
- Record home circumstances and social history.

Initial managment

- Pain relief (oral, parental, or nerve block)
- Intravenous fluids started in the emergency department
- Undertake routine biochemistry, haematology, and group and save
- ECG recorded
- Pressure relieving mattress used
- Chest x-ray presurgery if clinically indicated
- Nutritional support as indicated
- Thromboembolic prophylaxis
- Avoid excessive delays in transfer from the orthopaedic ward.

Surgical management

- If surgery is proposed, plan within 48h if possible
- Perioperative antibiotic prophylaxis
- Early and unrestricted mobilization after surgery
- Information for the patient and relatives and reassurance
- Early planning for rehabilitation and discharge.

Box 12.51.5 Acceptable reasons for delaying surgery include:

- Significant anaemia
- Hypovolaemia and/or severe dehydration
- Severe electrolyte imbalance
- Untreated cardiac failure
- Correctable cardiac arrhythmia
- Uncontrolled diabetes mellitus
- Severe hypertension
- Sepsis at the site of surgery.

- Through the artery of the ligamentum teres. This supplies a small area of bone around the insertion of the tendon at the fovea
- Via the retinacular vessels which are situated subperiostally along the femoral neck. This is the main supply with the majority of these vessels arising from the posterior medial and lateral femoral circumflex arteries (Figure 12.51.6).

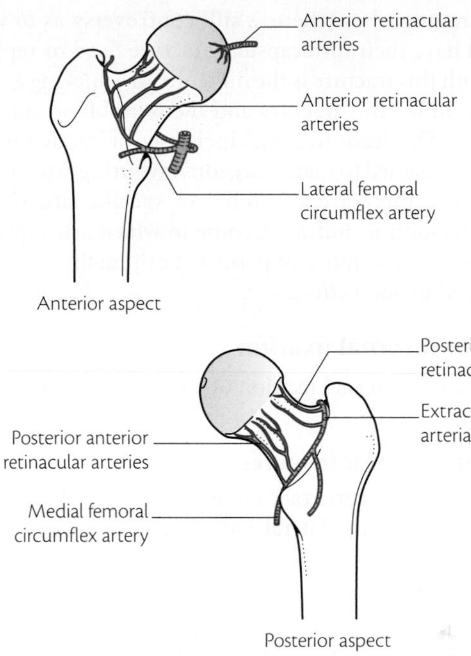

Fig. 12.51.6 Blood supply to the femoral head.

The main complication after internal fixation is non-union of the fracture which occurs in about a third of patients. Early redisplacement of the fracture is generally included within the term non-union. Avascular necrosis or late segmental collapse of the femoral head is caused by the damage to the blood supply to the femoral head and generally presents 1–2 years after the injury. Non-union is a more common complication in the elderly whilst avascular necrosis is more common in younger patients.

Operative versus conservative treatment

Undisplaced (including impacted Garden grade 1) intracapsular hip fractures may be managed conservatively. This entails a short period of bed rest followed by protected mobilization. The risk of the fracture displacing is markedly increased for conservative treatment compared with that after internal fixation (20–50% vs 5–10%). This increase is higher in the elderly and frail. Therefore non-operative treatment for an undisplaced fracture is only recommended if the patients several weeks after the episode of trauma or occasionally in younger individuals.

If a displaced intracapsular fracture is treated conservatively, non-union of the fracture is inevitable. This results in a painful hip with limited function. Conservative treatment may be used for those of limited life expectancy, but even for those of limited mobility, surgery is useful as it relieves pain, and provides a limb that can be used for walking and transfers. Excision arthroplasty, which is removing the femoral head, has been suggested as a means of providing pain relief for those that are immobile, but there is a limited published evidence to support such a method of treatment.

Osteosynthesis

Surgical treatment of an intracapsular hip fracture is either internal fixation to preserve the femoral head or a replacement arthroplasty.

This remains an area where there is still controversy as to which patients should have their intracapsular fracture fixed or replaced. The problem with this fracture is the difficulty in achieving a secure and stable fixation for this fracture and the poor blood supply of the femoral head. This leads to a high incidence of fracture healing complications and has led to many surgeons favouring arthroplasty. In clinical practice there are a number of specific situations in which internal fixation is indicated, some in which arthroplasty is appropriate, and for a number of patients both methods of treatment may be used to good effect.

Indications for internal fixation

The situations where internal fixation of a femoral neck fracture is appropriate are:

Undisplaced intracapsular fractures

The term undisplaced fractures refers to those fractures that show no displacement in the AP and lateral radiographs, but also includes those in which there is impaction of bone (see Figure 12.51.4). These fractures do not require any reduction at the time of surgery. Non-union of the fracture is the most common complication of this procedure with an expected incidence of 6%, although this will be influenced by the age and sex of the patient (Figure 12.51.7). Arthroplasty for an undisplaced intracapsular fracture is inappropriate as it is a more extensive procedure with a higher risk of complications.

Mildly displaced intracapsular fractures

Occasionally the clinician is presented with the radiographs of an intracapsular fracture in which the fracture is essentially undisplaced on one of the radiographs but is beginning to displace on the other view. This is normally the lateral view in which the fracture is beginning to 'open'. Such fractures are easily treated by internal fixation with an incidence of fracture healing complication only slightly more than that for an undisplaced fracture.

Displaced intracapsular fractures in the young

Two factors favour internal fixation in the young. Firstly the incidence of non-union of the fracture is lower in the younger patient (Figure 12.51.8). Secondarily the increased life expectancy of the patient means that if an arthroplasty is undertaken there is a definite possibility of the patient requiring a revision arthroplasty in the future. These two factors meant that reduction and internal fixation is the method of choice for the young patient. What constitutes a young patient is debatable with young being defined as somewhere between 60 and 70 years but others give a limit of up to 75 years. A physiological assessment may be more appropriate, rather than a chronological one. Both

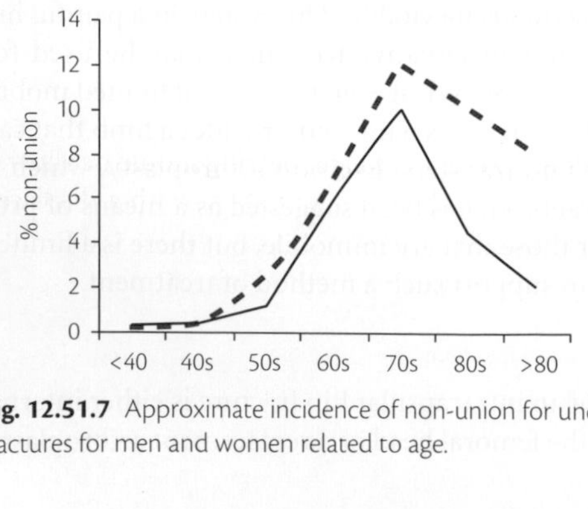

Fig. 12.51.7 Approximate incidence of non-union for undisplaced intracapsular fractures for men and women related to age.

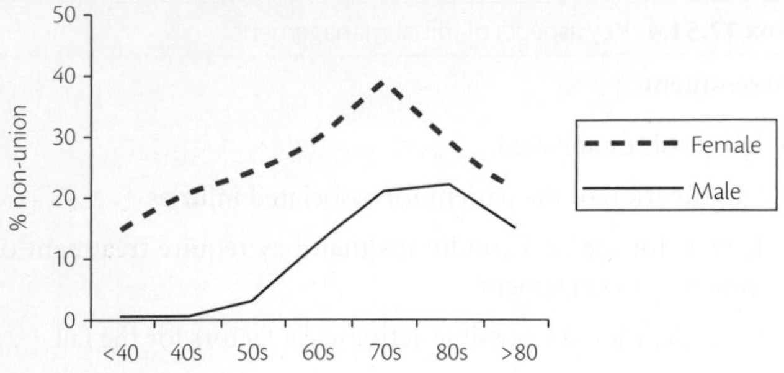

Fig. 12.51.8 Approximate incidence of non-union for displaced intracapsular fractures for men and women related to age.

fracture healing complications of non-union and avascular necrosis are less common in men compared to women.

Displaced intracapsular fractures in the very elderly

For the very frail elderly of limited life expectancy the lesser surgical procedure of reduction and internal fixation in comparison to arthroplasty may give a greater chance of the patient surviving. In addition, Figures 12.51.7 and 12.51.8 indicate that with increasing age the incidence of non-union falls. This is due to the death of patients before non-union occurs.

Displaced intracapsular fractures in specific situations

There may be a number of unusual but difficult situations in which reduction and fixation may be preferred to arthroplasty. Examples include a person with sepsis nearby. Internal fixation has a lower risk of sepsis. Patients with an increased risk of bleeding or wound haematoma may also be better treated with internal fixation.

Choice of implants

In 1931, Smith-Petersen described the technique of open reduction and fixation with a solid flanged nail. Johansson later improved the method by giving the nail a central channel which made it possible to position it over a guide wire. Since then, more than 100 different varieties of nails, screws, and pins have been used. Most implants consist or parallel pins or screws, inserted with the aid of the image intensifier.

Because of differences in patient selection and operative procedures, valid comparisons between different implants can only be made using a randomized controlled trial. All these studies to date have been summarized within the Cochrane review on the subject. This found that multiple parallel screws and the sliding hip screw were the most studied methods of fixation. The sliding hip screw was found to have a marginally lower risk of fracture healing complications to that of a multiple parallel screw technique (28% vs 33%), but requires a slightly larger surgical exposure to insert.

Timing of surgery

Debate exists as to how urgent surgery should be for a displaced femoral neck fracture. Early surgery may restore femoral head blood flow that was impeded by stretched vessels. Reports from one centre have supported early surgery within 6 hours of injury. However, other reports with large patient numbers, suggest that a delay of up to 7 days has only minimal effect on the incidence of fracture healing complications. After a delay of more than 1 week, closed reduction of the fracture becomes more difficult and an open reduction may be required.

Prediction of fracture healing complications

Various investigations have been used to try to predict the occurrence of fracture healing complications. To date, none have been shown to be reliable enough for routine clinical use. Preoperative scintimetry using $^{99}\mathrm{Tc}^{m}$ and postoperatively at 2–4 weeks postoperatively has been reported. If uptake on the fractured side is the same as than on the normal side, the fracture will heal without problems in over 90% of cases. More recently MRI has been used with a sensitivity of 81%. Other investigative methods that have been tried are intraosseous venography, intraosseous pressure measurement, arteriography, and injection of dye into the femoral head.

Surgical technique

The surgeon should supervise the transfer of the patient to the fracture table to guard against undue and excessive movements at the fracture site. The blood circulation to the femoral head via the capsular vessels along the femoral neck is vulnerable and could be impaired by sudden forceful movements of the hip during the reduction or by excessive traction causing fracture diastasis. Reduction is usually done in two stages. Firstly with the patient positioned in the fracture table, gentle traction is applied to the outstretched leg. Whilst this is done the fracture is screened with the image intensifier to ensure the leg is brought out to length. Traction is continued until the medial parts of the femoral neck (the calcar region) are approximated (Figure 12.51.9). Over-reduction must be avoided. Following this the fracture is reduced on the axial view by internal rotation (Figure 12.51.10). This part of the reduction can be looked upon as similar to closing a book. Full internal rotation may be required to complete this manoeuvre.

The goal is to restore the alignment of the femoral neck to an anatomical or slight valgus position. The ideal Garden alignment angle should be 160–170 degrees (Figure 12.51.9). On the lateral a straight line bisects the femoral head, the trochanteric region, and the shaft (Figure 12.51.10). After reduction, some slackening of the traction allows impaction to occur and reduces the risk of femoral head rotation during surgery. Failure to achieve an acceptable reduction by closed means may lead to an open reduction. This is achieved via a small anterior approach to the hip and reducing the fracture under direct vision.

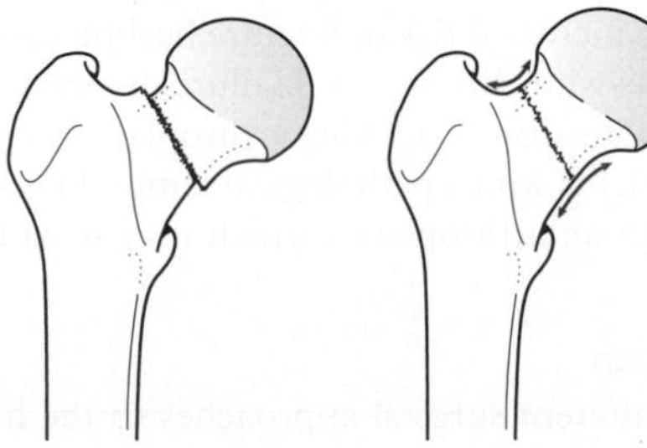

Fig. 12.51.9 Reduction on the AP view. Gentle traction is applied to restore femoral length. The ideal reduction trabeculae angle should be 160–170 degrees.

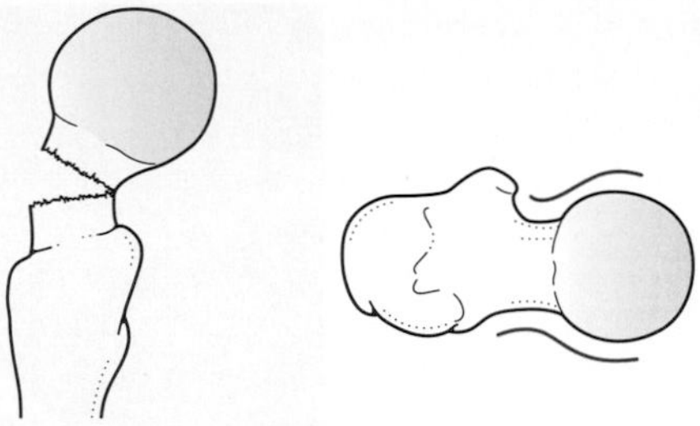

Fig. 12.51.10 Reduction on the lateral view. Internal rotation of the limb 'closes the book'. The ideal reduction angle should be 180 degrees.

Rarely for a late presentation (over 1 week from injury), in a young patient with a displaced cervical fracture, consideration should be given to undertaking open reduction and insertion of a vascularized pedicle graft to the fracture. The aim is not only to reduce the fracture but to restore the femoral head vascularity. A number of different grafts may be use. The most commonly reported method is a posterior approach to insert a graft based on quadratus femoris muscle.

The positioning of the implant used is the subject of more dogma than science. If a multiple pin or screw method is used, general advice is that the inferior screw or pin should rest along the calcar. The lateral insertion point on the femur should not be lower than the lower border of the lesser trochanter to reduced the risk of causing a subtrochanteric femur fracture. On the axial view, inferior calcar support is again recommended and there should be spread of the screws into different segments of the femoral head. The tips of the screws or pins should be 3–5mm from the subchondral bone to obtain the best purchase on the femoral head (Figure 12.51.11 and Box 12.51.6). Hammering to insert the implant or cause impaction of the fracture is not recommended.

Bleeding from a haematoma trapped inside the capsule can produce an increase in pressure sufficiently high to cause tamponade to those vessels located along the femoral neck and impede the circulation to the femoral head. Aspiration of the haematoma with a large-bore needle or even a limited open capsulotomy has been advocated. Clinical studies have indicated that this will reduce capsular pressures and improve femoral head circulation but it has yet to be proved that this leads to a reduced incidence of fracture healing complications.

Postoperative care

No restrictions on hip movements are necessary after internal fixation. Limited studies have addressed the role of restricted weight bearing, and to date no study has demonstrated any reduction in the occurrence of fracture healing complications with either non- or partial weight bearing. Therefore, weight bearing should be allowed after internal fixation, but for the younger patient with a displaced intracapsular fracture partial weight bearing may be recommended.

Complications of internal fixation

Early redisplacement of the fracture and non-union may be treated either by repeat internal fixation or arthroplasty. Repeat fixation is more likely to be used in the younger patient in which femoral

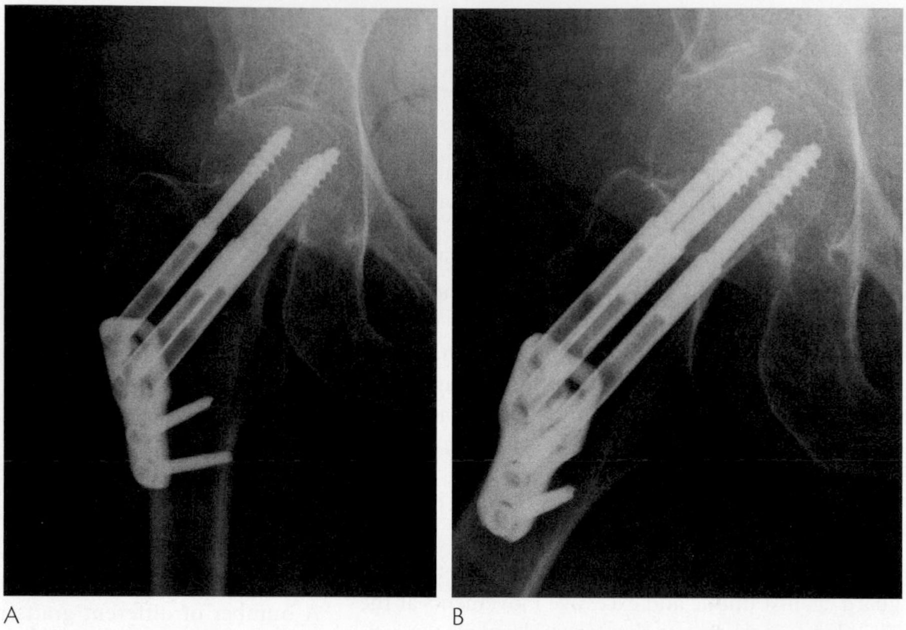

Fig. 12.51.11 AP and lateral view of a femoral neck fracture fixed with a screw and plate device.

Box 12.51.6 Femoral neck fractures: internal fixation
◆ Optimum reduction angle is 160–170 degrees on the AP and 180 degrees on the lateral radiograph ◆ Open reduction only required if unable to reduce fracture closed ◆ Lower screw or pin on the calcar on the AP view ◆ Implant tips must be close to the subchondral bone ◆ Reduction and implant positioning affect outcome ◆ Non-union is expected for 6% of undisplaced fractures and 33% of displaced fractures.

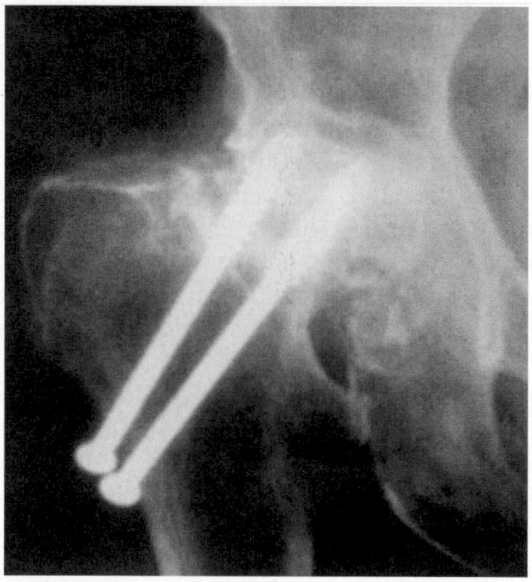

Fig. 12.51.12 Avascular necrosis after screw fixation. The fracture has healed but there is extensive collapse of the femoral head and damage to the joint.

head preservation is desired. An osteotomy such as that described by Pauwels may be used to increase the chance of the fracture healing. An alternative is a pedicle bone graft. For more elderly patients, replacement arthroplasty is generally recommended.

Avascular necrosis occurs in about 10% of undisplaced fractures and 12–16% for displaced fractures (Figure 12.51.12). However, it only causes sufficient symptoms to merit surgical intervention in about a third of cases. Treatment is generally with a replacement arthroplasty, although in the younger patient an osteotomy or revascularization procedure may be considered. The other complication after internal fixation is refracture of the femur below the implant. This has an incidence of approximately 1%.

Arthroplasty

Indications (Box 12.51.7)

Arthroplasty is only indicated for a displaced femoral neck fracture in specific situations. This includes the older patient (aged over 65–75 years). For these patients arthroplasty has a lower reoperation rate and better function outcomes. Patients with rheumatoid arthritis have an increased risk of fracture healing complications as do those patients with chronic renal failure, hyperparathyroidism, and metabolic bone disease, making arthroplasty the more favourable option. Patients with a pathological femoral neck fracture are best treated with an arthroplasty, which may need to be a long-stem implant.

Surgical approach

A number of different surgical approaches to the hip have been described. Most are divided into those via the posterior capsule

Box 12.51.7 Indications for arthroplasty (displaced fractures only)

- The elderly (aged over 65–75 years)
- Pathological fractures
- Fractures secondary to Paget's disease
- Metabolic bone disease
- Hyperparathyroidism
- Rheumatoid arthritis
- Symptomatic arthritis of the hip
- Delayed presentation.

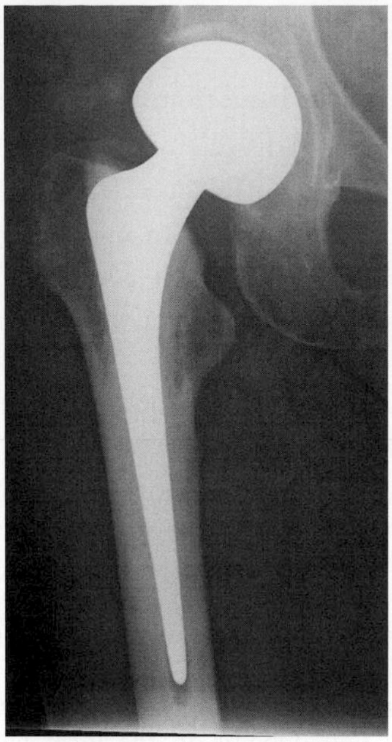

Fig. 12.51.13 Cemented hemiarthroplasty with a polished tapered stem.

(posterolateral exposure) and those via the anterior capsular (anterolateral and anterior). The anterolateral approach is generally favoured as there is a lower risk of postoperative dislocation (5% vs 2%) The anterolateral approach does have the disadvantages of requiring a greater tissue dissection with possible damage to the abductors, slightly larger blood loss, and more restricted access to the femoral canal. Regardless of the approach used, the hip joint capsule should always be preserved and repaired to reduce the risk of dislocation.

Cement

Cementing the stem leads to less residual pain and improved mobility; therefore, in general, all arthroplasties for hip fracture patients should be cemented in place. Cementing does add extra technical difficulties to the surgery and adds the risk of a major adverse reaction to the cement during surgery. Modern cementing techniques are recommended, particularly the use of the cement gun. For the very frail elderly in whom there are concerns about the safety of cement, consideration should be given to using either an uncemented prosthesis or undertaking reduction and internal fixation.

Unipolar, bipolar, or total hip arthroplasty

The most common types of hemiarthroplasty still used are those of Moore and Thompson, introduced in the 1950s. Many other stem types are now available including many of the stems used for total hip replacements. The early stems were designed before cement was introduced and generally have collars. The use of these older designs should be reduced in favour of the more modern stems (Figure 12.51.13).

More recently bipolar hemiarthroplasties have been introduced. They have a double articulating joint of an inner metal head on high-density polyethylene in addition to the outer metal shell articulating with the acetabulum. The intention is to decrease the movement between prosthesis and acetabular cartilage and thereby reduce the degree of acetabular wear and possible pain from this. Clinical studies to date have failed to demonstrate any benefit from this bipolar joint. The risk of dislocation is the same for a bipolar as compared with a unipolar prosthesis, but if a bipolar prosthesis dislocates it is more likely to require an open reduction. The bipolar prosthesis is also more expensive than the unipolar prosthesis. Therefore the use of a bipolar prosthesis cannot be justified.

Total hip replacement for hip fracture has been recently reported in a number of case series reports. These highlighted the increased risk of dislocation with this method of treatment with reported rates of about 10%. Recent randomized trials have, however, suggested improved functional outcomes and less residual pain for those treated by a total hip replacement in comparison to a hemiarthroplasty. Many of the patients in these studies were a slightly younger and fitter group of patients than the average hip fracture patient and therefore better able to recover from the more extensive operation of total hip replacement. It is likely that this method of treatment will become more extensively used in the future.

Postoperative care

Modern surgical techniques should allow early mobilization with full weight bearing. Repair of the capsule in combination with an anterolateral approach reduces the risk of dislocation, therefore restriction on hip movements and the use of abduction wedges is generally not necessary.

Complications of arthroplasty

Early surgical complications after arthroplasty are dislocation (2–5%), haematoma (2–10%), and wound sepsis (1–5%). Later complications are acetabular wear (5–40%), loosening of the prosthesis (2–20%), and fracture around or below the implant (1–5%). The complications of loosening and fracture around the implant are increased for an uncemented implant in comparison to a cemented implant. Acetabular wear and loosening are more common within the younger active group of patients. Revision arthroplasty to a total hip replacement is generally required for the late complications.

Rehabilitation

The goal is to rehabilitate the patient to the same functional level as before the hip fracture. An adequate operation is a prerequisite to achieving this. The main task of the orthopaedic surgeon is to perform an operation which gives the patient a hip that allows immediate postoperative weight bearing to start on the day after surgery.

Box 12.51.8 Different models of rehabilitation

- Admission to and discharge from an acute orthopaedic ward
- Admission to and discharge from a specialized hip fracture ward
- Admission to and discharge from an acute orthopaedic ward with geriatric support
- Admission to an acute orthopaedic ward and later transfer to a rehabilitation ward
- Admission to an acute orthopaedic ward and later transfer to a skilled nursing facility
- Early hospital discharge schemes with community rehabilitation.

The different models of rehabilitation that have been described are detailed in Box 12.51.8.

It remains unproven which model of care produces the foremost outcomes. Much will depend on the local facilities available. Transferring a patient to another ward will inevitably lead to a delay in the rehabilitation process, increase the length of hospital stay, and result in fragmented care. The optimum method of rehabilitation is therefore most likely admission to a specialized orthopaedic geriatric ward that is able to provide the acute care and the rehabilitation needed for these patients along with assessment for falls and further fracture prevention. Such a unit can be developed into a specialized hip fracture unit and be supported by additional community support teams to enable the early discharge of patients.

Secondary fracture prevention

A full description of the methods used for falls assessment and to reducing the occurrence of further fractures is beyond the scope of this article. The essence of this assessment is listed in Box 12.51.9.

The appropriate treatment of osteoporosis is still the subject of controversy. At present, the mainstay of treatment is the bisphosphonate drugs. These are being increasingly used in those patients over the age of 60 after a fall and fracture. A relative risk reduction of 45% and an absolute risk reduction of up to 6% may be expected. The role of these drugs in those aged over 80 years has not been so well evaluated and they may be less effective. The effectiveness of calcium and/or vitamin D remains controversial with some limited evidence suggesting that a combination of these drugs may be effective for the elderly living in institutional care. Hip protectors do not appear to be effective in reducing the incidence of hip fractures due to the problem of compliance with wearing them.

Box 12.51.9 Factors that may be used to reduce the risk of further fractures

- Home assessment for hazards
- Review of medications that may be implicated in falls or osteoporosis
- Review of medical conditions causing falls or osteoporosis
- Cardiovascular assessment
- Assessment of gait and balance
- Testing of vision and correction as indicated
- Provision of appropriate walking aids
- Provision of correct footwear
- Optimization of mobility
- Exercise and strength exercises
- Osteoporosis treatment
- Review of smoking habits
- Review of alcohol intake.

Prognosis

The reported mortality and morbidity after a hip fracture varies widely between different studies. This may be due to the different characteristics of patients within the different geographical areas or the different selection of patients to be included. Regarding mortality, this is generally reported as being between 20–30% at 1 year from injury. Most of these deaths are from other conditions associated with ageing, rather than the hip fracture itself.

For the survivors, most will be left with some degree of discomfort in the hip, although for the majority this will be fairly minimal. Whilst up to 80% of patients should eventually be able to return to the same residence as before the fracture, many will be more dependent on walking aids and require more assistance; 10–25% will need to a more supportive residence or require institutional care.

Further reading

Garden, R.S. (1961). Low-angle fixation in fractures of the femoral neck. *Journal of Bone and Joint Surgery*, **43B**, 647–63.

Parker, M.J. and Gurusamy, K. (2003). Internal fixation versus arthroplasty for intracapsular proximal femoral fractures in adults. *Cochrane Database of Systematic Reviews*, **4**, CD001708. DOI: 10.1002/14651858.CD001708.pub2. (www.thecochranelibrary.com).

Parker, M.J. and Gurusamy, K. (2010). Arthroplasties (with and without bone cement) for proximal femoral fractures in adults. *Cochrane Database of Systematic Reviews*, **6**, CD001706 10.1002/14651858.CD001706.pub4. (www.thecochranelibrary.com).

Scottish Intercollegiate Guidelines Network (SIGN). (2009). Management of hip fracture in older people. Number 111. Edinburgh: SIGN (www.sign.ac.uk).

Wells, G.A. Cranney, A. Peterson, J., *et al.* (2008). Alendronate for the primary and secondary prevention of osteoporotic fractures in postmenopausal women. *Cochrane Database of Systematic Reviews*, **1**, CD004523.

12.52

Trochanteric and subtrochanteric fractures

Martyn J. Parker

Summary points

- Traction is not useful for trochanteric fractures
- Surgery should not be delayed unless the medical condition of the patient can be improved
- Dynamic implants are best (sliding hip screw best)
- Early full weight bearing should be achieved
- Most patients return to their own home.

Epidemiology

In 1824, Sir Astley Cooper stated that trochanteric fractures occurred infrequently and mainly in adults under 50 years of age, whilst intracapsular hip fractures were more prevalent. Since that time there has been a progressive increase in the incidence of trochanteric fractures particularly in those aged over 70 years. Currently, approximately half of all hip fractures are extracapsular, with an incidence as high as 50 in 100 000 in some countries.

Imaging (Box 12.52.1)

The diagnosis of an extracapsular femoral fracture is invariably confirmed by radiography of the hip. Almost all extracapsular fractures are radiologically apparent but occasionally the diagnosis may be missed for one of the following reasons.

1) Failure to radiograph the hip because the patient experiences pain only in the knee. This is due to the shared sensory innervation of the hip and the knee
2) Failure to take radiographs in two planes. Both an anteroposterior and lateral view of the hip are essential
3) Inability to visualize the trochanteric or subtrochanteric region due to incorrect radiographic exposure. Occasionally repeat films with different exposures are necessary.

Only rarely are additional investigations required to establish the diagnosis of an extracapsular fracture. A magnetic resonance imaging (MRI) scan is the investigation of choice, with alternatives being an isotope bone scan or a computed tomography (CT) scan. These investigations, particularly the MRI scan may also reveal other cases for the hip pain such as an incomplete trochanteric fracture or other injuries in close proximity.

Box 12.52.1 Imaging

- Fracture almost always seen on radiograph unless:
  - Hip not radiographed (knee pain)
  - Radiograph not biplanar
  - Incorrect exposure
- Occasionally MRI or isotope scan to demonstrate fracture.

Classification (Box 12.52.2)

Extracapsular fractures may be subdivided into trochanteric and subtrochanteric fractures. The term 'intertrochanteric fracture', if used precisely, refers to a fracture running transversely in between (but not through) the lesser and greater trochanter, whilst the term 'pertrochanteric' pertains to a fracture running obliquely and through the greater to lesser trochanter. To avoid confusion the term trochanteric is easier to use. Basal fractures (also termed basicervical), relates to a two-part fracture in which the fracture line runs along the intertrochanteric line. They are considered by some as intracapsular fractures and others as extracapsular. As the treatment and prognosis of a basal fracture is akin to that of a trochanteric fracture they should be considered as extracapsular. Subtrochanteric fractures should only include those fractures in which the fracture line traversing the femur is predominately within the 5cm length of femur immediately distal to the lesser trochanter.

Numerous other methods of classifying and subdividing extracapsular fractures exist. The most frequently used is the Jensen–

Box 12.52.2 Classification

- Trochanteric, subdivided into two part (stable), comminuted (unstable), and reversed fracture line
- Subtrochanteric, distal to lesser trochanter, but within 5cm of it
- Fracture pattern determines treatment.

Michaelsen modification of the Evans classification of trochanteric fractures and the Seinsheimer classifications of subtrochanteric fractures. The more recently introduced AO classification of fractures may become more frequently used, but to date there is little published evidence of its reliability or effectiveness in determining treatment or prognosis.

For the orthopaedic surgeon it is important to recognize a number of specific fracture types (Figure 12.52.1), which will determine the choice of implant and surgical technique. Occasionally a fracture may show characteristics of more than one fracture type or the exact type of fracture may not be evident on the initial radiographs and only becomes apparent during surgery. This determination of the fracture pattern is the key to treatment.

Management

Operative versus conservative treatment

Treatment options for extracapsular fractures may be conservative or operative. Conservative treatment for an extracapsular fracture may take one of two forms.

'Skilful neglect'

This method of management is only appropriate for the patient who is completely immobile prior to the fracture. Such 'treatment' involves nursing the patient in bed with appropriate analgesia. The fracture will usually unite after a period of some months, albeit with considerable shortening and an external rotational deformity of the limb. Nursing care of such patients may be difficult, and there is a continued need for analgesia. These factors may mean that surgical fixation of the fracture is generally still indicated even for a completely immobile patient.

'Active' conservative treatment

This involves reducing the fracture by means of traction applied to the limb. Regular radiographs are required to check the fracture position whilst the traction is maintained for a period of 2–4 months. The only noteworthy randomized study to compare this method of treatment with a modern method of internal fixation showed no difference in mortality but a greatly increased proportion of patients who had a prolonged hospital stay (and presumably were unable to return home), following conservative treatment. A later study based on this evidence demonstrated clear cost/benefit advantages for operative treatment. Given this clear superiority of operative treatment, conservative treatment should be retained for only the following indications:

- Patient unfit for any form of anaesthesia
- Patient refuses to consent to surgery
- Lack of modern surgical facilities
- Lack of appropriate surgical implant
- Absence of experienced surgeon.

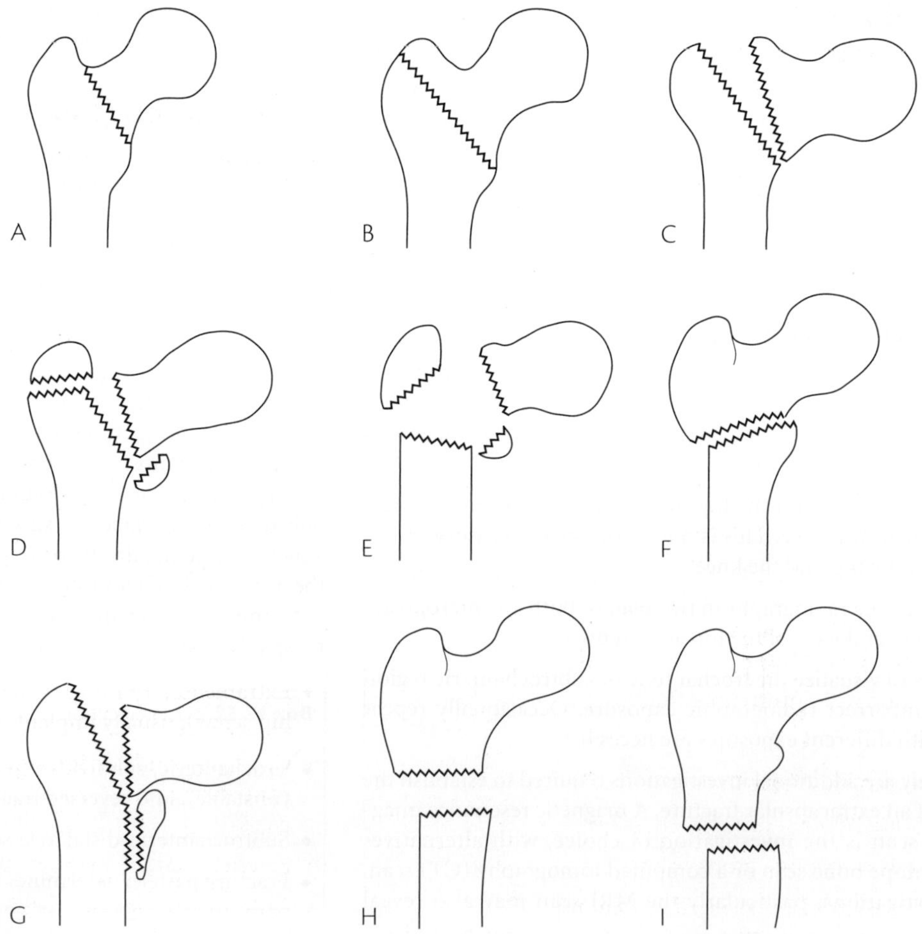

Fig. 12.52.1 Fracture patterns that dictate the method of treatment: A) basal; B) undisplaced two-part trochanteric; C) displaced two-part trochanteric; D) displaced and comminuted trochanteric; E) comminuted trochanteric with loss of lateral support; F) reversed fracture line; G) subtrochanteric extension; H) 'high' subtrochanteric; I) 'low' subtrochanteric.

The technique of conservative treatment entails applying traction to the leg using either a tibial pin or skin tapes and bandages. This may then be continued as simple traction over a pulley at the end of the bed or in the Hamilton Russell or 90 degree/90 degree traction. Alternatively, balanced traction with a Thomas splint may be used. A useful alternative form of skeletal traction is Perkins traction, which enables quadriceps power to be retained.

Operative treatment

Preoperative preparation (Box 12.52.3)

The majority of hip fractures occur in the frail elderly who invariably have many other medical problems associated with ageing. The medical assessment and management of these patients is therefore fraught with problems, yet this is an area that is frequently ignored by orthopaedic surgeons and delegated to the most junior member of the team. The optimum care of these patients is probably best served by having their medical care supervised by a specialist.

Preoperative assessment must include an assessment of associated medical conditions and medications. Resuscitation of all patients with an extracapsular fracture using intravenous fluids is essential. This should be started in the emergency room. Blood loss at the fracture site may exceed 1L, and in an elderly patient who is not drinking with impaired physiological response mechanisms, hypovolaemic shock is inevitable. Fluid correction should be adjusted to the patient's condition using crystalloids, colloid, and blood replacements. Monitoring of progress is essential to avoid precipitating cardiac failure.

Traction has not been shown to be of benefit for trochanteric fractures. The choice of thromboembolic prophylaxis is controversial and is still the subject of research. The most favoured pharmacological methods are either low-molecular-weight heparin or low-dose aspirin. The timing of surgery is important. It should be performed after the patient is resuscitated and a good urine output has been established but generally within 48h of admission. Only those patients in whom the medical condition can be further improved should have their surgery delayed (Box 12.52.4). For those patients in which surgery is delayed the haemoglobin will fall from continued blood loss at the fracture site and preoperative transfusion may be required.

Choice of implant (Box 12.52.5)

The implants available can be grouped into five types.

Extramedullary fixation

Extramedullary fixation refers to applying a side-plate to the proximal femur attached to a lag screw or pin which is passed proximally across the fracture site up the femoral neck. Such implants may be 'static' or 'dynamic'. Static implants have no capacity for sliding and therefore cannot allow for any bony collapse that occurs at the fracture site. Examples are the Jewett, Thornton, Holt, and McLaughlin nail plates. Dynamic implants have the capacity for sliding at the plate–screw junction and thereby allow for collapse at the fracture site. Examples of dynamic implants are the Pugh nail, the Massie nail, and the sliding hip screw (also termed the dynamic hip screw and the Ambi hip screw).

Static implants have been comprehensively demonstrated to be inferior to dynamic implants. The complications encountered with static implants were mainly related to penetration of the implant into the hip joint as the fracture collapsed, but in addition there were problems with breakage of the implant and loss of fracture position. Therefore static implants should not be used. Numerous reports, many of them randomized trials, have demonstrated dynamic implants to be the implant of choice for the fixation of the majority of extracapsular femoral fractures.

Cephalic–condylar intramedullary nails

This refers to an intramedullary implant that is passed distally within the femur from an insertion point in or near the greater trochanter. A cross-screw or blade is passed through or around the nail into the femoral neck and head. Early examples of one these nails are the Küntscher Y nail and the Zickle nail. There has been considerable development of these nails over recent years and the more recent designs include the Gamma nail, the proximal femoral nail, and the intramedullary hip screw.

A summary of the results of all randomized trials comparing intramedullary nails with the sliding hip screw for trochanteric hip

Box 12.52.3 Essential preoperative preparation

- Medical assessment
- Anaesthetic assessment
- Resuscitation with intravenous fluids
- Analgesia
- Thromboembolic prophylaxis
- Surgery with 48h of admission if possible
- Perioperative antibiotic prophylaxis
- Treatment of associated medical condition.

Box 12.52.4 Legitimate reasons for delaying surgery

- Hypovolaemia
- Acute dehydration
- Haemoglobin less than about 90–100g/L
- Severe electrolyte imbalance
- Congestive cardiac failure
- Uncontrolled hypertension
- Rectifiable cardiac arrhythmia
- Acute chest condition
- Unstable diabetes mellitus.

Box 12.52.5 Choice of implant

- Extramedullary implant: dynamic implant superior (sliding hip screw); usually implant of choice
- Cephalic–condylar intramedullary nails: higher failure rate than sliding hip screw but may be better for certain fracture types
- External fixation: may have a role in selected cases
- Arthroplasty: probably best reserved for revision surgery.

fractures found no major difference for blood transfusion requirements, length of surgery, lag screw cut-out rate, or mortality. However, there was an increased fixation failure rate and reoperation rate for the intramedullary nails because of the occurrence of secondary fractures around the nail. The controversy between intramedullary and extramedullary fixation is likely to continue with improvements in implant design and surgical technique. Until this issue is resolved it has to be concluded that the sliding hip screw has a lower incidence of complications and therefore is to be preferred for the majority of trochanteric fractures. The evidence in favour of the sliding hip screw hip screw applies for basal fractures and both stable and unstable trochanteric fractures. However, there are specific fracture types in which intramedullary fixation may have advantages and this is discussed next.

External fixation

A number of recent reports have described the use of an external fixator. This can if necessary be applied under local anaesthesia using two proximal pins in the femoral neck and head, and two pins distally. The frame is then retained for about 2–3 months. Complications relate to loss of fracture position and pin tract infection. This method may have a role for those who are very frail and considered at high risk from regional or general anaesthesia.

Arthroplasty

There have been a small number of reports using a long-stem cemented hemiarthroplasty for comminuted trochanteric fractures. Results appear to be comparable with those of internal fixation, but because the number of reports is limited, definite conclusions cannot be made on the place of arthroplasty for extracapsular fractures. At the present time arthroplasty is probably best reserved for revision surgery after failed internal fixation.

Condylar–cephalic intramedullary nails

The two types of condylocephalic nails that have been described are Ender nails and the Harris nail. Ender nails are prebent slightly flexible nails which are passed proximally from an entry point at the femoral condyle up the femur. The aim is to spread the tips of the nails out in the femoral head and stack the femur with three to five nails. The Harris nail is a single larger nail.

Numerous case series and randomized trials have consistently shown that these implants lead to problems with loss of fixation, fracture of the femur at the knee, residual pain at the knee, and an increased reoperation rate. Because of the clear superiority of other implants condylar–cephalic nails should no longer be used.

Surgical technique

The high prevalence of this condition in the elderly has dictated an evolution of treatment which enables immediate mobilization after surgery with full weight bearing. The current armament of implants and developments in surgical techniques allows this to be possible in the vast majority of cases, regardless of the extent of fracture comminution or the degree of osteoporosis. Immediate and unrestricted mobilization following surgery is therefore the aim of modern orthopaedic treatment.

The method of treatment will be determined primarily by the fracture types illustrated in Figure 12.52.1.

Basal fractures

These two-part fractures can be treated similarly to that of a two-part trochanteric fracture using a sliding hip screw. The only difference is that during surgery care should be taken to avoid rotating the femoral head. A supplementary guide wire may be placed across the fracture or an additional screw placed above the lag screw.

Undisplaced two-part trochanteric fractures

These account for approximately 5% of extracapsular fractures. The fracture line may be barely visible and result in the diagnosis initially being missed. The fracture pattern is stable and treatment may be either conservative or operative. For a fit person who is able to comply with a period of protected mobilization, conservative treatment may be considered. Careful follow-up is required and internal fixation is indicated if the fracture displaces, of if pain persists which restricts mobilization. Internal fixation is indicated for the elderly patient who is unable to comply with restricted mobilization.

Surgical treatment with a four-hole sliding hip screw is recommended. Surgical principles are simplified as the fracture need not be reduced.

Displaced two-part trochanteric fractures

These account for approximately 10% of extracapsular fractures. Again a sliding hip screw is the implant of choice. The fracture must first be reduced using the fracture table to either an anatomic position of a position of slight valgus. The most frequent mistake in surgical treatment is failure to reduce the fracture fully from a varus position. The best way to measure adequacy of reduction is using the trabeculae angle which must be between 160–175 degrees following fixation (Figure 12.52.2).

Comminuted trochanteric fractures

This is the most frequent fracture pattern accounting for approximately half of all extracapsular fractures. These fractures can be described as three-part fractures with loss of either lateral support (the greater trochanter), medial support (the lesser trochanter), or as four-part fractures (both the lesser and greater trochanters constitute separate fragments).

The sliding hip screw is again the implant of choice. The most important surgical principle is ensuring adequate fracture reduction. On the anteroposterior view the trabeculae angle must be between 165–170 degrees (Figure 12.52.2). The reduction of the fracture to a slight degree of valgus is recommended, as it offers mechanical advantages in creating stability and significantly reduces the chance of fixation failure. This valgus reduction is normally easily achieved by applying sufficient longitudinal traction to the limb using the fracture table. There is no indication for using an osteotomy with a sliding hip screw or for interoperative compression of the fracture.

A gap at the medial fracture margin may appear on the operative and immediate postoperative radiographs (Figure 12.52.3). This can worry surgeons who have been used to the concept of reconstituting medial bony support when using a fixed nail plate. When a modern dynamic implant is used, the controlled collapse of the fracture that occurs with weight-bearing rapidly results in the restoration of medial bony continuity. In addition a valgus reduction will reduce the chance of leg shortening as the fracture collapses.

On the lateral radiograph it is essential to reduce the fracture to enable the femoral head, neck, trochanteric region, and shaft to be in a straight line (Figure 12.52.4). Longitudinal traction is generally all that is required to achieve this although occasionally 'sag' at the fracture site needs to be corrected during surgery by open reduction.

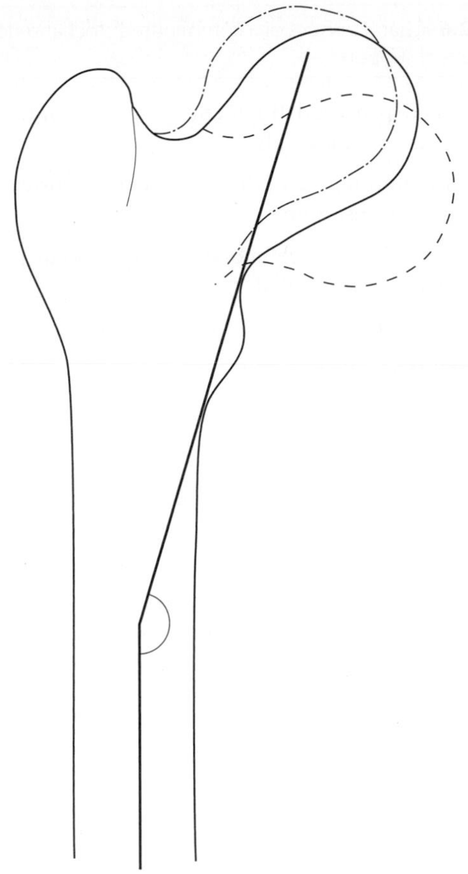

Fig. 12.52.2 Measurement of the trabeculae angle: – • –, valgus position (trabeculae angle more than 160 degrees); – – –, varus position (trabeculae angle less than 160 degrees); —–, normal position (trabeculae angle, 160 degrees). The fracture must never be fixed in a varus position. For a comminuted fracture a reduction angle of 165–170 degrees is recommended.

The position of the lag screw is important in reducing the risk of implant cut-out. All clinical studies on this issue indicate that the placement of the screw should be central/inferior on the anteroposterior radiograph and central on the lateral radiograph. It is essential that superior, anterior, or posterior placement of the screw is avoided at all times. The tip of the lag screw should be 3–7mm from the hip joint. This close placement to the joint ensures maximal hold on the stronger subchondral bone. An assessment of screw placement can be made by measuring the distance from the tip of the lag screw to the apex of the femoral head on both the anteroposterior and lateral radiographs. Cut-out is unlikely if the distance is less than 25mm after correction for magnification. A four-hole plate to achieve a hold on eight femoral cortices distal to the fracture is normally adequate for fixation of this fracture. A plate angle of 135 degrees appears to be optimum, with a higher risk of lag screw malpositioning and cut-out for the higher-angled plates.

Subsequent displacement of the fracture or cutting out of the implant will be rare if the following criteria for adequate fixation are satisfied:

- Reduce the fracture to a trabeculae angle of between 165–170 degrees on the anteroposterior radiograph

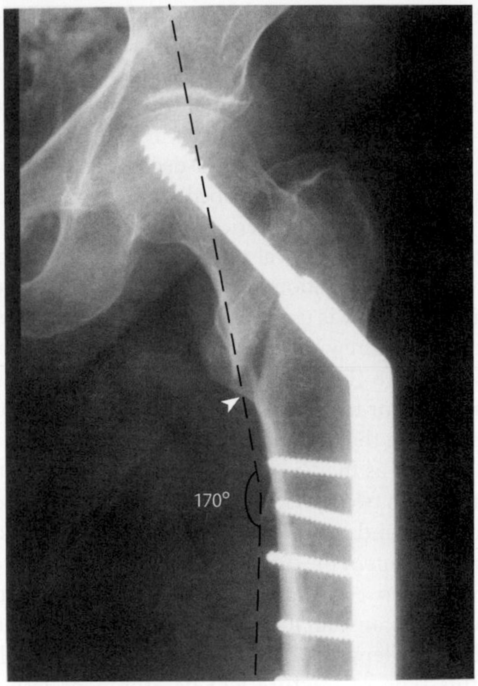

Fig. 12.52.3 A valgus reduction to a trabeculae angle of 170 degrees creates a gap at the medial side of the fracture (arrow), but bony continuity is rapidly restored as the fracture collapses.

- On the lateral radiograph align the femoral head, neck, and shaft in a straight line
- Place the lag screw centrally/inferior on the anteroposterior radiograph
- Place the lag screw centrally on the lateral radiograph
- Medial tip of lag screw should be 3–8mm from the joint
- Lag screw tip–apex distance less than 20mm
- A minimum of eight cortices fixed distal to the fracture.

Comminuted trochanteric fractures without lateral support (Box 12.52.6)

This type of fracture pattern is rare, accounting for approximately 5–10% of extracapsular fractures (Figure 12.52.5). Recognition of

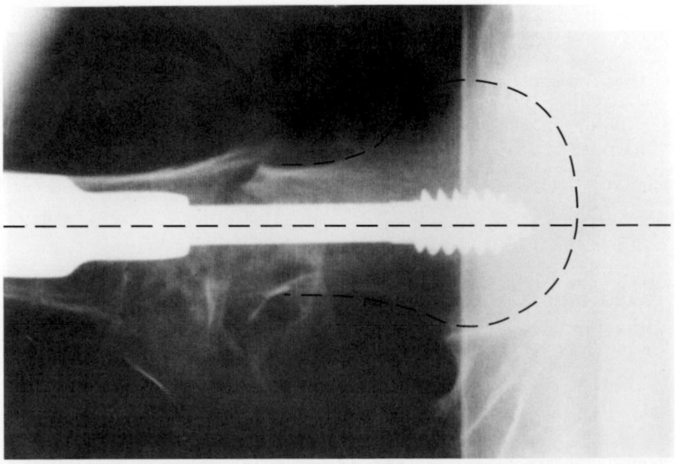

Fig. 12.52.4 On the lateral radiograph a straight line will bisect the femoral head, neck, trochanteric region, and femoral shaft with the lag screw placed centrally.

this fracture pattern may only be apparent during surgery, but there are a number of radiographic characteristics listed in Box 12.52.6, some of which may be apparent preoperatively. This fracture differs from a trochanteric fracture where the greater trochanter is a separate fragment (Jensen type 3), in that the lateral femoral cortex at the site of insertion of a 135-degree lag screw is also fractured. It has previously been described as an internal rotation fracture type or a type II trochanteric fracture. This fracture pattern presents considerable technical problems in treatment and unless special care is taken in fixation there is a high risk of fixation failure.

If a sliding hip screw is used to fix this fracture, at operation the guide wire and lag screw will be inserted directly into the proximal part of the fracture (Figure 12.52.6). There is no lateral femoral cortex to ream prior to insertion of the lag screw. On applying the plate and releasing the traction then the distal fragment invariably displaces medially as there is no lateral cortical support to prevent this. This results in two adverse effects. Firstly, the lag screw rapidly runs out of slide and may penetrate into the joint. Secondly, the medial displacement of the distal fragment reduces the area of bone to bone contact between fragments causing delayed fracture union. These two factors cause an increased incidence of fixation failure.

Invariably the length of lag screw of the sliding hip screw used for this type of fracture will be 80mm or less. If a long barrel (38mm) plate is used there is only 17mm of available slide. As this type of fracture rapidly collapses due to the lack of lateral support the standard sliding hip screw soon runs out of slide. If a sliding hip screw runs out of slide before fracture healing has occurred then invariably the lag screw will cut-out or the plate will come away from the femur. A short barrel (25mm) plate is recommended as it will increase the amount of available slide to 30mm (Figure 12.52.6).

Other than using a short barrel sliding hip screw the same surgical principles listed previously should be followed. Additional care needs to be taken as the lack of soft tissue attachment to the proximal fragment may allow this to rotate, leading to non-union or avascular necrosis. In order to prevent this rotation a supplementary guide wire across the fracture can be inserted during the operation.

Despite the use of this short barrel plate there is still a significant risk of fixation failure caused by the excessive medial displacement of the femur. Attempts have been made to prevent this femoral medialization with a number of new implants, but to date their effectiveness remains unproven. A trochanteric stabilizing plate is an add-on feature for the sliding hip screw plate. It clips over a standard sliding hip screw plate to provide additional lateral stability. In addition, a supplementary screw may be placed proximal to the lag screw to reduce the risk of rotation of the proximal fragment. The percutaneous compression plate (PCCP) is another alternative that has an extension of the side plate proximally to resist femoral medialization. A two-way sliding Medoff plate is another alternative implant with theoretical advantages as sliding can occur in a longitudinal direction.

Alternatively, a cephalic–condylar intramedullary nail has theoretical advantages in this type of fractures as the proximal portion of the nail will prevent the excessive medial displacement of

Box 12.52.6 Characteristics of a comminuted trochanteric fracture without lateral support

- A shortened proximal fragment lying horizontally on the anteroposterior radiograph
- Extensive comminution of the lateral femoral cortex at the site of the lag screw insertion
- Medial migration of the femoral shaft may occur particularly if a sliding hip screw is used
- Angulation at fracture site on the lateral radiograph
- Increases osteoporosis
- Technically harder fractures to achieve adequate fixation
- Greatly increased risk of fixation failure
- Comminuted fractures without lateral support.

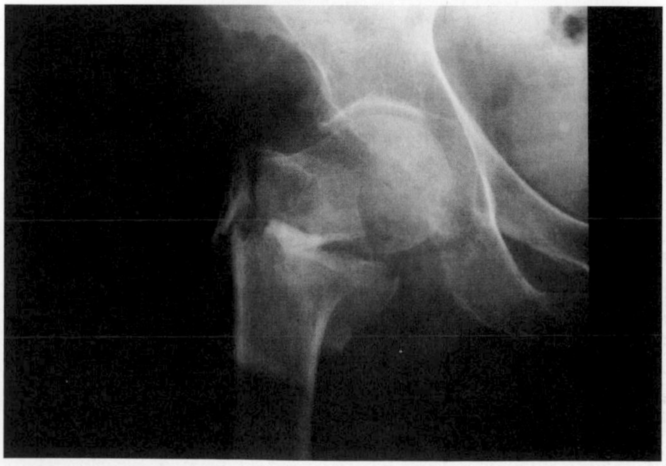

Fig. 12.52.5 A comminuted trochanteric fracture without lateral support.

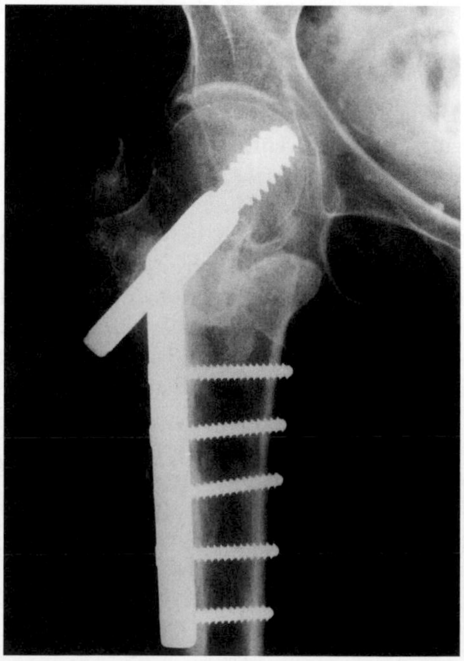

Fig. 12.52.6 Fixation of a comminuted trochanteric fracture with a sliding hip screw.

the femur. In addition, assuming the nail is not locked distally in a static mode, collapse and compression of the fracture can also occur in a longitudinal direction. Because of the increased risk of fixation failure for this particular fracture pattern, primary prosthetic replacement has even been advocated in a small number of studies. A long-stem cemented hemiarthroplasty is generally described as the implant of choice, reconstructing the greater trochanter with wires.

Reversed fracture line (Box 12.52.7)

This is also an unusual fracture pattern, accounting for less than 5% of extracapsular fractures, but recognition is important as it dictates the correct method of treatment. The fracture traversing the femur runs either transversely at the lever of the lesser trochanter or distally in a medial to lateral direction, in contrast to the normal lateral to medial direction of a trochanteric fracture. The fracture line may extend into the subtrochanteric zone. The nature of the fracture means that there is no bony support to prevent medialization of the femur due to the pull of the adductors. Therefore the problems encountered in fixation are similar to a trochanteric fracture with lack of lateral support.

Internal fixation with a sliding hip screw may still be used to good effect, but as the fracture line moves more distally the argument for using an intramedullary nail becomes more compelling. At present however there is inadequate evidence to suggest which method of fixation is best. The use of a static fixation implant such as a dynamic compression plate (DCP) or blade plate has been demonstrated to have a markedly increased risk of fixation failure in comparison to an intramedullary nail.

Trochanteric fracture with subtrochanteric extension

An extension of the fracture line from the trochanteric region to the subtrochanteric region occurs in approximately 5–10% of trochanteric fractures. In other respects this fracture may resemble one of the fracture types described and treatment should be as detailed earlier. The only difference is if a sliding hip screw is used then the length of the plate must be long enough to enable a minimum of eight cortices (four screws) to be anchored in the distal side of the fracture.

'High' subtrochanteric fractures

This fracture has an incidence of approximately 5% of extracapsular fractures. The essential point to differentiate this fracture from a 'low' subtrochanteric fracture is shown in Figure 12.52.7. If a sliding hip screw is used to fix a high subtrochanteric fracture then a dynamic fixation is normally achieved and the surgical principles listed above should be followed. The length of plate used should be sufficient to ensure that four screws are distal to the fracture. Static implants, such as the 95-degree AO blade plate or the dynamic condylar screw should be avoided because of the higher risk of fixation failure compared with the sliding hip screw.

Box 12.52.7 Reversed fracture line

- Less than 5% of extracapsular fractures
- Distal fragment may displace medially
- Increased rate of fixation failure.

More recently attention has been focused on intramedullary fixation of subtrochanteric fractures and as the fracture becomes more distal the argument for such a fixation becomes more convincing.

'Low' subtrochanteric fractures (Box 12.52.8)

These are infrequent fractures accounting for less than 5% of extracapsular fractures. Regardless of which method of treatment is chosen a significant incidence of healing complications including malunion, non-union, and implant breakage has been reported. This is because the bone in this area is subject of high mechanical forces with compressive stresses on the medial side and tensile stresses on the lateral side.

Conservative treatment has been described for this fracture. However, this involves a prolonged period of traction which, as previously discussed, reduces the prospect of successful rehabilitation. Therefore conservative treatment should be reserved only for those indications listed earlier. Operative treatment for this fracture may be either extramedullary or intramedullary fixation.

Extramedullary fixation of this type of fracture with a sliding hip screw will result in a 'static' fixation. The surgical principles of using a sliding hip screw for fixing this fracture therefore differ considerably from those listed previously. Valgus reduction of the fracture is not indicated as it results in a gap at the fracture site medially, which will not be closed by collapse at the fracture site, and an increased risk of non-union and fixation failure is to be expected. Therefore anatomic reduction of the fracture should be performed. It is essential that the sliding hip screw lag screw is

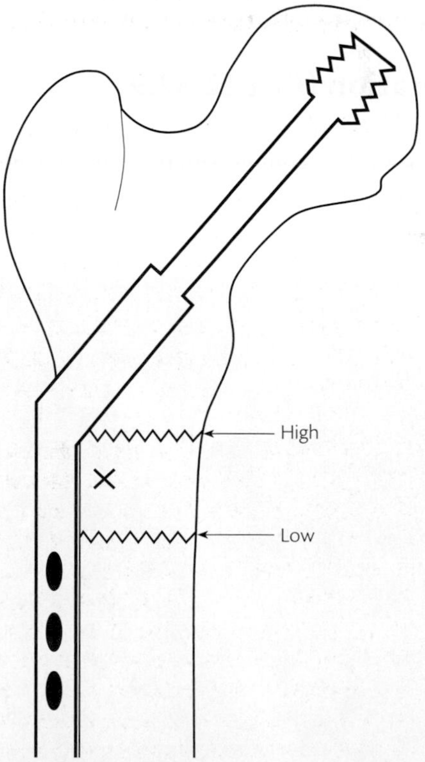

Fig. 12.52.7 Difference between a 'high' and 'low' subtrochanteric fracture. For a low fracture the bone in the proximal fragment in area X prevents the sliding hip screw acting as a dynamic implant. Using a sliding hip screw to fix a 'low' fracture results in a static fixation as opposed to a dynamic fixation with a high fracture.

Box 12.52.8 Low subtrochanteric fracture

- Are probably best treated with an intramedullary nail
- Closed reduction and fixation should normally be possible
- If fixed with an extramedullary implant needs an anatomic reduction.

inserted at exactly 135 degrees (or whichever angle of plate is used), otherwise the long sliding hip screw plate used will cause displacement at the fracture site. Supplementary fixation of additional fragments to restore medial bony support may not be necessary and may even delay healing by devascularizing bony fragments.

Intramedullary fixation of 'low' subtrochanteric fractures has now been well described. The Zickel nail was one of the earliest designs of such a nail but it has now been superseded by improved nail designs. It is essentially that any type of nail has adequate proximal fixation with a lag screw or pin passed up the femoral neck, instrumentation to assist fracture reduction and nail insertion and the capacity for distal locking.

If the lesser trochanter is intact and proximal to the fracture then the proximal femur will become flexed and externally rotated. This means that reduction of the fracture on the fracture table may not be fully possible and the limb may need to be placed in a position of slight external rotation, rather than the neutral position used for a trochanteric fracture. The insertion point on the tip of the greater trochanter for the nail may need to be of adjusted to compensate for this. Generally the fracture can be reduced by closed means using a reduction device or over the nail. The value of supplementary fixation to aid fracture reduction is unproven.

Rehabilitation (Box 12.52.9)

As discussed earlier, the elderly do not tolerate bed-rest well and neither are they able to comply with protected weight-bearing. The objective of any surgical fixation of a hip fracture is not just to stabilize the fracture, but to achieve a fixation that is sufficiently strong enough to allow full weight-bearing. This must be the aim at the outset of surgery and given the current options of modern surgical implants and operative techniques should be achieved in all cases. Failure to be confident enough to allow immediate and unrestricted mobilization following surgery should be considered as a failure of treatment.

Both pre- and postoperatively it is important to discuss rehabilitation and discharge arrangements immediately. Many elderly people on sustaining a hip fracture foresee either death or permanent disability. Patients should therefore be mobilized immediately and told that they cannot damage the security of the fixation. Goals of treatment and rehabilitation plans should be set with the aim for discharge back home as soon as is practicable. This rapid discharge of patients back to the community is to be pursued and has been shown to result in an improved outcome.

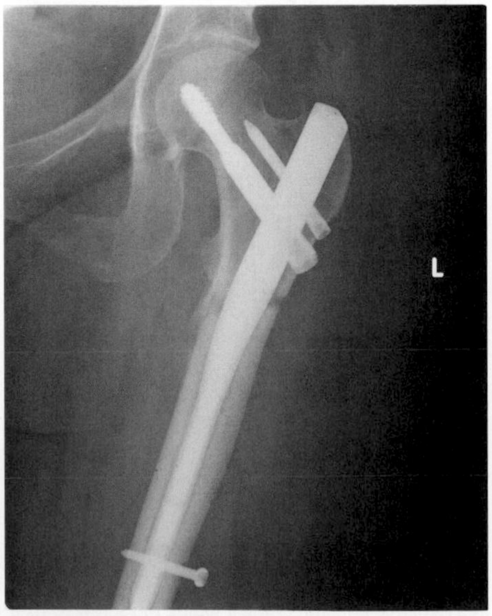

Fig. 12.52.8 Intramedullary nail used to fix a subtrochanteric fracture.

Complications

A number of complications related to fracture healing may be encountered after an extracapsular fracture:

- Limb shortening
- Rotational deformity
- Non-union
- Avascular necrosis
- Cut-out of the implant
- Refracture
- Detachment of the implant from the femur
- Breakage or disassembly of the implant
- Sepsis.

Limb-shortening

This is invariable after conservative treatment as the fracture will heal in a varus position. For operative treatment some collapse may occur at the fracture site as the fracture heals, resulting in about 1–2cm of shortening. This may be reduced if a valgus reduction has been performed. For those situations in which operative treatment fails to maintain fracture reduction, varus angulation will occur which will result in a more noticeable shortening in excess of 2cm.

Rotational deformity

An external rotational deformity is common after conservative treatment. Correct positioning of the patient on the fracture table with the patella lying horizontally should prevent this complication occurring with surgical treatment.

Box 12.52.9 Rehabilitation

- Fixation should allow full weight bearing
- Early mobilization
- Discharge planning on admission.

Non-union

Non-union should only be diagnosed in those fractures which show failure of radiographic union at least 6 months from injury. Before this time, failure for the fracture to unite should be termed delayed union. An increased risk of non-union is associated with subtrochanteric fractures and the use of a fixed nail plate. When a dynamic implant is used to treat a trochanteric fracture non-union is rare, occurring in about 1% of cases.

Non-union is generally symptomatic and should be treated by revision internal fixation and possible also bone grafting the fracture site.

Avascular necrosis

This is a rare complication of a trochanteric fracture in adults and tends to occur mainly in basal fractures in which damage of the blood supply to the femoral head has occurred. A possible iatrogenic cause of avascular necrosis is rotation of the femoral head during insertion of the lag screw. Overall the reported incidence is about 0.5% and treatment, if symptoms indicate, is generally by arthroplasty as for an intracapsular fracture.

Cut-out of the implant

This is the most common problem encountered by both extramedullary and intramedullary implants. It refers to both cut-out of the lag screw from the femoral head and screw penetration into the hip joint. The incidence is much higher for static implants (10–20%) than dynamic implants where, with the correct surgical technique and implant, the incidence should not exceed 3–4%.

Management of cut-out will depend on the degree of symptoms that the patient experiences. If the patient is able to continue to mobilize, the implant should be retained and then removed if necessary once the fracture has healed. Severe symptoms will necessitate surgical revision which may take the form of repeat internal fixation or replacement arthroplasty.

Refracture

This may take the form of fracture above, around, or below an implant or previous fracture. Fracture proximal to the lag screw is uncommon and in some cases has been attributed to failure to place the tip of the lag screw in the subchondral bone. Fracture immediately below an extramedullary fixation implant is rare. The use of a short intramedullary nail is, however, associated with an approximate risk of 2% for fracture around the distal part of the implant. Such fractures may be treated either conservatively with traction or, more commonly, with repeat internal fixation.

Detachment of the implant from the femur

This complication of extramedullary fixation has an incidence of about 1–3%. It is associated with either femoral medialization and consumption of lag screw slide, non-union of the fracture, or a subtrochanteric fracture extension.

Breakage or disassembly of the implant

Breakage of the older fixed nail plates such as the McLaughlin and Thornton nail plates is well documented with an incidence of 5–10%. Breakage of the newer implants is, however, rare and when it does occur it is invariably associated with delayed union of the fracture. Treatment is therefore similar to that for non-union of the fracture. Disassembly of the implant is rare with modern implants and is generally due to imperfect surgery.

Box 12.52.10 Outcome

- 1-year survival is 70%
- 10% mortality from hip fracture
- 80–90% of survivors return to original residence.

Sepsis

Sepsis is rare after conservative treatment. After internal fixation the incidence of deep sepsis (infection around the implant) is approximately 0.5% and that for superficial sepsis around 4%. There is no difference in the risk of sepsis between extramedullary and intramedullary fixation.

Superficial sepsis may be treated with antibiotics and wound debridement if indicated. Deep sepsis is a more devastating complication, but fortunately the hip joint is generally not affected and may be preserved. Occasionally the implant may be retained whilst the fracture heals, but generally it needs to be removed and the fracture left to heal by conservative methods.

Outcome (Box 12.52.10)

The prognosis after an extracapsular fracture is worse than after an intracapsular fracture. The reason for this is that patients with an extracapsular fracture tend to be older and frailer than those with an intracapsular fracture. Overall reports of mortality and morbidity after a hip fracture vary considerable. At 1 year from injury about 30% of patients will have died, but in many cases the death can be attributed to other causes associated with aging. The actual mortality attributed to the hip fracture will be about 10%.

Regarding morbidity, it should be possible for about 80–90% of the survivors to return to their original residence, albeit generally with increased social support and assistance. The remaining patients will need a change of accommodation to a more dependent environment. Long-term pain in the hip is uncommon and less prevalent with an extracapsular fracture compared with an intracapsular fracture.

Further reading

Chinoy, M.A., and Parker, M.J. (1999). Fixed nail plates versus sliding hip systems for the treatment of trochanteric femoral fractures: a meta-analysis of 14 comparative studies. *Injury*, **30**, 157–63.

Hornby, R., Grimley Evans, J. and Vardon, V. (1989). Operative or conservative treatment for trochanteric fractures of the femur: a randomised epidemiological trial in elderly patients. *Journal of Bone and Joint Surgery, British Volume*, **71B**, 619–23.

Keene, G.S., Parker, M.J and Pryor, G.A. (1993). Mortality and morbidity after hip fracture. *British Medical Journal*, **307**, 1248–50.

Parker, M.J., and Handoll, H.H.G. (2005). Gamma and other cephalocondylic intramedullary nails versus extramedullary implants for extracapsular hip fractures. *Cochrane Database of Systematic Reviews*, Issue 4. Chichester: Wiley.

Parker, M.J, and Handoll, H.H.G. (2006b). Replacement arthroplasty versus internal fixation for extracapsular hip fractures. *Cochrane Database of Systematic Reviews*, Issue 4. Chichester: Wiley

12.53

Femur shaft fractures

Thomas A. DeCoster and Zhiqing Xing

Summary points

- Intramedullary reamed nailing provides very good results
- Antegrade and retrograde nailing give similar results
- Associated injuries increase the risk of complications.

Incidence and prevalence

The incidence of femur shaft fractures in the United States of America is 1 per 10 000 population per year. They frequently result from high-energy trauma and associated injuries are common. With appropriate treatment, most patients are able to return to pre-injury function and long-term serious sequelae are uncommon.

Anatomy

The femur is the largest bone in the body. It functions mechanically to transmit load, maintain the length of the limb, and anchor muscles for weight bearing and locomotion. The shaft of the femur is that area distal to the lesser trochanter and proximal to the condyles.

The shaft contains the isthmus which is the narrowest portion of the medullary canal. The femoral shaft is bowed convex anteriorly by 10 degrees. There are several paths to the medullary canal proximally. The most direct is through a small fossa at the posteromedial base of the greater trochanter where the piriformis tendon inserts. Entry to the canal from the nearly subcutaneous tip of the greater trochanter is easier but offset from the medullary canal. Distally, direct access to the medullary canal can be obtained through the articular cartilage anterior to the intercondylar notch for rigid nails.

Associated pathology (Box 12.53.1)

When the femoral shaft fractures, it not only disrupts the skeletal integrity of the limb and precludes ambulating but also has major systemic consequences. These include blood loss, marrow embolization, and acute respiratory distress syndrome (ARDS). Femur shaft fractures are a common component of multiple trauma and the optimal treatment involves application of the principles of damage control.

Box 12.53.1 Associated pathology

- Frequently part of polytrauma
- Blood loss
- ARDS
- Embolization
- Neck of femur fractures (10%)
- Knee injuries (15–50%).

Associated injuries to the same limb are common. Communicating open wounds are present in about 10% of cases. Associated neurological and superficial or profunda femoral artery injuries are rare with an incidence of less than 1% and 1% respectively. Associated fractures in the same limb are common and the surgeon must be particularly aware of a 10% possibility of an ipsilateral femoral neck fracture. Thirty per cent of associated neck fractures are initially missed. Knee injuries occur in 15–50% of femoral shaft fractures. Injuries to other systems are also common. In prospective study the average Injury Severity Score in patients with femoral shaft fractures was 20.

Mechanism

Femur shaft fractures are major injuries. A large amount of force is required to break the thick cortical bone of the shaft which is covered circumferentially by muscles. Motor vehicle collisions and other high-energy mechanisms cause the vast majority of femur shaft fractures in Europe and North America. Falls may cause femur shaft fractures in the elderly.

Classification

The comprehensive classification of fractures published by the Orthopaedic Trauma Association (OTA) is the most logical system for classifying fractures of the femoral shaft.

Clinical evaluation

The history, physical examination, and early treatment should be dictated by ATLS® guidelines. Any patient who has sustained a femoral shaft fracture has experienced a high-energy injury that may involve multiple systems. Blood loss from a femur shaft fracture is considerable and it is possible to exsanguinate into the thigh. About one-third of patients with isolated femur shaft fractures require transfusion. However, it is dangerous and usually inappropriate to attribute hypotension to blood loss from a femur shaft fracture, other sources of bleeding must be excluded.

With regard to the femoral shaft fracture, the time and mechanism of injury, neurovascular function, and condition of the skin should all be determined and documented. Neurovascular status and integrity of the skin should be assessed and documented. Compartment syndrome of the thigh associated with a femoral shaft fracture is uncommon. Assessment for knee ligament injuries is difficult in the acute setting, but should be reassessed following stabilization.

Investigation

Plain x-rays should be obtained which show the hip and knee as well as the femoral shaft. Hip dislocation and femoral neck fractures should be identified. These patients will frequently have had computed tomography (CT) scans that include the femoral necks. Even under these circumstances some femoral neck fractures will be missed. An x-ray of the contralateral femur can be helpful in determining appropriate reduction length of the fractured femur when placing a static locked nail, especially in segmental multifragmentary fractures. More complex imaging studies are not usually necessary to manage routine femoral shaft fractures.

Management (Box 12.53.2)

Initial

It is advantageous to stabilize the fracture with internal or external fixation as soon as possible. However, initial emergency treatment of femoral shaft fractures should include splintage. When definitive treatment is delayed the patient will benefit from balanced suspension and proximal tibial skeletal traction with sufficient weight to slightly distract the fracture. Traction increases patient comfort, facilitates transfers during work-up and treatment of other injuries, partially immobilizes the fracture, and maintains length prior to definitive treatment. Distal femoral traction should be considered when there is clear evidence of a knee injury.

Box 12.53.2 Treatment

- ATLS®
- Splintage
- Early stabilization recommended
- Plating
- External fixation
- Intramedullary nail.

Definitive

Internal fixation by intramedullary nailing is currently the best treatment for the vast majority of femur shaft fractures. However, in certain situations, traction, plating, and external fixation can be considered

Traction

Traction may be appropriate when other techniques are not available or not possible. Approximately one-seventh body weight skeletal traction is applied through a pin placed transversely in the proximal tibial metaphysis. Balanced suspension of the lower extremity is achieved by use of a Thomas splint with a Pearson attachment with the hip and knee at 45 degrees of flexion. The traction needs to be adjusted and corrected daily. Reduction is checked weekly. Active range of motion of the hip and knee is encouraged as soon as the patient will tolerate it. Mobilization in a splint or cast brace with crutches is usually possible by 4–6 weeks.

Plating

Traditional femoral plating requires neither fluoroscopy nor as much other special instrumentation as medullary nailing. It is performed in the supine position on a regular operating table without traction. Classic plating requires extensive dissection resulting in blood loss and soft tissue injury. In most series, plating has a lower rate of union and higher rates of refracture, infection, and stiffness than nailing. Direct fracture visualization is detrimental to callus formation due to increased soft tissue stripping. However, it does simplify treatment, which may be particularly important in complex injuries such as fractures at multiple levels of the femur or when the medullary canal will not accept a nail. Plating in selected high-risk patients, may be associated with a lower incidence of pulmonary complications than medullary nailing. In these patients new techniques utilizing percutaneous submuscular locking plates have been described to minimize soft tissue dissection.

External fixation

Some multiple trauma patients appear to be harmed more than helped by early total care and damage control orthopaedics has been recommended. Staged use of external fixation is an effective component of damage control orthopaedics for severe multiple trauma cases. External fixation is effective initial treatment in severely injured patients, as it is applicable to nearly all fracture patterns with no special equipment requirements and can be applied rapidly. It allows access to the wound for debridement and ongoing care, and stabilizes the limb sufficiently to allow mobilization of the patient and an upright chest for better pulmonary function. After several days, when the patient's overall condition is more stable, the fixator is converted to a nail. Infection rates after early conversion to a nail are low.

The long-term use of external fixation in femur shaft fractures can be successful but is associated with pin track problems, delayed union, malunion, and knee stiffness. The large muscular soft tissue envelope of the thigh contributes to the pin track problem. The large forces across the femur during ambulation are difficult to control by a fixator. Instability of the construct contributes to the problems of delayed union and loss of reduction.

Intramedullary nailing: technique

A preoperative plan is developed including anticipated size and position of the implant (nail length and width, locking screw position), and to ensure that all necessary instrumentation and implants are available.

Antegrade supine position, piriformis entry site (Figure 12.53.1)

The procedure can be performed without traction on a radiolucent table or with traction on a fracture table.

If traction is used the patient is positioned supine and the legs are 'scissored' or the contralateral leg is placed with the hip and knee flexed and the hip abducted (Figure 12.53.2). Traction is applied to the injured limb through a boot or proximal tibial traction pin. A bar in the perineum provides counter traction. Rotation of the fluoroscopy C arm provides anteroposterior and lateral views. An incision is placed approximately 8cm proximal to the tip of the trochanter in line with the shaft of the femur. The desired entry point into the bone is the piriformis fossa, which is extracapsular and can be located at the junction of the trochanter and femoral neck just medial and posterior to the tip of the trochanter. A sharp awl or guide pin is placed and position is confirmed by biplanar image. The entry site is opened for 5cm in line with the shaft by a cannulated power reamer if a guide wire is used, or by an awl. A cannulated entry tool facilitates placement of subsequent instruments in the medullary canal, helps to remove medullary reamings and protects the soft tissues of the hip. If a cannulated nail or intramedullary reaming is planned, a guide wire is then passed down the medullary canal to the fracture site. Under fluoroscopic control, traction and manipulation are utilized to facilitate passage of the guide across the fracture into the medullary canal of the distal fragment.

If reaming is performed it proceeds sequentially initially in 1-mm and then in 0.5-mm increments. The first reamer is end-cutting for easier passage. The use of well-fluted sharp power reamers will minimize pressure on the medullary canal and embolization of medullary contents into the vascular system. Over-reaming by 1.0–1.5mm facilitates ease of nail insertion. Depending on the type

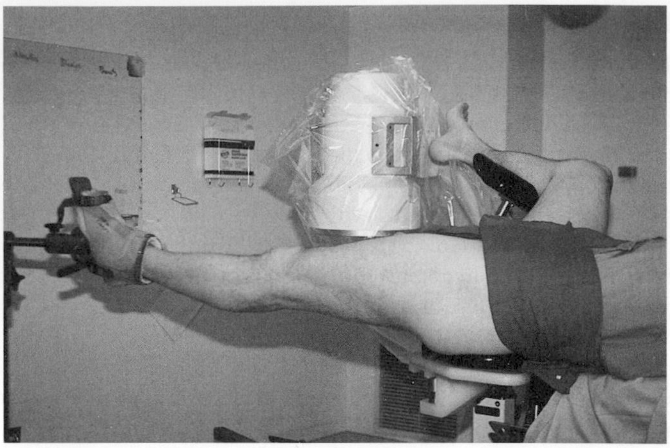

Fig. 12.53.2 Intraoperative position for antegrade left femoral nailing. The body is bent to the right and the left arm is held over the chest to avoid obstructing the instrumention.

of nail used, the proximal femur entry point may need to be further over-reamed. Since the introduction of interlocking, the most common nail diameters range between 11–12mm. There is no need for the routine use of very large nails with tight endosteal fit. Care is taken to match the anterior bow of the nail to that of the femur and to maintain rotation of both the fracture reduction and nail itself during insertion.

Proximal locking is through a nail-mounted guide and involves placement of one or two bicortical screws through the nail in the mid-coronal plane either transversely or obliquely between the greater and lesser trochanter. Reconstruction nails allow proximal locking into the femoral neck. Distal locking is achieved under image control by placing one or two screws in the coronal plane through the nail with bicortical purchase. A variety of techniques are described for accurate distal locking. Modern nails offer dynamic and static locking options.

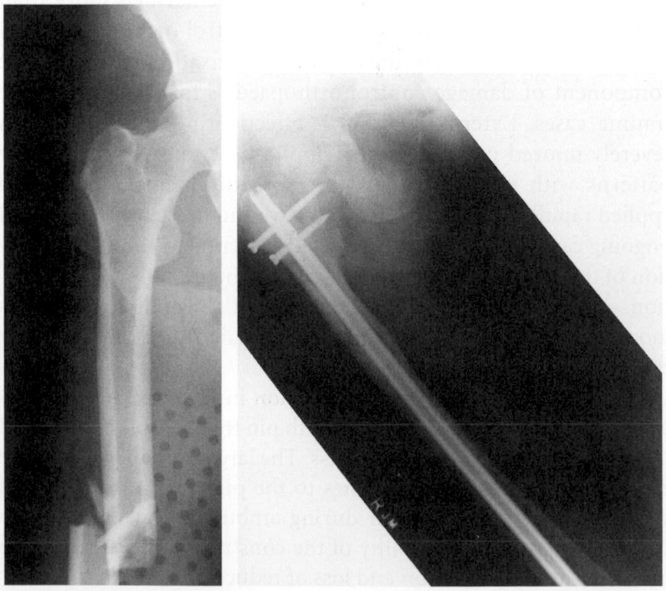

A B

Fig. 12.53.1 Antegrade femoral nail: A) AP radiograph of a right femoral shaft fracture; B) AP radiograph demonstrates healing after antegrade nailing of femoral shaft fracture with proximal interlocking.

Antegrade supine position, trochanteric entry

Because of difficulty with accessing the piriformis fossa as well as the occurrence of chronic hip pain and abductor weakness after antegrade nailing with a piriformis entry point, nailing systems have been developed to utilize a more lateral entry point on the greater trochanter. This entry point can be surgically accessed without muscle penetration and is much closer to the skin. The trochanteric entry site is lateral to the medullary canal of the femur and requires an additional coronal plane bend in the manufacturing of the nail. Studies have shown the trochanteric entry point nails can be associated with less blood loss and operative time and there is suggestion of improved function with less hip pain and abductor weakness. Healing rates and functional recovery from the fracture itself are equivalent to piriformis nailing.

The optimum position of the entry point is dependent on the coronal plane bend in the proximal nail and this varies depending on design and manufacturer. Failure to accurately place the entry point will result in varus/valgus malalignment. The majority of trochanteric entry point nails are designed to be inserted at the tip of the trochanter in the coronal plane. Varus malalignment is to be avoided and this is seen when a more lateral entry point is used. In the sagittal plane the entry point should be in line with the centre of the femoral canal. However, when using a cephalomedullary

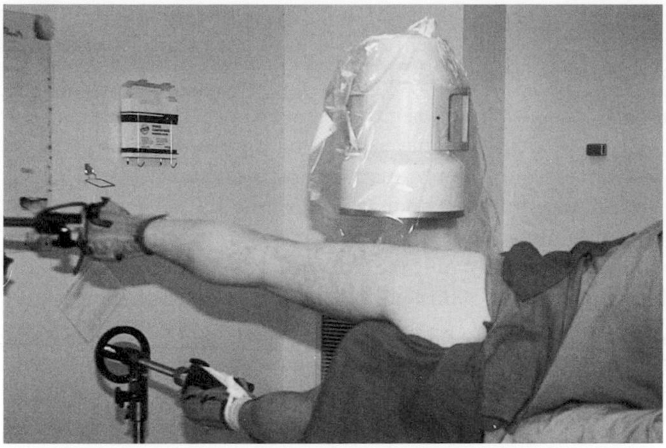

Fig. 12.53.3 Intraoperative position for lateral antegrade nailing is demonstrated with the patient on the fracture table with a bar between the thighs for counter traction and traction on the affected limb. The contralateral (down) limb is also supported and flexed at the hip to allow positioning of the C-arm.

device it has been recommended that the junction of the anterior third and posterior two-thirds of the greater trochanter facilitates alignment of the implant with the femoral neck.

Antegrade lateral position (Figure 12.53.3)

Intramedullary femoral nailing can also be performed in the lateral position where access to the piriformis fossa is much easier. This position is advantageous in large patients and proximal fracture patterns. Initial positioning is more time-consuming and there is an increased incidence of external rotation deformity.

Retrograde femoral nailing (Figure 12.53.4)

Retrograde nailing is performed with the patient supine on the radiolucent operating table with the lower extremity prepared and draped. Access to the knee joint is obtained through or medial to the patellar tendon. The entry site for a retrograde nail is at the top of the intercondylar notch through cartilage, which does not articulate with the patella. Retrograde femoral nailing offers the advantage of easier access to the starting point as the distal femur is not surrounded by muscle. In addition, patient positioning is easy since the fracture table is not used. There are a number of clinical situations in which retrograde nailing has apparent clinical advantages.

Positioning on the fracture table may not be well tolerated by patients with unstable pelvic ring or spine fractures. The proximal incision for antegrade nailing may compromise the approach for acetabular surgery. Set up time can be minimized for bilateral lower-extremity fractures requiring prompt fixation. Ipsilateral lower limb injuries (distal femur, tibia shaft or patella) in addition to the femoral shaft may be dealt with through a single knee incision. In patients with gross obesity positioning on the fracture table and the extensive mass of soft tissue at the hip are problems. In pregnancy there is theoretical reduction in the exposure to the fetus. The entry site problems (hip for antegrade and knee for retrograde) are equivalent. Early results with retrograde nailing suggested a higher non-union rate. However, small diameter and unreamed nails were initially used and more recent reports with standard diameter reamed nails show the union rates of antegrade and retrograde nails are similar.

There are concerns, with this technique, about direct damage to the knee joint, indirect damage from joint debris, and septic arthritis in open fractures. The significance of these problems has not been demonstrated in clinical studies.

Unreamed nailing

It is possible to treat femoral shaft fractures with smaller diameter nails inserted without reaming the canal. The results with this technique have not been as good as with standard nails inserted after reaming. Unreamed nails have higher rates of complications including malunion and delayed union, which are probably related

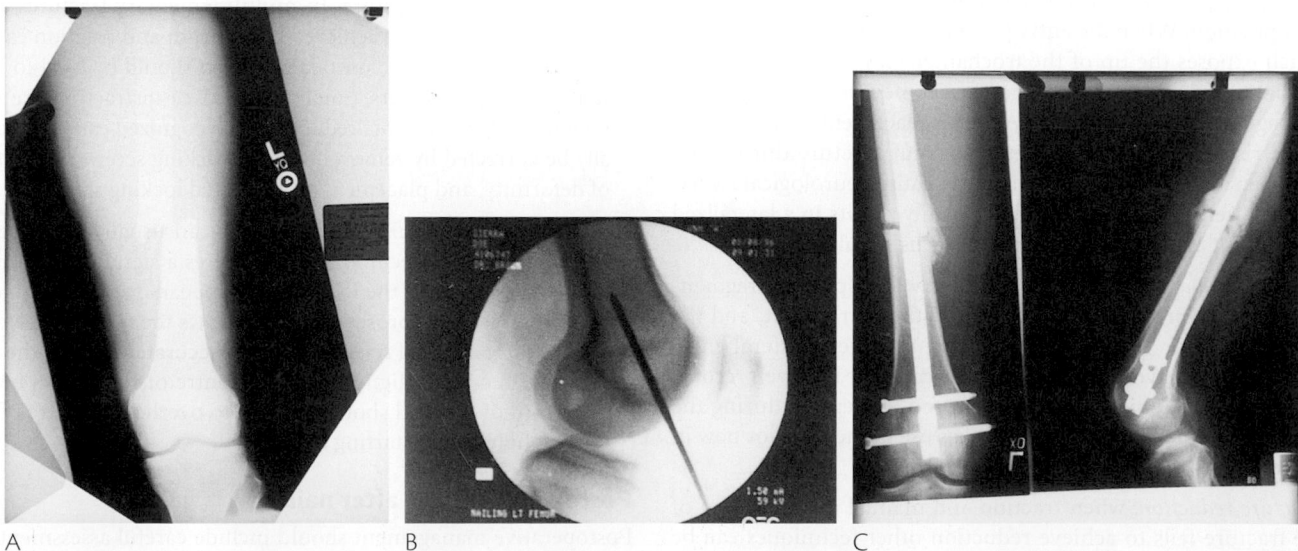

Fig. 12.53.4 Retrograde femoral nail. A) AP radiograph of a left femoral shaft fracture. B) Intraoperative lateral fluoroscopy demonstrating guide pin for starting position for retrograde femoral nailing technique. The entry point is in the middle of the femur on both the AP and lateral radiographic projection. C) Anteroposterior and lateral radiographs show partial healing 4 weeks after retrograde femoral nailing. Note the position of the nail seated 5mm beneath subchondral bone in the centre of the medullary canal.

Box 12.53.3 Femoral nail set-up

- Supine antegrade piriformis entry point:
  - Common set-up
  - Difficult access to piriformis fossa in large patients, optimize patient position
- Supine antegrade trochanteric entry point:
  - Easier access to entry point
  - Less damage to hip abductors
  - Be careful to avoid valgus malalignment
- Lateral, antegrade:
  - Easier access to trochanteric and piriformis entry points
  - Useful in large patients and proximal fractures
  - Associated with external rotation malalignment
- Retrograde:
  - Traction table not required
  - Useful in polytrauma and obese patients
  - Violates knee.

to the small size of the nail relative to the medullary canal and the tendency for excessive motion or overloading the implant prior to fracture healing. However, unreamed nails are quicker and avoid the high intramedullary pressures seen with reaming. This is considered by some to have advantages in the polytrauma patient.

Common technical problems

- *Patient positioning:* anticipation of problems related to the fracture pattern, body habitus, and fracture table helps to ensure appropriate positioning
- *Entry point:* the correct starting point is crucial to the success of the operation. When the entry point is difficult, a longer incision which exposes the tip of the trochanter may be necessary. The medial tip of the greater trochanter can be removed to prevent slippage of the insertion tool. Anterior placement of the starting point risks creation of a proximal femur fracture during nail insertion and posterior placement can cause neurological injury. Avoid eccentric reaming, this commonly results in a lateralized entry point and increases the risk of varus malalignment
- *Fracture propagation:* careful technique will help avoid fragmentation of the proximal femur, around the entry point, and the subtrochanteric medial cortex during passage of lateral entry point nails. To avoid the latter complication it has been recommended that the nail should be rotated 90 degrees during the early part of the insertion. This makes use of the anterior bow in the femoral nail
- *Fracture reduction:* when traction and manual manipulation of the fracture fails to achieve reduction other techniques can be used. The use of an external reduction clamp, F-tool, crutch or internal cannulated reduction tool have all been described. Direct manipulation of either fragment can be facilitated by placement of threaded pins proximal and distal to the fracture, using the pins as a joy stick to obtain reduction. As a last resort the fracture can be opened however the vast majority of femoral nails can be accomplished closed
- *Failure to advance reamer:* the reamer can become stuck and this can be prevented by never stopping the reamer while in bone, advancing only slowly, maintaining reduction while reaming, using deep fluted reamers and cleaning the flutes before they become impacted with bone, maintaining sharp reamers, and increasing size by only 0.5mm from the previous reamer. The reamer should be constantly moving to avoid thermal necrosis
- *Failure to advance nail:* this can be prevented by over-reaming the medullary canal by 1–2mm, maintaining reduction throughout the procedure, and utilization of the correct starting position. The nail should advance with each blow. If it does not, further insertion risks nail incarceration or fragment comminution. Nail removal and further reaming or use of a smaller nail is recommended
- *Accurate nail length:* following placement of the reduction guidewire, a measurement taken of a second guidewire, placed parallel with the tip at the greater trochanter, gives an accurate measurement. It is recommended that the tip of an antegrade nail should be distal to the superior pole of the patella and the tip of a retrograde nail should be proximal to the lesser trochanter. A nail cap is advisable to ease removal and has the limited ability to compensate for a nail that is too short
- *Malreduction:* assessment of length and rotation should be performed before and after nail placement and nail locking. In fractures of the proximal or distal fifth of the shaft, coronal malalignment is common since there is minimal contact between the medullary endosteum and the nail wall. It is important to centre the guide in the short fragment and maintain the reduction during reaming and nail insertion to avoid eccentric placement of the nail and coronal malreduction. This is uncommon in femoral mid-shaft fractures. For proximal fifth fractures, malposition of the entry point can also lead to apex anterior angulation of the nailed fracture. In multifragmentary fractures were direct reduction is not achieved both length and rotation can be difficult to judge. The contralateral limb should be used to help judge these parameters. Small amounts of distraction are well tolerated. Significant malreduction, if recognized early, can usually be corrected by removal of distal locking screws, correction of deformity, and placement of new distal locking screws
- *Difficulty distal locking:* distal locking can usually be achieved with the freehand technique but requires a significant learning curve. Ensuring that the locking hole appears perfectly round in the centre of the fluoroscopy screen allows the C arm to be used as a valuable external reference. When accurately set-up, the axis of the drill can be aligned with the centre of the C-arm beam. The point of the drill should be seen to overlie the centre of the locking hole before starting to drill.

Postoperative care after nailing

Postoperative management should include careful assessment for correct length and rotation. This should ideally be assessed when the patient is still in the operating room after removing the patient from traction, and again when the patient is mobilizing postoperatively. Rotation should be assessed by comparing the range of hip rotation between the injured and non-injured sides. Radiographs of the femur should be obtained to assess the position of the implant and locking screws, and as a basis of comparison for later films used to assess healing. Fixation is usually sufficient to allow early partial weight bearing as nails are load-sharing devices. Range of motion exercises for the hip and knee should be instituted early in the postoperative course.

Removal

The evidence suggests that retained nails do not cause predictable problems and that totally elective removal should be reserved for selected cases. Patients with specific symptoms like trochanteric bursitis over a prominent nail could expect their condition to improve after nail removal. Incomplete resolution of preoperative symptoms commonly occurs. Vague symptoms like 'cold intolerance' or 'thigh ache' often persist after nail removal and may relate to the healed fracture rather than the presence of the nail. Concerns about infection and fretting corrosion have so far proved unfounded. A variety of complications have been reported with nail removal including an increased cosmetic problem from using a larger incision than required for nail placement, haematoma, infection, femur fracture, and inability to extract the nail. The last problem is minimized by ensuring the correct equipment is available. Removal more than 2 years after implantation is particularly difficult due to bony ingrowth. If nail extraction is difficult, overdrilling locking screw paths or unfilled locking screw holes and passage of a driving guide inside the nail may break up a bone bridge, which is preventing nail removal. Enlarging the entry hole at the top of the femur by inserting narrow straight osteotomes along the proximal 3cm of the nail circumferentially is particularly important for removing 'shouldered' nails. Removal of titanium nails has not proved to be any more difficult than stainless steel nails despite the theoretical concern of bone ingrowth and difficult extraction.

Broken nails can generally be removed by placement of a ball-tipped guide out the distal end and gaining an interference fit by stacking additional guides inside the nail. Over-reaming of the proximal canal is helpful. A variety of other hooks have been described for removing broken nails. When other measures fail, a distal incision may be utilized to drive the nail from distal to proximal.

Post removal radiographic evaluation is important to detect femoral fractures and confirm implant removal.

Special circumstances

Multiple trauma

Early stabilization of long-bone fractures in patients with multiple trauma has been shown to increase patient survival and decrease pulmonary complications. Standard techniques can generally be utilized. In patients with severe multiple trauma damage control orthopaedic techniques with initial application of an external fixator and early exchange to a nail are popular as described in the section on external fixation. Other modifications of nailing technique that are used in damage control include second-stage placement of distal locking screws to avoid prolonged operative time, placement of smaller diameter nails with less reaming and retrograde nails. Percutaneous submuscular plating of femoral shaft fractures has also been advocated as a means of avoiding pulmonary complications from intramedullary nailing.

A variety of techniques have been recommended as alternatives to the use of a fracture table to simplify positioning in severely injured patients. Manual traction has been reported as successful in polytrauma patients. The authors emphasized the importance of an accurate preoperative plan for length. However this technique can be associated with a high incidence of non-anatomical reduction. The femoral distractor can be used to generate traction and improve alignment without the use of a fracture table. The proximal pin is placed into the lesser trochanter through the anterior thigh and medial to where the nail will be located. The distal pin is placed in the lateral femoral condyle anterior and distal to the nail.

Bifocal injuries

Combination neck and shaft fractures

Approximately 10% of femoral shaft fractures are associated with an ipsilateral fracture of the femoral neck. Many of these are not appreciated on initial evaluation and have been termed missed, occult, or iatrogenic. Femoral neck fractures which become apparent after nailing may have been present initially and subsequently displace as a result of the nailing or have been caused by the insertion of the nail.

A variety of treatments of these combination injuries have been suggested. Operative stabilization of both fractures is indicated. The complications associated with femoral neck fractures (avascular necrosis, non-union, malunion) are generally more severe and more difficult to treat than complications of the femoral shaft fracture; therefore, treatment of the shaft should not put the neck fracture at unnecessary risk. Multiple screws or dynamic hip screw and side plate is the standard treatment of femoral neck fractures in young adults. These typically block the proximal medullary canal preventing standard antegrade nailing. Plating or retrograde nailing are then the preferred alternate techniques to treat the femur shaft fracture. The reported results have been satisfactory. Antegrade nailing of the shaft with screws placed around the nail and then across the femoral neck fracture may be ideal for minimally displaced fractures which become apparent after nail placement. However, an 18% major complication rate when this technique was used routinely. Nails with proximal locking into the head and neck of the femur have been used for the combined neck shaft injury and reported to achieve good results. When using this technique it is important to obtain reduction of the femoral neck fracture and maintain it during the procedure (using a pin), and to obtain good fixation with screws well positioned in the head. Anatomical reduction of the femoral neck fracture should be confirmed radiographically and when in doubt by direct visualization. The canal must be over-reamed so the nail can be rotated freely to match the anteversion of the femoral neck. Only in this way will the proximal locking screws obtain central position in the femoral head. Fluoroscopic imaging is partially obscured by the nail, but confirmation of central placement is essential.

Shaft plus distal femur

Another type of bifocal femoral fracture is the shaft and distal femur. Operative stabilization of both fractures is recommended. A multitude of different techniques of internal fixation are available depending upon the fracture patterns. Antegrade nailing of the shaft fracture and lateral plating of the distal femur fracture have been the traditional treatments. Plating both fractures has also been reported, especially with a long lateral locking plate. Retrograde nailing as a single method for both fractures is a more recent development and results are generally good and superior to other techniques. The relative infrequency of this injury combination prevents definitive assessment of the optimal technique.

Ipsilateral tibia and femur (Figure 12.53.5)

The phrase 'floating knee' has been used to describe ipsilateral fractures of the tibia and femur shaft. Knee stiffness and delayed union of one or the other fracture were identified as common consequences of non-operative treatment. Operative stabilization of both fractures has given the best results. Retrograde nailing of the femur and nailing of the tibia have produced very good results. Many series have included various combinations of different major fractures of the femur and tibia. The intra-articular components of these fractures and the soft tissue injuries typically play a major role in determining outcome.

Femur shaft plus knee ligament

Following stabilization of a femur shaft fracture, ligamentous examination of the ipsilateral knee should always be performed. Ipsilateral knee ligament injuries occur commonly and are often missed. The femur shaft fracture may divert the patient and doctor from recognition of knee ligament injury. Until the fracture is stabilized physical examination of the knee is extremely difficult and unreliable. Early recognition and treatment of associated knee joint injuries will optimize outcome.

Open femoral shaft fractures

All femur shaft fractures have some degree of soft tissue injury even in the presence of intact skin but open femur shaft fractures have a higher complication rate, in particular infection and delayed union. Soft tissue management is the key to optimizing results and the type of skeletal fixation is of less importance. The classic treatment for most open femur fractures has been temporary or definitive external fixation and this remains a reasonable option, particularly for femur fractures associated with severe open wounds. Intramedullary nailing of many open femur fractures can be performed successfully and safely, and if infection can be avoided offers many advantages over external fixation, such as better alignment and less knee stiffness.

Grade 3C open femur shaft fractures are injuries which require repair of the femoral or popliteal artery. Although revascularization is usually possible, the functional outcome after this severe injury is often poor.

Special patients

Young patients

Avascular necrosis of the femoral head has been reported in children and adolescents treated with medullary nails and this is a devastating complication. The blood supply to the femoral head in a patient with an open physis is very dependent on the circumflex artery which runs along the posterior neck at the junction with the trochanter. This is very near the piriformis fossa, the classic starting point for femoral nailing. Trochanteric entry nails may avoid the blood supply to the femoral head and are now generally preferred to piriformis entry nails when rigid nailing of adolescent femur shaft fractures is chosen. The trochanteric apophysis may undergo premature closure but this is unlikely to cause any significant problem for patients older than the age of 10 years. The nail should stop proximal to the distal physis if it is still open.

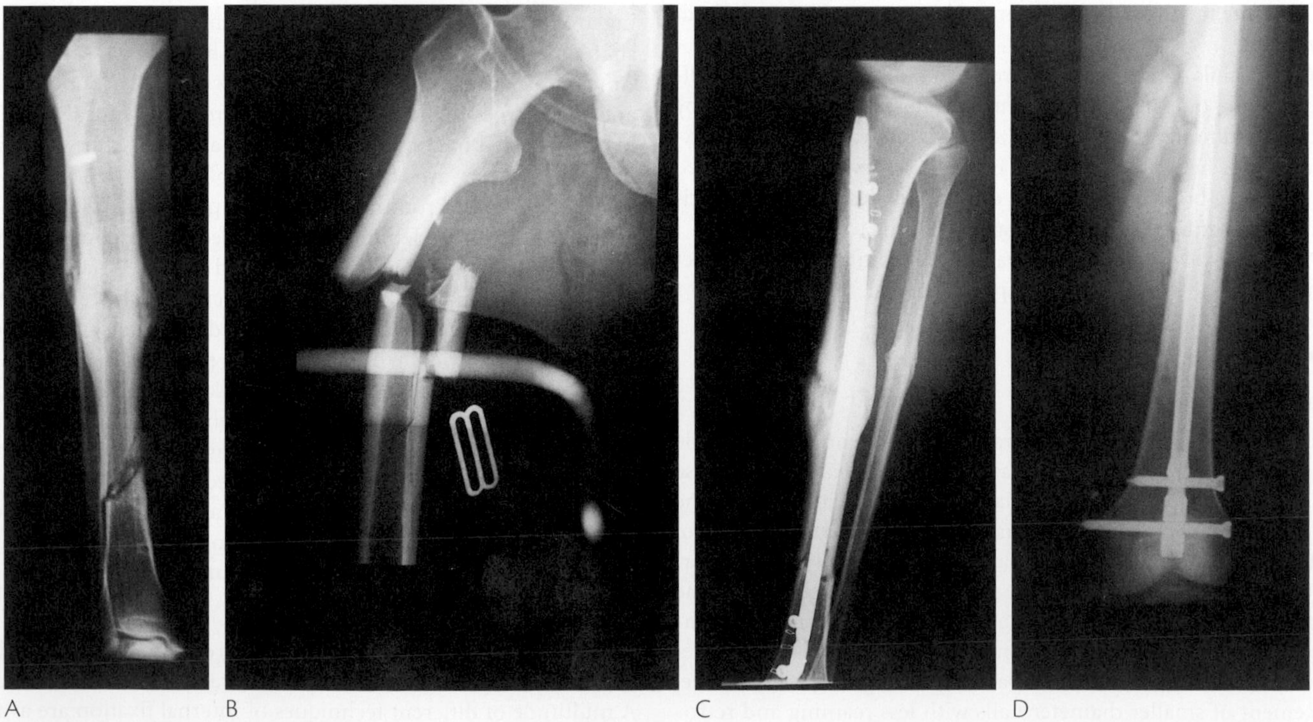

Fig. 12.53.5 Ipsilateral femur and tibia shaft fractures. A) and B) AP radiographs demonstrating ipsilateral fractures of the right femur and tibia shafts. Note that this patient had a healed tibia shaft fracture from a prior injury. C) and D) Radiographs after placement of tibia and retrograde femoral nails through a single incision at the knee shows good alignment of both fractures.

Box 12.53.4 Bifocal injuries

- Multiple implant combinations available
- Neck/shaft fractures—the neck fracture is the priority and treated with optimal fixation
- Examine under anaesthesia knee ligaments following stabilization of femoral shaft.

External fixation can be successful but has fallen out of favour. Non-operative treatment with traction, splints and casts is effective but has also fallen out of favour except in very young patients who heal within a month or two.

Elderly patients

Femoral shaft fractures in the elderly have recently received attention in the literature. One author reported a 10% mortality rate within 60 days of injury which was comparable to that of elderly patients with a proximal femur fracture. Only 39% returned to their pre-injury level of function. New postinjury medical problems were common and adversely affected outcome. In addition to operative stabilization they recommended close vigilance and ongoing medical evaluation. Among survivors, the rate of healing of the fracture was excellent.

Very large patients

In very large patients, positioning on the fracture table is difficult and access to the proximal femur through extensive soft tissue is fraught with a variety of complications including entry site malposition, malunion, increased blood loss, wound healing problems, and infection. Use of the femoral distractor instead of the fracture table has been reported, although the problems of the incision at the hip remain. Retrograde nailing has also been suggested as an effective means of overcoming both problems.

Pathological fractures

Pathological fractures of the femur shaft occur in an area of abnormal bone and typically have a high rate of non-union. Operative stabilization by intramedullary nail is generally indicated. With the use of interlocking, fixation is typically adequate and adjunctive use of methyl methacrylate is not required and often causes more problems than benefits. Owing to the limited demands of the patient, medullary fixation of shaft lesions or shaft fractures will typically provide adequate stabilization even if the fracture does not heal. However, extensive involvement of the proximal or distal femur may not be adequately stabilized by nailing and replacement arthroplasty may be preferred. Prophylactic nailing of lesions with high risk of fracture (greater than 50% of the cortex) is far easier and has a much lower complication rate than nailing after fracture has occurred. Consideration of life expectancy and quality of life should be discussed with the patient and family. Adjunctive use of radiation or chemotherapy is often helpful after the surgical incision has healed.

Results

Intramedullary nailing facilitates restoration of both form and function and achieves remarkably good short- and long-term results with low complication rates. Systemic complications and death rates have been lowered. The indirect reduction and splinting of the fracture achieved by closed nailing facilitates rather than retards natural healing by callous. Locked nailing accurately restores length and alignment which is important for the long-term function of the limb. Time lost from work has been dramatically reduced and patients are typically able to return to the most strenuous activities. However, patient based outcome studies demonstrate significant residual impact on patient's perception of their health and well being.

Complications (Box 12.53.5)

Complications of femur shaft fractures include non-union, malunion, infection, refracture, wound haematoma, neurological injury, vascular injury, deep venous thrombosis (DVT), compartment syndrome, heterotopic ossification, fracture comminution, implant breakage, implant malposition, haemorrhage, ARDS, stiffness, weakness, chronic pain, impaired ambulation, and death. Fortunately, the rate of these numerous complications is very low.

Deep venous thrombosis

Patients with femur shaft fractures are at risk for deep venous thrombosis. A 40% incidence of thrombosis in patients with femur shaft fractures has been reported, although there were no pulmonary emboli in this series. Early medullary nailing has helped reduce the incidence of thromboembolic problems in patients with femoral shaft fractures.

Marrow embolization and ARDS

Femur shaft fractures release medullary contents into the bloodstream which causes pulmonary dysfunction and increased capillary permeability with a variety of undesirable systemic consequences.

Medullary nailing of femur shaft fractures has both beneficial and deleterious effects on pulmonary function. Stabilization prevents motion at the fracture site and ongoing showering of medullary contents into the bloodstream. Stabilization also allows mobilization of the patient to an upright chest and reduces the pain of fracture motion which markedly improves pulmonary function in comparison to prolonged recumbency. However, each

Box 12.53.5 Complications

- 40% DVT incidence reported
- Fat embolus syndrome and ARDS
- Transient pudendal nerve dysfunction common
- Heterotopic ossification reported in up to 30% antegrade nails
- Iatrogenic fracture
- 1% non-union rate (union by 12 months)
- Malunion
- Infection
- Muscle weakness.

manipulation of the medullary canal causes particulate matter to enter the bloodstream with some pulmonary compromise results. Although this problem was greatly feared at the time of the introduction of intramedullary nailing the beneficial effects of nailing have been seen to far outweigh the detrimental effects. In a patient with near normal pulmonary function, the pulmonary consequences of medullary reaming are well tolerated. However, in patients with impaired pulmonary function it can cause major problems.

Heterotopic ossification

Heterotopic ossification after femoral nailing has been observed and although it may occur to some degree in up to 30% of patients it rarely is the cause of significant clinical symptoms. Three risk factors have been identified: male patient, more than 2 days between injury and nailing, and prolonged intubation for more than 4 days. Prevention of heterotopic ossification is best achieved by minimizing trauma to the gluteal muscles and by irrigation and debridement of devitalized reamings and muscle after nail insertion. Prophylactic radiation or indomethacin is not warranted.

Nerve injury

A15% incidence of pudendal nerve sensory disturbance has been reported as a result of pressure on the nerve between the countertraction post and pelvis. Spontaneous recovery is to be expected. Post-padding and the use of a large-diameter post are suggested ways to prevent this injury. The peroneal branch of the sciatic nerve can also be injured and there is a low incidence of injury to the tibial and femoral nerves.

Iatrogenic fractures

During femoral nailing, femoral neck fracture and other patterns of iatrogenic comminution have been observed. Careful instrumentation and the correct entry hole are critical in preventing iatrogenic fracture. Nail design is also important since more flexible nails are more forgiving of start points out of line with the medullary canal.

Delayed union and non-union

Delayed union has been defined as failure to achieve clinical and radiographic union by 4 months. The reported incidence is 10% although many of these patients will progress to full union without further treatment. Routine dynamization of statically locked nails is not necessary but may be advantageous in the presence of a delayed union or significant fracture distraction. Removal of the static locking screw is a simple procedure and is indicated as the first treatment of delayed union.

Non-union is defined as failure to achieve union by 12 months. The overall incidence is reported at 1%. In an aseptic non-union, exchange nailing with reaming and placement of a larger nail is usually successful. The reaming removes fibrous tissue that may have formed around the original nail and creates space for a larger diameter nail that has more stability. Open debridement of the fracture site is rarely required but drilling of the non-union site may be helpful to stimulate healing and create a space for reamings to function as bone graft. An 85% success rate has been reported with exchange nailing of aseptic femoral shaft non-unions. A very atrophic non-union with flail motion at the non-union site after removal of the initial internal fixation may require debridement of established scar tissue at the non-union site, freshening of the ends of the fragment and placement of cancellous bone graft or other biological stimulants to bone healing in addition to new osteosynthesis.

Recalcitrant femoral shaft non-unions are extremely difficult problems. Extensive debridement and reconstructive techniques have been described including the use of endosteal substitution or vascularized fibular grafts to obtain stability. Unfortunately, even these extensive techniques are not always successful and ablation may be required.

Malunion

A 20% incidence of angular malunion attributed to poor control of the distal fragment especially in more distal fracture patterns have been reported.

Infection

Infected unions are rare. Infections around an implant cannot be eradicated without implant removal. Since union has occurred the nail is no longer necessary or helpful. Typical treatment is removal of the nail, debridement of the surrounding tissue and medullary canal by reaming, and copious irrigation to dilute the residual bacteria. Temporary antibiotic-impregnated beads may be a useful way of delivering high levels of antibiotic to the medullary canal.

Infected non-unions require a careful assessment of the intensity of infection and relative benefits and problems with the fixation. Loose or broken implants that are not providing stability should be removed. The benefits of stable fixation on healing of the bone offset the foreign body effect that makes eradication of infection difficult. In general stable fixation in the face of infection should be retained until fracture healing while the infection is treated and suppressed. After fracture healing the implant can be removed and attempt at infection cure undertaken. When adequate debridement of infected bone creates a segmental bone defect extensive reconstructive techniques like vascularized fibula graft or bone transport distraction osteogenesis may be required.

Muscle weakness

Hip and thigh weakness has been considered usual for the first 4 months after nailing of femur shaft fractures. Chronic major weakness is unusual. Minor weakness of hip abduction strength at 2 years is prevalent. If present, hip abduction weakness correlated with symptoms of limp and discomfort. They recommended an aggressive strengthening program and careful monitoring of hip abductor function prior to release from care. Knee stiffness and weakness in the first two weeks after retrograde nailing is common but generally responds well to aggressive physical therapy and motion and strength return to near normal by 6–8 weeks.

Future directions

Continued refinement of medullary nailing will continue. Techniques to avoid pulmonary complications will be developed and the multiple trauma patients who benefit from damage control techniques will be more clearly identified to lower the death rate. Increased ease of insertion of the nail and placement of locking screws as well as other modifications of the technique, instruments and implants will be developed. The optimal entry site for trochanteric antegrade nails will be determined. Nail mounted guides for distal locking will become effective. Biological stimulation to speed healing and minimize soft tissue fracture disease may become available. With an aging population there will be more elderly patients with femur shaft fractures. Increased industrialization around the world will likely outpace any injury prevention advances and the incidence of femur shaft fractures will likely increase in the next 10 years.

Summary

Femoral shaft fractures are associated with high-energy mechanisms, polytrauma, bifocal injury and systemic complications. Early stabilization is important. Temporary stabilization techniques can be used in the physiologically unstable patient. Several definitive surgical stabilization techniques are available and they all have their relative merits and pitfalls. Careful planning and execution of the surgical strategy will minimize complication and is associated with high rates of success.

Further reading

Harwood, P.J., Giannoudis, P.V., van Griensven, M., Krettek, C., and Pape, H.C. (2005). Alterations in the systemic inflammatory response after early total care and damage control procedures for femoral shaft fracture in severely injured patients. *Journal of Trauma*, **58**(3), 446–52; discussion 452–4.

Morley, J.R., Smith, R.M., Pape, H.C., MacDonald, D.A., Trejdosiewitz, L.K., and Giannoudis, P.V. (2008). Stimulation of the local femoral inflammatory response to fracture and intramedullary reaming: a preliminary study of the source of the second hit phenomenon. *Journal of Bone and Joint Surgery*, **90B**(3), 393–9.

Pape, H.C., Rixen, D., Morley, J., *et al.*; EPOFF Study Group. (2007). Impact of the method of initial stabilization for femoral shaft fractures in patients with multiple injuries at risk for complications (borderline patients). *Annals of Surgery*, **246**(3), 491–9; discussion 499–501.

Tornetta, P. 3rd, Kain, M.S., and Creevy, W.R. (2007). Diagnosis of femoral neck fractures in patients with a femoral shaft fracture. Improvement with a standard protocol. *Journal of Bone and Joint Surgery*, **89A**(1), 39–43.

Zlowodzki, M., Vogt, D., Cole, P.A., and Kregor, P.J. (2007). Plating of femoral shaft fractures: open reduction and internal fixation versus submuscular fixation. *Journal of Trauma*, **63**(5), 1061–5.

12.54

Supracondylar fractures of the femur

Wingrove T. Jarvis and Ananda M. Nanu

Summary points

- Supracondylar fractures of the femur are seen in the young (high energy) and the old (low energy). Both groups have their own specific problems
- The advantages and disadvantages of each surgical option must be considered in relation to the individual patient and their fracture pattern.

Introduction

Supracondylar fractures in their true sense are non-articular distal metaphyseal femoral fractures. However, they may extend into the intercondylar (epiphyseal) region of the femur which in turn is usually intra-articular.

Results of treatment of these fractures are dictated by numerous factors, including pre-injury state of the knee, severity of the injury, and associated injuries. The presence of femoral implants such as intramedullary devices or total knee prosthesis also dictates management and outcome of these complex fractures.

Incidence and prevalence

The incidence of distal femoral fractures ranges from 4% of all femoral fractures in patients over 16 years, and 31% when hip fractures are excluded. These fractures predominantly occur in two patient groups: 84% mainly in elderly females with osteoporosis, average age 65 years and injury due to moderate-energy trauma; and the remainder mainly in young men due to high-energy trauma.

Anatomy

Normal anatomy

The detailed anatomy of the distal femur can be found in any standard textbook of anatomy. The transition zone between the distal diaphysis and the femoral condyles makes up the supracondylar area (Figure 12.54.1). At this point the metaphysis flares, especially on the medial side. Anteriorly, the patella articulates with the condyles in the trochlear groove. Between the two condyles posteriorly, there is the intercondyloid notch. On the medial aspect, there is the prominent adductor tubercle at the point of maximum flare of the metaphysis.

The distal femur serves as origin and insertion to several powerful muscles and ligaments. After a fracture these muscles usually cause characteristic deformities (Figure 12.54.1).

The mechanical and anatomical axes of the femur differ. The mechanical axis passes through the head of the femur and the middle of the knee joint, and subtends an angle of 3 degrees from the vertical. The anatomical axis is an average of 9 degrees valgus to the vertical axis. The axis of the knee joint is parallel to the horizontal (Figure 12.54.2). During fixation of these fractures all attempts should be made to restore these relationships. Approximately 10cm above the knee joint, the femoral artery passes into the popliteal fossa as it emerges from the adductor canal in the adductor magnus.

Pathological anatomy

Like any other bone in the body, the distal femur is also affected by osteoporosis which causes thinning of the cortices and expansion of the medullary cavity resulting in decreased bone stock and increased bone fragility. This is believed to contribute significantly to the age-related increase of distal femoral fractures, especially in elderly women, from minor trauma such as falls.

Associated pathology

Patients with supracondylar femur fractures who have been involved in high-energy trauma, frequently sustain both remote life-threatening (head, chest, and major vascular) and other local injuries. Soft tissue structures in and around the knee (skin, joint surface, menisci, cruciate, and collateral ligaments) are no exception. The incidence of associated vascular injury is low. The popliteal artery is more often at risk when an associated posterior dislocation of the knee occurs. Other associated fractures include condyles, tibial plateau, patella, ipsilateral femoral shaft and tibial shaft fracture creating a 'floating knee'. Ipsilateral acetabular, femoral head and neck fractures, and hip dislocation should be actively sought to avoid overlooking these frequently missed associated injuries.

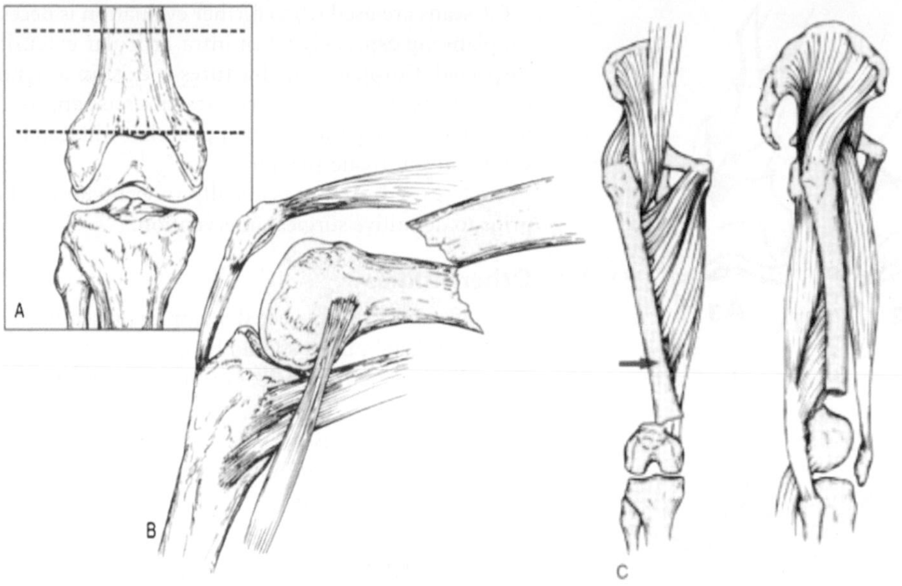

Fig. 12.54.1 Anatomic representation of the distal end of the femur and deformities resulting from unbalanced muscle action. A) Sketch of an anteroposterior radiograph of the metaphysis. The segment between the dashed lines is the supracondylar zone. B) Sketch of a lateral radiograph demonstrating muscle attachments and bone displacement. (Reproduced from Krettek and Helfet (2003)). C) Sketch of femur & muscle attachments. (Reproduced from Court-Brown et al. (2003)).

About 5–10% of these fractures are complicated by an open wound.

Mechanisms of injury

Most supracondylar fractures occur with the knee flexed. At low energy in the elderly, the patient usually stumbles and falls onto the knee. The high-energy injuries are usually dashboard injuries in motor vehicle collisions where the flexed knee impacts the dashboard. These high-energy injuries are often open and associated with a multiply injured young patient.

Figure 12.54.1 shows characteristic fracture displacement after injury.

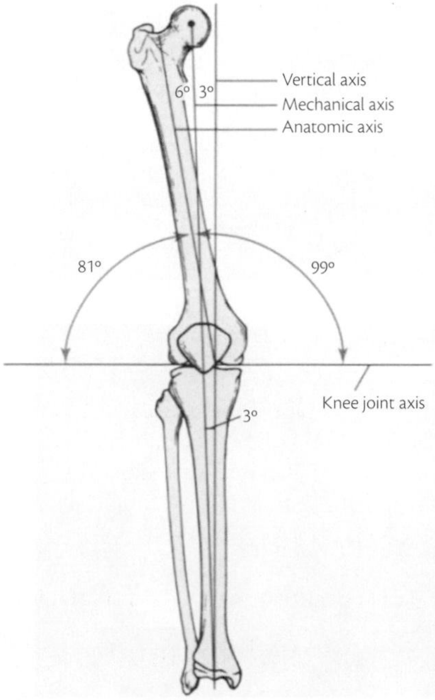

Fig. 12.54.2 Lower extremity axes. (Reproduced from Krettek and Helfet (2003).)

Classification

Several classification systems have been proposed, however, the AO/OTA classification is the most comprehensive. This classification is useful in determining treatment and prognosis. It is based on the location and pattern of the fracture and considers all fractures within the distal femur (Figure 12.54.3). Type A fractures involve the distal shaft only with varying degrees of comminution. Type B fractures are condylar fractures; type B1 is a sagittal split of the lateral condyle, type B2 is a sagittal split of the medial condyle, and type B3 is a coronal plane fracture. Type C fractures are T-condylar and Y-condylar fractures; type C1 fractures have no comminution, type C2 fractures have a comminuted shaft fracture with two principal articular fragments, and type C3 fractures have intra-articular comminution.

Clinical features

Initial evaluation is performed using ATLS® guidelines to ensure life-threatening injuries are identified and prioritized. The history of injury is usually either motor vehicle collision in a young person or a fall onto a flexed knee in an elderly person. The knee will be swollen and deformed. Evidence of neurological deficit, vascular injury, compartment syndrome, open fractures, and previous surgery (knee replacement in the elderly) should be identified.

Investigation

Imaging

Plain radiographs should include anteroposterior and lateral views of the entire limb, especially in high-energy trauma to rule out more proximal or distal associated fractures or dislocations. These should be repeated after initial reduction and application of traction or splint. The latter radiographs often supply more information about the anatomy of the fracture. Radiographs of the normal or uninvolved opposite femur may be taken for comparison to help in preoperative planning.

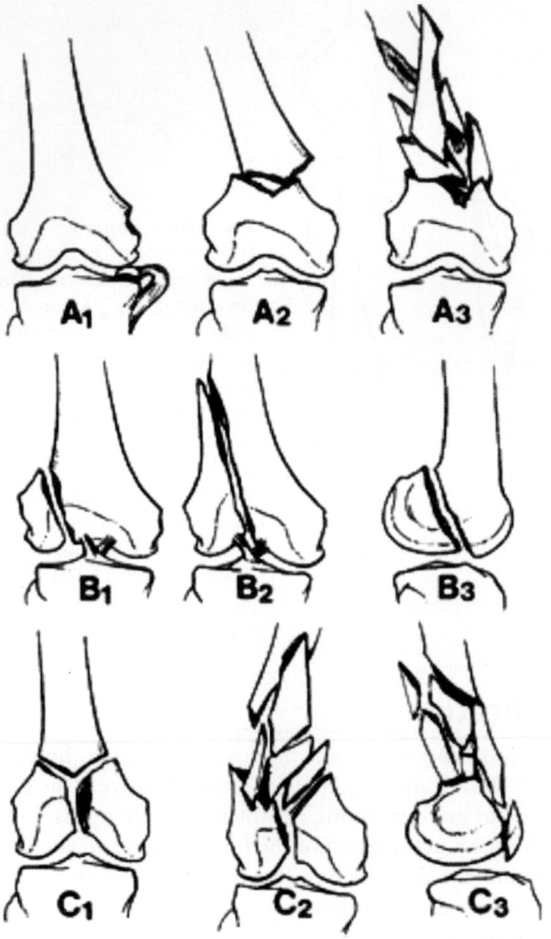

Fig. 12.54.3 Classification of fractures of distal femur described by Müller et al. (Reproduced from Whittle (2007).)

CT scans are used when further evaluation is necessary for surgical planning especially when intra-articular extension is noted or suspected. Coronal plane fractures coexist in a significant proportion of patients and if posterior fractures are approached through a medial or lateral parapatellar approach it will lead to extensive incisions and soft tissue stripping.

MRI is used only occasionally to evaluate the knee ligaments prior to definitive surgical intervention.

Other studies

If vascular injury is suspected, Doppler pulse recording of the popliteal and distal pulses should be documented. In dislocation and gross displacement, consideration should be given to performing arteriography.

Whenever there is a clinical suspicion of compartment syndrome, especially in an obtunded patient, compartment pressure monitoring is indicated.

Management

Initial

Primary

The femur should have been splinted prior to transportation. On arrival in the emergency department ATLS® guidelines dictate early prioritization and management of associated injuries. Following treatment of life threatening injuries, urgent limb-threatening injuries (vascular, compartment syndrome) are then managed. Management of open injuries is described in Chapter 12.7. In patients with severe multiple injuries, damage control orthopaedics may be appropriate. This usually entails using external fixators for the initial rapid stabilization of fractures, along with soft tissue care such as decompression of compartment syndrome and wound debridement (Figure 12.54.4). Definitive

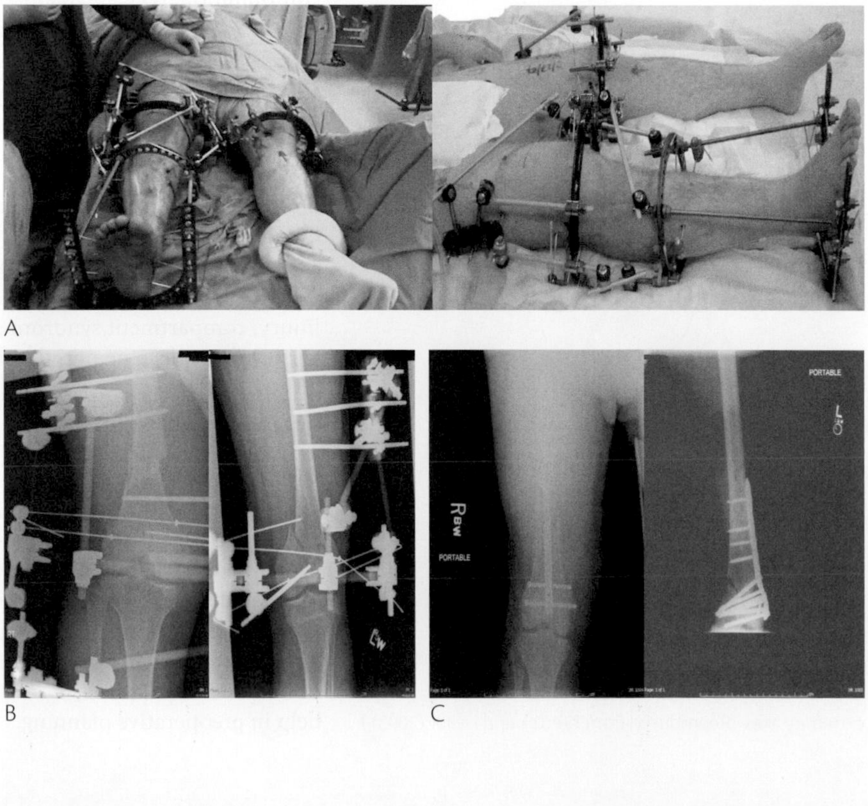

Fig. 12.54.4 'Damage control orthopaedics' (DCO). Lower extremity fractures of multiply injured young diabetic who had a hypoglycaemic episode while driving a car which then crossed the median and had a head-on collision with an on-coming car. He sustained: dislocated right shoulder, right supracondylar femoral and pilon fractures, left intra-condylar femoral fracture. A) Postoperative lower extremity temporary stabilization with external fixators. B) Radiographs of (A). C) Radiographs of definitive fixation carried out as staged procedure approximately 1 week later.

fracture fixation and complex reconstructive work can then be performed when the patient is physiologically stable.

Definitive treatment

Non-operative

Undisplaced fractures in elderly, high-risk patients may be treated in a cast brace. Subsequent displacement is an indication for fixation.

Operative

The principles of management of these injuries follows that of any long-bone fracture involving the metaphyseal region, namely anatomical reconstruction of the articular surface if involved and accurate realignment in all axes of the metadiaphyseal segment. The introduction of anatomical precontoured locking plates has greatly facilitated this task. The development of submuscular percutaneous plating, indirect reduction techniques, and limited arthrotomies allows the uninjured tissues to remain relatively inviolate (Figure 12.54.5).

Modern techniques require familiarity with all surgical options, see Box 12.54.1.

The priority flow of definitive management of these fractures begins with articular reduction and absolute stability of the joint reduction, and metaphyseal/diaphyseal bridging with either an intramedullary or extramedullary implant (relative stability), taking care to use a soft tissue sparing technique.

Box 12.54.1 Distal femur fixation options

- Antegrade intramedullary nailing (Figure 12.54.4C)
- Retrograde intramedullary nailing (see Chapter 12.53)
- Locked plating (Figure 12.54.4C)
- Conventional plating
- Circular frame (Figure 12.54.4A, B).

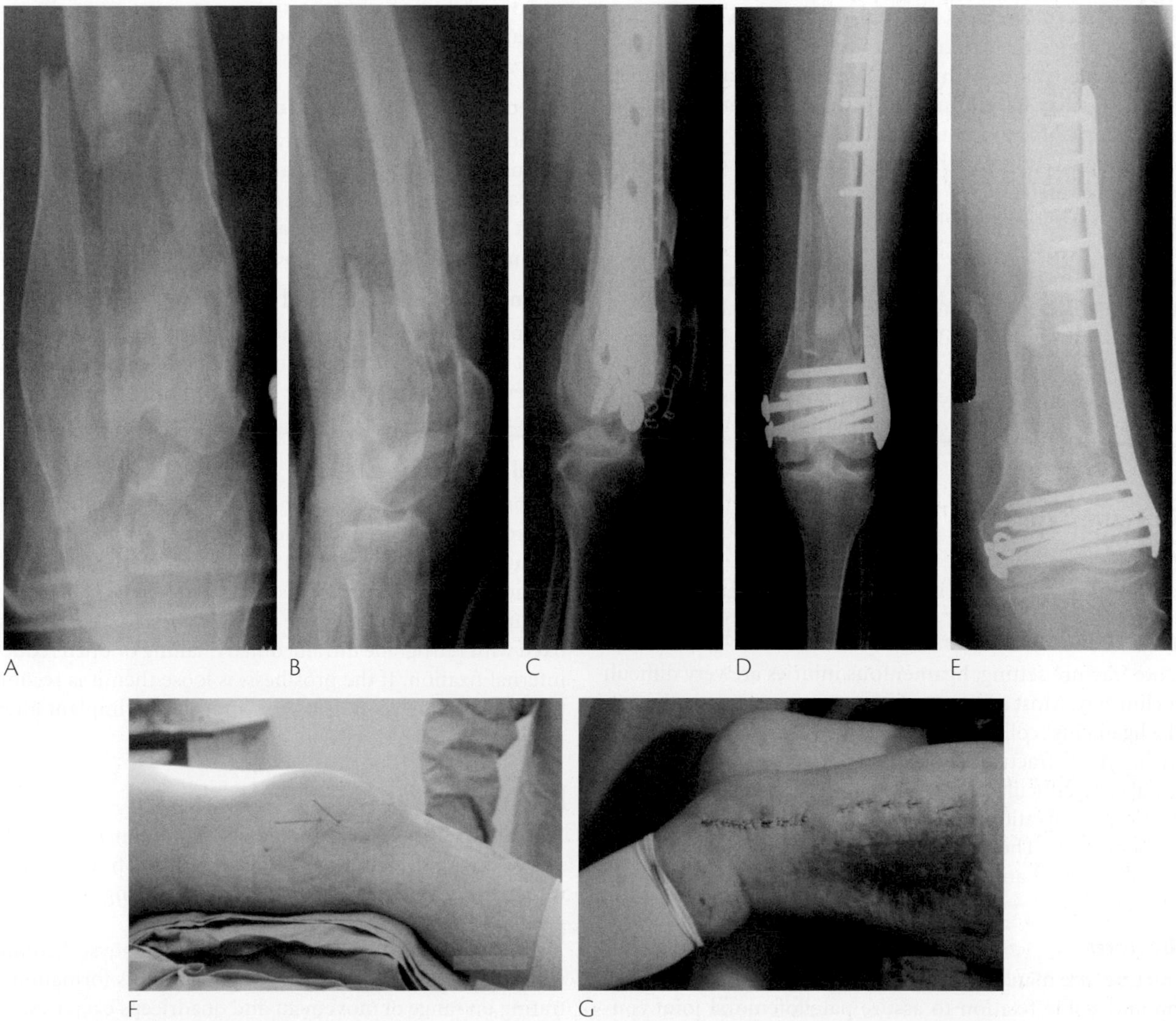

Fig. 12.54.5 A) and B) Preoperative radiographs of a C type distal femoral fracture. C) and D) Immediate postoperative radiographs of lateral locking plate and medial interfragmentary screw fixation. E) Healed fracture at 8 months postoperatively. F) Guide-wire placement for medial interfragmentary screws. G) Postoperative photograph showing incisions used for submuscular plating.

Antegrade and retrograde intramedullary nailing are usually preferred for A type fractures (extra-articular) or simple C fractures in the hands of enthusiastic proponents of nailing. Conventional plating using the blade plate, dynamic condylar screw, and condylar buttress plate have been reported extensively. The new millennium has seen several reports of the growing use of internal fixators or locked plates, coupled with minimally invasive techniques of application (Figure 12.54.5).

There is considerable confusion regarding the use of locked plates through open and percutaneous approaches, and the number, sequence, placement, and type of screws used in fixation of these fractures. The influence of permutations of these variables on the type of healing achieved is debated. Clarity is sought on the degree of construct stiffness required to optimize rapid callus formation, and the influence of screw type and position on the stiffness of the construct.

Alignment of the meta/diaphyseal segment remains of paramount importance, and single pass image intensifier screening is relatively inaccurate in judging long-bone alignment. The use of a 'horizontal plumb line' such as a diathermy cable or proprietary Perspex sheets with fine radio-opaque wires embedded helps get the 'big picture'.

Some locked internal fixators have cut-outs to allow screw placement to reconstitute the articular block. The placement of the screws requires meticulous planning. Despite this, certain complex fracture patterns may have bone loss/fracture lines in these locations, preventing optimum entry point use. An easy option is to introduce the lag screws from the medial side, taking care to avoid prominent medial metal.

Reduction is greatly aided by large pointed clamps. Special minimally invasive osteosynthesis instrument sets are commercially available to facilitate reduction and provisional stabilization. The large ball-pointed clamps from the pelvic and acetabular set are very useful in obtaining a hold on the articular block. Manual traction, the use of ankle strap distraction over a bolster, reduction triangles, and the use of completely radiolucent pelvic surgery table are invaluable in any attempt to obtain minimally invasive reduction and fixation.

Special circumstances

Open wounds

Management of open fractures is described in Chapter 12.7.

Ligamentous injuries

In the acute fracture setting, ligamentous injuries are very difficult to detect clinically. Most are due to fracture propagation with avulsion of the ligaments (collateral and cruciate) from the distal femur, especially in type C fractures. Magnetic resonance imaging (MRI) scans may also be difficult to interpret at this time. With good fracture reduction and fixation along with functional bracing, most of these ligaments heal. The knee is further evaluated at the time of fracture healing when any necessary ligament reconstruction can be undertaken.

Patella fractures

Patella fractures are managed in the standard fashion with accurate reduction and stable fixation to assure patellofemoral joint congruity. These are usually addressed at the same time as the fixation of the distal femur fracture. With extensive comminution of the patella, a partial or total patellectomy may have to be undertaken.

Associated fractures

An ipsilateral proximal femur fracture is also usually repaired at the same time. Most other associated fractures such as tibial plateau, tibial shaft, and ipsilateral acetabular fractures are usually repaired in a timely manner as patient fitness for surgery allows. In the case of a 'floating knee' (distal femur fracture and ipsilateral tibial shaft fracture) some surgeons may elect to fix both fractures under one anaesthesia or delay the tibial fixation depending on the patient's fitness.

Vascular and nerve injuries

A vascular injury is an emergency, and should therefore for treated well within 6h to avoid an ischaemic limb disaster. After repair of the vessels, a fasciotomy should be carried out to avoid compartment syndrome from reperfusion. Fracture stabilization is necessary to protect the repair.

Repair of nerve injuries if necessary should be undertaken as soon as possible, but is not an emergency.

Articular surface loss

Loss of articular cartilage is treated according to the patient's age and feasibility of carrying out a reconstruction. In the young patient, the defect, if large, should be reconstructed when the acute injury has settled.

Osteoporotic bone and the elderly

In the elderly, for a previously symptomatic arthritic knee that has sustained a complex articular fracture, a case can be made for a primary stemmed, stabilized, or partially constrained knee replacement. Multifragmentary metaphyseal fracture patterns (A3) can be spanned or replaced with modular segments.

Extensive comminution and bone loss

Extensive comminution of the metaphyseal region requires judgement to obtain accurate alignment in all three axes, as well as regain leg length. This may require screening the opposite leg to match the length.

Total knee prosthesis

Periprosthetic supracondylar femur fractures following total knee arthroplasty are an infrequent, but devastating, complication. Because of the poor results of non-operative management, internal fixation of these fractures is recommended. Depending on the fracture pattern and the type of prosthesis, these fractures may be fixed with retrograde intramedullary nailing or open reduction and internal fixation. If the prosthesis is loose then it is recommended to perform a revision using the appropriate implant after careful planning (Figure 12.54.6).

Post-treatment care

Internal fixation of type A fractures commences with immediate postoperative mobilization of the knee. In A1 fractures, early touch weight bearing progressing to weight bearing to tolerance over 4–6 weeks with the help of walking aids.

A2 and A3 fractures with significant metaphyseal comminution partially weight bear until early signs of callus formation, concentrating on range of movement and quadriceps exercises.

Articular fractures (B and C) are mobilized with immediate range of movement exercises and touch weight bearing for 10–12 weeks.

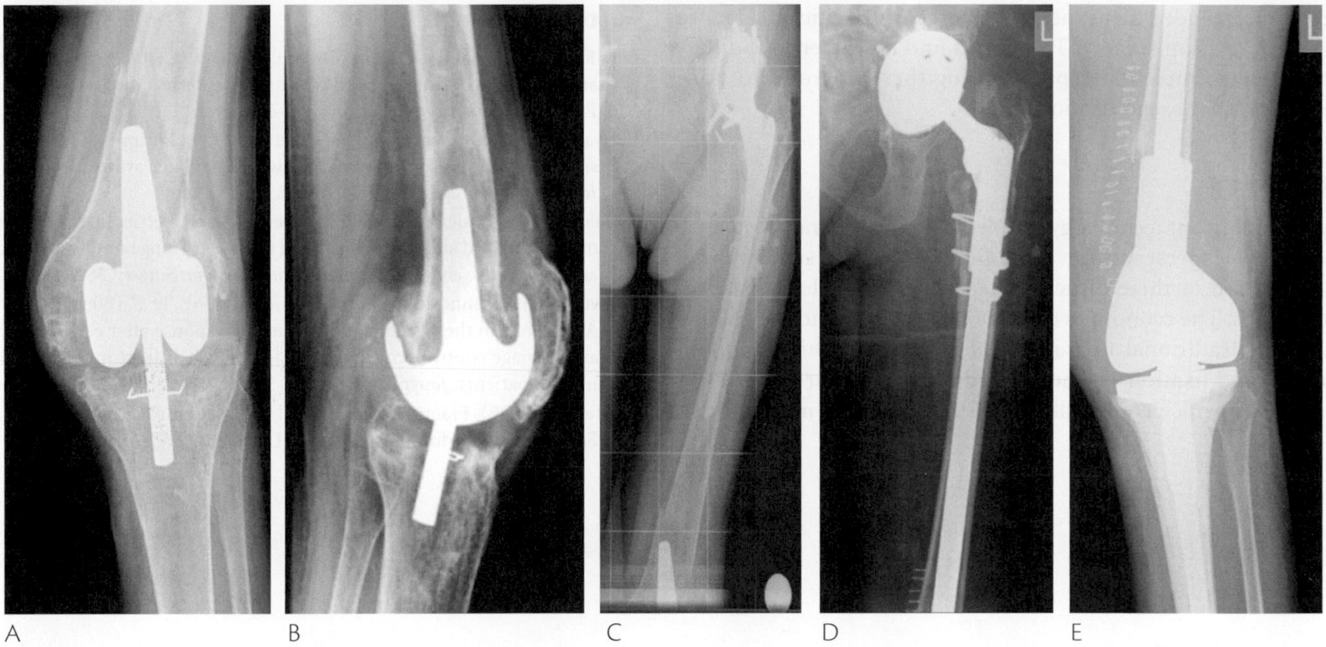

Fig. 12.54.6 A) and B) Supracondylar (S/C) periprosthetic fracture in rheumatoid arthritic patient. Loose, lytic SC area. C) Bad hip above (A) and (B). Patient had two attempts at revision. D) and E). Final hip and knee revised with interconnecting femoral segment.

Tenuous fixation leading to subsequent immobilization is likely to lead to stiffness and non-union, and is best revised early to allow compliance with immediate unrestrained access by the physiotherapist.

Complications

Failure to achieve pre-accident levels of form and function in the affected limb is partly determined by the nature of the injury. The iatrogenic component (Box 12.54.2) of this complication relates to infection, malunion, non-union, hardware failure, and stiffness.

All of these are directly related in some degree to imperfections in the treatment algorithm.

Early complications

This is a common injury in the fragile elderly population, and myocardial infarctions, chest infections, and deep wound infections are the commonest afflictions.

Box 12.54.2 Iatrogenic causes of poor outcome

- Injudicious exposure
- Imperfect timing of surgery
- Failure to recognize one's surgical limitations
- Failure to recognize and deal with axis orientation.
- Incorrect choice of implants
- Incorrect use of appropriate implant
- Lack of clarity of thought in determining method of healing to be desired.

Late complications

Malunion, non-union, and hardware failure may require reoperation.

Results

The outcome following treatment of supracondylar fractures of the femur is multifactorial (Box 12.54.3).

The authors could find only one randomized controlled trial of operative (dynamic condylar screw) versus non-operative management (Thomas' splint with a Pearson knee flexion attachment) of displaced fractures of the distal femur. Fewer complications, shorter length of stay, and better outcomes demonstrated the clear advantages of internal fixation.

Antegrade intramedullary nailing for supracondylar and intercondylar fractures is accomplished by either percutaneous or open reduction of the articular surface and fixation with screws followed by nailing. Ninety-four per cent good or excellent results are reported as is a good range of knee movement.

Retrograde nails are also extensively reported in these fractures with favourable results.

In a review of publications between 1989 and 2005 operative treatment results in a 32% reduction in the risk of a poor result.

Box 12.54.3 Outcome

- Initial injury severity
- Accuracy of articular reconstitution and axis realignment
- Maintenance of local tissue vascularity and viability
- The outcome measure chosen.

They also concluded that experienced surgeons significantly reduce the risk of revision surgery. They could find no evidence of difference between implants in predisposing these fractures to nonunions, infections, and fixation failures.

Summary

Improved implant technology coupled with the general acceptance of soft tissue preservation principles in trauma surgery have made fixation of these difficult fractures in a fragile population less onerous. The economics of today's health care and the gradual erosion of traditional nursing skills dictate that this trend will continue and fixation of undisplaced supracondylar fractures in elderly osteopenic people will pose a lesser risk than nursing them in bed.

Further reading

Bell, K.M., Johnstone, A.J., Court-Brown, A.M., *et al.* (1992). Primary knee arthroplasty for distal femoral fractures in elderly patients. *Journal of Bone and Joint Surgery*, **74B**(3), 400–2.

Bezwada, H.P., Neubauer, P., Baker, J., *et al.* (2004). Periprosthetic supracondylar femur fractures following total knee arthroplasty. *Journal of Arthroplasty*, **19**(4), 453–8.

Gustilo, R. B and Anderson, J.T. (1976). Prevention of infection in the treatment of one thousand and twenty-five open fractures of long bones: retrospective and prospective analyses. *Journal of Bone and Joint Surgery*, **58A**(4), 453–8.

Harwood, P.J., Giannoudis, P.V., van Griensven, M., *et al.* (2005). Alterations in the systemic inflammatory response after early total care and damage control procedures for femoral shaft fracture in severely injured patients. *Journal of Trauma*, **58**(3), 446-52; discussion 452–4.

Krettek, C. (2008). Fractures of the distal femur. In: Browner, B.D. (ed) *Skeletal Trauma*, fourth edition. St. Louis, MO: W.B. Saunders.

12.55

Patella fractures and dislocations

J.L. Marsh

Summary points

- Differentiate multipartite patella from fracture
- Non-operative treatment results satisfactory if extensor mechanism intact
- Avoid total patellectomy if possible
- Modified AO technique allows tension wires to be placed through cannulated screws
- Results of dislocation independent of duration of immobilization
- Osteochondral fractures should be either removed or internally fixed.

Introduction

Acute injuries to the extensor mechanism of the knee include patella fractures and dislocations and quadriceps and patella tendon ruptures. Despite their common occurrence, there is much controversy regarding the management of many aspects of patella injuries. Hardware irritation, loss of reduction, and recurrent dislocation continue to be common complications.

Anatomy

The patella, the largest sesamoid, is invested within the strong fascia of the extensor mechanism. Its shape is that of a pear turned upside down, with a broad proximal pole and narrower distal pole. The quadriceps insert into the proximal pole while the patella tendon originates from the inferior pole (Figure 12.55.1). The proximal three-quarters of the posterior patellar surface is composed of articular cartilage and articulates within the trochlear groove of the femur. The articular surface is divided by a vertical ridge into larger lateral and smaller medial facets. The inferior pole, which encompasses one-quarter of the patella, contains no articular surface. The patella serves four functions:

- Enhances the mechanical advantage of the quadriceps
- Protects the underlying femoral articular surface and knee joint
- Aids nourishment of the femoral articular surface
- Provides the bony contours for a 'normal' cosmetic appearance to the knee.

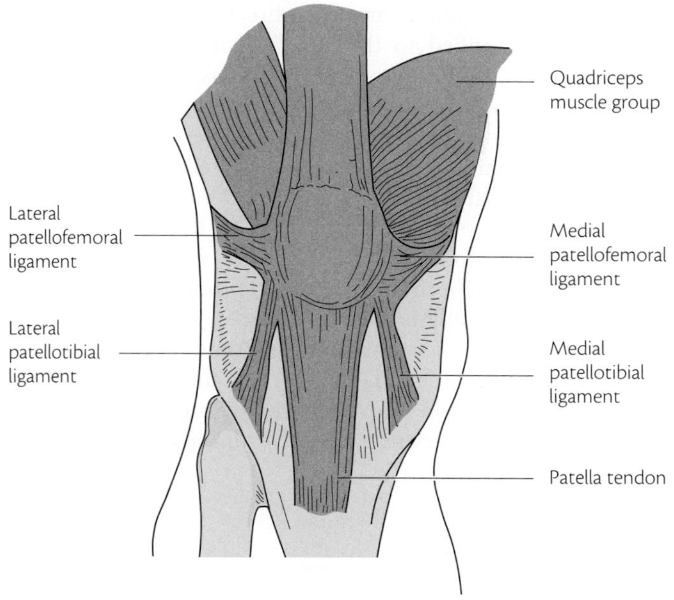

Fig. 12.55.1 Anatomy of the extensor mechanism of the knee.

Patella fractures

Incidence and prevalence

Patella fractures account for approximately 1% of fractures. Although they occur in patients of all ages, most occur in the third through fifth decades of life.

Pathological anatomy (Box 12.55.1)

The majority of patella fractures disrupt the extensor mechanism, albeit to varying degrees. With increasing amounts of fragment

Box 12.55.1 Patella fractures

- 1% of all fractures
- Usually disrupt knee extensor mechanism
- Assume articular cartilage injury with direct contact injuries.

Box 12.55.2 Injury mechanism in patella fractures

- Three-point bending—results in transverse fracture
- Direct contact—comminuted fracture
- Combines three-point bending and direct contact
- Knee flexed—proximal pole fracture
- Knee extended—distal pole fracture.

separation, there is greater injury to the adjacent medial and lateral retinacula signifying a greater disruption of the extensor mechanism. Direct contact injuries are undoubtedly associated with patellar and trochlear cartilage injury.

Mechanism of injury (Box 12.55.2)

Patella fractures result from both direct and indirect forces. A direct force applied to the anterior surface of the patella typically causes a comminuted, minimally displaced fracture pattern (Figure 12.55.2). Tensile and three-point bending forces indirectly produce patella fractures. With the knee in extension, the quadriceps transmits tensile forces to the patella. With increasing knee flexion, the patella engages in the trochlear groove. During a violent quadriceps contraction against a fixed, flexed lower extremity, as would occur from a fall from a height, the patella receives a combination of these indirect forces (tension and three-point bending) that typically creates a displaced, transverse fracture that may have a variable amount of comminution of the articular surface (Figures 12.55.3 and 12.55.4). The anterior surface fails in tension resulting in the transverse component while the posterior surface experiences compression accounting for the comminution.

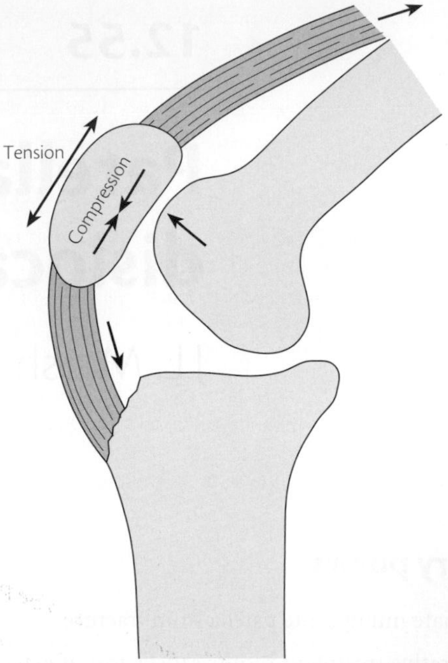

Fig. 12.55.3 Indirect forces causing patella fractures. With knee flexion, the femur applies an anteriorly directed force while the quadriceps and patella tendon provide posteriorly directed tension forces at the superior and inferior poles, respectively. This further increases tension along the anterior surface and creates compression along the articular surface.

A significant number of patella fractures occur as a result of combined direct and indirect forces (namely motor vehicle collisions—with the flexed knee striking the dashboard as the quadriceps contracts). These fractures also consist of both transverse and comminuted sections.

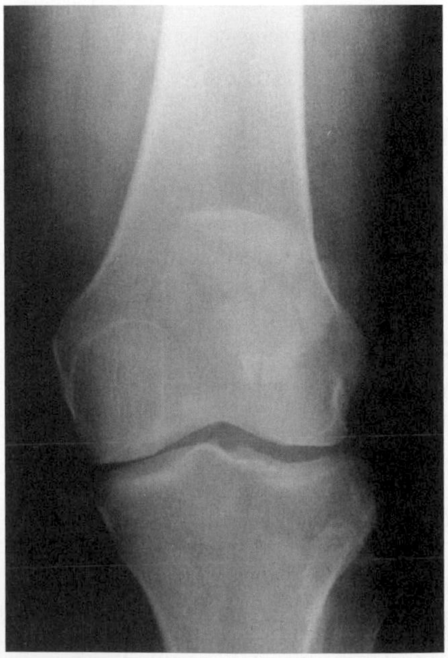

Fig. 12.55.2 A comminuted, minimally displaced patella fracture sustained from a fall onto a flexed knee (i.e. direct impact injury).

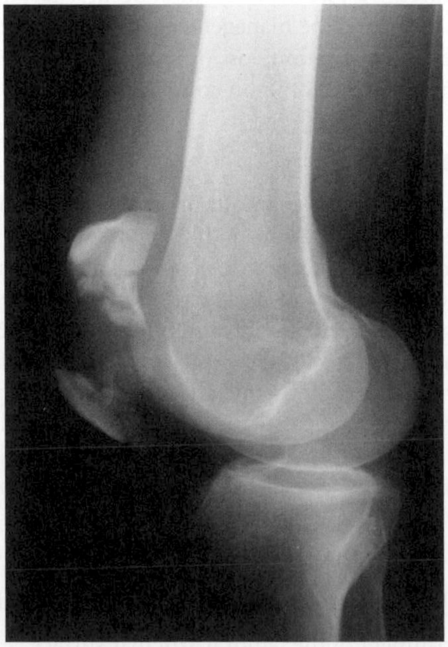

Fig. 12.55.4 A patella fracture caused by tension and three-point bending forces. Notice the transverse fracture at the anterior surface and comminution at the articular surface.

With increasing knee flexion, the patellar articular contact area shifts from distal to proximal. Therefore inferior pole fractures result from injuries that occur with the knee relatively extended and proximal fractures occur when the knee is in greater flexion.

Classification

Patella fractures are classified according to the morphology of the fracture pattern and the presence or absence of displacement. Common fracture patterns include transverse, vertical, comminuted or stellate, osteochondral, and sleeve fractures (Figure 12.55.5).

Clinical evaluation (Box 12.55.3)

The patient usually describes the acute onset of knee pain and swelling after a direct or indirect mechanism of injury, and is often unable to bear significant weight on the injured knee.

The patient's ability actively to extend the leg must be assessed, as the inability to extend the knee against gravity signifies a significant disruption of the extensor mechanism that may require surgical intervention. When pain is prohibitive, aspiration of fracture haematoma and intra-articular injection of local anaesthetic may be indicated to make the patient more comfortable and allow for a more accurate examination.

Investigation

Plain radiographs (anteroposterior, lateral, and Merchant (45-degree axial) views) are usually all that are needed to treat patella fractures. The anteroposterior view is assessed for patella position, displacement, and comminution. A bipartite or multipartite patella (Figure 12.55.6A) is distinguished from a fracture (Figure 12.55.6B) by its typical location (superolateral), smooth borders, and frequent bilateral occurrence. The lateral projection usually provides the best view of fracture lines and should be scrutinized for patella height, displacement, and comminution. The Merchant view (Figure 12.55.7) is often the only projection that will demonstrate vertical and osteochondral fractures.

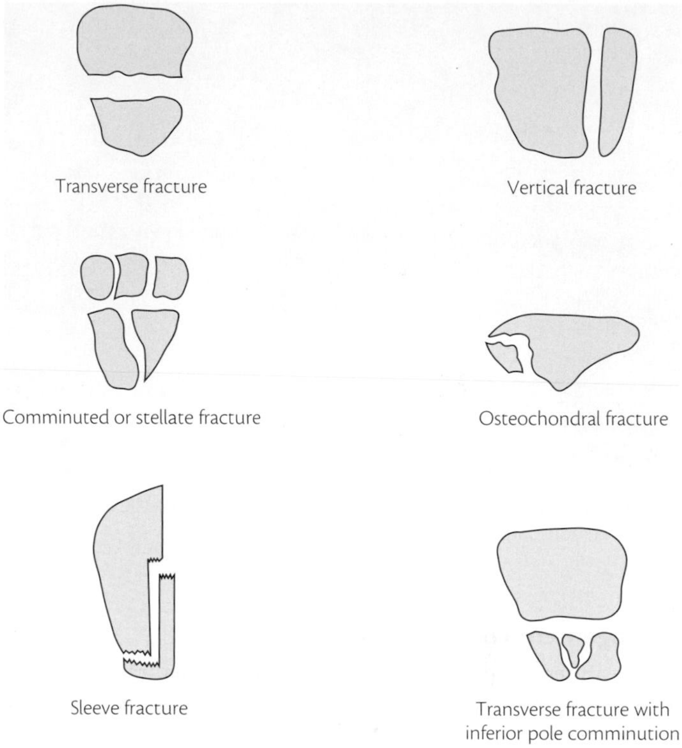

Fig. 12.55.5 Common patella fracture patterns.

Box 12.55.3 Evaluation of patella fractures
◆ Must assess ability to extend knee against gravity
◆ Anteroposterior, lateral, and Merchant radiographs.

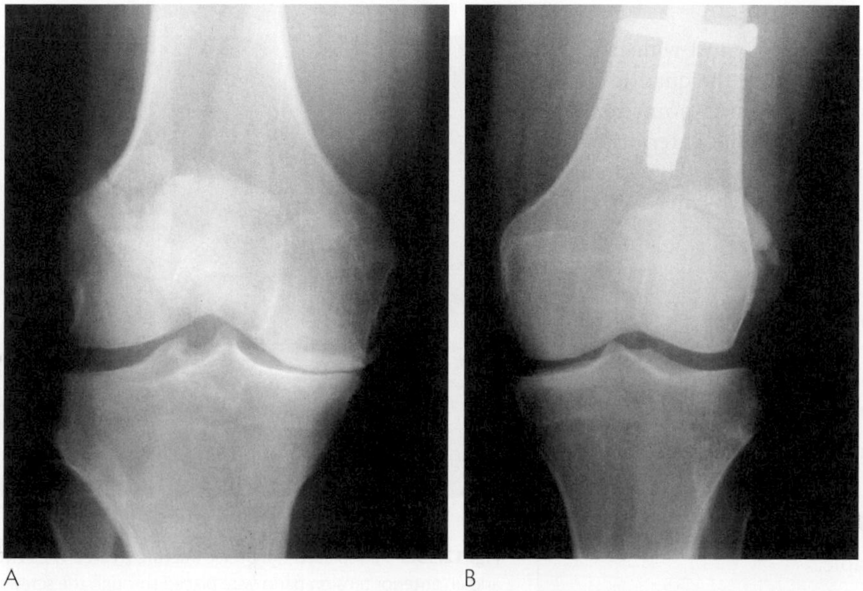

Fig. 12.55.6 A classic multipartite patella (A) is distinguished from an acute fracture (B) by the typical superolateral location and smooth borders of the fragments. An acute fracture (B) may occur in a similar location, but the borders are sharp and often associated with some degree of fracture comminution.

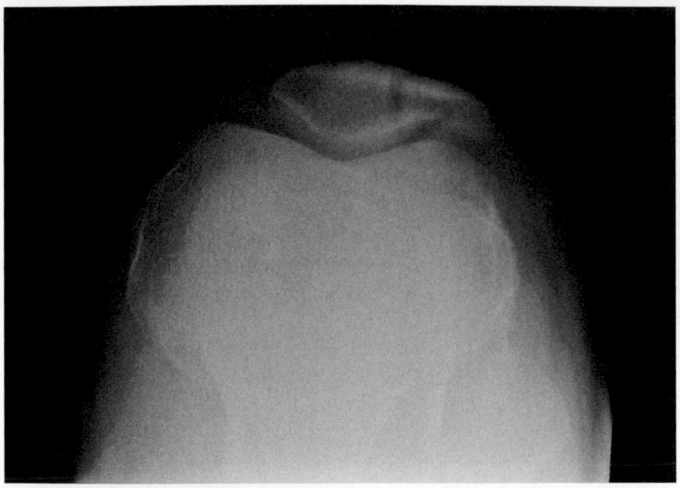

Fig. 12.55.7 The Merchant view (45-degree axial view) is often the only image that will demonstrate vertical and osteochondral fractures.

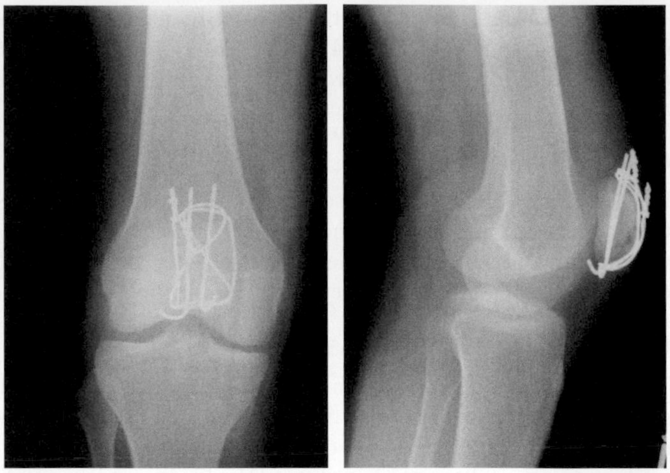

A B

Fig. 12.55.8 A displaced transverse fracture treated with the modified tension band wire technique. Both figure-of-eight and box-type anterior tension wires were placed. Notice that the wires are in direct contact with the superior and inferior poles of the patella.

Management (Box 12.55.4)

The treatment goals for most patients with patella fractures are to maintain or restore a stable extensor mechanism and a smooth articular surface.

Non-operative

Non-operative treatment produces excellent results in carefully selected patients; namely those with a functional extensor mechanism and minimal fracture displacement (Figure 12.55.8). The knee is immobilized in extension for 6 weeks followed by progressive active range of motion exercises. Full weight bearing and isometric quadriceps exercises are begun several days after injury. Radiographs must be obtained weekly for 3 weeks to rule out fracture displacement.

Operative

Displaced patella fractures with disrupted extensor mechanisms should be treated operatively with techniques ranging from reduction and fixation of all displaced fragments to total patellectomy.

Transverse fractures

Reduction and fixation of transverse fractures must withstand not only the considerable tension forces exerted by the quadriceps but also, if early knee motion is desired, the three-point bending forces which create additional tension along the anterior surface and compression along the articular surface. The modified tension band wiring technique as described by the AO group (Figure 12.55.8) has been clinically successful and is relatively simple and familiar to most surgeons. Two vertical 1.6-mm (0.062-inch) K-wires are placed parallel to each other across the reduced fracture. An 18-gauge wire is then placed directly posterior to the K-wires at their entrance into the superior pole, wrapped over the anterior surface of the patella in a figure-of-eight or box configuration, passed directly posterior to the K-wires at their point of exit at the inferior pole, and then twisted until appropriate compression is achieved across the fracture site.

The AO technique has been modified by replacing the K-wires with cannulated screws. The 18-gauge wire is threaded through the screws, rather than around the K-wires, before passing over the anterior surface of the patella in a similar figure-of-eight configuration (Figure 12.55.9). The screws produce interfragmentary compression across the fracture site while the wire neutralizes

Box 12.55.4 Treatment of patella fractures

- Non-operative (6 weeks immobilization) for intact extensor mechanism and <2–3mm fragment displacement
- Transverse tension band around parallel wires or through screws for transverse fractures
- One comminuted pole—partial patellectomy
- Avoid total patellectomy if possible.

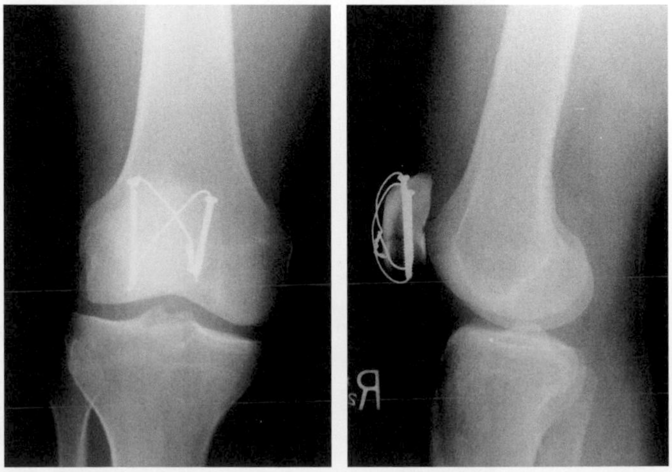

A B

Fig. 12.55.9 A displaced transverse fracture treated with two cannulated screws and an anterior tension band wire placed through the screws.

the tension forces across the anterior patellar surface. Mechanical testing has shown that this construct provides the strongest initial fixation. The use of an arthroscope to assess the reduction allows the possibility of a truly percutaneous approach to reduction and fixation. This technique needs further assessment but is attractive in cases where there are abrasions or other skin problems over the anterior surface of the patella.

Vertical fractures

Vertical fractures are rarely displaced. When displaced they are best treated with anatomical reduction and lag screw fixation.

Comminuted or stellate fractures

When possible, vertical fracture lines should be rigidly fixed with lag screws with the objective of creating two large pole fragments. These two fragments can then be fixed like a transverse fracture (Figure 12.55.10). When comminution severity precludes this technique, all attempts should be made to save some portion of the articular surface with the hope of maintaining patella function. This frequently involves partial patellectomy and reattachment of the patella or quadriceps tendon to the salvaged fragment (Figure 12.55.11). Total patellectomy is performed when there are no large articular surface fragments that can be congruently reconstructed.

Controversy exists regarding the proper site to reattach the patella tendon when inferior pole fragments are excised. Most authors have recommended that the tendon be reattached immediately adjacent to the articular surface in order to minimize the step-off between the tendon and articular cartilage, and prevent the posterior tilting and subsequent edge loading reported to occur with anterior reattachment. However, it has been demonstrated that when the tendon is reattached anteriorly there are smaller decreases in patellofemoral contact area and smaller increases in contact pressure compared to posterior reattachment. The author reattaches the patella tendon through drill holes in the central portion of the fracture surface of the residual proximal fragment.

Post-treatment care

The knee is immobilized and rehabilitated postoperatively based on fracture configuration and stability of fixation. Patients with severely comminuted fractures, tenuously fixed fractures, partial patellectomies, and total patellectomies are treated for 4–6 weeks with the knee immobilized in extension, followed by a gradual progressive range of motion and strengthening program.

For stable well-fixed transverse fractures, the current trend is to begin early active-assisted range of motion limited to 90 degrees. Gradual and progressive strengthening is begun at 6 weeks.

Special circumstances

Open fractures

Seven per cent of all patella fractures are open. Similar to other open fractures, antibiotics should be started and the fracture should be immediately irrigated, debrided, and rigidly internally fixed if the wound is clean. The wound should be closed or covered with a flap within 3–5 days of injury. The incidence of deep infection is correlated to the magnitude of soft-tissue injury with rates ranging from 0–10.7%.

Associated ipsilateral femoral shaft fracture

Ipsilateral femoral shaft and patella fractures are not uncommon. These tend to be high-energy injuries associated with more severe soft tissue trauma. Both fractures should be stably internally fixed to allow early knee motion and prevent quadriceps adherence at the femoral fracture site.

After bone–patellar tendon autograft anterior cruciate ligament reconstruction

Transverse patella fracture has been reported as a complication of bone–patellar tendon graft harvest. The fractures are usually associated with trauma and occur in the early months after the anterior cruciate ligament surgery. Standard treatment of the patella fracture leads to generally satisfactory results.

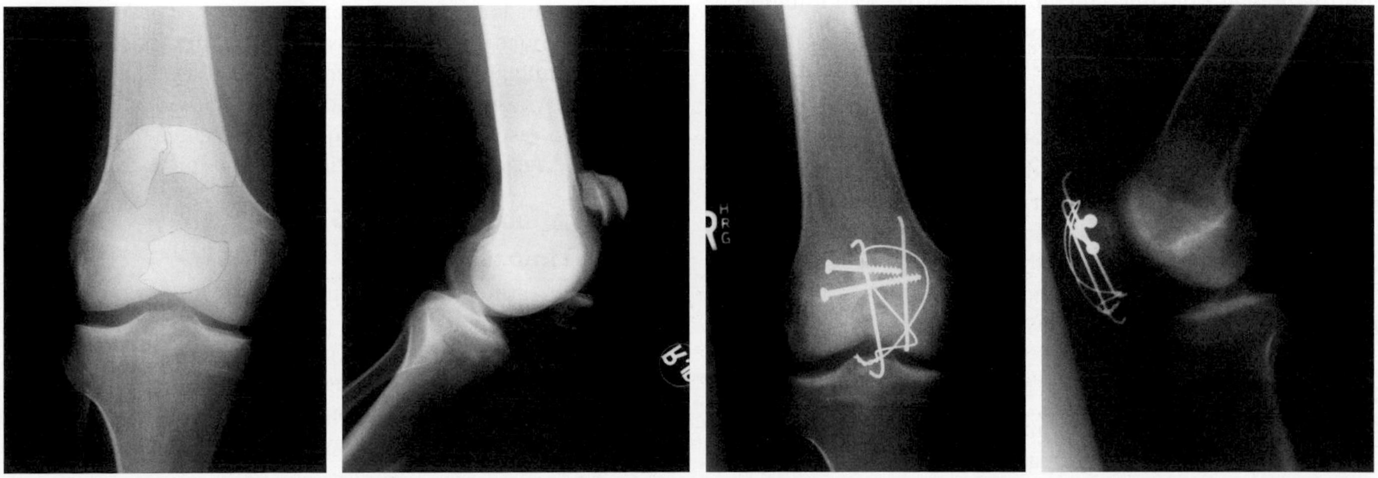
A B C D

Fig. 12.55.10 A) and B) A displaced comminuted fracture treated with lag screw fixation and C) and D) the modified tension band wire technique. The lag screws were used to fix the comminuted fractures, thus creating large superior and inferior pole fragments. These two fragments were then treated as a transverse fracture with the modified tension band wire technique.

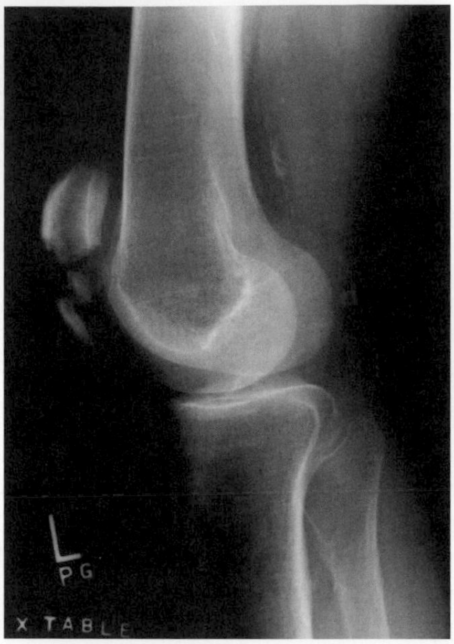

Fig. 12.55.11 A displaced comminuted fracture indicated for partial patellectomy. Attempts to fix the distal comminution would likely be fraught with complication. Excision of the distal comminution and reattachment of the patella tendon to the large proximal fragment is indicated.

Results (Box 12.55.5)

Non-operative treatment

Appropriately indicated patella fractures (namely those with minimal displacement and an intact extensor mechanism) have good results when treated non-operatively, with 99% good and excellent results (average 8.9-year follow-up) reported. In a study of 40 patients (average of 30.5 months after injury), 80% were pain free and 90% had full knee range of motion.

Operative treatment

The results of operatively-treated patella fractures are more related to the severity of injury and associated injuries than to the method of fixation. High-energy injuries, open fractures, comminution, and the presence of concomitant injuries have been found to be predictive of a poor result. Although residual articular displacement has also been associated with worse results, these findings have not been universal.

Open reduction and internal fixation

Most authors report 70–80% good and excellent results after open reduction and internal fixation of patella fractures. Perfect reduction has been found to be necessary to optimize outcomes. If precise reduction was not achieved, the results were better in patients treated with patellectomy. These results should be considered when attempting to fix comminuted cases internally. Good results after internal fixation have been reported even in elderly patients.

Partial patellectomy

Despite biomechanical studies which demonstrate decreased patellofemoral contact area and increased pressure after partial patellectomy, this procedure has resulted in outcomes comparable to those after open reduction and internal fixation, and the results appear to be maintained over time. At an average 8.4-year follow-up, 78% good and excellent results and an average quadriceps strength of 85% of the opposite side, has been reported. Partial patellectomy resulted in better outcomes than total patellectomy for the treatment of comminuted displaced fractures.

Box 12.55.5 Results of treatment of patella fractures

- Open fractures (Gustilo type 1 and 2): low infection rate when fixed
- Non-operative treatment (undisplaced/minimally displaced)
- 99% good/excellent results
- Poor results associated with:
  - High-energy injury
  - Open fractures
  - Concomitant injuries
  - Comminution
- Open reduction and internal fixation:
  - 80–90% good/excellent results
  - Precise reduction essential
- Partial patellectomy:
  - 78% good/excellent results
  - Quadriceps power, 85%
- Total patellectomy:
  - 60–80% good/excellent results
  - Quadriceps power, 50–75%
  - Functional limitations.

Total patellectomy

Patella fractures treated by total patellectomy have less predictable outcomes than after other treatments, with reports ranging from 61–88% good and excellent results. Pain has not been a major long-term problem, and patients continue to make functional improvements for up to 2–3 years postoperatively. Most patients have some quadriceps weakness (50–75%) and are functionally limited (running, squatting, ascending and descending stairs) after patellectomy. There is some evidence that newer operative techniques (e.g. vastus medialis obliquus advancement and cruciform repair) and aggressive rehabilitation result in improved outcomes.

Complications (Box 12.55.6)

Hardware irritation

Operative treatment of patella fractures is often complicated by hardware irritation because the patella is located subcutaneously and stabilized with wires that become prominent. Trimming excessive length from K-wires, bending prominent wire ends away from the subcutaneous tissues, and keeping suture and wire knots off the anterior surface of the patella may help to limit these problems.

Loss of fixation

Loss of fixation is usually related to poor patient compliance, unrecognized comminution, poor bone quality, or poor surgical technique (i.e. improper placement of the tension band wire).

Box 12.55.6 Complications of patellar fractures

- Prominent metalwork
- Loss of fixation:
  - 22% incidence of separation up to 2mm
    —imobilization may prevent loss of fixation
    —avoid fixing severely comminuted fractures
    —figure-of-eight wire contact with bone
- Arthritis—radiographic arthritis is relatively common
- Stiffness
- Infection is uncommon
- Non-union: 2–12%.

It has been reported that fracture fragments separated (up to 2mm) in 22% of transverse fractures treated with open reduction and internal fixation. Placing the non-compliant patient in a long leg cast for a limited period of time (3–4 weeks) may prevent fixation failure. Efforts to reconstruct severely comminuted fractures should be abandoned in favour of partial patellectomy. Tension band wires must be placed in direct contact with the patellar poles, posterior to longitudinal K-wires, and over the anterior surface of the patella. When fractures widely redisplace, they must be treated with repeat open reduction and internal fixation or partial patellectomy.

Post-traumatic osteoarthritis

In a 10- to 30-year follow-up, 45 of 64 injured knees had patellofemoral osteoarthritis compared to only 23 contralateral, uninjured knees. There is an increase in the frequency of osteoarthritis after high-energy injuries, open fractures, comminuted fractures, operatively treated fractures, and fractures with 1mm or more of articular incongruity. However, these radiographic findings often bear no relation to clinical results.

Knee stiffness/loss of range of motion

Fractures stabilized with current operative techniques and mobilized early in the postoperative period are generally considered to result in less knee stiffness and decreased range of motion. Some loss of flexion is expected after operative treatment, but is rarely of functional significance. When functionally limiting stiffness occurs, the knee should be aggressively rehabilitated. If it does not respond, it should be manipulated under anaesthesia and refractory cases should have adhesions lysed arthroscopically.

Infection

Infection following operatively-treated patella fractures is uncommon. Superficial infections should be treated with antibiotics and local wound care. Deep infections should be aggressively irrigated and debrided and the patient should be placed on intravenous antibiotics. All attempts should be made to preserve the patella, but patellectomy is inevitable is some cases of deep infection.

Non-union

Although patella non-unions are considered uncommon when fractures are treated with current techniques, reported rates have ranged from 2.7–12.5% of all fractures. Minimally symptomatic patients have been successfully treated non-operatively, accepting failure of fracture healing. Symptomatic non-unions can be expected to have improved knee function when treated with open reduction and internal fixation, partial patellectomy, or total patellectomy.

Future directions

Patella fractures have been treated using the same principles for the past three decades. The use of bioabsorbable implants may eliminate the need for hardware removal. The arthroscope has revolutionized surgery around the knee joint, allowing major surgery to be performed through small incisions in an almost percutaneous fashion and this technique may have increased use in fractures of the patella.

Summary

Patella fractures are common injuries caused by both direct and indirect trauma. They are classified based on the fracture pattern and presence of displacement. The status of the extensor mechanism is determined by physical examination and radiographic analysis. Surgical intervention is indicated for those patients with displaced fractures and disrupted extensor mechanisms. All attempts should be made to salvage a significant portion of the articular surface.

Patella dislocations (Box 12.55.7)

Incidence and prevalence

Acute lateral patella dislocations are relatively uncommon injuries. However, in many patients the patella relocates prior to presenting for medical care so the true incidence is unknown. Most dislocations occur in patients during their second and third decades of life and there is a slight female predominance.

Pathological anatomy

The patellofemoral joint is stabilized by both bony and soft tissue restraints. Bony stability is provided by the convex shape of the patellar articular surface as it articulates within the concave trough of the femoral trochlea. The quadriceps muscle group provides dynamic stability with an essential contribution from the vastus medialis obliquus. The medial and lateral retinacula along with their associated medial and lateral patellofemoral and tibiofemoral ligaments provide static stability (see Figure 12.55.1).

Many anatomical factors can predispose a patient to sustaining a patella dislocation (Table 12.55.1). Unfortunately, no single factor or combination of factors has been shown to be predictive of dislocation, redislocation, or poor outcome after dislocation.

Box 12.55.7 Acute patella dislocations

- Frequent predisposing anatomical factors
- Operative vs non-operative management controversial
- Look for osteochondral fractures—if present remove or internally fix
- Recurrent dislocation and persistent anterior knee pain are most frequent complications.

Table 12.55.1 Anatomic factors associated with patellofemoral instability and dislocation

Clinical findings
Q angle greater than 15°
Excessive femoral anteversion
Femoral torsion(internal)
Excessive genu valgum
Tibial torsion
Excessive ligamentous laxity
Lateral hypermobility of the patella
Tight lateral retinaculum
Abnormal patella tracking
Vastus medialis obliquus atrophy
Excessive hindfoot pronation
Radiographic findings
Patella alta
Patella tilt
Patella subluxation
Patella dysplasia
Hypoplastic lateral femoral condyle
Shallow femoral trochlea

The medial patellofemoral ligament is a major stabilizing component of the medial retinacular complex. Several studies have shown that there is a consistent injury to the medial patellofemoral ligament after dislocation. However, whether the major injury occurs at the patellar insertion, within the midsubstance, at the femoral origin, or some combination of locations continues to be a point of controversy and is a critical piece of knowledge if one is considering operative repair. Bony injuries of the medial border of the patella represent avulsions of the medial patellofemoral ligament. Other structures commonly injured during lateral dislocation include the vastus medialis obliquus and medial patellar and lateral trochlear articular surfaces.

Most patella dislocations occur as a result of a twisting injury. Internal rotation of the femur on a fixed lower extremity while the quadriceps contracts draws the patella out of the trochlea, resulting in a lateral patella dislocation. Less commonly, a direct force applied to the medial side of the patella causes lateral dislocation.

Box 12.55.8 Investigation of patella dislocation

- Radiograph (associated fractures)
- Joint aspiration:
  - Pain relief
  - Look for fat droplets
- MRI scan may be useful occasionally.

Classification

Superior, medial, lateral, and intra-articular dislocations have been described. Lateral dislocations represent the overwhelming majority of these injuries.

Clinical evaluation

The history is usually one of a twisting injury to the knee associated with collapse, acute pain, and swelling. A sensation that something 'popped' out of place is common. If the knee remains flexed, the patella will be visualized on the lateral side of the knee. With knee extension (by the patient or a bystander) the patella will relocate. A history of similar previous episodes along with a history of anterior knee symptoms may be elicited.

The injured knee is assessed for patella mobility and apprehension, to localize tenderness and identify tears of the medial retinaculum–vastus medialis obliquus complex, and to exclude cruciate and collateral ligament injuries. The uninjured knee is examined for anatomical factors associated with patellofemoral disorders (Table 12.55.1).

Investigation (Box 12.55.8)

Joint aspiration

Aspiration of the knee can serve three potential functions. Firstly, evacuation of the haematoma will provide pain relief for the patient. Secondly, fat droplets within the aspirate indicate the presence of an osteochondral fracture, a consideration for operative intervention. Thirdly, removal of the haematoma may aid reapproximation of the torn edges of the medial retinacular complex.

Radiographs

Standard plain radiographs (anteroposterior, lateral, and Merchant views) are required and should be scrutinized for osteochondral fractures and the presence of any factors known to be associated with patellofemoral disorders (Table12.55.1). Medial extra-articular capsular avulsion fractures are pathognomonic and should be differentiated from osteochondral fractures.

Some surgeons obtain MRI examinations after patella dislocations to document osteochondral and chondral injuries not seen on radiographs, detect bone bruises, and characterize the injury to the medial patellofemoral ligament. In rare instances, an MRI may be indicated for diagnostic purposes in a patient with a haemarthrosis and confusing physical examination.

Management

Initial

Patients presenting with the patella dislocated require a gentle, closed reduction as there is some evidence that the majority of osteochondral fractures occur with relocation. Using intravenous sedation to keep the quadriceps maximally relaxed, the leg is gradually extended passively until the patella reduces.

Definitive

Non-operative

Patella dislocations have traditionally been reduced and immobilized in extension for 6 weeks followed by quadriceps rehabilitation. However, several studies have shown the treatment results to be independent of the duration of immobilization. Based on these

Box 12.55.9 Osteochondral fractures of the patella

- Incidence 5–43% of all first-time patella dislocations
- 20–82% visible on radiograph
- Remove small fragments
- Internally fix large fragments.

Box 12.55.10 Results of treatment of patellar dislocation

- Many patients have persistent symptoms
- Medial retinacular repair reduces redislocation rate
- No advantage with surgery in long-term symptoms
- Conservative treatment probably as good as surgery.

data, many have decreased the period of immobilization and focused more on rehabilitation.

Operative

Operative procedures are most commonly indicated for patients with anatomical factors associated with patellofemoral instability (Table 12.55.1). Unfortunately, no single factor or group of factors have been shown to be highly predictive of future problems, and some patients respond well to conservative treatment despite having anatomical factors associated with instability.

Repair of the medial retinaculum–vastus medialis obliquus complex has been advocated by many, especially when a palpable defect is present on examination. The addition of a lateral release with or without a distal realignment has been advocated. An isolated lateral release can be performed arthroscopically. The indications for any one or more of these procedures are controversial and have been largely based on surgeon preference.

Post-treatment care

Post-treatment care focuses on regaining quadriceps strength, with special emphasis on the vastus medialis obliquus. This requires a prolonged rehabilitation program that lasts beyond symptomatic improvement.

Special circumstances

Osteochondral fractures (Box 12.55.9)

Osteochondral fractures have been estimated to occur in 5–43% of all first-time patella dislocations. Plain radiographs have been reported to detect 20–82% of these injuries. Although MRI would aid in detecting these fractures, no clear benefit has been reported to addressing fractures not appreciated on plain radiographs.

Small fragments should be excised and larger fragments with adequate subchondral bone internally fixed.

Results (Box 12.55.10)

Non-operative treatment

Redislocation rates for conservatively treated patients range from 22–44%. Forty to seventy-five per cent of patients have persistent symptoms related to the patellofemoral joint with 25% undergoing further surgical treatment. Approximately 65% of patients are satisfied with conservative treatment alone, although 40–50% will have some limitation of function.

Operative treatment

Arthroscopically assisted lateral release alone provides no benefit over conservative treatment. Other operative treatments (incorporating medial retinacular repair) have been reported to reduce redislocation rates to 0–10%. However, residual symptoms are common with 40–70% of patients having anterior knee pain and 20–30% having symptoms of instability. Patient satisfaction rates have been slightly higher (80–90%) with operative intervention, although there are no good controlled studies to provide definitive documentation.

Complications

Recurrent dislocations and persistent anterior knee symptoms are the major problems complicating first-time dislocation. Recurrent dislocation is associated with younger age at the time of first dislocation (less than 20 years old), non-operative treatment, and anatomical factors predisposing to instability. Surgery can reduce the rate of redislocation, but does not reduce residual symptoms of pain and instability. Furthermore, many patients with multiple predisposing factors respond well to conservative treatment alone.

Future directions

The debate between operative and non-operative management of first-time dislocators will likely continue. Future work will attempt to identify specific anatomical factors predictive of redislocation and methods to more effectively treat persistent symptoms of anterior knee pain and instability.

Summary

Acute patella dislocations occur primarily in patients with anatomical predisposition. Initial treatment involves a gentle reduction. Osteochondral fractures visible on plain radiographs should be removed or replaced, depending on the size of the fragment. Non-operative treatment is indicated for most patients, emphasizing the importance of a prolonged rehabilitation program. Operative intervention is considered in those patients with large palpable medial retinaculum–vastus medialis obliquus defects along with those with persistent symptoms of pain and instability after adequate rehabilitation.

Further reading

Carpenter, J.E., Kasman, R.A., Patel, N., Lee, M.L., and Goldstein, S.A. (1997). Biomechanical evaluation of current patella fracture fixation techniques. *Journal of Orthopaedic Trauma*, **11**(5), 351–6.

Christiansen, S.E., Jakobsen, B.W., Lund, B., and Lind, M. (2008). Isolated repair of the medial patellofemoral ligament in primary dislocation of the patella: a prospective randomized study. *Arthroscopy*, **24**(8), 881–7.

12.56

Tibial plateau fractures

Phil Walmsley and John Keating

Summary points

- Split depression pattern lateral plateau most common type
- Bicondylar and medial plateau fractures high energy injuries
- Compartment syndrome, vascular injury, and common peroneal palsy may occur with high energy patterns
- Internal fixation preferred treatment with good soft tissue envelope
- Limited internal fixation suitable for many simple patterns
- Plate fixation preferred for medial and bicondylar fractures
- External fixation used with poor soft tissues
- Fine wire external fixation should be considered for most complex patterns.

Introduction

Fractures of the proximal tibia present a challenging problem as the injury involves a principal weight-bearing joint and severe injuries can lead to functional impairment. A flexible approach is required to adapt treatment to the patient, fracture pattern, and clinical and radiological findings. The treatment options range from non-operative management through limited internal fixation to open reduction and internal fixation (ORIF) or external fixation. Regardless of the treatment method employed, the aim is to provide a stable, pain-free, and well-aligned joint whilst avoiding complications.

The aim of this chapter is to provide an overview of the injury, classification, management and technical tips in managing this type of fracture.

Epidemiology

In a consecutive series of 285 tibial plateau fractures treated at our institution, there were 168 female and 117 male patients giving a female: male ratio of 1.4:1. Most of these fractures were isolated injuries with multiple trauma accounting for only 1.4% of cases. There were 149 (49%) undisplaced fractures and 146 (51%) displaced fractures. Although the mean age of patients with plateau fractures was 58 years, there appeared to be a bimodal incidence with a peak of younger patients and a larger peak in the seventh and eighth decades of life (Figure 12.56.1). Simple falls and pedestrian accidents accounted for 70% of cases. Dogs running into their owners were a surprisingly common cause and accounted for 15% of fractures (Figure 12.56.2).

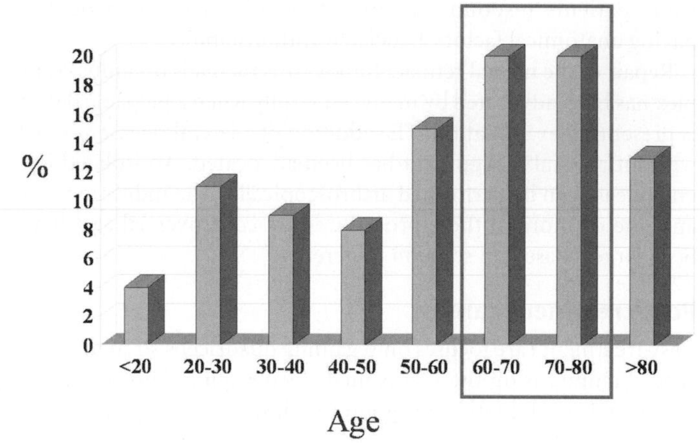

Fig. 12.56.1 Incidence of tibial plateau fractures.

Anatomy (Box 12.56.1)

The tibial plateau is formed by the medial and lateral condyles separated by the tibial (intercondylar) eminence. The intercondylar eminence is the site of attachment of the meniscal horns and the anterior cruciate ligament. There are important soft tissue structures that attach to the tibial plateau including the knee joint

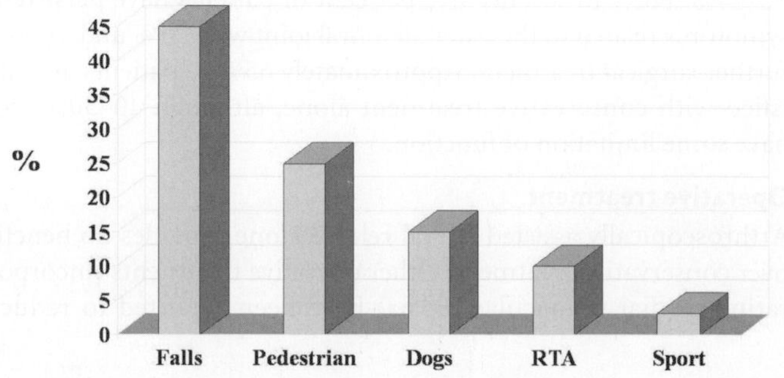

Fig. 12.56.2 Tibial plateau aetiology.

Box 12.56.1 Anatomy of tibial plateau

- 10-degree posterior slope
- Lateral plateau convex
- Medial plateau concave
- Subchondral bone higher on lateral side
- Load bearing on lateral side mainly through meniscus.

capsule, and the medial and lateral meniscotibial ligaments. The medial collateral ligament comprises a deep and superficial layer. The lateral collateral ligament is attached from the lateral epicondyle to the fibular head. The anterior cruciate ligament is attached to the intercondylar eminence between the tibial spines and the posterior cruciate ligament arises from the posterior aspect of the plateau in the midline. Further meniscal attachment is provided by the meniscotibial ligaments at the periphery of both sides. The attachment of the joint capsule can extend 1.5cm below the level of the joint margin, which has particular significance when using fine-wire external fixators, which are often situated, close to the joint. If they penetrate the capsule, pin track infection may result in septic arthritis.

Three additional structures have potential significance in assessment and management of tibial plateau fractures. The fascia lata attaches at Gerdy's tubercle, and is sometimes disrupted by the injury or requires to be released during the exposure and fixation of the fracture. The tendons of gracilis, sartorius, and semitendinosis are attached anteromedially at the pes anserinus and need to be reflected during exposure of the medial plateau.

The surface of the tibial plateau forms a 10-degree posterior slope in relation to the long axis of the tibia. The shape of the medial condyle is concave and has an average 3-mm thick hyaline cartilage articular surface that the medial meniscus covers about 50% from the periphery. It has less of a flare and as a result is less prone to the shear forces that render the lateral plateau more susceptible to fracture. The lateral plateau is convex with an average 4-mm thick hyaline cartilage that is almost completely covered by the lateral meniscus. Load bearing on the lateral plateau is transmitted mainly through the lateral meniscus, unlike the medial plateau where the load is distributed equally through the meniscus and the exposed articular surface.

The medial plateau surface is lower in the transverse plane than the lateral plateau and this can be easily seen on plain anteroposterior (AP) radiographs. This is significant when elevating a depressed segment of the plateau in assessing the accuracy of reduction and surgeons should be aware that the subchondral line on the lateral side should be higher than on the medial side. It is also important to appreciate that a screw or wire placed subchondrally on the lateral side proceeding medially, perpendicular to the tibial shaft, may penetrate the articular surface of the medial side if the location is very proximal. Ideal screw placement is in the subchondral bone just beneath the articular surface in a 'raft' construct.

Classification

Several classification systems of plateau fractures have been described. No one system provides a comprehensive description of all fracture patterns encountered. The Hohl and Moore, and Rasmussen systems are mainly of historical interest and no longer in widespread use. The Schatzker classification subdivides the plateau fractures into six groups and has been the most popular method of classifying tibial plateau fractures from plain radiographs and remains in common use today. However, it has some significant disadvantages. Medial plateau fractures are all classified as type IV injuries but there are a wide variety of these fractures. The oblique fractures which are a highly unstable pattern are not specifically covered by the classification (Figure 12.56.3). The type V fracture as originally described was a bicondylar fracture (Figure 12.56.4) with the interspinous eminence still in contact with the tibial diaphysis. However, this is actually a very rare pattern and in most bicondylar fractures the interspinous region is involved in the fracture and is not in continuity with the tibial shaft.

The more comprehensive classification is the AO/Orthopaedic Trauma Association (OTA) system which covers most fracture types and is now being used more commonly. It allows a more detailed description of fracture morphology including separate categories for oblique fractures and a number of categories for bicondylar fracture patterns. However, even this system does not describe the important posteromedial and anteromedial fractures as separate entities. It is worth noting that both classification systems are prone to inter- and intra-observer error.

AO/Orthopaedic Trauma Association classification

The AO/OTA classification is based on an alphanumeric system that assigns each major bone and the region of bone involved a number and then subdivides the injuries in that region based on severity. In the case of the tibial plateau, the bone is assigned the number 4 and proximal region is 1. Proximal tibial metaphyseal fractures, which are extra-articular, are classified as type A injuries. Type B fractures are partial articular fractures and type C fractures are complete articular fractures. All fractures involved the plateau are classified as 41 type B and C injuries. Type B1 fractures are simple splits, type B2 are pure depression, and type B3 are split

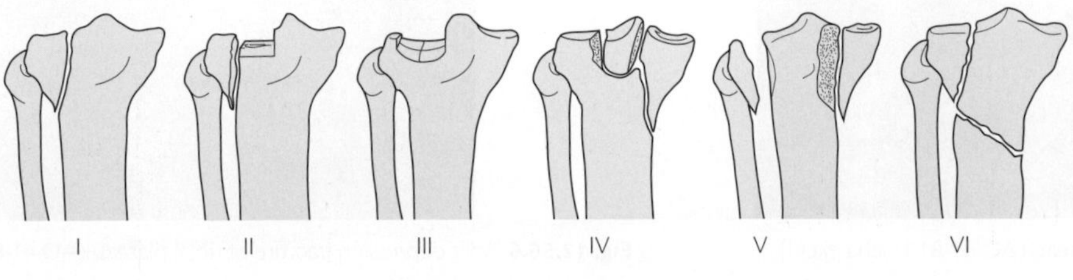

Fig. 12.56.3 Schatzker classification (Schatzker J., McBroom R., and Bruce D., (1979). The tibial plateau fracture. The Toronto experience 1968-1975. *Clinical Orthopaedics and Related Research*, **145**, 136–45).

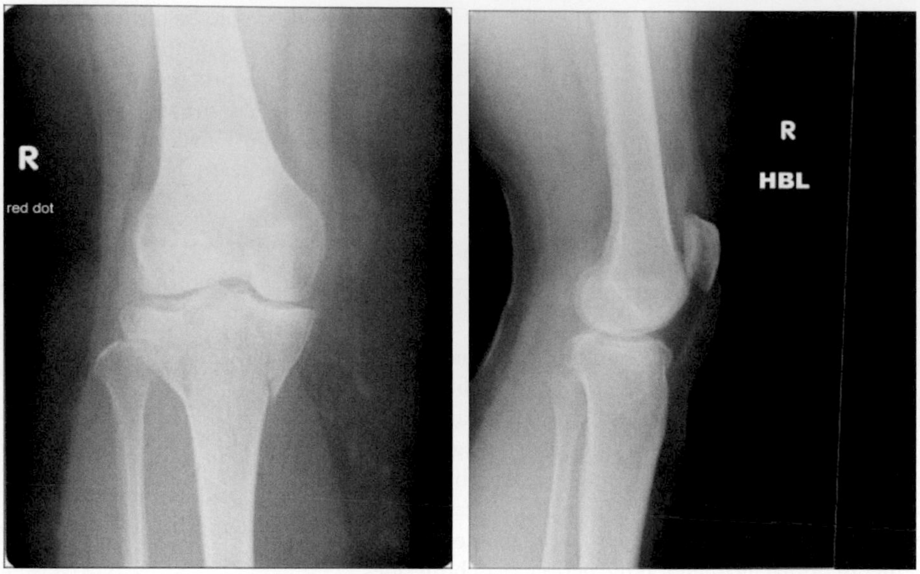

Fig. 12.56.4 AP and lateral x-rays of Schatzker V tibial plateau fracture.

depression fractures. Subdivisions of each category allow for description of whether the injury involves the medial or lateral plateau and the extent of involvement. The type C fractures are bicondylar fractures. Type C1 designates a fracture with a simple articular and metaphyseal configuration. Type C2 is a metaphyseal complex pattern with simple articular pattern and type C3 fractures are complex articular bicondylar plateau fractures.

Split fractures

- 41-B1.1 Lateral (Figure 12.56.5)
- 41-B1.2 Medial
- 41-B1.3 Oblique split.

These fractures are simple splits with no comminution or joint depression. They most commonly involve the lateral tibial plateau and usually occur in young patients with good bone stock. The most common mechanism of injury is axial loading coupled with a valgus force. The strong cancellous bone resists any surrounding articular depression that occurs in older or osteoporotic patients. Wide displacement of the split fracture may be associated with peripheral meniscal detachment and occasionally entrapment of the meniscus in the fracture may occur.

Split depression

- 41-B3.1 Lateral (Figure 12.56.6)
- 41-B3.2 Medial split depression
- 41-B3.3 Oblique split depression.

These fractures are intra-articular fractures of the tibial plateau but in addition have an adjacent area of articular depression.

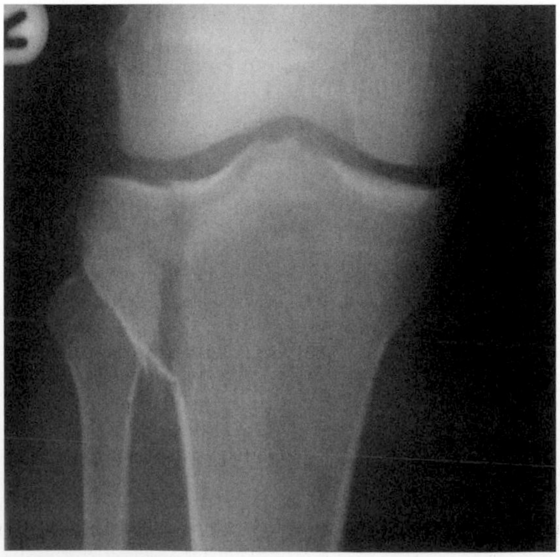

Fig. 12.56.5 Split fracture lateral tibial plateau (AO 41-B1.1/Schatzker I).

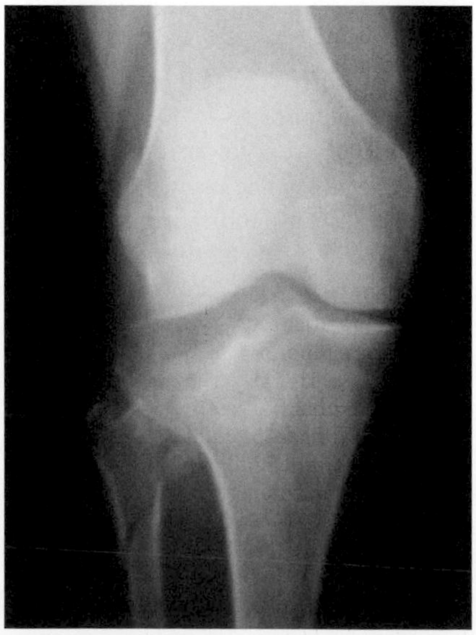

Fig. 12.56.6 Split depression fracture of tibial plateau (AO 41-B3.1/Schatzker II).

These are usually found in older patients or younger patients with higher-energy injuries. They occur when the surrounding cancellous bone is unable to withstand the axial load created by the lateral femoral condyle. The same associated soft tissue injuries occur as with the split fractures.

Depression fractures

- 41-B2.1 Lateral total depression
- 41-B2.2 Lateral limited depression (Figure 12.56.7).

This is a pure depression fracture of the lateral tibial plateau and principally occurs in older patients, again due to the weaker cancellous bone. Isolated depression fractures are actually quite uncommon—the majority have a split component which is undisplaced and is recognized only on computed tomography (CT) scan or at the time of surgery.

Medial fractures

- 41-B1.2 Medial split
- 41-B1.3 Oblique involving the tibial spines
- 41-B2.3 Medial depression
- 41-B3.2 Medial split depression
- 41-B3.3 Medial split depression, oblique (Figure 12.56.8).

Split or split depression fractures of the medial tibial plateau occur as a result of compression of the medial plateau by a varus force. Many of these are high-energy injuries and are associated with other soft tissue problems. Oblique medial plateau fractures that extend to the interspinous region or into the lateral plateau are fracture dislocations of the knee and are highly unstable injuries. Since all of these fractures involve application of varus force to the knee, there is a possibility of common peroneal nerve palsy.

Bicondylar fractures

- 41-C1.1–AO 41-C3.3 Complete articular (Figure 12.56.9).

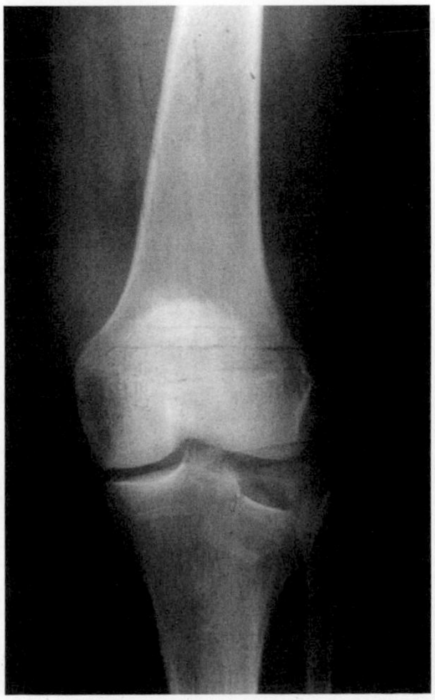

Fig. 12.56.7 Depression fracture of tibial plateau (AO 41-B2.2/Schatzker III).

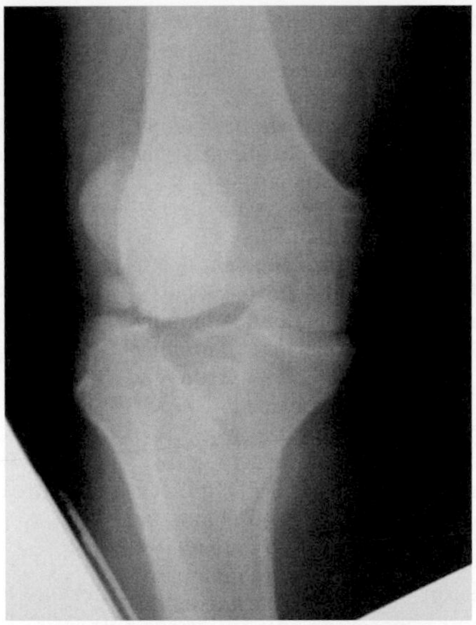

Fig. 12.56.8 Medial split depression oblique fracture of tibial plateau (AO 41-B3.3/Schatzker IV).

These fractures involve a bicondylar split with separation of the medial and lateral condyles and a variable involvement of the diaphysis. The proposed mechanism for this fracture is pure axial load on the extended knee. Bicondylar fractures account for 10–15% of all plateau fractures. The involvement of the intercondylar area in the fracture may compromise cruciate ligament attachments. The higher energy required to produce this fracture patterns means they are associated with greater soft tissue injury and an increased risk of compartment syndrome.

Clinical features

Mechanism of injury

The majority of tibial plateau fractures are isolated injuries but initial management involves careful general evaluation in line with

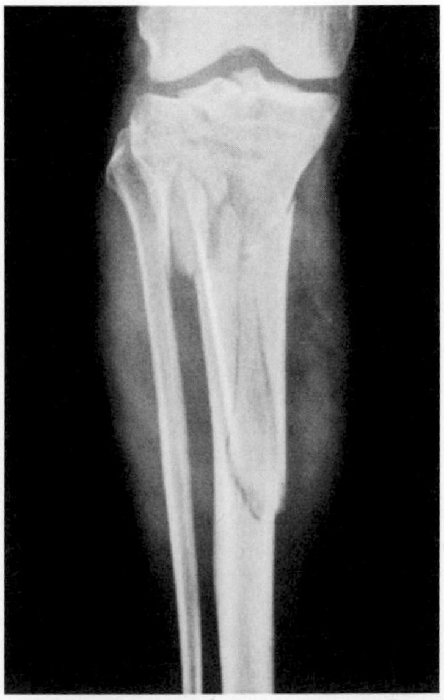

Fig. 12.56.9 Complete articular fracture of tibial plateau with multifragmentary metaphysis (AO 41-C2.3/Schatzker VI).

ATLS® principles to exclude other injuries. The most common mechanism of fracture is usually a combination of an axial load coupled with a valgus force. In this situation the medial collateral ligament acts as a hinge on the medial femoral condyle that then drives the lateral femoral condyle into the lateral tibial plateau. In patients with normal bone stock, this leads to a sagittal split of the lateral plateau. Damage to the articular surface of the lateral plateau with additional comminution is frequent, leading to a split depression fracture. Elderly patients with poorer bone stock often appear to have depression of the articular surface without a split fracture. However, pure depression fractures are uncommon and even patients who appear to have isolated depression usually have an undisplaced split component present.

Varus stress in combination with compression is a much less frequent mechanism of injury but can result in a fracture of the medial plateau. Progression of varus deformity may result in disruption of the posterolateral corner structures and subsequent traction injury or even avulsion of the common peroneal nerve. Occasionally a combination of hyperextension and varus deformity can occur and this leads typically to an anteromedial plateau fracture which may be associated with a posterior cruciate ligament and posterolateral corner ligament injury (Figure 12.56.10)

High-energy injuries with axial loads in addition to valgus or varus forces usually result in bicondylar plateau fractures. These fractures are often associated with a significant degree of soft tissue injury. As a consequence of the posterior slope of the tibia, the distal femoral condyles are subsequently directed posteriorly, leading to disruption of the joint capsule, cruciate and collateral ligaments and potential injury the neurovascular bundle.

Clinical assessment (Box 12.56.2)

Careful observation of the soft tissues is required in all cases, particularly to detect blisters, devitalized skin, and open fractures all of which will influence the clinical decisions regarding management.

An assessment of the neurovascular status of the limb should be performed and documented. If there is any doubt regarding the vascularity of the limb in high-energy fracture patterns angiography is required. Injury may take the form of a thrombus, occult intimal tear or, rarely, complete disruption of the artery. Either angiography or a CT angiogram should reveal these injuries. Fractures of the medial plateau may result in traction injury or avulsion of the common peroneal nerve and is present in 10% of these fractures. The neurological status of the limb should be examined and documented on admission.

Compartment syndrome is not commonly associated with the simpler fracture patterns (split, depression and split depression patterns). However it does occur in 5–10% of patients with bicondylar fractures and the high-energy oblique fractures and a high index of suspicion is warranted in these cases. Compartment pressure monitoring is advisable in these patients.

Box 12.56.2 Clinical assessment

- Examine soft tissue envelope of injured limb
- Careful neurological examination—common peroneal nerve
- Assess vascular supply of distal limb
- If any doubt over vascular supply obtain angiogram or CT angiography
- Assess for compartment syndrome.

Investigations (Box 12.56.3)

Plain AP and lateral radiographs of the tibial plateau are required in all cases. A 'Moore' view can be added, which is an AP view taken with 10–15-degree caudal tilt (Figure 12.56.11). This accounts for the posterior slope of the tibial plateau allowing a better evaluation of the joint surface. Oblique views taken at 45 degrees and plain tomography were commonly used in the past but have been superseded by CT scanning.

Modern CT scanning with sagittal, coronal, and three-dimensional reconstructions are not necessary for simpler fracture patterns but should be considered in more complex injuries, particularly bicondylar fractures. However, in some simple fracture

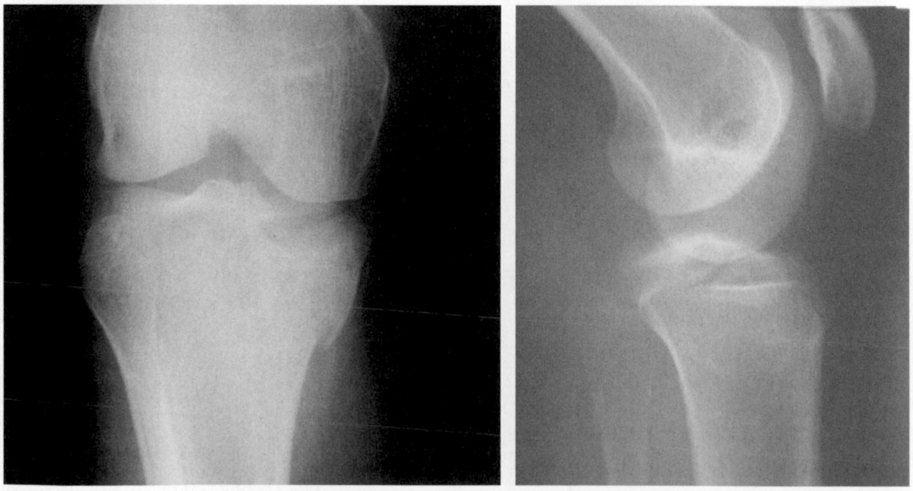

A B

Fig. 12.56.10 AP and lateral x-rays of anteromedial plateau fractures.

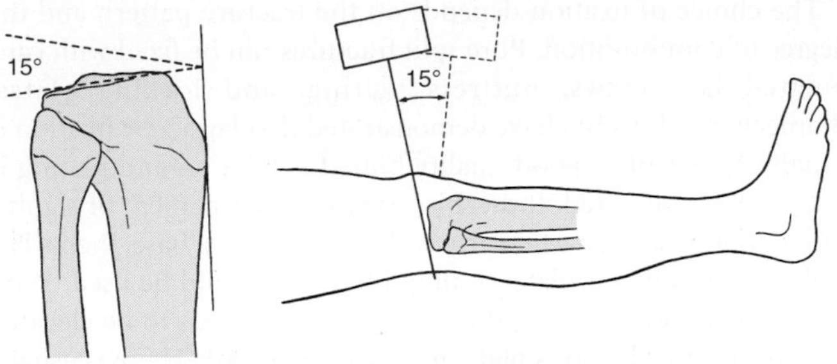

Fig. 12.56.11 Tibial plateau radiographic views.

patterns there may be some doubt about the diagnosis, the extent of plateau involvement or the degree of joint depression and CT scans are useful in these cases to determine the need for surgery. The coronal views show the size and location of all articular fragments. The use of CT reconstructions, as well as intraoperative CT has been shown to be superior to fluoroscopy in assessing fracture reduction. Magnetic resonance imaging (MRI) has been used, where available, to delineate occult fractures, soft tissue disruption and impaction of the articular surface. It is most useful in fracture patterns specifically associated with ligamentous injury, particularly anteromedial plateau fractures. In these cases the ligament injury is often impossible to diagnose clinically due to the presence of the unstable fracture.

If the fracture pattern involves the anteromedial portion of the tibial plateau then a careful examination of the posterolateral corner should be undertaken. Regardless of the mode of imaging employed, the objective is to provide a full assessment of the fracture pattern and any associated soft tissue disruption, which facilitates preoperative planning.

Management

The management of tibial plateau fractures is determined by the clinical evaluation of the patient and the limb, and the morphology of the fracture. Factors that will have a major influence on treatment choice are the presence of an open wound, a fracture dislocation, concurrent and pre-existing health or knee problems, age and activity level, bone quality, anticipated patient compliance with rehabilitation, and treatment expectations. The successful treatment of these injuries is a dependent on careful treatment selection and a properly structured rehabilitation programme. Even when this occurs many patients take over a year to recover knee muscle function and motion. Patients over 40 years of age recover significantly slower, and some have residual impairment of movement and muscle function.

Box 12.56.3 Investigations

- AP and lateral x-rays ± Moore view
- CT scan ± angiogram
- Angiography
- MRI
- Compartment pressure monitoring.

Any open fractures should be initially covered with a sterile dressing and administration of broad-spectrum intravenous antibiotics. The patient's tetanus status should be addressed. Initial debridement and irrigation with 10L of normal saline within 6h of injury is required.

If there is an associated vascular injury-requiring repair, then ideally the fracture should be stabilized first without delay. Complex fracture patterns may require temporary bridging external fixation across the knee joint. Pins should be placed as far as practical away from any future surgical incisions. Following a vascular repair, fasciotomies are commonly required, and definitive fracture fixation may be delayed 48–72h until the fasciotomies are closed.

Closed unstable fractures without vascular injury, can be fully evaluated clinically with appropriate imaging and preoperative planning prior to definitive surgery. During this time, the limb may be immobilized in a padded long leg splint. Deep vein thrombosis (DVT) prophylaxis should be prescribed and intermittent foot compression devices may be used on the contralateral foot as well.

Non-operative treatment (Box 12.56.4)

In the past this was a commonly employed treatment modality but with modern imaging techniques and a wider variety of surgical options, a smaller proportion of tibial plateau fractures are suitable for non-operative treatment in modern practice. Pure split, split depression, and depression fractures that are stable through 90 degrees of flexion with less than 3mm of articular depression are suitable. The bone quality, concomitant medical problems, and functional demands in elderly patients may also influence the decision to opt for non-operative treatment. If there is any doubt regarding the suitability of the fracture for non-operative treatment, a CT scan is the most helpful additional investigation to determine the extent of joint surface involvement and the degree of depression. Central depression fractures of the lateral plateau with minimal depression of the articular surface are suitable for non-operative treatment due to the load bearing nature of the lateral meniscus that protects the damaged articular surface.

If non-operative treatment is selected there are several forms of immobilization available. A full-length cast can be used but a cast braces with a hinge at the level of the knee to allow some knee motion is preferable. Removable hinged braces that do not enclose the foot are a good choice for stable fractures in compliant patients. Accurate placement of the brace by an orthotist or surgeon is essential and the patient, or carer, must be able to reproduce correct placement of the device for this to be successful.

Box 12.56.4 Indications for non-operative treatment

- <3mm articular depression
- Undisplaced fractures stable 0–90 degrees
- Poor bone quality
- Severe osteoarthritis (OA)
- Low demand elderly
- High American Society of Anaesthesiologists (ASA) grade.

Patients treated non-operatively should be allowed touch weight bearing for the first 6 weeks and progression to full weight bearing over the subsequent 6 weeks is allowed provided there is radiographic evidence of fracture healing. Radiographs are required in the first 2 weeks of treatment to check for loss of fracture position. If there is any loss of position, this may necessitate conversion to operative treatment.

Operative treatment (Box 12.56.5)

Operative treatment is indicated in unstable fracture patterns with joint surface displacement in excess of 3mm. Operative treatment is indicated in all open fractures, and those associated with significant soft tissue problems (compartment syndrome, ligament injury, common peroneal nerve palsy, and vascular injury).

Group 1: lateral split, split depression, and central depression fractures

A single linear anterior paramedian incision is suitable for access. It has the advantage of being used for a subsequent knee arthroplasty should one be required. A subperiosteal exposure of the lateral plateau is readily carried out. This approach allows excellent exposure of the lateral plateau fracture and facilitates reduction of the proximal tibial condyle prior to secure internal fixation. Direct visualization of the joint reduction is best achieved with an anterolateral arthrotomy. A plane is then developed between the capsule and edge of the lateral meniscus. The meniscus is then elevated to expose the plateau by incising the lateral meniscotibial ligaments. Some authors have proposed incising the lateral horn of the meniscus but we prefer to avoid this. A curved anterolateral incision can also be used. The main drawback of this exposure is that the curved portion is not suitable for use if knee arthroplasty is needed and may increase the risk of wound complications at subsequent surgery.

Box 12.56.5 Operative techniques

- Approach
  - Lateral—anterior paramedian or curved anterolateral
  - Medial—longitudinal posteromedial
  - Bicondylar—dual incisions
  - MIPO (minimally invasive plate osteosynthesis)
- Fixation:
  - Percutaneous screws
  - Raft screws
  - Buttress plates
  - Antiglide plates
  - Locking plates
  - Circular frame
- Surgical adjuncts:
  - Bone graft and bone graft substitute
  - Femoral distractor
  - Arthroscopy.

The choice of fixation depends on the fracture pattern and the degree of comminution. Pure split fractures can be fixed with cannulated lag screws, buttress plating, and locking plates. Biomechanical studies have demonstrated that lag screw fixation is usually sufficient in good quality bone for fixation and plating is not generally required. If there is a single large fragment or significant comminution, particularly at the metaphyseal base, then a laterally based buttress plate or antiglide plate should be used. With split depression fractures, the depressed area needs to be elevated and fixed with a buttress plate or periarticular raft. There is usually a subchondral defect once the joint surface is restored to the anatomical position. The addition of bone graft or bone substitutes is often required in addition to fixation to support the joint surface. Bone graft substitutes are a good choice in older patients where autogenous bone graft may be of poor quality.

Group 2: medial plateau and oblique fractures

Medial fractures are usually the result of high-energy injuries and frequently have associated soft tissue injuries. Almost all fractures of the medial plateau are unstable and require operative treatment, provided the patient is medically fit. Fractures which contain a predominantly split component, can usually be reduced indirectly with gentle traction or a femoral distractor. If the split is coronal then a posteromedial approach may be required. A vertical incision is employed starting posteroinferior to the adductor tubercle extending distal to the joint line by 6cm. The skin flaps are raised to expose the fascia. There is no true internervous plane and the saphenous nerve crosses the approach transversely and should be protected as it emerges between gracilis and sartorius muscles. Incise the fascia over the anterior border of the sartorius and retract this muscle posteriorly along with gracilis and semitendinosus. Separate the medial head of gastrocnemius from semimembranosus to expose the posteromedial corner of the tibial plateau. Further blunt dissection beneath the medial head of gastrocnemius is safe and allows access to the posterior tibia as far as the midline. Those with significant depression of the articular surface require open reduction. Fractures of the medial plateau usually have significant shear forces acting on them and as a result lag screws alone are not to provide enough stability. They require a medial buttress plate to counteract the shear forces acting.

Group 3: bicondylar fractures

Previously these fractures were treated with dual medial and lateral plates or by a combination of limited internal fixation and external fixation. Since the advent of locking plates, it is possible to fix the two condyles with 6.5-mm lag screws and stabilize the articular segment to the diaphysis with a lateral or medially placed locking plate. Having screws locked into the plate creates a fixed angle device with enough stability to counteract the forces acting on the contralateral tibial plateau. This obviates the need for a second plate with the additional soft tissue dissection this entails.

Fracture patterns that have dissociation of the metaphysis from the diaphysis, represent the most severe injuries. There is no consensus as to the definitive choice of fixation. In principle, however, they all require articular reconstruction and reconnection of the articular segment back to the tibial shaft. Most surgeons now use either locking plates or fine wire external fixation for these fracture patterns.

The method of fixation is influenced to a large extent by the status of the soft tissues. If the soft tissues are in good condition then a long locking plate after joint surface reconstruction is now probably the most popular method of treatment. If the soft tissues are extensively contused or there are fracture blisters then a more cautious approach is necessary. One option is the use of a temporary external fixator spanning the fracture until the soft tissue envelope has recovered and internal fixation can be safely undertaken. The alternative is to use fine wire external fixation as the definitive method of treatment. This may be the only choice if the soft tissue injury is extensive or the bone is of poor quality.

Results

It is difficult to compare the results of different treatments reported in the published literature. There are various reasons for this, including different classification systems and outcome scoring scales being routinely employed. In general, non-displaced fractures and lower-energy fractures such as split, split-depression, and central depression types have a better prognosis. A 20-year follow-up was performed on ten patients who underwent operative fixation. These patients were originally selected for surgery as they had greater than 10 degrees of coronal plane instability in full extension at examination under anaesthesia. Good to excellent results were found in 90% of patients. For the use of limited internal fixation combined with appropriate external support, reports show 90% good or excellent results. The higher energy, more complex fracture patterns present a greater challenge to manage. The Canadian Orthopaedic Trauma Society completed a multicentre, prospective, randomized clinical trial to compare ORIF with percutaneous, limited fixation and application of a circular fixator. The fracture patterns within this series were OTA types C1–3. The follow-up of this group is short term, but at 2 years showed no significant differences with respect to quality of reduction or functional outcome. However, there were a greater number of complications in the internal fixation group and a deep infection rate of 18%. Type C3 fractures treated with medial and lateral plates showed significant residual dysfunction in patients with greater than 2mm articular surface step. This is despite associations with patient age and presence of polytrauma.

Recently there has been increased use of locking plates to treat the more complex fractures, in particular osteoporotic fractures and those with extensive comminution. These devices minimize soft tissue injury by using minimally invasive approaches in conjunction with femoral distractors, K-wires, and percutaneously applied reduction forceps to control the major fragments. Results with this technique have shown a union rate of 96% and deep infection rate of 3.7%. However, malalignment has been reported in a significant number of cases. In comparison, dual plate techniques have been shown clinically to have less malalignment and less subsidence in cadaveric experiments. Although locking plates may provide a more biological solution to bicondylar plateau fractures it is clearly important to tailor the appropriate treatment to suit the patient's individual bony and soft tissue injuries.

Complications (Box 12.56.6)

Complications can occur with any of the described fracture patterns, but are more frequent with the higher energy injuries. Prevention, where possible, is the best treatment but in principle good surgical technique, limited incisions and careful tissue handling will reduce their incidence. The outcome of tibial plateau fractures following a complication is difficult to assess due to the heterogeneous nature of the groups reported in the published literature.

Compartment syndrome

This is not frequent in most plateau fractures but must be considered particularly in higher-energy patterns of bicondylar and medial plateau fractures. The most reliable method of diagnosis is by compartment pressure monitoring. Early fasciotomy to decompress the four compartments of the leg is required. This may influence selection of fixation method. However, it does not preclude using internal fixation with a plate, although difficulty may be encountered when attempting wound closure and use of a gastrocnemius flap is occasionally necessary to cover a plate on the medial or lateral plateau.

Deep vein thrombosis

Incidence of this complication following tibial plateau fractures is reported to be 5–10% and subsequent pulmonary embolus (PE) at 1–2%. Use of anticoagulant prophylaxis, compression pneumatic stockings, and early movement should be used to reduce this complication.

Infection

The incidence of this complication correlates well with the degree of soft tissues compromise and the amount of internal fixation required. Intravenous antibiotics should be used for closed fractures treated by internal fixation. Open fractures require adequate debridement, irrigation, antibiotics, and where appropriate soft tissue coverage within 7 days. Previous treatment strategies using large open approaches to implant metalware produced infection rates up to 80%. Modern techniques place greater emphasis on managing and handling the soft tissue envelope, combined with smaller incisions. This has led to a reduction of infection rates, in high-energy fractures, to approximately 10–18%.

Non-union

The metaphyseal bone of the proximal tibia usually heals without difficulty, resulting in a very low rate of non-union for tibial plateau fractures. When it occurs it is usually with the high-energy

Box 12.56.6 Complications

- Compartment syndrome
- DVT 5–10%
- PE 1–2%
- Infection 10–18% in high-energy fractures
- Malunion
  - Articular incongruity contributes to post-traumatic OA
  - Increased post-traumatic OA when malalignment > 5 degrees
- Reduced range of motion
- Post-traumatic OA
- Hardware irritation.

fractures and infection must be excluded as a cause. Most of these fractures heal within 6 months. Failure of progression to union at this stage may require revision of fixation with bone grafting of the metaphyseal non-union.

Malunion

Metaphyseal malunion generally occurs as a consequence of malreduction at the time of initial fixation. Loss of fixation leading to articular incongruity occurs if the articular surface is not adequately supported after reduction but may also occur in very osteoporotic bone. The fracture must be stable from 0–90 degrees with either operative or non-operative treatment. Accurate angular alignment is difficult to maintain in bicondylar fracture patterns and fractures with metaphyseal–diaphyseal dissociation. Patients with articular incongruity may develop painful post-traumatic OA at an early stage, often within 2 years of injury. In these circumstances conversion to total knee arthroplasty may be required. Revision implants are usually necessary due to loss of bone on the tibial side.

Reduced range of motion

The majority of knees regain a function range of movement following treatment of these fractures. Range of movement exercises should be commenced as soon as possible, irrespective of the treatment option selected, to try and prevent this problem. Low energy tibial plateau fractures treated surgically have a favourable outcome at 3–5 years. Recovery tends to be slower in patients over 40 years of age and patients can take over a year to rehabilitate. In general there is significant impairment of movement and muscle function after fracture of the tibial plateau and the majority of patients have not fully recovered 1 year after their injury.

Post-traumatic osteoarthritis

As a consequence of these fractures there is increased chance of damage to the articular surface that can lead to post-traumatic OA. This chance is increased with bicondylar fractures and those with increased comminution. Approximately one-third of patients will develop radiological changes following this fracture and the degree of arthritis is greater with malalignment of more than 5 degrees.

Prominent hardware

Care should be taken to limit the amount of hardware implanted where possible. Prominent screws should be avoided as painful bursae may form over them. In carefully selected patients removal of the prominent metalware can reduce symptoms. Before removing the metalware, other sources of pain such as occult infection, non-union, malunion, neuroma, and arthritis must be ruled out.

Summary

Tibial plateau fractures are complex problems associated with significant complication related to both the injury and treatment. In order to obtain good results, the associated injury to the soft tissue envelope must be taken into account.

Further reading

Barei, D.P., Nork, S.E., Mills, W.J., Coles, C.P., Henley, M.B., and Benirschke, S.K. (2006). Functional outcomes of severe bicondylar tibial plateau fractures treated with dual incisions and medial and lateral plates. *Journal of Bone and Joint Surgery*, **88A**, 1713–21.

Canadian Orthopaedic Trauma Society (2006). Open reduction and internal fixation compared with circular fixator application for bicondylar tibial plateau fractures. Results of a multicenter, prospective, randomized clinical trial. *Journal of Bone and Joint Surgery*, **88A**, 2613–23.

Gaston, P., Will, E., and Keating, J. (2005). Recovery of function following fracture of the tibial plateau. *Journal of Bone and Joint Surgery*, **87B**, 1233–6.

Keating, J.F., Hadjucka, C., and Harper, J. (2003). Minimal internal fixation and calcium-phosphate cement in the treatment of fractures of the tibial plateau. A pilot study. *Journal of Bone and Joint Surgery*, **85B**, 68–73.

Rademakers, M.V., Kerkhoffs, G.M., Sierevelt, I.N., Raaymakers, E.L., and Marti, R.K, (2007). Operative treatment of 109 tibial plateau fractures: five- to 27-year follow-up results. *Journal of Orthopedic Trauma*, **21**, 5–10.

12.57

Tibial shaft fractures

S. Naidu Maripuri and K. Mohanty

Summary points

- The tibia is the most commonly fractured long bone
- The orthopaedic surgeon needs to be familiar with all of the management options available in order to effectively manage the simple and complex cases
- Problems associated with the soft tissue envelope are frequently encountered.

Introduction (Box 12.57.1)

The tibia is the most commonly fractured long bone in the body. The majority of tibial shaft fractures result from high-energy road traffic and sports-related injuries. They tend to occur in the young, active, and economically productive population. The average age of the patients in a large published series was 37.2 years. Tibial fractures result in a significant number of hospital admissions and surgical operations. The goal of the treatment is to achieve union of the fracture with minimal complications and to help return the patients to the best possible functional state. The current trend is to treat most displaced tibial fractures by internal fixation.

Surgical anatomy

One-third of the tibia is subcutaneous in its entire length on the anteromedial surface. For this reason, it is more susceptible to open fractures than any other long bone. The posterior tibial artery through its nutrient branch is the main source of endosteal blood supply to the tibial shaft. The source of periosteal blood supply is from the anterior tibial artery. The blood flow through an uninjured tibia is centrifugal. After a fracture, the pressure head reverses to a centripetal flow. The periosteal vessels are therefore an important source of blood supply after displaced fracture of the tibia. The importance of preserving the soft tissue envelope at surgical fixation of the tibia cannot be overemphasized.

The tibial diaphysis is triangular in its cross-section with an anteriorly directed apex. The majority of the diaphyseal medullary canal is round and symmetric, a configuration amenable to intramedullary nailing. The medullary canal has a narrow isthmus in the middle third with a proximal and distal metaphyseal flares. An intramedullary nail used for either proximal or distal fractures has minimal cortical purchase in these locations, which contributes to high rates of malunion when nailing proximal or distal fractures.

The soft tissue envelope covering the tibia is divided by the interosseous membrane and the intermuscular septa into four closed osteofascial compartments (Figure 12.57.1). The anterior compartment contains tibialis anterior, extensor hallucis longus, extensor digitorum communis, and anterior tibial vessels. The deep peroneal nerve also courses through this compartment and supplies an autonomous sensory zone on the dorsum of the foot between the first and second toes. In the proximal third of the anterior compartment, the neurovascular bundle lies on the interosseous membrane and courses more anteriorly as it proceeds distally.

The lateral compartment envelops the fibula and contains the peroneus brevis and longus muscles. The common peroneal nerve runs under the peroneus longus, winds round the neck of the fibula and divides into superficial and deep branches. The superficial peroneal nerve lies within the lateral compartment.

The superficial posterior compartment contains gastrocnemius and soleus muscles and the sural nerve. The deep posterior compartment contains the tibialis posterior, flexor hallucis longus and flexor digitorum, and posterior tibial vessels and nerve. Each compartment contains a nerve with its own autonomous area of supply. Careful assessment of sensations in these autonomous zones may aid in diagnosing involvement of that particular compartment.

The thick interosseous membrane connects the posterolaterally oriented fibula to the tibia. The fibula also articulates with the tibia at the proximal and distal tibiofibular joints. The fibres of the interosseous membrane run downwards and laterally and are torn in major torsional fractures of the tibia and fibula.

The anterior tibial artery enters the anterior compartment at the superior margins of the interosseous membrane and is at risk of injury with proximal tibial fractures and proximal tibiofibular joint dislocations. The common peroneal nerve is also at risk with these fracture patterns, especially with fibular neck fractures. It is also vulnerable to direct blows or undue pressure from cast, splints, or constricting wraps.

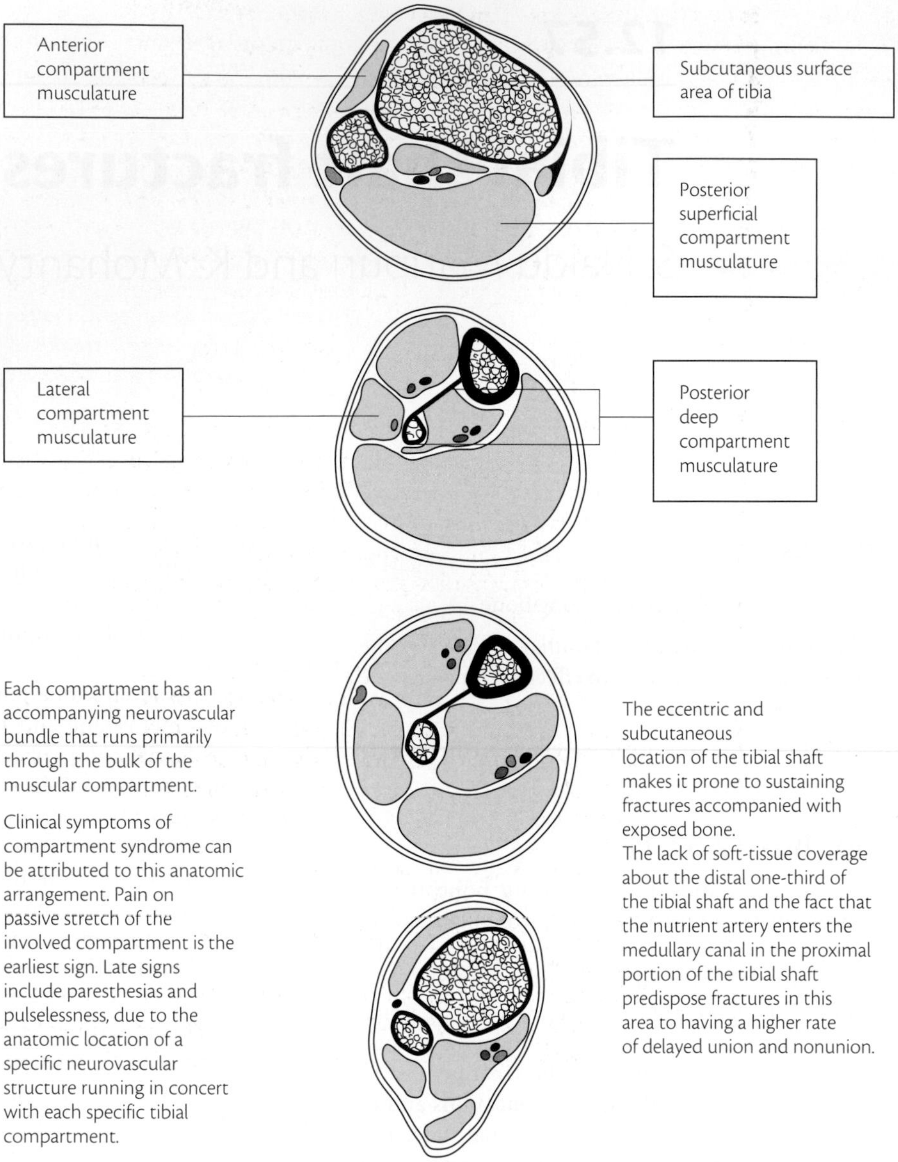

Anterior compartment musculature
Subcutaneous surface area of tibia
Posterior superficial compartment musculature
Lateral compartment musculature
Posterior deep compartment musculature
Each compartment has an accompanying neurovascular bundle that runs primarily through the bulk of the muscular compartment.
Clinical symptoms of compartment syndrome can be attributed to this anatomic arrangement. Pain on passive stretch of the involved compartment is the earliest sign. Late signs include paresthesias and pulselessness, due to the anatomic location of a specific neurovascular structure running in concert with each specific tibial compartment.
The eccentric and subcutaneous location of the tibial shaft makes it prone to sustaining fractures accompanied with exposed bone.
The lack of soft-tissue coverage about the distal one-third of the tibial shaft and the fact that the nutrient artery enters the medullary canal in the proximal portion of the tibial shaft predispose fractures in this area to having a higher rate of delayed union and nonunion.

Fig. 12.57.1 Anatomic cross-section of the tibia showing the compartmentalization of the lower leg.

The distal third of the tibial shaft has particularly poor soft tissue cover. The majority of the soft tissue in this area is tendinous and thus the extraosseous blood supply is minimal. The nutrient artery narrows as it reaches the distal third of the shaft and anastomoses with the distal metaphyseal endosteal vessels. If a displaced fracture occurs in this region, this small nutrient artery is often damaged resulting in loss of endosteal blood supply downstream from the site of injury. This lack of intramedullary blood supply combined with tenuous soft tissue envelope may account for delayed unions and non-unions, which occur frequently following high-energy distal-third tibial shaft fractures.

Associated pathology

The tibial shaft fractures are most commonly associated with open wounds and varying degrees of soft tissue injury. The degree and the extent of the soft tissue injury dictate the functional outcome. Fractures that present with high-grade soft tissue injuries, either open or closed, usually result from high-energy trauma. Up to 30% of tibial fractures occur in multiply injured patients. When evaluating these fractures the surgeon should carefully examine and record the neurovascular status of the limb and look for the presence of an associated compartment syndrome. Diligent clinical examination and compartment pressure monitoring in unresponsive or unconscious patients is essential to diagnose this devastating complication.

High-energy tibial fractures may also be associated with ipsilateral knee dislocations or femoral shaft fractures. The so-called 'floating-knee' injury (ipsilateral tibial and femoral fractures) can also occur in concert with ligamentous disruption about the knee. In addition, fractures and dislocations about the ankle may also occur in association with tibial shaft fractures, and therefore routine radiographs of the tibia should always include the knee and ankle.

Fractures at the diaphyseal–metaphyseal junction should be carefully evaluated for any extension into the articular surfaces. These fracture lines may be subtle and not readily apparent on standard anteroposterior (AP) and lateral radiographs. Preoperative computed tomography (CT) scanning may be helpful to identify an undisplaced fracture line, and assists in preventing displacement of such occult fracture during surgical intervention.

High-energy tibial shaft fractures are also associated with vascular injury. High index of suspicion is essential, particularly when evaluating tibial fractures in polytrauma patients. Early diagnosis and urgent involvement of vascular surgeon is essential for limb saving.

Mechanism of injury

Tibial shaft fractures associated with low-energy injury usually have little associated soft tissue injury and the interosseous membrane is intact and provides some degree of inherent stability, which may allow for conservative management.

Falls from a great height, direct blows, and motor vehicle-related injuries are high-energy mechanisms, which impart more kinetic energy in producing a fracture. The fracture patterns reflect this energy expenditure and have primarily a transverse orientation that may be accompanied by butterfly fragments or comminution, depending on the magnitude of the bending force. Fractures produced by crushing injuries or high-velocity gunshot projectiles are often the most severe. The fracture patterns are highly comminuted and may be segmental. The soft tissue component of the injury may be vastly underestimated, especially with crushing injuries, which often present as a closed de-gloving type of injury.

The level of the fibular fracture may indicate the type of injury mechanism, i.e. direct injury results in a fracture of both tibia and fibula at the same level, whereas fractures at a different level result from indirect forces or rotation.

'Stress' fractures are caused by repetitive stress, particularly in endurance athletes. Stress fracture management should take into consideration the injury site (low risk vs high risk), grade (extent of microdamage accumulation), and the individual's competitive situation. This separation into two groups is based on the biomechanical environment and natural history of the fracture. The anterior tibial shaft stress fractures are considered high-risk fractures. The undertreatment of high-risk stress fractures can lead to catastrophic bone failure and/or prolonged loss of playing time. Overtreatment of low-risk stress fractures can result in unnecessary loss of physical conditioning and activity.

Classification

Tibial fractures have been traditionally described in terms of their anatomical location—proximal, mid, or distal third fractures. The amount of initial displacement is recorded as a percentage of the diameter of the bone. The fracture pattern is described as spiral, oblique, or transverse with further description of the presence and extent of comminution, which correlates with absorbed energy and is an indicator of fracture severity.

The AO/Orthopaedic Trauma Association (OTA) comprehensive classification system (Figure 12.57.2) is commonly used to classify tibial fractures. This classification scheme does not account for the degree of soft tissue injury.

Unstable fractures are less conducive to non-operative management. Severe soft tissue injury, extension into or involvement of either the proximal or distal tibial articular surfaces, 100% initial displacement of the fracture, comminution of more than 50% of the bone circumference, and transverse fracture orientation are all hallmarks of an unstable fracture pattern. The presence of a fibular fracture in association with a tibial fracture at the same level often indicates an unstable injury from a high-energy mechanism (Figure 12.57.3).

Critical review of comparative studies reveals that non-operative treatment of high-energy tibial fractures is associated with high prevalence of malunion, stiffness of the knee and ankle joints, and poor functional outcome. Therefore classification of tibial shaft fractures into stable and unstable types may be more practical and useful when considering treatment options.

Box 12.57.1 Tibial shaft fractures

- Most commonly fractured long bone
- Most common open fracture among long bones
- Mostly involve young and productive population
- Majority result from road traffic accidents/sports related injuries.

Clinical evaluation

History

Determining the mechanism of injury is critical during the initial stages of patient evaluation. A cooperative conscious patient who

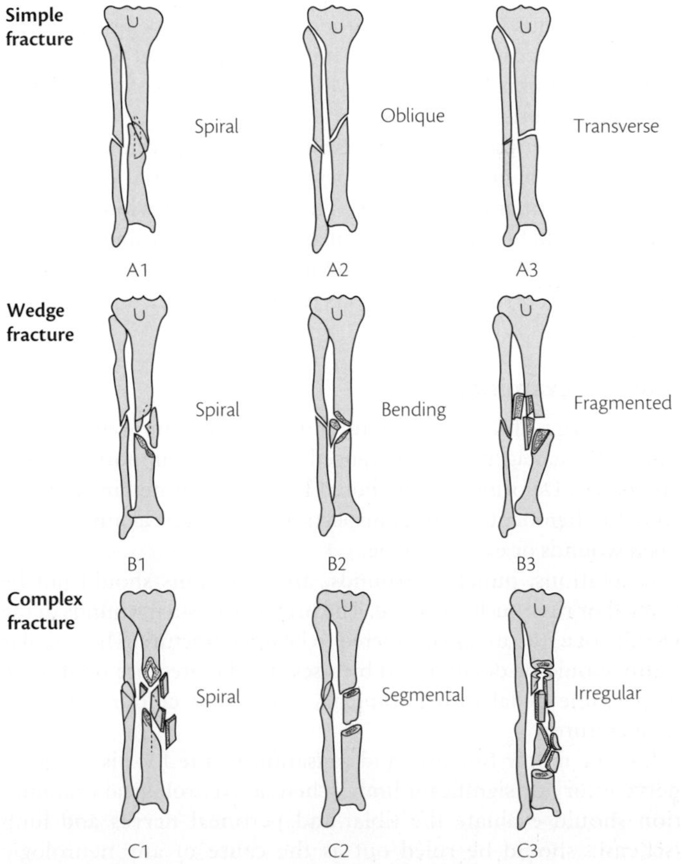

Fig. 12.57.2 AO classification of tibial shaft fractures. Classification is based on the orientation of the primary fracture line, the presence of associated butterfly fractures, and the presence of comminution.

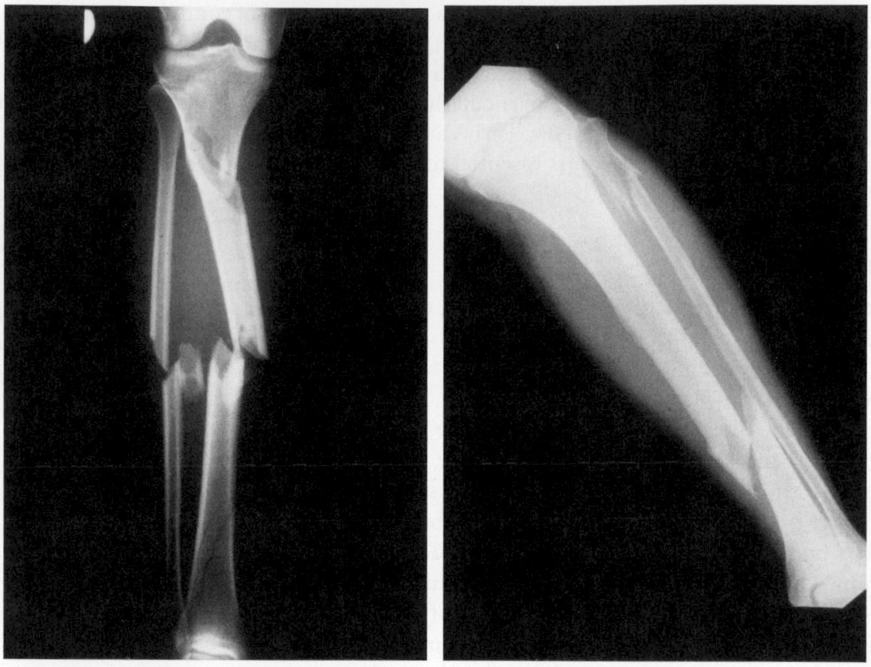

A B

Fig. 12.57.3 These fractures demonstrate the hallmarks of unstable fracture patterns, which typically will require fixation techniques: A) a segmental tibial fracture with a transverse fibular fracture at the same level as the more distal tibial fracture; B) a short oblique fracture pattern with 100 per cent displacement.

has had a minor slip-and-fall accident is managed differently from an unconscious victim of a motor vehicle versus pedestrian accident. In the face of a high-energy injury, the examiner will not only focus on the tibial fracture, but will evaluate the patient for other associated injuries

The time between injury and evaluation is important, especially for fractures associated with open wounds, arterial disruption, and compartment syndromes. The patient's previous medical history should be noted, in particular conditions causing immunocompromise. Social history including occupation, smoking, drug and alcohol use all affects treatment decisions and the outcome.

Physical examination

High-energy tibial shaft fractures in multiply injured patients should be managed as per Advanced Trauma life support (ATLS®) guidelines. Deformed limbs should be gently splinted in relatively straight alignment. A visual inspection should reveal any obvious open wounds or exposed bone.

Lacerations, puncture wounds, and abrasions should not be probed or rigorously explored. The presence of such wounds in the vicinity of a fracture is considered to be open fracture. The vascular status should be documented by assessing the presence or absence of palpable pedal pulses, capillary refill, skin colour, and skin temperature.

Loss of motor function and sensation to the foot is a sign of nerve injury or significant limb ischemia. Neurological examination should evaluate the tibial and peroneal nerves and limb ischemia should be ruled out as the cause of any neurologic dysfunction.

Compartment syndrome is common in all tibial fractures and should be assessed on a regular basis.

Mangled extremity severity score (MESS) or Ganga Hospital Injury severity score can be used to assess the open tibial shaft fractures. Ganga Hospital Injury severity score has been shown to be more sensitive and specific and help in determining treatment strategies (see Further reading).

Investigations

Imaging

Once the leg is splinted, an AP and lateral radiographs should be obtained for all tibias in which a fracture is suspected. The knee and ankle should be included to detect fracture–dislocations or articular extension.

Cone-down or magnification spot radiographs or CT scans are useful to evaluate subtle fracture lines, callus formation, or stress fractures.

CT scanning has been shown to be useful to determine the adequacy of fracture reduction, including rotational alignment as well as limb length. Additionally, CT imaging has been shown to be useful for those transitional injuries (junction of diaphysis and metaphysis) that present with extension into the articular regions. CT scanning has now replaced plain linear tomography for the routine evaluation of non-unions.

Other studies

If diminished pulses are present, the ankle pressure index has been shown to correlate highly with the presence or absence of arterial disruption. Doppler-assisted blood pressure is obtained at the ankle and brachial arteries. A ratio of ankle to brachial systolic pressure below 0.9 indicates a probable arterial injury.

Arteriography is indicated when arterial disruption is suspected. Direct compartment pressure monitoring is routinely performed, especially when patients are unable to cooperate with the physical examination or where the surgeon has a high index of suspicion.

Diagnostic ultrasound is used to assess the early presence of callus and is predictive of fracture healing in situations where hardware, such as intramedullary nails and complex external fixators, occlude adequate routine radiographic evaluation.

Management

All closed fractures are immobilized initially with an above the knee splint. Appropriate imaging is obtained in order to plan definitive treatment.

Non-operative treatment (Box 12.57.2)

Non operative treatment in the form of casting should be considered in all isolated tibial fractures which are either stable or undisplaced.

Fractures with stable configurations as seen on the initial radiographs merit treatment by closed reduction and application of a long leg cast. Careful and regular follow-up with serial weekly radiographs is essential to detect secondary displacement and angulation within the cast. Any residual angulation can be corrected to an acceptable degree by wedging of the plaster cast. A functional cast brace (patellar tendon bearing cast) and early weight bearing is encouraged when the fracture becomes 'sticky'.

If wide displacement or significant shortening is seen on initial screening radiographs, it is unlikely that even an anatomical initial reduction will be maintained throughout the course of treatment found that there was no difference between the amount of shortening seen on the initial versus final radiograph in over 80% of cases. There is experimental data to indicate that as the level of deformity approaches the distal one-third of the tibia, even a small degree of malalignment can affect the loading of the ankle joint. Most surgeons strive to achieve alignment with less than 5 degrees of angulation in any plane and 10 degrees of rotation. However, these values for acceptable reduction are not based on any hard data and good long term function has been reported with angulation of up to 10–15 degrees.

Excellent results have been reported with the use of closed reduction, casting, and subsequent functional bracing in over 1000 closed tibial fractures. Initial treatment was with closed reduction and long leg casting. Weight-bearing was permitted in the cast as tolerated. If length and alignment were acceptable and pain and swelling had subsided, patients were then converted to a fracture brace at an average of 3.7 weeks. In 95% of the fractures, the final amount of shortening was up to 12mm (average 4.28mm). Final angular deformity was less than 6 degrees in 90% of patients. In this series, the rate of non-union was less than 1.1%. This form of treatment was recommended for those closed injuries with no more than 15mm of initial shortening or stably reduced transverse fractures (Figure 12.57.4). Tibial fractures with an intact fibula were a relative contraindication to functional bracing because significant varus deformity (more than 5 degrees) was more likely to develop.

Other authors have noted the hazards of treating tibial shaft fractures with intact fibulae. Delayed or non-union was reported in 26% of adult patients with fractured tibia with intact fibula treated with cast immobilization. Sixty-one per cent experienced one or more complications during conservative treatment. The intact fibula prohibits axial loading of the tibia and therefore decreases the weight-bearing axial stimulus to healing (Figure 12.57.5).

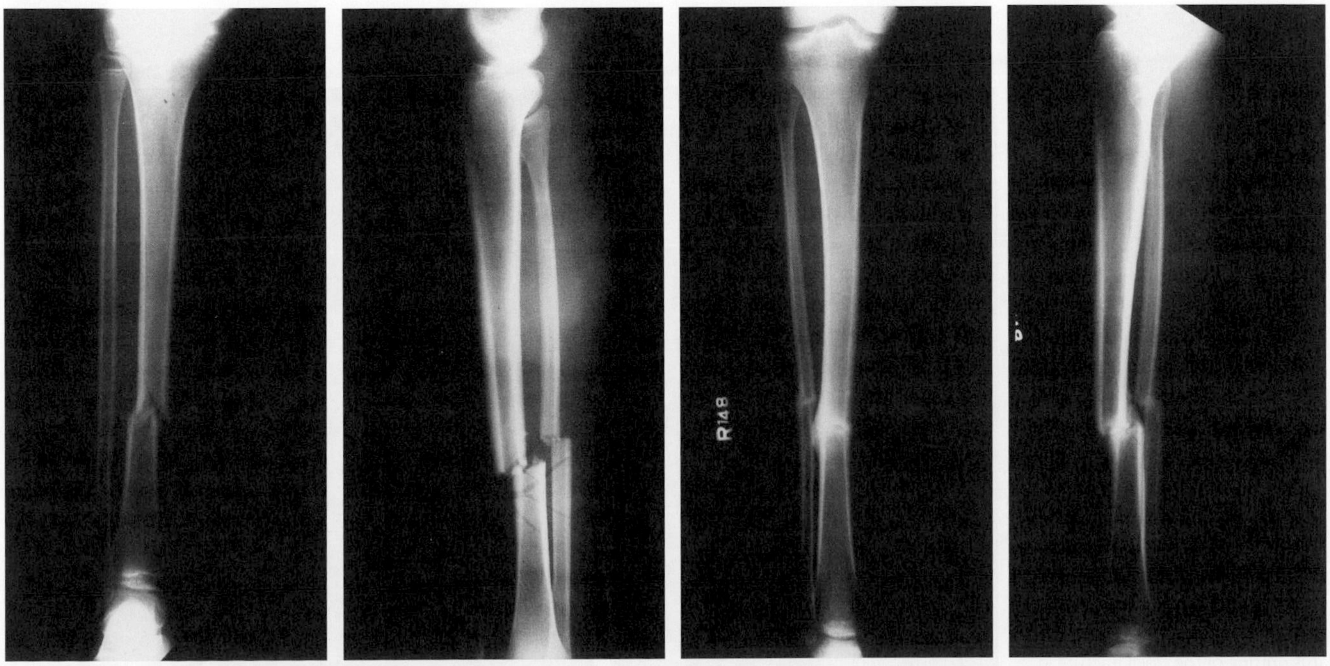

A B C D

Fig. 12.57.4 A), B) Anteroposterior and lateral views of a transverse tibial fracture with approximately 50 per cent displacement, as seen on the initial injury films. The fibula fracture is also minimally displaced. C), D) This stable fracture pattern healed uneventfully with nonoperative management.

A prospective randomized study has compared the results of application of the patellar ligament-bearing cast with those of operative treatment with closed interlocking intramedullary nailing. This study revealed longer healing times and increased residual angular deformity, limb shortening, and disability in the group treated conservatively. Hindfoot stiffness occurred in 15% of the patients treated in casts. Twenty-two per cent of patients in the closed-treatment group eventually underwent operative intervention for failure to maintain adequate reduction.

There are numerous limitations to the treatment with casts and functional braces. Loss of reduction as well as a residual limb length discrepancy is common. Prolonged treatment with a cast may result in excessive stiffness of the knee, ankle, hindfoot, or all three, which may require extended rehabilitation to regain the patient's pre-injury level of function. Even with earlier weight-bearing, residual joint stiffness has been reported in approximately 20–30% of patients treated conservatively.

Fractures that are associated with serious soft tissue compromise are not easily treated conservatively. Effective casting or bracing is highly dependent on the ability of the soft tissues to tolerate a well-contoured device. Limb oedema, contusions, abrasions, etc., may inhibit the early application of sufficient external support. Failure and complications of non-operative treatment indicate that there are many tibial fractures that benefit from operative treatment.

Some studies have suggested the benefit of pulsed, low-intensity ultrasound in shortening the time to healing in non operative treatment.

Box 12.57.2 Conservative treatment

- Undisplaced or stable tibial fractures without significant soft tissue injury
- Shortening on initial films usually predicts final shortening
- Intact fibula is a relative contraindication because of varus malunion
- Initial long leg cast followed by Sarmiento cast once fracture is 'sticky'
- Acceptable reduction:
  - Coronal plane <5 degrees
  - Sagittal plane <10 degrees
  - Rotation <10 degrees
  - >50% cortical contact in both AP and lateral views
- Serial wedging of cast may help correct the deformity.

Operative management

Unstable tibial shaft fractures, fractures with associated ipsilateral lower limb fractures, tibial shaft fractures in multiply injured patients, and fractures extending to either knee or ankle joints generally require surgical stabilization. Open tibial shaft fractures and fractures associated with neurovascular injury or impending compartment syndrome are dealt with emergency surgical management. Surgery should also be considered in fractures where attempts at non-operative management have failed and when secondary displacement and angulation occurs in follow-up radiographs. Occasionally, operative intervention is recommended for non-compliant patients. The goals of operative treatment should

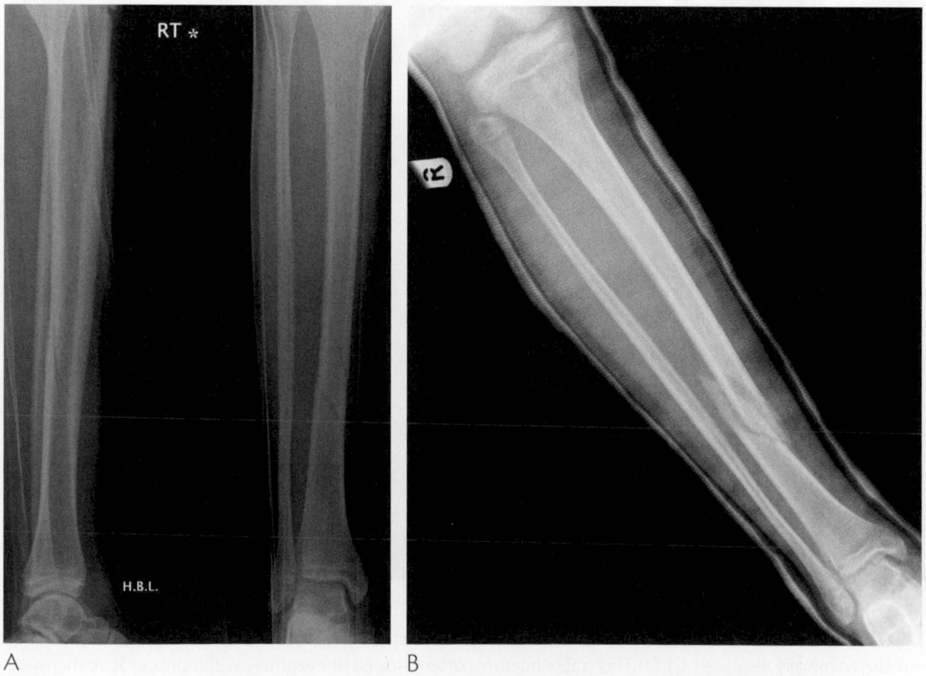

Fig. 12.57.5 A) Undisplaced tibial shaft fracture with intact fibula. B)Varus drifting of the tibial fracture in the plaster. Hence intact fibula is a relative contraindication for conservative treatment.

Box 12.57.3 Intramedullary nailing

- Most common operative treatment
- Best for unstable diaphyseal fractures
- Reaming has biomechanical and biological advantages and reduces non-union rates
- Newer-generation nails are effective in metaphyseal fractures.

be to restore the length and alignment of the limb, stable fixation to allow early mobilization, and rapid return to pre-injury function with no or minimal complications.

Intramedullary nailing (Box 12.57.3)

Locked intramedullary nailing has become the 'gold standard' treatment for most of the unstable tibial diaphyseal fractures. Interlocking intramedullary nails maintain axial alignment and provide rotational stability. The nails are either statically or dynamically locked depending on fracture configuration. The new-generation intramedullary nails that allow placement of distal locking screws near the end of the nail have helped extend the indications for nailing to metaphyseal fractures even with intra-articular extension (Figure 12.57.6). The current literature indicates high rates of fracture union in closed tibial diaphyseal fracture treated with intramedullary nailing.

Intramedullary nail insertion has traditionally involved the use of a fracture table to effect reduction. The time necessary for a fracture table set-up and correct positioning of the patient may be prohibitive when treating a multiply injured patient. In addition, complications such as nerve palsy and compartment syndrome have been related to the use of excessive traction.

Techniques have been developed to achieve and maintain reduction during intramedullary nailing when operating on a standard radiolucent orthopaedic table. Devices such as the femoral distractor or a temporary external fixator can serve this purpose. Accurate alignment without traction-related complications has been reported with the use of these reduction techniques (Figure 12.57.7).

The correct placement of the entry portal is an important technical consideration. It must be placed centrally in line with the medullary canal. Because of the wide discrepancy in tibial morphology, the centre of the tibial canal may be variable in its relationship to the patella and patellar tendon. The actual insertion site may be located lateral, medial, or directly posterior to the patellar tendon and should be verified with an image intensifier. Failure to place the entry portal centrally will result in varus or valgus malalignment. Entry portal can be placed either on the medial aspect of the patellar tendon or through a transpatellar tendon approach. Anterior knee pain is a common problem following intramedullary nailing with some reports showing an incidence of greater than 50%. In those patients whose work involves kneeling, consideration should be given to alternative methods of treatment. The relationship of the approach to postoperative anterior knee pain has been an area of controversy. However, recent randomized control studies have not demonstrated any correlation between the approach and anterior knee pain.

The major concern with operative management of tibial shaft fractures is the additional disruption of the blood supply caused by the operative procedure itself. Reaming the medullary canal devasularizes the inner two-thirds of the cortex, rendering the endosteal surface of the cortex ischaemic. Devascularization is reduced to one-third when the nail is inserted without reaming. Additional devascularization occurs through the entire cortex at the region of the fracture site. However, the relative avascularity is temporary and the medullary blood vessels regenerate after a relatively short time. Although reaming disrupts the blood flow to the

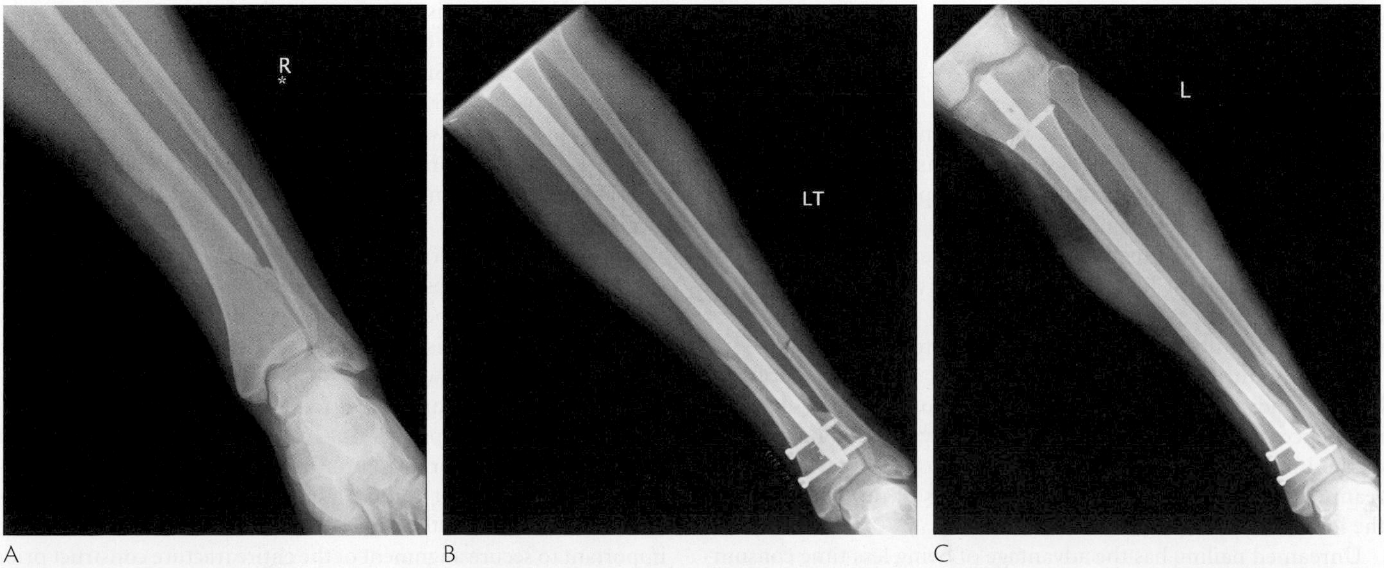

Fig. 12.57.6 A) Tibial shaft fracture extending very low in to the distal metaphysis. B) Fixed with a newer-generation nail with the distally placed screws. C) Healed fracture with no complications.

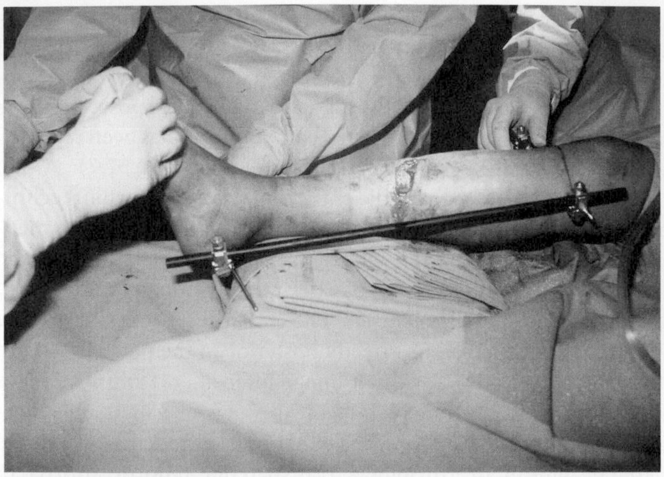

A

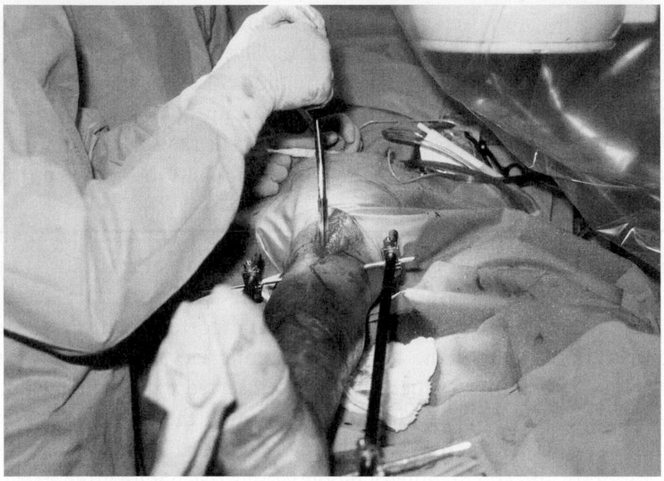

B

Fig. 12.57.7 A) A simple two-pin fixator is placed with one pin in the calcaneal tuberosity and an additional pin proximally at the level of the fibular head, posterior to the entrance point of the nail. B) Longitudinal distraction through the two radiolucent connecting bars reduces the fracture; once alignment and rotation is corrected, the nailing can proceed with the use of the awl positioned at the entry site.

cortex, reaming induces a sixfold increase in the periosteal blood flow. The periosteal blood supply compensates initially for the disruption of the intramedullary blood supply. Disruption of the intramedullary blood supply is usually not a concern for closed injuries that have a competent soft tissue envelope. However, in the treatment of open or high-energy fractures where the soft tissues including the periosteum may be completely disrupted, medullary reaming could further devascularize the fracture site.

Reaming during intramedullary nailing has biomechanical and biological advantages. Reaming allows insertion of a larger-diameter nail hence increasing its load sharing capacity. The biological effect of the increased periosteal vascularity is well known. Moreover, reaming has been shown to have faster rates of union and reduce the incidence of non-union.

Unreamed nailing has the advantage of being less time consuming offers advantages in the emergency setting for stabilizing polytrauma patients. Unreamed nails when used as a definitive method of fixation have a reduced incidence of reoperations, superficial infections, and malunions, when compared with external fixators.

Reaming allows the insertion of a bigger nail and locking bolts. Fatigue failure of small-diameter unreamed nails and/or interlocking screws has been reported in many series if union of the fracture is not achieved early. However failure of interlocking screws in some cases may facilitate fracture healing by autodynamization (Figure 12.57.8).

A recent large multicentre randomized study involving 1226 patients has compared reamed versus unreamed intramedullary nails. The study suggested that reamed nails offer a benefit in closed fractures with regard to further events (surgical intervention or autodynamization) within 1 year. Most of the difference was attributed to an excess of dynamizations (both surgical and autodynamization) in the unreamed group. A non-significant increase in number of postoperative events was noted in open fractures treated with a reamed nail. The authors note that overall the number of events for this study was less than previous randomized controlled trials. Previous grade II evidence, randomized controlled trials have shown that reamed nails have an advantage over unreamed nails with regard to rate of union and non-union.

Compartment syndrome has been reported following intramedullary nailing of the tibia. It is thought to be multifactorial and could be associated with excessive traction on the limb, limb tourniquet, and extravasation of the reamings. The type of anaesthesia and the postoperative analgesic regimen has been attributed to a delay in diagnosis of compartment syndrome.

The indications for intramedullary nailing have been extended to include very proximal and distal metaphyseal fractures. Nailing of proximal one-third tibial metaphyseal fractures are fraught with potential complications, primarily valgus malunion, anterior translation, and apex anterior deformities of the proximal segment. Review of proximal shaft fractures treated with intramedullary nailing found that 84% of these patients had residual angulation of more than 5 degrees and that 25% lost proximal fixation primarily related to the placement of a single proximal locking screw. Non-union rates have been reported as high as 26 %.

Surgical errors consisting of a medialized nail entry portal and a posterior and laterally directed nail insertion angle, all contribute to the malalignment. Suggested techniques for the successful nailing of proximal shaft fractures include a lateral entry portal, use of Poller's 'blocking screws' and adjunctive antiglide plates located at the level of the fracture apex. This small plate serves to prevent translation and apex anterior angulation of the proximal fragment (Figure 12.57.9).

Contiguous ipsilateral distal intra-articular fracture extension and non-contiguous ipsilateral ankle fractures in concert with diaphyseal injuries can be successfully treated with intramedullary nailing techniques. Distal articular extension displaced less than 5mm, may be treated with mini open reduction and internal fixation of the articular component followed by intramedullary nailing. Non-contiguous ipsilateral ankle fractures may be treated with fixation of the ankle prior to or after insertion of the intramedullary nail. Technically, it is important to keep the articular lag screws in subchondral bone to allow room for nail insertion. It is also important to secure alignment of the entire fracture construct prior to nail insertion using a two-pin fixator, a femoral distractor, or calcaneal pin traction (Fig. 10).

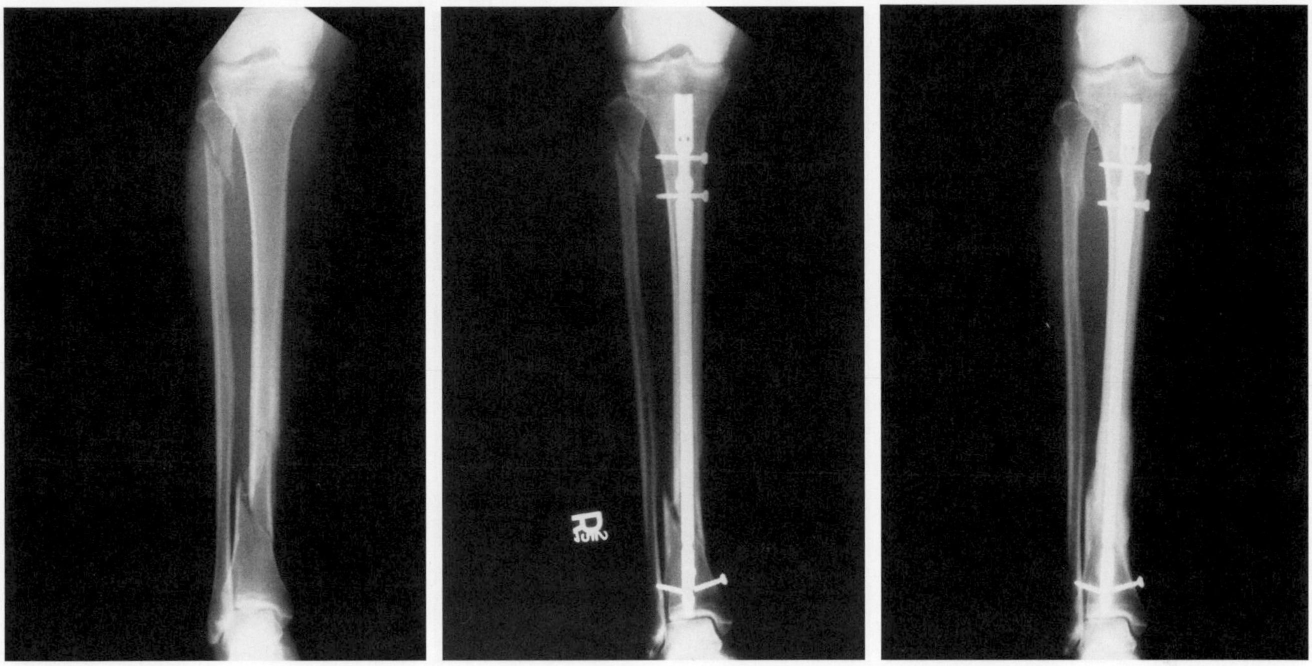

A B C

Fig. 12.57.8 A) A short oblique tibial shaft fracture treated with a small-diameter unreamed nail. B) The distal interlocking screw fractured allowing the nail to 'autodynamize' and compress the fracture site. C) Fortunately, the fracture healed prior to the small-diameter nail undergoing fatigue fracture.

Plate fixation (Box 12.57.4)

The traditional open reduction and internal fixation with plates and screws is not a preferred option for high-energy tibial shaft fractures. This method of fixation requires extensile exposure and additional soft tissue stripping resulting in secondary devascularization of the soft tissues and fracture fragments. Reports in the literature quote high rates of complications such as wound break down, infection, aseptic and septic non-union of the fracture.

With the advent of minimally invasive plate osteosynthesis (MIPO) using locking plates, plating has regained its popularity. This technique utilizes the principles of biological fixation. The fracture is realigned in all planes utilizing indirect reduction techniques. The adequacy of reduction and the plate position are confirmed by image intensifier. Depending upon the personality of the fracture the definitive fixation is planned. In simpler fracture configuration (AO/OTA 32A and B) primary fracture fixation is carried out by using lag screws through small incisions. A precontoured plate is then tunnelled extraperiostally along the medial aspect of the tibia through a small skin incision, distant from the zone of injury. This plate is then fixed with locking screws percutaneously through stab incisions and acts as a neutralization device. In complex fractures (AO/OTA 32C) only MIPO plating is performed without any attempt at direct reduction of the fracture fragments. Here the plate acts as a bridge bypassing the area of comminution whilst stabilizing the fracture (Figure 12.57.11). The MIPO technique can also be carried out with usage of low-profile standard plates in non-osteoporotic bones. The main advantage of MIPO is that the fracture haematoma and the soft tissue envelope around the fracture are not disturbed. This method of fixation results in secondary bone healing by callus response. Review of recent literature confirms the efficacy of this fixation method and encourages its usage. A recent comparative study has shown the that plate fixation in distal tibial shaft fractures (4–11cm above the plafond) produced better rate of union as compared to intramedullary nails. Complications such as delayed union, malunion, and secondary procedures were more frequent after nailing.

Indications for plate osteosynthesis has also extended to proximal tibial shaft fractures with or without intra-articular extension with the advent of angular stable device such as less invasive stabilization system (LISS).

External fixation (Box 12.57.5)

External fixation is carried out for both emergent and definitive management of tibial shaft fractures. In the initial management of open tibial fractures and in tibial fractures associated with polytrauma, skeletal stabilization is achieved in a rapid manner by using an external fixator assembly. This temporizing device is assembled with use of multiple Schanz pins inserted into the major fragments preferably outside the zone of injury. Such fixation allows wound care and subsequent reconstruction of the soft tissue envelope in open fractures. External fixation in multiply injured patients allows early mobilization and better nursing care and shown to have reduced mortality and morbidity. These devices can be exchanged to intramedullary nails within 2 weeks of index operation (Figure 12.57.12).

The use of an intramedullary nail following failed external fixation has demonstrated variable results. In general, if the external fixator is in place for less than 1–2 weeks, conversion to an intramedullary nail appears to have a low rate of associated infection. However, as the time period of external fixation increases, the risk of infection with immediate exchange to an intramedullary nail increases dramatically. Infection rates as high as 50% have

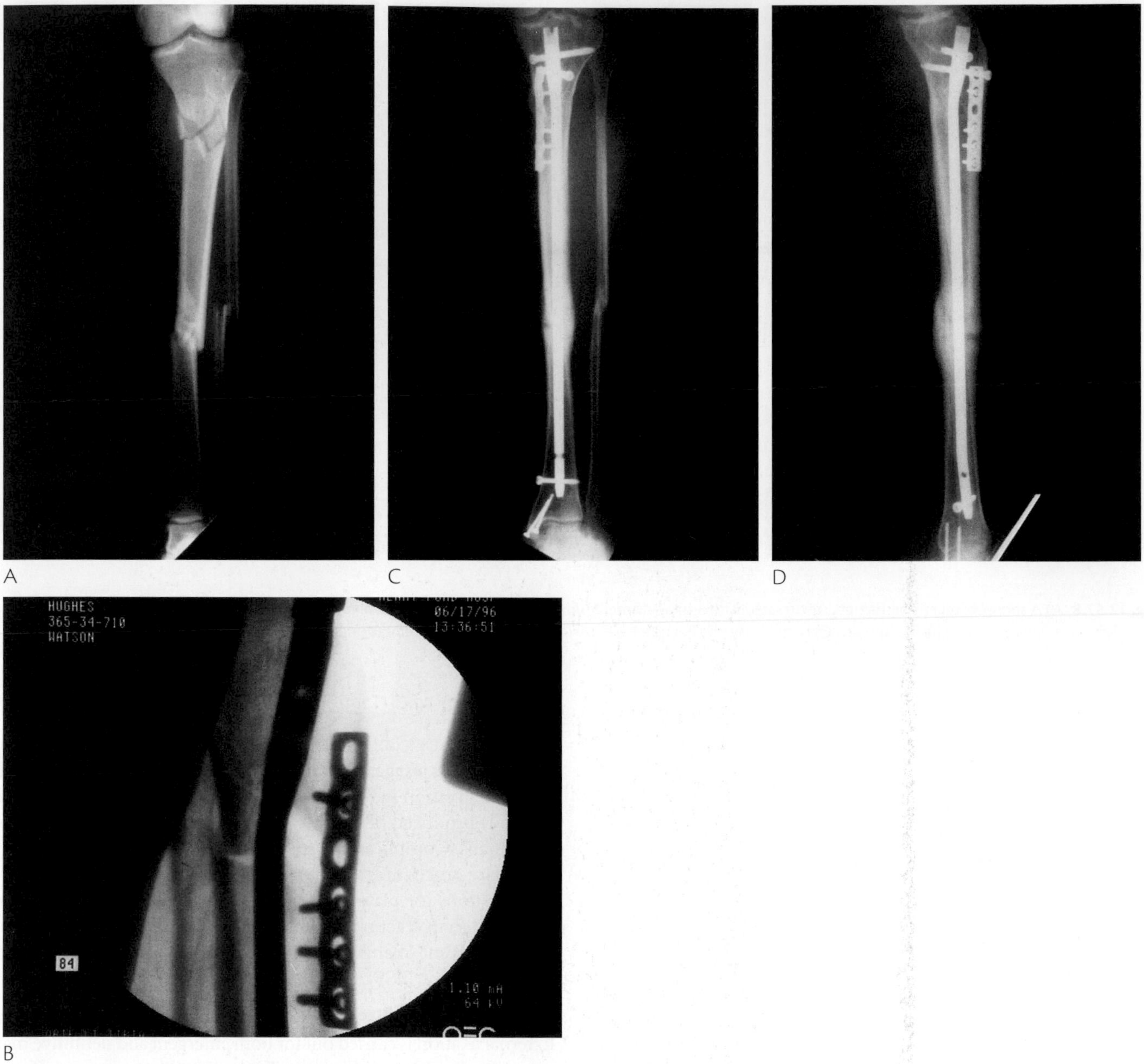

Fig. 12.57.9 A) Preoperative film of a segmental fracture. B) The plate blocks any anterior translation and angulation that can occur as the proximal curve of the intramedullary nail passes through and seats into the proximal fragment. C) Anteroposterior and D) lateral raidographs revealing complete healing and near anatomic alignment without any translation or angulation of the proximal fracture segment.

been reported for patients who have had this immediate exchange. If this type of treatment is contemplated, patients who have a latency period of more than 1 month following removal of the external fixator and prior to intramedullary nailing have a marked decrease in their rates of infection as well as increased rates of union. Although a delay of several weeks or months between fixator removal and nailing may decrease the risk of infection, there remains some elevated risk. Deep infection rates of 17% have been demonstrated in open tibial fractures treated with secondary intramedullary nailing (IMN) after external fixation (EF). All deep infections occurred in Gustilo type III fractures (22.6%, 7/31).They concluded that early skin closure within 1 week is the most important factor in preventing deep infections when treating open tibial fractures with secondary IMN after EF.

The external fixation techniques have been successfully used for definitive management of closed tibial fractures. External fixation does not cause additional disruption of the soft tissue envelope or the vascularity of the fracture fragments or other osseous structures. Axial and rotational stability can be achieved by using ring fixators, monoplanar or multiplanar external fixator constructs. In high-energy fractures, particularly with fractures associated with bone loss, an external fixator is used not only to acutely stabilize the fracture but also to aid in fracture union and bone transportation in restoring bone loss (Figure 12.57.13).

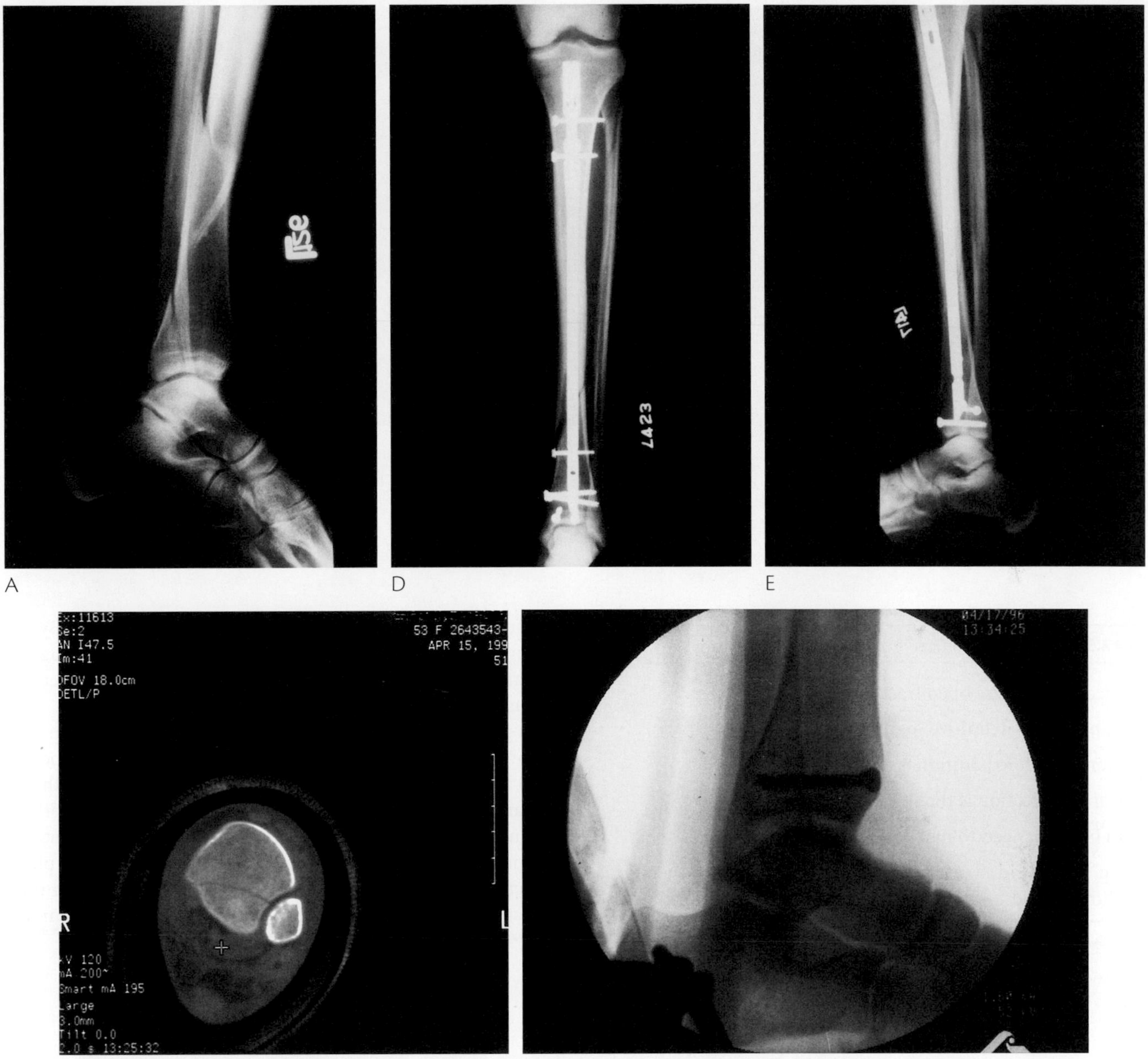

Fig. 12.57.10 A) Distal third shaft fracture with intra-articular extension and fracture through the posterior malleolus. B) CT scan through the distal tibial region reveals the posterior mallelor fracture. C) Lag screws are placed in a subchondral location prior to nail insertion in order to prevent displacement of these fracture lines during eventual nail seating. D), E) Initial postoperative radiographs reveal excellent position of the rod with no displacement of the intra-articular fracture lines.

Box 12.57.4 Plating

- Regained popularity with advent of MIPO
- Indicated for some metaphyseal fractures without severe soft tissue injury
- Good results in translated non-unions (not amenable to nailing) and after failed external fixation
- Good results in distal tibial metaphyseal fractures with MIPO.

With other fracture fixation methods, additional bracing or casting is often necessary to maintain a stable construct. With rigid internal fixation, primary bone healing demands that weight-bearing be delayed until full reconstitution of the cortex has been completed. Weight-bearing stimulates fracture healing. A major advantage of using adjustable external fixators is the ability to load the limb actively. Even in the most comminuted fractures, patients can begin at least partial weight bearing immediately after surgery without any supplementary casts or braces. Most frames allow for dynamization restoring cortical contact, achieving a more stable

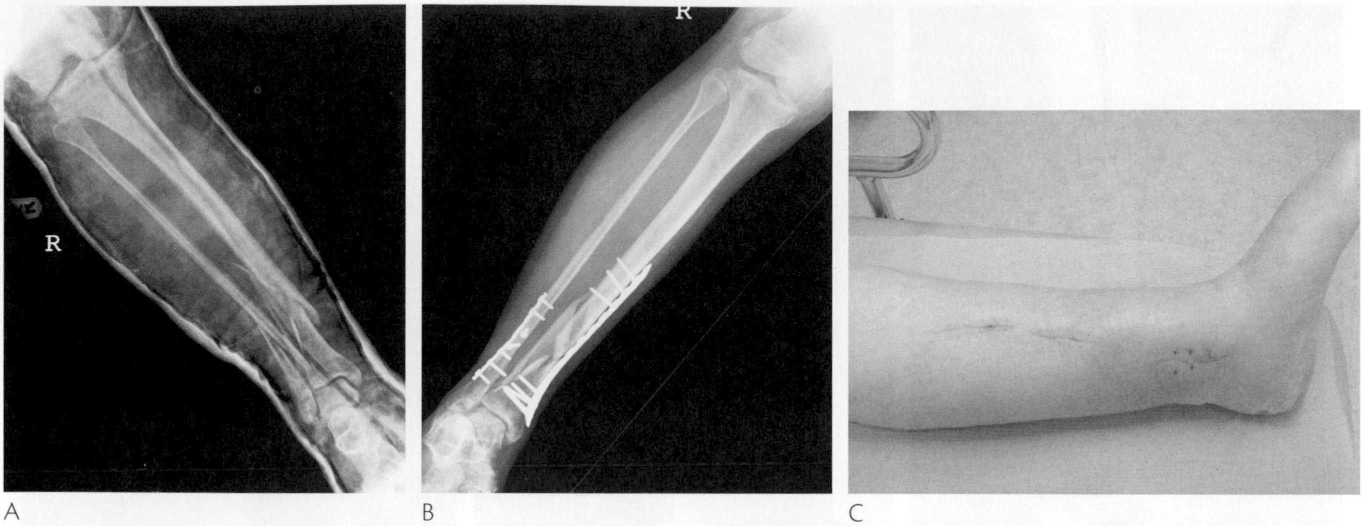

Fig. 12.57.11 A) Comminuted distal third tibial fracture. B) Fixed wth MIPO technique. C) Leg with healed incision wounds resulting from MIPO technique.

Box 12.57.5 External fixation

- Indicated in severe open fractures
- Temporary or definitive management
- Advantage of no additional soft tissue damage
- Pin track infection is the most common complication
- Can be exchanged to nail within 2 weeks
- Ring or hybrid fixator used in septic/aseptic non-union, malunion, and for bone transportation in case of bone loss.

fracture construct, and decreasing the pin/bone stresses. By subsequently disassembling external fixation frames, progressive dynamization leads to a less stiff frame, which facilitates secondary callus formation and bone healing.

In general, closed fractures heal with external fixation on average within 4 months. The rates of non-union have been reported as high as 5% for closed fractures. In most series, it was felt that early dynamization or gradual frame disassembly should be performed in an effort to load the fracture and promote secondary callus formation. The most common complication was minor pin tract infection, which is seen in the majority of patients. Major pin-site infections requiring secondary surgical procedures were noted to

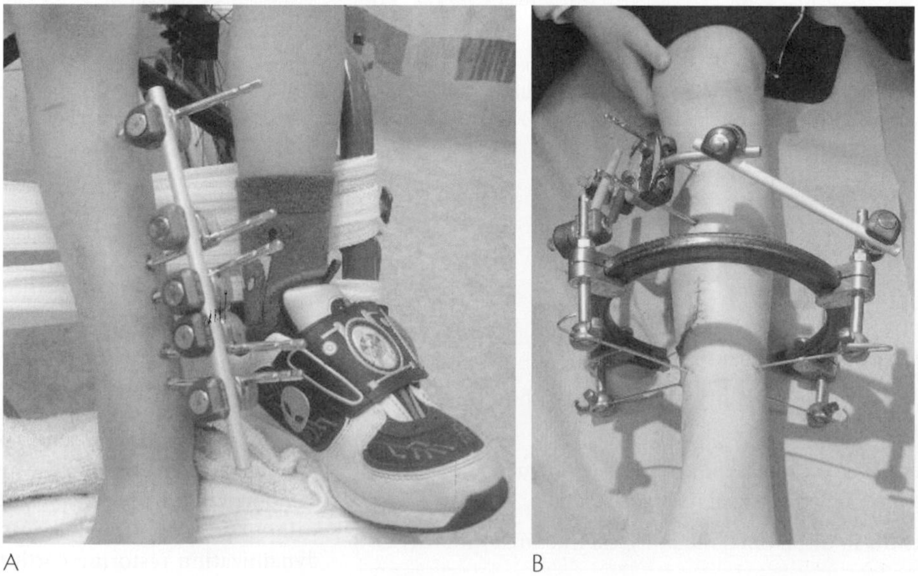

Fig. 12.57.12 A) Clinical photograph showing monolateral external fixator used for distal third tibial shaft fracture. Note the 'near- far' pin placement. B) Clinical photograph showing the hybrid external fixator used for open tibial shaft fracture.

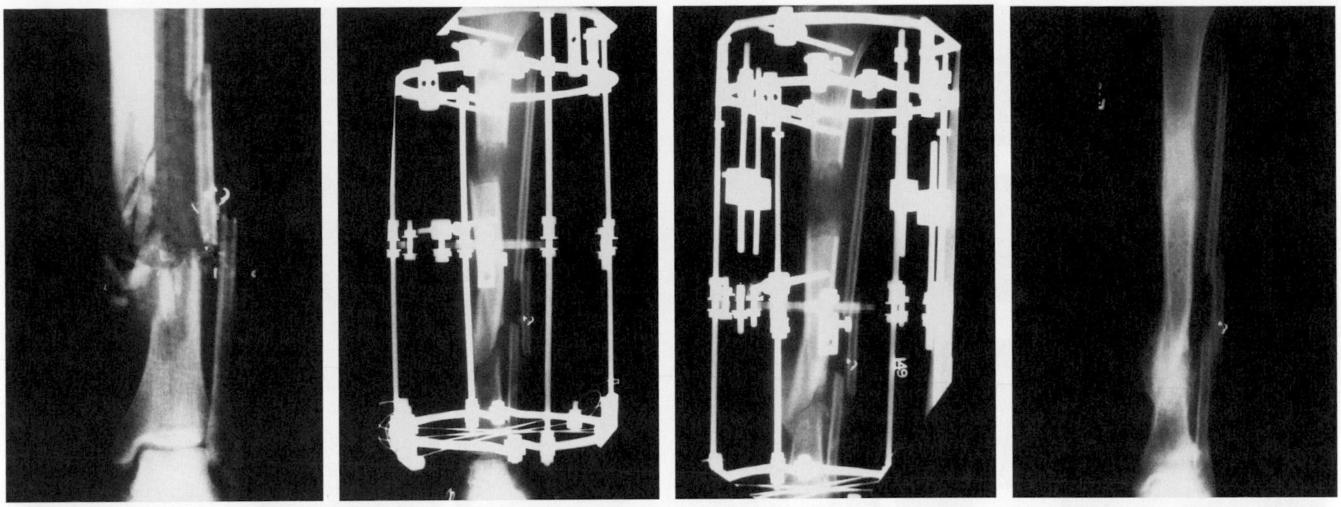

Fig. 12.57.13 A) Complex open tibia fracture with segmental bone loss. B), C) A circular small-wire external fixator facilitates stabilization and eventual bone transport through a proximal tibial corticotomy. Following distal docking, this region underwent a small bone graft to facilitate consolidation in this region. D) After frame removal, the segmental deficit has been bridged and leg length discrepancy resolved.

be less than 5% in most series and none appeared to have led to any serious sequelae. Most authors agree that although external fixation requires closer patient monitoring and pin care, external fixation is a safe and reliable device for treating tibial shaft fractures.

Open tibial shaft fractures (Box 12.57.6)

The tibial shaft is the most common site for open fractures of the long bones. Most of the open tibial shaft fractures occur in young and active population as a result of high-energy injury and are particularly associated with road traffic collisions. The standard treatment consists of: early debridement of the open wound; thorough surgical toilet; antibiotics; stabilization of the fracture; adequate and early soft tissue coverage; successful reconstruction of the limb and subsequent fracture healing (see Chapter 12.7).

Box 12.57.6 Open fractures

- Early debridement, skeletal fixation, and soft tissue cover
- Adequacy rather than time of debridement influences infection rates
- Primary closure is debatable. Closure within 1 week reduce infection rates
- Contraindications to primary closure:
  - Skin loss primarily or during debridement
  - Gross contamination with faeces, dirt, stagnant water
  - Farm-related injuries, fresh water-related accidents
  - Delay in antibiotic initiation >12h
  - Extensive tissue necrosis at debridement
- Secondary procedures frequently necessary.

It has been shown that definitive stabilization by reamed intramedullary nail for low-grade open fractures produces satisfactory outcomes. The infection rate has been shown to be less than 3% for grade I open fractures. However, when reamed intramedullary nailing was performed on severe open fractures (grade IIIB), the rate of infection has previously been reported as high as 23%. Open tibial fractures stabilized with unreamed interlocking nails have reported rates of union greater than 96%, a low rate of malunion, and rates of infection in the range of 4–8% for grade IIIB fractures. More recent studies have shown that results of reamed nailing for grade IIIB fractures are comparable to unreamed nails in terms of union rates and complications.

Randomized prospective studies have been performed comparing the results of unreamed interlocking nails with external fixation for the treatment of open fractures. All of these studies demonstrated similar rates of infection and non-union for both treatment modalities, but a significantly higher prevalence of malunion with external fixation. The major advantage to intramedullary nailing is that it facilitates soft-tissue procedures, and delayed bone and skin grafting without the hindrance of an external fixation device. Recent evidence supports the usage of unreamed solid nails in stabilizing open grade IIIb and IIIc fractures.

External fixation is still considered a good choice for highly contaminated open fractures or fractures associated with prolonged delay prior to operative intervention (Figure 12.57.14). Rates of infection with external fixation for grade III injures has ranged from 4–7%. This relatively low rate of infection has been offset by the increased rate of malunion that has been reported when treating open tibial shaft fractures to completion with an external fixator.

Postoperative care

When the tibial shaft fractures are treated conservatively, early weight bearing is encouraged. As soon as the patient is comfortable in the long leg cast and the swelling has subsided, conversion to a patellar tendon bearing cast is usually indicated. This will occur at

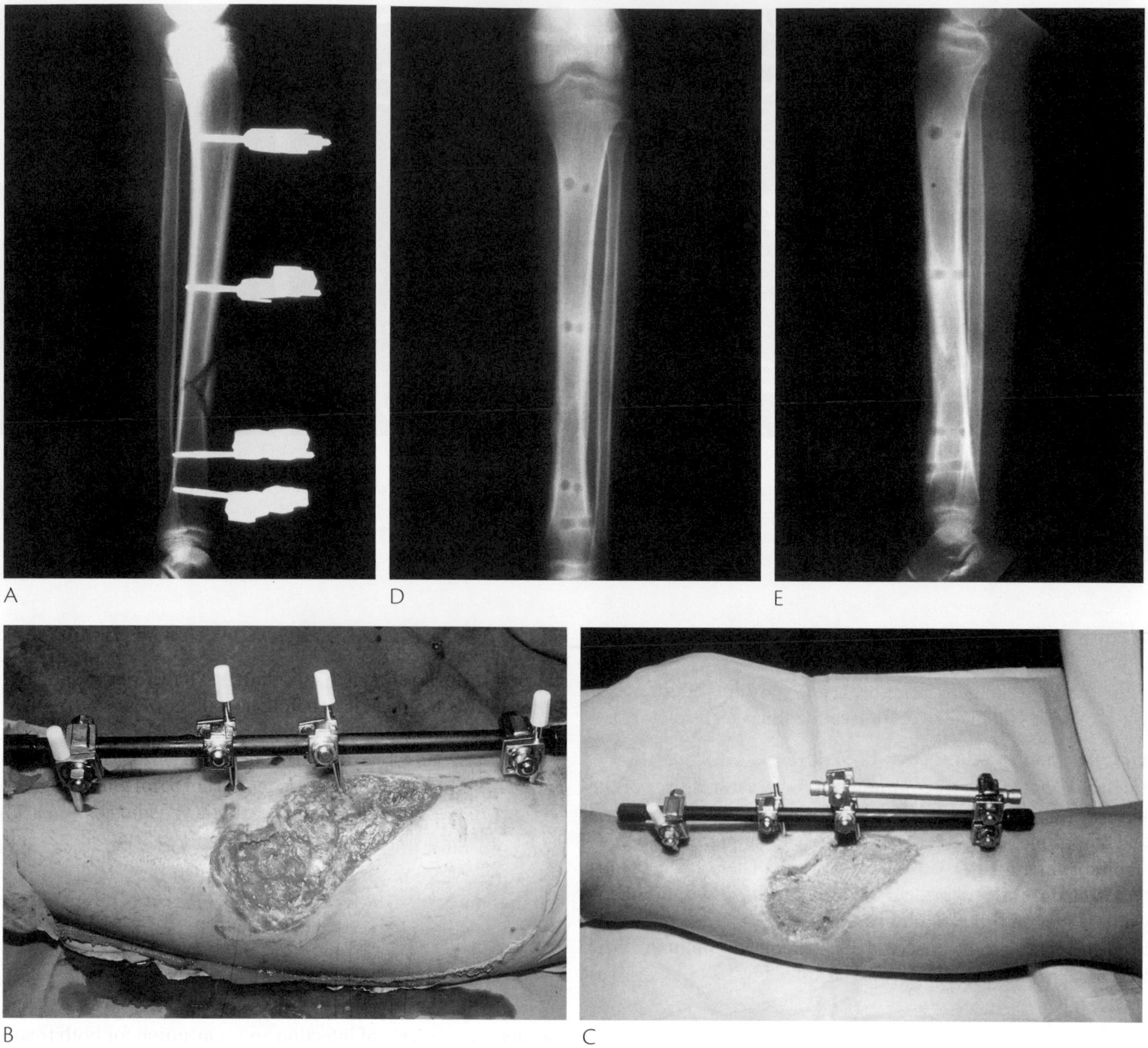

Fig. 12.57.14 A) Monolateral external fixation provides stabilization for this open tibia in an adolescent. B), C) Soft-tissue care and eventual skin grafting is facilitated using this simple external fixator. D), E) Frame dynamization should occur prior to frame removal to accentuate callus formation and facilitate load transfer. Anteroposterior and lateral radiographs show that uneventful union occurred, despite pin-bone interface lysis.

3–6 weeks. Following a short period of patellar tendon-bearing cast immobilization, the patient should be converted to a total-contact orthoses and full weight bearing encouraged.

The management of fractures treated with intramedullary nails can be varied depending on the fracture pattern, and configuration and morphology of the nail used. In general, reamed medullary nails are larger diameter and have bigger locking screws. When large locking screws are used the patient may be considered for early weight bearing. Regardless of the size of the nail and screws, if the fracture pattern is axially stable, the patient is allowed to progress to, at least, 50% weight bearing immediately after surgery. For fracture patterns with comminution or segmental injuries, which are axially unstable, then non-weight bearing should be maintained for at least 6 weeks. For the axially stable fracture patterns, full weight bearing can be initiated once progressive callus is seen on radiograph. For the axially unstable injuries, delaying full weight bearing for at least 3 months may need to be considered. Throughout the course of treatment, fracture healing should be monitored in order to avoid fatigue failure of the nail or locking bolts, especially for small nails. Early intervention is necessary to avoid these complications.

For tibial fractures treated with plate fixation, patients are usually immobilized either in a removable splint or cast until the incision heals. Soft tissue concerns are paramount in the early postoperative period to ensure that the wound heals without complications. Because the plate is a load-bearing device, weight bearing must be delayed. For the first 6–8 weeks, patients should be maintained as strict non-weight bearing, and if patient compliance is an issue, then long leg casting should be maintained with the knee flexed in order to prevent unrestricted weight-bearing. If the patient is reliable, then toe-touch non-weight bearing can be initiated immediately. In approximately 6–8 weeks when early cortical bridging and diminution of the fracture line is seen on radiograph, the patient can be advanced to 50% partial weight bearing. This may sometimes need to be augmented with a patellar tendon bearing orthosis or short-leg walking cast. When recorticalization is complete, the patient may progress to full unrestricted weight-bearing at approximately 4–6 months.

Postoperative management of external fixation is often problematic with respect to the management of the pin sites. In the case of circular small-wire external fixators for extra-articular injuries, full weight bearing may be initiated immediately after surgery. For most monolateral frames with dynamization capabilities, once early callus formation is noted the frames can be dynamized or sequentially disassembled to transfer more of the load to the fracture site itself and promote axial micromotion to facilitate healing. Following the removal of the external fixation device, a short period of orthotic management is required.

Regardless of the methodology of fracture fixation utilized, physical therapy should be initiated immediately to maintain knee and ankle range of motion. In cases of severe soft tissue injury and open fractures treated with external fixation, the foot should often be included in the fixation frame to avoid progressive equinus contracture due to the long period of non-weight bearing status necessary. Physical therapy should concentrate on maintaining a plantigrade foot. This is best established by allowing the patient to place the foot on the ground. This allows the foot to be placed in a plantigrade position while still avoiding full loading activities.

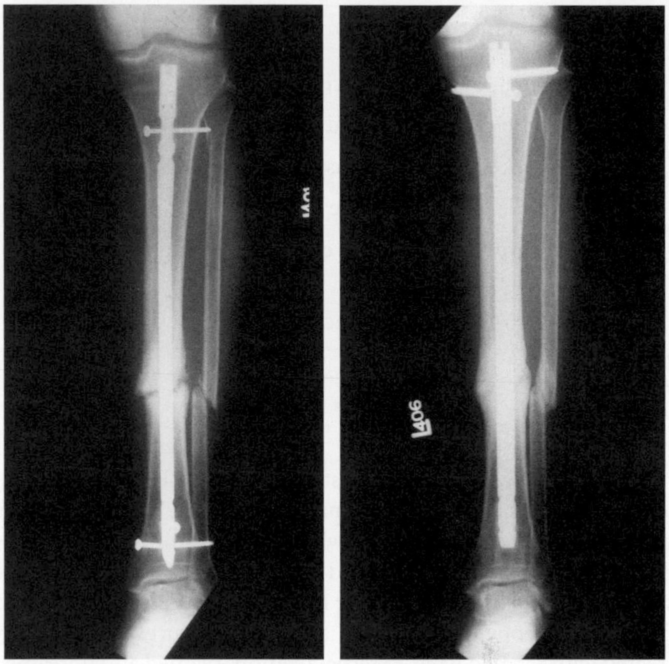

Fig. 12.57.15 A) This open fracture progressed to a nonunion after being treated with a statically locked unreamed nail. B) Following exchange nailing with a reamed nail of a larger diameter and a fibular osteotomy, complete healing occurred.

Complications (Box 12.57.7)

Complications of tibial shaft fractures include compartment syndrome, non-union, malunion, and infection. Arrest of the bony repair process with the formation of intervening fibrous or cartilaginous tissue is defined as a non-union. The usual time frame for this diagnosis is 6–8 months. Non-union most commonly occurs following open tibial shaft fractures, which have been treated with external fixation.

Secondary procedures have been advocated to promote union and avoid hardware failure in cases where delayed healing is likely. Nail dynamization, exchanged reamed nailing, open bone grafting, and fibular osteotomy all have been used alone or in combination to promote union (Figure 12.57.15).

Exchange nailing is a standard method of treatment for aseptic non-union. Progressive reaming until bone is seen on the flute of the reamer and exchange to a larger-diameter nail is recommended. Such nailing offers the unique biomechanical advantages of an intramedullary device, together with the osteoinductive stimulus of the by-products of reaming. A larger diameter nail also allows early weight-bearing and active rehabilitation. Following intervention it can be expected that 90% of non-unions will be united at an average of 3.5 months.

There is no consensus about the definition of malunion. The accepted arbitrary values for tibial shaft malunion are more than 10 degrees of angulation in sagittal plane, more than 5 degrees in coronal plane, and greater than 10 degrees of rotational malalignment. However, long-term follow-up studies have failed to establish any correlation between malunion and development of subsequent arthritis of ankle or subtalar joints. Established malunion is treated by corrective osteotomy along with refixation either by intramedullary or extramedullary devices.

Post-traumatic osteomyelitis occurs either after open fractures or surgically treated closed fractures. Treatment of an infected fracture utilizes a staged reconstruction protocol. If there is wound breakdown along with superficial infection, implants should be left in place in order to provide a stable fracture configuration. If the implant provides no stability at the time of debridement, all hardware should be removed. Furthermore, at debridement, all necrotic bone should be excised. Stabilization is necessary and is usually provided by external fixation. Serial debridements may be necessary to obtain a biologically sound wound. Dead-space is managed by using antibiotic beads or open-wound packing. Eventual soft tissue closure may be achieved with rotational flap or free-flap or coverage. Antibiotics directed at deep culture specimens should be administered for 4–6 weeks. Following resolution of the infection and healing of the soft tissues, delayed skeletal reconstruction is performed.

Overview

There are several well-accepted methods of treatment of tibial fractures. Orthopaedic surgeons tend to be preoccupied with the mechanics of fracture management and specifically with the implants to be utilized. However, there is no substitute for a thorough understanding of the so-called 'personality' of the fracture to help determine the best choice in treatment. Conservative management utilizing casts and functional orthoses is indicated for

Box 12.57.7 Compartment syndrome

- Maintain high index of suspicion
- Increased incidence associated with traction and reaming
- Extra vigilance in unconscious and unresponsive patients
- Look for serial rise in pressure
- Avoid postoperative patient-controlled analgesia to prevent delays in diagnosis
- Use long two-incision approach for release.

minimally displaced and axially stable fractures. Prospective studies indicate that intramedullary nailing with and without reaming both produce excellent results with high rates of union and low rates of occult infection. Reamed nailing has been shown to have shorter times to union and lower non union rates. Unstable closed fractures and open grades I, II, and IIIA fractures can be safely treated with reamed nails. External fixation, reamed and unreamed nails can be considered in grade IIIB fractures.

High-energy tibial shaft fractures pose a therapeutic challenge to the treating health-care professionals. These injuries are often seen in the context of polytrauma. Astute decision-making, collaboration with plastic surgeons, timely surgical intervention, and respect for soft tissue envelope of the leg will result in successful functional outcome. The recent development of minimally invasive fracture surgery will no doubt have a positive impact on the management of the tibial shaft fractures.

Further reading

Bhandari, M., Guyatt, G.H., Swiontkowski, M.F., *et al.* (2001). Surgeons' preferences for the operative treatment of fractures of the tibial shaft. An international survey. *Journal of Bone and Joint Surgery*, **83A**, 1746–52.

Bhandari, M., Guyatt, G., Tornetta, P., 3rd, *et al.* (2008). Randomized trial of reamed and unreamed intramedullary nailing of tibial shaft fractures. *Journal of Bone and Joint Surgery*, **90A**, 2567–78.

Rajasekaran, S., Naresh Babu, J., Dheenadhayalan, J., *et al.* (2006). A score for predicting salvage and outcome in Gustilo type-IIIA and type-IIIB open tibial fractures. *Journal of Bone and Joint Surgery*, **88B**, 1351–60.

Rhinelander, F. (1974). Tibial blood supply in relation to fracture healing. *Clinical Orthopaedic and Related Research*, **1053**, 4–40.

Sarmiento, A., Gersten, L., Sobol, P., Shankwiler, J., and Vangsness, C. (1989). Tibial shaft fractures treated with functional braces. Experience with 780 fractures. *Journal of Bone and Joint Surgery*, **71B**, 602–9.

SPRINT Investigators, Bhandari, M., Guyatt, G., *et al.* (2008). Study to prospectively evaluate reamed intramedually nails in patients with tibial fractures (S. P.R. I.N. T.): study rationale and design. *BMC Musculoskeletal Disorders*, **9**, 91.

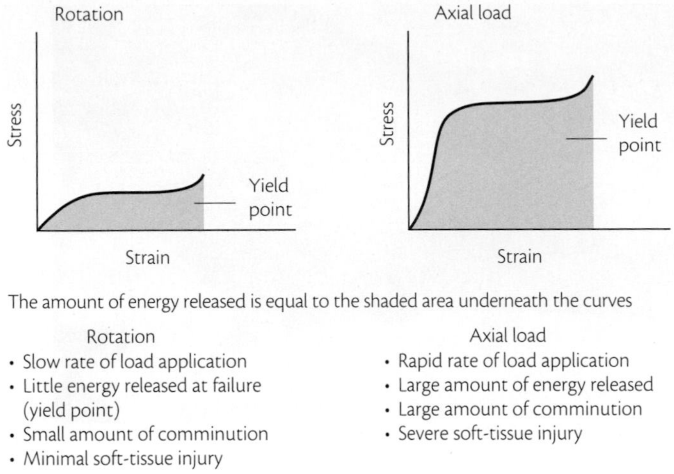

Rotation
Stress
Yield point
Strain
Axial load
Stress
Yield point
Strain
The amount of energy released is equal to the shaded area underneath the curves
Rotation
• Slow rate of load application
• Little energy released at failure (yield point)
• Small amount of comminution
• Minimal soft-tissue injury
Axial load
• Rapid rate of load application
• Large amount of energy released
• Large amount of comminution
• Severe soft-tissue injury

Fig. 12.58.5 Schematic stress–strain diagrams illustrate that the viscoelastic nature of bone leads to greater energy release after rapid axial load than slow rotational load.

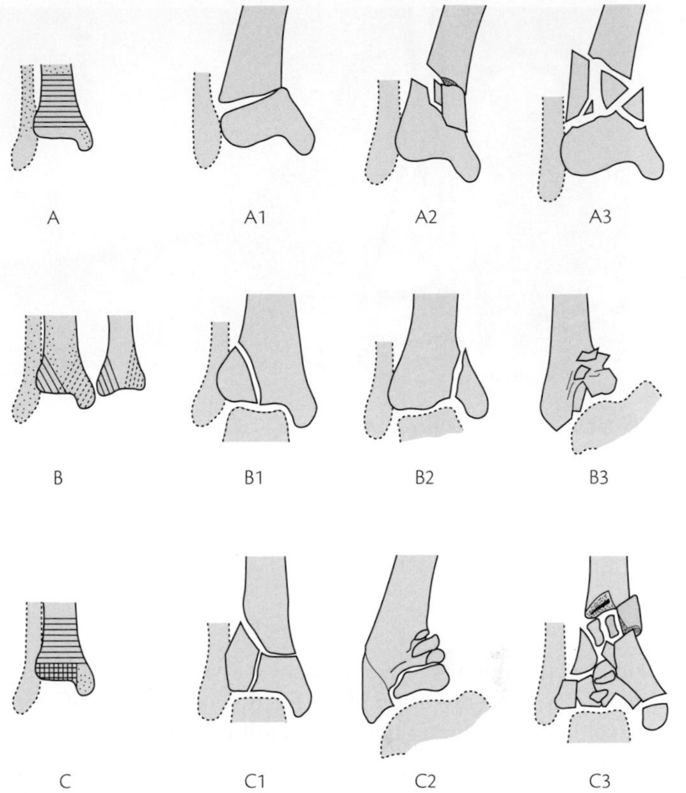

Fig. 12.58.6 The AO/OTA classification of distal tibia fractures. Type A fractures are extra-articular fractures of the distal tibia and are therefore not plafond fractures. Type B fractures involve only a portion of the articular surface, while the remaining articular surface has continuity with the tibial shaft. Type C fractures involve the entire articular surface and have increasing severity from group C1 to C3. http://www.ota.org/compendium/compendium.html

Classification

The AO/Orthopaedic Trauma Association (OTA) classification 2007 is the most complete and extensive classification of different subtypes of fractures of the plafond. This classification divides fractures of the distal tibia into groups A, B, and C, and then further subdivides them based on the amount of comminution (Figure 12.58.6). Group A consists of extra-articular fractures, group B of fractures involving part of the articular surface, and group C of fractures involving the entire articular surface. It is primarily the B3, C2, and C3 fracture types that are high-energy axial loading fractures and satisfy all definitions of a plafond fracture. B1, B2, and C1 fractures associated with marginal impaction can be considered to be plafond fractures. When combined with an assessment of the soft tissue injury, this classification may prove to be an aid to prognosis and allow comparison between patient groups.

Unfortunately, both this classification system and the Rüedi–Allgower system have been shown to have poor interobserver reliability and intraobserver reproducibility.

Treating these injuries requires accurate assessment of the soft tissue injury which is even more difficult to categorize accurately and reproducibly. Open fractures are classified based on the size of the wound using the criteria of Gustilo and Anderson, which do not address other components of the soft tissue injury or the majority of the fractures which are closed. The Tscherne–Goetzen classification assesses the grade and severity of the soft tissue injury in closed fractures. Although it is frequently cited in the literature, due to difficulties of clinical application, it has rarely been implemented in studies of plafond fractures. In addition, the full extent of swelling and local contusion can only be appreciated after several hours to days.

Clinical evaluation

History

The mechanism of injury provides insight into the amount of energy imparted to the bone and soft tissue at the time of fracture, which is crucial for surgical planning and for advising the patient on prognosis. In open fractures, assessing the environment in which the injury occurred will guide antibiotic treatment.

Examination

The neurological and vascular status of the foot must be evaluated. Absent pulses should be managed by realignment of the extremity and reassessment. Provisional splinting with the extremity aligned prevents further soft tissue trauma. Open wounds are inspected to determine their extent and evaluated for gross contamination. The condition of the skin, amount of swelling, and the presence of fracture blisters must be noted at initial evaluation as well as prior to surgical intervention.

Fracture blisters are common and can be divided into two types: clear-fluid filled and blood-filled. Histologically, both types are disruptions at the dermoepidermal junction, but the blood-filled blisters signify greater injury and have been associated with wound-healing complications when incisions are made through them (Figure 12.58.7).

Investigation

Standard imaging includes anteroposterior, lateral, and mortise views of the ankle. Repeat radiographs with the limb provisionally reduced provide useful information and should routinely be

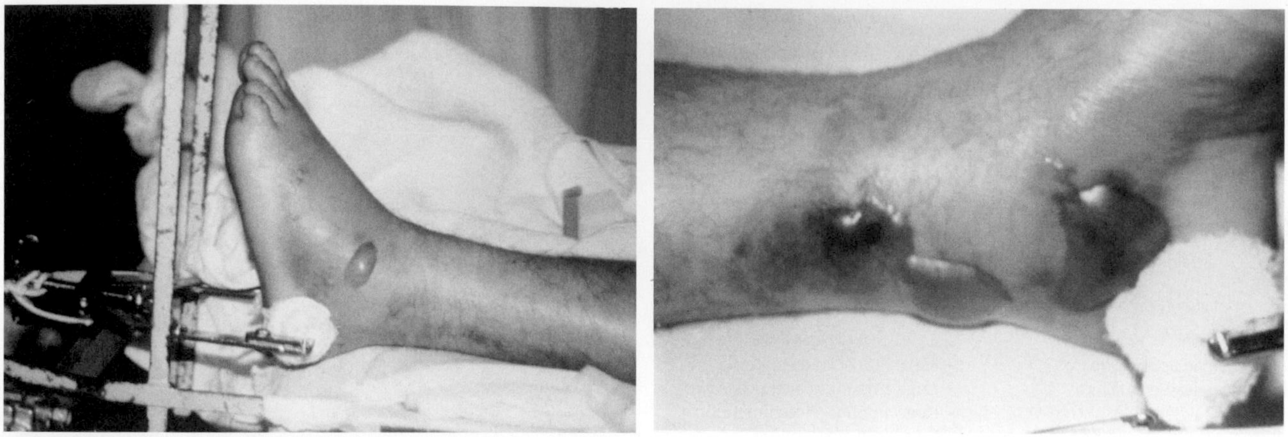

A B

Fig. 12.58.7 Fracture blisters are indicative of the severe soft tissue injury incurred in many tibial plafond fractures. There are blood-filled and clear-fluid-filled types. A) A single clear fluid-filled blister. B) Two blood-filled blisters and a single clear-fluid-filled blister.

obtained if the initial radiographs show the talus to be widely displaced. Proximal extension of the fracture or suspicion of more proximal injury mandates that full-length tibia and fibula radiographs be obtained. Some surgeons find views of the contralateral ankle helpful as a template for preoperative planning. Axial computed tomography (CT) scanning helps to define the severity of the injury and aids with surgical planning. The axial plane of the CT scan delineates the size and orientation of the articular fragments. This knowledge is crucial, especially for the less invasive approaches to articular reduction, where limited incisions are placed directly over fracture lines and implants are often applied percutaneously to limit the amount of soft tissue stripping. Coronal and sagittal reconstructions further delineate the fracture anatomy and assist in preoperative planning (Figure 12.58.8).

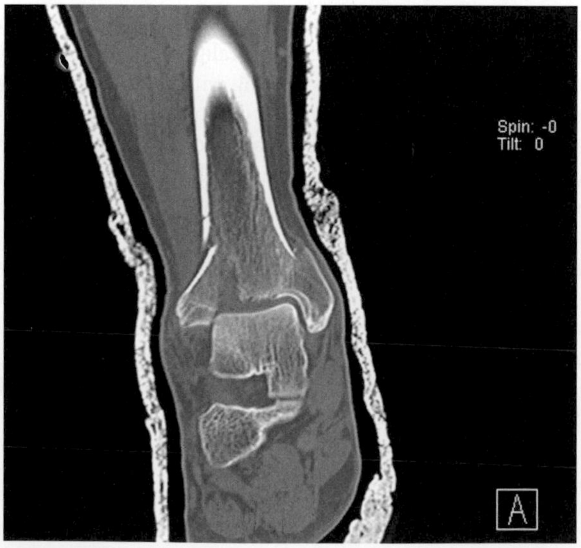

Fig. 12.58.8 A CT scans accurately depicts the major fracture lines and is an invaluable aid in preoperative planning as illustrated in this single coronal cut.

Management (Box 12.58.2)

Initial

Tibial plafond fractures are initially managed by provisional reduction, splinting, and elevation to minimize further soft tissue injury. A spanning external fixator with or without fibular fixation is used to maintain length and provisional reduction, and has been used as a means of portable traction prior to definitive treatment. This has the advantage of permitting mobilization. In patients with multiple injuries, open wounds, or compartment syndrome, application of a provisional spanning external fixator should always be part of the initial management.

Non-operative

Casting or splinting has generally been reserved for non-displaced fractures or as a treatment of default, when associated injuries or the severity of the fracture and soft tissue injury precluded any type of operative intervention.

Box 12.58.2 Treatment of tibial plafond fractures

- Soft tissues are the most important
- The complications of treatment are frequent and may be severe
- Optimal current treatment is controversial
- Internal and external fixation techniques are both utilized
- External fixation techniques decrease complication rate
- Temporary spanning external fixation allows soft tissue recovery
- Plating through limited approaches for some fracture patterns.

Open reduction and internal fixation

Current fixation of tibial plafond fractures by open reduction and internal fixation can be traced to the AO–ASIF group and their philosophy of obtaining anatomical reduction through wide operative approaches followed by rigid internal fixation to allow for early mobilization. Rüedi and Allgower reported good results with this technique and their method was widely adopted as the ideal form of treatment for this fracture type. A four-step protocol for open reduction and internal fixation was described (Figure 12.58.9):

- Reconstruct the fibula to restore length and to reduce articular fragments still attached to the distal fibula by intact ligaments
- Reconstruct the joint surface and obtain provisional fixation
- Apply cancellous bone graft to the metaphyseal defect
- Use a medial or anterior buttress plate on the distal tibia for definitive fixation.

Since the publication of Rüedi and Allgower's work, the technique for open reduction has been modified, but the four basic steps or tenets have remained unchanged. The modifications have centred around atraumatic soft tissue technique to avoid skin slough and wound breakdown. Delaying surgery for 7–21 days avoids the time period where interstitial oedema, tense swelling, and tissue ischaemia are most likely to lead to difficult wound closures and subsequent breakdown and infection. This may be the single most important principal that has decreased what was an unacceptably high complication rate. Fracture blisters are unroofed and sterile dressings used, and definitive surgery is delayed until it is clear that swelling is receding. Length and alignment are maintained with temporary joint spanning external fixation. This allows patient mobilization and facilitates subsequent joint reconstruction. The classic surgical approach is through two incisions, one lateral incision paralleling the posterior aspect of the fibula, and an anterior incision over the tibia that curves medially in its distal aspect. Flaps in the subcutaneous layer should not be elevated. If the paratenon of the anterior tibial tendon can be preserved a skin graft can be used, preventing a tight closure. Incisions directly over the anteromedial tibia are through poorly vascularized and damaged skin and may be directly over a location chosen for implant placement. A minimum of 7–12cm between the medial and lateral incisions has been recommended to retain the vascularity of the skin flap. Intraoperative use of a femoral distractor and indirect reduction techniques decrease the amount of stripping required to obtain reduction. The use of a precontoured plate assists in both reducing and internally fixing the fracture through more limited approaches. The wound closes more easily if small, low-profile implants are used.

Alternate approaches have been described and are now frequently used. The best approach is based on the fracture pattern and surgeon preference. The anterolateral tibia can be accessed through a lateral or anterolateral approach and specially countered plates are now available which have been designed for the anterolateral tibia. A posterolateral approach has been described and may have particular utility for posterior fracture patterns. This approach has a significant complication rate including infections and nonunions and it is recommended that it is not used for all fracture patterns. Percutaneous plating has been reported for pilon fractures. The easiest access to the tibia for percutaneous plating is the anteromedial surface. Through a small incision over the medial malleolus the plate is slid subcutaneously and fixed with proximal screws placed through stab wounds. A high secondary intervention

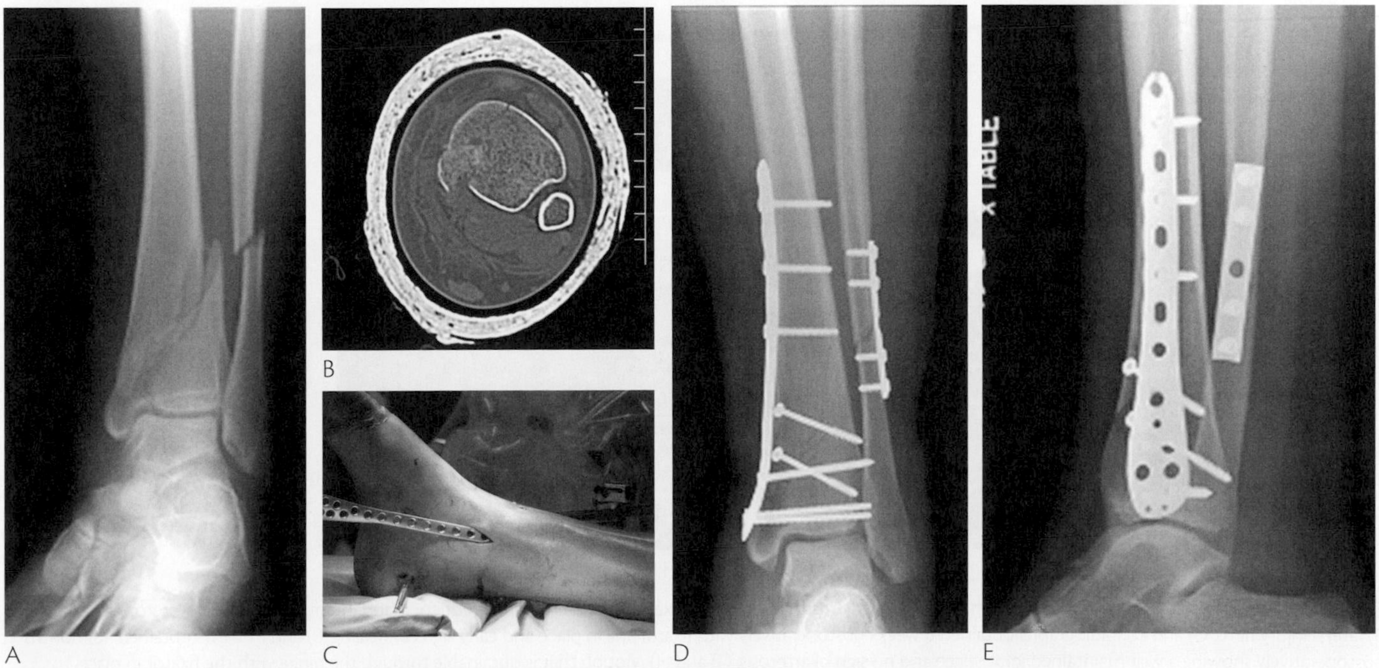

Fig. 12.58.9 A) Anteroposterior and B) an axial CT cut show a C1 tibial plafond fracture. C) An intraoperative photograph; D) postoperative anteroposterior; E) and lateral radiographs demonstrate treatment by percutaneous plating.

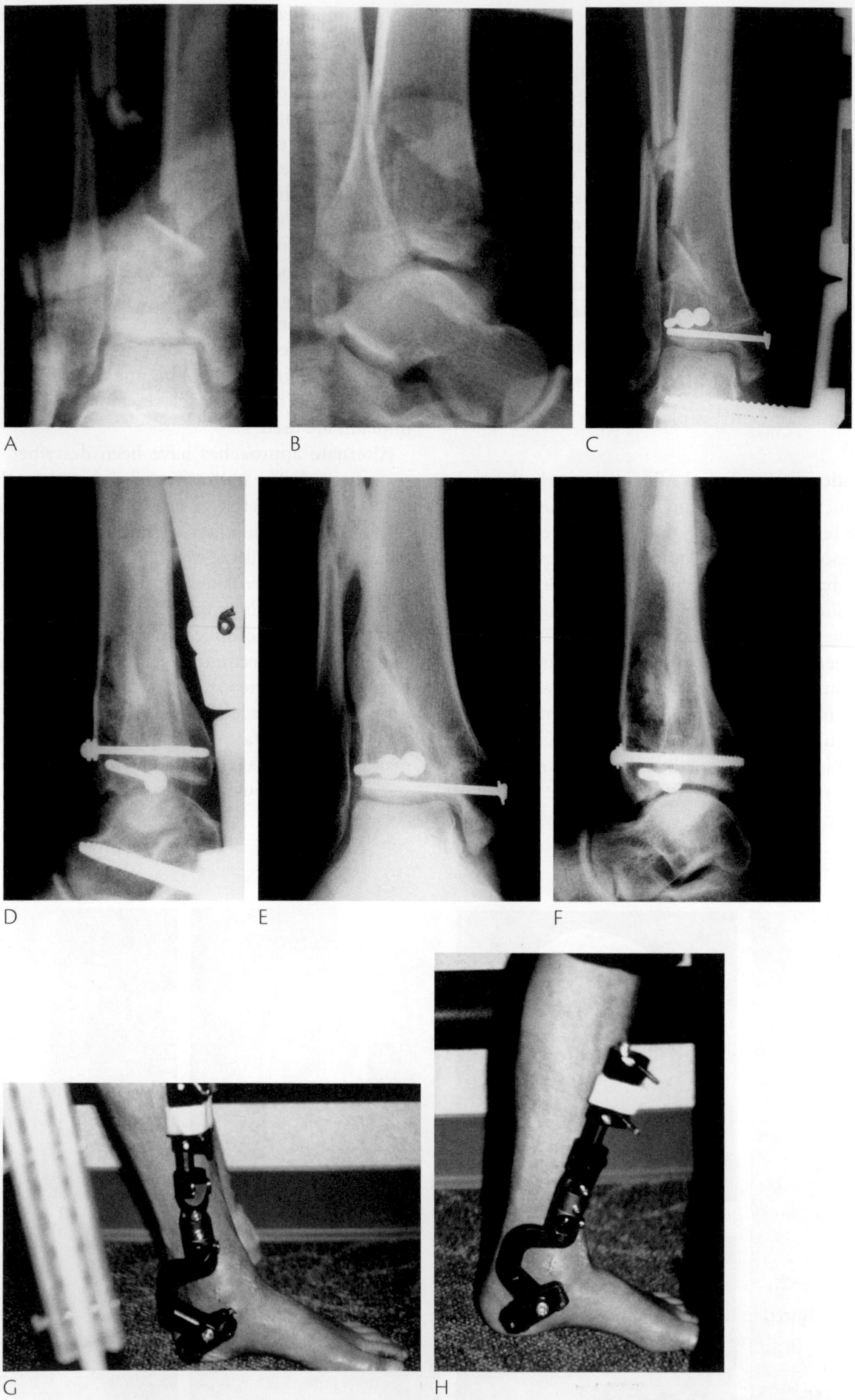

Fig. 12.58.10 Tibial plafond fracture treated with an articulated cross ankle external fixator and limited open reduction and internal fixation. A) Anteroposterior and B) lateral injury films. C) and D) Radiographs obtained 6 weeks postoperatively with fixator still in place and early signs of healing. E) and F) Views obtained 18 months postoperatively showing a well-maintained joint space and no sign of arthrosis. G) and H) Motion that is obtainable through the hinge with the fixator in place.

rate has been reported indicated that limited approach plating does not guarantee healing in all these fractures.

External fixation

Several methods of definitive external fixation have been advocated to decrease the complications associated with plates. These techniques all use one or more of three methods to reduce wound complications: limited surgical approaches to the injured area; limiting bulky internal implants; or stabilization that bridges the area of soft tissue injury. There are a variety of different frames and application techniques.

A fixator body spanning the ankle may be constructed using any of several different components and frame constructs including medial monolateral frames, delta frames, and small pin circular fixators. One technique spans the ankle but preserves ankle motion through an articulated hinge. These frames are applied as the first step in the procedure, distracted and the provisional reduction is assessed with fluoroscopic image intensification. The articular surface is reduced using percutaneous and indirect techniques. The fracture fragments are stabilized with small fragment or cannulated screws, often placed percutaneously. Plates are never used; the fixator provides axial stability. Grafting is rarely utilized.

Postoperatively the hinge is initially locked, but can be released during the postoperative course so the ankle moves with the fixator still in place. One study showed no advantage of early movement through the hinge over a rigidly locked hinge for 8 weeks. Partial weight bearing usually begins by 4–6 weeks postinjury. The average time until the frame is removed is 3 months.

External fixation which does not cross the ankle must obtain purchase in the bottom of the tibia. A variety of frame constructs have been utilized, most of which use tensioned wires attached to a ring for distal fixation. The ankle is free which preserves the possibility for ankle movements. The fibula, if broken, is stabilized with a one-third tubular plate and lag screws through a posterolateral incision. Through an incision over the major fracture line the articular surface is reduced and secured with lag screws. The reconstructed metaphysis and articular surface are secured to a semicircular ring with tensioned wires. The tensioned wire and ring construct is connected to a fixator body which spans the fracture and connects to the diaphysis with standard 5.0-mm half pins. A similar technique has been described utilizing pin fixators. The Ilizarov technique has frame modularity that allows the foot to be immobilized with a foot ring that can be removed at a time post injury dictated by the injury and other factors. Satisfactory results have been reported by many authors.

The most comminuted fractures and partial articular fractures are not amenable to this technique, since stable fixation of the distal tibia is not possible.

Postoperative management

The ankle should be splinted in the neutral position. The length of time for non-weight bearing must be tailored to the individual, the type of fixation, the characteristics of the fracture, and the personality of the patient.

Results (Box 12.58.3)

Interpreting the results of treatment of tibial plafond fractures is difficult at best. Recent studies incorporate patient perception of their outcome and have utilized validated outcome measuring tools. These studies have shown that these injuries have a profound effect on patient's general health status and result in long-term ankle pain and dysfunction. These results have been found in patients treated with plates, external fixators, and with both plates and fixators. Patients in the second 5 years after their injury still have decreased general health status. Better outcomes have been found in patients with college education and poorer outcomes in work related injuries.

> **Box 12.58.3** Outcome of tibial plafond fractures
>
> - Arthrodesis is unusual (<5%) in the absence of infection
> - Significant residual impairment 2 years after injury
> - Factors that produce optimal outcome are largely unknown
> - Complications of wound breakdown and infection must be avoided
> - Post-traumatic osteoarthritis common regardless of treatment technique.

Open reduction and internal fixation

Beginning in the late 1960s and early 1970s good results with open reduction and internal fixation were reported with 75–90% good or excellent clinical results and few complications. In contrast with these good results, there were a number of series which reported dismal results with open reduction and internal fixation. Most authors attributed their bad results, at least in part, to the higher number of 'high-energy' injuries in their patient groups. The high complication rates have led to modifications of techniques and in particular the practice of delays to definitive surgery to allow soft tissue recovery and the use of temporary spanning external fixation. Recent evidence indicates that the safety profile for treating these fractures with plates has improved significantly and current techniques are as safe as external fixation.

External fixation

Several authors have reported the results of treating open and severely comminuted plafond fractures with external fixators that spanned the ankle and in general, the results have been acceptable with 30–50% good or excellent and 10–25% poor outcomes. More importantly, in these injuries which were selected for their severity, all major complications were avoided. There were no infections or skin sloughs and only occasional minor pin or wire tract problems. Similar results have been reported when hybrid external fixators were used to treat selected tibial plafond fractures. Good or excellent results were obtained in 50–70% of cases treated. Complications were few and primarily related to pin sites, although each series had at least one deep infection or osteomyelitis.

In a prospective study of 49 displaced fractures of the tibial plafond managed using an articulated hinge fixator there was no tibial wound infections or osteomyelitis. At 2-year follow-up, 60% of the patients rated their result as excellent or satisfactory, 30% fair, and 10% were unsatisfied with the result.

In the most severe injuries, a substantial percentage (25–50%) of patients will continue to have pain or impaired function.

Comparative trials

There have been several comparative trials between external and internal fixation techniques. Higher rates of complication have been observed in patients treated with open reduction and internal fixation when compared to those treated with external fixation and limited open reduction and internal fixation. On the other hand, better outcomes have been identified in patients treated with plate fixation. It has been recommended that treatment should be based on the severity of the soft tissue injury with more severe injuries favouring external fixation.

Summary

The conclusions that can most readily be drawn from these studies are that both external fixation and open reduction and internal fixation can yield reasonable outcomes. Complications must be avoided. Regardless of the treatment method there is a subset of patients with severe injuries who have a poor outcome despite proper treatment that avoids complications and most patients continue to have some ankle symptoms. Table 12.58.1 summarizes the relative advantages and disadvantages of the current techniques that are most commonly utilized.

Complications

Postoperative complications may be divided into early and late by time of onset. Wound breakdown leading to osteomyelitis is the most troublesome, and an all too common early complication of tibial plafond fractures treated operatively. The incidence is quite variable ranging from none to 55%. The evidence indicates that the rate correlates with the severity of the injury and the operative technique (Table 12.58.2).

The high rate of infection is related to the tenuous soft tissue envelope about the distal tibia, which has inherent poor vascularity. Severe soft tissue damage results from the energy released by the fracture. This causes swelling and interstitial oedema resulting in relative tissue ischaemia. Surgical dissection, soft tissue stripping, and the use of large implants often tips the scales, resulting in the progression to skin slough, wound breakdown, and osteomyelitis. The best treatment is prevention which can be accomplished by delaying surgery until the initial swelling and oedema have diminished, using small implants, performing indirect reduction techniques and stabilizing with external fixation at least temporarily.

Once faced with wound breakdown and infection, treatment must be aggressive. All nonviable tissue must be debrided, loose hardware removed, and the fracture stabilized with an external fixator. A prolonged course of intravenous antibiotics is required. Free tissue transfer for soft tissue coverage is routinely necessary. Despite these aggressive measures, a long difficult treatment course may still result in arthrodesis or amputation.

The primary late complications are non-union, malunion, and post-traumatic arthrosis. The incidence of non-union and malunion has been reported to be as high as 18% and 42% respectively. Some authors have concluded that non-unions are not complications, but rather an expected outcome in a certain percentage of fractures. Aseptic non-unions may be treated with bone grafts and/or skeletal stabilization with a high degree of success. Non-unions complicated by infection pose a much greater problem. Treatment is prolonged and expensive often requiring multiple procedures with technically demanding techniques. Amputation may be required.

Post-traumatic arthrosis is a frequent sequelae of these severe injuries (54%). One study at 5–11 years of follow-up had fairly

Table 12.58.2 Incidence of complication of treatment

Nonunion	3–42%
Arthrosis	20–54%
Infection	0–55%
Amputation	0–15%

Table 12.58.1 Fixation techniques

Technique	Advantages	Disadvantages
Open reduction internal fixation	Wide exposure for articular reduction	Disrupts tenuous soft-tissue envelope
	Early motion of ankle joint	Multi-stage treatment necessary
	Temporary external fixation has decreased complications	Subcutaneous implants
Rigid cross-ankle external fixation	Minimal disruption of zone of injury	Rigidly immobilizes ankle
External fixation of same side of joint	Allows motion at the ankle	Cannot be used for all fractures
	Avoids large plates to stabilize metaphysis	Disrupts zone of injury
		Technically demanding
Articlated cross-ankle external fixation	Allows motion at the ankle (limited)	Hard to align axis of hinge with axis of ankle joint
	Technically easier to apply fixator	Value of motion through an articulated hinge is not proven
	Minimal disruption of zone of injury	

high-grade arthrosis in 26 out of 36 ankles studied. The relative role of the damage inflicted at the time of injury versus incomplete reduction is unclear. Radiographic arthrosis, or its absence, does not correlate well with clinical measures of outcome or patient satisfaction.

Treatment of arthrosis centres around symptomatic relief with non-steroidal anti-inflammatory drugs, braces, and shoe modifications. Once conservative treatment has been exhausted, arthrodesis is a reliable option for pain relief. Ankle fusion may become exceedingly difficult if early postoperative complications have resulted in infection, nonunion, or bone loss.

Future directions

The shortcomings seen in the current literature point out where future investigation and advancement is warranted. The inability to classify these fractures reliably and reproducibly makes comparison between any two series of patients extremely difficult. Comparison is further hampered by the multitude of scales used to measure outcome parameters. In order to become better at predicting the factors that are responsible for patient outcome, there needs to be some consensus on how to measure outcome. This problem is magnified by the relative rarity of this fracture, which ensures that no single surgeon or facility treats enough of these injuries to perform multiarmed studies comparing different treatment options. A goal of the future is to aim to decrease the incidence of complications and late sequelae of these injuries. Further advances in imaging such as intraoperative three-dimensional imaging may increase the use and utility of limited approaches.

Further reading

Harris, A.M., Patterson, B.M., Sontich, J.K., and Vallier, H.A. (2006). Results and outcomes after operative treatment of high-energy tibial plafond fractures. *Foot & Ankle International*, **27**(4), 256–65.

Howard, J.L., Agel, J., Barei, D.P., Benirschke, S.K., and Nork, S.E. (2008). A prospective study evaluating incision placement and wound healing for tibial plafond fractures. *Journal of Orthopaedic Trauma*, **22**(5), 299–305; discussion 305–6.

Marsh, J.L., Borrelli, J., Jr., Dirschl, D.R., and Sirkin, M.S. (2007). Fractures of the tibial plafond. *Instructional Course Lectures*, **56**, 331–52.

Marsh, J.L., Muehling, V., Dirschl, D., Hurwitz, S., Brown, T.D., and Nepola, J. (2006). Tibial plafond fractures treated by articulated external fixation: a randomized trial of postoperative motion versus nonmotion. *Journal of Orthopaedic Trauma*, **20**(8), 536–41.

Salton, H.L., Rush, S., and Schuberth, J. (2007). Tibial plafond fractures: limited incision reduction with percutaneous fixation. *Journal of Foot & Ankle Surgery*, **46**(4), 261–9.

12.59

Ankle fractures

R. Handley and A. Gandhe

Summary points

- Ankle fracture management is dependent on the patient, stability and congruence
- Comparative studies of treatment options should be interpreted with caution.

Introduction

Ankle fractures are often the first fractures treated operatively by trainees. Many principles of fracture fixation can be applied in the management of these fractures. The authors have developed an algorithm to apply to their management where possible. Otherwise, treatment decisions can be based on fundamental principles.

Normal and pathological anatomy of the ankle

It has probably been stated rather too readily that the aim of the treatment of ankle injuries is the restoration of normal anatomy and early function. Accepting this aim drives one toward operative intervention. The bulk of ankle injuries, including fractures, are treated non-operatively with good functional results. Therefore it is necessary to look critically at which anatomical features require restoration for satisfactory function and avoid unnecessary intervention.

The ankle is composed of joints between the tibia and fibula, the talus and tibia, and the talus and fibula, and their associated soft tissue structures. These joints have load-bearing surfaces to transmit the compressive forces. The bony contours and the soft tissue configuration of the joint maintain the load-bearing surfaces in the correct apposition to transmit the load without damage. Therefore skeletal injuries to the ankle region can be divided into two groups: those which directly affect the load-bearing surface, and those which damage the stability and alignment of the joints. The Comprehensive Classification of Fractures reflects this division by separating the load-bearing tibial plafond fractures or pilon-type fractures (AO/OTA 43) from a special group of malleolar segment fractures (AO/OTA 44). Tibial plafond fractures are discussed in Chapter 12.58.

The bony mortise of the ankle is formed from the distal tibia and fibula. The fibula sits posterolaterally in the incisura of the distal tibia. They are bound together by the five ligamentous components of the inferior tibiofibular joint. The strongest of these is the posterior tibiofibular ligament, which runs from the posterior fibula to the area of Volkman's triangle on the posterior aspect of the tibia. The anterior tibiofibular ligament is not as strong and runs from the fibula to the tubercle of Chaput. The talus fits snugly into this mortise. The collateral ligaments secure the talus in the mortise. The medial collateral ligament (deltoid ligament) comprises a superficial and a deep layer. The deep fibres are especially noteworthy for their short direct path and are said to be the most important component of this ligament. Their deep position, behind the anterior colliculus of the medial malleolus, renders them inaccessible to surgical repair.

Diagnosis (Box 12.59.1)

A careful assessment is necessary to avoid premature labelling as an 'ankle injury'. This will obscure diagnosis of one of the many other problems that can present around this region. The history must include the mechanism of the injury and the general features which may influence the choice of treatment, e.g. previous injury, mobility, anticoagulation, and diabetes. A history of weight bearing after the injury suggests a stable injury except in the neuropathic patient.

Dressings or splints should be removed to allow a full assessment by the person who will control management. Inspection will allow an assessment of swelling, wounds, or impending breakdown of skin. Palpation must be performed systematically to determine the precise location of tenderness. The examiner must have a mental picture of the structures being palpated and this should include the whole length of the fibula and the anterior tibiofibular syndesmosis. Random 'prodding' medially and laterally will lead to errors. The joint should be moved and note made of the range and confidence of the movement and the feel of the endpoint to help assess stability.

There are many pressures to order special investigations, particularly radiographs. Many departments have guidelines for the use of radiographs. Implementation of the Ottawa ankle rules can reduce the requests for ankle films and minimize the risk of missing

Box 12.59.1 Diagnosis

- History:
  - Mechanism
  - Postinjury weight bearing
  - Previous injury
  - Comorbidities
- Examination:
  - Assessment of the skin is important
  - Find the sites of maximal tenderness
  - Assess ankle stability
- Imaging:
  - Radiography only if clinically indicated
  - CT scan when indicated.

injuries. A mortise and a lateral view are usually required in the first instance. To obtain the mortise view the ankle needs to be internally rotated by 15 degrees; the anteroposterior view has little additional value. Indiscriminate use of ankle radiographs for all problems vaguely in that anatomical area with cursory scrutiny of the malleoli alone may lead to overlooking of subtalar dislocations, tarsometatarsal dislocations, talar fractures, and calcaneal fractures (Figure 12.59.1). A group of patients who require particular attention are those who have an emergency reduction of a clinically diagnosed ankle dislocation but then subsequent radiographs appear normal. In this group there may be occult subtalar dislocations, calcaneal and talar fractures. In our opinion they merit computed tomography (CT) examination.

The limitations of plain radiographs should be remembered and when the radiograph does not fit the clinical findings, think again. The radiograph in Figure 12.59.2 shows an apparently normal ankle in a patient with significant symptoms and local tenderness anterolaterally. Symptoms persisted and about 6 weeks later a scan demonstrated an intra-articular Tilleaux fracture. In this instance, even if a scan had not been available oblique views may well have demonstrated the injury. In fact, on closer inspection a depressed segment of the joint surface can be seen on the original lateral view. It may be helpful to look for a joint effusion analogous to the fat-pad sign at the elbow. The appearance of a joint effusion of more than 15mm on the lateral film indicates the presence of an occult fracture in 83% of cases and is an indication for further investigation.

Whilst soft tissue signs may prompt the diagnosis of a bony injury, the converse is also true. The soft tissue significance of bony abnormality should also be remembered. A vertically orientated fragment may be the marker of an avulsion of the peroneal sheath with dislocated or dislocatable peroneal tendons (Figure 12.59.3).

A two-dimensional picture of a three-dimensional structure can lead to confusion when estimating the shape and size of the posterior malleolar fragment. Plain radiograph measurements lead to very poor inter- and intra-examiner reliability. When compared with the CT scan measurement, 54% of the plain radiographic readings revealed more than 25% error. A further limitation of plain radiograph is the inability to demonstrate rotational abnormalities and relationships clearly. At other sites, rotational abnormalities of clinical importance can be assessed clinically however this is not possible when assessing fibular rotation.

Description and classification of injuries (Box 12.59.2)

Once the characteristics of an injury have been identified, it must be described and classified.

The Lauge-Hansen system is based on mechanism of injury. This system, which was introduced in the 1940s, has stood the test of time and is used in many papers on ankle injuries. For this reason alone, familiarity is required. However, as the terminology is difficult to remember and it is unusual for two people to both understand it adequately it is not very helpful in day-to-day communication.

Weber and Danis are credited with the basic classification of fibula fractures as A, B, or C depending on the relationship of the fracture to the inferior tibiofibular syndesmosis. It is easily remembered and understood, to the extent that it is used in plain speech. It is very limited in the other goals of a classification system, such as guiding treatment, prognosis, etc. However, it does provide the foundation to the malleolar segment injuries group in the Comprehensive Classification of Fractures. This more comprehensive system with its alphanumeric format is suited to use on computer-based systems for storage and retrieval. A comparison of the AO/OTA and Lauge-Hansen systems is shown in Figure 12.59.4.

Congruence and stability (Box 12.59.3)

Congruence

The articular surfaces of a normal ankle are congruent. The articular surface of the talus is not uniform and therefore to maintain full contact during the normal movements of flexion and extension the shape of the mortise must change, i.e. the fibula and tibia move relative to each other. Abnormal movements or displacements are likely to cause loss of congruence such that the load across the joint is spread unevenly, and the articular cartilage may be exposed to forces sufficient to cause it to fail. This potential cause of late degenerative arthritis following a displaced fracture has been recognized for a long time but attempts to quantify the forces and estimate their effects have given variable results. Interpreting clinical results is difficult because late degenerative changes may be the inevitable consequence of damage to the articular surfaces at the time of the original injury rather than any subsequent damage consequent upon instability or malunion. The difficulty in interpreting the results may lead one to the conclusion when treating ankle fractures: ‘If you don’t understand it, just put it back where it came from’.

Research has suggested that a 1-mm lateral shift in the talus caused a 42% decrease in contact area in the tibiotalar joint makes one wary of accepting any possibility of talar shift. In these experiments, talar shift was obtained by placing spacers of the appropriate width in the medial joint space. In this experiment, and others, the talus is noted to adopt its position of maximal congruence on loading, unless restrained. Mortise widening alone, with or without deltoid rupture, has not been seen to significantly affect contact area, centroid position, or joint contact pressure. Other experiments have suggested that lateral displacements of the talus and fibula up to 4mm

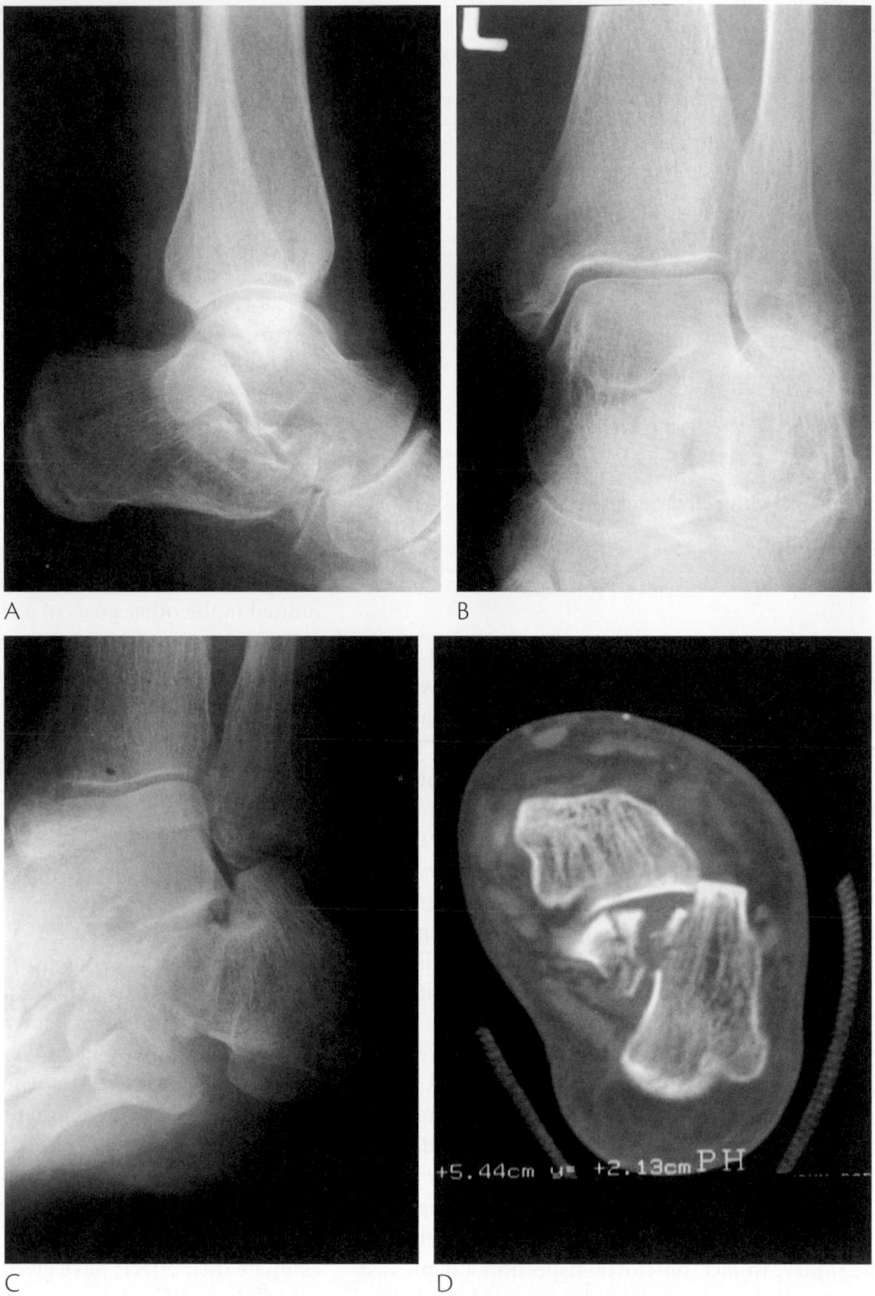

Fig. 12.59.1 A) and B) This ankle was originally described as normal, but closer scrutiny revealed a subtalar fracture dislocation. C) and D) Further imaging showed the true nature of the injury.

have not shown an increase in peak stress. It has been suggested that factors other than the magnitude of normal contact stresses are of greater importance in the pathogenesis of post-traumatic arthritis.

In the isolated Weber type B fibula fracture there is often the clear appearance of displacement of the lateral malleolar fragment on a plain radiograph. CT scans have been used for further delineation of the nature of this injury and the apparent external rotation of the lateral malleolus is relative only to the proximal fibula and is not associated with derangement of the talofibular articulation.

If the posterior malleolar fragment is sufficiently large and displaced, it will clearly affect the contact area and stability. As noted above, estimating the size of the fragment from plain films is inaccurate but it is usually all that is available. Experimentally produced posterior malleolar fracture fragments of 25%, 33%, and 50%, as visualized on lateral radiographs, lead to a corresponding decrease of 4%, 13%, and 22% in tibiotalar contact area.

Stability

Stability may be assessed in three ways.

1) Knowledge of the various injury patterns and their effects on the stabilizing structures of the ankle will allow an estimate of stability

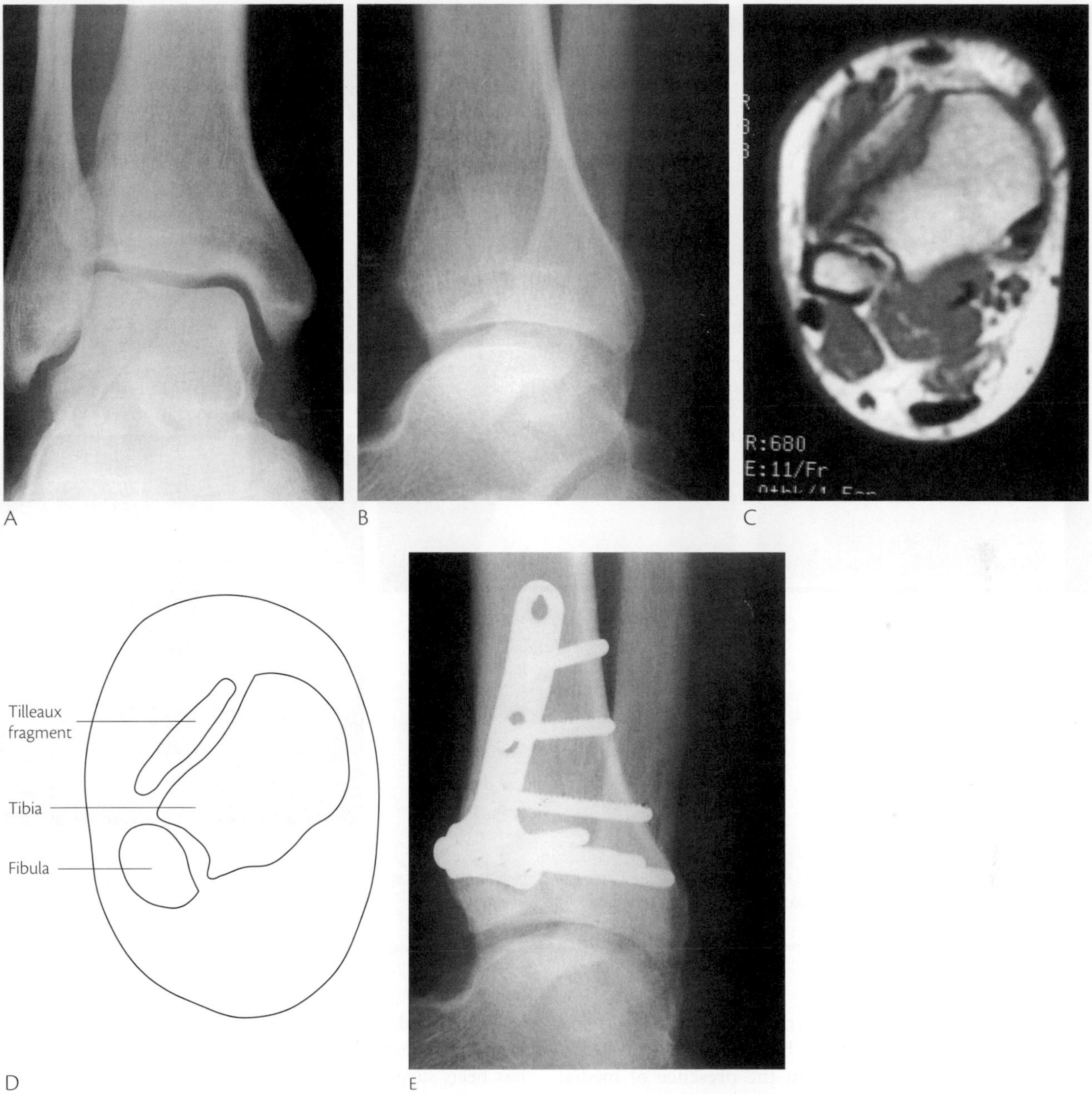

Fig. 12.59.2 A) Anteroposterior and B) lateral radiographs of a man with anterolateral tenderness after a fall. No abnormality was noted. C) An MRI obtained to investigate persisting pain revealed the fracture which is shown schematically on oblique view in (D). E) After operative fixation.

2) Direct observation may show the ankle to be displaced already
3) Stressing the ankle to observe for abnormal movements.

Assessment of the injury pattern is an attractive way of estimating stability as it would allow treatment decisions to be made on basis of fracture classification. Experimental destabilization of the ankle gives some insight into the importance of various components. Posterior malleolar fragments of up to 50% as seen on a lateral view are not necessarily associated with instability. Resection of the lateral malleolus causes greater instability than sectioning of the deltoid ligament. In clinical studies accurate reduction of the lateral malleolus has produced a satisfactory reduction of talus. In an experimental model of supination–external-rotation (type B) fractures, a significant increase in external rotation of the talus at maximum plantar flexion was seen with transection of the deep deltoid fibres. This was corrected incompletely by insertion of an anatomical fibular plate. Pronation–external-rotation (type C) fractures investigated in a similar fashion also noted the importance of an intact deep portion of the deltoid ligament.

These findings beg the question how to assess the integrity of the deep portion of the deltoid ligament. Demonstration of a medial diastasis of 4mm or more confirms rupture of the deltoid ligament.

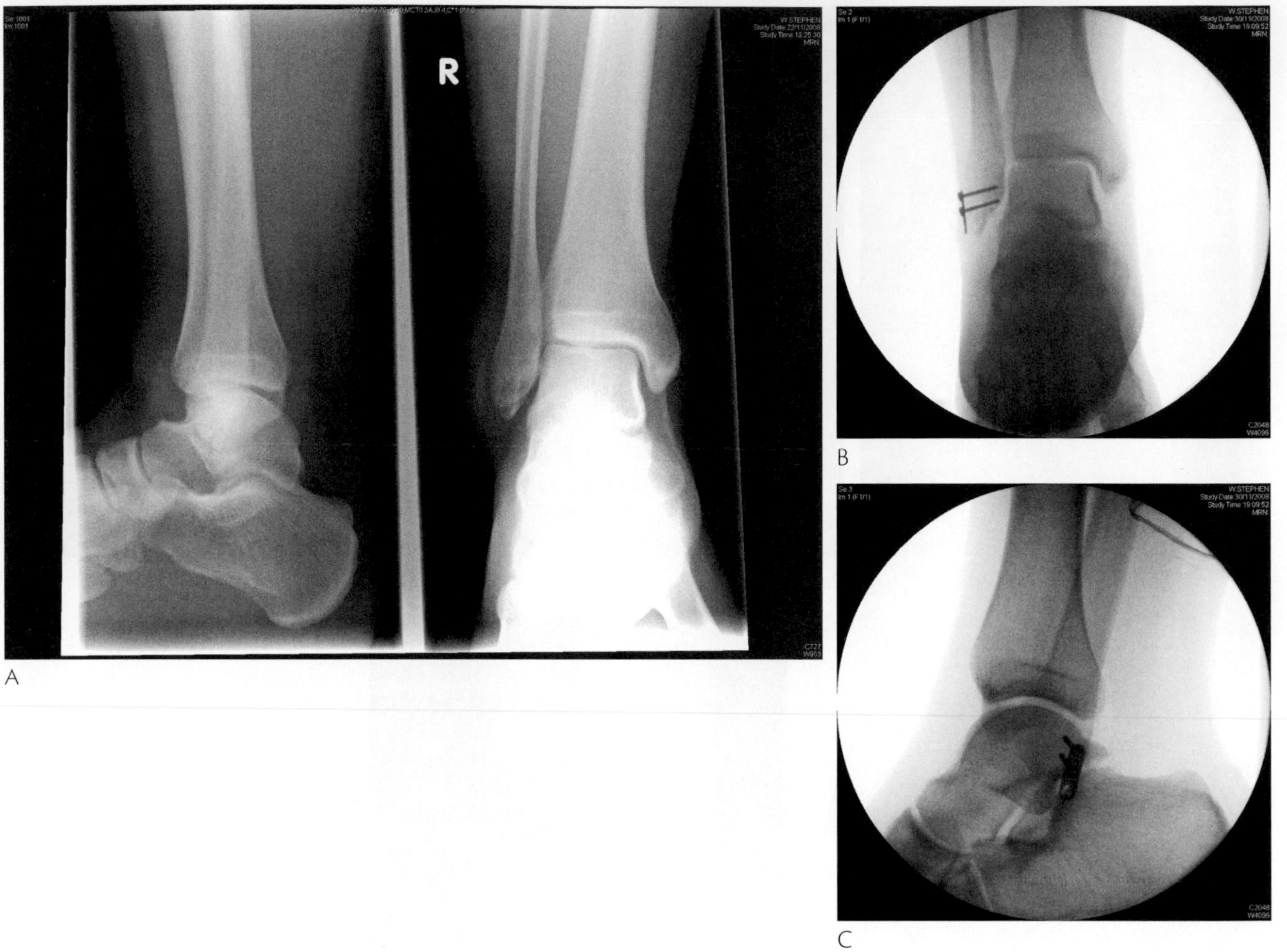

Fig. 12.59.3 A) These X-rays were initially reported as 'avulsion fracture of the lateral malleolus, treat as sprain'. However this represents an avulsion of the peroneal sheath. B) The bony fragment was of sufficient size that it could be fixed.

The finding of localized medial tenderness is less consistent and may suggest deltoid ligament rupture but can be present in the presence of incomplete disruption. In the presence of medial tenderness but no diastasis at rest, there may be an indication for a stress test under anaesthesia. Alternatively the consequences of physiological stresses may be monitored. Serial radiographic observation may be used to ensure bony alignment is maintained during the healing process.

The other aspect of stability which is often discussed relates to injuries of the tibiofibular syndesmosis and the need for placement of a diastasis screw. Not all fibula fractures above the syndesmosis require formal stabilization of the syndesmosis. Bimalleolar lesions where both fractures are fixed do not require a syndesmosis screw. It has been suggested that a syndesmosis screw is unnecessary in a type C fracture when the fibula break is within 3.5cm of the top of the syndesmosis with a medial ligamentous injury and within 15cm if a medial malleolar fragment was fixed. These recommendations are best confirmed by intraoperative assessment of the syndesmosis after the other bony injuries have been fixed. This is best achieved by taking a mortise view whilst the tibia is pushed with a screwdriver and the fibula is pulled with a bone hook (Figure 12.59.5). As most of the instability is in the sagittal plane it has been suggested that the fibula should be pulled in an anteroposterior direction.

Box 12.59.2 Injury classifications

- The Lauge-Hansen system is based on the mechanism of injury
- The Weber–Danis system is easy to remember and understand but is limited in guiding treatment
- The AO/OTA classification is useful for research.

General considerations in the treatment of ankle fractures

Initial treatment

The initial treatment of an ankle fracture is aimed at preventing further injury and keeping the patient comfortable. A grossly

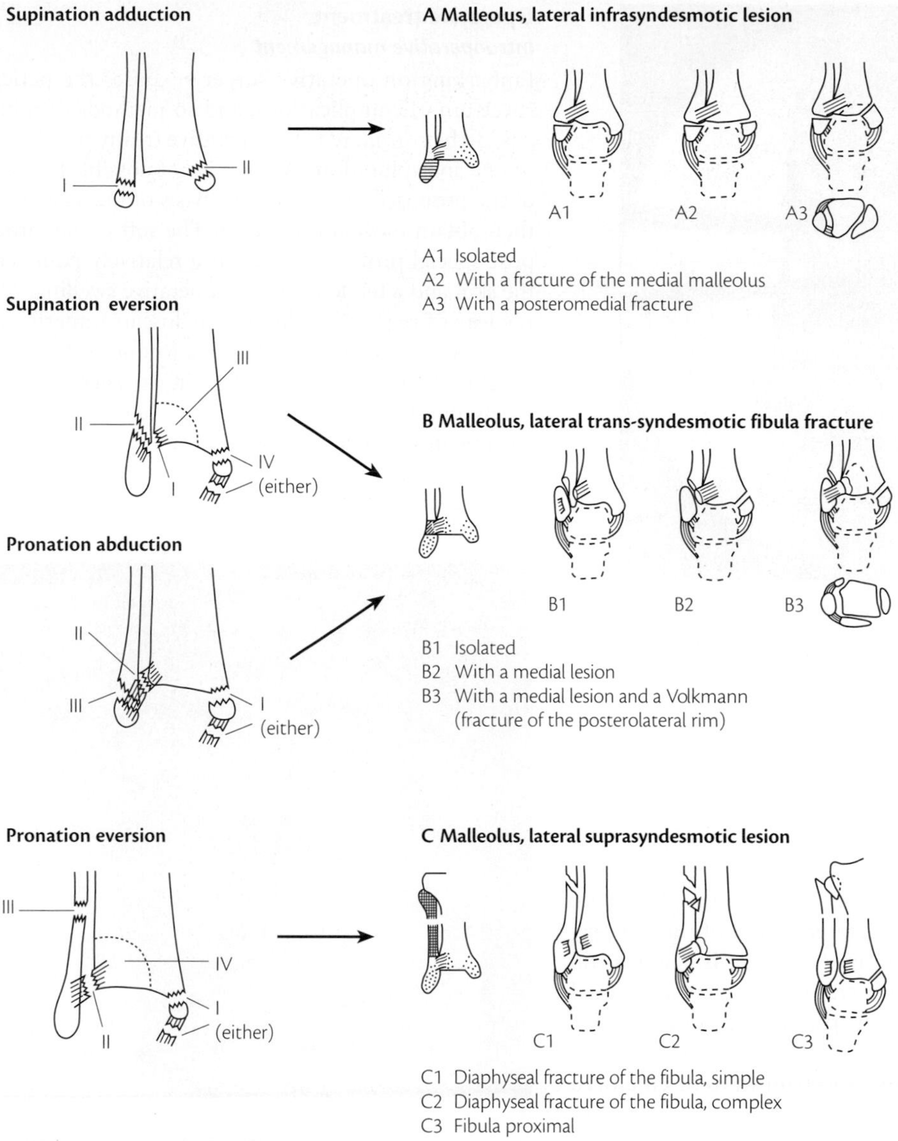

Fig. 12.59.4 Comparison of A) the Lauge-Hansen and B) the AO/OTA systems of ankle fracture classification.

Box 12.59.3 Congruence and stability

- In a type B fracture the talofibular relationship may be normal and any displacement may be of the proximal fragment
- Lateral displacement of the talus, up to 4mm, may not markedly affect peak joint stress
- Stability assessment:
  - Recognition of injury pattern
  - >4mm of static displacement
  - Stress test may displace the talus to an unacceptable position.

displaced fracture may compromise the overlying skin as well as deeper structures; prompt reduction and splintage is indicated. This is a clinical decision, and the procedure is generally carried out under sedation or with Entonox prior to any radiological examination. In these grossly unstable cases radiographs are taken with the splint in place. In other cases higher-quality images are obtained out of the splint.

Definitive treatment

Closed treatment

An injury deemed stable and in a satisfactory position does not require a fixed period of immobilization, multiple follow-up radiographs, or an operation. They may be treated symptomatically.

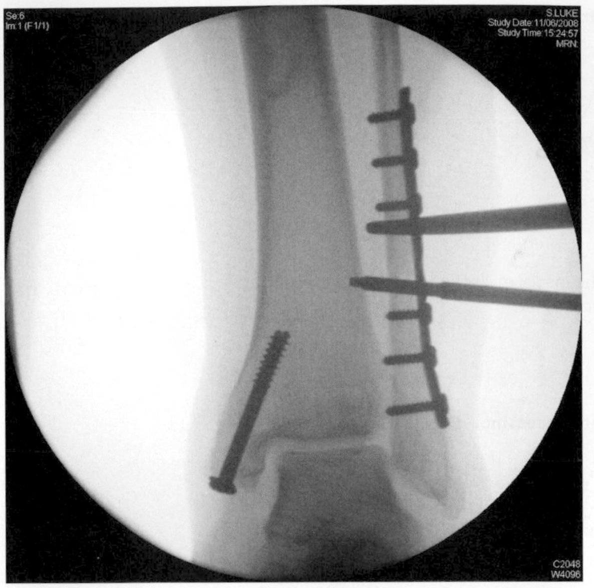

Fig. 12.59.5 Testing stability of a type C fracture intraoperatively using a screwdriver and bone hook.

The function of the injured part and the whole patient is important. Thus an identical physical injury may be treated with a Tubigrip bandage and crutches in one patient, but a mother with small children may require a short period in a cast or splint to allow her hands to be kept free.

Closed treatment of an unstable injury is not the simple option. More judgement is required over a greater period of time. A percentage of cases in which non-operative treatment is planned will at some stage need to be changed to operative management. Closed methods of treatment require the constructive use of the remaining intact soft tissue. Understanding the mechanism of the injury is helpful and allows the reversal of that mechanism to be employed in fracture reduction. Image intensifiers are of great benefit in facilitating reduction and determining how it will be maintained i.e. moulding and the need for an above- or below-knee cast. Managing an unstable fracture in cast requires skill (Figure 12.59.6), and a clear post-manipulative regimen must be prescribed by the surgeon dictating weight bearing and x-rays.

Box 12.59.4 General treatment of ankle fractures

- Reduce fracture–dislocations urgently
- Operate early on fractures which have been dislocated
- Stable fractures require little more than symptomatic treatment
- Control symptoms and maintain function
- Unstable fractures require close supervision.

Operative treatment

Intraoperative management

Embarking on operative surgery exposes the patient to a wider spectrum of complications, and so methods of minimizing these have to be considered. The operative treatment of a fracture should not be an exploration. When it is not possible to make a clear plan of the proposed surgery on the basis of the available information, then obtain more information. The soft tissues around the ankle pose special problems. There is a relatively poor blood supply to the skin and a tendency to postoperative swelling. There is little in the way of redundant skin so any loss or underlying swelling can lead to great difficulty in closing a wound. When a wound cannot be closed, the exposed underlying tissues are very frequently unsuitable for split-skin grafting. Therefore great care must be taken with soft tissue envelope.

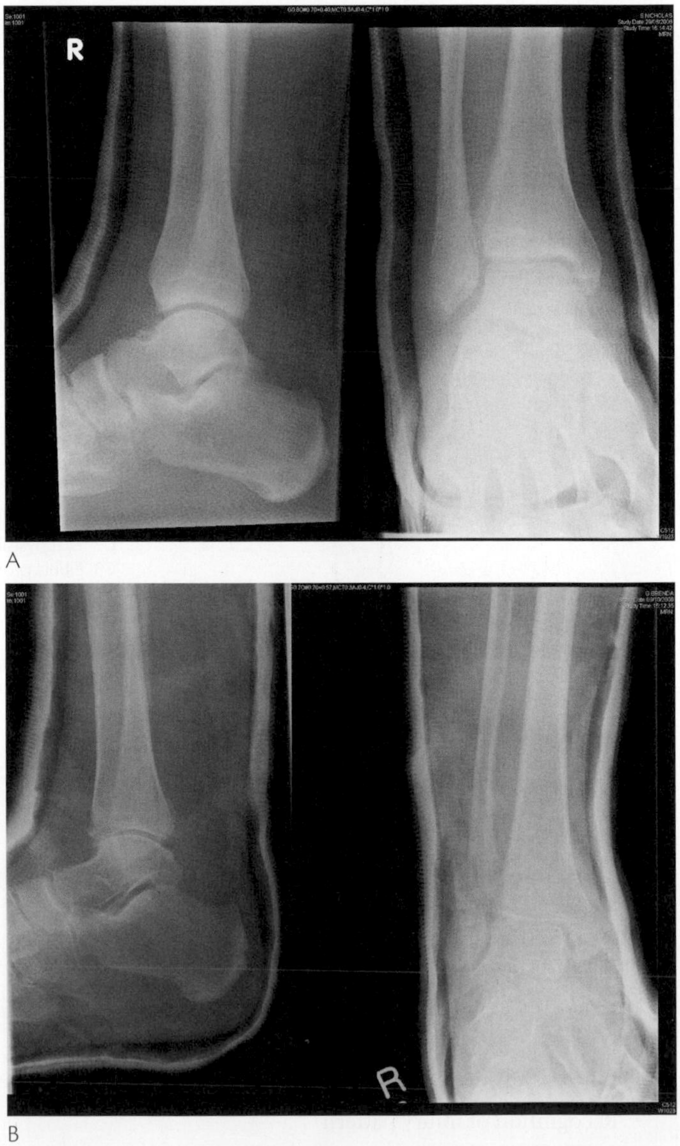

Fig. 12.59.6 A) Cast applied for symptomatic relief. B) Cast applied to control an unstable fracture. Note the difference in the closeness of fit and moulding of the casts.

Box 12.59.5 Considerations in operative treatment of ankle fracture

- Local cutaneous blood supply may be poor and may be compromised further by swelling
- Urgent fixation of fracture–dislocations reduces complications
- Do not use a tourniquet as routine but for a specific purpose
- Check radiographs before closure
- No conclusive evidence to support early mobilization.

The surgeon can control a number of factors which may affect the soft tissue outcome. The first is the timing of surgery. The actual manipulation and fixation of the fracture fragments is easier the sooner after the injury it is attempted. However, there are often pressures to delay surgery. The most common problem is the difficulty or inconvenience of gaining access to an operating room soon enough after the injury without the surgeon clearly designating it as an emergency. When there has been a fracture–dislocation there is good evidence to support emergency treatment. Major complications have been reported in 44% when surgery was delayed greater than 24h in comparison to 5.3% in those operated upon as emergencies.

Many surgeons routinely use a tourniquet when operating on ankle fractures. However, it is not always necessary and the period of tissue hypoxia and venous stasis caused by the use of a tourniquet has been shown to increase the incidence of soft tissue complications. It would seem appropriate to position a tourniquet but only inflate if required.

The patient should be positioned according to the planned procedure to facilitate access and instrumentation. It is recommended that the image intensifier and not the limb is moved to obtain the lateral view; this is particularly important when taking provisional views as the contortions required may displace a hard-won reduction.

The skin and soft tissues should be handled with care. To avoid damaging the skin's blood supply it should not be separated from the deep fascia. Straight incisions are easier to close and have less tension that curved incisions. Self retainers can be damaging and if they are used, do not over-tension them and move them from time to time.

The position of the fracture and the implant should be checked radiographically before closure so that any necessary alterations can be carried out easily.

Postoperative management

Postoperative management will naturally be tailored to the individual injury. In general the hours following operative treatment should be aimed primarily at making the patient comfortable. A backslab and elevation should provide such comfort and prevent the ankle resting in an equinus position.

When early range of motion is considered it is essential that stable fixation has been achieved and this needs to be assessed intraoperatively. As the deltoid ligament has been shown to be a significant component of stability, a lateral fracture associated with a major injury of the deltoid ligament may not be stable when treated with anatomical lateral fixation and may require a period of immobilization. Three quasi-randomized controlled studies have looked into the merits of early mobilization of surgically fixed ankles. All three have shown no difference in clinical scores at 12 weeks compared with immobilized ankles and only one demonstrated an earlier return to work if mobilized early. With regard to complication rates, the studies were too small to show any significant difference but infection rates appeared higher in the early mobilization group. The decision to mobilize early should therefore be made on an individual basis. Factors such as patient compliance, comorbidities that affect healing, occupation and the surgeon's confidence in the resulting construct should all be taken into account.

Fixation of specific bony injuries

Fibula

Type A fractures (Box 12.59.6)

Infrasyndesmotic fibula fractures tend to be transverse in orientation representing a failure in tension of the lateral malleolus. The majority will be suitable for non-operative treatment. When fixation is required it must be stable to tension loading, either using a third tubular plate placed or a tension band wire (Figure 12.59.7). When a wire construct is used, care should be taken to bury the longitudinal K-wires carefully under the lateral ligament. If soft tissues are caught in the crook of these wires, they will loosen, back out, and cause early problems. Furthermore, consideration should be given to the possibility that the wires will have to be removed and twists should be placed where they can be easily found.

Type B fractures (Box 12.59.7)

The most common fracture configuration is a spiral or long oblique with the apex of the distal fragment lying posteriorly. Soft tissue stripping including the periosteum should be kept to a minimum. Only the fracture site needs exposed. Reduction may be obtained directly by using reduction forceps; a small degree of shortening can be corrected by judicious rotation as shown in Figure 12.59.8. Excessive local force may lead to fragmentation and the creation of a more difficult fracture. When it is difficult to obtain length, traction may be applied indirectly via a sharp towel clip embedded in the cancellous bone of the distal fragment. The two common methods of fixation are a lag screw with a lateral plate or a posterolateral antiglide plate (Figure 12.59.9). When the bone is of good quality, either method can be used. The antiglide construct does not rely on screw fixation in the softer bone of the distal fragment. In addition it facilitates indirect reduction by a combination of longitudinal traction and tightening of the plate to the proximal fragment. The metalware is not placed laterally and so is more easily covered and less likely to require removal. The authors strongly favours the antiglide construct when there is any doubt about the bone quality.

Box 12.59.6 Type A fractures

- Usually transverse
- Fixation should use a tension band principle.

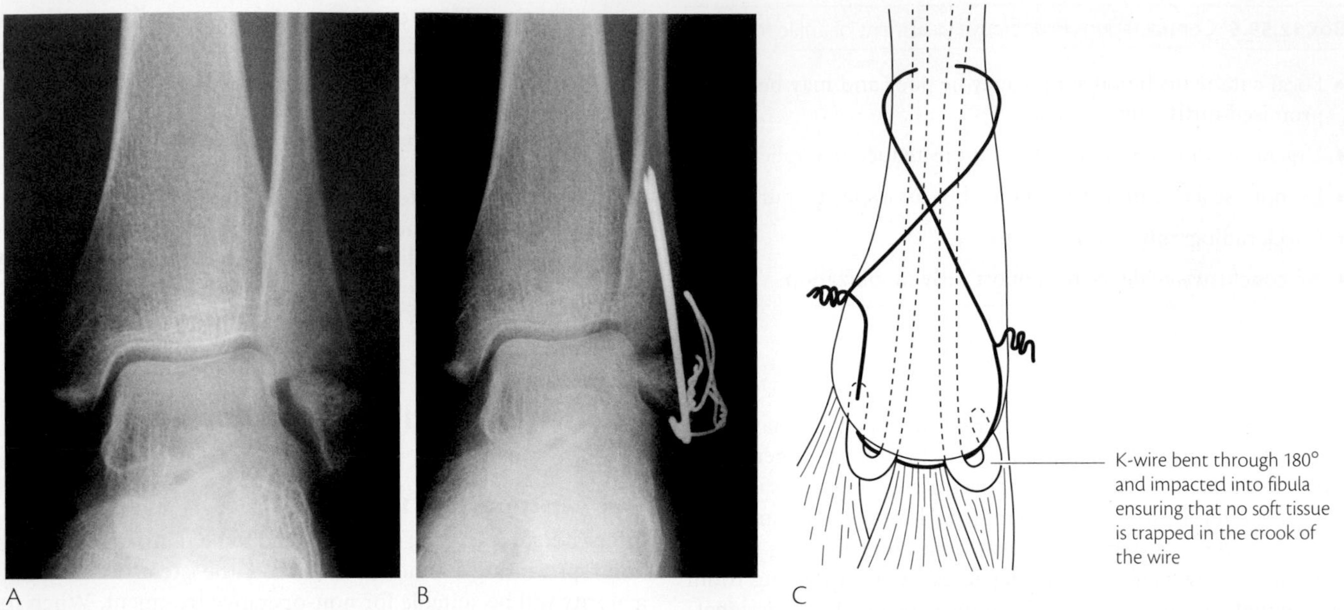

Fig. 12.59.7 A) Type A fracture; B) radiograph showing a tension band wire; C) schematic drawing of the K-wire position.

Type C fractures (Box 12.59.8)

With simple fractures a direct method should achieve an anatomical reduction, which is then often fixed with a lag screw neutralized with a one-third tubular plate. When the fracture is relatively distal the position of the plate should allow any diastasis screw which may be required to pass through the plate or at least not to be obstructed by it.

When there is fragmentation at the fracture site or there is a segmental injury judging reduction is much more difficult. It may help to key in small fragment, so long as this does not involve the sacrifice of soft tissues. When this cannot be done it is quite possible to greatly misjudge the adequacy of reduction, particularly the rotation of the fragments. Figure 12.59.10 shows the malrotation of a fixed fibula as seen on a postoperative CT scan. This problem is seen when a straight plate is used as it does not take into account the normal spiral arrangement of the fibulas lateral surface. The image intensifier can be used to compare the length and contour of the fibula with the uninjured leg. It may be necessary to expose the inferior tibiofibular joint to see whether the fibula is sitting in the incisura and, if not, whether it is blocked by debris in the joint or proximal malreduction. Even when it can be assessed, achieving a reduction may be awkward.

Where there is fragmentation it is preferable to bridge the damaged area, avoiding the temptation to fix the fragments. This requires the use of a plate stronger than the one-third tubular and a 3.5 mm reconstruction plate is usually sufficient. A precontoured plate can be used as a push plate. It is applied to one fragment and length is then obtained by using a small laminar spreader between the other end of the plate and a separate screw (Figure 12.59.11).

Box 12.59.7 Type B fractures

- Usually spiral with distal spike posteriorly
- Reduce with care and do not complicate the task by further fragmentation
- Consider bone quality when deciding on fixation technique: when poor bone quality use antiglide principle

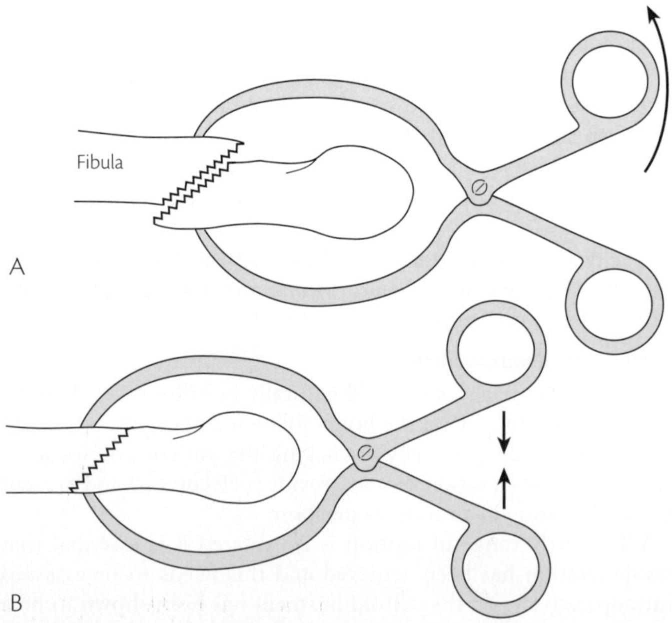

Fig. 12.59.8 Use of pointed reduction forceps to obtain a direct reduction of an oblique shortened fibula fracture. This direct technique is only suitable in good-quality bone as fracture propagation is a risk.

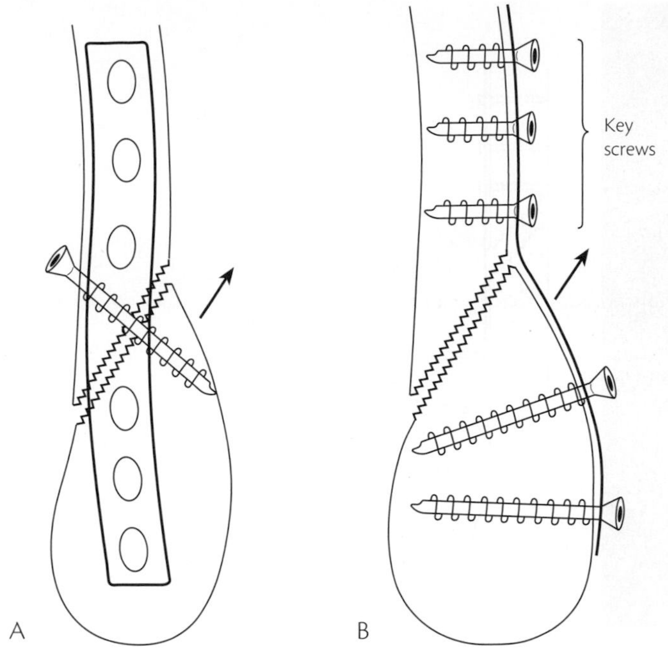

Fig. 12.59.9 Two methods of fixation of a type B malleolar fracture: A) lag screw and neutralization plate; B) antiglide plate. The direction in which the distal fragment will displace is shown by the arrows. The antiglide plate relies on the 'key' screws which are in the better cortical bone. The hold in the softer cancellous bone is not needed to maintain reduction. This is the preferred technique in poor-quality bone.

Box 12.59.8 Type C fractures

- Be prepared to use indirect reduction methods
- Simple fracture patterns—direct anatomical reduction
- Fragmented fracture patterns—consider indirect reduction and bridging the fragments.

Medial malleolar fractures (Box 12.59.9)

Medial malleolar fractures in combination with a diastasis or with fibular or posterior malleolar fractures require fixation owing to the unstable nature of the injury. However, controversy remains over the treatment of isolated medial 'unimalleolar' fractures. It has long been felt that non-operative treatment of displaced medial malleolar fractures may lead to painful non-union or osteoarthritis. However, a more recent study demonstrated a 96% union rate, and no post-traumatic arthritis at 3 years, in 57 cases treated non-operatively regardless of the degree of displacement

If operative treatment is decided, reduction of the medial malleolar fragment is usually under direct vision, and the fixation is most often placed from distal to proximal. This needs to be recalled when placing the incision, which frequently has a redundant proximal portion and needs distal extension.

During reduction there is a risk of fragmentation and it is safer to manipulate the fragment with a sharp instrument such as a dental pick. When cleaning the fracture site of soft bone avoid removing bone with instruments such as curettes and picks. Temporary reduction can be achieved with K-wires or a clamp. Drilling a location hole in the proximal fragment will help with clamp application.

Medial malleolar fractures have been classified by Herscovici and the method of fixation will depend on the fracture pattern (Figure 12.59.12). Type A is an avulsion of the tip of the anterior colliculus, thus leaving the deep deltoid ligament intact. Fixation of these would therefore not offer any benefit to stability. Types B and C are transverse fractures of the malleolus at the mid-portion and at the level of the plafond, respectively. These have usually failed in tension. Type D fractures are vertically orientated above the plafond.

The most common pattern is type C, where the bone has failed in tension. These together with type B fractures are often fixed with two partially threaded screws. The length of the screw required is determined by the length of shank needed to ensure that the threads

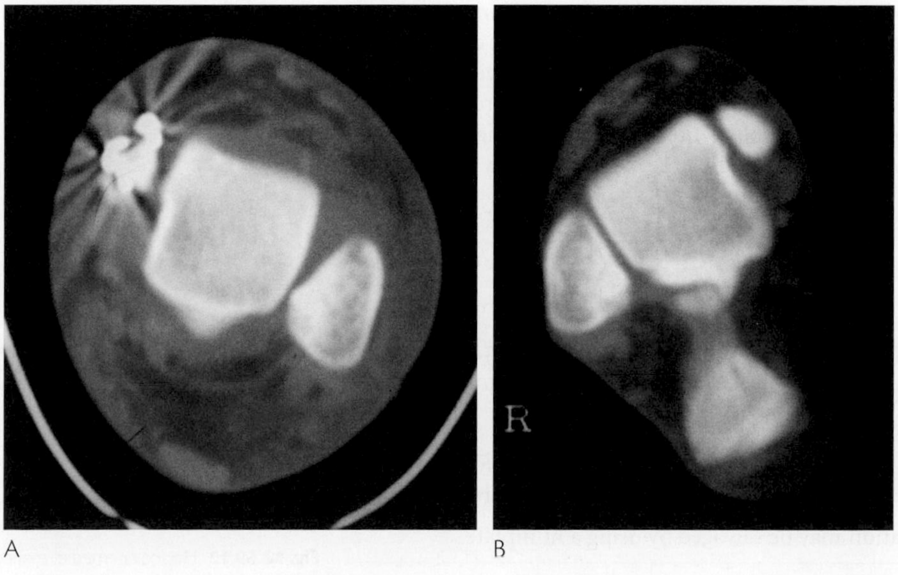

Fig. 12.59.10 A) Single-cut CT scans through the ankle after fixation of a type C fracture. The metalware in the medial malleolus is evident on the injured side. B) The malrotation of the poorly fixed fibula is clear when compared with the normal side.

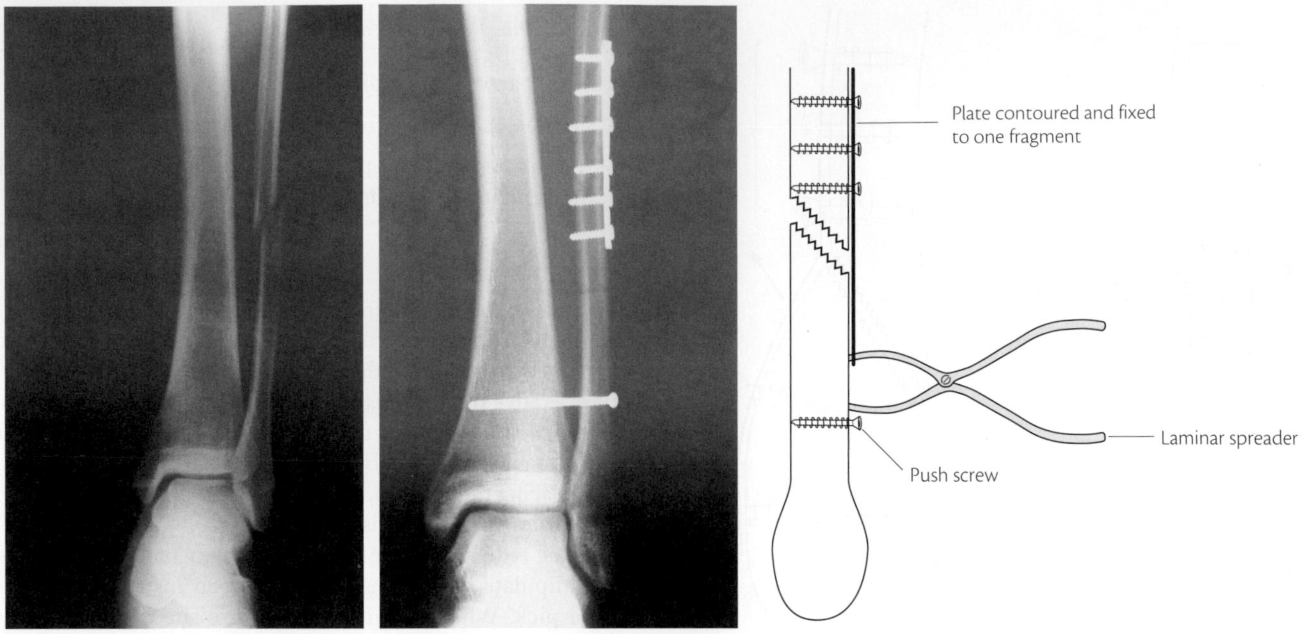

A B C

Fig. 12.59.11 A) A Weber type C fracture in an athlete in which length was difficult to achieve. B) On the postreduction film the hole distal to the plate is for the push screw. This indirect reduction method allows length to be regained without aggressive manipulation at the fracture site. C) Diagram showing the use of the push screw.

are passed fully across the fracture line. Unnecessarily long screws will result in the threads being in poorer-quality bone. Careful consideration should be made when placing the screws in order to avoid abutment of the posterior tibialis tendon.

Biomechanical tests demonstrated a fourfold increase in stiffness with tension band wiring compared to two cancellous screws. If a tension band is used, great care should be taken in burying the wires. Again, it is important to bury the K-wire ends into the deltoid ligament.

When the fracture is oblique (Type D), it is assumed that the failure was in compression. This compressive load may lead to impaction of the medial side of the tibial plafond thus obstructing any attempts at reducing the malleolus. A preoperative CT scan can thus prove very valuable if there is any suspicion of such an injury. If there is compression, the joint surface can be elevated and bone grafted. The malleolus itself may be fixed with partially threaded screws placed perpendicular to the fracture line. With larger fragments this is supplemented by using an antiglide plate at the apex of the fracture. Extending the plate all the way to the tip of the malleolus is not necessary.

Box 12.59.9 Medial malleolar fractures

- Gentle manipulation of the fragment to avoid fragmentation
- Lavage fracture site
- Beware of impaction of the medial edge of the plafond particularly when associated with a type A fibular fracture
- Fragmentation may be salvaged by using a miniplate.

When there is fragmentation of the medial malleolus, fixation with screws alone is not usually possible. A useful manoeuvre is to contour a mini fragment quarter tubular plate around the malleolus and pass the partially threaded 4.0-mm screws though it (Figure 12.59.13). The plate acts as a washer or artificial cortex binding the fragments together. Tension band wires are a useful alternative in these situations.

Posterior malleolar fragment (Box 12.59.10)

As discussed earlier, it often unnecessary to fix a posterior malleolar fracture. When fixation is required the first step is to have a mental image of where the fragment that needs fixing is located. It is usually posterolateral. Screws fixing the fragment need to run perpendicular to the fracture plane. The fixation may be placed from the front or the back. There are advantages to operating with

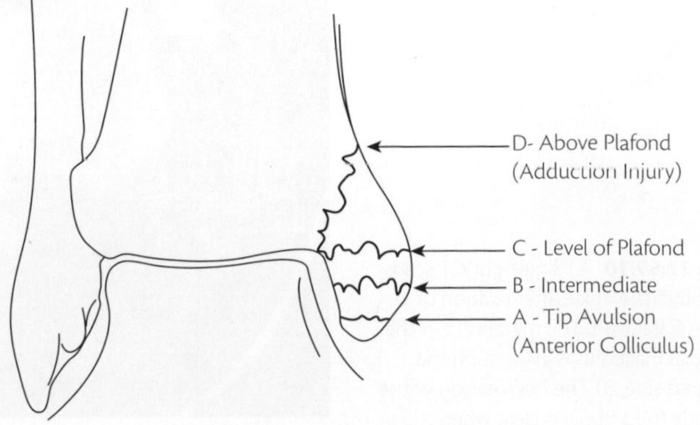

Fig. 12.59.12 Herscovici medial malleolar classification system.

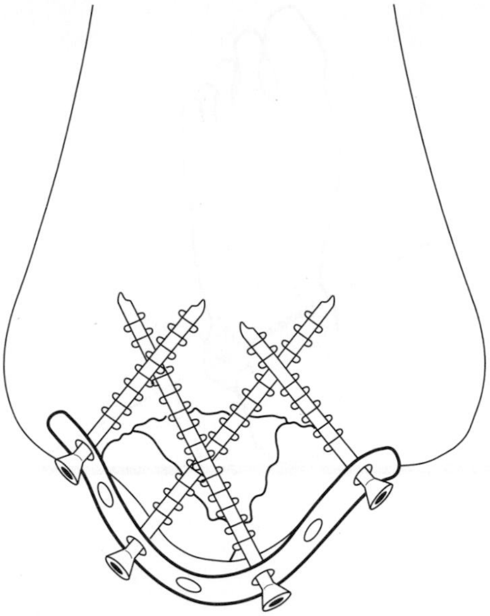

Fig. 12.59.13 Diagrammatic view of the medial malleolus from the medial aspect showing the use of a quarter tubular plate from the AO minifragment set.

the patient prone. Direct visualization of the fragment should allow a good reduction. When using a screw to fix a small to a large fragment, it is technically easier to pass through the smaller into the larger fragment. If compression screw fixation alone is inadequate it can be supplemented with an antiglide plate.

When the screw is placed from the front it is important that the threads only engage the posterior fragment to ensure both maximum hold and compression. In order to drill the two 3.5-mm gliding holes to the correct depth it is recommended to perform this step before reducing the fracture.

Diastasis fixation (Box 12.59.11)

A great deal has been written about the use of diastasis screws. Their indications have been discussed earlier.

Once again the treatment of an injured diastasis has two components: reduction and fixation. The objective is to hold the distal fibula in its correct position relative to the tibia, with the mortise neither too wide nor too narrow. The author uses a pelvic reduction clamp across the fibula to the medial aspect of the tibia applied at the level of the syndesmosis. The joint is viewed on an image intensifier. When compression is applied, the fibula should reduce into the incisura. If this does not happen the block to reduction should be sought, if necessary by opening the joint. If it looks 'odd' in some way, compare it with the normal side on image. Once reduction has been obtained, the foot is dorsiflexed during drilling and tapping as the talus is wider anteriorly. This is the conventional teaching to prevent overtightening of the syndesmosis. One study has suggested the position of the ankle during screw tightening does not affect maximal dorsiflexion. It is important to note that the study was performed on cadaveric models and so only passive and not active motion was evaluated.

If a screw is to be used, it should also be placed 1 cm proximal to the syndesmosis (4cm proximal to and parallel to the horizontal joint line). Placement distal to this may interfere with the interosseous ligament causing painful calcification. Too proximal placement can result in the lateral malleolus toeing outwards. The screw also needs to be angled anteriorly 25-30 degrees in order to obtain a good purchase of both fibular cortices and the tibia (Figure 12.59.14).

The diastasis stabilization has been an area of considerable debate. No biomechanical advantage has been demonstrated with 4.5 mm screws over 3.5mm screws and three cortex fixation has been shown to be as good as four. Many surgeons now feel that the need for planned screw removal is unnecessary as it rarely poses a clinical problem. The use of bio-absorbable screws also obviates the need for elective screw removal and some small studies have demonstrated no difference in terms of biomechanical and clinical outcomes. Another alternative is the use of a suture-button system passed through a 3.5mm drill hole placed 1.5cm proximal to and parallel to the horizontal joint line from fibula to tibia (Figure 12.59.15). Although biomechanical cadaveric studies have demonstrated inferior suture button strengths compared to tricortical screw pull-out strengths, some short-term clinical results have been promising.

Where possible the author places a diastasis screw through the fibula plate. When its placement is not associated with the operative fixation of a fibula fracture, for example, in a high fibular fracture (Masonneuve), it is sensible to place two screws for more adequate control of the fibula.

Box 12.59.10 Posterior malleolar fragment

- Consider whether it is necessary to fix the fragment
- If fixation is likely to be difficult, place the patient in the prone position
- If screws are placed from the front, be careful that the length is correct and threads are not across the fracture line.

Box 12.59.11 Diastasis screw

- Ensure that reduction is adequate
- Use one screw if the fibula is fixed
- Use two screws if the fibula is not fixed.

Outcome of ankle fractures (Box 12.59.12)

Some ankle fractures probably require nothing but symptomatic treatment. Lateral malleolar fractures with no medial injury (Type B, Lauge-Hansen SE stage II) managed by support in a cast without reduction demonstrate good long-term results. These injuries have also been successfully managed in just functional splints. Regardless of treatment, it is clear that anatomical reduction of the fibula fracture, in these injuries, is not required for good results.

What displacement is of clinical importance? A variety of radiographic markers have been said to be of importance in predicting outcome. Abnormal medial clear space, the presence of a large (>20%) posterior malleolar fracture, and an abnormal talocrural

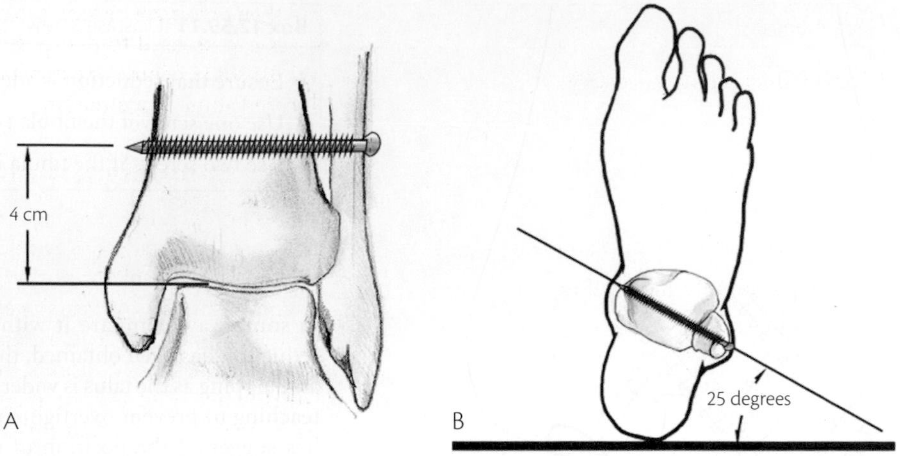

Fig. 12.59.14 Diastasis screw placement. A) Screw should be 1 cm proximal to the syndesmosis and 4 cm proximal to and parallel to the horizontal joint line. B) Screw should be angled anteriorly 25–30°.

angle have been reported as the most predictive of a poor outcome. Many studies comment that in effect better results are associated with the fractures which heal in a good position. Thus, with the exception of the isolated lateral malleolar fracture, it would seem that a key aim of treatment should be a good reduction.

How to achieve and maintain the adequate reduction of a displaced fracture is more debatable. When closed methods clearly fail to achieve a reduction, the need for an open procedure is agreed. However, assessing the adequacy of a closed reduction may not be easy, requiring judgment and good images. There are few prospective randomized studies to guide us in this field. There is some research to support both operative and non-operative treatment. The impact of age is becoming increasingly important. Data from the National Health Service in the United Kingdom (2005-6) show that 25% of ankle fractures occur in adults over 60. It has been noted that there is a high incidence of early complication in operated fractures of women over the age of 55 years. The problems are, mainly, twofold. Firstly, the fractures tend to occur in poor bone quality, often with large degrees of fragmentation, leaving the final bone-implant construct up to 10 times less effective than in younger patients. Secondly, this population often have comorbidities such as late onset diabetes, oedema from congestive cardiac failure, chronic venous insufficiency, and peripheral vascular disease that render the soft tissues less tolerant to wounds. Figure 12.59.16 illustrates the nature of the dilemma which may occur. Thus, if operative fixation is chosen, the mechanical construct should be considered even more carefully than usual. If the resulting construct is likely to be so fragile that the ankle requires protection from motion as well as weight bearing, the benefits of fixation allowing early ankle motion no longer apply. Indeed, the insult to the soft tissues may be the greater evil compared to a poorer functioning ankle joint.

The failed ankle fracture

Periodically a surgeon is confronted with a 'failed' ankle fracture. This may be the result of poor initial treatment, poor bone stock, infection, or comorbidities. A theme of all the treatments discussed

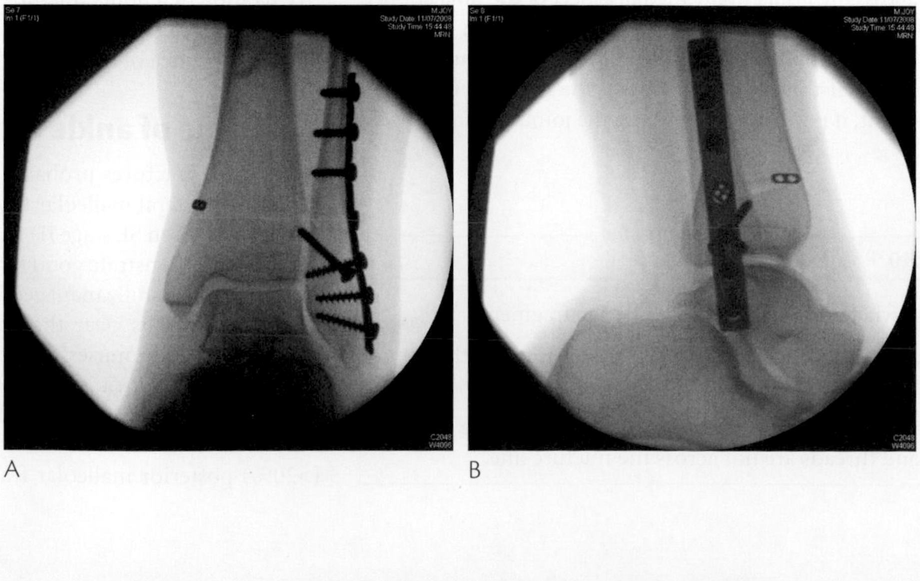

Fig. 12.59.15 A) and B) Syndesmotic stabilisation with suture button.

Box 12.59.12 Outcomes

- Anatomical fibula reduction not necessary
- Poor outcome if:
  - Large medial space
  - Large posterior malleolar fracture
- Best outcomes with reduced ankle displacement
- No definitive advantage to internal fixation
- Elderly females have less satisfactory results.

earlier in this chapter is that most ankle fractures, when reduced, require little force to hold them in place. Thus stabilization can generally be achieved with casting or metalware with a relatively low strength. When the fracture has demonstrated a tendency to fail then holding it becomes much more difficult. Three illustrative cases can be used to demonstrate this, see Figures 12.59.17–19). Whilst some failures are inevitable the clear message is to strive to succeed at the first attempt.

Treatment algorithm

The algorithm shown in Figure 12.59.20 summarizes the authors' treatment preferences. The major concern is to establish whether the fracture is stable or not. When the fracture is unstable, in the younger patient (<60 years) we prefer to offer operative fixation as we believe that this gives a greater chance of achieving and maintaining a satisfactory position. In the over sixties it remains unclear whether operative fixation is advantageous. The position at union seems to be the best predictor of a good result. The cost of achieving this improved position is the possibility of operative complications. Thus every effort must be made to minimize the risks. This involves the timing of the surgery, care of soft tissues, avoidance of tourniquets, and accommodation in the technique for poor-quality bone.

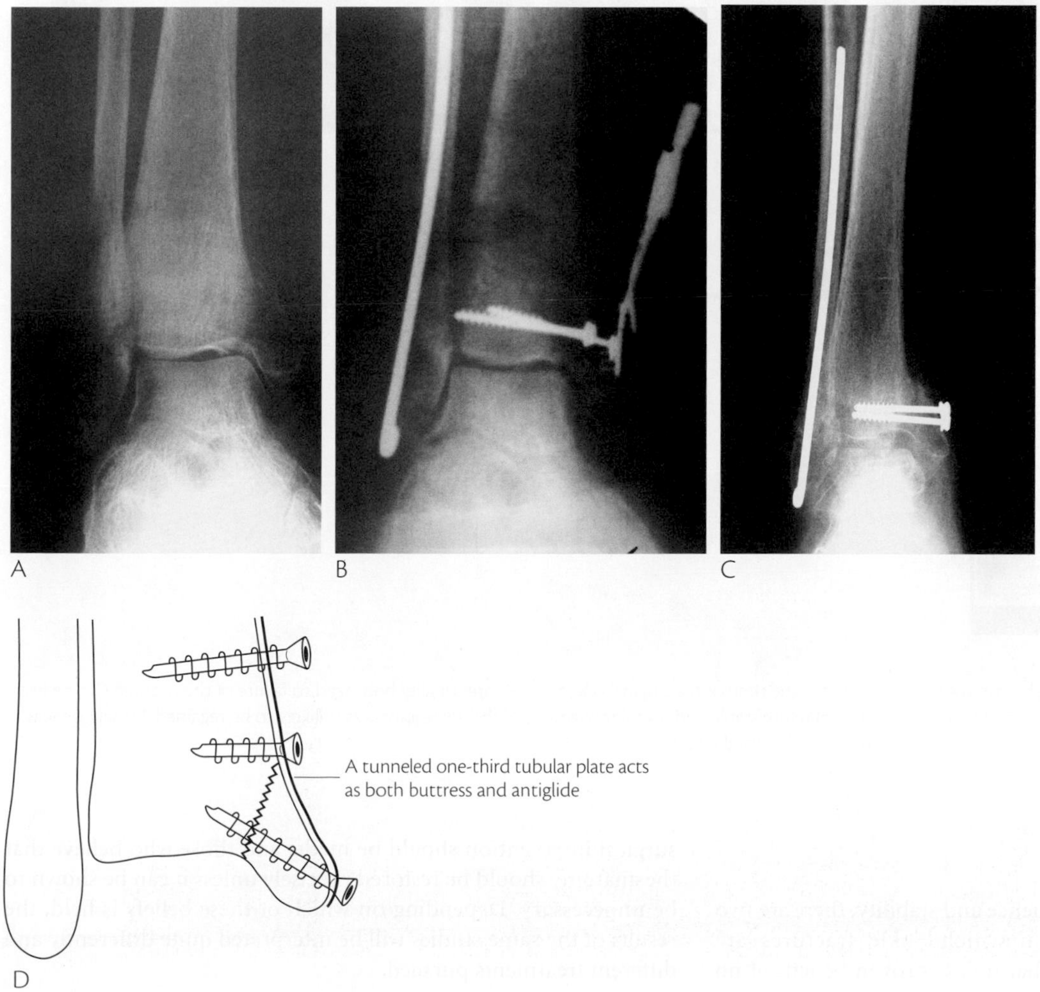
A
B
C
A tunneled one-third tubular plate acts as both buttress and antiglide
D

Fig. 12.59.16 Poor decision-making in an A-type fracture in osteoporotic bone. Because of problems with the skin, a minimally invasive approach was adopted. The construct asked too much of the screws on the medial side. A) Type A fracture in osteoporotic bone with medial impaction. B) Intraoperative view of fixation. C) Failure of the fixation. D) Thus if surgery was required for protection of the skin, the surgeon could have chosen a small plate as a buttress, rebated it to avoid prominence, and augmented with bone graft. Alternative option for the medial side; the other option is a cast.

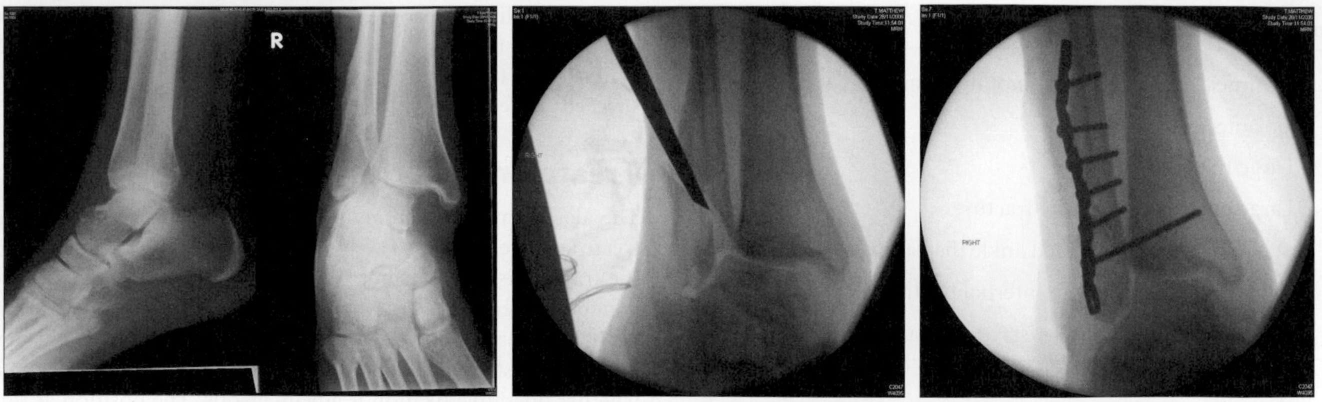

A B C

Fig. 12.59.17 A) Young adult with malunion evident at delayed presentation. B) The fracture was mobilized and the high-quality bone was harnessed using long screws, C), that were sufficient force to allow ankle joint mobilization.

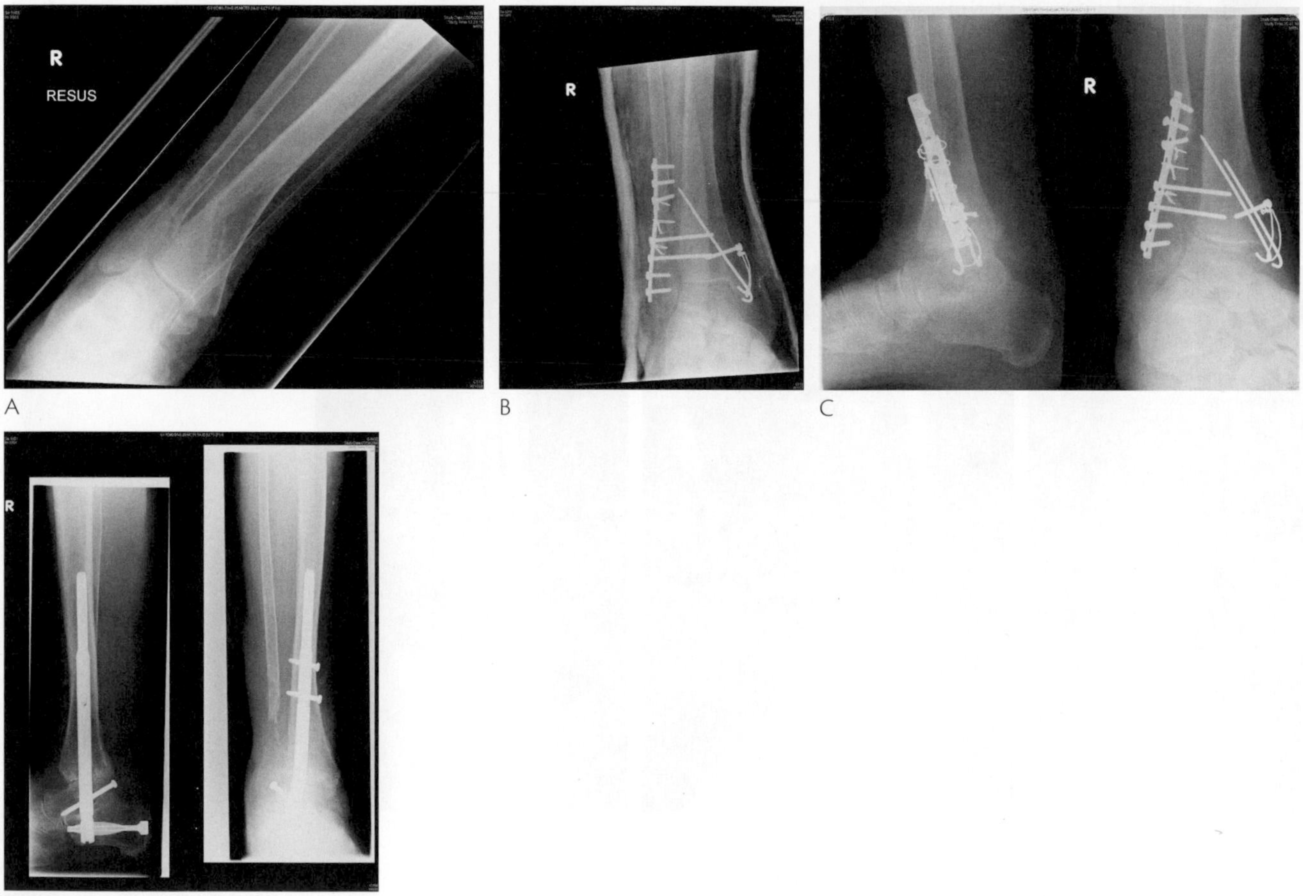

A B C D

Fig. 12.59.18 A) and B) Elderly patient with unstable fracture noted at the time of the original operation. Poorer quality bone lead to failure of the fixation. C) The loss of reduction had damaged the lateral side of the tibial plafond and therefore stable and useful movement of the ankle joint was unlikely to be regained. D) Salvage was obtained using a retrograde intramedullary nail arthrodesing the ankle and subtalar joint.

Summary

Despite all the discussion of congruence and stability, there are two basic surgical backgrounds from which ankle fractures are approached—those who believe that unless proven beneficial no surgical intervention should be made, and those who believe that the anatomy should be restored precisely unless it can be shown to be unnecessary. Depending on which of these beliefs is held, the results of the same studies will be interpreted quite differently and different treatments pursued.

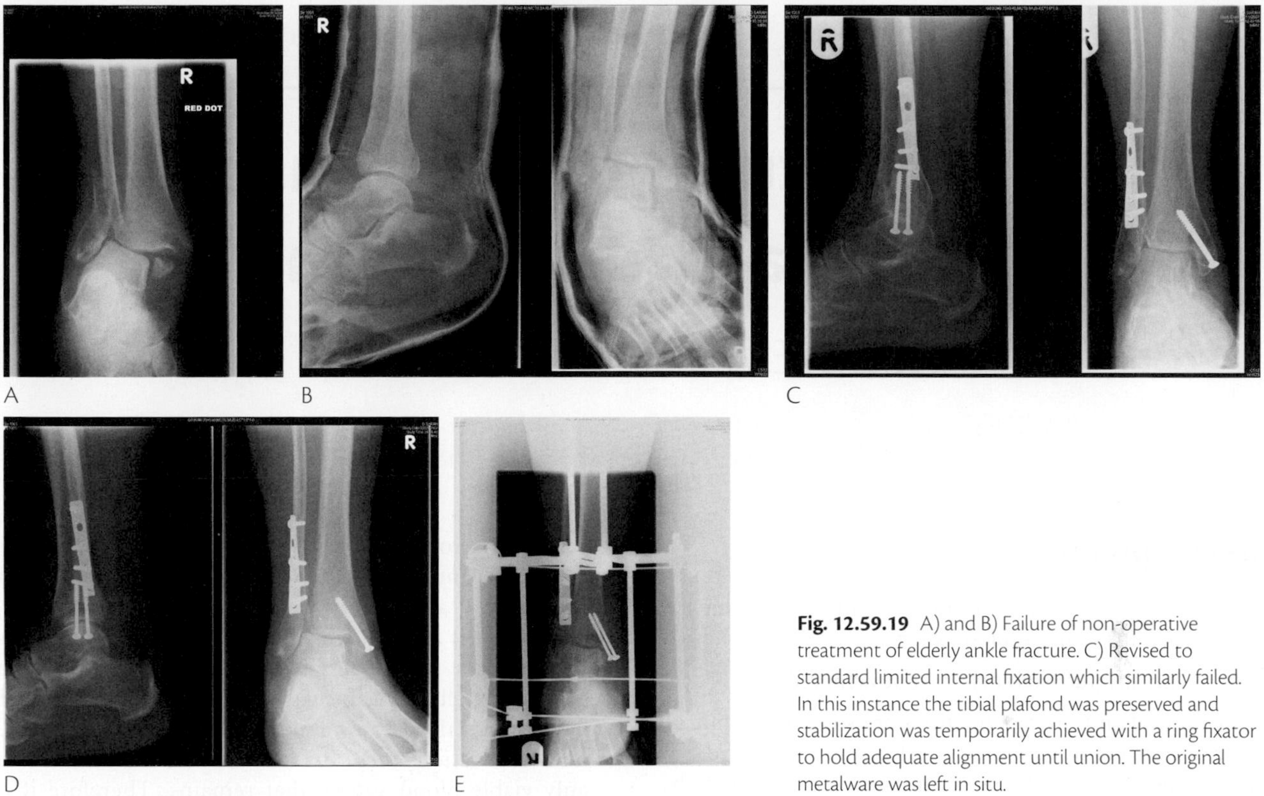

Fig. 12.59.19 A) and B) Failure of non-operative treatment of elderly ankle fracture. C) Revised to standard limited internal fixation which similarly failed. In this instance the tibial plafond was preserved and stabilization was temporarily achieved with a ring fixator to hold adequate alignment until union. The original metalware was left in situ.

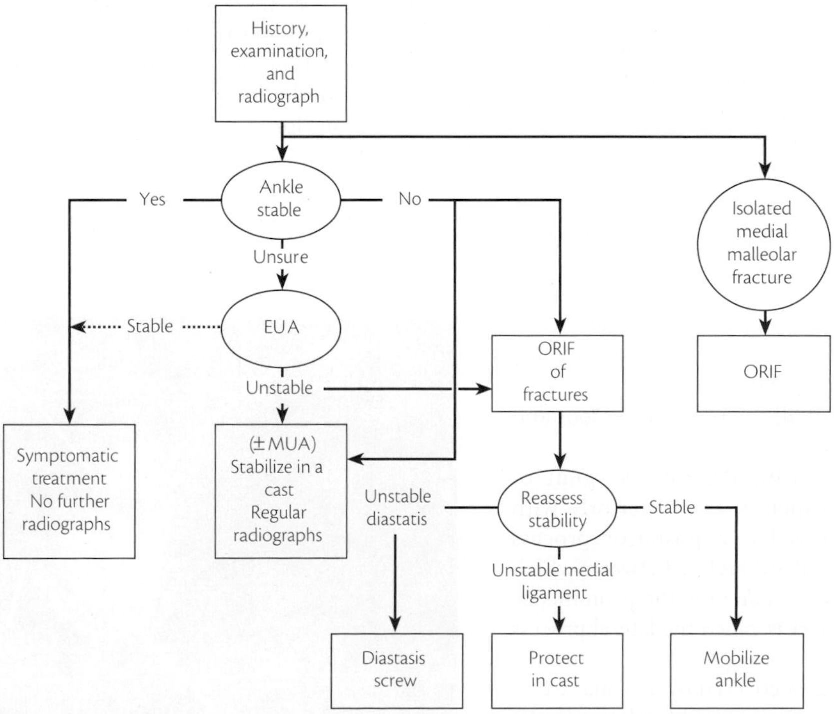

Fig. 12.59.20 Management of ankle fractures.

Further reading

Buckley, R. and Leung, F. (2006). Ankle fractures: early vs delayed motion following internal fixation. *Orthopaedic Trauma Directions*, **4**(4).

Charnley, J. (1999). *The Closed Treatment of Common Fractures.* Cambridge: Colt Books Ltd.

Moore, J.A. Jr., Shank, J.R., Morgan, S.J., and Smith, W.R. (2006). Syndesmosis fixation: a comparison of three and four cortices of screw fixation without hardware removal. *Foot & Ankle International*, **27**(8), 567–72.

Vioreanu, M., Brophy, S., and Dudeney, S. (2007). Displaced ankle fractures in the geriatric population: operative or non-operative treatment. *Foot & Ankle Surgery*, **13**(1), 10–14.

12.60

Fractures of the talus and peritalar dislocations

Stuart J.E. Matthews

Summary points

- Talar fractures are uncommon injuries and the outcome is very dependent on the tenuous blood supply
- Fixation with absolute stability must be achieved
- Osteochondral and process fractures are sometimes difficult to appreciate on plain x-rays. Clinical examination and a high degree of suspicion will help to identify these problems early.

Introduction

The talus is also known as the astragalus (see aviator's astragalus, discussed later). The ancient Grecian game of knuckle bones uses five taluses in which one is thrown up and the others are swept up in the hand in different combinations and the thrown talus is then caught before it hits the ground, in the same hand. Talus is the Latin name for the Greek Talos, the bronze giant portrayed in *Jason and the Argonauts* who was defeated by opening the porthole in his ankle and letting the liquor flow out.

The talus is a remarkable bone. Think of its small size in the context of its function. It has to transmit forces of 4g at heel strike at ordinary walking pace. Consider the forces it transmits when running and jumping. It is surprising that fractures are therefore rare accounting for between 3.4% of all fractures of the foot and only 0.32% of all fractures.

The talus articulates superiorly with the mortise joint of the ankle, inferiorly with the calcaneum, and anteriorly with the navicular. Posteriorly the talus has a posterior process comprised of the medial and lateral tubercles, between which runs the flexor hallucis longus tendon. Laterally the prominence of the lateral part of the posterior facet is called the lateral process (Figures 12.60.1–3.)

The talus has 60% of its surface area covered by articular cartilage and has limited soft tissue attachments and blood supply. An appreciation of the tenuous blood supply is important in understanding the disruption that occurs both at the time of injury and during surgical intervention (Figure 12.60.4). The head and neck of the talus are supplied by periosteal branches from the dorsalis pedis and peroneal arteries. Two-thirds of the body is supplied by the tarsal sinus and tarsal canal arteries. Laterally, the tarsal sinus artery arises from the perforating peroneal artery and dorsalis pedis artery. Medially, the tarsal canal artery arises from the posterior tibial artery within the deltoid below the medial malleolus. Deltoid (ligament) and posterior tubercle branches from the posterior tibial artery also supply the body of the talus. In fracture/subluxations these branches within the deltoid may be the only viable blood supply that remains. Therefore if a medial approach needs to be extended, a medial malleolar osteotomy should be used.

In 60% of cases there is a complete intraosseous anastomosis between all regions of the talus.

As a result of its unique anatomy, fractures of the talus have great potential for morbidity.

Investigations for talar and peritalar injuries are documented in Box 12.60.1.

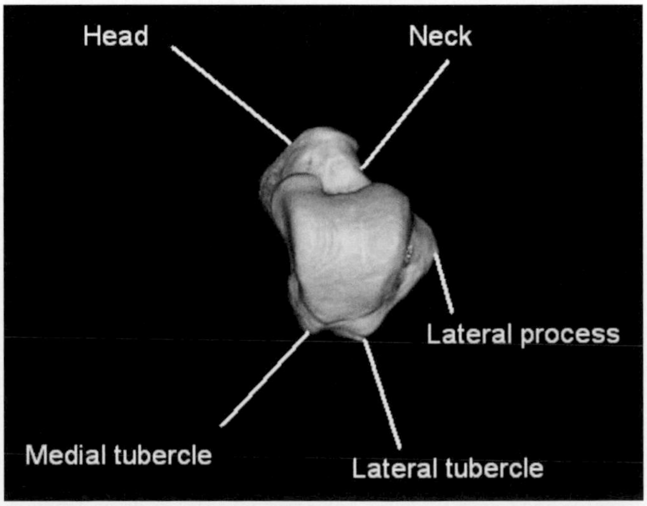

Fig. 12.60.1 Superior aspect of right talus.

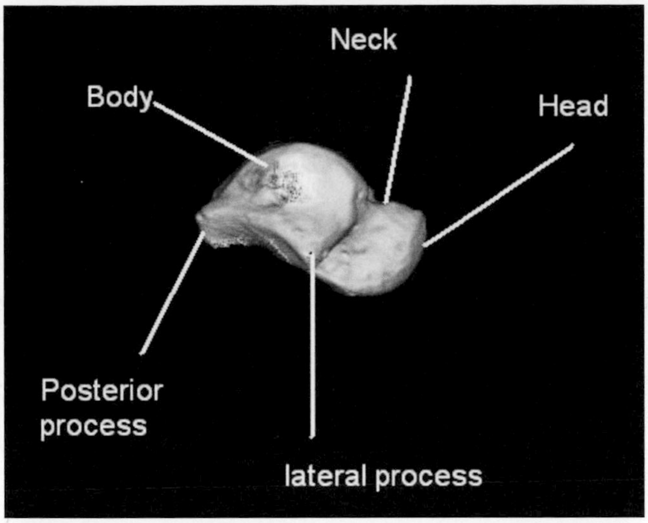

Fig. 12.60.2 Lateral aspect right talus.

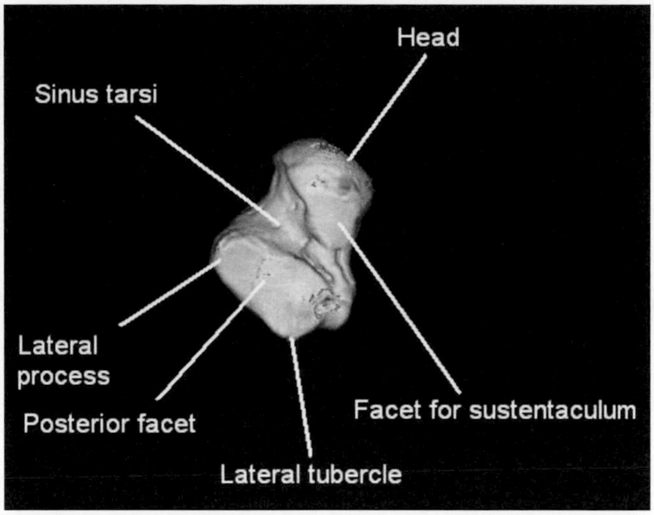

Fig. 12.60.3 Inferior aspect right talus.

Fractures of the talar neck are well described; however, the talus is prone to a number of other less well recognized fractures (Box 12.60.2).

Talar neck fractures

Aviator's astragalus (an anachronistic name for the talus) was a term used to describe talar neck fractures sustained by military glider pilots in crash landings. The Crawford-Adams arthrodesis, which he called the RAF arthrodesis, was developed as a consequence. It was postulated that hyperdorsiflexion of the ankle with impaction of the neck into the anterior lip of the tibia was a likely mechanism. Cadaveric work has demonstrated the role of focal loading of the talar neck and pre-impact bracing in the generation of these fractures.

Half of talar fractures appear in the neck and are basicervical. They usually have an oblique orientation and can be associated with disruption of the subtalar, tibiotalar, and talonavicular joints. Talar neck fractures are commonly described using the Hawkins classification (Table 12.60.1 and Figure 12.60.6). Not only does displacement increase the risk of avascular necrosis (AVN) but malunion will affect hindfoot function due to the complex relationship between subtalar, talonavicular, and calcaneocuboid function. Surgical reduction should be anatomical as malunion is associated with uniformly poor results.

Hawkins type I fractures are undisplaced (confirmed with computed tomography, CT) and can be treated non-operatively in a below-knee non-weight-bearing cast for 6 weeks. Fifty per cent of these injuries are not visible on presenting radiographs so the clinician must have a high level of suspicion. Full weight bearing is

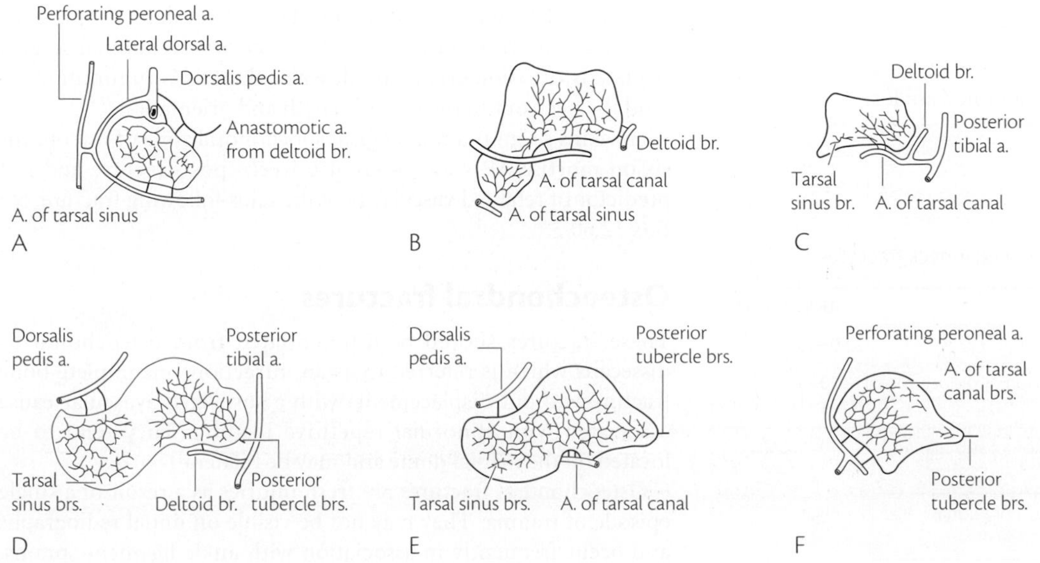

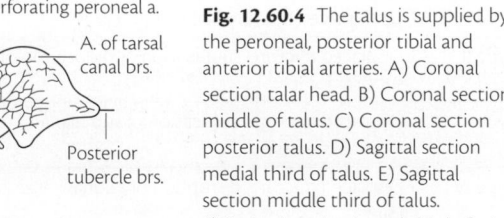

Fig. 12.60.4 The talus is supplied by the peroneal, posterior tibial and anterior tibial arteries. A) Coronal section talar head. B) Coronal section middle of talus. C) Coronal section posterior talus. D) Sagittal section medial third of talus. E) Sagittal section middle third of talus. F) Sagittal section lateral third of talus.

Box 12.60.1 Investigation of fractures of the talus and peritalar dislocations

- Radiographs:
  - Standard ankle and hindfoot views
  - Oblique views for posterior process fractures
  - Canale view to visualize talar neck (Figure 12.60.5)
- CT scan for talar body, neck, and head fractures
- MRI:
  - Osteochondral fractures
  - AVN.

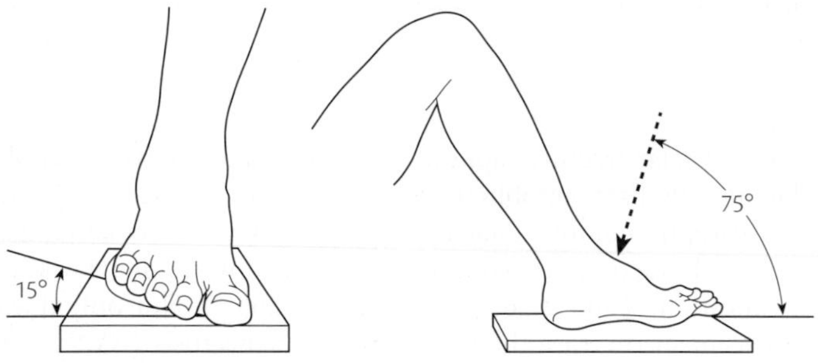

Fig. 12.60.5 The Canale view has been superseded by CT for preoperative assessment but is still useful for intraoperative views.

Box 12.60.2 Fractures of the talus

- Neck fractures—the commonest
- Osteochondral fractures of the dome
- Body fractures
- Lateral process fracture (snowboarder's fracture)
- Fractures of the posterior process
- Head fractures
- Avulsion fractures of the neck (sprained ankles).

Table 12.60.1 Hawkins classification of talar neck fractures

Type	Radiographic findings	Risk of AVN
Type I	Undisplaced fracture line	0–13%
Type II	Displaced fracture, subluxation or dislocation of subtalar joint	20–50%
Type III	Displaced fracture, dislocation of subtalar and tibiotalar joints	69–100%
Type IV	Displaced fracture, disruption of talonavicular joint	High

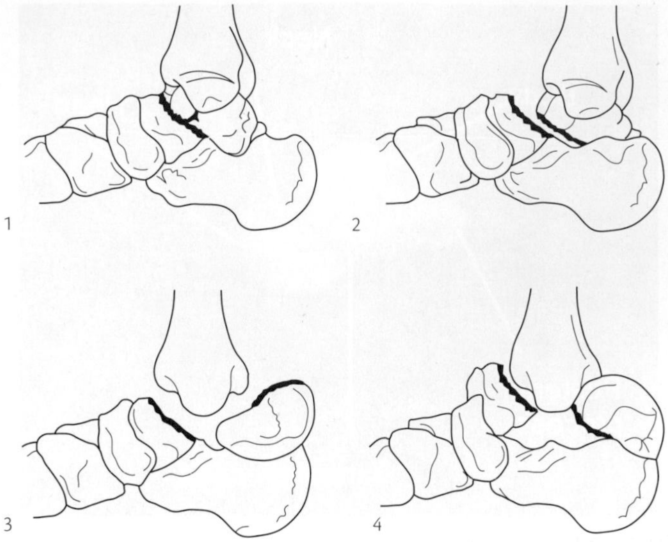

Fig. 12.60.6 The Hawkins–Canale classification of talar neck fractures.

permitted when radiological union is achieved (trabeculation crossing fracture site), usually 8–10 weeks.

In closed Hawkins type II fractures, closed reduction of the subtalar joint should be performed as a matter of urgency. If the surgeon waits until the swelling settles, reduction will be very difficult.

Surgery is indicated for all displaced fractures as it is associated with malunion and non-union. Malalignment of the talar neck has significant mechanical consequences and is associated with poor outcome. The approach must not further compromise vascularity and therefore the vascular anatomy must be clearly understood. The options involve anteromedial, anterolateral or posterolateral approaches. CT is mandatory and three-dimensional CT reconstruction can be very useful to determine the fracture plane and fragmentation. The anteromedial incision allows insertion of anterior to posterior longitudinal screws and can be extended to include a medial malleolus osteotomy. Reduction may be difficult to judge due to fragmentation and an additional anterolateral incision may be required to ensure reduction. The posterolateral approach allows the insertion of posterior to anterior longitudinal screws. A plate is occasionally required, when there is comminution, to hold the neck out to the correct length and orientation.

Hawkins's sign is a radiological subchondral zone of osteoporosis on mortise/AP views, seen at 6 weeks post-fracture and is a predictor of retained vascularity of the talus following fracture, see Box 12.60.3.

Osteochondral fractures

These fractures should be differentiated from osteochondritis dissecans which is referred to as an infraction (incomplete bone fracture without displacement) with a suspected avascular cause associated with abnormal repetitive loading. They tend to be located on the medial dome and may be bilateral.

Osteochondral fractures are fresh injuries as a result of a single episode of trauma. They may not be visible on initial radiographs and occur frequently in association with ankle ligament sprains.

Box 12.60.3 Avascular necrosis of the talus

- Hawkins sign:
  - Subchondral lucency implies intact blood supply
  - 4–5% false positive
  - Hawkins sign absent at 12 weeks—75% AVN
- MRI allows definitive diagnosis
- Treatment
  - Best managed expectantly
  - Arthroscopic debridement can help symptoms
  - Fusion should be considered for pain relief

Hence, if an ankle injury fails to settle within a reasonable period of time, further investigation with x-ray and magnetic resonance imaging (MRI) is indicated (Figure 12.60.7). Lesions may occur in up to 6.5% of ankle sprains.

An osteochondral fracture is essentially a divot of bone with overlying articular cartilage. The management depends on the size, location, and symptoms as well as general state of health considerations. The commonest location is the lateral dome and is a shear injury associated with an inversion which subluxes the talus in the mortise. Healing is an issue as the fragment has lost its blood supply and may act as a loose body. The separation may be incomplete or may in fact be a transchondral injury.

An undisplaced lesion may be stable or unstable and MRI scan may help to determine if there is a zone of lucency all around the lesion implying separation. The decision to fix *in situ* may then depend on whether the lesion is symptomatic or not.

Stability of a fragment offers the best chance of healing be that achieved in a cast or by internal fixation. The author uses CT with three-dimensional reconstruction to evaluate the size and position of the fragment as well as planning a surgical strategy in which it is important to determine if the fragment is to be reached via an arthrotomy (open or arthroscopic) or an osteotomy. The surgical options are to fix, excise, or drill the lesion.

Fixation depends on the size and when possible, the author favours 1-mm screws from the compact hand set. Internal fixation may need to be augmented with casting and protective weight bearing but if fixation is sound then non-weight-bearing range of movement exercises with a night resting splint to prevent equinus contracture, is to be preferred. A 2-month period of non-weight bearing is appropriate and sporting activities are not recommended for 1 year.

Salvage strategies may include drilling the defect to provoke healing with fibrocartilage together with loose body removal. Alternatively the defect can be grafted.

In 1959, Berndt and Harty proposed a staging system based on radiographic findings and Anderson et al. and Ferkel et al. used MRI to classify talar osteochondral injury. Pritsch et al. graded lesions according to articular injury visualized during ankle arthroscopy. These staging systems are summarized in Table 12.60.2

Talar body fractures:

These are intra-articular fractures that will usually require anatomical reduction of the articular surface with internal fixation. The dense trabecular bone frequently allows excellent screw purchase. Again CT scanning is mandatory and the author finds three-dimensional reconstruction useful to plan the approach and determine access to the fragments and hence the need for malleolar osteotomy (Figure 12.60.8).

The outcome of these fractures is generally poor with AVN rates similar to displaced neck of talus fractures. Post-traumatic arthritis is seen to occur frequently but does not always correlate with symptoms.

Snow boarder's fracture

These are fractures of the lateral process of the talus. The lateral talocalcaneal, cervical, bifurcate, and anterior talofibular ligaments

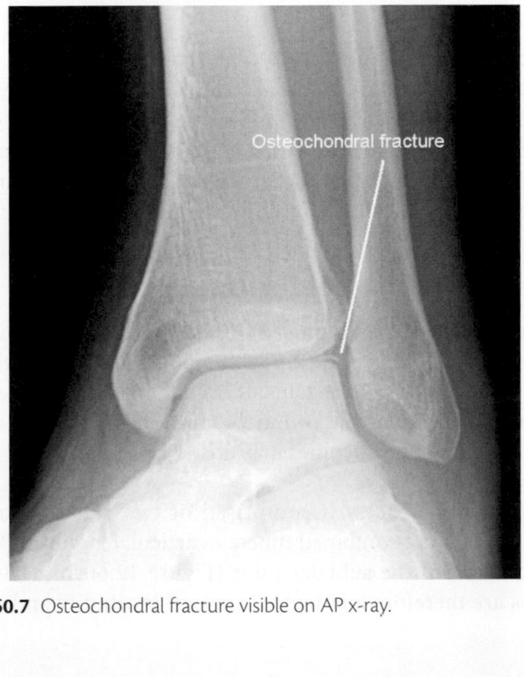

Fig. 12.60.7 Osteochondral fracture visible on AP x-ray.

Table 12.60.2 Classification of osteochondral fractures of the talar dome

Stage	Radiographs	MRI T_2WI	Arthroscopy
1	Normal	Diffuse, high-signal intensity	Normal, or softening of cartilage
2	Semicircular lucent line	Semicircular, low-signal line	Break in cartilage; fragment, no displacement
2a*	Subcortical round lucency	High-signal fluid within fragment	
3	Same as 2	High-signal fluid surrounds fragment	Displaceable fragment
4	Loose body	Defect talar dome, possibly loose body	Defect plus loose body

*Stage 2a is a variant in which a cyst forms in the subcortical bone

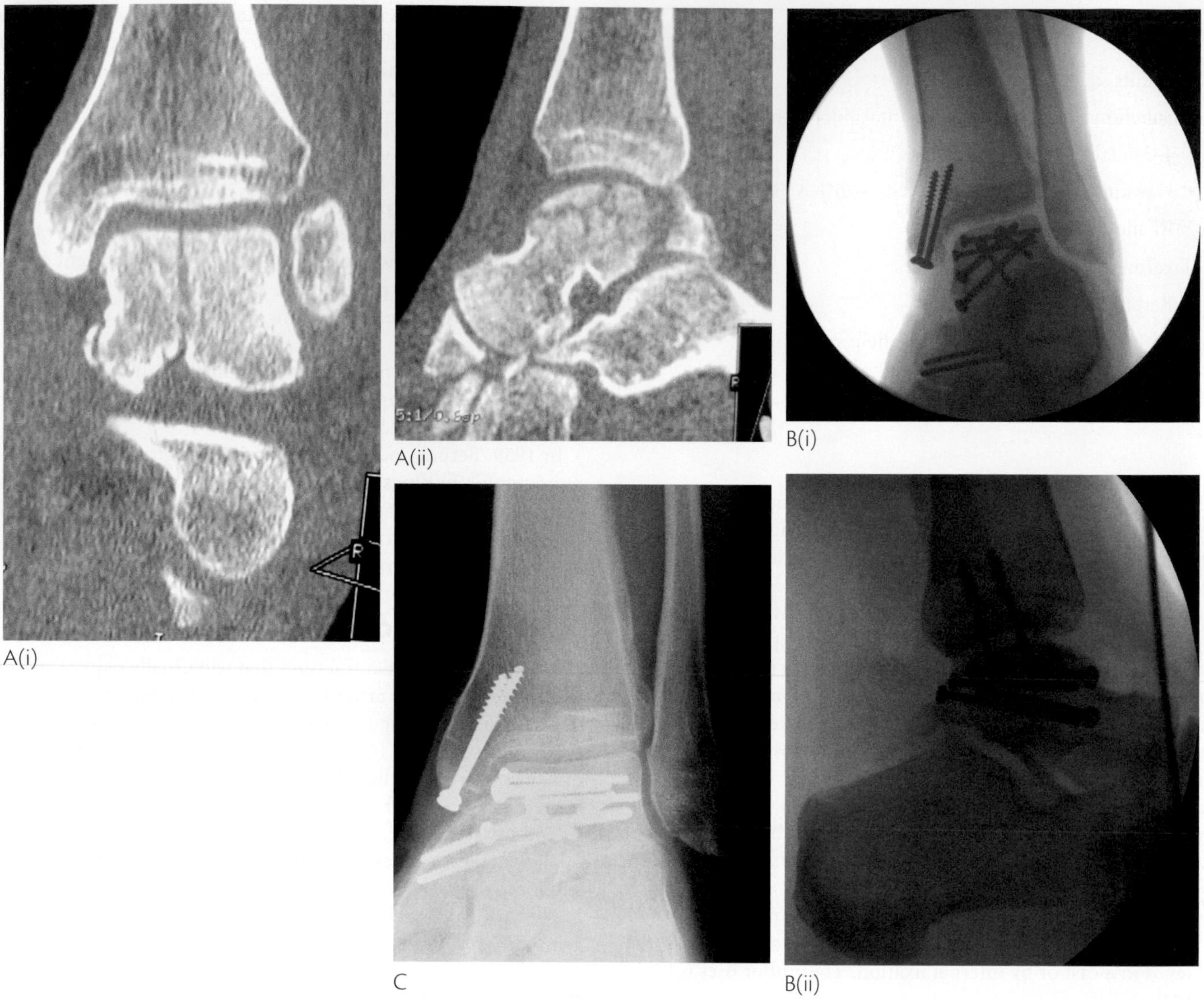

Fig. 12.60.8 A) Talar body fracture; B) treated with open reduction and internal fixation using medial malleolus osteotomy. C) Mortise view at 18 months.

originate from tip of this process. This fracture was seen rarely following falls and motor vehicle accidents but is now increasingly recognized and the incidence is rising. It is believed to occur as a result of dorsiflexion and eversion of an axially loaded ankle. It may mimic a lateral ankle ligament sprain and the injury may not be obvious on initial radiographs. Untreated it can be the cause of long-term disability. Primary surgical treatment may improve the outcome of this injury, reducing the risk of secondary subtalar joint osteoarthritis.

Any patient presenting following a snowboarding injury with lateral ankle pain, especially just distal to the tip of the lateral malleolus needs further investigation. Clinical suspicion of this injury mandates a CT scan (Figure 12.60.9). The author again favours three-dimensional reconstruction as well. This helps visualize the size, location, displacement, and degree of fragmentation of the fracture. This helps answer the question as to whether surgery is feasible.

Although these fractures may present late, the investigation and management are similar. Lateral process fractures are reported to have generally poor outcomes when treated in a cast alone. However, small (<1cm) minimally displaced (<2mm) fragments can be considered for non-weight bearing in a below-knee cast for 6–8 weeks. Large fragments should be stabilized with internal fixation unless truly undisplaced. Displaced multifragmentary fractures not amenable to fixation should be considered for excision.

Fractures of the posterior process

Fractures should not be confused with the os trigonum which is a secondary centre of ossification of the posterior process that has not fused to the body of the talus. It occurs in 7–10% of the population and is corticated and rounded. It can be fractured in its own right and diagnostic difficulties may arise which require CT or even MRI scanning to resolve.

The posterior process is comprised of two tubercles and the undersurface of the combined tubercles articulates with 25% of the posterior facet of the subtalar joint (Figure 12.60.10). Displaced fractures are therefore a potential cause of morbidity and oblique

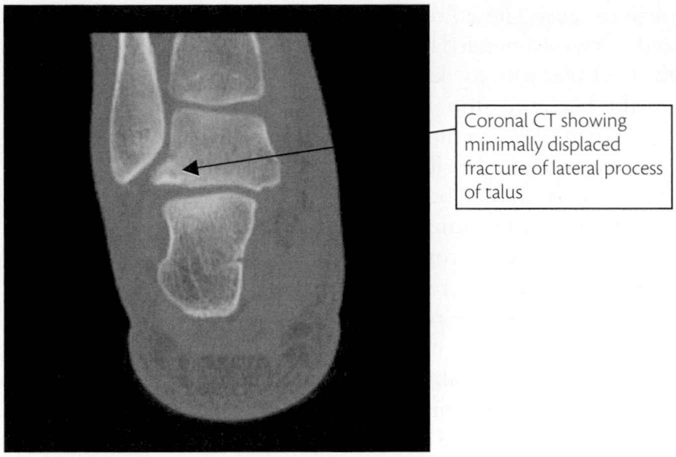

Coronal CT showing minimally displaced fracture of lateral process of talus

Fig. 12.60.9 Lateral process talar fracture.

views (30 degrees external rotation) or CT may be required to make the diagnosis.

Fractures of the lateral tubercle are known as Sheppard's fracture and may present clinically like an ankle sprain but may demonstrate tenderness posterolaterally with pain on movement of the subtalar joint and passive movement of flexor hallucis longus tendon.

Fractures of the medial tubercle, known as Cedell's fracture, will have a similar clinical presentation but may also present with a lump on palpation behind the medial malleolus.

Displaced fractures are best excised unless so large they can be reduced and fixed with small hand set screws (1-mm diameter). Undisplaced fractures may be treated in a cast, non-weight bearing for 6–8 weeks and although non-unions are rare, persistent painful non-union is best treated by excision of the fragment. Non-union may cause pain on subtalar movement or full plantar flexion.

Head fractures

The literature is limited largely to case reports and fractures are frequently associated with dislocations of the talonavicular joint. They represent less than 10% of talar fractures. The experience is that late presentation is common as the fracture may not be visible on plain radiographs. The consequence of late presentation is degenerative change. Diagnosis depends on a careful physical examination for pain, swelling and tenderness of the proximal medial column of the foot and CT scanning. Pain from degenerative changes may warrant fusion.

Accurate reduction and stable fixation should give rise to satisfactory results. Undisplaced fractures may be treated in a non-weight bearing below-knee cast for 8–10 weeks.

Avulsion fractures of the neck

These are small fractures that may be seen on lateral radiographs and are small irregular, often triangular fragments 2–3mm in size. They represent avulsions of the anterior talofibular ligament (ATFL) and are hence radiological signs of ankle sprains as the ATFL is the commonest ligament to be injured. The treatment is aimed at rapid restoration to function with elevation and compression and ice with early weight bearing with physiotherapy in the form of long extensor and proprioceptive retraining to prevent recurrent instability.

Caution is recommended to avoid missing associated undisplaced talar neck fractures.

Ankle dislocation

Dislocation of the tibiotalar joint, without associated ankle fracture, occurs infrequently. In 90% of cases the talus dislocates posteromedially and in 50% of cases there is an open anterolateral wound. In open injuries in addition to the standard management of an open wound the lateral ligaments can be repaired. In closed injuries reduction and immobilization in a below-knee cast for 6 weeks has been demonstrated to produce good to excellent results.

Subtalar dislocation

A subtalar dislocation involves disruption of both the talocalcaneal and talonavicular joints. The calcaneus and foot dislocate medially

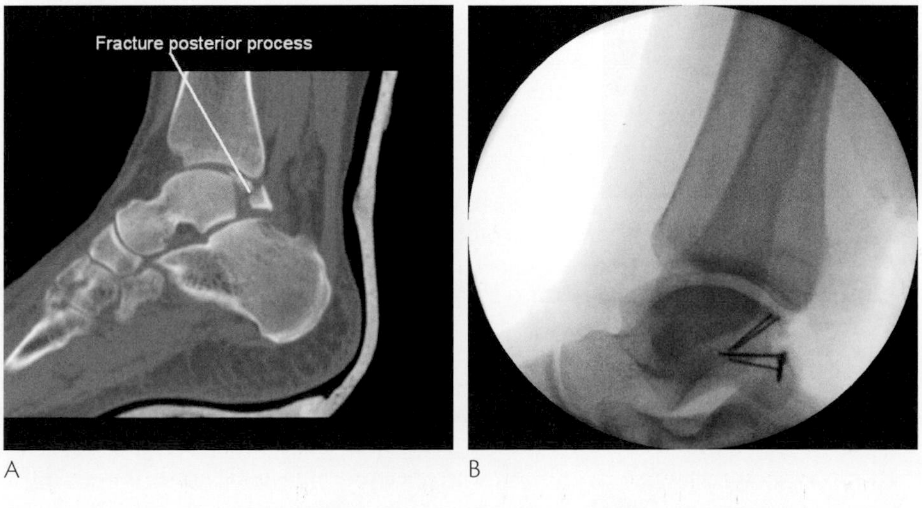

Fig. 12.60.10 A) Sagittal CT showing posterior process fracture involving posterior facet of subtalar joint. B) Fixation through posterolateral approach with compact hand set screws.

in 59%, laterally in 23%, posteriorly in 11%, and anteriorly in 7% (Figure 12.60.11). Subtalar dislocation is frequently associated with fractures of the foot (64%) and osteochondral fractures of the talus (47%). Many of these associated injuries will have an adverse effect on the outcome and may not be readily identifiable on plain x-rays.

Subtalar dislocations should be reduced as soon as possible to avoid further compromise of the soft tissue envelope. Reduction will frequently have been performed by emergency staff prior to the first x-rays and therefore subtalar dislocation should be considered in ankle injuries with a history of gross deformity without obvious cause. Closed reduction may require a general anaesthetic and it is recommended that it is performed by applying pressure to the navicular with the knee flexed and foot plantarflexed. Traction on the heel and initial exaggeration of the deformity may be required initially to unlock the talus and calcaneum. Closed reduction may not be possible due to entrapped tendons, ligament, capsule, retinaculum, bony impactions, or neurologic and vascular structures. It is recommended that postreduction CT scan is performed as a matter of routine. The subtalar joint is inherently stable and does not usually require internal fixation. In the absence of identifiable pathology requiring operative intervention, treatment involves a below-knee cast for 4–6 weeks depending on the initial instability. K-wire stabilization should be restricted to unstable injuries and it is important to use stout K-wires and strict non-weight bearing to avoid breakage. Assessment of stability should be performed after removal of the cast and in those cases demonstrating instability a further short period of immobilization is indicated.

The majority of patients will complain of subtalar stiffness and subtalar arthritis is common in the long term. AVN of the talus is rare.

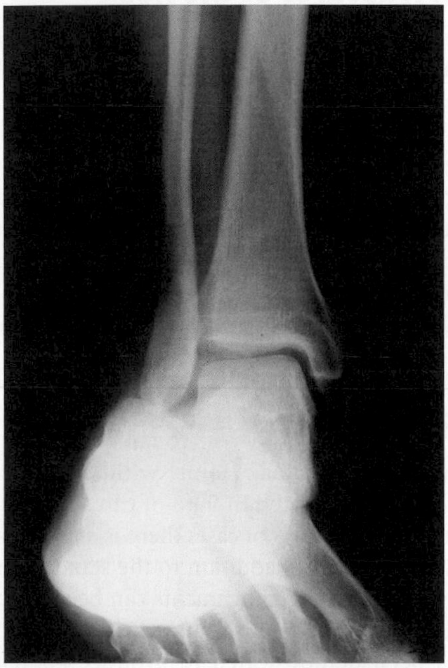

A

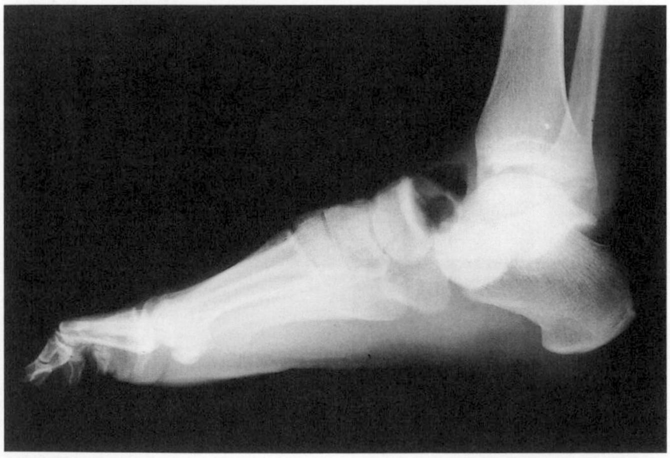

B

Fig. 12.60.11 These radiographs demonstrate a lateral subtalar dislocation.

Complete talar dislocation

Complete talar dislocation occurs very rarely and is associated with an open injury in approximately 75% of cases. In addition to standard treatment for open wounds, consideration can be given to reducing the talus and stabilising with K-wires. Although acceptable results have been reported, infection and AVN are common complications requiring secondary operative intervention. Alternatively, primary talectomy can be considered. Results of treatment for this injury are anecdotal.

Further reading

Rammelt, F. and Zwipp, H. (2009). Talar neck and body fractures. *Injury*, **40**, 120–35.

Valderrabano, V., Perren, T., Ryf, C., Rillmann, P., and Hintermann, B. (2005). Snowboarder's talus fracture: Treatment outcome of 20 cases after 3.5 years. *American Journal of Sports Medicine*, **33**(6), 871–80.

Veazey, B.L., Heckman, J.D., Galindo, M.J., and McGanity, P.L. (1992). Excision of ununited fractures of the posterior process of the talus: a treatment for chronic posterior ankle pain. *Foot and Ankle*, **13**, 453–7.

12.61

Fractures of the calcaneum

Roger M. Atkins

Summary points

- Surgical management of displaced fractures is becoming the norm
- Fixation and soft tissue procedures should allow early mobilization
- Subtalar fusion should not be used at the time of primary surgery
- In children minimal intervention indicated
- Abnormal hindfoot biomechanics frequent cause of long term disability.

Introduction

Calcaneal fractures account for 2% of fractures and 60% of tarsal bone injuries. Since the fracture usually occurs in the working population the economic cost is considerable.

Normal anatomy

Bone

The calcaneum is a box-like structure, squashed from superior to inferior anterior to posterior facet of subtalar joint (PFSTJ) by the sharp crucial angle of Gissane. Posteriorly, the superior surface is bare up to PFSTJ. This is quadrilateral in shape and orientated posteromedial to anterolateral. The bone behind and beneath PFSTJ is termed the *tuberosity* or *body* of the calcaneum (Figure 12.61.1A).

Anterior to PFSTJ, the bone is extended anteromedially as the sustentaculum tali (ST), which consists of two thick sheets of cortical bone with the middle facet of subtalar joint (STJ) on its superior surface. Anterior to ST a deep groove, the interosseous sulcus, passes laterally terminating as the crucial angle of Gissane, a sharp edge of thick cortical bone into which fits the anterolateral process of talus. The interosseous sulcus forms the inferior surface of the sinus tarsi which gives rise to the interosseous talocalcanean ligament and contains the artery of the sinus tarsi.

In front of the sinus tarsi, the calcaneum narrows. Medially, the superior surface contains the anterior facet of STJ (which may be confluent with the middle facet). It gives origin to three structures from medial to lateral, the bifurcate ligament, which inserts into the adjacent cuboid and navicular bones, the extensor digitorum brevis, and the inferior extensor retinaculum.

The lateral wall of the calcaneum is flat and is mainly thin cortical bone. Immediately anterior to the crucial angle of Gissane, the inferior peroneal retinaculum, through which run the peroneal tendons, is attached to the peroneal tubercle. The posterior calcaneofibular ligament arises from the lateral wall behind and below PFSTJ and immediately anterosuperior to this the capsule of STJ inserts, leaving a bare area posteroinferior to the lateral edge of the joint.

The medial wall is thicker than the lateral and is arched from posteroinferior to anterosuperior with its apex lateral from subcutaneous sustentaculum tali to the medial process inferiorly. The thick cortical sheets of ST are continued anteriorly as a strong anteromedial buttress and fuse with the medial aspect of the calcaneocuboid joint (CCJ).

The medial wall gives origin to the intrinsic muscles of the foot, which separate it from the posterior tibial neurovascular structures. Superiorly, the medial wall is grooved by the flexor hallucis tendon passing beneath ST.

The anterosuperior corner of the medial wall is intimately related to the talus and navicular.

The anterior wall of the calcaneum is the CCJ which is shield shaped with its point inferiorly (Figure 12.61.1B). The superior part of the joint is orientated in an oblique plane from posterolateral to anteromedial, while inferiorly the orientation is anterolateral to posteromedial. In addition, the superior edge lies anterior to the inferior. This complicated geometry makes reduction and fixation of the joint difficult.

The plantar surface of the calcaneum contains the medial and lateral processes, which give origin to the plantar fascia and the small muscles of the plantar aspect of the foot.

The posterior surface of the calcaneum contains the tendo Achilles (TA) insertion.

Soft tissues

Laterally, the calcaneum is subcutaneous and the sural nerve runs obliquely within the subcutaneous fat passing posterosuperior to anteroinferior with a variable course. It supplies the lateral border of the foot and is easily damaged in direct incisions over this area which may cause neuromas.

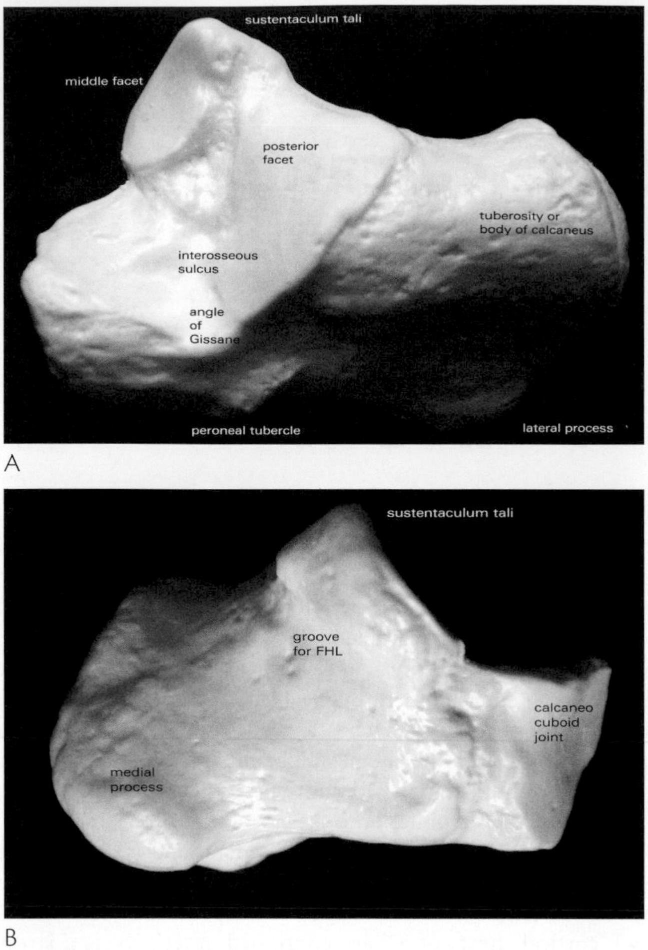

Fig. 12.61.1 Oblique views of the calcaneus showing important landmarks. A) Lateral oblique. B) Medial oblique.

Laterally above the calcaneum the soft tissues consist of superficial and deep triangles. The superficial triangle lies in the sagittal plane. Its boundaries are the superior border of the calcaneum inferiorly, anteriorly the peroneal muscles and tendons and posteriorly the TA. In the anterior wall of the superficial triangle, in the coronal plane is the deep triangle. It is bounded laterally by the peroneal tendons, inferiorly by the superior border of the calcaneum, just behind PFSTJ and medially by the flexor hallucis muscle covered by fascia. The floor from inferior to superior is PFSTJ, STJ capsule, talus, ankle joint capsule, and tibia. Surgical dissection of these triangles by the extended lateral approach gives massive access to the hindfoot.

The *posterior peroneal artery* is the artery of supply of the skin of the lateral aspect of the heel. It is usually the terminal branch of the peroneal artery and enters the deep triangle at its apex. It transits both triangles, anastomosing with the periarticular vascular ring around the ankle and crosses the superior border of the calcaneum behind PFSTJ in close proximity to the sural nerve, becoming an end artery. There are poor anastomoses between the posterior peroneal artery cutaneous angiosome and the posterior foot or the sole. Therefore a surgical approach to the lateral side of the hindfoot must dissect the angiosome or the wound is at high risk of breakdown.

Medially, the short abductor of the foot and flexor accessorius muscle separate the bone form the posterior tibial neurovascular bundle, which is in danger from medial incisions, lateral drills or instruments placed through the primary fracture line to reduce the body fragment (BF). It may also be damaged by the inferior spike of the sustentacular fragment (SF) which pierces the skin in an open fracture.

Anatomy of the fracture

Fractures of the calcaneum occur according to a series of readily definable patterns knowledge of which permits a logical approach to treatment.

The normal intra-articular fracture

This constitutes approximately 75% of cases and is usually caused by a fall from 6–12 feet (1.8–3.6m). It involves three fracture lines, the *primary fracture line (1#L)* and the *coronal (C2#L)* and *longitudinal secondary fracture lines (L2#L)* (Figure 12.61.2), modified from the original description of Essex-Lopresti.

1#L is the result of shearing forces between the heelstrike point and the mechanical axis of STJ (Figure 12.61.2). It splits the bone from posteromedial to anterolateral, crossing PFSTJ and usually CCJ creating a two-part fracture. The lateral fragment contains the lateral part of PFSTJ, the tuberosity or body of the calcaneum and the lateral part of CCJ while the medial fragment contains ST and the medial part of the subtalar and CCJ.

The two-part fracture is usually undisplaced, however the posterolateral fragment may dislocate lateral to the talus, either in a high-energy injury, or in middle aged females after a minor trip. As the lateral fragment is forced upwards, it escapes lateral to the talus and continues superiorly until stopped by the lateral malleolus, which sustains a small posterior fracture. The lateral fragment rebounds and pulls the lateral edge of the talus inferiorly, subluxing the ankle joint. This rare fracture is often missed and non-operative treatment leads to painful ankle and midfoot dysfunction which is difficult to salvage. Primary operative treatment through an extended lateral approach is straightforward.

Usually secondary fracture lines occur. C2#L runs along the sinus tarsi splitting the anterolateral fragment (ALF) from the posterolateral. Crossing 1#L in the majority of cases, it exits at the middle facet, splitting the medial fragment into an anteromedial fragment (AMF) and a posterior SF. L2#L arises on the lateral wall of the calcaneum and passes posteriorly splitting the residual posterolateral fragment into a lateral joint fragment (LJF) and a body fragment (BF). Usually it skirts PFSTJ creating a small semilunar, central joint depression LJF. Less frequently it passes directly posteriorly to the posterior aspect of the bone, creating a large, tongue type LJF.

Thus a four- or five-part fracture is created, depending on whether the coronal secondary line stops medially at 1#L.

Fragment description

- Body fragment (BF). Lateral to 1#L and below L2#L. It includes the heelstrike point, calcaneal tuberosities and TA insertion
- Sustentacular fragment (SF). Medial to 1#L and posterior to C2#L if this line crosses 1#L. It includes the medial part of PFSTJ,

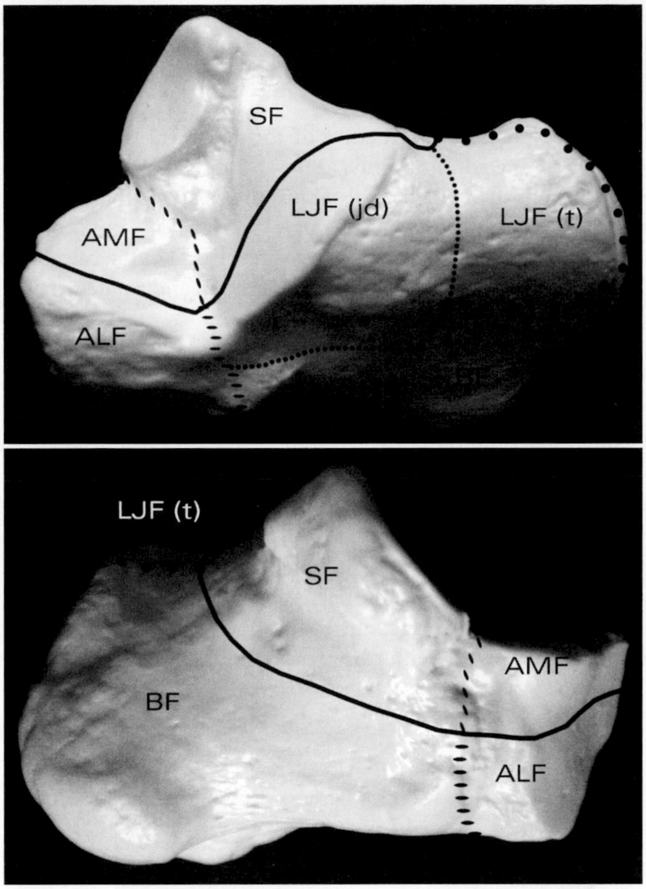

Fig. 12.61.2 The anatomy of the usual calcaneus fracture: A) lateral oblique view; B) medial oblique view. ALF, anterolateral fragment; AMF, anteromedial fragment; BF, body fragment; LJF (t) tongue type lateral joint fragment; LJF (jd), central joint depression type lateral joint fragment; SF, sustentacular fragment. Solid line, primary fracture line; dashed lines, coronal secondary fracture line; transverse dashes, lateral part; longitudinal dashes, medial part; small dots: longitudinal secondary fracture line forming a central joint depression type lateral joint fragment; large dots: longitudinal secondary fracture line where it separates to form a tongue type lateral joint fragment.

ST, and the superior part of medial wall of calcaneum. In a four-part fracture, where C2#L does not extend medial to 1#L, it also includes STJ middle and anterior facets and medial CCJ

- Lateral joint fragment (LJF). Lateral to 1#L, posterior to C2#L and above L2#L. It includes lateral PFSTJ
- Anterolateral fragment (ALF). Lateral to 1#L and anterior to C2#L, it includes the crucial angle of Gissane and lateral CCJ
- Anteromedial fragment (AMF). Medial to 1#L and anterior to C2#L. It contains the STJ middle and anterior facets and medial CCJ.

In a four-part fracture, where C2#L does not cross 1#L (approximately 30%), AMF remains part of SF. Open reduction and internal fixation (ORIF) is simple since the combined SF and AMF provides a large area for screw insertion. Occasionally, a four-part fracture is created by 1#L failing to pass anterior to C2#L. This leads to a combined ALF and AMF.

Fragment movement

The interaction of 1#L and C2#L usually produces a BF which has a sharp, wedge-shaped superior edge (Figure12.61.3). The injury forces BF superiorly and anteriorly, in a variable direction, sliding laterally on the oblique lateral surface of SF and tips into varus and internal rotation (Figure 12.61.3). The triangular upper surface of BF splits apart LJF and SF, tipping LJF into valgus and SF into varus. With increasing fragment displacement, the sharp inferior spike of SF becomes more medial, until it penetrates the skin causing an open fracture.

Occasionally, in high energy or osteoporotic fractures, the usual sharp triangular upper border of BF is absent. LJF is crushed into BF and may be captured within it causing true lateral joint fragment depression (Atkins type 3 fracture).

Displacements of AMF and ALF are less marked. AMF is undisplaced or shifted upwards. ALF rotates outward and upward filling

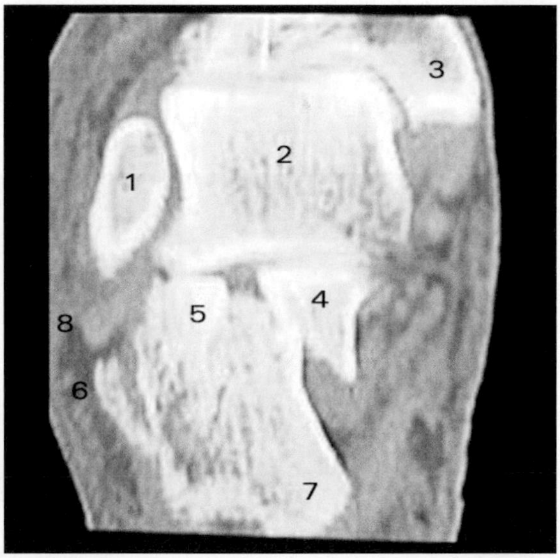

Fig. 12.61.3 Semicoronal reconstruction of an axial CT scan of a calcaneus fracture. This scan has been taken at the level of the lateral malleolus and posterior facet of subtalar joint. The posterior facet is disrupted into two main fragments with a primary fracture line in the middle of the posterior facet (a Sanders 2b fracture). The fractured lateral wall is comprised of the body fragment inferiorly and the lateral joint fragment superiorly (an Atkins type 2 fracture).

1. Lateral malleolus.
2. Body of talus.
3. Medial malleolus.
4. Sustentacular fragment and sustentaculum tali. Note that the fragment is rotated so that its inferior tip comes to lie more medial and that the tip of the sustentaculum is relatively undisplaced.
5. Lateral joint fragment and the lateral part of the posterior facet.
6. The lateral wall of the calcaneus which is pushed outwards and upwards broadening the heel and impinging on the lateral malleolus and the peroneal tendons.
7. The tuberosity of the calcaneus and the body fragment. The fragment is tipped into varus bringing the heel-strike point medially. The body fragment is also pushed upwards so that its superomedial corner moves up the medial oblique face of the sustentacular fragment and so causes the body fragment to move laterally. This broadens that heel.
8. The peroneal tendons which are closely applied to the displaced lateral wall.

in the crucial angle of Gissane. These displacements must be addressed in ORIF to prevent painful STJ impingement.

Fracture classification

A number of complementary fracture classifications are useful:

- Essex-Lopresti distinguished between central joint depression fractures and tongue-type fractures based on the course of L2#L
- Sanders classification depends on the number and position of fracture lines within PFSTJ
- The Zwipp and Tscherne system concentrates on the number of major fracture fragments (2 to 5) and the number of joints involved.
- The Atkins system is based on the composition of the residual lateral wall. In a type 1 fracture, the lateral wall is made up of LJF, in a type 2 it is formed of LJF above and BF below and in a type 3 fracture, LJF is captured within BF and the latter forms the entire lateral wall.

Tuberosity fractures

The classical tuberosity fracture is a TA avulsion in an osteoporotic bone.

The medial process fracture of the body of the calcaneum was originally described by Watson-Jones, as due to a fall with the foot in severe valgus and by Bohler, who considered it to be an avulsion of the plantar fascia.

We have identified a fracture of the calcaneal tuberosity that occurs in young adults (Figure 12.61.4). 1#L is replaced by a semi-coronal fracture line, which separates the posterosuperior part of the calcaneum. This fracture line may cross PFSTJ or pass posteriorly. The fracture line exits on the posterior wall of the calcaneum. The displaced fragment includes TA insertion and rotates upwards causing a heel boss.

Anterior process fracture

There are two different types, avulsion and compression.

The more common bony avulsion of the calcaneal origin either of the bifurcate ligament or of the extensor digitorum brevis is caused by forced inversion. There is tenderness on the lateral side of the hindfoot and the injury is usually obvious on the lateral x-ray. Non-operative treatment which may require cast immobilization gives good results although recovery may be slow.

The rare high violence compression fracture is caused by forced abduction of the foot with compression of the anterior part of the

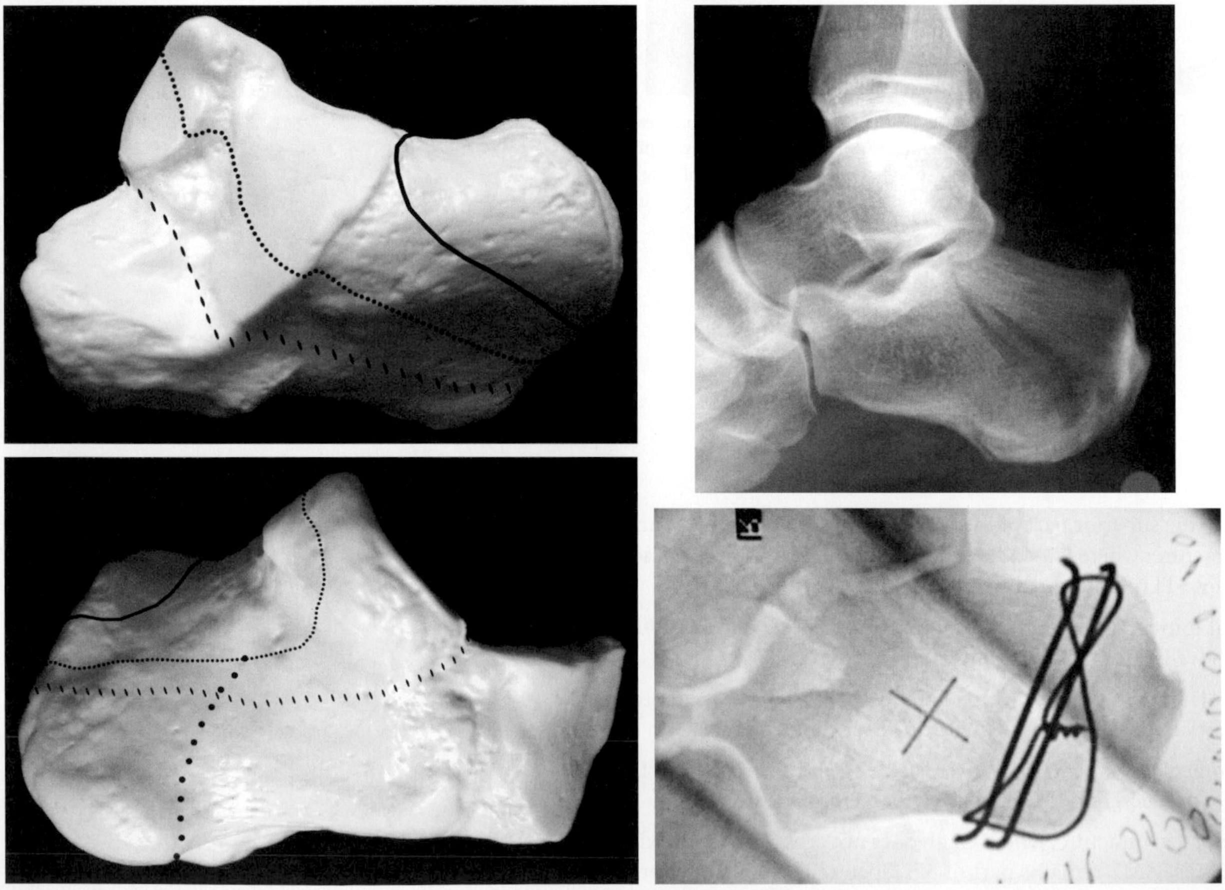

A B

Fig. 12.61.4 The anatomy of the tuberosity fracture of the calcaneus: A) lateral oblique view; B) medial oblique view. Solid line, an extra-articular fracture such as is seen in elderly or infirm patients; dotted line, a trans-articular fracture; dashed line, a total articular fracture; large dots (medial oblique view only), the outline of the small wedge-shaped body fragment.

calcaneum, classically either in motorcycle racing or waterskiing. The displaced fragment is larger than in the compression fracture and involves a significant portion of CCJ. Swelling is often considerable and CT scanning may demonstrate associated fractures of the calcaneum. Non-operative treatment gives poor results. Surgery is difficult and requires often involves stabilization of PFSTJ.

Sustentacular fracture

ST is small and fractures may be missed radiographically. ST is firmly attached to talus and medial malleolus, so fractures are rarely isolated and are associated with severe ligamentous and bony damage elsewhere and treatment is a part of treatment of the overall hindfoot injury. ST fractures are often associated with gross instability of PFSTJ.

Fractures in children

These are rare but easily missed. The usual mechanism is a jump or fall; however lawnmower accidents may directly involve the calcaneum. In younger children undisplaced extra-articular fractures predominate, with a high incidence of anterior process fractures. The prognosis is good with non-operative treatment. Adolescent fractures are rare, similar to adult fractures but simpler although occurring following greater falls (Figure 12.61.5).

Open fractures

Two types are seen. Type 1 is a standard highly displaced intra-articular fracture where the inferior border of SF penetrates the skin on the medial side of the foot beneath the medial malleolus.

A type 2 injury occurs in a high violence atypical fracture where random fracture fragments penetrate the skin. The open injury varies but is typically on the sole of the foot.

Clinical history (Box 12.61.1)

The majority of fractures occur in a fall from a height, usually more than 6 feet (1.8m). A two part fracture dislocation in a middle aged women or the avulsion fracture of the tuberosity in the elderly occur after a simple trip. Both open and bilateral fractures are associated with greater violence injuries and give poorer results. The other common cause for calcaneal fractures is a road traffic accident and in these cases atypical fractures, sometimes with dislocations are seen.

The patient experiences immediate hindfoot pain and cannot walk. Swelling soon follows. Initial clinical examination usually demonstrates swelling and tenderness of the heel. Very rarely, a calcaneal fracture with a dislocation will cause vascular compromise in the foot. Swelling increases over several days and bruising of the lateral side of the heel becomes obvious (the Battle sign). As the swelling subsides, the characteristic short, wide heel and poorly defined lateral malleolus become obvious.

The two part fracture dislocation of the body of the calcaneum presents a clinical trap. The x-ray may look deceptively normal and, because the calcaneum is impacted against the lateral malleolus, the patient may be able to walk with ease.

Radiographic assessment

Plain radiographs

Lateral and axial views of the heel will show most clinically significant fractures. Ankle and foot radiographs may also be performed. On the lateral radiograph assessment of Bohler's angle will give some indication of fracture displacement (Figure 12.61.6). The fracture may also be classified according to Essex-Lopresti into a tongue or central joint depression fracture. The axial view will demonstrate 1#L separating BF from SF and may give some indication of heel widening (Figure 12.61.7). Ankle radiographs will demonstrate subluxation with a dislocated calcaneal tuberosity in the case of a two-part fracture dislocation. Oblique radiographs of the foot demonstrate fractures of the anterior part of the calcaneum.

Computed tomography scanning

Fractures may easily be missed on plain radiographs and in case of doubt a computed tomography (CT) scan should be performed. CT scanning is essential to demonstrate fracture anatomy and displacement and for surgical planning. Using a spiral scanner, axial, sagittal and semi-coronal (normal to PFSTJ) views are obtained.

Semi-coronal scan (see Figure 12.61.3) shows the disposition of the fracture in the posterior part of the bone. PFSTJ is well demonstrated and BF displacement can be assessed. The composition of the fractured lateral wall can be determined. In the context of reconstruction of mal-union, impingement between displaced fracture fragments and the fibula can be assessed.

Axial scan (Figure 12.61.8) shows the fracture as it effects the anterior part of the bone well. Involvement of CCJ is clearly seen and fracture lines passing just anterior to ST can be visualized. In the posterior part of the bone, rotation of BF in the axial plane can be estimated. The scan will also show whether the fracture is an Essex-Lopresti tongue or central joint depression fracture, although this is normally readily seen on the lateral radiograph.

Treatment

Treatment remains controversial; however, with improved surgical understanding, anatomical approaches and implant technology, operative treatment is becoming the norm.

Non-operative treatment without reduction

Background

This should be reserved for undisplaced fractures or for cases unfit for operative treatment. After elevation to resolve swelling, the patient is mobilized non-weight bearing with physiotherapy. If this is too uncomfortable, a short period of initial immobilization is used. An elastic stocking aids resolution of swelling. The patient should be fully weight bearing by 12 weeks in a solid shoe with a permanent insole.

Open reduction and internal fixation

Background

There are four goals to calcaneal fracture fixation

1) Restoration of PFSTJ
2) Restoration of hindfoot biomechanics by reduction of the medial wall fracture line and realignment of BF
3) Reduction of the anterior part of the calcaneum in order to release STJ and reduce CCJ
4) Fixation and soft tissue procedures which allow early mobilization.

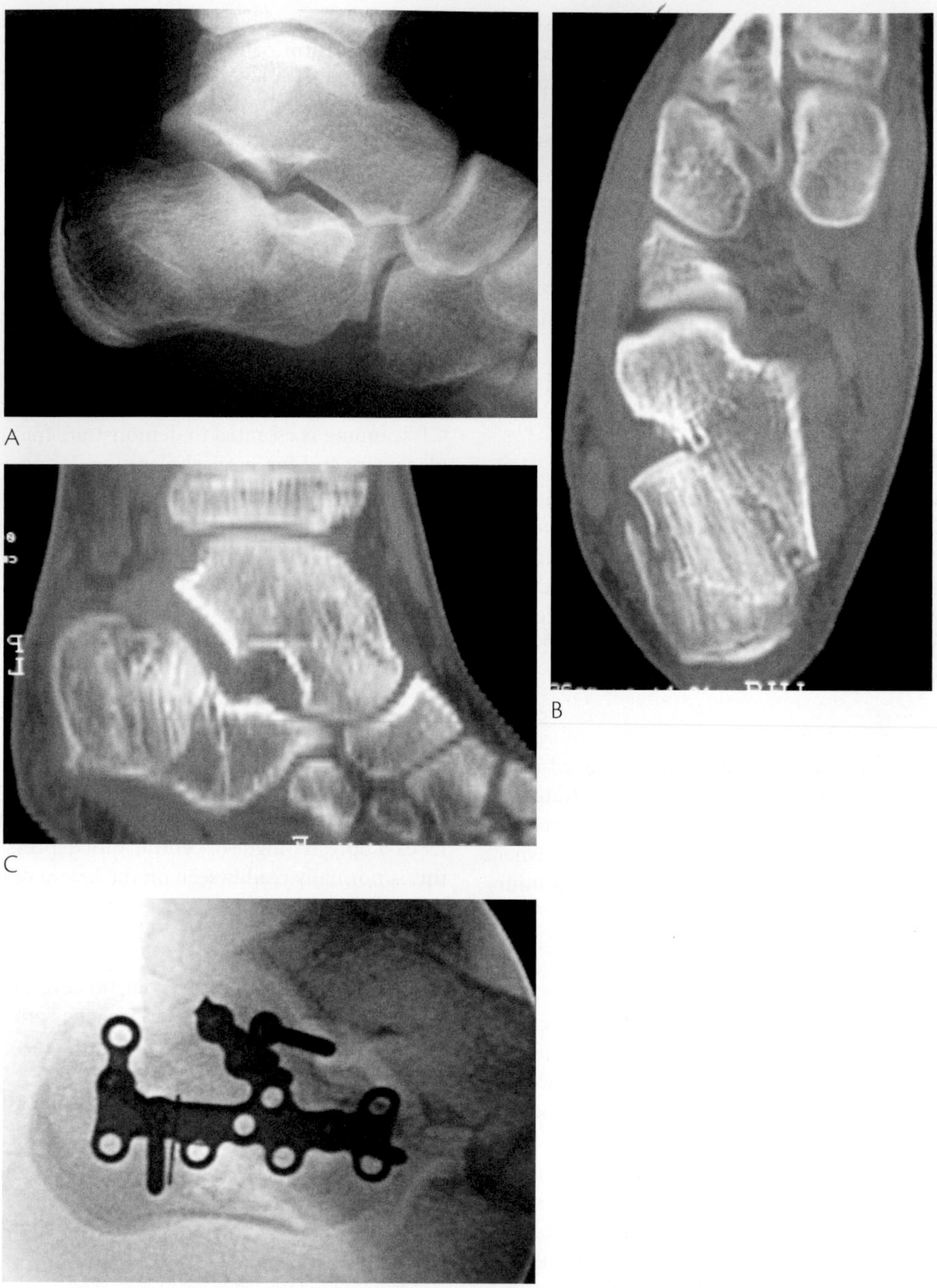

Fig. 12.61.5 Intra-articular calcaneal fracture in a mature child. The fracture is an Essex Lopresti central joint depression fracture. It is a Sanders 2b or 2c fracture, the exact place at which the primary fracture line crosses the posterior facet cannot be judged on these views. The posterior facet of the sub-talar joint is involved and probably the middle facet but the calcaneo-cuboid joint is intact. The primary fracture line does not extend anterior to the interosseous sulcus so that there is one large anterior fragment. It is therefore a Zwipp and Tscherne four part, two joint fracture.

A) Lateral radiograph. Bohler's angle is flattened indicating significant fracture displacement.

B) Axial CT scan. There is a large but incomplete lateral wall segment of bone suggesting an Atkins type 2 fracture, although this cannot be absolutely stated on these views. There is significant anterior movement of the body fragment on the sustentacular fragment. This would possibly remodel with time. A crack in the sustentaculum in visible.

C) This sagittal reconstruction CT scan shows severe derangement of the posterior facet of sub-talar joint which is unlikely to remodel.

D) Postoperative lateral radiograph. Bohler's angle is restored.

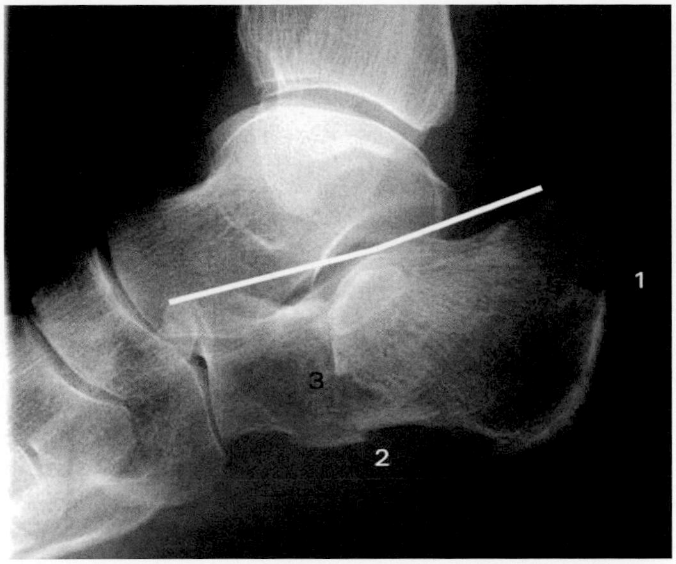

Fig. 12.61.6 Lateral view of a calcaneus showing an Essex–Lopresti tongue type fracture. Bohler's angle is outlined by the white line. Reversal of the angle, as here, suggests significant fracture fragment displacement and a poor prognosis following non-operative treatment. 1—the exit point of the longitudinal secondary fracture line on the posterior aspect of the bone. 2—the inferior part of the coronal splitting the bone into anterior and posterior parts. 3—the anterior corner of the posterior facet of the sub-talar joint on the lateral joint fragment. (Figures 12.61.6–8 show the same fracture.)

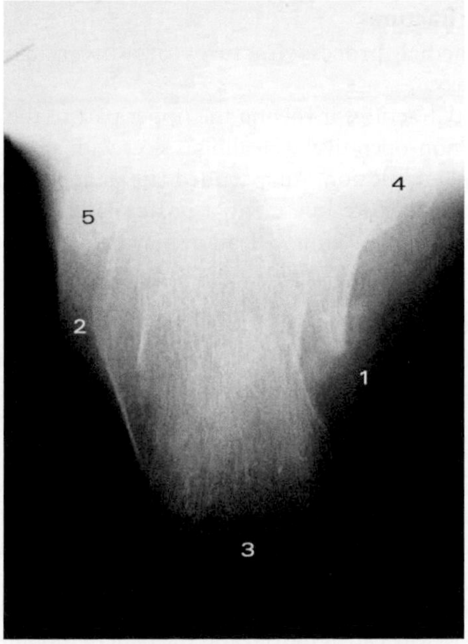

Fig. 12.61.7 Axial view of a fractured calcaneus.
1. The inferior tip of the sustentacular fragment.
2. The bulging lateral wall.
3. The tuberosity of the calcaneus, forming the body fragment, tipped into varus.
4. The sustentaculum tali.
5. The lateral malleolus.

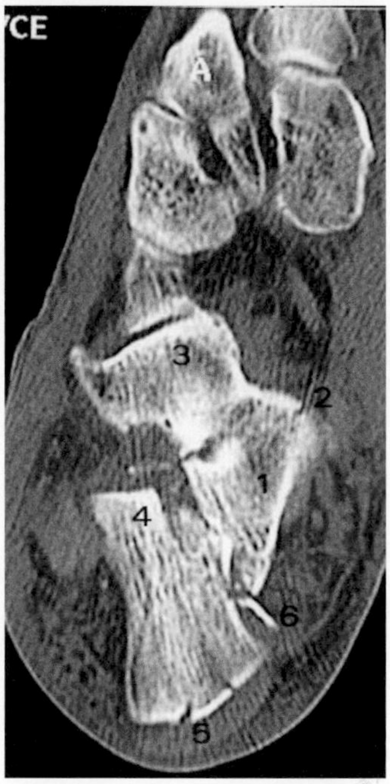

Fig. 12.61.8 Axial CT scan of a calcaneus fracture.
1. The sustentaculum tali and sustentacular fragment. This scan shows more clearly than the coronal scan the size of the fragment but does not demonstrate displacement.
2. The medial extension of the coronal secondary fracture line passing into the sustentaculum tali. This fracture line usually passes just anterior to the sustentaculum.
3. The anterior part of the calcaneus is in one piece in this fracture and the calcaneocuboid joint is not involved. This fracture is therefore a Zwipp and Tscherne 4 part 2 joint fracture. The fracture fragments are sustentacular, lateral joint, body and anterior. The two involved joints are the posterior and middle facets of the sub-talar joint.
4. The lateral joint fragment
5. The posterior extension of the longitudinal secondary fracture line. Since this exits the posterior rather than the superior aspect of the bone, the fracture is an Essex–Lopresti tongue type.
6. The posterior limit of the primary fracture line separating the sustentacular fragment antero-medially from the body fragment posterolaterally. The body fragment is displaced anteriorly compared to the sustentacular fragment.

The surgical approach is crucial and develops a fasciocutaneous flap based on the terminal branch of the peroneal artery. The incision heals well and allows early mobilization. The medial wall fracture line can be addressed through this lateral incision obviating the need for a medial approach.

Current surgical techniques (Fig. 12.61.9)

The usual intra-articular fracture

Preamble and positioning

Surgery is performed after the swelling has begun to subside and under general anaesthetic and antibiotic cover. The patient is placed in the lateral position and the foot prepared and draped free from the mid-calf.

Extended lateral approach to the hindfoot

The incision is in two parts joined at the posterior corner of the heel. The superior limb begins in the midline approximately 15cm

Box 12.61.1 Clinical assessment

History

- Falls from height—intra-articular fractures
- Low energy:
  - Two-part fracture dislocation, middle-aged women, x-rays deceptive
  - Tuberosity fracture, elderly
  - Avulsion anterior process, inversion injury

Examination

- Soft tissues:
  - Open injuries
  - Compartment syndrome
  - Suitability for ORIF
- Shape of foot:
  - Varus/valgus
  - Width

Investigations

- Lateral and axial hindfoot x-rays ± ankle and foot x-rays
- CT.

above the sole and passes inferiorly and anteriorly ending approximately 2cm anterior to the lateral corner of the heel. The inferior limb begins distally at the level of the base of the fifth metatarsal bone at the junction of the lateral side of the foot and the sole. It is below the bruised skin and separated from it by approximately 1cm. The two limbs meet at an angle of greater than 100 degrees in a gentle curve. The skin incision allows development of the cutaneous angiosome of the posterior peroneal artery. Flap elevation begins at the apex with dissection directly onto the calcaneum. Anteriorly, abductor digiti minimi is split and the entire lateral wall of the calcaneum is exposed subperiosteally as far as PFSTJ. The inferior peroneal retinaculum is dissected intact to expose of the crucial angle of Gissane and ALF. The lateral wall fragment is now removed and preserved for later reposition. This may require formal osteotomy.

Disimpaction of LJF and removal from STJ

LJF is rotated out of STJ. In a tongue type fracture the posterior soft tissues should be retained. In a central joint depression type fracture, the fragment will usually have been denuded of soft tissues and is removed. Exposure of the posterior aspect of STJ is improved by cutting directly through the superficial and deep triangles, avoiding damage to the peroneal tendons and flexor hallucis muscle.

Transcalcaneal reduction of BF and medial wall

This exposes the medial wall fracture line, between the apex of BF inferiorly and the lateral surface of SF medially and superiorly. A Steinman pin may be used for manipulative reduction of BF. I have not found this to be necessary.

A periosteal elevator is inserted gently between the visible apex of BF and the lateral edge of SF. Care is taken to avoid damage to the posterior tibial neurovascular bundle. The periosteal elevator is now rotated, levering BF downwards and medially, reducing the medial wall. The reduction may be held temporally with a K-wire.

Reconstruction of PFSTJ

The PFSTJ is now reconstructed anatomically and LJF is replaced. Fixation of intermediate fragments may require K-wires or Herbert screws. Temporary K-wire fixation is checked visually and radiographically. Definitive fixation is with a small fragment cortical lag screw into ST with a washer.

Reconstruction of the anterior part of the calcaneum

Subperiosteal dissection within the sinus tarsi allows reduction of ALF and AMF, which are stabilized with temporary K-wires. The lateral wall fragment is now replaced. If a good reduction has been obtained it fits well into the remaining lateral bone defect.

Plate fixation

The majority of standard calcaneal fractures do not require a locking plate. Once BF has been reduced beneath SF and PFSTJ stabilized by repositioning of LJF, the fracture is longitudinally stable and the plate serves to buttress BF against SF and to hold the anterior part of the bone in place. Union occurs rapidly possibly with a minor, irrelevant loss of height. Where significant bone crushing, comminution or osteoporosis renders the fracture longitudinally unstable, a locking plate is required. In these cases bone grafting may be advisable in order to enhance bone healing and prevent collapse.

Postoperatively ankle and subtalar joint exercises are begun immediately and the patient remains non-weight bearing until union is well advanced, usually at 6–8 weeks. Weight bearing is then gradually introduced.

Tuberosity fractures

Isolated medial process fractures are invariably managed conservatively.

Tuberosity fractures involving the upper part of the calcaneum fare poorly non-operatively. Healing is slow with a heel bump and weakened plantarflexion. An extended lateral approach is used to compress the fracture line using a posterolateral tension band. A short period of cast immobilization may be necessary; however, the patient can usually mobilize weight bearing and union is rapid.

Comminuted atypical cases

Comminuted fractures of the calcaneum fare poorly non-operatively but they are a daunting surgical prospect and will not be suitable for standard fixation. There is invariably at least one large fragment of bone, which usually contains the majority of PFSTJ and BF. ORIF using an extended lateral approach reduces the large fragment into its anatomic position beneath the talus and fixes it with K-wires into the talus. The remainder of the calcaneum is then fixed to this fragment. Non-weight-bearing cast immobilization is maintained until fracture healing is established, usually 6–8 weeks. The K-wires are removed and the patient mobilizes freely in a new cast until union is complete, after approximately a further 6–8 weeks. Treated thus, patients complain of few symptoms and revision to subtalar fusion is rare.

We do not advocate a subtalar fusion at the time of primary reduction. Subtalar fusion without prior reduction gives poor results.

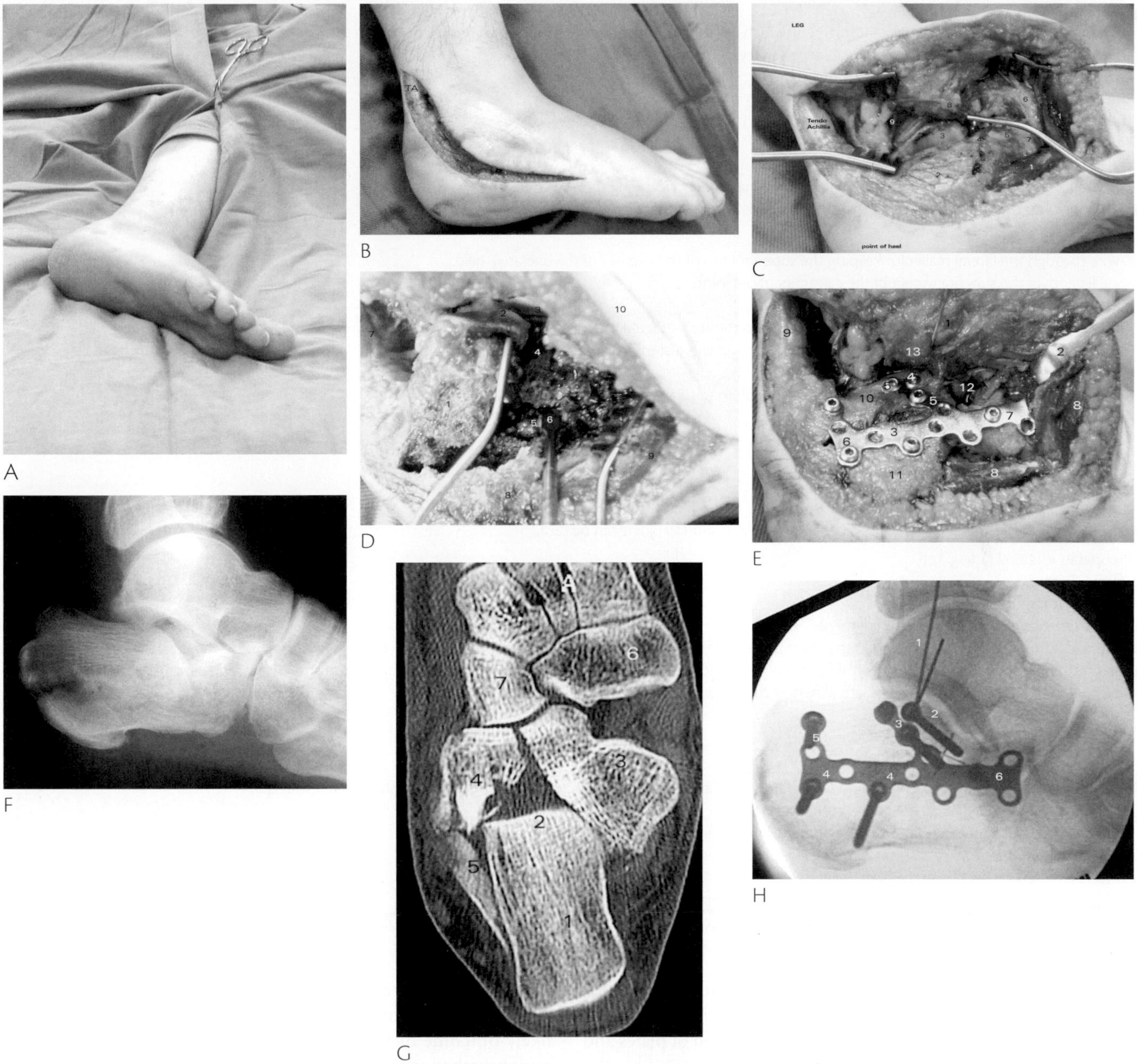

Fig. 12.61.9 Operative fixation of a calcaneus fracture. A) The patient is placed in the lateral position and the foot is draped free.
B) The extended lateral incision. The superior limb is in the midline superiorly, exposing the tendo Achilles (TA). The incision passes inferiorly and anteriorly curving along the apex of the heel.The inferior limb is placed at the inferolateral border of the hindfoot.
C) The full extent of the extended lateral dissection.
1. The abductor digiti minimi is split in the line of its fibres in order to maintain the blood supply to the overlying skin.
2. The visible lateral wall of the fractured calcaneus is comprised in part of the lateral joint fragment and in part of a thin shell of lateral cortex.
3. The inferior articular cartilage of the talus is displayed, demonstrating that the lateral joint fragment is displaced inferiorly.
4. The stout cortical bone of the crucial angle of Gissane which receives the lateral process of the talus.
5. The peroneal tubercle from which the peroneal tendons have been lifted by sub-periosteal dissection of the retinaculum.
6. The peroneal tendons have been lifted away from the calcaneus in order to display the anterior part of the bone.
7. The anterior limit of dissection is the calcaneal aspect of the calcaneo—cuboid joint.
8. The tip of the lateral malleolus, covered in soft tissue.
9. The posteroinferior part of the distal tibia.

D) The orientation is similar to (C). Fracture disimpaction and reduction. The lateral joint fragment has been rotated out of the sub-talar joint on its retained posterior soft tissues, revealing the entire medial wall. The periosteal elevator has been inserted into the medial wall fracture line between the sustentacular fragment superiorly and the body fragment inferiorly. By rotating the instrument handle downwards, the body fragment is moved inferiorly and laterally so reducing the medial wall and providing space into which the lateral joint fragment can be fitted.
1. The lateral wall of the lateral joint fragment. At this point, some of the lateral cortex is missing because it has been elevated from the lateral joint fragment during the fracture, forming the laterally displaced fractured lateral wall.

Fig. 12.61.9 (cont'd)
2. The articular cartilage of the lateral joint fragment which forms part of the calcaneal surface of the subtalar joint.
3. The subtalar joint articular cartilage of the inferior surface of the talus.
4. The lateral surface of the sustentacular fragment.
5. The apex of the body fragment.
6. The periosteal elevator is placed through the medial wall fracture line in order to reduce it.
7. The tendo Achilles.
8. The lateral surface of the body fragment.
9. The inferior fibres of the abductor digiti minimi, which has been split during the approach.
10. The lower arm of the superior flap of the extended lateral approach.

E) Final fixation
1. K-wire through the lateral malleolus keeping the superior limb of the flap out of the operative field.
2. Bone lever over the superior aspect of the calcaneocuboid joint.
3. Calcaneal fracture fixation plate.
4. Cortical lag screw through the lateral joint fragment into the sustentaculum tali part of the sustentacular fragment.
5. Neutralization screws through the lateral joint fragment and the sustentacular fragment.
6. Cancellous screws into the body fragment.
7. Cortical screw into the anterior aspect of the sustentaculum tali. Passing through the anterolateral fragment.
8. Abductor digiti minimi, split in the line of its fibres.
9. Tendo Achilles.
10. Lateral joint fragment.
11. Body fragment.
12. Lateral process of the talus.
13. Just below this, the lateral part of the posterior facet of the sub-talar joint can be seen.

F) Preoperative lateral radiograph.
G) Axial CT scan.
1. Lateral joint fragment
2. Articular cartilage of the lateral joint fragment
3. Sustentaculum tali, which is part of the sustentacular fragment. Note that in this case the coronal secondary fracture line does not pass medial to the primary fracture line so that there is no separate anteromedial fragment. The medial part of the calcaneo-cuboid joint is therefore part of the sustentacular fragment.
4. Anterolateral fragment containing the lateral part of the calcaneo-cuboid joint
5. Lateral wall
6. Navicular bone
7. Cuboid bone

H) Postoperative lateral image intensification radiograph at the time of surgery. Compare to (F). Bohler's angle has been restored.
1. Temporary K wire passing into the fibula (compare to (E)).
2. Lag screw passing through the lateral joint fragment into the sustentacular fragment.
3. Two neutralization screws passing through the lateral joint fragment and the sustentacular fragment.
4. Cancellous screws passing into the body fragment.
5. Cancellous screw passing into the posterior aspect of the lateral joint fragment.
6. Cortical screw passing through the anterolateral fragment into the anterior part of the combined sustentacular and anteromedial fragment.

Sometimes, a comminuted fracture combines features of a standard intra-articular fracture with those of a tuberosity fracture. In these cases, reduction is maintained by a combination of plates and screws and a tension band wire.

Open fractures

Type 1: the fracture is more displaced than the average and therefore untreated the outcome is poor. The open wound is debrided primarily and the foot elevated. By the time that the soft tissues have settled sufficiently to allow internal fixation, the open wound is usually healed and reduction and internal fixation are performed as outlined previously. Alternatively, ORIF may be performed at the time of initial wound debridement.

Type 2: these are among the most challenging hindfoot injuries to manage. Treated conservatively, the severe displacement leads to major disability and the combination of open wounds and unstable fracture fragments predisposes to chronic infection so that there is a high chance of late amputation. Operative treatment is very difficult and plastic surgical cover may be necessary. Surgical treatment may precipitate amputation but on balance it is the better option.

In all open cases and particularly where the open wound is more serious, the risks of ORIF must be carefully weighed against the likely outcome of non-operative management in order to determine whether operative management is indicated.

ST fractures

Treatment is determined by the associated injuries. ORIF may be with a lateral to medial lag screw through an extended lateral approach or from medial to lateral using a direct medial incision. However, the importance of the ST fracture is the instability which it confers on PFSTJ. It is often better to reduce PFSJT under direct vision and stabilize it with a 2mm K-wire. The patient is then mobilized non-weight bearing for 6 weeks in a cast and the wire is then removed.

Fractures in children

Calcaneal fractures in very young children heal uneventfully and treatment consists of immobilization until healing in a few weeks. In older children (see Figure 12.61.5), there is significant scope for remodelling of the hindfoot even after a displaced fracture. The aim of treatment is to provide a fully functional hindfoot with the minimum intervention possible. Minor joint and hindfoot malalignments even out with time but large displacements should be treated by operative reduction. Owing to the simple fracture pattern in adolescents, ORIF is straightforward and gives excellent results without damage to the calcaneal apophysis (Figure 12.61.5).

Compartment syndrome

Toe clawing is common after calcaneal fracture and while this may be due to a missed compartment syndrome, it is more likely to be the result of damage to the intrinsic muscles of the foot at the time of fracture. Foot compartment syndrome does occur and may be common after calcaneal fracture. This suggests that if the patient has clinical features of a compartment syndrome with excessive pain, sensory abnormalities, and raised compartment pressures, decompression should be performed if the patient has been evaluated within 24h. However, the open wounds of compartmental decompression may preclude subsequent ORIF because of the risk of infection. Therefore, either ORIF should be undertaken at the time of decompression or the morbidity of an unreduced calcaneal fracture will need to be traded against the disability of untreated compartment syndrome.

Techniques which avoid open surgery

In an attempt to avoid the massive exposure and consequent morbidity of the extended lateral approach, a number of different percutaneous methods of reduction and fixation have been devised. In some techniques an external fixator is used. They are applicable to a limited range of fractures and must be undertaken at an early stage. Perfect reduction is not obtained but the avoidance of the morbidity of open surgery may compensate for this. Early reports of these techniques are encouraging. It is important to note that the techniques all require a thorough knowledge of fracture anatomy and are generally undertaken by surgeons skilled in calcaneal fracture surgery.

Results

The results in some individual groups are outlined earlier. Despite a bewildering array of papers, the evidence base for calcaneal fracture treatment is unsatisfactory in that 'level 1 evidence' is not available as with much of orthopaedic surgery. The historic literature is difficult to interpret because it is impossible to know the exact nature of the fracture described and more modern studies are small or scientifically flawed or employ outmoded fixation techniques.

In general terms the evidence base for calcaneal fracture outcomes may be summarized as follows.

- Fractures which are initially undisplaced and unite in an undisplaced position fare well
- Displaced fractures give poor outcomes treated non-operatively. The more displaced the fracture the worse the outcome
- Modern operative treatment is safe but technically highly demanding
- An anatomical surgical reduction with stable internal fixation gives a better result than non-anatomical reduction
- The eventual disability may be predicted from the nature and displacement of the fracture.

Disability after fracture (Box 12.61.2)

Introduction

In deciding whether to treat a calcaneal fracture by ORIF, knowledge of the expected disability and management of a conservatively treated fracture is essential. The problem is that there are multiple causes of symptoms and overlapping disability syndromes. The patient will complain of a combination of pain, limitation of walking ability and derangement of their lifestyle and a superficial history and examination may give little indication of the true cause of the problem. In the past, excessive concentration on PFSTJ as the major cause of symptoms has clouded the issue. In a calcaneal malunion, careful assessment will usually reveal one or more of the following:

Subtalar joint derangement

Angular malalignment

Angular PFSTJ malalignment is invariable in a standard intra-articular calcaneal fracture. It may cause minimal early symptoms. The more severe the malalignment and the greater STJ comminution, the more likely is the development of painful arthritis later. This causes pain on walking particularly on uneven ground. Rest pain is a late feature.

In the presence of normal hindfoot biomechanics, subtalar joint symptoms are not usually a significant problem unless the patient in a heavy manual worker or regular rough ground walker. Therefore, isolated angular PFSTJ malalignment is not a strong indication for ORIF and symptoms may be treated with fusion. However, angular PFSTJ malalignment is usually associated with abnormalities of hindfoot biomechanics.

Subtalar joint depression

True lateral joint fragment depression invariably causes serious disability. There is a sense of insecurity and giving way within the foot with lateral pain on taking a step. With time rest pain occurs. Examination reveals tenderness laterally and a valgus hindfoot. This severe disability is an inevitable consequence of subtalar depression and this feature is a strong indication for ORIF.

Box 12.61.2 Disability after fracture

- Subtalar joint derangement:
    - Angular malalignment
    - Subtalar joint depression
- Abnormal hindfoot biomechanics:
    - Heelstrike medial
    - Heelstrike lateral
    - Short heel
- Anterior calcaneal syndromes
- Heelpad syndrome
- Fibular impingement.

Abnormal hindfoot biomechanics

This is due principally to BF displacement; this is a common cause of severe disability. Three syndromes occur: heelstrike medial, heelstrike lateral, and short heel.

Heelstrike medial

BF displacement has carried the heelstrike point medial to the axis of the hindfoot, the unloaded hindfoot lies in varus, accentuated on weight bearing. These patients complain of severe difficulty in walking or standing. There is a cavus midfoot and the medial ray is unloaded. At toe-off, the varus is accentuated because of TA medialization. Supination instability is common and the patient may walk on the outer border of the foot. FHL is often trapped in the fracture. Degenerative changes of the ankle and midfoot occur rapidly with increasing pain.

Conservative treatment of these feet is of little use. The only satisfactory solution is surgical reconstruction of the heel and this is made particularly difficult by the varus position of the hindfoot. Therefore, BF varus and internal rotation position, which will produce a heelstrike medial syndrome is a strong indication for ORIF.

Heelstrike lateral

This is more benign than heelstrike medial but less common. There is a valgus heel with fibular impingement and a planus midfoot, accentuated and painful on load bearing. Compensatory overactivity of tibialis posterior causes calf pain. However, resection of the lateral bony boss will make matters worse by allowing the heel to collapse further into valgus. Likewise, in situ fusion of STJ will destroy the compensatory effect of subtalar inversion and may make matters worse.

Treatment by a medial shoe-raise and supporting insole is often extremely effective in these cases. Operative treatment to reconstruct the hindfoot biomechanics and fuse STJ is easier than in the case of heelstrike medial.

Short heel

Following a calcaneal fracture, the heel is always shortened and broadened in relation to the extent of the displacement. However, when the heelstrike is displaced medially or laterally, the symptoms from this shortening are usually masked by those more intrusive problems.

The short broad heel causes problems with shoeware and sometimes the broadening is sufficient to cause lateral pain beneath the fibula. The major problem is, however, weakness of plantarflexion due to reduction of the moment arm of the gastrocnemius-soleus complex. In order to compensate for the short heel, the ankle is held in dorsiflexion and if the problem is severe, there may be an overall apparent equinus deformity of the foot. The abnormal posture of the ankle may lead to secondary arthritis. The patients characteristically complain of weakness of the foot and limping, while in a severe case, the equinus may lead to catching the foot. Later ankle arthritic pain becomes a feature.

Treatment is by a heel raise to restore the ankle to neutral and protect it; however, the patient often finds that this makes them symptomatically worse by exaggerating the weakness of the plantarflexors. Operative treatment is by hindfoot reconstruction. If treatment is delayed until ankle arthritis supervenes, the situation is difficult to recover.

Anterior calcaneal syndromes

Owing to its attachment to the bifurcate ligament, the anterior part of AMF is rarely displaced following a fracture. The posterior part is attached to the talus and may ride upwards compared to PFSTJ. The displacement is seldom great, however even this small malalignment may contribute to blocking subtalar joint movement. In contrast, ALF will often tip upwards because of its attachment to the inferior peroneal retinaculum. As it does so its posterosuperior border fills in the crucial angel of Gissane preventing eversion of heel and in severe cases causing a fixed inversion deformity. When this is combined with a medial translation of the heel due to BF movement, the resulting disability is severe.

ALF syndrome is seen in untreated isolated compression fractures or in inadequately treated fractures where the crucial angle of Gissane has not been correctly addressed. The patient complains of pain, initially only on attempted eversion. Gradually the pain becomes more intrusive, occurring first on walking on rough ground, then on any walking, on standing and finally as arthritic changes occur at rest. Rarely a late spontaneous fusion will occur. In my experience excision of the displaced fragment at a late stage does not relieve symptoms and fusion combined with reconstruction of the hindfoot is necessary.

These symptoms are an inevitable result of the displacement of LJF and I regard displacement of this fragment as a strong indication for ORIF of the fracture.

Heelpad syndrome

The specialized weight-bearing tissues of the heelpad are not permanently damaged in a calcaneal fracture and heelpad pain is rare after ORIF. However, in a displaced calcaneal fracture, shards of bone may penetrate the deep structures of the sole of the foot. If the fracture is treated conservatively, these pieces unite in their displaced position. These patients are always severely disabled clinically. They walk with a severe limp and great pain, although rest pain is rare. Treatment is very difficult. Thick insoles are of some help but reconstructive surgery is usually required and it is difficult to remove all the bone at this stage. Even a radical removal of the protruding bone combined with reconstruction does not relieve the heelpad pain. In contrast, acute fracture reduction removes the shards from the sole and heelpad pain does not occur. Therefore I regard bony protrusion in the heelpad as a strong indication for operative treatment of a fracture in the acute stage.

Fibular impingement (peroneal tendon impingement)

During a calcaneal fracture, lateral wall expansion closes the space between it and the fibula and compresses or even dislocates the peroneal tendons. In a severe case, the laterally displaced calcaneum will articulate with the lateral malleolus, defunctioning the ankle joint. Isolated lateral wall protrusion is effectively treated by simple resection. However, fibular impingement is usually associated with abnormal hindfoot biomechanics due to BF displacement. Simple lateral wall resection in these cases may cause further valgus collapse of the heel, worsening symptoms.

Late surgery in operated cases

After ORIF, metalwork removal is frequently necessary, which may be combined with arthrolysis of PFSTJ. This will often improve symptoms of apparent subtalar arthritis. It is therefore reasonable to do this surgery and defer fusion in a marginal case. *In situ* subtalar arthrodesis may be required for degenerative change but usually this is deferred to 2 years, since symptoms may settle for this period. It is performed either through the extended lateral incision or a sinus tarsi approach.

Reconstruction of calcaneal malunion

Calcaneal malunion surgery is technically highly demanding surgery. The case is analysed by careful clinical examination, plain radiology, and CT scanning. I do not find gait analysis or pedobarography of use. Non-operative treatment consists of modification of shoeware, the use of supportive and cushioning insoles and even a caliper, and change of lifestyle to cope with the disability. Some care must be exercised in pursuing a conservative course. Calcaneal malunion surgery is a major undertaking. There may well be morbidity from the bone graft donor site and if deep infection occurs, amputation is likely. However, a significantly misaligned calcaneum will cause a dorsiflexed talus leading in time to ankle arthritis, while bone beneath the lateral malleolus will eventually cause peroneal tendon dislocation or rupture. In addition, the hindfoot malalignment strains Chopart's joint causing arthritis. In these circumstances reconstruction needs to be performed early for optimal results. The problems that will be encountered include lateral impingement, peroneal tendon dislocation, PFSTJ arthritis, hindfoot malalignment, and bone in the sole of the foot.

The aim of surgical reconstruction is to restore the biomechanics and fuse degenerate joints. *In situ* subtalar fusion is ineffectual except rarely where there is symptomatic PFSTJ degeneration with normal hindfoot biomechanics.

Surgery is invariably performed through an extended lateral approach and proceeds stepwise, correcting only the necessary problems. The protruding lateral wall is resected. Dislocated peroneal tendons are located. PFSTJ is entered and laminar spreaders used to derotate the talus into correct orientation. PFSTJ is prepared and the talus held in its corrected position with a bone block from the ileac crest. An extra-articular calcaneal osteotomy is undertaken and used to place the heelstrike point in the correct place. If necessary, a bone block is used to hold the correction. The peroneal tendons are relocated in a new groove behind the lateral malleolus. The wound is sutured in three layers beginning with the periosteum.

In a two-part fracture dislocation, the reconstructive surgery is different. Through the extended lateral approach, the primary fracture line is found inferomedial to the talus. It is re-opened and the dislocated calcaneal body relocated. A PFSTJ fusion is undertaken if necessary.

Further reading

Eastwood, D.M., Gregg, P., and Atkins, R.M. (1993). Calcaneal fractures: pathological anatomy and classification. *Journal of Bone and Joint Surgery*, **75B**, 183–9.

Freeman, B.J., Duff, S., Allen, P.E., Nicholson, H.D., and Atkins, R.M. (1998). The extended lateral approach to the hindfoot. The anatomical basis and surgical implications. *Journal of Bone and Joint Surgery*, **80B**, 139–42.

Sanders, R. (2000). Current Concepts Review: Displaced Intra-articular fractures of the calcaneus. *Journal of Bone and Joint Surgery*, **82A**, 225–50.

Squires, B., Allen, P.E., Livingstone, J., and Atkins, R.M. (2001). Fractures of the tuberosity of the calcaneus. *Journal of Bone and Joint Surgery*, **83B**, 55–61.

Zwipp, H., Tscherne, H., Thermann, H., and Weber, T. (1993). Osteosynthesis of displaced intraarticular fractures of the calcaneus. *Clinical Orthopaedics and Related Research*, **290**, 76–86.

12.62

Midfoot and forefoot fractures and dislocations

Andrew Taylor

Summary points

- Mid- and forefoot injuries are common
- Minimally displaced and stable injuries allow early weight-bearing rehabilitation and lead to a good functional outcome
- Displaced and unstable injuries require restoration of the length, alignment, and joint congruency followed by stable fixation
- Respect the soft tissue element of the foot injury.

Introduction

Injuries to the mid- and forefoot are common. Many of these injuries are relatively benign. Fractures that are minimally displaced without significant soft tissue injury may be expected to give satisfactory clinical results with minimal intervention. However, a significant proportion of mid- and forefoot injuries can give rise to long-term impairment and disability, and require more careful attention.

Successful management of these injuries depends on recognizing the important distinction between the benign fracture and more significant fractures and dislocations that disrupt the normal form and function of the mid- and forefoot. Early functional rehabilitation is possible for minor fractures. More significant injuries require restoration of length and alignment of the columns of the mid- and forefoot, restoration of joint congruity, followed by stable fixation to achieve the best possible results. Even with optimum treatment of severe injuries, recovery may be incomplete. However, as close a restoration of normal anatomy as is possible is more likely to yield a more favourable outcome.

Functional anatomy

The foot may be considered as a tripod. The limbs are formed by the heel, with a medial column running from the talus through the cuneiforms, medial metatarsals, and toes and a lateral column running through the cuboid and lateral two metatar sals. Maintaining the relative length and alignment of these columns is a key element in treating mid- and forefoot injuries successfully.

It is convenient to consider the foot and ankle as units—ankle, hind-, mid-, and forefoot. Functionally, these units are integrated. Disruption of one unit may affect function throughout, and injuries commonly extend across more than one 'unit'.

The midfoot spans the area between Chopart's joint and Lisfranc's joint. It is formed by the navicular, three cuneiforms, and cuboid bones. Chopart's joint is formed by the talonavicular and calcaneocuboid articulations. With the hindfoot everted, the axis of these joints lie parallel, allowing maximum flexibility through the midfoot. With the hindfoot inverted, the joint axes converge thus locking the transverse tarsal joint and providing a more rigid lever for propulsion. Restricting movement at either joint limits movement at the other, as well as limiting movement at the subtalar joint by up to 50%.

Tibialis posterior provides the power to invert the subtalar joint and adduct the forefoot through its broad insertion on the navicular tuberosity and plantar aspect of the mid- and forefoot. It is opposed by the action of peroneus brevis that inserts on the base of the fifth metatarsal. Tibialis anterior inserts plantar medially on the medial cuneiform and base of the first metatarsal. Peroneus longus provides the antagonist.

There is little movement between the bones of the midfoot. Loss of motion between these joints is well tolerated.

Lisfranc's joint is formed between the base of the metatarsal bones distally and the three cuneiforms medially and cuboid laterally. In cross-section they resemble the form of a Roman arch, providing some inherent stability. They are held in place by strong plantar ligaments and weaker dorsal ligaments that are little more than the condensation of the joint capsule. Medially, the joint is relatively stable. The fourth and fifth tarsometatarsal joints permit significant motion, which allows the foot to adapt to uneven surfaces.

The base of the second metatarsal is recessed between the medial and lateral cuneiforms. Lisfranc's ligament extends between the plantar aspects of medial cuneiform and the base of the second metatarsal. Strong ligaments connect the second to fifth metatarsals, but there is no corresponding connection between the first and second metatarsal bases.

The first metatarsal is shorter and wider than the lesser metatarsals. The first metatarsal head bears twice the weight of each of the lesser metatarsals through the two subjacent hallucal sesamoids.

The lesser metatarsals demonstrate increasing sagittal mobility from medial to lateral. The only extrinsic attachments on the lesser metatarsals are the peroneus brevis and tertius muscles as they insert on the base and shaft of the fifth metatarsal, respectively.

An extension of the plantar aponeurosis, the deep transverse metatarsal ligament, serves as a transverse 'tether' between the metatarsal heads, except between the first and the second. This structure also limits excessive mobility in the sagittal plane.

The hallux has two phalanges, each with the insertion of a flexor and extensor tendon. The three phalanges of each lesser toe are similar. Flexor digitorum brevis attaches to each intermediate phalanx by way of two separate slips on either side of the flexor digitorum longus tendon. The distal phalanges are small and serve as attachments for the extensor digitorum longus and flexor digitorum longus.

The plantar aponeurosis runs from the tubercle of the calcaneum to the base of each proximal phalanx. It provides static support for the medial longitudinal arch of the foot. On dorsiflexion of the toes, the effective length of the aponeurosis shortens—the windlass effect—and further stabilizes the longitudinal arch.

Clinical evaluation

The majority of mid- and forefoot fractures occur in isolation. They are the result of low and medium energy trauma. Careful clinical examination for localizing tenderness will usually identify the anatomical location of the injury. Swelling and bruising develop rapidly, and may mask rather than reveal the exact site of injury.

The evaluation of high-energy injuries is more of a challenge. There may be other injuries that require immediate attention or distract from the 'minor' foot injury. In addition to identifying any fracture or dislocation, the soft tissue element must be considered. The presence of open injuries or devitalized skin from crush or degloving must be noted. Compartment syndrome should be excluded, although this can be more difficult to assess in the foot than the leg. The neurovascular status must be carefully evaluated and documented, especially after any manipulations.

Once assessed, the foot can be elevated and rested in a well-padded splint. A pneumatic compression device may be used in the case of severe, closed soft tissue injuries if tolerated by the patient.

Investigations

The majority of mid- and forefoot injuries can be diagnosed and managed on the basis of plain x-rays. The x-ray should be centred on the area of clinical concern. Standard dorsoplantar, lateral, and oblique views should be requested. Additional specific views, e.g. for the sesamoids or Lisfranc's joint, will be required on the basis of clinical examination.

When initial x-rays are normal or inconclusive, further imaging is required. Stress x-rays may be taken with the patient anaesthetized or with a more cooperative patient weight bearing after severe pain has resolved. However, computed tomography (CT) scan is the most useful additional investigation for diagnosing subtle injuries or defining the nature of complex injuries in greater detail. Appropriately directed requests and discussions with the radiologist are more likely to be fruitful than undirected scans.

Specific injuries

Navicular

The navicular is the keystone of the medial longitudinal arch of the foot—being wider dorsally than plantarwards. It is also wider medially than laterally. The proximal surface is concave and articulates with the head of the talus. This joint allows significant inversion and eversion as part of the subtalar–transverse tarsal articulation. Distally, it is relatively flat where it articulates with the cuneiforms. Little motion occurs at these joints.

Short dorsal and plantar ligaments support the naviculocuneiform joints. Proximally, the navicular is supported by the spring ligament and tendon of tibialis posterior. The dorsal and plantar talonavicular ligaments receive some reinforcement from the anterior deltoid ligament. Laterally, there is a variable articulation with the cuboid.

The central third of the navicular is relatively avascular. This may predispose to stress fractures of the central navicular and the risk of delayed healing or avascular collapse in acute injuries.

An accessory ossicle, the os tibialae externum, is present in up to 25% of the population. It lies in the insertion of the tibialis posterior to the navicular. It is bilateral 90% of the time. It is possible for adults to fracture the synchondrosis that exists between the ossicle and the navicular tuberosity.

Classification

Fractures of the navicular can be divided into fractures of the tuberosity, dorsal lip fractures, fractures of the body and stress fractures. Body fractures are subdivided into displaced and undisplaced. Displaced fractures may be further classified into Type I (coronal plane with large dorsal fragment), Type II (oblique dorsal plantar fragment with large medial fragment and Type III (comminuted). There may be associated injuries to the rest of the mid- and forefoot.

Management (Box 12.62.1)

Dorsal lip fractures are avulsion injuries resulting from forced plantar flexion. Other ligament injuries to the midfoot, subtalar and ankle joints should be excluded. They are stable injuries. They can be treated symptomatically with cast immobilization or bracing as required for 3–4 weeks. Prominent fragments that remain symptomatic may be excised.

Navicular tuberosity fractures are caused by forced abduction or eversion of the midfoot on the hindfoot. They should be differentiated from disruption of the synchondrosis of the accessory navicular. Associated fractures of the cuboid or forefoot may occur in association and so should be considered (Figure 12.62.1). Displacement is

Box 12.62.1 Management of navicular fractures

- Dorsal chip fractures and non-displaced tuberosity and body fractures are treated conservatively (6–8 weeks, below knee weight bearing cast)
- Undisplaced body fractures (6–8 weeks below knee non-weight bearing cast)
- Displaced body fractures are treated with open reduction and screw fixation
- Repetitive trauma (6–8 weeks below knee non-weight bearing cast).

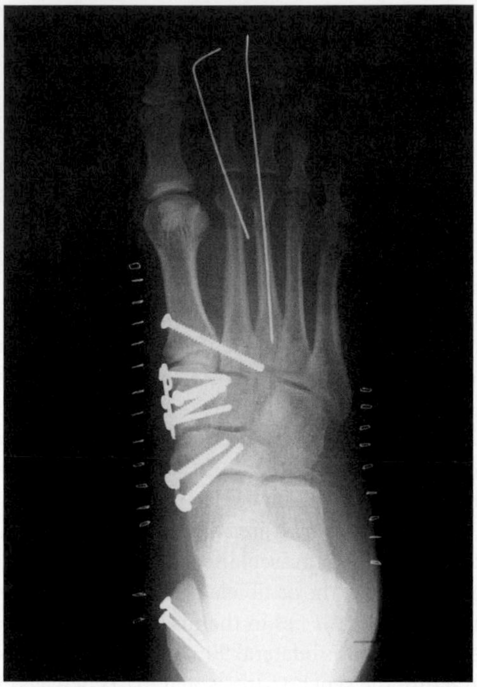

Fig. 12.62.1 This extensive medial column injury including a navicular tuberosity and medial cuneiform fracture, isolated first tarsometatarsal joint subluxation, and second and third metatarsal fractures, occurred in a motor vehicle accident. Multiple associated injuries in the forefoot are common.

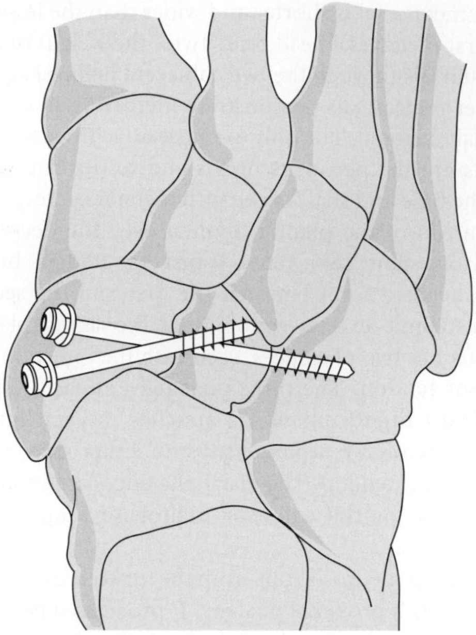

Fig. 12.62.2 Illustration of fixation of the navicular body fracture. Occasionally, screws need to be advanced into an adjacent bone to provide secure fixation. They are then removed after satisfactory bony healing has occurred. (Reproduced from Hansen and Swiontkowski (1993).)

uncommon, and may require open reduction and internal fixation with lag screws. The majority of tuberosity fractures can be managed in a supporting below-knee weight-bearing cast for 6–8 weeks. Occasionally, fibrous union occurs. If symptomatic, internal fixation should be considered. Where the fragment is too small, excision of the fragment and advancement and reattachment of the tibialis posterior tendon can be performed.

Fractures of the body are often the result of high-energy injuries. They may be isolated, but in all cases associated mid- and forefoot disruption should be considered and managed appropriately. Treatment is aimed at restoring the length, alignment, and stability of the medial column. Reconstruction of joint congruency, especially the talonavicular joint, should be achieved when possible. Specific complications of post-traumatic arthritis, deformity, and avascular necrosis may still occur.

Undisplaced navicular body fractures may be treated in a short-leg non-weight-bearing cast until radiographic healing is complete. This is usually 6–8 weeks. An orthotic device may be used thereafter to support the arch.

Displaced body fractures should be managed by open reduction and fixation when the soft tissues allow. Lag screw fixation is suitable for simple fracture patterns when anatomical reduction has been achieved. When comminution precludes this, the larger fragments may be reduced and fixed to the adjacent cuneiforms (Figure 12.62.2). Bridging the fracture with a plate or external fixator can maintain length and alignment while bone and ligament healing occurs. Any such bridging fixation will require removal before unprotected weight bearing is allowed, usually at 8–12 weeks. Bone graft is used when defects exist after reduction. Primary arthrodesis may be considered in cases where there is extensive destruction of the articular surfaces, taking care to maintain the length and alignment of the medial column.

Stress fractures of the navicular may occur following repetitive trauma, typically running. Symptoms of pain in the midfoot, aggravated by activity and relieved with rest should raise the suspicion of a stress fracture. Plain x-rays may be difficult to interpret, and CT or magnetic resonance imaging (MRI) scan may be required to make the diagnosis. Non-displaced (complete or incomplete) stress fractures should be treated in a short-leg non-weight-bearing cast for 6–8 weeks. Displaced injuries or fractures which did not unite with appropriate non-operative treatment should be treated with open reduction and lag screw fixation and bone grafting. This is followed by immobilization in a non-weight-bearing short-leg cast until union is complete.

Results

The more severe the injury the worse the outcome. In one study satisfactory reduction (defined as restoration of 60% of the joint surface) was achieved in all Type I fractures. In 67% of Type II fractures satisfactory reduction was achieved, and only 50% of Type III injuries were reduced satisfactorily. A satisfactory reduction was associated with a good clinical result (no restriction of daily living but pain associated with vigorous activities).

The majority of undisplaced stress fractures will heal when managed in a non-weight-bearing cast. However, displaced fractures treated by limited activity but persistent weight bearing are liable to result in pain associated with delayed union, non-union, or fracture recurrence. Therefore, operative treatment of navicular stress fractures is advised if radiographs show a wide fracture gap, cyst formation, delayed healing, or extension of an incomplete fracture. Recovery may take up to 12 months.

Complications

Avascular necrosis may follow either traumatic or stress fractures of the navicular body. If avascular necrosis involves only a small portion of the navicular, the patient may still have a satisfactory result. Larger areas of avascular necrosis often lead to collapse, arthrosis, and pain.

Malreduced or unreduced body fractures typically result in painful arthrosis. Persistent pain may accompany non-union of either body or tuberosity fractures (Figure 12.62.3).

Cuboid fractures

The cuboid occupies an important position in the lateral column of the foot. It articulates with the calcaneus, lateral cuneiform, fourth and fifth metatarsals, and sometimes the navicular. Injuries to this bone may alter articular relationships, which result in long-term deformity and disability.

Fortunately, most cuboid fractures are minimally displaced capsular avulsion fractures associated with inversion injuries and are treated symptomatically. Compressive forces typically produce higher-energy injuries resulting in more serious problems. The mechanism of injury involves forefoot abduction causing compression of the cuboid between the lateral two metatarsals and the calcaneus. Because of this mechanism, the cuboid body fracture has been called 'the nutcracker fracture'. Cuboid fractures often accompany other midfoot injuries, particularly tarsometatarsal joint injuries and navicular fractures.

Cuboid fractures may be difficult to image. Plain radiograph evaluations should include an oblique view. While plain films usually demonstrate this injury, the amount of intra-articular displacement and collapse is often underestimated. CT scan provides more accurate information about the magnitude of displacement and intra-articular incongruity as well as any associated medial column injury that may accompany cuboid fractures (Figure 12.62.4).

Classification

No meaningful classification system currently exists because of their infrequent occurrence. Cuboid fractures are typically referred to as capsular avulsion injuries, displaced or undisplaced body fractures.

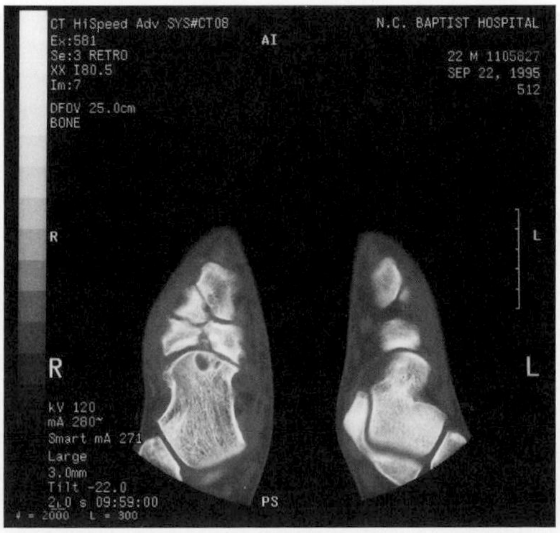

Fig. 12.62.3 CT scan demonstrates the origin of chronic midfoot pain in this runner to be both non-union of a navicular stress fracture and subsequent talonavicular and naviculocuneiform arthritis.

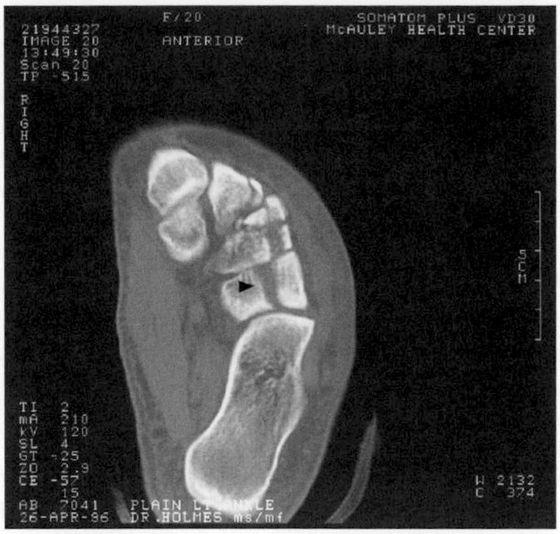

Fig. 12.62.4 This lateral column combination is well imaged on CT scan. Preoperative planning is greatly enhanced.

Management

Avulsion and undisplaced fractures may be treated in a short-leg weight-bearing cast with progressive weight bearing.

Treatment goals for displaced injuries should be those of any displaced intra-articular fracture: accurate anatomic reduction and stable fixation. A longitudinal dorsolateral incision is recommended. The extensor brevis is reflected medially and the peroneal tendons are protected. This approach provides exposure of both calcaneocuboid and cuboid-metatarsal joints. Impaction of the cuboid articular surface is frequently seen. A small distractor placed between the fifth metatarsal base and the calcaneus may be helpful in restoring cuboid length. Articular surfaces should be elevated and buttressed, with bone graft or substitutes. A plate spanning the cuboid from proximal to distal can be applied (Figure 12.62.5). If comminution of the fracture precludes stable fixation, a plate or external fixator may be applied as temporary bridging fixation of the calcaneocuboid or tarsometatarsal joints.

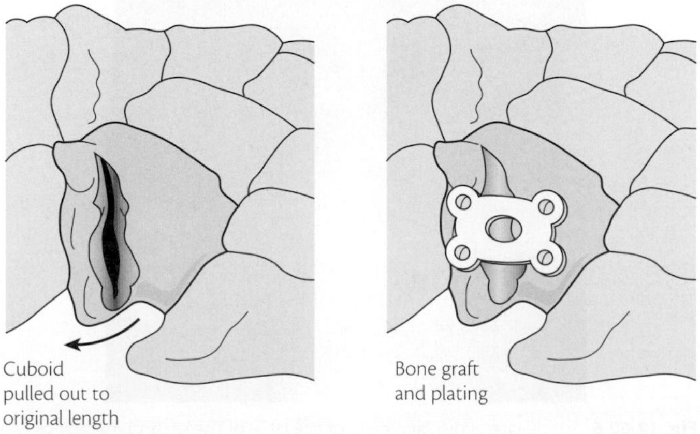

Fig. 12.62.5 Cuboid fracture reduced to restore length, bone grafted and plated. (Adapted from Hansen and Swiontkowski (1993).)

Results

Cuboid fractures are uncommon and so no large series have been reported. However, displaced fractures treated non-operatively tend to fair badly, often requiring late salvage by arthrodesis. In series where fractures have been reduced and fixed adequately, results tend to be better. Therefore, open reduction and stable fixation is recommended for displaced fractures.

Complications

Articular incongruity may result in degenerative arthritis and pain. Cuboid collapse will shorten the lateral column, and may result in medial or lateral foot pain.

Salvage

Fractures of the cuboid that result in post-traumatic arthritis of the calcaneocuboid joint or symptomatic shortening of the lateral column of the foot can be managed by arthrodesis. A tricortical iliac crest bone graft may be used to correct significant shortening.

Degenerative changes at the cuboid–fourth and fifth metatarsal articulation is a more difficult problem. Los of motion in these joints is more debilitating than on the medial side of the foot. Interposition arthroplasty has been described as a treatment for this difficult problem.

Tarsometatarsal (Lisfranc) injuries (Box 12.62.2)

Lisfranc injuries refers to any bony or ligamentous disruption of the tarsometatarsal complex. This covers a broad spectrum of injuries. A high proportion of injuries are overlooked, especially in multiply injured patients or in low-energy injuries. Associated midfoot injuries are common. Neglected injuries often result in long-term pain, deformity, and disability. Early recognition and appropriate management can reduce the risk of such complications.

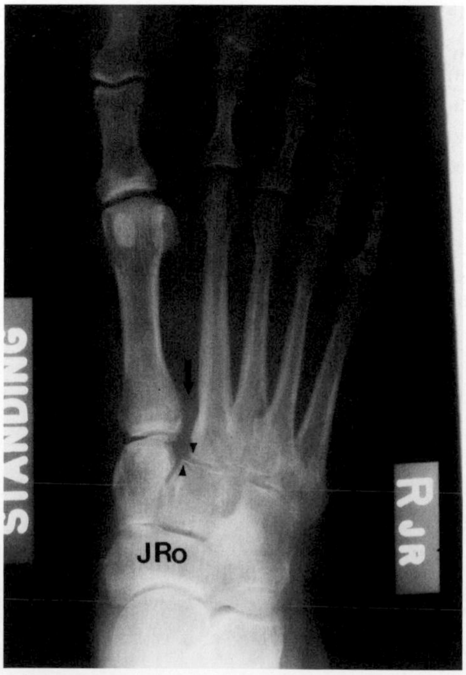

Fig. 12.62.6 Subtle lateral displacement of the base of the second metatarsal relative to the middle cuneiform. Equally, subtle lateral shift of first metatarsal base is also present.

Lisfranc injuries may be caused by direct or transmitted forces. Direct trauma may be applied as a dorsal crush or on the plantar aspect, for example through a car pedal (although it is difficult to determine whether an indirect load from the intruding foot well is the more likely mechanism) Longitudinal compressive forces applied to a plantar-flexed foot, as occurs in sport or even from simple falls down a step can be sufficient to disrupt a normal tarsometatarsal joint.

A high index of clinical suspicion is the key to avoid missing Lisfranc injuries. Significant midfoot pain, swelling and bruising, and an inability to weight bear merit active exclusion of a Lisfranc injury. Associated injuries should also be considered (e.g. intercuneiform disruption and cuboid fractures and calcaneocuboid joint injuries). Gentle manipulation of the distal metatarsals may provoke significant tarsometatarsal pain in individuals who have sustained this injury. The foot is usually too swollen at acute presentation to detect subtle instability, but this may become apparent after several days.

X-ray examination should focus on the tarsometatarsal joint. In subtle injuries, weight-bearing views taken after the acute pain has settled or after the administration of local nerve blocks can unmask an occult injury. A 20-degree sagittal oblique anteroposterior (AP) view, 45- degree coronal oblique view, and lateral view should be requested. On the AP view, the medial border of the base of the second metatarsal and the medial border of the medial cuneiform should be an unbroken line (Figure 12.62.6). Avulsion of the insertion of Lisfranc's ligament, the 'fleck sign', may be the only indication of a significant injury. Variants of the Lisfranc joint injury may also involve disruption of the cunieforms, (Figure 12.62.7). On the oblique projection, the medial base of the fourth metatarsal should line up with the medial border of the cuboid. Normal variations of 2–3mm have been described at this articulation. On the sagittal view, dorsal displacement of the metatarsal bases may be evident. On the lateral view, angular and/or translational abnormalities are often seen (Figure 12.62.8).

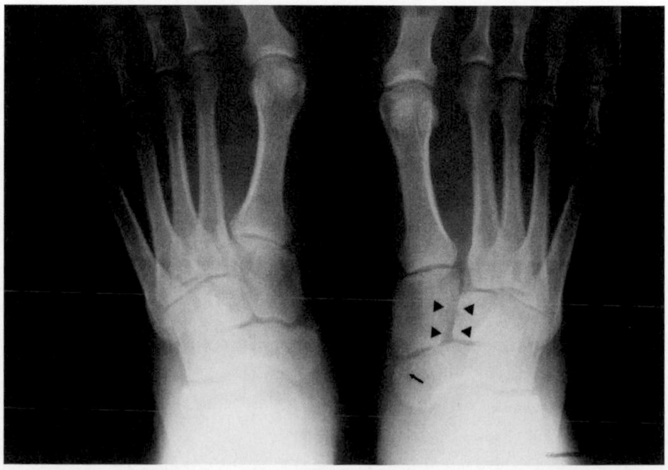

Fig. 12.62.7 Disruption between the medial and middle cuneiform represents a variant of the Lisfranc's joint injury. Note the navicular tuberosity fracture, often associated with this injury.

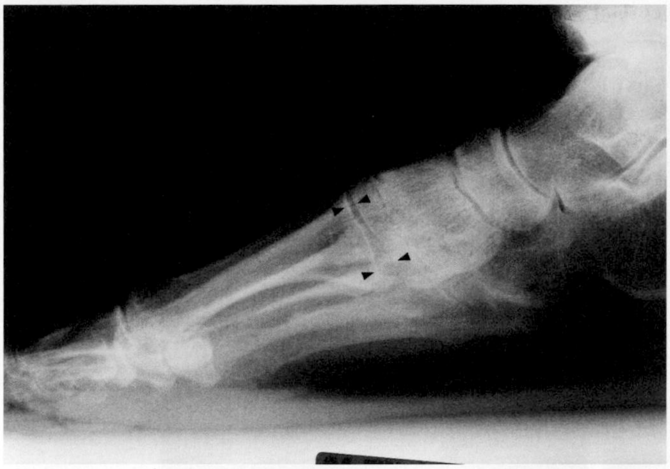

Fig. 12.62.8 Lateral radiograph demonstrates the first metatarsal to be dorsally translated and plantar widening of the joint.

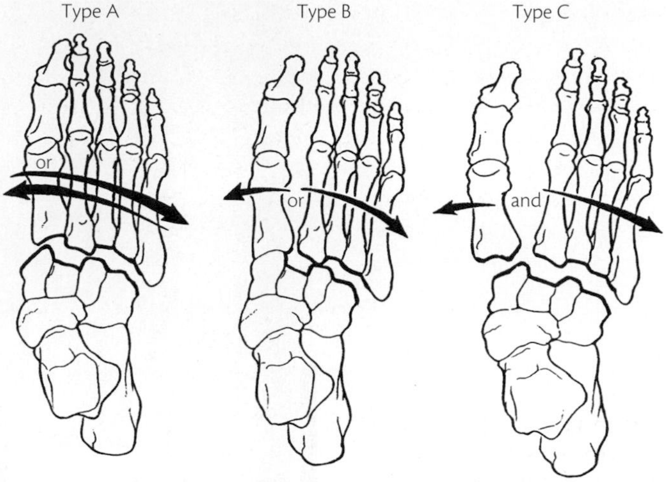

Fig. 12.62.10 Simplified classification of Lisfranc's fracture–dislocation: type A, complete homolateral dislocation; type B, partial dislocation (can be medial or lateral); type C, divergent dislocation. This system does not account for intercuneiform variations. (Reproduced from Hansen and Swiontkowski (1993).)

CT scanning is useful to pick up some occult injuries and to evaluate more complex injury patterns to aid in preoperative planning (Figure 12.62.9).

Classification

There are a number of classifications for tarsometatarsal injuries. None of these are comprehensive due to the diverse spectrum of injuries. Interobserver agreement is moderate at best. None of the classification systems have been shown to be prognostic. The outline of a popular system is reproduced in Figure 12.62.10.

Management

The goals of management of Lisfranc injuries are early recognition, anatomical reduction, and stable fixation. Closed reduction of grossly displaced injuries should be undertaken to reduce further soft tissue compromise. Temporary splintage, elevation, and the use of a foot pump aid the soft tissue management. Open reduction and internal fixation (ORIF) should be performed as soon as the soft tissues allow.

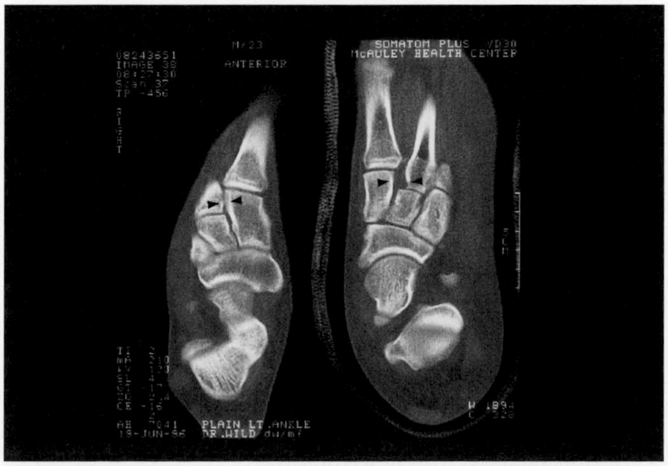

Fig. 12.62.9 Significant displacement of the base of the second metatarsal is easily seen on CT scans when plain radiographic interpretation is unclear.

Urgent fixation may be required in the presence of open fractures, compartment syndrome, or vascular injuries together with appropriate soft tissue management. In complex injuries, it is reasonable to stabilize the injury with temporary bridging fixation until the patient's general condition and soft tissue allow, and a suitably experienced team is available to perform definitive surgery.

ORIF is recommended for displaced tarsometatarsal joint injuries. Even if closed reduction can be accomplished, instability persists. Incisions must be planned to allow exposure of the relevant joints to confirm reduction. Fixation with a single positional screw of 3.5mm diameter is usually sufficient for the first to third tarsometatarsal joints (Figure 12.62.11). More complex fractures may require bridging with plates or external fixation.

More recently, it has been proposed that in patients with purely ligamentous injuries that fusion of the first to third tarsometatarsal joints is associated with a better outcome than open reduction and fixation alone. This has yet to receive acceptance across the board, but it has been my practice to consider arthrodesis in the older, low-demand patients with isolated Lisfranc's joint injuries.

Reduction and fixation of the fourth and fifth tarsometatarsal joints should be performed if displacement persists here after medial tarsometatarsal joint stabilization.

Protected weight bearing in a brace or cast may start at 8 weeks along with an active range of motion exercise programme for the hindfoot, ankle, and metatarsophalangeal joints. Hardware removal may be considered after 4 months. If the more mobile fourth and fifth tarsometatarsal joints have been stabilized, the lateral hardware should be removed before weight bearing.

Results

Better results are achieved when better reduction is achieved and maintained. Patients treated by open reduction and internal fixation do better than those treated by closed reduction and percutaneous pinning or closed reduction and plaster immobilization. Quality and maintenance of the initial reduction correlate with better clinical results.

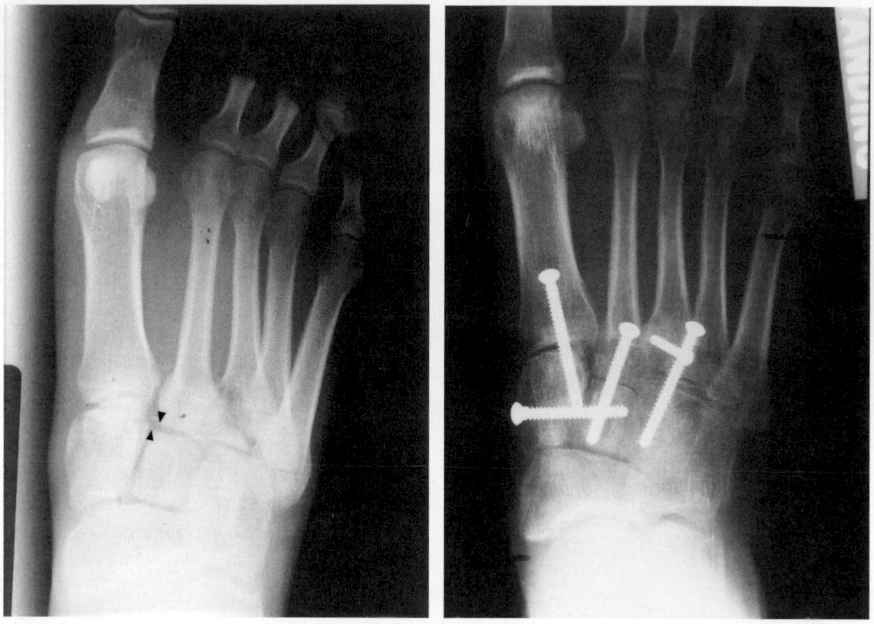

A B

Fig. 12.62.11 A) Lisfranc variant with subtle second tarsometatarsal disruption, third metatarsal base fracture, and intercuneiform disruption (discovered intraoperatively by stress testing and direct inspection). B) Fractures and ligamentous disruption have been reduced and stabilized.

However, patients defined as having good or excellent result often complain of residual symptoms. Those who do significant amounts of standing or walking are often not able to return to their pre-injury level of activity.

In patients with unrecognized or inadequately treated injuries pain and swelling and deformity often lead to significant impairment and disability.

Complications

Compartment syndromes may accompany Lisfranc joint injuries. This is discussed later.

Wound slough, particularly when using a two-incision technique, has been described. This problem can be minimized by waiting until the soft tissues are showing signs of wrinkling, no undermining of skin incisions and maintaining a skin bridge of at least 3cm.

Nerve injury, particularly the deep peroneal nerve and medial branches of the superficial peroneal nerve, can be minimized by careful dissection.

Hardware problems including screw breakage may also occur if the patient prematurely bears weight. Reflex sympathetic dystrophy may be the result of either the injury or surgical treatment. Early recognition and aggressive treatment can minimize any functional disability.

Salvage

Tarsometatarsal arthrodesis is indicated for patients with intractable pain following a Lisfranc's joint injury. Restoration of normal midfoot alignment should be the goal in addition to bony union of the affected joints.

Good pain relief may be expected, although a significant minority of patients may continue to complain of disabling pain despite successful fusion.

Midfoot sprains

The diagnosis of midfoot sprain should be one of exclusion. It may be applied to midfoot injuries when significant bony or ligament injury has been ruled out by appropriate clinical and radiological examination. As described earlier, midfoot fractures and dislocations may be subtle. Until these have been excluded, this diagnosis should not be used.

Radiographic evaluation

These injuries should be investigated as for suspected unstable injuries. Good quality plain x-rays are the mainstay. Weight bearing or stress views may be required to confirm stability. CT or MRI scans may be indicated if the diagnosis remains unclear.

Box 12.62.2 Tarsometatarsal injuries

- May be difficult to diagnose:
  - Routine x-rays
    - —20-degree sagittal oblique AP view
    - —45-degreecoronal oblique view
    - —Lateral view
  - Weight bearing or stress x-rays
  - CT
- Displaced and unstable injuries: ORIF ± arthrodesis
- Quality of reduction may relate to functional results
- Tarsometatarsal arthrodesis for salvage.

Management

Stable injuries may be managed by early functional rehabilitation. A failure to improve rapidly should prompt a review of the initial diagnosis, with repeat investigations if appropriate.

Results

With accurate diagnosis to exclude unstable injuries, the majority of patients make a good recovery. This may be prolonged, with return to sports taking up to 3 months.

Fractures of the medial four metatarsals

Fractures of the metatarsals are relatively common. Most authorities agree on early weight bearing for undisplaced fractures, although specific thresholds for reduction and fixation of displaced fractures are not established. However, relatively minor displacement and angulation can alter the distribution of weight across the forefoot, leading to intractable plantar keratosis or transfer metatarsalgia.

Classification

No specific classification system exists for all metatarsal fractures. Fifth metatarsal fracture classification and management are discussed separately.

Management

Undisplaced fractures may be treated by protected weight bearing in a cast or rigid soled shoe. The patient is allowed to weight bear once the acute pain has settled, and this may take 3–4 weeks.

The amount of displacement that can be accepted is not defined. However, most authorities suggest that more than 3mm of displacement or 10 degrees of angulation is likely to compromise forefoot function. In these cases, particularly in the more active patients, reduction and fixation may be required.

Closed reduction using Chinese finger traps can be attempted in cases of significant displacement. If a stable reduction is achieved, a short-leg cast is applied and progressive weight bearing initiated. If it is not possible to achieve a satisfactory and stable reduction, open reduction and internal fixation is required. First metatarsal fractures may require plate fixation, and there are many implants designed for use in the foot specifically. An external fixator may be used to reduce the fracture and maintain length and alignment as a definitive treatment (Figure 12.62.12). In the case of lesser metatarsal fractures, K-wire fixation may be sufficient, but for more unstable fracture patterns, plate fixation may be required (Figures 12.62.13 and 12.62.14).

Metatarsal neck fractures are more likely to angulate than shaft fractures. Therefore, ORIF is more likely to be required to achieve healing in a satisfactory position.

Displaced intra-articular metatarsal head fractures are uncommon. Displaced injuries should be reduced, with small fragments debrided. Fixation can be achieved with intramedullary K-wire fixation for about 3 weeks, or lag screw fixation of larger fragments. Avascular necrosis of smaller fragments doest not appear to be a significant problem.

Complications

Malunion is the most common complication. Shortening or elevation of a metatarsal, particularly the first, may lead to transfer metatarsalgia. Plantar displacement or angulation may cause an intractable plantar keratosis. Post-traumatic interdigital neuroma may accompany malalignment in the transverse plane. Non-union is rare.

Salvage

Orthotic management often provides satisfactory relief of transfer metatarsalgia in the majority of cases.

If non-operative measures have failed, surgery can be considered. The aim should be to restore relative length and alignment of the metatarsal heads. Osteotomy, with interposition structural

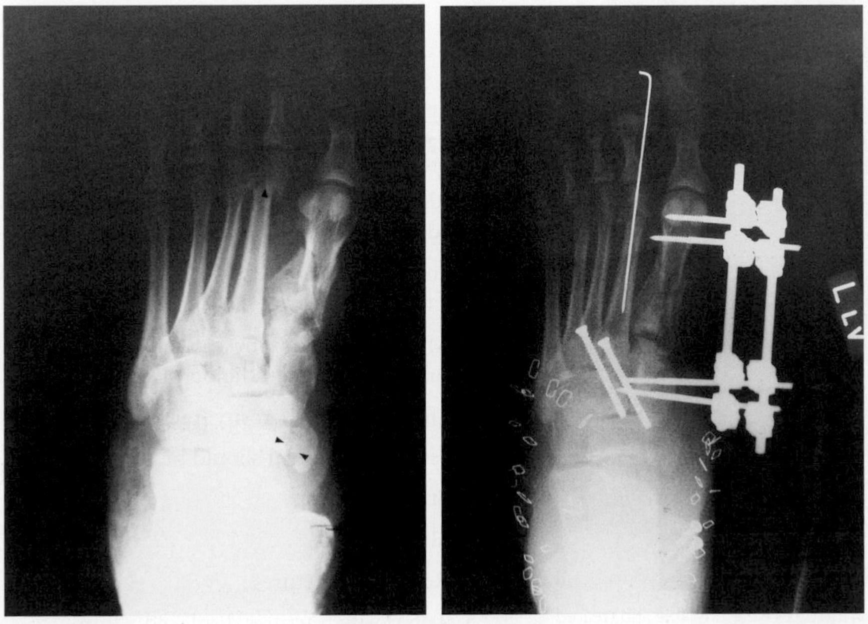

A B

Fig. 12.62.12 A) Comminuted short first metatarsal fracture associated with other forefoot trauma. B) The first metatarsal has been brought out to length and stabilized by an external fixator. Second metatarsal neck fracture and tarsometatarsal injury are also stabilized, restoring bony forefoot relationships.

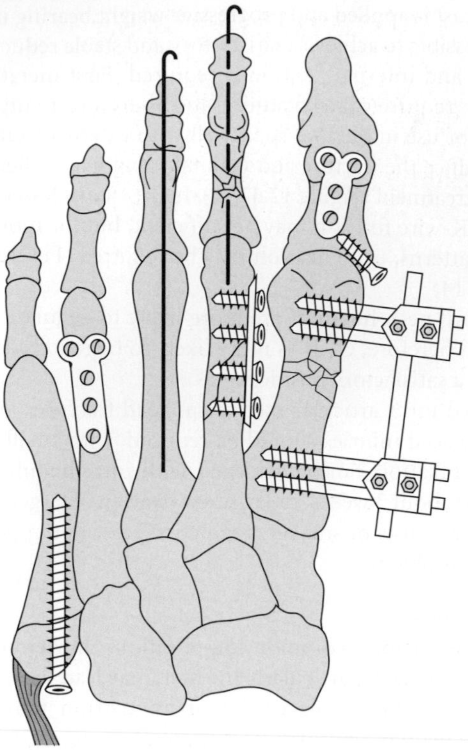

Fig. 12.62.13 Schematic diagram of fracture fixation options in the forefoot.

grafting can be effective in more severe cases. However, this may exacerbate pain and stiffness in the distal metatarsophalangeal joint. Where overload of a single metatarsal exists, osteotomy to shorten or elevate the metatarsal head can be undertaken. The patient should be warned that this might transfer load to an adjacent metatarsal. Diaphyseal shortening or dorsiflexion osteotomy of the overloaded metatarsal may be considered, but can result in subsequent overload of the adjacent metatarsal.

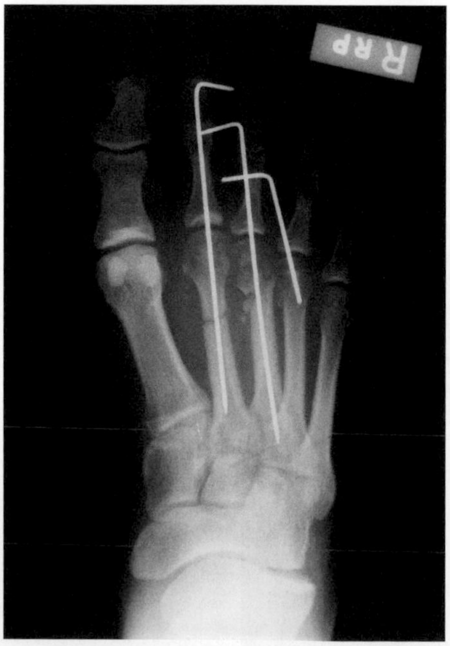

Fig. 12.62.14 Multiple displaced metatarsal fractures were unstable and treated with open reduction and intramedullary K-wire fixation.

Box 12.62.3 Medial four metatarsals

- Non-operative treatment with protective below knee splint weight bearing as tolerated if:
  - <10 degrees angulation
  - <3–4mm of shortening
- Otherwise consider closed/open reduction and internal fixation
- First metatarsal may require a plate or external fixator to maintain length
- Most common complication is malunion and subsequent abnormal load distribution.

Fractures of the fifth metatarsal (Box 12.62.4)

Fractures of the fifth metatarsal are the most common fracture in the forefoot. Fractures of the shaft should be evaluated and treated in the same manner as described for the medial four metatarsals. The mobility of the lateral tarsometatarsal joints does allow greater tolerance of malalignment. However, prominence of a lateral spike may require resection once the shaft fracture has united. Fractures of the proximal fifth metatarsal are considered separately.

Classification

Fractures of the base of the fifth metatarsal can be subdivided into fractures of the metaphyseal/diaphyseal junction (Type 1). These may be minimally displaced (Type IA) (Figure 12.62.15) or multi-fragmentary or displaced (Type IB). Stress fractures (Type II) may be more distal, and associated with a suggestive history including prodromal pain. X-rays may reveal sclerosis and or lucency around the fracture line, and a periosteal reaction. Type III fractures are those of the tuberosity or so-called 'avulsion' fractures. Type IIIA fractures are extra-articular and IIIB fractures extend into the fifth tarsometatarsal base.

Box 12.62.4 Fractures of the fifth metatarsal

- Mid-diaphyseal and distal fractures are treated similar to the medial metatarsals
- Non-operative treatment can be considered in undisplaced fractures:
  - Metaphyseal-diaphyseal fractures—non-weight bearing until evidence of radiological union
  - Undisplaced tuberosity fractures
- Operative treatment should be considered in:
  - Stress fractures
  - High demand
  - Recurrent fractures
  - Tuberosity fractures displaced >2mm.

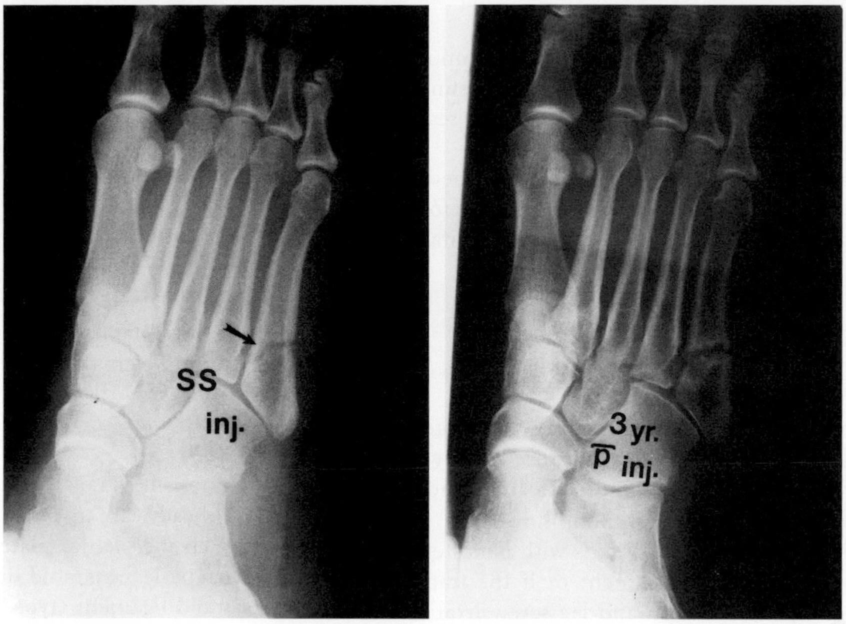

A B

Fig. 12.62.15 A) Acute type IA fracture. The patient refused treatment. B) The patient presented with persistent pain 3 years later. Non-union with significant intramedullary sclerosis is present.

Management

Acute Type I fractures are most commonly treated in a below-knee non-weight-bearing cast until signs of clinical and radiological union are well advanced. This may be up to 6 weeks. Premature weight bearing is associated with an increased risk of delayed or non-union.

Early operative treatment may be considered for patients with higher demand, recurrent fractures, or stress fractures. Surgery usually allows a more rapid functional recovery and return to pre injury activities. The majority of such injuries can be treated with intramedullary lag screw fixation alone (Figure 12.62.16). A 4.0-mm screw is often used, although depending on the size and contour of the fifth metatarsal, a 3.5- or 4.5-mm cortical screw may be appropriate. Protected weight bearing is allowed once symptoms allow. Occasionally, bone graft may be required.

Treatment of Type III tuberosity fractures is symptomatic. A cast is not required routinely. The threshold for open reduction and fixation of displaced intra-articular fractures has not been determined. Some authorities have suggested that fractures with more than 2 mm displacement should be considered for reduction and lag screw fixation.

Results

The majority of proximal fifth metatarsal fractures will heal when managed non-operatively and with good functional results. More rapid and reliable union has been reported in surgically treated zone II and zone III injuries.

Complications

Non-union and delayed union are well described complications of type I and II injuries (Figure 12.62.16). This may reflect the vascular watershed and the biomechanical stresses present at the metaphyseal-diaphyseal junction. Non-union of the tuberosity fractures are rarely symptomatic.

In surgically treated fractures, screw penetration through the distal cortex is usually asymptomatic. Screw breakage after may limit salvage options due to difficulty retrieving the distal portion of the screw. Prominent screw heads may require removal once the fracture has healed.

Salvage

Excision of small tuberosity fragments and reattachment of the peroneus brevis is recommended for the unusual case of symptomatic tuberosity non-union. Type I and II injuries that fail to unite can be treated by intramedullary screw fixation.

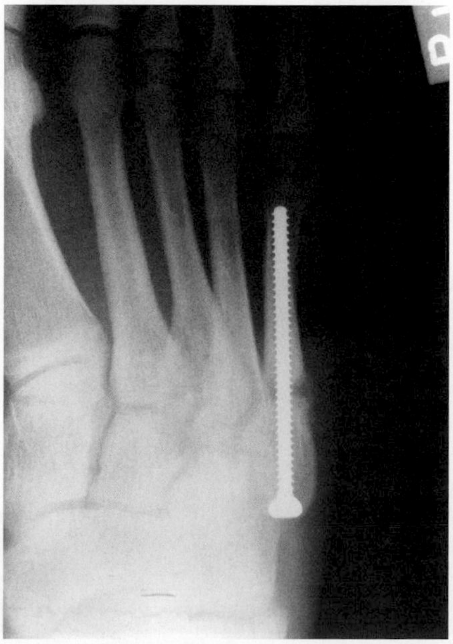

Fig. 12.62.16 Recurrent fifth metatarsal fracture stabilized with a 4.5-mm screw. Sclerotic bone has been debrided. Lateral bone graft can be seen.

Sesamoid fractures

Acute fractures of the sesamoid are rare. Bipartite sesamoids are common, with variable patterns. It can be difficult to distinguish a fracture from disruption of a synchondrosis of a bipartite sesamoid. Stress fractures of the sesamoids are well recognized.

Radiographic evaluation should include a tangential view of the sesamoids. An AP, lateral, and axial view of the opposite foot may be helpful in differentiating acute fracture from congenital partition (Figure 12.62.17).

Classification

Fractures may be displaced or undisplaced.

Management

The management of minimally displaced fractures is symptomatic. A well-padded cast with a recess for the sesamoids allows early mobilization. Patients with acute sesamoid fractures should be warned that symptoms might persist for months.

Surgery should be considered for patients with persistent pain after appropriate non-operative treatment or if the fracture is markedly displaced. Open reduction and lag screw fixation has been described, although excision of the smaller fragments and repair of the short flexors usually provides adequate pain relief.

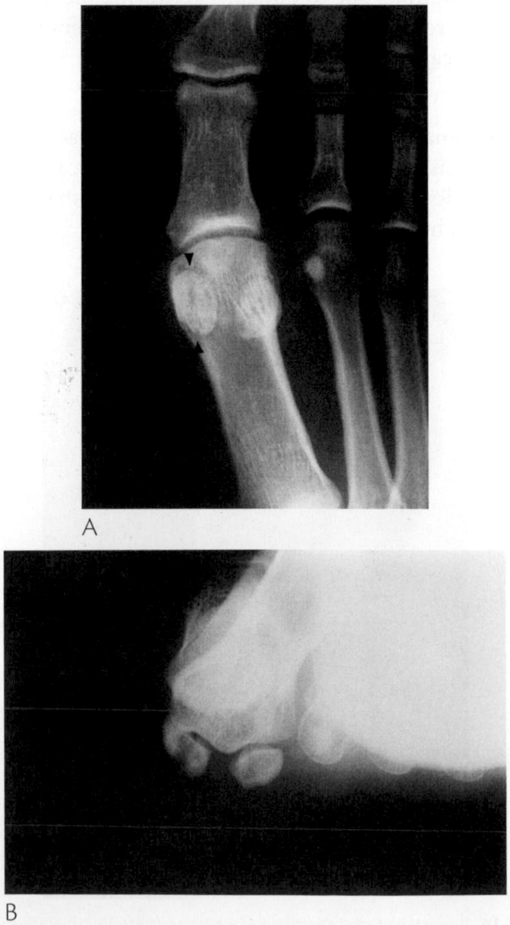

A

B

Fig. 12.62.17 A) Anteroposterior radiograph shows longitudinal lucency in medial sesamoid. B) A tangential view better demonstrates the fracture.

Complications

Symptomatic non-union or inflammation of the sesamoid–first metatarsal joint may follow appropriate treatment. Persistent pain, restricted dorsiflexion of the hallux metatarsophalangeal joint and plantar flexion weakness are common sequelae of sesamoidectomy. Disruption or imbalance of the short flexors may lead to a cock up toe deformity or hallux valgus or varus. Excision of both sesamoids is not recommended.

Metatarsophalangeal joint injuries

Injuries to the metatarsophalangeal joints range from mild sprains to dislocation. The majority are relatively mild injuries that follow a benign course.

Classification

Dislocation of first metatarsophalangeal joint usually forces the metatarsal head plantar wards. The metatarsal head may buttonhole through the plantar plate without disrupting the sesamoid complex (type I). Sesamoid disruption occurs by tearing of the intersesamoid ligament (type IIA) or a fracture through one or both sesamoids (type IIB).

Management

Sprains are managed symptomatically. After a period of rest, ice, elevation, and compression the patient is allowed to mobilize in a cast or rigid soled shoe. A prolonged recovery is not unusual, and it can take weeks for symptoms to resolve.

Dislocations of the first metatarsophalangeal joints should have a trial of closed reduction. However, interposition of the plantar plate will prevent reduction in Type 1 injuries. In such cases, open reduction through a dorsal approach is required. Sesamoid fractures usually reduce once the joint has been reduced. Loose fragments lying within the joint should be removed.

The first metatarsophalangeal joint is usually stable after reduction. Mobilization in a cast or rigid soled shoe can start as the patient's symptoms allow. Protected weight bearing for several weeks is advised.

Dislocation of the lesser metatarsophalangeal joints should undergo closed reduction and buddy taping to the adjacent toe until comfortable. Percutaneous pinning can be used to achieve stability in the unlikely event of residual instability.

Results

These are rare injuries, and so large series are not reported in the literature.

Complications

Instability is uncommon following reduction. Post-traumatic pain, from arthritis, loose body formation, or osteochondral injuries may all complicate recovery. Stiffness is common after metatarsophalangeal dislocations.

Salvage

Unstable joints should be reduced, ensuring no soft tissue interposition. If instability persists, transfixion with a K-wire for 2–3 weeks should be performed.

Post-traumatic arthrosis at the first metatarsophalangeal joint is managed by orthotics, injections and fusion when these measures fail.

Fractures of the phalanges

Fractures of the toes are the most common fracture in the forefoot. Phalangeal fractures and dislocations usually occur as a result of a direct blow. They are likely to be painful for 2–3 weeks but rarely cause long-term problems.

Classification

Phalangeal fractures are described as displaced or undisplaced.

Management

Undisplaced fractures or minimally displaced fractures are treated symptomatically. Displaced fractures that result in clinical deformity should be reduced and immobilized by neighbour strapping. Open reduction and K-wire fixation should be considered if a satisfactory closed reduction cannot be maintained.

Displaced intra-articular fractures involving the metatarsophalangeal joint may require ORIF. Displaced fractures that extend into the interphalangeal joints are less troublesome but may still result in joint incongruency and subsequent arthritis.

Complications

Significant malunion can cause localized pressure symptoms. Pain from arthritis or instability resulting from intra-articular fractures is relatively uncommon.

Salvage

Arthrodesis is a predictable salvage procedure for metatarsophalangeal or interphalangeal arthritis of the great toe. Malunion can be managed by resection arthroplasty or arthrodesis in the lesser toes.

Foot compartment syndrome

Compartment syndrome is defined by raised pressure in an osseofascial space leading to localized ischaemia. Once interstitial pressure rises above capillary closing pressure, occlusion of the capillary bed causes myoneural ischaemia. This is responsible for the intense pain of compartment syndrome. If unrelieved, necrosis followed by healing with fibrosis is the end result. These events usually occur in the presence of foot pulses and a warm foot, so an apparently well perfused foot does not preclude the presence of compartment syndrome. Compartment syndrome can develop in the presence of open foot fractures.

The foot has five major compartments that are clinically significant: the medial, central, lateral, interosseous, and calcaneal compartments. Communication between the compartments of the foot and leg may be demonstrated experimentally, but probably occur only under high pressures or following traumatic disruption of fascial membranes.

The diagnosis of compartment syndrome should be considered in any patient with a significant crush injury with or without fractures and dislocations. Massive swelling is usually apparent. Pain is unremitting and out of proportion to the severity of injury. Stretching the intrinsic muscles of the foot by dorsiflexion the toes exacerbates the pain. Other signs of altered sensation, pulses and capillary refill are not reliable indicators.

Compartment pressures may be monitored by passing a needle attached to a manometer under the base of the first metatarsal (medial and central compartments) or through the dorsal intermetatarsal approach (interosseous and central). The calcaneal compartment is reached by inserting the needle approximately 5cm distal and 2cm inferior to the medial malleolus.

Fasciotomy is indicated when the clinical diagnosis of compartment syndrome has been made or pressures reach 40mmHg or is within 30mmHg of the diastolic pressure. They should be performed as soon as possible, although a dilemma exists in patients

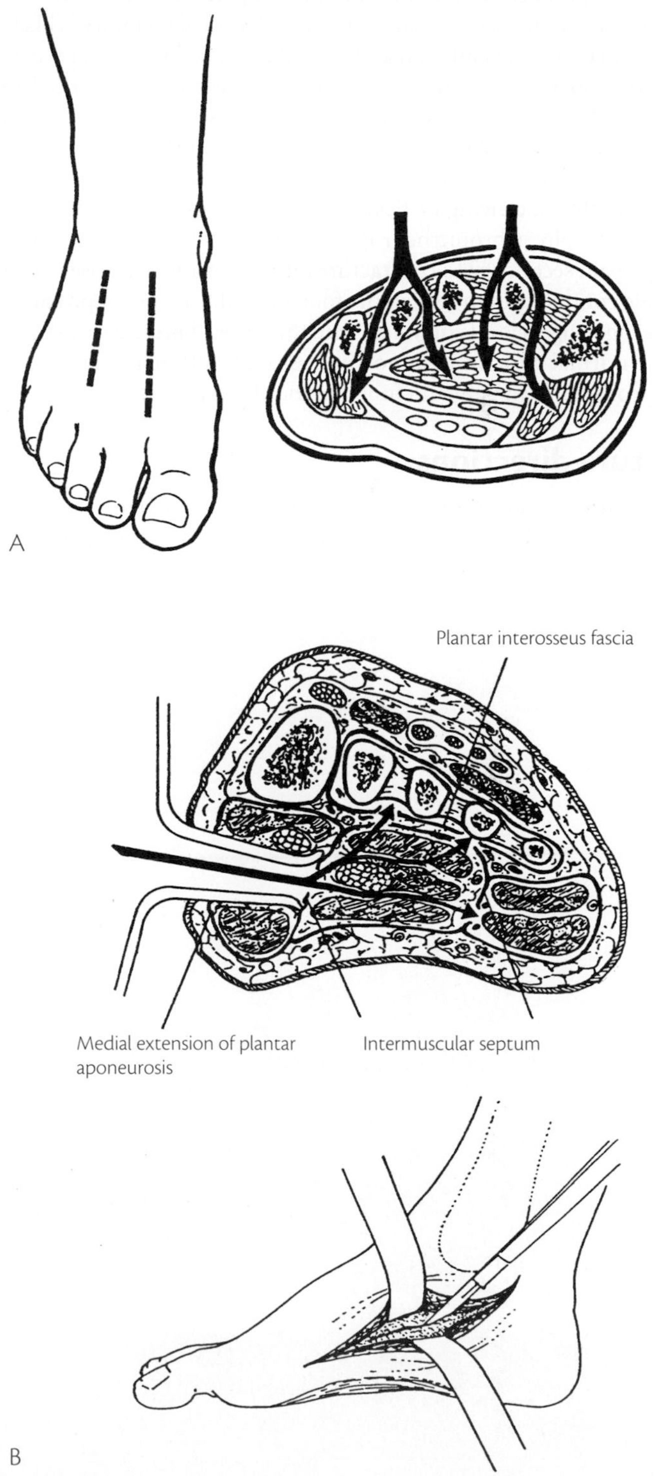

Fig. 12.62.18 Foot compartment release can be done through (A) two dorsal incisions and/or (B) a medial approach. Exposure needed for fixation of bony injuries may dictate the most appropriate approach.

presenting more than 24h following injury. Fasciotomy may expose necrotic muscle to an increased risk of infection. If surgery is required to reduce and fix the fractures, then decompression may be undertaken at the same time.

Fasciotomy technique is similar to elsewhere in the body. The skin is incised longitudinally without undermining. The muscle fascia is divided to expose the bulging muscle fibres. Dorsal or medial approaches or a combination may be used. Definitive or temporary reduction and stabilization of the skeletal injury is likely to reduce swelling and pain and should be considered if the expertise is available. Pneumatic compression devices can be used to aid swelling reduction. The wounds may be secondarily closed in 5–7 days. Split-thickness skin grafting may be required.

The sequelae of compartment syndrome can include chronic pain, stiffness, clawing or flexion deformities of the toes, and soft tissue atrophy. Chronic neuropathic pain should be distinguished from pain secondary to contractures and deformity. Release of soft tissue contractures to realign the foot and ankle fusion of proximal interphalangeal joints may help with the latter. It must be explained that normal function cannot be restored, although significant improvements in pain and function may be expected.

Future directions

A significant amount of foot trauma management is based upon our understanding of basic biomechanics and anatomy. Evidence based medicine in the form of clinical trials is starting to impact upon treatment. However, the evidence base remains thin with regard to tolerable degrees of malunion and optimum methods of operative treatment. In the current climate, it is difficult to see how the time and funding for such research is going to be made available.

Further reading

Coetzee, J.C. (2008). Making sense of Lisfranc injuries. *Foot and Ankle Clinics*, **13**(4), 695–704, ix. [Excellent overview of this under recognized injury.]

Hansen, S.T. Jr. (2000). *Functional Reconstruction of the Foot and Ankle.* Philadelphia, PA: Lippincot Williams and Wilkins. [If you like your evidence based on anecdote and experience (like me) this is for you.]

Pinzur, M.S. (ed) (2008). *Orthopaedic Knowledge Update: Foot and Ankle 4.* Rosemont, IL: American Academy of Orthopaedic Surgeons. [A concise summary of current knowledge.]

Rüedi, T.P., Buckley, R.E., and Moran, C.G. (eds) (2007). *AO Principles of Fracture Management*, Vol. 2, pp. 6–10. New York: Thieme. [Because principles will always matter]

SECTION 13

Paediatric Orthopaedics

13.1

Osteomyelitis and septic arthritis in children

J.S. Huntley and H. Crawford

Summary points

- *Staphylococcus aureus* is the commonest organism causing both septic arthritis and osteomyelitis
- There has been a decline in the number of infantile infections due to *Haemophilus influenzae* but both *Kingella kingae* and methicillin-resistant *Staphylococcus aureus* (MRSA) infections are increasing
- Early diagnosis and prompt treatment are key elements to the treatment of both conditions (Boxes 13.1.1 and 13.1.2).

Introduction

Although in the United Kingdom paediatric musculoskeletal infection is a diminishing problem, worldwide, bone and joint sepsis remains a common cause of morbidity. Despite improved imaging, delay to diagnosis remains common and treatment can be challenging. Nelson (1991) warns against 'a cookbook approach of standardized management for a disease with varied manifestations and a variable course'. With appropriate management, recurrence is unusual. Complications, however, are difficult to treat and constitute major morbidity. This chapter outlines the pathology, diagnosis, and treatment of paediatric musculoskeletal infections.

Aetiology, pathogenesis, and pathology

For osteomyelitis, infection usually occurs by the haematogenous route, with the metaphysis being the most common site for colonization; very rarely, osteomyelitis may involve an epiphysis. Trauma increases the likelihood of osteomyelitis subsequent to bacteraemia which may explain the increased incidence in males. Initially there is an acute inflammatory response in the cancellous bone. The formation of pus may lead to perforation of the metaphyseal cortex with subperiosteal accumulation of pus which in turn may breach the periosteum to track externally. A subperiosteal collection may also deprive some cortical bone of its blood supply; the dead cortical bone forms a sequestrum.

Although most bones in the body can be a focus for osteomyelitis, the commonest are the tibia and femur. Similarly, the commonest joints affected by septic arthritis are the knee and hip. The acute inflammatory response involves the influx of neutrophils into the synovial fluid and subsequent rapid destruction of the articular cartilage. Septic arthritis is, therefore, a surgical emergency and joint washout the key treatment.

In joints that have an intra-articular metaphysis (the femoral neck, proximal humerus, proximal radius, and distal lateral tibia), metaphyseal osteomyelitis can transgress directly into the joint. For these joints, particularly, an initial negative aspirate should not provide false reassurance. If the clinical picture deteriorates, secondary infection of the joint may have occurred.

In the neonate, bone and joint infection may present late because of the lack of clinical signs. Furthermore, transphyseal blood vessels allow epiphyseal extension of a metaphyseal osteomyelitis with a subsequent septic arthritis: 60–100% of neonates with septic arthritis have a contiguous osteomyelitis.

Osteomyelitis

The presentation and severity of acute haematogenous osteomyelitis (AHO) can vary considerably, sometimes making it difficult to

Box 13.1.1 Unwell and feverish? Bone pain and a limp? *Assume osteomyelitis*

- Investigations:
  - Blood tests: FBC, ESR, CRP, cultures
  - X-ray
  - Consider bone aspiration
  - MRI scan
  - Bone scan
- Management:
  - IV antibiotics
  - Rest/elevation
  - Reassess
  - Reimage further if condition declines
  - Consider surgical drainage
  - Modify antibiotics.

Box 13.1.2 'Septic' patient? Hot and swollen joint? *Assume septic arthritis*

- Investigations:
  - Blood tests: FBC, ESR, CRP, cultures
  - X-ray
  - MRI scan
  - Aspiration (must not be delayed by imaging)
    - —Microscopy (include Gram stain)
    - —Cell count
    - —Culture
- Management:
  - Joint washout
  - IV antibiotics
  - Rest/splintage
  - Reassess
  - Reimage if condition deteriorates
  - Modify antibiotics.

Box 13.1.3 Factors influencing the presentation of AHO

- The patient
- The organism
- The bone.

treat. Prompt diagnosis and appropriate intravenous (IV) antibiotics can lead to complete resolution with no sequelae. However multiple complications may occur, if diagnosis and treatment are delayed, or if the patient's response is poor. Three salient factors must be considered (see Box 13.1.3).

The patient

Bone infection occurs predominantly in lower socioeconomic classes where delayed presentation is common. As a result, the infection is well established within the bone before treatment commences and the subsequent clinical course is more likely to be complicated. Other patients also present late, including the immunocompromised, those with neuromuscular disabilities (whose 'bone pain' has been misdiagnosed as a fracture), and the neonate with a pseudoparalysis (Figure 13.1.1). If AHO is diagnosed 'early' when the infective organism is causing bone pain as a result of local inflammation, then prompt appropriate IV antibiotics will usually result in complete resolution. If there are significant comorbidities, the clinical course is less predictable and patients with diabetes mellitus, haemoglobinopathies, chronic renal disease, and rheumatoid arthritis will often require IV antibiotics for 2–3 months.

The organism

Staphylococcus aureus is the commonest infective organism in AHO but other organisms are relatively more common at specific ages and in certain patient groups. This knowledge influences antibiotic selection. Bactericidal levels of an appropriate antibiotic need to be delivered to the site of infection as swiftly as possible to halt progression (Table 13.1.1).

If the patient is slow to improve, other organisms like *Haemophilus influenza* and *Kingella kingae* need to be considered. In some areas, community-acquired methicillin resistant *Staphylococcus aureus* (CA-MRSA) is a significant cause of AHO

The bone

The most common sites of osteomyelitis are the proximal tibial and distal femoral metaphyses. Infection in these areas is relatively straightforward to diagnose and treat. Extension of the infection

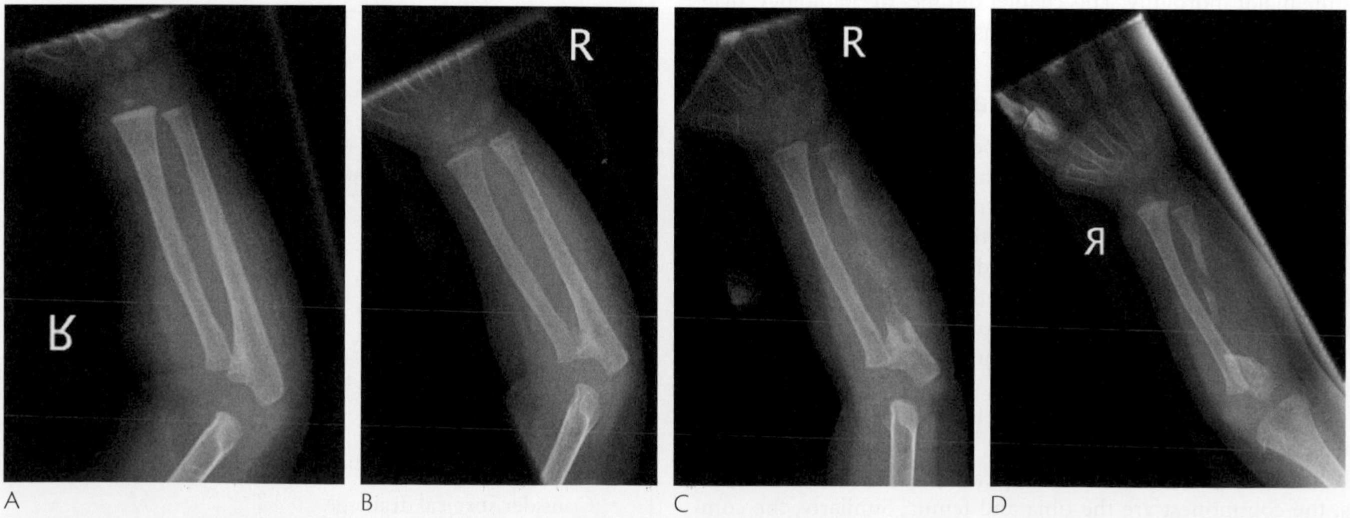

Fig. 13.1.1 Serial (monthly) radiographs right forearm. A 15-month-old boy had a delayed presentation for forearm tenderness and pseudoparalysis. Despite treatment, he developed whole bone ulna osteomyelitis.

Table 13.1.1 A summary of the most common pathogens and the most appropriate antibiotic

	Organism	Antibiotic
Neonate	*Group B Streptococcus* *Staphylococcus aureus* *Coliforms*	Cefotaxime, or oxacillin and gentamicin
Infant/child	*Staphylococcus aureus*	Oxacillin
Sickle cell disease	*Staphylococcus aureus* *Salmonella*	Oxacillin and ampicillin, *or* cefotaxime *or* chloramphenicol

along the diaphysis is uncommon if treated early, thus whole bone osteomyelitis and its sequelae are rare. Infection in the pelvis, clavicle, and calcaneus is less common, and therefore diagnosis is often delayed. These three bones are largely cancellous and eradication of the infection can take longer.

Clinical features

Bone pain, tenderness, and fever suggest osteomyelitis until proven otherwise. A painful limp and general malaise are also features. However, in immunocompromised and neonatal patients there may be few signs until the condition is well advanced. Pelvic osteomyelitis has a large differential diagnosis that includes psoas abscess, urinary tract infection, hip joint sepsis, appendicitis, and gynaecological conditions.

Clinical investigation

Blood investigations are: C-reactive protein (CRP), erythrocyte sedimentation rate (ESR), full blood count (FBC), and blood cultures. The CRP is raised in 98% of cases on admission). A normal value does not preclude infection especially in neonates, the immunocompromised or anaemic patients, or in sickle cell disease. The ESR is higher than 20mm/h in 70–90% of cases. The white blood cell count (WCC) may be useful when the differential shows a left shift but it is an unreliable indicator of bone infection, being elevated in only 35–40% of cases. In a young child with bone pain and fever, leukaemia is a possible diagnosis. A blood film and WCC will help determine this diagnosis. Blood cultures are only positive in 30–50% of patients with AHO.

Box 13.1.4 AHO: differential diagnosis

- Septic arthritis
- Ewing's sarcoma
- Langerhans cell hystiocytosis
- Leukaemia
- Metastatic neuroblastoma
- Sickle cell
- Fracture (e.g. in neuromuscular patient)
- Infarct
- Gaucher's disease
- Haemarthrosis (e.g. due to haemophilia).

Imaging includes plain radiographs and although these are normal in the initial 7–10 days of AHO, they help with the differential diagnosis (Box 13.1.4). After this early phase there may be periosteal elevation with underlying resorption and/or new bone formation. Other imaging options include the whole body bone scan: a cold scan may indicate early disease or hypoperfusion/osteonecrosis. Magnetic resonance imaging (MRI) is the most sensitive test for osteomyelitis (97–100%) and has a specificity of 73–92%. Furthermore it allows definition of soft tissue extension, intraosseous collection, joint involvement, and aids in planning the surgical approach (Figure 13.1.2).

Bone aspiration can identify the infecting organism accurately in 75–80% but reservations concerning this technique within the overall management are outlined in the following section.

Treatment and prognosis

The aims of AHO treatment are to treat promptly and appropriately with IV antibiotics in order to prevent overwhelming sepsis, to cure the local disease as rapidly as possible, and to prevent the secondary sequelae of growth plate damage, pathological fracture, osteonecrosis, deep vein thrombosis, and chronic osteomyelitis.

Antibiotics should be given on the assumption that osteomyelitis is present. It is controversial whether or not the bone should be aspirated first. Some surgeons advocate aspiration before starting parenteral antibiotics. However, aspiration usually involves sedation or a general anaesthetic which delays treatment. Therefore in our institution, we do not routinely aspirate bone before starting antibiotics. Antibiotics are given as soon as the diagnosis is presumed and the child is then investigated with either MRI or bone scan. The bone scan is especially useful if multiple sites of infection are present, or if the site is hard to localize. Beware the 'cold' scan which may represent early disease or the coexistence of infection

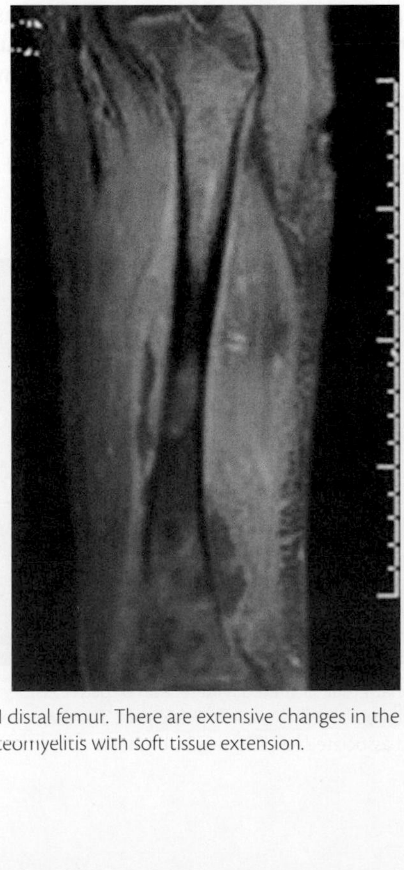

Fig. 13.1.2 MRI distal femur. There are extensive changes in the distal femur suggestive of osteomyelitis with soft tissue extension.

and osteonecrosis. If an abscess is present that requires surgical drainage, specimens are attained at that stage, acknowledging that antibiotic treatment may mean that the culture result is negative.

Conversely, in areas where AHO due to MRSA is common, bone aspiration may be useful. Initial treatment is with vancomycin, but subsequently, antibiotics can be modified if/when organisms other than MRSA are identified.

The patient needs to be monitored closely in a hospital environment and clinical improvement, in terms of vital signs, range of movement, and pain, assessed. Not all children respond well. The role of the orthopaedic surgeon is to establish why and reinvestigate. The patient may require repeat imaging, surgical debridement, or a change in antibiotics. In the situation where the infection is not resolving quickly and the child remains symptomatic, a repeat MRI is used to look for further collections (intraosseous or subperiosteal) or spread of infection. Ultrasound scans can also be useful. Infected deep vein thromboses may be visualized in vessels abutting AHO which may result in septic embolization and require anticoagulation (Figure 13.1.3).

The change in CRP values during treatment for AHO is useful in monitoring control of the infection. In conjunction with the clinical findings, a declining CRP can indicate when a change from IV to oral antibiotics is appropriate. For uncomplicated AHO, the CRP is likely to have normalized by day 9. IV antibiotics may be discontinued once the child has improved clinically and biochemically (often <5–7 days) although oral treatment should be continued for a total of at least 3–4 weeks.

The current controversies relate to duration of treatment and when to switch antibiotics to oral (Box 13.1.5). Prolonging IV therapy requires specialized 'long lines' that have their own inherent risks. Unless adequate home support is available the child has to remain an inpatient. Each patient with osteomyelitis is unique because of the factors outlined earlier. Therefore the clinical course must be closely monitored, with antibiotics and surgical interventions used appropriately. In resistant/intractable cases and compromised hosts, IV antibiotics should be continued until all clinical features are resolved (and total antibiotic treatment may need to be extended to 6–12 weeks).

The timing of surgical intervention is crucial to prevent secondary complications (Box 13.1.6). If pus is encountered on aspiration

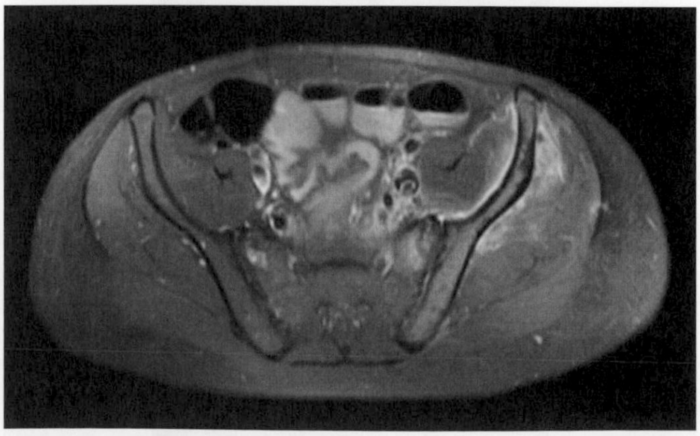

Fig. 13.1.3 Coronal T_1-fat saturated MRI section of pelvis. A 15-year-old boy with multifocal staphylococcal sepsis, and left pelvic pain. The scan shows extensive left ilium changes and associated left iliac vein thrombosis.

Box 13.1.5 Switching from IV to oral antibiotics? Factors to consider

- The patient—immuno-compromised vs. healthy
- The bone—proximal tibia vs. pelvis, clavicle, calcaneus
- The organism—Staph aureus vs. E coli, Pseudomonas, MRSA
- The clinical response—rapid improvement vs. repeat surgical debridement.

or an abscess localized by MRI (Figure 13.1.4), then surgical debridement is mandatory. Decisions concerning surgical approach are helped by accurate imaging. Occasionally small abscesses in difficult locations can be drained percutaneously with the help of ultrasound or computed tomography (CT) guidance. This is especially useful in pelvic osteomyelitis where, for example, a deep abscess in the iliacus muscle would otherwise require an extensive surgical approach. Rarely does the bone need to be 'drilled' as part of the surgical debridement, as the intraosseous collection has already decompressed itself into a subperiosteal collection. Following debridement, large drains are left in the wounds and the skin edges closed loosely with sutures. A 'second look',48h later, enables a repeat washout/debridement or definitive closure to be performed. If a large amount of pus is still present, the wound is left open and a suction dressing applied.

Depending on the clinical course, patients are seen regularly after discharge, for a clinical and radiographic review and blood tests (WCC, ESR, CRP). For patients on flucloxacillin, weekly liver function tests and neutrophil counts are advisable, as there can be a high rate of flucloxacillin-associated neutropenia (Box 13.1.7).

Septic arthritis

Clinical features

A patient with septic arthritis usually presents with signs of sepsis and a hot swollen joint with restricted movement due to pain. Swelling in some joints such as the hip is difficult to detect. For pyogenic septic arthritis the onset and progress is usually rapid and severe. The joint rests in the position of maximum capsular laxity. Such a picture is indicative of a septic arthritis until proven otherwise by appropriate investigations (usually aspiration and microscopy).

Box 13.1.6 Complications of osteomyelitis

- Chronic osteomyelitis
- Deep vein thrombosis
- Septic thrombus and pulmonary septic emboli
- Overwhelming sepsis
- Growth disturbance (Figure 13.1.5)
- Chronic osteomyelitis
- Pathological fracture
- Antibiotic complications—neutropenia.

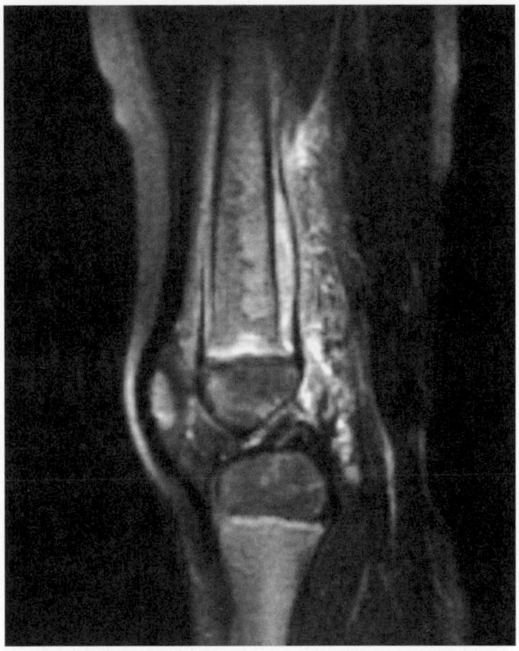

Fig. 13.1.4 Sagittal T_2-fat saturated MRI section of distal femur. A 3-year-old girl presented with 48h of fever and distal thigh pain with focal bony tenderness. The scan shows a distal femoral subperiosteal abscess.

The picture may be less overt if the patient is on steroids or has been on antibiotics. Limb pseudoparalysis in a neonate, often without overt signs of sepsis, is a typical presentation of septic arthritis.

Clinical investigations

Aspiration is the key to diagnosis with fluid being sent for microscopy, culture, and cell count. Preoperative investigations should include FBC, CRP, ESR, blood cultures, and plain radiographs. In certain circumstances, ancillary imaging (ultrasound, MRI, and bone scan) can help localization, indicate an effusion, or define an associated osteomyelitis. However, these tests should not delay aspiration. An ultrasound can confirm the presence of an effusion but cannot distinguish between infected and sterile fluid.

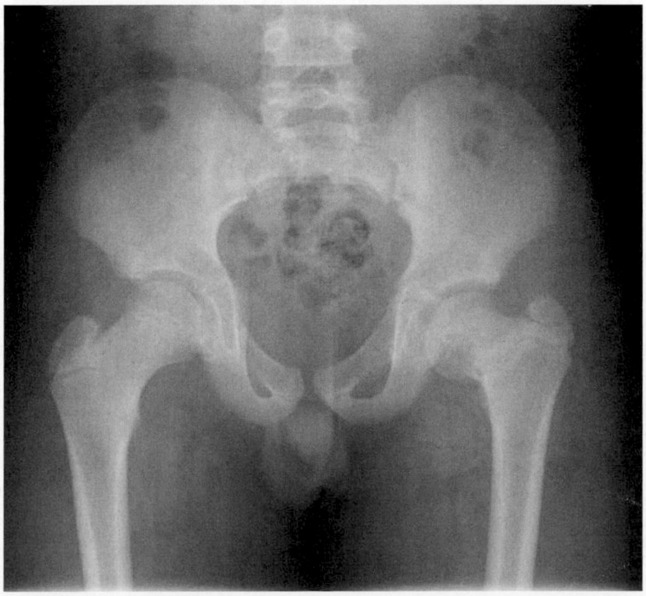

Fig. 13.1.5 AP pelvis radiograph. An 11-year-old boy with coxa vara after episode of neonatal left hip sepsis.

Box 13.1.7 Keeping out of trouble with osteomyelitis

1. Educate primary care physicians and paediatricians regarding early referral of patients with probable AHO
2. Suspect AHO in a child who is systemically unwell with associated bone pain
3. Aggressive IV antibiotic treatment appropriate to the child's age and the presumed organism
4. Radiological investigation, especially MRI, to localize collections of pus and to aid surgical debridement
5. Continue IV antibiotics until the clinical symptoms and signs and CRP have improved.

Criteria for diagnosis

Microscopy of the aspirated fluid may show organisms, confirming the diagnosis. If no organisms are seen, a WCC of more than 40.0×10^9/L has greater than 90% sensitivity and specificity in detecting a septic arthritis. However, WCC of greater than this value may be found in acute inflammatory arthritis. Furthermore, if the disease is detected early or has been partially treated with antibiotics, the WCC may be equivocal. If there is any doubt, proceed to immediate washout.

Differentiating between transient synovitis and septic arthritis can be difficult. Four factors are useful predictors to aid clinical judgement: history of fever, inability to weight-bear, ESR greater than 40mm/h, and WCC greater than 12.0×10^9/L. The CRP rises more rapidly than the ESR in early infection and therefore, is often preferred (Box 13.1.8).

Treatment

A septic joint must be washed out urgently by arthrotomy with high volumes of fluid. For the hip, a Smith–Petersen approach is preferred so that the posterior vessels supplying the femoral head are protected. Tissue biopsy should be performed for histology as

Box 13.1.8 Differential diagnosis of septic arthritis

- Osteomyelitis
- Transient synovitis
- Lyme arthritis
- Juvenile rheumatoid arthritis
- Leukaemia
- Avascular necrosis—Perthes disease, haemophilia
- Appendicitis
- Psoas abscess
- Gynaecological conditions.

well as microbial culture. Parenteral antibiotics, usually for 3–4 weeks, should cover the most likely organisms, and are then adjusted to culture results. The CRP is a useful guide to resolution. There is a trend towards a reduced duration of IV antibiotics.

Prognosis

Antibiotics have good joint penetration after surgical washout. If the condition is diagnosed and treated early, the prognosis is good. Neonatal sepsis, particularly of the hip, has a worse prognosis and may be complicated by limb length discrepancy, angular deformity, avascular necrosis, and joint dislocation.

Special cases

Osteomyelitis in sickle cell disease

Patients with sickle disease have an increased risk of osteomyelitis, and are more prone to complications. It can be difficult to distinguish a sickle crisis from AHO. Fever and raised ESR are suggestive of infection. *Staphylococcus aureus* remains the most common pathogen in sickle cell disease but *Salmonella* must also be covered.

Chronic osteomyelitis

Osteomyelitis is considered chronic if it has been present for more than 3 months. The definition of a sequestrum, by both CT and MRI scanning, is important with the aim of aggressive surgical debridement of infected material and sequestrectomy.

Epiphyseal osteomyelitis

Primary osteomyelitis of the epiphysis is rare and usually subacute. It presents with mild pain, minimal decrease in function, and little in the way of systemic reaction. The differential diagnosis is large and a gadolinium-enhanced MRI scan is useful in making the diagnosis, localizing and defining the extent of infection, and planning the surgical approach if required (Figure 13.1.6).

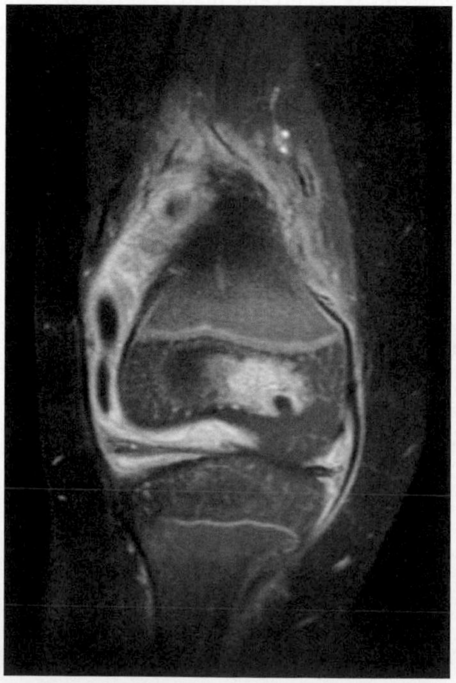

Fig. 13.1.6 MRI right knee. Appearances are of subacute epiphyseal osteomyelitis in a 21-month-old child. There is also a large effusion, which on aspiration was purulent, mandating knee arthrotomy and washout curettage of the epiphyseal abscess.

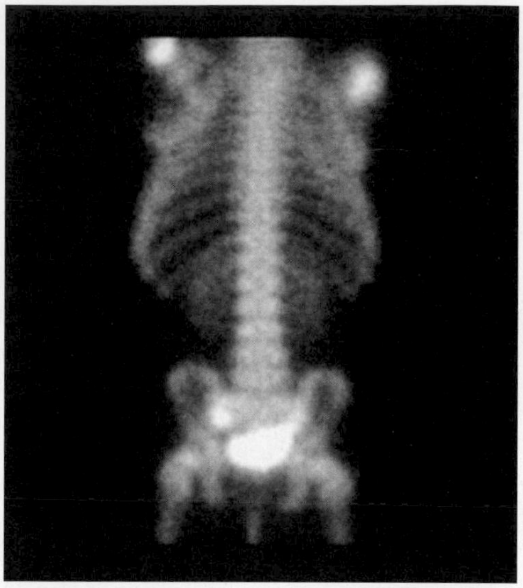

Fig. 13.1.7 Bone scan. Localizes pelvic pain to the right sacroiliac joint.

Gonococcal arthritis

Neisseria gonorrhoeae is a common cause of septic arthritis in the sexually active population. The major differential includes Reiter's disease. It is usual for more than one joint to be involved. The aspirate WCC is not as high as in pyogenic arthritis. Appropriate antibiotics are IV penicillin or third-generation cephalosporins for resistant strains.

Foot puncture wounds

This injury is common in children: washout, debridement, and tetanus prophylaxis are required. *Staphylococcus* is the commonest infecting organism. *Pseudomonas* which has a predilection for cartilage may also be involved, causing a stubborn infection that requires surgical debridement and IV antibiotics.

Sacroiliac joint infection

Infection of the sacroiliac joint presents with pain, abnormal gait, and pyrexia and may be mistaken for a variety of other conditions. Flexion–abduction–external rotation test and direct sacroiliac compression (with the patient prone) are useful in localizing pathology to the sacroiliac joint. A bone scan is also helpful (Figure 13.1.7). Blood, stool, and urine cultures should be obtained. Anti-staphylococcal IV antibiotics are the treatment of choice, and surgical debridement/drainage is not usually necessary.

Other issues

Panton–Valentine leukocidin (PVL) is a virulence factor secreted by certain strains of *Staphylococcus aureus*. PVL is capable of destroying host neutrophils, and has also been associated with increased intravascular coagulopathy. PVL is thought by some authorities to be responsible for increased severity of sepsis. In practice, PVL status has not yet been proven to be a useful guide to treatment.

Further reading

Arnold, S.R., Elias, D., Buckingham, S.C., *et al.* (2006). Changing patterns of acute hematogenous osteomyelitis and septic arthritis: emergence of community-associated methicillin-resistant Staphylococcus aureus. *Journal of Pediatric Orthopedics*, **26**, 703–8.

Hempfing, A., Placzek, R., Gottsche, T., and Meisss, A.L. (2003). Primary subacute epiphyseal and metaepiphyseal osteomyelitis in children. *Journal of Bone and Joint Surgery*, **81B**, 1029–34.

Kocher, M.S., Mandiga, R., Zurakowski, D., Barnewolt, C., and Kasser, J.R. (2004). Validation of a clinical prediction rule for the differentiation between septic arthritis and transient synovitis of the hip in children. *Journal of Bone and Joint Surgery*, **86A,** 1629–35.

McCarthy, J.J., Dormans, J.P., Kozin, S.H., and Pizzutillo, P.D. (2004). Musculoskeletal infections in children. Basic treatment principles and recent advancements. *Journal of Bone and Joint Surgery*, **86A**, 850–63.

Mitchell, P.D., Hunt, D.M., Lyall, H., Nolan, M., and Tudor-Williams, G. (2007). Panton-Valentine leukocidin-secreting *Staphylococcus aureus* causing severe musculoskeletal sepsis in children. A new threat. *Journal of Bone and Joint Surgery*, **89B**, 1239–42.

Nelson, J.D. (1991). Skeletal infections in children. *Advances in Pediatric Infectious Diseases*, **6**, 59–78.

Stott, N.S. (2001). Paediatric bone and joint infection. *Journal of Orthopedic Surgery (Hong Kong)*, **9**, 83–90.

Unkila-Kallio, L., Kallio, M.J., Eskola, J., and Peltola, H. (1994). Serum C-reactive protein, erythrocyte sedimentation rate, and white blood cell count in acute haematogenous osteomyelitis of children. *Pediatrics*, **93**, 59–62.

Whalen, J.L., Fitzgerald, Jr, R.H., and Morrissy, J.T. (1988). A histological study of acute hematogenous osteomyelitis following physeal injuries in rabbits. *Journal of Bone and Joint Surgery*, **70A**, 1383–92.

13.2a

Juvenile idiopathic arthritis: medical aspects

Clarissa Pilkington

Summary points

- Juvenile idiopathic arthritis is defined as an arthritis persisting for at least 6 weeks
- The cause may relate to the immune system response to a stimulus with a synovial or systemic manifestation
- Classification depends on the clinical picture and the immunological markers
- Joint sepsis is often a differential diagnosis
- Most cases respond to simple measures, a few need a structured medical management plan. Surgery is indicated in 10% of cases. All require physiotherapy
- Complications may occur secondary to the disease or its treatment.

Introduction

Juvenile idiopathic arthritis (JIA) comprises a group of diseases that are classified according to mode and age of onset. Their aetiopathogenesis is not understood. Initially, the classification criteria suffered because they had been adapted from adult criteria, and subsequently because the criteria developed differently across the continents. The current classification system is a research-based tool devised to ensure homogeneous groups of patients were being studied, both in the United States of America and Europe. It is used clinically but in a less rigorous manner and not all exclusion criteria are adhered to. The treatment principles for all forms of JIA are the same: to control completely the inflammation in the affected joint allowing normal growth, development, and function during childhood.

JIA is found worldwide with an incidence in the United Kingdom of 1:10 000 children. It is defined as an arthritis persisting for at least 6 weeks in a child under the age of 16. The arthritis itself is described as swelling of at least one peripheral joint or at least two of the following signs: limited range of movement; tenderness or pain on movement of a joint; or increased warmth of the skin overlying a joint (Box 13.2a.1). The cause may be a combination of genetic and environmental factors that relate to how the immune system responds to stimuli: the resultant inflammatory response may be limited to the synovium or manifested systemically.

There are a number of important conditions with an associated arthropathy that are *not* included within this classification system: inflammatory bowel disease, immune deficiencies and reactive arthritis.

Classification

Oligoarticular (oligo) juvenile inflammatory arthritis

Oligo JIA, previously known as pauciarticular JIA, is defined as involvement of up to four joints within the first 6 months of the disease. If more joints are involved after 6 months it becomes extended oligo JIA. Oligo JIA is the largest JIA subgroup accounting for 50% of cases. The disease onset is early (median age 5 years) and there is a female : male ratio of 5:1. The knee is the most commonly affected joint. If the child is anti-nuclear antibody (ANA) positive there is a strong association with uveitis. As the uveitis is asymptomatic, slit-lamp examination every 3 months for the first 2 years of the disease to screen for inflammation and thus prevent blindness is essential. Overall, 60% of cases are in remission by adulthood.

Patients with a family history of psoriasis, who are positive for rheumatoid factor (RF) or HLA-B27 or who have a HLA-B27 associated disease or an inflammatory bowel disease are excluded from a diagnosis of oligo JIA.

Box 13.2a.1 Definition of JIA

- JIA:
  - Arthritis persisting >6 weeks in a child <16 years
- Arthritis:
  - Swelling of at least one peripheral joint *or*
  - Two of the following criteria:
    - Limited range of joint movement
    - Pain or tenderness on movement
    - Increased warmth over the joint.

Polyarticular juvenile inflammatory arthritis

Rheumatoid factor negative

Poly JIA patients have more than five joints affected within 6 months of disease onset. It is the second most common subgroup and like oligo JIA, the age of onset is early (median age 6 years) and females are most commonly affected. The arthritis is symmetrical, often involving the wrists, metacarpophalangeal and proximal interphalangeal joint joints, the neck, and the temporomandibular joints (TMJs). If multiple joints are involved in one or more limbs, growth can be delayed.

Similar to oligo JIA, the child may be ANA positive and if so there is a risk of uveitis. Despite treatment, 10–15% of patients with RF-negative poly JIA will have severe functional limitation 10–15 years after disease onset.

Rheumatoid factor positive

RF positive poly patients comprise only 10% of the poly group and only 3% of all JIA cases. There is a marked female preponderance (female : male, 13:1) and the median age of onset is later at 9 years. The arthritis is aggressive, symmetrical, and similar to adult rheumatoid arthritis (Figure 13.2a.1).

The diagnosis of poly JIA (RF positive or negative) is *excluded* if the child is HLA-B27 positive.

Systemic onset juvenile inflammatory arthritis

This is the most severe form of the disease. It often presents as a pyrexia of unknown origin. There are three main criteria for diagnosis:

- *Fever*—classically, this daily (quotidian) or twice daily fever rises to more than 38 degrees centigrade and then falls back to or below baseline
- *Rash*—the salmon-pink maculopapular rash comes and goes with the fever (evanescent). It is rarely itchy.

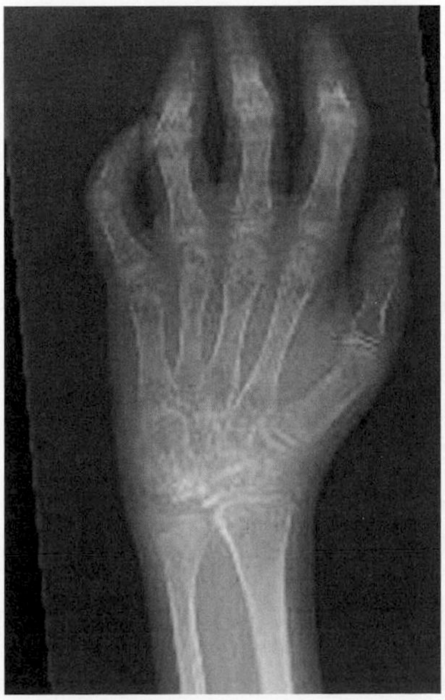

Fig. 13.2a.1 AP radiograph of a wrist showing gross joint destruction in a child with RF positive polyarticular JIA. Her other wrist was similarly involved.

- *Arthritis*—the arthritis may affect one or multiple joints but it may not appear for weeks or even months after the fever has subsided.

In contrast to the other JIA subgroups the female to male ratio is equal and there is no peak age of onset during the childhood years.

The systemic nature of the disease means that there is a generalized lymphadenopathy with hepatosplenomegaly and possibly a serositis (including pericarditis). Uncontrolled disease leads to osteoporosis and severe growth failure and causes a destructive arthritis in 30–60% of cases.

Patients who are RF or HLA-B27 positive are *excluded* from this diagnosis.

Psoriatic juvenile inflammatory arthritis

As the name implies, this subgroup of JIA patients must have an arthritis associated with nail pitting or dactylitis or have a first-degree relative with psoriasis. The condition is commoner in girls and the age of onset is between 7–11 years.

Patients *must* be RF and HLA B27 negative.

Enthesitis-related arthritis

This group of HLA-B27 positive patients used to be labelled as spondyloarthritis but the term is no longer used. It is the only subgroup of JIA that affects males more than females with a later median age of onset at 11 years. (Table 13.2a.1) Asymmetrical large peripheral joint arthritis is associated with enthesitis (inflammation of the muscular or tendinous attachment to bone) and tenosynovitis. Involvement of the axial skeleton is uncommon and usually a late feature.

All patients must be RF negative.

Other juvenile inflammatory arthritis

This research group is used to 'house' patients who can not be classified into any other category.

Investigations (Box 13.2a.2 and Box 13.2a.3)

Investigations should be used to help make a correct diagnosis and to exclude other similar conditions.

Haematology

Changes consistent with an inflammatory response such as anaemia, a raised platelet and white cell count, and a high erythrocyte sedimentation rate (ESR) and C-reactive protein (CRP). Patients with oligo JIA may have no such changes.

Biochemistry

Patients with systemic JIA may show a transaminitis.

Box 13.2a.2 Immunological markers in JIA

- ANA positive: check for uveitis
- RF positive: acts like adult rheumatoid arthritis
- HLA-B27 positive: enthesitis and tenosynovitis.

Table 13.2a.1 Differences between the various subtypes of JIA

	Enthesitis-related arthritis (ERA)	Systemic onset juvenile inflammatory arthritis (SOJIA)	Other JIA subtypes
HLA B27	Positive	Negative	Negative
Male (M): female (F)	M > F	M = F	F > M
Age of onset	Late	No peak age of onset	Early
Symptoms	Arthritis *and* enthesitis	Systemic illness *and* arthritis	Arthritis and possibly psoriasis or uveitis

Immunology (Box 13.2a.2)

A positive ANA or RF test clarifies diagnosis and influences prognosis. If the RF level is very high, a diagnosis of systemic lupus erythematosus (SLE) must be considered. HLA-B27 should be performed if the differential diagnosis includes psoriatic arthritis or ERA.

Microbiology

The presence of a fever may necessitate a septic screen, virological investigations, and a test to exclude *Borrelia*. If TB is suspected a Mantoux test (and a chest radiograph) should be performed.

Musculoskeletal imaging

Plain radiographs may show surprisingly little abnormality but in the more established case there may be periarticular osteoporosis, marginal erosions, and, at the wrist, carpal crowding. MRI will demonstrate synovial hypertrophy with contrast highlighting areas of active synovitis.

Others

Synovial biopsy is not required routinely but may be useful in excluding tuberculosis (TB) or sarcoidosis. Similarly, bone marrow aspirate (BMA) and measurement of urinary vanillyl mandelic acid (VMA) in patients with systemic disease excludes leukaemia and neuroblastomas (Box 13.2a.3).

Differential diagnosis

The list of differential diagnoses varies a little from subgroup to subgroup of JIA. A careful history and complete examination are essential prerequisites for a correct diagnosis and may influence the line of further investigation. Sepsis should always be considered when only one or two joints are affected (some cases of oligo JIA) but it is less likely in systemic JIA where the involvement (unlike with sepsis) is symmetrical. (Table 13.2a.2).

Box 13.2a.3 Investigation pitfalls

- RF very high: suspect SLE
- Synovial biopsy: not required routinely *but* excludes TB/sarcoid
- BMA/urinary VMA: excludes malignancy
- Transaminitis: systemic JIA
- Inflammatory markers: may be normal in oligo JIA.

Treatment

Patient and parent education is very important, as the diagnosis of 'arthritis' is often associated with incorrect preconceptions.

In some cases, all that is required for management is analgesic medication and relative rest. Non-steroidal anti-inflammatory drugs (NSAIDs) help pain, stiffness, and fever whilst physiotherapy maintains range of movement and muscle strength or helps rebuild muscle that may have wasted secondary to lack of activity and the release of inflammatory cytokines.

Other cases require a more structured medical management plan.

Steroids

If only a few joints are involved, intra-articular steroids may be used under general anaesthetic for children under 8 years and nitrous oxide for older patients. The steroid of choice is triamcinolone hexacetonide at a dose of 1mg/kg for each large joint.

Oral or intravenous steroids are used if systemic features are present or if there is multiple joint involvement.

Other drug therapies

- Methotrexate: this disease-modifying agent is used frequently but only in oligo JIA and if several joints are involved. If joints are not controlled by intra-articular steroids, methotrexate should be used promptly at a dose of 10–15mg/m2
- Sulphasalazine: used specifically in ERA patients
- Anti-TNF: antitumour necrosis factor drugs such as etanercept, infliximab or adalimumab are used if methotrexate fails to control the disease or the patient has axial ERA.

Occupational therapy has an important role particularly in patients with systemic disease or multiple joint involvement. Hand therapy is important but overall, joint splintage is not used frequently; the emphasis is on maintaining the activities of daily living with joint movement and normal weight-bearing activity when possible (physiotherapy).

Outcomes and complications

Failure of normal growth and development

A generalized growth failure may occur due to disease activity, more commonly in patients with systemic JIA than with poly JIA. However, a localized failure of growth may occur at any affected joint and premature fusion of a growth plate may lead to a clinically apparent limb length difference. Some patients demonstrate an overgrowth phenomenon secondary to the inflammatory response and the associated increase in blood flow. This too may

Table 13.2a.2 Differential diagnoses for some of the JIA subgroups

	Oligo	Poly	Systemic	ERA
Reactive arthritis	Yes	Yes	Yes (poststreptococcal)	Yes
Septic arthritis	Yes Consider TB if only one hip involved			
Infection		CRMO—non-infective osteomyelitis	PUO Viral, bacterial	CRMO SAPHO Sarcoidosis
Malignancy	Rare		Neuroblastoma Leukaemia	
Systemic lupus erythematosus		Yes	Yes	
JDM		Yes	Yes	
MPS		Yes—joints respond poorly to steroids		
Conditions associated with an arthropathy		Inflammatory bowel disease	Immune deficiencies	
'Trauma'	Yes			Mechanical pain syndromes
Others	Sickle cell disease PVNS Coagulation defects		Kawasaki's disease Haemophagiocytic lymphohistiocytosis	Sarcoidosis

CRMO: Chronic relapsing multifocal osteomyelitis; JDM: Juvenile dermatomyositis; MPS: mucopolysaccharoidoses; PUO: Pyrexia of unknown origin; PVNS: Pigmented villonodular synovitis; SAPHO: Synovitis, acne, pustulosis, hyperostosis, osteitis

lead to limb length inequality or an alteration in limb alignment: commonly increased knee valgus.

Pubertal delay is uncommon and seen only in severe disease.

Amyloidosis

Amyloidosis is only seen in some systemic JIA patients after years of uncontrolled inflammation documented by persistently elevated ESR/CRP levels. With improvements in medical therapy, the incidence of amyloidosis has fallen.

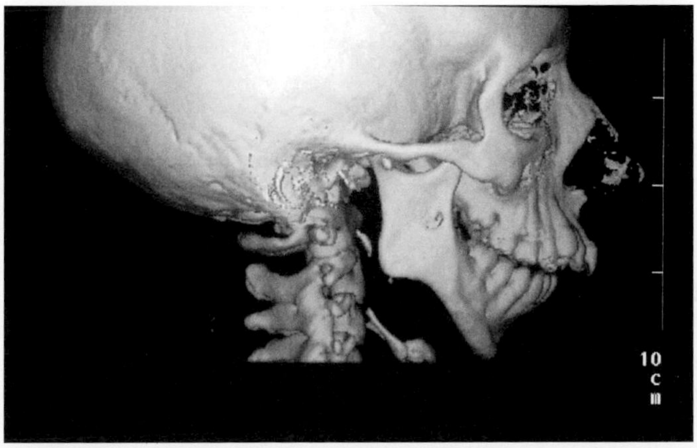

Fig. 13.2a.2 Three-dimensional CT scan of a child early onset JIA and temporomandibular joint involvement that led to reduced joint movement and micrognathia causing difficulties with anaesthetic intubation.

Macrophage activation syndrome

This can occur secondary to any systemic inflammatory disease. Macrophage activation within the bone marrow causes macrophages to ingest red blood cells, platelets and fibrinogen.

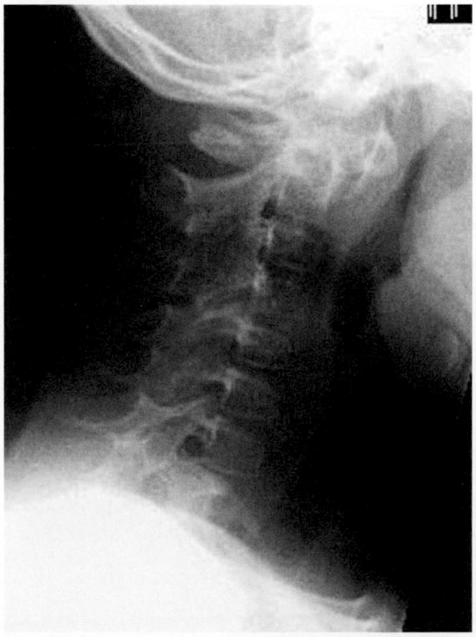

Fig. 13.2a.3 Lateral radiograph of a cervical spine showing posterior fusion from C2–C6 secondary to JIA.

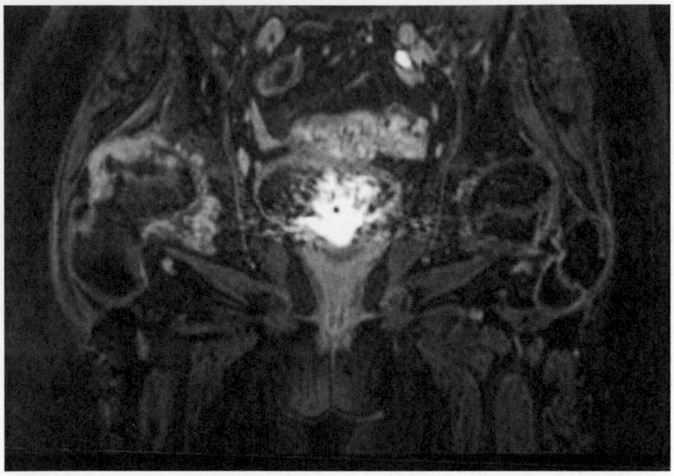

Fig. 13.2a.4 MRI scan of the pelvis showing avascular necrosis of the right femoral head and a joint effusion.

The patient becomes unwell acutely with a marked fall in platelets, fibrinogen, and ESR. The condition can be fatal.

Osteoporosis/fractures

Both complications can occur in patients with uncontrolled inflammation particularly in multiple joints and are thus more common in systemic JIA (and some poly JIA cases).

Joint damage

Restriction of joint movement secondary to pain and soft tissue contracture is common and all efforts must be taken to minimize this. Loss of cartilage leads to a reduction in joint space, problems with malalignment, and abnormal joint loading often requiring orthopaedic management (see Chapter 13.2b).

TMJ involvement in childhood may lead to micrognathia with dental and cosmetic consequences (Figure 13.2a.2). If associated with inflammation or fusion (Figure 13.2a.3) of the cervical spine there may be significant restriction of neck extension. Both problems may cause anaesthetic difficulties.

Atlantoaxial dislocation is rare but has been noted in patients with poly JIA and ligamentous laxity.

Avascular necrosis of the hips is not uncommon and may be related at least in part to treatment with steroids, or persistent active disease (Figure 13.2a.4).

13.2b

Juvenile idiopathic arthritis: surgical management

Nicholas D. Riley and A. Hashemi-Nejad

Summary points

- Approximately 10% of juvenile idiopathic arthritis cases will require a surgical procedure
- Non-operative management aims to prevent deformity, promote normal growth, and maintain function
- Perioperative problems must be anticipated and managed appropriately
- Deformity may be treated by soft tissue release and/or osteotomy
- Synovectomy may be useful if the articular surface is well-preserved
- Arthrodesis is rarely indicated except in the wrist/hand
- Arthroplasty is successful in restoring function.

Introduction

Juvenile idiopathic arthritis (JIA) is classified into three subtypes: systemic onset arthritis (10–20% of patients), typically involving fever and extra-articular manifestations, such as rash and myalgias; oligoarthritis (50–60% of patients) with four or fewer joints affected asymmetrically; and polyarthritis (20–30% of patients) characteristically involving multiple joints symmetrically. These are discussed in greater detail in Chapter 13.2a. The most common presentation to an orthopaedic surgeon is with subtalar arthritis and an associated valgus hindfoot but the most frequently involved joint is the knee.

As the aetiology and pathogenesis of JIA is unknown, treatment is supportive rather than curative, requiring specialist care from a multidisciplinary team. A holistic management plan to restore full function should include a rheumatologist, physiotherapist, occupational therapist, ophthalmologist, orthopaedic surgeon, and a psychologist for support and to ensure the child and their family cope optimally with the demands of JIA, enabling the child to integrate fully with their peer group.

Principles of management

Surgery now has a well-established role in the management of JIA with approximately 10% of children treated by a rheumatology unit requiring open surgical procedures. Short-term management is aimed principally at maintaining function, controlling inflammation, and reducing the resultant joint deformity, and thus in the long term, promoting normal growth and development and encouraging education and rehabilitation. The goal is to use the simplest, safest, and least invasive treatment strategy to maintain a normal lifestyle and to minimize morbidity and hospitalization.

Inflamed, arthritic joints will develop flexion deformities rapidly if managed inappropriately whilst prompt medical management, physiotherapy, and judicious splintage will maintain correct joint position and function. Should contracture occur despite this, the procedures to consider include intra-articular steroid injection, synovectomy, soft tissue release, epiphysiodesis, osteotomy, and arthroplasty. Arthrodesis is rarely indicated, other than in advanced disease of the hand or foot where splintage has failed.

Perioperative considerations (Box 13.2b.2)

The perioperative management of patients with JIA requires input from a multidisciplinary team. Anaesthesia can be problematic (Box 13.2b.1) due to the small airway, hypoplastic mandible, and stiff or unstable cervical spine and preoperative radiographic evaluation of the cervical spine is essential. Difficult airways may require malleable or fibreoptic intubation, or emergency tracheostomy. Laryngeal masks are useful in patients who cannot be intubated. To reduce the risk of postoperative infection, oral steroids should be stopped on the day of theatre; parenteral therapy is used during the perioperative period until the patient is able to tolerate oral medications.

Box 13.2b.1 Useful surgical procedures in JIA

- Intra-articular steroid injections
- Synovectomy
- Soft tissue release
- Epiphysiodesis—temporary/permanent
- Osteotomy
- Arthroplasty
- Arthrodesis—rarely in large joints.

Box 13.2b.2 Potential perioperative pitfalls for the JIA patient

- Stiff or unstable neck
- Micrognathia
- Inability to open mouth due to TMJ problems
- Side effects of steroid use
- Anaemia of chronic disease
- Osteoporosis.

Disease-associated hypervascularity in combination with disuse, means the bones of a JIA patient can be osteoporotic, especially when corticosteroids have been administered, so intraoperatively the limbs should be handled with care. Often the bones are smaller than normal due to growth retardation but, should JIA start in adolescence, bones may be of normal size with a large medullary cavity secondary to a thin cortical rim.

Postoperative rehabilitation can be hampered by general disease activity or more specifically adjacent joint disease activity. It is crucial to identify signs of JIA in adjacent joints preoperatively, as this will affect the success of the planned operation.

Intra-articular steroid injections

Due to their deleterious side effects, systemic steroids should be avoided where possible. Intra-articular injections of corticosteroid such as triamcinolone hexacetonide, have been shown to be safe and effective at controlling synovitis (see Chapter 13.2a). They provide rapid analgesia and facilitate physiotherapy allowing reduction or withdrawal of systemic therapy and a swifter return to normal activity than with systemic treatment alone. The early and repeated use of steroid injections reduces leg length discrepancy in oligoarthritis and prevents joint contractures. The joint effusion should be aspirated prior to injection and the fluid sent for microbiological analysis.

The post-injection regimen of rest, splintage, and physiotherapy remains controversial and has not been studied prospectively in children. It may be difficult to enforce rest in ambulatory children and whilst physiotherapy is helpful, splintage to prevent contractures is unnecessary given the efficacy of intra-articular steroids.

Outcome studies should be interpreted critically: there is inconsistency in the disease subtype studied and the time spans at which response is measured. In the largest published series to date (almost 1500 joint injections), the median duration of improvement was 74 weeks and the most effective injection was the first injection into a single joint.

The side effects of intra-articular steroid injections in JIA have not been studied prospectively but subcutaneous atrophy is a well-recognized complication. Infection rates following steroid injection are estimated at 1:100 000 with no reported cases of septic arthritis in the paediatric population. Damage to intra-articular structures has not been seen.

Synovectomy

Synovectomy is indicated when a persistent synovitis has not responded to medical management, in a joint with well-preserved articular cartilage. Given the high rate of spontaneous remission in children, judging the appropriate timing of surgical intervention can be difficult. Some units recommend waiting up to 18 months provided the joint space is maintained. Synovectomy is traumatic and can lead to a temporary increase in pain and this coupled with an uncooperative child can itself lead to stiffness and contracture. As joint damage is underestimated radiographically, MRI is recommended to assess the articular cartilage accurately prior to synovectomy (Figure 13.2b.1).

Historically, synovectomy was most commonly performed in the wrist and knee. Recently, the trend has been to avoid wrist synovectomy and to concentrate on intensive physiotherapy and

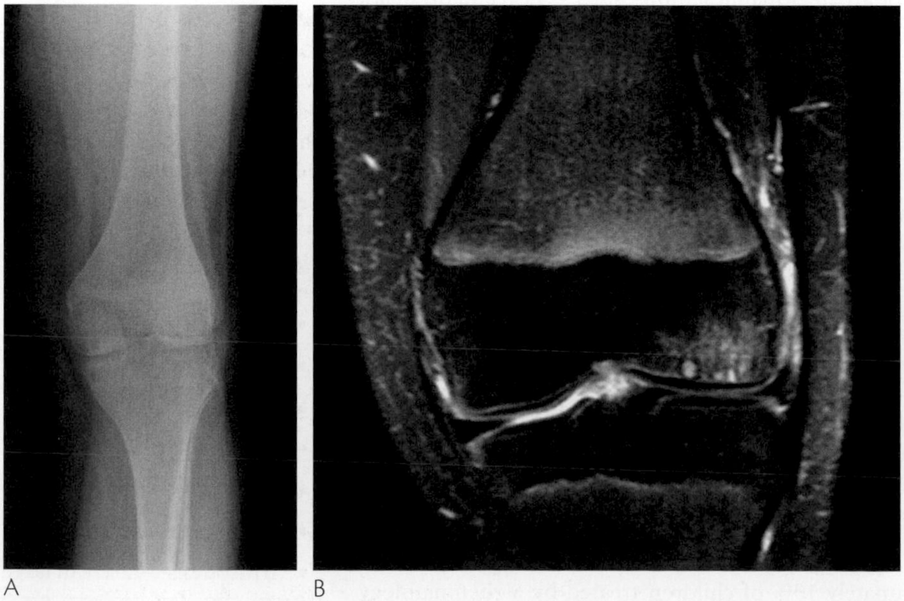

Fig. 13.2b.1 A) Plain AP radiograph of knee affected by JIA. Pain and stiffness can make it difficult to interpret the extent of the joint pathology. B) An MR image of the same knee showing bony changes particularly in the lateral femoral condyle but with relative preservation of the articular cartilage.

appropriate splintage. Should the wrist stiffen, maintaining an appropriate position will preserve function. Synovectomy of the knee is still accepted practice. Arthroscopic or open synovectomy can prevent the development of permanent contractures by relieving pain, conserving range of motion, and preventing articular damage. However, it will not improve range of motion or fixed deformity without associated corrective procedures.

There are few studies comparing open with arthroscopic synovectomy in the JIA patient. Open synovectomy requires a considerable incision and has a significant infection rate, whereas the arthroscopic procedure is less invasive and more accurate allowing early mobilization, preservation of range of motion, and reduced hospitalization. The recurrence rate for arthroscopic synovectomy is high (around 40%) and is more likely in patients who show systemic signs of disease progression. Synovectomy should not be delayed to allow systemic 'flares' to settle. The aim of synovectomy should be to lengthen the life span of articular cartilage and to remove pannus as once the articular cartilage is destroyed, articular function cannot be restored (Figure 13.2b.2).

Soft tissue release

The initial management of a soft tissue contracture should be physiotherapy and splintage. If this fails, soft tissue releases are often used especially for the hips and knees. Prior to release, joint decompression with or without synovectomy should be undertaken in order to reduce intra-articular pressure. Elevated pressure can lead to ischaemia, subluxation, porotic fractures, cartilage necrosis, and subarticular microfracture.

Fixed deformities lead to accelerated articular damage and secondary deformities in the ipsilateral adjacent joints and corresponding contralateral joint. As movement is restored after release, joint congruency and overall joint nutrition is improved. Should disease remission occur simultaneously, healing of the articular cartilage can occur and prevent more radical operations. If, conversely, the disease progresses then the subsequent prosthetic replacement is more straightforward as the soft tissue release has improved joint alignment Anterior hip and posterior knee releases are performed commonly. Hip involvement is the most important factor affecting mobility and independence and the typical deformity is that of fixed flexion and adduction. McCullough recommends the following algorithm:

1) Adductor and psoas tenotomy for a fixed flexion deformity (FFD) <25 degrees with an adduction contracture.
2) In addition to the previous step an anterior soft-tissue release with synovectomy for a FFD >25 degrees
3) Adductor and psoas release for an isolated adduction contracture with a laterally subluxed femoral head.

His colleagues report good short- to medium-term pain relief, improvement in gait, and reduction in fixed deformity with total hip replacement necessary in three of 17 patients at a mean 6.3 years after release.

Knee flexion contractures represent a major cause of disability in JIA patients. Soft tissue release can be considered as long as there is a joint space and the valgus deformity does not exceed 15 degrees. A particularly difficult problem is that of posterior subluxation of the proximal tibia, secondary to anterior cruciate ligament contracture; however, ligament resection still remains controversial. Soft tissue release of the knee is technically demanding and aims to release hamstrings, long head of biceps femoris, and the origin of gastrocnemius if required, correcting the flexion deformity and improving mobility. Intraoperative isolation of the common peroneal nerve is vital to reduce the risk of nerve injury. Good improvements in FFD and pain have been reported.

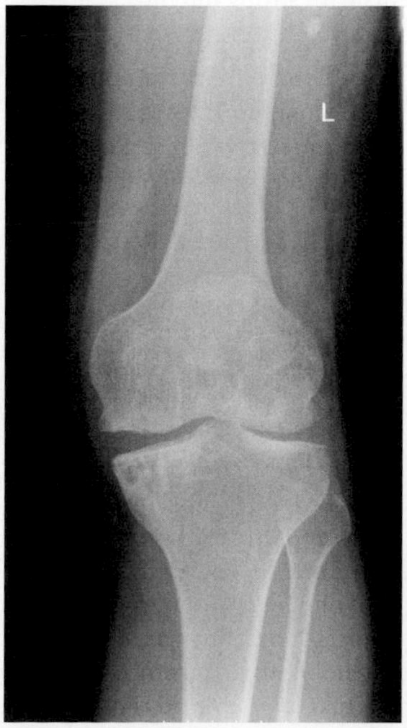

Fig. 13.2b.2 AP radiograph of a knee 7 years after synovectomy showing a preserved joint space.

Limb length discrepancy and angular deformity

Limb length inequality develops in JIA as a result of multiple local and systemic factors. Given the propensity for knee involvement in JIA, limb length discrepancy (LLD) most commonly occurs in the lower limb. The distal femoral and proximal tibial physes contribute around 2cm per year to limb length. As a result of the inflammatory process, the arthritic knee is hyperaemic adjacent to the physes causing accelerated growth. With oligoarticular disease, or early onset JIA, the medial and lateral aspects of the physis are usually affected equally, lengthening the limb symmetrically. Leg length can return to normal in 2 years with no intervention, either as the arthritis heals or the contralateral knee becomes involved. In a patient with polyarticular disease, a valgus deformity at the knee is common: this too tends to decrease with age. A LLD less than 2cm tends to be asymptomatic and should be treated conservatively with orthoses. If the LLD is due to a FFD that is not amenable to soft tissue release then osteotomy or physeal arrest is indicated. Examination of the ipsilateral hip and ankle is mandatory to ensure there is no other deformity present.

Temporary or permanent epiphysiodesis at the knee is a safe technique even in the immunocompromised child. In a child with JIA the traditional techniques of growth prediction, such as Greulich and Pyle atlas and the Eastwood and Cole graph, are less reliable due to systemic effects of corticosteroids limiting growth and local hyperaemia stimulating growth. Nevertheless, the aim is to achieve correction at skeletal maturity. This requires careful timing of surgery in addition to rigorous follow-up particularly if a temporary epiphysiodesis technique has been used. The possibility of rebound growth following staple removal or further growth of the arthritic joint must be taken into account.

The main indication for osteotomy is correction of an angular or a rotational deformity. Most commonly a supracondylar femoral osteotomy is undertaken to correct a valgus deformity at the knee. Care should be taken when performing the osteotomy as osteoporosis is common. Internal fixation is often difficult given the porotic nature of the bone and a plaster cast may be required for added stability and to maintain joint position. The plaster cast is usually removed at 1 month to enable early mobilization. Some patients require repeat osteotomies for recurrence of the deformity associated with excessive growth.

Arthrodesis

As the goal is to preserve range of motion, arthrodesis is rarely performed. However, arthrodesing a deformed wrist in a functional position is beneficial for hand function. This can be achieved by the use of a low profile arthrodesis plate or by intramedullary fixation with a Steinmann pin passed down the third metacarpal via the carpus into the distal radius.

Arthroplasty

Arthroplasty is reserved for those patients who have irreversible articular damage with associated restriction of movement, deformity, and significant pain. The choice of treatment and the timing may be influenced by the overall pattern of joint involvement (Figure 13.2b.3). Arthroplasty in a patient with JIA requires care pre-, intra-, and post-operatively to ensure that potential pitfalls specific to the patient group are avoided. Other treatments should be pursued prior to arthroplasty and whilst they may only delay prosthetic replacement, improvement in systemic symptoms and increased growth may be vital for the success of an arthroplasty. The survival rate of total hip arthroplasty (THA) and total knee arthroplasty (TKA) improves with increasing patient age. Currently, joint replacements are undertaken for the hip, knee, shoulder, elbow, wrist, and ankle.

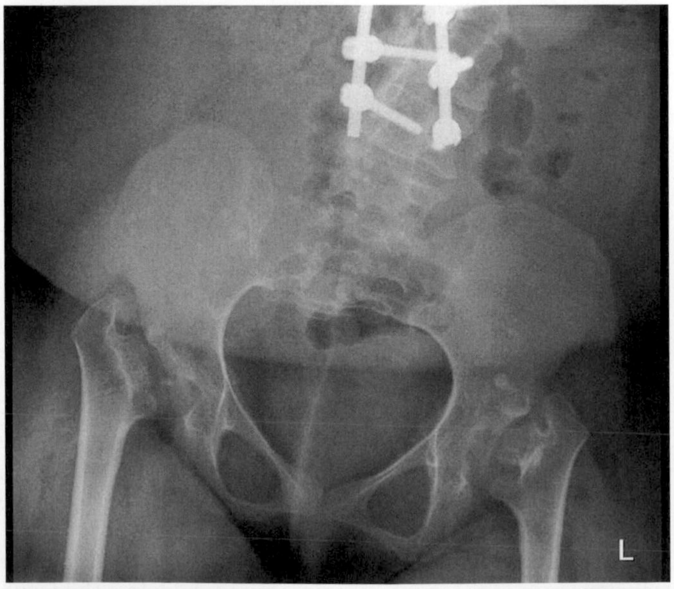

Fig. 13.2b.3 AP radiograph of the pelvis and lower lumbar spine. The patient has already undergone a spinal fusion and has bilateral hip destruction. The stiffness from all 3 sites has severely limited the patient's ability to mobilize. Bilateral hip joint arthroplasties were performed.

Hip arthroplasty

In JIA patients, THA has been used successfully, in terms of functional recovery, for 40 years. The main indications for THA in addition to those mentioned earlier are subluxation/dislocation and protrusio acetabuli. THA is usually undertaken once skeletal maturity has been reached. However, an open physis is only a relative contraindication to surgery as the proximal femoral physis only contributes 15% to limb length and is often damaged by JIA. There is a slightly higher rate of acetabular failure with an open triradiate physis and in our opinion THA should be performed when the triradiate is fused (which may be early as a result of JIA). The relationship between diaphyseal expansion of the femur and the longevity of a cemented or uncemented femoral prosthesis in a growing patient is still unknown. JIA patients are protected by their low weight and low activity but still experience significant rates of aseptic loosening. The growing, remodelling skeleton, associated osteopenia and steroid treatment may contribute to early prosthetic loosening. Component wear rates are low in JIA populations because of their low demand.

Should hip and knee arthroplasty be indicated, then the THA should precede the TKA. THA is less painful than TKA and rehabilitation post-THA is possible in the presence of stiff knees. Hip deformity can contribute to knee deformity and correction of the former may suffice. Conservative management of knee contractures are possible with a THA *in situ* and the best TKA outcomes are seen in patients with strong hip muscles.

In young patients, THA will not usually last a lifetime: the current consensus is, where possible, to use uncemented components. With cemented femoral prostheses, it is difficult to centralize the prosthesis and obtain an adequate cement mantle. Subsequent cement fracture, subsidence, osteolysis, and reduction in bone stock lead to failure. Although cementless stems are technically challenging, careful, gradual reaming and the use of longer modular stems helps preserve bone stock. In early press-fit design stems there was a higher failure rate due to a lack of early fixation. With the advent of porous and hydroxyapatite coating, the results of uncemented femoral components have improved. Despite the characteristics of JIA bone, rapid osteointegration has been demonstrated.

Early to mid-term function is improved in the JIA patient regardless of the fixation method. Postoperatively, function improves more slowly than in patients with other pathologies because of the polyarticular nature of the disease and systemic treatment but both sitting and activities of daily life show marked improvement. In one study, 94% of THA patients were wheelchair bound preoperatively but 88% were still ambulatory at 11-year follow up. Survival at 15 years for cemented THA in JIA is approximately 70% and 90% acetabular and 100% femoral component survival rates for uncemented prostheses have been reported at 13 years.

Knee arthroplasty

TKA is indicated in JIA patients with marked functional impairment or disabling pain from advanced joint involvement. As with THA, skeletal immaturity is only a relative contraindication. However, incomplete distal femoral physeal closure can lead to progressive angular deformity and arthroplasty should be delayed in those patients with significant growth potential. Contraindications to arthroplasty include systemic or local knee infection, hyperextension deformity, quadriceps weakness, and Charcot neuropathic arthropathy.

Preoperative physiotherapy and serial casting should be employed to minimize flexion contractures and facilitate the surgery. Postoperative bracing and manipulation to maintain or regain ranges of motion are preferable to increasing the distal femoral excision to accomplish intraoperative correction of deformity. This allows the knee to function more naturally and reduces the propensity to raise the joint line. As little bone as possible should be removed and bone graft used to address bony defects. At the time of TKA, JIA is usually burnt out; however any remaining synovium should be excised. The patella, which is frequently small, deformed, laterally subluxed, and high riding, should be resurfaced and the osteophytes excised.

In the presence of severe flexion contracture or posterior tibial subluxation, the posterior cruciate ligament (PCL) must be sacrificed to achieve optimal soft tissue balancing and alignment. Proponents of the PCL sacrificing prosthesis argue that it allows improved deformity correction, increases joint congruency, and reduces polyethylene wear. However, cruciate retaining prostheses preserve bone stock, allow femoral roll-back, facilitate stair climbing, and absorb shear forces better. There are no long-term studies comparing cruciate retaining or sacrificing prostheses in the JIA patient.

Potential long-term cement failure with component loosening and osteolysis has led to increased interest in uncemented prostheses. As JIA patients are young, uncemented prostheses have obvious benefits; maintenance of bone stock for revision, lack of biological response to polymethylmethacrylate, reduced operating time, no cement extrusion and associated wear debris. There are no long-term results for uncemented TKA and as cement is tolerated better in the knee than the hip, there is less urgency to abandon its use in younger patients.

Radiolucent lines are common and remain a concern: the majority are asymptomatic and their clinical significance remains to be established. Regular and long-term follow-up of this young patient group is essential.

The literature indicates that TKA in JIA patients with severe and disabling knee joint involvement provides predictably good pain relief and functional improvement. Survival rates ranging from 100% at 4 years to 77% at 10 years have been reported.

Shoulder hemiarthroplasty

Shoulder involvement is seen later in the course of systemic or polyarticular JIA, with an incidence of 15% at 15 years. Indications for shoulder arthroplasty are pain, reduced function and joint destruction in patients who have failed more conservative treatments. Significant improvement in joint movement has been reported.

Elbow arthroplasty

Encouraging results have been reported following total elbow arthroplasty with 87% of joints showing increased function and a reduction in pain at 2 years postoperatively. Indications include destruction of the ulnohumeral joint with gross restriction of movement (<30 degrees) and pain.

Further reading

Breit, W., Frosch, M., Meyer, U., Heinecke, A., and Ganser, G. (2000). A subgroup-specific evaluation of the efficacy of intraarticular triamcinolone hexacetonide in juvenile chronic arthritis. *Journal of Rheumatology*, **27**, 2696–702.

Cage, D.J., Granberry, W.M., and Tullos, H.S. (1992). Long-term results of total arthroplasty in adolescents with debilitating polyarthropathy. *Clinical Orthopaedics and Related Research*, **283**, 156–62.

Davidson, J. (2000). Juvenile idiopathic arthritis: a clinical overview. *European Journal of Radiology*, **33**, 128–34.

Dell'Era, L., Facchini, R., and Corona, F. (2008). Knee synovectomy in children with juvenile idiopathic arthritis. *Journal of Pediatric Orthopedics*, **17**, 128–30.

Iesaka, K., Kubiak, E.N., Bong, M.R., Su, E.T., and Di Cesare, P.E. (2006). Orthopedic surgical management of hip and knee involvement in patients with juvenile rheumatoid arthritis. *American Journal of Orthopedics*, **35**, 67–73.

Kitsoulis, P.B., Stafilas, K.S., Siamopoulou, A., Soucacos, P.N., and Xenakis, T.A. (2006). Total hip arthroplasty in children with juvenile chronic arthritis: long-term results. *Journal of Pediatric Orthopedics*, **26**, 8–12.

McCullough, C.J. (1994). Surgical management of the hip in juvenile chronic arthritis. *British Journal of Rheumatology*, **33**, 178–83.

Simmons, B.P., Nutting, J.T., and Bernstein, R.A. (1996). Juvenile rheumatoid arthritis. *Hand Clinics*, **12**, 573–89.

Swann, M. (1990). The surgery of juvenile chronic arthritis. An overview. *Clinical Orthopaedics and Related Research*, **259**, 70–5.

Woo, P. (2006). Systemic juvenile idiopathic arthritis: diagnosis, management, and outcome. *Nature Clinical Practice. Rheumatology*, **2**, 28–34.

13.3

An overview of cerebral palsy

Lucinda J. Carr

Summary points

- Cerebral palsy is a permanent disorder of movement or posture due to non-progressive lesions of the immature brain
- Magnetic resonance imaging is generally recommended and can provide important prognostic information
- Only a minority of cases are due to birth trauma
- Modern classification systems incorporate function as well as anatomical involvement
- Management aims to maximize a child's potential both as an individual and within society. Other associated conditions may impact on quality of life and participation
- Multidisciplinary involvement is essential with use of physiotherapy, orthotics, and tone management (focal and systemic) as necessary.

Definition and introduction

Cerebral palsy is a descriptive umbrella term describing a permanent disorder of movement or posture due to non-progressive lesions of the immature brain. It is the most common childhood movement disorder with an incidence of around 1:400 live births (2–2.5/1000 live births). Despite improvements in obstetric and perinatal care, the incidence has not changed significantly over recent decades.

Although the cerebral lesion is itself static, the clinical manifestations typically evolve over time and with growth. For example, the abnormal movements of dyskinetic cerebral palsy are rarely seen in infancy and the full clinical picture is often only established by the second year. Children with a moderate diplegia often deteriorate during adolescence and become non-ambulant.

Cerebral palsy is defined as a motor disorder but there are often associated conditions, such as perceptual and sensory changes, disturbances of feeding and communication, cognitive and behavioural difficulties, and seizures. This has led to recent calls for a more inclusive definition that acknowledges the wider functional effects of cerebral palsy.

Aetiology

Over recent years a better understanding of the causes of cerebral palsy has been reached due largely to detailed epidemiological studies that have included neuroimaging. Magnetic resonance imaging (MRI) is the more sensitive tool. It allows assessment of the aetiology and timing of the cerebral insult and can provide important prognostic information for families, not just for the affected child but also for future pregnancies. A recent review identified abnormal neuroimaging in 80–90% of children with cerebral palsy. Scan abnormalities may be summarized into three main types as follows.

Brain malformations

Malformations most commonly result from disruption in normal neuronal migration during early pregnancy (<20 weeks' gestation). They account for around 10% of imaging abnormalities seen in children with cerebral palsy. Whilst the majority of these defects are sporadic, there are a number of recognized genetic, infective, and metabolic causes that should be excluded. Typically neuronal migration disorders result in the abnormal development of the gyral and sulcal patterns as in lissencephaly (Figure 13.3.1), pachygyria, and polymicrogyria, or in the periventricular heterotopic collection of abnormal neurones. Occasionally, an early destructive process impedes migration resulting in parenchymal clefts or cysts lined with heterotopic grey matter and often associated with cortical dysplasia (e.g. schizencephaly (Figure 13.3.2) and porencephaly). Infants are usually born at term with no obvious risk factors. The clinical features vary from mild hemiplegia to severe quadriplegia. Epilepsy is particularly common in these conditions.

Grey and white matter damage

White matter abnormalities represent damage occurring before 34 weeks' gestation. They are most common in premature infants. The classical pattern is one of a loss of periventricular white matter (PVL, periventricular leucomalacia, Figure 13.3.3) associated with signal change on T_1- and T_2-weighted images. Changes generally affect the posterior ventricular regions in diplegia and are more extensive in quadriplegia. Characteristically there is associated

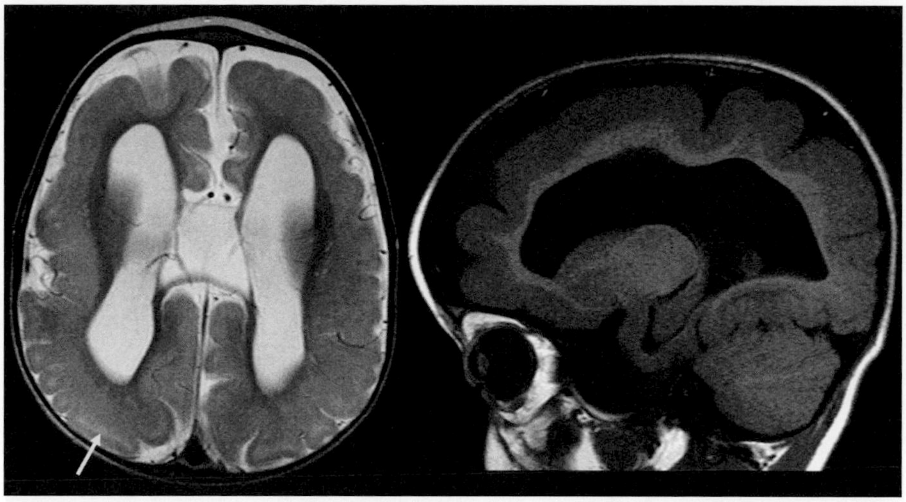

Fig. 13.3.1 Lissencephaly type 1 (Classical): the term means 'smooth brain' and the MRI shows a thickened and poorly convoluted cortex with lack of sulci and gyri. There is reduced volume of white matter without gliosis. The characteristic cell sparse zone is identified by the arrow.

irregular enlargement of the lateral ventricles and thinning of the corpus callosum. If the damage is more extensive, both cortical and subcortical changes may result (multicystic encephalomalacia) and a more severe clinical picture is seen.

Damage confined to grey matter is uncommon but is seen in children with dystonic cerebral palsy.

Focal infarcts may also extend into grey and white matter. They are almost exclusively seen in children with hemiplegia, involving middle cerebral artery territory.

Ventriculomegaly, atrophy, and cerebrospinal fluid abnormalities

Hydrocephalus is not uncommon in cerebral palsy, particularly following intraventricular haemorrhage related to prematurity. This is distinct from secondary ventriculomegaly due to the volume loss of cerebral atrophy.

The causes of cerebral palsy are often multifactorial. It was once considered that the majority of cases were due to birth trauma but in term infants with cerebral palsy, the current consensus is that less than 10% are due to birth asphyxia itself. Infants that are already compromised *in utero* are likely to be more vulnerable during the delivery itself. As discussed later, different causal factors are implicated in the different forms of cerebral palsy.

Risk factors

Risk factors are generally divided into prenatal, perinatal (from labour to the end of the first week of life), and postnatal factors. In most term infants, the origins of cerebral palsy can be traced back to the prenatal period, whilst in preterm infants, damage usually occurs perinatally (Table 13.3.1).

Prematurity and low birthweight

Cerebral palsy risk increases with decreasing gestation and birthweight. Studies consistently show that prematurity (<37 completed weeks' gestation) is the single most important risk factor for

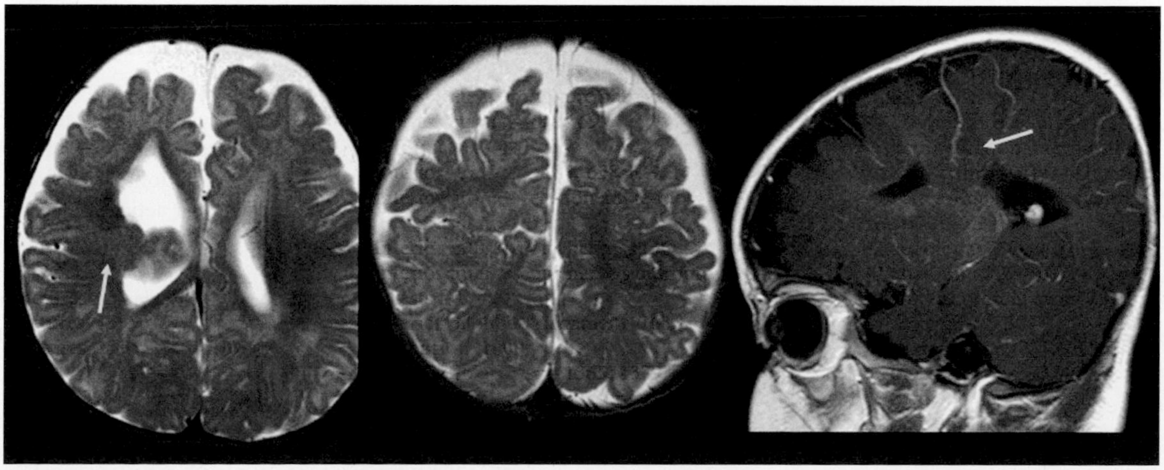

Fig. 13.3.2 Schizencephaly (unilateral, close-lipped): the term means 'split' brain and the condition is characterized by deep slits and clefts in the cerebral hemispheres. The scan shows a deep cleft in the right frontal lobe, lined by abnormal (polymicrogyric) grey matter (arrows). The cortex elsewhere is normal. The white matter is reduced in volume without gliosis.

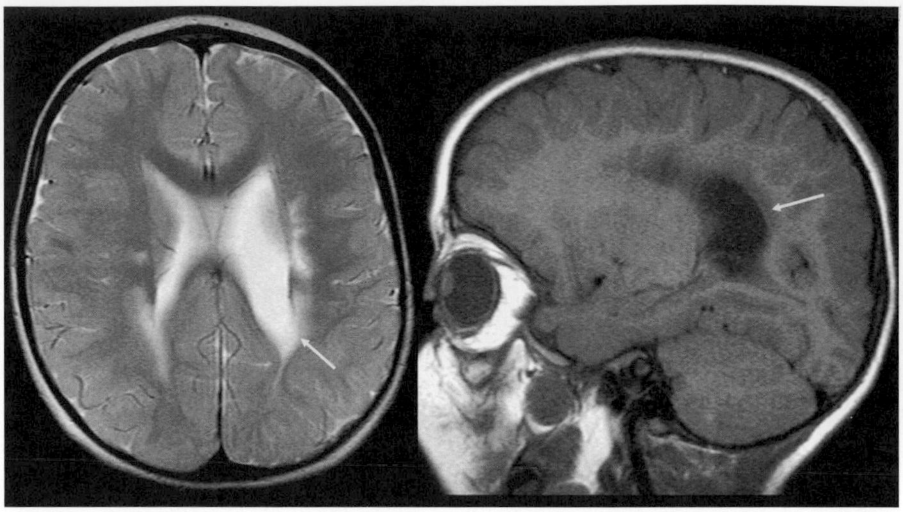

Fig. 13.3.3 Periventricular leucomalacia (PVL): the ischaemic changes are seen in the white matter around the lateral ventricles. Gliosis and atrophy of the periventricular white matter is demonstrated by the arrow. The cortex is normal.

cerebral palsy; the risk being approximately eight times higher than in term infants. With intrauterine growth retardation (IUGR) where birthweight is significantly less than that expected for the gestational age, the risk of cerebral palsy is increased further. Although improvements in neonatal intensive care have increased the survival rate of extreme preterm infants, the risk of significant complications remains high, particularly in those of very low birthweight (≤1500g). Around 15% of infants of very low birthweight will suffer severe intraventricular haemorrhage or PVL, the majority of whom will go on to develop cerebral palsy. Other major complications such as chronic lung and bowel disease (bronchopulmonary dysplasia and necrotizing enterocolitis) are common in this group. Overall, these children account for only 2.2% of all live births, but they comprise almost 40% of the cases of children diagnosed with cerebral palsy each year in the United States of America.

Table 13.3.1 Risk factors for the development of cerebral palsy

Prenatal	Perinatal	Postnatal
Intrauterine growth retardation	Vascular event	Infection (particularly CNS)
Maternal chorioamnionitis	Birth asphyxia	Head injury (accidental or non-accidental)
Congenital infection (TORCH*)	Sepsis/meningitis	Vascular event (spontaneous or postoperative)
Toxin exposure (recreational/iatrogenic)	Metabolic derangement including kernicterus	
Vascular event		
Fetal malformation		
Neuronal migration disorder		

*TORCH infections: Toxoplasmosis, other infections (HIV, syphilis), Rubella, Cytomegalovirus, Herpes simplex virus. Adapted from Swaiman and Wu, 2006.

Multiple births

A multiple pregnancy increases the risk of premature delivery, intrapartum complications, and low birthweight. In itself it is an independent risk for cerebral palsy, particularly where there is fetal or infant death of a twin and this is probably due to monochorionic placentation resulting in twin-to-twin transfusion.

Postnatal factors

Postnatal factors are generally defined as events occurring outside the neonatal period (>28 days postdelivery) and distinguish acquired from congenital cerebral palsy. There is poor agreement as to the upper age limit for this definition which in different studies varies from 2–10 years. Postnatal causes account for 10% of cases of cerebral palsy and despite an improved understanding of the underlying causes in this group, the incidence has not changed significantly recently. The causes in order of frequency are listed in Table 13.3.1. The acquired injuries most commonly result in hemiplegic or four-limb cerebral palsy. An acquired diplegia is very rare.

Classification of cerebral palsy (Box 13.3.1)

Cerebral palsy syndromes are generally classified by the clinical nature of the motor disorder, namely the tonal abnormalities and the anatomical distribution of these abnormalities. There have been many attempts to refine this traditional classification that fails to consider underlying pathological or aetiological factors and any of the associated impairments. The clinical groups are themselves ill-defined: the distinction between asymmetric diplegia and hemiplegia, and between diplegia and quadriplegia is often inconsistent. By convention the predominant tonal abnormality is reported, but in reality, tone is often mixed with both pyramidal and extrapyramidal components.

Surprisingly, there is no measure of function within the current classification system but increasingly physicians are adding some measure of functional grading to the clinical description of cerebral palsy. The Gross Motor Function Classification System (GMFCS) is the most widely used validated measure that can be used as a

Box 13.3.1 Types of cerebral palsy

- Spastic motor disorders—approximately 60–70%:
  - Diplegia 33%
  - Hemiplegia 25%
  - Total body involvement <10%
- Extrapyramidal/dyskinetic—approximately 15%:
  - Dystonic 10%
  - Hyperkinetic 5%
- Ataxic <10%
- Unclassified—approximately 10%

basis for prognostic counselling and planning management. It is based on longitudinal observations and provides a description of the pattern of gross motor development by severity and age (Figure 13.3.4).

For the practising clinician, the traditional definitions (as described by Hagberg and Hagberg, 1993) still apply and are described here.

Spastic motor disorders

The spastic motor disorders are the most common and seen in 60–70% of children with cerebral palsy. Spasticity is just one feature of a wider 'upper motorneuron syndrome' and these other factors should also be considered when managing a child with spasticity. They comprise both positive and negative features as illustrated in Table 13.3.2.

Bilateral spastic cerebral palsy

Diplegia

This is the most common cerebral palsy syndrome accounting for around 33% of cases. Clinically, it is characterized by increased muscle tone with legs more affected than arms. Walking is often delayed but more than 50% of affected children will eventually walk. It is the most common consequence of preterm delivery; around 70% of children with diplegia having been born before 36 weeks gestation. The classical pathology of diplegia relates to the PVL seen in preterm infants. This damage typically affects motor fibres to the lower limbs. The nearby optic radiations are also vulnerable accounting for the visual difficulties and strabismus often seen in diplegia. Other associated conditions include epilepsy in around 15% of children and mild to moderate learning difficulties in 30%.

Quadriplegia (also known as tetraplegia, four-limb cerebral palsy, or total body involvement)

It is seen in less than 10% of children with cerebral palsy but these children are likely to have multiple difficulties and significant functional impairment. Damage may result from a variety of cortical and subcortical lesions particularly multicystic encephalomalacia but also from severe PVL and brain malformations. Tone is increased in both upper and lower limbs and often involves bulbar musculature so that typically these children show extensive feeding and communication difficulties. Only the minority will walk. Over 80% will have microcephaly and significant learning difficulties. Epilepsy is present in more than 50%.

Unilateral spastic cerebral palsy

Hemiplegia

Manifest as a unilateral paresis with spasticity, hemiplegia is the second most common cerebral palsy syndrome. It is seen in around 25% of children with cerebral palsy. It is often congenital and without any clear prenatal event. Focal ischaemic lesions and subcortical periventricular lesions are the most common causes. Unilateral brain malformations may be seen in term infants. Congenital hemiplegia often has an apparent 'silent period' with the absence of clinical signs in the first 4–5 months. The appearance of strong hand preference around this time may be the first sign of an abnormality. Fifty percent of children with hemiplegia will walk at the appropriate time and most are ambulant by age 2 years. Comorbid features are common, particularly undergrowth of the affected side with abnormal sensation. Visual problems in terms of hemianopia should be looked for. Epilepsy, which is strongly associated with learning difficulties, is present in 30% of cases and subtle behavioural problems are common.

Extrapyramidal/dyskinetic cerebral palsy

Extrapyramidal cerebral palsy

The abnormal movements or postures result from defective coordination and/or regulation of muscle tone. The group is subdivided into dystonic and hyperkinetic forms. In dystonic cerebral palsy (10% of cases), there are slow sustained tonic contractions of limbs or axial musculature, which are often provoked by emotion and effort and associated with persisting primitive reflexes, particularly the asymmetric tonic neck reflex. In hyperkinetic cerebral palsy (5% of cases) movements are purposeless and involuntary and may comprise athetoid movements that are slow, writhing, and distal, or jerky, more proximal choreic movements. There is often some associated spasticity. In the older child, the repeated, uncontrolled neck flexion and extension may lead to a secondary spinal cord myelopathy.

Dyskinetic cerebral palsy

Typically, the child with dyskinetic cerebral palsy is initially hypotonic before the classical features emerge by the second year of life. Dyskinetic cerebral palsy is seen in both term and preterm infants. In the term infant it is most often the result of acute severe peripartum hypoxia. In the preterm infant, it is associated with more prolonged severe hypoxia and/or hyperbilirubinaemia, where neonatal jaundice has led to kernicterus, defined as dyskinetic cerebral palsy associated with sensorineural deafness, abnormal dentition, and supranuclear ophthalmoplegia. Neuroimaging commonly shows basal ganglia changes, sometimes in conjunction with more widespread cortical damage.

Ataxic cerebral palsy

This is the least common subgroup (<10%) of cerebral palsy. The predominant clinical features are those of a non-progressive cerebellar ataxia with poor balance and coordination and intention tremor. The diagnosis is made with caution as there are a number of very slowly progressive disorders, such as Pelizeus–Merzbacher disease that can mimic this clinically. Neuroimaging should always be performed.

GMFCS for children aged 6–12 years: Descriptors and illustrations

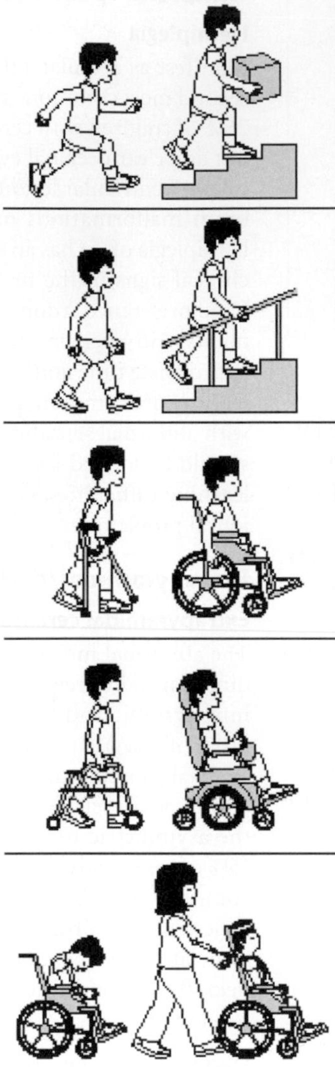

GMFCS Level I
Children walk indoors and outdoors and climb stairs without limitation. Children perform gross motor skills including running and jumping, but speed, balance and co-ordination are impaired.

GMFCS Level II
Children walk indoors and outdoors and climb stairs holding onto a railing but experience limitations walking on uneven surfaces and inclines and walking in crowds or confined spaces.

GMFCS Level III
Children walk indoors or outdoors on a level surface with an assistive mobility device. Children may climb stairs holding onto a railing. Children may propel a wheelchair manually or are transported when traveling for long distances or outdoor on uneven terrain.

GMFCS Level IV
Children may continue to walk for short distances on a walker or rely more on wheeled mobility at home and schoold and in the community.

GMFCS Level V
Physical impairment restricts voluntary control of movement and the ability to maintain antigravity head and trunk postures. All areas of motor function are limited. Children have no means of independent mobility and are transported.

Fig. 13.3.4 The Gross Motor Function Classification System (GMFCS). This system classifies the gross motor function of children with cerebral palsy at various age ranges on the basis of their self-initiated movement with particular emphasis on sitting (truncal control), walking, and wheeled mobility. The example shown is for children between the ages of 6–12 years. It is a classification system not an outcome measure. Palisano, RJ, *et al* (2003). Effect of environmental setting on mobility methods of children with cerebal palsy. *Dev Med Child Neurol*, **45**, 113–120. With permission.

Table 13.3.2 Positive and negative effects of the upper motorneuron syndrome

Positive features	Negative features
Spasticity: Dynamic hypertonus Hyperreflexia Clonus Abnormal cocontraction	Loss of dexterity
Increased flexor reflexes: Babinski response Mass synergy patterns	Weakness (distal): Inadequate force generation Slow movements
	Loss of selective control

Making the diagnosis

History and examination

From the history, a child may already be identified as 'high risk' for cerebral palsy, namely through antenatal detection or through perinatal events and such children should be assessed regularly and early intervention offered if/when physical signs emerge. In many children the diagnosis of cerebral palsy is not suspected initially but even in these cases a careful history may reveal risk factors, not previously recognized and on assessment 'warning signs' of neurological abnormality may be detected (Box 13.3.2). The child who is labelled with cerebral palsy is presumed to have a static motor disorder. However, motor abnormalities may be the earliest signs of a

Box 13.3.2 Early warning signs for the development of cerebral palsy

- In high-risk neonate:
  - Abnormal tone
  - Irritability and/or seizures
  - Poor feeding
  - Abnormal head growth
- Later signs:
  - Delayed or deviant milestones
  - Persisting primitive reflexes
  - Abnormal tone
  - Microcephaly
  - Comorbid signs (e.g. abnormal visual behaviour).

neurodegenerative disorder (genetic or metabolic disease) or they may be an early manifestation of more global developmental delay. The clinician should always consider an alternative diagnosis if the child with 'cerebral palsy' has a strong family history of motor disorder, or if history and investigation fail to provide an underlying explanation. Suspicions should also be raised if the physical signs themselves are unusual, such as clearly progressive or fluctuating in nature.

Investigation

To establish the diagnosis of cerebral palsy, further investigation should be considered: neuroimaging is now widely available and is generally advised. It enables clarification of aetiology and more accurate discussion of the likely neurodevelopmental outcome. Neuroimaging will show characteristic abnormalities in approximately 85% of children with cerebral palsy. Many of the neurodegenerative conditions have distinct and characteristic scan abnormalities. Further genetic, metabolic, and neurophysiological tests are indicated if the diagnosis of cerebral palsy is not established or if an alternative diagnosis is suspected.

There are some rare conditions where diagnosis is best established by a 'trial of treatment'. This is particularly true when despite investigation, cerebral palsy remains unexplained and is associated with a dystonia. There is a spectrum of dystonias which are partially or fully responsive to dopamine. The best described, Segawa syndrome, is often diagnosed initially as a spastic/dystonic diplegia. Children classically present with an abnormal gait that worsens through the day and is improved by sleep. Diagnosis is confirmed by genetic testing and measurement of cerebrospinal fluid (CSF) neurotransmitters. The presentation of the dopa-responsive dystonias is highly variable so that where there is uncertainty, paediatric neurologists advocate a 3–6 month trial of high dose L-dopa.

Principles of management

In 2001, the World Health Organization revised their classifications of impairment, disability, and handicap suggesting that classification should now be based on functioning and disability from the perspectives of the individual (structure and function) and society (activities and participation). The principal aim of management is to maximize a child's potential both as an individual and within society. This requires a holistic approach that is responsive to the specific difficulties of each child and his/her family. For children in the United Kingdom with cerebral palsy, care is generally delivered through a multidisciplinary Child Development Team often coordinated by a key worker (Figure 13.3.5).

In the child with cerebral palsy, mobility and posture will be of particular concern but other associated conditions should always be considered and indeed there may be times when they are functionally more significant then the motor difficulties themselves. These may include aspects of feeding and communication and medical issues, such as epilepsy, the management of hydrocephalus, and visual problems. Support around behaviour, social care, and education is also essential and often, in more severely involved children, a large team of professionals is involved.

With respect to management, problems and priorities should be agreed between the child, parents, and therapists. Any intervention undertaken should have a clear aim and where possible the outcome measured objectively. In terms of physical management the aims are to maximize function and prevent the complications that result from abnormal tone. Physiotherapy is the first line of intervention and may be delivered through many different techniques. To date, no one method has proven superior. Physiotherapy generally includes muscle stretching and strengthening, to encourage the maintenance of active and passive ranges of joint movements and, where necessary, positioning and seating are addressed. Orthotics are often used to support this.

Systemic or focal medications may be indicated if abnormal tone is clearly affecting function and/or delivery of care. The means of administration and any potential side effects should be carefully considered. The goals of treatment should be agreed and re-evaluated after treatment and where possible objective measures taken.

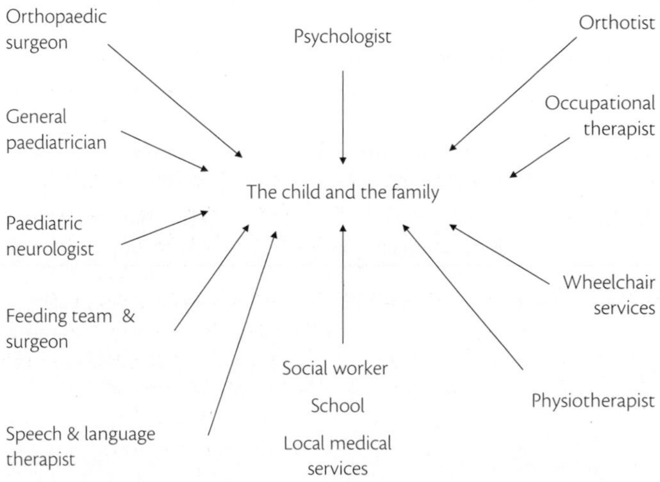

Fig. 13.3.5 The multidisciplinary team may involve all or some of the people listed and may require input from others depending on the individual needs of the child and their family. The figure depicts all arrows focusing on the family but the team and the system relies on communication both forward and backward (and sideways) between all members of the team. A lead clinician or team member should be identified to ensure that all care and communication is coordinated appropriately.

Table 13.3.3 summarizes the oral drugs most commonly used in the treatment of spasticity. In the United Kingdom, baclofen is the drug most widely used in children with spasticity. Baclofen can also be of benefit for dystonia but the anticholinergic drugs, particularly trihexyphenidyl, are the mainstay of treatment. In a minority of patients a trial of L-dopa is indicated.

Oral baclofen has poor CSF penetration but baclofen can be administered directly into the CNS using an indwelling intrathecal catheter and implanted intra-abdominal reservoir. Thus effective drug doses are delivered to the target areas minimizing systemic side effects. Although the treatment is expensive and specialized, its benefits in spasticity management are well described. It is not yet widely available in the United Kingdom.

To target treatment to more focal areas of spasticity or dystonia, intramuscular injections with botulinum toxin (BTA) should be considered (see Chapter 13.4). BTA injections can be a valuable adjunct in the management of children with cerebral palsy, not just in improving function but also for comfort, cosmesis, and for ease of care.

For comprehensive management, specialist clinics for children with cerebral palsy play a valuable role; in particular combined neurology/orthopaedic clinics, feeding clinics, and clinics assessing and augmenting communication. Close working with Education and Social Services is crucial in supporting the child and family and furthering participation. In the United Kingdom, a Statement of Special Educational Needs provides an individual statutory assessment and agreed care package for the child within an Educational Setting. There are ongoing government initiatives looking at improving the integration of these services.

Table 13.3.3 Oral drug treatments for spasticity

Drug	Mechanism	Side effects
Baclofen	$GABA_B$ agonist	Sedation Weakness
Diazepam	$GABA_{A\ \&\ B}$ agonist	As above + tolerance
Tizanidine	α adrenergic agonist	Dry mouth Tiredness Hepatotoxicity
Dantrolene	Inhibits calcium release in muscle	Weakness Hepatotoxicity
Gabapentin	GABA analogue Mechanism unknown	Behavioural change Dry mouth

There are many alternative therapies on offer for families and children and with the increasing use of the Internet this is an area many families will explore. Information online is not always accurate and claims are not always realistic. Ideally this can be discussed openly with the doctors and therapists and advice and information shared. Support groups, in particular SCOPE, offer factsheets about many standard and more alternative treatments. They also run a helpline for children and families.

Transition into adult medical services can be difficult for the child and family and needs careful preplanning. Adult services do not offer the inclusive service seen in paediatric practice and care can often become fragmented.

Conclusion

Cerebral palsy remains a common condition. Whilst recent studies have improved our understanding of the associated risks and underlying causes we are still a long way from preventing its occurrence. It is important that clinical and scientific data can be shared between centres and increasingly, clinicians recognize that an agreed systematic approach to describing the clinical and scientific data collected is needed. This will allow further clarification of the causes and better evaluation of any management interventions.

Further reading

Albright, A.L., Barron, W.B., Fusik, M.P., *et al* (1993). Continuous intrathecal baclofen infusion for spasticity of cerebral origin. *Journal of the American Medical Association,* **270**, 2475–7.

Bax, M., Goldstein, M., Rosenbaum, P., Leviton, A., and Paneth, N. (2005). Proposed definition and classification of cerebral palsy April 2005. *Developmental Medicine and Child Neurology*, **47**, 571–6.

Hagberg, B. and Hagberg, G. (1993). The origins of cerebral palsy. In David, T.J. (ed) *Recent Advances in Paediatrics* Vol. 11, pp. 67–83. Edinburgh: Churchill Livingstone.

Mutch, L.W., Alberman, E., Hagberg, B., Kodama, K., and Perat, M.V. (1992). Cerebral palsy epidemiology: where are we now, where are we going. *Developmental Medicine and Child Neurology*, **34**, 547–55.

Rosenbaum, P.L., Walter, S.D., Hanna, S.E., *et al* (2002). Prognosis for gross motor function in cerebral palsy: Creation of motor development curves. *Journal of the American Medical Association,* **288**, 1357–63.

Swaiman, K.F. and Yu, Y. (2006). Cerebral palsy. In Swaiman, K., Ashwal, S., and Ferriero, D.M. (eds) *Pediatric Neurology: Principles and Practice,* fourth edition, pp.491–504. Philadelphia, PA: Mosby, Elsevier.

World Health Organization. (2001). *The International Classification of Functioning, Disability and Health (ICF)*. Geneva: World Health Organization.

13.4

Lower limb management in cerebral palsy

Tim Theologis and J.M.H. Paterson

Summary points

- All patients with cerebral palsy have lower limb involvement
- Determination of the pattern of neurological involvement and the degree of selective muscle control is important when considering orthopaedic intervention
- The neurological insult is non-progressive but the musculoskeletal effects do progress.
- Specific treatment aims must be identified and realistic targets defined
- The appropriate treatment must be selected for the child's age and stage of development
- It is important to differentiate between dynamic and fixed contractures
- Surgery is only one of the management options and is rarely successful if considered in isolation.

Introduction

Lower limb involvement is universal in the group of disorders of posture and movement that come under the general heading of cerebral palsy. The clinical features of cerebral palsy may closely resemble those seen in older patients with traumatic head injury, stroke and near-drowning events, and the orthopaedic management of all such patients is governed by similar treatment philosophies. The aetiology of cerebral palsy is discussed in Chapter 13.3.

Classification (see Chapter 13.3)

Patients with cerebral palsy may be grouped according to which part of the body is affected. Thus, *hemiplegia* indicates involvement of the ipsilateral upper and lower limbs whereas *diplegia* means that although both sides of the body are involved, the lower limbs are most affected. The term *quadriplegia* has been replaced by *total body involvement*, reflecting the fact that those patients in whom all four limbs are affected also invariably demonstrate axial problems such as scoliosis and central problems with the bulbar musculature.

Cerebral palsy is also classified by the predominant nature of the underlying disturbance to the motor system remembering that mixed patterns are common.

- *Spasticity*, the most common abnormality and the one around which orthopaedic management is focused, is an increase in muscle tone that occurs as a response to hypersensitive stretch reflexes that a damaged cerebral cortex is no longer able to control
- *Rigidity* is characterized by an involuntary sustained muscle contraction that does not depend on stretching
- *Dyskinetic (choreoathetoid or dystonic)* cerebral palsy reflects damage to the basal ganglia, and is characterized by involuntary movements
- *Ataxic* cerebral palsy is due to cerebellar damage and features problems with balance and limb placement.

Determination of the neurological pattern is important when considering orthopaedic intervention. In general, the responses in patients displaying predominantly spastic patterns are more predictable and reproducible than those involving dyskinetic types. Impairment of selective muscle control in ataxia may limit the success of surgical procedures.

This chapter concerns patients with diplegia and the lower limb problems faced by hemiplegic patients. The hip dislocations encountered in severe total body involvement patients are covered in Chapter 13.6.

Natural history

Although the incidence of cerebral palsy is not decreasing, the prevalence of different types of cerebral palsy is changing. Spastic cerebral palsy is becoming more common and athetosis less so. Furthermore, severe total body involvement cerebral palsy related to prematurity and low birth weight appears to be becoming more common than diplegia due to perinatal asphyxia.

Motor development is delayed in cerebral palsy. Children may be late in reaching motor milestones or fail to develop some skills entirely. Furthermore, they often develop abnormal motor patterns. The persistence of primitive reflexes and the absence of postural reactions at the age of 2 years are associated with a poor prognosis for future walking ability, whereas a child who is able to sit without support by the age of 2 years is likely to be able to learn to walk.

Stretching is necessary for normal muscle growth but spastic muscle resists stretching and consequently, affected muscles become relatively short during skeletal growth. Unless treated, this leads to muscle and joint contractures in the limbs, which in turn contribute to abnormal loading of the skeleton and the development of bone deformity. This deterioration is exacerbated by abnormal postures and movement control problems resulting directly from the central brain lesion. Muscle and joint contractures often deteriorate rapidly during growth spurts. The sequence of events is shown in Figure 13.4.1.

From the management point of view, it is important to differentiate between dynamic and fixed contractures as well as between mobile and fixed deformities. The term 'dynamic contracture' indicates that the muscle or joint in question functions through a restricted range of motion during activity while it still maintains adequate passive range. Similarly, a mobile deformity is one that can be passively corrected. Fixed contractures and deformities are not correctable passively.

Although the neurological lesion is non-progressive, the musculoskeletal consequences of cerebral palsy often change during the growing years. Dynamic contractures and mobile deformities may deteriorate and become fixed. Spastic muscle is not necessarily powerful muscle and muscle weakness is a common associated factor that will compromise function over time as both height and weight increase with growth.

Associated problems

Individuals with cerebral palsy often have other problems which not only influence their motor development, but which should also inform surgical management decisions. Seizure disorder, learning disability, behavioural problems, and abnormal visual perception are common. Impaired cognition may make rehabilitation from surgery difficult and prejudice the outcome of such interventions. However, it is important to remember that many people with severe cerebral palsy have average or above-average intelligence.

Central balance problems cannot be addressed by treating peripheral limb deformity; indeed, some children with severe balance problems may choose to adopt a crouched wide-based externally-rotated gait in order to lower their centre of gravity and achieve better stability.

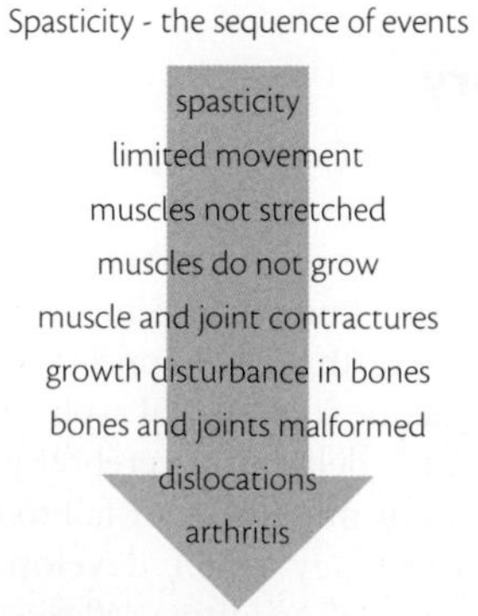

Fig. 13.4.1 The sequence of events affecting joints in a patient with a neuromuscular condition.

Inherent muscle weakness has already been mentioned: any assault on spastic muscle will result in further weakening, even if (as in the case of myoneural blockade) this is temporary.

In their efforts to overcome some of their limitations, children with cerebral palsy use various compensatory mechanisms. Hemiplegic children, for example, often vault during walking to obtain clearance of their equinus foot. From the management point of view, it is important to recognize compensations. True primary problems that generate compensations should be addressed. Compensations themselves do not necessarily require treatment but if used over a prolonged period they can lead to secondary deformities.

Overview of clinical management

As mentioned in previous chapters, the care of a child with cerebral palsy is complex and challenging. Parents and other carers devote huge parts of their lives to looking after such children, for whom a mundane event such as feeding or dressing may represent a difficult and time-consuming activity. They are often determined and single-minded in their search for treatments, a wide variety of which are advertised on the Internet although they are often scientifically unsubstantiated.

The management of children with cerebral palsy requires a multidisciplinary approach because of the wide-ranging nature of their problems (see Chapter 13.3, Figure 13.3.4). It must be remembered that musculoskeletal problems are only one aspect of these children's lives. Coordination between the various disciplines is important, as families may receive conflicting advice or information regarding therapy: a further source of frustration for the family.

Setting up priorities and defining realistic targets is crucial in the management of children with cerebral palsy. Indications for orthopaedic treatment are not always clear. Therefore, when approaching a child and their family it is important to clarify the family's perceptions of the child's orthopaedic problems, their priorities in his or her management, and their expectations from treatment.

History

The diagnosis of cerebral palsy is usually made before a child is referred for an orthopaedic opinion. However, occasionally, the orthopaedic surgeon will have the opportunity to make the diagnosis. The possibility of cerebral palsy should always be considered in a child presenting as a toe-walker or with a limp.

It is important to obtain as full a perinatal history as possible. In particular, it is essential to know the neurological type of cerebral palsy as this helps determine orthopaedic management. It is helpful if the child has already been seen and investigated by a paediatric neurologist.

The date at which motor milestones have been attained should be recorded as these give some indication as to what future achievements are possible. A child who cannot sit unsupported at 2 years of age or who has not walked by 4 years is unlikely to walk.

The current walking status should be noted (Box 13.4.1). It is important to establish how well they walk and whether this is stable, improving, or deteriorating. Community walkers can walk

Box 13.4.1 Questions to ask the walking patient

- What aids do they use?
  - Frames, crutches, sticks
  - Orthoses
- How good are they?
  - Community walker
  - Household walker
  - Therapeutic walker
- What progress are they making?
  - Improving, static, deteriorating.

reasonable distances outdoors and the approximate walking distance or time should be recorded. Household walkers only walk indoors. Therapeutic walkers walk only limited distances under supervision and do not use walking as their main means of mobility. The use of any walking aids or orthoses is noted. Current or previous therapy and its frequency should be recorded, together with the use of postural management devices such as sleep management systems and standing frames. At the end of this assessment it should be possible to assign a Gross Motor Function Classification System (GMFCS) level to the child (see Chapter 13.3, Figure 13.3.3). This is a useful, clinically validated indicator of motor function that assesses the child's progress during growth.

The history should also include the presence of associated conditions and details of any previous treatments and their outcomes (Box 13.4.2). It is important to maintain respect for the patient: whenever age and cognition allow, questions should be addressed to the child by name.

Clinical examination

The effect of an unfamiliar or uncomfortable environment and a rushed consultation will be to increase spasticity and make meaningful examination difficult.

Box 13.4.2 Associated difficulties—do they influence choice of treatment?

- Increased perioperative risk:
  - Poorly controlled epilepsy
  - Gastro-oesophageal reflux
  - Absent gag reflex
- Problems with rehabilitation:
  - Limited cognitive function
  - Visual/perceptual difficulties
  - Poor balance.

The clinical examination starts with an observation of posture: standing, sitting, and lying. Head and trunk control and limb posture will give an impression of the child's level of motor development. Balance reactions and primary reflexes may be observed and involuntary movements and obvious skeletal deformities recorded.

Lower limb examination assesses the passive range of motion of all joints and the presence of any fixed contractures (Box 13.4.3). Thomas's test detects a fixed flexion contracture of the hip but if a knee contracture is also present, the test should be performed with the patient's pelvis at the end of the table. Alternatively, Staheli's test is used, where prone hip extension is tested with the patient's pelvis at the edge of the couch.

Femoral anteversion is measured clinically with the patient prone and the knee flexed at 90 degrees. The hip is rotated until the greater trochanter reaches maximum prominence laterally. The angle between the tibia and the vertical is then equal to the femoral anteversion. From this position, the total arc of hip rotation can be assessed.

Hip abduction should be tested first with both hips and knees in maximum extension. Phelp's test differentiates limited abduction due to adductor tightness from that due to hamstring (mainly gracilis) tightness. Abduction is tested with the knees extended and then with knee flexion: if flexion improves abduction the limitation in abduction is due mainly to hamstring tightness.

The popliteal angle assesses hamstring tightness. With the patient supine, both hip and knee are flexed to 90 degrees, the knee is then brought to maximum extension: the angle between the tibia and the vertical line is the popliteal angle. Normal subjects have a popliteal angle of less than 30 degrees. In the same position, fast extension of the knee is attempted. Spasticity of the hamstrings will prevent extension before the maximum 'passive' popliteal angle is reached. This test measures dynamic hamstring spasticity.

Spasticity of the rectus femoris muscle can prevent knee flexion in the swing phase of gait. It is assessed by the Duncan–Ely test. With the patient supine, the knee is flexed rapidly. If the rectus is spastic, it will contract, flexing the hip joint and causing the patient's buttock to lift off the couch. If the same is observed with slow knee flexion of the knee, a fixed contracture of the rectus is present.

A shortened calf complex (gastrocnemius and soleus) presents as reduced ankle dorsiflexion. Silverskjold's test involves assessing dorsiflexion with the ipsilateral knee flexed and extended. As the muscle origins of gastrocnemius and soleus originate above and below the knee respectively, this test differentiates between shortening in the two muscles. In estimating dorsiflexion it is important not to allow any hindfoot valgus (as this creates a spurious correction of equinus).

Lower limb examination also includes measurement of muscle power. This can be particularly difficult in the presence of spasticity and impaired selective muscle control. However, measurement of the main muscle groups should be attempted using the Medical Research Council scale. If selective muscle control is so poor that voluntary contraction of major muscle groups, such as the hip or knee extensors is impossible, this should be recorded.

An appropriate neurological examination of the child with cerebral palsy should be performed. The modified Ashworth scale (Table 13.4.1) is used to assess spasticity and the confusion test measures selective muscle control. A child without selective control

Box 13.4.3 Assessment of joint range—the use of eponymous tests

- Thomas's test: hip flexion supine
- Staheli's test: hip extension prone
- Phelps test: hip abduction
- Duncan–Ely test: rectus femoris
- Silverskjold's test: gastrocsoleus complex.

of ankle dorsiflexion shows contraction of the tibialis anterior muscle when asked to flex the hip against resistance: a positive confusion test.

Gait analysis

Cerebral palsy is a disorder of movement and posture; in the ambulant child, examination of the lower limb is incomplete without an assessment of walking. The conventional static physical examination often fails to reveal the dynamic posturing adopted as soon as a child assumes an upright weight-bearing position: in the past, failure to appreciate the variable and dynamic nature of these postures has resulted in inappropriate surgery. Mistakes have also been made as a result of considering one joint segment in isolation and from failing to realize that the effects of muscle activity at one level (e.g. the ankle) have consequences at distant sites (e.g. the hip). Such relationships can be appreciated only through evaluation of an individual's gait pattern. A knowledge of normal gait is essential before one can appreciate the errors that occur in cerebral palsy (Figure 13.4.2).

Gait analysis involves the systematic study of the body's mobile segments and joints during locomotion. Movement is studied separately in the three orthogonal planes, namely sagittal, coronal, and transverse. Observational gait analysis employs video recordings in normal and slow motion to obtain qualitative information about gait. Instrumented gait analysis requires sophisticated laboratory equipment. Kinematic information on the three-dimensional movement of body segments and joints is derived from data generated from cameras tracking markers placed on anatomical landmarks.

Table 13.4.1 The Modified Ashworth Scale (Bohannon and Smith 1987)

Grade	Description
0	No increase in muscle tone
1	Slight increase in muscle tone, manifested by a catch and release or by minimal resistance at the end of the range of motion when the affected part(s) is(are) moved in flexion or extension
1a	Slight increase in muscle tone, manifested by a catch followed by minimal resistance through the remainder of the range of motion but the affected part(s) is(are) easily moved
2	More marked increase in muscle tone through most of the range of movement, but the affected part(s) is (are) easily moved
3	Considerable increases in muscle tone, passive movement difficult
4	Affected part(s) is (are) rigid in flexion or extension

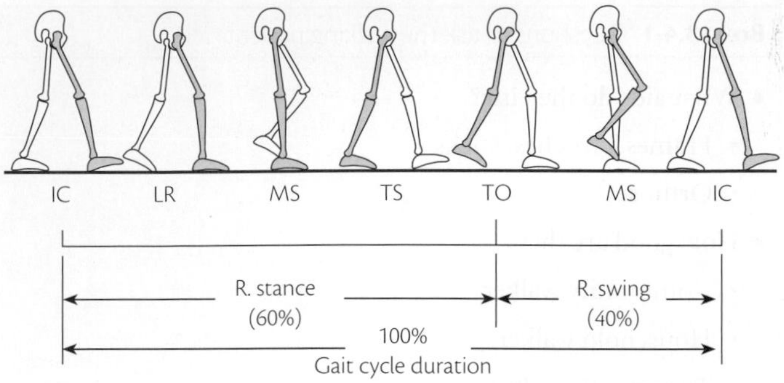

Fig. 13.4.2 The gait cycle and its subdivisions. IC, initial contact; LR loading response; MS, mid stance; TS, terminal stance; TO, toe-off; MS, mid-swing; IC, initial contact.

Data from force platforms relates forces occurring during gait to the kinematic data in order to produce information on moments and powers around joints during gait: kinetic information. Dynamic electromyography via surface electrodes or fine wires provides information on the pattern of muscle activity during gait. This is significantly deranged in many people with cerebral palsy. Energy expenditure is estimated by measuring oxygen consumption.

The information obtained during observational and instrumented gait analysis, combined with the clinical history and examination, aids the understanding of gait deviations and helps plan management. The reliability and reproducibility of gait data have been demonstrated and gait analysis is used in most centres that treat children with diplegic cerebral palsy (Figure 13.4.3). It is also

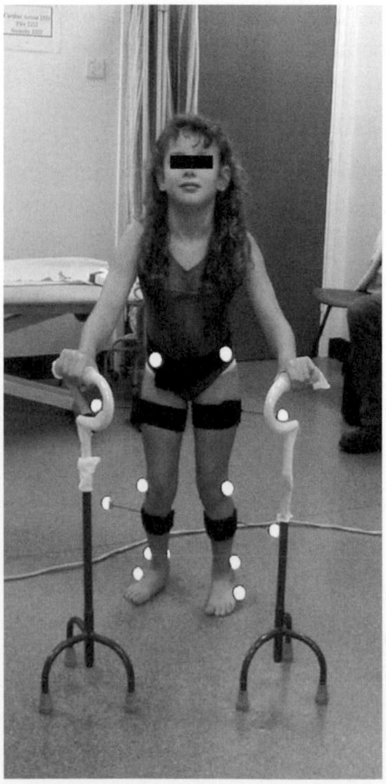

Fig. 13.4.3 Photograph of a child with diplegic cerebral palsy who is about to undergo an instrumented gait analysis. She walks with tripods as walking aids.

a well-established outcome measure. However, instrumented gait analysis is only a tool that guides management: it should not be used as a prescriptive device that ignores the many other considerations surrounding surgical management of cerebral palsy.

Treatment modalities

Different treatments or management regimens are appropriate for different children at different stages of their growth and development.

From the musculoskeletal viewpoint, the priority in the early years is to maintain muscle length and promote muscle growth in order to minimize risk of contracture and deformity. Muscle grows rapidly in the early years of life, doubling its length in the first 4 years. It takes another 12 years to double again. It is thus sensible, if possible, to avoid surgical interference during these critical early years.

Physiotherapy

Physiotherapy has a central role in the management of young children with cerebral palsy. It focuses on assisting motor development whilst preventing the development of deformity and contractures. Serial casting to improve passive range may augment joint range and muscle stretching regimens.

There are many different schools of physiotherapy and related techniques such as conductive education that will not be discussed in this chapter. Claims that one method is better than another are all hampered by a lack of randomized controlled trials. However, it is reasonable to accept that some form of structured physical therapy is of importance in the child with cerebral palsy.

Orthoses

Orthoses are used in children with cerebral palsy to aid function and prevent deformity. Immobilizing a muscle in an elongated position provides passive stretching and enhances its longitudinal growth. Orthoses also provide joint stability during gait. Ankle–foot orthoses (AFOs) stabilize the ankle and foot from the early stages of motor development (Figure 13.4.4). An orthosis can also use the ground reaction force during weight bearing to stabilize more proximal joints. Thus, the ground reaction AFO (GRAFO) aids knee extension. This rigid orthosis transfers the ground reaction force applied at the forefoot area to the pretibial area, encouraging extension of the knee (Figure 13.4.5).

Orthoses are used for the postural management of non-ambulant patients. Hip orthoses provide hip abduction in patients at risk of hip dislocation. Standing frames of various designs are used to support patients in the upright position. This is thought to help with the prevention of contractures and osteoporosis. The upright posture is also beneficial for gastrointestinal and urinary tract function, as well as morale.

Nerve blocks and botulinum toxin

Spasticity can be reduced by blocking the reflex arc. The previous practice of efferent nerve destruction using agents such as phenol has been abandoned in favour of localized interruption at the motor endplate (myoneural blockade). Although this can be done successfully with diluted (50%) ethanol, it is more commonly performed using botulinum toxin-A (BTA), a neurotoxin derived from *Clostridium botulinum*.

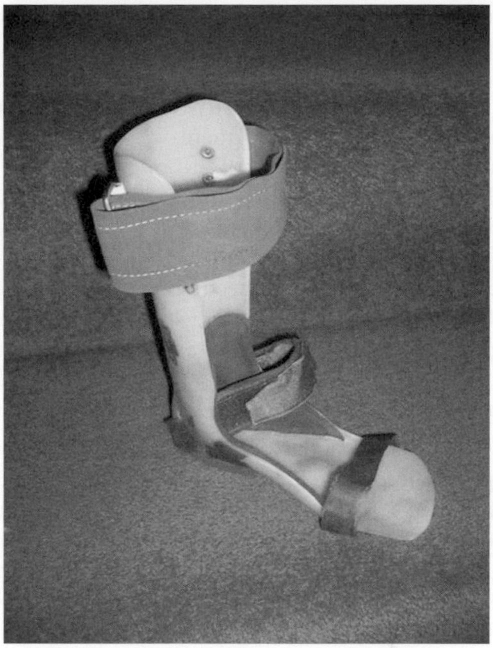

Fig. 13.4.4 AFO (ankle-foot orthosis).

BTA prevents the release of acetylcholine at the motor endplate which results in reduced neural stimulation of the muscle. Over a period of 3–6 months new nerve ends sprout that allow the muscle function to return.

BTA is given as an intramuscular injection into the region of the muscle where the motor end plates are concentrated. Local anaesthetic, often combined with sedation, is used for the injection. Reduced spasticity should be noticed within a few days. BTA is

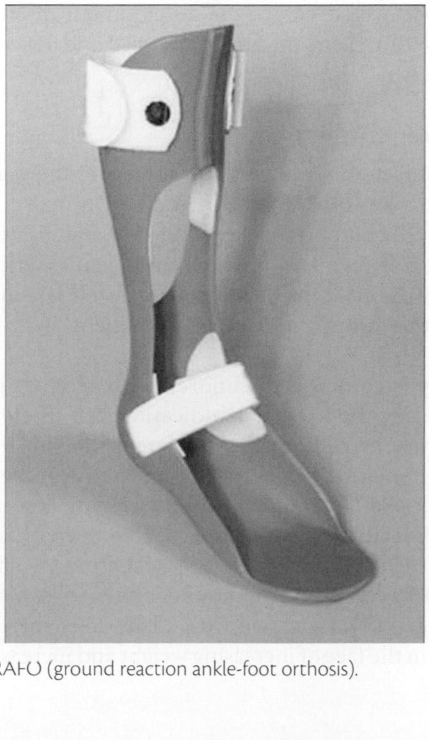

Fig. 13.4.5 GRAFO (ground reaction ankle-foot orthosis).

effective in the presence of dynamic rather than fixed contractures: it has been shown to be effective in the treatment of dynamic equinus and is often combined with serial casting for more resistant contractures but there is no supportive evidence for this practice.

The long-term effects of treatment with BTA are unknown, although isolated histological studies of muscle that has been repeatedly treated with BTA are showing evidence of long-term damage and atrophy. To date, treatment has not been shown to prevent fixed contractures or delay the need for surgery. Views on optimal dose and frequency of injections vary. Potential complications, although rare, include local or generalized allergic reaction, fatigue, gastric dilatation, and temporary urinary incontinence.

Intrathecal baclofen

Baclofen is used as a systemic drug to control spasticity. However, the dosage required to reduce spasticity is often high leading to undesirable effects, such as drowsiness and confusion. Intrathecal use was introduced for patients with predominant lower limb spasticity. Low doses of baclofen are administered intrathecally via an implanted catheter and pump usually sited in the right iliac fossa (see Chapter 13.6, Figure 13.6.4). A test dose precedes implantation to confirm that the drug is effective for the individual patient at a reasonable dosage. Recharging of the pump or modification of the rate of drug delivery is possible on an outpatient basis. Close patient monitoring and a well-organized team are necessary. Potential complications include leakage of cerebrospinal fluid, migration of the catheter, and infection. The method does reduce lower limb spasticity in children with cerebral palsy.

Selective dorsal rhizotomy

This neurosurgical procedure reduces lower limb spasticity in diplegic patients. The operation involves partial (25–40%) division of the posterior nerve roots from L1 to S1. Functional improvement has been documented in the short term.

Patient selection is important and those with neurological involvement other than spasticity must be excluded. Rhizotomy should be performed before the development of any significant contractures. Muscle weakness is unmasked and a secondary spinal deformity may develop.

Orthopaedic surgery

The main indication for lower-limb surgery in the walking child is preservation or improvement of walking function. Unlike the totally involved child with a dislocating hip, pain is not a common problem apart from a group with intransigent anterior knee pain. Similarly, cosmetic considerations are rarely an indication for surgery in this group in contrast to patients with upper limb problems.

Deformity is common in children with cerebral palsy and its presence is not, in itself, an indication for intervention. The deformity must be responsible for current functional impairment or at risk of impairing future function if left unchecked.

The ability to walk and to continue walking is seen by parents and some clinicians as the ultimate goal but overall, patients themselves do not rank the ability to walk as highly as the ability to communicate effectively or to be independently mobile. Many teenagers are encouraged to struggle on with a laborious energy-inefficient assisted gait in the face of increasing weight and increasing demands on their time from other sources when they would be able to lead a more fulfilling and independent life as chair-users.

During the process of defining targets of treatment and planning intervention the potential risks and complications of any procedures should also be discussed as these can outweigh any potential benefit.

Hemiplegia

The vast majority of children with hemiplegic cerebral palsy maintain their ability to walk into adulthood. Orthopaedic referral is usually related to gait abnormalities: delayed or asymmetric walking, leg-length discrepancy, or unilateral equinus deformity. Hypertonia, brisk reflexes, and ipsilateral upper limb involvement lead to the diagnosis of hemiplegia. Posturing of the ipsilateral upper limb by flexing the elbow during gait is a subtle but important sign of a mild hemiplegia (Figure 13.4.6).

Winters *et al.* (1987) attempted to classify hemiplegic gait according to severity of involvement (Table 13.4.2). They suggested treatment choices for the four different types of hemiplegic gait in their classification. AFOs help with type 1 and some type 2, for fixed equinus in types 2, 3, and 4 surgery may be indicated but in types 3 and 4 management must address problems around the hip and knee simultaneously.

More recently, Hullin *et al.* described another classification of hemiplegic gait based on kinematic and kinetic gait data. The aim of this classification was to highlight the aetiology of various gait deviations (Table 13.4.3).

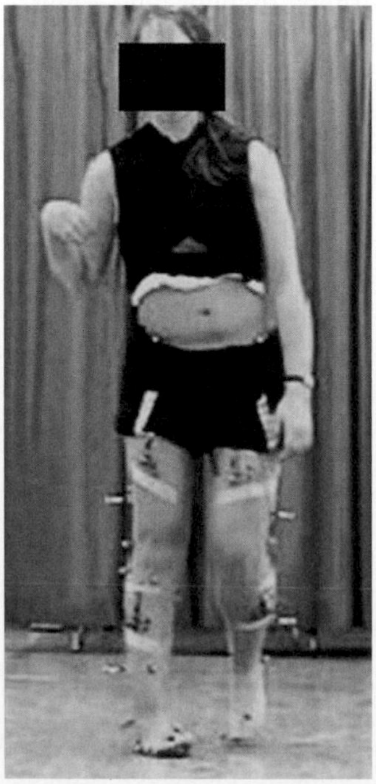

Fig. 13.4.6 A child with a right hemiplegia undergoing an instrumented gait analysis. The lower limb abnormalities are minor but the right upper limb posture is distinctive.

Table 13.4.2 Winter's classification of the hemiplegic gait

Type	Description
1	Equinus in swing phase of gait only (e.g. a foot drop). This can be treated with an AFO
2	Equinus throughout the gait cycle, with either toe contact only or toe–heel contact and compensatory hyperextension of the ipsilateral knee
3	Involvement of the hamstrings and rectus is observed and there is increased knee flexion throughout the gait cycle
4	The hip flexors and adductors are affected and internal hip rotation is observed

Foot deformity

The most common foot deformities in hemiplegia are equinus and equinovarus. Spasticity of the gastrocnemius is the primary cause but weakness of the dorsiflexors and the peronei often contributes. Spasticity of the tibialis posterior muscle may also be present. Planovalgus deformity with persistent hindfoot equinus and a collapsed midfoot is much more commonly seen in diplegia.

Clinical examination identifies the muscles responsible for the deformity and distinguishes between the hindfoot varus caused by an overactive tibialis posterior and the forefoot adductus and supination caused by an unopposed tibialis anterior.

Equinovarus foot deformity causes clearance problems during the swing phase of gait as well as stance phase instability as the foot turns into varus and inversion. Furthermore, the ipsilateral knee is subjected to abnormal loading and a tendency to hyperextension. Compensatory hip flexion may be observed.

The severity of the deformity depends on the age of the patient and the degree of involvement. A flexible deformity in young patients becomes more rigid with age although the true natural history is unknown. Some hemiplegic patients develop a fixed equinovarus foot deformity before skeletal maturity. Weight-bearing on a deformed foot should lead to degenerative changes in adult life but there are no long-term studies to confirm this.

The flexible deformity can be treated conservatively. Treatment aims are to improve gait and prevent a fixed deformity. Physiotherapy stretching regimens are used and an AFO maintains the foot in the neutral position, improving gait whilst protecting hip and knee from abnormal loading. BTA injections in the gastrocnemius and the tibialis posterior reduce spasticity. The treatment of fixed deformities may involve surgical lengthening of contracted muscles. In principle, simple Z-lengthening of the tendon should be avoided as this allows further contraction of the muscle belly with consequently reduced power and reduced stimulus to grow. When possible the muscle–tendon unit is lengthened as a whole by means of aponeurotic or intramuscular lengthening techniques.

Table 13.4.3 Hullin classification of hemiplegic gait

Type	Description
I	A drop-foot pattern associated with weak anterior tibial muscles
II	Characterized by knee flexion throughout stance due to a functionally tight gastrocnemius with normal hip extension
III	Persistent knee and hip flexion due to functionally tight gastrocnemius and hip flexors
IV	Knee hyperextension and 'tibial arrest' associated with a functionally tight soleus
V	Persistent ankle dorsiflexion with knee hyperextension, the latter compensates for weak or spastic quadriceps

In addition to muscle lengthening, tendon transfer surgery is frequently performed to achieve a longer lasting balance to muscle action around the foot. Depending on the major source of deformity, either the tibialis anterior or posterior tendons can be transferred laterally. Tibialis anterior is often transferred in its entirety whilst split tendon transfers work well for both tibialis anterior and posterior with the split tendons acting like the reins on a horse to control the mid/fore foot. The split anterior tibial transfer is popular: the lateral half of the tendon is sutured to the intact peroneus brevis or transferred more distally via a bone tunnel. This operation works well in conjunction with simple lengthening of the tibialis posterior and gastrocnemius muscles.

Muscle/tendon lengthening is not recommended in early life when rapid muscle growth is occurring: failure to heed this advice results in a high recurrence rate. If surgery is delayed until the age of 7–8 years, the risk of recurrent equinus is minimal.

In the older child with significant fixed deformities, bony surgery may be necessary. This should be combined with lengthening of the deforming muscles. Hindfoot varus is addressed with a calcaneal osteotomy whilst additional deformity may require appropriate midfoot osteotomies. Triple fusion should be reserved only for the severe, symptomatic and rigid equinovarus foot

The hip and knee

Hip dysplasia is uncommon in hemiplegia and dislocation rare.

Femoral derotation to correct anteversion and internal rotation of the leg during gait can be rewarding. It improves gait and prevents excessive knee loading. Extension and valgus can be included in the osteotomy to correct flexion and adduction at the hip. Most hemiplegic patients have a degree of pelvic rotation during gait, with the affected side retracted. This persists following derotation femoral osteotomy and can lead to unacceptable external rotation of the leg postoperatively if the femoral anteversion was corrected fully.

Operations around the knee are rarely indicated. Hamstring lengthening to correct flexion contracture can sometimes be combined with equinus foot correction. As in diplegia (see below) spasticity of the rectus and patella alta may contribute to anterior knee pain. Treatment is challenging and in most cases is for symptoms only. Interference with the quadriceps-patellar mechanism invites many problems including failure to relieve pain and exposing underlying weakness of the knee extensors.

Leg-length discrepancy

Neurological involvement of the affected lower limb results in reduced growth and a leg length difference is common. The discrepancy is rarely more than 1–2cm and can work to the child's advantage aiding clearance of the equinus foot in swing phase. For this reason, correction of the equinus deformity may need to be followed by provision of a shoe raise.

When the leg length discrepancy is more marked, gait compensations may be seen. These include increased hip and knee flexion on the unaffected side and pelvic obliquity. A shoe raise is usually all that is necessary, with contralateral epiphysiodesis being reserved for patients with marked discrepancies and relatively mild involvement.

Diplegia

The orthopaedic management of children with diplegia relates mainly to problems with their gait. Diplegic patients often have mild upper limb involvement affecting their ability to use walking aids (Figure 13.4.3).

At the severe end of the diplegic spectrum, lower limb involvement is marked, primitive reflex patterns persist, and upper limb involvement is pronounced. This group of patients (resembling the milder end of quadriplegic cerebral palsy) may lose their ability to walk as growth progresses and contractures develop. In contrast, the gait pattern of a child with mild spastic diplegia may seem normal to the casual observer, their problems limited to minor problems with tripping, balance and endurance. It has been suggested that 85% of children with diplegia maintain their ability to walk in the long term but this probably excludes many of the more severely involved children at the poorly defined interface between diplegia and total body involvement.

Diplegic gait is complex. The child with diplegia is delayed in acquiring standing and walking skills. Initially, an extensor pattern of activity is common, featuring a combination of adducted hips ('scissoring'), stiff extended knees, and ankle equinus (toe-walking). As the child grows, the biarticular muscles (hamstrings, rectus femoris, and gastrocnemius) are the prime targets of impaired control and increased tone, leading to hip and knee flexion contractures and increasingly fixed equinus. The hips become increasingly internally rotated. The equinus is followed by a progressive planovalgus deformity, collapse of the longitudinal arch, and forefoot abduction: the so-called 'mid-foot break' (Figure 13.4.7). However, gait variation is infinite, and a classification of diplegic gait has not yet been possible.

Early treatment

The general principles of spasticity management apply. Joint ranges and muscle length are maintained, encouraging the acquisition of assisted standing and walking skills, with the help of orthoses. AFOs control equinus and improve limb stability. Myoneural blocks of the gastrocnemius reduce dynamic equinus and encourage a heel-toe gait pattern.

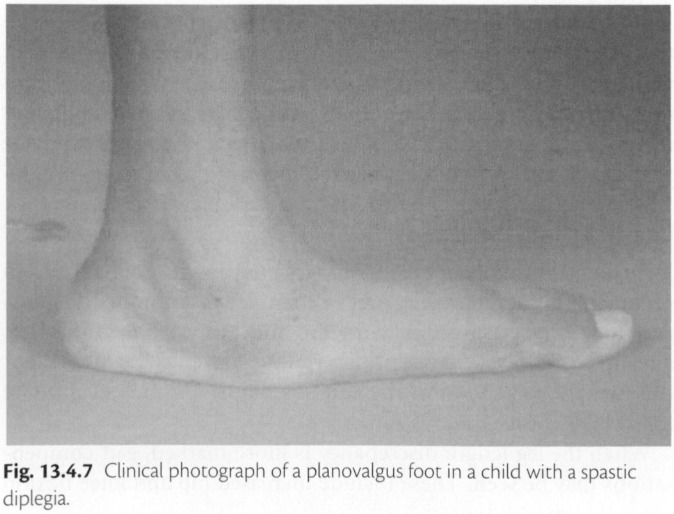

Fig. 13.4.7 Clinical photograph of a planovalgus foot in a child with a spastic diplegia.

As with hemiplegic patients, surgery should be deferred when possible until the child is 7–8 years old as the risk of recurrent contracture following muscle lengthening at this age is low and any alteration in neural patterning ('neuroplasticity') that might have compensated for some of the centrally-mediated gait problems has been exhausted. Lastly, at this age, the concept of extensive surgery and rehabilitation can be explained and understood and some degree of cooperation expected.

Single-event multilevel surgery

In the past, poor understanding of the diplegic gait pattern compounded by an inappropriate reliance on static as opposed to dynamic assessment, frequently led to young children undergoing repeated operations each followed by an extensive period of rehabilitation.

The development of gait analysis has led to a much better understanding of the problems faced in spastic diplegia, and in particular how it is inappropriate to consider a joint or limb segment in isolation. This improved understanding, led to the concept of single-event multilevel surgery (SEMLS) in which, following detailed preoperative gait analysis, all gait abnormalities are treated in a single operative procedure with a single period of rehabilitation. This principle has been developed over the past three decades and has changed the management approach to children with diplegic cerebral palsy.

Multilevel surgery includes a variety of procedures tailored for the individual patient. Soft tissue procedures to correct fixed or dynamic contractures are guided by the principle of 'lengthening without weakening'. Extensive soft tissue releases are avoided. Judicious lengthening is performed, usually at the musculotendinous junction. The muscles crossing two joints appear to be more affected in cerebral palsy, probably because of their different function at each joint and thus inevitably more complex neurological control. These biarticular muscles frequently require surgical intervention (Box 13.4.4).

Calculations of muscle length based on gait-analysis models can assist surgical decision-making. For example, the hamstrings in crouched gait are more often than not relatively long, not short.

Another biarticular muscle, the rectus femoris, is also often affected: activity of the spastic rectus in swing prevents adequate knee flexion and causes foot clearance problems. A positive Duncan–Ely test, together with reduced sagittal knee movement and electromyographic confirmation of rectus activity in swing characterizes this problem which can be dealt with by posterior transfer of the rectus to the sartorius or gracilis.

Excessive hip internal rotation results in the knee and ankle acting across the direction of body movement, which often causes a valgus thrust at the knee. Femoral derotation osteotomy either proximally or distally restores alignment. Compensatory external tibial torsion can be addressed by a simple supramalleolar derotation osteotomy.

Knee flexion contracture is a major problem in the older child with diplegia. Soft tissue surgery alone is unlikely to give good results and enthusiasm for bony surgery to address residual flexion contractures has been revived. Supracondylar knee extension

Box 13.4.4 Site of muscle lengthening: biarticular muscles

- Iliopsoas: over the pelvic brim
- Medial hamstrings:
  - Fractional lengthening
  - Mid/distal thigh
- Gastrosoleus complex: aponeurotic lengthening
- Rectus femoris: release and transfer.

osteotomies with or without accompanying distal transfer of the tibial tuberosity have been recommended. In the skeletally immature child the same result can be obtained safely and simply by anterior hemieiphysiodesis of the distal femoral physis. This has the advantage of a slow correction, allowing the soft tissues to adapt to both sides of the gradually extending knee (Figure 13.4.8).

Osteotomies to correct rotational malalignment of the leg and resulting abnormal moments across joints are included as necessary. Femoral anteversion affects the lever arm of the abductors and often causes a valgus thrust at the knee. Tibial derotation may be indicated in some children.

Surgery to correct foot deformity is indicated in a number of children. As a rule, there is no place for muscle lengthening or tendon transfer surgery in the valgus foot in diplegia, with the exception of the gastrocnemius, whose contracture may be responsible for exacerbating the valgus. Severe hindfoot valgus that is impeding gait and causing pain may be treated by extra-articular subtalar arthrodesis. A calcaneal lengthening osteotomy treats the valgus foot with a collapsed longitudinal arch and forefoot abduction. The operation offers good correction of all three elements of the deformity in the reasonably flexible foot and can be combined, if necessary, with a subtalar arthrodesis. Gastrocnemius lengthening to correct equinus may be necessary. Triple fusion is reserved for the severely deformed, rigid, and symptomatic foot. Hallux valgus is treated by arthrodesis of the first metatarsophalangeal joint with recognition that the deformity is often secondary to more proximal midfoot deformity which may need addressing.

Multilevel operations should be planned and performed in centres where there is an appropriate interest and expertise and multidisciplinary approach. Careful assessment of potential patients, carers, and local support services is needed to ensure good patient selection and detailed planning is essential to ensure that there is a seamless transition from hospital to community care for rehabilitation. Experienced paediatric anaesthetists, postoperative epidural analgesia, and pain teams are essential to ensure that the patient does not enter into the pain/spasm/pain spiral that causes so much distress and which is responsible for many poor operative results. A comfortable, confident child is able to mobilize quickly, be discharged promptly and continue rehabilitation at home. Rehabilitation may continue for as long as 12–18 months.

Midterm results of multilevel surgery or of specific procedures are encouraging but studies into adult life are required to establish the long-term results. Such studies are difficult to conduct due to the inherent variability in patient characteristics, use of other treatment modalities and ethical issues over the use of control groups.

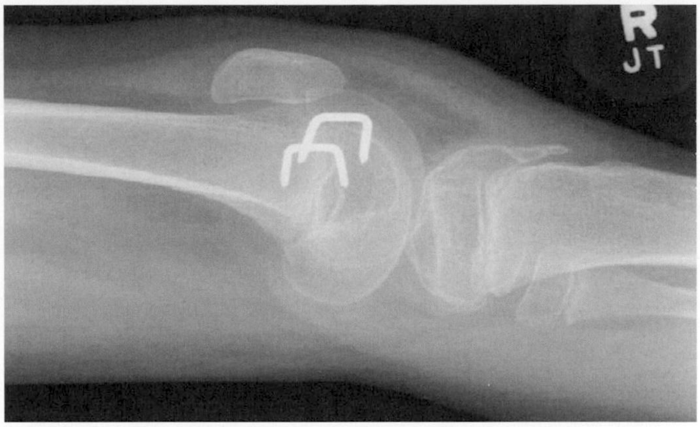

Fig. 13.4.8 Lateral radiograph of the knee showing staples inserted anteriorly at the level of the distal femoral physis to give a gradual correction of the knee flexion posture.

Hip dysplasia

Mild hip dysplasia is common in diplegic cerebral palsy. As before, the incidence is difficult to ascertain due to the difficulty with diagnostic labelling at the severe end of the diplegia spectrum. The ability to walk does not exclude the possibility of progressive hip subluxation and hip monitoring should be part of the regular follow-up of these patients. The management of hip subluxation and dislocation is considered in the following section on the management of patients with total body involvement.

Lower limb management in the adult

Increasing height and weight in the teenager expose underlying problems with muscle weakness. Those who as younger children coped well, 'walking on their spasticity', find to their frustration and disappointment that despite maintenance of joint ranges their exercise tolerance decreases significantly in early adult life. Major surgical interventions are not generally indicated for fear of contributing further to the weakness. Appropriate management involves advice regarding regular exercise (in gyms and swimming pools), with occasional courses of physiotherapy to target specific problems. Increasing crouch posture with a contracted and weak quadriceps leads to a high-riding patella and patellofemoral joint problems. This in turn leads to increasing reliance on walking aids. There is no reliable operative solution. Degenerative hip disease occurs in the older physically active patient with diplegia and this is best treated with total hip replacement. Overall, the natural history of diplegia in adult life is unclear. Moreover, the influence of orthopaedic treatment on the long-term walking potential of diplegic patients is unknown.

Further reading

Bleck, E.E. (2007). *Orthopaedic management in cerebral palsy*. Clinics in Developmental Medicine Nos. 173/4. London: Mac Keith Press

Browne, A.O. and McManus, F. (1987). One session surgery for bilateral correction of lower limb deformities in spastic diplegia. *Journal of Pediatric Orthopedics*, **7**, 259–61.

Hullin, M.G., Robb, J.E., and Loudon, I.R. (1996). Gait patterns in children with hemiplegic spastic cerebral palsy. *Journal of Pediatric Orthopedics, Part B*, **5**, 247–51.

Jenter, M., Lipton, G.E., and Miller, F. (1998). Operative treatment of hallux valgus in children with cerebral palsy. *Foot and Ankle International*, **19**, 830–5.

Mosca, V.S. (1995). Calcaneal lengthening for valgus deformity of the hindfoot. *Journal of Bone and Joint Surgery, American Volume*, **77A**, 500–12.

Nene, A.V., Evans, G.A., and Patrick, J.H. (1993). Spastic diplegia: a functional assessment of simultaneous multiple surgical procedures to assist walking. *Journal of Bone and Joint Surgery*, **75B**, 488–94.

Skaggs, D.L., Rethlefsen, S.A., Kay, R.M., Dennis, S.W., Reynolds, R.A.K., and Tolo, V.T. (2000). Variability in gait analysis interpretation. *Journal of Pediatric Orthopedics*, **20**, 759–64.

Winters, T.F., Gage, J.R., and Hicks, R. (1987). Gait patterns in spastic hemiplegia in children and young adults. *Journal of Bone and Joint Surgery*, **69A**, 437–41.

13.5

Upper limb management in cerebral palsy

Rachel Buckingham

Summary points

- Evaluation of the upper limb must assess all aspects of sensation, motor control, and function. Will the hand be used for bimanual activities?
- Individual treatment goals must be established
- Non-operative treatment may encourage use and awareness of the more affected limb
- Many muscles cross two joints and therefore the limb must be considered as a whole and not as a series of isolated joints.

Introduction

The upper extremity is involved in all varieties of cerebral palsy. These limbs display the 'positive' features of the upper motor neuron syndrome—spasticity, hyper-reflexia, clonus, and co-contraction—but they also demonstrate the negative features including weakness, sensory deficit, poor selective, motor control (see Chapter 13.3, Table 13.3.2), as well as dystonia, which further influence the fine motor skills. Upper limbs perform a multitude of tasks and must work together, although they have differing functions depending on dominance. Whereas children need both lower limbs to walk, many upper-limb tasks can be performed single-handedly, and neglect or 'learned non-use' of the other hand can be a problem. Management of the upper limb in cerebral palsy involves detailed assessment by a multidisciplinary team (see Chapter 13.3, Figure 13.3.4) and careful planning.

Classification (see Chapter 13.3)

Cerebral palsy is classified by the predominant type of movement disorder: spasticity is present in 85% of those affected and is the most amenable to treatment. It is also classified by topographical involvement. Those with total body involvement have the greatest problems with motor control, spasticity, sensory deficit, and contractures leading to poor function. Goals of treatment are usually to improve hygiene and ease of dressing for these patients. Spastic diplegic patients have meagre involvement of the upper extremity and so rarely require intensive upper limb therapy or surgery. Hemiplegic patients can be helped most in terms of function and cosmesis.

Clinical evaluation

A careful and repeated evaluation should be performed evaluating the factors listed in Box 13.5.1.

Sensation

Sensory status is a predictor of the degree of spontaneous use of the limb.

Light touch, pain, and temperature sensations are present in cerebral palsy, but whether they are 'normal' is difficult to determine. They are 'normal' for that patient who will report them as such. Proprioception is measured objectively and tends to be more affected distally. Stereognosis is the child's ability to recognize objects by feel, and its reduction correlates with a decrease in limb size. Graphesthesia is the recognition of pictures or letters drawn on the palm. Two-point discrimination is considered satisfactory if less than 5–10mm.

Spasticity

Resting posture gives an idea of the amount of spasticity present. It tends to cause shoulder adduction and internal rotation, elbow flexion, forearm pronation, and wrist flexion. Fingers are flexed or show swan-neck deformity. The thumb may be adducted, or adducted and flexed, the so called 'thumb-in-palm' deformity. Stretching of the affected muscles meets with resistance which is velocity dependent and correlates with the degree of spasticity present. This can be assessed further with the Modified Ashworth and the Modified Tardieu Scales.

Box 13.5.1 Important factors in assessing the upper limb

- Sensation
- Spasticity
- Motor ability
- Contractures
- Function.

Motor ability

Spasticity often predominates in the shoulder adductors, elbow flexors, pronators, wrist, and finger flexors, and these muscles often overpower their antagonist muscles. The wrist and finger extensors, supinators, and abductor pollicis longus can be weak with poor voluntary control. Assessment of their power may only be possible after spasticity in other muscle groups has been reduced (by motor blocks or botulinum toxin A).

Contractures

Spasticity, fibrous contractures within spastic muscles, and joint contractures can be difficult to distinguish. It is usually possible to overcome spasticity, unless severe. Fibrous contractures cannot be overcome by passive movement, but can sometimes be distinguished from joint contractures by altering joint positions when testing muscles that cross more than one joint. For example, if finger flexors are tight, passive finger extension may only be possible with wrist flexion. Joint contractures such as elbow and wrist flexion and a pronation contracture due to shortening of the intra-osseous membrane may develop in adolescence or adulthood. Occasionally the radial head may dislocate.

Function

A number of objective, reproducible, validated tests, such as the Melbourne Unilateral Upper Limb Assessment, the Quality of Upper Extremity Skills Test (QUEST), the Assisting Hand Assessment (AHA), and the Shriners Hospital Upper Extremity Evaluation (SHUEE) can help assess and score the child's functional ability. Functional tests should be recorded on video and form a useful outcome measure after surgery. Bi-manual tests which measure what the child actually does rather than what he or she is capable of (the performance gap) will give a better measure of actual function. The chosen test needs to be responsive to change in order to be a good measure of outcome. In addition, the Manual Ability Classification System (MACS) reports the child's ability to handle objects in daily life. It does not assess the hands independently of each other. It gives a score of I–V and correlates well with Gross Motor Function Classification System (GMFCS) level ratings. The House score assesses the affected limb (Table 13.5.1).

Wrist flexion and thumb deformities have been shown to be major contributors to functional problems and in fact the House score was originally used to assess function before and after thumb surgery (Figure 13.5.1).

Table 13.5.1 The House functional classification system

Class	Designation	Activity level
0	Does not use	Does not use
1	Poor passive assist	Uses as a stabilizing weight only
2	Fair passive assist	Can hold onto object placed in hand
3	Good passive assist	Can hold onto object and stabilize it for use by other hand
4	Poor active assist	Can actively grasp object and hold it weakly
5	Fair active assist	Can actively grasp object and stabilize it well
6	Good active assist	Can actively grasp object and manipulate it against other hand
7	Spontaneous use, partial	Can perform bimanual activities easily and occasionally uses hand spontaneously
8	Spontaneous use, complete	Uses hand completely independently without reference to the other hand

Investigations

Three-dimensional motion analysis for the upper limb is in its infancy and not yet standardized between different centres. Electromyography may help determine which muscles are used in grasp and which in release, but is not widely used. Radiographs are rarely necessary.

Treatment

Goals

The treatment goals must be realistic and clearly defined by patient, carers, therapists, and surgeon together. In the severely affected quadriplegic patient, the goals may be to improve hygiene and ease of dressing. In many hemiplegic patients it is possible to improve function. Older children may simply seek an improvement in appearance but often do not admit to this unless directly questioned. Treatment must be individualized.

Non-operative treatment

Physiotherapy and occupational therapy

A number of treatments are available. Splinting to serially stretch contractures or to position the limb to its biomechanical advantage; stretching spastic muscles or strengthening weak ones; neurodevelopmental therapy to encourage functional movement patterns and inhibit primitive posturing; conductive education which practises motor skills for functional use and constraint induced movement therapy to encourage use and awareness of the more affected limb by restricting the more able hand, in much the same way as eye patches are used over a good eye to help train the 'lazy' eye.

Botulinum toxin A

Botulinum toxin blocks the presynaptic release of acetyl choline at the neuromuscular junction. The dose is calculated according to the patient's bodyweight, and each target muscle should be located with a nerve stimulator or ultrasound probe to ensure accurate drug placement. Splinting and stretching as well as strengthening programmes for weak antagonists should be implemented following injections.

Operative treatment

Many muscles of the upper limb cross more than one joint and therefore the limb must be considered as a whole and not as individual joints in isolation (Table 13.5.2). For example, a flexor–pronator slide will release the tight pronator, finger and wrist flexors, but will also slightly improve elbow extension. A flexor carpi ulnaris to extensor carpi radialis brevis transfer will augment wrist extension, but will also significantly increase active supination. Equally, a wrist should not be arthrodesed in a neutral position without addressing tight finger flexors or the patient will no

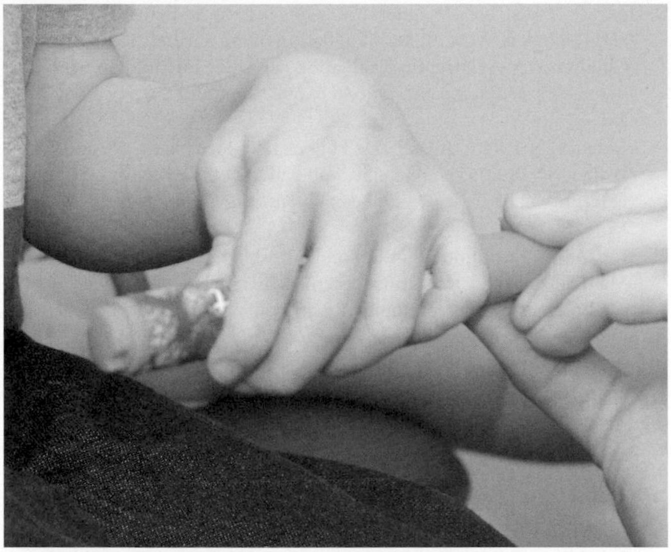

A

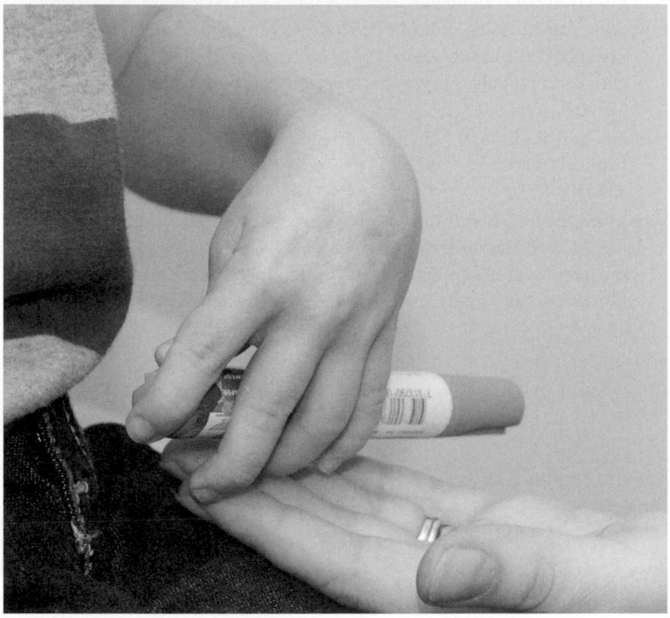

B

Fig. 13.5.1 A) Grasp. During grasp the wrist is flexed rather than extended. This slackens the finger flexors, making grasp more difficult. The thumb metacarpal is adducted, and to increase span the interphalangeal joint has become hyperextended. B) Attempted release. The wrist flexes further to aid finger extension. Swan necking of the fingers becomes evident as the extensors contract. The thumb is still unable to abduct and so release is not successful.

longer be able to release their grasp. It is also important to remember that the primary issue is with brain function and not to see the problem as a purely biomechanical one. A neglected limb is unlikely to gain function despite surgery. Generally, the surgeon has the following options for treatment:

- Spastic or contracted muscles may be released, either at their origin, or at the musculotendinous junction, or within the tendinous portion

Table 13.5.2 Common surgical procedures

Indication	Procedure
Elbow flexion	Lengthening or release of: Biceps Brachialis Brachioradialis
Forearm pronation	Release of pronator teres Rerouting of pronator teres to change its action to one of supination
Wrist flexion	Lengthening or release of wrist flexors Transfer of FCU to ECRB to augment weak extensors
Finger flexion	Lengthening or release of: FDS FDP FDS to FDP transfer FCU to ED transfer to augment weak finger extensors This often improves if wrist extension is augmented to prevent recruitment of finger extensors during wrist extension.
Swan neck deformity	Central extensor slip tenotomy with temporary K wire stabilization FDS slip tenodesis
'Thumb-in-palm' deformity	Release of adductor pollicis Double Z-plasty first web Rerouting of EPL to augment abduction
Thumb MCPJ	Sesamoid arthrodesis

ECRB, extensor carpi radialis brevis; ED, extensor digitorum; EPL, extensor pollicis longus; FCU, flexor carpi ulnaris: FDP, flexor digitorum profundus; FDS, flexor digitorum superficialis; MCPJ metacarpophalangeal joint.

- These muscles may be transferred in order to augment the function of a weak antagonist
- Joints may require release, or stabilization by capsulodesis, or occasionally arthrodesis.

Motor nerves may be divided, partially resected at the neuromuscular junction, or injected with phenol.

If possible, all the applicable procedures should be performed in one sitting (multilevel surgery for the upper limb).

Postoperatively the arm is immobilized in a cast, the position dependent on which procedures have been carried out. This is maintained for 6 weeks and then replaced with a thermoplastic splint to be worn at night time for 3 months or more to prevent recurrence of contractures. Movement is commenced on the non-immobilized joints immediately postoperatively, and therapy is intensified once the cast comes off. Occupational and physiotherapy are essential adjuncts to medical and surgical treatment.

Results

A systematic review of the literature on BTA identified 12 studies of high methodological quality. Six of ten that measured spasticity showed improvement; three of ten showed increased range of movement and six of ten showed improvement in function. The authors concluded, however, that due to differences in treatment goals, invalid assessment instruments and insufficient statistical power there was insufficient evidence to state that injections were beneficial.

Although there are no prospective randomized controlled trials assessing the efficacy of surgical treatment for the upper limb in cerebral palsy, from the large retrospective studies, the literature would seem to support surgery for improvement in function, cosmesis, and hygiene. A review of the literature from 1966–2006 concluded that surgery improved the position of the hand and there are indications that it might improve hand function.

Future directions

Prospective studies using validated outcome measures and long-term follow-up of treated patients, as well as the development of valid three-dimensional upper-limb modelling, will enhance our understanding of the effect of interventions on the upper limb in cerebral palsy.

Conclusions

Management of the upper limb in cerebral palsy requires assessment by a multidisciplinary team with an understanding of neuromuscular disability and of anatomy. Realistic goals need to be agreed with the patient and family, and validated outcome measures need to be documented. This is an exciting field for clinicians and researchers, with ample scope for future development and research.

Further reading

Chin, T.Y.P., Selber, P., Nattrass, G.R., and Graham, H.K. (2005). Accuracy of intramuscular injection of botulinum toxin: a comparison between manual needle placement and electrical stimulation. *Journal of Pediatric Orthopedics,* **25**(3), 286–91.

Davids, J.R., Peace, L.C., Wagner, L.V., Gidewall, M.A., Blackhurst, D.W., and Roberson, W.M. (2006). Validation of the Shriners Hospital for Children Upper Extremity Evaluation (SHUEE) for children with hemiplegic cerebral palsy. *Journal of Bone and Joint Surgery,* **88A**, 326–33.

De Matteo, C., Law, M., Russell, D., Pollock, N., Rosenbaum, P., and Walter, S. (1993). The reliability and validity of the Quality of Upper Extremity Skills Test. *Physical & Occupational Therapy in Pediatrics,* **13**, 1–18.

Eliasson, A.-C., Krumlinde-Sundholm, L., Rösblad, B., *et al.* (2006). The Manual Ability Classification System (MACS) for children with cerebral palsy: Scale development and evidence of validity and reliability. *Developmental Medicine and Child Neurology,* **48**, 549–54.

House, J.H., Gwathmey, F.W., and Fiddler, M.O. (1981). A dynamic approach to the thumb-in-palm deformity in cerebral palsy. *Journal of Bone and Joint Surgery,* **63A**, 216–25.

Johnstone, B.R., Richardson, P.W.F., Coombs, C.J., and Duncan, J.A. (2003). Functional and cosmetic outcome of surgery for cerebral palsy in the upper limb. *Hand Clinics,* **19**, 679–86.

Randall, M., Carlin, J.B., Chondros, P., and Reddihough, D. (2001). Reliability of the Melbourne Assessment of Unilateral Upper Limb Function. *Developmental Medicine and Child Neurology,* **43**, 761–7.

Reeuwijk, A., van Schie, P.E.M., Becher, J.G., and Kwakkel, G. (2006). Effects of botulinum toxin type A on upper limb function in children with cerebral palsy: a systematic review. *Clinical Rehabilitation,* **20**, 375–87.

Van Heest, A.E., House, J.H., and Cariello, C. (1999). Upper extremity surgical treatment of cerebral palsy. *Journal of Hand Surgery,* **24**, 323–30.

Van Munster, J.C., Maathius, K.G.B., Haga, N., Verheij, N.P., Nicolai, J.-P.A., and Hadders-Algra, M. (2007). Does surgical management of the hand in children with spastic unilateral cerebral palsy affect functional outcome? *Developmental Medicine and Child Neurology,* **49**, 385–9.

13.6

Management of the child with total body involvement

Tim Theologis

Summary points

- The most common musculoskeletal problems in TBI are scoliosis and hip dislocation
- Hip screening is necessary in young non-ambulant children
- The role of soft tissue surgery to prevent hip displacement is unclear
- Bony surgery offers more predictable results but complications are frequent
- Spinal stabilization should be considered for curves exceeding 50 degrees.

Introduction

This group includes children with severe motor disability that affects control and posture of all four limbs, the trunk, and the head. The majority of children are non-ambulant or therapeutic/household walkers (Gross Motor Function Classification System (GMFCS) IV or V). As a result of the severity of their neurological condition and their limited mobility most develop a variety of secondary musculoskeletal deformities but deformity in itself is not an indication for orthopaedic treatment. Management of the child with total body involvement cerebral palsy (TBI CP) should have well-defined aims and targets. Parents/carers as well as a multidisciplinary team of health professionals involved in the care of the child should take part in the decision-making process (see Chapter 13.3, Figure 13.3.5). Orthopaedic interventions are indicated to relieve or prevent pain, to improve quality of life, and to maintain or improve function.

Prevention of musculoskeletal deformity is an essential part of the management of these children. The treatment modalities that are used have been discussed in the preceding chapters and include physiotherapy, postural management, orthotics, casts, and botulinum toxin injections. The use of intrathecal baclofen treatment may also have a place in the management of intractable spasticity that affects the lower body predominantly. Dorsal rhizotomy is usually restricted to those children with spastic diplegia.

The most common musculoskeletal deformities requiring orthopaedic treatment in the TBI CP child are scoliosis and hip displacement (subluxation or dislocation). Indications for other orthopaedic interventions are less common and require careful, individual consideration.

Hip displacement

Hip displacement in CP is a common problem, particularly in non-ambulant patients. Depending on age and severity of involvement, the incidence of hip displacement varies from 10–70%. Lack of weight-bearing stimulation to the femoral head and acetabulum, muscle spasticity, and asymmetrical posture may explain the higher incidence of displacement in the non-ambulant children. The displacement is gradual and secondary changes occur on both sides of the joint. The femoral head becomes oval-shaped while acetabular dysplasia develops gradually with the formation of a groove-shaped deficiency. In the majority of patients, the direction of displacement is superoposterior. Posterior acetabular defects are more often seen in patients who progress to subluxation, while global defects are more common in patients with fully dislocated hips.

Both the Reimers migration percentage and the acetabular index can be used to quantify the severity of the displacement but problems with the reliability of both measurements have been reported (Figure 13.6.1). Three-dimensional imaging, particularly as part of preoperative planning may be appropriate in determining the direction of instability and the site of acetabular deficiency.

Indications for treatment of hip displacement in CP include pain during the displacement process and prevention of pain from the secondary degenerative changes that develop with chronic, established displacement. Correction of posture and improvement in the range of hip movement facilitate better sitting as well as easier care and hygiene.

Management

There are several areas of controversy in the management of hip displacement in TBI CP that will hopefully become clearer over years to come with a better understanding of the outcome of intervention in various subgroups of CP.

Screening for hip displacement

The indications for early screening and any preventative interventions are unclear.

The acetabular index represents the single most important predictor of hip dislocation in children with CP. A normal index at

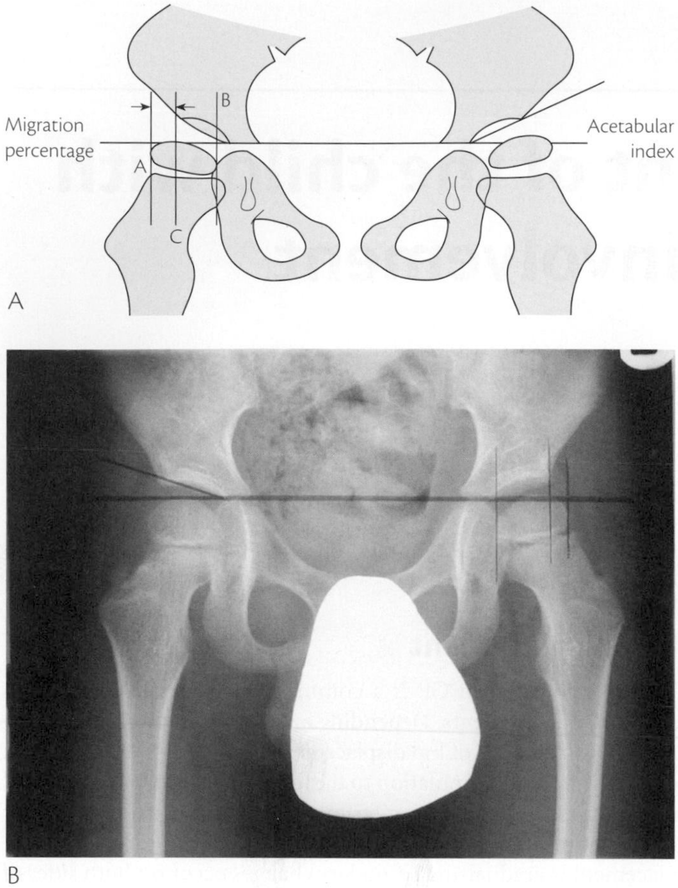

Fig. 13.6.1 A) Diagrammatic representation of an AP pelvic radiograph: the migration percentage (MP) is measured as shown on the right hip. MP = AC/AB x 100. The acetabular index is illustrated on the left hip. B) AP radiograph with AI (on the right hip) and migration percentage illustrated on the left hip.

the age of 3 years predicts normal hip development, provided that the clinical examination remains normal and that no scoliosis develops. Similarly, it has been suggested that the migration percentage is the best guide for hip surveillance. A population study has recommended that all children with bilateral CP should undergo a standardised position AP pelvic radiograph at the age of 30 months, in order to predict the risk of dislocation. Another population-based study in southern Sweden claimed that, with adequate screening and early intervention, the incidence of dislocation dropped significantly, when compared with historical controls. The screening was based on a register of children with CP and relied on this for its validity.

Overall the existing literature suggests that all children with bilateral CP should undergo an anteroposterior (AP) pelvic radiograph around the age of 2–3 years in order to assess the risk of hip dislocation (Box 13.6.1). The presence of an abnormal acetabular index (> 30 degrees) or an abnormal migration percentage (>15%) would indicate a significant risk of dislocation (Figure 13.6.2). A normal radiograph at this age would be reassuring but ongoing clinical surveillance is still essential. There is consensus in the literature that non-ambulant children (GMFCS IV and V) are at higher risk and should be screened regularly.

Box 13.6.1 CP hip surveillance—pelvic radiograph age 2–3 years

High risk:

- Acetabular index > 30 degrees
- Migration percentage >15%
- GMFCS IV or V.

Natural history and indications for treatment

Hip displacement in CP is a slow process that allows secondary structural changes in the femoral head and the acetabulum to develop. These secondary changes occur early and, in some cases, before the evolution of hip instability.

Poor sitting balance as well as prevention of windswept posture and the resulting pain have been suggested as indications for treatment of the displaced hip in CP. Loss of mobility in ambulant children as well as decubitus ulceration and secondary deformity of the spine in the non-ambulant patients have also been suggested as indications. However, a comparison between quadriplegic children with scoliosis *and* hip displacement and similar children with spinal deformity *but no* hip displacement showed no effect of hip displacement on the progression of the spinal curvature, despite the higher incidence of pelvic obliquity in the group with hip displacement (Box 13.6.2).

Pain in the non-ambulant child and loss of mobility in the ambulant one are suggested as the main indications for treatment. Posture, care, and hygiene are secondary indications.

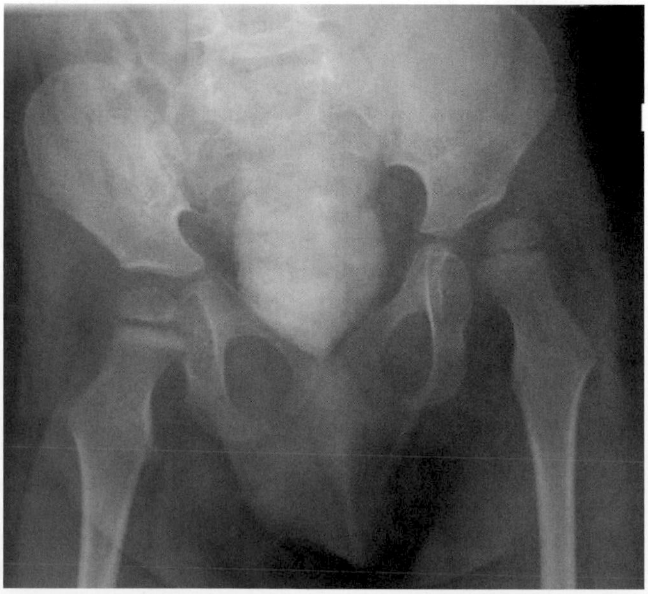

Fig. 13.6.2 AP radiograph of a 3-year-old child with TBI CP. The left AI is 28 degrees and the migration percentage is 55%. Treatment is indicated but bony surgery is required: a femoral varus/derotation osteotomy may suffice as there is little evidence of acetabular dysplasia.

Box 13.6.2 Hips and spines

Hip dislocation does *not* increase the risk of scoliosis progression.

Prevention of hip displacement

The role of soft tissue surgery (Box 13.6.3)

The role of soft tissue surgery around the hips in the prevention of hip displacement in children with bilateral disease is controversial. Some have suggested that such surgery can result in long-term radiographic stability in previously displaced hips in approximately 65% of treated patients but the effectiveness of adductor tenotomy alone in comparison with more extensive releases and obturator neurectomy is unclear. There is agreement that a preoperative migration percentage of less than 40% predicts a successful outcome and early surgery, before the age of 6 years, with postoperative bracing leads to good results. Approximately two-thirds of patients maintain hip stability at 8–10 years from surgery.

An American Academy of Cerebral Palsy and Developmental Medicine (AACPDM) evidence report concluded that the published evidence on the effects of adductor surgery in CP should be 'regarded as preliminary at best'. The lack of long-term studies and comparison with controls was highlighted, as was the need to study the reliability and validity of the radiographic methods used.

Other measures

In a Swedish population-based study, it was shown that the introduction of preventative measures to treat spasticity or dystonia reduced the incidence of hip dislocation compared with historical controls. Preventative measures included selective dorsal rhizotomy, continuous intrathecal baclofen infusion, botulinum toxin injections, and non-surgical treatment of contractures.

Bone procedures for hip displacement and dislocation

Choice and results (Box 13.6.4)

Surgical correction of hip displacement in CP may include a combination of femoral and/or pelvic procedures. The choice of surgical procedure to treat displacement or to salvage the painful chronically dislocated hip remains controversial. Furthermore, there is also the question of whether or not to treat the contralateral hip.

Femoral varus/derotation osteotomy used in isolation for the treatment of the displaced hip in CP is associated with a relatively high risk (10–40%) of redislocation, particularly if acetabular dysplasia is already present when treatment is undertaken (Figure 13.6.2 and Figure 13.6.3).

A variety of procedures have been suggested to treat the acetabular deformity and deficiency. The Salter and Pemberton osteotomies, designed for the treatment of developmental dysplasia, offer improved anterolateral cover that may not be appropriate in CP hip displacement. Results with the Chiari osteotomy have also been unsatisfactory. The triple pelvic osteotomy offers good stability but adds significantly to the complexity of the surgical procedure.

The Dega osteotomy and its modifications address posterolateral instability and may carry advantages over conventional pelvic osteotomies performed for developmental hip dysplasia. The common principle of these procedures is that they leave the medial cortex of the ilium intact and centre the osteotomy on the triradiate cartilage. The claim is that they reduce the volume of the acetabulum and provide posterolateral articular cartilage cover whilst maintaining some stability by preserving the medial wall of the ilium. Such an acetabular procedure, in combination with femoral varus shortening derotation osteotomy, provides more consistent satisfactory results in the treatment of CP hip displacement with improvement in pain, hip mobility, and sitting balance (Figure 13.6.3). Additional soft tissue releases may be required. Satisfactory clinical and radiographic results in over 90% of patients at 5–10 years of follow-up have been reported from retrospective reviews.

In children with TBI CP, by definition, both hips are at risk of displacement and dislocation. In two retrospective studies, unilateral surgery to treat hip displacement in non-ambulant CP patients was shown to be associated with progressive deformity and displacement of the contralateral non-operated hip in over 50% of cases. Bilateral pelvic and femoral osteotomies were shown to carry similar perioperative risks as unilateral or staged surgery.

Box 13.6.3 Soft tissue surgery

- Prevents hip displacement in approximately 2/3 of young children
- Good results with migration index <40% and age <6 years.

Box 13.6.4 Bony surgery: hip reconstruction

- Combined femoral and pelvic osteotomies lead to better results
- Beware the contralateral hip: treat appropriately
- Surgery is associated with a high complication rate.

Windswept hips

Patients with TBI CP may demonstrate significant asymmetry and develop a windswept posture with one hip lying abducted and the other adducted. This posture is frequently associated with pelvic obliquity. The pseudo-Galeazzi sign identifies apparent shortening of the thigh; due more to a fixed abduction of one hip and an associated pelvic tilt rather than a true discrepancy in femoral length. The abducted hip may benefit from release of the gluteus maximus and tensor fascia lata with or without preventative bony surgery as discussed earlier. If there is clinical subluxation with a femoral head palpable in the groin, a hip reconstruction including a varus/derotational femoral osteotomy and acetabuloplasty is indicated (Figure 13.6.4).

Established dislocation

The established hip displacement in CP may develop secondary degenerative changes and pain, which may result in further functional compromise affecting the patient and carer's quality of life (see Figure 13.6.4). Hip reconstruction can still be considered if there is a reasonable chance of creating an acetabulum to contain the femoral head which is often deformed and degenerate but the recovery period is prolonged and the outcome variable. Hip replacement

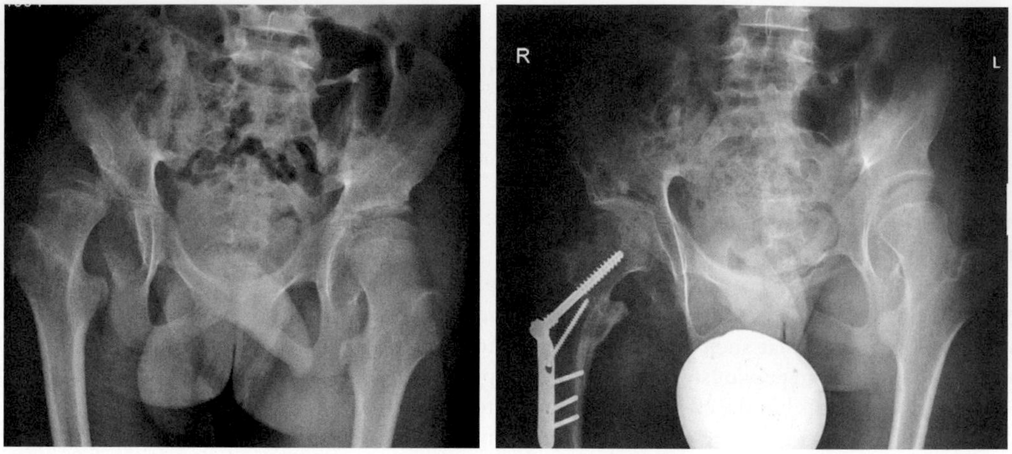

A B

Fig. 13.6.3 AP radiograph of a teenager with a painful subluxation of the right hip A) which was treated by hip reconstruction involving a soft tissue release, a shortening varus/derotation femoral osteotomy and modified Dega acetabuloplasty B).

surgery, excision/interposition arthroplasty with or without valgus femoral osteotomy and hip arthrodesis have all been suggested as treatment methods. However, the existing literature reports a limited follow-up on small numbers of patients with no control group. If an excision arthroplasty is considered this should be performed as a proximal femoral excision below the lesser trochanter with a repair of the soft tissues over the acetabulum (Figure 13.6.5).

Complications

Non ambulant patients with CP often suffer with reflux, absent gag reflex, epilepsy, and respiratory problems. Therefore there is a small but significant mortality rate and they are more at risk of perioperative complications, particularly respiratory problems. It has been suggested that 25% of CP patients undergoing hip osteotomies suffer at least one complication. Surgical complications of hip reconstruction include infection, skin sores, metalwork failure, heterotopic ossification, femoral head osteonecrosis, redislocation, persistent pain, and loss of ambulation. Some studies suggest that many of these complications are more frequent in patients who were casted following surgery compared to those who were not.

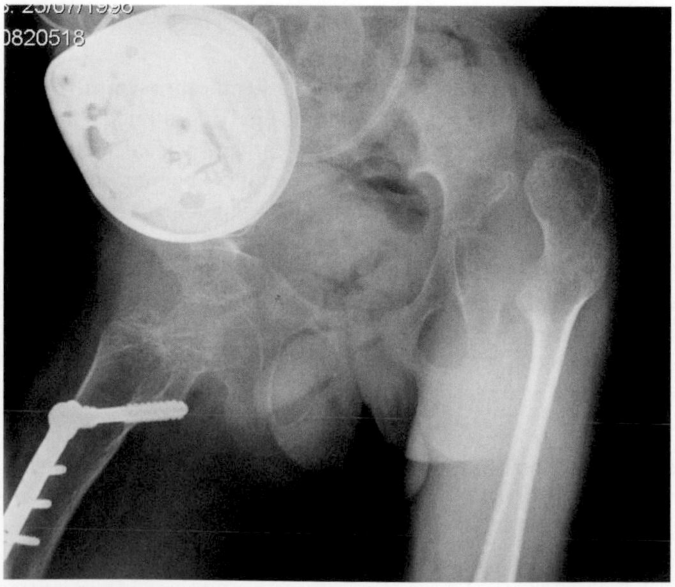

Fig. 13.6.4 AP pelvic radiograph showing pelvic obliquity and a posterior dislocation of the left hip. Despite previous surgery to the right hip there is a windswept posture and clinically anterior subluxation of the femoral head. A baclofen pump is sited in the right iliac fossa.

Anterior dislocation

Whilst most CP hips displace in a posterolateral direction, some hips lie in abduction, extension, and external rotation and are at risk of anterior subluxation or dislocation. This may result in painful restriction of hip flexion which has a significant effect on sitting ability and thus quality of life (Figure 13.6.6).

An early soft tissue release (as mentioned previously for the abducted side in windswept hips), often combined with femoral shortening varus derotation osteotomy may help in maintaining a balanced sitting posture. Treatment of the established anterior dislocation is difficult and salvage with proximal femoral resection may become necessary.

Spinal deformity

A large number of patients with TBI CP develop a scoliosis and once it has developed it does tend to progress. The curve pattern is classically a long 'C'-shaped curve. The pelvis frequently becomes part of the curve and the subsequent pelvic obliquity leads to an unstable sitting base which may cause more functional problems than the curve itself. Children with low-toned CP develop a thoracic kyphosis (Figure 13.6.7).

Severe curves may lead to back pain and respiratory compromise but the main problems are associated with an unstable sitting posture which often limits upper-limb function if one arm is needed to support the body position. Abdominal discomfort secondary to chest wall impingement on the pelvis is common.

Curve prevention and control

There is no good evidence that spinal deformity can be prevented but care with seating and posture is considered good practice.

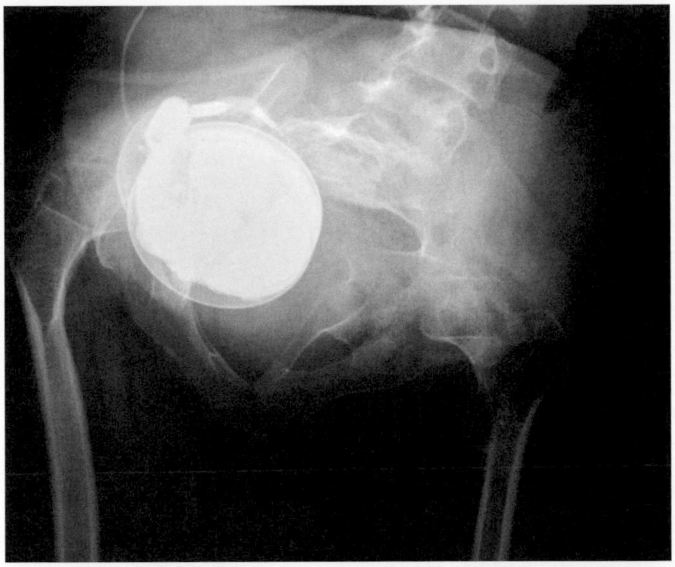

A

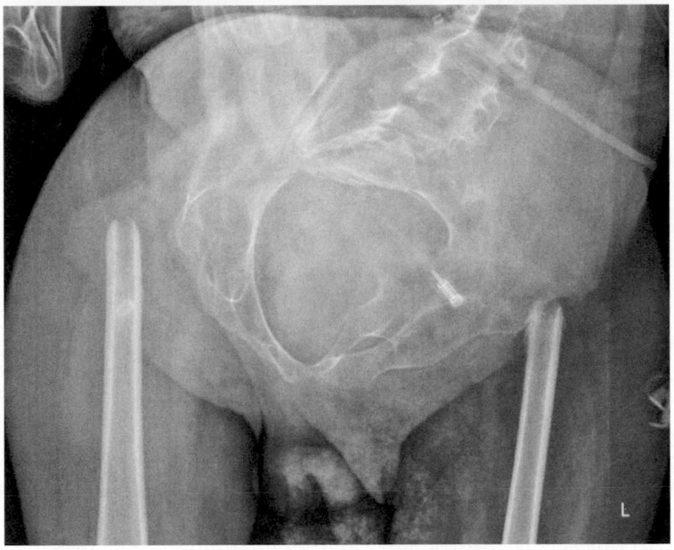

B

Fig. 13.6.5 AP pelvic radiograph demonstrating bilateral long standing posterior dislocations (A) that were treated by bilateral proximal femoral excisions. The baclofen pump has been removed, there is still some pelvic obliquity but seating is easier and more comfortable.

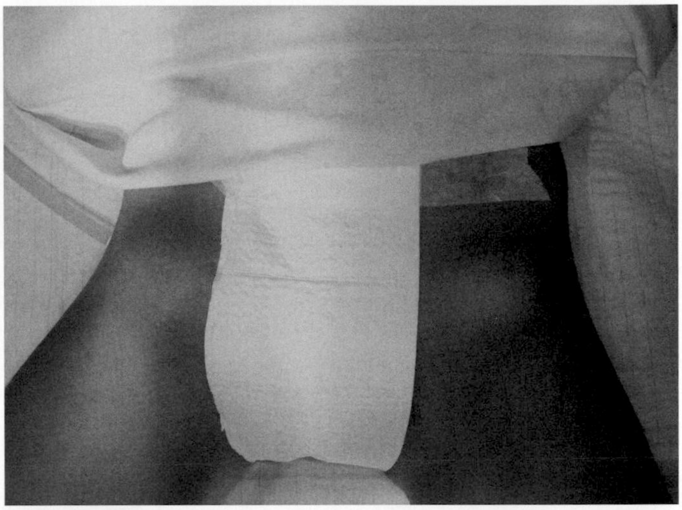

A

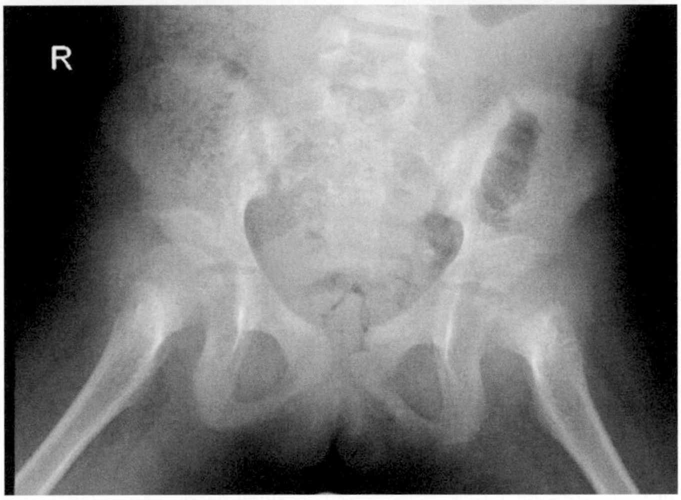

B

Fig. 13.6.6 Clinical photograph of a child with bilateral anterior hip dislocations (A) noticeable as 'lumps' in the groin with the femoral artery prominent over the femoral head. The accompanying pelvic radiograph (B) looks surprisingly normal.

Seating with adequate trunk and pelvic control may delay the onset of scoliosis. Deformity often becomes clinically apparent between the ages of 5–10 years and once progression has been documented, brace wear should be considered. Spinal braces are often poorly tolerated particularly in these children with multiple other problems and who are 'peg fed' in which case reliance on adapted seating with a tilt-in-space facility and good lateral supports may be more appropriate. The aim of bracing is to delay the progression of deformity rather than to halt it: allowing surgical correction to be delayed until sufficient spinal growth has taken place.

Curve correction

Untreated curves do tend to progress throughout adulthood and may leave the patient in a position where they are unable to sit and must be cared for in bed. Thus, once the curve has reached a Cobb angle of approximately 50 degrees, surgical correction should be considered and a full explanation of the risks and benefits of the procedure given to the parents.

Spinal fusion is usually undertaken posteriorly from T2–pelvis using a segmental instrumentation system. It is important to correct pelvic obliquity and to recreate a normal lumbar lordosis (see Figure 13.6.7). A failure to do so may exacerbate rather then relieve seating problems. As the spinal fixation is usually secure, prompt mobilization is possible. In these children, there are frequently associated hip problems and postoperative rehabilitation may be hampered initially by increased stiffness and discomfort at hip level, particularly if the pelvic position and effective hamstring length have been altered.

Preoperative assessment must pay close attention to the patient's nutritional status as well as to respiratory compromise. A poor swallowing reflex combined with the supine position and potential ileus postoperatively mean that oral feeding should be delayed

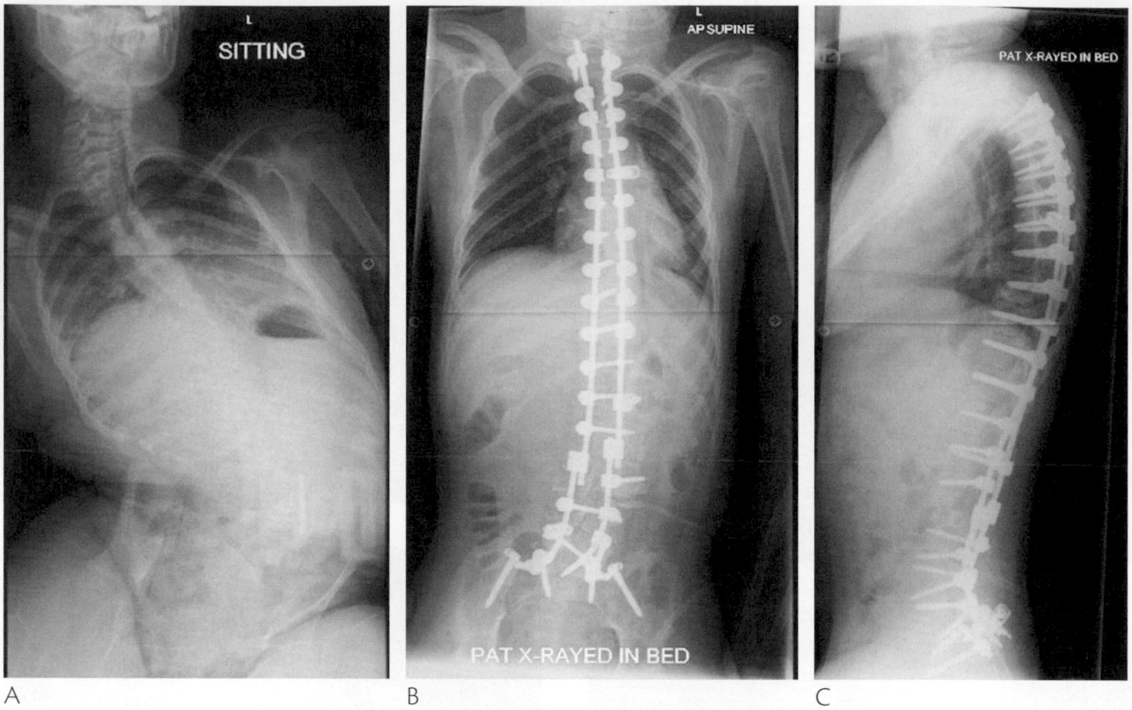

Fig. 13.6.7 A) AP radiograph showing a severe scoliosis with pelvic obliquity pre-operatively. B) AP and C) lateral views of the same spine following posterior instrumentation. Fixation is to the pelvis. The pelvic obliquity has been corrected and the lumbar lordosis restored.

until the patient is able to be in a more upright position and swallow safely.

Other considerations

The ability to perform a weight-bearing transfer is a significant factor in maintaining quality of life and a degree of independence. Patients who can perform such transfers or have the potential to achieve this may be candidates for correction of knee contractures over 15–20 degrees. Hamstring lengthening should provide enough correction for this purpose (Box 13.6.5) and supracondylar femoral extension osteotomies are rarely indicated. Lengthening of the hamstrings may also improve sitting posture by reducing posterior pelvic tilt.

Box 13.6.5 Hamstring lengthening
Be careful not to stretch the sciatic nerve.

Foot deformities may also require correction to aid standing transfers or simply to accommodate the feet more comfortably on the foot-plates of the wheelchair. Severe foot deformities may also merit treatment if they risk skin ulceration over prominent bones or due to external pressure. In addition, severe upper or lower limb contractures may require treatment to facilitate care and hygiene. Any upper limb interventions should be carefully considered to avoid compromise of existing function, such as the use of an electric wheelchair control (the 'joystick'), computer keyboards or communication devices.

Further reading

Leet, A.I., Chhor, K., Launay, F., Kier-York, J., and Sponseller, P.D. (2005). Femoral head resection for painful hip subluxation in cerebral palsy: Is valgus osteotomy in conjunction with femoral head resection preferable to proximal femoral head resection and traction? *Journal of Pediatric Orthopedics*, **25**(1), 70–3.

Gordon, G.S. and Simkiss, D.E. (2006). A systematic review of the evidence for hip surveillance in children with cerebral palsy. *Journal of Bone and Joint Surgery*, **88B**, 1492–6.

13.7

The orthopaedic management of myelomeningocoele

Philip Henman

Summary points

- Myelomeningocoele is a congenital failure of neural tube development
- Hydrocephalus is a common association
- Multidisciplinary management is important
- An alteration in neurological status requires further investigation
- Beware the insensate skin
- A supple plantigrade foot aids independence.

Introduction

Myelomeningocoele or spina bifida is a congenital condition in which the embryological development of the neural tube is incomplete. The neurological effects are due to the combination of the absent or damaged neural elements at birth and the secondary effects of tethering of the spinal cord at the site of the lesion during growth.

For the orthopaedic surgeon, the main challenges are the position and stability of the hip joints and the management of foot deformities. The management of the spine itself in patients with myelomeningocoele is dealt with in Chapter 13.8.

Incidence

The incidence in the United Kingdom is currently approximately 1:1000 live births. It has fallen over the last three decades particularly in Wales and Northern Ireland. This fall is probably attributable to the routine use of folate supplements in pregnancy, improved prenatal diagnosis, and the termination of affected pregnancies.

General principles of management

The neurological effects of a myelomeningocoele are not restricted to the musculoskeletal system. Many patients develop a hydrocephalus that requires a ventriculoperitoneal (VP) shunt and neurosurgical monitoring. Bowel and bladder function is also often abnormal and appropriate medical and surgical care essential. Hence, many centres employ a multidisciplinary approach to the management of these complex cases.

The orthopaedic goal of management is to optimize the patient's comfort and mobility while avoiding overtreatment. Surgical treatment must be planned in the context of the individual's abilities and circumstances; the number of surgical episodes should be minimized, and postoperative immobilization must be as brief as possible. Latex allergy has been reported in patients with spina bifida and latex-free equipment should be used in areas such as the operating theatre suite.

Whilst a rough prediction of lower limb function can be made by assessment of the level of the neurological lesion, it is not possible to make absolute or accurate forecasts of future mobility for any individual infant. Many other factors influence function. The asymmetric and often 'patchy' nature of the peripheral neurological lesion, the variability of the effects on the central nervous system, individual personality and drive, the possible effects of spinal cord tethering with growth, weight gain, and bone fragility are just some of these factors. Many children require the aid of orthotic devices to stabilize and support joints to achieve independent mobility and many are predominantly wheelchair users (Figure 13.7.1).

As a general rule it makes sense to treat identifiable musculoskeletal problems as simply and effectively as possible in the infant, then tailor future treatment to the individual as their particular pattern of involvement and development unfolds. In practice this involves early, minimally invasive treatment of selected hip dislocations and foot deformities in the young child, and more complex surgery where needed in older patients. It is true that with growth and associated weight changes, the child's function may change but a change in their neurological status must also be considered and excluded by appropriate investigation (Box 13.7.1).

Box 13.7.1 Changing Neurological Status?

Consider:

- Developing hydrocephalus
- Blocked VP shunt
- Tethered cord.

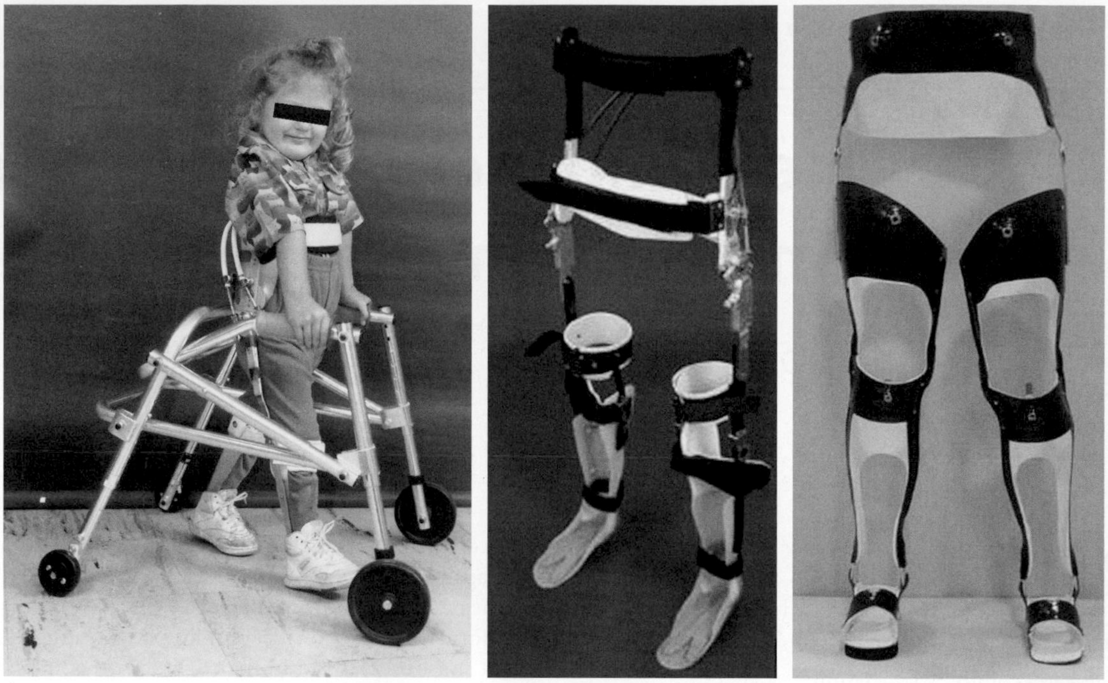

A B C

Fig. 13.7.1 A) A child with spina bifida who achieves independent mobility with the aid of a reciprocating gait orthosis (RGO) and a Kaye walker. B) Photograph of a RGO. C) Photograph of a HKAFO (hip–knee–ankle-foot orthosis).

The hip

Hip deformities in spina bifida are associated with lesions at all neurological levels but are more common with higher lesions. An absence of muscular control appears to be the major influence on hip stability rather than muscular imbalance across the joint. Hip dislocation alone has not been shown to influence gait efficiency, sitting balance, or the formation of pressure areas around the pelvis. The hip joint may have sensation even in high lumbar lesions, however, and these patients may develop pain in subluxated or dislocated joints.

Hip flexion contracture

Hip flexion contractures are more troublesome in thoracic and high lumbar neurosegmental patients. In non-ambulant patients with a thoracic lesion, a progressive deformity develops which has a tendency to recur after surgical release. Well-controlled seating following surgery may be effective in younger children but a progressive deformity in the older child or adolescent is difficult to reverse.

A hip flexion deformity of more than 30 degrees in the ambulant child, with or without orthoses, is best managed with a soft tissue release to allow an upright stance and comfort when using orthotic supports and walking aids (see Figure 13.7.1B,C).

Hip dislocation

Hip dislocation, noted at birth, in lumbar and sacral neurosegmental patients can, as a rule, be reduced surgically though a medial approach in early infancy. There is no benefit to reducing the hips in patients with a definite thoracic neurosegmental lesion.

Surgery for subsequent or later subluxation or dislocation remains the subject of debate in the high lumbar neurosegmental group. No clear benefits have been demonstrated from surgical relocation in terms of gait, standing ability, or sitting balance, even for unilateral dislocations. In the event of a painful subluxation or dislocation, joint stabilization is indicated. Children with low neurosegmental levels are better candidates for surgery. Typically, this involves osteotomies above and below the joint in addition to soft tissue surgery. Unfortunately, the results of surgery are unpredictable and recurrent subluxation and dislocation does occur (Figure 13.7.2).

Muscle balancing surgery is less commonly performed now but some centres still advocate muscle transfers around the hip in association with bony surgery in patients with a low lumbar level (Figure 13.7.3 and Box 13.7.2).

The knee

Flexion deformity

As with the hip, the more severe knee flexion deformities are associated with high neurosegmental lesions and are not directly related to muscle imbalance. The late onset of a knee flexion deformity

Box 13.7.2 Joint stability
Absence of muscle control is more important than *muscle imbalance.*

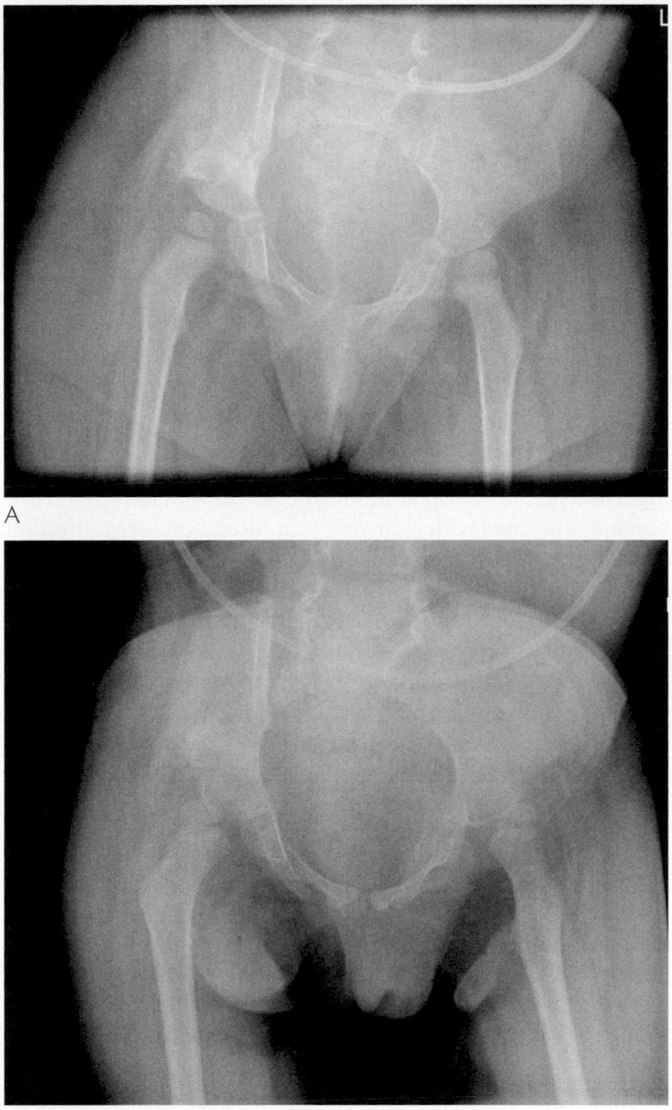

A

B

Fig. 13.7.2 A) AP pelvic radiograph of a child with spina bifida 6 months after successful open reduction of the right hip with an acetabuloplasty and associated soft tissue release. Note the presence of a VP shunt. B) AP pelvic radiograph 12 months later shows that the right hip has redislocated and the left hip has also dislocated.

with associated hamstring tightness or an unexpected deterioration in an existing deformity should raise the possibility of a tethered spinal cord.

A knee flexion deformity of more than 30 degrees in a potential walker is an indication for soft tissue release in children below the age of 7 or 8 years. In older children, surgery is best delayed to closer to skeletal maturity at which time anterior hemiepiphyseodesis or extension osteotomies can be used to correct residual flexion. (see Chapter 13.4, Figure 13.4.8)

Extension deformity

This is a much less common deformity. In the neonate, manipulation and serial splints or casts will achieve adequate correction in many cases. Surgical treatment can involve quadriceps lengthening

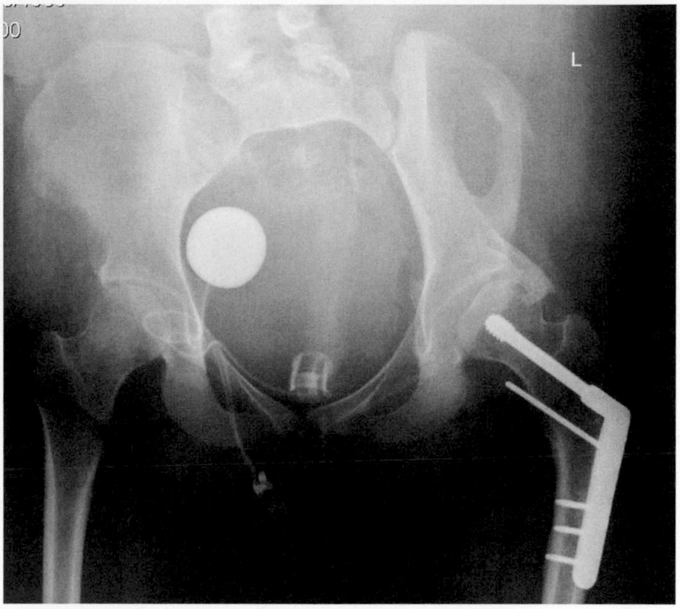

Fig. 13.7.3 AP pelvic radiograph of an adult patient with spina bifida who was treated as a child for a dislocated left hip. Note the hole in the iliac wing which denotes the site of a previous psoas transfer.

with relocation of the hamstrings in patients with low lesions, or tenotomy of the patella tendon in those with no quadriceps function.

Torsional deformities

Both external and internal deformities are recognized and may be treated by derotational osteotomies. It is essential that prior to surgery any existing ankle deformity is identified.

The foot

The goal of treatment is a supple plantigrade foot: whatever the function of the patient, stiffness and deformity increase the risk of skin ulceration in a foot with impaired or absent sensation.

The principles of Ponseti's method of foot deformity treatment (see Chapter 13.21) can be applied to the foot in spina bifida, much as they can in idiopathic cases and in arthrogryposis. Where surgery is judged inadvisable, adaptive footware can allow continued ambulation. Development of new deformities throughout childhood should raise the possibility of a tethered spinal cord.

Equinovarus deformity

Treatment in the neonatal period begins with manipulations and serial casts complemented where appropriate with minimal surgery to release tight tendons. Some children present with a rigid foot deformity similar to that seen in arthrogryposis, and can be treated similarly with a more prolonged series of gradual manipulations and casts. An Achilles tenotomy is usual and may need to be performed earlier than with the idiopathic foot. Relapsed or resistant deformities may be treated with more extensive surgery but at the risk of causing more stiffness in the long term. In older children, equinovarus deformities can be corrected with osteotomies, whilst many surgeons consider a triple arthrodesis as the definitive salvage procedure suitable for use from adolescence onwards.

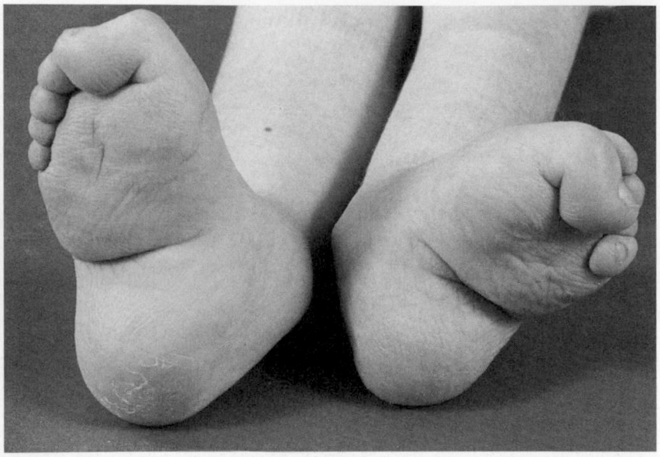

Fig. 13.7.4 Calcaneus feet. Note the prominent heel pad which helps protect the foot from damage but the presence of insensate skin means that ulcer formation is still a risk.

An alternative in severe deformity is the Ilizarov method of gradual correction using an external fixator. This is surprisingly well tolerated in this patient group and may avoid the problems associated with a rigid insensate foot following arthrodesis.

Vertical talus

This foot deformity traditionally required extensive open surgery to correct the troublesome rigid rocker-bottom foot. Recently the Iowa group have described a method of serial manipulations and casts complemented by minimal surgery, derived from the Ponseti clubfoot treatment. This method has the advantages of less extensive surgery and a reduced risk of significant stiffness.

Cavovarus deformity

A progressive cavus deformity may indicate a tethered spinal cord and this possibility must be investigated before surgery to the foot is performed. Molded insoles can accommodate minor deformities but prominence of the metatarsal heads combined with impaired sensation is a common cause of skin breakdown and recurrent infection. Metatarsal and calcaneal osteotomies may be needed to realign the foot. Severe deformities may require triple arthrodesis or correction using the Ilizarov method.

Calcaneus deformity

This troublesome deformity gives an unstable base for stance and causes point-loading on the prominent calcaneum with associated risks to the skin. Management consists of serial manipulations and casts to relax the dorsal structures followed by dorsal soft tissue release and osteotomies of the mid-foot and calcaneum (Figure 13.7.4).

Amputation

Rigid foot deformities in an ambulant patient with impaired sensation are associated with recurrent skin ulceration, deep infection, and osteomyelitis. In intractable cases, amputation may be a robust practical solution, particularly where the prosthesis loads through a sensate area, such as a patellar-tendon-bearing socket in a patient with a low lumbar lesion. Amputation should be delayed where possible till skeletal maturity to avoid the complication of appositional bone growth.

Further reading

Broughton, N.S. and Menelaus, M.B. (1998). *Menelaus' Orthopaedic Management of Spina Bifida Cystica*, third edition. London: W.B. Saunders.

Crandall, R.C., Birkebak, R.C., and Winter, R.B. (1989). The role of hip location and dislocation in the functional status of the myelodysplastic patient. A review of 100 patients. *Orthopaedics*, **12**, 675–84.

Lorente Molto, F.J. and Martinez Garrido, I. (2005). Retrospective review of L3 myelomeningocele in three age groups: should posterolateral iliopsoas transfer still be indicated to stabilize the hip? *Journal of Pediatric Orthopedics*, **14**, 177–84.

Thompson, D. (2000). Hairy backs, tails and dimples. *Current Paediatrics*, **10**, 177–83.

13.8

Neurological aspects of spinal disorders in children

Najma Farooq, S.K. Tucker, and D. Thompson

Summary points

- Spinal neurological problems may be a focal anomaly or part of a systemic disorder
- The neuro-orthopaedic syndrome should be considered in any dysraphic patient with a changing clinical picture—urological symptoms respond well to prompt untethering
- Ten per cent of central nervous system tumours originate in the spinal cord—they may be intramedullary, intradural extramedullary, or extradural.

Introduction

Spinal neurological conditions in the paediatric population can be part of a systemic disorder or a focal abnormality within the spine and neural axis (Table 13.8.1). When a child presents with signs and symptoms of possible underlying neurosurgical pathology, both developmental and acquired aetiologies must be considered.

Spinal dysraphism

Normal spinal cord development can be divided broadly into three processes. Aberrations at each of these stages may be responsible for clinical disorders that are included under the broad term spinal dysraphism

The first stage in development of the neuraxis is *gastrulation.* It is during this stage that the germ cell layers of the embryo are established: these comprise ectoderm, mesoderm, and endoderm. Anomalies that have their origins early in development will commonly affect each of these layers. This is exemplified with neurenteric cysts where there is a persistent connection between the gut epithelium and the nervous system or split cord malformations where there is duplication of the spinal cord and vertebral body defects.

By the end of gastrulation the ectodermal plate has been formed and soon after the process of *neurulation* begins.

In *primary neurulation* a midsagittal groove is seen in the neuroectodermal plate. As this deepens, the edges of the groove fold towards each other and eventually join to form the neural tube. This process forms the brain and the spinal cord as far as the conus medullaris.

Secondary neurulation describes the process by which the terminal components of the CNS are formed: the tip of the conus medullaris, the cauda equina, and the filum terminale. This involves tissues located within the tail bud, caudal to the neural tube, known as the caudal cell mass. Vacuoles form within the caudal cell mass. These cavities become confluent with the central canal of the neural tube. This terminal dilatation forms the distal neural tube. Much of the dilatation regresses in a process termed caudal regression or retrogressive differentiation. The associated differential growth of vertebral column and neural tube results in a more cranial placement of the conus. The filum terminale remains as a connection between the conus and its original caudal attachment.

Spinal dysraphism is a term encompassing a broad spectrum of spinal anomalies arising from any disturbance during any of the stages of neural development and categorized broadly into open and closed neural tube defects.

Table 13.8.1 Aetiology of paediatric spinal neurological conditions

Congenital	Spinal dysraphism: Diastematomyelia Sacral agenesis Meningomyelocoele
Infection	Viral poliomyelitis Pyogenic Tuberculosis
Tumours	Extradural Intradural Intramedullary Metastatic
Vascular	Arterio-venous malformations type 3
Skeletal dysplasias	Chromosomal syndromes Metabolic disorders, e.g. mucopolysaccharidoses
Autoimmune	Guillain–Barré syndromes
Inherited	Charcot–Marie–Tooth Friedreich's ataxia Neurofibromatosis
Trauma	

Open neural tube defects

Failure of the neural tube to fuse leads to open defects such as myelocoeles and meningomyelocoeles. Neural tissue is exposed or covered by a thin meningeal layer. Neurulation is a process that is in part dependent on folate metabolism and folate deficiency is a major aetiological factor in open neural tube defects. Supplementation of the diet with folate prior to conception significantly reduces the risk of an open neural tube defect. Antenatal diagnosis can be made on ultrasound examination, by a raised maternal serum alpha feta-protein (AFP), or by amniocentesis measuring AFP and acetylcholinesterase.

Developments in the management of prenatally identified meningomyelocoeles include *in utero* repair of the defect. The benefits of this intervention compared to early postnatal closure are still undergoing evaluation through a randomized controlled trial. Some of the perceived advantages of *in utero* surgery are reduced hindbrain herniation (Arnold–Chiari II malformation) and a reduced need for a ventriculoperitoneal (VP) shunt.

A multidisciplinary approach is required to manage open neural tube defects and this should be undertaken in a unit with appropriate expertise.

Initial management

Following delivery, it important to maintain a sterile environment for the exposed tissues and a sterile, moist, non-adhesive dressing which prevents pressure on the neural sac should be applied to the open defect. The child is nursed prone. There is a high incidence of latex allergy and latex exposure should be avoided.

Surgical closure of the defect is usually required within the first few days of life after appropriate imaging for brain ventricular size and following a thorough evaluation to assess the neurological level of the lesion and exclude associated cardiac and renal anomalies. In the perioperative period, the clinician should look for cerebrospinal fluid (CSF) leaks, superficial or deep wound infection, deterioration of neurological level, or the development of acute hydrocephalus. Shunt placement to control hydrocephalus is required in between 50–70% of cases.

Later management

Open neural defects are associated with significant long-term implications in respect of urological function, mobility, spinal deformity, and cognitive development. Minimizing the risk of urinary tract infections during infancy and the early introduction of clean intermittent catheterization helps reduce the incidence of renal scarring. Long-term mobility is strongly correlated with the neurological level of the lesion: lower lesions resulting in better prospects for independent ambulation. Lower limb treatment may involve surgical correction of deformity and the use of orthotic supports (see Chapter 13.9). Comorbidities such as respiratory compromise and weight gain contribute to the loss of mobility seen in adulthood.

Closed neural tube defects

Closed neural tube defects include a group of anomalies of caudal spinal cord development in which the neural tissues, in contrast to myelomeningocoele, are covered by overlying skin. The term occult spinal dysraphism or spina bifida occulta is used to describe this group. The term occult is a misnomer as in many instances there is some feature of the overlying skin that signifies an underlying anomaly: such features are known as the cutaneous stigmata of spinal dysraphism. The following conditions are included under the term spina bifida occulta.

Diastematomyelia

The split cord malformation can occur with or without the presence of a dividing bony, cartilage, or fibrous septum. The two cords may lie within the same dural sac or separately. The two hemicords are often asymmetric with the smaller cord usually on the side of a smaller limb or foot. A focal hairy patch is the cutaneous stigmata commonly associated with this condition (Figure 13.8.1).

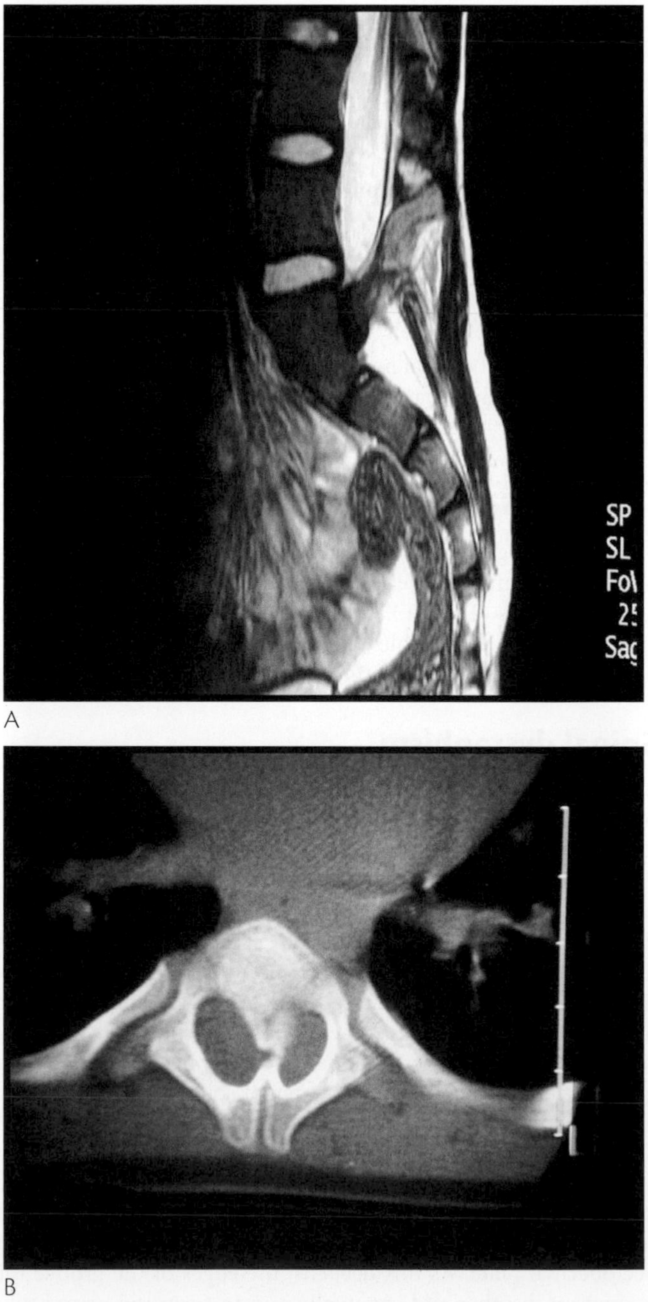

Fig. 13.8.1 Transverse and sagittal images showing a type 1 split cord malformation with a bony dividing bar.

Lumbosacral lipomas

Most commonly a subcutaneous lipoma passes through a defect in the lumbosacral fascia, the posterior bony elements and the dura to be attached to the terminal spinal cord (Figure 13.8.2). Various anatomical forms are recognized depending on the point of attachment of the lipoma in relation to the conus. For practical purposes, the terms lipomyelomeningocoele, lipomyelocoele, and spinal lipoma are synonymous. These are complex developmental malformations which may or may not be associated with neurological or urological symptoms at the time of presentation. Symptoms may occur as a result of primary neuronal dysgenesis or as a result of mechanical stretching (tethering) as the child grows.

Thickened filum terminale

This is perhaps the mildest of the dysraphic states. It is thought to result from a developmental defect of secondary neurulation and regression of the caudal cell mass. The filum terminale is shortened resulting in a low conus and thickened (>2mm diameter) by abnormal fatty or fibrous infiltration that affects its viscoelastic nature (Figure 13.8.3). This may result in undue traction on the conus during flexion and extension of the spine.

Dermal sinus tracts

These are remnants of the embryological connection between the skin (cutaneous ectoderm) and nervous tissue (neuroectoderm). An epithelial lined, midline tract extends from the skin surface through the subcutaneous tissue and spinal coverings to the intradural compartment where the tract terminates usually on the dorsum of the spinal cord. These tracts are significant as they can act as a portal for infection (spinal abscess or meningitis) or as a nidus for intraspinal dermoid formation.

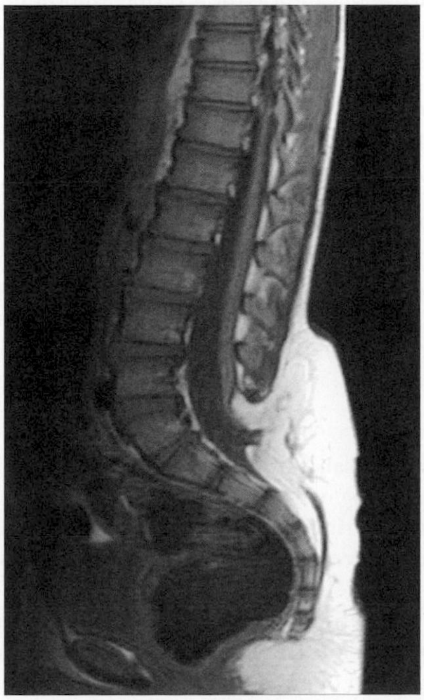

Fig. 13.8.2 Sagittal image demonstrating a lipomyelomeningocoele.

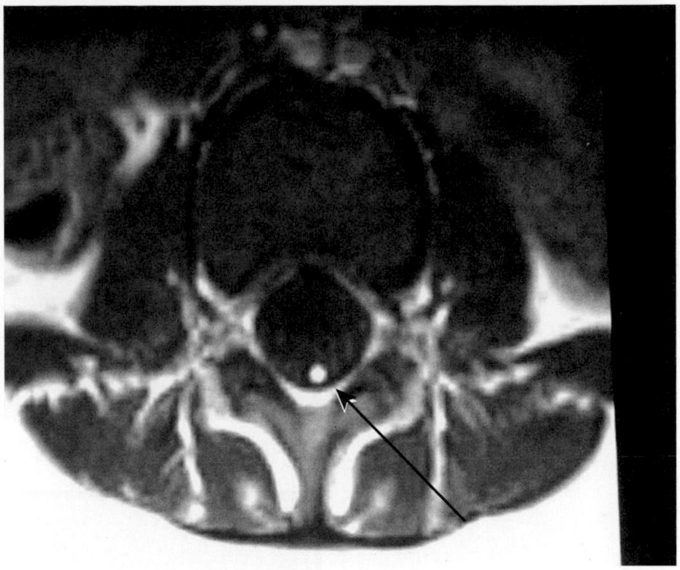

Fig. 13.8.3 Axial MRI demonstrating a thickened filum terminale. Arrow points to the filum.

Neurenteric cyst

These intraspinal cysts of endodermal origin are thought to represent a persistent communication between the ectoderm and the underlying endoderm. They have a lining of mucus secreting or gut epithelium. There is commonly a ventral defect through the vertebral body connecting to a cyst in the retroperitoneum or posterior mediastinum.

Tethered cord syndrome

Any of the anomalies described earlier can be associated with the tethered cord syndrome. This is not a pathological entity in itself but rather a clinical syndrome that results from traction on the spinal cord or nerves as the child grows.

Experimental studies on the pathophysiology of tethered cord syndrome suggest that excessive traction on the spinal cord can produce impaired oxidative metabolism in the spinal cord, diminished blood flow, and local ischaemic changes. The severity and reversibility of these changes probably relate to duration and magnitude of the traction highlighting the importance of identifying this condition early.

Clinical symptoms and signs

The clinical syndrome of tethering is sometimes referred to as the neuro-orthopaedic syndrome and comprises a variety of symptoms that might be orthopaedic, urological, or neurological. It should be considered in *any* dysraphic patient presenting with new, changing or progressive symptoms.

Midline cutaneous stigmata

A subcutaneous lipoma, midline cutaneous punctum (particularly if associated with a history of discharge) lumbosacral appendage, or focal hairy patch is highly suggestive of occult spinal dysraphism (Figure 13.8.4). Lower-risk lesions include very low, sacrococcygeal dimples and gluteal crease deviation. Diffuse hypertrichosis, haemangioma, and naevi, if found in isolation, are of less concern.

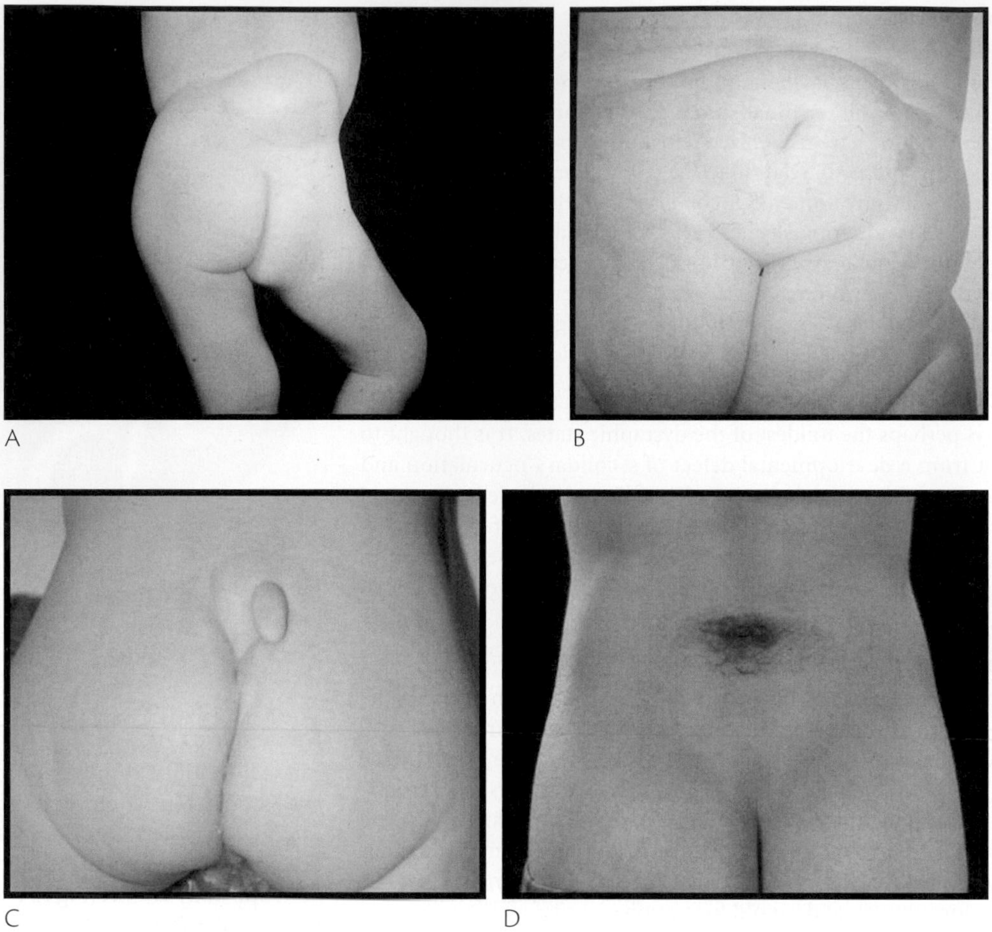

Fig. 13.8.4 Cutaneous stigmata of spinal dysraphism. A) Subcutaneous lipoma; B) midline cutaneous punctum; C) lumbosacral appendage; D) focal hairy patch.

Growth discrepancies/deformities

The development of foot deformity (pes cavus, claw toes) or a rapidly progressive scoliosis may indicate a tethered cord or a recurrence following initial release. Asymmetry in foot size or a leg length discrepancy may also indicate tethering.

Sphincter dysfunction

A spectrum of abnormalities can occur including a neurogenic bladder, faecal and urinary incontinence, and frequent urinary tract infections. A formal assessment with urodynamic studies is essential.

Neurological signs and symptoms

There may be upper or lower motor neuron signs or a combination of both. Asymmetrical weakness may present as decreased leg movements in the infant whilst the older child may present with delayed ambulation and gait abnormalities. Trophic ulceration of the feet may occur as a result of sensory deficits.

Back/leg pain

Classically the pain worsens on spinal flexion or with vigorous exercise. The pain is often poorly localized and usually does *not* have the typical features of sciatica.

Imaging

A clinical suspicion of tethered cord syndrome should be confirmed by further investigations.

Ultrasound

This has limited application as the acoustic window into the lumbar spine closes after 2–3 months of age: in the infant it is a useful technique to assess the level of the conus.

Plain radiographs

These are of little diagnostic help and their role is primarily in the monitoring of spinal deformity.

Magnetic resonance imaging

This is the imaging modality of choice in dysraphic disorders. It has a very high specificity and sensitivity and permits evaluation of the position of the spinal cord, the anatomical features of the dysraphic anomaly and any associated abnormalities such as syringomyelia.

Treatment

Surgical treatment can halt the progression of established neurological deficits in the majority of patients. Symptoms vary in their response to untethering, pain will commonly resolve after successful untethering whereas foot weakness or deformity is less likely to improve.

Numerous clinical studies have demonstrated that patients with urological dysfunction fare better with prompt detethering. An objective assessment of urological function can be made using urodynamic measurements. Postoperative measurements can be useful during long-term surveillance demonstrating early recurrence of cord tethering and the need for further intervention.

Although the role of surgery in symptomatic patients appears clear, in asymptomatic patients, it remains controversial. Many clinicians will advocate prophylactic surgery in order to prevent the development of neurological deficits that may not recover with therapeutic surgery. The exception to this is dermal sinus tract where the perceived natural history and risk of infective complications make prophylactic surgical intervention essential in the majority of cases.

Other considerations with tethered cord syndrome are the associated spinal and foot deformities. Studies suggest that detethering procedures in patients with a myelomeningocoele, tethered cord and scoliosis measuring less than 40 degrees will produce a plateau in curve progression. Larger curves will continue to progress necessitating operative correction and ultimately fusion.

Spinal tumours

Although central nervous tumours are the second most common type of childhood neoplasia, tumours of the spinal cord are relatively rare. The majority of central nervous tumours are intracranial and only 10% are located in the spine. Spinal tumours are classified into three broad groups.

Intramedullary

Intramedullary lesions (Figure 13.8.5) make up 40% of spinal cord tumours, the most common types being astrocytomas and ependymomas. Although 10–15% of astrocytomas are high-grade malignant tumours, the majority of these intramedullary lesions are low grade and present in an insidious manner.

Clinical features

Pain

Characteristically, the pain is a diffuse axial pain that worsens at night secondary to venous congestion and the associated dural distension. Pain usually precedes the onset of neurological symptoms.

Neurological dysfunction

This is of gradual onset. As intramedullary tumours are usually centrally located, dorsal column abnormalities are uncommon, motor signs appear early whereas sphincter dysfunction tends to develop late.

Hydrocephalus

May occur in the context of intramedullary spinal neoplasms and is thought to be related to the high protein concentration in the CSF.

Spinal deformity/torticollis

Pain and an abnormal posture or deformity should raise the suspicion of a spinal tumour.

Management

Surgical excision is the mainstay of treatment for intramedullary spinal tumours. The degree of surgical clearance possible will be governed by the tumour type. Infiltrative astrocytomas are less amenable to radical excision and high-grade tumours have a poor prognosis with median survival of 6–12 months. Removal of ependymomas is often curative. Patients should be monitored for development of postlaminectomy spinal deformity. The laminoplasty approach, which preserves the posterior tension band of the vertebral column, reduces this risk.

Intradural extramedullary

This group (Figure 13.8.6) comprising 20% of spinal cord tumours includes meningiomas and peripheral nerve sheath tumours.

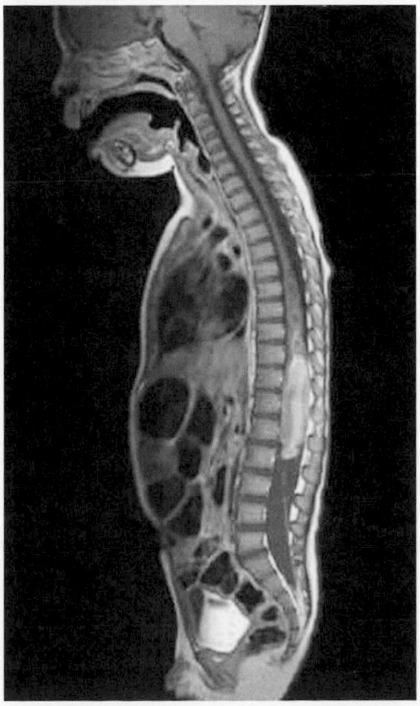

Fig. 13.8.5 Sagittal MRI showing an intramedullary spinal tumour.

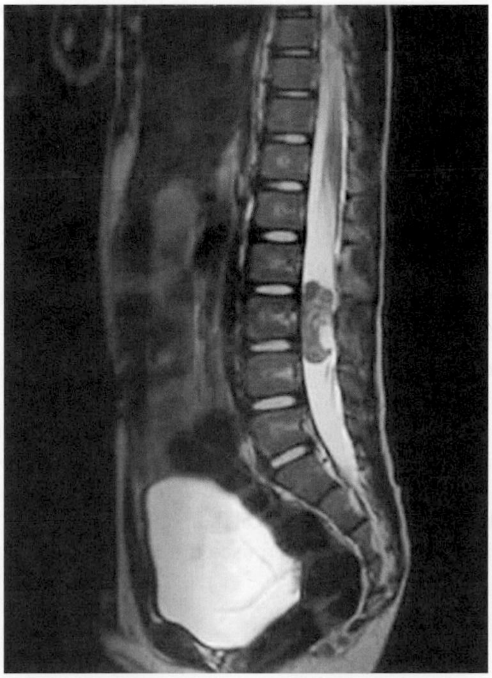

Fig. 13.8.6 Sagittal MRI demonstrating an intradural extramedullary tumour.

Again the most common feature is pain followed by neurological dysfunction. Both tumour types are associated with neurofibromatosis.

Magnetic resonance imaging (MRI) of the whole neural axis will help distinguish between solitary lesions and those arising from metastatic spread from an intracranial primary. Peripheral nerve sheath tumours produce characteristic erosion and enlargement of the neural foramina seen on plain radiographs.

The treatment of choice is surgical excision. Incomplete excisions run a high risk of recurrence. Malignant transformation of peripheral nerve sheath tumours is also a concern, especially in patients with NF-1 and those treated with adjuvant radiation.

Extradural

Primary or metastatic extradural tumours make up 40% of spinal cord neoplasms. Metastatic lesions from a systemic malignancy can produce spinal cord compression in up to 5% of cases. Primary extradural lesions originate from various structures.

The bony structures of the spinal column

Ewings sarcoma

This is the sarcoma that most frequently affects the paediatric spine. The lytic lesions within the vertebral body are often associated with soft tissue masses, the commonest site being the sacrum. The recent improved chemotherapeutic agents have produced better 5–10-year survival rates.

Osteoid osteoma and osteoblastoma

These are histologically similar lesions, differentiated on size. Osteoblastomas are larger than 1.5cm in diameter. The lumbar spine is a common site with the posterior elements more frequently affected than the vertebral bodies. Patients may present with a painful scoliosis, the lesion being located on the apex of the curve convexity. The pain is classically worse at night and relieved by non-steroidal anti-inflammatory drugs. The typical appearance of the central nidus can be identified on computed tomography (CT) scanning. Radionucleotide bone scans and MRI are also helpful. Although osteoid osteomas usually run a self-limiting course, osteoblastomas often require surgical intervention.

Eosinophilic granuloma

Otherwise known as Langerhans cell histiocytosis, can produce either solitary or multiple lytic lesions in the spine. Pathological fractures of the vertebral body may result in a vertebra plana deformity. There may also be an intraspinal extension of the soft tissue tumour. The usually self-limiting nature of this condition makes it amenable to symptomatic management with a period of spinal bracing. More aggressive lesions may require surgery, chemotherapy and low dose radiation.

Aneurymal bone cysts

Approximately one-third of aneurymal bone cysts (ABCs) are found in the spine, most frequently the posterior elements. They are expansile thin-walled lesions with a multiloculated appearance and fluid-fluid levels on MRI or CT imaging. Pain, a palpable mass, spinal deformity, and neurological deficits are common presenting features. Embolization has been used both as a treatment modality and preoperatively to reduce bleeding during surgical excision. Recurrence rates are almost 30% and tend to occur within the first year.

Osteochondromas

Osteochondromas are benign cartilage capped bony protuberances. Five per cent of cases are located in the spine, commonly affecting either the transverse or the spinous process. Multiple lesions can be found in hereditary multiple exostosis. In those patients with multiple lesions, the risk of malignant transformation to a chondrosarcoma is higher. In solitary lesions the risk is less than 1%. Surgical excision is the treatment of choice.

The paravertebral tissues

Neuroblastoma is an embryonal tumour originating from neural crest cell precursors. It is the fourth most common paediatric malignancy. Half of these cases will occur before the age of 2 years. The majority will be located in the abdomen either in the adrenals or in the paraspinal sympathetic chain. Most will have raised serum and urinary VMA (vanillylmandelic acid) and HVA (homovanillic acid) levels. Treatment options include chemotherapy, radiation, steroids, and surgery depending on whether the tumour is localized or disseminated.

Within the epidural space

Lymphomas and *leukaemia* usually occur in the spine as a result of metastatic spread but rarely the spine may be the primary tumour site. In general these tumours are very sensitive to chemotherapy and radiotherapy. Surgical decompression should only be considered if these treatments fail or if the neurological state is deteriorating rapidly.

Summary

The combination of a varied clinical presentation and the diverse nature of the conditions producing neurological abnormalities in the paediatric patient can pose a clinical challenge. A multidisciplinary approach that allows for a thorough assessment and investigation of the paediatric patient with axial pain and neurological signs is essential.

Further reading

Adzick, N.S. and Walsh, D.S: (2003). Myelomeningocele: Prenatal diagnosis, pathophysiology and management. *Seminars in Pediatric Surgery*, **12**, 168–74.

Binning, M., Klimo, P. Jr, Gluf, W., and Goumnerova, L. (2007). Spinal tumors in children. *Neuroimaging Clinics of North America*, **18**, 31–58.

Bruner, J.P. (2007). Intrauterine surgery in myelomeningocoele. *Seminars in Fetal & Neonatal Medicine*, **12**, 471–6.

Lew, S.M. and Kothbauer, K.F. (2007). Tethered cord syndrome: an updated review. *Pediatric Neurosurgery*, **43**, 236–48.

Rossi, A., Gandolfo, C., Morana, G., and Tortori-Donati, P. (2007). Tumors of the spine in children. *Neuroimaging Clinics of North America*, **17**, 17–35.

Thompson, D. (2009). Postnatal management and outcome for neural tube defects including spina bifida and encephalocoeles. *Prenatal Diagnosis*, **29**, 412.

13.9

Arthrogryposis

Roderick Duncan

Summary points

- A rare condition with the potential to cause serious physical disability
- Early recognition and treatment reduces the impact of the condition on the individual
- Physiotherapists, occupational therapists, and orthotists play a pivotal role in patient management and a coordinated multidisciplinary team is required
- Many children need orthopaedic surgery but the treatment principles differ from those applied to unaffected children with similar individual deformities
- Prolonged postoperative splinting reduces the risk of recurrent deformities
- Individuals with amyoplasia or distal arthrogryposis often have normal intelligence and great potential to cope with their physical disability.

Introduction

Arthrogryposis, or arthrogryposis multiplex congenital (AMC), is purely a descriptive term: it means 'hooked or curved joints present at birth'. If a child has joint contractures present in two or more different body areas associated with muscle wasting, then the child can be said to have arthrogryposis but there are over 300 different, specific conditions that present in such a way. The clinical features, inheritance patterns, and prognoses of these conditions vary considerably, so an accurate diagnosis is imperative. Three broad groups have been identified which occur with approximately equal incidence (Box 13.9.1). Firstly, there are those with primarily joint involvement. Secondly, there is a group that includes children with involvement of another body system as well as their limbs. The third group includes those with limb and central nervous system involvement in which there is a high mortality in early life.

This discussion relates principally to children with amyoplasia and distal arthrogryposis but the principles are common to all those with multiple congenital contractures.

Aetiology, pathogenesis, and pathology

The joint contractures are caused by limb deformation *in utero*. The deformities are not a result of primary limb malformations. A lack of fetal movement, or fetal akinesia, is thought to be the final common pathway in the development of the clinical picture but many other factors may play a role and both myopathic and neuropathic aetiologies have been implicated. The lack of joint movement leads to extra connective tissue around the joint, shortened tendons, and modelling of joint surfaces. Although the contractures are not progressive they have a tendency to recur rapidly after correction. Correction can be difficult because the tissue planes encountered during surgery are significantly less well defined than normal as are the individual muscles. Muscles are generally weak, sometimes profoundly so, but the pattern and extent of muscle weakness is very variable. Preservation of muscle strength is an important principle of treatment.

Epidemiology and genetics

Multiple congenital contractures occur in 1 in 3000–5000 live births but true amyoplasia is less frequent (1 in 10 000). Most case series in the literature report on less than 20 patients. Amyoplasia is a sporadic condition whilst at least one form of distal arthrogryposis is inherited in an autosomal dominant fashion with the defect mapped to the short arm of chromosome 9.

Box 13.9.1 The three 'groupings' of arthrogryposis

- Joint involvement alone:
  - Amyoplasia *or* classical arthrogryposis
  - Distal arthrogryposis
- With involvement of another body system:
  - Freeman–Sheldon syndrome
  - Osteochondrodysplasias
- With central nervous system involvement: high early mortality rate.

Clinical features (Box 13.9.2)

A child with amyoplasia will usually have symmetrical limb deformities and the majority have all four limbs affected (Figure 13.9.1). Birth fractures may be identified in one in five children. The skin is shiny and joint creases are reduced or absent in affected limbs. The deformities are symmetrical with severe equinovarus (CTEV) deformities of the feet and extended elbows; 10% have abdominal wall defects. The limb deformities are most severe at birth and often quite alarming. However, some of the deformities are positional and will respond to treatment in the neonatal period. Resistant deformities will require more intensive therapy or surgery.

Distal arthrogryposis is characterized by medial deviation of the digits, camptodactyly, clenched fists, and foot contractures. Mild proximal joint involvement can occur. Problems related to each joint or region will be discussed in the following sections.

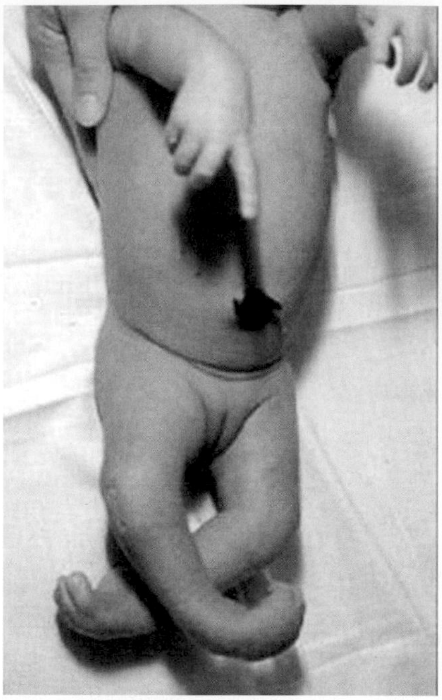

Fig. 13.9.1 Clinical photograph of a child with amyoplasia. All four limbs are affected. The symmetrical involvement of the lower limbs is obvious.

Prognosis

Most families will not have heard of arthrogryposis but most adapt well to the diagnosis. Organizations such as The Arthrogryposis Group (TAG) in the United Kingdom can provide invaluable support for families of affected children. Childhood can be challenging because of the intensive treatment required in the early years of life and the considerable effort required to ensure that the child functions safely in his/her environment. Although they may be affected profoundly by multiple joint contractures, they do not have the same communication problems, sensory abnormalities, perceptual, and balance problems that affect children with cerebral palsy and spina bifida. The prognosis for walking, without treatment, is poor particularly in the amyoplasia group. With treatment, the majority of children with amyoplasia should be able to walk in childhood but they may lose this ability as they pass through adolescence into adult life. The children have near-normal or normal levels of intelligence and tend to be very determined: described by their mothers as 'kind, social, attractive but more persistent or even stubborn than their siblings'. The life expectancy for those with distal arthrogryposis is thought to be normal and for those with amyoplasia a survival rate of 94% at 20 years has been reported.

As far as personal and social development are concerned, one demographic study reported that 64% of older children in one series were in an educational setting appropriate for their age with 75% independent for feeding, 20% for grooming, 10% for dressing, 35% for toileting, and 25% for bathing. Another study found that half of their adult patients were employed, a third were married, half were independently mobile (with wheelchairs as necessary), and 70% had no limitations in activities of daily living. Their conclusion was that their dependence upon others 'was not related to physical deformity but to their personality, their education and to their coping skills'. Clearly orthopaedic surgery is only one aspect of the care needed by these children and their families.

Box 13.9.2 Clinical features

- Symmetrical involvement
- Smooth 'featureless' joints
- Rigid deformities.

Treatment

General principles (Box 13.9.3)

Coordination between health professionals is essential in managing these children and a multidisciplinary team (MDT) approach is recommended. Treatment must be directed at enhancing function and independence throughout their lifetime. It is therefore important that treatment interferes as little as possible with the child's normal development, education, and family life. Treatment should begin as soon after birth as possible. Serial casting and orthoses are used to correct the positional deformities of the limbs, reassuring the parents that the deformities are always the most severe at birth. Most authors recommend correcting fixed deformities in infancy

Box 13.9.3 Management principles

- Overall: retain joint movement
- Lower limb:
  - Facilitate standing and walking where possible
  - Plantigrade, stable feet
  - Extended knees
- Upper limb:
  - Functional grip
  - Adequate ranges of joint movement at shoulder and elbow to enable activities of daily living.

with 'fine tuning' procedures later in life and the Seattle group have recommended the following approach to treatment:

1) *Infancy* is the time for surgical correction of most fixed contractures. Surgery should be decisive and achieve permanent correction. The worst outcome from surgery is incomplete correction with recurrent contracture
2) During *early childhood* it is important to prevent recurrence following surgery by splinting at night and encouraging play and independence during the day. This will also help to preserve muscle strength
3) In *later childhood*, education and the development of skills for life are more important and few if any interventions should be undertaken during this period
4) *Adolescence* is a time for education, vocational planning, socialization, independence, and preparation for adult life, when one should correct any residual disabilities caused by deformity.

Children with arthrogryposis can present significant problems for the anaesthetists. It may be extremely difficult to secure venous access and mouth opening may be restricted, making tracheal intubation difficult. An increased risk of malignant hyperpyrexia and aspiration has been reported.

Orthoses are an essential part of the management of arthrogryposis. They are used to maintain correction of deformities and to facilitate standing in cases of muscle weakness and joint contracture. They must fit well and make a significant difference to function otherwise the child is likely to reject the splints. A great deal of parents' energy can be used trying to get their child to wear splints: these children can be very strong willed! The team must be prepared to offer the families as much support as they need (Figure 13.9.2).

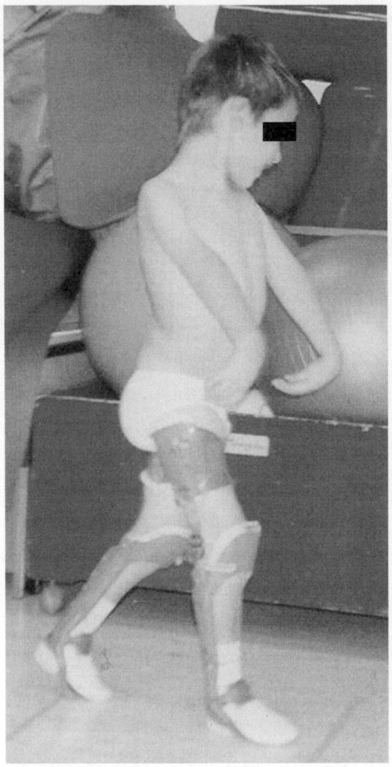

Fig. 13.9.2 Clinical photograph of a child with amyoplasia. He is only able to walk with the aid of KAFOs (knee ankle foot orthoses). Note upper limb involvement which can affect balance and influence gait.

Upper limbs

Upper limb involvement is common in amyoplasia. The classic posture is of internal rotation of the shoulders, extension of the elbows, and flexion and ulnar deviation of the wrists and fingers (Figure 13.9.3). The degree of muscle weakness in the upper limbs is variable but may be profound. Generally, the elbow extensors are stronger than the flexors and the wrist flexors are stronger than the extensors. Some children have very little movement in the hands. The management of these deformities should be directed towards independence in adult life. The MDT must promote the skills necessary not only for activities of daily living, such as eating, dressing, and toileting, but also for vocational skills such as the use of a computer keyboard. The child may also need to use crutches for walking, or to use their upper limbs for operating a wheelchair. The aims are to help the child to hold objects with as functional a hand as possible, and also to be able to position that hand in space appropriately. One simple philosophy is that the child should have one hand available for hand-to-mouth activities, such as eating and drinking, and the other able to help with perineal hygiene or with pushing themselves up out of a chair. Others prefer a more individualized treatment programme based on the child's needs and abilities. There is no doubt that stretching, casting, and the use of orthotics are very effective for upper limb deformities. However, for them to be most effective, they must be started as soon after birth as practically possible, and the involvement of a hand therapist is recommended. Most authors recommend that surgical treatment for upper limb problems should be performed either in infancy or early childhood with later secondary procedures if required.

Shoulders

The shoulders are internally rotated and the profile of the shoulder is down-sloping. It is rare for the fixed internal rotation contracture to cause a functional problem but occasional derotation osteotomies of the humerus have been performed.

Elbows

The elbows may be fixed in flexion or extension but extension is more common. A fixed elbow contracture is the deformity likely to produce most disability. The range of motion is variable and usually the triceps is much stronger than the biceps. It is important to achieve as much passive movement as possible to enable the hand to reach the face, but ideally this should not be at the expense of losing strong elbow extension which is necessary for getting out of a chair or for using crutches. There needs to be a compromise. Stretching and splinting can increase the range of movement in

Box 13.9.4 Useful hand function?

Bad prognostic signs at birth:

- A complete lack of finger flexion creases
- No active motion
- Extremely stiff joints.

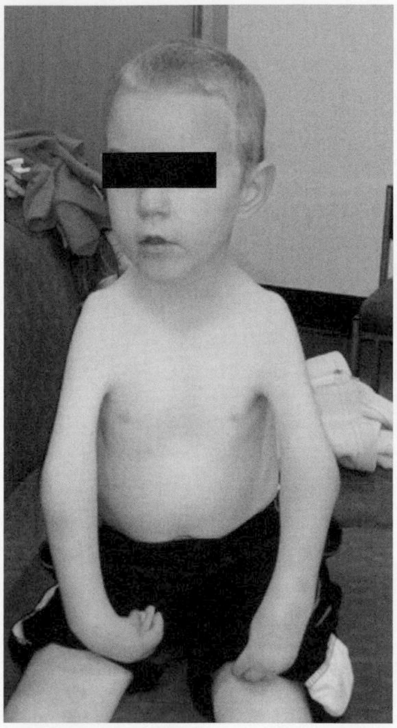

Fig. 13.9.3 Clinical photograph that demonstrates the classical pattern of upper limb involvement: downward sloping shoulders, internally rotated arms, extended elbows and flexed wrists.

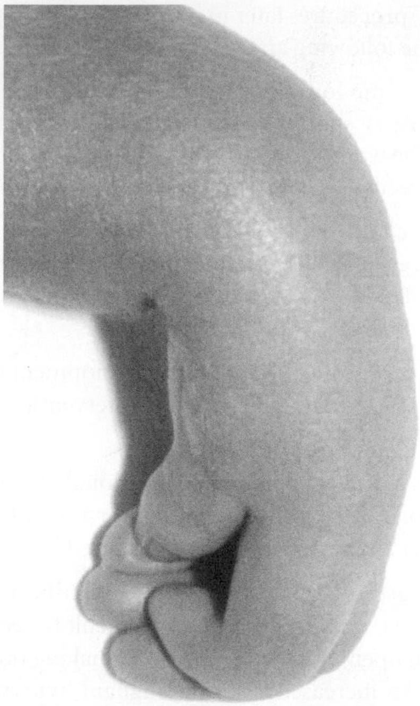

Fig. 13.9.4 Clinical photograph of a hand/wrist deformity demonstrating the featureless appearance of the soft tissues and the absence of joint creases.

infants. If there is less than 90 degrees of elbow flexion then a posterior release and triceps lengthening will increase the passive range of movement. There is more controversy about the role of muscle transfers to restore active elbow flexion. The pattern of muscle involvement is variable. Triceps transfer is the most widely used but pectoralis major, latissimus dorsi, and proximal transfer of the common flexor origin have also been described. The risk with these procedures is that a fixed flexion contracture may develop and all muscle transfers will result in decreased function elsewhere.

Wrists and hands

In both amyoplasia and distal arthrogryposis, the classic deformities of the hand and wrist are flexion and ulnar deviation of the wrists and curved flexed fingers (Figures 13.9.3 and 13.9.4). The thumb is often tucked in the palm. This posture makes prehension and grip difficult and the problems are compounded by forearm and intrinsic muscle weakness. The use of neonatal serial casting is extremely effective in improving wrist position, particularly in distal arthrogryposis. Casting should be followed by the use of lightweight custom-made orthoses, worn principally at night, to enable the child to use the hand during the day. This splinting regimen is supplemented with a regular stretching programme. The orthoses need to be replaced regularly as the child grows. There does not appear to be a consensus on the indications and timing for wrist surgery but, on average, only one-third of those with upper limb involvement undergo surgical treatment. Surgery can either be performed within the first year of life or at a later age. Those who advocate early surgery do so because they claim that surgery is more difficult after the first year of life: the contractures are more severe in the older child, the joint surfaces will have remodelled with intra-articular adhesions, and the skin has become less elastic. They claim that there is a more rapid recovery with less scarring and a greater remodelling potential when surgery is performed in infancy. Others suggest that surgery should not be undertaken early but only after the wrist position that will give best function has been identified. This needs to take into account finger flexor power, extension power, and the child's specific functional requirements (Box 13.9.4). Each child develops their own coping strategies for dealing with the activities of daily living: surgical intervention must be sure to improve the situation rather than simply altering it (Figure 13.9.5). Surgery may involve a volar capsular release, a trapezoidal dorsally-based wedge carpectomy, and tendon transfers to act as check reins.

There can be a significant improvement in finger position and function after the correction of wrist deformities, as the resection of a trapezoidal wedge reduces tension in the contracted finger flexors. Surgical correction of finger deformities is rarely required. When they are refractory to splinting, thumb contractures may be treated by adductor release or, in older children, by metacarpophalangeal fusion and brachioradialis transfer. Web-deepening procedures may also be necessary to improve grasp particularly for the first web space.

Lower limbs

Almost 90% of children with amyoplasia will have lower limb deformities. Rigid equinovarus deformities and flexed knees are the commonest pattern accompanied by flexed and abducted hips (see Figure 13.9.1). Sometimes the lower limb deformities at birth can be quite bizarre but these tend to be postural deformities that respond well to careful stretching and splinting. The goals of lower limb management are to provide stability and symmetry to maximize the potential for walking. Surgery for lower limb deformities should be deferred until it is clear whether the child is likely to

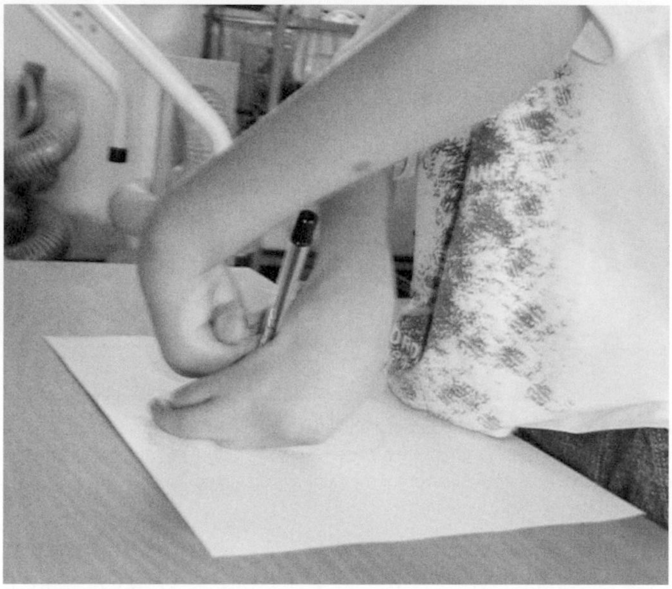

Fig. 13.9.5 The reverse grip that is used by many children with arthrogryposis looks awkward but functions well.

walk, which can be exceedingly difficult to judge. Preoperative assessment must take into account not only the degree of joint deformity and muscle strength, particularly of the hip extensors and quadriceps, but also the extent of upper limb involvement. A child who is likely to spend most of their time sitting needs symmetrical lower limbs with plantigrade feet. When surgery is required it is better to do simultaneous procedures on different joints, in order to reduce the immobilization time and the time spent in hospital during childhood.

Hips

Soft tissue contractures around the hip are common. Most positional deformities respond to careful stretching and splinting. Flexion contractures in excess of 30 degrees are likely to impair walking and those over 45 degrees are likely to require surgical release.

Hip dislocation occurs in almost a half of all children with amyoplasia and is usually bilateral A unilateral dislocation will affect standing, gait, and sitting balance and should be reduced (Figure 13.9.6). Closed reduction is usually unsuccessful in arthrogryposis. There is still debate about what should be done with bilateral hip dislocations—some believe they should be left untreated, particularly if stiff, but the balance of opinion is tending to swing towards reduction in those who are likely to walk. Reduction of bilateral dislocated hips is said to provide a better-looking and more efficient gait. Some recommend the medial approach for hip reduction because the soft tissue dissection is minimal and there is little blood loss. This is important if the feet and knees are being treated in the same operating session. It is also claimed that there is less stiffness following reduction through a medial approach than after an anterolateral approach but success has been reported with both techniques. In older children concomitant pelvic surgery or femoral shortening may be required. The threshold for treating residual acetabular dysplasia is higher in children with arthrogryposis than without.

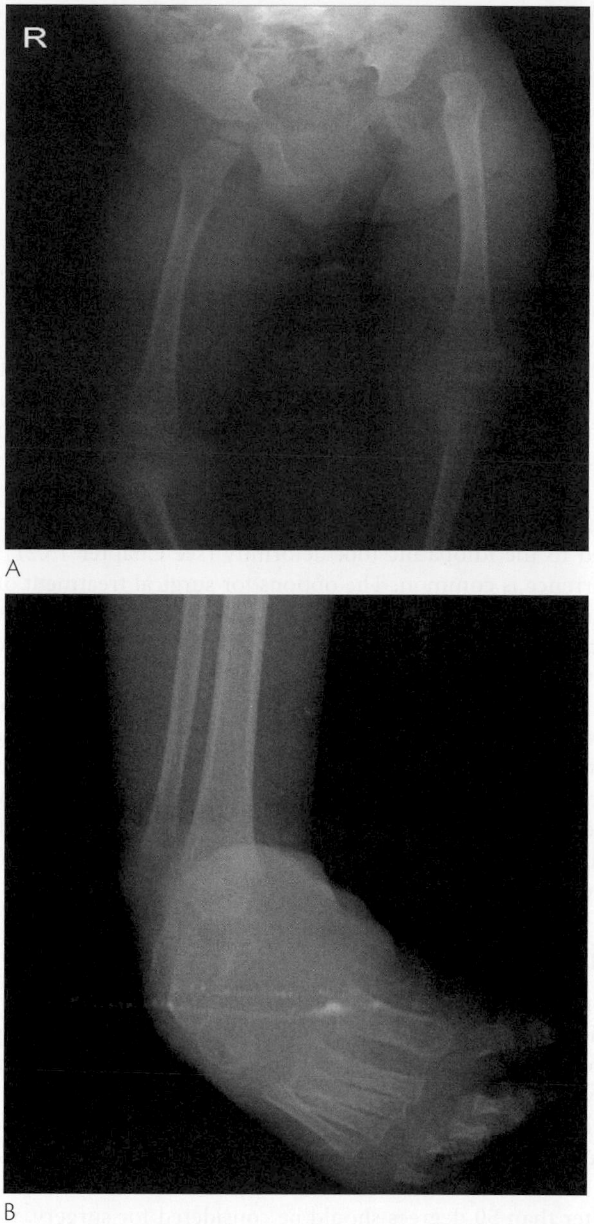

Fig. 13.9.6 A) AP radiograph demonstrating a unilateral (left) hip dislocation. The contralateral (right) knee is in fixed extension and there were bilateral severe TEV deformities (B, right foot). The management of the left hip dislocation must take into account the other joint deformities. The hip was reduced and both feet treated with talectomies.

Knees

Knee involvement is present in 70% children with amyoplasia. The common patterns are fixed flexion, fixed extension, or, less frequently, hyperextension. Fixed flexion of greater than 20 degrees makes standing difficult whilst conversely sitting is difficult with fixed extension (Figure 13.9.6). Patients with extended knees are more likely to be community walkers in the long term but may be at a higher risk of degenerative joint disease. An arc of movement between 15–60 degrees is the ideal. Flexion can be gained with a quadricepsplasty but, in the child with significant quadriceps weakness, this may make it less likely that they will be able to stand. Extension can be achieved by a soft tissue release (with femoral shortening in severe cases), a supracondylar femoral osteotomy, or through the use of a ring fixator. Recurrent deformities are common and splintage is essential after surgery to reduce this risk (Figure 13.9.2). Straightening out flexed knees is the only procedure in paediatric orthopaedics that makes a child walk (Staheli 1993).

Feet

The vast majority of children with arthrogryposis have foot deformities, most commonly a rigid equinovarus (Figure 13.9.6). Occasionally they may have congenital vertical talus (Figure 13.9.7). Recurrence is the main problem following surgery and many children will require second procedures despite long-term postoperative splinting. The aim of surgery is to produce a rigid plantigrade platform which can be accommodated in normal shoes. Ponseti-style serial casting has been tried and although early reports are favourable, to date, there are no published series available with satisfactory follow-up. More casts are required for correction compared to the idiopathic foot deformity (see Chapter 13.21) and recurrence is common. The options for surgical treatment of the equinovarus foot are either a radical soft tissue release or primary talectomy (see Figure 13.9.6). Most authors recommend a radical soft tissue release as the primary procedure but the recurrence rate may be up to 73%. Recurrences can respond to serial casting or secondary soft tissue surgery and satisfactory results can be achieved in over 90%. There is no doubt that talectomy is a valuable salvage procedure, provided the bone is completely excised and the foot is placed in the correct position after surgery. The Ilizarov method has been used to treat recurrences with good results reported from some specialist centres.

Spine

Approximately 20–30% of children with amyoplasia will develop scoliosis. This may affect sitting balance and interfere with upper limb function. The most common curve pattern is thoracolumbar. Curves that develop in early childhood tend to become the most severe. Some, but not all, curves progress relentlessly even after skeletal maturity. Bracing should be used to contain progression and to treat curves less than 30 degrees. Children with curves greater than 50 degrees should be considered for surgery, with a combined anterior and posterior instrumented correction appearing to produce the most reliable results.

Summary

Arthrogryposis is uncommon, but needs to be recognized early in life so that treatment can be started, and positional deformities corrected. In the next 5–10 years, there are likely to be great advances in the understanding of the conditions of which multiple congenital contractures are a feature. There are many controversies regarding the timing and nature of surgical treatment and very little evidence upon which to base management. More children are being managed in specialist centres by MDTs and it is to be hoped that collaborative research will lead to better outcomes for these children in the future.

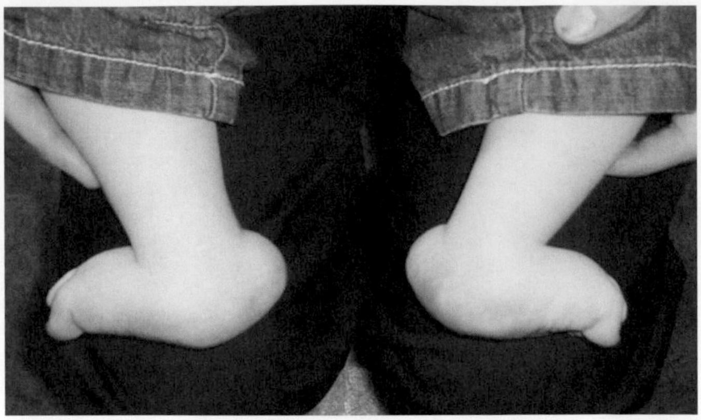

Fig. 13.9.7 Clinical photograph of a child with distal arthrogryposis and bilateral vertical tali. The feet demonstrate a 'rocker-bottom' deformity with hindfoot equinus and a dorsal subluxation of the talonavicular joint.

Further reading

Axt, M., Niethard, F., Doderlein, L., and Weber, M. (1997). Principles of treatment of the upper extremity in arthrogryposis multiplex congenital type I. *Journal of Pediatric Orthopaedics, Part B*, **6**, 179–85.

Bevan, W.P., Hall, J.G., Bamshad, M., Staheli, L.T., Jaffe, K.M., and Song, K. (2007). Arthrogryposis multiplex congenita (amyoplasia): an orthopaedic perspective. *Journal of Pediatric Orthopedics*, **27**, 594–600.

Carlson, W., Speck, G., Vicari, V., and Wenger, D. (1985). Arthrogryposis multiplex congenita – a long-term follow-up study. *Clinical Orthopaedics and Related Research*, **194**, 115–23.

Lahoti, O. and Bell, M.J. (2005). 'Transfer of pectoralis major in arthrogryposis to restore elbow flexion: deteriorating results in the long term'. *Journal of Bone and Joint Surgery*, **87B**, 858–60.

Mennen, U., van Heest, A., Ezaki, M.B., Tonkin, M., and Gericke, G. (2005). Arthrogryposis multiplex congenita. *Journal of Hand Surgery*, **30B**, 468–74.

Sells, J.M., Jaffe, K.M., and Hall, J.G. (1996). Amyoplasia, the most common type of arthrogryposis: the potential for good outcome. *Pediatrics*, **97**, 225–31.

Staheli, L., Hall, J. Jaffe, K., and Paholke, D. (eds) (1998). *Arthrogryposis: A Text Atlas.* Cambridge: Cambridge University Press.

13.10

Common disorders of the lower limb

Tim Theologis

Summary points

- Most torsional or angular deviations are physiological and resolve with time
- Ensure the child has normal growth parameters
- Take care to exclude the rare underlying condition that will require treatment
- Coronal knee deformities may be due to a systemic or local bone dysplasia.

Introduction

Abnormalities of lower-limb alignment, particularly during walking, often cause parental concern and require assessment in the paediatric orthopaedic clinic. Rotational deviations that lead to in-toeing or out-toeing gait, coronal plane knee deformities (genu varum or valgum), and pes planovalgus are the most common causes of parental concern. In the majority of these children, deviations are physiological and of no functional consequence. However, in a small number of children, these abnormalities may be representative of an underlying condition that requires treatment. Therefore, careful clinical assessment of these children is necessary before adequate reassurance can be offered to the parents.

Gait abnormalities

An assessment of gait must include watching the child stand, walk, and run. Many children are on 'best behaviour' in the consulting room and parents are frequently concerned that the doctor has not seen their child's 'normal' walk. Every effort must be made to ensure that the child is as relaxed as possible before the assessment is made: often more can be learnt from watching the child leave the room than watching them come in.

Observational (clinical) gait analysis skills must be used to exclude a generalized problem such as a neuromuscular abnormality or skeletal dysplasia before a more specific assessment of their walking pattern is made. Assessment of the child's torsional profile may help determine where the main deformity lies and reveal the extent of any compensatory deformity (Box 13.10.1 and Figure 13.10.1).

In-toeing gait

The foot progression angle is defined as the angle between the longitudinal axis of the foot and the line of progression of walking. The average foot progression angle in the adult healthy population is approximately 10 degrees external, with a range between 5 degrees internal and 20 degrees external being considered as normal. Mild deviations from the norm are well tolerated and do not cause functional problems or symptoms. Significant deformities may cause frequent tripping and falling, particularly when children are tired and their compensatory mechanisms are failing. It is not known how significant these deviations need be before they cause abnormal joint loading and moments that may lead to long-term joint degeneration. Measurement of joint moments through instrumented gait analysis may have a role in assessing children with significant deviations who are candidates for treatment. This can establish if these deviations are purely cosmetic or likely to cause long-term clinical problems (Figure 13.10.2).

Femoral anteversion

Femoral anteversion is the angle between the longitudinal axis of the femoral neck and the frontal plane of the femur defined by the transcondylar axis and the femoral diaphysis. Femoral anteversion is approximately 40 degrees at birth and gradually remodels to the average adult 15 degrees, usually within the first 3–4 years of life. Little remodelling is expected after the age of 8 years. Early remodelling occurs as a result of pressure on the anterior femoral neck by the soft tissues, particularly the ligaments and the joint capsule, which results from the upright human posture. Conditions preventing upright posture or associated with ligament laxity or joint instability are usually associated with failure of remodelling and

Box 13.10.1 Torsional profile

- Foot progression angle
- Prone hip internal rotation range
- Prone thigh–foot axis
- Foot deformity.

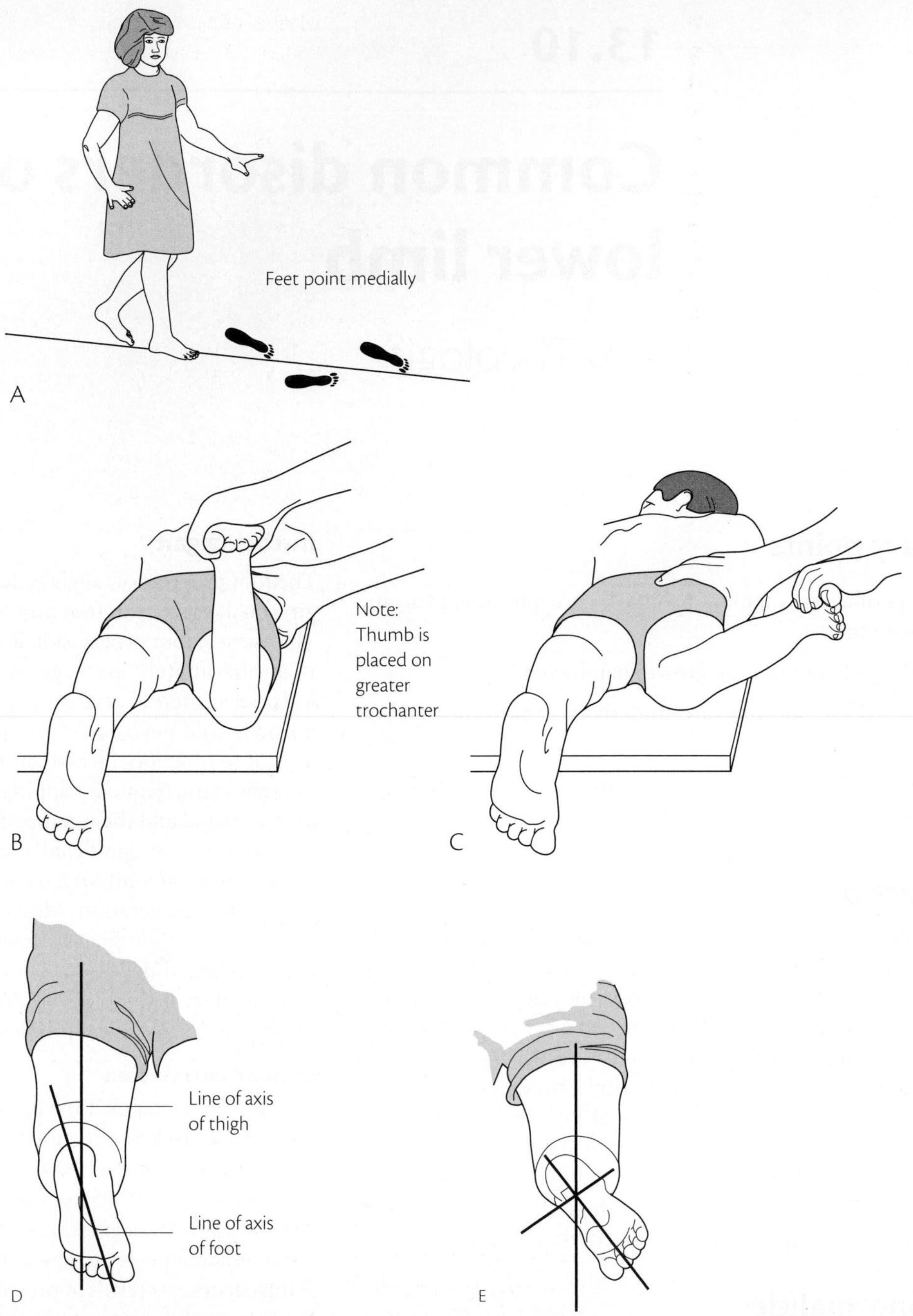

Fig. 13.10.1 Assessment of torsional profile. A) As the child walks, look at the angle the feet make with the imaginary line of forward progression. This is the foot progression angle. B) With the patient prone and the knee flexed to 90 degrees place your thumb on the greater trochanter then C) internally rotate the leg. When the trochanter reaches its most lateral position, the angle between the tibia and the vertical is equal to the femoral anteversion. D) With the patient prone and the knee flexed to 90 degrees, allow the hindfoot to be in a relaxed position. The angle between the longitudinal axis of the hindfoot is the thigh–foot angle. Be careful to 'ignore' forefoot deformity. E) In the same position, the angle between the transcondylar axis of the proximal tibia and the transmalleolar axis of the ankle is also a measure of tibial torsion.

persistent femoral anteversion. However, persistent femoral anteversion is also present in a significant number of normal children. In addition to their in-toeing gait, children often have a typical running pattern with their lower legs swinging out to the side and they are able to 'W' sit comfortably (Figure 13.10.3).

Clinical assessment of femoral anteversion is performed with the child in the prone position and the knee in 90 degrees of flexion. The hip is rotated until the most prominent part of the greater trochanter is palpated in the mid-lateral position. In this position, the angle between the tibia and the vertical is equal to the femoral anteversion (see Figure 13.10.1B,C). The range of hip rotation is often affected and excessive internal rotation is present, at the expense of external rotation. During walking or running, the knees are facing inwards and, as the tibia flexes, the visual impression of genu valgum is often present. Computed tomography (CT) scan or, preferably, the radiation-free magnetic resonance imaging (MRI) scan can be used for a more accurate measurement of anteversion, particularly when surgical correction is contemplated.

In the absence of any underlying or associated conditions, persistent femoral anteversion rarely requires treatment. Whilst increased femoral anteversion is often present in developmental hip dysplasia, patients with the condition would rarely present with in-toeing as their main complaint. It is important to ensure that examination of the hips is normal in children who present with

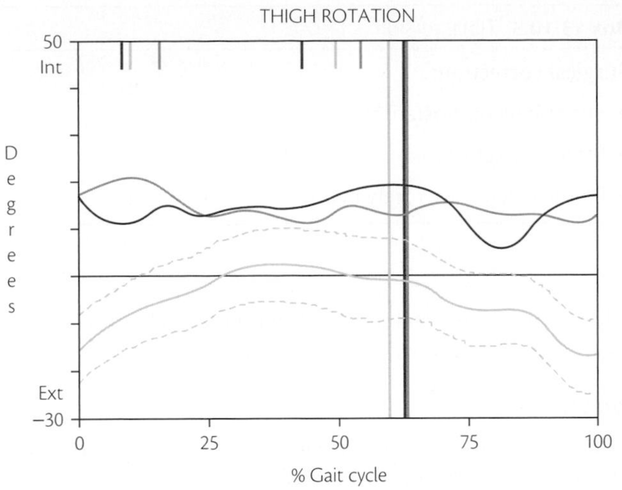

Fig. 13.10.2 This graph from a gait analysis report demonstrates the internal and external rotation that occurs at thigh level during the stance and swing phases of gait. The light grey band represents the mean and 2 standard deviations either side of the mean values whilst the dashed and black lines represent the right and left legs respectively. Both show significant internal rotation.

increased femoral anteversion and, if necessary, a pelvic radiograph should be taken to exclude hip dysplasia. Reassurance can be offered to parents of children under the age of 8 years as in the majority of cases the deformity is likely to remodel spontaneously. Non-surgical treatment does not influence the rate of remodelling. Significant anteversion causing functional problems and persisting beyond the age of 8 years may require surgical correction. Given the potential risks and complications involved in bilateral femoral derotation osteotomies, patients should be carefully selected and treatment indications discussed thoroughly with their families.

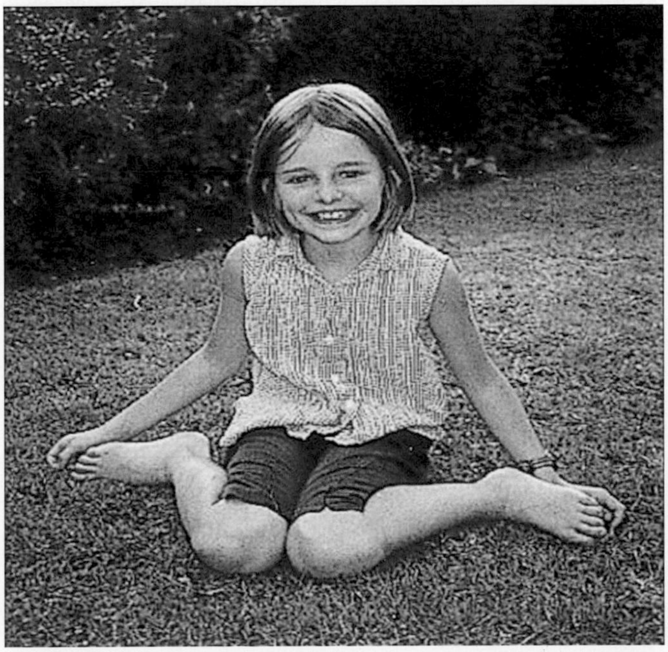

Fig. 13.10.3 Young child sitting in the 'W' position—easily achievable because she has significant femoral neck anteversion. She is asymptomatic.

Internal tibial torsion

Tibial torsion is defined as the angle between the transcondylar axis of the proximal tibia and the transmalleolar axis of the ankle (Figure 13.10.1E). The normal adult average is approximately 20 ±10 degrees of external torsion. Clinically tibial torsion is measured by palpating the above landmarks, defining the axes and using a goniometer to measure the angle. The thigh–foot angle is also used as an estimate of tibial torsion. This is the angle between the longitudinal axis of the foot and the femur assessed in the prone position with the knee flexed at 90 degrees (Figure 13.10.1D). Both clinical measurements can be inaccurate, the former because of the difficulty in defining the transcondylar axis and the latter because of knee rotation and foot deformity compromising the measurement. During walking, the knees are facing forward but the foot progression is internal. In the absence of foot deformity this clinical picture would suggest that internal tibial torsion is present. CT or MRI scan can be used for the accurate measurement of tibial torsion, particularly in surgical candidates.

Internal tibial torsion is probably caused by moulding *in utero* and resolves spontaneously in the vast majority of infants within the first few years of life. When the deformity is purely torsional, reassurance can be offered to parents of young children. Tibial bowing associated with torsion may require further investigation with radiographs, particularly if it persists after the age 3 years, in order to rule out underlying pathology. If the deformity persists after the age of 6–8 years it is unlikely to remodel spontaneously. Surgical treatment may be appropriate in a small minority of selected cases with significant deformity and functional problems. A supramalleolar tibial derotation osteotomy is undertaken and stabilized, often with internal fixation. A concomitant fibular osteotomy is usually unnecessary.

Metatarsus adductus

Adduction of the forefoot with a normal hindfoot is present in approximately 1:1000 newborn infants and is probably caused by moulding *in utero*. It can be associated with hip dysplasia and careful assessment of the hips should be undertaken. The deformity is usually observed immediately after birth but a significant number of children present later with parental concerns over in-toeing. Older children may complain of pain from excessive pressure over the lateral plantar area and/or difficulty with shoe fitting.

Clinical examination reveals a curved lateral border of the foot with a normally aligned hindfoot and sometimes a mild degree of forefoot supination. When the deformity is flexible, the forefoot can be manipulated easily to the neutral position or beyond. When the deformity is rigid, further assessment is required to rule out a congenital skeletal abnormality or a varus deformity of the hindfoot that would suggest a mild form of congenital talipes equinovarus.

Dynamic adduction and supination of the forefoot in toddlers with a normal but immature gait pattern can sometimes be confused with metatarsus adductus. This is caused by the predominant use of tibialis anterior tendon for foot dorsiflexion during the swing phase of gait while the peronei are silent. The foot assumes normal alignment at rest and clinical examination is entirely normal. This should be considered as a normal stage of gait maturation that will resolve spontaneously over time.

Flexible metatarsus adductus deformity usually resolves spontaneously within the first 1–2 years of life. Rigid deformity should be treated with early serial above-knee casting. The role of orthotic management and/or splinting in older children is unclear as evidence on the effectiveness of such treatment is lacking. Persistent symptomatic deformity may require surgical treatment in a minority of patients. Relatively mild deformity in younger children responds to soft tissue surgery, including medial capsular release of the appropriate joint(s) at the apex of the deformity (usually navicular–cuneiform or cuneiform–first metatarsal). Lengthening of the abductor hallucis may also be necessary. When forefoot supination is present, lengthening or transfer of tibialis anterior tendon may be appropriate. Rigid deformity in older children requires bony procedures in the form of basal metatarsal or midtarsal osteotomies: this is very rarely necessary and should not be undertaken without considerable thought.

Out-toeing gait (Box 13.10.2)

Common causes of external foot progression include external tibial torsion, planovalgus foot deformity (see Chapter 13.22) or more rarely, external hip rotation due to femoral neck retroversion.

External tibial torsion

This may be present at birth or may develop overtime as compensation for increased femoral anteversion. Planovalgus foot deformity may further compromise the rotational alignment of the foot in relation to the knee. As a result of this malalignment, the physiological knee extension moment generated by the foot plantarflexors, using the foot as the lever-arm, is compromised. This, in turn, causes excessive strain on the knee and particularly, the patellofemoral joint.

Mild deviations of external tibial torsion are usually asymptomatic, at least during childhood, and cause no functional problems. Significant rotational anomalies may cause symptoms at the knee and/or the foot. Spontaneous correction can only be expected in young infants and toddlers with congenital deviations. Acquired or persistent deformity causing symptoms or functional problems after the age of 5 years is unlikely to remodel and may require surgical treatment. As with deformity due to internal torsion a supramalleolar derotational tibial osteotomy is performed and stabilized with internal fixation. Again a fibular osteotomy is seldom necessary (Box 13.10.3).

Relative femoral neck retroversion

Predominant external rotation at the hips due to reduced femoral anteversion or retroversion is a rare cause of out-toeing gait. Children with the condition walk with knees facing outwards and an external foot progression. Clinical examination reveals excessive external rotation of the hips at the expense of internal rotation. Usually the condition is idiopathic and of no functional consequence in childhood, therefore no treatment is indicated. Coxa vara can be an underlying cause in younger children while chronic bilateral slipped upper femoral epiphysis should be considered in

Box 13.10.2 Out-toeing gait

- External tibial torsion
- Planovalgus (flat foot) deformity
- Femoral neck retroversion.

Box 13.10.3 Tibial torsion

Surgical correction:

- Supramalleolar osteotomy
- Internal fixation
- Fibula osteotomy rarely necessary

children of prepubertal age. Radiographic evaluation should be undertaken when these diagnoses are considered.

Toe walking

Walking on tip-toes is a normal stage in the development of a mature gait pattern but by the age of 3 a child should have outgrown this phase. Most children with idiopathic toe walking (ITW) can get their heel to the ground and will do so when standing but when walking or running there is a toe–toe or toe–heel pattern. In both situations there is disturbance of the ankle rockers (Box 13.10.4). The aetiology of ITW is not known but it may be due to an undefined and minor 'error' in the central nervous system (CNS).

A full history and examination is required as it is imperative to distinguish ITW from mild cerebral palsy, muscular dystrophy, or other neurological disorders. It is particularly important to clarify if toe walking developed late in children who had previously walked normally as this would suggest a progressive neurological disorder. The foot may be triangular in shape with a splayed forefoot and a relatively under-developed heel. Neurological examination is essentially normal but there may be some symmetrical loss of ankle dorsiflexion. Formal gait analysis distinguishes ITW from mild cerebral palsy but this is rarely necessary.

Many children stop toe walking spontaneously over time and perhaps with an increase in body mass and compensatory external tibial torsion. Persistent ITW with maintenance of 5 degrees of dorsiflexion is unlikely to cause any functional problems. Treatment with Achilles tendon stretches and dorsiflexion strengthening exercises may help improve gait pattern. Serial casting and/or botulinum toxin injections may be successful but if there is significant tightness of the Achilles tendon a surgical lengthening will be necessary. Although the operation itself is simple and reliable, the procedure changes the gait pattern dramatically and the parents must be forewarned. The gait improves in the rehabilitation phase as the plantar flexors regain their strength. Recurrent toe walking is not uncommon perhaps because the cause lies in the CNS. Toe walking in children with behavioural problems or autistic syndrome disorders should be distinguished from ITW as it is rarely associated

Box 13.10.4 Three ankle rockers of normal gait

- 1st—plantarflexion in early stance between heel strike and foot flat
- 2nd—dorsiflexion in mid stance as the leg moves over the foot
- 3rd—plantarflexion in terminal stance for push off.

Box 13.10.5 Unilateral toe walking

Is not ITW—so look for another cause:

- A late diagnosed developmental dysplasia of the hip or other hip pathology
- A leg length discrepancy
- Neurological problem.

with tightness of the Achilles tendon and responds less well to surgical treatment (Box 13.10.5).

Angular deformity

Genu varum and valgum

The coronal alignment of the knee changes in the first 6–7 years of life. These changes can cause parental concerns, particularly at times of development when they reach peak values. Knowledge of the physiological evolution of the coronal knee alignment is therefore important when advising parents about the natural history of the deformity.

At birth and during the first year of life the knee alignment is 15 degrees (±5 degrees) varus. It remodels to neutral alignment during the second year of life, presumably as the result of weight bearing. After the age of 2 years the knee progresses to valgus alignment to reach a maximum of 10 degrees (±5 degrees) valgus at the age of 3–4 years. From there it gradually remodels to the average adult value of 7 degrees valgus by the age of 6–7 years (Figure 13.10.4).

A wide variety of conditions, including metabolic bone diseases, bone dysplasias, and Blount's disease, can lead to coronal plane knee deformity. Consideration should be given to those conditions if knee alignment deviates from the pattern described earlier. While varus knee alignment at the age of 18 months is likely to be physiological, if it deteriorates overtime or persists after the age of 3 years it may require further investigation. Similarly, the combination of significant tibial torsion with a varus deformity raises concern regarding underlying pathology.

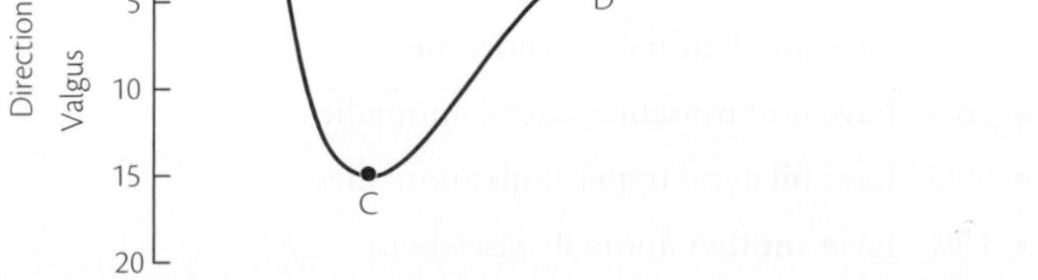

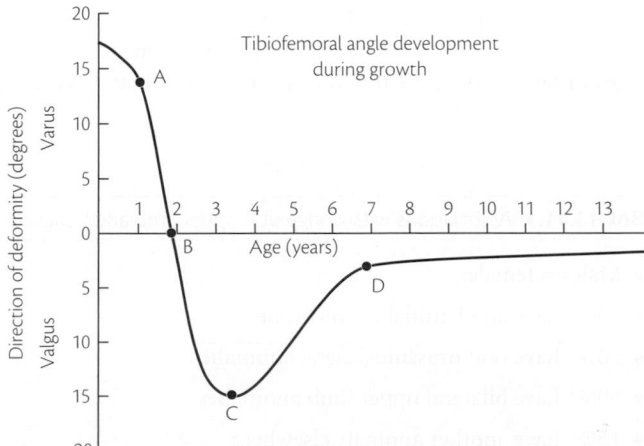

Fig. 13.10.4 Graph to show the evolution of physiological angular lower limb alignment with time. The line represents the mean values. A child may be 2 standard deviations away from this line and still be within normal limits.

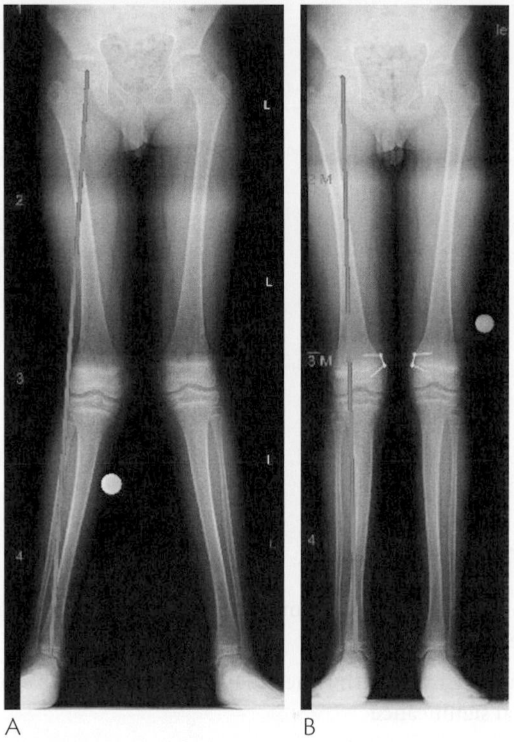

Fig. 13.10.5 A) Leg alignment radiographs showing bilateral genu valgum. The mechanical axis of the right leg has been drawn and shows the line passing through the lateral aspect of the knee. The patient was treated by temporary hemiepiphysiodesis of the medial distal femoral physis. B) 13 months later the axis had improved significantly. (At 18 months, the axes were normal and the plates were removed.)

Persistent varus or valgus alignment of the knee after the age of 8 years is unlikely to remodel spontaneously. Although there are no long-term studies to substantiate this, it is logical to assume that significant coronal knee deviations will lead to degenerative arthropathy, particularly if the mechanical axis lies outside the joint. Therefore, severe deformity may be an indication for surgical correction, particularly if symptomatic. It is essential to establish the level of the deformity with appropriate radiographs: is it in the distal femur or the proximal tibia? Furthermore, it is important to confirm that the deformity is truly and entirely in the coronal plane as increased femoral anteversion combined with external tibial torsion may give the false impression of genu valgum. During growth, coronal knee alignment can be corrected with temporary hemiepiphyseodesis at the appropriate level (Figure 13.10.5). After the end of growth, osteotomy of the distal femur or proximal tibia would be necessary.

Further reading

Salenius, P. and Vankka, E. (1975). The development of the tibiofemoral angle in children. *Journal of Bone and Joint Surgery*, **57A**, 259–61.

Staheli, L.T. (1990). Lower positional deformity in infants and children: a review. *Journal of Pediatric Orthopedics*, **10**, 559–63.

13.11

Congenital upper limb anomalies

Benjamin J. Hudson and Deborah M. Eastwood

Summary points

- Anomalies are common but often minor and of little functional concern
- Often associated with other manifestations that are of greater clinical significance
- A knowledge of embryological development allows a better understanding of the clinical picture and informs management plans.

Incidence and aetiology

The term *congenital upper limb anomaly* is used to describe all hand and upper limb abnormalities that arise as a result of an error of normal embryological development. This error can either be environmental or genetic in aetiology.

A good knowledge of these anomalies is important as not only can they have a profound impact on the functional and cosmetic condition of the child affected but they may also have important psychological consequences for both the child and parents. It is often the position of the surgeon to relay information regarding the aetiological and embryological basis for these disorders to the parents as well as to discuss the prognosis and possible management strategies.

These anomalies are common: they may be obvious at birth if severe or they may present when the child is older, becoming more apparent with growth. They are often very visible and identifiable as a result of this but equally many anomalies are minor and interfere little with upper limb function.

Most epidemiological studies regarding upper limb anomalies are based on relative frequency, as opposed to true incidence and prevalence rates. In a recent study in Western Australia, upper limb anomalies were reported in 1:506 live births but this reduced to 1:610 at the time of presentation due to neonatal or infant deaths perhaps with conditions related to the upper limb anomaly. Previous studies have reported an overall incidence of any congenital anomaly as 1:100–200 live births and as 10% of these were upper limb abnormalities, the incidence for upper limb anomalies was given as 1:1000–2000. Many upper limb problems are associated with non-musculoskeletal problems. There is no evidence that anomaly rates are higher in monozygotic rather than dizygotic twins but rates are higher in mothers who are either old or young and babies born both pre- and post-term (Box 13.11.1).

Upper limb anomalies can be the result of either a malformation or a deformation. A malformation is described as an abnormality of primary structural development whereas deformation is the result of secondary change in a part which was previously developing normally.

Whilst upper limb anomalies do occur in isolation, they may well be associated with other systemic disorders or syndromes. These associated conditions are often of more clinical importance to the health of the child than the musculoskeletal abnormality. It is therefore important to be aware of these disorders so that the patient is evaluated properly.

The aetiology of congenital upper limb anomalies is incompletely understood. The accepted classification of this group of anomalies is based on clinical diagnosis and according to our understanding of where and when the failure took place during fetal development. There is no good evidence to link congenital upper limb anomalies to specific environmental agents although the use of thalidomide was associated with phocomelia. Some studies have shown an association with the use of antiepileptic agents in the early gestational period. The causative environmental agent or genetic abnormality can impact upon development at various stages of fetal development and a specific insult may have a very

Box 13.11.1 Associations with congenital upper limb anomalies

- Males = females
- 20%* have an identifiable syndrome
- 50%* have non musculoskeletal anomalies
- 50%* have bilateral upper limb anomalies
- 15%* have another anomaly elsewhere
- 15%* have multiple separate hand anomalies.

*approximate percentages

different effect if it is given at different stages of development. Similarly, seemingly very different insults given at a specific stage of development can cause the same anomaly.

Overall, duplications and failures of differentiation and formation account for the majority of the upper limb anomalies identified.

Embryology

The upper limb bud appears on the lateral aspect of the embryo 24h before the lower limb bud around 26 days postfertilization. There is then rapid progress with upper limb development and the process is complete by 8 weeks (Figure 13.11.1). Therefore it holds that congenital upper limb anomalies are most likely to occur during this short time period of development.

Three areas of signalling have been discovered which guide the development of the embryonic upper limb. Firstly, the apical ectodermal ridge (AER) which overlies the limb bud, guides the mesoderm to differentiate by the medium of fibroblast growth factors. Differentiation occurs in a proximal to distal direction; thereby the upper arm will differentiate prior to the forearm which develops prior to the hand. It is this mechanism that allows the webbed hand to develop by way of dorsal grooving and interdigital necrosis regulated by apoptosis (programmed cell death) separates the digits between weeks 7–8.

The second mechanism is the zone of polarizing activity (ZPA), located on the posterior aspect of the limb bud. This activity is mediated by the Sonic hedgehog (SHH) protein and its function is to signal radio–ulnar development and orientate the limb.

The final mechanism of upper limb embryonic development is through the Wingless-type (Wnt) signalling centre. This centre is located in the dorsal ectoderm and it controls dorsoventral differentiation and limb rotation by secreting factors that influence mesodermal development around week 7.

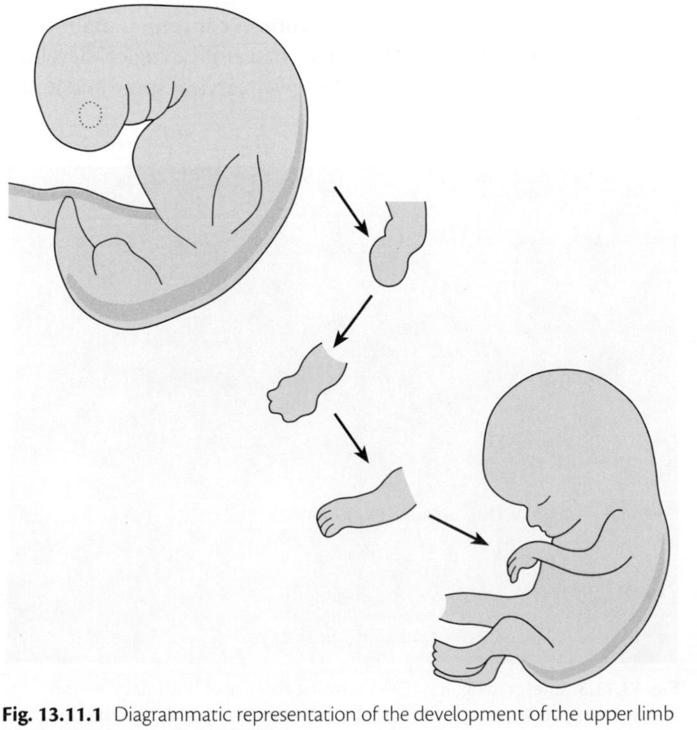

Fig. 13.11.1 Diagrammatic representation of the development of the upper limb bud between weeks 4–8 of fetal life.

The HOX (homeobox containing) genes also play an important role in limb development as their genetic expression controls growth by regulating mesenchymal cell function.

Thus, any abnormality in the function of any of these mechanisms could result in a specific and possibly predictable upper limb anomaly; for example, failure of the AER can lead to a failure of distal limb development including syndactyly. In experimental situations, transplantation of the AER has led to duplication of the limb or the development of supernumerary digits.

By the end of week 5, the majority of the skeletal limb has differentiated, as well as the brachial plexus. More distal neurological branches are complete at the end of week 6, with musculature defined at the end of week 8.

Other systems are also developing between weeks 4–8 and therefore a more general embryological insult, genetic or environmental, can result in abnormalities elsewhere in the developing embryo. Specifically the gastrointestinal, cardiovascular, and neurological systems are all also developing rapidly at this time. Therefore it is important for the clinician to consider the possibility of a wider and potentially more clinically serious disorder than the musculoskeletal anomaly alone and to investigate and refer as appropriate.

Classification

Currently the most widely accepted classification for congenital upper limb anomalies is the Swanson classification which has been adopted by the International Federation of Surgical Societies of the Hand and known now as the IFSSH classification (see Table 13.11.1, and Chapter 13.13). It is based on the specific developmental failure and relies on clinical diagnosis of the anomaly.

Often, as shown in epidemiological studies, more than one anomaly may be present in more than one area of the limb and with this current embryological classification of upper limb anomalies it is not possible to classify all hand anomalies. For example, brachysyndactyly may fit in either of two categories, failure of formation and failure of differentiation.

Anomalies of the shoulder

Congenital pseudarthrosis of the clavicle

Congenital pseudarthrosis of the clavicle is a rare condition. Less than 200 cases have been reported in the English literature.

Table 13.11.1 Classification of Sprengel deformity

Grade	Description
I	Mild deformity where shoulder girdles are at the same level. The deformity is not visible in the dressed patient
II	Slight deformity still present, where shoulder joints are almost level, but superomedial portion of scapula visible as a lump
III	Moderate shoulder joint deformity with scapula visibly elevated 2–5cm
IV	Severe deformity with scapula angle close to the occiput with webbing of the neck

The majority of cases are right sided and the common presentation is that of a painless, non-tender, and mobile mass at the centre of the clavicle identified soon after birth. The clavicle begins to ossify at 8 weeks and is the first bone to do so. It normally develops from two separate intramembranous centres of ossification which go on to unite. In pseudarthrosis of the clavicle this process fails due either to a mechanical or an environmental insult: it may be caused by an intrinsic primary failure of development or because of external compression. The two parts of the clavicle form a fibrous bridge which then goes onto develop into a true pseudarthrosis. Histologically, each clavicular end is capped with cartilage tissue and they are joined by dense fibrous or fibrocartilaginous tissue. Generally, radiographs show that the medial part of the clavicle sits anteriorly and superior to the lateral acromial section of the pseudarthrosis (Figure 13.11.2). A birth fracture is the most common differential diagnosis but the lack of callus formation over time excludes this diagnosis. Occasionally neurofibromatosis or cleidocranial dysostosis may be considered.

It is postulated that pressure from the subclavian artery which runs posterior to the clavicle on the right accounts for the fact that the right clavicle is much more commonly affected. In accordance with this theory, left-sided cases are found almost exclusively in individuals with dextrocardia or situs inversus.

There is usually no significant functional deficit of the shoulder. The natural history is not known as most reported cases have undergone operative treatment. The aesthetic appearance worsens with time as the pseudarthrosis becomes more prominent, tenting the skin on movement. There may be pain on certain activities or with compression.

The indications for treatment are often aesthetic and surgical treatment is usually advocated between the ages of 3–5 years. Treatment involves surgical excision of the pseudarthrosis, remembering that approximation of the bone ends followed by bone grafting and stable internal fixation is essential if union is to be achieved. Some authors emphasize the importance of maintaining the periosteal sleeve. Currently, plate and screw fixation is recommended. The major complication of this surgery is non-union but overall, reported union rates are high and the cosmetic appearance is improved.

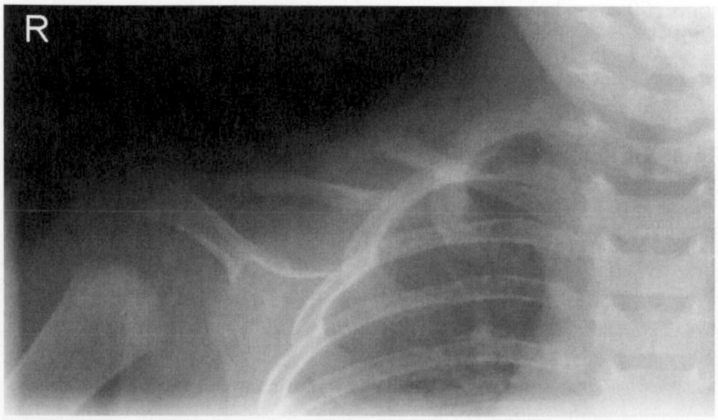

Fig. 13.11.2 Anteroposterior radiograph of the right clavicle in a 16-month-old child showing a pseudarthrosis. The bone ends are often bulbous and bony sclerosis obliterates the medullary cavity.

Cleidocranial dysostosis

This skeletal dysplasia affects the development of many bones, primarily those of membranous origin. As the name implies, the bones most significantly affected are the clavicles and the skull although there is also delayed ossification and underdevelopment of the pelvis (including the hips) and the spine. The clavicles can be hypoplastic or absent and in the skull, there is delayed closure of the cranial sutures and the fontanelles with maxillary hypoplasia and dental abnormalities (Figures 13.11.3 and 13.11.4).

Recently, genetic studies have concluded that the disorder is inherited in an autosomal dominant fashion with an increase in mutations of the *CBFA1* gene located on the short arm of chromosome 6.

Clinically the patient has bilateral 'drooping' shoulders, often with the ability to oppose the shoulders anteriorly, due to the profound hypoplasia or absence of the clavicles. This can lead to difficulty with coordination of arm movements and a theoretical potential for brachial plexus injury. Abnormalities of the musculature can also occur depending on which part of the clavicle is deficient. If lateral, deltoid and trapezius muscles can be affected but if the medial end is affected problems with the pectoralis major and sternocleidomastoid muscles can occur.

Other associations include hypoplastic scapulae, hypoplasia of the iliac wings, joint laxity, and dislocations and abnormalities of hands and feet. The patient is often of short stature and he may walk with a Trendelenburg gait secondary to the associated coxa vara.

Management involves genetic testing and counselling. Specific orthopaedic intervention at the shoulder is only indicated if the hypoplastic ends of the clavicles compress the subclavian vessels or the brachial plexus or to prevent secondary complications of pressure on the overlying skin. Treatment is usually by excision of the hypoplastic clavicle. Craniofacial surgery and surgical correction of the concomitant coxa vara or scoliosis may be required.

Sprengel deformity

A Sprengel deformity is the most common congenital malformation of the shoulder girdle. During normal embryological development the scapula arises opposite the lower cervical spine and in the

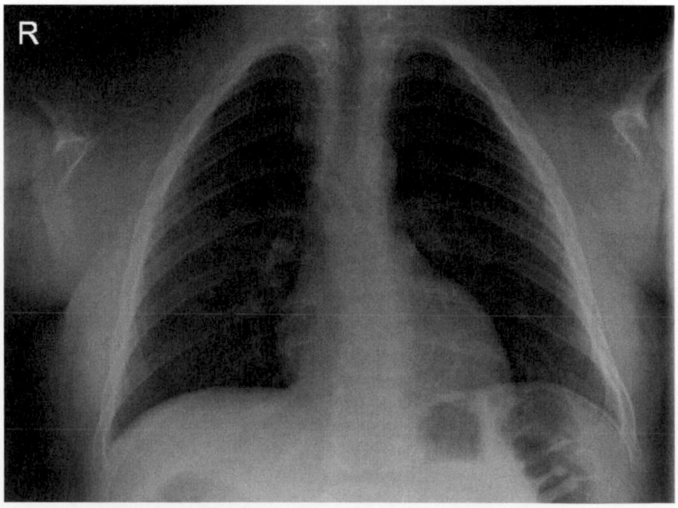

Fig. 13.11.3 Chest radiograph (CXR) showing absence of both clavicles: this occurs in only 10% of cases. The scapulae were also hypoplastic and the child went on to develop a scoliosis (a minor curve is visible on this CXR).

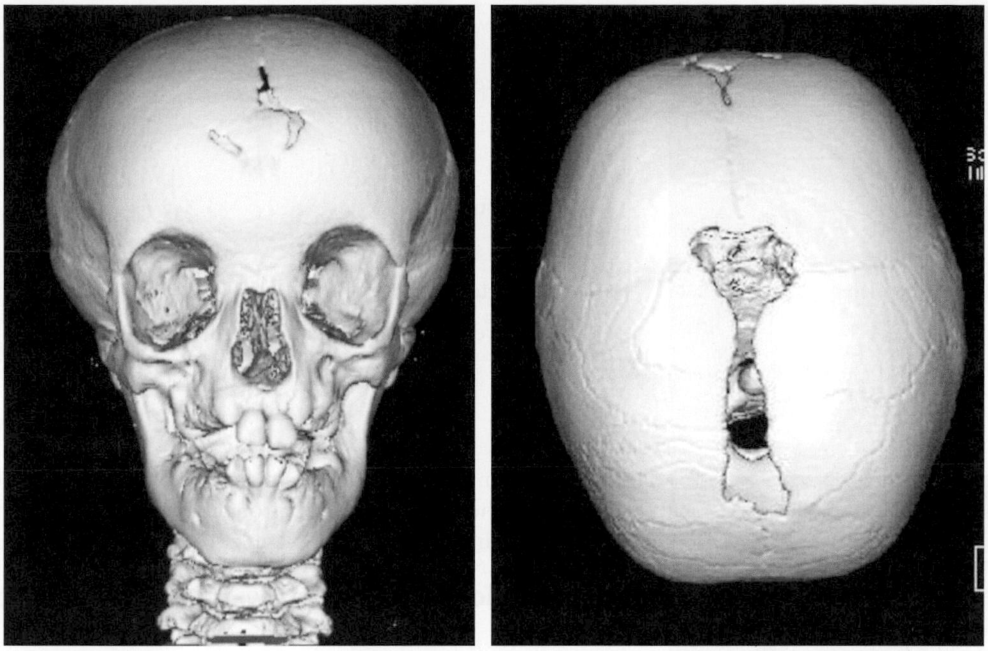

Fig. 13.11.4 A) Frontal and B) superior views of a three-dimensional CT reconstruction of the skull of a 12-year-old child with cleidocranial dysostosis showing that the sutures and fontanelles remain open.

third month of gestation it descends caudally to the thorax. Failure of this normal migration leads to a hypoplastic, undescended, and hence malpositioned scapula. Associated with this bony abnormality are abnormalities of the surrounding musculature: pectoralis major, trapezius, rhomboids, and latissimus dorsi may be hypoplastic, absent, or weak. A weak serratus anterior can lead to a winged scapula.

The condition is three times more common in males than females but it affects both left and right sides equally. It can occur sporadically but sometimes there is an autosomal dominant inheritance pattern.

Clinically there is an asymmetrical shoulder line (Figure 13.11.5). The scapula can sit up to 10cm more superiorly than normal as well as more medially. The inferior pole is medially rotated which in turn points the glenoid fossa inferiorly. Patients often complain most about a 'lump' in the web of the neck where the superior pole of the scapula bends anteriorly over the top of the thorax (Figure 13.11.6).

Movements of the glenohumeral joint are often normal but scapulothoracic movement is limited and thus there is a restriction of shoulder abduction (Figure 13.11.7). Rotation and forward flexion may also be limited.

The deformity can be classified in rudimentary terms (Table 13.11.1) and the more severe the deformity the greater the restriction in joint movement and the more likely there are to be associated developmental anomalies (Box 13.11.2).

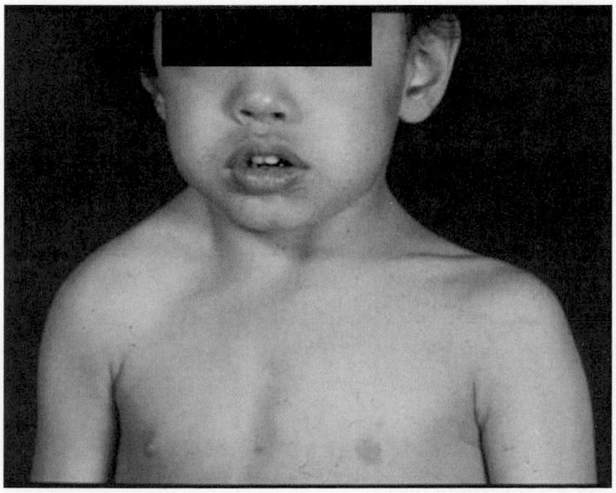

Fig. 13.11.5 Clinical photograph of a child with a unilateral Sprengel deformity.

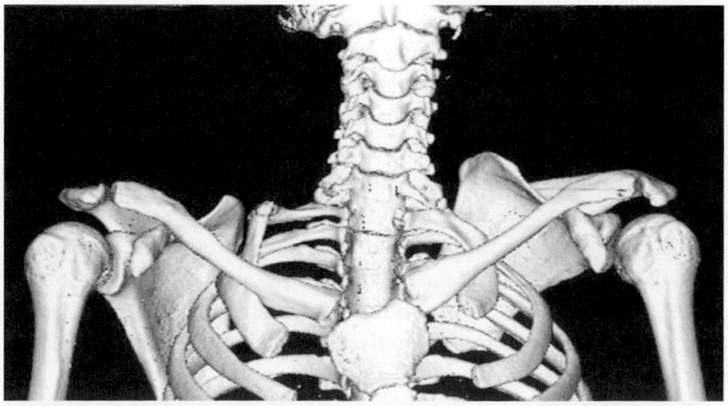

Fig. 13.11.6 Three-dimensional CT scan showing a left Sprengel shoulder and highlighting the abnormal shape, position, and orientation of the scapula. It resembles an 'equilateral triangle' and there is no long medial border. No bony omovertebral bar is seen and there are no anomalies of the cervical spine. Excision of the superomedial corner of the scapula in the base of the neck can improve the cosmetic appearance.

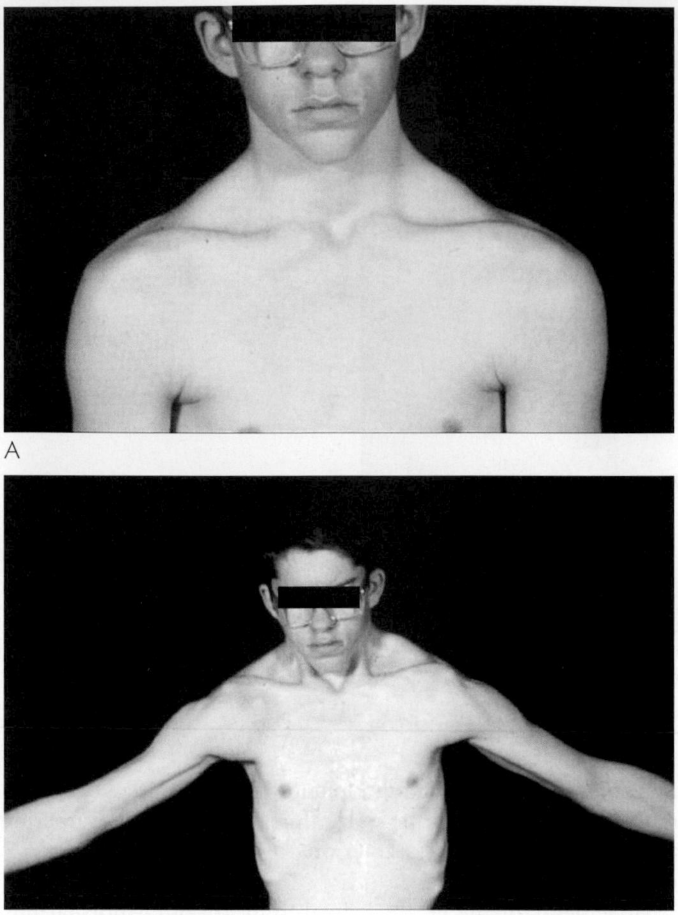

A

B

Fig. 13.11.7 Clinical photograph of an adolescent with bilateral Sprengel deformities. He was a talented badminton player but had an unorthodox service action perhaps because of the limited shoulder abduction. Only 10–30% of cases are bilateral.

An omovertebral connection is present in up to 50% of cases: this may consist of a fibrous, cartilaginous, or bony bar and it may contribute adversely to the cosmetic appearance.

Treatment for a Sprengel deformity is based on the severity of the functional loss and to some extent cosmesis. Passive stretching exercises are recommended in less severe cases to increase the range of movement and strengthen the surrounding muscles. If surgery is required it should be carried out before 8 years of age to reduce the risk of complications such as a brachial plexus neuropathy. Many of the operations described can leave an unsightly scar and therefore careful consideration should be given to the cosmetic benefits of such surgery. In mild cases, an extraperiosteal resection of the superior pole of the scapula and any associated omovertebral tissue may provide significant cosmetic improvement with little risk of morbidity.

In more severe cases, the aim of surgical treatment is to improve the range of functional abduction by relocating and repositioning the scapula and hence the glenoid. Several surgical options are essentially soft tissue releases involving resection of the omovertebral bone with division of the trapezius, rhomboids, levator scapula, and parascapular muscles from either their spinal or scapular origins. The muscles are then reattached via various suture techniques once the scapula has been brought distally. Another popular technique involves a vertical scapular osteotomy.

Box 13.11.2 Malformations associated with a sprengel deformity

- Musculoskeletal:
  - Klippel–Feil syndrome
  - Scoliosis
  - Absent/fused ribs
  - Cervical spina bifida
  - Omovertebral bar
- Systemic: renal and pulmonary disorders.

Other developmental anomalies of the shoulder region

Phocomelia

Phocomelia is rare but in such cases there is often glenoid aplasia as there is in amelia. The management is non-operative. Prosthetic limbs are not often a good functional solution.

Glenoid dysplasia

In this uncommon condition, the glenoid is flat and shallow. It can be found in association with a malformed proximal humerus (which may be an aetiological factor) and may develop secondary to a neonatal brachial plexus lesion (see Chapter 13.12). Clinically the patient may complain of instability and/or dysfunction but often the condition is entirely asymptomatic. If the deformity is severe enough to cause loss of function, operative management involves a glenoplasty using iliac crest graft.

Glenoid dysplasia is often an isolated condition but it can be part of other more general conditions (Box 13.11.3).

Holt–Oram syndrome is an autosomal dominant condition resulting in a complex of cardiac defects and skeletal malformations. The genetic defect is in a transcription factor *TBX5*. All cases have abnormalities of the carpal bones and the most severe cases will have a phocomelia. In between, manifestations include a rotated, hypoplastic scapula with associated wrist and forearm problems (see Chapter 13.13).

Os acromiale is a disorder where there is a non-union between one, two, or all of the three normal ossification centres of the acromium with the rest of the scapula. The condition is not inherited (Box 13.11.4). It is often an incidental finding on plain radiographs but symptoms may be similar to those of subacromial impingement syndrome. Initial treatment is conservative but occasionally,

Box 13.11.3 Conditions associated with glenoid dysplasia

- Apert's syndrome
- Mucopolysaccharoidoses such as Hurler's syndrome
- Holt–Oram syndrome

Box 13.11.4 The bipartite acromium

- Failure of fusion of the three ossification centres
- Present in 1–15% of patients
- Approximately 50% are bilateral

surgical excision or fixation of the fragment is required and subacromial decompression may be necessary.

Humeral dysplasia

Congenital humerus varus is analogous to coxa vara. It may be due to medial epiphyseal damage of the humeral head. Often it is asymptomatic but severe cases demonstrate a limitation of abduction.

Humeral head retroversion develops in response to abnormal pressures on the shoulder: it is commonly associated with a neonatal brachial plexus palsy. Movements of abduction, external rotation, and adduction are limited. Treatment, if necessary, is by anterior capsular release. If the deformity and decreased function are severe, a proximal derotation osteotomy can be performed but only after careful assessment of shoulder congruity.

Poland's syndrome (Box 13.11.5)

Poland's syndrome is a sporadic, uncommon, unilateral congenital disorder characterized by underdevelopment or absence of the chest wall and scapula muscles and the breast tissue with associated rib cage defects and hand anomalies (see Chapter 13.13). Not all features need be present to constitute a diagnosis of Poland's syndrome and subtle cases may be missed. Girls may present in puberty due to the unilateral failure of breast development.

Like congenital pseudarthrosis of the clavicle it is thought to arise from an abnormality in the development of the subclavian artery. Non-musculoskeletal manifestations of Poland's syndrome include dextrocardia, diaphragmatic hernia, and gastrointestinal abnormalities.

Functional impairment in Poland's syndrome is rare and surgical management is often primarily to improve appearance. Syndactyly is usually treated prior to school age.

Anomalies around the elbow

Abnormalities of the elbow joint can be overlooked particularly in the patient with normal function in the joints above and below (the shoulder and wrist/hand) and when the elbow is essentially asymptomatic. Congenital disorders of the elbow can involve bone and joint or soft tissues.

Box 13.11.5 Poland's syndrome

- Males 3:1 females
- Right 2:1 left
- Incidence 1:10–50 000.

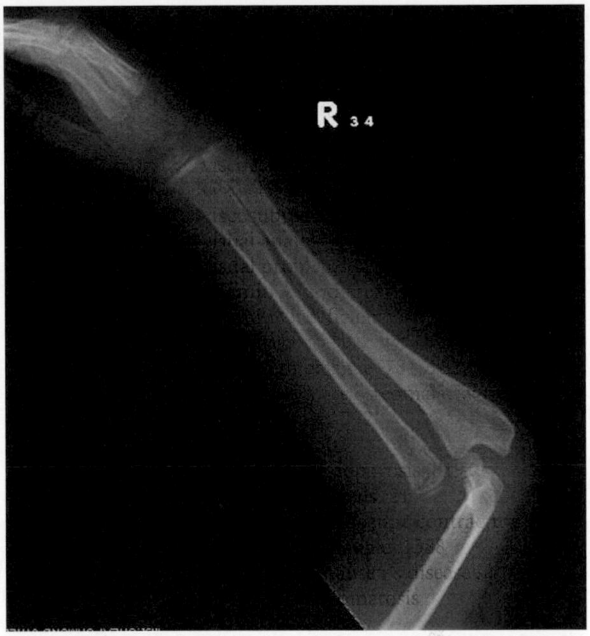

Fig. 13.11.8 Lateral radiograph of the forearm of a 4.5-year-old child. There was no history of trauma, simply a lump in the antecubital fossa. The ulna is bowed and the direction of radial head dislocation is anterior: usually traumatic rather than congenital in origin.

Radial head subluxation and dislocation

Radial head subluxation or dislocation is the most frequently occurring congenital abnormality of the elbow; 60% of cases are bilateral. The pathology is thought to be due to a hypoplastic capitellum allowing the radius to dislocate. In about one-third of patients, there will be another anomaly elsewhere in the upper limb. The forearm is often hypoplastic, and the ulna may be short with a negative variance at the distal radioulnar joint. Acquired dislocations can occur in infancy. It is, however, the hypoplastic nature of the capitellum on radiography or arthrography or other imaging that help distinguish a congenitally dislocated radial head from an acquired one (Figure 13.11.8).

Congenital radial head dislocation often presents at ages 3–5 years. There is usually no functional loss of movement but clinically the patient may have reduced supination with an inability to achieve full extension. Pain or clicking is not usually a major feature but many patients or their parents notice a lump on the lateral side of the elbow.

Three types of isolated congenital dislocation are described: type 1 is the least frequently occurring, but is associated with pain (Table 13.11.2). Radial head dislocations can also be classified

Table 13.11.2 Classification of severity of radial head subluxation/dislocation

Type	Description
1	Subluxation
2	Posterior dislocation with minor displacement
3	Posterior dislocation with proximal radial migration.

Table 13.11.3 Classification of radial head dislocation according to direction of displacement

Direction of dislocation	Frequency	Problems
Posterior	65%	May restrict extension, head thin
Anterior	18%	May erode humerus and restrict flexion, head round
Lateral	17%	Usually asymptomatic but more obvious

according to the direction of dislocation (Table 13.11.3). Radial head dislocation is associated with a variety of conditions: in some such as diaphyseal aclasis, the dislocation develops over time as a result of the abnormal forces that growth places on the developing forearm structures (Figure 13.11.9 and Box 13.11.6).

Treatment

Management in most cases is to reassure and observe. Analgesia may be required. Surgical treatment is indicated when the patient has significant symptoms of pain. Occasionally, surgery is advised for deformity (with growth the dislocated radial head may become more obvious) and to try and improve movement *if* there is severe restriction.

Due to the hypoplastic capitellum and reciprocal changes in the radial head, relocation of the congenitally dislocated radial head is not a very successful option. For acquired dislocations, most frequently seen secondary to a missed or late diagnosis of a Monteggia fracture dislocation of the forearm, relocation of the radial head is advisable and usually successful. This involves an open reduction of the joint in combination with a reconstruction of the annular ligament with a triceps fascial sling and an ulnar osteotomy to restore length and correct the bowing deformity.

Excision of the congenitally dislocated radial head invariably reduces symptoms of pain but it is less likely to improve the patient's range of movement. This can be performed safely at any age if symptoms are severe (Box 13.11.7).

Box 13.11.6 Conditions associated with radial head dislocation

- Ehlers–Danlos syndrome
- Klinefelter's syndrome
- Arthrogryposis
- Diaphyseal aclasis.

Prevention of dislocation/subluxation

Diaphyseal aclasis (hereditary multiple exostoses)

Classically, the exostoses around the distal ulna lead to differential growth rates in the foream bones. The ulna is short and the radius becomes progressively bowed leading to radial head dislocation in a significant number of cases (see Figure 13.11.9). Surgery designed to prevent this complication has been advised. This involves excision of the prominent exostoses, correction of the radial deformity and lengthening of the short ulna. Whilst this approach may keep the radial head in joint, it risks decreased function due to an increase in forearm stiffness with further limitation of pronation/supination.

Congenital radioulnar synostosis

This abnormality is a congenital osseous or fibrous union between the radius and ulna. It is generally sporadic but occasionally autosomal dominant inheritance can occur with incomplete penetrance and variable expression. It is a rare disorder demonstrating an equal sex distribution.

During the sixth week of gestation, the cartilage anlage of the humerus, ulna, and radius starts to separate. An abnormality in this separation can cause a synostosis to occur. The union may be complete or more commonly partial. Over half of patients will have bilateral synostoses. The most common site for partial synostosis is the proximal radius and ulna and the proximal radius is often hypoplastic. Radioulnar synostosis is associated with a large range of limb and other congenital anomalies and some syndromes.

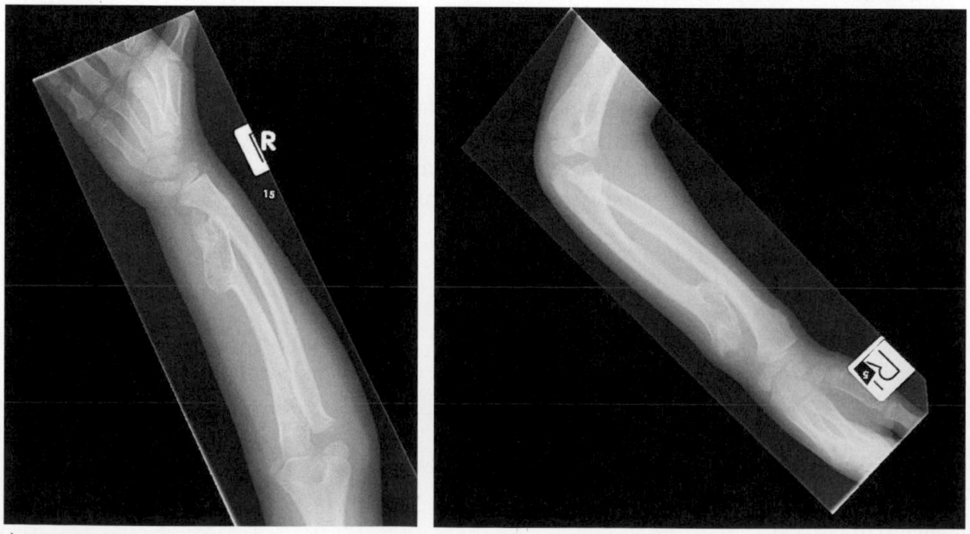

A B

Fig. 13.11.9 Anteroposterior and lateral views of a forearm with diaphyseal aclasis. The ulna is short and the radius bowed and the radial head is at risk of subluxation.

Box 13.11.7 Radial head excision

- For congenital dislocations: at any age *if* symptomatic
- Following trauma: delay until skeletal maturity to reduce complication rate.

The clinical problem is loss of forearm rotation but presentation may not be until late childhood. There is usually a fixed pronation position that most patients adapt to by extending their range of movement at the radiocarpal joint so that, overall, there is little functional loss. There is no association between forearm position and level of the synostosis or between forearm position and function. The condition has been classified into four types (Table 13.11.4 and Figure 13.11.10).

Treatment

Indications for operative treatment usually include bilateral synostoses with a severe degree of functional loss and fixed pronation deformity of both forearms. The shoulder and wrist joints can compensate, to a certain extent, for loss of forearm supination and pronation. If required, a derotational osteotomy is performed designed to improve the fixed forearm position: attempts to restore range of movement by excision of the synostosis and/or silastic or tissue interposition have been unsuccessful. Even in bilateral cases, a position of 10–20 degrees pronation is usually preferred although an individual decision may be required to take into account particular cultural or social requirements. Although various osteotomy levels have been described, some have a high complication rate and simple methods are often the most reliable. Vascular compromise is a particular risk if the correction is greater than 45 degrees.

Table 13.11.4 Classification of radioulnar synostosis according to Cleary and Omer

Type	Description	Radial head anatomy
I	Fibrous synostosis	Normal but small
II	Osseous synostosis	Normal but small
III	Osseous synostosis	Posterior dislocation, hypoplastic radial head
IV	Osseous synostosis	Anterior dislocation, hypoplastic radial head

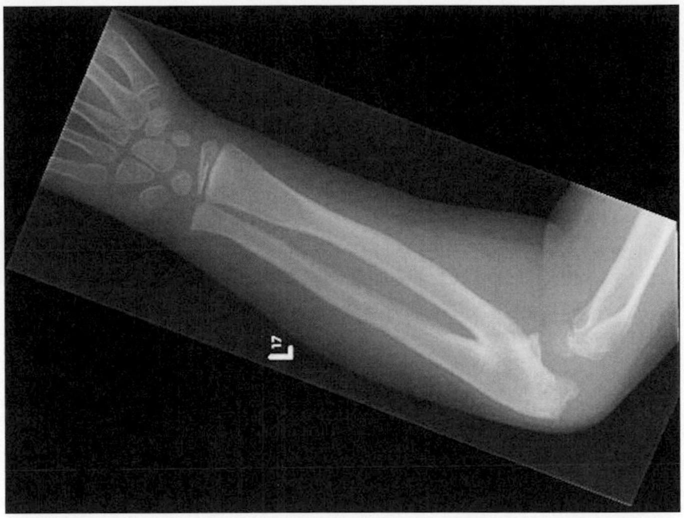

Fig. 13.11.10 Lateral radiograph of a forearm showing a type 3 synostosis of the proximal radius and ulna. The radial head remnant is lying posterolaterally.

Pseudarthrosis of the forearm

Congenital pseudarthrosis most commonly affects the tibia but it has been documented in all the long bones. In the forearm, the ulna is more frequently affected. The reported incidence of associated neurofibromatosis is higher with forearm pseudarthrosis than with tibial pseudarthrosis. As with tibial pseudarthrosis, surgical management is often required but frequently fraught with difficulties. The use of a vascularized fibula graft is perhaps the most popular and successful technique reported but in severe cases the creation of a single bone forearm may be most realistic solution.

Further reading

Borges, J.L., Shah, A., Torres, B.C., and Bowen, J.R. (1996). Modified Woodward procedure for Sprengel deformity of the shoulder: long-term results. *Journal of Pediatric Orthopedics*, **16**, 508–13.

Cleary, J.E. and Omer, G.E. (1985). Congenital proximal radio-ulnar synostosis. *Journal of Bone and Joint Surgery*, **67A**, 539–45.

Cooper, S.C., Flaitz, C.M., Johnston, D.A., Lee, B., and Hecht, J.T. (2001). A natural history of cleidocranial dysplasia. *American Journal of Medical Genetics*, **104**, 1–6.

Gupta, A., Kay, S.P.J., and Scheker, L.R. (eds) (2000). *The Growing Hand. Diagnosis and management of the upper extremity in children*. London: Mosby.

Ramachandran, M., Lau, K., and Jones, D.H. (2005). Rotational osteotomies for congenital radioulnar synostosis. *Journal of Bone and Joint Surgery*, **87B**, 1406–10.

13.12

Congenital brachial plexus palsy

Marco Sinisi

Summary points

- The congenital brachial plexus palsy is significantly different from the adult injury
- The mechanism of injury is invariably traction
- Classifying the lesion at 1–2 weeks of age aids with prognosis and management
- Surgical exploration and repair is indicated early in selected cases
- Good shoulder function is essential for a useful upper limb
- Recovery of hand function is slow and may continue until age 5 years.

Introduction

Congenital brachial plexus palsy (CBPP) is very different from the adult injury. The main difference between the two is that the neonatal nervous system is still immature and capable of repair. In the immature system, the position and form of the 'transitional zone', the interface between central nervous system (CNS) and peripheral nervous system (PNS), oscillates. In neonatal nerves, there is a greater density of neural fibres with a relative paucity of collagen fibres and this might contribute to their mechanical vulnerability. The nerve blood flow is also highest in the first weeks of life and then declines so that during this time, the immature nervous system might be more susceptible to ischaemia and anoxic conduction block. Once axonotomy occurs, chromatolysis starts and this can lead to neuronal death. Moreover, the developing neuron does depend upon neurotrophic factors produced by the target tissues.

It is therefore clear that a CBPP does not inevitably undergo a spontaneous recovery and equally clear, that such a vulnerable system might be susceptible to a 'second injury' such as occurs with a surgical resection of the neuroma and subsequent nerve graft.

Incidence

The reported incidence of CBPP varies from 0.6–2.6 per 1000 live births and there has been one study from an area of Sweden that has documented an increasing incidence of CBPP (from 1.4 per 1000 live births in 1980 to 2.3 in 1994).

Risk factors

In almost all cases the mechanism of injury is traction pulling the upper limb away from the axial skeleton as delivery of the baby is 'obstructed' at the narrowest point of the birth canal. This trauma is not necessarily excessive or inappropriate. Intrauterine causes have also been described such as oligohydramnios and the umbilical cord wrapped around the neck. Muscular denervation has been reported within days of birth implying intrauterine development of the lesion.

A strong relationship between birth weight and CBPP has been noted and there is an associated shoulder dystocia in more than 60%. Breech presentation with vaginal delivery is another risk factor and associated with more severe, and often bilateral, lesions with a high percentage of avulsions. Delivery by Caesarean section appears to be protective against the development of CBPP with the incidence of Caesarean section delivery being only 2% in patients with a CBPP compared to 18% in the general population.

Natural history

The study of the natural history of these lesions must start with the classification proposed by Narakas in 1987 as it offers a good guide to management. It should be used 1–2 weeks after birth by which time a simple conduction block should be showing signs of recovery.

Group 1

There is paralysis of the shoulder muscles specifically deltoid, supra- and infraspinatus, and of biceps (which influences elbow function). This implies a lesion of C5/C6 only. Complete recovery is seen in 90% of cases. Hand activity is not affected directly but the degree of shoulder recovery can influence hand function.

Group 2

One more nerve, C7, is affected and thus a lack of wrist extension on top of shoulder and elbow impairment. Full recovery is still possible in about 70% of children but the process is much slower than in group I.

Group 3

This is a complete brachial plexus lesion involving all nerve roots. At birth, paralysis of shoulder, elbow, wrist, and hand is complete. Within a few days some recovery in finger flexion may be apparent but less than 50% of cases show a good functional recovery and 25% do not recover finger and wrist extension.

Group 4

This is the most severe lesion with a Bernard–Horner syndrome (damage to the cervical sympathetic trunk) accompanying the complete brachial plexus palsy. Few children demonstrate good spontaneous functional recovery but, surprisingly, many do show a satisfying degree of recovery in the hand—a fact that must be remembered when considering surgical repair of the lower trunk lesion. In most children, shoulder and elbow function does not recover as well as forearm pronation/supination. Sometimes even after many years the Bernard–Horner signs are still present. In all these children the nerve lesion affects growth and development of the upper limb. This is particularly evident at the shoulder and elbow level where the degree of growth inhibition is related to the severity of the lesion at birth.

Clinical evaluation

After a difficult delivery or a shoulder dystocia, difficulty in moving the affected limb may be obvious straight away but sometimes it is not noticed for several days and the possibility of trauma or joint infection must be considered (Box 13.12.1). Depending on the severity of the injury the child's arm movement may be simply limited or completely absent. The characteristic posture of Narakas group 1 and 2 with the shoulder adducted and medially rotated, the elbow extended, forearm pronated, and wrist and fingers flexed compares with a completely flaccid arm in group 3 which is associated with a Bernard–Horner syndrome in group 4. In some, the phrenic nerve is paralyzed with obvious breathing problems.

On first assessment, a complete history of risk factors, mode of delivery, and progress to date is taken. As a matter of simplicity it is better to think of the different roots in terms of their main muscle innervation. The clinical examination must focus on *evaluation of shoulder function*, particularly active abduction and lateral rotation, because pectoralis major can supply forward flexion; *elbow function*, examining biceps and triceps; and *wrist function* looking at wrist extensors and *hand function* looking at finger flexors. In this way the recovery of individual nerve roots can be assessed more accurately allowing a management plan to be instigated promptly. In many children the recovery starts within a few days of birth and by the time they are seen in the specialist clinic, considerable improvement in upper limb function is obvious. Nevertheless, it is important to ask what muscle activity was at one week of age (Box 13.12.2).

With *early recovery*, physiotherapy must be started as soon as possible to avoid the development of contractures and to maximize functional recovery. If there is *no recovery* in any nerve root at 1 month then electrophysiological assessment is required urgently. If there is *some recovery* in some muscles, the investigation focuses on the roots which do not show recovery and can be performed between 2–3 months. Records are made of active and passive ranges at glenohumeral, thoracoscapular, and radioulnar joints: the difference between passive and active ranges defines the presence of contractures in muscles, capsules, and ligaments. These records and the modified Mallett score for shoulder, the Raimondi score for the hand, and Raimondi and Gilbert for the elbow, quantify recovery, progression of deformities, and response to treatment.

Investigations

Neurophysiology

Neurophysiological tests are important in defining the prognosis of a CBPP and thus help the surgeon to identify which cases would be helped by a surgical procedure. Nerve action potentials (NAPs) are measured from the median and ulnar nerves by stimulating at the wrist and recording at the elbow. The deltoid for C5, biceps for C6, wrist extensors and triceps for C7, wrist flexors for C8 and first interosseous for T1 are sampled by electromyography (EMG). For each nerve root, the lesion is then graded according to the degree of reduction of the NAP and amount of spontaneous and volitional activity in the muscles:

- Grade A: NAP normal or near normal. EMG normal units, no spontaneous activity
- Grade B favourable: NAP ≥50% of normal. EMG mild axonal injury with copious recruitment
- Grade B unfavourable: NAP absent or ≤50%. EMG limited recruitment, moderate axonal injury. Collateral reinnervation present
- Grade C: NAP present in some cases (predictive of avulsion), but more often absent. EMG poor recruitment, fibrillations, nascent units. Severe axonal injury.

Neurophysiological evaluation of a slowly recovering CBPP lesion can predict correctly the nature of the lesion and help in defining the indication for brachial plexus exploration. The importance of identifying the cases of prolonged conduction block has been emphasized as, clinically, these babies may be indistinguishable from those with more severe lesions. At the Peripheral Nerve

Box 13.12.1 Differential diagnosis of a CBPP

- Clavicular fracture
- Physeal separation of the proximal humerus
- Sepsis of the glenohumeral joint
- Ischaemic cord injury
- Arthrogryposis.

Box 13.12.2 Nerve roots related to muscle innervation.

- C5: shoulder activity
- C6: elbow flexion
- C7: wrist extension
- C8-T1: hand function.

Injury Unit at the Royal National Orthopaedic Hospital, 56% of patients who had no/minimal recovery at 3 months had favourable neurophysiological investigations and therefore no operative procedure was performed even when there was no recognizable clinical activity in biceps. Outcomes based on this neurophysiological prediction were found reliable in 92% for C5 and 96% for C7. Predictions for C5 were confirmed in only 76%. The inability to record NAP for C5 and the high incidence of posterior dislocation of the shoulder probably accounts for this.

Imaging

Magnetic resonance imaging is useful in severe cases of CBPP to identify nerve root avulsion and is preferred to contrast computed tomography or myelography.

Management

Physiotherapy/occupational therapy

These treatment methods are the mainstays of CBPP management. Parents play a major role in caring for their child as regular, gentle stretching exercises are essential to prevent fixed deformity and should be started within a few weeks of birth. Specific stretches for medial and lateral shoulder rotation are required with the arm at their side (elbow flexed) and at 90 degrees of abduction. Holding the scapula fixed to the chest wall whilst the arm is abducted, stretches the inferior scapulohumeral angle abduction of the arm and with forward flexion and medial rotation of the arm, the stretch is to the posterior glenohumeral angle.

Surgical management

Indication for surgical treatment of a nerve lesion

Surgical exploration is reserved for:

1) Group 4 lesions where neurophysiology and radiological evidence suggest avulsion
2) Lesions secondary to breech position when the complete lesion of the plexus is associated with phrenic nerve palsy

With both these indications, an operation is performed early, ideally by 8 weeks of age.

3) Group 1, 2, and 3 patients in whom there is failure of recovery of shoulder abduction and lateral rotation and elbow flexion by 3 months of age or even later.

Operations on the brachial plexus

After induction of anaesthesia, recording electrodes are placed on the neck and scalp and sensory evoked potentials (SEPs) are recorded from median and ulnar nerves bilaterally. After a suitable exposure, the brachial plexus lesion can be dissected and neurophysiological assessment performed to identify the type of the lesion (Table 13.12.1).

Good shoulder function is essential for a useful upper limb—poor shoulder recovery is thus more of a concern than poor elbow flexion. Muscle transfers around the shoulder are less useful than those around the elbow and hand, so every effort must be made to define prognosis for the C5 nerve root and particularly for the suprascapular nerve. At shoulder level, the author prefers to leave the upper trunk neuroma alone and perform a spinal accessory to suprascapular nerve transfer. At times it is impossible to say how much lack of function in the shoulder is due to the nerve injury itself and how much is due to subluxation or even dislocation of the glenohumeral joint and it is very important that the mechanical status of the joint is known. When indicated, relocation of the shoulder joint should accompany nerve repair/transfer.

To restore elbow function, a graft can be used to reconstruct the nerve root rupture but fascicles from the ulnar nerve can be implanted on to the nerve to biceps and selective reinnervation of the avulsed ventral root are very valuable procedures particularly for group 4 lesions.

To restore partial hand activity, repair of the nerve root rupture is not the only possibility. With avulsion of C7, C8, and T1, the hand can be reinnervated using the proximal stumps of the ruptured C5 and C6 roots or with selective reinnervation of the ventral roots of the avulsed nerves by transfer of the spinal accessory. It is important to remember that good functional recovery is

Table 13.12.1 Type of nerve lesion identified on neurophysiological testing

Type	Lesion	Neurophysiological evaluation preoperative	Intraoperative SSEP *foramen*	Intraoperative SSEP *distal*	Muscle response *foramen*	Appearance
1	Intact	A	Normal	Normal	Strong	Normal
2	Recovering rupture	B Favourable	Normal	>50%	Strong	Fusiform neuroma (normal nerve proximally)
3	Rupture	B Unfavourable	Normal	<50%	Weak	Hard 'double humped' neuroma
4	Rupture with preganglionic	B Unfavourable or C	Diminished	Dimished or absent	Weak	Diffuse longitudinal fibrosis
5	Preganglionic with no displacement	C	Absent	Absent	Absent	Atrophy at foramen
6	Incomplete preganglionic	B Unfavourable or C	Diminished or absent	Diminished or absent	Weak or absent	Atrophy at foramen
7	Preganglionic with displacement	C	Absent	Absent	Absent	Visible DRG

observed in about one half of the group 4 lesions without surgical intervention.

Postoperative care

Following nerve repair, a 3–4-week period of immobilization is necessary and after that gentle stretching of joints can be resumed.

Results from repair

Recovery is very slow and in the hand may take many years. The PNI unit results show that only one-third of C5 lesions had a good result with a worse mean Mallett score in children who had shoulder relocation performed at a later stage. C6 repair was associated with a good result in just over 50% and C7 repair was disappointing with less than one in three children regaining wrist and finger extension. Results for reinnervation of proven avulsion of C8 and T1 were good in 57%. Table 13.12.2 reports these results.

Deformity

The main causes of deformity associated with CBPP are direct damage to the shoulder and proximal humerus, occurring at the time of the difficult delivery but unrecognized and hence untreated. Atrophy of denervated target organs and persisting muscular imbalance from incomplete neurological recovery are also common. Muscle imbalance is the underlying cause of many shoulder dislocations. Supination and ulnar deviation deformities of the forearm and hand are often present. Deformity can be induced by over stretching incongruent joints and/or by performing muscle transfers on them.

Shoulder

Shoulder deformity is frequent and if not recognized leads to a progressive deterioration in function not only of the joint itself but of the whole upper limb. Whilst the deformity can be observed as a progression from medial contracture to subluxation and then dislocation, it is present in the perinatal period in 25% of patients referred to our unit (Figure 13.12.1). These cases showed extreme glenoid dysplasia, muscular fibrosis and humeral head retroversion. A further 21% subluxed/dislocated by 12 months and the remaining 54% presented later. The shoulder subluxation/dislocation occurred after neurological recovery was established in approximately 25%. The incidence of shoulder problems is higher in the Narakas group 3 and 4 where muscular imbalance around the shoulder is greater. Altered muscle pull also affects growth and development and it is likely that the shortening of the clavicle is implicated in abnormal shoulder growth.

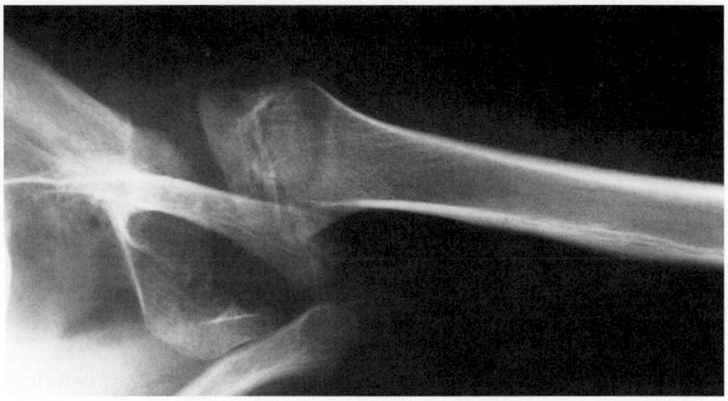

Fig. 13.12.1 Radiograph showing a dislocated shoulder with a retroverted glenoid and a deformed humeral head.

Diagnosis

To the experienced clinician, diagnosis is straightforward. The posture of the arm with fixed internal rotation and limited elevation associated with a humeral head palpable posterior to the glenoid and a forearm lying in full pronation is indicative of a dislocated shoulder. The diagnosis of subluxation is based on the same findings but is more subtle and relies more on the restriction of passive external rotation beyond 10 degrees and on the prominent head of the humerus.

Surgical treatment

Surgical treatment used to be delayed until the child was of walking age but recently early relocation is advised and may, if indicated, take place at the time of nerve repair. Early relocation facilitates greater remodelling of both the glenoid and the humeral retroversion. Subscapularis recession has been associated with a high recurrence rate and has therefore been abandoned. Whilst some surgeons favour a lateral rotation osteotomy, this does increase humeral head retroversion which is a major contribution to the recurrence of shoulder dislocation.

Two relatively minor procedures are useful in the treatment of contractures in congruent shoulders: release of the coracoacromial and coracohumeral ligaments and shortening of the coracoid process increase lateral rotation whilst release of the tight axillary fascia improves abduction.

The procedure to deal with an incongruent shoulder is more complex and it is defined by several sequential steps (Box 13.12.3). At the end of each step the passive lateral rotation and the position of the head of the humerus are checked. The shoulder joint is

Table 13.12.2 Results of nerve repair by root level

Results	C5	C6	C7	C8–T1
Good	Mallett ≥ 13, Gilbert 4+*33%	Full elbow flexion Full supination Biceps MRC 5*>50%	Full extension wrist*<33%	Raimondi 4 or 5*57%
Fair	Mallett 11 or 12 Gilbert 3+	Functional flexion MRC 3 Supination to 45°	Wrist extension MRC 3	Raimondi 3
Poor	Less than above	Less than above	Less than above	Less than above

Box 13.12.3 Steps in surgical management of an incongruent shoulder

After each step check passive lateral rotation and the position of the humeral head:

1. Expose the coracoid process and section the ligaments with basal osteotomy of coracoid process if necessary
2. Z-lengthening of the subscapularis muscle with preservation of the capsule
3. Correct humeral head retroversion
4. Correct glenoid dysplasia with a glenoplasty (not a posterior bone block).

always inspected even in those cases where a complete elongation of the subscapularis muscle is not performed.

Postoperative care

The child is immobilized in a full plaster jacket with the arm abducted 30 degrees and externally rotated 2–30 degrees for a period of time: 6 weeks (simple cases of medial contracture) to 12 weeks (complex dislocation). Physiotherapy is recommenced after the cast is removed.

Elbow and forearm

Flexion deformity of the elbow is common and may be minimized by gentle, continuous stretching exercises and splinting and occasionally by serial casting. Surgical release provides only a modest improvement and recurrent contracture is common. Forearm rotation is usually reduced if not completely lost when the shoulder is dislocated—treatment of the latter improves supination. Supination deformity is associated with ulnar deviation of the hand and can be treated by rotation osteotomy of the radius repeated as necessary as the child grows.

Hand

The recovery of hand function is very slow and can continue until the age of 5 years. Careful and prolonged functional splinting of wrist and thumb is essential in order to maximize neurological improvement. All candidates for a muscle transfer must use a functional splint for 1 year and in many cases, at the end of this period, the operation is not required because of significant improvement in function. In a few selected patients flexor to extensor transfers are performed. Thumb abduction is essential for hand function.

Conclusion

The treatment of CBBP does not end with neurological repair/reconstruction. The deformities during growth, particularly around the shoulder, can downgrade a potentially excellent neurological recovery. Recognition and treatment of a shoulder dislocation is of primary importance and a greater understanding of the deformities and their development is required. Further advances in the performance and interpretation of intraoperative neurophysiology will help the surgeon choose the most appropriate treatment for the nerve lesion.

Further reading

Birch, R., Ahad, N., Kono, H., and Smith, S. (2005). Repair of obstetric brachial plexus palsy. Results in 100 children. *Journal of Bone and Joint Surgery*, **87B**, 1089–95.

Bisinella, G., Birch, R., and Smith, S. (2003). Neurophysiological prediction of outcome in obstetric lesions of the brachial plexus. *Journal of Hand Surgery*, **28B**, 148–152.

Carlstedt, T.P., Grane, P., Hallin, R.G., and Noren, G. (1995). Return of function after spinal cord implantation of avulsed spinal nerve roots. *Lancet*, **346**, 1323–5.

Goldie, B. and Coates, C.J. (1991). Brachial plexus injuries: a survey of incidence and referral patterns. *Journal of Bone and Joint Surgery*, **74B**, 86–8.

Ross, A. and Birch, R. (1991). Reconstruction of the paralysed shoulder after brachial plexus injuries. In Tubiana, R. (ed) *The Hand* Vol. III, pp. 126–33. Philadelphia, PA: W.B. Saunders.

Smith, N.J, Rowan, P., Benson, L., Ezaki, M., and Carter, P. (2004). Neonatal brachial plexus palsy. Outcome of absent biceps function at three months of age. *Journal of Bone and Joint Surgery*, **86A**, 2163–70.

13.13

Malformations of the hand and wrist

Henk Giele

Summary points

- Malformations of the upper limb are amongst the most common anomalies seen in surgical practice
- Recognition and awareness of the varied diagnoses, their significance, and their impact on the child and family are vital to help these children and improve their function.

Introduction

Congenital upper limb anomalies are common with an incidence of 1:506 live births but the variety of anomalies is huge and many are subtle. Approximately 25% of anomalies are syndromic and the variation in hand anomalies helps geneticists identify individual syndromes. The child usually adapts easily to the problem but the impact of anomalies on the parents can be more significant. Despite this adaptation, the surgeon has much to offer in terms of diagnosis, advice, and treatment to improve the function and aesthetics of the hand and upper limb. This chapter gives some general information, a classification of anomalies, and a brief description of the commoner conditions and their treatment. See also Chapter 13.11.

Knowledge of the general principles of upper limb embryology helps in understanding the pattern of some anomalies. Males are more affected than females and although 50% of problems are bilateral, the severity of the condition may differ from side to side. The aetiology is unknown in most cases but in the isolated anomaly genetic causes are unlikely. Often, it is difficult to determine the cause as several aetiologies may result in a similar appearance. Gene defects have been identified for some conditions.

Antenatal diagnosis of some defects, particularly failure of formation, is now common and the surgeon may be called upon for advice at this early stage.

Assessment of the child is based mainly on observation: paying particular attention to features like flexion creases that indicate joint movement. Observe the child's hand movement and correlate it to normal development. Feel for the presence of bones and move joints to assess passive mobility. Take a family history and assess the whole child and their family to detect inherited conditions.

The timing of surgery in congenital hand anomalies is controversial and as good evidence is lacking, decisions are based on personal preference. Generally, the earlier the reconstruction the better the cortical integration of the reconstructed part and the better the anatomical adaptation. Growth potential is maximized and physical and psychological scarring is minimized.

It is important to emphasize to the parents that they were not responsible for the anomaly and explain briefly why such anomalies have occurred. Reassure the parents that even with the most severe anomalies children adapt amazingly well. Offer psychological and genetic counselling, if you feel it is appropriate. For complex conditions it is wise to watch development over several consultations, to help decide the appropriate intervention and prepare the parents for surgery. Treatment is designed to improve function and allow growth and development. Dysfunction often draws attention to the hand anomaly and conversely improved function often renders the anomaly less noticeable. Functional requirements generally centre on thumb function and its ability to oppose with stability and strength (Box 13.13.1).

Classification

The classification of congenital upper limb anomalies is based on current beliefs of their embryological derivation. It was adopted by the International Federation of Surgical Societies of the Hand and is called the IFSSH or Swanson classification. The main categories are divided further according to descriptive or site characteristics (Table 13.13.1).

I Failure of formation

This group shows arrested limb development. The pattern can be transverse, or longitudinal (Figure 13.13.1). The longitudinal patterns are named according to the affected side.

Box 13.13.1 Hand development

- 0–3 months: ulnar sided grasp
- 3–6 months: palmar grasp
- 6–9 months: extends wrist
- 9–12 months: palmar pinch, pinch, uses thumb for adduction.

Table 13.13.1 Swanson/IFSSH classification of congenital upper limb anomalies (examples of old terminology are in parentheses)

I	**Failure of formation** Transverse (reduction defect, congenital amputation): Description of level (e.g. mid forearm reduction defect) Longitudinal: Radial (radial dysplasia, radial club hand) Central (typical cleft hand, lobster claw hand) Ulnar (ulna dysplasia, ulna club hand) Intercalated (phocomelia)
II	**Failure of differentiation** Soft tissue: Syndactyly Trigger digit Camptodactyly Clasp thumb Skeletal: Clinodactyly Tumerous
III	**Duplication (polydactyly)** Preaxial (thumb) Central Postaxial (little finger)
IV	**Undergrowth (hypoplasia)** Brachydactyly Symbrachydactyly (atypical cleft hand)
V	**Overgrowth** Level of involvement of macrodactyly/gigantism
VI	**Amniotic band syndrome/constriction ring**
VII	**Generalized conditions** Achondroplasia, dyschondroplasia, Madelung's

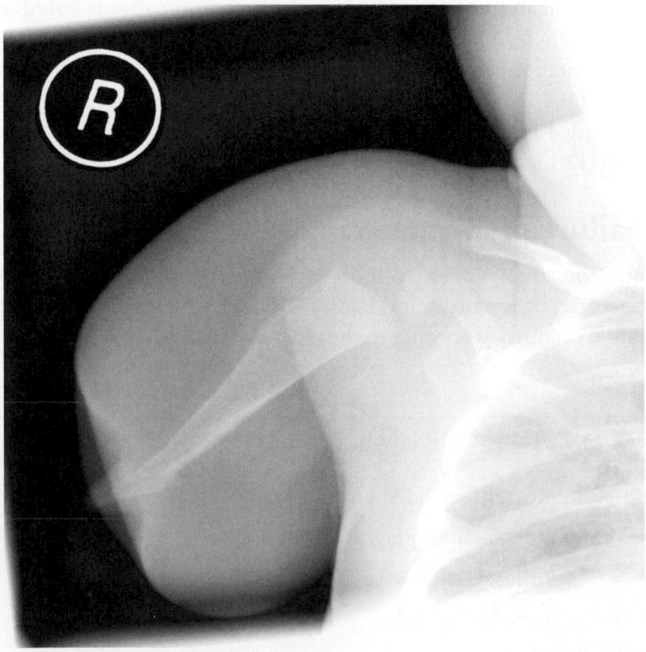

Fig. 13.13.1 Radiograph showing a transverse arrest of the upper limb.

Radial dysplasia

Radial dysplasia (radial club hand) is the congenital failure of formation in a longitudinal distribution affecting all preaxial or radial structures, resulting most obviously in radial deviation of the wrist. It is defined by the most obvious skeletal deficiency.

The incidence of radial dysplasia is 1:30 000–100 000 live births. Fifty to sixty-six per cent of cases are bilateral but the dysplasia is usually not symmetrical. Right-sided involvement is most frequent and males are twice as commonly affected as females. Radial anomalies are always associated with thumb hypoplasia (except in TAR (thrombocytopenia with absent radius) syndrome) but only 50% of thumb hypoplasia cases are associated with an anomaly of radius.

The aetiology is unknown, and most cases are sporadic. Some are syndromal and some linked to teratogens such as thalidomide, valproeic acid, or radiation. Due to the presumed timing of the congenital insult (the cardiac septum and radius both form in the fifth week), there are many associated disorders (Box 13.13.2).

Pathology

The pathology of radial dysplasia is well described. The humerus is shorter then normal with distal defects of coronoid, capitellum, and medial condyle that reduce elbow flexion. Most commonly there is complete absence or absence of the distal third of the radius. The fibrous anlage or mesenchymal 'scar' that replaces the deficient radius tethers growth producing progressive deformity that includes curvature of the ulna and forearm shortening. The radial carpal bones are absent, hypoplastic or coalesced, especially the scaphoid and trapezium.

The soft tissues are as severely affected as the skeleton with hypoplastic, fused, or absent radial wrist and thumb, extensors, and flexors. In severe cases, the finger flexors/extensors are also affected. The fingers are stiff and this determines the outcome of thumb reconstruction by pollicization. The ulnar digits are less affected.

Box 13.13.2 Disorders commonly associated with radial dysplasia

- VACTERL or VATER: vertebral, anal, cardiac, tracheo-oesophageal, renal and limb anomalies
- Cardiac: Holt–Oram syndrome (familial, with atrial septal defect)
- Gastrointestinal
- Haemopoietic:
  - Thrombocytopenia (TAR syndrome)
  - Fanconi anaemia (with renal anomalies and pancytopenia)
- Skeletal:
  - Syndactyly
  - Scoliosis
  - Sprengel's
  - Knee deformity (tibia)
- Craniofacial: Nager, Rothmund–Thompson.

Table 13.13.2 Types of radial dysplasia (Bayne and Klug 1987)

Type	Radius	Treatment
I	Short but normal radius (2nd commonest type)	Do nothing or lengthen radius
II	Hypoplastic radius (rarest)	lengthen radius
III	Partial absence, usually distal portion	Centralization/radialization with or without prior distraction
IV	Complete absence (commonest)	Centralization/radialization with or without prior distraction

The radial artery is absent as are several nerves (superficial radial, musculocutaneous, lateral cutaneous nerve of forearm). The median nerve is abnormal, lying quite radial and supplying areas normally supplied by the radial and musculocutaneous nerves.

Classification

The classification of radial dysplasia relates to the severity of skeletal involvement but the soft tissue deficiencies are correlated, for example, the absent radius is usually associated with a Blauth type 4 or 5 hypoplastic thumb (except in TAR syndrome). (Table 13.13.2 and Figure 13.13.2).

Presentation

The clinical presentation is usually obvious at birth: 'isolated' thumb anomalies may alert the surgeon to look at the forearm. The hand and wrist are flexed, pronated, palmar subluxed, and radially displaced. The thumb is hypoplastic or absent and the radial digits absent or stiff.

Management

Initial management consists of careful evaluation of the whole child and a passive stretching and splintage regime for the wrist/hand. At this age most postural deformity can be corrected and maintained providing the wrist is splinted continuously. This makes subsequent surgery easier. In all but type 1 and mild type 2 cases, surgery is indicated to stabilize the wrist and later to reconstruct the thumb. Wrist stabilization improves hand position, allows more effective use of the thumb and improves finger flexion strength. There is the additional benefit of improved aesthetics, easier care, and potentially improved ulnar physeal growth. Thumb reconstruction depends on the exact anomaly. Contraindications to surgery include bilateral radial dysplasia, lack of elbow flexion, a very short forearm, severe systemic illness (or an adult who has adjusted to the deformity).

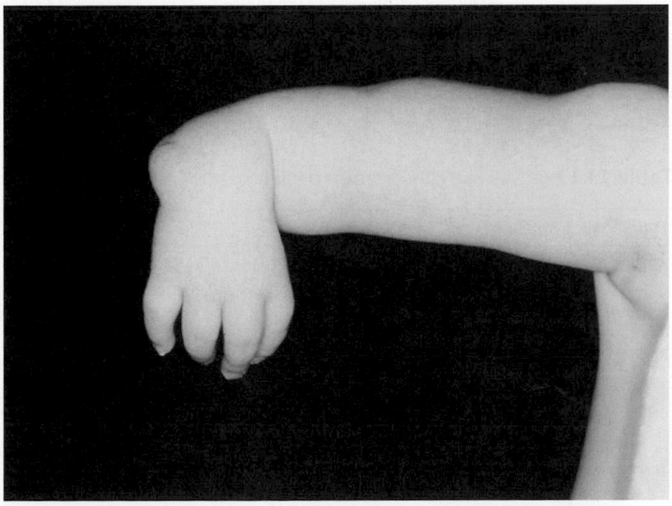

Fig. 13.13.2 Clinical photograph of a child with radial dysplasia: there are four digits, the wrist is radially deviated and the distal ulnar is prominent.

Surgical (Box 13.13.3)

Understandably there are variations in operative technique: some surgeons believe in soft tissue distraction prior to operative reduction and this may be necessary if operative reduction is delayed. If soft tissue distraction is used, apply the distractor at 6–9 months, distract slowly over 2 months, stabilize and then proceed with the definitive operation.

The two definitive wrist procedures are: centralization or radialization.

- In *centralization* the wrist is reduced and stabilized by placing the distal ulna into a surgically created carpal slot, avoiding injury to the ulnar physis. This results in a well-aligned but stiffer and shorter limb
- In *radialization*, no carpal bones are excised. Full passive correction is a prerequisite for surgery. Tendons are released and the ulna is placed radial to carpus, overcorrecting the wrist. Tendon transfers maximize their lever arm and create an ulnar force. The position is maintained by temporary pin fixation for 2–12months. Radialization results in better motion and possibly less disturbance to growth.

Correction of the ulna bow may be performed simultaneously or later with forearm lengthening (if required).

The outcome of these procedures should be a short forearm with a neutral stable wrist and prehensile grasp (Figures 13.13.3 and 13.13.4). Complications are common including skin necrosis, pin breakage or infection, recurrent deformity especially carpal subluxation, premature distal ulnar physeal closure, wrist stiffness.

Cleft hand (Box 13.13.4)

Cleft hand is defined as a congenital longitudinal failure of formation of the central portion of the hand and forearm. It has a very variable presentation from the classic V-shaped central cleft to a

Box 13.13.3 Management of radial dysplasia: surgical principles

- Before 6-9 months:
  - Correct wrist alignment and stabilise the joint
  - Rebalance deforming forces with tendon transfers
  - Correct ulnar bow
- At 9-18 months: thumb reconstruction
- Later:
  - Oppensplasty
  - Ulna osteotomy ± distraction lengthening.

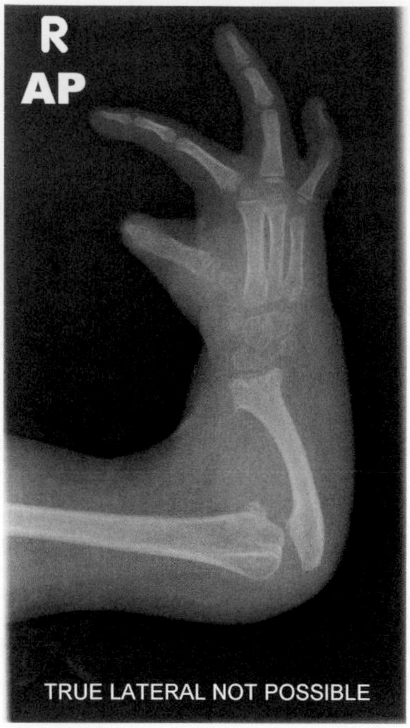

Fig. 13.13.3 Radiograph of a type IV radial dysplasia following surgical reconstruction.

single ulnar digit hand (Figure 13.13.5). The incidence is estimated at 1:30 000–100 000 live births. Fifty per cent are bilateral and involve the feet as well. These bilateral cases are familial: autosomal dominant with high penetrance. The aetiology of cleft hand is unknown. The interdigital spaces should form between days 39–50. When this process fails osseous syndactyly occurs whereas if necrosis occurs in the middle of a digit, there is polydactyly and if excess necrosis occurs then a cleft results. Thus cleft hands are frequently seen with syndactyly, polydactyly, osseous fusions, as well as cleft feet (Box 13.13.5).

This category used to include both typical and atypical cleft hands. The latter group are now best classified with symbrachydactyly in the hypoplasia category.

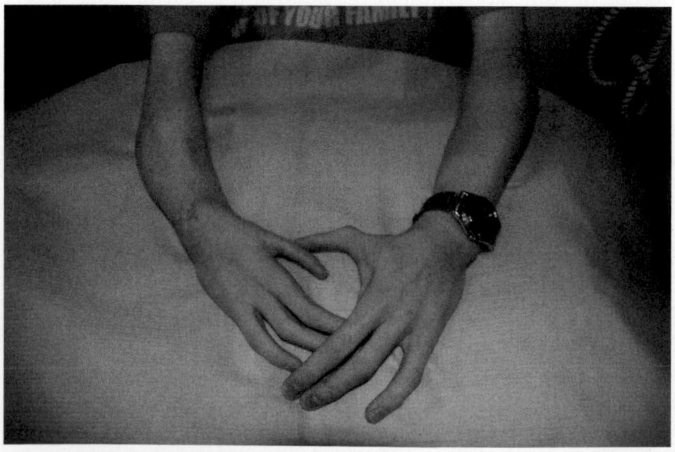

Fig. 13.13.4 Clinical photograph of bilateral radial dysplasia following surgical reconstruction including pollicizations. The wrist is in neutral and stable. There is good thumb function.

Box 13.13.4 Cleft hand synonyms

- Ectrodactyly
- Lobster claw hand
- Split hand
- Median hypoplasia.

Box 13.13.5 Cleft hand associations

- EEC syndrome: ectrodactyly, ectodermal dysplasia and cleft lip/palate
- Poland's syndrome
- Deafness
- Ocular anomalies
- VSD.

Cleft hands are classified according to their description and the number of digits remaining or by the quality of the thumb and first web as these are important in determining hand function (Manske's classification) (Tables 13.13.3 and 13.13.4).

Presentation

Cleft hand presents with absence of the middle finger and to varying degrees the middle metacarpal. Adjacent digits may be absent or present: if present they are often large, frequently syndactylized,

Table 13.13.3 Classification of cleft hands

Type	Description
Type 1	Central V-shaped cleft with absent middle finger
Type 2	Central V-shaped cleft with absent middle and index
Type 3	V shaped cleft with absent middle, index and ring
Type 4	Absent thumb, index, middle
Type 5	Monodactylous—little finger only
Subtype s	Syndactyly
Subtype p	Polydactyly

Table 13.13.4 Manske classification of cleft hands

Type	Web space	Treatment
1	Normal	Close cleft, excise extra bone, reconstruct transverse metacarpal ligament
2	Narrowed—mild	Close cleft + web plasty
2	Narrowed—severe	Close cleft + flap
3	Syndactylized	Close cleft, release syndactyly, + flaps or excise index
4	Merged as missing index	No treatment, stabilize MCP joint
5	No thumb	Toe transfer

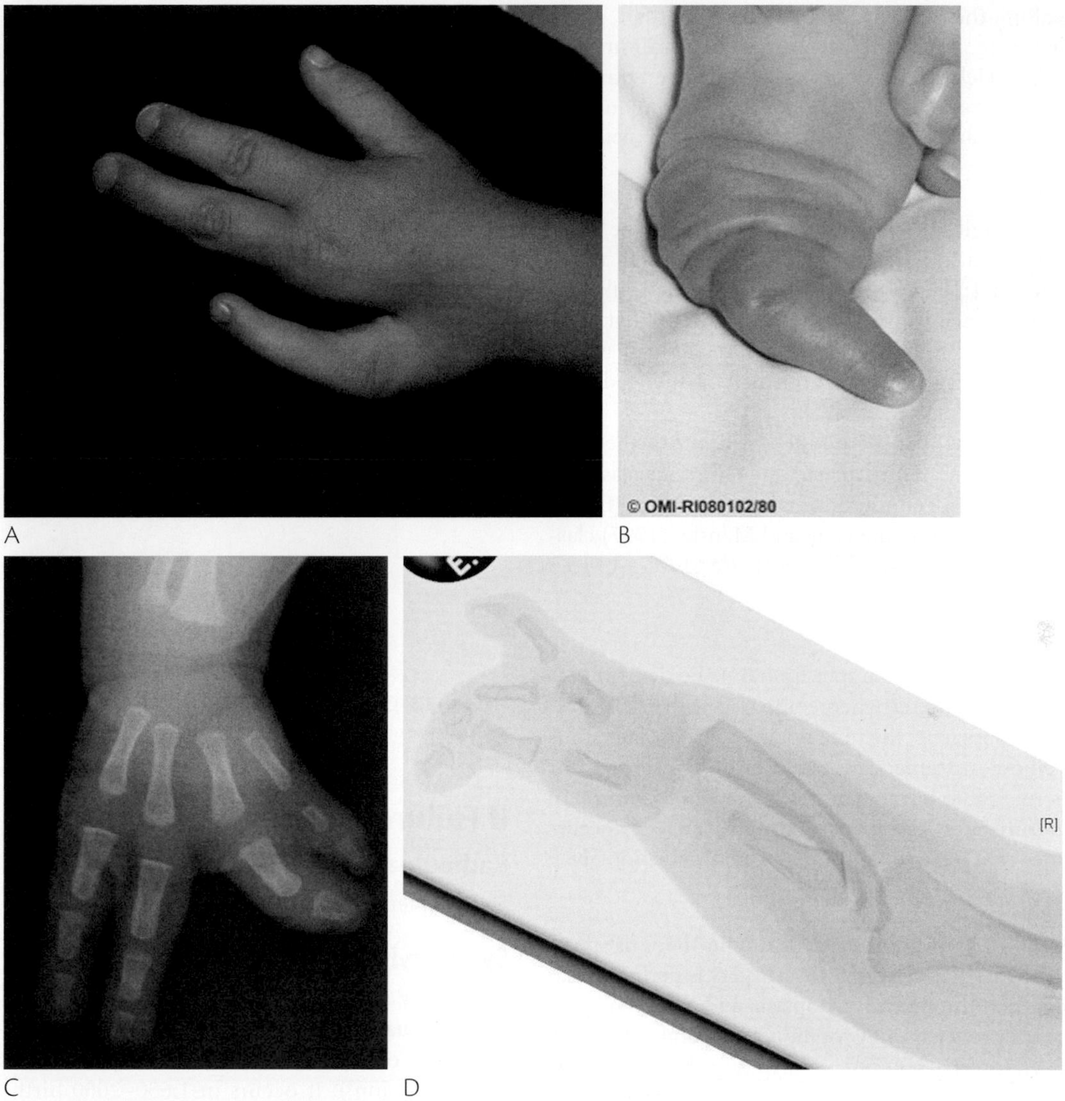

Fig. 13.13.5 A, B) Clinical pictures of cleft hands of varying severity. In (B) there is a single ulnar digit (Type 5). C, D) Radiographs that show a cleft hand can be associated with significant abnormalities of bone development more proximally (D).

and with camptodactyly. With increasing severity the radial side of the cleft becomes absent eventually leaving only the single little finger (Figure 13.13.5B), or in worst cases no digits at all (peromelia). Fusions are often present in the palm but usually there are no carpal anomalies. The intrinsic muscles and long tendons are present but insert anomalously.

Box 13.13.6 Ulnar dysplasia associations

- Musculoskeletal anomalies:
  - Fibular hemimelia
  - Proximal focal deficiency
  - Phocomelia
  - Scoliosis
- No systemic anomalies

Management

Cleft hands are often described as having good function but poor aesthetics. Function can be improved by increasing the first web space, releasing any syndactyly, improving motion at metacarpophalangeal (MCP) joints by excision or release of cross bones, releasing proximal interphalangeal (PIP) joint contractures, performing osteotomies of the metacarpals to align the digits, improving abduction and opposition of the thumb, and providing opposition posts or digits when these are absent. Occasionally straightening and covering a cross bone can create a digit. Aesthetics are improved by the closure of the cleft.

Several techniques exist to create a first web space and close the cleft simultaneously by transposing the cleft skin to the first web and the border digit into the cleft. The Snow–Littler technique uses a palmar-based flap from the cleft transposed to widen the first web space and simultaneously transposing the index finger at the metacarpal base onto the middle finger metacarpal base. The Miura–Komada technique uses the same index transposition but with an incision along the web space and around the digit, and a dorsal extension for access to the metacarpal base minimizing wound problems. The Ueba technique uses the same digit transposition but the flaps lie transverse with the dorsal flap from one side of the cleft and the palmar flap from the other side of the cleft.

Ulnar dysplasia

Ulnar dysplasia is a longitudinal failure of formation of the ulnar portion of the hand and forearm. It is less common than radial dysplasia occurring in 1:100 000 live births. Most are unilateral with no sex preponderance. It is more common on the left. Half are associated with other musculoskeletal anomalies but unlike radial dysplasia, ulnar dysplasia is not normally associated with systemic anomalies (Box 13.13.6).

Ulnar dysplasia is thought to be due to an injury to the zone of polarizing activity (ZPA). The forearm anomalies are classified according to the ulna and elbow anomalies (Bayne or Baur). Whereas the hand is defined by the Cole and Mansky (1997) classification based on the thumb and first web space (Tables 13.13.5 and 13.13.6) (Figure 13.13.6).

Presentation

Ulnar dysplasia affects the whole upper limb but the deformity is less obvious and function better when compared with radial dysplasia. The limb is hypoplastic, the ulna possibly absent, the radius bowed, and the elbow unstable. The radial head is dislocated or fused to the humerus (radio humeral synostosis, Figure 13.13.7). In the hand, the digits are hypoplastic or absent and syndactyly occurs in 30%. Seventy per cent have some thumb or first web anomaly.

Management

Splinting and stretches help improve or maintain the wrist position: wrist surgery is rarely indicated. Most surgery is performed to release syndactyly, treat the thumb hypoplasia and first web space deficiency to provide prehension. A rotational humeral osteotomy can help the marked internal rotation deformity and radial osteotomy/lengthening can improve radial curvature if required. Early excision of the fibrous ulnar anlage can prevent progressive bowing of the radius and may result in better growth.

Table 13.13.5 Classification of forearm anomalies in ulna dysplasia

Type	Description
I	Hypoplastic ulna
II	Partial absence ulna
III	Absence ulna
IV	Humeroradial synostosis

Table 13.13.6 Classification of the hand anomalies in ulna dysplasia

Type	Description
A	Normal
B	Mild first web and thumb deficiency (narrow)
C	Moderate–severe (syndactyly of thumb to index, thumb in palmar plane, lack of opposition, absence of thumb extension, hypoplastic thumb)
D	Absent thumb

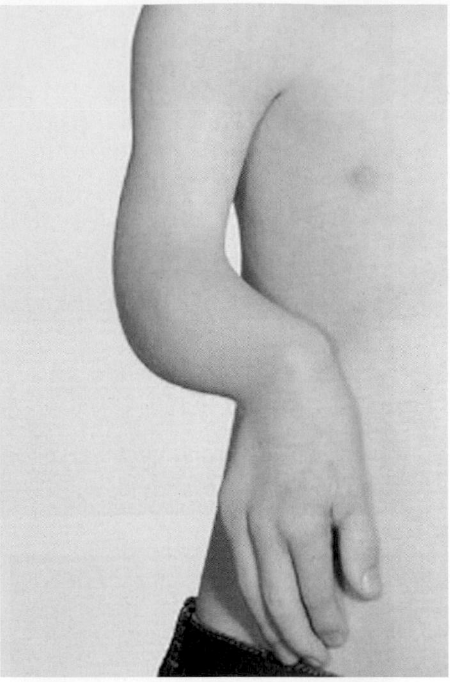

Fig. 13.13.6 Clinical photograph of an ulnar dysplasia showing a short arm and forearm and ulnar deviation of the wrist/hand.

II Failure of differentiation

Radioulnar synostosis

See Chapter 13.11.

Syndactyly

Syndactyly is one of the two most common hand anomalies. The term is usually used to describe conjoined digits due to a congenital failure of separation (but it can apply to post-burn or post-trauma 'fusion'). It occurs in 1:650–2000 births and is twice as common in men as women. Half affect the third web space and only 5% involve the first web space (Figure 13.13.8).

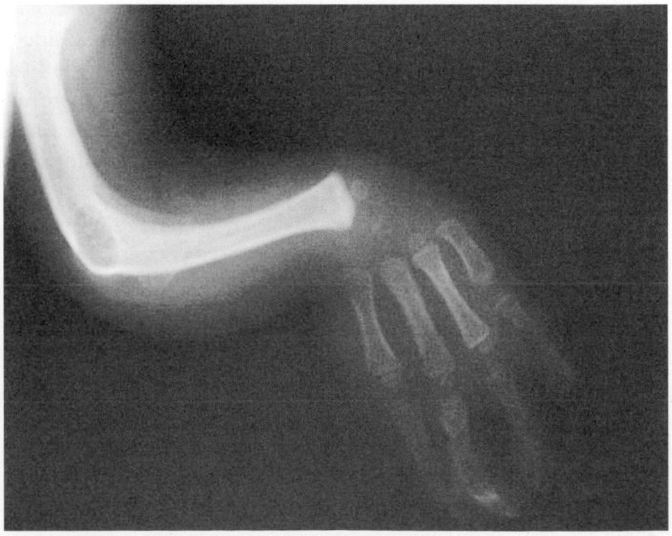

Fig. 13.13.7 Radiograph of a type IV ulnar dysplasia.

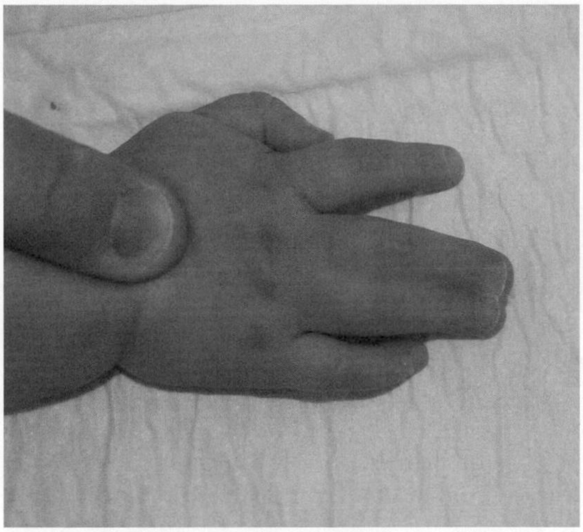

Fig. 13.13.8 Clinical photograph of a complete type 2 syndactyly affecting the middle/ring fingers.

The aetiology is unknown, but 20% are familial usually displaying autosomal dominant inheritance with incomplete penetration and variable expression.

Failure of separation is linked to steroid use in early pregnancy and also fibroblast growth factor receptor deficiency. Some congenital cases are due to trauma and healing as in amniotic band/constriction ring syndrome. Many cases of syndactyly are associated with other syndromes and chromosomal disorders such as Apert's, Poland's, symbrachydactyly, and Aarskog's.

Syndactyly is classified according to site and degree (Table 13.13.7 and Box 13.13.7).

Presentation

Syndactyly is present at birth although occasionally not noticed until later in life. Assess the web involved: does the failure of separation involve soft tissue, nail, and/or bone. Is the syndactyly causing a deformity?

Hand development occurs rapidly between 6–24 months so it can be important to separate the syndactyly before this period especially if the involved digits are of different lengths.

Management

Surgery involves separation of the digits, creation of a web space and resurfacing of the digits: the circumference of two separate digits is 22% greater than the circumference of conjoined fingers. Problems may arise from the fascial, neurovascular, or tendinous connections running transversely between the digits. The aim is to create a web space sloping at 45 degrees from dorsal to palmar, with a free transverse distal edge, and an aesthetic shape, with minimal scarring on the dorsum of the hand and fingers, no scar contracture, and no longitudinal scars on the digits. In general, avoid separating an adjacent syndactyly simultaneously: staged procedures pose less risk to the vascular supply.

Table 13.13.7 Temtamy and McKusick classification for syndactyly

Type	Description
I	Second postaxial web syndactyly
II	Synpolydactyly (third web syndactyly and duplication finger 3 or 4).
III	Ring and little finger syndactyly
IV	Complete syndactyly all fingers
V	Syndactyly associated with metacarpal/tarsal synostosis.

Box 13.13.7 Classification of syndactyly

- Complete (extends to tips) or incomplete
- Simple (soft tissues only) or complex (bone involved)
- Acrosyndactyly (digit tips fused, bases free)
- Single or multiple
- Unilateral or bilateral
- Hand or foot or both
- Isolated anomaly or part of a syndrome.

Digital separation is by a zig-zag design, creating interdigitating triangular skin flaps of varying width from the dorsum and palmar aspects of the digits to cover the sides of the separated digits. These flaps avoid longitudinal digital scars that may cause flexion contracture. In digits with symphalangism (such as in Apert's syndrome) simple longitudinal division is permissible, as flexion contractures cannot occur.

Web reconstruction has many more surgical options: most require full thickness skin grafts to fill the defect created by formation of the web. Most surgeons use a modification of the Bauer design (1956), which creates a dorsal rectangular flap to recreate the web space, or opposing palmar and dorsal triangles, or an omega and anchor design. There are also techniques that avoid skin grafts by redistributing the dorsal digital skin. For complicated syndactyly some surgeons have attempted using distraction of the digital skeleton laterally from the involved web or tissue expansion of the dorsal skin but neither technique is popular due to the high complication rate. Reconstruction of the lateral nail folds is by Buck–Gramcko triangular pulp flaps (Figure 13.13.9).

Complications

Injury to digital neurovascular bundles leading to an inability to separate the digits or digital necrosis is the most feared but also the rarest complication.

Distal web creep due to digital scarring and growth is more common in complex syndactyly.

Deformity of the digit usually a flexion and lateral curvature due to scarring and growth disturbance from the length inequality between the syndactylized digits is common particularly in border digit involvement.

When skin grafts are used there is the risk of hyperpigmentation or hair growth of the skin graft. Skin graft loss or flap necrosis can lead to delayed healing and scarring.

Camptodactyly

Camptodactyly is defined as a congenital flexion deformity of the PIP joint. It affects 1% of the population but is under-reported. It can be subtle and is sometimes only noticed late, giving two peaks of presentation: early childhood and adolescence. In adolescence it often presents after trauma although this is *not* the cause. There is a female preponderance in the adolescent group. Camptodactyly is

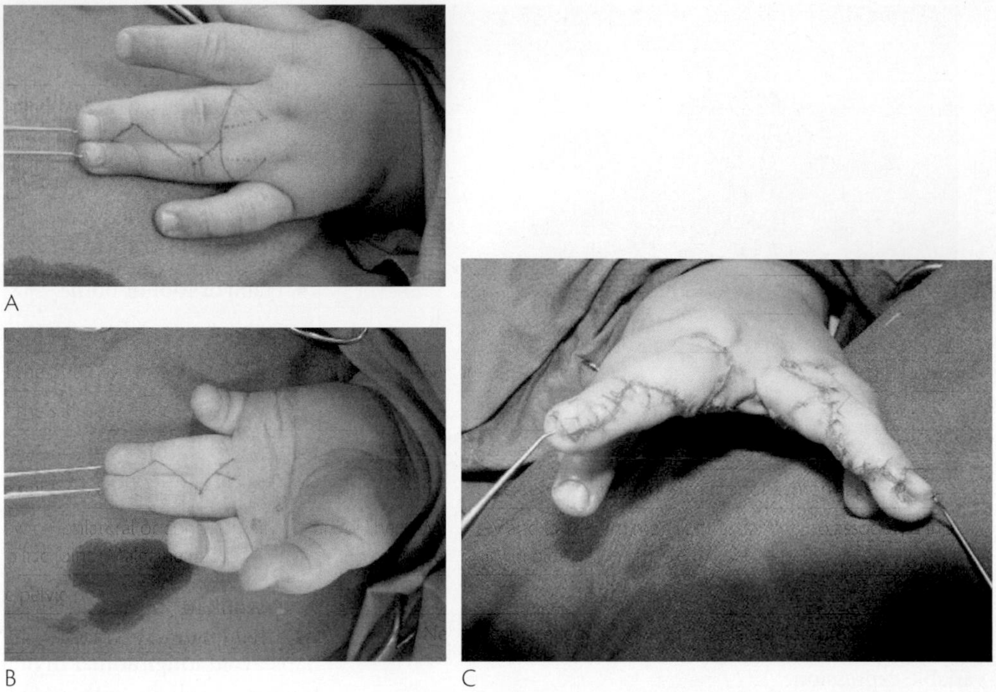

Fig. 13.13.9 Clinical photographs showing the Giele design for dorsal and palmar skin flaps for release of a syndactyly and the postoperative result.

most frequent in the little finger. Some cases are familial (autosomal dominant).

Camptodactyly results from a congenital imbalance of the flexion and extension forces at the PIP joint. The theories of causation include abnormal intrinsics, anomalous finger flexors or extensors.

Presentation

Camptodactyly presents with a flexion deformity at the PIP joint but from this position, full flexion is possible. Rarely the deformity is fixed. A history of preceding trauma is common but unrelated. Lateral x-rays in adolescents show characteristic changes at the PIP joint (Figure 13.13.10). In addition on the anteroposterior view the PIP joint slopes to the ulnar aspect and clinically a 'ulnar drift' of the middle and distal phalanges is noted. Though rarely found, always check for dysfunction of the ulnar nerve, intrinsic muscles, and the flexor digitorum superficialis (FDS).

Management

Splinting and stretches are used first. In most cases this improves the contracture sufficiently. If conservative therapy fails and the contracture is greater than 50–70 degrees then surgery can be considered. The principles of surgery involve release of the skin, soft tissues, and joint, an attempt to rebalance flexor and extensor forces, and reconstruction of the skin defect. The options are: exploration for specific anomalies, resection and/or release of the anomaly and then splintage, or tendon transfers to augment extension at the central slip utilizing the lumbrical, FDS, extensor indicis profundus (EIP), or extensor plication. Alternatively the FDS lasso procedure can increase MCP flexion, helping transfer some of the extensor pull to the central slip.

In older patients with established PIP joint changes not amenable to soft tissue correction an osteotomy can be performed at the proximal phalangeal neck to correct flexion and inclination.

Congenital trigger digit

A discrepancy between the size of the pulley and the size of the flexor tendon leads to a flexion contracture of the digit or less commonly triggering as seen in adults. Thumbs are most commonly affected. The aetiology is unknown.

It is not usually apparent at birth but becomes noticeable in the first year of age, or occasionally later.

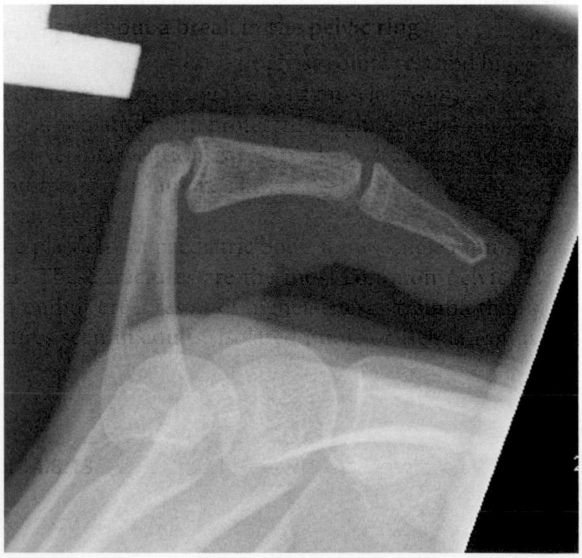

Fig. 13.13.10 Lateral radiograph of a camptodactyly showing abnormalities at the PIPJ: an anvil or wedged shaped head of the proximal phalanx with a divot in the articular base of the middle phalanx and an exaggerated sub condylar recess (Drucker's space).

The child presents with a digit locked in flexion or extension and a palpable nodule on the flexor tendon may be felt called Notta's node.

Reports suggest that 33% of trigger thumbs resolve with stretches and splinting if the tendon is mobile (triggering) on presentation but they do not improve sufficiently to allow normal interphalangeal (IP) joint hyperextension. Operative release of the A1 pulley should be performed. Finger triggering does not resolve spontaneously and should be treated operatively. Steroid injections are not indicated unless there is other pathology such as diabetes or inflammatory arthritis.

Clasp thumb

An anomaly where the thumb is flexed into the palm and no active extension is seen. The clasp thumb can be passively extended. This is normal behaviour in babies under 6 weeks and should not be confused with the fixed thumb-in-palm deformity.

The incidence is unknown as is the aetiology. Some cases are due to hypoplasia of extensor pollicis longus (EPL). It can occur in association with Digitotalar syndrome, Freeman–Sheldon 'whistling face syndrome' and arthrogryposis or it may be the first presentation of thumb hypoplasia or mild radial club hand.

Clasp thumb was classified by Weckesser according to severity or clumped together by McCarroll into supple (having an absent EPL) or complex (an absent EPL with a flexion contracture of the MCP joint and thumb hypoplasia) (Table 13.13.8).

Management

If the child is young, reassure the parents that this is probably normal and reflects a mild imbalance of flexor and extensor development. Initially it is treated by splinting the thumb in extension. This is usually successful. In resistant or complex cases surgical management may be needed with tendon transfer to reconstruct the absent EPL. The EIP is often absent and cannot be used. Complex thumbs may need extensive palmar skin release, and thumb hypoplasia reconstruction as well.

III Duplication

Polydactyly

Polydactyly is the formation of all or a part of an extra digit. It is the commonest congenital upper limb anomaly (Figure 13.13.11). The aetiology is unknown. It can be hereditary especially when the little finger is involved. Polydactyly is associated with many syndromes (Table 13.13.9 and Box 13.13.8).

Management

- *Type A:* sometimes the polydactyly is 'strangulated' by ligating the base with a suture. This may leave a tender nodule on the ulnar border of the little finger due to the underlying neuroma. Alternatively, excision, under local or general anaesthesia, can be done soon after childbirth. Dissect out and divide the neurovascular bundle deep to avoid a neuroma
- *Type B* polydactyly cannot be excised under local anaesthetic due to the bone reduction required. Leave more skin than first appearances suggests, as the resulting defect is often large. In central polydactyly, correction of adjacent bone or soft tissue anomalies may avoid problems with further growth
- *Type C* polydactyly requires excision of the whole ray, closure of the space, and creation of the intermetacarpal ligament. Try to excise a central rather than a border ray if there is no obvious choice, as the result will be more stable but may leave some widening of the interdigital space and scissoring (Figure 13.13.12).

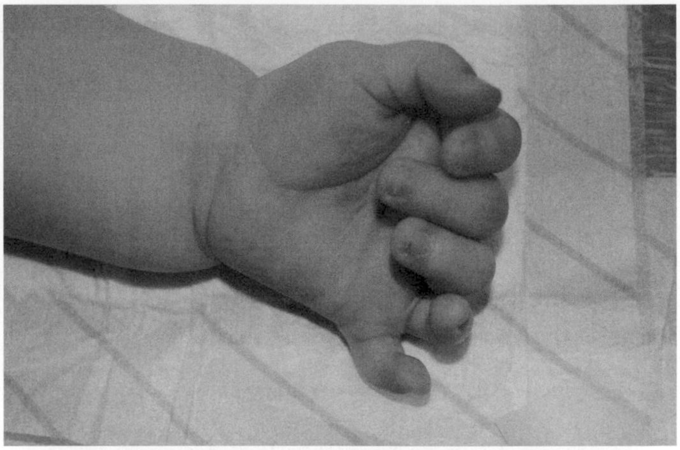

Fig. 13.13.11 Clinical photograph of ulnar sided polydactyly.

Thumb duplication

Thumb duplication is common, it differs from other digital polydactyly in the complexity of the duplication, the functional importance of the thumb, and hence the reconstruction.

Wassel based his classification of thumb duplication on the most proximal extent of the duplication (Table 13.13.10 and Figure 13.13.13). The commonest type is type 4, next commonest is type 2, then type 6. Note that types with even numbers are duplications which extend to joint level. A Stelling A polydactyly-type duplication of the thumb where there is a small nubbin of a thumb connected by a thin soft tissue pedicle (usually at the level of the metacarpophalangeal joint) is not covered adequately by this classification, but is sometimes described as a rudimentary thumb.

Table 13.13.8 Classification of clasp thumb (Weckesser)

Type	Description
1	Deficient extension
2	Flexion contracture combined with deficient extension
3	Hypoplasia of the thumb
4	Others

Table 13.13.9 Stelling classification of polydactyly

Type	Description
A	Incomplete digit, soft tissue only, often attached by small pedicle
B	Complete digit
C	Complete digit and metacarpal

Box 13.13.8 Polydactyly associated syndromes

- Ellis van Creveld
- Lawrence–Moon–Bardet–Biedl
- Trisomy 13.

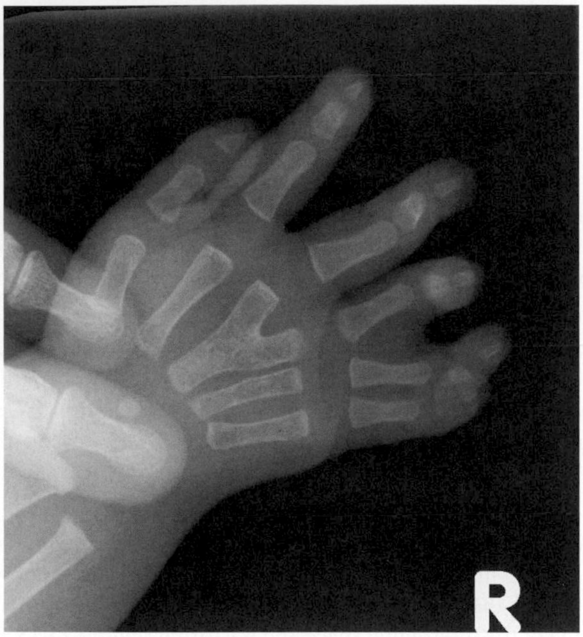

Fig. 13.13.12 Radiograph showing a central polydactyly with partial duplication of the metacarpal.

Table 13.13.10 Wassell classification of thumb duplication

Type	Level
1	Duplication of distal phalanx
2	Duplication to IP joint
3	Duplication proximal phalanx
4	Duplication to MCP joint
5	Duplication metacarpal
6	Duplication to CMC joint
7	Triphalangeal thumb

Management

Treatment does *not* consist of simple excision of the extra thumb. Prior to excision assess the level of the duplication, the development and stability of the joints, and the degree of axial deviation of each element. Excision of the most hypoplastic thumb is combined with osteotomies, and reconstruction of the collateral ligaments. Osteotomies are needed to align the joint surfaces, the axis of the phalanges and to thin the widened metacarpal or phalangeal head. Division of intertendinous connections and realignment of the flexor and extensor tendon may also be needed.

In many cases the remaining thumb is smaller then the opposite thumb, and stiffer. This does not substantially affect function, but should be pointed out to the parents pre-operatively. It is common to reoperate for a subsequent zigzag deformity if initial osteotomies are not performed.

IV Undergrowth (hypoplasia)

Brachydactyly

Brachydactyly describes short fingers usually due to an autosomally dominant inherited condition. These are sometimes syndromic

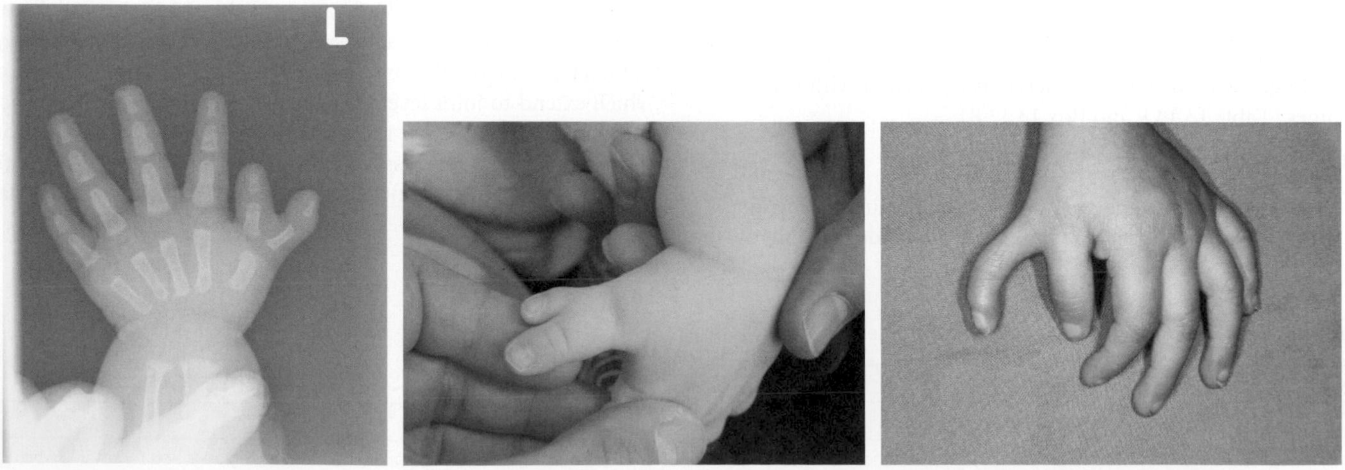

A B C

Fig. 13.13.13 A) AP radiograph showing a type 4 duplication of the thumb. B) Clinical photograph of a type 3 duplication. C) Clinical photograph of a type 7 duplication.

such as in achondroplasia, or part of a systemic condition like pseudohypoparathyroidism (with short metacarpals), but most commonly are asymptomatic and often unnoticed such as little finger clinodactyly.

Management

Good function means intervention is usually not required. Associated conditions such as syndactyly will need treatment. Occasionally a functional problem such as a palpable and painful short metacarpal head in palmar grip or a finger deformity that impacts on function will require surgery. Longitudinally bracketed epiphyses in delta phalanges may benefit from epiphyseolysis. Mature deformities causing functional problems can be corrected by osteotomies. Lengthening is rarely indicated.

Symbrachydactyly

Symbrachydactyly, translated as short fingers joined together, represents a spectrum of failure of digital development with a tendency to preserve the thumb (in contrast to a similar spectrum of cleft hand which preserves the little finger).

The incidence of symbrachydactyly is 1:10 000. The inheritance is mostly sporadic. The aetiology is unknown but thought to be a mesodermal defect of vascular origin leaving ectodermal remnants such as skin and nails as nubbins. It usually affects the left side but when associated with Poland's syndrome affects the right.

Presentation

Symbrachydactyly has a spectrum of severity: the best cases have all digits and all phalanges present but the fingers are slightly shorter and stiffer whilst at the other extreme, in essence there is a transverse failure of formation that may be through the level of the forearm. The rudimentary digital remnants suggest a symbrachydactyly rather than a reduction defect.

In between these two extremes there are reducing patterns of digital loss described as a teratologic sequence starting with loss of the middle phalanges, then the distal phalanges, then the metacarpals as well. The pattern of loss tends to be more severe on the ulnar side sparing the thumb initially. The pattern with short/absent middle fingers preserving the thumb and little finger was called an atypical or U-shaped cleft hand, as compared to the classical V-shaped cleft pattern (Figure 13.13.14).

Management

In symbrachydactyly with short fingers no intervention is indicated, as function is good. Where digits are absent, the number of remaining digits and their function determines treatment. The quality of the thumb and first web space determine the final functional outcome.

Operatively consider whether the hand would benefit from first web space release/deepening, would lengthening of the thumb or other digits improve grasp and pinch? Methods of achieving the latter include vascularized or non-vascularized toe transplant and distraction lengthening of existing parts.

Non-vascularized toe phalanx transfer is very much a second choice option. The donor site leaves an ugly defect once growth occurs as the growth in the remaining middle and distal phalanx is reduced by 50%. The donor defect can be minimized by suturing the flexor to extensor tendons or by bone graft from iliac crest. One expects growth of approximately 1mm per year, eventually achieving approximately 78% of the length of contralateral toe phalanx, or 52% of opposite digital phalanx. This type of transfer results in better growth if performed before 15 months of age.

Thumb hypoplasia

Congenital hypoplasia or aplasia of the thumb may be categorized either in the failure of formation or in the hypoplasia category of

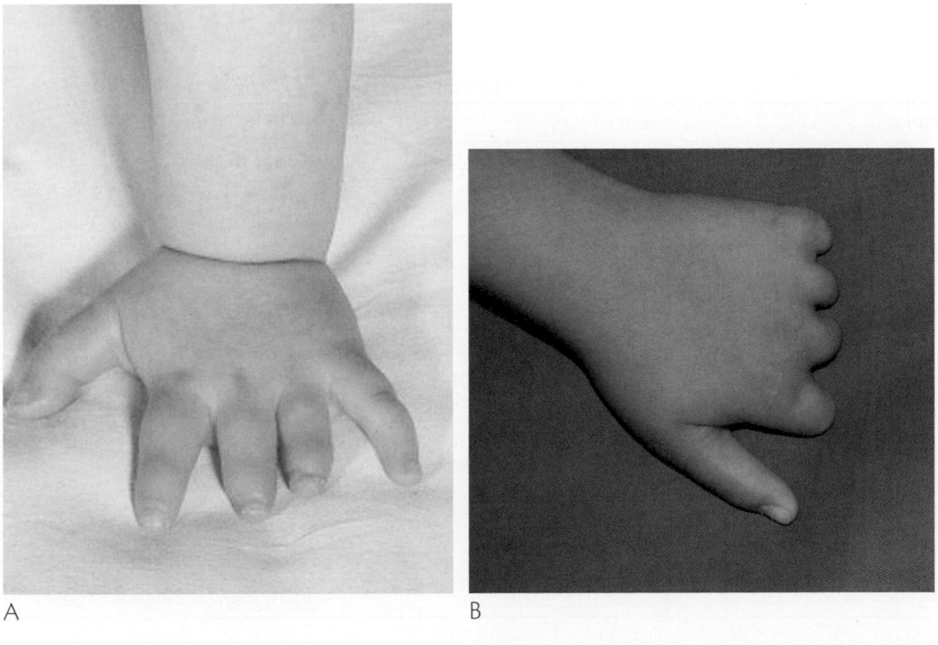

A B

Fig. 13.13.14 Clinical examples of symbrachydactyly. A) atypical cleft type B) adactylous type.

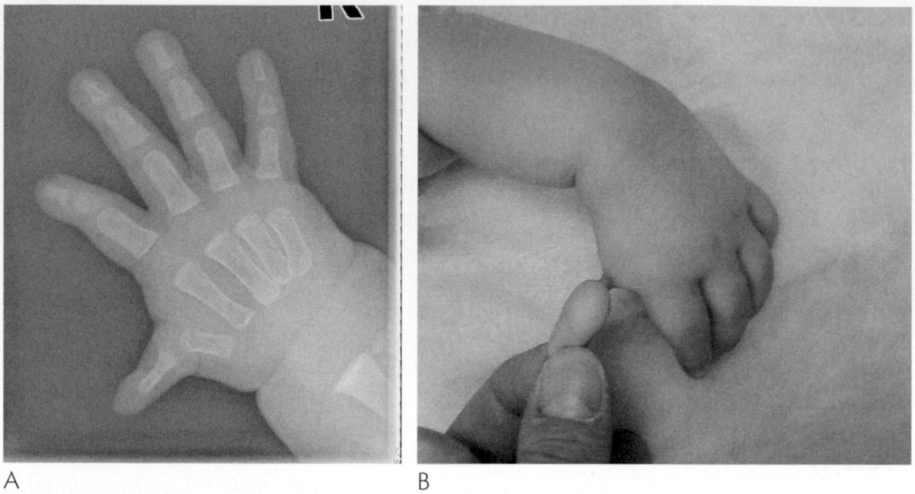

Fig. 13.13.15 A) Radiograph of a type 3a thumb hypoplasia. B) Clinical photograph of a pouce flottant thumb hypoplasia.

the IFSSH classification. It is common and may be an isolated phenomenon or part of a radial dysplasia, cleft hand, or symbrachydactyly. The aetiology is unknown but has been linked to fetal neurogenic injury and thalidomide.

Thumb hypoplasia presents with a very predictable pattern and is classified according to Blauth (1967). This classification does not cover transverse absences of the thumb due to different pathologies (Figure 13.13.15 and Table 13.13.11).

Management

Surgery aims to increase function and appearance of the hand. Try to reconstruct all the deficiencies in one operation and do this before 1 year of age to encourage full thumb function (Box 13.13.9).

The MCP joint stabilization and UCL reconstruction is achieved by UCL plication or soft tissue gubbinsoplasty where tissue allows or, if necessary, with a tendon graft (palmaris longus or extensor digiti minimi) or use the end of the tendon used for the opponensplasty.

Pollicization creates a thumb by the transposition, stabilizing and shortening of a finger ray (usually the index). The index MCP joint becomes the basal joint of the new thumb, the PIP joint becomes the new MCP joint, and the DIP joint becomes the new IP joint. A first web space must also be created.

The outcome of pollicization depends more on the quality of the index finger and the presence of intrinsics and other musculotendinous structures than the surgical procedure. Complications include overgrowth of the trapezium due to persistence of the physis, stiffness, instability usually due to hyperextension of the new carpometacarpal (CMC) joint, lack of flexion or extension due to tendon imbalance, poor opposition either due to inadequate rotation or poor intrinsics, poor position of thumb and skin flap necrosis.

Table 13.13.11 Blauth's classification of the hypoplastic thumb

Type	Anatomy or subtype	Anatomy	Surgery
I	Smaller thumb, all structures present		No intervention
II	Hypoplastic thenar muscles, There is also hypoplasia of thumb metacarpal, phalanges and radial carpal bones. There may be only one neurovascular bundle. Narrow first web space. Instability of MCP joint especially UCL		Increase the first web space, stabilize the MCP joint, improve opposition, and improve flexion and extension at the IP joint
III	Absent thenar muscles, very reduced first web space, ulnar collateral ligament instability of the MCP joint. Varying degrees of partial aplasia of the proximal thumb metacarpal, and thumb extrinsic muscles (EPL, APL, EPB, FPL)		
IIIa		With a CMC joint, and hypoplastic extrinsic muscles	As type II
IIIb		Without a CMC joint, and thumb extrinsic extensors absent	Debatable: some argue for reconstruction, others for removal and pollicization
IV	Pouce flottant, (floating thumb or pendel daumen). No metacarpal or musculo-tendinous structures		Pollicization of the index finger
V	Absent thumb		Pollicization of the index finger

Box 13.13.9 Thumb reconstruction

- First web space—improve width and depth
- MCP joint stabilization (occasionally fusion)
- UCL reconstruction
- Oppensplasty
- EIP or EDM transfer for thumb extension/flexion *or*
- Pollicization

Poland's syndrome

Pectoral and hand anomalies were described in 1841 by Alfred Poland, a medical student at Guy's Hospital, London. With an incidence of 1:20 000–30 000 the condition is rare but well known. The sex ratio is equal but the right side is affected twice as commonly as the left. The aetiology is unknown but there are a few families identified with an inherited form. Left-sided Poland's syndrome is also linked with leukaemia, non-Hodgkin's lymphoma, and dextrocardia. The current theory is that the musculoskeletal malformations seen in Poland's and symbrachydactyly stem from a disrupted subclavian artery occurring in the sixth week of gestation as the ribs grow forward and medially causing a subclavian artery kink and the subclavlan artery supply disruption sequence.

In Poland's syndrome the hand anomaly is the most obvious defect. It varies from syndactyly and symbrachydactyly to amputation. The upper limb girdle and chest anomalies are less obvious but consist of a hypoplastic forearm or arm, an absent sternal (and sometimes clavicular) head of pectoralis major, deficiency or absence of pectoralis minor, latissimus dorsi, serratus anterior and other shoulder muscles, hypoplastic breast and nipple, abnormal ribs and costal cartilages with deficient subcutaneous fat and axillary hair, and the sternum may rotate to the involved side causing a contralateral carinatum deformity.

The hand conditions are treated appropriately by syndactyly correction or by deepening the webs to create the illusion of longer fingers. The first web often needs a flap to deepen and widen it. The deformity of the rib cage occasionally requires surgical correction. The anterior axillary fold is reconstructed by using a latissimus dorsi transposition by detaching its insertion and transferring it forward on the humerus or by contralateral latissimus dorsi free flap transfer if the muscle is absent.

Females may need tissue expansion of their breast through puberty, followed by a permanent implant. The thin chest subcutaneous tissue will need simultaneous latissimus dorsi transfer. There are autologous tissue alternatives.

V Overgrowth

Macrodactyly

Congenital overgrowth of a digit is rare (2:100 000 live births, 1% of all congenital anomalies). It may be a component of other hypertrophic conditions or gigantism. Ninety per cent are unilateral but involving more than one digit. The index and middle digits are most commonly affected: distally more than proximally (Figure 13.13.16). The cause is unknown but probably varies with the type of overgrowth. There is a theory that the commonest type 'progressively growing lipofibromatous nerve overgrowth' is related to neural growth factors (Box 13.13.10).

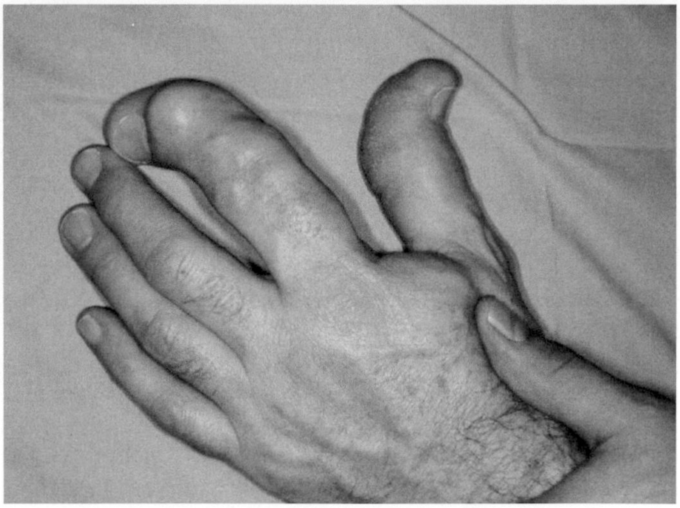

Fig. 13.13.16 Macrodactyly of the thumb and index finger in an adult.

Primary macrodactyly has generalized soft tissue enlargement of lipofibromatous tissue. This follows a nerve-like distribution and so often affects one side of a digit or ray, frequently following the median nerve.

Secondary macrodactyly may occur with a variety of conditions.

Pathologically four types have been described: lipofibromatous, neurofibromatous, hyperostotic, hemihypertrophy or Proteus syndrome.

Management

Surgery is indicated for poor function or cosmetic concerns. Surgery aims to create a relatively normal sized digit with some function. The operative options are amputation; reduction (by combination of bone excision, osteotomies to correct angulation and soft tissue excision perhaps including the nerve); epiphysiodesis (if at age 10 the digit is already the size of the parents). Reduction of a macrodactyly is performed through a midlateral incision on the convex side of the digit, extending in an L-shaped pattern at the pulp. Excise the fat, enlarged digital nerve, and the

Box 13.13.10 Macrodactyly

- Primary (non-syndromic)
- Secondary (associated conditions), e.g.:
  - Neurofibromatosis
  - Vascular malformations
  - Proteus syndrome
  - Ollier's enchondromatosis
  - Albright's polyostotic fibrous dysplasia
- Static or progressive.

overlying skin. Perform a closing wedge osteotomy of the proximal phalanx and excise sufficient middle and distal phalanx to shorten the digit and fuse the DIP joint. A nail partial excision to reduce the length and width of the nail will complete the procedure. Secondary surgery is often required.

VI Amniotic band syndrome/ constriction ring

Amniotic band syndrome (also known as constriction ring syndrome)

Amniotic band syndrome is a congenital disorder mostly affecting the limbs but occasionally seen around the trunk and face. It is thought to be caused by amniotic bands that wind around extremities, possibly related to perforation of the amniotic sac but alternative theories do exist. Interestingly 50% have more than one limb affected. It occurs in 1:2000–15 000 births. There is an association with oligohydramnios, cleft lip and palate, and talipes. The central digits and the hands are most commonly affected (Table 13.13.12).

Clinically, the appearances are diagnostic for types 1, 2, and 3. With amputation the diagnosis is more difficult, though unlike symbrachydactyly there is tapering of the stumps and there are no nail remnants. X-rays show amputation occurring through bone or joint and the remaining part is not hypoplastic. The proximal soft tissue structures are all present, influencing reconstruction. The band if deep may involve or divide major nerves or vessels resulting in altered sensibility or a temperature difference below the band even after treatment.

Treatment involves multiple Z-plasties around the band releasing the constriction and flattening the depression by re-distribution of periband fat. Release of any acrosyndactyly should be done before any growth disturbance occurs. In cases with amputation consider lengthening the thumb by distraction, toe transfer or on-top plasty (extending the length of the thumb by moving the index stump on top).

Surgery should be preformed very early if there is any vascular compromise, severe lymphoedema or acrosyndactyly affecting development. Late treatment of distal lymphoedema or macrodactyly may be needed.

VII Generalized conditions

Arthrogryposis (see Chapter 13.9)

The management of arthrogryposis is multidisciplinary. Initially stretches and splinting aim to maintain joint movement with the ultimate goal for the hands to be used at the desk top rather than the traditional aim of one hand extended for toileting and the other flexed for feeding. Management is influenced by the fact that sensation is normal and the patient is usually well motivated.

Table 13.13.12 Classification of amniotic band syndrome (Patterson)

Type	Description
1	Circular groove
2	With distal oedema
3	With acrosyndactyly: Normal web, joined tips Incomplete web, joined tips Fenestration between digits
4	With intrauterine amputation

Madelung's deformity

In 1878, Madelung described a congenital 'dinner-fork' deformity of the distal radius and wrist but credited Dupuytren. This is an inheritable, autosomal dominant condition with incomplete penetrance. It is usually bilateral affecting females more than males. The anomaly occurs on the ulnar palmar aspect of the distal radial growth plate such that the radial side grows but an abnormal bone bar on the ulnar side tethers growth. This leads to early closure of ulnar aspect of distal radial physis. The tether is thought to be an abnormal radiolunate ligament. Madelung's deformity is associated with achondroplasia, Turner's, nail-patella syndrome, Leri–Weill mesomelic dwarfism, dyschondrostosis, and with the *SHOX* (short stature homeobox) gene. This gene affects the mid portion of the limbs, so sitting height is near normal.

Presentation

Madelung's presents usually at age 8–12 years with a spontaneous palmar subluxation of the wrist with increasing radiopalmar and ulnar tilt due to abnormal growth forces, producing a dinner fork-like deformity. Radiographically there is a short bowed radius whose articular surface is inclined in a palmar and ulnar direction. The ulna head is prominent dorsally and a triangular-shaped proximal carpus has the lunate apparently retracted in between the radius and ulna leading to ulna carpal impingement (Figure 13.13.17).

Management

Observation and reassurance is the main method of management as most patients have excellent function. Surgery is considered if there is pain secondary to impingement, degeneration, or gross deformity.

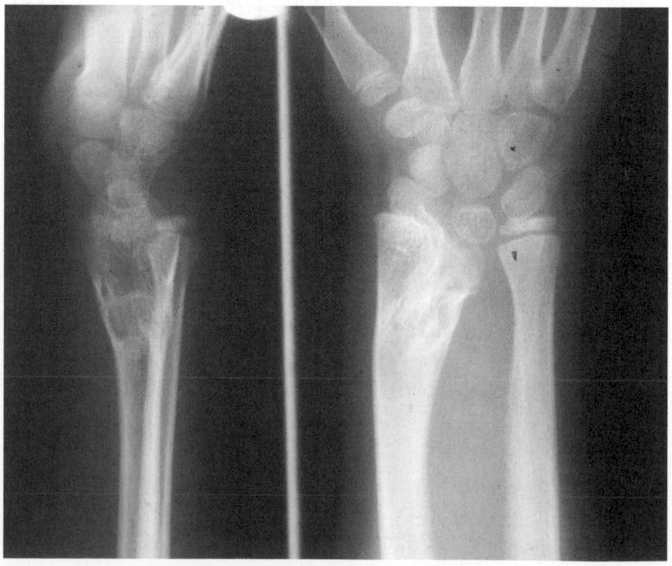

A B

Fig. 13.13.17 AP and lateral radiographs of a wrist demonstrating the classical features associated with a Madelung's deformity.

If the patient presents before skeletal maturity consider an epiphysiolysis and release of the tight tethering radiolunate ligament. After skeletal maturity consider a volar approach releasing the pronator quadratus and radiolunate ligament, followed by a dome osteotomy of the radius to rotate the distal radius into a better position. An ulnar shortening may also be necessary.

Further reading

Buck-Gramcko, D. (1998). *Congenital Malformations of the Hand and Forearm.* London: Churchill Livingston.

Flatt, A. (1994). *The Care of Congenital Hand Anomalies.* St Louis: Quality Medical Publishing.

Gupta, A., Kay, S., and Scheker, L. (2000). *The Growing Hand.* London: Mosby.

Patterson, T.J.S. (1961). Congenital ring-constrictions. *British Journal of Plastic Surgery,* **14**, 1–8.

Rayan, G.M. and Frey, B. (2001). Ulnar polydactyly. *Plastic and Reconstructive Surgery,* **107**, 1449–54.

Swanson A (1976). A classification for congenital limb malformation. *Journal of Hand Surgery,* **1**, 8–22.

Wassel, H.B. (1969). The results of surgery for polydactyly of the thumb. *Clinical Orthopaedics,* **64**, 175–93.

13.14

Management of the limb deficient child

Peter Calder and Rajiv S. Hanspal

Summary points

- The majority of congenital limb defects are sporadic and unilateral
- The skeletal deficiency is described as transverse or longitudinal
- A multidisciplinary approach to management is required
- The balance between surgical reconstruction of the limb vs primary amputation is difficult to find.

Introduction

Congenital limb deficiency is rare, with an overall incidence of 1:2000 live births. In 2005/2006, there were 95 new upper limb and 68 new lower limb referrals to United Kingdom Prosthetic Rehabilitation Centres. Upper limb congenital absence is commoner than lower limb absence with fingers, hands, and forearms most affected. The majority of children will develop coping strategies to deal with their deficiency with many benefiting from prostheses or appliances and a few from surgical intervention. In 2005/2006, only 17% of congenital abnormalities required a surgical amputation, the majority of which involved the lower limb. These procedures usually aid prosthetic fitting or improve cosmetic appearance. Sometimes limb lengthening and/or reconstruction procedures must be considered.

Normal limb development

Limb development begins during the fourth week after fertilization. Thickening of the lateral plate mesoderm occurs opposite the cervicothoracic and lumbosacral segments. The overlying ectoderm differentiates into a ridge known as the apical ectodermal ridge (AER). This controls the proximodistal limb growth by keeping the cells beneath the ridge in a continuous proliferating state. As the limb grows away from the trunk these cells stabilize and differentiate. The femur and humerus are both patterned before cell differentiation; however, formation of the remaining bones and digits depends upon the AER. The lower limb lags behind the upper limb by 1–2 days.

Further control of development in an anteroposterior direction (radial to ulnar) is by the zone of polarizing activity (ZPA), a small area of mesoderm along the posterior border of the limb. The limb development from the dorsal to ventral surface is controlled by the dorsal ectoderm. Ossification begins around the seventh week with vascular invasion and creation of the primary ossification centres within the cartilage anlage model by the process of endochondral ossification.

Control of limb development involves factors such as fibroblast growth factors (FGF)-4 and -8. FGF-4 is present after the AER has been induced; FGF-8 is present before and therefore may be involved in the initiation process. Overexpression of FGF-8 in chick embryos has resulted in limb anomalies: truncations, deletions, and extra digits. The action of the ZPA is related to a protein produced by the sonic hedgehog gene (*SHH*). Other genes involved include the *Wnt-7a*, that controls dorsoventral development, and the *Hox* (homeobox containing) genes that influence proximodistal and anteroposterior patterning.

Aetiology of congenital limb deficiency

The majority of limb defects are unilateral and sporadic. In 60–70% of cases the cause is unknown. Some are associated with known genetic changes resulting in specific syndromes (Table 13.14.1). Chromosomal abnormalities can lead to limb deficiency, for example, trisomy 18 may be associated with a central ray deficiency.

Table 13.14.1 Examples of syndromes associated with limb deficiencies

Syndrome	Main features
TAR	Thrombocytopaenia Absent radius
Fanconi	Upper limb deficiencies (thumb/radius) Occasional hip dysplasia Pancytopaenia—predisposition to leukaemia Cardiac, ophthalmic and urogenital anomalies
Holt–Oram	Cardiac anomalies (ASD) Absent radius or more severe upper limb deficiencies
Roberts	Craniofacial abnormalities Limb deficiencies of varying severity May affect all 4 limbs

Maternal drug ingestion, including both alcohol and smoking, during the first trimester can lead to limb anomalies. In the recent past, thalidomide, prescribed as an antiemetic, resulted in severe multiple limb deficiencies.

Vascular disruption at a critical stage of limb development can result in birth defects. Poland's syndrome presents with unilateral absence of the sternocostal head of pectoralis major muscle, ipsilateral hypoplasia (or absence) of the breast with absence or hypoplasia of the fingers, hand, and occasionally the forearm. It is hypothesized that these deficiencies occur following an interruption of the early embryonic blood supply in the subclavian, vertebral, and/or branch arteries.

True intrauterine amputation in association with amniotic bands is very uncommon. The amnion becomes disrupted resulting in mesenchymal tissue developing fine hair-like structures that wrap around the limbs resulting in amputation or a constriction requiring emergency release soon after delivery.

Classification

Traditionally surgical classifications describe the affected bone and its deficiency, for example fibula hemimelia and proximal femoral focal deficiency (PFFD). While these remain convenient terms for clinical practice, the accepted classification is the International Standards Organization's *Method of Describing Limb Deficiencies at Birth* (ISO 8548-1, 1989). The system describes the skeletal element deficiency as either transverse or longitudinal.

- *Transverse deficiencies* resemble surgical amputations and are described by the level at which the limb ends. If a long bone is partially deficient the level is quantified, for example, 'transverse deficiency, forearm, upper third'. If the deficiency is at the elbow level the classification is 'transverse deficiency, forearm total'. Vestigial digital buds may be present (Figure 13.14.1)
- *Longitudinal deficiencies* are described by naming the absent or deficient bones. The description passes proximal to distal describing partial or complete absence. For example, PFFD is 'longitudinal deficiency femur, partial upper third' (Figure 13.14.2).

Principles of management

The birth of a child with congenital limb deficiency is a cause of great anxiety to the family. They require support along with adequate explanation of the condition and its management and with reassurance that experts are available for advice and assistance. Information given to parents and family should be accurate and avoid unrealistic expectations and if an antenatal diagnosis has been made on fetal ultrasound, an early referral to a Prosthetic Rehabilitation Centre could be considered.

Provided there are no associated congenital abnormalities, these children are expected to develop normally until they are old enough to compare themselves to their peers. The lifelong management of patients with congenital limb deficiencies may involve different professional disciplines at different stages. The emphasis of management is on the needs of the child and thus as the needs change with growth from childhood to adulthood so does the management. Good liaison between the Paediatric Services, Limb Deficiency and Prosthetic Clinics, and the orthopaedic or plastic surgeons is vital. Combined clinics are recommended to facilitate management plans.

The child with a limb deficiency requires a multidisciplinary approach for both the child's clinical condition and the psychological support for the family. In the lower limb, our treatment algorithm (Figure 13.14.3) always raises the question of possible limb reconstruction. For the lower limb, the aim is that at skeletal maturity, the legs will be of equal length with a stable foot and good, pain-free function. Upper limb reconstruction may involve procedures such as pollicization in cases of absent thumbs, carpal centralization in radial hemimelia, or ulna lengthening in ulna hemimelia to provide support for the carpus. (For further details see Chapter 13.13.)

In cases where limb reconstruction is considered unachievable, treatment concentrates on providing support and improving function. This may consist of simple advice, appliances (e.g. to hold cutlery), orthotics, or prostheses. Surgical intervention is indicated in only a minority of cases. Procedures are performed for cosmesis or to improve prosthetic fitting, the latter by removal of obstructing

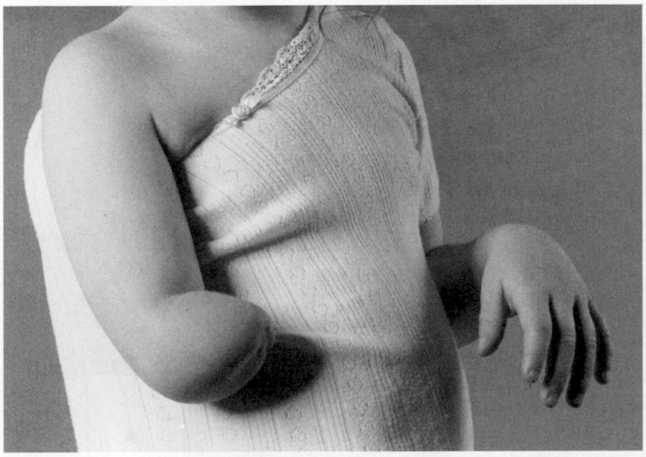
A

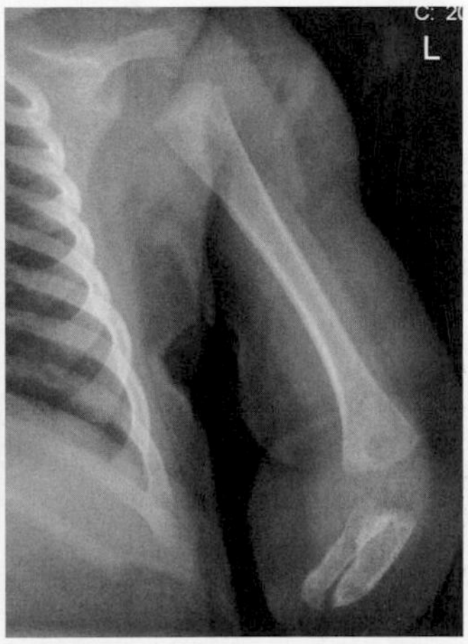

B

Fig. 13.14.1 A) Child with a right transverse deficiency of the forearm, upper third. B) Radiograph of an infant's left upper limb demonstrating the same type of transverse upper limb deficiency as in (A).

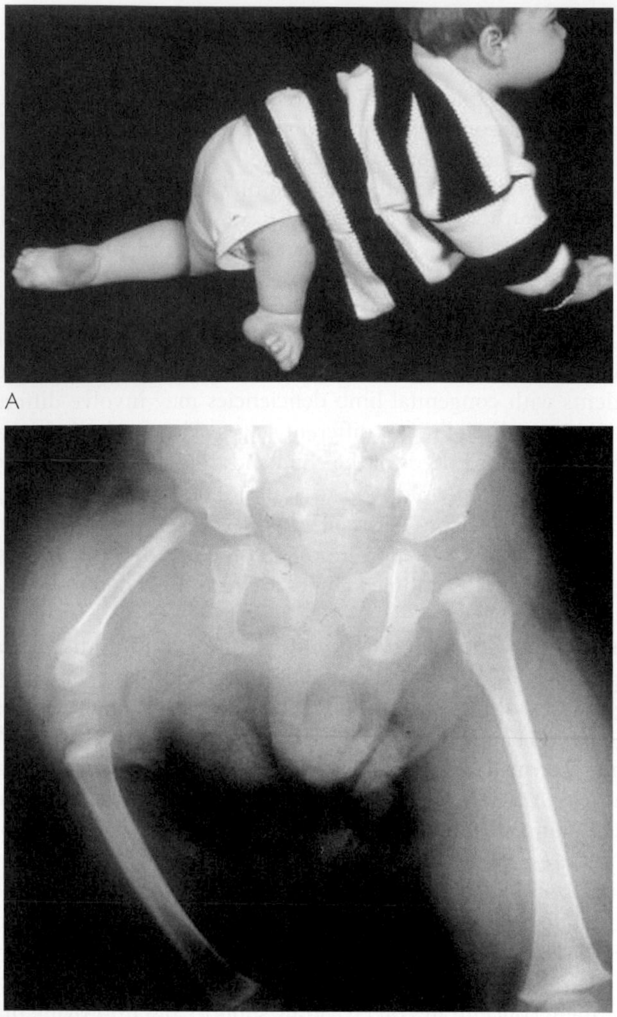

Fig. 13.14.2 A) Clinical photograph of an infant with a Right PFFD. The length of the whole right leg equals the length of the thigh on the normal side—posing no problem to crawling! B) AP radiograph of the same child showing a right PFFD with a poor quality hip joint—a predictor of final function.

appendages (Syme's disarticulation) or correction of deformity (lateral femoral hypoplasia creating genu valgum or significant tibial bowing in complete fibula absence).

In the growing child, the optimal level for a surgical amputation is a disarticulation (or a 'through joint' amputation).This reduces the risk of bone overgrowth: a common complication of diaphyseal amputations particularly with transtibial or transhumeral levels where the growing end of the bone is retained in the residual limb. The overgrowth can result in pain, bursa formation, and skin ulceration often requiring surgical revision. Through joint amputation or disarticulation also offers a larger end-bearing surface and better proprioreceptive properties. The malleolar or condylar flare also aids suspension and rotational control of the prosthesis.

Specific treatments

Upper limb deficiencies

Transverse

Transverse radial deficiency is the commonest level of congenital limb loss in children (see Figure 13.14.1). The management is prosthetic replacement, as part of an overall rehabilitation programme, with virtually no place for surgical intervention. As children are generally likely to benefit from prostheses, they should be introduced to them early. This allows the child to learn and make valid choices, based on personal experience. However, many children prefer not to use any prostheses at all, or opt to use it part time for specific tasks or for cosmetic purposes.

The rehabilitation programme starts with a simple cosmetic arm (Figure 13.14.4) first provided when independent sitting balance is achieved at 6 months. A functioning prosthesis, either body powered (Figure 13.14.5) or with electric controls (Figure 13.14.6) can be introduced at 18–24 months of age, when the child is better established with walking. The first powered prostheses use switch controls incorporated in a shoulder loop. Later, surface electrodes are used to pick up signals from extensor and flexor muscles for opening and closing myoelectric hands. The increased weight of these prostheses may limit their use in younger children. With increasing maturity (and as required) more complicated control

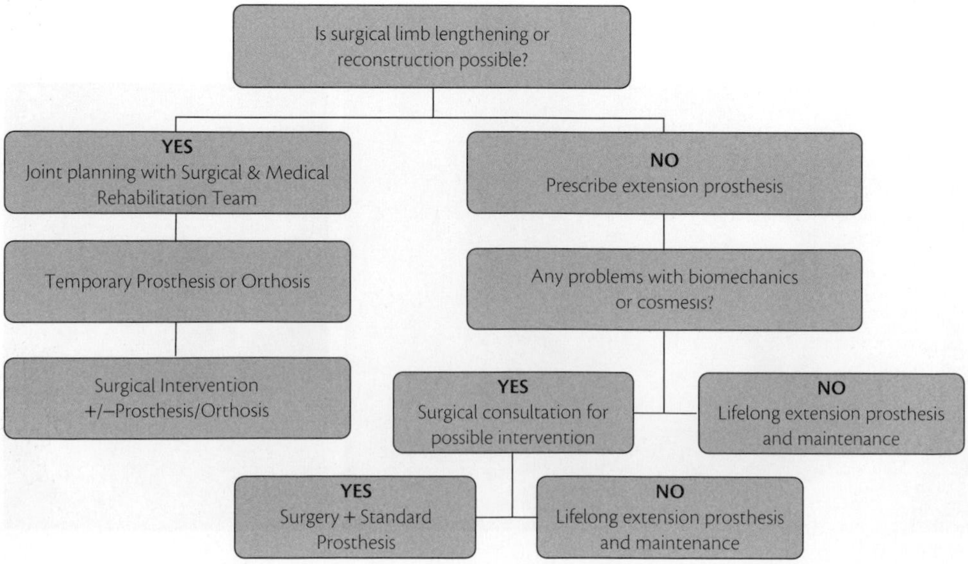

Fig. 13.14.3 Algorithm for management of congenital limb deficiency (Calder and Hanspal).

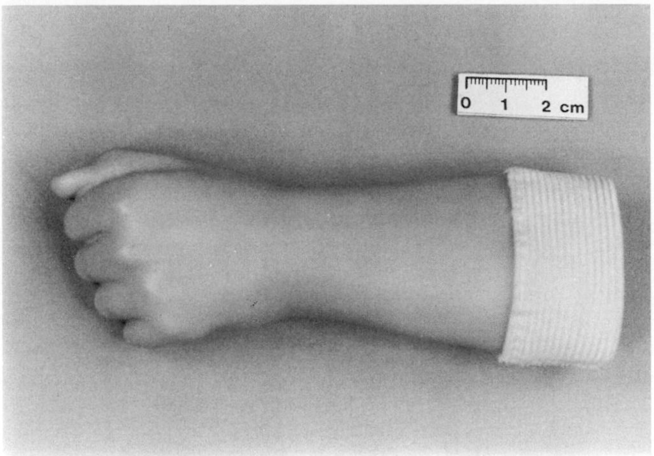

Fig. 13.14.4 A simple cosmetic infant arm, often termed a 'crawling hand' prosthesis.

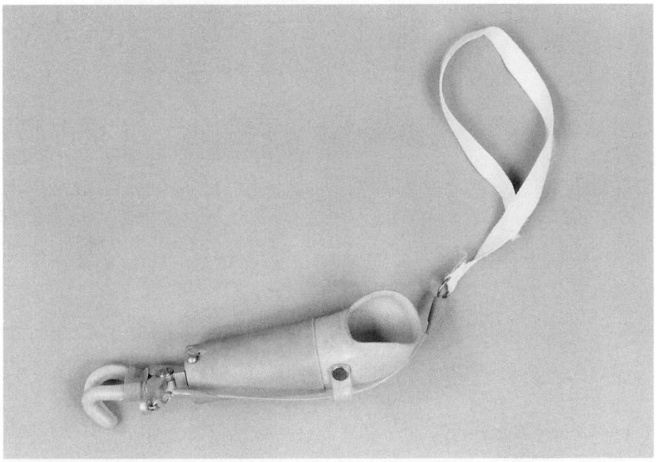

Fig. 13.14.5 Exoskeletal prosthesis for transverse deficiency of the forearm with a split hoot 'hand' and an operating cord.

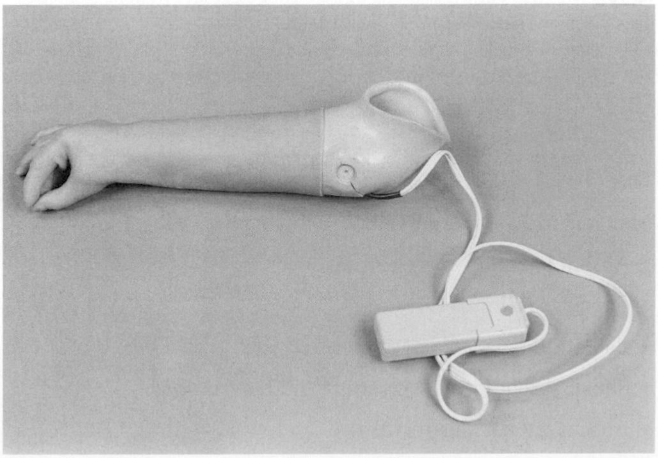

Fig. 13.14.6 Myoelectric prosthesis for transverse deficiency of the forearm. Note the electrode on the socket and the remote battery. This would be incorporated within the forearm of a larger child.

mechanisms and additional tasks can be added to the limb. A specialist occupational therapist is crucial in training the patient how to use the limb and for advice on the use of other appliances, aids or 'gadgets' and how to manage one-handed activities.

Prostheses for more proximal levels of limb deficiencies (through elbow or transhumeral) are appreciably more difficult to use because of the need to control the prosthetic elbow. A figure-of-eight harness is required for suspension and control and the electric prostheses are heavy. 'Hybrid' prostheses may be required. Many patients opt for a passive function or cosmetic prosthesis and even those who have a functioning prosthesis often use them simply as a cosmetic arm. A comprehensive review of the literature over the past 25 years showed that there is a rejection rate of 45% in body-powered and 35% in myoelectric prostheses in children, although, worldwide, a wide variance is reported.

Children with distal limb loss (partial hand or transcarpal), if unilateral, generally function very well without active prosthetic intervention. However 'appliances' or orthoses in the form of simple leather gauntlets with pockets to hold cutlery or cup sockets for cycle handle bars or other activities need to be considered as part of the rehabilitation and management. Recently, myoelectric prostheses have been made available for transcarpal or partial hand levels of limb loss.

Longitudinal (see Chapter 13.13)

These deficiencies are less common and tend to be bilateral. They sometimes occur as part of various syndromes, for example VATER (vertebral defects, imperforate anus, tracheo-oesophageal fistula, radial and renal dysplasia), Holt–Oram syndrome, Fanconi syndrome, TAR (thrombocytopaenia and absent radius) syndrome, etc. (see Table 13.14.1).

Unlike transverse deficiencies, surgical reconstruction has a major role in maintaining optimum hand function in longitudinal limb deficiencies (Box 13.14.1). Radial longitudinal deficiency is commoner than ulnar longitudinal deficiency. Centralization of the hand or 'radialization' have been recommended but results are not always encouraging in the long term. Pollicization is generally recommended after these procedures to establish pinch grip. However these procedures are contraindicated in the presence of severe restriction of elbow function because the repositioned hand is unable to reach the face.

Longitudinal ulnar deficiency is associated with variable degrees of deficiencies in the hand on the ulnar side. The radius is short and associated with a functionless elbow and possible fusion of the radius with the humerus. Function is often better than expected. Various surgical procedures have been attempted but radical surgery is best avoided. Function is assisted by use of various aids, appliances, and other forms of orthoses.

Box 13.14.1 Surgical options (see Chapter 13.13)

- Absent thumb—consider pollicization
- Cleft hand—consider closure
- Syndactyly—consider release
- Finger deficiencies—reconstruction for pinch grip.

Congenital deficiencies in the hand may be an absence of the thumb, central hand deficiency (cleft hand), syndactyly, or absence of a number of digits.

Cleft hand function is usually good without surgery and syndactyly can be released if felt appropriate. With severe finger deficiencies, reconstruction or rarely finger prostheses are used to provide a pinch grip.

Lower limb deficiencies

Transverse

Transverse lower limb deficiencies are rare and surgical intervention is usually unnecessary. This type of limb loss is managed with a prosthesis, just like an acquired amputation at the same level. When limb loss is unilateral, they are well tolerated with good function.

For forefoot absence or complete metatarsal loss, a total contact silicone prosthetic foot may be provided. If the residual limb is hypoplastic or there is a Chopart-type amputation (partial tarsal) additional support will be required above the ankle such as a plastic or leather bootee with an ankle–foot orthosis. Alternatively, a Syme's disarticulation may be indicated with an appropriate appliance and later the possibility of revising this to a standard transtibial prosthesis. Total absence of the foot will require similar prostheses. A Syme's appliance in children does not have the same problem of poor cosmesis as for adults, because as the child grows, the malleoli tend to be hypoplastic and a standard below knee prostheses can be used.

Transverse limb loss at a higher level requires a standard lower limb prosthesis to compensate for the partial or complete tibial deficiency or the partial femoral loss (Figure 13.14.7). Treatment should start when the child begins to show signs of standing independently. For above knee levels, the introduction of a flexible knee unit may need to be delayed. Unilateral complete absence of the lower limb is worth treating with a prosthesis but the prosthetic socket encompasses both hips and presents practical problems in daily living. Regular follow-up is essential to allow modifications or replacement to the prostheses to accommodate for growth.

Longitudinal

Fibula hemimelia (Box 13.14.2)

This is the most common congenital lower limb deficiency. The diagnosis covers a spectrum of limb deformities often involving proximal and distal anomalies both in the femur and in the foot, such as tarsal coalition and absence of the lateral ray. The fibula itself can simply be smaller in size but in the most severe cases it may be completely absent (Table 13.14.2).

Treatment guidelines were highlighted by Birch et al. (1998) in their 'Functional classification of fibular deficiency' (Table 13.14.3). Patients are divided by possessing a functional foot or a non-functional foot, and further divided by leg length discrepancy: minor discrepancies may be considered for equalization but a discrepancy of 30% or more would require multiple lengthenings and could be considered for amputation (Box 13.14.3).

Our preferred amputation for a severe Type I is the modified Syme's disarticulation (Figure 13.14.8). The remaining stump acts as a below-knee level amputation at skeletal maturity and is fitted with the corresponding type of prosthesis. The Boyd type amputation may be considered but difficulties in placing the calcaneum

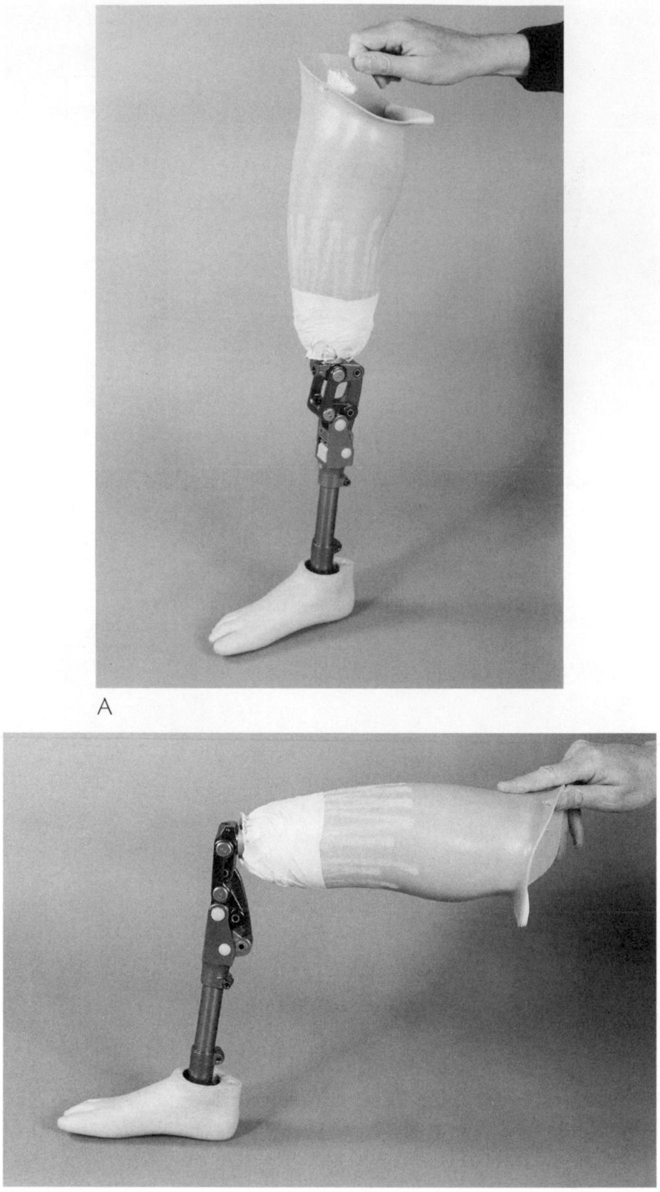

A

B

Fig. 13.14.7 A) Endoskeletal prosthesis, at fitting stage and without cosmetic cover, for transverse deficiency of the leg, total ('transverse loss at knee level') with an ischial bearing socket. Note the polycentric knee joint that allows a stable free-knee gait. B) Same prosthesis with polycentric knee in flexed position for sitting.

Box 13.14.2 Fibula hemimelia

May include some or all of the following features:

- Absent lateral rays of the foot
- Tarsal coalition
- Ball and socket ankle joint
- Short, absent fibula with short and bowed tibia
- Absent cruciate ligaments
- Deficient lateral femoral condyle
- Short, externally rotated femur.

Table 13.14.2 Classification of fibula hemimelia (Achterman and Kalamchi)

Type	Description
I	Fibula present
Ia	Proximal fibula below the proximal tibial physis and distal fibula above the talar dome
Ib	Fibula much shorter than in Ia
II	Fibula absent

Table 13.14.3 Functional classification of fibula hemimelia

Type	Description
I	Functional foot (3 rays or more)
Ia	0–5% LLD
Ib	6–10% LLD
Ic	11–30% LLD
Id	>30% LLD
II	Non-functional foot
IIa	Functional proximal limb component

Box 13.14.3 Functional classification of fibular deficiency

- How good is the foot?
- How big is the limb length discrepancy?

below the tibia can be encountered as the calcaneum is often in significant equinus and adherent to the posterior cortex of the tibial shaft.

Type II cases with a non-functional foot are further subdivided into IIA with a functional proximal component of the limb, treated with amputation as described earlier and IIB with a non-functional proximal part. In these cases salvage procedures are considered as the foot may become important for function.

Other surgical interventions may be necessary for associated femoral deformity such as the genu valgum secondary to lateral femoral hypoplasia (Figure 13.14.8B).

Tibial hemimelia

This uncommon condition is characterized by complete or partial loss of the tibia but usually with the presence of a normal fibula. Clinically, there is anterolateral bowing of the lower leg with equinovarus position of the foot. There may be duplication of the toes and associated hand anomalies. Jones classified tibial deficiency into four types (Table 13.14.4 and Figure 13.14.9).

Classic recommendations dictate knee disarticulation for types 1a and 3, and below-knee amputation for types 1b and 2. Reconstruction may be considered in types 1b, 2, and 4 either by limb lengthening or consideration of ipsilateral fibula transfer using Brown's procedure.

Femoral deficiency

Femoral deficiency may present with subtotal absence of the femur, true PFFD (see Figure 13.14.2), or simple femoral hypoplasia, with a femur that is normal anatomically but simply smaller than the contralateral bone. There are several classifications in the literature describing the spectrum of radiological appearances that can be seen.

Radiographs alone may, however, be misleading of the actual femoral length, especially if the film is taken with the limb in its

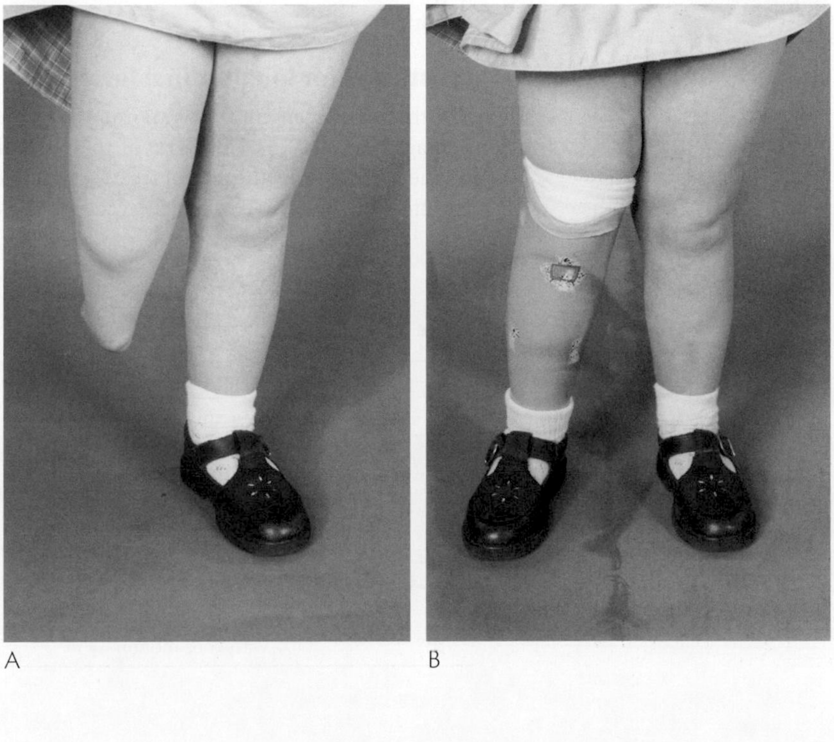
A B

Fig. 13.14.8 A) Child with a Syme's amputation for longitudinal deficiency of fibula, total, tarsus partial, rays 4 and 5 total (Type 1d fibula hemimelia, Table 13.14.2). B) Same child wearing her prosthesis. Note genu valgum which is part of the anomaly.

characteristic resting posture of hip flexion, abduction, and external rotation. Although radiographs obviously aid in management decisions, they should be used in conjunction with a full clinical assessment of the limb. The function and possible fixed contractures of the hip and knee joints will impact on surgical intervention (see Figure 13.14.2B).

Gillespie and Torode initially recognized two broad groups—true PFFD and congenital short femur. Later a change was proposed that would take into account the clinical features. Group A consist of congenital short femur with no hip instability and minimal fixed flexion of hip and knee. By extending the limb the foot lies opposite the mid part of the contralateral tibia or lower. The shortening will be 20% or less. Group B are an exaggeration of group A, the thigh is short and bulbous with the hip in flexion, abduction and external rotation. There is a sense of proximal instability with 'pistoning' of the proximal femur. When the limb is pulled down into extension the foot lies at the level of the opposite knee or shorter, the knee fixed flexion persists. Group C represents those patients with a subtotal loss of the femur. There is marked proximal instability with a similar clinical appearance to group B.

Table 13.14.4 Classification of tibial hemimelia

Type	Description
1a	Absent tibia
1b	Rudimentary tibia
2	Ossified proximal tibia, distal portion absent
3	Proximal tibia absent Diaphysis and distal tibia present
4	Shortened tibia with diastasis of the distal tibiofibular joint

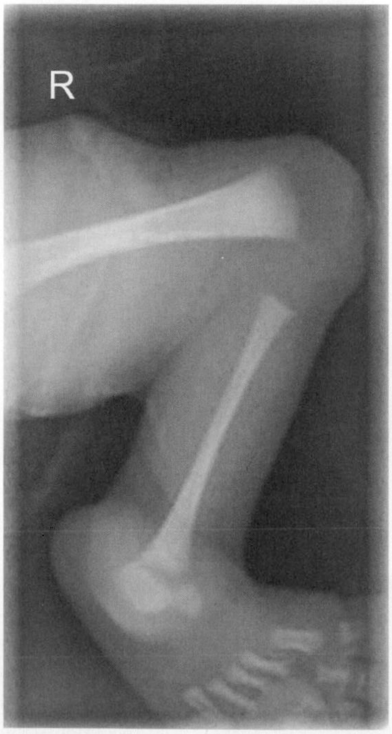

Fig. 13.14.9 Lateral radiograph of a child with a type 1a tibial dysplasia: note the well formed foot, the seemingly 'normal' fibula and the absence of a normal contour to the 'knee'.

In *group B* the proximal femur tends to flex anteriorly during weight bearing. This makes prosthetic fitting difficult: treatment options include performing an arthrodesis of the knee in combination with an ankle disarticulation. This produces a single lever arm with the aim of leaving the end of the limb slightly proximal to the opposite knee and allowing an above knee prosthesis to be fitted.

In *group C* patients, due to the femur being so much shorter, anterior displacement of the thigh segment does not occur and therefore knee fusion may not be required as an ischial bearing prosthesis can be fitted more easily.

An alternative procedure is the van Nes rotationplasty, described in 1950. The aim with this procedure is to fuse the knee as above whilst rotating the foot 180 degrees to leave the ankle lying at the level of the opposite knee. The gastrocnemius and soleus muscles then act as 'knee' extensors and a below-knee type prosthesis may be fitted. We have no experience of this technique. A comparison between the two procedures emphasized the need for individual treatment plans. With a good hip and adequate ankle function then the rotationplasty allows more 'normal' function as judged clinically, but there can be a psychological price to pay due to the abnormal cosmetic appearance.

Recently, authors have emphasized again the importance of knee mobility and knee deficiency in patient management and some feel that knee function is of greater importance than hip stability (Table 13.14.5).

The strategy of Paley's treatment algorithm is for reconstruction from proximal to distal thus ultimately reconstructing a functional limb of equal length. He does accept that amputation may be the preferred option in type 3 cases.

Finally, the Steel femoropelvic fusion is a procedure that may be considered in those severe cases of significant diaphyseal femoral loss (Gillespie Group C, Paley Type 3). The femur is fused to the pelvis in a flexed position to allow the knee to act as the 'hip'. A good result allows the patient to function as an above-knee amputee.

Prostheses for longitudinal lower limb deficiencies

Prosthetic replacement forms an important and integral part of the management of PFFD. Because of the inevitable limb shortening on the affected side, the aim of treatment is to equalize limb length for effective gait. This can be achieved by simple devices like heel or

Table 13.14.5 Paley classification of PFFD

Type	Description
1	Intact femur, mobile hip and knee
2	Mobile pseudarthrosis of the proximal femur
2a	with a mobile femoral head in the acetabulum
2b	with a stiff hip
3	Diaphyseal femoral deficiency
3a	with knee motion >45°
3b	with knee motion <45°

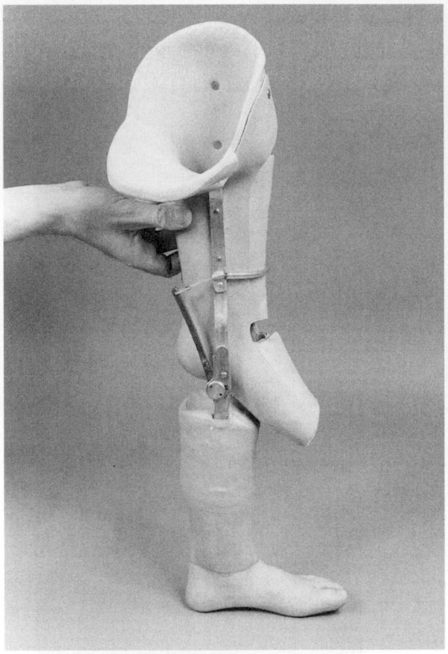
A
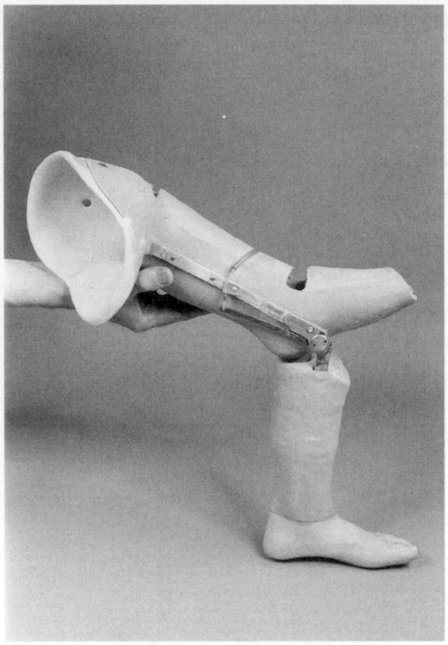
B

Fig. 13.14.10 A) Exoskeletal extension prosthesis for young child with longitudinal deficiency of femur, partial, upper third (PFFD) with external knee hinges and knee lock and an ischial bearing socket. B) Same prosthesis flexed in the sitting position: the lower part of the socket which accommodates the natural foot, projects awkwardly.

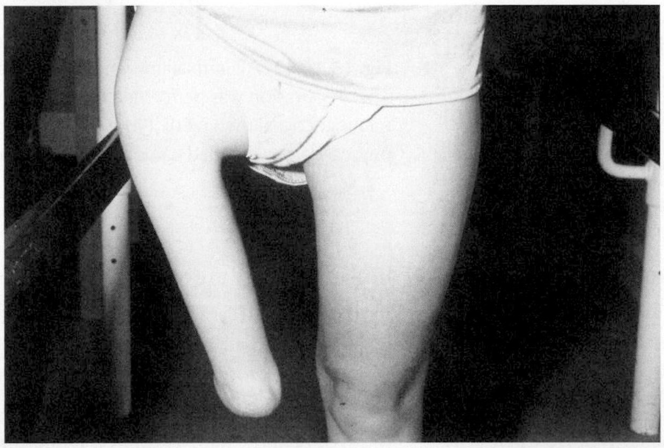
A
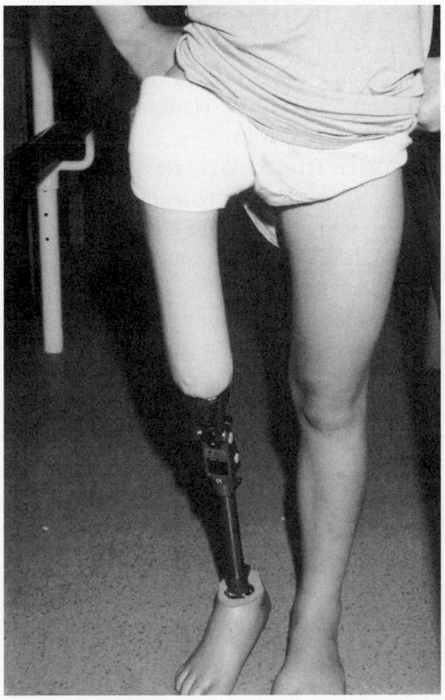
B
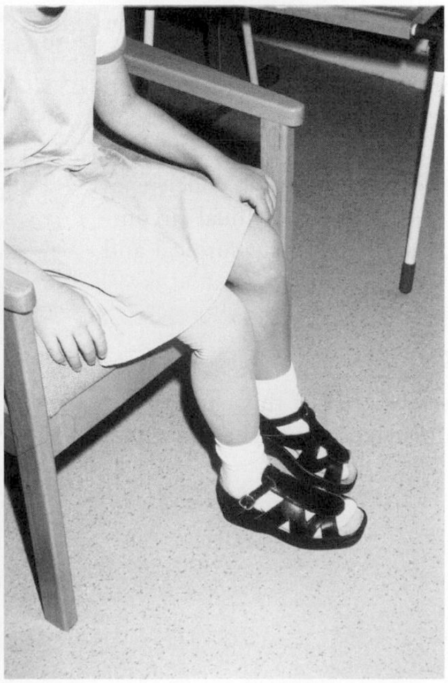
C

Fig. 13.14.11 A) Child with a right longitudinal deficiency of the femur, partial upper third (PFFD) following a Syme's amputation. The end of the stump approximates to the level of the contralateral knee. B) Same child wearing an endoskeletal prosthesis at fitting stage with polycentric knee. She walks with a free knee gait. C) Same child sitting, wearing her completed prosthesis. Foot amputation and the use of a polycentric prosthetic knee has much improved the cosmesis compared with an extension prosthesis as seen in Figure 13.14.9.

shoe raises if the shortening is minimal. If the shortening is significant and greater than that which can be managed reasonably with a shoe raise, an 'extension prostheses' is used. This is essentially a prostheses accommodated distally to the end of the short limb, effectively 'extending' it to the ground level and attached proximally to the short limb by enclosing it in the prosthetic socket. The design and construction varies, dependant on the deformity including shape and size of the residual limb and joint function and understandably they are not particularly aesthetic (Figure 13.14.10). Sometimes, surgical intervention may be advisable, to improve function and appearance by facilitating use of standard below or above-knee prostheses. Thus, a Syme's disarticulation in a child with fibular hemimelia or PFFD with a stable hip joint may allow use of a cosmetically more acceptable, standard transtibial or transfemoral prosthesis (Figure 13.14.11).

All categories of patients with femoral shortening should initially be treated with extension prostheses to allow them to stand up when they are ready to do so, generally around the ages of 12–18 months. In patients with a severe form of PFFD with no true hip joint and the knee virtually at the hip level and with associated fixed contracture, the prostheses needs to be ischial tuberosity bearing. Rarely, they may need to enclose the whole pelvis. If the foot is a significant cosmetic problem, a Syme's disarticulation should be recommended. With an intermediate degree of PFFD and minor loss of hip extension, an arthrodeses of the knee joint and Syme's amputation may allow the use of standard transfemoral prostheses if the resultant stump length is approximately equal to the contralateral femur. In practice, this is most effective and appropriate in those patients who have associated distal limb deficiencies in the fibula and foot.

The principles for prosthetic prescription for distal deficiencies are similar. An extension prosthesis is provided for limb shortening, if it is too great to be overcome conveniently with an orthosis or shoe raise. However, the extension prostheses may not need to extend proximal to the knee joint. If a Syme's disarticulation has been performed, a standard transtibial prosthesis will be appropriate, and cosmetically preferred. Good function is achieved. If a knee disarticulation has been performed, a standard prosthesis for the appropriate level is prescribed. It should be noted that a transfemoral prosthesis is often appropriate for a knee disarticulation because of the associated minor femoral shortening and knee clearance available.

Prosthetic management for longitudinal lower limb deficiencies is challenging. Each case has to be assessed on individual circumstances and management planned jointly with the surgical and medical rehabilitation teams.

Acquired limb deficiency

Discussion of this topic is outside the remit of this chapter but many of the principles that govern management of the congenital limb deficiency are applied to patients with acquired limb deficiency: in both groups, consideration must always be given to possible problems with the opposite lower limb (Figure 13.14.12).

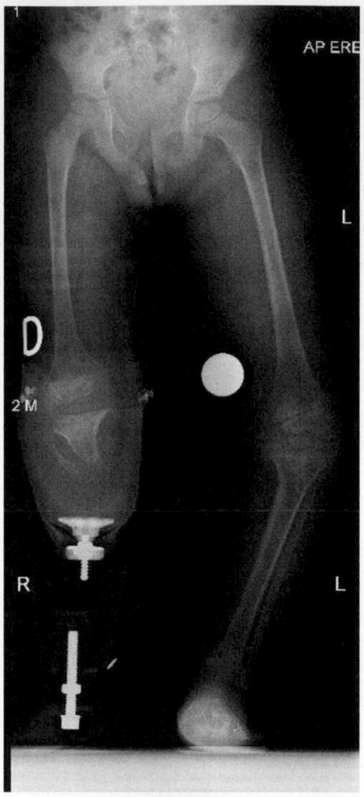

Fig. 13.14.12 AP limb alignment radiograph of a child with a right BK prosthesis. The amputation was performed following complications associated with meningococcal meningitis. Note that the left leg has also been affected and the physeal damage has led to both shortening and angulation.

Further reading

Biddiss, E. and Chau, T. (2007). Upper limb prosthetic use and abandonment: A survey of the last 25 years. *Prosthetics and Orthotics International*, **31**(3), 236–57.

British Society of Rehabilitation Medicine (2003). Amputee and Prosthetic Rehabilitation – Standards and Guidelines, second edition; Report of the Working Party (Chair: Hanspal, RS). London: British Society of Rehabilitation Medicine.

Day, H.J.B. (1991). The ISO/ISPO classification of congenital limb deficiency. *Prosthetics and Orthotics International*, **15**, 67–9.

Herring, J.A. and Birch, J.G. (1998). *The Child With a Limb Deficiency.* Rosemont, IL: American Academy of Orthopaedic Surgeons.

Jones, D., Barnes, J., and Lloyd-Roberts, G. (1978). Congenital aplasia and dysplasia of the tibia with intact fibula: classification and management. *Journal of Bone and Joint Surgery*, **60B**, 31–9.

13.15

The management of limb length inequality

Fergal Monsell

Summary points

- Limb length inequality is common: prediction of the final discrepancy at skeletal maturity is important to allow appropriate management plans to be made
- Knowledge of the underlying cause helps with prognosis
- Management is influenced by various factors including age and height and often involves a combination of treatment methods.

Introduction

Limb length inequality occurs as a result of a spectrum of musculoskeletal conditions. The degree of asymmetry ranges from a subtle difference without functional consequence, to major congenital reduction deformities (see Chapter 13.14). These patients present in general orthopaedic practice and a robust knowledge of the natural history and an appreciation of the likely short- and long-term functional consequences of each condition is essential for sensible management. This chapter discusses diagnosis, clinical and radiological assessment, including methods of prediction of final discrepancy, and management strategies that include various treatment options.

Aetiology

Length discrepancy occurs acutely due to fracture malunion or because of retardation or stimulation of limb growth in childhood. Growth retardation may be secondary to congenital reduction syndromes, growth plate injury or neurological abnormality. Shapiro *et al.* recognized that specific patterns of retardation were a function of the causative pathology. Identification of the cause allows prediction of final discrepancy, particularly in conditions where this evolves at a constant rate. Growth stimulation may be a feature of conditions such as juvenile idiopathic arthritis, trauma, vascular malformation syndromes, and neurofibromatosis.

In the major congenital reduction syndromes, the discrepancy increases in proportion to longitudinal limb growth. The evolution of the discrepancy has been demonstrated using antenatal ultrasonography and with serial radiographs in childhood. It remains constant from the time of fetal limb formation until skeletal maturity.

Physeal injury following acute fracture, local infection or generalized septicaemia has a profound affect on growth, particularly around the knee. As the rate of growth at each site is known, the limb length discrepancy at skeletal maturity can be predicted. These growth plate injuries, when incomplete, are often associated with additional sagittal, coronal, and rotational deformities. Neurological conditions including hemiplegic cerebral palsy and poliomyelitis also cause a predictable reduction in leg length related to the degree of involvement in cerebral palsy and the age of onset and extent of involvement in poliomyelitis. Variable overgrowth related to age of onset, extent of synovial involvement, and response to therapy complicates inflammatory conditions such as juvenile idiopathic arthritis. Other conditions that cause a discrepancy by stimulation include some vascular malformation syndromes and neurofibromatosis. All tend to increase in proportion to normal growth. Overgrowth following fracture does occur but unpredictably. The common causes of limb length inequality are outlined in Table 13.15.1.

Clinical assessment

Initial clinical assessment involves visual analysis of the pattern of walking, barefoot and with shoes/orthotics, to identify compensatory strategies. Long-standing minor discrepancies may produce no more than a subtle abnormality in the gait pattern.

The patient is examined standing comfortably to attention and features such as dipping of the short side pelvis, flexion of the long side knee, and equinus of the short side ankle noted (Box 13.15.1). Active and passive joint ranges of movement are assessed for all lower limb joints and fixed deformity and contractures identified.

Clinical measurement of limb length discrepancy is imprecise, particularly in the presence of long bone deformity and joint contracture, although measurement between bony points can help document an evolving discrepancy. A simple and reasonably accurate method of assessment uses graduated wooden blocks under the short limb to balance the pelvis until the anterior superior iliac spines are on the same horizontal line. Clinical assessment must include the spine to identify a coexisting postural or structural scoliosis and the upper limbs to identify involvement in congenital reduction and hemiasymmetry syndromes.

It can be surprisingly difficult to define the degree of leg length discrepancy accurately and investigations including plain x-rays may be necessary.

Table 13.15.1 Causes of leg-length inequality

Cause	Shortening	Lengthening
Congenital	Skeletal anomalies (PFFD and dysplasia of tibia and fibula	Partial giantism (Klippel–Trenaunay syndrome)
	Dyschondroplasias	Arteriovenous fistula
	DDH	Congenital hemihypertrophy
	TEV	
	Generalized congenital hemiatrophy	
Infection	Physeal damage	Diaphyseal osteomyelitis
	Tuberculous joints	
	Septic 'arthritis'	
Neurological	Poliomyelitis	
	Cerebral palsy	
	Spinal dysraphism	
Trauma	Physeal damage	Diaphyseal fracture
	Diaphyseal fracture	
Tumours		Neurofibromatosis
		Hemangioma
Other	SUFE	
	Perthes disease	
	Physeal damage from radiation	
	Surgical (e.g. osteotomy)	

DDH, developmental dysplasia of the hip; PFFD, proximal femoral focal deficiency; SUFE, slipped upper femoral epiphysis; TEV, talipes equinovarus.

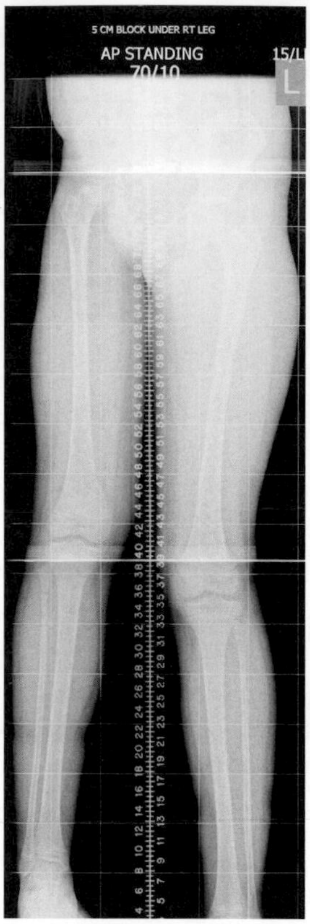

Fig. 13.15.1 Long leg alignment view—the patellae are facing anteriorly and a 5cm block has been placed under the short right leg to balance the pelvis.

Radiological investigations

The bench mark of limb length discrepancy assessment is clinical, with radiographs as necessary to ensure an appropriate degree of accuracy.

The most useful radiograph is the standing long leg alignment view (Figure 13.15.1). The patient is positioned with blocks to accommodate the limb length discrepancy and the limb is aligned with the patella facing anteriorly to produce a reproducible radiograph that allows comparison over time. This is also useful for assessing associated sagittal plane malalignment. With this technique, there is the disadvantage of parallax error due to the single beam.

Box 13.15.1 Leg length discrepancy

In stance:

- Dipping of the short side pelvis
- Flexion of the long leg knee
- Equinus of the short side ankle
- Are there fixed contractures or deformity?

Prediction of final discrepancy

Accurate prediction of the discrepancy at skeletal maturity is of fundamental importance in planning the type and timing of corrective surgery. A number of popular methods of assessment rely on historical growth data. This data was used by Paley to calculate the proportion of final growth of the femur and tibia and he produced the multiplier method of assessment for children of all ages. The product of the measured difference in bone length and the relevant multiplier for age, sex, and site determined the maturity discrepancy for that segment. The information is presented in tabular form and allows straightforward, accurate prediction of leg length discrepancy at maturity.

Estimation of skeletal age

Conventional methods of skeletal maturity assessment use the Greulich and Pyle radiographic atlas and more recently the method of assessment described by Dimeglio (see Chapter 13.23). Recent studies demonstrate that skeletal and chronological ages do not diverge significantly until the later part of skeletal growth. This allows prediction of final discrepancy to be conducted with some confidence without a radiological assessment of skeletal maturity.

The patient's height must be related to that of their parents and an estimation of their pubertal stage made. A simple, additional question as part of the history asks whether the child is tall or short compared to their classmates. For those at the extremes, more care needs to be taken but those in the middle can be assumed to fall within two standard deviations of normal with concordant skeletal and chronological age up until the age of 13 years in girls and 14 years in boys.

Consequences of limb length discrepancy

Conventional wisdom dictates that limb length inequality up to 2.0cm is tolerated without compensatory mechanisms, symptoms or long-term disability. Greater discrepancies lead to secondary compensation and in the short term, the functional leg length is equalized with an equinus posture of the short leg/ankle, a flexion posture of the long leg knee, or a combination of both.

In the longer term, this leads to an oblique pelvis with the potential for 'long leg acetabular dysplasia' and an increased incidence of low back pain and a non-progressive scoliosis. This eventually leads to a loss of spinal mobility with a fixed scoliosis and later radiological abnormalities that include disc space asymmetry, marginal osteophyte formation, and wedging of the vertebral bodies. There is, however, no good statistical correlation between the degree of limb length discrepancy and the incidence of low back pain.

Management

The initial management involves reassurance and a cogent treatment plan made soon after diagnosis. The parents of children born with congenital abnormalities are often distraught. The initial consultation frequently includes questions about the cause, the role of avoidable factors, and the risk to future pregnancies. Unfounded statements at this stage often cause long-standing management difficulties.

It is possible to estimate the final discrepancy in the major congenital abnormalities and this determines whether long-term management should involve surgical or prosthetic reconstruction (Box 13.15.2). The decision is difficult, particularly with recent advances in surgical reconstruction techniques, but in general, a reduction deformity greater than 20–30% with instability of the adjacent joints signifies a very difficult reconstruction with the potential for a functionally poor result in the longer term. Following a decision to manage the deformity with a prosthesis, the purpose of surgery is to improve prosthetic wear and function: procedures include hip reconstruction and amputation of the foot to allow for a more cosmetic prosthesis (see Chapter 13.14).

Box 13.15.2 An example strategy for 20cm predicted leg length discrepancy

- Age 1 year: Femoral valgus/derotation osteotomy, Millis acetabuloplasty
- Age 5 years: soft tissue knee reconstruction
- Age 6 years: lengthen 5cm
- Age 8 years: lengthen 5cm
- Age 10–15 years: lengthen 5cm
- Age 12 years: contralateral epiphysiodesis.

For less significant reduction deformities, surgical limb lengthening is often appropriate but must be embarked upon with caution and it is often only part of the overall operative strategy.

In a long-standing minor discrepancy, surgical correction should be prefaced with a shoe raise to simulate the post operative result. Continuing low back pain after a period of 3–6 months of functional limb equality implies that surgical equalization may not relieve this symptom. The options for treatment in the skeletally immature patient are dependant on the degree of growth remaining and predicted final discrepancy. Epiphysiodesis is relevant for correction of differences up to 5cm. After skeletal maturity, diaphyseal resection of bone with internal fixation allows equalization of between 3–5cm. More aggressive shortening leads to long-standing muscle weakness particularly in the quadriceps and hamstrings with an associated extensor leg which may not recover.

In patients with a congenital deformity, an early decision needs to be made regarding whether it is in the patients' best interest to consider surgical reconstruction or if long term, prosthetic management is the preferred option.

Surgery

Epiphysiodesis

Epiphysiodesis is the conventional approach for equalization of a discrepancy of up to 5cm. There are numerous descriptions of the technique but the Canale percutaneous approach is technically straight forward and should be within the remit of the general orthopaedic surgeon.

The distal femoral and proximal tibial physes are visualized using an image intensifier. A lateral stab incision is made at the level of the physis and using a single entry point in the perichondral ring, a hemiepiphysiodesis is performed with a 3.5mm drill with multiple passes, fanning towards the mid line (Figure 13.15.2).

The target area is the resting zone of the physis and therefore the drill should pass close to the epiphyseal/physeal junction to increase the likelihood of growth arrest: the epiphysiodesis is completed

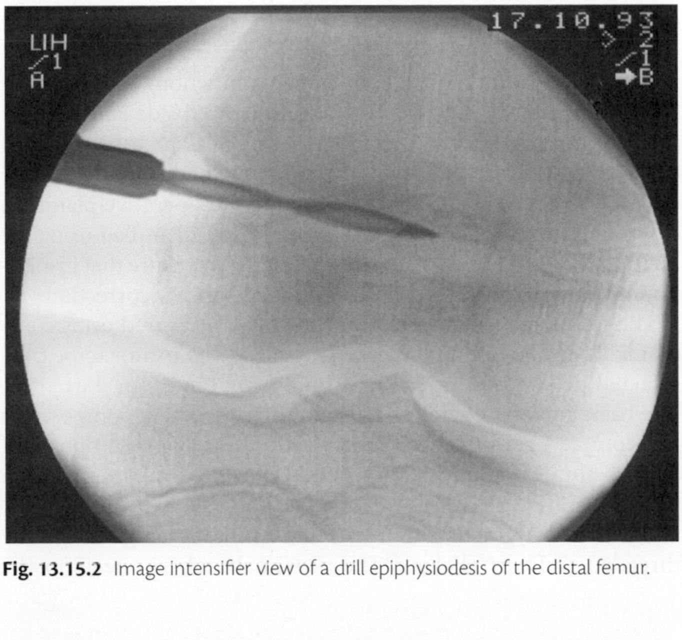

Fig. 13.15.2 Image intensifier view of a drill epiphysiodesis of the distal femur.

with a curette. The procedure is repeated from the medial side in an identical fashion. The fibula is approached under direct vision using a hand held burr, due to the proximity of the common peroneal nerve.

Postoperatively, full weight bearing is encouraged but contact sports prohibited for 6 weeks. Clinical and radiographic follow-up is to ensure that there has been successful, symmetrical growth arrest. Any signs of differential growth mean the procedure must be redone.

Timing

Determination of the optimum time for surgery is crucial. The author's preferred method involves prediction of the final discrepancy using the Paley multiplier method and timing of surgery using the Eastwood-Cole chart. This chart is a graphic representation of a simple arithmetic method for predicting future growth and hence the timing of an epiphysiodesis described by Menalaus and Westh. It relies on the assumption that the distal femoral and proximal tibial growth plates make a predictable contribution (10mm femur, 6mm tibia) to longitudinal growth with boys reaching skeletal maturity at 16 and girls at 14 years of age.

Shortening

After skeletal maturity, segmental shortening of up to 5cm can be performed using a step-cut osteotomy of the proximal femur, stabilized with a blade plate or similar device. Alternatively, closed shortening over an intramedullary nail affords the most rapid return to normal activity with a limited approach and more cosmetically acceptable scarring (Figure 13.15.3).

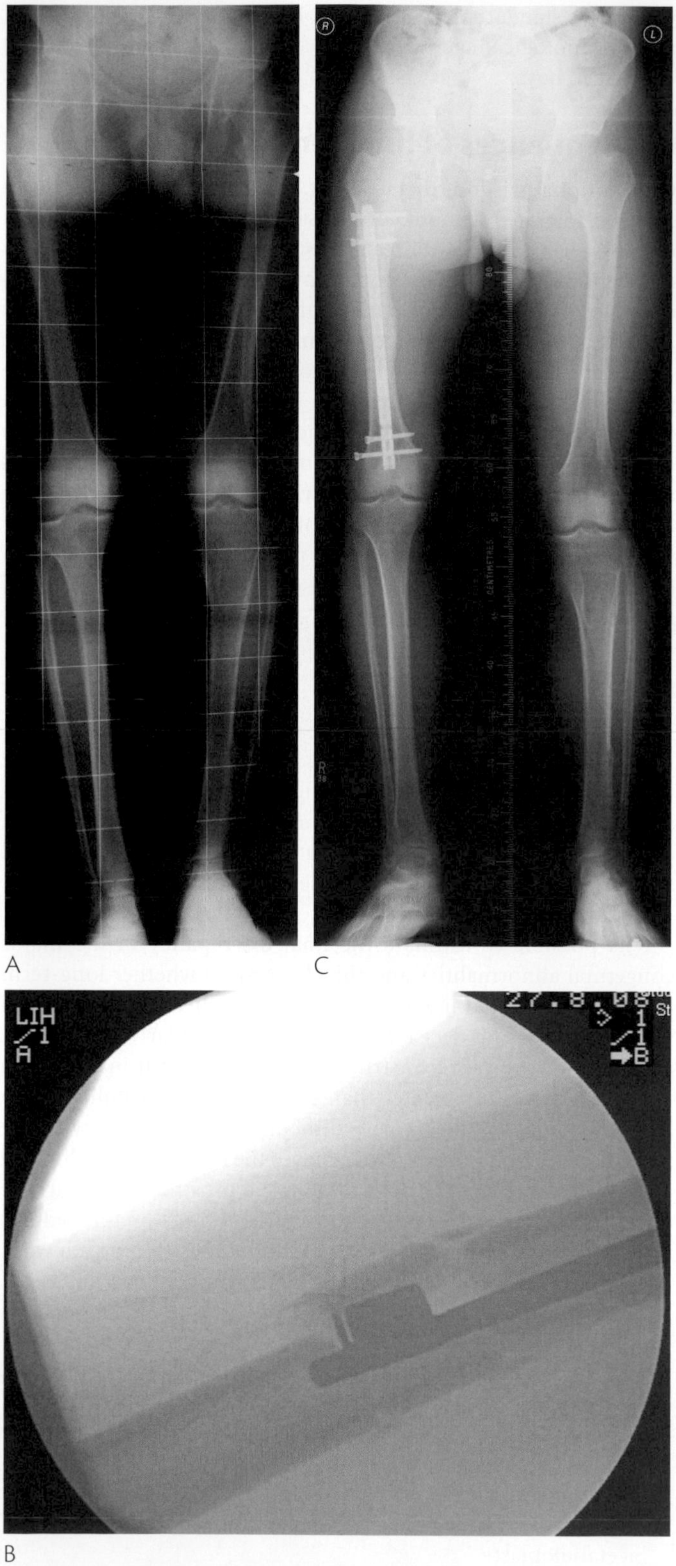

Fig. 13.15.3 A) Leg alignment radiograph showing a short left leg. B) Diaphyseal femoral shortening of 4cm using an intramedullary saw. C) Leg alignment radiographs showing a balanced pelvis and with a right intramedullary nail in situ following diaphyseal shortening.

Lengthening

Modified Ilizarov technique for femoral lengthening

The following description is the author's preferred method of lengthening the femur and combines the classic technique described by Ilizarov (1992) with techniques modified by Catagni and others (1998). This description is of the technique used to lengthen the femur but it can be modified to address any three-dimensional long bone deformity. Recent advances in computerized hexapod external fixators have simplified femoral lengthening and deformity correction but this description highlights the essential mechanical principles that need to be understood, irrespective of the hardware used.

This procedure is suitable for patients in whom the predicted length discrepancy is 20–30% of the uninvolved side and assumes that the hip and knee are intrinsically stable. The assessment of current length discrepancy and prediction of final discrepancy described above are essential for accurate pre-operative planning. Coexisting coronal and sagittal deformities are identified using the methods popularized by Paley and colleagues to ensure that in addition to limb lengthening there is accurate deformity correction.

The soft tissue dimensions of the thigh are measured using commercially available templates and this allows the fixator to be constructed prior to the operation, simplifying the surgical exercise. The basic construct involves a distal fixation segment composed of two complete rings. The proximal fixation segment is composed of an arch support and these are connected using a floating or force transmission ring (Figure 13.15.4).

The distal segment connects to the floating ring using four threaded rods, or clickers. The proximal arch connects to the

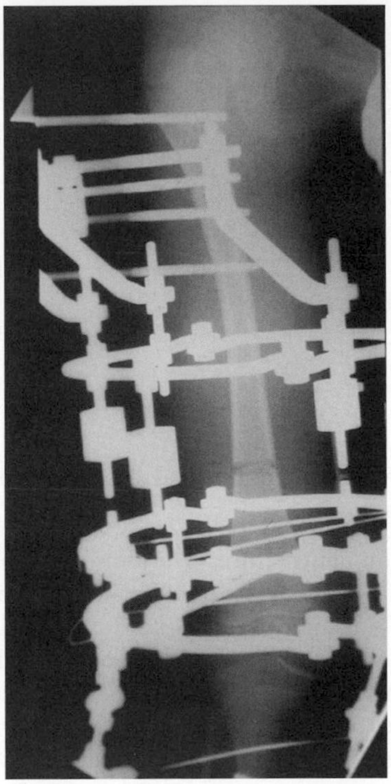

Fig. 13.15.4 AP radiograph of the femur during femoral lengthening. A proximal arch, two distal rings and a floating, force transmission ring are noted. The fixator crosses the knee to prevent posterior subluxation of the tibia.

floating ring using three oblique supports. The device is constructed using the smallest ring that allows adequate soft tissue clearance, 1–1.5 finger breaths clearance circumferentially is the usual requirement.

Procedure

The procedure is performed under general anaesthesia, without neuromuscular blockade or non-steroidal anti-inflammatory medication. The patient is supine on a radiolucent operating table; the entire limb is draped after skin preparation from the toes to above the iliac crest. The ipsilateral buttock and flank are raised with a pillow or large sandbag to enhance access to the proximal femur and allow flexion of the hip and knee during wire and pin placement. An operating table with a detachable segment also allows satisfactory access to the leg, with the tibia supported on a Mayo table.

Using an image intensifier, a 1.8-mm reference wire is inserted into the distal femur, parallel to the joint line from lateral to medial, at the level of the distal metaphyseal flare. The fixator must be placed parallel to the mechanical axis of the femur to prevent medialization of the knee during lengthening. The joint line is approximately perpendicular with the mechanical axis and therefore provides a good point of reference (Box 13.15.3).

Careful attention to detail is required during wire placement to minimize subsequent pin site infection and allow maximum excursion of the knee and hip joints.

The knee is passively flexed and extended, and the skin over the lateral aspect of distal femur is observed. There is a consistent area of skin that does not move during knee excursion and this is the optimum entry point for the wire. The knee is fully flexed before

Box 13.15.3 Fixator 'rules' for femoral lengthening

- Fixator parallel to mechanical (not anatomical) axis
- Adequate soft tissue clearance around all rings/arches
- Transfix muscles at their maximal length
- Ensure that the bone is in the middle of the frame
- Precise technique for the insertion/placement of pins/wires.

the wire penetrates the lateral quadriceps and this transfixes the muscle at its maximum length, preventing a tether that will restrict knee motion. The wire is inserted into the femur at its maximum diameter, avoiding high-speed insertion, which will generate intense heat, causing a ring sequestrum and early loosening. The wire can be cooled, sterilized, and controlled using an alcohol-soaked swab. The knee is fully extended and the wire advanced through the medial hamstring muscles using a mallet. Power insertion is to be avoided on the distant side to minimize the risk of neurovascular damage. At this point, the range of knee movement is checked and any skin tethering is released with a scalpel.

A 6-mm hydroxyapatite (HA) coated half pin is inserted into the proximal femur at the level of the lesser trochanter. The image intensifier is used to insert this pin parallel to the line that joins the tip of the greater trochanter to the centre of the femoral head, provided the morphology of the proximal femur is normal. If there is a significant abnormality, the pin is inserted 7 degrees to the anatomical axis of the femur, perpendicular to the mechanical axis.

The fixator is attached to the proximal pin and distal wire, ensuring that the femoral diaphysis is centred in the rings in the anteroposterior and mediolateral planes, with adequate soft tissue clearance. The fixator has now been positioned parallel to the mechanical axis of the femur, with the femur in the centre of the frame.

The distal wire is tensioned to 110–130kg and the proximal pin is attached to the arch using the appropriate pin holder.

Distal fixation is secured using two further tensioned wires or HA coated half pins, with the greatest possible crossing angle that does not jeopardize other structures. Again a careful insertion technique is required for each wire or pin.

Proximal fixation is completed using two further 6-mm HA coated half pins, inserted above and below the reference pin, with the maximum crossing angle that is allowed by the dimensions of the arch.

The method and site of femoral osteotomy is a controversial subject. In general there is agreement that the femur should be divided in the metaphyseal region using a low energy technique: the author prefers a distal osteotomy.

A 2-cm longitudinal incision is made in the mid lateral line. The iliotibial band is identified and its anterior and posterior limits dissected. It is then divided transversely under direct vision. The vastus lateralis muscle is defined and reflected anteriorly using a bone lever placed over the anterior surface of the femoral shaft. The periosteum is identified and incised longitudinally. Periosteal stripping has a negative effect on bone formation and should be avoided. Using a sharp osteotome, the anterior and posterior cortices are divided completely, leaving the posteromedial corner undivided. The osteotome is rotated 45 degrees in either direction, completing the osteotomy.

Usually the periosteum can not be closed but a careful, layered wound closure is performed. The pin and wires are dressed with alcohol-soaked sponges and stoppers.

Femoral lengthening using a computerized hexapod fixator is more straightforward and can be accomplished with a two-ring fixator. The ring placement is not as critical, but the position of the rings in relation to the bone must be accurately determined with postoperative radiographs.

Postoperative management

The patient is encouraged to put 25% body weight through the limb as soon as comfort allows, graduating to full weight over a period of several weeks. Distraction commences after a latent period of 5–7 days depending on the age of the patient and the bone pathology. It continues at a rate of 0.25mm every 6h or according to the computer-generated prescription, until the target length (and deformity correction) has been achieved.

The patient attends for follow-up on a regular basis, with radiographs to assess the quality and quantity of new bone formation. The rate of distraction may be altered to prevent premature consolidation or incomplete regenerate formation.

Complications

Surgical limb lengthening is associated with a high, but not necessarily prohibitive, complication rate. The knowledge that complication rates can approach 100% should not lead to a feeling of inevitability or complacency. The detailed description of wire/pin insertion techniques, pin-site care, and postoperative management is deliberate and leads to a substantial reduction of the frequency and severity of these complications.

Infection. Pin site infection is a common consequence of prolonged external fixation. Careful attention to detail during pin and wire insertion and good postoperative pin-site care reduces but does not abolish this complication. Pain and erythema usually herald infection. The use of broad-spectrum antibiotics, in appropriate doses for patient body weight is often effective. If rapid resolution does not occur, hospital admission may be necessary for parenteral antibiotics, according to microbiological culture. The majority of infections will resolve if treated promptly but it is occasionally necessary to remove the infected fixation and very rarely to abandon the procedure.

Pain. Pain is often associated with infection. Neurogenic pain may be associated with the lengthening process and may limit the rate of lengthening. Instability due to improper fixator construction or loosening must also be considered and appropriate adjustments made.

Problems with the regenerate bone. The quality of the new bone depends on a number of mechanical and biological factors. An excessive rate of distraction may lead to deficient regenerate whilst premature consolidation is associated with slow distraction. Bone formation is monitored with frequent radiographs and, in some centres, with ultrasound and computed tomography. There is poor correlation between radiological and mechanical parameters of bone 'strength' and decisions relating to consolidation of the regenerate are usually based on plain radiographs in two planes. The optimum time for fixator removal is difficult to predict. Premature removal is complicated by regenerate failure, with deformity or fracture.

Joint subluxation/contracture. The joint laxity that is commonly encountered in congenital femoral deficiency or fibular hemimelia predisposes to joint subluxation and dislocation. An early sign is a loss of joint movement with a flexion adduction deformity at the hip or a flexion contracture at the knee causing concern. If joint subluxation does occur, the lengthening and deformity correction may have to be stopped and the fixator extended to incorporate the knee before the programme can be continued. Careful preoperative assessment, surgical reconstruction of the joints before lengthening and aggressive physical therapy during lengthening is important to prevent this complication.

Box 13.15.4 Before lengthening

- Careful assessment of the problem and the child/family
- Plan and agree aims of treatment
- Reconstruct unstable joints first
- Consider spanning the neighbouring joint
- Ensure that the need for a postoperative rehabilitation programme is understood.

Summary

Discrimination between conditions that are due to overgrowth or reduction in growth and an estimation of the compounding effect of future growth during childhood allows a rational approach to limb equalization. Whilst the current enthusiasm for surgical limb lengthening is appropriate in carefully assessed patients, the importance of shortening by acute resection or epiphysiodesis should not be underrated. The aim should be for limb equalization by the simplest and most appropriate method (Box 13.15.4).

Further reading

Catagni, M., Malzev, V., Kirienko, A. (1998). *Advances in Ilizarov Apparatus Assembly. Fracture Treatment, Pseudarthroses, Lengthening, Deformity Correction.* Milan: Il Quadratino.

Diméglio, A., Charles, Y., Daures, J.-P., de Rosa, V., and Boniface, K. (2005). Accuracy of the Sauvegrain method in determining skeletal age during puberty. *Journal of Bone and Joint Surgery*, **87**, 1689–96.

Eastwood, D. and Cole W. (1995). A graphic method for timing the correction of leg-length discrepancy. *Journal of Bone and Joint Surgery*, **77B**, 743–7.

Ilizarov G. and Ledyaev V. (1992). The replacement of long tubular bone defects by lengthening distraction osteotomy of one of the fragments. *Clinical Orthopaedics and Related Research*, **280**, 7–10.

Paley, D., Herzenberg, J., Tetsworth, K., McKie, J., and Bhave, A. (1994). Deformity planning for frontal and sagittal plane corrective osteotomies. *Orthopedic Clinics of North America*, **25**, 425–65.

Paley, D. Bhave, A., Herzenberg, J., and Bowen, J (2000). Multiplier method for predicting limb-length discrepancy. *Journal of Bone and Joint Surgery*, **82A**, 1432–46.

13.16

Developmental deformities of the lower limbs

Andrew Wainwright

Summary points

- Some rare angular deformities of the lower limbs must be recognized early
- Most deteriorate with time and cause significant functional problems
- With tibial bowing, description of the apex of the bow determines prognosis and management
- Surgical management of these conditions can be difficult: multiple procedures may be required during the growth period.

Introduction

There are a group of rare angular deformities of the lower limbs such as coxa vara, congenital dislocation of the knee, tibia vara, and two types of tibial bowing, posteromedial and anterolateral, that may present at birth or at walking age. All can lead to problems with function in the long term; and all but one (posteromedial bow) deteriorate without intervention.

Coxa vara

Infantile coxa vara is a rare condition that causes the femoral neck-shaft angle to be reduced (<125 degrees), associated with a characteristic defect in the femoral neck (Figure 13.16.1).

Incidence

The quoted incidence is 1:25 000 births. However, the condition is not evident at birth and although often noticed when the child begins walking, in half of the cases it is not recognized until age 5 years. There is an equal sex distribution, little geographical variation and, in up to a third of cases, both hips are affected.

Anatomy

Normal

Radiographically, the normal neck shaft angle increases from 130 degrees in the newborn to 145 degrees by 1 year of age. It then decreases to 125 degrees by adulthood. Microscopically, the femoral neck physis is typical of other long bone growth plates.

Pathological

Radiographs show a decreased neck-shaft angle (typically 85–115 degrees initially) and a short femoral neck but with a normal head and a straight shaft. In 25% hips the neck–shaft angle worsens with time. There is a characteristic triangular osseous fragment (Fairbanks' triangle) at the inferomedial corner of the metaphysis (Figure 13.16.1) and abnormal irregular ossification of the femoral neck metaphysis. The physis is wide and vertical with disturbance of the normal cellular organization. The affected growth plate closes early, usually at the age of 10 years.

Classification

Infantile coxa vara should be differentiated from other causes of coxa vara, including congenital dysplasias and acquired abnormalities (Box 13.16.1).

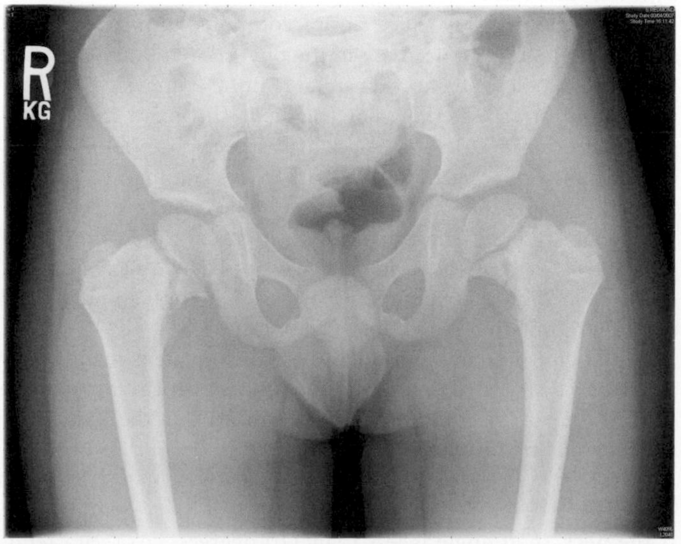

Fig. 13.16.1 AP radiograph of the pelvis showing bilateral coxa vara. Both femoral necks show the characteristic Fairbanks triangle at the inferior metaphyseal margin where there is defective ossification.

Box 13.16.1 Causes of a radiological coxa vara

- Congenital/developmental:
  - Infantile
  - Congenital dysplasia–PFFD
- Acquired:
  - Post-traumatic
  - Osteomyelitis
  - Avascular necrosis
  - Osteogenesis imperfecta/other bone softening disorders.

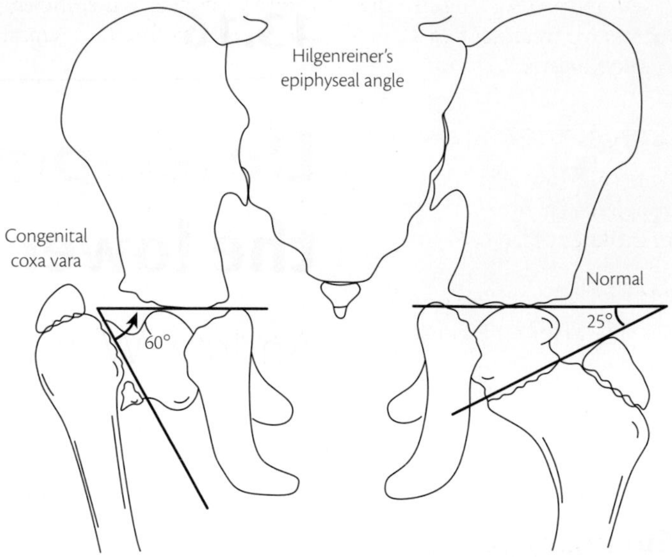

Fig. 13.16.2 The Hilgenreiner–epiphyseal (HE) angle lies on the medial side from a horizontal line that joins the triradiate cartilages, and line that runs through the proximal femoral physis.

Clinical

History

A limp is noticed as the child begins to walk or in early childhood. Children may complain of stiffness after resting and pain after walking.

Physical examination

Examination identifies a short leg with a high trochanter. Hip abduction is significantly reduced but the adduction range is maintained. There is often a fixed flexion deformity of the hip associated with a lumbar lordosis. The poor lever-arm of the hip abductors leads to a Trendelenburg gait.

Investigation

Pelvic x-rays show the characteristic features outlined earlier. Imaging of other bones may be needed to rule out a generalized skeletal dysplasia. Two radiographic lines are commonly used to assess the deformity the neck–shaft angle and the Hilgenreiner–epiphyseal (HE) angle (Figure 13.16.2). Both angles may be affected by lower limb rotation.

In some cases of isolated coxa vara, computed tomography (CT) studies have shown a decrease in the physeal–femoral neck angle (as seen in adolescent slipped capital femoral epiphysis). The epiphysis and attached triangular fragment slip from the normal superoanterior portion of the neck in an inferioposterior direction. Often, in severe congenital coxa vara, there is a marked femoral retroversion.

Magnetic resonance imaging (MRI) studies in patients with congenital coxa vara reveal a widened growth plate with expansion of cartilage mediodistally between the capital femoral epiphysis and metaphysis but do not identify a true slip.

Histological studies have found the growth plate is made of few irregularly distributed germinal cells. Similar changes found in the growth zone of the iliac bone seem to indicate that the ossification disturbances are multifocal.

Natural history

If the neck-shaft angle is less than 110 degrees, coxa vara tends to worsen with time. Hips with HE angles less than 45 degrees will usually correct spontaneously without surgery. Those with HE angles of 45–60 degrees represent a 'grey zone' and should be observed. However, progression of deformity is the rule if the HE angle is greater than 60 degrees. Progression is often accompanied by other problems such as a pseudarthrosis at the site of the defect, leg length differences, mechanical axis deviation, and rotational deformity. There are associated dysplastic changes in the acetabulum.

Management

Operative

The indications for surgery are a Trendelenburg gait and a HE angle greater than 60 degrees, or evidence of progressive deformity. The conventional operative procedure is a valgus extension proximal femoral osteotomy, as described by Pauwels. The aim of surgery is to correct varus to a HE angle less than 45 degrees, equalize leg lengths, and normalize abductor muscle length. However, these operations are often technically difficult and may lead to joint stiffness without sufficient correction of the coxa vara or associated deformities.

The valgus osteotomy may be combined with a greater trochanter epiphysiodesis or trochanteric advancement if the trochanter is high. Circular fixators can also be used to correct the deformity.

Results/complications

In some series recurrence rates of up to 50% are seen following a valgus extension osteotomy. However, when the HE angle is well-corrected (<38 degrees), the recurrence rate is only 5%. If deformity correction is achieved and maintained before age 10 years, 87% of children have excellent acetabular depth, spherical congruency, no pain, and a correction of Trendelenburg gait in the short to medium term. The triangular defect closes within 6 months of surgery.

Premature capital femoral physeal closure is frequent, leading to relative overgrowth of the greater trochanter and, in unilateral cases, unequal leg lengths. The leg length discrepancy is sufficient to require treatment in 40% of cases, usually with contralateral epiphysiodesis.

Congenital dislocation of the knee

This spectrum of hyperextension disorders of the knee includes congenital genu recurvatum (CGR) and congenital dislocation of the knee (CDK) (Figure 13.16.3).

Incidence

The incidence is estimated to be 2:100 000 with equal sex distribution.

Anatomy

Normal

Cadaver studies of neonatal knees demonstrate that 5–15 degrees of hyperextension is normal which could be increased by 10 degrees with prolonged pressure. By 3 months, fixed flexion of 5 degrees develops. Extension can be achieved with prolonged pressure but at this age, hyperextension does not occur.

Pathological

Knee hyperextension greater than 30 degrees is demonstrated with associated limited flexion. There are two groups: those involving anomalies of the elastic tissues and those with a postural deformity secondary to intrauterine problems. In 60% of children with CGR/CDK there are other anomalies, including hip dysplasia, foot deformities, cleft lip and palate, chest wall deformities, and elbow dislocation. CDK is commonly seen in conditions such as arthrogryposis, spina bifida, and syndromes associated with joint laxity, such as Down syndrome. The combination of CDK or joint laxity with other malformations should raise the possibility of a chromosomal abnormality.

At operation, an absent cruciate ligament is a common finding. Other aetiological theories include fetal molding or quadriceps contracture.

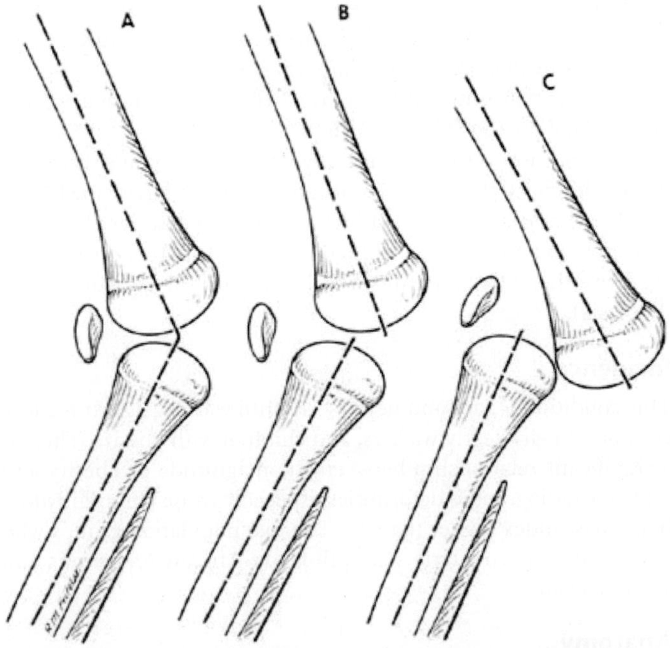

Fig. 13.16.3 Diagram to illustrate Table 13.16.1 and the types of congenital hyperextension of the knee. A) congenital hyperextension, B) Subluxation of knee, and C) dislocation of knee (from Curtis, B.H. and Fisher, R.L. (1969). Congenital hyperextension with anterior subluxation of the knee. Surgical treatment and long-term observations. *Journal of Bone and Joint Surgery*, **51A**, 255–69.

Classification

The classification system by Leveuf and Pais (1946) has been used to determine management. Essentially these types are: hyperextension of the knee, anterior subluxation of the tibia, or anterior dislocation of the tibia (Table 13.16.1) (Figure 13.16.3).

Clinical

The diagnosis is usually obvious at birth: 30% are associated with a breech delivery.

Physical examination

The knee appears 'back to front' (Figure 13.16.4). There is a deep anterior skin fold and the femoral condyles are easily palpable in the popliteal fossa. The patella is deep and often difficult to feel. As the child lies flat, the hyperextension tends to externally rotate the leg giving an impression of valgus.

Investigation

The diagnosis may be made on antenatal ultrasound. After birth, ultrasound can be used to follow the progress of the condition; radiographs are less helpful due to the cartilaginous nature of the neonatal knee joint.

Management

Initial

As the deformity is often very striking in the newborn, the parents need prompt reassurance that most children can be treated successfully by conservative means. The aim of treatment is to gain a range of movement adequate for activities of daily living. Other associated conditions such as developmental dysplasia of the hip and talipes equinovarus should be treated as appropriate: most authors suggest that the knee be treated first. The presence of associated deformities, delay in treatment, and generalized joint laxity adversely affect the prognosis.

Table 13.16.1 Classification of congenital hyperextension of the knee

Grade	Passive flexion	Hyperextension at rest	Tibia:femur
1	45–60°	10–20°	Minimal subluxation
2	Neutral	20–40°	Moderate
3	Hyperextension only	>40°	Dislocation

From: Leveuf, J. and Pais C (1946). Les dislocations congenitales du genou. *Revue d'Orthopedie*, **32**, 313.

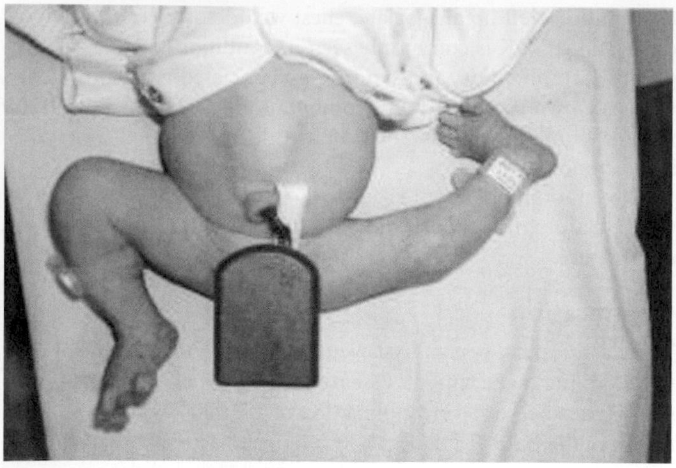

Fig. 13.16.4 An infant with congenital hyperextension of the left knee.

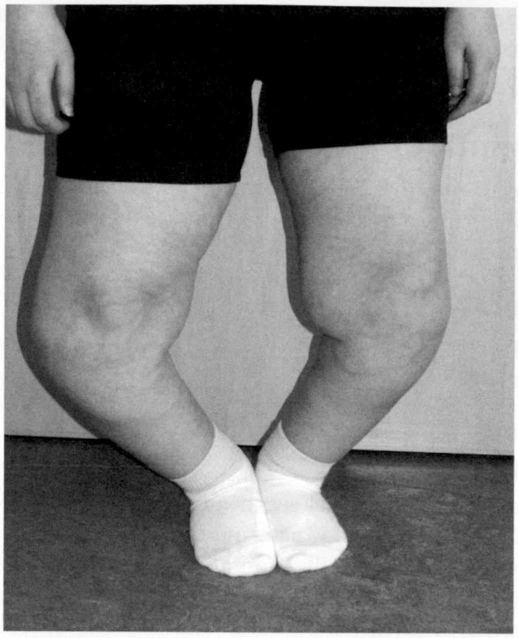

Fig. 13.16.5 Clinical photograph of a heavy child with bilateral tibia vara.

Non-operative

Immediate reduction or serial casting should be tried when the patient is seen within the first week or so of life. In the infant, it is important to ensure that the manipulation and casting is performed in the correct direction: the limb lies in external rotation and there is a tendency to 'flex' the knee into valgus. The deep anterior skin crease helps in orientation of the limb. Flattening of the tibial plateau and anterior bowing of the tibia is common after prolonged conservative treatment but remodels eventually. If the patient is seen late and serial casting proves to be unsuccessful, traction in the Bryant position or in a prone position should be used for 1–2 weeks, and then gentle closed reduction of the CDK can be tried with or without anaesthesia.

Operative

Not all children respond to serial casting. Those with fibrous changes in the quadriceps muscles often require operative treatment, (10–50%). This is performed with an arthrogram to assess the knee, a V–Y plasty of the quadriceps and anterior release of the adherent capsule. This allows the collaterals, the iliotibial band, and the hamstrings to return from the extensor to the flexor side of the knee axis. Intraoperatively the aim is to achieve 90 degrees of flexion and this is maintained with a cast in 90 degrees of flexion for 6 weeks. An operation at age 9 months appears to be optimal, enabling the children to walk and function normally.

Results

Non-operative correction appears to be most effective if it starts immediately after birth. This may restore complete function and joint range, although some children may lack full flexion.

In patients with valgus alignment and hyperlaxity, ongoing bracing or even a corrective osteotomy may be required. Selected patients may benefit from transposition of the pes anserinus and the tibial insertion of the medial collateral ligament to reinforce the medial aspect of the knee joint.

Good results are more difficult to achieve in children with Larsen's syndrome and arthrogryposis: conservative treatment usually fails and operative treatment may need to be more aggressive. Indications for surgery need to be considered carefully.

Tibia vara

Infantile tibia vara is characterized by an acute varus angulation of the tibia just below the knee joint, secondary to disturbance of the posteromedial proximal tibial physis (Figure 13.16.5). This is a multiplanar deformity with proximal tibial varus, procurvatum, and internal torsion (Figure 13.16.6).

The condition is most commonly known as Blount's disease as Blount described the first series of cases, although he acknowledged that Erlacher described it first in 1922. He also described a similar deformity in adolescence that is considered a different disorder (as are two other types: late onset tibia vara and fibrocartilagenous dysplasia).

Incidence

This condition is rare and never seen until walking age. It is more common in girls, early walkers, and children with obesity. There is a significant relationship between the magnitude of obesity and biplanar radiographic deformities especially those children with a body mass index higher than 40. The two population groups who appear to be particularly susceptible are African Americans and Scandinavians.

Anatomy

Normal

The normal lower limb alignment of a child under the age of 2 years is of knee varus ('bow-legs') that normally progresses to maximum knee valgus ('knock-knees') by the age of 5 years (see Chapter 13.10).

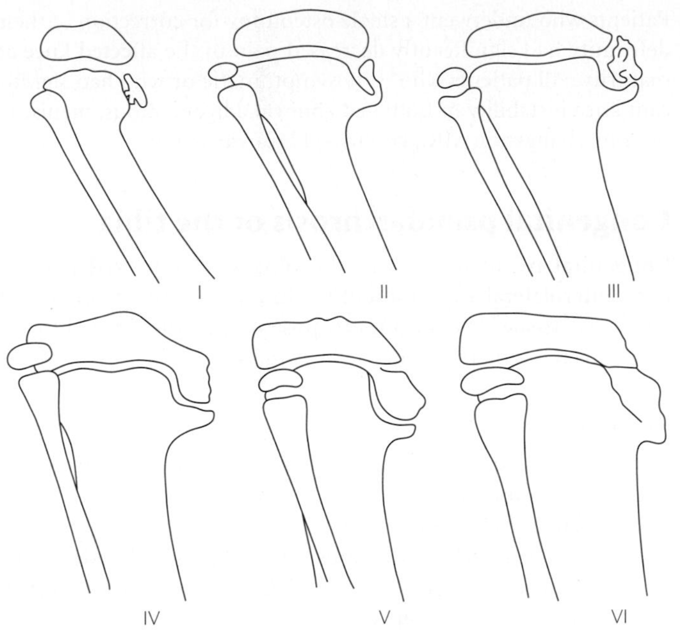

Fig. 13.16.6 Langenskiold's six-stage classification of tibia vara.

Box 13.16.2 Differential diagnosis of Blount's disease

- Physiological bowing
- Congenital bowing
- Rickets
- Trauma
- Osteomyelitis
- Skeletal dysplasia:
  - Metaphyseal chondrodysplasia
  - Ollier's disease.

Pathological

If a child walks early, whilst they are in varus alignment, their mechanical axis will fall medial to the knee and put pressure on the medial growth plate. If there is excessive varus or excessive force (related to body mass) going through the medial growth plate then this may damage the growth plate. There is also tension on the convex side. According to the principles of Heuter, Volkmann, and Delpech, this encourages increased growth laterally. In turn this leads to a positive feedback phenomenon of worsening varus deformity, leading to even further force medially.

Histological examination of tibia vara in 6–7-year-olds shows widening and depression of the medial growth plate, small and deep intrusions of cartilage into the metaphysis, oedema of the medial tibial epiphysis, medial and lateral metaphysis; widening of the lateral growth plate, hypertrophy of the medial meniscus and focal bone bridging. Patients with infantile tibia vara have normal alignment of the distal femur unlike adolescent tibia vara.

Classification

Langenskiöld described a classification system that is based on stages of progression with age, *not* prognosis. The stages, from I to VI, show progressively increasing deformity with bone bridge formation between the tibial epiphysis and metaphysis (see Figure 13.16.6).

Clinical

History

Many young children are referred to orthopaedic clinics with bowlegs. Predicting whether these deformities will progress can be challenging. There is no consensus as to whether children with radiographic medial tibial beaking should all be classified as having Blount's disease.

Physical examination

As noted earlier these children have varus alignment of one or both knees, and are often obese. A differential diagnosis must be considered (Box 13.16.2).

Investigation

Imaging

Radiographs of the knees show the deformity with medial tibial depression and beaking progressing onto physeal bridging, as described by Langenskiöld.

Levine and Drennan described the tibial metaphyseal-diaphyseal angle (TMDA) (Figure 13.16.7). An angle greater than 11 degrees can distinguish between physiological and pathological varus. Subsequent work shows that there is a grey area between 9–16 degrees, where there is some overlap between physiological and pathological. The epiphyseal–metaphyseal angle (EMA) is also helpful under the age of 3 years. Children with TMDA above 9 degrees and EMA over 20 degrees are at greater risk for Blount's disease and should be followed closely. A combination of a body mass index higher than 22 and a TMDA greater than 10 degrees has a high predictive value for tibia vara in children between 2–4 years.

MRI has been used to confirm the pathological changes and to plan surgical management (Figure 13.16.8B).

Management

Initial

Bracing (knee–ankle–foot–orthoses, KAFOs) has been used for children with a significant degree of varus before the age of 3 years. There is an overlap between toddlers with a marked physiological varus and those with a mild tibia vara and thus debate as to whether bracing works. It is agreed that bracing is only effective in Langenskiöld stages I and II, and in half of those treated.

Operative

The conventional operation that has been used for tibia vara is a proximal tibial valgus osteotomy often combined with external rotation. It is important to avoid damaging the apophysis, and to aim for some overcorrection into overall valgus alignment. Such surgery, performed early (under 4 years of age) may prevent

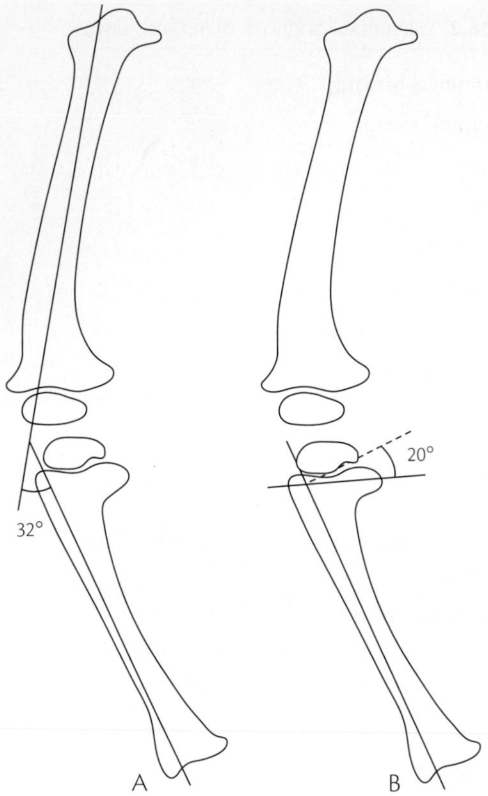

Fig. 13.16.7 A) shows the anatomical femoro-tibial angle and B) demonstrates the TMDA (with the dotted line being perpendicular to the long axis of the tibia shaft). The Levine and Drennan tibial metaphyseal–diaphyseal angle (TMDA) is created by the intersection of a line perpendicular to the longitudinal axis of the tibial diaphysis and another line drawn through the transverse axis of the tibial metaphysis.

recurrence of varus deformity in Blount's disease at long-term follow-up. On its own, a lateral staple physeodesis does not seem to be effective although recently, encouraging results have been seen following the use of a physeal plate that acts as a tension band tether to physeal growth.

Elevation of the medial hemi-plateau of the tibia for correction of severe varus deformity secondary to Blount's disease produces satisfactory results but a tibial osteotomy may also be required for full correction (Figure 13.16.8C). On the basis of knee arthrograms and MRIs, there is some disagreement as to whether the medial tibial plateau is truly depressed or simply filled with unossified cartilage (Figure 13.16.8B).

Circular frames have been used effectively to treat the combined problem of a complex tibial deformity and leg length difference in older children.

Results and complications

The most significant early complication of a proximal tibial osteotomy is compartment syndrome or neurological damage and close postoperative monitoring is essential.

Recurrence of deformity requiring repeated osteotomy occurred more frequently in children who underwent a late (>4 years of age) initial osteotomy and/or were Langenskiöld stage III or more. Patients who underwent a single osteotomy for correction of their deformity had significantly decreased pain in the affected knee at maturity. All patients who were symptomatic or who had significant knee instability or both had abnormal ligamentous, meniscal, or bony changes on MRI, confirmed by arthroscopy.

Congenital pseudarthrosis of the tibia

Congenital pseudarthrosis of the tibia is characterized by an apex anterolateral angulation of the lower leg through an area of abnormal tissue. It continues to pose one of the most difficult problems in paediatric orthopaedic surgery.

Incidence

Congenital pseudarthrosis of the tibia is rare with an incidence of 1: 250 000 live births.

The pseudarthrosis is usually not present at birth (and therefore not truly congenital) but develops during the first decade of life. The male: female ratio is 3:2, left and right sides are equally affected, but only 1% of cases are bilateral.

Anatomy

Pathological

Most of the lesions are initially found in the middle or distal third of the tibia. In 29% the localization changes during the course of the disease. The fibula is also affected.

Associated pathology

Signs and symptoms of neurofibromatosis (NF) are present in 55%. It has also been noted that many have curly or overlapping toes on the affected leg. Screening for the NF gene is advised.

Classification

Various morphologic classification systems have been proposed but because the appearance changes during the course of the disease, all classification systems have some limitation. The most common classification is that by Boyd (Table 13.16.2).

Clinical

History

Presentation depends on degree of tibial deformity and the presence of a fracture.

Physical examination

Typically there is bowing of the tibia, apex anterolateral. This must be differentiated from posteromedial bowing (see later). The affected segment is short and there may be the scars of previous operations (Figure 13.16. 9). Stigmata of NF should be sought.

Investigation

Imaging

X-ray changes as described previously are seen depending on type (see Table 13.16.2).

MRI of congenital pseudarthrosis allows assessment of the type and extent of the disease. It is especially recommended for the evaluation of periosteal and soft tissue changes near the pseudarthrosis.

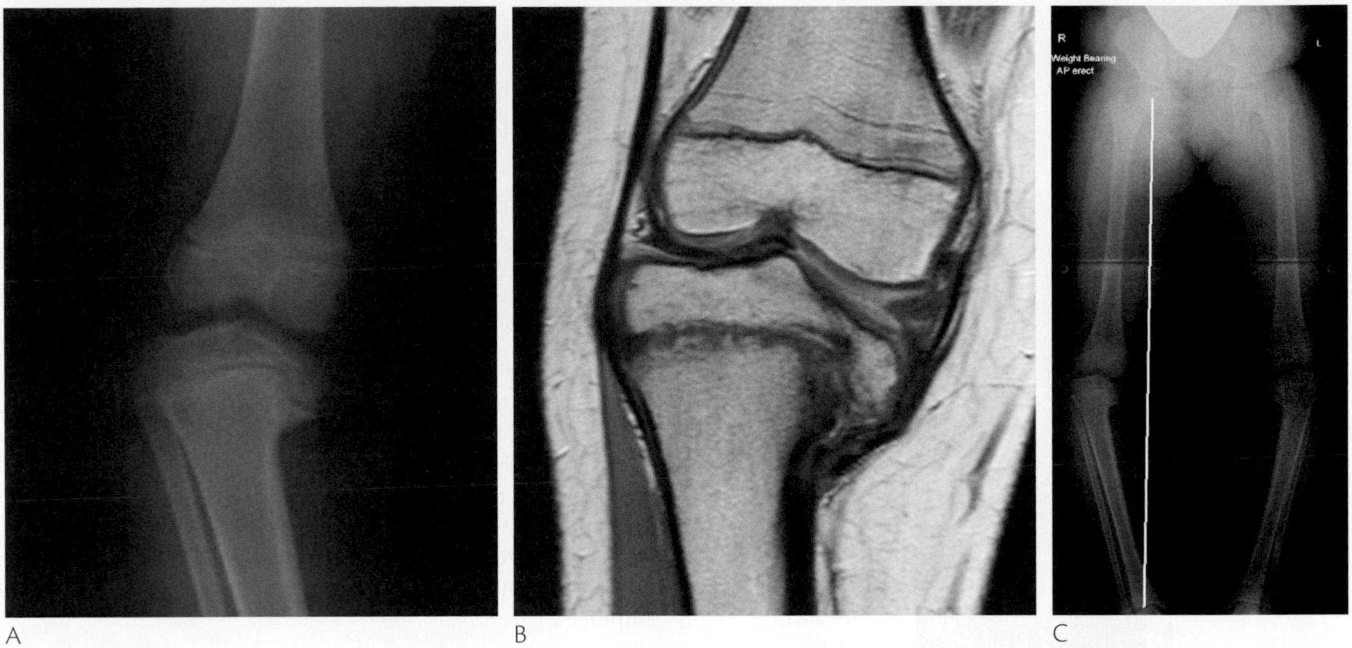

Fig. 13.16.8 A) AP radiograph of a knee showing the changes associated with tibia vara (Blount's disease). B) Corresponding MR image highlighting the changes in the physeal cartilage. C) Long-leg radiographs of the same child. She has bilateral disease. The mechanical axis of her right leg lies medial to the joint. There is significant deformity of the right tibial plateau and 'compensatory' distal femoral valgus. The left leg shows a lesser deformity: there is evidence of previous treatment (hemiplateau elevation and a distal fibula osteotomy).

Table 13.16.2 Boyd classification of congenital pseudarthrosis of the tibia

Type	Description
I	Anterior bow and defect in tibia
II	Anterior bow and hourglass constriction, spontaneous fracture <2 years
III	Bone cyst at junction of distal and middle thirds of tibia
IV	Sclerotic segment with insufficiency fracture developing
V	Dysplastic fibula
VI	Intraosseous neurofibroma

Histopathology

Histological examination shows a non-specific fibrous appearance in 45%; in 16% the ultrastructure resembles fibrous dysplasia; and in 39% there is evidence of NF1.

Histological comparison of the pathologic samples of patients with and without NF reveals no significant differences. The pseudarthrosis gap is continuous with periosteal soft tissues and filled by fibrous tissue, fibrocartilage, and hyaline cartilage with features of enchondral ossification.

A single pathologic process appears to occur in all cases: growth of an abnormal, fibromatosis-like tissue either within the periosteum or within the endosteal or marrow tissues. This may represent a skeletal expression of NF, either within the fully expressed syndrome (patients with known NF) or as isolated lesion (patients with unknown/cryptic NF). Fibrous hamartoma cells maintain some of the mesenchymal lineage cell phenotypes but do not undergo osteoblastic differentiation in response to bone morphogenic protein.

Management

Initial

Once the condition has been diagnosed, protective bracing should be started usually with a KAFO or clamshell orthosis. If the tibia remains intact surgery may be avoided.

Operative

There is debate about surgical intervention; in particular regarding the age at first operation, whether the resection should be conservative or radical and whether reconstruction or amputation would be the better option.

Reconstructive

The aim of reconstructive surgery is to manage the biological and mechanical abnormality by:

- Resecting the pseudarthrosis to provide stability, the basic requirement for bony consolidation
- Correcting length discrepancy and axial deformity (including consideration of the hind foot)
- Achieving fusion/fracture union.

The surgical techniques most frequently used for treating congenital pseudarthrosis of the tibia are intramedullary nailing associated with bone grafting, vascularized fibular grafting, and the Ilizarov circular external fixator device for stabilization and correction of deformity.

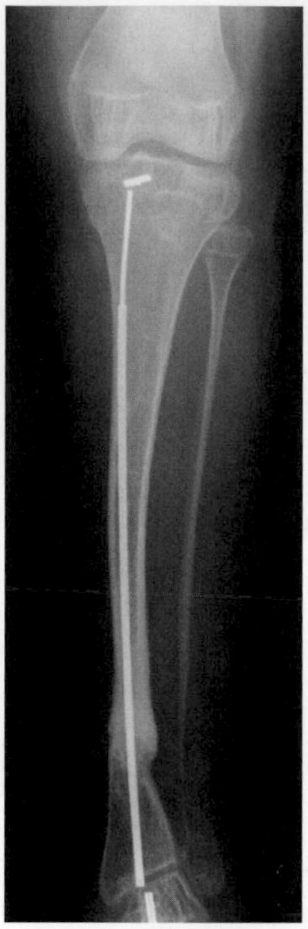

Fig. 13.16.9 AP view left tibia. An expanding intramedullary nail has been used to treat the tibial pseudarthrosis. The pseudarthrosis has healed but the nail has broken. There is residual ankle deformity. The fibula is also involved.

Recent studies using an intramedullary rod suggest that the best results are seen in children under 3 years of age at surgery: this contradicts the previous belief that surgery should be deferred until after 3 years.

Ipsilateral or contralateral vascularized fibular grafts are effective treatments and can be considered as a primary option. Both techniques involve resection of the abnormal tissue with transfer of normal living tissue into the defect and stabilization of the bone and the ankle joint.

Circular frames have become increasingly popular in the management of this condition. The technique may be used in various ways: for acute compression and stabilization after resection, for simple longitudinal compression of the 'non-union', side to side compression of over-riding atrophic bone ends or segmental bone transport to fill a bone defect.

For all of these techniques, a brace is advocated until the end of growth and often beyond.

Amputation

An alternative approach to reconstruction is amputation. Following Syme's amputation, a solid union may be seen across the pseudarthrosis site, even without internal fixation or bone grafting. Healing is achieved by vertical alignment of the limb in a total contact prosthesis, along with the compressive forces of weight bearing (Box 13.16.3).

Results

A multicentre study by the European Paediatric Orthopaedic Society found that the Ilizarov technique had the highest rate of fusion (75.5%) of the pseudarthrosis and the best success in correcting the associated deformities. The Japanese multicentre study showed that the Ilizarov method with a vascularized fibular graft provided the best results. The worst outcomes seem to occur in patients with an associated fibular pseudarthrosis.

Box 13.16.3 Indications for amputation

- Failure to achieve bony union after 3 surgical attempts
- Limb length discrepancy > 5cm
- Development of a significant foot deformity distal to the pseudarthrosis
- Concerns regarding the functional loss due to prolonged medical care and hospitalization.

Despite good anatomical results, gait and muscle strength of patients with 'healed' congenital pseudarthrosis of the tibia are markedly disturbed. Early onset of disease, early surgery, and transankle fixation lead to an inefficient gait, comparable to that of amputees.

Complications

Even when union is achieved, the residual deformities in the affected limb often result in significant disability. These deformities include leg-length discrepancy, angular tibial deformities, ankle valgus and fibular non-union. Refracture is common. Factors predisposing to non-union/refracture are distal location of the tibial pseudarthrosis and the presence of concomitant pseudarthrosis of the fibula (Figures 13.16.9 and 13.16.10).

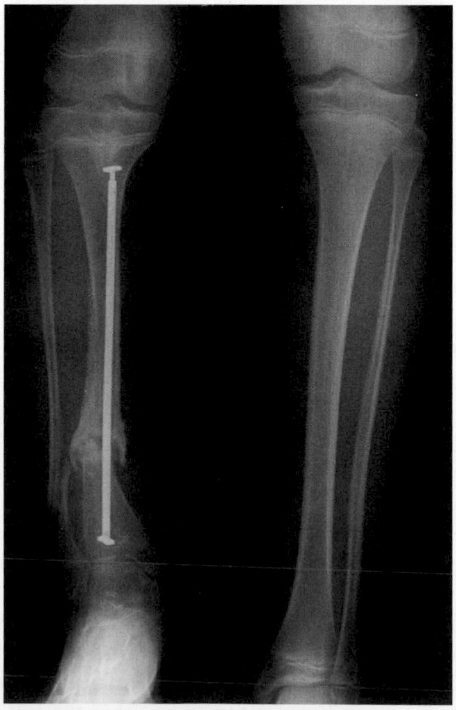

Fig. 13.16.10 AP view of both tibiae. The right tibial pseudarthrosis has recurred following insertion of an expanding intramedullary nail. The tibia is short but the nail has maintained satisfactory alignment. Resection of the pseudarthrosis and bone transport using an external fixator is planned.

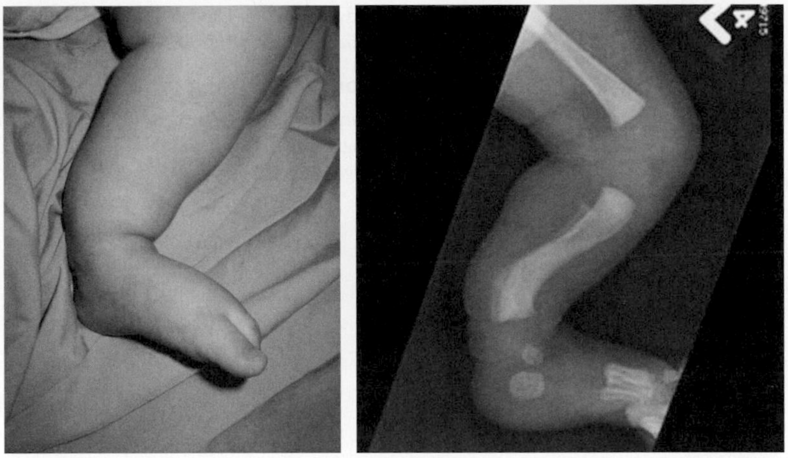

A B

Fig. 13.16.11 Clinical (A) and radiological (B) features of a congenital posteromedial bow of the tibia.

Future directions

Various adjuvant treatments such as bone morphogenic protein and bisphosphonates have been tried and although early results suggest that bone healing may be enhanced, none have yet documented a reduction in the refracture rate.

Box 13.16.4 Tibial bowing?

Direction determines prognosis and management:

- Posteromedial: benign' with spontaneous improvement
- Anteromedial: consider fibular hemimelia
- Anterolateral:
  - Associated with congenital
  - Pseudarthrosis of the tibia.

Congenital posteromedial tibial bow

This variety of bowed tibia is usually associated with a dimple at the apex and with a calcaneovalgus foot (Figure 13.16.11A).

Incidence

The deformity is very rare and much less common than an anterolateral bow. There is equal sex distribution.

Clinical

History/physical examination

This is alarming to parents as the acute angular deformity of the lower leg is obvious at birth. There is usually a skin dimple at the site of the bow and an associated calcaneovalgus foot deformity.

Investigation

It may be detected on the antenatal ultrasound scan and spontaneous correction starting before birth has been noted. X-rays show sclerosis at the site of the bow with the deformity as seen clinically (Figure 13.16.11B).

Histology has been performed in one case of an aborted fetus and this demonstrated evidence of amniotic perforation, abnormal periosteal ossification, and remodeling.

Management

Initial

The natural history is of resolution but this may be incomplete (Box 13.16.4).

Non-operative

Serial casting is often advocated but there are no studies of the effectiveness of this compared to the natural history. The process of spontaneous resolution may continue for several years and a conservative approach to treatment is recommended.

Operative

Tibial osteotomy to correct deformity is not usually required but there is always an associated leg length discrepancy which averages 3cm (2–6cm) at maturity. The degree of leg length difference and difference in calf size appears to be related to the degree of deformity. Operative techniques described elsewhere may be needed to correct this leg length discrepancy.

Complications

The degree of limitation of ankle movement is related directly to the severity of the initial deformity and the subsequent leg length discrepancy. It is probably due to a contracture of the heel cord and posterior capsule resulting from chronic use of an abnormally short limb.

Further reading

Coxa vara

Weinstein, J.N., Kuo, K.N., and Millar, E.A. (1984). Congenital coxa vara. A retrospective review. *Journal of Pediatric Orthopedics*, **4**, 70–7.

Congenital dislocation of the knee

Ko, J.Y., Shih, C.H., and Wenger, D.R. (1999). Congenital dislocation of the knee. *Journal of Pediatric Orthopedics*, **19**, 252–9.

Blount's disease

Doyle, B.S., Volk, A.G., and Smith, C.F (1996). Infantile Blount disease: long-term follow-up of surgically treated patients at skeletal maturity. *Journal of Pediatric Orthopedics*, **16**(4), 469–76.

Congenital pseudarthrosis of the tibia

Grill, F., Bollini, G., Dungl, P., *et al.* (2000). Treatment approaches for congenital pseudarthrosis of tibia: results of the EPOS multicenter study. European Paediatric Orthopaedic Society (EPOS). *Journal of Pediatric Orthopedics*, **9**(2), 75–89.

Posteromedial bowing

Hofmann, A. and Wenger, D.R. (1981). Posteromedial bowing of the tibia. Progression of discrepancy in leg lengths. *Journal of Bone and Joint Surgery*, **63A**, 384–8.

13.17

Developmental dysplasia of the hip

Anish Sanghrajka and Deborah M. Eastwood

Summary points

- Developmental dysplasia of the hip represents a spectrum of hip pathology with or without hip instability
- Controversy continues regarding the relative roles of clinical and ultrasound screening programmes
- Early diagnosis and prompt, appropriate treatment is important
- All treatment methods risk compromising the vascularity of the developing femoral head
- Residual dysplasia may require an aggressive surgical approach.

Introduction

Developmental dysplasia of the hip (DDH) is an umbrella term encompassing many different clinical presentations of disordered hip development, ranging from a deficiency in acetabular coverage of the femoral head (dysplasia), through instability of the femoral head (dislocatable hip), to displacement of the femoral head from the acetabulum. This displacement may be partial (subluxation) or complete (dislocation) and either reversible or irreversible on examination. Whilst gross hip instability is found only in the neonate and infant, dysplasia and complete dislocations present at any age.

Anatomical dysplasia is defined as inadequate development of the acetabulum and/or the proximal femur. Radiographically, the integrity of Shenton's line distinguishes between dysplasia and subluxation: it is intact in dysplasia and disrupted with subluxation (Figure 13.17.1).

'Teratologic' dislocations are a separate entity. They are often associated with neuromuscular conditions and dislocated in utero. Consequently they are stiff and frequently irreducible.

Embryology and pathoanatomy

An understanding of normal hip development, the pathological processes that affect it, and the resultant anatomical malformations helps explain the clinical presentation and the rationale for management.

At 8 weeks postfertilization, a cleft develops between the femoral head and the acetabulum, the joint forms, and the labrum can be distinguished as a distinct entity.

Normal hip development occurs with balanced growth of the proximal femoral and triradiate cartilages. An imbalance in this system may be a genetically determined cause for DDH but, at the outset, the only anatomical abnormalities identified are an elongation of the hip capsule and ligamentum teres; the acetabulum, labrum, and femur are usually normal.

The relative capacity of the normally developing acetabulum decreases over the last 3 months of gestation becoming smallest around birth. Neonates of African origin have deeper acetabulae: a possible explanation for their significantly lower incidence of DDH.

DDH may, therefore, be the result of capsular laxity that allows the femoral head to escape from a normal acetabulum that happens to be at its shallowest around birth. Coexistent adverse intrauterine factors and the hormonal changes during birth may promote this pathological process.

An unstable hip at birth may either stabilize spontaneously and continue normal development or, if instability persists, develop progressive subluxation or complete dislocation with predictable secondary anatomical changes. Initially, these abnormalities are reversible but with time, the anatomic malformations become irreversible. Unfortunately, the fate of any individual hip is unpredictable.

Femoral head instability results in a ridge of hypertrophied acetabular cartilage on the posterior wall that Ortolani referred to as the neolimbus. It is the movement of the femoral head over this ridge that produces the 'clunk' of the Ortolani sign.

The primary stimulus for acetabular development is the presence of a spherical femoral head. In its absence, the acetabular floor becomes thickened and the acetabulum aspherical, shallow, and anteverted as the anterosuperior wall fails to develop. Over time, a pseudoacetabulum forms in response to the abnormal femoral head position either within the superior portion of the true acetabulum or above it.

The predominantly cartilaginous proximal femur may undergo compressive ischaemic injury as a consequence of its displacement, resulting in segmental flattening or increased anteversion. The greater trochanteric region is unaffected and may demonstrate relative overgrowth.

As well as osseous abnormalities, DDH is associated with specific soft tissue changes. The labrum together with its capsular attachment and adjacent acetabular ring epiphysis (the 'limbus')

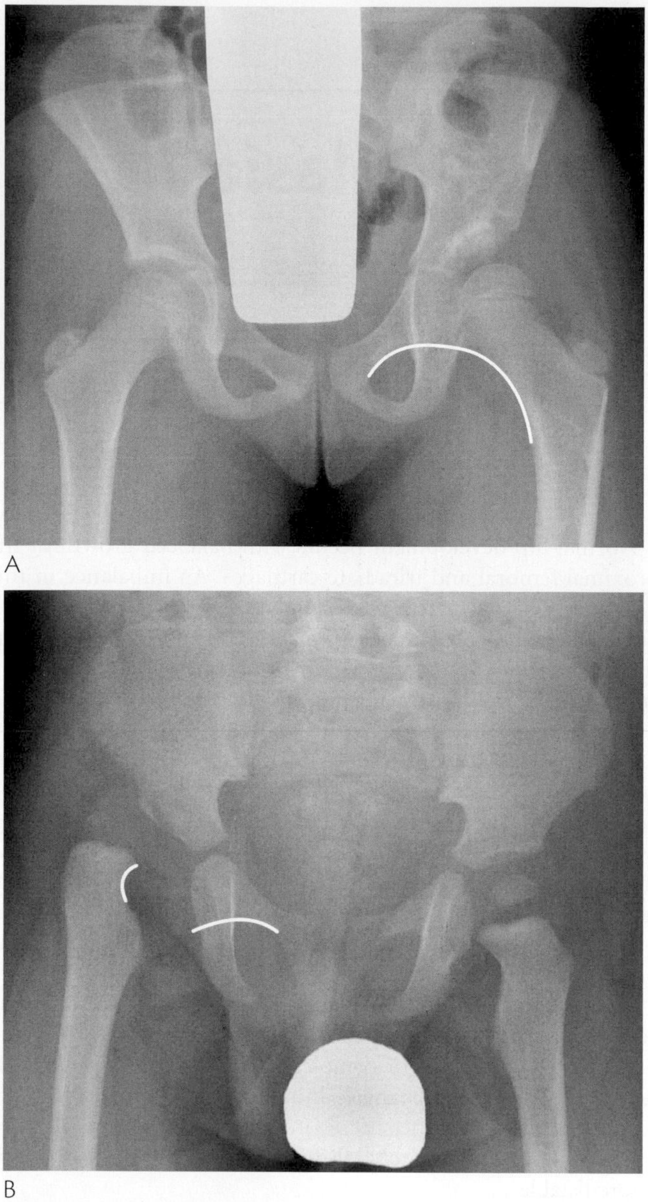

Fig. 13.17.1 A) AP radiograph of the pelvis showing an intact Shenton's line in the presence of left-sided acetabular dysplasia. There is evidence of a previous left femoral osteotomy. B) AP pelvic radiograph showing a disrupted Shenton's line in the presence of right sided acetabular dysplasia. This hip has progressed from subluxation to frank dislocation (See also Figure 13.17.3 for explanation.)

becomes distorted. The fibrofatty tissue in the acetabular floor ('pulvinar'), the ligamentum teres and the transverse acetabular ligament all hypertrophy and encroach into the empty acetabulum. The capsule is pulled upwards by the femoral head, causing the inferior capsule to cover the mouth of the acetabulum. Muscles spanning the hip joint shorten, most significantly the iliopsoas whose tendon crosses the anterior aspect of the capsule leading to an hourglass capsular constriction that keeps the femoral head in its displaced position.

Incidence, epidemiology, and aetiology

Given the different clinical pictures and detection methods, an accurate determination of the incidence and prevalence of the DDH spectrum is difficult: estimates have ranged from 1:1000 to 1:50 live births. The incidence of actual hip dislocation is 1–1.5:1000. Several risk factors have well-recognized associations with DDH but it is unlikely that any single factor is responsible.

Box 13.17.1 Familial incidence suggests genetic link

- Identical twins: 34% concordance
- Fraternal twins: 3%
- Parents of patients: 5–10× increased incidence
- Siblings: 7× increased incidence.

The incidence of DDH varies considerably with both location and race; the former Yugoslavia had an incidence 50 times greater than other parts of Europe. The incidence in North American Indians has been reported to be as high as 1:50, whilst it is 0.1:1000 in the Hong Kong Chinese and essentially not seen in African Bantu babies. Eighty per cent of cases are female.

Twin studies have demonstrated a tenfold increased incidence of DDH in identical twins compared to fraternal twins suggesting that there is a genetic basis for the familial tendency (Box 13.17.1).

The intrauterine environment has also been implicated as a risk factor. There are associations with increased birth weight, oligohydramnios, and the other 'packaging disorders' (metatarsus adductus, torticollis), suggesting that intrauterine crowding may be involved in the pathogenesis. The risk of DDH in a child with metatarsus adductus is approximately 10% and double this with torticollis. The left hip is more frequently affected than the right, perhaps because in the most common fetal position, the left hip is adducted by pressure against the sacrum. Over half of all DDH cases are in firstborn children, related to the increased abdominal and uterine muscle tone of the nulliparous woman restricting fetal movement.

There is a strong association between breech presentation in the last month of pregnancy and DDH: the incidence is 20% with the extended breech position. Although overall, less than 5% of babies are breech, 15% of DDH cases were breech. It is the prolonged effect of the intrauterine environment that is responsible for DDH, thus the method of delivery (vaginal or Caesarean) may have no significant independent effect.

Neonatal positioning also influences the incidence of DDH. Swaddling babies with their hips extended increases the incidence whilst carrying babies with hips abducted is protective.

Capsular laxity is a key finding in DDH and a unifying hypothesis that explains many of the epidemiological characteristics of the condition is a connective tissue abnormality resulting in generalized ligamentous laxity. Studies have demonstrated higher ratios of type III to type I collagen and increased laxity of the symphysis pubis in neonates with DDH. Joint laxity can be inherited and so could account for the recognized familial tendency of DDH. Laxity also follows the same racial predilections that DDH does. Maternal relaxin hormone crosses the placenta and induces laxity in the fetus. The effect is greater in the female explaining the gender association. However, there is no increased incidence of DDH in some of the conditions characterized by hyperlaxity such as Ehlers–Danlos or Marfan syndrome (Box 13.17.2).

Box 13.17.2 Risk factors for DDH

- Female gender
- First born
- Family history
- Breech presentation
- Race/ethnic origin
- Oligohydramnios—associated packaging anomalies.

Natural history

Course in newborns

In his classic paper, Barlow reported that 1:60 infants have unilateral or bilateral hip instability. Untreated, more than 60% stabilized during the first week and 88% within the first 2 months. Other studies have also demonstrated that a significant proportion of unstable hips, including Ortolani-positive hips, will become normal over time.

Course in adults

The outlook differs between the subluxed hip and the dislocated hip. Counterintuitively, patients with subluxed hips usually experience symptoms of degenerative disease at a younger age than those with untreated dislocations. Degenerative disease is related to increased point-loading and contact stresses between the articular surfaces of the dysplastic hip, and is an inevitable consequence of subluxation. Radiographic parameters of dysplasia, such as the centre-edge angle (CEA) of Wiberg and the acetabular angle of Sharp do not act as predictors of degenerative disease. The rate of degeneration is related to the severity of subluxation, with the most severe cases developing symptoms in the second decade of life and those with minimal subluxation affected during the fifth decade.

The prognosis for a dislocated hip depends on the formation of a false acetabulum: in its absence, the hip maintains a good range of movement and a better chance of a good clinical outcome (52% vs 24%).

In addition to osteoarthritis, unilateral dislocations are associated with limb length discrepancy, valgus knee deformity and scoliosis whilst bilateral dislocation causes hyperlordosis of the spine and back pain.

Clinical presentation

The presentation of DDH depends on the age of the child. It is important to identify the unstable hip before irreversible anatomical changes develop, as these reduce the likelihood of success with non-operative measures.

In early life, there are few clinical signs, all of which may be subtle. Most cases are diagnosed through clinical screening but parental concerns regarding hip movements should always be taken seriously.

The second peak for presentation is significantly later, after the child begins to walk. Contrary to popular belief there is no significant delay in walking age but the family may notice an abnormal gait, classically described as 'waddling': a combination of a Trendelenburg and short-leg gait. The child with bilateral hip dislocations will walk with a bilateral Trendelenburg gait and a hyperlordosis secondary to hip flexion contractures. Unfortunately, as gait abnormalities are common in the toddler, unsuspecting physicians often falsely reassure parents.

Neonatal hip examination should follow a systematic approach, adhering to Apley's basic tenets of 'look, feel, move'. The clinical signs vary with age and depend on the exact nature of the hip pathology. In unilateral dislocations, asymmetry is an important feature. Asymmetry may be identified as a discrepancy in length (Galeazzi test) and an external rotation deformity but *limitation of abduction in flexion* is regarded as the most reliable sign of DDH. Asymmetrical thigh creases will be found in the dislocated hip but the sign has low specificity and many children with normal hips demonstrate the same feature.

In the neonate the dislocated head may be palpable in the buttock but in the older child with hip dysplasia the uncovered femoral head can be felt as a lump in the groin.

All of these signs rely on asymmetry that makes it more difficult to identify the child with bilateral hip dislocations. The Klisic test is helpful in these circumstances; a line from the greater trochanter to the ASIS should point to the umbilicus, but in a dislocated hip, in which the trochanter lies more proximally, this line will point halfway between the umbilicus and pubis.

The *Ortolani test* reduces the dislocated hip. Having identified that the hip has limited abduction in flexion, the examiner holds the thigh between the index finger and thumb, and uses the middle finger to lift the greater trochanter 'up'. When positive, the femoral head is felt to reduce into the acetabulum with a 'clunk'.

The *Barlow manoeuvre* attempts to sublux or dislocate an enlocated hip, by applying a gentle posteriorly-directed axial force to the adducted and flexed hip. In a positive test, the examiner will feel the femoral head sliding out of the acetabulum posteriorly.

By the age of 3–6 months, the anatomic changes associated with DDH, particularly the soft tissue contractures mean that these tests will no longer be useful.

Screening

Von Rosen introduced routine clinical screening in Sweden in 1957 and now most countries have some form of neonatal screening programme for DDH. Universal clinical examination forms the bedrock of all these programmes: good quality screening performed by experienced practitioners reduces the rates of late-presenting DDH but may not abolish it (Box 13.17.3).

Box 13.17.3 Questions to ask on clinical examination of the newborn

- Is the hip dislocated?
  - If, so is it reducible?
- If the hip is not dislocated—is it dislocatable?
- If the hip is neither of these—is it clinically normal?
  - If so, does it have the risk factors that mandate an ultrasound scan?

In order to improve detection, ultrasound imaging of the hip has been adopted widely albeit with significant differences in protocols for its use. In North America and most of the United Kingdom, selective ultrasound screening is used to investigate those hips that are clinically suspicious and/or the at-risk groups (e.g. family history, breech). In Austria, Germany, and a single district in England, universal ultrasound screening takes place in the neonatal period.

In the United Kingdom, the SMAC guidelines advocate additional clinical assessment of the hips at 6–8 weeks and 8 months of age.

Recently, some have questioned the validity of DDH screening. Proponents of screening argue that earlier detection makes a clear difference to management allowing the early use of effective non-operative treatment methods. The strongest argument against screening is the lack of knowledge regarding the natural history of DDH and the over-treatment that screening may encourage. A proportion of unstable hips will stabilize spontaneously requiring no treatment but as they are unidentifiable, it is likely that some hips are treated unnecessarily.

Ultrasound imaging complicates things further as it detects anatomically abnormal hips that may not be unstable. Universal screening as practised in Coventry (United Kingdom) has eliminated late-presenting DDH and proven to be cost-effective. Other reports have highlighted an increase in treatment rates with universal ultrasound. Prospective longitudinal studies that chart the outcomes of minor sonographic abnormalities may allow us to refine treatment criteria. Selective ultrasound screening intuitively sounds an attractive compromise but the evidence suggests that it does not reduce the incidence of late-presenting DDH more than competent clinical screening alone.

Another controversy is whether some late-presenting cases may in fact be a separate entity: they could develop *after* birth and so would be undetected by neonatal screening.

Ultrasound examination

Graf introduced neonatal hip ultrasound over 30 years ago to assess hip joint morphology by evaluating two specific anatomic features (Figure 13.17.2):

- *Alpha angle*: measures inclination of the superior aspect of the bony acetabulum
- *Beta angle*: evaluates the cartilaginous component of the acetabulum.

With increasing dysplasia and subluxation, the alpha angle decreases and the beta angle increases. Graf has created a classification system based on these parameters (Table 13.17.1). Put simply, class I hips are normal and class III/IV hips require treatment. Class II is a grey area for which the optimal management is unclear.

The methods of both Terjesen and Morin measure femoral head coverage by the bony acetabular roof but in different anatomical planes. Morin failed to find abnormalities in any hips that had more than 58% femoral head coverage. The normal values for Terjesen's method are 55% and 57% in girls and boys, respectively.

Harcke described the use of real-time dynamic screening that allows direct visualization of femoral head instability and displacement from the acetabulum during the Barlow manoeuvre: minor subluxation can be detected. This dynamic assessment of hip stability is often considered to be of greater value in the management decision-making process than static images of morphology.

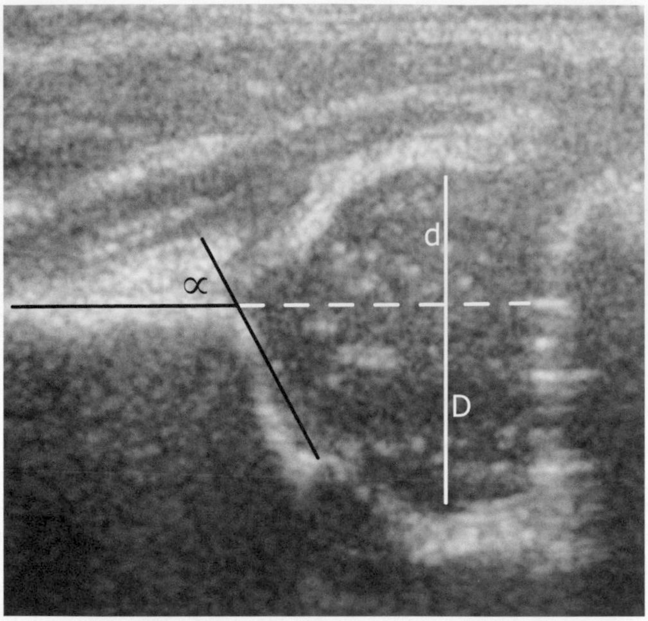

Fig. 13.17.2 An ultrasound scan showing a femoral head located within a well formed acetabulum. The α angle is 62 degrees. Femoral head coverage is assessed as a percentage by D/D+d x100.

Imaging

Radiographs are of limited use as they demonstrate only the ossified portion of the pelvis and proximal femur: an imperfect indicator of the mainly cartilaginous hip joint. A femoral head uncovered on a radiograph may be well covered by the cartilaginous acetabular anlage. However, even if this is the case, failure of the cartilage to ossify results in dysplasia and possibly subluxation.

There are three primary lines that are of use in evaluating the hip on an anteroposterior radiograph (Figure 13.17.3A). The medial beak of the femoral metaphysis, or once present, the ossific nucleus, should lie in the inferomedial quadrant of the four quadrants produced by Perkin's and Hilgenreiner's lines. The femur of a dislocated hip joint will lie lateral to Perkin's line.

The acetabular index (AI) estimates acetabular dysplasia (Figure 13.17.3B). The normal limit for the AI is 30 degrees at birth: decreasing to less than 20 degrees by the age of 2 years. The acetabular angle of Sharp is a useful alternative once the triradiate cartilages have closed.

Normally, the U-shaped acetabular teardrop appears between 6–24 months of age. The teardrop is absent or its appearance

Table 13.17.1 A simplified description of the Graf ultrasound classification of DDH

Class	Alpha angle	Beta angle	Description	Treatment
I	>60	<55	Normal	None
II	43–60	55–77	Delayed ossification	? Harness
III	<43	>77	Lateralization	Pavlik harness
IV		Unmeasurable	Dislocated	Pavlik harness

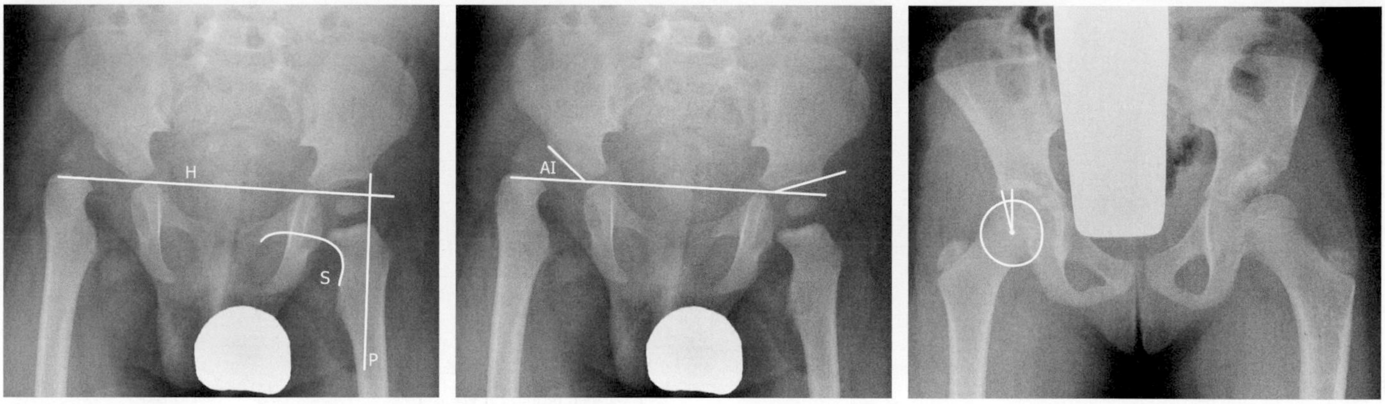

A B C

Fig. 13.17.3 A) Hilgenreiner's line (H) is a horizontal line through the two triradiate cartilages. Perkin's line (P) is a perpendicular to Hilgenreiner's line, drawn at the lateral margin of the acetabulum. Shenton's line (S) is formed by tracing the inferior margin of the femoral neck and continuing along the inferior border of the superior pubic ramus. This should produce a smooth curved line on any view of the hip, and if disrupted, a subluxation or dislocation should be suspected (see also Figure 13.17.1). The femoral head should lie in the inner medial quadrant defined by the H and P lines. The left hip is in joint, the right hip is dislocated. B) The AI is the angle formed between Hilgenreiner's line and a line following the acetabular roof. The AI is significantly increased on the right side where the hip is dislocated. In the older child once the tri-radiate cartilages have fused, Sharp's angle is measured using a horizontal between the inferior edges of the teardrops instead of Hilgenreiner's line. C) The CEA of Wiberg is the angle subtended between a line through the centre of the femoral head, parallel to Perkin's line, and a line from the centre of the femoral head to the lateral edge of the acetabulum. The right hip has a normal angle of 23 degrees. The left hip has a dysplastic acetabulum.

delayed with a dislocated hip. A V-shaped teardrop is associated with dysplasia and a poor outcome. Following joint reduction, the acetabulum remodels and the teardrop narrows. The gap between the acetabular floor and femoral head should not exceed 5mm on a standardized radiograph. DDH can be classified according to the radiological appearance (Table 13.17.2).

The femoral head ossific nucleus should appear between 3–6 months of age, characteristically its appearance is delayed in the dislocated hip. The CEA becomes a useful measure of acetabular coverage of the femoral head after 5 years (Figure 13.17.3C). In childhood this angle should measure at least 15 degrees, reaching 25 degrees by maturity.

Treatment

In all patients, the primary aim of treatment is to obtain and maintain reduction of the hip providing an optimal environment for future development. The method by which this can be achieved depends on the chronicity of the dislocation, and thus on the age of the patient. A simple algorithm is shown in Figure 13.17.4.

Table 13.17.2 The Hartofilakidis classification of hip dysplasia

Type		Description
A	Dysplasia	Femoral head contained within original acetabulum
B	Low dislocation	Femoral head articulates with a false acetabulum which partially covers the true acetabulum
C	High dislocation	Femoral head has migrated superiorly and posteriorly to the hypoplastic true acetabulum

Non-operative

A clinically unstable hip (either Barlow or Ortolani-positive) that persists at the age of 2–3 weeks should be treated with full-time splintage in flexion and abduction, maintaining it in a reduced position. As discussed previously, the management of clinically normal hips with sonographic evidence of dysplasia remains unclear as some spontaneous improvement in acetabular morphology is likely. The more severely dysplastic hips (Graf III and IV) are less likely to demonstrate spontaneous improvement particularly if associated with instability on ultrasound or clinical assessment: our personal protocol is to treat these with splintage from 2–3 weeks of age. As the Graf II hip is most likely to normalize spontaneously, our management is initially expectant. If a repeat ultrasound before the age of 6 weeks shows persistent dysplasia, treatment should be considered particularly in the presence of instability.

The Pavlik harness is the most commonly used DDH splint. It prevents dislocation by limiting hip extension and adduction whilst allowing some movement to encourage joint development (Figure 13.17.5). Other splints such as the Van Rosen splint also have high success rates with few complications.

All splints must be applied appropriately. In the Pavlik harness, the hips should be flexed no more than 100 degrees, and the posterior strap adjusted to allow comfortable abduction within the safe zone (the arc of abduction/adduction that is between redislocation and unforced abduction). If the hip cannot be placed in this position, treatment with the harness is less likely to be successful. However, even hips that are irreducible at the start of treatment can be successfully managed with a harness.

Our protocol is to review the infant at fortnightly intervals. Hip development is assessed both clinically and ultrasonographically. It is also important to review the harness to ensure that it remains appropriately fitted. Strap adjustments may be necessary to accommodate growth of the child, as otherwise the hips will gradually become over-flexed.

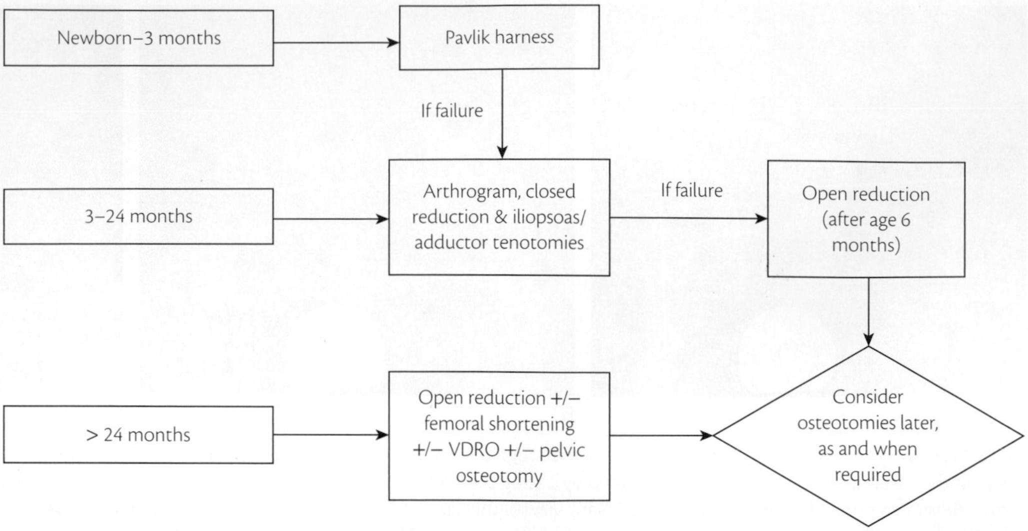

Fig. 13.17.4 A suggested algorithm for the principles of management of DDH. The ages given are a guideline only and management of the individual hip may be influenced by many factors.

If the dislocated hip remains irreducible after 2 weeks of treatment, the harness is unlikely to be successful and should be discontinued. Persisting with treatment risks damage to both the femoral head and the posterior acetabular wall.

The minimum treatment advised is 6 weeks from the time the hip reduced. If at this time, the hip is found to be both stable and anatomically normal on ultrasound, the harness can be discontinued. The child should be reviewed at 4–6 months of age with a pelvic radiograph and again at 1 year of age with further follow-up as required.

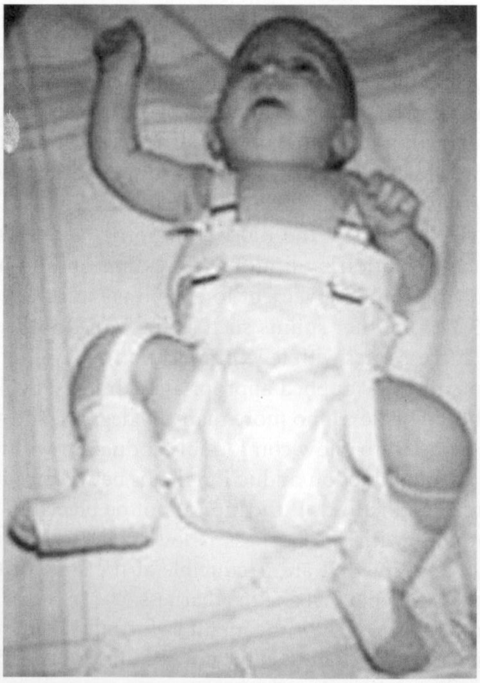

Fig. 13.17.5 The Pavlik harness must be applied properly both to achieve reduction and prevent complications. The chest strap should be at nipple level, the shoulder straps in the anterior axillary line and the posterior 'abduction' strap at the level of the scapulae.

The success rate of Pavlik harness treatment has been reported as 95% for the Ortolani-positive hip and 80% for dislocated hips that are not initially reducible. The failure rate increases in children older than 7 weeks of age at the start of treatment reaching 50% after the age of 6 months: primarily because of the difficulty in keeping the larger child compliant with harness wear. Bilateral hip dislocations are associated with higher failure rates (Box 13.17.4).

A number of different splint complications have been reported, most associated with improper application or use. The most serious complication is avascular necrosis (AVN) of the femoral head due to excessive pressure from incomplete reduction or excessive abduction, with an incidence of 2.4% in one series. Femoral nerve palsy also occurs and quadriceps function should be checked during treatment. Prolonged excessive hip flexion may lead to inferior dislocation of the femoral head. Other problems include skin rashes, foot deformities, brachial plexus palsy, and knee subluxation.

Closed reduction

Closed reduction of the hip is indicated in those who either fail conservative treatment or for whom it would be inappropriate due to age or associated disorders.

Arthrography

A closed reduction should always be performed under general anaesthesia and include a hip arthrogram. The arthrogram provides a dynamic examination of hip morphology: identifying obstacles to reduction and defining the position of 'best fit'. Only a small amount of contrast medium is required otherwise anatomical detail is obscured.

Box 13.17.4 Pavlik harness

Less suitable for patients with:

- Significant muscle imbalance (myelodysplasia)
- Joint stiffness (arthrogryposis)
- Excessive ligamentous laxity (Ehlers–Danlos syndrome).

The arthrogram demonstrates the extent of the cartilaginous roof and the labrum. When the head is appropriately covered by the labrum, a 'rose-thorn' is seen, representing a recess lateral to the labrum. This thorn will not be seen with a subluxed femoral head because the labrum is deformed (Figure 13.17.6).

If the head is concentric within the acetabulum, then a narrow rim of contrast will outline the femoral head in all positions. With femoral head subluxation, dye pools medially. If there is associated acetabular insufficiency, this pool will move superiorly as the femoral head reduces with abduction and flexion.

The hip is reduced by the Ortolani test and then screened clinically and radiographically to determine the range over which the hip remains reduced. The 'safe zone' as described by Ramsay is the arc of abduction/adduction that is between redislocation and unforced abduction: a relatively wide zone implies a stable reduction, whereas a narrow zone in which wide abduction is required, is considered unstable.

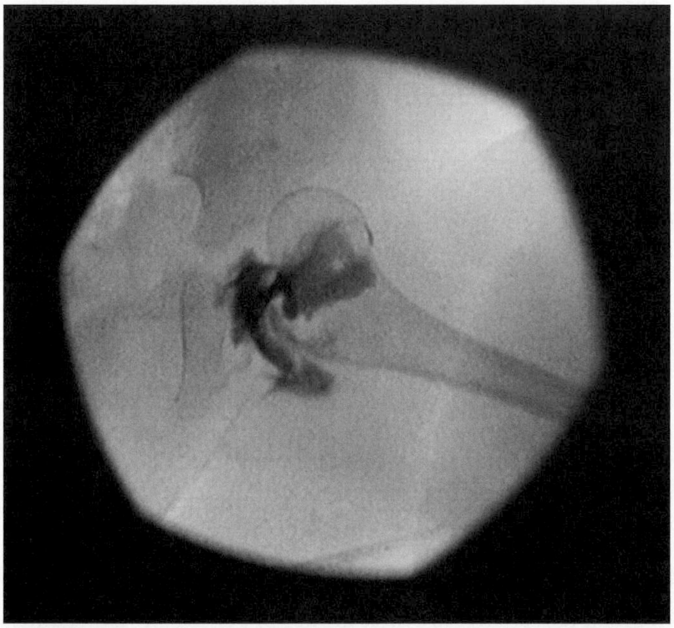

A

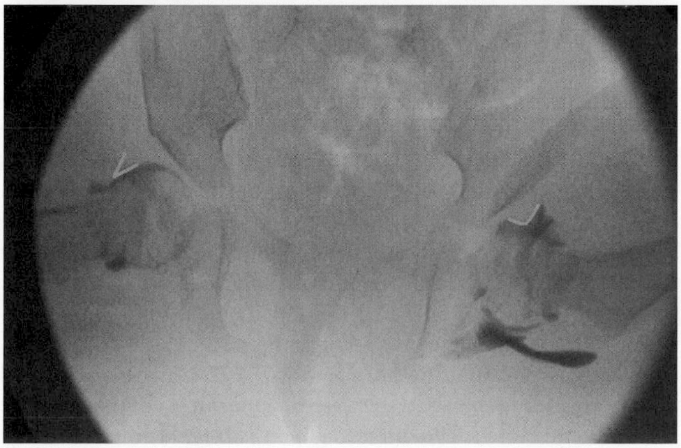

B

Fig. 13.17.6 A) Arthrogram of the left hip showing a dislocated femoral head. The femoral head outline is overlapping the acetabulum and the infolded labrum can be seen. B) Bilateral hip arthrograms. The patient's right hip is essentially normal. The rose thorn of the normal labrum has been accentuated by added lines. On the left side, the femoral head has been reduced underneath the labrum which is still deformed (as outlined by the heavy line). The labral shape improves with time once the head is reduced.

If an adduction contracture is limiting abduction, an adductor tenotomy should be performed concomitantly with the closed reduction. This increases the range of hip movement and the safe zone, thereby helping to obtain and maintain joint reduction. The adductor tenotomy also reduces pressure on the reduced femoral head. An iliopsoas tenotomy can be performed through the same incision for the same reasons.

If despite soft tissue releases, the closed reduction is difficult to maintain, it should not be forced, for fear of avascular necrosis.

Our policy is to use a short leg (above-knee) spica cast after closed reduction, as rotation is not usually required to hold the reduction. The hip spica plaster should be applied with the hips flexed to at least 90 degrees and in safe abduction. The cast is completely responsible for holding the reduction so it must be well moulded, especially dorsal to the greater trochanters.

Plain radiographs of the pelvis can be used to confirm satisfactory reduction but limited multiplanar CT scans and MRI are perhaps more helpful.

Treatment times vary: our protocol involves a total treatment time of 4.5 months with 3 months in a cast and 6 weeks full-time in an abduction brace. If indicated, hip stability and morphology can be checked with a repeat arthrogram to ensure that satisfactory progress is occurring.

Open reduction

Open reduction is indicated in cases in which closed reduction has failed or not been possible. It is often the treatment of choice for teratologic dislocations. Irrespective of the approach, the surgeon must address all soft tissue obstacles to reduction (Box 13.17.5).

Medial approach

The medial approach is considered most appropriate for the child under or around walking age. The approach can be either in the plane between adductor brevis and adductor magnus (after Ferguson) or in the interval between iliopsoas and the pectineus (after Ludloff, and modified by Weinstein and Ponseti). The medial approaches are associated with higher rates of AVN than the anterior approach partly because of injury to the medial circumflex artery. Advantages include preservation of the iliac apophysis and reduced blood loss. Bilateral dislocations can be

Box 13.17.5 Soft tissue blocks to reduction

- Adductor muscles
- Iliopsoas tendon
- Capsular constriction
- Deformed/infolded labrum
- Hypertrophied ligamentum teres
- Pulvinar
- Thickened transverse acetabular ligament.

addressed at the same operation. The medial approach does not allow any other concomitant surgical procedures such as capsulorrhaphy to be performed although the ligamentum teres can be shortened and anchored to the inferior acetabular margin to aid hip stability.

Anterior approach

The anterior approach uses the interval between tensor fascia lata and sartorius. Traditionally performed through the longitudinal Smith–Petersen approach, most surgeons now use a bikini-line incision below the inguinal ligament. The capsule is opened with a T-shaped incision: the long arm passing along the femoral neck to allow a capsular reefing at the end of the procedure, with or without excision of redundant capsule superiorly. Bilateral open reductions should be staged.

The medial approach allows the adductor and iliopsoas tendons to be divided through the same incision whilst with the anterior approach, an intramuscular lengthening of the psoas tendon is performed at the pelvic brim. A separate medial incision is required for an adductor tenotomy.

Following an anterior approach, the ligamentum teres is divided at its femoral head attachment. The ligament is followed to its inferior attachment to identify the true acetabulum and then excised. The transverse acetabular ligament is divided. The pulvinar, if excessive, can be removed. The limbus must be preserved as excising it endangers the lateral acetabular epiphysis with adverse affects on later acetabular development.

In longstanding dislocation, the superior capsule must be freed from its adhesions to the iliac wing above the true acetabulum and the inferior capsule released fully to allow the femoral head to reduce. Every effort is made to preserve the posterior capsule but in some instances, such as revision surgery, this is not possible. In these cases, the capsule must be released carefully at the acetabular margin to minimize vascular injury.

The acetabular floor is often thickened in DDH, and may limit deep seating of the otherwise reduced femoral head. Maintaining the head within the acetabulum will encourage further acetabular development and 'thinning' of its floor.

With the anterior approach and a capsulorrhaphy, our protocol is to apply a 'one-and-a-half' spica cast for 8–10 weeks. As a capsulorrhaphy cannot be performed with the medial approach, the cast is usually maintained for 12 weeks.

At the time of open reduction, an associated pelvic or femoral osteotomy may be required to either obtain the reduction or to provide the stability to maintain the reduction.

The role of osteotomies

As detailed previously, subluxation that has progressed to an established dislocation results in a shallow and anteverted acetabulum, often associated with an anteverted and valgus femoral neck. Following hip reduction, these abnormalities can remodel but the potential for this depends on the age of the patient. Several schools of thought exist regarding the indications for additional osteotomies (Box 13.17.6).

Box 13.17.6 Questions regarding the role of osteotomy in the initial management of DDH

- Are they needed?
  - Or will the hip remodel with time?
- Above the joint or below?
  - Femoral – varus ± derotation ± shortening
  - Pelvic – redirectional or reshaping
- At the time of open reduction or as a staged procedure?

Some surgeons believe that children older than 18 months have poor potential for acetabular development and must undergo a pelvic osteotomy with their open reduction. Others believe that in children younger than 3years, the acetabulum has significant development potential for 5 years following reduction. In most cases, the acetabulum is not actually deficient but its cartilage has failed to ossify. Thus, if the reduction is stable, normal acetabular development can be expected and observed radiographically. With time the acetabular cartilage ossifies thereby correcting the dysplasia. The majority of this occurs during the first 12–18 months.

Radiographic indicators of adequate development include a decreasing AI and an improvement in teardrop morphology. The development of the superolateral acetabular margin, (the 'sourcil' or eyebrow) is also regarded as a reliable indicator of acetabular development. If significant acetabular dysplasia persists beyond the age of 5 years, a pelvic osteotomy is required.

Another area of controversy is whether the osteotomy should be performed on the femur or the pelvis. As the primary abnormality lies within the acetabulum, some surgeons will always direct their attention to the pelvis, in the knowledge that femoral neck anteversion will often correct spontaneously. Others will perform a varus derotation osteotomy on the dysplastic proximal femur to redirect the femoral head towards the centre of the acetabulum and stimulate normal acetabular development. In this situation, the femoral osteotomy should be performed before the age of 4 years.

Pelvic osteotomies

In broad terms, there are three groups of pelvic osteotomy, differentiated by indication and by the manner in which they improve femoral head coverage (Table 13.17.3).

Redirectional procedures

The prerequisite for considering a redirectional acetabular osteotomy is that the subluxed hip can be placed in a position where the joint is congruent throughout a useful range of motion. This 'best-fit' position must then be recreated by the osteotomy. In such cases, the acetabulum is essentially an appropriate size and shape but it is facing the wrong way. Acetabular orientation is changed by the osteotomy, which improves anterosuperior cover in the weight bearing position.

The Salter innominate osteotomy is the classic example of a redirectional pelvic osteotomy. A transverse osteotomy is performed through the ilium, between the anterior inferior iliac spine and the greater sciatic notch. The distal fragment is rotated anterolaterally: the osteotomy must remain closed posteriorly and the resultant anterior gap is filled with a triangular bone graft from the iliac crest. Threaded wires are used to stabilize the osteotomy. It provides anterior cover at the expense of posterior cover and if a derotation femoral osteotomy is performed concurrently there is a risk that the femoral head will sublux posteriorly. Redirection is achieved by rotation of the acetabulum around the symphysis pubis.

Table 13.17.3 Types of pelvic osteotomy that could be considered in cases of DDH

Redirectional	Reshaping	Salvage
Salter	Pemberton	Shelf
Triple	Dega	Chiari
Periacetabular		Colonna interpositional arthroplasty

With skeletal maturity such rotation is impossible and thus osteotomies of the pubic ramus and the ischium are required (Sutherland double and Steel triple osteotomies). Perhaps the best correction is achieved with the technically more complex periacetabular osteotomy.

Reshaping procedures

This group of acetabuloplasties, including those described by Pemberton and Dega, reshape the acetabulum. Their 'volume-reducing' effect makes them most useful when the dyplastic acetabulum appears too capacious for the femoral head and hence these hips do not show a congruent 'best-fit' position on arthrogram. An open triradiate cartilage is a prerequisite for this procedure as it acts as the fulcrum upon which to hinge the acetabular correction. Injury to the triradiate cartilage is a serious but uncommon complication that could result in premature physeal fusion.

Pemberton's pericapsular osteotomy is an incomplete curvilinear iliac osteotomy that follows the contour of the acetabular roof inferomedially to the triradiate cartilage. The acetabular roof is then levered downwards to improve anterolateral cover, and a graft placed into the gap that is created. The Dega osteotomy is similar in principle: it is perhaps used most frequently for hip dysplasia secondary to neuromuscular disorders where the primary acetabular deficiency is more commonly posterior.

Salvage procedures

These procedures augment acetabular cover and hence support of the femoral head by placing bone over the hip capsule and inducing fibrocartilaginous metaplasia within the capsule. These procedures are used in circumstances in which the there is irreducible subluxation or if the other osteotomies cannot be performed due to previous surgical interventions.

The Shelf procedures improve femoral head coverage in cases with mild to moderate acetabular insufficiency. Various techniques have been reported, but common features are the use of a slab or strips of cortical graft taken from the ilium and placed on top of the hip capsule (the 'shelf'), which is then buttressed from above by a bone graft that is supported proximally against the ilium. Over time and in response to loading from the femoral head, the shelf hypertrophies and remodels.

If acetabular insufficiency is associated with pronounced lateralization of the femoral head, the joint should be medialized. The Chiari osteotomy is performed through the ilium, allowing medial displacement of the acetabular fragment with its attached hip capsule.

The interpositonal arthroplasty described by Colonna, is suitable in cases of severe femoroacetabular incongruity but when the femoral head is still spherical. The capsule is divided circumferentially at its acetabular insertion, and oversewn over the femoral head. The acetabulum is then enlarged using serial reamers until it can provide a stable articulation for the capsule-enveloped femoral head.

Treatment in later childhood

Occasionally, children present later in life with established DDH. The surgeon must note that the untreated child is unlikely to develop pain before adolescence, whilst the unsuccessfully treated child will do. The remodelling potential of those over 3 years is limited, so as well as a femoral shortening ostetomy, a concomitant corrective acetabular and femoral procedure must be considered. Unilateral dislocations are more likely to affect gait and function and so treatment is recommended up to the age of 10 years. Surgical reduction is not recommended for bilateral dislocations after the age of 6–8 years as the complication rate is higher and the surgical outcomes inferior to the natural history of the condition.

Late complications

The two most common late complications are residual dysplasia and AVN of the proximal femur. Thus regular follow-up until skeletal maturity is advised for all children who undergo operative treatment for DDH.

Residual dysplasia

Deficiency of the anterior acetabular wall is one of the primary anatomic abnormalities in early childhood but by adolescence the deficiency is often more global. Late-onset femoral dysplasia is usually secondary to AVN. Treatment of the dysplastic young adult hip is a subspecialty in its own right.

In cases of unilateral DDH, the opposite hip may show subtle signs of acetabular dysplasia that are exacerbated by a leg length discrepancy. Follow-up should include assessment of both hips.

Avascular necrosis of the proximal femur

AVN is potentially disabling and difficult to manage successfully. It is not a feature of the natural history of DDH and is therefore regarded as a consequence of treatment. Some controversy exists over the term 'AVN': there is little histological evidence that this is the underlying pathology and 'proximal femoral growth disturbance' may be a better term.

Several factors have been implicated in the development of AVN, including forced reduction, and the use of extreme positions of abduction and/or internal rotation. The femoral head has a rich blood supply, predominantly endarteries arising from the medial and lateral circumflex branches of the profunda femoris. Extremes in hip positioning can result in compression of the medial femoral circumflex artery. In order to reduce the incidence of AVN, certain management strategies have been adopted but their role remains controversial.

The protective role of the ossific nucleus

Until the ossific nucleus appears, the femoral head has a cartilaginous structure that can be deformed when it is forcibly reduced or held in an extreme position. This, together with its poor vascular anastomoses, makes the cartilaginous femoral head particularly vulnerable to infarction. A recent meta-analysis found that the presence of the ossific nucleus reduced the probability of AVN by 60% after closed reduction but its presence had no significant protective effect following open reduction. The results also suggested that the ossific nucleus protects against the higher grades of AVN. The possible protective effects of the ossific nucleus have to be weighed against the pathological changes that develop the longer the hip is left dislocated and that may reduce the likelihood of a successful closed reduction.

Traction versus femoral shortening

In the older child with a longstanding high dislocation and soft tissue contractures, reduction of the hip can be considerably more difficult with concerns about the effects of excessive forces acting on the newly-reduced femoral head. Several studies have demonstrated that preoperative traction does not reduce the rate of avascular necrosis. Femoral shortening prevents excessive compression of the proximal epiphysis and has been shown to reduce the rates of AVN more significantly than pre-operative traction.

A diagnosis of AVN is made when the femoral head is not seen to ossify or grow within a year of reduction. The variable extent of the subsequent growth disturbance forms the basis of the Bucholz–Ogden classification system (Table 13.17.4). Type II is most common and may not be manifest until after the age of 12 years, making long-term follow-up of all patients essential. In type III, the entire metaphysis is affected, resulting in a very short femoral neck. The greater trochanter remains unaffected in AVN and develops normally leading to relative overgrowth compared to the stunted femoral head and neck in types III–IV (Figure 13.17.7).

Surgical treatment for AVN is aimed at correcting the resultant anatomical abnormalities including any leg length discrepancy. Epiphysiodesis of the opposite distal femoral physis may be considered to equalize leg lengths and trochanteric epiphysiodesis could prevent trochanteric overgrowth. In late cases, trochanteric advancement can restore normal abductor function and improve the Trendelenburg gait. Valgus and varus deformities of the femoral neck can be addressed by corrective osteotomies but femoral neck length must also be considered when planning these procedures.

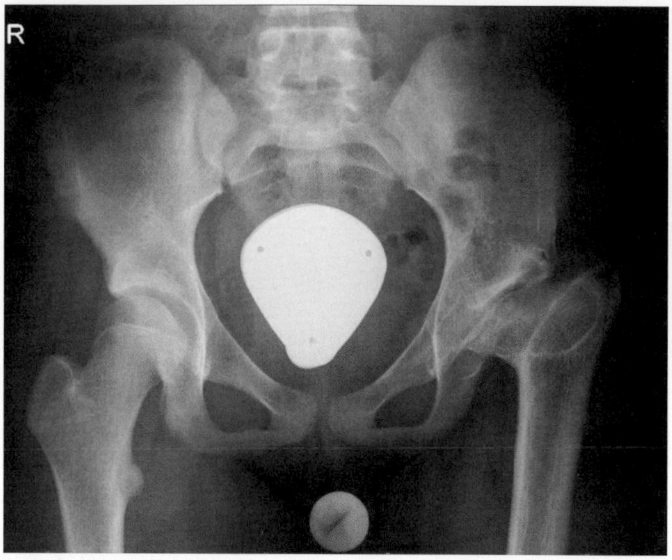

Fig. 13.17.7 AP pelvic radiograph demonstrating severe AVN of the left femoral head with a short femoral neck. In contrast, trochanteric growth is unaffected and the greater trochanter is 'high-riding'.

Outcomes

Few papers look at the long-term outcomes and most have significant methodological differences, making objective comparisons impossible. Most studies use the Severin classification for radiographic outcome of treated DDH (Table 13.17.5) despite its low levels of inter- and intraobserver reliability and there is little uniformity in the literature with respect to the use of functional measures. Excellent functional outcomes in the short to medium term are reported with poorer radiological outcomes although the latter are more accurate predictors of long-term outcome.

A recent series looking at the natural history after treatment with a Pavlik harness found a late dysplasia rate of 3.5% and AVN rate of 1%. Importantly, they found no significant differences in development between normal hips and those treated successfully with the harness. Another study investigating long-term outcomes after similar treatment found good or excellent radiological outcomes in 90%, but an AVN rate of 12.3%. Contrary to contemporary practice, the mean time spent in the harness was 6 months.

The published results for closed reduction have varied with a recent long-term study of closed reduction finding excellent or good radiological outcomes in only 46% of cases. There was some evidence of AVN in 60%, degenerative joint disease in 43%, and residual subluxation in 36%. Contemporary belief is that current results are better than this.

Table 13.17.4 The Bucholz–Ogden classification for AVN

Type	Description	Effect
I	Changes limited to the capital epiphysis	No significant growth disturbance
II	Injury to the lateral physis and metaphysis	Premature closure of the lateral physis with formation of a valgus femoral neck
III	Entire metaphysis and physis affected	Short femoral neck
IV	Injury to the medial physis with radiolucent defect in the medial metaphysis	Varus deformity of the femoral neck

Table 13.17.5 The Severin classification for radiographic outcome after treatment for DDH

Type	Description
I	Normal
II	Moderate deformity of femoral head/neck or acetabulum
III	Dysplasia without subluxation
IVa	Moderate subluxation
IVb	Severe subluxation
V	Femoral head articulates with a pseudoacetabulum related to the original acetabulum
VI	Complete redislocation

Medium term outcome studies of open reduction via the medial approaches have reported AVN rates that vary from 16–43% with residual dysplasia requiring surgical intervention in almost a third. A skeletal maturity review of 95 hips treated by anterior open reduction and concomitant pelvic or femoral osteotomy as indicated by the 'test of stability' showed 86% of hips were Severin I/II. AVN was associated with a poorer outcome and treatment under the age of 2 with a better result.

Most recently, the Toronto group have presented the outcomes after open reduction, capsulorrhaphy and inominate osteotomy at a mean follow-up of 45 years: 35% had good function, 13.5% had definite osteoarthritis, and 46% of patients had undergone arthroplasty.

In summary, various treatment methods result in good functional outcomes for the first two decades of life. The radiological outcomes are not of a similar high standard and consequently a substantial proportion develops premature osteoarthritis. There is some evidence that treatment at an earlier age and by closed methods leads to a better outcome.

Edgar Somerville wrote that 'in the treatment of congenital dislocation of the hip it is our successors who will judge our results rather than ourselves'. Good quality, objective, long-term studies are required to evaluate those results, in order to improve the outcomes for tomorrow's patient.

Further reading

Jones, D.H., Dezateaux, C.A., Danielsson, L.G., Paton, R.W., and Clegg, J. (2000). At the crossroads – neonatal detection of developmental dysplasia of the hip. *Journal of Bone and Joint Surgery*, **82B**, 160–64.

MacNicol, M. (1995). *Color Atlas and Text of Osteotomy of the Hip*. London: Mosby-Wolfe.

Mahan, S.T., Katz, J.N., and Kim, Y.-J. (2009). To screen or not to screen A decision analysis of the utility of screening for developmental dysplasia of the hip. *Journal of Bone and Joint Surgery*, **91A**, 1705–19.

Pavlik, A. (1992). The functional method of treatment using a harness with stirrups as the primary method of conservative therapy for infants with congenital dislocation of the hip. *Clinical Orthopaedics and Related Research*, **281**, 4–10.

Roposch, A., Stohr, K.K., and Dobson, M. (2009). The effect of the femoral head ossific nucleus in the treatment of developmental dysplasia of the hip, A meta-analysis. *Journal of Bone and Joint Surgery*, **91A**, 911–8.

Thomas, S.R., Wedge, J.H., and Salter, R.B. (2007). Outcome at forty-five years after open reduction and innominate osteotomy for late presenting developmental dislocation of the hip. *Journal of Bone and Joint Surgery*, **89A**, 2341–50.

Zadeh, H.G., Catterall, A., Hashemi-Nejad, A., and Perry, R.E. (2000). Test of stability as an aid to decide the need for ostetomy in association with open reduction in developmental dysplasia of the hip. *Journal of Bone and Joint Surgery*, **82B**, 17–27.

13.18

Legg–Calve–Perthes disease

Colin Bruce

Summary points

- Avascular necrosis of the femoral head initiated by unknown factors is followed by gradual restoration of blood supply and regeneration
- Current treatment methods aim to prevent development of an aspherical and incongruent femoral head and acetabulum
- Treatment should be offered to the child with a poor prognosis so that the natural history of the condition can be improved: identification of such cases is difficult
- Early and late management strategies differ significantly.

Introduction

The radiological changes of Legg–Calve–Perthes disease were identified soon after the development of x-ray machines for clinical use. In 1909, Waldenström was the first to publish a description of the radiological changes seen in the condition but his name is not credited to the disease because he considered the appearances to be a form of tuberculosis of the hip.

In 1910, Legg, Calve, and Perthes secured their place in history when each published observations distinguishing the condition from tuberculosis, reflecting a more benign clinical course and dissimilar radiological progression. Perthes original description (1913) is still valid today:

> *a self-limiting, non-inflammatory condition, affecting the capital femoral epiphysis with stages of degeneration and regeneration, leading to a restoration of the bone nucleus*

Currently it is accepted that the series of changes described by Perthes are initiated by events that lead to avascular necrosis (AVN) of the ossific nucleus followed by gradual restoration of the blood supply and subsequent regeneration. The underlying aetiology of these events remains elusive and so the condition cannot be prevented. Management is focused on trying to limit progressive femoral head deformity after the AVN has occurred.

Epidemiology

Perthes disease occurs worldwide. The incidence is relatively low in black populations (0.45/100 000), intermediate in Asians (3.8/100 000), and high in Caucasians (15.4/100 000). Within populations, the incidence varies from region to region and reports from the United Kingdom and South India suggest an association with deprivation. Most clinicians will be aware of patients with a family history of the disease but the evidence for a genetic predisposition is unclear. Some studies show little support for a genetic aetiology whilst others suggest a multifactorial inheritance pattern.

The condition is four to five times more common in boys than girls. Eighty per cent of children present between 4–9 years of age. Patients may share some typical characteristics and the notion of the 'susceptible child' has emerged (Box 13.18.1).

Pathology

The blood supply of the child's femoral epiphysis is vulnerable. No blood reaches the epiphysis from the metaphysis because the physeal plate presents a complete barrier and the blood supply from the ligamentum teres is negligible. The primary supply to the femoral epiphysis is derived from the medial femoral circumflex artery which pierces the capsule of the hip joint in the posterior trochanteric fossa and becomes the lateral ascending cervical artery (Figure 13.18.1).

Effectively, a single trunk vessel supplies the epiphysis which makes it vulnerable to ischaemic necrosis. The anteromedial part of the femoral epiphysis is furthest from the main trunk and this may explain why it is the first area to show evidence of AVN in Perthes disease and why the posterolateral portion, closer to the trunk vessel, is sometimes preserved.

Box 13.18.1 The susceptible child

- Male
- Aged 4–9 years
- Delayed bone age
- Family of low socioeconomic status
- Disproportionate short stature: distal limb segments predominantly.

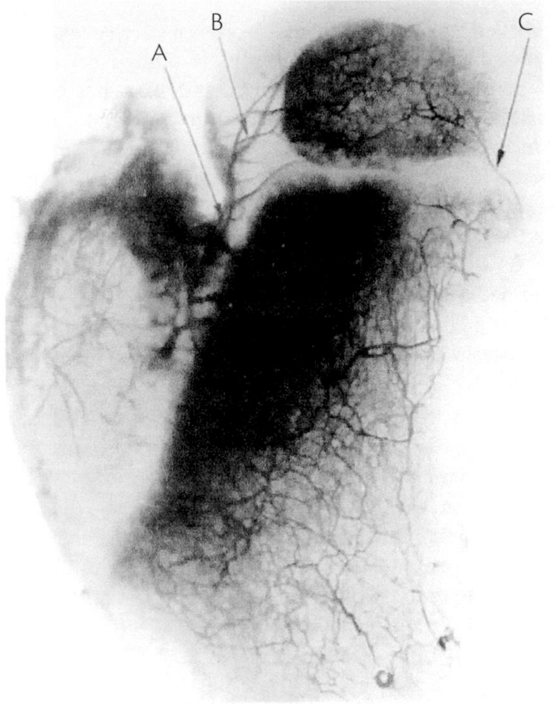

Fig. 13.18.1 The blood supply of the immature femoral head: The lateral ascending cervical artery (A) and the epiphyseal branches of both the lateral (B) and medial (C) ascending cervical arteries pass through the perichondral ring and not the epiphyseal plate. Reproduced with permission from Chung, S.M. (1976). The arterial supply of the developing proximal end of the human femur. *Journal of Bone and Joint Surgery*, **58A**, 961–70.

The nature and cause of the disturbance in the blood supply in Perthes disease is uncertain. A single infarct of the femoral epiphysis does not necessarily lead to the radiological changes seen in the disease. Most reports to date support the notion that recurrent infarcts are necessary to cause the typical radiological features. Once AVN is established, progressive changes may occur. The current working hypothesis suggests that a fracture develops in the weakened avascular bone which is unable to unite until it is revascularized. As revascularization ensues, the repair process results in the characteristic radiological changes, as dead bone trabeculae are slowly removed and replaced. This process can take years to complete and during this time the cartilaginous femoral head, devoid of its internal supporting structure, can become deformed.

Why an infarct should occur is still unknown. Reports have implicated disturbances on both the arterial and the venous side of the femoral head circulation. Trauma has been postulated as a potential explanation as has transient synovitis: both may tamponade the circulation but although symptoms of synovitis are often the first presentation of the disease, most studies do not support a causal relationship between transient synovitis and Perthes disease. More recent reports implicated various abnormalities of the plasma proteins involved in the coagulation cascade. Some are associated with a predisposition to clot formation (thrombophilia) and others are associated with a limited potential to 'lyse' clots once formed (hypofibrinolysis). To date no single explanation for the aetiology has been identified and it may be that Perthes disease is simply the final common pathway of a variety of circumstances, environmental and/or genetic, that leads to AVN of the femoral epiphysis.

Radiological stages and pathological correlation

Perthes disease occurs in healthy children and therefore there are few accounts where the sequential radiological changes have been correlated with the histological morphology (Figure 13.18.2).

Early stage

In the early stages following infarction, there is a growth disturbance. The bony epiphysis, devoid of its blood supply, stops growing but the cartilage does not and this relative overgrowth, particularly on the medial and lateral aspects of the femoral head, results in a cartilaginous coxa magna. Thus, in the early stages of Perthes disease, radiographs sometimes reveal a smaller bony epiphysis on the affected side although the apparent joint space is wider (Figure 13.18.2A).

Sclerotic stage

It is postulated that recurrent infarction within the epiphysis eventually weakens the bony epiphysis and trabecular fractures and collapse occur. Radiographically, this leads to loss of bony epiphyseal height and increased density (Figure 13.18.2B). Catterall has shown that the density noted on fine-detail radiography during the stage of sclerosis is, in part, due to mechanical compression of the fractured necrotic trabeculae but, in the main, is due to calcification of the necrotic marrow within the epiphysis. During this stage, the growth plate becomes abnormal with distortion of the cell columns and an increase in the quantity of calcified cartilage in the primary spongiosa.

Fragmentation stage

Once infarction has occurred, a process of repair becomes established to revascularize the avascular area. A process of creeping substitution slowly removes the necrotic bone and replaces it with fibrocartilage (Figure 13.18.2C). This repair process produces the radiological appearance of fragmentation. Islands of new bone formation in the thickened anterior and lateral articular cartilage gradually enlarge and coalesce. These islands appear radiologically as areas of calcification lateral to the epiphysis and reveal the extent to which the cartilaginous femoral epiphysis has been extruded outside the confines of the acetabulum. In the growth plate, areas of unossified cartilage extend down into the metaphyseal region producing the radiological appearance of a metaphyseal cyst. If these are large, the normal architecture of the growth plate is lost. It has been postulated that such an area might act as a tether to further growth in the anterolateral part of the neck, leading to tilting of the femoral head on the long axis of the neck. In the long term, this process might explain the radiological transcervical line described as the sagging rope sign. This radiological appearance is the result of superimposition of the anterolateral part of the femoral head overhanging the femoral neck, like the head of a mushroom overhanging its stalk (see Figure 13.18.14).

Healing and late stage

In the healing phase of the disease the necrotic trabeculae have been removed and replaced by fibrocartilage which is progressively reossified. The last portion to reform is the anterosuperior portion of the epiphysis and this is seen as a residual central lucency on the anteroposterior (AP) radiograph (Figure 13.18.2D). As the structural function of the epiphysis to maintain the femoral head shape is lost during the stages of sclerosis and fragmentation, the cartilaginous femoral head becomes flatter and broader under load, and

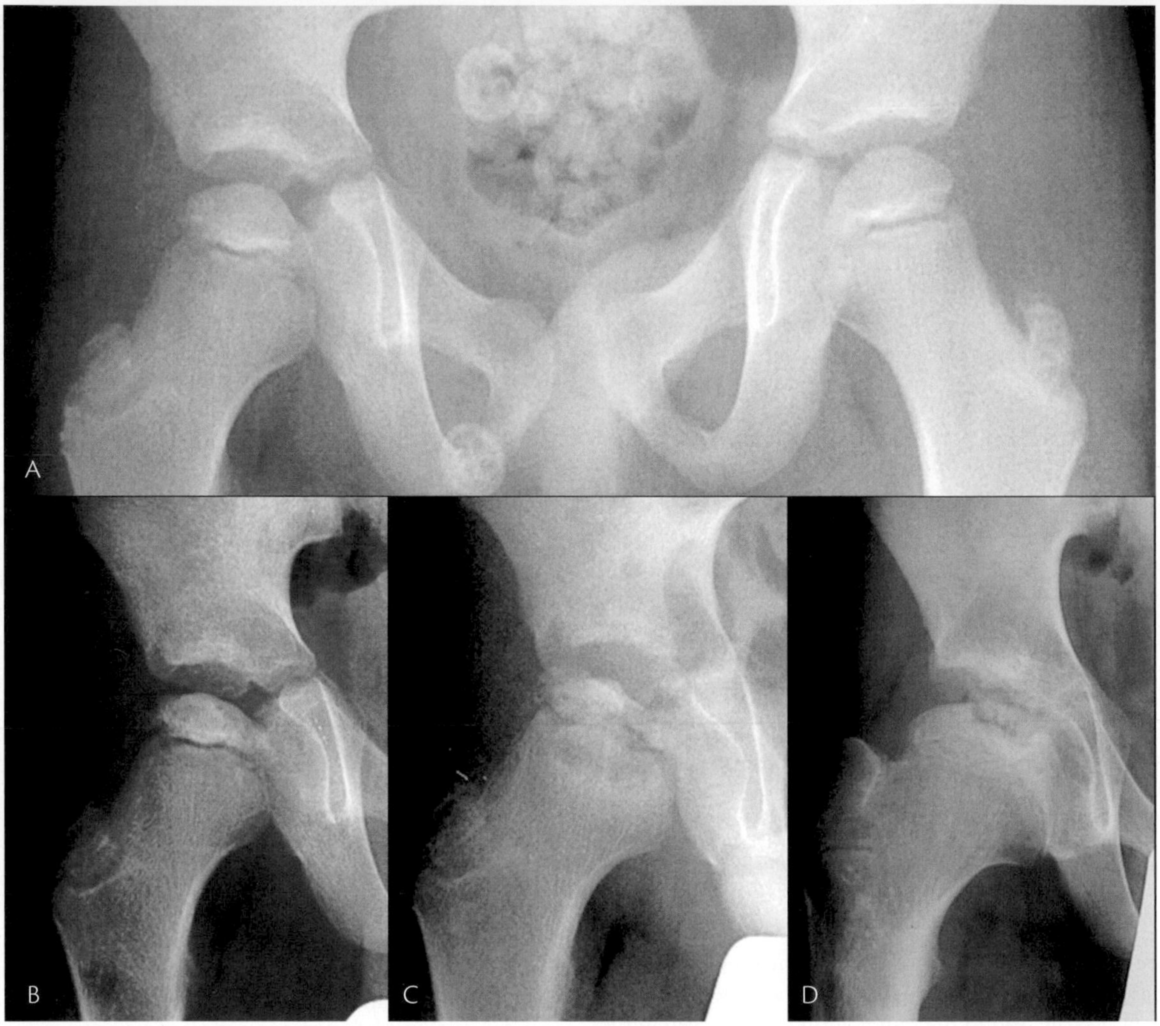

Fig. 13.18.2 Radiological stages of Perthes disease. A) Early stage. B) Sclerotic stage. C) Fragmentation stage. D) Healing and late stage. See text for explanation.

when the healing process is complete the femoral head is ovoid rather than spherical. Clearly the extent to which the shape changes, depends on how much or how little of the epiphyseal support is affected by the disease.

Clinical presentation, differential diagnosis, and investigation

Early Perthes disease typically presents with groin, thigh, or referred knee pain and an antalgic limp. This is the clinical picture of an irritable hip. On examination the most sensitive sign of hip irritability is discomfort with internal rotation, but as irritability increases abduction becomes limited and eventually an external rotation, adduction, flexion posture develops. When a child presents with an irritable hip, ultrasound identification of a joint effusion is the key investigation to confirm the clinical suspicion that the hip joint is the source of the problem. Perthes disease is but one cause of hip irritability and other differential diagnoses must be considered depending on the age of the child at presentation (Box 13.18.2). The most common explanation for an irritable hip is transient synovitis. Septic arthritis is an important differential diagnosis in any child and must always be considered. In older children a slipped upper femoral epiphysis is possible.

At initial presentation there may be no radiological evidence of Perthes disease and the condition is difficult to differentiate from transient synovitis. If a patient's symptoms do not resolve within a week or two of presentation then a diagnosis of transient synovitis should be questioned.

Box 13.18.2 Irritable hip: differential diagnosis

- Transient synovitis (commonest)
- Septic arthritis
- Perthes disease
- Slipped capital femoral epiphysis (>10 years)
- Juvenile idiopathic arthritis.

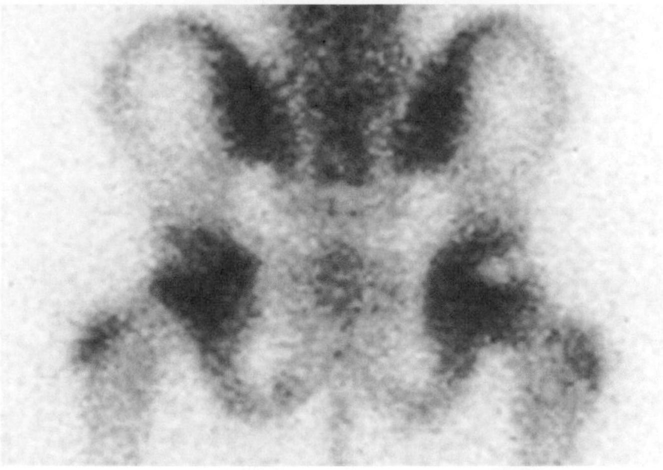

Fig. 13.18.3 Radionuclide bone scan: Scan shows a 'cold' area of decreased uptake in the ischaemic area of epiphyseal bone in Perthes disease.

A radionuclide bone scan is a useful investigation because it will show a 'cold' area of decreased uptake in Perthes disease which distinguishes the condition from most other differential diagnoses (Figure 13.18.3).

Magnetic resonance imaging (MRI) scanning may help identify altered signal from the epiphyseal marrow in Perthes disease but, in the author's opinion, offers little advantage over bone scanning (Figure 13.18.4).

Eventually radiological changes will be apparent. While Perthes disease is the most common explanation for the radiological appearance of epiphyseal AVN of the hip in children, other known causes of AVN will give a similar appearance. Conditions including systemic corticosteroid therapy, sickle cell disease, other haemoglobinopathies, and storage diseases (Gaucher's) should be considered. Bilateral Perthes disease is unusual but when present it is asymmetrical with each affected hip at a different stage. Bilateral symmetrical disease should raise suspicion of bony dysplasias such as multiple epiphyseal dysplasia.

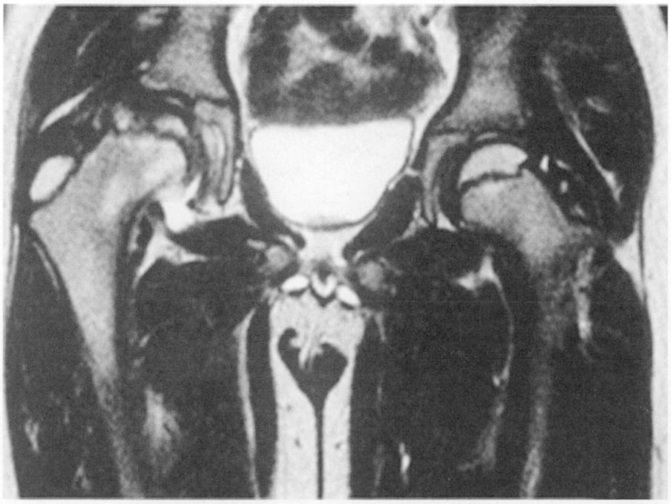

Fig. 13.18.4 MRI scan: scan shows altered signal from the epiphyseal marrow in a case of Perthes disease.

Classification and prognosis

Classification

The Stulberg classification

Premature degeneration of the hip joint due to joint deformity is the potential consequence of Perthes disease. Eighty-six per cent of patients will develop osteoarthritis by the age of 65, but in the majority symptoms will not become a problem until the fifth or sixth decade (Figure 13.18.5).

It is important to understand why some hips have a better long-term prognosis than others and Stulberg's work gives some insight into the explanation (Box 13.18.3). If the femoral head remains spherical and the acetabulum matches, the hip is termed spherical and congruent. Although this outcome is relatively uncommon such hips show no propensity to long-term degeneration. If the femoral head becomes ovoid and the acetabulum grows to match then the hip is aspherical and congruent. Such hips develop mild to moderate arthritis in late adult life. Finally, if the femoral head becomes ovoid or flattened and the acetabulum does not grow to match then the hip is aspherical and incongruent. Such hips develop severe arthritis before the age of 50. Current treatment methods focus on preventing the development of an aspherical and incongruent hip.

The Catterall classification

An early report on Perthes disease described a favourable outcome when only the anterior half of the epiphysis was involved and Catterall later published a milestone paper introducing a classification of Perthes disease which separated patient groups based on how much of the epiphysis was involved by the condition (Figure 13.18.6). The findings of this study reflect the findings of the majority of published works both past and present. Children with limited involvement of the epiphysis (group I) were shown to have a

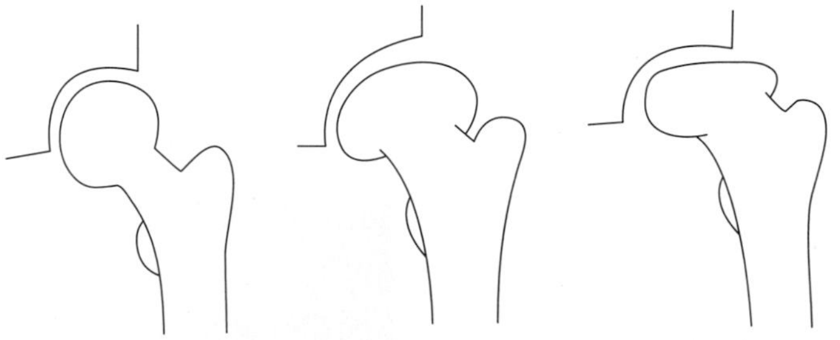

Fig. 13.18.5 Stulberg et al. (1981) classified hips according to the final shape of the femoral head and acetabulum. Hips were considered spherical if the femoral head could be fitted onto the circumference of the same circle on anteroposterior and lateral radiographs. There are three functional outcomes. 1) A head that is spherical with a congruent acetabulum. There may be some coxa magna or femoral neck shortening but spherical and congruent hips show no propensity to premature degeneration. 2) A head that is aspherical, often ovoid in shape, with a congruent acetabulum that has grown to match the femoral head. Again there may be some coxa magna or neck shortening or acetabular dysplasia. Such hips do degenerate prematurely but usually after middle adult life. 3) A head that is aspherical and flattened but the acetabulum remains round and thus the joint is incongruent. Such hips degenerate prematurely often before middle adult life.

Box 13.18.3 The Stulberg concept—does the femoral head match the acetabulum?

- The spherical and congruent hip
- The aspherical but congruent hip
- The aspherical and incongruent hip.

favourable prognosis irrespective of treatment. Children with onset below the age of 4 years also had a favourable prognosis irrespective of treatment and girls had a worse prognosis than boys. The recognition that a subset of patients might have a favourable outcome without treatment spared many children from the blanket application of the treatment regimens such as prolonged recumbency, weight relief, and bracing that were popular at the time.

Catterall further described five head at risk signs that might give an early indication of a potentially unfavourable outcome (Figure 13.18.7).

The Herring lateral pillar classification

The lateral pillar classification recognizes the importance of the integrity of the lateral part of the femoral epiphysis (Figure 13.18.8). If the lateral portion is intact it functions like a strut, column, or pillar, bearing the load transmitted to the femoral head from the acetabular roof. The remaining medial and central parts of the epiphysis are thus protected from load bearing and epiphyseal collapse is prevented. Increasing fragmentation and collapse of the lateral pillar is associated with a worsening prognosis. This concept was first observed by Ferguson but recognition that changes in the lateral epiphysis are a bad prognostic sign was also embodied in some of Catterall's head at risk signs.

Herring's classification divides the femoral epiphysis into a lateral third, a central third and a medial third. Changes seen in the lateral pillar at the end of the fragmentation stage determine the group (Table 13.18.1). The Herring classification is reported to have lower intra- and interobserver variability compared to the Catterall classification.

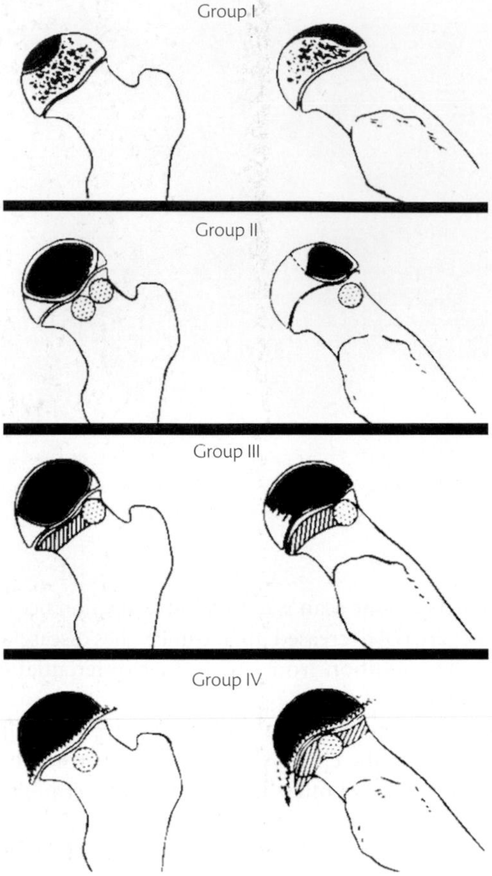

Fig. 13.18.6 Diagrams representing anteroposterior and lateral views of the Catterall classification of Perthes disease into four groups. Dark shading represents the area of ischaemic necrosis. The dotted circular areas represent metaphyseal involvement and the diagonal hatching demonstrates that the physis is also affected.

The Salter and Thompson classification

Classification of the extent of femoral epiphyseal involvement using either the Catterall or the Herring system can only be established at the end of the fragmentation stage. Consequently neither

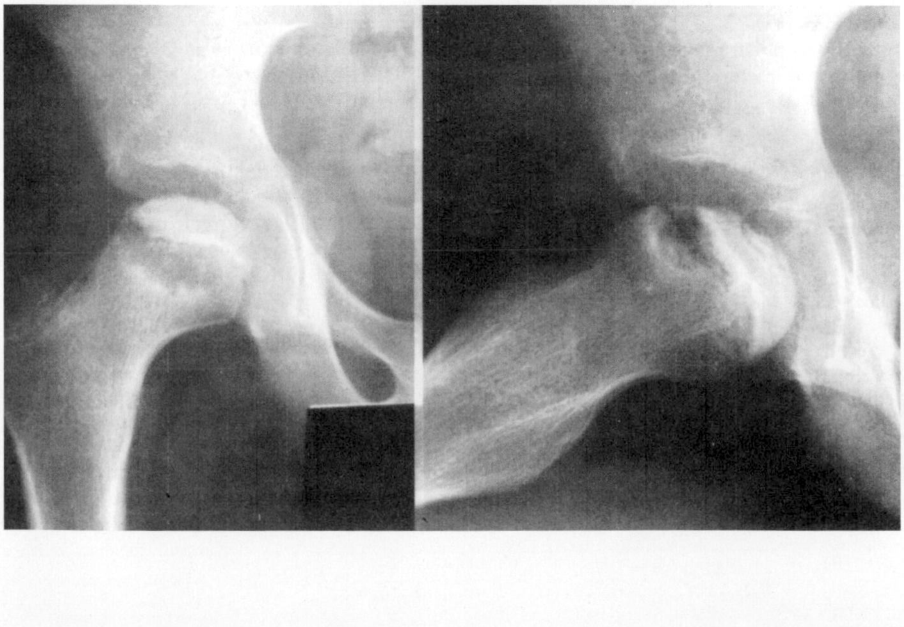

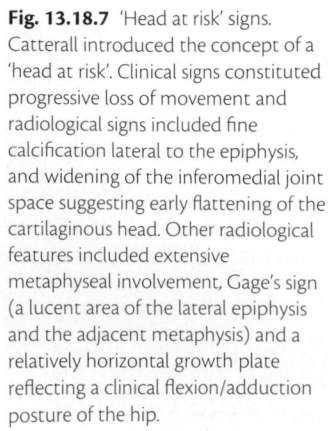

Fig. 13.18.7 'Head at risk' signs. Catterall introduced the concept of a 'head at risk'. Clinical signs constituted progressive loss of movement and radiological signs included fine calcification lateral to the epiphysis, and widening of the inferomedial joint space suggesting early flattening of the cartilaginous head. Other radiological features included extensive metaphyseal involvement, Gage's sign (a lucent area of the lateral epiphysis and the adjacent metaphysis) and a relatively horizontal growth plate reflecting a clinical flexion/adduction posture of the hip.

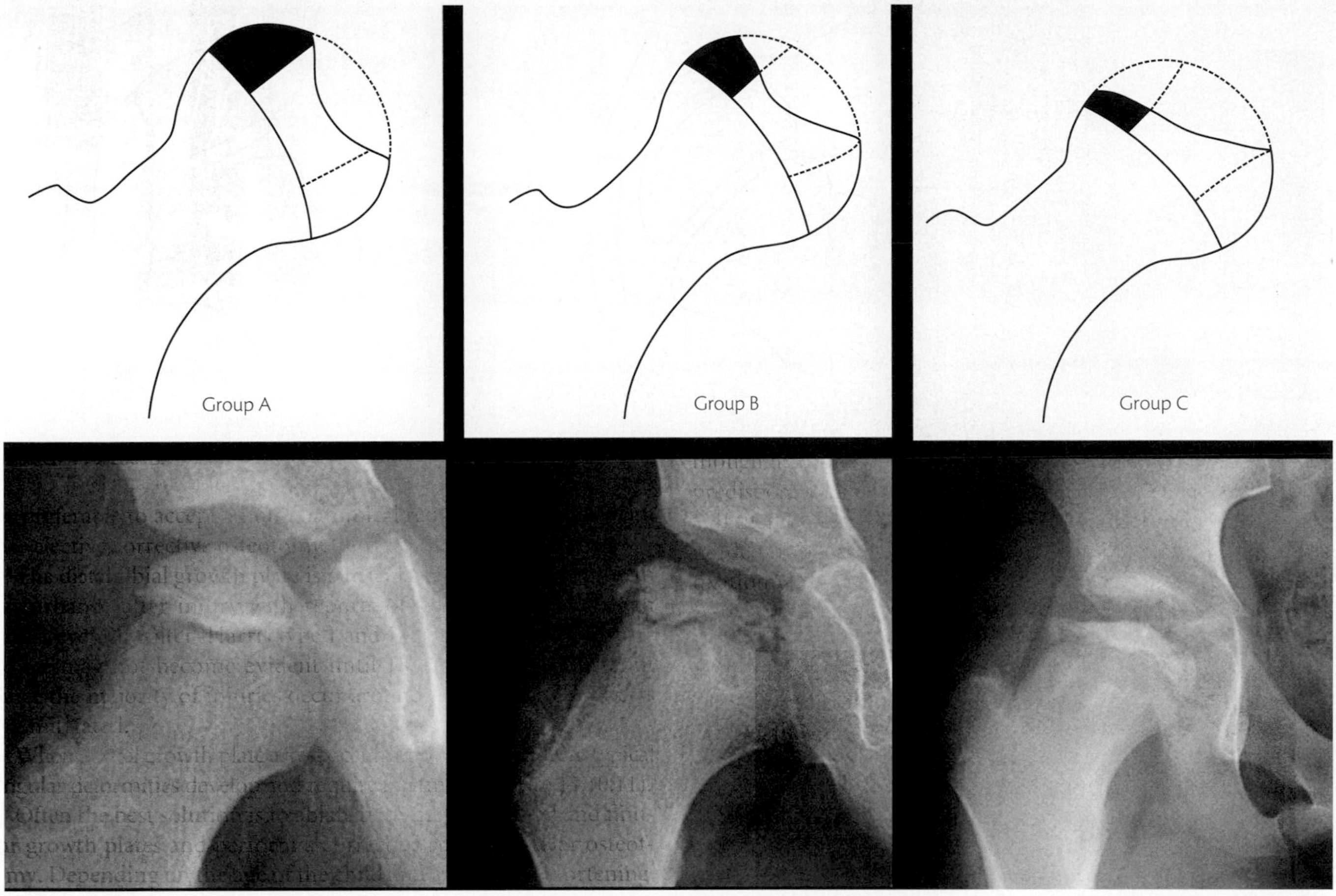

Fig. 13.18.8 Diagrams and radiographs illustrating the lateral pillar classification of Perthes disease into groups. Dark shading illustrates the remaining height of the lateral pillar or column of the epiphysis. See text for explanation.

system is able to predict how much collapse will develop until the collapse has actually occurred. This limits the usefulness of the two systems for determining who might do badly and therefore who might benefit from early treatment aimed at prevention or limitation of femoral head deformation. Salter and Thompson observed a subchondral crescentic radiolucent line early in the disease process. They believed that the line represented a pathological fracture and that the fracture was responsible for the onset of pain and clinical symptoms. It was observed that only the portion of the epiphysis underlying the subchondral fracture was affected by the avascular process. A simple classification that would predict the extent of the collapse was proposed. In Group A the fracture extended for less than half of the head and the prognosis was relatively good and in Group B (Figure 13.18.9) it extended over more than half of the head and the prognosis was relatively poor.

Table 13.18.1 Description of the lateral pillar classification

Group	Description of lateral pillar	Prognosis
A	Little or no density change with no loss of height	Good
B	Lucency and loss of height that is <50%	Intermediate
C	Loss of height >50%	Poor

Unfortunately the subchondral fracture was apparent in less than 33% of the patients studied.

Determinants of prognosis

Historically, patients have been enrolled into a variety of treatment programmes as soon as Perthes disease was recognized and it has therefore been difficult to unravel the natural history of the condition from the effect of treatment. Nevertheless most studies suggest that age, extent of epiphyseal involvement, and gender each influence the prognosis.

Age

The prognosis is better for the younger child. The remaining growth potential is at least part of the explanation for this phenomenon. Even if a young patient's femoral head becomes deformed and aspherical there is still time for the immature acetabulum to grow to match the femoral head and the long-term result is an aspherical congruent joint with a fair prognosis. In an older patient the more mature acetabulum has already grown to match a spherical femoral head: if the femoral head then deforms, the mature acetabulum is unable to remodel because remaining growth is limited and the result is an aspherical and incongruent joint with a relatively poor prognosis. Nevertheless, being young at disease onset does not guarantee a good outcome and up to 20% of cases

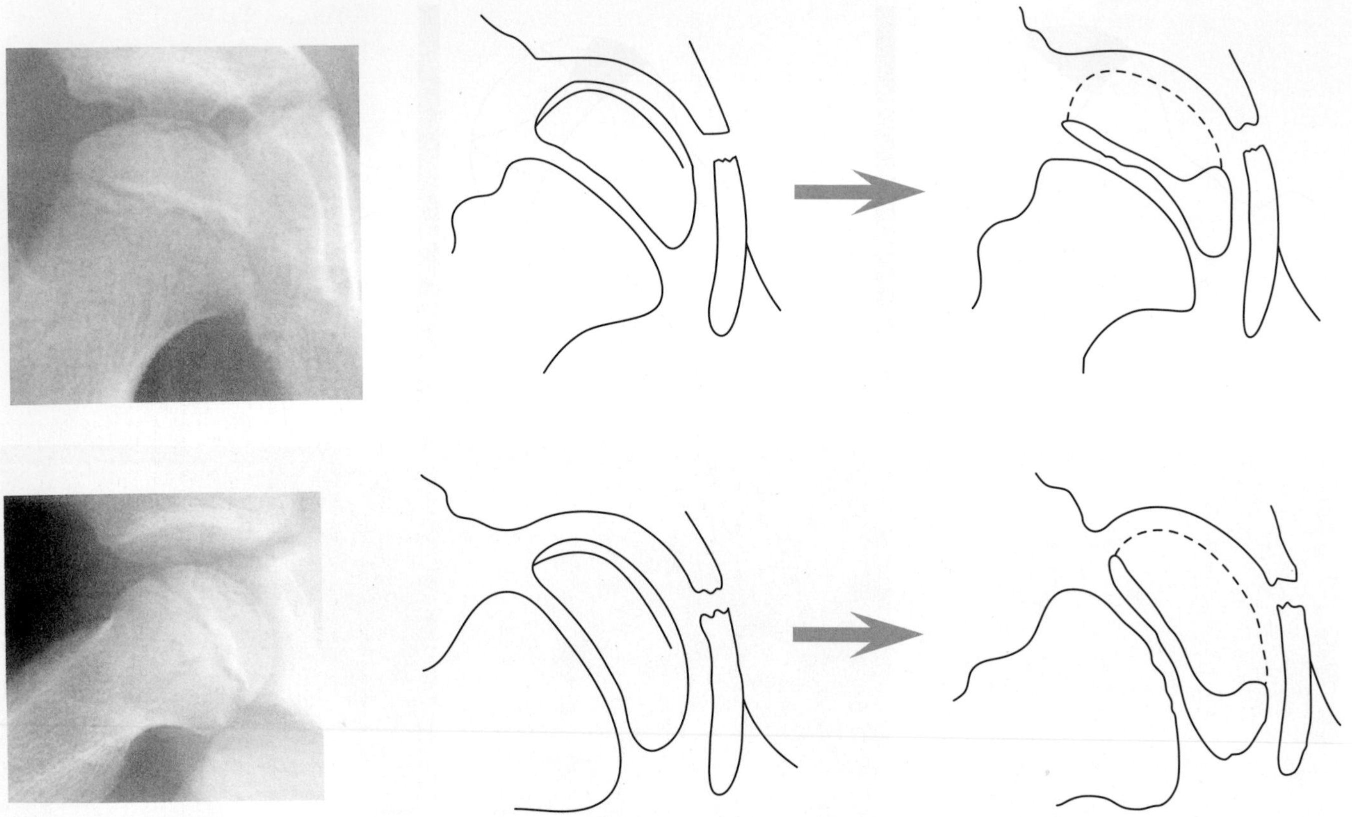

Fig. 13.18.9 AP and frog leg lateral radiographs illustrating a subchondral fracture line. Salter and Thompson (1984) observed that only the portion of the epiphysis underlying the subchondral fracture would collapse as illustrated in the diagrams. A simple classification was devised. In Group A the fracture extended less than halfway across the epiphysis and the prognosis was relatively good while in Group B it extended more than halfway across the epiphysis and the prognosis was relatively poor.

in young children can ultimately reach a poor outcome, even with adequate treatment. Nonetheless most children who develop long-term poor results have disease starting over the age of 8 years.

Extent of epiphyseal involvement and stage at diagnosis

The extent of epiphyseal involvement is defined by the Catterall, Salter and Thompson, and Herring classification systems. The prognosis for an individual case is proportional to the degree of the radiological involvement. It is also accepted that early treatment, before significant deformity has occurred, is likely to deliver a better outcome.

Gender

Most series reveal that girls have a worse outcome than boys. The reason for this is not entirely clear but some reports show that, although the condition is much less frequent in girls, a greater proportion of girls present with more extensive epiphyseal involvement than boys.

Defining early and late disease

If there is extensive epiphyseal involvement during the early stages of Perthes disease, the cartilaginous femoral head loses its internal bony support and its spherical shape may not be maintained because living cartilage is a plastic material. During this period of plasticity the ultimate shape of the femoral will be influenced by the external mechanical forces applied to it. Later in the disease process when the femoral head is healing or healed, a new bony epiphysis is in place and the cartilaginous femoral head is again supported by an internal bony structure, albeit often a different shape from the original. At this stage, the femoral head is no longer plastic and the shape is fixed. Thus, once radiological healing is established there will be no further deterioration in femoral head shape and its shape cannot be influenced by the external mechanical environment. The management approach to these two periods is thus quite different. The approach to the early plastic stage requires strategies that attempt to keep the cartilaginous femoral head as spherical as possible by altering its external mechanical environment; in contrast, the approach to the late non-plastic stage must accommodate the new shape by orientating it into a congruent position, relative to the acetabulum, whilst maintaining a functional arc of movement.

Management

Early (plastic phase) Perthes disease

Review of current management approaches

The femoral head remains plastic over a prolonged period (1–2 years) until there is radiological evidence of healing. Consequently, unless the physiological processes at the root of fragmentation can be stopped or reversed, any treatment directed at changing the external mechanical environment of the cartilaginous femoral head, in order to influence shape, must be equally prolonged.

Non-weight bearing

When Perthes disease was discovered, the initial management approach was similar to that used for tuberculosis of the hip joint. Programmes of prolonged non-weight bearing, including hospitalization and enforced recumbency or via the use of crutches or weight-relieving calipers were adopted. From the outset the efficacy of such treatment methods was questioned and gradually the approach was superseded by the development of newer strategies. Currently, it is accepted that non-weight bearing alone is ineffective: it does not succeed in unloading the femoral head. Indeed biomechanical studies suggest that an ischial bearing caliper might actually increase hip joint loading because of compressive muscle forces acting across the joint.

Containment

When the hip is in the anatomical position, the lateral part of the epiphysis is directly below, or just outside, the lateral rim of the bony acetabulum. In the absence of hip movement, compression forces will tend to flatten the superior part of a plastic femoral head while the uncovered anterolateral part is pushed outwards. Hip abduction brings the lateral epiphysis under the cover of the bony acetabulum redirecting the forces applied to the femoral head. The '*containment*' hypothesis suggests that the femoral head should then become the same shape as the surrounding acetabulum, like jelly poured into a mould. This hypothesis has been adopted widely and is the principle behind most current treatment approaches.

Containment can be achieved by a number of means. The hip can be abducted, the epiphysis can be realigned surgically to face into the acetabulum by means of a femoral osteotomy, or the acetabulum can be redirected or extended over the femoral epiphysis by various pelvic osteotomies. At presentation, many patients have significant limitation of abduction usually as a consequence of synovitis and muscle spasm but occasionally due to a true mechanical limitation of abduction because of established femoral head deformity. It is self-evident that abduction must be restored before any containment approach can be applied. Methods for restoration of abduction include bed rest, traction, serial abduction casting, or even tenotomy, but if abduction cannot be restored then the epiphysis cannot be contained and treatment following the containment concept is futile.

Abduction bracing

Initially, good results were reported using bilateral above knee cylinder casts with broomsticks applied to hold each leg abducted to 45 degrees and internally rotated to 5–10 degrees for around 18 months. The Petrie cast, like many subsequent braces, is a restrictive device not conducive to 'a normal life'. Such treatment methods have become unacceptable and a plethora of ambulatory braces such as the Atlanta Scottish Rite brace were developed to maintain abduction whilst preserving mobility. Although bracing is still used, its efficacy compared to the surgical alternatives is questioned.

Femoral osteotomy

A femoral osteotomy aims to redirect the lateral or sometimes the anterolateral epiphysis inside the confines of the lateral rim of the bony acetabulum. An intertrochanteric osteotomy is performed and then fixed in varus angulation. On occasion, some internal rotation or extension of the proximal fragment is included and some advocate simultaneous trochanteric growth arrest to limit the high trochanter that commonly occurs in this condition. Before embarking on surgery, it must be documented that the affected hip will abduct sufficiently to contain the epiphysis and that the patient will be left with some residual abduction range after the osteotomy has been performed. These prerequisites are usually confirmed by examination under anaesthesia and arthrography. If they are not met a varus osteotomy will only serve to put the affected leg into an adducted posture and the epiphysis will not be contained. Children who are treated between the ages of 5–8 years, when the disease is in the early or fragmentation stages and before significant femoral head deformity has developed, have the best outcome. Femoral osteotomy is not without its side effects and reported problems include failure of the varus to remodel, especially in the older patient, limb shortening, increased abductor lurch, trochanteric overgrowth, and the need to remove the fixation device.

Salter osteotomy

While the femoral osteotomy moves the uncovered epiphysis under the acetabulum, the Salter innominate osteotomy does the reverse. The prerequisites for the procedure with regard to range of movement and epiphyseal containment are thus the same and again are often confirmed with an examination under anaesthesia and arthrography. Advantages of the Salter osteotomy include the absence of the iatrogenic varus and consequent limb shortening that is associated with femoral osteotomy. The Salter osteotomy typically leads to modest limb lengthening which may be advantageous given that Perthes disease usually leads to limb shortening. However, relative overlengthening tends to offset the containment effect by adducting the limb slightly when the patient bears weight. Nevertheless comparative studies show little difference between the outcome of Salter versus femoral varus osteotomy.

Shelf osteotomy

The Shelf osteotomy is a form of acetabular augmentation which extends the acetabular roof to cover the uncovered anterolateral femoral epiphysis. Once again the procedure has the advantage of avoiding iatrogenic varus and limb shortening from a femoral osteotomy. This can be important in the older patient who may not have the growth potential to remodel a varus alignment. This procedure is used less frequently than the femoral or Salter osteotomies but encouraging reports of its use, especially in the older patient, are growing.

Bisphosphonates

If the structural integrity of the femoral epiphysis could be maintained during the revascularization of the epiphysis then femoral head collapse and deformity might be prevented. It is on these grounds that some groups are attempting to treat Perthes disease with bisphosphonates

Joint distraction

Some authors postulate that joint distraction in early Perthes disease may prevent collapse and enhance recovery by unloading the femoral epiphysis. A few studies report the use of external fixators to distract the joint in this way but again the efficacy of this approach remains uncertain.

Decision-making in early disease

The clinician faces the challenge of identifying the patient who is likely to benefit from intervention and then choosing the appropriate intervention. In 1971, Catterall wrote 'the reported results of treatment are so variable that it is difficult to be sure that the (published) series are strictly comparable'. More than two decades later Herring wrote 'it is difficult if not impossible to compare the results of these (published) studies'. To date, no adequate prospective randomized controlled trial has compared the outcome of untreated cases of Perthes disease against similar cases treated by various means.

Herring and associates studied prospectively the outcome of Perthes disease in children over 6 years of age who had been managed by various means. The outcome of physiotherapy and several containment methods (surgical and non-surgical) were compared. The study identified a group of patients who benefit from containment treatment and showed that surgical containment methods (both femoral varus osteotomy and Salter innominate osteotomy) led to a better outcome that non surgical containment by abduction bracing but only some patients benefited (Table 13.18.2).

When the lateral pillar was completely preserved (Herring A) all patients did well and treatment, by any means, made little difference. Therefore if a Group A patient could be identified accurately, treatment could be withheld safely. When the lateral pillar collapsed completely (Herring C) the outcome was poor and treatment by any means made little difference. This implies that it is futile to offer such patients any of the containment methods studied. Unfortunately the clinician managing a patient who presents with early disease is unable to foretell whether the presenting hip will remain a Herring A or become a Herring C and it is therefore difficult (or impossible) to decide to withhold treatment for a particular patient on radiological grounds alone. Moreover it is accepted that treatment before deformation occurs is preferable and it is therefore difficult to deliberately delay treatment, and risk compromising the outcome, while waiting for the hip to declare itself.

It is apparent that although the Catterall and Herring radiological classification systems are useful as research tools to ensure that studies can compare like patients at final review, they cannot be used to determine which patients should be treated in the early stages of the disease. With this backdrop how can the clinician make rational management choices?

Table 13.18.2 Summary of results from Herring et al.'s prospective study into the outcome of the most common treatment approaches to Perthes disease

Herring grade	Age in years (S—skeletal age; C—chronological age)	Outcome
A	All ages	All do well, even without treatment (rare)
B	Age ≤6(S) or 8(C)	Favourable outcome irrespective of type treatment
B and B/C border	Age ≥6(S) or 8(C)	Benefit from femoral or Salter osteotomy > benefit from brace treatment > benefit from no treatment
C	All ages	Poor outcome irrespective of type of treatment

Author's approach

The concept of passive and active containment

How can current knowledge regarding Perthes disease be resolved into a useable clinical management approach? The clinician manages patients not radiographs and the author's philosophy is a clinical rather than a radiological approach (Figure 13.18.10).

All patients who develop Perthes disease must contain the vulnerable epiphysis. Some patients achieve this containment for themselves by maintaining a full range of movement, especially abduction. The author refers to this circumstance as passive containment and the patient simply requires observation not intervention.

Clinical evaluation of abduction is therefore the most important decision making assessment. During the clinical examination it is important to abduct the unaffected hip maximally and flex the knee over the edge of the examination couch to lock the pelvis before measuring abduction on the affected side otherwise unconsciously rolling or tilting of the pelvis means that abduction of the affected hip can appear spuriously good.

Passive containment is most apparent in the young patient (under age 4). Clinical experience shows that many young patients maintain an excellent range of movement with modest symptoms. These favourable clinical findings do not always match the sometimes unfavourable extent of radiological epiphyseal involvement but may explain why the outlook is often good for younger patients. The bony nucleus of the young epiphysis only represents a small proportion of the whole cartilaginous head and its contribution to maintenance of femoral head shape is modest in the younger (and lighter) patient. In older patients extensive femoral epiphyseal involvement is typically matched by significant clinical symptoms and loss of movement, especially abduction.

If a patient begins to lose range of movement, particularly with abduction less than 20 degrees, then the lateral femoral epiphysis will not move in and out of the acetabulum during normal activity. Such patients are unable to contain their own epiphysis adequately. This loss of clinical abduction is the cue that the patient needs help in containing the epiphysis and the clinician must intervene. The author refers to this circumstance as active or interventional containment. This approach is inclusive to all patients, even for the rare case of a young patient who presents with such loss of abduction. It is possible that the small proportion of young patients who present in this way are likely to represent the young patients whose outcome is unexpectedly poor when managed passively. Given current evidence it seems reasonable to expect interventional containment in such children to improve the outcome, although there is no study to date to support this notion.

Based on current evidence, the author's preferred interventional containment procedure for children under 8 years of age is a femoral varus osteotomy (Figure 13.18.11).

Following the surgical procedure the patient is immobilized in a spica cast for 6–8 weeks to maintain abduction. Experience has shown that without the cast, movement is lost and the hip adducts.

Femoral varus osteotomy in the child over age 8 years has some distinct disadvantages. There may not be enough growth

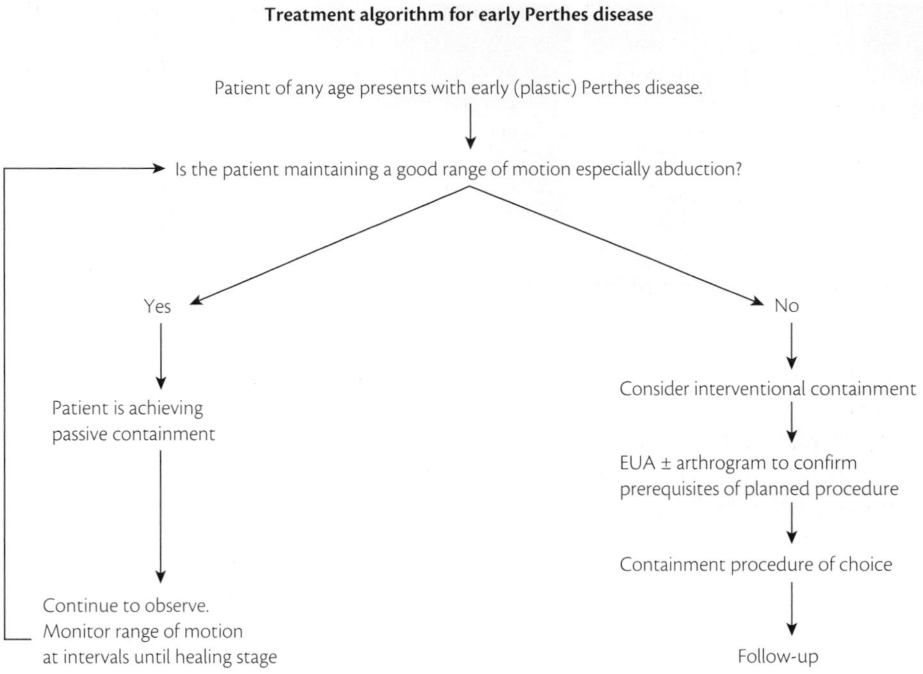
Treatment algorithm for early Perthes disease
Patient of any age presents with early (plastic) Perthes disease.
Is the patient maintaining a good range of motion especially abduction?
Yes
No
Patient is achieving passive containment
Continue to observe. Monitor range of motion at intervals until healing stage
Consider interventional containment
EUA ± arthrogram to confirm prerequisites of planned procedure
Containment procedure of choice
Follow-up

Fig. 13.18.10 Author's treatment algorithm for any patient presenting with Perthes disease in the early (plastic) phase of the condition. See text for detailed explanation.

remaining for the iatrogenic varus deformity to remodel with time and if the deformity persists it leads to limb shortening and a Trendelenburg lurch. The author's preferred method of interventional containment for the older patient is the shelf osteotomy (Figure 13.18.12).

This procedure has none of the disadvantages of the varus osteotomy and increasingly, reports show its efficacy as a containment procedure. The author has found that postoperative immobilization with a spica cast is unnecessary. Partial weight bearing is allowed with increase of the load allowed over a period of 12 weeks.

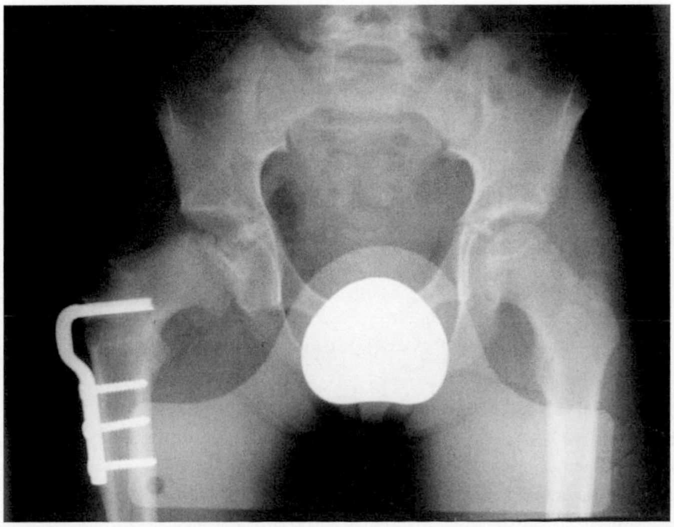

Fig. 13.18.11 Radiograph of 7-year-old boy with Perthes disease of the right hip, 9 months following a femoral varus osteotomy.

Arthrography

Before embarking on an interventional containment approach the prerequisites of the chosen method must be met. Examination under anaesthetic and arthrography confirms that containment is possible and sufficient abduction is available. Early flattening of the cartilaginous femoral head is acceptable provided the lateral part of the epiphysis comes under the cover of the bony acetabulum (Figure 13.18.13A).

According to the author, interventional containment is indicated because the patient has lost abduction in the outpatient setting. This loss of abduction is present only when the patient is conscious: it is usually the result of muscle spasm secondary to synovitis and pain. Once the patient is under general anaesthetic the spasm is overcome and most patients then have an adequate range of abduction and a containable epiphysis. If abduction is limited, even

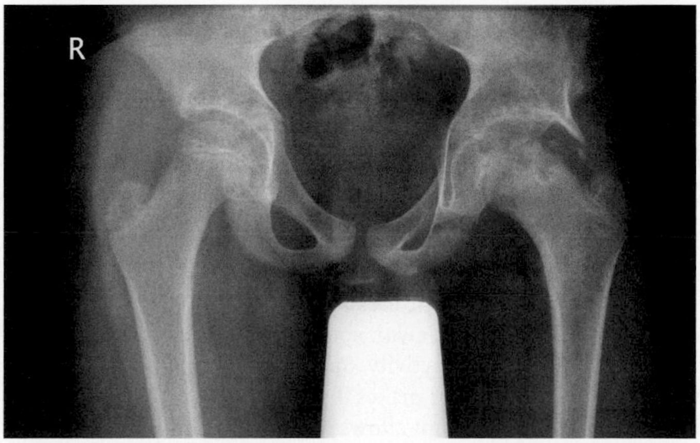
R

Fig. 13.18.12 Radiograph of 9-year-old boy with Perthes disease of the left hip, 8 months following a shelf osteotomy.

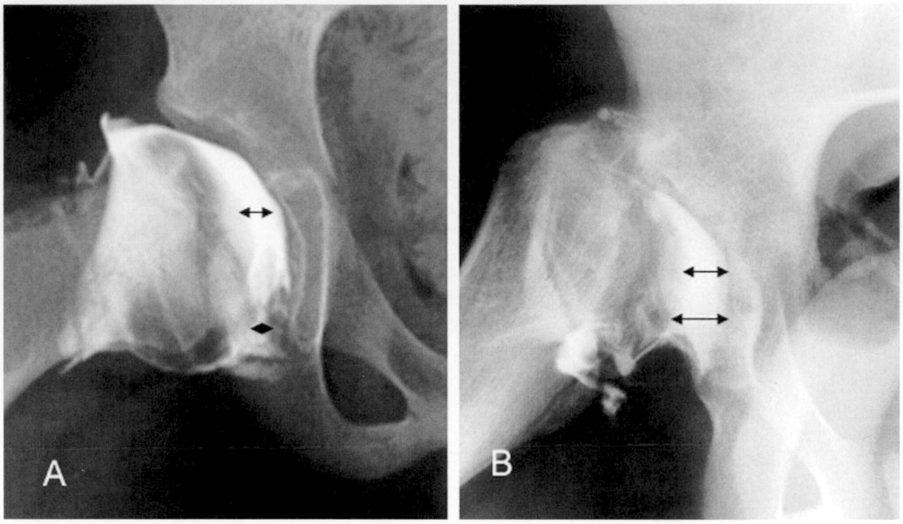

Fig. 13.18.13 Arthrogram images illustrating two hips in abduction. The femoral head in image A is flattened but is nevertheless containable. The lateral pillar of the epiphysis comes under the lateral edge of acetabular roof. The contrast pool reveals middle column flattening at the level of the upper arrow but the medial column still touches the floor of the acetabulum near the teardrop at the lower arrow. In contrast the femoral head in image B is too deformed to enter the acetabulum in abduction and demonstrates so called 'hinge abduction'. The lateral column does not come under the roof of the acetabulum but impinges at its edge acting as the fulcrum for further abduction. Consequently the femoral head is levered from the acetabular floor. The middle column does not touch the floor and the medial column is pulled further away from the floor adjacent to the teardrop figure. Arrows illustrate the widening contrast pool.

under anaesthetic, it may sometimes be restored by serial casting, or tenotomy, but if the restriction is mechanical because of hinge abduction (Figure 13.18.13B) then the epiphysis is not containable and interventional containment is contraindicated.

Follow-up

The author believes that patient follow-up following the management of Perthes disease should be continued until they reach skeletal maturity. Patients rarely develop symptoms that require attention in their childhood or early adult life but most do develop a modest shortening on the affected side of about 10–15mm. Although this rarely requires intervention, limb length monitoring is the primary reason for follow-up. If the discrepancy is greater than expected or if symptoms develop, then monitoring during growth will facilitate limb length equilibration using a well timed epiphysiodesis.

Late non-plastic Perthes disease

Many childhood hip disorders leave a deformed femoral head in their wake. If a patient develops an aspherical and incongruent joint then symptoms of discomfort can present as early as the late teens or early twenties. The typical anatomy of the deformed hip includes a short broad femoral neck with a high greater trochanter and a large broad aspherical (flattened) femoral head (Figure 13.18.14). The acetabulum may match the femoral head shape or not and the severely deformed femoral head develops a saddle-shaped depression under the region of the bony acetabular rim.

These anatomical deformities present clinically as a short limb and a Trendelenburg lurch with abductor fatigue and discomfort in the gluteal muscles after activity. Superior flattening and increasing width of the femoral head makes the head ovoid rather than spherical. While a spherical joint allows easy movement in all directions the ovoid head behaves more like a roller with its long axis in the coronal plane. There is usually good flexion but limited rotation and abduction. Although patients often have good flexion they cannot always achieve full flexion with the leg in the sagittal plane. As flexion proceeds the bulge of the deformed anterolateral part of the femoral head will not fit under the anterior lip of the acetabulum. To achieve further flexion the patient's leg (and femur) must externally rotate to direct the bulge around the anterolateral rim of the acetabulum: the classical sign of a deformed femoral head.

In the worst cases the superior surface of the femoral head is flat or even concave and abduction is severely limited because the deformed femoral head will not fit under the lateral rim of the acetabulum when abducted. If the hip is forced into abduction, the

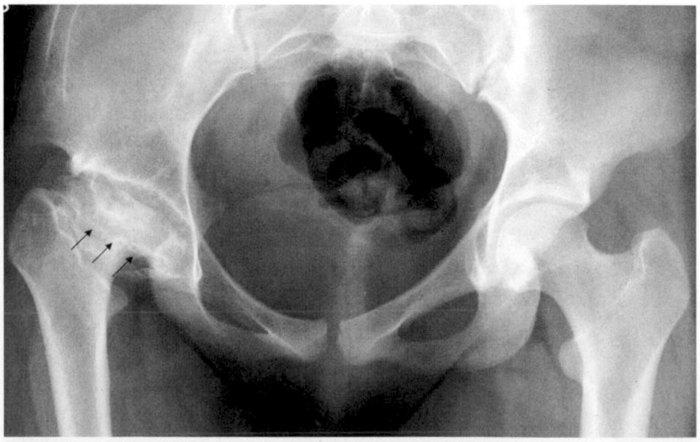

Fig. 13.18.14 Sagging rope sign: radiograph of a broad and flattened femoral head following Perthes disease. The trochanter is high, the neck short and broad, and there is a coxa magna. Arrows highlight a sagging rope sign. The outcome was poor with restricted 'hinge' abduction in this girl with onset age 11; in spite of a shelf osteotomy performed 2 years before the current radiograph. She subsequently underwent a valgus osteotomy.

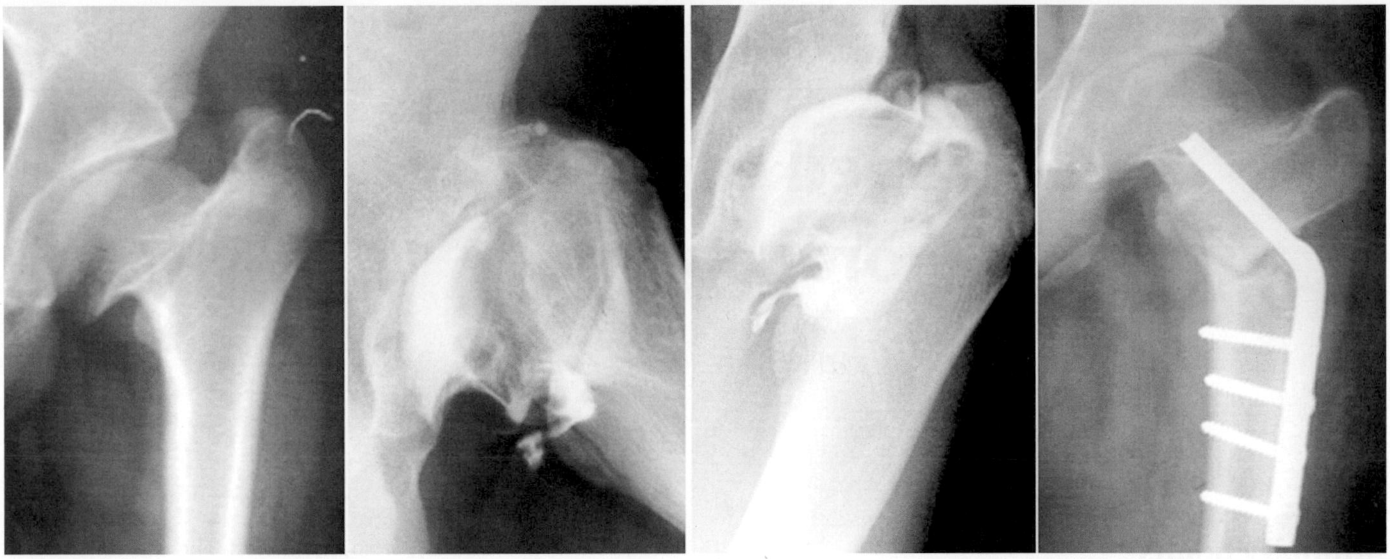

Fig. 13.18.15 An ovoid femoral head with a broad, short neck and a high trochanter is illustrated (A). The arthrogram illustrates hinge abduction (B), in this case primarily because of impingement of the high trochanter, although the impingement is usually secondary to an extruded lateral part of a flattened epiphysis in Perthes disease. When the hip is held in adduction the arthrogram reveals a reasonably congruent position of 'best fit' (C). A valgus osteotomy can reproduce the position of 'best fit' (D) restoring a functional range of abduction.

lateral part of the head impinges on the lateral rim of the acetabulum. Further abduction causes the hip to be levered from the medial floor of the acetabulum with the fulcrum or '*hinge*' of the lever at the point of impingement. This is so called '*hinge abduction*'. A patient whose hip hinges will not allow any abduction when conscious because it is too painful. Under anaesthetic the hip can be forced into abduction and the hinging demonstrated on an arthrogram (Figure 13.18.13B).

Once the femoral head has reached the healing stage its shape is fixed and cannot be further influenced by containment. The objective now is to accept the shape and align the femoral head with the acetabulum in a congruent position that also offers the patient a functional arc of movement. The management principle is the '*position of best fit*' and can be applied to any deformed femoral head.

Dynamic arthrography is the key investigation for evaluation of the deformed hip. In the typical case, following Perthes disease the arthrogram often demonstrates a congruent fit when the hip is adducted. In these circumstances a proximal femoral valgus osteotomy will reproduce the congruent alignment when the patient is standing (Figure 13.18.15).

The valgus osteotomy will allow some clinical abduction before the point of impingement is reached. Furthermore the osteotomy can sometimes lengthen the short leg and the greater trochanter will be brought to a lower and more lateral position, lengthening the abductor lever arm and improving the Trendelenburg lurch and abductor fatigue. The procedure reduces symptoms and can extend the lifespan of the patient's hip joint before interventions such as joint replacement become necessary.

Further reading

Catterall, A. (1971). The natural history of Perthes' disease. *Journal of Bone and Joint Surgery*, **53B**, 37–53.

Catterall, A., Pringle, J., Byers, P.D., *et al.* (1982). A review of the morphology of Perthes' disease. *Journal of Bone and Joint Surgery*, **64B**, 269–75.

Chung, S.M. (1976). The arterial supply of the developing proximal end of the human femur. *Journal of Bone and Joint Surgery*, **58A**, 961–70.

Herring, J.A. (1994). The treatment of Legg–Calve–Perthes disease. A critical review of the literature. *Journal of Bone and Joint Surgery*, **76**, 448–58.

Herring, J.A., Kim, H.T., and Browne, R. (2004). Legg–Calve–Perthes disease. Part II: Prospective multicenter study of the effect of treatment on outcome. *Journal of Bone and Joint Surgery*, **86A**, 2121–34.

Myers, G.J., Mathur, K., and O'Hara, J. (2008). Valgus osteotomy: a solution for late presentation of hinge abduction in Legg–Calve–Perthes disease. *Journal of Pediatric Orthopedics*, **28**, 169–72.

Stulberg, S.D., Cooperman, D.R., and Wallensten, R. (1981). The natural history of Legg–Calve–Perthes disease. *Journal of Bone and Joint Surgery*, **63A**, 1095–108.

13.19

Slipped capital femoral epiphysis

N.M.P. Clarke

Summary points

- Slipped capital femoral epiphysis occurs during rapid growth periods of adolescence
- Delay in diagnosis remains a major problem
- Acute, severe, and unstable slips are an orthopaedic emergency: the preferred treatment option remains controversial.

Introduction

Slipped capital femoral epiphysis (SCFE) is a condition that occurs during a period of rapid growth in adolescence, when shear forces, particularly in the obese individual, increase across the proximal femoral growth plate resulting in a posteromedial displacement of the epiphysis relative to the femoral metaphysis.

Delay in diagnosis remains the major problem because of the failure to associate knee and thigh pain in the adolescent with hip pathology. AP pelvic radiographs are easily misinterpreted in the early stages.

Most slips can be treated by cannulated single screw stabilization. There is continuing debate about the necessity for prophylactic contralateral fixation and the management of the acute unstable slip.

Incidence and aetiology

The reported incidence varies from 1–7 per 100 000. Males are affected three times more than females. Bilateral slips occur in approximately 20% of cases.

The typical phenotype of obesity and possible hypogonadism implicates an endocrine cause. There is a clear association with hypothyroidism and with growth hormone treatment and pathological values of follicle stimulating hormone, luteinizing hormone, and testosterone have been identified. Cases are also seen in association with metabolic bone disease such as renal rickets and in survivors of childhood malignancy who had received chemo- or radiotherapy. Perhaps more worryingly, recent evidence has highlighted a close correlation between rising childhood obesity and increasing incidence of SCFE. There is also a link between SCFE and femoral retroversion.

Ultrastructural studies of SCFE growth plates have shown diminished cellularity and marked distortion of the architecture in both the proliferative and hypertrophic zones. The diminished cell number has been shown to be due to abnormal frequency and distribution of chondrocytes undergoing apoptosis. In this context the concept of 'preslip' has been confirmed by magnetic resonance imaging.

Classification (Box 13.19.1)

There are various classifications related to onset of symptoms (*temporal*), ability to weight bear (*functional*), and extent of epiphyseal displacement relative to the neck (*morphological*).

Temporal

An *acute* SCFE is one that occurs in a patient with prodromal symptoms of 3 weeks or less followed by an acute event often after minor trauma, considered to be too insignificant to cause a type I physeal fracture.

The *chronic* SCFE is the more common presentation. There is usually several months' history of vague groin, thigh, and knee pain with increasing limp and out-toeing gait. Radiographs reveal signs of remodelling.

In the *acute-on-chronic slip*, there has been a history of prodromal symptoms for more than 3 weeks followed by a sudden exacerbation of pain.

Functional

The concept of stability popularized by Loder relates to the patient's ability to weight bear after the acute event. Both acute and acute-on-chronic slips may be categorized further in this way. Patients with an unstable slip are in such severe pain that they are unable to weight bear.

Box 13.19.1 Classification systems for SCFE

- *Temporal* according to onset of symptoms: acute, acute-on-chronic, chronic
- *Functional* according to ability to bear weight: stable, unstable
- *Morphological* according to extent of epiphyseal displacement relative to the neck: mild, moderate, or severe.

Morphological

The degree of displacement is assessed on radiographs. Lines are drawn corresponding to the axis of the femoral shaft and the base of the capital epiphysis. It is not necessary to obtain a computed tomography scan. A grade I slip is 0–30°, grade II 30–60° and grade III 60–90+°.

Diagnosis and imaging

The symptoms and physical findings vary according to the type of slip. In a stable chronic SCFE the presenting complaint is usually of groin pain and/or vague anteromedial thigh and knee pain. This localization of the pain continues to cause diagnostic delay and confusion. The relationship between delay in diagnosis and increased slip severity has been confirmed and there have been calls for a more robust educational strategy, particularly for allied health professionals.

The early physical signs are perhaps subtle, with loss of internal rotation of the hip progressing to limb shortening and external rotation deformity. Acute unstable or acute-on-chronic slips will usually present with sudden pain and inability to bear weight.

The standard radiographs of an anteroposterior (AP) pelvis and lateral views of the hips are usually sufficient for diagnosis. The earliest sign is a widening of the physis (pre-slip). The diagnosis may be difficult to detect on the AP view. A line drawn parallel to the superior femoral neck (Klein's line) will intersect the lateral portion of the epiphysis but not in an early slip (Trethowan's sign). Steel described the 'metaphyseal blanch sign' that corresponds to increased density caused by overlapping of the femoral head and displaced epiphysis (Figure 13.19.1 and Box 13.19.2). An ultrasound scan may demonstrate an effusion and confirm an early/mild slip.

Treatment

The primary aims of treatment are to stabilize the epiphysis and prevent further slip. Prevention of avascular necrosis (AVN) and chondrolysis are secondary aims. A treatment algorithm is presented in Figure 13.19.2 (and see Figure 13.19.1).

The chronic slip

The majority of slips are chronic and can be treated with single cannulated screw fixation. The screw thread should traverse the physis into the centre of the epiphysis. Recent biomechanical studies have indicated that there should be equal distribution of threads across the physis for optimum stability. Joint penetration should be avoided to reduce the risk of chondrolysis. It is not necessary to employ a reverse cutting thread to facilitate screw removal, since there is now a consensus that screws should not be removed because of the associated morbidity.

Box 13.19.2 Radiographic features of a SCFE

- Widened physis
- Klein's line
- Trethowan's sign
- Metaphyseal blanch sign.

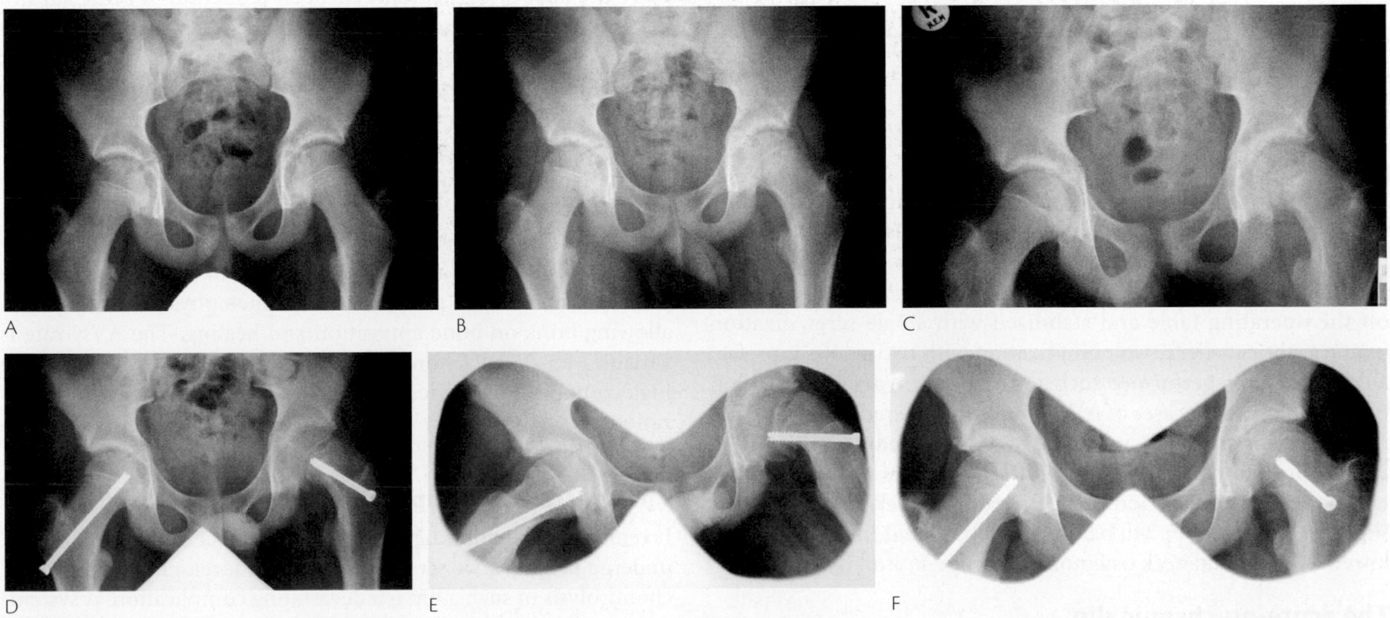

Fig. 13.19.1 Radiographic series depicting natural history of an evolving slip, surgical treatment and remodelling. A) Radiographic appearances of a 'pre-slip' on the left in a 13-year-old boy with thigh pain. There is widening of the growth plate and metaphyseal blanch. B) Twelve months later continuing symptoms. Trewthowan's sign is present (see text). C) After a further 2 months there are signs of advanced chronic slip with remodelling on the left and possible displacement on the right (Klein's line, see text). D, E) Appearances post screw stabilization. Note the differing screw entry points (anterior on the left) necessary to engage the epiphysis. F) Eleven months postoperation there is evidence of remodelling.

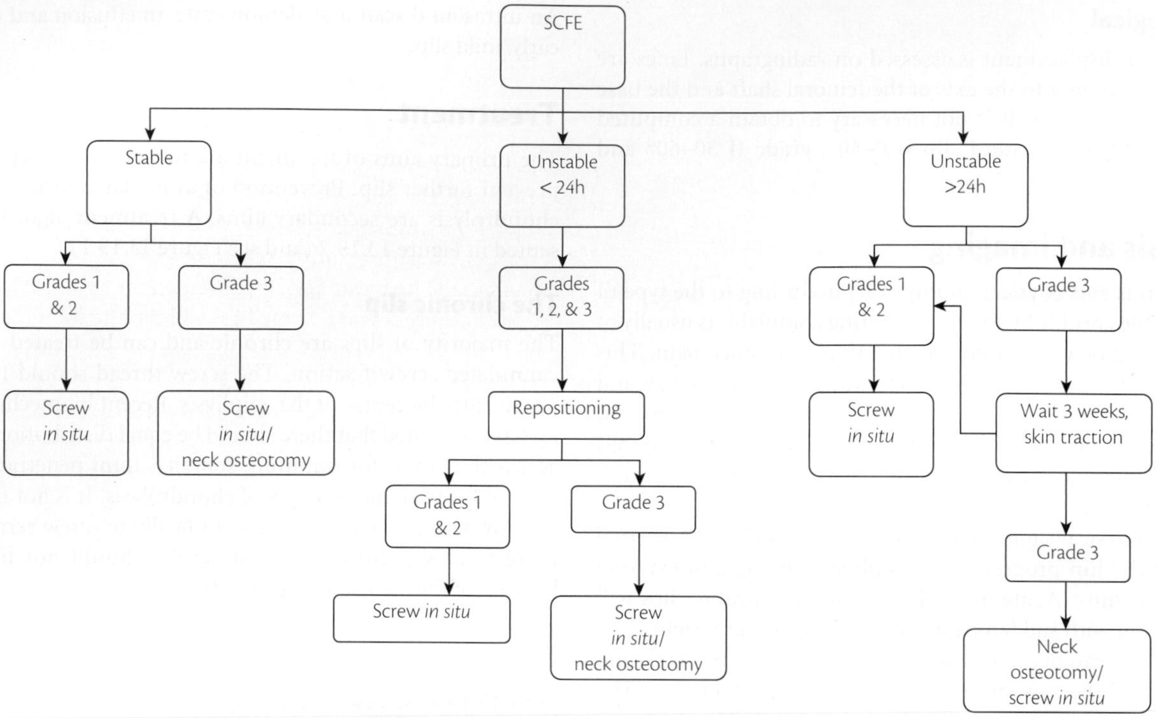

Fig. 13.19.2 A suggested treatment for SCFE. Reproduced with permission and copyright © of the British Editorial Society of Bone and Joint Surgery.

Single screw fixation is reliable but in the more severely displaced slips, knowledge of the pathoanatomy is required for accurate anterior placement of the screw. Remodelling will occur and often the external rotation deformity will resolve but there is concern among some about long-term femoroacetabular impingement.

In younger patients with endocrine disease, smooth pins may be inserted and subsequently removed if it is anticipated that healing will occur with endocrine replacement therapy, for example in hypothyroidism.

The acute unstable slip

The primary treatment of the acute unstable slip remains controversial mainly because of the incidence of AVN as a consequence of the injury to the epiphyseal blood supply. Many support the proposition that the displaced epiphysis should be gently repositioned on the operating table and stabilized with single screw fixation (some authors believe two point fixation with two screws is preferable). One study performed such a manoeuvre in acute slips within the first 24h and no cases of AVN were encountered whilst another report documented a 7% incidence of AVN for reductions less than 24h from presentation, but 20% if treatment was delayed. This author advocates a period of traction for 3 weeks in those acute slips that present after 24h before any subsequent intervention followed by a femoral neck osteotomy or screw *in situ* if possible.

The acute-on-chronic slip

In acute on-chronic slips no attempt should be made to reposition the epiphysis beyond its acute displacement and full correction should be avoided. *In situ* screw fixation is used.

The severely displaced slip

There are protagonists who believe that anatomical realignment of the capital epiphysis should be attempted in severe slips in order to improve function and to reduce the risk of later osteoarthritis. They therefore advocate osteotomy or open reduction in acute slips to correct the deformity with single or double screw stabilization.

Reference has already been made to the capacity for femoral neck remodelling but recent studies have drawn attention to femoroacetabular impingement as a cause of early structural abnormalities in the acetabular rim and late osteoarthritis.

Some surgeons advocate surgical dislocation of the hip and osteochondroplasty at the femoral neck junction, even for minor slips but conventionally, neck osteotomies at the level of the physis are performed. The cuneiform neck osteotomy of Fish results in complete excision of the physis from the metaphysis and epiphysis allowing bone on bone apposition and healing. The AVN rate is variable (4.5–35%). Chondrolysis has an incidence of 10–30%. The high complication rate leads many to advise primary screw stabilization and a subsequent osteotomy to correct deformity if necessary (vide infra).

The contralateral slip

It remains debatable whether the contralateral normal hip should undergo prophylactic screw fixation. The development of AVN or chondrolysis in such a hip is a devastating complication. A systematic review of the literature identified the probability of contralateral SCFE occurring as 19%. They concluded that the overall optimum decision path is observation. When the probability of contralateral slip exceeds 27%, for example in endocrinopathies, or

Box 13.19.3 Complications of SCFE

- Of the condition?
- Of the management?
- AVN:
  - Open reduction
  - Femoral neck osteotomy
  - Manipulation of stable slips
  - Late/forcible manipulation of unstable slips
  - Down syndrome
- Chondrolysis:
  - Hip spica treatment (rarely used)
  - Pin penetration?

when reliable follow-up is not feasible, screw stabilization is favoured.

Delayed bone age does *not* appear to be a predictor for a contralateral slip.

Salvage

Residual deformity can be managed by subsequent intertrochanteric osteotomy. Southwick described a triplane osteotomy at the level of the lesser trochanter. It is technically difficult and corrects the deformity a long distance from the site of the deformity. The osteotomy described by Dunn (and that by Fish) is performed at the site of deformity but the complication rate is higher. Such osteotomies do increase hip range of movement but may not provide improvement in functional outcome. Furthermore the influence of such osteotomies on late onset osteoarthritis, and the ease with which subsequent arthroplasties can be performed, remains uncertain.

Complications (Box 13.19.3)

AVN is the most common complication but radiological changes may take 18 months to become evident. The acute unstable slip has a relatively high incidence (up to 35%). The risk factors for AVN include open reduction, femoral neck osteotomies, manipulation of stable slips, forcible manipulation (late) of unstable hips and Down syndrome. Many hips with AVN will require early arthroplasty.

Chondrolysis is defined as narrowing of greater than 50% of the joint space. Hip spica cast treatment increases the incidence. The aetiology is not exactly known but appears to be related to immune system activation. Historically, there may be an association with joint penetration of implants. Maximum joint space narrowing occurs in the first year and improvement in up to 50% of cases can occur for up to 3 years. Some hips will require joint replacement.

Further reading

Adamczyk, M.J., Weiner, D.S., Nugent, A., McBurney, D., and Horton, W.E. Jr. (2005). Increased chondrocyte apoptosis in growth plates from children with slipped capital femoral epiphysis. *Journal of Pediatric Orthopedics*, **25**, 440–4.

Diab, M., Daluvoy, S., Snyder, B.D., and James, R. (2006). Osteotomy does not improve early outcome after slipped capital femoral epiphysis. *Journal of Pediatric Orthopedics*, **15**, 87–92.

Fraitzl, C.R., Käfer, W., Nelitz, M., Reichel, H. (2007). Radiological evidence of femoroacetabular impingement in mild slipped capital femoral epiphysis: a mean follow-up of 14.4 years after pinning in situ. *Journal of Bone and Joint Surgery*, **89B**, 1592–6.

Kocher, M.S., Bishop, J.A., Hresko, M.T., Millis, M.B., Kim, Y-J, and Kasser, J.R. (2004). Prophylactic pinning of the contralateral hip after unilateral slipped capital femoral epiphysis. *Journal of Bone and Joint Surgery*, **86A**, 2658–65.

Kordelle, J., Mills, M., Jolesz, F.A., Kikinis, R., and Richolt, J.A. (2001). Three-dimensional analysis of the proximal femur in patients with slipped capital femoral epiphysis based on computed tomography. *Journal of Pediatric Orthopedics*, **21**, 179–82.

Murray, A.W. and Wilson, N.I.L. (2008). Changing incidence of slipped capital femoral epiphysis: a relationship with obesity? *Journal of Bone and Joint Surgery*, **90B**, 92–4.

Papavasiliou, K.A., Kirkos, J.M., Kapetanos, G.A., and Pournaras, J. (2007). Potential influence of hormones in the development of slipped capital femoral epiphysis: a preliminary study. *Journal of Pediatric Orthopedics*, **16**, 1–5.

Rahme, D., Comley, A., Foster, B., and Cundy, P. (2006). Consequences of diagnostic delays in slipped capital femoral epiphysis. *Journal of Pediatric Orthopedics*, **15**, 93–7.

Southwick, W.O. (1973). Compression fixation after biplane intertrochanteric osteotomy for slipped capital femoral epiphysis. A technical improvement. *Journal of Bone and Joint Surgery*, **55**, 1218–24.

13.20

Common knee conditions

Shahryar Noordin and Andrew Howard

Summary points

- All children who complain of knee symptoms must be assessed for ipsilateral hip and spine pathology
- Congenital or persistent lateral dislocation of the patella and obligatory dislocation of the patella have two different clinical presentations: surgical treatment (if required) is often complex
- The natural history of stable osteochondritis dissecans lesions is generally favourable in a child with open physes.

Introduction

The knee is one of the most common joints that paediatric orthopaedic surgeons are asked to evaluate. All children who complain of knee symptoms also need to be assessed for ipsilateral hip and lumbar spine disorders. This chapter will discuss common knee conditions seen in the paediatric population. Knee disorders specific to young athletes will be reviewed in the section on sports medicine (see Chapter 13.23). The adolescent patellofemoral joint has also been covered in Chapter 8.10.

Congenital and habitual dislocation of the patella

The patellofemoral articulation is a complex joint that relies on bony conformity as well as on static and dynamic soft tissue components for stability. Any disturbance of the normal anatomical relations due to dysplasia, malalignment, or trauma can affect this balance and lateral subluxation and dislocation are common.

The patella forms during the seventh week of embryonic life. The cells develop deep to the patellar tendon as an uncalcified cartilaginous anlage that grows over time, ossifying between 4–6 years. The soft tissues surrounding the patella contribute significantly to patellofemoral joint stability. More specifically, the medial patellofemoral ligament (MPFL) and the vastus medialis obliquus (VMO) provide the greatest restraints to excessive lateral patellar displacement. The MPFL crosses the anteromedial aspect of the knee from the adductor tubercle of the femoral epicondyle to the superomedial aspect of the patella (Figure 13.20.1). It has been estimated to provide 50–80% of the restraining force to lateral translation and isolated release of the MPFL increases lateral displacement of the patella by 50%. The VMO is important as the primary dynamic medial stabilizer and is intimately associated with the MPFL.

With the knee in full extension, the patella naturally rests superolateral to the femoral sulcus. Engagement between the patella and trochlea does not occur until the knee flexes about 10–30 degrees. This can be affected by changes in patellar tendon length. Patients with patella alta, for instance, engage the trochlea at greater flexion angles, leading to less bony constraint at earlier degrees of flexion, theoretically increasing the risk for dislocation (Figure 13.20.2). Trochlear dysplasia has also been identified as a contributing factor to patellar instability. Broadly defined as flattening of the trochlear sulcus, dysplasia has been seen in 29–85% of patients with patellofemoral instability (Figure 13.20.3). Various torsional deformities of both the femur and tibia have also been implicated in this disorder. Historically, increased Q angles have been considered a risk factor for patellar instability: larger Q angles subject the patella to a larger overall lateral force vector (Box 13.20.1). Recent reports, however, question the significance of this finding. Generalized ligamentous laxity has been implicated in as many as two-thirds of patients with patellar instability but again the relevance of this has been queried recently.

Congenital dislocation of the patella is uncommon and two clinical syndromes have been described. One is referred to as a fixed lateral dislocation of the patella and the second described as habitual dislocation of the patella. Others have used the term obligatory dislocation of the patella to describe habitual, acquired, or atraumatic dislocation. Congenital or persistent lateral dislocation of the patella and obligatory dislocation of the patella have two different clinical presentations as shown in Table 13.20.1.

The child with congenital lateral dislocation of the patella presents with a knee flexion contracture and no patella palpable anterior to the femoral condyles. Palpation of the hypoplastic patella in its lateral position is difficult. A magnetic resonance

Box 13.20.1 Q angle

- The angle formed by a line from the ASIS to the centre of the patella and a line from there to the tibial tubercle
- Normal = 14 degrees in males, 17 degrees in females.

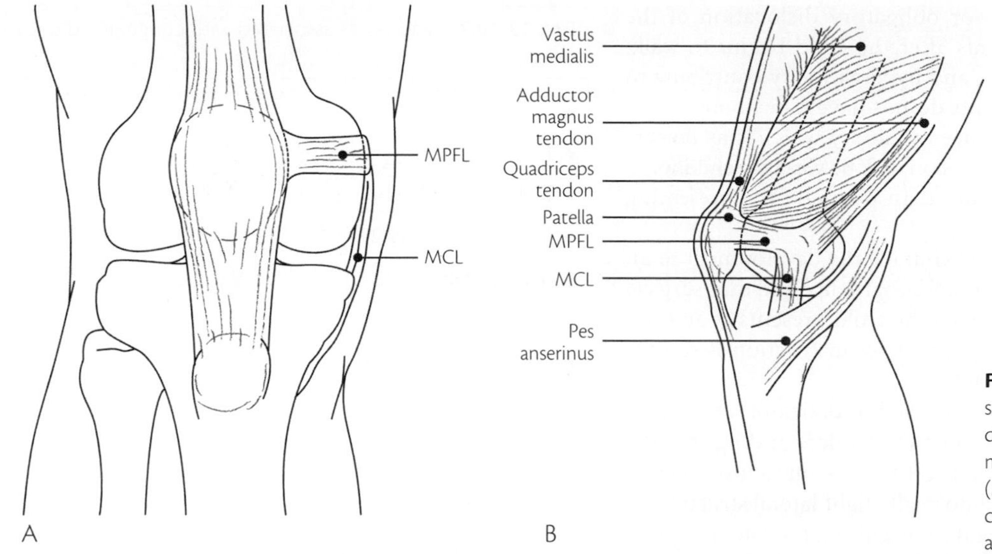

Fig. 13.20.1 A) AP and B) lateral simplified line diagrams of the knee demonstrating the position of the medial patellofemoral ligament (MPFL) with relation to the medial collateral ligament (MCL) and the pes anserinus.

imaging (MRI) scan may be necessary to ascertain the location of the cartilaginous patella. This child may present with a delay in the ability to walk independently or with an abnormal gait related to a knee flexion contracture and the associated external tibial torsion. Affected patients may have a musculoskeletal syndrome of which the patella dislocation is one feature. Congenital dislocation of the patella may occur bilaterally but more commonly it is unilateral (Box 13.20.2).

The pathoanatomy of congenital patellar dislocation always includes a joint contracture, with contracted posterior capsule and hamstring tendons, and may include congenital absence of the cruciate ligaments. In addition, there are varying degrees of contracture of the lateral retinaculum, iliotibial band, vastus lateralis, rectus femoris, vastus intermedius, and also the lateral patellofemoral, patellotibial, and patellomeniscal ligaments. In cases of fixed lateral dislocation of the patella, the extensor mechanism becomes a flexor and external rotator of the knee, leading to progressive genu valgum.

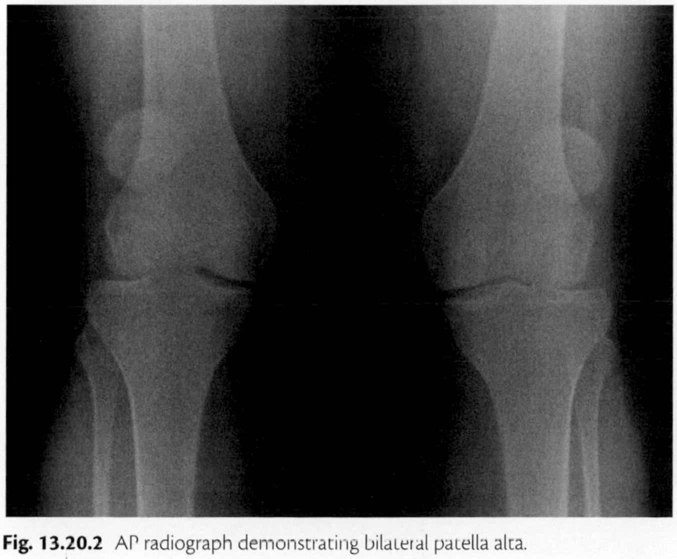

Fig. 13.20.2 AP radiograph demonstrating bilateral patella alta.

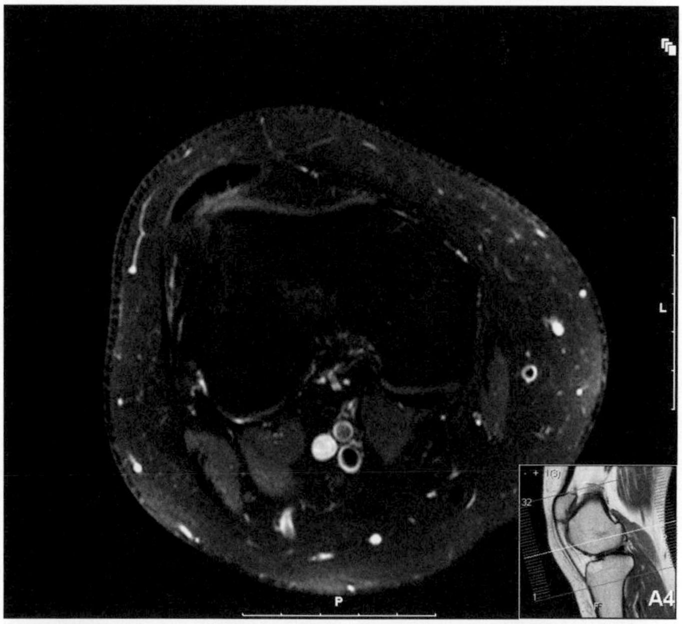

Fig. 13.20.3 MRI showing that the patella is subluxed laterally with a shallow, dysplastic trochlear groove.

Table 13.20.1 The differing clinical presentations of congenital and obligatory patella dislocation

Congenital dislocation	Obligatory dislocation
Patella dislocated laterally—fixed	Patella dislocates and reduces spontaneously with knee flexion and extension
Often obvious in infancy	Usually present with deformity at 5–10 years
Usually part of a generalized syndrome	Usually an isolated anomaly
Flexion contracture	Knee ROM normal
Frequently present with functional difficulty	Often well tolerated with little functional disability
Early surgical correction	Surgery delayed until symptomatic

Acute atraumatic, habitual, or obligatory dislocation of the patella characteristically presents after the child begins to walk. Patella alta, trochlear dysplasia, and hyperelasticity contribute to the pathoanatomy. These patients do not have a flexion contracture but they do complain of knee instability which may be surprisingly well tolerated. Knee extension may be weak. In childhood, dysfunction and deformity, rather than pain, are the presenting complaints (Figure 13.20.4).

Relocation of the patella can encourage the development of an adequate trochlea and patellofemoral congruence and thus surgical intervention is recommended when the child presents at an early age. For the adolescent, reduction and reconstruction is recommended only if symptoms warrant.

Whether the patella dislocation is fixed or obligatory, the surgical management can be quite complex. Understanding that the pathoanatomy includes significant soft tissue contractures is critical. An extensive release of all abnormally tight lateral structures is necessary: this includes the lateral retinaculum, the lateral capsule with the imbedded patellofemoral ligaments, and the lateral patellomeniscal ligaments found within the fat pad of the knee. The retinaculum is repaired in a lengthened position after the patella has been realigned. The vastus lateralis is also invariably involved and either shortened or abnormally adherent to the iliotibial band or lateral intermuscular septum. To avoid overcorrection, lengthening of the vastus lateralis after release from surrounding adhesions is preferred to release alone.

After an extensive lateral release, the patella should lie well-centered within the trochlea. However, in most cases, there is still a contracture of the central portion of the quadriceps mechanism which must be lengthened if the patella stability is to be maintained as the knee flexes. In the presence of an arthrogrypotic like flexion contracture of the knee, a formal posterior approach may be required for a hamstring lengthening and release of the posterior capsule.

The medial retinaculum with the inclusion of the MPFL is always severely attenuated with congenital patellar dislocations. In the fixed type, the retinaculum may be adherent to the underlying medial femoral condyle and requires a careful dissection to free it from the underlying joint surface. After appropriate lateral releases and lengthenings have allowed the patella to be reduced, the medial retinaculum is repaired and the MPFL is reconstructed. In older patients, additional augmentation of the medial repair vector is required. Transferring the semitendinosus tendon into the patella accomplishes this.

Box 13.20.2 Syndromes associated with congenital dislocation of the patella

- Arthrogryposis
- Larsen's
- Rubinstein–Taybi
- Downs (trisomy 21)
- Nail–patella
- Ellis–van Creveld
- Dyschondrosteosis.

In obligatory atraumatic dislocation, the contractures are generally not severe. Lengthening rather than release of the lateral retinaculum is performed to prevent overcorrection and to maintain the positive effect of the lateral retinaculum on patellar stability. MPFL reconstruction can be included if it is not associated with hyperelasticity and/or significant trochlear dysplasia.

Adolescent acute traumatic patella dislocation

The mean annual incidence of acute traumatic lateral patellar dislocation is 5.8:100 000 increasing to 29:100 000 in the subgroup of

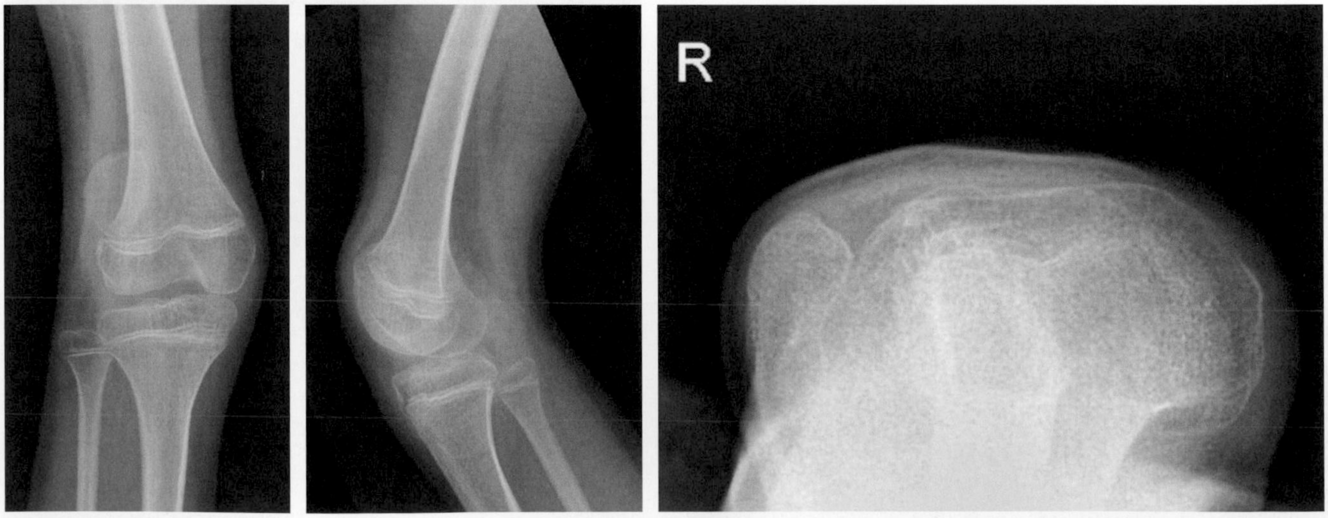

A B C

Fig. 13.20.4 A) AP, B) lateral, and C) axial views of the knee demonstrating a long-standing, obligatory dislocation of the patella in an older child.

10–17-year-olds. Contrary to previous beliefs, the most commonly affected person is not an obese, sedentary female but rather a young athlete of either gender. Two common mechanisms of traumatic patellar dislocation are sports (61%) and dance (9%) injuries (Box 13.20.3). Dislocation may result from a non-contact injury with a mechanism similar to that responsible for anterior cruciate ligament injuries or it may be a result of blunt trauma producing either a valgus/external rotation moment about the knee or a laterally directed force on the patella that exceeds the tensile strength of the MPFL in patients predisposed to dislocation. Particular care should be taken to determine whether the patient has had a previous patellar dislocation on the index or contralateral knee. A history of contralateral patellar dislocation increases the risk of recurrence sixfold: as much as a previous dislocation event on the index knee. A family history of patellar dislocation can be elicited in 9–15% of patients (Box 13.20.3).

A significant number of patients with acute traumatic patellar instability will experience chronic instability or chronic patellofemoral pain. Reported redislocation rates range from 15–44% but perhaps more troublesome is that at least 30–50% of patients can be expected to have anterior knee pain more than 2 years after injury.

Medial dislocations are uncommon and almost universally iatrogenic: secondary to overzealous release of the lateral patellar retinaculum in the treatment of lateral instability. Intra-articular dislocations are exceedingly rare.

Physical examination for patellar instability should include assessment of resting position of the patella standing and in extension and tracking of the patella from flexion into extension looking for lateral translation (J sign) and from extension into flexion looking for capture into the trochlea. More than 50% passive lateral translation of the patella is abnormal, more so if it is accompanied by apprehension. Knee hyperextension and signs of general laxity should be sought and the strength and tightness of hamstrings and quadriceps should be assessed. A rotational profile often reveals internal femoral torsion and external tibial torsion, 'squinting knees', which may predispose to lateral subluxation of the patella.

Traditionally, plain radiographs have been the standard form of initial radiographic assessment to document patellar location and identify osteochondral fractures (Box 13.20.4). MRI may delineate the pathology further: it is 85% sensitive and 70% accurate in the diagnosis of MPFL ligament injury. The sensitivity for chondral injuries is variable but improves with specific cartilage imaging sequences. In addition, ultrasound has recently been reported to detect MPFL injury reliably in addition to identifying bony avulsions.

For patients with acute traumatic patellar dislocation *without* osteochondral injury, the knee should be immobilized, following reduction, with a compressive dressing and a knee immobilizer. Weight bearing as tolerated is allowed, with the assistance of crutches. At first review, a failure to improve, as evidenced by persistent pain, swelling, and limited motion, heralds more significant intra-articular pathology which should prompt further radiographic investigation and/or arthroscopy. Early operative intervention should be considered in patients with associated osteochondral injuries, defects of the MPFL–VMO complex, and in children with high-level athletic demands. Damage to critical weight-bearing articular surfaces may require repair, debridement, or one of the many types of cartilage restoration procedures. These can be performed open or arthroscopically, depending on the size and condition of the lesion.

Box 13.20.3 Injury mechanisms for acute traumatic patella dislocations

- *Non contact*: valgus/abduction moment about the knee combined with internal rotation of the femur and/or external rotation of the tibia
- *Blunt trauma*: valgus/external rotation moment about the knee or a laterally directed blow to the patella.

Box 13.20.4 Radiographic knee series

4 views:
AP, lateral, notch and skyline/axial (Merchant).

In children with recurrent atraumatic dislocation or persistent patellar instability despite a well-controlled rehabilitation programme, operative management should be considered to prevent progressive articular damage. Invariably the underlying aetiology is due to fixed pathoanatomy, which may be bony (trochlear dysplasia, increased Q angle, increased tibial tuberosity:trochlear groove distance). Many different surgical techniques for the treatment of patellar instability have been described (Box 13.20.5).

These can be grouped broadly into soft tissue balancing and realignment or bony procedures. In children with open growth plates, procedures such as the Elmslie-Trillat technique are contraindicated because damage to the growth plate risks subsequent deformity. Proximal or distal soft tissue realignment procedures, with or without tibial tuberosity transfer have had limited success in patients with trochlear dysplasia. In these knees, ligamentous insufficiency is not a cause, but rather a consequence of recurrent dislocation. Different surgical techniques have been described in an attempt to correct trochlear dysplasia and femoral or tibial osteotomies may be necessary to correct the overall limb alignment.

Osteochondritis dissecans

This is an acquired condition affecting subchondral bone that manifests as a pathological spectrum ranging from softening of the overlying articular cartilage with an intact articular surface, through early articular cartilage separation, with or without partial detachment of an articular lesion, to osteochondral separation with loose body formation. The prevalence of osteochondritis dissecans (OCD) is 15–29:100 000 individuals with males affected in a ratio of 5:3. The increasing participation of young children in competitive sports has led to a decrease in the mean age of presentation and an increased prevalence amongst girls. The site of the lesion in the femoral condyles does not differ between age groups, and more than 70% of lesions are found in the 'classic' area of the posterolateral aspect of the medial femoral condyle (Box 13.20.6 and Figure 13.20.5). Patellar involvement is uncommon.

Idiopathic OCD must be differentiated from similar lesions resulting from avascular necrosis associated with chemotherapy, haemoglobinopathy, and steroid use. Several causes of OCD have

Box 13.20.5 Surgical treatment of patella instability

- Soft tissue balancing procedures:
  - Proximal or distal (Roux–Goldthwait) realignment
  - Alone or in combination
- Bony procedures: Elmslie–Trillat (contraindicated with open physes).

been postulated, including inflammation, genetic influences, ischaemia, and defects in ossification but there is insufficient evidence to support any single factor. Histologically, the typical OCD lesion of the medial femoral condyle resembles a subchondral stress fracture. Lesions are typically associated with osteoid production and giant cell resorption and generally appear avascular. Fairbanks in 1933 suggested that OCD was the result of violent inwards rotation of the tibia, driving the tibial spine against the inner aspect of the MFC. Repetitive trauma may also induce a stress fracture within the underlying subchondral bone and if repetitive loading persists and prevents the subchondral bone from healing (non-union), necrosis of the fragment may occur and lead to fragment dissection and separation. External tibial torsion is increased in patients with bilateral OCD and even more so in patients with persisting complaints which suggests that tibial torsion has a role in the development of OCD of the knee.

Box 13.20.6 Site of OCD lesions

- Femoral condyles:
  - MFC—posterolateral 70%
  - LFC—inferocentral 15–20%
  - Trochlear 1%
- Patella:
  - Inferomedial 5–10%.

OCD is traditionally divided into juvenile (open physes) and adult (closed physes) based on skeletal maturity. This distinction is useful because higher rates of healing have been seen in juvenile OCD than in the adult form. Juvenile OCD is seen more frequently in athletic children. Symptoms are preceded by a history of trauma to the knee in 40–60% of cases. It typically presents as anterior knee pain: worse with activity and improved by rest. Patients with early, intact OCD lesions, present with vague symptoms of poorly localized knee pain, stiffness with or after activities, and occasional swelling after activity. Mechanical symptoms such as grinding, locking, and catching are more commonly associated with the late stages of OCD where loose or detached OCD lesions are present.

An initial physical finding is tenderness over the involved condyle with the knee flexed. Later, patients develop a joint effusion and a decreased range of motion. The child may limp and the involved leg may be externally rotated to prevent impingement of the tibial spine on the MFC. Pain may be elicited with internal rotation of the tibia (Wilson's sign) but this sign lacks sensitivity. In stable lesions, there is usually no effusion, crepitus or pain through a range of normal motion. Quadriceps atrophy may be noted in long standing cases.

Mechanical symptoms are pronounced with unstable lesions. An antalgic gait is common and there is usually a knee effusion, possibly associated with crepitus with motion. Both knees should be examined since the condition is bilateral in 20–25% of cases. If bilateral disease is present, lesions are typically asymmetrical in terms of size and symptoms.

Initial investigations include standing AP and lateral radiographs. If OCD is suspected 'notch' or 'tunnel' views should be requested to localize and characterize the lesion, rule out additional bony pathology, and evaluate skeletal maturity. In children less than 7 years of age, irregularities of the distal femoral epiphyseal

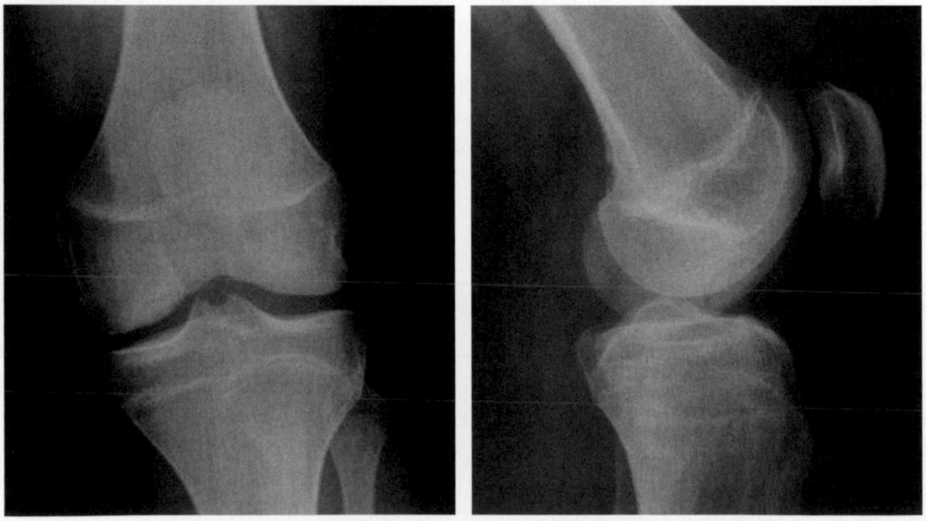

A B

Fig. 13.20.5 A) AP and B) lateral radiographs of an adolescent knee demonstrating an OCD lesion on the lateral aspect of the MFC – it is perhaps not posterior enough to be called the 'classic' site.

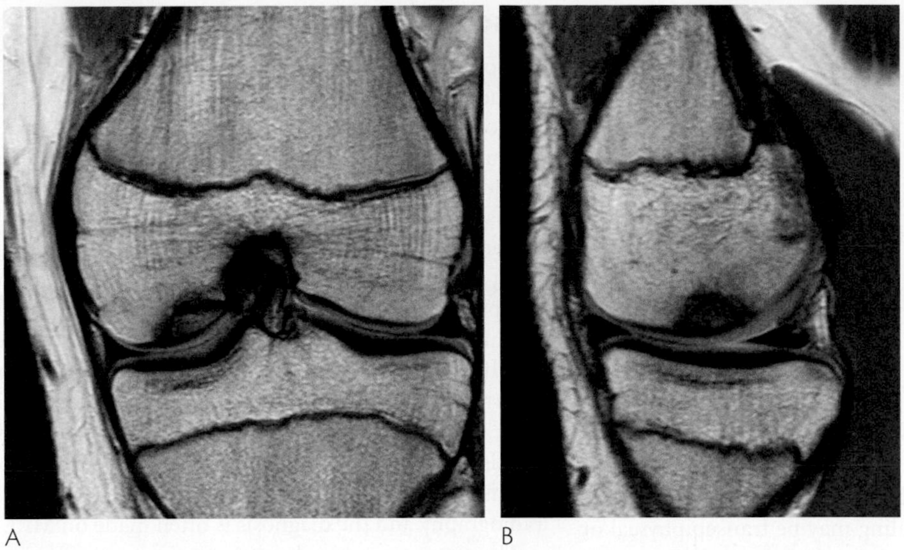

Fig. 13.20.6 A) AP and B) lateral MRI of the same knee as in Figure 13.20.5 demonstrating the OCD lesion.

ossification centre may simulate OCD but these asymptomatic sites are anatomic variants of normal ossification. The location of the lesion can be described and an estimate of size obtained from the radiographs (Figure 13.20.5). Characteristic findings include a well-circumscribed area of subchondral bone separated by a crescent-shaped sclerotic radiolucent outline of the fragment.

OCD of the knee can be diagnosed using plain radiographs alone but they are poor at establishing the stability of the lesion or the state of the overlying cartilage. MRI is considered the gold standard for evaluation of OCD. MRI can give an accurate estimate of the size of the lesion and status of cartilage and subchondral bone (Figure 13.20.6). The extent of bony oedema, the appearance of a high signal zone beneath the fragment, and presence of loose bodies are additional important MRI findings (Table 13.20.2). The most useful diagnostic feature of MRI is its ability to distinguish between stage II and III lesions. The presence of synovial fluid or granulation tissue at the interface between the fragment and the parent bone, manifested as increased signal intensity on T_2-weighted spin echo MRIs, generally indicates an unstable lesion. Conversely, the absence of a zone of high signal at this interface is a reliable sign of lesion stability. In stage II OCD lesions, the low signal in the interface indicates fibrous attachment stabilizing the lesion. In contrast, stage III lesions will show high signal intensity at the interface, indicating synovial fluid between the fragment and underlying parent bone.

As the natural history of stable OCD lesions is generally favourable in a child with open physes, there is widespread agreement that initial non-operative treatment is indicated.

Kocher advocates a three-phase non-operative management protocol (Box 13.20.7). At the end of phase 1, the child should be pain-free, and repeat radiographs should be obtained. In phase 2, weight bearing as tolerated is permitted without immobilization. A rehabilitation programme is initiated emphasizing knee range of motion and low-impact quadriceps and hamstring strengthening exercises. Sports and repetitive impact activities are restricted. If there are radiographic and clinical signs of healing at 3–4 months after the diagnosis, phase 3 can begin. This phase includes supervised initiation of running, jumping, and cutting sports readiness activities. A gradual return to sports with increasing intensity is allowed in the absence of knee symptoms. An MRI may be repeated in phase 3 to assess healing. If symptoms return or follow-up radiographs show recurrence, repeat non-operative treatment can be considered.

Operative treatment should be considered in patients with detached or unstable lesions (stage III and IV) regardless of the age of the child and in those patients approaching physeal closure whose lesions have been unresponsive to non-operative management (Box 13.20.8). In general, unstable lesions require partial takedown with debridement to remove fibrous tissue and restore vascularity. These techniques are based on the premise that the

Table 13.20.2 MRI classification of juvenile OCD lesions

Stage	Description
I	Small change of signal without clear margins of fragment
II	Osteochondral fragment with clear margins without fluid between fragment and underlying bone
III	Fluid is partially visible between fragment and underlying bone
IV	Fluid completely surrounds the fragment but the fragment is *in situ*
V	Fragment is completely detached and displaced (loose body)

Box 13.20.7 Three-phase non-operative management protocol

1. Knee immobilization 4–6 weeks, partial weight bearing (PWB) with crutches
2. Weeks 6–12, weight bearing as tolerated without immobilization and commencement of a rehabilitation programme
3. Months 3–4, if healing, staged return to sporting activity.

Table 13.20.3 Arthroscopic staging of OCD lesions

Stage	Description
I	Irregularity and softening of articular cartilage. No definable fragment
II	Articular cartilage breached, definable fragment, not displaceable
III	Articular cartilage breached, definable fragment, displaceable but attached by some overlying articular cartilage
IV	Loose body

lesion is essentially a fracture non-union and rely on the penetration of subchondral bone to promote vascular ingrowth into the non-union site. Guhl described the system for arthroscopic staging of the lesions (Table 13.20.3).

Arthroscopic drilling of juvenile OCD to create channels for potential revascularization and healing may be transepiphyseal or transarticular. Antegrade drilling through the epiphysis avoids damage to the articular surface but is associated with technical challenges of maintaining accurate drill placement and depth. On the other hand, retrograde transarticular drilling is relatively straightforward, although the channels it creates through the articular cartilage heal with fibrocartilage. If partially unstable lesions have subchondral bone loss, autogenous bone graft is packed into the crater before fragment reduction and fixation.

Mechanical stabilization of unstable OCD lesions increases the likelihood of maintaining joint congruity postoperatively, and allows for the potential of early joint motion. Stabilization can be performed using a variety of implants including Kirschner wires, low-profile compression screws, cannulated screws, bone pegs, bioabsorbable fixation, or fibrin glue. A variety of treatments have evolved over the past few years aimed at addressing irreparable chondral defects and OCD lesions. Interventions include perichondral/periosteal autografts, autologous chondrocyte implantation (ACI) and matrix-induced ACI techniques, abrasion chondroplasty, microfracture, osteochondral autograft transplantation (OAT—mosaicplasty), and osteochondral allografts. Most of these treatment options result in the formation of fibrocartilage covering the exposed defect rather than true hyaline cartilage. The long-term results from these procedures have yet to be clearly determined. A completely separated OCD fragment in a skeletally immature person may be treated by arthroscopic or open excision, or by reduction and fixation. Recent separation and a larger bony fragment favour an attempt at reduction and fixation into the debrided defect. Failure to of the fragment to heal, or a chronic separation, favour excision with debridement of the defect: this itself will result in substantial fibrocartilage healing.

Box 13.20.8 Goals of operative treatment of OCD lesions

- Maintenance of joint congruity
- Rigid fixation of unstable fragments
- Repair/reconstruction of osteochondral defects.

Discoid meniscus

Discoid menisci invariably affect the lateral meniscus and the overall incidence is 3–5% with up to one-fifth of cases being bilateral. Although the condition is a congenital anomaly, or perhaps simply an anatomical variant, no explanation for its occurrence has been found. Discoid menisci are more likely to tear due to the increased stresses on their larger surface area. The meniscus is also often hypermobile. The Watanabe classification (Table 13.20.4) is used most frequently. Type III lesions often present at a young age with symptoms of a 'snapping knee' and unexplained falls due to giving way. Pain is not a feature. Physical examination may elicit a reproducible 'clunk' on the lateral side of the knee as the flexed and externally rotated knee is brought into extension and internal rotation. Type I and II lesions present in later childhood, following a meniscal tear, with symptoms and signs similar to other types of meniscal injury. A widened lateral joint space may be seen on plain radiography and the diagnosis is often made on MRI.

The asymptomatic discoid meniscus requires no treatment. A torn meniscus may have a stable rim in which case the central portion is simply 'saucerized'. If there is instability or peripheral detachment of the remaining meniscus, meniscal suturing should be performed (see Chapter 13.23).

Meniscal cysts

As in adults, torn menisci can lead to the formation of meniscal cysts (Figure 13.20.7). Treatment is directed at the meniscal tear and the cyst will usually drain and close spontaneously.

Anterior knee pain

Osgood–Schlatter disease and Sinding–Larsen–Johansson syndrome are typically overuse injuries causing apophysitis of the anterior tibial tubercle and inferior pole of the patella respectively. They are common in active adolescents and associated with local tenderness and palpable swelling. Symptoms are often bilateral but both symptoms and signs may be markedly asymmetrical. Often a history of increased use, rapid growth, or jumping/landing sports accompanies the onset of pain. Repetitive small injuries to the tendon insertion are believed to be important in the aetiology of this condition. Growing children are particularly vulnerable because growth leads to tight muscles especially those, such as rectus femoris, which cross two joints. A tight rectus femoris (positive Ely–Duncan test) can often be elicited among adolescents with Osgood–Schlatter disease or jumper's knee. Radiographs confirm fragmentation of the apophysis and in such cases other differential diagnoses for unilateral bony pain and swelling in this age group such as a malignancy become much less likely.

Table 13.20.4 Classification of discoid menisci (after Watanabe)

Type	Description
I	Meniscus covers the entire tibial plateau Intact peripheral attachments
II	Meniscus covers 80% of the plateau
III	Meniscus covers 75–80% of the plateau with a thick posterior horn and abnormal peripheral attachments

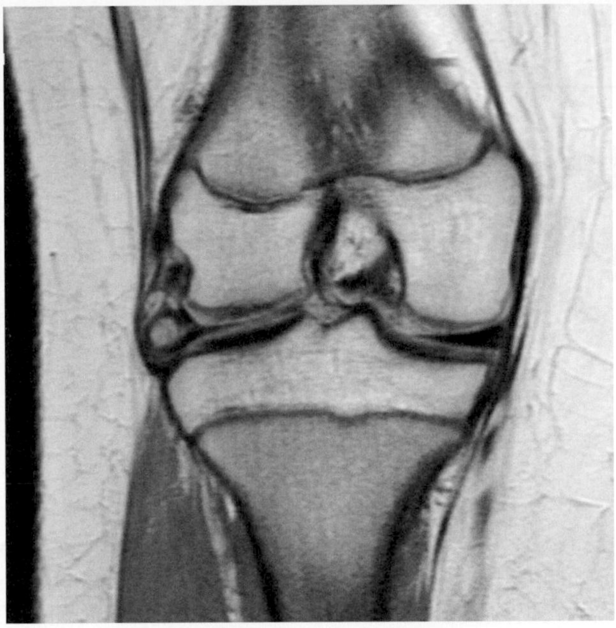

Fig. 13.20.7 MRI of a right knee showing a lateral meniscal cyst that was associated with a meniscal tear.

Management is conservative with physiotherapy indicated to address tight hamstrings or quadriceps and general advice on the use of cushioned insoles and restriction of sporting activity but only if symptoms warrant this. Attention to jumping and landing technique, or play on soft surfaces, may be useful adjuncts. Most cases of Osgood–Schlatter disease have resolved by skeletal maturity when the apophysis fuses with the rest of the tibial tubercle. For the small minority of cases that continue with symptoms, surgical excision of a painful residual ossicle(s) with decompression of the patella tendon may give dramatic symptom relief.

Further reading

Bahr, R., Fossan, B., Loken, S., and Engebretsen, L. (2006). Surgical treatment compared with eccentric training for patellar tendinopathy (jumper's knee). A randomized, controlled trial. *Journal of Bone and Joint Surgery*, **88A**, 1689–98.

Kelly, B.T. and Green, D.W. (2002). Discoid lateral meniscus in children. *Current Opinion in Pediatrics*, **14**, 54–61.

Kocher, M.S., Czarnecki, J.J., Andersen, J.S., and Micheli, L.J. (2007). Internal fixation of juvenile osteochondritis dissecans lesions of the knee. *American Journal of Sports Medicine*, **35**(5), 712–18.

MacIntyre, N.J., Hill, N.A., Fellows, R.A., Ellis, R.E., and Wilson, D.R. (2006). Patellofemoral joint kinematics in individuals with and without patellofemoral pain syndrome. *Journal of Bone and Joint Surgery*, **88A**, 2596–605.

Smirk, C. and Morris, H. (2003). The anatomy and reconstruction of the medial patellofemoral ligament. *Knee*, **10**(3), 221–7.

13.21

Congenital talipes equinovarus

Michael Uglow

Summary points

- Aetiology of idiopathic congenital talipes equinovarus remains unknown
- Antenatal diagnosis is common with good differentiation of the idiopathic from the syndromic foot
- The Ponseti method is the treatment of choice: results are poorer in the atypical and syndromic feet
- Surgery is required in selected cases as the primary treatment and in others, as treatment for residual and/or recurrent deformity.

Introduction

The treatment of patients with clubfeet in the twenty-first century has gone through a revolution pioneered in the mid-twentieth century: the primary treatment was surgical but now serial manipulation and casting is the mainstay of management. Surgery still has a role in the management of older children with relapsed deformities and especially for recalcitrant and teratologic feet.

Aetiology

The incidence of talipes equinovarus (TEV) varies with ethnicity: 0.4 (Chinese)–1.2 (Caucasians)–6.8 (Polynesians) per 1000 births. The male to female ratio is 2.5:1. Fifty per cent of cases show bilateral involvement and in 24% there is a positive family history. These factors indicate a polygenic inheritance. See Box 13.21.1.

Although the aetiology of idiopathic clubfoot remains unknown, there are numerous theories regarding its development. Intrauterine moulding as a cause of clubfoot was first proposed by Hippocrates and whilst it may play a role in some cases, the evidence from antenatal ultrasound scans is that most TEV deformities are identifiable early in pregnancy in the presence of adequate amniotic fluid.

Histological studies have identified abnormalities both in the muscles and in the medial ligaments with an increase in connective tissue content and a greater number of myofibroblasts. A higher prevalence of type 1 muscle fibres in affected feet compared to unaffected feet has been noted. One study found a significant reduction in the number of anterior horn cells in the affected side of stillborn fetuses with unilateral clubfoot but as with much of this work it does not distinguish between cause and effect. Subtle abnormalities have been identified on neurophysiological testing.

Contrary to popular belief, there is no known association with hip dysplasia.

Investigations into the genetic influences on TEV have progressed rapidly and are based on Hox genes involved in limb bud development. Chromosomal deletions (2q31–33) and candidate genes such as *CASP8* and *10*, and *CFLAR* that encode protein regulators of apoptosis during growth and development have been associated with clubfoot.

TEV found in association with other conditions is referred to as teratologic or syndromic TEV rather than idiopathic (Box 13.21.2).

Anatomy

The essential deformities are a displacement of the navicular, os calcis, and cuboid around the talus, characterized by hindfoot equinus, internal rotation with varus and adduction, and supination of the forefoot (Figure 13.21.1).

The key to understanding the TEV deformity is to consider that the talus is firmly held by the ankle mortise and to assess the remainder of the foot in relation to the talus. Thus, the essential deformity is that the os calcis is internally rotated beneath the talus. In order to achieve this position it must assume an equinus and varus posture. The remainder of the foot is attached to the os calcis through the cuboid and the navicular allows rotation of the forefoot around the talar head. With the os calcis internally rotated, the

Box 13.21.1 Demographics of TEV deformity

- Incidence: 1:1000 live births
- Males > females: 2.5:1
- Bilateral: 50%
- Family history: 24%
- Sibling risk: 3–7%.

Box 13.21.2 Syndromes associated with TEV deformities

- Larsen's syndrome
- Diastrophic dwarfism
- Freeman–Sheldon syndrome
- Arthrogryposis multiplex congenital
- Spinal dysraphism.

forefoot must be in an adducted and supinated position. The metatarsals are joined in the transverse plane but there is independence of the medial and lateral columns in the sagittal plane and the first metatarsal often adopts a plantar flexed posture which explains the cavus deformity of the medial foot.

In addition to the abnormal bony architecture, the soft tissues are frequently abnormal and vascular studies have identified abnormalities in the arterial supply in patients with TEV.

The limb below the knee is thinner than normal and both the foot and the lower leg are usually short. The degree of shortening reflects the severity of the initial deformity.

Classification

Classification systems are of value in providing a prognosis to parents and for comparing the results of treatment between centres. There have been numerous attempts to classify clubfeet but the most popular in use today are those described by Pirani and Dimeglio. The Pirani system is based on 6 criteria: 3 each from the hindfoot and forefoot. Each criteria is graded 0, 0.5 or 1, giving a maximum score of 6 for each foot. The Dimeglio system scores each foot out of 20 points and then assigns it a grade. Both systems can be used for sequential assessments to monitor treatment and to predict the need for tenotomy when using the Ponseti method of treatment.

Treatment

The earliest documented treatment for TEV, in 1000BC, was massage and Hippocrates (circa 400BC) recommended treating the foot as near to birth as possible using gentle serial manipulations and fixation, aiming for over-correction. Special shoes were worn afterwards to help prevent relapse and maintain correction.

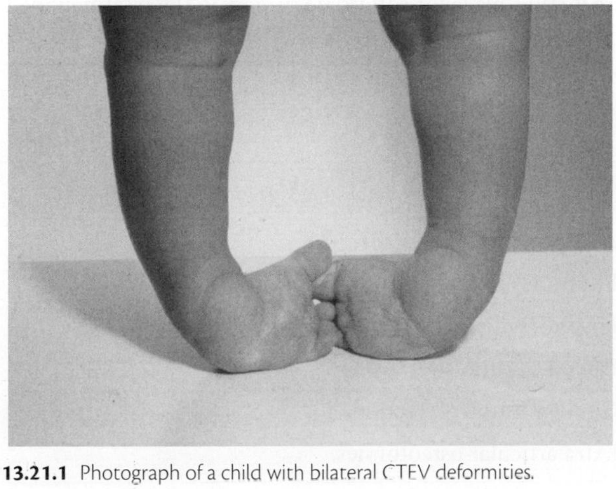

Fig. 13.21.1 Photograph of a child with bilateral CTEV deformities.

Surgery became a part of treatment in the eighteenth century and became increasingly common and increasingly aggressive during the twentieth century due to disillusionment with the protracted nature of the contemporary casting techniques such as that advocated by Kite. In time, however, it became apparent that the results following an aggressive surgical approach were also disappointing and a resurgence of the conservative management of TEV has been seen.

Kite's view was that the fulcrum for correction of the clubfoot was the calcaneocuboid joint but correction at this site results in a midfoot break through the metatarsal–tarsal articulation. Ponseti has shown clearly that the fulcrum for correction is the lateral head of the talus and hence he developed his method of correcting a clubfoot by serial stretching and casting according to the principles of Hippocrates. The description was first published in 1963 but it took over 30 years for the method to be adopted by other surgeons.

The Ponseti method (Box 13.21.3)

The method consists of weekly manipulations during which the foot is stretched gently according to a well-defined sequence. After stretching, the foot is placed in a plaster cast to maintain the position that has been achieved. The procedure is repeated until correction is achieved. This takes approximately 6 weeks but varies depending on the flexibility of the foot (Figure 13.21.2).

Firstly the cavus of the first ray is elevated and the foot assumes a supinated position. This ensures that the metatarsals are in the same plane. The foot is then progressively abducted in the plane of the metatarsals, the effect of which is to correct the adduction deformity of the forefoot and additionally the internal rotation of the os calcis. As the abduction progresses the forefoot drives the os calcis from its position of internal rotation beneath the talus to its reduced position thus correcting the varus and part of the equinus deformity.

It is important to over correct the forefoot to 70 degrees of abduction to ensure accurate reduction of the hindfoot. As the forefoot abducts it adopts a more pronated position because of the change in position of the os calcis relative to the talus. Forced pronation should never be used as it recreates the original cavus deformity by plantar flexing the first ray thus locking the foot and preventing hindfoot correction.

The final correction required is the residual ankle equinus. Approximately 25% of feet correct completely with further stretching but most will not. If ankle dorsiflexion of 10–15 degrees cannot be achieved, a tenotomy is required. This can be done simply in the clinic under local anaesthesia. In 5% of cases insufficient dorsiflexion

Box 13.21.3 Sequential correction of deformities with the Ponseti method

- First ray elevation
- Forefoot abduction
- Ankle dorsiflexion.

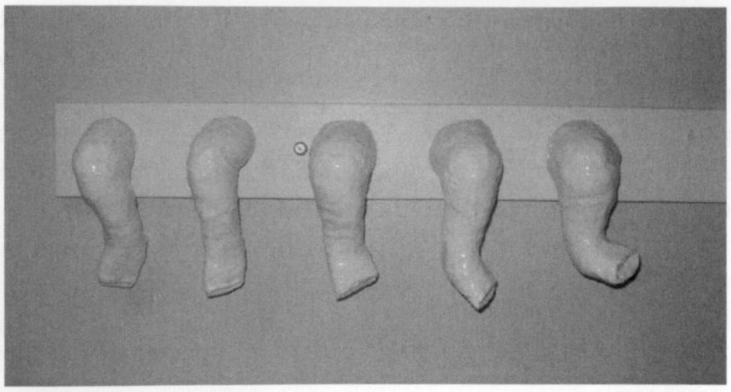

Fig. 13.21.2 Examples of sequential casts used to correct a CTEV deformity by the Ponseti method.

is achieved and surgery is required to gain complete correction. This can usually be achieved by a posterior release of the ankle capsule but in a few feet more radical soft tissue surgery is required. Following complete correction, the foot is held in a final cast for 3 weeks and then the child is treated with boots on a bar to maintain the correction (Figure 13.21.3). For the first 3 months, the boots are worn for 23 hours a day and then at 'night time and nap time' until the age of 4 years.

Pirani's elegant MRI study showed that the cartilaginous deformities of the clubfoot correct with progressive manipulation and casting.

Results using Ponseti's method

Cooper and Dietz published a 30-year follow up on 29 of Ponseti's original group of 45 patients. The functional results did deteriorate over time but at 30 years, 78% of feet were rated as excellent/good with a supple, plantigrade foot. Relapse occurred in 50% overall but was treatable by repeated casting, with or without a further Achilles tenotomy and with a transfer of the anterior tibialis tendon in those feet with a supination deformity. Long-term results are better in those with a sedentary occupation and who are not overweight.

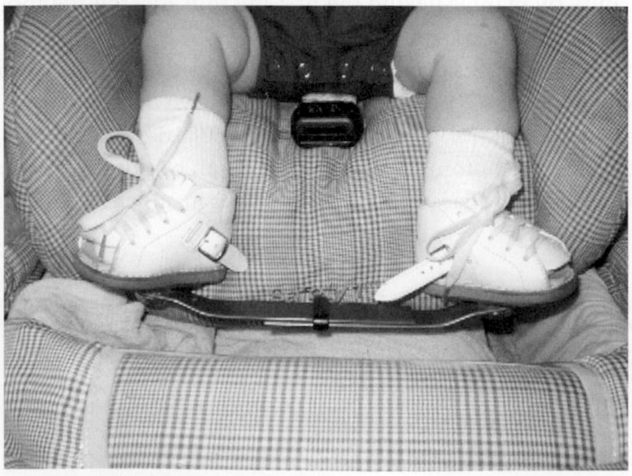

Fig. 13.21.3 Child using 'Boots and Bars' to maintain correction of deformity. Feet are held shoulder width apart with the foot externally rotated.

The true success of a procedure is whether the results can be repeated by others: initial reports failed to produce satisfactory results, invariably due to inaccurate casting techniques; however, with strict adherence to the Ponseti method, good results have been published from many centres. Relapse rates are significantly higher with poor brace compliance and although they may be treated by reapplication of the Ponseti method, compliance may still be a problem and open surgery is often necessary. A complete correction of the deformities is essential to ensure accurate brace fitting which is important to optimize brace compliance. In a series of 62 patients with 3-year follow-up from Southampton the author reports an initial failure rate of 5% and a subsequent relapse rate of 21% successfully treated with repeat casting, Achilles tenotomy or tibialis anterior transfer. All of the relapses occurred in patients with an initial hindfoot Pirani score of 2.5 or 3.0.

The Ponseti method has also been shown to be an effective means of treating clubfeet when performed by non-medical personnel such as physiotherapists and clinical officers in the developing world where facilities for surgery are less established. However, the involvement of a paediatric orthopaedic surgeon is essential to ensure continuity of care and to manage the early failures and recurrences.

The atypical or complex idiopathic clubfoot

Ponseti and others have identified certain atypical feet that behave differently to the standard idiopathic clubfoot. Clinically, they are defined as having rigid equinus, severe plantar flexion of all metatarsals, a deep crease above the heel, a transverse crease in the sole of the foot, and a short and hyperextended first toe. The Achilles tendon is exceptionally tight and fibrotic up to midcalf. In such patients, correction can be achieved by modifying the Ponseti technique and performing an Achilles tenotomy earlier than usual, prior to full correction of the forefoot. This has the effect of releasing the os calcis from under the talus. Casting may then proceed as usual but a further tenotomy may be required as little as 3 weeks later if the equinus cannot be corrected.

The syndromic foot

With teratologic or syndromic foot deformities, the Ponseti method is less likely to succeed, but it should be attempted and it may reduce the extent of the subsequent surgical release.

The role of surgery (Box 13.21.4)

There is still a place for soft tissue surgery in the treatment of TEV. All published reports of the Ponseti method have a small, early failure rate and these feet will require a limited posterior or full

Box 13.21.4 The role of surgery in TEV

- Achilles tenotomy
- Posterior release
- Posteromedial release
- Lateral column shortening
- Circular frame correction
- Extra articular osteotomies.

posteromedial release. In addition there are some families for whom the Ponseti method will not be suitable for logistical reasons. For some, the use of the boots and bar present a major problem and poor compliance amongst certain population groups has been noted. In these patients surgery may be advocated to provide a traditional complete correction with no need for on going orthotic use.

Surgery also has a role in the treatment of relapses. As discussed previously the initial approach to a relapse is to repeat the Ponseti method. If the forefoot is supinating then a transfer of the anterior tibialis muscle is required. On occasion these steps are insufficient and more extensive surgery may be required. If the child is less than 5 years old, a posteromedial release can be performed to restore the orientation of the os calcis beneath the talus. Shortening of the lateral column can be very effective in correcting the adductus deformity that occurs. Several methods are described and include resecting part of the anterior os calcis or cuboid, or fusing the calcaneocuboid joint.

Relapse following surgical release is common: a 9–16-year follow-up study found that almost 80% of Dimeglio grade 4 feet had relapsed. With increasing age and increasingly rigid deformities, the prospect of further open surgery becomes less attractive due to the inevitable increased stiffness and scarring associated with it. For those feet that do require surgical intervention to obtain a plantigrade foot, the use of gradual correction using the principles of Ilizarov avoids the need to perform extensive soft tissue dissection. By using circular frames the complex deformities can be corrected gradually with distraction and fixed or virtual hinges. The Taylor Spatial Frame (TSF) is a circular frame device where the correction is calculated using a web-based software program. Using the principles of the Ponseti method, an olive wire inserted into the head of the talus can be used as a fulcrum to correct the deformity in the same way as the thumb is used in a standard manipulation.

Summary

TEV is relatively common affecting approximately 1 in 1000 live births. The optimal contemporary management is the Ponseti method of sequential manipulation and casting followed by maintenance of the correction by boots and bar for approximately 4 years. Ideally, treatment starts as soon after birth as possible but it can still be used for delayed presentations. The same approach is used for relapses that occur in approximately 20–30% of cases and a transfer of the anterior tibialis muscle may be required to treat supination of the forefoot. Soft tissue surgery may still be necessary for initial failures, for relapses and teratologic feet. Gradual correction using circular frames is one method of treating difficult deformities without the need for open surgery and the risk of associated fibrosis.

Further reading

Cooper, D.M. and Dietz, F.R. (1995). Treatment of idiopathic clubfoot. A thirty-year follow-up note. *Journal of Bone and Joint Surgery*, **77A**, 1477–89.

Dimeglio, A., Bensahel, H., Souchet, P.H., Mazeau, P.H., and Bonnet, F. (1995). Classification of clubfoot. *Journal of Pediatric Orthopedics*, **4**, 129–36.

Dyer, P.J. and Davis, N. (2006). The role of the Pirani scoring system in the management of club foot by the Ponseti method. *Journal of Bone and Joint Surgery*, **88B**, 1082–4.

Heck, A., Bray, M., Scott, A., Blanton, S., and Hecht, J. (2005). Variation in CASP10 gene is associated with idiopathic talipes equinovarus. *Journal of Pediatric Orthopedics*, **25**(5), 598–602.

Kite, J. (1972). Non-operative treatment of congenital clubfoot. *Clinical Orthopedics*, **84**, 29–38.

Pirani, S., Zeznik, L., and Hodges, D. (2001). Magnetic resonance imaging study of the congenital clubfoot treated with the Ponseti method. *Journal of Pediatric Orthopedics*, **21**, 719–6.

Ponseti, I. (1992). Current concepts review. Treatment of congenital clubfoot. *Journal of Bone and Joint Surgery*, **74A**, 448–54.

Ponseti, I.V., Zhivkov, M., Davis, N., Sinclair, M., Dobbs, M.B., and Morcuende, J.A. (2006). Treatment of the complex idiopathic clubfoot. *Clinical Orthopaedics and Related Research*, **451**, 171–6.

Uglow, M.G., Senbaga, N., Pickard, R., and Clarke, N.M.P. (2007). Relapse rates following staged surgery in the treatment of recalcitrant talipes equinovarus: 9 to 16 year outcome study. *Journal of Children's Orthopaedics*, **1**, 115–19.

13.22

The foot in childhood

Manoj Ramachandran

Summary points

- Congenital foot anomalies are common: most are minor and do not affect function
- Postural problems must be differentiated from structural anomalies
- An underlying neuromuscular aetiology should be considered
- A pain-free, functional foot is the goal of treatment.

Foot development

The limb buds appear 4 weeks after fertilization and form rapidly over the next few weeks. By 10 weeks, joint cavitation has occurred and ligaments and capsule have developed with forefoot ossification. Ossification proceeds progressively to the hindfoot and at birth, ossification centres are seen throughout the forefoot, the calcaneum, cuboid, and talus. The navicular ossifies last between 2–5 years. An additional ossification centre develops in the posterior aspect of the calcaneum at approximately 6 years and numerous other accessory ossification centres may be noted with growth (Box 13.22.1).

It is not uncommon for a problem to occur during fetal maturation. Failure of formation may be complete or partial and the anomalies classified as terminal transverse or longitudinal deficiencies involving either the preaxial or postaxial border. The foot anomaly may simply be part of a more generalized limb deficiency, such as fibular dysplasia, or it may be restricted to the foot but associated with similar anomalies in the hand. Such foot deformities include ectrodactyly (or lobster claw foot), absent or short metatarsals, syndactyly, and polydactyly (Figure 13.22.1).

The most significant congenital foot abnormality is the clubfoot or talipes equinovarus deformity which is discussed separately (see Chapter 13.21).

Box 13.22.1 Foot size and shape

- At 12 months (girls)–18 months (boys) the foot is half its adult size
- Longitudinal arch appears by 2 years: best observed in the moving foot
- At 14 years (girls)–16 years (boys) the foot is mature adult size.

Genetic abnormalities

Genetic disorders can be inherited in either dominant or recessive modes and the associated anomalies may affect the foot alone or be part of a more generalized condition. Polydactyly and syndactyly are common examples of inherited conditions (Figure 13.22.2). Minor genetic variations, such as the number of phalanges in the fifth toe, often have little clinical significance. The common major chromosomal malformations are associated with foot abnormalities (Box 13.22.2).

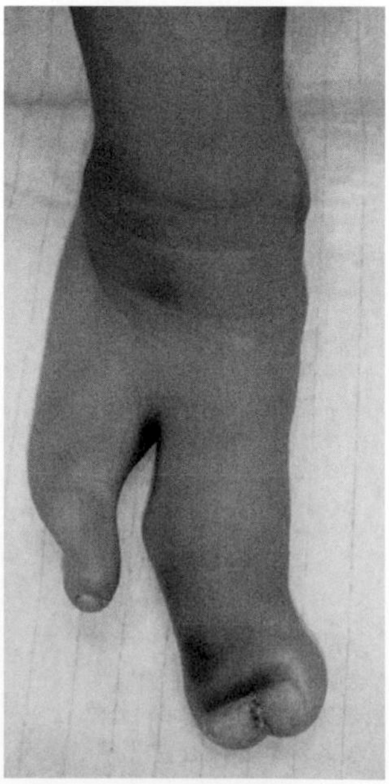

Fig. 13.22.1 Clinical photograph of an ectrodactyly or cleft foot.

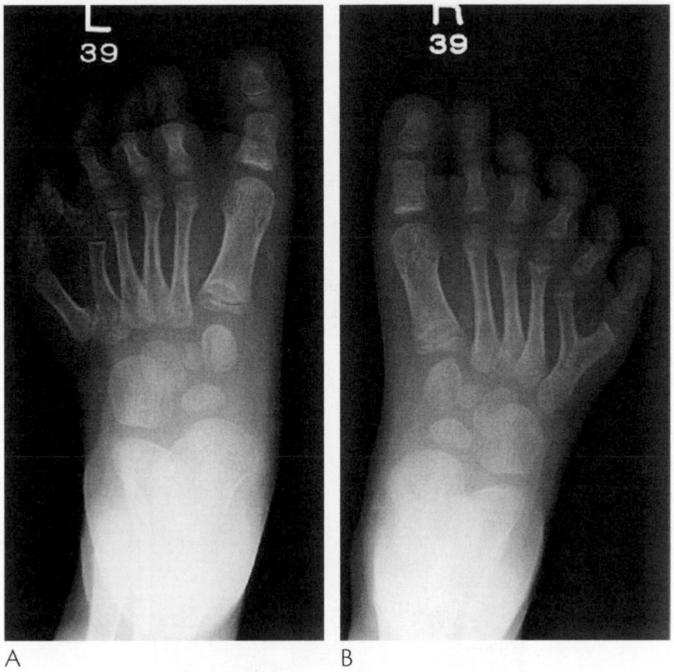

Fig. 13.22.2 AP radiographs demonstrating bilateral polydactyly. Both hands were also affected and the condition was familial.

Clinical evaluation

Many conditions seen during the neonatal period are inherited and appropriate genetic counselling helps with management. In the older child, the history of onset of symptoms and deformity becomes more important. Clinical photographs and standard radiographs may help in documenting progression of deformity.

Pain becomes a more common complaint with increasing age. Severe unremitting night pain suggests a serious pathology. Pain occurring in a specific area during a specific activity suggests a mechanical cause whilst a burning pain in association with swelling may indicate an inflammatory condition. In children, the report of pain is often second hand and the parents' and the child's interpretation of the pain may be different. A child who truly has severe pain, even intermittently, is unlikely to behave normally at other times of the day.

At all ages, it may be difficult to conduct an adequate foot examination but the standing posture, gait, and function should be observed with a particular focus on lower limb alignment and asymmetry. A generalized neuromuscular examination should be performed in addition to a survey of all lower limb joints and the spine.

The simplest active movements of the foot and ankle are dorsiflexion and plantar flexion but this movement is not confined to one standard axis. In the hindfoot joints, all movement is around an oblique axis such that dorsiflexion includes elements of both external rotation (motion around a vertical axis) and pronation (motion around a longitudinal axis). Plantar flexion includes an element of internal rotation and supination. Inversion as an active movement not only has supination but also plantar flexion and internal rotation; eversion includes mainly pronation, dorsiflexion, and external rotation (Figure 13.22.3). All hindfoot joints contribute to these movements and loss of movement at one joint is often disguised by increased movement at another neighbouring joint. Assessment of the passive joint ranges at differing levels helps identify this.

The neonatal foot may be relatively easy to examine but careful observation is necessary to assess muscle activity and power. The neonate and young infant are best examined in an informal manner with the child supported on the parent's knee and distracted by suitable activity. In the older child, a more formal structured examination becomes feasible.

Box 13.22.2 Chromosomal malformations

- Trisomy 21:
  - Flexible planovalgus
  - Metatarsus adductus
  - Hallux varus *or* valgus
- Trisomy 18:
  - Talipes equinovarus *or*
  - Vertical talus
- Trisomy 13 or 15:
  - Polydactyly
  - Syndactyly
  - Midtarsal subluxations
- Trisomy 8:
  - Great toe clawing
  - Talipes equinovarus.

Investigation

Children over the age of 4 years can generally stand for AP and lateral weight-bearing radiographs that allow the foot to be seen in its fully loaded position. The site of deformity can be identified and measurements made with reference to the weight-bearing surface

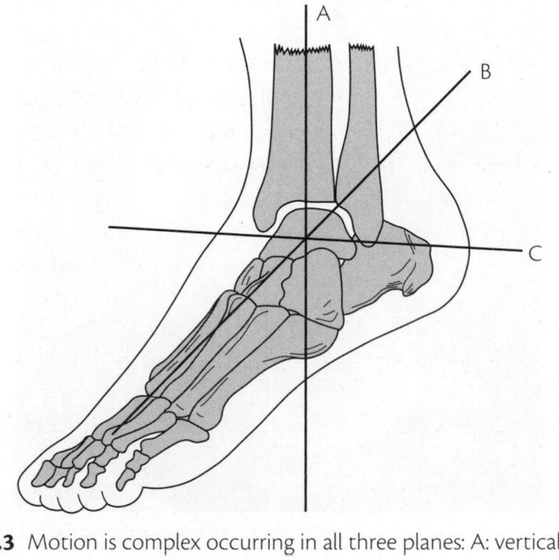

Fig. 13.22.3 Motion is complex occurring in all three planes: A: vertical axis; B: transverse axis; C: longitudinal axis. See text for details.

to document progressive deformity. Under this age, non-weight-bearing films are accepted. An oblique view may demonstrate abnormalities of the midtarsal and tarsometatarsal regions identifying accessory ossicles or coalitions.

In the child, bone scans can be helpful in isolating inflammatory and infective aetiologies, while computed tomography (CT) and magnetic resonance (MR) scans are useful in the diagnosis and assessment of anatomic abnormalities such as coalitions (Figure 13.22.4) and soft tissue disorders. Three-dimensional CT imaging has a potential role in planning surgical intervention (Figure 13.22.5).

Postural foot deformities

These deformities arise in late pregnancy, in an otherwise normal limb, and are generally due to fetal crowding and consequent moulding secondary to oligohydramnios or a twin pregnancy. They are characterized by the lack of significant structural changes and the ease with which they correct, usually spontaneously, soon after birth. Their greatest significance lies in the increased joint laxity with which they may be associated.

Talipes calcaneovalgus (Box 13.22.3)

This condition, the most common postural foot deformity, is associated with other postural deformities such as torticollis, plagiocephaly, infantile skeletal skew, developmental hip dysplasia, and hyperextension deformity of the knee. It is more common in girls. The foot is dorsiflexed with a variable degree of eversion. Most feet are passively correctible and improve promptly but if the soft tissues over the dorsum of the ankle are tight, stretching exercises are advocated.

Metatarsus adductus

Metatarsus adductus is a common benign postural deformity. It is often bilateral and associated with DDH as part of fetal moulding.

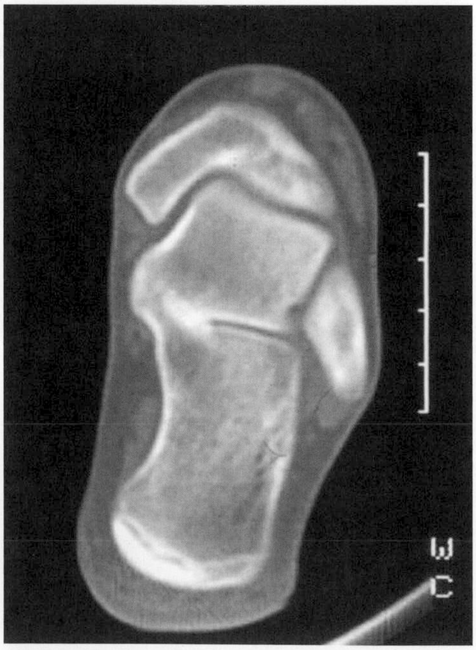

Fig. 13.22.4 Coronal CT scan showing a talocalcaneal coalition involving the sustentaculum tali and the medial portion of the posterior facet.

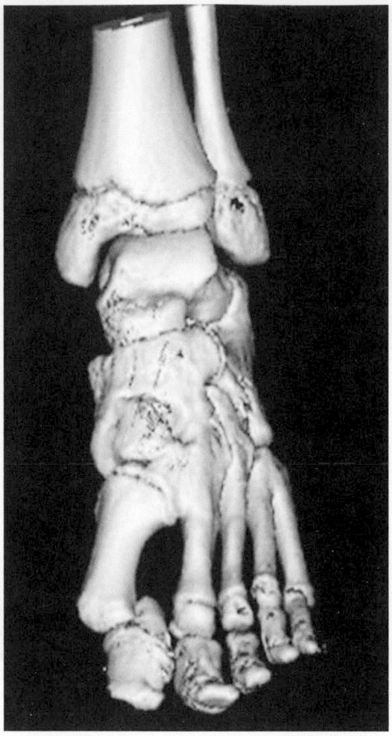

Fig. 13.22.5 Three-dimensional CT scan demonstrating a variety of foot abnormalities in a child with Apert's syndrome

The child often presents with an in-toeing gait with the abnormality confined to the forefoot. The metatarsals are adducted at the level of the tarsometatarsal joint and the severity of the deformity is assessed by the curvature of the medial border and whether the deformity is correctible or not (Table 13.22.1) (Figure 13.22.6). The forefoot may be supinated as well as adducted. A stiff foot with a deep medial sulcus represents a severe deformity.

Plain radiographs of the foot are rarely needed but demonstrate the abnormal alignment of the forefoot compared to the hindfoot.

The vast majority of cases resolve by the age of 3 years. Although widely advocated, stretching exercises probably make little difference to the long-term outcome. Straight or reverse-last shoes have been recommended in children with flexible deformities and serial casting may be helpful in rigid deformities.

Significant persistent deformity beyond the age of 4 years may warrant surgical treatment. Up to the age of 6 years, soft tissue procedures (abductor hallucis recession, medial release, and tarsometatarsal release) may suffice. In older children with more rigid deformities, osteotomy of either the metatarsals or preferably the midfoot (lateral closing, medial opening wedge osteotomies) should be considered.

Box 13.22.3 Talipes calcaneovalgus deformity

- Exclude associated conditions such as developmental dysplasia of the hip
- Differentiate this postural deformity from structural vertical talus with equinovalgus position.

Table 13.22.1 Classification of metatarsus adductus

Group	Description
I	Flexible deformity: active correction beyond neutral
II	Flexible deformity, passive correction beyond neutral
III	Rigid deformity, passive correction to neutral not possible

Structural foot deformities

Isolated forefoot anomalies may occur but they are often associated with more proximal problems and the foot must be examined carefully to identify them. The most frequent hindfoot and midfoot abnormalities lead to a position that is planus (flatfooted) and valgus, or cavus (high arched) and varus.

The planovalgus foot

The flexible flat foot

Flexible flat feet are found in up to 30% of the adult population so it is important to differentiate between the healthy 'normal' flatfoot and the 'pathological' flat foot that becomes mechanically inefficient and therefore symptomatic.

Pathological anatomy

The characteristic feature of the flatfoot is loss of the medial longitudinal arch. In the hindfoot there is plantar flexion and medial rotation of the talus that almost certainly becomes pathological at the point when the calcaneonavicular (spring) ligament fails, perhaps due to increasing laxity. This change in alignment has secondary effects: the calcaneum moves into valgus altering the line of pull of the Achilles tendon. This then becomes tight in its laterally displaced position limiting the ability of the heel to return to a neutral or varus position. In the normal foot the calcaneocuboid joint (CCJ) movement is approximately half that of the talonavicular joint, primarily because of its more complex anatomical shape.

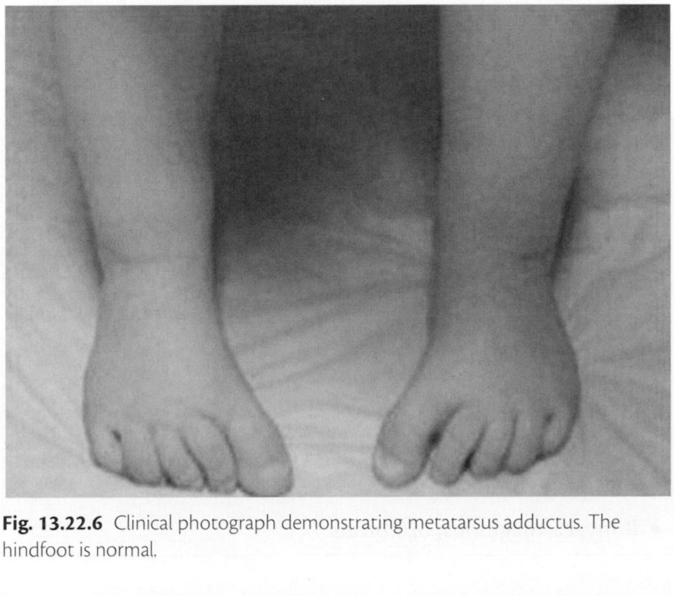

Fig. 13.22.6 Clinical photograph demonstrating metatarsus adductus. The hindfoot is normal.

With hindfoot deformity, the CCJ becomes subluxed, effectively fixing the position of the forefoot; further deformity of forefoot abduction and supination can occur and if secondary contractures develop the deformity becomes fixed.

It is useful to consider whether the foot is primarily rigid or flexible. The 'surgical sieve' can be considered for each category. Asymmetry can indicate unilateral pathology as in the unusual event of a laceration of the tibialis posterior tendon or involvement of the subtalar joint with an inflammatory arthritis. The flexible foot may be normal or associated with excessive and generalized joint laxity commonly seen in conditions such as Ehlers–Danlos, Marfan, trisomy 21, and osteogenesis imperfecta. Other causes of acquired flatfoot are muscle imbalance, contractures, and arthritic conditions.

Clinical evaluation

Flat feet may present with problems due to ill-fitting shoes or with concerns about abnormal shoewear. As the child progresses into puberty, particularly if he or she is obese, there may be aching discomfort. These minor problems settle at maturity. The flexibility of the foot is determined by watching the behaviour of the longitudinal arch in walking and during tip-toe standing. The latter should improve the longitudinal arch whilst the calcaneum swings into varus. Passive dorsiflexion of the first toe as the child stands (Jack's test) should produce the same appearance.

Investigation

Standing anteroposterior and lateral films identify the site of joint subluxation. Primary and secondary deformity can occur at any joint along the medial column but the talonavicular joint is the most common level. The navicular becomes abducted and dorsiflexed relative to the talus. Although the overall appearance is one of a pronated foot, differential dorsiflexion of the first ray and plantar flexion of the fifth ray may produce relative supination of the forefoot with respect to the hindfoot. The overall alignment of bones and joints can be measured and compared both with normal values and on serial films. Although these angles may illustrate the severity of the deformity, their main purpose is in monitoring its progression.

Treatment

Several factors should be considered before treatment is advocated.

Non-operative

Treatment of the asymptomatic mobile flat foot is unnecessary. These children have a normal exercise tolerance. If abnormal shoewear is causing problems, insoles may improve matters.

Box 13.22.4 Should flat feet be treated?

Consider:

- Age
- Severity and rate of progression of the deformity
- Shoewear
- Symptoms—the most important factor.

Some flat feet, despite having mobile joints, are functionally rigid because of the severity of their joint laxity or because the muscles have undergone secondary contracture. Exercises that stretch the gastrocsoleus complex and strengthen the tibialis posterior muscle may be important: once the foot regains its flexibility, orthotic supports can be used to maintain the neutral foot position. This may prevent symptoms and the tendency for contractures to occur which place an increasing pressure on the foot to deform as it grows. Evidence suggests that a variety of customized devices can control foot position and some studies have shown additional benefits including pain relief and improvement in gait pattern. Other studies suggest that such benefits are only seen in the more severely deformed feet. It is probable that if this form of symptomatic treatment is to be successful, it must continue throughout the adolescent growth spurt.

Operative

It is inappropriate to consider surgery in the vast majority of children with a flexible flat foot. The small group of children who have a functionally rigid foot associated with increased joint laxity may be suitable for surgical treatment if their deformity becomes progressive and there is a functional deficit with symptoms. Pain is often felt medially due to strain of the tibialis posterior and the medial capsular structures or laterally secondary to impingement in the sinus tarsi or between the lateral malleolus and the calcaneum. Operative treatment should only be considered if all conservative methods have failed to relieve symptoms or prevent progressive deformity. Surgery may involve soft tissue procedures, osteotomies or fusion of selected joints.

In planning surgical management, several factors must be considered. Soft tissue procedures include those that aim to reef or tighten the medial ligamentous structures and those which seek to redirect the pull of various tendons in the foot, but they are rarely performed in isolation. Osteotomies correct the valgus position of the calcaneum or lengthen the functionally short lateral border of the foot. Arthrodesis of one or more of the hindfoot joints is a last resort.

Box 13.22.5 Surgery for the flexible flat foot

- Options:
  - Soft tissue release/rebalancing
  - Osteotomy
  - Arthrodesis: hindfoot or midfoot or triple
- Factors to be considered:
  - Heel position
  - TA contracture
  - Severity of joint involvement:
    —Subluxation of midfoot
    —Presence/rigidity of forefoot supination
    —Degenerative change.

The rigid flat foot

Congenital tarsal coalition (Box 13.22.6)

The overall incidence of this condition is less than 1%. Occasionally they are associated with carpal coalitions. There is evidence to support an autosomal dominant inheritance for calcaneonavicular bars.

Coalitions are classified according to the site of involvement and whether they are part of a complex malformation or not. Coalitions may be complete or incomplete, or may be bony (synostosis), cartilaginous (synchondrosis) or fibrous (syndesmosis).

Clinical evaluation

Although present from birth, they are rarely recognized before the adolescent growth spurt when the coalition becomes partially or completely ossified. This leads to a reduction in hindfoot movement that may be associated with pain, especially if the coalition is fibrous. Patients may also present with deformity. A planovalgus foot may be associated with peroneal muscle spasm (peroneal spastic flatfoot) whilst a heel with mild varus and reduced subtalar movement may present with symptoms of ankle instability.

As a simple screening test, the lack of a longitudinal arch when the flat-footed child stands on tip-toe is highly suggestive of a coalition. In the presence of a coalition, inversion/eversion may appear to be preserved but in reality the movement is often occurring at ankle level.

Investigation

Initial anteroposterior, lateral, and oblique views may show talonavicular and calcaneocuboid coalitions (Figure 13.22.7). Talocalcaneal bars are the most difficult to diagnose radiologically: they may be seen on an axial view of the calcaneum and by the 'C' sign on a lateral view of the hindfoot (Figure 13.22.8). Imaging techniques such as CT and MRI scanning (Figure 13.22.4) are more helpful and will also reveal incomplete and fibrous coalitions.

Treatment

Initially, activity restriction or a period of cast immobilization may help but if symptoms persist then surgical treatment is warranted (Box 13.22.7). The nature of the surgery will depend on the age of presentation and the type, site and extent of the coalition. The options lie between bar excision and fusion. Arthrodesis should only be considered for non-resectable bars, for joints with extensive involvement or in the older patient where there is evidence of

Box 13.22.6 Tarsal coalition

- Common:
  - Talocalcaneal
  - Calcaneonavicular
- Rare:
  - all others
- 50% are bilateral
- More than one coalition may be present per foot
- Complete or incomplete
- Bony, cartilaginous, or fibrous.

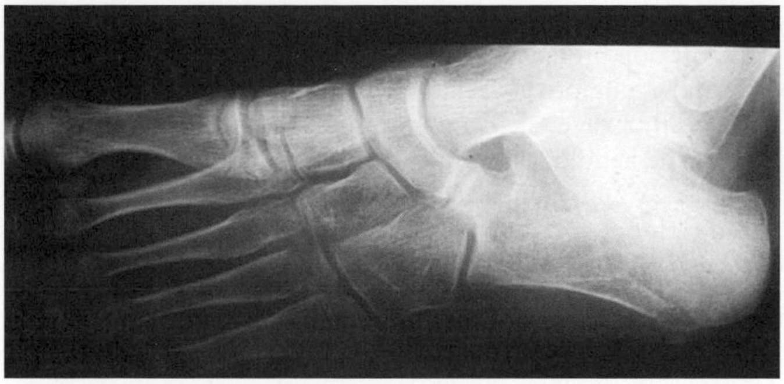

Fig. 13.22.7 Oblique view of the foot showing a calcaneonavicular coalition.

Box 13.22.7 Surgery for tarsal coalition

If conservative treatment fails:

- Excision:
  - Relieves pain
  - Does not restore movement
- Arthrodesis:
  - For extensive talocalcaneal bars
  - Greater than 50% of the posterior facet of the subtalar joint on CT
  - If degenerative change present.

joint degeneration. Bar excision results in good relief of pain but surgery does not usually lead to a significant improvement in joint motion.

Congenital vertical talus (Box 13.22.8)

This rare disorder has an equal sex distribution and the majority of cases occur bilaterally. It may occur as an isolated deformity or in combination with other congenital malformations.

The primary deformity is a dorsal dislocation of the navicular onto the talar neck effectively locking the talus in the vertical position. The secondary deformities of hindfoot equinus and forefoot dorsiflexion and eversion arise from this producing the typical rocker-bottom foot (Figure 13.22.9).

Clinical evaluation

The sole of the foot is convex with the talar head prominent on its medial aspect. The forefoot is abducted and dorsiflexed while the hindfoot is in equinovalgus. The muscles of the anterior and lateral compartments are tight. The deformity is rigid such that there is no restoration of the longitudinal arch with any foot position. Passive correction of the deformity is not possible.

Investigation

On plain lateral radiographs the talus lies vertically with its axis parallel to that of the tibia. The calcaneus is in equinus and the forefoot is dorsiflexed. In infancy, the cartilaginous navicular is not visible but later, when ossified, it can be seen lying on the dorsum of the neck of the talus (Figure 13.22.10).

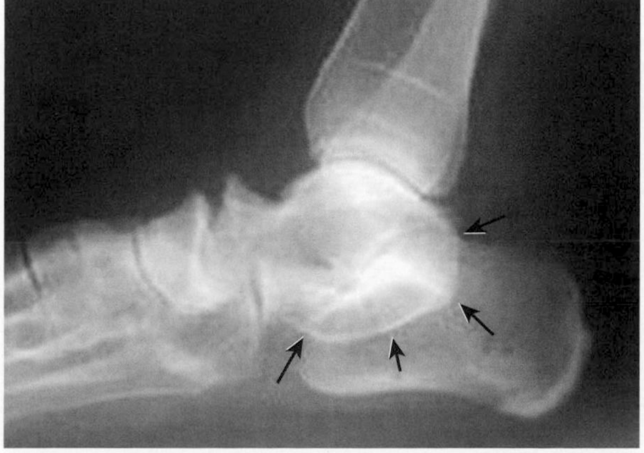

Fig. 13.22.8 Lateral view of the ankle of a skeletally mature adolescent. The arrows outlie a 'C' sign suggestive of a talocalcaneal coalition.

Treatment

The aim of treatment is to reduce the talonavicular joint dislocation and restore normal alignment of the forefoot on the hindfoot and the hindfoot on the tibia.

Non-operative treatment is with passive stretching, which should be started as soon as possible after birth. The principles of the Ponseti management of the talipes equinovarus deformity have been 'reversed' and used with some success for this equinovalgus deformity. Once the talonavicular joint has been reduced, it is stabilized with a K-wire. A tenotomy of the Achilles tendon is then performed to achieve ankle dorsiflexion. Foot abduction orthoses ('boots and bars') are used and supplemented with AFOs once the child is able to weight-bear.

If these measures fail to reduce the dislocation, operative management will be necessary. A full peritalar release is often required. Many surgeons transfer the tibialis anterior tendon to the talar neck in addition to reefing the tibialis posterior tendon and the stretched capsular tissues on the inferior aspect of dislocated joint. In syndromic cases, talectomy may need to be performed as a primary procedure although usually it has been reserved for management of the relapsed foot with significant recurrent deformity.

In older children, soft tissue procedures alone are unlikely to be successful, and excision of the navicular has been advocated. After the age of 6, open reduction is associated with a significant risk of avascular necrosis of the talus, and in children presenting at this late stage, it is better to delay surgery until a triple fusion is appropriate.

Box 13.22.8 Congenital vertical talus

- Isolated
- Syndromic:
  - Myelomeningocoele
  - Arthrogryposis
  - Trisomy 18.

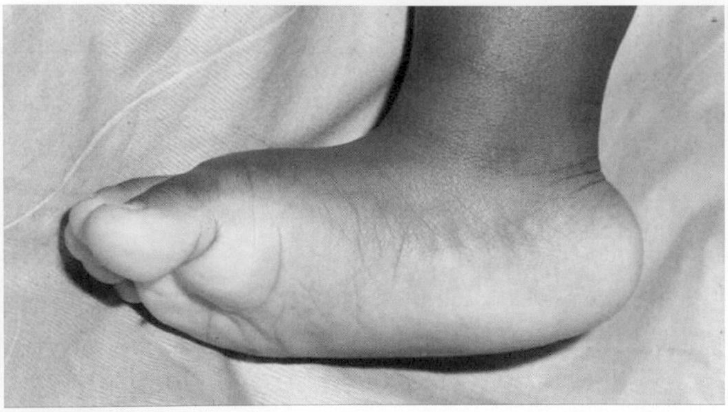

Fig. 13.22.9 Clinical photograph of an infant with a vertical talus. The hindfoot is in equinus and there is a 'rocker-bottom' appearance to the sole of the foot.

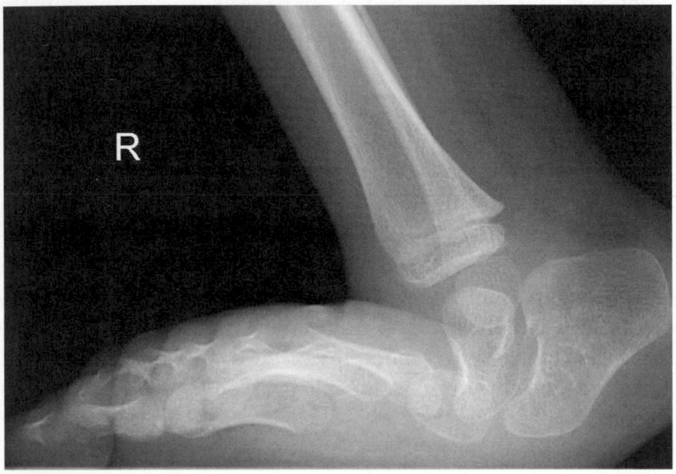

Fig. 13.22.10 Weight-bearing lateral radiograph demonstrating a vertical talus. The navicular is displaced dorsally and is 'articulating' with the talar neck.

The cavovarus foot

A variety of foot deformities present with a high longitudinal arch. This may be due to abnormalities in the hindfoot, the forefoot, or both and a significant number of children will have an underlying neurological abnormality.

Pes cavus

Pes cavus is a high arched foot where the longitudinal arch fails to flatten with weight-bearing. A high arched foot has an angle of 150 degrees or less between the long axes of the first metatarsal and calcaneum on a standing lateral radiograph.

Pathological anatomy

The calcaneum is dorsiflexed and often in varus. The forefoot deformity varies but frequently involves a degree of plantar flexion of the metatarsals. Claw toes are commonly seen in the cavus foot along with tightness of the plantar fascia. At the metatarsophalangeal joints (MTPJs), there is a range of deformity from fully mobile claw toes to toes that are dorsally dislocated.

The hindfoot varus may be due primarily to a stiff subtalar joint or, more commonly, it may be secondary to plantarflexion of the medial metatarsals relative to the lateral rays. This differential plantarflexion pronates the forefoot which can only be accommodated if the hindfoot goes into varus.

Feet with a cavus deformity can be classified according to the level of the aetiological insult within the neuromuscular system (Table 13.22.2). In children, dysraphism, cerebral palsy, undercorrected clubfoot, and arthrogryposis are the most common causes of cavus feet.

Clinical evaluation

In children, the family history is crucial. The age of onset of the deformity may indicate the likely cause and predict the rate of progression. Evidence of progression must always be documented carefully. Each component of the foot (hindfoot, midfoot, forefoot) must be examined in turn to define the deformity and ascertain whether it is flexible or fixed. The Coleman block test is particularly important when assessing hindfoot varus. It tests the flexibility of the hindfoot in the presence of fixed forefoot deformity. The neurological examination must include assessment of the spine especially when there is asymmetrical foot involvement.

Investigation (Box 13.22.9)

Standard weight-bearing radiographs are important in assessing the degree of deformity, monitoring its progression and planning treatment. If the calcaneal pitch, (the angle between the plantar surface of the calcaneum and the weight-bearing surface) is greater than 30 degrees, the calcaneum is excessively dorsiflexed. Spinal radiographs supplemented with MRI are often required to identify treatable causes of a progressive neurological lesion.

Other investigations may be necessary to identify the neurological cause.

Management

Non-operative

Stretching exercises for the Achilles tendon, other long tendons, and plantar structures should be performed regularly. A flexible deformity can be held with an AFO or balanced with outside wedges on the shoes or by posting the outer border of an insole. Appropriate, customized shoewear can be used to accommodate a fixed deformity. The aim of treatment is reduce pain and prevent progression of deformity.

Table 13.22.2 The causes of a pes cavus deformity

Site of abnormality	Example
Cerebral–supratentorial	Hysterical foot deformity
Pyramidal	Cerebral palsy
Extrapyramidal	Friedrich's ataxia
Spinal cord	Tethered cord, spinal dysraphism Tumours Poliomyelitis
Peripheral nerve	HSMN
	Sciatic nerve injury
Muscle	Muscular dystrophy
Trauma	Ischaemic contractures secondary to compartment syndromes

Box 13.22.9 Pes cavus—investigations

- Plain radiographs and MRI spine
- Biopsy of nerve and/or muscle
- Nerve conduction studies
- Gait analysis.

Operative (Box 13.22.10)

In childhood the deformity is usually mobile. Release of the soft tissues of the longitudinal arch in combination with tendon transfers may help to correct deformities and rebalance muscle pulls which should reduce recurrence.

Correction of claw toes can be achieved by soft tissue surgery in children. In the younger child with significant growth potential, the great toe can be corrected by a modified Jones procedure where the long extensor is used both to elevate the first metatarsal by transfer to the neck of the metatarsal and to tenodese the interphalangeal joint (IPJ). Alternatively, the long extensor can be transferred to peroneus tertius. The older child may undergo a more traditional Jones procedure where the IPJ is fused. The lesser toes can be treated by a variety of methods including tendon transfer although IPJ fusions are often required eventually.

Box 13.22.10 Tendon transfers for the cavovarus foot

- *Correct fixed deformity first*
- Peroneus longus to brevis
- Tibialis posterior to PB or to the lateral border
- Transfer toe extensors to peroneus tertius or the metatarsal necks.

If the deformity is fixed, bony surgery is usually necessary. In general, arthrodesis should not be performed in a growing foot. Midfoot and hindfoot osteotomies can be performed. Metatarsal or midfoot osteotomies may correct fixed plantar flexion. A calcaneal osteotomy will correct a varus heel. In adolescence, a triple arthrodesis can be considered in order to stabilize the foot in a plantigrade position.

The skew foot

This uncommon deformity is characterized by hindfoot valgus and forefoot adduction and supination. Historically, many such feet were a result of aggressive surgery for a congenital talipes equinovarus deformity. The primary deformity is felt to be medial subluxation of the tarsometatarsal joints leading to fixed forefoot adduction. The talonavicular joint is subluxed dorsolaterally.

In infancy, this condition must be differentiated from congenital talipes equinovarus and metatarsus adductus which both have an adducted forefoot with a medial skin crease. The distinguishing features are in the midfoot and hindfoot. In talipes equinovarus, the hindfoot is fixed in equinus and varus but in the skew foot the hindfoot is in valgus although this may be difficult to appreciate in the newborn. The midfoot changes differentiate skew foot from metatarsus adductus: the medial border of the foot is concave in metatarsus adductus but in the skew foot, there is a medial convexity at the level of the talonavicular joint proximal to the forefoot concavity (Figure 13.22.11).

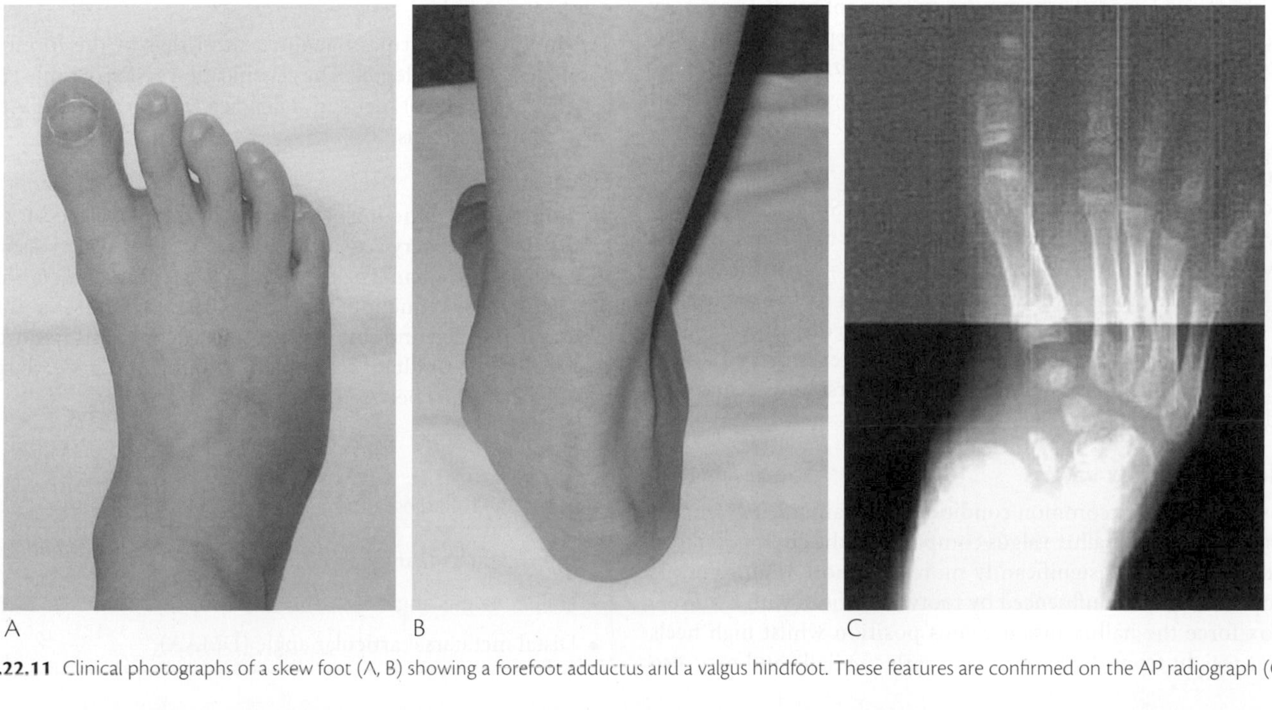

Fig. 13.22.11 Clinical photographs of a skew foot (A, B) showing a forefoot adductus and a valgus hindfoot. These features are confirmed on the AP radiograph (C).

Investigation

Weight-bearing anteroposterior and lateral views reveal the hindfoot valgus and the forefoot adductus. The midfoot is shifted laterally with respect to the hindfoot. The lateral view may show a degree of midfoot cavus.

Management

The natural history of the skew foot is unclear. While some may correct either spontaneously or with simple measures such as serial casting, others persist to cause long-term disability. Casting may correct the forefoot adductus, but will have limited effect on the hindfoot valgus. If the Achilles tendon shortens, the hindfoot valgus is accentuated.

Symptomatic skew feet generally require operative treatment. Stretching the Achilles tendon may benefit those with plantar heel pain. All components of the deformity must be addressed. A calcaneal lengthening osteotomy to correct hindfoot valgus has good long-term results but should be combined with a forefoot correction, which might entail a medially based opening wedge osteotomy of the medial cuneiform and a closing wedge of the cuboid. The Achilles tendon may need lengthening to allow full correction of the hindfoot deformity.

Forefoot abnormalities

Congenital hallux varus

The hallux is in varus. It is important to establish whether this is an isolated abnormality or part of a more generalized condition. There is medial deviation of the proximal phalanx of the hallux.

Pathological anatomy

Three types of hallux varus can be recognized. The first is an isolated or local type where the primary abnormality is a tight band of tissue extending along the medial side of the foot. The effect of this band is to pull the great toe further into varus with growth. A second group relates to patients who have a set of congenital deformities including a marked varus of the first metatarsal, which is also short and broad. There may be an adjacent medial accessory bone. This type may be due to a longitudinal epiphyseal bracket. Finally, it can occur in more generalized conditions such as diastrophic dysplasia. Plain radiographs will distinguish the different types of the condition.

Management

Non-operative treatment has little or no effect. Surgical correction involves lengthening the tight medial structures and stabilizing the first MTPJ. Temporary K-wire fixation of the joint is needed. If there is varus deviation of the first metatarsal, a metatarsal osteotomy is indicated. In the second type, the growth disturbance of the first metatarsal may contribute to recurrence after surgery. In these cases, it may be necessary to syndactylize the first and second toes in order to prevent progressive deformity.

Adolescent hallux valgus

This is a relatively uncommon condition. The familial incidence is higher in adolescent hallux valgus compared to the adult onset type of hallux valgus. It is significantly more common in girls and its development may be influenced by footwear. Shoes with a narrow toe box force the hallux into a valgus position whilst high heels transfer weight from the lesser metatarsals medially and may also contribute to the deformity. There may be an associated primary varus angulation of the first metatarsal.

Clinical evaluation

The foot should be examined weight-bearing to determine the true degree of valgus and pronation. As with all childhood foot deformities, a neurological cause must be excluded.

Investigation (Box 13.22.11)

Weight-bearing anteroposterior radiographs are essential and various angular measurements should be made.

Management

Initial management should be non-operative with shoewear modification. If the deformity is progressive or symptoms are severe, surgery may be warranted. Soft-tissue procedures alone are frequently unsuccessful. If the intermetatarsal angle between the first and second metatarsals is 15–20 degrees (metatarsus primus varus), a distal metatarsal osteotomy may suffice. Larger intermetatarsal angles require a more proximal osteotomy such as the Scarf combined with distal soft tissue realignment. Recurrence rates are higher than in mature feet.

Congenital hallux valgus interphalangeus

This is a congenital, often bilateral, condition where there is marked lateral deviation at the IPJ of the hallux. In young children, the condition is generally asymptomatic. Local irritation over the IPJ may cause problems in adolescence in which case a medial closing-wedge osteotomy of the proximal phalanx will correct the deformity.

Congenital cleft foot

This rare congenital anomaly is characterized by absence of two or three of the central rays of the foot and inherited as an autosomal dominant trait with incomplete penetrance. It is bilateral and often associated with cleft hand and other anomalies. Unilateral cases are sporadic in nature. The incidence is reported to be 1: 90 000 live births (see Figure 13.22.1).

Clinical evaluation

The hindfoot is normal but the central rays of the forefoot are absent to a variable degree. The classification system (Table 13.22.3) is based on degree of metatarsal deficiency. Types IV and V are the most common forms.

Management

The foot usually functions well and no surgery is necessary in the milder forms. Surgery is usually indicated for cosmetic reasons and to improve shoe wear. The foot is narrowed by basal metarsal osteotomies and/or reduction of subluxed tarsometatarsal joints with closure of the cleft and soft tissue reconstruction. It is important to ensure that the resultant foot is supple and plantigrade. Surgery is usually performed between 1–2 years of age.

Box 13.22.11 Radiographic assessment of hallux valgus

- Intermetatarsal angle (<12 degrees)
- Hallux valgus angle
- Distal metatarsal articular angle (DMAA).

Table 13.22.3 Classification of cleft foot anomalies (Blauth and Borisch 1990)

Type	Description
I	Minor deficiencies only
II	Central metatarsals hypoplastic
III	Four metatarsals only
IV	Three metatarsals only
V	Two metatarsals only
VI	One metatarsal only

Lesser ray problems

Curly toes

This common congenital condition affects one or more toes. It is usually bilateral, symmetrical and often familial. The affected toes (usually third and/or fourth) curl medially and tend to lie under the neighbouring toe. A tenotomy of all flexor tendons to the affected toe is often recommended for cosmetic reasons. An osteotomy performed later may be more effective in producing a lasting result.

Congenital overriding little (fifth) toe (Box 13.22.12)

This common familial abnormality is often bilateral. The toe is dorsiflexed and adducted, overlying the fourth toe. The MPTJ is subluxed due to capsular contracture. Symptoms develop in about 50% of cases. Non-operative treatment methods (stretching, strapping) are rarely successful. Surgical treatment is warranted for symptom relief or for cosmesis and is usually successful. Recurrence may occur but bony surgery such as proximal phalangectomy is rarely indicated and never in a child.

Macrodactyly

This is a rare deformity that may be secondary to neurofibromatosis (NF), haemangiomatosis, or congenital hyperplasia of the lymphatic and adipose tissue. The diagnosis of NF must be excluded by careful clinical examination. In true gigantism, there is an increase in size of all the elements of the toe. The degree of hypertrophy is variable: sometimes the deformity is static in that the increase in size is proportionate to growth but in others there is progressive disproportionate growth. If the appearance is unacceptable, surgery is indicated. Several procedures have been described, none of which is very successful. Simple debulking and epiphysiodesis is frequently followed by recurrence. Ray amputation may be indicated in severe cases of recurrence but may be complicated by the development of hallux valgus.

Box 13.22.12 The overriding fifth toe—surgical management

- Soft tissue release: V–Y plasty
- Extensor tendon lengthening
- Circumferential MTP joint capsulotomy.

Polydactyly

Polydactyly is a common deformity occurring in 2:1000 live births (see Figure 13.22.2). It is often inherited in an autosomal dominant fashion but sporadic cases do occur. There may be associated polydactyly of the hand or other major congenital malformations such as tibial aplasia. It is also seen in syndromes such as Ellis–van Creveld syndrome and chondroectodermal dysplasia.

The extra toe may be preaxial (15%), postaxial (80%), or central. The child must be assessed thoroughly to look for associated malformations. The extra digit may be either fully formed or rudimentary. Plain radiographs will show the level and extent of bony duplication.

The extra toe should be excised both for cosmetic reasons and for shoe fitting although some cultures are opposed to this. The operation is best performed when the child is around 9–12 months old. Generally the most peripheral toe is excised, although radiographic appearances must be considered.

Miscellaneous conditions

Osteochondroses

Osteochondroses affect active growth areas and involve a defect in ossification in either an epiphysis or an apophysis. They generally occur soon after the ossific nucleus has appeared when the epiphysis is growing rapidly. Most are more common in boys.

Kohler's disease

Osteochondritis of the navicular occurs predominantly in children aged 3–6 years. Boys are more commonly affected and up to 33% are bilateral. The navicular is the last bone of the foot to ossify and may be subjected to significant pressures while still cartilaginous as it is the keystone to the longitudinal arch. Histologically, avascular necrosis is seen.

Clinically, there is pain, swelling, and tenderness around the navicular and the child limps. There may be surrounding warmth and erythema but the normal movement at the mid-tarsal and subtalar joints distinguishes this from inflammatory arthritides.

Radiographs show a small, sclerotic ossific nucleus and diagnosis rests on the combination of radiographic appearances and the clinical picture (Figure 13.22.12).

The condition is self-limiting and the prognosis good. Symptomatic improvement usually occurs within a few months. If symptoms are severe, a period of immobilization in a cast may be warranted.

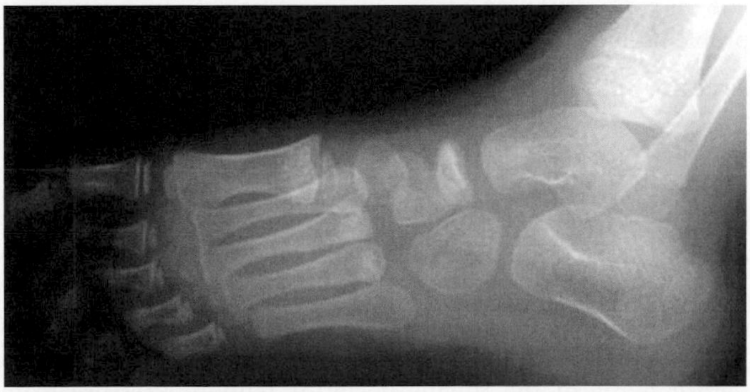

Fig. 13.22.12 Kohler's disease of the navicular. The radiograph shows a sclerotic ossific nucleus.

Sever's disease

Osteochondritis of the calcaneal apophysis affects boys predominantly between the ages of 8, when the apophysis first appears, and 12 years, when it fuses with the parent bone. It is a common cause of heel pain in the immature athlete, probably related to overuse. The diagnosis rests on clinical symptoms and signs. There is pain and tenderness around the insertion of the Achilles tendon to the calcaneum. Radiographs show sclerosis and fragmentation of the calcaneal apophysis, features which are consistent with normal apophyseal development.

Like the other osteochondritides, this is a self-limiting condition and symptoms abate once the apophysis has fused. Stretching the gastrocnemius and soleus with strengthening of the anterior muscles helps to reduce symptoms and activity should be reduced. A period of rest in plaster may be necessary to control symptoms.

Freiberg's disease

Infraction of the metatarsal head occurs in adolescents, mainly girls, and may be bilateral. Although any metatarsal can be affected, it is most frequently the second, perhaps because it is the longest and subject to overloading of the MTP joint. Clinically, there is pain under the metatarsal head with swelling, tenderness and restriction of MTPJ movement particularly dorsiflexion. Radiographs shows flattening and irregularity of the metatarsal head with sclerosis and metatarsal shaft hypertrophy.

Initial treatment is conservative. Often all that is required is modification of shoewear and activity levels. A metatarsal bar may offload the joint. If symptoms persist, curettage and bone grafting of the defect is indicated. At skeletal maturity, if there are ongoing severe symptoms, a dorsiflexion osteotomy may be necessary. Debridement of the metatarsal head or resection of the base of the proximal phalanx is a salvage procedure.

Congenital constriction bands

Congenital constriction band syndrome (Streeter's dysplasia) is believed to be due to constriction of the limb by amniotic bands. The bands may be either partial or complete. The clinical picture is variable but includes congenital amputations, syndactyly and equinovarus foot deformities (Figure 13.22.13). The bands can cause obstruction to venous and lymphatic drainage and Z-plasties may be required urgently in the neonatal period. The clubfoot deformity may be resistant to conservative treatment.

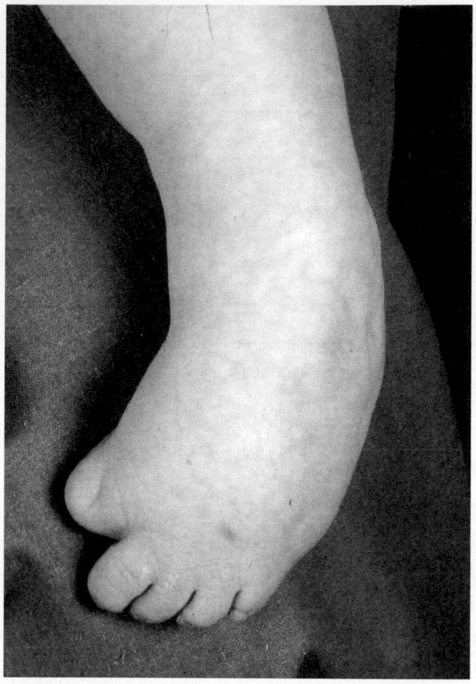

Fig. 13.22.13 Talipes equinovarus deformity with amniotic band syndrome affecting the toes.

Accessory ossific centres

Almost a quarter of children have one or more accessory bones visible on radiographs. Many are unimportant but some may cause problems in childhood.

Accessory navicular (Box 13.22.13)

The accessory navicular represents a separate ossification centre for the navicular tuberosity. Three types have been described (see Table 13.22.4). Generally, the accessory centre fuses with the main ossific nucleus but in about 2% of people it remains as a separate ossicle. The tendon of tibialis posterior is therefore attached to the medial aspect rather than the inferior aspect of the navicular, weakening the support for the longitudinal arch, and the foot becomes planovalgus. Midfoot pain may develop after activity, together with tenosynovitis of the tibialis posterior tendon. Pressure from shoewear may lead to local pain, swelling and tenderness.

Anteroposterior and external oblique radiographs reveal the accessory navicular located on the proximal medial aspect of the navicular. Its smooth outline distinguishes it from a fracture (Figure 13.22.14). The bipartite navicular appears on the dorsal surface of the navicular as a separate comma-shaped segment and is a separate entity from the accessory navicular.

Non-operative treatment is indicated initially. An orthosis may be useful if there is a flexible hindfoot valgus. A short period in a plaster cast with or without a local anaesthetic injection of the synchondrosis may settle acute symptoms. Persistent symptoms may warrant surgery. The Kidner procedure involves excision of the accessory navicular and advancement of the tibialis posterior tendon onto the plantar surface of the navicular but simple excision of the accessory navicular with trimming of any residual prominence is a simpler and equally reliable alternative.

Os trigonum

An os trigonum is seen in nearly 10% of the population. It represents failure of fusion of the posterolateral tubercle of the talus with the main ossific centre. Repetitive minor trauma may be an aetiological factor.

The main clinical features are pain around the posterior aspect of the ankle and limitation of plantar flexion and it is frequently

Box 13.22.13 Accessory navicular

- Seen in 10% of children
- Often bilateral
- Girls >boys.

Table 13.22.4 Classification of an accessory navicular

Type	Description
I	A separate ossicle within the tibialis posterior tendon
II	An ossicle connected to the navicular via a synchondrosis
III	A cornuate navicular after a synostosis between the accessory and main ossific nucleus

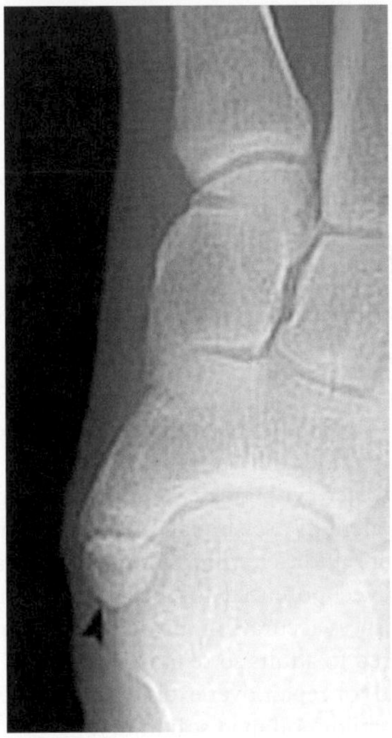

Fig. 13.22.14 Radiograph of a foot demonstrating an accessory navicular.

seen in ballet dancers and gymnasts. It must be distinguished from flexor hallucis longus tendinitis, although the two conditions coexist. Radiographs reveal an ossicle at the posterior aspect of the talus. Non-operative treatment consists of limiting ankle plantar flexion. Local steroid injections may help control symptoms and open excision may be warranted for persistent symptoms.

Further reading

Coleman, S.S. and Chesnut, W.J. (1977). A simple test for hindfoot flexibility in the cavovarus foot. *Clinical Orthopaedics and Related Research*, **123**, 60–2.

Dobbs, M.B., Purcell, D.B., Nunley, R. and Morcuende, J.A. (2006). Early results of a new method of treatment for idiopathic congenital vertical talus. *Journal of Bone and Joint Surgery*, **88A**, 1192–200.

Gonzalez, P. and Kumar, S.I. (1990). Calcaneonavicular coalition treated by resection and interposition of the extensor digitorum brevis muscle. *Journal of Bone and Joint Surgery*, **72A**, 71–7.

Mosca, V.S. (1995). Calcaneal lengthening for valgus deformity of the hindfoot. *Journal of Bone and Joint Surgery*, **77A**, 500–11.

Rose, G.K., Welton, E.A., and Marshall, T. (1985). The diagnosis of flatfoot in the child. *Journal of Bone and Joint Surgery*, **67B**, 71–8.

13.23

Sports injuries and syndromes

Simon Thomas and Michael Walton

Summary points

- Paediatric sports medicine is an evolving multidisciplinary specialty with increasing rates of injury in paediatric athletes:
  - Injury prevention programmes are important
  - Training regimes must be adapted to the age group and the sport
- Sports injuries to the immature skeleton require different treatment approaches to those in adults even when injury patterns appear similar
- The knee is the most commonly injured region—anterior cruciate ligament ruptures in children and adolescents are higher than previously appreciated
- Upper limb paediatric sports injuries are more commonly secondary to overuse than acute injury—physiotherapy and activity modification are the mainstays of treatment.

Introduction

As a truly multidisciplinary specialty, sports medicine crosses traditional medical boundaries. The focus of this chapter is on sports-related injuries, rather than injuries from accidents but the epidemiological data for such injuries are sparse for some disciplines and studies use varying definitions and methodology. Nonetheless, it is clear that the majority of children and adolescents aged 5–17 years participate in organized sport in both the United Kingdom and United States of America that accounts for a significant proportion of injuries in this age group. For most sports, the knee is the most common site of injury. Increased participation in competitive sport is reflected in a 15% increase in reported knee injuries in the under 17-year age group between 1996 and 2001 despite increased injury prevention programmes.

Injuries in children secondary to sports trauma are modulated by the unique properties of the growing musculoskeletal system with vulnerable epiphyseal and apophyseal cartilage plates but with greater capacity for healing and remodelling than in adults.

Lower limb injuries

Knee injuries

Meniscal injury

If discoid menisci and other congenital malformations are excluded, meniscal injuries in the immature athlete are uncommon, particularly under the age of 10 years. Their incidence is on the increase, however, with greater and more vigorous sports participation. The menisci are similar in structure and function to those in the adult but differ critically in their increased vascularity and thus improved potential for healing. Magnetic resonance imaging (MRI) is less accurate in the diagnosis of meniscal tears in children compared to adults so reliance on clinical evaluation and a lower threshold for repair over excision are the key differences in management of childhood meniscal injury.

The anxious child or apparently indifferent adolescent may not recall a twisting injury or varus/valgus strain and decreasing age and increasing time from the relevant injury further diminish the value of direct questioning. Key features in the clinical examination are the presence of focal joint line tenderness and the presence of an effusion. In the acute setting, this indicates a likely haemarthrosis (Box 13.23.1).

Box 13.23.1 Differential diagnosis of a haemarthrosis

- Meniscal tear:
  - 47% of preadolescents (aged 7–12 years)
  - 45% of adolescents (aged 13–18 years)
- ACL rupture:
  - 47% of preadolescents
  - 65% of adolescents
- Osteochondral fracture: 7% overall
- Extensor mechanism rupture: rare.

There is a high rate of concomitant meniscal and anterior cruciate ligament (ACL) injury in children with haemarthrosis, especially adolescents. With chronic tears, intermittent locking, clicking, or 'popping' and the presence of an effusion and quadriceps wasting are common findings.

Despite reports of improved specificity and sensitivity in the diagnosis of meniscal tears using contemporary MRI sequences, this modality is less accurate in children, especially those aged less than 12 years, in part because of differing patterns of vascularity. The presence of joint line tenderness and a modified McMurray's test in the clinic is at least as accurate for diagnosis as MRI, with arthroscopic evaluation the gold standard for assessment of tear morphology. The majority are vertical longitudinal ('bucket-handle') type; oblique, radial, and degenerative tear patterns are seen less commonly than in adults. Standard plain orthogonal radiographs form part of the diagnostic work-up to exclude occult pathology such as infection or bone tumour as a cause for symptoms. Additional skyline patella and tunnel or notch views are helpful to search for osteochondral defects or patellofemoral incongruity.

Short (<10mm) longitudinal tears that are stable when probed can be left to heal. A hinged knee brace permitting 0–60 degrees of flexion restricts activity for 4–6 weeks. All other unstable and arthroscopically reducible tears should undergo repair, particularly if anterior cruciate ligament reconstruction is also required. A combined repair is associated with improved healing rates, most likely reflecting an enhanced vascular response. Similarly, in chronic tears, local preparation of the tear site with an arthroscopic shaver or rasp is advisable to promote vascular ingress. Early meniscal resection causes increased joint contact stresses which are associated with osteoarthritis. Adult guidelines for repair versus excision, based on tear location in relation to centrally decreasing zones of vascularity, are less relevant in children with greater healing capacity, except perhaps for very central tears which can be debrided back to a stable rim.

Arthroscopic techniques for meniscal repair include placement of 'inside-out' or 'outside-in' sutures, employing posteromedial or posterolateral incisions to protect the saphenous and peroneal nerves for posterior horn tears. The latest generation of 'all-inside' suture passing kits with an appropriate tissue-guard and straight and curved needle tips are increasingly favoured over the 'inside-out' technique for most tears. Exceptions include anterior horn tears which are difficult to access and are an indication for 'outside-in' suture placement. Similarly, concerns about the 'all-inside' needle damaging structures behind the capsule in a small knee mean the 'inside-out' technique is preferred with posterior horn tears in younger children. A hinged knee brace restricted to 60 degrees of flexion should be worn for 6 weeks after meniscal repair, followed by a gradual return to sport once a full range of knee motion has been restored. Larger and more chronic tears may benefit from a period of partial weight bearing postoperatively but clear guidance regarding rehabilitation is lacking.

Anterior cruciate ligament injuries

ACL injuries in the skeletally immature knee are currently a focus for debate. It is increasingly clear that ACL deficiency in this age group is associated with high rates of symptomatic instability and secondary osteochondral and meniscal damage. Techniques for anatomical placement of a tunnelled, intra-articular graft reconstruction have been refined in the last 20 years for adult injuries. In children and adolescents, the open physes around the knee account for two-thirds of lower limb growth. Damaging either risks limb length discrepancy or angular deformity that may be difficult to manage. With an increasing incidence of immature ACL injury, especially in female adolescents, interest has focused on whether, when and by what means tunnels can be placed safely around the immature knee. Similarly, older techniques such as non-anatomical reconstruction and primary repair have been revisited.

Below the age of 12 years, ACL failure by tibial spine fracture is much more common than intrasubstance rupture: after this the relative likelihood of these injury patterns is reversed. Meniscal tear is the commonest associated injury but physeal fracture, patellar dislocation, and posterior cruciate ligament injury are also reported.

The hallmark clinical features in the history of a 'pop' at the time of injury (sustained during a sudden deceleration, pivoting movement or awkward landing) followed by an immediate haemarthrosis, inability to complete the game, and subsequent instability with a return to cutting sports are much harder to elicit in this younger age group. The Lachman and anterior drawer tests should be performed but the pivot shift test is the best predictor of symptomatic ACL insufficiency although it requires optimal relaxation in the conscious child. Signs of an effusion or meniscal injury should be sought. As mentioned previously, standard radiographs with additional tunnel/notch and skyline patella views may be required to exclude bony injury such as tibial spine avulsion and associated osteochondral lesions. MRI may delineate primary, high signal and/or ligament discontinuity, and secondary, bone bruising, signs of ACL injury. Overall, this modality is less accurate in children and is considered an adjunct to clinical diagnosis determining the presence of associated injuries.

ACL injury in the immature athlete does not require urgent operative intervention in the absence of an associated tibial spine fracture or incarcerated meniscus. A phased non-operative programme of rest followed by restoration of range of movement and strengthening exercises and finally sports rehabilitation is indicated. Recurrent instability with ongoing risk of cumulative damage to the knee should prompt consideration of surgical intervention (Box 13.23.2).

The physeal-sparing iliotibial band technique is well described for preadolescent children (Tanner Stage 2 or less) with ACL rupture.

Box 13.23.2 Reconstructive options for ACL injury

- Direct repair
- Physeal sparing techniques:
  - *Non-anatomical* (non-isometric) with iliotibial band graft taken 'over the top' and under transverse inter-meniscal ligament
  - *Anatomical* using 'all epiphyseal' tunnels for graft placement and fixation
- Partial trans-physeal—such as 'over the top' femoral attachment and transtibial tunnel
- Transphyseal—adult-type surgery but with more centrally placed, vertically orientated tunnels.

The iliotibial band is detached proximally but left attached at Gerdy's tubercle and brought into the knee through the 'over the top' position of the femur. It then passes out under the intermeniscal ligament and is secured in a groove in the anteromedial aspect of the proximal tibial epiphysis. Non-anatomical reconstructions such as this are unlikely to be isometric throughout the range of knee motion, predisposing to graft failure and suboptimal function. Furthermore, iatrogenic injury to the perichondrial ring of the distal femoral physis, which is in close proximity to the over-the-top position, predisposes to growth arrest with angular deformity.

Technically challenging, 'all epiphyseal' reconstructions involve the placement of short tunnels within the confines of the epiphysis. The undulating femoral physis provides resistance to shear but the projections into the epiphysis increase the risk of damage.

The literature in adult knee ACL reconstruction emphasizes the importance of anatomical tunnel placement to ensure isometric graft function. Animal studies indicate a low risk of growth arrest with violation of up to 7% of the total cross-sectional area of a physis. Six to nine-mm centrally placed tunnels, in the femur or tibia, damage less than 5% of the physis. They have not been associated with angular deformity or limb length discrepancy except when material other than a soft tissue graft is placed across the defect. Hence the consensus recommendation for ACL rupture in the skeletally immature is increasingly for adult-type surgery using soft tissue graft fixation techniques that avoid bone plugs or screws across the physis. Nonetheless this remains an area of controversy. Historically, direct repair has been associated with poor outcomes although there are obvious advantages to this procedure in the immature knee. Interest is now centred on attempts to produce a biological scaffold to augment the repair.

Any consideration of surgical reconstruction requires a careful assessment of skeletal age and development. Growth rate peaks during puberty between 13–15 years bone age in boys and 11–13 years in girls; after this lower limb growth is virtually complete with remaining growth occurring simply through the spine. Chronological age is generally a good guide to skeletal age, but this generalization cannot be applied to individual cases (Box 13.23.3).

Box 13.23.3 Methods of assessment of skeletal maturity

- Chronological age
- Gruelich–Pyle atlas comparative method using hand/wrist radiographs to derive bone age
- Sauvegrain method or simplified olecranon method using lateral elbow radiograph
- Tanner and Whitehouse classification of sexual maturity stage
- Patency of triradiate cartilage (closure occurs half way up the accelerating phase of the pubertal growth spurt).

The Gruelich–Pyle atlas method for determining skeletal maturity derives from old population data which may no longer be applicable and bone age determinations for the hand do not always coincide with growth remaining at the knee. Secondary sexual characteristics are staged in the Tanner classification and provide a guide to skeletal growth remaining but these milestones are not familiar to most orthopaedic surgeons and are rarely used. The Sauvegrain or simplified olecranon method of assessment is perhaps the most useful (Figure 13.23.1). At the beginning of puberty, there are two olecranon centres of ossification visible on a lateral elbow radiograph marking the start of the accelerating phase of pubertal growth. Two years later, the olecranon apophysis appears fused and growth decelerates. During the intervening period, morphology of the olecranon ossification centre(s) is a reliable staging guide to the accelerating phase of growth with closure of the triradiate cartilage occurring half way through this phase.

Therefore in adolescents approaching skeletal maturity with a fused olecranon and bone age greater than 15 in boys and greater than 13 in girls, adult-type ACL reconstructive surgery is to be preferred when indicated. The same recommendation can be applied to younger adolescents providing the physeal tunnels are no greater than 9mm in diameter and bridged by soft tissue graft only.

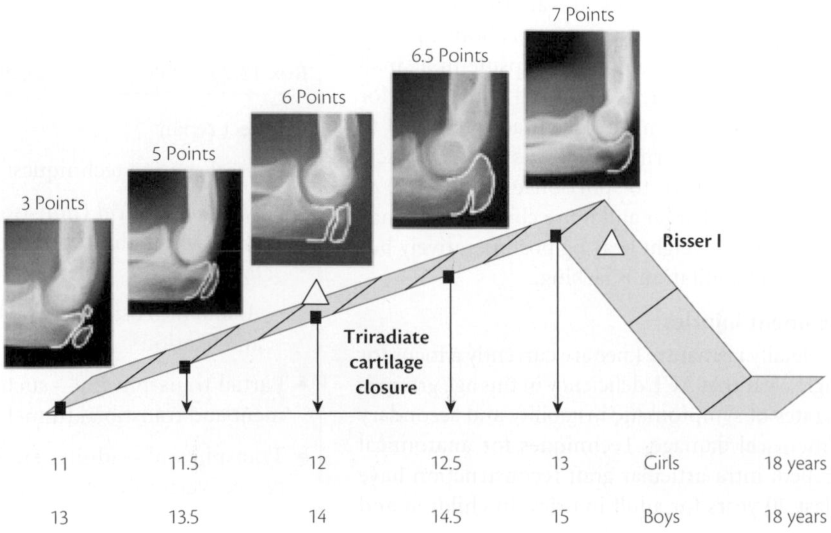

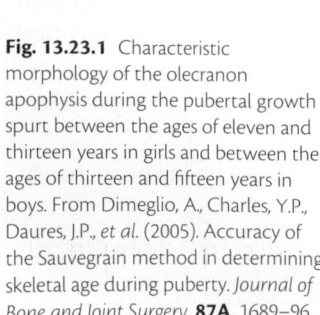

Fig. 13.23.1 Characteristic morphology of the olecranon apophysis during the pubertal growth spurt between the ages of eleven and thirteen years in girls and between the ages of thirteen and fifteen years in boys. From Dimeglio, A., Charles, Y.P., Daures, J.P., *et al.* (2005). Accuracy of the Sauvegrain method in determining skeletal age during puberty. *Journal of Bone and Joint Surgery*, **87A**, 1689–96.

Although tunnelled ACL reconstruction is reported in prepubertal children without secondary growth arrest, this remains controversial and non-anatomical reconstruction avoiding physeal graft placement should be considered even if only as a temporizing measure.

Avulsion fractures of the ACL

This injury pattern is seen mainly in 8–14-year-olds whose ACL is attached to the chondroepiphyses of the distal femur and proximal tibia. These attachments are relatively weak compared to the adult fibrocartilaginous insertions into bone and so, in this age group, 'the bone 'fails' before the (midsubstance) ligament'. Femoral fractures are rare; most are an avulsion of the tibial spine (also known as the tibial eminence).

The mechanism of injury is commonly a valgus force to the knee with rotation or forced flexion. The patient presents with a tense haemarthrosis, reluctance to weight bear, and restricted motion. Anteroposterior and lateral radiographs are indicated (Figure 13.23.2A). Computed tomography (CT) scans are reserved for evaluation of fracture displacement either at presentation or after manipulation. The fractures are classified as a guide to treatment (Table 13.23.1).

Casting after closed reduction is recommended: the cast position of hyperextension, extension, or flexion 20 degrees does not affect outcome. Entrapment of meniscus or the intermeniscal ligament may block closed reduction. A range of open (mini-arthrotomy) and arthroscopic reduction and fixation methods are reported. There are case reports of anterior physeal arrest with screw fixation

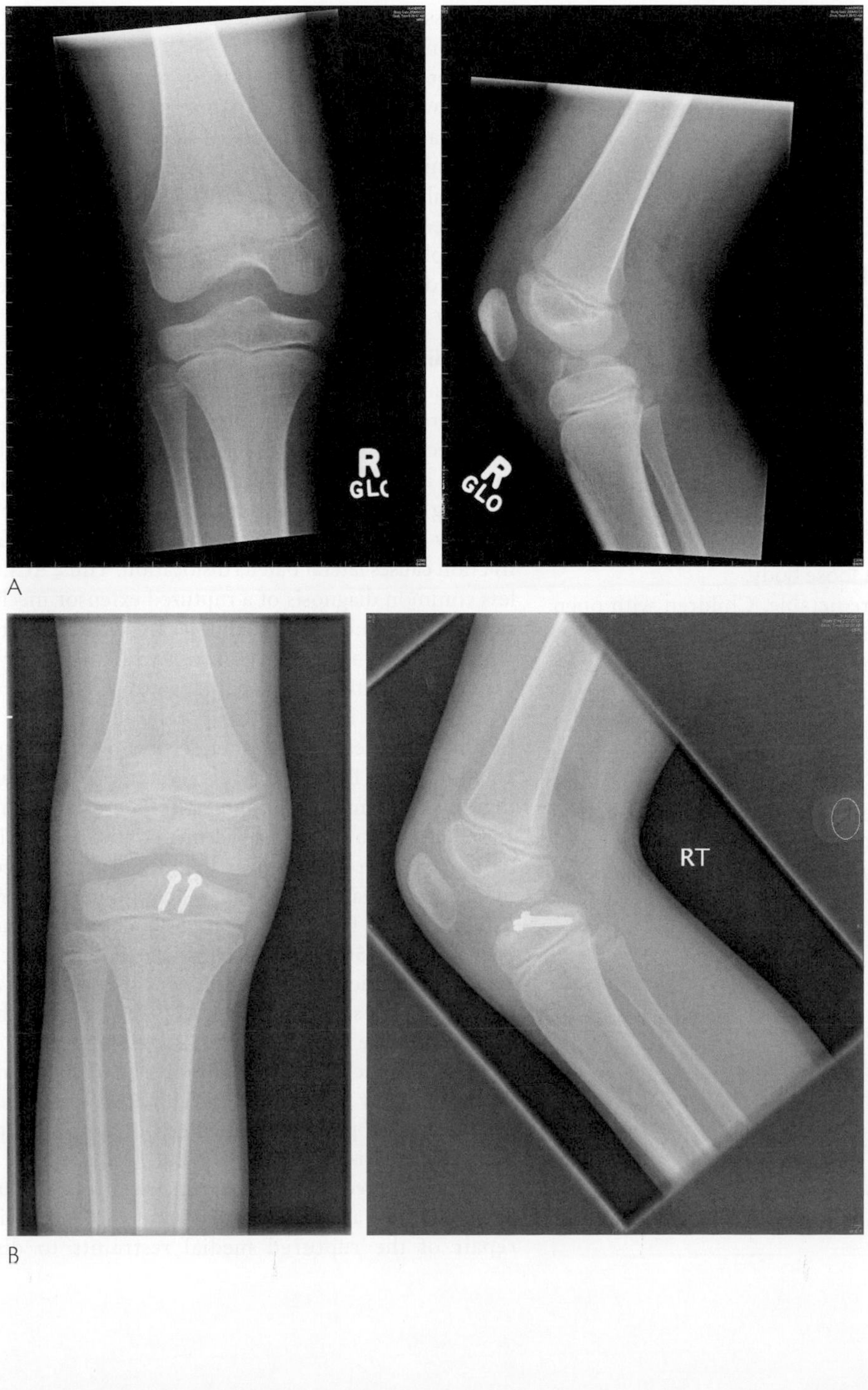

Fig. 13.23.2 A) AP and lateral radiographs of the right knee in a 9-year-old patient demonstrating a type 3 avulsion fracture of the tibial spine. B) AP and lateral radiographs of the same patient following open reduction and screw fixation of the fracture.

Table 13.23.1 Myers and McKeever classification of tibial spine fractures

Type	Description	Treatment
I	Undisplaced	Cast in extension for 6–8 weeks
II	Anterior half of fragment displaced superiorly, hinging posteriorly	Closed reduction and cast if position acceptable, otherwise as Type III
III	Entire fragment separates and rotates superiorly	Open or arthroscopic reduction and fixation

across the physis; hence cannulated all-epiphyseal screws are to be preferred (Figure 13.23.2B). Fixation techniques using smooth wires or heavy sutures, which can be passed across the physis via cannulae, are also described.

Slight reduction in motion, with loss of hyperextension and deep flexion, is common but rarely symptomatic: arthrofibrosis is rare. During the original injury, it is postulated that the ligament substance stretches prior to the bone failing and this may be the cause of subsequent knee laxity after the fracture has healed. A study comparing treated tibial spine fractures with ACL deficient and reconstructed knees indicated that reduction with fixation restored both adequate stability and proprioception to the knee after fracture.

Osteochondritis dissecans of the knee (see also Chapter 13.20)

This Latin name describes the tendency of articular cartilage to separate from subchondral bone. The aetiology is unknown but currently the theory of a primary, ischaemic defect of subchondral bone secondary to repetitive microtrauma is popular. The bone then offers inadequate support to the overlying cartilage which subsequently accrues damage.

Presentation is with activity related knee pain and ache postexercise. Local palpation may indicate the site of the lesion. An effusion may indicate an unstable lesion and mechanical symptoms of locking or giving way, the presence of a loose body.

Healing of these lesions is unpredictable. Children with open physes around the knee have much greater potential for spontaneous healing but larger defects are more likely to fail non-operative treatment. Plain radiographs, including notch and skyline views, will show the majority of significant lesions. The lateral aspect of the medial femoral condyle is the commonest location which is well visualized on the notch view. Additional imaging modalities such as MRI are often used to diagnose and stage the lesion and to predict the likelihood of healing or the requirement for surgical intervention. A breach in the overlying cartilage and high signal behind the lesion on MRI are the most reliable indicators of a poor prognosis (Box 13.23.4).

Box 13.23.4 Features of a poor prognosis

- Large lesion
- Break in the surface of the articular cartilage
- High signal beneath the lesion on MRI
- No increase in blood flow on serial technetium bone scans.

Given the good prognosis for children with open physes, initial management for early stage lesions should be non-operative. A short period of restricted weight bearing in a slightly flexed cylinder cast, or a knee brace is followed by physiotherapy to restore motion. Once symptoms have resolved, a graduated return to sports begins: the timing may be influenced by further imaging.

Operative management should be considered for larger lesions in older children that fail to heal following non-operative management and with MRI signs of ongoing bone oedema or a break in the articular cartilage. Drilling with K-wires is appropriate for early lesions with intact overlying cartilage or early separation. This can be done arthroscopically in a retrograde fashion. Alternatively a marker wire can be placed percutaneously under image intensifier guidance into the centre of the lesion: the position is confirmed arthroscopically and then multiple passes of a second wire parallel and circumferential to the first are made. These passes abut but do not cross the articular surface allowing containment of the reparative haematoma.

Larger, unstable lesions can be pinned *in situ* by a variety of techniques with favourable outcomes. These techniques include the use of variable pitch cannulated screws or bioabsorbable implants.

Techniques to reconstruct full thickness cartilage defects, either from unhealed Stage IV osteochondritis dissecans (OCD) or previous osteochondral fracture (see below), include the techniques of mosaicplasty and autologous chondrocyte implantation and are mainly described for adults. Good results have been reported in younger patients (see Chapter 13.20).

Acute dislocation of the patellofemoral joint

Acute patellar dislocation is the most common acute knee disorder in children and adolescents with a peak age incidence of 15 years. The mechanism of injury for the first episode can be identical to that for an ACL rupture. In changing direction whilst running or pivoting the femur rotates internally relative to the tibia which is fixed by a planted foot. This in association with quadriceps contraction causes lateral patella dislocation. Thus, ACL injury and the less common diagnosis of a ruptured extensor mechanism (quadriceps insertion or patella tendon) are included in the differential diagnosis of an acute haemarthrosis with this history.

Relocation often occurs spontaneously on the sports field making the diagnosis less obvious in the Emergency Department. Examination demonstrates tenderness over the ruptured medial patellofemoral ligament (MPFL) or retinaculum and a haemarthrosis, confirmed on aspiration. There is often considerable apprehension to lateral displacement of the patella. There may also be tenderness palpable over the lateral femoral condyle or the medial patella facet which are the common sites for an associated osteochondral fracture. As an osteochondral fracture may be present in 25–50% cases, skyline patella and notch view radiographs in addition to standard films are essential. If an osteochondral fracture is suspected, an MRI is indicated to characterize the fragment: large fragments with sufficient subchondral bone to facilitate reattachment should be repaired, smaller fragments or those with only a sliver of bone should be removed arthroscopically. Arthroscopic reattachment is difficult in the patellofemoral joint and a mini-arthrotomy is usually required.

The rate of recurrent patellar instability after acute dislocation may be as high as 60% in children and adolescents and immediate repair of the ruptured medial restraints to dislocation has been advocated. However, in the acute setting, it can be difficult to delineate the MPFL clearly and to repair it in a durable fashion. A recent study showed that, compared to non-operative management, MPFL repair did not reduce the redislocation rate and therefore in the absence of a significant osteochondral fracture, conservative management with a period of immobilization followed by restoration of motion and quadriceps strength remains the treatment of choice. This rationale accepts a high rate of recurrent instability and the need for a secondary stabilizing procedure in some cases (see Chapter 13.20).

Osteochondral fracture

The relatively high incidence of this injury in adolescents reflects the transition period from the juvenile joint, in which the chondral surface is anchored to the underlying bone by interdigitations of cartilage, and the adult joint in which the bond is formed orthogonally to this at the calcified cartilage layer (cement line or tidemark). During this period, the knee is at risk of osteochondral fractures. The commonest locations are the medial patella facet and the lateral femoral condyle, reflecting a strong association with acute patella dislocation. For these and other anatomical areas of involvement, the injury is often a direct blow or a twisting mechanism about a fixed foot.

Diagnostic work-up is similar to that for acute patella dislocation, with a low threshold for additional MRI studies. The false negative rate for osteochondral fracture may be over a third with plain radiographs alone. Large fragments should be reattached if possible, particularly when from a weight-bearing area of cartilage. The detached fragment may imbibe joint fluid and swell considerably, particularly if fixation is delayed, such that it must be trimmed to fit back into the defect. Smaller defects with a thin cortical fragment should be removed. Microfracture is indicated for the remaining defect if it is significant and involves a weight-bearing region (Box 13.23.5).

Osgood–Schlatter disease and Sinding–Larsen–Johansson syndrome

Osgood-Schlatter disease and Sinding-Larsen Johansson syndrome are typical overuse injuries causing apophysitis of the anterior tibial tubercle and inferior pole of the patella respectively. They are common in active adolescents and associated with local tenderness and palpable swelling (see Chapter 13.20).

Hip injuries and syndromes

Avulsion fractures

Avulsion fractures around the pelvis are common injuries in football, gymnastics, and track and field. They are usually visible on a plain radiograph and are caused by the sudden contraction of powerful muscles against an apophysis. If presentation is delayed, radiographs may demonstrate a large ossified area and clinical examination may reveal an obvious 'lump'. The possibility of a tumour must be considered but the classic history usually ensures that the avulsion fracture is correctly diagnosed (Figure 13.23.3 and Box 13.23.6).

The vast majority can be managed non-operatively with rest until symptoms subside. Repair may occasionally be indicated in high-demand athletes with symptomatic weakness or pain. Ruptures at the musculotendinous junction of the same muscle groups, particularly the quadriceps, are associated with weakness during kicking and visible bunching of the muscle belly on resisted motion. Repair may be attempted even after delayed presentation, with MRI or ultrasound useful to confirm the diagnosis and location of the rupture.

'Snapping' hip

A 'popping' or 'snapping' hip, often reported by the patient or family as one which goes in and out of joint, should provoke consideration of an 'internal' snapping psoas tendon or 'external' snapping iliotibial band at the lesser and greater trochanters respectively. The Ganz test of snapped adduction in hip flexion can help differentiate these from a labral tear: injection of contrast into the joint for magnetic resonance arthrogram (MRA) is uncomfortable and best avoided. Physiotherapy is the mainstay of treatment, with injection of local anaesthetic and steroid for refractory cases. Surgical release should only be performed as a last resort: results are often disappointing.

Slipped epiphysis

Any child complaining of groin, thigh, or knee pain should undergo thorough clinical examination, in particular to assess range of hip rotation in flexion. There should be a low threshold for anteroposterior and cross table lateral views of the hip. Slipped capital femoral

Box 13.23.5 Radiographic 'work-up' of a knee injury

- AP and lateral plain radiographs
- Tunnel/notch views
- Skyline views of the patella
- MRI to characterize cartilage injury.

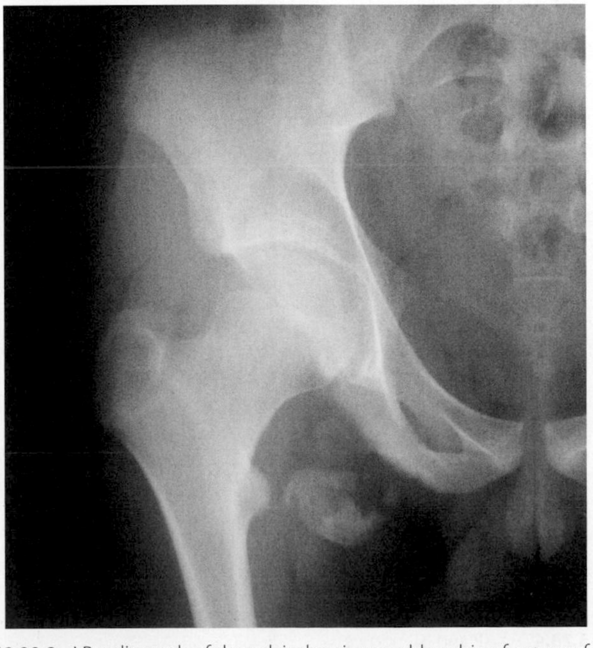

Fig. 13.23.3 AP radiograph of the pelvis showing an old avulsion fracture of the right ischial tuberosity.

Box 13.23.6 Common sites for pelvic avulsion fractures

- Anterior superior iliac spine: sartorius
- Anterior inferior iliac spine: rectus femoris (direct head)
- Ischial tuberosity: hamstrings and adductors.

epiphysis can present with a sports injury and may be misdiagnosed as a 'groin strain': the consequences of missing this diagnosis or making a late diagnosis can be significant. See Chapter 13.19.

Ankle injuries and syndromes

Osteochondral lesions of the talus

Osteochondral lesions of the talus are uncommon but can be a cause of persistent ankle pain in children. In an adult study, lesions of the talar dome were slightly more common on the medial side with lateral lesions occurring more anteriorly and more commonly associated with trauma (see Chapter 14.11) (Figure 13.23.4). The staging system of Berndt and Harty is a useful guide to prognosis and treatment (Table 13.23.2). Lesions up to Stage 3 can be managed non-operatively with a period of immobilization and a good result expected with open physes. Stage 4 lesions and symptomatic Stage 2/3 lesions that fail to respond to non-operative management can be considered for arthroscopic debridement, drilling, or microfracture. ACI and mosaicplasty is also described but is rarely indicated in the paediatric sports-injured population.

Ankle sprains and instability

Inversion injuries to the ankle are very common. In the paediatric population this can result in injuries to the lateral ligament complex, in particular the anterior talofibular ligament (ATFL), local bony avulsions, and fibular fractures including Salter–Harris injuries of the distal fibular physis. Diagnosis of a soft tissue sprain can be made by eliciting localized tenderness over the ATFL without bony or physeal tenderness. All are managed non-operatively and the vast majority have no persistent symptoms. Chronic pain may be related to instability or non-union of small fracture fragments. Examination may demonstrate a positive anterior drawer sign, indicative of ATFL incompetence, and varus stress radiographs may uncover talar tilt. Again, initial management should be with intensive physiotherapy to restore stability. Good results have been reported with a variety of procedures to repair, reconstruct or otherwise advance the capsular condensations which form the lateral ligament complex in children and adolescents with persistent and symptomatic ankle instability.

Table 13.23.2 Berndt and Harty classification of OCD of the talus

Stage	Description
I	Small area of subchondral compression
II	Partially detached fragment
III	Completely detached fragment with a crater
IV	Loose fragment within the joint

Upper limb injuries

Most upper limb sports injuries are subacute and related to overuse. Their increased incidence reflects the earlier and more intensive sports training now seen in the paediatric population. The predominant mechanism is the repetitive overhead motion of the throwing action. This is best characterized for the sport of baseball; however, the biomechanical science is applicable to other disciplines such as tennis and swimming. Gymnastic sports have a particular range of injuries as the upper limbs are required to weight bear for many activities.

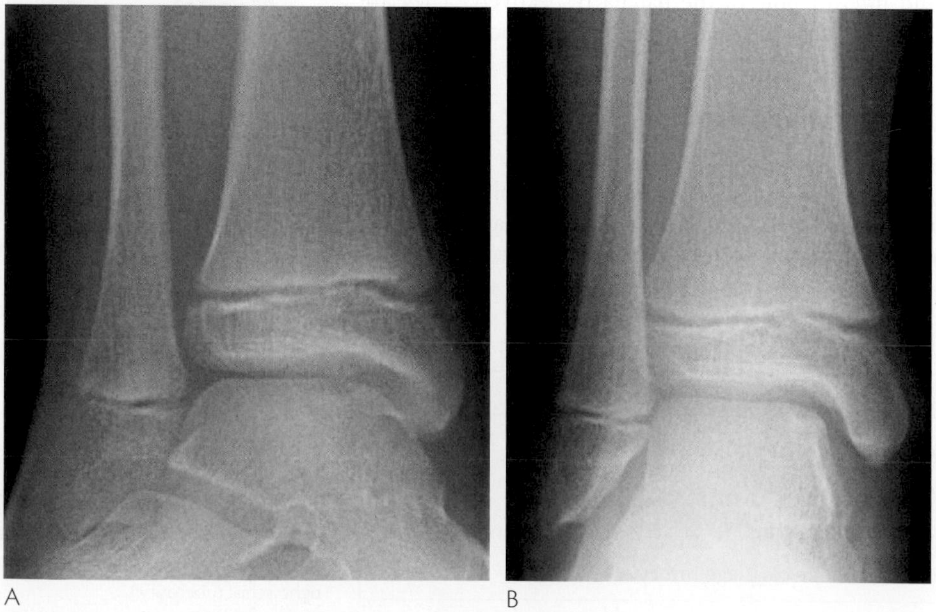

Fig. 13.23.4 A) AP and B) mortice views of an ankle showing an OCD lesion of the medial talus.

The throwing action

The throwing action can be divided into distinct phases; wind-up, early and late cocking, acceleration, deceleration, and follow-through. Most injuries are related to the late cocking and acceleration phases due to the extreme range of motion and forces generated in these actions. The late cocking phase places the shoulder in abduction and maximal external rotation generating large shear forces across the rotator cuff muscles and anterior structures. In the acceleration phase the forward force is generated by shoulder internal rotation and adduction combined with rapid elbow extension. This results in a valgus force across the elbow with tension across the medial compartment and compression in the radio-capitellar joint. Forceful triceps contraction in elbow extension generates tensile stress at the triceps insertion.

Shoulder injuries

'Little League' shoulder

Repetitive microtrauma, secondary to rotational torque forces with overhead activity and throwing, can lead to epiphysiolysis of the proximal humeral physis. This is most common in the 11–13-year age group and is often associated with poor technique. The athlete presents with diffuse shoulder pain, exacerbated by the throwing action and often with characteristic radiographic features. MRI may demonstrate signal change in both the proximal humeral metaphysis and the epiphysis.

Treatment is with rest from throwing (which should be prolonged if radiographic changes exist—Box 13.23.7) followed by action modification and a gradual return to sport.

Shoulder instability

Anterior glenohumeral instability following acute traumatic dislocation is by far the commonest form of shoulder instability seen in the paediatric athlete. Reported recurrent instability approaches a rate of 100% in children with open physes, but in a 25-year prospective series it was only 50% in the 12–16-year age group. Initial management is typically non-operative. Surgery, in the form of an open or arthroscopic repair of the anteroinferior glenoid labrum (Bankart repair), is reserved for those with ongoing instability and the desire to continue with a sport that causes symptoms. There is good evidence of a reduced recurrence risk in young adults immobilized in external rotation for 3 weeks after the primary dislocation but, to date, there is little enthusiasm for this management. Otherwise there is no evidence to recommend immobilization beyond that limited by pain. A good randomized controlled trial of arthroscopic Bankart repair versus arthroscopic lavage alone performed in young adults (under age 30 years) after primary anterior dislocation, demonstrated a 76% reduction in risk of recurrent instability after immediate Bankart repair with better function, satisfaction and rate of return to competitive sports. Despite these results, the authors did not recommend primary operative stabilization for *all* first time dislocations in this age group because of the risk of over-treatment. However, the primary surgical management of choice would be an arthroscopic Bankart repair.

Multidirectional instability is typically seen in adolescents with underlying generalized hyperlaxity, compounded by an acute traumatic event or repetitive microtrauma. Physical examination of the glenohumeral joint will show increased translation in many planes; however, determining the direction of symptomatic subluxation is crucial as an athlete may display mulitdirectional laxity *without* instability. The diagnosis is clinical. Management is with intensive physiotherapy to address altered scapulothoracic biomechanics and dynamic glenohumeral stabilization. Occasionally, MRI or arthroscopy may be helpful to assess cuff or labral damage and to demonstrate redundant capsule.

The immature shoulder may undergo adaptive changes with repetitive overhead activity. Repeated maximal external rotation, particularly in late cocking, causes microtrauma to the anterior capsule and ligament complex creating anterior laxity. This is often associated with posterior capsular hypertrophy and contraction leading to a glenohumeral internal rotation deficit (GIRD). Secondary anterior instability and translation may follow together with internal impingement of the rotator cuff tendon at the posterosuperior rim on the glenoid. The presence of GIRD and anterior hyperlaxity is associated with a significantly increased risk of injury and with secondary adaptive bony changes such as a retroverted glenoid.

Box 13.23.7 Radiographic features of epiphysiolysis (epiphyseal stress reaction)

- Physeal irregularity and/or widening
- Metaphyseal demineralization and fragmentation or cystic changes
- Local periosteal reaction.

Impingement

Rotator cuff impingement in the subacromial space, generally a degenerative condition of early middle age, can occur in the young throwing athlete. Altered scapulothoracic biomechanics lead to a laterally placed, downwardly rotated, and protracted scapula secondary to repetitive overhead activity. The imbalanced scapulothoracic musculature fatigues easily and is often painful. This position of the scapula, particularly in association with GIRD, predisposes to rotator cuff impingement in the subacromial space. Management is with rest and anti-inflammatory medication followed by physiotherapy to address scapulothoracic biomechanics and modification of overhead throwing technique. Subacromial decompression is seldom if ever required in the paediatric athlete.

Elbow injuries

Little Leaguers' elbow

Some 18–69% of players in the United States of America report some degree of elbow pain, most commonly in pitchers aged 8–16 years. The term 'Little Leaguers' elbow' initially described an avulsion fracture of the medial epicondyle but now encompasses a combination of elbow complaints that occur due to repeated rapid extension in the acceleration phase of throwing leading to valgus strain across the elbow joint. This strain causes tension in the medial structures and compression in the lateral joint. Forceful extension in the acceleration phase and locked extension in the deceleration and follow-through place significant stress on the triceps insertion and olecranon apophysis (Box 13.23.8).

Initial symptoms of pain and reduced elbow function relate to inflammation of the common flexor mass or medial apophysitis,

Box 13.23.8 Conditions associated with Little Leaguer's elbow

- Medial epicondyle apophysitis
- Medial epicondyle epiphysiolysis
- Medial epicondyle fragmentation and avulsion
- OCD of capitellum, trochlear, and radial head
- Hypertrophy of the ulna.
- Olecranon apophysitis.

progressing to irregular ossification and enlargement of the medial apophysis which may separate and eventually fragment. Younger players tend to develop apophysitis whereas similar valgus stresses in an adolescent may result in complete or partial avulsion of the medial epicondyle. On the lateral side, repetitive compression leads to radial head hypertrophy or OCD of the capitellum. In the posterior compartment, repetitive extension may lead to the development of olecranon apophysitis, ulna hypertrophy, and traction spur formation. After treatment with rest, anti-inflammatory medication and physiotherapy a cautious return to sport may require specific limitation in the number of throws or pitches per session.

Osteochondritis dissecans of the elbow

Repetitive compression within the radiocapitellar joint causes articular cartilage to separate from subchondral bone secondary to ischaemic micro-trauma resulting in an OCD lesion (Table 13.23.3). This is distinct from the condition of Panner's disease that has a presumed temporary avascular aetiology similar to that of Perthes disease of the hip. Panner's disease has a defined clinical course: revascularization is to be expected with return of normal appearance and function to the radiocapitellar joint. (This differs from Perthes disease, presumably because the hip is a weight-bearing joint.) (Table 13.23.4).

OCD usually develops in adolescence with well-demarcated areas of cartilage damage that may progress to osteochondral fragmentation and loose body formation (Figure 13.23.5). Pain may be marked, particularly with ongoing sports participation, and mechanical locking may occur if loose bodies are present. As for the knee, treatment depends upon the size, stability, and articular continuity of the lesion and the state of the physis. Stable, continuous lesions may be managed non-operatively and loose bodies may be amenable to arthroscopic removal. Unstable, discontinuous lesions that restrict elbow motion, in the presence of a closed physis, may be suitable for subchondral drilling, open fragment fixation or osteochrondral plug grafting. These procedures are technically difficult to perform arthroscopically and a mini-arthrotomy through a posterolateral approach with the elbow flexed is often useful.

Table 13.23.3 Staging of osteochondritis dissecans of the elbow (based on Ewing and Voto scheme)

Stage	Description
I	Subchondral bone oedema, overlying cartilage softened but intact
II	Fissuring of overlying cartilage
III	Fragment of bone or cartilage partially attached, or 'detached *in situ*'
IV	Detached fragment or loose body with crater

Table 13.23.4 Differing characteristics of OCD and Panner's disease of the elbow

	OCD	Panner's disease
Age	12–15 years	<10 years
Aetiology	Related to overuse	Idiopathic
Extent	Localized fragmentation of the capitellum	Osteonecrosis and fragmentation of entire capitellum
Natural history	Minimal remodelling	Revascularization occurs leading to minimal residual deformity
Management	Loose body removal and articular surface reconstruction if lesions unstable	Non-operative

Hand and wrist

Gymnast's wrist

Wrist pain can affect up to 80% of elite gymnasts in whom wrist loads may regularly exceed twice body weight and peak to 16 times this level. Repetitive compressive forces at the distal radial physis cause a stress reaction (Box 13.23.7) (Figure 13.23.6) that can culminate in premature closure of the distal radial physis and positive ulna variance. Avascular necrosis of the lunate (Keinbock's disease) has been noted in some athletes (Figure 13.23.7). Secondary overload of the ulna side of the carpus and wrist joint is a cause of degenerative

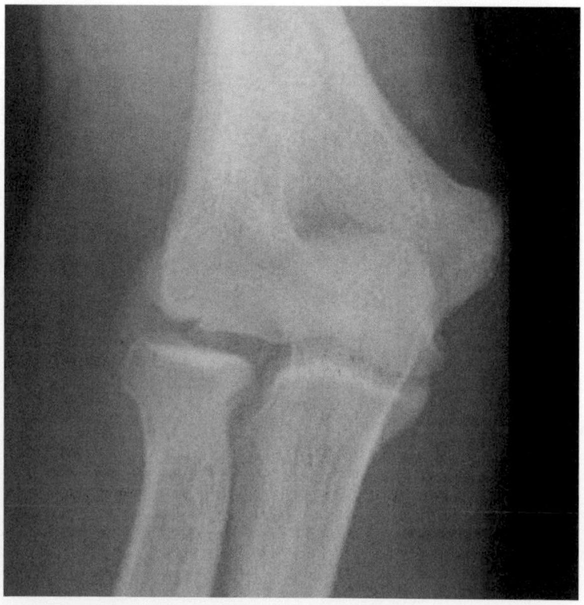

Fig. 13.23.5 AP radiograph of the distal humerus showing an OCD lesion of the capitellum.

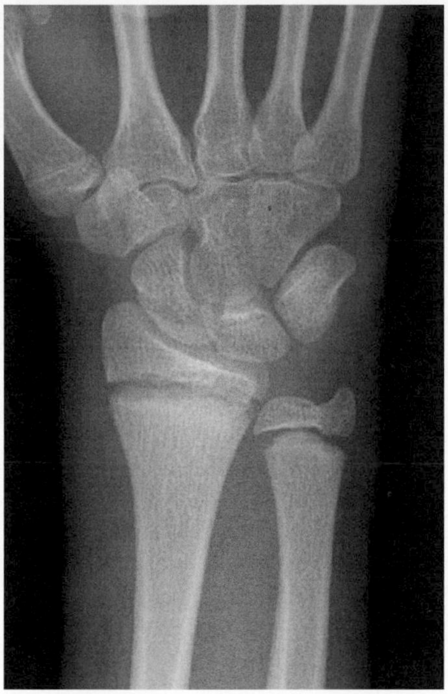

Fig. 13.23.6 AP radiograph of a gymnast's wrist showing physeal change in keeping with a stress reaction.

changes and potentially long-term disability. The weight bearing upper limb position also places the elbow under valgus stress which can lead to a similar pattern of injury to that seen in the overhead athlete. Radiographic follow-up is required in children and adolescents with a pattern of physeal stress injury because of the risk of premature physeal closure.

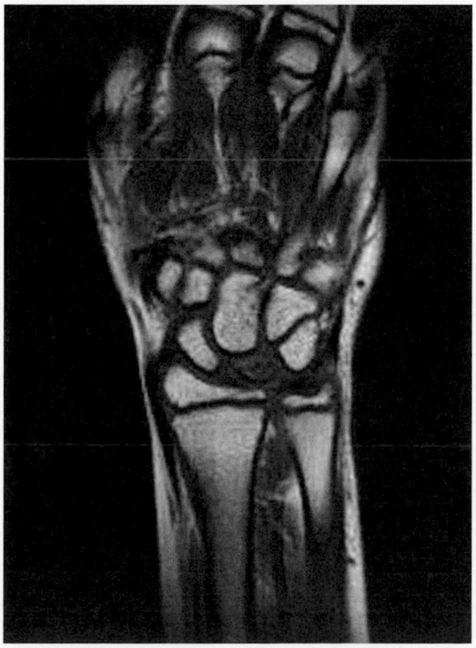

Fig. 13.23.7 MR image of the wrist of an elite adolescent swimmer showing decreased vascularity of the lunate in Keinbock's disease.

Other injuries or syndromes

'Shin splints'

This term has been applied to almost any type of lower leg pain that results from overuse in the teenage athlete, most commonly after running or hiking. The pain is usually felt on the posteromedial border of the tibia and may correspond with the medial origin of the soleus muscle. Pain may be exacerbated by resisted plantar flexion or toe raises. The differential diagnosis should include a stress fracture and an exercise-induced compartment syndrome whilst the possibility of infection or a benign or malignant bone tumour must also be considered.

An exercise-induced compartment syndrome should be confirmed with pressure studies both at rest and after exercise. The compartments most frequently affected are the deep posterior and the anterior compartments: numbness in the sole or on the dorsum of the foot may be part of the clinical picture. A careful surgical fasciotomy is the treatment of choice. The procedure can be performed through limited skin incisions to improve the cosmetic appearance.

Stress fractures

Stress fractures are increasingly common in those children and adolescents participating in sports involving running. True stress fractures (defined as abnormal stresses applied to normal bone) are rare in children who are active but *not* involved in training programmes. Training, particularly after a period of inactivity such as after an injury or a long vacation, leads to a stimulation of both osteoblastic activity *and* osteoclastic activity and perhaps an increased tendency to fracture. In adolescents, the combination of ligamentous laxity, muscle tightness, and relative muscle weakness are relative risk factors for a stress fracture and the risk may be increased if the athlete is tall and heavy and involved in a sport which requires bursts of explosive activity.

Fractures are often diagnosed on careful history taking and examination. Radiographic features may take some time to develop and imaging techniques such as MR and bone scans are often useful.

Treatment will depend on the age of the child, the site of injury and the severity of the symptoms but usually involves relative rest from the sporting activity and the use of a brace, orthotics, or a cast until symptoms resolve. Surgical treatment is sometimes required for fractures affecting the femoral neck and the medial malleolus (Box 13.23.9).

Box 13.23.9 Common sites for stress fractures

- Proximal tibia
- Femur:
  - Neck
  - Diaphysis
  - Distal metaphysis
- Medial malleolus
- Metatarsals.

Future developments

Sports participation in children and adolescents is on the increase and is to be encouraged for the control of body weight, development of peak bone mass, and instilling the virtues of teamwork and discipline. Ongoing analysis of the environment and specific sports situations in which critical injuries occur will lead to better information for the development of injury prevention programmes for paediatric athletes. Greater recognition of particular injury patterns through ever-improving imaging techniques and better data collection with a denominator of hours and type of sports played will occur. The development of increasingly sophisticated techniques and instruments for arthroscopic management of osteochondral and meniscal injuries may improve outcomes and there is the potential for stem cell manipulation to aid reconstruction of damaged tissue.

Further reading

Caine, D., Maffulli, N., and Caine, C. (2008). Epidemiology of injury in child and adolescent sports: injury rates, risk factors and prevention. *Clinics in Sports Medicine*, **27**, 19–50.

Stanitski, C., Harvell, J., and Fu, F. (1993). Observations on acute hemarthrosis in children and adolescents. *Journal of Pediatric Orthopedics*, **3**, 506–10.

Kocher, M.S., Smith, J.T., Zoric, B.J., Lee, B., and Micheli, L.J. (2007). Transphyseal anterior cruciate ligament reconstruction in skeletally immature pubescent adolescents. *Journal of Bone and Joint Surgery*, **89A**, 263–9.

Palmu, S., Kallio, P., Donell, S., Helenius, I., and Nietosvaara, Y. (2008). Acute patella dislocation in children and adolsescents: a randomised clinical trial. *Journal of Bone and Joint Surgery*, **90A**, 463–70.

Robinson, M., Jenkins, P., White, T., Ker, A., and Will, E. (2008). Primary arthroscopic stabilization for a first-time anterior dislocation of the shoulder. A randomized, double-blind trial. *Journal of Bone and Joint Surgery*, **90A**, 708–21.

SECTION 14

Paediatric Trauma

14.1

Musculoskeletal injuries in children

Tim Theologis

Summary points

- In children, bone is more flexible and heals faster than in adults but is at risk of growth disturbance. It is also capable of remodelling
- The physis is weaker than the structures around it and therefore is liable to disruption in trauma
- The possibility of injuries as a result of abuse must be considered in children and have a characteristic pattern
- In poly trauma, children are more susceptible to hypothermia. Abdominal viscera and the cranium are more vulnerable. However, the central nervous system has more scope for recovery, and the cardiovascular system has an excellent capacity for coping with hypovolaemic shock
- A reliable specific paediatric score should be used to plan treatment
- The management of fractures is more likely to involve traction, plaster, and K-wires.

Introduction (Box 14.1.1)

Musculoskeletal injuries in children have some unique characteristics and differences from those in adults. Injury to the growing skeleton may cause growth disturbance. While the injured adult has to recover from the trauma itself, children also need to cope with any implications of trauma to their growth.

Bone healing is faster in children and complications affecting bone healing rarer than in adults because the bone is more biologically active with a thick vascular periosteum.

The biomechanical characteristics of the growing skeleton are also different. Bone is more elastic and incomplete fractures, that are rare in the adult, often occur. The periosteum is loosely attached to bone while tendons, ligaments, and muscles are firmly attached to the periosteum. As a result, children suffer fractures more often than sprains, ligament ruptures, and joint dislocations. The biomechanical properties change with age and there are characteristic injury patterns for different age groups. Fractures involving the physis only occur in children.

The property of growing bone to remodel by asymmetric growth at the physes is also unique and age dependent. Overgrowth may complicate long-bone fractures in children.

Management of the multiply injured child follows adult principles but there are some differences that are essential for the treating physician to recognize. This also applies to the surgical treatment of children's fractures: while some general principles are similar to those in the adult, certain characteristics exist which may often be crucial for the optimal management of young patients.

Finally, child abuse is discussed—a clinical entity unique in children. Suspecting and diagnosing child abuse is essential for the safety and future development of infants and young children.

Structure of the growing bone—physeal injuries (Box 14.1.2)

Long bones begin to ossify *in utero* when the primary bone collar appears in the middle of the cartilage anlage. This region of primary endochondral ossification then expands and progresses towards the bone ends, establishing primary ossification fronts, the physes or growth plates, in both directions.

Vascular invasion of the hypertrophic cartilage inside this primary bone collar results in either direct cartilage resorption or a transient stage of endochondral bone formation followed by osteoclasis. The medullary canal and an endosteal surface are thus established.

The entire anlage continues to grow in length by the proliferation and ossification of cartilage at the physis. Further growth and development of the diaphysis are achieved by direct bone apposition and resorption on the periosteal and endosteal surfaces, respectively.

Box 14.1.1 Musculoskeletal injuries in children

- May affect growth
- Incomplete fractures common
- Physeal fractures common.

Therefore there are two different processes that contribute to the final structure of a typical long bone: appositional cortical bone formation, mainly in the diaphysis, and progressive endochondral ossification at the physes, leading to cancellous bone formation. Only after birth (with the exception of the distal femoral epiphysis) will secondary centres of ossification form at a time characteristic for each epiphysis.

These processes lead to the development of the final structure of the growing long bone: the tubular diaphysis in the middle is made of cortical bone, the conical metaphyses on either side of the diaphysis, and the epiphyses at both ends consist of cancellous bone; the cartilaginous physes separate the metaphyses from the epiphyses.

Injuries involving the physis occur as a result of the unique structure of bone during childhood. The physis is biomechanically the weakest structure of the growing bone, particularly when shear forces are applied, and is therefore the most vulnerable to injury. Physeal injuries, their treatment, and their complications are discussed in Chapter 14.2.

Box 14.1.2 Physeal injuries

- Physis is weakest part.

Biology and biomechanics of injury to the growing skeleton

Biology (Box 14.1.3)

Box 14.1.3 Biology

- Healing is rapid
- Fewer complications until adolescence
- Open upper-limb fractures more commonly complicated.

Bone in children is biologically more active than in adults. Apart from the activity at the growth plate, the modelling process, where bone is continuously absorbed and replaced by new bone, is more active in children. These processes of growth and modelling are genetically determined but are also influenced by complex factors including circulating hormones, nutritional intake, mechanical influences, and disease. At the age of skeletal maturity, bone growth is completed but the modelling process—frequently referred to as remodelling in adults—continues at a slower rate. Overall the biological activity of bone reduces after skeletal maturity.

The periosteum plays an important role in the biology of the growing bone. It shows greater osteogenic potential in younger children and has increased vascularity compared to adult periosteum. This contributes to the overall increased vascularity of the growing bone.

Healing capacity

As a result of the increased biological activity of the growing bone, fractures in children heal rapidly. This healing capacity is significantly dependent on age: fractures heal very rapidly in the newborn, less so in childhood, and reaches adult rates during adolescence. This generally accepted knowledge was confirmed in a clinical study in which the time required for union of fractures of the femoral diaphysis in children followed a log-normal distribution and the increment in mean time to union was 0.7 weeks for every year of age.

Bone healing and callus formation in children may follow a slightly different pattern compared to the adult. A study of the external periosteal callus using a scanning electron microscope, a transmission electron microscope, and a radiograph microdiffractometer, demonstrated that the rapid fracture healing in children is related mostly to brushite mineral deposition among the collagen fibres, while hydroxyapatite deposition is insufficient. In the adult, fracture repair relies on hydroxyapatite deposition among the collagen fibres. Deposition of brushite minerals in external periosteal callus in children may be compensating for the insufficient hydroxyapatite mineralization, thereby making fracture repair more rapid in children than in adults.

When radiological fracture union criteria and staging are used, the pattern of healing in children is similar to that in the adult. Radiographic criteria can be used to date fractures. The length that each stage takes is age dependent but not sex dependent.

Complications of bone healing

Increased biological activity of the growing bone leads to a lower incidence of complications related to fracture healing. Delayed union, infection, and non-union have all been reported as a result of high-energy trauma and open injuries. Furthermore, displaced intra-articular fractures and/or soft tissue interposition within the fracture may lead to delayed or non-union.

The incidence of these complications in adolescents is similar to that in adults. Children under 12 years of age are at lower risk of developing any of these complications. The actively osteogenic periosteum and the overall increased vascularity of the growing bone account for this.

Current knowledge and understanding of fracture-healing complications in children is based on a number of clinical studies. In the absence of segmental bone loss or extensive soft tissue loss requiring major reconstruction, healing in children can be expected within 6 months after open lower-limb fracture, with younger children healing more quickly. Union times for open tibial fractures are prolonged relative to closed injuries in similarly aged children, but bone grafting is seldom required. Delayed union is often a problem in children older than 11 years, while leg length discrepancy can complicate tibial fractures in children under the age of 11 years.

When a delayed or non-union occurs they are often associated with infection. The incidence of infection is also age related, being a rare complication in young children. Chronic osteomyelitis following acute wound infection after an open fracture in the lower limbs is also rare in children, and its incidence has been reported at 2–3%. The prevention of wound infection should follow the same principles as in adults: thorough immediate and, if necessary, repeated debridement and irrigation of the wound, stabilization of the fracture, and intravenous administration of antibiotics. Primary wound closure in the treatment of selected non-contaminated open fractures has been suggested, although the issue remains controversial.

Compartment syndrome following open injuries of the lower extremity is less frequent in children than in adults but it is important to recognize that it may occur in 2–4% of cases. Early fascial release is necessary to prevent the long-term consequences of unrecognized compartment syndrome.

Open fractures of the forearm and humerus in children are more frequently associated with healing-related complications. Delayed union, non-union, refracture, and malunion complicate about 25% of cases. Open type II and III fractures of the radius and ulna are at the highest risk. Excellent or good long-term results can be anticipated in 90% of all open fractures of the arm.

Biomechanics (Box 14.1.4)

There are several structural differences between growing and mature bone that account for their differences in biomechanical behaviour. Mature bone has a higher density, and growing bone more porosity due in part to increased vascularity. The increased porosity may be one of the reasons why fracture propagation is less likely to occur in growing bone and fracture comminution is more common in adults than in children.

Woven bone predominates in the neonate and is gradually replaced by lamellar bone as haversian systems develop and osteons assume a longitudinal orientation. The stiffness, strength, and resistance to stress of bone increases with increasing age.

In the metaphyseal area, the cortex is thinner and perforated with more vessels, while the haversian systems develop close to skeletal maturity. This area can fail under either tension or compression in children, while in adults it is much more resistant to compression forces.

The epiphysis becomes increasingly stiffer as secondary ossification centres develop and its response to stress and strain alters with age. The development of subchondral bone over the physis changes the biomechanical characteristics of the area even further. This explains why different patterns of epiphyseal fractures occur in different age groups.

The periosteum is thicker and stronger in children. It is loosely attached to the diaphysis and separates from it easily in the case of a fracture. For this reason, complete circumferential rupture of the periosteum is rare in children and usually a significant part of the periosteum remains intact. This remaining periosteal 'hinge' prevents severe displacement of the fracture and aids reduction. The periosteum is more firmly attached to the metaphysis where it blends into the perichondrial ring that surrounds the physis.

Muscles are attached to the periosteum, while tendons and ligaments blend into the fibrous regions of the metaphysis, perichondrial ring, and epiphysis. With few exceptions, no soft tissue structures are directly attached onto bone. The periosteum, together with all its soft tissue attachments, adds significantly to the overall stability of the bone. The loose attachment of periosteum to bone, the intrinsic mechanical weakness of the physis, and the firm attachment of ligaments, tendons, and muscles to periosteum, all contribute to the fact that sprains, ligament injuries, and joint dislocations are rare in children, while physeal injuries are common.

There is experimental evidence that children's bone have a lower modulus of elasticity, a lower bending strength, and a lower mineral content. However, children's bone can deflect and absorb more energy before breaking by undergoing plastic rather than elastic deformation. The considerable plastic deformation occurring before the fracture starts may be due to multiple shear cracks opening up within the bone.

Furthermore, children's bone breaks at a lower load than adult bone and so the stress in the bone is less. The energy required for the fracture to be propagated through the bone comes mainly from the strain energy. Children's bone undergoes plastic deformation prior to fracturing, and therefore the bone in the region of the fracture will have yielded and have little strain energy.

Both of these factors—the small amount of strain energy available at the beginning of fracture and the difficulty a fracture has in propagating straight across the bone—tend to produce incomplete fractures in children.

Specific fractures (Box 14.1.5)

Greenstick fracture

Greenstick fractures are incomplete fractures produced by angulatory forces. The periosteum and cortex on the tension side are disrupted, while on the opposite side the cortex may be compressed or bent but remains in continuity. Greenstick fractures usually occur in the metaphyseal region of long bones but can occur in the

Box 14.1.4 Biomechanics

- Epiphysis becomes stiffer with age
- Periosteum thick and strong
- Periosteum rarely completely divided
- Bone has lower modulus of elasticity and bending strength
- Plastic deformation high before fracture.

Box 14.1.5 Specific fractures

Greenstick fractures

- Bending injuries
- Usually metaphyseal
- May require completion during manipulation

Torus fractures

- Axial compression
- Young children

Plastic deformation

- Paired bones
- May be difficult to correct

Stress fractures

- Adolescents
- Repetitive activity
- Heal rapidly.

diaphysis of long bones in neonates and young children (typically in the forearm).

Completion of the fracture with manipulation as well as simple manipulation to correct the angulation have keen supporters. This is a subject of debate since both methods have disadvantages. Completion of the fracture produces instability, makes immobilization more difficult, and increases the risk of late displacement. Simple manipulation of greenstick fractures of the diaphysis can lead to incomplete consolidation on the tension side of the injury, which may lead to refracture.

Buckle (torus) fracture

These are incomplete fractures of the metaphyseal region due to axial compression forces. The metaphyseal cortex, which is thin in childhood, gives way usually on one side. The fracture appears as a 'kink' in the cortex and minimal angulation may also occur. Typical sites include the distal forearm and the tibia. Buckle fractures occur in young children only. In older children similar injuries produce compression metaphyseal fractures. Treatment may be required to correct any significant angulation.

Plastic deformation

Angulatory or longitudinal forces applied to the immature bone may cause deformation beyond the limit of elasticity but below the fracture point. Plastic deformation then occurs without an apparent macroscopic fracture. Microfractures may occur on the tension side but are not apparent on radiographs. This type of injury occurs in young children and typically in paired bones. Usually one of the bones fractures and the other deforms. Plastic deformation may be missed but should be suspected when one of the paired bones is fractured and the other is apparently intact. Periosteal reaction does not usually follow plastic deformation.

Correction of the deformity with manipulation is difficult and may result in a complete fracture but is often necessary in order to reduce a fracture or dislocation of the paired bone.

Stress fracture

Stress fractures may occur in older children and adolescents. They are usually associated with increased and repetitive physical activity and typically occur in the tibia, fibula, and femur. They heal quickly, with modification of activities and immobilization, by extensive periosteal reaction and abundant callus formation. Careful history, physical examination, and radiographs can help diagnose most common stress fractures and differentiate them from infection or neoplasm that would need aggressive treatment. Magnetic resonance imaging (MRI) scanning can also help establish the diagnosis and negate the need for histological diagnosis.

Epidemiology and age characteristics (Box 14.1.6)

In developed countries, injury has become a leading cause of childhood morbidity and mortality. Musculoskeletal injury is one of the more important groups associated with high morbidity and mortality. The overall estimated annual incidence of limb fractures requiring hospital treatment in the age group up to 16 years is 0.5–1%. The age group of 4–11 years is at the highest risk. The sex distribution shows a male predominance in the range of 2–3:1 which increases with age and becomes 5.5:1 in adolescence.

Epidemiological studies on fracture incidence from different parts of the world show considerable variation because of cultural, socioeconomic, demographic, and other population characteristics. Despite this variation, there is overall agreement that the pattern, site, and frequency of childhood fractures all depend on age.

During birth, fractures of the clavicle, skull, and proximal humerus can occur. Fractures within the first 2 years of life are rare and should raise suspicion of metabolic disease or non-accidental injury. Greenstick and torus fractures occur in early childhood while fractures in adolescence follow a more adult pattern.

The secondary ossification centres appear at an age characteristic for each epiphysis, the increasing size changes the biomechanical characteristics of the epiphysis, making it stiffer. As a result, different epiphyseal fractures occur at different ages.

Upper-limb injuries in children are more common than lower-limb ones and the non-dominant side is at higher risk. Fractures of the forearm are the most common in all age groups with a peak between the years of 8–16. Clavicle fractures as well as hand and phalangeal fractures are frequent in all age groups. Supracondylar fractures of the humerus usually occur between the ages of 4–7 years. Tibial fractures occur in all age groups but the pattern of fracture is different: toddlers' fracture between the ages of 2–5 years, and spiral or physeal fractures in the older age groups.

Multiple, high-energy, and open fractures are relatively rare in children compared to adults, and they usually result from road traffic collisions. Seasonal variations are also noted with summer usually being the peak period for childhood trauma. The relatively high prevalence of fractures resulting from bicycle or pedestrian injuries in adolescents has been highlighted recently.

Joint and soft tissue injuries (Box 14.1.7)

Ligament injuries and joint dislocations are rare in young children but reach adult frequency close to skeletal maturity.

In the growing skeleton, ligaments, tendons, and muscles are firmly attached to the periosteum. In the epiphyseal region and particularly around the physis periosteum is firmly attached on bone. Tensile forces to ligaments and tendons in this region lead to the failure of the weakest biomechanical structure, namely the physis. With this mechanism of injury, therefore, whereas an adult

Box 14.1.6 Epidemiology of fractures

- 1 per cent per year
- Male predominance up to 5.5:1
- Adolescent fractures follow adult patterns
- Nondominant/upper limb more at risk
- Peak incidence in summer
- High-energy/multiple injuries from motor vehicle accidents.

Box 14.1.7 Joint and soft-tissue injuries

- Uncommon
- Dislocation is rare
- Fractures usually rather than ligament injuries
- Joint stiffness rare.

would suffer a ligament rupture or joint dislocation, a child sustains a physeal fracture.

Dislocations can occur in children. The elbow or the radiocapitellar joint is the most frequently affected joint; other joints include the hip, knee and the proximal tibiofibular joint.

Ligament injuries around the ankle are rare, while physeal fractures are more common. The ligaments of the knee are also infrequently injured and tibial spine avulsion rather than anterior cruciate ligament rupture is a typical example. Also characteristic of the different behaviour of the growing skeleton is the low incidence of 4% of knee ligamentous instability associated with femoral fracture; in the adult this incidence is in the range of 40–70%.

Children tend to regain full range of movement quickly after removal of casts and splints and physiotherapy is rarely needed. However, some particular types of intra-articular or physeal fractures in children may lead to permanent loss of full range joint motion despite treatment.

Articular cartilage in children does not differ from the adult. The superficial layers of the growing epiphyseal cartilage develop into adult-type hyaline cartilage and lose the ability to transform into bone or heal after injury. The recovery expected following damage to the articular cartilage should therefore be similar to that in adults.

There is no documented evidence that healing of soft tissues following penetrating or blunt trauma is faster in children than in adults or that complications after such injuries are rarer. Musculoskeletal injuries should always raise suspicion of neurovascular damage and this usually responds better to early intervention. Compartment syndrome is also associated with some paediatric fractures and decompression may be needed to avoid Volkmann's ischaemic contracture.

Remodelling of the growing bone (Box 14.1.8)

Fractures may heal in a non-anatomical position. It is well recognized that the growing skeleton has, to a certain extent, the capacity to correct residual deformities after a fracture has healed and this process is usually referred to as remodelling. The remodelling potential differs according to the location of the fracture, the severity of its residual deformity after healing, and the skeletal age of the patient. Decisions upon the acceptability of a residual deformity have to be based on knowledge of the remodelling potential of the individual fracture so that unnecessary treatment or acceptance of a malunion should be avoided.

During fracture healing and remodelling in children, bone growth acceleration may occur. This overgrowth phenomenon has to be taken into account when treating fractures, particularly those in the lower limb.

Mechanisms of remodelling

Remodelling of adult fractures occurs at the site of the fracture and follows Wolf's law: alteration in the mechanical environment, as a result of bone deformity, leads to new bone formation on the concave side (compression) and bone resorption in the convex side (tension). In adults this is a slow process and little correction of deformity can be expected.

The Heuter–Volkmann law suggests that, in children, the physis tends to align itself perpendicular to the resultant force acting across it by a mechanism of asymmetric growth. In the presence of an angulatory deformity, therefore, the physis would grow faster on the concave side of the fracture and would reorientate the joint and, eventually, the fracture.

The hypothesis of asymmetric physeal growth has been confirmed in animal experiments including radiological and histological studies. The overall alignment of the malunited bone corrects rapidly as a result of asymmetric growth at the epiphyseal plates. The joints at both bone ends regain their normal alignment with this mechanism. The angulation at the fracture site corrects slowly as a result of both asymmetric physeal growth and local remodelling at the fracture, following Wolf's law. Local remodelling accounts for only 25% of the correction at the fracture site, the remaining 75% of correction being achieved by asymmetric physeal growth (Figure 14.1.1).

The exact mechanism of deformity correction by asymmetric physeal growth is not known. The role of the periosteum has been investigated but results were discouraging: experimental periosteal division to release tension has little effect on deformity correction. Mechanical factors may play a role but do not solely control the mechanism of correction: experimental studies demonstrated femoral overgrowth in animals with tibial fractures, suggesting a systemic factor contributing to the correction mechanism.

Box 14.1.8 Remodeling

- Asymmetric physeal growth mainly corrects angulation
- Periosteum is important
- Helical growth may correct torsion
- Little remodeling after age of 11 years
- Metaphyseal fractures close to joints remodel well
- Epiphyseal and intra-articular fractures have little ability to remodel
- Deformities in plane of movement of joint remodel well
- Remodeling is diffcult to predict.

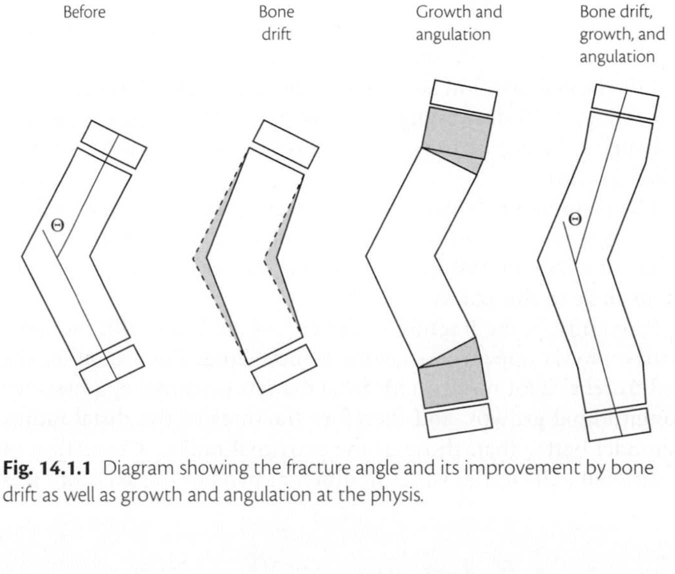

Fig. 14.1.1 Diagram showing the fracture angle and its improvement by bone drift as well as growth and angulation at the physis.

Rotational moments applied on the physis may induce helical growth, which in turn may be responsible for the correction of torsional deformities following fractures. The same mechanism may be responsible for the development of late secondary torsional deformities following fractures healed with angulation.

Experimental findings on asymmetric physeal growth in malunited fractures are supported by clinical evidence. Measurements on radiographs of malunited forearm fractures showed most of the angular correction to occur at the growth plate. Furthermore, children over the age of 11 years do not show the same potential for correction of deformities and are closer to adult patterns of remodelling. The physis still shows some potential in correcting the orientation of the joint but this does not contribute substantially to the correction of the fracture angulation.

Expectations for remodelling

In clinical practice, knowledge of the remodelling potential of the specific fracture concerned is important. Precise guidelines are not available and, in clinical practice, a lot relies on the personal experience and training of the treating surgeon. This may lead to overtreatment of some fractures with good remodelling potential, or acceptance of deformities that are not going to remodel and may cause functional problems. Some attempts have been made to determine the factors that influence the remodelling potential in general and also to define guidelines for some specific fractures.

The age of the patient influences the potential for remodelling. In young children under the age of 2 years, angulations of up to 90 degrees in femoral fractures remodel well. This potential decreases with age to the degree that little remodelling should be expected after the age of 11 years. Since correction of deformity relies mainly on asymmetric physeal growth it is only logical that the younger and more active the physis, the greater the potential for remodelling.

The distance of the fracture from the physis also influences remodelling potential. Metaphyseal fractures remodel better than diaphyseal ones. Radiographic studies of malunited forearm fractures have confirmed that midshaft radial fractures have less potential for correction than distal radial ones. Epiphyseal fractures, and particularly intra-articular ones, have little potential for deformity correction.

The severity of the residual deformity once fracture healing has been accomplished also plays an important role. The more severe the deformity, the less potential it has for complete remodelling. With the exception of some fractures that present late with deformity, the healed position is similar to the one accepted at the end of treatment. A 20-degree angulation of a femoral fracture is acceptable up to the age of 13 years, but this would not be the case for a tibial fracture.

The plane of movement of the adjacent joint in relation to fracture angulation also influences remodelling. Deformities in the plane of movement of the adjacent joint remodel better than ones at an angle to this plane.

Proximity of the fracture to the end of the bone with the most active physis appears to favour remodelling. For example, the radius relies a lot more on its distal than its proximal epiphysis for longitudinal growth, and therefore fractures of the distal radius remodel better than those of the proximal radius. Correction of rotational deformities varies in different parts of the skeleton. It is generally less optimal than angular remodelling, despite experimental evidence of helical growth of the epiphyseal plate under rotational moments. The proximity of the fracture to a joint with multiplanar movement may be playing a role. Proximal humeral fractures appear to remodel their rotational deformities well. The question, however, is whether the humerus shows true rotational improvement or the rotational malalignment is compensated for at the glenohumeral joint.

Overgrowth (Box 14.1.9)

Acceleration of growth following long-bone fractures in children is a well-recognized phenomenon. There is experimental evidence that this overgrowth occurs at the epiphyseal plates but the exact mechanism of physeal stimulation is unknown. Femoral fracture in the rabbit also stimulates ipsilateral tibial overgrowth. At the end of this process the femur is overgrown by 2% of its length and the tibia by 1%.

Radiographic measurements show that, in femoral fractures, growth acceleration reaches its maximum at about 3 months after the fracture. It is significantly higher than normal for about 2 years and then slows down but is still higher than normal until about 4–5 years after the fracture. The uninjured ipsilateral tibia follows the same time-pattern but overall its overgrowth is slower. A fractured tibia shows growth acceleration but does not influence the ipsilateral femur. Bone scintigraphy studies have demonstrated increased growth plate activity in the distal femoral and proximal tibial growth plates following femoral fracture. Recent evidence suggests that this may be due to increased mitotic activity at the growth plate, rather than increased vascularity as it was initially thought.

Growth acceleration is higher when there is overlap of the fracture ends. When there is little or no overlap between fragments the increase of the growth rate is minimal and results can be predictably good with leg-length discrepancy of 0.5cm or less at the end of growth. The average overgrowth following femoral fractures—with or without overlap of the fracture ends—is less than 1cm but can reach 2.5cm in some cases.

Overgrowth is also age dependent, with the 4- to 7-year-old age group being most likely to show significant growth acceleration. An increased effect on boys has been reported but a much larger proportion of boys than girls in the 4- to 7-year-old age group were included in this study.

The multiply injured child (Box 14.1.10)

Injury is the leading cause of children's morbidity and mortality in developed countries. Road traffic collisions and falls account for

Box 14.1.9 Overgrowth

- 1.25 cm for femur
- Maximal between 4 and 7 years of age
- Avoid distraction
- Overlaps should be less than 1 cm
- Upper-limb overgrowth in 20 per cent of fractures.

Box 14.1.10 Multiple injuries

- Head injury
- Fractures often absent in visceral injuries
- Large cardiac and pulmonary reserve
- Use Pediatric Trauma Score/Coma Scale
- Vital signs are age dependent
- Intraosseous infusion under the age of 6 years
- Early diagnosis/treatment reduces mobidity/mortality.

80% of childhood trauma. Multiple injuries and multisystem involvement is frequent because of the small size of the young patients. The order and priorities in the assessment and management of the multiply injured child are the same as in the adult. However, there are unique characteristics in children that require particular attention and these are analysed in the following section.

Priority should be given to the treatment of life-threatening injuries and limb-threatening injuries should follow. Errors in the management of ventilation and circulation, or failure to detect hidden injuries, are the most common causes of preventable death.

Special considerations in children

Size and shape

Because of the small body mass in children, there is a greater force per unit of body area during injury. Furthermore, because of the proximity of multiple organs, multiple system injury is frequent. This is often the case with the abdominal viscera which are not well protected by the poorly developed abdominal musculature. The head is large relative to the trunk; therefore it is injured in 80% of multiply injured children and is often the leading contact point.

Age- and size-appropriate equipment is also needed for the treatment of injured children. Drug doses and some equipment size determination are based on body weight.

Elasticity

The skeleton in children contains less mineral than in the adult and is therefore more elastic. In multiply injured children, soft tissue and visceral injuries may occur without concomitant bony injuries. For example, the thoracic cage is very elastic and rib fractures are rare. Lung injury with little external evidence may occur and mediastinal injury is not uncommon.

Surface area

Children have a higher ratio of body surface area to body volume. As a result, they are more prone to thermal energy loss, particularly in the presence of hypovolaemia.

Psychological status

The emotional instability of the injured child, together with difficulty in interacting with unfamiliar individuals makes communication difficult. Obtaining a history of the injury may be a challenge and cooperation of the young patient is not always available. Psychological and emotional support in the acute phase as well as during recovery are important in order to prevent long-term effects of psychological injury.

Beneficial features

Some of the beneficial features in children with multiple injuries include the low incidence of pre-existing disease, the high capacity for recovery from central nervous system injury, and the larger cardiac and pulmonary reserves. Their vascular system can maintain normal systolic pressure despite significant hypovolaemia by reflex tachycardia and vasoconstriction. However, with ongoing blood loss the body can no longer maintain normal blood pressure and haemodynamic deterioration in children is usually rapid.

Long-term effects

Injury may have long-term effects on growth and development. Unlike in the adult, the child's temporary disability as a result of trauma may lead to long-term disability as a result of growth disturbance or abnormal development. Treatment should aim at helping the child not only to recover from the injury but also to continue the normal process of growth.

Management and outcome

Transport and triage in multiply injured children follows the same principles as in adults. Paediatric trauma scores have been developed to facilitate triage and offer a prediction of outcome (Table 14.1.1). The Revised Trauma Score, often used in adults, is not applicable in children, particularly young ones whose verbal communication is poor. The Paediatric Trauma Score is often used in trauma centres and is presented here.

Each variable is given one of three scores and the total score can vary between –6 and +12. Children with a score higher than 8 have better prognosis with usually preventable mortality, morbidity, and disability. Ideally, children with a score below 8 should be triaged to specialized centres with experience and facilities for paediatric trauma. The Paediatric Trauma Score has been evaluated and has been found to be predictive of outcome in multiply injured children.

Resuscitation of the multiply injured child

The same principles of resuscitation as in the adult apply in children and Advanced Trauma Life Support methodology is used in most major trauma centres.

Table 14.1.1 Pediatric trauma score

	+2	+1	–1
Weight (kg)	>20	10–20	<10
Airway patency	Normal	Maintained with oral or nasal airway	Unmaintained: tracheostomy or other invasive technique
Systolic blood pressure (mmHg)	>90	50–90	<50
Level of consciousness	Completely awake	Obtunded or any loss of consciousness	Comatose
Open wound fractures	None	Minor	Major or penetrating
Total score	None	Minor	Open or multiple

Cervical spine control during this is important. The incidence of cervical injury in children is lower than that in the adult. However, children have a larger occiput, and lying on a spinal board may produce significant flexion of their cervical spine and/or obstruct their airway. Modified spinal boards with a recess for the occiput or a pad to raise the chest have been suggested. Orotracheal intubation in children is usually performed using an uncuffed tube. A guide for the size of the appropriate tube is the size of the little finger.

Managing circulation also follows the adult principles. It is useful to remember that the circulating blood volume of a child is 80mL/kg body weight. An estimate of the child's weight is given by the following equation:

$$(\text{age in years} \times 2) + 8\text{kg}$$

In children, hypotension occurs when blood volume loss is in excess of 45% and the patient can rapidly deteriorate and become comatose. It is important to remember that vital signs are age dependent: an infant can normally have a pulse rate of 160 beats per minute, a blood pressure of 80mmHg, and 40 respirations per minute, while for an older child these values would correspond to hypovolaemia and shock.

An alternative method for fluid resuscitation in children under the age of 6 years is intraosseous infusion. The proximal tibial or distal femoral metaphysis can be accessed but infusion in the proximity of fractures should be avoided. Infusion rate is similar to intravenous rate.

Urine output is age dependent and this should be remembered when assessing circulation in the injured child. Output is 1–2mL/kg/h in infants, 0.5–1mL/kg/h in children, and 0.5mL/kg/h in adolescents.

Part of the resuscitation protocol includes assessing the neurological status of the patient. A paediatric modification of the Glasgow Coma Scale is used for this purpose (Table 14.1.2). The 'best verbal response' part of the scoring is the only variable which has been modified.

Musculoskeletal injuries are common in the multiply injured child, with fractures of the long bones of the lower limb and the humerus being the most frequent. About 10% of the fractures in polytrauma are open. Central musculoskeletal injuries, involving the clavicle, scapula, spine, or pelvis, are more often associated with low trauma scores, long hospital admission, complications, and mortality. Early diagnosis helps in reducing the morbidity and mortality of these injuries.

Musculoskeletal injuries can be missed in the early stages of resuscitation and management. The priority of treating potentially life-threatening conditions is often the reason for overlooking skeletal trauma. Furthermore, imaging of the immature skeleton may often be more challenging.

Table 14.1.2 Glasgow Coma Scale—children's best verbal response

Variable	Score
Smiler, oriented to sound, follows objects, interacts	5
Consolable when crying, interacts inappropriately	4
Inconsistently consolable, moans	3
Inconsolable, irritable, restless	2
No response	1

Treatment

Options

Treatment options in children are largely similar to those in the adult. External immobilization or internal fixation are the two main forms of treatment and each has a variety of alternative methods available.

Traction, skin or skeletal, using different frames and devices has been the treatment of choice for many fractures. However, this requires prolonged hospital admission and close supervision, both clinical and radiographic. The impact of the prolonged hospital admission on the young patient's psychology, the family implications, and other socioeconomic factors have now made traction a less favoured form of treatment.

Plaster cast immobilization, with or without previous manipulation and reduction of the fracture, is the treatment of choice for a large number of paediatric fractures. Immobilization of adjacent non-injured joints has very low morbidity in children who, almost without exception, recover full movement soon after removal of casts. Loss of fracture position ischaemia due to soft tissue swelling, and poor cast application are potential complications.

Functional bracing is an alternative external immobilization method for some fracture types. This allows joint movement while providing some stability to the fracture. Functional braces for the long bones of the upper as well as the lower extremity have been suggested.

A number of fractures in children are optimally treated with K-wire fixation following closed or open reduction. While this method is often insufficient for fixation of adult fractures, it works well in children where deforming forces are weaker and fractures heal faster. K-wire fixation is often supplemented by plaster casts. Wires are left prominent through the skin and do not usually require a second anaesthetic for removal. Potential complications include pin tract infection, ectopic ossification, and migration. Biodegradable pin fixation has been suggested as an alternative to avoid these complications. Polyglycolic acid pins are buried into bone and the risk of infection, ectopic ossification, or the need for further anaesthesia are much lower. They offer similar quality of fixation with ordinary K-wires but their insertion is technically more demanding.

Flexible intramedullary nails have become the treatment of choice for most long-bone fractures in children. The fracture site is not exposed, periosteal stripping is avoided, and stability is adequate for the low level of loading that is present in children. Overgrowth or malunion have not been observed and the only reported complication is skin ulceration at the ends of prominent nails, requiring early removal. Flexible nails offer optimal treatment for multiply injured children where fast and adequate early stabilization is essential. The use of external fixation devices is indicated mostly in open fractures with extensive soft tissue damage and/or bone loss. Open reduction and internal fixation with plate and screws is indicated in intra-articular and metaphyseal/epiphyseal injuries where anatomical reduction is essential.

Indications for surgical treatment

Absolute and relative indications for surgical treatment of children's fractures vary between centres. Specific experience with paediatric fractures is necessary for correct decision-making upon surgical treatment. Absolute and relative indications for surgical treatment are shown in Table 14.1.3 and discussed in the following sections.

Absolute indications

Open fractures require surgical exploration and debridement to prevent infection. All grades require attention and intervention. Grade I fractures with minimal skin laceration may be complicated by anaerobic infection or compartment syndrome and need prompt exploration. Stabilization of the fracture and soft tissue coverage where appropriate are also essential.

Multiply injured children with multiple long-bone fractures require surgical stabilization. This makes nursing and rehabilitation easier and facilitates treatment of other systemic injuries.

Neurovascular damage to the fractured limb, requiring repair, is an indication for surgical treatment to provide stability and facilitate repair. Vascular supply to the limb may be obstructed by the displaced fracture and limb oedema, without vascular injury. Fracture reduction facilitates blood flow through the vessel. At times, however, a vessel or nerve may be trapped into the fracture and attempts at closed reduction may cause further neurovascular injury.

Relative indications

Displaced intra-articular fractures do not remodel and require anatomical reduction and stabilization. Furthermore, the majority of these fractures in children are at the same time complex physeal fractures (type III or IV) which carry the potential of growth disturbance. This adds to the indication for anatomical reduction and stable fixation.

Older children who are close to skeletal maturity and have little remodelling potential should be treated as adults. When all the indications for surgery listed here are considered, the age of the child should be taken into account first as it represents the single most important factor influencing the final decision.

Children with conditions such as neuromuscular disorders which result in muscle spasticity, fracture immobilization, and maintenance of reduction may often be a challenge. Fixation of the fracture may offer an uneventful recovery and rehabilitation. Children with metabolic bone disease or skeletal dysplasias may also require particular attention and conservative treatment may be inadequate.

Late intervention may be required when early conservative treatment has failed. Failure of the fracture to produce early callus may be due to soft tissue interposition and may require surgical intervention.

There are fractures in specific locations in the skeleton that are prone to non-union. Furthermore, fractures at sites of muscle or tendon attachment may be inherently unstable and often require fixation.

Pathological fractures may need excision of the bone lesion and grafting, depending on the underlying pathology. Fixation may also be required in cases of instability or in high stress areas. Histological diagnosis is essential before proceeding with fracture fixation.

Table 14.1.3 Indications for surgical treatment in children's fractures

Indication	Conditions
Absolute	Open fractures
	Polytrauma/multiple fractures
	Neurovascular damage
Relative	Displaced intra-articular/complex physeal fracture
	Older children/adolescents
	Pre-existing disorder (neurologic, metabolic, bone dysplasia)
	Failed conservative treatment
	Specific fractures/delayed union
	Pathologic fractures

Non-accidental injury

Physicians involved in the care of children at any level should be aware of the possible diagnosis of non accidental injury and have a high index of suspicion when infants and young children are involved. In cases where the diagnosis of child abuse is missed and patients are discharged from hospital care, the risk of further non accidental injury is 20% with a 5% risk of lethal injury. The majority of deaths from injury under the age of 1 year are the result of child abuse.

In order to avoid missing the diagnosis or overdiagnosing child abuse, standard hospital, regional, and national protocols and guidelines for suspected child abuse that involve senior medical personnel with experience in children from the early stages of the procedure are necessary. All health care professionals who interact with children should be aware of these protocols and report any suspected cases of non-accidental injury through the appropriate channels.

Risk factors and presentation

An unsettled family environment with immaturity or emotional instability of the parent(s), failure to cope with the crying baby, failure to establish bonding, drug and alcohol abuse, and social deprivation may increase the likelihood of non-accidental injury. However, it is not necessary for any of these factors to be present and incidents of child abuse may present in apparently settled and happy families. In an analysis of non-accidental injuries leading to death, no risk factors within the families could be identified. There was no recognizable pattern in the age and sex of the abusers, nor their ethnic origin and social and marital status.

Indications in the presentation and history of the injury may raise a suspicion of child abuse. The mechanism of injury as described by the parents/guardians may not fit with the degree and nature of the resulting injury. The history may differ between parents/guardians or discrepancies may exist when the history is repeated. A significant delay in seeking medical advice should raise suspicions. This is not necessarily true with subtle injuries, such as undisplaced greenstick fractures, but it is unusual for complete long-bone fractures not to be noticed.

Box 14.1.11 Child abuse—diagnosis

- Document
- Clinical photographs
- Exclude leukemia, osteogenesis, etc.

Repeated injuries in the same child, particularly when treated at different places, poor compliance with treatment, and non-attendance at follow-up appointments may be indicative of abuse.

Injury patterns

The typical 'battered child syndrome', as described by Caffey, includes a combination of multiple fractures at various stages of healing, subdural haematoma, failure to thrive, soft tissue swellings, and skin bruising. Some of the musculoskeletal injuries, although not unique, may be characteristic of the abused child and raise suspicions. Since the original recognition and description of child abuse, the patterns have changed with subdural haematomas and fractures being present in a smaller percentage of patients. In a recent epidemiological study, however, the most common non-orthopaedic injury was found to be the injury to the head, with or without skull fracture. The most common fractures were those of the femur and humerus.

Fractures

Fractures occur in a relatively small percentage of abused children, probably in the range of 10–15%.

Characteristic metaphyseal injuries include the chip fracture with periosteal avulsion and irregular/diffuse metaphyseal changes, while complete physeal separation is rare. Impaction and buckle fractures may occur, but these are also common in accidental injuries.

Metaphyseal injuries in children occur from indirect shear forces applied when the extremity is pulled, pushed or twisted, or when the infant is shaken. The fracture occurs proximally to the physis and a disk of bone is avulsed from the metaphysis. This disk has a peripheral margin that is thicker and denser than its central part, as a result of its protection by the subperiosteal bone collar at the chondro-osseous junction. The peripheral margin is therefore the most conspicuous component of the fracture which, when viewed tangentially, results in a corner-fracture (chip fracture) appearance and when viewed obliquely results in a bucket-handle appearance.

Diaphyseal fractures and spiral humeral fractures under 2 years are highly suspicious; the most common and transverse ones may be more common than spiral. Abundant callus formation, with or without gross deformity, is often seen due to the lack of fracture immobilization. Furthermore, several fractures at different stages of healing are characteristic.

Periosteal elevation is often seen in the metaphysis or diaphysis of long bones. However, normal infants may have symmetric long-bone periosteal elevation with double-cortex appearance persisting up to the age of 2 years.

Rib fractures, otherwise uncommon in children, may be seen in cases of abuse. Skull fractures and widened sutures are characteristic and spinal injuries may be observed.

Soft tissue injuries

The vast majority of abused children have soft tissue injuries. The age of the child is an important parameter when studying soft tissue injuries. Infants rarely present with soft tissue injuries after accidents. Abused infants have at least one major soft tissue injury at presentation, the head and face being the most common location. Abused children over the age of 3 years usually present with three or more soft tissue injuries. Head and face injuries, and particularly perioral trauma, are also common in this age group.

Burns should also raise suspicions, particularly the round, sharply demarcated burns from cigarettes or third-degree burns in areas that are not usually exposed. Rope marks or linear ecchymoses are also characteristic. Visceral rupture without a history of major blunt trauma and trauma to the perineum and genitalia should also alarm the physician.

Diagnosis (Box 14.1.11)

History and clinical examination is the cornerstone of diagnosis of child abuse. If suspicion is raised, a senior physician with experience in children, usually a paediatrician, should be involved as part of a standard hospital procedure. All injuries should be recorded carefully and clinical photographs should be obtained for any external injuries. An impression of the family background and the rapport between child and parents/guardians should be established.

Further investigations may include radiographs and blood tests. Radiographic examination of clinically suspicious areas for new or old fractures is often sufficient. A complete skeletal survey is needed in cases of uncertainty and often in young infants. Isotope bone scans can create confusion because of the presence of the physes.

Determining the age of fractures and soft-tissue injuries is often important in order to establish the diagnosis of non-accidental injury. The radiographic appearance of a healing fracture depends on the age of the fracture and the age of the patient. Knowledge of the expected speed of healing and the corresponding radiographic appearance is important. Furthermore, the degree of soft tissue swelling at first presentation indicates how recent the injury is and may indicate delay in seeking medical advice.

A full blood count is necessary to exclude iron-deficient anaemia, leukaemia, and other haematological conditions that may cause bruising and petechiae. Coagulation tests to exclude haemophilia may also be needed. Copper level in serum can be ordered when multiple epiphyseal spurs are observed on radiographs. The differential diagnosis of child abuse is summarized in Table 14.1.4. Child abuse should be differentiated from conditions that cause multiple fractures or multiple soft tissue bruising.

Type IV osteogenesis imperfecta remains the most difficult type to differentiate because of its mild clinical presentation and the absence of blue sclerae. Collagen testing is available in specialized centres and can sometimes be helpful.

The diagnosis of one of the discussed conditions does not necessarily exclude child abuse, as these may coexist.

Table 14.1.4 Differential diagnosis of child abuse

Condition	Common characteristics	Differential diagnosis
Hemophillia, purpura, leukemia	Bruising, petechiae, periosteal reaction	Family history Blood tests
Copper deficiency	Metaphyseal spurs osteoporotic fractures	Serum copper
Osteogenesis imperfecta	Diaphyseal fractures	Family history, wormian bone (skull), blue sclerae
Neurologic/ neuromuscular conditions	Osteoporotic fractures	Clinical examination

Further reading

Loder, R.T. and Feinberg, J.R. (2007). Orthopaedic injuries in children with nonaccidental trauma: demographics and incidence from the 2000 kids' inpatient database. *Journal of Pediatric Orthopedics,* **27,** 421–6.

McCollough, N.C., Vinsant, J.E., and Sarmiento, A. (1978). Functional fracture bracing of long-bone fractures of the lower extremity in children. *Journal of Bone and Joint Surgery,* **60A**, 314–19.

Murray, D.M., Wilson-MacDonald, J., Morscher, E., Rahn, B.A., and Kaslin, M. (1996). Bone growth and remodelling after fracture. *Journal of Bone and Joint Surgery,* **78B**, 42–50.

Rennie, L., Court-Brown, C.M., Mok, J.Y., and Beattie, T.F. (2007). The epidemiology of fractures in children. *Injury,* **38,** 913–22.

Witherow, P.J. (1994). Non-accidental injury. In: Benson, M.K.D., Fixsen, J.A., and Macnicol, M.F. (eds) *Children's Orthopaedics and Fractures* pp. 749–53. Edinburgh: Churchill Livingstone.

14.2

Physeal injuries

G. Spence and Deborah M. Eastwood

Summary points

- Damage to the physis may lead to slowing or angulation of growth, especially if a bone bar forms
- Fractures involving the physis may be difficult to diagnose on x-ray
- The Salter–Harris classification is commonly used
- Fixation of fractures should not cross the physis if it can be avoided
- Partial growth arrest may be best treated with a complete epiphysiodesis followed by reconstruction.

Essentials

The primary role of the physis is coordinated, longitudinal growth. An injury to the physis may recover without adverse effect, or it may go on to cause a growth disturbance. This may take the form of a slow-down in the rate of growth or an angular deformity, although an increase in the rate of growth is also seen after some injuries. Physeal fracture is the most common, but not the only cause of a physeal injury; many authors use these terms interchangeably. Although progress has been made in understanding the nature and types of physeal injuries, much remains unknown.

Introduction

The anatomy of the physis and its relation to function is largely understood; however, less is known of the physiology of the physis and its response to injury. It is known to respond to the genetic, hormonal, and nutritional environment as well as to the local influences of blood supply, innervation, and mechanical stress. Thus the physis is not just an area of supportive tissue like the rest of the growing skeleton, but a responsive, specialized organ with a function (growth) that is subject to a range of pathological 'injuries' including endocrinopathy, ischaemia, autoimmune disease, and of course trauma. The various causes of physeal injury are listed in Table 14.2.1. Meningococcal disease is a particularly potent cause of multiple severe growth arrests in survivors. The physis is characteristically resistant to infiltration by malignant tumours, but some benign tumours are associated with disturbance of physeal function with deformity.

Anatomy and pathology

The rates of growth of the different physes vary (Figure 14.2.1), fast in some (the distal femur for example) and slow in others. Histologically, the physis is a layered structure. In humans this layered appearance is only easily seen in fast growing physes. Different authors variously subdivide them into three, four, or five zones. The main zones are the germinal layer (or resting zone) from which the cellular columns originate and which is critical to physeal function; the proliferative zone, the hypertrophic zone, and the zone of calcification (Figure 14.2.2) (see also Chapter 1.3).

The physis is surrounded by the perichondrial ring which is contiguous with the articular cartilage of the epiphysis and to which the metaphyseal periosteum is firmly attached. It encircles the physis just as periosteum encircles the bone. As well as contributing cells to the germinal layer for latitudinal growth (the zone of Ranvier), the perichondrial ring plays an important role in

Table 14.2.1 Causes of physeal injury

	Examples
Traumatic	
Direct	Physeal fracture
Indirect (trauma elsewhere)	Overgrowth after diaphyseal fracture
Iatrogenic	Transphyseal trauma implants
Non-traumatic	
Infection	Disseminated meningococcal disease
Tumour	Ollier's disease, osteochondroma
Endocrinopathy	Acromegaly, hypothyroidism
Vascular	AV fistula causing overgrowth
Neurological	Shortening after poliomyelitis
Developmental	Madelung deformity, Blount's disease
Idiopathic	Hemihypertrophy, hemiatrophy

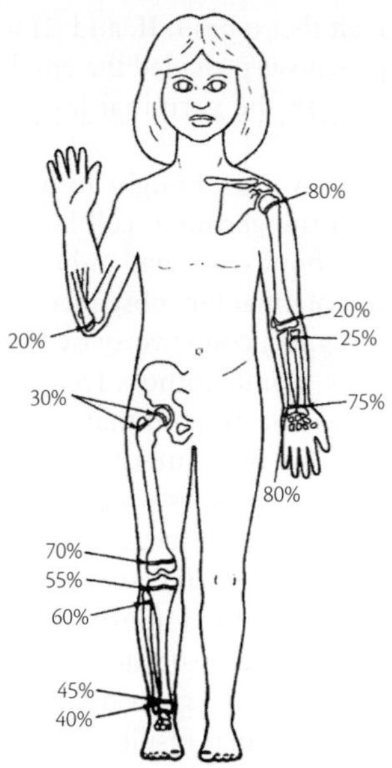

Fig. 14.2.1 The relative contribution to the longitudinal growth of the different physes of the long tubular bones. Reproduced from Skak, S.V. and Macnicol, M.F. (2000). A clinical approach to the assessment of physeal injuries. *Current Orthopaedics*, **14**, 267–77. With permission from Elsevier.

maintaining the structural integrity of the physis, in particular its resistance to shear and tensile forces. Logically a fracture line should take the path of least resistance and traverse the weakest of the layers, the hypertrophic zone, which is characterized by large voids occupied by apoptotic cells and relatively little supporting matrix. However, experimental studies suggest that in practice the fracture line propagates variably through the physis and can involve all layers.

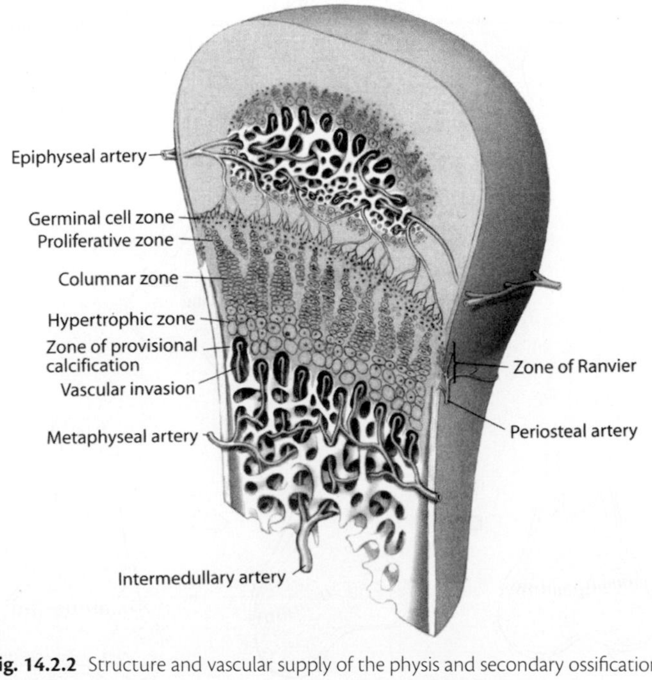

Fig. 14.2.2 Structure and vascular supply of the physis and secondary ossification centre. Reprinted from Peterson, H.A. (ed) (2007). *Epiphyseal Growth Plate Fractures*. Berlin Heidelberg. Springer-Verlag. With permission from Springer.

Although the physis itself is devoid of vascular channels, it receives a blood supply via three separate sources (see Figure 14.2.2). Arterioles descending from the epiphyseal vessels supply the dividing cells of the germinal layer of the physis, periosteal vessels nourish the perichondrial ring and the peripheral part of the physis, whilst the nutrient artery via its branches supplies the majority of the metaphyseal side of the physis. Damage to the epiphyseal vessels, which directly affects the nutrition of the germinal layer, is usually permanent and the consequences are severe. The damage prevents cell division in the region supplied by the vessel leading to differential physeal growth. Angular and/or longitudinal growth deformity may result. The central area of the physis appears more susceptible to vascular damage than the peripheral portion. By contrast, disruption of the metaphyseal circulation is usually transient. It does not affect chondrogenesis in the germinal cell layer or its maturation, but it does temporarily hinder the subsequent transformation of cartilage to bone.

Epidemiology

Little data is available on the incidence of physeal injuries in general. As regards fracture, if the data from three large recent studies are amalgamated, physeal fractures account for 24.8% of childhood fractures.

The much quoted Olmsted County study, which used a meticulously documented database and a stable population, reported an incidence of 279.2 acute physeal fractures per 100 000 person-years as well as a 2:1 male to female ratio and a peak incidence that corresponded to pubescence (age 14 in boys, 11–12 in girls). The latter might have a hormonal basis which results in a relative weakness of the physis at this time, although the frequency of fracture-prone behaviour at these ages may also be a factor.

Clinical features

Bone fracture is usually followed by pain and loss of function and the same features are apparent with physeal fractures. In a young child it may be difficult to localize the site of the injury and therefore careful examination is essential. Swelling, tenderness, abnormal movement, and crepitus are the cardinal signs of an acute injury. Do not forget to consider non-accidental injury as a possible aetiological factor, particularly in the case of fractures involving the entire distal humeral physis.

The gradual development of limb length discrepancy with or without angular deformity may be the late presenting features of trauma that is occult or has been overlooked. Other causes of physeal injury aside from trauma also typically present in this way (see Table 14.2.1).

Clinical investigation (Box 14.2.1)

Plain radiographs are the basic means of investigation of physeal injuries and the accurate interpretation of radiographic features is required if acute physeal fractures are to be classified. However, the physis itself is radiolucent and assessment of the injury involves looking at the adjacent radiodense epiphysis and metaphysis. A single radiograph provides only a one-dimensional view of the complex three-dimensional structure that comprises the physis and even with two views at right angles to each other, only a limited appreciation of the injury is achieved. Radiographs should be

Box 14.2.1 Investigations

- Plain radiographs
  - At least two views
  - Standing long leg (for assessing late deformity)
- CT
- Ultrasound
- Arthrography.

taken at right angles to the physis (rather than the diaphysis). Supplementary oblique views are often necessary when assessing physeal fractures around the knee and ankle, and stress views can be useful in injures around a uniplanar joint. For assessing late deformity following physeal injury, plain radiographs are crucial for determining the location, extent, and progression of the problem. Standing long leg films, with the patellae pointing forwards and the pelvis level (by placing the shorter leg on blocks if necessary), require a similar radiation dose to a computerized tomography (CT) scanogram and have the advantage of imaging the weight-bearing position. The advent of digital imaging and viewing has made these films far more manageable for measurement purposes.

CT is useful to identify the degree of fragmentation and the orientation of the pieces, particularly in complex fracture patterns such as Tillaux or triplane injuries. Reconstructed images can be particularly helpful. In late cases, it can be used to image osseous bars. Although magnetic resonance imaging (MRI) has theoretical advantages with its ability to demonstrate cartilage and soft tissue, the severity of the bone and soft tissue oedema which accompanies the injury limits its use and its exact role has not yet been determined.

In very young children with small secondary ossification centres, ultrasound is occasionally used for diagnostic purposes; similarly arthrography can be useful for diagnosis and guiding treatment when the injury pattern is unclear.

Classification

Classification systems of acute physeal injuries are based on radiographic appearances. The Salter-Harris classification remains the most popular (Box 14.2.2). This defines five patterns of physeal injury. The authors felt that types I, II, and III were generally associated with a good prognosis provided the epiphyseal blood supply remained intact, because the germinal layer in theory remains largely undisturbed.

The uncommon type V was thought to involve a longitudinal compression injury to the germinal cell layer which showed no visible discontinuity of bone ('normal' radiographs in two planes) but which had a high potential for subsequent growth disturbance. There has been considerable controversy over the nature and incidence of type V injury. Some authors feel that the true isolated type V injury may indeed be rare but that a crushing element may be associated with other fracture patterns and that this may account for the unexpectedly bad outcomes which are known to occur, on occasion, even with type II or III fractures.

Rang extended the Salter–Harris classification to include a sixth category where there was localized injury to the perichondrial ring (Figure 14.2.3). The injury was associated with a high risk of subsequent growth disturbance and angular deformity, though whether this was due to localized vascular insult or crushing of physeal cells is unclear. Although the original description was of a direct blow to the perichondrial ring, many authors have interpreted this to include avulsion injuries of the ring and open injuries where portions of the metaphysis, physis, and epiphysis are lost or damaged. Such patterns have been described classically in association with lawnmower injuries and those that occur as a result of burns, frostbite, or extravasation injuries.

Box 14.2.2 Salter–Harris classification

- Type I: through the physis
- Type II: through the physis with metaphyseal fracture
- Type III: epiphyseal fracture
- Type IV: epiphyseal fracture extending across the physis to the metaphysis
- Type V: crush
- Type VI: perichondral ring injury – addition by Rang (1969).

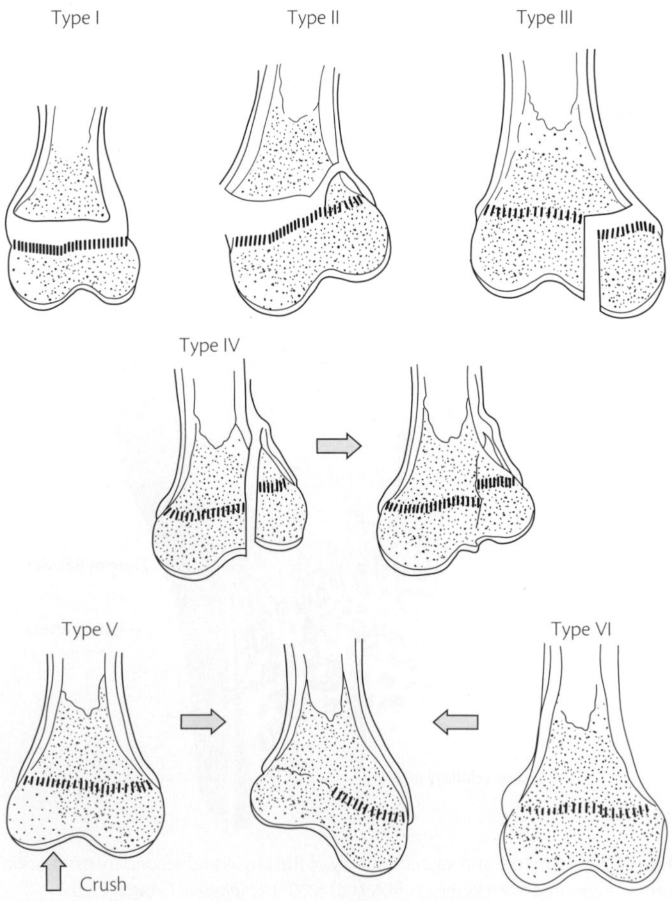

Fig. 14.2.3 Rang's modification of the Salter–Harris classification.

The relationship of this classification system to outcome is less predictable than was originally implied by Salter and Harris. Fracture line propagation is not as constant as was once thought and outcome is known to vary with many other factors including age, site, mechanism of injury, degree of displacement, and method of treatment as well as fracture type.

Other classification systems exist. With the shortcomings of the Salter–Harris classification in mind and based on the Olmsted County epidemiological study, Peterson has recently described a new classification system (Figure 14.2.4).

The advantages of this system are that it has an anatomical basis and depicts physeal injury as a continuum from relatively minor damage (Type I), through complete transphyseal involvement (Type III), to disruption of the physis with loss of some of the physeal cartilage (Type VI). It has an epidemiological basis as well, as the fracture types occur with decreasing frequency from Type II to Type VI. It includes two 'new' injury patterns not included in the Salter–Harris system; the Type I fracture (which is essentially a transverse metaphyseal fracture which extends to the physis), and the Type VI injury which occurs only in open injuries and involves loss of physeal cartilage and usually some epiphysis and metaphysis as well. There is also prognostic significance to this classification, in that from Type I to Type VI the need for immediate and late surgery goes up.

Some physeal fractures do not fit neatly into these classifications systems; examples are the Tilleaux and triplane fractures, which are multiplanar intra-articular fractures of the distal tibia occurring exclusively in patients close to skeletal maturity through a partially closed physis. For this reason they rarely cause significant growth arrest in practice, despite their anatomical similarities to physeal injuries of poor prognosis.

Treatment

In acute injuries, the aim of management is to reduce pain, regain function, and preserve growth potential if possible. These goals are most likely achieved by obtaining and maintaining an anatomical reduction of all components of the injury, especially the physeal plate and the articular surface, by open or closed means. A large gap between separated physeal layers tends to fill in with fibrous tissue which has the potential to become ossified and lead to growth disturbance given time and an adequate blood supply. Although the particular methods chosen will vary according to individual fracture patterns, fixation from epiphysis to epiphysis or metaphysis to metaphysis is preferred. Transfixation of the physis itself may cause further damage, but is sometimes unavoidable. Multiple passes across the physis should be avoided, and smooth removable metallic wires are ideal. Treatment needs to be prompt as physeal fractures heal in about half the time of the metaphysis of the corresponding bone.

For the late sequelae of physeal injury the focus is on preventing worsening deformity, and restoring function usually by restoring the correct anatomical relationships between body segments (see later).

Prognosis

The outcome of physeal injury is dependent on a number of variables (Box 14.2.3).

Of these, only the first (the anatomical extent of the lesion and displacement) can be influenced by medical treatment, which can 'reduce' it to some degree. However, even then the prognosis must be guarded. Severe growth disturbance can still result from seemingly benign fracture patterns, for example in Salter–Harris Type I and II distal femoral physeal fractures. This probably reflects the magnitude of the energy inflicted on the physis during the injury, and the tendency of the straight fracture line to cut across the undulating growth plate, thus involving all layers including the germinal layer. Intra-articular fractures of the femoral or radial neck often cause severe growth disturbance even in 'favourable' fracture types because the epiphyseal blood supply is frequently interrupted.

Complications

The two major complications are joint incongruity and growth disturbance and the two are often interrelated. Joint incongruity can follow the malunion of displaced intra-articular physeal fractures.

Box 14.2.3 Influences on the outcome of physeal injury

- Anatomical extent of the lesion (classification) and displacement
- Age at time of injury
- Type of physis (slow- or fast-growing, see Figure 14.2.1)
- Effect upon rate of growth (increase, decrease, arrest)
- Duration of growth disturbance (temporary, permanent).

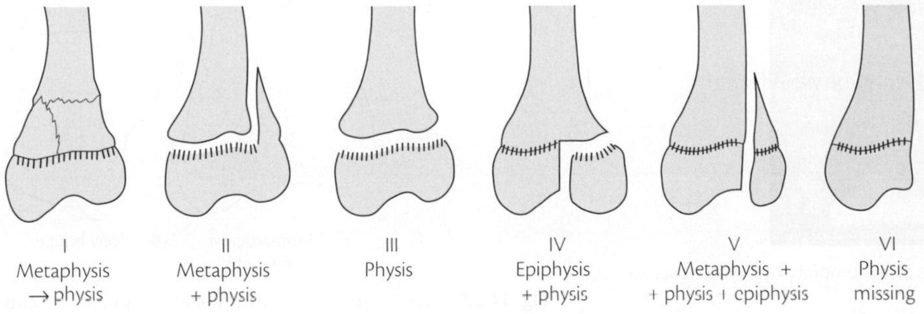

Fig. 14.2.4 Classification system according to Peterson. Reproduced fromPeterson, H.A., Madhok, R., Benson, J.T., et al. (1994). Physeal fractures: Part 1. Epidemiology in Olmsted County, Minnesota. *Journal of Pediatric Orthopedics*, **14**, 423–30.

Such fractures are often associated with displacement at the level of the physis and thus the effects of the joint incongruity become worse with time as the associated growth arrest increases the degree of the deformity. In theory, degenerative change will occur but there is little evidence to support this in the literature.

The physeal response to injury varies. Minor trauma to the physis, such as that arising in association with a diaphyseal fracture, can cause a temporary and usually benign overgrowth. With increasing energy of the insult the cellular response in the physis shifts from hyperactivity to necrosis and the rate of growth slows. Growth disturbance of this type is called a growth arrest, which may be partial or complete.

Complete arrest is uncommon but usually results in a progressive limb length discrepancy, the effect of which varies with the age at which the arrest occurs (Figure 14.2.5). Additional problems arise if the bone affected is one of a pair, for example the radius and ulna.

Temporary cessation of longitudinal growth following trauma is marked by the appearance of a so-called Harris line in the adjacent metaphysis (Figure 14.2.6). The Harris line will appear to 'migrate' away from the physis on sequential radiographs once growth resumes, and it should remain parallel to it. If the Harris line and the physis appear to converge however, then a partial growth arrest is occurring.

Partial arrest is more common, and usually results from trauma. The size and location of the bony tether determine the clinical deformity, though all are associated with a degree of shortening. The age at injury and remaining growth potential define the ultimate severity. Three basic categories have been described: central, peripheral, and elongated (Figure 14.2.7). Central arrests tend to cause so-called 'fishtail' deformities of the articular surface (Figure 14.2.8).

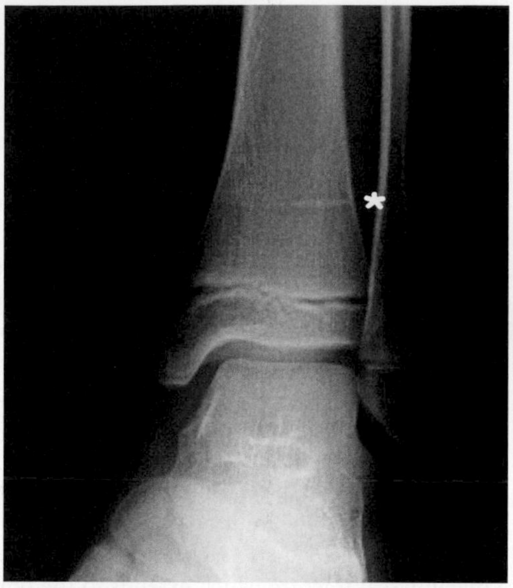

Fig. 14.2.6 Harris line (asterisk) in the distal tibia. The patient had a road traffic collision 3 years previously, without a fracture; normal growth has proceeded.

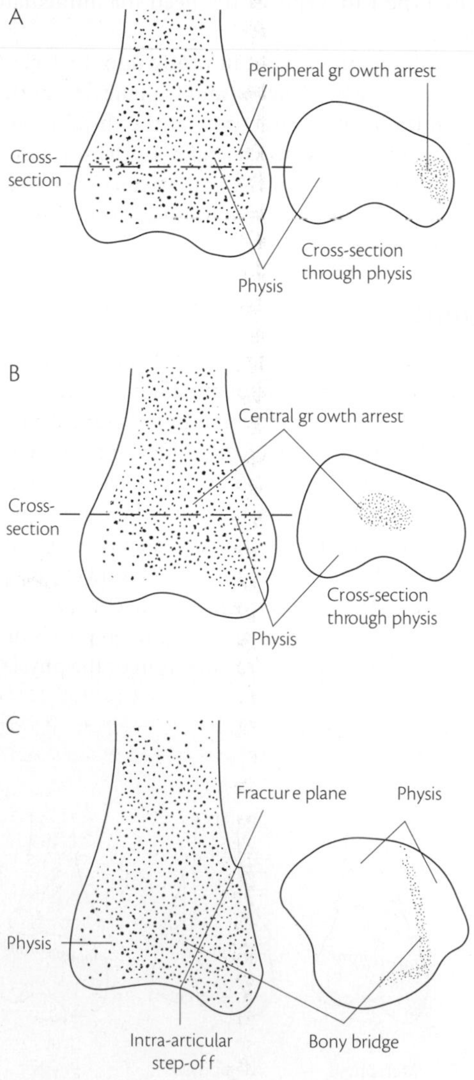

Fig. 14.2.7 Types of partial growth arrest: A) peripheral; B) central; C) elongated.

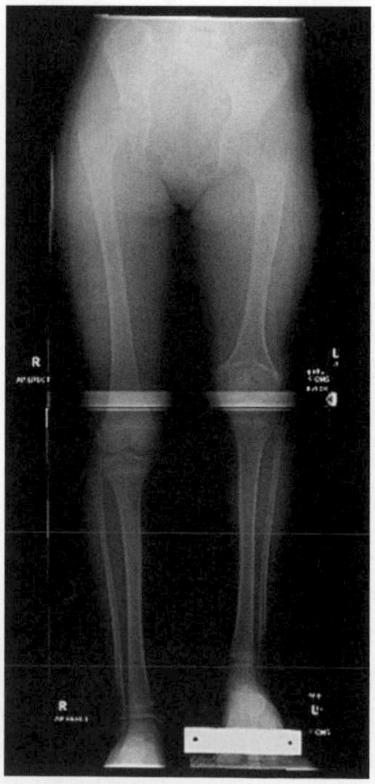

Fig. 14.2.5 Complete growth arrest of the distal femoral physis secondary to trauma in infancy.

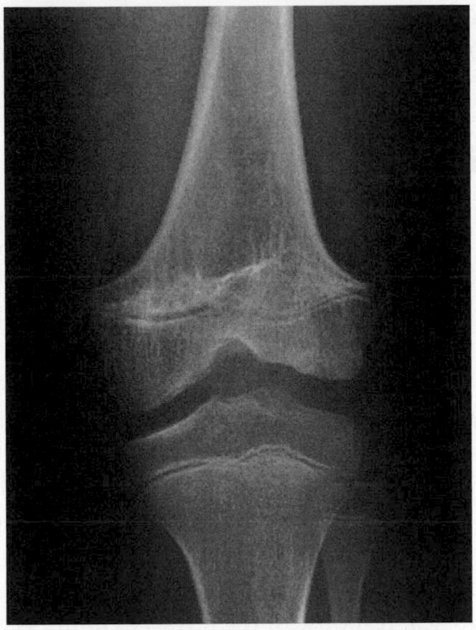

Fig. 14.2.8 'Fishtail' deformity of the distal femur due to a central growth arrest.

Peripheral arrests cause angular deformity (Figure 14.2.9). Elongated arrests commonly develop after Salter–Harris III or IV fractures of the medial malleolus or lateral humeral condyle. Partial arrests may be associated with a bony bar, but not invariably so; similarly, a radiographically open physis does not guarantee that normal growth will proceed.

Once identified, partial growth arrest may be treated in various ways and a combination of treatments may be necessary, including epiphysiodesis of the contralateral limb, ipsilateral leg lengthening, corrective osteotomy, acute shortening, and bony bar excision depending on the existing clinical problem and the predicted problem at skeletal maturity. It may be better to convert a partial arrest into a complete arrest by surgical epiphysiodesis, and deal with the resulting leg length discrepancy later as in general this is an easier option than correcting major angular deformity.

Apophyseal injuries

The apophysis is associated with a major muscle attachment and linked to the shaft of the bone by a physeal plate. This traction physis is subjected to tensile forces which serve to shape the bone (Box 14.2.4). In contrast to other physes, these plates are not usually perpendicular to the long axis of the bone and only in certain sites do they contribute to joint congruity (proximal ulna, periacetabular, and periglenoid areas). Injury is caused by direct trauma or by a sudden major muscular contraction which disrupts the tendon–physis–bone unit when physeal injury is more likely than tendon rupture. The physeal vascular supply is via its muscle attachments and damage is unusual. If it does occur, the germinal layer of the physis is affected leading to plate closure. Most injuries happen around the time of physiological plate closure; between the ossification and fusion of the apophysis and the peak incidence for injuries is in the adolescent years. The radiological appearances of healing apophyseal fractures can be quite alarming, characterized by florid callus which can take on the appearance of an osteogenic sarcoma. Biopsy of such a lesion is not reassuring as large numbers of mitotic osteogenic cells will be seen, hence the importance of a careful history if diagnostic confusion is to be avoided. At this age, significant growth disturbance does not occur. The major apophyses are listed in Box 14.2.5.

The outcome of these injuries is dependent on the degree of displacement of the apophysis and the muscles attached to it. It is thought that muscle strength is reduced when displacement is greater than 1cm although there is little scientific evidence to support this argument and thus open reduction and internal fixation is advocated in certain cases. A symptomatic non-union or malunion is treated similarly or by excision.

Future directions

New or improved imaging modalities may identify new physeal injury patterns which may in turn lead to a new classification

Box 14.2.4 Traction physis (apophysis)

- Associated with muscle attachments
- Injury
  - Direct trauma
  - Muscle contraction
- Peak incidence in adolescence.

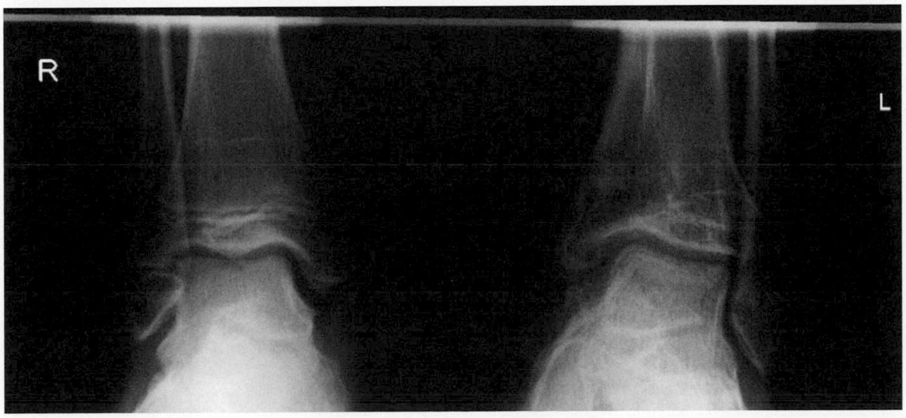

Fig. 14.2.9 Angular deformity of the left distal tibia due to a peripheral partial growth arrest. Note the Harris line in the contralateral distal tibia.

Box 14.2.5 Apophyses which may be subject to injury

- Upper limb:
  - Coracoid
  - Olecranon
  - Medial humeral epicondyle
  - Coronoid process of the ulna
- Lower limb:
  - Greater and lesser trochanters
  - Calcaneal apophysis
  - Tibial tuberosity
- Pelvis:
  - Anterosuperior and anteroinferior iliac spines
  - Iliac crest
  - Periacetabular rim
  - Ischial tuberosity.

system that might predict prognosis more accurately than current systems and therefore guide treatment more appropriately.

Distraction osteogenesis can address shortening and angular deformity, and this technique can also be applied across the physis to distract it and encourage new bone formation. It has recently been used to treat physeal bars, with or without excision. However it tends to be reserved for older children as although considerable length can be gained, the physis tends to fuse once treatment has stopped.

Replacing physeal cartilage by transplantation of physeal tissue or iliac apophysis has been attempted with some success in the experimental and clinical settings, but the technique is hampered by a lack of donor sites. Therefore considerable work is now being directed experimentally at attempts to regenerate physeal tissue. So-called mesenchymal 'stem' cells harvested from periosteum and embedded in a biocompatible scaffold have been shown to correct leg length discrepancy and angular deformity in an experimental model of a physeal defect in rabbits. The effects of the biological manipulation of physeal cells with cytokines such as osteogenic protein-1 (OP-1) are also under investigation, with some favourable results.

Conclusions

Physeal fractures usually heal quickly. For acute injuries the aim of treatment is the prompt anatomical reduction of the injured physis in the hope that normal growth will resume after healing. Predicting whether a problem will arise is not easy, although classification systems give a guide. The ultimate outcome of a physeal injury depends on many factors besides the fracture type including the age of the patient and the rate of growth of the physis concerned, and most of these factors are not under the control of the surgeon.

Whilst physeal fractures are common, permanent physeal injury resulting from them is fortunately relatively rare except in certain subtypes (e.g. Salter–Harris IV injuries). There are many other less common causes of physeal injury apart from trauma. The pathophysiological response of the physis to injury is incompletely understood but various responses have been observed including overgrowth, slow-down, growth arrest, and angular deformity. Treatment of these problems involves a variety of techniques to attempt to restore normal anatomy. Regeneration of injured physeal tissue may be available to clinicians in the future.

Further reading

Peterson, H.A. (2007). *Epiphyseal Growth Plate Fractures.* Berlin Heidelberg: Springer-Verlag.

Peterson, H.A., Madhok, R., Benson, J.T., *et al.* (1994). Physeal fractures: Part 1. Epidemiology in Olmsted County, Minnesota. *Journal of Pediatric Orthopedics*, **14**, 423–30.

Rathjen, K.E. and Birch, J.G. (2006). Physeal injuries and growth disturbances. In: Beaty, J.H. and Kasser, J.R. (eds) *Rockwood and Wilkins' Fractures in Children*, sixth edition, pp.99–131. Philadelphia, PA: Lippincott Williams and Wilkins.

Salter, R. B. and W. R. Harris (1963). Injuries involving the epiphyseal plate. *Journal of Bone and Joint Surgery*, **45**, 587–621.

Skak, S.V. and Macnicol, M.F. (2000). A clinical approach to the assessment of physeal injuries. *Current Orthopaedics*, **14**, 267–77.

Xian, C.J. and Foster, B.K. (2006). The biologic aspects of children's fractures. In: Beaty, J.H. and Kasser, J.R. (eds) *Rockwood and Wilkins' Fractures in Children*, sixth edition, pp.21–50. Philadelphia, PA: Lippincott Williams and Wilkins.

14.3

Fractures of the spine in children

James Wilson-MacDonald and Colin Nnadi

Summary points

- Spinal injuries in children are rare
- Pseudosubluxation above C4 is common in healthy children so the sign needs careful interpretation
- Epiphyseal plates and a high incidence of skeletal variability make the interpretation of spinal x-rays in children difficult. Anterior wedging is also normal as is interpedicular widening
- Spinal cord injury without radiographic abnormality (SCIWORA) may occur for up to one-third of spinal injuries in children
- Deformity secondary to trauma tends to deteriorate with growth.

Introduction

Fractures of the spine are rare in skeletally immature children and represent only 2–5% of all spinal injuries (7 per 100 000 population annually). There are characteristic features of spinal injuries in children because of the mechanisms involved and certain predisposing factors. The mechanism of injury usually involves recreational activities. There are also injuries which may occur at birth or secondary to congenital conditions. Non-accidental causes are a very important differential in this age group.

There are ossification centres and synchondroses which have not fused. The paraspinal soft tissue envelope is undergoing development as well. There is differential growth between the soft tissue element of the spinal column and the bony element. The net effect is a bony column which is capable of stretching beyond the limits of the spinal cord and causing injury. There are also the physes of the vertebral bodies which are susceptible to injury. Physeal damage can result in growth deformities that affect canal dimensions and spinal symmetry. The spinal canal reaches adult size in the first decade. There can be neurological compromise from displaced cartilaginous fragments which are not seen on plain radiographs.

Normal anatomical variations in children

There is a larger head to body ratio in children. It is also common for pseudosubluxation to occur in children above the C4 level. Pseudosubluxation can easily be interpreted as instability and is relatively common in children. About 9% of children between the ages of 1–7 years demonstrate pseudosubluxation between C2 and C3 normally.

Vertebral body translation of up to 4mm is acceptable. Forty per cent of children show excessive anterior displacement between C2 and C3 or between C3 and C4. The spinolaminar line posteriorly should remain intact. There may also be widening of the atlantodens interval when compared to adults. Up to 20% of children aged 1–7 years demonstrate overriding of the atlas on the odontoid process, seen in extension radiography. This may also be defined when more than two-thirds of the anterior arch of the atlas lies above the odontoid.

The prevertebral soft tissue mass should not exceed more than two-thirds of the width of the vertebral body on lateral views in the upper cervical spine. In the lower cervical spine the tissue dimensions can be up to twice as thick. Occasionally a synchondrosis of the odontoid can be misinterpreted as a fracture. Anatomical variations in the lumbosacral region are not uncommon. There is an abnormal lumbosacral transition in a significant number of patients. This can be in the form of lumbarization of the first sacral vertebra or sacralization of the fifth lumbar vertebra. There can also be segmentation anomalies between the transverse processes of L5 and the ilium. Another incidental finding is spina bifida occulta.

Abnormal anatomical variation in children

The C1–C2 articulation is the most mobile and lies between two relatively stiff joints. This is probably why it is prone to injury. More than 10 degrees of angulation or an atlantodens interval of more than 5mm is considered abnormal in a child. The definition of instability of the lower cervical spine is not well defined in children. In general an interspinous distance greater than 1.5 times normal is considered pathological. Other abnormal signs on radiography include divergence of the articular processes and widening of the posterior disc space.

The immature spine

It is important to recognize the physes in the spine because they can resemble fractures. The atlas and axis vertebrae have their own special physes; C3 and below are all similar.

The atlas has three ossification centres, one anteriorly for the body and two for the two neural arches (Figure 14.3.1). Sometimes the ring is bifid anteriorly. The posterior arch closes during the third year of life, although occasionally it can remain open into adult life. The axis has four ossification centres. Like the atlas it has one for the body and one each for the neural arches, but it also has one for the dens. When viewed anteriorly this resembles the letter H. Occasionally the body has two ossification centres. The physis between the odontoid and the body fuses between the ages of 3–6 years and can resemble a type 2 odontoid fracture. However, it lies well below the level of the articular facets. The lower ring apophysis ossifies in late childhood and does not close until early adult life. The tip of the odontoid has a 'summit' ossification centre, which appears between the ages of 3–6 years and fuses by the age of 12. It may persist as an 'ossiculum terminale' and should be not confused with an os odontoidenum which is a separation of the odontoid from the body of the axis.

In hyperextension the arch of C1 may appear to be in the foramen magnum on computed tomography (CT) scan in children under the age of 2. The posterior aspect of the dens may have a defect which is the remnant of the right and left growth centres. This may be seen up to the age of 7.

The lower cervical spine ossifies from three centres, one from the body and one from each of the neural arches. These fuse between the third and sixth years. Each vertebra has cartilage endplates which contribute to growth as in a long bone, and these can fracture across. The inferior endplate is most prone to fracture because the uncinate processes protect the upper growth plate.

The apophyseal rings ossify in late childhood and fuse to the vertebral body at about the age of 25.

It is important to note that surgical intervention may disrupt open physis or synchondroses thereby resulting in asymmetrical growth.

Aetiology

The pattern of injury in children under the age of 10 is quite different from that in older children. The characteristic anatomical features of the upper cervical spine in this age group means that most injuries occur above C4. While injuries in those aged 10 or under are less common, cord injury and death are more common in this group.

The pattern of injury in children over the age of 10 is similar to that in adults, and in general the management is similar. Most of these injuries are caused by high-energy trauma. A less common but significant cause is non-accidental trauma.

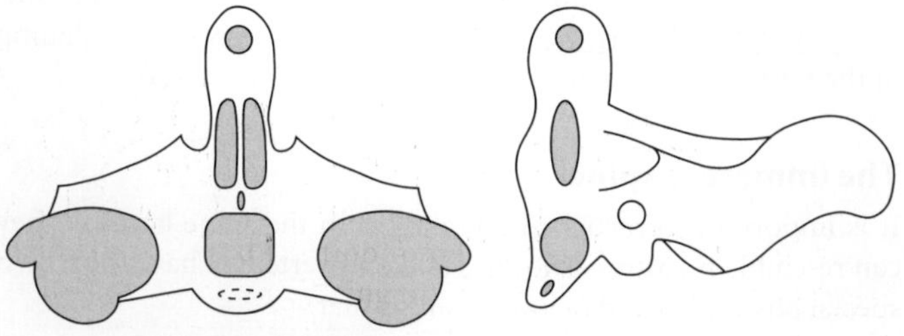

Fig. 14.3.1 Atlas ossification centres.

Box 14.3.1 Problems in diagnosing spinal injuries in children

- Spinal column injuries are rare in children
- Variations in anatomy exist
- Injuries can arise from differential lengthening of the spinal column.

Clinical features

It is important to establish the mechanism of injury and assess for other life-threatening trauma. Where there is no obvious cause, non-accidental injury should be suspected. It is often very difficult to establish a mechanism of injury from a child who is either very distressed or comatose. A history should be obtained from the ambulance crew, relatives, or eyewitnesses at the scene of the accident. It is important to elicit any history of sustained or transient motor dysfunction as this may be indicative of instability. These children should be immobilized on a specially adapted spinal board avoiding hyperflexion of the neck. An initial ABC assessment should be performed. Any child with major trauma should be suspected of having a spinal cord injury. A neurological examination is done as part of the secondary survey. In the conscious child the presence or absence of limb movement should be noted. Light touch and pin prick sensation should be quantified. A log roll is performed to assess skin integrity, bruising, tenderness, and increased interspinous process gapping. A rectal examination should be performed and the bulbocavernosus reflex assessed for spinal shock.

In the comatose child with a suspicion of spinal cord injury, imaging of the whole spine should be obtained. In the conscious child radiological investigation is directed by clinical examination if the child is fully awake and cooperative.

Assessment of the infant for spinal trauma is an even more challenging prospect. On the whole, a thorough and repeated evaluation is required.

Radiological evaluation

Plain radiography in most centres remains the initial screening method of choice. The views are taken of the whole spine. The cervical views consist of anteroposterior, lateral, and open mouth views. Oblique views may also be appropriate. The lateral view should incorporate occiput to the cervicothoracic junction. The lateral views are also used to determine the Powers ratio although this formula has its shortcomings. Although a single lateral radiograph is sensitive for isolating injuries, 25% of injuries will be missed. Flexion–extension views may help to isolate an area of instability, but should only be carried out under supervision in a cooperative child. The bony articulations and soft tissues from the occiput to the cervicothoracic junction should be carefully assessed. Multiple-level injuries in the cervical spine are common in children (24%) and radiography should be scrutinized carefully for other injuries. In the thoracolumbar spine both the anterior and posterior columns are carefully assessed for loss of alignment and deformity. Vertebral body height may cause confusion as there is often normal anterior wedging in the immature spine.

Secondary ossification centres may look like avulsion fractures. Interpedicular widening should also be noted.

Assessment of radiographs should include the following:

- Interspinous distances
- Spinolaminar line
- The funnel shape made by the spinal canal.

Radiography is not necessary if the following features are present:

- Alert and cooperative child
- No neck pain
- Normal neck and neurological examination
- No head, face, or neck trauma.

In all other cases cervical immobilization should be used until the neck has been cleared radiographically.

CT scan is used to assess the extent of bony injury and canal compromise. It can therefore be used to predict stability and guide treatment interventions. In one study two out of 112 patients studied prospectively had injuries which were missed on all examinations except for CT. Children under 4 years of age may require sedation for CT.

Magnetic resonance imaging (MRI) is used to assess for neural and discoligamentous injury. A general anaesthetic may be necessary for children. Three types of MRI change are described in the spinal cord:

- Type I—decreased signal (haemorrhage)
- Type II—increased signal (oedema)
- Type III—mixed signal (contusion).

Patients with type II and III changes have a better chance of recovery.

Differential diagnosis

Congenital defects, skeletal dysplasias, infection, tumours, metabolic, and inflammatory conditions may also present with features similar to a spinal injury.

General principles of management of paediatric cervical spine trauma

Immediate immobilization of those suspected of having a cervical injury is mandatory, as the consequences of missed injury can be catastrophic. Even if the child is able to give a history, this combined with clinical examination can be inaccurate.

Box 14.3.2 General principles of management in spinal injuries in children

- Under the age of 10 most injuries occur above C4
- Exclude other life-threatening injuries
- Appropriate investigations to confirm diagnosis
- Clinical examination can exclude spinal injury in alert and cooperative child.

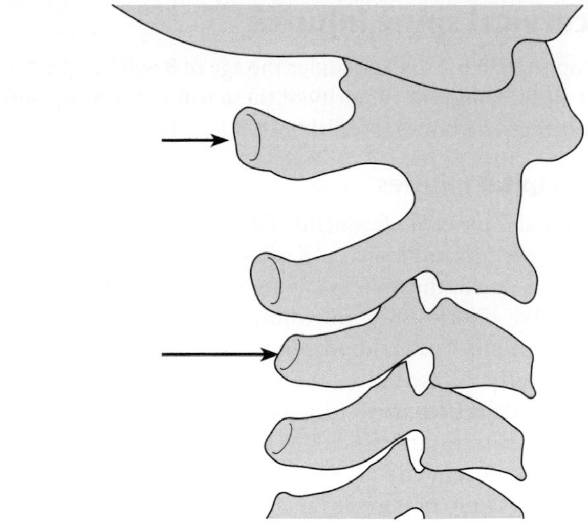

Fig. 14.3.2 Posterior cervical line: arrows indicate the points from which the line is drawn to assess any displacement of the axis.

Paediatric cervical braces are available but should be supplemented with tape and sandbags in order to adequately immobilize the cervical spine. Establishing an airway in the comatose patient can be difficult due to the inherent dangers of further spinal injury. The cervical spine can be immobilized with a brace or with in-line traction. Braces do not provide secure immobilization and there is a risk of over-distraction with the in-line method. This is a controversial topic. Children under 6 years of age have a relatively large head, and a split mattress technique is best to elevate the thorax and lower the head (Figure 14.3.3). A Minerva jacket has been used in the past for long-term cervical immobilization. Nowadays halo traction and halo jackets are more commonly used, but there is a significant incidence of pin loosening and infection. Lower torque pressures are used and in children less than age 7, 8–10 pins may be used. The halo should be applied under general anaesthetic, and a custom halo vest used. Dural tear can occur with skull perforation. If this occurs the screw should be replaced elsewhere, and usually the perforation will heal within a few days.

On the whole, apart from very unstable injuries, the majority of cases are treated non-operatively because of concerns regarding growth potential and long-term deformity.

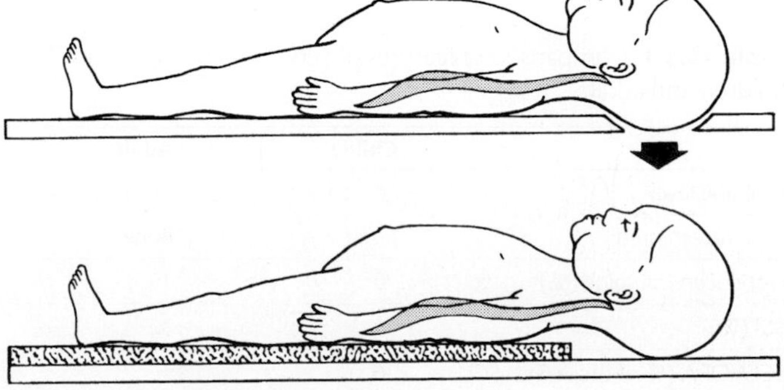

Fig. 14.3.3 Modified backboard.

Upper cervical spine injuries

Injuries in up to 87% of children under the age of 8 will be between the occiput and C3, and the majority of these will occur to the soft tissues rather than the bones (see Table 14.3.1).

Atlanto-occipital injuries

Atlanto-occipital injuries are frequently fatal and usually occur as a result of high-energy trauma such as a motor vehicle collision. The high mortality is due to the accompanying spinal cord, brain stem, and cranial nerve injuries. Recently, however, there has been an increase in the number of children surviving this injury, possibly due to better early resuscitation measures. The injury may go unrecognized initially because dislocations often reduce and radiographs will be normal or are difficult to interpret. There are useful radiographic measurements which are useful in assessing the injury. The Powers ratio represents the distance between the basion of the skull and the posterior arch of C1 divided by the distance between the opisthion and the anterior arch of C1. Abnormality is indicated by a ratio of more than 1. This ratio has its limitations in that whilst it is useful in assessing anterior dislocations it does not have the same accuracy in identifying posterior dislocations. In the presence of a fracture of C1 or a congenital anomaly of the base of skull the Powers ratio is invalid. Symptoms and signs include respiratory distress, cranial nerve lesions, and spinal cord dysfunction. Treatment can be operative by occipitocervical fusion usually down to C2 or non-operative with immobilization in a halo jacket. Reduction by traction is contraindicated.

Occipital condyle fractures are rare. Diagnosis can only be completed with CT scanning, preferably with multiplanar reconstruction. The Anderson–Montesano classification is described in Chapter 12.39.

Fractures of the atlas

Fractures of the atlas are rare in children. They are usually caused by axial forces transmitted through the occipital condyles to the lateral masses of the atlas. The synchondroses of C1 remain open up to the age of 10 and can fail under stress. The transverse ligament may rupture or avulse from its attachment. Neurological deficits rarely occur. Radiographically, open-mouth views should show symmetry of the C1 lateral masses both in relation to the odontoid process and to the lateral masses of C2. CT scanning is essential for diagnosis. Halo-jacket immobilization is usually adequate and surgery is rarely indicated.

Table 14.3.1 Comparison of features of cervical spine injuries in children and adults

	Child	Adult
Multiple level	Less common	Common
Structure injured	Ligament	Bone
Upper cervical spine (%)	70	15
SCI (%)	10	30
SCIWORA (% of those with SCI)	16	7

SCI, spinal cord injury.

Table 14.3.2 Causes of atlantoaxial instability

Down syndrome
Larsen syndrome
Reiter syndrome
Juvenile rheumatoid arthritis
Bone dysplasias (e.g. mucopolysaccharidoses)
Multiple epiphyseal dysplasia
Achondroplasia
Pseudoachondroplasia
Kneist syndrome

Atlantoaxial injuries

These injuries can be traumatic but rare giving rise to transverse ligament deficiencies or atraumatic due to developmental conditions such as Down syndrome, skeletal dysplasia, Klippel–Feil syndrome or os odontidenum (Table 14.3.2). These children in the last group are at increased risk of neurological compromise with minor trauma. Neurological signs such as change in physical tolerance, incontinence, and long-tract or cranial nerve signs should be investigated. Fifty per cent of normal cervical rotation takes place between C1 and C2. The joint surfaces are relatively flat, and stability depends mainly on the ligaments. The spinal canal is relatively large, and Steel's rule of thirds applies. The spinal canal at C1 is occupied equally by the odontoid process, the spinal cord, and free space. The course of the vertebral artery between C1 and C2 is relatively fixed and therefore excessive movement at this level is liable to compromise blood supply to neural tissue.

Treatment decisions are based on the space available for the cord and the anatomy of the posterior arch of C1. The presence of an excessive atlantodens interval or hypoplastic posterior arch increases the likelihood of neurological injury.

Reduction in extension is recommended. Observation is adequate where the atlantodens interval is less than 10mm, but where this is greater than 10mm, or where there are neurological symptoms or signs, spinal fusion from C1 to C2 is recommended. Immobilization for 8–12 weeks is necessary postoperatively.

Atlantoaxial rotary subluxation

Atlantoaxial rotary subluxation is seen commonly in children. It can occur secondary to local infection, inflammation (e.g. respiratory infection), rheumatoid disease, or trauma.

Atlantoaxial rotary subluxation often occurs after minor trauma and symptoms vary from mild to severe pain. Neurological injury

Box 14.3.3 Cervical spine injuries in children

- Avoid over-distraction with immobilization
- Most injuries in this area are soft tissue injuries
- Radiographs may be difficult to interpret
- Most injuries treated non-operatively.

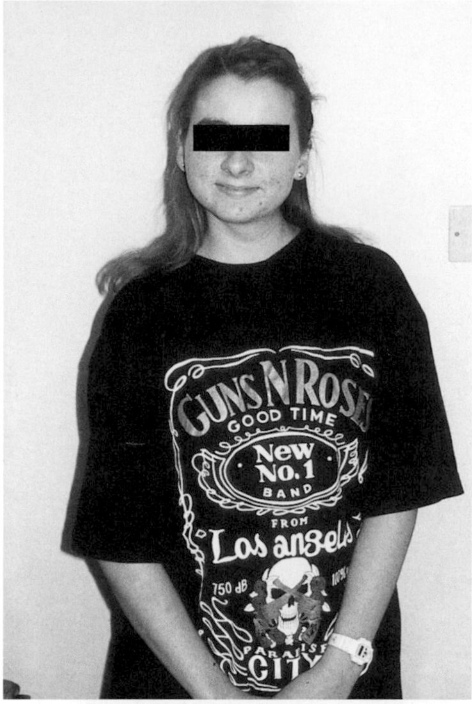

Fig. 14.3.4 Cock robin position.

or death is rare. The child may wake with a 'crick' in the neck and this sometimes resolves spontaneously. The 'cock robin' position is typical (Figure 14.3.4). The chin points in the direction of the side with muscle spasm.

Radiographic changes are difficult to interpret on plain films (Figure 14.3.5) and dynamic CT scanning is essential. The head is turned maximally to either side. A positive test shows loss of normal rotation between C1 and C2. Plain anteroposterior radiographs show a wider C1 lateral mass on the side which has moved forwards, a narrower C1 lateral mass on the side which has moved backwards, and an obscured facet joint on one side. Plain lateral radiographs show that the wedge-shaped lateral mass lies anteriorly and that posterior arches are not superimposed.

If symptoms are mild and of less than a week's duration, a soft collar alone may be adequate treatment. If symptoms are more severe or long-standing, but of less than a month's duration, halter traction and sedation for a few days usually results in reduction. Some authors recommend Minerva immobilization for 6 weeks if the atlas is displaced anteriorly on the axis. If the condition has been present for 1–3 months it is described as fixed rotatory fixation. Halo traction may achieve reduction. Failure of traction or a history longer than 3 months will usually require open reduction followed by fusion and immobilization. If reduction is not possible, fusion *in situ* is acceptable. There are various instrumented techniques that have been described.

Odontoid fractures

Odontoid fractures are the most common cervical injuries in children, occurring at an average age of 4 years. They really represent physeal injuries through the growth plate between the odontoid and body of the axis. The growth plate closes at the age of 3–6 years. The injury may follow trivial head trauma or a severe fall or road traffic accident and is almost never associated with any neurological injury. The child will often resist extension of the neck.

Lateral radiographs are usually diagnostic and the angulation is usually anterior. Posterior angulation of the odontoid is seen in 4% of normal children and should not be confused with a fracture. Dynamic CT or MRI scanning in flexion and extension will usually clarify the situation where the diagnosis is in doubt. Diagnosis can be particularly difficult in children with congenital abnormalities, for example in osteogenesis imperfecta or Morquio's syndrome where the odontoid is dysplastic.

Treatment consists of reduction in extension either simply by head positioning or by halter traction. This should be followed by Minerva or halo-vest immobilization for 6–12 weeks. The results are universally good. Fractures of the odontoid in older children usually behave in a similar manner to adults.

Os odontoideum

Os odontoideum probably represents non-union of an odontoid fracture which has gone unrecognized. It is usually asymptomatic but can be a cause of neck pain, or even occasionally of instability and spinal cord compression. If instability is present, posterior C1–C2 fusion is the treatment of choice.

Hangman's fracture

Hangman's fracture (fracture of the pedicle of C2) is unusual in children. Neurological deficit is rare. There are two major causes for confusion in making a diagnosis. Firstly, the synchondroses between the body of C2 and the pedicle ossification centres can be mistaken for a fracture. The synchondrosis normally closes by the age of 7. Secondly, pseudosubluxation of C2 on C3 occurs in up to 50% of children under the age of 8 years. Therefore the lateral radiographs must be properly assessed and, if necessary, further imaging obtained. Reduction should be achieved by positioning; immobilization in a Minerva cast for 6–12 weeks usually results in union. Surgery in the form of spinal fusion is only used if there is non-union or instability. Traction should be avoided because the risk of over-distraction.

Lower cervical spine injuries (C3–C7)

These injuries are not common in children. They can present as injuries to the growth plates which can be difficult to identify on plain radiographs. In the older child they present a similar picture to adults.

Salter–Harris type injuries can occur when the endplate separates from the vertebral body at the level of the physis. These injuries can cause neurologic deficit. Type I SalterHarris injuries are unstable and require surgical stabilization while type III injuries are stable and can be managed in a halo. Compression fractures are

Box 14.3.4 Lower cervical spine injuries in children

- Uncommon injuries in children under 10 years
- Fractures can occur through physis
- Cartilaginous material can cause neurological injury
- Surgical treatment similar to adults.

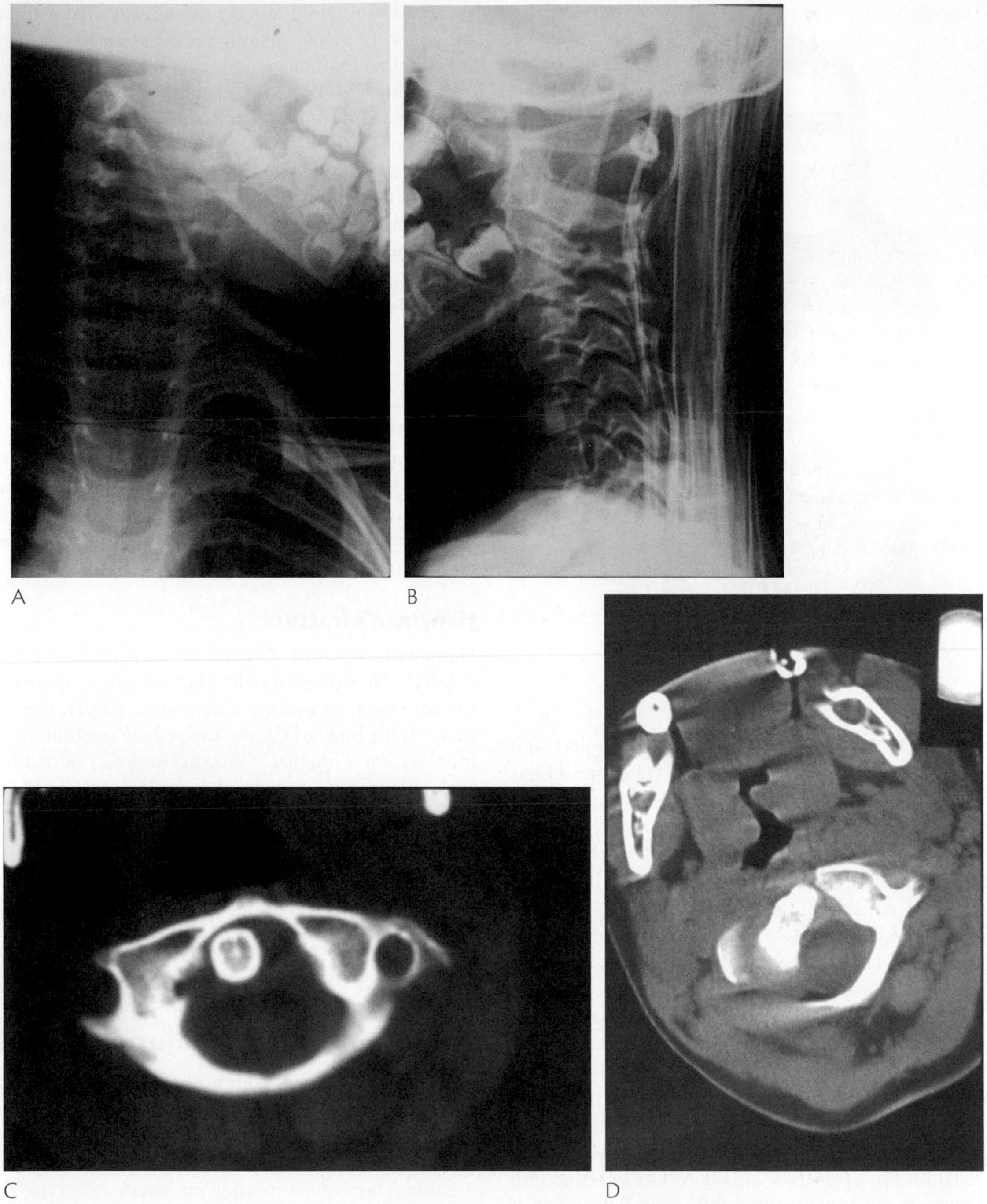

Fig. 14.3.5 C1–C2 rotation.

the most commonly occurring injury. Other types of injury seen are fracture dislocations, bifacetal dislocations, unifacetal dislocation, burst fractures, and posterior ligament ruptures. A description of the individual injury patterns and their treatment follows.

Wedge compression fractures

Wedge compression fractures are the most common subaxial fractures. They are stable fractures which heal rapidly in children. They may be difficult to recognize because of varying ossification patterns, and because the vertebrae tend to look wedged normally in children. Fracture healing time is 3–6 weeks, and immobilization in a collar for 2–4 weeks is usually adequate. There may be associated fractures such as anterior teardrop fracture, laminar fracture, or spinous process fracture.

Distraction shear fracture injuries

Distraction shear fracture injuries are rare. They occur through the endplate and they may be associated with birth trauma. Associated quadriplegia is not uncommon. Where neurological deficit is present, reduction and surgical stabilization is advised.

Fracture dislocation injuries

Fracture dislocation injuries are similar to those occurring in adults. They are usually high-velocity injuries. Treatment is by early reduction and stabilization. Late deformity may occur.

Facet dislocation injuries

Facet dislocation injuries are relatively uncommon. The patterns of injury are similar to those in adults, and they occur in adolescents. Dislocations can usually be reduced with traction. Some authors recommend non-operative management in a brace for 6 weeks, whereas others recommend surgical stabilization. If a unifacet dislocation is irreducible or if there is a bifacet dislocation, surgical stabilization with instrumentation and bone grafting is recommended. In children there is a high incidence of fusion extension, when extra laminae or spinous processes are exposed. The surgical exposure should be confined to the area being fused to avoid this. Whereas wire techniques tend to be inadequate in adults, in children the small forces exerted on the fixation and rapid healing make wire techniques more acceptable (Figure 14.3.6).

General principles of management of fractures of the thoracic and lumbar spine

Thoracolumbar fractures in infants can be caused by child abuse. Children in the first decade usually sustain injuries as passengers or pedestrians in motor collisions. Beware the seatbelt bruise on the abdominal wall which is usually indicative of major spinal trauma in association with a visceral injury. In children over the age of 10 years, sport and recreational activities are the most common causes.

Clinical assessment is difficult in the very young and in those with multiple injuries. The child may not be able to isolate the site of pain and examination is difficult. A significant fracture may be overlooked. In the emergency department initial trauma resuscitation protocol is carried out to avoid mortality from these other injuries. A thorough secondary survey is carried out to inspect the soft tissues over the front and back of the trunk. Abdominal bruising or the presence of a defect or step posteriorly may point to a thoracolumbar fracture. Serious abdominal injury occurs in 20% of children (50–90% of those with Chance fractures). Signs and symptoms of prolapsed intervertebral disc should alert the clinician to the possibility of slipping of the vertebral apophysis.

The presence of a neurological injury should be established. Where a deficit is present, an assessment to determine whether the injury is complete or incomplete is necessary as incomplete injuries will have a better prognosis. During resuscitation, attention to spine immobilization should be observed at all times to prevent further injury. Further evaluation with plain radiographs is performed although CT is increasingly being used as a first choice investigation. Where there is evidence of neurological injury an MRI scan should be done. Treatment for stable injuries can be with a plaster jacket or orthosis usually fitted to hold the trunk in extension. Unstable injuries require surgical stabilization. Modern instrumentation allows for preservation of more motion segments by using shorter constructs and thereby avoiding the pitfalls of stabilization across several segments. Fracture patterns in the thoracolumbar spine are caused the injury mechanism involved. This is reflected in the classification systems which describe these injuries. Unfortunately these classifications do not serve as a guide for treatment but do allude to injury severity and likelihood of neurological compromise.

Classification of thoracic and lumbar fractures

Fractures are classified by mechanism of injury. As in adult fractures, they can be divided into three broad groups:

- Compression
- Distraction
- Rotation.

The three groups have an increasing incidence of neurological injury and other complications.

Compression

As in adults, *flexion injuries* are the most common. The discs are more resistant to vertical compression than the bones. The nucleus of the disc causes the endplate to fracture, and nuclear material herniates into the vertebral body. In older children the nucleus of the disc is more viscous and the compression forces are dissipated peripherally; either the annulus is torn and the sides of the vertebrae buckle, or a marginal fracture occurs. More severe forces cause burst fractures similar to those in adults. Flexion injuries commonly occur at multiple levels in children.

Slipping of the vertebral apophysis occurs most commonly in teenage boys. This causes traumatic displacement of the ring apophysis into the spinal canal and disc protrusion. The most commonly injured level is L4. The injury resembles slipped epiphysis of the hip. The symptoms resemble those of disc herniation, and can be acute or chronic. This injury may be associated with Scheuermann's disease.

Distraction

Chance fractures (Figure 14.3.7) occur with hyperflexion and distraction in the posterior column. A fracture occurs across the osseous or posterior ligamentous (soft tissue Chance fracture) elements of a vertebra. The fracture is propagated anteriorly through the anterior and middle columns or in the case of the soft tissue Chance injury through the disc. The most common mechanism is a lap seatbelt injury in a motor vehicle collision. Bony Chance fractures can be treated non-operatively in a plaster jacket or thoracolumbosacral orthosis (TLSO). However, if there is severe kyphosis at presentation or neurological deficit at presentation surgery should be considered. The soft tissue Chance fracture generally has poorer healing capacity if treated non-operatively and therefore surgery should be considered as first choice treatment.

Rotation

These injuries usually occur in motor vehicle collisions. The injury passes through the endplate apophysis. Traumatic spondylolisthesis can occur.

Box 14.3.5 Thoracolumbar spine injuries in children

- Suspect visceral injury with seatbelt bruising
- Stable injuries treated in orthosis
- Surgical stabilization for unstable injuries
- Preserve motion segments.

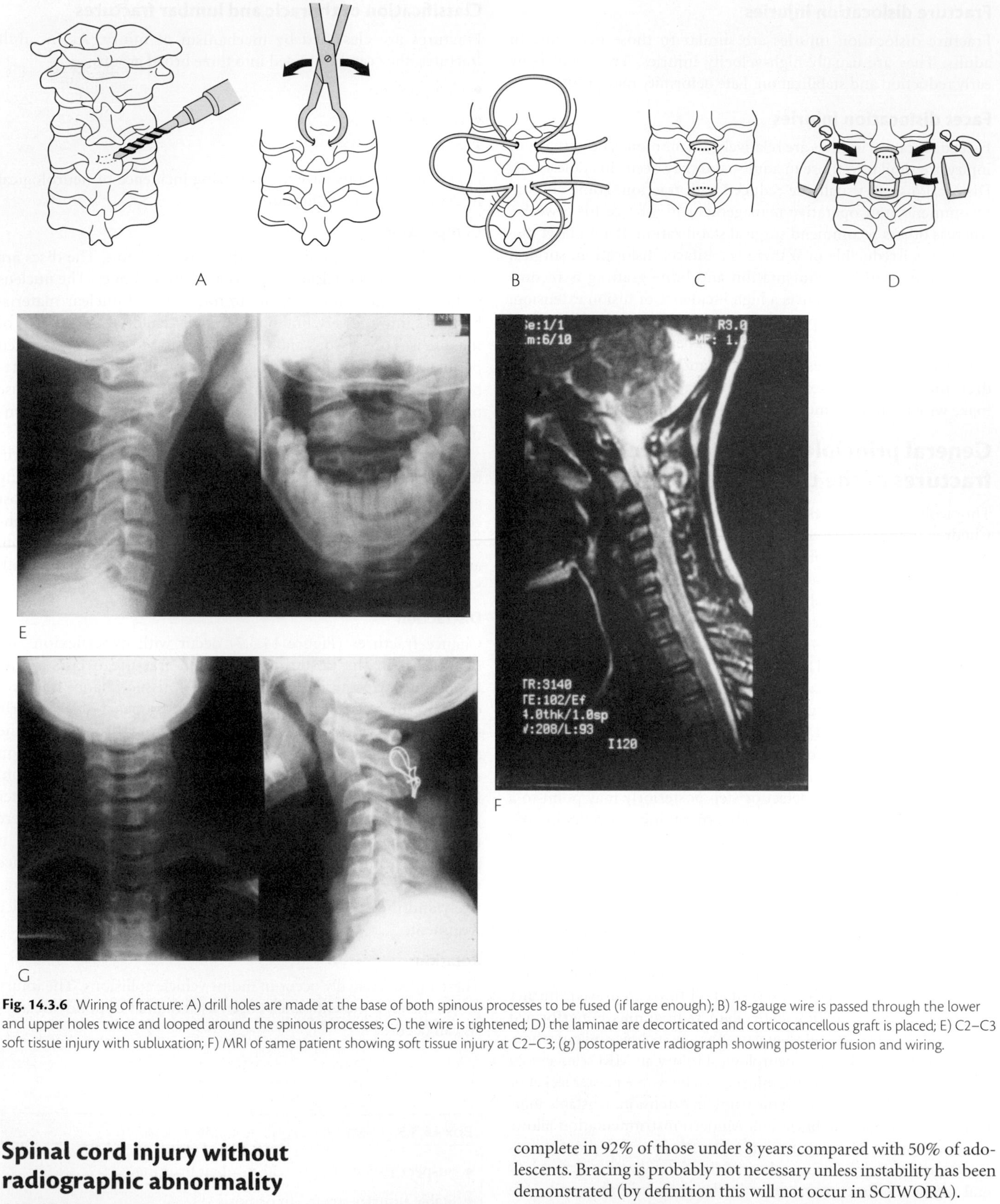

Fig. 14.3.6 Wiring of fracture: A) drill holes are made at the base of both spinous processes to be fused (if large enough); B) 18-gauge wire is passed through the lower and upper holes twice and looped around the spinous processes; C) the wire is tightened; D) the laminae are decorticated and corticocancellous graft is placed; E) C2–C3 soft tissue injury with subluxation; F) MRI of same patient showing soft tissue injury at C2–C3; (g) postoperative radiograph showing posterior fusion and wiring.

Spinal cord injury without radiographic abnormality

SCIWORA occurs in about 7% of children with spinal cord injury although it has been said to account for up to a third of spinal cord injuries in children. Neurological loss is more commonly complete in younger children and in thoracic injuries. Thoracic lesions are complete in 92% of those under 8 years compared with 50% of adolescents. Bracing is probably not necessary unless instability has been demonstrated (by definition this will not occur in SCIWORA).

When this condition was originally described, MRI scan was unavailable which has now made the diagnosis somewhat controversial. However, the absence of abnormal cord signal on MRI may indicate good prospects for recovery.

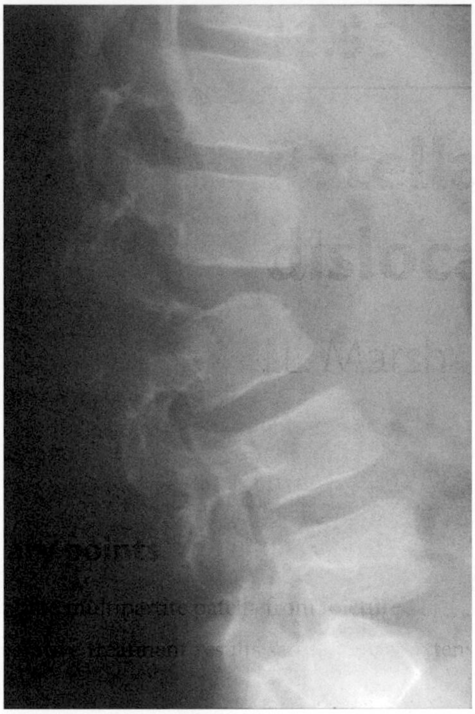

Fig. 14.3.7 Chance fracture.

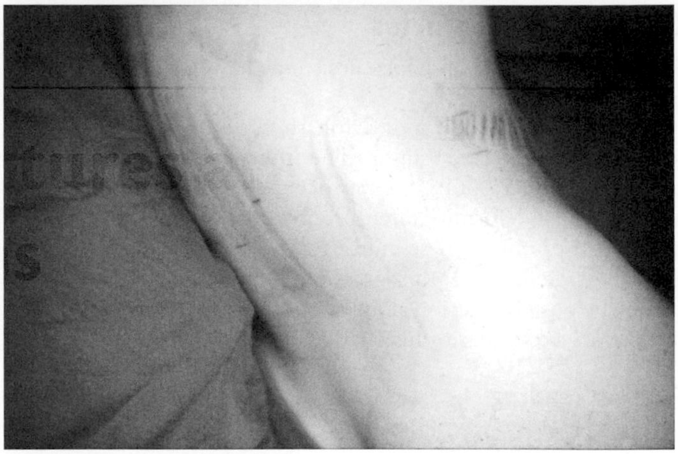

Fig. 14.3.8 Abdominal bruising.

Neonatal injuries

Neonatal injuries are seldom reported, possibly because the spine is difficult to assess radiographically as most of it is still cartilage. In traumatic vaginal delivery, neck hyperextension ('stargazing fetus') with breech presentation is associated with a high incidence of cord transection (25%). Treatment is usually limited to a neck support or orthosis, and bone injury rapidly heals.

Child abuse can occasionally cause spinal fracture or spinal cord injury, and is associated with intracranial and intraocular haemorrhages. This has been called 'shaken infant syndrome'.

Complications

Post-traumatic deformity

The same complications arise as in adults after spinal cord injury (see Chapter 12.45), such as pressure sores, renal tract infection and stones, contractures, etc.

Spinal deformity commonly occurs in children following spinal cord injury. The incidence of scoliosis is related to the age of the child at the time of injury. Ninety-seven per cent of those presenting before the growth spurt may develop scoliosis, compared with 52% presenting after. The onset of scoliosis has been reported in children as young as 3 years. Progression potential depends on the following:

- Age of the patient
- Level of the lesion
- Severity of the spinal cord injury.

Scoliosis is known to deteriorate with growth. The majority of these children will deteriorate and require surgical stabilization in the form of a spinopelvic fusion. Many of them will have seating problems and pressure sores due to pelvic obliquity which is corrected at the time of surgery. Up to 68% of children may require surgical stabilization.

A post-traumatic syringomyelia may develop which manifests as pain, deteriorating neurological function and deformity. Surgical drainage may be required.

Neurological injury

Neurological injury may occur in up to 45% of children with spinal injury, but in general this has a better prognosis than in adults

Partial or complete injuries must not be overlooked. Serial observations are useful if neurological status is in doubt. The single most important finding is of a neurological level. Boys are twice as commonly affected as girls, and those aged 10–15 years are at most risk. Ten to fifteen per cent of spinal cord injuries occur in children. In newborn children, neurological injury should be suspected in a floppy infant following a difficult delivery.

Delayed-onset paraplegia has a very poor prognosis.

Growth arrest

Significant growth arrest in the spine is rare. The vertebral bodies have great remodelling potential, especially in children under the age of 10 years. Asymmetric damage to the growth plates seldom causes scoliosis because the adjacent vertebrae adapt. Occasionally kyphosis will occur when the endplates are damaged. Spontaneous interbody fusion is rare.

Box 14.3.6 Special features in recovery from spinal injury in children

- Post-traumatic deformity common in prepubertal spinal injury
- SCIWORA present in a third of cases
- Syringomyelia can cause progressive deformity
- Growth arrest rare.

Other spinal injuries

Spondylolysis and spondylolisthesis may have a traumatic aetiology in children.

Acute spondylolytic spondylolisthesis is a rare occurrence following high-energy trauma. The injury usually occurs in the pars interarticularis of L5 but may occur elsewhere in the posterior elements. The deformity often progresses and may cause neurological compromise. These injuries should be treated surgically at an early stage to prevent progression. Grade I deformities can be treated by posterior fusion alone; more severe slips are best treated by anterior and posterior fusion.

Further reading

Anderson, P.A., Henley, B., Rivara, F.P., and Maier, R.V. (1991). Flexion distraction and Chance injuries to the thoracolumbar spine. *Journal of Orthopaedic Trauma*, **5**, 153–60.

Caffey, J. (1974). The whiplash shaken infant syndrome. *Pediatrics*, **54**, 396–403.

Cattell, S. and Filtzer, D.L. (1965). Pseudosubluxation and other normal variations in the cervical spine in children. *Journal of Bone and Joint Surgery*, **47A**, 1295–309.

Hamilton, M.G. and Myles, S.T. (1992). Paediatric spinal injury: review of a 174 hospital admissions. *Journal of Neurosurgery*, **77**, 700–4.

McGrory, B.J., Klassen, R.A., Chao, E.Y.S., Staeheli, J.W., and Weaver, A.L. (1993). Acute fractures and dislocations of the cervical spine in children. *Journal of Bone and Joint Surgery*, **75A**, 988–95.

14.4

Injuries around the shoulder in children

Tanaya Sarkhel and Jonathan Clasper

Summary points

- Dislocation of the shoulder is rare in children but may be mimicked by epiphyseal disruption
- Midshaft clavicle fractures are common and have great powers of remodelling
- Proximal humeral fractures commonly involve the physis and lead to shortening although this is rarely apparent to the patient.

Introduction

Children cannot be considered as small adults, and this is especially true when dealing with injuries around the shoulder. Although one of the most common fractures in both is the clavicle fracture, this is where the similarity ends. Physeal involvement is a factor and the potential for remodelling is considerable. In particular, the pattern and behaviour of fractures of the proximal humerus in children is completely different from that in adults. Shoulder dislocation, a common adult condition, is very uncommon in children. Often epiphyseal fractures in children may appear as joint dislocations.

Anatomy

The three bones of the shoulder girdle—the clavicle, scapula, and humerus—connect with the torso via the sternoclavicular joint. The flat, triangular scapula provides attachment for 17 muscles, and expands into the acromion, which articulates with the clavicle, the coracoid, and the glenoid, which articulates with the humerus. The adult proximal humerus is considered in four parts: the articular head, the greater and lesser tuberosities, and the proximal shaft. In children, the most commonly injured site is the growth plate, and a fracture in the child rarely consists of more than two parts (Figure 14.4.1). In adults, the bony architecture cannot be considered in isolation from the soft tissues, especially the rotator cuff. In children, the growth plates and epiphyses must also be considered, and the rotator cuff is of less importance.

Ossification

The scapula, formed by membranous ossification, is largely present at birth. The coracoid ossifies from two separate centres, fusing by the fifteenth year. By puberty, between two and five ossification centres form the acromion (Figure 14.4.2), which fuses by 20–22 years. Failure of acromial fusion, resulting in an os acromiale, occurs in about 5% of the population, visible on axial view. It may be confused with fracture.

The clavicle develops two ossification centres around weeks 5–6 of fetal life. These fuse within a few weeks of their appearance; failure of this may produce a congenital pseudarthrosis of the clavicle. A secondary ossification centre appears in the medial end of the clavicle in the late teens and fuses by about the age of 25 years. The lateral end occasionally develops a secondary ossification centre at the age of 18–20 years. This is usually small and rapidly fuses to the shaft.

The shaft of the humerus is evident at birth, with the head appearing at 6 months. The greater and lesser tuberosities appear between 2–5 years, fusing by 6 years to produce a conical growth plate with a posteromedial apex, which accounts for 80% of the humeral growth. In children under 6 years, fracture through this growth plate is usually a Salter–Harris type I injury, as before the

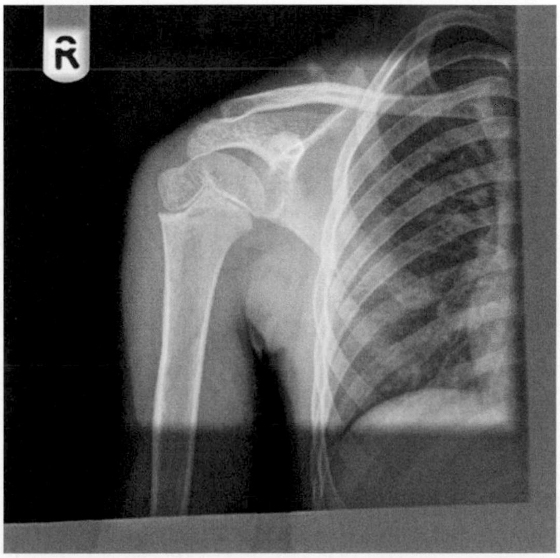

Fig. 14.4.1 Normal appearance of the growth plate in an 8-year-old boy.

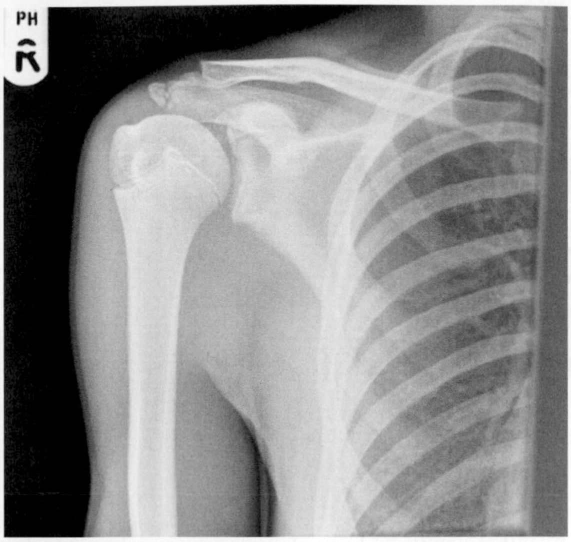

Fig. 14.4.2 Normal acromial appearance in a 14-year-old boy.

tuberosities fuse the growth plate is more transverse. In the older child, a Salter–Harris type II fracture occurs through the conical growth plate, retaining the posteromedial metaphysic.

General principles

Falls, traffic accidents, and sports are the commonest cause of shoulder girdle injury. However, with any childhood injury the possibility of child abuse must always be considered. In general, most shoulder injuries occur in children over 5 years old, an age at which child abuse resulting in fractures is uncommon. In the under 5s a proximal humerus fracture is rarely due to child abuse, although all scapular fractures and clavicle fractures in those under 18 months old should be viewed with suspicion. Many of the other fractures seen around the shoulder occur after major trauma, and an appropriate history is available. However, if the mechanism of injury does not fit the history given or there was a significant delay in presentation, child abuse should be considered.

Children under 5 years have tremendous potential to remodel, and significant deformity can be accepted, especially in the proximal humerus. Given the malalignment and shortening that can be accepted even in adults, few of these fractures in children will need operative intervention.

Adolescents should be considered as adults if they are reaching skeletal maturity. The management of their injuries, including the indications for operative treatment, should be the same as those in an adult. In a child of any age, an open fracture must be treated by operative debridement, and stabilization of the fracture site. In children as in adults, polytrauma is a relative indication for surgical treatment.

High-energy trauma around the shoulder is very uncommon in children, so that examples of injuries such as scapulothoracic dissociation, or intrathoracic dislocations in children exist only as isolated case reports in the literature. They will not be considered further in this chapter.

Epidemiology

The risk of at least one fracture up to the age of 16 years in a boy is 42%, and 27% in girls. Of these fractures, the clavicle is involved in 8–15.5%, the fourth most common site of fracture in children. Fractures of the proximal humerus account for less than 5%, the fourth most frequent epiphyseal injury. Other fractures around the shoulder account for less than 1% of all childhood fractures.

Infants of 4kg or more are at increased risk of fracture during birth. Ninety-five per cent% of birth fractures involve the clavicle by pressure from the symphysis pubis on the anterior shoulder in a cephalic presentation, and heal rapidly. Salter–Harris type I affect the proximal humerus if the arm becomes hyperextended or rotated during delivery.

Specific injuries

Sternoclavicular joint

Dislocations of this joint are rare in children and most apparent dislocations, even in adults up to the age of 25 years, represent epiphyseal separations. True dislocations and epiphyseal injuries can be manipulated closed and are often stable. Even if unstable, metalwork is avoided as disastrous results have been reported, including pin migration and infection. Sutures or repair of the periosteal sleeve are sufficient, with 3–4 weeks of sling immobilization as rapid healing and remodelling will occur. Anterior displacement is more common, whilst posterior displacement may be a surgical emergency if vital structures are compromised.

Clavicle

Fractures of the medial end of the clavicle were considered earlier.

Midshaft fractures account for 88% of children's clavicle injuries (Figure 14.4.3), with a mean age of 8 years. The mechanism is a fall directly on to the shoulder with the arm at the side. A direct blow or a fall on the outstretched hand can rarely produce this injury. Greenstick fractures commonly occur, requiring temporary rest in a sling for a short period. Displaced clavicle fractures are very common, but rarely require reduction (Figure 14.4.1). A broad arm sling for 2–3 weeks until comfortable is all that is required. Malunion is very common but rarely causes a functional problem; non-union is very rare in children. Parents should be reassured that the prominent callus will usually resolve over the subsequent months; pressure to remove this 'unsightly' lump surgically should be strongly resisted.

Open reduction and fixation with wires or a plate may be occasionally required. The indications are similar to those in the adult: open fracture, skin compromise, vascular injury, etc.

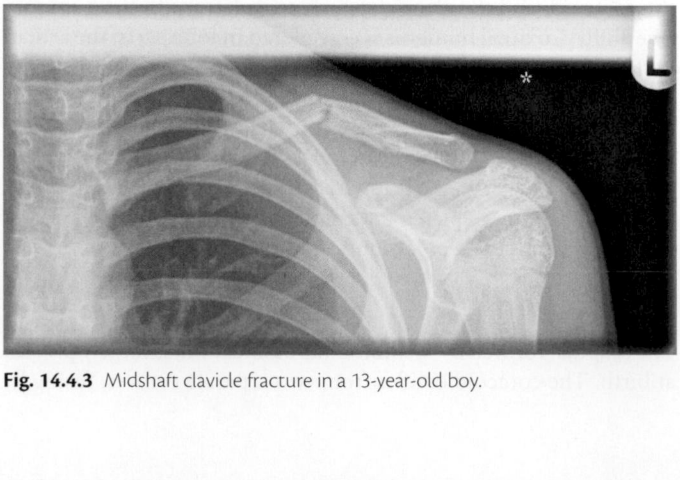

Fig. 14.4.3 Midshaft clavicle fracture in a 13-year-old boy.

Fractures of the lateral end of the clavicle may also be confused with joint dislocations, as discussed later.

Acromioclavicular joint

True dislocations of this joint are unusual in children, especially in the younger child. The ligaments around the joint are very strong, and more often the lateral end of the clavicle will fracture, herniating through the thick periosteal sleeve although this may not be apparent on radiographs if it is unossified. The inferior periosteum is left behind, with the conoid and trapezoid components of the coracoclavicular ligament intact, producing a 'pseudo-dislocation'. This will heal and remodel with conservative treatment, a sling for comfort followed by early mobilization. Rockwood *et al.* (1984) have classified these injuries.

Coracoid

Fractures of the coracoid are usually an epiphyseal separation. In combination with a lateral clavicle fracture, this constitutes a childhood equivalent of an acromioclavicular dislocation and represents failure through the epiphyseal plate before ligamentous injury.

Acromion

Acromion fractures are rare in children and are often due to direct violence. An os acromiale may be confused with a fracture. Treatment depends on displacement, and other injuries around the shoulder. Wires, screws, tension band wiring, and plate fixation have all been used and non-union has not been reported in children.

Scapula body

These are uncommon injuries and usually represent direct violence. The significance of this injury is the possibility of underlying chest wall and pulmonary contusion rather than the scapula fracture itself. These injuries will almost always be treated conservatively with analgesia, and a sling for comfort. The arm should be mobilized as comfort allows.

Glenoid

Glenoid fractures are rare and represent a fracture dislocation of the shoulder. The size and displacement of the fragment must be assessed, and this is best achieved by computed tomography. Minimally displaced fractures respond to sling immobilization, rarely for more than 3 weeks. Indications for internal fixation, usually by a lag screw technique, include large displaced fragments, and an unstable shoulder. Operative approach, method of fixation, and postoperative mobilization will be determined by the fracture pattern and fixation achieved at surgery.

Glenohumeral joint

Shoulder dislocation in pre-teen children is unusual, as the ligaments are stronger than the epiphysis; more commonly a Salter–Harris fracture of the proximal humerus will occur. In adolescents as in adults, glenohumeral dislocation is frequently due to a sporting injury. Treatment is along adult lines, with early closed reduction using standard techniques. The recurrence rate is age related, highest in 14–17-year-olds, with a recurrent dislocation rate of 92%, in comparison with 33% for those under 12 years. When traumatic dislocations occur, Bankart lesions are found in 80%, leading to suggestions of prophylactic stabilizing surgery. This is controversial, but if recurrence does happen, surgery is indicated. Surgical patients are less likely to have recurrent instability, but in a study of 66 adolescents, stability improved anyway over 2 years with 90% performing at the same or higher levels of sport and work in both operative and non-operative groups. Another study has found no significant difference was found in functional outcomes between patients who had undergone surgical stabilization and those treated non-operatively.

Atraumatic dislocations can occur in children with joint laxity or connective tissue disorders and can be produced by voluntary muscle activity. Posterior glenohumeral dislocations in children have been reported as case reports.

Proximal humerus

Most fractures of the proximal humerus usually occur in the older child or adolescent. Not only are accidents more common at this age, but the perichondral ring may be weaker just before skeletal maturity. The majority of injuries occur through the growth plate; Salter–Harris type II in the older child, and type I in the younger child. Salter–Harris types III and IV are very uncommon injuries of the proximal humerus. No cases were reported in three of the largest series, which in total comprised over 200 patients.

Neer and Horowitz (1965) graded fracture displacement into four groups: group I, less than 3mm; group II, up to 33% of the shaft diameter; group III, up to 67% of the shaft; group IV, more than 67% displacement of the shaft. No specific grading of angulation was made, though noted to be always present in groups III and IV. Varus displacement is most common and is due to the pull of the pectoralis major attaching to the distal fragment which tends to pull it anteriorly and medially. Neer and Horowitz noted residual shortening in nearly 10% of patients of groups I and II at an average follow-up of 4.8 years. This figure rose to 33% of those in group IV, all treated by reduction, nine by open reduction and nine by closed reduction. Despite this, all patients had satisfactory functional results.

Baxter and Wiley (1986) in a review of the treatment of 57 patients, reported that manipulation of a displaced fresh fracture did not improve the final outcome, when humeral growth or function were assessed. Ninety per cent of the 30 patients they assessed more than 2 years after injury had measurable shortening; however, the maximum was 2cm, and none of their patients were aware of the shortening.

Conservative treatment is generally acceptable, not only because of the remodelling potential but also because some degree of malalignment can be accepted around the shoulder. An angulation of 45 degrees and 50% of displacement can be accepted (Figure 14.4.4). In the younger child, 70% angulation and any bony contact should heal with good functional results. The fracture is usually treated in a collar and cuff sling, although rarely a hanging cast may be used in the older child with significant shortening or angulation.

If the position is unacceptable, closed reduction is attempted and the fracture held with two or three wires (Figure 14.4.5). These wires can be removed after 3 weeks. The use of cannulated screws instead of wires allows earlier and unimpaired mobilization. Premature closure of the growth plate will occur, but this method of treatment will usually be used in the adolescent approaching skeletal maturity Figure 14.4.6).

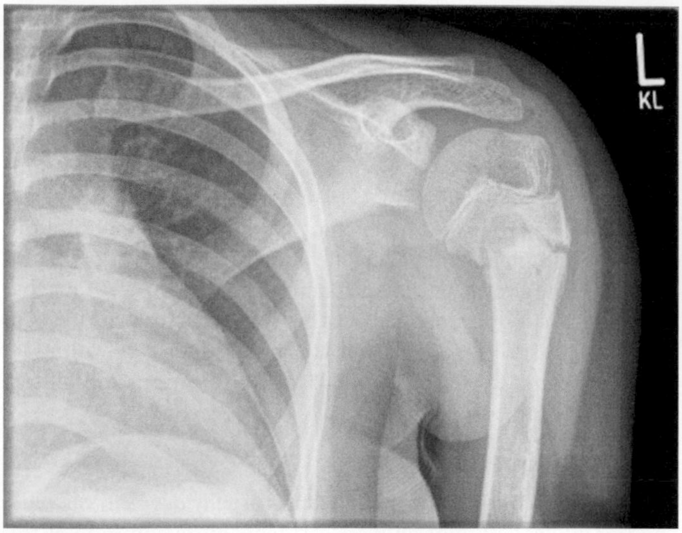

Fig. 14.4.4 Proximal humeral fracture in typical varus.

Open reduction may occasionally be required for soft tissue interposition often the biceps tendon, and this can be achieved through a standard deltopectoral approach (Figure 14.4.7). Fracture stabilization is carried out as described earlier.

Metaphyseal fracture

This may occur with direct trauma, or may occur as a pathological fracture, classically through a unicameral bone cyst (Figure 14.4.8). Displacement is not usually significant; angulation may occur but rarely produces a functional problem. The fractures usually heal rapidly with conservative treatment in a sling. The proximal humerus is the only common site for pathologic fractures around the shoulder.

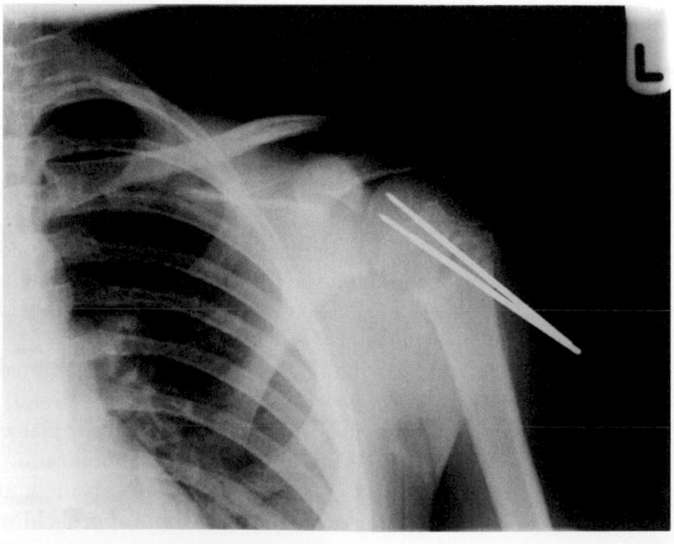

Fig. 14.4.5 Percutaneous fixation with wires.

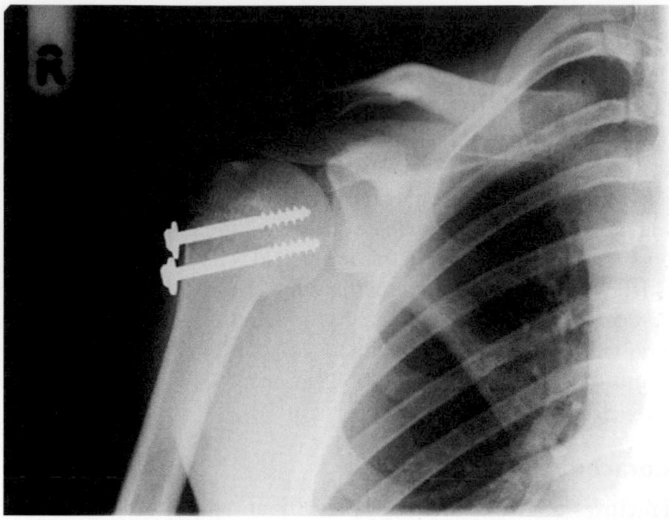

Fig. 14.4.6 Fixation with screws; closure of growth plate occurring.

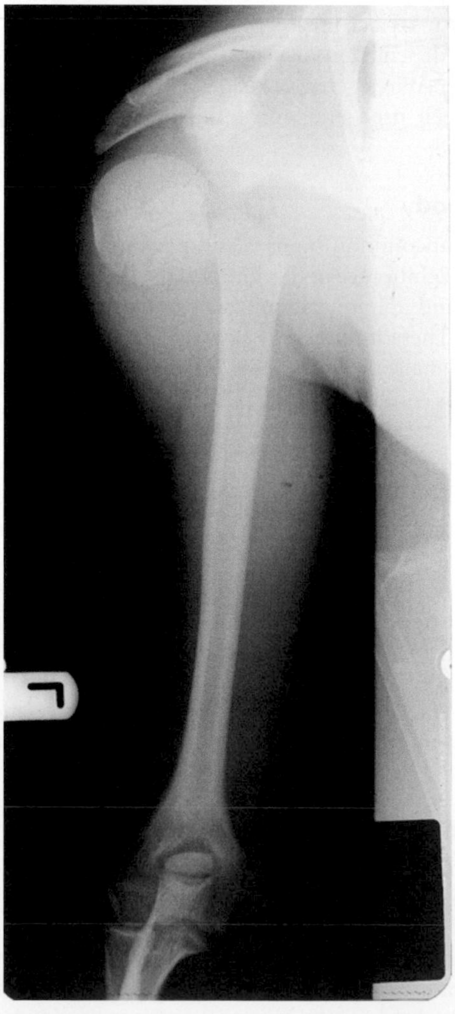

Fig. 14.4.7 Totally displaced proximal humerus fracture; the biceps tendon was interposed.

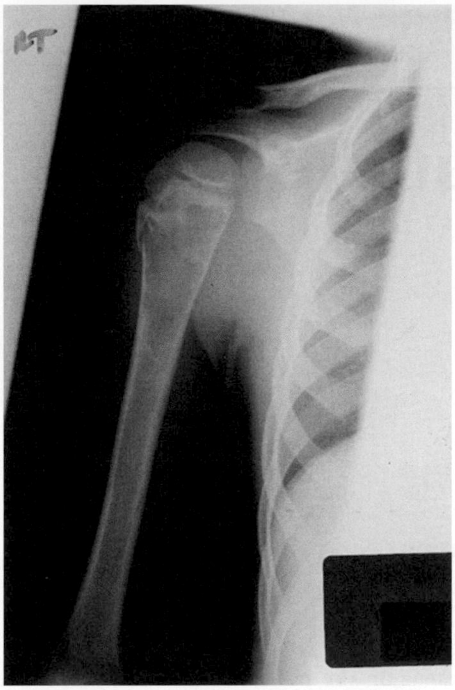

Fig. 14.4.8 Fracture through a unicameral bone cyst.

Summary

Fractures of the clavicle or proximal humerus are relatively common injuries in childhood; most can be treated conservatively with excellent functional recovery.

Other fractures are uncommon and an awareness of the basic ossification patterns will further inform a radiographic abnormality. Joint dislocations are very rare in a child; injury usually occurs through an epiphysis near to the joint. Again, a good result can be expected with conservative treatment.

High-energy shoulder trauma or polytrauma need to be treated on an individual basis, following the basic principles of trauma care.

Further reading

Baxter, M.P. and Wiley, J.J. (1986). Fractures of the proximal humeral epiphysis: their influence on humeral growth. *Journal of Bone and Joint Surgery,* **68B**, 570–3.

Landin, L.A. (1994). *Fracture Epidemiology from Children's Orthopaedics and Fractures.* Edinburgh: Churchill Livingstone.

Neer, C.S. and Horwitz, B.S. (1965). Fractures of the proximal humeral epiphyseal plate. *Clinical Orthopaedics and Related Research,* **41**, 24–31.

Rockwood, C.A., Wilkins, K.E., and King, R.E. (eds) (1984). *Fractures in children,* Vol. 3. Philadelphia, PA: J.B. Lippincott.

Sanders, J.O. and Cermak, M.B. (2004). Fractures, dislocations and acquired problems of the shoulder in children. In: Rockwood, C.A, Matsen, F.A, Wirth, M.A and Lippitt, S.B (eds) *The Shoulder,* third edition. Philadelphia, PA: Saunders.

Worlock, P., Stower, M., and Barbor, P. (1986). Patterns of fractures in accidental and non-accidental injury in children: a comparative study. *British Medical Journal,* **293**, 100–2.

14.5

Fractures about the elbow in children

J. Chell

Summary points

- Fractures around the elbow are a common occurrence in childhood
- Closed fracture reduction is best supplemented with percutaneous wires
- Damage to nerves and vessels (less common) are associated with these fractures
- The index of suspicion for compartment syndrome should always be high
- The transcondylar fracture has a high association with non-accidental injury.

Introduction

Fractures around the elbow are a common occurrence in childhood; however, these fractures require careful assessment and treatment if complications are to be avoided.

Supracondylar humeral fractures

These are the most common elbow fractures in children. Although they can occur throughout childhood there is a peak incidence between the ages of 5–8 years. A review of supracondylar humeral fractures noted that the average age was 6.7 years, 60.8% were on the left, 62.8% were in boys, and 1% were open. The usual mechanism of injury is a fall on the outstretched hand with the elbow locked in hyperextension. The natural predisposition to ligamentous laxity in this age group allows this increased hyperextension to cause the olecranon to lever in the olecranon fossa creating a stress concentration at the supracondylar area resulting in the typical extension fracture pattern.

Two per cent of these injuries have a flexion pattern and typically are caused by a direct blow to the posterior aspect of the elbow. Careful consideration of the distal humeral anatomy is needed for recognition since these fractures can be subtle. Displaced flexion fractures have a high incidence of ulnar nerve injury from where it is stretched over the posterior edge of the proximal fragment. Fracture displacement tends to be valgus, in contrast with extension supracondylar fractures which may heal in varus.

Classification

The classification described by Gartland (1959) and modified by Wilkins *et al.* (1996) is the most commonly used (Table 14.5.1); this is based on the degree and direction of displacement of the distal fragment on the initial x-rays. In approximately 75% of supracondylar fractures, the displacement of the distal fragment is posteromedial and the lateral spike of the proximal humeral shaft may injure the radial nerve. Whereas when the distal fragment is displaced posterolaterally, the brachial artery is at risk along with the median nerve. The direction of displacement also influences management by either pronating (posteromedial displacement) or supinating (posterolateral displacement) the forearm will help maintain fracture stability from the intact periosteal hinge prior to wiring of the fracture.

Clinical evaluation

In completely displaced fractures there will be swelling, bruising, and crepitus apparent and an S-shaped deformity of the elbow may be present. The carrying angle is approximately 15 degrees of valgus but should be compared to the other side as it can vary from 0–25 degrees. Whereas with undisplaced or minimally displaced fractures, swelling and point tenderness may be the only clinical signs present. Puckering of the skin indicates penetration of the brachialis muscle by the proximal end of the humerus which increases the possibility of an open reduction being required.

Associated injuries

Nerve injuries have been reported to occur in up to 7% of patients with supracondylar humeral fractures and all the nerves passing across the elbow should be carefully assessed. The most commonly injured is the anterior interosseous nerve since its fibres make up

Table 14.5.1 Classification of supracondylar fractures

Type I	Undisplaced
Type II	Displaced, with intact posterior cortex
Type III	Displaced, no cortical contact
	Posteromedial
	Posterolateral

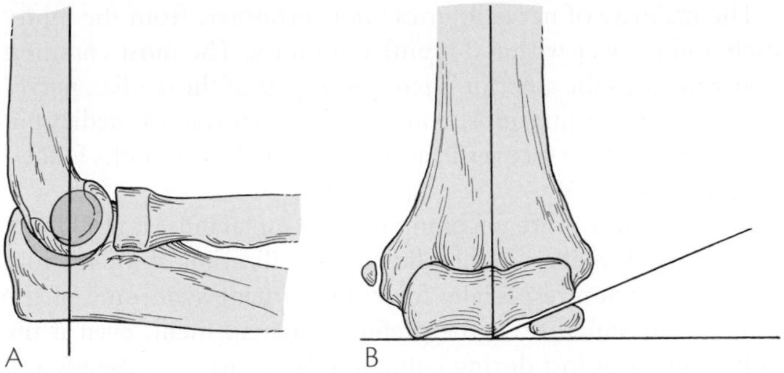

Fig. 14.5.1 Anterior humeral line (A) and shaft-physeal angle (B). Baumann described the orientation of the shaft and physis of the lateral condyle and observed a normal range of 75–80 degrees; this should be compared to the other side. In addition the integrity of the olecranon fossa needs to be considered.

the part of the median nerve closest to the bone; testing for this by flexion of the index finger and thumb into an 'O' shape should be undertaken.

The distal circulation of the arm should also be assessed. If a radial pulse is not palpable further investigation can be performed using Doppler or pulse oximetry to assess this but this should not delay the time of operative intervention. Evaluation for compartment syndrome is needed both pre and postoperatively even when there has been no vascular compromise.

Ipsilateral forearm injuries occur in about 5–10% of patients, but the supracondylar fractures should be treated operatively and stabilized, before treatment of the other fractures.

Radiographic evaluation

When determining the degree of displacement of the fracture on x-ray, several features should be identified (Figure 14.5.1 and Box 14.5.1).

Treatment

Treatment of supracondylar fractures is based upon their classification. Type I (undisplaced) fractures need only simple immobilization in a collar and cuff under the clothes for two to three weeks then with advice for mobilization. Swelling can be significant and application of any rigid splintage can create pressure problems and is to be avoided. Complications particularly medial collapse or impaction can occur, leading to varus malunion, and so follow-up evaluation is recommended.

The treatment of type II fractures is by reduction of the extension deformity. Due to the significant incidence of instability then it is the author's preferred technique for stabilization of these with percutaneous pins.

In type III fractures olecranon screw traction can be undertaken, but this is now rarely used because of the lengthy hospital admission required. Traction is however useful where condition of the skin precludes the presence of wires or where fracture comminution is so severe as to prevent an acceptable reduction being maintained with percutaneous pinning.

Closed reduction and percutaneous pinning

Gentle longitudinal traction should be applied followed by closed reduction of the fracture with flexion and the appropriate forearm rotation under image intensifier control is initially performed. The adequacy of the reduction needs to be assessed using shoot through (Jones view), oblique and lateral views (the latter, particularly in unstable fractures, may demonstrate rotational malalignment but is useful for assessing displacement). Numerous variations of pinning techniques have been described in an attempt to minimize complications. The two most stable constructs consist of medial and lateral pins placed through the supracondylar ridges and into the opposite cortex or two lateral divergent pins. Stabilization using the former technique involves insertion of the lateral wire in full flexion, extending the arm and inserting the medial wire (utilizing a small incision to protect the ulnar nerve) (Figure 14.5.2). Both techniques have their advocates and the main complications of loss of reduction and iatrogenic ulnar nerve injury are technique dependent.

Once stabilized, the elbow can then be assessed for stability and reduction. Radiographic and clinical assessment, as described earlier, should be used.

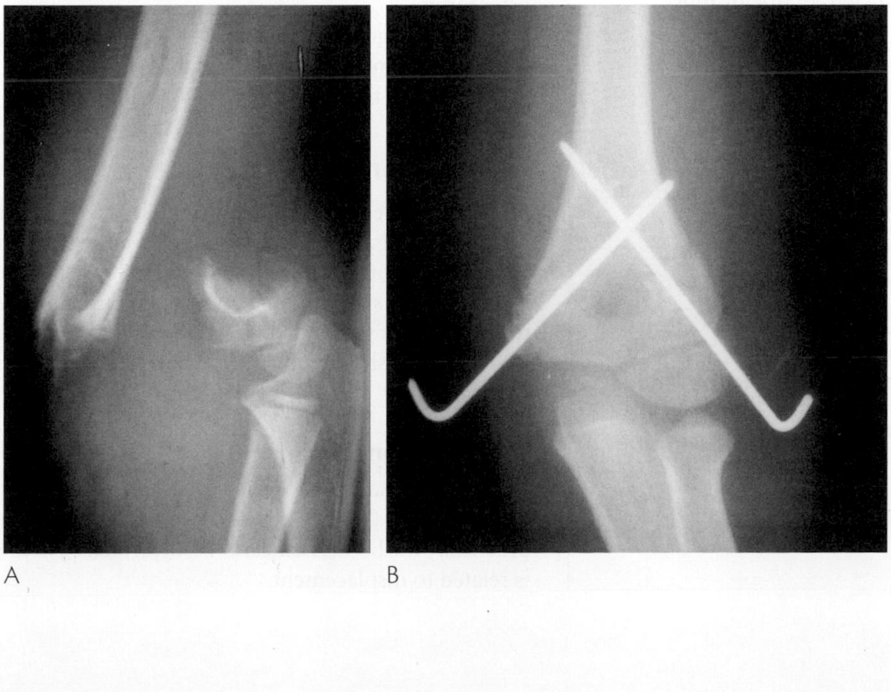

Fig. 14.5.2 A) Type III supracondylar humeral fracture. B) After closed reduction and fixation with medial and lateral K-wires.

Box 14.5.1 Assessment of reduction of supracondylar humeral fracture

- Anterior humeral line
- Shaft–physeal angle
- Restoration of olecranon fossa
- Comparison with other side.

After closed reduction and pinning, a wool and crepe dressing and non-removable collar-and-cuff sling are worn for 3–4 weeks. Then the pins are removed and an active range-of-motion rehabilitation programme is begun.

Open reduction

Open reduction is required for fractures that cannot be reduced by closed means, open fractures, and in some cases of fractures with vascular compromise. This allows the soft tissue interposition to be treated, following which stabilization can be undertaken in the same manner as for closed reduction with the benefit of direct visualization. Approaches from all directions have been described, the commonest being anteromedial or anterolateral depending upon fracture displacement. Approaching from the same side as the displacement of the proximal fragment, often allows a direct 'cortical read' and does not add significantly to the periosteal stripping. Where vascular compromise requires intervention an anterior approach is preferable. Delayed open reduction beyond 10 days has an increased risk of myositis ossificans.

Complications (Box 14.5.2)

Supracondylar humeral fracture complications can be either functional or cosmetic. Functional complications relate to nerve and vessel injury and elbow stiffness. Cosmetic complications are related to inadequate reduction creating malunion.

Box 14.5.2 Complications of supracondylar fractures

- Nerve damage:
  - ulnar nerve—may be caused by percutaneous pins
  - median nerve—may mask compartment syndrome
  - anterior interosseous nerve—most common
- Vascular system:
  - loss of radial pulse with good capillary return and careful observation
  - poor capillary return—urgent exploration
  - loss of circulation after reduction—urgent exploration
- Avascular necrosis of trochlea—produces fishtail deformity of humerus
- Stiffness
- Myositis ossificans
- Deformity
- Cubitus varus (gunstock deformity)
- May have rotatory component.

The majority of nerve injuries are neuropraxic from the injury itself and recover within 3 months of injury. The most common injury involves the anterior interosseous part of the median nerve.

Ulnar nerve injury most commonly occurs due to medial pin insertion but these recover in almost all cases by 3 months following pin removal.

Vascular injuries are uncommon. If the radial pulse is absent but there is good capillary refill following stabilization of the fracture then observation, especially for compartment syndrome of the forearm musculature, is the preferred management, even if the radial pulse was lost during reduction. If the arm is pulseless and capillary refill is poor the fracture should be stabilized and the situation reassessed, and if persistent, observation can still be undertaken since the vast majority of pulses return within 24h without detriment. Close observation should be undertaken with a low threshold to return the child to theatre for release of compartment syndrome and arterial exploration if necessary. The child should be transferred to a unit where facilities exist for vascular surgery.

Avascular necrosis of the trochlear has been reported from vascular injury leading to a fishtail deformity of the distal humerus, symptoms from which are delayed.

Elbow stiffness after this fracture may result in loss of terminal elbow extension. Most patients regain almost complete elbow motion, although this may require several months. Elbow stiffness also can occasionally be caused by myositis ossificans, which usually occurs after delayed open reduction or too vigorous rehabilitation.

Angular deformities result from inaccurate reduction or subsequent displacement producing a malunion. Cubitus varus ('gunstock') deformity is most common. The deformity remains static occurring at the fracture site rather than the joint and there are minimal functional deficits but often a considerable cosmetic deformity. Rarely this can occur in undisplaced fractures which may be a feature of vascular compromise to the lateral condyle.

Correction of cubitus varus is directed at the coronal plane deformity with various techniques having been described (Figure 14.5.3). The commonest technique of a lateral closing-wedge osteotomy may produce a lateral prominence and apparent persistence of the deformity, whereas other techniques attempt to avoid this problem using a dome osteotomy or step-cut lateral closing-wedge osteotomy.

Cubitus valgus deformity is rare. Hyperextension occurs when the lateral humeral capitellar angle is not corrected at the time of reduction and this does not improve with growth.

Lateral condylar fracture

Fractures of the lateral humeral condyle account for approximately 15% of distal humeral fractures in children, occurring most commonly around the age of 6 years. They can be easily missed radiologically since the metaphyseal fragment appears small but the presence of point tenderness over the lateral condyle with localized swelling should alert the clinician to the possibility of this injury.

Classification

Lateral condylar fractures classically were classified by the fracture pattern; Milch (1964) described two types of fracture direction; but practically the best classification is described by Wilkins (1996) and is related to displacement.

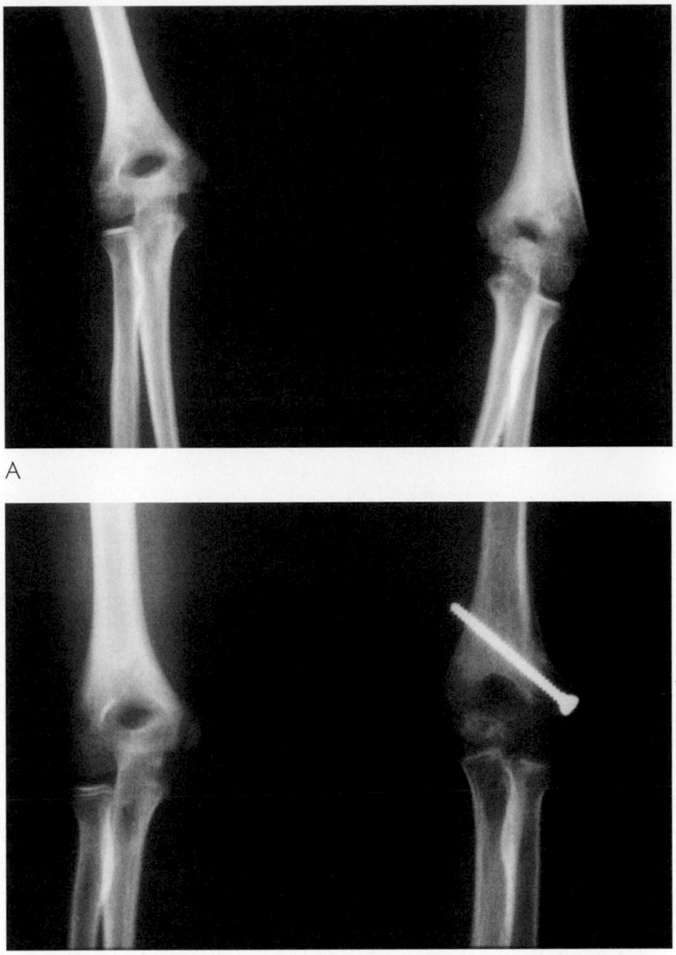

A

B

Fig. 14.5.3 Residual cubitus varus deformity: A) after closed treatment of a type III supracondylar humeral fracture, and B) after osteotomy and screw fixation.

Mechanism of injury

Two mechanisms of injury have been proposed for fractures of the lateral humeral condyle fracture: a 'push-off' mechanism where a fall onto the hand with the elbow flexed causes the radius to push off the lateral condyle; and a 'pull-off' mechanism which is more common and occurs when a fall on the outstretched hand with an extended elbow creates a varus moment and the lateral condyle is pulled by the extensor muscles.

Radiographic evaluation

In undisplaced or minimally displaced fractures a 'fat-pad' sign is present. The metaphyseal fragment is difficult to visualize on the anteroposterior view and on the lateral view will appear falsely small since it is being viewed in profile. In displaced fractures the capitellar ossification centre and the radial head are not aligned, distinguishing this from a supracondylar type fracture where this is maintained. Close monitoring of these fractures is required since with displacement operative treatment is required and it is difficult to assess whether there is an intact periosteal hinge stabilizing a minimally displaced fracture.

Box 14.5.3 Key features of lateral condyle fractures

- Common but easily missed
- Fracture line hidden in epiphysis and physis
- Muscles attached to distal fragment may increase displacement
- Local tenderness and swelling over lateral epicondyle is diagnostic
- Fat-pad sign commonly visible on radiograph.

Treatment

Fractures with less than 2mm displacement can be treated conservatively by immobilization; however they need monitoring to exclude late displacement, in which case fixation will be required. Immobilization is continued until radiographic healing is present.

Fractures with less than 4mm of displacement can be treated by closed reduction and percutaneous pinning with care not to cross the fixation wires at the site of the fracture and a degree of wire divergence is preferable.

For significantly displaced or unstable fractures, open reduction and internal fixation is required. A posterolateral approach in the brachioradialis–triceps interval presents the fracture which is reduced by extension and the metaphyseal fragment is always larger than expected from radiology and can be stabilized with a cannulated small fragment screw into the metaphysis. Excellent results with no complications have been reported with screw fixation. Alternatively two K-wires can be utilized.

Complications

The commonest complications of lateral condylar fractures relate to problems of union. In undisplaced fractures treated conservatively delayed union is frequent. Possible causes are poor vascularity of the fragment, synovial fluid in the fracture preventing fracture healing, and the muscle pull of the common extensors.

Non-union is usually due to incomplete reduction of fracture fragments. Non-unions without angulation are usually asymptomatic; however, where angulation remains, a cubitus valgus deformity develops which can lead to a tardy ulnar nerve palsy. Treatment of a non-union depends on functional problems as well as progressive deformity but open reduction with bone graft and internal fixation is required (Figure 14.5.4) and ulna nerve transposition may also be indicated.

Avascular necrosis of the lateral condyle fragment can occur from open reduction; however, when union is achieved the fragment revascularizes and long-term functional deficit is rare.

Transcondylar fracture

Transcondylar fractures of the humerus are a physeal separation of the whole of the distal humerus and occur prior to ossification, typically under 3 years of age (Figure 14.5.5). Since this area is cartilaginous, no fracture may be apparent on x-ray and a misdiagnosis of an elbow dislocation is made. These is a rare injury infrequently reported in the literature. These fractures have also been

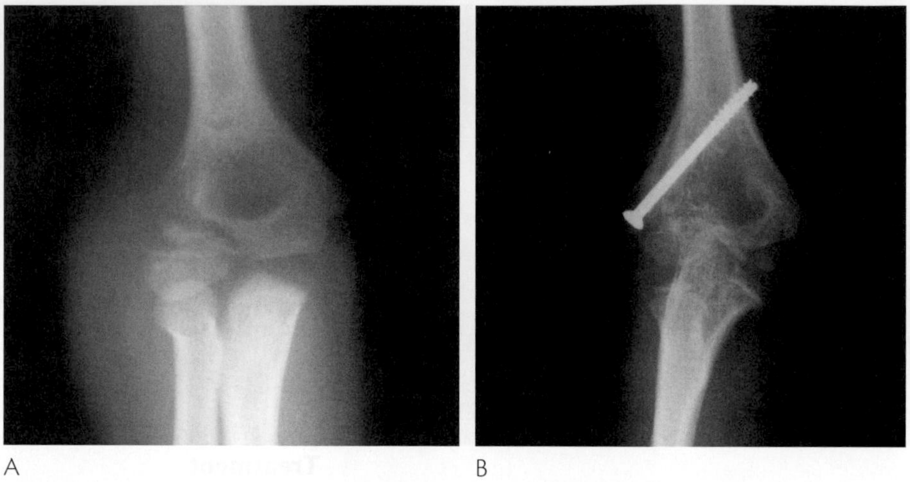

Fig. 14.5.4 A) Non-union of lateral condylar fracture. B) After extra-articular screw fixation and bone grafting.

reported as birth injuries following difficult deliveries and also in child abuse cases.

Clinical and radiographic evaluation

Swelling and hypermobility may be present or in the very young pseudoparalysis of the limb may be the presenting complaint. Assessment of the relationship of the medial and lateral epicondyles and the olecranon as an equilateral triangle exclude the diagnosis of dislocation and should alert the clinician to the possibility of a transcondylar fracture. Radiologically there may be loss of alignment between the radius and ulna and the humerus and the displacement is usually posteromedially. Arthrography or ultrasound may be required to confirm the diagnosis in the operating theatre prior to intervention.

Classification

Three groups are described depending on the degree of ossification present. In group A fractures (up to 12 months of age), the lateral condyle secondary ossification centre is not present and there is no visible metaphyseal fragment. In group B fractures (1–3 years) the capitellar ossification centre is present; a metaphyseal fragment, if present, is very small. Group C fractures (3–7 years) have a well-developed capitellar ossification centre and a large metaphyseal fragment.

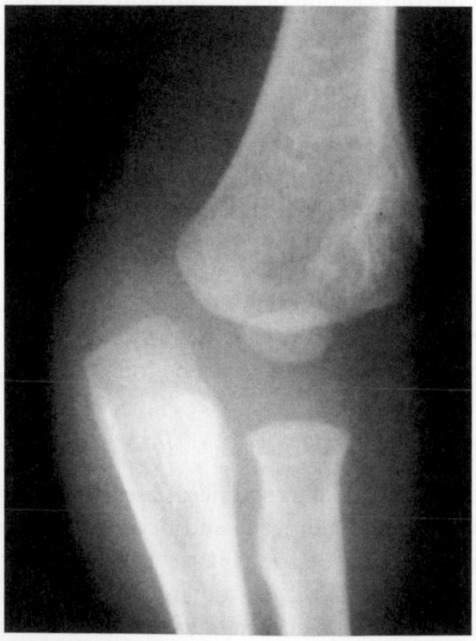

Fig. 14.5.5 Transepiphyseal fracture–separation of distal humerus.

Treatment

The recognition of the fracture and its association with child abuse in children under 2 years is mandatory, up to 38% in this age group have been reported to have this mechanism of injury. The fracture is reduced by elbow flexion and pronation of the forearm should then be stabilized using two divergent lateral wires (cross K-wires are difficult to insert medially due to the cartilaginous medial epicondyle) and then immobilized but the adequacy of reduction may require arthrographic assessment. Postoperatively a supportive dressing is required with the limb held flexed by a collar and cuff worn under the clothes for 3 weeks and then mobilization following wire removal. If the fracture has been missed and is more than 5 or 6 days old it will be irreducible and is better left to heal and corrected by osteotomy at a later date if necessary.

Complications

Neurovascular complications are infrequent but cubitus varus is common although generally minor (less than 15 degrees) and is related to the difficulty of assessment of reduction in the absence of ossification of the physeal fragment. This degree of cubitus varus deformity rarely causes functional problems and rarely requires

Box 14.5.4 Key features of transcondylar fractures

- Easily confused with dislocated elbow
- Associated with nonaccidental injury
- Arthrogram or ultrasound may be needed for diagnosis
- Best fixed with two lateral pins
- Most common complication is cubitus varus.

corrective osteotomy. Avascular necrosis of the trochlea can occur after this fracture and tends to occur early with a subsequent varus or fishtail deformity.

Medial humeral condylar fracture

Medial humeral condylar fractures are rare, occurring around 8–14 years of age. The fracture involves the trochlea and the distal humeral metaphysis, with the attached medial epicondyle, and is inherently unstable. Up to 40% are associated with elbow dislocations.

The fracture can either enter the elbow medial to the lateral crista of the trochlea or pass directly through the medial condylar ossific nucleus. Due to the presence of the attached medial epicondyle the fracture is rotated by the common flexors so that the fracture surface presents anteromedially and the articular surface faces posterolaterally (Figure 14.5.6A).

Mechanism of injury

Medial condylar fractures are caused by a direct blow on the flexed causing the olecranon to split the trochlea or where a fall is associated with a valgus stress and the forearm flexor muscles avulse the condyle.

Clinical and radiographic evaluation

Clinically there is medial swelling and tenderness and varus instability. Ulnar nerve function should be carefully assessed. After ossification of the trochlea and medial epicondyle the fracture is apparent on standard radiology and a fat pad sign is also present but before ossification a high index of suspicion is required and alternative techniques such as magnetic resonance imaging (MRI) may be required.

Treatment

Undisplaced fractures can be treated by immobilization in a backslab but must be regularly assessed for displacement. For displaced fractures the preferred option is open reduction and internal fixation via a posteromedial approach decompressing the ulnar nerve, limiting dissection to avoid avascular necrosis. The medial condyle should be stabilized with two parallel pins or a screw (Figure 14.5.6B). Post operatively due to swelling a supportive bandage or back slab is required with immobilization in a collar and cuff for 3 weeks and then mobilization.

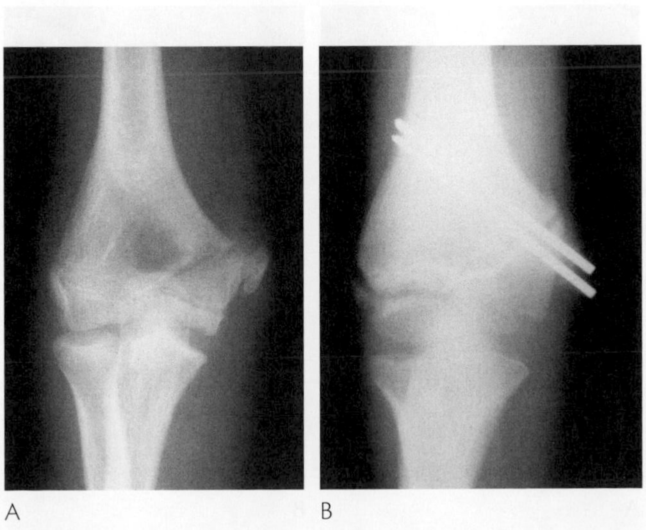

Fig. 14.5.6 A) Medial condylar fracture. B) After open reduction and K-wire fixation.

Box 14.5.5 Key features of medial condyle fractures

- Rare
- Elbow may be unstable
- Associated with dislocated elbow and ulnar nerve palsy
- Easy to confuse with medial epicondyle fracture
- Difficult to visualize without arthrogram or MRI.

Complications

The common complications are non-union, avascular necrosis of the trochlea causing a 'fishtail' growth deformity, and stiffness. Restriction of extension is the most frequent problem. Non-union is usually secondary to delayed diagnosis and treatment or inadequate fixation. Treatment of established non-union requires bone grafting and internal fixation.

Fractures of the capitellum

Fractures of the capitellum are a rare injury at any age, but especially in children. Anterior sleeve fractures have been reported in 8-year-old patients, but capitellar fractures are usually in older adolescents.

These fractures occur following a fall on the outstretched hand, where shear forces are transmitted through the radial head, injuring all or part of the capitellum. Recurvatum and cubitus valgus deformities may be predisposing factors.

The diagnosis of this fracture may be difficult and easily missed, particularly since they can be associated with radial head fractures. Swelling is often minimal about the elbow, with tenderness over the capitellum. A positive fat-pad sign is usually present on standard radiographs. Oblique radiographs or an MRI may necessary for diagnosis.

Two fracture patterns are described (Figure 14.5.7). Type I is a complete fracture of the capitellum, which has a portion of

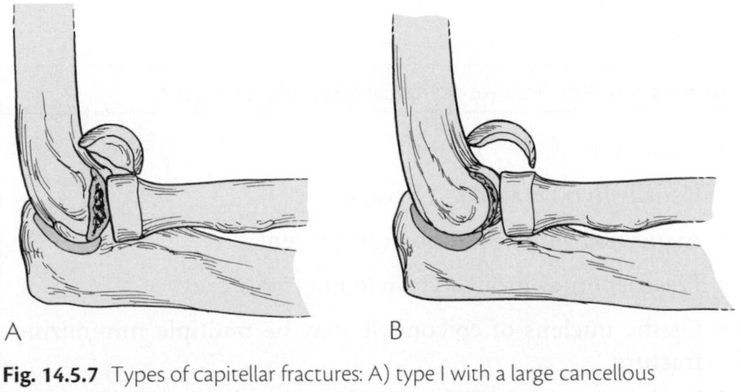

Fig. 14.5.7 Types of capitellar fractures: A) type I with a large cancellous fragment; B) type II, almost a pure articular fracture with little or no subchondral bone.

cancellous bone attached to the distal fragment. Type II fractures involve mainly articular cartilage with only a thin margin of subchondral bone.

Treatment

Open reduction is necessary, if the metaphyseal fragment is large enough this can be reattached and secured with Herbert type screws, via a posterior approach through the lateral condyle but careful dissection is required to avoid avascular necrosis of the lateral condyle. Smaller fragments should be excised and early range of motion exercises undertaken. The complications of capitellar fractures are avascular necrosis of the fracture fragment, loss of motion about the elbow, and early degenerative arthritis.

Medial epicondylar fractures

Medial epicondylar fractures are the third most common fracture of the elbow in children, accounting for 11% of fractures about the elbow. This injury most frequently occurs between 9–14 years of age, and is four times more common in boys than in girls. Elbow dislocation occurs in approximately 30% of cases and in half of these the medial epicondylar fragment will be incarcerated in the elbow joint after reduction of the dislocation leading to a block to elbow extension.

Anatomy

The medial epicondyle is a traction apophysis with the forearm common flexor muscles arising from its anterior surface and the ulnar collateral ligament also being attached. Ossification of the medial epicondyle begin at 4–6 years of age, and it fuses with the distal humerus by the age of 15 years. Irregularity of ossification can give the nucleus a fragmented appearance, which can be mistaken for a fracture. In younger children some capsular attachments may remain and a positive fat-pad sign may be seen, but in older children the epicondyle is extra-articular.

Mechanism of injury

Medial epicondylar fractures can be caused by a direct blow, an avulsion injury due to the pull of the common flexor muscles of the forearm, or with an elbow dislocation where under hyperextension and valgus stress the ulnar collateral ligament avulses the epicondylar. This dislocation may spontaneously reduce prior to presentation. This mechanism of injury also may produce associated injuries to the radial neck and the olecranon.

This fracture can be produced by a sudden isolated muscle contraction, such as the simple act of throwing a baseball (which can also be a chronic condition termed Little Leaguer's elbow where elbow extension is lost and pain is reproduced by valgus stress, x-rays revealing an irregular and widened physis).

Clinical and radiographic evaluation

The elbow is swollen and tender medially and if the medial epicondyle is displaced, it may be palpable and freely moveable. X-rays of minimally displaced fractures may show changes to the smooth physeal edges or a widened physis. In displaced fractures, if the fragment appears at the level of the joint, an oblique radiograph should be performed to exclude incarceration of the fragment within the elbow joint.

Classification

Wilkins *et al.* combined several classification systems and divided medial epicondylar injuries into acute and chronic injuries. Acute injuries are further divided into (a) undisplaced or minimally displaced; (b) displaced by more than 5mm but proximal to the joint line; (c) incarcerated with no elbow dislocation; and (d) incarcerated with elbow dislocation.

Treatment

Undisplaced or minimally displaced fractures should be treated with immobilization followed by early range of motion of the elbow. For displaced fractures proximal to the joint line good results with non-operative treatment are reported. Although healing in a displaced position occurs this does not lead to any functional deficit or any instability of the elbow joint. In children with high functional demands and a fracture of the dominant arm, fixation can be considered but it is debatable whether this affords any long term benefit.

The only absolute indication for operative treatment is incarceration of the fragment in the joint (Figure 14.5.8). Although successful extraction of the fragment from the joint can be achieved

Box 14.5.6 Key features of medial epicondyle fractures

- Common
- Usually in boys aged 9–14 years
- Associated with dislocation (30 per cent)
- Fragment may incarcerate in joint (15 per cent)
- Ossific nucleus of epicondyle may be multiple minimizing fracture
- Commonly avulsion of common flexor origin.

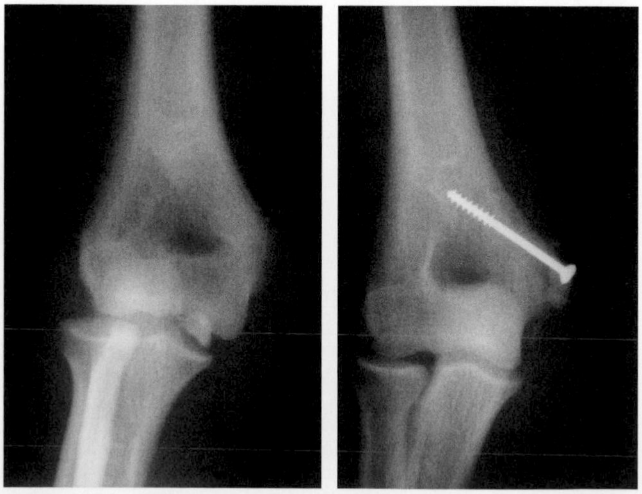

A B

Fig. 14.5.8 A) Medial epicondylar fracture entrapped in elbow joint. B) After open reduction and screw fixation.

by manipulation in up to 40% by placing a valgus stress on the elbow while supinating the forearm and dorsiflexing the wrist, it is more likely than not that there has been a significant injury to the elbow joint to allow incarceration to occur and that this has been a dislocation that has spontaneously reduced and the fragment is better secured by open fixation affording an element of stability to the elbow joint.

Operatively the fragment is exposed via a medial approach protecting the ulnar nerve. The fragment is always larger than is apparent radiologically and can be secured with a single cannulated screw which will afford sufficient stability to allow early graduated mobilization. If ulnar nerve symptoms are present at the time of fixation, decompression of the nerve should also be performed and this is present in up to 50% of incarcerated cases.

Complications

The most serious complication of this fracture is an unrecognized incarcerated fracture fragment within the elbow joint, this becomes adherent blocking elbow motion. In patients with chronic incarceration of medial epicondylar fractures a thick fascial band binds the ulnar nerve to the underlying muscle causing ulnar nerve dysfunction. Once identified, it should be removed.

Lateral epicondylar fracture

Fracture of the lateral epicondyle is rare, occurring as a traction injury from the pull of the common extensor origin. Localized swelling and tenderness are present and the only treatment required is immobilization and early mobilization; functional deficit rarely occurs. Incarceration of the fragment in the elbow joint has been reported and is the only indication for operative management to reattach the extensor origin.

T-condylar fractures

T-condylar fractures occur in adolescents and have an adult fracture pattern with the fracture starting in the trochlea propagating and dividing the medial and lateral columns. This is caused by the wedge effect of the olecranon splitting the humerus following axial compression or a direct blow on the flexed elbow. Displacement of the fragments occur secondary to the pull of the forearm muscles rotating the fragments in two planes.

Gross swelling is present due to the unstable nature of the fracture and radiologically displaced fractures are readily apparent. Undisplaced fractures need careful evaluation to differentiate these from the other forms of distal humeral injury.

Classification

The classification described by Wilkins is well recognized: type I, minimally displaced; type II, displaced with no comminution; type III, displaced and comminuted.

Treatment

Whilst each case should have its treatment determined by the fracture pattern the basic principles of treating this intra-articular fracture should be applied. The articular surface should be restored to congruency; the medial and lateral columns should be restored and stabilized to allow early mobilization because the attached muscles will increase displacement if adequate stability is not achieved.

Type I fractures can be treated with percutaneous pinning. Type II and III fractures require open reduction and internal fixation. The fracture needs adequate exposure by either a triceps-splitting approach, an olecranon osteotomy, or an extensile approach. Initial reduction of the articular surface is performed with stabilization using transverse fixation with subsequent reduction of the medial and lateral columns using wires is the younger adolescents or reconstruction plates at 90 degrees to each other in the older child. In Type III fractures where comminution of the columns is severe the joint surface can be reconstructed and the extra-articular fracture treated by traction to maintain alignment.

Complications

The commonest complications are elbow stiffness and loss of motion, and a degree of this is the usual outcome so the parents should be advised of this. Non-union, avascular necrosis of the trochlea, and failure of internal fixation have all been reported.

Elbow dislocation

Elbow dislocations accounts for 6% of all elbow injuries in children, most commonly occurring once the physes have closed at 13–14 years of age. Up to 50% of elbow dislocations have an associated fracture, typically the medial epicondyle, the lateral condyle, and the radial head and neck.

The presence of an elbow dislocation is readily apparent as the deformity, depending on the direction of displacement and swelling, is usually significant. A detailed neurological examination should always be performed and any deficit documented prior to reduction.

Anatomy

The elbow has little bony stability except when fully extended. The majority of its stability is provided by the collateral ligaments and the joint capsule. The medial collateral ligament consists of anterior (taut in extension) and posterior (taut in flexion) bands. Lateral stability is provided by the radial collateral ligament and the radial head also provides stability to valgus stress. Dynamic stabilizers of the elbow are the forearm flexors and extensor muscles. The brachialis muscle protects the brachial artery and median nerve from injury during elbow dislocation.

Classification

Elbow dislocations are classified according to the direction of dislocation and the status of the proximal radioulnar joint (Table 14.5.2). When the proximal radioulnar joint is intact, the elbow can be dislocated in five directions, the commonest being posterolateral. Disruption of the proximal radioulnar joint leading to a divergent dislocation or radioulnar translocation is rare.

Box 14.5.7 Key features of T-condylar fractures

- Grossly unstable elbow
- Both columns must be stabilized
- Joint surface must be congruent
- Open reduction is needed for displaced fractures.

Table 14.5.2 Classification of elbow dislocations

Type I	Proximal radio-ulnar joint intact
	A Posterior
	1. Posteromedial
	2. Posterolateral
	B Anterior
	C Medial
	D Lateral
Type II	Proximal radio-ulnar joint disrupted
	A Divergent
	1. Anteroposterior
	2. Mediolateral
	B Radio-ulnar translocation

Treatment

In uncomplicated elbow dislocations closed reduction followed by short-term (10–14 days) immobilization is the treatment of choice. Reduction is obtained by one of two methods. In the 'push' technique the surgeons thumb pushes on the olecranon tip causing reduction. In the alternative 'pull' technique the elbow is flexed 70 to 80 degrees traction applied longitudinally to the forearm reducing the dislocation. Placing the arm in supination avoids translocation of the radius and ulna during reduction.

Open reduction is indicated for (a) failed closed reduction, (b) open dislocation, (c) fractures requiring open fixation, or (d) bony fragment incarceration in the joint.

Complications

The most common complication is elbow stiffness which can be minimized by early mobilization, but there is usually a minor loss of extension. Nerve injury occurs in 10%, of which in the majority a neuropraxia and a full recovery is the norm. The ulnar nerve is the most commonly involved, particularly when the dislocation is associated with a medial epicondylar fracture, and exploration of the affected nerve should be considered at the time of fracture stabilization.

Myositis ossificans can occur typically in the brachialis muscle. Its incidence is reduced by prompt reduction, the avoidance of hyperextension, and passive mobilization.

Proximal radioulnar translocation may be unnoticed after closed reduction of a dislocated elbow. In this situation, the radius articulates with the trochlea and the olecranon articulates with the capitellum. In a posterolateral dislocation, if the forearm is hyperpronated at the same time as traction is applied, the radial head can easily pass anterior to the ulna and cause the translocation. Treatment of the translocation requires surgery open reduction.

Recurrent dislocation has either soft tissue or bony components causing the instability. Surgical stabilization using an anterior bone block or transfer of the medial epicondyle proximally to tighten the medial restraining structures can be performed for bone defects. In soft tissue instability triceps tendon transfer or lateral capsular plication are the options of choice.

Box 14.5.8 Elbow dislocation

- 50 per cent have other fractures around the elbow
- Neurologic deficit common
- Elbow should be reduced with forearm supinated to unlock radial head
- Early mobilization reduces stiffness.

Divergent elbow dislocation

With the elbow in extension and a high-energy proximally directed force being applied through the forearm a divergent dislocation can occur. The radius displaces laterally and the olecranon medially. Closed reduction usually can be easily obtained due to the degree of the soft tissue injury, by longitudinal traction releasing the humerus and then compressing the radius and ulna together before flexing the elbow where stability is maintained.

Pulled elbow syndrome

The classical history is of a sudden longitudinal pull being applied to a child's wrist or hand (under 4 years of age) with forearm pronation and elbow extension resulting in radial head subluxation. Following this episode the child will be reluctant to use the limb, local tenderness over the radial head and annular ligament is present but swelling is rarely a feature. Supination and flexion movements of the elbow are painful but necessary to reduce the subluxation. If supination alone does not reduce the subluxation then maximal flexion followed by supination should be performed and will usually be accompanied by a characteristic snapping reduction.

Further reading

Kalenderer, O., Reisoglu, A., Surer, L., and Agus, H. (2008). How should one treat iatrogenic ulnar injury after closed reduction and percutaneous pinning of paediatric supracondylar humeral fractures? *Injury*, **39**(4), 463–6.

Loizou, C.L., Simillis, C., and Hutchinson, J.R. (2009). A systematic review of early versus delayed treatment for type III supracondylar humeral fractures in children. *Injury*, **40**(3), 245–8.

Omid, R., Choi, P.D., and Skaggs, D.L. (2008). Supracondylar humeral fractures in children. *Journal of Bone and Joint Surgery*, **90A**, 1121–32.

Song, K.S., Kang, C.H., Min, B.W., Bae, K.C., and Cho, C.H. (2007). Internal oblique radiographs for diagnosis of nondisplaced or minimally displaced lateral condylar fractures of the humerus in children. *Journal of Bone and Joint Surgery*, **89A**, 58–63.

Yen, Y.M. and Kocher, M.S. (2008). Lateral entry compared with medial and lateral entry pin fixation for completely displaced supracondylar humeral fractures in children. Surgical technique. *Journal of Bone and Joint Surgery*, **90A**, 20–30 [erratum **90A**, 1337].

14.6

Fractures and dislocations about the paediatric forearm

A. Bass

Summary points

- Growth plate fractures are common and of these the commonest is a Salter–Harris type II through the distal radial physis. There is considerable capacity for remodelling so reduction may not be needed. Remodelling capacity is inversely proportional to age
- Elastic intramedullary nails are valuable in the forearm
- Complications of fractures include malunion, refracture, and cross union.

Distal physeal injuries (Box 14.6.1)

Incidence

Growth-plate fractures comprise 10–25% of all forearm fractures in the paediatric population. When all physeal injuries are studied, the distal radius is considered the most frequently injured single growth plate comprising 17.9–29.7% of all physeal fractures. The distal ulna is less commonly injured and consists of 2.5–4.5% of all physeal fractures. Although radial physeal fractures may occur without visible injury to the ulna, the vast majority of ulnar physeal fractures are associated with a distal radius metaphyseal or growth-plate fracture. The average age of children with distal physeal fractures varies with gender; the peak age of injury in females is at 10–11 years of age while in males it is 12–13 years of age. This disparity is likely due to differences in the age of maximal mean peak growth velocity.

Management

The most common type of growth-plate fracture encountered at the distal radius results in a Salter–Harris type II fracture. The majority of these fractures are minimally angulated and are immobilized without reduction. Gentle closed reduction under adequate anaesthesia is usually successful for displaced fractures sufficient to cause clinical deformity on examination. Treatment guidelines reflect the large capacity for remodelling at the distal radial physis. Fifty per cent apposition is acceptable but may compromise maintenance of reduction. Dorsal–volar tilt of 20 degrees and radial angulation of 15 degrees will remodel as long as 2 years of growth remain and the physis does not close prematurely. The results of treatment are uniformly good given the substantial capacity for remodelling, particularly under ten years of age.

The long-term prognosis into adulthood is also excellent with almost all patients functioning normally even with radioulnar shortening of up to 1cm or an ulnar styloid non-union. If the fracture redisplaces after 7 days, further attempts at reduction should be avoided as evidence suggest that this can result in damage to the physis and subsequent shortening and deformity. Fractures are immobilized in a long arm cast or a well-fitted short arm cast for 3–4 weeks and protected activities are instituted after cast removal. It is recommend that percutaneous pinning after closed reduction, is considered, in cases of instability and severe soft tissue injury resulting in swelling or neurovascular compromise.

Distal ulnar physeal fractures are uncommon and may be difficult to diagnose as the secondary centre of ossification does not appear radiographically prior to the age of 6 years. Ulnar physeal injuries are more likely to result in premature growth arrest than radial physeal injuries. Treatment of these fractures depends on the associated radial injury as well as the ulnar fracture. It has been reported that up to 50% of distal ulna physeal injuries result in growth arrest. However only rarely does this result in symptoms or functional disability.

Distal radius fractures (Box 14.6.2)

Incidence, classification, and diagnosis

Distal radius fractures represent the commonest fracture occurring in the forearm, and there is some evidence that this incidence may be increasing. The peak incidence in boys is 11–14 and in girls 8–11 years of age.

Box 14.6.1 Distal physeal fractures

- 80% of growth at distal physis
- With 2 years growth remaining, up to 20 degrees dorsal angulation and 15 degrees radial deviation is acceptable
- Ulnar physeal fractures have a high incidence of premature growth arrest.

Box 14.6.2 Distal radius fractures

- In isolated fractures of distal radius consider Galeazzi and pseudo-Galeazzi fractures
- Loss of reduction more common in:
  - Apex–volar angulation
  - Complete vs greenstick
  - Apposition <50%
- With 2 years growth remaining, up to 20 degrees dorsal angulation and 15 degrees radial deviation is acceptable.

These fractures are classified by type, displacement, and associated fractures. The type is dependent on the predominant force producing the fracture.

A compression force will result in a torus fracture, whereas a bending force will result in a greenstick or complete fracture. This is important as the former is an inherently stable pattern and it has been shown that they can be safely and effectively treated by a simple 'futura' type wrist brace and discharged after the initial visit. Displacement in the majority of cases is dorsal displacement with apex volar angulation where the periosteum is intact dorsally. Fractures of the distal third of the radius are usually associated with an ulna metaphyseal fracture or avulsion fracture of the ulna styloid. Rarely there is no obvious associated fracture of the ulna. Such a fracture is a Galeazzi fracture. However it has been shown that in many cases such a pattern in children would be better referred to as a 'Galeazzi equivalent' or 'pseudo Galeazzi' fracture with a radius fracture associated with a fracture occurring through the ulna physis in a bone in which the ulna epiphyseal ossification centre has not yet appeared. These injuries are difficult to diagnose and are missed in up to 41% of cases. The outcome of such an injury has been shown to be poor and if recognized should be treated in a supination cast.

Mechanism of injury

Distal radius fractures with an intact ulna usually follow a fall on an outstretched hand; resultant angulation may also be accompanied with rotational deformity. Apex–volar angulation (the most common deformity) is produced by forced supination and apex–dorsal angulation with forced pronation. Galeazzi fractures usually follow a fall on an outstretched hand with hyperpronation of the forearm.

Management

Distal radius fractures have significant remodelling capacity in the sagittal plane but less so in the coronal plane. Many authors have suggested widely varying limits of acceptable deformity with good outcomes; however, it is our experience that if the arm appears clinically deformed or there is greater than 10 degrees of angulation, reduction is necessary.

Fractures are reduced with a combination of traction, angulation, and rotation of the palm in the direction of the angulation. The fracture is brought out to length, deformity exaggeration and rotation may produce end-to-end contact. If this fails then percutaneous methods using a dorsally inserted pin into the fracture site and levering the distal fragment of the fracture into position may be successful. Typically these fractures are immobilized in short arm casts moulded to produce three-point fixation as they have been shown to be as effective as long arm casts.

Relatively high rates of reangulation in distal radius fractures from 11–62.5% have been reported. Higher rates of reangulation are noted in fractures with apex–volar angulation (supination injuries) and complete fractures versus greenstick fractures. In addition, redisplacement is also commonly seen where bony apposition following reduction is less than 50% or the fracture was initially completely displaced. Although remodelling is substantial (Figure 14.6.1), it is our recommendation that completely displaced fractures should be reduced and plaster cast immobilization should be

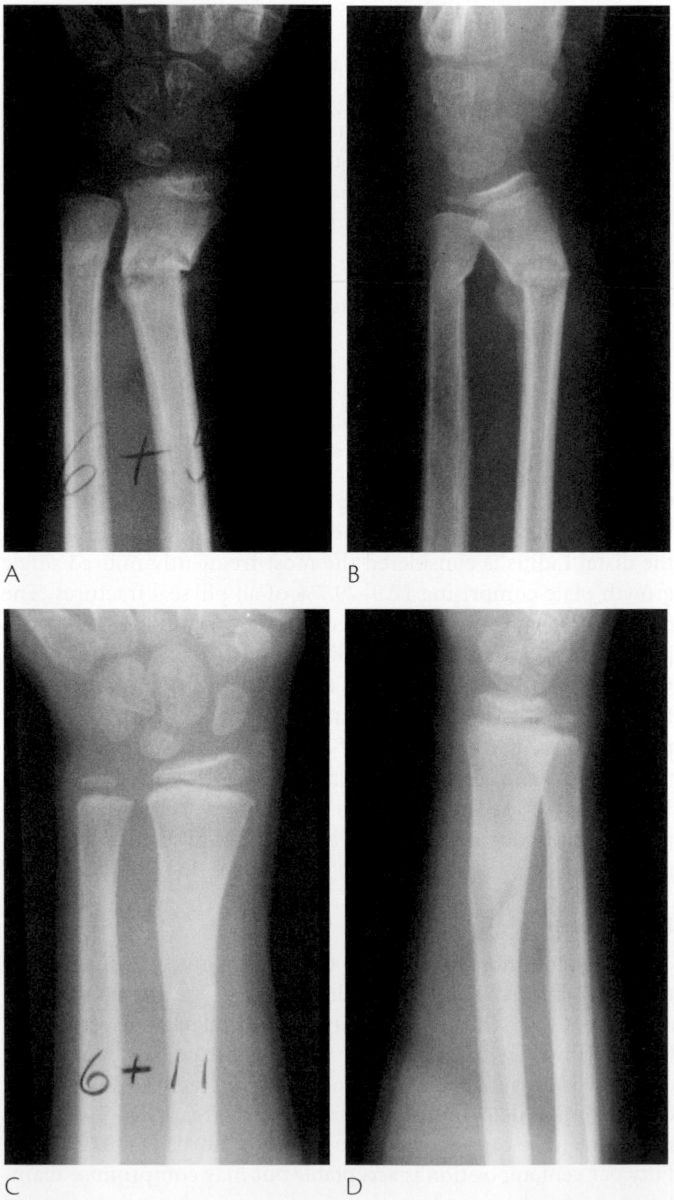

Fig. 14.6.1 A) and B) Radiographs of a boy aged 6 years and 5 months 3 weeks after distal radius and ulna fracture. This angulatory deformity was determined to be acceptable in light of early callus formation. C) and D) Radiographs 6 months later demonstrating nearly complete remodelling.

supplemented with percutaneous K-wire fixation as this reduces the risk of subsequent redisplacement requiring further treatment.

Both-bone forearm fractures (Box 14.6.3)

Introduction

Historically, adult forearm fractures treated non-operatively had poor results from non-union or malalignment and stiffness due to lengthy immobilization required for union. In paediatric fractures, treatment is primarily non-operative due to uniformly rapid healing, the potential for remodelling of residual deformity, and the inherent stability of the fractures once reduced.

Pertinent anatomy and physiology

The radius and ulna are stabilized by the interosseous membrane and by the triangular fibrocartilage complex distally and the annular ligament proximally. The pronator quadratus (distally) and pronator teres (inserting on the mid radius) actively pronate the forearm while the biceps and supinator (proximal insertions) provide supination. The insertion of these four muscles can partially account for fragment position in complete fractures. In complete distal third fractures, the proximal fragment will be in neutral to slight supination while the weight of the hand combined with the pronator quadratus tends to pronate the distal fragment. In complete proximal third fractures the proximal fragment is usually supinated.

Normal growth and implications for remodelling

The distal radial and ulnar growth plates are responsible for 75% and 81% of the longitudinal growth of each respective bone. This is consistent with the often made observation that distal forearm fractures have greater potential for remodelling than do more proximal fractures. Additional remodelling can also be attributed to elevation of the thick osteogenic periosteum after fracture. This periosteal sleeve aids remodelling of residual diaphyseal deformity.

Mechanism of injury

An understanding of the forces leading to forearm fracture is important as reductions are often performed opposite the direction of initial injury. Paediatric forearm fractures typically follow indirect trauma, such as a fall on an outstretched hand. Direct trauma may additionally account for open fractures, severely displaced fractures, and those seen in the proximal forearm. While the final degree of fragment displacement following indirect trauma varies between greenstick and complete fractures, the initial mechanism of injury is usually the same.

In cases where sufficient force does not completely displace the fracture, an incomplete or greenstick fracture results. A greenstick fracture in one bone may accompany a complete fracture in the other. Radiographically, greenstick fractures demonstrate two-dimensional angulation which in reality is a rotational displacement. Fractures with apex–volar angulation result from an axial force applied with the forearm in supination, those fractures with apex–dorsal angulation result from an axial force applied in pronation. Reducing a greenstick fracture usually requires rotation opposite the direction of the deforming force.

When significant indirect or direct trauma exceeds the resistance of the forearm, complete fractures of both bones will follow. When completely broken by either indirect or direct forces the bones shorten, angulate, and rotate within the confines of the surrounding periosteum, interosseous membrane, and muscle attachments.

Box 14.6.3 Both-bone forearm fracture

- Acceptable reduction
  - <9 years—complete displacement, 15 degrees angulation
  - >9 years—10 degrees proximal angulation or 15 degrees distal angulation
  - Approaching skeletal maturity—no angulation
- Reduce greenstick fractures by rotating in direction of angulation
- Complications: malunion, refracture, cross union, compartment syndrome (rare).

Clinical evaluation

The diagnosis of forearm fractures is usually self-evident based upon history and obvious deformity. Radiographic evaluation should include anteroposterior and lateral views of the forearm. If the elbow and wrist are not adequately visualized, corresponding views are obtained to rule out radial head dislocation, supracondylar fractures and distal radioulnar joint injury.

Malrotation in complete fractures can be difficult to detect and assess. Malrotation is suspected when cortical, medullary, or bone diameters of adjacent fragments are not equal. Alternatively, malrotation can be gauged from deviations of normal orientation of proximal and distal bony prominences on radiographic analysis.

On standard anteroposterior views, the radial tuberosity is seen in profile on the medial side, while the radial styloid and thumb are seen on the opposite side. On the same view, the ulnar styloid and coronoid process are not seen. On standard lateral views the ulnar styloid is seen pointing posterior and the coronoid process pointing directly anterior; the aforementioned radial prominences will not be seen. Another useful method for determining rotation of the proximal fragment utilizes the 'tuberosity view'. This technique uses a calibration chart to determine the rotation of the proximal radius. The distal fragment can then be manipulated and rotated into a corresponding position.

Adequacy of reduction and results of closed treatment

It is uniformly understood that post-traumatic paediatric angular deformities have a variable remodelling potential; however, it has not been consistently proven that rotational malalignment will also remodel. Many studies have documented better radiographic remodelling in fractures that are distal and in patients less than 9 or 10 years of age. It is important to realize that fracture location and age may not be independent variables.

It is unclear from clinical studies how much malalignment can be accepted. Studies in cadavers have demonstrated clinically significant loss of forearm rotation with residual deformities in the midshaft of the radius and ulna angulation of greater than 10 degrees.

Although several authors have demonstrated decreased remodelling potential in proximal fractures 'marked loss of function' is reported infrequently. Some authors have demonstrated little functional loss with decreases of forearm rotation of 35–40 degrees. It must, however, be remembered that loss of pronation can be compensated for by shoulder abduction but supination loss is not well tolerated.

The literature regarding acceptable limits of alignment is confusing and contradictory. It is our view that given the unpredictable nature of remodelling, the unclear relationship between deformity and loss of motion and the difficulty in the assessment of rotation on radiographs that the acceptable limits for alignment in both bone forearm fractures are thus. In fractures at any level in children less then 9 years of age we will accept complete displacement and 15 degrees of angulation. In children older then 9 years of age we will accept angulation in proximal fractures of 10 degrees while more distally it remains 15 degrees. However once a child approaches skeletal maturity no angulation should be considered acceptable.

Management

Greenstick fractures (Box 14.6.4)

Historically, incomplete fractures were treated by completing the fracture and then manipulating the bones into an acceptable position. This approach has the theoretical advantage of increasing the size of the fracture callus and decreasing the risk of refracture. Currently, it is recognized that residual angulation is a result of malrotation and should be reduced with rotation opposite the deforming force. Traction and manipulation of the apex while rotating will often assist in the reduction. The majority of greenstick fractures are supination injuries with apex–volar angulation, and these are reduced with variable degrees of pronation. It can be difficult to remember whether to pronate or supinate the hand based on the direction of the angulation. Most fractures reduce by rotating the palm towards the direction of the deformity. Those fractures with apex–volar angulation are a result of axial load in supination, therefore rotate the palm volarly (pronation). Fractures with apex–dorsal angulations are a result of pronation force, therefore rotate the palm dorsally (supination). It is not uncommon to see a greenstick fracture of one bone and a complete fracture of the other. In these cases we use the same principles of reduction by rotation. After reduction the forearm should be immobilized in the same position that reduced the fracture. Studies have documented redisplacement of 10–16% in greenstick fractures that were not adequately rotated in the cast.

Complete fractures

Complete both-bone forearm fractures are reduced with a combination of sustained traction and manipulation. The fingers are taped to prevent sores and placed in fingertraps with the elbow at 90 degrees of flexion, counter traction is provided with 4.5–6.75kg (10–15lb) suspended from a sling over the distal humerus. The fracture and soft tissues are slowly brought out to length for 10–15min, the arm is allowed to find its own rotation. End-to-end apposition is then attempted with deformity exaggeration and direct manipulation. If attempts to achieve bony apposition are unsuccessful, complete over-riding of fracture fragments is accepted as long as rotation and angulation is within guidelines (Figure 14.6.2).

Fracture alignment in traction is assessed with fluoroscopy or plain radiographs; if adequate, the distal part of the long arm cast is applied and moulded while still in traction. Residual malrotation is addressed prior to cast application by rotating the forearm. Because most displaced both-bone fractures are in the middle region, the hand is placed in a neutral or slightly supinated position; this usually accommodates rotation and angulation. This approach has been supported in other studies that demonstrate little correlation between position of immobilization and end result. Pronation is rarely employed for complete fractures and may result in a functional loss of supination due to soft tissue contracture. Recent studies suggest that immobilizing the forearm in a cast with the elbow extended may result in a lower rate of redisplacement.

Meticulous casting is critical as several studies have documented reangulation in approximately 8–14% of cases. Some have blamed poor cast technique while others have attributed this to residual rotational malalignment. Forearm anteroposterior and lateral radiographs are taken after reduction and immobilization, minimal improvements of residual angulation can be corrected by wedging the cast.

After an adequate reduction and immobilization, patients typically return for a follow-up radiograph at 1–2 weeks after injury. Several studies have documented reangulation during the first 2 weeks. If reangulation is documented, cast removal and rereduction is recommended. Good results of rereduction have been documented if performed within a few weeks of the initial fracture. If no reangulation is appreciated, the cast is continued for 6–8 weeks or until radiographic healing. Patients are released to all activities 3–4 months after injury.

Box 14.6.4 Greenstick fracture

- Rotate palm in direction of angulation
- Higher rate of refracture until 6 months after injury
- Beware plastic deformation without fracture

Operative indications and technique

Indications for surgical intervention in paediatric forearm fractures include:

- Open fractures
- Fractures shortly before skeletal maturity
- Irreducible/unstable fractures
- Unacceptable closed reduction
- Failure to maintain a closed reduction
- Multiple trauma/floating elbow.

Several different techniques are available but the two most commonly applied are open reduction and internal fixation with plates and closed intramedullary nailing of either one or both bones.

As anatomical reduction is usually not needed, we prefer closed intramedullary fixation of one or both bones. Elastic stable intramedullary nailing is now the treatment of choice using a nail 0.4 times the diameter of the medullary canal.

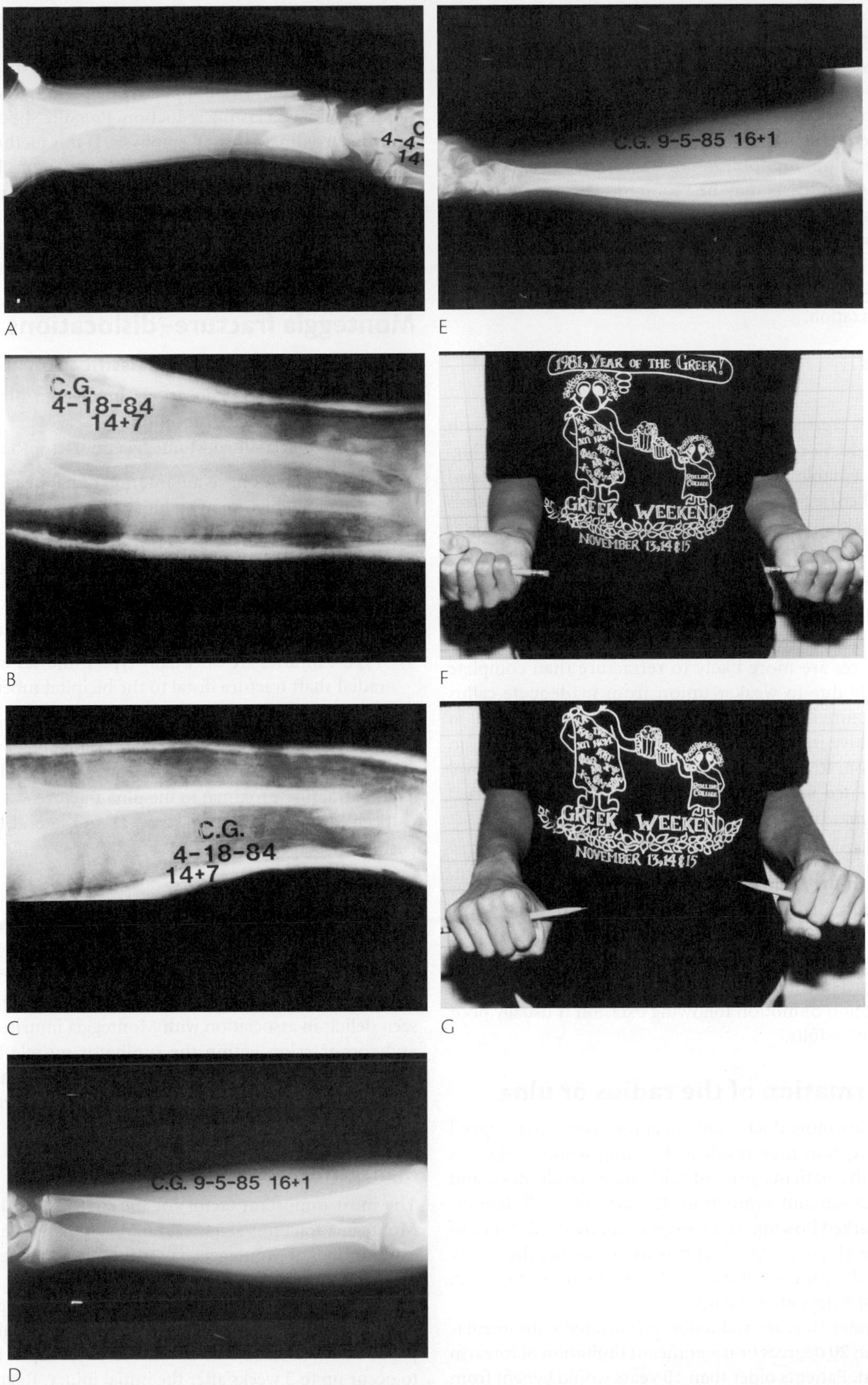

Fig. 14.6.2 A) Forearm radiograph of a boy aged 14 years and 7 months with completely displaced distal radius and ulna shaft fracture. B) and C) Radiographs in a cast demonstrates acceptable alignment with residual complete displacement and radial translation of the distal fragments. This reduction was accepted. D) and E) Radiographs 18 months after fracture demonstrate almost complete remodeling. F) and G) Clinical photographs demonstrating symmetrical pronation and supination.

This is introduced into the radius through an oblique drill hole in the distal metaphysis, taking care to avoid the superficial branch of the radial nerve, and through the posterolateral part of the olecranon (Figure 14.6.3). It is considered important to pre-bend the nails so that the maximum curvature occurs at the level of the fracture. Limited open reduction may be required in order to pass the intramedullary fixation. Immobilization with supplemental plaster or fibreglass long arm casts may be required. The advantages of nailing include simplicity of the procedure, union with minimal stress shielding by hardware, easier hardware removal and a better cosmetic result. Studies have shown this procedure is successful and associated with a low rate of complications compared with plate and screw fixation.

Complications

Malunion

Forearm fractures treated conservatively will rarely present with significant malreduction that precludes activities of daily living. In cases of unacceptable malunion or loss of functional forearm rotation, surgical correction can be obtained with drill osteoclasis and casting or open osteotomy and plating. Both techniques will increase motion; better results are obtained when surgical correction is performed without delay.

Refracture

Refracture can occur up to 9 months after original injury. Greenstick fractures are more likely to refracture than complete fractures, possibly due to weaker union from inadequate callus formation. Refracture is associated with poor clinical outcome. In these cases operative intervention may be indicated to ensure an adequate reduction. Refractures have also followed plate removal in those cases treated with primary open reduction and internal fixation and this may be lower for nail fixation.

Cross-union

Synostosis between the radius and ulna is very rare, but can compromise the results in cases of fracture from very high-energy injury. It is associated with fixation of both bones through a single incision and therefore this should be avoided. Extensive bone formation that restricts pronation and supination can be surgically removed. Restoration of motion following excision is usually poor in comparison with adults.

Plastic deformation of the radius or ulna

Children's bones are more ductile and an appropriate force applied in the proper direction may result in bending without obvious fracture. Clinically, patients present with pain, tenderness, and diminished pronation and supination. Radiographs will demonstrate slight to marked bowing which extends along the distance of the affected bone (Figure 14.6.4). If bowing is subtle, the injury may be diagnosed with comparison radiographs or a bone scan performed at least 3 days after the injury.

For children under 10 years, reduction is indicated if the angulation is greater than 20 degrees or if significant limitation of forearm rotation is present. Patients older than 10 years would benefit from reduction for deformity greater than 15 degrees or when limited forearm rotation is present. Additionally, plastic deformation must be reduced when the radial head is dislocated (Monteggia equivalent) or redislocation will occur.

Treatment consists of closed reduction under general anaesthesia. A described technique of reduction involves applying a force directly over the apex of the deformity with a sandbag or rolled towel. The force must be applied for a period of several minutes in order to achieve a lasting reduction. Pressure should not be applied over the proximal or distal epiphysis. If this method is not successful, it may be worthwhile to consider open or closed osteoclasis. Following reduction, patients are typically immobilized for 6–8 weeks. This extended period of immobilization may be required due to slightly slower healing resulting from the lack of a significant periosteal reaction.

Monteggia fracture–dislocations

Mechanism of injury and classification

Monteggia fracture–dislocations involve an ulna fracture combined with radial head dislocation.

Bado (1967) classified Monteggia injuries into four types:

1) Type 1 injuries have an anterior radial head dislocation with anterior angulation of an ulnar fracture.
2) Type 2 injuries have posterior or posterolateral dislocations of the radial head with concordant ulnar fracture angulation.
3) Type 3 injuries have lateral or anterolateral radial head dislocations with radial angulation of the ulna fracture.
4) Type 4 injuries are essentially type 1 injuries with an associated radial shaft fracture distal to the bicipital tuberosity.

Monteggia equivalent injuries were also described and include plastic deformation of the ulna with radial head dislocation, ulna fracture with radial neck fracture, and radial head dislocation with a radial fracture proximal to the ulna fracture.

In children the anterior (type 1) and lateral (type 3) fracture patterns predominate.

Clinical evaluation

It is important to identify nerve deficits as they occur more commonly in Monteggia type injuries. Clinically evident nerve dysfunction has been documented in all major nerves in 3–24% of fractures. Posterior interosseous nerve palsy is the most commonly seen deficit in association with Monteggia injuries due to tethering and compression within the supinator muscle by the arcade of Frohse. The majority of these palsies recover spontaneously within 3–6 months. Exploration may be indicated if no recovery is identified within this time frame.

Management

The most important factor for the successful outcome following Monteggia fractures (Figure 14.6.5) is its early diagnosis. A significant number of Monteggia patterns of fracture are missed resulting in pain and loss of function. This is particularly true with greenstick fractures of the ulna which may recoil to a position of minimal displacement that masks the significant initial energy that also produces radial head dislocation and dislocations have been shown to occur up to 3 weeks after the initial injury. Regular radiographic review is necessary for up to 3–4 weeks following such injuries.

It is essential to assess the radiohumeral integrity on all radiographic views. Regardless of radiographic projection, a line drawn down the shaft of the radius should intersect the centre of

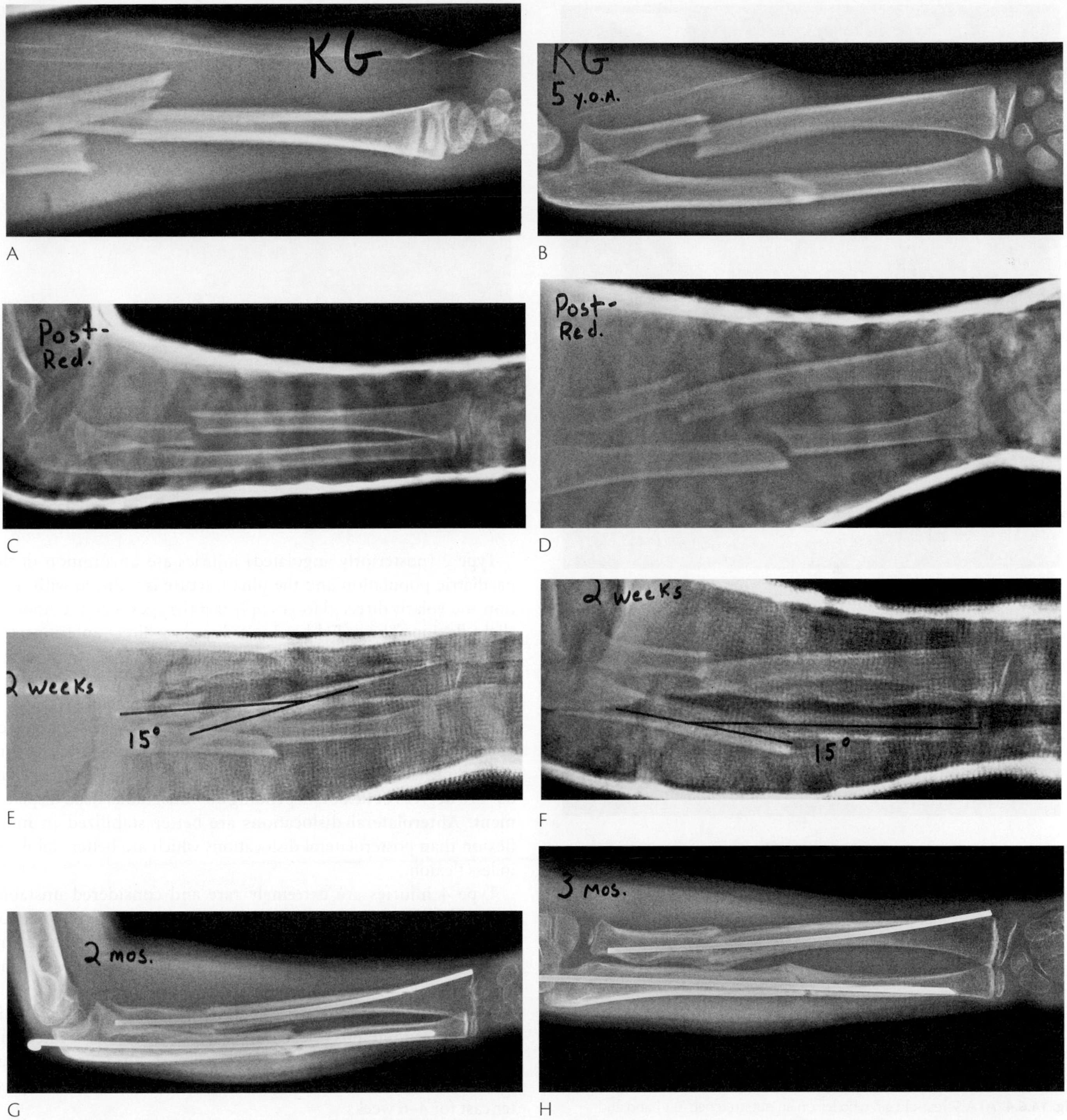

Fig. 14.6.3 A) and B) Radiographs of a 5-year-old girl with a proximal both-bone forearm fracture. C) and D) Following closed reduction under general anaesthesia minimal angulation and moderate displacement is noted. This was accepted. E) and F) Due to soft-tissue swelling her cast was split and 2 weeks after closed manipulation she was noted to have loss of reduction with angulation greater than 15 degrees. This was not accepted. G) and H) She underwent open reduction and intramedullary pinning with good alignment and callus formation at 2 and 3 months.

the capitellum. Deviation from this relationship indicates dislocation or subluxation and therefore merits intervention.

Most authors believe that in children less than 9 years of age Monteggia injuries should be managed with initial attempted closed reduction. Successful management requires firstly reduction of the ulna fracture, secondly the reduction of the radial head and finally the alleviation of deforming forces.

Therefore type 1(anteriorly angulated) injuries are reduced by first correcting ulna length by traction and angulation by elbow hyperflexion. Secondly, gentle direct pressure over the radial head

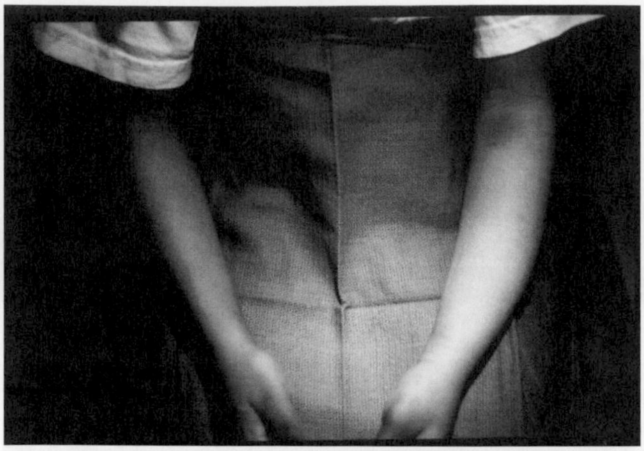

A

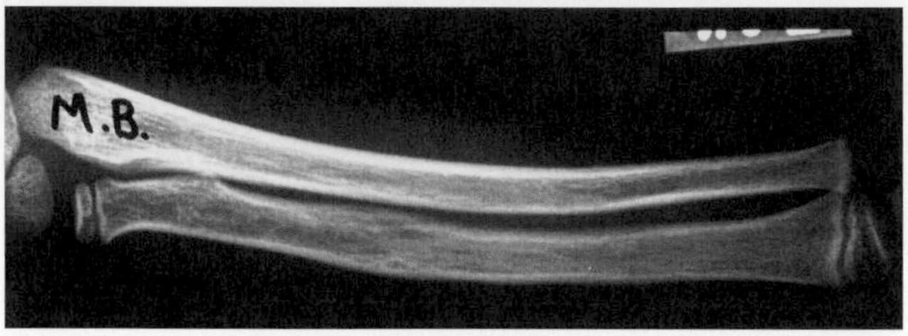

B

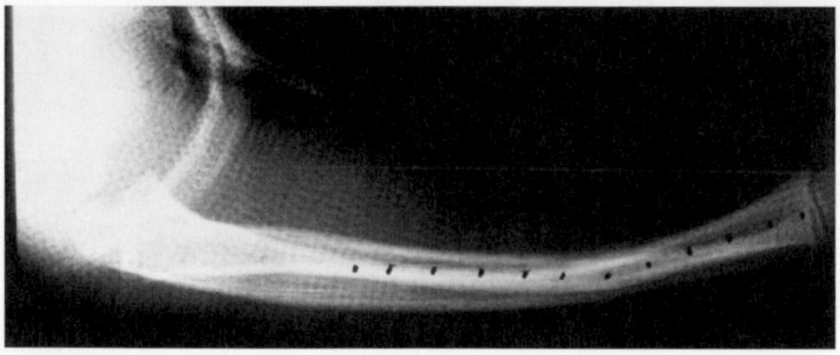

C

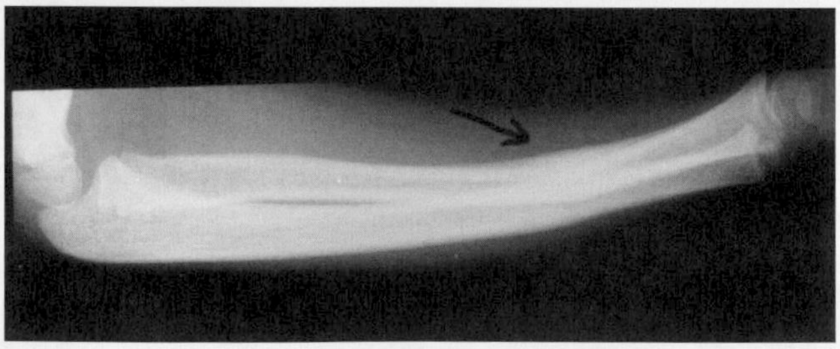

D

Fig. 14.6.4 A) A 5-year-old girl who fell on an outstretched left hand and presented to the emergency room with pain and clinical deformity. B) and C) Radiographs demonstrated dorsal-radial bowing and she was immobilized in a long arm cast without reduction. D) Three months later she was non-tender and had decreased pronation and supination of 20 degrees in each direction. Radiographs demonstrated periosteal reaction.

may facilitate reduction that is heralded by a gentle snap and placing the hand in supination may stabilize it. Finally these injuries are immobilized in well-moulded long arm cast in supination at 100–110 degrees of flexion. This positioning relaxes the biceps which may be a factor in late anterior radial head subluxation.

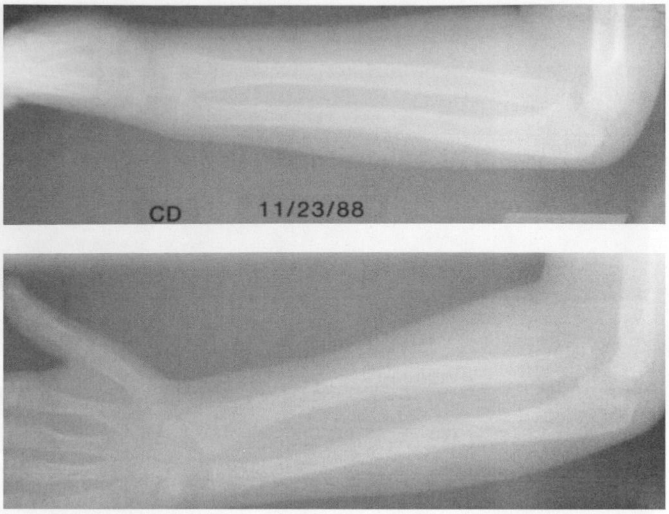

Fig. 14.6.5 Radiographs of the forearm obtained 5 weeks after a non-displaced greenstick fracture of the ulna. Dislocation of the radial head had gone unnoticed. A line down the shaft of the radius should intersect the capitellum on all views.

Type 2 (posteriorly angulated) injuries are uncommon in the paediatric population and the ulna fracture is reduced with traction and volarly directed force applied at the apex with the elbow in slight flexion. The radial head is reduced by direct anterior pressure and finally these fractures are immobilized in extension following reduction of ulnar alignment and restoration of normal radiohumeral articulation to prevent redisplacement.

Type 3 (lateral angulation) are reduced with a valgus force applied to the apex of the ulna fracture and direct lateral pressure on the radial head. Once reduced, the arm is immobilized in 60–110 degrees of flexion depending on initial radial head displacement. Anterolateral dislocations are better stabilized in more flexion than posterolateral dislocations which are better stabilized in less flexion.

Type 4 injuries are extremely rare and considered unstable. Closed reduction in a manner similar to type 1 injuries may be attempted but these injuries should be considered unstable and operative stabilization is probably needed to prevent radial head instability.

Regardless of injury type, patients should return to the clinic weekly for radiographs to ensure that the radius is still located and the deformity of the ulna has not recurred resulting in redislocation of the radial head. The patient should be maintained in a plaster cast for 4–6 weeks.

Operative intervention will be required in those injuries where the ulnar reduction is unstable, or the radial head is irreducible due to ulnar malreduction or an interposed annular ligament. Type 4 injuries and Monteggia equivalent injuries with radial neck fractures are relatively unstable and require operative stabilization of both radial and ulna fractures in the majority of cases. The ulna is managed with closed reduction and intramedullary fixation using a flexible nail passed distally from the olecranon. The radial head is then checked radiographically for reduction. Open reduction and ligament reconstruction or repair is recommended when the radial head will not reduce in the face of good ulnar alignment. Following repair or reconstruction of the annular ligament, the proximal radius may be further stabilized by K-wire pinning if it continues to be unstable. Because of the risk of pin failure, transcapitellar pinning of the radius has been abandoned in favour of pinning the radius to the ulna directly. The postoperative care of Monteggia fractures is similar to that for cases that are successfully managed via closed reduction. Good clinical results can be expected in paediatric patients with Monteggia injuries diagnosed within 2 weeks of injury and treated with surgery.

Radial neck and head fractures (Box 14.6.5)

Incidence

Proximal radius injuries in children usually result in fracture of the radial neck. Radial head fractures have been reported in the paediatric population but are considered to be rare entities. As such, this chapter will not focus on these injuries except to point out that they are usually Salter–Harris type III or IV fractures with potentially higher rates of growth abnormalities and attendant concerns for joint incongruity. Radial neck fractures in children accounted for 5.8% and 8.5% of all elbow fractures. Radial neck fractures are rarely diagnosed prior to age 4 or 5 years as the epiphysis does not ossify until after this. Radial neck fractures typically occur at two different levels—either through the physis with or without an attached metaphyseal fragment (Salter–Harris type I and II respectively) or 3–4mm distal to the physis in the anatomic radial neck.

Classification

Type 1 fractures usually result in lateral displacement of the proximal fragment with angulation that varies in direction and magnitude. The direction of angulation and displacement of the radial fragment is always lateral in relationship to the humerus; however, its angulation relative to the radius depends on the degree of hand rotation upon impact. Type 2 fractures are posteriorly displaced and result from posterior dislocation of the elbow (Figure 14.6.6). In these cases, the radial neck may be fractured following spontaneous elbow reduction or secondary to attempted closed reduction. These fractures are exceedingly rare but are important to recognize as the radial head may be rotated 180 degrees following reduction.

Management

The majority of authors agree that angulation less than 30 degrees in the paediatric population is acceptable and should be immobilized without attempts at closed or open reduction. Translocation may be accepted when the radial head is less than 4mm displaced.

Box 14.6.5 Radial neck fractures

- Angulation <30 degrees is acceptable
- Progressive treatment if >30 degrees
  - Direct pressure ± forearm rotation
  - Percutaneous manipulation
  - Metaizeau technique
  - Open reduction + stabilization (NB avoid damaging blood supply in intact periosteal hinge).

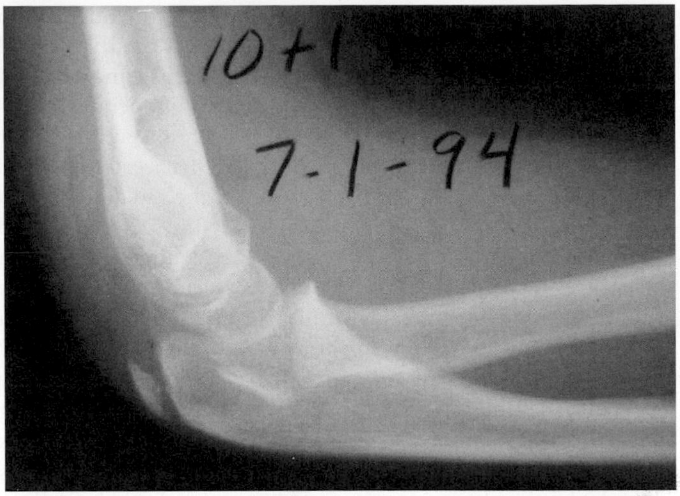

Fig. 14.6.6 Type 2 fracture of the radial neck. This is easily missed and usually follows spontaneous reduction of a posterior dislocation of the elbow. Closed reduction is attempted by recreating the dislocation followed by distraction and reduction.

Once a decision has been made to reduce the radial neck fracture we follow a treatment algorithm until the fracture has been adequately reduced and stabilized. Initially we attempt direct pressure over the radial head under fluoroscopy control. Direct pressure is applied to the radial head as the elbow is placed into varus while partially extended. An alternative manoeuvre involves placing the elbow in 90 degrees of flexion with the elbow fully supinated. Pressure is applied to the radial head and the arm is gently pronated to reduce the fracture. If this fails, manipulation is facilitated with the use of a percutaneously placed Steinmann pin into the head of the radius or the fracture site. The pin is then used like a crow bar to lever the radial head into an acceptable position.

If closed reductions fail then we employ the technique described by Metaizeau. This involves the insertion of an intramedullary wire from distal to proximal in the radius; it is passed into the radial head which is disimpacted and by rotating the wire it reduces the fracture. The wire is left in position to stabilize the reduction.

Only if all these methods fail would we consider open reduction. Open reduction is performed through a lateral Kocher approach and caution is directed towards avoiding extensive exposure distally on the neck of the radius. Dissection in this area may disrupt the blood supply which enters proximal to the neck resulting in delayed or non-union and risking the development of avascular necrosis, or may injure the posterior interosseous nerve as it courses through the supinator muscle. Sectioning of the annular ligament may be used to facilitate reduction; however, this structure should also be repaired. If the reduction appears unstable the fracture may be stabilized with an intramedullary wire as for the Metaizeau technique, patients should be immobilized for 3–4 weeks in a long arm cast or splint.

Results and complications

Diminished rotation is more commonly seen in children with more severe displacement and angulation, fracture comminution, concurrent associated elbow injury, and in older patients when compared to younger patients.

Some reports have demonstrated poorer results in patients who undergo operative intervention than in those treated via closed means. These studies imply that it is better to accept some degree of malalignment rather than accept the problems of operative treatment in order to achieve an anatomical result. However, superior results have been obtained with the use of the Metaizeau technique.

Complications include aseptic necrosis of the radial head with the majority of series reporting incidences around 5%. Radial head excision in cases of aseptic necrosis may be required due to pain and loss of motion. Occasionally excessive cubitus valgus may follow excision; however, deformity is rarely associated with significant increases in pain, functional limitations, or tardy ulnar nerve palsy. Radial head enlargement has also been commonly reported in several series and may present with pain or clicking during forearm rotation. Proximal cross-union between the radius and ulna has similarly been noted in approximately 3–4% of cases with a higher incidence in patients with associated proximal ulnar injury.

Further reading

Evans, E.M. (1945). Rotational deformity in the treatment of fractures of both bones of the forearm. *Journal of Bone and Joint Surgery, British Volume*, **27B**, 373–9.

Flynn, J.M. (2002). Pediatric forearm fractures: decision making, surgical techniques, and complications. *Instructional Course Lectures*, **51**, 355–60.

Gibbons, C.L.M.H., Woods, D.A., Pailthorpe, C., Carr, A.J., and Worlock, P. (1994, 1991). The management of isolated distal radius fractures in children. *Journal of Pediatric Orthopedics*, **14**, 207–10.

Holdsworth, B.J. and Sloan, J.P. (1982). Proximal forearm fractures in children: residual disability. *Injury*, **14**, 174–9.

Ploegmakers, J.J. and Verheyen, C.C. (2006). Acceptance of angulation in the non-operative treatment of paediatric forearm fractures. *Journal of Pediatric Orthopaedics*, **15**(6), 428–32.

14.7

Children's hand trauma

Henk Giele

Summary points

- This chapter reinforces that children are not small adults and the management of these injuries must consider the effect on growth and development
- Nail bed injuries require microsurgical repair if permanent deformity is to be avoided
- Every attempt should be made to replace amputated digits, whatever the level of amputation
- Good results are the common outcome in children's fractures unless complicated by surgical intervention or infection. However, angulation, rotation, and intra-articular deformities should be corrected where possible
- All children with deep lacerations of the upper limb should have a general anaesthetic for adequate exploration and repair of the wound
- A high index of suspicion of nerve injury should exist when assessing hand lacerations, and the outcome of early surgical repair is good.

Incidence and epidemiology

Soft tissue injuries and lacerations are the most common paediatric hand injuries, most of which are the result of the fingertip being crushed. Fractures, followed by burns, bites, and infections are the next most frequent.

The incidence of the various injuries and subtypes of injuries varies with age. Babies suffer scalds, toddlers from soft tissue injuries and crush injuries, with burns also being common in this age group. Older age groups have a higher incidence of fractures, and to a lesser extent lacerations with damage to the underlying longitudinal structures.

Injuries usually occur at home, with a higher incidence in boys.

Examination of children with hand injuries

In young children, it is important to gain the confidence of the child and parents. Time should be taken to allow the child time to look and assess you, whilst you look and assess them. Speak to both the child and parents to obtain the history and establish rapport. It helps to bring a toy, penlight, or other distraction device to draw the attention of the child. If the child is sitting on a parent's lap, examine them there. Crouch down to their level rather than standing over them.

When possible avoid causing the child any pain. A history of the accident may at times provide sufficient independent reason for surgical exploration making it unnecessary to examine the hand or view the wound prior to theatre. Although wound examination may allow better assessment of injured structures and hence communication, it will not usually change the decision to operate. If a dressing must be removed do this after as much of the examination has already been completed. Examination may require heavy reliance on observation and indirect methods such as the tenodesis effect. Consider examining the child's unaffected hand to gain their confidence. Much of the examination can be done by observation of the child playing or trying to hold objects. Observe their hand's posture and movement. Ask them to open or close their fingers of both their hands together. Sensation is extremely difficult to assess even in older children, as they will believe they are feeling something even if they cannot. Trying to assess sensation with them blinded is difficult and unreliable. The wrinkling test following water immersion (denervated areas fail to wrinkle) may be useful, but is time consuming in the clinic. It is much better to observe the hand immediately after any dressing has been removed, as many hands will be moist beneath their dressings and will demonstrate the wrinkling sign. Dryness and sheen of the skin as determined by palpation or by the tactile adhesion test (gently slide a pen against their skin and assess the degree of friction), are often later signs of denervation and may not be that useful in the acute setting.

Movement often provokes pain, hence leave this component of the examination until last. Children can often be encouraged to open and close their fingers. If children are uncooperative then compression of the forearm musculature produces movement of the digits. Failure of movement may indicate a tendon injury. Partial injury can be suspected when there is painful movement. If the injury is distal to the wrist then the tenodesis effect of differential digital tendon gliding on passive wrist flexion and extension can provide evidence of tendon injury or continuity. If there is any doubt then surgical exploration is indicated, as the long-term consequences may be severe.

Dressings

Where dressings are indicated in younger children, it is usually easier to dress the whole hand in a boxing glove type bandage, as this is more difficult for children to remove. Usually, it is not necessary to extend the dressings above the elbow or to plaster them. The additional weight and discomfort of a plaster cast gives the child extra incentive to wriggle out of these extended dressings. A boxing glove bandage wrapped with tape preventing use of the fingers is very effective. To prevent the bandage becoming dirty, wet, or removed, the parents may apply a sock over the bandage, which can be changed as required.

When suturing children's skin always use absorbable sutures, as this obviates the need to distress the child further by suture removal and avoids an additional anaesthetic. 5/0 or 6/0 Vicryl Rapide is usually rubbed away within several weeks, but may last longer.

Prevention

Accident awareness and prevention should be an important part of general health care. Several projects increasing such education are proving successful in reducing injuries.

Child abuse

Non-accidental injury (NAI) to children's hands should be suspected when the pattern of injury does not seem to follow the explanation given by the parents or differs from the explanation given by the child or changes with each telling. Burns are the commonest presentation of NAI in the hand. Recurrent presentations or admissions should alert one to the possibility of NAI.

The consequences of such an accusation are severe, so do seek further opinions, and repeat the history and examination several times over the ensuing days as well as reviewing the records and relevant x-rays before making a diagnosis of NAI.

Fingertip injuries

Crush injuries and distal fingertip amputations

Crush injuries to the fingertip are extremely common injuries, often occurring when the fingertips of toddlers and younger children become jammed in the hinge side of a closing door. The mechanism is an off-step crushing force that presses on the nail plate on one side and on the pulp on the other. The usual result is a fracture or avulsion of the nail plate, associated with an underlying nail bed laceration, lateral perionychial lacerations, and an underlying tuft fracture of the distal phalanx or a Salter–Harris type I fracture of the distal phalanx physis (Seymour's lesion). Different patterns of the injury depend on the distribution of the force. Crush injuries most commonly involve the longer ring or middle fingers; however any finger may be injured. Complete amputation including bone is uncommon, but tip avulsion is common.

Deformity of the nail and fingertip is common following conservative therapy (Figure 14.7.1A,B). Operative treatment requires local or general anaesthesia depending on the age of the patient. The operation involves removal of the damaged nail and meticulous repair of the lacerated nail bed and surrounding skin. The nail bed is repaired with the finest absorbable sutures available, usually 7/0 or 8/0 Vicryl, using microsurgical instruments and loupe magnification. Where nail bed loss is present the defect can be closed by excision and direct suture or by using a graft. The graft may be nail bed graft harvested from the adjacent remaining nail bed, from a toe nail bed, or may be a dermal graft. Once repaired the previously removed nail, silicon sheeting, or piece of foil suture packet is applied as a nail splint, covering the nail bed and maintaining the nail fold. Dressings are applied and left for 2 weeks, following which no dressings are needed. Nail growth will take around 6 months before the result can be assessed (Figure 14.7.1C).

Where avulsion of the fingertip has occurred, the tip frequently contains one or more tiny fragments of distal phalanx tuft. These should be debrided, as if they remain they frequently become infected or resorb. If the avulsed segment is still tenuously attached or is brought in with the patient, it should be replaced. This should be performed within 5h of injury for the maximal chance of success. Once the delay is greater than 5h, the pulp portion should be defatted prior to replacement, returning it as a full thickness graft. It is important to debride the recipient bed thoroughly, particularly removing any damaged fat to enhance revascularization of the restored part. When the amputated portion is not retained the defect may be treated conservatively with dressings, by the application of split, full thickness, or composite toe pulp grafts, or by the use of flaps. The indications for these various treatments are similar to those in adults; however, the greater regenerative potential in children dictates a greater dependence on conservative measures. In the case of failure of revascularization of the replaced avulsed segment it should be retained as a biological dressing until healing occurs underneath and the dry eschar separates (Figure 14.7.1D,E).

Fingertip injuries with an underlying distal phalanx fracture should be thoroughly washed under anaesthesia, prior to reduction of the fracture. These fractures are sufficiently stable following the soft tissue repair not to require further stabilization. Wiring may damage the epiphysis, and serve as a portal for infection in these open fractures. A mid shaft distal phalanx fracture is uncommon in children, as the points of weakness produces tuft or proximal physeal fractures. In the under 5s the commonest distal phalanx physeal fracture is a Salter–Harris type I pattern, eponymously described by Seymour. The child presents with avulsion of the nail plate from the nail fold. The injury appears innocuous but is an open fracture. Seymour fractures should not be treated conservatively as they may become infected leading to destruction of the physis, leading to growth disturbance. Seymour fractures are frequently missed until they present as a paronychial infection. A good lateral x-ray at the time of the original assessment is mandatory, but the only radiological clue may be a widening of the physeal line (Figure 14.7.1F,G).

Amputations

Amputated digits occur infrequently in children. Unlike adults every attempt should be made to replant amputated parts irrespective of the level of the injury or the involvement of a single digit, within limits of technical ability. The outcome of replants in children is more favourable than in adults. With due care to the epiphyses, even growth of the replanted digit can be normal.

Tip amputations are treated depending on the degree, direction, and salvage of the loss. Complete tip amputations at the level of the proximal nail fold should be replanted if the part is salvaged. If replantation fails or should the part be not suitable or unavailable,

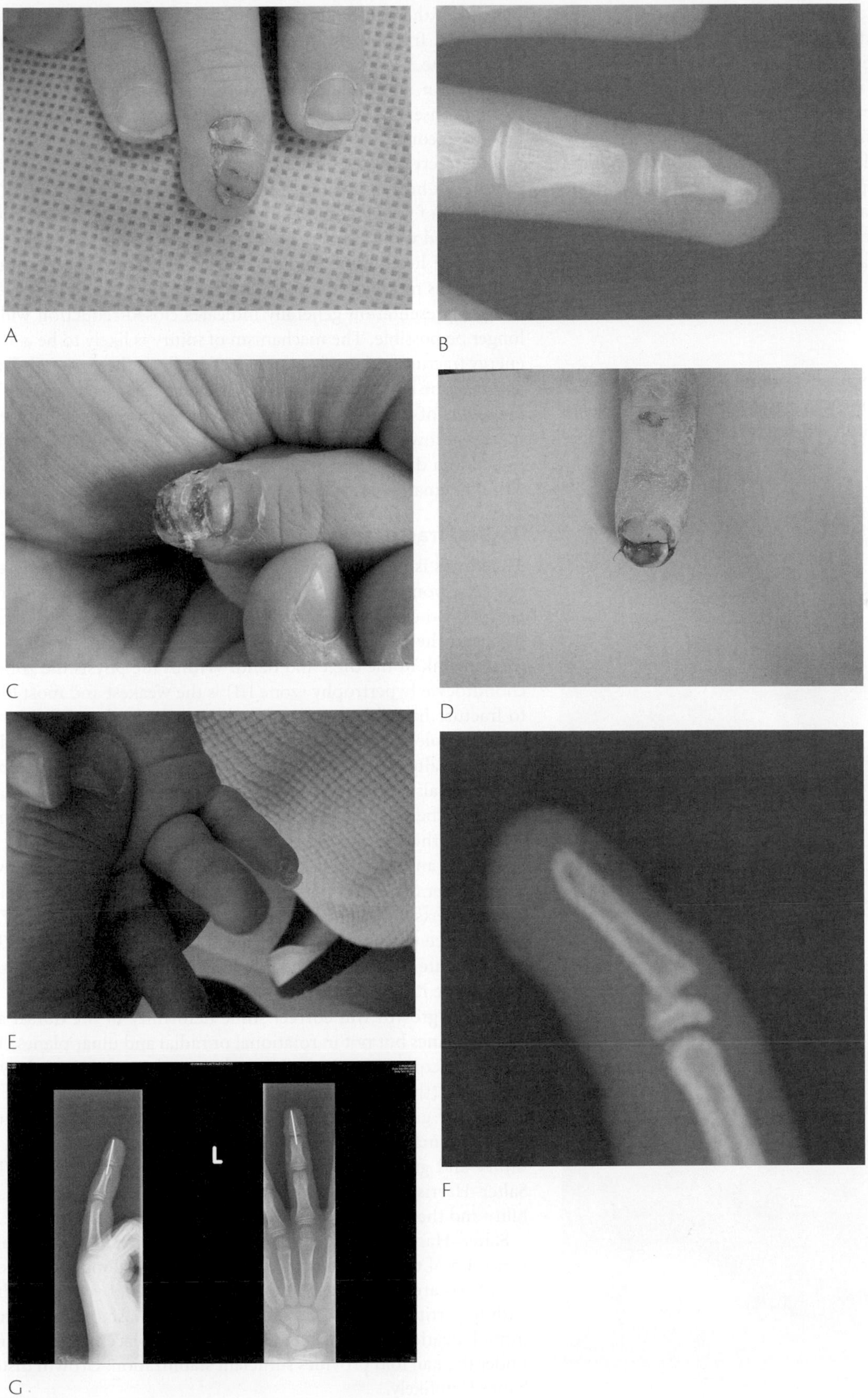

Fig. 14.7.1 Fingertip injuries. A) Nail deformity after conservative treatment trapped fingertip injury. B) Distal phalanx deformity after conservative treatment. C) Nail regeneration after nail bed repair. D) Trapped finger injury with the amputated part replaced as a composite graft. E) Trapped finger injury left to heal by secondary intention. F) X-ray of Seymour fracture. G) Seymour fracture reduced and fixed with a K-wire.

the tip should be reconstructed making every attempt to maintain length. All the methods used in adults may be used. The results from many procedures is better in children due to greater digit flexibility, a lower tendency to joint contractures, better sensory restoration even in non innervated flaps or grafts, and better cortical re-orientation in neurotized switch flaps. One reconstructive technique that works particularly well in children when the amputated part includes the nail apparatus and revascularization is not possible, is to retain the nail and surrounding skin but discard the phalanx and pulp, replace the nail portion on the end of the finger and revascularize it with a palmar flap such as a cross finger flap (Figure 14.7.2).

Fractures

Hand fractures are one of the most common presenting problems in children, occurring at a rate of 26.4 fractures per 10 000. Hand fractures form 25% of all childhood fractures, with the proximal phalanx of the border digits the most affected. One-third of paediatric hand fractures involve the physis, with 78% being Salter–Harris type II, 13% type III, and 7% type I. Dislocations are uncommon. Although most paediatric hand fractures can be treated conservatively, it is important not to completely depend on growth to correct all displacement.

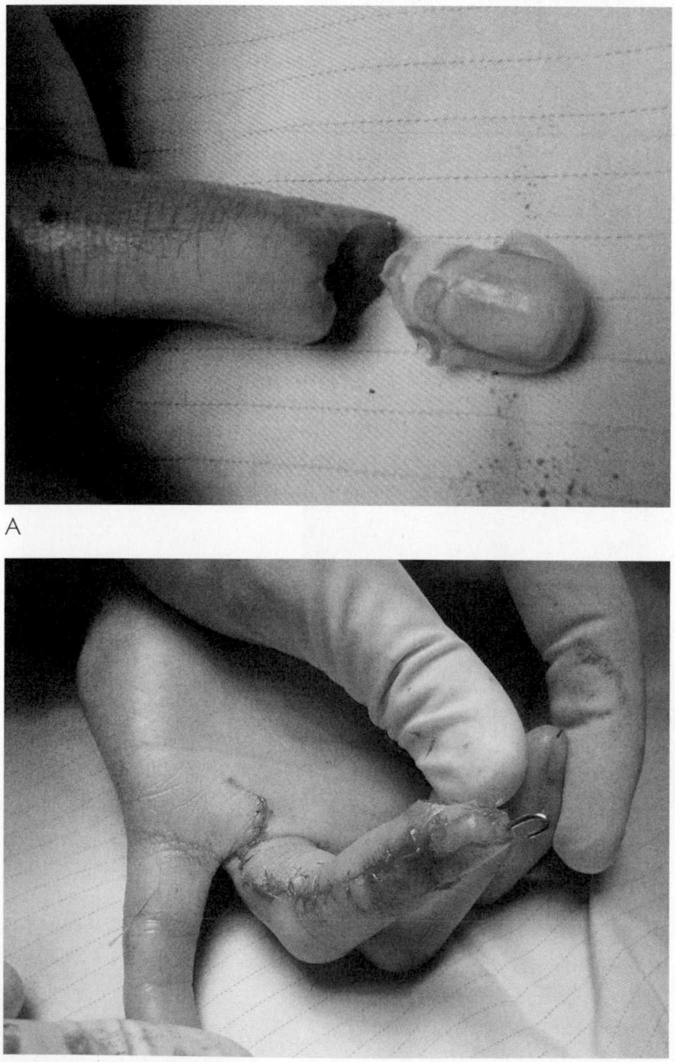

A

B

Fig. 14.7.2 Amputations—fingertip reposition flap technique. A) Fingertip amputation. B) The nail and surrounding peionychium removed and reattached to the finger and supported by a neurovascular island advancement flap.

The differences between adult and child hand fractures include rapidity of healing, pattern of fracture related to the mechanism and zones of weakness along the physis, tolerance of displacement, growth, and variation in the risk of stiffness.

Fracture healing in children occurs in about half the time of adults. This means shorter periods of immobilization but also that delayed presentation generally indicates closed reduction will no longer be possible. The mechanism of injury is likely to be a lower energy fracture and the fracture pattern reflects the greater deformability of the bone and thickness of the periosteum in children. The incidence of open fractures other than trapped finger injuries is markedly lower in children. Stiffness is less commonly a problem in children due not only to the reduced period of immobility but also the remarkable tolerance of the tissues.

Physeal fractures

The physis is the cartilage plate between the metaphysis and epiphysis responsible for longitudinal growth. It is found at the distal end of the metacarpals except the thumb metacarpal, which has its physis at the proximal end like the phalanges. The physis is the weakest link in the digit and hand. Within the physis the zone of chondrocyte hypertrophy (zone III) is the weakest and most likely to fracture in children giving Salter–Harris type I and II injuries. During adolescence, the physeal zones become less distinct leading to more Salter–Harris type III and IV fractures. The pattern of fracture is also influenced by the attachments of the ligaments and tendons. The collateral ligaments of the interphalangeal (IP) joints attach to the epiphysis and the metaphysis at the base of the phalanges, and this protects the physis form lateral forces. However, in the finger metacarpophalangeal (MCP) joints the collateral ligaments inserts only onto the epiphysis of the proximal phalanx, so lateral force produces a Salter–Harris type II or III fracture. The palmar plate inserts into the epiphysis so injury causes a Salter–Harris type III avulsion fracture of the epiphysis.

Physeal growth will correct some deformity in the dorsal and palmar planes but not in rotational or radial and ulnar planes. The degree of correction depends on the proximity of the injury to the physis (the closer the better), the degree of deformity, and the amount of growth potential remaining. Injury to the physis may lead to premature arrest of growth or growth deformity should the injury and growth arrest only involve a part of the physis. The Salter–Harris classification of physeal injuries predicts fracture stability and the potential for growth disturbance (see Chapter 14.2).

Salter–Harris type I injuries (see Figure 14.7.1F) with a transverse slip of the metaphysis from the epiphysis along the plane of the physis are commonest in the distal phalanx of young children with fingertip crush injuries. Reduction after wash out and simple immobilization may be all that is required. Replacement of the nail under the nail fold provides sufficient stabilization. Growth disturbance is unlikely.

Salter–Harris type II injuries with physeal separation and a fragment of metaphysis, is the commonest form of physeal hand injury. These frequently present at the bases of the proximal phalanges with bruising, pain, and deformity. These are generally easy to reduce and are stable after reduction. Reduction can be aided by the use of a pencil placed in the web space to provide a fulcrum on which to exert the reducing force or by flexing the MCP joinys to tighten the collateral ligaments and stabilize the proximal segment. Buddy splinting may be all the immobilization required. Growth disturbance is unusual (Figure 14.7.3A).

Salter–Harris type III injuries are physeal separation with a fracture fragment of the epiphysis. These are intra-articular and hence require careful reduction and frequently fixation for a short period, as they may be unstable. Fixation is usually by fine K-wires. These are more commonly seen at the distal phalanx in adolescents and present as mallet finger injuries, or less commonly at the middle phalanx as a central slip type injury causing boutonnière deformity, or of the proximal phalanx of the thumb presenting as a 'bony game keeper's thumb avulsion'.

Salter–Harris type IV injuries extend through the physis and are associated with a potential for growth disturbance. These are also intra-articular and careful reduction and fixation is required.

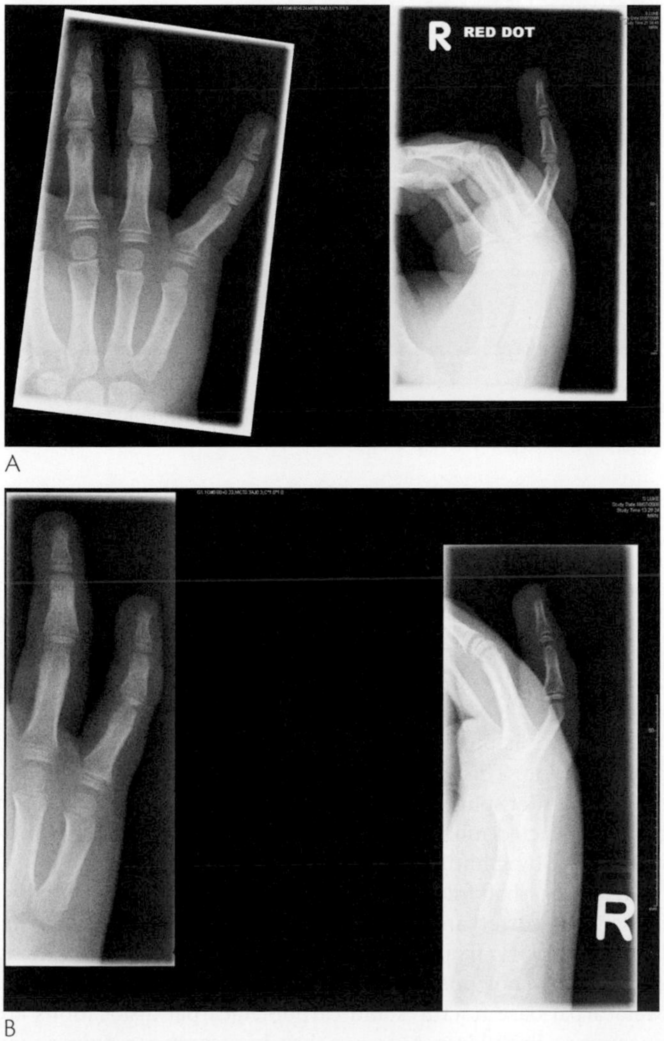

Fig. 14.7.3 Salter–Harris type II fracture. A) Before reduction. B) After reduction and buddy splinting.

Salter–Harris type V injuries are rare and are a crush injury of the physis. They are often not diagnosed until the growth arrest is noted.

What the Salter–Harris classification does not consider is the degree of displacement of the fracture fragments. Growth allows spontaneous correction of some displacement, see Box 14.7.1.

Non-physeal fractures

Paediatric hand fractures become increasingly common with adolescence, in association with increasing activity and skeletal maturity. The commonest fractures are fractures of the phalangeal shaft, particularly the proximal phalanx. As mentioned previously, minor angulation (up to 30 degrees up to 10 years of age, and less than 20 degrees in those older) in a palmar or dorsal plane will remodel; however, angulation in lateral planes or rotational deformity will not remodel and thus must be reduced and stabilized, if clinically indicated. Phalangeal fractures without gross displacement are frequently stable postreduction due to the thicker periosteum in children. In these cases 2–4 weeks of buddy strapping or splintage with the hand in an intrinsic plus position is sufficient. However, very displaced fractures indicating a greater degree of periosteal disruption will commonly require fixation. Fixation by closed reduction and fine percutaneous Kirschner wires is adequate (Figure 14.7.4). Additional support by buddy strapping will allow early mobilization. Wires are removed at 3 or 4 weeks, once clinical union is achieved. Wires that are left exposed through the skin can be removed in the outpatient clinic without anaesthesia; however, care must be taken during their tenure that the tips are well protected to prevent injury.

Intra-articular fractures

Intra-articular fractures must be carefully reduced and fixed to prevent long-term problems. These fractures are often condylar fractures of the head of the proximal phalanx. These are easily missed and can result in reduced flexion of the proximal interphalangeal (PIP) joint as the proximal fragment blocks the subcondylar recess. Closed reduction should be attempted to minimize the risk of avascular necrosis of the small fragments. Reduction must restore correct alignment of the articular surface and ensure the subcondylar recess is restored. Occasionally, these fractures are best reduced under direct vision. Accurate relatively stable fixation with minimal trauma to the tiny bony fragments is usually best achieved with small K-wires. With open reduction care must be

Box 14.7.1 Remodelling potential in the paediatric hand

- <10 years old:
  - 20–30 degrees sagittal displacement
  - 10–12 degrees coronal displacement
- >10 years old:
  - 10–20 degrees sagittal displacement
  - 5–10 degrees coronal displacement
- Rotation will not remodel.

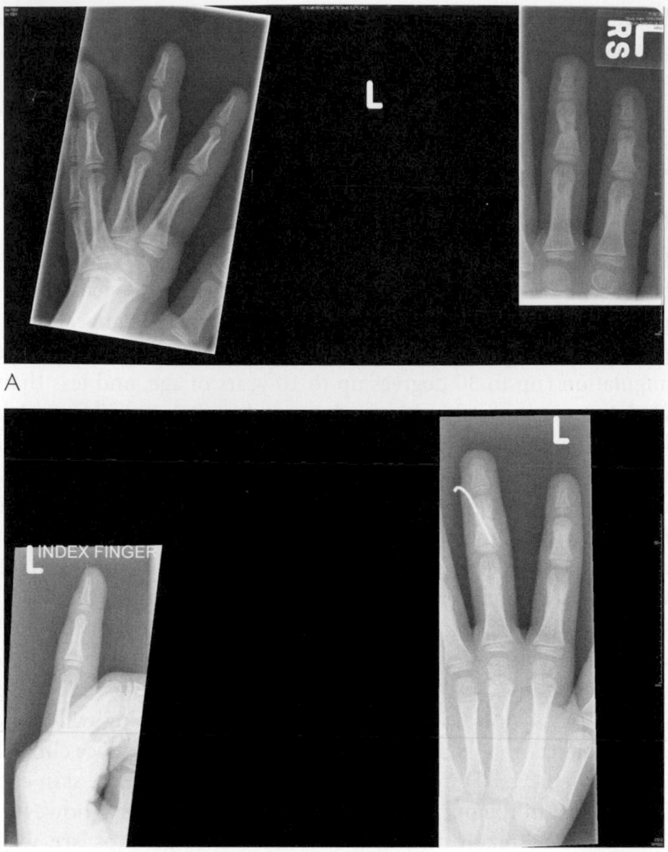

A

B

Fig. 14.7.4 Midshaft middle phalanx fracture. A) Middle finger middle phalanx fracture and index finger neck fracture. B) Postreduction and K-wire fixation.

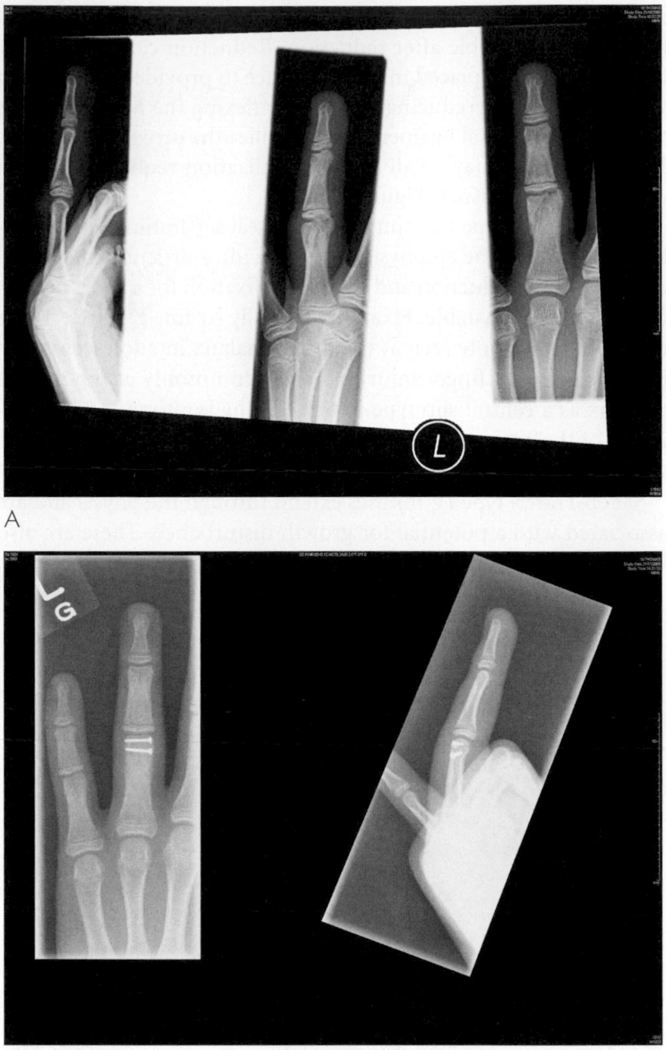

A

B

Fig. 14.7.5 Proximal phalanx condylar fracture. A) Prereduction. B) Following reduction and fixation with lag screws.

taken not to devascularize the fragments by preserving any soft tissue attachments (Figure 14.7.5).

Phalangeal neck fractures

Fractures of the neck of the proximal or middle phalanges are often hardest to diagnose and extension of the head or even 180 degrees of rotation may not be appreciated. These fractures need to be reduced and K-wired. The technique involves inserting a wire longitudinally down the distal phalanx, then hyperextend the distal interphalangeal (DIP) joint and pick up the displaced head of the proximal phalanx, then reduce the fracture and pin to the shaft of the middle phalanx (Figure 14.7.6).

Metacarpal fractures

Metacarpal fractures are common in late adolescents. The mechanisms and patterns of injury are similar to those in adults. See Box 14.7.2 for acceptable metacarpal position.

If an unacceptable degree of angulation exists clinically and radiologically, then reduce the fracture using the Jahss manoeuvre. This consists of flexing the MCP joints and IP joints then pushing dorsally on the PIP joint, whilst pushing down on the metacarpal shaft. Once the fracture is reduced, stabilize it using K-wires or plaster of Paris. Wires are much more difficult to insert into the metacarpals of children due to the lack of metacarpal head collateral ligament recesses and hence the lack of 'shoulders' on which to aim the wires. Consequently there is a much greater risk in children of the wires impinging on the extensor tendons or the MCP joint. This is not too great a problem provided the MCP joint is kept in a flexed position and the wires removed within 3 weeks. As children will tolerate immobilization of their IP joints in a flexed position for 2–3 weeks, maintenance of the reduced metacarpal neck fracture is possible by bandaging the ulnar two digits in a fisted position. This maintains the fracture in a more stable position than gutter splinting. Three weeks is adequate immobilization before protected mobilization is commenced. Protection is provided either by splinting or by buddy strapping.

Metacarpal shaft fractures are treated as in adults, mainly needing reduction to correct any severe angulation and rotational deformity. Intra-medullary fixation techniques such as Bouquet wiring are generally not possible due to the narrowness of the canal. Metacarpal base fractures and carpometacarpal dislocations are uncommon in children, but when they do occur they require closed reduction and K-wire fixation.

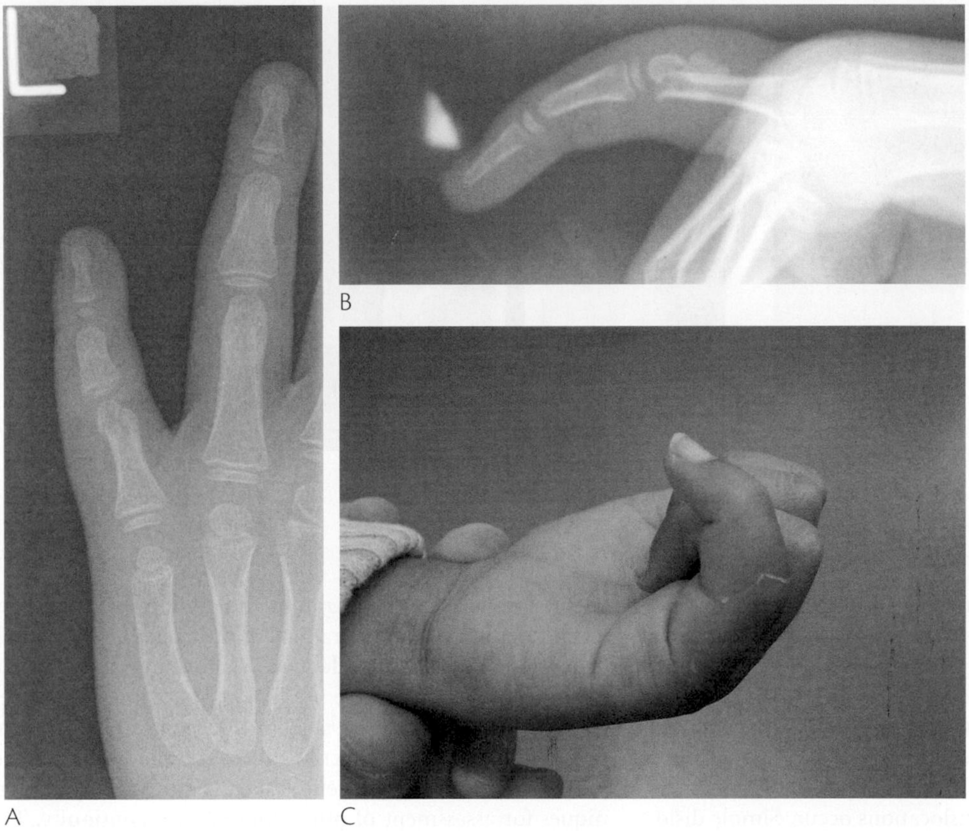

Fig. 14.7.6 Proximal phalanx neck fracture. A) Undisplaced and treated conservatively. B) Displaced and neglected. C) Loss of the retro condylar recess limits.

Thumb metacarpal fractures

Thumb metacarpal fractures are frequent and are usually found at the proximal metaphysis or physis (Figure 14.7.7). Epiphyseal fractures are usually Salter–Harris type II, with the small Thurston–Holland metaphyseal fragment usually found on the radial aspect. Reduction of these fractures is easy but they are often difficult to stabilize without using K-wires due to the displacing forces. These forces are the radial pull of the abductor pollicis longus on the proximal fragment and the ulnar deviating force of the adductor on the distal fragment.

Outcomes in children's hand fracture

Good results are almost inevitable in children's fractures unless complicated by surgical intervention or infection. Avoidance of angulation, rotation, and intra-articular deformities leads to good results in paediatric hand fractures. Malunion is the commonest complication albeit uncommon. If detected before 2 weeks the malunion may still be amenable to closed manipulation. Beyond this period, open exposure and careful unpicking of the malunion should be possible up to the 6- or 8-week stage. Subsequently they should be treated as in adults with opening or closing wedge osteotomies or rotational osteotomies either at the site or distant to the site of the malunion. Care must be taken to avoid damage to any physis. In cases of intra-articular malunion all attempts at intra-articular realignment should be made. Failing that, a pseudarthrosis usually gives adequate function. It is exceptional to consider procedures such as arthrodeses, or arthroplasty.

Box 14.7.2 Acceptable metacarpal position

- Younger children <60 degrees of apex dorsal angulation of fourth and fifth metacarpal neck fractures
- Older adolescents < 40 degrees
- Index and middle metacarpals only 10–20 degrees of angulation is tolerated due to the relative stiffness of the carpometacarpal joints.

Joint dislocations in the fingers and thumb

PIP joint dislocations are usually dorsal. Reduction is usually easily achieved and following this the PIP joint is usually stable, requiring only buddy strapping or an extension-blocking splint for 2–4 weeks. Rarely collateral ligament ruptures result in gross lateral instability and require repair. Open reduction may be required in cases of irreducible dislocations due to interposition of soft tissue such as an articular flap or the button holing of the proximal phalanx head between the palmar plate and the flexor tendon.

MCP joint dislocations are rare other than in the thumb. The index fingers are the next most commonly affected, and in this case are often irreducible due to the button holing of the metacarpal

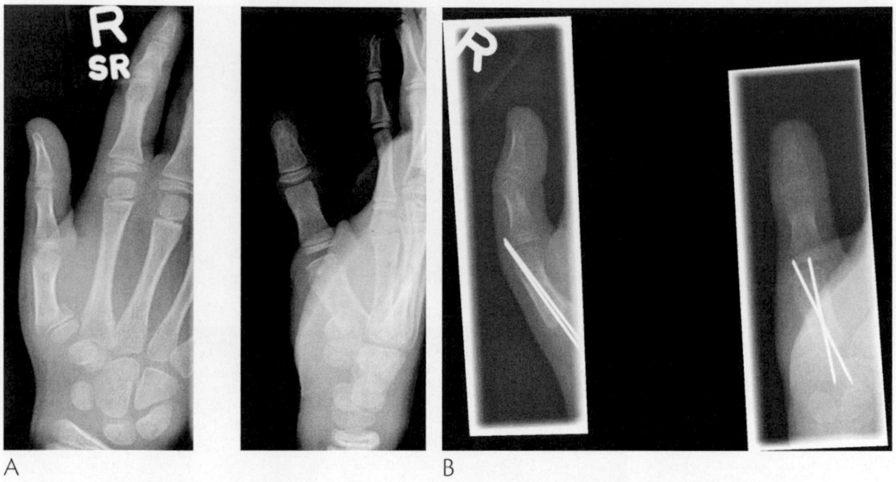

Fig. 14.7.7 A) Thumb metacarpal fracture. B) After reduction and K-wire fixation.

head between the flexor tendons and the lumbrical. Open reduction can be performed from either a palmar or dorsal approach, though one must be wary of the displaced digital nerves when approaching from the palmar aspect.

Thumb MCP joint dislocations are less common in children than adults due to the relative strengths of the soft tissues to the epiphysis. When they do occur however the pattern is similar to adults. Both simple and complex dislocations occur. Simple dislocations are amenable to closed reduction by hyperextension of the MCP joint and then with pressure on the base of the dorsum of the proximal phalanx a longitudinal traction and flexion force is gently applied. Complex dislocations require open reduction to free the palmar plate, or the entrapment of the head of the metacarpal between the volar plate and the flexor tendons. The x-ray signs of the proximal phalanx lying almost parallel in line with the metacarpal (as opposed to lying angulated in simple dislocations) or the presence of a widened joint space or with the sesamoid bone lying interposed can predict complex dislocations.

Tendon injuries

These injuries become more frequent with increasing age. The mechanism of these injuries differs from those in adults—most are clean, tidy sharp injuries caused by glass. As the principles of the treatment, particularly the surgical technique of these, are similar to those in adults already presented in previous chapters, this section will concentrate on the differences and special features of these injuries in children.

The major difference is the growth potential and the reduced cooperation with rehabilitation. Growth can be inhibited by lack of movement and scar, and to a larger extent by denervation. Postoperative care is affected by the age and cooperation of the child and rehabilitation is generally limited. However, tendon healing occurs faster and with fewer adhesions than in adults. Hence the results are frequently better, and the complications fewer. The operative techniques and principles are the same, keeping in mind the increased fragility of the structures such as the pulleys. Children's flexor tendon repairs require special care in their assessment and examination, postoperative care and rehabilitation, and operative indications when complications arise.

Due to the lack of cooperation and compromised examination, all children with deep lacerations of the upper limb should have a general anaesthetic for adequate exploration and repair of the wound. Some preoperative prediction of the injuries can be made by observant examination skills including specialist examination techniques, such as the tactile adherence and immersion test for sensory assessment, and tenodesis and forearm squeezing techniques for assessment of musculotendinous continuity. This will permit discussion with the parents and theatre staff about the likely operative procedure and timing.

Flexor tendon injuries

Children's flexor tendon injuries should be explored as soon as possible, though a delay of a few days is unlikely to affect the outcome. The tendon should be repaired primarily. The mechanism of injury is usually a fall onto glass or whilst clutching a glass, meaning that more frequently than in adults the distal tendon end is found at the level of the laceration making the exposure and repair easier. The smaller tendon structure may prevent the use of a multiple strand core suture tendon repair technique, though this may still be possible if a smaller gauge of suture such as 4/0 is used. The tendon repair strength may be less important in children if immobilization rather than active motion techniques are used for postoperative rehabilitation. Immobilization following repair is the usual postoperative regimen due to the lack of cooperation with exercises and because although children do develop tendon adhesions, once formed the adhesions seem to be more responsive to manipulation and therapy. There is a tendency for long-term absorbable sutures such as PDS to be used rather than non-absorbable sutures, though there is no scientific evidence to support or refute this practise.

In zone 1 injuries, care must be taken not to injure the distal phalanx physis when reinserting the tendon. In zone 2 injuries every attempt should be made to repair both flexor tendons. In situations of delayed repair or untidy injuries requiring debridement of the tendon endsn significant tendon shortening can occur. This would preclude primary tendon repair in adults so as to prevent the quadriga effect, in which one tendon is out of synchronization with the others leading to reduced movement. However, shortened tendon repair is possible in children, as musculotendinous lengthening and readjustment of tension occurs more readily and is far more forgiving. Flexor sheath closure and pulley preservation or reconstruction, are as important as in adults.

Postoperative rehabilitation differs depending on the age and understanding of the child and their parents. Immobilization for 3–4 weeks is as effective in the final outcome. This is probably because complete immobilization is impossible and these children move within the confines of their protective splint or bandage, thereby performing their own protected active mobilization programme. Results deteriorate if they are immobilized for longer than 4 weeks. Children are more likely to spontaneously use their hands once their splints are removed and require less directed therapy to achieve function. Botulinum toxin can be used to weaken the affected muscles so as to reduce the risk of tendon rupture, though rupture can still occur with unintended extension.

The results of flexor tendon repairs in children are generally better than those achieved in adults. However, tendon ruptures and adhesions preventing movement do occur. Tendon rerupture is difficult to assess in children. Assessment is dependent on history, palpation of the tendon, assessment of active and tenodesis movement, and ultrasound examination. An acute rerupture detected early may be amenable to direct rerepair. Frequently the tendon rupture is not detected until a later stage (beyond 2 months) and direct repair is not possible. The situation is then similar to delayed detection of a tendon injury.

The use of immediate or staged tendon grafting techniques is controversial in children. Some believe tendon grafting procedures should only be performed once the child is old enough to participate in rehabilitation programmes. There is little evidence on this subject however, and it is reasonable to perform the tendon graft regardless of age, in order to obtain better function. Children develop hand use patterns during early years, and further digital growth and development are dependent on function, so all attempts should be made for reconstruction of normal anatomy and function in children. Alternatives to tendon repair such as tenodesis or arthrodesis of the DIP joint are contraindicated due to the potential to interfere with growth.

Tendon adhesions are uncommon in children. Indications for tenolysis are similar to adults though the timing of the operation is disputed. Tenolysis is recommended when the child is old enough to understand and participate in the rehabilitation programme.

Extensor tendon injuries

Closed extensor tendon injuries are rare in children. When they do occur it is essential to exclude epiphyseal fractures, particularly in the closed mallet finger. These are usually Salter–Harris type I in younger children and type III in older children, the latter mimicking the bony avulsion injury seen in adults. Treatment of these is identical to adults, though the challenges involved in maintaining a splint on the child may increase the number that are pinned in extension rather than just splinted. The period of splintage can be reduced by 2 weeks in children.

Delay in the diagnosis of extensor tendon injuries is common in children. Despite the delay the treatment is the same and good results can be obtained in mallet and boutonniere injuries with splintage. Splinting periods in the treatment of delayed extensor tendon injuries in zones 1–5 are 2–4 weeks greater than when treating the acute injury.

Open extensor tendon injuries are more common, usually associated with a crush injury. When there is associated nail bed or epiphyseal injury, operative treatment is indicated. When the injury is a clean tidy laceration over the middle phalanx or the IP joints (extensor tendon zones 1–4), then tendon approximation is possible solely by splinting the finger in extension for 4–6 weeks. The extensor tendon does not retract like the flexor due to the anatomical structure of the extensor tendon at this level. This feature allows direct repair even in cases of delayed detection of extensor tendon division. Where direct repair is not possible all methods of adult reconstruction can be used in the child, with a preference for those that reconstruct the normal anatomy and interfere least with growth and development.

Rehabilitation of extensor tendon repairs depends on the level of the repair. Digital injuries should be splinted for 4 weeks, whereas hand and forearm injuries should be mobilized earlier. Where pins or K-wires have been used for internal splinting, these are carefully protected to prevent them being pulled out or causing injury, early mobilization in a removable splint can be used in cooperative children. Once the splint is removed, the children are allowed to use their hand normally.

Extensor tendon adhesions causing poor movement should be tenolysed following a lengthy trial of mobilization. The results of extensor tendon surgery in children are poorly reported but generally believed to be better than those in adults. Some extensor lag or loss of flexion may occur in 22%.

Nerve injuries

A high index of suspicion of nerve injury should exist when assessing hand lacerations. Examination of nerve injuries in children is even harder than tendon injuries. If any doubt exists, lacerations should be explored under general anaesthesia. The operative techniques are identical to those previously described for adults. The peripheral nerves are more mobile in children and so less tension is present at the repair site. Consequently, less post operative immobilization is required. Two weeks should be sufficient, if there are no other injuries. The results of nerve repair are much better in children, and this is rewarding surgery. Better results are attributed to better regenerative ability of the nervous system, better neural ingrowth from surrounding areas, and better central cortical reorientation. Children's superior cerebral ability to develop and adapt probably accounts for a large proponent of their better outcomes. Nerve injuries complicating fractures or tendon lacerations are associated with worse outcomes of all the involved injuries. Tendon transfers of functioning muscles following identical principles used in adult transfers can treat failure of motor recovery. During neural recovery the child will need protection from injuring the insensate portion of the hand.

Burns (Box 14.7.3)

Hand and upper limb burns are amongst the commonest injuries presenting in children. The mechanism is usually a scald caused by the child pulling a cup of hot liquid off the table. Almost all scald hand burns heal spontaneously, requiring little more than assessment, analgesia, reassurance, dressings, and follow-up. However, not all burns are that simple. The outcome and management depend on the depth and size of the burn. Assessment of burns is based on

Box 14.7.3 Burn thickness and healing potential

- Superficial/epidermal—healed within 48h
- Superficial partial thickness—healed within 2 weeks
- Deep partial thickness—months, leaving scarring and contracture
- Full thickness—will not heal except from edges leaving bad scars/contractures.

history and examination. The size of the burn is measured and recorded as a percentage of body surface area and the depth is assessed using the same principles described in Chapter 12.24.

Treatment

Immediate first aid and resuscitation

Remove the heat source and cool the burn with running water for 20min. Resuscitation should be given in accordance with Advanced Paediatric Life Support (APLS®) protocols.

Superficial and superficial dermal burns

Blisters should be debrided as they contain eiconasoids and prostaglandins detrimental to healing and which deepen the burn. Once debrided, desiccation and infection must be avoided, as these will also deepen the burn. Dressings such as paraffin gauze and absorbent gauze are useful in the first few days when the burns are quite productive of ooze. Dressings should be made as light as possible to allow some movement. Once the ooze has diminished, the burn can be dressed with a retention dressing such as Hypafix, Mefix, or Fixomull, adhered directly onto the burn. This dressing can be washed, allows almost normal mobility, and is easily removed, as the adhesive is oil soluble.

Deep dermal and full thickness burns

The general rule is that if burns heal within 10–14 days then hypertrophic scarring is unlikely. However, deeper burns that remain unhealed at 14 days have a high risk of developing contractures and hypertrophic scarring. If the burn is obviously deep or fails to heal within 2 weeks then the burn should be debrided and skin grafted. Debridement should aim to remove all dead tissue but preserve as much dermis as possible. Dermis preservation or reconstruction is the key factor in outcome in terms of scarring and contracture.

Severe burns should be admitted for analgesia, splinting into a functional position, assessment, elevation to reduce oedema, and preparation for surgery.

Children should be followed as they grow, as scars that initially were non-contracting may become tight and cause functionally limiting contractures. These may require surgical revision by excision and grafting, local flaps, or Z-plasties.

Bites and infections

Dogs and cats cause most bites in children. The principles of assessment of underlying structures, exploration if indicated coupled with good surgical excision, and primary closure is as true in children as in adults. The infecting organism is usually *Pasturella multocida* or mixed organisms, sensitive to penicillin or co-amoxiclav.

Conclusions

Children's hand injuries are extremely common but most are easily primarily treated with excellent outcomes to be expected. The greatest error is in underestimating the degree of injury. Failure to recognize and treat the injury or failure of treatment can lead to devastating loss of function and growth, which may not be immediately apparent.

Further reading

Elhassan, B., Moran, S.L., Bravo, C., and Amadio, P. (2006). Factors that influence the outcome of zone I and zone II flexor tendon repairs in children. *Journal of Hand Surgery*, **31A**(10), 1661–6.

Fitoussi, F., Badina, A., Ilhareborde, B., Morel, E., Ear, R., and Penneßot, G.F. (2007). Extensor tendon injuries in children. *Journal of Pediatric Orthopedics*, **27**(8), 863–6.

Fischer, M.D. and McElfresh, E.C. (1994). Physeal and periphyseal injuries of the hand. Patterns of injury and results of treatment. *Hand Clinics*, **10**(2), 287–301.

Havenhill, T.G. and Birnie, R. (2005). Pediatric flexor tendon injuries. *Hand Clin*, **21**(2), 253-6.

Vadivelu, R., Dias, J.J., Burke, F.D., and Stanton, J. (2006). Hand injuries in children: a prospective study. *Journal of Pediatric Orthopedics*, **26**(1), 29–35.

14.8

Injuries of the pelvis and hip in children

Jon D. Hop and J.L. Marsh

Summary points

- Displaced cervical fractures must be reduced and then fixed with lag screws
- Avascular necrosis remains a significant problem
- Intertrochanteric fractures may be treated closed with traction if an adequate reduction can be obtained and held
- Dislocated hips should be reduced as soon as possible, open if necessary
- Pelvic fractures are associated with a high mortality not so much from bleeding from pelvic veins as from accompanying major trauma to the rest of the body
- The elasticity of children's bones allows for single breaks in the pelvic ring.

Hip fracture

Incidence (Box 14.8.1)

Paediatric hip fractures are rare, comprising less than 1% of all paediatric fractures. These severe injuries frequently have complications that have lifelong significance for the patient.

Anatomy (Box 14.8.2)

The proximal femoral physis contributes the majority of metaphyseal growth in the neck of the femur and to a lesser degree to the appositional growth of the femoral head. The trochanteric apophysis contributes mostly to the appositional growth of the greater trochanter and to a lesser degree to metaphyseal growth.

Box 14.8.1 Injuries of pelvis and hip

- Rare
- Complications frequent
- Management difficult
- Associated injuries are common
- Associated with high-energy trauma.

The metaphyseal and epiphyseal blood supplies of the proximal femur in children are functionally separate until physeal closure (usually at age 14–17 years) except for small penetrating vessels. The terminal branch of the medial femoral circumflex artery, the lateral epiphyseal artery, supplies the majority of the femoral head from childhood into adult life. The anterior portion of the femoral head receives a significant portion of its blood supply from branches of the lateral femoral circumflex artery until age 5–6 years. The obturator artery system supplies a minor contribution to the femoral head through the artery of the ligamentum teres. The dominance of the medial femoral circumflex arterial system makes the child's femoral head vulnerable for avascular necrosis following femoral neck fracture. Fractures closer to the physis and fractures with greater displacement are at greater risk for arterial disruption and subsequent necrosis.

Classification

The most widely utilized classification of paediatric hip fractures is based on the anatomical location of the fracture. The classification divides children's hip fractures as follows (Figure 14.8.1).

- Type I: transepiphyseal fracture (with or without dislocation of the femoral head from the acetabulum)
- Type II: transcervical fractures (displaced or non-displaced)
- Type III: cervicotrochanteric fractures (displaced or non-displaced)
- Type IV: intertrochanteric fractures.

Clinical evaluation (Box 14.8.3)

The patient presenting with a displaced proximal femoral fracture will show a shortened, externally rotated extremity with pain

Box 14.8.2 Anatomy

- Growth-plate injuries may affect growth
- Terminal branch of medial circumflex artery supplies most of the femoral head
- Lateral circumflex artery important until age 6 years.

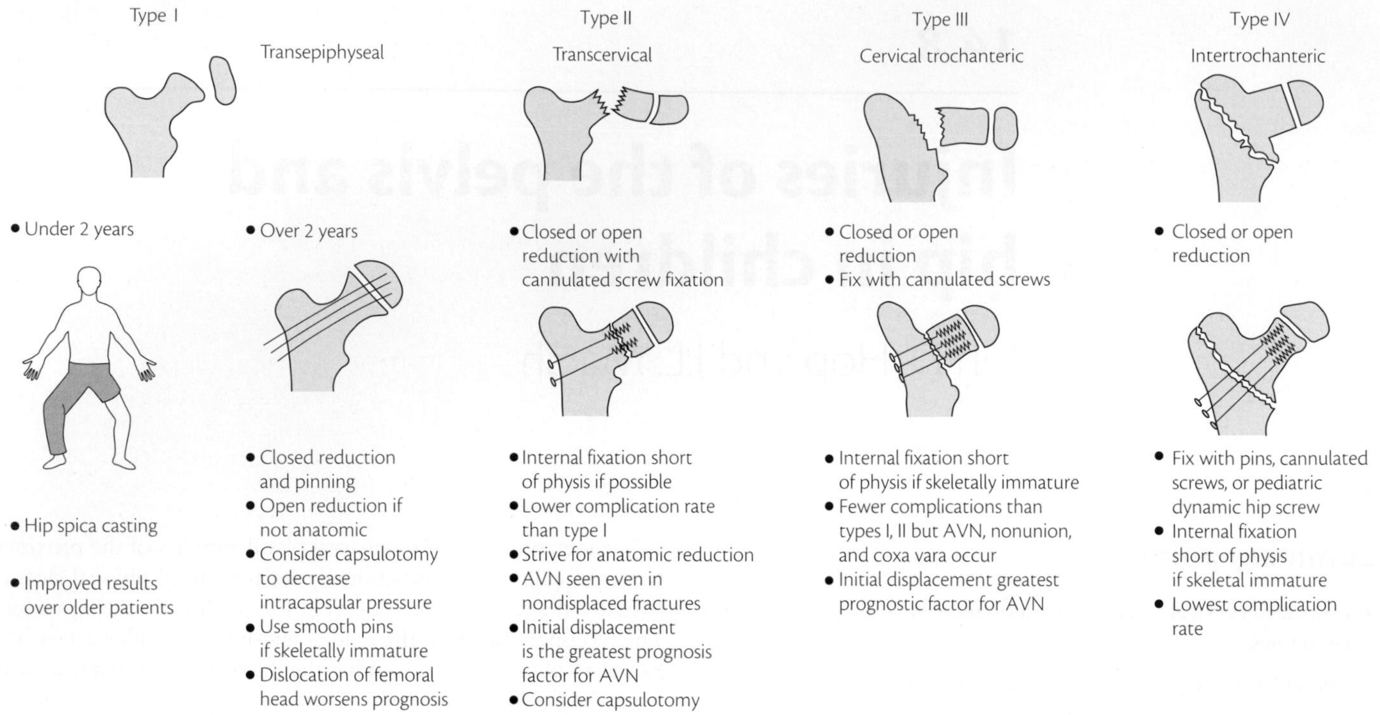

Fig. 14.8.1 Classification of children's hip fractures: AVN, avascular necrosis.

on movement. The symptoms of pain in the hip along with restricted motion should alert the physician to the possibility of a non-displaced fracture.

Investigation (Box 14.8.4)

An anteroposterior pelvis radiograph is standard for the evaluation of a child involved in a major trauma. If a hip fracture is suspected on history/examination or seen on the screening film, further plain radiographs (anteroposterior and lateral views of the hip) are recommended.

Magnetic resonance imaging (MRI) may be helpful in delineating an occult fracture. Ultrasound followed by hip aspiration with or without arthrography can be used to differentiate between fracture and other potential pathology such as hip joint sepsis or synovitis. The aspiration should yield bloody fluid in the presence of fracture.

Management (Box 14.8.5)

Controversy exists over the need for routine anterior capsulotomy and there are differing opinions on whether this procedure decreases the incidence of avascular necrosis.

Type I—transepiphyseal

These fractures can be managed with closed reduction and application of a hip spica cast with the hip in an abducted and externally rotated position. An anatomical reduction must be achieved unless the child is under the age of 2 years, when remodelling of the femoral neck can be anticipated (Figure 14.8.2). In children over the age of 2, if an anatomical reduction cannot be achieved closed, the fracture should be stabilized with percutaneous pins or cannulated screws. Smooth pins are preferred over threaded pins or screws, especially in children with significant growth remaining. If an anatomical reduction cannot be obtained by closed means, open reduction through an anterolateral approach should be performed followed by insertion of pins or cannulated screws. Fixation should be protected with a postoperative hip spica cast.

Type II—transcervical

Type II fractures have been treated with closed reduction and casting with some success but this should be reserved for only truly non-displaced type II fractures. Most of these fractures should be treated operatively. Closed reduction, or an open reduction if an

Box 14.8.3 Clinical evaluation

- Undisplaced—pain without deformity
- Displaced short and externally rotated
- Look for associated injuries.

Box 14.8.4 Investigation

- Anteroposterior pelvic radiograph
- Anteroposterior/lateral radiograph of hip where injury suspected
- Bone scan/MRI if occult fracture suspected
- Ultrasound aspiration/arthrogram sometimes in very young.

Box 14.8.5 Management

- Need for urgent capsulotomy controversial
- Is there displacement requiring reduction?
- Should reduction be done open or closed?
- Is internal fixation required?

anatomical reduction cannot be obtained closed, is followed by fixation with two to three lag screws placed into the femoral neck short of the proximal femoral physis (Figure 14.8.3). Cannulated or solid screws ranging from 4.0–6.5mm are appropriate depending on the size of the child. Fixation may be supplemented with a hip spica cast.

Type III—cervicotrochanteric

Non-displaced type III fractures can be treated by application of a hip spica cast depending on the age of the patient. Close follow-up in the cast is mandatory to avoid loss of reduction and resultant coxa vara deformity. Operative treatment is preferred for most type III cervicotrochanteric fractures. The fixation of choice are lag screws inserted short of the proximal femoral physis unless physeal closure has occurred or is imminent in which case the physis may be crossed. Open reduction must be performed if a satisfactory reduction cannot be obtained closed. A supplementary hip spica cast may be used.

Type IV—intertrochanteric fractures

Some intertrochanteric fractures, particularly in younger patients, can be treated with skin or skeletal traction followed by application of a hip spica cast. Close follow-up is necessary to detect loss of reduction. Polytrauma patients, those who fail to obtain an adequate reduction in traction or those who lose reduction, and most patients older than 6 years of age should be managed with operative fixation. Closed reduction is frequently possible, but if a satisfactory reduction cannot be obtained, open reduction and internal fixation is required. In children under the age of 6 years, fixation is with threaded pins or lag screws. If the child is 6–12 years of age, lag screws are recommended or if the patient is large enough a paediatric sliding hip screw can be placed short of the proximal femoral physis (Figure 14.8.4). Children older than 12 years of age should be managed with a sliding hip screw or an angled blade plate short of the physis. Patients treated with only pin or screw fixation need supplemental immobilization in a hip spica cast.

Results (Box 14.8.6)

Type I—transepiphyseal

The results of treatment of type I fractures are generally poor secondary to the frequent development of complications such as avascular necrosis, non-union, and premature physeal closure. Many type I fractures are accompanied by dislocation of the head from the acetabulum and dislocation further worsens the prognosis.

Type II—transcervical

The results of treatment for type II fractures is more favourable than type I but significant numbers will have complications, such as premature proximal femoral physeal closure, non-union, and avascular necrosis Urgent open reduction and internal fixation with capsulotomy may favourably influence the results, but it appears that the initial displacement of the fracture is the greatest determinant in the development of avascular necrosis.

Type III—cervical trochanteric

Improved results with fewer complications can be expected with type III fractures, although avascular necrosis (30% of cases), non-union, and coxa vara can all occur.

Type IV—intertrochanteric

Avascular necrosis and premature physeal closure are rare in type IV fractures. The quality of reduction obtained will be the largest determinant of the incidence of malunion which is the most common problem following intertrochanteric fractures. Non-anatomical reductions and non-operatively treated fractures have a greater likelihood of developing coxa vara.

Complications (Box 14.8.7)

Avascular necrosis

The rate of avascular necrosis depends on the fracture type. Between 80 and 100% of type I fractures (depending on whether

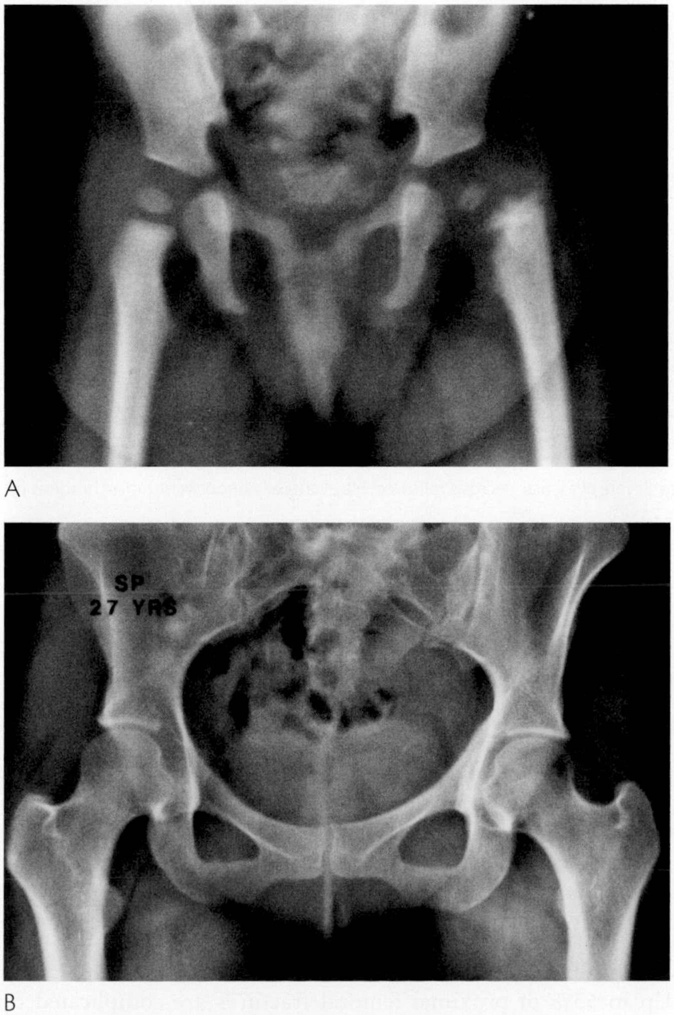

Fig. 14.8.2 This 18-month-old patient sustained a type I proximal femoral fracture of the left hip. Treatment consisted of hip spica casting without reduction. A 27-year follow-up shows excellent results. (Courtesy of Dr S.L. Weinstein.)

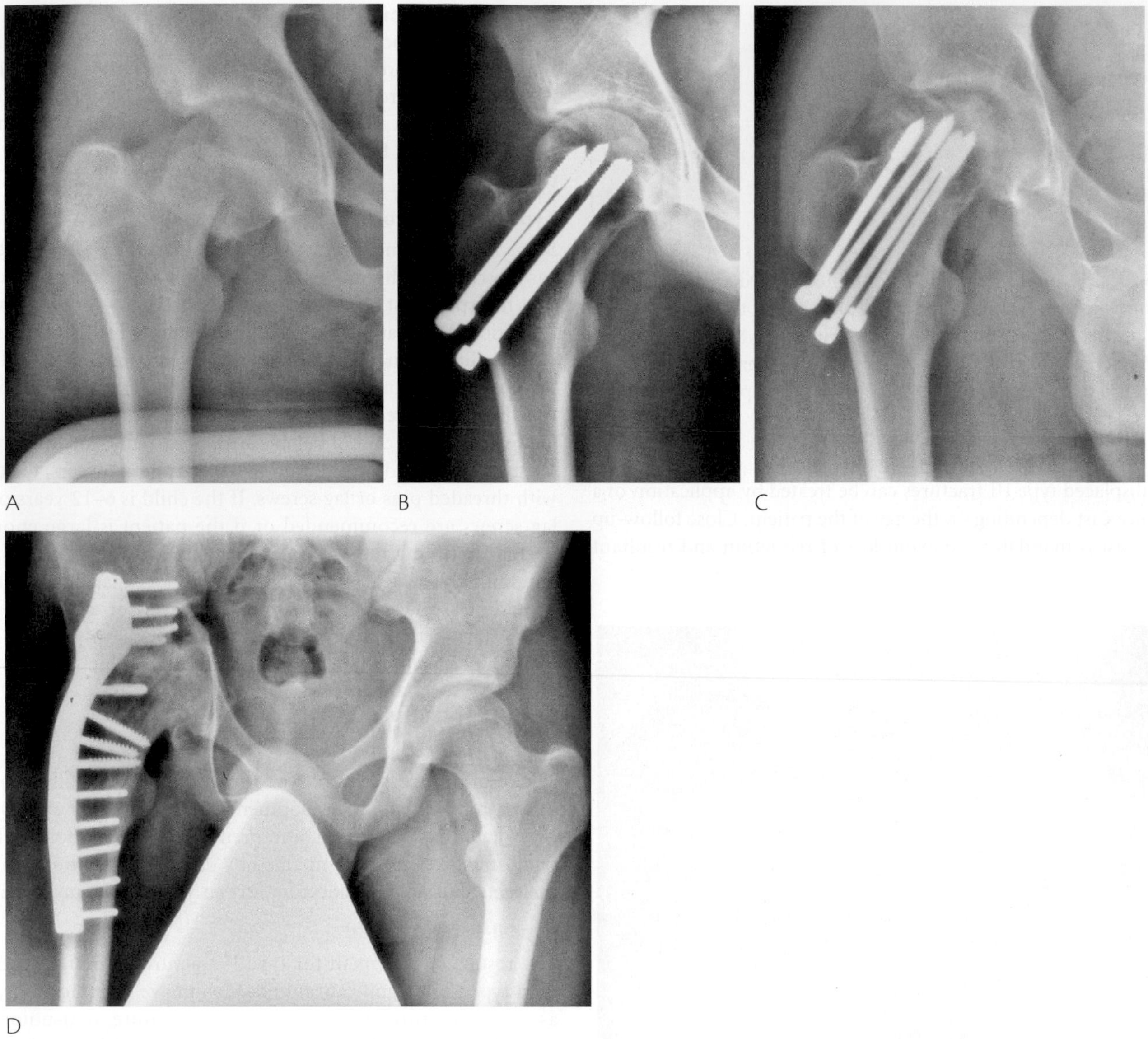

Fig. 14.8.3 This 14-year-old patient underwent multiple pin fixation of a type II fracture. Severe avascular necrosis followed. He eventually underwent hip arthrodesis for severe hip pain. (Courtesy of Dr S.L. Weinstein.)

the head is dislocated), 60% of type II fractures, and 30% of type III fractures develop this severe complication. Three patterns of avascular necrosis following paediatric hip fractures have been described (Figure 14.8.5).

- Type I: diffuse sclerosis and total femoral head involvement followed by complete collapse of the head
- Type II: sclerosis localized to a portion of the epiphysis which is accompanied by minimal collapse
- Type III: sclerosis within the metaphyseal portion of the femoral neck from the fracture line to the physis. The femoral head is spared.

The initial fracture displacement is the critical determinant for the development of necrosis. Patients with avascular necrosis fare poorly at long-term follow-up. There are no predictable treatments for avascular necrosis other than hip arthrodesis or arthroplasty when the patient's symptoms become severe enough.

Non-union

Non-union is more common in neck than intertrochanteric fractures. If non-union is associated with varus deformity, valgus osteotomy is indicated. If the neck–shaft alignment is normal, bone grafting and internal fixation is indicated. This complication can be minimized by obtaining good fixation at the time of initial treatment.

Premature physeal closure

Up to 65% of proximal femoral fractures are complicated by physeal closure. The proximal femoral physis contributes 30% to overall femoral growth and limb-length discrepancy may be more than 2cm.

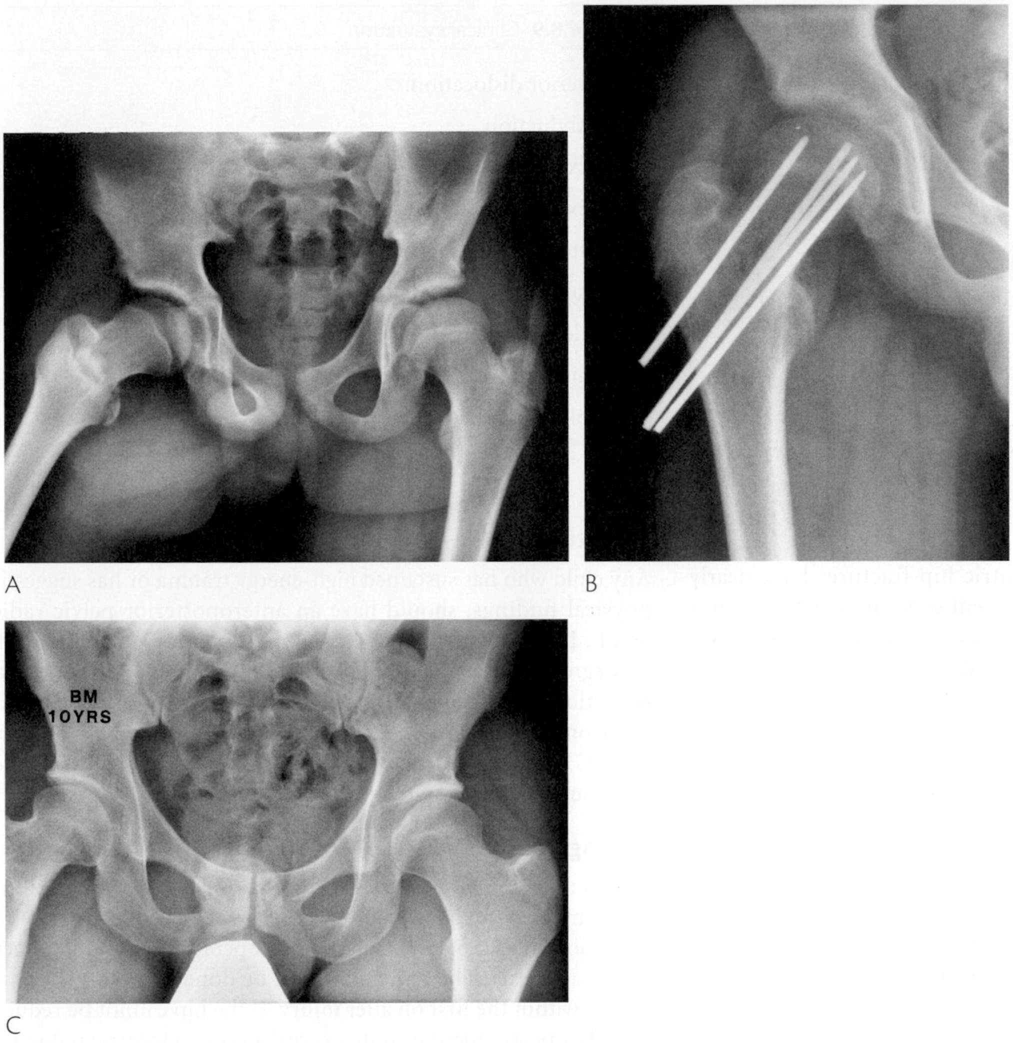

Fig. 14.8.4 A) This 13-year-old male sustained a type IV fracture which was B) treated with multiple pins crossing the physis as he was near skeletal maturity. The 10-year follow-up shows mild coxa vara but otherwise excellent radiographic results. C) Clinical results were also excellent. (Courtesy of Dr S.L. Weinstein.)

Box 14.8.6 Results

- Type I:
  - Avascular necrosis common (80–100%)
  - Dislocation high chance of avascular necrosis
- Type II:
  - Premature physical closure
  - Avascular necrosis (60%)
  - Non-union
  - Initial displacement main prognostic factor
- Type III:
  - Results better than types I and II
  - Avascular necrosis 30%
- Type IV:
  - Malunion most common complication
  - Other complications rare.

Box 14.8.7 Complications

- Avascular necrosis:
  - Displacement is risk factor
  - Urgent capsulotomy and fixation may reduce incidence of avascular necrosis
  - Two-thirds have poor long-term results
- Non-union:
  - Type II: 10%
  - Type III: 15%
  - Type IV: rare
  - Treat with valgus osteotomy
- Premature physeal closure:
  - 65%
  - Limb-height discrepancy
- Coxa vara: up to 32% of patients.

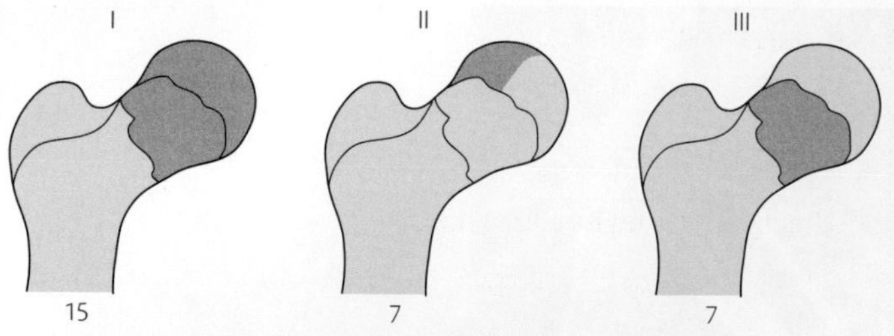

Fig. 14.8.5 Types of avascular necrosis. (Reproduced from Ratliff (1962).)

Coxa vara

The use of internal fixation decreases the incidence and severity of coxa vara.

Future directions

Historically, treatments for paediatric hip fractures have nearly always been non-operative. More recent series in which operative treatment has been more prevalent, have shown decreased incidence of complications and improved results. Future treatment should focus on anatomical reductions of these fractures and utilization of open approaches if necessary.

Hip dislocations

Incidence and prevalence (Box 14.8.8)

Although the incidence is estimated to be higher than paediatric hip fractures, traumatic hip dislocation in children is rare and comprises about 5% of paediatric dislocations. Posterior hip dislocations comprise the majority of dislocations, although anterior dislocations have been described.

Associated pathology

Patients with a high-energy mechanism of injury must be closely examined and monitored for associated injuries involving the chest, abdomen, and head.

Classification

The dislocation can be generally classified into anterior (obturator, anterosuperior, anteroinferior) or posterior.

Clinical evaluation (Box 14.8.9)

A patient presenting with an anterior hip dislocation will have abduction, external rotation, and extension at the hip while a posterior dislocation will present with adduction, internal rotation, and flexion. Function of the sciatic nerve should be documented prior to reduction of the hip.

Box 14.8.8 Hip dislocations in children

- Rare
- High and low energy
- Usually posterior.

Box 14.8.9 Clinical evaluation

- Anterior dislocation:
  - Abduction
  - Extension
  - External rotation
- Posterior dislocation:
  - Adduction
  - Flexion
  - Internal rotation
- Look for sciatic nerve injury.

Investigation

Any child who has sustained high-energy trauma or has suggestive physical findings, should have an anteroposterior pelvic radiograph. If a fracture of the acetabulum is seen or suspected, Judet 45-degree oblique radiographs should be obtained. If a concentric reduction is not achieved (suggested by widening of the hip joint space on postreduction films) a postreduction computed tomography (CT) scan or MRI is indicated to evaluate for incarcerated osteocartilaginous fragments or soft tissues.

Management (Box 14.8.10)

Closed reduction of the hip should be performed in the emergency department if adequate sedation can be achieved, otherwise the reduction should be performed in the operating room under general anaesthesia. The reduction must be done on an urgent basis, ideally within the first 6h after injury. If the hip cannot be reduced closed or postreduction studies reveal a non-concentric reduction, an open reduction must be performed. A posterior approach is indicated for a posterior dislocation while an anterior approach is best for an anterior dislocation. The obstacle to reduction is usually a button hole through the capsule, interposed piriformis tendon, or osteocartilaginous fragments.

Young children and those with questionable compliance should be managed in a one and one half hip spica cast. Older children can be managed with mobilization when the hip is comfortable with crutch ambulation for 3–4 weeks.

Box 14.8.10 Hip dislocation—management

- Radiographs:
  - Anteroposterior
  - Judet views if fracture suspected
  - CT scan if non-concentric reduction
- Urgent closed reduction within 6h
- Open reduction if irreducible or if closed reduction is non-concentric
- Hip spica or traction/crutches for 3–4 weeks.

Results (Box 14.8.11)

Traumatic hip dislocations without associated fractures generally do well. Higher-energy injuries, associated fractures, and delayed reduction all contribute to a higher number of poor results.

Complications

Avascular necrosis

The incidence of avascular necrosis following traumatic hip dislocation in children is 10% or less and is more common in older children. Reduction of the hip as soon as possible and preferably within 6h of injury should remain the goal to minimize the chances of this complication.

Neurological injury

Injury to the sciatic nerve or its peroneal division is not uncommon. Unfortunately not all of these nerves recover completely and the rate of recovery may not be better than that reported for adults which is only in roughly one-third of cases.

Osteoarthritis

Early degenerative disease after hip dislocation is usually secondary to necrosis. Osteoarthritis is felt to be infrequent in the absence of avascular necrosis, but no good long-term studies on children's hip dislocations have been done.

Recurrent dislocation

Recurrent dislocation following traumatic hip dislocation in a patient without a hyperlaxity syndrome such as Down syndrome is quite rare. Plication of the posterior capsule should be reserved for patients who fail 6 weeks of hip spica casting after their first episode of recurrent dislocation.

Pelvis fractures (Box 14.8.12)

Incidence and prevalence

Pelvic fractures in children are uncommon. The majority are stable injuries and acetabular fractures are rare.

Anatomy

The anatomy of the pelvis in children differs from the adult secondary to the presence of the triradiate acetabular cartilage complex and the many extra-articular apophyses. The biomechanical properties of the child's pelvis are also different. The child's pelvis is more malleable, absorbs more energy prior to fracture, and therefore requires higher-energy trauma to produce a fracture. Even innocent fractures may be caused by high forces and have a significant incidence of associated injuries. The more ductile nature of paediatric bone and the increased elasticity of the joints allows for a single break in the pelvic ring in contrast to the adult where a double break is almost always present. Injury to the triradiate cartilage can result in growth arrest and a deficient acetabulum.

Box 14.8.11 Hip dislocation—results

- Poor results:
  - High energy
  - Fracture dislocations
  - Delay in reduction
- Avascular necrosis 8–10%:
  - Children over 5 years of age
  - Common if reduction delayed
- Neurological injury—20%
- Osteoarthritis—usually secondary to avascular necrosis
- Recurrent dislocation—rare unless hyperlaxity syndrome.

Box 14.8.12 Pelvic fractures

- Usually stable
- Acetabular fractures rare
- Almost always high-energy injuries
- Injury to triradiate cartilage:
  - May be difficult to diagnose
  - May cause growth arrest
- Mortality rate 9–18% (associated injuries)
- Genitourinary injuries common
- Haemorrhage from fracture unusual—look for other sources of blood loss
- Open fracture must be excluded if significant rami displacement
- Vaginal/rectal examination with sedation/general anaesthetic.

Associated pathology

Because of the high-energy trauma required to produce a paediatric pelvic fracture, associated injuries are common. Mortality rates of 9–18% have been reported. Mortality and morbidity are highly related to associated injuries to the head, chest, and abdomen. Genitourinary injuries including urethral injury, bladder rupture, and vaginal lacerations occur more commonly in the more severe pelvic injuries.

Significant haemorrhage from paediatric pelvic fractures is not as common as in adults. This indicates that other sources for excessive bleeding should be sought. Management of haemorrhage from the pelvic fracture requires resuscitation, stabilization of the pelvis, and, if necessary, selective arteriography and embolization.

Classification

The system of Key and Conwell is commonly used and will be the classification system further described here (Table 14.8.1).

Although the system of Key and Conwell includes acetabular fractures, the classification system of Judet and Letournel devised for adult acetabular fractures should also be applied to delineate further the extent of the injury and treatment needed.

Clinical evaluation

Paediatric pelvic ring injuries most commonly result from motor vehicle collisions or falls from a height. Pelvic injuries sustained in

Table 14.8.1 Key and Conwell pelvic fracture classification

Type			Comments
I	**Fracture of the pelvis without a break in the ring**		Symptomatic treatment
	A	Avulsion fractures: iliac spine, ischial tuberosity, lesser trochanter, iliac crest	Excellent results
	B	Fractures of the pubis or ischium	
	C	Fractures of the iliac wing	
	D	Fractures of the sacrum or coccyx	
II	**Single break in the pelvic ring**		Symptomatic treatment
	A	Fracture of two ipsilateral rami	Excellent results
	B	Fracture near or subluxation of the pubic symphysis	Beware of associated injuries
	C	Fracture near or subluxation of the sacroiliac joint	
III	**Double break in the pelvic ring**		Beware of severe associated life-threatening injuries
	A	Double vertical fractures of the pubis (straddle fracture)	Consider external fixation for significant haemorrhage
	B	Fracture of two ipsilateral rami with ipsilateral or contralateral fracture of the ilium or dislocation of the sacroiliac joint (Malgaine fracture)	Mortality and long-term morbidity secondary to associated injuries or deformity in older children
	C	Severe multiple fractures of the pelvic ring	
IV	**Fractures of the acetabulum**		Needs accurate reduction when displaced fracture present in weight-bearing portion of acetabulum Beware of triradiate injuries
	A	Small fragment associated with dislocation of the hip	
	B	Linear fracture associated with non-displaced pelvic fracture	
	C	Linear fracture associated with hip instability	
	D	Fracture secondary to central dislocation of the hip	

sports competition are usually avulsion fractures. Anterior muscle contraction with the hip in extension and the knee in flexion can result in avulsion fracture of the anterosuperior or anteroinferior iliac spine, whereas avulsion fracture of the ischial tuberosity occurs after maximal contraction of the hamstrings. The patient will complain of pain localized to the area of the injured apophysis.

A thorough general physical examination must be performed secondary to the high incidence of associated injuries. Once the general examination is complete and resuscitation initiated, the bony pelvic landmarks are evaluated for asymmetry and the stability of the pelvis is tested. Range of both hips should be tested. If a pelvic fracture with significant displacement of the rami is present, digital vaginal and rectal examination under sedation or general anaesthesia should be performed to rule out occult open fracture. The neurovascular examination must carefully assess the sciatic, femoral, and obturator nerves, and lumbosacral plexus.

Investigation

Pelvic ring fractures should be evaluated with an anteroposterior pelvic radiograph as well as 40-degree caudad inlet–40-degree cephalad outlet pelvic views. If an acetabular fracture is present, Judet 45-degree oblique views should be obtained. If further detail on an acetabular, sacral, or sacroiliac joint injury is needed a CT scan is the study of choice and the common use of CT in trauma assessment may eliminate the need for pelvic radiographs in some cases.

Management (Boxes 14.8.13 and 14.8.14)

Initial management of the child with a pelvic fracture is directed at haemodynamic resuscitation and treatment of associated life-threatening injuries. Although massive haemorrhage from pelvic fractures is uncommon in children, if an alternative source for blood loss cannot be found, pelvic external fixation to decrease the pelvic volume and control fracture movement and selective angiography with embolization is indicated. Provisional stabilization of the injured pelvis with a pelvic binder has decreased the need for acute external fixation.

Fractures without a break in the pelvic ring

Avulsion fractures about the pelvis require rest and hip positioning to decrease stretch on the involved muscle group. A short period of crutch ambulation with protected weight bearing may be required. Operative intervention is reserved for fractures which result in symptomatic non-union. The results of conservative treatment are generally good.

The plasticity of paediatric bone allows single ramus fractures to occur. These fractures are the most common pelvic fractures in children but are a result of higher-energy trauma than the ramus fractures seen in adults. Isolated pubic or ischial ramus fractures

Box 14.8.13 Pelvic fractures—initial management

- Resuscitate
- Treat life-threatening conditions
- Associated injuries common in single/double breaks of pelvic ring.

Box 14.8.14 Management of pelvic fractures

- Fractures without break in pelvic ring:
  - Rest
  - Progressive rehabilitation
  - Surgery for symptomatic non-union
- Single break in pelvic ring:
  - Short-term bed rest
  - Protected weight bearing/spica cast
  - Symphysis injuries may be plated
- Double break in pelvic ring:
  - Pubic rami—non-operative treatment
  - Malgaine fracture—traction or surgery
  - Severe multiple—traction or bilateral spica
  - Internal fixation preferable if significantly displaced in older child
- Acetabular fractures:
  - Skeletal traction
  - Displaced fractures require open reduction and internal fixation
- Note few outcome studies.

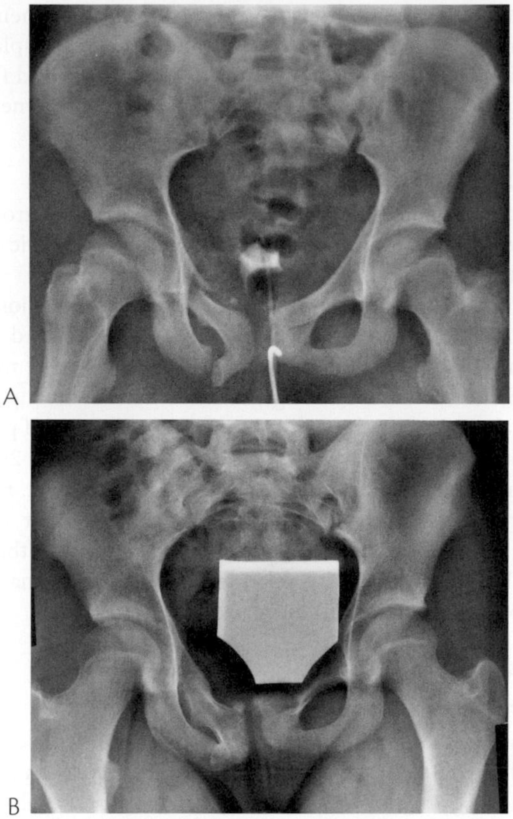

Fig. 14.8.6 This 12-year-old patient sustained fractures of the ipsilateral rami which healed with protected weight bearing. No posterior injury was present making this a single break in the pelvic ring.

should be treated with bed rest followed by progressive ambulation when symptoms subside.

Fractures of the iliac wing often are accompanied by other fractures in the pelvis which may dictate the treatment required. The isolated iliac wing fracture can be treated with bed rest until comfortable with the hip abducted to relieve stretch on the hip abductor muscles. Once symptoms subside, a programme of progressive weight bearing is followed.

Fractures of the sacrum or coccyx should be treated by ambulation with progressive weight bearing as pain allows. Manual reductions should be avoided since reduction is often lost and there is a risk of rectal tearing with the technique of reduction during digital rectal examination.

Single break in the pelvic ring

The elasticity of the child's sacroiliac joints and symphysis pubis allow for fractures which constitute a single break in the pelvic ring. Single breaks in the pelvic ring usually have minimal or no displacement. Although single breaks in the pelvic ring are stable and often look benign, the physician must remember that significant energy is required to produce these fractures, and associated injuries are not uncommon and must not be missed.

Fracture of the superior and inferior pubic rami on the same side, symphysis disruption, or fracture of the pubis near the symphysis constitute a break in the pelvic ring. These patterns are stable and require only short-term bed rest followed by protected, progressive weight-bearing on the affected side (Figure 14.8.6).

If significant symphysis displacement is present there must be posterior injury at the anterior sacroiliac joint. Widely displaced (over 3cm) symphysis disruptions of the 'open book' type are rotationally unstable injuries. Some authors feel the symphysis should be reduced with either external fixation or internal fixation with a plate. Plating is particularly efficacious if laparotomy is performed for abdominal injuries. Some of these disruptions will partially reduce spontaneously during conservative treatment. There is insufficient data about which disruptions will benefit from surgical reduction.

Double breaks in the pelvic ring

Double breaks in the pelvic ring are less common than single breaks. They are inherently unstable and usually the result of higher-energy trauma than single breaks. Associated injuries are common.

In double vertical fractures of the pubic rami (straddle fracture) there is often significant superior displacement of the free floating fragment created by the fracture of the bilateral superior and inferior pubic rami. This fracture does not involve the weight-bearing portion of the pelvis and does not require reduction via manipulation or traction. The fracture will usually heal and remodel even when significant displacement is present. Bed rest as necessary for comfort followed by progressive crutch ambulation.

Fracture of the ipsilateral pubic rami with ipsilateral/contralateral fracture of the ilium or dislocation/subluxation of the sacroiliac joint (Malgaine fracture) is a more severe injury. If significantly displaced, similar to adults, these injuries are commonly treated with reduction and internal fixation of the unstable hemipelvis. There are no good studies to determine how much displacement will lead to a poor outcome without being reduced and fixed. To avoid significant deformities more than 1cm of displacement of the posterior pelvic ring should be considered for surgery.

Acetabular fractures

Injury to the triradiate cartilage can cause acetabular growth disturbance which should always be considered in paediatric acetabular fractures.

Small posterior wall fractures that do not result in hip joint instability can be treated with bed rest followed by protected ambulation. Since these usually occur with hip dislocation, the main goal of treatment is to ensure a congruent reduction of the hip.

Skeletal traction can be utilized to obtain reduction of paediatric acetabular fractures. If an adequate reduction (less than 2mm) can be obtained, traction can be used as definitive treatment. However, more frequently children with displaced acetabular fractures through the superior part of the acetabulum or through the triradiate cartilage are treated with open reduction and internal fixation using approaches similar to those used in adults.

Results (Box 14.8.15)

Pelvic fractures without a break in the ring

Avulsions of the anterosuperior or anteroinferior iliac spine do well with rest and conservative treatment followed by a progressive strengthening programme prior to return to sport. Results of treatment of ischial spine avulsions have not been quite as predicable since persistent symptoms at the site are possible.

Single ramus fractures heal reliably. Despite the common presence of comminution or wide displacement fractures of the iliac wing, whether isolated or combined with other fractures, heal with conservative therapy and residual symptoms are rare.

Box 14.8.15 Pelvic fracture—results

Type of fracture (pelvic ring)

- Without break:
  - Usually heal without complications
  - Occasionally some limitation of athletic ability
- Single break: usually heal with good function
- Double break:
  - Usually heal well
  - Long-term morbidity due to associated injuries (genitourinary/neurological/vascular/abdominal)
  - Avoid deformities in older children
- Acetabular:
  - Usually satisfactory with traction/open reduction and internal fixation
  - Poor results—non-congruent reduction
  - Type V triradiate fractures.

Sacrum and coccyx fractures in children heal without long-term impairment in contrast to the frequent persistent symptoms seen in adults.

Single breaks in the pelvic ring

Fractures of two ipsilateral rami, isolated subluxation of the pubic symphysis, and fracture near the pubic symphysis can be expected to have excellent results with a short period of bed rest and progressive protected weight bearing. Isolated fracture near the sacroiliac joint or subluxation of the sacroiliac joint should result in good function after conservative treatment.

Double breaks in the pelvic ring

The results of double breaks in the pelvic ring are not as encouraging as those of single breaks in the ring. This is largely related to the energy of the injury and associated injuries. There is higher morbidity and mortality related to associated genitourinary, neurological, vascular, and abdominal injuries. Straddle fractures generally heal well without sequelae when treated conservatively. Operative treatment to prevent permanent deformity may be chosen particularly in older children

Acetabular fractures

Conservative treatment of non-displaced acetabular fractures and fractures that reduced acceptably in traction can be good. Poor results are seen in those with non-congruent reductions and type V Salter–Harris triradiate injuries. Operative treatment of displaced transverse fractures of the acetabulum in children can lead to excellent outcomes if a satisfactory reduction is obtained.

Complications (Box 14.8.16)

Many of the complications of paediatric pelvic fractures are related to concomitant injuries to the head, chest, abdomen, long bones, and genitourinary system.

Delayed union and non-union may occur. Non-unions of the rami are frequently asymptomatic. If symptomatic non-union is present, open reduction and internal fixation and bone grafting are appropriate treatments.

Malunion of pelvic fractures may occur including limb-length discrepancy secondary to cephalad displacement of the hemipelvis. Malunion can be prevented by obtaining and maintaining adequate reduction of the fracture.

Injury to the triradiate cartilage is a rare complication of acetabular injury which may result in premature closure of the physis and

Box 14.8.16 Pelvic fracture complications

- Majority due to associated injuries
- Delayed union/non-union up to 5%
- Malunion rarely symptomatic (leg-length discrepancy)
- Triradiate injury:
  - Rare
  - Salter–Harris type I, II, or V
  - Require long-term follow-up
- Incongruity can cause osteoarthritis.

resultant acetabular dysplasia. Classifying triradiate injuries can be difficult, especially in type V injuries which are often not detected until physeal growth abnormality is present. Patients with documented or suspected triradiate injury need long-term follow-up to assess for the development of acetabular dysplasia. If dysplasia is seen consideration should be given to acetabular osteotomy or bar resection to prevent subluxation or degenerative changes.

Incongruity of the acetabulum following acetabular fracture can lead to osteoarthritis of the hip. This complication can best be prevented by accurate reduction of the acetabular fracture utilizing open reduction and internal fixation when necessary.

Conclusion

Paediatric pelvic fractures are usually secondary to high-energy trauma and carry a high risk of associated injury. The treating physician must be aware of this potential and look for other injuries when a pelvic fracture is seen. The majority of pelvic fractures in children can be treated non-operatively with the exception of widely displaced ring fractures and displaced acetabular fractures.

Further reading

Boardman, M.J., Herman, M.J., Buck, B., and Pizzutillo, P.D. (2009). Hip fractures in children. *Journal of the American Academy of Orthopaedic Surgeons,* **17**(3), 162–73.

Banerjee, S., Barry, M.J., and Paterson, J.M. (2009). Paediatric pelvic fractures: 10 years experience in a trauma centre. *Injury,* **40**(4), 410–13.

Herrera-Soto, J.A. and Price, C.T. (2009). Traumatic hip dislocations in children and adolescents: pitfalls and complications. *Journal of the American Academy of Orthopaedic Surgeons,* **17**(1), 15–21.

Shrader, M.W., Jacofsky, D.J., Stans, A.A., *et al.* (2007). Femoral neck fractures in pediatric patients: 30 years experience at a level 1 trauma center. *Clinical Orthopaedics and Related Research,* **454**, 169–73.

Smith, W., Shurnas, P., Morgan, S., Aqudelo, J., Luszko, G., Knox, E.C., and Georgopoulos, G. (2005). Clinical outcomes of unstable pelvic fractures in skeletally immature patients. *Journal of Bone and Joint Surgery,* **87A**, 2423–31.

14.9

Injuries of the femur and patella in children

David Hollinghurst

Summary points

- There is considerable scope for remodelling in the child's femur
- Significant overgrowth may correct shortening after a fracture
- Below the age of 5 years femoral fractures may be treated non-operatively in a spica or with traction; above the age of 11 years surgical stabilization of the fracture will normally be needed
- Flexible intramedullary nails have largely replaced external fixators
- Fractures involving the distal femoral physis need careful treatment and follow-up as they may lead to significant growth arrest
- Osteochondral fractures accompany a proportion of acute patella dislocations.

Introduction

Fractures of the femoral shaft represent 1–2% of all childhood fractures (Box 14.9.1) demonstrating a bimodal age distribution. Incidence peaks around 2–3 years and with a further peak in adolescence. The rapid increase in cortical thickness from age 5 may account for the reduced incidence. Non-accidental injury should be considered in all age groups but is most likely in younger children. After the exclusion of obvious causes such as car accidents, child abuse has been identified in up to 65% of femoral shaft fractures in children under 1 year old. Towards the end of the first decade, bicycle accidents account for 50% of fractures with the majority caused by car and motorbike collisions in adolescence. Higher energy trauma increases the risk of associated injuries such as hip dislocation or femoral neck fracture, pelvic and knee injuries, or thoracoabdominal trauma. Haemodynamic instability should not be attributed to an isolated femur fracture without careful assessment to exclude other injuries.

Acceptable deformity, femoral regrowth, and overgrowth

The degree of acceptable deformity at union is in part determined by the anatomical location of the fracture and the age at time of injury (Figure 14.9.1). Girls under the age of 10 and boys less than 12 years generally have significant growth remaining and a long-term study has suggested that up to 25 degrees of midshaft angulation in any plane can remodel in children under 13 years. Generally more than 15 degrees in the coronal plane and 20 degrees in the sagittal plane should not be accepted. Deformity will be more apparent in distal femoral fractures. Remodelling can continue for up to 5 years after fracture union with the majority of deformity correction occurring from physeal reorientation and longitudinal growth, compared to remodelling at the fracture site itself. Rotational deformity is usually well tolerated even with failure to remodel. Absolute values for acceptable angular deformity are not well documented but surgeons should aim for less than 20 degrees of malrotation.

Increased growth after femoral shaft fracture is frequently seen, particularly in children aged 3–9 years. The absolute value of overgrowth reported in studies is unclear with the difference between true overgrowth and compensatory growth in the face of shortening often not clearly differentiated. Stimulation of growth is most prominent in the first 18 months, lasting up to 5 years after fracture and is in the region of 1–1.5cm. Fractures of the femur on the non-dominant side of the body have been reported to show statistically greater overgrowth. Opinion suggests fracture overlap no greater than 2cm is desirable in the age group 3–9 years. Older children have less growth remaining to resolve shortening and hence fractures should be stabilized out to length. Younger children with malunited fractures and shortening greater than 2cm can be observed for a significant period as there will be ample time to perform a contra lateral epiphysiodesis to equalize limb length.

Box 14.9.1 Paediatric femur fractures—general

- Consequence of child abuse in 30% under 4 years of age
- 1.0–1.5cm overgrowth anticipated ages 3–10 years
- Can accept up to 15 degrees coronal, 20 degrees sagittal malalignment
- The significance of rotational malunion is controversial.

Management guidelines and techniques

Union of the femoral shaft fractures in childhood is almost inevitable for closed low-energy injuries and a variety of management options can be employed from the non-operative methods of traction and cast immobilization to various forms of surgical stabilization. Complications related to the injury and treatments include infection, compartment syndrome, neurovascular injuries, and fracture non-union with high-energy or open injuries. The commonest problem is that of malunion which may or may not be associated with a limb-length discrepancy. In younger children this complication can resolve with growth.

Multiply injured children, head injuries, open fractures and simultaneous ipsilateral fractures of femur and tibia, and the floating knee, are all good indications for surgical stabilization.

The age, weight, and maturity of the child are some of the important factors in deciding the method of fracture stabilization. Presuming children are of average weight and maturity, guidelines are given on the basis of age with a subsequent discussion of the techniques.

Birth to 1 year (Box 14.9.2)

Fractures can occur from birth trauma, abuse including neglect, or can be the presenting feature of osteogenesis imperfecta and other metabolic disorders. A Pavlik harness may be used in the majority of children up the age of 6 months with thick periosteum and rapid fracture healing reducing the risk of significant malunion. The potential for remodelling is sufficient to accept up to 3cm of shortening or 30 degrees of angulation. Spica casts are more suitable in children over 6 months and retained for 4–6 weeks in this age group.

1 year to preschool (Figure 14.9.3)

The majority of fractures can be treated with early spica immobilization within 48h of injury and the spica retained for approximately 8 weeks. Temporary splintage or traction may be used prior to spica application. With shortening in excess of 2cm or significant telescoping of the fracture under anaesthetic an initial period in traction to correct length and alignment may be appropriate. A spica can be applied after fracture haematoma consolidation. Alternatively, incorporation of a traction pin into the spica to maintain length and alignment has been proposed.

5–11 years

Hip spica remains an acceptable treatment of low-energy injuries without significant displacement in young patients. However, the loss of independence whilst in a spica combined with the longer time to fracture healing increase the benefits of surgical stabilization. Many schools will not accept a child in a spica, causing a significant interruption in the child's education. Internal or external fixation techniques are appropriate, with flexible intramedullary nails becoming the usual practice. This facilitates early mobilization and a return to school or social activities for this and older age groups with likely psychological benefits for the child and family. Unstable fragmented fractures can be treated with submuscular bridge plating.

11 years to adult

Surgical stabilization is usually indicated. Fractures have a more limited ability to remodel and early mobilization and rapid progression to unsupported weight bearing is desirable. Methods of treatment should aim for less than 10 degrees of deformity in

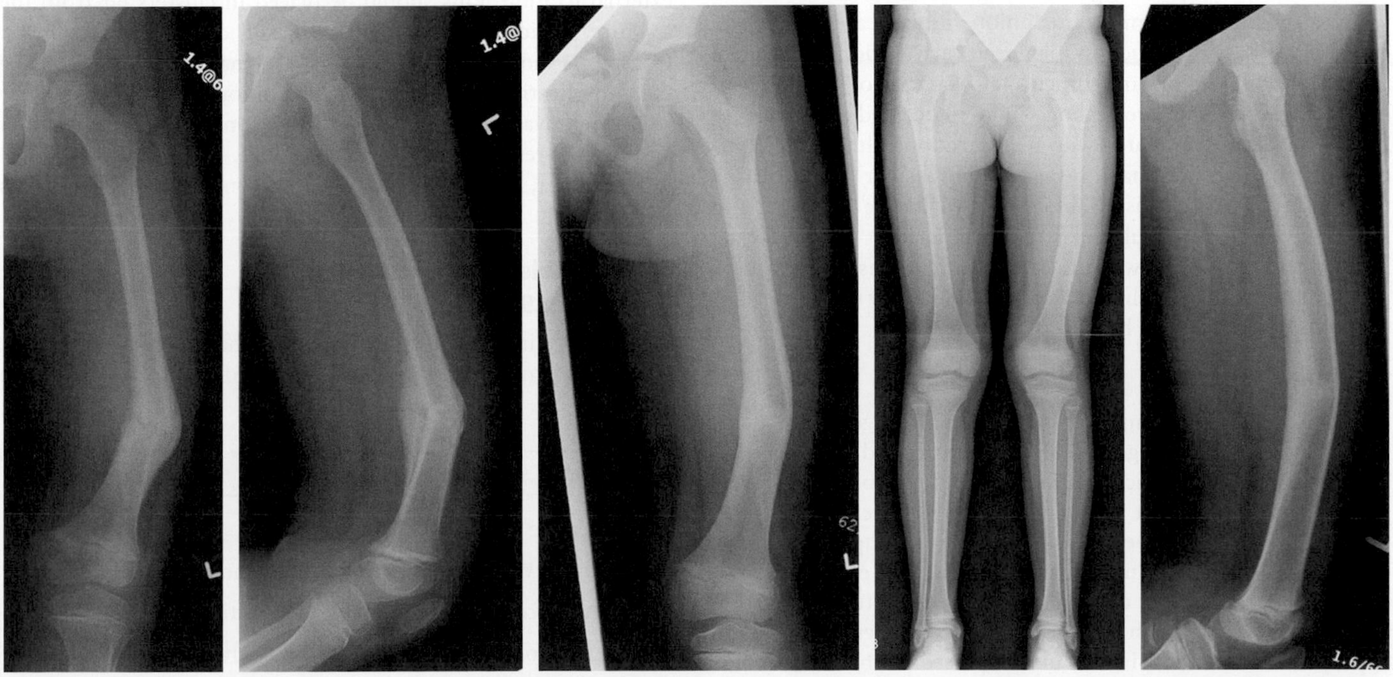

A B C D E

Fig. 14.9.1 A) and B) An 8.5-year-old patient with a diaphyseal femur fracture treated non-operatively with approximately 25-degree malunion in the coronal and sagittal planes; C) 1 year and D, E) 3 years postinjury showing satisfactory alignment and limb length.

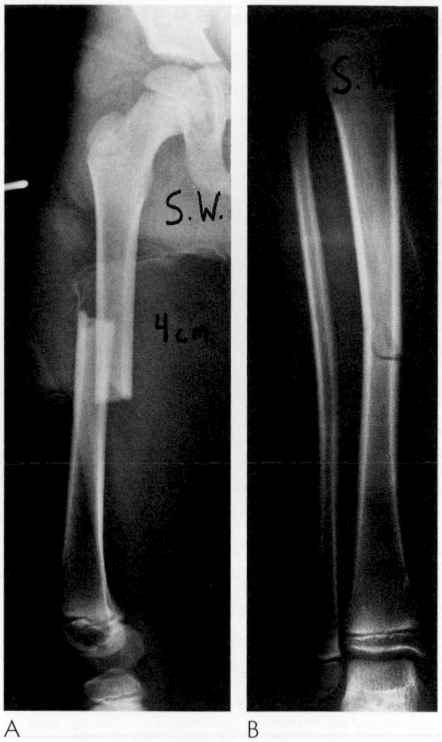

Fig. 14.9.2 A 7-year-old patient with ipsilateral tibia and femur fracture. Floating-knee injuries are a relative indication for operative stabilization of the femur. (Courtesy of P. Nourbash.)

coronal and/or sagittal planes with less than 1.5cm of shortening. Younger, lighter children are still suitable for flexible intramedullary nails, usually up to weights of 50kg. However, older children with less potential to remodel malunion and increase weight predisposing to loss of reduction may need early periods of bed rest prior to mobilization and functional bracing to help prevent deformity during fracture healing. Children deemed unsuitable for flexible nails can be treated with plate fixation. Although technically demanding, minimally invasive submuscular bridge plating techniques avoid the disadvantages of soft tissue stripping and large incisions. Successful use of anterograde adult pattern locked intramedullary nails is well described but even using the lateral aspect of the greater trochanter for entry point may not completely avoid the risk of femoral head avascular necrosis.

Traction

Skin or skeletal traction may be used although it is generally a temporary measure as younger children can be treated in a spica and older children with surgical stabilization. Bryant's or gallows overhead skin traction is not recommended for children over 11kg in weight. Risks include peroneal nerve palsy, compartment syndrome, and skin blistering necessitating frequent examination of the neurovascular status of the limb. Simple longitudinal traction or balanced traction with the knee flexed 45 degrees is often more appropriate. Traction pins should be placed in the distal femur 2cm proximal to the physis under fluoroscopy from a medial to lateral direction to avoid injury to the femoral vessels. The proximal tibia should not used because of the risk of causing growth arrest and subsequent tibial recuvatum. If skeletal traction is used as a definitive treatment then radiographs should be obtained periodically to adjust the weight and direction of traction in order to maintain fracture alignment. When adequate callus formation is evident the patient can be mobilized in a cast or function brace.

Hip spica

Prior to spica application femoral shortening is assessed by longitudinal compression to confirm the fracture does not shorten by more than 3cm. This has been referred to as the telescope test. The fracture is reduced with traction applied manually directly to the calf and reduction confirmed with fluoroscopy. The popliteal fossa and all bony prominences must be well padded and one and half limb spica applied. Flexion of the hip and knee to approximately 45 degrees is usually adequate to control the fracture position with appropriate moulding of the thigh. Some authors recommend hip and knee flexion of 90 degrees in the spica. Whilst this has undoubtedly been used many times without adverse outcome, there are reports of catastrophic complications with full thickness skin loss and leg compartment syndrome. Initial application of a long leg cast and subsequent completion of the spica may be helpful, but the cast should not be used to apply traction to the leg. Maintenance of fracture reduction should be confirmed at 1 and 2 weeks. Angular deformity can often be treated with appropriate wedging of the cast.

External fixation (Box 14.9.3)

External fixation was previously popular in children inappropriate for spica casts but has been largely superseded by flexible intramedullary nails. There is still a role in patients with fragmented and unstable fracture patterns where control of length and alignment is difficult. Open fractures, significant soft tissue injury such as burns, or the multiplied injured patient may be relative indications for external fixation. Pins should be placed in clusters far from the fracture, avoiding the femoral neck and distal femoral physis. Constructs should not be too rigid and dynamized early to reduce the complications of delayed or non-union and refracture after fixator removal. Pin site infection is the commonest complication and usually responsive to oral antibiotics. The need for surgical debridement, intravenous antibiotics, and fixator removal is uncommon.

Elastic stable intramedullary nailing (Figures 14.9.5, 14.9.6)

Elastic stable intramedullary nails (ESIN) have become the mainstay of treatment to stabilize fractures of the femur from the

Box 14.9.2 Closed treatment

- Immediate spica:
  - Up to 2 years of age is treatment of choice
  - Beware comminution or excessive initial shortening
- Traction followed by spica (3 weeks average):
  - Split Russell skin traction in young children
  - Skeletal in older children.

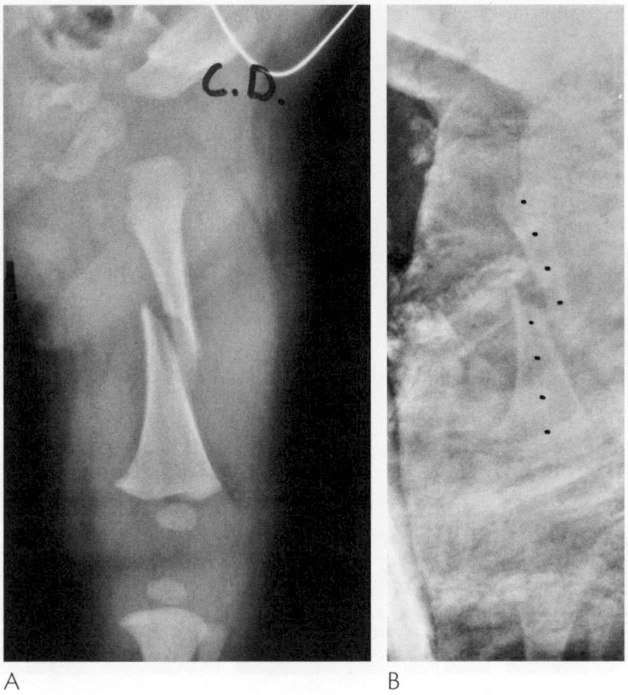

Fig. 14.9.3 A) Femoral fracture in a 4-month-old male. Injuries such as this in non-ambulating patients should be considered a consequence of child abuse. B) Fractures in this age group may be treated with immediate spica cast immobilization with excellent results.

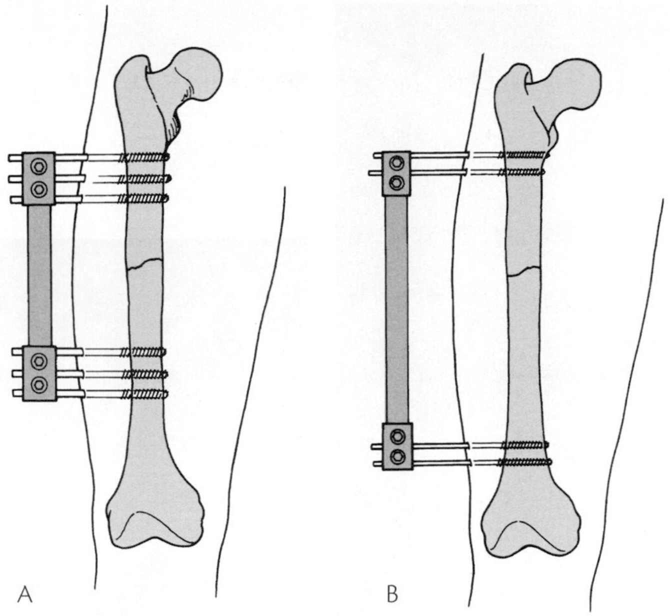

Fig. 14.9.4 External fixation of paediatric femur fractures should be performed with 'flexible frame constructs'. A) Large-diameter pins (more than two pins per cluster) with wide pin clusters and close approximation to the fracture increase the structural stiffness of the construct. Smaller-diameter pins placed in narrow clusters away from the fracture site are preferable. B) The second construct and lateral displacement of the fixator may diminish the risk of delayed union and refracture.

subtrochanteric region to the distal quarter of the shaft. Advantages include avoidance of injury to the blood supply of the trochanter, femoral neck, or head. Limited incisions are used provided the fracture can be reduced by closed methods, using either the nails directly at the fracture site to guide reduction, a traction table, or radiolucent reduction tools applied to the thigh.

The majority of fractures are stabilized with two C-shaped nails inserted retrograde from medial and lateral starting points approximately 2cm proximal to the growth plate. Each nail is 40% of the diameter of the femoral canal at the isthmus and prebent to an identical curvature, approximately three times the diameter of the isthmus, to achieve a stable construct. Nails should cross each other far from the fracture site and not pass around each other in the manner of a corkscrew. Nails are inserted to the level of the lesser trochanter, although subtrochanteric fractures may require nail passage into the femoral neck to achieve stability or an alternative method of stabilization. The fracture is impacted and rotational alignment is compared to the contralateral limb prior to final nail insertion. Leaving 1cm of nail outside the bone facilitates removal and nails should lie flush to the bone to avoid soft tissue irritation. Distal fractures can be treated with a C- and S-shaped nail passed anterograde from below the level of the lesser trochanter. Entry points are on the lateral aspect of the femur with one nail starting slightly distal and anterior to the other. Patients are mobilized protected or non-weight bearing depending on fracture configuration and stability. Full weight bearing is allowed when good callus is present, usually around 6–8 weeks.

The largest elastic nail available is 4mm in diameter; hence femora up to 10–12mm in diameter at the isthmus can be treated using this method. However, consensus suggests that 50–60kg in weight represents an upper limit. The incidence of malunion rises significantly with increasing patient weight and older or heavier children may require either a period of postoperative bed rest and/or bracing to supplement fracture fixation. Additionally, older children will have less growth remaining so are less tolerant of fracture malunion. Flexible nails that allow proximal and distal interlocking screws have been reported but are not in widespread use. There is continued debate over the use of stainless steel or titanium implants. An incidence of malunion with titanium of 23% compared with 6% for stainless steel suggests titanium may be too flexible a material for nails particularly in older or heavier children.

Implants are generally removed after fracture union and consolidation, usually at least 6 months postinjury. Refracture after implant removal is uncommon.

Plate fixation (Figure 14.9.7)

Open reduction and dynamic compression plates allow anatomical reduction of fractures without the aid of fluoroscopy and have relative indications in the case of proximal fractures, head injury, or multiply injured patients allowing simultaneous surgery to other injuries. However, this comes at the expense of large incisions and significant soft tissue stripping. Hence flexible nails are more commonly used. Submuscular bridge plating combined with minimally invasive techniques avoids many of the disadvantages of open plate fixation. In association with locking compression plates this technique is an alternative to a locked anterograde nail in adolescents considered too heavy for flexible nails but with an open proximal femoral physis. The technique is demanding particularly as these

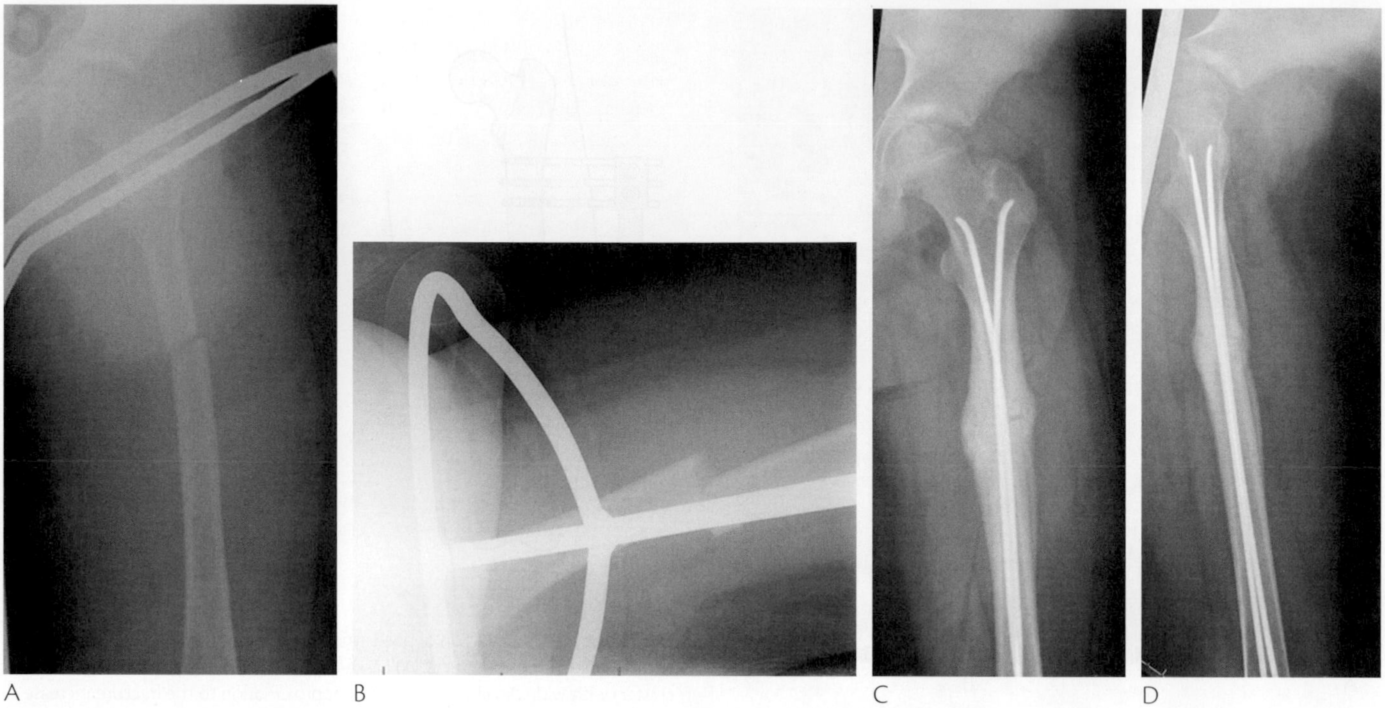

Fig. 14.9.5 A) and B) Transverse fracture patterns are ideal for treatment with ESIN, allowing early weight bearing in this 12-year-old patient and encouraging union (C, D).

older patients have a greater need for anatomical reduction of length and alignment. Screw placement is based on similar principles to that of external fixation with six cortices either side of the fracture. The fracture is indirectly reduced by the plate and no interfragmentary compression is applied. Patients can usually bear weight unsupported by 10 weeks. Implants can be removed using the same minimal incisions around 6–8 months after injury depending on fracture consolidation.

Rigid locked intramedullary nails

There is continued controversy over the safety of adult pattern anterograde femoral nails in the treatment of femoral shaft fractures in older or heavier children where there are clear biomechanical advantages. Nails implanted through the piriform fossa have been associated with avascular necrosis of the femoral head at a rate of around 2%. Prior to physeal closure the femoral head blood supply is almost entirely dependant on the lateral ascending branch of the medial circumflex artery. The artery is at risk from nails using a piriformis fossa entry point or the medial aspect of the greater trochanter, including inadvertent entry by reaming out the medial trochanter wall from trochanter tip entry. This is a devastating complication with no satisfactory reconstructive option. Coxa valga and thinning of the femoral neck is also reported, which also is likely to represent a vascular insult. Modern nail designs allow a lateral trochanteric entry which avoids dissection near to the artery. Several large series have reported good maintenance of alignment and length with this technique but numbers studied are probably too small to report the true incidence of avascular necrosis with a suitably narrow confidence interval. Overall this remains a controversial device to stabilize the adolescent femur, despite reports of safe usage. Therefore a 1–2% risk of avascular necrosis of the femoral head should be clearly stated if this method is used.

Distal femur fractures

Supracondylar fractures involving the metaphysis but not the physis are relatively uncommon. The gastrocnemius muscle can pull the distal fragment into flexion making it difficult to maintain a reduction with cast alone. Patients can be managed in traction, but usual treatment involves closed reduction using longitudinal traction with the knee flexed and placement of crossed percutaneous pins to stabilize the fracture. Initially a long leg cast is used to stabilize the fracture with possible transfer to a cast brace when

Box 14.9.3 Operative treatment—indications

- Strong:
  - Head injury
  - Multiple trauma
  - Ipsilateral tibia
  - Open fractures
- Relative:
  - Age and patient size
  - Psychosocial and economic considerations
  - Unacceptable alignment.

Box 14.9.4 Operative treatment—techniques

- Plate fixation—disadvantages include extensive scarring or the technical demands of minimally invasive submuscular techniques, possible delayed weight bearing
- Rigid/reamed nails—disadvantages include trochanteric arrest, 1–2% femoral head avascular necrosis
- Flexible nails—disadvantages include length instability, pin migration, supplemental immobilization
- External fixation—disadvantages include pin infection, delayed union, refracture.

early callus is seen. Ideally pins should not cross the physis but it may be necessary to achieve fracture stability. There is a low risk of growth disturbance with smooth pins for approximately 4 weeks.

Distal femoral physeal fractures

Physeal injuries of the distal femur represent 5% of physeal injuries and require significant trauma to disrupt the complex shape of the growth plate which is securely fixed to the metaphysis. The distal femoral physis contributes approximately 40% of the total leg length and 70% of femoral growth at maturity. Fractures with any displacement are at significant risk of growth plate arrest with resultant limb-length discrepancy and angular deformity. Minimally displaced fractures can be confused with knee ligamentous injuries but maximal tenderness to palpation is remote from the joint line. Physeal displacement usually follows the direction of applied force either by direct impact or via ligamentous structures; for example, medial femoral condyle fractures results from a valgus force applied via the medial collateral ligament. It is presumed that less energy is required to cause the fracture than disrupt the cruciate or collateral ligaments.

Distal femoral fractures are seen following obstetric trauma and deformity can usually be expected to remodel with a low incidence of growth arrest. The majority of injuries occur in the age group 11–13 years following sports or road traffic collisions and are Salter–Harris type I or II. Most studies demonstrate worse outcomes in young patients with the greatest fracture displacement and failure to achieve an anatomical fracture reduction. The Salter–Harris grade does not seem to correlate with the risk of growth arrest and type I and II injuries have shown a 50% incidence of growth arrest. Careful follow-up is advised to detect partial or complete growth arrest. Other complications include knee stiffness, ligamentous laxity, and neurovascular injury. Popliteal vessel injury is rare and peroneal nerve neurapraxia generally resolves spontaneously.

Cast immobilization for 4 weeks is usually sufficient for undisplaced, stable fractures although radiographic surveillance for late displacement is required. For displaced fractures a gentle closed reduction is attempted under general anaesthesia. Indications for open reduction include failure to achieve reduction due to muscle or periosteal interposition, open injuries, associated neurovascular injury, and intra articular fracture extension. Salter–Harris type III and IV injuries require anatomical reduction to reduce the risk of bony bar formation and growth arrest. Surgical approaches should be from the tension side of the fracture (Figure 14.9.10),

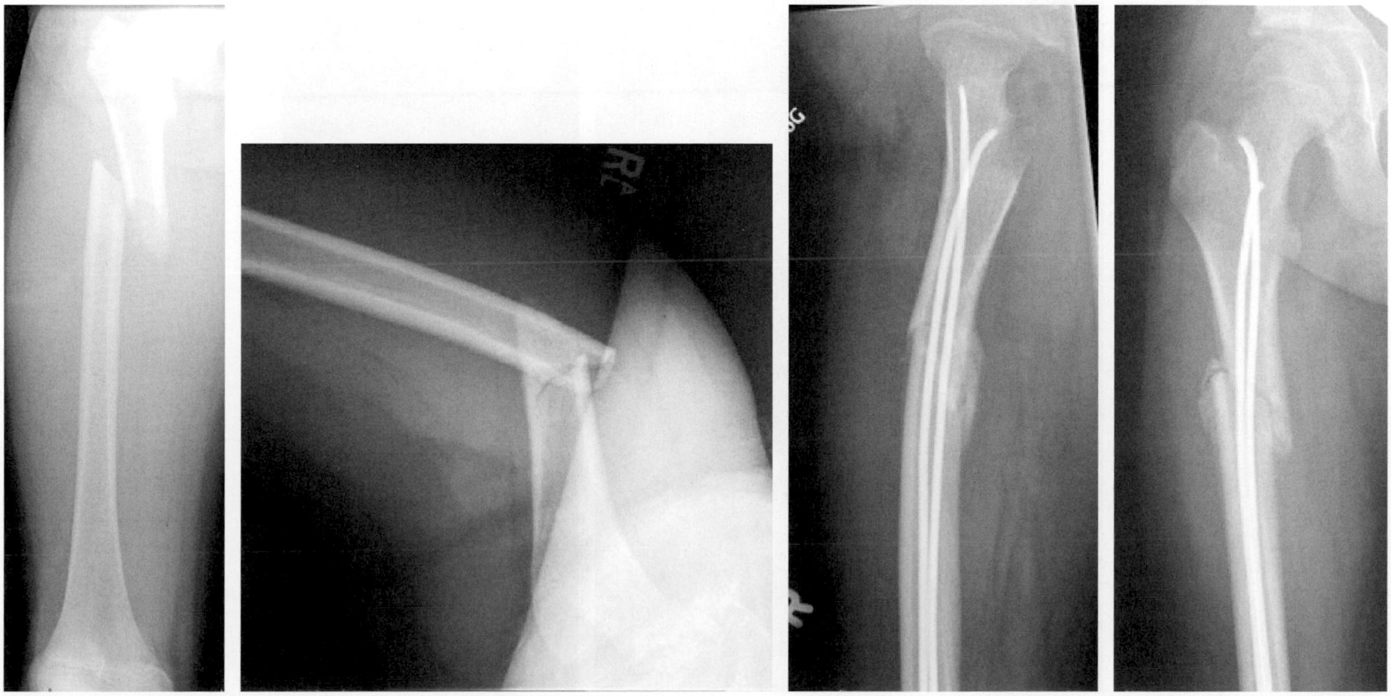

A B C D

Fig. 14.9.6 A) and B) Proximal fractures towards the subtrochanteric region show flexion of the proximal fragment which is difficult to control in a spica. C) and D) Fracture stability was enhanced by passing nails above the lesser trochanter in this 12-year-old patient.

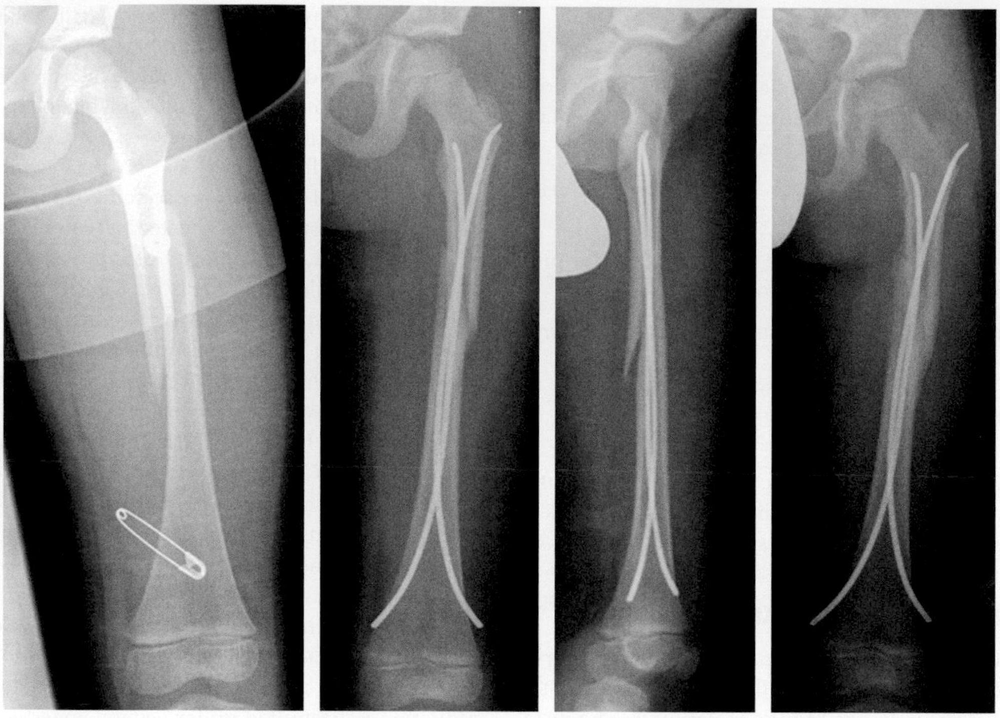

A B C D

Fig. 14.9.7 A) Spiral fractures can be length unstable and anatomical reduction more difficult to achieve (B, C). Shortening at fracture union is likely to be compensated for in this 7 year old boy (D).

A B C

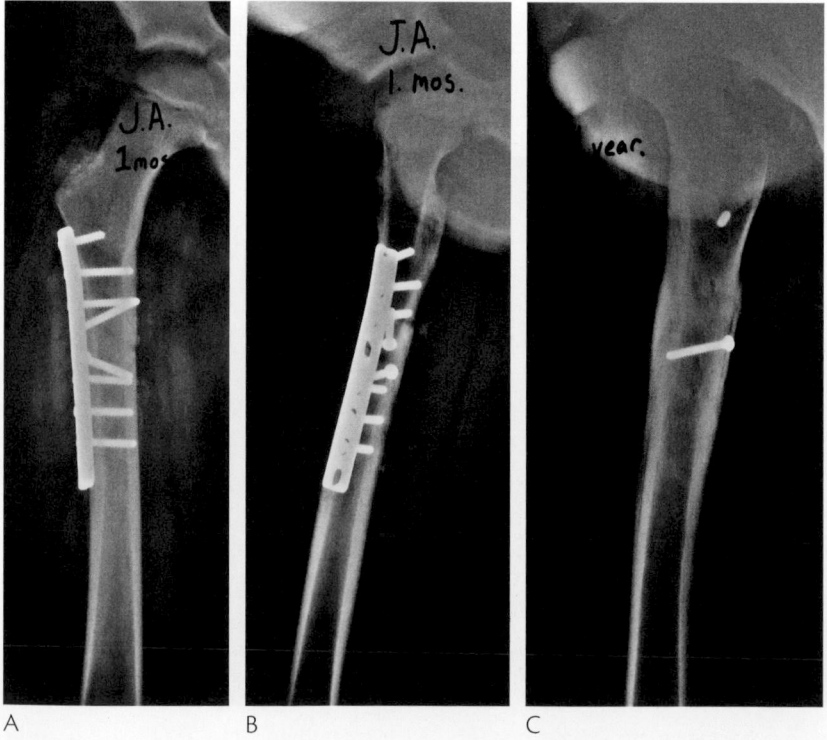

Fig. 14.9.8 A) A 7-year-old patient with a comminuted subtrochanteric femur fracture associated with closed cranial trauma. B) and C) Fracture stabilization was accomplished with osteosynthesis. D) At 1 year the difficulty in routine hardware removal is evident. (Courtesy of P. Nourbash.)

Box 14.9.5 Distal femoral physeal fractures

- Distal femoral physis contributes 40% of total leg length and 70% of femoral length
- Average age 11–13 years
- Leg-length discrepancy and/or angular deformity in up to 55%
- Reduction and fixation under general anaesthesia
- Open reduction common in Salter–Harris types III and IV and may be necessary in types I and II.

where the block to reduction is most likely to be encountered. Reduction is stabilized with crossed K-wires (Figure 14.9.9). Placement from proximal to distal avoids transgressing the knee joint. Screw fixation through the Thurston–Holland metaphyseal fragment avoids hardware crossing the growth plate when the fragment is of sufficient size. A long leg cast then applied for 4 weeks.

Clinical evaluation after injury screens for signs of growth disturbance and ligamentous laxity until skeletal maturity. Magnetic resonance scans can identify early signs of physeal arrest 3–6 months postinjury. Predicted limb length discrepancy of more than 1cm is an indication for contralateral epiphysiodesis in adolescent patients. Bar excision should be considered with growth arrest in younger age groups.

Patella fractures (Box 14.9.6 and Figure 14.9.12)

Fractures of the patella in children and adolescents are uncommon representing 1% and 8% of patella fractures overall. The predominance of fibrocartilaginous tissue and relative increased mobility of the patella probably account for the rarity of this injury. These differences can make diagnosis of a patella fracture more difficult and there is often a tense haemarthrosis preventing palpation of a defect. Abnormal action of the extensor mechanism and loss of function may indicate an injury. Bipartite patella, classically with a superolateral defect, can be painful mimicking a minimally displaced fracture, particularly with incomplete ossification. Sleeve fractures describe an avulsion fracture of the distal cartilaginous part of the patella from the ossification centre, with a significant proportion of the articular surface attached to the distal fragment. The injury is best identified on the lateral radiograph which may merely show patella alta and a small distal avulsion fragment.

Undisplaced fractures with an intact extensor mechanism can be immobilized in extension for 4–6 weeks. Displaced fractures require open reduction to achieve articular congruity and fixation using tension band techniques with wire or non-absorbable suture. Fixation can be supplemented with cerclage techniques and repair of the retinaculum is important. Partial and total patellectomy is described for severely fragmented injuries but should be avoided if at all possible. After suitable cast immobilization, range of motion and muscle strengthening exercises are commenced. Growth disturbance is uncommon after injury with the patella a sesamoid bone, hence growing by apposition.

Acute patella dislocation

Acute dislocations of the patella are generally seen in adolescents and high-level athletes with a significant number having anatomical variation predisposing to the injury. Recurrent or habitual dislocation associated with patella alta, generalized laxity, and genu valgum is discussed elsewhere. Injury commonly occurs from indirect trauma with foot planted and the knee flexed in valgus causing an internal rotation moment. Direct trauma to either the medial aspect of the patella or laterally resulting in knee valgus can cause injury.

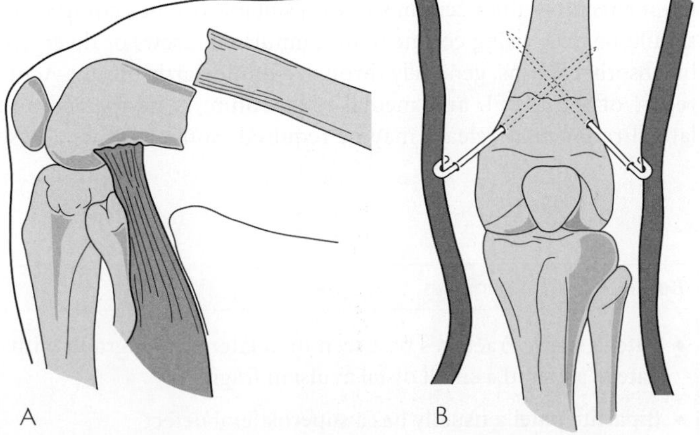

Fig. 14.9.9 A) Distal femoral metaphyseal fractures are prone to malalignment secondary to gastrocnemius pull. B) Fractures are best treated with closed reduction percutaneous pinning and cast immobilization.

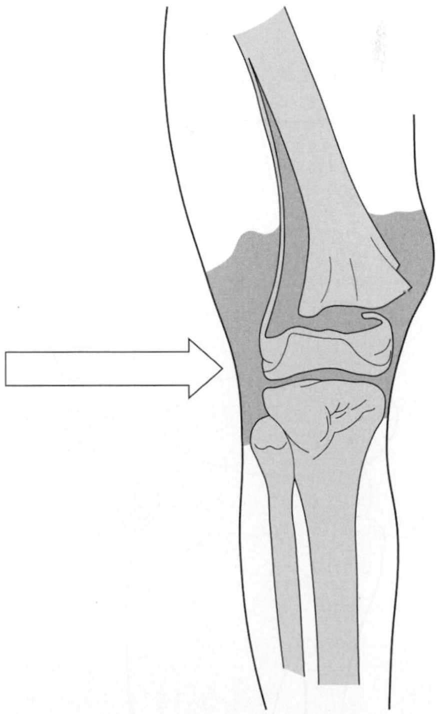

Fig. 14.9.10 Salter–Harris type I fracture may follow an excessive lateral force. Fracture reduction may be difficult secondary to interposed periosteum. Failure to achieve a closed reduction warrants an open approach in order to remove any obstacles including interposed periosteum.

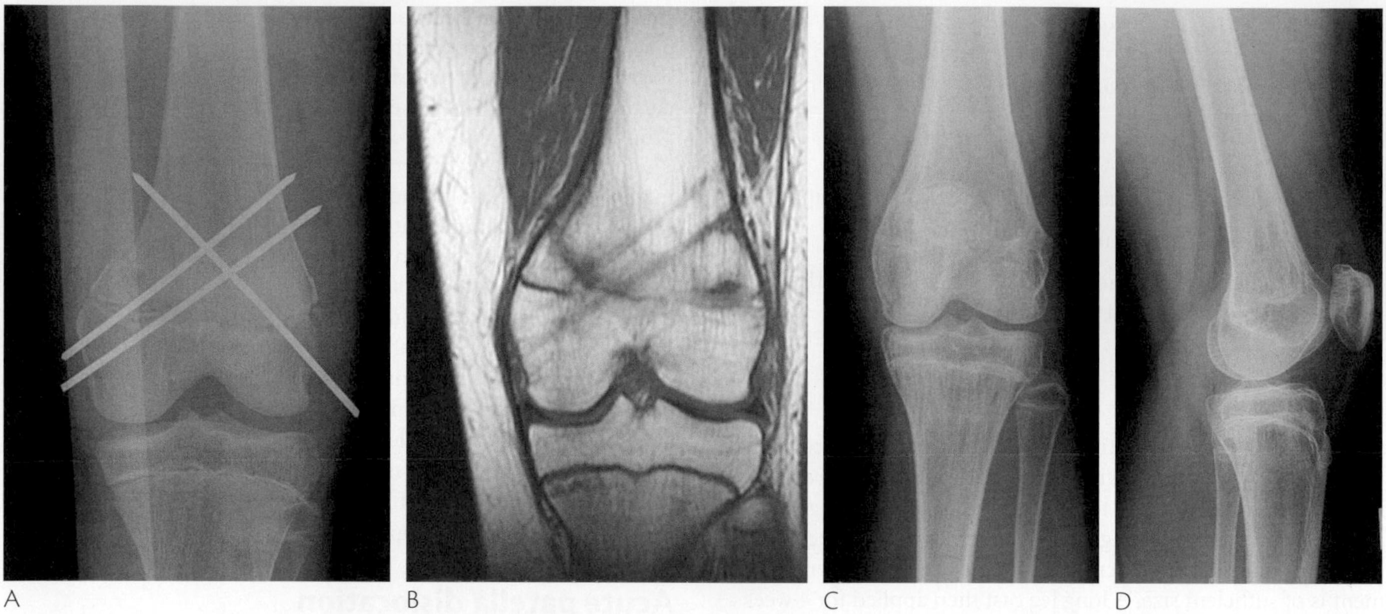

Fig. 14.9.11 A) Salter-Harris II fracture treated with closed reduction and percutaneous fixation. Non-anatomical reduction may have contributed to the subsequent growth arrest (B) and mild angular deformity (C, D).

This damages the medial structures involving the sartorius fascia in the superficial layer, medial patellofemoral ligament (MPFL), and patella retinaculum in the middle layer and medial collateral ligament and joint capsule deep. The MPFL provides between 50–80% of the restraining force to lateral patellar displacement, originating at the adductor tubercle and inserting into the superior half of the medial patella border.

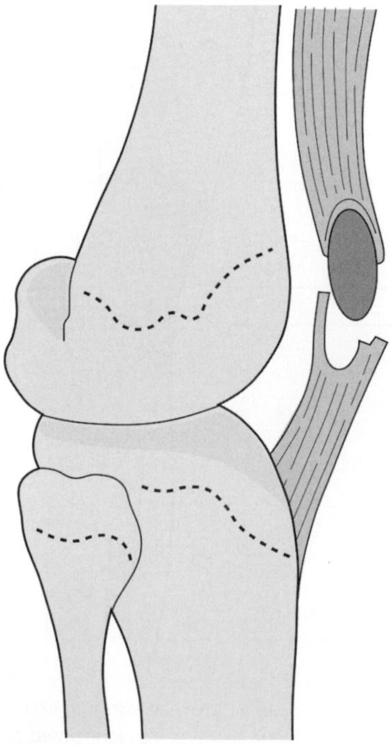

Fig. 14.9.12 Patellar sleeve fractures are operatively stabilized when the extensor mechanism is disrupted and to reduce the articular incongruity.

After injury the patella is often relocated otherwise the knee will still be flexed with the patella palpable to one side of the lateral femoral condyle. After suitable analgesia and sedation the knee is extended and gentle medial pressure reduces the patella. Turning onto a prone position helps relax the hamstrings if difficulty is encountered. Considering the similarity in mechanism of injury and likelihood of a large haemarthrosis; the patient should be evaluated for a tear of the anterior cruciate ligament. Radiographs including a skyline view should be assessed for the quality of reduction and the presence of an osteochondral fragment. Damage to the medial retinaculum and the haemarthrosis can cause significant patella tilt on skyline views which reduces as knee swelling resolves.

Osteochondral fractures are reported in 5–50% of acute patella dislocations and their presence may necessitate arthroscopy and evaluation. If radiographs or clinical assessment are unclear then magnetic resonance imaging should be undertaken. Osteochondral fragments more than 2cm in size with suitable osseous component should be fixed using countersunk cannulated screws or divergent bioabsorbable pins, generally through a limited arthrotomy. Acute repair of the MPFL and medial retinaculum is performed and lateral retinacular release may be required. Some authors advise

Box 14.9.6 Patella injuries

- Patella sleeve fractures best seen on a lateral radiograph with patella alta and a small distal avulsion fragment
- Bipartite patella usually has a superolateral defect
- Osteochondral fractures greater than 2cm should undergo fixation ± repair of medial structures.

correction of significant predisposing anatomical variants at the same time. In absence of an osteochondral fracture repair of the medial structures is probably unnecessary and doesn't seem to reduce the risk of further instability compared to non-operative management. Up to 60% of patients over 10 years old have no recurrence of instability after their first dislocation.

Conclusions

Femoral shaft fractures in children can be successfully managed using all the methods previously discussed. Fracture pattern, associated injuries, the age, maturity, and the weight of the child influence the choice of management. Ultimately the preferences of the surgeon and family may dominate. Children of 5 years or less can usually be managed in a hip spica and older children with flexible intramedullary nails unless fracture pattern, weight, or maturity makes this method unsuitable. Submuscular plate fixation can be used for most patients unsuitable for flexible nails. The use of adult pattern intramedullary nails inserted through the greater trochanter remains controversial and the risk of femoral head avascular necrosis is approximately 1–2%. Reconstruction following this devastating complication is often unsatisfactory.

Displaced distal femoral physeal fractures require anatomical reduction by either gentle closed manoeuvres or open techniques and stabilization. Surveillance for post-traumatic growth arrest is important.

Patella fractures can often be managed in a similar fashion to adult injuries with tension band and cerclage techniques. Patella injuries should be evaluated for osteochondral fractures presenting as sleeve fractures or avulsion injuries following patella dislocation.

Further reading

Arkader, A., Warner, W.C., Horn, D., Shaw, R.N., and Wells, L. (2007). Predicting the outcome of physeal fractures of the distal femur. *Journal of Paediatric Orthopedics*, **27**, 703–8.

Gordon, J.E., Khanna, N., Luhmann, S.J., Dobbs, M.B., Ortman, M.R., and Schoenecker, P.L. (2004). Intramedullary nailing of femoral fractures in children through the lateral aspect of the greater trochanter using a modified rigid humeral intramedullary nail. *Journal of Orthopedic Trauma*, **18**, 416–22.

Hedequist, D., Bishop, J., and Hresko, T. (2008). Locking plate fixation for paediatric femur fractures. *Journal of Paediatric Orthopedics*, **28**, 6–9.

Mubarak, S., Frick, S., Sink, E., *et al.* (2006). Compartment syndromes and Volkmanns contractures resulting from femur fractures treated by 90/90 spica cast. *Journal of Paediatric Orthopedics*, **26**, 567–72.

Sink, E., Gralla, J., and Repine, M. (2005). Complications of paediatric femur fractures treated with titanium elastic nails. *Journal of Paediatric Orthopedics*, **25**, 577–80.

Sink, E., Hedequist, D., Morgan, S., and Hresko, T. (2006). Results and technique of unstable paediatric femoral fractures treated with submuscular bridge plating. *Journal of Paediatric Orthopedics*, **26**, 177–81.

Wall, E.J., Jain, V., Vora, V., Mehlman, C.T., and Crawford, A.H. (2008). Complications of titanium and stainless steel elastic nail fixation of paediatric fractures. *Journal of Bone and Joint Surgery*, **90A**, 1305–13.

Wright, J., Wang, E., Owen, J., *et al.* (2005). Treatments for paediatric femoral fractures: a randomised trail. *Lancet*, **365**, 1153–8.

14.10

Tibial and ankle fractures in children

B.W. Scott and P.A. Templeton

Summary points

- After forearm and digital injuries, tibial and ankle fractures are the commonest fractures in the immature skeleton and the majority of these involve the diaphysis or ankle
- Compared to the morbidity seen in adults these are relatively forgiving injuries in children as the healing rate of bone and soft tissues is rapid and remodelling will occur
- It is wise, however, to guard against overconfidence in the remodelling potential of certain injuries; for example, angulated mid-diaphyseal fractures, rotational malalignment, and metaphyseal fractures within 2 years of skeletal maturity
- Children will tolerate manipulative/cast treatment better than adults as the duration of treatment is usually shorter and rapid rehabilitation is almost the norm with or without physiotherapy
- Postfracture overgrowth does occur but is less than that following femoral fractures and seldom clinically significant (over 10mm)
- Isolated fibular fractures are of minor importance but need to be taken into account in managing complex injuries involving the distal tibia
- It is convenient to discuss injuries according to three anatomical sections: proximal, diaphyseal, and distal.

Proximal tibial injuries

Tibial spine (intercondylar eminence/tubercle)

This is the commonest proximal fracture and is associated with sports injuries, particularly boarding, skiing, and cycling and is, in effect, the child equivalent of an anterior cruciate ligament rupture (Figure 14.10.1). Pain and an acute effusion (lipohaemarthrosis) are characteristic. X-ray classification and treatment is according to displacement (Box 14.10.2).

Open reduction through a 3cm anteromedial arthrotomy is a straightforward procedure.

With the knee flexed the fracture is easily reduced under direct vision and is held with an absorbable transepiphyseal suture. In the older child, which most are, the fracture is easily secured with a short cannulated screw taking care not to cross the growth plate. The screw head does not impinge on the notch and does not require removal.

The attached anterior cruciate ligament is almost certainly stretched immediately prior to the avulsion fracture and though residual laxity may be clinically evident, symptomatic late instability is rare.

Tibial tubercle

Avulsion fractures are uncommon but when acute mechanical failure of the extensor apparatus occurs it tends to do so distally in children (Figure 14.10.2). This is in contrast to patellar and quadriceps injury seen in adults. There is no relationship to Osgood–Schlatter disease though x-rays may confuse the inexperienced.

Rarely the fracture extends into the knee joint as a type III Salter–Harris growth plate injury. The fracture is usually displaced.

Treatment is by open reduction and fixation with screws. Growth disturbance is unusual but to minimize the risk of late damaging recurvatum metalwork should be removed after the fracture has healed unless the child is close to skeletal maturity.

Proximal tibial physeal injuries

Salter–Harris type II are rare in the proximal tibia. When complete separations do occur there is a reported 10% risk of neurovascular damage to the sciatic nerve and the popliteal artery trifurcation akin to knee dislocations in adults.

Proximal metaphyseal (Cozen) fractures (Box 14.10.1)

If undisplaced, an above-knee cast in 10 degrees flexion for 5–6 weeks is effective (Figure 14.10.3). Angulated fractures require initial manipulation under general anaesthesia to within 5 degrees of normal alignment. Interposition of the pes anserinus can prevent closed reduction and open reduction may be needed combined with fixation with crossed 2-mm K-wires in small children or a plate in older children. Above-knee casting is also required.

As for physeal injuries, the popliteal artery trifurcation is at risk in high-energy displaced injuries so the distal pulses should be checked and the child monitored for compartment syndrome.

Cozen described late valgus deformity developing following early uneventful healing of this fracture. Spontaneous correction may occur though this may take years. Late recurrence of valgus even after corrective osteotomy has been reported and generally it is

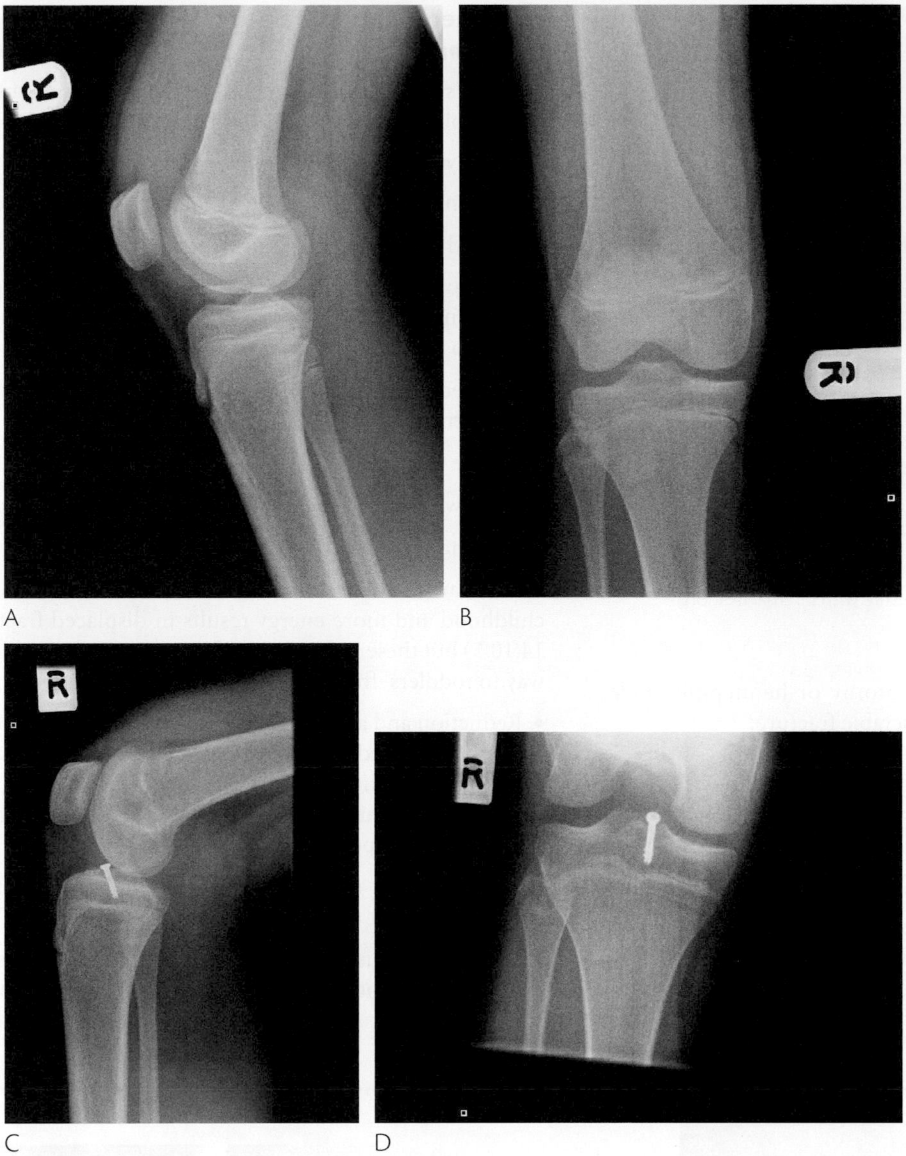

Fig. 14.10.1 Type II tibial spine fracture. A) and B) Displaced tibial spine fracture. C) and D) Post-fixation tibial spine fracture.

Box 14.10.1 Relevant physeal anatomy

- Growth of tibia: proximal physis 60%
- Ankle ligaments attach to epiphysis:
  - Physis weak in comparison to ligament
  - Physeal fractures rather than sprains
- Distal tibial physeal closure begins centrally then medially and lastly anterolaterally
- Beware of vascular injuries in proximal tibial physeal injury.

Box 14.10.2 Classification of tibial spine fractures

- Type 1: minimally displaced: requires immobilization in an above-knee cast in slight flexion for 5–6 weeks
- Type 2: posteriorly hinged: trial of a fully extended above-knee cast and if radiological reduction demonstrated continue with 5–6 weeks of immobilization. If reduction doubtful treat as type 3
- Type 3: completely displaced: associated with a broad 'angel wing' epiphyseal attachment which is held irreducibly displaced by the underlying intact menisci. It can be difficult to distinguish types 2 and 3. Attempts at reduction of displaced fractures in an extension cast are seldom successful and open reduction is needed.

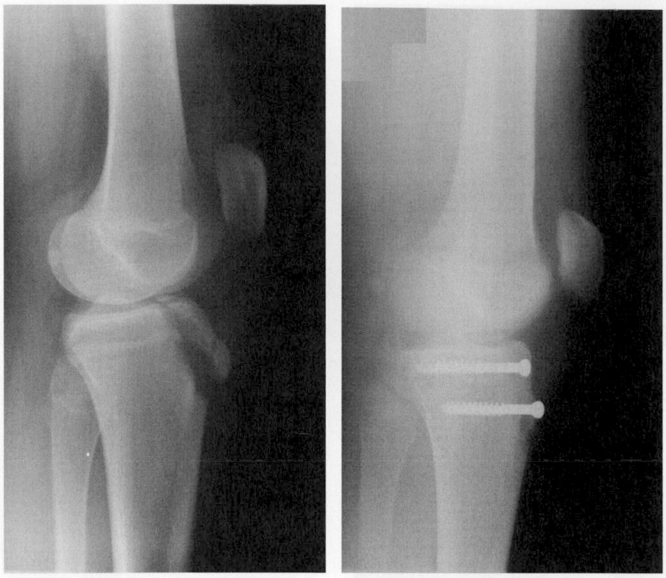

Fig. 14.10.2 Displaced tibial tuberosity fracture with internal fixation.

better to defer correction by osteotomy or hemiepiphysiodesis until late childhood in this unpredictable fracture.

Diaphyseal injuries

In this heterogeneous group, management is strongly influenced by the amount of energy causing the injury and the age of the patient. For example, management of a 14-year-old close to skeletal maturity with multiple injuries including an open multifragmentary tibial fracture will be very different compared to a 3-year-old with a toddler's fracture, and therefore this section has been subdivided into low-energy closed injuries and high-energy open injuries.

Low-energy closed fractures—non-operative management

Toddler's fractures (Figure 14.10.4) are common and characterized as follows:

- Usually found at 1–3 years
- Low-energy spiral fractures of the distal tibial diametaphysis
- Caused indirectly by simple trips and twisting injuries
- Diagnosis delayed as the clinical presentation is unimpressive with an otherwise well toddler simply reluctant to weight bear and no traumatic episode recalled
- Delayed presentation and inadequate history may give rise to concern about non-accidental injury
- Degree of displacement and angulation minor
- Treat with above-knee walking cast in 10 degrees of knee flexion
- Predictably good prognosis.

Falls and road traffic collisions are common throughout childhood and more energy results in displaced fractures (Figure 14.10.5) but these isolated closed injuries can be treated in a similar way to toddlers' fractures.

- Reduction and application of an acceptable full-leg cast can usually be achieved in the Emergency Department using sedation and/or inhalational analgesia. This will stabilize the fracture better and minimizes handling of the injured limb in a frightened or uncooperative child
- Complete cast acceptable if child admitted for elevation and observation for compartment syndrome
- Ankle equinus is unimportant in children's fractures as late ankle stiffness will not be a problem and may help maintain reduction

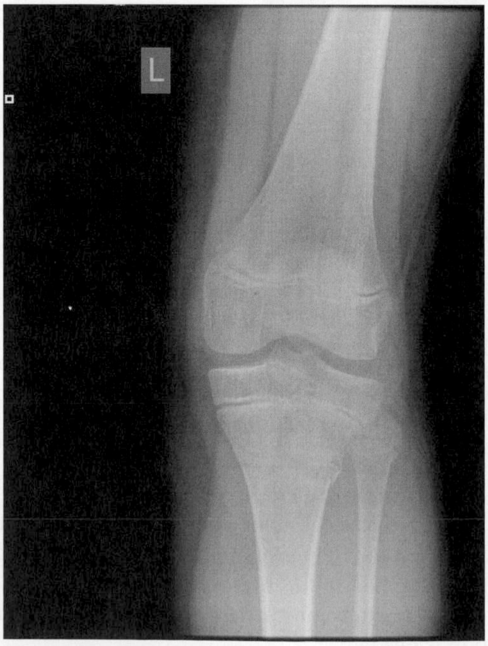

Fig. 14.10.3 Minimally displaced proximal tibial metaphyseal fracture.

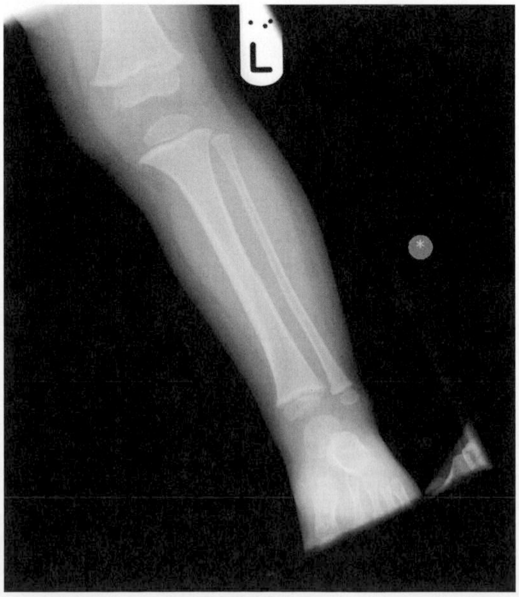

Fig. 14.10.4 Toddlers fracture. Can be radiologically subtle. May be missed or misinterpreted as vascular marking. Callus at 2 weeks is the giveaway.

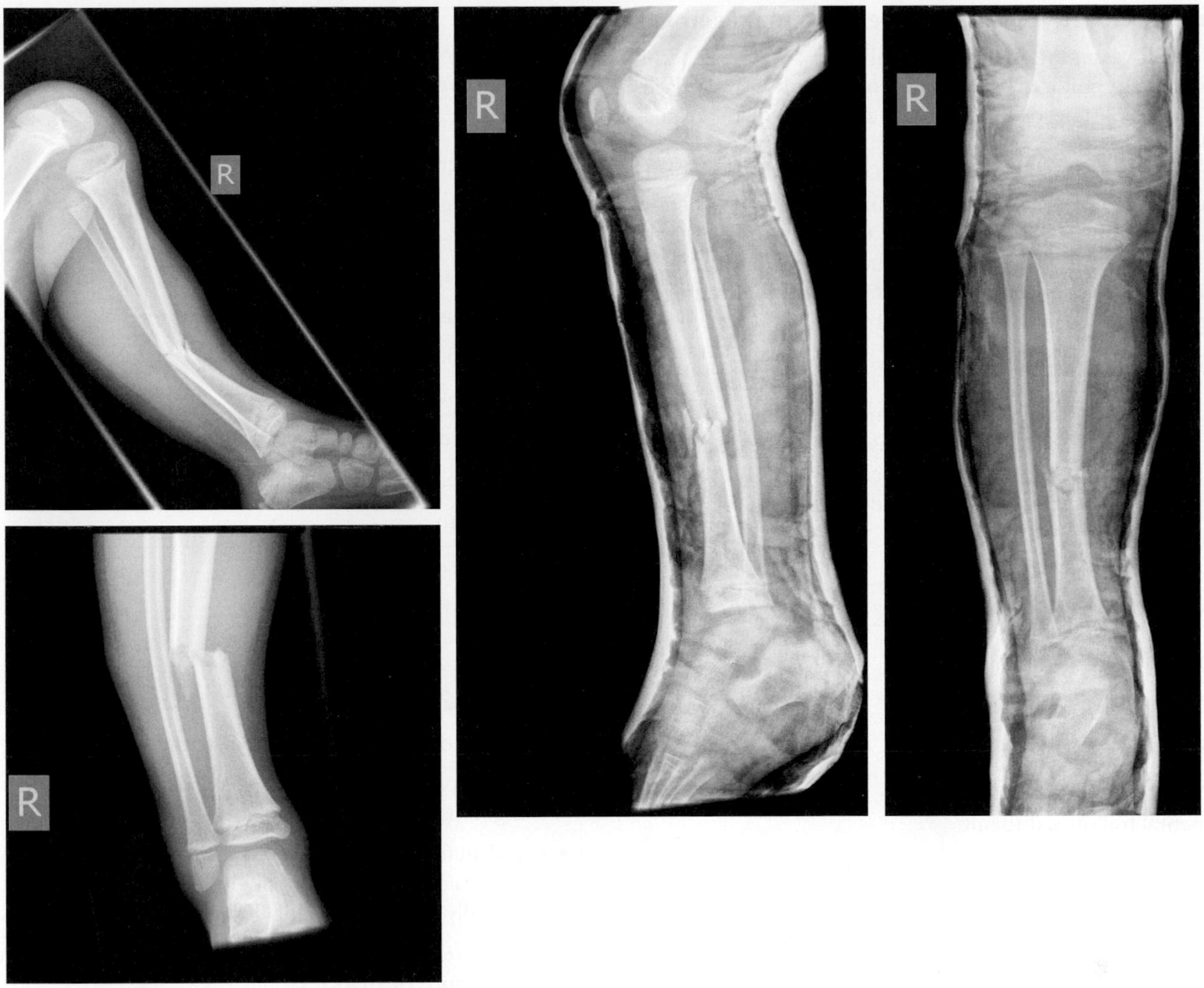

Fig. 14.10.5 Displaced tibial shaft fracture manipulated into acceptable position and held in an above-knee cast.

- Check radiographs at 1, 2, and even 3 weeks postinjury are needed as late displacement may occur. Plaster wedging can correct angular deformity but it is often better to reapply and mould a fresh cast under general anaesthetic
- Surgery is the better option when casting fails to achieve or maintain satisfactory alignment. A guide to the amount of displacement and angulation permissible is shown in Table 14.10.1.

Table 14.10.1 Suggested acceptable limits in childrens' tibial shaft fractures

	< 8 years	**>8 years**
Valgus	5°	5°
Varus	10°	5°
Apex anterior angulation	10°	5°
Apex posterior angulation	5°	5°
Shortening	10mm	5mm
Rotation	5°	5°

Reproduced from Heinrich, S.D. (2001). Fractures of the shaft of the tibia. In: Beaty, J.H. and Kasser, J.R. (eds) *Rockwood and Wilkins' Fractures in Children*, Vol. III, fifth edition, pp.1077–19. Philadelphia, PA: Lippincott Williams & Wilkins.

It may be argued that these criteria are strict but orthogonal anteroposterior (AP) and lateral x-rays may underestimate the degree of deformity if it lies in an oblique plane.

Advice about weight bearing is often ignored and if children can weight bear they tend to do so. Children younger than school age struggle with crutches but cope with a small walking frame or simply use a buggy. It is worth considering reducing an above-knee cast to a below-knee one when fracture callus is visible on radiographs. This will help older children who appreciate a lighter, less restrictive cast but young children dislike such interventions and are better left to heal in their existing cast which in most cases would be removed 2 or 3 weeks hence.

As a rule-of-thumb, most low energy, closed children's diaphyseal fractures require 6–8 weeks' cast splintage though toddlers' fractures are usually sufficiently healed in about 4 weeks. Seeing the child walking comfortably in clinic in the cast and fracture callus on x-ray indicates that the cast can be removed.

It is important to warn parents that it takes a few days for confidence to be regained and for weight bearing to resume.

Knee and ankle stiffness seldom occur and formal rehabilitation is not needed. Sport should be prohibited until the child can walk normally and run with confidence, perhaps a further 6 weeks.

Low-energy closed fractures—operative management

In the last 20 years, intramedullary nailing in adults has become very popular. In children, however, proximal physeal damage at the nail entry point needs to avoided as anterior growth arrest and tibial recurvatum may result.

When closed treatment has already failed or is not a practical proposition, for example, in multiply injured patients, there is a variety of fixation devices that can be used. The role of each is dependent on the fracture type and the surgeon's training and experience. Relative indications, advantages and disadvantages of each are summarized in Boxes 14.10.3–14.10.6.

High energy, open injury

After open finger injuries this is the commonest open fracture in children. The Gustilo and Anderson classification helps define the prognosis and is useful for communication. The full extent of injury may only be apparent at formal debridement. High-energy

Box 14.10.3 Elastic intramedullary nailing (Figure 14.10.6)

- Over 7 years
- Minimal intervention
- Quick to insert (with experience)
- Very good fracture control
- Segmental fractures difficult
- May well require removal especially if nails ends palpable/irritate
- Infection rare and usually minor/superficial
- Supplementary below-knee cast for 4 weeks.

Box 14.10.4 External fixation, monolateral fixator (Figure 14.10.7)

- Minimal intervention
- Easy technique to learn, very quick to apply
- Good fracture control
- Adjustable (general anaesthetic)
- Requires 3–4cm diaphysis/metaphysis proximally and distally for screw fixation
- Infection at screw sites common but superficial
- Pock mark scarring at screw sites
- Can remove in clinic
- Difficult to know when to remove
- Stress shielding and late fracture rate
- Malunion.

Box 14.10.5 External fixation—circular frame

- Complex devices, more time to assemble and apply
- Minimal proximal/distal bone needed to obtain sound fixation using transfixation wires
- Excellent fracture control, even segmental fragments, and possibility to adjust incrementally in all planes in clinic/at home (especially the Taylor Spatial Frame)
- Usually reserved for complex/high energy/revision surgery cases (Figure 14.10.8).

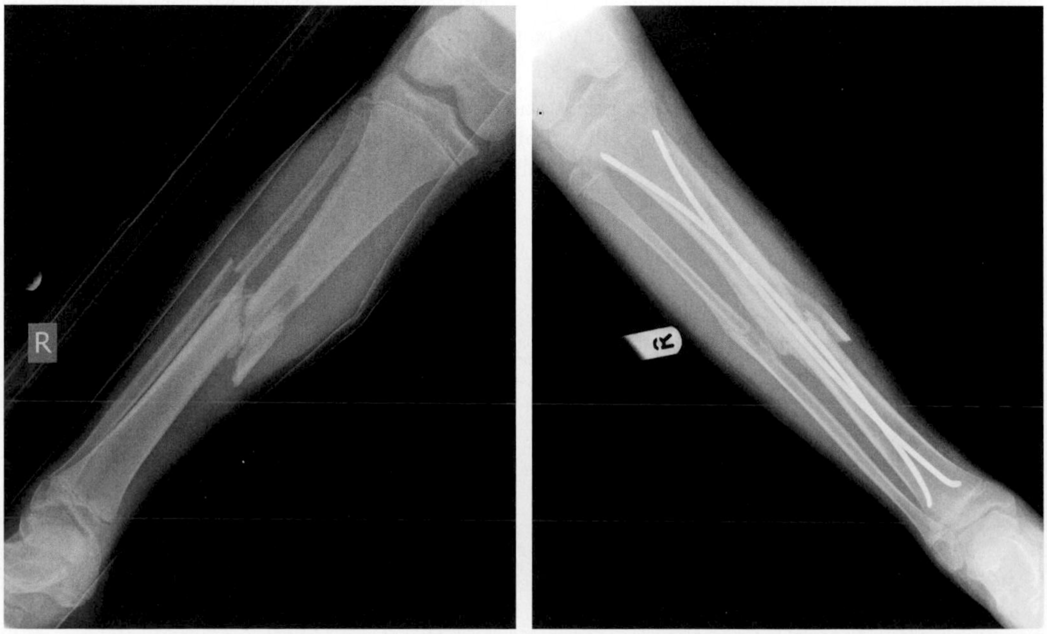

(A) (B)

Fig. 14.10.6 Displaced tibial shaft fracture (A)treated with flexible intramedullary nails (B).

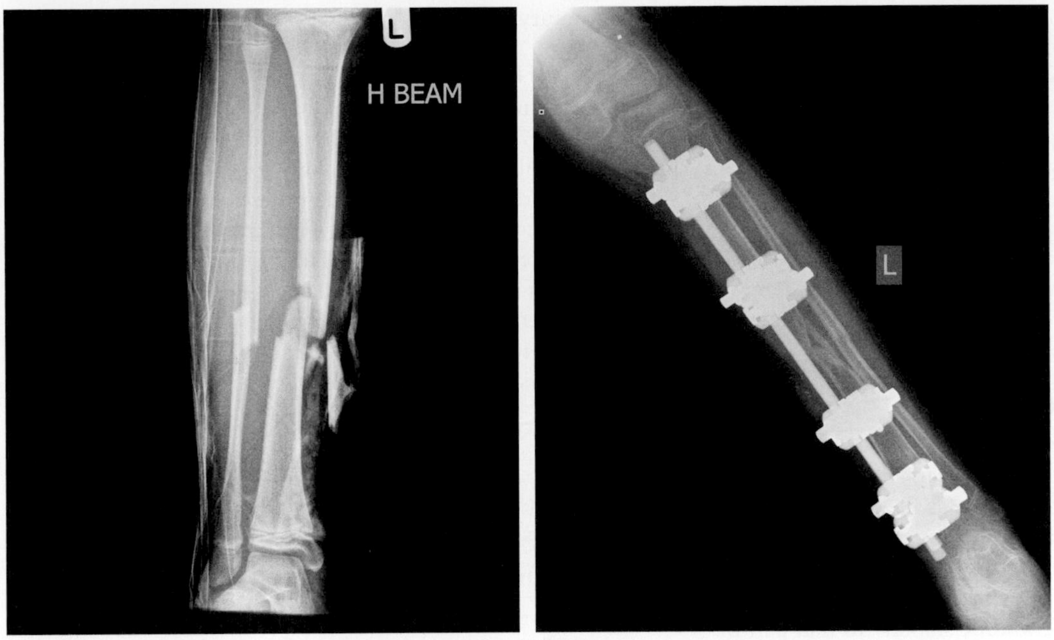

(A) (B)

Fig. 14.10.7 Open multifragmentary diaphyseal fracture with bone loss (A). Primary stabilization in a monolateral fixator (B).

Box 14.10.6 Plating
◆ When used usually applied for metaphyseal injuries but possible in the diaphysis ◆ Unpopular in diaphyseal fractures as other methods less invasive.

unstable ipsilateral tibial and femoral fractures ('floating knee') injuries are difficult to manage without surgical stabilization of one or, preferably, both.

Grades 1 and possibly 2 can be treated without surgical stabilization but where facilities and expertise exist, surgical stabilization is preferable. The management strategy is the same as for adult open fractures, except:

- Adult type transphyseal intramedullary nailing contraindicated
- Superior age-related healing of soft tissues and bone
- Less debridement may be required in children
- In younger children judicious use of a windowed cast is adequate.

Distal tibial and ankle injuries

Distal tibial metaphysis

Fractures are usually greenstick pattern and the large majority are minimally displaced. Closed reduction and immobilization in a

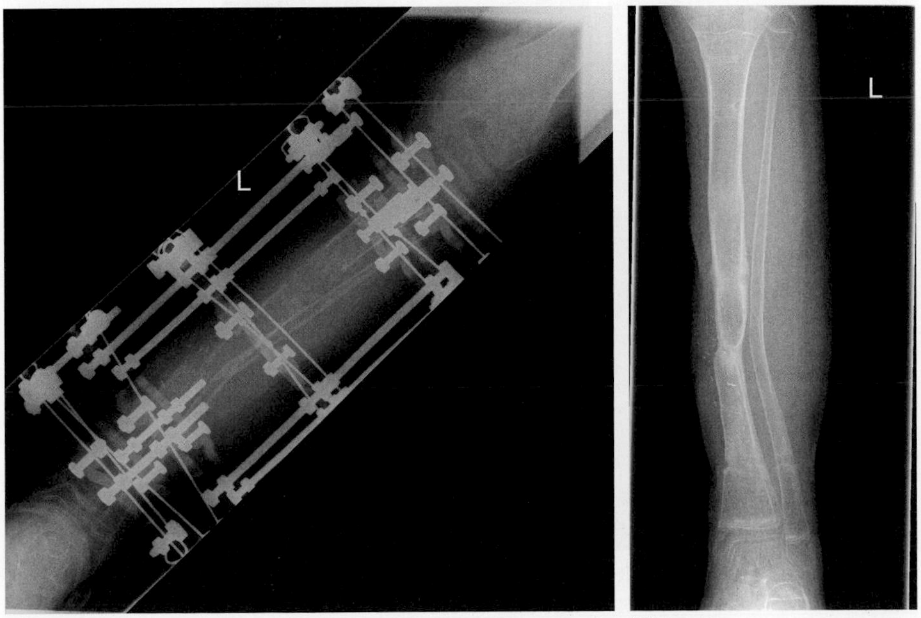

(A) (B)

Fig. 14.10.8 Open multifragmentary diaphyseal fracture with bone loss (same case as Figure 14.10.7). Failure to consolidate in a monolateral fixator treated by segmental bone excision and bone transport using a circular frame (A) resulting in union (B).

long leg cast allows correction of any deformity. High-energy displaced injuries with soft tissue compromise may require stabilization with crossed percutaneous wires (2mm), external fixation or even plating (Figure 14.10.9).

Severe open injuries including open 'grinding' injuries from road abrasion require plastic surgical assessment and the circular frame is a useful stabilizing device.

Remodelling will correct minor translational deformities; rotation, however, will not and angular deformities should not exceed 10 degrees.

These injuries merge with those described in the following section on ankle and growth plate injuries.

Ankle and distal growth plate injuries

These are injuries of older children and adolescents. The predictable way the tibial physis fuses in the last 2 years of growth dictates injury patterns around the immature ankle as the open part of the physis is more vulnerable than adjacent bone (and ligaments). Fusion begins centrally then medially and lastly anterolaterally. It is also thought that the characteristic medial prominence seen on AP x-rays ('Kump's bump') confers some stability to that part of the physis and also modifies fracture patterns.

Injuries involving a partially fused physis are sometimes referred to as transitional fractures.

These distal injuries are the most complex group to consider and in an attempt to clarify discussion is in terms of:

- Mechanism of injury
- Salter–Harris type (intra- vs extra-articular)
- Adolescent Tillaux fracture
- Triplane fracture
- Fibular injury.

Mechanism of injury

A modified Lauge–Hansen classification was devised by Dias and Tachdjian (1978) (Figure 14.10.10), to describe mechanisms of injury and resulting characteristic x-ray appearances.

Children seldom report anything other than a twist or fall and the value of recognition of the x-ray appearance is that it allows the fracture to be reduced by reversal of the injuring force. This is helpful in children as closed treatment and splintage of the foot and ankle in an over-corrected non-plantigrade position is much better tolerated than in adults where a policy of open reduction/internal fixation renders such fracture pattern analysis largely redundant.

Salter–Harris type I and II injuries

- Salter-Harris type I and II tibial injuries do not cross the weight-bearing joint surface and are non-articular. Manipulation under general anaesthetic is usually easy
- Stable reduction held in an above-knee cast for about 5 weeks
- Check x-ray at 1 week. Patients are allowed to weight bear when comfortable.

Interposition of the thick and elastic periosteum is a well-recognized cause of failure of closed reduction and requires open reduction. At surgery it is simple to split the infolded periosteum longitudinally and lift it out of the fracture gap.

Where there is doubt about stability or the ability of a cast to maintain reduction, crossed transphyseal 2mm K-wires can be used.

Healing is rapid and a delay of more than 1–2 weeks risks physeal damage if a forcible reduction is then attempted. In this case it may

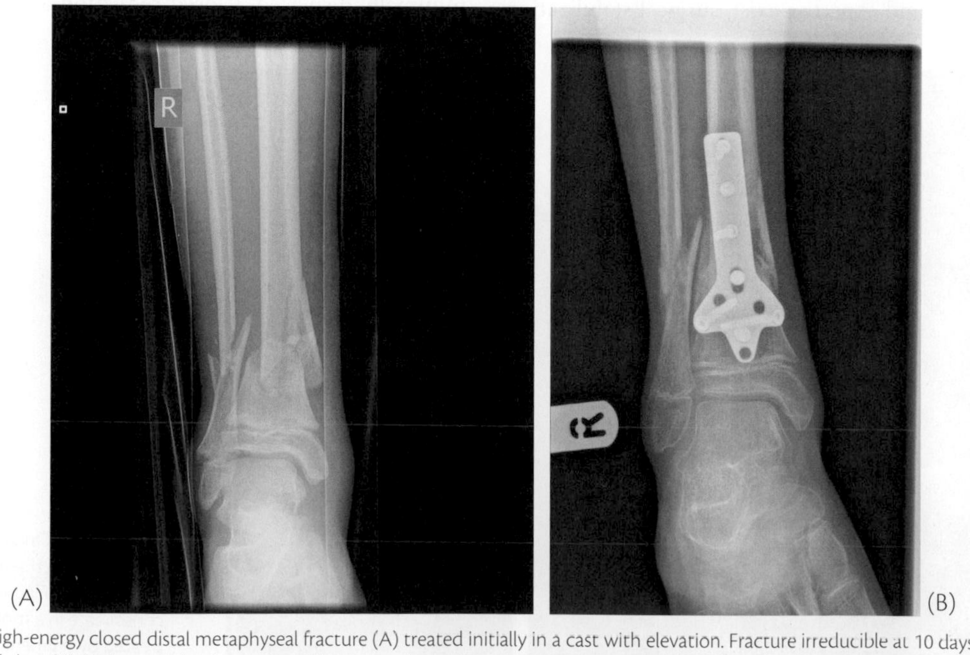

Fig. 14.10.9 Displaced high-energy closed distal metaphyseal fracture (A) treated initially in a cast with elevation. Fracture irreducible at 10 days and treated by open reduction with clover leaf plate (B). (Primary reduction and stabilization with K-wires or spanning external fixator would have been a better option.)

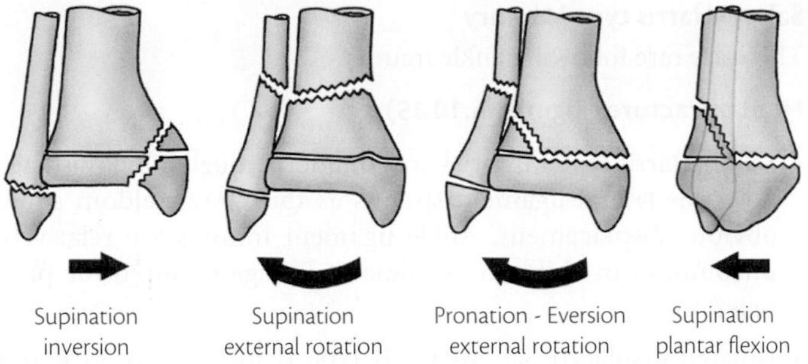

Fig. 14.10.10 Mechanism of ankle injury and typical fracture line pattern—Dias and Tachdjian ankle fracture classification. Supination: inversion (SH 3 or 4 tibia); supination: external rotation; pronation–eversion: external rotation (SH 2); supination: plantarflexion (SH 2). Reproduced from Dias, L.S. and Tachdjian, M.O. (1978). Physeal injuries of the ankle in children. *Clinical Orthopaedics and Related Research*, **136**, 230–3.

be preferable to accept a non-anatomical reduction and consider a late elective corrective osteotomy.

The distal tibial growth plate is particularly vulnerable to growth disturbance after injury with reports of up to 50% late growth arrest even in Salter–Harris type I and II injuries. Growth disturbance may not become evident until 18 months postinjury but since the majority of injuries occur around adolescence the effects are mitigated.

When partial growth plate arrest occurs in younger children, typical angular deformities develop and require treatment (Figure 14.10.11).

Often the best solution is to ablate both the distal tibial and fibular growth plates and perform a corrective supramalleolar osteotomy. Depending on the age of the child and amount of shortening, some lengthening may be required. This may be done as a secondary procedure towards skeletal maturity or as part of a one-stage reconstruction using a lengthening device.

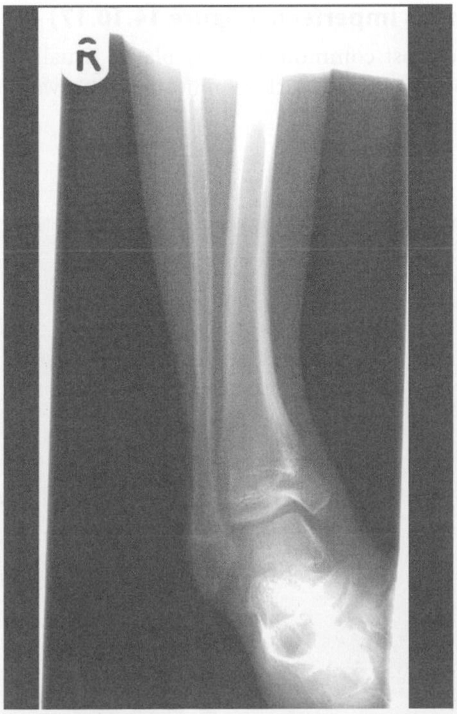

Fig. 14.10.11 Partial distal tibial growth arrest resulting in a varus ankle and relative fibular overgrowth.

Medial malleolar fracture/Salter–Harris type III or IV injury (Figure 14.10.12)

- Supination–inversion injures before the medial physis has fused
- Aim is anatomical reduction of joint surfaces
- Reduction of the closely adjacent physis is important to reduce the risk of growth disturbance by a physeal bar
- Open mini-arthrotomy/closed reduction of displaced fractures and stabilization with percutaneous cannulated 4.0-mm screw(s).

Whilst there is a generally held view that the intra-articular reduction should be within 2mm at most (the authors included) there is little clinical evidence to support this '2mm displacement rule'.

It is unclear whether a gap is of greater significance than a step though it would seem intuitive that a step would be more likely to predispose to late joint degenerative change than a 'level' gap.

If there is doubt or difficulty in reduction then open reduction is needed. If the fracture line is steeply oblique then intraepiphyseal fixation with a 4.0-mm cannulated screw is an excellent method.

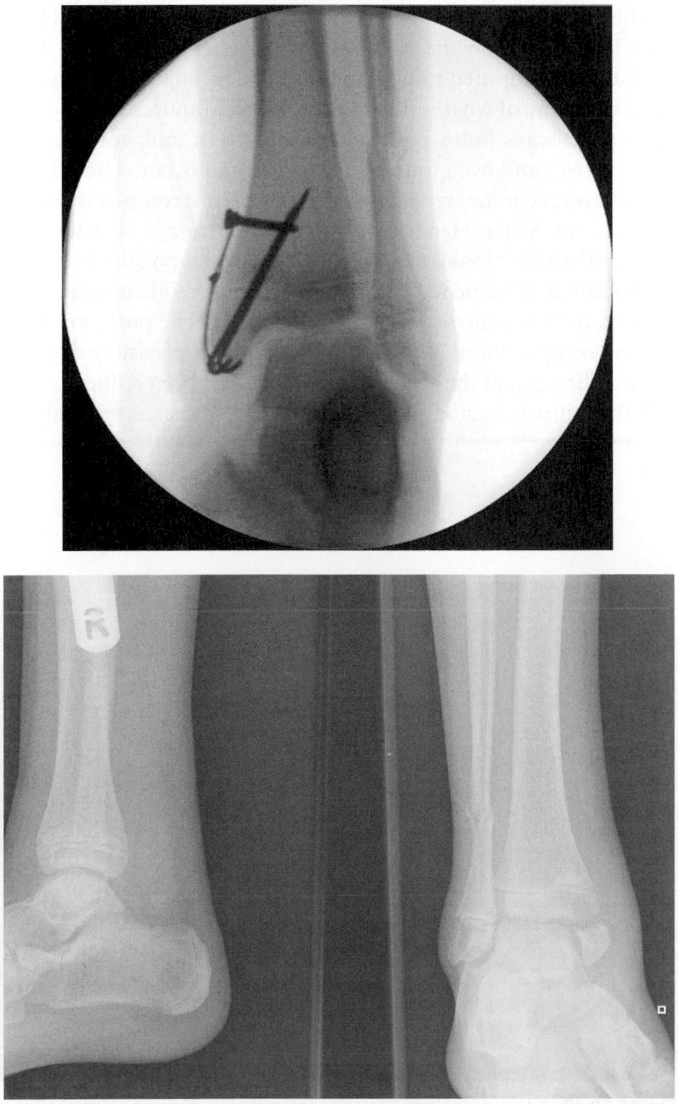

Fig. 14.10.12 Medial malleolar fracture.

More horizontal fracture lines require transphyseal fixation into the metaphysis. Tension band wiring is a useful option for smaller fragments or when the malleolus has split during attempted screw fixation.

Occasionally diagnostic confusion arises from an accessory area of ossification at the tip of the medial malleolus.

Adolescent Tillaux fracture/Salter–Harris type III injury (Figure 14.10.13)

Similar management as for type III medial malleolar fracture.

This is a Salter–Harris type III avulsion injury of the anterolateral portion of the epiphysis. They tend to occur in older adolescents shortly before the end of growth as this portion of the epiphysis is the last to fuse. External rotation of the talus in the mortise puts tension on the anterior tibiofibular ligament which avulses a substantial intra-articular fragment of the epiphysis.

Triplane fracture/Salter–Harris type IV injury (Figure 14.10.14)

This describes the sagittal, axial, and coronal planes that the fracture line follows. The mechanism is as for Tillaux fractures but a more complex pattern occurs because the patient is younger and a larger part of the lateral physis remains open and vulnerable to injury.

This injury pattern is typified on plain x-rays by a Salter–Harris type III fracture on the AP view and a Salter–Harris type II on the lateral. Computed tomography (CT) scanning has clarified the pathoanatomy of what is in reality a group of injuries with fracture lines not always following the typical pattern and, for example, two-, three-, and even four-part fractures can occur. The CT scan also allows accurate preoperative planning for screw placement.

As for the Salter–Harris type III and IV intra-articular fractures described earlier, closed manipulative treatment is possible but where significant displacement (>2mm) persists, open reduction and screw fixation of the epiphyseal fracture is indicated. The posterior metaphyseal component is, of itself, unimportant but persisting displacement indicates that the articular surface has not been reduced.

If the injury is treated closed a check CT at 1 week is preferable to plain x-rays.

Salter–Harris type V injury

These are rare following ankle trauma.

Fibular fracture (Figure 14.10.15)

- Salter–Harris type I injuries are common though often misdiagnosed as lateral ligament sprains as the x-rays seldom show obvious displacement. Ankle ligament injuries are relatively uncommon in children. Minimal splintage required for pain relief
- Isolated displaced Salter–Harris type II injuries are rare and probably merit closed reduction and below-knee cast
- Displaced fractures associated with tibial fractures usually reduce when the tibia is reduced
- High-energy complex metaphyseal injuries with residual fibular shortening and ankle incongruence may require open reduction and fixation.

Miscellaneous conditions

Corner or 'bucket handle' fractures (Figure 14.10.16)

These are subtle but important injuries to recognize. These represent small avulsion fractures of either the proximal or distal metaphyses and are usually seen in infants subject to violent twisting injuries. They are generally recognized as a strong indicator, some say pathognomonic, of non-accidental injury.

Tibial pseudarthrosis/prepseudarthrosis

Rare, associated with neurofibromatosis, typical anterolateral bow and radiological features. Simple splintage is used before fracture. Complex surgery always required for fracture, sometimes Symes amputation needed.

Osteogenesis imperfecta (Figure 14.10.17)

One of the most common bone dysplasias usually with typical 'gracile' bones on x-ray. Fractures unite in normal way but repeated

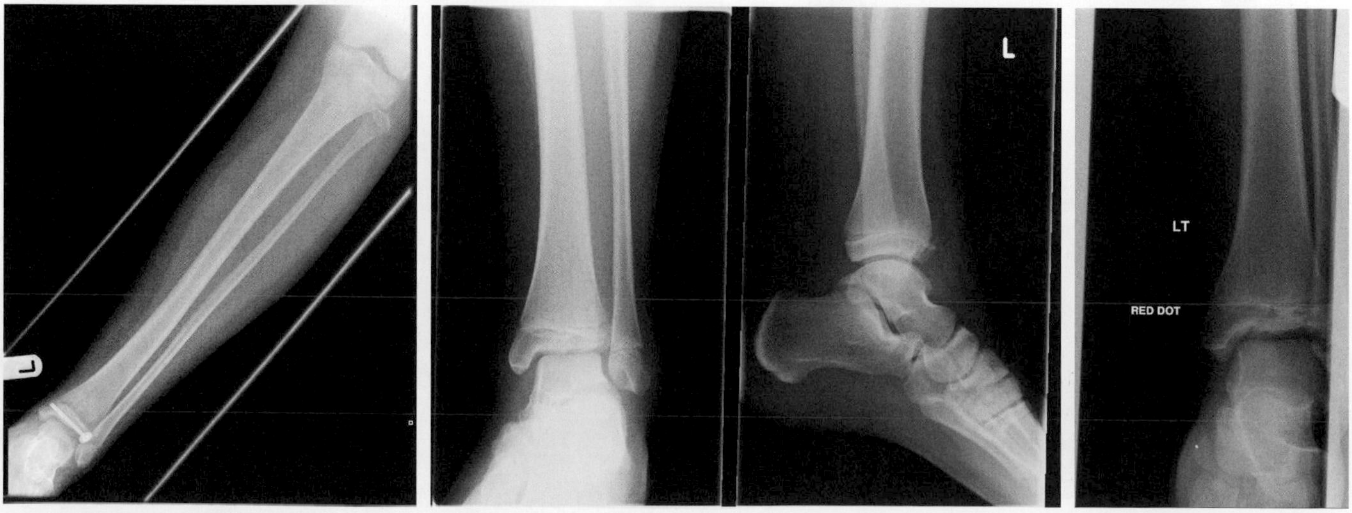

Fig. 14.10.13 Adolescent Tillaux treated conservatively (1) and operatively (2&3).

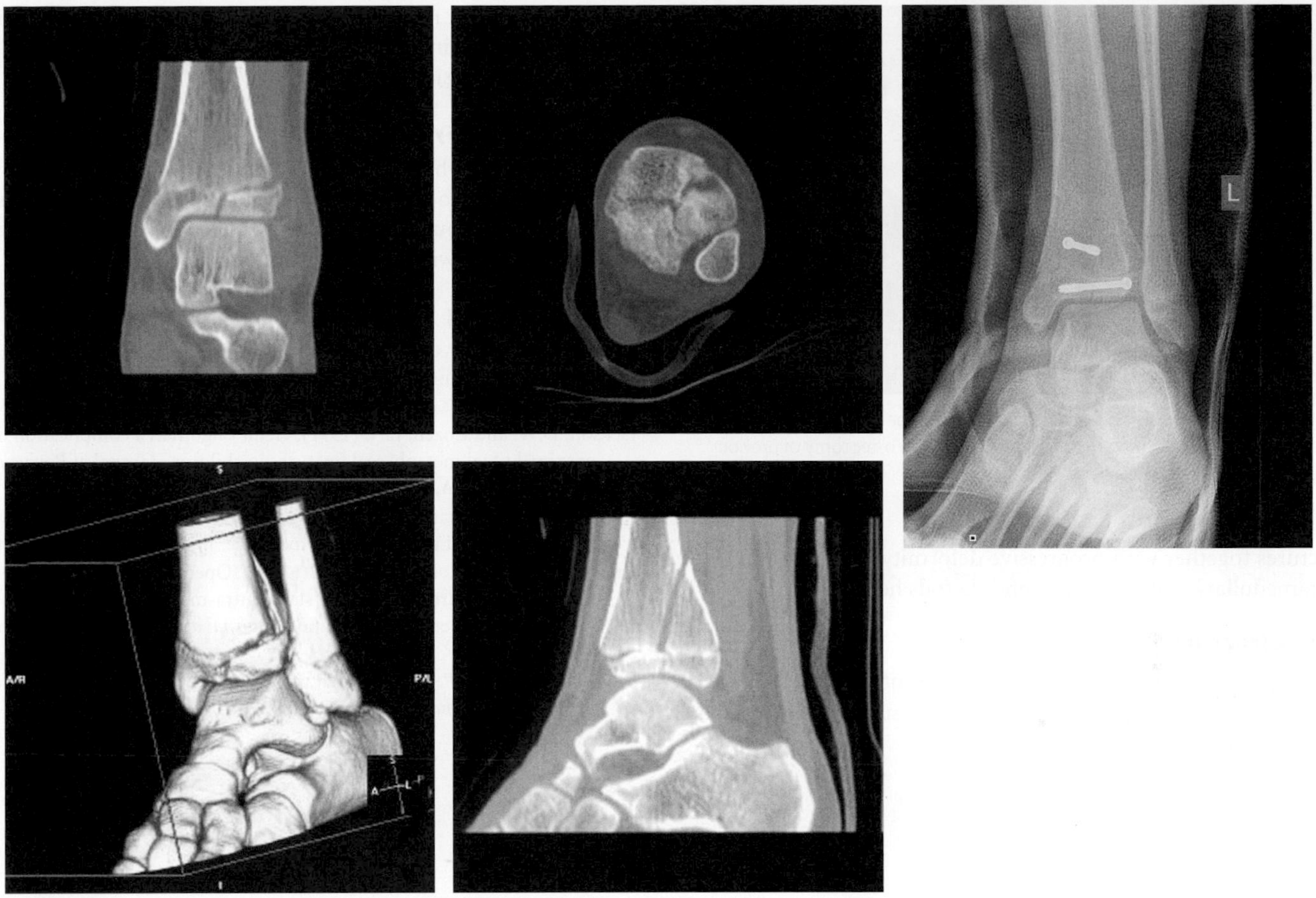

Fig. 14.10.14 T imaging in three planes and three-dimensional reconstruction helps understanding of this three-part triplane fracture and screw placement.

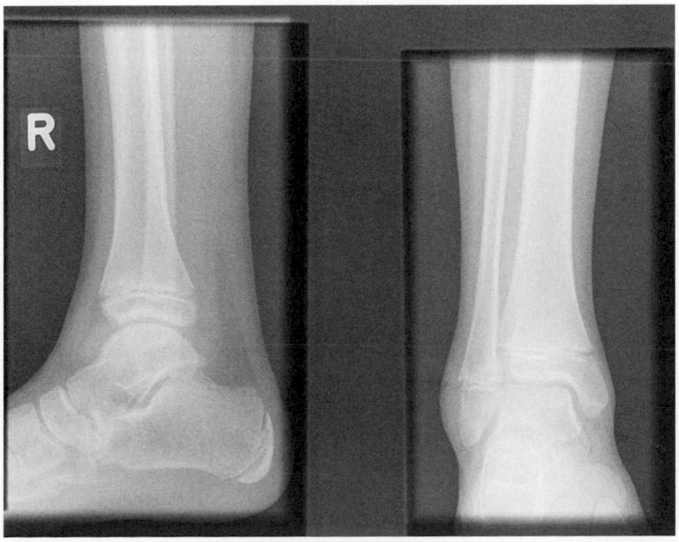

Fig. 14.10.15 SH type 2 distal fibular physeal injury, minimally displaced and easily overlooked, especially SH type 1.

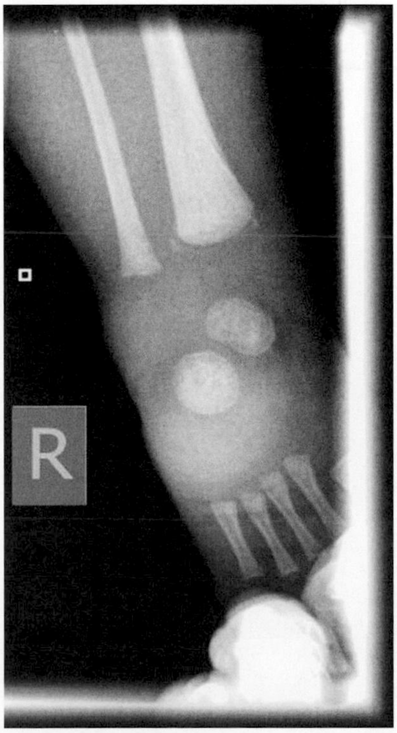

Fig. 14.10.16 Bucket handle/corner fractures distal tibia in an infant.

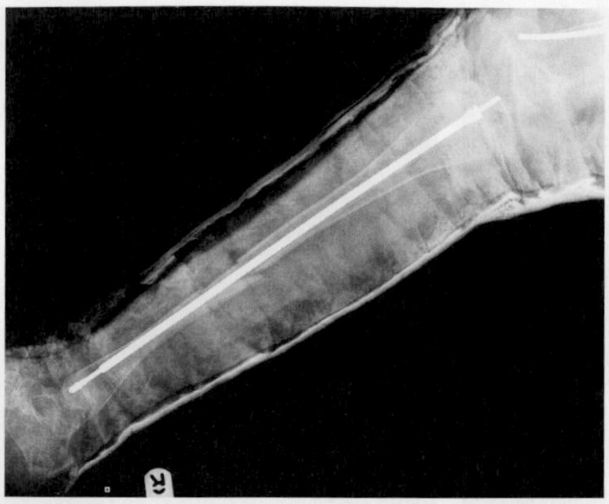

Fig. 14.10.17 Child with osteogenesis imperfecta (type 1). Extending intramedullary nail stabilizing fresh fracture. Corrective osteotomy of previous malunion just distal to realign and pass nail.

fractures together with progressive deformity hinder mobility and intramedullary nailing with extending rods helps.

Stress fracture

Rare and sometimes bilateral. Subtle presentation and may cause concern initially because of x-ray appearance suggestive of tumour or infection. Magnetic resonance imaging is both sensitive and specific. Consider 'shin splints' or chronic compartment syndrome in the differential diagnosis.

Compartment syndrome

Always consider when pain is out of proportion to injury even in open fractures. Proceed to emergency pressure measurements in theatre and wide four compartment fasciotomies if pressure greater than 30mmHg or within 20mmHg of diastolic.

Further reading

British Orthopaedic Association and British Association of Plastic Surgeons (1997). Publications to download. http://www.boa.ac.uk/site/showpublications.aspx?ID=59

Jackson, D.W. and Cozen, L.N. (1971). Genu valgum as a complication of proximal tibial metaphyseal fractures in children. *Journal of Bone and Joint Surgery*, **53A**, 1571–8.

Jones, B.G. and Duncan, R.D. (2003). Open tibial fractures in children under 13 years of age – 10-year experience. *Injury*, **34**(10), 776–80.

Kubiak, E., Egol, K.A., Scher, D., *et al.* (2005). Operative treatment of tibial fractures in children: Are elastic stable intra-medullary nails an improvement over external fixation? *Journal of Bone and Joint Surgery*, **87A**, 1761–8.

Schmittembecher, P.P. (2005). What must we respect in articular fractures in childhood? *Injury*, **36**, S-A35–S-A43.

14.11

Foot injuries in children

Michael J. Oddy and Deborah M. Eastwood

Summary points

- The child's foot is very supple but when injuries do occur conventional imaging is not as valuable as it should be because of the late ossification. Accessory centres of ossification complicate matters
- Transchondral fractures are not easily seen on conventional x-rays
- Lawnmower injuries (shredding of the forefoot) should have a slightly more tissue-preserving approach than in adults
- Lacerated tendons in the hindfoot need repairing if foot growth is to be normal.

Introduction

Children's feet are very supple and consist mainly of soft non-osseous tissues. Significant injuries are rare, as forces applied to the foot are invariably transmitted up the limb leading to a fracture more proximally. With growth and ossification of the skeleton, the stiffness of the foot increases and fractures occur more regularly.

A thorough assessment of an injury requires a full clinical history, a careful physical examination, and appropriate investigations. Interpretation of children's radiographs may be difficult without a full understanding of the array of minor growth variants and the multitude of sesamoids which may occur (Figure 14.11.1). It is important to appreciate the potential damage that might arise from an injury and ensure that the clinical site of tenderness is correlated with the abnormality on the radiograph.

Subtle radiographic abnormalities may hide a serious injury to the soft tissues which could have a devastating effect on the development of the foot and its function. Recent advances in imaging techniques have improved our understanding of these injuries but they are an adjunct to, not a substitute for, good clinical judgement.

Calcaneum (Box 14.11.1)

Until recently, calcaneal fractures in children have been reported infrequently and in general terms it was felt that the injury was benign, required minimum treatment, and was invariably associated with a good outcome. In the adult population, computed tomography (CT) scans are considered essential for the thorough assessment of calcaneal fractures and they have become an important influence on the choice of treatment and the assessment of outcome. In the child over 10 years of age, fracture patterns are similar to those in adults (see Chapter 12.56) and appropriate management can be instigated (Figure 14.11.2).

In the young child, the ossific nucleus of the calcaneum is not the same shape as the cartilage anlage and the lateral process of the talus is underdeveloped. Thus the forces applied to the immature calcaneum cause fracture patterns which differ from those seen in the adult. The anatomical differences also account for the smaller Bohler's angle found in the uninjured child. Many fractures in this age group are extra-articular. Involvement of the anterior process may be difficult to identify on plain radiographs. Unfortunately, delay in diagnosis is common and a high index of suspicion is required.

Conservative treatment is usually recommended with good results reported for both intra- and extra-articular fractures. Displaced avulsion fractures of the tuberosity or indeed of the apophysis itself, particularly when associated with soft tissue compromise or loss of Achilles tendon function should be treated by closed or open reduction and internal fixation.

Talus (Box 14.11.2)

The cartilaginous structure of the young child's talus is resistant to compression and this combined with the lower body mass of a child means that injuries to the talus are rare. They usually occur through the neck of the talus and are thus extra-articular injuries (Figure 14.11.3A). A high index of suspicion is required in this as in many other injuries in childhood as the initial radiographs may seem normal. Forced dorsiflexion is the mechanism of injury and even in undisplaced fractures there will be tenderness distal to the anterior ankle joint. If there is less than 5mm displacement and less than 5 degrees malalignment the position can be accepted. If displacement is greater than this then reduction by either closed or open means should be performed with internal fixation from the posterior aspect.

The risk of avascular necrosis is the major concern with fractures of the talus and the risk is related to the site of the fracture and the

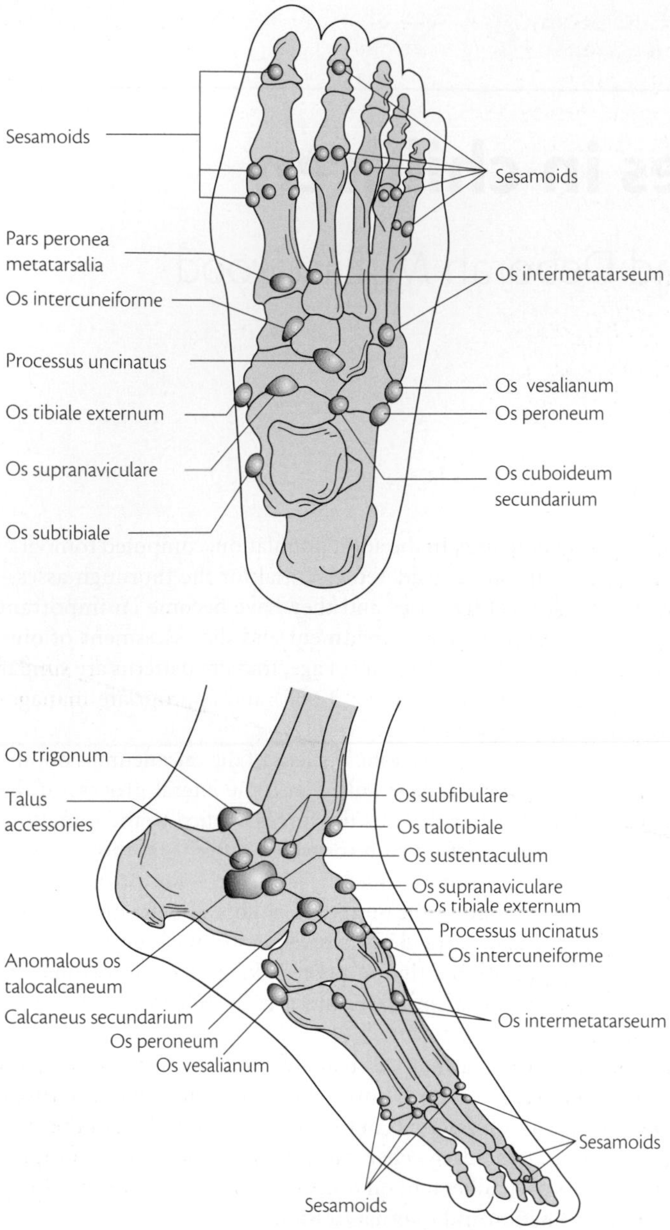

Fig. 14.11.1 Accessory ossicles and sesamoid bones of the foot and ankle. (Reproduced from Mann and Coughlin (1993).)

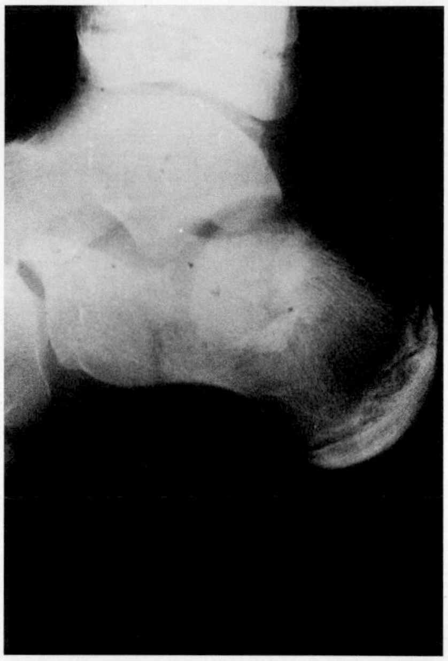

A

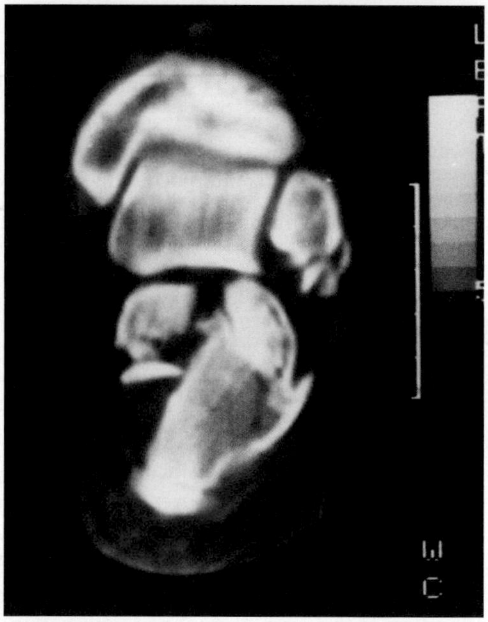

B

Fig. 14.11.2 A) Lateral radiograph showing a joint depression type of calcaneal fracture. B) Coronal CT scan showing the displacement of the three main fragments in an adult configuration.

Box 14.11.1 Calcaneal fractures

- Different fracture patterns in young children
- Adolescents follow adult patterns—consider fixation
- Young children:
  - Fractures usually extra-articular
  - Fractures often involve the anterior process of the calcaneum
  - Delay in diagnosis is common
  - High index of suspicion required
  - Good results with conservative treatment.

degree of displacement. The risk should be low in undisplaced fractures. However, avascular changes can occur even in undisplaced fractures. Weight bearing may have been detrimental in these cases and indeed, restricted weight bearing is recommended for all cases where avascular change is suspected. In adults the presence of the 'Hawkins sign', a subchondral lucency in the dome of the talus, is a good indicator of bone viability. The absence of the Hawkins sign in children may not necessarily be indicative of avascular necrosis. Magnetic resonance imaging (MRI) is the method of choice for the detection and definition of avascular change.

Box 14.11.2 Talar fractures

- Fractures usually occur through the neck
- Initial radiographs may be normal
- Mechanism of injury is forced dorsiflexion
- If <5mm, displacement treat conservatively
- Greater displacement requires reduction
- Major risk is avascular necrosis:
  - Related to site and displacement of fracture
  - Related to early weight bearing
  - Absence of Hawkins sign not indicative of avascular necrosis in children.

Other fractures of the talus are rare. Anatomically, fractures of the talar body should be associated with a worse prognosis but there is little evidence to support this statement. Basic principles of fracture management should be applied as they would in an adult.

The os trigonum is an accessory centre of ossification for the posterior process of the talus which first appears in girls aged 8–10 and in boys aged 11–13 years. It usually fuses to the talar body approximately a year after its appearance but if it fails to do so it may be mistaken for a fracture of the posterior talar process.

Transchondral fractures of the talus

Various terms such as osteochondritis dissecans and osteochondral fracture have been used to describe this condition which presents in adolescents as a chronic ankle sprain or activity-related stiffness. The lesions occur either on the posteromedial or anterolateral aspects of the talar dome. Most studies report a predominance of medial lesions in approximately 75% of cases but those on the lateral side are often associated with an injury with a torsional component to it. The posteromedial lesion is often deeper and cup-shaped compared with the thinner, more wafer-shaped anterolateral lesion. The fracture is unlikely to heal if the fragment is displaced from the talar body as fibrous tissue becomes interposed between the two injured surfaces. The cartilage, nourished by the synovial fluid, grows whilst the osseous fragment becomes avascular and dies.

Anderson *et al.* have modified Berndt and Harty's staging system for transchondral fractures of the talar dome based on the MRI findings in such injuries (Table 14.11.1 and Figure 14.11.4). Initial radiographs may be normal so if a transchondral injury is suspected further investigation must take place. An isotope bone scan will confirm damage in the region of the talus. Helical CT scans visualize bone damage well and are useful in detecting acute transchondral fractures and MRI highlights areas of soft tissue injury. MRI identifies the stage of the lesion which in turn dictates which treatment is most appropriate. Anatomical variants can be confusing and lead to the appearances of pseudodefects. In the presence of an abnormal radiograph, further investigation is unnecessary. Arthroscopy is useful in differentiating between incomplete and complete separation of the fragment.

Treatment aims to achieve stable union of the fracture, and if this appears unlikely, excision of the fragment and healing of the defect with fibrocartilage is allowed. In early cases, symptomatic relief and occasionally healing can be obtained by immobilization in either a weight-bearing or a non-weight-bearing plaster cast. Arthroscopic assessment and management of the lesion has become popular but a child's ankle is small and care must be taken not to inflict further damage with the instruments. Arthrotomy is still preferred by some, especially for the posteromedial lesion, although care must be taken with the transmalleolar approach in the

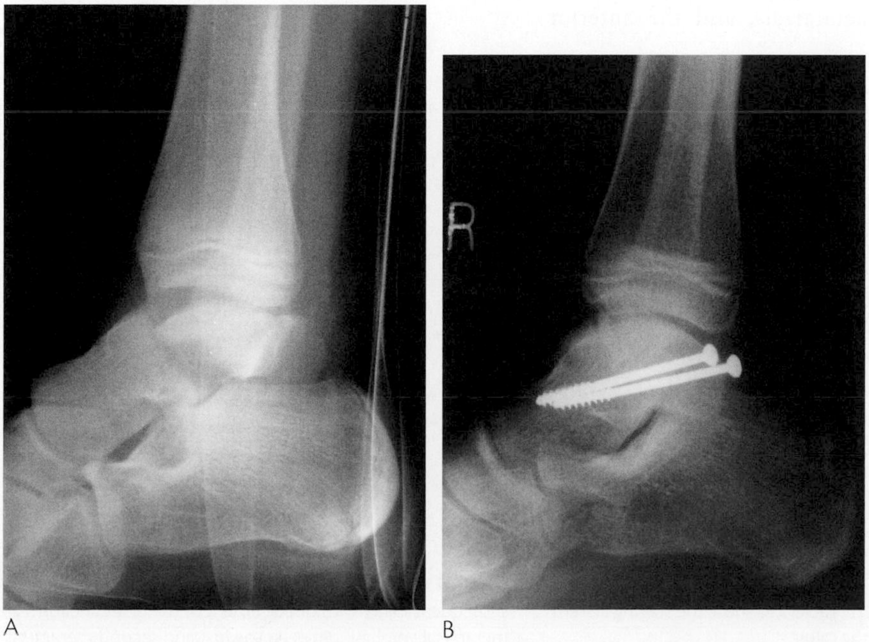

A B

Fig. 14.11.3 A) Lateral radiograph showing a displaced fracture of the talar neck. B) Postoperative lateral radiograph of the same case showing the fracture reduced and held with screws placed from the posterior aspect.

Table 14.11.1 Staging system for transchondral fractures of the dome of the talus

Stage 1	Subchondral trabecular compression—seen on MRI only
Stage 2	Incomplete separation of fragment
Stage 2a	Formation of a subchondral cyst
Stage 3	Fragment detached but undisplaced
Stage 4	Fragment displaced

skeletally immature patient in order that physeal damage does not occur. Stage 2a and 3 lesions may be treated by drilling of the fragment whilst in stage 4 lesions the loose fragment is excised, the defect debrided, and the base curetted or drilled. Some advocate direct autogenous bone grafting of the symptomatic medial lesion to replace the necrotic subchondral bone and promote the ingrowth of viable bone to support the talar surface. Postoperative rehabilitation depends on the procedure performed as does the outcome. In general terms, lateral lesions are associated with more persistent symptoms than the medial lesions. Degenerative change occurs in approximately 50% of cases.

Other tarsal bones

Significant fractures rarely occur other than in association with major foot injuries. Minor fractures are seen more commonly and may divert attention from the more subtle radiographic features which might indicate a major injury such as a peritalar dislocation.

The *accessory navicular* is a congenital anomaly in which the tuberosity of the navicular develops from a separate ossification centre. The radiographic appearances can be of a synchondrosis, an isolated ossicle, or an elongated cornuate process. The accessory navicular may be mistaken for a fracture and can be associated with localized pain and flat feet in the adolescent when the cartilaginous synchondrosis is subjected to tensile forces and fails.

The *cuboid* is susceptible to a crushing abduction mechanism between the fourth and fifth metatarsals, and the anterior calcaneum—the nutcracker fracture. This seldom occurs in isolation, and the coexistence of other midfoot injuries should be sought. Untreated, the shortened lateral column can result in an acquired flatfoot deformity. Non-operative treatment is acceptable in the majority of cases; however, displaced fractures require reduction and bone grafting.

Tarsometatarsal injuries

Such injuries do occur in the paediatric population and although overall they are of lesser severity due to the smaller applied forces, the mechanisms of injury are similar to those in adults. Wiley has described the pathoanatomy associated with these injuries and highlighted the significance of the ligament which runs from the medial cuneiform to the base of the second metatarsal, which is important in maintaining the metatarsal within the mortise formed by the cuneiforms. Anatomical reduction is essential and must be achieved by either closed or open means with suitable fixation as indicated. The apparently undisplaced joint injury should be assessed for stability but in suitable cases conservative management can be used.

A variation of the classic Lisfranc injury may occur in younger children when a plantarflexion force wedges the oblique first cuneiform–first metatarsal epiphysis between the first and second metatarsals. This has been termed the 'bunk bed' injury (Figure 14.11.5). Radiological changes are subtle in the young child and buckling of the cortex of the first metatarsal may be the only sign.

Forefoot fractures

Metatarsal fractures

These injuries are relatively common and conservative treatment is the rule. However, although children have extensive capabilities of remodelling this is not infinite and some fractures will require

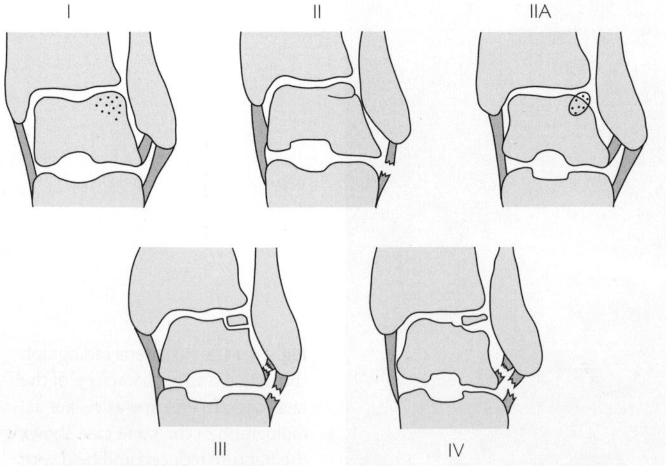

Fig. 14.11.4 Diagrammatic representation of Table 1 to show the staging system for transchondral fractures of the dome of the talus.

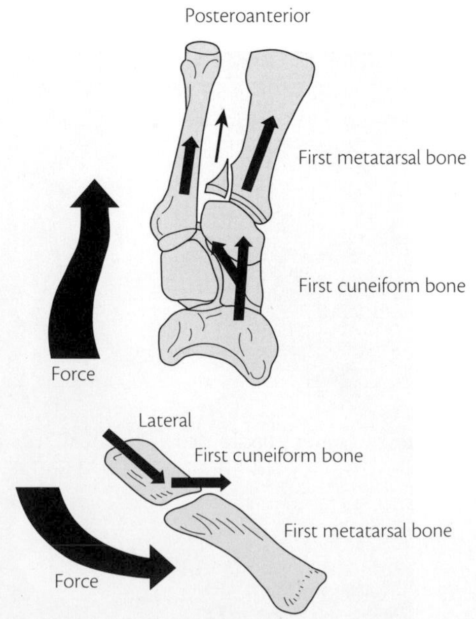

Fig. 14.11.5 'Bunk-bed' fracture. Diagram to show the direction of force and the subsequent injury with displacement of the first cuneiform and part of the first metatarsal epiphysis between the first and second metatarsal.

more aggressive management with the use of finger traps for a manipulative reduction and the use of K-wires for fixation. Open reduction is rarely indicated. Soft tissue swelling or injury may necessitate hospital admission with monitoring of the compartment pressures as appropriate. An apparently solitary fracture of the base of the second metatarsal should raise the possibility of a paediatric Lisfranc injury where the subluxation has reduced spontaneously.

Non-accidental injury

Fractures of the metatarsals and the phalanges consistent with a mechanism of forced hyperextension are subtle but important injuries in children who have been abused.

Fractures of the fifth metatarsal base

Avulsion fractures of the base of the fifth metatarsal occur relatively frequently and this is the classical site where radiological variants are confused with fracture patterns. The diagnosis is confirmed on radiograph where the fracture line is noted to be perpendicular to the long axis of the bone. The attachment of the peroneus brevis tendon is often blamed for the avulsion injury but the tendinous portion of abductor digiti minimi and the lateral cord of the plantar aponeurosis may also be implicated in the pathology. Treatment is a weight-bearing cast for a time appropriate to the child's age. The fracture must be distinguished from sesamoids, within the tendons of peroneus brevis and longus (see Figure 14.11.1), and from the apophysis which lies parallel to the shaft of the metatarsal and is not apparent before the age of 8 years. The apophysis unites to the metatarsal shaft by the age of 12 in girls and 15 in boys.

Fractures at the junction of the proximal diaphysis with the metaphysis occur in the adolescent. A stress injury often predates the fracture in which case operative reduction and fixation with bone grafting may be required.

Phalangeal injuries

Fractures and joint dislocations do occur and treatment is based on clinical grounds. Reduction may be required particularly with the proximal phalanx of the great toe. Rotational deformity should be prevented. The ossification centre of the proximal phalanx of the hallux is frequently bipartite and may be mistaken for an intra-articular fracture.

Stress fractures

With the current trend for an increasingly active lifestyle, stress fractures are becoming more common in the paediatric population. They occur most frequently in the metatarsals. An appreciation of this injury and its frequency is important otherwise the clinical and radiological signs can be worrying and biopsy will be necessary to exclude a neoplastic growth. Localized tenderness without obvious bruising or swelling is observed and a high index of suspicion is necessary. The stress fracture itself is a relatively benign lesion and the aim is to restore the child to his or her normal activity level. There is rarely any concern regarding growth disturbance. Fractures are most common in the adolescent with the relatively less flexible foot who is beginning to participate in intensive sports training. Treatment varies with the duration and severity of symptoms. A simple restriction of activities may be all that is necessary or a plaster cast may be applied. Operative treatment may be necessary if there is an underlying abnormality.

Soft tissue involvement

Open fractures

The principles of management for open foot fractures in childhood are the same as those for the adult and for open fractures at any site. Fractures involving the physis should be anatomically reduced. This is easier to achieve at the initial visit to the operating room for wound debridement but should not be performed if the risk of osteomyelitis is high.

Lawnmower injuries

These are any injury where there is significant damage to both the soft tissues and the bones associated with a crushing force. It may be difficult to judge the extent of the soft tissue damage at the time of injury and the decision whether to amputate an injured extremity or to save it requires considerable experience. A thorough debridement of dead tissue at the time of injury is essential although a conservative approach to tissue of doubtful viability is justified in children. A plastic surgical opinion should be sought as many of the advances in the management of these devastating injuries have occurred due to advances in plastic surgical techniques; particularly in the choice and timing of soft-tissue reconstruction. At the initial assessment it is important to document the extent of the injuries and the anticipated problems such as physeal or joint damage and loss of tendon function in order that treatment can consider both short-term goals and long-term development and function. Broad-spectrum antibiotic cover is required as wound contamination is inevitable with multiple organisms which are similar to those seen in farmyard accidents. Wounds must be examined every 48–72h and intra-articular and transphyseal injuries reduced and stabilized.

In general terms, shredding injuries and injuries to the posterior and plantar surfaces do less well. Amputation of at least part of the forefoot or toes is common with amputation rates varying from 39–67%. Limb salvage must always be considered and the decision to amputate can often be delayed until the second visit to the operating room, when the viability of previously doubtful tissue can be reassessed. Split-skin grafting is the most common method of achieving soft tissue cover. Even on weight-bearing areas such grafts do surprisingly well. In cases where there are exposed bone, tendon or neurovascular structures a rotational or more commonly a free vascularized flap must be considered. The long-term outcome of free flap reconstruction in 91 cases has shown a lower incidence of trophic ulcers in muscle flaps with a cutaneous component compared with skin-grafted muscle flaps, and overall flap survival of 95%. Immediate tendon reconstruction can be successful and lead to fewer overall operations.

Soft tissue lacerations

The Achilles tendon and the tendons of tibialis anterior, tibialis posterior, and peroneus longus are important for foot shape and function. Damage to these tendons often leads to a severe and progressive deformity with foot dysfunction. Such damage should be recognized promptly and treated by appropriate tendon repair and postoperative splinting. Lacerated flexor or extensor tendons to the toe may not be repaired but in such cases the affected toe should be strapped to its neighbour to prevent deformity. Satisfactory function usually returns. Most surgeons feel that tidy lacerations to extensor hallucis longus should also be repaired.

Compartment syndrome

Compartment syndrome is not a common problem in children but the diagnosis should be considered in any child who has had a crush injury to the foot with swelling and pain on passive motion. The potential morbidity of chronic pain and loss of protective sensation in the foot following an unrecognized compartment syndrome is a high price to pay for poor clinical judgement. Adults with a compartment syndrome are expected to have a concomitant serious bony injury but in children this is rarely the case. In suspected cases, pressure measurements should be made in the central and interosseous compartments and the readings related to the child's diastolic blood pressure. Treatment of an established compartment syndrome is prompt decompression of all nine compartments of the foot via either a dorsal or medial approach (Figure 14.11.6).

Non-traumatic causes of foot pain

In addition to the above injuries, non-traumatic causes of foot pain in the active child must always be considered (Box 14.11.3).

Box 14.11.3 Other causes of foot pain
◆ Infection: • Puncture wounds • Calcaneal osteomyelitis • Tuberculosis ◆ Tumours ◆ Plantar fasciitis ◆ Tarsal coalition ◆ Calcaneal apophysitis ◆ Juvenile inflammatory arthritis ◆ Osteochondroses: • Kohler's—navicular • Freiberg's infraction—metatarsal heads.

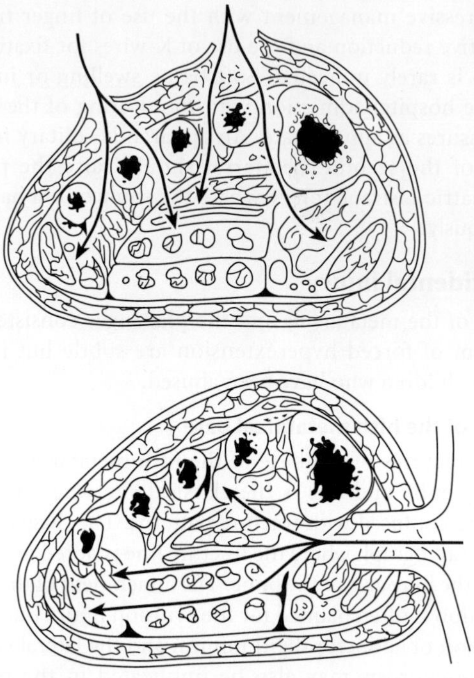

Fig. 14.11.6 Dorsal and medial surgical approaches for fasciotomy of the foot. The dorsal incisions are more suitable for injuries of the forefoot or midfoot whilst the medial approach is more applicable for injuries of the hindfoot. (Reproduced from Rockwood *et al.* (1996).)

Further reading

Anderson, I.F., Crichton, K.J., Grattan-Smith, T., Cooper, R.A., and Brazier, D. (1989). Osteochondral fractures of the dome of the talus. *Journal of Bone and Joint Surgery*, **71A,** 1143–52.

Berndt, A.L. and Harty, M. (1959). Transchondral fractures (osteochondritis dissecans) of the talus. *Journal of Bone and Joint Surgery*, **41A**, 988–1020.

Canale, S.T. and Kelly, F.B. (1978). Fractures of the neck of the talus. *Journal of Bone and Joint Surgery, American Volume*, **60A**, 143–55.

Ribbans, W.J., Natarajan, R., and Alavala, S. (2005). Paediatric foot fractures. *Clinical Orthopaedics and Related Research*, **432**, 107–15.

Rockwood, C.A., Wilkins, K.E., and Beaty, J.H. (ed.) (1996). *Fractures in Children*, third edition, pp. 1449, 1488. Philadelphia, PA: Lippincott-Raven.

Index

Page numbers in *italics* represent figures and/or tables.